2008

USP 31
THE UNITED STATES PHARMACOPEIA

NF 26
Volume 3

THE NATIONAL FORMULARY

By authority of the United States Pharmacopeial Convention, meeting at Washington, D.C., March 9–13, 2005. Prepared by the Council of Experts and published by the Board of Trustees

Official from May 1, 2008

The designation on the cover of this publication, "USP NF 2008," is for ease of identification only. The publication contains two separate compendia: *The United States Pharmacopeia*, Thirty-First Revision, and *The National Formulary*, Twenty-Sixth Edition.

THE UNITED STATES PHARMACOPEIAL CONVENTION
12601 Twinbrook Parkway, Rockville, MD 20852

SIX-MONTH IMPLEMENTATION GUIDELINE

The *United States Pharmacopeia–National Formulary* and its *Supplements* become official **six months** after being released to the public. The *USP–NF*, which is released on November 1 of each year, becomes official on May 1 of the following year.

This change was adopted to give users more time to bring their methods and procedures into compliance with new and revised *USP–NF* requirements.

The table below describes the new official dates. The 2007 *USP30–NF25*, and the *Supplements* and *Interim Revision Announcements (IRAs)* to that edition, will be official until May 1, 2008, at which time the *USP31–NF26* becomes official.

Publication	Release Date	Official Date	Official Until
USP31–NF26	Nov. 1, 2007	May 1, 2008	May 1, 2009 (except as superceded by *Supplements, IRAs,* and *Revision Bulletins*)
First Supplement	Feb. 1, 2008	Aug. 1, 2008	May 1, 2009 (except as superceded by *Second Supplement, IRAs,* and *Revision Bulletins*)
Second Supplement	June 1, 2008	Dec. 1, 2008	May 1, 2009 (except as superceded by *IRAs* and *Revision Bulletins*)
USP32–NF27	Nov. 1, 2008	May 1, 2009	May 1, 2010 (except as superceded by *Supplements, IRAs,* and *Revision Bulletins*)

IRAs will continue to become official on the first day of the second month of the *Pharmacopeial Forum (PF)* issue in which they are published as final. For instance, *IRAs* published as final in the May-June *PF* (issue 3) will become official on June 1. This table gives the details of the *IRAs* that will apply to *USP30–NF25* and *USP31–NF26*.

IRA*	Release Date	Official Date	Revises
Jan. 1, 2008 *IRA, PF* 34(1)	Jan. 1, 2008	Feb. 1, 2008	*USP30–NF25* and its *Supplements*
Mar. 1, 2008 *IRA, PF* 34(2)	Mar. 1, 2008	April 1, 2008	*USP30–NF25* and its *Supplements*
May 1, 2008 *IRA, PF* 34(3)	May 1, 2008	June 1, 2008	*USP31–NF26*
July 1, 2008 *IRA, PF* 34(4)	July 1, 2008	Aug. 1, 2008	*USP31–NF26* and *First Supplement*
Sept. 1, 2008 *IRA, PF* 34(5)	Sept. 1, 2008	Oct. 1, 2008	*USP31–NF26* and *First Supplement*
Nov. 1, 2008 *IRA, PF* 34(6)	Nov. 1, 2008	Dec. 1, 2008	*USP31–NF26* and its *Supplements*
Jan. 1, 2009 *IRA, PF* 35(1)	Jan. 1, 2009	Feb. 1, 2009	*USP31–NF26* and its *Supplements*
Mar. 1, 2009 *IRA, PF* 35(2)	Mar. 1, 2009	April 1, 2009	*USP31–NF26* and its *Supplements*

*NOTE—Beginning January 1, 2007, USP ceased identifying *IRAs* numerically (*First, Second,* etc.) and instead now designates them by the date on which they are published.

Revision Bulletins published on the USP website will continue to become official immediately upon publication, unless the *Revision Bulletin* specifies otherwise.

Revisions that contain a specific official date shall continue to become official upon such specified date, which supercedes the general official date for the publication.

For more information about the change in official dates, please visit the USP website at http://www.usp.org.

NOTICE AND WARNING

Concerning U.S. Patent or Trademark Rights
The inclusion in *The United States Pharmacopeia* or in the *National Formulary* of a monograph on any drug in respect to which patent or trademark rights may exist shall not be deemed, and is not intended as, a grant of, or authority to exercise, any right or privilege protected by such patent or trademark. All such rights and privileges are vested in the patent or trademark owner, and no other person may exercise the same without express permission, authority, or license secured from such patent or trademark owner.

Concerning Use of USP *or* NF *Text*
Attention is called to the fact that *USP* and *NF* text is fully copyrighted. Authors and others wishing to use portions of the text should request permission to do so from the Secretary of the USPC Board of Trustees.

Copyright © 2007 The United States Pharmacopeial Convention
12601 Twinbrook Parkway, Rockville, MD 20852
All rights reserved.
ISSN 0195-7996
ISBN 1-889788-53-8
Printed in the United States by Port City Press, Baltimore

USP 31   *Contents*   iii

Contents

VOLUME 1

Mission Statement and Preface v

People xi

    Officers (2005–2010) xi

    Board of Trustees (2005–2010) xi

    Council of Experts (2005–2010) xi

    Council of Experts Executive Committee (2005–2010) xii

    Expert Committees (2005–2010) xii

    Information Expert Committees (2005–2010) xiv

    Ad Hoc Advisory Panels (2005–2010) xv

    Members of the United States Pharmacopeial Convention as of June 1, 2007 xviii

Articles of Incorporation xxiii

USP Governance xxiv

    Constitution and Bylaws xxiv

    Rules and Procedures xxiv

    USP Policies xxiv

Admissions xxvii

    Articles Admitted to *USP 31* by Supplement xxvii

    Changes in Official Titles xxviii

    Revisions Appearing in *USP 31* That Were Not Included in *USP 30* Including Supplements xxix

    Articles Included in *USP 30* but Not Included in *USP 31* xxx

Commentary xxxi

Notices

    USP General Notices and Requirements 1

General Chapters

    See page 29 for detailed contents

    General Tests and Assays 33

    General Requirements for Tests and Assays 33

    Apparatus for Tests and Assays 59

    Microbiological Tests 67

    Biological Tests and Assays 91

    Chemical Tests and Assays 126

    Physical Tests and Determinations 209

    General Information 375

    Dietary Supplement 717

Reagents, Indicators, and Solutions 747

    Reagent Specifications 751

    Indicators and Indicator Test Papers 808

    Chromatographic Reagents 810

    Solutions 813

        Buffer Solutions 813

        Colorimetric Solutions 814

        Test Solutions 814

        Volumetric Solutions 821

Reference Tables

    Containers for Dispensing Capsules and Tablets 831

    Description and Relative Solubility of *USP* and *NF* Articles 840

    Approximate Solubilities of *USP* and *NF* Articles 886

    Atomic Weights 895

    Alcoholometric Table 900

    Intrinsic Viscosity Table 902

    Thermometric Equivalents 905

Dietary Supplements

Official Monographs 907

NF 26

Admissions

Articles Admitted to *NF 26* by Supplement 1056

Revisions Appearing in *NF 26* That Were
Not Included in *NF 25* Including
Supplements............................. 1056

Excipients

USP and *NF* Excipients, Listed by
Category 1057

Notices

NF General Notices and Requirements 1062

Monographs

Official Monographs for *NF 26* 1063

Index

Combined Index to *USP 31* and *NF 26* I-1

VOLUME 2

Guide to General Chapters v

Notices

USP General Notices and Requirements ix

USP 30

Monographs

Official Monographs for *USP 31*, A–L 1265

Index

Combined Index to *USP 31* and *NF 26* I-1

VOLUME 3

Guide to General Chapters v

Notices

USP General Notices and Requirements ix

USP 31

Monographs

Official Monographs for *USP 31*, M–Z 2561

Index

Combined Index to *USP 31* and *NF 26* I-1

Guide to General Chapters

(For complete alphabet list of all general chapters in this Pharmacopeia, see under "General chapters" in the index.)

General Tests and Assays

General Requirements for Tests and Assays

⟨1⟩ Injections 33
⟨11⟩ USP Reference Standards 37

Apparatus for Tests and Assays

⟨16⟩ Automated Methods of Analysis 59
⟨21⟩ Thermometers 66
⟨31⟩ Volumetric Apparatus 66
⟨41⟩ Weights and Balances 67

Microbiological Tests

⟨51⟩ Antimicrobial Effectiveness Testing 67
⟨55⟩ Biological Indicators—Resistance Performance Tests 69
⟨61⟩ Microbial Limit Tests 71
⟨61⟩ Microbiological Examination of Nonsterile Products: Microbial Enumeration Tests (Harmonized Chapter, Official May 1, 2009) 76
⟨62⟩ Microbiological Examination of Nonsterile Products: Tests for Specified Microorganisms (Harmonized Chapter, Official May 1, 2009) 81
⟨71⟩ Sterility Tests 85

Biological Tests and Assays

⟨81⟩ Antibiotics—Microbial Assays 91
⟨85⟩ Bacterial Endotoxins Test 98
⟨87⟩ Biological Reactivity Tests, In Vitro 102
⟨88⟩ Biological Reactivity Tests, In Vivo 104
⟨91⟩ Calcium Pantothenate Assay 107
⟨111⟩ Design and Analysis of Biological Assays 108
⟨115⟩ Dexpanthenol Assay 120
⟨121⟩ Insulin Assays 121
⟨141⟩ Protein—Biological Adequacy Test 122
⟨151⟩ Pyrogen Test 123
⟨161⟩ Transfusion and Infusion Assemblies and Similar Medical Devices 124
⟨171⟩ Vitamin B_{12} Activity Assay 125

Chemical Tests and Assays

IDENTIFICATION TESTS

⟨181⟩ Identification—Organic Nitrogenous Bases 126
⟨191⟩ Identification Tests—General 127
⟨193⟩ Identification—Tetracyclines 129
⟨197⟩ Spectrophotometric Identification Tests 129
⟨201⟩ Thin-Layer Chromatographic Identification Test 130

LIMIT TESTS

⟨206⟩ Aluminum 131
⟨211⟩ Arsenic 131
⟨221⟩ Chloride and Sulfate 132
⟨223⟩ Dimethylaniline 132
⟨226⟩ 4-Epianhydrotetracycline 133
⟨231⟩ Heavy Metals 133
⟨241⟩ Iron 135
⟨251⟩ Lead 135
⟨261⟩ Mercury 136
⟨271⟩ Readily Carbonizable Substances Test 137
⟨281⟩ Residue on Ignition 137
⟨291⟩ Selenium 138

OTHER TESTS AND ASSAYS

⟨301⟩ Acid-Neutralizing Capacity 138
⟨311⟩ Alginates Assay 139
⟨331⟩ Amphetamine Assay 140
⟨341⟩ Antimicrobial Agents—Content 140
⟨345⟩ Assay for Citric Acid/Citrate and Phosphate 142
⟨351⟩ Assay for Steroids 143
⟨361⟩ Barbiturate Assay 143
⟨371⟩ Cobalamin Radiotracer Assay 143
⟨381⟩ Elastomeric Closures for Injections 144
⟨391⟩ Epinephrine Assay 145
⟨401⟩ Fats and Fixed Oils 145
⟨411⟩ Folic Acid Assay 149
⟨425⟩ Iodometric Assay—Antibiotics 150
⟨429⟩ Light Diffraction Measurement of Particle Size 150
⟨431⟩ Methoxy Determination 153
⟨441⟩ Niacin or Niacinamide Assay 154
⟨451⟩ Nitrite Titration 156
⟨461⟩ Nitrogen Determination 157
⟨466⟩ Ordinary Impurities 157
⟨467⟩ Organic Volatile Impurities 158
⟨467⟩ Residual Solvents (Harmonized Chapter, Official July 1, 2008) 170
⟨471⟩ Oxygen Flask Combustion 181
⟨481⟩ Riboflavin Assay 182
⟨501⟩ Salts of Organic Nitrogenous Bases 182
⟨511⟩ Single-Steroid Assay 183

⟨521⟩ Sulfonamides 183
⟨531⟩ Thiamine Assay 184
⟨541⟩ Titrimetry 185
⟨551⟩ Alpha Tocopherol Assay 187
⟨561⟩ Articles of Botanical Origin 188
⟨563⟩ Identification of Articles of Botanical Origin 195
⟨565⟩ Botanical Extracts 201
⟨571⟩ Vitamin A Assay 203
⟨581⟩ Vitamin D Assay 204
⟨591⟩ Zinc Determination 208

Physical Tests and Determinations

⟨601⟩ Aerosols, Nasal Sprays, Metered-Dose Inhalers,
and Dry Powder Inhalers 209
⟨611⟩ Alcohol Determination 230
⟨616⟩ Bulk Density and Tapped Density 231
⟨621⟩ Chromatography 232
⟨631⟩ Color and Achromicity 243
⟨641⟩ Completeness of Solution 244
⟨643⟩ Total Organic Carbon 244
⟨645⟩ Water Conductivity 245
⟨651⟩ Congealing Temperature 247
⟨660⟩ Containers—Glass 248
⟨661⟩ Containers—Plastic 251
⟨671⟩ Containers—Performance Testing 255
⟨681⟩ Repackaging into Single-Unit Containers and
Unit-Dose Containers for Nonsterile Solid
Liquid Dosage Forms 258
⟨691⟩ Cotton 259
⟨695⟩ Crystallinity 260
⟨696⟩ Crystallinity Determination by Solution
Calorimetry 261
⟨698⟩ Deliverable Volume 262
⟨699⟩ Density of Solids 265
⟨701⟩ Disintegration 266
⟨711⟩ Dissolution 267
⟨721⟩ Distilling Range 274
⟨724⟩ Drug Release 275
⟨726⟩ Electrophoresis 278
⟨727⟩ Capillary Electrophoresis 281
⟨729⟩ Globule Size Distribution in Lipid Injectable
Emulsions 285
⟨730⟩ Plasma Spectrochemistry 287
⟨731⟩ Loss on Drying 292
⟨733⟩ Loss on Ignition 293
⟨736⟩ Mass Spectrometry 293
⟨741⟩ Melting Range or Temperature 297
⟨751⟩ Metal Particles in Ophthalmic Ointments 298
⟨755⟩ Minimum Fill 298
⟨761⟩ Nuclear Magnetic Resonance 298
⟨771⟩ Ophthalmic Ointments 304
⟨776⟩ Optical Microscopy 304
⟨781⟩ Optical Rotation 306
⟨785⟩ Osmolality and Osmolarity 307
⟨786⟩ Particle Size Distribution Estimation by Analytical
Sieving 308
⟨788⟩ Particulate Matter in Injections 311
⟨789⟩ Particulate Matter in Ophthalmic Solutions 313
⟨791⟩ pH 314
⟨795⟩ Pharmaceutical Compounding—Nonsterile
Preparations 315
⟨797⟩ Pharmaceutical Compounding—Sterile
Preparations 319
⟨801⟩ Polarography 337
⟨811⟩ Powder Fineness 339
⟨821⟩ Radioactivity 340
⟨823⟩ Radiopharmaceuticals for Positron Emission
Tomography—Compounding 347
⟨831⟩ Refractive Index 351
⟨841⟩ Specific Gravity 351
⟨846⟩ Specific Surface Area 352
⟨851⟩ Spectrophotometry and Light-Scattering 355

⟨861⟩ Sutures—Diameter 360
⟨871⟩ Sutures—Needle Attachment 360
⟨881⟩ Tensile Strength 360
⟨891⟩ Thermal Analysis 362
⟨905⟩ Uniformity of Dosage Units 363
⟨911⟩ Viscosity 369
⟨921⟩ Water Determination 370
⟨941⟩ X-Ray Diffraction 372

General Information

⟨1005⟩ Acoustic Emission 375
⟨1010⟩ Analytical Data—Interpretation and
Treatment 378
⟨1015⟩ Automated Radiochemical Synthesis
Apparatus 389
⟨1031⟩ The Biocompatibility of Materials Used in Drug
Containers, Medical Devices, and Implants 390
⟨1035⟩ Biological Indicators for Sterilization 399
⟨1041⟩ Biologics 402
⟨1043⟩ Ancillary Materials for Cell, Gene, and Tissue-
Engineered Products 403
⟨1045⟩ Biotechnology-Derived Articles 409
⟨1046⟩ Cell and Gene Therapy Products 419
⟨1048⟩ Quality of Biotechnological Products: Analysis
of the Expression Construct in Cells Used for
Production of r-DNA Derived Protein
Products 449
⟨1049⟩ Quality of Biotechnological Products: Stability
Testing of Biotechnological/Biological
Products 450
⟨1050⟩ Viral Safety Evaluation of Biotechnology
Products Derived from Cell Lines of Human
or Animal Origin 453
⟨1051⟩ Cleaning Glass Apparatus 462
⟨1052⟩ Biotechnology-Derived Articles—Amino Acid
Analysis 463
⟨1053⟩ Biotechnology-Derived Articles—Capillary
Electrophoresis 471
⟨1054⟩ Biotechnology-Derived Articles—Isoelectric
Focusing 475
⟨1055⟩ Biotechnology-Derived Articles—Peptide
Mapping 477
⟨1056⟩ Biotechnology-Derived Articles—Polyacrylamide
Gel Electrophoresis 481
⟨1057⟩ Biotechnology-Derived Articles—Total Protein
Assay 486
⟨1061⟩ Color—Instrumental Measurement 489
⟨1065⟩ Ion Chromatography 490
⟨1070⟩ Emergency Medical Services Vehicles and
Ambulances—Storage of Preparations 493
⟨1072⟩ Disinfectants and Antiseptics 493
⟨1074⟩ Excipient Biological Safety Evaluation
Guidelines 497
⟨1075⟩ Good Compounding Practices 500
⟨1078⟩ Good Manufacturing Practices for Bulk
Pharmaceutical Excipients 503
⟨1079⟩ Good Storage and Shipping Practices 512
⟨1080⟩ Bulk Pharmaceutical Excipients—Certificate of
Analysis 517
⟨1081⟩ Gel Strength of Gelatin 523
⟨1086⟩ Impurities in Official Articles 523
⟨1087⟩ Intrinsic Dissolution 526
⟨1088⟩ In Vitro and In Vivo Evaluation of Dosage
Forms 527
⟨1090⟩ In Vivo Bioequivalence Guidances 532
⟨1091⟩ Labeling of Inactive Ingredients 572
⟨1092⟩ The Dissolution Procedure: Development
and Validation 573
⟨1101⟩ Medicine Dropper 578
⟨1111⟩ Microbiological Attributes of Nonsterile
Pharmaceutical Products 578

⟨1111⟩ Microbiological Examination of Nonsterile Products: Acceptance Criteria for Pharmaceutical Preparations and Substances for Pharmaceutical Use (Harmonized Chapter, Official May 1, 2009) 579
⟨1112⟩ Application of Water Activity Determination to Nonsterile Pharmaceutical Products 580
⟨1116⟩ Microbiological Evaluation of Clean Rooms and Other Controlled Environments 582
⟨1117⟩ Microbiological Best Laboratory Practices 589
⟨1118⟩ Monitoring Devices—Time, Temperature, and Humidity 593
⟨1119⟩ Near-Infrared Spectrophotometry 595
⟨1120⟩ Raman Spectrophotometry 599
⟨1121⟩ Nomenclature 605
⟨1136⟩ Packaging—Unit-of-Use 607
⟨1146⟩ Packaging Practice—Repackaging a Single Solid Oral Drug Product into a Unit-Dose Container 609
⟨1150⟩ Pharmaceutical Stability 613
⟨1151⟩ Pharmaceutical Dosage Forms 615
⟨1160⟩ Pharmaceutical Calculations in Prescription Compounding 626
⟨1163⟩ Quality Assurance in Pharmaceutical Compounding 634
⟨1171⟩ Phase-Solubility Analysis 638
⟨1174⟩ Powder Flow 639
⟨1176⟩ Prescription Balances and Volumetric Apparatus 642
⟨1177⟩ Good Packaging Practices 643
⟨1178⟩ Good Repackaging Practices 645
⟨1181⟩ Scanning Electron Microscopy 646
⟨1184⟩ Sensitization Testing 650
⟨1191⟩ Stability Considerations in Dispensing Practice 656
⟨1196⟩ Pharmacopeial Harmonization 659
⟨1207⟩ Sterile Product Packaging—Integrity Evaluation 664
⟨1208⟩ Sterility Testing—Validation of Isolator Systems 665

⟨1209⟩ Sterilization—Chemical and Physicochemical Indicators and Integrators 668
⟨1211⟩ Sterilization and Sterility Assurance of Compendial Articles 670
⟨1216⟩ Tablet Friability 675
⟨1217⟩ Tablet Breaking Force 676
⟨1221⟩ Teaspoon 678
⟨1222⟩ Terminally Sterilized Pharmaceutical Products— Parametric Release 678
⟨1223⟩ Validation of Alternative Microbiological Methods 681
⟨1225⟩ Validation of Compendial Procedures 683
⟨1226⟩ Verification of Compendial Procedures 687
⟨1227⟩ Validation of Microbial Recovery from Pharmacopeial Articles 687
⟨1230⟩ Water for Health Applications 690
⟨1231⟩ Water for Pharmaceutical Purposes 691
⟨1241⟩ Water–Solid Interactions in Pharmaceutical Systems 710
⟨1251⟩ Weighing on an Analytical Balance 712
⟨1265⟩ Written Prescription Drug Information— Guidelines 714

Dietary Supplements

⟨2021⟩ Microbial Enumeration Tests—Nutritional and Dietary Supplements 717
⟨2022⟩ Microbiological Procedures for Absence of Specified Microorganisms—Nutritional and Dietary Supplements 721
⟨2023⟩ Microbiological Attributes of Nonsterile Nutritional and Dietary Supplements 724
⟨2030⟩ Supplemental Information for Articles of Botanical Origin 727
⟨2040⟩ Disintegration and Dissolution of Dietary Supplements 732
⟨2091⟩ Weight Variation of Dietary Supplements 736
⟨2750⟩ Manufacturing Practices for Dietary Supplements 736

…

General Notices and Requirements

Applying to Standards, Tests, Assays, and Other Specifications of the United States Pharmacopeia

Title xi

"Official" and "Official Articles" xi
    Designating Conformance with Official Standards xi
    Products Not Marketed in the United States xi
    Nutritional and Other Dietary Supplements xi

Atomic Weights and Chemical Formulas xi

Abbreviations xii
    Abbreviated Statements in Monographs xii

Significant Figures and Tolerances xii
    Equivalence Statements in Titrimetric Procedures xii
    Tolerances xii
    Interpretation of Requirements xii

General Chapters xiii

Pharmacopeial Forum xiii
    Interim Revision Announcement xiii
    In-Process Revision xiii
    Pharmacopeial Previews xiii
    Stimuli to the Revision Process xiii
    Nomenclature xiii
    Official Reference Standards xiii

Supplements xiii

Reagent Standards xiii

Reference Reagents xiii

USP Reference Standards xiii

Units of Potency xiii

Ingredients and Processes xiii
    Water xiv
    Alcohol xiv
    Alcohol xiv
    Dehydrated Alcohol xiv
    Denatured Alcohol xiv
    Added Substances xiv
    Nutritional and Dietary Supplements xiv
    Additional Ingredients xiv
    Inert Headspace Gases xiv
    Colors xiv
    Ointments and Suppositories xiv

Tests and Assays xiv
    Apparatus xiv
    Steam Bath xiv
    Water Bath xv
    Foreign Substances and Impurities xv
    Other Impurities xv
    Residual Solvents xv
    Procedures xv
    Blank Determination xvi
    Desiccator xvi
    Dilution xvi
    Drying to Constant Weight xvi
    Filtration xvi
    Identification Tests xvi
    Ignition to Constant Weight xvi
    Indicators xvi
    Logarithms xvi
    Microbial Strains xvi
    Negligible xvi
    Odor xvi
    Pressure Measurements xvi
    Solutions xvi
    Specific Gravity xvi
    Temperatures xvi
    Time Limit xvi
    Vacuum xvi
    Water xvi
    Water and Loss on Drying xvi
    Test Results, Statistics, and Standards xvii
    Description xvii

x *General Notices* USP 31

Solubility xvii
Interchangeable Methods xvii

Prescribing and Dispensing xvii

Preservation, Packaging, Storage, and Labeling xvii
Containers xvii
Tamper-Evident Packaging xvii
Light-Resistant Container xvii
Well-Closed Container xvii
Tight Container xviii
Hermetic Container xviii
Single-Unit Container xviii
Single-Dose Container xviii
Unit-Dose Container xviii
Unit-of-Use Container xviii
Multiple-Unit Container xviii
Multiple-Dose Container xviii
Poison Prevention Packaging Act xviii
Storage Temperature and Humidity xviii
Freezer xviii
Cold xviii
Cool xviii
Controlled Cold Temperature xviii
Room Temperature xviii
Controlled Room Temperature xviii
Warm xviii
Excessive Heat xviii
Protection from Freezing xviii

Dry Place xviii
Storage under Nonspecific Conditions xix
Labeling xix
Amount of Ingredient per Dosage Unit xix
Use of Leading and Terminal Zeros xix
Labeling of Salts of Drugs xix
Labeling Vitamin-Containing Products xix
Labeling Botanical-Containing Products xix
Labeling Parenteral and Topical Preparations xix
Labeling Electrolytes xix
Labeling Alcohol xix
Special Capsules and Tablets xix
Expiration Date and Beyond-Use Date xix
Pharmaceutical Compounding xx
Guidelines for Packaging and Storage Statements in *USP–NF* **Monographs** xx

Vegetable and Animal Substances xx
Foreign Matter xx
Preservation xx

Weights and Measures xxi

Concentrations xxi
Percentage Measurements xxi
Percent Weight in Weight xxi
Percent Weight in Volume xxi
Percent Volume in Volume xxi

absorbances of the *Assay preparation* and the *Standard preparation*, respectively.

Magaldrate and Simethicone Tablets

(Current title—not to change until February 1, 2010)
Monograph title change—to become official February 1, 2010 See Magaldrate and Simethicone Chewable Tablets

» Magaldrate and Simethicone Tablets contain not less than 90.0 percent and not more than 110.0 percent of the labeled amount of magaldrate [$Al_5Mg_{10}(OH)_{31}(SO_4)_2$], and an amount of polydimethylsiloxane [$-(CH_3)_2SiO-$]$_n$ that is not less than 85.0 percent and not more than 115.0 percent of the labeled amount of simethicone.

Packaging and storage—Preserve in well-closed containers.
Labeling—Label the Tablets to indicate that they are to be chewed before being swallowed.
USP Reference standards ⟨11⟩—USP Magaldrate RS. USP Polydimethylsiloxane RS.
Identification—
A: Transfer a quantity of powdered Tablets, equivalent to about 2 g of magaldrate, to a 100-mL centrifuge tube. Add about 60 mL of water, cap, and shake for 3 minutes. Centrifuge the suspension, and discard the supernatant. Repeat the washing with three more 60-mL portions of water. Transfer the residue to a 250-mL beaker, and heat on a steam bath to dryness: the residue so obtained meets the requirements of the *Identification* tests under *Magaldrate*.
B: The IR absorption spectrum, in the 7- to 11-μm region, determined in a 0.5-mm cell, of the *Assay preparation* prepared as directed in the *Assay for polydimethylsiloxane*, exhibits maxima only at the same wavelengths as that of the *Standard preparation* containing about 2 mg of USP Polydimethylsiloxane RS per mL prepared as directed in the *Assay for polydimethylsiloxane*.
Microbial limits ⟨61⟩—Tablets meet the requirements of the test for absence of *Escherichia coli*.
Uniformity of dosage units ⟨905⟩: meet the requirements for *Weight Variation* with respect to magaldrate.
Acid-neutralizing capacity—Proceed as directed under *Acid-Neutralizing Capacity* ⟨301⟩. The acid consumed by the minimum single dose recommended in the labeling is not less than 5 mEq, and not less than the number of mEq calculated by the formula:

$$0.8(0.0282M)$$

in which 0.0282 is the theoretical acid-neutralizing capacity, in mEq per mg, of magaldrate; and *M* is the quantity, in mg, of the labeled amount of magaldrate.
Defoaming activity—
Foaming solution and *System suitability tests*—Proceed as directed in the test for *Defoaming activity* under *Magaldrate and Simethicone Oral Suspension*.
Procedure—[NOTE—For each test use a clean 250-mL cylindrical jar (50-mm internal diameter × 110-mm internal height) with a 50-mm opening fitted with a tight cap with an inert liner.] Transfer a quantity of finely powdered Tablets, equivalent to 20 mg of simethicone, to a 250-mL cylindrical jar containing 50 mL of 0.6 N hydrochloric acid that has been warmed to 37°, and proceed as directed in the test for *Defoaming activity* under *Magaldrate and Simethicone Oral Suspension*, beginning with "Cap the jar." Record the time, in seconds, for the foam to collapse to the extent that its thickness, measured from the surface of the liquid, is 1.0 cm. The defoaming activity time does not exceed 45 seconds.
Magnesium hydroxide content—
Test preparation—Weigh and finely powder not fewer than 20 Tablets. Transfer an accurately weighed portion of the powder, equivalent to about 1 g of magaldrate, to a 100-mL volumetric flask, add 30 mL of dilute hydrochloric acid (1 in 10), shake for 15 minutes, dilute with water to volume, and mix.

Procedure—Transfer 10.0 mL of *Test preparation* to a 400-mL beaker, and proceed as directed in the test for *Magnesium hydroxide content* under *Magaldrate*, beginning with "and dilute with water to about 200 mL." Not less than 492 mg and not more than 666 mg of magnesium hydroxide [$Mg(OH)_2$] per g of the labeled amount of magaldrate is found.
Aluminum hydroxide content—
Edetate disodium titrant—Prepare and standardize as directed in the *Assay* under *Ammonium Alum*.
Test preparation—Prepare as directed in the test for *Magnesium hydroxide content*.
Procedure—Transfer 10.0 mL of *Test preparation* and 20 mL of water to a 250-mL beaker, and proceed as directed for *Procedure* in the test for *Aluminum hydroxide content* under *Magaldrate*, beginning with "Add, with stirring, 25.0 mL of *Edetate disodium*." Not less than 321 mg and not more than 459 mg of aluminum hydroxide [$Al(OH)_3$] per g of the labeled amount of magaldrate is found.
Assay for magaldrate—Weigh and finely powder not fewer than 20 Tablets. Transfer an accurately weighed portion of the powder, equivalent to about 6 g of magaldrate, to a 200-mL volumetric flask. Add 100.0 mL of 2 N hydrochloric acid VS, and swirl by mechanical means for 30 minutes. Dilute with water to volume, mix, and filter. Transfer 100.0 mL of the filtrate to a beaker. Titrate the excess acid with 1 N sodium hydroxide VS to a pH of 3.0, determined potentiometrically. Perform a blank determination (see *Residual Titrations* under *Titrimetry* ⟨541⟩). Each mL of 2 N hydrochloric acid is equivalent to 70.80 mg of $Al_5Mg_{10}(OH)_{31}(SO_4)_2$.
Assay for polydimethylsiloxane—Weigh and finely powder not fewer than 20 Tablets. Transfer an accurately weighed portion of the powder, equivalent to about 20 mg of simethicone, to a 60-mL separator. Add 10.0 mL of hexanes and 25 mL of 6 N hydrochloric acid, cap the separator, and shake by mechanical means for not less than 2 hours. Allow to stand for about 10 minutes, and drain off as much of the lower, aqueous layer as possible without removing any of the unseparated interphase. Add 25 mL of 4 N sodium hydroxide to the separator, cap it, and shake by mechanical means for 1 hour. Transfer the mixture from the separator to a 50-mL centrifuge tube, cap, and centrifuge to obtain clear layers. Transfer not less than 5 mL of the clear upper hexanes layer to a test tube containing about 0.5 g of anhydrous sodium sulfate. Cap the tube, shake vigorously, and allow to stand to obtain a clear supernatant (*Assay preparation*). Prepare three *Standard preparations* in hexanes having known concentrations of about 1.6, 2.0, and 2.4 mg of USP Polydimethylsiloxane RS per mL, respectively. Concomitantly determine the absorbances of the *Assay preparation* and the *Standard preparations* in a 0.5-mm cell at the wavelength of maximum absorbance at about 1260 cm^{-1} with an IR spectrophotometer, using hexanes as the blank. [NOTE—Between each measurement, rinse the cell with heptane, empty, and dry it.] Plot the absorbances for the *Standard preparations* versus concentration, in mg per mL, of USP Polydimethylsiloxane RS, and draw the straight line best fitting the three plotted points. From the graph so obtained, determine the concentration, *C*, in mg per mL, of polydimethylsiloxane in the *Assay preparation*. Calculate the quantity, in mg, of [$-(CH_3)_2SiO-$]$_n$ in the portion of Tablets taken by multiplying *C* by 10.

Magaldrate and Simethicone Chewable Tablets

(Monograph under this new title—to become official February 1, 2010)
(Current monograph title is Magaldrate and Simethicone Tablets)

» Magaldrate and Simethicone Chewable Tablets contain not less than 90.0 percent and not more than 110.0 percent of the labeled amount of magaldrate [$Al_5Mg_{10}(OH)_{31}(SO_4)_2$], and an amount of polydimethylsiloxane [$-(CH_3)_2SiO-$]$_n$ that is not less than 85.0 per-

Magaldrate and Simethicone Oral Suspension

» Magaldrate and Simethicone Oral Suspension contains not less than 90.0 percent and not more than 110.0 percent of the labeled amount of magaldrate [$Al_5Mg_{10}(OH)_{31}(SO_4)_2$], and an amount of polydimethylsiloxane [$-(CH_3)_2SiO-$]$_n$ that is not less than 85.0 percent and not more than 115.0 percent of the labeled amount of simethicone.

Packaging and storage—Preserve in tight containers, and keep from freezing.

USP Reference standards ⟨11⟩—USP Magaldrate RS. USP Polydimethylsiloxane RS.

Identification—

A: Dissolve an amount of Oral Suspension, equivalent to about 800 mg of magaldrate, in 20 mL of 3 N hydrochloric acid, dilute with water to about 50 mL, add 3 drops of methyl red TS, and proceed as directed in *Identification* test A under *Magaldrate*, beginning with "and heat to boiling."

B: Wash the precipitate obtained in *Identification* test A with hot ammonium chloride solution (1 in 50), and dissolve the precipitate in hydrochloric acid. Divide this solution into two portions: the dropwise addition of 6 N ammonium hydroxide to one portion yields a gelatinous white precipitate, which does not dissolve in an excess of 6 N ammonium hydroxide. The dropwise addition of 1 N sodium hydroxide to the other portion yields a gelatinous white precipitate, which dissolves in an excess of 1 N sodium hydroxide, leaving some turbidity.

C: Transfer an amount of Oral Suspension, equivalent to about 1 g of magaldrate, to a 100-mL centrifuge tube. Add about 60 mL of water, insert the cap, and shake for 3 minutes. Centrifuge the suspension, and discard the supernatant. Repeat the washing of the residue with three 60-mL portions of water. Transfer the residue to a 250-mL beaker, and heat on a steam bath to dryness: the X-ray diffraction pattern (see *X-ray Diffraction* ⟨941⟩), in the d-spacings region below 2.57 angstrom units, of the residue so obtained conforms to that of USP Magaldrate RS.

D: The IR absorption spectrum, in the 7- to 15-μm region, determined in a 0.1-mm cell, of the *Assay preparation* prepared as directed in the *Assay for polydimethylsiloxane* exhibits maxima only at the same wavelengths as that of the *Standard preparation* prepared as directed in the *Assay for polydimethylsiloxane*.

Microbial limits ⟨61⟩—Its total aerobic microbial count does not exceed 100 cfu per mL, and it meets the requirements of the test for absence of *Escherichia coli*.

Acid-neutralizing capacity ⟨301⟩—The acid consumed by the minimum single dose recommended in the labeling is not less than 5 mEq, and not less than the number of mEq calculated by the formula:

$$0.8(0.0282M)$$

in which 0.0282 is the theoretical acid-neutralizing capacity, in mEq per mg, of magaldrate; and M is the quantity, in mg, of the labeled amount of magaldrate.

Defoaming activity—

Foaming solution—Dissolve 5 mg of FD&C Blue No. 1 and 10 g of polyoxyethylene (23) lauryl ether in 1000 mL of water. Warm to 37° before use.

Procedure—[NOTE—For each test use a clean 250-mL cylindrical jar (50-mm internal diameter × 110-mm internal height) with a 50-mm opening fitted with a tight cap with an inert liner.] Transfer a volume of well-mixed Oral Suspension, equivalent to 20 mg of simethicone, to a 250-mL cylindrical jar containing 50 mL of 0.6 N hydrochloric acid that has been warmed to 37°. Cap the jar, and clamp it in an upright position on a wrist-action shaker. Employing a radius of 13.3 ± 0.4 cm (measured from the center of shaft to center of bottle), shake for 30 seconds through an arc of 10 degrees at a frequency of 300 ± 30 strokes per minute. Uncap the jar, add 50 mL of *Foaming solution*, recap the jar, and shake for 10 seconds using the conditions specified above. Record the time required for the foam to collapse. The time, in seconds, for foam collapse is determined at the instant the first portion of foam-free liquid surface appears, measured from the end of the shaking period. The defoaming activity time does not exceed 45 seconds.

System suitability tests—[NOTE—For each of the following tests use a separate clean 250-mL cylindrical jar having the dimensions specified for *Procedure*.] Transfer 50 mL of *Foaming solution* to a 250-mL cylindrical jar containing 50 mL of 0.6 N hydrochloric acid that has been warmed to 37°. Cap the jar, and shake it for 10 seconds using the conditions specified for *Procedure*: the foam layer remains intact for not less than 5 minutes. Transfer 0.15 mL of simethicone and 50 mL of *Foaming solution* to a second 250-mL cylindrical jar containing 50 mL of 0.6 N hydrochloric acid that has been warmed to 37°. Cap the jar, and shake it for 10 seconds using the conditions specified for *Procedure*: the time required for the foam to collapse does not exceed 45 seconds.

Magnesium hydroxide content—

Test preparation—Transfer an accurately measured quantity of Oral Suspension, equivalent to about 1 g of magaldrate, to a 100-mL volumetric flask, add 30 mL of dilute hydrochloric acid (1 in 10), shake to dissolve, dilute with water to volume, and mix.

Procedure—Transfer 10.0 mL of *Test preparation* to a 400-mL beaker, and proceed as directed in the test for *Magnesium hydroxide content* under *Magaldrate*, beginning with "and dilute with water to about 200 mL." Not less than 492 mg and not more than 666 mg of magnesium hydroxide [$Mg(OH)_2$] per g of the labeled amount of magaldrate is found.

Aluminum hydroxide content—

Edetate disodium titrant—Prepare and standardize as directed in the *Assay* under *Ammonium Alum*.

Test preparation—Prepare as directed in the test for *Magnesium hydroxide content*.

Procedure—Transfer 10.0 mL of *Test preparation* and 20 mL of water to a 250-mL beaker, and proceed as directed for *Procedure* in the test for *Aluminum hydroxide content* under *Magaldrate*, beginning with "Add, with stirring, 25.0 mL of *Edetate disodium titrant*." Not less than 321 mg and not more than 459 mg of aluminum hydroxide [$Al(OH)_3$] per g of the labeled amount of magaldrate is found.

Other requirements—Evaporate a volume of Oral Suspension, equivalent to about 5 g of magaldrate, on a steam bath to dryness: the residue so obtained meets the requirements of the tests for *Arsenic* and *Heavy metals* under *Magaldrate*.

Assay for magaldrate—Transfer an accurately measured quantity of Oral Suspension, equivalent to about 3 g of magaldrate, to a beaker. Add 100.0 mL of 1 N hydrochloric acid VS, and mix, using a magnetic stirrer to achieve dissolution. Titrate the excess acid with 1 N sodium hydroxide VS to a pH of 3.0, determined potentiometrically. Perform a blank determination (see *Residual Titrations* under *Titrimetry* ⟨541⟩). Each mL of 1 N hydrochloric acid is equivalent to 35.40 mg of magaldrate [$Al_5Mg_{10}(OH)_{31}(SO_4)_2$].

Assay for polydimethylsiloxane—Transfer an accurately measured quantity of Oral Suspension, equivalent to about 250 mg of simethicone, to a 200-mL centrifuge bottle. Add an equal volume of hydrochloric acid, swirl to dissolve the Oral Suspension, add 25.0 mL of hexanes, and immediately close the bottle securely with a cap having an inert liner. Shake the bottle for 30 minutes, and centrifuge the mixture until a clear supernatant layer is obtained (*Assay preparation*). Prepare a *Standard preparation* of USP Polydimethylsiloxane RS in hexanes having a known concentration of about 10 mg per mL. Concomitantly determine the absorbances of the *Assay preparation* and the *Standard preparation* in 0.1-mm cells at the wavelength of maximum absorbance at about 7.9 μm and at the wavelengths of minimum absorbance at about 7.5 μm and 8.3 μm, with a suitable IR spectrophotometer, using hexanes as the blank. Draw a linear baseline between the two minima, and determine the absorbances for the *Standard preparation* and the *Assay preparation* with respect to the baseline, making any necessary correction for the blank. Calculate the quantity, in mg, of [$-(CH_3)_2SiO-$]$_n$ in the portion of Oral Suspension taken by the formula:

$$25C(A_U / A_S)$$

in which C is the concentration, in mg per mL, of USP Polydimethylsiloxane RS in the *Standard preparation*; and A_U and A_S are the

Titrimetry ⟨541⟩). Each mL of 1 N hydrochloric acid is equivalent to 35.40 mg of Al$_5$Mg$_{10}$(OH)$_{31}$(SO$_4$)$_2$.

Magaldrate Oral Suspension

» Magaldrate Oral Suspension contains not less than 90.0 percent and not more than 110.0 percent of the labeled amount of magaldrate [Al$_5$Mg$_{10}$(OH)$_{31}$(SO$_4$)$_2$].

Packaging and storage—Preserve in tight containers.
USP Reference standards ⟨11⟩—*USP Magaldrate RS*.
Identification—
A: Dissolve an amount of Oral Suspension, equivalent to about 800 mg of magaldrate, in 20 mL of 3 N hydrochloric acid, dilute with water to about 50 mL, add 3 drops of methyl red TS, and proceed as directed in *Identification* test A under *Magaldrate*, beginning with "and heat to boiling."
B: It responds to *Identification* test B under *Magaldrate*.
C: Transfer an amount of Oral Suspension, equivalent to about 1 g of magaldrate, to a 100-mL centrifuge tube. Add about 60 mL of water, cap, and shake for 3 minutes. Centrifuge the suspension, and discard the supernatant. Repeat the washing of the residue with three 60-mL portions of water. Transfer the residue to a 250-mL beaker, and heat on a steam bath to dryness: the X-ray diffraction pattern (see *X-ray Diffraction* ⟨941⟩), in the d-spacings region below 2.57 angstrom units, of the residue so obtained conforms to that of USP Magaldrate RS.
Microbial limits ⟨61⟩—Its total aerobic microbial count does not exceed 100 cfu per mL, and it meets the requirements of the test for absence of *Escherichia coli*.
Acid-neutralizing capacity ⟨301⟩—The acid consumed by the minimum single dose recommended in the labeling is not less than 5 mEq, and not less than the number of mEq calculated by the formula:

$$0.8(0.0282M)$$

in which 0.0282 is the theoretical acid-neutralizing capacity, in mEq per mg, of magaldrate, and M is the quantity, in mg, of the labeled amount of magaldrate.
Magnesium hydroxide content—
Test preparation—Transfer an accurately measured quantity of Oral Suspension, equivalent to about 1 g of magaldrate, to a 100-mL volumetric flask, add 30 mL of dilute hydrochloric acid (1 in 10), shake to dissolve, dilute with water to volume, and mix.
Procedure—Transfer 10.0 mL of *Test preparation* to a 400-mL beaker, and proceed as directed in the test for *Magnesium hydroxide content* under *Magaldrate*, beginning with "and dilute with water to about 200 mL." Not less than 492 mg and not more than 666 mg of magnesium hydroxide [Mg(OH)$_2$] per g of the labeled amount of magaldrate is found.
Aluminum hydroxide content—
Edetate disodium titrant—Prepare and standardize as directed in the *Assay* under *Ammonium Alum*.
Test preparation—Prepare as directed in the test for *Magnesium hydroxide content*.
Procedure—Transfer 10.0 mL of *Test preparation* and 20 mL of water to a 250-mL beaker, and proceed as directed for *Procedure* in the test for *Aluminum hydroxide content* under *Magaldrate*, beginning with "Add, with stirring, 25.0 mL of *Edetate disodium titrant*." Not less than 321 mg and not more than 459 mg of aluminum hydroxide [Al(OH)$_3$] per g of the labeled amount of magaldrate is found.
Other requirements—Evaporate a volume of Oral Suspension, equivalent to about 5 g of magaldrate, on a steam bath to dryness: the residue so obtained meets the requirements of the tests for *Arsenic* and *Heavy metals* under *Magaldrate*.
Assay—Transfer an accurately measured quantity of Oral Suspension, equivalent to about 3 g of magaldrate, to a beaker. Add 100.0 mL of 1 N hydrochloric acid VS, and mix, using a magnetic stirrer to achieve dissolution. Titrate the excess acid with 1 N sodium hydroxide VS to a pH of 3.0, determined potentiometrically. Perform a blank determination (see *Residual Titrations* under *Titrimetry* ⟨541⟩). Each mL of 1 N hydrochloric acid is equivalent to 35.40 mg of Al$_5$Mg$_{10}$(OH)$_{31}$(SO$_4$)$_2$.

Magaldrate Tablets

» Magaldrate Tablets contain not less than 90.0 percent and not more than 110.0 percent of the labeled amount of magaldrate [Al$_5$Mg$_{10}$(OH)$_{31}$(SO$_4$)$_2$].

Packaging and storage—Preserve in well-closed containers.
Labeling—Label the Tablets to indicate whether they are to be swallowed or to be chewed.
USP Reference standards ⟨11⟩—*USP Magaldrate RS*.
Identification—Transfer a quantity of powdered Tablets, equivalent to about 2 g of magaldrate, to a 100-mL centrifuge tube. Add about 60 mL of water, cap, and shake for 3 minutes. Centrifuge the suspension, and discard the supernatant. Repeat the washing with three more 60-mL portions of water. Transfer the residue to a 250-mL beaker, and heat on a steam bath to dryness: the residue so obtained meets the requirements of the *Identification* tests under *Magaldrate*.
Microbial limits ⟨61⟩—Tablets meet the requirements of the test for absence of *Escherichia coli*.
Disintegration ⟨701⟩: 2 minutes, for Tablets labeled to be swallowed.
Uniformity of dosage units ⟨905⟩: meet the requirements for *Weight Variation*.
Acid-neutralizing capacity—Proceed as directed under *Acid-Neutralizing Capacity* ⟨301⟩. The acid consumed by the minimum single dose recommended in the labeling is not less than 5 mEq, and not less than the number of mEq calculated by the formula:

$$0.8(0.0282M)$$

in which 0.0282 is the theoretical acid-neutralizing capacity, in mEq per mg, of magaldrate; and M is the quantity, in mg, of the labeled amount of magaldrate.
Magnesium hydroxide content—
Test preparation—Weigh and finely powder not fewer than 20 Tablets. Transfer an accurately weighed portion of the powder, equivalent to about 1 g of magaldrate, to a 100-mL volumetric flask, add 30 mL of dilute hydrochloric acid (1 in 10), shake for 15 minutes, dilute with water to volume, and mix.
Procedure—Transfer 10.0 mL of *Test preparation* to a 400-mL beaker, and proceed as directed in the test for *Magnesium hydroxide content* under *Magaldrate*, beginning with "and dilute with water to about 200 mL." Not less than 492 mg and not more than 666 mg of magnesium hydroxide [Mg(OH)$_2$] per g of the labeled amount of magaldrate is found.
Aluminum hydroxide content—
Edetate disodium titrant—Prepare and standardize as directed in the *Assay* under *Ammonium Alum*.
Test preparation—Prepare as directed in the test for *Magnesium hydroxide content*.
Procedure—Transfer 10.0 mL of *Test preparation* and 20 mL of water to a 250-mL beaker, and proceed as directed for *Procedure* in the test for *Aluminum hydroxide content* under *Magaldrate*, beginning with "Add, with stirring, 25.0 mL of *Edetate disodium titrant*." Not less than 321 mg and not more than 459 mg of aluminum hydroxide [Al(OH)$_3$] per g of the labeled amount of magaldrate is found.
Assay—Weigh and finely powder not fewer than 20 Tablets. Transfer an accurately weighed portion of the powder, equivalent to about 6 g of magaldrate, to a 200-mL volumetric flask. Add 100.0 mL of 2 N hydrochloric acid VS, and swirl by mechanical means for 30 minutes. Dilute with water to volume, mix, and filter. Transfer 100.0 mL of the filtrate to a beaker. Titrate the excess acid with 1 N sodium hydroxide VS to a pH of 3.0, determined potentiometrically. Perform a blank determination (see *Residual Titrations* under *Titrimetry* ⟨541⟩). Each mL of 2 N hydrochloric acid is equivalent to 70.80 mg of Al$_5$Mg$_{10}$(OH)$_{31}$(SO$_4$)$_2$.

is about 1.0 mL per minute. Chromatograph the *Standard preparation*, and record the peak responses as directed for *Procedure:* the relative standard deviation for replicate injections is not more than 2.0%.

Procedure—Separately inject equal volumes (about 20 µL) of the *Standard preparation* and the *Assay preparation* into the chromatograph, record the chromatograms, and measure the responses for the major peaks. Calculate the quantity, in mg, of mafenide acetate ($C_7H_{10}N_2O_2S \cdot C_2H_4O_2$) in the portion of the constituted Topical Solution taken by the formula:

$$25C(r_U / r_S)$$

in which C is the concentration, in mg per mL, of USP Mafenide Acetate RS in the *Standard preparation;* and r_U and r_S are the peak responses obtained from the *Assay preparation* and the *Standard preparation*, respectively.

Magaldrate

Aluminum magnesium hydroxide sulfate ($Al_5Mg_{10}(OH)_{31}(SO_4)_2 \cdot xH_2O$).
Aluminum magnesium hydroxide sulfate, hydrate [74978-16-8].
Anhydrous 1097.38

» Magaldrate is a chemical combination of aluminum and magnesium hydroxides and sulfate, corresponding approximately to the formula:

$$Al_5Mg_{10}(OH)_{31}(SO_4)_2 \cdot xH_2O.$$

It contains the equivalent of not less than 90.0 percent and not more than 105.0 percent of $Al_5Mg_{10}(OH)_{31}(SO_4)_2$, calculated on the dried basis.

Packaging and storage—Preserve in well-closed containers.

USP Reference standards ⟨11⟩—USP Magaldrate RS.

Identification—

A: Dissolve about 600 mg in 20 mL of 3 N hydrochloric acid, add 3 drops of methyl red TS and about 30 mL of water, and heat to boiling. Add 6 N ammonium hydroxide until the color just changes to yellow, continue boiling for 2 minutes, and filter: the filtrate responds to the tests for *Magnesium* ⟨191⟩.

B: Wash the precipitate obtained in *Identification* test A with 50 mL of hot ammonium chloride solution (1 in 50), then dissolve the precipitate in 15 mL of 3 N hydrochloric acid: the solution responds to the tests for *Aluminum* ⟨191⟩.

C: Its X-ray diffraction pattern (see *X-ray Diffraction* ⟨941⟩) in the d-spacings region below 0.257 nm (2.57 angstrom units) conforms to that of USP Magaldrate RS.

Microbial limits ⟨61⟩—It meets the requirements of the test for absence of *Escherichia coli*.

Loss on drying ⟨731⟩—Dry it at 200° for 4 hours: it loses between 10.0% and 20.0% of its weight.

Soluble chloride—Boil 1 g of it, accurately weighed, with 50.0 mL of water for 5 minutes, cool, add water to restore the original volume, mix, and filter. To 25.0 mL of the filtrate add 0.1 mL of potassium chromate TS, and titrate with 0.10 N silver nitrate until a persistent pink color is obtained: not more than 5.0 mL of 0.10 N silver nitrate is required (3.5%).

Soluble sulfate ⟨221⟩—A 2.5-mL portion of the filtrate obtained in the test for *Soluble chloride* shows no more sulfate than corresponds to 1.0 mL of 0.020 N sulfuric acid (1.9%).

Sodium—Transfer 2 g of it, accurately weighed, to a 100-mL volumetric flask, place in an ice bath, add 5 mL of nitric acid, and swirl to dissolve. Allow to warm to room temperature, dilute with water to volume, and mix. Filter, if necessary, to obtain a clear solution. Dilute 10.0 mL of the filtrate with water to 100.0 mL: the emission intensity of this solution, determined with a suitable flame photometer at 589 nm and corrected for background transmission at 580 nm, is not greater than that produced by a standard containing 2.2 µg of Na per mL, similarly measured (0.11%).

Arsenic, *Method I* ⟨211⟩: 8 ppm.

Heavy metals ⟨231⟩—Dissolve 330 mg in 10 mL of 3 N hydrochloric acid, filter if necessary to obtain a clear solution, and dilute with water to 25 mL: the limit is 0.006%.

Organic volatile impurities, *Method V* ⟨467⟩: meets the requirements.

Solvent—Use dimethyl sulfoxide.

(Official until July 1, 2008)

Magnesium hydroxide content—Dissolve about 100 mg, accurately weighed, in 3 mL of dilute hydrochloric acid (1 in 10), and dilute with water to about 200 mL. Add, with stirring, 1 g of ammonium chloride, 20 mL of triethanolamine, 10 mL of ammonia–ammonium chloride buffer TS, and 0.1 mL of eriochrome black TS, and titrate with 0.05 M edetate disodium VS to a blue color. Perform a blank determination, and make any necessary correction. Each mL of 0.05 M edetate disodium is equivalent to 2.916 mg of $Mg(OH)_2$: between 49.2% and 66.6% of $Mg(OH)_2$ is found, calculated on the dried basis.

Aluminum hydroxide content—

Edetate disodium titrant—Prepare and standardize as directed in the *Assay* under *Ammonium Alum*.

Procedure—Dissolve about 100 mg of Magaldrate, accurately weighed, in 3 mL of dilute hydrochloric acid (1 in 10), and dilute with water to about 30 mL. Add, with stirring, 25.0 mL of *Edetate disodium titrant*, mix, and allow to stand for 5 minutes. Then add 20 mL of acetic acid-ammonium acetate buffer TS, 60 mL of alcohol, and 2 mL of dithizone TS, and titrate with 0.05 M zinc sulfate to a bright rose-pink color. Perform a blank determination, and make any necessary correction. Each mL of 0.05 M *Edetate disodium titrant* is equivalent to 3.900 mg of $Al(OH)_3$: between 32.1% and 45.9% of $Al(OH)_3$ is found, calculated on the dried basis.

Sulfate content—

Chromatographic column—Transfer 15 mL of strongly acidic 50- to 100-mesh styrene-divinylbenzene cation-exchange resin to a 1-cm inside diameter glass column. Wash the resin with 30 mL of water.

Indicator solution—Prepare a solution in water containing 2 mg of sodium alizarinsulfonate per mL.

Magnesium acetate solution—Dissolve 26.8 g of magnesium acetate in 500 mL of water.

0.05 M Barium chloride—Dissolve 12.2 g of barium chloride in about 900 mL of water, adjust with 1 N hydrochloric acid to a pH of 3.0, dilute with water to 1000 mL, and mix. Standardize this solution as follows: Transfer 10.0 mL of 0.1 N sulfuric acid VS to a 125-mL conical flask. Adjust by adding *Magnesium acetate solution* to a pH of 3.0. Add 25 mL of methanol and 3 or 4 drops of *Indicator solution*. Add from a buret an accurately measured volume of 8 to 9 mL of 0.05 M barium chloride. Add an additional 4 drops of *Indicator solution*, and titrate slowly until the yellow color disappears and a pink tinge is visible. Calculate the molarity of the barium chloride titrant taken by the formula:

$$5(N / V)$$

in which N is the normality of the sulfuric acid; and V is the volume, in mL, of titrant consumed.

Test preparation—Transfer about 875 mg of Magaldrate, accurately weighed, to a 25-mL volumetric flask. Dissolve in 10 mL of water and 5 mL of glacial acetic acid, dilute with water to volume, and mix. Transfer 5.0 mL of this solution to the chromatographic column and wash the column with 15 mL of water, collecting the eluate in a 125-mL conical flask (*Test preparation*).

Procedure—Add to the *Test preparation* 5 mL of *Magnesium acetate solution*, 32 mL of methanol, and 3 or 4 drops of *Indicator solution*. Add from a buret an accurately measured volume of 5.0 to 5.5 mL of 0.05 M barium chloride. Add an additional 3 drops of *Indicator solution*, and titrate slowly until the yellow color disappears and a pink tinge is visible. Each mL of 0.05 M barium chloride is equivalent to 4.803 mg of sulfate (SO_4): between 16.0% and 21.0% of SO_4 is found, calculated on the dried basis.

Assay—Transfer about 3 g of Magaldrate, accurately weighed, to a 250-mL beaker, add 100.0 mL of 1 N hydrochloric acid VS, and stir until the solution becomes clear. Titrate the excess acid with 1 N sodium hydroxide VS to a pH of 3.0, determined potentiometrically. Perform a blank determination (see *Residual Titrations* under flask, add 1 mL of 1 N hydrochloric acid, add water to volume, and mix.

Procedure—Concomitantly determine the absorbances of the *Standard preparation* and the *Assay preparation* in 1-cm cells at the wavelength of maximum absorbance at about 267 nm, with a suitable spectrophotometer, using 0.01 N hydrochloric acid as the blank. Calculate the quantity, in mg, of $C_7H_{10}N_2O_2S \cdot C_2H_4O_2$ in the portion of Cream taken by the formula:

$$0.5C(A_U / A_S)$$

in which C is the concentration, in µg per mL, of USP Mafenide Acetate RS in the *Standard preparation*, and A_U and A_S are the absorbances of the solutions from the *Assay preparation* and the *Standard preparation*, respectively.

Mafenide Acetate for Topical Solution

» Mafenide Acetate for Topical Solution contains not less than 98.0 percent and not more than 102.0 percent of mafenide acetate ($C_7H_{10}N_2O_2S \cdot C_2H_4O_2$), calculated on the anhydrous basis.

Packaging and storage—Preserve in tight, light-resistant containers, at controlled room temperature. For prepared solutions, use within 48 hours of preparation.

USP Reference standards ⟨11⟩—*USP Mafenide Acetate RS. USP Mafenide Related Compound A RS.*

Identification—
 A: *Infrared Absorption ⟨197K⟩.*
 B: The retention time of the major peak in the chromatogram of the *Assay preparation* corresponds to that in the chromatogram of the *Standard preparation,* as obtained in the *Assay.*

Chromatographic purity—
 Ion-pairing solution and *Mobile phase*—Proceed as directed in the *Assay.*
 Concentrated standard solution—Prepare a solution of USP Mafenide Related Compound A RS in *Mobile phase* having a known concentration of about 25 µg per mL. [NOTE—USP Mafenide Related Compound A RS is 4-formylbenzenesulfonamide.]
 Working standard solution—Pipet 10.0 mL of *Concentrated standard solution* into a 50-mL volumetric flask, dilute with *Mobile phase* to volume, and mix.
 System suitability solution—Transfer about 10 mg of USP Mafenide Acetate RS, accurately weighed, to a 10-mL volumetric flask, and dissolve by sonication in about 2 mL of *Mobile phase*. Pipet 4.0 mL of *Concentrated standard solution* into the same flask, dilute with *Mobile phase* to volume, and mix.
 Standard solution—Pipet 10.0 mL of *Working standard solution* into a 50-mL volumetric flask, dilute with *Mobile phase* to volume, and mix.
 Test solution—Use the *Assay preparation.*
 Chromatographic system—Prepare as directed in the *Assay.* Chromatograph the *System suitability solution,* and record the peak responses as directed for *Procedure:* the resolution, *R,* between mafenide acetate and mafenide related compound A is not less than 3.0; and the tailing factor is not more than 2.0. Chromatograph the *Working standard solution,* and record the peak responses as directed for *Procedure:* the relative standard deviation for replicate injections is not more than 2.0%. Chromatograph the *Standard solution,* and record the peak responses as directed for *Procedure:* adjust the integration parameters so that the response is between 5% and 15% of full-scale deflection.
 Procedure—Separately inject equal volumes (about 20 µL) of the *Mobile phase,* the *Working standard solution,* and the *Test solution* into the chromatograph, allowing the *Test solution* to elute for a period of not less than three times the retention time of mafenide acetate; record the chromatograms, and measure the responses for the major peaks, disregarding the peaks corresponding to those obtained from the *Mobile phase.* Calculate the percentage of each impurity in the portion of the constituted Topical Solution taken by the formula:

$$100C(r_i / r_S)$$

in which C is the concentration, in mg per mL, of USP Mafenide Related Compound A RS in the *Working standard solution;* r_i is the peak response for each impurity obtained from the *Test solution;* and r_S is the peak response of mafenide related compound A obtained from the *Working standard solution:* not more than 0.5% of any individual impurity is found; and not more than 1.0% of total impurities is found.

Content of acetic acid—
 Internal standard solution—Dissolve 0.5 mL of propionic acid in 100.0 mL of water.
 Standard solution—Transfer about 50 mL of water to a 100-mL volumetric flask, insert a stopper, and weigh. Add 0.5 mL of glacial acetic acid to the flask, insert the stopper, weigh, and calculate, by difference, the amount of acetic acid added. Dilute with water to volume, and mix.
 Test solution—Constitute the Topical Solution as directed in the labeling. Transfer an accurately measured volume of the constituted Topical Solution, equivalent to about 200 mg of mafenide acetate, to a 100-mL volumetric flask containing 200 mg of oxalic acid. Pipet 10.0 mL of *Internal standard solution* into the flask, dilute with water to volume, and mix.
 Chromatographic system (see *Chromatography ⟨621⟩*)—The gas chromatograph is equipped with a flame-ionization detector and a 0.25-mm × 60-m fused-silica capillary column coated with a 0.5-µm layer of acid-deactivated phase G35. The carrier gas is helium, flowing at a rate of 40 cm per second. The column temperature is programmed as follows. It is maintained at 150° for 11 minutes; then increased at a rate of 25° per minute to 240°; maintained for 10 minutes; then decreased at a rate of 25° per minute to 150°; and maintained for 1 minute prior to the next injection. The detector and the injection port temperatures are maintained at 250°. Chromatograph the *Standard solution,* and record the peak responses as directed for *Procedure:* the resolution, *R,* between acetic acid and propionic acid is not less than 3.0; and the relative standard deviation of the peak response ratios for replicate injections is not more than 6.0%.
 Procedure—Separately inject equal volumes (about 1 µL) of the *Test solution* and the *Standard solution* into the chromatograph, record the chromatograms, and measure the responses for all the peaks. Calculate the quantity, in mg, of acetic acid in the portion of the constituted Topical Solution taken by the formula:

$$200C(R_U / R_S)$$

in which C is the concentration, in mg per mL, of acetic acid in the *Standard solution;* and R_U and R_S are the peak response ratios of acetic acid to propionic acid obtained from the *Test solution* and the *Standard solution,* respectively.

Other requirements—It meets the requirements for *pH* and *Water* under *Mafenide Acetate.*

Assay—
 Ion-pairing solution—Dissolve 6.8 g of monobasic potassium phosphate and 1.0 g of sodium 1-hexanesulfonate in about 800 mL of water. Adjust with phosphoric acid to a pH of 2.5, dilute to 1000 mL, and mix.
 Mobile phase—Prepare a filtered and degassed mixture of *Ion-pairing solution* and acetonitrile (9 : 1). Make adjustments if necessary (see *System Suitability* under *Chromatography ⟨621⟩*).
 Standard preparation—Transfer about 25 mg of USP Mafenide Acetate RS, accurately weighed, to a 25-mL volumetric flask. Add about 12 mL of *Mobile phase,* and dissolve by sonication. Dilute with *Mobile phase* to volume, and mix.
 Assay preparation—Constitute the Topical Solution as directed in the labeling. Transfer an accurately measured volume of the constituted Topical Solution, equivalent to about 25 mg of mafenide acetate, to a 25-mL volumetric flask. Using sonication, dissolve in about 12 mL of *Mobile phase.* Dilute with *Mobile phase* to volume, and mix.
 Chromatographic system (see *Chromatography ⟨621⟩*)—The liquid chromatograph is equipped with a 267-nm detector and a 4.6-mm × 15-cm column that contains 5-µm packing L1. The flow rate

Mafenide Acetate

$C_7H_{10}N_2O_2S \cdot C_2H_4O_2$ 246.28
Benzenesulfonamide, 4-(aminomethyl)-, monoacetate.
α-Amino-*p*-toluenesulfonamide monoacetate   [13009-99-9].

» Mafenide Acetate contains not less than 98.0 percent and not more than 102.0 percent of $C_7H_{10}N_2O_2S \cdot C_2H_4O_2$, calculated on the anhydrous basis.

Packaging and storage—Preserve in tight, light-resistant containers.

USP Reference standards ⟨11⟩—*USP Mafenide Acetate RS. USP Mafenide Related Compound A RS.*

Identification—
 A: *Infrared Absorption* ⟨197K⟩.
 B: The R_F value of the principal spot in the chromatogram of the *Identification solution* corresponds to that in the chromatogram of *Standard solution A*, as obtained in the test for *Chromatographic purity*.

Melting range ⟨741⟩:   between 162° and 171°, but the range between beginning and end of melting does not exceed 4°.

pH ⟨791⟩:   between 6.4 and 6.8, in a solution (1 in 10).

Water, *Method I* ⟨921⟩:   not more than 1.0%.

Residue on ignition ⟨281⟩:   not more than 0.2%.

Selenium ⟨291⟩:   0.003%, a 200-mg test specimen being used.

Heavy metals, *Method II* ⟨231⟩:   0.002%.

Chromatographic purity—
 Standard solutions—Dissolve USP Mafenide Acetate RS in methanol, mix to obtain *Standard solution A* having a known concentration of 500 µg per mL, dissolve USP Mafenide Related Compound A RS in methanol, and mix to obtain *Standard solution D* having a known concentration of 500 µg per mL. [NOTE—USP Mafenide Related Compound A RS is 4-formylbenzenesulfonamide.] Quantitatively dilute portions of these solutions with methanol to obtain *Standard solutions* having the following compositions:

Standard solution	Dilution	Concentration (µg RS per mL)	Percentage (%, for comparison with test specimen)
A	(undiluted)	500	1.0
B	5 in 10	250	0.5
C	1 in 5	100	0.2
D	(undiluted)	500	1.0
E	5 in 10	250	0.5
F	1 in 5	100	0.2

Test solution—Dissolve an accurately weighed quantity of Mafenide Acetate in methanol to obtain a solution containing 50 mg per mL.

Identification solution—Quantitatively dilute a portion of the *Test solution* with methanol to obtain a solution containing 500 µg per mL.

Ninhydrin solution—Dissolve 300 mg of ninhydrin in 100 mL of butyl alcohol, add 3 mL of glacial acetic acid, and mix.

Procedure—Apply separately 5 µL of the *Test solution*, 5 µL of the *Identification solution*, and 5 µL of each *Standard solution* to a suitable thin-layer chromatographic plate (see *Chromatography* ⟨621⟩) coated with a 0.25-mm layer of chromatographic silica gel mixture. Position the plate in a chromatographic chamber, and develop the chromatograms in a solvent system consisting of a mixture of ethyl acetate, methanol, and isopropylamine (77 : 20 : 3) until the solvent front has moved about three-fourths of the length of the plate. Remove the plate from the developing chamber, mark the solvent front, and allow the solvent to evaporate in warm, circulating air. Examine the plate under short-wavelength UV light, and compare the intensities of any secondary spots observed in the chromatogram of the *Test solution* at the R_F value corresponding to those of the principal spots in the chromatograms of *Standard solutions D, E,* and *F*. Spray the plate with the *Ninhydrin solution,* heat the plate at 105° for 5 minutes, and examine the plate. Compare the intensities of any secondary spots observed in the chromatogram of the *Test solution* to those of the principal spots in the chromatograms of *Standard solutions A, B,* and *C*. No secondary spot, observed by both visualizations, from the chromatogram of the *Test solution* is larger or more intense than the principal spots obtained from *Standard solution B* (0.5%) and *Standard solution E* (0.5%), and the sum of the intensities of all secondary spots obtained from the *Test solution* corresponds to not more than 1.0%.

Organic volatile impurities, *Method V* ⟨467⟩:   meets the requirements.
                                          (Official until July 1, 2008)

Assay—Transfer about 100 mg of Mafenide Acetate, accurately weighed, to a 50-mL volumetric flask, dissolve in about 20 mL of water, dilute with water to volume, and mix. Pipet 10 mL of this solution into a 100-mL volumetric flask containing 1 mL of 1 N hydrochloric acid, dilute with water to volume, and mix. Dissolve an accurately weighed quantity of USP Mafenide Acetate RS in 0.01 N hydrochloric acid, and dilute quantitatively and stepwise with the same solvent to obtain a Standard solution having a known concentration of about 200 µg per mL. Concomitantly determine the absorbance of both solutions in 1-cm cells at the wavelength of maximum absorbance at about 267 nm, with a suitable spectrophotometer, using 0.01 N hydrochloric acid as the blank. Calculate the quantity, in mg, of $C_7H_{10}N_2O_2S \cdot C_2H_4O_2$ in the portion of Mafenide Acetate taken by the formula:

$$0.5C(A_U / A_S)$$

in which C is the concentration, in µg per mL, of USP Mafenide Acetate RS in the Standard solution; and A_U and A_S are the absorbances of the solution of Mafenide Acetate and the Standard solution, respectively.

Mafenide Acetate Cream

» Mafenide Acetate Cream is Mafenide Acetate in a water-miscible, oil-in-water cream base, containing suitable preservatives. It contains not less than 90.0 percent and not more than 110.0 percent of mafenide acetate ($C_7H_{10}N_2O_2S \cdot C_2H_4O_2$) in terms of the labeled amount of mafenide ($C_7H_{10}N_2O_2S$).

Packaging and storage—Preserve in tight, light-resistant containers, and avoid exposure to excessive heat.

USP Reference standards ⟨11⟩—*USP Mafenide Acetate RS.*

Identification—
 A: *Ultraviolet Absorption* ⟨197U⟩—
  Solution: *Assay preparation*.
 B: Place about 1 g in a beaker, warm to melt the cream, add about 25 mL of water, and mix: the solution responds to the tests for *Acetate* ⟨191⟩.

Assay—
 Standard preparation—Dissolve an accurately weighed quantity of USP Mafenide Acetate RS in 0.01 N hydrochloric acid, and dilute quantitatively and stepwise with the same solvent to obtain a solution having a known concentration of about 200 µg per mL.

 Assay preparation—Transfer a quantity of Cream, equivalent to about 100 mg of mafenide acetate and accurately weighed, to a 60-mL separator, and add 20 mL of chloroform to dissolve it. Add 20 mL of water, shake for 2 minutes, allow the layers to separate completely, and discard the lower, chloroform layer. Repeat this washing with two separate 20-mL portions of chloroform, and discard the chloroform washings. Filter the aqueous phase through a dry filter into a 100-mL volumetric flask. Rinse the separator and the filter with water, passing all rinses through the filter, add water to volume, and mix. Centrifuge about 30 mL of the *Assay preparation,* then pipet 20 mL of the clear, supernatant into a 100-mL volumetric

WEIGHTS AND MEASURES

The International System of Units (SI) is used in this Pharmacopeia. The SI metric and other units, and the symbols commonly employed, are as follows.

Bq = becquerel	L = liter
kBq = kilobecquerel	mL = milliliter,[‡]
MBq = megabecquerel	µL = microliter
GBq = gigabecquerel	Eq = gram-equivalent weight
Ci = curie	mEq = milliequivalent
mCi = millicurie	mol = gram-molecular weight (mole)
µCi = microcurie	Da = dalton (relative molecular mass)
nCi = nanocurie	mmol = millimole
Gy = gray	Osmol = osmole
mGy = milligray	mOsmol = milliosmole
m = meter	Hz = hertz
dm = decimeter	kHz = kilohertz
cm = centimeter	MHz = megahertz
mm = millimeter	V = volts
µm = micrometer (0.001mm)	MeV = million electron volts
nm = nanometer [*]	keV = kilo-electron volt
kg = kilogram	mV = millivolt
g = gram[**]	psi = pounds per square inch
mg = milligram	Pa = pascal
µg; mcg = microgram[†]	kPa = kilopascal
ng = nanogram	g = gravity (in centrifugation)
pg = picogram	
fg = femtogram	
dL = deciliter	

[*]Formerly the symbol mµ (for millimicron) was used.

[**]The gram is the unit of mass that is used to measure quantities of materials. Weight, which is a measure of the gravitational force acting on the mass of a material, is proportional to, and may differ slightly from, its mass because of the effects of factors such as gravity, temperature, latitude, and altitude. The difference between mass and weight is considered to be insignificant for compendial assays and tests, and the term "weight" is used throughout USP and NF.

[†]Formerly the abbreviation mcg was used in the Pharmacopeial monographs; however, the symbol µg now is more widely accepted and thus is used in this Pharmacopeia. The term "gamma," symbolized by γ, is frequently used for microgram in biochemical literature. [NOTE—The abbreviation mcg is still commonly employed to denote microgram(s) in labeling and in prescription writing. Therefore, for purposes of labeling,"mcg" may be used to denote microgram(s).]

[‡]One milliliter (mL) is used herein as the equivalent of 1 cubic centimeter (cc).

CONCENTRATIONS

Molal, molar, and normal solution concentrations are indicated throughout this Pharmacopeia for most chemical assay and test procedures (see also *Volumetric Solutions* in the section *Reagents, Indicators, and Solutions*). Molality is designated by the symbol m preceded by a number that is the number of moles of the designated solute contained in 1 kilogram of the designated solvent. Molarity is designated by the symbol M preceded by a number that is the number of moles of the designated solute contained in an amount of the designated solvent that is sufficient to prepare 1 L of solution. Normality is designated by the symbol N preceded by a number that is the number of equivalents of the designated solute contained in an amount of the designated solvent that is sufficient to prepare 1 L of solution.

Percentage Measurements—Percentage concentrations are expressed as follows:

Percent Weight in Weight—(w/w) expresses the number of g of a constituent in 100g of solution or mixture.

Percent Weight in Volume—(w/v) expresses the number of g of a constituent in 100mL of solution, and is used regardless of whether water or another liquid is the solvent.

Percent Volume in Volume—(v/v) expresses the number of mL of a constituent in 100mL of solution.

The term *percent* used without qualification means, for mixtures of solids and semisolids, percent weight in weight; for solutions or suspensions of solids in liquids, percent weight in volume; for solutions of liquids in liquids, percent volume in volume; and for solutions of gases in liquids, percent weight in volume. For example, a 1 percent solution is prepared by dissolving 1 g of a solid or semisolid, or 1 mL of a liquid, insufficient solvent to make 100 mL of the solution.

In the dispensing of prescription medications, slight changes in volume owing to variations in room temperatures may be disregarded.

on taking into account the foregoing, place on the label of a multiple-unit container a suitable beyond-use date to limit the patient's use of the article. Unless otherwise specified in the individual monograph, or in the absence of stability data to the contrary, such beyond-use date shall be not later than (a) the expiration date on the manufacturer's container, or (b) 1 year from the date the drug is dispensed, whichever is earlier. For nonsterile solid and liquid dosage forms that are packaged in single-unit and unit-dose containers, the beyond-use date shall be 1 year from the date the drug is packaged into the single-unit or unit-dose container or the expiration date on the manufacturer's container, whichever is earlier, unless stability data or the manufacturer's labeling indicates otherwise.

The dispenser must maintain the facility where the dosage forms are packaged and stored, at a temperature such that the mean kinetic temperature is not greater than 25°. The plastic material used in packaging the dosage forms must afford better protection than polyvinyl chloride, which does not provide adequate protection against moisture permeation. Records must be kept of the temperature of the facility where the dosage forms are stored, and of the plastic materials used in packaging.

Pharmaceutical Compounding—The label on the container or package of an official compounded preparation shall bear a beyond-use date. The beyond-use date is the date after which a compounded preparation is not to be used. Because compounded preparations are intended for administration immediately or following short-term storage, their beyond-use dates may be assigned based on criteria different from those applied to assigning expiration dates to manufactured drug products.

The monograph for an official compounded preparation typically includes a beyond-use requirement that states the time period following the date of compounding during which the preparation, properly stored, is to be used. In the absence of stability information that is applicable to a specific drug and preparation, recommendations for maximum beyond-use dates have been devised for nonsterile compounded drug preparations that are packaged in tight, light-resistant containers and stored at controlled room temperature unless otherwise indicated (see *Stability Criteria and Beyond-Use Dating* under *Stability of Compounded Preparations* in the general tests chapter *Pharmaceutical Compounding—Nonsterile Preparations* ⟨795⟩).

Guidelines for Packaging and Storage Statements in *USP–NF* Monographs—In order to provide users of the *USP–NF* with proper guidance on how to package and store compendial articles, every monograph in the *USP–NF* is required to have a packaging and storage specification.

For those instances where, for some reason, storage information is not yet found in the *Packaging and storage* specification of a monograph, the section *Storage Under Nonspecific Conditions* is included in the *General Notices* as interim guidance. The *Storage Under Nonspecific Conditions* statement is not meant to substitute for the inclusion of proper, specific storage information in the *Packaging and storage* statement of any monograph.

For the packaging portion of the statement, the choice of containers is given in the *General Notices* and includes *Light-Resistant Container, Well-Closed Container, Tight Container, Hermetic Container, Single-Unit Container, Single-Dose Container, Unit-Dose Container,* and *Unit-of-Use Container.* For most preparations, the choice is determined by the container in which it is to be dispensed (e.g., tight, well-closed, hermetic, unit-of-use, etc). For active pharmaceutical ingredients (APIs), the choice would appear to be tight, well-closed, or, where needed, a light-resistant container. For excipients, given their typical nature as large-volume commodity items, with containers ranging from drums to tank cars, a well-closed container is an appropriate default. Therefore, in the absence of data indicating a need for a more protective class of container, the phrase "Preserve in well-closed containers" should be used as a default for excipients.

For the storage portion of the statement, the choice of storage temperatures presented in the *General Notices* includes *Freezer, Cold, Cool, Controlled Cold Temperature, Room Temperature, Controlled Room Temperature, Warm, Excessive Heat,* and *Protection from Freezing.* The definition of a dry place is provided if protection from humidity is important.

For most preparations, the choice is determined by the experimentally determined stability of the preparation and may include any of the previously stated storage conditions as determined by the manufacturer. For APIs that are expected to be retested before incorporation into a preparation, a more general and nonrestrictive condition may be desired. In this case, the specification "room temperature" (the temperature prevailing in a working area) should suffice. The use of the permissive room temperature condition reflects the stability of an article over a wide temperature range. For excipients, the phrase "No storage requirements specified" in the *Packaging and storage* statement of the monograph would be appropriate.

Because most APIs in the *USP–NF* have associated Reference Standards, special efforts should be considered to ensure that the Reference Standards' storage conditions correspond to the conditions indicated in the *USP–NF* monographs.

The Packaging and Storage Expert Committee may review questionable *Packaging and storage* statements on a case-by-case basis. In cases where the *Packaging and storage* statements are incomplete, the monographs would move forward to publication while the *Packaging and storage* statements are temporarily deferred.

VEGETABLE AND ANIMAL SUBSTANCES

The requirements for vegetable and animal substances apply to the articles as they enter commerce; however, lots of such substances intended solely for the manufacture or isolation of volatile oils, alkaloids, glycosides, or other active principles may depart from such requirements.

Statements of the distinctive microscopic structural elements in powdered substances of animal or vegetable origin may be included in the individual monograph as a means of determining identity, quality, or purity.

Foreign Matter—Vegetable and animal substances are to be free from pathogenic organisms (see *Microbiological Attributes of Nonsterile Pharmaceutical Products* ⟨1111⟩), and are to be as free as reasonably practicable from microorganisms, insects, and other animal contamination, including animal excreta. They shall show no abnormal discoloration, abnormal odor, sliminess, or other evidence of deterioration.

The amount of foreign inorganic matter in vegetable or animal substances, estimated as *Acid-insoluble ash,* shall not exceed 2 percent of the weight of the substance, unless otherwise specified in the individual monograph.

Before vegetable substances are ground or powdered, stones, dust, lumps of soil, and other foreign inorganic matter are to be removed by mechanical or other suitable means.

In commerce it is seldom possible to obtain vegetable substances that are without some adherent or admixed, innocuous, foreign matter, which usually is not detrimental. No poisonous, dangerous, or otherwise noxious foreign matter or residues may be present. Foreign matter includes any part of the plant not specified as constituting the substance.

Preservation—Vegetable or animal substances may be protected from insect infestation or microbiological contamination by means of suitable agents or processes that leave no harmful residues.

Storage under Nonspecific Conditions—Where no specific directions or limitations are provided in the *Packaging and storage* section of individual monographs or in the article's labeling, the conditions of storage shall include storage at controlled room temperature, protection from moisture, and, where necessary, protection from light. Articles shall be protected from moisture, freezing, and excessive heat, and, where necessary, from light during shipping and distribution. Active pharmaceutical ingredients are exempt from this requirement.

Labeling—The term "labeling" designates all labels and other written, printed, or graphic matter upon an immediate container of an article or upon, or in, any package or wrapper in which it is enclosed, except any outer shipping container. The term "label" designates that part of the labeling upon the immediate container.

A shipping container containing a single article, unless such container is also essentially the immediate container or the outside of the consumer package, is labeled with a minimum of product identification (except for controlled articles), lot number, expiration date, and conditions for storage and distribution.

Articles in this Pharmacopeia are subject to compliance with such labeling requirements as may be promulgated by governmental bodies in addition to the Pharmacopeial requirements set forth for the articles.

Amount of Ingredient per Dosage Unit—The strength of a drug product is expressed on the container label in terms of micrograms or milligrams or grams or percentage of the therapeutically active moiety or drug substance, whichever form is used in the title, unless otherwise indicated in an individual monograph. Both the active moiety and drug substance names and their equivalent amounts are then provided in the labeling.

Pharmacopeial articles in capsule, tablet, or other unit dosage form shall be labeled to express the quantity of each active ingredient or recognized nutrient contained in each such unit; except that, in the case of unit-dose oral solutions or suspensions, whether supplied as liquid preparations or as liquid preparations that are constituted from solids upon addition of a designated volume of a specific diluent, the label shall express the quantity of each active ingredient or recognized nutrient delivered under the conditions prescribed in *Deliverable Volume* ⟨698⟩. Pharmacopeial drug products not in unit dosage form shall be labeled to express the quantity of each active ingredient in each milliliter or in each gram, or to express the percentage of each such ingredient (see *Percentage Measurements*), except that oral liquids or solids intended to be constituted to yield oral liquids may, alternatively, be labeled in terms of each 5-mL portion of the liquid or resulting liquid. Unless otherwise indicated in a monograph or chapter, such declarations of strength or quantity shall be stated only in metric units (see also *Units of Potency* in these *General Notices*).

Use of Leading and Terminal Zeros—In order to help minimize the possibility of errors in the dispensing and administration of drugs, the quantity of active ingredient when expressed in whole numbers shall be shown without a decimal point that is followed by a terminal zero (e.g., express as 4 mg [not 4.0 mg]). The quantity of active ingredient when expressed as a decimal number smaller than 1 shall be shown with a zero preceding the decimal point (e.g., express as 0.2 mg [not .2mg]).

Labeling of Salts of Drugs—It is an established principle that Pharmacopeial articles shall have only one official name. For purposes of saving space on labels, and because chemical symbols for the most common inorganic salts of drugs are well known to practitioners as synonymous with the written forms, the following alternatives are permitted in labeling official articles that are salts: HCl for hydrochloride; HBr for hydrobromide; Na for sodium; and K for potassium. The symbols Na and K are intended for use in abbreviating names of the salts of organic acids; but these symbols are not used where the word Sodium or Potassium appears at the beginning of an official title (e.g.,Phenobarbital Na is acceptable, but Na Salicylate is not to be written).

Labeling Vitamin-Containing Products—The vitamin content of an official drug product shall be stated on the label in metric units per dosage unit. The amounts of vitamins A, D, and E may be stated also in USP Units. Quantities of vitamin A declared in metric units refer to the equivalent amounts of retinol (vitamin A alcohol).The label of a nutritional supplement shall bear an identifying lot number, control number, or batch number.

Labeling Botanical-Containing Products—The label of an herb or other botanical intended for use as a dietary supplement bears the statement, "If you are pregnant or nursing a baby, seek the advice of a health professional before using this product."

Labeling Parenteral and Topical Preparations—The label of a preparation intended for parenteral or topical use states the names of all added substances (see *Added Substances* in these *General Notices and Requirements*, and see *Labeling* under *Injections* ⟨1⟩), and, in the case of parenteral preparations, also their amounts or proportions, except that for substances added for adjustment of pH or to achieve isotonicity, the label may indicate only their presence and the reason for their addition.

Labeling Electrolytes—The concentration and dosage of electrolytes for replacement therapy (e.g., sodium chloride or potassium chloride) shall be stated on the label in milliequivalents (mEq). The label of the product shall indicate also the quantity of ingredient(s) in terms of weight or percentage concentration.

Labeling Alcohol—The content of alcohol in a liquid preparation shall be stated on the label as a percentage (v/v) of C_2H_5OH.

Special Capsules and Tablets—The label of any form of Capsule or Tablet intended for administration other than by swallowing intact bears a prominent indication of the manner in which it is to be used.

Expiration Date and Beyond-Use Date—The label of an official drug product or nutritional or dietary supplement product shall bear an expiration date. All articles shall display the expiration date so that it can be read by an ordinary individual under customary conditions of purchase and use. The expiration date shall be prominently displayed in high contrast to the background or sharply embossed, and easily understood (e.g., "EXP 6/89," "Exp. June 89," or "Expires 6/89"). [NOTE—For additional information and guidance, refer to the Nonprescription Drug Manufacturers Association's *Voluntary Codes and Guidelines of the OTC Medicines Industry*.]

The monographs for some preparations state how the expiration date that shall appear on the label is to be determined. In the absence of a specific requirement in the individual monograph for a drug product or nutritional supplement, the label shall bear an expiration date assigned for the particular formulation and package of the article, with the following exception: the label need not show an expiration date in the case of a drug product or nutritional supplement packaged in a container that is intended for sale without prescription and the labeling of which states no dosage limitations, and which is stable for not less than 3 years when stored under the prescribed conditions.

Where an official article is required to bear an expiration date, such article shall be dispensed solely in, or from, a container labeled with an expiration date, and the date on which the article is dispensed shall be within the labeled expiry period. The expiration date identifies the time during which the article may be expected to meet the requirements of the Pharmacopeial monograph, provided it is kept under the prescribed storage conditions. The expiration date limits the time during which the article may be dispensed or used. Where an expiration date is stated only in terms of the month and the year, it is a representation that the intended expiration date is the last day of the stated month. The beyond-use date is the date after which an article must not be used. The dispenser shall place on the label of the prescription container a suitable beyond-use date to limit the patient's use of the article based on any information supplied by the manufacturer and the *General Notices and Requirements* of this Pharmacopeia. The beyond-use date placed on the label shall not be later than the expiration date on the manufacturer's container.

For articles requiring constitution prior to use, a suitable beyond-use date for the constituted product shall be identified in the labeling.

For all other dosage forms, in determining an appropriate period of time during which a prescription drug may be retained by a patient after its dispensing, the dispenser shall take into account, in addition to any other relevant factors, the nature of the drug; the container in which it was packaged by the manufacturer and the expiration date thereon; the characteristics of the patient's container, if the article is repackaged for dispensing; the expected storage conditions to which the article may be exposed; any unusual storage conditions to which the article may be exposed; and the expected length of time of the course of therapy. The dispenser shall,

Tight Container—A tight container protects the contents from contamination by extraneous liquids, solids, or vapors; from loss of the article; and from efflorescence, deliquescence, or evaporation under the ordinary or customary conditions of handling, shipment, storage, and distribution; and is capable of tight reclosure. Where a tight container is specified, it may be replaced by a hermetic container for a single dose of an article.

A gas cylinder is a metallic container designed to hold a gas under pressure. As a safety measure, for carbon dioxide, cyclopropane, helium, nitrous oxide, and oxygen, the Pin-Index Safety System of matched fittings is recommended for cylinders of Size E or smaller.

NOTE—Where packaging and storage in a *tight container* or a *well-closed container* is specified in the individual monograph, the container used for an article when dispensed on prescription meets the requirements under *Containers—Permeation* ⟨671⟩.

Hermetic Container—A hermetic container is impervious to air or any other gas under the ordinary or customary conditions of handling, shipment, storage, and distribution.

Single-Unit Container—A single-unit container is one that is designed to hold a quantity of drug product intended for administration as a single dose or a single finished device intended for use promptly after the container is opened. Preferably, the immediate container and/or the outer container or protective packaging shall be so designed as to show evidence of any tampering with the contents. Each single-unit container shall be labeled to indicate the identity, quantity and/or strength, name of the manufacturer, lot number, and expiration date of the article.

Single-Dose Container (see also *Containers for Injections* under *Injections* ⟨1⟩)—A single-dose container is a single-unit container for articles intended for parenteral administration only. A single-dose container is labeled as such. Examples of single-dose containers include prefilled syringes, cartridges, fusion-sealed containers, and closure-sealed containers when so labeled.

Unit-Dose Container—A unit-dose container is a single-unit container for articles intended for administration by other than the parenteral route as a single dose, direct from the container.

Unit-of-Use Container—A unit-of-use container is one that contains a specific quantity of a drug product and that is intended to be dispensed as such without further modification except for the addition of appropriate labeling. A unit-of-use container is labeled as such.

Multiple-Unit Container—A multiple-unit container is a container that permits withdrawal of successive portions of the contents without changing the strength, quality, or purity of the remaining portion.

Multiple-Dose Container (see also *Containers for Injections* under *Injections* ⟨1⟩)—A multiple-dose container is a multiple-unit container for articles intended for parenteral administration only.

Poison Prevention Packaging Act—This act (see the Website, www.cpsc.gov/businfo/pppa.html) requires special packaging of most human oral prescription drugs, oral controlled drugs, certain nonoral prescription drugs, certain dietary supplements, and many over-the-counter (OTC) drug preparations in order to protect the public from personal injury or illness from misuse of these preparations (16 CFR § 1700.14).

The immediate packaging of substances regulated under the PPPA must comply with the special packaging standards (16 CFR § 1700.15 and 16 CFR § 1700.20). The PPPA regulations for special packaging apply to all packaging types including reclosable, nonclosable, and unit-dose types.

Special packaging is not required for drugs dispensed within a hospital setting for inpatient administration. Manufacturers and packagers of bulk-packaged prescription drugs do not have to use special packaging if the drug will be repackaged by the pharmacist. PPPA-regulated prescription drugs may be dispensed in nonchild-resistant packaging upon the request of the purchaser or when directed in a legitimate prescription (15 U.S.C. § 1473).

Manufacturers or packagers of PPPA-regulated OTC preparations are allowed to package one size in nonchild-resistant packaging as long as popular-size, special packages are also supplied. The nonchild-resistant package requires special labeling (18 CFR § 1700.5).

Various types of child-resistant packages are covered in ASTM International Standard D-3475, Standard Classification of Child-Resistant Packaging. Examples are included as an aid in the understanding and comprehension of each type of classification.

Storage Temperature and Humidity—Specific directions are stated in some monographs with respect to the temperatures and humidity at which Pharmacopeial articles shall be stored and distributed (including the shipment of articles to the consumer) when stability data indicate that storage and distribution at a lower or a higher temperature and a higher humidity produce undesirable results. Such directions apply except where the label on an article states a different storage temperature on the basis of stability studies of that particular formulation. Where no specific storage directions or limitations are provided in the individual monograph, but the label of an article states a storage temperature that is based on stability studies of that particular formulation, such labeled storage directions apply (see also *Pharmaceutical Stability* ⟨1150⟩). The conditions are defined by the following terms.

Freezer—A place in which the temperature is maintained thermostatically between −25° and −10° (−13° and 14 °F).

Cold—Any temperature not exceeding 8° (46 °F). A *refrigerator* is a cold place in which the temperature is maintained thermostatically between 2° and 8° (36° and 46°F).

Cool—Any temperature between 8° and 15° (46° and 59 °F). An article for which storage in a *cool place* is directed may, alternatively, be stored and distributed in a *refrigerator*, unless otherwise specified by the individual monograph.

Controlled Cold Temperature—This temperature is defined as the temperature maintained thermostatically between 2° and 8° (36° and 46 °F), that allows for excursions in temperature between 0° and 15° (32° and 59 °F) that may be experienced during storage, shipping, and distribution such that the allowable calculated MKT is not more than 8° (46°F). Transient spikes up to 25° (77 °F) may be permitted if the manufacturer so instructs and provided that such spikes do not exceed 24 hours unless supported by stability data or the manufacturer instructs otherwise.

Room Temperature—The temperature prevailing in a working area.

Controlled Room Temperature—A temperature maintained thermostatically that encompasses the usual and customary working environment of 20° to 25° (68° to 77 °F); that results in a mean kinetic temperature calculated to be not more than 25°; and that allows for excursions between 15° and 30° (59° and 86 °F) that are experienced in pharmacies, hospitals, and warehouses. Provided the mean kinetic temperature remains in the allowed range, transient spikes up to 40° are permitted as long as they do not exceed 24 hours. Spikes above 40° may be permitted if the manufacturer so instructs. Articles may be labeled for storage at "controlled room temperature" or at "up to 25°", or other wording based on the same mean kinetic temperature. The mean kinetic temperature is a calculated value that may be used as an isothermal storage temperature that simulates the nonisothermal effects of storage temperature variations. (See also *Pharmaceutical Stability* ⟨1150⟩.)

An article for which storage at *Controlled Room Temperature* is directed may, alternatively, be stored and distributed in a *cool place*, unless otherwise specified in the individual monograph or on the label.

Warm—Any temperature between 30° and 40° (86° and 104 °F).

Excessive Heat—Any temperature above 40° (104°F).

Protection from Freezing—Where, in addition to the risk of breakage of the container, freezing subjects an article to loss of strength or potency, or to destructive alteration of its characteristics, the container label bears an appropriate instruction to protect the article from freezing.

Dry Place—The term "dry place" denotes a place that does not exceed 40% average relative humidity at *Controlled Room Temperature* or the equivalent water vapor pressure at other temperatures. The determination may be made by direct measurement at the place or may be based on reported climatic conditions. Determination is based on not less than 12 equally spaced measurements that encompass either a season, a year, or, where recorded data demonstrate, the storage period of the article. There may be values of up to 45% relative humidity provided that the average value is 40% relative humidity.

Storage in a container validated to protect the article from moisture vapor, including storage in bulk, is considered a dry place.

erally given under the heading *Loss on drying*. However,*Loss on drying* is most often given as the heading where the loss in weight is known to represent residual volatile constituents, including organic solvents as well as water.

Test Results, Statistics, and Standards—Interpretation of results from official tests and assays requires an understanding of the nature and style of compendial standards, in addition to an understanding of the scientific and mathematical aspects of laboratory analysis and quality assurance for analytical laboratories.

Confusion of compendial standards with release tests and with statistical sampling plans occasionally occurs. Compendial standards define what is an acceptable article and give test procedures that demonstrate that the article is in compliance. These standards apply at any time in the life of the article from production to consumption. The manufacturer's release specifications, and compliance with good manufacturing practices generally, are developed and followed to ensure that the article will indeed comply with compendial standards until its expiration date, when stored as directed. Thus, when tested from the viewpoint of commercial or regulatory compliance, any specimen tested as directed in the monograph for that article shall comply.

Tests and assays in this Pharmacopeia prescribe operation on a single specimen, that is, the singlet determination, which is the minimum sample on which the attributes of a compendial article should be measured. Some tests, such as those for *Dissolution* and *Uniformity of dosage units*, require multiple dosage units in conjunction with a decision scheme. These tests, albeit using a number of dosage units, are in fact the singlet determinations of those particular attributes of the specimen. These procedures should not be confused with statistical sampling plans. Repeats, replicates, statistical rejection of outliers, or extrapolations of results to larger populations are neither specified nor proscribed by the compendia; such decisions are dependent on the objectives of the testing. Commercial or regulatory compliance testing, or manufacturer's release testing, may or may not require examination of additional specimens, in accordance with predetermined guidelines or sampling strategies. Treatments of data handling are available from organizations such as ISO, IUPAC, and AOAC.

Where the *Content Uniformity* determinations have been made using the same procedure specified in the *Assay*, the average of all of the individual *Content Uniformity* determinations may be used as the *Assay* value.

Description—Information on the "description" pertaining to an article, which is relatively general in nature, is provided in the reference table *Description and Relative Solubility of USP and NF Articles* in this Pharmacopeia for those who use, prepare, and dispense drugs and/or related articles, solely to indicate properties of an article complying with monograph standards. The properties are not in themselves standards or tests for purity even though they may indirectly assist in the preliminary evaluation of an article.

Solubility—The statements concerning solubilities given in the reference table *Description and Relative Solubility of USP and NF Articles* for Pharmacopeial articles are not standards or tests for purity but are provided primarily as information for those who use, prepare, and dispense drugs and/or related articles. Only where a quantitative solubility test is given, and is designated as such, is it a test for purity.

The approximate solubilities of Pharmacopeial substances are indicated by the descriptive terms in the accompanying table.

Descriptive Term	Parts of Solvent Required for 1 Part of Solute
Very soluble	Less than 1
Freely soluble	From 1 to 10
Soluble	From 10 to 30
Sparingly soluble	From 30 to 100
Slightly soluble	From 100 to 1000
Very slightly soluble	From 1000 to 10,000
Practically insoluble, or Insoluble	Greater than or equal to 10,000

Soluble Pharmacopeial articles, when brought into solution, may show traces of physical impurities, such as minute fragments of filter paper, fibers, and other particulate matter, unless limited or excluded by definite tests or other specifications in the individual monographs.

Interchangeable Methods—Certain general chapters contain a statement that the text in question is harmonized with the corresponding text of the *European Pharmacopoeia* and/or the *Japanese Pharmacopoeia* and that these texts are interchangeable. Therefore, if a substance or preparation is found to comply with a requirement using an interchangeable method from one of these pharmacopeias, it should comply with the requirements of the *United States Pharmacopeia*. However, where a difference appears, or in the event of dispute, only the result obtained by the procedure given in this Pharmacopeia is conclusive.

PRESCRIBING AND DISPENSING

Prescriptions for compendial articles shall be written to state the quantity and/or strength desired in metric units unless otherwise indicated in the individual monograph (see also *Units of Potency* in these *General Notices*). If an amount is prescribed by any other system of measurement, only an amount that is the metric equivalent of the prescribed amount shall be dispensed.

PRESERVATION, PACKAGING, STORAGE, AND LABELING

Containers—The *container* is that which holds the article and is or may be in direct contact with the article. The *immediate container* is that which is in direct contact with the article at all times. The *closure* is a part of the container.

Prior to being filled, the container should be clean. Special precautions and cleaning procedures may be necessary to ensure that each container is clean and that extraneous matter is not introduced into or onto the article.

The container does not interact physically or chemically with the article placed in it so as to alter the strength, quality, or purity of the article beyond the official requirements.

The Pharmacopeial requirements for the use of specified containers apply also to articles as packaged by the pharmacist or other dispenser, unless otherwise indicated in the individual monograph.

Tamper-Evident Packaging—The container or individual carton of a sterile article intended for ophthalmic or otic use, except where extemporaneously compounded for immediate dispensing on prescription, shall be so sealed that the contents cannot be used without obvious destruction of the seal.

Articles intended for sale without prescription are also required to comply with the tamper-evident packaging and labeling requirements of the FDA where applicable.

Preferably, the immediate container and/or the outer container or protective packaging used by a manufacturer or distributor for all dosage forms that are not specifically exempt is designed so as to show evidence of any tampering with the contents.

Light-Resistant Container (see *Light Transmission* under *Containers* ⟨661⟩)—A light-resistant container protects the contents from the effects of light by virtue of the specific properties of the material of which it is composed, including any coating applied to it. Alternatively, a clear and colorless or a translucent container may be made light-resistant by means of an opaque covering, in which case the label of the container bears a statement that the opaque covering is needed until the contents are to be used or administered. Where it is directed to "protect from light" in an individual monograph, preservation in a light-resistant container is intended.

Where an article is required to be packaged in a light-resistant container, and if the container is made light-resistant by means of an opaque covering, a single-use, unit-dose container or mnemonic pack for dispensing may not be removed from the outer opaque covering prior to dispensing.

Well-Closed Container—A well-closed container protects the contents from extraneous solids and from loss of the article under the ordinary or customary conditions of handling, shipment, storage, and distribution.

signifies that the substance is to be dried as directed under *Loss on drying* or *Water* (gravimetric determination).

Unless otherwise directed in the test or assay in the individual monograph or in a general chapter, USP Reference Standards are to be dried before use, or used without prior drying, specifically in accordance with the instructions given in the chapter *USP Reference Standards* ⟨11⟩, and on the label of the Reference Standard. Where the label instructions differ in detail from those in the chapter, the label text is determinative.

In stating the appropriate quantities to be taken for assays and tests, the use of the word "about" indicates a quantity within 10% of the specified weight or volume. However, the weight or volume taken is accurately determined, and the calculated result is based upon the exact amount taken. The same tolerance applies to specified dimensions.

Where the use of a pipet is directed for measuring a specimen or an aliquot in conducting a test or an assay, the pipet conforms to the standards set forth under *Volumetric Apparatus* ⟨31⟩, and is to be used in such manner that the error does not exceed the limit stated for a pipet of its size. Where a pipet is specified, a suitable buret, conforming to the standards set forth under *Volumetric Apparatus* ⟨31⟩, may be substituted. Where a "to contain" pipet is specified, a suitable volumetric flask may be substituted.

Expressions such as "25.0 mL" and "25.0 mg," used with respect to volumetric or gravimetric measurements, indicate that the quantity is to be "accurately measured" or "accurately weighed" within the limits stated under *Volumetric Apparatus* ⟨31⟩ or under *Weights and Balances* ⟨41⟩.

The term "transfer" is used generally to specify a quantitative manipulation.

The term "concomitantly," used in such expressions as "concomitantly determine" or "concomitantly measured," in directions for assays and tests, is intended to denote that the determinations or measurements are to be performed in immediate succession. See also *Use of Reference Standards* under *Spectrophotometry and Light-Scattering* ⟨851⟩.

Blank Determination—Where it is directed that "any necessary correction" be made by a blank determination, the determination is to be conducted using the same quantities of the same reagents treated in the same manner as the solution or mixture containing the portion of the substance under assay or test, but with the substance itself omitted.

Desiccator—The expression "in a desiccator" specifies the use of a tightly closed container of suitable size and design that maintains an atmosphere of low moisture content by means of silica gel or other suitable desiccant.

A "vacuum desiccator" is one that maintains the low-moisture atmosphere at a reduced pressure of not more than 20 mm of mercury or at the pressure designated in the individual monograph.

Dilution—Where it is directed that a solution be diluted "quantitatively and stepwise," an accurately measured portion is to be diluted by adding water or other solvent, in the proportion indicated, in one or more steps. The choice of apparatus to be used should take into account the relatively larger errors generally associated with using small-volume volumetric apparatus (see *Volumetric Apparatus* ⟨31⟩).

Drying to Constant Weight—The specification "dried to constant weight" means that the drying shall be continued until two consecutive weighings do not differ by more than 0.50 mg per g of substance taken, the second weighing following an additional hour of drying.

Filtration—Where it is directed to "filter," without further qualification, the intent is that the liquid be passed through suitable filter paper or equivalent device until the filtrate is clear.

Identification Tests—The Pharmacopeial tests headed *Identification* are provided as an aid in verifying the identity of articles as they are purported to be, such as those taken from labeled containers. Such tests, however specific, are not necessarily sufficient to establish proof of identity; but failure of an article taken from a labeled container to meet the requirements of a prescribed identification test indicates that the article may be mislabeled. Other tests and specifications in the monograph often contribute to establishing or confirming the identity of the article under examination.

Ignition to Constant Weight—The specification "ignite to constant weight" means that the ignition shall be continued, at 800 ±25° unless otherwise indicated, until two consecutive weighings do not differ by more than 0.50 mg per g of substance taken, the second weighing following an additional 15-minute ignition period.

Indicators—Where the use of a test solution ("TS") as an indicator is specified in a test or an assay, approximately 0.2 mL, or 3 drops, of the solution shall be added, unless otherwise directed.

Logarithms—Logarithms used in the assays are to the base 10.

Microbial Strains—Where a microbial strain is cited and identified by its ATCC catalog number, the specified strain shall be used directly or, if subcultured, shall be used not more than five passages removed from the original strain.

Negligible—This term indicates a quantity not exceeding 0.50 mg.

Odor—Terms such as "odorless," "practically odorless," "a faint characteristic odor," or variations thereof, apply to examination, after exposure to the air for 15 minutes, either of a freshly opened package of the article (for packages containing not more than 25 g) or (for larger packages) of a portion of about 25 g of the article that has been removed from its package to an open evaporating dish of about 100-mL capacity. An odor designation is descriptive only and is not to be regarded as a standard of purity for a particular lot of an article.

Pressure Measurements—The term "mm of mercury" used with respect to measurements of blood pressure, pressure within an apparatus, or atmospheric pressure refers to the use of a suitable manometer or barometer calibrated in terms of the pressure exerted by a column of mercury of the stated height.

Solutions—Unless otherwise specified in the individual monograph, all solutions called for in tests and assays are prepared with *Purified Water*.

An expression such as "(1 in 10)" means that 1 part *by volume* of a liquid is to be diluted with, or 1 part *by weight* of a solid is to be dissolved in, sufficient of the diluent or solvent to make the volume of the finished solution 10 parts *by volume*.

An expression such as "(20 : 5 : 2)" means that the respective numbers of parts, by volume, of the designated liquids are to be mixed, unless otherwise indicated.

The notation "VS" after a specified volumetric solution indicates that such solution is standardized in accordance with directions given in the individual monograph or under *Volumetric Solutions* in the section *Reagents, Indicators, and Solutions*, and is thus differentiated from solutions of approximate normality or molarity.

Where a standardized solution of a specific concentration is called for in a test or an assay, a solution of other normality or molarity may be used, provided allowance is made for the difference in concentration and provided the error of measurement is not increased thereby.

Specific Gravity—Unless otherwise stated, the specific gravity basis is 25°/25°, i.e., the ratio of the weight of a substance in air at 25° to the weight of an equal volume of water at the same temperature.

Temperatures—Unless otherwise specified, all temperatures in this Pharmacopeia are expressed in centigrade (Celsius) degrees, and all measurements are made at 25°. Where moderate heat is specified, any temperature not higher than 45° (113° F) is indicated. See *Storage Temperature* under *Preservation, Packaging, Storage, and Labeling* for other definitions.

Time Limit—In the conduct of tests and assays, 5 minutes shall be allowed for the reaction to take place unless otherwise specified.

Vacuum—The term "in vacuum" denotes exposure to a pressure of less than 20 mm of mercury unless otherwise indicated.

Where drying in vacuum over a desiccant is directed in the individual monograph, a vacuum desiccator or a vacuum drying pistol, or other suitable vacuum drying apparatus, is to be used.

Water—Where water is called for in tests and assays, *Purified Water* is to be used unless otherwise specified. For special kinds of water such as "carbon dioxide–free water," see the introduction to the section *Reagents, Indicators, and Solutions*. For *High-Purity Water* see *Containers* ⟨661⟩.

Water and Loss on Drying—Where the water of hydration or adsorbed water of a Pharmacopeial article is determined by the titrimetric method, the test is generally given under the heading *Water*. Monograph limits expressed as a percentage are figured on a weight/weight basis unless otherwise specified. Where the determination is made by drying under specified conditions, the test is gen-

Water Bath—Where the use of a water bath is directed without qualification with respect to temperature, a bath of vigorously boiling water is intended.

Foreign Substances and Impurities—Tests for the presence of foreign substances and impurities are provided to limit such substances to amounts that are unobjectionable under conditions in which the article is customarily employed (see also *Impurities in Official Articles* ⟨1086⟩).

While one of the primary objectives of the Pharmacopeia is to assure the user of official articles of their identity, strength, quality, and purity, it is manifestly impossible to include in each monograph a test for every impurity, contaminant, or adulterant that might be present, including microbial contamination. These may arise from a change in the source of material or from a change in the processing, or may be introduced from extraneous sources. Tests suitable for detecting such occurrences, the presence of which is inconsistent with applicable good manufacturing practice or good pharmaceutical practice, should be employed in addition to the tests provided in the individual monograph.

Other Impurities—Official substances may be obtained from more than one process, and thus may contain impurities not considered during preparation of monograph assays or tests. Wherever a monograph includes a chromatographic assay or purity test based on chromatography, other than a test for organic volatile impurities, and that monograph does not detect such an impurity, solvents excepted, the impurity shall have its amount and identity, where both are known, stated under the heading *Other Impurity(ies)* by the labeling (certificate of analysis) of the official substance.

The presence of any unlabeled impurity in an official substance is a variance from the standard if the content is 0.1% or greater. Tests suitable for detecting and quantitating unlabeled impurities, when present as the result of process change or other identifiable, consistent occurrence, shall be submitted to the USP for inclusion in the individual monograph. Otherwise, the impurity shall be identified, preferably by name, and the amount listed under the heading *Other Impurity(ies)* in the labeling (certificate of analysis) of the official substance. The sum of all *Other Impurities* combined with the monograph-detected impurities does not exceed 2.0% (see *Ordinary Impurities* ⟨466⟩), unless otherwise stated in the monograph.

Categories of drug substances excluded from *Other Impurities* requirements are fermentation products and semi-synthetics derived therefrom, radio pharmaceuticals, biologics, biotechnology-derived products, peptides, herbals, and crude products of animal or plant origin. Any substance known to be toxic must not be listed under *Other Impurities*.

Residual Solvents—The requirements are stated in *Residual Solvents* ⟨467⟩ together with information in *Impurities in Official Articles* ⟨1086⟩. Thus all drug substances, excipients, and products are subject to relevant control of residual solvents, even when no test is specified in the individual monograph. The requirements have been aligned with the ICH guideline on this topic. If solvents are used during production, they are of suitable quality. In addition, the toxicity and residual level of each solvent are taken into consideration, and the solvents are limited according to the principles defined and the requirements specified in *Residual Solvents* ⟨467⟩, using the general methods presented therein or other suitable methods. (Official July 1, 2008•₅)

Procedures—Assay and test procedures are provided for determining compliance with the Pharmacopeial standards of identity, strength, quality, and purity.

In performing the assay or test procedures in this Pharmacopeia, it is expected that safe laboratory practices will be followed. This includes the use of precautionary measures, protective equipment, and work practices consistent with the chemicals and procedures used. Prior to undertaking any assay or procedure described in this Pharmacopeia, the individual should be aware of the hazards associated with the chemicals and the procedures and means of protecting against them. This Pharmacopeia is not designed to describe such hazards or protective measures.

Every compendial article in commerce shall be so constituted that when examined in accordance with these assay and test procedures, it meets all the requirements in the monograph defining it. However, it is not to be inferred that application of every analytical procedure in the monograph to samples from every production batch is necessarily a prerequisite for ensuring compliance with Pharmacopeial standards before the batch is released for distribution. Data derived from manufacturing *process validation* studies and from *in-process controls* may provide greater assurance that a batch meets a particular monograph requirement than analytical data derived from an examination of finished units drawn from that batch. On the basis of such assurances, the analytical procedures in the monograph may be omitted by the manufacturer in judging compliance of the batch with the Pharmacopeial standards.

Automated procedures employing the same basic chemistry as those assay and test procedures given in the monograph are recognized as being equivalent in their suitability for determining compliance. Conversely, where an automated procedure is given in the monograph, manual procedures employing the same basic chemistry are recognized as being equivalent in their suitability for determining compliance. Compliance may be determined also by the use of alternative methods, chosen for advantages in accuracy, sensitivity, precision, selectivity, or adaptability to automation or computerized data reduction or in other special circumstances. Such alternative or automated procedures or methods shall be validated. However, Pharmacopeial standards and procedures are interrelated; therefore, where a difference appears or in the event of dispute, only the result obtained by the procedure given in this Pharmacopeia is conclusive.

In the performance of assay or test procedures, not fewer than the specified number of dosage units should be taken for analysis. Proportionately larger or smaller quantities than the specified weights and volumes of assay or test substances and Reference Standards may be taken, provided the measurement is made with at least equivalent accuracy and provided that any subsequent steps, such as dilutions, are adjusted accordingly to yield concentrations equivalent to those specified and are made in such manner as to provide at least equivalent accuracy. To minimize environmental impact or contact with hazardous materials, apparatus and chemicals specified in Pharmacopeial procedures also may be proportionally changed.

Where it is directed in an assay or a test that a certain quantity of substance or a counted number of dosage units is to be examined, the specified quantity or number is a minimal figure (the singlet determination) chosen only for convenience of analytical manipulation; it is not intended to restrict the total quantity of substance or number of units that may be subjected to the assay or test or that should be tested in accordance with good manufacturing practices.

Where it is directed in the assay of Tablets to "weigh and finely powder not fewer than" a given number, usually 20, of the Tablets, it is intended that a counted number of Tablets shall be weighed and reduced to a powder. The portion of the powdered tablets taken for assay is representative of the whole Tablets and is, in turn, weighed accurately. The result of the assay is then related to the amount of active ingredient per Tablet by multiplying this result by the average Tablet weight and dividing by the weight of the portion taken for the assay.

Similarly, where it is directed in the assay of Capsules to remove, as completely as possible, the contents of not fewer than a given number, usually 20, of the Capsules, it is intended that a counted number of Capsules should be carefully opened and the contents quantitatively removed, combined, mixed, and weighed accurately. The portion of mixed Capsules contents taken for the assay is representative of the contents of the Capsules and is, in turn, weighed accurately. The result of the assay is then related to the amount of active ingredient per Capsule by multiplying this result by the average weight of Capsule content and dividing by the weight of the portion taken for the assay.

Where the definition in a monograph states the tolerances as being "calculated on the dried (or anhydrous or ignited) basis," the directions for drying or igniting the sample prior to assaying are generally omitted from the *Assay* procedure. Assay and test procedures may be performed on the undried or unignited substance and the results calculated on the dried, anhydrous, or ignited basis, provided a test for *Loss on drying,* or *Water,* or *Loss on ignition,* respectively, is given in the monograph. Results are calculated on an "as-is" basis unless otherwise specified in the monograph. Where the presence of moisture or other volatile material may interfere with the procedure, previous drying of the substance is specified in the individual monograph and is obligatory.

Throughout a monograph that includes a test for *Loss on drying* or *Water,* the expression "previously dried" without qualification processes or methods of compounding, though not from the ingredients or proportions thereof, provided the finished preparation conforms to the relevant standards laid down herein and to preparations produced by following the specified process.

The tolerances specified in individual monographs and in the general chapters for compounded preparations are based on attributes of quality such as might be expected to characterize an article compounded from suitable bulk drug substances and ingredients in accordance with the procedures provided or under recognized principles of good pharmaceutical practice as described in this Pharmacopeia (see *Pharmaceutical Compounding—Nonsterile Preparations* ⟨795⟩) and elsewhere.

Monographs for preparations intended to be compounded pursuant to prescription may contain assay methods. Assay methods are not intended for evaluating a compounded preparation prior to dispensing. Assay methods are intended to serve as the official test methods in the event of a question or dispute as to whether the compounded preparation complies with official standards.

Where a monograph on a preparation calls for an ingredient in an amount expressed on the dried basis, the ingredient need not be dried prior to use if due allowance is made for the water or other volatile substances present in the quantity taken.

Unless specifically exempted elsewhere in this Pharmacopeia, the identity, strength, quality, and purity of an official article are determined by the definition, physical properties, tests, assays, and other specifications relating to the article, whether incorporated in the monograph itself, in the *General Notices*, or in the section *General Chapters*.

Water—Water used as an ingredient of official preparations meets the requirements for *Purified Water,* for *Water for Injection,* or for one of the sterile forms of water covered by a monograph in this Pharmacopeia.

Potable water meeting the requirements for drinking water as set forth in the regulations of the U.S. Environmental Protection Agency may be used in the preparation of official substances.

Alcohol—All statements of percentages of alcohol, such as under the heading *Alcohol content,* refer to percentage, by volume, of C_2H_5OH at 15.56°. Where reference is made to "C_2H_5OH," the chemical entity possessing absolute (100 percent) strength is intended.

Alcohol—Where "alcohol" is called for in formulas, tests, and assays, the monograph article *Alcohol* is to be used.

Dehydrated Alcohol—Where "dehydrated alcohol" (absolute alcohol) is called for in tests and assays, the monograph article *Dehydrated Alcohol* is to be used.

Denatured Alcohol—Specially denatured alcohol formulas are available for use in accordance with federal statutes and regulations of the Internal Revenue Service. A suitable formula of specially denatured alcohol may be substituted for Alcohol in the manufacture of Pharmacopeial preparations intended for internal or topical use, provided that the denaturant is volatile and does not remain in the finished product. A finished product that is intended for topical application to the skin may contain specially denatured alcohol, provided that the denaturant is either a normal ingredient or a permissible added substance; in either case the denaturant must be identified on the label of the topical preparation. Where a process is given in the individual monograph, the preparation so made must be identical with that prepared by the given process.

Added Substances—An official substance, as distinguished from an official preparation, contains no added substances except where specifically permitted in the individual monograph. Where such addition is permitted, the label indicates the name(s) and amount(s) of any added substance(s).

Unless otherwise specified in the individual monograph, or elsewhere in the *General Notices,* suitable substances such as antimicrobial agents, bases, carriers, coatings, colors, flavors, preservatives, stabilizers, and vehicles may be added to an official preparation to enhance its stability, usefulness, or elegance or to facilitate its preparation. Such substances are regarded as unsuitable and are prohibited unless (a) they are harmless in the amounts used, (b) they do not exceed the minimum quantity required for providing their intended effect, (c) their presence does not impair the bioavailability or the therapeutic efficacy or safety of the official preparation, and (d) they do not interfere with the assays and tests prescribed for determining compliance with the Pharmacopeial standards.

Nutritional and Dietary Supplements—Unless otherwise specified in the individual monograph, or elsewhere in the *General Notices,* consistent with applicable regulatory requirements, suitable added substances such as bases, carriers, coatings, colors, flavors, preservatives, and stabilizers may be added to a nutritional supplement preparation to enhance its stability, usefulness, or elegance, or to facilitate its preparation. Such added substances shall be regarded as suitable and shall be permitted unless they interfere with the assays and tests prescribed for determining compliance with Pharmacopeial standards.

Additional Ingredients—Additional ingredients, including excipients, may be added to nutritional supplement preparations containing recognized nutrients, consistent with applicable regulatory requirements, provided that they do not interfere with the assays and tests prescribed for determining compliance with Pharmacopeial standards.

Inert Headspace Gases—The air in a container of an article for parenteral use may be evacuated or be replaced by carbon dioxide, helium, or nitrogen, or by a mixture of these gases, which fact need not be declared in the labeling.

Colors—Added substances employed solely to impart color may be incorporated into official preparations, except those intended for parenteral or ophthalmic use, in accordance with the regulations pertaining to the use of colors issued by the FDA, provided such added substances are otherwise appropriate in all respects. (See also *Added Substances* under *Injections* ⟨1⟩.)

Ointments and Suppositories—In the preparation of ointments and suppositories, the proportions of the substances constituting the base may be varied to maintain a suitable consistency under different climatic conditions, provided the concentrations of active ingredients are not varied and the bioavailability, therapeutic efficacy, or safety of the preparation is not impaired.

Change to read:

TESTS AND ASSAYS

Apparatus—A specification for a definite size or type of container or apparatus in a test or assay is given solely as a recommendation. Where volumetric flasks or other exact measuring, weighing, or sorting devices are specified, this or other equipment of at least equivalent accuracy shall be employed. (See also *Thermometers* ⟨21⟩, *Volumetric Apparatus* ⟨31⟩, and *Weights and Balances* ⟨41⟩.) Where low-actinic or light-resistant containers are specified, clear containers that have been rendered opaque by application of a suitable coating or wrapping may be used.

Where an instrument for physical measurement, such as a spectrophotometer, is specified in a test or assay by its distinctive name, another instrument of equivalent or greater sensitivity and accuracy may be used. In order to obtain solutions having concentrations that are adaptable to the working range of the instrument being used, solutions of proportionately higher or lower concentrations may be prepared according to the solvents and proportions thereof that are specified for the procedure.

Where a particular brand or source of a material, instrument, or piece of equipment, or the name and address of a manufacturer or distributor, is mentioned (ordinarily in a footnote), this identification is furnished solely for informational purposes as a matter of convenience, without implication of approval, endorsement, or certification. Items capable of equal or better performance may be used if these characteristics have been validated.

Where the use of a centrifuge is indicated, unless otherwise specified, the directions are predicated upon the use of apparatus having an effective radius of about 20 cm (8 inches) and driven at a speed sufficient to clarify the supernatant layer within 15 minutes.

Unless otherwise specified, for chromatographic tubes and columns the diameter specified refers to internal diameter (ID); for other types of tubes and tubing the diameter specified refers to outside diameter (OD).

Steam Bath—Where the use of a steam bath is directed, exposure to actively flowing steam or to another form of regulated heat, corresponding in temperature to that of flowing steam, may be used.

GENERAL CHAPTERS

Each general chapter is assigned a number that appears in brackets adjacent to the chapter name (e.g., ⟨621⟩ *Chromatography*). Articles recognized in these compendia must comply with the official standards and tests and assays in the *General Notices*, relevant monographs, and General Chapters numbered below 1000. General Chapters numbered above 1000 are considered interpretive and are intended to provide information on, give definition to, or describe a particular subject. They contain no official standards, tests, assays, or other mandatory requirements applicable to any Pharmacopeial article unless specifically referenced in a monograph or elsewhere in the Pharmacopeia.

The use of the general chapter numbers is encouraged for identification of and rapid access to general tests and information. It is especially helpful where monograph section headings and chapter names are not the same (e.g., *Ultraviolet Absorption* ⟨197U⟩ in a monograph refers to method ⟨197U⟩ under general tests chapter ⟨197⟩ *Spectrophotometric Identification Tests*; *Specific rotation* ⟨781S⟩ in a monograph refers to method ⟨781S⟩ under general tests chapter ⟨781⟩ *Optical Rotation*; and *Calcium* ⟨191⟩ in a monograph refers to the tests for *Calcium* under general tests chapter ⟨191⟩ *Identification Tests—General*).

PHARMACOPEIAL FORUM

Pharmacopeial Forum (PF) is the USP journal of standards development and official compendia revision. *Pharmacopeial Forum* is the working document of the USP Council of Experts. It is intended to provide public portions of communications within the General Committee of Revision and public notice of proposed new and revised standards of the *USP* and *NF* and to afford opportunity for comment thereon. The organization of *PF* includes, but is not limited to, the following sections. Subsections occur where needed for Drugs and Pharmaceutic Ingredients (Excipients) and for Dietary Supplements.

Interim Revision Announcement (if present)—Official revisions and their effective dates, announcement of the availability of new USP Reference Standards, and announcement of assays or tests that are held in abeyance pending availability of required USP Reference Standards.

In-Process Revision—New or revised monographs or chapters that are proposed for adoption as official *USP* or *NF* standards.

Pharmacopeial Previews—Possible revisions or new monographs or chapters that are considered to be in a preliminary stage of development.

Stimuli to the Revision Process—Reports, statements, articles, or commentaries relating to compendial issues.

Nomenclature—Articles and announcements relevant to compendial nomenclature issues and listings of suggested and new United States Adopted Names (USAN) and International Nonproprietary Names (INN).

Official Reference Standards—Catalog of current lots of USP Reference Standards with ordering information and names and addresses of worldwide suppliers.

SUPPLEMENTS

Supplements to official text are published periodically and include text previously published in *PF*, which is ready to be made official.

REAGENT STANDARDS

The proper conduct of the Pharmacopeial tests and assays and the reliability of the results depend, in part, upon the quality of the reagents used in the performance of the procedures. Unless otherwise specified, reagents are to be used that conform to the specifications set forth in the current edition of *Reagent Chemicals* published by the American Chemical Society. Where such ACS reagent specifications are not available or where for various reasons the required purity differs, compendial specifications for reagents of acceptable quality are provided (see *Reagents, Indicators, and Solutions*). Listing of these reagents, including the indicators and solutions employed as reagents, in no way implies that they have therapeutic utility; furthermore, any reference to USP or NF in their labeling shall include also the term "reagent" or "reagent grade."

REFERENCE REAGENTS

Some compendial tests or assays require the use of specific reagents. These are supplied by USP when they might not be generally commercially available or because they are necessary for the testing and are available only to the originator of the tests or assay.

USP REFERENCE STANDARDS

USP Reference Standards are authentic specimens that have been approved by the USP Reference Standards Committee as suitable for use as comparison standards in *USP* or *NF* tests and assays. (see *USP Reference Standards* ⟨11⟩.) Currently official lots of USP Reference Standards are published in *Pharmacopeial Forum*.

Where a USP Reference Standard is referred to in a monograph or chapter, the words "Reference Standard" are abbreviated to "RS" (see *USP Reference Standards* ⟨11⟩).

Where a test or an assay calls for the use of a compendial article rather than for a USP Reference Standard as a material standard of reference, a substance meeting all of the compendial monograph requirements for that article is to be used.

The requirements for any new *USP* or *NF* standards, tests, or assays for which a new USP Reference Standard is specified are not in effect until the specified USP Reference Standard is available. The availability of new USP Reference Standards and the official dates of the *USP* or *NF* standards, tests, or assays requiring their use are announced via *Supplements* or *Interim Revision Announcements*.

UNITS OF POTENCY

For substances that cannot be completely characterized by chemical and physical means, it may be necessary to express quantities of activity in biological units of potency, each defined by an authoritative, designated reference standard.

Units of biological potency defined by the World Health Organization (WHO) for International Biological Standards and International Biological Reference Preparations are termed International Units (IU). Units defined by USP Reference Standards are USP Units, and the individual monographs refer to these. Unless otherwise indicated, USP Units are equivalent to the corresponding International Units, where such exist. Such equivalence is usually established on the basis solely of the compendial assay for the substance.

For biological products, whether or not International Units or USP Units do exist (see *Biologics* ⟨1041⟩), units of potency are defined by the corresponding U.S. Standard established by the FDA.

INGREDIENTS AND PROCESSES

Official drug products and finished devices are prepared from ingredients that meet the requirements of the compendial monographs for those individual ingredients for which monographs are provided (see also *NF 26*). Generally, nutritional and dietary supplements are prepared from ingredients that meet requirements of the compendial monographs for those ingredients for which monographs are provided, except that substances of acceptable food grade quality may be used in the event of a difference.

Official substances are prepared according to recognized principles of good manufacturing practice and from ingredients complying with specifications designed to ensure that the resultant substances meet the requirements of the compendial monographs (see also *Foreign Substances and Impurities* under *Tests and Assays*).

Preparations for which a complete composition is given in this Pharmacopeia, unless specifically exempted herein or in the individual monograph, are to contain only the ingredients named in the formulas. However, there may be deviation from the specified

ABBREVIATIONS

The term RS refers to a USP Reference Standard as stated under *Reference Standards* in these *General Notices* (see also *USP Reference Standards* ⟨11⟩ for a comprehensive discussion of reference materials).

The terms CS and TS refer to Colorimetric Solution and Test Solution, respectively (see under *Reagents, Indicators, and Solutions*). The term VS refers to Volumetric Solution as stated under *Solutions* in the *General Notices*.

The term PF refers to *Pharmacopeial Forum*, the journal of standards development and official compendia revision (see *Pharmacopeial Forum* in these *General Notices*).

Abbreviations for the names of many institutions, organizations, and publications are used for convenience throughout *USP* and *NF*. An alphabetized tabulation follows.

Abbreviation	Institution, Organization, or Publication
AAMI	Association for the Advancement of Medical Instrumentation
ACS	American Chemical Society
ANSI	American National Standards Institute
AOAC	AOAC International (formerly Association of Official Analytical Chemists)
ASTM	American Society for Testing and Materials
ATCC	American Type Culture Collection
CAS	Chemical Abstracts Service
CFR	U.S. Code of Federal Regulations
EP	European Pharmacopoeia
EPA	U.S. Environmental Protection Agency
FCC	Food Chemicals Codex
FDA	U.S. Food and Drug Administration
HIMA	Health Industry Manufacturers Association
ISO	International Organization for Standardization
IUPAC	International Union of Pure and Applied Chemistry
JP	Japanese Pharmacopoeia
NIST	National Institute of Standards and Technology
USAN	United States Adopted Names
WHO	World Health Organization

Abbreviated Statements in Monographs—Incomplete sentences are employed in various portions of the monographs for directness and brevity. Where the limit tests are so abbreviated, it is to be understood that the chapter numbers (shown in angle brackets) designate the respective procedures to be followed, and that the values specified after the colon are the required limits.

SIGNIFICANT FIGURES AND TOLERANCES

Where limits are expressed numerically herein, the upper and lower limits of a range include the two values themselves and all intermediate values, but no values outside the limits. The limits expressed in monograph definitions and tests, regardless of whether the values are expressed as percentages or as absolute numbers, are considered significant to the last digit shown.

Equivalence Statements in Titrimetric Procedures—The directions for titrimetric procedures conclude with a statement of the weight of the analyte that is equivalent to each mL of the standardized titrant. In such an equivalence statement, it is to be understood that the number of significant figures in the concentration of the titrant corresponds to the number of significant figures in the weight of the analyte. Blank corrections are to be made for all titrimetric assays where appropriate (see *Titrimetry* ⟨541⟩).

Tolerances—The limits specified in the monographs for Pharmacopeial articles are established with a view to the use of these articles as drugs, nutritional or dietary supplements, or devices, except where it is indicated otherwise. The use of the molecular formula for the active ingredient(s) named in defining the required strength of a Pharmacopeial article is intended to designate the chemical entity or entities, as given in the complete chemical name of the article, having absolute (100 percent) purity.

A dosage form shall be formulated with the intent to provide 100 percent of the quantity of each ingredient declared on the label. The tolerances and limits stated in the Definitions in the monographs for Pharmacopeial articles allow for analytical error, for unavoidable variations in manufacturing and compounding, and for deterioration to an extent considered acceptable under practical conditions. Where the minimum amount of a substance present in a nutritional or dietary supplement is required to be higher than the lower tolerance limit allowed for in the monograph because of applicable legal requirements, then the upper tolerance limit contained in the monograph shall be increased by a corresponding amount.

The specified tolerances are based upon such attributes of quality as might be expected to characterize an article produced from suitable raw materials under recognized principles of good manufacturing practice.

The existence of compendial limits or tolerances does not constitute a basis for a claim that an official substance that more nearly approaches 100 percent purity "exceeds" the Pharmacopeial quality. Similarly, the fact that an article has been prepared to closer tolerances than those specified in the monograph does not constitute a basis for a claim that the article "exceeds" the Pharmacopeial requirements.

Interpretation of Requirements—Analytical results observed in the laboratory (or calculated from experimental measurements) are compared with stated limits to determine whether there is conformance with compendial assay or test requirements. The observed or calculated values usually will contain more significant figures than there are in the stated limit, and a reportable result is to be rounded off to the number of places that is in agreement with the limit expression by the following procedure. Intermediate calculations (e.g., slope for linearity in *Validation of Compendial Procedures* ⟨1225⟩) may be rounded for reporting purposes, but the original value (not rounded) should be used for any additional required calculations. Rounding off should not be done until the final calculations for the reportable value have been completed. [NOTE—Limits, which are fixed numbers, are not rounded off.]

A reportable value is often a summary value for several individual determinations. It is the end result of a completed measurement method, as documented. It is the value compared with the acceptance criterion. In most cases, the reportable value is used as documentation for internal or external users.

When rounding off is required, consider only one digit in the decimal place to the right of the last place in the limit expression. If this digit is smaller than 5, it is eliminated and the preceding digit is unchanged. If this digit is greater than 5, it is eliminated and the preceding digit is increased by one. If this digit equals 5, the 5 is eliminated and the preceding digit is increased by one.

Illustration of Rounding Numerical Values for Comparison with Requirements			
Compendial Requirement	Unrounded Value	Rounded Result	Conforms
Assay limit ≥98.0%	97.96%	98.0%	Yes
	97.92%	97.9%	No
	97.95%	98.0%	Yes
Assay limit ≤101.5%	101.55%	101.6%	No
	101.46%	101.5%	Yes
	101.45%	101.5%	Yes
Limit test ≤0.02%	0.025%	0.03%	No
	0.015%	0.02%	Yes
	0.027%	0.03%	No
Limit test ≤3ppm	0.00035%	0.0004%	No
	0.00025%	0.0003%	Yes
	0.00028%	0.0003%	Yes

The *General Notices and Requirements* (hereinafter referred to as the *General Notices*) and general requirements appearing in *General Chapters* provide in summary form the basic guidelines for the interpretation and application of the standards, tests, assays, and other specifications of the *United States Pharmacopeia* and eliminate the need to repeat throughout the book those requirements that are pertinent in numerous instances. Where no specific language is given to the contrary, the requirements under the *General Notices* and *General Chapters* apply.

Where exceptions to the *General Notices* or *General Chapters* are made, the wording in the individual monograph takes precedence and specifically indicates the directions or the intent. To emphasize that such exceptions do exist, the *General Notices* or *General Chapters* in some places employ where indicated a qualifying expression such as "unless otherwise specified." In the individual monographs, it is understood that the specific wording of standards, tests, assays, and other specifications is binding wherever deviations from the *General Notices* or *General Chapters* exist whether or not a statement of exception is made.

TITLE

The full title of this publication, including its supplements, is *The Pharmacopeia of the United States of America*, Thirtieth Revision. This title may be abbreviated to *United States Pharmacopeia*, Thirtieth Revision, or to *USP 30*. The *United States Pharmacopeia*, Thirtieth Revision, supersedes all earlier revisions. Where the term "USP" is used, without further qualification, during the period in which this Pharmacopeia is official, it refers only to *USP 30* and any supplement(s) thereto. The same titles, with no further distinction, apply equally to print or electronic presentation of these contents.

"OFFICIAL" AND "OFFICIAL ARTICLES"

The word "official", as used in this Pharmacopeia or with reference hereto, is synonymous with "Pharmacopeial", with "USP", and with "compendial".

The designation "USP" in conjunction with the official title or elsewhere on the label of an article indicates that a monograph is included in the *USP* and that the article purports to comply with all applicable USP standards. The designation "USP" on the label may not and does not constitute a representation, endorsement, or incorporation by the manufacturer's labeling of the informational material contained in the USP monograph, nor does it constitute assurance by USP that the article is known to comply with USP standards. An article may purport to comply with a USP standard or other requirements only when the article is recognized in the *USP*. The standards apply equally to articles bearing the official titles or names derived by transposition of the definitive words of official titles or transposition in the order of the names of two or more active ingredients in official titles, whether or not the added designation "USP" is used. Names considered to be synonyms of the official titles may not be used for official titles.

Although both compendia, the *United States Pharmacopeia* and the *National Formulary*, currently are published under one cover, they remain separate compendia. The designation *USP–NF* or similar combination may be used on the label of an article, provided the label also bears a statement such as "Meets *NF* standards as published by the USP," indicating the particular compendium to which the article purports to apply.

Where an article differs from the standards of strength, quality, and purity, as determined by the application of the assays and tests set forth for it in the Pharmacopeia, its difference shall be plainly stated on its label. Where an article fails to comply in identity with the identity prescribed in the *USP*, or contains an added substance that interferes with the prescribed assays and tests, such article shall be designated by a name that is clearly distinguishing and differentiating from any name recognized in the Pharmacopeia.

Articles listed herein are official and the standards set forth in the monographs apply to them only when the articles are intended or labeled for use as drugs, as nutritional or dietary supplements, or as medical devices and when bought, sold, or dispensed for these purposes or when labeled as conforming to this Pharmacopeia.

An article is deemed to be recognized in this Pharmacopeia when a monograph for the article is published in it, including its supplements, addenda, or other interim revisions, and an official date is generally or specifically assigned to it.

The following terminology is used for distinguishing the articles for which monographs are provided: an *official substance* is an active drug entity, a recognized nutrient, a dietary supplement ingredient, or a pharmaceutical ingredient (see also *NF 26*) or a component of a finished device for which the monograph title includes no indication of the nature of the finished form; an *official preparation* is a *drug product*, a *nutritional supplement, dietary supplement*, or a *finished device*. It is the finished or partially finished (e.g., as in the case of a sterile solid to be constituted into a solution for administration) preparation or product of one or more official substances formulated for use on or for the patient or consumer; an *article* is an item for which a monograph is provided, whether an official substance or an official preparation.

Designating Conformance with Official Standards—When the letters "USP" or "NF" or "USP–NF" are used on the label of an article to indicate compliance with compendial standards, the letters shall appear in conjunction with the official title of the article or when appropriate, with the ingredients contained therein. The letters are not to be enclosed in any symbol such as a circle, square, etc., and must appear in block capital letters.

If a dietary supplement purports to be or is represented as an official product and such claim is determined by the USP not to be made in good faith, it is the policy of the USP to seek appropriate legal redress.

Products Not Marketed in the United States—Interest in the USP outside the United States has always existed. From time to time, monographs may be adopted for articles not legally marketed in the United States as a service to authorities in other countries where USP standards are recognized and applied. Appearance of any such monograph does not grant any marketing rights whatsoever, and the status of the article in the United States must be checked with the U.S. Food and Drug Administration in the event of any question.

Nutritional and Other Dietary Supplements—The designation of an official preparation containing one or more recognized nutrients or dietary supplement ingredients as "USP" or the use of the designation "USP" in conjunction with the title of such nutritional or dietary supplement preparation may be made only if the preparation meets all the applicable requirements contained in the individual monograph and general chapters. Any language modifying or limiting this representation shall be accompanied by a statement indicating that the article is "not USP", and indicating how the article differs from the standards of strength, quality, or purity as determined by the application of the tests and assays set forth in the compendia. Any additional ingredient in such article that is not recognized in the Pharmacopeia and for which nutritional value is claimed shall not be represented nor imply that such ingredient is of USP quality or recognized by USP. If a preparation does not comply with all applicable requirements but contains nutrients or dietary supplement ingredients that are recognized in the *USP*, the article may not designate the individual nutrients or ingredients as complying with USP standards or being of USP quality without designating on the label that the article itself does not comply with USP standards.

ATOMIC WEIGHTS AND CHEMICAL FORMULAS

The atomic weights used in computing molecular weights and the factors in the assays and elsewhere are those recommended in 1997 by the IUPAC Commission on Atomic Weights and Isotopic Abundances. Chemical formulas, other than those in the Definitions, tests, and assays, are given for purposes of information and calculation. The format within a given monograph is such that after the official title, the primarily informational portions of the text appear first, followed by the text comprising requirements, the latter section of the monograph being introduced by a boldface double-arrow symbol ». (Graphic formulas and chemical nomenclature provided as information in the individual monographs are discussed in the *Preface*.)

cent and not more than 115.0 percent of the labeled amount of simethicone.

Packaging and storage—Preserve in well-closed containers.
Labeling—Label the Chewable Tablets to indicate that they are to be chewed before being swallowed.
USP Reference standards ⟨11⟩—*USP Magaldrate RS. USP Polydimethylsiloxane RS.*
Identification—
  A: Transfer a quantity of powdered Chewable Tablets, equivalent to about 2 g of magaldrate, to a 100-mL centrifuge tube. Add about 60 mL of water, cap, and shake for 3 minutes. Centrifuge the suspension, and discard the supernatant. Repeat the washing with three more 60-mL portions of water. Transfer the residue to a 250-mL beaker, and heat on a steam bath to dryness: the residue so obtained meets the requirements of the *Identification* tests under *Magaldrate*.
  B: The IR absorption spectrum, in the 7- to 11-μm region, determined in a 0.5-mm cell, of the *Assay preparation* prepared as directed in the *Assay for polydimethylsiloxane*, exhibits maxima only at the same wavelengths as that of the *Standard preparation* containing about 2 mg of USP Polydimethylsiloxane RS per mL prepared as directed in the *Assay for polydimethylsiloxane*.
Microbial limits ⟨61⟩—Chewable Tablets meet the requirements of the test for absence of *Escherichia coli*.
Uniformity of dosage units ⟨905⟩: meet the requirements for *Weight Variation* with respect to magaldrate.
Acid-neutralizing capacity—Proceed as directed under *Acid-neutralizing Capacity* ⟨301⟩. The acid consumed by the minimum single dose recommended in the labeling is not less than 5 mEq, and not less than the number of mEq calculated by the formula:

$$0.8(0.0282 M)$$

in which 0.0282 is the theoretical acid-neutralizing capacity, in mEq per mg, of magaldrate, and M is the quantity, in mg, of the labeled amount of magaldrate.
Defoaming activity—
  Foaming solution and *System suitability tests*—Proceed as directed in the test for *Defoaming activity* under *Magaldrate and Simethicone Oral Suspension*.
  Procedure—[NOTE—For each test use a clean 250-mL cylindrical jar (50-mm internal diameter × 110-mm internal height) with a 50-mm opening fitted with a tight cap with an inert liner.] Transfer a quantity of finely powdered Chewable Tablets, equivalent to 20 mg of simethicone, to a 250-mL cylindrical jar containing 50 mL of 0.6 N hydrochloric acid that has been warmed to 37°, and proceed as directed in the test for *Defoaming activity* under *Magaldrate and Simethicone Oral Suspension*, beginning with "Cap the jar." Record the time, in seconds, for the foam to collapse to the extent that its thickness, measured from the surface of the liquid, is 1.0 cm. The defoaming activity time does not exceed 45 seconds.
Magnesium hydroxide content—
  Test preparation—Weigh and finely powder not fewer than 20 Chewable Tablets. Transfer an accurately weighed portion of the powder, equivalent to about 1 g of magaldrate, to a 100-mL volumetric flask, add 30 mL of dilute hydrochloric acid (1 in 10), shake for 15 minutes, dilute with water to volume, and mix.
  Procedure—Transfer 10.0 mL of the *Test preparation* to a 400-mL beaker, and proceed as directed in the test for *Magnesium hydroxide content* under *Magaldrate*, beginning with "and dilute with water to about 200 mL." Not less than 492 mg and not more than 666 mg of magnesium hydroxide [Mg(OH)$_2$] per g of the labeled amount of magaldrate is found.
Aluminum hydroxide content—
  Edetate disodium titrant—Prepare and standardize as directed in the *Assay* under *Ammonium Alum*.
  Test preparation—Prepare as directed in the test for *Magnesium hydroxide content*.
  Procedure—Transfer 10.0 mL of *Test preparation* and 20 mL of water to a 250-mL beaker, and proceed as directed for *Procedure* in the test for *Aluminum hydroxide content* under *Magaldrate*, beginning with "Add, with stirring, 25.0 mL of *Edetate disodium*." Not less than 321 mg and not more than 459 mg of aluminum hydroxide [Al(OH)$_3$] per g of the labeled amount of magaldrate is found.

Assay for magaldrate—Weigh and finely powder not fewer than 20 Chewable Tablets. Transfer an accurately weighed portion of the powder, equivalent to about 6 g of magaldrate, to a 200-mL volumetric flask. Add 100.0 mL of 2 N hydrochloric acid VS, and swirl by mechanical means for 30 minutes. Dilute with water to volume, mix, and filter. Transfer 100.0 mL of the filtrate to a beaker. Titrate the excess acid with 1 N sodium hydroxide VS to a pH of 3.0, determined potentiometrically. Perform a blank determination (see *Residual Titrations* under *Titrimetry* ⟨541⟩). Each mL of 2 N hydrochloric acid is equivalent to 70.80 mg of Al$_5$Mg$_{10}$(OH)$_{31}$(SO$_4$)$_2$.

Assay for polydimethylsiloxane—Weigh and finely powder not fewer than 20 Chewable Tablets. Transfer an accurately weighed portion of the powder, equivalent to about 20 mg of simethicone, to a 60-mL separator. Add 10.0 mL of hexanes and 25 mL of 6 N hydrochloric acid, cap the separator, and shake by mechanical means for not less than 2 hours. Allow to stand for about 10 minutes, and drain off as much of the lower, aqueous layer as possible without removing any of the unseparated interphase. Add 25 mL of 4 N sodium hydroxide to the separator, cap it, and shake by mechanical means for 1 hour. Transfer the mixture from the separator to a 50-mL centrifuge tube, cap, and centrifuge to obtain clear layers. Transfer not less than 5 mL of the clear upper hexanes layer to a test tube containing about 0.5 g of anhydrous sodium sulfate. Cap the tube, shake vigorously, and allow to stand to obtain a clear supernatant (*Assay preparation*). Prepare three *Standard preparations* in hexanes having known concentrations of about 1.6, 2.0, and 2.4 mg of USP Polydimethylsiloxane RS per mL, respectively. Concomitantly determine the absorbances of the *Assay preparation* and the *Standard preparations* in a 0.5-mm cell at the wavelength of maximum absorbance at about 1260 cm^{-1} with an IR spectrophotometer, using hexanes as the blank. [NOTE—Between each measurement, rinse the cell with heptane, empty, and dry it.] Plot the absorbances for the *Standard preparations* versus concentration, in mg per mL, of USP Polydimethylsiloxane RS, and draw the straight line best fitting the three plotted points. From the graph so obtained, determine the concentration, *C,* in mg per mL, of polydimethylsiloxane in the *Assay preparation.* Calculate the quantity, in mg, of [–(CH$_3$)$_2$SiO–]$_n$ in the portion of Chewable Tablets taken by multiplying *C* by 10.

(Official February 1, 2010)

Milk of Magnesia

Mg(OH)$_2$ 58.32
Magnesium hydroxide.
Magnesium hydroxide   [*1309-42-8*].

» Milk of Magnesia is a suspension of Magnesium Hydroxide. Milk of Magnesia, Double-Strength Milk of Magnesia, and Triple-Strength Milk of Magnesia contain not less than 90.0 percent and not more than 115.0 percent of the labeled amount of Mg(OH)$_2$, the labeled amount being 80, 160, and 240 mg of Mg(OH)$_2$ per mL, respectively. It may contain not more than 0.05 percent of a volatile oil or a blend of volatile oils, suitable for flavoring purposes.

Packaging and storage—Preserve in tight containers, preferably at a temperature not exceeding 35°. Avoid freezing.
Labeling—Double- or Triple-Strength Milk of Magnesia is so labeled, or may be labeled as 2× or 3× Concentrated Milk of Magnesia, respectively.
Identification—A solution of the equivalent of 1 g of regular-strength Milk of Magnesia in 2 mL of 3 N hydrochloric acid meets the requirements of the tests for *Magnesium* ⟨191⟩.
Microbial limits ⟨61⟩—Its total aerobic microbial count does not exceed 100 cfu per mL, and it meets the requirements of the test for absence of *Escherichia coli*.

Acid-neutralizing capacity ⟨301⟩—Not less than 5 mEq of acid is consumed by the minimum single dose recommended in the labeling, and not less than the number of mEq calculated by the formula:

$$0.8(0.0343M)$$

in which 0.0343 is the theoretical acid-neutralizing capacity, in mEq, of Mg(OH)$_2$; and M is the quantity, in mg, of Mg(OH)$_2$ in the specimen tested, based on the labeled quantity.
Soluble alkalies—Centrifuge about 50 mL of Milk of Magnesia. Dilute 5.0 mL of the clear supernatant with 40 mL of water. Add 1 drop of methyl red TS, and titrate the solution with 0.10 N sulfuric acid to the production of a persistent pink color: not more than 1.0 mL of the acid is required. Where the specimen is Double- or Triple-Strength Milk of Magnesia, not more than 2.0 or 3.0 mL of the acid is required, respectively.
Carbonate and acid-insoluble matter—To the equivalent of 1 g of regular-strength Milk of Magnesia add 2 mL of 3 N hydrochloric acid: not more than a slight effervescence occurs, and the solution is not more than slightly turbid.
Assay—Transfer an accurately measured quantity of Milk of Magnesia, previously shaken in its original container, equivalent to about 800 mg of magnesium hydroxide, to a 250-mL volumetric flask. Dissolve in 30 mL of 3 N hydrochloric acid, dilute with water to volume, and mix. Filter, if necessary, and transfer 25.0 mL of the filtrate to a beaker containing 75 mL of water, and mix. Adjust the reaction of the solution with 1 N sodium hydroxide to a pH of 7 (using pH indicator paper; see *Indicator and Test Papers* under *Reagents*, in the section *Reagents, Indicators, and Solutions*), add 5 mL of ammonia–ammonium chloride buffer TS and 0.15 mL of eriochrome black TS, and titrate with 0.05 M edetate disodium VS to a blue endpoint. Each mL of 0.05 M edetate disodium is equivalent to 2.916 mg of Mg(OH)$_2$.

Magnesia Tablets

» Magnesia Tablets contain not less than 93.0 percent and not more than 107.0 percent of the labeled amount of magnesium hydroxide [Mg(OH)$_2$].

Packaging and storage—Preserve in well-closed containers.
Identification—Crush several Tablets, and dissolve 1 g of the powder in 20 mL of 3 N hydrochloric acid: the solution responds to the tests for *Magnesium* ⟨191⟩.
Disintegration ⟨701⟩: 10 minutes, simulated gastric fluid TS being substituted for water in the test.
Uniformity of dosage units ⟨905⟩: meet the requirements.
Acid-neutralizing capacity ⟨301⟩—Not less than 5 mEq of acid is consumed by the minimum single dose recommended in the labeling, and not less than the number of mEq calculated by the formula:

$$0.8(0.0343M)$$

in which 0.0343 is the theoretical acid-neutralizing capacity, in mEq, of Mg(OH)$_2$; and M is the quantity, in mg, of Mg(OH)$_2$ in the specimen tested, based on the labeled quantity.
Assay—Weigh and finely powder not fewer than 20 Tablets. Transfer an accurately weighed portion of the powder, equivalent to about 250 mg of magnesium hydroxide, to a 100-mL volumetric flask, and proceed as directed in the *Assay* under *Milk of Magnesia* beginning with "Dissolve in 10 mL of 3 N hydrochloric acid."

Magnesium Carbonate

Carbonic acid, magnesium salt, basic; or, Carbonic acid, magnesium salt (1 : 1), hydrate
Magnesium carbonate, basic; or, Magnesium carbonate (1 : 1) hydrate [23389-33-5].
Anhydrous 84.31 [546-93-0].

» Magnesium Carbonate is a basic hydrated magnesium carbonate or a normal hydrated magnesium carbonate. It contains the equivalent of not less than 40.0 percent and not more than 43.5 percent of magnesium oxide (MgO).

Packaging and storage—Preserve in well-closed containers.
Identification—When treated with 3 N hydrochloric acid, it dissolves with effervescence, and the resulting solution meets the requirements of the tests for *Magnesium* ⟨191⟩.
Microbial limits ⟨61⟩—It meets the requirements of the test for absence of *Escherichia coli*.
Soluble salts—Mix 2.0 g with 100 mL of a mixture of equal volumes of *n*-propyl alcohol and water. Heat the mixture to the boiling point with constant stirring, cool to room temperature, dilute with water to 100 mL, and filter. Evaporate 50 mL of the filtrate on a steam bath to dryness, and dry at 105° for 1 hour: the weight of the residue does not exceed 10 mg (1.0%).
Acid-insoluble substances—Mix 5.0 g with 75 mL of water, add hydrochloric acid in small portions, with agitation, until no more of the magnesium carbonate dissolves, and boil for 5 minutes. If an insoluble residue remains, filter, wash well with water until the last washing is free from chloride, and ignite: the weight of the ignited residue does not exceed 2.5 mg (0.05%).
Arsenic, *Method I* ⟨211⟩—Prepare the *Test Preparation* by dissolving 750 mg in 25 mL of 3 N hydrochloric acid. The limit is 4 ppm.

Change to read:
Limit of calcium—▲[NOTE—A commercially available atomic absorption standard solution for calcium may be used where preparation of a calcium standard stock solution is described below. Concentrations of the *Standard preparations* and the *Test preparation* may be modified to fit the linear or working range of the instrument.]▲USP31
Dilute hydrochloric acid—Dilute 100 mL of hydrochloric acid with water to 1000 mL.
Lanthanum solution—To 58.65 g of lanthanum oxide add 400 mL of water, and add, gradually with stirring, 250 mL of hydrochloric acid. Stir until dissolved, dilute with water to 1000 mL, and mix.
Standard preparations—Transfer 249.7 mg of calcium carbonate, previously dried at 300° for 3 hours and cooled in a desiccator for 2 hours, to a 100-mL volumetric flask, dissolve in a minimum amount of hydrochloric acid, dilute with water to volume, and mix. Transfer ▲1.0,▲USP315.0, 10.0, and 15.0 mL of this stock solution to separate 1000-mL volumetric flasks, each containing 20 mL of *Lanthanum solution* and 40 mL of *Dilute hydrochloric acid*, add water to volume, and mix. These *Standard preparations* contain ▲1.0,▲USP315.0, 10.0, and 15.0 μg of calcium in each mL, respectively.
Blank solution—Transfer 4 mL of *Lanthanum solution* and 10 mL of *Dilute hydrochloric acid* to a 200-mL volumetric flask, dilute with water to volume, and mix.
Test preparation—Transfer 250 mg of Magnesium Carbonate to a beaker, add 30 mL of *Dilute hydrochloric acid*, and stir until dissolved, heating if necessary. Transfer the solution so obtained to a 200-mL volumetric flask containing 4 mL of *Lanthanum solution*, dilute with water to volume, and mix.
Procedure—Concomitantly determine the absorbances of the *Standard preparations* and the *Test preparation* at the calcium emission line at 422.7 nm with a suitable atomic absorption spectrophotometer (see *Spectrophotometry and Light-Scattering* ⟨851⟩) equipped with a calcium hollow-cathode lamp and ▲a nitrous oxide-acetylene▲USP31flame, using the *Blank solution* as the blank. ▲Determine the concentration, *C*, in μg per mL, of calcium in the *Test preparation* using the calibration graph. Calculate the content of calcium, in percentage, in the portion of Magnesium Carbonate taken by the formula:

$$100(0.001CV/W)$$

in which *C* is as defined above; the multiplier of 0.001 is for conversion of μg per mL to mg per mL; *V* is the volume, in mL, of the *Test preparation*; and *W* is the amount of Magnesium Carbonate, in mg, taken to prepare the *Test preparation*:▲USP31the limit is 0.45%.

Heavy metals, *Method I* ⟨231⟩—Dissolve 0.67 g in 10 mL of 3 N hydrochloric acid in a suitable crucible, and evaporate the solution on a steam bath to dryness. Ignite at 550 ± 25° until all carbonaceous material is consumed. Dissolve the residue in 15 mL of water and 5 mL of hydrochloric acid, and evaporate to dryness. Toward the end of the evaporation, stir frequently to disintegrate the residue so that finally a dry powder is obtained. Dissolve the residue in 20 mL of water, and evaporate in the same manner as before to dryness. Redissolve the residue in 20 mL of water, filter, if necessary, and add to the filtrate 2 mL of 1 N acetic acid and water to make 25 mL: the limit is 0.003%.

Iron ⟨241⟩—Boil 50 mg with 5 mL of 2 N nitric acid for 1 minute. Cool, dilute with water to 45 mL, add 2 mL of hydrochloric acid, and mix: the limit is 0.02%.

Change to read:

Assay—Dissolve about 1 g of Magnesium Carbonate, accurately weighed, in 30.0 mL of 1 N sulfuric acid VS, add methyl orange TS, and titrate the excess acid with 1 N sodium hydroxide VS. ▲Record the volume, V_A, in mL, of 1 N sodium hydroxide consumed. Perform the blank determination, and record the volume, V_B, in mL, of 1 N sodium hydroxide consumed. Calculate the volume, V_S, of 1 N sulfuric acid, in mL, consumed by the sample, by the formula:

$$(V_B - V_A) \times N_{NaOH}$$

in which N_{NaOH} is the exact normality of the sodium hydroxide solution. Calculate the volume of 1 N sulfuric acid, V_{Ca}, in mL, consumed by calcium which is present in the portion of Magnesium Carbonate taken for the *Assay*, by the formula:

$$(W \times L_{Ca})/(100 \times 20.04)$$

in which W is the weight, in mg, of Magnesium Carbonate taken; L_{Ca} is the content of calcium, in percentage, as determined in the test for *Limit of calcium;* and 20.04 is the weight, in mg, of Ca that is equivalent to each mL of 1 N sulfuric acid.

Calculate the percentage of MgO in the portion of Magnesium Carbonate taken by the formula:

$$100(V_S - V_{Ca}) \times 20.15/W$$

in which 20.15 is the weight, in mg, of MgO that is equivalent to each mL of 1 N sulfuric acid; and the other terms are as defined above.▲USP31

Magnesium Carbonate and Citric Acid for Oral Solution

» Magnesium Carbonate and Citric Acid for Oral Solution contains a dry mixture of Magnesium Carbonate and Citric Acid that when constituted as directed in the labeling yields a solution that contains not less than 90.0 percent and not more than 110.0 percent of the labeled amount of magnesium citrate ($C_{12}H_{10}Mg_3O_{14}$).

Packaging and storage—Preserve in tight containers.
Labeling—The label contains directions for constitution of the powder and states the equivalent amount of magnesium citrate ($C_{12}H_{10}Mg_3O_{14}$) in a given volume of the Oral Solution obtained after constitution.
USP Reference standards ⟨11⟩—*USP Citric Acid RS.*
(Official January 1, 2009)
Microbial limits ⟨61⟩—It meets the requirements of the test for absence of *Escherichia coli* and *Salmonella* species.
Uniformity of dosage units ⟨905⟩: meets the requirements.
Content of anhydrous citric acid—
Cation-exchange column—Mix 10 g of styrene-divinylbenzene cation-exchange resin with 50 mL of water in a beaker. Allow the resin to settle, and decant and discard the supernatant until a slurry of resin remains. Pour the slurry into a 15-mm × 30-cm glass chromatographic tube having a pledget of glass wool in the bottom and a stopcock, and allow to settle as a homogeneous bed. Place a pledget of glass wool on the top of the bed. Wash the resin bed with about 100 mL of water, closing the stopcock when the water level has just entered the glass wool pledget on the surface above the resin bed.

Test solution—Transfer an accurately measured volume of the constituted Oral Solution, equivalent to about 9 g of anhydrous citric acid, to a 100-mL volumetric flask, dilute with water to volume, and mix.

Procedure—Transfer 5.0 mL of the *Test solution* carefully onto the top of the resin bed in the cation-exchange column. Place a 250-mL volumetric flask below the column, open the stopcock, and allow to flow until the solution has entered the resin bed. Elute the column with 70 mL of water at a rate of about 5 mL per minute, collecting the eluate in a beaker. Boil the eluate for 1 minute, cool, and add 5 drops of phenolphthalein TS. Titrate with 0.1 N sodium hydroxide VS to a pink endpoint. Each mL of 0.1 N sodium hydroxide is equivalent to 6.404 mg of anhydrous citric acid ($C_6H_8O_7$). The content of anhydrous citric acid is between 76.6% and 107.8% of the labeled amount of magnesium citrate.
(Official until January 1, 2009)

Content of anhydrous citric acid—
Mobile Phase, Standard Preparation 1, and *Chromatographic System*—Proceed as directed under *Assay for Citric Acid/Citrate and Phosphate* ⟨345⟩.

Assay preparation—Transfer an accurately measured volume of the constituted Oral Solution, equivalent to about 9 g of anhydrous citric acid into a suitable volumetric flask, and proceed as directed for *Assay Preparation for Citric Acid/Citrate Assay* under *Assay for Citric Acid/Citrate and Phosphate* ⟨345⟩.

Procedure—Proceed as directed for *Procedure* under ⟨345⟩, and calculate the quantity, in mg, of anhydrous citric acid ($C_6H_8O_7$) in the volume of constituted Oral Solution taken by the formula:

$$0.001(192.12/189.10)C_S D(r_U / r_S)$$

in which 192.12 is the molecular weight of anhydrous citric acid; 189.10 is the molecular weight of citrate ($C_6H_5O_7$); C_S is the concentration, in μg per mL, of citrate in *Standard Preparation 1; D* is the dilution factor; and r_U and r_S are the citrate peak areas obtained from the *Assay preparation* and *Standard Preparation 1,* respectively. The content of anhydrous citric acid is between 76.6% and 107.8% of the labeled amount of magnesium citrate.
(Official January 1, 2009)

Other requirements—Constitute Magnesium Carbonate and Citric Acid for Oral Solution as directed in the labeling: it responds to the *Identification* tests and meets the requirements for *Chloride, Sulfate,* and *Tartaric acid* under *Magnesium Citrate Oral Solution.*

Assay—Transfer an accurately measured volume of constituted Oral Solution, equivalent to about 18.7 g of magnesium citrate ($C_{12}H_{10}Mg_3O_{14}$), to a 1000-mL volumetric flask. Add 200 mL of 1 N hydrochloric acid, swirl, and allow to stand for about 10 minutes. Dilute with water to volume, and mix. Stir by mechanical means for about 30 minutes. Transfer 10.0 mL of this solution to a 250-mL beaker. Add 10 mL of ammonia–ammonium chloride buffer TS, 5 mL of triethanolamine, 0.3 mL of eriochrome black TS, and titrate with 0.05 M edetate disodium VS until the last hint of violet disappears (blue endpoint). Each mL of 0.05 M edetate disodium is equivalent to 7.520 mg of magnesium citrate ($C_{12}H_{10}Mg_3O_{14}$).

Magnesium Carbonate, Citric Acid, and Potassium Citrate for Oral Solution

» Magnesium Carbonate, Citric Acid, and Potassium Citrate for Oral Solution contains a dry mixture of Magnesium Carbonate, Citric Acid, and Potassium Citrate that when constituted as directed in the labeling yields a solution that contains not less than 90.0 percent and not more than 110.0 percent of the labeled amount of magnesium citrate ($C_{12}H_{10}Mg_3O_{14}$).

Packaging and storage—Preserve in tight, single-dose containers. Store at controlled room temperature.
Labeling—The label specifies the directions for the constitution of the powder and states the equivalent amount of magnesium citrate ($C_{12}H_{10}Mg_3O_{14}$).
USP Reference standards ⟨11⟩—*USP Citric Acid RS.*
Microbial limits ⟨61⟩—The total aerobic microbial count does not exceed 1000 cfu per g, and the total combined molds and yeasts count does not exceed 100 cfu per g. It meets the requirements of the test for absence of *Escherichia coli*.
Uniformity of dosage units ⟨905⟩: meets the requirements.
pH ⟨791⟩: between 3.3 and 4.3, determined in a solution constituted as directed in the labeling.
Content of anhydrous citric acid—
Mobile Phase and *Chromatographic System*—Proceed as directed under *Assay for Citric Acid/Citrate and Phosphate* ⟨345⟩.
Standard preparation—Dissolve USP Citric Acid RS in a freshly prepared 1 mM sodium hydroxide to obtain a solution having a known concentration of about 0.02 mg of anhydrous citric acid per mL.
Assay preparation—Constitute the Oral Solution as directed in the labeling. Transfer the amount of the constituted Oral Solution, equivalent to about 500 mg of magnesium citrate, to a suitable volumetric flask, and dilute quantitatively, and stepwise if necessary, with a freshly prepared 1 mM sodium hydroxide to obtain a solution having a concentration of about 0.02 mg of magnesium citrate per mL, based on the label claim. Pass the resulting solution through a filter having a 0.5-μm or finer porosity, and use the filtrate.
Procedure—Proceed as directed for *Procedure* under *Assay for Citric Acid/Citrate and Phosphate* ⟨345⟩, and calculate the content, in g, of anhydrous citric acid ($C_6H_8O_7$) by the formula:

$$0.001(C_S D V_T / V)(r_U / r_S)$$

in which 0.001 is the conversion factor from mg to g; C_S is the concentration, in mg per mL, of anhydrous citric acid in the *Standard preparation*; D is the dilution factor for the *Assay preparation*; V_T is the total volume of constituted Oral Solution, as measured, when constituted as directed; V is the volume, in mL, of the constituted Oral Solution taken to prepare the *Assay preparation*; and r_U and r_S are the citrate peak areas obtained from the *Assay preparation* and the *Standard preparation*, respectively. The content of anhydrous citric acid is between 126.1% and 154.4% of the labeled amount of magnesium citrate.
Other requirements—Constitute as directed in the labeling: it meets the requirements of the tests for *Identification, Chloride, Sulfate,* and *Tartaric acid* under *Magnesium Citrate Oral Solution*.
Assay—Transfer an accurately measured volume of the constituted Oral Solution, equivalent to about 0.5 g of magnesium oxide, to a 100-mL volumetric flask, dilute with water to volume, and mix. Transfer 10.0 mL of this solution to a beaker. While stirring, add 10 mL of ammonia–ammonium chloride buffer TS, 5 mL of triethanolamine, 0.3 mL of eriochrome black TS, and titrate with 0.05 M edetate disodium VS until the last hint of violet disappears (blue endpoint). Each mL of 0.05 M edetate disodium is equivalent to 7.520 mg of magnesium citrate ($C_{12}H_{10}Mg_3O_{14}$).

Magnesium Carbonate and Sodium Bicarbonate for Oral Suspension

» Magnesium Carbonate and Sodium Bicarbonate for Oral Suspension contains not less than 90.0 percent and not more than 110.0 percent of the labeled amounts of $MgCO_3$ and $NaHCO_3$. It may contain suitable flavors.

Packaging and storage—Preserve in tight containers.
Identification—
A: Place about 1 g in a flask equipped with a stopper and glass tubing, the tip of which is immersed in calcium hydroxide TS in a test tube. Add 5 mL of 3 N hydrochloric acid to the flask, and immediately insert the stopper: gas evolves in the flask and a precipitate is formed in the test tube.
B: The solution remaining in the flask responds to the tests for *Magnesium* ⟨191⟩ and for *Sodium* ⟨191⟩.
Minimum fill ⟨755⟩: meets the requirements.
Acid-neutralizing capacity ⟨301⟩—Not less than 5 mEq of acid is consumed by the minimum single dose recommended in the labeling, and not less than the number of mEq calculated by the formula:

$$0.8(0.024M) + 0.8(0.0119S)$$

in which 0.024 and 0.0119 are the theoretical acid-neutralizing capacities, in mEq, of $MgCO_3$ and $NaHCO_3$, respectively; and M and S are the quantities, in mg, of $MgCO_3$ and $NaHCO_3$ in the specimen tested, based on the labeled quantities.
Assay for magnesium carbonate—Transfer an accurately weighed portion of Magnesium Carbonate and Sodium Bicarbonate for Oral Suspension, equivalent to about 4.2 g of $MgCO_3$, to a 500-mL volumetric flask. Add 200 mL of 1 N hydrochloric acid, and mix. When dissolved, dilute with water to volume, and mix. Transfer 10.0 mL of this stock solution to a suitable container, dilute with water to 100 mL, add 10 mL of ammonia–ammonium chloride buffer TS, 5 mL of triethanolamine, and 0.3 mL of eriochrome black TS, and titrate with 0.05 M edetate disodium VS to a blue endpoint. Each mL of 0.05 M edetate disodium consumed is equivalent to 4.216 mg of $MgCO_3$.
Assay for sodium bicarbonate—
Standard preparations—Dissolve a suitable quantity of sodium chloride, previously dried at 125° for 30 minutes and accurately weighed, in water, and dilute quantitatively with water to obtain a solution having a known concentration of about 600 μg per mL. On the day of use, further dilute this solution quantitatively with water to obtain three solutions containing 6.0, 12.0, and 18.0 μg of sodium chloride per mL, respectively.
Assay preparation—Transfer an accurately measured volume of the stock solution remaining from the *Assay for magnesium carbonate*, equivalent to about 180 mg of $NaHCO_3$, to a 100-mL volumetric flask, dilute with water to volume, and mix. Transfer 10.0 mL of the resulting solution to a 1000-mL volumetric flask, dilute with water to volume, and mix.
Procedure—Concomitantly determine the absorbances of the *Standard preparations* and the *Assay preparation* at the sodium emission line at about 589.0 nm, with a suitable atomic absorption spectrophotometer (see *Spectrophotometry and Light-scattering* ⟨851⟩) equipped with a sodium hollow-cathode lamp and an air–acetylene flame, using water as the blank. Plot the absorbances of the *Standard preparations* versus concentration, in μg of sodium chloride per mL, and draw the straight line best fitting the three plotted points. From the graph so obtained, determine the concentration, in μg per mL, of sodium chloride equivalent in the *Assay preparation*. Calculate the quantity, in g, of $NaHCO_3$ in the portion of Magnesium Carbonate and Sodium Bicarbonate for Oral Suspension taken by the formula:

$$(84.01 / 58.44)(5C / V)$$

in which 84.01 and 58.44 are the molecular weights of sodium bicarbonate and sodium chloride, respectively; C is the concentration, in μg per mL, of sodium chloride equivalent in the *Assay preparation*; and V is the volume, in mL, of the stock solution remaining from the *Assay for magnesium carbonate* taken.

Magnesium Chloride

$MgCl_2 \cdot 6H_2O$ 203.30
Magnesium chloride, hexahydrate
Magnesium chloride hexahydrate   [7791-18-6].
Anhydrous   95.21   [7786-30-3].

» Magnesium Chloride contains not less than 98.0 percent and not more than 101.0 percent of MgCl$_2 \cdot$ 6H$_2$O.

Packaging and storage—Preserve in tight containers.
Labeling—Where Magnesium Chloride is intended for use in hemodialysis, it is so labeled.
Identification—A solution (1 in 20) responds to the tests for *Magnesium* ⟨191⟩ and for *Chloride* ⟨191⟩. [NOTE—When performing the test for *Chloride*, acidify the sample solution with diluted nitric acid prior to adding 6 N ammonium hydroxide.]
pH ⟨791⟩: between 4.5 and 7.0, in a 1 in 20 solution in carbon dioxide-free water.
Insoluble matter—Dissolve 20 g, accurately weighed, in 200 mL of water, heat to boiling, and digest in a covered beaker on a steam bath for 1 hour. Filter through a tared filtering crucible, wash thoroughly, dry at 115°, and determine the weight of the residue: not more than 0.005% is found.
Sulfate ⟨221⟩—A 10-g portion shows no more sulfate than corresponds to 0.50 mL of 0.020 N sulfuric acid (0.005%).
Barium—Dissolve 1 g in 10 mL of water, and add 1 mL of 2 N sulfuric acid: no turbidity is produced within 2 hours.

Change to read:
Limit of calcium—
Dilute hydrochloric acid, Lanthanum solution, Standard preparations, and *Blank solution*—Proceed as directed in the test for *Limit of calcium* under *Magnesium Carbonate*.
Test preparation—Transfer 10.0 g of Magnesium Chloride to a 200-mL volumetric flask, add water to dissolve it, add 4 mL of *Lanthanum solution*, dilute with water to volume, and mix.
Procedure—Proceed as directed for *Procedure* in the test for *Limit of calcium* under *Magnesium Carbonate*. ▲Determine the concentration, *C*, in μg per mL, of calcium in the *Test preparation* using the calibration graph. Calculate the content of calcium, in percentage, in the portion of Magnesium Chloride taken by the formula:

$$100(0.001CV/W)$$

in which *C* is as defined above; the multiplier of 0.001 is for conversion of μg per mL to mg per mL; *V* is the volume, in mL, of the *Test preparation;* and *W* is the amount of Magnesium Chloride, in mg, taken to prepare the *Test preparation*:▲USP31 the limit is 0.01%.
Potassium—Dissolve 5 g in 5 mL of water, and add 0.2 mL of sodium bitartrate TS: no turbidity is produced within 5 minutes.
Aluminum ⟨206⟩ (where it is labeled as intended for use in hemodialysis)—Proceed as directed, using 2.0 g of Magnesium Chloride to prepare the *Test Preparation*: the limit is 1 μg per g.
Heavy metals ⟨231⟩—Dissolve 2 g in water to make 25 mL: the limit is 0.001%.
Organic volatile impurities, *Method I* ⟨467⟩: meets the requirements.

(Official until July 1, 2008)
Assay—Accurately weigh about 450 mg of Magnesium Chloride, dissolve in 25 mL of water, add 5 mL of ammonia–ammonium chloride buffer TS and 0.1 mL of eriochrome black TS, and titrate with 0.05 M edetate disodium VS to a blue endpoint. Each mL of 0.05 M disodium edetate is equivalent to 10.17 mg of MgCl$_2 \cdot$ 6H$_2$O.

Magnesium Citrate

C$_{12}$H$_{10}$Mg$_3$O$_{14}$ 451.11
1,2,3-Propanetricarboxylic acid, hydroxy-, magnesium salt (2 : 3).
Magnesium citrate (3 : 2)   [3344-18-1].

» Magnesium Citrate contains not less than 14.5 percent and not more than 16.4 percent of magnesium (Mg), calculated on the dried basis.

Packaging and storage—Preserve in tight containers.
Labeling—Magnesium Citrate that loses not more than 2.0% of its weight in the test for *Loss on drying* may be labeled as Anhydrous Magnesium Citrate.
Identification—
   A: A solution (10 mg per mL) responds to the tests for *Magnesium* ⟨191⟩.
   B: A solution (80 mg per mL) responds to the tests for *Citrate* ⟨191⟩.
pH ⟨791⟩: between 5.0 and 9.0, in a suspension (50 mg per mL).
Loss on drying ⟨731⟩—Dry 1 g in a mechanical convection oven at 135° for 16 hours, then to constant weight: it loses not more than 29% of its weight, except that where it is labeled as anhydrous, it loses not more than 2.0% of its weight.
Chloride ⟨221⟩—A 300-mg portion shows no more chloride than corresponds to 0.20 mL of 0.020 N hydrochloric acid (0.05%).
Sulfate ⟨221⟩—A 100-mg portion shows no more sulfate than corresponds to 0.20 mL of 0.020 N sulfuric acid (0.2%).
Arsenic, *Method I* ⟨211⟩:   3 μg per g.
Heavy metals, *Method I* ⟨231⟩—Dissolve 0.4 g in 25 mL of water, and proceed as directed for *Test Preparation*, except to use glacial acetic acid to adjust the pH: the limit is 50 μg per g.
Iron ⟨241⟩—Boil 50 mg with 5 mL of 2 N nitric acid for 1 minute. Cool, dilute with water to 45 mL, add 2 mL of hydrochloric acid, and mix: the limit is 200 μg per g.
Limit of calcium—
Dilute hydrochloric acid, Lanthanum solution, Standard preparations, and *Blank solution*—Prepare as directed in the test for *Calcium* under *Magnesium Carbonate*.
Test preparation—Transfer 250 mg of Magnesium Citrate to a beaker, add 30 mL of *Dilute hydrochloric acid*, and stir until dissolved. Transfer the solution so obtained to a 200-mL volumetric flask containing 4 mL of *Lanthanum solution*, dilute with water to volume, and mix.
Procedure—Proceed as directed in the test for *Calcium* under *Magnesium Carbonate*: the limit is 1.0%, calculated on the dried basis.
Organic volatile impurities, *Method IV* ⟨467⟩: meets the requirements.

(Official until July 1, 2008)
Assay—Weigh accurately about 400 mg of Magnesium Citrate, dissolve in 50 mL of water, add 20 mL of ammonia–ammonium chloride buffer TS and 0.1 mL of eriochrome black TS, and titrate with 0.05 M edetate disodium VS to a blue endpoint. Perform a blank determination, and make any necessary correction. From the volume of 0.05 M edetate disodium consumed, deduct the volume of 0.05 M edetate disodium corresponding to the amount of calcium in the portion of Magnesium Citrate taken, based on the amount of calcium found in the test for *Limit of calcium*. Each mg of calcium (Ca) is equivalent to 0.25 mL of 0.05 M edetate disodium. The difference is the volume of 0.05 M edetate disodium consumed by the magnesium. Each mL of 0.05 M edetate disodium is equivalent to 1.215 mg of magnesium (Mg).

Magnesium Citrate Oral Solution

C$_{12}$H$_{10}$Mg$_3$O$_{14}$ 451.11
1,2,3-Propanetricarboxylic acid, hydroxy-, magnesium salt (2 : 3).
Magnesium citrate (3 : 2)   [3344-18-1].

» Magnesium Citrate Oral Solution is a sterilized or pasteurized solution containing, in each 100 mL, not less than 7.59 g of anhydrous citric acid ($C_6H_8O_7$) and an amount of magnesium citrate equivalent to not less than 1.55 g and not more than 1.9 g of magnesium oxide (MgO).

Magnesium Citrate Oral Solution may be prepared as follows:

Magnesium Carbonate	15 g
Anhydrous Citric Acid	27.4 g
Syrup	60 mL
Talc	5 g
Lemon Oil	0.1 mL
Potassium Bicarbonate	2.5 g
Purified Water, a sufficient quantity, to make	350 mL

Dissolve the anhydrous Citric Acid in 150 mL of hot Purified Water in a suitable dish, slowly add the Magnesium Carbonate, previously mixed with 100 mL of Purified Water, and stir until it is dissolved. Then add the Syrup, heat the mixed liquids to the boiling point, immediately add the Lemon Oil, previously triturated with the Talc, and filter the mixture, while hot, into a strong bottle (previously rinsed with boiling Purified Water) of suitable capacity. Add boiled Purified Water to make the product measure 350 mL. Use Purified Cotton as a stopper for the bottle, allow to cool, add the Potassium Bicarbonate, and immediately insert the stopper in the bottle securely. Finally, shake the solution occasionally until the Potassium Bicarbonate is dissolved, cap the bottle, and sterilize or pasteurize the solution.

NOTE—An amount (30 g) of citric acid containing 1 molecule of water of hydration, equivalent to 27.4 g of anhydrous citric acid, may be used in the foregoing formula. In this process the 2.5 g of potassium bicarbonate may be replaced by 2.1 g of sodium bicarbonate, preferably in tablet form. The Oral Solution may be further carbonated by the use of carbon dioxide under pressure.

Packaging and storage—Preserve at controlled room temperature or in a cool place, in bottles containing not less than 200 mL.

USP Reference standards ⟨11⟩—*USP Citric Acid RS.*
(Official January 1, 2009)

Identification—
A: It responds to the tests for *Magnesium* ⟨191⟩.
B: To 5 mL of Oral Solution add 1 mL of potassium permanganate TS and 5 mL of mercuric sulfate TS, and heat the solution: a white precipitate is formed.
Chloride ⟨221⟩—A 2.0-mL portion shows no more chloride than corresponds to 0.30 mL of 0.020 N hydrochloric acid (0.01%).
Sulfate ⟨221⟩—A 2.0-mL portion shows no more sulfate than corresponds to 0.30 mL of 0.020 N sulfuric acid (0.015%).
Tartaric acid—To 10 mL in a test tube add 1 mL of glacial acetic acid and 3 mL of a solution of potassium acetate (1 in 2), shake the mixture vigorously, then gently rub the inner wall of the test tube with a glass rod for a few minutes, and allow to stand for 1 hour: no white, crystalline precipitate soluble in 6 N ammonium hydroxide is formed.
Assay for anhydrous citric acid—Measure accurately 10 mL of Oral Solution, which previously has been freed from excessive carbon dioxide by repeated pouring, into a 250-mL beaker, and add 30 mL of water. Then add phenolphthalein TS and just enough 1 N sodium hydroxide to give the liquid a persistent pink color, and acidify with 4 drops of 1 N hydrochloric acid. Add 20 mL of calcium chloride TS, and concentrate, by boiling, to about 30 mL, stirring constantly with a rubber-tipped glass rod during the boiling. Completely transfer the precipitate from the hot mixture to a filter from 9 to 11 cm in diameter with the aid of small quantities of boiling water, then wash the precipitate five times with boiling water. Collect the filtrate and washings in a 150-mL beaker, and concentrate the solution, by boiling, to about 20 mL. Add sufficient 6 N ammonium hydroxide, dropwise, to give the liquid a distinct red color, and then concentrate to about 10 mL. Transfer the precipitate completely from the hot mixture to a filter from 7 to 9 cm in diameter with the aid of small quantities of boiling water, and wash the precipitate six times with 5-mL portions of boiling water.

Dry the two filters with the precipitates, and incinerate them together in a loosely covered platinum crucible, heating first at a low temperature until the precipitates are well charred, and then removing the cover and raising the temperature until the residue is nearly white. If a gas flame is used, prevent its contact with the mass in the crucible. Cool, place the crucible with its contents in a suitable beaker, and add about 30 mL of water and then 50.0 mL of 0.5 N hydrochloric acid VS. When the residue has dissolved, remove the crucible, rinsing it well with water into the beaker. Add 100 mL of water, cover the beaker with a watch glass, and boil gently for 10 minutes. Cool, and titrate the excess acid with 0.5 N sodium hydroxide VS, using phenolphthalein TS as the indicator. Each mL of 0.5000 N hydrochloric acid is equivalent to 32.02 mg of $C_6H_8O_7$.
(Official until January 1, 2009)

Assay for anhydrous citric acid—
Mobile Phase, Standard Preparation 1, and *Chromatographic System*—Proceed as directed under *Assay for Citric Acid/Citrate and Phosphate* ⟨345⟩.

Assay preparation—Measure accurately 10 mL of Oral Solution that previously has been freed from excessive carbon dioxide by repeated pouring, into a suitable volumetric flask, and proceed as directed for *Assay Preparation for Citric Acid/Citrate Assay* under *Assay for Citric Acid/Citrate and Phosphate* ⟨345⟩.

Procedure—Proceed as directed for *Procedure* under ⟨345⟩, and calculate the quantity, in mg, of anhydrous citric acid ($C_6H_8O_7$) in the volume of Oral Solution taken by the formula:

$$0.001(192.12 / 189.10)C_S D(r_U / r_S)$$

in which 192.12 is the molecular weight of anhydrous citric acid; 189.10 is the molecular weight of citrate ($C_6H_5O_7$); C_S is the concentration, in µg per mL, of citrate in *Standard Preparation 1*; D is the dilution factor; and r_U and r_S are the citrate peak areas obtained from the *Assay preparation* and *Standard Preparation 1*, respectively.
(Official January 1, 2009)

Assay for magnesium oxide—Transfer to a 100-mL volumetric flask 50.0 mL of Oral Solution that has been previously freed from excessive carbon dioxide by repeated pouring. Dilute with water to volume, and mix. Transfer 5.0 mL of this solution to a beaker containing 150 mL of water heated to 70° to 80°, and add 1 mL of ammonium chloride TS and then 3 mL of ammonium hydroxide. Mix, and add slowly, with stirring, 8 mL of 8-hydroxyquinoline TS. After standing for 30 minutes, filter through a sintered-glass crucible, previously dried and weighed, and wash the precipitate with ten 10-mL portions of water. Dry the crucible and contents at 105° for 3 hours, cool, and weigh. Determine the equivalent of MgO in 100 mL of the Oral Solution by multiplying the weight of $C_{18}H_{12}MgN_2O_2 \cdot 2H_2O$ so obtained by 4.624.

Magnesium Citrate for Oral Solution

» Magnesium Citrate for Oral Solution, when constituted as directed in the labeling, yields a solution that contains not less than 90.0 percent and not more than 110.0 percent of the labeled amount of magnesium citrate ($C_{12}H_{10}Mg_3O_{14}$).

Packaging and storage—Preserve in tight containers.
Labeling—The label contains directions for constitution of the powder and states the equivalent amount of magnesium citrate ($C_{12}H_{10}Mg_3O_{14}$) in a given volume of the Oral Solution obtained after constitution.
USP Reference standards ⟨11⟩—*USP Citric Acid RS*.

(Official January 1, 2009)
Microbial limits ⟨61⟩—It meets the requirements of the test for absence of *Escherichia coli* and *Salmonella* species.
Uniformity of dosage units ⟨905⟩: meets the requirements.
Content of anhydrous citric acid—
Cation-exchange column, Test solution, and *Procedure*—Proceed as directed in the test for *Content of anhydrous citric acid* under *Magnesium Carbonate and Citric Acid for Oral Solution*. The content of anhydrous citric acid is between 76.6% and 93.7% of the labeled amount of magnesium citrate.

(Official until January 1, 2009)
Content of anhydrous citric acid—
Mobile Phase, Standard Preparation 1, and *Chromatographic System*—Proceed as directed under *Assay for Citric Acid/Citrate and Phosphate* ⟨345⟩.
Assay preparation—Transfer an accurately measured volume of the constituted Oral Solution, equivalent to about 9 g of anhydrous citric acid into a suitable volumetric flask, and proceed as directed for *Assay Preparation for Citric Acid/Citrate Assay* under *Assay for Citric Acid/Citrate and Phosphate* ⟨345⟩.
Procedure—Proceed as directed for *Procedure* under ⟨345⟩, and calculate the quantity, in mg, of anhydrous citric acid ($C_6H_8O_7$) in the volume of constituted Oral Solution taken by the formula:

$$0.001(192.12 / 189.10) C_S D(r_U / r_S)$$

in which 192.12 is the molecular weight of anhydrous citric acid; 189.10 is the molecular weight of citrate ($C_6H_5O_7$); C_S is the concentration, in μg per mL, of citrate in *Standard Preparation 1; D* is the dilution factor; and r_U and r_S are the citrate peak areas obtained from the *Assay preparation* and *Standard Preparation 1*, respectively. The content of anhydrous citric acid is between 76.6% and 93.7% of the labeled amount of magnesium citrate.

(Official January 1, 2009)
Other requirements—Constitute Magnesium Citrate for Oral Solution as directed in the labeling: it responds to the *Identification* tests and meets the requirements for *Chloride, Sulfate,* and *Tartaric acid* under *Magnesium Citrate Oral Solution*.
Assay—Transfer an accurately measured volume of constituted Oral Solution, equivalent to about 18.7 g of magnesium citrate ($C_{12}H_{10}Mg_3O_{14}$), to a 1000-mL volumetric flask. Add 200 mL of 1 N hydrochloric acid, swirl, and allow to stand for about 10 minutes. Dilute with water to volume, and mix. Stir by mechanical means for about 30 minutes. Transfer 10.0 mL of this solution to a 250-mL beaker. Add 10 mL of ammonia–ammonium chloride buffer TS, 5 mL of triethanolamine, 0.3 mL of eriochrome black TS, and titrate with 0.05 M edetate disodium VS until the last hint of violet disappears (blue endpoint). Each mL of 0.05 M edetate disodium is equivalent to 7.520 mg of magnesium citrate ($C_{12}H_{10}Mg_3O_{14}$).

Magnesium Gluconate

$C_{12}H_{22}MgO_{14} \cdot xH_2O$ (anhydrous) 414.60
D-Gluconic acid, magnesium salt (2 : 1), hydrate.
Magnesium D-gluconate (1 : 2) hydrate.
Magnesium D-gluconate (1:2) dihydrate 450.64 [59625-89-7].
Anhydrous [3632-91-5].

» Magnesium Gluconate contains not less than 98.0 percent and not more than 102.0 percent of $C_{12}H_{22}MgO_{14}$, calculated on the anhydrous basis.

Packaging and storage—Preserve in well-closed containers.
USP Reference standards ⟨11⟩—*USP Potassium Gluconate RS*.
Identification—
A: A solution (1 in 10) responds to the tests for *Magnesium* ⟨191⟩.
B: It responds to *Identification* test B under *Calcium Gluconate*.
pH ⟨791⟩: between 6.0 and 7.8, in a solution (1 in 20).
Water, *Method Ib* ⟨921⟩: between 3.0% and 12.0%, 30 minutes being allowed for solubilization of the specimen and for the reaction to reach completion, and a blank determination being performed with the same volume of *Reagent* but without the specimen. Calculate the water content of the specimen, in mg, taken by the formula:

$$F(X_b - X)R,$$

in which X_b is the volume, in mL, of standardized *Water-Methanol Solution* required to neutralize the unconsumed *Reagent* in the blank determination; and the other terms are as defined therein.
Chloride ⟨221⟩—A 1.0-g portion shows no more chloride than corresponds to 0.70 mL of 0.020 N hydrochloric acid (0.05%).
Sulfate ⟨221⟩—A 2.0-g portion shows no more sulfate than corresponds to 1.0 mL of 0.020 N sulfuric acid (0.05%).
Heavy metals ⟨231⟩—Dissolve 1.0 g in 10 mL of water, add 6 mL of 3 N hydrochloric acid, and dilute with water to 25 mL: the limit is 0.002%.
Reducing substances—Transfer 1.0 g to a 250-mL conical flask, dissolve in 10 mL of water, and add 25 mL of alkaline cupric citrate TS. Cover the flask, boil gently for 5 minutes, accurately timed, and cool rapidly to room temperature. Add 25 mL of 0.6 N acetic acid, 10.0 mL of 0.1 N iodine VS, and 10 mL of 3 N hydrochloric acid, and titrate with 0.1 N sodium thiosulfate VS, adding 3 mL of starch TS as the endpoint is approached. Perform a blank determination, omitting the specimen, and note the difference in volumes required. Each mL of the difference in volume of 0.1 N sodium thiosulfate consumed is equivalent to 2.7 mg of reducing substances (as dextrose): the limit is 1.0%.
Organic volatile impurities, *Method I* ⟨467⟩: meets the requirements.

(Official until July 1, 2008)
Assay—Weigh accurately about 800 mg of Magnesium Gluconate, dissolve in 20 mL of water, add 5 mL of ammonia-ammonium chloride buffer TS and 0.1 mL of eriochrome black TS, and titrate with 0.05 M edetate disodium VS to a blue endpoint. Each mL of 0.05 M edetate disodium is equivalent to 20.73 mg of $C_{12}H_{22}MgO_{14}$.

Magnesium Gluconate Tablets

» Magnesium Gluconate Tablets contain not less than 95.0 percent and not more than 105.0 percent of the labeled amount of magnesium gluconate ($C_{12}H_{22}MgO_{14}$).

Packaging and storage—Preserve in well-closed containers.
USP Reference standards ⟨11⟩—*USP Potassium Gluconate RS*.
Identification—A filtered solution of Tablets, equivalent to magnesium gluconate solution (1 in 10), diluted with water where necessary, responds to the *Identification* tests under *Magnesium Gluconate*.
Dissolution ⟨711⟩—
Medium: water; 900 mL.
Apparatus 2: 50 rpm.
Time: 30 minutes.
Procedure—Determine the amount of $C_{12}H_{22}MgO_{14}$ dissolved, employing atomic absorption spectrophotometry at a wavelength of about 285.2 nm, in filtered portions of the solution under test, suitably diluted with water, in comparison with a Standard solution having a known concentration of magnesium in the same *Medium*.
Tolerances—Not less than 80% *(Q)* of the labeled amount of $C_{12}H_{22}MgO_{14}$ is dissolved in 30 minutes.
Uniformity of dosage units ⟨905⟩: meet the requirements.
Assay—Weigh and finely powder not fewer than 20 Tablets. Weigh accurately a portion of the powder, equivalent to about 800 mg of

magnesium gluconate, transfer to a suitable crucible, and ignite, gently at first, until free from carbon. Cool the crucible, add 25 mL of water and 5 mL of hydrochloric acid, and stir. Heat on a steam bath for 5 minutes, and filter, rinsing the filter with several portions of water. Dilute the combined filtrate and washings with water to about 150 mL. Add ammonia–ammonium chloride buffer TS until the solution is neutral to litmus. Add 5 mL of ammonia–ammonium chloride buffer TS and 0.1 mL of eriochrome black TS, and titrate with 0.05 M edetate disodium VS to a blue endpoint. Each mL of 0.05 M edetate disodium is equivalent to 20.73 mg of magnesium gluconate ($C_{12}H_{22}MgO_{14}$).

Magnesium Hydroxide

$Mg(OH)_2$ 58.32
Magnesium hydroxide.
Magnesium hydroxide   [1309-42-8].

» Magnesium Hydroxide, dried at 105° for 2 hours, contains not less than 95.0 percent and not more than 100.5 percent of $Mg(OH)_2$.

Packaging and storage—Preserve in tight containers.
Identification—A 1 in 20 solution in 3 N hydrochloric acid responds to the tests for *Magnesium* ⟨191⟩.
Microbial limits ⟨61⟩—It meets the requirements of the test for absence of *Escherichia coli*.
Loss on drying ⟨731⟩—Dry it at 105° for 2 hours: it loses not more than 2.0% of its weight.
Loss on ignition ⟨733⟩—Ignite it at 800°, increasing the heat gradually, to constant weight: it loses between 30.0% and 33.0% of its weight.
Soluble salts—Boil 2.0 g with 100 mL of water for 5 minutes in a covered beaker, filter while hot, cool, and dilute the filtrate with water to 100 mL. Titrate 50 mL of the diluted filtrate with 0.10 N sulfuric acid, using methyl red TS as the indicator: not more than 2.0 mL of the acid is consumed. Evaporate 25 mL of the diluted filtrate to dryness, and dry at 105° for 3 hours: not more than 10 mg of residue remains.
Carbonate—Boil a mixture of 0.10 g with 5 mL of water, cool, and add 5 mL of 6 N acetic acid: not more than a slight effervescence is observed.
Limit of calcium—
  Dilute hydrochloric acid, Lanthanum solution, Standard preparations, and *Blank solution*—Prepare as directed in the test for *Limit of calcium* under *Magnesium Carbonate*.
  Test preparation—Transfer 250 mg of Magnesium Hydroxide, previously dried, to a beaker, add 30 mL of *Dilute hydrochloric acid*, and stir until dissolved, heating if necessary. Transfer the solution so obtained to a 200-mL volumetric flask containing 4 mL of *Lanthanum solution*, dilute with water to volume, and mix.
  Procedure—Proceed as directed in the test for *Limit of calcium* under *Magnesium Carbonate*: the limit is 1.5%.
Heavy metals, *Method I* ⟨231⟩—Dissolve 1.0 g in 15 mL of 3 N hydrochloric acid, and evaporate the solution on a steam bath to dryness. Toward the end of the evaporation, stir the residue frequently, disintegrate it so that finally a dry powder is obtained, dissolve the residue in 20 mL of water, and filter. To the filtrate, which should be neutral to litmus, add 2 mL of 1 N acetic acid, and dilute with water to 25 mL: the limit is 20 μg per g.
Limit of lead—[NOTE—When water is specified as a diluent, use deionized ultra-filtered water.]
  Blank solution—Transfer 3.0 mL of nitric acid to a 50-mL volumetric flask, and dilute with water to volume.
  Thallium internal standard 20 ppb—[NOTE—Use this solution only if an ICP–MS instrument is used. This internal standard is added in-line via a mixing block between the sample probe and the spray chamber.] Dilute 20.0 mL of a commercially prepared thallium ICP standard solution (1000 ppb) with water to 1 L.
  Dilute nitric acid—Dilute 2.0 mL of nitric acid with water to 100 mL.
  Standard stock solution 100 ppb—Prepare this solution fresh every two months. Quantitatively dilute an accurately measured volume of a commercially prepared lead ICP standard (1000 ppm) with *Dilute nitric acid* to obtain a solution containing 10 ppm of lead. Further dilute this solution with *Dilute nitric acid* to obtain a solution containing 1000 ppb of lead. Transfer 10.0 mL of this solution to a separate 100-mL volumetric flask, add 2.0 mL of nitric acid, and dilute with water to volume.
  Standard solutions—Prepare these solutions fresh weekly. [NOTE—The concentrations specified below are recommended if an ICP–MS instrument is used. If an ICP–AES instrument is used, the concentrations of the *Standard solutions* may be modified to adapt to the working range of the instrument.] Transfer 5.0 mL of the *Standard stock solution 100 ppb* to a 50-mL volumetric flask, add 3.0 mL of nitric acid, and dilute with water to volume *(Standard lead solution 10 ppb)*. Transfer 5.0 mL of *Standard lead solution 10 ppb* to a 50-mL volumetric flask, add 3.0 mL of nitric acid, and dilute with water to volume *(Standard lead solution 1 ppb)*.
  Test solution—[NOTE—The concentration specified below is recommended if an ICP–MS instrument is used. If an ICP–AES instrument is used, the concentration of the *Test solution* may be modified to adapt to the working range of the instrument.] Accurately weigh about 0.25 g of Magnesium Hydroxide. Cautiously add 3.0 mL of nitric acid, and mix until the sample is dissolved. Accurately transfer this solution to a 50-mL volumetric flask, and dilute with water to volume.
  Procedure (see *Plasma Spectrochemistry* ⟨730⟩)—The inductively coupled plasma–mass spectrometer (ICP–MS) is equipped with a quadrupole mass spectrometer and an ion detector maintained under vacuum. The instrument should read all isotopes for lead (206, 207, and 208 amu) and the thallium internal standard (205 amu), and should report the total lead content using the most naturally abundant isotope at 208 amu. Alternatively, lead could be determined using an inductively coupled plasma–atomic emission spectrometer (ICP–AES) by measuring the emission at 220.353 nm, with the settings optimized as directed by the manufacturer. [NOTE—To minimize matrix interference when using an ICP–AES instrument, it is recommended that the method of standard additions be used.]
  Instrument performance must be verified to conform to the manufacturer's specifications for resolution and sensitivity. Before analyzing samples, the instrument must pass a suitable performance check. Generate the calibration curve using the *Blank solution*, *Standard lead solution 1 ppb*, and *Standard lead solution 10 ppb*: a linear regression coefficient is not less than 0.999.
  Aspirate the *Test solution*, at least in duplicate, and calculate the amount of lead using the calibration curve. Report the average reading as the lead content of the sample. Calculate the content of lead in the portion of Magnesium Hydroxide taken: not more than 0.00015% (1.5 ppm) is found.
Assay—Transfer about 75 mg of Magnesium Hydroxide, previously dried and accurately weighed, to a conical flask. Add 2 mL of 3 N hydrochloric acid, and swirl to dissolve. Add 100 mL of water, adjust the reaction of the solution to a pH of 7 (using pH indicator paper; see *Indicator and Test Papers* under *Reagents* in the section *Reagents, Indicators, and Solutions*) with 1 N sodium hydroxide, add 5 mL of ammonia-ammonium chloride buffer TS and 0.15 mL of eriochrome black TS, and titrate with 0.05 M edetate disodium VS to a blue endpoint. Each mL of 0.05 M edetate disodium is equivalent to 2.916 mg of $Mg(OH)_2$.

Magnesium Hydroxide Paste

» Magnesium Hydroxide Paste is an aqueous paste of Magnesium Hydroxide. It contains not less than 93.0 percent and not more than 107.0 percent of the labeled amount of magnesium hydroxide [$Mg(OH)_2$], the labeled amount being not less than 28.0 percent and not more than 70.0 percent of magnesium hydroxide.

Packaging and storage—Preserve in tight containers.
Identification—One g of Paste dissolved in 10 mL of 3 N hydrochloric acid responds to the tests for *Magnesium* ⟨191⟩.
Microbial limits ⟨61⟩—Its total aerobic microbial count does not exceed 400 cfu per g, and it meets the requirements of the test for absence of *Escherichia coli*.
Soluble alkalies—Accurately weigh a portion of Paste, equivalent to about 7.75 g of magnesium hydroxide, and mix with 75.0 mL of water. Transfer about 25 mL of this diluted Paste to a filter, and reject the first 5 mL of the filtrate. [NOTE—Retain the remaining diluted Paste for the tests for *Carbonate and acid-insoluble matter* and *Heavy metals*.] Dilute 5 mL of the clear filtrate with 40 mL of water. Add 1 drop of methyl red TS, and titrate the solution with 0.10 N sulfuric acid to the production of a persistent pink color: not more than 1.0 mL of the acid is required.
Soluble salts—To 5.0 mL of the clear filtrate obtained in the test for *Soluble alkalies* add 3 drops of sulfuric acid, evaporate on a steam bath to dryness, and ignite gently to constant weight: the residue weighs not more than 12 mg.
Carbonate and acid-insoluble matter—To 1 mL of the diluted Paste obtained in the test for *Soluble alkalies* add 2 mL of 3 N hydrochloric acid: not more than a slight effervescence occurs, and the solution is not more than slightly turbid.
Limit of calcium—
Dilute hydrochloric acid, Lanthanum solution, Standard preparations, and *Blank solution*—Prepare as directed in the test for *Limit of calcium* under *Magnesium Carbonate*.
Test preparation—Transfer a portion of the Paste, equivalent to 250 mg of Mg(OH)$_2$, to a beaker, add 30 mL of *Dilute hydrochloric acid*, and stir until dissolved, heating if necessary. Transfer the solution so obtained to a 200-mL volumetric flask containing 4 mL of *Lanthanum solution*, dilute with water to volume, and mix.
Procedure—Proceed as directed in the test for *Limit of calcium* under *Magnesium Carbonate*: the limit is 1.5%.
Heavy metals, *Method I* ⟨231⟩—To 4.0 mL of the diluted Paste obtained in the test for *Soluble alkalies* add 6 mL of 3 N hydrochloric acid, and evaporate the solution on a steam bath to dryness, with frequent stirring. Dissolve the residue in 20 mL of water, and evaporate to dryness in the same manner as before. Redissolve in 20 mL of water, filter if necessary, and dilute with water to 25 mL: the limit is 5 ppm, based on the amount of diluted Paste taken.
Limit of lead—
Blank solution, Thallium internal standard 20 ppb, Dilute nitric acid, Standard stock solution 100 ppb, and *Standard solutions*—Proceed as directed in the test for *Limit of lead* under *Magnesium Hydroxide*.
Test solution—Accurately weigh an amount of Paste equivalent to 0.25 g of magnesium hydroxide. Cautiously add 3.0 mL of nitric acid, and mix until the sample is dissolved. Accurately transfer this solution to a 50-mL volumetric flask, and dilute with water to volume. [NOTE—This concentration is recommended if an ICP–MS instrument is used. If an ICP–AES instrument is used, the concentration of the *Test solution* may be modified to adapt to the working range of the instrument.]
Procedure—Proceed as directed in the test for *Limit of lead* under *Magnesium Hydroxide*. Calculate the content of lead in the portion of Paste taken based on the content of magnesium hydroxide in the Paste, as determined in the *Assay:* not more than 0.00015% (1.5 ppm) is found.
Assay—Transfer an accurately weighed portion of Paste, equivalent to about 250 mg of magnesium hydroxide, to a 100-mL volumetric flask. Dissolve in 10 mL of 3 N hydrochloric acid, dilute with water to volume, and mix. Filter, if necessary, and transfer 25.0 mL of the filtrate to a beaker containing 75 mL of water, and mix. Adjust the reaction of the solution to a pH of 7 (using pH indicator paper; see *Indicator and Test Papers* under *Reagents* in the section *Reagents, Indicators, and Solutions*) with 1 N sodium hydroxide, add 5 mL of ammonia–ammonium chloride buffer TS and 0.15 mL of eriochrome black TS, and titrate with 0.05 M edetate disodium VS to a blue endpoint. Each mL of 0.05 M edetate disodium is equivalent to 2.916 mg of magnesium hydroxide [Mg(OH)$_2$].

Magnesium Oxide

MgO   40.30
Magnesium oxide.
Magnesium oxide   [*1309-48-4*].

» Magnesium Oxide, after ignition, contains not less than 96.0 percent and not more than 100.5 percent of MgO.

Packaging and storage—Preserve in tight containers.
Labeling—Label it to indicate its bulk density. The indicated density may be in the form of a range.
Identification—A solution in diluted hydrochloric acid meets the requirements of the tests for *Magnesium* ⟨191⟩.
Loss on ignition ⟨733⟩—Transfer to a tared platinum crucible about 500 mg, weigh accurately, and ignite at 800 ± 25° to constant weight: it loses not more than 10.0% of its weight.
Free alkali and soluble salts—Boil 2.0 g with 100 mL of water for 5 minutes in a covered beaker, and filter while hot. To 50 mL of the cooled filtrate add methyl red TS, and titrate with 0.10 N sulfuric acid: not more than 2.0 mL of the acid is consumed. Evaporate 25 mL of the remaining filtrate to dryness, and dry at 105° for 1 hour: not more than 10 mg of residue remains (2.0%).
Acid-insoluble substances—Mix 2 g with 75 mL of water, add hydrochloric acid in small portions, with agitation, until no more dissolves, and boil for 5 minutes. If an insoluble residue remains, filter, wash well with water until the last washing is free from chloride, and ignite: the weight of the ignited residue does not exceed 2 mg (0.1%).

Change to read:
Limit of calcium—
Dilute hydrochloric acid, Lanthanum solution, Standard preparations, and *Blank solution*—Prepare as directed in the test for *Limit of calcium* under *Magnesium Carbonate*.
Test preparation—Transfer 250 mg of Magnesium Oxide, freshly ignited, to a beaker, add 30 mL of *Dilute hydrochloric acid,* and stir until dissolved, heating if necessary. Transfer the solution so obtained to a 200-mL volumetric flask containing 4 mL of *Lanthanum solution,* dilute with water to volume, and mix.
Procedure—Proceed as directed in the test for *Limit of calcium* under *Magnesium Carbonate*. ▲Determine the concentration, *C*, in µg per mL, of calcium in the *Test preparation* using the calibration graph. Calculate the content of calcium, in percentage, in the portion of Magnesium Oxide taken by the formula:

$$100(0.001CV/W)$$

in which *C* is as defined above; the multiplier of 0.001 is for conversion of µg per mL to mg per mL; *V* is the volume, in mL, of the *Test preparation;* and *W* is the amount of Magnesium Oxide, in mg, taken to prepare the *Test preparation:*▲$_{USP31}$ the limit is 1.1%.
Heavy metals ⟨231⟩—Dissolve 2.0 g in 35 mL of 3 N hydrochloric acid, and evaporate on a steam bath to dryness. Toward the end of the evaporation, stir frequently to disintegrate the residue so that finally a dry powder is obtained. Dissolve the residue in 20 mL of water, and evaporate to dryness in the same manner as before. Redissolve the residue in 20 mL of water, filter if necessary, and dilute with water to 40 mL. To 20 mL add water to make 25 mL: the limit is 20 µg per g.
Iron ⟨241⟩—Boil 40 mg with 5 mL of 2 N nitric acid for 1 minute. Cool, dilute with water to 50 mL, and mix. Dilute 25 mL of this solution with water to 45 mL, and add 2 mL of hydrochloric acid: the limit is 0.05%.
Bulk density, *Method I* ⟨616⟩—Using the procedure specified in the chapter, determine the bulk density of Magnesium Oxide.

Change to read:
Assay—Ignite about 500 mg of Magnesium Oxide to constant weight in a tared platinum crucible, weigh the residue accurately, dissolve it in 30.0 mL of 1 N sulfuric acid VS, add methyl orange TS, and titrate the excess acid with 1 N sodium hydroxide VS. ▲Record the volume, *V$_A$*, in mL, of 1 N sodium hydroxide con-

sumed. Perform the blank determination, and record the volume, V_B, in mL, of 1 N sodium hydroxide consumed. Calculate the volume, V_S, of 1 N sulfuric acid, in mL, consumed by the sample, by the formula:

$$(V_B - V_A) \times N_{NaOH}$$

in which N_{NaOH} is the exact normality of the sodium hydroxide solution. Calculate the volume of 1 N sulfuric acid, V_{Ca}, in mL, consumed by calcium that is present in the Magnesium Oxide taken for the *Assay*, by the formula:

$$(W \times L_{Ca}) / (100 \times 20.04)$$

in which W is the weight, in mg, of Magnesium Oxide taken; L_{Ca} is the content of calcium, in percentage, as determined in the test for *Limit of calcium;* and 20.04 is the weight, in mg, of Ca that is equivalent to each mL of 1 N sulfuric acid.

Calculate the percentage of MgO in the portion of Magnesium Oxide taken by the formula:

$$100(V_S - V_{Ca}) \times 20.15/W$$

in which 20.15 is the weight, in mg, of MgO that is equivalent to each mL of 1 N sulfuric acid; and the other terms are as defined above.▲USP31

Magnesium Oxide Capsules

» Magnesium Oxide Capsules contain not less than 90.0 percent and not more than 110.0 percent of the labeled amount of magnesium oxide (MgO).

Packaging and storage—Preserve in well-closed containers.
Identification—Transfer the contents of 1 Capsule to a beaker, add 10 mL of 3 N hydrochloric acid and 5 drops of methyl red TS, heat to boiling, add 6 N ammonium hydroxide until the color of the solution changes to deep yellow, then continue boiling for 2 minutes, and filter: the filtrate so obtained responds to the tests for *Magnesium* ⟨191⟩.
Dissolution ⟨711⟩—
  Medium: 0.1 N hydrochloric acid; 900 mL.
  Apparatus 1: 100 rpm.
  Time: 45 minutes.
  Procedure—Determine the amount of MgO dissolved, employing atomic absorption spectrophotometry at a wavelength of about 285.2 nm using filtered portions of the solution under test, suitably diluted with *Medium* if necessary, in comparison with a Standard solution having a known concentration of magnesium in the same *Medium*.
  Tolerances—Not less than 75% (*Q*) of the labeled amount of MgO is dissolved in 45 minutes.
Uniformity of dosage units ⟨905⟩: meet the requirements.
Acid-neutralizing capacity ⟨301⟩: not less than 5 mEq of acid is consumed by the minimum single dose recommended in the labeling, and not less than 85.0% of the expected mEq value calculated from the results of the *Assay* is obtained. Each mg of MgO has an expected acid-neutralizing capacity value of 0.0492 mEq.
Assay—Weigh accurately the contents of not fewer than 20 Capsules, and mix. Transfer an accurately weighed portion of the powder, equivalent to about 500 mg of magnesium oxide, to a beaker, add 20 mL of water, and slowly add 40 mL of 3 N hydrochloric acid, with mixing. Heat the mixture to boiling, cool, and filter into a 200-mL volumetric flask. Wash the beaker with water, adding the washings to the filter. Add water to volume, and mix. Transfer 20.0 mL of this solution to a 400-mL beaker, add 180 mL of water and 20 mL of triethanolamine, and stir. Add 10 mL of ammonia–ammonium chloride buffer TS and 3 drops of an eriochrome black indicator solution prepared by dissolving 200 mg of eriochrome black T in a mixture of 15 mL of triethanolamine and 5 mL of dehydrated alcohol, and mix. Cool the solution to between 3° and 4° by immersion of the beaker in an ice bath, then remove, and titrate with 0.05 M edetate disodium VS to a blue endpoint. Perform a blank determination, substituting 20 mL of water for the assay solution, and make any necessary correction. Each mL of 0.05 M edetate disodium consumed is equivalent to 2.015 mg of magnesium oxide (MgO).

Magnesium Oxide Tablets

» Magnesium Oxide Tablets contain not less than 90.0 percent and not more than 110.0 percent of the labeled amount of magnesium oxide (MgO).

Packaging and storage—Preserve in well-closed containers.
Dissolution ⟨711⟩—
  Medium: 0.1 N hydrochloric acid; 900 mL.
  Apparatus 2: 75 rpm.
  Time: 45 minutes.
  Procedure—Determine the amount of MgO dissolved, employing atomic absorption spectrophotometry at a wavelength of about 285.2 nm using filtered portions of the solution under test, suitably diluted with *Medium* if necessary, in comparison with a standard solution having a known concentration of magnesium in the same *Medium*.
  Tolerances—Not less than 75% (*Q*) of the labeled amount of MgO is dissolved in 45 minutes.
Uniformity of dosage units ⟨905⟩: meet the requirements.
Acid-neutralizing capacity ⟨301⟩ (where Tablets are labeled as intended for antacid use): not less than 5 mEq of acid is consumed by the minimum single dose recommended in the labeling, and not less than 85.0% of the expected mEq value calculated from the results of the *Assay* is obtained. Each mg of MgO has an expected acid-neutralizing capacity value of 0.0492 mEq.
Other requirements—One powdered Tablet responds to the *Identification* test under *Magnesium Oxide Capsules*.
Assay—Weigh and finely powder not fewer than 20 Tablets. Transfer an accurately weighed portion of the powder, equivalent to about 500 mg of magnesium oxide, to a beaker. Proceed as directed in the *Assay* under *Magnesium Oxide Capsules* beginning with "add 20 mL of water." Each mL of 0.05 M edetate disodium consumed is equivalent to 2.015 of mg of magnesium oxide (MgO).

Magnesium Phosphate

$Mg_3(PO_4)_2 \cdot 5H_2O$ 352.93
Phosphoric acid, magnesium salt (2 : 3), pentahydrate.
Magnesium phosphate (3 : 2) pentahydrate   [10233-87-1].
Anhydrous   262.86   [7757-87-1].

» Magnesium Phosphate, ignited at 425° to constant weight, contains not less than 98.0 percent and not more than 101.5 percent of $Mg_3(PO_4)_2$.

Packaging and storage—Preserve in well-closed containers.
Identification—
  A: Dissolve about 200 mg in 10 mL of 2 N nitric acid, and add, dropwise, ammonium molybdate TS: a greenish yellow precipitate of ammonium phosphomolybdate is formed and it is soluble in 6 N ammonium hydroxide.
  B: Dissolve 0.1 g in 0.7 mL of 1 N acetic acid and 20 mL of water. Add 1 mL of ferric chloride TS, allow to stand for 5 minutes, and filter: 5 mL of the filtrate responds to the test for *Magnesium* ⟨191⟩.
Microbial limits ⟨61⟩—It meets the requirements of the test for absence of *Escherichia coli*.
Loss on ignition ⟨733⟩—Ignite it at 425° to constant weight: it loses between 20.0% and 27.0% of its weight.
Acid-insoluble substances—If an insoluble residue remains in the test for *Carbonate*, filter the solution, wash well with hot water until the last washing is free from chloride, and ignite the residue: the weight of the residue does not exceed 4 mg (0.2%).

Soluble substances—Digest 2.0 g with 100 mL of water on a steam bath for 30 minutes, cool, add sufficient water to restore the original volume, mix, and filter. Evaporate 50 mL of the filtrate to dryness, and ignite gently to constant weight: the weight of the residue does not exceed 15 mg (1.5%).

Carbonate—Mix 2.0 g with 20 mL of water, and add hydrochloric acid, dropwise, to effect solution: no effervescence occurs when the acid is added.

Chloride ⟨221⟩—Dissolve 0.50 g in 50 mL of 2 N nitric acid, and add 1 mL of silver nitrate TS: the turbidity does not exceed that produced by 1.0 mL of 0.020 N hydrochloric acid (0.14%).

Limit of nitrate—Mix 0.20 g with 5 mL of water, and add just sufficient hydrochloric acid to effect solution. Dilute with water to 10 mL, add 0.1 mL of indigo carmine TS, then add, with stirring, 10 mL of sulfuric acid: the blue color persists for not less than 5 minutes.

Sulfate ⟨221⟩—Dissolve 0.50 g in the smallest possible amount of 3 N hydrochloric acid, dilute with water to 48 mL, and add 2 mL of barium chloride TS: the turbidity does not exceed that produced by 3.0 mL of 0.020 N sulfuric acid (0.6%).

Arsenic, *Method I* ⟨211⟩—Prepare a *Test Preparation* by dissolving 1.0 g in just sufficient 3 N hydrochloric acid (about 9 mL) to dissolve the specimen. The limit is 3 ppm.

Barium—Mix 2.0 g with 40 mL of water, heat, add hydrochloric acid, dropwise, to effect solution, and then add 1 mL of acid in excess. Cool, dilute with water to 50 mL, and filter. To 5 mL of the filtrate add 1 mL of potassium sulfate TS: no turbidity is produced within 15 minutes.

Calcium—Mix 0.50 g with 15 mL of water, heat, and add sufficient hydrochloric acid, in small portions, to effect solution. Cool, add 6 N ammonium hydroxide, in small portions, to produce a slight permanent precipitate, then add 2 mL of 6 N acetic acid. Dilute with water to 25 mL, and filter. To 10 mL of the filtrate add 2 mL of ammonium oxalate TS: not more than a slight turbidity is produced within 5 minutes.

Dibasic salt and magnesium oxide—Ignite about 2.5 g to constant weight. Weigh accurately about 2 g of ignited salt, and dissolve it by warming with 50.0 mL of 1 N hydrochloric acid VS. Cool, add 1 or 2 drops of methyl orange TS, and slowly titrate the excess 1 N hydrochloric acid VS with 1 N sodium hydroxide VS to a yellow color, vigorously shaking the mixture during the titration. Between 14.8 and 15.4 mL of 1 N hydrochloric acid is consumed for each g of the ignited salt.

Lead ⟨251⟩—Prepare a *Test Preparation* by dissolving 1.0 g in 20 mL of 3 N hydrochloric acid, evaporating on a steam bath to about 10 mL, diluting with water to about 20 mL, and cooling. Use 5 mL of *Diluted Standard Lead Solution* (5 μg of Pb) for the test: the limit is 5 ppm.

Heavy metals, *Method I* ⟨231⟩—Dissolve 0.67 g in 4.5 mL of 3 N hydrochloric acid, and dilute with water to 25 mL: the limit is 0.003%.

Assay—Weigh accurately about 200 mg of Magnesium Phosphate, previously ignited at 425° to constant weight, and dissolve in a mixture of 25 mL of water and 10 mL of 2 N nitric acid. Filter, if necessary, wash any precipitate, add sufficient 6 N ammonium hydroxide to the filtrate to produce a slight precipitate, and then dissolve the precipitate by the addition of 1 mL of 2 N nitric acid. Adjust the temperature to about 50°, add 75 mL of ammonium molybdate TS, and maintain the temperature at about 50° for 30 minutes, stirring occasionally. Wash the precipitate once or twice with water by decantation, using from 30 to 40 mL each time and passing the washings through a filter. Transfer the precipitate to the filter, and wash with potassium nitrate solution (1 in 100) until the last washing is not acid to litmus. Transfer the precipitate and filter to the precipitation vessel, add 50 mL of water and 40.0 mL of 1 N sodium hydroxide VS, agitate until the precipitate is dissolved, add phenolphthalein TS, and then titrate the excess alkali with 1 N sulfuric acid VS. Each mL of 1 N sodium hydroxide is equivalent to 5.716 mg of $Mg_3(PO_4)_2$.

Magnesium Salicylate

$C_{14}H_{10}MgO_6 \cdot 4H_2O$ 370.59
Magnesium, bis(2-hydroxybenzoato-O^1,O^2)-, tetrahydrate.
Magnesium salicylate (1 : 2), tetrahydrate   [18917-95-8].
Anhydrous   298.54   [18917-89-0].

» Magnesium Salicylate contains not less than 98.0 percent and not more than 103.0 percent of $C_{14}H_{10}MgO_6 \cdot 4H_2O$.

Packaging and storage—Store in tight containers.
USP Reference standards ⟨11⟩—*USP Magnesium Salicylate RS. USP Salicylic Acid RS.*
Identification—
  A: *Infrared Absorption* ⟨197K⟩: previously dried at 105° for 4 hours.
  B: *Ultraviolet Absorption* ⟨197U⟩—
    Solution: 20 μg per mL.
    Medium: water.
  C: It responds to the test for *Magnesium* ⟨191⟩.
Water, *Method I* ⟨921⟩:   between 17.5% and 21.0%.
Heavy metals, *Method I* ⟨231⟩:   0.004%.
Magnesium content—Transfer about 800 mg, accurately weighed, to a 200-mL volumetric flask. Dissolve in and dilute with water to volume, and mix. Stir the resulting solution continuously for about 15 minutes and filter, discarding the first 10 mL of the filtrate, into a flask. Transfer 50.0 mL of the filtrate to a 250-mL conical flask, add 50 mL of water, 5 mL of ammonia–ammonium chloride buffer TS, and 0.15 mL of eriochrome black TS, and titrate with 0.05 M edetate disodium VS to a blue endpoint. Each mL of 0.05 M edetate disodium is equivalent to 1.215 mg of magnesium: between 6.3% and 6.7% of magnesium is found.
Organic volatile impurities, *Method I* ⟨467⟩:   meets the requirements.
(Official until July 1, 2008)
Assay—Transfer 3.0 mL of the filtrate prepared in the test for *Magnesium content* to a 500-mL volumetric flask, dilute with water to volume, and mix. Concomitantly determine the absorbances of this solution and a solution of USP Salicylic Acid RS in water having a known concentration of about 18 μg per mL, in 1-cm cells at the wavelength of maximum absorbance at about 296 nm, with a suitable spectrophotometer, using water as the blank. Calculate the quantity, in mg, of $C_{14}H_{10}MgO_6 \cdot 4H_2O$ in the Magnesium Salicylate taken in the test for *Magnesium content* by the formula:

$$(370.59 / 276.24)(33.3C)(A_U / A_S)$$

in which 370.59 is the molecular weight of magnesium salicylate tetrahydrate; 276.24 is twice the molecular weight of salicylic acid; *C* is the concentration, in μg per mL, of USP Salicylic Acid RS in the Standard solution; and A_U and A_S are the absorbances of the test solution and the Standard solution, respectively.

Magnesium Salicylate Tablets

» Magnesium Salicylate Tablets contain an amount of magnesium salicylate ($C_{14}H_{10}MgO_6 \cdot 4H_2O$) equivalent to not less than 95.0 percent and not more than 105.0 percent of the labeled amount of $C_{14}H_{10}MgO_6$.

Packaging and storage—Preserve in tight containers.
USP Reference standards ⟨11⟩—*USP Magnesium Salicylate RS. USP Salicylic Acid RS.*

Identification—
A: The IR absorption spectrum of a potassium bromide dispersion of a quantity of finely powdered Tablets exhibits maxima at the same wavelengths as that of a similar preparation of USP Magnesium Salicylate RS.
B: A filtered solution of Tablets, equivalent to magnesium salicylate solution (1 : 20), responds to the test for *Magnesium* ⟨191⟩.

Dissolution ⟨711⟩—
Medium: water; 900 mL.
Apparatus 2: 50 rpm.
Time: 120 minutes.
Procedure—Determine the amount of $C_{14}H_{10}MgO_6$ dissolved from UV absorbances at the wavelength of maximum absorbance at about 296 nm of filtered portions of the solution under test, suitably diluted with water, in comparison with a Standard solution having a known concentration of USP Salicylic Acid RS in the same medium, using water as the blank. Calculate the quantity of magnesium salicylate ($C_{14}H_{10}MgO_6$), dissolved by the formula:

$$(298.54 / 276.24)(900C)(A_U / A_S)$$

in which the terms are as defined in the *Assay*.
Tolerances—Not less than 80% (*Q*) of the labeled amount of $C_{14}H_{10}MgO_6$ is dissolved in 120 minutes.

Uniformity of dosage units ⟨905⟩: meet the requirements.
Assay—Weigh and finely powder not fewer than 20 Tablets. Weigh accurately a portion of the powder, equivalent to about 500 mg of magnesium salicylate, and transfer to a 250-mL volumetric flask. Dilute with water to volume, mix, and filter, discarding the first 20 mL of the filtrate. Dilute an accurately measured portion of the filtrate quantitatively and stepwise, if necessary, to obtain a final concentration of about 20 μg per mL. Dissolve an accurately weighed quantity of USP Salicylic Acid RS in water, and dilute quantitatively and stepwise, if necessary, with water to obtain a Standard solution having a known concentration of about 18 μg per mL. Concomitantly determine the absorbances of both solutions in 1-cm cells at the wavelength of maximum absorbance at about 296 nm, with a suitable spectrophotometer, using water as the blank. Calculate the quantity, in mg, of $C_{14}H_{10}MgO_6$ in the portion of Tablets taken by the formula:

$$(298.54 / 276.24)(L / D)(C)(A_U / A_S)$$

in which 298.54 is the molecular weight of anhydrous magnesium salicylate; 276.24 is twice the molecular weight of salicylic acid; *L* is the labeled quantity, in mg, of magnesium salicylate in each Tablet; *D* is the concentration, in mg per mL, of magnesium salicylate in the solution from the Tablets, based on the labeled quantity per Tablet and the extent of dilution; *C* is the concentration, in mg per mL, of USP Salicylic Acid RS in the Standard solution; and A_U and A_S are the absorbances of the solution from the Tablets and the Standard solution, respectively.

Magnesium Sulfate

$MgSO_4 \cdot xH_2O$
Sulfuric acid magnesium salt (1 : 1), hydrate.
Magnesium sulfate (1 : 1) monohydrate   138.36
Magnesium sulfate (1 : 1) heptahydrate   246.48   [10034-99-8].
Anhydrous   120.37   [7487-88-9].

» Magnesium Sulfate, rendered anhydrous by ignition, contains not less than 99.0 percent and not more than 100.5 percent of $MgSO_4$.

Packaging and storage—Preserve in well-closed containers.
Labeling—The label states whether it is the monohydrate, the dried form, or the heptahydrate. Magnesium Sulfate intended for use in preparing parenteral dosage forms is so labeled. Magnesium Sulfate not intended for use in preparing parenteral dosage forms is so labeled; in addition, it may be labeled also as intended for use in preparing nonparenteral dosage forms.
Identification—A solution (1 in 20) responds to the tests for *Magnesium* ⟨191⟩ and for *Sulfate* ⟨191⟩.

pH ⟨791⟩: between 5.0 and 9.2, in a solution (1 in 20).
Loss on drying ⟨731⟩—Dry it at 105° for 2 hours: the anhydrous form loses not more than 2% of its weight.
Loss on ignition ⟨733⟩—Weigh accurately about 1 g in a crucible, heat at 105° for 2 hours, then ignite in a muffle furnace at 450 ± 25° to constant weight: the monohydrate loses between 13.0% and 16.0% of its weight, the dried form loses between 22.0% and 28.0% of its weight, and the heptahydrate loses between 40.0% and 52.0% of its weight.
Chloride ⟨221⟩—A 1.0-g portion shows no more chloride than corresponds to 0.20 mL of 0.020 N hydrochloric acid (0.014%).
Iron ⟨241⟩—
FOR MAGNESIUM SULFATE INTENDED FOR USE IN PREPARING NONPARENTERAL DOSAGE FORMS—Dissolve 0.50 g in 40 mL of water and proceed as directed in the test for *Iron* ⟨241⟩: the limit is 20 μg per g.
FOR MAGNESIUM SULFATE INTENDED FOR USE IN PREPARING PARENTERAL DOSAGE FORMS—[NOTE—Rinse all glassware used in this test with *Dilute hydrochloric acid*.]
Dilute hydrochloric acid—Dilute 1 mL of hydrochloric acid to 1000 mL with water, and mix.
Ammonium acetate solution—Transfer 250 g of ammonium acetate to a 500-mL volumetric flask, dissolve in and dilute with water to volume, and mix.
Ascorbic acid solution—Transfer 1.34 g of ascorbic acid to a 100-mL volumetric flask, dissolve in and dilute with water to volume, and mix. Use this solution on the day prepared.
Color reagent—Transfer 380 mg of 3-(2-pyridyl)-5,6-di-(2-furyl)-1,2,4-triazine-5′,5″-disulfonic acid, disodium salt to a 100-mL volumetric flask, dissolve in *Ammonium acetate solution*, shaking by mechanical means if necessary, dilute with *Ammonium acetate solution* to volume, and mix. Use this solution on the day prepared.
Standard iron solution—Transfer 5.0 mL of *Standard Iron Solution* to a 50-mL volumetric flask, dilute with *Dilute hydrochloric acid* to volume, and mix. This solution contains 1.0 μg of iron per mL.
Standard preparations—To three separate 50-mL volumetric flasks transfer 2.0, 5.0, and 10.0 mL of *Standard iron solution*, and dilute each to 35 mL with *Dilute hydrochloric acid*. These solutions contain 2.0, 5.0, and 10.0 μg of iron, respectively.
Test preparation—Transfer 10.0 g of Magnesium Sulfate to a 50-mL volumetric flask, add *Dilute hydrochloric acid* to 35 mL, and sonicate, if necessary, to achieve complete dissolution.
Blank—Transfer 35 mL of *Dilute hydrochloric acid* to a 50-mL volumetric flask.
Procedure—To each of the flasks containing the *Standard preparations*, the *Test preparation*, and the *Blank*, add 5 mL of *Ascorbic acid solution* and 5 mL of *Color reagent*. Dilute each solution with *Dilute hydrochloric acid* to volume, mix, and allow to stand for 10 minutes. Concomitantly determine the absorbances of the solutions from the *Standard preparations* and the *Test preparation* at the wavelength of maximum absorbance at about 594 nm, with a suitable spectrophotometer, using the solution from the *Blank* to set the instrument to zero. Plot the absorbance values of the solutions from the *Standard preparations* versus their iron contents, in μg per 50-mL volumetric flask, and draw the straight line best fitting the three plotted points. From the graph so obtained determine the iron content, *C*, in μg per 50-mL volumetric flask, of the solution from the *Test preparation*. Calculate the content, in ppm, of iron in the portion of Magnesium Sulfate taken by multiplying *C* by 0.1: the limit is 0.5 μg per g.
Heavy metals ⟨231⟩—Dissolve 2 g in 25 mL of water: the limit is 0.001%.
Selenium ⟨291⟩—Dissolve 200 mg in 50 mL of 0.25 N nitric acid to obtain the *Test Solution*. The limit is 0.003%.
Organic volatile impurities, *Method I* ⟨467⟩: meets the requirements.

(Official until July 1, 2008)
Assay—Weigh accurately about 250 mg of the ignited Magnesium Sulfate obtained in the test for *Loss on ignition*, and dissolve in 100 mL of water and the minimum amount of 3 N hydrochloric acid required for a clear solution. Adjust the reaction of the solution (using pH indicator paper; see *Indicator and Test Papers* under *Reagents* in the section *Reagents, Indicators, and Solutions*) with 1 N

sodium hydroxide to a pH of 7, add 5 mL of ammonia–ammonium chloride buffer TS and 0.15 mL of eriochrome black TS, and titrate with 0.05 M edetate disodium VS to a blue endpoint. Each mL of 0.05 M edetate disodium is equivalent to 6.018 mg of MgSO$_4$.

Magnesium Sulfate Injection

» Magnesium Sulfate Injection is a sterile solution of Magnesium Sulfate in Water for Injection. It contains magnesium sulfate equivalent to not less than 93.0 percent and not more than 107.0 percent of the labeled amount of MgSO$_4$ · 7H$_2$O.

Packaging and storage—Preserve in single-dose or multiple-dose containers, preferably of Type I glass.
Labeling—The label states the total osmolar concentration in mOsmol per L. Where the contents are less than 100 mL, or where the label states that the Injection is not for direct injection but is to be diluted before use, the label alternatively may state the total osmolar concentration in mOsmol per mL.
USP Reference standards ⟨11⟩—*USP Endotoxin RS*.
Identification—It responds to the tests for *Magnesium* ⟨191⟩ and for *Sulfate* ⟨191⟩.
Bacterial endotoxins ⟨85⟩—It contains not more than 0.09 USP Endotoxin Unit per mg of magnesium sulfate.
pH ⟨791⟩: between 5.5 and 7.0, when diluted to a concentration of 5% (w/v).
Particulate matter ⟨788⟩: meets the requirements for small-volume injections.
Other requirements—It meets the requirements under *Injections* ⟨1⟩.
Assay—Transfer to a beaker an accurately measured volume of Injection, equivalent to about 250 mg of anhydrous magnesium sulfate, and dilute with water to 100 mL. Adjust the reaction of the solution to a pH of 7 (using pH indicator paper; see *Indicator and Test Papers* under *Reagents* in the section *Reagents, Indicators, and Solutions*) with 1 N sodium hydroxide, add 5 mL of ammonia–ammonium chloride buffer TS and 0.15 mL of eriochrome black TS, and titrate with 0.05 M edetate disodium VS to a blue endpoint. Each mL of 0.05 M edetate disodium is equivalent to 12.32 mg of MgSO$_4$ · 7H$_2$O.

Magnesium Sulfate in Dextrose Injection

» Magnesium Sulfate in Dextrose Injection is a sterile solution of Magnesium Sulfate and Dextrose in Water for Injection. It contains not less than 93.0 percent and not more than 107.0 percent of the labeled amount of magnesium sulfate (MgSO$_4$ · 7H$_2$O) and not less than 90.0 percent and not more than 110.0 percent of the labeled amount of dextrose (C$_6$H$_{12}$O$_6$ · H$_2$O).

Packaging and storage—Preserve in single-dose glass or plastic containers. Glass containers are preferably of Type 1 or Type II glass.
USP Reference standards ⟨11⟩—*USP Endotoxin RS*.
Identification—It responds to the *Identification* test under *Dextrose*, and to the tests for *Magnesium* ⟨191⟩.
Bacterial endotoxins ⟨85⟩—It contains not more than 0.039 USP Endotoxin Unit per mg of magnesium sulfate.
pH ⟨791⟩: between 3.5 and 6.5.
Limit of 5-hydroxymethylfurfural and related substances—Dilute an accurately measured volume of Injection, equivalent to 1.0 g of C$_6$H$_{12}$O$_6$ · H$_2$O, with water to 500.0 mL. Determine the absorbance of this solution in a 1-cm cell at 284 nm with a spectrophotometer, using water as the blank: the absorbance is not more than 0.25.
Other requirements—It meets the requirements under *Injections* ⟨1⟩.
Assay for magnesium sulfate—Proceed with Injection as directed in the *Assay* under *Magnesium Sulfate Injection*.
Assay for dextrose—Proceed with Injection as directed in the *Assay* under *Dextrose Injection*.

Magnesium Trisilicate

2MgO · 3SiO$_2$ · xH$_2$O(anhydrous)   260.86
Silicic acid (H$_4$Si$_3$O$_8$), magnesium salt (1 : 2), hydrate.
Magnesium silicate hydrate (Mg$_2$Si$_3$O$_8$ · xH$_2$O)   [39365-87-2].
Anhydrous   [14987-04-3].

» Magnesium Trisilicate is a compound of Magnesium Oxide and silicon dioxide with varying proportions of water. It contains not less than 20.0 percent of magnesium oxide (MgO) and not less than 45.0 percent of silicon dioxide (SiO$_2$).

Packaging and storage—Preserve in well-closed containers.
Identification—
A: Mix about 500 mg with 10 mL of 3 N hydrochloric acid, filter, and neutralize the filtrate to litmus paper with 6 N ammonium hydroxide: the neutralized filtrate responds to the tests for *Magnesium* ⟨191⟩.
B: Prepare a bead by fusing a few crystals of sodium ammonium phosphate on a platinum loop in the flame of a Bunsen burner. Place the hot, transparent bead in contact with Magnesium Trisilicate, and again fuse: silica floats about in the bead, producing, upon cooling, an opaque bead with a web-like structure.
Water, *Method III* ⟨921⟩—Weigh accurately about 1 g in a tared platinum crucible provided with a cover. Gradually apply heat to the crucible at first, then strongly ignite to constant weight: it loses between 17.0% and 34.0% of its weight.
Soluble salts—Boil 10.0 g with 150 mL of water for 15 minutes. Cool to room temperature, allow the mixture to stand for 15 minutes, filter with the aid of suction, transfer the filtrate to a 200-mL volumetric flask, dilute with water to volume, and mix. Evaporate 50.0 mL of this solution, representing 2.5 g of the Trisilicate, in a tared platinum dish to dryness, and ignite gently to constant weight: the weight of the residue does not exceed 38.0 mg (1.5%).
Chloride ⟨221⟩—A 20-mL portion of the diluted filtrate prepared in the test for *Soluble salts*, representing 1 g of Magnesium Trisilicate, shows no more chloride than corresponds to 0.75 mL of 0.020 N hydrochloric acid (0.055%).
Sulfate—Treat the residue obtained in the test for *Soluble salts* with 2 mL of hydrofluoric acid, and evaporate on a steam bath to dryness. Mix the residue with water, transfer to a filter, and wash, using approximately 50 mL of water for the complete procedure. Heat the filtrate to boiling, and add 0.1 mL of hydrochloric acid and 5 mL of barium chloride TS. Maintain the mixture near its boiling point for 1 hour, filter, wash the precipitate thoroughly with water, dry, and ignite to constant weight: the weight of the residue does not exceed 30 mg (0.5%).
Free alkali—Add 2 drops of phenolphthalein TS to 20 mL of the diluted filtrate prepared in the test for *Soluble salts*, representing 1 g of the Trisilicate: if a pink color is produced, not more than 1.0 mL of 0.10 N hydrochloric acid is required to discharge it.
Arsenic, *Method I* ⟨211⟩: 8 ppm.
Heavy metals ⟨231⟩—Boil 2.67 g with a mixture of 50 mL of water and 5 mL of hydrochloric acid for 20 minutes, adding water to maintain the volume during the boiling. Add ammonium hydroxide until the mixture is only slightly acid to litmus paper. Filter with the aid of suction, and wash with 15 to 20 mL of water, combining the washing with the original filtrate. Add 2 drops of phenolphthalein TS, then add a slight excess of 6 N ammonium hydroxide. Discharge the pink color with dilute hydrochloric acid (1 in 100), then add 8 mL of dilute hydrochloric acid (1 in 100). Dilute with water

to 100 mL, and use 25 mL of the solution for the test: the limit is 0.003%.

Acid-consuming capacity—Weigh accurately about 200 mg into a glass-stoppered, 125-mL conical flask. Add 30.0 mL of 0.1 N hydrochloric acid VS and 20.0 mL of water. Place the flask in a bath maintained at 37°, and shake the mixture occasionally during a period of 4 hours but leave the mixture undisturbed during the last 15 minutes of the heating period. Cool to room temperature. To 25.0 mL of the supernatant add methyl red TS, and titrate the excess acid with 0.1 N sodium hydroxide VS. One g of Magnesium Trisilicate, calculated on the anhydrous basis, consumes not less than 140 mL and not more than 160 mL of 0.10 N hydrochloric acid.

Assay for magnesium oxide—Weigh accurately about 1.5 g, and transfer to a 250-mL conical flask. Add 50.0 mL of 1 N sulfuric acid VS, and digest on a steam bath for 1 hour. Cool to room temperature, add methyl orange TS, and titrate the excess acid with 1 N sodium hydroxide VS. Each mL of 1 N sulfuric acid is equivalent to 20.15 mg of MgO.

Assay for silicon dioxide—Transfer about 700 mg of Magnesium Trisilicate, accurately weighed, to a small platinum dish. Add 10 mL of 1 N sulfuric acid, and heat on a steam bath to dryness, leaving the dish uncovered. Treat the residue with 25 mL of water, and digest on a steam bath for 15 minutes. Decant the supernatant through an ashless filter paper, with the aid of suction, and wash the residue, by decantation, three times with hot water, passing the washings through the filter paper. Finally transfer the residue to the filter, and wash thoroughly with hot water. Transfer the filter paper and its contents to the platinum dish previously used. Heat to dryness, incinerate, ignite strongly for 30 minutes, cool, and weigh. Moisten the residue with water, and add 6 mL of hydrofluoric acid and 3 drops of sulfuric acid. Evaporate to dryness, ignite for 5 minutes, cool, and weigh: the loss in weight represents the weight of SiO_2.

Ratio of SiO_2 to MgO—Divide the percentage of SiO_2 obtained in the *Assay for silicon dioxide* by the percentage of MgO obtained in the *Assay for magnesium oxide*: the quotient obtained is between 2.10 and 2.37.

Magnesium Trisilicate Tablets

» Magnesium Trisilicate Tablets contain not less than 90.0 percent and not more than 110.0 percent of the labeled amount of $Mg_2Si_3O_8$.

Packaging and storage—Preserve in well-closed containers.
Identification—
  A: Powder 1 Tablet, add 10 mL of 3 N hydrochloric acid and 5 drops of methyl red TS, heat to boiling, add 6 N ammonium hydroxide until the color of the solution changes to deep yellow, then continue boiling for 2 minutes, and filter: the filtrate so obtained responds to the tests for *Magnesium* ⟨191⟩.
  B: Wash the solids on the filter obtained in *Identification* test *A* with hot ammonium chloride solution (1 in 50), add 10 mL of 3 N hydrochloric acid, and filter. Transfer the filter paper and contents to a small platinum dish, ignite, cool in a desiccator, and weigh. Moisten the residue with water, and add 6 mL of hydrofluoric acid. Evaporate to dryness, ignite for 5 minutes, cool in a desiccator, and weigh: a loss of more than 10% in relation to the weight of the residue from the initial ignition indicates SiO_2.

Disintegration ⟨701⟩: 10 minutes, simulated gastric fluid TS being substituted for water in the test.
Uniformity of dosage units ⟨905⟩: meet the requirements.
Acid-neutralizing capacity ⟨301⟩—Not less than 5 mEq of acid is consumed by the minimum single dose recommended in the labeling.
Assay—Weigh and finely powder not fewer than 20 Tablets. Transfer an accurately weighed portion of the powder, equivalent to about 1 g of magnesium trisilicate, to a beaker, add 20 mL of water, and slowly add 40 mL of 3 N hydrochloric acid, with mixing. Heat the mixture to boiling, cool, and filter into a 200-mL volumetric flask. Wash the beaker with water, adding the washings to the filter. Add water to volume, and mix. Transfer 20.0 mL of this solution to a 400-mL beaker, add 180 mL of water and 20 mL of triethanolamine, and stir. Add 10 mL of ammonia–ammonium chloride buffer TS and 3 drops of an eriochrome black indicator solution prepared by dissolving 200 mg of eriochrome black T in a mixture of 15 mL of triethanolamine and 5 mL of dehydrated alcohol, and mix. Cool the solution to between 3° and 4° by immersion of the beaker in an ice bath, then remove, and titrate with 0.05 M edetate disodium VS to a blue endpoint. Perform a blank determination, substituting 20 mL of water for the assay solution, and make any necessary correction. Each mL of 0.05 M edetate disodium consumed is equivalent to 6.521 mg of $Mg_2Si_3O_8$.

Malathion

$C_{10}H_{19}O_6PS_2$ 330.36
Butanedioic acid, [(dimethoxyphosphinothioyl)-thio], diethyl ester, (±)-.
Diethyl (±)-mercaptosuccinate, S-ester with O,O-dimethyl phosphorodithioate [121-75-5].

» Malathion contains not less than 98.0 percent and not more than 102.0 percent of $C_{10}H_{19}O_6PS_2$.

Packaging and storage—Preserve in tight, light-resistant containers.
USP Reference standards ⟨11⟩—USP Isomalathion RS. USP Malathion RS.
Identification, *Infrared Absorption* ⟨197F⟩.
Specific gravity ⟨841⟩: between 1.220 and 1.240.
Water, *Method I* ⟨921⟩: not more than 0.1%.
Limit of isomalathion—
  Mobile phase—Prepare a suitable degassed solution of methanol and water (50:30). Make adjustments if necessary (see *System Suitability* under *Chromatography* ⟨621⟩).
  Standard preparation—Dissolve an accurately weighed quantity of USP Isomalathion RS in methanol to obtain a solution having a known concentration of about 0.1 mg per mL.
  Test preparation—Dissolve an accurately weighed quantity of Malathion in methanol to obtain a solution having a known concentration of about 20 mg per mL.
  Chromatographic system (see *Chromatography* ⟨621⟩)—The liquid chromatograph is equipped with a 210-nm detector and a 4-mm × 30-cm column that contains 10-µm packing L1. The flow rate is about 1 mL per minute. Chromatograph the *Standard preparation*, and record the peak responses as directed for *Procedure*: the relative retention times are about 0.5 for isomalathion and 1.0 for malathion; and the relative standard deviation for replicate injections is not more than 2.0%.
  Procedure—Separately inject equal volumes (about 20 µL) of the *Standard preparation* and the *Test preparation* into the chromatograph, record the chromatograms, and measure the responses of the major peaks. Calculate the percentage of isomalathion in the Malathion taken by the formula:

$$(C_S / C_U)(P)(r_U / r_S)$$

in which C_S is the concentration, in mg per mL, of USP Isomalathion RS in the *Standard preparation*; C_U is the concentration, in mg per mL, of specimen in the *Test preparation*; P is the stated purity, in percentage, of the USP Isomalathion RS; and r_U and r_S are the isomalathion peak responses obtained from the *Test preparation* and the *Standard preparation*, respectively: not more than 0.3% of isomalathion is found.

Assay—

Mobile phase—Prepare a suitable degassed solution of methanol and water (50:30). Make adjustments if necessary (see *System Suitability* under *Chromatography* ⟨621⟩).

Internal standard solution—Dissolve propylparaben in *Mobile phase* to obtain a solution containing about 0.6 mg per mL.

Standard preparation—Transfer about 100 mg of USP Malathion RS, accurately weighed, to a 10-mL volumetric flask, add 1.0 mL of *Internal standard solution*, dilute with methanol to volume, and mix.

Assay preparation—Transfer about 500 mg of Malathion, accurately weighed, to a 50-mL volumetric flask, add 5.0 mL of *Internal standard solution*, dilute with methanol to volume, and mix.

Chromatographic system (see *Chromatography* ⟨621⟩)—The liquid chromatograph is equipped with a 254-nm detector and a 4-mm × 30-cm column that contains 10-μm packing L1. The flow rate is about 1 mL per minute. Chromatograph the *Standard preparation*, and record the peak responses as directed for *Procedure*: the relative retention times are about 0.6 for propylparaben and 1.0 for malathion; and the resolution, R, of the propylparaben and malathion peaks is not less than 4, and the relative standard deviation for replicate injections is not more than 2.0%.

Procedure—Separately inject equal volumes (about 20 μL) of the *Standard preparation* and the *Assay preparation* into the chromatograph, record the chromatograms, and measure the responses for the major peaks. Calculate the quantity, in mg, of $C_{10}H_{19}O_6PS_2$ in the portion of Malathion taken by the formula:

$$50C(R_U / R_S)$$

in which C is the concentration, in mg per mL, of USP Malathion RS in the *Standard preparation*; and R_U and R_S are the ratios of the peak responses of malathion to propylparaben obtained from the *Assay preparation* and the *Standard preparation*, respectively.

Malathion Lotion

» Malathion Lotion is Malathion in a suitable isopropyl alcohol vehicle. It contains not less than 90.0 percent and not more than 110.0 percent of the labeled amount of malathion ($C_{10}H_{19}O_6PS_2$).

Packaging and storage—Preserve in tight, glass containers.
Labeling—The labeling states the percentage (v/v) of isopropyl alcohol in the Lotion.
USP Reference standards ⟨11⟩—*USP Malathion RS*.
Identification—The chromatogram of the *Assay preparation* obtained as directed in the *Assay* exhibits a major peak for malathion, the retention time of which corresponds to that exhibited in the chromatogram of the *Standard preparation*, both relative to the internal standard, obtained as directed in the *Assay*.
Isopropyl alcohol content—

Internal standard solution—Mix 4 volumes of ethyl acetate and 1 volume of dehydrated alcohol.

Standard preparation—Transfer 2.0 mL of isopropyl alcohol and 5.0 mL of *Internal standard solution* to a 200-mL volumetric flask, dilute with ethyl acetate to volume, and mix.

Test preparation—Transfer an accurately measured volume of Malathion Lotion, equivalent to about 2.0 mL of isopropyl alcohol, to a 200-mL volumetric flask. Add 5.0 mL of *Internal standard solution*, dilute with ethyl acetate to volume, and mix.

Chromatographic system (see *Chromatography* ⟨621⟩)—The gas chromatograph is equipped with a flame-ionization detector and contains a 2-mm × 1.8-m glass column packed with 110- to 120-mesh support S2. Maintain the temperatures of the column, the injector port, and the detector block at 130°, 200°, and 220°, respectively. Use dry nitrogen as the carrier gas at a flow rate of about 7 mL per minute. Chromatograph the *Standard preparation*, and record the peak responses as directed for *Procedure*: the relative standard deviation of the ratio of the isopropyl alcohol peak response to the internal standard peak response for replicate injections is not more than 2.0%.

Procedure—Separately inject equal volumes (about 1 μL) of the *Standard preparation* and the *Test preparation* into the gas chromatograph, record the chromatograms, and measure the areas for the major peaks. Calculate the percentage of isopropyl alcohol (C_3H_8O) in the Lotion by the formula:

$$(200 / V)(R_U / R_S)$$

in which V is the volume, in mL, of Lotion taken; and R_U and R_S are the ratios of the peak responses of isopropyl alcohol to internal standard obtained from the *Test preparation* and the *Standard preparation*, respectively: between 90% and 110% of the labeled amount of C_3H_8O is found.

Assay—

Solvent mixture—Mix 4 volumes of methyl ethyl ketone and 1 volume of *n*-hexane.

Internal standard solution—Prepare a solution of parathion in *Solvent mixture* containing about 2 mg per mL.

Standard preparation—Dissolve an accurately weighed quantity of USP Malathion RS in *Solvent mixture* to obtain a solution having a known concentration of about 2 mg per mL. Transfer 5.0 mL of this solution to a 25-mL volumetric flask, add 5.0 mL of *Internal standard solution*, dilute with *Solvent mixture* to volume, and mix.

Assay preparation—Transfer an accurately measured volume of Lotion, equivalent to about 10 mg of malathion, to a 25-mL volumetric flask, add 5.0 mL of *Internal standard solution*, dilute with *Solvent mixture* to volume, and mix.

Chromatographic system (see *Chromatography* ⟨621⟩)—The gas chromatograph is equipped with a flame-ionization detector and contains a 2-mm × 1.8-m glass column packed with 5% G6 liquid phase on 110- to 120-mesh support S1A. Maintain temperatures of the column, the injector port, and the detector block at 190°, 230°, and 250°, respectively. Use dry nitrogen as the carrier gas at a flow rate of about 15 mL per minute. Chromatograph the *Standard preparation*, and record the peak responses as directed for *Procedure*: the relative retention times are 1.0 for malathion and about 1.3 for parathion; the resolution, R, between the malathion and parathion peaks is not less than 3.0; and the relative standard deviation for replicate injections is not more than 2.0%.

Procedure—Separately inject equal volumes (about 1 μL) of the *Standard preparation* and the *Assay preparation* into the chromatograph, record the chromatograms, and measure the responses of the major peaks. Calculate the quantity, in mg, of malathion ($C_{10}H_{19}O_6PS_2$) in each mL of the Lotion taken by the formula:

$$25(C / V)(R_U / R_S)$$

in which C is the concentration, in mg per mL, of USP Malathion RS in the *Standard preparation*; V is the volume, in mL, of Lotion taken; and R_U and R_S are the ratios of the peak responses of malathion to parathion obtained from the *Assay preparation* and the *Standard preparation*, respectively.

Mangafodipir Trisodium

$C_{22}H_{27}MnN_4Na_3O_{14}P_2$ 757.33
Trisodium trihydrogen (*OC*-6-13)-[[*N,N*′-1,2-ethanediylbis[*N*-[[3-hydroxy-2-methyl-5-[(phosphonooxy)methyl]-4-pyridinyl]methyl]glycinato]](8-)]manganate(6-).
Trisodium trihydrogen (*OC*-6-13)-[[*N,N*′-ethylenebis[*N*-[[3-hydroxy-5-(hydroxymethyl)-2-methyl-4-pyridyl]methyl]glycine] 5,5′-bis(phosphato)](8-)]manganate(6-) [*140678-14-4*].

» Mangafodipir Trisodium contains not less than 97.0 percent and not more than 103.0 percent of

$C_{22}H_{27}MnN_4Na_3O_{14}P_2$, calculated on the anhydrous basis.

Packaging and storage—Preserve in well-closed containers. Store in a cold place.

USP Reference standards ⟨11⟩—USP Endotoxin RS. USP Mangafodipir Related Compound A RS. USP Mangafodipir Related Compound B RS. USP Mangafodipir Related Compound C RS. USP Mangafodipir Trisodium RS.

Identification—
 A: *Infrared Absorption* ⟨197K⟩.
 B: It meets the requirements of the tests for *Sodium* ⟨191⟩ and *Manganese* ⟨191⟩.

Microbial limits ⟨61⟩—The total aerobic microbial count is not more than 500 cfu per g.

Bacterial endotoxins ⟨85⟩: not more than 0.13 USP Endotoxin Unit per mg.

pH ⟨791⟩: between 5.5 and 7.0, in a solution (1 in 100).

Water, *Method I* ⟨921⟩: not more than 20%.

Limit of residual solvents—
 Internal standard solution—Transfer 600 µL of methyl ethyl ketone to a 100-mL volumetric flask, dilute with water to volume, and mix to obtain a solution having a concentration of about 5 mg per mL. Transfer 2 mL of this solution to a 100-mL volumetric flask, dilute with water to volume, and mix to obtain a solution having a known concentration of about 0.1 mg per mL.
 Standard stock solution—Transfer about 1 g of dehydrated alcohol and 1 g of acetone, both accurately weighed, to a 100-mL volumetric flask, and dilute with water to volume. Transfer 10.0 mL of this solution to a 100-mL volumetric flask, dilute with water to volume, and mix to obtain a solution having a known concentration of about 1 mg each of alcohol and acetone per mL.
 Standard solutions—Transfer 10.0 mL of *Internal standard solution* to each of four 100-mL volumetric flasks. Separately add 0 mL, 1.0 mL, 5.0 mL, and 10.0 mL of *Standard stock solution* to the volumetric flasks, and dilute each with water to volume to obtain solutions having known concentrations of 0.0 µg per mL and about 10 µg per mL, 50 µg per mL, and 100 µg per mL each of alcohol and acetone, respectively. Add 7.0 mL of each *Standard solution* to separate headspace sample vials, and cap.
 Test solution—Transfer about 1 g of Mangafodipir Trisodium, accurately weighed, to a sample vial, add 7.0 mL of the *Standard solution* having a concentration of 0.0 µg per mL, cap, and swirl to dissolve.
 Chromatographic system (see *Chromatography* ⟨621⟩)—The gas chromatograph is equipped with a flame-ionization detector, a 0.32-mm × 30-m fused silica column coated with 1.8-µm G43 stationary phase. The carrier gas is helium, flowing at a rate of 1.5 mL per minute. The temperatures of the injection port and the oven are maintained at 150° and 50°, respectively. The bath temperature for the headspace sample vials is maintained at 90°, the valve/loop temperature is maintained at 130°, and the sample thermostating time is 15 minutes. Chromatograph the *Standard solutions,* and record the peak responses as directed for *Procedure:* the resolution, *R,* between alcohol and acetone is not less than 5; and the relative standard deviation for replicate injections of the *Standard solution* having a concentration of 100 µg per mL, determined from the peak response ratios of the analyte to the internal standard, is not more than 2.0%. Calculate the peak response ratios of the analyte to the internal standard, and plot the results. Determine the linear regression equation of the standards by the mean-square method, and record the linear regression equation and the correlation coefficient. A suitable system is one that yields a line having a correlation coefficient of not less than 0.990.
 Procedure—Separately inject equal volumes (about 1 mL) of the gaseous headspace of each of the *Standard solutions* and the *Test solution* into the chromatograph, record the chromatograms, and measure the peak responses. Calculate the percentages (w/w) of alcohol and acetone in the portion of Mangafodipir Trisodium taken by the formula:

$$(7/10{,}000)(C/W)$$

in which *C* is the concentration, in µg per mL, of alcohol or acetone in the *Test solution,* as determined from the relevant standard response line; and *W* is the weight, in g, of Mangafodipir Trisodium taken: not more than 0.1% of alcohol is found; and not more than 0.01% of acetone is found, both calculated on the anhydrous basis.

Limit of free manganese and free fodipir—
 Ascorbic acid solution—Dissolve 0.5 g of ascorbic acid in 10 mL of water.
 Manganese solution—Transfer about 3.6 g of manganese chloride, accurately weighed, to a 1000-mL volumetric flask, dissolve in and dilute with 0.1 N hydrochloric acid to volume, and mix. Transfer 100.0 mL of this solution to a 500-mL volumetric flask, dilute with water to volume, and mix.
 Edetate titrant solution—Transfer about 37 g of edetate disodium, accurately weighed, to a 1000-mL volumetric flask, dilute with water to volume, and mix. Transfer 36 mL of this solution to a 1000-mL volumetric flask, dilute with water to volume, and mix to obtain a solution having a concentration of 0.0036 moles per L.
 STANDARDIZATION OF 0.0036 M EDETATE TITRANT SOLUTION—Accurately weigh about 200 mg of chelometric standard calcium carbonate, previously dried at 110° for 2 hours and cooled in a desiccator, transfer to a 100-mL volumetric flask, and add 10 mL of water and about 4 mL of diluted hydrochloric acid. Swirl the flask to dissolve, dilute with water to volume, and mix. Transfer 5.0 mL of this solution to a beaker while stirring, preferably with a magnetic stirrer; and add about 15 mL of sodium hydroxide TS and enough hydroxynaphthol blue indicator to achieve a percent transmission of about 95%, using a suitable autotitrator at a wavelength of 620 nm, calibrated to 100% transmission with water. Add 20.0 mL of *Edetate titrant solution,* and continue to titrate until 3 mL of titrant have been added beyond the sharp break point, as determined from the titration curve obtained by plotting relative transmittance versus volume, in mL, of titrant added. Determine the endpoint volume from the titration curve. The final titration volume is the sum of the endpoint volume and the 20.0 mL of *Edetate titrant solution* initially added. Calculate the molarity of the *Edetate titrant solution* by the formula:

$$(5/100.09)(W)/(100V)$$

in which 100.09 is the molecular weight of calcium carbonate; *W* is the weight, in mg, of the calcium carbonate taken; and *V* is the final titration volume, in mL, of *Edetate titrant solution.*
 Procedure—Transfer about 1 g of Mangafodipir Trisodium, accurately weighed, to a suitable beaker, add about 100 mL of water, 1.0 mL of *Ascorbic acid solution,* 10 mL of ammonia–ammonium chloride buffer TS, 0.1 mL of eriochrome black TS, and 1.0 mL of *Manganese solution,* and record the color. If the color is yellow to green, add additional 1.0-mL increments of *Manganese solution* until the color is red. Record the volume added. Titrate with the *Edetate titrant solution,* determining the endpoint photometrically. Perform a blank determination, and make any necessary correction (see *Titrimetry* ⟨541⟩). Calculate the percentage of free manganese in the portion of Mangafodipir Trisodium taken by the formula:

$$5.49V(M/W)$$

in which *V* is the volume, in mL, of the *Edetate titrant solution; M* is the molarity of the *Edetate titrant solution;* and *W* is the weight, in g, of Mangafodipir Trisodium taken. Calculate the percentage of free fodipir in the portion of Mangafodipir Trisodium taken by the formula:

$$63.85V(M/W)$$

in which *V, M,* and *W* are as defined herein: not more than 0.03% of free manganese is found; and not more than 0.5% of free fodipir is found, both calculated on the anhydrous basis.

Related compounds—
 Ascorbic acid solution—Dissolve 0.4 g of ascorbic acid in 100 mL of water.
 Phosphate buffer—Prepare as directed in the *Assay.*
 Mobile phase—Prepare as directed in the *Assay.* [NOTE—Increasing the proportion of acetonitrile will decrease the retention times.]
 System suitability stock solution—Prepare as directed for *Standard stock preparation* in the *Assay.*
 System suitability solution 1—Prepare a solution of USP Mangafodipir Trisodium RS having a known concentration of about 4.0 mg per mL. Transfer 5.0 mL of this solution to a 50-mL volumetric

flask, add 5.0 mL of *System suitability stock solution,* 5.0 mL of *Phosphate buffer,* and 5.0 mL of *Ascorbic acid solution.* Dilute with nitrogen-purged water to volume, and mix to obtain a solution having a concentration of about 0.4 mg of USP Mangafodipir Trisodium RS, and about 0.01 mg each of USP Mangafodipir Related Compound A RS and USP Mangafodipir Related Compound B RS per mL. [NOTE—Store in a refrigerator and under nitrogen to avoid excessive exposure to heat, air, and light.]

System suitability solution 2—Transfer about 10 mg of USP Mangafodipir Related Compound C RS to a 100-mL volumetric flask, dilute with water to volume, and mix. Transfer 5.0 mL of this solution to a 50-mL volumetric flask, and add 5.0 mL of *Phosphate buffer.*

Test solution—Transfer an accurately weighed quantity of Mangafodipir Trisodium, equivalent to about 100 mg of mangafodipir trisodium, to a 50-mL volumetric flask, dilute with water to volume, and mix. Transfer 10.0 mL of this solution to a second 50-mL volumetric flask, add 5.0 mL of *Phosphate buffer,* dilute with water to volume, and mix. [NOTE—Store in a refrigerator and under nitrogen to avoid excessive exposure to heat, air, and light.]

Chromatographic system (see *Chromatography* ⟨621⟩)—Prepare as directed in the *Assay.* Chromatograph *System suitability solution 2,* and record the peak responses as directed for *Procedure:* note the elution time to identify the mangafodipir related compound C peak, if present, in the chromatogram of *System suitability solution 1.* Chromatograph *System suitability solution 1,* and record the peak responses as directed for *Procedure:* the retention time for mangafodipir is between 18 and 30 minutes. The peak area for mangafodipir related compound C is less than 0.1%. [NOTE—If the peak area is more than 0.1% of the total of all peak areas, prepare fresh quantities of *Ascorbic acid solution* and *System suitability solution 1,* and repeat the test. If the peak area of mangafodipir related compound C is still greater than 0.1%, repeat the test using another column. A contaminated column can result in oxidation of Mn(II) to Mn(III), forming related compound C.] The tailing factor for the mangafodipir peak is not more than 2.3; the column efficiency is not less than 1000 theoretical plates; the resolution, *R,* between mangafodipir related compound B and mangafodipir is not less than 1.5; and the relative standard deviation for replicate injections is not more than 10% for each peak. [NOTE—If the resolution is less than 1.5, adjust the *Mobile phase* by increasing the concentration of tetrabutylammonium hydrogen sulfate.]

Procedure—Inject about 10 µL of the *Test solution* into the chromatograph, record the chromatogram, and measure the areas for all the major peaks. The relative retention times for ascorbic acid, mangafodipir related compound A, Mn(II)-5-methyl dipyridoxal monophosphate (Mn(II)-5-methyl DPMP) if present, mangafodipir related compound C, mangafodipir related compound B, and mangafodipir are about 0.1, 0.3, 0.4, 0.6, 0.8, and 1.0, respectively. Calculate the percentages of mangafodipir related compound A, mangafodipir related compound B, mangafodipir related compound C, and Mn(II)-5-methyl DPMP in the portion of Mangafodipir Trisodium taken by the formula:

$$100(r_i / r_s)$$

in which r_i is the peak area of each impurity; and r_s is the sum of the areas of all of the peaks: not more than 0.5% each of mangafodipir related compound A and mangafodipir related compound B is found; not more than 0.6% of mangafodipir related compound C is found; not more than 0.3% of Mn(II)-5-methyl DPMP is found; not more than 0.3% of any other impurity is found; not more than a total of 0.5% of other impurities is found; and not more than a total of 2.0% of impurities is found.

Assay—

Phosphate buffer—Transfer about 26.8 g of dibasic sodium phosphate to a 1000-mL volumetric flask, add 900 mL of water, and adjust with 1 N sodium hydroxide or 1 N hydrochloric acid to a pH of about 8.0. Dilute with water to volume, filter, and degas.

Mobile phase—Transfer about 0.61 g of boric acid and 9.2 g of tetrabutylammonium hydrogen sulfate to a 1000-mL volumetric flask, add 640 mL water, and mix. Adjust with 3 N sodium hydroxide to a pH of about 9.3, add 250 mL of acetonitrile, dilute with water to volume, and mix. Adjust with 3 N hydrochloric acid or 3 N sodium hydroxide to a pH of about 10.5, filter, and degas. Make adjustments if necessary (see *System Suitability* under *Chromatography* ⟨621⟩).

Standard stock preparation—Transfer about 10 mg each of USP Mangafodipir Related Compound A RS and USP Mangafodipir Related Compound B RS, both accurately weighed, to a 100-mL volumetric flask, dilute with water to volume, and mix.

Standard preparation—Transfer about 100 mg of USP Mangafodipir Trisodium RS to a 50-mL volumetric flask, dilute with water to volume, and mix. Transfer 10.0 mL of this solution to a 50-mL volumetric flask, add 5.0 mL of *Standard stock preparation* and 5.0 mL of *Phosphate buffer,* dilute with water to volume, and mix. [NOTE—Store in a refrigerator and under nitrogen to avoid exposure to excessive heat, air, or light.]

Assay preparation—Transfer an accurately measured quantity of Mangafodipir Trisodium, equivalent to about 100 mg of mangafodipir trisodium, to a 50-mL volumetric flask, dilute with water to volume, and mix. Transfer 10.0 mL of this solution to a 50-mL volumetric flask, add 5.0 mL of *Phosphate buffer,* dilute with water to volume, and mix. [NOTE—Store in a refrigerator and under nitrogen to avoid exposure to excessive heat, air, or light.]

Chromatographic system (see *Chromatography* ⟨621⟩)—The liquid chromatograph is equipped with a 310-nm detector and a 4.6-mm × 15-cm column that contains 5-µm packing L21. The chromatograph is maintained at about 20°. The flow rate is 0.8 mL per minute. Chromatograph the *Standard preparation,* and record the peak responses as directed for *Procedure:* the resolution, *R,* between mangafodipir related compound A and mangafodipir related compound B is not less than 1.5; the column efficiency is not less than 1000 theoretical plates; and the tailing factor is not more than 2.3.

Procedure—Separately inject equal volumes (about 10 µL) of the *Standard preparation* and the *Assay preparation* into the chromatograph, record the chromatograms, and measure the responses for the major peaks. Calculate the percentage of $C_{22}H_{27}MnN_4Na_3O_{14}P_2$ in the portion of Mangafodipir Trisodium taken by the formula:

$$25{,}000(C/W)(r_U / r_S)$$

in which *C* is the concentration, in mg per mL, of USP Mangafodipir Trisodium RS in the *Standard preparation;* *W* is the weight, in mg, of the Mangafodipir Trisodium taken; and r_U and r_S are the peak responses obtained from the *Assay preparation* and the *Standard preparation,* respectively.

Mangafodipir Trisodium Injection

» Mangafodipir Trisodium Injection is a sterile solution of Mangafodipir Trisodium in Water for Injection. It contains not less than 94.0 percent and not more than 106.0 percent of the labeled amount of mangafodipir trisodium ($C_{22}H_{27}MnN_4Na_3O_{14}P_2$). It may contain stabilizers and buffers. It contains no antimicrobial agents.

Packaging and storage—Preserve in single-dose containers of Type I glass. Store at controlled room temperature, with containers on their sides in the original carton.

USP Reference standards ⟨11⟩—*USP Endotoxin RS. USP Mangafodipir Trisodium RS.*

Identification—
A: The retention time of the major peak in the chromatogram of the *Assay preparation* corresponds to that in the chromatogram of the *Standard preparation,* as obtained in the *Assay.*
B: It meets the requirements of the tests for *Manganese* ⟨191⟩.

Bacterial endotoxins ⟨85⟩: not more than 0.66 USP Endotoxin Unit per mg of mangafodipir trisodium.

pH ⟨791⟩: between 8.4 and 9.2.

Osmolarity ⟨785⟩: between 244 and 330 mOsmol per kg of water.

Other requirements—It meets the requirements under *Injections* ⟨1⟩.

Mangafodipir

Assay—
Phosphate buffer and *Mobile phase*—Proceed as directed in the *Assay* under *Mangafodipir Trisodium*.

Standard preparation—Prepare a solution of USP Mangafodipir Trisodium RS in water having a known concentration of about 2 mg per mL. Transfer 10.0 mL of this solution to a 50-mL volumetric flask, add 5.0 mL of *Phosphate buffer,* dilute with water to volume, and mix. [NOTE—Store under nitrogen to avoid excessive exposure to air and light.]

Assay preparation—Transfer an accurately measured volume of Injection, equivalent to about 100 mg of mangafodipir trisodium, to a 50-mL volumetric flask, dilute with water to volume, and mix. Transfer 10.0 mL of this solution to a 50-mL volumetric flask, add 5.0 mL of *Phosphate buffer,* dilute with water to volume, and mix. [NOTE—Store under nitrogen to avoid excessive exposure to air and light.]

Chromatographic system—Prepare as directed in the *Assay* under *Mangafodipir Trisodium.* Chromatograph the *Standard preparation,* and record the peak responses as directed for *Procedure:* the column efficiency is not less than 1000 theoretical plates; and the tailing factor is not more than 2.3.

Procedure—Separately inject equal volumes (about 10 µL) of the *Standard preparation* and the *Assay preparation* into the chromatograph, record the chromatograms, and measure the responses for the major peaks. Calculate the quantity, in mg, of mangafodipir trisodium ($C_{22}H_{27}MnN_4Na_3O_{14}P_2$) in each mL of the Injection taken by the formula:

$$250(C/V)(r_U / r_S)$$

in which C is the concentration, in mg per mL, of USP Mangafodipir Trisodium RS in the *Standard preparation;* V is the volume, in mL, of Injection taken to prepare the *Assay preparation;* and r_U and r_S are the mangafodipir peak responses obtained from the *Assay preparation* and the *Standard preparation,* respectively.

Manganese Chloride

$MnCl_2 \cdot 4H_2O$ 197.90
Manganese chloride ($MnCl_2$) tetrahydrate.
Manganese (2+) chloride tetrahydrate   [13446-34-9].
Anhydrous   125.84   [7773-01-5].

» Manganese Chloride contains not less than 98.0 percent and not more than 101.0 percent of $MnCl_2$, calculated on the dried basis.

Packaging and storage—Preserve in tight containers.
Identification—
  A: *Chloride* ⟨191⟩—Yields white, curdy precipitate of silver chloride with silver nitrate TS, which is insoluble in nitric acid. After being washed with water, this precipitate is soluble in a slight excess of 6 N ammonium hydroxide.
  B: It meets the requirements of the test for *Manganese* ⟨191⟩.
pH ⟨791⟩:   between 3.5 and 6.0, 10 g dissolved in 200 mL of carbon dioxide- and ammonia-free water being used.
Loss on drying ⟨731⟩—Dry it at 50° for 2 hours, then raise the temperature to 150° for 24 hours: it loses between 36.0% and 38.5% of its weight.
Insoluble matter—Transfer 10 g to a 250-mL beaker, add 150 mL of water, cover the beaker, and heat to boiling. Digest the hot solution on a steam bath for 1 hour, and pass through a tared, fine-porosity filtering crucible. Rinse the beaker with hot water, passing the rinsings through the filter, and finally wash the filter with additional hot water. Dry the filter at 105°: the residue weighs not more than 0.5 mg (0.005%).
Sulfate ⟨221⟩—A 2.0 g portion shows no more sulfate than corresponds to 0.10 mL of 0.020 N sulfuric acid (0.005%).
Substances not precipitated by ammonium sulfide—Dissolve 2.0 g in about 90 mL of water, add 5 mL of ammonium hydroxide, and warm the solution to about 80°. Pass a stream of hydrogen sulfide through the solution for 30 minutes. Dilute with water to 100 mL, mix, and allow the precipitate to settle. Decant the supernatant through a fine-porosity filter, and transfer 50.0 mL to an evaporating dish that previously has been ignited and tared. Evaporate the filtrate to dryness, cool, add 0.5 mL of sulfuric acid, heat gently to remove the excess acid, and ignite at 800 ± 25° for 15 minutes: the weight of the residue is not greater than 2.0 mg (0.2% as sulfate).
Iron ⟨241⟩—Dissolve 2.0 g in 40 mL of water: the limit is 5 µg per g.
Zinc—Dissolve 1 g in a mixture of 48 mL of water and 2 mL of sulfuric acid, and add, slowly and with constant agitation, 1 mL of potassium ferrocyanide solution (1 in 100): no turbidity is produced within 5 minutes.
Heavy metals, *Method I* ⟨231⟩—Dissolve 6.0 g in 30 mL of water. Use 25 mL of this solution in the *Test Preparation*, and use the remaining 5.0 mL in preparing the *Standard Preparation:* the limit is 5 µg per g.
Organic volatile impurities, *Method I* ⟨467⟩:   meets the requirements.

(Official until July 1, 2008)
Assay—Transfer about 425 mg of Manganese Chloride, accurately weighed, to a 400-mL beaker, dissolve in about 25 mL of water, add 300 mg of ammonium chloride and 0.5 g of hydroxylamine hydrochloride, and swirl to dissolve. Warm slightly on a hot plate, and dilute with water to 100 mL. Add about 3 mL of triethanolamine, stir the solution, using, preferably, a magnetic stirrer, begin the titration by adding about 25 mL of 0.05 M edetate disodium VS, using a suitable buret, then add 10 mL of ammonia–ammonium chloride buffer TS, and 1 mL of eriochrome black TS, and complete the titration with 0.05 M edetate disodium VS to a blue endpoint. Each mL of 0.05 M edetate disodium is equivalent to 6.292 mg of $MnCl_2$.

Manganese Chloride Injection

» Manganese Chloride Injection is a sterile solution of Manganese Chloride in Water for Injection. It contains not less than 90.0 percent and not more than 110.0 percent of the labeled amount of manganese (Mn).

Packaging and storage—Preserve in single-dose or in multiple-dose containers, preferably of Type I or Type II glass.
Labeling—Label the Injection to indicate that it is to be diluted to the appropriate strength with Sterile Water for Injection or other suitable fluid prior to administration.
USP Reference standards ⟨11⟩—*USP Endotoxin RS*.
Identification—The *Assay preparation,* prepared as directed in the *Assay,* exhibits an absorption maximum at about 279 nm when tested as directed for *Procedure* in the *Assay.*
Bacterial endotoxins ⟨85⟩—It contains not more than 0.45 USP Endotoxin Unit per µg of manganese.
pH ⟨791⟩:   between 1.5 and 2.5.
Particulate matter ⟨788⟩:   meets the requirements for small-volume injections.
Other requirements—It meets the requirements under *Injections* ⟨1⟩.
Assay—
  Sodium chloride solution—Dissolve 1.8 g of sodium chloride in water, dilute with water to 2000 mL, and mix.
  Manganese stock solution—Transfer 1.000 g of manganese to a 1000-mL volumetric flask, dissolve in 20 mL of nitric acid, dilute with 0.1 N hydrochloric acid to volume, and mix. This solution contains 1000 µg of manganese per mL. Store in a polyethylene bottle.
  Standard preparations—Pipet 10 mL of the *Manganese stock solution* into a 500-mL volumetric flask, dilute with water to volume, and mix. Transfer 4.0, 5.0, and 6.0 mL, respectively, of this solution to separate 50-mL volumetric flasks, containing 10 mL of *Sodium chloride solution,* dilute the contents of each flask with water to volume, and mix. These *Standard preparations* contain, respectively, 1.6, 2.0, and 2.4 µg of manganese per mL.
  Assay preparation—Transfer an accurately measured volume of Injection, equivalent to about 1 mg of manganese, to a 100-mL volumetric flask, dilute with water to volume, and mix. Pipet 10 mL of

this solution into a 50-mL volumetric flask. From the labeled amount of sodium chloride, if any, in the Injection, calculate the amount, in mg, of sodium chloride in the initial dilution, and add sufficient *Sodium chloride solution* to bring the total sodium chloride content in this flask to 9 mg. Dilute with water to volume, and mix.

Procedure—Concomitantly determine the absorbances of the *Standard preparations* and the *Assay preparation* at the manganese emission line of 279 nm, with a suitable atomic absorption spectrophotometer (see *Spectrophotometry and Light-scattering* ⟨851⟩) equipped with a manganese hollow-cathode lamp and an air–acetylene flame, using a dilution of *Sodium chloride solution* (1 : 5) as the blank. Plot the absorbances of the *Standard preparations* versus concentration, in µg per mL, of manganese, and draw the straight line best fitting the three plotted points. From the graph so obtained, determine the concentration, in µg per mL, of manganese in the *Assay preparation*. Calculate the quantity, in mg, of manganese in each mL of the Injection taken by the formula:

$$0.5C / V$$

in which *C* is the concentration, in µg per mL, of manganese in the *Assay preparation*; and *V* is the volume, in mL, of Injection taken.

Manganese Chloride for Oral Solution

» Manganese Chloride for Oral Solution contains not less than 90.0 percent and not more than 110.0 percent of the labeled amount of manganese (Mn). It may contain one or more suitable flavors, sweetening agents, thickening agents, and stabilizers.

Packaging and storage—Preserve in tight, light-resistant, single-dose containers.
Labeling—The label contains directions for constitution of the powder and states the amount of manganese in a given volume of the Oral Solution obtained after constitution.
Identification—It meets the requirements of the tests for *Chloride* ⟨191⟩ and for *Manganese* ⟨191⟩.
Uniformity of dosage units ⟨905⟩—
FOR POWDER PACKAGED IN SINGLE-UNIT CONTAINERS: meets the requirements.
Deliverable volume ⟨698⟩—
FOR POWDER PACKAGED IN MULTIPLE-UNIT CONTAINERS: meets the requirements.
pH ⟨791⟩: between 6.0 and 8.0, when constituted to 300 mL with water.
Osmolarity ⟨785⟩: 230 mOsmol pH 6.0 to 8.0.
Assay—
Sodium chloride solution, Manganese stock solution, and *Standard preparations*—Prepare as directed in the *Assay* under *Manganese Chloride Injection*.
Assay preparation—Constitute the Manganese Chloride for Oral Solution as directed in the labeling. Transfer about 25 mL, accurately measured, of the constituted Manganese Chloride for Oral Solution to a 100-mL volumetric flask, dilute with water to volume, and mix. Proceed as directed for *Assay preparation* in the *Assay* under *Manganese Chloride Injection*, beginning with "Pipet 10 mL of this solution."
Procedure—Proceed as directed in the *Assay* under *Manganese Chloride Injection*. Calculate the quantity, in µg, of manganese in each mL of the constituted for Oral Solution taken by the formula:

$$500C/V$$

in which *C* is the concentration, in µg per mL, of the manganese in the *Assay preparation;* and *V* is the volume, in mL, of the constituted Manganese Chloride for Oral Solution taken.

Manganese Gluconate

$C_{12}H_{22}MnO_{14}$ (anhydrous)   445.23
Bis(D-gluconato-O^1,O^2) manganese.
Manganese D-gluconate (1 : 2).
Dihydrate   481.27

» Manganese Gluconate is dried or contains two molecules of water of hydration. It contains not less than 98.0 percent and not more than 102.0 percent of $C_{12}H_{22}MnO_{14}$, calculated on the anhydrous basis.

Packaging and storage—Preserve in well-closed containers.
Labeling—The label indicates whether it is the dried or the dihydrate form.
USP Reference standards ⟨11⟩—*USP Potassium Gluconate RS.*
Identification—
A: A solution (1 in 20) responds to the tests for *Manganese* ⟨191⟩.
B: It responds to *Identification* test B under *Calcium Gluconate*.
Water, *Method I* ⟨921⟩ *(where labeled as the dried form)*: between 3.0% and 9.0%, the determination being performed by stirring the mixture containing the *Test preparation*, maintained at a temperature of 50°, for 30 minutes before titrating with the *Reagent:* where labeled as the dihydrate it is between 6.0% and 9.0%.
Chloride ⟨221⟩—A 1.0-g portion shows no more chloride than corresponds to 0.70 mL of 0.020 N hydrochloric acid (0.05%).
Sulfate ⟨221⟩—A 2.0-g portion shows no more sulfate than corresponds to 4.0 mL of 0.020 N sulfuric acid (0.2%).
Limit of lead—[NOTE—For the preparation of all aqueous solutions and for the rinsing of glassware before use, employ water that has been passed through a strong-acid, strong-base, mixed-bed ion-exchange resin before use. Select all reagents to have as low a content of lead as practicable, and store all reagent solutions in containers of borosilicate glass. Cleanse glassware before use by soaking in warm 8 N nitric acid for 30 minutes and by rinsing with deionized water.]
Ascorbic acid–sodium iodide solution—Dissolve 20 g of ascorbic acid and 38.5 g of sodium iodide in water in a 200-mL volumetric flask, dilute with water to volume, and mix.
Trioctylphosphine oxide solution—[*Caution*—*This solution causes irritation. Avoid contact with eyes, skin, and clothing. Take special precautions in disposing of unused portions of solutions to which this reagent is added.*] Dissolve 5.0 g of trioctylphosphine oxide in 4-methyl-2-pentanone in a 100-mL volumetric flask, dilute with the same solvent to volume, and mix.
Standard solution and *Blank*—Transfer 5.0 mL of *Lead Nitrate Stock Solution,* prepared as directed in the test for *Heavy Metals* ⟨231⟩, to a 100-mL volumetric flask, dilute with water to volume, and mix. Transfer 2.0 mL of the resulting solution to a 50-mL volumetric flask. To this volumetric flask and to a second, empty 50-mL volumetric flask (*Blank*) add 10 mL of 9 N hydrochloric acid and about 10 mL of water. To each flask add 20 mL of *Ascorbic acid–sodium iodide solution* and 5.0 mL of *Trioctylphosphine oxide solution,* shake for 30 seconds, and allow to separate. Add water to bring the organic solvent layer into the neck of each flask, shake again, and allow to separate. The organic solvent layers are the *Blank* and the *Standard solution,* and they contain 0.0 µg and 2.0 µg of lead per mL, respectively.
Test solution—Add 1.0 g of Manganese Gluconate, 10 mL of 9 N hydrochloric acid, about 10 mL of water, 20 mL of *Ascorbic acid–sodium iodide solution,* and 5.0 mL of *Trioctylphosphine oxide solution* to a 50-mL volumetric flask, shake for 30 seconds, and allow to separate. Add water to bring the organic solvent layer into the neck of the flask, shake again, and allow to separate. The organic solvent layer is the *Test solution.*

Procedure—Concomitantly determine the absorbances of the *Blank, Standard solution,* and *Test solution* at the lead emission line at 283.3 nm, with a suitable atomic absorption spectrophotometer (see *Spectrophotometry and Light-Scattering* ⟨851⟩) equipped with a lead hollow-cathode lamp and an air–acetylene flame, using the *Blank* to set the instrument to zero. In a suitable analysis, the absorbance of the *Standard solution* and the absorbance of the *Blank* are significantly different: the absorbance of the *Test solution* does not exceed that of the *Standard solution*(0.001%).

Heavy metals ⟨231⟩—Dissolve 1 g in 10 mL of water, add 6 mL of 3 N hydrochloric acid, and dilute with water to 25 mL: the limit is 20 µg per g.

Reducing substances—Transfer 1.0 g to a 250-mL conical flask, dissolve in 10 mL of water, and add 25 mL of alkaline cupric citrate TS. Cover the flask, boil gently for 5 minutes, accurately timed, and cool rapidly to room temperature. Add 25 mL of 0.6 N acetic acid, 10.0 mL of 0.1 N iodine VS, and 10 mL of 3 N hydrochloric acid, and titrate with 0.1 N sodium thiosulfate VS, adding 3 mL of starch TS as the endpoint is approached. Perform a blank determination, omitting the specimen, and note the difference in volumes required. Each mL of the difference in volume of 0.1 N sodium thiosulfate consumed is equivalent to 2.7 mg of reducing substances (as dextrose): the limit is 1.0%.

Organic volatile impurities, *Method I* ⟨467⟩: meets the requirements.

(Official until July 1, 2008)

Assay—Dissolve about 700 mg of Manganese Gluconate, accurately weighed, in 50 mL of water. Add 1 g of ascorbic acid, 10 mL of ammonia–ammonium chloride buffer TS, and 0.1 mL of eriochrome black TS, and titrate with 0.05 M edetate disodium VS until the solution is deep blue in color. Each mL of 0.05 M edetate disodium is equivalent to 22.26 mg of $C_{12}H_{22}MnO_{14}$.

Manganese Sulfate

$MnSO_4 \cdot H_2O$ 169.02
Sulfuric acid, manganese(2+) salt (1:1) monohydrate.
Manganese(2+) sulfate (1:1) monohydrate   [10034-96-5].
Anhydrous   151.00   [7785-87-7].

» Manganese Sulfate contains not less than 98.0 percent and not more than 102.0 percent of $MnSO_4 \cdot H_2O$.

Packaging and storage—Preserve in tight containers. Store at 25°, excursions permitted between 15° and 30°.

Identification—A solution (1 in 10) responds to the tests for *Manganese* ⟨191⟩ and for *Sulfate* ⟨191⟩.

Loss on ignition ⟨733⟩—Ignite it at 450° to constant weight: it loses between 10.0% and 13.0% of its weight.

Substances not precipitated by ammonium sulfide—Dissolve 2.0 g in 90 mL of water, add 5 mL of ammonium hydroxide, warm the solution, and pass hydrogen sulfide through the solution for about 30 minutes. Dilute with water to 100 mL, mix, and allow the precipitate to settle. Decant the supernatant through a filter, transfer 50 mL of the clear filtrate to a tared dish, evaporate to dryness, and ignite, gently at first and finally at 800 ± 25°: the weight of the residue does not exceed 5 mg (0.5%).

Organic volatile impurities, *Method I* ⟨467⟩: meets the requirements.

(Official until July 1, 2008)

Assay—Dissolve about 350 mg of Manganese Sulfate, accurately weighed, in 200 mL of water. Add about 10 mg of ascorbic acid, begin the titration by adding about 25 mL of 0.05 M edetate disodium VS, using a suitable buret, then add 10 mL of ammonia–ammonium chloride buffer TS, and about 0.15 mL of eriochrome black TS, and complete the titration with 0.05 M edetate disodium VS to a blue endpoint. Each mL of 0.05 M edetate disodium is equivalent to 8.451 mg of $MnSO_4 \cdot H_2O$.

Manganese Sulfate Injection

» Manganese Sulfate Injection is a sterile solution of Manganese Sulfate in Water for Injection. It contains not less than 90.0 percent and not more than 110.0 percent of the labeled amount of manganese (Mn).

Packaging and storage—Preserve in single-dose or in multiple-dose containers, preferably of Type I or Type II glass.

Labeling—Label the Injection to indicate that it is to be diluted to the appropriate strength with Sterile Water for Injection or other suitable fluid prior to administration.

USP Reference standards ⟨11⟩—*USP Endotoxin RS.*

Identification—The *Assay preparation*, prepared as directed in the *Assay*, exhibits an absorption maximum at about 279 nm when tested as directed for *Procedure* in the *Assay*.

Bacterial endotoxins ⟨85⟩—It contains not more than 0.45 USP Endotoxin Unit per µg of manganese.

pH ⟨791⟩:   between 2.0 and 3.5.

Particulate matter ⟨788⟩:   meets the requirements for small-volume injections.

Other requirements—It meets the requirements under *Injections* ⟨1⟩.

Assay—

Sodium chloride solution, Manganese stock solution, and *Standard preparations*—Prepare as directed in the *Assay* under *Manganese Chloride Injection*.

Assay preparation—Transfer an accurately measured volume of Injection, equivalent to about 1 mg of manganese, to a 100-mL volumetric flask, dilute with water to volume, and mix. Pipet 10 mL of this solution into a 50-mL volumetric flask, dilute with water to volume, and mix.

Procedure—Proceed as directed for *Procedure* in the *Assay* under *Manganese Chloride Injection*.

Mannitol

$C_6H_{14}O_6$ 182.17
D-Mannitol.
D-Mannitol   [69-65-8].

» Mannitol contains not less than 96.0 percent and not more than 101.5 percent of $C_6H_{14}O_6$, calculated on the dried basis. The amounts of total sugars, other polyhydric alcohols, and any hexitol anhydrides, if detected, are not included in the requirements nor the calculated amount under *Other Impurities*.

Packaging and storage—Preserve in well-closed containers.

USP Reference standards ⟨11⟩—*USP Mannitol RS.*

Identification, *Infrared Absorption* ⟨197K⟩.

Melting range ⟨741⟩:   between 164° and 169°.

Specific rotation ⟨781S⟩:   between +137° and +145°.

Test solution—Transfer about 1 g of Mannitol, accurately weighed, to a 100-mL volumetric flask, and add 40 mL of ammonium molybdate solution (1 in 10), which previously had been filtered if necessary. Add 20 mL of 1 N sulfuric acid, dilute with water to volume, and mix.

Acidity—Dissolve 5.0 g in 50 mL of carbon dioxide-free water, add 3 drops of phenolphthalein TS, and titrate with 0.020 N sodium hydroxide to a distinct pink endpoint: not more than 0.30 mL of 0.020 N sodium hydroxide is required for neutralization.

Loss on drying ⟨731⟩—Dry it at 105° for 4 hours: it loses not more than 0.3% of its weight.

Chloride ⟨221⟩—A 2.0-g portion shows no more chloride than corresponds to 0.20 mL of 0.020 N hydrochloric acid (0.007%).
Sulfate ⟨221⟩—A 2.0-g portion shows no more sulfate than corresponds to 0.20 mL of 0.020 N sulfuric acid (0.01%).
Arsenic, *Method II* ⟨211⟩: 1 ppm.
Reducing sugars—To 5 mL of alkaline cupric citrate TS add 1 mL of a saturated solution of Mannitol (about 200 mg). Heat for 5 minutes in a boiling water bath: not more than a very slight precipitate is formed. The amount determined in this test is not included in the calculated amount under *Other Impurities.*
Assay—
 Mobile phase—Use degassed water.
 Resolution solution—Dissolve sorbitol and USP Mannitol RS in water to obtain a solution having concentrations of about 4.8 mg per mL of each.
 Standard preparation—Dissolve an accurately weighed quantity of USP Mannitol RS in water, and dilute quantitatively with water to obtain a solution having a known concentration of about 4.8 mg per mL.
 Assay preparation—Transfer about 0.24 g of Mannitol, accurately weighed, to a 50-mL volumetric flask, dissolve in 10 mL of water, dilute with water to volume, and mix.
 Chromatographic system (see *Chromatography* ⟨621⟩)—The liquid chromatograph is equipped with a refractive index detector that is maintained at a constant temperature and a 4-mm × 25-cm column that contains packing L19. The column temperature is maintained at a temperature between 30° and 85° controlled within ±2° of the selected temperature, and the flow rate is about 0.5 mL per minute. Chromatograph the *Standard preparation,* and record the peak responses as directed for *Procedure:* the relative standard deviation for replicate injections is not more than 2.0%. In a similar manner, chromatograph the *Resolution solution:* the resolution, *R,* between the sorbitol and mannitol peaks is not less than 2.0.
 Procedure—Separately inject equal volumes (about 20 μL) of the *Assay preparation* and the *Standard preparation* into the chromatograph, record the chromatograms, and measure the responses for the major peaks. Calculate the quantity, in mg, of $C_6H_{14}O_6$, in the Mannitol taken by the formula:

$$50C(r_U / r_S)$$

in which *C* is the concentration, in mg per mL, of USP Mannitol RS in the *Standard preparation*; and r_U and r_S are the peak responses obtained from the *Assay preparation* and the *Standard preparation,* respectively.

Mannitol Injection

» Mannitol Injection is a sterile solution, which may be supersaturated, of Mannitol in Water for Injection. It may require warming or autoclaving before use if crystallization has occurred. It contains not less than 95.0 percent and not more than 105.0 percent of the labeled amount of mannitol ($C_6H_{14}O_6$). It contains no antimicrobial agents.

Packaging and storage—Preserve in single-dose glass or plastic containers. Glass containers are preferably of Type I or Type II glass.
Labeling—The label states the total osmolar concentration in mOsmol per L. Where the contents are less than 100 mL, or where the label states that the Injection is not for direct injection but is to be diluted before use, the label alternatively may state the total osmolar concentration in mOsmol per mL.
USP Reference standards ⟨11⟩—*USP Endotoxin RS. USP Mannitol RS.*
Identification—
 A: Evaporate a portion of Injection on a steam bath to dryness, and dry the residue at 105° for 4 hours. To 3 mL of freshly prepared solution of catechol in water (1 in 10) add 6 mL of sulfuric acid with cooling. Place 3 mL of this solution in each of two separate test tubes. To one tube add 0.3 mL of water (reagent blank) and to the other add 0.3 mL of a solution of it in water (1 in 10). Heat the tubes over an open flame for about 30 seconds: the solution in the tube containing mannitol is dark pink or wine red, and the solution in the tube containing the reagent blank is light pink.
 B: The retention time for the major peak in the chromatogram of the *Assay preparation* corresponds to that in the chromatogram of the *Standard preparation,* as obtained in the *Assay.*
Specific rotation ⟨781⟩—Transfer an accurately measured volume of Injection, equivalent to about 1 g of mannitol as determined by the *Assay,* to a 100-mL volumetric flask: it meets the requirements of the test for *Specific rotation* under *Mannitol.*
Bacterial endotoxins ⟨85⟩—It contains not more than 0.04 USP Endotoxin Unit per mg of mannitol where the labeled amount of mannitol in the Injection is 10% or less, and not more than 2.5 USP Endotoxin Units per g of mannitol where the labeled amount of mannitol in the Injection is greater than 10%.
pH ⟨791⟩: between 4.5 and 7.0, determined potentiometrically, on a portion to which 0.30 mL of saturated potassium chloride solution has been added for each 100 mL, and which previously has been diluted with water, if necessary, to a concentration of not more than 5% of mannitol.
Particulate matter ⟨788⟩: meets the requirements for small-volume injections.
Other requirements—It meets the requirements under *Injections* ⟨1⟩.
Assay—
 Mobile phase, Resolution solution, and *Chromatographic system*—Proceed as directed in the *Assay* under *Mannitol.*
 Standard preparation—Dissolve an accurately weighed quantity of USP Mannitol RS in water, and dilute quantitatively with water to obtain a solution having a known concentration of about 5 mg per mL.
 Assay preparation—Transfer an accurately measured volume of Injection, equivalent to about 500 mg of mannitol, to a 100-mL volumetric flask, dilute with water to volume, and mix.
 Procedure—Proceed as directed for *Procedure* in the *Assay* under *Mannitol.* Calculate the quantity, in mg, of mannitol ($C_6H_{14}O_6$) in each mL of the Injection taken by the formula:

$$100(C/V)(r_U / r_S)$$

in which *V* is the volume, in mL, of Injection taken; and the other terms are as defined therein.

Mannitol in Sodium Chloride Injection

» Mannitol in Sodium Chloride Injection is a sterile solution of Mannitol and Sodium Chloride in Water for Injection. It contains not less than 95.0 percent and not more than 105.0 percent of the labeled amounts of $C_6H_{14}O_6$ and NaCl. It contains no antimicrobial agents.

Labeling—The label states the total osmolar concentration in mOsmol per L. Where the contents are less than 100 mL, or where the label states that the Injection is not for direct injection but is to be diluted before use, the label alternatively may state the total osmolar concentration in mOsmol per mL.
USP Reference standards ⟨11⟩—*USP Mannitol RS. USP Endotoxin RS.*
Identification—
 A: Evaporate a portion of Injection on a steam bath to dryness, and dry the residue at 105° for 4 hours: the residue responds to the *Identification* tests under *Mannitol Injection.*
 B: It responds to the tests for *Sodium* ⟨191⟩ and for *Chloride* ⟨191⟩.
Bacterial endotoxins ⟨85⟩—It contains not more than 0.04 USP Endotoxin Unit per mg of mannitol.

pH ⟨791⟩: between 4.5 and 7.0.
Other requirements—It meets the requirements for *Packaging and storage* under *Mannitol Injection*. It meets also the requirements under *Injections* ⟨1⟩.
Assay for mannitol—Proceed with Injection as directed in the *Assay* under *Mannitol Injection*.
Assay for sodium chloride—Proceed with Injection as directed in the *Assay* under *Sodium Chloride Injection*.

Maprotiline Hydrochloride

$C_{20}H_{23}N \cdot HCl$ 313.86

9,10-Ethanoanthracene-9(10H)-propanamine, N-methyl-, hydrochloride.
N-Methyl-9,10-ethanoanthracene-9(10H)-propylamine hydrochloride [10347-81-6].

» Maprotiline Hydrochloride contains not less than 99.0 percent and not more than 101.0 percent of the labeled amount of $C_{20}H_{23}N \cdot HCl$, calculated on the dried basis.

Packaging and storage—Preserve in tight containers.
USP Reference standards ⟨11⟩—*USP Maprotiline Hydrochloride RS.*
Identification—
  A: *Infrared Absorption* ⟨197K⟩.
  B: *Ultraviolet Absorption* ⟨197U⟩—
  Solution: 100 μg per mL.
  Medium: methanol.
  Absorptivities at 266 nm and 272 nm, calculated on the dried basis, do not differ by more than 3.0%.
  C: A solution (1 in 200) responds to the tests for *Chloride* ⟨191⟩, when tested as specified for alkaloidal hydrochlorides.
Loss on drying ⟨731⟩—Dry it in vacuum at 80° to constant weight: it loses not more than 1.0% of its weight.
Residue on ignition ⟨281⟩: not more than 0.1%.
Heavy metals, *Method II* ⟨231⟩: 0.001%.
Chromatographic purity—
  Standard solutions—Dissolve USP Maprotiline Hydrochloride RS in methanol, and mix to obtain a stock standard solution having a known concentration of 20 mg per mL. Dilute quantitatively with methanol to obtain *Standard solution* having a known concentration of 0.10 mg per mL. Dilute quantitatively with methanol to obtain *Standard solutions*, designated below by letter, having the following compositions:

Standard solution	Dilution	Concentration (μg RS per mL)	Percentage (%) for comparison with test specimen)
A	(undiluted)	100	0.5
B	(4 in 5)	80	0.4
C	(3 in 5)	60	0.3
D	(2 in 5)	40	0.2
E	(1 in 5)	20	0.1

  Test solution—Dissolve an accurately weighed quantity of Maprotiline Hydrochloride in methanol to obtain a solution containing 20 mg per mL.
  Procedure—In a suitable chromatographic chamber (see *Chromatography* ⟨621⟩), place a volume of a solvent system consisting of a mixture of secondary butyl alcohol, ethyl acetate, and 2 N ammonium hydroxide (6 : 3 : 1) sufficient to develop a chromatogram. Place a beaker containing 25 mL of ammonium hydroxide in the bottom of the chamber, and allow it to equilibrate for 1 hour. Apply 5-μL portions of the *Test solution*, the stock standard solution, and each of the *Standard solutions* to a suitable thin-layer chromatographic plate coated with a 0.25-mm layer of chromatographic silica gel that has been pre-washed with chloroform by allowing chloroform to move the full length of the plate, and dried at 100° for 30 minutes, and allow the spots to dry. Develop the chromatograms until the solvent front has moved about three-fourths of the length of the plate, remove the plate from the developing chamber, mark the solvent front, and allow the solvent to evaporate. Expose the plate to hydrogen chloride vapor for 30 minutes, expose it to a high-intensity UV light irradiator (1000 to 1600 watts) *[Caution—UV irradiators emit UV radiation that is harmful to eyes and skin.]* until the spot in the chromatogram of *Standard solution E* is clearly visible, and compare the chromatograms under long-wavelength UV light: the R_F value of the principal spot obtained from the *Test solution* corresponds to that obtained from the stock standard solution; and the sum of the intensities of all secondary spots obtained from the *Test solution*, compared with those of the principal spots obtained from the *Standard solutions*, corresponds to not more than 1.0%.
Organic volatile impurities, *Method V* ⟨467⟩: meets the requirements.
  Solvent—Use dimethyl sulfoxide.

(Official until July 1, 2008)

Assay—Dissolve about 600 mg of Maprotiline Hydrochloride, accurately weighed, in 25 mL of mercuric acetate TS, and titrate with 0.1 N perchloric acid VS, determining the endpoint potentiometrically, using a glass electrode and a calomel electrode containing saturated lithium chloride in glacial acetic acid (see *Titrimetry* ⟨541⟩). Perform a blank determination, and make any necessary correction. Each mL of 0.1 N perchloric acid is equivalent to 31.39 mg of $C_{20}H_{23}N \cdot HCl$.

Maprotiline Hydrochloride Tablets

» Maprotiline Hydrochloride Tablets contain not less than 90.0 percent and not more than 110.0 percent of the labeled amount of maprotiline hydrochloride ($C_{20}H_{23}N \cdot HCl$).

Packaging and storage—Preserve in well-closed containers.
USP Reference standards ⟨11⟩—*USP Maprotiline Hydrochloride RS.*
Identification—
  A: *Standard solution*—Dissolve 20 mg of USP Maprotiline Hydrochloride RS in 1.0 mL of methanol.
  Test solution—Transfer a portion of powdered Tablets, equivalent to about 100 mg of maprotiline hydrochloride, to a glass-stoppered centrifuge tube. Add 5.0 mL of methanol to the tube, sonicate for 10 minutes, shake by mechanical means for 10 minutes, and centrifuge.
  Procedure—In a suitable chromatographic chamber (see *Chromatography* ⟨621⟩), place a volume of a solvent system consisting of a mixture of secondary butyl alcohol, ethyl acetate, and 2 N ammonium hydroxide (6 : 3 : 1) sufficient to develop a chromatogram. Place a beaker containing 25 mL of ammonium hydroxide in the bottom of the chamber, and allow it to equilibrate for 1 hour. Apply 5-μL portions of the *Test solution* and the *Standard solution* to a suitable thin-layer chromatographic plate, coated with a 0.25-mm layer of chromatographic silica gel that has been prewashed with chloroform by allowing chloroform to travel the full length of the plate and dried at 100° for 30 minutes, and allow the spots to dry. Develop the chromatogram until the solvent front has moved about three-fourths of the length of the plate, remove the plate from the developing chamber, mark the solvent front, and allow the solvent to evaporate. Expose the plate to hydrogen chloride vapor for 30 minutes, expose it to a high-intensity UV light irradiator (1000 to 1600 watts) *[Caution—UV irradiators emit UV radiation that is*

harmful to eyes and skin.] for 5 minutes, and compare the chromatograms under long-wavelength UV light: the R_F value of the principal spot obtained from the *Test solution* corresponds to that obtained from the *Standard solution*.

B: The retention time of the major peak in the chromatogram of the *Assay preparation* corresponds to that of the *Standard preparation*, as obtained in the *Assay*.

Dissolution ⟨711⟩—

Medium: dilute hydrochloric acid (7 in 1000); 900 mL.

Apparatus 2: 50 rpm.

Time: 60 minutes.

Procedure—Determine the amount of $C_{20}H_{23}N \cdot HCl$ dissolved from UV absorbances, using the difference between the absorbance maximum at about 272 nm and the absorbance minimum at about 268 nm, of filtered portions of the solution under test, suitably diluted with dilute hydrochloric acid (7 in 1000), in comparison with a Standard solution having a known concentration of USP Maprotiline Hydrochloride RS in the same *Medium*.

Tolerances—Not less than 75% (*Q*) of the labeled amount of $C_{20}H_{23}N \cdot HCl$ is dissolved in 60 minutes.

Uniformity of dosage units ⟨905⟩: meet the requirements.

Assay—

Mobile phase—Dissolve 4 g of tetramethylammonium chloride in 495 mL of water, add 500 mL of acetonitrile and 1 mL of phosphoric acid, mix, filter, and degas. Make adjustments if necessary (see *System Suitability* under *Chromatography* ⟨621⟩).

Standard preparation—Transfer an accurately weighed quantity of USP Maprotiline Hydrochloride RS to a suitable volumetric flask, and prepare a solution having a known concentration of about 0.75 mg per mL in a mixture of water, methanol, and 0.1 N hydrochloric acid (80 : 10 : 10) by sonicating the Reference Standard in the methanol and 0.1 N hydrochloric acid for 5 minutes to dissolve, diluting with water to volume, and mixing.

Assay preparation—Transfer not fewer than 15 Tablets to a 500-mL volumetric flask, add 100 mL of 0.1 N hydrochloric acid, sonicate, and shake occasionally for 5 minutes to disintegrate the Tablets. Add 100 mL of methanol, shake, and sonicate for 5 minutes. Dilute with water to volume, mix, and centrifuge. Dilute a portion of the supernatant quantitatively, and stepwise if necessary, with water to obtain a solution having a concentration of about 0.75 mg per mL. [NOTE—Filtration through commonly available filters may result in unsatisfactory drug adsorption.]

Chromatographic system (see *Chromatography* ⟨621⟩)—The liquid chromatograph is equipped with a 272-nm detector and an 8-mm × 10-cm column that contains 10-μm packing L10. The flow rate is about 2.0 mL per minute. Chromatograph the *Standard preparation*, and record the peak responses as directed for *Procedure*: the column efficiency, determined from the analyte peak, is not less than 1500 theoretical plates; the tailing factor is not more than 2.0; and the relative standard deviation of the major peak response from replicate injections is not more than 2.0%.

Procedure—Separately inject equal volumes (about 20 μL) of the *Standard preparation* and the *Assay preparation* into the chromatograph, record the chromatograms, and measure the areas for the major peaks. Calculate the quantity, in mg, of $C_{20}H_{23}N \cdot HCl$ in the portion of Tablets taken by the formula:

$$(L/D)C(r_U/r_S)$$

in which L is the labeled amount, in mg, of maprotilene hydrochloride in each Tablet; D is the concentration, in mg per mL, of maprotilene hydrochloride in the *Assay preparation*, based on the labeled quantity per Tablet and the extent of dilution; C is the concentration, in mg per mL, of USP Maprotiline Hydrochloride RS in the *Standard preparation*; and r_U and r_S are the maprotilene peak responses obtained from the *Assay preparation* and the *Standard preparation*, respectively.

Mazindol

$C_{16}H_{13}ClN_2O$ 284.74

3*H*-Imidazo[2,1-a]isoindol-5-ol, 5-(4-chlorophenyl)-2,5-dihydro-, (±)-.

(±)-5-(*p*-Chlorophenyl)-2,5-dihydro-3*H*-imidazo[2,1-a]isoindol-5-ol [22232-71-9].

» Mazindol contains not less than 98.0 percent and not more than 102.0 percent of $C_{16}H_{13}ClN_2O$, calculated on the dried basis.

Packaging and storage—Preserve in tight containers.

USP Reference standards ⟨11⟩—*USP Mazindol RS.*

Clarity and color of solution—A 1 in 100 solution of Mazindol in a mixture of chloroform and methanol (9 : 1) is clear and not darker in color than a solution prepared by mixing equal volumes of *Matching Fluid C* (see *Color and Achromicity* ⟨631⟩) and water.

Identification—

A: *Infrared Absorption* ⟨197K⟩.

B: *Ultraviolet Absorption* ⟨197U⟩—

Solution: 10 μg per mL.

Medium: 0.6 N hydrochloric acid.

Absorptivities at 272 nm, calculated on the dried basis, do not differ by more than 3.0%.

Loss on drying ⟨731⟩—Dry it in vacuum at 60° for 2 hours: it loses not more than 0.5% of its weight.

Residue on ignition ⟨281⟩: not more than 0.1%.

Heavy metals, *Method II* ⟨231⟩: 0.002%.

Sulfate ⟨221⟩—Triturate a 500-mg portion with 10 mL of water in a mortar. Filter the suspension through a water-washed filter, and rinse the mortar and filter with 30 mL of water, collecting the combined filtrate and washings in a 50-mL color-comparison tube. The filtrate shows no more sulfate than corresponds to 0.20 mL of 0.020 N sulfuric acid (0.04%).

Chromatographic purity—Dissolve 10 mg in 2.0 mL of a mixture of chloroform and methanol (9 : 1) to obtain the test solution. Dissolve a suitable quantity of USP Mazindol RS in a mixture of chloroform and methanol (9 : 1) to obtain a Standard solution having a concentration of 5.0 mg per mL. Dilute portions of this solution quantitatively and stepwise with the mixture of chloroform and methanol (9 : 1) to obtain a series of diluted standard solutions having concentrations of 0.100, 0.050, 0.025, and 0.0125 mg per mL, respectively. Separately apply a 20-μL portion of the test solution and 20-μL portions of the Standard solution and each diluted standard solution to a suitable thin-layer chromatographic plate (see *Chromatography* ⟨621⟩) coated with a 0.25-mm layer of chromatographic silica gel mixture. Allow the spots to dry, and develop the chromatogram in a solvent system consisting of a mixture of chloroform, alcohol, and ammonium hydroxide (80 : 20 : 1) until the solvent front has moved about three-fourths of the length of the plate. Remove the plate from the developing chamber, mark the solvent front, and allow the solvent to evaporate. Locate the spots on the plate by examination under short-wavelength UV light: the chromatograms show principal spots at about the same R_F value. Estimate the concentration of any secondary spots present in the chromatogram from the test solution by comparison with the diluted standard solutions: the principal spots from the 0.100, 0.050, 0.025, and 0.0125 mg per mL dilutions are equivalent to 2.0%, 1.0%, 0.50%, and 0.25% of impurities, respectively. No individual impurity is greater than 1.0%, and the sum of the impurities is not greater than 2.0%.

Assay—Transfer about 230 mg of Mazindol, accurately weighed, to a suitable flask, dissolve in 40 mL of glacial acetic acid, add 3 drops of crystal violet TS, and titrate with 0.1 N perchloric acid VS to an emerald-green endpoint. Perform a blank determination, and make any necessary correction. Each mL of 0.1 N perchloric acid is equivalent to 28.47 mg of $C_{16}H_{13}ClN_2O$.

Mazindol Tablets

» Mazindol Tablets contain not less than 90.0 percent and not more than 110.0 percent of the labeled amount of mazindol ($C_{16}H_{13}ClN_2O$).

Packaging and storage—Preserve in tight containers, at a temperature not exceeding 25°.

USP Reference standards ⟨11⟩—USP Mazindol RS.

Identification—Place a portion of powdered Tablets, equivalent to about 1 mg of mazindol, in a suitable flask. Add 40 mL of methanol, shake by mechanical means for not less than 5 minutes, and heat for several minutes on a steam bath to boiling. Cool, dilute with methanol to about 100 mL, and filter. Separate the filtrate into two approximately equal portions, add 2 drops of hydrochloric acid to one portion, and mix: the UV absorption spectra of the solutions so obtained exhibit maxima and minima at the same wavelengths as those of similar solutions prepared from USP Mazindol RS, concomitantly measured.

Dissolution ⟨711⟩—

Medium: 0.01 N hydrochloric acid; 500 mL.
Apparatus 2: 50 rpm.
Time: 120 minutes.

Determine the amount of $C_{16}H_{13}ClN_2O$ dissolved by employing the following method.

Mobile phase—Mix 11.50 g of monobasic ammonium phosphate and 1.32 g of dibasic ammonium phosphate with water to obtain 1000 mL of an ammonium phosphate buffer. The *Mobile phase* is a suitably filtered and degassed mixture of the ammonium phosphate buffer and acetonitrile (55 : 45). Make adjustments if necessary (see *System Suitability* under *Chromatography* ⟨621⟩).

Chromatographic system (see *Chromatography* ⟨621⟩)—The liquid chromatograph is equipped with a 271-nm detector and a 4-mm × 30-cm column that contains packing L7. The flow rate is about 2 mL per minute. Chromatograph three replicate injections of the Standard solution, and record the peak responses as directed for *Procedure:* the relative standard deviation is not more than 3.0%.

Procedure—Inject an appropriate volume (50 μL to 500 μL) of a filtered portion of the solution under test into the chromatograph, record the chromatogram, and measure the response for the major peak. Calculate the quantity of $C_{16}H_{13}ClN_2O$ dissolved in comparison with a Standard solution having a known concentration of USP Mazindol RS in the same *Medium* and similarly chromatographed.

Tolerances—Not less than 80% (Q) of the labeled amount of $C_{16}H_{13}ClN_2O$ is dissolved in 120 minutes.

Uniformity of dosage units ⟨905⟩: meet the requirements.

PROCEDURE FOR CONTENT UNIFORMITY—

Dye solution—Dissolve 100 mg of bromocresol purple in 1000 mL of 0.33 N acetic acid, and mix.

Standard solution—Dissolve an accurately weighed quantity of USP Mazindol RS in 0.33 N acetic acid, and dilute quantitatively and stepwise with 0.33 N acetic acid to obtain a solution having a known concentration of about 20 μg per mL.

Test solution—Mix 1 finely powdered Tablet with an accurately measured volume of 0.33 N acetic acid, sufficient to provide a solution having a concentration of about 20 μg of mazindol per mL, shake by mechanical means for 30 minutes, and filter, discarding the first few mL of the filtrate.

Procedure—Transfer 25.0 mL each of the *Standard solution*, the *Test solution*, and 0.33 N acetic acid to provide the blank, to individual 125-mL separators. Add 30 mL of *Dye solution* and 50.0 mL of chloroform to each, and shake by mechanical means for 15 minutes. Allow the layers to separate, and filter the chloroform layers. Concomitantly determine the absorbances of the filtered solutions obtained from the *Test solution* and the *Standard solution* at the wavelength of maximum absorbance at about 420 nm, using the blank to set the instrument. Calculate the quantity, in mg, of mazindol ($C_{16}H_{13}ClN_2O$) in the Tablet by the formula:

$$(TC/D)(A_U/A_S)$$

in which T is the labeled quantity, in mg, of mazindol in the Tablet; C is the concentration, in μg per mL, of USP Mazindol RS in the *Standard solution*; D is the concentration, in μg per mL, of mazindol in the *Test solution*, based on the labeled quantity per Tablet and the extent of dilution; and A_U and A_S are the absorbances of the solutions from the *Test solution* and the *Standard solution*, respectively.

Assay—

Internal standard solution—Dissolve 50 mg of amitriptyline hydrochloride in 250 mL of methanol, and mix.

Standard preparation—Transfer about 32 mg of USP Mazindol RS, accurately weighed, to a 100-mL volumetric flask, add about 50 mL of *Internal standard solution*, and shake by mechanical means for 30 minutes. Dilute with *Internal standard solution* to volume, and mix.

Assay preparation—Weigh and finely powder not fewer than 20 Tablets. Transfer an accurately weighed portion of the powder, equivalent to about 8 mg of mazindol, to a suitable flask, add 25.0 mL of *Internal standard solution*, and shake by mechanical means for 30 minutes. Pass through a fine-porosity, sintered-glass filter, discarding the first few mL of the filtrate.

Mobile phase—Transfer 200 mL of aqueous 0.01 M dibasic ammonium phosphate to a 1000-mL volumetric flask, dilute with methanol to volume, and mix. Pass through a 0.5-μm porosity polytef filter, and degas under vacuum. Protect this solution from light.

Chromatographic system (see *Chromatography* ⟨621⟩)—The liquid chromatograph is equipped with a 254-nm detector and a 4-mm × 30-cm column that contains packing L10. Inject three replicate portions of the *Standard preparation*, and record the peak responses as directed for *Procedure:* the resolution, R, is not less than 2.0: and the relative standard deviation is not more than 3.0%.

Procedure—Separately inject equal volumes (about 20 μL) of the *Standard preparation* and the *Assay preparation* into the chromatograph, record the chromatograms, and measure the peak responses for mazindol and amitriptyline hydrochloride. Calculate the quantity, in mg, of mazindol ($C_{16}H_{13}ClN_2O$) in the portion of Tablets taken by the formula:

$$25C(R_U/R_S)$$

in which C is the concentration, in mg per mL, of USP Mazindol RS in the *Standard preparation*; and R_U and R_S are the peak response ratios of mazindol to amitriptyline hydrochloride obtained from the *Assay preparation* and the *Standard preparation*, respectively.

Measles Virus Vaccine Live

» Measles Virus Vaccine Live conforms to the regulations of the FDA concerning biologics (630.30 to 630.37) (see *Biologics* ⟨1041⟩). It is a bacterially sterile preparation of live virus derived from a strain of measles virus tested for neurovirulence in monkeys, for safety, and for immunogenicity, free from all demonstrable viable microbial agents except unavoidable bacteriophage, and found suitable for human immunization. The strain is grown for purposes of vaccine production on chicken embryo primary cell tissue cultures derived from pathogen-free flocks and meets the requirements of the specific safety tests in adult and suckling mice; the requirements of the tests in monkey kidney, chicken embryo and human tissue cell cultures and embryonated eggs; and the requirements of the tests for absence of *Mycobacterium tuberculosis* and of avian leucosis, unless the production cultures were derived from certified avian leucosis-free sources and the control fluids were tested for avian leucosis. The strain cultures are treated to remove all intact tissue cells. The Vaccine meets the requirements of the specific tissue culture test for live virus titer, in a single immunizing dose, of not less than the equivalent of 1000 TCID$_{50}$ (quantity of virus estimated to infect 50% of inoculated cultures × 1000) when tested in parallel with the U. S. Reference Measles Virus, Live Attenuated. It may contain suitable antimicrobial agents.

Packaging and storage—Preserve in single-dose containers, or light-resistant, multiple-dose containers, at a temperature between 2° and 8°. Multiple-dose containers for 50 doses are adapted for use only in jet injectors, and those for 10 doses for use by jet or syringe injection.
Expiration date—The expiration date is 1 to 2 years, depending on the manufacturer's data, after date of issue from manufacturer's cold storage (−20°, 1 year).
Labeling—Label the Vaccine in multiple-dose containers to indicate that the contents are intended solely for use by jet injector or for use by either jet or syringe injection, whichever is applicable. Label the Vaccine in single-dose containers, if such containers are not light-resistant, to state that it should be protected from sunlight. Label it also to state that constituted Vaccine should be discarded if not used within 8 hours.

Measles, Mumps, and Rubella Virus Vaccine Live

» Measles, Mumps, and Rubella Virus Vaccine Live conforms to the regulations of the FDA concerning biologics (see *Biologics* ⟨1041⟩). It is a bacterially sterile preparation of a combination of live measles virus, live mumps virus, and live rubella virus such that each component is prepared in conformity with and meets the requirements for Measles Virus Vaccine Live, for Mumps Virus Vaccine Live, and for Rubella Virus Vaccine Live, whichever is applicable. Each component provides an immunizing dose and meets the requirements of the corresponding Virus Vaccine in the total dosage prescribed in the labeling. It may contain suitable antimicrobial agents.

Packaging and storage—Preserve in single-dose containers, or light-resistant, multiple-dose containers, at a temperature between 2° and 8°. Multiple-dose containers for 50 doses are adapted for use only in jet injectors, and those for 10 doses for use by jet or syringe injection.
Expiration date—The expiration date is 1 to 2 years, depending on the manufacturer's data, after date of issue from manufacturer's cold storage (−20°, 1 year).
Labeling—Label the Vaccine in multiple-dose containers to indicate that the contents are intended solely for use by jet injector or for use by either jet or syringe injection, whichever is applicable. Label the Vaccine in single-dose containers, if such containers are not light-resistant, to state that it should be protected from sunlight. Label it also to state that constituted Vaccine should be discarded if not used within 8 hours.

Measles and Rubella Virus Vaccine Live

» Measles and Rubella Virus Vaccine Live conforms to the regulations of the FDA concerning biologics (see *Biologics* ⟨1041⟩). It is a bacterially sterile preparation of a combination of live measles virus and live rubella virus such that each component is prepared in conformity with and meets the requirements for Measles Virus Vaccine Live and for Rubella Virus Vaccine Live, whichever is applicable. Each component provides an immunizing dose and meets the requirements of the corresponding Virus Vaccine in the total dosage prescribed in the labeling. It may contain suitable antimicrobial agents.

Packaging and storage—Preserve in single-dose containers, or light-resistant, multiple-dose containers, at a temperature between 2° and 8°. Multiple-dose containers for 50 doses are adapted for use only in jet injectors, and those for 10 doses for use by jet or syringe injection.
Expiration date—The expiration date is 1 to 2 years, depending on the manufacturer's data, after date of issue from manufacturer's cold storage (−20°, 1 year).
Labeling—Label the Vaccine in multiple-dose containers to indicate that the contents are intended solely for use by jet injector or for use by either jet or syringe injection, whichever is applicable. Label the Vaccine in single-dose containers, if such containers are not light-resistant, to state that it should be protected from sunlight. Label it also to state that constituted Vaccine should be discarded if not used within 8 hours.

Mebendazole

$C_{16}H_{13}N_3O_3$ 295.29
Carbamic acid, (5-benzoyl-1*H*-benzimidazol-2-yl), methyl ester.
Methyl 5-benzoyl-2-benzimidazolecarbamate   [*31431-39-7*].

» Mebendazole contains not less than 98.0 percent and not more than 102.0 percent of $C_{16}H_{13}N_3O_3$, calculated on the dried basis.

Packaging and storage—Preserve in well-closed containers.
USP Reference standards ⟨11⟩—*USP Mebendazole RS*.
Identification, *Infrared Absorption* ⟨197K⟩.
Loss on drying ⟨731⟩—Dry it at 105° for 4 hours: it loses not more than 0.5% of its weight.
Residue on ignition ⟨281⟩:   not more than 0.1%.
Heavy metals, *Method II* ⟨231⟩:   0.002%.
Chromatographic purity—Dissolve 50 mg in 1.0 mL of 96 percent formic acid in a 10-mL volumetric flask, add chloroform to volume, and mix. Similarly prepare a solution of USP Mebendazole RS in the same medium having a concentration of 5 mg per mL. Transfer 1.0 mL of this Standard solution to a 200-mL volumetric flask, add a mixture of chloroform and 96 percent formic acid (9 : 1) to volume, and mix (diluted Standard solution). Apply 10-µL portions of the test solution, the Standard solution, and the diluted Standard solution to a suitable thin-layer chromatographic plate (see *Chromatography* ⟨621⟩) coated with a 0.25-mm layer of chromatographic silica gel mixture. Allow the spots to dry, and develop the chromatogram in a solvent system consisting of a mixture of chlo-

roform, methanol, and 96 percent formic acid (90 : 5 : 5) until the solvent front has moved about three-fourths of the length of the plate. Remove the plate from the developing chamber, mark the solvent front, allow the solvent to evaporate, and examine the plate under short-wavelength UV light: the R_F value of the principal spot obtained from the test solution corresponds to that obtained from the Standard solution, and no spot, other than the principal spot, in the chromatogram of the test solution is larger or more intense than the principal spot obtained from the diluted Standard solution.

Assay—Dissolve about 225 mg of Mebendazole, accurately weighed, in 30 mL of glacial acetic acid. Titrate with 0.1 N perchloric acid VS, determining the endpoint potentiometrically, using a calomel-glass electrode system. Perform a blank determination, and make any necessary correction. Each mL of 0.1 N perchloric acid is equivalent to 29.53 mg of $C_{16}H_{13}N_3O_3$.

Mebendazole Oral Suspension

» Mebendazole Oral Suspension is Mebendazole in an aqueous vehicle. It contains not less than 90.0 percent and not more than 110.0 percent of the labeled amount of mebendazole ($C_{16}H_{13}N_3O_3$).

Packaging and storage—Preserve in tight containers at controlled room temperature.

Labeling—Label it to indicate that it is for veterinary use only.

USP Reference standards ⟨11⟩—*USP Mebendazole RS*.

Identification—Mix a quantity of Oral Suspension, equivalent to about 200 mg of mebendazole, with 20 mL of a mixture of chloroform and 96 percent formic acid (19 : 1). Proceed as directed for *Identification* under *Mebendazole Tablets*, beginning with "Warm the suspension on a water bath for a few minutes." The specified result is obtained.

pH ⟨791⟩: between 6.0 and 7.0.

Assay—

Standard preparation—Transfer about 10 mg of USP Mebendazole RS, accurately weighed, to a 100-mL volumetric flask, and add 90 mL of chloroform, 7 mL of isopropyl alcohol, and 2 mL of 96 percent formic acid. Agitate until the solid has dissolved, add isopropyl alcohol to volume, and mix. Transfer 5.0 mL of this solution to a second 100-mL volumetric flask, dilute with isopropyl alcohol to volume, and mix to obtain a solution having a known concentration of about 5 µg per mL.

Assay preparation 1—Transfer an accurately measured quantity of Oral Suspension, equivalent to about 1000 mg of mebendazole, to a 100-mL volumetric flask, dilute with 96 percent formic acid to volume, and mix. Transfer 10.0 mL of this mixture to a second 100-mL volumetric flask, add 40 mL of 96 percent formic acid, and heat in a water bath at a temperature of 50° for 15 minutes. Cool, add water to volume, mix, and pass through a medium-porosity, sintered-glass filter. Transfer 10.0 mL of the filtrate to a 250-mL separator, and add 50 mL of water and 50 mL of chloroform. Shake for about 2 minutes, allow the phases to separate, and transfer the chloroform layer to a second 250-mL separator. Wash the aqueous layer with two 10-mL portions of chloroform, add the chloroform washings to the second separator, and discard the aqueous layer. Wash the combined chloroform solutions with a mixture of 4 mL of 1 N hydrochloric acid and 50 mL of a 1 in 10 solution of 96 percent formic acid in water, and transfer the chloroform layer to a 100-mL volumetric flask. Extract the aqueous washing with two 10-mL portions of chloroform, add these chloroform extracts to the chloroform solution in the volumetric flask, add 2 mL of 96 percent formic acid and 7 mL of isopropyl alcohol, dilute with chloroform to volume, and mix. Transfer 5.0 mL of this solution to another 100-mL volumetric flask, dilute with isopropyl alcohol to volume, and mix.

Assay preparation 2 (where the Oral Suspension is packaged in syringes calibrated to deliver stated increments of mebendazole)—Express an increment of Oral Suspension to a volumetric flask of an appropriate nominal volume so that when diluted with 96 percent formic acid to volume a mixture containing about 10 mg of mebendazole per mL is obtained. Transfer 10.0 mL of this mixture to a 100-mL volumetric flask, add 40 mL of 96 percent formic acid, and heat in a water bath at a temperature of 50° for 15 minutes. Proceed as directed for *Assay preparation 1* beginning with "Cool, add water to volume."

Procedure—Mix 90 mL of chloroform with 2 mL of 96 percent formic acid in a 100-mL volumetric flask, add isopropyl alcohol to volume, and mix. Transfer 5.0 mL of this solution to a second 100-mL volumetric flask, dilute with isopropyl alcohol to volume, and mix to obtain a reagent blank. Concomitantly determine the absorbances of the relevant *Assay preparation* and the *Standard preparation* at the wavelength of maximum absorbance at about 247 nm with a spectrophotometer, using the reagent blank to set the instrument. Calculate the quantity, in mg, of mebendazole ($C_{16}H_{13}N_3O_3$) in the portion of Oral Suspension taken to prepare *Assay preparation 1* by the formula:

$$200C(A_U / A_S)$$

in which C is the concentration, in µg per mL, of USP Mebendazole RS in the *Standard preparation*; and A_U and A_S are the absorbances of *Assay preparation 1* and the *Standard preparation*, respectively. Where appropriate, calculate the quantity, in mg, of mebendazole ($C_{16}H_{13}N_3O_3$) in the increment of Oral Suspension taken to prepare *Assay preparation 2* by the formula:

$$20{,}000(C / V)(A_U / A_S)$$

in which V is the volume, in mL, of the volumetric flask into which the increment of Oral Suspension was expressed; A_U is the absorbance of *Assay preparation 2*; and the other terms are as defined above.

Mebendazole Tablets

» Mebendazole Tablets contain not less than 90.0 percent and not more than 110.0 percent of the labeled amount of mebendazole ($C_{16}H_{13}N_3O_3$).

Packaging and storage—Preserve in well-closed containers.

USP Reference standards ⟨11⟩—*USP Mebendazole RS*.

Identification—Finely powder a quantity of Tablets, equivalent to about 200 mg of mebendazole, and mix the powder with 20 mL of a mixture of chloroform and 96 percent formic acid (19 : 1). Warm the suspension on a water bath for a few minutes, cool, and filter through a medium-porosity, sintered-glass filter. Apply 10 µL of this solution and 10 µL of a Standard solution of USP Mebendazole RS in a mixture of chloroform and 96 percent formic acid (19 : 1) containing 10 mg per mL to a suitable thin-layer chromatographic plate (see *Chromatography* ⟨621⟩) coated with a 0.25-mm layer of chromatographic silica gel mixture. Allow the spots to dry, and develop the chromatogram in a solvent system consisting of a mixture of chloroform, methanol, and 96 percent formic acid (90 : 5 : 5) until the solvent front has moved about three-fourths of the length of the plate. Remove the plate from the developing chamber, mark the solvent front, allow the solvent to evaporate, and examine the plate under short-wavelength UV light: the R_F value of the principal spot obtained from the test solution corresponds to that obtained from the Standard solution.

Dissolution ⟨711⟩—

Medium: 0.1 N hydrochloric acid containing 1.0% sodium lauryl sulfate; 900 mL.

Apparatus 2: 75 rpm.

Time: 120 minutes.

Determine the amount of $C_{16}H_{13}N_3O_3$ dissolved by employing the following method.

Buffer solution—Dissolve 8.0 g of sodium hydroxide in 2 L of water, add 3.0 g of sodium lauryl sulfate, and mix; then add 20 mL of phosphoric acid, and adjust with phosphoric acid to a pH of 2.5.

Mobile phase—Prepare a filtered and degassed mixture of acetonitrile and *Buffer solution* (3 : 7). Make adjustments if necessary (see *System Suitability* under *Chromatography* ⟨621⟩).

Standard solution—Transfer 25 mg of USP Mebendazole RS to a 50-mL volumetric flask, add 10.0 mL of formic acid and dissolve, dilute with methanol to volume, and mix. Dilute a portion of this solution quantitatively and stepwise with *Dissolution Medium* to obtain a solution having a known concentration similar to the expected concentration in the solution under test.

Chromatographic system (see *Chromatography* ⟨621⟩)—The liquid chromatograph is equipped with a 254-nm detector and a 4.6-mm × 3-cm column that contains packing L7. The flow rate is about 1 mL per minute. Chromatograph the *Standard solution*, and record the peak responses as directed for *Procedure*: the relative standard deviation for replicate injections is not more than 2.0%.

Procedure—Separately inject equal volumes (about 10 μL) of filtered portions of the *Standard solution* and the solution under test into the chromatograph, record the chromatograms, and measure the responses for the major peaks.

Tolerances—Not less than 75% (*Q*) of the labeled amount of $C_{16}H_{13}N_3O_3$ is dissolved in 120 minutes.

Uniformity of dosage units ⟨905⟩: meet the requirements.

PROCEDURE FOR CONTENT UNIFORMITY—

Standard preparation—Transfer about 20 mg of USP Mebendazole RS, accurately weighed, to a 10-mL volumetric flask, add 4 mL of 96 percent formic acid, and mix to dissolve. Add isopropyl alcohol to volume, and mix. Pipet 0.5 mL of this solution into a 100-mL volumetric flask, dilute with isopropyl alcohol to volume, and mix.

Test preparation—Mix 1 Tablet with 20 mL of 96 percent formic acid in a 100-mL volumetric flask, and heat on a steam bath for 15 minutes. Cool, add isopropyl alcohol to volume, mix, and pass through a medium-porosity, sintered-glass filter. Transfer an accurately measured portion of the filtrate, equivalent to 1 mg of mebendazole, to a 100-mL volumetric flask, dilute with isopropyl alcohol to volume, and mix.

Procedure—Concomitantly determine the absorbances of the *Standard preparation* and the *Test preparation* in 1-cm cells at the wavelength of maximum absorbance at about 310 nm, with a suitable spectrophotometer, using a 1 in 500 solution of 96 percent formic acid in isopropyl alcohol as the blank. Calculate the quantity, in mg, of $C_{16}H_{13}N_3O_3$ in the Tablet taken by the formula:

$$(TC/D)(A_U/A_S)$$

in which *T* is the labeled quantity, in mg, of mebendazole in the Tablet; *C* is the concentration, in μg per mL, of USP Mebendazole RS in the *Standard preparation*; *D* is the concentration, in μg per mL, of mebendazole in the *Test preparation*, based upon the labeled quantity per Tablet and the extent of dilution; and A_U and A_S are the absorbances of the solutions from the *Test preparation* and the *Standard preparation*, respectively.

Assay—

Mobile phase—Prepare a mixture of methanol and 0.05 M monobasic potassium phosphate (60 : 40), adjust with 0.1 M phosphoric acid or 1 N sodium hydroxide to a pH of 5.5, filter, and degas. Make adjustments if necessary (see *System Suitability* under *Chromatography* ⟨621⟩).

Standard preparation—Transfer about 25 mg of USP Mebendazole RS, accurately weighed, to a 100-mL volumetric flask. Add 10 mL of formic acid, and heat in a water bath at 50° for 15 minutes. Shake by mechanical means for 5 minutes, add 90 mL of methanol, and allow to cool. Dilute with methanol to volume, and mix. Transfer 5.0 mL of this solution to a 25-mL volumetric flask, dilute with *Mobile phase* to volume, mix, and filter through a filter having a porosity of 0.5 μm or finer.

Assay preparation—Weigh and finely powder not fewer than 20 Tablets. Transfer an accurately weighed portion of the powder, equivalent to about 500 mg of mebendazole, to a 100-mL volumetric flask. Add 50 mL of formic acid, and heat in a water bath at 50° for 15 minutes. Shake by mechanical means for 1 hour, dilute with water to volume, mix, and filter. Transfer 5.0 mL of the filtrate to a 100-mL volumetric flask, dilute with a solution of formic acid in methanol (1 : 9) to volume, and mix. Transfer 5.0 mL of this solution to a 25-mL volumetric flask, dilute with *Mobile phase* to volume, mix, and pass through a filter having a porosity of 0.5 μm or finer.

Chromatographic system (see *Chromatography* ⟨621⟩)—The liquid chromatograph is equipped with a 247-nm detector, a precolumn that contains packing L1, and a 3.9-mm × 30-cm analytical column that contains packing L1 and is maintained at about 30°. The flow rate is about 1.5 mL per minute. Chromatograph the *Standard preparation*, and record the peak responses as directed for *Procedure*: the tailing factor is not more than 2.0, the column efficiency is not less than 2500 theoretical plates, and the relative standard deviation for replicate injections is not more than 1%.

Procedure—Separately inject equal volumes (about 15 μL) of the *Standard preparation* and the *Assay preparation* into the chromatograph, record the chromatograms, and measure the responses for the major peaks. Calculate the quantity, in mg, of mebendazole ($C_{16}H_{13}N_3O_3$) in the portion of Tablets taken by the formula:

$$10,000C(r_U/r_S)$$

in which *C* is the concentration, in mg per mL, of USP Mebendazole RS in the *Standard preparation*; and r_U and r_S are the mebendazole peak responses obtained from the *Assay preparation* and the *Standard preparation*, respectively.

Mebrofenin

$C_{15}H_{19}BrN_2O_5$ 387.23

Glycine, *N*-[2-[(3-bromo-2,4,6,-trimethylphenyl)amino]-2-oxoethyl]-*N*-(carboxymethyl)-.

[[[(3-Bromomesityl)carbamoyl]methyl]imino]diacetic acid [78266-06-5].

» Mebrofenin contains not less than 97.0 percent and not more than 101.0 percent of $C_{15}H_{19}BrN_2O_5$, calculated on the dried basis.

Packaging and storage—Preserve in tight containers. Store at 25°, excursions permitted between 15° and 30°.

USP Reference standards ⟨11⟩—*USP Mebrofenin RS*.

Identification, *Infrared Absorption* ⟨197K⟩.

Melting range, *Class I* ⟨741⟩: between 185° and 200°, but the range between beginning and end of melting does not exceed 4°.

Loss on drying ⟨731⟩—Dry it in vacuum at 100° for 3 hours: it loses not more than 0.3% of its weight.

Residue on ignition ⟨281⟩: not more than 0.1%.

Heavy metals, *Method II* ⟨231⟩: 0.003%.

Limit of nitrilotriacetic acid—

Mobile phase—Add 10 mL of a 1 in 4 solution of tetrabutylammonium hydroxide in methanol to 200 mL of water, and adjust with 1 M phosphoric acid to a pH of 7.5 ± 0.1. Transfer this solution to a 1000-mL volumetric flask, add 90 mL of methanol, dilute with water to volume, mix, pass through a filter having a 0.5-μm or finer porosity, and degas. Make adjustments if necessary (see *System Suitability* under *Chromatography* ⟨621⟩).

Cupric nitrate solution—Prepare a solution containing about 10 mg of cupric nitrate per mL.

Standard stock solution—Transfer about 25 mg of nitrilotriacetic acid, accurately weighed, to a 50-mL volumetric flask, dilute with dilute ammonium hydroxide (1 in 20) to volume, and mix.

Standard solution—Transfer 10 mL of the *Standard stock solution* to a 100-mL volumetric flask, and dilute with *Cupric nitrate solution* to volume. [NOTE—Prepare fresh on the day of use.]

Test solution—Transfer about 250 mg of Mebrofenin, accurately weighed, to a 25-mL volumetric flask, dilute with *Cupric nitrate solution* to volume, and mix. Sonicate, if necessary, to achieve complete solution. [NOTE—Prepare fresh on the day of use.]

Chromatographic system (see *Chromatography* ⟨621⟩)—The liquid chromatograph is equipped with a 254-nm detector and a 4.6-mm × 25-cm column that contains packing L7. The flow rate is about 0.8 mL per minute. Chromatograph the *Standard solution*, and record the peak responses as directed for *Procedure:* the resolution, *R*, between the major peak and any other peak is not less than 1.7. [NOTE—Peaks containing copper may be present.] The relative standard deviation for replicate injections is not more than 2.0%.

Procedure—Separately inject equal volumes (about 20 µL) of the *Standard solution* and the *Test solution* into the chromatograph, and record the chromatograms. Measure the responses for the peaks in each chromatogram at the locus for copper nitrilotriacetic acid. Calculate the quantity, in mg, of nitrilotriacetic acid in the portion of Mebrofenin taken by the formula:

$$25C(r_U / r_S)$$

in which *C* is the concentration, in mg per mL, of nitrilotriacetic acid in the *Standard solution;* and r_U and r_S are the peak responses obtained from the *Test solution* and the *Standard solution*, respectively: not more than 0.1% is found.

Chromatographic purity—

Mobile phase—Prepare a mixture of equal volumes of 0.025 M monobasic potassium phosphate and 0.025 M dibasic sodium phosphate. To 400 mL of this solution add 600 mL of methanol. Adjust the volume to 1000 mL with water, and adjust with 1 N hydrochloric acid to a pH of 5.0 ± 0.1. Make adjustments if necessary (see *System Suitability* under *Chromatography* ⟨621⟩). Pass through a filter having a 0.45-µm porosity, and degas.

Test solution—Transfer about 12.5 mg of Mebrofenin, accurately weighed, to a 25-mL volumetric flask, dilute with *Mobile phase* to volume, and mix.

Chromatographic system (see *Chromatography* ⟨621⟩)—The liquid chromatograph is equipped with a 220-nm detector and a 4.6-mm × 25-cm column containing packing L1. The flow rate is about 1 mL per minute. Chromatograph about 20 µL of the *Test solution*, and record the peak responses. The capacity factor, *k'*, is not less than 1.2; and the effective plate number, n_{eff}, calculated by the formula $16[(t - t_a)/W]^2$, in which the terms are as defined under *Chromatography* ⟨621⟩, is not less than 200. The tailing factor is not more than 4.0, and the relative standard deviation of the mebrofenin peak responses for replicate injections is not more than 2.0%.

Procedure—Chromatograph about 20 µL of the *Test solution*, run the chromatogram for twice the elution time of the mebrofenin peak, and record the peak response for individual impurities and the total response for the entire chromatogram. Calculate the percentage of chromatographic impurities taken by the formula:

$$100(r_s / r_t)$$

in which r_s is the sum of the peak responses of the individual impurities; and r_t is the total of all of the peak responses in the chromatogram: not more than 3% is found.

Assay—Dissolve about 100 mg of Mebrofenin, accurately weighed, in about 40 mL of dimethylformamide in a conical flask, with the aid of sonication if necessary. Add 3 drops of thymol blue TS, and titrate with 0.1 N sodium methoxide (in toluene) VS to a blue endpoint while flushing the flask with a gentle stream of nitrogen. Perform a blank determination, and make any necessary correction. Each mL of 0.1 N sodium methoxide is equivalent to 19.36 mg of $C_{15}H_{19}BrN_2O_5$.

Mecamylamine Hydrochloride

$C_{11}H_{21}N \cdot HCl$ 203.75

Bicyclo[2.2.1]heptan-2-amine, *N*,2,3,3-tetramethyl-, hydrochloride.
N,2,3,3-Tetramethyl-2-norbornanamine hydrochloride   [826-39-1]

» Mecamylamine Hydrochloride contains not less than 98.0 percent and not more than 100.5 percent of $C_{11}H_{21}N \cdot HCl$, calculated on the dried basis.

Packaging and storage—Preserve in tight containers.

USP Reference standards ⟨11⟩—*USP Mecamylamine Hydrochloride RS. USP Mecamylamine Related Compound A RS.*

Identification—

A: *Infrared Absorption* ⟨197K⟩.

B: It responds to the tests for *Chloride* ⟨191⟩.

Acidity—Dissolve 5.0 g in 100 mL of methanol, and titrate potentiometrically with 0.10 N alcoholic potassium hydroxide to an apparent pH of 5.5, using a calomel-glass electrode system and a potentiometer previously standardized with pH 5.0 neutralized phthalate buffer (see *Solutions* in the section *Reagents, Indicators, and Solutions*): after correction for the volume of alkali consumed by 100 mL of methanol, not more than 0.55 mL of 0.10 N alcoholic potassium hydroxide is required.

Loss on drying ⟨731⟩—Dry it at a pressure not exceeding 5 mm of mercury at 105° for 1 hour: it loses not more than 1.0% of its weight.

Residue on ignition ⟨281⟩:   not more than 0.5%.

Heavy metals, *Method I* ⟨231⟩—Dissolve 400 mg in 20 mL of water, add 2 mL of 1 N acetic acid, and dilute with water to 25 mL: the limit is not more than 50 ppm.

Limit of residual solvents—

Diluent—Prepare a mixture of dimethyl sulfoxide and water (2 : 1).

Internal standard solution—Prepare a solution of absolute alcohol in *Diluent* having a known concentration of about 15 µL per mL.

Standard stock solution—Transfer 50 mL of the *Diluent* to a 100-mL volumetric flask, add 0.64 mL of isopropyl alcohol, dilute with *Diluent* to volume, and mix.

Standard solution—Pipet 1.0 mL of the *Standard stock solution* into a 25-mL volumetric flask, dilute with *Diluent* to volume, and mix (*Solution 1*). Transfer about 500 mg of sodium chloride, accurately weighed, to a headspace vial, add 1.5 mL of *Solution 1* and 1.5 mL of the *Internal standard solution*, and mix.

Test solution—Transfer about 150 mg of Mecamylamine Hydrochloride, accurately weighed, to a headspace vial, add about 500 mg of sodium chloride, 1.5 mL of *Diluent*, and 1.5 mL of the *Internal standard solution*, and mix.

Chromatographic system (see *Chromatography* ⟨621⟩)—The gas chromatograph is equipped with a flame-ionization detector and a 0.53-mm × 30-m capillary column whose internal wall is coated with a 1.0-µm film of liquid phase G16. This column is joined with a 0.53-mm × 25-m capillary column whose internal wall is coated with a 5.0-µm film of liquid phase G1. The G16 column is connected to the detector, and the G1 column is connected to the injector. The injection port temperature is maintained at about 100°; the detector temperature is maintained at about 210°; and the column temperature is maintained at 50° for 10 minutes, then increased at a rate of 5° per minute to 110°, then increased at a rate of 30° per minute to 210°, and maintained for 5 minutes at 210°. Nitrogen is used as the carrier gas, flowing at a rate of about 6.5 mL per minute. The split flow is 15 mL per minute.

Procedure—Allow the *Standard solution*, the *Internal standard solution*, and the *Test solution* to stand for 20 minutes at 90°. Separately inject equal volumes (about 1 mL) of the headspace of the *Standard solution*, the *Internal standard solution*, and the *Test solution* into the gas chromatograph, record the chromatograms, and measure the peak responses of the internal standard and isopropyl alcohol. Calculate the quantity, in ppm, of isopropyl alcohol in the portion of Mecamylamine Hydrochloride taken by the formula:

$$150(R_U)(W_S) / (R_S)(W_U)$$

in which W_S is the amount, in ppm, of isopropyl alcohol in the *Standard solution;* W_U is the weight, in mg, of Mecamylamine Hydrochloride taken to prepare the *Test solution;* and R_U and R_S are the peak response ratios of isopropyl alcohol to the internal standard obtained from the *Test solution* and the *Standard solution*, respectively: not more than 2000 ppm of isopropyl alcohol is found.

Related compounds—

Internal standard solution—Proceed as directed in the *Assay*.

Solution 1—Prepare a solution of *dl*-camphene and USP Mecamylamine Related Compound A RS in the *Internal standard solution* containing 625 µg of each per mL.

System suitability solution—Transfer about 125 mg of USP Mecamylamine Hydrochloride RS, accurately weighed, to a 50-mL volumetric flask, add 1 mL of *Solution 1*, dilute with *Internal standard solution* to volume, and mix.

Test solution—Use the *Assay preparation*.

Chromatographic system—Prepare as directed in the *Assay*. Chromatograph the *System suitability solution*, and record peak responses as directed for *Procedure*: the resolution, *R*, between the mecamylamine and mecamylamine related compound A is not less than 5; the column efficiency is not less than 4000 theoretical plates; the tailing factor is not more than 1.5; and the relative standard deviation for replicate injections is not more than 2.0%.

Procedure—Inject a volume (about 1 μL) of the *Test solution* into the chromatograph, record the chromatogram, and measure all the peak responses. Calculate the percentage of each impurity in the portion of Mecamylamine Hydrochloride taken by the formula:

$$100(r_i / r_s)$$

in which r_i is the peak response for each impurity; and r_s is the sum of the responses for all the peaks: not more than 0.5% of mecamylamine related compound A is found; not more than 0.5% of *dl*-camphene is found; and not more than 1.0% of total impurities is found.

Chloride content—Dissolve about 500 mg, accurately weighed, in 5 mL of water. Add 5 mL of glacial acetic acid, 50 mL of methanol, and 1 drop of eosin Y TS, and titrate with 0.1 N silver nitrate VS. Each mL of 0.1 N silver nitrate is equivalent to 3.545 mg of Cl: the content is between 17.0% and 17.8%.

Assay—

Internal standard solution—Transfer about 600 mg of sodium hydroxide pellets to a 1 L volumetric flask, dissolve in about 800 mL of methanol. Add an accurately weighed quantity of about 1.7 g of biphenyl to the flask, and dilute with methanol to volume.

Standard preparation—Dissolve an accurately weighed quantity of USP Mecamylamine Hydrochloride RS in *Internal standard solution*, and dilute with *Internal standard solution*, quantitatively and stepwise if necessary, to obtain a solution having a known concentration of about 2.5 mg per mL.

Assay preparation—Transfer about 125 mg of Mecamylamine Hydrochloride, accurately weighed, to a 50-mL volumetric flask, dissolve in and dilute with *Internal standard solution* to volume, and mix.

Chromatographic system (see *Chromatography* ⟨621⟩)—The gas chromatograph is equipped with a flame-ionization detector connected to a 0.53-mm × 30-m capillary column, coated with a 1.5-μm film of liquid phase G27. The injection port temperature is maintained at about 200°, the detector temperature is maintained at about 280°, and the column temperature is at 120° for 15 minutes then increased at 25° per minute to 250° and maintained for 7 minutes at 250°. Nitrogen is used as the carrier gas at 7.4 mL per minute. Chromatograph the *Standard preparation*, and record the peak responses as directed for *Procedure*: the column efficiency is not less than 4000 theoretical plates; the tailing factor is not more than 1.5; and the relative standard deviation for replicate injections is not more than 2.0%.

Procedure—Inject equal volumes (about 1 μL) of the *Assay preparation* and the *Standard preparation* into the gas chromatograph, record the chromatogram, and measure the responses for the major peaks. Calculate the quantity, in mg, of $C_{11}H_{21}N \cdot HCl$ in the portion of Mecamylamine Hydrochloride taken by the formula:

$$50C(R_U / R_S)$$

in which *C* is the concentration of USP Mecamylamine Hydrochloride RS, in mg per mL, in the *Standard preparation*; and R_U and R_S are the peak response ratios of mecamylamine hydrochloride to the internal standard biphenyl obtained from the *Assay preparation* and the *Standard preparation*, respectively.

Mecamylamine Hydrochloride Tablets

» Mecamylamine Hydrochloride Tablets contain not less than 90.0 percent and not more than 110.0 percent of the labeled amount of mecamylamine hydrochloride ($C_{11}H_{21}N \cdot HCl$).

Packaging and storage—Preserve in well-closed containers.

USP Reference standards ⟨11⟩—*USP Mecamylamine Hydrochloride RS*.

Identification—

A: To a quantity of powdered Tablets, equivalent to about 75 mg of mecamylamine hydrochloride, add 50 mL of chloroform, and triturate the mixture for 5 minutes. Filter, and evaporate the filtrate on a steam bath with the aid of a current of air to dryness: the IR absorption spectrum of a potassium bromide dispersion of a portion of the residue so obtained exhibits maxima only at the same wavelengths as that of a similar preparation of USP Mecamylamine Hydrochloride RS.

B: A portion of the residue obtained in *Identification* test *A* responds to the tests for *Chloride* ⟨191⟩.

Dissolution ⟨711⟩—

Medium: water; 750 mL.
Apparatus 2: 50 rpm.
Time: 30 minutes.

Determine the amount of $C_{11}H_{21}N \cdot HCl$ dissolved using the following procedure.

Diluent—Prepare a solution of triethylamine in alcohol (1 : 100).

Internal standard solution—Prepare a solution of biphenyl in *Diluent* having a concentration of 82.5 μg per mL.

Standard solution—Prepare a solution of USP Mecamylamine Hydrochloride RS and biphenyl in *Diluent* having concentrations of 8.25 μg per mL of each.

Test solution—[NOTE—Condition the solid-phase extraction column specified in this procedure in the following manner. Wash the column with 5 mL of water, then with 5 mL of *Diluent*, and finally with two 5-mL portions of water.] Transfer by pipetting 25.0 mL of the solution under test through a freshly conditioned solid-phase extraction column containing L1 packing with a sorbent-mass to column volume ratio of 360 mg per 5 mL, or equivalent. Wash the pipet and the solid-phase extraction column with two 5-mL portions of water. Discard the filtrate. Elute the solid-phase extraction column with two 4-mL portions of *Diluent*, and collect the eluate in a 10-mL volumetric flask containing 1.0 mL of *Internal standard solution*. Dilute with *Diluent* to volume, and mix.

Chromatographic system (see *Chromatography* ⟨621⟩)—The gas chromatograph is equipped with a flame-ionization detector, a splitless injection system, and a 0.53-mm × 30-m analytical column coated with a 1-5-μm layer of phase G27. The carrier gas is helium at a flow rate of 5.2 mL per minute. The detector and column temperatures are maintained at 250° and 150°, respectively. Chromatograph replicate injections of the *Standard solution*, and record the peak responses as directed for *Procedure*: the column efficiency is not less than 4000 theoretical plates, the tailing factor is not more than 2, and the relative standard deviation is not more than 2.0%.

Procedure—Separately inject equal volumes (about 2 μL) of the *Standard solution* and the *Test solution* into the chromatograph, record the chromatograms, and measure the responses for the major peaks. Calculate the amount in mg, of $C_{11}H_{21}N \cdot HCl$ dissolved by the formula:

$$0.3C(R_U / R_S)$$

in which *C* is the concentration, in μg per mL, of USP Mecamylamine Hydrochloride RS in the *Standard solution*; and R_U and R_S are the peak response ratios of the mecamylamine hydrochloride peak to the internal standard peak obtained from the *Test solution* and *Standard solution*, respectively.

Tolerances—Not less than 75% (*Q*) of the labeled amount of $C_{11}H_{21}N \cdot HCl$ is dissolved in 30 minutes.

Uniformity of dosage units ⟨905⟩: meet the requirements.

Procedure for content uniformity—Place 1 Tablet in the digestion flask, and proceed as directed under *Nitrogen Determination, Method II* ⟨461⟩. Each mL of 0.01 N sulfuric acid is equivalent to 2.038 mg of mecamylamine hydrochloride.

Assay—Weigh and finely powder not fewer than 30 Tablets. Transfer an accurately weighed portion of the powder, equivalent to about 50 mg of mecamylamine hydrochloride, to a glass-stoppered, 125-mL conical flask. Add about 25 mL of water, insert the stopper in the flask, and shake by mechanical means for 20 minutes. Transfer the contents of the flask to a 250-mL separator with the aid of small portions of water. Add 1 mL of 1 N sodium hydroxide and 5 g of sodium chloride, and extract the mixture successively with two 50-mL and three 25-mL portions of ether. Wash the combined ether extracts with three 10-mL portions of water, and wash, in turn, the combined water washes with a 10-mL portion of ether, adding it to the washed combined ether extracts. Transfer the ether phase to a 250-mL conical flask containing 25.0 mL of 0.02 N sulfuric acid VS, and evaporate the ether on a steam bath. Cool the solution, add methyl red TS, and titrate the excess acid with 0.02 N sodium hydroxide VS. Each mL of 0.02 N sulfuric acid is equivalent to 4.075 mg of mecamylamine hydrochloride ($C_{11}H_{21}N \cdot HCl$).

Mechlorethamine Hydrochloride

$C_5H_{11}Cl_2N \cdot HCl$ 192.51
Ethanamine, 2-chloro-*N*-(2-chloroethyl)-*N*-methyl-, hydrochloride.
2,2'-Dichloro-*N*-methyldiethylamine hydrochloride   [55-86-7].

» Mechlorethamine Hydrochloride contains not less than 97.5 percent and not more than 100.5 percent of $C_5H_{11}Cl_2N \cdot HCl$, calculated on the anhydrous basis.

Packaging and storage—Preserve in tight, light-resistant containers.
Labeling—The label bears a warning that great care should be taken to prevent inhaling particles of Mechlorethamine Hydrochloride and exposing the skin to it.
USP Reference standards ⟨11⟩—*USP Mechlorethamine Hydrochloride RS*.
Identification—
  A: *Infrared Absorption* ⟨197K⟩.
  B: Transfer 100 mg to a test tube containing 1 mL of sodium thiosulfate solution (prepared by dissolving 1 g of sodium thiosulfate and 100 mg of sodium carbonate in 40 mL of water), shake, allow to stand for 2 hours, then add 1 drop of iodine TS: the color of free iodine remains.
Melting range ⟨741⟩: between 108° and 111°.
pH ⟨791⟩: between 3.0 and 5.0, in a solution (1 in 500).
Water, *Method I* ⟨921⟩: not more than 0.4%.
Ionic chloride content—Dissolve about 30 mg, accurately weighed, in 30 mL of water contained in a beaker. Add 5 mL of nitric acid and stir. Titrate with 0.02 N silver nitrate VS to a potentiometric endpoint, using a silver combination electrode. Perform a blank determination (see *Titrimetry* ⟨541⟩), and make any necessary correction. Each mL of 0.02 N silver nitrate is equivalent to 0.709 mg of ionic chloride: not less than 18.0% and not more than 19.3% of ionic chloride is found.
Assay—Transfer about 100 mg of Mechlorethamine Hydrochloride, accurately weighed, to a 125-mL conical flask. Add 100 mg of sodium bicarbonate and 20.0 mL of 0.1 N sodium thiosulfate VS. Allow to stand for 2½ hours, add 3 mL of starch TS, and titrate the excess sodium thiosulfate with 0.1 N iodine VS. Each mL of 0.1 N sodium thiosulfate is equivalent to 9.626 mg of $C_5H_{11}Cl_2N \cdot HCl$.

Mechlorethamine Hydrochloride for Injection

» Mechlorethamine Hydrochloride for Injection is a sterile mixture of Mechlorethamine Hydrochloride with Sodium Chloride or other suitable diluent. It contains not less than 90.0 percent and not more than 110.0 percent of the labeled amount of mechlorethamine hydrochloride ($C_5H_{11}Cl_2N \cdot HCl$).

Packaging and storage—Preserve in *Containers for Sterile Solids* as described under *Injections* ⟨1⟩.
Labeling—It meets the requirements for *Labeling* under *Injections* ⟨1⟩. The label bears a warning that great care should be taken to prevent inhaling particles of Mechlorethamine Hydrochloride for Injection and exposing the skin to it.
USP Reference standards ⟨11⟩—*USP Endotoxin RS. USP Mechlorethamine Hydrochloride RS*.
Completeness of solution ⟨641⟩—A 0.10-g portion dissolves in 10 mL of carbon dioxide-free water to yield a clear solution.
Constituted solution—At the time of use, it meets the requirements for *Constituted Solutions* under *Injections* ⟨1⟩.
Identification—It meets the requirements of the *Identification* tests under *Mechlorethamine Hydrochloride*.
Bacterial endotoxins ⟨85⟩—It contains not more than 12.5 USP Endotoxin Units per mg of mechlorethamine hydrochloride.
pH ⟨791⟩: between 3.0 and 5.0, in a solution (1 in 50).
Water, *Method I* ⟨921⟩: not more than 1.0%.
Particulate matter ⟨788⟩: meets the requirements for small-volume injections.
Other requirements—It meets the requirements for *Sterility Tests* ⟨71⟩ and *Uniformity of Dosage Units* ⟨905⟩.
Assay—
  Assay preparation—Select a counted number of not fewer than 10 containers of Mechlorethamine Hydrochloride for Injection, equivalent to about 100 mg of mechlorethamine hydrochloride. Dissolve the contents of each container in water, and transfer the resulting solutions to a 250-mL conical flask.
  Procedure—Immediately proceed as directed in the *Assay* under *Mechlorethamine Hydrochloride*, beginning with "Add 100 mg of sodium bicarbonate." Calculate the average content, in mg, of mechlorethamine hydrochloride ($C_5H_{11}Cl_2N \cdot HCl$) per container of Mechlorethamine Hydrochloride for Injection taken by the formula:

$$9.626(V/N)$$

in which V is the volume, in mL, of 0.1 N sodium thiosulfate consumed; and N is the number of containers selected to prepare the *Assay preparation*.

Meclizine Hydrochloride

$C_{25}H_{27}ClN_2 \cdot 2HCl \cdot H_2O$ 481.88
Piperazine, 1-[(4-chlorophenyl)phenylmethyl]-4-[(3-methylphenyl)methyl]-, dihydrochloride, monohydrate.
1-(*p*-Chloro-α-phenylbenzyl)-4-(*m*-methylbenzyl)piperazine dihydrochloride monohydrate   [31884-77-2].
Anhydrous   463.88   [1104-22-9].

» Meclizine Hydrochloride contains not less than 97.0 percent and not more than 100.5 percent of $C_{25}H_{27}ClN_2 \cdot 2HCl$, calculated on the anhydrous basis.

Packaging and storage—Preserve in tight containers.
USP Reference standards ⟨11⟩—*USP Meclizine Hydrochloride RS*.

Identification—
A: *Infrared Absorption* ⟨197K⟩.
B: *Ultraviolet Absorption* ⟨197U⟩—
Solution: 10 µg per mL.
Medium: dilute hydrochloric acid (1 in 100).
C: Dissolve 25 mg in a mixture of 3 mL of 2 N nitric acid and 5 mL of alcohol: the solution responds to the tests for *Chloride* ⟨191⟩.
Water, *Method I* ⟨921⟩: not more than 5.0%.
Residue on ignition ⟨281⟩: not more than 0.1%.
Chromatographic purity—
Mobile phase—Dissolve 1.5 g of sodium 1-heptanesulfonate in 300 mL of water, and mix this solution with 700 mL of acetonitrile. Adjust with 0.1 N sulfuric acid to a pH of 4, filter, and degas. Make adjustments if necessary (see *System Suitability* under *Chromatography* ⟨621⟩).
Standard solution—Dissolve an accurately weighed quantity of USP Meclizine Hydrochloride RS in *Mobile phase*, and dilute quantitatively, and stepwise if necessary, with *Mobile phase* to obtain a solution having a known concentration of about 2.5 µg per mL.
Test solution—Prepare a solution of Meclizine Hydrochloride in *Mobile phase* having a known concentration of about 0.5 mg per mL.
System suitability solution—Prepare a solution in *Mobile phase* containing about 0.01 mg of USP Meclizine Hydrochloride RS and 0.01 mg of 4-chlorobenzophenone per mL.
Chromatographic system (see *Chromatography* ⟨621⟩)—The liquid chromatograph is equipped with a 230-nm detector and a 4.6-mm × 25-cm column that contains 10-µm packing L1. The flow rate is about 1.3 mL per minute. Chromatograph the *System suitability solution*, and record the peak responses as directed for *Procedure:* the relative retention times are about 0.8 for meclizine hydrochloride and 1.0 for 4-chlorobenzophenone; and the resolution, *R*, between the 4-chlorobenzophenone and meclizine hydrochloride peaks is not less than 2.0. Chromatograph the *Standard solution*, and record the peak responses as directed for *Procedure:* the tailing factor for the analyte peak is not more than 1.5; the column efficiency, *N*, determined from the analyte peak is not less than 1800 theoretical plates; and the relative standard deviation for replicate injections is not more than 1.5%.
Procedure—Separately inject equal volumes (about 20 µL) of the *Standard solution* and the *Test solution* into the chromatograph. Allow the *Test solution* to elute for not less than three times the retention time of meclizine hydrochloride. Record the chromatograms and measure all of the peak areas: the sum of the peak responses, excluding that of meclizine hydrochloride, from the *Test solution* is not more than two times the meclizine hydrochloride response from the *Standard solution* (1.0%), and no single peak response is greater than that of the meclizine hydrochloride response from the *Standard solution* (0.5%).
Organic volatile impurities, *Method IV* ⟨467⟩: meets the requirements.

(Official until July 1, 2008)

Assay—Dissolve about 350 mg of Meclizine Hydrochloride, accurately weighed, in about 50 mL of chloroform. Add 50 mL of glacial acetic acid, 5 mL of acetic anhydride, and 10 mL of mercuric acetate TS, and titrate with 0.1 N perchloric acid VS, determining the endpoint potentiometrically, using a calomel-glass electrode system (see *Titrimetry* ⟨541⟩). Perform a blank determination, and make any necessary correction. Each mL of 0.1 N perchloric acid is equivalent to 23.19 mg of $C_{25}H_{27}ClN_2 \cdot 2HCl$.

Meclizine Hydrochloride Tablets

» Meclizine Hydrochloride Tablets contain not less than 95.0 percent and not more than 110.0 percent of the labeled amount of meclizine hydrochloride ($C_{25}H_{27}ClN_2 \cdot 2HCl$).

Packaging and storage—Preserve in well-closed containers.
USP Reference standards ⟨11⟩—*USP Meclizine Hydrochloride RS.*
Identification—
A: Tablets meet the requirements under *Identification—Organic Nitrogenous Bases* ⟨181⟩.
B: *Thin-Layer Chromatographic Identification Test* ⟨201⟩—
Adsorbent: 0.5-mm layer of chromatographic silica gel mixture.
Test solution—Extract a quantity of finely powdered Tablets, equivalent to about 125 mg of meclizine hydrochloride, by shaking for 15 minutes with 50 mL of methanol.
Standard solution—Prepare a solution of USP Meclizine Hydrochloride RS in methanol, containing 2.5 mg per mL.
Application volume: 50 µL.
Developing solvent system: a mixture of cyclohexane, toluene, and diethylamine (15 : 3 : 2).
Procedure—Proceed as directed in the chapter, except to place the plate in a developing chamber that contains and has been equilibrated with *Developing solvent system*.
Dissolution, *Procedure for a Pooled Sample* ⟨711⟩—
Medium: 0.01 N hydrochloric acid; 900 mL.
Apparatus 1: 100 rpm.
Time: 45 minutes.
Determine the amount of $C_{25}H_{27}ClN_2 \cdot 2HCl$ dissolved by employing the following method.
Mobile phase—Prepare a suitable degassed and filtered mixture of water and methanol (55 : 45) that contains 0.69 g of monobasic sodium phosphate in each 100 mL and is adjusted with phosphoric acid, if necessary, to a pH of 4.0.
Chromatographic system (see *Chromatography* ⟨621⟩)—The liquid chromatograph is equipped with a 230-nm detector, a 4.6-mm × 25-cm precolumn positioned between the pump and the injection valve that contains packing L27, and a 4.6-mm × 25-cm analytical column that contains packing L9. The flow rate is about 2 mL per minute. Chromatograph replicate injections of the Standard solution, and record the peak responses as directed for *Procedure:* the relative standard deviation is not more than 2.0%.
Procedure—Inject about 100 µL of a filtered portion of the solution under test, suitably diluted with *Mobile phase*, if necessary, into the chromatograph, record the chromatogram, and measure the response for the major peak. Determine the amount of $C_{25}H_{27}ClN_2 \cdot 2HCl$ dissolved from the peak response obtained in comparison with the peak response obtained from a Standard solution having a known concentration of USP Meclizine Hydrochloride RS in a mixture of *Medium* and *Mobile phase* (1 : 1), similarly chromatographed. An amount of alcohol not to exceed 1% of the total volume of the Standard solution may be used to dissolve USP Meclizine Hydrochloride RS prior to dilution.
Tolerances—Not less than 75% (*Q*) of the labeled amount of $C_{25}H_{27}ClN_2 \cdot 2HCl$ is dissolved in 45 minutes.
Uniformity of dosage units ⟨905⟩: meet the requirements.
Procedure for content uniformity—Place 1 Tablet in a 100-mL volumetric flask, add 50 mL of dilute hydrochloric acid (1 in 100), shake by mechanical means for 30 minutes, add the dilute acid to volume, and filter, discarding the first 20 mL of the filtrate. Dilute quantitatively and stepwise with the same acid to obtain a solution having a concentration of about 15 µg of meclizine hydrochloride per mL. Similarly, prepare a Standard solution of USP Meclizine Hydrochloride RS in dilute hydrochloric acid (1 in 100) having a known concentration of about 15 µg per mL. Concomitantly determine the absorbances of the solution from the Tablet and the Standard solution in 1-cm cells at the wavelength of maximum absorbance at about 232 nm, with a suitable spectrophotometer, using dilute hydrochloric acid (1 in 100) as the blank. Calculate the quantity, in mg, of meclizine hydrochloride ($C_{25}H_{27}ClN_2 \cdot 2HCl$) in the Tablet taken by the formula:

$$(T/D)C(A_U/A_S)$$

in which *T* is the quantity, in mg, of meclizine hydrochloride in the Tablet; *D* is the concentration, in µg per mL, of meclizine hydrochloride in the solution from the Tablet, on the basis of the labeled quantity per Tablet and the extent of dilution; *C* is the concentration, in µg per mL, of USP Meclizine Hydrochloride RS in the

Standard solution; and A_U and A_S are the absorbances of the solution from the Tablet and the Standard solution, respectively.

Assay—

Mobile phase—Prepare a filtered and degassed mixture of methanol and water (65 : 35) that contains 0.69 g of monobasic sodium phosphate in each 100 mL, and adjust with phosphoric acid, if necessary, to a pH of 4.0. Make adjustments if necessary (see *System Suitability* under *Chromatography* ⟨621⟩).

Solvent mixture—Prepare a mixture of 0.1 N hydrochloric acid and *Mobile phase* (1 : 1).

Standard preparation—Dissolve an accurately weighed quantity of USP Meclizine Hydrochloride RS in *Solvent mixture* to obtain a solution having a known concentration of about 0.25 mg per mL.

Assay preparation—Weigh and finely powder not fewer than 20 Tablets. Transfer an accurately weighed portion of the powder, equivalent to about 25 mg of meclizine hydrochloride, to a 100-mL volumetric flask. Add about 60 mL of *Solvent mixture*, sonicate for about 10 minutes, and shake by mechanical means for about 30 minutes. Dilute with *Solvent mixture* to volume, mix, and filter a portion of this solution, discarding the first 5 mL of the filtrate.

Chromatographic system (see *Chromatography* ⟨621⟩)—The liquid chromatograph is equipped with a 230-nm detector, a 4.6-mm × 25-cm precolumn (positioned between the pump and the injection valve) that contains packing L27, and a 4.6-mm × 25-cm analytical column that contains packing L9. The flow rate is about 1.6 mL per minute. Chromatograph the *Standard preparation*, and record the peak responses as directed for *Procedure*: the tailing factor for the analyte peak is not more than 2.0; and the relative standard deviation for replicate injections is not more than 2.0%.

Procedure—Separately inject equal volumes (about 25 μL) of the *Standard preparation* and the *Test preparation* into the chromatograph, record the chromatograms, and measure the responses for the major peaks. Calculate the quantity, in mg, of meclizine hydrochloride ($C_{25}H_{27}ClN_2 \cdot 2HCl$) in the portion of Tablets taken by the formula:

$$100C(r_U / r_S)$$

in which C is the concentration, in mg per mL, of USP Meclizine Hydrochloride RS in the *Standard preparation*; and r_U and r_S are the peak responses obtained from the *Assay preparation* and the *Standard preparation*, respectively.

Meclocycline Sulfosalicylate

$C_{22}H_{21}ClN_2O_8 \cdot C_7H_6O_6S$ 695.05

2-Naphthacenecarboxamide, 7-chloro-4-(dimethylamino)-1,4,4a,5,5a,6,11,12a-octahydro-3,5,10,12,12a-pentahydroxy-6-methylene-1,11-dioxo-, [4S-(4α,4aα,5α,5aα,12aα)]-, mono(2-hydroxy-5-sulfobenzoate) (salt).

(4S,4aR,5S,5aR,12aS)-7-Chloro-4-(dimethylamino)-1,4,4a,5,5a,6,11,12a-octahydro-3,5,10,12,12a-pentahydroxy-6-methylene-1,11-dioxo-2-naphthacene carboxamide mono(5-sulfosalicylate) (salt)   [73816-42-9].

» Meclocycline Sulfosalicylate has a potency equivalent to not less than 620 μg of meclocycline ($C_{22}H_{21}ClN_2O_8$) per mg.

Packaging and storage—Preserve in tight containers, protected from light.

USP Reference standards ⟨11⟩—*USP Meclocycline Sulfosalicylate RS.*

Identification, *Infrared Absorption* ⟨197K⟩.

Crystallinity ⟨695⟩:   meets the requirements.

pH ⟨791⟩:   between 2.5 and 3.5, in a solution containing 10 mg per mL.

Water, *Method I* ⟨921⟩:   not more than 4.0%.

Assay—

0.001 M Ammonium edetate—Transfer 293 mg of edetic acid, accurately weighed, to a 1000-mL volumetric flask, add 1 mL of methanol and 7 mL of ammonium hydroxide, and shake to dissolve the edetic acid. Add 900 mL of water, adjust with glacial acetic acid to a pH of 6.6, dilute with water to volume, and mix.

Mobile phase—Prepare a solution of *0.001 M Ammonium edetate* and tetrahydrofuran (85 : 15). Filter and degas the solution before use.

Standard preparation—Transfer 36 mg of USP Meclocycline Sulfosalicylate RS, accurately weighed, to a 50-mL volumetric flask, dilute with methanol to volume, and mix. Transfer 3.0 mL of this solution to a 25-mL volumetric flask, dilute with *Mobile phase* to volume, and mix to obtain a solution having a known concentration of about 60 μg of meclocycline per mL.

Assay preparation—Using 36 mg of Meclocycline Sulfosalicylate, accurately weighed, prepare as directed for *Standard preparation*.

Procedure—Introduce equal volumes (about 10 μL) of the *Assay preparation* and the *Standard preparation* into a high-pressure liquid chromatograph (see *Chromatography* ⟨621⟩), operated at room temperature, by means of a suitable microsyringe or sampling valve, adjusting the specimen size and other operating parameters such that the peak obtained from the *Standard preparation* is about 0.6 full-scale. Typically, the apparatus is fitted with a 25-cm × 4-mm column packed with packing L1 and is equipped with an UV detector capable of monitoring absorption at 340 nm, and a suitable recorder. In a suitable chromatogram the coefficient of variation for replicate injections of the *Standard preparation* is not more than 3.0%. Measure the peak responses at equivalent retention times, obtained from the *Assay preparation* and the *Standard preparation*, and calculate the quantity, in mg, of $C_{22}H_{21}ClN_2O_8$ in the portion of Meclocycline Sulfosalicylate taken by the formula:

$$(1.25 / 3)(C)(r_U / r_S)$$

in which C is the equivalent, in μg per mL, of meclocycline from the USP Meclocycline Sulfosalicylate RS in the *Standard preparation*; and r_U and r_S are the peak responses obtained from the *Assay preparation* and the *Standard preparation*, respectively.

Meclocycline Sulfosalicylate Cream

» Meclocycline Sulfosalicylate Cream contains the equivalent of not less than 90.0 percent and not more than 125.0 percent of the labeled amount of meclocycline ($C_{22}H_{21}ClN_2O_8$).

Packaging and storage—Preserve in tight containers, protected from light.

USP Reference standards ⟨11⟩—*USP Meclocycline Sulfosalicylate RS.*

Minimum fill ⟨755⟩:   meets the requirements.

Assay—

Mobile phase—Prepare as directed in the *Assay* under *Meclocycline Sulfosalicylate*.

Standard preparation—Transfer 36 mg of USP Meclocycline Sulfosalicylate RS, accurately weighed, to a 50-mL volumetric flask, dilute with methanol to volume, and mix. Transfer 2.0 mL of this solution to a 100-mL volumetric flask, dilute with *Mobile phase* to volume, and mix to obtain a solution having a known concentration of about 10 μg of meclocycline per mL.

Assay preparation—Transfer an accurately weighed quantity of Cream, equivalent to about 5 mg of meclocycline, to a glass-stoppered, 50-mL centrifuge tube, add 20 mL of methanol and 20 mL of 0.025 N sulfuric acid, and shake vigorously for 15 minutes. Transfer the solution to a 50-mL volumetric flask, rinsing the centrifuge tube with two 5-mL portions of methanol and adding the rinsings to the flask, dilute with methanol to volume, and mix. Centrifuge a portion of this solution for 5 minutes, transfer 5 mL of the supernatant to a 50-mL volumetric flask, dilute with *Mobile phase* to volume, mix, and filter.

Procedure—Proceed as directed in the *Assay* under *Meclocycline Sulfosalicylate*. Calculate the quantity, in mg, of meclocycline ($C_{22}H_{21}ClN_2O_8$) in the portion of Cream taken by the formula:

$$0.5C(r_U / r_S)$$

in which C is the concentration, in µg per mL, of meclocycline in the *Standard preparation*; and r_U and r_S are the peak responses obtained from the *Assay preparation* and the *Standard preparation*, respectively.

Meclofenamate Sodium

$C_{14}H_{10}Cl_2NNaO_2 \cdot H_2O$ 336.15
Benzoic acid, 2-[(2,6-dichloro-3-methylphenyl)amino]-, monosodium salt, monohydrate.
Monosodium *N*-(2,6-dichloro-*m*-tolyl)anthranilate monohydrate [6385-02-0].
Anhydrous 318.13

» Meclofenamate Sodium contains not less than 97.0 percent and not more than 103.0 percent of $C_{14}H_{10}Cl_2NNaO_2$, calculated on the anhydrous basis.

Packaging and storage—Preserve in tight, light-resistant containers.
USP Reference standards ⟨11⟩—*USP Meclofenamate Sodium RS*.
Identification—
  A: *Infrared Absorption* ⟨197K⟩.
  B: *Ultraviolet Absorption 1* ⟨197U⟩—
  Solution: 25 µg per mL.
  Medium: 0.01 N hydrochloric acid in methanol.
  Absorptivities at 242 nm, 279 nm, and 336 nm, calculated on the anhydrous basis, do not differ by more than 3.0%.
  C: *Ultraviolet Absorption 2* ⟨197U⟩—
  Solution: 1 in 40,000.
  Medium: 0.1 N sodium hydroxide.
  Absorptivities at 279 nm and 317 nm, calculated on the anhydrous basis, do not differ by more than 3.0%.
Water, Method I ⟨921⟩: between 4.8% and 5.8%.
Copper—
  Standard copper solution—Dissolve 1000 mg of copper wire in 6 mL of nitric acid in a 1 L volumetric flask. Add 8 mL of hydrochloric acid, dilute with water to volume, and mix. Dilute this solution quantitatively and stepwise with water to obtain a *Standard copper solution* having a known concentration of 0.6 µg per mL.
  Test solution—Transfer 2 g of Meclofenamate Sodium, accurately weighed, to a 100-mL volumetric flask, and add 1 drop of ammonium hydroxide. Dissolve in water, dilute with water to volume, and mix.
  Procedure—Concomitantly determine the absorbances of the *Standard copper solution* and the *Test solution* at the copper emission line at about 325 nm, with a suitable atomic absorption spectrophotometer (see *Spectrophotometry and Light-scattering* ⟨851⟩) equipped with a copper hollow-cathode lamp, using water as the blank. Adjust the operating conditions to obtain about 70% full-scale detector response with the *Standard copper solution*. The detector response obtained with the *Test solution* is not greater than that obtained with the *Standard copper solution* (0.003%).
Chromatographic purity—
  Standard solutions—Dissolve an accurately weighed quantity of USP Meclofenamate Sodium RS in methanol to obtain a solution containing 20 mg per mL (*Standard solution A*). Dilute 1.0 mL of *Standard solution A* with sufficient methanol to obtain 200 mL of solution (*Standard solution B*).
  Test solution—Dissolve 200 mg of Meclofenamate Sodium in 10.0 mL of methanol.
  Procedure—Apply 10-µL portions of *Standard solution A*, *Standard solution B*, and the *Test solution* to a suitable thin-layer chromatographic plate (see *Chromatography* ⟨621⟩) coated with a 0.25-mm layer of chromatographic silica gel mixture. Allow the spots to dry, and develop the chromatogram in a solvent system consisting of a mixture of methylene chloride, methyl ethyl ketone, and glacial acetic acid (50 : 48 : 2) until the solvent front has moved about eight-tenths of the length of the plate. Remove the plate from the developing chamber, mark the solvent front, and allow the solvent to evaporate. Examine the plate under short-wavelength UV light: the chromatograms show a principal spot at about the same R_F value, and any secondary spot, if present in the chromatogram from the *Test solution* is not more intense than the principal spot obtained from *Standard solution B* (0.5%).
Organic volatile impurities, *Method I* ⟨467⟩: meets the requirements.
  (Official until July 1, 2008)
Assay—Transfer about 350 mg of Meclofenamate Sodium, accurately weighed, to a 125-mL separator, add 10 mL of water, and mix to dissolve. To this solution add 3 mL of 3 N hydrochloric acid, shake, and extract with three 30-mL portions of chloroform, collecting the chloroform extracts in an evaporating flask. Evaporate the chloroform extracts to dryness. Dissolve the residue in 5 mL of dimethyl sulfoxide and 25 mL of methanol. Mix, add 5 drops of phenolphthalein TS, and titrate the mixture with 0.1 N sodium hydroxide VS. Each mL of 0.1 N sodium hydroxide is equivalent to 31.81 mg of $C_{14}H_{10}Cl_2NNaO_2$.

Meclofenamate Sodium Capsules

» Meclofenamate Sodium Capsules contain an amount of $C_{14}H_{10}Cl_2NNaO_2$ equivalent to not less than 90.0 percent and not more than 110.0 percent of the labeled amount of meclofenamic acid ($C_{14}H_{11}Cl_2NO_2$).

Packaging and storage—Preserve in tight, light-resistant containers.
USP Reference standards ⟨11⟩—*USP Meclofenamate Sodium RS*.
Identification—Prepare a solution of Capsule contents in methanol containing 20 mg per mL, and filter. The clear filtrate so obtained meets the requirements of the *Thin-Layer Chromatographic Identification Test* ⟨201⟩, the solvent mixture consisting of methylene chloride, methyl ethyl ketone, and glacial acetic acid (50 : 48 : 2).
Dissolution ⟨711⟩—
  Medium: 0.05 M pH 7.5 phosphate buffer (see under *Buffer Solutions* in the section *Reagents, Indicators, and Solutions*); 900 mL.
  Apparatus 2: 50 rpm.
  Time: 45 minutes.
  Procedure—Determine the amount of meclofenamic acid ($C_{14}H_{11}Cl_2NO_2$) dissolved from UV absorbances at the wavelength of maximum absorbance at about 279 nm of filtered portions of the solution under test, suitably diluted with *Medium*, if necessary, in comparison with a Standard solution having a known concentration of USP Meclofenamate Sodium RS in the same *Medium*.
  Tolerances—Not less than 75% (*Q*) of the labeled amount of $C_{14}H_{11}Cl_2NO_2$ is dissolved in 45 minutes.
Uniformity of dosage units ⟨905⟩: meet the requirements.
Assay—Remove, as completely as possible, the contents of not fewer than 20 Capsules, and weigh accurately. Mix the combined contents, and transfer an accurately weighed quantity of the powder, equivalent to about 50 mg of meclofenamic acid, to a 200-mL volumetric flask. Add 0.01 N hydrochloric acid in methanol to volume, and mix. Filter, discarding the first 20 mL of the filtrate. Transfer 10.0 mL of the filtrate to a 100-mL volumetric flask, add 0.01 N hydrochloric acid in methanol to volume, and mix. Dissolve an accurately weighed quantity of USP Meclofenamate Sodium RS

in 0.01 N hydrochloric acid in methanol to obtain a solution having a known concentration of about 27 µg per mL. Concomitantly determine the absorbances of both solutions in 1-cm cells at the wavelength of maximum absorbance at about 336 nm, with a suitable spectrophotometer, using 0.01 N hydrochloric acid in methanol as the blank. Calculate the quantity, in mg, of meclfenamic acid ($C_{14}H_{11}Cl_2NO_2$) in the portion of Capsule contents taken by the formula:

$$2C(296.15/318.13)(A_U/A_S)$$

in which C is the concentration, in µg per mL, of USP Meclofenamate Sodium RS in the Standard solution; 296.15 and 318.13 are the molecular weights of meclofenamic acid and meclofenamate sodium, respectively; and A_U and A_S are the absorbances of the solution from the Capsule contents and the Standard solution, respectively.

Medroxyprogesterone Acetate

$C_{24}H_{34}O_4$ 386.53

Pregn-4-ene-3,20-dione, 17-(acetyloxy)-6-methyl-, (6α)-.
17-Hydroxy-6α-methylpregn-4-ene-3,20-dione acetate   [71-58-9].

» Medroxyprogesterone Acetate contains not less than 97.0 percent and not more than 103.0 percent of $C_{24}H_{34}O_4$, calculated on the dried basis.

Packaging and storage—Preserve in tight, light-resistant containers. Store at 25°, excursions permitted between 15° and 30°.

USP Reference standards ⟨11⟩—USP Medroxyprogesterone Acetate RS. USP Medroxyprogesterone Acetate Related Compound A RS.

Identification—
  A: Infrared Absorption ⟨197K⟩.
  B: Ultraviolet Absorption ⟨197U⟩—
    Solution: 10 µg per mL.
    Medium: alcohol.
  Absorptivities at 241 nm, calculated on the dried basis, do not differ by more than 2.0%.

Specific rotation ⟨781S⟩: between +45° and +51°.
  Test solution: 10 mg per mL, in dioxane.

Loss on drying ⟨731⟩—Dry it at 105° for 3 hours: it loses not more than 1.0% of its weight.

Limit of medroxyprogesterone acetate related compound A—
  Adsorbent: a suitable thin-layer chromatographic plate (see Chromatography ⟨621⟩) coated with a 0.25-mm layer of chromatographic silica gel mixture.
  Test solution—Dissolve an accurately weighed amount of Medroxyprogesterone Acetate in methylene chloride to obtain a solution having a concentration of about 20 mg per mL.
  Standard solution—Prepare a solution of USP Medroxyprogesterone Acetate RS and USP Medroxyprogesterone Acetate Related Compound A RS in methylene chloride containing 20 mg per mL and 0.1 mg per mL, respectively.
  Application volume: 10 µL.
  Developing solvent system: a mixture of hexanes, tert-butyl methyl ether, and tetrahydrofuran (45 : 45 : 10).
  Spray reagent—Prepare a solution of 20 g of p-toluenesulfonic acid in 100 mL of alcohol.
  Procedure—Proceed as directed for Thin-Layer Chromatography under Chromatography ⟨621⟩. Develop the chromatogram until the solvent front has moved about 10 cm. Allow the plate to air-dry, and develop the chromatogram again until the solvent front has moved about 10 cm. Allow the plate to dry at 120° for 10 minutes. Spray the plate with Spray reagent. Heat the plate for 10 minutes at 120°, and examine the plate under UV light at 365 nm. Any blue fluorescent spot with an R_F value higher than that of the principal spot due to medroxyprogesterone acetate in the chromatogram obtained from the Test solution is not more intense than the corresponding blue fluorescent spot in the chromatogram obtained from the Standard solution: not more than 0.5% is found.

Chromatographic purity—
  Mobile phase—Prepare a filtered and degassed mixture of acetonitrile and water (3 : 2). Make adjustments if necessary (see System Suitability under Chromatography ⟨621⟩).
  Standard solution—Dissolve an accurately weighed quantity of USP Medroxyprogesterone Acetate RS in Mobile phase, and dilute quantitatively, and stepwise if necessary, with Mobile phase to obtain a solution having a known concentration of about 50 µg per mL.
  System suitability solution—Dissolve suitable quantities of megestrol acetate and USP Medroxyprogesterone Acetate RS in Mobile phase to obtain a solution containing about 40 µg of each per mL.
  Test solution—Transfer about 62.5 mg of Medroxyprogesterone Acetate, accurately weighed, to a 25-mL volumetric flask, dissolve in and dilute with Mobile phase to volume, and mix.
  Chromatographic system (see Chromatography ⟨621⟩)—The liquid chromatograph is equipped with a 254-nm detector and a 4.6-mm × 25-cm column that contains packing L1. The flow rate is about 1 mL per minute. Chromatograph the System suitability solution, and record the peak responses as directed for Procedure: the resolution, R, between megestrol acetate and medroxyprogesterone acetate is not less than 1.5. Chromatograph the Standard solution, and record the peak responses as directed for Procedure: the relative standard deviation for replicate injections is not more than 3.0%.
  Procedure—Inject a volume (about 20 µL) of the Test solution into the chromatograph, record the chromatogram, and measure the peak responses. Calculate the percentage of each impurity in the portion of Medroxyprogesterone Acetate taken by the formula:

$$2500(C/W)(r_i/r_S)$$

in which C is the concentration, in mg per mL, of USP Medroxyprogesterone Acetate RS in the Standard solution; W is the weight, in mg, of Medroxyprogesterone Acetate taken to prepare the Test solution; r_i is the peak response for each impurity obtained from the Test solution; and r_S is the response from the major peak obtained from the Standard solution: not more than 1.0% of any individual impurity is found; and not more than 1.5% of total impurities is found.

Assay—
  Mobile phase—Prepare a filtered and degassed mixture of water and acetonitrile (60 : 40). Make adjustments if necessary (see System Suitability under Chromatography ⟨621⟩).
  Standard preparation—Dissolve an accurately weighed quantity of USP Medroxyprogesterone Acetate RS in acetonitrile to obtain a solution having a known concentration of about 1 mg per mL.
  Assay preparation—Dissolve about 25 mg of Medroxyprogesterone Acetate, accurately weighed, in 25.0 mL of acetonitrile, and mix.
  Chromatographic system (see Chromatography ⟨621⟩)—The liquid chromatograph is equipped with a 254-nm detector and a 4-mm × 30-cm column that contains packing L1. The flow rate is about 2 mL per minute. Chromatograph the Standard preparation, and record the peak responses as directed for Procedure: the tailing factor is not more than 2; and the relative standard deviation of the peak responses for replicate injections is not more than 2.0%.
  Procedure—Separately inject equal volumes (about 10 µL) of the Standard preparation and the Assay preparation into the chromatograph, record the chromatograms, and measure the responses for the major peaks. Calculate the quantity, in mg, of $C_{24}H_{34}O_4$ in the portion of Medroxyprogesterone Acetate taken by the formula:

$$25C(r_U/r_S)$$

in which C is the concentration, in mg per mL, of USP Medroxyprogesterone Acetate RS in the Standard preparation; and r_U and r_S

are the peak responses obtained from the *Assay preparation* and the *Standard preparation*, respectively.

Medroxyprogesterone Acetate Injectable Suspension

» Medroxyprogesterone Acetate Injectable Suspension is a sterile suspension of Medroxyprogesterone Acetate in a suitable aqueous medium. It contains not less than 90.0 percent and not more than 110.0 percent of the labeled amount of medroxyprogesterone acetate ($C_{24}H_{34}O_4$).

Packaging and storage—Preserve in single-dose or multiple-dose containers, preferably of Type I glass.

USP Reference standards ⟨11⟩—*USP Medroxyprogesterone Acetate RS*.

Identification—Transfer a volume of Injectable Suspension, equivalent to about 50 mg of medroxyprogesterone acetate, to a centrifuge tube, centrifuge, decant the supernatant, and wash the solids with two 15-mL portions of water, discarding the water washings. Dissolve the solids in 10 mL of chloroform, transfer to a small beaker, evaporate the chloroform on a steam bath, and dry at 105° for 3 hours: the residue so obtained responds to *Identification* test A under *Medroxyprogesterone Acetate*.

pH ⟨791⟩: between 3.0 and 7.0.

Other requirements—It meets the requirements under *Injections* ⟨1⟩.

Assay—

Mobile phase—Mix 700 mL of butyl chloride, 300 mL of hexane, both previously saturated with water, and 80 mL of acetonitrile. The acetonitrile concentration may be varied to meet system suitability requirements and to provide elution times of about 12 and 15 minutes for progesterone and medroxyprogesterone acetate, respectively. Pass the solution through a membrane filter (1 µm or finer porosity).

Internal standard solution—Prepare a solution of progesterone in *Mobile phase* containing 0.25 mg per mL.

Standard preparation—Dissolve about 8 mg of USP Medroxyprogesterone Acetate RS, accurately weighed, in 20.0 mL of *Internal standard solution*.

Assay preparation—Transfer to a suitable container an accurately measured volume of Injectable Suspension, equivalent to about 50 mg of medroxyprogesterone acetate. Pipet 25 mL of chloroform into the container, shake for about 20 minutes, and centrifuge. Pipet 4 mL of the chloroform layer into a suitable container, and evaporate to dryness. Pipet 20 mL of *Internal standard solution* into the container to dissolve the residue.

Chromatographic system—The liquid chromatograph is equipped with a 254-nm detector and a 2-mm × 25-cm column that contains 5-µm packing L3. The flow rate is about 2 mL per minute. Chromatograph the *Standard preparation*, and record the peak responses as directed for *Procedure:* the resolution of progesterone and medroxyprogesterone is not less than 5.0, and the relative standard deviation of the peak responses for replicate injections is not more than 2.0%.

Procedure—Proceed as directed in the *Assay* under *Medroxyprogesterone Acetate*. Calculate the quantity, in mg, of medroxyprogeterone acetate ($C_{24}H_{34}O_4$) in each mL of the Injectable Suspension taken by the formula:

$$125(C/V)(R_U/R_S)$$

in which C is the concentration, in mg, of USP Medroxyprogesterone Acetate RS in the *Standard preparation*; V is the volume, in mL, of Injectable Suspension taken; and R_U and R_S are the ratios of peak areas of medroxyprogesterone acetate peak to internal standard peak obtained from the *Assay preparation* and the *Standard preparation*, respectively.

Medroxyprogesterone Acetate Tablets

» Medroxyprogesterone Acetate Tablets contain not less than 93.0 percent and not more than 107.0 percent of the labeled amount of medroxyprogesterone acetate ($C_{24}H_{34}O_4$).

Packaging and storage—Preserve in well-closed containers.

USP Reference standards ⟨11⟩—*USP Medroxyprogesterone Acetate RS*.

Identification—Triturate a number of Tablets, equivalent to about 25 mg of medroxyprogesterone acetate, with 15 mL of chloroform, filter, evaporate the chloroform on a steam bath, and dry the residue at 105° for 3 hours: the residue so obtained responds to *Identification* test A under *Medroxyprogesterone Acetate*.

Dissolution ⟨711⟩—

Medium: 0.5% sodium lauryl sulfate; 900 mL.
Apparatus 2: 50 rpm.
Time: 45 minutes.

Determine the amount of $C_{24}H_{34}O_4$ dissolved by employing the following method.

Sodium lauryl sulfate stock solution—Transfer 180.0 g of sodium lauryl sulfate to a 2000-mL volumetric flask. Add 1500 mL of water, and stir until dissolved. [NOTE—Several hours of stirring are required.] Dilute with water to volume.

Standard stock solution—Dissolve about 70 mg of USP Medroxyprogesterone Acetate RS, accurately weighed, in 140 mL of *Sodium lauryl sulfate stock solution*, and dilute with water to 250 mL. [NOTE—It may be necessary to sonicate the solution to bring the Reference Standard into solution prior to dilution with water. Prepare this *Standard stock solution* fresh daily.]

Standard solution—Pipet a 20-mL aliquot of *Standard stock solution* into a 1 L volumetric flask. Add 40 mL of *Sodium lauryl sulfate stock solution*, and dilute with water to volume. This solution is stable for up to 7 days.

Test solution—Withdraw 15 mL of the solution under test, and filter, discarding the first 5 mL of the filtrate.

Mobile phase—Prepare a filtered and degassed solution of acetonitrile and water (60 : 40). Make adjustments if necessary (see *System Suitability* under *Chromatography* ⟨621⟩).

Chromatographic system (see *Chromatography* ⟨621⟩)—The liquid chromatograph is equipped with a 254-nm detector and a 4-mm × 8-cm column that contains packing L7. The flow rate is about 1.5 mL per minute. Chromatograph the *Standard solution*, and record the peak responses as directed for *Procedure:* the tailing factor for the analyte peak is not more than 1.2; and the relative standard deviation for replicate injections is not more than 2.0%.

Procedure—Separately inject equal volumes (about 20 µL) of the *Standard solution* and the *Test solution* into the chromatograph, record the chromatograms, and measure the responses for the major peaks. Calculate the percentage of $C_{24}H_{34}O_4$ dissolved from the peak responses so obtained.

Tolerances—Not less than 50% (Q) of the labeled amount of $C_{24}H_{34}O_4$ is dissolved in 45 minutes.

Uniformity of dosage units ⟨905⟩: meet the requirements.

Procedure for content uniformity—Dissolve an accurately weighed portion of USP Medroxyprogesterone Acetate RS in a mixture of alcohol and water (3 : 1) to obtain a solution having a known concentration of about 15 µg per mL. Transfer 1 Tablet to a volumetric flask, add a mixture of alcohol and water (3 : 1) to volume, and shake for about 15 minutes. Filter, and quantitatively dilute a portion of the filtrate as required to obtain a final solution containing about 15 µg per mL. Concomitantly determine the absorbances of this solution and the Standard solution in 1-cm cells at the wavelength of maximum absorbance at about 242 nm. Calculate the quantity, in mg, of $C_{24}H_{34}O_4$ in the Tablet taken by the formula:

$$(T/D)C(A_U/A_S)$$

in which T is the labeled quantity, in mg, of medroxyprogesterone acetate in the Tablet; D is the concentration, in µg per mL, of medroxyprogesterone acetate in the solution from the Tablet; C is the concentration, in µg per mL; of USP Medroxyprogesterone Acetate

RS in the Standard solution, and A_U and A_S are the absorbances of the solution from the Tablet and the Standard solution, respectively.

Assay—

Mobile phase, Standard preparation, and *Chromatographic system—*Prepare as directed in the *Assay* under *Medroxyprogesterone Acetate.*

*Assay preparation—*Weigh and finely powder not fewer than 20 Tablets. Weigh accurately a portion of the powder, equivalent to about 25 mg of medroxyprogesterone acetate, into a 50-mL glass centrifuge tube. Pipet 25 mL of acetonitrile into the tube, shake to wet the powder thoroughly, and sonicate for not less than 10 minutes, and centrifuge. Use the clear supernatant as the *Assay preparation.*

*Procedure—*Proceed as directed for *Procedure* in the *Assay* under *Medroxyprogesterone Acetate.* Calculate the quantity, in mg, of medroxyprogesterone acetate ($C_{24}H_{34}O_4$) in the portion of Tablets taken by the formula:

$$25C(r_U/r_S)$$

in which C is the concentration, in mg per mL, of USP Medroxyprogesterone Acetate RS in the *Standard preparation*; and r_U and r_S are the peak responses obtained from the *Assay preparation* and the *Standard preparation,* respectively.

Mefenamic Acid

$C_{15}H_{15}NO_2$ 241.29
Benzoic acid, 2-(2,3-dimethylphenyl)amino-.
N-2,3-Xylylanthranilic acid   [61-68-7].

» Mefenamic Acid contains not less than 98.0 percent and not more than 102.0 percent of $C_{15}H_{15}NO_2$, calculated on the dried basis.

Packaging and storage—Preserve in tight, light-resistant containers.

USP Reference standards ⟨11⟩—*USP Mefenamic Acid RS.*
Identification—
  A: *Infrared Absorption* ⟨197K⟩.
  B: The retention time of the major peak in the chromatogram of the *Assay preparation* corresponds to that in the chromatogram of the *Standard preparation,* as obtained in the *Assay.*
Loss on drying ⟨731⟩—Dry it at 105° for 4 hours: it loses not more than 1.0% of its weight.
Residue on ignition ⟨281⟩: not more than 0.1%.
Heavy metals ⟨231⟩: 0.002%.
Chromatographic purity—
Buffer solution, Mobile phase, and *Chromatographic system—*Proceed as directed in the *Assay.*
*Standard solution—*Dissolve an accurately weighed quantity of USP Mefenamic Acid RS in *Mobile phase* to obtain a solution having a known concentration of about 10 μg per mL.
*Test solution—*Transfer about 100 mg of Mefenamic Acid, accurately weighed, to a 100-mL volumetric flask, dissolve in and dilute with *Mobile phase* to volume, and mix.
*Procedure—*Separately inject equal volumes (about 10 μL) of the *Standard solution* and the *Test solution* into the chromatograph, record the chromatograms, and measure the responses for the major peaks. Calculate the percentage of each impurity in the portion of Mefenamic Acid taken by the formula:

$$100(C_S/C_U)(r_i/r_S)$$

in which C_S is the concentration, in μg per mL, of USP Mefenamic Acid RS in the *Standard solution*; C_U is the concentration, in μg per mL, of Mefenamic Acid in the *Test solution*; r_i is the peak response for each impurity obtained from the *Test solution*; and r_S is the peak response for mefenamic acid obtained from the *Standard solution*: not more than 0.1% of any individual impurity is found; and not more than 0.5% of total impurities is found.

Assay—

*Buffer solution—*Prepare a 50 mM solution of monobasic ammonium phosphate, and adjust with 3 M ammonium hydroxide to a pH of 5.0.

*Mobile phase—*Prepare a filtered and degassed mixture of acetonitrile, *Buffer solution,* and tetrahydrofuran (23 : 20 : 7). Make adjustments if necessary (see *System Suitability* under *Chromatography* ⟨621⟩).

*Standard preparation—*Dissolve an accurately weighed quantity of USP Mefenamic Acid RS in *Mobile phase,* and dilute quantitatively, and stepwise if necessary, with *Mobile phase* to obtain a solution having a known concentration of about 0.2 mg per mL.

*Assay preparation—*Transfer about 100 mg of Mefenamic Acid, accurately weighed, to a 500-mL volumetric flask, dissolve in and dilute with *Mobile phase* to volume, and mix.

Chromatographic system (see *Chromatography* ⟨621⟩)—The liquid chromatograph is equipped with a 254-nm detector and a 4.6-mm × 25-cm column that contains packing L1. The flow rate is about 1 mL per minute. Chromatograph the *Standard preparation,* and record the peak responses as directed for *Procedure*: the column efficiency is not less than 8200 theoretical plates; the tailing factor for the analyte peak is not more than 1.6; and the relative standard deviation for replicate injections is not more than 1.0%.

*Procedure—*Separately inject equal volumes (about 10 μL) of the *Standard preparation* and the *Assay preparation* into the chromatograph, record the chromatograms, and measure the responses for the major peaks. Calculate the quantity, in mg, of $C_{15}H_{15}NO_2$ in the portion of Mefenamic Acid taken by the formula:

$$500C(r_U/r_S)$$

in which C is the concentration, in mg per mL, of USP Mefenamic Acid RS in the *Standard preparation*; and r_U and r_S are the mefenamic acid peak responses obtained from the *Assay preparation* and the *Standard preparation,* respectively.

Mefenamic Acid Capsules

» Mefenamic Acid Capsules contain not less than 90.0 percent and not more than 110.0 percent of the labeled amount of mefenamic acid ($C_{15}H_{15}NO_2$).

Packaging and storage—Preserve in tight containers.

USP Reference standards ⟨11⟩—*USP Mefenamic Acid RS.*
Identification—
  A: Place a portion of Capsule contents, equivalent to about 250 mg of mefenamic acid, in a 250-mL volumetric flask, add about 100 mL of a mixture of chloroform and methanol (3 : 1), and shake vigorously. Dilute with a mixture of chloroform and methanol (3 : 1) to volume, mix, and filter: the filtrate so obtained responds to the *Thin-layer Chromatographic Identification Test* ⟨201⟩, a solvent system consisting of a mixture of chloroform, ethyl acetate, and glacial acetic acid (75 : 25 : 1) and the *Ordinary Impurities* ⟨466⟩ visualization technique 17 being used.
  B: The retention time of the major peak in the chromatogram of the *Assay preparation* corresponds to that of the *Standard preparation,* obtained as directed in the *Assay.*
Dissolution ⟨711⟩—

*0.05 M Tris buffer—*Dissolve 60.5 g of tris(hydroxymethyl)aminomethane in 6 L of water, and dilute with water to 10 L. Adjust with phosphoric acid to a pH of 9.0 ± 0.05. To a second container, transfer about 6 liters of this solution, add 100 g of sodium lauryl sulfate, and mix to dissolve the solid material. Transfer this solution back into the first container, and mix.

USP 31

Official Monographs / **Megestrol** 2603

Medium: 0.05 M Tris buffer; 900 mL.
Apparatus 1: 100 rpm.
Time: 45 minutes.
Procedure—Determine the amount of $C_{15}H_{15}NO_2$ dissolved, employing the procedure set forth in the *Assay*, making any necessary volumetric adjustments.
Tolerances—Not less than 75% (*Q*) of the labeled amount of $C_{15}H_{15}NO_2$ is dissolved in 45 minutes.
Uniformity of dosage units ⟨905⟩: meet the requirements.
Assay—
Mobile phase, Standard preparation, and *Chromatographic system*—Proceed as directed in the *Assay* under *Mefenamic Acid.*
Assay preparation—Remove, as completely as possible, the contents of not fewer than 20 Capsules. Weigh the contents, and determine the average weight per capsule. Mix the combined contents, and transfer an accurately weighed quantity of the powder, equivalent to about 100 mg of mefenamic acid, to a 500-mL volumetric flask. Add 10.0 mL of tetrahydrofuran, and sonicate for about 5 minutes with occasional mixing. Dilute with *Mobile phase* to volume, mix, and filter.
Procedure—Proceed as directed for *Procedure* in the *Assay* under *Mefenamic Acid.* Calculate the quantity, in mg, of $C_{15}H_{15}NO_2$ in the portion of Capsules taken by the formula:

$$500C(r_U / r_S)$$

in which the terms are as defined therein.

Mefloquine Hydrochloride

$C_{17}H_{16}F_6N_2O \cdot HCl$ 414.77
4-Quinolinemethanol, α-2-piperidinyl-2,8-bis(trifluoromethyl)-, monohydrochloride, (*R*,S**)-(±)-.
DL-*erythro*-α-2-Piperidyl-2,8-bis(trifluoromethyl)-4-quinolinemethanol monohydrochloride   [51773-92-3].

» Mefloquine Hydrochloride contains not less than 99.0 percent and not more than 101.0 percent of $C_{17}H_{16}F_6N_2O \cdot HCl$, calculated on the anhydrous basis.

Packaging and storage—Preserve in tight, light-resistant containers. Store between 15° and 30°.
USP Reference standards ⟨11⟩—*USP Mefloquine Hydrochloride RS. USP Mefloquine Related Compound A RS.*
Identification—
  A: *Infrared Absorption* ⟨197K⟩.
  B: It responds to the tests for *Chloride* ⟨191⟩.
Specific rotation ⟨781⟩: between −0.2° and +0.2°. Use a solution prepared by dissolving about 2.5 g in methanol, and dilute with methanol to 50.0 mL.
Water, *Method I* ⟨921⟩: not more than 3.0%.
Residue on ignition ⟨281⟩: not more than 0.1%.
Heavy metals, *Method II* ⟨231⟩: 0.002%.
Related compounds—
  Mobile phase—Dissolve 1 g of tetraheptylammonium bromide in a 1-L mixture of a 1.5 g per L solution of sodium hydrogen sulfate, acetonitrile, and methanol (2 : 2 : 1). Make adjustments if necessary (see *System Suitability* under *Chromatography* ⟨621⟩).
  System suitability solution—Transfer about 4 mg of USP Mefloquine Hydrochloride RS and 4 mg of USP Mefloquine Related Compound A RS to a 50-mL volumetric flask, dissolve in and dilute with *Mobile phase* to volume, and mix. [NOTE—Mefloquine related compound A is *threo*-mefloquine.] Transfer 5.0 mL of this solution to a 100-mL volumetric flask, dilute with *Mobile phase* to volume, and mix.

Test solution—Transfer about 0.10 g of Mefloquine Hydrochloride, accurately weighed, to a 25-mL volumetric flask, dissolve in and dilute with *Mobile phase* to volume, and mix.
Diluted test solution—Transfer 1.0 mL of the *Test solution* to a 50-mL volumetric flask, dilute with *Mobile phase* to volume, and mix. Transfer 1.0 mL of this solution to a 20-mL volumetric flask, dilute with *Mobile phase* to volume, and mix.
Chromatographic system (see *Chromatography* ⟨621⟩)—The liquid chromatograph is equipped with a 280-nm detector, a 4-mm × 2.5-cm precolumn, and a 4.0-mm × 25-cm column, both containing 5-μm packing L1. The flow rate is about 0.8 mL per minute. Chromatograph the *System suitability solution*, and record the peak responses as directed for *Procedure:* the relative retention times are about 0.7 for mefloquine related compound A and 1.0 for mefloquine; the resolution, *R*, between mefloquine related compound A and mefloquine is not less than 2.0; and the relative standard deviation for replicate injections is not more than 2.0%.
Procedure—Equilibrate the column with *Mobile phase* at a flow rate of about 0.8 mL per minute for about 30 minutes. Inject 20 μL of *Diluted test solution*. Adjust the sensitivity of the system so that the height of the major peak is at least 50% of the full scale of the recorder. Separately inject equal volumes (about 20 μL) of the *Test solution* and *Diluted test solution* into the chromatograph, record the chromatogram for a time that is 10 times the retention time of the main peak, and measure the responses of all the peaks, excluding the main peak and any other peak producing a response of less than 0.2 times (0.02%) of the main peak in the chromatogram of the *Diluted test solution*. The response of the mefloquine related compound A peak in the *Test solution* with a relative retention time of about 0.7, with reference to the main peak, is not more than twice the area of the main peak in the chromatogram of the *Diluted test solution* (0.2%). The response of any other individual peak, other than the main peak, in the chromatogram of the *Test solution,* is not greater than that of the main peak in the chromatogram of the *Diluted test solution* (0.1%); and the sum of the responses of any such peaks in the chromatogram of the *Test solution* is not greater than five times the response of the main peak in the chromatogram of the *Diluted test solution* (0.5%).
Assay—Dissolve about 0.35 g, accurately weighed, in 15 mL of anhydrous formic acid, and add 40 mL of acetic anhydride. Titrate with 0.1 N perchloric acid VS, and determine the endpoint potentiometrically. Perform a blank determination, and make any necessary correction. Each mL of 0.1 N perchloric acid is equivalent to 41.48 mg of $C_{17}H_{16}F_6N_2O \cdot HCl$.

Megestrol Acetate

$C_{24}H_{32}O_4$ 384.51
Pregna-4,6-diene-3,20-dione, 17-(acetyloxy)-6-methyl-.
17-Hydroxy-6-methylpregna-4,6-diene-3,20-dione acetate   [595-33-5].

» Megestrol Acetate contains not less than 97.0 percent and not more than 103.0 percent of $C_{24}H_{32}O_4$, calculated on the anhydrous basis.

Packaging and storage—Preserve in well-closed containers, protected from light.
USP Reference standards ⟨11⟩—*USP Megestrol Acetate RS.*
Completeness of solution ⟨641⟩: meets the requirements, 500 mg being dissolved in 10 mL of acetone.

Identification, Infrared Absorption ⟨197K⟩.
Melting range ⟨741⟩: between 213° and 220°, but the range between beginning and end of melting does not exceed 3°.
Specific rotation ⟨781S⟩: between +8.8° and +12.0° ($t = 20°$).
  Test solution: 20 mg per mL, in chloroform.
Water, Method I ⟨921⟩: not more than 0.5%.
Residue on ignition ⟨281⟩: not more than 0.2%, a platinum dish being used, with ignition at 600 ± 25°.
Heavy metals, Method II ⟨231⟩: not more than 0.002%.
Organic volatile impurities, Method IV ⟨467⟩: meets the requirements.

(Official until July 1, 2008)

Assay—
  *Mobile phase—*Prepare a solution of acetonitrile and water (55 : 45), mix, and degas. The acetonitrile concentration may be varied slightly to meet system suitability test requirements and to provide a suitable elution time.
  *Solvent mixture—*Mix 60 volumes of water and 40 volumes of acetonitrile.
  *Internal standard solution—*Transfer about 80 mg of propylparaben to a 100-mL volumetric flask, dissolve in acetonitrile, add acetonitrile to volume, and mix.
  *Standard preparation—*Using an accurately weighed quantity of USP Megestrol Acetate RS, prepare a solution in acetonitrile containing about 1 mg per mL. Transfer 4.0 mL of this solution and 5.0 mL of *Internal standard solution* to a 50-mL volumetric flask, dilute with *Solvent mixture* to volume, and mix. The *Standard preparation* has a known concentration of about 80 µg of megestrol acetate per mL.
  *Assay preparation—*Transfer about 100 mg of Megestrol Acetate, accurately weighed, to a 100-mL volumetric flask. Dissolve in acetonitrile, add acetonitrile to volume, and mix. Transfer 4.0 mL of this solution and 5.0 mL of *Internal standard solution* to a 50-mL volumetric flask, dilute with *Solvent mixture* to volume, and mix.
  Chromatographic system (see Chromatography ⟨621⟩*)—*The liquid chromatograph is equipped with an UV detector that monitors absorption at 280 nm and 3.9-mm × 30-cm column containing packing L1. The flow rate is about 1 mL per minute. Chromatograph the *Standard preparation*, and record the peak responses as directed for *Procedure*: the relative retention times are about 0.4 for propylparaben and 1.0 for megestrol acetate; the resolution factor, R (see *Chromatography* ⟨621⟩), between the peaks for propylparaben and megestrol acetate is not less than 8.0; and the relative standard deviation of the peak response ratio, R_S, for replicate injections is not more than 2.0%.
  *Procedure—*Separately inject equal volumes (about 25 µL) of the *Standard preparation* and the *Assay preparation* into the chromatograph, record the chromatograms, and measure the peak responses of the major peaks. Calculate the quantity, in mg, of $C_{24}H_{32}O_4$ in the portion of Megestrol Acetate taken by the formula:

$$1.25C(R_U / R_S)$$

in which C is the concentration, in µg per mL, of USP Megestrol Acetate RS in the *Standard preparation*; and R_U and R_S are the ratios of the peak responses of megestrol acetate and propylparaben obtained from the *Assay preparation* and the *Standard preparation*, respectively.

Megestrol Acetate Oral Suspension

» Megestrol Acetate Oral Suspension contains not less than 90.0 percent and not more than 110.0 percent of the labeled amount of megestrol acetate ($C_{24}H_{32}O_4$).

Packaging and storage—Preserve in well-closed, light-resistant containers.
Labeling—When more than one test for *Dissolution* is given, the labeling states the test used only if *Test 1* is not used.

USP Reference standards ⟨11⟩*—USP Megestrol Acetate RS.*
Thin-layer chromatographic identification test ⟨201⟩**—**
  *Test solution—*Transfer an accurately measured volume of Oral Suspension, equivalent to about 160 mg of megestrol acetate, to a separatory funnel, add 50 mL of water and 40 mL of chloroform, and shake. Allow the phases to separate, and discard the aqueous layer.
  *Standard solution—*Prepare a solution containing about 4.0 mg of USP Megestrol Acetate RS per mL of chloroform.
  Developing solvent system: a mixture of chloroform and ethyl acetate (4 : 1).
Dissolution ⟨711⟩**—**
  TEST 1—
  Medium: 0.5% sodium lauryl sulfate in water; 900 mL.
  Apparatus 2: 25 rpm.
  Time: 30 minutes.
  *Standard solution—*Transfer about 45 mg, accurately weighed, of USP Megestrol Acetate RS to a 250-mL volumetric flask, add about 12 mL of methanol, and place the flask in a warm water bath until the solid is dissolved. Dilute with *Medium* to volume. The final concentration is about 180 µg of megestrol acetate per mL.
  *Procedure—*Transfer to the surface of the *Medium* in the dissolution vessel an accurately measured volume of Oral Suspension, freshly mixed and free from air bubbles, equivalent to about 160 mg of megestrol acetate. Determine the amount of $C_{24}H_{32}O_4$ dissolved by employing UV absorption at the wavelength of maximum absorbance at about 292 nm on filtered portions of the solution under test, in comparison with the *Standard solution*. Calculate the percentage of megestrol acetate ($C_{24}H_{32}O_4$) released by the formula:

$$\frac{A_U \times C_S \times 900 \times 100}{A_S \times V \times LC}$$

in which A_U and A_S are the absorbances obtained from the solution under test and the *Standard solution*, respectively; C_S is the concentration, in mg per mL, of the *Standard solution*; V is the sample volume, in mL, of Oral Suspension taken; 900 is the volume, in mL, of *Medium*; 100 is the conversion factor to percentage; and LC is the label claim, in mg per mL.
  *Tolerances—*Not less than 80% *(Q)* of the labeled amount of $C_{24}H_{32}O_4$ is dissolved in 30 minutes.
  TEST 2—If the product complies with this test, the labeling indicates that it meets USP Dissolution Test 2.
  Medium: 0.5% sodium lauryl sulfate in water; 900 mL.
  Apparatus 2: 25 rpm.
  Time: 30 minutes.
  *Standard solution—*Transfer about 45 mg, accurately weighed, of USP Megestrol Acetate RS to a 250-mL volumetric flask. Add about 5 mL of methanol, and mix. Dilute with *Medium* to volume. Transfer 10 mL of this solution to a 100-mL volumetric flask, and dilute with *Medium* to volume. The final concentration is about 18 µg per mL.
  Test solution—[NOTE—Use a separate syringe for each vessel.] Withdraw more than 10 mL of the Oral Suspension, using a 10-mL syringe with a long cannula. Remove air bubbles from the syringe. Adjust the volume to the 10-mL mark on the syringe, and remove the needle. Wipe the tip of the syringe, and accurately weigh (gross weight). Operate the apparatus, and rapidly dispense the Oral Suspension to the side of the vessel at about halfway from the bottom. Similarly dispense the Oral Suspension into other vessels. Accurately weigh each syringe after dispensing the sample (tare weight). Record sample weights. After completion of the dissolution, pass an aliquot through a nylon filter having a 0.45-µm porosity, and dilute 2.0 mL of the filtrate with *Medium* to 50.0 mL to obtain a solution having a theoretical concentration of about 18 µg per mL.
  *Procedure—*Determine the amount of $C_{24}H_{32}O_4$ dissolved by employing UV absorption at the wavelength of maximum absorbance at about 292 nm, using 0.5-cm pathlength cuvettes, on the *Test solution* in comparison with the *Standard solution*. Calculate the percentage of megestrol acetate ($C_{24}H_{32}O_4$) released by the formula:

$$\frac{A_U \times C_S \times 900 \times d \times 100}{A_S \times W_U \times LC}$$

in which A_U and A_S are the absorbances obtained from the *Test solution* and the *Standard solution*, respectively; C_S is the concentration, in mg per mL, of the *Standard solution*; *d* is the density, in mg per mL, of the Oral Suspension obtained by dividing the weight of Oral Suspension taken by 10 mL; W_U is the weight, in mg, of Oral Suspension taken; 900 is the volume, in mL, of *Medium*; 100 is the conversion factor to percentage; and LC is the label claim, in mg per mL.

Tolerances—Not less than 80% (Q) of the labeled amount of $C_{24}H_{32}O_4$ is dissolved in 30 minutes.

TEST 3—If the product complies with this test, the labeling indicates that it meets USP *Dissolution Test 3*.

Medium: 0.5% sodium lauryl sulfate in degassed water; 900 mL. Use ultrapure sodium lauryl sulfate with an assay content of not less than 99.0%.

Apparatus 2: 50 rpm.
Time: 30 minutes.

Determine the amount of $C_{24}H_{32}O_4$ dissolved by employing the following method.

Mobile phase—Proceed as directed in the *Assay*.

Standard solution—Transfer about 11.5 mg, accurately weighed, of USP Megestrol Acetate RS to a 25-mL volumetric flask, and dilute with *Mobile phase* to volume.

Test solution—Proceed as directed for *Test 2*, introducing the sample into the vessel over a 10- to 15-second period (about 1 mL per second).

Chromatographic system (see *Chromatography* ⟨621⟩)—Proceed as directed in the *Assay*.

Procedure—Separately inject equal volumes (about 10 μL) of the *Standard solution* and the *Test solution* into the chromatograph, record the chromatograms, and measure the responses for the major peaks. Calculate the percentage of megestrol acetate ($C_{24}H_{32}O_4$) released by the formula:

$$\frac{r_U \times C_S \times 900 \times d \times 100}{r_S \times W_U \times LC}$$

in which r_U and r_S are the peak responses obtained from the *Test solution* and the *Standard solution*, respectively; C_S is the concentration, in mg per mL, of the *Standard solution*; *d* is the density, in mg per mL, of the Oral Suspension obtained by dividing the weight of Oral Suspension taken by 10 mL; W_U is the weight, in mg, of Oral Suspension taken; 900 is the volume, in mL, of *Medium*; 100 is the conversion factor to percentage; and LC is the label claim, in mg per mL.

Tolerances—Not less than 80% (Q) of the labeled amount of $C_{24}H_{32}O_4$ is dissolved in 30 minutes.

Deliverable volume ⟨698⟩: meets the requirements.
pH ⟨791⟩: between 3.0 and 4.7.
Assay—

Mobile phase—Prepare a filtered and degassed mixture of acetonitrile and water (11:9). Make adjustments if necessary (see *System Suitability* under *Chromatography* ⟨621⟩).

Standard preparation—Dissolve an accurately weighed quantity of Megestrol Acetate RS in *Mobile phase*, and dilute quantitatively, and stepwise if necessary, with *Mobile phase* to obtain a solution having a known concentration of about 80 μg per mL.

Assay preparation—Transfer an accurately measured volume of Oral Suspension, equivalent to about 160 mg of megestrol acetate, to a 100-mL volumetric flask, and dissolve in and dilute with *Mobile phase* to volume. Transfer 5.0 mL of the solution so obtained to a 100-mL volumetric flask, dilute with *Mobile phase* to volume, and mix.

Chromatographic system (see *Chromatography* ⟨621⟩)—The liquid chromatograph is equipped with a 280-nm detector and a 3.9-mm × 30-cm column that contains packing L1. The flow rate is about 1.5 mL per minute. Chromatograph the *Standard preparation*, and record the peak responses as directed for *Procedure*: the column efficiency is not less than 2500 theoretical plates; the tailing factor is not more than 1.4; and the relative standard deviation for replicate injections is not more than 2.0%.

Procedure—Separately inject equal volumes (about 25 μL) of the *Standard preparation* and the *Assay preparation* into the chromatograph, record the chromatograms, and measure the responses for the major peaks. Calculate the quantity, in mg, of megestrol acetate ($C_{24}H_{32}O_4$) in the portion of Oral Suspension taken by the formula:

$$2C(r_U / r_S)$$

in which C is the concentration, in μg per mL, of USP Megestrol Acetate RS in the *Standard preparation*; and r_U and r_S are the peak responses obtained from the *Assay preparation* and the *Standard preparation*, respectively.

Megestrol Acetate Tablets

» Megestrol Acetate Tablets contain not less than 93.0 percent and not more than 107.0 percent of megestrol acetate ($C_{24}H_{32}O_4$).

NOTE—Megestrol Acetate Tablets labeled solely for veterinary use are exempt from the requirements of the test for *Dissolution*.

Packaging and storage—Preserve in well-closed containers.
Labeling—Tablets intended solely for veterinary use are so labeled.
USP Reference standards ⟨11⟩—*USP Megestrol Acetate RS*.
Identification—Grind a suitable number of Tablets in a known volume of chloroform, not less than 10 mL, to obtain a solution containing about 4 mg of megestrol acetate per mL. Filter into a beaker. Introduce 0.6 mL of the filtrate via a transfer pipet into a stainless steel grinding vial containing 500 mg of potassium bromide, dry with a current of air, grind, pellet, and record the IR spectrum: the IR absorption spectrum of the potassium bromide dispersion so obtained exhibits maxima only at the same wavelengths as that of a similar preparation of USP Megestrol Acetate RS.
Disintegration ⟨701⟩: Tablets labeled solely for veterinary use; proceed as directed for film-coated Tablets, 30 minutes.
Dissolution ⟨711⟩—

Medium: 1% sodium lauryl sulfate; 900 mL.
Apparatus 2: 75 rpm.
Time: 60 minutes.

Procedure—Determine the amount of $C_{24}H_{32}O_4$ dissolved from UV absorbances at the wavelength of maximum absorbance at about 292 nm of filtered portions of the solution under test, suitably diluted with 1% sodium lauryl sulfate, if necessary, in comparison with a Standard solution having a known concentration of USP Megestrol Acetate RS in the same *Medium*.

Tolerances—Not less than 75% (Q) of the labeled amount of $C_{24}H_{32}O_4$ is dissolved in 60 minutes.

Uniformity of dosage units ⟨905⟩: meet the requirements.

Procedure for content uniformity—Place 1 Tablet in a volumetric flask of suitable size so that the final expected solution concentration is between about 0.2 and 1.0 mg of megestrol acetate per mL. Add 1 mL of water, and gently shake until the Tablet has disintegrated. Fill the flask to three-quarters of its nominal capacity with methanol, and shake by mechanical means for 20 minutes. Dilute with methanol to volume, mix, and filter, discarding the first 15 mL of the filtrate. Dilute 5.0 mL of the subsequent filtrate quantitatively with methanol to obtain a solution containing about 10 μg of megestrol acetate per mL. Prepare a Standard solution of USP Megestrol Acetate RS in the same medium having a known concentration of about 10 μg per mL. Record the absorbances of the solutions in 1-cm cells, against a blank of methanol, scanning from 350 nm to 260 nm. Measure the absorbances at the wavelength of maximum absorbance at about 288 nm. Calculate the quantity, in mg, of $C_{24}H_{32}O_4$ in the Tablet taken by the formula:

$$(TC / D)(A_U / A_S)$$

in which T is the labeled quantity, in mg, of megestrol acetate in the Tablet; C is the concentration, in μg per mL of USP Megestrol Acetate RS in the Standard solution; D is the concentration, in μg per mL, of the solution from the Tablet, based upon the labeled quantity per Tablet and the extent of dilution; and A_U and A_S are the absorbances of the solution from the Tablet and the Standard solution, respectively.

Assay—

Mobile phase, Solvent mixture, Internal standard solution, Standard preparation, and *Chromatographic system*—Prepare as directed in the *Assay* under *Megestrol Acetate.*

Assay preparation—Weigh and finely powder not fewer than 20 Tablets. Transfer an accurately weighed portion of the powder, equivalent to about 80 mg of megestrol acetate, to a 100-mL volumetric flask. Add about 10 mL of water, and shake for 10 minutes. Add 75 mL of acetonitrile, and shake for 30 minutes, then dilute with acetonitrile to volume, and mix. Place a 25-mL aliquot in a glass-stoppered, 35-mL centrifuge tube, insert the stopper, and centrifuge for 10 minutes. Transfer 5.0 mL of the supernatant and 5.0 mL of *Internal standard solution* to a 50-mL volumetric flask, dilute with *Solvent mixture* to volume, and mix.

Procedure—Proceed as directed for *Procedure* in the *Assay* under *Megestrol Acetate.* Calculate the quantity, in mg, of megestrol acetate ($C_{24}H_{32}O_4$) in the portion of Tablets taken by the formula:

$$C(R_U / R_S)$$

in which the terms are as defined therein.

Meglumine

$C_7H_{17}NO_5$ 195.21

D-Glucitol, 1-deoxy-1-(methylamino)-.
1-Deoxy-1-(methylamino)-D-glucitol   [6284-40-8].

» Meglumine contains not less than 99.0 percent and not more than 100.5 percent of $C_7H_{17}NO_5$, calculated on the dried basis.

Packaging and storage—Preserve in well-closed containers.

Completeness and color of solution—A solution (1 in 5) is clear, and its absorbance, determined in a 1-cm cell at 420 nm, with a suitable spectrophotometer, water being used as the blank, is not greater than 0.030.

Identification—Transfer about 250 mg to a dry, 50-mL centrifuge tube, add 500 mg of sodium metaperiodate, then add 5 mL of water rapidly in one portion. Allow to stand undisturbed: the solution instantly turns yellow and heat is produced. The color then changes from deep yellow to orange-brown (rust), and after 20 minutes, the rust-colored solution is cloudy. Then add 2 mL of 2.5 N sodium hydroxide: the mixture turns bright yellow and becomes clear.

Melting range ⟨741⟩: between 128° and 132°.

Specific rotation ⟨781S⟩: between −15.7° and −17.3°.

  Test solution: 100 mg, undried, per mL, in water.

Loss on drying ⟨731⟩—Dry about 1 g at 105° to constant weight: it loses not more than 1.0% of its weight.

Residue on ignition ⟨281⟩: not more than 0.1%.

Heavy metals ⟨231⟩—Dissolve 1 g in 20 mL of water, add phenolphthalein TS, neutralize with 3 N hydrochloric acid, and dilute with water to 25 mL. The limit is 0.002%.

Absence of reducing substances—To 5 mL of a solution (1 in 20) add 5 mL of alkaline cupric tartrate TS, and heat to boiling: the color of the solution does not change.

Assay—Transfer about 500 mg of Meglumine, accurately weighed, to a conical flask, dissolve in about 40 mL of water, add 2 drops of methyl red TS, and titrate with 0.1 N hydrochloric acid VS. Each mL of 0.1 N hydrochloric acid is equivalent to 19.52 mg of $C_7H_{17}NO_5$.

Melengestrol Acetate

$C_{25}H_{32}O_4$ 396.52

Pregna-4,6-diene-3,20-dione, 17-(acetyloxy)-6-methyl-16-methylene-.
17-Hydroxy-6-methyl-16-methylenepregna-4,6-diene-3,20-dione acetate   [2919-66-6].

» Melengestrol Acetate contains not less than 97.0 percent and not more than 103.0 percent of $C_{25}H_{32}O_4$, calculated on the dried basis.

Packaging and storage—Preserve in tight, light-resistant containers, and store at controlled room temperature.

Labeling—Label it to indicate that it is for veterinary use only.

USP Reference standards ⟨11⟩—*USP Melengestrol Acetate RS. USP Melengestrol Acetate Related Compound A RS. USP Melengestrol Acetate Related Compound B RS.*

Identification—

  A: *Infrared Absorption* ⟨197K⟩.

  B: *Ultraviolet Absorption* ⟨197U⟩—

  Solution: 10 μg per mL.

  Medium: alcohol.

  C: The retention time of the melengestrol acetate peak in the chromatogram of the *Assay preparation* corresponds to that in the chromatogram of the *Standard preparation,* as obtained in the *Assay.*

Melting temperature ⟨741⟩: between 219° and 226°.

Specific rotation ⟨781S⟩: between −132.0° and −122.0°, at 20°.

  Test solution: 10.0 mg per mL, in chloroform.

Loss on drying ⟨731⟩—Dry it at 105° for 3 hours: it loses not more than 0.5% of its weight.

Heavy metals, *Method II* ⟨231⟩: not more than 0.001%.

Related compounds—

  Mobile phase—Prepare a mixture of acetonitrile and water (50 : 50).

  Standard solution—Dissolve an accurately weighed quantity of USP Melengestrol Acetate RS, USP Melengestrol Acetate Related Compound A RS, and USP Melengestrol Acetate Related Compound B RS in methanol to obtain a solution having known concentrations of about 0.005 mg of each per mL.

  Test solution—Use the *Assay preparation.*

  Chromatographic system (see *Chromatography* ⟨621⟩)—The liquid chromatograph is equipped with a multiwavelength detector set at 240 and 262 nm and a 4.6-mm × 25-cm column that contains 5-μm packing L7. The flow rate is about 1.0 mL per minute. Chromatograph the *Standard solution,* and record the peak responses as directed for *Procedure* [NOTE—Melengestrol acetate and melengestrol related compound B will generate larger peak areas at 262 nm than at 240 nm; melengestrol acetate related compound A will generate a larger peak area at 240 nm than at 262 nm]: the relative retention times are about 0.78, 1.0, and 1.05 for melengestrol acetate related compound A, melengestrol acetate, and melengestrol acetate related compound B, respectively; the resolution, *R,* between melengestrol acetate related compound A and melengestrol acetate related compound B is not less than 5.0; the column efficiency for the melengestrol acetate related compound A peak is greater than 1500 theoretical plates; the tailing factor is less than 2.0; and the relative standard deviation for replicate injections is not more than 5.0%.

  Procedure—Separately inject equal volumes (about 20 μL) of the *Standard solution* and the *Test solution* into the chromatograph, record the chromatograms, identify the peaks, and determine which detector wavelength generates the larger peak area for each impurity.

Using the larger peak area, calculate the percentage of each impurity in the portion of Melengestrol Acetate taken by the formula:

$$100(C_S / C_U)(r_i / r_S)$$

in which C_S is the concentration, in mg per mL, of either melengestrol related compound A or melengestrol related compound B in the *Standard solution* [NOTE—If using the impurity peak area generated at 240 nm, C_S is the concentration of melengestrol related compound A; if using the impurity peak area generated at 262 nm, C_S is the concentration of melengestrol related compound B]; C_U is the concentration, in mg per mL, of melengestrol acetate in the *Test solution*; r_i is the peak area of each impurity obtained from the *Test solution*; and r_S is the peak area of either melengestrol related compound A or melengestrol related compound B obtained from the *Standard solution* [NOTE—If using the impurity peak area generated at 240 nm, r_S is the peak area of melengestrol related compound A; if using the impurity peak area generated at 262 nm, C_S is the peak area of melengestrol related compound B]: not more than 0.5% of any identified impurity is found; not more than 0.2% of any unidentified impurity is found; and not more than 1.0% of total impurities is found.

Assay—
*Mobile phase—*Prepare a mixture of acetonitrile and water (50 : 50).

*Standard preparation—*Dissolve an accurately weighed quantity of USP Melengestrol Acetate RS in methanol to obtain a solution having a known concentration of about 0.5 mg per mL.

*Assay preparation—*Transfer about 50 mg of Melengestrol Acetate, accurately weighed, to a 100-mL volumetric flask, and dissolve in and dilute with methanol to volume.

Chromatographic system (see *Chromatography* ⟨621⟩)—The liquid chromatograph is equipped with a 287-nm detector and a 4.6-mm × 25-cm column that contains 5-μm packing L7. The flow rate is about 1.0 mL per minute. Chromatograph the *Standard preparation* as directed for *Procedure:* the column efficiency is not less than 1500 theoretical plates; the tailing factor is not more than 2; and the relative standard deviation for replicate injections is not more than 2.0%.

*Procedure—*Separately inject equal volumes (about 20 μL) of the *Standard preparation* and the *Assay preparation* in duplicate into the chromatograph, record the chromatograms, and measure the areas for the major peaks. Calculate the quantity, in mg, of $C_{25}H_{32}O_4$ in the portion of Melengestrol Acetate taken by the formula:

$$2CW(r_U / r_S)$$

in which C is the concentration, in mg per mL, of the *Standard preparation*; W is the weight, in mg, of Melengestrol Acetate used to prepare the *Assay preparation*; r_U is the average peak area of the melengestrol acetate peak obtained from the *Assay preparation*; and r_S is the average peak area of the melengestrol acetate peak obtained from the *Standard preparation*.

Meloxicam

$C_{14}H_{13}N_3O_4S_2$ 351.40
4-Hydroxy-2-methyl-*N*-(5-methyl-2-thiazolyl)-2*H*-1,2-benzothiazine-3-carboxamide 1,1-dioxide   [71125-38-7].

» Meloxicam contains not less than 99.0 percent and not more than 100.5 percent of $C_{14}H_{13}N_3O_4S_2$, calculated on the dried basis.

Packaging and storage—Preserve in well-closed containers. Store at room temperature.

Labeling—The labeling states with which *Related compounds* test the article complies if a test other than *Test 1* is used.

USP Reference standards ⟨11⟩—*USP Meloxicam RS. USP Meloxicam Related Compound A RS. USP Meloxicam Related Compound B RS. USP Meloxicam Related Compound C RS. USP Meloxicam Related Compound D RS.*

Identification—
A: *Infrared Absorption* ⟨197K⟩.
B: *Ultraviolet Absorption* ⟨197U⟩.
Spectral range: 240 to 450 nm.
Solution: 10 μg per mL.
Medium: methanol.

Loss on drying ⟨731⟩—Dry it at 105° for 4 hours: it loses not more than 0.5% of its weight.

Residue on ignition ⟨281⟩:   not more than 0.1%.

Heavy metals, *Method II* ⟨231⟩:   not more than 0.001%.

Related compounds—[NOTE—Perform either *Test 1* or *Test 2* depending on the manufacturing process used.]

TEST 1—
Solution A: a 0.1% (w/v) solution of monobasic potassium phosphate adjusted with 1 N sodium hydroxide to a pH of 6.0.
Solution B: methanol.
*Mobile phase—*Use variable mixtures of *Solution A* and *Solution B* as directed for *Chromatographic system*. Make adjustments if necessary (see *System Suitability* under *Chromatography* ⟨621⟩).

*System suitability solution—*Transfer about 4 mg of USP Meloxicam RS and about 4 mg each of USP Meloxicam Related Compound A RS and USP Meloxicam Related Compound B RS into a 50-mL volumetric flask, dissolve in 5 mL of methanol and 0.3 mL of 1 N sodium hydroxide, dilute with methanol to volume, and mix.

*Standard solution—*Transfer about 12 mg of USP Meloxicam RS, accurately weighed, to a 20-mL volumetric flask, dissolve in 5 mL of methanol and 0.3 mL of 1 N sodium hydroxide, dilute with methanol to volume, and mix. Transfer 2 mL of this solution to a 100-mL volumetric flask, dilute with methanol to volume, and mix.

*Test solution—*Transfer about 80 mg of Meloxicam, accurately weighed, to a 20-mL volumetric flask, dissolve in 5 mL of methanol and 0.3 mL of 1 N sodium hydroxide, dilute with methanol to volume, and mix.

Chromatographic system (see *Chromatography* ⟨621⟩)—The liquid chromatograph is equipped with a variable wavelength or multi-wavelength UV detector and a 4.6-mm × 15-cm column that contains 5-μm packing L1. The column temperature is maintained at 45°. The flow rate is about 1 mL per minute, and the detection wavelengths are 260 nm and 350 nm. The chromatograph is programmed as follows.

Time (minutes)	Solution A (%)	Solution B (%)	Elution
0–2	60	40	isocratic
2–10	60→30	40→70	linear gradient
10–15	30	70	isocratic
15–15.1	30→60	70→40	linear gradient
15.1–18	60	40	equilibration

Chromatograph the *System suitability solution,* and record the peak responses as directed for *Procedure:* the relative retention times based on the meloxicam peak at about 7 minutes are listed in *Table 1.* At 350 nm, the resolution, *R*, between meloxicam related compound A and meloxicam is not less than 3.0; at 260 nm, the resolution, *R*, between meloxicam related compound B and meloxicam is not less than 3.0. Chromatograph the *Standard solution,* and record the peak responses as directed for *Procedure:* the relative standard deviation for replicate injections is not more than 10%.

*Procedure—*Separately inject equal volumes (about 5 μL) of the *Standard solution* and the *Test solution* into the chromatograph, record the chromatograms at detection wavelengths of 260 nm and 350 nm, and measure the peak responses. Calculate the percentage of each impurity in the portion of Meloxicam taken by the formula:

$$100(C_S / C_T)(1 / F)(r_U / r_S)$$

in which C_S is the concentration, in mg per mL, of USP Meloxicam RS in the *Standard solution*; C_T is the concentration, in mg per mL, of Meloxicam in the *Test solution*; *F* is the relative response factor (see *Table 1*); r_U is the peak response of each impurity obtained from the *Test solution*; and r_S is the peak response of meloxicam at 350 nm obtained from the *Standard solution*. [NOTE—For the specified impurities, calculate the percentage content of each impurity, using the *Test solution* peak responses recorded at the detection wavelength given in *Table 1*. For an unknown impurity, calculate the percentage content, using peak responses recorded at the wavelength that gives the greater response.]

TEST 2—If an article complies with this test, the labeling indicates that it meets the requirements of *Related compounds Test 2*.

Solution A and *Solution B*—Prepare as directed in *Test 1*.

Mobile phase—Use variable mixtures of *Solution A* and *Solution B* as directed for *Chromatographic system*. Make adjustments if necessary (see *System Suitability* under *Chromatography* ⟨621⟩).

Diluent A: a mixture of *Diluent B* and 0.4 N sodium hydroxide (50 : 3).

Diluent B: a mixture of water and methanol (60 : 40).

Standard stock solution 1—Prepare a solution having a known concentration of about 50 µg per mL of USP Meloxicam RS in *Diluent A*. Transfer 2 mL of the solution to a 10-mL volumetric flask, dilute with *Diluent B* to volume, and mix.

Standard stock solution 2—Transfer about 5 mg each of USP Meloxicam Related Compound B RS, USP Meloxicam Related Compound C RS, and USP Meloxicam Related Compound D RS into a 100-mL volumetric flask, add 6 mL of 0.4 N sodium hydroxide, and sonicate for about 2 minutes. Add 40 mL of methanol to the resulting solution, sonicate for about 2 minutes, dilute with water to volume, and mix.

Standard solution—Transfer 1 mL each of *Standard stock solution 1* and *Standard stock solution 2* into a 10-mL volumetric flask, dilute with *Diluent B* to volume, and mix.

System suitability stock solution—Prepare a solution containing about 2 mg per mL of USP Meloxicam RS in *Diluent A*.

System suitability solution—Transfer 5 mL of *System suitability stock solution* and 1 mL of *Standard stock solution 2* into a 10-mL volumetric flask, dilute with *Diluent B* to volume, and mix.

Test solution—Transfer about 20 mg of Meloxicam, accurately weighed, to a 20-mL volumetric flask, dissolve in 10 mL of *Diluent A*, dilute with *Diluent B* to volume, and mix.

Chromatographic system (see *Chromatography* ⟨621⟩)—The liquid chromatograph is equipped with a variable wavelength or multiwavelength UV detector and a 4.6-mm × 25-cm column that contains 5-µm packing L1. The column temperature is maintained at 45°. The flow rate is about 1 mL per minute and the detection wavelengths are 260 nm and 350 nm. The chromatograph is programmed as follows.

Time (minutes)	Solution A (%)	Solution B (%)	Elution
0–25	45	55	isocratic
25–30	45→30	55→70	linear gradient
30–40	30	70	isocratic
40–45	30→45	70→55	linear gradient
45–50	45	55	equilibration

Chromatograph the *System suitability solution*, and record the peak responses as directed for *Procedure*: the relative retention times based on the meloxicam peak at about 5 minutes are listed in *Table 2*; and the resolution, *R*, between meloxicam related compound D and meloxicam at 350 nm is not less than 5.0. Chromatograph the *Standard solution*, and record the peak responses as directed for *Procedure*: the relative standard deviation for replicate injections is not more than 5.0% for meloxicam related compound C and for meloxicam related compound D at 350 nm; and not more than 5.0% for meloxicam related compound B at 260 nm.

Procedure—Separately inject equal volumes (about 20 µL) of the *Standard solution* and *Test solution* into the chromatograph, record the chromatograms at detection wavelengths of 260 nm and 350 nm, and measure the peak responses. Calculate the percentage of each impurity in the portion of Meloxicam taken by the formula:

$$100(C_S / C_T)(r_U / r_S)$$

in which C_S is the concentration, in mg per mL, of the corresponding USP Related Compound RS in the *Standard solution* [NOTE—Use the concentration of the USP Meloxicam RS for unknown impurities.]; C_T is the concentration, in mg per mL, of Meloxicam in the *Test solution*; r_U is the peak response of each impurity obtained from the *Test solution*; and r_S is the peak response of the corresponding related compound obtained from the *Standard solution*. [NOTE—Use the peak response of the USP Meloxicam RS for unknown impurities; for the specified impurities, calculate the percentage content of each impurity using the *Test solution* peak responses recorded at the detection wavelength given in *Table 2*. For an unknown impurity, calculate the percentage content using peak responses recorded at the wavelength that gives the greater response.]

Table 2

Compound	Approximate Relative Retention Time	Wavelength (nm)	Limit (w/w, %)
2-Amino-5-methyl-thiazole (meloxicam related compound B)	0.8	260	0.1
Isopropyl-4-hydroxy-2-methyl-2*H*-1,2-benzothiazine-3-carboxylate-1,1-dioxide (meloxicam related compound C)	3.2	350	0.1
4-Methoxy-2-methyl-*N*-(5-methyl-1,3-thiazol-2yl)-2*H*-1,2-benzothiazine-3-carboxamide-1,1-dioxide (meloxicam related compound D)	2.4	350	0.1
Individual unknown impurity	—	260/350	0.1
Total impurity	—	—	0.3

Assay—

Buffer solution: a mixture of a 0.1% (w/v) solution of ammonium acetate adjusted with 10% ammonia solution to a pH of 9.1.

Mobile phase—Prepare a filtered and degassed mixture of *Buffer solution* and methanol (58 : 42). Make adjustments if necessary (see *System Suitability* under *Chromatography* ⟨621⟩).

System suitability solution—Transfer about 4 mg of USP Meloxicam RS and about 4 mg of USP Meloxicam Related Compound A RS into a 50-mL volumetric flask, dissolve in 25 mL of methanol and 0.1 mL of 1 N sodium hydroxide, dilute with water to volume, and mix.

Standard preparation—Transfer about 20 mg of USP Meloxicam RS, accurately weighed, into a 100-mL volumetric flask, dissolve in 50 mL of methanol and 0.2 mL of 1 N sodium hydroxide, dilute with water to volume, and mix.

Assay preparation—Transfer about 20 mg of Meloxicam, accurately weighed, into a 100-mL volumetric flask, dissolve in 50 mL of methanol and 0.2 mL of 1 N sodium hydroxide, dilute with water to volume, and mix.

Chromatographic system (see *Chromatography* ⟨621⟩)—The liquid chromatograph is equipped with a 360-nm detector and a 4.6-mm × 15-cm column that contains packing L1. The column temperature is maintained at 45°. The flow rate is about 1.0 mL per minute. Chromatograph the *System suitability solution,* and record the peak responses as directed for *Procedure:* the relative retention times are about 0.7 for related compound A and 1.0 for meloxicam; the resolution, *R*, between the two peaks is not less 3.0; the tailing factor for the meloxicam peak is not more than 2.0; and the relative standard deviation for replicate injections, calculated for the meloxicam peak, is not more than 2.0%.

Procedure—Separately inject equal volumes (about 10 µL) of the *Standard preparation* and the *Assay preparation* into the chromatograph, record the chromatograms, and measure the responses for the meloxicam peak. Calculate the quantity, in mg, of $C_{14}H_{13}N_3O_4S_2$ in the portion of Meloxicam taken by the formula:

$$100C(r_U / r_S)$$

in which *C* is the concentration, in mg per mL, of USP Meloxicam RS in the *Standard preparation;* and r_U and r_S are the peak responses obtained from the *Assay preparation* and the *Standard preparation,* respectively.

Table 1

Compound	Approximate Relative Retention Time	Wavelength (nm)	Relative Response Factor (*F*)	Limit (w/w, %)
4-Hydroxy-2-methyl-2*H*-1,2-benzothiazine-3-carboxylic acid ethylester 1,1-dioxide (meloxicam related compound A)	1.4	350	0.5	0.1
2-Amino-5-methyl-thiazole (meloxicam related compound B)	0.4	260	1.0	0.1
4-Hydroxy-2-methyl-*N*-(*N*′-methyl-5-methyl-2-thiazolyl)-2*H*-1,2-benzothiazine-3-carboxamide-1,1-dioxide	1.9	350	1.0	0.05
4-Hydroxy-2-methyl-*N*-(*N*′-ethyl-5-methyl-2-thiazolyl)-2*H*-1,2-benzothiazine-3-carboxamide-1,1-dioxide	1.7	350	1.0	0.05
Individual unknown impurity	—	260/350	1.0	0.1
Total impurity	—	—	—	0.3

Add the following:

▲Meloxicam Oral Suspension

» Meloxicam Oral Suspension contains not less than 90.0 percent and not more than 110.0 percent of the labeled amount of meloxicam ($C_{14}H_{13}N_3O_4S_2$).

Packaging and storage—Preserve in well-closed containers. Store at 25°, excursions permitted between 15° and 30°.

USP Reference standards ⟨11⟩—USP Meloxicam RS. USP Meloxicam Related Compound B RS.

Identification—

A: *Thin-Layer Chromatographic Identification Test* ⟨201⟩—

Test solution—Transfer a volume of Oral Suspension, equivalent to about 2.5 mg of meloxicam, to a 10-mL volumetric flask. Dilute with acetone to volume, and mix for 10 minutes. If necessary, pass through fluted filter paper.

Standard solution: 0.25 mg per mL, prepared by dissolving USP Meloxicam RS in 1 mL of water and diluting with acetone to volume.

Developing solvent solution: a mixture of chloroform, methanol, and ammonium hydroxide (80 : 20 : 1)

Procedure—Proceed as directed in the chapter. After removing the plate from the chamber and drying, examine the chromatograms under UV light at 254-nm: the R_F value (approximately 0.45) of the principal dark spot obtained from the *Test solution* corresponds to that obtained from the *Standard solution*.

B: The retention time of the major peak in the chromatogram of the *Assay preparation* corresponds to that in the chromatogram of the *Standard preparation,* as obtained in the *Assay.*

pH ⟨791⟩: between 3.5 and 4.5.

Viscosity ⟨911⟩—Determine using a shear rate programmable rotational viscometer: between 40 and 100 centipoises, determined at 20°.

Dissolution ⟨711⟩—

Medium: pH 7.5 phosphate buffer; 900 mL.
Apparatus 2: 25 rpm.
Time: 15 minutes.

Determine the amount of $C_{14}H_{13}N_3O_4S_2$ dissolved by employing the following method.

Standard solution—Transfer about 20.83 mg of USP Meloxicam RS, accurately weighed, into a 100-mL volumetric flask. Dissolve in 5 mL of methanol and 1 mL of 0.1 M sodium hydroxide, and dilute with *Medium* to volume. Dilute with *Medium* to a final concentration of about 8.3 µg per mL of meloxicam.

Test solution—Shake each sample for 15 minutes. Weigh six portions, equivalent to 7.5 mg of the Oral Suspension, into separate tared 10-mL beakers, and record each weight. Introduce each of the samples to the middle of the dissolution vessels, and rinse each beaker with about 20 mL of the *Medium* withdrawn from the vessel. Carefully lower the paddle to the appropriate height and start the rotation. After completion of the dissolution, pass a 20-mL aliquot through a nylon filter having a 0.45-µm porosity, discarding the first 3 mL of the filtrate.

Procedure—Determine the amount of $C_{14}H_{13}N_3O_4S_2$ dissolved by employing UV absorption at the wavelength of maximum absorbance at about 362 nm on the *Test solution* in comparison with the *Standard solution,* using *Medium* as the blank. Calculate the percentage of $C_{14}H_{13}N_3O_4S_2$ released by the formula:

$$\frac{A_U \times C_S \times 900 \times d \times 100}{A_S \times W_U \times LC}$$

in which A_U and A_S are the absorbances obtained from the *Test solution* and the *Standard solution,* respectively; C_S is the concentration, in mg per mL, of the *Standard solution;* *d* is the density, in g per mL, of the Oral Suspension; W_U is the weight, in mg, of the Oral Suspension taken; 900 is the volume, in mL of the *Medium;* 100 is the conversion factor to percentage; and *LC* is the label claim, in mg per mL.

Tolerances—Not less than 75% (*Q*) of the labeled amount of $C_{14}H_{13}N_3O_4S_2$ is dissolved in 15 minutes.

Microbial limits ⟨61⟩—The total aerobic microbial count does not exceed 100 cfu per g or 100 cfu per mL. The total yeasts and molds count does not exceed 50 cfu per g or 50 cfu per mL. It meets the requirements of the test for the absence of *Escherichia coli.*

Chromatographic purity—

Buffer, Mobile phase, and *Diluent*—Proceed as directed in the *Assay.*

Related compound standard stock solution—Proceed as directed for *Related compound standard stock preparation* in the *Assay.*

Sensitivity solution—Dilute the *Related compound standard stock solution* with *Diluent* to a final concentration of about 0.08 µg per mL.

Related compound standard solution—Dilute *Related compound standard stock preparation* with *Diluent* to a final concentration of about 0.5 µg per mL.

Test solution—Proceed as directed for *Assay preparation* in the *Assay.*

Chromatographic system (see *Chromatography* ⟨621⟩)—Proceed as directed in the *Assay.* Chromatograph the *Sensitivity solution* (about 10 µL), and record the peak responses as directed for *Procedure* at 260 nm: the relative standard deviation of three replicate injections is not more than 10% for meloxicam related compound B. Chromatograph the *Related compound standard solution* (about 10 µL), and record the peak responses as directed for *Procedure* at 260 nm: the tailing factor for meloxicam related compound B is not more than 2.0.

Procedure—Separately inject equal volumes (about 10 µL) of the *Related compound standard solution* and the *Test solution* into the chromatograph, record the chromatograms, and record the peak areas at 260 nm and 360 nm. The run time is about 20 minutes or two times the retention time of meloxicam. Calculate the percentage of meloxicam related compound B in the portion of Oral Suspension taken by the formula:

$$(5000/L)(C/V)(r_U / r_S)$$

in which L is the label claim, in mg per mL; C is the concentration, in mg per mL, of USP Meloxicam Related Compound B RS in the *Related compound standard solution;* V is the volume, in mL, of Oral Suspension taken to prepare the *Test solution;* r_U is the peak area obtained for meloxicam related compound B in the *Test solution* at 260 nm; and r_S is the peak area for meloxicam related compound B in the *Related compound standard solution* at 260 nm. Calculate the percentage of each unknown degradation product in the portion of Oral Suspension taken by the formula:

$$100(r_i / r_s)$$

in which r_i is the area of any unknown degradant at 360 nm; r_s is the sum of areas of meloxicam and all impurities in the *Test solution* at 360 nm. Not more than 0.15% of meloxicam related compound B is found; not more than 0.2% of any individual unknown degradation product is found; and not more than 0.5% of total degradation products is found.

Assay—

Buffer—Dissolve 2 g of monohydrate citric acid and 2 g of boric acid in 1000 mL of water, and adjust with dihydrate trisodium citrate to a pH of 2.9.

Mobile phase—Mix 565 mL of *Buffer,* 260 mL of methanol, and 200 mL of acetonitrile. Degas the solution, and then dissolve 200 mg of sodium dodecyl sulfate in 1000 mL of the resulting solution.

Diluent—Dissolve 3 g of boric acid and 1.5 g of dihydrate trisodium citrate in 1000 mL of water, and adjust with 2 M sodium hydroxide to a pH of 8.3. Mix 420 mL of the resulting buffer with 420 mL of methanol and 160 mL of acetonitrile.

Standard stock preparation—Transfer about 67 mg of USP Meloxicam RS, accurately weighed, into a 100-mL volumetric flask. Add 3.0 mL of dimethylformamide. Swirl the flask, and allow to stand for about 5 minutes. Add 15 mL of methanol. Dilute with *Diluent* to just below volume. Sonicate for 30 minutes, and mix until dissolved. Cool to room temperature. Dilute with *Diluent* to volume.

Standard preparation—Dilute *Standard stock preparation* with *Diluent* to a final concentration of about 0.27 mg per mL.

Related compound standard stock preparation—Transfer about 21 mg of USP Meloxicam Related Compound B RS, accurately weighed, into a 100-mL volumetric flask. Add 3.0 mL of dimethylformamide, 15 mL of methanol, and about 60 mL of *Diluent.* Sonicate, and mix until dissolved. Cool to room temperature. Dilute with *Diluent* to volume. Dilute further with *Diluent* to a concentration of about 8.4 µg per mL.

System suitability solution—Transfer a volume of Oral Suspension, equivalent to about 15 mg of meloxicam, accurately weighed, to a 50-mL volumetric flask. Add 3.0 mL of *Related compound standard stock preparation.* Add 3.0 mL of dimethylformamide. Swirl the flask, and allow to stand for about 5 minutes. Add 15 mL of methanol. Dilute with *Diluent* to just below volume. Sonicate for 30 minutes, mixing the flask vigorously about every 5 minutes. Cool to room temperature. Dilute with *Diluent* to volume. Mix, and allow particulates to settle. Pass through a 0.45-µm membrane filter with a fiberglass prefilter.

Assay preparation—Transfer an accurately meaured volume of Oral Suspension, equivalent to about 15 mg of meloxicam, to a 50-mL volumetric flask. Add 3.0 mL of dimethylformamide. Swirl the flask, and allow to stand for about 5 minutes. Add 15 mL of methanol. Dilute with *Diluent* to just below volume. Sonicate for 30 minutes, mixing the flask vigorously about every 5 minutes. Cool to room temperature. Dilute with *Diluent* to volume. Mix, and allow particulates to settle. Pass through a 0.45-µm membrane filter with a fiberglass prefilter.

Chromatographic system (see *Chromatography* ⟨621⟩)—The liquid chromatograph is equipped with a programmable dual wavelength detector, a single wavelength detector in series, or a photodiode array detector capable of detecting wavelengths from 190 nm to 400 nm, or equivalent, and a 4-mm × 12.5-cm analytical column that contains 5-µm packing L1. The column temperature is maintained at 40°. The flow rate is about 1.0 mL per minute. The run time is about 20 minutes or two times the retention time of meloxicam. Chromatograph the *System suitability solution* (about 10 µL), and record the peak responses as directed for *Procedure* at 360 nm and 260 nm: at 360 nm the resolution, R, between meloxicam and any other adjacent peak is not less than 1.5. The tailing factor for the meloxicam peak is not more than 2.0. Chromatograph the *Standard preparation,* and record the peak responses as directed for *Procedure* at 360 nm: the relative standard deviation for replicate injections of the *Standard preparation* is not more than 1.5%.

Procedure—Separately inject equal volumes (about 10 µL) of the *Standard preparation* and the *Assay preparation* into the chromatograph, record the chromatograms, and record the peak areas at 360 nm. Calculate the amount of meloxicam ($C_{14}H_{13}N_3O_4S_2$), in mg per mL, in the portion of Oral Suspension taken by the formula:

$$50(C/V)(r_U / r_S)$$

in which C is the concentration, in mg per mL, of USP Meloxicam RS in the *Standard preparation;* V is the volume, in mL, of Oral Suspension taken to prepare the *Assay preparation;* r_U is the peak area obtained for meloxicam in the *Assay preparation* at 360 nm; and r_S is the peak area for meloxicam in the *Standard solution* at 360 nm.▲USP31

Meloxicam Tablets

» Meloxicam Tablets contain not less than 90.0 percent and not more than 110.0 percent of the labeled amount of meloxicam ($C_{14}H_{13}N_3O_4S_2$).

Packaging and storage—Preserve in well-closed containers. Store at 25°, excursions permitted between 15° and 30°.

USP Reference standards ⟨11⟩—*USP Meloxicam RS.*

Identification—

A: *Thin-Layer Chromatographic Identification Test* ⟨201⟩—

0.1 N Methanolic sodium hydroxide—Dilute 100 mL of 1 N sodium hydroxide with methanol to 1000 mL.

Test solution—Transfer a portion of finely powdered Tablets, equivalent to about 50 mg of meloxicam, to a suitable flask. Add 5 mL of *0.1 N Methanolic sodium hydroxide,* and mix. Add 20 mL of methanol, and stir for about 15 minutes. Filter the mixture to remove insoluble material, and use the filtrate.

Standard solution—Transfer about 20 mg of USP Meloxicam RS, accurately weighed, to a 10-mL volumetric flask, dissolve in 2 mL of *0.1 N Methanolic sodium hydroxide,* dilute with methanol to volume, and mix.

Developing solvent system—Prepare a mixture of chloroform, methanol, and ammonia water (25%) (80 : 20 : 1).

Procedure—Proceed as directed in the chapter.

B: The retention time of the major peak in the chromatogram of the *Assay preparation* corresponds to that in the chromatogram of the *Standard preparation,* as obtained in the *Assay.*

Uniformity of dosage units ⟨905⟩: meet the requirements.

Related compounds—

Solution A, Solution B, and *Mobile phase*—Proceed as directed in the *Assay.*

Standard solution—Use the *Standard preparation* from the *Assay.*

System sensitivity solution—Transfer 4 mL of the *Standard solution* to a 100-mL volumetric flask, dilute with methanol to volume, and mix. Transfer 5 mL of the resulting solution to a 50-mL volumetric flask, add 5 mL of 1 N sodium hydroxide, and dilute with methanol to volume.

Test solution—Use the *Assay preparation* from the *Assay.*

Chromatographic system (see *Chromatography* ⟨621⟩)—Proceed as directed in the *Assay,* except to chromatograph the *Standard solution* and the *System sensitivity solution:* the tailing factor for the meloxicam peak is not more than 2.0; the relative standard deviation for replicate injections of the *Standard solution* is not more than 2.0%; and the signal-to-noise ratio of the meloxicam peak in the chromatogram of the *System sensitivity solution* is not less than 10.

Procedure—Separately inject equal volumes (about 25 µL) of the *Standard solution* and the *Test solution* into the chromatograph, record the chromatograms, and measure the peak responses. Determine the relative retention times for the impurity peaks relative to that of the meloxicam peak. Calculate the percentage of each impurity in the portion of Tablets taken by the formula:

$$(5000/3)(1/F)(C/W)(A/L)(r_i / r_S)$$

in which F is the relative response factor for each impurity and is equal to 2.7 for the impurity with a relative retention time of about 0.5 (meloxicam related compound B [2-amino-5-methylthiazole]) and 1.0 for all other impurities; *C* is the concentration, in mg per mL, of USP Meloxicam RS in the *Standard solution; W* is the weight, in mg, of powdered Tablets taken to prepare the *Test solution; A* is the average weight of a Tablet; *L* is the labeled amount, in mg, of meloxicam in each Tablet; r_i is the peak response obtained for each impurity in the *Test solution;* and r_S is the peak response for meloxicam in the *Standard solution:* not more than 0.15% of meloxicam related compound B is found; not more than 0.2% of any individual unknown impurity is found; and not more than 0.5% of total impurities is found.

Assay—

Solution A—Dissolve 2.0 g of dibasic ammonium phosphate in 1 L of water, and adjust with phosphoric acid to a pH of 7.0 ± 0.1.

Solution B—Mix 650 mL of methanol and 100 mL of isopropyl alcohol.

Mobile phase—Prepare a filtered and degassed mixture of *Solution A* and *Solution B* (63 : 37). Make adjustments if necessary (see *System Suitability* under *Chromatography* ⟨621⟩).

Standard stock preparation—[NOTE—The *Standard stock preparation* is prepared so that the final concentration of meloxicam, in mg per mL, is approximately equivalent to the concentration of the *Assay stock preparation.*] Transfer a suitable quantity of USP Meloxicam RS, accurately weighed, to a 50-mL volumetric flask, dissolve in 1 mL of 1 N sodium hydroxide and 30 mL of methanol, and dilute with methanol to volume. Transfer 10 mL of the resulting solution to a 100-mL volumetric flask, add 10 mL of 1 N sodium hydroxide, and dilute with methanol to volume.

Standard preparation—Transfer 15 mL of the *Standard stock preparation* to a 25-mL volumetric flask, and dilute with water to volume.

Assay stock preparation—Transfer 10 Tablets to a 1000-mL volumetric flask, add about 100 mL of 1 N sodium hydroxide, shake to disperse the Tablets, and add 800 mL of methanol. Sonicate the solution for about 15 minutes, then stir for 30 minutes. Dilute with methanol to volume, and mix. Filter the resulting solution, and use the filtrate.

Assay preparation—Transfer 15 mL of the *Assay stock preparation* to a 25-mL volumetric flask, and dilute with water to volume.

Chromatographic system (see *Chromatography* ⟨621⟩)—The liquid chromatograph is equipped with a 254-nm detector, a guard column that contains packing L1, and a 4-mm ×10-cm column that contains packing L1. The flow rate is about 0.8 mL per minute. The column temperature is maintained at 40°. Chromatograph the *Standard preparation,* and record the peak responses as directed for *Procedure:* the tailing factor for the meloxicam peak is not more than 2.0; and the relative standard deviation for replicate injections is not more than 2.0%.

Procedure—Separately inject equal volumes (about 25 µL) of the *Standard preparation* and the *Assay preparation* to the chromatograph, record the chromatograms, and measure the responses for the meloxicam peak. Calculate the quantity, in mg, of meloxicam ($C_{14}H_{13}N_3O_4S_2$) in the portion of Tablets taken by the formula:

$$5000(C/3)(r_U / r_S)$$

in which C is the concentration, in mg per mL, of USP Meloxicam RS in the *Standard preparation;* and r_U and r_S are the peak responses obtained from the *Assay preparation* and the *Standard preparation,* respectively.

Melphalan

$C_{13}H_{18}Cl_2N_2O_2$ 305.20
L-Phenylalanine, 4-bis(2-chloroethyl)amino]-.
L-3-[*p*-[Bis(2-chloroethyl)amino]phenyl]alanine   [148-82-3].

» Melphalan contains not less than 93.0 percent and not more than 100.5 percent of $C_{13}H_{18}Cl_2N_2O_2$, calculated on the dried and ionizable chlorine-free basis.

Caution—Handle Melphalan with exceptional care because it is a highly potent agent.

Packaging and storage—Preserve in tight, light-resistant, glass containers.

USP Reference standards ⟨11⟩—USP Melphalan Hydrochloride RS.

Identification—

A: *Ultraviolet Absorption* ⟨197U⟩—
Solution: 5 µg per mL.
Medium: methanol.

B: To 1 mL of 1 in 10,000 solution in alcohol in a glass-stoppered test tube add 1 mL of pH 4.0 acid phthalate buffer (see under *Solutions* in the section *Reagents, Indicators, and Solutions*), 1 mL of a 1 in 20 solution of 4-(*p*-nitrobenzyl)pyridine in acetone, and 1 mL of saline TS. Heat on a water bath at 80° for 20 minutes, and cool quickly. Add 10 mL of alcohol and 1 mL of 1 N potassium hydroxide: a violet to red-violet color is produced.

C: Heat 100 mg with 10 mL of 0.1 N sodium hydroxide on a water bath for 10 minutes: the resulting solution, after acidification with 2 N nitric acid, responds to the tests for *Chloride* ⟨191⟩.

Specific rotation ⟨781S⟩: between −30° and −36°.
Test solution: 7 mg per mL, in methanol, prepared with the aid of gentle heating.

Loss on drying ⟨731⟩: Dry it in vacuum at 105° to constant weight: it loses not more than 7.0% of its weight.

Residue on ignition ⟨281⟩: not more than 0.3%.

Ionizable chlorine—Dissolve about 500 mg of Melphalan, accurately weighed, in a mixture of 75 mL of water and 2 mL of nitric acid, allow to stand for 2 minutes, and titrate with 0.1 N silver nitrate VS, determining the endpoint potentiometrically: not more than 1.0 mL of 0.1 N silver nitrate is required for each 500 mg of test specimen.

Nitrogen content ⟨461⟩—Determine the nitrogen content as directed under *Method II*, using about 325 mg of Melphalan, accurately weighed, and 0.1 N sulfuric acid VS for the titration: not less than 8.90% and not more than 9.45% of N is found, calculated on the dried basis.

Organic volatile impurities, *Method IV* ⟨467⟩: meets the requirements.

(Official until July 1, 2008)

Assay—Transfer to a beaker about 200 mg of Melphalan, accurately weighed, and dissolve in 20 mL of 0.5 N sodium hydroxide. Cover the beaker with a watch glass, and boil the solution for 30 minutes, adding water as necessary to maintain the volume. Cool, neutralize to phenolphthalein TS with acetic acid, and add 1 mL of acetic acid in excess. Titrate with 0.1 N silver nitrate VS, determining the endpoint potentiometrically, using silver and calomel electrodes, the latter modified to contain saturated potassium sulfate solution. From the results obtained in the test for *Ionizable chlorine*, calculate the volume, in mL, of 0.1 N silver nitrate that is equivalent to the ionizable chlorine in the quantity of Melphalan taken for the *Assay*, and subtract it from the *Assay* titration volume. Each mL of 0.1 N silver nitrate is equivalent to 15.26 mg of $C_{13}H_{18}Cl_2N_2O_2$.

Melphalan Tablets

» Melphalan Tablets contain not less than 90.0 percent and not more than 110.0 percent of the labeled amount of melphalan ($C_{13}H_{18}Cl_2N_2O_2$).

Packaging and storage—Preserve in well-closed, light-resistant, glass containers.

USP Reference standards ⟨11⟩—*USP Melphalan Hydrochloride RS.*

Identification—
A: The retention time of the major peak in the chromatogram of the *Assay preparation* corresponds to that in the chromatogram of the *Standard preparation*, as obtained in the *Assay*.
B: Shake a portion of finely powdered Tablets, equivalent to about 2 mg of melphalan, with 20 mL of alcohol, and filter: a 1-mL portion of the solution so obtained responds to *Identification* test B under *Melphalan*.

Dissolution ⟨711⟩—
Medium: 0.1 N hydrochloric acid; 900 mL.
Apparatus 2: 50 rpm.
Time: 30 minutes.
Determine the amount of $C_{13}H_{18}Cl_2N_2O_2$ dissolved by employing the following method.
Mobile phase—Prepare a filtered and degassed mixture of water, acetonitrile, ammonium acetate, glacial acetic acid, and triethylamine (1500 : 500 : 2 : 2 : 0.4). Make adjustments if necessary (see *System Suitability* under *Chromatography* ⟨621⟩).
Chromatographic system (see *Chromatography* ⟨621⟩)—The liquid chromatograph is equipped with a 254-nm detector and a 4.6-mm × 5-cm column that contains packing L7. The flow rate is about 1.5 mL per minute. Chromatograph replicate injections of the *Standard solution*, and record the peak responses as directed for *Procedure:* the relative standard deviation is not more than 3.0%.
Procedure—Inject a volume (about 50 µL) of a filtered portion of the solution under test into the chromatograph, record the chromatogram, and measure the response for the major peak. Calculate the quantity of $C_{13}H_{18}Cl_2N_2O_2$ dissolved in comparison with a Standard solution having a known concentration of USP Melphalan Hydrochloride RS in the same *Medium* and similarly chromatographed.

Tolerances—Not less than 80% *(Q)* of the labeled amount of $C_{13}H_{18}Cl_2N_2O_2$ is dissolved in 30 minutes.

Uniformity of dosage units ⟨905⟩: meet the requirements.

Procedure for content uniformity—Place 1 Tablet in a 200-mL volumetric flask, add 10 mL of water and 10 mL of alcohol, sonicate to dissolve the soluble components in the mixture, dilute with alcohol to volume, mix, and filter to obtain a clear solution. Dissolve an accurately weighed quantity of USP Melphalan Hydrochloride RS in alcohol to obtain a Standard solution having a known concentration of about 10 µg per mL. Concomitantly determine the absorbances of the solution from the Tablet and the Standard solution in 1-cm cells at the wavelength of maximum absorbance at about 260 nm, with a suitable spectrophotometer, using alcohol as the blank. Calculate the quantity, in mg, of melphalan ($C_{13}H_{18}Cl_2N_2O_2$) in the Tablet taken by the formula:

$$(305.20/341.66)(T/D)C(A_U/A_S)$$

in which 305.20 and 341.66 are the molecular weights of melphalan and melphalan hydrochloride, respectively; *T* is the labeled quantity, in mg, of melphalan in the Tablet; *D* is the concentration, in µg per mL, of melphalan in the solution from the Tablet, on the basis of the labeled quantity per Tablet and the extent of dilution; *C* is the concentration, in µg per mL, of USP Melphalan Hydrochloride RS in the Standard solution; and A_U and A_S are the absorbances of the solution from the Tablet and the Standard solution, respectively.

Assay—
Mobile phase—Prepare a solution of 0.025 M diethylamine in a mixture of methanol and water (1 : 1), adjust with 3.5 N hydrochloric acid to a pH of 5.5, filter, and degas. Make adjustments if necessary (see *System Suitability* under *Chromatography* ⟨621⟩).
Standard preparation—Dissolve an accurately weighed quantity of USP Melphalan Hydrochloride RS in alcohol, and quantitatively dilute with alcohol to obtain a solution having a known concentration of about 0.9 mg of melphalan hydrochloride per mL. Pipet 10 mL of this solution into a 100-mL volumetric flask containing 75 mL of alcohol and 2.0 mL of glacial acetic acid, dilute with alcohol to volume, and mix to obtain a *Standard preparation* having a known concentration of about 90 µg of USP Melphalan Hydrochloride RS per mL (equivalent to about 80 µg of melphalan per mL).
Assay preparation—Weigh and finely powder not fewer than 20 Tablets. Transfer an accurately weighed portion of the powder, equivalent to 8 mg of anhydrous melphalan, to a 100-mL volumetric flask. Add about 75 mL of alcohol and 2.0 mL of glacial acetic acid to the flask, and sonicate for 15 minutes. Cool, dilute with alcohol to volume, and mix. Filter through a medium-porosity, sintered-glass funnel, discarding the first few mL of the filtrate, and use the remainder of the filtrate as the *Assay preparation*.
Chromatographic system (see *Chromatography* ⟨621⟩)—The liquid chromatograph is equipped with a 254-nm detector and a 4.2-mm × 25-cm column that contains packing L7. The flow rate is about 1 mL per minute. Chromatograph the *Standard preparation*, and record the peak responses as directed for *Procedure*: the tailing factor for the analyte peak is not more than 2.0; and the relative standard deviation for replicate injections is not more than 2.0%.
Procedure—Separately inject equal volumes (between 10 and 20 µL) of the *Standard preparation* and the *Assay preparation* into the chromatograph, record the chromatograms, and measure the responses for the major peaks. Calculate the quantity, in mg, of melphalan ($C_{13}H_{18}Cl_2N_2O_2$) in the portion of Tablets taken by the formula:

$$(305.20/341.67)(0.1C)(r_U/r_S)$$

in which 305.20 and 341.67 are the molecular weights of melphalan and melphalan hydrochloride, respectively; *C* is the concentration, in µg per mL, of melphalan hydrochloride in the *Standard preparation*; and r_U and r_S are the peak responses obtained from the *Assay preparation* and the *Standard preparation*, respectively.

Menadiol Sodium Diphosphate

$C_{11}H_8Na_4O_8P_2 \cdot 6H_2O$ 530.17

1,4-Naphthalenediol, 2-methyl-, bis(dihydrogen phosphate), tetrasodium salt, hexahydrate.
2-Methyl-1,4-naphthalenediol bis(dihydrogen phosphate) tetrasodium salt, hexahydrate [6700-42-1].
Anhydrous 422.09 [131-13-5].

» Menadiol Sodium Diphosphate contains not less than 97.5 percent and not more than 102.0 percent of $C_{11}H_8Na_4O_8P_2$, calculated on the anhydrous basis.

Packaging and storage—Preserve in tight, light-resistant containers, and store in a cold place.

Identification—
  A: Dissolve about 200 mg of Menadiol Sodium Diphosphate in 10 mL of water, add 10 mL of 2 N sulfuric acid, 10 mL of 0.1 N ceric sulfate, and 1 mL of 30 percent hydrogen peroxide previously diluted with 5 mL of water, and extract the solution with two 10-mL portions of chloroform. Gently evaporate the clear chloroform solution on a steam bath to dryness, and dry the residue at 80° for 1 hour: the menadione so obtained melts between 104° and 107°.
  B: To 50 mg of the dried residue obtained in *Identification* test A add 5 mL of water, then add 75 mg of sodium bisulfite, and heat on a steam bath, shaking vigorously until the substance is dissolved and the solution is practically colorless. Dilute with water to 50 mL, and mix. To 2 mL of the solution add 2 mL of alcoholic ammonia (prepared by mixing equal volumes of alcohol and ammonium hydroxide), shake, and add 3 drops of ethyl cyanoacetate: a deep purplish blue color is produced, and on the addition of 1 mL of sodium hydroxide solution (1 in 3), it changes to green and then to yellow.
  C: To about 20 mg contained in a small beaker add 1 mL of water, 2 drops of nitric acid, and 1 mL of sulfuric acid, and heat slowly to the evolution of white fumes. Cool, cautiously dilute with water to about 10 mL, and filter if not clear. Render the filtrate slightly alkaline to litmus with 6 N ammonium hydroxide, then render it acid with nitric acid, and add to the warm solution 3 mL of ammonium molybdate TS: a yellow precipitate is formed within a few minutes.

Water, *Method I* ⟨921⟩: between 19.0% and 21.5%.

Assay—Dissolve about 100 mg of Menadiol Sodium Diphosphate, accurately weighed, in 25 mL of water, and add 25 mL of glacial acetic acid and 25 mL of 3 N hydrochloric acid. Titrate the solution with 0.02 N ceric sulfate VS, determining the endpoint potentiometrically using a calomel-platinum electrode system. Each mL of 0.02 N ceric sulfate is equivalent to 4.221 mg of $C_{11}H_8Na_4O_8P_2$.

Menadiol Sodium Diphosphate Injection

» Menadiol Sodium Diphosphate Injection is a sterile solution of Menadiol Sodium Diphosphate in Water for Injection. It contains not less than 95.0 percent and not more than 110.0 percent of the labeled amount of $C_{11}H_8Na_4O_8P_2 \cdot 6H_2O$.

Packaging and storage—Preserve in single-dose, light-resistant containers, preferably of Type I glass.

USP Reference standards ⟨11⟩—*USP Endotoxin RS. USP Menadione RS.*

Identification—
  A: Transfer a volume of Injection, equivalent to about 100 mg of menadiol sodium diphosphate, to a separator, add 10 mL of 2 N sulfuric acid, and extract with six 25-mL portions of ether, discarding the ether extracts. To the aqueous solution add 1 mL of 0.5 N ceric sulfate and 1 mL of 30 percent hydrogen peroxide, and extract with two 10-mL portions of chloroform. Evaporate the combined chloroform extracts on a steam bath just to dryness, then dry at 80° for 1 hour: the IR absorption spectrum of a potassium bromide dispersion of the menadione so obtained exhibits maxima at the same wavelengths as that of a similar preparation of USP Menadione RS. The solid also responds to *Identification* test B under *Menadiol Sodium Diphosphate*.
  B: Adjust, if necessary, a volume of Injection, equivalent to about 20 mg of menadiol sodium diphosphate, by evaporation or dilution with water, as required, to 2 mL: the solution responds to *Identification* test C under *Menadiol Sodium Diphosphate*.

Bacterial endotoxins ⟨85⟩—It contains not more than 25.0 USP Endotoxin Units per mg of menadiol sodium diphosphate.

pH ⟨791⟩: between 7.5 and 8.5.

Other requirements—It meets the requirements under *Injections* ⟨1⟩.

Assay—Transfer an accurately measured volume of Injection, equivalent to about 50 mg of menadiol sodium diphosphate, to a 125-mL separator, and extract with three 25-mL portions of chloroform, discarding the chloroform extracts. Transfer the aqueous solution to a 250-mL beaker, add 25 mL of glacial acetic acid and 25 mL of 3 N hydrochloric acid, vigorously bubble nitrogen through this solution for not less than 15 minutes, and titrate with 0.01 N ceric sulfate VS, determining the endpoint potentiometrically using a calomel-platinum electrode system. Each mL of 0.01 N ceric sulfate is equivalent to 2.651 mg of $C_{11}H_8Na_4O_8P_2 \cdot 6H_2O$.

Menadiol Sodium Diphosphate Tablets

» Menadiol Sodium Diphosphate Tablets contain not less than 95.0 percent and not more than 110.0 percent of the labeled amount of $C_{11}H_8Na_4O_8P_2 \cdot 6H_2O$.

Packaging and storage—Preserve in well-closed, light-resistant containers.

USP Reference standards ⟨11⟩ —*USP Menadione RS.*

Identification—
  A: Triturate a quantity of powdered Tablets, equivalent to about 100 mg of menadiol sodium diphosphate, with a mixture of 10 mL of water and 10 mL of 2 N sulfuric acid, centrifuge the mixture, and filter the supernatant. To the filtrate add 1 mL of 0.5 N ceric sulfate, mix, extract with 10 mL of chloroform, and centrifuge. Evaporate the chloroform extract on a steam bath just to dryness, then dry at 80° for 1 hour: the IR absorption spectrum of a potassium bromide dispersion of the menadione so obtained exhibits maxima at the same wavelengths as that of a similar preparation of USP Menadione RS.
  B: To 50 mg of the menadione obtained in *Identification* test A add 5 mL of water, then add 75 mg of sodium bisulfite, and heat on a steam bath, shaking vigorously until the substance is dissolved and the solution is almost colorless. Add water to make 50 mL, and mix. To 2 mL of the solution add 2 mL of alcoholic ammonia (prepared by mixing equal volumes of alcohol and ammonium hydroxide), shake, and add 3 drops of ethyl cyanoacetate: a deep purplish blue color is produced, and, on the addition of 1 mL of sodium hydroxide solution (1 in 3), it changes to green and then to yellow.
  C: Triturate a quantity of powdered Tablets, equivalent to about 20 mg of menadiol sodium diphosphate, with 10 mL of water, centrifuge the mixture, filter the supernatant, and evaporate to a volume of about 2 mL. Add 2 drops of nitric acid and 1 mL of sulfuric acid, and heat slowly to the evolution of white fumes. Cool, cautiously dilute with water to about 10 mL, and filter if not clear. Render the filtrate slightly alkaline to litmus with 6 N ammonium hydroxide, then render it acid with nitric acid, and add to the warm

solution 3 mL of ammonium molybdate TS: a yellow precipitate is formed within a few minutes.

Dissolution ⟨711⟩—
Medium: 0.1 N hydrochloric acid; 900 mL.
Apparatus 1: 100 rpm.
Time: 30 minutes.
Procedure—Determine the amount of $C_{11}H_8Na_4O_8P_2 \cdot 6H_2O$ dissolved from UV absorbances at the wavelength of maximum absorbance at about 227 nm on filtered portions of the solution under test, suitably diluted with *Medium*, in comparison with a standard solution prepared by dissolving in the same *Medium* an accurately weighed quantity of Menadiol Sodium Diphosphate, previously dried in vacuum over phosphorus pentoxide for 4 hours, the dried sample having a known concentration determined by titration with 0.01 N ceric sulfate VS as directed in the *Assay*.
Tolerances—Not less than 75% (*Q*) of the labeled amount of $C_{11}H_8Na_4O_8P_2 \cdot 6H_2O$ is dissolved in 30 minutes.

Uniformity of dosage units ⟨905⟩: meet the requirements.
Procedure for content uniformity—[NOTE—Use low-actinic glassware.] Transfer 1 finely powdered Tablet to a glass-stoppered centrifuge tube, add 25 mL of pH 8.0 phosphate buffer (see under *Solutions* in the section *Reagents, Indicators, and Solutions*), and shake vigorously for several minutes. Filter into a 50-mL volumetric flask, rinse the centrifuge tube, and filter with three 5-mL portions of pH 8.0 phosphate buffer, adding the rinsings to the volumetric flask, dilute with pH 8.0 phosphate buffer to volume, and mix. Dilute a portion of this solution quantitatively and stepwise, if necessary, with pH 8.0 phosphate buffer to provide a solution containing approximately 40 μg of menadiol sodium diphosphate per mL. Concomitantly determine the absorbances of this solution and of a solution of Menadiol Sodium Diphosphate, previously dried in vacuum over phosphorus pentoxide for 4 hours, in the same *Medium* having a known concentration of about 40 μg per mL, at the wavelength of maximum absorbance at about 297 nm, with a suitable spectrophotometer, using pH 8.0 phosphate buffer as the blank. Calculate the quantity, in mg, of $C_{11}N_8Na_4O_8P_2 \cdot 6H_2O$ in the Tablet taken by the formula:

$$(TC/D)(A_U/A_S)$$

in which *T* is the labeled quantity, in mg, of menadiol diphosphate in the Tablet, *C* is the concentration, in μg per mL, of $C_{11}H_8Na_4O_8P_2 \cdot 6H_2O$ in the Standard solution, *D* is the concentration, in μg per mL, of menadiol sodium diphosphate in the test solution, based upon the labeled quantity per Tablet and the extent of dilution, and A_U and A_S are the absorbances of the solution from the Tablet and the standard solution, respectively.

Assay—Weigh and finely powder not less than 20 Tablets. Transfer an accurately weighed portion of the powder, equivalent to about 50 mg of menadiol sodium diphosphate, to a 250-mL beaker. Moisten the powder with a few mL of glacial acetic acid, and then add sufficient of the acid to make 25 mL. Add 25 mL of 3 N hydrochloric acid and 25 mL of water, mix, and titrate with 0.01 N ceric sulfate VS, determining the endpoint potentiometrically using a calomel-platinum electrode system. Each mL of 0.01 N ceric sulfate is equivalent to 2.651 mg of $C_{11}H_8Na_4O_8P_2 \cdot 6H_2O$.

Menadione

$C_{11}H_8O_2$ 172.18
1,4-Naphthalenedione, 2-methyl-.
2-Methyl-1,4-naphthoquinone   [58-27-5].

» Menadione contains not less than 98.5 percent and not more than 101.0 percent of $C_{11}H_8O_2$, calculated on the dried basis.

Caution—Menadione powder is irritating to the respiratory tract and to the skin, and a solution of it in alcohol is a vesicant.

Packaging and storage—Preserve in well-closed, light-resistant containers. Store at 25°, excursions permitted between 15° and 30°.

USP Reference standards ⟨11⟩—*USP Menadione RS.*

Identification—
A: *Infrared Absorption ⟨197K⟩.*
B: *Ultraviolet Absorption ⟨197U⟩*—
Solution: 5 μg per mL.
Medium: alcohol.
Absorptivities at 250 nm, calculated on the dried basis, do not differ by more than 3.0%.

Melting range, Class I ⟨741⟩: between 105° and 107°.

Loss on drying ⟨731⟩—Dry it over silica gel for 4 hours: it loses not more than 0.3% of its weight.

Residue on ignition ⟨281⟩: not more than 0.1%.

Ordinary impurities ⟨466⟩—
Test solution: methanol.
Standard solution: methanol.
Eluant: chloroform.
Visualization: 1.

Assay—Accurately weigh about 150 mg of Menadione, and transfer to a 150-mL flask. Add 15 mL of glacial acetic acid and 15 mL of 3 N hydrochloric acid, and rotate the flask until the Menadione is dissolved. Then add about 3 g of zinc dust, close the flask with a stopper bearing a Bunsen valve, shake, and allow to stand in the dark for 1 hour, with frequent shaking. Rapidly decant the solution through a pledget of cotton into another flask, immediately wash the reduction flask with three 10-mL portions of freshly boiled and cooled water, add 0.1 mL of orthophenanthroline TS, and immediately titrate the combined filtrate and washings with 0.1 N ceric sulfate VS. Perform a blank determination, and make any necessary correction. Each mL of 0.1 N ceric sulfate is equivalent to 8.609 mg of $C_{11}H_8O_2$.

Menadione Injection

» Menadione Injection is a sterile solution of Menadione in oil. It contains not less than 90.0 percent and not more than 120.0 percent of the labeled amount of $C_{11}H_8O_2$.

Packaging and storage—Preserve in single-dose or in multiple-dose containers, preferably of Type I glass.

USP Reference standards ⟨11⟩—*USP Menadione RS. USP Endotoxin RS.*

Bacterial endotoxins ⟨85⟩—It contains not more than 58.3 USP Endotoxin Units per mg of menadione.

Other requirements—It meets the requirements under *Injections ⟨1⟩*.

Assay—[NOTE—Avoid exposing Menadione and its solutions to light throughout the *Assay*.]

Standard preparation—Transfer about 25 mg of USP Menadione RS, accurately weighed, to a 100-mL volumetric flask, dissolve in a mixture of equal volumes of alcohol and ether, dilute with the same mixture to volume, and mix. Keep the solution tightly closed in a dark, cool place, and use it within 7 days.

Assay preparation—Transfer an accurately measured volume of Injection, equivalent to about 25 mg of menadione, to a 100-mL volumetric flask, dilute with a mixture of equal volumes of ether and alcohol to volume, and mix.

Procedure—Transfer 1.0 mL each of the *Standard preparation* and the *Assay preparation* to separate 50-mL volumetric flasks, add to each 4 mL of alcohol, and mix. Then to each flask add 1.0 mL of a solution prepared by dissolving 50 mg of 2,4-dinitrophenylhydrazine in 20 mL of a mixture of 2 volumes of 3 N hydrochloric acid and 1 volume of water. Place the flasks in a bath maintained at 70° to 75° for 15 minutes, shaking vigorously every 2 to 3 minutes. Immediately after the heating, cool the flasks to about 25°; then add to each 5 mL of alcoholic ammonia, prepared by mixing equal volumes of alcohol and ammonium hydroxide. Shake the flasks thoroughly, add alcohol to make 50.0 mL, mix, allow to stand for 15 minutes, and decant from any separated oil. Determine the absorbances of the solutions, in 1-cm cells at the wavelength of maximum absorbance at about 635 nm, with a suitable spectrophotometer, using a reagent blank to set the instrument. Calculate the quantity, in mg, of $C_{11}H_8O_2$ in each mL of the Injection taken by the formula:

$$(0.1C/V)(A_U/A_S)$$

in which C is the concentration, in µg per mL, of USP Menadione RS in the *Standard preparation*, V is the volume, in mL, of Injection taken, and A_U and A_S are the absorbances of the solutions from the *Assay preparation* and the *Standard preparation*, respectively.

Menotropins

» Menotropins is an extract of human post-menopausal urine containing both follicle-stimulating hormone and luteinizing hormone, having the property in females of stimulating growth and maturation of ovarian follicles and the properties in males of maintaining and stimulating testicular interstitial cells (Leydig tissue) related to testosterone production and of being responsible for the full development and maturation of spermatozoa in the seminiferous tubules. It has a potency of not less than 40 USP Follicle-Stimulating Hormone Units and not less than 40 USP Luteinizing Hormone Units per mg, and it contains not less than 80 percent and not more than 125 percent of each of the hormone potencies stated on the label. The ratio of Units of Follicle-Stimulating Hormone to Units of Luteinizing Hormone is approximately 1. When necessary, Chorionic Gonadotropin obtained from the urine of pregnant women may be added to achieve this ratio. Not more than 30 percent of the luteinizing hormone activity is contributed by Chorionic Gonadotropin, as determined by a validated method.

Packaging and storage—Preserve in tight containers, preferably of Type I glass, and store in a refrigerator.

USP Reference standards ⟨11⟩—*USP Endotoxin RS. USP Human Chorionic Gonadotropin RS. USP Menotropins RS.*

Bacterial endotoxins ⟨85⟩—It contains not more than 2.5 Endotoxin Units per USP Follicle-Stimulating Hormone Unit.

Safety—Prepare a test solution of it in *Sodium Chloride Injection* containing 75 USP Follicle-Stimulating Hormone Units per mL. Select five healthy mice, each weighing between 18 g and 22 g. Inject intravenously one dose of 1.0 mL of the test solution into each of the mice. Observe the animals over the 48 hours following the injection. If, at the end of 48 hours, not more than 1 of the animals shows outward symptoms of a toxic reaction, the requirements of the test are met. If 1 or 2 of the animals die, repeat the test on 10 additional, similar animals; if all of the animals survive for 48 hours and show no symptoms of a toxic reaction, the requirements of the test are met.

Water, *Method I* ⟨921⟩: not more than 5.0%.

Assay for luteinizing hormone—

Diluent—Dissolve 10.75 g of dibasic sodium phosphate, 7.6 g of sodium chloride, and 1.0 g of bovine serum albumin in 1 L of freshly distilled water. Adjust with 1 N sodium hydroxide or dilute with 20% phosphoric acid to a pH of 7.2 ± 0.2.

Standard preparations—Dissolve an accurately weighed quantity of USP Menotropins RS in the *Diluent* to obtain solutions having known concentrations of about 8.75, 17.5, and 35.0 USP Luteinizing Hormone Units per mL.

Assay preparations—Following the procedure given under the *Standard preparations*, use Menotropins in place of the USP Reference Standard to obtain similar solutions.

Control solution—Use the *Diluent* as the control solution. Store all solutions at 5 ± 3° for the duration of the assay and properly dispose of any unused portions.

Test animals—Select 20- to 21-day old male rats with weights within a 10 g range of each other. House the animals under uniform conditions of temperature, light, food, and water. Mark the animals for identification, and divide them at random into 7 groups of the same number, having not less than 6 animals per group. Assign one group to each *Standard preparation*, one group to each *Assay preparation*, and one group to the *Control solution*.

Dose determination trial—Use the method described for *Procedure* to determine a 3-dose range in which the lowest dose produces a definite response in some of the rats in the low-dose group (as compared with the control group) and the highest dose produces a submaximal to maximal response in the high-dose group. Doses must be established in a geometric progression. The normal dose response range will occur between 3.5 and 28 USP Luteinizing Hormone Units total dose per rat. Useful dose ranges will vary with the sensitivity of the rat strain selected.

Procedure—Inject each rat of each group subcutaneously in the dorsal area with 0.2 mL of the solution to which it was assigned. For the *Dose determination trial* only, similarly inject each rat in the control group with 0.2 mL of the *Control solution*. Repeat these injections at approximately the same time of day after 24, 48, and 72 hours. Twenty-four hours after the last injection, weigh each rat, sacrifice the animals, and carefully dissect out the seminal vesicle of each rat, removing any fat and fibrous tissue. Thoroughly dry the vesicles by pressing against absorbent paper, avoiding damage to the vesicles, and immediately weigh them to the nearest 0.2 mg, using a suitable balance.

Calculation—Tabulate the observed seminal vesicle weights (*y*) for each dosage group of *f* rats. For apparently outlying seminal vesicle weights, an attempt may be made to correct the organ mass relative to the mass of the rat from which it was taken. For the *y*-value in question, calculate for each of the *f* rats in the appropriate group the ratio of seminal vesicle weight to total body weight. Reject the *y*-value if its corresponding ratio differs from the rest of the group by more than 1.5 standard deviations.

If the data from one or more rats are missing, adjust to groups of equal size by suitable means (see *Replacement of Missing Values* under *Design and Analysis of Biological Assays* ⟨111⟩). Total the values of *y* in each group, and designate each total as *T*, using subscripts 1 to 3 for the three successive dosage levels and subscripts *S* and *U* for the Standard and the material under test, respectively. Test both the agreement in slope of the dosage–response lines for the Standard and for the material under test, and the lack of curvature as directed for a 3-dose balanced assay (see *Tests of Assay Validity* under *Design and Analysis of Biological Assay* ⟨111⟩). If the combined discrepancy as measured by F_3 exceeds its tabular value in *Table 9*, repeat the assay.

Determine the logarithm of luteinizing hormone potency of the Menotropins taken by the formula:

$$M = (4iT_A/3T_B) + \log R,$$

in which $T_A = \Sigma(T_U - T_S)$; $T_B = \Sigma(T_3 - T_1)$; *i* is the interval between successive log doses of both the *Standard preparation* and the *Assay preparation;* and $R = v_S/v_U$ is the ratio of the high dose of the Standard in USP Luteinizing Hormone Units (v_S) to the high dose of the Menotropins in mg (v_U). Compute the log confidence interval (see *Design and Analysis of Biological Assays* ⟨111⟩).

Replication—Repeat the entire determination at least once. Test the agreement among the two or more independent determinations, and compute the weight for each (see *Combination of Independent Assays* ⟨111⟩). Calculate the weighted mean log-potency *M* and its confidence interval, L_C (see *Confidence Intervals for Individual Assays* ⟨111⟩). The potency, P_*, is satisfactory if P_* = antilog *M* is not less than 80% and not more than 125% of the labeled potency and if the confidence interval does not exceed 0.18.

Assay for follicle-stimulating hormone—
Diluting solution—Using the *Diluent* under *Assay for luteinizing hormone,* dissolve an accurately weighed quantity of USP Human Chorionic Gonadotropin RS to obtain a solution having a concentration of 70 USP Chorionic Gonadotropin Units per mL, readjusting the pH, if necessary, to 7.2 ± 0.2.

Standard preparations—Dissolve an accurately weighed quantity of USP Menotropins RS in the *Diluting solution* to obtain solutions having known concentrations of about 2.5, 5.0, and 10.0 USP Follicle-Stimulating Hormone Units per mL.

Assay preparations—Following the procedure given under the *Standard preparations,* use Menotropins in place of the USP Reference Standard to obtain similar solutions.

Control solution—Use the *Diluting solution* as the control solution. Store all solutions at 5 ± 3° for the duration of the assay, and properly dispose of any unused portions.

Test animals—Select 20- to 21-day old female rats with weights within a 10-g range of each other. Proceed as directed under *Test animals* in the *Assay for luteinizing hormone* beginning with "House the animals."

Dose determination trial—Use the method described for *Procedure* to determine a 3-dose range in which the lowest dose produces a definite response in some of the rats in the low-dose group (as compared with the control group) and the highest dose produces a submaximal to maximal response in the high-dose group. Doses must be established in a geometric progression. The normal dose response range will occur between 0.5 and 6.0 USP Follicle-Stimulating Hormone Units total dose per rat. Useful dose ranges will vary with the sensitivity of the rat strain selected.

Procedure—Inject each rat of each group subcutaneously in the dorsal area with 0.2 mL of the solution to which it was assigned. For *Dose determination trial* only, similarly inject each rat in the control group with 0.2 mL of the *Control solution.* Repeat these injections at approximately the same time of day after 24 hours and 48 hours. Twenty-four hours after the last injection, weigh each rat, sacrifice the animals, and carefully dissect out the ovaries of each rat, removing any fat and fibrous tissue. Thoroughly dry the ovaries by pressing against absorbent paper, avoiding damage to follicles on the ovary surface, and immediately weigh them to the nearest 0.2 mg, using a suitable balance.

Calculation—Tabulate the observed ovarian pair weight for each rat designated by the symbol y, for each dosage group of f rats. For apparently outlying ovarian weight gain, an attempt may be made to correct the organ mass relative to the mass of the rat from which it was taken. For the y-value in question, calculate for each of the f rats in the appropriate group the ratio of ovarian weight to the total body weight. Reject the y-value if its corresponding ratio differs from the rest of the group by more than 1.5 standard deviations.

If the data from one or more rats are missing, adjust to groups of equal size by suitable means (see *Replacement of Missing Values* under *Design and Analysis of Biological Assays* ⟨111⟩). Total the values of y in each group, and designate each total as T, using subscripts 1 to 3 for the three successive dosage levels and subscripts S and U for the Standard and the material under test, respectively. Test both the agreement in slope of the dosage-response lines for the Standard and for the material under test, and the lack of curvature as directed for a 3-dose balanced assay (see *Tests of Assay Validity* under *Design and Analysis of Biological Assays* ⟨111⟩). If the combined discrepancy as measured by F_3 exceeds its tabular value in *Table 9* (see *Combination of Independent Assays* under *Design and Analysis of Biological Assays* ⟨111⟩), regard these data as preliminary, and repeat the assay.

Determine the logarithm of follicle-stimulating hormone potency of the Menotropins taken by the formula:

$$M = (4iT_A / 3T_B) + \log R,$$

in which $T_A = \Sigma(T_U - T_S)$; $T_B = \Sigma(T_3 - T_1)$; i is the interval between successive log doses of both the *Standard preparation* and *Assay preparation;* and $R = v_S / v_U$ is the ratio of the high dose of the Standard in USP Units (v_S) to the high dose of the Menotropins in mg (v_U). Compute the log confidence interval (see *Design and Analysis of Biological Assays* ⟨111⟩).

Replication—Repeat the entire determination at least once. Test the agreement among the two or more independent determinations, and compute the weights/mean log-potency M and its confidence interval, L_C (see *Confidence Intervals for Individual Assays* under *Design and Analysis of Biological Assays* ⟨111⟩). If this exceeds 0.18, repeat the assay until the confidence interval of the combined results is 0.18 or less.

The potency P_* is satisfactory if $P_* =$ antilog M is not less than 80% and not more than 125% of the labeled potency and if the log confidence interval does not exceed 0.18.

Menotropins for Injection

» Menotropins for Injection is a sterile, freeze-dried mixture of menotropins and suitable excipients. Its potency is not less than 80 percent and not more than 125 percent of each of the Follicle-stimulating Hormone and Luteinizing Hormone potencies stated on the label. It may contain an antimicrobial agent.

Packaging and storage—Preserve in *Containers for Sterile Solids* as described under *Injections* ⟨1⟩.

USP Reference standards ⟨11⟩—*USP Endotoxin RS. USP Human Chorionic Gonadotropin RS. USP Menotropins RS.*

Constituted solution—At the time of use, it meets the requirements for *Constituted Solutions* under *Injections* ⟨1⟩.

Bacterial endotoxins ⟨85⟩—It contains not more than 2.5 USP Endotoxin Units per USP Follicle-stimulating Hormone Unit.

pH ⟨791⟩: between 6.0 and 7.0, in the solution constituted as directed in the labeling.

Uniformity of dosage units ⟨905⟩—Open 10 containers and accurately weigh each individual container and its contents, taking care to preserve the identity of each container. Remove the contents of each container by rinsing thoroughly with water, dry at 105° to constant weight, and reweigh. Calculate for each container the net weight of its contents by subtracting the weight of the dry, empty container from its initial gross weight. Determine the average weight of the contents and the relative standard deviation (see *Calculation of the Relative Standard Deviation* under *Uniformity of Dosage Units* ⟨905⟩). The requirements are met if the weight of the contents of each container does not deviate from the average weight by more than 5.0% and the relative standard deviation of the 10 containers is not greater than 3.0%. If the requirements of the test are not met, test 20 additional containers. The requirements are met if the net weight of not more than 1 container of the 30 deviates by more than 7.5% from the average weight of the contents of the 30 containers and the relative standard deviation of the 30 containers is not greater than 3.3%.

Other requirements—It meets the requirements for *Sterility Tests* ⟨71⟩ and *Labeling* under *Injections* ⟨1⟩.

Assay—Using an *Assay preparation* obtained by diluting a portion of the solution constituted as directed in the labeling, proceed with Menotropins for Injection as directed in the *Assay for luteinizing hormone* and the *Assay for follicle-stimulating hormone* under *Menotropins.*

Menthol

$C_{10}H_{20}O$ 156.27
Cyclohexanol, 5-methyl-2-(1-methylethyl)-   [1490-04-6].

» Menthol is an alcohol obtained from diverse mint oils or prepared synthetically. Menthol may be levorotatory (*l*-Menthol), from natural or synthetic sources, or racemic (*dl*-Menthol).

Packaging and storage—Preserve in tight containers, preferably at controlled room temperature.

Labeling—Label it to indicate whether it is levorotatory or racemic.

Identification—When it is triturated with about an equal weight of camphor, of chloral hydrate, or of phenol, the mixture liquefies.

Melting range of *l*-Menthol ⟨741⟩: between 41° and 44°.

Congealing range of *dl*-Menthol ⟨651⟩—[NOTE—Perform this test preferably in a room having a temperature below 30° and a relative humidity below 50%.] Place about 10 g of racemic Menthol, previously dried in a desiccator over silica gel for 24 hours, in a dry test tube of from 18- to 20-mm internal diameter, and melt the contents at a temperature of about 40°. Suspend the test tube in water having a temperature of 23° to 25°, and stir the contents of the tube continually with a thermometer, keeping the bulb of the thermometer immersed in the liquid. Racemic Menthol congeals at a temperature between 27° and 28°. Shortly after the temperature has stabilized at the congealing point, add a few mg of dried racemic Menthol to the congealed mass, and continue the stirring: after a few minutes the temperature of the mass quickly rises to 30.5° to 32.0°.

Specific rotation ⟨781S⟩: between −45° and −51° for *l*-Menthol; between −2° and +2° for *dl*-Menthol.

Test solution: 100 mg per mL, in alcohol.

Limit of nonvolatile residue—Volatilize 2 g, accurately weighed, in a tared open porcelain dish on a steam bath, and dry the residue at 105° for 1 hour: the residue weighs not more than 1 mg (0.05%).

Chromatographic purity—

System suitability preparation—Dissolve decanol and Menthol in ether to obtain a solution having concentrations of about 0.05 mg of each per mL.

Test preparation—Dissolve 10 mg of Menthol in 50 mL of ether, and mix. Dilute 25 mL of this solution with ether to 100 mL, and mix.

Chromatographic system—The gas chromatograph is equipped with a flame-ionization detector and contains a 1.8-m × 2-mm column packed with 10% phase G16 on support S1AB. The column is maintained at about 170°, the injection port is maintained at about 260°, and the detector block is maintained at about 240°. Dry helium is used as the carrier gas at a flow rate of about 50 mL per minute. Chromatograph the *System suitability preparation*, and record the peak responses as directed under *Procedure:* the retention time of menthol is about 0.7 relative to decanol. In a suitable chromatogram, the resolution, *R*, of the 2 peaks is not less than 2.5, and the relative standard deviation of the ratio of the peak response obtained with menthol to that obtained with decanol is not more than 2%.

Procedure—Inject about 2 µL of the *Test preparation* into the gas chromatograph, and measure the peak responses. The peak response due to menthol is not less than 97% of the sum of all the peak responses, excluding any due to the ether.

Readily oxidizable substances in *dl*-Menthol—Place 500 mg of *dl*-Menthol in a clean, dry test tube, add 10 mL of a solution of potassium permanganate, prepared by diluting 3 mL of 0.1 N potassium permanganate with water to 100 mL, and place the test tube in a beaker of water at a temperature between 45° and 50°. Remove the tube from the bath at intervals of 30 seconds, and mix quickly by shaking: the purple color of potassium permanganate is still apparent after 5 minutes.

Organic volatile impurities, *Method V* ⟨467⟩: meets the requirements.

Solvent—Use dimethyl sulfoxide.

(Official until July 1, 2008)

Menthol Lozenges

» Menthol Lozenges contain not less than 90.0 percent and not more than 125.0 percent of the labeled amount of $C_{10}H_{20}O$, in a suitable molded base.

Packaging and storage—Preserve in well-closed containers.

USP Reference standards ⟨11⟩—*USP Menthol RS.*

Identification—The retention time of the menthol peak in the chromatogram of the *Assay preparation* corresponds to that in the chromatogram of the *Standard preparation*, obtained as directed in the *Assay*.

Assay—

Sodium chloride solution—Dissolve 250 g of sodium chloride in water to make 1000 mL.

Internal standard solution—Dissolve suitable quantities of anethole in hexanes to obtain a solution having a concentration of about 2 mg per mL.

Standard preparation—Dissolve an accurately weighed quantity of USP Menthol RS in *Internal standard solution* to obtain a solution having a known concentration of about 0.20*L* mg per mL, *L* being the labeled quantity, in mg, of menthol in each Lozenge.

Assay preparation—Transfer 20 Lozenges to a 1-liter screw-capped conical flask. [NOTE—Use caps with inert white rubber liners.] Add 200 mL of water, 260 mL of *Sodium chloride solution*, and 100.0 mL of *Internal standard solution*, and shake by mechanical means for 30 minutes. Allow the phases to separate, and transfer a portion of the hexanes phase to a suitable container.

Chromatographic system (see *Chromatography* ⟨621⟩)—The gas chromatograph is equipped with a flame-ionization detector, a split injection system with a split ratio of about 10 : 1, and a 0.53-mm × 30-m fused silica column coated with a 1-µm layer of G16 stationary phase. The column is maintained isothermally at about 125°, and the injection port and the detector block are maintained at about 250°. The carrier gas is helium at a flow rate of about 10 mL per minute. Chromatograph the *Standard preparation*, and record the peak responses as directed for *Procedure:* the relative retention times are about 0.5 for menthol and 1.0 for anethole, the resolution, *R*, between the menthol and the anethole peaks is not less than 15, the tailing factor for the menthol and anethole peaks is not more than 2.0, and the relative standard deviation for replicate injections is not more than 2.0%.

Procedure—Separately inject equal volumes (about 1 µL) of the *Standard preparation* and the *Assay preparation* into the gas chromatograph, and measure the responses for the menthol and anethole peaks. Calculate the quantity, in mg, of $C_{10}H_{20}O$ in each Lozenge taken by the formula:

$$5C(R_U / R_S)$$

in which *C* is the concentration, in mg per mL, of USP Menthol RS in the *Standard preparation*, and R_U and R_S are the ratios of the menthol peak to the anethole peak obtained from the *Assay preparation* and the *Standard preparation*, respectively.

Meperidine Hydrochloride

$C_{15}H_{21}NO_2 \cdot HCl$ 283.79

4-Piperidinecarboxylic acid, 1-methyl-4-phenyl-, ethyl ester, hydrochloride.

Ethyl 1-methyl-4-phenylisonipecotate hydrochloride [*50-13-5*].

» Meperidine Hydrochloride contains not less than 98.0 percent and not more than 102.0 percent of $C_{15}H_{21}NO_2 \cdot$ HCl, calculated on the dried basis.

Packaging and storage—Preserve in well-closed, light-resistant containers, and store at room temperature.

USP Reference standards ⟨11⟩—*USP Meperidine Hydrochloride RS.*

Identification—

A: It meets the requirements under *Identification—Organic Nitrogenous Bases* ⟨181⟩.

B: A solution (1 in 100) responds to the tests for *Chloride* ⟨191⟩.

C: The retention time of the major peak in the chromatogram of the *Assay preparation* corresponds to that in the chromatogram of the *Standard preparation*, as obtained in the *Assay*.

Melting range ⟨741⟩: between 186° and 189°, determined after drying in vacuum at 80° for 4 hours.

Loss on drying ⟨731⟩—Dry it in vacuum at a pressure between 20 to 40 mm of mercury at 80° for 4 hours: it loses not more than 1.0% of its weight.

Residue on ignition ⟨281⟩: not more than 0.1%.

Chromatographic purity—Dissolve it in water to obtain a solution containing about 10 mg per mL. Inject 2.0 µL of the solution into a suitable gas chromatograph equipped with a flame-ionization detector. Under typical conditions, the instrument contains a 2-mm × 2-m glass column packed with 10% phase G3 on support S1A. Maintain the temperature of the column at 190°, the injection port at 255°, and the detector at 280°. Use helium as the carrier gas at a flow rate of 28 mL per minute. Calculate the area percentage of each peak observed in the chromatogram. No peak, other than the principal peak (except for the solvent peak), constitutes more than 1.0% of the total area.

Organic volatile impurities, *Method I* ⟨467⟩: meets the requirements.

(Official until July 1, 2008)

Chloride content—Accurately weigh about 500 mg, previously dried, and transfer to a 250-mL conical flask. Add 15 mL of water, 5 mL of glacial acetic acid, 50 mL of methanol, and 0.2 mL of eosin Y TS, and titrate with 0.1 N silver nitrate VS to a rose-colored endpoint. Each mL of 0.1 N silver nitrate is equivalent to 3.545 mg of Cl. Not less than 12.2% and not more than 12.7% of Cl is found.

Assay—

Buffer solution—Transfer about 6.8 g of monobasic potassium phosphate to a 1000-mL volumetric flask. Dissolve in and dilute with water to volume. Add 10 mL of triethylamine, and mix. Adjust with phosphoric acid to a pH of 7.0, and filter.

Mobile phase—Prepare a filtered and degassed mixture of acetonitrile and *Buffer solution* (55 : 45). Make adjustments if necessary (see *System Suitability* under *Chromatography* ⟨621⟩).

Standard preparation—Transfer an accurately weighed quantity of about 30 mg of USP Meperidine Hydrochloride RS to a 50-mL volumetric flask, dissolve in and dilute with water to volume, and mix. Transfer 5.0 mL of this solution to a 25-mL volumetric flask, dilute with *Mobile phase* to volume, and mix.

Assay preparation—Transfer an accurately weighed quantity of about 30 mg of Meperidine Hydrochloride to a 50-mL volumetric flask, dissolve in and dilute with water to volume, and mix. Transfer 5.0 mL of this solution to a 25-mL volumetric flask, dilute with *Mobile phase* to volume, and mix.

Chromatographic system (see *Chromatography* ⟨621⟩)—The liquid chromatograph is equipped with a 230-nm detector and a 3.9-mm × 30-cm column that contains packing L1. The flow rate is about 1 mL per minute. Chromatograph the *Standard preparation*, and record the peak responses as directed for *Procedure*: the column efficiency is not less than 2000 theoretical plates; the tailing factor for the meperidine peak is not more than 2; and the relative standard deviation for replicate injections is not more than 2%.

Procedure—Separately inject equal volumes (about 20 µL) of the *Standard preparation* and the *Assay preparation* into the chromatograph, record the chromatograms, and measure the peak responses. Calculate the quantity, in mg, of $C_{15}H_{21}NO_2 \cdot HCl$ in the portion of Meperidine Hydrochloride taken by the formula:

$$250C(r_U/r_S)$$

in which C is the concentration, in mg per mL, of USP Meperidine Hydrochloride RS in the *Standard preparation*; and r_U and r_S are the meperidine peak responses obtained from the *Assay preparation* and the *Standard preparation*, respectively.

Meperidine Hydrochloride Injection

» Meperidine Hydrochloride Injection is a sterile solution of Meperidine Hydrochloride in Water for Injection. It contains not less than 95.0 percent and not more than 105.0 percent of the labeled amount of $C_{15}H_{21}NO_2 \cdot HCl$.

Packaging and storage—Preserve in single-dose or in multiple-dose containers, preferably of Type I glass.

USP Reference standards ⟨11⟩—*USP Endotoxin RS. USP Meperidine Hydrochloride RS.*

Identification—

A: It meets the requirements under *Identification—Organic Nitrogenous Bases* ⟨181⟩.

B: The retention time of the major peak in the chromatogram of the *Assay preparation* corresponds to that obtained from the *Standard preparation* obtained in the *Assay*.

Bacterial endotoxins ⟨85⟩—It contains not more than 2.4 USP Endotoxin Units per mg of meperidine hydrochloride.

pH ⟨791⟩: between 3.5 and 6.0.

Other requirements—It meets the requirements under *Injections* ⟨1⟩.

Assay—

Buffer solution, Mobile phase, Chromatographic system, and *Standard preparation*—Proceed as directed in the *Assay* under *Meperidine Hydrochloride*.

Assay preparation—Transfer an accurately measured volume of Injection, equivalent to about 300 mg to a 100-mL volumetric flask, dilute with water to volume, and mix. Transfer 1.0 mL of this solution to a 25-mL volumetric flask, dilute with *Mobile phase* to volume, and mix.

Procedure—Separately inject equal volumes (about 20 µL) of the *Standard preparation* and the *Assay preparation* into the chromatograph, record the chromatograms, and measure the peak responses. Calculate the quantity, in mg, of $C_{15}H_{21}NO_2 \cdot HCl$ in the volume of Injection taken by the formula:

$$2500Cr_U/r_S$$

in which C is the concentration, in mg per mL, of USP Meperidine Hydrochloride RS in the *Standard preparation*, and r_U and r_S are the meperidine peak responses obtained from the *Assay preparation* and the *Standard preparation*, respectively.

Meperidine Hydrochloride Oral Solution

» Meperidine Hydrochloride Oral Solution contains not less than 95.0 percent and not more than 105.0 percent of the labeled amount of meperidine hydrochloride ($C_{15}H_{21}NO_2 \cdot HCl$).

Packaging and storage—Preserve in tight, light-resistant containers.

USP Reference standards ⟨11⟩—*USP Meperidine Hydrochloride RS.*

Identification—Transfer a volume of Oral Solution, equivalent to about 100 mg of meperidine hydrochloride, to a 125-mL separator, add 40 mL of water and 3 mL of 1 N sodium hydroxide, and extract with three 25-mL portions of *n*-hexane. Wash the combined extracts with two 20-mL portions of water, discard the water, and then extract with three 25-mL portions of 0.1 N hydrochloric acid. Transfer the extracts to a 100-mL volumetric flask, dilute with 0.1 N hydrochloric acid to volume, and mix: the UV absorption spectrum of this solution exhibits maxima and minima at the same wavelengths as that of a similar preparation of USP Meperidine Hydrochloride RS, concomitantly measured.

Uniformity of dosage units ⟨905⟩—
FOR ORAL SOLUTION PACKAGED IN SINGLE-UNIT CONTAINERS: meets the requirements.
Deliverable volume ⟨698⟩—
FOR ORAL SOLUTION PACKAGED IN MULTIPLE-UNIT CONTAINERS: meets the requirements.
pH ⟨791⟩: between 3.5 and 4.1.
Assay—Transfer an accurately measured volume of Oral Solution, equivalent to about 250 mg of meperidine hydrochloride, to a separator, and add 3 mL of 1 N sodium hydroxide. Extract with five 20-mL portions of chloroform, and filter the extracts through a pledget of cotton into a 250-mL conical flask. Wash the cotton with 5 mL of chloroform, and add the washing to the combined filtrates. Add 10 mL of glacial acetic acid and 2 drops of crystal violet TS, and titrate with 0.1 N perchloric acid VS to a blue endpoint. Perform a blank determination, and make any necessary correction. Each mL of 0.1 N perchloric acid is equivalent to 28.38 mg of meperidine hydrochloride ($C_{15}H_{21}NO_2 \cdot HCl$).

Meperidine Hydrochloride Tablets

» Meperidine Hydrochloride Tablets contain not less than 95.0 percent and not more than 105.0 percent of the labeled amount of $C_{15}H_{21}NO_2 \cdot HCl$.

Packaging and storage—Preserve in well-closed, light-resistant containers.

USP Reference standards ⟨11⟩—*USP Meperidine Hydrochloride RS.*

Identification—
  A: Transfer a quantity of powdered Tablets, equivalent to about 50 mg of meperidine hydrochloride, to a separator, add 10 mL of water, and shake. Add 5 mL of saturated sodium chloride solution and 1 mL of sodium hydroxide solution (1 in 25). Extract with three 20-mL portions of chloroform, filtering the extracts through cotton overlaid with anhydrous sodium sulfate. Evaporate the chloroform on a steam bath, and dissolve the residue in 4 mL of carbon disulfide. In a second separator, prepare a similar solution, using 50 mg of USP Meperidine Hydrochloride RS. Proceed as directed under *Identification—Organic Nitrogenous Bases* ⟨181⟩, beginning with "Determine the absorption spectra."
  B: The retention time of the major peak in the chromatogram of the *Assay preparation* corresponds to that obtained in the *Standard preparation* obtained in the *Assay.*

Dissolution ⟨711⟩—
  Medium: water; 500 mL.
  Apparatus 1: 100 rpm.
  Time: 45 minutes.
  Procedure—Determine the amount of $C_{15}H_{21}NO_2 \cdot HCl$ dissolved employing the procedure set forth in the *Assay*, using filtered portions of the solution under test, suitably diluted with *Dissolution Medium*, if necessary, in comparison with a Standard solution having a known concentration of USP Meperidine Hydrochloride RS in the same *Medium.*
  Tolerances—Not less than 75% (*Q*) of the labeled amount of $C_{15}H_{21}NO_2 \cdot HCl$ is dissolved in 45 minutes.

Uniformity of dosage units ⟨905⟩—meet the requirements.

Assay—
  Buffer solution, Mobile phase, Chromatographic system, and *Standard preparation*—Proceed as directed in the *Assay* under *Meperidine Hydrochloride.*
  Assay preparation—Weigh and grind not less than 20 Tablets to a fine powder. Transfer an accurately weighed portion of the powder, equivalent to about 60 mg of meperidine hydrochloride, to a 100-mL volumetric flask, add about 70 mL of *Mobile phase*, and sonicate for 10 minutes with occasional shaking. Shake by mechanical means for about 30 minutes, dilute with *Mobile phase* to volume, mix, and filter. Transfer 5.0 mL of the filtered solution to a 25-mL volumetric flask, dilute with *Mobile phase* to volume, and mix.
  Procedure—Proceed as directed for *Procedure* in the *Assay* under *Meperidine Hydrochloride.* Calculate the quantity, in mg, of $C_{15}H_{21}NO_2 \cdot HCl$ in the portion of Tablets taken by the formula:

$$500C(r_U / r_S)$$

in which *C* is the concentration, in mg per mL, of USP Meperidine Hydrochloride RS in the *Standard preparation*, and r_U and r_S are the meperidine peak responses obtained from the *Assay preparation* and the *Standard preparation,* respectively.

Mephenytoin

$C_{12}H_{14}N_2O_2$ 218.26
2,4-Imidazolidinedione, 5-ethyl-3-methyl-5-phenyl-, (±)-.
(±)-5-Ethyl-3-methyl-5-phenylhydantoin   [50-12-4].

» Mephenytoin contains not less than 98.0 percent and not more than 102.0 percent of $C_{12}H_{14}N_2O_2$, calculated on the dried basis.

Packaging and storage—Preserve in tight containers, and store at controlled room temperature.

USP Reference standards ⟨11⟩—*USP Mephenytoin RS.*

Identification—
  A: *Infrared Absorption* ⟨197K⟩.
  B: *Ultraviolet Absorption* ⟨197U⟩—
  Solution: 1 mg per mL.
  Medium: methanol.

Melting range ⟨741⟩: between 136° and 140°.
Loss on drying ⟨731⟩—Dry it at 105° for 4 hours: it loses not more than 1.0% of its weight.
Residue on ignition ⟨281⟩: not more than 0.1%.
Heavy metals, *Method II* ⟨231⟩: 0.002%.

Chromatographic purity—
  Mobile phase and *System suitability solution*—Proceed as directed in the *Assay.*
  Test preparation—Use the *Assay preparation.*
  Chromatographic system—Proceed as directed in the *Assay* except to use a 225-nm detector.
  Procedure—Inject a volume (about 10 µL) of the *Test preparation* into the chromatograph, record the chromatogram, and measure the peak responses. Calculate the percentage of each impurity in the portion of Mephenytoin taken by the formula:

$$100(Fr_i / r_s)$$

in which *F* is the relative response factor and is equal to 1.16 for any peak with a relative retention time of 0.66, 0.37 for propiophenone, and 1.0 for all other peaks; r_i is the peak response for each impurity; and r_s is the sum of the responses of all of the peaks, adjusted for the relative response factor: not more than 1.0% of any individual impurity is found, and not more than 1.5% of total impurities is found.

Organic volatile impurities, *Method V* ⟨467⟩: meets the requirements.
  Solvent: dimethyl sulfoxide.

(Official until July 1, 2008)

Assay—
  Mobile phase—Prepare a filtered and degassed mixture of water, methanol, and acetonitrile (52 : 38 : 10). Make adjustments if necessary (see *System Suitability* under *Chromatography* ⟨621⟩).
  System suitability solution—Transfer about 7.5 mg of propiophenone, accurately weighed, to a 50-mL volumetric flask, dissolve in and dilute with *Mobile phase* to volume, and mix. Transfer 1.0 mL of this solution to a 10-mL volumetric flask, add about 15 mg of Mephenytoin, dissolve in *Mobile phase*, sonicate, dilute with *Mobile phase* to volume, and mix.

Standard preparation—Dissolve an accurately weighed quantity of USP Mephenytoin RS in *Mobile phase*, sonicate, and dilute quantitatively, and stepwise if necessary, with *Mobile phase* to obtain a solution having a known concentration of about 5.0 mg per mL.

Assay preparation—Transfer about 125.0 mg of Mephenytoin, accurately weighed, to a 25-mL volumetric flask, dissolve in *Mobile phase*, sonicate, dilute with *Mobile phase* to volume, and mix.

Chromatographic system (see *Chromatography* ⟨621⟩)—The liquid chromatograph is equipped with a 257-nm detector and a 3.9-mm × 15-cm column that contains packing L7. The flow rate is about 1 mL per minute. Chromatograph the *System suitability solution*, and record the peak responses as directed for *Procedure*: the relative retention times are about 1.0 for mephenytoin and 1.5 for propiophenone; the column efficiency is not less than 4000 theoretical plates for the mephenytoin peak; and the relative standard deviation for replicate injections for the mephenytoin peak is not more than 2.0%.

Procedure—Separately inject equal volumes (about 10 µL) of the *Standard preparation* and the *Assay preparation* into the chromatograph, record the chromatograms, and measure the responses for the major peaks. Calculate the quantity, in mg, of $C_{12}H_{14}N_2O_2$ in the portion of Mephenytoin taken by the formula:

$$25C(r_U/r_S)$$

in which C is the concentration, in mg per mL, of USP Mephenytoin RS in the *Standard preparation*; and r_U and r_S are the peak responses obtained from the *Assay preparation* and the *Standard preparation*, respectively.

Mephenytoin Tablets

» Mephenytoin Tablets contain not less than 90.0 percent and not more than 110.0 percent of the labeled amount of mephenytoin ($C_{12}H_{14}N_2O_2$).

Packaging and storage—Preserve in tight containers, and store at controlled room temperature.

USP Reference standards ⟨11⟩—*USP Mephenytoin RS.*
Dissolution ⟨711⟩—
  Medium: water; 500 mL.
  Apparatus 2: 75 rpm.
  Time: 60 minutes.
  Procedure—Determine the amount of $C_{12}H_{14}N_2O_2$ dissolved by employing UV absorption at the wavelength of maximum absorbance at about 257 nm on filtered portions of the solution under test, suitably diluted with *Dissolution Medium*, if necessary, in comparison with a Standard solution having a known concentration of USP Mephenytoin RS in the same *Medium*.
  Tolerances—Not less than 70% (Q) of the labeled amount of $C_{12}H_{14}N_2O_2$ is dissolved in 60 minutes.
Uniformity of dosage units ⟨905⟩: meet the requirements.
Chromatographic purity—
  Mobile phase and *System suitability solution*—Proceed as directed in the *Assay* under *Mephenytoin*.
  Test preparation—Use the *Assay preparation*.
  Chromatographic system—Proceed as directed in the *Assay* under *Mephenytoin* except to use a 225-nm detector.
  Procedure—Inject a volume (about 10 µL) of the *Test preparation* into the chromatograph, record the chromatogram, and measure the peak responses. Calculate the percentage of each impurity in the portion of Tablets taken by the formula:

$$100(Fr_i/r_s)$$

in which F is the relative response factor and is equal to 1.16 for any peak with a relative retention time of 0.66, 0.37 for propiophenone, and 1.0 for all other peaks; r_i is the peak response for each impurity; and r_s is the sum of the responses of all of the peaks, adjusted for the relative response factor: not more than 1.0% of any individual impurity is found, and not more than 2.0% of total impurities is found.

Assay—
  Mobile phase, *System suitability solution*, *Standard preparation*, and *Chromatographic system*—Proceed as directed in the *Assay* under *Mephenytoin*.
  Assay preparation—Weigh and finely powder not fewer than 20 Tablets. Transfer an amount of powder, equivalent to about 500 mg of mephenytoin, accurately weighed, to a 100-mL volumetric flask, add about 60 mL of *Mobile phase*, sonicate for 10 minutes, and shake by mechanical means for 30 minutes. Dilute with *Mobile phase* to volume, mix, and filter, discarding a suitable portion of the filtrate.
  Procedure—Separately inject equal volumes (about 10 µL) of the *Standard preparation* and the *Assay preparation* into the chromatograph, record the chromatograms, and measure the responses for the major peaks. Calculate the quantity, in mg, of mephenytoin ($C_{12}H_{14}N_2O_2$) in the portion of Tablets taken by the formula:

$$25C(r_U/r_S)$$

in which C is the concentration, in mg per mL, of USP Mephenytoin RS in the *Standard preparation*; and r_U and r_S are the peak responses obtained from the *Assay preparation* and the *Standard preparation*, respectively.

Mephobarbital

$C_{13}H_{14}N_2O_3$ 246.26
2,4,6(1H,3H,5H)-Pyrimidinetrione, 5-ethyl-1-methyl-5-phenyl-.
5-Ethyl-1-methyl-5-phenylbarbituric acid   [115-38-8].

» Mephobarbital contains not less than 98.0 percent and not more than 100.5 percent of $C_{13}H_{14}N_2O_3$, calculated on the dried basis.

Packaging and storage—Preserve in well-closed containers.

USP Reference standards ⟨11⟩—*USP Mephobarbital RS.*
Identification—
  A: *Infrared Absorption* ⟨197M⟩.
  B: Boil about 200 mg with 10 mL of 1 N sodium hydroxide: ammonia is evolved.
  C: Shake about 60 mg with 5 mL of sodium hydroxide solution (1 in 500), and filter. To a 1-mL portion of the filtrate add 3 drops of mercuric nitrate TS: a white precipitate is formed, and it is soluble in 6 N ammonium hydroxide. To another 1-mL portion of the filtrate add silver nitrate TS, dropwise: a white precipitate is formed, and it dissolves readily in 6 N ammonium hydroxide.
Melting range, *Class I* ⟨741⟩:   between 176° and 181°.
Loss on drying ⟨731⟩—Dry it at 105° for 4 hours: it loses not more than 1.0% of its weight.
Residue on ignition ⟨281⟩:   not more than 0.1%.
Organic volatile impurities, *Method IV* ⟨467⟩:   meets the requirements.

(Official until July 1, 2008)

Assay—Dissolve about 500 mg of Mephobarbital, accurately weighed, in 50 mL of dimethylformamide in a 200-mL flask. Add 4 drops of thymolphthalein TS, and titrate with 0.1 N lithium methoxide in toluene VS, using a magnetic stirrer and a cover for the flask to protect against atmospheric carbon dioxide. Perform a blank determination, and make any necessary correction. Each mL of 0.1 N lithium methoxide is equivalent to 24.63 mg of $C_{13}H_{14}N_2O_3$.

Mephobarbital Tablets

» Mephobarbital Tablets contain not less than 95.0 percent and not more than 110.0 percent of the labeled amount of mephobarbital ($C_{13}H_{14}N_2O_3$).

Packaging and storage—Preserve in well-closed containers.
USP Reference standards ⟨11⟩—*USP Mephobarbital RS.*
Identification—The mephobarbital obtained in the *Assay* melts between 174° and 181° (see *Melting Range or Temperature* ⟨741⟩) and meets the requirements for *Identification*test A under *Mephobarbital.*
Dissolution ⟨711⟩—
  Medium: a 1% solution of 3-(dodecyldimethylammonio) propanesulfonate in pH 8.0 phosphate buffer (prepared by dissolving 10.0 g of 3-(dodecyldimethylammonio) propanesulfonate in 400 mL of warm water, and adding 250 mL of 0.2 M monobasic potassium phosphate and about 220 mL of 0.2 M sodium hydroxide; the solution is then cooled to room temperature, and adjusted with 0.2 M sodium hydroxide to a pH of 8.0, followed by diluting with water to 1000 mL, mixing, and degassing); 900 mL.
  Apparatus 2: 75 rpm.
  Time: 75 minutes.
  Procedure—Determine the amount of $C_{13}H_{14}N_2O_3$ dissolved by employing UV absorption at the wavelength of maximum absorbance at about 244 nm on portions of the solution under test passed through 0.45-µm nylon filters, suitably diluted with *Medium,* if necessary, in comparison with a Standard solution having a known concentration of USP Mephobarbital RS in the same *Medium.*
  Tolerances—Not less than 70% *(Q)* of the labeled amount of $C_{13}H_{14}N_2O_3$ is dissolved in 75 minutes.
Uniformity of dosage units ⟨905⟩: meet the requirements.
  PROCEDURE FOR CONTENT UNIFORMITY—
  Alkaline borate solution—Dissolve 6.2 g of boric acid and 7.45 g of potassium chloride in 500 mL of water, add 210 mL of sodium hydroxide solution (1 in 25), and mix. Add water to make 2000 mL of solution, and mix.
  Standard solution—[NOTE—Prepare the *Standard solution* and the *Test solution* concomitantly.] Dissolve an accurately weighed quantity of USP Mephobarbital RS in *Alkaline borate solution* to obtain a solution having a concentration of about 10 mg per mL, and quantitatively dilute with water to obtain a solution having a known concentration of about 1.5 mg per mL.
  Test solution—Transfer 1 Tablet to a glass-stoppered centrifuge tube, crush the tablet, and add 25.0 mL of *Alkaline borate solution.* Insert the stopper, shake for 10 minutes, and centrifuge until clear, filtering the supernatant, if necessary. Dilute a portion of the subsequent liquid quantitatively, and stepwise if necessary, with water to obtain a solution having a concentration of about 1.5 mg of mephobarbital per mL.
  Procedure—Transfer 3.0 mL each of the *Standard solution* and the *Test solution* to separate 200-mL volumetric flasks, dilute each with a 1 in 3 solution of *Alkaline borate solution* in water to volume, and mix. Concomitantly determine the absorbances of the solutions in 1-cm cells at the wavelength of maximum absorbance at about 245 nm, with a suitable spectrophotometer, using a 1 in 3 solution of *Alkaline borate solution* in water as the blank. Calculate the quantity, in mg, of $C_{13}H_{14}N_2O_3$ in the Tablet taken by the formula:

$$(TC/D)(A_U / A_S)$$

in which T is the labeled quantity, in mg, of mephobarbital in the Tablet; C is the concentration, in mg per mL, of USP Mephobarbital RS in the *Standard solution;* D is the concentration, in mg per mL, of mephobarbital in the *Test solution,* based upon the labeled quantity per Tablet and the extent of dilution; and A_U and A_S are the absorbances of the solutions from the *Test solution* and the *Standard solution,* respectively.
Assay—Weigh and finely powder not fewer than 20 Tablets. Transfer an accurately weighed portion of the powder, equivalent to about 300 mg of mephobarbital, to an extraction thimble. Extract with 15 mL of solvent hexane, allow the thimble to drain, transfer to a continuous-extraction apparatus provided with a tared flask, and extract the mephobarbital with chloroform for 2 hours. Evaporate the chloroform on a steam bath with the aid of a current of air, cool, dissolve the residue in about 10 mL of alcohol, evaporate, dry the residue at 105° for 1 hour, cool, and weigh. The weight of the residue represents the weight of mephobarbital ($C_{13}H_{14}N_2O_3$) in the portion of Tablets taken.

Mepivacaine Hydrochloride

$C_{15}H_{22}N_2O \cdot HCl$ 282.81
2-Piperidinecarboxamide, *N*-(2,6-dimethylphenyl)-1-methyl-, monohydrochloride, (±)-.
(±)-1-Methyl-2′,6′-pipecoloxylidide monohydrochloride   [1722-62-9].

» Mepivacaine Hydrochloride contains not less than 98.0 percent and not more than 102.0 percent of $C_{15}H_{22}N_2O \cdot HCl$, calculated on the dried basis.

Packaging and storage—Preserve in well-closed containers.
USP Reference standards ⟨11⟩—*USP Mepivacaine Hydrochloride RS.*
Identification—
  A: *Infrared Absorption* ⟨197K⟩.
  B: Dissolve about 250 mg in 10 mL of water, render slightly alkaline with sodium carbonate TS, extract the precipitate with ether, evaporate the ether extract on a steam bath to dryness, and dry the residue in vacuum at 60° for 1 hour: the mepivacaine so obtained melts between 149° and 153°.
  C: A solution (1 in 100) responds to the tests for *Chloride* ⟨191⟩.
Loss on drying ⟨731⟩—Dry it at 105° for 4 hours: it loses not more than 1.0% of its weight.
Residue on ignition ⟨281⟩: not more than 0.1%.
Chromatographic purity—Mix about 500 mg with 10 mL of water to obtain a test solution. Inject about 1 µL of this solution into a suitable gas chromatograph (see *Chromatography* ⟨621⟩), equipped with a flame-ionization detector. Under typical conditions, the instrument contains a 1.8-m × 4-mm glass column packed with 3 percent phase G19 on packing S1A. The column is maintained at about 230°, and dry helium, flowing at the rate of about 40 mL per minute, is used as the carrier gas. Similarly inject about 1 µL of a Standard solution of USP Mepivacaine Hydrochloride RS in water having a concentration of about 5 mg per mL. Locate the mepivacaine peak in each chromatogram. The total area of all extraneous peaks (except that of the solvent peak) recorded for the test solution, over a time span of not less than 1.3 × the retention time for mepivacaine, relative to the total area of all peaks does not exceed 0.4%.
Assay—Transfer about 550 mg of Mepivacaine Hydrochloride, accurately weighed, to a 200-mL beaker, and dissolve in 50 mL of glacial acetic acid, heating if necessary. Add 10 mL of mercuric acetate TS and 1 drop of crystal violet TS, and titrate with 0.1 N perchloric acid VS to a green endpoint. Perform a blank determination, and make any necessary correction. Each mL of 0.1 N perchloric acid is equivalent to 28.28 mg of $C_{15}H_{22}N_2O \cdot HCl$.

Mepivacaine Hydrochloride Injection

» Mepivacaine Hydrochloride Injection is a sterile solution of Mepivacaine Hydrochloride in Water for Injection. It contains not less than 95.0 percent and not more than 105.0 percent of the labeled amount of mepivacaine hydrochloride ($C_{15}H_{22}N_2O \cdot HCl$).

Packaging and storage—Preserve in single-dose or multiple-dose containers, preferably of Type I glass. Injection labeled to contain 2% or less of mepivacaine hydrochloride may be packaged in 50-mL multiple-dose containers.

USP Reference standards ⟨11⟩—*USP Endotoxin RS. USP Mepivacaine Hydrochloride RS.*

Identification—
A: It meets the requirements under *Identification—Organic Nitrogenous Bases* ⟨181⟩.
B: Extract a volume of Injection, equivalent to about 200 mg of mepivacaine, with two 10-mL portions of ether, and discard the ether extracts: the remaining solution meets the requirements for *Identification* test B under *Mepivacaine Hydrochloride*.

Bacterial endotoxins ⟨85⟩—It contains not more than 0.8 USP Endotoxin Unit per mg of mepivacaine hydrochloride.

pH ⟨791⟩: between 4.5 and 6.8.

Other requirements—It meets the requirements under *Injections* ⟨1⟩.

Assay—
pH 6.3 Phosphate buffer—Dissolve 3.40 g of monobasic potassium phosphate and 4.35 g of dibasic potassium phosphate in 1000 mL of water, and adjust, if necessary, with potassium hydroxide or phosphoric acid to a pH of 6.3.

Mobile phase—Prepare a filtered and degassed mixture of *pH 6.3 Phosphate buffer* and acetonitrile (65 : 35). Make adjustments if necessary (see *System Suitability* under *Chromatography* ⟨621⟩).

System suitability preparation—Dissolve suitable amounts of methylparaben and USP Mepivacaine Hydrochloride RS in an appropriate volume of *Mobile phase* to obtain a solution containing about 0.05 mg per mL and 1.0 mg per mL, respectively.

Standard preparation—Dissolve an accurately weighed quantity of USP Mepivacaine Hydrochloride RS in *Mobile phase*, and dilute quantitatively, and stepwise if necessary, with *Mobile phase* to obtain a solution having a known concentration of about 1.0 mg per mL.

Assay preparation—Transfer a volume of Injection, equivalent to about 100 mg of mepivacaine hydrochloride, to a 100-mL volumetric flask, dilute with *Mobile phase* to volume, and mix.

Chromatographic system (see *Chromatography* ⟨621⟩)—The liquid chromatograph is equipped with a 263-nm detector and a 4.6-mm × 25.0-cm column that contains 5-μm packing L1.[*] The flow rate is about 1.0 mL per minute. The column temperature is maintained at 40°. Chromatograph the *System suitability preparation*, and record the peak responses as directed for *Procedure*: the relative retention times are about 1.4 for methylparaben and 1.0 for mepivacaine; the resolution, *R*, between methylparaben and mepivacaine is not less than 2.0; the capacity factor, *k′*, for the mepivacaine peak is not less than 1.0; and the tailing factor for the mepivacaine peak is not more than 2.0. Chromatograph the *Standard preparation*, and record the peak responses as directed for *Procedure*: the relative standard deviation for replicate injections is not more than 2.0%.

Procedure—Separately inject equal volumes (about 10 μL) of the *Standard preparation* and the *Assay preparation* into the chromatograph, record the chromatograms, and measure the responses for the mepivacaine peaks. Calculate the quantity, in mg, of mepivacaine hydrochloride ($C_{15}H_{22}N_2O \cdot HCl$) in the volume of Injection taken by the formula:

$$100C(r_U / r_S)$$

in which *C* is the concentration, in mg per mL, of USP Mepivacaine Hydrochloride RS in the *Standard preparation*; and r_U and r_S are the peak responses obtained from the *Assay preparation* and the *Standard preparation*, respectively.

---

[*] A Whatman Partisphere RTF C18 brand of L1 column has been shown to be an appropriate column.

Mepivacaine Hydrochloride and Levonordefrin Injection

» Mepivacaine Hydrochloride and Levonordefrin Injection is a sterile solution of Mepivacaine Hydrochloride and Levonordefrin in Water for Injection. It contains not less than 95.0 percent and not more than 105.0 percent of the labeled amount of mepivacaine hydrochloride ($C_{15}H_{22}N_2O \cdot HCl$) and not less than 90.0 percent and not more than 110.0 percent of the labeled amount of levonordefrin ($C_9H_{13}NO_3$).

Packaging and storage—Preserve in single-dose or multiple-dose containers, preferably of Type I glass.

Labeling—The label indicates that the Injection is not to be used if its color is pinkish or darker than slightly yellow or if it contains a precipitate.

USP Reference standards ⟨11⟩—*USP Endotoxin RS. USP Levonordefrin RS. USP Mepivacaine Hydrochloride RS.*

Color and clarity—
Standard solution—Transfer 2.0 mL of 0.100 N iodine VS to a 500-mL volumetric flask, dilute with water to volume, and mix.

Procedure—Visually examine a portion of the Injection (*Test solution*) in a suitable clear glass test tube against a white background: it is not pinkish and it contains no precipitate. If any yellow color is observed in the *Test solution*, concomitantly determine the absorbances of the *Test solution* and the *Standard solution* in 1-cm cells with a suitable spectrophotometer set at 460 nm: the absorbance of the *Test solution* does not exceed that of the *Standard solution*.

Identification—
A: Extract a volume of Injection, equivalent to about 200 mg of mepivacaine, with two 10-mL portions of ether, and discard the ether extracts. Render slightly alkaline with sodium carbonate TS, extract the precipitate with ether, evaporate the ether extract on a steam bath to dryness, and dry the residue in vacuum at 60° for 1 hour: the mepivacaine so obtained melts between 149° and 153°.
B: It meets the requirements of the tests for *Chloride* ⟨191⟩.

Bacterial endotoxins ⟨85⟩—It contains not more than 0.8 USP Endotoxin Unit per mg of mepivacaine hydrochloride.

pH ⟨791⟩: between 3.3 and 5.5.

Other requirements—It meets the requirements under *Injections* ⟨1⟩.

Assay for mepivacaine hydrochloride—Proceed as directed for the *Assay* under *Mepivacaine Hydrochloride Injection*.

Assay for levonordefrin—
Ferro-citrate Solution and *Buffer Solution*—Prepare as directed under *Epinephrine Assay* ⟨391⟩.

Standard preparation—With the aid of 20 mL of sodium bisulfite solution (1 in 50), transfer about 25 mg of USP Levonordefrin RS, accurately weighed, to a 50-mL volumetric flask, dilute with water to volume, and mix. Transfer 5 mL of this solution to a 50-mL volumetric flask, dilute with sodium bisulfite solution (1 in 500) to volume, and mix to obtain a solution having a known concentration of about 50 μg per mL. [NOTE—Make the final dilution at the time the assay is to be carried out.]

Assay preparation—Use the Injection, diluting, if necessary, to obtain a concentration of about 50 μg of levonordefrin per mL.

Procedure—Proceed as directed under *Epinephrine Assay* ⟨391⟩, except to read levonordefrin wherever epinephrine (base) is called for. When the *Ferro-citrate Solution* and the *Buffer Solution* are mixed with the *Assay preparation*, a fine precipitate may be formed. Remove this precipitate by centrifugation or by passing through dry filter paper before the colorimetric measurements are taken. Calculate the quantity, in mg, of levonordefrin ($C_9H_{13}NO_3$) in each mL of the Injection taken by the formula:

$$C(V_F / V_T)(A_U / A_S)$$

in which *C* is the concentration, in mg per mL, of USP Levonordefrin RS in the *Standard preparation*; V_F is the final volume of the *Assay preparation* after dilution; V_T is the volume of Injection taken

Meprednisone

$C_{22}H_{28}O_5$ 372.45

Pregna-1,4-diene-3,11,20-trione, 17,21-dihydroxy-16-methyl-, (16β)-.
17,21-Dihydroxy-16β-methylpregna-1,4-diene-3,11,20-trione [1247-42-3].

» Meprednisone contains not less than 97.5 percent and not more than 102.5 percent of $C_{22}H_{28}O_5$, calculated on the dried basis.

Packaging and storage—Preserve in tight, light-resistant containers, and avoid exposure to excessive heat.

USP Reference standards ⟨11⟩—*USP Meprednisone RS*.
Identification—
  A: *Infrared Absorption* ⟨197M⟩.
  B: *Ultraviolet Absorption* ⟨197U⟩—
  Solution: 10 μg per mL.
  Medium: methanol.
  Absorptivities at 238 nm, calculated on the dried basis, do not differ by more than 3.0%.
  C: *Thin-Layer Chromatographic Identification Test* ⟨201⟩—
  Test solution: 20 mg per mL, in a mixture of toluene and alcohol (1 : 1).
  Spray reagent: 10% (v/v) sulfuric acid in alcohol solution.
  Procedure—Proceed as directed in the chapter. Locate the spots on the plate by spraying with *Spray reagent* and heating at 105° for 10 minutes.
Specific rotation ⟨781S⟩: between +180° and +188°.
  Test solution: 10 mg per mL, in dioxane.
Loss on drying ⟨731⟩—Dry it at 105° for 3 hours: it loses not more than 1.0% of its weight.
Residue on ignition ⟨281⟩: not more than 0.1%.
Assay—
  Standard preparation—Prepare as directed under *Single-Steroid Assay* ⟨511⟩, using USP Meprednisone RS.
  Assay preparation—Accurately weigh about 20 mg of Meprednisone, previously dried, dissolve it in a sufficient quantity of a mixture of alcohol and chloroform (1 : 1) to make 10.0 mL, and mix.
  Procedure—Proceed as directed for *Procedure* under *Single-Steroid Assay* ⟨511⟩, using a solvent system consisting of chloroform, methanol, and water (180 : 15 : 1), through the fourth sentence of the second paragraph under *Procedure*. Then centrifuge the tubes for 5 minutes, and determine the absorbances of the supernatants in 1-cm cells at the wavelength of maximum absorbance at about 238 nm, with a suitable spectrophotometer, against the blank. Calculate the quantity, in mg, of $C_{22}H_{28}O_5$ in the portion of Meprednisone taken by the formula:

$$10C(A_U / A_S)$$

in which C is the concentration, in mg per mL, of USP Meprednisone RS in the *Standard preparation*; and A_U and A_S are the absorbances of the solutions from the *Assay preparation* and the *Standard preparation*, respectively.

Meprobamate

$C_9H_{18}N_2O_4$ 218.25
1,3-Propanediol, 2-methyl-2-propyl-, dicarbamate.
2-Methyl-2-propyl-1,3-propanediol dicarbamate [57-53-4].

» Meprobamate contains not less than 97.0 percent and not more than 101.0 percent of $C_9H_{18}N_2O_4$, calculated on the dried basis.

Packaging and storage—Preserve in tight containers.
USP Reference standards ⟨11⟩—*USP Meprobamate RS*.
Identification—
  A: The IR absorption spectrum of a potassium bromide dispersion of it (about 1 mg in 200 mg), previously dried, exhibits maxima only at the same wavelengths as that of a similar preparation of USP Meprobamate RS. If a difference appears, dissolve portions of both the test specimen and the Reference Standard in acetone at a concentration of 8 mg per mL. Dilute 0.1-mL portions of the acetone solutions with 1 mL of *n*-heptane, and remove the solvents by evaporation under nitrogen at a temperature of about 30°. Dry the residues in vacuum at room temperature for 30 minutes, and repeat the test on the residues.
  B: The R_F value of the principal spot in the chromatogram of the *Identification preparation* corresponds to that of *Standard preparation A* as obtained in the test for *Chromatographic purity*.
Melting range ⟨741⟩: between 103° and 107°, but the range between beginning and end of melting does not exceed 2°.
Loss on drying ⟨731⟩—Dry it in vacuum at 60° for 3 hours: it loses not more than 0.5% of its weight.
Chromatographic purity—
  Standard preparations—Dissolve USP Meprobamate RS in alcohol, and mix to obtain *Standard preparation A* having a known concentration of 1.0 mg per mL. Dilute quantitatively with alcohol to obtain *Standard preparations*, designated below by letter, having the following compositions:

Standard preparation	Dilution	Concentration (mg RS per mL)	Percentage (%, for comparison with test specimen)
A	(undiluted)	1.0	1.0
B	(4 in 5)	0.8	0.8
C	(3 in 5)	0.6	0.6
D	(2 in 5)	0.4	0.4
E	(1 in 5)	0.2	0.2

  Test preparation—Dissolve an accurately weighed quantity of Meprobamate in alcohol to obtain a solution containing 100 mg per mL.
  Identification preparation—Dilute a portion of the *Test preparation* quantitatively with alcohol to obtain a solution containing 1.0 mg per mL.
  Procedure—Apply separately 2 μL of the *Test preparation*, 2 μL of the *Identification preparation*, and 2 μL of each *Standard preparation* to a suitable thin-layer chromatographic plate (see *Chromatography* ⟨621⟩) coated with a 0.25-mm layer of chromatographic silica gel. Position the plate in a chromatographic chamber, and develop the chromatograms in a solvent system consisting of a mixture of hexane, acetone, and pyridine (7 : 3 : 1) until the solvent front has moved about three-fourths of the length of the plate. Remove the plate from the developing chamber, mark the solvent front, and air-dry the plate for 15 minutes. Heat the plate at 100° for 15 minutes, cool, and spray with a solution prepared by dissolving 1 g of vanillin in a cooled mixture of sulfuric acid and alcohol (160 :

40). Heat the plate at 110° for 15 to 20 minutes, cool, and allow the plate to develop blue-purple spots at room temperature. [NOTE—Color development requires approximately 30 to 60 minutes.] Examine the plate, and compare the intensities of any secondary spots observed in the chromatogram of the *Test preparation* with those of the principal spots in the chromatograms of the *Standard preparations*. No secondary spot from the chromatogram of the *Test preparation* is larger or more intense than the principal spot obtained from *Standard preparation A* (1.0%), and the sum of the intensities of all secondary spots obtained from the *Test preparation* corresponds to not more than 2.0%.

Limit of methyl carbamate—
Mobile phase—Use filtered and degassed water.
Standard preparation—Dissolve an accurately weighed quantity of methyl carbamate in water to obtain a solution having a known concentration of 1.0 mg per mL.
Test preparation—Transfer 1.0 g of finely powdered Meprobamate, accurately weighed, to a beaker, add 5.0 mL of water, and stir to wet the powder completely. Filter the slurry through a small plug of glass wool in the stem of a glass funnel. Use the clear filtrate as the *Test preparation*.
Chromatographic system (see *Chromatography* ⟨621⟩)—The liquid chromatograph is equipped with a 200-nm detector and a 3.9- to 4.6-mm × 25- to 30-cm column that contains packing L1. The flow rate is about 1 mL per minute. Chromatograph replicate injections of the *Standard preparation*, and record the peak responses as directed for *Procedure*: the relative standard deviation is not more than 2.0%.
Procedure—Separately inject equal volumes (about 50 μL) of the *Standard preparation* and the *Test preparation* into the chromatograph, record the chromatograms, and measure the responses for the methyl carbamate peaks: the peak response obtained from the *Test preparation* is not greater than that obtained from the *Standard preparation*, corresponding to not more than 0.5% of methyl carbamate.

Organic volatile impurities, *Method V* ⟨467⟩: meets the requirements.
Solvent—Use dimethyl sulfoxide.

(Official until July 1, 2008)
Assay—Transfer about 400 mg of Meprobamate, accurately weighed, to a conical flask, add 40 mL of hydrochloric acid and several boiling chips, and reflux for 90 minutes. Remove the condenser, and continue boiling until the volume is reduced to between 5 and 10 mL. Cool the flask to room temperature, add 50 mL of water and 1 drop of methyl red TS, and, while cooling the flask continuously, cautiously neutralize the acid with 10 N sodium hydroxide until the indicator begins to change color. If necessary, add 1 N hydrochloric acid to restore the pink color, and carefully neutralize with 0.1 N sodium hydroxide VS. Add a mixture of 15 mL of formaldehyde TS and 15 mL of water, which previously has been neutralized with 0.1 N sodium hydroxide VS to phenolphthalein TS, and titrate with 0.1 N sodium hydroxide VS to a yellow endpoint. Add 0.2 mL of phenolphthalein TS, and continue the titration with 0.1 N sodium hydroxide VS to a distinct pink color. Perform a blank determination, and make any necessary correction. Each mL of the total volume of 0.1 N sodium hydroxide consumed after the addition of formaldehyde TS is equivalent to 10.91 mg of $C_9H_{18}N_2O_4$.

Meprobamate Oral Suspension

» Meprobamate Oral Suspension contains not less than 95.0 percent and not more than 110.0 percent of the labeled amount of $C_9H_{18}N_2O_4$.

Packaging and storage—Preserve in tight containers.
Identification—Mix 2 mL of Oral Suspension with 2 mL of acetone and 2 mL of a 1 in 100 solution of furfural in glacial acetic acid, add 5 mL of hydrochloric acid, and shake: a purple color is produced, and, on standing, it changes to blue, then to blue-black, and finally to black-brown.

Uniformity of dosage units ⟨905⟩—
FOR ORAL SUSPENSION PACKAGED IN SINGLE-UNIT CONTAINERS: meets the requirements.
Deliverable volume ⟨698⟩—
FOR ORAL SUSPENSION PACKAGED IN MULTIPLE-UNIT CONTAINERS: meets the requirements.
Assay—Transfer an accurately measured volume of Oral Suspension, equivalent to about 400 mg of meprobamate, to a separator, and completely extract the meprobamate with 20-mL portions of chloroform, filtering the extracts through a pledget of cotton enclosed in glass wool that previously has been moistened with chloroform. Collect the filtrate in a conical flask, add several glass beads to the flask, and evaporate on a steam bath to dryness. To the residue add 20 mL of water, heat on a steam bath for several minutes, then add 40 mL of hydrochloric acid, and reflux for 90 minutes. Remove the condenser, and continue boiling until the volume is reduced to about 20 mL. Cool to room temperature, add 50 mL of water, and cool in an ice bath. Add 1 drop of methyl red TS, and, while cooling continuously, cautiously neutralize with sodium hydroxide solution (4 in 10) until the indicator begins to change color. Add hydrochloric acid, if necessary, to restore the pink color, then carefully neutralize with 0.1 N sodium hydroxide VS. Add 30 mL of neutral formaldehyde solution (18% w/w), and titrate with 0.1 N sodium hydroxide VS until the solution becomes yellow. Add 0.2 mL of phenolphthalein TS, and continue the titration with 0.1 N sodium hydroxide VS to a distinct pink color. Perform a blank determination, and make any necessary correction. Each mL of the total volume of 0.1 N sodium hydroxide consumed after the addition of the formaldehyde solution is equivalent to 10.91 mg of $C_9H_{18}N_2O_4$.

Meprobamate Tablets

» Meprobamate Tablets contain not less than 90.0 percent and not more than 110.0 percent of the labeled amount of $C_9H_{18}N_2O_4$.

Packaging and storage—Preserve in well-closed containers.

USP Reference standards ⟨11⟩—*USP Meprobamate RS.*
Identification—
A: To a portion of finely powdered Tablets, equivalent to about 800 mg of meprobamate, add 5 mL of dehydrated alcohol, and heat just below the boiling temperature for about 5 minutes, with occasional swirling. Cool, filter into 15 mL of solvent hexane, and mix. With the aid of suction, filter the crystals that form, and dry at 60°: the crystals of meprobamate so obtained melt between 103° and 107°, but the range between beginning and end of melting does not exceed 2°.
B: A portion of the crystals obtained in *Identification* test A responds to *Identification* test A under *Meprobamate*.
Dissolution, *Procedure for a Pooled Sample* ⟨711⟩—
Medium: deaerated water; 900 mL.
Apparatus 1: 100 rpm.
Time: 30 minutes.
Procedure—Determine the amount of $C_9H_{18}N_2O_4$ dissolved using the method set forth for the *Assay*, making any necessary volumetric adjustments.
Tolerances—Not less than 75% (*Q*) of the labeled amount of $C_9H_{18}N_2O_4$ is dissolved in 30 minutes.
Uniformity of dosage units ⟨905⟩: meet the requirements.
Assay—
Mobile phase—Prepare a filtered and degassed mixture of water and acetonitrile (7 : 3), making adjustments if necessary (see *System Suitability* under *Chromatography* ⟨621⟩).
Phenacetin stock solution—Dissolve phenacetin in acetonitrile to obtain a solution having a concentration of about 125 μg per mL. Pipet 20 mL of this solution into a 100-mL volumetric flask, add 30 mL of acetonitrile, dilute with water to volume, and mix.
Standard preparation—Transfer about 50 mg of USP Meprobamate RS, accurately weighed, to a 10-mL volumetric flask, add 3 mL of acetonitrile, and shake to dissolve. Dilute with water to vol-

ume, and mix to obtain a solution having a known concentration of about 5 mg of USP Meprobamate RS per mL.

Resolution solution—Transfer 25 mg of meprobamate to a 5-mL volumetric flask, add 1 mL of acetonitrile, and shake to dissolve. Add 1 mL of *Phenacetin stock solution*, dilute with water to volume, and mix.

Assay preparation—Weigh and finely powder not less than 20 Tablets. Transfer an accurately weighed portion of the powder, equivalent to about 250 mg of meprobamate, to a 50-mL volumetric flask, add 15 mL of acetonitrile, and shake to dissolve. Dilute with water to volume, mix, and filter, discarding the first 10 mL of the filtrate.

Chromatographic system (see *Chromatography* ⟨621⟩)—The liquid chromatograph is equipped with a 200-nm detector and a 3.9- to 4.6-mm × 25- to 30-cm column that contains packing L1. The flow rate is about 1 mL per minute. Chromatograph the *Resolution solution*, and record the peak responses as directed for *Procedure:* the resolution, *R*, between the meprobamate and the phenacetin peaks is not less than 2.0, and the area of the phenacetin peak is not less than 65.0% and not more than 100.0% of the meprobamate peak area. The relative retention times are about 0.7 for meprobamate and 1.0 for phenacetin. Chromatograph the *Standard preparation*, and record the peak responses as directed for *Procedure:* the relative standard deviation for replicate injections is not more than 2.0%.

Procedure—Separately inject equal volumes (about 20 µL) of the *Standard preparation* and the *Assay preparation* into the chromatograph, record the chromatograms, and measure the responses for the major peaks. Calculate the quantity, in mg, of $C_9H_{18}N_2O_4$ in the portion of Tablets taken by the formula:

$$50C(r_U / r_S)$$

in which *C* is the concentration, in mg per mL, of USP Meprobamate RS in the *Standard preparation*, and r_U and r_S are the meprobamate peak responses obtained from the *Assay preparation* and the *Standard preparation*, respectively.

Meradimate

$C_{17}H_{25}NO_2$ 275.39
Menthyl-*O*-aminobenzoate.
Anthranilic acid, *p*-menth-3-yl ester   [*134-09-8*].

» Meradimate contains not less than 95.0 percent and not more than 105.0 percent of $C_{17}H_{25}NO_2$.

Packaging and storage—Preserve in tight containers.
USP Reference standards ⟨11⟩—*USP Meradimate RS*.
Identification—
  A: *Infrared Absorption* ⟨197F⟩.
  B: *Ultraviolet Absorption* ⟨197U⟩—
  Solution: 5.0 µg per mL.
  Medium: alcohol.
  Absorptivities, calculated on the as-is basis, do not differ by more than 3.0%.
Specific rotation ⟨781S⟩:   between −4° and +4°.
  Test solution: 10 mg per mL, in alcohol.
Refractive index ⟨831⟩:   between 1.540 and 1.544 at 20°.
Acidity—Transfer 50 mL of alcohol to a suitable container, add 1 mL of phenolphthalein TS, and add sufficient 0.1 N sodium hydroxide to obtain a persistent pink color. Transfer 50 mL of this solution to a suitable container, add about 5.0 mL of Meradimate, accurately measured, mix, and titrate with 0.1 N sodium hydroxide: not more than 0.2 mL of titrant per mL of Meradimate is necessary.

Chromatographic purity—
Test solution—Use the *Assay preparation*.
Chromatographic system—Proceed as directed in the *Assay*. To evaluate the system suitability requirements, use the *Standard preparation* prepared as directed in the *Assay*.
Procedure—Inject a volume (about 1 µL) of the *Test solution* into the chromatograph, record the chromatogram, and measure all of the peak responses. Calculate the percentage of each impurity in the portion of Meradimate taken by the formula:

$$100(r_i / r_s)$$

in which r_i is the peak response for each impurity; and r_s is the sum of the responses of all the peaks: not more than 0.1% of any individual impurity is found; and not more than 2.0% of total impurities is found.

Assay—
Standard preparation—Dissolve an accurately weighed quantity of USP Meradimate RS in *tert*-butyl methyl ether, and dilute quantitatively, and stepwise if necessary, with *tert*-butyl methyl ether to obtain a solution having a known concentration of about 20.0 mg per mL.

Assay preparation—Transfer about 2 g of Meradimate, accurately weighed, to a 100-mL volumetric flask, dilute with *tert*-butyl methyl ether to volume, and mix.

Chromatographic system (see *Chromatography* ⟨621⟩)—The gas chromatograph is equipped with a flame-ionization detector and a 0.32-mm × 25-m column coated with a 0.1-µm film of G1. The carrier gas is helium, flowing at a rate of about 6 mL per minute. The chromatograph is programmed as follows. Initially the temperature of the column is equilibrated at 60°, then the temperature is increased at a rate of 8° per minute to 240°, and is maintained at 240° for 10 minutes. The injection port temperature is maintained at 240°, and the detector temperature is maintained at 260°. Chromatograph the *Standard preparation*, and record the peak responses as directed for *Procedure:* the resolution, *R*, between meradimate and any other peak is not less than 1.0; and the relative standard deviation for replicate injections is not more than 2.0%.

Procedure—Separately inject equal volumes (about 1 µL) of the *Standard preparation* and the *Assay preparation* into the chromatograph, record the chromatograms, and measure the responses for the major peaks. Calculate the quantity, in mg, of $C_{17}H_{25}NO_2$ in the portion of Meradimate taken by the formula:

$$100C(r_U / r_S)$$

in which *C* is the concentration, in mg per mL, of USP Meradimate RS in the *Standard preparation;* and r_U and r_S are the peak responses obtained from the *Assay preparation* and the *Standard preparation*, respectively.

Mercaptopurine

$C_5H_4N_4S \cdot H_2O$ 170.19
6*H*-Purine-6-thione, 1,7-dihydro-, monohydrate.
Purine-6-thiol monohydrate   [*6112-76-1*].
Anhydrous   152.18   [*50-44-2*].

» Mercaptopurine contains not less than 97.0 percent and not more than 102.0 percent of $C_5H_4N_4S$, calculated on the anhydrous basis.

Mercaptopurine / Official Monographs

Packaging and storage—Preserve in well-closed containers.

USP Reference standards ⟨11⟩—USP Mercaptopurine RS.

Identification—

A: *Ultraviolet Absorption* ⟨197U⟩—
Solution: 5 µg per mL.
Medium: 0.1 N hydrochloric acid.
Absorptivities at 325 nm, calculated on the anhydrous basis, do not differ by more than 3.0%. The ratio A_{255}/A_{325} does not exceed 0.06.

B: To a solution of 600 mg in 6 mL of sodium hydroxide solution (1 in 33) add slowly, with shaking, 0.5 mL of methyl iodide. Allow the mixture to stand for 2 hours at room temperature, cool in an ice bath, and adjust with acetic acid to a pH of about 5. Collect the crystals, and recrystallize from hot water: the methylmercaptopurine trihydrate so obtained, dried at 120° for 30 minutes, melts between 218° and 222°, with decomposition.

Water, *Method I* ⟨921⟩: not more than 12.0%.

Phosphorus—Digest 200 mg with 2 mL of 15 N sulfuric acid in a large test tube, periodically adding nitric acid, dropwise and with caution. Continue heating until practically all of the liquid has evaporated and the residue is colorless. Transfer the residue, with the aid of small portions of water, to a 25-mL volumetric flask, add 1 mL of 15 N sulfuric acid, 0.5 mL of nitric acid, 0.75 mL of ammonium molybdate TS, and 1 mL of aminonaphtholsulfonic acid TS, then dilute with water to volume, and mix. Allow to stand for 5 minutes, and determine the absorbance of this solution at 750 nm, with a suitable spectrophotometer, using as a blank a solution of the same quantities of the same reagents, prepared in the same manner. The absorbance of this solution is not greater than that of a solution obtained by treating as directed above, beginning with "add 1 mL of 15 N sulfuric acid," a 2-mL portion of a standard phosphate solution prepared to contain, in each mL, 43.96 µg of dried monobasic potassium phosphate, equivalent to 10 µg of P (0.010%).

Organic volatile impurities, *Method V* ⟨467⟩: meets the requirements.
Solvent—Use dimethyl sulfoxide.

(Official until July 1, 2008)

Assay—Dissolve about 300 mg of Mercaptopurine, accurately weighed, in 80 mL of dimethylformamide. Add 5 drops of a 1 in 100 solution of thymol blue in dimethylformamide, and titrate with 0.1 N sodium methoxide VS, using a magnetic stirrer and taking precautions against absorption of atmospheric carbon dioxide. Perform a blank determination, and make any necessary correction. Each mL of 0.1 N sodium methoxide is equivalent to 15.22 mg of $C_5H_4N_4S$.

Mercaptopurine Tablets

» Mercaptopurine Tablets contain not less than 93.0 percent and not more than 110.0 percent of the labeled amount of mercaptopurine ($C_5H_4N_4S \cdot H_2O$).

Packaging and storage—Preserve in well-closed containers.

Labeling—When more than one *Dissolution* test is given, the labeling states the *Dissolution* test used only if *Test 1* is not used.

USP Reference standards ⟨11⟩—USP Mercaptopurine RS.

Identification—

A: The UV absorption spectrum of the solution of Tablets employed for measurement of absorbance in the *Assay* exhibits a maximum at 325 ± 2 nm, and the ratio A_{255}/A_{325} does not exceed 0.09.

B: Triturate a quantity of finely powdered Tablets, equivalent to about 600 mg of mercaptopurine, with three 25-mL portions of hot alcohol. Filter the hot alcohol extracts, and evaporate the filtrate on a steam bath to dryness. Add to the residue 5 mL of sodium hydroxide solution (1 in 33), agitate well, and filter: the clear filtrate so obtained responds to *Identification* test *B* under *Mercaptopurine*.

Dissolution ⟨711⟩—
TEST 1—
Medium: 0.1 N hydrochloric acid; 900 mL.
Apparatus 2: 50 rpm.
Time: 60 minutes.
Determine the amount of mercaptopurine ($C_5H_4N_4S$) dissolved by employing the following method.
Mobile phase—Prepare a filtered and degassed solution of 0.1% acetic acid in water. Make adjustments if necessary (see *System Suitability* under *Chromatography* ⟨621⟩).
Chromatographic system (see *Chromatography* ⟨621⟩)—The liquid chromatograph is equipped with a 230-nm detector and a 3.9-mm × 15-cm column that contains packing L1. The flow rate is about 2.5 mL per minute. Chromatograph replicate injections of the Standard solution prepared as described below for *Procedure*, and record the peak responses as directed for *Procedure*: the retention time for mercaptopurine is not less than 4 minutes, and the relative standard deviation is not more than 2.0%.
Procedure—Inject a volume (about 10 µL) of a filtered portion of the solution under test into the chromatograph, record the chromatogram, and measure the response for the major peak. Calculate the quantity of $C_5H_4N_4S$ dissolved in comparison with a Standard solution having a known concentration of USP Mercaptopurine RS in the same *Medium* and similarly chromatographed.
Tolerances—Not less than 80% *(Q)* of the labeled amount of $C_5H_4N_4S$ is dissolved in 60 minutes.

TEST 2—If the product complies with this test, the labeling indicates that it meets USP *Dissolution Test 2*.
Medium, Apparatus, Chromatographic system, and *Procedure*—Proceed as directed for *Test 1*.
Time: 120 minutes.
Tolerances—Not less than 80% *(Q)* of the labeled amount of $C_5H_4N_4S$ is dissolved in 120 minutes.

Uniformity of dosage units ⟨905⟩: meet the requirements.

Assay—Weigh and finely powder not fewer than 20 Tablets. Accurately weigh a portion of the powder, equivalent to about 50 mg of mercaptopurine, and transfer to a 100-mL volumetric flask. Add 20 mL of water and 1.5 mL of 1 N sodium hydroxide, and swirl for not more than 5 minutes. Dilute with water to volume, mix, and filter, discarding the first 20 mL of the filtrate. Dilute an accurately measured portion of the filtrate quantitatively and stepwise with 0.1 N hydrochloric acid to give a final concentration of about 5 µg per mL. Dissolve an accurately weighed quantity of USP Mercaptopurine RS in a mixture of 10 mL of water and 1 mL of 1 N sodium hydroxide contained in a 100-mL volumetric flask, dilute with water to volume, and mix. Dilute an aliquot of this solution quantitatively and stepwise with 0.1 N hydrochloric acid to obtain a Standard solution having a known concentration of about 5 µg per mL. Concomitantly determine the absorbances of both solutions in 1-cm cells at the wavelength of maximum absorbance at about 325 nm, with a suitable spectrophotometer, using 0.1 N hydrochloric acid as the blank. Calculate the quantity, in mg, of mercaptopurine ($C_5H_4N_4S \cdot H_2O$) in the portion of Tablets taken by the formula:

$$(170.19/152.18)10C(A_U/A_S)$$

in which 170.19 and 152.18 are the molecular weights of mercaptopurine monohydrate and anhydrous mercaptopurine, respectively; *C* is the concentration, in µg per mL, of USP Mercaptopurine RS in the Standard solution; and A_U and A_S are the absorbances of the solution from Tablets and the Standard solution, respectively.

Ammoniated Mercury

$Hg(NH_2)Cl$ 252.07
Mercury amide chloride.
Mercury amide chloride   [10124-48-8].

» Ammoniated Mercury contains not less than 98.0 percent and not more than 100.5 percent of $Hg(NH_2)Cl$.

Packaging and storage—Preserve in well-closed, light-resistant containers.

Identification—
A: A 0.1-g portion is soluble, with the evolution of ammonia, in a cold solution of 1 g of sodium thiosulfate in 2 mL of water. When this solution is heated gently, a rust-colored mixture is formed, from which a red precipitate is obtained on centrifugation. If the solution is strongly heated, a black mixture forms.

B: When heated with 1 N sodium hydroxide, it becomes yellow, and ammonia is evolved.

C: A solution in warm acetic acid yields with potassium iodide TS a red precipitate, which is soluble in an excess of the reagent. The solution yields a white precipitate with silver nitrate TS.

Residue on ignition ⟨281⟩: not more than 0.2%.

Mercurous compounds—Dissolve 2.5 g in 25 mL of warm hydrochloric acid, filter through a tared filtering crucible, wash with water, and dry at 60° to constant weight: the weight of the residue does not exceed 5 mg (0.2%).

Assay—Mix about 0.25 g of Ammoniated Mercury, accurately weighed, with about 10 mL of water. Add 3 g of potassium iodide, mix occasionally until dissolved, and add about 40 mL of water. Add methyl red TS, and titrate with 0.1 N hydrochloric acid VS. Perform a blank determination, and make any necessary correction. Each mL of 0.1 N hydrochloric acid is equivalent to 12.60 mg of Hg(NH$_2$)Cl.

Meropenem

$C_{17}H_{25}N_3O_5S \cdot 3H_2O$ 437.52

1-Azabicyclo[3.2.0]hept-2-ene-2-carboxylic acid, 3-[[5-[(dimethylamino)carbonyl]-3-pyrrolidinyl]thio]-6-(1-hydroxyethyl)-4-methyl-7-oxo, trihydrate, [4R-[3(3S*,5S*),4α,5β,6β(R*)]]-.
(4R,5S,6S)-3-[[(3S,5S)-5-(Dimethylcarbamoyl)-3-pyrrolidinyl]thio]-6-[(1R)-1-hydroxyethyl]-4-methyl-7-oxo-1-azabicyclo[3.2.0]hept-2-ene-carboxylic acid, trihydrate   [119478-56-7].
Anhydrous   383.47   [96036-03-2].

» Meropenem contains not less than 98.0 percent and not more than 101.0 percent of $C_{17}H_{25}N_3O_5S$, calculated on the anhydrous basis.

Packaging and storage—Preserve in tight containers. Store the dry powder at controlled room temperature.

Labeling—Where it is intended for use in preparing injectable dosage forms, the label states that it is sterile or must be subjected to further processing during the preparation of injectable dosage forms.

USP Reference standards ⟨11⟩—USP Endotoxin RS. USP Meropenem RS.

Identification—
A: *Infrared Absorption* ⟨197K⟩.
B: *Ultraviolet Absorption* ⟨197U⟩—
  Solution: 30 μg per mL.
  Medium: water.

Specific rotation ⟨781⟩: between −17° and −21°, measured at 20°.
  Test solution: 5 mg per mL, in water.

pH ⟨791⟩: between 4.0 and 6.0, in a solution (1 in 100).

Water, *Method Ic* ⟨921⟩: between 11.4% and 13.4%.

Residue on ignition ⟨281⟩: not more than 0.1%, igniting at 500 ± 50°, instead of at 800 ± 25°. Use a desiccator containing silica gel.

Heavy metals—
Sodium sulfide reagent—Dissolve 5 g of sodium sulfide in a mixture of 10 mL of water and 30 mL of glycerin. Preserve in well-filled, light-resistant bottles, and use within 3 months.

Test solution—Transfer 1.0 g of Meropenem to a quartz or porcelain crucible, cover loosely with a lid, and carbonize by gentle ignition. After cooling, add 2 mL of nitric acid and 5 drops of sulfuric acid, heat cautiously until white fumes evolve, and incinerate by ignition at 500° to 600°. Cool, add 2 mL of hydrochloric acid, and evaporate on a water bath to dryness. Moisten the residue with 3 drops of hydrochloric acid, add 10 mL of hot water, and warm for 2 minutes. Add 1 drop of phenolphthalein TS, add ammonia TS, dropwise, until the solution develops a pale red color, and add 2 mL of 1 N acetic acid. Filter, if necessary, to obtain a clear solution, washing the filter with 10 mL of water. Transfer the filtrate and the washing to a 50-mL color-comparison tube, and add water to obtain a volume of 50 mL.

Standard solution—Evaporate a mixture of 2 mL of nitric acid, 5 drops of sulfuric acid, and 2 mL of hydrochloric acid on a water bath, further evaporate to dryness on a hot sand bath, and moisten the residue with 3 drops of hydrochloric acid. Proceed as directed for *Test solution*, beginning with "add 10 mL of hot water," except add water to obtain a volume of 49 mL. Add 1.0 mL of *Standard Lead Solution* (see *Heavy Metals* ⟨231⟩).

Procedure—To the tubes containing the *Test solution* and the *Standard solution*, add 1 drop of *Sodium sulfide reagent*, mix, and allow to stand for 5 minutes. The color in the tube containing the *Test solution* is not darker than the color in the tube containing the *Standard solution* (0.001%).

Limit of acetone—
Internal standard solution—Prepare a solution in dimethylformamide containing 0.05 μL of ethyl acetate per mL.

Standard solution—Transfer about 50 mg of acetone, accurately weighed, to a 100-mL volumetric flask, dilute with dimethylformamide to volume, and mix. To 1.0 mL of this solution, add 10.0 mL of the *Internal standard solution*, and mix.

Test solution—Dissolve 100 mg of Meropenem, accurately weighed, in 0.2 mL of dimethylformamide and 2.0 mL of *Internal standard solution*.

Chromatographic system (see *Chromatography* ⟨621⟩)—The gas chromatograph is equipped with a flame-ionization detector and a 3-mm × 2-m column that contains support S2 and is maintained at a constant temperature of about 150°. The injection port temperature is maintained at about 170°. Nitrogen is the carrier gas, with the flow rate adjusted so that the retention time for acetone is about 3 minutes.

Procedure—Separately inject equal volumes (about 2 μL) of the *Standard solution* and the *Test solution* into the chromatograph, record the chromatograms, and measure the peak responses for the acetone peak and the internal standard peak. Calculate the percentage of acetone in the portion of Meropenem taken by the formula:

$$(W_A/5W_U)(R_U/R_S)$$

in which W_A is the weight, in mg, of acetone in the *Standard solution*; W_U is the quantity, in mg, of Meropenem in the *Test solution*; and R_U and R_S are the peak area ratios of acetone to the internal standard obtained from the *Test Solution* and the *Standard solution*, respectively. Not more than 0.05% is found.

Chromatographic purity—
Diluted phosphoric acid—Dilute 10 mL of phosphoric acid with water to make 100 mL of solution.

Solvent—Transfer 1.0 mL of triethylamine to a 1000-mL volumetric flask containing 900 mL of water. Adjust with *Diluted phosphoric acid* to a pH of 5.0 ± 0.1, dilute with water to volume, and mix.

Mobile phase—Transfer 1.0 mL of triethylamine to a 1000-mL volumetric flask containing 900 mL of water. Adjust with *Diluted phosphoric acid* to a pH of 5.0 ± 0.1, dilute with water to volume, and mix. Mix this solution with 70 mL of acetonitrile. Make adjustments if necessary (see *System Suitability* under *Chromatography* ⟨621⟩).

Standard solution—Prepare a solution of USP Meropenem RS in *Solvent* having a known concentration of about 0.025 mg of USP Meropenem RS per mL. [NOTE—Immediately after preparation, store this solution in a refrigerator and use within 24 hours.]

Test solution—Dissolve an accurately weighed quantity of Meropenem quantitatively in *Solvent* to obtain a solution having a known concentration of about 5 mg per mL. Use this *Test solution* immediately.

Chromatographic system (see *Chromatography* ⟨621⟩)—The liquid chromatograph is equipped with a 220-nm detector and a 4.6-

mm × 25-cm column that contains 5-µm packing L1 and is maintained at a constant temperature of about 40°. The flow rate is about 1.6 mL per minute, and is adjusted so that the retention time of meropenem is between 5 and 7 minutes. Chromatograph the *Standard solution*, and record the peak responses as directed for *Procedure:* the column efficiency is not less than 2500 theoretical plates; the tailing factor is not more than 1.5; and the relative standard deviation for replicate injections is not more than 2.0%.

Procedure—Separately inject equal volumes (about 10 µL) of the *Standard solution* and the *Test solution* into the chromatograph, record the chromatograms, using a period of chromatography for the *Test solution* that is about 3 times the retention time of meropenem, and measure the peak responses. Major impurity peaks may be observed at retention times of about 0.45 and 1.9 in relation to the retention time of meropenem. Calculate the percentage of each impurity in the chromatogram obtained from the *Test solution* by the formula:

$$(C_S / C_U)(P)(r_i / r_S)$$

in which C_S is the concentration, in mg per mL, of USP Meropenem RS in the *Standard solution*; C_U is the concentration, in mg per mL, of Meropenem in the *Test solution*; P is the stated percentage, calculated on the anhydrous basis, of meropenem in USP Meropenem RS; r_i is the peak response of any individual impurity obtained from the *Test solution*; and r_S is the peak response of meropenem obtained from the *Standard solution*. Not more than 0.3% of any of two major impurities is found, calculated on the anhydrous basis; not more than 0.1% of any other impurity is found, calculated on the anhydrous basis; and the sum of all such other impurities is not more 0.3%.

Other requirements—Where the label states that Meropenem is sterile, it meets the requirements for *Sterility* ⟨71⟩ and for *Bacterial endotoxins* under *Meropenem for Injection*. Where the label states that Meropenem must be subjected to further processing during the preparation of injectable dosage forms, it meets the requirements for *Bacterial endotoxins* under *Meropenem for Injection*.

Assay—

Diluted phosphoric acid—Dilute 10 mL of phosphoric acid with water to make 100 mL of solution.

Solvent—Transfer 1.0 mL of triethylamine to a 1000-mL volumetric flask containing 900 mL of water. Adjust with *Diluted phosphoric acid* to a pH of 5.0 ± 0.1, dilute with water to volume, and mix.

Mobile phase—Prepare a mixture of *Solvent* and methanol (5 : 1). Make adjustments if necessary (see *System Suitability* under *Chromatography* ⟨621⟩).

Standard preparation—Transfer about 25 mg of USP Meropenem RS, accurately weighed, to a 50-mL volumetric flask, add *Solvent*, swirl to dissolve, dilute with *Solvent* to volume, and mix. [NOTE—Immediately after preparation, store this solution in a refrigerator. It may be used for 24 hours.]

Assay preparation—Transfer about 25 mg of Meropenem, accurately weighed, to a 50-mL volumetric flask, add *Solvent*, swirl to dissolve, dilute with *Solvent* to volume, and mix. Use this solution immediately after preparation.

Chromatographic system (see *Chromatography* ⟨621⟩)—The liquid chromatograph is equipped with a 300-nm detector and a 4.6-mm × 25-cm column that contains 5-µm packing L1. Adjust the flow rate so that the retention time for meropenem is about 6 to 8 minutes. The flow rate is about 1.5 mL per minute. Chromatograph the *Standard preparation*, and record the peak responses as directed for *Procedure:* the column efficiency is not less than 2500 theoretical plates; the tailing factor is not more than 1.5; and the relative standard deviation for replicate injections is not more than 2.0%.

Procedure—Separately inject equal volumes (about 5 µL) of *Standard preparation* and *Assay preparation* into the chromatograph, record the chromatograms, and measure the areas for the major peaks. Calculate the quantity, in mg, of $C_{17}H_{25}N_3O_5S$ in the portion of Meropenem taken by the formula:

$$(W_S/W_U)(P)(r_U / r_S)$$

in which W_S is the weight, in mg, of USP Meropenem RS taken to prepare the *Standard preparation*, calculated on the anhydrous basis; W_U is the weight, in mg, of Meropenem taken to prepare the *Assay preparation*; P is the stated percentage, calculated on the anhydrous basis, of meropenem in USP Meropenem RS; and r_U and r_S are the meropenem peak responses obtained from the *Assay preparation* and the *Standard preparation*, respectively.

Meropenem for Injection

» Meropenem for Injection is a sterile dry mixture of Meropenem and Sodium Carbonate. It contains not less than 90.0 percent and not more than 120.0 percent of the labeled amount of meropenem ($C_{17}H_{25}N_3O_5S$).

Packaging and storage—Preserve in tight *Containers for Sterile Solids* as described under *Injections* ⟨1⟩. Store at controlled room temperature.

Labeling—It meets the requirements for *Labeling* under *Injections* ⟨1⟩. Label it to state the quantity, in mg, of sodium (Na) in a given dosage of meropenem.

USP Reference standards ⟨11⟩—*USP Endotoxin RS. USP Meropenem RS.*

Constituted solution—At the time of use, it meets the requirements for *Constituted Solutions* under *Injections* ⟨1⟩.

Identification—The retention time for the meropenem peak in the chromatogram of the *Assay preparation* corresponds to that in the chromatogram of the *Standard preparation*, as obtained in the *Assay*.

Bacterial endotoxins ⟨85⟩—It contains not more than 0.125 USP Endotoxin Unit per mg of meropenem.

Sterility ⟨71⟩—It meets the requirements when tested as directed for *Membrane Filtration* under *Test for Sterility of the Product to be Examined*.

Uniformity of dosage units ⟨905⟩: meets the requirements.

pH ⟨791⟩: between 7.3 and 8.3, in a solution (1 in 20).

Loss on drying ⟨731⟩—Dry it in vacuum at 65° for 6 hours: it loses between 9.0% and 12.0% of its weight.

Particulate matter ⟨788⟩: meets the requirements for small-volume injections.

Chromatographic purity—

Diluted phosphoric acid, *Solvent*, *Mobile phase*, and *Chromatographic system*—Proceed as directed in the test for *Chromatographic purity* under *Meropenem*.

Standard solution—Prepare a solution of USP Meropenem RS in *Solvent* having a known concentration of about 0.029 mg of USP Meropenem RS per mL. [NOTE—Immediately after preparation, store this solution in a refrigerator. It may be used for 24 hours.]

Test solution—Transfer an accurately weighed portion of Meropenem for Injection, equivalent to about 50 mg of meropenem, based on the labeled amount, to a 10-mL volumetric flask, dilute with *Solvent* to volume, and mix. Use this *Test solution* immediately.

Procedure—Proceed as directed in the test for *Chromatographic purity* under *Meropenem*. Calculate the percentage of each impurity in the portion of Injection taken by the formula:

$$10(CP/m)(r_i / r_S)$$

in which C is the concentration, in mg per mL, of USP Meropenem RS in the *Standard solution*; P is the stated percentage, calculated on the anhydrous basis, of meropenem in USP Meropenem RS; m is the amount, in mg, of meropenem in the portion of Injection taken to prepare the *Test solution*, based on the label claim; r_i is the peak response of any individual impurity obtained from the *Test solution*; and r_S is the peak response of meropenem obtained from the *Standard solution*. Not more than 0.8% of the impurity, if any, with a retention time of about 0.45 relative to that of meropenem, is found; and not more than 0.6% of the impurity, if any, with a retention time of about 1.9 relative to that of meropenem, is found.

Content of sodium—

Potassium chloride solution—Transfer 38.1 g of potassium chloride to a 1000-mL volumetric flask, dissolve in and dilute with water to volume, and mix.

Standard sodium solution—Dissolve 25.42 mg of sodium chloride, previously dried at 105° for 2 hours and accurately weighed, quantitatively in water to obtain a solution having a concentration of 25.42 µg of sodium chloride per mL. Transfer 5.0 mL of this solution to a 50-mL volumetric flask, add 5.0 mL of *Potassium chloride solution*, dilute with water to volume, and mix.

Test solution—Transfer an accurately measured volume of the stock solution used to prepare *Assay preparation 1* or *Assay preparation 2*, as appropriate, equivalent to about 25 mg of meropenem, to a 200-mL volumetric flask, dilute with water to volume, and mix. Transfer 5.0 mL of this solution to a 50-mL volumetric flask, add 5.0 mL of *Potassium chloride solution*, dilute with water to volume, and mix.

Blank solution—Transfer 5.0 mL of *Potassium chloride solution* to a 50-mL volumetric flask, dilute with water to volume, and mix.

Procedure—Concomitantly determine the absorbances of the *Standard sodium solution* and the *Test solution* at the sodium emission line at 589.6 nm with an atomic absorption spectrophotometer (see *Spectrophotometry and Light-Scattering* ⟨851⟩), equipped with a sodium hollow-cathode lamp and a single-slot burner, using an air–acetylene flame and the *Blank solution* as the blank. Calculate the quantity, in mg, of sodium (Na) in the constituted Meropenem for Injection by the formula:

$$(22.99/58.44)(C)(2000V/vM)(A_U/A_S)$$

in which 22.99 and 58.44 are the atomic weight of sodium and the molecular weight of sodium chloride, respectively; C is the concentration, in µg per mL, of sodium chloride in the *Standard sodium solution*; V is the volume, in mL, of the stock solution obtained in *Assay preparation 1* or *Assay preparation 2*, as appropriate; v is the volume, in mL, of the portion of the stock solution taken to prepare the *Test solution*; M is the total quantity, in mg, of meropenem in the stock solution obtained in *Assay preparation 1* or *Assay preparation 2*, as appropriate, based on the result of the *Assay*; and A_U and A_S are the absorbances of the *Test solution* and the *Standard sodium solution*, respectively: it contains between 80% and 120% of the labeled amount of sodium.

Change to read:
Assay—
Mobile phase—Dilute 15 mL of tetrabutylammonium hydroxide solution (25% in water) with water to 750 mL. Adjust with dilute phosphoric acid (1 in 10) to a pH of 7.5 ± 0.1. Add 150 mL of acetonitrile and 100 mL of methanol, mix, and degas. Make adjustments if necessary (see *System Suitability* under *Chromatography* ⟨621⟩).

Standard preparation—Dissolve an accurately weighed portion of USP Meropenem RS quantitatively in *Mobile phase* to obtain a solution having a known concentration of about 0.11 mg per mL. This solution contains the equivalent of about 0.1 mg of meropenem per mL. [NOTE—Immediately after preparation, store this solution in a refrigerator and use within 24 hours.]

Assay preparation 1 (where it is represented as being a single-dose container)—Constitute a container of Meropenem for Injection with a volume of water, accurately measured, corresponding to the amount of solvent specified in the labeling. Withdraw all of the withdrawable contents, using a suitable hypodermic needle and syringe, and transfer to a 100-mL volumetric flask. Dilute with water to volume, and mix. Dilute an accurately measured volume of this stock solution quantitatively with *Mobile phase* to obtain a solution having a concentration of about 0.1 mg of meropenem per mL. Hold this *Assay preparation 1* for 2 hours at 25 ± 1° before testing.

Assay preparation 2 (where the label states the quantity of meropenem in a given volume of constituted solution)—Constitute a container of Meropenem for Injection with a volume of water, accurately measured, corresponding to the amount of solvent specified in the labeling. Transfer an accurately measured volume of the constituted solution, equivalent to about 100 mg of meropenem to a 100-mL volumetric flask, ▲and dilute with water to volume.▲*USP31* Transfer 5.0 mL of this stock solution to a 50-mL volumetric flask, dilute with *Mobile phase* to volume, and mix. Hold this *Assay preparation 2* for 2 hours at 25 ± 1° before testing.

Chromatographic system (see *Chromatography* ⟨621⟩)—The liquid chromatograph is equipped with a 300-nm detector and a 4.6-mm × 25-cm column that contains 5-µm packing L1. The flow rate is about 1.5 mL per minute. Adjust the flow rate to obtain a retention time for meropenem of about 6 to 8 minutes. Chromatograph the *Standard preparation*, and record the peak responses as directed for *Procedure*: the column efficiency is not less than 2500 theoretical plates; the tailing factor is not more than 1.5; and the relative standard deviation for replicate injections is not more than 2.0%.

Procedure—Separately inject equal volumes (about 20 µL) of *Standard preparation*, *Assay preparation 1*, and *Assay preparation 2* into the chromatograph, record the chromatograms, and measure the areas for the major peaks. Calculate the quantity, in mg, of meropenem ($C_{17}H_{25}N_3O_5S$) withdrawn from the container or in the portion of constituted solution taken by the formula:

$$100(L/D)(CP)(r_U/r_S)$$

in which L is the labeled quantity, in mg, of meropenem in the container or in the volume of constituted solution taken; D is the concentration, in mg per mL, of meropenem in *Assay preparation 1* or *Assay preparation 2*, based on the labeled quantity in the container or in the portion of constituted solution taken, respectively; C is the concentration, in mg per mL, of USP Meropenem RS in the *Standard preparation*, calculated on the anhydrous basis; P is the stated percentage, on the anhydrous basis, of meropenem in USP Meropenem RS; and r_U and r_S are the peak responses of meropenem obtained from *Assay preparation 1* or *Assay preparation 2*, as appropriate, and the *Standard preparation*, respectively.

Mesalamine

$C_7H_7NO_3$ 153.14
Benzoic acid, 5-amino-2-hydroxy-.
5-Aminosalicylic acid   [89-57-6].

» Mesalamine contains not less than 98.5 percent and not more than 101.5 percent of $C_7H_7NO_3$, calculated on the dried basis.

Packaging and storage—Preserve in tight, light-resistant containers.
USP Reference standards ⟨11⟩—USP Mesalamine RS.
Clarity of solution—A freshly prepared solution of 0.25 g of it in 10 mL of 1 N hydrochloric acid is clear.
Identification—
   A: *Infrared Absorption* ⟨197K⟩.
   B: *Ultraviolet Absorption* ⟨197U⟩—
   Solution: 12 µg per mL.
   Medium: 0.1 N hydrochloric acid.
   Absorptivities at 230 nm do not differ by more than 3.0%.
   C: Dissolve about 100 mg of it in 5 mL of 0.1 N hydrochloric acid, and add 1 drop of ferric chloride TS: a purplish-violet color is produced.
pH ⟨791⟩: between 3.5 and 4.5, in a suspension (1 in 40).
Loss on drying ⟨731⟩—Dry it in vacuum at 105° for 3 hours: it loses not more than 0.5% of its weight.
Residue on ignition ⟨281⟩: not more than 0.2%.
Chloride ⟨221⟩—Disperse 500 mg in 40 mL of water, sonicate for 5 minutes, and filter the dispersion. To the filtrate add 1 mL of nitric acid: the solution shows no more chloride than corresponds to 0.7 mL of 0.020 N hydrochloric acid (0.1%).
Heavy metals, *Method II* ⟨231⟩: 0.002%.
Hydrogen sulfide and sulfur dioxide—Dissolve about 500 mg in 5 mL of 1 N sodium hydroxide, add 6 mL of 3 N hydrochloric acid, and stir vigorously. A piece of moistened lead acetate test paper held over the mixture does not become discolored.
Sulfate—Proceed as directed in the test for *Sulfate* ⟨221⟩: a 500-mg portion shows no more sulfate than corresponds to 1.0 mL of 0.02 N sulfuric acid (0.2%).

Related compounds—
TEST 1 (*for 3-aminosalicylic acid and other related impurities*)—[NOTE—Use *Test 1* to measure 3-aminosalicylic acid and other related impurities not measured in *Test 2*.]

Mobile phase—Dissolve 1.36 g of monobasic potassium phosphate and 2.2 g of sodium 1-octanesulfonate in 890 mL of water, and adjust with phosphoric acid to a pH of 2.2. Pass through a filter having a 0.5-μm or finer porosity. To the filtrate add 80 mL of methanol and 30 mL of acetonitrile. Make adjustments if necessary (see *System Suitability* under *Chromatography* ⟨621⟩).

Standard solution—Quantitatively dissolve accurately weighed quantities of USP Mesalamine RS and 3-aminosalicylic acid in *Mobile phase* to obtain a solution having known concentrations of about 1 μg of each per mL.

Test solution—Transfer about 50 mg of Mesalamine, accurately weighed, to a 100-mL volumetric flask, add about 75 mL of *Mobile phase*, and sonicate briefly to dissolve. Dilute with *Mobile phase* to volume, and mix.

Chromatographic system (see *Chromatography* ⟨621⟩)—The liquid chromatograph is equipped with a 220-nm detector and a 4.6-mm × 15-cm column that contains 5-μm packing L7. The flow rate is about 1.2 mL per minute. Chromatograph the *Standard solution*, and record the peak responses as directed for *Procedure*: the relative retention times are about 1.0 for mesalamine and 1.3 for 3-aminosalicylic acid; and the resolution, R, between mesalamine and 3-aminosalicylic acid is not less than 2.

Procedure—Separately inject equal volumes (about 20 μL) of the *Standard solution* and the *Test solution* into the chromatograph, record the chromatograms for a period of time that is three times the retention time of mesalamine, and measure the peak area responses. Calculate the percentage of 3-aminosalicylic acid by the formula:

$$0.2C_3(r_3/r_{S3})$$

in which C_3 is the concentration, in μg per mL, of 3-aminosalicylic acid in the *Standard solution*; r_3 is the response of the 3-aminosalicylic acid peak in the chromatogram obtained from the *Test solution*; and r_{S3} is the response of the 3-aminosalicylic acid peak in the chromatogram obtained from the *Standard solution*. Calculate the percentage of each other impurity by the formula:

$$0.2C_m(r_i/r_{Sm})$$

in which C_m is the concentration, in μg per mL, of USP Mesalamine RS in the *Standard solution*; r_i is the response of the individual impurity peak in the chromatogram obtained from the *Test solution*; and r_{Sm} is the response of the mesalamine peak in the chromatogram obtained from the *Standard solution*: not more than 0.2% of 3-aminosalicylic acid is found; not more than 0.2% of any other impurity, expressed in terms of mesalamine equivalent, is found; and the total of all impurities found is not more than 1.0%.

TEST 2 (*for aniline, 2-aminophenol, and 4-aminophenol*)—

Standard solution—Prepare a solution of aniline, 2-aminophenol, and 4-aminophenol in methanol having concentrations of 0.05, 2, and 2 mg per mL, respectively; and dilute quantitatively, and stepwise if necessary, with methylene chloride to obtain a solution having concentrations of 0.5, 20, and 20 μg per mL, respectively.

Test solution—Mix 1.0 g of Mesalamine with 10.0 mL of methylene chloride. Allow to settle, and use the clear methylene chloride solution as the *Test solution*.

Chromatographic system (see *Chromatography* ⟨621⟩)—The gas chromatograph is equipped with a flame-ionization detector and a 0.53-mm × 10-m fused-silica capillary column coated with a 2.65-μm film of stationary phase G27. The carrier gas is helium flowing at a rate of 15 mL per minute. The injection port and the detector temperatures are maintained at about 280° and 300°, respectively. The column temperature is programmed according to the following steps: the starting column temperature is 70°; after injection it is held at 70° for 2 minutes, then increased to 150° at a rate of 30° per minute, then held for 1 minute. Chromatograph the *Standard solution*, and record the peak responses as directed for *Procedure*: the relative retention times are about 0.5 for aniline, 0.9 for 2-aminophenol, and 1.0 for 4-aminophenol; and the peaks are baseline separated.

Procedure—Separately inject equal volumes (about 2 μL) of the *Standard solution* and the *Test solution* into the chromatograph, record the chromatograms, and measure the peak area responses. Identify by retention time any peaks present in the chromatogram of the *Test solution* that correspond to those in the chromatogram obtained from the *Standard solution*. Calculate the quantities, in μg per g, of aniline, 2-aminophenol, and 4-aminophenol in the portion of Mesalamine taken by the formula:

$$10C(r_a/r_{Sa})$$

in which C is the concentration, in μg per mL, of the relevant analyte in the *Standard solution*; r_a is the response of the relevant analyte in the chromatogram obtained from the *Test solution*; and r_{Sa} is the response of the relevant analyte in the chromatogram obtained from the *Standard solution*: not more than 5 μg of aniline, 200 μg of 2-aminophenol, and 200 μg of 4-aminophenol per g are found.

Assay—
Buffer solution—Transfer 7.1 g of anhydrous dibasic sodium phosphate and 6.9 g of monobasic sodium phosphate to a 1000-mL volumetric flask, add 500 mL of water, and swirl to dissolve. Add 7.5 mL of a solution of tetrabutylammonium hydroxide in methanol (1 in 4), dilute with water to volume, and mix.

Mobile phase—Prepare a suitable degassed mixture of *Buffer solution* and methanol (85 : 15). Make adjustments if necessary (see *System Suitability* under *Chromatography* ⟨621⟩).

Resolution solution—Prepare a solution in *Mobile phase* containing about 0.25 mg of 4-aminosalicylic acid and 0.4 mg of USP Mesalamine RS per mL.

Standard preparation—Quantitatively dissolve an accurately weighed quantity of USP Mesalamine RS in *Mobile phase* to obtain a solution having a known concentration of about 1 mg per mL. Transfer 10.0 mL of this solution to a 25-mL volumetric flask, dilute with *Mobile phase* to volume, and mix. This solution contains about 0.4 mg of USP Mesalamine RS per mL.

Assay preparation—Transfer about 50 mg of Mesalamine, accurately weighed, to a 50-mL volumetric flask, dissolve in and dilute with *Mobile phase* to volume, and mix. Transfer 10.0 mL of this solution to a 25-mL volumetric flask, dilute with *Mobile phase* to volume, and mix.

Chromatographic system (see *Chromatography* ⟨621⟩)—The liquid chromatograph is equipped with a 254-nm detector and a 4-mm × 30-cm column that contains packing L1. The flow rate is about 2 mL per minute. Chromatograph the *Resolution solution*, and record the peak responses as directed for *Procedure*: the resolution, R, between 4-aminosalicylic acid and mesalamine is not less than 2.0. Chromatograph the *Standard preparation*, and record the peak responses as directed for *Procedure*: the tailing factor is not more than 2.5; and the relative standard deviation for replicate injections is not more than 2.0%.

Procedure—Separately inject equal volumes (about 15 μL) of the *Standard preparation* and the *Assay preparation* into the chromatograph, record the chromatograms, and measure the responses for the major peaks. Calculate the quantity, in mg, of $C_7H_7NO_3$ in the portion of Mesalamine taken by the formula:

$$125C(r_U/r_S)$$

in which C is the concentration, in mg per mL, of USP Mesalamine RS in the *Standard preparation*; and r_U and r_S are the responses of the mesalamine peaks obtained from the *Assay preparation* and the *Standard preparation*, respectively.

Mesalamine Extended-Release Capsules

» Mesalamine Extended-Release Capsules contain not less than 90.0 percent and not more than 110.0 percent of the labeled amount of mesalamine ($C_7H_7NO_3$).

Packaging and storage—Preserve in tight, light-resistant containers.

USP Reference standards ⟨11⟩—*USP Mesalamine RS.*
Identification, *Infrared Absorption* ⟨197K⟩**:** the powdered, undried Capsule contents being used, and the spectra being recorded in the range between 2000 cm⁻¹ and 1240 cm⁻¹.
Dissolution ⟨711⟩—
Medium: 0.05 M pH 7.5 phosphate buffer prepared by dissolving 6.8 g of monobasic potassium phosphate and 1 g of sodium hydroxide in water to make 1000 mL of solution, and adjusting with 10 N sodium hydroxide to a pH of 7.50 ± 0.05; 900 mL.
Apparatus 2: 100 rpm.
Times: 1, 2, 4, and 8 hours.
Procedure—Determine the amount of $C_7H_7NO_3$ dissolved from UV absorbances at the wavelength of maximum absorbance at about 330 nm on filtered portions of the solution under test suitably diluted with *Medium,* if necessary, in comparison with a Standard solution having a known concentration of USP Mesalamine RS in the same *Medium.*
Tolerances—The percentages of the labeled amount of $C_7H_7NO_3$ dissolved at the times specified conform to *Acceptance Table 2.*

Time (hours)	Amount dissolved
1	between 5% and 25%
2	between 30% and 50%
4	between 60% and 90%
8	not less than 85%

Uniformity of dosage units ⟨905⟩**:** meet the requirements.
Assay—
Buffer—Dissolve 6.8 g of monobasic potassium phosphate and 1.65 g of sodium hydroxide in 800 mL of water, adjust with 1 N sodium hydroxide to a pH of 7.5, dilute with water to 1000 mL, and mix.
Mobile phase A—Dissolve 3.4 g of tetrabutylammonium hydrogen sulfate and 1.4 g of sodium acetate trihydrate in 1000 mL of water, and adjust with 1 N sodium hydroxide to a pH of 6.6. Add 200 mL of acetonitrile, mix, and pass through a filter having a 0.5-μm or finer porosity. Make any necessary adjustments (see *System Suitability* under *Chromatography* ⟨621⟩). [NOTE—Increasing the proportion of acetonitrile decreases the retention times. Prepare fresh daily.]
Mobile phase B—Dissolve 4.6 g of tetrabutylammonium hydrogen sulfate and 1.9 g of sodium acetate trihydrate in 1000 mL of water, and adjust with 1 N sodium hydroxide to a pH of 6.6. Add 650 mL of acetonitrile, mix, and pass through a filter having a 0.5-μm or finer porosity. Make any necessary adjustments (see *System Suitability* under *Chromatography* ⟨621⟩). [NOTE—Prepare fresh daily.]
Internal standard solution—Prepare a solution in *Buffer* containing about 35 mg of sodium benzoate per mL.
Standard preparation—Transfer about 50 mg of USP Mesalamine RS, accurately weighed, to a 100-mL volumetric flask, add 4.0 mL of *Internal standard solution,* mix, dilute with *Buffer* to volume, and mix. Transfer 5.0 mL of this solution to a 25-mL volumetric flask, dilute with *Buffer* to volume, and mix.
Assay preparation—Transfer, as completely as possible, the contents of not fewer than 20 Capsules to a suitable tared container, and determine the average weight of the contents of a Capsule. Finely powder the Capsule contents so that the powder thus obtained passes through a No. 40 sieve (see *Powder Fineness* ⟨811⟩). Transfer an accurately weighed portion of the powder, equivalent to about 250 mg of mesalamine, to a 500-mL volumetric flask, add 20.0 mL of *Internal standard solution* and about 300 mL of *Buffer,* and shake by mechanical means for 1 hour. Dilute with *Buffer* to volume, and mix. Transfer 5.0 mL of this solution to a 25-mL volumetric flask, dilute with *Buffer* to volume, mix, and pass about 10 mL of this solution through a filter having a 0.5-μm or finer porosity. Use the filtrate as the *Assay preparation.*
Chromatographic system (see *Chromatography* ⟨621⟩)—The liquid chromatograph is equipped with a 240-nm detector and a 4.6-mm × 25-cm column that contains 5-μm packing L1, and is programmed to provide variable mixtures of *Mobile phase A* and *Mobile phase B.* The flow rate is about 1.5 mL per minute. The system is equilibrated with *Mobile phase A.* Five minutes after the injection of the *Standard preparation* and the *Assay preparation,* the proportion of *Mobile phase B* is increased linearly from 0% to 100% over a period of 2 minutes, and held for 8 minutes. The proportion of *Mobile phase A* is then increased linearly from 0% to 100% over a period of 2 minutes and held for 3 minutes. Chromatograph the *Standard preparation,* and record the peak responses as directed for *Procedure:* the relative retention times are about 0.6 for mesalamine and 1.0 for sodium benzoate, the resolution, *R*, between mesalamine and sodium benzoate; is not less than 2.5; and the relative standard deviation for replicate injections is not more than 2.0%.
Procedure—Separately inject equal volumes (about 10 μL) of the *Standard preparation* and the *Assay preparation* into the chromatograph, record the chromatograms, and measure the responses for the major peaks. Calculate the quantity, in mg, of mesalamine ($C_7H_7NO_3$) in the portion of Capsule contents taken by the formula:

$$2500C(R_U / R_S)$$

in which *C* is the concentration, in mg per mL, of USP Mesalamine RS in the *Standard preparation;* and R_U and R_S are the peak response ratios of the mesalamine peak to the sodium benzoate peak obtained from the *Assay preparation* and the *Standard preparation,* respectively.

Mesalamine Rectal Suspension

» Mesalamine Rectal Suspension is a suspension of Mesalamine in a suitable aqueous vehicle. It contains not less than 90.0 percent and not more than 110.0 percent of the labeled amount of mesalamine ($C_7H_7NO_3$). It contains one or more suitable preservatives.

Packaging and storage—Preserve in tight, light-resistant containers.

USP Reference standards ⟨11⟩—*USP Mesalamine RS.*
Identification—The retention time of the major peak in the chromatogram of the *Assay preparation* corresponds to that in the chromatogram of the *Standard preparation,* as obtained in the *Assay.*
Uniformity of dosage units ⟨905⟩: meets the requirements.
PROCEDURE FOR CONTENT UNIFORMITY—
Buffer solution, Mobile phase, Resolution solution, and *Chromatographic system*—Proceed as directed in the *Assay* under *Mesalamine.*
Standard solution—Transfer about 100 mg of USP Mesalamine RS, accurately weighed, to a 50-mL volumetric flask, add 15 mL of 2 N hydrochloric acid, and dissolve by swirling. Dilute with 2 N hydrochloric acid to volume, and mix. Transfer 5.0 mL of this solution to a 25-mL volumetric flask, add 5 mL of 2 N sodium hydroxide, dilute with *Mobile phase* to volume, and mix. Pass this solution through a suitable filter having a 0.5-μm or finer porosity.
Test solution—Transfer, with the aid of 2 N hydrochloric acid, the contents of a container of Rectal Suspension to a 200-mL volumetric flask. Add 2 N hydrochloric acid to obtain about 160 mL of solution, and shake for about 10 minutes. Dilute with 2 N hydrochloric acid to volume, and mix. Transfer an accurately measured volume of this stock solution, equivalent to about 40 mg of mesalamine, to a 100-mL volumetric flask, add a volume of 2 N hydrochloric acid, equal to the added stock solution volume, dilute with *Mobile phase* to volume, and mix. Pass this solution through a suitable filter having a 0.5-μm or finer porosity.
Procedure—Proceed as directed in the *Assay.* Calculate the quantity, in g, of $C_7H_7NO_3$ in the container of Rectal Suspension taken by the formula:

$$20(C / V)(r_U / r_S)$$

in which *V* is the volume, in mL, of stock solution taken to prepare the *Test solution;* and the other terms are as defined therein.

pH ⟨791⟩: between 3.5 and 5.5, when diluted 1 to 10 with water.

Related compounds—

Mobile phase, Standard solution, and *Chromatographic system*—Proceed as directed in *Test 1* for *Related compounds* under *Mesalamine.*

Test solution—Transfer an accurately measured volume of Rectal Suspension, previously well shaken, equivalent to 100 mg of mesalamine, to a beaker, add water to give a volume of about 80 mL, adjust with phosphoric acid to a pH of 2.0, sonicate briefly to dissolve, transfer to a 100-mL volumetric flask, dilute with water to volume, and mix.

Procedure—Proceed as directed in the test for *Related compounds* under *Mesalamine.* Calculate the percentage of each impurity in the Rectal Suspension taken by the formula:

$$0.1 C_M (r_i / r_{SM})$$

in which the terms are as defined therein. Not more than 0.2% of any individual impurity is found; and not more than 1.0% of total impurities is found.

Content of sodium benzoate *(if present)*—

Mobile phase—Transfer 390 mg of ammonium acetate to a 1000-mL volumetric flask, add 100 mL of water, and dissolve by swirling. Add 6 mL of glacial acetic acid and 300 mL of methanol, dilute with water to volume, and mix. Pass this solution through a filter having a 0.5-μm or finer porosity. Make adjustments if necessary (see *System Suitability* under *Chromatography* ⟨621⟩).

Standard solution—Transfer about 100 mg of sodium benzoate, accurately weighed, to a 100-mL volumetric flask, dissolve in and dilute with water to volume, and mix. Transfer 5.0 mL of this solution to a second 100-mL volumetric flask, add 40 mL of methanol, dilute with water to volume, and mix. Pass this solution through a filter having a 0.5-μm or finer porosity.

Test solution—Transfer about 5 g of well-shaken Rectal Suspension, accurately weighed, to a 100-mL volumetric flask, add 40 mL of methanol, dilute with water to volume, and mix. Pass this solution through a filter having a 0.5-μm or finer porosity.

Chromatographic system—The liquid chromatograph is equipped with a 254-nm detector and a 4.6-mm × 25-cm column that contains packing L7. The flow rate is about 1.5 mL per minute. Inject the *Standard solution* into the chromatograph, and record the peak responses as directed for *Procedure:* the tailing factor is not more than 2.5; and the relative standard deviation for replicate injections is not more than 2.0%.

Procedure—Separately inject equal volumes (about 15 μL) of the *Standard solution* and the *Test solution* into the chromatograph, record the chromatograms, and measure the responses for the major peaks. Calculate the percentage (w/w) of sodium benzoate in the Rectal Suspension taken by the formula:

$$10(C / W)(r_U / r_S)$$

in which *C* is the concentration, in mg per mL, of sodium benzoate in the *Standard solution; W* is the weight, in g, of the Rectal Suspension taken; and r_U and r_S are the responses obtained from the *Test solution* and the *Standard solution,* respectively: it contains between 0.05% and 0.125% of sodium benzoate.

Assay—

Buffer solution, Mobile phase, Resolution solution, Standard preparation, and *Chromatographic system*—Proceed as directed in the *Assay* under *Mesalamine.*

Assay preparation—Transfer an accurately measured, well-shaken quantity of Rectal Suspension, equivalent to about 100 mg of mesalamine, to a 100-mL volumetric flask, add 55 mL of *Mobile phase,* and dissolve by shaking for about 10 minutes. Dilute with *Mobile phase* to volume, and mix. Transfer 10.0 mL of this solution to a 25-mL volumetric flask, dilute with *Mobile phase* to volume, and mix. Pass this solution through a suitable filter having a 0.5-μm or finer porosity, and use the filtrate as the *Assay preparation.*

Procedure—Proceed as directed in the *Assay* under *Mesalamine.* Calculate the quantity, in mg, of mesalamine ($C_7H_7NO_3$) in the portion of Rectal Suspension taken by the formula:

$$250 C (r_U / r_S)$$

in which the terms are as defined therein.

Mesalamine Delayed-Release Tablets

» Mesalamine Delayed-Release Tablets contain not less than 90.0 percent and not more than 110.0 percent of the labeled amount of mesalamine ($C_7H_7NO_3$).

Packaging and storage—Preserve in tight containers.

USP Reference standards ⟨11⟩—*USP Mesalamine RS. USP Salicylic Acid RS.*

Identification, *Infrared Absorption* ⟨197K⟩—

Test specimen—To about 50 mL of water add a quantity of finely powdered Tablets, equivalent to about 800 mg of mesalamine. Boil the mixture for about 5 minutes, with constant stirring. Filter the hot solution, and allow the filtrate to cool. Collect the precipitated crystals, and dry at about 110°.

Dissolution ⟨711⟩—

pH 6.0 Phosphate buffer—Transfer about 43.35 g of monobasic potassium phosphate and 1.65 g of sodium hydroxide to a 2-L volumetric flask. Dissolve in and dilute with water to volume, and mix. Adjust with 1 N sodium hydroxide or phosphoric acid to a pH of 6.0, and mix.

Sodium hydroxide solution—Transfer 133.6 g of sodium hydroxide to a 2-L volumetric flask, dissolve in and dilute with water to volume, and mix.

Media: 0.1 N hydrochloric acid, 500 mL for *Acid stage;* pH 6.0 *Phosphate buffer,* 900 mL for *Buffer stages.*

Apparatus 2: 100 rpm for *Acid stage* and for *Buffer stage 1;* 50 rpm for *Buffer stage 2.*

Times: 2 hours for *Acid stage;* 1 hour for *Buffer stage 1;* 90 minutes for *Buffer stage 2.*

ACID STAGE—After 2 hours of operation, withdraw an aliquot of the fluid, discard the remaining solution, and retain the Tablets in proper order, so that each will be returned to its respective vessel later on. Blot the Tablets with a paper towel to dry, and proceed immediately as directed for *Buffer stage 1.*

Procedure—Determine the amount of $C_7H_7NO_3$ dissolved by employing UV absorption at the wavelength of maximum absorbance at about 302 nm on filtered portions of the solution under test, suitably diluted with *Medium,* if necessary, in comparison with a Standard solution having a known concentration of USP Mesalamine RS, equivalent to about 1% of the labeled amount of $C_7H_7NO_3$, in the same *Medium.*

Tolerances—The percentage of the labeled amount of $C_7H_7NO_3$ dissolved from the units tested conforms to the *Acceptance Table* shown below. Continue testing through all levels unless the results conform at an earlier level.

BUFFER STAGE 1—[NOTE—Use buffer that has been equilibrated to a temperature of 37 ± 0.5°.] Transfer *pH 6.0 Phosphate buffer* to each of the dissolution vessels, and place each Tablet from the *Acid stage* into its respective vessel. After 1 hour remove a 50-mL aliquot, and proceed immediately as directed for *Buffer stage 2.*

Procedure—Determine the amount of $C_7H_7NO_3$ dissolved by employing UV absorption at the wavelength of maximum absorbance at about 330 nm on filtered portions of the solution under test, suitably diluted with *Medium,* if necessary, in comparison with a Standard solution having a known concentration of USP Mesalamine RS, equivalent to about 1% of the labeled amount of $C_7H_7NO_3$, in the same *Medium.*

Tolerances—The percentage of the labeled amount of $C_7H_7NO_3$ dissolved from the units tested conforms to the *Acceptance Table* shown below. Continue testing through all levels unless the results conform at an earlier level.

Acceptance Table

Level	Number Tested	Criteria
L_1	6	No individual value exceeds 1% dissolved.
L_2	6	Average of the 12 units (L_1 + L_2) is not more than 1% dissolved, and no individual unit is greater than 10% dissolved.
L_3	12	Average of the 24 units (L_1 + L_2 + L_3) is not more than 1% dissolved, and not more than one individual unit is greater than 10% dissolved.

BUFFER STAGE 2—Add 50 mL of *Sodium hydroxide solution* to each dissolution vessel to adjust to a pH of 7.2, and continue the run.

Procedure—Determine the amount of $C_7H_7NO_3$ dissolved by employing UV absorption at the wavelength of maximum absorbance at about 332 nm on filtered portions of the solution under test, suitably diluted with *Medium*, if necessary, in comparison with a Standard solution having a known concentration of USP Mesalamine RS in the same *Medium*.

Tolerances—Not less than 80% (*Q*) of the labeled amount of $C_7H_7NO_3$ is dissolved. The requirements are met if the quantities dissolved from the product conform to *Acceptance Table 4*. Continue testing through all levels unless the results conform at an earlier level.

Uniformity of dosage units ⟨905⟩: meet the requirements for *Weight Variation*.

Chromatographic purity—
Mobile phase—Proceed as directed in the *Assay*.
Chromatographic system—Proceed as directed in the *Assay*. To evaluate the system suitability requirements, use the *System suitability preparation*, *Standard stock preparation*, and the *Standard preparation* prepared as directed in the *Assay*.
Test solution—Weigh and finely powder not fewer than 20 Tablets. Transfer an accurately weighed portion of the powder, equivalent to about 400 mg of mesalamine, to a 500-mL volumetric flask. Add 50 mL of 1 N hydrochloric acid, and sonicate to dissolve. Shake by mechanical means for 10 minutes, dilute with water to volume, mix, and pass through a filter having a 0.5-μm or finer porosity. [NOTE—Use an aliquot of this solution for the *Assay preparation*.]
Procedure—Inject a volume (about 20 μL) of the *Test solution* into the chromatograph, record the chromatogram, and measure the areas for all the peaks. Calculate the percentage of each impurity in the portion of Tablets taken by the formula:

$$100(r_i / r_s)$$

in which r_i is the peak response for each impurity; and r_s is the sum of the responses of all the peaks: the largest secondary peak is not more than 1.0% of the total area; not more than 0.5% of any other individual impurity is found; and not more than 2.0% of total impurities is found.

Assay—
Mobile phase—Dissolve 4.3 g of sodium 1-octanesulfonate in 1 L of water. Adjust with phosphoric acid to a pH of 2.15, pass through a filter having a 0.45-μm or finer porosity, and degas.
System suitability preparation—Transfer about 20 mg each of 3-aminosalicylic acid and USP Salicylic Acid RS, accurately weighed, to a 200-mL volumetric flask. Dissolve in 50 mL of 1 N hydrochloric acid, sonicating to dissolve, dilute with water to volume, and mix. Dilute the solution so obtained quantitatively and stepwise with water, and mix to obtain a solution having known concentrations of about 0.01 mg each of 3-aminosalicylic acid and salicylic acid per mL.
Standard stock preparation—Transfer about 25 mg of USP Mesalamine RS, accurately weighed, to a 25-mL volumetric flask. Dissolve in 5 mL of 0.25 N hydrochloric acid, sonicating to dissolve, dilute with water to volume, and mix.

Standard preparation—Transfer 10.0 mL of *Standard stock preparation* and 5.0 mL of *System suitability preparation* to a 50-mL volumetric flask. Dilute with water to volume, mix, and pass through a filter having a 0.5-μm or finer porosity.
Assay preparation—Pipet a 25.0-mL aliquot of the *Test solution*, obtained as directed for the *Chromatographic purity* test, into a 100-mL volumetric flask, dilute with water to volume, mix, and pass through a filter having a 0.5-μm or finer porosity.
Chromatographic system (see *Chromatography* ⟨621⟩)—The liquid chromatograph is equipped with a 230-nm detector, a 4.6-mm × 3.3-cm analytical column that contains 3-μm base-deactivated packing L1, and two 4.6-mm × 3.0-cm precolumns, each containing 10-μm packing L1 and being located between the pump and the injector. The flow rate is about 2 mL per minute. Chromatograph the *Standard preparation*, and record the peak responses as directed for *Procedure*: the resolution, *R*, between mesalamine and salicylic acid or 3-aminosalicylic acid is not less than 2; the tailing factor is not more than 2; and the relative standard deviation for replicate injections is not more than 2.0%.
Procedure—Separately inject equal volumes (about 20 μL) of the *Standard preparation* and the *Assay preparation* into the chromatograph, record the chromatograms, and measure the responses for the major peaks. Calculate the quantity, in mg, of mesalamine ($C_7H_7NO_3$) in the portion of Tablets taken by the formula:

$$2000C(r_U / r_S)$$

in which *C* is the concentration, in mg per mL, of USP Mesalamine RS in the *Standard preparation*; and r_U and r_S are the mesalamine peak responses obtained from the *Assay preparation* and the *Standard preparation*, respectively.

Mesoridazine Besylate

$C_{21}H_{26}N_2OS_2 \cdot C_6H_6O_3S$ 544.75

10*H*-Phenothiazine, 10-[2-(1-methyl-2-piperidinyl)ethyl]-2-(methylsulfinyl)-, (±)-, monobenzenesulfonate.
(±)-10-[2-(1-Methyl-2-piperidyl)ethyl]-2-(methylsulfinyl)phenothiazine monobenzenesulfonate [32672-69-8].

» Mesoridazine Besylate contains not less than 98.0 percent and not more than 102.0 percent of $C_{21}H_{26}N_2OS_2 \cdot C_6H_6O_3S$, calculated on the dried basis.

Packaging and storage—Preserve in tight, light-resistant containers.

USP Reference standards ⟨11⟩—*USP Mesoridazine Besylate RS*.
NOTE—Throughout the following procedures, protect test or assay specimens, the USP Reference Standard, and solutions containing them, by conducting the procedures without delay, under subdued light, or using low-actinic glassware.

Identification—
A: *Infrared Absorption* ⟨197M⟩.
B: *Ultraviolet Absorption* ⟨197U⟩—
Solution: 10 μg per mL.
Medium: methanol.
Absorptivities at 263 nm, calculated on the dried basis, do not differ by more than 3.0%.

pH ⟨791⟩: between 4.2 and 5.7, in a freshly prepared solution (1 in 100).

Loss on drying ⟨731⟩—Dry it at 105° for 4 hours: it loses not more than 0.5% of its weight.

Residue on ignition ⟨281⟩: not more than 0.2%.
Heavy metals, *Method II* ⟨231⟩: 0.002%.
Selenium ⟨291⟩—The absorbance of the solution from the *Test Solution*, prepared with 100 mg of Mesoridazine Besylate and 100 mg of magnesium oxide, is not greater than one-half that from the *Standard Solution* (0.003%).
Ordinary impurities ⟨466⟩—
  Test solution: a solution in methanol having a known concentration of 14.1 mg per mL equivalent to 10 mg of mesoridazine per mL.
  Standard solution: methanol.
  Eluant: a mixture of chloroform, isopropyl alcohol, and ammonium hydroxide (87 : 12 : 1).
  Visualization: 3, followed by spraying with 3% (v/v) aqueous hydrogen peroxide.
  Application volume: 10 µL.
  Limit: 3.0%.
Organic volatile impurities, *Method I* ⟨467⟩: meets the requirements.
(Official until July 1, 2008)
Assay—Dissolve about 150 mg of Mesoridazine Besylate, accurately weighed, in 70 mL of acetic anhydride, and titrate with 0.1 N perchloric acid VS, determining the endpoint potentiometrically. Perform a blank determination, and make any necessary correction. Each mL of 0.1 N perchloric acid is equivalent to 27.24 mg of $C_{21}H_{26}N_2OS_2 \cdot C_6H_6O_3S$.

Mesoridazine Besylate Injection

» Mesoridazine Besylate Injection is a sterile solution of Mesoridazine Besylate in Water for Injection. It contains mesoridazine besylate ($C_{21}H_{26}N_2OS_2 \cdot C_6H_6O_3S$) equivalent to not less than 90.0 percent and not more than 110.0 percent of the labeled amount of mesoridazine ($C_{21}H_{26}N_2OS_2$).

Packaging and storage—Preserve in single-dose containers, preferably of Type I glass, protected from light.
USP Reference standards ⟨11⟩—USP Endotoxin RS. USP Mesoridazine Besylate RS.
  NOTE—Throughout the following procedures, protect test or assay specimens, the Reference Standard, and solutions containing them, by conducting the procedures without delay, under subdued light, or using low-actinic glassware.
Identification—Dilute a volume of Injection, equivalent to about 50 mg of mesoridazine besylate, with 0.01 N hydrochloric acid to 25 mL, and proceed as directed under *Identification—Organic Nitrogenous Bases* ⟨181⟩, beginning with "Transfer the liquid to a separator": the Injection meets the requirements of the test.
Bacterial endotoxins ⟨85⟩—It contains not more than 7.0 USP Endotoxin Units per mg of mesoridazine besylate.
pH ⟨791⟩: between 4.0 and 5.0.
Other requirements—It meets the requirements under *Injections* ⟨1⟩.
Assay—[NOTE—Conduct this procedure with minimum exposure to light.] Proceed with Injection as directed under *Salts of Organic Nitrogenous Bases* ⟨501⟩, except to use 1.0 mL each of the *Standard Preparation* and the *Assay Preparation* in the *Procedure*, and determine the absorbances at the wavelength of maximum absorbance at about 262 nm. Calculate the quantity, in mg, of $C_{21}H_{26}N_2OS_2$ in each mL of the Injection taken by the formula:

$$(386.59 / 544.75)(0.05C / V)(A_U / A_S)$$

in which 386.59 and 544.75 are the molecular weights of mesoridazine and mesoridazine besylate, respectively; C is the concentration, in µg per mL, of USP Mesoridazine Besylate RS in the *Standard Preparation*; and V is the volume, in mL, of Injection taken.

Mesoridazine Besylate Oral Solution

» Mesoridazine Besylate Oral Solution contains not less than 90.0 percent and not more than 110.0 percent of the labeled amount of mesoridazine ($C_{21}H_{26}N_2OS_2$).

Packaging and storage—Preserve in tight, light-resistant containers, and store at a temperature not exceeding 25°.
Labeling—Label it to indicate that it is to be diluted to the appropriate strength with water or other suitable fluid prior to administration.
USP Reference standards ⟨11⟩—USP Mesoridazine Besylate RS.
  NOTE—Throughout the following procedures, protect test or assay specimens, the USP Reference Standard, and solutions containing them, by conducting the procedures without delay, under subdued light, or using low-actinic glassware.
Identification—[NOTE—Conduct this test without exposure to daylight and with the minimum necessary exposure to artificial light.]
  Standard solution—Prepare a solution of USP Mesoridazine Besylate RS in methanol to contain 14 mg per mL.
  Test solution—Transfer 4.0 mL of the Oral Solution into a separator, add 6 mL of 1 N sodium hydroxide and 10 mL of chloroform, shake for 2 minutes, and filter the chloroform layer through anhydrous sodium sulfate into a small, glass-stoppered conical flask.
  Developing solvent—To a separator add benzene, alcohol, and ammonium hydroxide (10 : 2 : 1), shake, and allow the layers to separate. Use the upper layer.
  Procedure—Into a suitable chromatographic chamber arranged for thin-layer chromatography, place a volume of *Developing solvent* sufficient to develop the chromatogram, and allow to equilibrate. Apply separate 10-µL portions of the *Test solution* and the *Standard solution* to a suitable thin-layer chromatographic plate coated with a 0.25-mm layer of chromatographic silica gel mixture. Allow the spots to dry, and develop the chromatogram until the solvent front has moved about three-fourths of the length of the plate. Remove the plate from the developing chamber, mark the solvent front, and allow the solvent to evaporate in a fume hood. Spray the plate with a solution prepared by diluting 15 mL of perchloric acid with water to 100 mL, and heat at 80° for 2 minutes: the principal spot obtained from the *Test solution* corresponds in R_F value and color to that of the *Standard solution*.
Alcohol content, *Method I* ⟨611⟩: between 0.25% and 1.0% of C_2H_5OH.
Uniformity of dosage units ⟨905⟩—
  FOR ORAL SOLUTION PACKAGED IN SINGLE-UNIT CONTAINERS: meets the requirements.
Deliverable volume ⟨698⟩—
  FOR ORAL SOLUTION PACKAGED IN MULTIPLE-UNIT CONTAINERS: meets the requirements.
Assay—[NOTE—Conduct this procedure with the minimum necessary exposure to light.]
  Standard preparation—Transfer about 14 mg of USP Mesoridazine Besylate RS, accurately weighed, to a 125-mL separator containing 30 mL of water. Render the solution alkaline with 10 mL of 1 N sodium hydroxide, and extract with three 30-mL portions of chloroform. Filter the extracts through anhydrous sodium sulfate into a 100-mL volumetric flask. Rinse the filter with small portions of chloroform, collecting the rinsings in the volumetric flask, dilute with chloroform to volume, and mix. Dilute 10.0 mL of this solution with chloroform to 100.0 mL, and mix.
  Assay preparation—Pipet a volume of Oral Solution, equivalent to about 100 mg of mesoridazine, into a separator containing 30 mL of water. Proceed as directed under *Standard preparation*, beginning with "Render the solution alkaline." Pipet 10.0 mL of this solution into a third 100-mL volumetric flask, dilute with chloroform to volume, and mix.
  Procedure—Concomitantly determine the absorbances of the *Standard preparation* and the *Assay preparation* in 1-cm cells at the wavelength of maximum absorbance at about 267 nm, with a suitable spectrophotometer, using chloroform as the blank. Calculate

the quantity, in mg, of mesoridazine ($C_{21}H_{26}N_2OS_2$) in each mL of the Oral Solution taken by the formula:

$$(386.59/544.75)(10C/V)(A_U/A_S)$$

in which 386.59 and 544.75 are the molecular weights of mesoridazine and mesoridazine besylate, respectively; C is the concentration, in μg per mL, of USP Mesoridazine Besylate RS in the *Standard preparation*; V is the volume, in mL, of Oral Solution taken; and A_U and A_S are the absorbances of the *Assay preparation* and the *Standard preparation*, respectively.

Mesoridazine Besylate Tablets

» Mesoridazine Besylate Tablets contain mesoridazine besylate ($C_{21}H_{26}N_2OS_2 \cdot C_6H_6O_3S$) equivalent to not less than 90.0 percent and not more than 110.0 percent of the labeled amount of mesoridazine ($C_{21}H_{26}N_2OS_2$).

Packaging and storage—Preserve in well-closed, light-resistant containers. Preserve Tablets having an opaque coating in well-closed containers.

USP Reference standards ⟨11⟩—*USP Mesoridazine Besylate RS*.
NOTE—Throughout the following procedures, protect test or assay specimens, the Reference Standard, and solutions containing them, by conducting the procedures without delay, under subdued light, or using low-actinic glassware.

Identification—Tablets meet the requirements under *Identification—Organic Nitrogenous Bases* ⟨181⟩.

Dissolution ⟨711⟩—
Medium: 0.01 N hydrochloric acid; 1000 mL.
Apparatus 2: 100 rpm.
Time: 60 minutes.
Procedure—Determine the amount of $C_{21}H_{26}N_2OS_2$ dissolved by employing UV absorption at the wavelength of maximum absorbance at about 261 nm on filtered portions of the solution under test, suitably diluted with *Medium*, if necessary, in comparison with a Standard solution having a known concentration of USP Mesoridazine Besylate RS in the same *Medium*. [NOTE—A volume of methanol not exceeding 1% of the final total volume may be used to prepare the Standard solution.]
Tolerances—Not less than 80% (*Q*) of the labeled amount of $C_{21}H_{26}N_2OS_2$ is dissolved in 60 minutes.

Uniformity of dosage units ⟨905⟩: meet the requirements.

Assay—
Mobile phase—Prepare a filtered and degassed mixture of acetonitrile, water, and triethylamine (850 : 150 : 1). Make adjustments if necessary (see *System Suitability* under *Chromatography* ⟨621⟩).
Standard preparation—Dissolve an accurately weighed quantity of USP Mesoridazine Besylate RS in methanol, and dilute quantitatively, and stepwise if necessary, with methanol to obtain a solution having a known concentration of about 0.35 mg per mL.
Assay preparation—Weigh and finely powder not fewer than 20 Tablets. Transfer an accurately weighed portion of the powder, equivalent to about 50 mg of mesoridazine, to a 200-mL volumetric flask. Add about 150 mL of methanol, shake by mechanical means for about 15 minutes, dilute with methanol to volume, and mix. Sonicate for 30 minutes, and allow dispersed material to settle. Filter through a 0.25-μm disk, discarding the first 20 mL of the filtrate.
System suitability preparation—Dissolve a suitable quantity of thioridazine hydrochloride in a portion of the *Standard preparation*, and mix to obtain a solution containing 0.025 mg of thioridazine hydrochloride per mL.
Chromatographic system (see *Chromatography* ⟨621⟩)—The liquid chromatograph is equipped with a 265-nm detector and a 4.6-mm × 25-cm column that contains packing L1. The flow rate is about 2.5 mL per minute. Chromatograph the *Standard preparation* and the *System suitability preparation*, and record the peak areas as directed for *Procedure*: the resolution, *R*, between mesoridazine besylate and thioridazine hydrochloride is not less than 1.0; the column efficiency determined from the analyte peak is not less than 750 theoretical plates; and the relative standard deviation for replicate injections of the *Standard preparation* is not more than 2.0%.
Procedure—Separately inject equal volumes (about 10 μL) of the *Standard preparation* and the *Assay preparation* into the chromatograph, record the chromatograms, and measure the areas for the major peaks. Calculate the quantity, in mg, of mesoridazine ($C_{21}H_{26}N_2OS_2$) in the portion of Tablets taken by the formula:

$$(386.59/544.75)(200C)(r_U/r_S)$$

in which 386.59 and 544.75 are the molecular weights of mesoridazine and mesoridazine besylate, respectively; C is the concentration, in mg per mL, of USP Mesoridazine Besylate RS in the *Standard preparation*; and r_U and r_S are the peak areas obtained from the *Assay preparation* and the *Standard preparation*, respectively.

Mestranol

$C_{21}H_{26}O_2$ 310.43
19-Norpregna-1,3,5(10)-trien-20-yn-17-ol, 3-methoxy-, (17α)-.
3-Methoxy-19-nor-17α-pregna-1,3,5(10)-trien-20-yn-17-ol   [72-33-3].

» Mestranol contains not less than 97.0 percent and not more than 102.0 percent of $C_{21}H_{26}O_2$, calculated on the dried basis.

Packaging and storage—Preserve in well-closed, light-resistant containers.

USP Reference standards ⟨11⟩—*USP Mestranol RS*.

Identification—
A: *Infrared Absorption* ⟨197K⟩.
B: *Ultraviolet Absorption* ⟨197U⟩—
Solution: 100 μg per mL.
Medium: methanol.
C: Prepare a solution in chloroform to contain 1 mg of mestranol per mL. Apply 10 μL of this solution and 10 μL of a solution of USP Mestranol RS in chloroform containing 1 mg per mL to a line parallel to and about 2.5 cm from the bottom edge of a thin-layer chromatographic plate (see *Chromatography* ⟨621⟩) coated with a 0.25-mm layer of chromatographic silica gel mixture. Place the plate in a developing chamber containing and equilibrated with a mixture of 29 volumes of chloroform and 1 volume of dehydrated alcohol. Develop the chromatogram until the solvent front has moved about 15 cm above the line of application. Remove the plate, allow the solvent to evaporate, and spray with *Methanol–sulfuric acid* prepared as described in the *Assay*. Heat the plate in an oven at 105° for 5 minutes, and observe under long-wavelength UV light: the R_F value of the principal spot obtained from the solution under test corresponds to that obtained with the Standard solution.

Melting range ⟨741⟩: between 146° and 154°, but the range between beginning and end of melting does not exceed 4°.

Specific rotation ⟨781S⟩: between +2° and +8°.
Test solution: 20 mg, previously dried, per mL, in dioxane.

Loss on drying ⟨731⟩—Dry it at 105° for 3 hours: it loses not more than 1.0% of its weight.

Assay—
Methanol–sulfuric acid—Pipet 30 mL of methanol into a 100-mL volumetric flask contained in an ice bath. Add slowly and cautiously, and with continuous stirring, about 65 mL of sulfuric acid, taking care that the temperature remains below 15°. Allow the solution to warm to room temperature, and dilute with sulfuric acid to 100 mL.
Standard preparation—Dissolve a suitable quantity of USP Mestranol RS, accurately weighed, in chloroform, and dilute quantita-

tively and stepwise with chloroform to obtain a solution having a known concentration of about 5 µg per mL.

Assay preparation—Weigh accurately about 20 mg of Mestranol, dissolve in chloroform to make 200.0 mL, and mix. Pipet 5 mL of this solution into a 100-mL volumetric flask, add chloroform to volume, and mix.

Procedure—Pipet 4 mL each of the *Standard preparation* and the *Assay preparation* into separate glass-stoppered, 25-mL conical flasks. Evaporate the solutions under a slow stream of air, without the aid of heat, to dryness. Dissolve the residue in 0.3 mL of methanol. Place the flasks in a water bath maintained at a temperature of 25°, and pipet into each, with constant swirling, 10 mL of *Methanol–sulfuric acid*. Insert the stoppers in the flasks. At 6 minutes, accurately timed, after the addition of the *Methanol–sulfuric acid*, concomitantly determine the absorbances of the solutions obtained from the *Assay preparation* and the *Standard preparation* at the wavelength of maximum absorbance at about 545 nm, with a suitable spectrophotometer, using *Methanol–sulfuric acid* as the blank. Calculate the quantity, in mg, of $C_{21}H_{26}O_2$ in the Mestranol taken by the formula:

$$4C(A_U / A_S)$$

in which C is the concentration, in µg per mL, of USP Mestranol RS in the *Standard preparation*; and A_U and A_S are the absorbances of the solutions from the *Assay preparation* and the *Standard preparation*, respectively.

Metacresol

C_7H_8O 108.14
3-Methylphenol.
3-Hydroxytoluene   [108-39-4].

» Metacresol contains not less than 95.0 percent and not more than 101.0 percent of C_7H_8O.

Packaging and storage—Preserve in tight, light-resistant containers.

Clarity of solution—
   A: Add 10 mL of it to 10 mL of solvent hexane, and mix: a clear solution is obtained.
   B: Add 1.0 mL of it to 20 mL of 1 N sodium hydroxide, and mix: a clear solution is obtained.

Identification—Shake 10 mL of it with 30 mL of water in a separator, and allow to separate. The lower layer is clear; the upper layer clears slowly. To 5 mL of the upper layer add a drop of ferric chloride TS: a bluish color is produced. To a separate 5-mL portion of the upper layer add bromine TS dropwise: a white precipitate is obtained.

Assay—Transfer about 10 drops of Metacresol to an accurately tared 100-mL volumetric flask, and weigh to determine the amount, in mg, added. Add about 50 mL of 1 N sodium hydroxide, shake to dissolve, dilute with 1 N sodium hydroxide to volume, and mix. Transfer 10.0 mL of this solution to an iodine flask, add about 50 mL of water and sufficient 18 N sulfuric acid to neutralize the solution to litmus, and cool to 20°. Add 25.0 mL of 0.1 N bromine VS and 15 mL of hydrochloric acid, and immediately insert the stopper. Shake the flask, and cool under running water. Allow to stand in a cool, dark place for 30 minutes, shaking every 10 minutes. Cool to 20°, quickly add 5 mL of potassium iodide solution (1 in 5) to the collar of the flask, gently lift the stopper momentarily, and allow the solution to be drawn into the flask, shake thoroughly, remove the stopper, and rinse it and the inside neck of the flask with a small quantity of water so that the washings flows into the flask. Add 1 mL of chloroform, shake, and titrate the liberated iodine with 0.1 N sodium thiosulfate VS, adding 3 mL of starch TS as the endpoint is approached. Perform a blank determination (see *Residual Titrations* under *Titrimetry* ⟨541⟩). Each mL of 0.1 N bromine is equivalent to 1.802 mg of C_7H_8O.

Metaproterenol Sulfate

$(C_{11}H_{17}NO_3)_2 \cdot H_2SO_4$ 520.59
1,3-Benzenediol, 5-[1-hydroxy-2-(1-methylethyl)amino]ethyl-, (±)-, sulfate (2 : 1) (salt).
(±)-3,5-Dihydroxy-α-[(isopropylamino)methyl]benzyl alcohol sulfate (2 : 1)   [5874-97-5].

» Metaproterenol Sulfate contains not less than 98.0 percent and not more than 102.0 percent of $(C_{11}H_{17}NO_3)_2 \cdot H_2SO_4$, calculated on the anhydrous, isopropyl alcohol-free, and methanol-free basis.

Packaging and storage—Preserve in tight, light-resistant containers.

USP Reference standards ⟨11⟩—USP Metaproterenol Sulfate RS.

Identification—
   A: *Infrared Absorption* ⟨197K⟩.
   B: To a solution of 10 mg in 1 mL of water add 1 drop of ferric chloride TS: a violet color is produced.
   C: It responds to the tests for *Sulfate* ⟨191⟩.
   D: The chromatogram of the *Assay preparation* obtained as directed in the *Assay* exhibits a major peak for metaproterenol, the retention time of which corresponds with that exhibited in the chromatogram of the *Standard preparation* obtained as directed in the *Assay*.

pH ⟨791⟩: between 4.0 and 5.5, in a solution containing 100 mg per mL.

Water, *Method I* ⟨921⟩: not more than 2.0%.

Residue on ignition ⟨281⟩: not more than 0.1%.

Heavy metals, *Method II* ⟨231⟩: 0.001%.

Iron ⟨241⟩—Dissolve 2.0 g in 45 mL of water, add 2 mL of hydrochloric acid, and mix: the limit is 5 ppm.

Limit of metaproterenone sulfate—Its absorptivity (see *Spectrophotometry and Light-Scattering* ⟨851⟩) at 328 nm, determined in an aqueous solution containing 9.0 mg per mL, is not more than 0.009 (0.1%).

Isopropyl alcohol and methanol—

Isopropyl alcohol standard solution—Transfer about 0.3 g of isopropyl alcohol, accurately weighed, to a 100-mL volumetric flask containing about 10 mL of water, dilute with water to volume, and mix. Pipet 10 mL of the resulting solution into a 100-mL volumetric flask, add about 85 mL of pyridine, mix, and allow to stand for 1 hour. Dilute with pyridine to volume, and mix. Pipet 5 mL of this solution to a 50-mL volumetric flask, dilute with pyridine to volume, and mix. The solution so obtained contains about 30 µg of isopropyl alcohol per mL.

Methanol standard solution—Prepare as directed for *Isopropyl alcohol standard solution*, using about 0.1 g of methanol, accurately weighed. The resulting solution contains about 10 µg of methanol per mL.

Test preparation—Transfer about 1 g of Metaproterenol Sulfate, accurately weighed, to a 100-mL volumetric flask, dissolve in about 2 mL of water, dilute with pyridine to volume, and mix.

Chromatographic system—The gas chromatograph is equipped with a flame-ionization detector and contains a 2-m × 2-mm column packed with 0.1% liquid phase G25 on 80- to 100-mesh support S7. The injection port is maintained at a temperature of about 150°; the column is programmed for 2 minutes at 40°, to increase at a rate of about 15° per minute to 200°, and for 10 minutes at 200°; the detector is maintained at about 250°; and helium is used as the carrier gas at a flow rate of about 15 mL per minute.

Procedure—Inject equal volumes (about 2 µL) of the *Test preparation*, the *Isopropyl alcohol standard solution*, and the *Methanol standard solution* successively into the gas chromatograph. Measure the responses of the isopropyl alcohol peak and the methanol peak in each chromatogram. Determine the quantities, in mg, of isopropyl alcohol and methanol in the portion of Metaproterenol Sulfate taken by the formula:

$$0.1C(r_U / r_S)$$

in which C is the concentration, in µg per mL, of isopropyl alcohol or methanol in the *Isopropyl alcohol standard solution* or the *Methanol standard solution*; and r_U and r_S are the responses of the respective analytes in the *Test preparation* and of the corresponding *Isopropyl alcohol standard solution* or *Methanol standard solution*: not more than 0.3% of isopropyl alcohol and not more than 0.1% of methanol are found.

Organic volatile impurities, *Method IV* ⟨467⟩: meets the requirements.

(Official until July 1, 2008)

Assay—
Mobile phase—Dissolve 11.9 g of anhydrous dibasic sodium phosphate in water to make 1000 mL of solution, and mix (*Solution A*). Dissolve 9.1 g of monobasic potassium phosphate in water to make 1000 mL of solution, and mix (*Solution B*). Mix 735 mL of *Solution A* and 140 mL of *Solution B*, add 125 mL of methanol, and mix. Filter and degas this solution before use.

Standard preparation—Dissolve an accurately weighed quantity of USP Metaproterenol Sulfate RS in 0.01 N hydrochloric acid to obtain a solution having a known concentration of about 2 mg per mL.

Assay preparation—Transfer about 100 mg of Metaproterenol Sulfate, accurately weighed, to a 50-mL volumetric flask, dilute with 0.01 N hydrochloric acid to volume, and mix.

Chromatographic system (see *Chromatography* ⟨621⟩)—The liquid chromatograph is equipped with a 278-nm detector and a 4.6-mm × 5-cm guard column that contains packing L7 and a 4.6-mm × 25-cm analytical column that contains 10-µm packing L7. The flow rate is about 2 mL per minute. Chromatograph the *Standard preparation*, and record the peak responses as directed for *Procedure*: the column efficiency determined from the analyte peak is not less than 500 theoretical plates, the tailing factor for the analyte peak is not more than 3.0, and the relative standard deviation for replicate injections is not more than 2.0%.

Procedure—Separately inject equal volumes (about 10 µL) of the *Standard preparation* and the *Assay preparation* into the chromatograph, record the chromatograms, and measure the responses for the major peaks. Calculate the quantity, in mg, of $(C_{11}H_{17}NO_3)_2 \cdot H_2SO_4$ in the portion of Metaproterenol Sulfate taken by the formula:

$$50C(r_U / r_S)$$

in which C is the concentration, in mg per mL, of USP Metaproterenol Sulfate RS in the *Standard preparation*, and r_U and r_S are the peak responses from the *Assay preparation* and the *Standard preparation*, respectively.

Metaproterenol Sulfate Inhalation Aerosol

» Metaproterenol Sulfate Inhalation Aerosol is a suspension of microfine Metaproterenol Sulfate in fluorochlorohydrocarbon propellants in a pressurized container. It contains not less than 90.0 percent and not more than 110.0 percent of the labeled amount of metaproterenol sulfate [$(C_{11}H_{17}NO_3)_2 \cdot H_2SO_4$].

Packaging and storage—Preserve in small, nonreactive, light-resistant aerosol containers equipped with metered-dose valves and provided with oral inhalation actuators.

USP Reference standards ⟨11⟩—*USP Metaproterenol Sulfate RS*.
Identification—The UV absorption spectrum of the solution from the *Assay preparation*, obtained as directed in the *Assay*, exhibits maxima and minima at the same wavelengths as that of the *Standard preparation* prepared as directed in the *Assay*.

Delivered dose uniformity over the entire contents: meets the requirements for *Metered-Dose Inhalers* under *Aerosols, Nasal Sprays, Metered-Dose Inhalers, and Dry Powder Inhalers* ⟨601⟩.

PROCEDURE FOR DOSE UNIFORMITY—
Standard preparation—Using a suitable quantity of USP Metaproterenol Sulfate RS, accurately weighed, prepare a solution in 0.01 N hydrochloric acid to obtain a solution having a known concentration of 0.05 mg per mL.

Test preparation—Discharge the minimum recommended dose into the sampling apparatus and detach the inhaler as directed. Rinse the apparatus (filter and interior) with four 5.0-mL portions of 0.01 N hydrochloric acid, and quantitatively transfer the rinsings to a 25-mL volumetric flask. Dilute with 0.01 N hydrochloric acid to volume, and mix.

Procedure—Transfer 20.0 mL portions of the *Standard preparation*, the *Test preparation*, and 0.01 N hydrochloric acid to serve as a blank to separate centrifuge tubes. Add 10.0 mL of chloroform to each, shake by mechanical means for 5 minutes, and separate the layers by centrifuging for 5 minutes. Determine the absorbances of the respective aqueous layers in 1-cm cells, at the wavelength of maximum absorbance at about 276 nm, with a suitable spectrophotometer, against the blank. Calculate the quantity, in mg, of metaproterenol sulfate [$(C_{11}H_{17}NO_3)_2 \cdot H_2SO_4$] contained in the minimum dose taken by the formula:

$$12.5CN(A_U / A_S)$$

in which C is the concentration, in mg per mL, of USP Metaproterenol Sulfate RS in the *Standard preparation*; N is the number of sprays discharged to obtain the minimum dose; and A_U and A_S are the absorbances of the solutions from the *Test preparation* and the *Standard preparation*, respectively.

Particle size—Prime the valve of an Inhalation Aerosol container by alternately shaking and firing it several times, and then actuate one measured spray onto a clean, dry microscope slide held 5 cm from the end of the oral inhalation actuator, perpendicular to the direction of the spray. Carefully rinse the slide with about 2 mL of chloroform, and allow to dry. Examine the slide under a microscope equipped with a calibrated ocular micrometer, using 450× magnification. Focus on the particles of 25 fields of view near the center of the test specimen pattern, and note the size of the great majority of individual particles: they are less than 5 µm along the longest axis. Record the number and size of all individual crystalline particles (not agglomerates) more than 10 µm in length measured along the longest axis: not more than 10 such particles are observed.

Water—Transfer the contents of a weighed container to the titration vessel by attaching the valve stem to an inlet tube. Weigh the empty container and determine the weight of the specimen taken. The water content, determined by *Method I* under *Water Determination* ⟨921⟩, is not more than 0.075%.

Assay—Cool an accurately weighed Inhalation Aerosol container for 10 minutes in a bath consisting of a mixture of acetone and solid carbon dioxide. Cut the valve from the aerosol container and allow the container to warm to room temperature. When most of the propellants have evaporated, transfer the residue in the container to a 250-mL separator with the aid of 30 mL of chloroform and 50 mL of 0.01 N hydrochloric acid. Reserve the valve and the empty container. Shake the separator for 1 minute and allow the phases to separate. Transfer the chloroform phase to a second 250-mL separator and the aqueous phase to a 250-mL volumetric flask. Wash the chloroform phase with two 50-mL portions of 0.01 N hydrochloric acid, add the washings to the 250-mL volumetric flask, dilute with 0.01 N hydrochloric acid to volume, and mix. Transfer an accurately measured volume of this stock solution, equivalent to about 10 mg of metaproterenol sulfate, to a 100-mL volumetric flask, dilute with 0.01 N hydrochloric acid to volume, and mix. Dissolve an accurately weighed quantity of USP Metaproterenol Sulfate RS in 0.01 N hydrochloric acid, and dilute quantitatively and stepwise with the same solvent to obtain a Standard solution having a known concentration of about 100 µg per mL. Concomitantly determine the absorbances of both solutions at the wavelength of maximum absorbance at about 276 nm, with a suitable spectrophotometer, using 0.01 N hydrochloric acid as the blank. Rinse the empty aerosol container and the valve with water and dry them at 105° for 10 minutes, allow to cool, and weigh. Subtract the weight thus obtained from the original weight of the Inhalation Aerosol container to obtain the weight of the Inhalation Aerosol taken. Calculate the quantity, in mg, of metaproterenol sulfate [$(C_{11}H_{17}NO_3)_2 \cdot H_2SO_4$] in each mL of the Inhalation Aerosol taken by the formula:

$$25(C/V)(d/W)(A_U/A_S)$$

in which C is the concentration, in μg per mL, of USP Metaproterenol Sulfate RS in the Standard solution, V is the volume, in mL, of stock solution taken, W is the weight, in g, of the Inhalation Aerosol taken, and A_U and A_S are the absorbances of the solution from the Inhalation Aerosol and the Standard solution, respectively. [The density, d, is determined as follows: Weigh a known volume (v) of the Inhalation Aerosol in a suitable 5-mL gas-tight syringe equipped with a linear valve. Calibrate the volume of the syringe by filling to the 5-mL mark with dichlorotetrafluoroethane withdrawn from a plastic-coated glass vial sealed with a neoprene multiple-dose rubber stopper and an aluminum seal, using 1.456 g per mL as the density of the calibrating liquid. Maintain the dichlorotetrafluoroethane, the Inhalation Aerosol sample, and the syringe (protected from becoming wet) at 25° in a water bath. Obtain the sample, equivalent to the same volume as that obtained during the sampling procedure, from the Inhalation Aerosol by means of a sampling device consisting of a replaceable rubber septum engaged in the plate threads at one end of a threaded fitting, the opposite end of which contains a sharpened tube capable of puncturing the aerosol container, and a rubber gasket around the tube to prevent leakage of the container contents after puncture.* Calculate the density taken by the formula:

$$w/v$$

in which w is the weight of the volume, v, of the Inhalation Aerosol taken.]

Metaproterenol Sulfate Inhalation Solution

» Metaproterenol Sulfate Inhalation Solution is a sterile solution of Metaproterenol Sulfate in Purified Water. It may contain Sodium Chloride. It contains not less than 90.0 percent and not more than 110.0 percent of the labeled amount of metaproterenol sulfate [$(C_{11}H_{17}NO_3)_2 \cdot H_2SO_4$].

Packaging and storage—Store in small, tight containers that are well-filled or otherwise protected from oxidation. Protect from light.
Labeling—Label it to indicate that the Inhalation Solution is not to be used if its color is pinkish or darker than slightly yellow or if it contains a precipitate.
USP Reference standards ⟨11⟩—*USP Metaproterenol Sulfate RS.*
Color and clarity—
Standard solution—Transfer 2.0 mL of 0.100 N iodine VS to a 500-mL volumetric flask, dilute with water to volume, and mix.
Procedure—Visually examine a portion of the Inhalation Solution (*Test solution*) in a suitable clear glass test tube against a white background: it is not pinkish, and it contains no precipitate. If any yellow color is observed in the *Test solution*, concomitantly determine the absorbances of the *Test solution* and the *Standard solution* in 1-cm cells with a suitable spectrophotometer set at 460 nm: the absorbance of the *Test solution* does not exceed that of the *Standard solution*.

---
*A suitable sampling system is available from Alltek Associates, P. O. Box 498, Arlington Heights, IL 60006.

Identification—
A: Apply 4 μL of the Inhalation Solution and 4 μL of an aqueous solution of USP Metaproterenol Sulfate RS containing about 50 mg per mL to a suitable thin-layer chromatographic plate (see *Chromatography* ⟨621⟩) coated with a 0.25-mm layer of chromatographic silica gel mixture. Allow the spots to dry, and develop the chromatogram in a solvent system consisting of the upper layer of a freshly prepared mixture of butyl alcohol, water, and formic acid (50 : 25 : 7) until the solvent front has moved about three-fourths of the length of the plate. Remove the plate from the developing chamber, mark the solvent front, and allow the solvent to evaporate. Locate the spots on the plate by examination under short-wavelength UV light: the R_F value of the principal spot obtained from the Inhalation Solution corresponds to that obtained from the *Standard solution*.
B: The chromatogram of the *Assay preparation* obtained as directed in the *Assay* exhibits a major peak for metaproterenol, the retention time of which corresponds to that exhibited in the chromatogram of the *Standard preparation* obtained as directed in the *Assay*.
Sterility ⟨71⟩: meets the requirements.
pH ⟨791⟩: between 2.8 and 4.0.
Assay—
Mobile phase, Standard preparation, and *Chromatographic system*—Prepare as directed in the *Assay* under *Metaproterenol Sulfate*.
Assay preparation—Transfer an accurately measured volume of Inhalation Solution, equivalent to about 200 mg of metaproterenol sulfate, to a 100-mL volumetric flask, dilute with 0.01 N hydrochloric acid to volume, and mix.
Procedure—Proceed as directed for *Procedure* in the *Assay* under *Metaproterenol Sulfate*. Calculate the quantity, in mg, of metaproterenol sulfate [$(C_{11}H_{17}NO_3)_2 \cdot H_2SO_4$] in each mL of the Inhalation Solution taken by the formula:

$$100(C/V)(r_U/r_S)$$

in which V is the volume, in mL, of Inhalation Solution taken; and $C, r_U,$ and r_S are as defined therein.

Metaproterenol Sulfate Oral Solution

» Metaproterenol Sulfate Oral Solution contains not less than 90.0 percent and not more than 110.0 percent of the labeled amount of metaproterenol sulfate [$(C_{11}H_{17}NO_3)_2 \cdot H_2SO_4$].

Packaging and storage—Preserve in tight, light-resistant containers.
USP Reference standards ⟨11⟩—*USP Metaproterenol Sulfate RS.*
Identification—
A: Transfer a portion of Oral Solution, equivalent to about 10 mg of metaproterenol sulfate, to a separator, and extract with four 30-mL portions of ether, discarding the ether extracts. Apply 10 μL of the extracted portion of Oral Solution to the lower right corner of a suitable thin-layer chromatographic plate (see *Chromatography* ⟨621⟩) coated with a 0.25-mm layer of chromatographic silica gel mixture, and allow to dry. Develop the chromatogram in a solvent system consisting of the lower layer of a well-shaken mixture of dioxane, methylene chloride, alcohol, and ammonium hydroxide (4 : 4 : 1 : 1). Allow the solvent front to move about three-fourths of the length of the plate. Remove the plate from the developing chamber, mark the solvent front, and dry in vacuum at 35° to 40° for 30 minutes. Rotate the plate 90°. At a point about four-fifths of the distance between the initial application of the Oral Solution extract and the solvent front, apply 10 μL of a Standard solution of USP Metaproterenol Sulfate RS in water containing about 2 mg per mL. Proceed as directed in *Identification* test A under *Metaproterenol Sulfate Inhalation Solution*, beginning with "Allow the spots to dry": the R_F value of the principal spot obtained from the Oral Solution corresponds to that obtained from the Standard solution.

B: The retention time of the major peak for metaproterenol in the chromatogram of the *Assay preparation* corresponds to that in the chromatogram of the *Standard preparation*, as obtained in the *Assay*.

pH ⟨791⟩: between 2.5 and 4.0, in a solution obtained by mixing 1 volume of Oral Solution and 4 volumes of water.

Assay—
Mobile phase—Mix 10 mL of formic acid and water to make 1000 mL of solution. Filter and degas this solution before use. Make adjustments if necessary (see *System Suitability* under *Chromatography* ⟨621⟩).

Standard preparation—Dissolve an accurately weighed quantity of USP Metaproterenol Sulfate RS in water to obtain a solution having a known concentration of about 0.2 mg per mL.

Assay preparation—Transfer an accurately measured volume of Oral Solution, equivalent to about 20 mg of metaproterenol sulfate, to a 100-mL volumetric flask, dilute with water to volume, and mix.

Chromatographic system (see *Chromatography* ⟨621⟩)—The liquid chromatograph is equipped with a 278-nm detector, a 4.6-mm × 5-cm guard column that contains packing L2, and a 3.9-mm × 30-cm analytical column that contains packing L1. [NOTE—After use, rinse the analytical column with water and store with water in it.] The flow rate is about 2 mL per minute. Chromatograph the *Standard preparation*, and record the peak responses as directed for *Procedure*: the tailing factor for the analyte peak is not more than 3.0; and the relative standard deviation for replicate injections is not more than 2.0%.

Procedure—Separately inject equal volumes (about 100 μL) of the *Standard preparation* and the *Assay preparation* into the chromatograph, record the chromatograms, and measure the responses for the major peaks. Calculate the quantity, in mg, of metaproterenol sulfate [$(C_{11}H_{17}NO_3)_2 \cdot H_2SO_4$] in each mL of the Oral Solution taken by the formula:

$$100(C/V)(r_U/r_S)$$

in which C is the concentration, in mg per mL, of USP Metaproterenol Sulfate RS in the *Standard preparation*; V is the volume, in mL, of Oral Solution taken; and r_U and r_S are the peak responses from the *Assay preparation* and the *Standard preparation*, respectively.

Metaproterenol Sulfate Tablets

» Metaproterenol Sulfate Tablets contain not less than 92.0 percent and not more than 108.0 percent of the labeled amount of metaproterenol sulfate [$(C_{11}H_{17}NO_3)_2 \cdot H_2SO_4$].

Packaging and storage—Preserve in well-closed, light-resistant containers.

USP Reference standards ⟨11⟩—*USP Metaproterenol Sulfate RS*.

Identification—
A: Powder a number of Tablets, equivalent to about 100 mg of metaproterenol sulfate, add 10 mL of water, stir for about 3 minutes, and centrifuge. Use the clear solution so obtained as the *Test solution*. Dissolve a suitable quantity of USP Metaproterenol Sulfate RS in water to obtain a Standard solution having a concentration of 10 mg per mL. Apply separate 10-μL portions of the *Test solution* and the Standard solution to a thin-layer chromatographic plate (see *Chromatography* ⟨621⟩) coated with a 0.25-mm layer of chromatographic silica gel mixture. Proceed as directed in *Identification* test A under *Metaproterenol Sulfate Inhalation Solution*, beginning with "Allow the spots to dry": the R_F value of the principal spot obtained from the *Test solution* corresponds to that obtained from the Standard solution.

B: Mix a quantity of powdered Tablets, equivalent to about 20 mg of metaproterenol sulfate, with 5 mL of water, and filter: the filtrate responds to the tests for *Sulfate* ⟨191⟩.

C: The chromatogram of the *Assay preparation* obtained as directed in the *Assay* exhibits a major peak for metaproterenol, the retention time of which corresponds to that exhibited in the chromatogram of the *Standard preparation* obtained as directed in the *Assay*.

Dissolution ⟨711⟩—
Medium: water; 500 mL.
Apparatus 2: 50 rpm.
Time: 30 minutes.
Procedure—Determine the amount of $(C_{11}H_{17}NO_3)_2 \cdot H_2SO_4$ dissolved from UV absorbances at the wavelength of maximum absorbance at about 276 nm of filtered portions of the solution under test, suitably diluted with *Dissolution Medium*, if necessary, in comparison with a Standard solution having a known concentration of USP Metaproterenol Sulfate RS in the same *Medium*.

Tolerances—Not less than 70% (*Q*) of the labeled amount of $(C_{11}H_{17}NO_3)_2 \cdot H_2SO_4$ is dissolved in 30 minutes.

Uniformity of dosage units ⟨905⟩: meet the requirements.

Assay—
Mobile phase, Standard preparation, and *Chromatographic system*—Prepare as directed in the *Assay* under *Metaproterenol Sulfate*.

Assay preparation—Transfer 20 Tablets to a 500-mL conical flask. Add an accurately measured volume of 0.01 N hydrochloric acid sufficient to yield a solution containing about 2 mg of metaproterenol sulfate per mL, shake by mechanical means for 30 minutes, and filter. Use the filtrate so obtained as the *Assay preparation*.

Procedure—Proceed as directed for *Procedure* in the *Assay* under *Metaproterenol Sulfate*. Calculate the quantity, in mg, of metaproterenol sulfate [$(C_{11}H_{17}NO_3)_2 \cdot H_2SO_4$] in each Tablet taken by the formula:

$$(CV/20)(r_U/r_S)$$

in which V is the volume, in mL, of 0.01 N hydrochloric acid added; and C, r_U, and r_S are as defined therein.

Metaraminol Bitartrate

$C_9H_{13}NO_2 \cdot C_4H_6O_6$ 317.29

Benzenemethanol, α-(1-aminoethyl)-3-hydroxy-, [*R*-(*R**,*S**)]-, [*R*-(*R**,*R**)]-2,3-dihydroxybutanedioate (1 : 1) (salt).

(−)-α-(1-Aminoethyl)-*m*-hydroxybenzyl alcohol tartrate (1 : 1) (salt)   [*33402-03-8*].

» Metaraminol Bitartrate contains not less than 99.0 percent and not more than 100.5 percent of $C_9H_{13}NO_2 \cdot C_4H_6O_6$, calculated on the dried basis.

Packaging and storage—Preserve in well-closed containers. Store at 25°, excursions permitted between 15° and 30°.

USP Reference standards ⟨11⟩—*USP Metaraminol Bitartrate RS*.

Identification—
A: *Infrared Absorption* ⟨197K⟩.
B: To 0.5 mL of a solution (1 in 2000) add 1 mL of Folin-Ciocalteu phenol TS, then add 5 mL of sodium carbonate solution (1 in 10), mix, and allow to stand for 5 minutes: an intense blue color appears (*presence of a phenol*).
C: To 4 mL of a solution (1 in 2000) add 5 mL of pH 9.6 alkaline borate buffer (see *Buffer Solutions* in the section *Reagents, Indicators, and Solutions*), then add about 5 mg of β-naphthoquinone-4-sodium sulfonate, mix until dissolved, and allow to stand for 5 minutes. Add 0.2 mL of benzalkonium chloride solution (1 in 100), mix, add 5 mL of toluene, and shake: the toluene layer turns purple immediately (*distinction from phenylephrine*).

Melting range ⟨741⟩: between 171° and 175°.

Specific rotation ⟨781S⟩: between −31.5° and −33.5° (λ = 405 nm).

2640 Metaraminol / *Official Monographs*

Test solution: 100 mg per mL, in 0.5 N hydrochloric acid.
pH ⟨791⟩: between 3.2 and 3.5, in a solution (1 in 20).
Loss on drying ⟨731⟩—Dry it at 105° for 2 hours: it loses not more than 1.0% of its weight.
Residue on ignition ⟨281⟩: not more than 0.1%.
Heavy metals, *Method I* ⟨231⟩: 0.002%.
Assay—Dissolve about 600 mg of Metaraminol Bitartrate, accurately weighed, in 20 mL of glacial acetic acid, warming slightly to effect solution. Cool the solution to room temperature, add 2 drops of crystal violet TS, and titrate with 0.1 N perchloric acid VS to an emerald-green color. Perform a blank determination, and make any necessary correction. Each mL of 0.1 N perchloric acid is equivalent to 31.73 mg of $C_9H_{13}NO_2 \cdot C_4H_6O_6$.

Metaraminol Bitartrate Injection

» Metaraminol Bitartrate Injection is a sterile solution of Metaraminol Bitartrate in Water for Injection. It contains, in each mL, an amount of metaraminol bitartrate equivalent to not less than 9.0 mg and not more than 11.0 mg of metaraminol ($C_9H_{13}NO_2$).

Packaging and storage—Preserve in single-dose or in multiple-dose containers, preferably of Type I glass, protected from light.
USP Reference standards ⟨11⟩—*USP Endotoxin RS. USP Metaraminol Bitartrate RS.*
Identification—
 A: Evaporate a 1-mL portion to dryness: the residue so obtained meets the requirements for *Identification* test A under *Metaraminol Bitartrate*.
 B: It meets the requirements for *Identification* tests B and C under *Metaraminol Bitartrate*.
Bacterial endotoxins ⟨85⟩—It contains not more than 3.5 USP Endotoxin Units per mg of metaraminol.
pH ⟨791⟩: between 3.2 and 4.5.
Particulate matter ⟨788⟩: meets the requirements for small-volume injections.
Other requirements—It meets the requirements under *Injections* ⟨1⟩.
Assay—
 0.0032 M Hexanesulfonate buffer—Mix 600 mg of sodium 1-hexanesulfonate with water to obtain 1000 mL of solution, adjust with phosphoric acid to a pH of 3.0 ± 0.05, and filter.
 Mobile phase—Prepare a suitable degassed and filtered mixture of methanol and *0.0032 M Hexanesulfonate buffer* (7 : 3). Make adjustments if necessary (see *System Suitability* under *Chromatography* ⟨621⟩).
 Standard preparation—Dissolve an accurately weighed quantity of USP Metaraminol Bitartrate RS in water to obtain a solution having a known concentration of about 0.2 mg of metaraminol per mL.
 Assay preparation—Transfer an accurately measured volume of Injection, equivalent to about 20 mg of metaraminol, to a 100-mL volumetric flask, dilute with water to volume, and mix.
 System suitability preparation—Prepare a solution of propylparaben in alcohol containing 0.4 mg per mL. Mix 1 volume of this solution with 99 volumes of the *Standard preparation*.
 Chromatographic system (see *Chromatography* ⟨621⟩)—The liquid chromatograph is equipped with a 264-nm detector and a 4-mm × 25-cm column that contains packing L7. The flow rate is about 1 mL per minute. Chromatograph the *System suitability preparation* and the *Standard preparation*, and record the peak responses as directed for *Procedure*: the column efficiency is not less than 2600 theoretical plates, the resolution, R, between the metaraminol bitartrate and propylparaben peaks is not less than 3.0 with propylparaben eluting first, and the relative standard deviation for replicate injections is not more than 2.0%.
 Procedure—Separately inject equal volumes (about 10 µL) of the *Standard preparation* and the *Assay preparation* into the chromatograph, record the chromatograms, and measure the responses for the major peaks. Calculate the quantity, in mg, of metaraminol ($C_9H_{13}NO_2$) in each mL of the Injection taken by the formula:

$$100(C/V)(r_U/r_S)$$

in which C is the concentration, in mg per mL, of metaraminol represented by the USP Metaraminol Bitartrate RS in the *Standard preparation*; V is the volume, in mL, of Injection taken; and r_U and r_S are the peak responses obtained from the *Assay preparation* and the *Standard preparation*, respectively.

Metformin Hydrochloride

[Structure of metformin hydrochloride shown]

$C_4H_{11}N_5 \cdot HCl$ 165.62
Imidodicarbonimidic diamide, *N,N*-dimethyl-, monohydrochloride.
1,1-Dimethylbiguanide monohydrochloride   [*1115-70-4*].

» Metformin Hydrochloride contains not less than 98.5 percent and not more than 101.0 percent of $C_4H_{11}N_5 \cdot HCl$, calculated on the dried basis.

Packaging and storage—Preserve in well-closed containers. Store at room temperature.
USP Reference standards ⟨11⟩—*USP Metformin Hydrochloride RS. USP Metformin Related Compound A RS.*
Identification—
 A: *Infrared Absorption* ⟨197K⟩.
 B: It meets the requirements of the tests for *Chloride* ⟨191⟩.
Loss on drying ⟨731⟩—Dry it at 105° for 5 hours: it loses not more than 0.5% of its weight.
Residue on ignition ⟨281⟩: not more than 0.1%.
Heavy metals, *Method I* ⟨231⟩: 0.001%.
Related compounds—
 Mobile phase—Prepare a solution in water, containing 17 g of monobasic ammonium phosphate per L, adjust with phosphoric acid to a pH of 3.0, and mix.
 Standard solution—Prepare a solution of USP Metformin Related Compound A RS in water having a known concentration of about 0.2 mg per mL. Transfer 1.0 mL of this solution to a 200-mL volumetric flask, dilute with *Mobile phase* to volume, and mix. [NOTE—Metformin related compound A is 1-cyanoguanidine.]
 Test solution—Transfer about 500 mg of Metformin Hydrochloride, accurately weighed, to a 100-mL volumetric flask, dissolve in and dilute with *Mobile phase* to volume, and mix.
 Diluted test solution—Transfer 1.0 mL of the *Test solution* to a 10-mL volumetric flask, dilute with *Mobile phase* to volume, and mix. Transfer 1.0 mL of this solution to a 100-mL volumetric flask, dilute with *Mobile phase* to volume, and mix.
 Resolution solution—Prepare a solution in water containing about 0.25 mg of metformin hydrochloride and about 0.1 mg of melamine per mL. Transfer 1.0 mL of this solution to a 50-mL volumetric flask, dilute with *Mobile phase* to volume, and mix.
 Chromatographic system (see *Chromatography* ⟨621⟩)—The liquid chromatograph is equipped with a 218-nm detector and a 4.6-mm × 25-cm column containing packing L9. The flow rate is about 1.0 to 1.7 mL per minute. Chromatograph the *Resolution solution*, and record the peak responses as directed for *Procedure*: the resolution, R, between melamine and metformin is not less than 10.
 Procedure—Separately inject equal volumes (about 20 µL) of the *Test solution,* the *Standard solution,* and the *Diluted test solution* into the chromatograph, record the chromatograms for not less than twice the retention time of metformin, and measure the peak areas.

Calculate the percentage of metformin related compound A in the portion of Metformin Hydrochloride taken by the formula:

$$10C/W(r_U/r_S)$$

in which C is the concentration, in µg per mL, of USP Metformin Related Compound A RS in the *Standard solution*; W is the weight, in mg, of Metformin Hydrochloride taken to prepare the *Test solution*; and r_U and r_S are the metformin related compound A peak responses obtained from the *Test solution* and the *Standard solution*, respectively: not more than 0.02% of metformin related compound A is found.

Calculate the percentage of any other impurity in the portion of Metformin Hydrochloride taken by the formula:

$$0.1(r_i/r_S)$$

in which r_i is the peak response for an individual impurity obtained from the *Test solution*; and r_S is the metformin peak response obtained from the *Diluted test solution*: not more than 0.1% of any other impurity is found; and not more than 0.5% of total impurities is found.

Assay—[NOTE—To avoid overheating of the reaction medium, mix thoroughly throughout the titration, and stop the titration immediately after the endpoint has been reached.] Dissolve about 60 mg of Metformin Hydrochloride, accurately weighed, in 4 mL of anhydrous formic acid. Add 50 mL of acetic anhydride. Titrate with 0.1 N perchloric acid VS, determining the endpoint potentiometrically. Perform a blank determination, and make any necessary correction (see *Titrimetry* ⟨541⟩). Each mL of 0.1 N perchloric acid is equivalent to 8.28 mg of $C_4H_{11}N_5 \cdot HCl$.

Metformin Hydrochloride Tablets

» Metformin Hydrochloride Tablets contain not less than 95.0 percent and not more than 105.0 percent of metformin hydrochloride ($C_4H_{11}N_5 \cdot HCl$).

Packaging and storage—Preserve in tight containers. Store at controlled room temperature.
Labeling—When more than one *Dissolution* test is given, the labeling states the *Dissolution* test used only if *Test 1* is not used.
USP Reference standards ⟨11⟩—USP Metformin Hydrochloride RS.
Identification—
  A: *Infrared Absorption* ⟨197K⟩.
  Test specimen—Transfer a quantity of powdered Tablets, equivalent to about 20 mg of metformin hydrochloride, to a suitable flask, add 20 mL of dehydrated alcohol, and shake. Filter, evaporate the filtrate on a water bath to dryness, and dry the residue at 105° for 2 hours.
  B: Triturate a quantity of the powdered Tablets, equivalent to about 50 mg of metformin hydrochloride, with 10 mL of water, and filter. To 5 mL of the filtrate add 1.5 mL of 5 N sodium hydroxide solution and 1 mL of a 1-naphthol solution, prepared by dissolving 1 g of 1-naphthol in a solution containing 6 g of sodium hydroxide and 16 g of anhydrous sodium carbonate in 100 mL of water. Add 0.5 mL of sodium hypochlorite TS, dropwise, and with shaking: an orange-red color is produced that darkens on standing.
  C: Triturate a quantity of the powdered Tablets, equivalent to about 50 mg of metformin hydrochloride, with 10 mL of water, and filter. The filtrate meets the requirements of the tests for *Chloride* ⟨191⟩.
Dissolution ⟨711⟩—
  TEST 1—
  Medium: pH 6.8 phosphate buffer; 1000 mL.
  Apparatus 1: 100 rpm.
  Time: 45 minutes.
  Procedure—Determine the amount of $C_4H_{11}N_5 \cdot HCl$ dissolved by employing UV absorption at the wavelength of maximum absorbance at about 233 nm on filtered portions of the solution under test, suitably diluted with *Medium*, if necessary, in comparison with a *Standard solution* having a known concentration of USP Metformin Hydrochloride RS in the same *Medium*.
  Tolerances—Not less than 70% (Q) of the labeled amount of $C_4H_{11}N_5 \cdot HCl$ is dissolved in 45 minutes.
  TEST 2—If the product complies with this test, the labeling indicates that it meets USP *Dissolution Test 2*.
  FOR PRODUCTS LABELED TO CONTAIN 500 MG OF METFORMIN—
  Medium: pH 6.8 phosphate buffer; 1000 mL.
  Apparatus 2: 50 rpm.
  Time: 30 minutes.
  Procedure—Proceed as directed for *Test 1*.
  Tolerances—Not less than 80% (Q) of the labeled amount of $C_4H_{11}N_5 \cdot HCl$ is dissolved in 30 minutes.
  FOR PRODUCTS LABELED TO CONTAIN 850 MG OR 1000 MG OF METFORMIN—
  Medium: pH 6.8 phosphate buffer; 1000 mL.
  Apparatus 2: 75 rpm.
  Time: 30 minutes.
  Procedure—Proceed as directed for *Test 1*.
  Tolerances—Not less than 75% (Q) of the labeled amount of $C_4H_{11}N_5 \cdot HCl$ is dissolved in 30 minutes.
Uniformity of dosage units ⟨905⟩: meet the requirements.
Related compounds—
  Mobile phase, Resolution solution, and *Chromatographic system*—Proceed as directed in the test for *Related compounds* under Metformin Hydrochloride.
  Test solution—Weigh and finely powder not fewer than 20 Tablets. Transfer a portion of the powder, equivalent to about 500 mg of metformin hydrochloride, to a 100-mL volumetric flask, dissolve in *Mobile phase*, with shaking, dilute with *Mobile phase* to volume, and mix. Filter, and use the filtrate.
  Diluted test solution—Proceed as directed in the test for *Related compounds* under Metformin Hydrochloride, except to use the *Test solution* prepared as described herein.
  Procedure—Separately inject equal volumes (about 20 µL) of the *Test solution* and the *Diluted test solution* into the chromatograph, record the chromatograms for not less than twice the retention time of metformin, and measure the peak areas.
  Calculate the percentage of each impurity in the portion of Tablets taken by the formula:

$$0.1(r_i/r_S)$$

in which r_i is the peak response for each individual impurity obtained from the *Test solution*; and r_S is the metformin peak response obtained from the *Diluted test solution*: not more than 0.1% of any impurity is found; and not more than 0.6% of total impurities is found.
Assay—
  Standard preparation—Prepare a solution of USP Metformin Hydrochloride RS in water having a known concentration of about 10 µg per mL.
  Assay preparation—Weigh and finely powder not fewer than 20 Tablets. Transfer an accurately weighed portion of the powder, equivalent to about 100 mg of metformin hydrochloride, to a 100-mL volumetric flask. Add 70 mL of water, shake by mechanical means for 15 minutes, dilute with water to volume, and filter, discarding the first 20 mL of the filtrate. Dilute 10.0 mL of the filtrate with water to 100.0 mL, and dilute 10.0 mL of the resulting solution with water to 100.0 mL.
  Procedure—Concomitantly determine the absorbances of the *Standard preparation* and the *Assay preparation*, in 1-cm cells, at the wavelength of maximum absorbance at about 232 nm, with a suitable spectrophotometer, using water as a blank. Calculate the quantity, in mg, of metformin hydrochloride ($C_4H_{11}N_5 \cdot HCl$) in the portion of Tablets taken by the formula:

$$10C(A_U/A_S)$$

in which C is the concentration, in µg per mL, of USP Metformin Hydrochloride RS in the *Standard preparation*; and A_U and A_S are the absorbances obtained from the *Assay preparation* and the *Standard preparation*, respectively.

Add the following:

▲Metformin Hydrochloride Extended-Release Tablets

» Metformin Hydrochloride Extended-Release Tablets contain not less than 90.0 percent and not more than 110.0 percent of the labeled amount of metformin hydrochloride ($C_4H_{11}N_5 \cdot HCl$).

Packaging and storage—Preserve in well-closed, light-resistant containers, and store at controlled room temperature.

Labeling—When more than one *Dissolution Test* is given, the labeling states the *Dissolution Test* used only if *Test 1* is not used.

USP Reference standards ⟨11⟩—*USP Metformin Hydrochloride RS. USP Metformin Related Compound B RS. USP Metformin Related Compound C RS.*

Identification—The retention time of the major peak in the chromatogram of the *Assay preparation* corresponds to that in the chromatogram of the *Standard preparation*, as obtained in the *Assay*.

Dissolution ⟨711⟩—

TEST 1—

Medium: pH 6.8 phosphate buffer prepared by dissolving 6.8 g of monobasic potassium phosphate in 1000 mL of water and adjusting with 0.2 N sodium hydroxide to a pH of 6.8 ± 0.1; 1000 mL.

Apparatus 2: 100 rpm, for Tablets labeled to contain 500 mg.

Apparatus 1: 100 rpm, for Tablets labeled to contain 750 mg.

Times: 1, 3, and 10 hours.

Procedure—Determine the amount of $C_4H_{11}N_5 \cdot HCl$ dissolved by UV absorption at the wavelength of maximum absorbance at about 232 nm on portions of the solution under test passed through a 0.45-μm hydrophilic polyethylene filter, suitably diluted with *Medium*, if necessary, in comparison with a *Standard solution* having a known concentration of USP Metformin Hydrochloride RS in the same *Medium*. Calculate the amount of metformin hydrochloride ($C_4H_{11}N_5 \cdot HCl$), in percentage, released at each time point by the formula:

$$\frac{[C \times (A_U/A_S) \times (V - V_S) + (C_{60} \times V_S) + (C_{180} \times V_S)] \times 100}{L}$$

in which C is the concentration, in mg per mL, of the Standard solution; A_U and A_S are the absorbances of the solution under test and the Standard solution, respectively; V is the initial volume, in mL, of *Medium* in the vessel; V_S is the volume, in mL, withdrawn from the vessel for previous samplings; C_{60} is the concentration, in mg per mL, of metformin hydrochloride in the *Medium* determined at 1 hour; C_{180} is the concentration, in mg per mL, of metformin hydrochloride in the *Medium* determined at 3 hours; 100 is the conversion factor to percentage; and L is the Tablet label claim, in mg.

Tolerances—The percentages of the labeled amount of $C_4H_{11}N_5 \cdot HCl$ dissolved at the times specified conform to *Acceptance Table 2*.

Time (hours)	500-mg Tablet, Amount dissolved	750-mg Tablet, Amount dissolved
1	between 20% and 40%	between 22% and 42%
3	between 45% and 65%	between 49% and 69%
10	not less than 85%	not less than 85%

TEST 2—If the product complies with this test, the labeling indicates that it meets USP *Dissolution Test 2*.

Medium: Prepare as directed for *Medium* in *Test 1*; 1000 mL.

Apparatus 2: 100 rpm.

Times: 1, 2, 6, and 10 hours.

Procedure—Determine the amount of $C_4H_{11}N_5 \cdot HCl$ dissolved by UV absorption at the wavelength of maximum absorbance at about 232 nm on portions of the solution under test passed through a 0.45-μm polyethylene filter, suitably diluted with *Medium*, if necessary, in comparison with a *Standard solution* having a known concentration of USP Metformin Hydrochloride RS in the same *Medium*. Calculate the content of metformin hydrochloride ($C_4H_{11}N_5 \cdot HCl$), C_t, in mg per mL, in the *Medium* at each time point, t, by the formula:

$$\frac{A_U \times C_s \times D_U}{A_s}$$

in which A_U and A_S are the absorbances of the solution under test and the Standard solution, respectively; C_S is the concentration of metformin hydrochloride, in mg per mL, in the Standard solution; and D_U is the dilution factor of the solution under test. Calculate the percentage of metformin hydrochloride ($C_4H_{11}N_5 \cdot HCl$) dissolved at each time point by the following formulas:

Percentage dissolved at the first time point (1 hour):

$$\frac{C_1 \times 1000 \times 100}{L}$$

in which C_1 is the content of metformin hydrochloride, in mg per mL, in the *Medium* at the first time interval; 1000 is the volume, in mL, of *Medium*; 100 is the conversion factor to percentage; and L is the Tablet label claim, in mg.

Percentage dissolved at the second time point (2 hours):

$$\frac{C_2 \times (1000 - SV_1) + C_1 \times SV_1 \times 100}{L}$$

in which C_2 is the content of metformin hydrochloride, in mg per mL, in the *Medium* at the second time interval; 1000 is the volume, in mL, of *Medium*; SV_1 is the volume, in mL, of the sample withdrawn at 1 hour; C_1 is the content of metformin hydrochloride, in mg per mL, in the *Medium* at 1 hour; 100 is the conversion factor to percentage; and L is the Tablet label claim, in mg.

Percentage dissolved at the nth time point:

$$\frac{C_n \times [1000 - (n-1)SV] + (C_1 + C_2 + \ldots + C_{n-1}) \times SV \times 100}{L}$$

in which C_n is the content of metformin hydrochloride, in mg per mL, in the *Medium* at the nth time interval; n is the time interval of interest; SV is the volume, in mL, of sample withdrawn at each time interval; $C_1, C_2, C_3, \ldots C_{n-1}$ is the content of metformin hydrochloride, in mg per mL, in the *Medium* at each time interval; 100 is the conversion factor to percentage; and L is the Tablet label claim, in mg.

Tolerances—The percentages of the labeled amount of $C_4H_{11}N_5 \cdot HCl$ dissolved at the times specified conform to *Acceptance Table 2*.

Time (hours)	Amount dissolved
1	between 20% and 40%
2	between 35% and 55%
6	between 65% and 85%
10	not less than 85%

TEST 3—If the product complies with this test, the labeling indicates that it meets USP *Dissolution Test 3*.

Medium, Apparatus, and *Procedure*—Proceed as directed for *Test 1*.

Times: 1, 2, 5, and 12 hours for Tablets labeled to contain 500 mg; and 1, 3, and 10 hours for Tablets labeled to contain 750 mg.

Procedure—Determine the amount of $C_4H_{11}N_5 \cdot HCl$ dissolved by UV absorption at the wavelength of maximum absorbance at about 232 nm on portions of the solution under test passed through a 0.45-μm hydrophilic polyethylene filter, suitably diluted with *Medium*, if necessary, in comparison with a *Standard solution* having a known concentration of USP Metformin Hydrochloride RS in the same *Medium*. Calculate the amount of metformin hydrochloride ($C_4H_{11}N_5 \cdot HCl$), in percentage, released at each time point by the formula:

$$\frac{[C \times (A_U/A_S) \times (V - V_S) + (C_{60} \times V_S) + (C_{120} \times V_S) + (C_{300} \times V_S)] \times 100}{L}$$

in which C is the concentration, in mg per mL, of the Standard solution; A_U and A_S are the absorbances of the solution under test and the Standard solution, respectively; V is the initial volume, in mL, of Medium in the vessel; V_S is the volume, in mL, withdrawn from the vessel for previous samplings; C_{60} is the concentration, in mg per mL, of metformin hydrochloride in the Medium determined at 1 hour; C_{120} is the concentration, in mg per mL, of metformin hydrochloride in the Medium determined at 2 hours; C_{300} is the concentration, in mg per mL, of metformin hydrochloride in the Medium determined at 5 hours; 100 is the conversion factor to percentage; and L is the Tablet label claim, in mg.

Tolerances—The percentages of the labeled amount of $C_4H_{11}N_5 \cdot HCl$ dissolved at the times specified conform to *Acceptance Table 2*.

FOR TABLETS LABELED TO CONTAIN 500 MG:

Time (hours)	Amount dissolved
1	between 20% and 40%
2	between 35% and 55%
5	between 60% and 80%
12	not less than 85%

FOR TABLETS LABELED TO CONTAIN 750 MG:

Time (hours)	Amount dissolved
1	between 22% and 42%
3	between 49% and 69%
10	not less than 85%

TEST 4—If the product complies with this test, the labeling indicates that it meets USP *Dissolution Test 4*.
Medium: Prepare as directed for *Medium* in *Test 1*; 1000 mL.
Apparatus 2: 100 rpm.
Times: 1, 3, 6, and 10 hours.
Procedure—Determine the amount of $C_4H_{11}N_5 \cdot HCl$ dissolved by UV absorption at the wavelength of maximum absorbance at about 250 nm (shoulder) on portions of the solution under test passed through a 0.45-μm polyethylene filter, suitably diluted with *Medium*, if necessary, in comparison with a Standard solution having a known concentration of USP Metformin Hydrochloride RS in the same *Medium*. Calculate the content of metformin hydrochloride ($C_4H_{11}N_5 \cdot HCl$), C_t, in mg per mL, in the *Medium* at each time point, t, by the formulas specified in *Test 2*.

Tolerances—The percentages of the labeled amount of $C_4H_{11}N_5 \cdot HCl$ dissolved at the times specified conform to *Acceptance Table 2*.

Time (hours)	Amount dissolved
1	between 20% and 40%
3	between 45% and 65%
6	between 65% and 85%
10	not less than 85%

TEST 5—If the product complies with this test, the labeling indicates that it meets USP *Dissolution Test 5*.
Medium: pH 6.8 phosphate buffer prepared by dissolving 6.8 g of monobasic potassium phosphate in 1000 mL of water and adjusting with 0.2 N sodium hydroxide to a pH of 6.8 ± 0.1; 900 mL, deaerated.
Apparatus 1: 100 rpm, with the vertical holder described below.
Times: 2, 8, and 16 hours.
Procedure—Place a vertical sample holder into each basket (see *Figures 1* and *2*). Place one Tablet inside the sample holder, making sure that the Tablets are vertical at the bottom of the baskets. Determine the amount of $C_4H_{11}N_5 \cdot HCl$ dissolved by UV absorption at the wavelength of maximum absorbance at about 250 nm on portions of the solution under test passed through a 0.45-μm polyethylene filter, suitably diluted with *Medium*, if necessary, in comparison with a Standard solution having a known concentration of USP Metformin Hydrochloride RS in the same *Medium*. Calculate the content of metformin hydrochloride ($C_4H_{11}N_5 \cdot HCl$), C_t, in mg per mL, in the *Medium* at each time point, t, by the formulas specified in *Test 2*.

Tolerances—The percentages of the labeled amount of $C_4H_{11}N_5 \cdot HCl$ dissolved at the times specified conform to *Acceptance Table 2*.

Time (hours)	500-mg Tablet, Amount dissolved	1000-mg Tablet, Amount dissolved
2	not more than 30%	not more than 30%
8	between 60% and 85%	between 65% and 90%
16	not less than 90%	not less than 90%

TEST 6—If the product complies with this test, the labeling indicates that it meets USP *Dissolution Test 6*.
Medium: pH 6.8 phosphate buffer prepared by dissolving 6.8 g of monobasic potassium phosphate in 1000 mL of water and adjusting with 0.2 N sodium hydroxide to a pH of 6.8 ± 0.05; 1000 mL, deaerated.
Apparatus 2: 100 rpm, with USP sinker, if necessary.
Procedure—Determine the amount of $C_4H_{11}N_5 \cdot HCl$ dissolved by UV absorption at the wavelength of maximum absorbance at about 233 nm on portions of the solution under test passed through a 0.45-μm hydrophilic polyethylene filter, suitably diluted with *Medium*, if necessary, in comparison with a Standard solution having a known concentration of USP Metformin Hydrochloride RS in the same *Medium*. Calculate the amount of metformin hydrochloride ($C_4H_{11}N_5 \cdot HCl$), in percentage, released at each time point by the formula:

$$\frac{[C \times (A_U/A_S) \times (V - V_S) + (C_{60} \times V_S) + (C_{180} \times V_S) + (C_{600} \times V_S)] \times 100}{L}$$

in which C is the concentration, in mg per mL, of the Standard solution; A_U and A_S are the absorbances of the solution under test and the Standard solution, respectively; V is the initial volume, in mL, of Medium in the vessel; V_S is the volume, in mL, withdrawn from the vessel for previous samplings; C_{60} is the concentration, in mg per mL, of metformin hydrochloride in the Medium determined at 1 hour; C_{180} is the concentration, in mg per mL, of metformin hydrochloride in the Medium determined at 3 hours; C_{600} is the concentration, in mg per mL, of metformin hydrochloride in the Medium determined at 10 hours; 100 is the conversion factor to percentage; and L is the Tablet label claim, in mg.

Tolerances—The percentages of the labeled amount of $C_4H_{11}N_5 \cdot HCl$ dissolved at the times specified conform to *Acceptance Table 2*.

Time (hours)	500-mg Tablet, Amount dissolved	750-mg Tablet, Amount dissolved
1	between 20% and 40%	between 20% and 40%
3	between 45% and 65%	between 45% and 65%
10	not less than 85%	not less than 85%

TEST 7—If the product complies with this test, the labeling indicates that it meets USP *Dissolution Test 7*.
Medium—Prepare as directed for *Medium* in *Test 1*; 1000 mL.
Apparatus 2: 50 rpm, with USP sinker, for Tablets labeled to contain 500 mg.
Apparatus 1: 100 rpm, for Tablets labeled to contain 750 mg.
Times: 1, 3, and 10 hours.
Procedure—Determine the amount of $C_4H_{11}N_5 \cdot HCl$ dissolved by UV absorption at the wavelength of maximum absorbance at about 232 nm on portions of the solution under test passed through a suitable 0.45-μm filter, suitably diluted with *Medium*, if necessary, in comparison with a Standard solution having a known con-

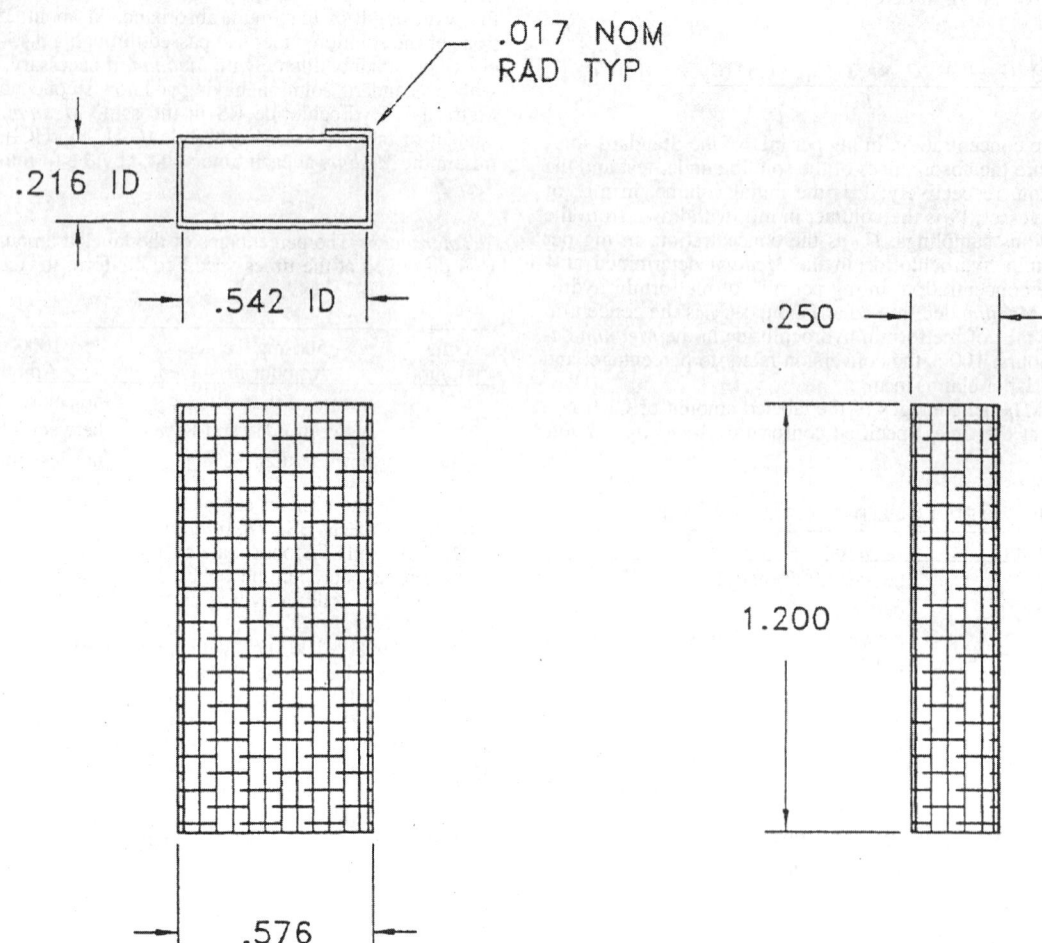

NOTES:
1. MATERIAL: 316SS OR EQUIVALENT .017 WIRE VERTICAL MEAS SQUARE WEAVE WITH .039 SQUARE OPENINGS.
2. ALL DIMENSIONS ARE IN INCHES. TOLERANCES TO BE +/-.010

Figure 1

centration of USP Metformin Hydrochloride RS in the same *Medium*. Calculate the amount of metformin hydrochloride ($C_4H_{11}N_5 \cdot HCl$), in percentage, released at each time point by the formula:

$$\frac{[C \times (A_U / A_S) \times (V - V_S) + (C_{60} \times V_S) + (C_{180} \times V_S) + (C_{600} \times V_S)] \times 100}{L}$$

in which C is the concentration, in mg per mL, of the Standard solution; A_U and A_S are the absorbances of the solution under test and the Standard solution, respectively; V is the initial volume, in mL, of *Medium* in the vessel; V_S is the volume, in mL, withdrawn from the vessel for previous samplings; C_{60} is the concentration, in mg per mL, of metformin hydrochloride in the *Medium* determined at 1 hour; C_{180} is the concentration, in mg per mL, of metformin hydrochloride in the *Medium* determined at 3 hours; C_{600} is the concentration, in mg per mL, of metformin hydrochloride in the *Medium* determined at 10 hours; 100 is the conversion factor to percentage; and L is the Tablet label claim, in mg.

Tolerances—The percentages of the labeled amount of $C_4H_{11}N_5 \cdot HCl$ dissolved at the times specified conform to *Acceptance Table 2*.

Time (hours)	500-mg Tablet, Amount dissolved	750-mg Tablet, Amount dissolved
1	between 20% and 40%	between 20% and 40%
3	between 45% and 65%	between 40% and 60%
10	not less than 85%	not less than 80%

TEST 8—If the product complies with this test, the labeling indicates that it meets USP *Dissolution Test 8*.

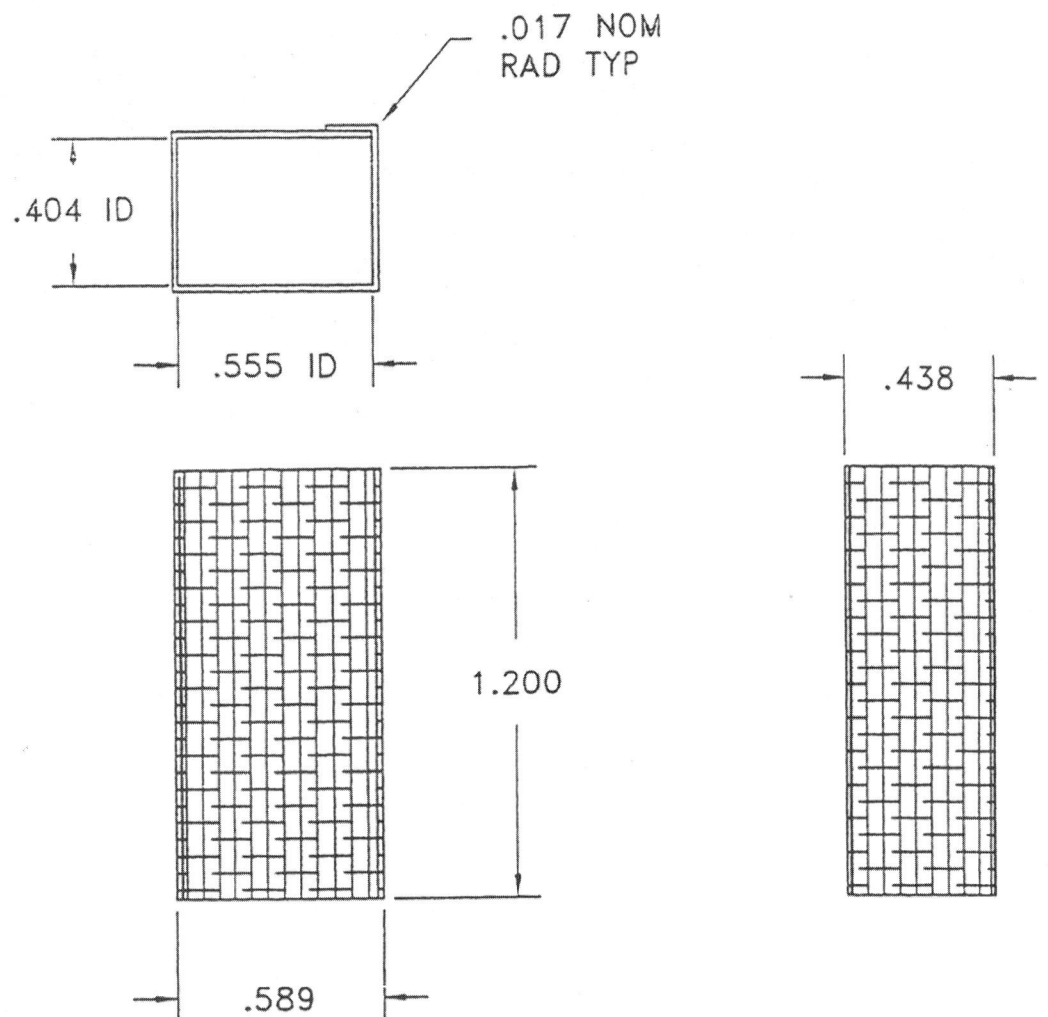

NOTES:
1. MATERIAL: 316SS OR EQUIVALENT .017 WIRE VERTICAL MEAS SQUARE WEAVE WITH .039 SQUARE OPENINGS.
2. ALL DIMENSIONS ARE IN INCHES. TOLERANCES TO BE +/-.010

Figure 2

Medium—Prepare as directed for *Medium* in *Test 1;* 1000 mL.

Apparatus 2: 100 rpm, with sinker, for Tablets labeled to contain 500 mg.

Apparatus 1: 100 rpm, for Tablets labeled to contain 750 mg.

Times: 1, 2, 6, and 10 hours

Procedure—Determine the amount of $C_4H_{11}N_5 \cdot HCl$ dissolved by UV absorption at the wavelength of maximum absorbance at about 232 nm on portions of the solution under test passed through a suitable 0.45-μm filter, suitably diluted with *Medium*, if necessary, in comparison with a Standard solution having a known concentration of USP Metformin Hydrochloride RS in the same *Medium*. Calculate the amount of metformin hydrochloride ($C_4H_{11}N_5 \cdot HCl$), in percentage, released at each time point by the formula (1): in which C is the concentration, in mg per mL, of the Standard solution; A_U and A_S are the absorbances of the solution under test and the Standard solution, respectively; V is the initial volume, in mL, of *Medium* in the vessel; V_S is the volume, in mL, withdrawn from the vessel for previous samplings; C_{60} is the concentration, in mg per mL, of metformin hydrochloride in the *Medium* determined at 1 hour; C_{120} is the concentration, in mg per mL, of metformin hydrochloride in the *Medium* determined at 2 hours; C_{360} is the concentration, in mg per mL, of metformin hydrochloride in the *Medium* determined at 6 hours; C_{600} is the concentration, in mg per mL, of metformin hydrochloride in the *Medium* determined at 10 hours; 100 is the conversion factor to percentage; and L is the tablet label claim, in mg.

Tolerances—The percentages of the labeled amount of $C_4H_{11}N_5 \cdot HCl$ dissolved at the times specified conform to *Acceptance Table 2*.

2646 Metformin / Official Monographs

Time (hours)	500-mg Tablet, Amount dissolved	750-mg Tablet, Amount dissolved
1	between 20% and 40%	between 20% and 40%
2	between 30% and 50%	between 35% and 55%
6	between 65% and 85%	between 75% and 95%
10	not less than 85%	not less than 85%

Uniformity of dosage units ⟨905⟩: meet the requirements.

Chromatographic purity—
Mobile phase and *Chromatographic system*—Prepare as directed in the *Assay*.
Test solution—Use the *Assay preparation*, prepared as directed in the *Assay*.
Procedure—Inject a volume (about 10 µL) of the *Test solution* into the chromatograph, record the chromatogram, and measure all of the peak responses. Calculate the percentage of each impurity in the portion of Tablets taken by the formula:

$$100(r_i / r_s)$$

in which r_i is the peak response for each impurity, and r_s is the sum of the responses of all the peaks: not more than 0.1% of any individual impurity is found, and not more than 0.6% of total impurities is found. Disregard any peak less than 0.05%, and disregard any peak observed in the blank.

Assay—
Buffer solution—Transfer 1.0 g each of sodium heptanesulfonate and sodium chloride to a 2000-mL volumetric flask, add 1800 mL of water, and mix. Adjust with 0.06 M phosphoric acid to a pH of 3.85, and dilute with water to volume.
Mobile phase—Prepare a filtered and degassed mixture of *Buffer solution* and acetonitrile (90 : 10). Make adjustments if necessary (see *System Suitability* under *Chromatography* ⟨621⟩). [NOTE—To improve the separation, the composition may be changed to 95 : 5, if necessary.]
Diluent—Use a 1.25% solution of acetonitrile in water.
Standard preparation—Dissolve an accurately weighed quantity of USP Metformin Hydrochloride RS in *Diluent*, and dilute quantitatively, and stepwise if necessary, with *Diluent* to obtain a solution having a known concentration of about (L/4000) mg per mL, where L is the labeled quantity, in mg, of metformin hydrochloride in each Tablet.
System suitability preparation—Dissolve suitable quantities of USP Metformin Related Compound B RS and USP Metformin Related Compound C RS in *Diluent* to obtain a solution containing about 12.5 µg of each per mL. Pipet 0.5 mL of this solution into a 50-mL volumetric flask, and dilute with the *Standard preparation* to volume.
Assay stock preparation—Weigh and finely powder not fewer than 10 Tablets. Transfer an accurately weighed portion of the powder, equivalent to the average Tablet weight, to a homogenization vessel, and accurately add 500 mL of 10% acetonitrile solution. Alternately, homogenize and allow to soak until the sample is fully homogenized. [NOTE—A suggested homogenization sequence is as follows: Homogenize the sample using 5 pulses, each of 5 second, at about 20,000 rpm; allow to soak for 2 minutes. Repeat these steps a further two times.]
Assay preparation—Pass a portion of the *Assay stock preparation* through a filter having a 0.45-µm porosity, discarding the first 3 mL of filtrate. Transfer 25 mL of the filtrate to a 200-mL volumetric flask, and dilute with water to volume.
Chromatographic system (see *Chromatography* ⟨621⟩)—The liquid chromatograph is equipped with a 218-nm detector and a 3.9-mm × 30-cm column that contains 10-µm packing L1. The flow rate is about 1.0 mL per minute. The column temperature is maintained at 30°. Chromatograph the *System suitability preparation*, and record the peak responses as directed for *Procedure*: the relative retention times are about 0.86 for metformin related compound B, 1.0 for metformin, and about 2.1 to 2.3 for metformin related compound C [NOTE—This impurity can have a variable retention time; the composition of the *Mobile phase* may be changed to 95 : 5, if metformin related compound C elutes at a relative retention time of less than 2.1.]; the resolution, R, between peaks due to metformin related compound B and metformin is not less than 1.5; the tailing factor for the metformin peak is not less than 0.8 and not more than 2.0; and the relative standard deviation for replicate injections is not more than 1.5% for the metformin peak and not more than 10% for each of the peaks due to metformin related compound B and metformin related compound C.

Procedure—Separately inject equal volumes (about 10 µL) of the *Standard preparation* and the *Assay preparation* into the chromatograph, carrying out the run until after the elution locus of metformin related compound C; record the chromatograms; and measure the responses for the major peaks. Calculate the quantity, in mg per Tablet, of metformin hydrochloride ($C_4H_{11}N_5 \cdot HCl$) by the formula:

$$C(V/W)TD(r_U / r_S)$$

in which C is the concentration, in mg per mL, of USP Metformin Hydrochloride RS in the *Standard preparation*; V is the volume, in mL, of the *Assay stock preparation*; W is the weight, in mg, of sample used to prepare the *Assay stock preparation*; T is the average Tablet weight, in mg; D is the dilution factor of the *Assay preparation*; and r_U and r_S are the peak responses obtained from the *Assay preparation* and the *Standard preparation*, respectively. ▲USP31

Methacholine Chloride

$C_8H_{18}ClNO_2$ 195.69
1-Propanaminium, 2-(acetyloxy)-N,N,N-trimethyl-, chloride, (±)-.
(±)-(2-Hydroxypropyl)trimethylammonium chloride acetate [62-51-1].

» Methacholine Chloride, dried at 105° for 4 hours, contains not less than 98.0 percent and not more than 101.0 percent of $C_8H_{18}ClNO_2$.

Packaging and storage—Preserve in tight containers.
Identification—
A: Dissolve about 100 mg in about 2 mL of water on a watch glass, and add 3 mL of platinic chloride TS: small rhombohedric plates are formed, which melt between 220° and 225° (see *Melting Range or Temperature* ⟨741⟩) (*distinction from acetylcholine chloride, which forms needles radiating from a central point, and from choline chloride, which forms no crystals*).
B: To 1 mL of a solution (1 in 10) add 1 mL of alcohol and 1 mL of sulfuric acid, and heat gently: the odor of ethyl acetate is perceptible.
C: To 5 mL of a solution (1 in 10) add 2 g of potassium hydroxide and heat gently: the odor of trimethylamine is perceptible.
D: A solution (1 in 50) responds to the tests for *Chloride* ⟨191⟩.
Melting range ⟨741⟩—Dissolve about 100 mg in 2 to 3 mL of chloroform in a small beaker. Heat at 110° for 1 hour. While the test specimen is still hot, quickly powder the dry residue with a glass rod, and transfer to a melting point tube in the usual manner. Determine the melting range without delay. It melts between 170° and 173°.
Loss on drying ⟨731⟩—Dry it at 105° for 4 hours: it loses not more than 1.5% of its weight.
Residue on ignition ⟨281⟩: not more than 0.1%.
Acetylcholine chloride—To 2 mL of a solution (1 in 10) add 3 mL of a solution of sodium perchlorate (1 in 5), shake, and immerse in ice water for 5 minutes: no precipitate is formed.

$$\frac{[C \times (A_U / A_S) \times (V - V_S) + (C_{60} \times V_S) + (C_{120} \times V_S) + (C_{360} \times V_S) + (C_{600} \times V_S)] \times 100}{L} \quad (1)$$

Heavy metals, *Method II* ⟨231⟩: 0.002%.
Assay—Transfer to a conical flask about 400 mg of Methacholine Chloride, previously dried and accurately weighed (because it is very hygroscopic, store the dried material in a vacuum desiccator), dissolve it in 50 mL of glacial acetic acid, add 10 mL of mercuric acetate TS and 1 drop of crystal violet TS, and titrate with 0.1 N perchloric acid VS to a blue-green endpoint. Perform a blank determination, and make any necessary correction. Each mL of 0.1 N perchloric acid is equivalent to 19.57 mg of $C_8H_{18}ClNO_2$.

Methacycline Hydrochloride

$C_{22}H_{22}N_2O_8 \cdot HCl$ 478.88

2-Naphthacenecarboxamide, 4-(dimethylamino)-1,4,4a,5,5a, 6,11,12a-octahydro-3,5,10,12,12a-pentahydroxy-6-methylene-1,11-dioxo-, monohydrochloride, [4S-(4α,4aα,5α,5aα,12aα)]-.

4-(Dimethylamino)-1,4,4a,5,5a,6,11,12a-octahydro-3,5,10,12,12a-pentahydroxy-6-methylene-1,11-dioxo-2-naphthacenecarboxamide monohydrochloride   [3963-95-9].

» Methacycline Hydrochloride has a potency equivalent to not less than 832 μg and not more than 970 μg of methacycline ($C_{22}H_{22}N_2O_8$) per mg.

Packaging and storage—Preserve in tight, light-resistant containers.
USP Reference standards ⟨11⟩—*USP Doxycycline Hyclate RS. USP Methacycline Hydrochloride RS.*
Identification, *Ultraviolet Absorption* ⟨197U⟩—
 Solution: 20 μg per mL.
 Medium: hydrochloric acid in methanol (1 in 1200).
 Absorptivity at 345 nm, calculated on the dried basis, is between 88.4% and 96.4% of the USP Methacycline Hydrochloride RS, the potency of the Reference Standard being taken into account.
Crystallinity ⟨695⟩: meets the requirements.
pH ⟨791⟩: between 2.0 and 3.0, in a solution containing 10 mg of methacycline per mL.
Water, *Method I* ⟨921⟩: not more than 2.0%.
Assay—
 Mobile phase—Prepare a mixture of 0.2 M ammonium oxalate, dimethylformamide, and 0.1 M edetate disodium (11 : 5 : 4), adjust with tetrabutylammonium hydroxide, 40 percent in water, to a pH of 7.0, and filter. Make adjustments, if necessary (see *System Suitability* under *Chromatography* ⟨621⟩).
 System suitability preparation—Prepare a solution of USP Methacycline Hydrochloride RS and USP Doxycycline Hyclate RS in *Mobile phase* containing about 0.5 mg of each per mL.
 Standard preparation—Quantitatively dissolve an accurately weighed quantity of USP Methacycline Hydrochloride RS in *Mobile phase* to obtain a solution having a known concentration of about 0.5 mg per mL.
 Assay preparation—Transfer about 50 mg of Methacycline Hydrochloride, accurately weighed, to a 100-mL volumetric flask, dilute with *Mobile phase* to volume, and mix.
 Chromatographic system (see *Chromatography* ⟨621⟩)—The liquid chromatograph is equipped with a 354-nm detector and a 4.6-mm × 15-cm column that contains 3.5-μm packing L1. The flow rate is about 1 mL per minute. Chromatograph the *System suitability preparation*, and record the peak responses as directed for *Procedure*: the relative retention times are about 0.75 for methacycline and 1.0 for doxycycline; and the resolution, *R*, between methacycline and doxycycline is not less than 1.5. Chromatograph the *Standard preparation*, and record the peak responses as directed for *Procedure*: the tailing factor is not more than 1.5; and the relative standard deviation for replicate injections is not more than 1.0%.

 Procedure—Separately inject equal volumes (about 20 μL) of the *Standard preparation* and the *Assay preparation* into the chromatograph, record the chromatograms, and measure the areas for the major peaks. Calculate the quantity, in μg, of methacycline ($C_{22}H_{22}N_2O_8$) in each mg of Methacycline Hydrochloride taken by the formula:

$$100(CE/W)(r_U/r_S)$$

in which *C* is the concentration, in mg per mL, of USP Methacycline Hydrochloride RS in the *Standard preparation*; *E* is the methacycline content, in μg per mg, of *USP Methacycline Hydrochloride RS*; *W* is the quantity, in mg, of Methacycline Hydrochloride taken to prepare the *Assay preparation*; and r_U and r_S are the methacycline peak areas obtained from the *Assay preparation* and the *Standard preparation*, respectively.

Methacycline Hydrochloride Capsules

» Methacycline Hydrochloride Capsules contain the equivalent of not less than 90.0 percent and not more than 120.0 percent of the labeled amount of methacycline ($C_{22}H_{22}N_2O_8$).

Packaging and storage—Preserve in tight, light-resistant containers.
USP Reference standards ⟨11⟩—*USP Doxycycline Hyclate RS. USP Methacycline Hydrochloride RS.*
Identification—Shake a suitable quantity of Capsule contents with methanol to obtain a solution containing the equivalent of about 1 mg of methacycline per mL, and filter. Using the filtrate as the *Test Solution*, proceed as directed for *Method II* under *Identification—Tetracyclines* ⟨193⟩.
Dissolution ⟨711⟩—
 Medium: water; 900 mL.
 Apparatus 1: 100 rpm.
 Time: 60 minutes.
 Procedure—Determine the amount of $C_{22}H_{22}N_2O_8 \cdot HCl$ dissolved from UV absorbances at the wavelength of maximum absorbance at about 345 nm of filtered portions of the solution under test, suitably diluted with water, in comparison with a Standard solution having a known concentration of USP Methacycline Hydrochloride RS in the same *Medium*.
 Tolerances—Not less than 70% (*Q*) of the labeled amount of $C_{22}H_{22}N_2O_8 \cdot HCl$ is dissolved in 60 minutes.
Uniformity of dosage units ⟨905⟩: meet the requirements.
Water, *Method I* ⟨921⟩: not more than 7.5%.
Assay—
 Mobile phase, System suitability preparation, and *Chromatographic system*—Proceed as directed in the *Assay* under *Methacycline Hydrochloride*.
 Standard preparation—Transfer about 28 mg of USP Methacycline Hydrochloride RS, accurately weighed, to a 50-mL volumetric flask, add 10 mL of water, dilute with *Mobile phase* to volume, and mix.
 Assay preparation—Place no fewer than 5 Capsules in a high-speed, glass blender jar containing an accurately measured volume of water, and blend for 3 to 5 minutes to obtain a stock solution having a concentration of about 2.5 mg of methacycline ($C_{22}H_{22}N_2O_8$) per mL. Filter, transfer 10.0 mL of the filtrate to a 50-mL volumetric flask, add 10 mL of water, dilute with *Mobile phase* to volume, and mix.
 Procedure—Proceed as directed in the *Assay* under *Methacycline Hydrochloride*. Calculate the quantity, in mg, of methacycline ($C_{22}H_{22}N_2O_8$) in each Capsule taken by the formula:

$$5(CE/1000)(V/N)(r_U/r_S)$$

in which *V* is the volume, in mL, of water used to prepare the stock solution for the *Assay preparation*; *N* is the number of Capsules taken to prepare the stock solution for the *Assay preparation*; and the other terms are as defined therein.

Methacycline Hydrochloride Oral Suspension

» Methacycline Hydrochloride Oral Suspension contains the equivalent of not less than 90.0 percent and not more than 125.0 percent of the labeled amount of methacycline ($C_{22}H_{22}N_2O_8$). It contains one or more suitable and harmless buffers, colors, diluents, dispersants, flavors, and preservatives.

Packaging and storage—Preserve in tight, light-resistant containers.

USP Reference standards ⟨11⟩—*USP Doxycycline Hyclate RS. USP Methacycline Hydrochloride RS.*

Identification—To an accurately measured volume of Oral Suspension, equivalent to about 50 mg of methacycline, add 50 mL of methanol, shake, and allow the mixture to settle. Using the clear supernatant as the *Test Solution*, proceed as directed for *Method II* under *Identification—Tetracyclines* ⟨193⟩.

Uniformity of dosage units ⟨905⟩—
FOR SUSPENSION PACKAGED IN SINGLE-UNIT CONTAINERS: meets the requirements.

Deliverable volume ⟨698⟩: meets the requirements.

pH ⟨791⟩: between 6.5 and 8.0.

Assay—
Mobile phase, System suitability preparation, and *Chromatographic system*—Proceed as directed in the *Assay* under *Methacycline Hydrochloride.*

Standard preparation—Transfer about 28 mg of USP Methacycline Hydrochloride RS, accurately weighed, to a 50-mL volumetric flask, add 10 mL of water, dilute with *Mobile phase* to volume, and mix.

Assay preparation—Transfer an accurately measured quantity of Oral Suspension, freshly mixed and free from air bubbles, equivalent to about 50 mg of methacycline ($C_{22}H_{22}N_2O_8$), to a 100-mL volumetric flask, dilute with *Mobile phase* to volume, mix, and filter.

Procedure—Proceed as directed in the *Assay* under *Methacycline Hydrochloride*. Calculate the quantity, in mg, of methacycline ($C_{22}H_{22}N_2O_8$) in each mL of the Oral Suspension taken by the formula:

$$100(CE/1000V)(r_U/r_S)$$

in which V is the volume, in mL, of Oral Suspension taken to prepare the *Assay preparation;* and the other terms are as defined therein.

Methadone Hydrochloride

$C_{21}H_{27}NO \cdot HCl \quad 345.91$

3-Heptanone, 6-(dimethylamino)-4,4-diphenyl-, hydrochloride.
6-(Dimethylamino)-4,4-diphenyl-3-heptanone hydrochloride [1095-90-5].

» Methadone Hydrochloride contains not less than 98.5 percent and not more than 100.5 percent of $C_{21}H_{27}NO \cdot HCl$, calculated on the dried basis.

Packaging and storage—Preserve in tight, light-resistant containers. Store at 25°, excursions permitted between 15° and 30°.

USP Reference standards ⟨11⟩—*USP Methadone Hydrochloride RS.*

Identification—
A: *Infrared Absorption* ⟨197K⟩.
B: A solution of it responds to the tests for *Chloride* ⟨191⟩.

pH ⟨791⟩: between 4.5 and 6.5, in a solution (1 in 100).

Loss on drying ⟨731⟩—Dry about 500 mg, accurately weighed, at 105° for 1 hour: it loses not more than 0.3% of its weight.

Residue on ignition ⟨281⟩: not more than 0.1%.

Ordinary impurities ⟨466⟩—
Test solution: alcohol.
Standard solution: alcohol.
Eluant: a mixture of methanol and ammonium hydroxide (100 : 1.5).
Visualization: 3.
Limits—The sum of the intensities of all secondary spots obtained from the *Test solution* corresponds to not more than 1.0%.

Organic volatile impurities, *Method I* ⟨467⟩: meets the requirements.
(Official until July 1, 2008)

Assay—Dissolve about 500 mg of Methadone Hydrochloride, accurately weighed, in a mixture of 10 mL of glacial acetic acid and 10 mL of mercuric acetate TS, warming slightly if necessary to effect solution. Cool the solution to room temperature, add 10 mL of dioxane, then add crystal violet TS, and titrate rapidly with 0.1 N perchloric acid VS. Perform a blank determination, and make any necessary correction. Each mL of 0.1 N perchloric acid is equivalent to 34.59 mg of $C_{21}H_{27}NO \cdot HCl$.

Methadone Hydrochloride Oral Concentrate

» Methadone Hydrochloride Oral Concentrate contains, in each mL, not less than 9.0 mg and not more than 11.0 mg of methadone hydrochloride ($C_{21}H_{27}NO \cdot HCl$). It contains a suitable preservative and may contain suitable coloring, flavoring, and surface-active agents.

Packaging and storage—Preserve in tight containers, protected from light, at controlled room temperature.

Labeling—Label it to indicate that it is to be diluted with water or other liquid to 30 mL or more prior to administration.

USP Reference standards ⟨11⟩—*USP Methadone Hydrochloride RS.*

Identification—
A: Shake a volume of Oral Concentrate, equivalent to about 5 mg of methadone hydrochloride, with 5 mL of sodium carbonate TS, and extract with 5 mL of chloroform: the extract so obtained responds to the *Thin-layer Chromatographic Identification Test* ⟨201⟩, a solvent mixture of alcohol, glacial acetic acid, and water (5 : 3 : 2) being used for development and iodoplatinate TS being used to visualize the spots.
B: It responds to the tests for *Chloride* ⟨191⟩.

pH ⟨791⟩: between 1.0 and 6.0.

Assay—
Mobile phase—Prepare a suitable mixture of 0.033 M monobasic potassium phosphate and acetonitrile (60 : 40), adjust with phosphoric acid to a pH of 4.0, filter, and degas. Make adjustments if necessary (see *System Suitability* under *Chromatography* ⟨621⟩).

Standard preparation—Dissolve an accurately weighed quantity of USP Methadone Hydrochloride RS in *Mobile phase* to obtain a solution having a known concentration of about 0.4 mg per mL.

Assay preparation—Transfer an accurately measured volume of Oral Concentrate, equivalent to about 50 mg of methadone hydrochloride, to a 50-mL volumetric flask, dilute with *Mobile phase* to volume, and mix. Transfer 10.0 mL of this solution to a 25-mL volumetric flask, dilute with *Mobile phase* to volume, and mix.

Chromatographic system (see *Chromatography* ⟨621⟩)—The liquid chromatograph is equipped with a 254-nm detector and a 3.9-

mm × 30-cm column that contains packing L11. The flow rate is about 2 mL per minute. Chromatograph the *Standard preparation*, and record the peak responses as directed for *Procedure:* the column efficiency determined from the analyte peak is not less than 1500 theoretical plates, the tailing factor for the analyte peak is not more than 2.0, and the relative standard deviation for replicate injections is not more than 2.0%.

Procedure—Separately inject equal volumes (about 10 µL) of the *Standard preparation* and the *Assay preparation* into the chromatograph, record the chromatograms, and measure the responses for the major peaks. Calculate the quantity, in mg, of methadone hydrochloride ($C_{21}H_{27}NO \cdot HCl$) in each mL of the Oral Concentrate taken by the formula:

$$125(C/V)(r_U/r_S)$$

in which C is the concentration, in mg per mL, of USP Methadone Hydrochloride RS in the *Standard preparation*; V is the volume, in mL, of Oral Concentrate taken; and r_U and r_S are the peak responses obtained from the *Assay preparation* and the *Standard preparation*, respectively.

Methadone Hydrochloride Injection

» Methadone Hydrochloride Injection is a sterile solution of Methadone Hydrochloride in Water for Injection. It contains, in each mL, not less than 9.5 mg and not more than 10.5 mg of methadone hydrochloride ($C_{21}H_{27}NO \cdot HCl$).

Packaging and storage—Preserve in single-dose or in multiple-dose, light-resistant containers, preferably of Type I glass.
USP Reference standards ⟨11⟩—*USP Endotoxin RS. USP Methadone Hydrochloride RS.*
Identification—It meets the requirements under *Identification—Organic Nitrogenous Bases* ⟨181⟩.
Bacterial endotoxins ⟨85⟩—It contains not more than 8.8 USP Endotoxin Units per mg of methadone hydrochloride.
pH ⟨791⟩: between 3.0 and 6.5.
Other requirements—It meets the requirements under *Injections* ⟨1⟩.
Assay—
Internal standard solution—Weigh about 100 mg of procaine, and dissolve in 20 mL of methylene chloride.
Standard preparation—Weigh accurately about 10 mg of USP Methadone Hydrochloride RS, transfer to a 60-mL separator, add 1 mL of water and 2 mL of 0.5 N sodium hydroxide, and proceed as directed for *Assay preparation*, beginning with "extract with three 10-mL portions of chromatographic grade methylene chloride."
Assay preparation—Transfer 1.0 mL of Injection, equivalent to 10 mg of methadone hydrochloride, to a 60-mL separator, add 2 mL of 0.5 N sodium hydroxide, and extract with three 10-mL portions of chromatographic grade methylene chloride, combining the extracts in a vessel containing about 3 g of anhydrous sodium sulfate. Transfer 2.0 mL of *Internal standard solution* to the vessel containing the extracts, insert the stopper, and mix. Decant about 15 mL of the methylene chloride solution to a test tube, and evaporate to a volume of 2 to 3 mL, using vacuum or a stream of nitrogen.
Procedure—Use a suitable gas chromatograph equipped with a flame-ionization detector and a glass column 1.2-m long and 4-mm in diameter, packed with 3% phase G2 on 100- to 200-mesh support S1A. Maintain the column temperature at 170°, the injection port at 225°, and the detector at 240°. Use dry helium as the carrier gas, at a flow rate of about 55 mL per minute. In a suitable chromatogram, six replicate injections of the *Standard preparation* show a coefficient of variation of not more than 1% in the ratios of the peak areas of methadone to the peak area of procaine, and the resolution factor is not less than 5. Inject, separately, suitable volumes of the *Assay preparation*, containing about 5 µg of methadone, and of the *Standard preparation*. Calculate the quantity, in mg, of methadone hydrochloride ($C_{21}H_{27}NO \cdot HCl$) in each mL of the Injection taken by the formula:

$$W(R_U/R_S)$$

in which W is the weight, in mg, of USP Methadone Hydrochloride RS in the *Standard preparation*; and R_U and R_S are the ratios of the peak areas of methadone to the peak area of procaine in the *Assay preparation* and the *Standard preparation*, respectively.

Methadone Hydrochloride Oral Solution

» Methadone Hydrochloride Oral Solution contains not less than 90.0 percent and not more than 110.0 percent of the labeled amount of methadone hydrochloride ($C_{21}H_{27}NO \cdot HCl$).

Packaging and storage—Preserve in tight containers, protected from light, at controlled room temperature.
USP Reference standards ⟨11⟩—*USP Methadone Hydrochloride RS.*
Identification—
A: Shake a volume of Oral Solution, equivalent to about 5 mg of methadone hydrochloride, with 5 mL of sodium carbonate TS, and extract with 5 mL of chloroform: the extract so obtained responds to the *Thin-layer Chromatographic Identification Test* ⟨201⟩, a solvent mixture of alcohol, glacial acetic acid, and water (5 : 3 : 2) being used for development and iodoplatinate TS being used to visualize the spots.
B: It responds to the tests for *Chloride* ⟨191⟩.
Uniformity of dosage units ⟨905⟩—
FOR ORAL SOLUTION PACKAGED IN SINGLE-UNIT CONTAINERS: meets the requirements.
Deliverable volume ⟨698⟩—
FOR ORAL SOLUTION PACKAGED IN MULTIPLE-UNIT CONTAINERS: meets the requirements.
pH ⟨791⟩: between 1.0 and 4.0.
Alcohol content, *Method II* ⟨611⟩*(if present):* between 90.0% and 115.0% of the labeled amount of C_2H_5OH, determined by the gas-liquid chromatographic procedure, acetone being used as the internal standard.
Assay—
Mobile phase—Prepare a solution containing about 40 volumes of acetonitrile and 60 volumes of 0.033 M monobasic potassium phosphate adjusted, dropwise, with phosphoric acid to a pH of 4.0.
Internal standard solution—Prepare a solution of pyrilamine maleate in water containing 250 µg per mL.
Standard preparation—Transfer about 20 mg of USP Methadone Hydrochloride RS, accurately weighed, to a 25-mL volumetric flask, add 2.0 mL of *Internal standard solution*, dilute with water to volume, and mix.
Assay preparation—Transfer an accurately measured volume of Oral Solution, equivalent to about 20 mg of methadone hydrochloride, to a 125-mL separator. Extract the specimen with two 50-mL portions of ether, collecting the ether extracts in a second separator. Wash the combined ether extracts with 2 mL of water, and discard the ether extract. Transfer the aqueous wash and the aqueous specimen to a 25-mL volumetric flask, add 2.0 mL of *Internal standard solution*, dilute with water to volume, and mix. Pass the solution through a 5-µm filter.
Chromatographic system (see *Chromatography* ⟨621⟩)—The liquid chromatograph is equipped with a 254-nm detector and a 3.9-mm × 30-cm column that contains packing L11. The flow rate is about 1.3 mL per minute. Chromatograph five replicate injections of the *Standard preparation*, and record the peak responses as directed for *Procedure:* the relative standard deviation is not more than 2.0%.
Procedure—Separately inject equal volumes (about 10 µL) of the *Standard preparation* and the *Assay preparation* into the chromatograph by means of a suitable microsyringe or sampling valve, rec-

ord the chromatograms, and measure the responses for the major peaks. The relative retention times are about 5.5 minutes for the internal standard and 9 minutes for methadone hydrochloride. Calculate the quantity, in mg, of methadone hyrdrochloride ($C_{21}H_{27}NO \cdot HCl$) in each mL of the Oral Solution taken by the formula:

$$25(C/V)(R_U / R_S)$$

in which C is the concentration, in mg per mL, of USP Methadone Hydrochloride RS in the *Standard preparation*; V is the volume, in mL, of Oral Solution taken; and R_U and R_S are the peak response ratios of the methadone hydrochloride to the internal standard peaks obtained from the *Assay preparation* and the *Standard preparation*, respectively.

Methadone Hydrochloride Tablets

» Methadone Hydrochloride Tablets contain not less than 93.0 percent and not more than 107.0 percent of the labeled amount of methadone hydrochloride ($C_{21}H_{27}NO \cdot HCl$).

Packaging and storage—Preserve in well-closed containers.

USP Reference standards ⟨11⟩—*USP Methadone Hydrochloride RS*.

Identification—A quantity of powdered Tablets, equivalent to about 5 mg of methadone hydrochloride, responds to *Identification* test A under *Methadone Hydrochloride Oral Solution*.

Dissolution ⟨711⟩—
  Medium: water; 500 mL.
  Apparatus 1: 100 rpm.
  Time: 45 minutes.
  Procedure—Filter a portion of the solution under test, and pipet a volume of the filtrate, equivalent to about 400 µg of methadone hydrochloride, into a suitable separator. Add 1 mL of glacial acetic acid and 20 mL of a solution of bromocresol purple, prepared by dissolving 200 mg of bromocresol purple in 1000 mL of dilute glacial acetic acid (1 in 50), mix, and extract with 20.0 mL of chloroform. Determine the amount of $C_{21}H_{27}NO \cdot HCl$ dissolved from visible absorbances at the wavelength of maximum absorbance at about 405 nm of the chloroform extract so obtained in comparison with the chloroform extract similarly prepared from a Standard solution having a known concentration of USP Methadone Hydrochloride RS in water.
  Tolerances—Not less than 75% (*Q*) of the labeled amount of $C_{21}H_{27}NO \cdot HCl$ is dissolved in 45 minutes.

Uniformity of dosage units ⟨905⟩: meet the requirements.

Assay—
  Mobile phase—Prepare a filtered and degassed mixture of 0.03 M monobasic potassium phosphate and acetonitrile (60 : 40). Adjust with phosphoric acid to a pH of 3.2. Make adjustments if necessary (see *System Suitability* under *Chromatography* ⟨621⟩).
  Standard preparation—Dissolve an accurately weighed quantity of USP Methadone Hydrochloride RS in *Mobile phase* to obtain a solution having a known concentration of about 0.4 mg per mL.
  Assay preparation—Weigh and finely powder not fewer than 20 Tablets. Transfer an accurately weighed portion of the powder, equivalent to about 10 mg of methadone hydrochloride, to a 25-mL volumetric flask. Add 10 mL of *Mobile phase*, and sonicate briefly. Shake by mechanical means for 15 minutes, dilute with *Mobile phase* to volume, mix, and filter.
  Chromatographic system (see *Chromatography* ⟨621⟩)—The liquid chromatograph is equipped with a 254-nm detector and a 3.9-mm × 30-cm column that contains packing L11. The flow rate is about 1.5 mL per minute. Chromatograph the *Standard preparation*, and record the peak responses as directed for *Procedure*: the tailing factor is not more than 2.0, and the relative standard deviation is not more than 2.0%.
  Procedure—Separately inject equal volumes (about 10 µL) of the *Standard preparation* and the *Assay preparation* into the chromatograph, record the chromatograms, and measure the responses for the major peaks. Calculate the quantity, in mg, of methadone hydrochloride ($C_{21}H_{27}NO \cdot HCl$) in the portion of Tablets taken by the formula:

$$25C(r_U / r_S)$$

in which C is the concentration, in mg per mL, of USP Methadone Hydrochloride RS in the *Standard preparation*; and r_U and r_S are the peak responses obtained from the *Assay preparation* and the *Standard preparation*, respectively.

Methadone Hydrochloride Tablets for Oral Suspension

» Methadone Hydrochloride Tablets for Oral Suspension contain not less than 93.0 percent and not more than 107.0 percent of the labeled amount of methadone hydrochloride ($C_{21}H_{27}NO \cdot HCl$).

Packaging and storage—Preserve in well-closed containers.

Labeling—Label the Tablets for Oral Suspension to indicate that they are intended for dispersion in a liquid prior to oral administration of the prescribed dose.

USP Reference standards ⟨11⟩—*USP Methadone Hydrochloride RS*.

Identification—A quantity of powdered Tablets for Oral Suspension, equivalent to about 5 mg of methadone hydrochloride, responds to *Identification* test A under *Methadone Hydrochloride Oral Solution*.

Disintegration ⟨701⟩: 15 minutes.

Uniformity of dosage units ⟨905⟩: meet the requirements.

Assay—
  Mobile phase—Prepare a filtered and degassed mixture of 0.03 M monobasic potassium phosphate and acetonitrile (60 : 40). Adjust with phosphoric acid to a pH of 3.2. Make adjustments if necessary (see *System Suitability* under *Chromatography* ⟨621⟩).
  Standard preparation—Dissolve an accurately weighed quantity of USP Methadone Hydrochloride RS in *Mobile phase* to obtain a solution having a known concentration of about 0.4 mg per mL.
  Assay preparation—Weigh and finely powder not fewer than 20 Tablets for Oral Suspension. Transfer an accurately weighed portion of the powder, equivalent to about 10 mg of methadone hydrochloride, to a 25-mL volumetric flask. Add 10 mL of *Mobile phase*, and sonicate briefly. Shake by mechanical means for 15 minutes, dilute with *Mobile phase* to volume, mix, and filter.
  Chromatographic system (see *Chromatography* ⟨621⟩)—The liquid chromatograph is equipped with a 254-nm detector and a 3.9-mm × 30-cm column that contains packing L11. The flow rate is about 1.5 mL per minute. Chromatograph the *Standard preparation*, and record the peak responses as directed for *Procedure*: the tailing factor is not more than 2.0, and the relative standard deviation is not more than 2.0%.
  Procedure—Separately inject equal volumes (about 10 µL) of the *Standard preparation* and the *Assay preparation* into the chromatograph, record the chromatograms, and measure the responses for the major peaks. Calculate the quantity, in mg, of methadone hydrochloride ($C_{21}H_{27}NO \cdot HCl$) in the portion of Tablets for Oral Suspension taken by the formula:

$$25C(r_U / r_S)$$

in which C is the concentration, in mg per mL, of USP Methadone Hydrochloride RS in the *Standard preparation*; and r_U and r_S are the peak responses obtained from the *Assay preparation* and the *Standard preparation*, respectively.

Methamphetamine Hydrochloride

$C_{10}H_{15}N \cdot HCl$ 185.70
Benzeneethanamine, N, α-dimethyl-, hydrochloride, (S)-.
(+)-(S)-N, α-Dimethylphenethylamine hydrochloride   [51-57-0].

» Methamphetamine Hydrochloride contains not less than 98.5 percent and not more than 100.5 percent of $C_{10}H_{15}N \cdot HCl$, calculated on the dried basis.

Packaging and storage—Preserve in tight, light-resistant containers.

USP Reference standards ⟨11⟩—*USP Methamphetamine Hydrochloride RS*.

Identification—
  A: *Infrared Absorption* ⟨197K⟩.
  B: It responds to the tests for *Chloride* ⟨191⟩.

Melting range ⟨741⟩: between 171° and 175°.

Specific rotation ⟨781S⟩: between +16° and +19°.
  Test solution: 20 mg per mL, in water.

Loss on drying ⟨731⟩—Dry it at 105° for 2 hours: it loses not more than 0.5% of its weight.

Residue on ignition ⟨281⟩: not more than 0.1%.

Ordinary impurities ⟨466⟩—
  Test solution: chloroform.
  Standard solution: chloroform.
  Eluant: a mixture of chloroform, cyclohexane, and diethylamine (5 : 4 : 1).
  Visualization: 1.

Organic volatile impurities, *Method I* ⟨467⟩: meets the requirements.

(Official until July 1, 2008)

Assay—
  Mobile phase—Prepare a degassed solution of 1.1 g of sodium 1-heptanesulfonate in a mixture of water, methanol, and diluted glacial acetic acid (7 in 50) (575 : 400 : 25). Adjust with the addition of acetic acid to a pH of 3.3 ± 0.1, if necessary. Filter through a 0.5-μm disk. Make adjustments if necessary (see *System Suitability* under *Chromatography* ⟨621⟩).
  Standard preparation—Dissolve an accurately weighed quantity of USP Methamphetamine Hydrochloride RS in 0.12 M phosphoric acid, and dilute quantitatively and stepwise, with the aid of sonication if necessary, with 0.12 M phosphoric acid to obtain a solution having a known concentration of about 0.2 mg per mL.
  Assay preparation—Transfer about 20 mg of Methamphetamine Hydrochloride, accurately weighed, to a 100-mL volumetric flask, dissolve in and dilute with 0.12 M phosphoric acid to volume, and mix.
  Chromatographic system (see *Chromatography* ⟨621⟩)—The liquid chromatograph is equipped with a 257-nm detector and a 3.9-mm × 30-cm column that contains packing L1. The flow rate is about 2 mL per minute. Chromatograph the *Standard preparation*, and record the peak responses as directed for *Procedure*: the column efficiency determined from the analyte peak is not less than 1000 theoretical plates; the tailing factor for the analyte peak is not more than 1.5; and the relative standard deviation for replicate injections is not more than 2.0%.
  Procedure—Separately inject equal volumes (about 20 μL) of the *Standard preparation* and the *Assay preparation* into the chromatograph, record the chromatograms, and measure the responses for the major peaks. Calculate the quantity, in mg, of $C_{10}H_{15}N \cdot HCl$ in the portion of Methamphetamine Hydrochloride taken by the formula:

$$100C(r_U / r_S)$$

in which *C* is the concentration, in mg per mL, of USP Methamphetamine Hydrochloride RS in the *Standard preparation*; and r_U and r_S are the peak responses obtained from the *Assay preparation* and the *Standard preparation*, respectively.

Methamphetamine Hydrochloride Tablets

» Methamphetamine Hydrochloride Tablets contain not less than 90.0 percent and not more than 110.0 percent of the labeled amount of methamphetamine hydrochloride ($C_{10}H_{15}N \cdot HCl$).

Packaging and storage—Preserve in tight, light-resistant containers.

USP Reference standards ⟨11⟩—*USP Methamphetamine Hydrochloride RS*.

Identification—The UV absorption spectrum of the *Test preparation* prepared as described in *Procedure for content uniformity* under *Uniformity of dosage units*, exhibits maxima and minima at the same wavelengths as that of the *Standard preparation*, concomitantly measured.

Dissolution ⟨711⟩—
  Medium: water; 900 mL.
  Apparatus 2: 50 rpm.
  Time: 45 minutes.
  Determine the amount of $C_{10}H_{15}N \cdot HCl$ dissolved by employing the following method.
  Mobile phase—Prepare a filtered and degassed mixture of dilute perchloric acid (1 in 20) and acetonitrile (7 : 3).
  Standard solution—Dissolve an accurately weighed quantity of USP Methamphetamine Hydrochloride RS in water to obtain a solution having a known concentration similar to the one expected in the *Test solution*. Dilute 2 : 1 with 0.15 M perchloric acid.
  Test solution—Use filtered aliquots of the solution under test. Dilute 2 : 1 with 0.15 M perchloric acid.
  Procedure—The liquid chromatograph is equipped with a 211-nm detector and a 3.9-mm × 30-cm column that contains packing L1. The flow rate is about 2.5 mL per minute. Chromatograph the *Standard solution* (about 100 μL), record the chromatogram, and measure the response for the major peak: the tailing factor is not more than 1.5; and the relative standard deviation for replicate injections is not more than 3.0%. Inject an equal volume of the *Test solution* into the chromatograph, record the chromatogram, and measure the response of the major peak. Calculate the quantity of $C_{10}H_{15}N \cdot HCl$ dissolved by comparison with the Standard solution.
  Tolerances—Not less than 75% (*Q*) of the labeled amount of $C_{10}H_{15}N \cdot HCl$ is dissolved in 45 minutes.

Uniformity of dosage units ⟨905⟩: meet the requirements.

  PROCEDURE FOR CONTENT UNIFORMITY—
  Chloroform-saturated 0.1 N sulfuric acid—Shake 250 mL of 0.1 N sulfuric acid with 25 mL of chloroform for 10 minutes. Allow to stand for 1 hour with occasional shaking. Drain off the chloroform, and retain the chloroform-saturated sulfuric acid in a stoppered flask.
  Standard preparation—Dissolve an accurately weighed quantity of USP Methamphetamine Hydrochloride RS in *Chloroform-saturated 0.1 N sulfuric acid*, and mix to obtain a solution having a known concentration of about 0.5 mg per mL.
  Test preparation—Place 1 Tablet in a 125-mL separator, add 15 mL of water, and shake by mechanical means for 15 minutes to dissolve. Add 2.5 mL of 1 N sodium hydroxide, and shake. Extract the liberated methamphetamine with four 10-mL portions of chloroform, collecting the chloroform extracts in a second 125-mL separator. Transfer 10.0 mL of *Chloroform-saturated 0.1 N sulfuric acid* to the second separator, and shake by mechanical means for 10 minutes. Allow the layers to separate, and collect the aqueous layer.
  Procedure—Concomitantly determine the absorbances of the *Test preparation* and the *Standard preparation* in 1-cm cells, at the wavelength of maximum absorbance at about 257 nm, with a suitable spectrophotometer, using *Chloroform-saturated 0.1 N sulfuric*

acid as the blank. Calculate the quantity, in mg, of $C_{10}H_{15}N \cdot HCl$ in the Tablet taken by the formula:

$$10C(A_U/A_S)$$

in which C is the concentration, in mg per mL, of USP Methamphetamine Hydrochloride RS in the *Standard preparation*; and A_U and A_S are the absorbances of the *Test preparation* and the *Standard preparation*, respectively.

Assay—
Mobile phase, Standard preparation, and *Chromatographic system—*Proceed as directed in the *Assay* under *Methamphetamine Hydrochloride*.

*Assay preparation—*Weigh and finely powder not fewer than 20 Tablets. Transfer an accurately weighed portion of the powder, equivalent to about 10 mg of methamphetamine hydrochloride, to a 50-mL volumetric flask. Add 20 mL of 0.12 M phosphoric acid, and sonicate for 5 minutes. Dilute with 0.12 M phosphoric acid to volume, mix, and filter.

*Procedure—*Separately inject equal volumes (about 20 µL) of the *Standard preparation* and the *Assay preparation* into the chromatograph, record the chromatograms, and measure the responses for the major peaks. Calculate the quantity, in mg, of methamphetamine hydrochloride ($C_{10}H_{15}N \cdot HCl$) in the portion of Tablets taken by the formula:

$$50C(r_U/r_S)$$

in which C is the concentration, in mg per mL, of USP Methamphetamine Hydrochloride RS in the *Standard preparation*; and r_U and r_S are the peak responses obtained from the *Assay preparation* and the *Standard preparation*, respectively.

Methazolamide

$C_5H_8N_4O_3S_2$ 236.27
Acetamide, N-[5-(aminosulfonyl)-3-methyl-1,3,4-thiadiazol-2(3H)-ylidene]-.
N-(4-Methyl-2-sulfamoyl-Δ^2-1,3,4-thiadiazolin-5-ylidene)-acetamide [*554-57-4*].

» Methazolamide contains not less than 98.0 percent and not more than 102.0 percent of $C_5H_8N_4O_3S_2$, calculated on the dried basis.

Packaging and storage—Preserve in well-closed, light-resistant containers.

USP Reference standards ⟨11⟩—*USP Methazolamide RS.*
Identification—
  A: *Infrared Absorption* ⟨197K⟩.
  B: *Ultraviolet Absorption* ⟨197U⟩—
  Solution: 10 µg per mL.
  Medium: sodium hydroxide solution in water (1 in 250).
Loss on drying ⟨731⟩—Dry it at 105° for 2 hours: it loses not more than 0.5% of its weight.
Residue on ignition ⟨281⟩: not more than 0.1%.
Selenium ⟨291⟩: 0.003%, a 200-mg specimen being used.
Heavy metals, *Method II* ⟨231⟩: 0.002%.
Organic volatile impurities, *Method V* ⟨467⟩: meets the requirements.
  *Solvent—*Use dimethyl sulfoxide.

(Official until July 1, 2008)

Assay—
*Buffer solution—*Dissolve 1.80 g of anhydrous sodium acetate in 1 L of water. Adjust, if necessary, with glacial acetic acid to a pH of 4.5 ± 0.2.

*Mobile phase—*Prepare a filtered and degassed mixture of *Buffer solution* and acetonitrile (86 : 14). Make adjustments if necessary (see *System Suitability* under *Chromatography* ⟨621⟩).

*Standard preparation—*Dissolve about 20 mg of USP Methazolamide RS, accurately weighed, in 20 mL of acetonitrile contained in a 200-mL volumetric flask. Dilute with *Buffer solution* to volume, and mix. Quantitatively dilute an accurately measured volume of this solution with *Buffer solution* to obtain a solution having a known concentration of about 50 µg of USP Methazolamide RS per mL.

*Resolution solution—*Prepare a solution of acetaminophen and USP Methazolamide RS in acetonitrile containing 0.3 mg of acetaminophen and 0.5 mg of methazolamide per mL. Quantitatively dilute an accurately measured volume of this solution with *Buffer solution* to obtain a solution containing 30 µg of acetaminophen and 50 µg of methazolamide per mL.

*Assay preparation—*Transfer about 100 mg of Methazolamide, accurately weighed, to a 200-mL volumetric flask, dissolve in 20 mL of acetonitrile, dilute with *Buffer solution* to volume, and mix. Quantitatively dilute an accurately measured volume of this solution with *Buffer solution* to obtain a solution having a known concentration of about 50 µg per mL.

Chromatographic system (see *Chromatography* ⟨621⟩)—The liquid chromatograph is equipped with a 265-nm detector and a 3.9-mm × 15.0-cm column containing packing L1. The flow rate is about 1.5 mL per minute. Chromatograph the *Resolution solution*, and record the peak responses as directed for *Procedure*: the relative retention times are about 0.6 for acetaminophen and 1.0 for methazolamide, the resolution, R, between the acetaminophen peak and the methazolamide peak is not less than 4.0, and the tailing factor is not more than 2.0. Chromatograph the *Standard preparation*, and record the peak responses as directed for *Procedure*: the relative standard deviation for replicate injections is not more than 2%.

*Procedure—*Separately inject equal volumes (about 10 µL) of the *Standard preparation* and the *Assay preparation* into the chromatograph, record the chromatograms, and measure the areas of the responses for the major peaks. Calculate the quantity, in mg, of $C_5H_8N_4O_3S_2$ in the portion of Methazolamide taken by the formula:

$$2C(r_U/r_S)$$

in which C is the concentration, in µg per mL, of USP Methazolamide RS in the *Standard preparation*; and r_U and r_S are the peak responses obtained from the *Assay preparation* and the *Standard preparation*, respectively.

Methazolamide Tablets

» Methazolamide Tablets contain not less than 90.0 percent and not more than 110.0 percent of the labeled amount of methazolamide ($C_5H_8N_4O_3S_2$).

Packaging and storage—Preserve in well-closed containers.

USP Reference standards ⟨11⟩—*USP Methazolamide RS.*
Identification—
  A: Extract a quantity of finely powdered Tablets, equivalent to about 250 mg of methazolamide, with about 50 mL of acetone. Filter, and add solvent hexane until a heavy white precipitate is formed. Collect the solid on a filter, and dry: the IR absorption spectrum of a potassium bromide dispersion of the methazolamide so obtained exhibits maxima only at the same wavelengths as that of a similar preparation of USP Methazolamide RS.
  B: Dissolve about 100 mg of the dried solid obtained in *Identification test A* in 5 mL of 1 N sodium hydroxide, and add 5 mL of a mixture of 1 g of hydroxylamine hydrochloride and 500 mg of cupric sulfate in 100 mL of water. Heat the solution on a steam bath for 15 minutes: the solution turns dark amber, then a black precipitate is formed.
  C: The retention time of the major peak in the chromatogram of the *Assay preparation* corresponds to the chromatogram of the *Standard preparation*, as obtained in the *Assay*.

Dissolution ⟨711⟩—
Medium: pH 4.5 acetate buffer, prepared by mixing 2.99 g of sodium acetate and 1.66 mL of glacial acetic acid with water to obtain 1000 mL of a solution having a pH of 4.5; 900 mL.
Apparatus 2: 75 rpm.
Time: 45 minutes.
*Procedure—*Determine the amount of $C_5H_8N_4O_3S_2$ dissolved from UV absorbances at the wavelength of maximum absorbance at about 252 nm of filtered portions of the solution under test, suitably diluted with pH 4.5 acetate buffer, in comparison with a Standard solution having a known concentration of USP Methazolamide RS in the same *Medium*.
*Tolerances—*Not less than 75% (*Q*) of the labeled amount of $C_5H_8N_4O_3S_2$ is dissolved in 45 minutes.

Uniformity of dosage units ⟨905⟩: meet the requirements.

Assay—
*pH 2.5 Buffer—*Transfer 16.8 mL of dibutylamine to a beaker containing 70 mL of water. Adjust with phosphoric acid to a pH of 2.5, dilute with water to 100 mL, and mix.
*Mobile phase—*Prepare a mixture of water, methanol, and *pH 2.5 Buffer* (375 : 15 : 6). Make adjustments if necessary (see *System Suitability* under *Chromatography* ⟨621⟩).
*pH 4.5 Acetate buffer—*Dissolve 2.99 g of sodium acetate and 1.66 mL of glacial acetic acid in water, dilute with water to 1000 mL, and mix. Adjust, if necessary, with glacial acetic acid or sodium hydoxide to a pH of 4.5.
*Standard preparation—*Dissolve an accurately weighed quantity of USP Methazolamide RS in methanol to obtain a solution having a concentration of about 0.5 mg per mL. Dilute this solution quantitatively, and stepwise if necessary, with *pH 4.5 Acetate buffer* to obtain a solution having a known concentration of about 50 μg per mL.
*Assay preparation—*Weigh and finely powder not fewer than 20 Tablets. Transfer an accurately weighed portion of the powder, equivalent to about 50 mg of methazolamide, to a 250-mL volumetric flask, add 65 mL of *pH 4.5 Acetate buffer*, and sonicate to dissolve. Add 65 mL of methanol, and sonicate again until dissolved. Dilute with *pH 4.5 Acetate buffer* to volume, mix, and filter. Dilute an accurately measured volume of the filtrate with *pH 4.5 Acetate buffer* to obtain a solution having a concentration of about 50 μg of methazolamide per mL.
Chromatographic system (see *Chromatography* ⟨621⟩)—The liquid chromatograph is equipped with a 252-nm detector and an 8-mm × 10-cm column that contains packing L10. The flow rate is about 2 mL per minute. Chromatograph the *Standard preparation,* and record the peak responses as directed for *Procedure:* the tailing factor is not more than 1.5; and the relative standard deviation for replicate injections is not more than 3.0%.
*Procedure—*Separately inject equal volumes (about 25 μL) of the *Standard preparation* and the *Assay preparation* into the chromatograph, record the chromatograms, and measure the areas for the major peaks. Calculate the quantity, in mg, of methazolamide ($C_5H_8N_4O_3S_2$) in the portion of Tablets taken by the formula:

$$C(r_U / r_S)$$

in which *C* is the concentration, in μg per mL, of USP Methazolamide RS in the *Standard preparation;* and r_U and r_S are the peak responses obtained from the *Assay preparation* and the *Standard preparation,* respectively.

Methdilazine Hydrochloride

$C_{18}H_{20}N_2S \cdot HCl$ 332.89
10*H*-Phenothiazine, 10-[(1-methyl-3-pyrrolidinyl)methyl]-, monohydrochloride.
10-[(1-Methyl-3-pyrrolidinyl)methyl]phenothiazine monohydrochloride [1229-35-2].

» Methdilazine Hydrochloride contains not less than 97.0 percent and not more than 103.0 percent of $C_{18}H_{20}N_2S \cdot HCl$, calculated on the dried basis.

Packaging and storage—Preserve in tight, light-resistant containers.

USP Reference standards ⟨11⟩—*USP Methdilazine Hydrochloride RS.*
NOTE—Throughout the following procedures, protect test or assay specimens, the Reference Standard, and solutions containing them, by conducting the procedures without delay, under subdued light, or using low-actinic glassware.

Identification—
A: *Infrared Absorption* ⟨197K⟩.
B: *Ultraviolet Absorption* ⟨197U⟩—
Solution: 5 μg per mL.
Medium: water.
C: A solution of it responds to the tests for *Chloride* ⟨191⟩.

Melting range, *Class I* ⟨741⟩:   between 184° and 190°.

pH ⟨791⟩: between 4.8 and 6.0, in a solution (1 in 100).

Loss on drying ⟨731⟩—Dry it in vacuum at 65° for 16 hours: it loses not more than 1.0% of its weight.

Residue on ignition ⟨281⟩: not more than 0.5%.

Selenium ⟨291⟩—The absorbance of the solution from the *Test Solution*, prepared with 100 mg of Methdilazine Hydrochloride and 100 mg of magnesium oxide, is not greater than one-half that from the *Standard Solution* (0.003%).

Heavy metals, *Method II* ⟨231⟩:   0.002%.

Ordinary impurities ⟨466⟩—
Test solution: methanol.
Standard solution: methanol.
Application volume: 10 μL.
Eluant: a mixture of toluene, isopropyl alcohol, and ammonium hydroxide (70 : 29 : 1), in a nonequilibrated chamber.
Visualization: 5.

Organic volatile impurities, *Method I* ⟨467⟩:   meets the requirements.
(Official until July 1, 2008)

Assay—Transfer about 100 mg of Methdilazine Hydrochloride, accurately weighed, to a 1000-mL volumetric flask, add water to volume, and mix. Transfer 5.0 mL of this solution to a 100-mL volumetric flask, dilute with water to volume, and mix. Concomitantly determine the absorbances of this solution and of a Standard solution of USP Methdilazine Hydrochloride RS in the same medium having a known concentration of about 5 μg per mL, in 1-cm cells at 252 and 275 nm, with a suitable spectrophotometer, using water as the blank. Calculate the quantity, in mg, of $C_{18}H_{20}N_2S \cdot HCl$ in the portion of Methdilazine Hydrochloride taken by the formula:

$$20C(A_{252} - A_{275})_U / (A_{252} - A_{275})_S$$

in which *C* is the concentration, in μg per mL, of USP Methdilazine Hydrochloride RS in the Standard solution; and the parenthetic expressions are the differences in the absorbances of the two solutions at the wavelengths indicated by the subscripts, for the solution of Methdilazine Hydrochloride (*U*) and the Standard solution (*S*), respectively.

Methdilazine Hydrochloride Oral Solution

» Methdilazine Hydrochloride Oral Solution contains not less than 93.0 percent and not more than 107.0 percent of the labeled amount of methdilazine hydrochloride ($C_{18}H_{20}N_2S \cdot HCl$).

Packaging and storage—Preserve in tight, light-resistant containers.

USP Reference standards ⟨11⟩—*USP Methdilazine Hydrochloride RS.*
NOTE—Throughout the following procedures, protect test or assay specimens, the USP Reference Standard, and solutions containing them, by conducting the procedures without delay, under subdued light, or using low-actinic glassware.

Identification—Transfer a volume of Oral Solution, equivalent to about 4 mg of methdilazine hydrochloride, to a 60-mL separator, add 5 mL of 0.1 N hydrochloric acid, and extract with 10 mL of ether, discarding the extract. Add 10 mL of sodium bicarbonate solution (1 in 10) to the separator, and extract with 3 mL of chloroform. Filter the extract through a pledget of cotton. Evaporate the chloroform, carefully removing the last trace of solvent in a small vacuum flask: the IR absorption spectrum of a potassium bromide dispersion of the methdilazine so obtained exhibits maxima only at the same wavelengths as that of a similar preparation of USP Methdilazine Hydrochloride RS that has been treated in the same manner.

pH ⟨791⟩: between 3.3 and 4.1.

Alcohol content, *Method II* ⟨611⟩: between 6.5% and 7.5% of C_2H_5OH.

Assay—
Standard preparation—Dissolve a suitable quantity of USP Methdilazine Hydrochloride, accurately weighed, in chloroform, and quantitatively dilute with chloroform to obtain a solution having a known concentration of about 400 µg per mL.

Assay preparation—Transfer a volume of Oral Solution, equivalent to about 4 mg of methdilazine hydrochloride, to a 60-mL separator, add 10 mL of a saturated solution of sodium chloride, and extract with three 10-mL portions of chloroform, transferring the extracts to a 100-mL volumetric flask.

Procedure—Transfer 10.0 mL of *Standard preparation* to a 100-mL volumetric flask, and add 20 mL of chloroform. To this flask and to the flask containing the *Assay preparation* add 4.0 mL of buffered palladium chloride TS, dilute with alcohol to volume, and mix. Concomitantly determine the absorbances of the solutions in 1-cm cells at the wavelength of maximum absorbance at about 460 nm, with a suitable spectrophotometer, using a mixture of 30 mL of chloroform, 4 mL of palladium chloride TS, and 66 mL of alcohol as the blank. Calculate the quantity, in mg, of methdilazine hydrochloride ($C_{18}H_{20}N_2S \cdot HCl$) in each mL of the Oral Solution taken by the formula:

$$(0.01C / V)(A_U / A_S)$$

in which *C* is the concentration, in µg per mL, of USP Methdilazine Hydrochloride RS in the *Standard preparation*; *V* is the volume, in mL, of Oral Solution taken; and A_U and A_S are the absorbances of the solutions from the *Assay preparation* and the *Standard preparation*, respectively.

Methdilazine Hydrochloride Tablets

» Methdilazine Hydrochloride Tablets contain not less than 93.0 percent and not more than 107.0 percent of the labeled amount of methdilazine hydrochloride ($C_{18}H_{20}N_2S \cdot HCl$).

Packaging and storage—Preserve in tight, light-resistant containers.

USP Reference standards ⟨11⟩—*USP Methdilazine Hydrochloride RS*.
NOTE—Throughout the following procedures, protect test or assay specimens, the Reference Standard, and solutions containing them, by conducting the procedures without delay, under subdued light, or using low-actinic glassware.

Identification—Transfer a portion of finely powdered Tablets, equivalent to about 8 mg of methdilazine hydrochloride, to a 60-mL separator, add 10 mL of sodium bicarbonate solution (1 in 10), and extract with 3 mL of chloroform. Filter the extract through a pledget of cotton. Evaporate the chloroform, carefully removing the last trace of solvent in a small vacuum flask: the IR absorption spectrum of a potassium bromide dispersion of the methdilazine so obtained exhibits maxima only at the same wavelengths as that of a similar preparation of USP Methdilazine Hydrochloride RS, similarly treated and measured.

Dissolution ⟨711⟩—
Medium: water; 900 mL.
Apparatus 1: 100 rpm.
Time: 45 minutes.
Procedure—Determine the amount of $C_{18}H_{20}N_2S \cdot HCl$ dissolved from UV absorbances at the wavelength of maximum absorbance at about 252 nm of filtered portions of the solution under test, suitably diluted with *Dissolution Medium*, if necessary, in comparison with a Standard solution having a known concentration of USP Methdilazine Hydrochloride RS in the same *Medium*.
Tolerances—Not less than 75% *(Q)* of the labeled amount of $C_{18}H_{20}N_2S \cdot HCl$ is dissolved in 45 minutes.

Uniformity of dosage units ⟨905⟩: meet the requirements.

Assay—
Standard preparation—Dissolve a suitable quantity of USP Methdilazine Hydrochloride RS, accurately weighed, in chloroform, and dilute quantitatively with chloroform to obtain a solution having a known concentration of about 400 µg per mL.

Assay preparation—Weigh and finely powder not fewer than 20 Tablets, and transfer an accurately weighed portion of the powder, equivalent to about 80 mg of methdilazine hydrochloride, to a 200-mL volumetric flask. Add 60 mL of chloroform, shake for 20 minutes, dilute with chloroform to volume, and mix. Filter, discarding the first 15 mL of the filtrate. Use the subsequent filtrate as directed in the *Procedure*.

Procedure—Into three separate 100-mL volumetric flasks transfer 10.0 mL each of the *Standard preparation*, the *Assay preparation*, and chloroform to provide the blank. To each flask add 20 mL of chloroform and 4.0 mL of buffered palladium chloride TS, dilute with alcohol to volume, and mix. Concomitantly determine the absorbances of the solutions in 1-cm cells at the wavelength of maximum absorbance at about 460 nm, with a suitable spectrophotometer, using the blank to set the instrument. Calculate the quantity, in mg, of methdilazine hydrochloride ($C_{18}H_{20}N_2S \cdot HCl$) in the portion of Tablets taken by the formula:

$$0.2C(A_U / A_S)$$

in which *C* is the concentration, in µg per mL, of USP Methdilazine Hydrochloride RS in the *Standard preparation*; and A_U and A_S are the absorbances of the solutions from the *Assay preparation* and the *Standard preparation*, respectively.

Methenamine

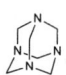

$C_6H_{12}N_4$ 140.19
1,3,5,7-Tetraazatricyclo[3.3.1.1^{3,7}]decane.
Hexamethylenetetramine   [*100-97-0*].

» Methenamine, dried over phosphorus pentoxide for 4 hours, contains not less than 99.0 percent and not more than 100.5 percent of $C_6H_{12}N_4$.

Packaging and storage—Preserve in well-closed containers.

USP Reference standards ⟨11⟩—*USP Methenamine RS*.
Identification—
A: *Infrared Absorption* ⟨197K⟩.
B: Heat a solution (1 in 10) with 2 N sulfuric acid: formaldehyde is liberated, recognizable by its odor and by its darkening of paper moistened with silver ammonium nitrate TS. On the subsequent addition of an excess of 1 N sodium hydroxide to the solution, ammonia is evolved.

Loss on drying ⟨731⟩—Dry it over phosphorus pentoxide for 4 hours: it loses not more than 2.0% of its weight.
Residue on ignition ⟨281⟩: not more than 0.1%.
Chloride ⟨221⟩—A 1.0-g portion shows no more chloride than corresponds to 0.20 mL of 0.020 N hydrochloric acid (0.014%).

Sulfate—To 10 mL of a solution (1 in 50), acidified with 5 drops of hydrochloric acid, add 5 drops of barium chloride TS: no turbidity is produced within 1 minute.

Ammonium salts—To 10 mL of a solution (1 in 20) add 1 mL of alkaline mercuric-potassium iodide TS: the mixture is not darker in color than a mixture of 1 mL of the reagent and 10 mL of water.

Heavy metals, *Method I* ⟨231⟩—Dissolve 2 g in 10 mL of water, add 2 mL of 3 N hydrochloric acid, and dilute with water to 25 mL. Proceed as directed, except to use glacial acetic acid to adjust the pH: the limit is 0.001%.

Organic volatile impurities, *Method I* ⟨467⟩: meets the requirements.

(Official until July 1, 2008)

Assay—

Chromotropic acid spot test solution—Suspend 100 mg of chromotropic acid in 2 mL of water, and *cautiously* add 3 mL of sulfuric acid. Allow to cool. Add 25 mL of sulfuric acid, and mix. [NOTE—If excessive heat generated during mixing causes a violet color to appear in the solution, discard the solution and prepare another, taking precautions to avoid excessive heat.]

Procedure—Transfer about 1 g of Methenamine, previously dried and accurately weighed, to a beaker. Add 40.0 mL of 1 N sulfuric acid VS, and heat to a gentle boil, adding water from time to time if necessary, until the formaldehyde has been expelled. Test for the absence of formaldehyde by adding a drop of the assay solution to a glass fiber filter disk, on a watch glass, on which has previously been placed 3 or 4 drops of *Chromotropic acid spot test solution*. Formaldehyde produces a violet color with this reagent; repeat the test until no violet color is obtained on the warmed test filter disk upon comparison with a blank filter disk to which no assay specimen is added. Cool, add 20 mL of water, then add methyl red TS, and titrate the excess acid with 1 N sodium hydroxide VS. Perform a blank determination (see *Residual Titrations* under *Titrimetry* ⟨541⟩). Each mL of 1 N sulfuric acid is equivalent to 35.05 mg of $C_6H_{12}N_4$.

Methenamine Oral Solution

» Methenamine Oral Solution contains not less than 90.0 percent and not more than 110.0 percent of the labeled amount of methenamine ($C_6H_{12}N_4$).

Packaging and storage—Preserve in tight containers.

USP Reference standards ⟨11⟩—*USP Methenamine RS*.

Identification—Heat a volume of Oral Solution, equivalent to about 1 g of methenamine, with 10 mL of 2 N sulfuric acid: formaldehyde is liberated, recognizable by its odor and by its darkening of paper moistened with silver ammonium nitrate TS. On the subsequent addition of an excess of 1 N sodium hydroxide to the solution, ammonia is evolved.

Uniformity of dosage units ⟨905⟩—
  FOR ORAL SOLUTION PACKAGED IN SINGLE-UNIT CONTAINERS: meets the requirements.

Deliverable volume ⟨698⟩—
  FOR ORAL SOLUTION PACKAGED IN MULTIPLE-UNIT CONTAINERS: meets the requirements.

Alcohol content, *Method I* ⟨611⟩: between 90.0% and 110.0% of the labeled amount of C_2H_5OH.

Assay—

Chromotropic acid solution—Mix 100 mg of chromotropic acid with 50 mL of water in a 100-mL volumetric flask. Cool in an ice bath and, while cooling, cautiously and slowly add 50 mL of sulfuric acid, and mix. Allow the solution to reach room temperature, and add dilute sulfuric acid (1 in 2) to volume. [NOTE—If excessive heat generated during mixing causes a violet color to appear in the solution, discard the solution, and prepare another, taking precautions to avoid excessive heat.]

Standard preparation—Transfer about 50 mg of USP Methenamine RS, accurately weighed, to a 1000-mL volumetric flask, dissolve in and dilute with water to volume, and mix. Proceed as directed for *Assay preparation*, beginning with "Transfer a 2.0-mL portion of this stock solution to a 100-mL volumetric flask." The concentration of USP Methenamine RS in the *Standard preparation* is about 1 µg per mL.

Assay preparation—Transfer an accurately measured volume of Oral Solution, equivalent to about 1.5 g of methenamine, to a 500-mL volumetric flask, dissolve in and dilute with water to volume, and mix. Transfer 2.0 mL of this solution to a 100-mL volumetric flask, dilute with water to volume, and mix to obtain the stock solution. Transfer a 2.0-mL portion of this stock solution to a 100-mL volumetric flask, add 25 mL of *Chromotropic acid solution* and 50 mL of dilute sulfuric acid (1 in 2), and mix. Transfer another 2.0-mL portion of the stock solution to a second 100-mL volumetric flask to provide a blank, add 75 mL of dilute sulfuric acid (1 in 2), and mix. Place the two 100-mL flasks in a boiling water bath for 30 minutes, accurately timed, then remove them from the bath, cool immediately to room temperature, add dilute sulfuric acid (1 in 2) to volume, and mix.

Procedure—Concomitantly determine the absorbances of the solutions in 1-cm cells at the wavelength of maximum absorbance at about 570 nm, with a suitable spectrophotometer, using dilute sulfuric acid (1 in 2) to set the instrument. Calculate the quantity, in mg, of methenamine ($C_6H_{12}N_4$) in each mL of the Oral Solution taken by the formula:

$$(1250C/V)[(A_U - B_U) / (A_S - B_S)]$$

in which C is the concentration, in µg per mL, of USP Methenamine RS in the *Standard preparation*; V is the volume, in mL, of Oral Solution taken; A_U and A_S are the absorbances of the *Assay preparation* and the *Standard preparation*, respectively; and B_U and B_S are the absorbances of the blanks from the *Assay preparation* and the *Standard preparation*, respectively.

Methenamine Tablets

» Methenamine Tablets contain not less than 95.0 percent and not more than 105.0 percent of the labeled amount of methenamine ($C_6H_{12}N_4$).

Packaging and storage—Preserve in well-closed containers.

USP Reference standards ⟨11⟩—*USP Methenamine RS*.

Identification—Dissolve about 500 mg of powdered Tablets in 10 mL of water, add 10 mL of 2 N sulfuric acid, and heat: formaldehyde is liberated, recognizable by its odor and by its darkening of paper moistened with silver ammonium nitrate TS. On the subsequent addition of an excess of 1 N sodium hydroxide to the solution, ammonia is evolved.

Dissolution, *Procedure for a Pooled Sample* ⟨711⟩—
  Medium: water; 900 mL.
  Apparatus 1: 100 rpm.
  Time: 45 minutes.
  Procedure—Determine the amount of $C_6H_{12}N_4$ dissolved, employing the procedure set forth in the *Assay*, making any necessary modifications.
  Tolerances—Not less than 75% (*Q*) of the labeled amount of $C_6H_{12}N_4$ is dissolved in 45 minutes.

Uniformity of dosage units ⟨905⟩: meet the requirements.

Assay—

Chromotropic acid solution and *Standard preparation*—Prepare as directed in the *Assay* under *Methenamine Oral Solution*.

Assay preparation—Weigh and finely powder not fewer than 20 Tablets. Transfer an accurately weighed portion of the powder, equivalent to about 500 mg of methenamine, to a 250-mL volumetric flask, dilute with water to volume, mix, and filter, discarding the first 20 mL of the filtrate. Transfer 25.0 mL of the subsequent filtrate to a 1000-mL volumetric flask, dilute with water to volume, and mix. Proceed as directed for *Assay preparation* in the *Assay* under *Methenamine Oral Solution*, beginning with "Transfer a 2.0-mL portion of this stock solution."

Procedure—Proceed as directed for *Procedure* in the *Assay* under *Methenamine Oral Solution.* Calculate the quantity, in mg, of methenamine ($C_6H_{12}N_4$) in the portion of Tablets taken by the formula:

$$500C[(A_U - B_U)/(A_S - B_S)]$$

in which C is the concentration, in µg per mL, of USP Methenamine RS in the *Standard preparation*; and A_U, A_S, B_U, and B_S are as defined therein.

Methenamine Hippurate

$C_6H_{12}N_4 \cdot C_9H_9NO_3$ 319.36
Glycine, *N*-benzoyl, compd. with 1,3,5,7-tetraazatricyclo[3.3.1.1^{3,7}]
    decane (1 : 1).
Hexamethylenetetramine monohippurate   [5714-73-8].

» Methenamine Hippurate, dried in vacuum at 60° for 1 hour, contains not less than 95.5 percent and not more than 102.0 percent of $C_6H_{12}N_4 \cdot C_9H_9NO_3$, and contains not less than 54.0 percent and not more than 58.0 percent of hippuric acid ($C_9H_9NO_3$).

Packaging and storage—Preserve in well-closed containers.

USP Reference standards ⟨11⟩—*USP Methenamine Hippurate RS.*
Identification, *Infrared Absorption* ⟨197M⟩.
Loss on drying ⟨731⟩—Dry it in vacuum at 60° for 1 hour: it loses not more than 1.0% of its weight.
Residue on ignition ⟨281⟩: not more than 0.1%.
Sulfate—Dissolve 200 mg in 10 mL of water, and add 5 drops of 3 N hydrochloric acid and 5 drops of barium chloride TS: no turbidity appears within 1 minute.
Heavy metals, *Method II* ⟨231⟩: 0.0015%.
Organic volatile impurities, *Method I* ⟨467⟩: meets the requirements.

(Official until July 1, 2008)
Hippuric acid content—Transfer about 1 g, accurately weighed, to a 250-mL conical flask, and add 50 mL of water. When solution is complete, add phenolphthalein TS, and titrate with 0.1 N sodium hydroxide VS. Each mL of 0.1 N sodium hydroxide is equivalent to 17.92 of $C_9H_9NO_3$.
Assay—Dissolve about 700 mg of Methenamine Hippurate, accurately weighed, in 50 mL of glacial acetic acid, and titrate with 0.1 N perchloric acid VS, determining the endpoint potentiometrically. Perform a blank determination, and make any necessary correction. Each mL of 0.1 N perchloric acid is equivalent to 31.94 mg of $C_6H_{12}N_4 \cdot C_9H_9NO_3$.

Methenamine Hippurate Tablets

» Methenamine Hippurate Tablets contain not less than 95.0 percent and not more than 105.0 percent of the labeled amount of methenamine hippurate ($C_6H_{12}N_4 \cdot C_9H_9NO_3$).

Packaging and storage—Preserve in well-closed containers.
Labeling—When more than one *Dissolution* test is given, the labeling states the *Dissolution* test used only if *Test 1* is not used.
USP Reference standards ⟨11⟩—*USP Methenamine Hippurate RS.*
Identification—A portion of finely powdered Tablets responds to the *Identification* test under *Methenamine Hippurate.*

Dissolution ⟨711⟩—
TEST 1—
    Medium: water; 900 mL.
    Apparatus 2: 100 rpm.
    Time: 30 minutes.
    Standard solution—Dissolve an accurately weighed quantity of USP Methenamine Hippurate RS in water to obtain a solution having a known concentration of about 22 µg per mL.
    Procedure—Determine the amount of $C_6H_{12}N_4 \cdot C_9H_9NO_3$ dissolved by employing UV absorption, using a suitable spectrophotometer, at the wavelength of maximum absorbance at about 227 nm on filtered portions of the solution under test, suitably diluted with water, if necessary, in comparison with the *Standard solution*.
    Tolerances—Not less than 80% *(Q)* of the labeled amount of $C_6H_{12}N_4 \cdot C_9H_9NO_3$ is dissolved in 30 minutes.
    TEST 2—If the product complies with this test, the labeling indicates that it meets USP *Dissolution Test 2*.
    Medium: water; 900 mL.
    Apparatus 2: 50 rpm.
    Time: 60 minutes.
    Standard solution and *Procedure*—Proceed as directed for *Test 1*.
    Tolerances—Not less than 80% *(Q)* of the labeled amount of $C_6H_{12}N_4 \cdot C_9H_9NO_3$ is dissolved in 60 minutes.
Uniformity of dosage units ⟨905⟩: meet the requirements.
Assay—Weigh and finely powder not fewer than 20 Tablets. Transfer an accurately weighed portion of the powder, equivalent to about 700 mg of methenamine hippurate, to a 250-mL conical flask. Add 50 mL of alcohol, then add thymolphthalein TS, and titrate with 0.1 N sodium hydroxide VS. Perform a blank determination on a mixture of 50 mL of alcohol and 20 mL of water, and make any necessary correction. Each mL of 0.1 N sodium hydroxide is equivalent to 31.94 mg of methenamine hippurate ($C_6H_{12}N_4 \cdot C_9H_9NO_3$).

Methenamine Mandelate

$C_6H_{12}N_4 \cdot C_8H_8O_3$ 292.33
Benzeneacetic acid, α-hydroxy-, (±)-, compd. with 1,3,5,7-tetraazatricyclo[3.3.1.1^{3,7}]decane (1 : 1).
Hexamethylenetetramine mono-(±)-mandelate   [587-23-5].

» Methenamine Mandelate contains not less than 95.5 percent and not more than 102.0 percent of $C_6H_{12}N_4 \cdot C_8H_8O_3$, and contains not less than 50.0 percent and not more than 53.0 percent of mandelic acid ($C_8H_8O_3$), calculated on the dried basis.

Packaging and storage—Preserve in well-closed containers.

USP Reference standards ⟨11⟩—*USP Methenamine Mandelate RS.*
Identification, *Infrared Absorption* ⟨197K⟩.
Loss on drying ⟨731⟩—Dry it over silica gel for 18 hours: it loses not more than 1.5% of its weight.
Residue on ignition ⟨281⟩: not more than 0.1%.
Chloride ⟨221⟩—Dissolve 1.0 g in 10 mL of water, and add gradually 500 mg of anhydrous sodium carbonate. Evaporate to dryness, and ignite the residue at a dull-red heat. Add 20 mL of 2 N nitric acid, stir gently, and filter: the filtrate shows no more chloride than corresponds to 0.15 mL of 0.020 N hydrochloric acid (0.01%).
Sulfate—Dissolve 0.20 g in 10 mL of water, and add 5 drops of 3 N hydrochloric acid and 5 drops of barium chloride TS: no turbidity appears within 1 minute.
Heavy metals ⟨231⟩—Dissolve 1.3 g in 10 mL of water, add 2 mL of 3 N hydrochloric acid, and dilute with water to 25 mL: the limit is 0.0015%.

Organic volatile impurities, *Method I* ⟨467⟩: meets the requirements.

(Official until July 1, 2008)

Mandelic acid content—Transfer about 90 mg, accurately weighed, to a 250-mL conical flask containing 50 mL of water. When solution is complete, titrate the magnetically stirred solution with 0.05 N ceric ammonium nitrate VS, determining the endpoint potentiometrically. Each mL of 0.05 N ceric ammonium nitrate is equivalent to 3.804 mg of $C_8H_8O_3$.

Assay—

0.05 N Silver nitrate in dehydrated alcohol—Dissolve, by stirring, about 8.5 g of silver nitrate in 1000 mL of dehydrated alcohol. Transfer about 100 mg, accurately weighed, of sodium chloride, previously dried at 110° for 2 hours, to a 100-mL beaker, and dissolve in 50 mL of water. Titrate with the silver nitrate solution to the potentiometric endpoint, using a silver billet indicator electrode and a silver-silver chloride double-junction reference electrode containing a potassium nitrate salt bridge. Calculate the normality of the titrant.

Procedure—Transfer about 60 mg of Methenamine Mandelate, accurately weighed, to a 250-mL conical flask. Add 15 mL of dehydrated alcohol, stir to dissolve, and add 40 mL of chloroform. Titrate with *0.05 N Silver nitrate in dehydrated alcohol*, determining the endpoint potentiometrically, using a silver billet indicator electrode and a silver-silver chloride double-junction reference electrode containing a potassium nitrate salt bridge. Each mL of 0.05 N silver nitrate is equivalent to 7.308 mg of $C_6H_{12}N_4 \cdot C_8H_8O_3$.

Methenamine Mandelate for Oral Solution

» Methenamine Mandelate for Oral Solution contains not less than 90.0 percent and not more than 110.0 percent of the labeled amount of methenamine mandelate ($C_6H_{12}N_4 \cdot C_8H_8O_3$).

Packaging and storage—Preserve in well-closed containers.

Labeling—Label Methenamine Mandelate for Oral Solution that contains insoluble ingredients to indicate that the aqueous constituted Oral Solution contains dissolved methenamine mandelate, but may remain turbid because of the presence of added substances.

USP Reference standards ⟨11⟩—*USP Methenamine Mandelate RS*.

Identification—A finely powdered portion, equivalent to about 100 mg of methenamine mandelate, responds to the *Identification* test under *Methenamine Mandelate Oral Suspension*.

Uniformity of dosage units ⟨905⟩—

FOR POWDER PACKAGED IN SINGLE-UNIT CONTAINERS: meets the requirements.

Deliverable volume ⟨698⟩

FOR POWDER PACKAGED IN MULTIPLE-UNIT CONTAINERS: meets the requirements.

pH ⟨791⟩: between 4.0 and 4.5, in a mixture of 1 g with 30 mL of water.

Water, *Method I* ⟨921⟩: not more than 0.5%.

Assay—Accurately weigh the contents of not fewer than 10 containers of Methenamine Mandelate for Oral Solution, and reduce to a fine powder. Transfer an accurately weighed portion of the powder, equivalent to about 60 mg of methenamine mandelate, to a 150-mL beaker. Add 15 mL of dehydrated alcohol, stir to dissolve, and proceed as directed in the *Assay* under *Methenamine Mandelate,* beginning with "add 40 mL of chloroform."

Methenamine Mandelate Oral Suspension

» Methenamine Mandelate Oral Suspension is Methenamine Mandelate suspended in vegetable oil. It contains not less than 90.0 percent and not more than 110.0 percent of the labeled amount of methenamine mandelate ($C_6H_{12}N_4 \cdot C_8H_8O_3$).

Packaging and storage—Preserve in tight containers.

USP Reference standards ⟨11⟩—*USP Methenamine Mandelate RS*.

Identification—Triturate a quantity, equivalent to about 100 mg of methenamine mandelate, with 10 mL of chloroform, and pass through a 0.45-μm membrane filter. Evaporate the solvent, wash the residue with 5 small portions of ether, and allow it to air-dry: the IR absorption spectrum of a potassium bromide dispersion of the residue so obtained exhibits maxima only at the same wavelengths as that of a potassium bromide dispersion of USP Methenamine Mandelate RS.

Uniformity of dosage units ⟨905⟩—

FOR ORAL SUSPENSION PACKAGED IN SINGLE-UNIT CONTAINERS: meets the requirements.

Deliverable volume ⟨698⟩—

FOR ORAL SUSPENSION PACKAGED IN MULTIPLE-UNIT CONTAINERS: meets the requirements.

Water, *Method I* ⟨921⟩: not more than 0.1%.

Assay—Shake the Oral Suspension, then pipet, using a "to contain" pipet, an amount equivalent to 1 g of methenamine mandelate, into a 100-mL volumetric flask. Add 5.0 mL of dehydrated alcohol, mix, and add methylene chloride to volume. Pipet 5 mL of this solution into a 250-mL conical flask. Add 15 mL of dehydrated alcohol, and proceed as directed in the *Assay* under *Methenamine Mandelate,* beginning with "add 40 mL of chloroform."

Methenamine Mandelate Tablets

» Methenamine Mandelate Tablets contain not less than 95.0 percent and not more than 105.0 percent of the labeled amount of methenamine mandelate ($C_6H_{12}N_4 \cdot C_8H_8O_3$).

Packaging and storage—Preserve in well-closed containers.

USP Reference standards ⟨11⟩—*USP Methenamine Mandelate RS*.

Identification, *Infrared Absorption* ⟨197⟩—Obtain the test specimen as follows. Triturate a quantity of finely powdered Tablets, equivalent to about 5.0 mg of methenamine mandelate, with 5 mL of chloroform, and pass through a 0.45-μm membrane filter. Evaporate the solvent, and allow the residue to air-dry.

Dissolution ⟨711⟩—

FOR UNCOATED OR PLAIN COATED TABLETS—

Medium: water; 900 mL.

Apparatus 1: 100 rpm.

Time: 45 minutes.

Procedure—Determine the amount of $C_6H_{12}N_4 \cdot C_8H_8O_3$ dissolved from UV absorbances at the wavelength of maximum absorbance at about 257 nm of portions of the solution under test, filtered through a 0.45-μm filter and suitably diluted with *Medium*, if necessary, in comparison with a Standard solution having a known concentration of USP Methenamine Mandelate RS in the same *Medium*.

Tolerances—Not less than 75% (*Q*) of the labeled amount of $C_6H_{12}N_4 \cdot C_8H_8O_3$ is dissolved in 45 minutes.

Uniformity of dosage units ⟨905⟩: meet the requirements.

Assay—Weigh and finely powder not fewer than 20 Tablets. Weigh accurately a portion of the powder, equivalent to about 60 mg of methenamine mandelate, and transfer to a 250-mL conical flask.

Proceed as directed in the *Assay* under *Methenamine Mandelate*, beginning with "Add 15 mL of dehydrated alcohol."

Methenamine Mandelate Delayed-Release Tablets

» Methenamine Mandelate Delayed-Release Tablets contain not less than 95.0 percent and not more than 105.0 percent of the labeled amount of methenamine mandelate ($C_6H_{12}N_4 \cdot C_8H_8O_3$).

Packaging and storage—Preserve in well-closed containers.

USP Reference standards ⟨11⟩—*USP Methenamine Mandelate RS*.

Disintegration ⟨701⟩: 2 hours and 30 minutes, determined as directed under *Delayed-release (enteric coated) Tablets*.

Other requirements—Delayed-release Tablets respond to the *Identification* test and meet the requirements for *Uniformity of dosage units* and *Assay* under *Methenamine Mandelate Tablets*.

Methimazole

$C_4H_6N_2S$ 114.17
2*H*-Imidazole-2-thione, 1,3-dihydro-1-methyl-.
1-Methylimidazole-2-thiol   [60-56-0].

» Methimazole contains not less than 98.0 percent and not more than 101.0 percent of $C_4H_6N_2S$, calculated on the dried basis.

Packaging and storage—Preserve in well-closed, light-resistant containers.

USP Reference standards ⟨11⟩—*USP Methimazole RS*.
Identification—
  A: *Infrared Absorption* ⟨197K⟩.
  B: Mercuric chloride TS produces in a solution (1 in 200) a white precipitate, but no precipitation is produced by trinitrophenol TS. The solution is colored intensely blue by molybdophosphotungstate TS.

Melting range ⟨741⟩: between 143° and 146°.
Loss on drying ⟨731⟩—Dry it at 105° for 2 hours: it loses not more than 0.5% of its weight.
Residue on ignition ⟨281⟩: not more than 0.1%.
Selenium ⟨291⟩: 0.003%, a 200-mg specimen being used.
Ordinary impurities ⟨466⟩—
  Test solution: ethyl acetate.
  Standard solution: ethyl acetate.
  Eluant: a mixture of toluene, isopropyl alcohol, and ammonium hydroxide (70 : 29 : 1), in a nonequilibrated chamber.
  Visualization: 2.
Organic volatile impurities, *Method I* ⟨467⟩: meets the requirements.

(Official until July 1, 2008)

Assay—Dissolve about 250 mg of Methimazole, accurately weighed, in 75 mL of water. Add from a buret 15 mL of 0.1 N sodium hydroxide VS, mix, and add, with agitation, about 30 mL of 0.1 N silver nitrate. Add 1 mL of bromothymol blue TS, and continue the titration with the 0.1 N sodium hydroxide VS until a permanent, blue-green color is produced. Each mL of 0.1 N sodium hydroxide is equivalent to 11.42 mg of $C_4H_6N_2S$.

Methimazole Tablets

» Methimazole Tablets contain not less than 94.0 percent and not more than 106.0 percent of the labeled amount of methimazole ($C_4H_6N_2S$).

Packaging and storage—Preserve in well-closed, light-resistant containers.

USP Reference standards ⟨11⟩—*USP Methimazole RS*.
Identification—Digest a quantity of powdered Tablets, equivalent to about 10 mg of methimazole, with 10 mL of warm chloroform for 20 minutes, filter, and evaporate the filtrate on a steam bath to dryness: the residue responds to the *Identification* tests under *Methimazole*.

Dissolution ⟨711⟩—
  Medium: water; 500 mL.
  Apparatus 1: 100 rpm.
  Time: 30 minutes.
  Procedure—Determine the amount of $C_4H_6N_2S$ dissolved from UV absorbances at the wavelength of maximum absorbance at about 252 nm of filtered portions of the solution under test, suitably diluted with *Medium*, if necessary, in comparison with a Standard solution having a known concentration of USP Methimazole RS in the same *Medium*.
  Tolerances—Not less than 80% (*Q*) of the labeled amount of $C_4H_6N_2S$ is dissolved in 30 minutes.

Uniformity of dosage units ⟨905⟩: meet the requirements.
  Procedure for content uniformity—Place 1 Tablet, previously crushed or finely powdered, in a 100-mL volumetric flask, add 50 mL of water, and shake by mechanical means for 30 minutes. Dilute with water to volume, mix, and filter, discarding the first 20 mL of filtrate. Dilute a portion of the subsequent filtrate quantitatively and stepwise with water so that the assumed concentration of methimazole is about 5 μg per mL. Dissolve an accurately weighed quantity of USP Methimazole RS in water, and dilute quantitatively and stepwise with water to obtain a Standard solution having a known concentration of about 5 μg per mL. Concomitantly determine the absorbances of both solutions in 1-cm cells at the wavelength of maximum absorbance at about 252 nm, with a suitable spectrophotometer, using water as the blank. Calculate the quantity, in mg, of methimazole ($C_4H_6N_2S$) in the Tablet taken by the formula:

$$(T/5)C(A_U/A_S)$$

in which *T* is the labeled quantity, in mg, of methimazole in the Tablet; *C* is the concentration, in μg per mL, of USP Methimazole RS in the Standard solution; and A_U and A_S are the absorbances of the solution from the Tablet and the Standard solution, respectively.

Assay—Weigh and finely powder not fewer than 20 Tablets. Weigh accurately a portion of the powder, equivalent to about 120 mg of methimazole, and place in a 100-mL volumetric flask. Add about 80 mL of water, insert the stopper, and shake by mechanical means or occasionally by hand during 30 minutes. Dilute with water to volume, and mix. Filter, and transfer 50.0 mL of the filtrate to a 125-mL conical flask. Add from a buret 3.5 mL of 0.1 N sodium hydroxide VS, mix, and add, with agitation, about 7 mL of 0.1 N silver nitrate. Add 1 mL of bromothymol blue TS, and continue the titration with the 0.1 N sodium hydroxide VS until a permanent, blue-green color is produced. Each mL of 0.1 N sodium hydroxide is equivalent to 11.42 mg of $C_4H_6N_2S$.

Methionine

$C_5H_{11}NO_2S$ 149.21
L-Methionine.
L-Methionine [63-68-3].

» Methionine contains not less than 98.5 percent and not more than 101.5 percent of $C_5H_{11}NO_2S$, as L-methionine, calculated on the dried basis.

Packaging and storage—Preserve in well-closed containers.

USP Reference standards ⟨11⟩—*USP L-Methionine RS. USP L-Serine RS.*

Identification, *Infrared Absorption* ⟨197K⟩.

Specific rotation ⟨781S⟩: between +22.4° and +24.7°.
  Test solution: 20 mg per mL, in 6 N hydrochloric acid.

pH ⟨791⟩: between 5.6 and 6.1 in a solution (1 in 100).

Loss on drying ⟨731⟩—Dry it at 105° for 3 hours: it loses not more than 0.3% of its weight.

Residue on ignition ⟨281⟩: not more than 0.4%.

Chloride ⟨221⟩—A 0.73-g portion shows no more chloride than corresponds to 0.50 mL of 0.020 N hydrochloric acid (0.05%).

Sulfate ⟨221⟩—A 0.33-g portion shows no more sulfate than corresponds to 0.10 mL of 0.020 N sulfuric acid (0.03%).

Iron ⟨241⟩: 0.003%.

Heavy metals, *Method I* ⟨231⟩: 0.0015%.

Chromatographic purity—
  Adsorbent: 0.25-mm layer of chromatographic silica gel mixture.
  Test solution—Dissolve an accurately weighed quantity of Methionine in 0.3 M hydrochloric acid to obtain a solution having a concentration of 10 mg per mL. Apply 5 µL.
  Standard solution—Dissolve an accurately weighed quantity of USP L-Methionine RS in 0.3 M hydrochloric acid to obtain a solution having a known concentration of about 0.05 mg per mL. Apply 5 µL. [NOTE—This solution has a concentration equivalent to about 0.5% of that of the *Test solution.*]
  System suitability solution—Prepare a solution in 0.3 N hydrochloric acid containing 0.4 mg each of USP L-Methionine RS and USP L-Serine RS per mL. Apply 5 µL.
  Spray reagent—Dissolve 0.2 g of ninhydrin in 100 mL of a mixture of butyl alcohol and 2 N acetic acid (95 : 5).
  Developing solvent system—Prepare a mixture of butyl alcohol, glacial acetic acid, and water (60 : 20 : 20).
  Procedure—Proceed as directed for *Thin-Layer Chromatography* under *Chromatography* ⟨621⟩. After air-drying the plate, spray with *Spray reagent*, and heat between 100° and 105° for about 15 minutes. Examine the plate under white light. The chromatogram obtained from the *System suitability solution* exhibits two clearly separated spots. Any secondary spot in the chromatogram obtained from the *Test solution* is not larger or more intense than the principal spot in the chromatogram obtained from the *Standard solution*: not more than 0.5% of any individual impurity is found; and not more than 2.0% of total impurities is found.

Organic volatile impurities, *Method I* ⟨467⟩: meets the requirements.

(Official until July 1, 2008)

Assay—Transfer about 140 mg of Methionine, accurately weighed, to a 125-mL flask, dissolve in a mixture of 3 mL of formic acid and 50 mL of glacial acetic acid, and titrate with 0.1 N perchloric acid VS, determining the endpoint potentiometrically. Perform a blank determination, and make any necessary correction. Each mL of 0.1 N perchloric acid is equivalent to 14.92 mg of $C_5H_{11}NO_2S$.

Methocarbamol

$C_{11}H_{15}NO_5$ 241.24
1,2-Propanediol, 3-(2-methoxyphenoxy)-, 1-carbamate, (±)-.
(±)-3-(*o*-Methoxyphenoxy)-1,2-propanediol 1-carbamate [532-03-6].

» Methocarbamol contains not less than 98.5 percent and not more than 101.5 percent of $C_{11}H_{15}NO_5$, calculated on the dried basis.

Packaging and storage—Preserve in tight containers.

USP Reference standards ⟨11⟩—*USP Guaifenesin RS. USP Methocarbamol RS.*

Identification—
  A: *Infrared Absorption* ⟨197K⟩.
  B: *Ultraviolet Absorption* ⟨197U⟩—
  Solution: 40 µg per mL.
  Medium: alcohol.

Loss on drying ⟨731⟩—Dry it at 60° for 2 hours: it loses not more than 0.5% of its weight.

Residue on ignition ⟨281⟩: not more than 0.1%.

Heavy metals, *Method I* ⟨231⟩—Dissolve 1.0 g in a mixture of 7 mL of methanol and 3 mL of 1 N acetic acid, and dilute with water to 25 mL. The limit is 0.002%.

Organic volatile impurities, *Method V* ⟨467⟩: meets the requirements.
  Solvent—Use dimethyl sulfoxide.

(Official until July 1, 2008)

Chromatographic purity—
  pH 4.5 Buffer solution—Dissolve 6.8 g of monobasic potassium phosphate in 1000 mL of water. Adjust with 18 N phosphoric acid or 10 N potassium hydroxide to a pH of 4.5 ± .05.
  Mobile phase—Prepare a suitably filtered and degassed solution of *pH 4.5 Buffer solution* and methanol (about 75 : 25) (see *System suitability*).
  Guaifenesin solution—Transfer 20.0 mg of USP Guaifenesin RS to a 50-mL volumetric flask. Dissolve in and dilute with methanol to volume, and mix.
  Standard solution—Transfer 20.0 mg of USP Methocarbamol RS, accurately weighed, to a 10-mL volumetric flask. Add 1.0 mL of *Guaifenesin solution* and 2.0 mL of methanol to dissolve the methocarbamol. Dilute with *pH 4.5 Buffer solution* to volume, and mix. Use this solution within 24 hours.
  Test solution—Transfer about 100 mg of Methocarbamol, accurately weighed, to a 50-mL volumetric flask, add 13 mL of methanol to dissolve, dilute with *pH 4.5 Buffer solution* to volume, and mix. Use this solution within 24 hours.
  Chromatographic system (see *Chromatography* ⟨621⟩)—The liquid chromatograph is equipped with a 274-nm detector and a 4-mm × 25-cm column that contains packing L1. Adjust the operating conditions so that *System suitability* requirements are met.
  System suitability—Chromatograph three replicate 20-µL portions of the *Standard solution* as directed for the *Test solution* under *Procedure*. The analytical system is suitable for use if the peak area percentage of guaifenesin is 2.4 ± 1.0, the relative standard deviation for the peak area percentage is not greater than 4.0%, and the resolution, *R*, between guaifenesin and methocarbamol is not less than 2.0.
  Procedure—By means of a suitable microsyringe or sampling valve, inject about 20 µL of the *Test solution* into the chromatograph. Determine the peak areas of the methocarbamol peak and all extraneous peaks having a retention time greater than 0.5 of the retention time of methocarbamol. The relative retention times are

about 0.8 for guaifenesin and 1.0 for methocarbamol. Calculate the percentage of related impurities taken by the formula:

$$100(2.4/G)(P_E/P_T)$$

in which G is the area percentage of the guaifenesin peak in the chromatogram of the *Standard solution* determined under *System suitability*; P_E is the peak area of all extraneous peaks; and P_T is the total of the peak areas of all extraneous peaks and the methocarbamol. The limit is 2.0%.

Assay—Transfer about 100 mg of Methocarbamol, accurately weighed, to a 100-mL volumetric flask, add methanol to volume, and mix. Transfer 4.0 mL of this solution to a second 100-mL volumetric flask, dilute with methanol to volume, and mix. Concomitantly determine the absorbances of this solution and a Standard solution of USP Methocarbamol RS in methanol having a known concentration of about 40 μg per mL at the wavelength of maximum absorbance at about 274 nm in 1-cm cells, using methanol as the blank. Calculate the quantity, in mg, of $C_{11}H_{15}NO_5$ in the portion of Methocarbamol taken by the formula:

$$2.5C(A_U/A_S)$$

in which C is the concentration, in μg per mL, of USP Methocarbamol RS in the Standard solution; and A_U and A_S are the absorbances of the *Assay solution* and the *Standard solution*, respectively.

Methocarbamol Injection

» Methocarbamol Injection is a sterile solution of Methocarbamol in an aqueous solution of Polyethylene Glycol 300. It contains not less than 95.0 percent and not more than 105.0 percent of the labeled amount of methocarbamol ($C_{11}H_{15}NO_5$).

Packaging and storage—Preserve in single-dose containers, preferably of Type I glass.
USP Reference standards 〈11〉—*USP Endotoxin RS. USP Methocarbamol RS.*
Identification—Mix a volume of Injection, equivalent to about 500 mg of methocarbamol, with 40 mL of water in a small separator. Extract with 10 mL of ethyl acetate, and dry the ethyl acetate layer over anhydrous sodium sulfate. Evaporate the ethyl acetate with the use of a water bath maintained at 40° under a stream of nitrogen to dryness: the residue so obtained meets the requirements for *Identification* test A under *Methocarbamol*.
Bacterial endotoxins 〈85〉—It contains not more than 0.2 USP Endotoxin Unit per mg of methocarbamol.
pH 〈791〉: between 3.5 and 6.0.
Particulate matter 〈788〉: meets the requirements for small-volume injections.
Aldehydes—Transfer to a 25-mL volumetric flask an accurately measured volume of Injection, equivalent to 400 mg of methocarbamol, add 2.0 mL of a filtered 1 in 100 solution of phenylhydrazine hydrochloride in dilute alcohol (1 in 5), and allow to stand for 10 minutes. Add 1 mL of potassium ferricyanide solution (1 in 100), and allow to stand for 5 minutes. Add 4 mL of hydrochloric acid, dilute with alcohol to volume, and mix. Determine the absorbance of this solution in a 1-cm cell at the wavelength of maximum absorbance at about 515 nm, with a suitable spectrophotometer, using a reagent blank to set the instrument: the absorbance is not greater than that produced by 4 mL of formaldehyde solution (1 in 100,000), treated in the same manner as the portion of Injection taken and similarly measured, corresponding to not more than 0.01%, as formaldehyde, based upon the content of $C_{11}H_{15}NO_5$ as determined in the *Assay*.
Other requirements—It meets the requirements under *Injections* 〈1〉.
Assay—
pH 4.5 Buffer solution—Dissolve 6.8 g of monobasic potassium phosphate in 1000 mL of water. Adjust with 18 N phosphoric acid or 10 N potassium hydroxide to a pH of 4.5 ± 0.05.

Mobile phase—Prepare a suitable filtered and degassed solution of *pH 4.5 Buffer solution* and methanol (about 70 : 30) (see *System Suitability* under *Chromatography* 〈621〉).
Standard preparation—Dissolve an accurately weighed quantity of USP Methocarbamol RS in *Mobile phase* to obtain a solution having a known concentration of about 1 mg per mL.
Assay preparation—Transfer an accurately measured volume of Injection, equivalent to 100 mg of methocarbamol, to a 100-mL volumetric flask. Dilute with *Mobile phase* to volume, and mix.
Chromatographic system (see *Chromatography* 〈621〉)—The liquid chromatograph is equipped with a 274-nm detector and a 4.6-mm × 10-cm column that contains 3- or 5-μm packing L1, operated at 30°. The flow rate is 1 mL per minute. Chromatograph the *Standard preparation*, and record the peak responses as directed for *Procedure*: the relative standard deviation for replicate injections is not more than 2.0%.
Procedure—Separately inject equal volumes (about 20 μL) of the *Standard preparation* and the *Assay preparation* into the chromatograph, record the chromatograms, and measure the responses for the major peaks. Calculate the quantity, in mg, of methocarbamol ($C_{11}H_{15}NO_5$) in each mL of the Injection taken by the formula:

$$(100C/V)(r_U/r_S)$$

in which C is the concentration, in mg per mL, of USP Methocarbamol RS in the *Standard preparation*; V is the volume, in mL, of Injection taken; and r_U and r_S are the peak responses of methocarbamol obtained from the *Assay preparation* and the *Standard preparation*, respectively.

Methocarbamol Tablets

» Methocarbamol Tablets contain not less than 95.0 percent and not more than 105.0 percent of the labeled amount of methocarbamol ($C_{11}H_{15}NO_5$).

Packaging and storage—Preserve in tight containers.
USP Reference standards 〈11〉—*USP Methocarbamol RS.*
Identification—Mix a portion of finely powdered Tablets, equivalent to about 1 g of methocarbamol, with 25 mL of water in a separator, and extract with 25 mL of chloroform. Filter the extract, and evaporate to dryness: the residue of methocarbamol so obtained responds to *Identification* test A under *Methocarbamol*.
Dissolution, *Procedure for a Pooled Sample* 〈711〉—
   Medium: water; 900 mL.
   Apparatus 2: 50 rpm.
   Time: 45 minutes.
   Procedure—Determine the amount of $C_{11}H_{15}NO_5$ dissolved, employing the procedure set forth in the *Assay*, making any necessary modifications.
   Tolerances—Not less than 75% (*Q*) of the labeled amount of $C_{11}H_{15}NO_5$ is dissolved in 45 minutes.
Uniformity of dosage units 〈905〉: meet the requirements.
Assay—
pH 4.5 Buffer solution, Mobile phase, and *Chromatographic system*—Proceed as directed in the *Assay* under *Methocarbamol Injection*.
Internal standard solution—Prepare a solution of caffeine in methanol containing about 3 mg per mL.
Standard preparation—Transfer about 100 mg of USP Methocarbamol RS, accurately weighed, to a 100-mL volumetric flask. Dissolve in about 50 mL of *pH 4.5 Buffer solution* and 25 mL of methanol. Add 5.0 mL of *Internal standard solution*, dilute with *pH 4.5 Buffer solution* to volume, and mix.
Assay preparation—Weigh and powder not less than 10 Tablets. Transfer an accurately weighed portion of the powder, equivalent to 100 mg of methocarbamol, to a 100-mL volumetric flask. Add about 50 mL of *pH 4.5 Buffer solution*, 25 mL of methanol, and 5.0 mL of *Internal standard solution*. Shake vigorously for 10 minutes, dilute with *pH 4.5 Buffer solution* to volume, and mix. Filter, discarding the first 20 mL of the filtrate.

Procedure—Proceed as directed for *Procedure* in the *Assay* under *Methocarbamol Injection*. Calculate the quantity, in mg, of methocarbamol ($C_{11}H_{15}NO_5$) in the portion of Tablets taken by the formula:

$$100C(R_U / R_S)$$

in which C is the concentration, in mg per mL, of USP Methocarbamol RS in the *Standard preparation*; and R_U and R_S are the peak response ratios of methocarbamol and caffeine obtained from the *Assay preparation* and the *Standard preparation*, respectively.

Methohexital

$C_{14}H_{18}N_2O_3$ 262.30
2,4,6(1*H*,3*H*,5*H*)-Pyrimidinetrione, 1-methyl-5-(1-methyl-2-pentynyl)-5-(2-propenyl)-, (±)-.
(±)-5-Allyl-1-methyl-5-(1-methyl-2-pentynyl)barbituric acid [*18652-93-2*].

» Methohexital contains not less than 98.0 percent and not more than 101.0 percent of $C_{14}H_{18}N_2O_3$, calculated on the anhydrous basis.

Packaging and storage—Preserve in well-closed containers.
USP Reference standards ⟨11⟩—*USP Methohexital RS*.
Identification, *Infrared Absorption* ⟨197S⟩—
  Solution: 1 in 100.
  Medium: chloroform.
Melting range ⟨741⟩: between 92° and 96°, but the range between beginning and end of melting does not exceed 3°.
Water, *Method I* ⟨921⟩: not more than 2.0%.
Chloride ⟨221⟩—Dissolve 200 mg in a mixture of 75 mL of ether and 25 mL of water, agitate, and allow to separate: the water solution shows no more chloride than corresponds to 0.17 mL of 0.010 N hydrochloric acid (0.03%).
Heavy metals, *Method II* ⟨231⟩: 0.001%.
Ordinary impurities ⟨466⟩—
  Test solution: methanol.
  Standard solution: methanol.
  Eluant: a mixture of chloroform and acetone (7 : 3).
  Visualization—Expose the plate to chlorine gas for 1 minute, and air-dry the plate at room temperature for 2 minutes. Prepare a solution of 0.5 g of potassium iodide in 50 mL of water, and prepare a solution of 1.5 g of soluble starch in 50 mL of hot water. Mix 10 mL of each solution with 4 mL of alcohol to obtain the *Detection reagent*. [NOTE—The *Detection reagent* so obtained may be used for up to 3 or 4 days.] Spray the plate with the *Detection reagent*.
Assay—Dissolve about 100 mg of Methohexital, accurately weighed, in chloroform, and dilute quantitatively and stepwise with chloroform to obtain a solution having a concentration of about 10 mg per mL. Dissolve an accurately weighed quantity of USP Methohexital RS in chloroform, and dilute quantitatively and stepwise with chloroform to obtain a Standard solution having a known concentration of about 10 mg per mL. Concomitantly determine the absorbances of both solutions in 0.1-mm cells at the wavelength of maximum absorbance at about 5.93 μm, with a suitable spectrophotometer, using chloroform as the blank. Calculate the quantity, in mg, of $C_{14}H_{18}N_2O_3$ in the portion of Methohexital taken by the formula:

$$10C(A_U / A_S)$$

in which C is the concentration, in mg per mL, of USP Methohexital RS in the *Standard solution*; and A_U and A_S are the absorbances of the solution of Methohexital and the *Standard solution*, respectively.

Methohexital Sodium for Injection

$C_{14}H_{17}N_2NaO_3$ 284.29
2,4,6(1*H*,3*H*,5*H*)-Pyrimidinetrione, 1-methyl-5-(1-methyl-2-pentynyl)-5-(2-propenyl)-, (±)-, monosodium salt.
Sodium 5-allyl-1-methyl-5-(1-methyl-2-pentynyl)barbiturate [*309-36-4; 22151-68-4*].

» Methohexital Sodium for Injection is a freeze-dried, sterile mixture of methohexital sodium and anhydrous Sodium Carbonate as a buffer, prepared from an aqueous solution of Methohexital, Sodium Hydroxide, and Sodium Carbonate. It contains not less than 90.0 percent and not more than 110.0 percent of the labeled amount of methohexital sodium ($C_{14}H_{17}N_2NaO_3$).

Packaging and storage—Preserve in tight *Containers for Sterile Solids* as described under *Injections* ⟨1⟩. Store at controlled room temperature. Injection may be packaged in 50-mL multiple-dose containers.
USP Reference standards ⟨11⟩—*USP Endotoxin RS. USP Methohexital RS*.
Completeness of solution—Mix 1 g with 20 mL of carbon dioxide–free water: after 1 minute, the solution is clear and free from undissolved solid.
Constituted solution—At the time of use, it meets the requirements for *Constituted Solutions* under *Injections* ⟨1⟩.
Identification—
  A: Dissolve about 500 mg in 10 mL of water in a separator, add 10 mL of 3 N hydrochloric acid, and extract the liberated methohexital with two 25-mL portions of chloroform. Evaporate the combined chloroform extracts to dryness, add 10 mL of ether, evaporate again, and dry the residue in vacuum at 80° for 4 hours. Dissolve 50 mg of the residue so obtained in 5 mL of chloroform: the solution exhibits IR absorption maxima at the same wavelengths as that of a similar preparation of USP Methohexital RS.
  B: The methohexital obtained and dried as directed for *Identification* test A melts between 92° and 96°.
Bacterial endotoxins ⟨85⟩—It contains not more than 0.5 USP Endotoxin Unit per mg of methohexital sodium.
Uniformity of dosage units ⟨905⟩: meets the requirements.
  Procedure for content uniformity—
  Standard solution—Transfer about 23 mg of USP Methohexital RS, accurately weighed, to a 250-mL volumetric flask, add 50 mL of water, 0.5 mL of sodium hydroxide solution (1 in 10), and 1.5 mL of sodium carbonate solution (1 in 1000), and mix. Dilute with water to volume, and mix. Transfer 20.0 mL of this solution to a 100-mL volumetric flask, dilute with water to volume, and mix.
  Test solution—Transfer the contents of 1 vial of Methohexital Sodium for Injection with the aid of water to a 1000-mL volumetric flask, dilute with water to volume, and mix. Transfer an accurately measured volume of this solution, equivalent to about 100 mg of methohexital sodium, to a 1000-mL volumetric flask, add about 200 mL of water and 2.0 mL of sodium hydroxide solution (1 in 10), mix, dilute with water to volume, and again mix. Transfer 20.0 mL of the resulting solution to a 100-mL volumetric flask, dilute with water to volume, and mix.
  Procedure—Concomitantly determine the absorbances of the *Standard solution* and the *Test solution* in 1-cm cells at the wavelength of maximum absorbance at about 247 nm, with a suitable spectrophotometer, using water as the blank. Calculate the quantity, in mg, of $C_{14}H_{17}N_2NaO_3$ in the Methohexital Sodium for Injection taken by the formula:

$$(284.29/262.30)(TC/D)(A_U / A_S)$$

in which 284.29 and 262.30 are the molecular weights of methohexital sodium and methohexital, respectively; T is the labeled quantity, in mg, of methohexital sodium in the Methohexital Sodium for Injection; C is the concentration, in μg per mL, of USP Methohexital RS in the *Standard solution*; D is the concentration, in μg per mL, of methohexital sodium in the *Test solution* based on the labeled quantity per container and the extent of dilution; and A_U and

2662 Methohexital / *Official Monographs*

A_S are the absorbances of the *Test solution* and the *Standard solution*, respectively.

pH ⟨791⟩: between 10.6 and 11.6 in the solution prepared in the test for *Completeness of solution*.

Loss on drying ⟨731⟩—Dry it at 105° for 4 hours: it loses not more than 2.0% of its weight.

Heavy metals, *Method II* ⟨231⟩: 0.001%.

Other requirements—It meets the requirements under *Injections* ⟨1⟩.

Assay—

Internal standard solution—Dissolve aprobarbital in chloroform to obtain a solution having a concentration of about 1.35 mg per mL.

Standard preparation—Dissolve an accurately weighed quantity of USP Methohexital RS in chloroform to obtain a solution having a known concentration of about 0.46 mg per mL. Transfer 5.0 mL of the resulting solution to a 10-mL volumetric flask, add 2.0 mL of *Internal standard solution*, dilute with chloroform to volume, and mix to obtain a *Standard preparation* having a known concentration of about 230 µg per mL.

Assay preparation—Combine and mix the constituted solutions prepared from the contents of 5 vials of Methohexital Sodium for Injection. Transfer an accurately measured volume of the resulting solution, equivalent to about 50 mg of methohexital sodium, to a 125-mL separator containing 25 mL of water, and mix. Add 0.2 mL of dilute hydrochloric acid (1 in 2), and mix. Extract with three 25-mL portions of chloroform, shaking each extraction for 2 minutes and filtering the extracts through about 15 g of anhydrous sodium sulfate, that previously has been washed with about 5 mL of chloroform, into a 100-mL volumetric flask. Wash the sodium sulfate with several small portions of chloroform, collecting the washings in the 100-mL volumetric flask. Dilute with chloroform to volume, and mix. Transfer 5.0 mL of this solution to a 10-mL volumetric flask, add 2.0 mL of *Internal standard solution*, dilute with chloroform to volume, and mix.

Chromatographic system (see *Chromatography* ⟨621⟩)—The gas chromatograph is equipped with a flame-ionization detector and contains a 1.2-m × 4-mm column packed with 3% phase G10 on support S1AB. The column is maintained at about 230°, the injection port at about 265°, and the detector block at about 265°. Dry helium is used as the carrier gas at a flow rate of about 60 mL per minute. Chromatograph replicate injections of the *Standard preparation*, and record the peak responses as directed for *Procedure*: the resolution, *R*, between methohexital and aprobarbital is not less than 4.0, and the relative standard deviation is not more than 2.0%.

Procedure—Separately inject equal volumes (about 2 µL) of the *Assay preparation* and the *Standard preparation* into the gas chromatograph, and measure the peak responses for the major peak. The relative retention times are about 0.6 for methohexital and 1.0 for aprobarbital. Calculate the quantity, in mg, of methohexital sodium ($C_{14}H_{17}N_2NaO_3$) in the portion of Methohexital Sodium for Injection taken by the formula:

$$(284.29/262.30)(0.2C)(R_U/R_S)$$

in which 284.29 and 262.30 are the molecular weights of methohexital sodium and methohexital, respectively; *C* is the concentration, in µg per mL, of USP Methohexital RS in the *Standard preparation*; and R_U and R_S are the peak response ratios obtained from the *Assay preparation* and the *Standard preparation*, respectively.

Methotrexate

$C_{20}H_{22}N_8O_5$ 454.44

L-Glutamic acid, *N*-[4[[-(2,4-diamino-6-pteridinyl)methyl]-methylamino]benzoyl]-.
L-(+)-*N*-[*p*-[[(2,4-Diamino-6-pteridinyl)methyl]methylamino]-benzoyl]glutamic acid [59-05-2].

» Methotrexate is a mixture of 4-amino-10-methylfolic acid and closely related compounds. It contains not less than 98.0 percent and not more than 102.0 percent of $C_{20}H_{22}N_8O_5$, calculated on the anhydrous basis.

Caution—Great care should be taken to prevent inhaling particles of Methotrexate and exposing the skin to it.

Packaging and storage—Preserve in tight, light-resistant containers.

USP Reference standards ⟨11⟩—*USP Methotrexate RS*.
Identification—
  A: *Infrared Absorption* ⟨197K⟩—Do not dry specimens.
  B: *Ultraviolet Absorption* ⟨197U⟩—
  Solution: 10 µg per mL.
  Medium: 0.1 N hydrochloric acid.
Specific rotation ⟨781S⟩: between +19° and +24°, 2-dm polarimeter tube being used.
  Test solution: 10 mg per mL, in 0.05 M sodium carbonate.
Water, *Method I* ⟨921⟩: not more than 12.0%.
Residue on ignition ⟨281⟩: not more than 0.1%.
Chromatographic purity—
  pH 6.0 Buffer solution, Mobile phase, System suitability solution, and *Chromatographic system*—Proceed as directed in the *Assay*.
  Standard preparation—Dissolve an accurately weighed quantity of USP Methotrexate RS in *Mobile phase* to obtain a solution having a known concentration of about 5 µg per mL.
  Test preparation—Transfer about 100 mg of Methotrexate, accurately weighed, to a 100-mL volumetric flask, dissolve in *Mobile phase*, with the aid of sonication or shaking if necessary, dilute with *Mobile phase* to volume, and mix.
  Procedure—[NOTE—Use peak areas where peak responses are indicated.] Separately inject equal volumes (about 10 µL) of the *Standard preparation* and the *Test preparation* into the chromatograph, and allow the *Test preparation* to elute for not less than three times the retention time of methotrexate. Record the chromatograms, and measure the peak responses. The sum of all of the peak responses, other than that of methotrexate, is not more than four times the methotrexate response from the *Standard preparation* (2.0%), and no single peak response is greater than that of the methotrexate response from the *Standard preparation* (0.5%).
Organic volatile impurities, *Method V* ⟨467⟩: meets the requirements.
  Solvent: dimethyl sulfoxide.

(Official until July 1, 2008)

Assay—
  pH 6.0 Buffer solution—Prepare a mixture of 0.2 M dibasic sodium phosphate and 0.1 M citric acid (630 : 370). Adjust if necessary with 0.1 M citric acid or 0.2 M dibasic sodium phosphate to a pH of 6.0.
  Mobile phase—Prepare a filtered and degassed solution of *pH 6.0 buffer solution* and acetonitrile (90 : 10). Make adjustments if necessary (see *System Suitability* under *Chromatography* ⟨621⟩).
  Standard preparation—Dissolve an accurately weighed quantity of USP Methotrexate RS in *Mobile phase* to obtain a solution having a known concentration of about 100 µg per mL.

Assay preparation—Transfer about 25 mg of Methotrexate, accurately weighed, to a 250-mL volumetric flask, dissolve in *Mobile phase*, dilute with *Mobile phase* to volume, and mix.

System suitability solution—Prepare a solution in *Mobile phase* containing about 0.1 mg per mL each of USP Methotrexate RS and folic acid.

Chromatographic system (see *Chromatography* ⟨621⟩)—The liquid chromatograph is equipped with a 302-nm detector and a 4.6-mm × 25-cm column that contains packing L1. The flow rate is about 1.2 mL per minute. Chromatograph the *System suitability solution*, and record the peak responses as directed for *Procedure*: the relative retention times are about 0.35 for folic acid and 1.0 for methotrexate, the resolution, *R*, between the folic acid and methotrexate peaks is not less than 8.0, and the relative standard deviation for replicate injections is not more than 2.5% for methotrexate.

Procedure—Separately inject equal volumes (about 10 μL) of the *Assay preparation* and the *Standard preparation* into the chromatograph, record the chromatograms, and measure the responses for the major peaks. Calculate the quantity, in mg, of $C_{20}H_{22}N_8O_5$ in the portion of Methotrexate taken by the formula:

$$(0.25C)(r_U / r_S)$$

in which *C* is the concentration, in μg per mL, of USP Methotrexate RS in the *Standard preparation*; and r_U and r_S are the peak responses obtained from the *Assay preparation* and the *Standard preparation*, respectively.

Methotrexate Injection

» Methotrexate Injection is a sterile solution of Methotrexate in Water for Injection prepared with the aid of Sodium Hydroxide. It contains not less than 90.0 percent and not more than 110.0 percent of the labeled amount of methotrexate ($C_{20}H_{22}N_8O_5$).

Packaging and storage—Preserve in single-dose or in multiple-dose containers, preferably of Type I glass, protected from light.

USP Reference standards ⟨11⟩—*USP Endotoxin RS. USP Methotrexate RS.*

Identification—Dilute, if necessary, a volume of Injection, equivalent to about 25 mg of methotrexate, with water to obtain a solution having a concentration of about 2.5 mg per mL. Adjust with 0.1 N hydrochloric acid to a pH of 4.0. Place the slurry in a 50-mL centrifuge tube, and centrifuge. Decant the supernatant, add 25 mL of acetone, shake, and filter through a solvent-resistant, membrane filter of 0.45-μm pore size. Air-dry the filtered precipitate: the methotrexate so obtained responds to *Identification* test *A* under *Methotrexate*.

Bacterial endotoxins ⟨85⟩—It contains not more than 0.4 USP Endotoxin Unit per mg of methotrexate sodium.

pH ⟨791⟩: between 7.0 and 9.0.

Other requirements—It meets the requirements under *Injections* ⟨1⟩.

Assay—
pH 6.0 Buffer solution, Mobile phase, System suitability preparation, System suitability test, and *Standard preparation*—Proceed as directed in the *Assay* under *Methotrexate*.

Assay preparation—Transfer an accurately measured volume of Injection, equivalent to about 25 mg of methotrexate, to a 250-mL volumetric flask, dilute with *Mobile phase* to volume, and mix.

Procedure—Proceed as directed for *Procedure* in the *Assay* under *Methotrexate*. Calculate the quantity, in mg, of methotrexate ($C_{20}H_{22}N_8O_5$) in each mL of the Injection taken by the formula:

$$250(C/V)(P_U/P_S)$$

in which *C* is the concentration, in mg per mL, of USP Methotrexate RS in the *Standard preparation*; *V* is the volume, in mL, of Injection taken; and P_U and P_S are the peak responses obtained from the *Assay preparation* and the *Standard preparation*, respectively.

Methotrexate for Injection

» Methotrexate for Injection is a sterile, freeze-dried preparation of methotrexate sodium with or without suitable added substances, buffers, and/or diluents. It contains not less than 95.0 percent and not more than 115.0 percent of the labeled amount of methotrexate ($C_{20}H_{22}N_8O_5$).

Caution—Great care should be taken to prevent inhaling particles of methotrexate sodium and exposing the skin to it.

Packaging and storage—Preserve in *Containers for Sterile Solids* as described under *Injections* ⟨1⟩, protected from light.

USP Reference standards ⟨11⟩—*USP Endotoxin RS. USP Methotrexate RS.*

Constituted solution—At the time of use, it meets the requirements for *Constituted Solutions* under *Injections* ⟨1⟩.

Identification—Dissolve a sufficient quantity in water to obtain a solution having a concentration of about 2.5 mg per mL. Adjust with 0.1 N hydrochloric acid to a pH of 4.0. Place the slurry in a 50-mL centrifuge tube, and centrifuge. Decant the supernatant, add 25 mL of acetone, shake, and filter through a solvent-resistant, membrane filter having a porosity of 0.45 μm. Air-dry the filtered precipitate: the methotrexate so obtained responds to *Identification* test *A* under *Methotrexate*.

Bacterial endotoxins ⟨85⟩—It contains not more than 0.4 USP Endotoxin Unit per mg of methotrexate sodium.

pH ⟨791⟩: between 7.0 and 9.0 in a solution constituted as directed in the labeling, except that water is used as the diluent.

Other requirements—It meets the requirements for *Labeling* under *Injections* ⟨1⟩, for *Sterility Tests* ⟨71⟩, and for *Uniformity of Dosage Units* ⟨905⟩.

Assay—
pH 6.0 Buffer solution, Mobile phase, System suitability preparation, System suitability test, and *Standard preparation*—Proceed as directed in the *Assay* under *Methotrexate*.

Assay preparation—Dissolve the contents of 1 container of Methotrexate for Injection in an accurately measured volume of *Mobile phase* to obtain a solution having a known concentration of about 0.1 mg per mL.

Procedure—Proceed as directed for *Procedure* in the *Assay* under *Methotrexate*. Calculate the quantity, in mg, of methotrexate ($C_{20}H_{22}N_8O_5$) in the container of Methotrexate for Injection taken by the formula:

$$C(L/D)(r_U/r_S)$$

in which *C* is the concentration, in mg per mL, of USP Methotrexate RS, corrected for water content, in the *Standard preparation*; *L* is the labeled quantity of Methotrexate in the container; *D* is the concentration, in mg per mL, of Methotrexate in the *Assay preparation* on the basis of the labeled quantity in the container and the extent of dilution; and r_U and r_S are the peak responses obtained from the *Assay preparation* and the *Standard preparation*, respectively.

Methotrexate Tablets

» Methotrexate Tablets contain not less than 90.0 percent and not more than 110.0 percent of the labeled amount of methotrexate ($C_{20}H_{22}N_8O_5$).

Packaging and storage—Preserve in well-closed containers. A unit-of-use container contains a quantity of Tablets sufficient to provide one week's therapy as indicated in the labeling.

Labeling—When packaged in a unit-of-use container, the label indicates the total amount of methotrexate present as one week's supply.

USP Reference standards ⟨11⟩—*USP Methotrexate RS*.

Identification—Dissolve 1 Tablet in 100 mL of dilute hydrochloric acid (1 in 100), and filter the solution: the UV absorption spectrum of the filtrate exhibits maxima and minima at the same wavelengths as that of a solution containing about 2.5 mg of USP Methotrexate RS in 100 mL of dilute hydrochloric acid (1 in 100).

Dissolution ⟨711⟩—
  Medium: 0.1 N hydrochloric acid; 900 mL.
  Apparatus 2: 50 rpm.
  Time: 45 minutes.
  Procedure—Determine the amount of $C_{20}H_{22}N_8O_5$ dissolved from UV absorbances at the wavelength of maximum absorbance at about 306 nm of filtered portions of the solution under test, suitably diluted with *Dissolution Medium*, in comparison with a Standard solution having a known concentration of USP Methotrexate RS in the same *Medium*.
  Tolerances—Not less than 75% (*Q*) of the labeled amount of $C_{20}H_{22}N_8O_5$ is dissolved in 45 minutes.

Uniformity of dosage units ⟨905⟩: meet the requirements.

Assay—
  pH 6.0 Buffer solution, Mobile phase, System suitability preparation, System suitability test, and *Standard preparation*—Proceed as directed in the *Assay* under *Methotrexate*.
  Assay preparation—Weigh and finely powder not less than 20 Tablets. Weigh accurately a portion of the powder, equivalent to about 25 mg of methotrexate, and transfer to a 250-mL volumetric flask. Add about 200 mL of *Mobile phase*, and dissolve the methotrexate using a mechanical shaker or ultrasonic bath. Dilute with *Mobile phase* to volume, and mix.
  Procedure—Proceed as directed for *Procedure* in the *Assay* under *Methotrexate*. Calculate the quantity, in mg, of methotrexate ($C_{20}H_{22}N_8O_5$) in the portion of Tablets taken by the formula:

$$250C(P_U / P_S)$$

in which *C* is the concentration, in mg per mL, of USP Methotrexate RS in the *Standard preparation;* and P_U and P_S are the peak responses obtained from the *Assay preparation* and the *Standard preparation,* respectively.

Methotrimeprazine

$C_{19}H_{24}N_2OS$ 328.47
10*H*-Phenothiazine-10-propanamine, 2-methoxy-*N,N,β*-trimethyl-, (−)-.
(−)-10-[3-(Dimethylamino)-2-methylpropyl]-2-methoxyphenothiazine [60-99-1].

» Methotrimeprazine contains not less than 98.0 percent and not more than 101.0 percent of $C_{19}H_{24}N_2OS$, calculated on the dried basis.

Packaging and storage—Preserve in well-closed, light-resistant containers. Store at 25°, excursions permitted between 15° and 30°.

USP Reference standards ⟨11⟩—*USP Methotrimeprazine RS*.
  NOTE—Throughout the following procedures, protect test or assay specimens, the USP Reference Standard, and the solutions containing them, by conducting the procedures without delay, under subdued light, or using low-actinic glassware.

Identification—
  A: *Infrared Absorption* ⟨197K⟩.
  B: *Ultraviolet Absorption* ⟨197U⟩—
  Solution: 7 µg per mL.
  Medium: alcohol.
  Absorptivities at 255 nm, calculated on the dried basis, do not differ by more than 3.0%.

Specific rotation ⟨781S⟩: between −15° and −18°.
  Test solution: 50 mg per mL, in chloroform.

Loss on drying ⟨731⟩—Dry it at 100° for 3 hours: it loses not more than 0.5% of its weight.

Selenium ⟨291⟩—The absorbance of the solution from the *Test Solution,* prepared with 100 mg of Methotrimeprazine and 100 mg of magnesium oxide, is not greater than one-half that from the *Standard Solution* (0.003%).

Assay—Dissolve about 700 mg of Methotrimeprazine, accurately weighed, in 100 mL of chloroform, add 1 drop of a 1 in 500 solution of crystal violet in chloroform, and titrate with 0.1 N perchloric acid VS to the first disappearance of the violet tinge. Perform a blank determination, and make any necessary correction. Each mL of 0.1 N perchloric acid is equivalent to 32.85 mg of $C_{19}H_{24}N_2OS$.

Methotrimeprazine Injection

» Methotrimeprazine Injection is a sterile solution of Methotrimeprazine in Water for Injection, prepared with the aid of hydrochloric acid. It contains not less than 90.0 percent and not more than 110.0 percent of the labeled amount of methotrimeprazine ($C_{19}H_{24}N_2OS$), as the hydrochloride.

Packaging and storage—Preserve in single-dose or in multiple-dose containers, preferably of Type I glass, protected from light.

USP Reference standards ⟨11⟩—*USP Endotoxin RS. USP Methotrimeprazine RS*.
  NOTE—Throughout the following procedures, protect test or assay specimens, the Reference Standard, and solutions containing them, by conducting the procedures without delay, under subdued light, or using low-actinic glassware.

Identification—Place 1 mL of Injection in a 125-mL separator, and add 1 N sodium hydroxide dropwise until the solution becomes opaque white. Extract with 50 mL of ether, wash the ether extract with 25 mL of water, and discard the washing. Filter the ether extract through a layer of anhydrous sodium sulfate into a beaker, evaporate the filtrate by means of a stream of nitrogen to complete dryness, and dry at 100° for 3 hours: the methotrimeprazine so obtained responds to *Identification* test A under *Methotrimeprazine*.

Bacterial endotoxins ⟨85⟩—It contains not more than 17.9 USP Endotoxin Units per mg of methotrimeprazine.

pH ⟨791⟩: between 3.0 and 5.0.

Other requirements—It meets the requirements under *Injections* ⟨1⟩.

Assay—
  20% Phosphoric acid—Transfer 23.5 mL of 85% phosphoric acid into a 100-mL volumetric flask containing water, and dilute with water to volume.
  Mobile phase—Prepare a filtered and degassed mixture of water, acetonitrile, *20% Phosphoric acid,* and triethylamine by using the following procedure. Add 20 mL of *20% Phosphoric acid* to 450 mL of water, to this solution add 5 mL of triethylamine, and adjust with 1 N sodium hydroxide to a pH of 3.0. Add 500 mL of acetonitrile, and dilute with water to 1000 mL. Make adjustments if necessary (see *System Suitability* under *Chromatography* ⟨621⟩).
  Standard preparation—Dissolve an accurately weighed quantity of USP Methotrimeprazine RS in *Mobile phase,* and dilute quantitatively, and stepwise if necessary, with *Mobile phase* to obtain a solution having a known concentration of about 0.1 mg per mL.
  System suitability preparation—Dissolve or add suitable quantities of 1% benzyl alcohol in *Mobile phase* and USP Methotrimep-

razine RS in *Mobile phase* to obtain a solution containing about 2.0 and 0.1 mg per mL, respectively.

Assay preparation—Transfer an accurately measured amount of Injection, equivalent to about 20 mg of methotrimeprazine, accurately weighed, to a 200-mL volumetric flask, dissolve in and dilute with *Mobile phase* to volume, and mix.

Chromatographic system (see *Chromatography* ⟨621⟩)—The liquid chromatograph is equipped with a 254-nm detector and a 4.6-mm × 25-cm column that contains packing L7. The flow rate is about 1 mL per minute. Chromatograph the *System suitability preparation*, and record the peak responses as directed for *Procedure*: the resolution, R, between benzyl alcohol and methotrimeprazine is not less than 4.0; and the tailing factor is not more than 1.2. Chromatograph the *Standard preparation*, and record the peak responses as directed for *Procedure*: the relative standard deviation for replicate injections is not more than 1.5%.

Procedure—Separately inject equal volumes (about 20 µL) of the *Standard preparation* and the *Assay preparation* into the chromatograph, record the chromatograms, and measure the responses for the major peaks. Calculate the quantity, in mg, of methotrimeprazine ($C_{19}H_{24}N_2OS$) in the portion of Injection taken by the formula:

$$200C(r_U/r_S)$$

in which C is the concentration, in mg per mL, of USP Methotrimeprazine RS in the *Standard preparation*; and r_U and r_S are the peak responses obtained from the *Assay preparation* and the *Standard preparation*, respectively.

Methoxsalen

$C_{12}H_8O_4$ 216.19
7H-Furo[3,2-g][1]benzopyran-7-one, 9-methoxy-.
9-Methoxy-7H-furo[3,2-g][1]benzopyran-7-one   [298-81-7].

» Methoxsalen contains not less than 98.0 percent and not more than 102.0 percent of $C_{12}H_8O_4$, calculated on the anhydrous basis.

Caution—Avoid contact with the skin.

Packaging and storage—Preserve in well-closed, light-resistant containers.
USP Reference standards ⟨11⟩—*USP Methoxsalen RS*.
Identification, *Infrared Absorption* ⟨197K⟩.
Melting range, *Class I* ⟨741⟩:   between 143° and 148°.
Water, *Method I* ⟨921⟩:   not more than 0.5%.
Residue on ignition ⟨281⟩:   not more than 0.1%, a 1-g specimen being used.
Heavy metals, *Method II* ⟨231⟩:   0.002%.
Chromatographic impurities—Prepare a solution of it in chloroform containing about 20 mg per mL (*Solution A*). Dilute 1.0 mL of it with chloroform to 100.0 mL (*Solution B*). Apply 5-µL portions of both solutions at points along a line about 2.5 cm from one edge of a thin-layer chromatographic plate coated with a 0.25-mm layer of chromatographic silica gel mixture and previously dried at 105° for 30 minutes. Develop the plate in a suitable chamber, without previous equilibration, using a mixture of 9 volumes of benzene and 1 volume of ethyl acetate, until the solvent front has moved to about 15 cm above the line of application. Remove the plate from the chamber, air-dry, and observe under long-wavelength UV light: any spot in the chromatogram from *Solution A*, other than the principal spot, is not more intense than the spot from *Solution B* (1.0%).
Organic volatile impurities, *Method V* ⟨467⟩:   meets the requirements.
Solvent—Use dimethyl sulfoxide.

(Official until July 1, 2008)

Assay—
Mobile phase—Prepare a solution of acetonitrile in water (35 in 100). Make adjustments if necessary (see *System Suitability* under *Chromatography* ⟨621⟩).
Internal standard preparation—Dissolve trioxsalen in alcohol to obtain a solution containing about 0.2 mg per mL.
Standard preparation—Using an accurately weighed quantity of USP Methoxsalen RS, prepare a solution in alcohol having a known concentration of about 0.2 mg per mL. Transfer 2.0 mL of this solution to a 100-mL volumetric flask, add 2.0 mL of *Internal standard preparation*, dilute with *Mobile phase* to volume, and mix to obtain a *Standard preparation* having a known concentration of about 4 µg of USP Methoxsalen RS per mL. Pass through a 0.45-µm disk before using.
Assay preparation—Using 20 mg of Methoxsalen, accurately weighed, proceed as directed for *Standard preparation*.
Chromatographic system (see *Chromatography* ⟨621⟩)—The liquid chromatograph is equipped with a 254-nm detector and a 4-mm × 30-cm column that contains packing L1. The flow rate is about 1.5 mL per minute. Chromatograph the *Standard preparation*, and record the peak responses as directed for *Procedure*: the resolution, R, between the analyte and internal standard peaks is not less than 4.0, and the relative standard deviation for replicate injections is not more than 2.0%.
Procedure—Separately inject equal volumes (about 20 µL) of the *Standard preparation* and the *Assay preparation* into the chromatograph, record the chromatograms, and measure the responses for the major peaks. The relative retention times are about 2.1 for trioxsalen and 1.0 for methoxsalen. Calculate the quantity, in mg, of $C_{12}H_8O_4$, in the portion of Methoxsalen taken by the formula:

$$5C(R_U/R_S)$$

in which C is the concentration, in µg per mL, of USP Methoxsalen RS in the *Standard preparation*; and R_U and R_S are the ratios of the peak responses of methoxsalen to the internal standard obtained from the *Assay preparation* and the *Standard preparation*, respectively.

Methoxsalen Capsules

» Methoxsalen Capsules contain not less than 90.0 percent and not more than 110.0 percent of the labeled amount of methoxsalen ($C_{12}H_8O_4$).

Packaging and storage—Preserve in tight, light-resistant containers.
Labeling—Label the Capsules to state that Methoxsalen Hard Gelatin Capsules may not be interchangeable with Methoxsalen Soft Gelatin Capsules without retitration of the patient.
USP Reference standards ⟨11⟩—*USP Methoxsalen RS*.
Identification—
A: The retention time exhibited by methoxsalen in the chromatogram of the *Assay preparation* corresponds to that of methoxsalen in the chromatogram of the *Standard preparation* as obtained in the *Assay*.
B: Place one capsule in 50 mL of alcohol contained in a high-speed glass blender jar and blend thoroughly until the shell is completely dispersed. Dilute a portion quantitatively with alcohol to obtain a solution having a concentration of about 4 µg per mL: the UV absorption spectrum of the solution so obtained exhibits maxima and minima at the same wavelengths as that of a similar solution of USP Methoxsalen RS, concomitantly measured.
Dissolution ⟨711⟩—
FOR SOFT GELATIN CAPSULES—
Medium: water; 900 mL.
Apparatus 2:   50 rpm.
Time: 45 minutes.
Procedure—Determine the amount of $C_{12}H_8O_4$ dissolved from UV absorbances at the wavelength of maximum absorbance at about 300 nm using filtered portions of the solution under test, suitably diluted with water, if necessary, in comparison with a Standard

2666 Methoxsalen / *Official Monographs*

solution having a known concentration of USP Methoxsalen RS in the same *Medium*. [NOTE—An amount of alcohol not to exceed 1% of the total volume of the Standard solution may be used to bring the Reference Standard into solution prior to dilution with *Medium*.]
Tolerances—Not less than 75% *(Q)* of the labeled amount of $C_{12}H_8O_4$ is dissolved in 45 minutes.
FOR HARD GELATIN CAPSULES—
Medium: water; 900 mL.
Apparatus 1: 150 rpm.
Time: 90 minutes.
Procedure—Determine the amount of $C_{12}H_8O_4$ dissolved from UV absorbances at the wavelength of maximum absorbances at about 252 nm of filtered portions of the solution under test in comparison with a Standard solution having a known concentration of USP Methoxsalen RS prepared in alcohol and diluted with water.
Tolerances—Not less than 75% *(Q)* of the labeled amount of $C_{12}H_8O_4$ is dissolved in 90 minutes.
Uniformity of dosage units ⟨905⟩: meet the requirements.
Assay—
Mobile phase—Prepare a filtered and degassed mixture of acetonitrile and water (65 : 35). Make adjustments if necessary (see *System Suitability* under *Chromatography* ⟨621⟩).
Internal standard solution—Prepare a solution of trioxsalen in alcohol having a known concentration of 0.2 mg per mL.
Standard preparation—Prepare a solution in alcohol having an accurately known concentration of 0.2 mg of USP Methoxsalen RS per mL. Pipet 2.0 mL of this solution into a 100-mL volumetric flask containing 2.0 mL of *Internal standard solution*, dilute with *Mobile phase* to volume, and mix.
Assay preparation—Place not less than 10 Capsules in a high-speed glass blender jar containing 100.0 mL of alcohol, and blend thoroughly. Transfer an accurately measured volume of the aliquot from the blender jar, equivalent to about 2 mg of Methoxsalen, to a 50-mL volumetric flask containing 10.0 mL of *Internal standard solution*, dilute with alcohol to volume, mix, and filter. Transfer 5.0 mL of this solution to a 50-mL volumetric flask, dilute with *Mobile phase* to volume, mix, and filter.
Chromatographic system (see *Chromatography* ⟨621⟩)—The liquid chromatograph is equipped with a 254-nm detector and a 4-mm × 30-cm column that contains packing L1. The flow rate is about 1.5 mL per minute. Chromatograph the *Standard preparation*, and record the peak responses as directed for *Procedure*: the resolution, *R*, between the analyte peak and internal standard peak is not less than 4.0, and the relative standard deviation for replicate injections is not more than 2.0%.
Procedure—Separately inject equal volumes (about 20 µL) of the *Standard preparation* and the *Assay preparation* into the chromatograph, record the chromatograms, and measure the responses for the major peaks. The relative retention times are about 0.5 for Methoxsalen and 1.0 for Trioxsalen. Calculate the quantity, in mg, of methoxsalen ($C_{12}H_8O_4$) per Capsule taken by the formula:

$$500(C/V)(R_U/R_S)$$

in which *C* is the concentration, in mg per mL, of USP Methoxsalen RS in the *Standard preparation*; *V* is the volume, in mL, of *Assay preparation* taken; and R_U and R_S are the peak response ratios obtained from the *Assay preparation* and the *Standard preparation*, respectively.

Methoxsalen Topical Solution

» Methoxsalen Topical Solution is a solution of Methoxsalen in a suitable vehicle. It contains not less than 9.2 mg and not more than 10.8 mg of methoxsalen ($C_{12}H_8O_4$) per mL.

Packaging and storage—Preserve in tight, light-resistant containers.
USP Reference standards ⟨11⟩—*USP Methoxsalen RS*.
Identification—Transfer a volume of Topical Solution to a 100-mL volumetric flask, and dilute quantitatively and stepwise with alcohol to obtain a concentration of about 8 µg per mL: the UV absorption spectrum of this solution exhibits maxima and minima at the same wavelengths as that of a similar solution of USP Methoxsalen RS, concomitantly measured.
Alcohol content (if present) ⟨611⟩: between 66.5% and 77.0% of C_2H_5OH.
Assay—
Mobile phase, Internal standard preparation, Standard preparation, and *Chromatographic system*—Prepare as directed in the *Assay* under *Methoxsalen*.
Assay preparation—Transfer an accurately measured volume of Topical Solution, equivalent to about 20 mg of methoxsalen, to a 100-mL volumetric flask. Dilute with alcohol to volume, and mix. Transfer 2.0 mL of this solution and 2.0 mL of *Internal standard preparation* to a 100-mL volumetric flask. Dilute with *Mobile phase* to volume, and mix. Pass through a 0.45-µm disk before using.
Procedure—Proceed as directed for *Procedure* in the *Assay* under *Methoxsalen*. Calculate the quantity, in mg, of methoxsalen ($C_{12}H_8O_4$) in each mL of the Topical Solution taken by the formula:

$$5(C/V)(R_U/R_S)$$

in which *V* is the volume, in mL, of Topical Solution taken, and the other terms are as defined therein.

Methoxyflurane

$C_3H_4Cl_2F_2O$ 164.97
Ethane, 2,2-dichloro-1,1-difluoro-1-methoxy-.
2,2-Dichloro-1,1-difluoroethyl methyl ether   [76-38-0].

» Methoxyflurane contains not less than 99.9 percent and not more than 100.0 percent of $C_3H_4Cl_2F_2O$. It may contain a suitable stabilizer.

Packaging and storage—Preserve in tight, light-resistant containers, and avoid exposure to excessive heat.
USP Reference standards ⟨11⟩—*USP Methoxyflurane RS*.
Identification—
A: The IR absorption spectrum of a 1 in 20 solution in chloroform exhibits maxima only at the same wavelengths as that of a similar solution of USP Methoxyflurane RS.
B: To 1 mL in a test tube add 1 mL of sulfuric acid: the specimen forms a layer over the acid (*distinction from halothane*).
C: Cautiously heat the contents of the test tube from *Identification* test B with agitation: the interface disappears, and hydrofluoric acid is evolved (*distinction from chloroform, trichloroethylene, and halothane*).
Specific gravity ⟨841⟩: between 1.420 and 1.425.
Acidity—Shake 25 mL with 25 mL of carbon dioxide-free water for 2 minutes, and allow the layers to separate. Add 1 drop of methyl red TS to the water extract, boil for 1 minute, and titrate with 0.010 N sodium hydroxide: not more than 0.50 mL of 0.010 N sodium hydroxide is required to produce a distinct yellow color.
Water, *Method I* ⟨921⟩: not more than 0.1%.
Limit of nonvolatile residue—Allow 50 mL to evaporate at room temperature in a tared evaporating dish, and dry the residue at 105° for 1 hour: the weight of the residue does not exceed 1 mg.
Assay—Inject a volume of Methoxyflurane (30 µL or less) into a suitable gas chromatograph (see *Chromatography* ⟨621⟩) equipped with a thermal conductivity detector. Under typical conditions, the instrument contains a 4-mm × 3-m stainless steel column packed with liquid phase G11 on support S1A, the column is maintained at a temperature of 100° to 110°, the injection port is maintained at about 150°, and dry helium is used as the carrier gas at a flow rate of about 60 mL per minute. Calculate the percentage purity by di-

viding 100 times the area of the methoxyflurane peak by the sum of all the areas in the chromatogram.

Methscopolamine Bromide

$C_{18}H_{24}BrNO_4$ 398.29

3-Oxa-9-azoniatricyclo[3.3.1.0^{2,4}]nonane, 7-(3-hydroxy-1-oxo-2-phenylpropoxy)-9,9-dimethyl-, bromide, [7(S)-(1α,2β,4β,5α,7β)]-

6β,7β-Epoxy-3α-hydroxy-8-methyl-1αH,5αH-tropanium bromide (−)-tropate   [155-41-9].

» Methscopolamine Bromide contains not less than 97.0 percent and not more than 103.0 percent of $C_{18}H_{24}BrNO_4$, calculated on the dried basis.

Packaging and storage—Preserve in tight, light-resistant containers, and store at room temperature.
USP Reference standards ⟨11⟩—*USP Methscopolamine Bromide RS. USP Scopolamine Hydrobromide RS.*
Identification—
  A: *Infrared Absorption* ⟨197K⟩.
  B: A solution (1 in 20) meets the requirements of the tests for *Bromide* ⟨191⟩.
Specific rotation ⟨781⟩: between −21° and −25°, determined in a solution containing 500 mg in each 10 mL.
Loss on drying ⟨731⟩—Dry it at 105° for 2 hours: it loses not more than 2.0% of its weight.
Residue on ignition ⟨281⟩: not more than 0.1%.
Chromatographic purity—
  Buffer solution, Solution A, Solution B, and *Mobile phase*—Proceed as directed in the *Assay*.
  Standard solution—Prepare as directed for the *Standard preparation* in the *Assay*.
  Diluted standard solution—Dilute 5 μL of the *Standard solution* with *Solution A* to 10.0 mL.
  Test solution—Prepare as directed for the *Assay preparation*.
  Scopolamine hydrobromide solution—Dissolve an accurately weighed quantity of USP Scopolamine Hydrobromide RS in *Solution A* to obtain a solution having a known concentration of about 0.05 mg per mL.
  System suitability solution—Dissolve about 50 mg of USP Methscopolamine Bromide RS in *Solution A*, add 1.0 mL of *Scopolamine hydrobromide solution*, and dilute with *Solution A* to 50.0 mL. This solution contains about 0.1% of scopolamine hydrobromide.
  Chromatographic system (see *Chromatography* ⟨621⟩)—Proceed as directed in the *Assay*. In addition, chromatograph the *System suitability solution*, and record the peak responses as directed for *Procedure:* the resolution, *R*, between methscopolamine and scopolamine is not less than 1.5; and the tailing factor for the methscopolamine peak is not more than 2.0.
  Procedure—Separately inject equal volumes (about 5 μL) of the *Diluted standard solution* and the *Test solution* into the chromatograph, record the chromatogram for four times the retention time of methscopolamine, and measure the responses for the major peaks. Disregard any peak with an area less than that of the methscopolamine peak in the chromatogram obtained from the *Diluted standard solution*, and disregard any peak that is due to *Solution A*. Calculate the percentage of each impurity in the portion of Methscopolamine Bromide taken by the formula:

$$100F(r_i / r_S)$$

in which *F* is the relative response factor for the methscopolamine bromide impurities (see *Table 1*); r_i is the peak area of any impurity obtained from the *Test solution;* and r_S is the peak area of methscopolamine obtained from the chromatogram of the *Test solution*: not more than 0.1% of any individual impurity is found; and not more than 0.5% of total impurities is found.

Table 1

Name	Relative Retention Time	Relative Response Factor (*F*)
Tropic acid	0.4	0.4
Scopolamine hydrobromide	0.9	1.0
Methylatropine bromide	1.2	1.0
Apomethscopolamine bromide	3.5	0.6
Any other impurity	—	1.0

Assay—
  Buffer solution—Prepare a solution containing 5.16 g of sodium 1-hexanesulfonate monohydrate and 3.40 g of monobasic potassium phosphate in 1000 mL of water, adjust with 1 M phosphoric acid to a pH of 2.8, and mix.
  Solution A—Mix 850 mL of *Buffer solution* and 150 mL of acetonitrile, filter, and degas.
  Solution B—Mix 500 mL of *Buffer solution* and 500 mL of acetonitrile, filter, and degas.
  Mobile phase—Use variable mixtures of *Solution A* and *Solution B* as directed for *Chromatographic system*. Make adjustments if necessary (see *System Suitability* under *Chromatography* ⟨621⟩).
  Standard preparation—Dissolve an accurately weighed quantity of USP Methscopolamine Bromide RS in *Solution A* to obtain a solution having a known concentration of about 1.0 mg per mL.
  Assay preparation—Transfer about 50 mg of Methscopolamine Bromide, accurately weighed, to a 50-mL volumetric flask, dissolve in and dilute with *Solution A* to volume, and mix.
  Chromatographic system (see *Chromatography* ⟨621⟩)—The liquid chromatograph is equipped with a 210-nm detector and a 4.6-mm × 10-cm column that contains packing L1. The flow rate is about 3 mL per minute. The column temperature is maintained at 50°. The chromatograph is programmed as follows.

Time (minutes)	Solution A (%)	Solution B (%)	Elution
0–3	100	0	isocratic
3–10	100→85	0→15	linear gradient
10–10.1	85→100	15→0	linear gradient
10.1–13	100	0	re-equilibration

Chromatograph the *Standard preparation,* and record the peak responses as directed for *Procedure:* the relative standard deviation for six replicate injections is not greater than 1%.
  Procedure—Separately inject equal volumes (about 5 μL) of the *Standard preparation* and the *Assay preparation* into the chromatograph, record the chromatograms, and measure the peak area responses. Calculate the quantity, in mg, of $C_{18}H_{24}BrNO_4$ in the portion of Methscopolamine Bromide taken by the formula:

$$50C(r_U / r_S)$$

in which *C* is the concentration, in mg per mL, of USP Methscopolamine Bromide RS in the *Standard preparation;* and r_U and r_S are the peak area responses of methscopolamine obtained from the *Assay preparation* and the *Standard preparation*, respectively.

Methscopolamine Bromide Tablets

» Methscopolamine Bromide Tablets contain not less than 93.0 percent and not more than 107.0 percent of the labeled amount of methscopolamine bromide ($C_{18}H_{24}BrNO_4$).

Packaging and storage—Preserve in tight containers, and store at controlled room temperature.

USP Reference standards ⟨11⟩—*USP Methscopolamine Bromide RS*.

Identification—
  A: *Thin-Layer Chromatographic Identification Test* ⟨201⟩—
  pH 7.3 Dye-buffer solution—Prepare a solution containing, in each 500 mL, 200 mg of bromothymol blue, 3.2 mL of 0.1 N sodium hydroxide, 577.5 mg of citric acid monohydrate, and 6.3 mg of anhydrous dibasic sodium phosphate.
  Test solution—Finely powder 1 Tablet, and transfer an amount, equivalent to about 0.5 mg of methscopolamine bromide, to a suitable container. Add 20 mL of water, heat for 5 minutes on a steam bath with frequent agitation, and centrifuge to obtain a clear supernatant. Transfer 10 mL of the supernatant to a vessel containing 10 mL of chloroform and 10 mL of *pH 7.3 Dye-buffer solution*. Shake vigorously for 3 minutes, centrifuge, and transfer 8 mL of the chloroform layer to a suitable container. Evaporate to dryness, and dissolve the residue in 1 mL of chloroform.
  Standard solution—Prepare a solution in water containing about 0.025 mg of USP Methscopolamine Bromide RS per mL, and treat as directed above, beginning with "Transfer 10 mL of the supernatant."
  Application volume: 50 µL.
  Developing solvent system—In a suitable container, mix water, butyl alcohol, and glacial acetic acid (5 : 4 : 1), then transfer a measured volume of the upper organic layer to a suitable container, and mix with a volume of alcohol equivalent to 20% of the volume of the organic layer.
  Procedure—Allow the solvent front to move about three-fourths of the length of the plate, remove the plate from the developing chamber, mark the solvent front, and dry the plate under a current of air for 30 minutes. Spray the plate evenly with potassium–bismuth iodide TS: the chromatogram of the *Test solution* shows a bright orange spot on a yellow background corresponding in R_F value (about 0.25) to that in the chromatogram obtained from the *Standard solution*. [NOTE—Bromothymol blue produces a dark yellow spot at an R_F value of about 0.8.]
  B: Powder a number of Tablets, equivalent to about 5 mg of methscopolamine bromide, digest with 5 mL of water for 10 minutes, and filter: a portion of the clear solution so obtained responds to the test for *Bromide* ⟨191⟩.

Dissolution ⟨711⟩—
  Medium: 0.1 N hydrochloric acid; 500 mL.
  Apparatus 2: 50 rpm.
  Time: 30 minutes.
  Determine the percentage of the labeled amount of methscopolamine bromide dissolved using the following method.
  pH 3.0 Phosphate buffer—Dissolve 5.44 g of monobasic potassium phosphate in 1 L of water. Adjust with 1 N phosphoric acid to a pH of 3.0.
  Mobile phase—Prepare a filtered and degassed mixture of *pH 3.0 Phosphate buffer* and methanol (3 : 1). Make adjustments if necessary (see *System Suitability* under *Chromatography* ⟨621⟩).
  Standard solution—Dissolve an accurately weighed quantity of USP Methscopolamine Bromide RS in *Medium*, and dilute quantitatively, and stepwise if necessary, with *Medium* to obtain a solution having a known concentration similar to the one expected in the *Test solution*.
  Test solution—Use portions of the solution under test that have been passed through a 0.45-µm PTFE filter.
  Chromatographic system (see *Chromatography* ⟨621⟩)—The liquid chromatograph is equipped with a 204-nm detector and a 4.6-mm × 15-cm column that contains packing L1. The flow rate is about 1.0 mL per minute. The column temperature is maintained at 30°. Chromatograph the *Standard solution*, and record the peak responses as directed for *Procedure*: the tailing factor is not more than 2.0; and the relative standard deviation for replicate injections is not more than 2.0%.
  Procedure—Separately inject equal volumes (about 25 µL) of the *Standard solution* and the *Test solution* into the chromatograph, record the chromatograms, and measure the responses for the major peaks. Calculate the percentage of methscopolamine bromide dissolved by the formula:

$$\frac{r_U \times C_S \times 500 \times 100}{r_S \times LC}$$

in which r_U and r_S are the peak responses obtained from the *Test solution* and the *Standard solution*, respectively; C_S is the concentration, in mg per mL, of USP Methscopolamine Bromide RS in the *Standard solution;* 500 is the volume, in mL, of *Medium;* 100 is the factor for conversion to percentage; and *LC* is the tablet label claim, in mg.
  Tolerances—Not less than 80% (*Q*) of the labeled amount of $C_{18}H_{24}BrNO_4$ is dissolved in 30 minutes.

Uniformity of dosage units ⟨905⟩: meet the requirements.

Assay—
  Mobile phase—Prepare a solution containing 2.6 g of decyl sodium sulfate in 450 mL of water. Add 550 mL of methanol, adjust with 1 N sulfuric acid to a pH of 3.5, mix, filter, and degas.
  Standard preparation—Transfer about 25 mg of USP Methscopolamine Bromide RS, accurately weighed, to a 100-mL volumetric flask, dissolve in and dilute with *Mobile phase* to volume, and mix.
  Assay preparation—
  FOR TABLETS THAT CONTAIN 2.5 MG OF METHSCOPOLAMINE BROMIDE—Place 10 Tablets in a 100-mL volumetric flask, add about 50 mL of *Mobile phase*, and sonicate for 30 minutes. Shake by mechanical means for 30 minutes, dilute with *Mobile phase* to volume, and mix. Pass a portion through a 0.45-µm PTFE filter, discarding the first 2 to 3 mL of the filtrate.
  FOR TABLETS THAT CONTAIN 5 MG OF METHSCOPOLAMINE BROMIDE—Place 10 Tablets in a 200-mL volumetric flask, add about 100 mL of *Mobile phase*, and sonicate for 30 minutes. Shake by mechanical means for 30 minutes, dilute with *Mobile phase* to volume, and mix. Pass a portion through a 0.45-µm PTFE filter, discarding the first 2 to 3 mL of the filtrate.
  Chromatographic system (see *Chromatography* ⟨621⟩)—The liquid chromatograph is equipped with a 254-nm detector and a 4.6-mm × 25-cm column that contains packing L1. Chromatograph the *Standard preparation*, and record the peak responses as directed for *Procedure:* the relative standard deviation for replicate injections is not more than 2.0%.
  Procedure—Separately inject a volume (about 50 µL) of the *Standard preparation* and the *Assay preparation* into the chromatograph, record the chromatogram, and measure the peak responses. Calculate the quantity, in mg, of methscopolamine bromide ($C_{18}H_{24}BrNO_4$) in the portion of Tablets taken by the formula:

$$100C(r_U / r_S)$$

in which *C* is the concentration, in mg per mL, of USP Methscopolamine Bromide RS in the *Standard preparation;* and r_U and r_S are the peak responses of the methscopolamine bromide obtained from the *Assay preparation* and the *Standard preparation*, respectively.

Methsuximide

$C_{12}H_{13}NO_2$ 203.24
2,5-Pyrrolidinedione, 1,3-dimethyl-3-phenyl-, (±)-.
(±)-*N*,2-Dimethyl-2-phenylsuccinimide   [77-41-8].

» Methsuximide contains not less than 97.0 percent and not more than 103.0 percent of $C_{12}H_{13}NO_2$, calculated on the dried basis.

Packaging and storage—Preserve in tight containers.
USP Reference standards ⟨11⟩—*USP Methsuximide RS.*
Identification—
  A: *Infrared Absorption* ⟨197K⟩.
  B: *Ultraviolet Absorption* ⟨197U⟩—
  Solution: 350 µg per mL.
  Medium: alcohol.
Melting range ⟨741⟩: between 50° and 56°, determined by a *Class I* procedure, except that the test specimen is inserted into the bath at about room temperature.
Loss on drying ⟨731⟩—Dry it over phosphorus pentoxide for 16 hours: it loses not more than 0.5% of its weight.
Residue on ignition ⟨281⟩: not more than 0.2%.
Limit of cyanide—Dissolve 1.0 g in 10 mL of alcohol, and add 3 drops of ferrous sulfate TS, 1 mL of 1 N sodium hydroxide, and a few drops of ferric chloride TS. Warm gently, and finally acidify with 2 N sulfuric acid: no blue precipitate or blue color develops within 15 minutes.
Chromatographic purity—
  Mobile phase and *Chromatographic system*—Proceed as directed in the *Assay*. To evaluate the system suitability requirements, use the *Standard preparation* as prepared in the *Assay*.
  Standard solution—Dissolve an accurately weighed quantity of USP Methsuximide RS in *Mobile phase*, and dilute quantitatively, and stepwise if necessary, with *Mobile phase* to obtain a solution having a known concentration of about 6.0 µg per mL.
  Test solution—Transfer about 300 mg of Methsuximide, accurately weighed, to a 50-mL volumetric flask, dissolve in and dilute with *Mobile phase* to volume, and mix.
  Procedure—Separately inject equal volumes (about 20 µL) of the *Standard solution* and the *Test solution* into the chromatograph, record the chromatograms, and measure all of the peak responses. Calculate the percentage of each impurity in the portion of Methsuximide taken by the formula:

$$0.1(C_S/C_U)(r_i/r_S)$$

in which C_S is the concentration, in µg per mL, of USP Methsuximide RS in the *Standard solution*; C_U is the concentration, in mg per mL, of Methsuximide in the *Test solution*; r_i is the peak response for each impurity obtained from the *Test solution*; and r_S is the peak response for methsuximide obtained from the *Standard solution*: not more than 0.1% of any individual impurity is found; and not more than 2.0% of total impurities is found.
Organic volatile impurities, *Method V* ⟨467⟩: meets the requirements.
  Solvent—Use dimethyl sulfoxide.

(Official until July 1, 2008)

Assay—
  Mobile phase—Prepare a filtered and degassed mixture of water and acetonitrile (11 : 9). Make adjustments if necessary (see *System Suitability* under *Chromatography* ⟨621⟩).
  Standard preparation—Dissolve an accurately weighed quantity of USP Methsuximide RS in *Mobile phase*, and dilute quantitatively, and stepwise if necessary, with *Mobile phase* to obtain a solution having a known concentration of about 0.6 mg per mL.
  Assay preparation—Transfer about 120 mg of Methsuximide, accurately weighed, to a 200-mL volumetric flask, dissolve in and dilute with *Mobile phase* to volume, and mix.
  Chromatographic system—The liquid chromatograph is equipped with a 254-nm detector and a 3.9-mm × 30-cm column that contains packing L1. The flow rate is about 1 mL per minute. Chromatograph the *Standard preparation*, and record the peak responses as directed for *Procedure*: the column efficiency is not less than 5800 theoretical plates; the tailing factor is not more than 1.3; and the relative standard deviation for replicate injections is not more than 0.6%.
  Procedure—Separately inject equal volumes (about 20 µL) of the *Standard preparation* and the *Assay preparation* into the chromatograph, record the chromatograms, and measure the responses for the major peaks. Calculate the quantity, in mg, of $C_{12}H_{13}NO_2$ in the portion of Methsuximide taken by the formula:

$$200C_S(r_U/r_S)$$

in which C_S is the concentration, in mg per mL, of USP Methsuximide RS in the *Standard preparation*; and r_U and r_S are the peak responses obtained from the *Assay preparation* and the *Standard preparation*, respectively.

Methsuximide Capsules

» Methsuximide Capsules contain not less than 92.0 percent and not more than 108.0 percent of the labeled amount of methsuximide ($C_{12}H_{13}NO_2$).

Packaging and storage—Preserve in tight containers, and avoid exposure to excessive heat.
USP Reference standards ⟨11⟩—*USP Methsuximide RS.*
Identification—
  A: Mix a portion of the contents of Capsules, equivalent to about 200 mg of methsuximide, with 25 mL of water in a separator, extract with 50 mL of ether, and discard the aqueous layer. Wash the ether extract with 25 mL of water, and discard the water. Filter the extract, evaporate with the aid of a current of warm air to dryness, and dry the methsuximide over phosphorus pentoxide for 16 hours: the residue so obtained responds to *Identification* test A under *Methsuximide*.
  B: The retention time exhibited by methsuximide in the chromatogram of the *Assay preparation* corresponds to that of methsuximide in the chromatogram of the *Standard preparation* as obtained in the *Assay*.
Dissolution ⟨711⟩—
  Medium: water; 900 mL.
  Apparatus 1: 100 rpm.
  Time: 120 minutes.
  Procedure—Determine the amount of $C_{12}H_{13}NO_2$ dissolved, employing the procedure set forth in the *Assay*, making any necessary modifications.
  Tolerances—Not less than 75% (*Q*) of the labeled amount of $C_{12}H_{13}NO_2$ is dissolved in 120 minutes.
Uniformity of dosage units ⟨905⟩: meet the requirements.
Assay—
  Mobile phase—Prepare a filtered and degassed mixture of water and acetonitrile (55 : 45). Make adjustments if necessary (see *System Suitability* under *Chromatography* ⟨621⟩).
  Standard preparation—Dissolve an accurately weighed quantity of USP Methsuximide RS in *Mobile phase* to obtain a solution having a known concentration of about 0.6 mg per mL.
  Assay preparation—Place 10 Capsules in a 500-mL volumetric flask, and add 280 mL of water. Sonicate in a water bath at 40° to 50°, with occasional shaking, until the Capsules have broken, and cool to room temperature. Dilute with acetonitrile to volume, mix, and filter. Transfer an accurately measured volume of this specimen solution, equivalent to about 30 mg of methsuximide, to a 50-mL volumetric flask, dilute with *Mobile phase* to volume, and mix.
  Chromatographic system (see *Chromatography* ⟨621⟩)—The liquid chromatograph is equipped with a 254-nm detector and a 3.9-mm × 30-cm column that contains packing L1. The flow rate is about 1 mL per minute. Chromatograph the *Standard preparation*, and record the peak responses as directed under *Procedure*: the column efficiency determined from the analyte peak is not less than 2100 theoretical plates, and the relative standard deviation for replicate injections is not more than 1.5%.
  Procedure—Separately inject equal volumes (about 20 µL) of the *Standard preparation* and the *Assay preparation* into the chromatograph, record the chromatograms, and measure the responses for the

major peaks. Calculate the quantity, in mg, of methsuximide ($C_{12}H_{13}NO_2$) per Capsule taken by the formula:

$$2500(C/V)(r_U/r_S)$$

in which C is the concentration, in mg per mL, of USP Methsuximide RS in the *Standard preparation*; V is the volume, in mL, of specimen solution taken for the *Assay preparation*; and r_U and r_S are the methsuximide peak responses obtained from the *Assay preparation* and the *Standard preparation*, respectively.

Methyclothiazide

$C_9H_{11}Cl_2N_3O_4S_2$ 360.24
2*H*-1,2,4-Benzothiadiazine-7-sulfonamide, 6-chloro-3-(chloromethyl)-3,4-dihydro-2-methyl-, 1,1-dioxide, (±)-.
(±)-6-Chloro-3-(chloromethyl)-3,4-dihydro-2-methyl-2*H*-1,2,4-benzothiadiazine-7-sulfonamide 1,1-dioxide   [135-07-9].

» Methyclothiazide contains not less than 97.0 percent and not more than 102.0 percent of $C_9H_{11}Cl_2N_3O_4S_2$, calculated on the dried basis.

Packaging and storage—Preserve in well-closed containers.
USP Reference standards ⟨11⟩—*USP Methyclothiazide RS. USP Methyclothiazide Related Compound A RS.*
Identification—
  A: *Infrared Absorption* ⟨197K⟩.
  B: *Ultraviolet Absorption* ⟨197U⟩—
   Solution: 20 µg per mL.
   Medium: methanol.
  C: Fuse about 100 mg of it with a pellet of sodium hydroxide: the ammonia fumes produced turn moistened red litmus paper blue. The fused mixture responds to the test for *Sulfite* ⟨191⟩.
Loss on drying ⟨731⟩—Dry it at 105° for 4 hours: it loses not more than 0.5% of its weight.
Residue on ignition ⟨281⟩: not more than 0.2%.
Chloride ⟨221⟩—Shake 750 mg with 25 mL of water for 2 minutes, filter through a suitable membrane filter, and add 4 or 5 drops of 2 N nitric acid: the acidified filtrate shows no more chloride than corresponds to 0.20 mL of 0.020 N hydrochloric acid (0.02%).
Selenium ⟨291⟩: 0.003%.
Heavy metals, *Method II* ⟨231⟩: 0.002%.
Diazotizable substances—
  Standard preparation—Transfer about 10 mg of USP Methyclothiazide Related Compound A RS, accurately weighed, to a 50-mL volumetric flask, dilute with acetonitrile to volume, and mix. Pipet 25 mL of the solution into a 100-mL volumetric flask, dilute with acetonitrile to volume, and mix. Each mL of *Standard preparation* contains about 50 µg of the Reference Standard.
  Test preparation—Transfer about 500 mg of Methyclothiazide, accurately weighed, to a 100-mL volumetric flask, dissolve in and dilute with acetonitrile to volume, and mix.
  Procedure—Pipet 2 mL each of the *Standard preparation* and the *Test preparation* into separate 50-mL volumetric flasks. Pipet 2 mL of acetonitrile into a third 50-mL flask to provide the blank. To each flask add 4 mL of 0.1 N hydrochloric acid, and mix. Add 3.0 mL of sodium nitrite solution (1 in 200) to each flask, mix, and place the flasks in an ice bath for 5 minutes, shaking occasionally. Add to each flask 3.0 mL of ammonium sulfamate solution (1 in 50), mix, and allow the flasks to remain in the ice bath for 1 additional minute. Remove the flasks from the ice bath, add 1.0 mL of N-(1-naphthyl)ethylenediamine dihydrochloride solution (1 in 1000), and mix. Allow the flasks to stand at room temperature for 1 minute, then dilute with water to volume, and mix. Concomitantly determine the absorbances of the solutions obtained from the *Standard preparation* and the *Test preparation* in 1-cm cells at 525 nm, with a suitable spectrophotometer, using the reagent blank to set the instrument. The absorbance of the solution from the *Test preparation* does not exceed that of the solution from the *Standard preparation*, corresponding to not more than 1.0% of diazotizable substances.
Assay—Transfer about 350 mg of Methyclothiazide, accurately weighed, to a 250-mL conical flask, add 40 mL of a 1 in 20 solution of potassium hydroxide in methanol, and reflux at full boil for 1 hour. Cool, rinse the inner walls of the condenser with 20 mL of water and two 20-mL portions of methanol, add 10 mL of glacial acetic acid and 2 drops of eosin Y TS, and titrate with 0.1 N silver nitrate VS to the first appearance of a definite pink color. Each mL of 0.1 N silver nitrate is equivalent to 36.02 mg of $C_9H_{11}Cl_2N_3O_4S_2$.

Methyclothiazide Tablets

» Methyclothiazide Tablets contain not less than 90.0 percent and not more than 110.0 percent of the labeled amount of methyclothiazide ($C_9H_{11}Cl_2N_3O_4S_2$).

Packaging and storage—Preserve in well-closed containers.
USP Reference standards ⟨11⟩—*USP Methyclothiazide RS.*
Identification, *Ultraviolet Absorption* ⟨197U⟩—
  Solution—Powder a number of Tablets, equivalent to about 50 mg of methyclothiazide, and transfer to a 100-mL volumetric flask with the aid of methanol. Add about 60 mL of methanol, and shake the flask for 1 hour. Dilute with methanol to volume, mix, and centrifuge a portion of the solution. Pipet 2 mL of the clear supernatant into a second 100-mL volumetric flask, dilute with methanol to volume, and mix: the UV absorption spectrum of this solution exhibits maxima and minima only at the same wavelengths as that of a similar solution of USP Methyclothiazide RS.
Dissolution ⟨711⟩—
  Medium: 0.01 N hydrochloric acid; 900 mL.
  Apparatus 2: 50 rpm.
  Time: 60 minutes.
  Procedure—Determine the amount of $C_9H_{11}Cl_2N_3O_4S_2$ dissolved by employing UV absorption at the wavelength of maximum absorbance at about 270 nm on filtered portions of the solution under test, suitably diluted with *Dissolution Medium*, if necessary, in comparison with a Standard solution having a known concentration of USP Methyclothiazide RS in the same *Medium*. An amount of alcohol not to exceed 1% of the total volume of the Standard solution may be used to dissolve USP Methyclothiazide RS prior to dilution with *Dissolution Medium*.
  Tolerances—Not less than 70% (*Q*) of the labeled amount of $C_9H_{11}Cl_2N_3O_4S_2$ is dissolved in 60 minutes.
Uniformity of dosage units ⟨905⟩: meet the requirements.
  Procedure for content uniformity—Transfer 1 finely powdered Tablet to a 50-mL volumetric flask, add about 30 mL of methanol, and shake by mechanical means for 1 hour. Dilute with methanol to volume, mix, and centrifuge a portion of the mixture. Dilute quantitatively with methanol to obtain a solution containing approximately 10 µg per mL of methyclothiazide. Concomitantly determine the absorbances of this solution and a Standard solution of USP Methyclothiazide RS in the same medium, having a known concentration of about 10 µg per mL, in 1-cm cells at the wavelength of maximum absorbance at about 267 nm, with a suitable spectrophotometer, using methanol as the blank. Calculate the quantity, in mg, of $C_9H_{11}Cl_2N_3O_4S_2$ in the Tablet taken by the formula:

$$(TC/D)(A_U/A_S)$$

in which T is the labeled quantity, in mg, of methyclothiazide in the Tablet; C is the concentration, in µg per mL, of USP Methyclothiazide RS in the Standard solution; D is the concentration, in µg per mL, of methyclothiazide in the solution from the Tablet, based upon the labeled quantity per Tablet and the extent of dilution; and A_U and A_S are the absorbances of the solution from the Tablet and the Standard solution, respectively.

Assay—

Standard preparation—Transfer about 20 mg of USP Methyclothiazide RS, accurately weighed, to a 100-mL volumetric flask, add methanol to volume, and mix. Transfer 10.0 mL of this solution to a 200-mL volumetric flask, add chloroform to volume, and mix.

Assay preparation—Weigh and finely powder not fewer than 20 Tablets. Transfer an accurately weighed portion of the powder, equivalent to about 2 mg of methyclothiazide, to a 150-mL beaker, add 2.0 mL of methanol, mix, allow the mixture to stand for 30 minutes while taking precautions against loss of solvent, add 2.0 mL of 0.1 M sodium bicarbonate, and mix.

Procedure—[NOTE—Use water-saturated solvents throughout this procedure.] Mix about 3 g of chromatographic siliceous earth with 2.0 mL of 0.1 M sodium bicarbonate in a 150-mL beaker. Pack the mixture into a 25- × 200-mm chromatographic column. Add 4 g of chromatographic siliceous earth to the *Assay preparation*, mix, transfer the mixture to the column, and pack. Dry-wash the beaker with 1 g of the siliceous earth mixed with 3 drops of water, and transfer to the column. Place a small pad of glass wool above the column packing, pass 75 mL of a mixture of isooctane and ether (9 : 1) through the column, and discard the eluate. Using a 200-mL volumetric flask as a receiver, pass 100 mL of chloroform through the column, wash the tip of column with ether, add 10.0 mL of methanol, dilute with chloroform to volume, and mix. Concomitantly determine the absorbances of this solution and the *Standard preparation* at the wavelength of maximum absorbance at about 268 nm, with a suitable spectrophotometer, using chloroform as the blank. Calculate the quantity, in mg, of methyclothiazide ($C_9H_{11}Cl_2N_3O_4S_2$) in the portion of Tablets taken by the formula:

$$0.2C(A_U / A_S)$$

in which C is the concentration, in µg per mL, of USP Methyclothiazide RS in the *Standard preparation;* and A_U and A_S are the absorbances of the solution from the *Assay preparation* and the *Standard preparation*, respectively.

Methylbenzethonium Chloride

$C_{28}H_{44}ClNO_2 \cdot H_2O$ 480.12
Benzenemethanaminium, *N,N*-dimethyl-*N*-[2-[2-[methyl-4-(1,1,3,3-tetramethylbutyl)phenoxy]ethoxy]ethyl]-, chloride, monohydrate.
Benzyldimethyl[2-[2-[[4-(1,1,3,3-tetramethylbutyl)tolyl]oxy]ethoxy]ethyl]ammonium chloride monohydrate   [*1320-44-1*].
Anhydrous   462.12   [*25155-18-4*].

» Methylbenzethonium Chloride contains not less than 97.0 percent and not more than 103.0 percent of $C_{28}H_{44}ClNO_2$, calculated on the dried basis.

Packaging and storage—Preserve in tight containers.
Identification—
  A: To 1 mL of a solution (1 in 100) add 2 mL of alcohol, 0.5 mL of 2 N nitric acid, and 1 mL of silver nitrate TS: a white precipitate, which is insoluble in 2 N nitric acid and soluble in 6 N ammonium hydroxide, is formed.
  B: Treat separate portions of a solution (1 in 100) with 2 N nitric acid and with mercuric chloride TS, respectively: precipitates are formed that dissolve upon the addition of alcohol.
  C: To 10 mL of a solution (1 in 20,000) add 0.1 g of sodium carbonate, 1 mL of bromophenol blue TS, and 10 mL of chloroform, and shake the mixture: the chloroform layer is blue.
  D: Dissolve 100 mg in 1 mL of sulfuric acid, add 1.0 g of potassium nitrate, and heat on a steam bath for 3 minutes. Cautiously dilute the solution with water to 10 mL, add 0.5 g of granulated zinc, and warm the mixture for 10 minutes. Cool, add 0.2 g of sodium nitrite to 1 mL of the clear liquid, and add this mixture to 20 mg of naphthol dipotassium disulfonate or naphthol disodium disulfonate in 1 mL of ammonium hydroxide: the solution turns orange-red, and a brown precipitate may be formed.

Melting range ⟨741⟩:   between 159° and 163°, the specimen having been previously dried.
Loss on drying ⟨731⟩—Dry it at 105° for 4 hours: it loses not more than 5.0% of its weight.
Residue on ignition ⟨281⟩:   not more than 0.1%.
Limit of ammonium compounds—To 5 mL of a solution (1 in 50) add 3 mL of 1 N sodium hydroxide, and heat to boiling: the odor of ammonia is not perceptible.
Assay—Accurately weigh a quantity of Methylbenzethonium Chloride, equivalent to about 500 mg of dried methylbenzethonium chloride, and transfer, with the aid of 35 mL of water, to a glass-stoppered, 250-mL conical separator containing 25 mL of chloroform. Add 10.0 mL of freshly prepared potassium iodide solution (1 in 20), insert the stopper in the separator, shake, allow the layers to separate, and discard the chloroform layer. Wash the aqueous layer with three 10-mL portions of chloroform, and discard the washings. Transfer the aqueous layer to a glass-stoppered, 250-mL conical flask, and rinse the separator with three 5-mL portions of water, adding the washings to the flask. Add 40 mL of cold hydrochloric acid to the flask, mix, and titrate with 0.05 M potassium iodate VS until the solution becomes light brown in color. Add 5 mL of chloroform, insert the stopper in the flask, and shake vigorously. Continue the titration, dropwise, with shaking after each addition, until the chloroform layer becomes colorless and the aqueous layer is clear yellow. Perform a blank determination, using 20 mL of water as the test specimen (see *Residual Titrations* under *Titrimetry* ⟨541⟩). Each mL of 0.05 M potassium iodate is equivalent to 46.21 mg of $C_{28}H_{44}ClNO_2$.

Methylbenzethonium Chloride Lotion

» Methylbenzethonium Chloride Lotion is an emulsion containing not less than 90.0 percent and not more than 110.0 percent of the labeled amount of methylbenzethonium chloride ($C_{28}H_{44}ClNO_2 \cdot H_2O$).

Packaging and storage—Preserve in tight containers.

USP Reference standards ⟨11⟩—*USP Docusate Sodium RS*.
Identification—Suspend about 0.5 mL of Lotion in 20 mL of water, add 0.1 g of sodium carbonate, 1 mL of bromophenol blue TS, and 10 mL of chloroform, and shake the mixture: the chloroform layer is blue.
pH ⟨791⟩:   between 5.2 and 6.0.
Assay—
  0.0001 N Docusate sodium—Dissolve an accurately weighed quantity of USP Docusate Sodium RS in isopropyl alcohol, and dilute quantitatively with isopropyl alcohol to obtain a solution having a concentration of 4.446 mg of anhydrous docusate sodium per mL. Store this solution in a tightly stoppered glass container. On the day of use, pipet 10 mL of this solution into a 1000-mL volumetric flask, add water to volume, and mix to obtain a 0.0001 N solution.
  Procedure—Transfer an accurately weighed portion of Lotion, equivalent to about 0.5 mg of methylbenzethonium chloride, to a glass-stoppered, 50-mL cylinder. Add 5 mL of chloroform (freshly purified by shaking 100 mL with 10 g of silica gel, allowing to settle, and withdrawing the supernatant), 5 mL of phosphoric acid solution (1 in 10), and 1 mL of safranin O solution (1 in 20,000). Titrate with *0.0001 N Docusate sodium* until about 1 mL from the endpoint, then shake the stoppered tube vigorously for about 2 minutes, and continue the titration in 0.1-mL increments, shaking vigorously after each addition, until a pink color appears in the chloroform layer. Perform a blank determination, and make any necessary correction. Each mL of *0.0001 N Docusate sodium* is equivalent to 48.01 µg of methylbenzethonium chloride ($C_{28}H_{44}ClNO_2 \cdot H_2O$).

Methylbenzethonium Chloride Ointment

» Methylbenzethonium Chloride Ointment contains not less than 90.0 percent and not more than 110.0 percent of the labeled amount of methylbenzethonium chloride ($C_{28}H_{44}ClNO_2 \cdot H_2O$).

Packaging and storage—Preserve in collapsible tubes or in tight containers.
USP Reference standards ⟨11⟩—*USP Docusate Sodium RS*.
Identification—Suspend about 0.5 g of Ointment in 10 mL of water, add 0.1 g of sodium carbonate, 1 mL of bromophenol blue TS, and 10 mL of chloroform, and shake: the chloroform layer is blue.
pH ⟨791⟩: between 5.0 and 7.0, in a dispersion of it in carbon dioxide-free water (1 in 100).
Assay—
0.0001 N Docusate sodium—Prepare as directed for *0.0001 N Docusate sodium* in the *Assay* under *Methylbenzethonium Chloride Lotion*.
Procedure—Transfer an accurately weighed portion of Ointment, equivalent to about 0.5 mg of methylbenzethonium chloride, to a glass-stoppered, 50-mL cylinder, and proceed as directed in the *Assay* under *Methylbenzethonium Chloride Lotion*, beginning with "Add 5 mL of chloroform."

Methylbenzethonium Chloride Topical Powder

» Methylbenzethonium Chloride Topical Powder contains not less than 85.0 percent and not more than 115.0 percent of the labeled amount of methylbenzethonium chloride ($C_{28}H_{44}ClNO_2 \cdot H_2O$) in a suitable fine powder base, free from grittiness.

Packaging and storage—Preserve in well-closed containers.
USP Reference standards ⟨11⟩—*USP Docusate Sodium RS*.
Identification—Suspend about 0.1 g in 10 mL of water, add 0.1 g of sodium carbonate, 1 mL of bromophenol blue TS, and 10 mL of chloroform, and shake the mixture: the chloroform layer is blue.
pH ⟨791⟩: between 9.0 and 10.5, in a dispersion of it in carbon dioxide-free water (1 in 100).
Other tests—Not less than 99% of it passes through a No. 200 sieve (see *Powder Fineness* ⟨811⟩).
Assay—
0.0001 N Docusate sodium—Prepare as directed for *0.0001 N Docusate sodium* in the *Assay* under *Methylbenzethonium Chloride Lotion*.
Procedure—Transfer an accurately weighed portion of Topical Powder, equivalent to about 0.5 mg of methylbenzethonium chloride, to a glass-stoppered, 50-mL cylinder, and proceed as directed in the *Assay* under *Methylbenzethonium Chloride Lotion*, beginning with "Add 5 mL of chloroform."

Methylcellulose

Cellulose, methyl ether.
Cellulose methyl ether   [9004-67-5].

» Methylcellulose is a methyl ether of cellulose. When dried at 105° for 2 hours, it contains not less than 27.5 percent and not more than 31.5 percent of methoxy (OCH_3) groups.

Packaging and storage—Preserve in well-closed containers.
Labeling—Label it to indicate its viscosity type [viscosity of a solution (1 in 50)].
Identification—
A: Gently add 1 g to the top of 100 mL of water in a beaker, and allow to disperse over the surface, tapping the top of the container to ensure an even dispersion of the test specimen. Allow the beaker to stand until the specimen becomes transparent and mucilaginous (about 5 hours), and swirl the beaker to wet the remaining substance, add a stirring bar, and stir until solution is complete: the mixture remains stable when an equal volume of 1 N sodium hydroxide or 1 N hydrochloric acid is added.
B: Heat a few mL of the solution prepared for *Identification* test *A*: the solution becomes cloudy and a flaky precipitate, which redissolves as the solution cools, appears.
C: Pour a few mL of the solution prepared for *Identification* test *A* onto a glass plate, and allow the water to evaporate: a thin, self-sustaining film results.
Apparent viscosity—Place a quantity, accurately weighed, equivalent to 2 g of solids on the dried basis, in a tared, wide-mouth 250-mL centrifuge bottle, and add 98 g of water previously heated to 80° to 90°. Stir with a propeller-type stirrer for 10 minutes, place the bottle in an ice-bath, continue the stirring, and allow to remain in the ice-bath for 40 minutes to ensure that hydration and solution are complete. Adjust the weight of the solution to 100 g, if necessary, and centrifuge the solution to expel any entrapped air. Adjust the temperature of the solution to 20 ± 0.1°, and determine the viscosity in a suitable viscosimeter of the Ubbelohde type as directed for *Procedure for Cellulose Derivatives* under *Viscosity* ⟨911⟩. Its viscosity is not less than 80.0% and not more than 120.0% of that stated on the label for viscosity types of 100 centipoises or less, and not less than 75.0% and not more than 140.0% of that stated on the label for viscosity types higher than 100 centipoises.
Loss on drying ⟨731⟩—Dry it at 105° for 2 hours: it loses not more than 5.0% of its weight.
Residue on ignition ⟨281⟩: not more than 1.5%.
Heavy metals, *Method II* ⟨231⟩: 0.001%, adding 1 mL of hydroxylamine hydrochloride solution (1 in 5) to the solution of the residue.
Organic volatile impurities, *Method V* ⟨467⟩: meets the requirements.
Solvent—Use dimethyl sulfoxide.

(Official until July 1, 2008)

Assay—[*Caution—Perform all steps involving hydriodic acid carefully, in a well-ventilated hood. Use goggles, acid-resistant gloves, and other appropriate safety equipment. Be exceedingly careful when handling the hot vials, since they are under pressure. In the event of hydriodic exposure, wash with copious amounts of water, and seek medical attention at once.*]
Hydriodic acid—Use a reagent having a specific gravity of at least 1.69, equivalent to 55% HI.
Internal standard solution—Transfer about 2.5 g of toluene, accurately weighed, to a 100-mL volumetric flask containing 10 mL of *o*-xylene, dilute with *o*-xylene to volume, and mix.
Standard preparation—Into a suitable serum vial weigh about 135 mg of adipic acid, add 4.0 mL of *Hydriodic acid*, then pipet 4 mL of *Internal standard solution* into the vial, and close the vial securely with a suitable septum stopper. Weigh the vial and contents accurately, add 90 µL of methyl iodide with a syringe through the septum, again weigh, and calculate the weight of methyl iodide added, by difference. Shake, and allow the layers to separate.
Assay preparation—Transfer about 0.065 g of dried Methylcellulose, accurately weighed, to a 5-mL thick-walled reaction vial equipped with a pressure-tight septum closure, add an amount of adipic acid equal to the weight of the test specimen, and pipet 2 mL of *Internal standard solution* into the vial. Cautiously pipet 2 mL of *Hydriodic acid* into the mixture, immediately secure the closure, and weigh it accurately. Shake the vial for 30 seconds, heat at 150° for 20 minutes, using a heating block or a protective wrapping, remove it from the source of heat, shake it again, using extreme caution, and heat it as before at 150° for an additional 40 minutes. Allow the vial to cool for about 45 minutes, and again weigh it. If the weight loss is greater than 10 mg, discard the mixture, and prepare another *Assay preparation*.

Chromatographic system—Use a gas chromatograph equipped with a thermal conductivity detector. Under typical conditions, the instrument contains a 1.8-m × 4-mm glass column packed with 10% liquid phase G1 on 100- to 120-mesh support S1A, the column is maintained at 100°, the injection port and the detector are maintained at 200°, and helium is used as the carrier gas at a flow rate of 20 mL per minute.

Calibration—Inject about 2 µL of the upper layer of the *Standard preparation* into the gas chromatograph, and record the chromatogram. The retention times for methyl iodide, toluene, and *o*-xylene are approximately 3, 7, and 13 minutes, respectively. Calculate the relative response factor, F_{mi}, of equal weights of toluene and methyl iodide taken by the formula:

$$Q_{smi} / A_{smi}$$

in which Q_{smi} is the quantity ratio of methyl iodide to toluene in the *Standard preparation*, and A_{smi} is the peak area ratio of the methyl iodide to toluene obtained from the *Standard preparation*.

Procedure—Inject about 2 µL of the upper layer of the *Assay preparation* into the gas chromatograph, and record the chromatogram. Calculate the percentage of methoxy in the Methylcellulose taken by the formula:

$$2(31 / 142) F_{mi} A_{umi} (W_t / W_u)$$

in which 31/142 is the ratio of the formula weights of methoxy and methyl iodide; F_{mi} is defined under *Calibration*, A_{umi} is the ratio of the area of the methyl iodide peak to that of the toluene peak obtained from the *Assay preparation*; W_t is the weight, in g, of toluene in the *Internal standard solution*; and W_u is the weight, in g, of Methylcellulose taken for the *Assay*.

Methylcellulose Ophthalmic Solution

» Methylcellulose Ophthalmic Solution is a sterile solution of Methylcellulose. It contains not less than 85.0 percent and not more than 115.0 percent of the labeled amount of methylcellulose. It may contain suitable antimicrobial, buffering, and stabilizing agents.

Packaging and storage—Preserve in tight containers.
Identification—
  A: Heat a few mL of Ophthalmic Solution: the solution becomes cloudy and a flaky precipitate, which redissolves as the solution cools, appears.
  B: Pour a few mL of Ophthalmic Solution onto a glass plate, and allow the water to evaporate: a thin, self-sustaining film results.
Sterility ⟨71⟩: meets the requirements.
pH ⟨791⟩: between 6.0 and 7.8.
Assay—To boiling flask *A*, as described under *Methoxy Determination* ⟨431⟩, pipet a quantity of Ophthalmic Solution, equivalent to 50 mg of methylcellulose. Evaporate on a steam bath to dryness, cool the flask in an ice bath, add the specified amount of hydriodic acid, and proceed as directed under *Methoxy Determination* ⟨431⟩. Each mL of 0.1 N sodium thiosulfate is equivalent to 1.753 mg of methylcellulose.

Methylcellulose Oral Solution

» Methylcellulose Oral Solution is a flavored solution of Methylcellulose. It contains not less than 85.0 percent and not more than 115.0 percent of the labeled amount of methylcellulose.

Packaging and storage—Preserve in tight, light-resistant containers, and avoid exposure to direct sunlight and to excessive heat. Avoid freezing.
Identification—
  A: Heat a few mL of Oral Solution: the solution becomes cloudy and a flaky precipitate, which redissolves as the solution cools, appears.
  B: Pour a few mL of Oral Solution onto a glass plate, and allow the water to evaporate: a thin, self-sustaining film results.
Microbial limits ⟨61⟩—Its total aerobic microbial count does not exceed 100 cfu per mL, and it meets the requirements of the test for the absence of *Escherichia coli*.
Alcohol content, *Method II* ⟨611⟩: between 3.5% and 6.5% of C_2H_5OH.
Assay—To boiling flask *A*, as described under *Methoxy Determination* ⟨431⟩, transfer an accurately measured volume of Oral Solution, equivalent to 50 mg of methylcellulose. Evaporate on a steam bath to dryness, cool the flask in an ice bath, add the specified amount of hydriodic acid, and proceed as directed under *Methoxy Determination* ⟨431⟩. Each mL of 0.1 N sodium thiosulfate is equivalent to 1.753 mg of methylcellulose.

Methylcellulose Tablets

» Methylcellulose Tablets contain not less than 90.0 percent and not more than 110.0 percent of the labeled amount of methylcellulose.

Packaging and storage—Preserve in well-closed containers.
Identification—
  A: Gently add about 250 mg of the residue obtained in the *Assay* to the top of 25 mL of water in a beaker, and allow to disperse over the surface, tapping the top of the container to ensure an even dispersion of the test specimen. Allow the beaker to stand until the specimen becomes transparent and mucilaginous (about 5 hours), swirl the beaker to wet the remaining substance, add a stirring bar, and stir until dissolved: the mixture remains stable when an equal volume of 1 N sodium hydroxide or 1 N hydrochloric acid is added.
  B: Heat a few mL of the solution prepared for *Identification* test *A*: the solution becomes cloudy, and a flaky precipitate, which redissolves as the solution cools, appears.
  C: Pour a few mL of the solution prepared for *Identification* test *A* onto a glass plate, and allow the water to evaporate: a thin, self-sustaining film results.
Disintegration ⟨701⟩: 30 minutes.
Uniformity of dosage units ⟨905⟩: meet the requirements.
Assay—Weigh and finely powder not less than 20 Tablets. Weigh accurately a portion of the powder, equivalent to about 500 mg of methylcellulose, and transfer to a tared, fine fritted-glass, low-form, 30-mL crucible having a fitted crucible lid. Add 20 mL of alcohol, and macerate the solid for about 5 minutes, mixing intermittently with a glass stirring rod. Repeat the extraction with ten consecutive 10-mL portions of alcohol. Test for completeness of extraction by evaporating the last alcohol extract on a steam bath to dryness, taking up the residue in about 1 mL of water, and adding this to 5 mL of hot alkaline cupric tartrate TS (no red precipitate of cuprous oxide is formed within 5 minutes). If a precipitate is formed, continue with the alcohol extractions until the test is negative. Wash the completely extracted residue with a 10-mL portion of ether, using suction to drain off the liquid. Dry the residue in the crucible in a drying oven at 105° to constant weight. Weigh the crucible with the crucible lid in place. The weight of residue is the weight of methylcellulose present in the portion of powdered Tablets taken.

Methyldopa

$C_{10}H_{13}NO_4 \cdot 1\frac{1}{2}H_2O$ 238.24
L-Tyrosine, 3-hydroxy-α-methyl-, sesquihydrate.
L-3-(3,4-Dihydroxyphenyl)-2-methylalanine sesquihydrate [41372-08-1].
Anhydrous   211.22   [555-30-6].

» Methyldopa contains not less than 98.0 percent and not more than 101.0 percent of $C_{10}H_{13}NO_4$, calculated on the anhydrous basis.

Packaging and storage—Preserve in well-closed, light-resistant containers.

USP Reference standards ⟨11⟩—*USP Methyldopa RS. USP 3-O-Methylmethyldopa RS.*

Identification—
 A: *Infrared Absorption* ⟨197M⟩.
 B: *Ultraviolet Absorption* ⟨197U⟩—
  Solution: 40 μg per mL.
  Medium: 0.1 N hydrochloric acid.
  Absorptivities at 280 nm, calculated on the anhydrous basis, do not differ by more than 3.0%.
 C: To 10 mg add 0.15 mL of a solution of ninhydrin in sulfuric acid (1 in 250): a dark purple color is produced within 5 to 10 minutes. Add 0.15 mL of water: the color changes to pale brownish yellow.

Specific rotation ⟨781S⟩: between −25° and −28°.
 Test solution: 44 mg per mL, in a solvent that is a solution of aluminum chloride in water (2 in 3) which previously has been treated with activated charcoal, filtered, and adjusted with 0.25 N sodium hydroxide to a pH of 1.5.

Acidity—Dissolve 1.0 g in carbon dioxide-free water with the aid of heat, add 1 drop of methyl red TS, and titrate with 0.10 N sodium hydroxide to a yellow endpoint: not more than 0.50 mL is required.

Water, *Method I* ⟨921⟩: between 10.0% and 13.0%.
Residue on ignition ⟨281⟩: not more than 0.1%.
Heavy metals, *Method II* ⟨231⟩: 0.001%.

Limit of 3-O-methylmethyldopa—
 Developing solvent—Mix 65 parts by volume of butyl alcohol, 15 parts by volume of glacial acetic acid, and 25 parts by volume of water. Prepare this mixture fresh.
 Chromatographic plate—Prepare a thin-layer chromatographic plate with a suitable grade of cellulose, 250 μm thick, prewashed with the *Developing solvent*. Wash the plate by placing it in a tank containing the solvent system and allowing the solvent to rise to the top of the plate. Dry with the aid of a current of dry air.
 Spray solution 1—Dissolve 300 mg of *p*-nitroaniline in 100 mL of 10 N hydrochloric acid (*Solution A*). Dissolve 2.5 g of sodium nitrite in 50 mL of water (*Solution B*). Mix 90 mL of *Solution A* and 10 mL of *Solution B* (*Spray solution 1*). Prepare all solutions fresh, just before spraying.
 Spray solution 2—Dissolve 25 g of sodium carbonate in 100 mL of water, and mix.
 Test solution—Dissolve 100 mg of Methyldopa in methanol, and dilute with methanol to 10.0 mL.
 Standard solution—Dissolve 5.0 mg of USP 3-O-Methylmethyldopa RS in methanol, and dilute with methanol to 50.0 mL to obtain a Standard solution having a known concentration of 100 μg per mL.
 Procedure—Apply 20 μL of the *Test solution* in two 10-μL increments and 10 μL of the *Standard solution* to the *Chromatographic plate*, so that the spots are not larger than 0.5 cm in diameter. Develop the chromatogram using the *Developing solvent* until the solvent front has moved about 10 cm from the origin. Remove the plate from the chamber, and dry with the aid of a current of dry air until no odor of acetic acid is perceptible. Place the plate in a vertical position, and evenly spray with *Spray solution 1* until the adsorbent layer is uniformly soaked down to the glass (do not overspray). Place the plate in a horizontal position, and dry as completely as possible with the aid of a current of warm dry air (no odor of hydrochloric acid is perceptible). Place the plate in a vertical position, and evenly spray with *Spray solution 2* until the plate is uniformly wet (do not overspray). The major methyldopa spot is black on a pale pink or orange background at an R_F value of about 0.50, and the 3-O-methylmethyldopa spot is dark on a similar background at an R_F value of about 0.65. The area and intensity of any 3-O-methylmethyldopa spot from the *Test solution* are not greater than those from the *Standard solution* (0.5%).

Organic volatile impurities, *Method V* ⟨467⟩: meets the requirements.
 Solvent—Use dimethyl sulfoxide.
 (Official until July 1, 2008)

Assay—Dissolve about 200 mg of Methyldopa, accurately weighed, in 25 mL of glacial acetic acid, with the aid of heat. Cool to room temperature, and add 0.1 mL of crystal violet TS and 50 mL of acetonitrile. Titrate with 0.1 N perchloric acid VS to a blue endpoint. Perform a blank determination, and make any necessary correction. Each mL of 0.1 N perchloric acid is equivalent to 21.12 mg of $C_{10}H_{13}NO_4$.

Methyldopa Oral Suspension

» Methyldopa Oral Suspension is an aqueous suspension of Methyldopa. It contains one or more suitable flavors, wetting agents, and preservatives, and it may contain Sucrose. It contains not less than 90.0 percent and not more than 110.0 percent of the labeled amount of $C_{10}H_{13}NO_4$.

Packaging and storage—Preserve in tight, light-resistant containers, and store at a temperature not exceeding 26°.

USP Reference standards ⟨11⟩—*USP Methyldopa RS.*

Identification—Apply 10-μL portions of the *Assay preparation* and the *Standard preparation* prepared as directed in the *Assay* to a suitable thin-layer chromatographic plate (see *Chromatography* ⟨621⟩) coated with a 0.25-mm layer of chromatographic silica gel mixture. Allow to dry, develop the chromatogram in a solvent system consisting of equal volumes of acetone, butyl alcohol, glacial acetic acid, toluene, and water until the solvent front has moved about three-fourths of the length of the plate. Remove the plate from the developing chamber, mark the solvent front, and allow the solvent to evaporate. Locate the spots by staining the plate with iodine vapor for about 50 minutes, then view the plate under short-wavelength UV light: the R_F value of the principal spot obtained from the *Assay preparation* corresponds to that obtained from the *Standard preparation*.

Uniformity of dosage units ⟨905⟩—
 FOR ORAL SUSPENSION PACKAGED IN SINGLE-UNIT CONTAINERS: meets the requirements.

Deliverable volume ⟨698⟩—
 FOR ORAL SUSPENSION PACKAGED IN MULTIPLE-UNIT CONTAINERS: meets the requirements.

pH ⟨791⟩: between 3.0 and 5.0; between 3.2 and 3.8 if sucrose is present.

Assay—
 Mobile phase—To 6.8 g of monobasic potassium phosphate add 750 mL of water, and stir until solution is complete. Adjust with 1 M phosphoric acid to a pH of 3.5, dilute with water to 1000 mL, mix, and pass through a filter having a 10-μm or finer porosity.
 Standard preparation—Dissolve an accurately weighed quantity of USP Methyldopa RS in 0.1 N sulfuric acid to obtain a solution having a known concentration of about 1 mg of anhydrous methyldopa per mL.
 Assay preparation—Transfer an accurately measured volume of Oral Suspension, freshly mixed, equivalent to about 250 mg of methyldopa, to a 250-mL volumetric flask, dilute with 0.1 N sul-

furic acid to volume, and mix to dissolve the methyldopa. Pass the solution through a 0.45-µm membrane filter before using.

Chromatographic system (see *Chromatography* ⟨621⟩)—The liquid chromatograph is equipped with a 280-mm detector and a 3.9-mm × 30-cm column that contains packing L1. The flow rate is about 1 mL per minute. Chromatograph three replicate injections of the *Standard preparation,* and record the peak responses as directed for *Procedure:* the relative standard deviation is not more than 2.0%.

Procedure—Separately inject equal volumes (about 50 µL) of the *Standard preparation* and the *Assay preparation* into the chromatograph by means of a suitable microsyringe or sampling valve, record the chromatograms, and measure the responses for the major peaks. Calculate the quantity, in mg, of $C_{10}H_{13}NO_4$ in each mL of the Oral Suspension taken by the formula:

$$250(C/V)(r_U/r_S)$$

in which C is the concentration, in mg per mL, of USP Methyldopa RS in the *Standard preparation;* V is the volume, in mL, of Oral Suspension taken; and r_U and r_S are the peak responses obtained from the *Assay preparation* and the *Standard preparation,* respectively.

Methyldopa Tablets

» Methyldopa Tablets contain not less than 90.0 percent and not more than 110.0 percent of the labeled amount of $C_{10}H_{13}NO_4$.

Packaging and storage—Preserve in well-closed containers.
USP Reference standards ⟨11⟩—*USP Methyldopa RS.*
Identification—
  A: To about 10 mg of finely ground Tablets add 3 drops of a solution of ninhydrin in sulfuric acid (1 in 250): a dark purple color is produced within 5 to 10 minutes. Add 3 drops of water: the color changes to pale brownish yellow.
  B: To about 10 mg of finely ground Tablets add 2 mL of 0.1 N sulfuric acid and 2 mL of *Ferrous tartrate solution* prepared as directed in the *Assay,* then add 0.25 mL of 6 N ammonium hydroxide, and mix: a dark purple color is produced immediately.
Dissolution ⟨711⟩—
  Medium: 0.1 N hydrochloric acid; 900 mL.
  Apparatus 2: 50 rpm.
  Time: 20 minutes.
  Procedure—Determine the amount of $C_{10}H_{13}NO_4$ dissolved from UV absorbances at the wavelength of maximum absorbance at about 280 nm of filtered portions of the solution under test, suitably diluted with *Medium,* if necessary, in comparison with a Standard solution having a known concentration of USP Methyldopa RS in the same medium.
  Tolerances—Not less than 80% (*Q*) of the labeled amount of $C_{10}H_{13}NO_4$ is dissolved in 20 minutes.
Uniformity of dosage units ⟨905⟩: meet the requirements.
Assay—
  Ferrous tartrate solution—Dissolve 1 g of ferrous sulfate, 2 g of potassium sodium tartrate, and 100 mg of sodium bisulfite in water to make 100 mL. Prepare this solution fresh.
  Buffer solution—Dissolve 50 g of ammonium acetate in 1000 mL of 20 percent alcohol. Adjust with 6 N ammonium hydroxide to a pH of 8.5.
  Standard preparation—Dissolve a suitable quantity of USP Methyldopa RS in 0.1 N sulfuric acid to obtain a solution having a known concentration of about 1 mg of anhydrous methyldopa per mL.
  Assay preparation—Weigh and finely powder not less than 20 Tablets. Transfer an accurately weighed portion of the powder, equivalent to about 100 mg of methyldopa, to a 100-mL volumetric flask, add 50 mL of 0.1 N sulfuric acid, agitate by mechanical means for 15 minutes, add the dilute acid to volume, and mix. Filter the solution, rejecting the first 20 mL of the filtrate.

Procedure—Pipet 5 mL each of the *Assay preparation* and *Standard preparation* into separate 100-mL volumetric flasks. To a third 100-mL volumetric flask add 5 mL of water to provide a blank. Add to each flask 5 mL of *Ferrous tartrate solution,* and dilute with *Buffer solution* to volume. Determine the absorbances of both solutions at the wavelength of maximum absorbance at about 520 nm, with a suitable spectrophotometer, using the blank in the reference cell. Calculate the quantity, in mg, of $C_{10}H_{13}NO_4$ in the portion of Tablets taken by the formula:

$$100C(A_U/A_S)$$

in which C is the concentration, in mg per mL, of USP Methyldopa RS in the Standard solution; and A_U and A_S are the absorbances of the solutions from the *Assay preparation* and the *Standard preparation,* respectively.

Methyldopa and Chlorothiazide Tablets

» Methyldopa and Chlorothiazide Tablets contain not less than 90.0 percent and not more than 110.0 percent of the labeled amounts of methyldopa ($C_{10}H_{13}NO_4$) and chlorothiazide ($C_7H_6ClN_3O_4S_2$).

Packaging and storage—Preserve in well-closed containers.

SUSP Reference standards ⟨11⟩—*USP Chlorothiazide RS. USP Methyldopa RS.*
Identification—Transfer the finely ground contents of 1 Tablet to a test tube, add 10 mL of dilute alcohol (1 in 2), shake for 5 minutes, and centrifuge. Use the clear supernatant as the Test solution. Prepare a solution of alcohol and 0.1 N sodium hydroxide (1 : 1) containing in each mL about 10 mg of USP Methyldopa RS and 10 mg of USP Chlorothiazide RS. Apply 20 µL of the Test solution on a line parallel to and about 2 cm from the bottom edge of a 20-cm × 10-cm thin-layer chromatographic plate (see *Chromatography* ⟨621⟩) coated with chromatographic silica gel mixture, and apply 20 µL of the Standard solution separately on the starting line. Allow the spots to dry, develop the chromatogram in a solvent system consisting of equal volumes of glacial acetic acid, acetone, butyl alcohol, toluene, and water until the solvent front has moved about three-fourths of the length of the plate. Remove the plate from the developing tank, and allow the solvent to evaporate. View the plate under short-wavelength UV light: the solution under test exhibits two major spots having R_F values corresponding to those of the two major spots obtained with the Standard solution.
Dissolution ⟨711⟩—
  PROCEDURE FOR METHYLDOPA—
  Medium: 0.1 N hydrochloric acid; 900 mL.
  Apparatus 2: 75 rpm.
  Time: 30 minutes.
  Standard preparation—Dissolve an accurately weighed quantity of USP Methyldopa RS in *Medium,* and dilute quantitatively with the same solvent to obtain a solution having a known concentration of about 275 µg of anhydrous methyldopa per mL.
  Ferrous tartrate solution—Dissolve 1 g of ferrous sulfate, 2 g of potassium sodium tartrate, and 100 mg of sodium bisulfite in water to make 100 mL, and mix. Use a freshly prepared solution.
  Buffer solution—Dissolve 50 g of ammonium acetate in 1000 mL of dilute alcohol (1 in 5). Adjust with 6 N ammonium hydroxide to a pH of 8.5.
  Procedure—Filter 35 mL of the solution under test, and transfer an aliquot estimated to contain between 2 mg and 3 mg of methyldopa to a 100-mL volumetric flask. Adjust the final volume, if necessary, with *Medium* to 10 mL. To a second 100-mL volumetric flask add 10.0 mL of *Standard preparation,* and to a third 100-mL volumetric flask add 10.0 mL of *Medium* to provide a blank. Pipet 5.0 mL of *Ferrous tartrate solution* into each flask, dilute with *Buffer solution* to volume, and mix. Concomitantly determine the absorbances of the treated *Standard preparation* and test solution at the wavelength of maximum absorbance at about 520 nm, with a

suitable spectrophotometer, against the reagent blank. Calculate the amount of $C_{10}H_{13}NO_4$ dissolved, in mg, taken by the formula:

$$9(C/V)(A_U/A_S)$$

in which C is the concentration, in μg of anhydrous methyldopa per mL, of USP Methyldopa RS in the *Standard preparation*; V is the volume, in mL, of the aliquot of test solution used; and A_U and A_S are the absorbances of the solutions from the test solution and the *Standard preparation*, respectively.

Tolerances—Not less than 80% *(Q)* of the labeled amount of $C_{10}H_{13}NO_4$ is dissolved in 30 minutes.

PROCEDURE FOR CHLOROTHIAZIDE—

Medium: 0.05 M, pH 8.0 phosphate buffer (see *Buffer Solutions* in the section *Reagents, Indicators, and Solutions*) containing sodium sulfite (1 in 5000); 900 mL.

Apparatus 2: 75 rpm.

Time: 60 minutes.

Procedure—Determine the amount of $C_7H_6ClN_3O_4S_2$ dissolved from UV absorbances of the solution under test, suitably diluted with *Medium*, if necessary, at the wavelength of maximum absorbance at about 317 nm in comparison with a Standard solution having a known concentration of USP Chlorothiazide RS in the same *Medium*.

Tolerances—Not less than 75% *(Q)* of the labeled amount of $C_7H_6ClN_3O_4S_2$ is dissolved in 60 minutes.

Uniformity of dosage units ⟨905⟩: meet the requirements with respect to methyldopa and to chlorothiazide.

Assay—

Mobile phase—Prepare a filtered and degassed mixture of 0.08 M monobasic sodium phosphate and methanol (95 : 5). Adjust by the addition of phosphoric acid to a pH of 2.8. Make adjustments if necessary (see *System Suitability* under *Chromatography* ⟨621⟩).

Standard preparation—Transfer to a 100-mL volumetric flask accurately weighed quantities of USP Methyldopa RS and USP Chlorothiazide RS, equivalent to one-fifth of their labeled amounts, in mg, per Tablet. Add 15 mL of water and 5 mL of 1 N hydrochloric acid, and sonicate for about 3 minutes. Add 10 mL of acetonitrile, and sonicate for 2 minutes. Dilute with water to volume, and mix.

Assay preparation—Weigh and finely powder not less than 10 Tablets. Transfer an accurately weighed portion of the powder, equivalent to the weight of 1 Tablet, to a 500-mL volumetric flask. Add 75 mL of water and 25 mL of 1 N hydrochloric acid, and sonicate for about 5 minutes. Add 50 mL of acetonitrile, and sonicate for 10 minutes. Dilute with water to volume, and mix. Filter through a 0.45- to 2.0-μm membrane filter, discarding the first 10 mL.

Chromatographic system (see *Chromatography* ⟨621⟩)—The liquid chromatograph is equipped with a 280-nm detector and a 3.9-mm × 30-cm column that contains packing L1. The flow rate is about 2 mL per minute. Chromatograph the *Standard preparation*, and record the peak responses as directed under *Procedure:* the column efficiency determined from the chlorothiazide peak is not less than 1300 theoretical plates, the tailing factor for chlorothiazide peak is not more than 2, the resolution, *R*, between the chlorothiazide and methyldopa peaks is not less than 7, and the relative standard deviation for replicate injections is not more than 2.0%.

Procedure—Separately inject equal volumes (about 10 μL) of the *Standard preparation* and the *Assay preparation* into the chromatograph, record the chromatograms, and measure the responses for the major peaks. The relative retention times are about 1.0 for methyldopa and 2.5 for chlorothiazide. Calculate the quantity, in mg, of chlorothiazide ($C_6H_6ClN_3O_4S_2$) in the portion of Tablets taken by the formula:

$$500C(r_U/r_S)$$

in which C is the concentration, in mg per mL, of USP Chlorothiazide RS in the *Standard preparation*; and r_U and r_S are the peak responses of the chlorothiazide peak obtained from the *Assay preparation* and the *Standard preparation*, respectively. Calculate the quantity, in mg, of methyldopa ($C_{10}H_{13}NO_4$) taken by the same formula, reading "methyldopa" instead of "chlorothiazide."

Methyldopa and Hydrochlorothiazide Tablets

» Methyldopa and Hydrochlorothiazide Tablets contain not less than 90.0 percent and not more than 110.0 percent of the labeled amounts of methyldopa ($C_{10}H_{13}NO_4$) and hydrochlorothiazide ($C_7H_8ClN_3O_4S_2$).

Packaging and storage—Preserve in well-closed containers.

USP Reference standards ⟨11⟩—*USP Hydrochlorothiazide RS. USP Methyldopa RS.*

Identification—

A: The retention times of the 2 major peaks in the chromatogram of the *Assay preparation* correspond to those in the chromatogram of the *Standard preparation* as obtained in the *Assay*.

B: A portion of crushed Tablets, equivalent to about 10 mg of methyldopa, responds to *Identification* test C under *Methyldopa*.

Dissolution ⟨711⟩—

Medium: 0.1 N hydrochloric acid; 900 mL.

Apparatus 2: 50 rpm.

Times: 30 minutes; 60 minutes.

PROCEDURE FOR METHYLDOPA—

Standard preparation—Dissolve an accurately weighed quantity of USP Methyldopa RS in *Medium*, and dilute quantitatively with the same solvent to obtain a solution having a known concentration of about 275 μg of anhydrous methyldopa per mL.

Ferrous tartrate solution—Dissolve 1 g of ferrous sulfate, 2 g of potassium sodium tartrate, and 100 mg of sodium bisulfite in water to make 100 mL. Use a freshly prepared solution.

Buffer solution—Dissolve 50 g of ammonium acetate in 1000 mL of dilute alcohol (1 in 5). Adjust with 6 N ammonium hydroxide to a pH of 8.5.

Procedure—Filter 35 mL of the solution under test through paper, and transfer an aliquot estimated to contain between 2 mg and 3 mg of methyldopa into a 100-mL volumetric flask. Adjust the final volume, if necessary, with *Medium* to 10 mL. To a second 100-mL volumetric flask add 10.0 mL of *Standard preparation*, and to a third 100-mL volumetric flask add 10.0 mL of *Medium* to provide a blank. Treat each flask as follows: Add by pipet 5 mL of *Ferrous tartrate solution* and, dilute with *Buffer solution* to volume. Concomitantly determine the absorbances of the treated *Standard preparation* and test solution in 1-cm cells at the wavelength of maximum absorbance at about 520 nm, with a suitable spectrophotometer, against the reagent blank. Calculate the amount of $C_{10}H_{13}NO_4$ dissolved, in mg, taken by the formula:

$$9(C/V)(A_U/A_S)$$

in which C is the concentration, in μg of anhydrous methyldopa per mL, of USP Methyldopa RS in the *Standard preparation*; V is the volume, in mL, of the aliquot of test solution used; and A_U and A_S are the absorbances of the solutions from the test solution and the *Standard preparation*, respectively.

PROCEDURE FOR HYDROCHLOROTHIAZIDE—Determine the amount of $C_7H_8ClN_3O_4S_2$ dissolved from UV absorbances at the wavelength of maximum absorbance at about 317 nm in 1-cm cells, of filtered portions of the solution under test, suitably diluted with *Dissolution Medium*, in comparison with a Standard solution having a known concentration of USP Hydrochlorothiazide RS in the same medium.

Tolerances—Not less than 80% *(Q)* of the labeled amount of methyldopa ($C_{10}H_{13}NO_4$) is dissolved in 30 minutes, and not less than 80% *(Q)* of the labeled amount of hydrochlorothiazide ($C_7H_8ClN_3O_4S_2$) is dissolved in 60 minutes.

Uniformity of dosage units ⟨905⟩: meet the requirements with respect to methyldopa and to hydrochlorothiazide.

Procedure for content uniformity—Proceed as directed in the *Assay*, except use the following *Test preparation* instead of the *Assay preparation*.

Test preparation—Transfer 1 Tablet to a 250-mL volumetric flask, add 50 mL of water, and shake gently, if necessary, to disintegrate the tablet. Do not sonicate. After the tablet has completely disintegrated, add 25 mL of acetonitrile, and shake by mechanical means for 30 minutes. Add 13 mL of 1 N hydrochloric acid, and shake by mechanical means for an additional 5 minutes. Dilute with water to volume, and mix.

Assay—
*pH 2.8 Sodium phosphate solution—*Dissolve 11.04 g of monobasic sodium phosphate in 950 mL of water. Adjust this solution with phosphoric acid to a pH of 2.8. Transfer the solution to a 1-liter volumetric flask, add water to volume, and mix. Filter through a membrane filter.

*Mobile phase—*Prepare a solution containing 95 volumes of *pH 2.8 Sodium phosphate solution* and 5 volumes of methanol.

*Standard preparation—*Transfer a suitable quantity of USP Methyldopa RS to a 100-mL volumetric flask to obtain a solution having a known concentration of about 1 mg of anhydrous methyldopa per mL. Add an accurately weighed quantity of USP Hydrochlorothiazide RS that corresponds to the ratio of hydrochlorothiazide to methyldopa in the Tablets. Dissolve in 10 mL of water, 10 mL of acetonitrile, and 5 mL of 1 N hydrochloric acid. Dilute with water to volume, and mix.

*Assay preparation—*Weigh and finely powder not less than 20 Tablets. Transfer an accurately weighed portion of the powder, equivalent to about 250 mg of methyldopa, to a 250-mL volumetric flask, and add 50 mL of water, 25 mL of acetonitrile, and 13 mL of 1 N hydrochloric acid. Shake the flask for 5 minutes, dilute with water to volume, and mix.

Chromatographic system (see *Chromatography* ⟨621⟩)—The liquid chromatograph is equipped with a 270-nm detector and a 3.9-mm × 30-cm column that contains packing L1. The flow rate, about 2 mL per minute, is adjusted until the relative retention times for methyldopa and hydrochlorothiazide are about 0.38 and 1.0, respectively. Chromatograph five replicate injections of the *Standard preparation*, and record the peak responses as directed under *Procedure:* the relative standard deviation is not more than 2.0%, and the resolution factor between methyldopa and hydrochlorothiazide is not less than 6.

*Procedure—*Separately inject equal volumes (about 10 µL) of the *Standard preparation* and the *Assay preparation* into the chromatograph by means of a suitable microsyringe or sampling valve. Record the chromatograms, and measure the responses for the major peaks. Calculate the quantity, in mg, of methyldopa ($C_{10}H_{13}NO_4$) in the portion of Tablets taken by the formula:

$$250C(r_U / r_S)$$

in which *C* is the concentration, in mg per mL, of USP Methyldopa RS in the *Standard preparation;* and r_U and r_S are the responses of the methyldopa peak obtained from the *Assay preparation* and the *Standard preparation*, respectively. Calculate the quantity, in mg, of hydrochlorothiazide ($C_7H_8ClN_3O_4S_2$) in the portion of Tablets taken by the same formula, reading "hydrochlorothiazide" instead of "methyldopa."

Methyldopate Hydrochloride

$C_{12}H_{17}NO_4 \cdot HCl$ 275.73

L-Tyrosine, 3-hydroxy-α-methyl-, ethyl ester, hydrochloride.
L-3-(3,4-Dihydroxyphenyl)-2-methylalanine ethyl ester hydrochloride [5123-53-5; 2508-79-4].

» Methyldopate Hydrochloride contains not less than 98.0 percent and not more than 101.0 percent of $C_{12}H_{17}NO_4 \cdot HCl$, calculated on the dried basis.

Packaging and storage—Preserve in well-closed containers. Store at 25°, excursions permitted between 15° and 30°.

USP Reference standards ⟨11⟩—*USP Methyldopate Hydrochloride RS.*

Identification—
A: Infrared Absorption ⟨197M⟩.
B: Ultraviolet Absorption ⟨197U⟩—
Solution: 50 µg per mL.
Medium: 0.1 N hydrochloric acid.
Absorptivities at 280 nm, calculated on the dried basis, do not differ by more than 3.0%.
C: It responds to *Identification* test C under *Methyldopa.*
D: It responds to the tests for *Chloride* ⟨191⟩, except that on the addition of the slight excess of 6 N ammonium hydroxide a brown precipitate is formed.

Specific rotation ⟨781S⟩: between −13.5° and −14.9° (λ= 405 nm).
Test solution: 40 mg per mL, in 0.1 N hydrochloric acid.

pH ⟨791⟩: between 3.0 and 5.0, in a solution (1 in 100).

Loss on drying ⟨731⟩—Dry it at 100° and at a pressure not exceeding 5 mm of mercury for 2 hours: it loses not more than 0.5% of its weight.

Residue on ignition ⟨281⟩: not more than 0.1%.

Heavy metals, *Method II* ⟨231⟩: 0.001%.

Assay—
*Mobile solvent—*Prepare a suitable solution of 0.02 M monobasic sodium phosphate and 0.015 M phosphoric acid in a water and methanol solution (approximately 15.5 : 4.5) such that the retention time of methyldopate hydrochloride is approximately 6.5 minutes.

*Standard preparation—*Dissolve an accurately weighed quantity of USP Methyldopate Hydrochloride RS in the *Mobile solvent* to obtain a solution containing about 1 mg per mL.

*Assay preparation—*Transfer about 50 mg of Methyldopate Hydrochloride, accurately weighed, to a 50-mL volumetric flask, dissolve in and dilute with *Mobile solvent* to volume.

*Procedure—*Introduce separately 20-µL portions of the *Assay preparation* and the *Standard preparation* into a high-pressure liquid chromatograph (see *Chromatography* ⟨621⟩) operated at 25°, by means of a suitable microsyringe or sampling valve, adjusting the operating parameters such that the peak obtained with the *Standard preparation* is 100% full-scale. Typically, the apparatus is fitted with a 4-mm × 30-cm column that contains packing L1, is equipped with an UV detector capable of monitoring absorption at 280 nm and a suitable recorder, and is capable of operating at a column pressure between 700 and 1700 psi. In a suitable chromatogram, three replicate injections of the *Standard preparation* show a relative standard deviation of not more than 1.5%. Determine the peak areas, at equivalent retention times, obtained with the *Assay preparation* and the *Standard preparation,* and calculate the quantity, in mg, of $C_{12}H_{17}NO_4 \cdot HCl$ in the portion of Methyldopate Hydrochloride taken by the formula:

$$50C(A_U / A_S)$$

in which *C* is the concentration, in mg per mL, of USP Methyldopate Hydrochloride RS in the *Standard preparation;* and A_U and A_S are the peak areas obtained from the *Assay preparation* and the *Standard preparation*, respectively.

Methyldopate Hydrochloride Injection

» Methyldopate Hydrochloride Injection is a sterile solution of Methyldopate Hydrochloride in Water for Injection. It contains not less than 90.0 percent and not more than 110.0 percent of the labeled amount of methyldopate hydrochloride ($C_{12}H_{17}NO_4 \cdot HCl$).

Packaging and storage—Preserve in single-dose containers, preferably of Type I glass.

USP Reference standards ⟨11⟩—*USP Endotoxin RS. USP Methyldopate Hydrochloride RS.*

Identification—
A: Dilute a volume of Injection with a mixture of chloroform and methanol (1 : 1), if necessary, to obtain a solution containing about 5 mg of methyldopate hydrochloride per mL. Apply separ-

ately 10 µL of this solution and 10 µL of a Standard solution of USP Methyldopate Hydrochloride RS in a solvent mixture of chloroform and methanol (1 : 1) containing 5 mg per mL to a suitable thin-layer chromatographic plate (see *Chromatography* ⟨621⟩) coated with a 0.25-mm layer of chromatographic silica gel. Allow the spots to dry, and develop the chromatogram in a saturated chamber with a solvent system consisting of a mixture of butyl alcohol, water, and formic acid (7 : 2 : 1), until the solvent front has moved about three-fourths of the length of the plate. Remove the plate from the developing chamber, mark the solvent front, and allow the solvent to evaporate. Locate the spots on the plate by lightly spraying with Folin-Ciocalteu phenol TS followed by spraying with sodium carbonate solution (1 in 10): the R_F value of the principal spot obtained from the test solution corresponds to that obtained from the Standard solution.

B: It responds to the tests for *Chloride* ⟨191⟩, with the exception that the 6 N ammonium hydroxide is omitted.

Bacterial endotoxins ⟨85⟩—It contains not more than 0.5 USP Endotoxin Unit per mg of methyldopate hydrochloride.

pH ⟨791⟩: between 3.0 and 4.2.

Particulate matter ⟨788⟩: meets the requirements under small-volume injections.

Other requirements—It meets the requirements under *Injections* ⟨1⟩.

Assay—

Buffer solution—To 214 g of monobasic potassium phosphate add 700 mL of water, and stir. Cautiously add 75 mL of sodium hydroxide solution (1 in 2), and stir until solution is complete. Adjust with sodium hydroxide solution (1 in 2) to a pH of 8.0, and dilute with water to 1000.0 mL.

Water-saturated tributyl phosphate—Shake 800 mL of tributyl phosphate with 100 mL of water, and discard the lower, aqueous phase. Filter the upper phase.

Standard preparation—Transfer about 25 mg of USP Methyldopate Hydrochloride RS, accurately weighed, to a 25-mL volumetric flask, add water to volume, and mix. Transfer 5 mL of this solution to a 100-mL volumetric flask, add 0.1 N sulfuric acid to volume, and mix. Use a freshly prepared solution. The *Standard preparation* contains about 50 µg per mL.

Assay preparation—Transfer to a 50-mL volumetric flask an accurately measured volume of Injection, equivalent to about 50 mg of methyldopate hydrochloride, add water to volume, and mix. Transfer a 5.0-mL aliquot of the solution to a 60-mL separator, add 15 mL of *Buffer solution* and 10 mL of *Water-saturated tributyl phosphate*, and shake for about 1 minute. Allow the phases to separate, and transfer the lower, aqueous phase to a second 60-mL separator. To this separator add a second 10-mL portion of *Water-saturated tributyl phosphate*, shake for about 1 minute, allow the phases to separate, discard the lower, aqueous phase, and add the upper tributyl phosphate phase to the phase retained in the first separator. Rinse the second separator with about 2 mL of *Water-saturated tributyl phosphate*, and add the rinsing to the first separator. Extract the phase contained in the first separator with two 25-mL portions of 0.1 N sulfuric acid. Collect the acid extracts in a 100-mL volumetric flask, add 0.1 N sulfuric acid to volume, and mix. Filter, if necessary, to obtain a clear solution.

Procedure—Concomitantly determine the absorbances of the *Assay preparation* and the *Standard preparation* in 1-cm cells at the wavelength of maximum absorbance at about 283 nm, with a suitable spectrophotometer, using 0.1 N sulfuric acid as the blank. Calculate the quantity, in mg, of methyldopate hydrochloride ($C_{12}H_{17}NO_4 \cdot HCl$) in each mL of the Injection taken by the formula:

$$(C / V)(A_U / A_S)$$

in which C is the concentration, in µg per mL, of USP Methyldopate Hydrochloride RS in the *Standard preparation*; V is the volume, in mL, of Injection taken; and A_U and A_S are the absorbances of the *Assay preparation* and the *Standard preparation*, respectively.

Methylene Blue

$C_{16}H_{18}ClN_3S \cdot 3H_2O$ 373.90
Phenothiazin-5-ium, 3,7-bis(dimethylamino)-, chloride, trihydrate.
C.I. Basic Blue 9 trihydrate   [7220-79-3].
Anhydrous   319.86   [61-73-4].

» Methylene Blue contains not less than 98.0 percent and not more than 103.0 percent of $C_{16}H_{18}ClN_3S$, calculated on the dried basis.

Packaging and storage—Preserve in well-closed containers. Store at 25°, excursions permitted between 15° and 30°.

USP Reference standards ⟨11⟩—*USP Methylene Blue RS*.

Identification, *Infrared Absorption* ⟨197K⟩.

Loss on drying ⟨731⟩—Dry it at 75° and at a pressure not exceeding 5 mm of mercury for 4 hours: it loses between 8.0% and 18.0% of its weight.

Residue on ignition ⟨281⟩: not more than 1.2%.

Arsenic, *Method I* ⟨211⟩—Prepare the *Test Preparation* by mixing 0.375 g with 10 mL of water in the arsine generator flask. Add 15 mL of nitric acid and 5 mL of perchloric acid, mix, and heat cautiously to the production of strong fumes of perchloric acid. Cool, wash down the sides of the flask with water, and again heat to strong fumes. Again cool, wash down the sides of the flask, and heat to fumes. Cool, dilute with water to 52 mL, and add 3 mL of hydrochloric acid: the resulting solution meets the requirements of the test, the addition of 20 mL of 7 N sulfuric acid specified for *Procedure* being omitted. The limit is 8 ppm.

Copper or zinc—Ignite 1.0 g in a porcelain crucible, using as low a temperature as practicable, until all of the carbon is oxidized. Cool the residue, add 15 mL of 2 N nitric acid, and boil for 5 minutes. Filter the cooled solution, and wash any residue with 10 mL of water. To the combined filtrate and washing add an excess of 6 N ammonium hydroxide, and filter the solution into a 50-mL volumetric flask. Wash the precipitate with small portions of water, adding the washings to the filtrate, dilute the solution with water to volume, and mix. To 25 mL of the solution add 10 mL of hydrogen sulfide TS: no turbidity is produced within 5 minutes (*absence of zinc*). Any dark color produced does not exceed that of a control prepared by boiling a quantity of cupric sulfate, equivalent to 200 µg of copper, with 15 mL of 2 N nitric acid for 5 minutes and by treating this solution as directed above, beginning with "Filter the cooled solution" (0.02% of copper).

Chromatographic purity—Quantitatively dissolve an accurately weighed quantity of Methylene Blue in methanol to obtain a *Test solution* containing 1.0 mg per mL. Dissolve a suitable quantity of USP Methylene Blue RS in methanol to obtain a *Standard solution* having a concentration of 100 µg per mL. Quantitatively dilute a portion of this solution with methanol to obtain a *Diluted standard solution* having a concentration of 10 µg per mL. Apply 5 µL each of the *Test solution*, the *Standard solution*, and the *Diluted standard solution* to a suitable thin-layer chromatographic plate (see *Chromatography* ⟨621⟩) coated with a 0.25-mm layer of octadecylsilanized chromatographic silica gel. Allow the spots to dry, and develop the chromatogram in a chromatographic chamber with a solvent system consisting of a mixture of the upper layer separated from a well-shaken mixture of water, *n*-butanol, and glacial acetic acid (100 : 80 : 20), until the solvent front has moved about three-fourths of the length of the plate. Remove the plate from the chamber, allow the solvent to evaporate, and visually locate the spots on the plate: the R_F value of the principal spot in the chromatogram from the *Test solution* corresponds to that from the *Standard solution*, and other spots, if present in the chromatogram from the *Test solution*, consist of a secondary spot that does not exceed in size or intensity, the principal spot obtained from the *Standard solution* (10%), and not more than two additional spots, neither of which exceeds in size or intensity the principal spot from the *Diluted standard solution* (1%).

Organic volatile impurities, *Method I* ⟨467⟩: meets the requirements.

(Official until July 1, 2008)

Assay—Transfer about 100 mg of Methylene Blue, accurately weighed, to a 250-mL volumetric flask, dissolve in and dilute with diluted alcohol to volume, and mix. Transfer 5.0 mL of this solution to a 100-mL volumetric flask, dilute with diluted alcohol to volume, and mix. Transfer 5.0 mL of this solution to a 50-mL volumetric flask, dilute with diluted alcohol to volume, and mix. This solution contains about 2 μg per mL. Dissolve an accurately weighed quantity of USP Methylene Blue RS in diluted alcohol, and dilute quantitatively and stepwise with diluted alcohol to obtain a Standard solution having a known concentration of about 2 μg per mL. Concomitantly determine the absorbances of both solutions in 1-cm cells at the wavelength of maximum absorbance at about 663 nm, with a suitable spectrophotometer, using diluted alcohol as the blank. Calculate the quantity, in mg, of $C_{16}H_{18}ClN_3S$ in the Methylene Blue taken by the formula:

$$50C(A_U / A_S)$$

in which C is the concentration, in μg per mL, of anhydrous methylene blue in the Standard solution; and A_U and A_S are the absorbances of the solution of Methylene Blue and the Standard solution, respectively.

Methylene Blue Injection

» Methylene Blue Injection is a sterile solution of Methylene Blue in Water for Injection. It contains, in each mL, not less than 9.5 mg and not more than 10.5 mg of methylene blue ($C_{16}H_{18}ClN_3S \cdot 3H_2O$).

Packaging and storage—Preserve in single-dose containers, preferably of Type I glass.

USP Reference standards ⟨11⟩—*USP Endotoxin RS. USP Methylene Blue RS.*

Identification—

A: The visible absorption spectrum of the solution employed for measurement of absorbance in the *Assay* exhibits maxima and minima at the same wavelengths as that of the Standard solution employed in the *Assay*, concomitantly measured.

B: Dilute a portion of the Injection with an equal volume of methanol. Dissolve 5 mg of USP Methylene Blue RS in 1 mL of a mixture of equal volumes of methanol and water. Apply 1 μL of each solution to a thin-layer chromatographic plate, coated with a 0.25-mm layer of chromatographic silica gel, allow the spots to dry, and develop the chromatogram, using a mixture of water, alcohol, and acetic acid (4 : 3 : 3) as the solvent system, until the solvent front has moved about 10 cm above the line of application. Remove the plate from the developing chamber, and allow the solvent to evaporate: the R_F value of the principal spot obtained from the Methylene Blue corresponds to that obtained from the Reference Standard.

Bacterial endotoxins ⟨85⟩—It contains not more than 2.5 USP Endotoxin Units per mL.

pH ⟨791⟩: between 3.0 and 4.5.

Other requirements—It meets the requirements under *Injections* ⟨1⟩.

Assay—Dilute an accurately measured volume of Injection, equivalent to about 100 mg of methylene blue trihydrate to a 200-mL volumetric flask, dissolve in and dilute with diluted alcohol to volume, and mix. Transfer 5.0 mL of this solution to a 100-mL volumetric flask, dilute with diluted alcohol to volume, and mix. Transfer 5.0 mL of this solution to a 50-mL volumetric flask, dilute with diluted alcohol to volume, and mix. This solution contains about 2.4 μg of methylene blue trihydrate (2 μg of anhydrous methylene blue) per mL. Prepare a Standard solution of USP Methylene Blue RS as directed in the *Assay* under *Methylene Blue*. Concomitantly determine the absorbance of both solutions in 1-cm cells at the wavelength of maximum absorbance at about 663 nm, with a suitable spectrophotometer, using diluted alcohol as the blank. Calculate the quantity, in mg, of methylene blue ($C_{16}H_{18}ClN_3S \cdot 3H_2O$) in each mL of the Injection taken by the formula:

$$(373.90 / 319.86)(40C / V)(A_U / A_S)$$

in which 373.90 and 319.86 are the molecular weights of methylene blue trihydrate and anhydrous methylene blue, respectively; C is the concentration, in μg per mL, of USP Methylene Blue RS in the Standard solution; V is the volume, in mL, of Injection taken; and A_U and A_S are the absorbances of the solution from the Injection and the Standard solution, respectively.

Methylergonovine Maleate

$C_{20}H_{25}N_3O_2 \cdot C_4H_4O_4$ 455.50

Ergoline-8-carboxamide, 9,10-didehydro-N-[1-(hydroxymethyl)propyl]-6-methyl-, [8β(S)]-, (Z)-2-butenedioate (1 : 1) (salt).

9,10-Didehydro-N-[(S)-1-(hydroxymethyl)propyl]-6-methylergoline-[8β-carboxamide maleate (1 : 1) (salt)   [7054-07-1].

» Methylergonovine Maleate contains not less than 97.0 percent and not more than 103.0 percent of $C_{20}H_{25}N_3O_2 \cdot C_4H_4O_4$, calculated on the dried basis.

Packaging and storage—Preserve in tight, light-resistant containers, and store in a cold place.

USP Reference standards ⟨11⟩—*USP Methylergonovine Maleate RS.*

Identification—

A: *Infrared Absorption* ⟨197K⟩.

B: The R_F values of the principal fluorescent spot and the principal blue spot obtained from the *Test preparation* correspond to those obtained from *Standard preparation A* in the chromatogram prepared as directed in the test for *Related alkaloids*.

Specific rotation ⟨781S⟩: between +44° and +50°.

Test solution: 5 mg per mL, in water.

pH ⟨791⟩: between 4.4 and 5.2, in a solution (1 in 5000).

Loss on drying ⟨731⟩—Dry it in vacuum at 80° to constant weight: it loses not more than 2.0% of its weight.

Residue on ignition ⟨281⟩: not more than 0.1%.

Related alkaloids—Proceed as directed for *Related alkaloids* under *Ergonovine Maleate*, using Methylergonovine Maleate in place of Ergonovine Maleate.

Assay—[NOTE—Conduct this procedure with a minimum exposure to light.]

Mobile phase—Prepare a filtered and degassed mixture of 0.015 M monobasic potassium phosphate and acetonitrile (4 : 1). Make adjustments if necessary (see *System Suitability* under *Chromatography* ⟨621⟩).

Solvent mixture—Transfer 2.5 g of tartaric acid to a 1000-mL volumetric flask, add 500 mL of water, and mix with shaking. Dilute with methanol to volume, and allow the mixture to cool before use.

Standard preparation—Transfer about 20 mg of USP Methylergonovine Maleate RS, accurately weighed, to a 200-mL volumetric flask. Add 150 mL of *Solvent mixture*, and shake by mechanical means for 15 minutes. Dilute with *Solvent mixture* to volume, and mix. Quantitatively dilute a portion of this solution with *Solvent mixture* to obtain a solution having a known concentration of about 4 μg of USP Methylergonovine Maleate RS per mL.

Assay preparation—Transfer about 100 mg of Methylergonovine Maleate, accurately weighed, to a 500-mL volumetric flask. Add 300 mL of *Solvent mixture*, and shake by mechanical means for 15 minutes or until completely dissolved. Dilute with *Solvent mixture* to volume, and mix. Quantitatively dilute a portion of this solution with *Solvent mixture* to obtain the *Assay preparation* having a known concentration of about 4 μg of Methylergonovine Maleate per mL.

Chromatographic system (see *Chromatography* ⟨621⟩)—The liquid chromatograph is equipped with a fluorometric detector set at an excitation wavelength of 315 nm, and an emission wavelength that is set to zero, using a cutoff filter that passes light from about 418 to 700 nm, and a 4.6-mm × 25-cm column that contains packing L7 maintained at 30°. The flow rate is about 2 mL per minute. Chromatograph the *Standard preparation*, and record the peak responses as directed under *Procedure*: the column efficiency is not less than 1000 theoretical plates, the tailing factor is not more than 2.0, and the relative standard deviation for replicate injections is not more than 2.0%.

Procedure—Separately inject equal volumes (about 20 μL) of the *Standard preparation* and the *Assay preparation* into the chromatograph, record the chromatograms, and measure the responses for the major peaks. Calculate the quantity, in mg, of $C_{20}H_{25}N_3O_2 \cdot C_4H_4O_4$ in the Methylergonovine Maleate taken by the formula:

$$25C(r_U/r_S)$$

in which C is the concentration, in μg per mL, of USP Methylergonovine Maleate RS in the *Standard preparation*, and r_U and r_S are the fluorescence intensity responses obtained from the *Assay preparation* and the *Standard preparation*, respectively.

Methylergonovine Maleate Injection

» Methylergonovine Maleate Injection is a sterile solution of Methylergonovine Maleate in Water for Injection. It contains, in each mL, not less than 90.0 percent and not more than 110.0 percent of the labeled amount of methylergonovine maleate ($C_{20}H_{25}N_3O_2 \cdot C_4H_4O_4$).

Packaging and storage—Preserve in single-dose, light-resistant containers, preferably of Type I glass.

USP Reference standards ⟨11⟩—USP Endotoxin RS. USP Methylergonovine Maleate RS.

Identification—
A: The R_F values of the principal fluorescent spot and the principal blue spot in the chromatogram of the *Test preparation* correspond to those in the chromatogram of the *Standard preparation*, as obtained in the test for *Related alkaloids* under *Ergonovine Maleate*, using the Injection instead of Ergonovine Maleate.

B: Dilute a volume of Injection with water to obtain a solution having a concentration of about 0.67 mg per mL: the solution exhibits a bluish fluorescence under UV light. To this solution, add 2 mL of a solution of glacial acetic acid in ethyl acetate (1 in 2), and stratify 2 mL of sulfuric acid, by pipetting, under the solution: a bluish purple ring appears at the interface of the two liquids.

Bacterial endotoxins ⟨85⟩—It contains not more than 1.7 USP Endotoxin Units per μg of methylergonovine maleate.

pH ⟨791⟩: between 2.7 and 3.5.

Related alkaloids—[NOTE—Conduct this test without exposure to daylight and with minimum exposure to artificial light.]

Solvent mixture—Mix 9 volumes of alcohol with 1 volume of ammonium hydroxide.

Test preparation—Transfer a volume of Injection, equivalent to about 5 mg of methylergonovine maleate, to a separator, and extract with three 5-mL portions of chloroform. Discard the chloroform extracts. Render alkaline to litmus with 6 N ammonium hydroxide, and extract with three 5-mL portions of chloroform. Evaporate the combined extracts with the aid of a current of air, but without heat, to dryness. Dissolve the residue so obtained in 0.5 mL of *Solvent mixture*.

Standard preparation and *Standard dilutions*—Prepare a solution of USP Methylergonovine Maleate RS in *Solvent mixture* to contain 10 mg per mL (*Standard preparation*). Prepare a series of dilutions of the *Standard preparation* in *Solvent mixture* to contain 0.50 mg, 0.20 mg, 0.10 mg, and 0.05 mg per mL (*Standard dilutions*).

Procedure—In a suitable chromatographic chamber arranged for thin-layer chromatography place a volume of a solvent system consisting of a mixture of chloroform, methanol, and water (75 : 25 : 3) sufficient to develop the chromatogram, cover, and allow to equilibrate for 30 minutes. Apply 5-μL portions of the *Test preparation*, the *Standard preparation*, and each of the three *Standard dilutions* to a suitable thin-layer chromatographic plate (see *Chromatography* ⟨621⟩) coated with a 0.25-mm layer of chromatographic silica gel. Allow the spots to dry, and develop the chromatogram until the solvent front has moved about three-fourths of the length of the plate. Remove the plate from the developing chamber, mark the solvent front, and allow the solvent to evaporate. Locate the spots on the plate by spraying thoroughly and evenly with a solution prepared by dissolving 1 g of *p*-dimethylaminobenzaldehyde in a cooled mixture of 50 mL of alcohol and 50 mL of hydrochloric acid: the R_F value of the principal spot obtained from the *Test preparation* corresponds to that obtained from the *Standard preparation*. Estimate the concentration of any other spots observed in the lane for the *Test preparation* by comparison with the *Standard dilutions*: the spots from the 0.50-, 0.20-, 0.10-, and 0.05-mg-per-mL dilutions are equivalent to 5.0%, 2.0%, 1.0%, and 0.50% of impurities, respectively. The sum of the impurities is not greater than 5.0%.

Other requirements—It meets the requirements under *Injections* ⟨1⟩.

Assay—[NOTE—Conduct this procedure with a minimum of exposure to light.]

Mobile phase—Prepare a filtered and degassed mixture of 800 mL of monobasic potassium phosphate solution (1 in 500) and 200 mL of acetonitrile. Make adjustments if necessary (see *System Suitability* under *Chromatography* ⟨621⟩).

Extraction solvent—Dissolve 5 g of tartaric acid in 500 mL of water. Add 500 mL of methanol, and mix.

Standard preparation—Transfer about 20 mg of USP Methylergonovine Maleate RS, accurately weighed, to a 200-mL volumetric flask. Add 150 mL of *Extraction solvent*, and shake by mechanical means for 15 minutes. Dilute with the *Extraction solvent* to volume, and mix to obtain the *Standard preparation* having a known concentration of about 100 μg of USP Methylergonovine Maleate RS per mL.

Assay preparation—Transfer an accurately measured volume of Injection, equivalent to about 10 mg of methylergonovine maleate to a 100-mL volumetric flask. Dilute with *Extraction solvent* to volume, and mix.

Chromatographic system (see *Chromatography* ⟨621⟩)—The liquid chromatograph is equipped with a 240-nm detector, and a 4-mm × 25-cm column that contains packing L7 maintained at 30°. The flow rate is about 2 mL per minute. Chromatograph the *Standard preparation*, and record the peak responses as directed for *Procedure*: the column efficiency determined from the analyte peak is not less than 1000 theoretical plates, the tailing factor is not more than 2.0, and the relative standard deviation for replicate injections is not more than 2.0%.

Procedure—Separately inject equal volumes (about 20 μL) of the *Standard preparation* and the *Assay preparation* into the chromatograph, record the chromatograms, and measure the responses for the major peaks. Calculate the quantity, in mg, of methylergonovine maleate ($C_{20}H_{25}N_3O_2 \cdot C_4H_4O_4$) in each mL of the Injection taken by the formula:

$$0.1(C/V)(r_U/r_S)$$

in which C is the concentration, in μg per mL, of USP Methylergonovine Maleate RS in the *Standard preparation*; V is the volume, in mL, of Injection taken; and r_U and r_S are the peak responses obtained from the *Assay preparation* and the *Standard preparation*, respectively.

peak response ratios of the analyte to the internal standard for replicate injections is not more than 2.0%.

Procedure—Separately inject equal volumes (about 50 µL) of the *Standard preparation* and the *Assay preparation* into the chromatograph, record the chromatograms, and measure the responses for the major peaks. Calculate the quantity, in mg, of methylphenidate hydrochloride ($C_{14}H_{19}NO_2 \cdot HCl$) in the portion of Tablets taken by the formula:

$$100C(R_U / R_S)$$

in which C is the concentration, in mg per mL, of USP Methylphenidate Hydrochloride RS in the standard stock solution used to prepare the *Standard preparation;* and R_U and R_S are the peak response ratios of the analyte to the internal standard obtained from the *Assay preparation* and the *Standard preparation*, respectively.

Methylphenidate Hydrochloride Extended-Release Tablets

» Methylphenidate Hydrochloride Extended-Release Tablets contain not less than 90.0 percent and not more than 110.0 percent of the labeled amount of methylphenidate hydrochloride ($C_{14}H_{19}NO_2 \cdot HCl$).

Packaging and storage—Preserve in tight containers.

USP Reference standards ⟨11⟩—*USP Methylphenidate Hydrochloride RS.*

Identification—Place a portion of powdered Tablets, equivalent to about 100 mg of methylphenidate hydrochloride, in a 100-mL beaker. Add 20 mL of chloroform, stir for 5 minutes, and filter, collecting the filtrate. Evaporate the filtrate to about 5 mL. Add ethyl ether slowly, with stirring, until crystals form. Filter the crystals, wash with ethyl ether, and dry at 80° for 30 minutes: the IR absorption spectrum of a mineral oil dispersion of the crystals so obtained exhibits maxima only at the same wavelengths as that of a similar preparation of USP Methylphenidate Hydrochloride RS.

Dissolution ⟨711⟩—

Medium: water; 500 mL.

Apparatus 2: 50 rpm.

Times: 1, 2, 3.5, 5, and 7 hours.

Test solution—Use portions of the solution under test passed through a 0.45-µm polypropylene filter. [NOTE—Do not use glass fiber filters.]

Procedure—Determine the amount of $C_{14}H_{19}NO_2 \cdot HCl$ dissolved, employing the procedure set forth in the *Assay*, making any necessary volumetric adjustments.

Tolerances—The percentages of the labeled amount of $C_{14}H_{19}NO_2 \cdot HCl$ dissolved at the times specified conform to *Acceptance Table 2*.

Time (hours)	Amount dissolved
1	between 25% and 45%
2	between 40% and 65%
3.5	between 55% and 80%
5	between 70% and 90%
7	not less than 80%

Uniformity of dosage units ⟨905⟩: meet the requirements.

Assay—Proceed as directed in the *Assay* under *Methylphenidate Hydrochloride Tablets*, using Extended-Release Tablets.

Methylprednisolone

$C_{22}H_{30}O_5$ 374.48

Pregna-1,4-diene-3,20-dione, 11,17,21-trihydroxy-6-methyl-, (6α,11β)-.

11β,17,21-Trihydroxy-6α-methylpregna-1,4-diene-3,20-dione [83-43-2].

» Methylprednisolone contains not less than 97.0 percent and not more than 103.0 percent of $C_{22}H_{30}O_5$, calculated on the dried basis.

Packaging and storage—Preserve in tight, light-resistant containers.

USP Reference standards ⟨11⟩—*USP Methylprednisolone RS.*

Identification—

A: *Infrared Absorption* ⟨197K⟩.

B: *Ultraviolet Absorption* ⟨197U⟩—

Solution: 10 µg per mL.

Medium: alcohol.

Absorptivities at 243 nm, calculated on the dried basis, do not differ by more than 3.0%.

C: Dissolve about 5 mg in 2 mL of sulfuric acid: a red color is produced.

Specific Rotation ⟨781S⟩: between +79° and +86°.

Test solution: 5 mg per mL, in dioxane.

Loss on drying ⟨731⟩—Dry it at 105° for 3 hours: it loses not more than 1.0% of its weight.

Residue on ignition ⟨281⟩: not more than 0.2%.

Chromatographic purity—

Mobile phase—Prepare a filtered and degassed mixture of water, tetrahydrofuran, dimethylsulfoxide, and butanol (149 : 40 : 10 : 1). Make adjustments if necessary (see *System Suitability* under *Chromatography* ⟨621⟩).

Diluting solution—Prepare a filtered mixture of water, tetrahydrofuran, and glacial acetic acid (72 : 25 : 3).

Standard solution—Dissolve an accurately weighed quantity of USP Methylprednisolone RS in *Diluting solution*. Dilute quantitatively, and stepwise if necessary, with *Diluting solution* to obtain a solution having a known concentration of about 0.01 mg per mL.

Test solution—Transfer about 25 mg of Methylprednisolone, accurately weighed, to a 25-mL volumetric flask, dissolve in and dilute with *Diluting solution* to volume, and mix.

Chromatographic system (see *Chromatography* ⟨621⟩)—The liquid chromatograph is equipped with a 254-nm detector and a 4.6-mm × 20-cm column that contains packing L1. The flow rate is about 1 mL per minute. Chromatograph the *Standard solution*, and record the peak responses as directed for *Procedure:*the column efficiency is not less than 800 theoretical plates; and the relative standard deviation for replicate injections is not more than 5.0%.

Procedure—Separately inject equal volumes (about 10 µL) of the *Standard solution* and the *Test solution* into the chromatograph, record the chromatograms, and measure the peak responses. Calculate the percentage of each impurity in the portion of Methylprednisolone taken by the formula:

$$25 \times 100(C/W)(r_i / r_S)$$

in which C is the concentration, in mg per mL, of USP Methylprednisolone RS in the *Standard solution;* W is the weight, in mg, of the sample taken to prepare the *Test solution;* r_i is the peak response for each impurity obtained from the *Test solution;* and r_S is the peak response for methylprednisolone in the *Standard solution:* not more than 1.0% of any individual impurity is found, and not more than 2.0% of total impurities is found.

2684 Methylprednisolone / Official Monographs

Assay—
Mobile phase—Prepare a solution containing a mixture of butyl chloride, water-saturated butyl chloride, tetrahydrofuran, methanol, and glacial acetic acid (475 : 475 : 70 : 35 : 30).
Internal standard solution—Dissolve prednisone in a 3 in 100 solution of glacial acetic acid in chloroform to obtain a solution having a concentration of about 0.2 mg per mL.
Standard preparation—Dissolve an accurately weighed quantity of USP Methylprednisolone RS in *Internal standard solution* to obtain a solution having a known concentration of about 0.2 mg per mL.
Assay preparation—Using about 10 mg of Methylprednisolone, accurately weighed, proceed as directed for *Standard preparation*.
Chromatographic system (see *Chromatography* ⟨621⟩)—The liquid chromatograph is equipped with a 254-nm detector and a 4-mm × 25-cm column that contains packing L3. The flow rate is about 1 mL per minute. Chromatograph the *Standard preparation*, and record the peak responses as directed for *Procedure*: the resolution, *R*, between the methylprednisolone and internal standard peaks is not less than 4.0; and the relative standard deviation for replicate injections is not more than 2.0%.
Procedure—Separately inject equal volumes (about 10 μL) of the *Standard preparation* and the *Assay preparation* into the chromatograph, record the chromatograms, and measure the responses for the major peaks: the relative retention times are about 0.7 for prednisone and 1.0 for methylprednisolone. Calculate the quantity, in mg, of $C_{22}H_{30}O_5$ in the portion of Methylprednisolone taken by the formula:

$$50C(R_U/R_S)$$

in which *C* is the concentration, in mg per mL, of USP Methylprednisolone RS in the *Standard preparation;* and R_U and R_S are the ratios of the peak responses for the methylprednisolone peak and the internal standard peak obtained from the *Assay preparation* and the *Standard preparation*, respectively.

Methylprednisolone Tablets

» Methylprednisolone Tablets contain not less than 92.5 percent and not more than 107.5 percent of the labeled amount of methylprednisolone ($C_{22}H_{30}O_5$).

Packaging and storage—Preserve in tight containers.
USP Reference standards ⟨11⟩—*USP Methylprednisolone RS.*
Identification—Powder a number of Tablets, equivalent to about 40 mg of methylprednisolone, and digest with 25 mL of solvent hexane for 15 minutes. Filter, and discard the filtrate. Digest the residue with 25 mL of chloroform for 15 minutes. Filter, evaporate the filtrate to dryness, and dry at 105° for 2 hours: the residue so obtained responds to *Identification* tests *A* and *C* under *Methylprednisolone.*
Dissolution ⟨711⟩—
Medium: water; 900 mL.
Apparatus 2: 50 rpm.
Time: 30 minutes.
Procedure—Measure the UV absorption of filtered aliquots removed from the *Dissolution Medium* and suitably diluted, if necessary, in 1-cm cells at 246 nm, with a suitable spectrophotometer, using water as the blank and utilizing a standard curve, representing the absorbance versus concentration of USP Methylprednisolone RS. [NOTE—Dissolve about 20 mg of USP Methylprednisolone RS, accurately weighed, in 1 mL of alcohol, dilute in a 1000-mL volumetric flask with water to volume, and mix. Prepare quantitative dilutions of this solution for the development of a standard curve.]
Tolerances—Not less than 70% (*Q*) of the labeled amount of $C_{22}H_{30}O_5$ is dissolved in 30 minutes.
Uniformity of dosage units ⟨905⟩: meet the requirements.
PROCEDURE FOR CONTENT UNIFORMITY—
Mobile phase, Internal standard solution, Standard preparation, and *Chromatographic system*—Proceed as directed in the *Assay* under *Methylprednisolone.*

Test preparation—Place 1 Tablet in a suitable container. For tablet labeled strengths of 10 mg or less, add 0.5 mL of water. For tablet labeled strengths greater than 10 mg, add 1.0 mL of water. Allow the tablet to stand for about 2 minutes, then swirl the container to disperse the tablet. Add 5.0 mL of *Internal standard solution* for each mg of labeled tablet strength, shake for 15 minutes, and filter or centrifuge a portion of the test specimen. Analyze the clear solution as directed under *Procedure.*
Procedure—Proceed as directed for *Procedure* in the *Assay* under *Methylprednisolone.* Calculate the quantity, in mg, of $C_{22}H_{30}O_5$ in the Tablet taken by the formula:

$$(FW_S)(R_U/R_S)$$

in which *F* is the ratio of the volume of *Internal standard preparation*, in mL, in the *Test preparation* to the volume, in mL, of the *Internal standard preparation* in the *Standard preparation*; W_S is the weight, in mg, of USP Methylprednisolone RS taken for the *Standard preparation*; and the other terms are as defined for *Procedure* in the *Assay* under *Methylprednisolone.*
Assay—
Mobile phase, Internal standard solution, Standard preparation, and *Chromatographic system*—Proceed as directed in the *Assay* under *Methylprednisolone.*
Assay preparation—Accurately weigh 20 Tablets, and grind to a fine powder in a mortar and pestle. Accurately weigh a portion of the powder, equivalent to about 10 mg of methylprednisolone, and transfer to a suitable container. Add 2.5 mL of water to the ground tablet material and swirl to form a fine slurry. Add 50.0 mL of *Internal standard solution*, and shake for 15 minutes. Filter or centrifuge a portion of the liquid so obtained, if necessary, and analyze the clear solution as directed under *Procedure.*
Procedure—Proceed as directed for *Procedure* in the *Assay* under *Methylprednisolone.* Calculate the quantity, in mg, of $C_{22}H_{30}O_5$ in the portion of Tablets taken by the formula:

$$50C(R_U/R_S)$$

in which the terms are as defined therein.

Methylprednisolone Acetate

$C_{24}H_{32}O_6$ 416.51
Pregna-1,4-diene-3,20-dione, 21-(acetyloxy)-11,17-dihydroxy-6-methyl-, (6α,11β)-.
11β,17,21-Trihydroxy-6α-methylpregna-1,4-diene-3,20-dione 21-acetate   [53-36-1].

» Methylprednisolone Acetate contains not less than 97.0 percent and not more than 103.0 percent of $C_{24}H_{32}O_6$, calculated on the dried basis.

Packaging and storage—Preserve in tight, light-resistant containers. Store at 25°, excursions permitted between 15° and 30°.
USP Reference standards ⟨11⟩—*USP Methylprednisolone Acetate RS.*
Identification—
A: Infrared Absorption ⟨197K⟩.
B: Ultraviolet Absorption ⟨197U⟩—
Solution: 10 μg per mL.
Medium: alcohol.
Absorptivities at 243 nm, calculated on the dried basis, do not differ by more than 3.0%.
Specific rotation ⟨781S⟩: between +97° and +105°.
Test solution: 10 mg per mL, in dioxane.
Loss on drying ⟨731⟩—Dry it at 105° for 3 hours: it loses not more than 1.0% of its weight.
Residue on ignition ⟨281⟩: not more than 0.2%.
Chromatographic purity—
Mobile phase—Prepare a filtered and degassed mixture of water and tetrahydrofuran (149 : 51). Make adjustments if necessary (see *System Suitability* under *Chromatography* ⟨621⟩).
Diluting solution—Prepare a mixture of water, tetrahydrofuran, acetonitrile, and glacial acetic acid (499 : 250 : 250 : 1).

Standard solution—Dissolve an accurately weighed quantity of USP Methylprednisolone Acetate RS, sonicate if necessary, in *Diluting solution*, and dilute quantitatively, and stepwise if necessary, with *Diluting solution* to obtain a solution having a known concentration of about 20 µg per mL.

Test solution—Transfer about 20 mg of Methylprednisolone Acetate, accurately weighed, to a 20-mL volumetric flask, dissolve in *Diluting solution*, sonicate if necessary, dilute with *Diluting solution* to volume, and mix.

Chromatographic system (see *Chromatography* ⟨621⟩)—The liquid chromatograph is equipped with a 254-nm detector and a 4.6-mm × 25-cm column that contains packing L1. The flow rate is about 1 mL per minute. Chromatograph the *Standard solution*, and record the peak responses as directed for *Procedure*: the relative standard deviation for replicate injections is not more than 5.0%.

Procedure—Inject equal volumes (about 20 µL) of the *Standard solution* and the *Test solution* into the chromatograph, record the chromatograms, and measure the peak responses. Calculate the percentage of each impurity in the portion of Methylprednisolone Acetate taken by the formula:

$$2000(C/W)(r_i/r_S)$$

in which C is the concentration, in mg per mL, of USP Methylprednisolone Acetate RS in the *Standard solution*; W is the weight, in mg, of Methylprednisolone Acetate taken in the *Test solution*; r_i is the peak response for each impurity; and r_S is the peak response of methylprednisolone in the *Standard solution*: not more than 1.0% of any individual impurity is found; and not more than 2.0% of total impurities is found.

Assay—

Mobile phase—Prepare a mixture of n-butyl chloride, water-saturated n-butyl chloride, tetrahydrofuran, methanol, and glacial acetic acid (475 : 475 : 70 : 35 : 30). Make adjustments if necessary (see *System Suitability* under *Chromatography* ⟨621⟩).

Internal standard solution—Prepare a solution containing about 6 mg per mL of prednisone in a mixture of chloroform and glacial acetic acid (97 : 3) by first adding the entire amount of glacial acetic acid to the prednisone contained in a 100-mL volumetric flask, followed by sonication. Then slowly add the chloroform, using sonication and shaking to dissolve the material. Dilute with chloroform to volume, and mix.

Standard preparation—Transfer about 20 mg of USP Methylprednisolone Acetate RS, accurately weighed, and 5.0 mL of the *Internal standard solution* to a 100-mL volumetric flask. Dilute with chloroform to volume, and shake to dissolve the specimen.

Assay preparation—Prepare a solution of Methylprednisolone Acetate as directed under *Standard preparation*.

Chromatographic system (see *Chromatography* ⟨621⟩)—The liquid chromatograph is equipped with a 254-nm detector and a 4-mm × 25-cm column that contains packing L3. The flow rate is about 1 mL per minute. Chromatograph the *Standard preparation*, and record the peak responses as directed for *Procedure*: the relative retention times are about 1.3 for prednisone and 1.0 for methylprednisolone acetate; the resolution, R, between the analyte and internal standard peaks is not less than 2.5; and the relative standard deviation for replicate injections is not more than 2.0%.

Procedure—Separately inject equal volumes (about 10 µL) of the *Standard preparation* and the *Assay preparation* into the chromatograph, record the chromatograms, and measure the responses for the major peaks. Calculate the quantity, in mg, of $C_{24}H_{32}O_6$ in the portion of Methylprednisolone Acetate taken by the formula:

$$100C(R_U/R_S)$$

in which C is the concentration, in mg per mL, of USP Methylprednisolone Acetate RS in the *Standard preparation*; and R_U and R_S are the peak height response ratios of the methylprednisolone acetate peak and the internal standard peak obtained from the *Assay preparation* and the *Standard preparation*, respectively.

Methylprednisolone Acetate Cream

» Methylprednisolone Acetate Cream contains not less than 90.0 percent and not more than 110.0 percent of the labeled amount of methylprednisolone acetate ($C_{24}H_{32}O_6$).

Packaging and storage—Preserve in collapsible tubes or in tight containers, protected from light.

USP Reference standards ⟨11⟩—*USP Methylprednisolone Acetate RS*.

Identification—In the thin-layer chromatogram, prepared as directed in the *Assay*, the R_F value of the principal spot obtained from the *Assay preparation* corresponds to that obtained from the *Standard preparation*, prepared as directed in the *Assay*.

Minimum fill ⟨755⟩: meets the requirements.

Assay—

Standard preparation—Dissolve an accurately weighed quantity of USP Methylprednisolone Acetate RS in a mixture of equal volumes of alcohol and chloroform, and dilute quantitatively with the same solvent to obtain a solution having a known concentration of about 500 µg per mL.

Assay preparation—Transfer an accurately weighed quantity of Cream, equivalent to about 5 mg of methylprednisolone acetate, to a 125-mL separator, add 50 mL of solvent hexane, and mix. Extract with three 10-mL portions of acetonitrile, and evaporate the combined extracts on a steam bath with the aid of a current of air nearly to dryness. Transfer the residue to a 10-mL volumetric flask with the aid of one 5-mL portion and two 2-mL portions of a mixture of equal volumes of alcohol and chloroform, dilute with the same solvent to volume, and mix.

Procedure—Divide the area of a suitable thin-layer chromatographic plate (see *Chromatography* ⟨621⟩) coated with a 0.5-mm layer of chromatographic silica gel mixture, into three equal sections, the left and right sections to be used for the *Assay preparation* and the *Standard preparation*, respectively, and the center section for the blank. Apply 250 µL each of the *Assay preparation* and of the *Standard preparation* as streaks 2.5 cm from the bottom of the designated section of the plate, and dry the streaks with the aid of a current of air. Develop the chromatogram in a solvent system consisting of a mixture of ethyl acetate and chloroform (7 : 5) until the solvent front has moved about three-fourths of the length of the plate. Remove the plate from the developing chamber, mark the solvent front, and allow the solvent to evaporate. Locate the principal bands occupied by the *Standard preparation* and the *Assay preparation* (see also the *Identification* test) by viewing under short-wavelength UV light. Mark these bands and the corresponding band in the section of the plate representing the blank. Quantitatively remove the silica gel containing these bands, and transfer to separate glass-stoppered, 50-mL centrifuge tubes. Add 25.0 mL of alcohol to each tube, shake for 2 minutes, and centrifuge at about 1500 rpm for 5 minutes. Transfer 20.0 mL of each supernatant to separate glass-stoppered, 50-mL conical flasks, add 2.0 mL of blue tetrazolium TS to each solution, mix, and to each flask add 2.0 mL of a mixture of 1 volume of tetramethylammonium hydroxide TS and 9 volumes of alcohol. Mix, and allow the solutions to stand in the dark for 90 minutes. Concomitantly determine the absorbances of the solutions in 1-cm cells at the wavelength of maximum absorbance at about 525 nm, with a suitable spectrophotometer, against the blank. Calculate the quantity, in mg, of methylprednisolone acetate ($C_{24}H_{32}O_6$) in the portion of Cream taken by the formula:

$$0.01C(A_U/A_S)$$

in which C is the concentration, in µg per mL, of USP Methylprednisolone Acetate RS in the *Standard preparation*; and A_U and A_S are the absorbances of the solutions from the *Assay preparation* and the *Standard preparation*, respectively.

Methylprednisolone Acetate Injectable Suspension

» Methylprednisolone Acetate Injectable Suspension is a sterile suspension of Methylprednisolone Acetate in a suitable aqueous medium. It contains not less than 90.0 percent and not more than 110.0 percent of the labeled amount of methylprednisolone acetate ($C_{24}H_{32}O_6$).

Packaging and storage—Preserve in single-dose or in multiple-dose containers, preferably of Type I glass.

USP Reference standards ⟨11⟩—*USP Methylprednisolone Acetate RS.*

Identification, *Infrared Absorption* ⟨197K⟩—Obtain the test specimen as follows. Filter a volume of Injectable Suspension, equivalent to about 100 mg of methylprednisolone acetate, through paper. Wash the residue with several 5-mL portions of water, and dry at 105° for 3 hours.

Uniformity of dosage units ⟨905⟩: meets the requirements.

pH ⟨791⟩: between 3.0 and 7.0.

Particle size—Transfer 1 drop to a microscope slide, and spread evenly, diluting with water, if necessary, to decrease the density of the field. Examine the slide under a microscope, equipped with a calibrated ocular micrometer, using about 400× magnification. Scan the entire slide, and note the size of the individual particles: not less than 99% of the particles are less than 20 μm in length when measured along the longest axis, and not less than 75% of the particles are less than 10 μm.

Other requirements—It meets the requirements under *Injections* ⟨1⟩.

Assay—

Mobile phase, Internal standard solution, Standard preparation, and *Chromatographic system*—Proceed as directed in the *Assay* under *Methylprednisolone Acetate.*

Assay preparation—Swirl the Injectable Suspension to ensure uniformity prior to analysis. Transfer an accurately measured volume of Injectable Suspension, equivalent to about 40 mg of methylprednisolone acetate, to a 25-mL volumetric flask, add 10.0 mL of *Internal standard solution*, dilute with chloroform to volume, and shake for about 15 minutes or until the aqueous layer is clear. Transfer 4.0 mL of the chloroform layer to a suitable vial, add 30 mL of chloroform and a small quantity (about 400 mg) of anhydrous sodium sulfate, shake for 5 minutes, and use the clear solution.

Procedure—Proceed as directed for *Procedure* in the *Assay* under *Methylprednisolone Acetate.* Calculate the quantity, in mg, of methylprednisolone acetate ($C_{24}H_{32}O_6$) in each mL of the Injectable Suspension taken by the formula:

$$(200C / V)(R_U / R_S)$$

in which V is the volume, in mL, of Injectable Suspension taken, and the other terms are as defined therein.

Methylprednisolone Hemisuccinate

$C_{26}H_{34}O_8$ 474.54

Pregna-1,4-diene-3,20-dione, 21-(3-carboxy-1-oxopropoxy)-11,17-dihydroxy-6-methyl-, (6α,11β)-.

11β,17,21-Trihydroxy-6α-methylpregna-1,4-diene-3,20-dione 21-(hydrogen succinate)   [2921-57-5].

» Methylprednisolone Hemisuccinate contains not less than 97.0 percent and not more than 103.0 percent of $C_{26}H_{34}O_8$, calculated on the dried basis.

Packaging and storage—Preserve in tight containers.

USP Reference standards ⟨11⟩—*USP Fluorometholone RS. USP Methylprednisolone Hemisuccinate RS.*

Identification—

A: *Infrared Absorption* ⟨197M⟩.

B: *Ultraviolet Absorption* ⟨197U⟩—

Solution: 20 μg per mL.

Medium: alcohol.

Absorptivities at 243 nm, calculated on the dried basis, do not differ by more than 3.0%.

Specific rotation ⟨781S⟩: between +87° and +95°.

Test solution: 10 mg per mL, in dioxane.

Loss on drying ⟨731⟩—Dry it at 105° for 3 hours: it loses not more than 1.0% of its weight.

Residue on ignition ⟨281⟩: not more than 0.2%.

Chromatographic purity—

Diluent—Prepare a mixture of water, tetrahydrofuran, acetonitrile, and acetic acid (47 : 25 : 25 : 3).

Mobile phase—Prepare a filtered and degassed mixture of water, tetrahydrofuran, and formic acid (745 : 255 : 1). Make adjustments if necessary (see *System Suitability* under *Chromatography* ⟨621⟩).

Standard solution—Dissolve an accurately weighed quantity of USP Methylprednisolone Hemisuccinate RS in *Diluent* to obtain a solution having a final concentration of about 0.02 mg per mL.

Test solution—Prepare a solution of Methylprednisolone Hemisuccinate in *Diluent* containing about 1 mg per mL. Shake or sonicate to aid in solubilization.

Chromatographic system (see *Chromatography* ⟨621⟩)—The liquid chromatograph is equipped with a 254-nm detector and a 4.6-mm × 20-cm column that contains 5-μm packing L1. The flow rate is about 1.0 mL per minute. Chromatograph the *Standard solution*, and record the peak responses as directed for *Procedure:* the column efficiency determined from the methylprednisolone hemisuccinate peak is not less than 5000; and the relative standard deviation for replicate injections is not more than 5.0%.

Procedure—Separately inject equal volumes (about 20 μL) of the *Standard solution* and the *Test solution* into the chromatograph, record the chromatograms, and measure all of the peak areas. Calculate the percentage of each impurity in the portion of Methylprednisolone Hemisuccinate taken by the formula:

$$100(C_S / C_U)(r_i / r_S)$$

in which C_S is the concentration, in mg per mL, of USP Methylprednisolone Hemisuccinate RS in the *Standard solution;* C_U is the concentration, in mg per mL, of Methylprednisolone Hemisuccinate in the *Test solution;* r_i is the peak area for each impurity obtained from the *Test solution;* and r_S is the peak area of methylprednisolone hemisuccinate obtained from the *Standard solution:* not more than 1.0% of any individual impurity is found, and not more than 2.0% of total impurities is found.

Assay—

Internal standard solution—Dissolve USP Fluorometholone RS in tetrahydrofuran to obtain a solution containing about 6 mg per mL.

Mobile phase—Prepare a solution containing a mixture of butyl chloride, water-saturated butyl chloride, tetrahydrofuran, methanol, and glacial acetic acid (475 : 475 : 70 : 35 : 30).

Standard preparation—Transfer about 40 mg of USP Methylprednisolone Hemisuccinate RS, accurately weighed, to a 100-mL volumetric flask. Add 5.0 mL of *Internal standard solution.* Dilute with chloroform containing 3% glacial acetic acid to volume, and mix to dissolve the powder.

Assay preparation—Using about 40 mg of Methylprednisolone Hemisuccinate, accurately weighed, prepare as directed for *Standard preparation.*

Procedure—Using a suitable microsyringe or sampling valve, inject separately suitable portions, between 4 and 8 μL, of the *Standard preparation* and the *Assay preparation* into a suitable high-pressure liquid chromatograph (see *Chromatography* ⟨621⟩) of the general type equipped with a detector for monitoring UV absorption at about 254 nm, equipped with a suitable recorder, capable of providing column pressure up to about 1000 psi and fitted with a 4-mm × 30-cm stainless steel column that contains packing L3. In a suitable chromatogram, the resolution, R, between methylprednisolone hemisuccinate and the internal standard is not less than 2.0; and six replicate injections of the *Standard preparation* show a coefficient of variation of not more than 2.0%. Calculate the quantity, in mg, of

$C_{26}H_{34}O_8$ in the portion of Methylprednisolone Hemisuccinate taken by the formula:

$$100C(R_U/R_S)$$

in which C is the concentration, in mg per mL, of USP Methylprednisolone Hemisuccinate RS in the *Standard preparation*; and R_U and R_S are the peak area ratios of methylprednisolone hemisuccinate to the internal standard obtained from the *Assay preparation* and the *Standard preparation*, respectively.

Methylprednisolone Sodium Succinate

$C_{26}H_{33}NaO_8$ 496.53

Pregna-1,4-diene-3,20-dione, 21-(3-carboxy-1-oxopropoxy)-11,17-dihydroxy-6-methyl-, monosodium salt, (6α,11β)-.
11β,17,21-Trihydroxy-6α-methylpregna-1,4-diene-3,20-dione 21-(sodium succinate)   [2375-03-3].

» Methylprednisolone Sodium Succinate contains not less than 97.0 percent and not more than 103.0 percent of $C_{26}H_{33}NaO_8$, calculated on the dried basis.

Packaging and storage—Preserve in tight, light-resistant containers.
USP Reference standards ⟨11⟩—*USP Methylprednisolone Hemisuccinate RS.*
Identification—
A: Transfer about 100 mg to a separator, dissolve in 10 mL of water, add 1 mL of 3 N hydrochloric acid, and extract immediately with 50 mL of chloroform. Filter the chloroform extract through cotton, evaporate on a steam bath to dryness, and dry in vacuum at 60° for 3 hours: the IR absorption spectrum of a mineral oil dispersion of the residue so obtained exhibits maxima only at the same wavelengths as that of a similar preparation of USP Methylprednisolone Hemisuccinate RS.
B: *Ultraviolet Absorption* ⟨197U⟩—
Solution: 20 µg per mL.
Medium: methanol.
Absorptivities at 243 nm, calculated on the dried basis, do not differ by more than 3.0%.
C: It responds to the flame test for *Sodium* ⟨191⟩.
Specific rotation ⟨781S⟩: between +96° and +104°.
Test solution: 10 mg per mL, in alcohol.
Loss on drying ⟨731⟩—Dry it at 105° for 3 hours: it loses not more than 3.0% of its weight.
Sodium content—Dissolve, with gentle heating, about 1 g of it, accurately weighed, in 75 mL of glacial acetic acid. Add 20 mL of dioxane, then add 1 drop of crystal violet TS, and titrate with 0.1 N perchloric acid VS to a blue-green endpoint. Perform a blank determination, and make any necessary correction. Each mL of 0.1 N perchloric acid is equivalent to 2.299 mg of Na. Not less than 4.49% and not more than 4.77%, calculated on the dried basis, is found.
Assay—
Standard preparation—Proceed as directed under *Assay for Steroids* ⟨351⟩, using USP Methylprednisolone Hemisuccinate RS to obtain a solution having a known concentration of about 12.5 µg per mL.
Assay preparation—Weigh accurately about 100 mg of Methylprednisolone Sodium Succinate, dissolve it in alcohol to make 200.0 mL, and mix. Pipet 5 mL of this solution into a 200-mL volumetric flask, add alcohol to volume, and mix. Pipet 20 mL of the resulting solution into a glass-stoppered, 50-mL conical flask.
Procedure—To each of the flasks containing the *Assay preparation* and the *Standard preparation*, and to a similar flask containing 20.0 mL of alcohol, to provide the blank, add 2.0 mL of a solution prepared by dissolving 50 mg of blue tetrazolium in 10 mL of alcohol, and mix. Then to each flask add 4.0 mL of a mixture of 1 volume of tetramethylammonium hydroxide TS and 9 volumes of alcohol. Mix, allow to stand in the dark for 90 minutes, add 1.0 mL of glacial acetic acid, mix, and proceed as directed under *Procedure* under *Assay for Steroids* ⟨351⟩, beginning with "Concomitantly determine the absorbances." Calculate the quantity, in mg, of $C_{26}H_{33}NaO_8$ in the portion of Methylprednisolone Sodium Succinate taken by the formula:

$$8.37C(A_U/A_S).$$

Methylprednisolone Sodium Succinate for Injection

» Methylprednisolone Sodium Succinate for Injection is a sterile mixture of Methylprednisolone Sodium Succinate with suitable buffers. It may be prepared from Methylprednisolone Sodium Succinate or from Methylprednisolone Hemisuccinate with the aid of Sodium Hydroxide or Sodium Carbonate. It contains the equivalent of not less than 90.0 percent and not more than 110.0 percent of the labeled amount of methylprednisolone ($C_{22}H_{30}O_5$) in the volume of constituted solution designated on the label.

Packaging and storage—Preserve in *Containers for Sterile Solids* as described under *Injections* ⟨1⟩.
USP Reference standards ⟨11⟩—*USP Endotoxin RS. USP Fluorometholone RS. USP Methylprednisolone RS. USP Methylprednisolone Hemisuccinate RS.*
Constituted solution—At the time of use, it meets the requirements for *Constituted Solutions* under *Injections* ⟨1⟩.
Identification—It meets the requirements of *Identification* test A under *Methylprednisolone Sodium Succinate*.
Bacterial endotoxins ⟨85⟩—It contains not more than 0.17 USP Endotoxin Unit per mg of methylprednisolone.
pH ⟨791⟩: between 7.0 and 8.0, in a solution containing about 50 mg of methylprednisolone sodium succinate per mL.
Loss on drying ⟨731⟩—Dry it at 105° for 3 hours: it loses not more than 2.0% of its weight.
Particulate matter ⟨788⟩: meets the requirements for small-volume injections.
Free methylprednisolone—Using the chromatograms obtained in the *Assay*, measure the areas of the peaks from the internal standard and free methylprednisolone. Calculate the ratio of the area of the free methylprednisolone peak to that of the internal standard in the chromatogram obtained from the *Standard preparation*, S_S, and the same ratio in the chromatogram obtained from the *Assay preparation*, S_U. Calculate the quantity, in mg, of free methylprednisolone in the *Assay preparation* taken by the formula:

$$100C(S_U/S_S)$$

in which C is the concentration, in mg per mL, of USP Methylprednisolone RS in the *Standard preparation*; and S_U and S_S are the ratios as defined above. The amount of free methylprednisolone is not more than 6.6% of the labeled amount of methylprednisolone.
Other requirements—It meets the requirements for *Sterility Tests* ⟨71⟩, *Uniformity of Dosage Units* ⟨905⟩, and *Labeling* under *Injections* ⟨1⟩.
Assay—
Internal standard solution—Prepare a solution of USP Fluorometholone RS in tetrahydrofuran containing about 3 mg per mL.
Mobile phase—Prepare a filtered mixture of butyl chloride, water-saturated butyl chloride, tetrahydrofuran, methanol, and glacial acetic acid (95 : 95 : 14 : 7 : 6). Make adjustments if necessary (see *System Suitability* under *Chromatography* ⟨621⟩).
Standard preparation—Weigh accurately about 32.5 mg of USP Methylprednisolone Hemisuccinate RS, and transfer it to a 50-mL volumetric flask. Add by pipet 5.0 mL of *Internal standard solution* and 5.0 mL of a solution of glacial acetic acid in chloroform (3 in 100) containing in each mL an accurately known quantity of about 0.30 mg of USP Methylprednisolone RS. Dilute with glacial acetic acid in chloroform (3 in 100) to volume, and mix.

Assay preparation—Mix the constituted solutions prepared from the contents of 10 vials of Methylprednisolone Sodium Succinate for Injection. Transfer an accurately measured volume of the resulting constituted solution, equivalent to about 50 mg of methylprednisolone, to a suitable flask containing 10.0 mL of *Internal standard solution*, and dilute with glacial acetic acid in chloroform (3 in 100) to 100.0 mL. Shake thoroughly for 5 minutes, then allow the phases to separate, discarding the upper phase.

Chromatographic system (see *Chromatography* ⟨621⟩)—The liquid chromatograph is equipped with a 254-nm detector and a 3.9-mm × 30-cm column that contains packing L3. The flow rate is about 1.0 mL per minute. Chromatograph the *Standard preparation*, and record the peak responses as directed for *Procedure*: the order of elution of peaks is the internal standard peak, methylprednisolone hemisuccinate peak, and successive smaller peaks of free methylprednisolone and methylprednisolone 17-hemisuccinate.

Procedure—Separately inject equal volumes (about 6 µL) of the *Standard preparation* and the *Assay preparation* into the chromatograph, record the chromatograms, and measure the peak areas for the internal standard, methylprednisolone hemisuccinate, and methylprednisolone 17-hemisuccinate. Calculate the quantity, in mg, of methylprednisolone ($C_{22}H_{30}O_5$) in the portion of constituted solution taken by the formula:

$$0.789(100C)(R_U/R_S)$$

in which 0.789 is the ratio of the molecular weight of methylprednisolone to that of methylprednisolone hemisuccinate; C is the concentration, in mg per mL, of USP Methylprednisolone Hemisuccinate RS in the *Standard preparation*; and R_U and R_S are the ratios of the sum of the peak areas for methylprednisolone hemisuccinate and methylprednisolone 17-hemisuccinate to the peak area of the internal standard obtained from the *Standard preparation* and the *Assay preparation*, respectively. To this quantity add the amount, in mg, of free methylprednisolone found in the test for *Free methylprednisolone*.

Methyltestosterone

$C_{20}H_{30}O_2$ 302.45
Androst-4-en-3-one, 17-hydroxy-17-methyl-, (17β)-.
17β-Hydroxy-17-methylandrost-4-en-3-one   [58-18-4].

» Methyltestosterone contains not less than 97.0 percent and not more than 103.0 percent of $C_{20}H_{30}O_2$, calculated on the dried basis.

Packaging and storage—Preserve in well-closed, light-resistant containers.

USP Reference standards ⟨11⟩—*USP Methyltestosterone RS. USP Testosterone RS*.
Identification—
  A: *Infrared Absorption* ⟨197K⟩.
  B: *Ultraviolet Absorption* ⟨197U⟩—
    Solution: 10 µg per mL.
    Medium: alcohol.
Melting range ⟨741⟩: between 162° and 167°.
Specific rotation ⟨781S⟩: between +79° and +85°.
  Test solution: 10 mg per mL, in alcohol.
Loss on drying ⟨731⟩—Dry it at 105° for 4 hours: it loses not more than 2.0% of its weight.
Chromatographic purity—
  Solution A—Prepare a filtered and degassed mixture of methanol and water (55 : 45).
  Solution B—Use methanol.
  Mobile phase—Use variable mixtures of *Solution A* and *Solution B* as directed for *Chromatographic system*. Make adjustments if necessary (see *System Suitability* under *Chromatography* ⟨621⟩).
  System suitability solution—Dilute a volume of the *Test solution* quantitatively, and stepwise if necessary, with methanol to obtain a solution having a concentration of about 0.005 mg of methyltestosterone per mL.
  Test solution—Dissolve an accurately weighed quantity of Methyltestosterone in methanol to obtain a solution containing about 0.5 mg per mL.
  Chromatographic system (see *Chromatography* ⟨621⟩)—The liquid chromatograph is equipped with a 254-nm detector and a 4.6-mm × 25-cm column that contains 5-µm packing L1. The flow rate is 1 mL per minute. The chromatograph is programmed as follows.

Time (minutes)	Solution A (%)	Solution B (%)	Elution
0	100	0	equilibration
0–20	100→60	0→40	linear gradient
20–40	60→0	40→100	linear gradient
40–45	0	100	isocratic
45–60	0→100	100→0	re-equilibration

Chromatograph the *Test solution* and the *System suitability solution*, and record the peak responses as directed for *Procedure*: the column efficiency is not less than 33,000 theoretical plates; and the relative standard deviation for replicate injections for the methyltestosterone peak in the chromatogram of the *Test solution* is not more than 2.0%; and the signal-to-noise ratio of the methyltestosterone peak in the chromatogram of the *System suitability solution* is not less than 100.

Procedure—Inject a volume (about 5 µL) of the *Test solution* into the chromatograph, record the chromatogram, and measure all of the peak areas. Calculate the percentage of each impurity in the portion of Methyltestosterone taken by the formula:

$$100(r_i/r_s)$$

in which r_i is the peak response for each impurity; and r_s is the sum of the responses of all the peaks, disregarding any impurity having a peak less than 0.05%. Not more than 0.5% of any individual impurity is found, and not more than 1.0% of total impurities is found.

Organic volatile impurities, *Method V* ⟨467⟩: meets the requirements.
  Solvent: dimethyl sulfoxide.

(Official until July 1, 2008)

Assay—
  Mobile phase—Prepare a filtered and degassed mixture of acetonitrile and water (55 : 45). Make adjustments if necessary (see *System Suitability* under *Chromatography* ⟨621⟩).
  Standard preparation—Transfer about 25 mg of USP Methyltestosterone RS, accurately weighed, to a 100-mL volumetric flask, dilute with methanol to volume, and mix. Pipet 8 mL of this solution into a 100-mL volumetric flask, dilute with *Mobile phase* to volume, and mix to obtain the *Standard preparation* having a known concentration of about 20 µg per mL.
  Assay preparation—Transfer about 50 mg of Methyltestosterone, accurately weighed, to a 100-mL volumetric flask, dilute with methanol to volume, and mix. Pipet 8 mL of this solution to a 200-mL volumetric flask, dilute with *Mobile phase* to volume, and mix.
  System suitability preparation—Prepare a solution of testosterone in methanol containing about 250 µg per mL. Dilute 4 mL of this solution with the *Standard preparation* to 50 mL, and mix.
  Chromatographic system (see *Chromatography* ⟨621⟩)—The liquid chromatograph is equipped with a 241-nm detector and a 4-mm × 25-cm column that contains packing L1. The flow rate is about 1 mL per minute. Chromatograph the *Standard preparation* and the *System suitability preparation*, and record the peak responses as directed for *Procedure*: the relative retention times are about 0.8 for testosterone and 1.0 for methyltestosterone; the resolution, R, between testosterone and methyltestosterone is not less than 2.0; the column efficiency determined from the analyte peak is not less than

2000 theoretical plates; the tailing factor for the analyte peak is not more than 2.7; and the relative standard deviation for replicate injections is not more than 2.0%.

Procedure—Separately inject equal volumes (about 50 µL) of the *Standard preparation* and the *Assay preparation* into the chromatograph, record the chromatograms, and measure the responses for the major peaks. Calculate the quantity, in mg, of $C_{20}H_{30}O_2$ in the portion of Methyltestosterone taken by the formula:

$$2500C(r_U / r_S)$$

in which C is the concentration, in mg per mL, of USP Methyltestosterone RS in the *Standard preparation*; and r_U and r_S are the peak responses obtained from the *Assay preparation* and the *Standard preparation*, respectively.

Methyltestosterone Capsules

» Methyltestosterone Capsules contain not less than 90.0 percent and not more than 110.0 percent of the labeled amount of methyltestosterone ($C_{20}H_{30}O_2$).

Packaging and storage—Preserve in well-closed containers.
USP Reference standards ⟨11⟩—*USP Methyltestosterone RS*.
Identification—Evaporate 25 mL of the first alcohol solution of methyltestosterone obtained in the *Assay* to dryness: the IR absorption spectrum of a potassium bromide dispersion of the residue so obtained exhibits maxima at the same wavelengths as that of a similar preparation of USP Methyltestosterone RS.
Dissolution ⟨711⟩—
 Medium: water; 900 mL.
 Apparatus 1: 100 rpm.
 Time: 45 minutes.
 Procedure—Determine the amount in solution on filtered portions of the *Medium*, suitably diluted quantitatively and stepwise with water to obtain a solution containing about 10 µg of methyltestosterone per mL at the wavelength of maximum absorbance at about 248 nm, with a suitable spectrophotometer, in comparison with a solution of USP Methyltestosterone RS in the same medium at the same concentration, water being used as the blank.
 Tolerances—Not less than 70% (*Q*) of the labeled amount of $C_{20}H_{30}O_2$ is dissolved in 45 minutes.
Uniformity of dosage units ⟨905⟩: meet the requirements.
 Procedure for content uniformity—Transfer the contents of 1 Capsule to a 100-mL volumetric flask, add 50 mL of methanol, and shake by mechanical means for 60 minutes. Dilute with methanol to volume, and filter, discarding the first 20 mL of the filtrate. Dilute a portion of the subsequent filtrate quantitatively and stepwise, if necessary, with methanol to obtain a solution containing about 10 µg of methyltestosterone per mL. Concomitantly determine the absorbances of this solution and a Standard solution of USP Methyltestosterone RS in the same medium having a known concentration of about 10 µg per mL, in 1-cm cells at the wavelength of maximum absorbance at about 241 nm, with a suitable spectrophotometer, using methanol as the blank. Calculate the quantity, in mg, of $C_{20}H_{30}O_2$ in the Capsule taken by the formula:

$$(T/D)C(A_U / A_S)$$

in which T is the labeled quantity, in mg, of methyltestosterone in the Capsule; D is the concentration, in µg per mL, of methyltestosterone in the solution from the Capsule, based on the labeled quantity per Capsule and the extent of dilution; C is the concentration, in µg per mL, of USP Methyltestosterone RS in the Standard solution; and A_U and A_S are the absorbances of the solution from the Capsule and the Standard solution, respectively.
Assay—Remove as completely as possible and weigh the contents of not less than 20 Capsules, and mix. Transfer an accurately weighed portion of the powder, equivalent to about 10 mg of methyltestosterone, to a 125-mL separator with the aid of about 5 mL of water. Extract with four 20-mL portions of chloroform, filtering each through chloroform-washed cotton. Evaporate the combined extracts on a steam bath, with the aid of a current of air, to dryness. Dissolve the residue in alcohol, transfer to a 50-mL volumetric flask, add alcohol to volume, and mix. Pipet a 5-mL aliquot into a 100-mL volumetric flask, add alcohol to volume, and mix. Concomitantly determine the absorbances of this solution and a Standard solution of USP Methyltestosterone RS in the same medium having a known concentration of about 10 µg per mL, in 1-cm cells at the wavelength of maximum absorbance at about 241 nm, with a suitable spectrophotometer, using alcohol as the blank. Calculate the quantity, in mg, of methyltestosterone ($C_{20}H_{30}O_2$) in the portion of Capsules contents taken by the formula:

$$C(A_U / A_S)$$

in which C is the concentration, in µg per mL, of USP Methyltestosterone RS in the Standard solution; and A_U and A_S are the absorbances of the solution from the Capsules and the Standard solution, respectively.

Methyltestosterone Tablets

» Methyltestosterone Tablets contain not less than 90.0 percent and not more than 110.0 percent of the labeled amount of methyltestosterone ($C_{20}H_{30}O_2$).

Packaging and storage—Preserve in well-closed containers.
USP Reference standards ⟨11⟩—*USP Methyltestosterone RS*.
Identification—Evaporate to dryness 25 mL of the first alcohol solution of methyltestosterone obtained in the *Assay*: the IR absorption spectrum of a potassium bromide dispersion of the residue so obtained exhibits maxima at the same wavelengths as that of a similar preparation of USP Methyltestosterone RS.
Disintegration ⟨701⟩: 30 minutes. Tablets intended for buccal administration meet the requirements for *Buccal Tablets*.
Uniformity of dosage units ⟨905⟩: meet the requirements.
 Procedure for content uniformity—Transfer 1 finely powdered Tablet to a 100-mL volumetric flask, add 50 mL of methanol, and shake by mechanical means for 60 minutes. Dilute with methanol to volume, and filter, discarding the first 20 mL of the filtrate. Dilute a portion of the subsequent filtrate quantitatively and stepwise, if necessary, with methanol to provide a solution containing about 10 µg of methyltestosterone per mL. Concomitantly determine the absorbances of this solution and a solution of USP Methyltestosterone RS in the same medium having a known concentration of about 10 µg per mL, in 1-cm cells at the wavelength of maximum absorbance at about 241 nm, with a suitable spectrophotometer, using methanol as the blank. Calculate the quantity, in mg, of $C_{20}H_{30}O_2$ in the Tablet taken by the formula:

$$(T/D)C(A_U / A_S)$$

in which T is the labeled quantity, in mg, of methyltestosterone in the Tablet; D is the concentration, in µg per mL, of methyltestosterone in the solution from the Tablet, based on the labeled quantity per Tablet and the extent of dilution; C is the concentration, in µg per mL, of USP Methyltestosterone RS in the Standard solution; and A_U and A_S are the absorbances of the solution from the Tablet and the Standard solution, respectively.
Assay—Weigh and finely powder not less than 20 Tablets. Weigh accurately a portion of the powder, equivalent to about 10 mg of methyltestosterone, and transfer to a 125-mL separator with the aid of about 5 mL of water. Extract with four 25-mL portions of chloroform, filtering each through chloroform-washed cotton. Evaporate the combined extracts on a steam bath, with the aid of a current of air, to dryness. Dissolve the residue in alcohol, transfer to a 50-mL volumetric flask, add alcohol to volume, and mix. Pipet a 5-mL aliquot into a 100-mL volumetric flask, add alcohol to volume, and mix. Concomitantly determine the absorbances of this solution and a solution of USP Methyltestosterone RS in the same medium having a known concentration of about 10 µg per mL, in 1-cm cells at the wavelength of maximum absorbance at about 241 nm, with a suitable spectrophotometer, using alcohol as the blank. Calculate

the quantity, in mg, of methyltestosterone ($C_{20}H_{30}O_2$) in the portion of Tablets taken by the formula:

$$C(A_U/A_S)$$

in which C is the concentration, in µg per mL, of USP Methyltestosterone RS in the Standard solution; and A_U and A_S are the absorbances of the solution from the Tablets and the Standard solution, respectively.

Methysergide Maleate

$C_{21}H_{27}N_3O_2 \cdot C_4H_4O_4$ 469.53

Ergoline-8-carboxamide, 9,10-didehydro-N-[1-(hydroxymethyl)propyl]-1,6]-dimethyl-, (8β)-, (Z)-2-butenedioate (1 : 1) (salt).
9,10-Didehydro-N-[1-(hydroxymethyl)propyl-1,6]-dimethylergoline-8β-carboxamide maleate (1 : 1) (salt)   [129-49-7].

» Methysergide Maleate contains not less than 97.0 percent and not more than 103.0 percent of $C_{21}H_{27}N_3O_2 \cdot C_4H_4O_4$, calculated on the dried basis.

Packaging and storage—Preserve in tight, light-resistant containers, in a cold place.

USP Reference standards ⟨11⟩—*USP Methysergide Maleate RS*.
Identification—
   A: *Infrared Absorption* ⟨197K⟩.
   B: [NOTE—Conduct this test without exposure to daylight, and with the minimum exposure to artificial light.] In a suitable chromatographic chamber, arranged for thin-layer chromatography (see *Chromatography* ⟨621⟩), place a volume of a solvent system consisting of a mixture of chloroform and methanol (20 : 1) sufficient to develop the chromatogram. Place a beaker containing 25 mL of ammonium hydroxide in the chamber, cover, and allow to equilibrate for 30 minutes. Prepare a test solution of Methysergide Maleate in methanol containing 5 mg per mL. Apply 25 µL of this solution and 25 µL of a Standard solution of USP Methysergide Maleate RS in methanol containing 5 mg per mL to a suitable thin-layer chromatographic plate (see *Chromatography* ⟨621⟩) coated with a 0.25-mm layer of chromatographic silica gel. Develop the chromatogram until the solvent front has moved about three-fourths of the length of the plate. Remove the plate from the developing chamber, mark the solvent front, and allow the solvent to evaporate. Locate the spots on the plate by lightly spraying with a solution prepared by dissolving 800 mg of *p*-dimethylaminobenzaldehyde in a cooled mixture of 80 mL of alcohol and 20 mL of sulfuric acid, allow the plate to dry, then expose it briefly to fumes of a mixture of nitric and hydrochloric acids: the R_F value of the principal spot obtained from the test solution corresponds to that obtained from the Standard solution.

Specific rotation ⟨781S⟩:   between +35° and +45°.
   Test solution: 2.5 mg per mL, in water.
pH ⟨791⟩:   between 3.7 and 4.7, in a 1 in 500 solution in carbon dioxide-free water.
Loss on drying ⟨731⟩—Dry it in vacuum at 120° for 2 hours: it loses not more than 7.0% of its weight.
Ordinary impurities ⟨466⟩—
   Test solution: methanol.
   Standard solution: methanol.
   Eluant: prepare as directed under *Identification* test B.
   Visualization: 1.
Assay—Dissolve about 200 mg of Methysergide Maleate, accurately weighed, in 30 mL of glacial acetic acid, add 1 drop of crystal violet TS, and titrate with 0.1 N perchloric acid VS to a blue endpoint. Perform a blank determination, and make any necessary correction. Each mL of 0.1 N perchloric acid is equivalent to 46.95 mg of $C_{21}H_{27}N_3O_2 \cdot C_4H_4O_4$.

Methysergide Maleate Tablets

» Methysergide Maleate Tablets contain not less than 90.0 percent and not more than 110.0 percent of the labeled amount of methysergide maleate ($C_{21}H_{27}N_3O_2 \cdot C_4H_4O_4$).

Packaging and storage—Preserve in tight containers.

USP Reference standards ⟨11⟩—*USP Methysergide Maleate RS*.
Identification—To a portion of finely powdered Tablets, equivalent to about 10 mg of methysergide maleate, add 50 mL of tartaric acid solution (1 in 100) and 4 drops of benzalkonium chloride solution (1 in 10), and shake vigorously by mechanical means for 30 minutes. Filter the mixture. To 5 mL of the filtrate add 10 mL of *p*-dimethylaminobenzaldehyde TS: a violet-blue color develops.
Dissolution ⟨711⟩—
   Medium: tartaric acid solution (1 in 200); 900 mL.
   Apparatus 2: 100 rpm.
   Time: 30 minutes.
   Procedure—Filter a portion of the solution under test into a flask. Concomitantly determine the fluorescence intensity of this solution in comparison with a Standard solution of USP Methysergide Maleate RS in the same medium having a known concentration of about 2.2 µg per mL in a fluorometer at an excitation wavelength of about 327 nm and an emission wavelength of about 428 nm, using tartaric acid solution (1 in 200) as the blank.
   Tolerances—Not less than 70% (*Q*) of the labeled amount of $C_{21}H_{27}N_3O_2 \cdot C_4H_4O_4$ is dissolved in 30 minutes.
Uniformity of dosage units ⟨905⟩:   meet the requirements.
Assay—[NOTE—Conduct this procedure with a minimum exposure to light.]
   Mobile phase—Dissolve 6.8 g of monobasic potassium phosphate in 700 mL of water, add 300 mL of acetonitrile, and mix. Filter through a 0.45-µm membrane, and degas under vacuum. Make adjustments if necessary (see *System Suitability* under *Chromatography* ⟨621⟩).
   Solvent mixture—Dissolve 10 g of tartaric acid in 1 L of water, add 1 L of methanol, and mix.
   Standard preparation—Dissolve an accurately weighed quantity of USP Methysergide Maleate RS in *Solvent mixture* with the help of sonication, and dilute quantitatively, and stepwise if necessary, with the same solvent to obtain a solution having a known concentration of about 0.1 mg per mL.
   Assay preparation—Weigh and finely powder not less than 20 Tablets. Transfer an accurately weighed portion of the powder, equivalent to about 10 mg of methysergide maleate, to a 100-mL volumetric flask. Add 75 mL of *Solvent mixture*, and shake by mechanical means for 60 minutes. Add *Solvent mixture* to volume, mix, and filter through a 0.45-µm membrane, discarding the first 20 mL of the filtrate.
   Chromatographic system (see *Chromatography* ⟨621⟩)—The liquid chromatograph is equipped with a 318-nm detector and a 4.6-mm × 15-cm column that contains packing L7. The flow rate is about 2 mL per minute. Chromatograph the *Standard preparation*, and record the peak responses as directed for *Procedure*: the column efficiency determined from the analyte peak is not less than 1000 theoretical plates, the tailing factor for the analyte peak is not more than 2.5, the resolution, *R*, between the analyte and the closest adjacent peak is not less than 1.0, and the relative standard deviation for replicate injections is not more than 2.0%.
   Procedure—Separately inject equal volumes (about 20 µL) of the *Standard preparation* and the *Assay preparation* into the chromatograph, record the chromatograms, and measure the responses for the major peaks. Calculate the quantity, in mg, of methysergide maleate

($C_{21}H_{37}N_3O_2 \cdot C_4H_4O_4$) in the portion of Tablets taken by the formula:

$$(100C)(r_U / r_S)$$

in which C is the concentration, in mg per mL, of USP Methysergide Maleate RS in the *Standard preparation;*, and r_U and r_S are the peak responses obtained from the *Assay preparation* and the *Standard preparation*, respectively.

Metoclopramide Hydrochloride

$C_{14}H_{22}ClN_3O_2 \cdot HCl \cdot H_2O$ 354.27
Benzamide, 4-amino-5-chloro-*N*-[2-(diethylamino)ethyl]-2-methoxy-, monohydrochloride, monohydrate.
4-Amino-5-chloro-*N*-[2-(diethylamino)ethyl]-*o*-anisamide monohydrochloride monohydrate [*54143-57-6*].

» Metoclopramide Hydrochloride contains not less than 98.0 percent and not more than 101.0 percent of $C_{14}H_{22}ClN_3O_2 \cdot HCl$, calculated on the anhydrous basis.

Packaging and storage—Preserve in tight, light-resistant containers.
USP Reference standards ⟨11⟩—*USP Metoclopramide Hydrochloride RS.*
Identification—
  A: *Infrared Absorption* ⟨197M⟩.
  B: Dissolve 50 mg in 5 mL of water, and add 5 mL of a 1 in 100 solution of *p*-dimethylaminobenzaldehyde in 1 N hydrochloric acid: a yellow-orange color is produced.
  C: The R_F value of the principal spot in the chromatogram of the *Identification preparation* corresponds to that of *Standard preparation A*, as obtained in the test for *Chromatographic purity*.
Water, *Method I* ⟨921⟩: between 4.5% and 6.0%.
Residue on ignition ⟨281⟩: not more than 0.1%.
Chromatographic purity—
  Standard preparations—Dissolve USP Metoclopramide Hydrochloride RS in methanol, and mix to obtain a solution having a known concentration of 1 mg per mL. Dilute quantitatively with methanol to obtain three *Standard preparations*, designated below by letters, having the following compositions:

Standard preparation	Dilution	Concentration (µg RS per mL)	Percentage (%, for comparison with test specimen)
A	(1 in 4)	250	0.5
B	(3 in 20)	150	0.3
C	(1 in 20)	50	0.1

  Test preparation—Dissolve an accurately weighed quantity of Metoclopramide Hydrochloride in methanol to obtain a solution containing 50 mg per mL.
  Identification preparation—Dilute a portion of the *Test preparation* quantitatively with methanol to obtain a solution containing 250 µg per mL.
  Procedure—Apply separately 10 µL of the *Test preparation*, 10 µL of the *Identification preparation*, and 10 µL of each *Standard preparation* to a suitable thin-layer chromatographic plate (see *Chromatography* ⟨621⟩) coated with a 0.25-mm layer of chromatographic silica gel mixture. Allow the spots to dry, position the plate in a chromatographic chamber, and develop the chromatograms in a solvent system consisting of a mixture of chloroform, methanol, toluene, and ammonium hydroxide (140 : 60 : 20 : 1) until the solvent front has moved about three-fourths of the length of the plate. Remove the plate from the developing chamber, mark the solvent front, and allow the solvent to evaporate. Examine the plate under short-wavelength UV light, and compare the intensities of any secondary spots observed in the chromatogram of the *Test preparation* with those of the principal spots in the chromatograms of the *Standard preparations*. [NOTE—Disregard any spots observed at the origins of the chromatograms.] No secondary spot from the chromatogram of the *Test preparation* is larger or more intense than the principal spot obtained from *Standard preparation A* (0.5%), and the sum of the intensities of all secondary spots obtained from the *Test preparation* corresponds to not more than 1.0%.
Organic volatile impurities, *Method I* ⟨467⟩: meets the requirements.

(Official until July 1, 2008)
Assay—Transfer about 300 mg of Metoclopramide Hydrochloride, accurately weighed, to a stoppered, 125-mL flask, add 10 mL of mercuric acetate TS and 2 mL of acetic anhydride, and allow to stand for 3 hours. Add 80 mL of glacial acetic acid, and titrate with 0.1 N perchloric acid VS, determining the endpoint potentiometrically (see *Titrimetry* ⟨541⟩). Perform a blank determination, and make any necessary correction. Each mL of 0.1 N perchloric acid is equivalent to 33.63 mg of $C_{14}H_{22}ClN_3O_2 \cdot HCl$.

Metoclopramide Injection

» Metoclopramide Injection is a sterile solution of Metoclopramide Hydrochloride in Water for Injection. It contains the equivalent of not less than 90.0 percent and not more than 110.0 percent of the labeled amount of metoclopramide ($C_{14}H_{22}ClN_3O_2$).

Packaging and storage—Preserve in single-dose or in multiple-dose containers, preferably of Type I glass, protected from light. [NOTE—Injection containing an antioxidant agent does not require protection from light.]
USP Reference standards ⟨11⟩—*USP Endotoxin RS. USP Metoclopramide Hydrochloride RS.*
Identification—
  A: The retention time of the major peak in the chromatogram of the *Assay preparation* corresponds to that of the *Standard preparation* as obtained in the *Assay*.
  B: Mix a volume of Injection, equivalent to about 50 mg of metoclopramide, with 5 mL of water and 5 mL of a 1 in 100 solution of *p*-dimethylaminobenzaldehyde in 1 N hydrochloric acid: a yellow-orange color is produced.
Bacterial endotoxins ⟨85⟩—It contains not more than 2.5 USP Endotoxin Units per mg of metoclopramide.
pH ⟨791⟩: between 2.5 and 6.5.
Particulate matter ⟨788⟩: meets the requirements under small-volume injections.
Other requirements—It meets the requirements under *Injections* ⟨1⟩.
Assay—
  Mobile phase—Dissolve 2.7 g of sodium acetate in 500 mL of water, add 500 mL of acetonitrile, 2 mL of tetramethylammonium hydroxide solution in methanol (1 in 5), mix, adjust with glacial acetic acid to a pH of 6.5, filter, and degas. Make adjustments if necessary (see *System Suitability* under *Chromatography* ⟨621⟩).
  Standard preparation—Dissolve an accurately weighed quantity of USP Metoclopramide Hydrochloride RS in 0.01 M phosphoric acid to obtain a stock solution having a known concentration of about 0.9 mg of anhydrous metoclopramide hydrochloride per mL. Dilute quantitatively, and stepwise if necessary, a volume of this stock solution with 0.01 M phosphoric acid to obtain a *Standard preparation* having a known concentration of about 45 µg of USP Metoclopramide Hydrochloride RS, on the anhydrous basis, per mL (equivalent to about 40 µg of anhydrous metoclopramide per mL).
  System suitability solution—Transfer about 12.5 mg of benzenesulfonamide to a 25-mL volumetric flask, add 15 mL of methanol, and shake to dissolve. Dilute with 0.01 M phosphoric acid to volume, and mix. Pipet 5 mL of this solution and 5 mL of

the stock solution used to prepare the *Standard preparation* into a 100-mL volumetric flask, dilute with 0.01 M phosphoric acid to volume, and mix.

Assay preparation—Transfer an accurately measured volume of Injection, equivalent to about 40 mg of metoclopramide, to a 100-mL volumetric flask, dilute with 0.01 M phosphoric acid to volume, and mix. Transfer 10.0 mL of this solution to a 100-mL volumetric flask, dilute with 0.01 M phosphoric acid to volume, and mix.

Chromatographic system (see *Chromatography* ⟨621⟩)—The liquid chromatograph is equipped with a 215-nm detector and a 4.6-mm × 25-cm column that contains packing L1. The flow rate is about 1.5 mL per minute. Chromatograph the *System suitability solution*, and record the peak responses as directed under *Procedure:* the relative retention times are about 0.7 for benzenesulfonamide and 1.0 for metoclopramide, and the resolution, *R*, between the benzenesulfonamide peak and the metoclopramide peak is not less than 1.5. Chromatograph the *Standard preparation*, and record the peak responses as directed under *Procedure:* the tailing factor for the metoclopramide peak is not more than 2.0, and the relative standard deviation for replicate injections is not more than 2.0%.

Procedure—Separately inject equal volumes (about 20 μL) of the *Standard preparation* and the *Assay preparation* into the chromatograph, record the chromatograms, and measure the responses for the major peaks. Calculate the quantity, in mg, of $C_{14}H_{22}ClN_3O_2$ in each mL of the Injection taken by the formula:

$$(299.80 / 336.26)(C / V)(r_U / r_S)$$

in which 299.80 and 336.26 are the molecular weights of metoclopramide and anhydrous metoclopramide hydrochloride, respectively; *C* is the concentration, in μg per mL, of USP Metoclopramide Hydrochloride RS, on the anhydrous basis, in the *Standard preparation*; *V* is the volume, in mL, of Injection taken; and r_U and r_S are the peak responses of metoclopramide obtained from the *Assay preparation* and the *Standard preparation*, respectively.

Metoclopramide Oral Solution

» Metoclopramide Oral Solution contains an amount of Metoclopramide Hydrochloride ($C_{14}H_{22}ClN_3O_2 \cdot$ HCl · H_2O) equivalent to not less than 90.0 percent and not more than 110.0 percent of the labeled amount of metoclopramide ($C_{14}H_{22}ClN_3O_2$).

Packaging and storage—Preserve in tight, light-resistant containers, and store at controlled room temperature. Protect from freezing.

USP Reference standards ⟨11⟩—*USP Metoclopramide Hydrochloride RS*.
Identification—The retention time of the major peak in the chromatogram of the *Assay preparation* corresponds to that in the chromatogram of the *Standard preparation*, as obtained in the *Assay*.
Uniformity of dosage units ⟨905⟩—
FOR ORAL SOLUTION PACKAGED IN SINGLE-UNIT CONTAINERS: meets the requirements.
Deliverable volume ⟨698⟩—
FOR ORAL SOLUTION PACKAGED IN MULTIPLE-UNIT CONTAINERS: meets the requirements.
pH ⟨791⟩: between 2.0 and 5.5.
Assay—
Mobile phase—Dissolve 2.7 g of sodium acetate in 600 mL of water, add 400 mL of acetonitrile, and 4 mL of tetramethylammonium hydroxide solution in methanol (25%), and mix. Adjust with glacial acetic acid to a pH of 6.5, filter, and degas. Make adjustments if necessary (see *System Suitability* under *Chromatography* ⟨621⟩).
Standard stock solution—Dissolve an accurately weighed quantity of USP Metoclopramide Hydrochloride RS in 0.01 M phosphoric acid to obtain a stock solution having a known concentration of about 9 mg of anhydrous metoclopramide hydrochloride per mL.

System suitability solution—Transfer about 125 mg of benzenesulfonamide to a 25-mL volumetric flask, add 15 mL of methanol, and shake to dissolve. Dilute with 0.01 M phosphoric acid to volume, and mix. Pipet 15 mL of this solution and 5 mL of the *Standard stock solution* into a 250-mL volumetric flask, dilute with 0.01 M phosphoric acid to volume, and mix.

Standard preparation—Transfer 5.0 mL of the *Standard stock solution* to a 250-mL volumetric flask, dilute with 0.01 M phosphoric acid to volume, and mix to obtain a solution having a known concentration of about 180 μg of USP Metoclopramide Hydrochloride RS, on the anhydrous basis, per mL (equivalent to about 160 μg of anhydrous metoclopramide per mL).

Assay preparation—Transfer an accurately measured volume of Oral Solution, equivalent to about 4 mg of metoclopramide, to a 25-mL volumetric flask, dilute with 0.01 M phosphoric acid to volume, and mix.

Chromatographic system (see *Chromatography* ⟨621⟩)—Prepare as directed in the *Assay* under *Metoclopramide Injection*. The relative retention times are about 0.2 for benzenesulfonamide and 1.0 for metoclopramide.

Procedure—Separately inject equal volumes (about 20 μL) of the *Standard preparation* and the *Assay preparation* into the chromatograph, record the chromatograms, and measure the responses for the major peaks. Calculate the quantity, in mg, of metoclopramide ($C_{14}H_{22}ClN_3O_2$) in each mL of the Oral Solution taken by the formula:

$$(299.80/336.26)(25C/V)(r_U / r_S)$$

in which 299.80 and 336.26 are the molecular weights of metoclopramide and anhydrous metoclopramide hydrochloride, respectively; *C* is the concentration, in mg per mL, of USP Metoclopramide Hydrochloride RS, on the anhydrous basis, in the *Standard preparation;* *V* is the volume, in mL, of Oral Solution taken; and r_U and r_S are the peak responses of metoclopramide obtained from the *Assay preparation* and the *Standard preparation*, respectively.

Metoclopramide Tablets

» Metoclopramide Tablets contain an amount of metoclopramide hydrochloride ($C_{14}H_{22}ClN_3O_2 \cdot$ HCl · H_2O) equivalent to not less than 90.0 percent and not more than 110.0 percent of the labeled amount of metoclopramide ($C_{14}H_{22}ClN_3O_2$).

Packaging and storage—Preserve in tight, light-resistant containers.

USP Reference standards ⟨11⟩—*USP Metoclopramide Hydrochloride RS*.
Identification—
A: The retention time of the major peak in the chromatogram of the *Assay preparation* corresponds to that of the *Standard preparation* as obtained in the *Assay*.
B: Transfer a quantity of finely ground Tablets, equivalent to about 50 mg of metoclopramide, to a suitable flask, add 5 mL of water, shake by mechanical means, and filter. Add to the filtrate 5 mL of a 1 in 100 solution of *p*-dimethylaminobenzaldehyde in 1 N hydrochloric acid: a yellow-orange color is produced.
Dissolution ⟨711⟩—
Medium: water; 900 mL.
Apparatus 1: 50 rpm.
Time: 30 minutes.
Procedure—Determine the amount of $C_{14}H_{22}ClN_3O_2$ dissolved from UV absorbances at the wavelength of maximum absorbance at about 309 nm of filtered portions of the solution under test, suitably diluted with water, if necessary, in comparison with a Standard solution having a known concentration of USP Metoclopramide Hydrochloride RS in the same medium.
Tolerances—Not less than 75% (*Q*) of the labeled amount of $C_{14}H_{22}ClN_3O_2$ is dissolved in 30 minutes.

Uniformity of dosage units ⟨905⟩: meet the requirements.
Assay—
Mobile phase, Standard preparation, System suitability solution, and *Chromatographic system*—Prepare as directed in the *Assay* under *Metoclopramide Injection*.

Assay preparation—Weigh and finely powder not less than 20 Tablets. Transfer an accurately weighed portion of the powder, equivalent to about 40 mg of metoclopramide, to a 100-mL volumetric flask, add about 70 mL of 0.01 M phosphoric acid, and sonicate for 5 minutes. Cool to room temperature, dilute with 0.01 M phosphoric acid to volume, and mix. Filter the solution through a 0.45-µm filter, discarding the first portion of the filtrate. Transfer 10.0 mL of this solution to a 100-mL volumetric flask, dilute with 0.01 M phosphoric acid to volume, and mix.

Procedure—Proceed as directed for *Procedure* in the *Assay* under *Metoclopramide Injection*. Calculate the quantity, in mg, of metoclopramide ($C_{14}H_{22}ClN_3O_2$) in the portion of Tablets taken by the formula:

$$(299.80 / 336.26)C(r_U / r_S)$$

in which 299.80 and 336.26 are the molecular weights of metoclopramide and anhydrous metoclopramide hydrochloride, respectively; C is the concentration, in µg per mL, of USP Metoclopramide Hydrochloride RS, on the anhydrous basis, in the *Standard preparation*; and r_U and r_S are the peak responses of metoclopramide obtained from the *Assay preparation* and the *Standard preparation*, respectively.

Metolazone

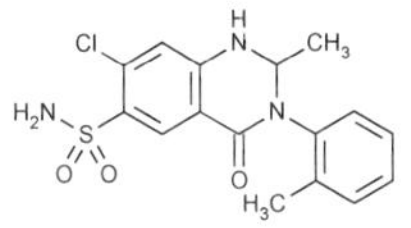

$C_{16}H_{16}ClN_3O_3S$ 365.84
6-Quinazolinesulfonamide, 7-chloro-1,2,3,4-tetrahydro-2-methyl-3-(2-methylphenyl)-4-oxo-.
7-Chloro-1,2,3,4-tetrahydro-2-methyl-4-oxo-3-*o*-tolyl-6-quinazolinesulfonamide [*17560-51-9*].

» Metolazone contains not less than 97.0 percent and not more than 102.0 percent of $C_{16}H_{16}ClN_3O_3S$, calculated on the dried basis.

Packaging and storage—Preserve in tight, light-resistant containers.
USP Reference standards ⟨11⟩—*USP Metolazone RS*.
Identification—
   A: *Infrared Absorption* ⟨197K⟩.
   B: *Ultraviolet Absorption* ⟨197U⟩—
   Solution: 5 µg per mL.
   Medium: methanol.
Loss on drying ⟨731⟩—Dry it at 105° for 2 hours: it loses not more than 1.0% of its weight.
Residue on ignition ⟨281⟩: not more than 0.1%.
Heavy metals, *Method II* ⟨231⟩: 0.0015%.
Chromatographic purity—[NOTE—Protect Metolazone solutions from light.]
   Standard preparations—Dissolve an accurately weighed quantity of USP Metolazone RS in tetrahydrofuran and mix to obtain *Standard preparation A* having a known concentration of 0.50 mg per mL. Dilute a portion of *Standard preparation A* quantitatively with tetrahydrofuran to obtain *Standard preparation B* having a known concentration of 0.25 mg per mL.
   Test preparation—Dissolve an accurately weighed quantity of Metolazone in tetrahydrofuran to obtain a solution containing 50 mg per mL.
   Procedure—Separately apply 10 µL of the *Test preparation* and each of the two *Standard preparations* to a suitable thin-layer chromatographic plate (see *Chromatography* ⟨621⟩) coated with a 0.25-mm layer of chromatographic silica gel mixture. Allow the spots to dry, and develop the chromatogram in a solvent system consisting of a mixture of chloroform, ethyl acetate, and formic acid (55 : 40 : 5) until the solvent front has moved about three-fourths of the length of the plate. Remove the plate from the developing chamber, mark the solvent front, air-dry, examine the plate under short-wavelength UV light, and compare the intensities of any secondary spots observed in the chromatogram of the *Test preparation* with those of the principal spots in the chromatograms of the *Standard preparations*: no secondary spot from the chromatogram of the *Test preparation* is larger or more intense than the principal spot obtained from *Standard preparation B* (0.5%) and the sum of the intensities of the secondary spots obtained from the *Test preparation* corresponds to not more than 1.0%.
Assay—[NOTE—Use low-actinic glassware throughout the *Assay*.]
   Standard preparation—Dissolve an accurately weighed quantity of USP Metolazone RS in methanol to obtain a solution having a known concentration of about 40 µg per mL.
   Assay preparation—Transfer about 50 mg of Metolazone, accurately weighed, to 100-mL volumetric flask, dilute with methanol to volume, and mix. Pipet 20 mL into 250-mL volumetric flask, dilute with methanol to volume, and mix.
   Procedure—Concomitantly determine the absorbances of the solutions at the wavelength of maximum absorbance at about 343 nm, with a suitable spectrophotometer, using methanol as the blank. Calculate the quantity, in mg, of $C_{16}H_{16}ClN_3O_3S$ in the portion of Metolazone taken by the formula:

$$1.25C(A_U / A_S)$$

in which C is the concentration, in µg per mL, of USP Metolazone RS in the *Standard preparation;* and A_U and A_S are the absorbances of the *Assay preparation* and the *Standard preparation*, respectively.

Add the following:

▲Metolazone Oral Suspension

» Metolazone Oral Suspension contains not less than 90.0 percent and not more than 110.0 percent of the labeled amount of metolazone ($C_{16}H_{16}ClN_3O_3S$). Prepare Metolazone Oral Suspension 1 mg per mL as follows (see *Pharmaceutical Compounding—Nonsterile Preparations* ⟨795⟩):

Metolazone	100 mg
Vehicle: a mixture of Vehicle for Oral Solution, (regular or sugar-free), *NF* and Vehicle for Oral Suspension, *NF* (1 : 1),	
a sufficient quantity to make	100 mL

If using Tablets, place the Metolazone Tablets in a suitable mortar, and comminute to a fine powder, or add Metolazone powder to the mortar. Add about 20 mL of the Vehicle, and mix to a uniform paste. Add the Vehicle in small portions, and transfer the contents of the mortar, stepwise and quantitatively, to a calibrated bottle. Add sufficient Vehicle in portions to rinse the mortar, add sufficient Vehicle to final volume, and mix well.

Packaging and storage—Preserve in tight, light-resistant containers. Store at controlled room temperature, or in a cold place.
Labeling—Label it to state that it is to be well shaken, and to state the beyond-use date.
USP Reference standards ⟨11⟩—USP Metolazone RS.
pH ⟨791⟩: between 3.6 and 4.6.
Beyond-use date: 60 days after the day on which it was compounded.
Assay—
  Mobile phase—Prepare a suitable filtered and degassed mixture of 700 mL of methanol, 300 mL of 1.5 g ammonium acetate, and 1 mL of diisopropylamine. Make adjustments if necessary (see *System Suitability* under *Chromatography* ⟨621⟩).
  Standard preparation—Dissolve USP Metolazone RS in water to obtain a solution having a known concentration of 1.0 µg per mL.
  Assay preparation—Agitate the container of Oral Suspension for 30 minutes on a rotating mixer, remove a 5-mL sample, and store in a clear glass vial at –70° until analyzed. At the time of analysis, remove the sample from the freezer, allow it to reach room temperature, and mix with a vortex mixer for 30 seconds. Pipet 1.0 mL of the sample into a 1000-mL volumetric flask, and dilute with *Mobile phase* to volume.
  Chromatographic system (see *Chromatography* ⟨621⟩)—The liquid chromatograph is equipped with a 254-nm detector and a 4.6-mm × 20-cm analytical column that contains 5-µm packing L3. The flow rate is about 1.0 mL per minute. Chromatograph the *Standard preparation*, and record the peak responses as directed for *Procedure*: the retention time for metolazone is about 6.0 minutes, and the relative standard deviation for replicate injections is not more than 2.2%.
  Procedure—Separately inject equal volumes (about 20 µL) of the *Standard preparation* and the *Assay preparation* into the chromatograph, record the chromatograms, and measure the responses for the major peaks. Calculate the quantity, in mg, of metolazone ($C_{16}H_{16}ClN_3O_3S$) in the volume of Oral Suspension taken by the formula:

$$1000(C/V)(r_U/r_S)$$

in which C is the concentration, in µg per mL, of USP Metolazone RS in the *Standard preparation*; V is the volume, in mL, of Oral Suspension taken; and r_U and r_S are the peak responses obtained from the *Assay preparation* and the *Standard preparation*, respectively. ▲USP31

Metolazone Tablets

» Metolazone Tablets contain not less than 90.0% and not more than 110.0% of the labeled amount of metolazone ($C_{16}H_{16}ClN_3O_3S$).

Packaging and storage—Preserve in tight, light-resistant containers, and store below 30°.
USP Reference standards ⟨11⟩—USP Metolazone RS.
Identification, *Ultraviolet Absorption* ⟨197U⟩—
  Solution—Pipet 3 mL of the *Assay preparation* into a 25-mL volumetric flask, dilute with methanol to volume, and mix.
Uniformity of dosage units ⟨905⟩: meet the requirements.
Assay—[NOTE—Use low-actinic glassware throughout the *Assay*.]
  Mobile phase—Dissolve 1.38 g of monobasic potassium phosphate monohydrate in about 900 mL of water, adjust with phosphoric acid to a pH of 3.0, and dilute with water to 1000 mL. Prepare a filtered and degassed mixture of this buffer solution, methanol, and acetonitrile (65 : 28 : 7). Make adjustments if necessary (see *System Suitability* under *Chromatography* ⟨621⟩).
  Standard preparation—Dissolve an accurately weighed quantity of USP Metolazone RS in methanol to obtain a solution having a known concentration of about 5 µg per mL.
  Assay preparation—Transfer 10 Tablets to a 200-mL volumetric flask, and add 3 mL of water and about 100 mL of methanol. Sonicate for 30 minutes. If disintegration is not complete, sonicate for an additional 30 minutes. Shake by mechanical means for about 30 minutes. Dilute with methanol to volume, and mix. Transfer an accurately measured volume of this stock solution, equivalent to about 0.25 mg of metolazone, to a 50-mL volumetric flask, dilute with methanol to volume, and mix.
  Chromatographic system (see *Chromatography* ⟨621⟩)—The liquid chromatograph is equipped with a 235-nm detector and a 3.9-mm × 15-cm column that contains packing L1. The flow rate is about 1.1 mL per minute. Chromatograph the *Standard preparation*, and record the peak responses as directed for *Procedure*: the relative standard deviation for replicate injections is not more than 2.0%.
  Procedure—Separately inject equal volumes (about 100 µL) of the *Standard preparation* and the *Assay preparation* into the chromatograph, record the chromatograms, and measure the responses for the metolazone peak. Calculate the quantity, in mg, of metolazone ($C_{16}H_{16}ClN_3O_3S$) in the portion of Tablets taken by the formula:

$$50C(r_U/r_S)$$

in which C is the concentration, in mg per mL, of USP Metolazone RS in the *Standard preparation*; and r_U and r_S are the peak responses obtained from the *Assay preparation* and the *Standard preparation*, respectively.

Metoprolol Fumarate

$(C_{15}H_{25}NO_3)_2 \cdot C_4H_4O_4$ 650.80
2-Propanol, 1-[4-(2-methoxyethyl)phenoxy]-3-[(1-methylethyl)amino]-, (±)-, (E)-2-butanedioate (2 : 1) (salt).
(±)-1-(Isopropylamino)-3-[p-(2-methoxyethyl)-phenoxy]-2-propanol fumarate (2 : 1) (salt)   [119637-66-0].

» Metoprolol Fumarate contains not less than 99.0 percent and not more than 100.5 percent of $(C_{15}H_{25}NO_3)_2 \cdot C_4H_4O_4$, calculated on the dried basis.

Packaging and storage—Preserve in tight, light-resistant containers.
USP Reference standards ⟨11⟩—USP Metoprolol Fumarate RS.
Identification—
  A: *Infrared Absorption* ⟨197K⟩.
  B: Prepare a test solution in methanol containing 10 mg per mL. Separately apply 20 µL of the test solution and 20 µL of a Standard solution of USP Metoprolol Fumarate RS containing 10 mg per mL to a thin-layer chromatographic plate (see *Chromatography* ⟨621⟩) coated with a 0.25-mm layer of chromatographic silica gel mixture. Allow the spots to dry, and develop the chromatogram in an unsaturated chamber with a solvent system consisting of a mixture of alcohol, water, and ammonium hydroxide (8 : 1 : 1) until the solvent front has moved about three-fourths of the length of the plate. Remove the plate from the chamber, mark the solvent front, dry at 110° for 30 minutes, and spray the plate with bromocresol purple TS. Examine the chromatograms: the R_F value of the yellow spot obtained from the test solution corresponds to that obtained from the Standard solution.
Melting range ⟨741⟩: between 145° and 148°.
pH ⟨791⟩: between 5.5 and 6.5, in a solution (1 in 10).
Loss on drying ⟨731⟩—Dry it in vacuum at 60° for 4 hours: it loses not more than 0.5% of its weight.
Residue on ignition ⟨281⟩: not more than 0.1%.
Heavy metals, *Method I* ⟨231⟩:   0.001%.
Organic volatile impurities, *Method I*   ⟨467⟩: meets the requirements.
            (Official until July 1, 2008)
Chromatographic purity—
  Diluent—Prepare a mixture of methanol and water (10 : 1).
  Standard dilutions—Dissolve a suitable quantity of USP Metoprolol Fumarate RS, accurately weighed, in *Diluent*, and dilute quantitatively with *Diluent* to obtain solutions having known concentrations of 1.0, 0.5, 0.2, and 0.1 mg per mL, respectively.
  Test solution—Dissolve a quantity of Metoprolol Fumarate in *Diluent* to obtain a solution containing 100 mg per mL.

Chromatographic chamber and *Detecting reagent*—Prepare as directed in the test for *Chromatographic purity* under *Metoprolol Tartrate*.

Procedure—Proceed as directed for *Procedure* in the test for *Chromatographic purity* under *Metoprolol Tartrate*: the specified results are obtained.

Assay—Dissolve about 325 mg of Metoprolol Fumarate, accurately weighed, in 20 mL of glacial acetic acid, and titrate with 0.1 N perchloric acid VS, determining the endpoint potentiometrically, using a glass electrode and a calomel electrode containing glacial acetic acid saturated with lithium chloride (see *Titrimetry* ⟨541⟩). Perform a blank determination, and make any necessary correction. Each mL of 0.1 N perchloric acid is equivalent to 32.54 mg of $(C_{15}H_{25}NO_3)_2 \cdot C_4H_4O_4$.

Metoprolol Succinate

$(C_{15}H_{25}NO_3)_2 \cdot C_4H_6O_4$ 652.81

2-Propanol, 1-[4-(2-methoxyethyl)phenoxy]-3-[(1-methylethyl)amino]-, (±)-, butanedioate (2 : 1) (salt).

(±)-1-(Isopropylamino)-3-[*p*-(2-methoxyethyl)phenoxy]-2-propanol succinate (2 : 1) (salt)   [98418-47-4].

» Metoprolol Succinate contains not less than 98.0 percent and not more than 102.0 percent of $(C_{15}H_{25}NO_3)_2 \cdot C_4H_6O_4$, calculated on the dried basis.

Packaging and storage—Preserve in tight containers at controlled room temperature.

USP Reference standards ⟨11⟩—*USP Metoprolol Succinate RS. USP Metoprolol Related Compound A RS. USP Metoprolol Related Compound B RS. USP Metoprolol Related Compound C RS. USP Metoprolol Related Compound D RS.*

Clarity and color of solution—A solution of Metoprolol Succinate having a concentration of 20 mg per mL is not less clear than an equal volume of water in a test tube of similar size. The absorbance of the solution determined at 440 nm in a 5-cm cell, using water as the blank, is not more than 0.1.

Identification, *Infrared Absorption* ⟨197K⟩.

pH ⟨791⟩: between 7.0 and 7.6, in a solution containing 65 mg per mL.

Loss on drying ⟨731⟩—Dry it in vacuum at 60° for 4 hours: it loses not more than 0.2% of its weight.

Residue on ignition ⟨281⟩: not more than 0.1%.

Heavy metals, *Method I* ⟨231⟩: 0.001%.

Related compounds—

TEST 1—

Adsorbent: 0.25-mm layer of chromatographic silica gel mixture.

Test solution—Dissolve an accurately weighed quantity of Metoprolol Succinate in methanol to obtain a solution containing 50 mg per mL.

Standard solution—Dilute the *Test solution* quantitatively, and stepwise if necessary, with methanol to obtain a solution having a concentration of 0.1 mg per mL.

Application volume: 10 μL.

Developing solvent system: a mixture of ethyl acetate and methanol (80 : 20).

Procedure—Proceed as directed for *Thin-Layer Chromatography* under *Chromatography* ⟨621⟩. Place two 50-mL beakers, each containing 30 mL of ammonium hydroxide, on the bottom of a chromatographic chamber that is lined with filter paper and contains the *Developing solvent system,* and allow to equilibrate for 1 hour. Position the plate in the chromatographic chamber, and develop the chromatogram until the solvent front has moved about two-thirds of the length of the plate. Remove the plate from the chamber, mark the solvent front, and dry the plate for 3 hours in a current of warm air. Place the plate in a chamber containing iodine vapor, and allow to react for at least 15 hours. Compare the intensities of the brown spots appearing on the chromatogram: any secondary spot obtained from the *Test solution* is not more intense than the corresponding spot obtained from the *Standard solution*. Not more than 0.2% is found.

TEST 2—

Sodium dodecyl sulfate solution, Mobile phase, and *Resolution solution*—Prepare as directed in the *Assay*.

Standard solution—Dissolve an accurately weighed quantity of USP Metoprolol Succinate RS in *Mobile phase*, and dilute quantitatively, and stepwise if necessary, with *Mobile phase* to obtain a solution having a known concentration of about 1.0 μg per mL.

Test solution—Transfer about 50 mg of Metoprolol Succinate, accurately weighed, to a 50-mL volumetric flask, dissolve in and dilute with *Mobile phase* to volume, and mix.

Chromatographic system (see *Chromatography* ⟨621⟩)—Prepare as directed in the *Assay*. Chromatograph the *Resolution solution,* and record the peak responses as directed for *Procedure:* the resolution, *R,* between metoprolol related compound A and metoprolol related compound B is not less than 1.5; and the resolution, *R,* between metoprolol related compound B and metoprolol related compound C is not less than 2.5. [NOTE—The relative retention times are about 0.6 for metoprolol related compound C, 0.7 for metoprolol related compound B, 0.8 for metoprolol related compound A, 1.0 for metoprolol, and 5.0 and 5.2 for the two diastereomers of metoprolol related compound D.] Chromatograph the *Standard solution,* and record the peak responses as directed for *Procedure:* the relative standard deviation for replicate injections is not more than 5.0%.

Procedure—Inject equal volumes (about 10 μL) of the *Standard solution* and the *Test solution* into the chromatograph, record the chromatograms, and measure the peak responses. Calculate the percentage of each impurity in the portion of Metoprolol Succinate taken by the formula:

$$100(C_S / C_T)(r_i / r_S)$$

in which C_S is the concentration, in mg per mL, of USP Metoprolol Succinate RS in the *Standard solution*; C_T is the concentration of metoprolol succinate in the *Test solution*; r_i is the individual peak response of related impurities; and r_S is the peak response obtained from the *Standard solution*: not more than 0.1% of any single impurity is found, and not more than 0.5% of total impurities is found. [NOTE—The sum of the peak responses for the two diastereomers of metoprolol related compound D is used in the above calculation to report the amount of metoprolol related compound D.]

Assay—

Sodium dodecyl sulfate solution—Add 1.3 g of sodium dodecyl sulfate to 1 L of aqueous phosphoric acid, 0.1% (w/v).

Mobile phase—Prepare a filtered and degassed mixture of *Sodium dodecyl sulfate solution* and acetonitrile (60 : 40). Make adjustments if necessary (see *System Suitability* under *Chromatography* ⟨621⟩).

Resolution solution—Prepare a solution in *Mobile phase* containing about 5 μg each of USP Metoprolol Succinate RS, USP Metoprolol Related Compound A RS, USP Metoprolol Related Compound B RS, USP Metoprolol Related Compound C RS, and USP Metoprolol Related Compound D RS per mL.

Standard preparation—Dissolve an accurately weighed quantity of USP Metoprolol Succinate RS in *Mobile phase*, and dilute quantitatively, and stepwise if necessary, with *Mobile phase* to obtain a solution having a known concentration of about 0.08 mg per mL.

Test preparation—Transfer about 80 mg of Metoprolol Succinate, accurately weighed, to a 100-mL volumetric flask, dissolve in and dilute with *Mobile phase* to volume, and mix. Transfer 5.0 mL of this solution to a 50-mL volumetric flask, dilute with *Mobile phase* to volume, and mix.

Chromatographic system (see *Chromatography* ⟨621⟩)—The liquid chromatograph is equipped with a 223-nm detector and a 4-mm × 12.5-cm column that contains 4-μm packing L7. The column temperature is maintained at 30°. The flow rate is about 0.9 mL per minute. Chromatograph the *Resolution solution,* and record the peak responses as directed for *Procedure:* the resolution, *R,* between metoprolol related compound A and metoprolol related compound B is not less than 1.5; and the resolution, *R*, between metoprolol related compound B and metoprolol related compound C is not less than 2.5. [NOTE—The relative retention times are about 0.6 for metoprolol related compound C, 0.7 for metoprolol related compound B, 0.8 for metoprolol related compound A, 1.0 for metoprolol, and 5.0 and 5.2 for the two diastereomers of metoprolol related compound D.] Chromatograph the *Standard preparation,* and record the peak responses as directed for *Procedure:* the relative standard deviation for replicate injections is not more than 2.0%.

Procedure—Inject equal volumes (about 10 μL) of the *Standard preparation* and the *Test preparation* into the chromatograph, record the chromatograms for at least 1.5 times the retention of the metoprolol peak, and measure the peak responses. Calculate the quantity, in mg, of $(C_{15}H_{25}NO_3)_2 \cdot C_4H_6O_4$ in the portion of Metoprolol Succinate taken by the formula:

$$1000C(r_U / r_S)$$

in which *C* is the concentration, in mg per mL, of USP Metoprolol Succinate RS in the *Standard preparation;* and r_U and r_S are the peak responses obtained from the *Test preparation* and the *Standard preparation,* respectively.

Metoprolol Succinate Extended-Release Tablets

» Metoprolol Succinate Extended-Release Tablets contain not less than 90.0 percent and not more than 110.0 percent of the labeled amount of metoprolol succinate $[(C_{15}H_{25}NO_3)_2 \cdot C_4H_6O_4]$.

Packaging and storage—Preserve in tight containers, and store at controlled room temperature.

Labeling—Label it to indicate the content of metoprolol succinate and its equivalent, expressed as metoprolol tartrate $(C_{15}H_{25}NO_3 \cdot C_4H_6O_6)$.

USP Reference standards ⟨11⟩—*USP Metoprolol Succinate RS.*
Identification—
  A: *Infrared Absorption* ⟨197K⟩—
  Test specimen—Transfer one or more Tablets, equivalent to about 200 mg of metoprolol succinate, to a stoppered centrifuge tube. Add about 40 mL of pH 6.8 phosphate buffer (see *Buffer Solutions* in the section *Reagents, Indicators, and Solutions*) and 40 mL of methylene chloride, and shake for 5 minutes. Centrifuge, filter, and use the aqueous phase as the *Test solution.* Transfer 3 mL of the *Test solution* to a separator, add 2 mL of ammonium hydroxide, and extract with 20 mL of methylene chloride. Filter the methylene chloride phase. Grind 1 mL of the filtrate with 300 mg of potassium bromide, dry in a current of warm air, and prepare a disk: the IR spectrum of the *Test specimen* exhibits maxima only at the same wavelengths as that obtained from a similar preparation of USP Metoprolol Succinate RS (*presence of metoprolol*).
  B: *Infrared Absorption* ⟨197K⟩—
  Test specimen—Transfer 5 mL of the *Test solution* prepared as directed for *Identification* test A to a glass-stoppered test tube, add 2 mL of 5 N hydrochloric acid, and extract with 5 mL of ether. Filter the ether phase. Grind 2 mL of the filtrate with 300 mg of potassium bromide, dry in a current of warm air, and prepare a disk: the IR spectrum of the *Test specimen* exhibits maxima only at the same wavelengths as that obtained from a similar preparation of succinic acid (*presence of succinate*).
Dissolution ⟨711⟩—
  Medium: pH 6.8 phosphate buffer (see *Buffer Solutions* in the section *Reagents, Indicators, and Solutions*); 500 mL.
  Apparatus 2: 50 rpm.
  Times: 1, 4, 8, and 20 hours.
  Determine the amount of $(C_{15}H_{25}NO_3)_2 \cdot C_4H_6O_4$ dissolved by employing the following method.

pH 3.0 Phosphate buffer, Mobile phase, and *Standard solution*—Proceed as directed in the test for *Uniformity of dosage units.*

Procedure—Proceed as directed in the test for *Uniformity of dosage units,* except to use 5.0 mL of a filtered portion of the solution under test as the *Test solution,* and *Medium* as the blank, in comparison with a *Standard solution* having a known concentration of USP Metoprolol Succinate RS in the same *Medium.*

Tolerances—The percentages of the labeled amount of $(C_{15}H_{25}NO_3)_2 \cdot C_4H_6O_4$ dissolved at the times specified conform to Acceptance Table 2.

Time (hours)	Amount dissolved
1	not more than 25%
4	between 20% and 40%
8	between 40% and 60%
20	not less than 80%

Uniformity of dosage units ⟨905⟩:   meet the requirements.

PROCEDURE FOR CONTENT UNIFORMITY—

pH 3.0 Phosphate buffer—Mix 50 mL of 1 M monobasic sodium phosphate and 8.0 mL of 1 M phosphoric acid, and dilute with water to 1000 mL. If necessary, adjust with 1 M monobasic potassium phosphate or 1 M phosphoric acid to a pH of 3.0.

Mobile phase—Prepare a filtered and degassed mixture of *pH 3.0 Phosphate buffer* and acetonitrile (375 : 125). Make adjustments if necessary (see *System Suitability* under *Chromatography* ⟨621⟩).

Standard solution—Dissolve a quantity of USP Metoprolol Succinate RS, accurately weighed, in *Mobile phase* to obtain a solution having a known concentration of about 0.05 mg per mL.

Test stock solution—Transfer 1 Tablet, accurately weighed, to a volumetric flask of suitable capacity to obtain a solution having a concentration of about 1 mg per mL of metoprolol succinate. Add about 5 mL of water, and allow the Tablet to disintegrate. Add a volume of alcohol such that when diluted to volume, the concentration of alcohol is 30%. Shake for 30 minutes. Add a portion of 0.1 N hydrochloric acid equivalent to about one half of the flask volume, and shake for 30 minutes. Dilute with 0.1 N hydrochloric acid to volume, and mix.

Test solution—Filter the *Test stock solution,* and discard the first 10 mL of the filtrate. Dilute the filtrate quantitatively with *Mobile phase* to obtain a solution containing about 0.05 mg per mL of metoprolol succinate.

Chromatographic system (see *Chromatography* ⟨621⟩)—The liquid chromatograph is equipped with a 280-nm detector and a 4-mm × 12.5-cm column that contains packing L7. The flow rate is about 1 mL per minute. Chromatograph the *Standard solution,* and record the peak responses as directed for *Procedure:* the relative standard deviation for replicate injections is not more than 2.0%.

Procedure—Separately inject equal volumes (about 40 μL) of the *Standard solution* and the *Test solution* into the chromatograph, record the chromatograms, and measure the responses for the major peaks. Calculate the quantity, in mg, of metoprolol succinate $(C_{15}H_{25}NO_3)_2 \cdot C_4H_6O_4$ in the Tablet taken by the formula:

$$20CV(r_U / r_S)$$

in which *C* is the concentration, in mg per mL, of USP Metoprolol Succinate RS in the *Standard solution;* *V* is the volume of the *Test stock solution* used to prepare the *Test solution;* and r_U and r_S are the peak responses obtained from the *Test solution* and the *Standard solution,* respectively.

Assay—Determine the mean value of the quantity, in mg, of metoprolol succinate $[(C_{15}H_{25}NO_3)_2 \cdot C_4H_6O_4]$ in the Tablets analyzed in the test for *Uniformity of dosage units.*

Metoprolol Tartrate

$(C_{15}H_{25}NO_3)_2 \cdot C_4H_6O_6$ 684.81

2-Propanol, 1-[4-(2-methoxyethyl)phenoxy]-3-[(1-methylethyl)amino]-, (±)-, [R-(R*,R*)]-2,3-dihydroxybutanedioate (2 : 1) (salt).
(±)-1-(Isopropylamino)-3-[p-(2-methoxyethyl)phenoxy]-2-propanol L-(+)-tartrate (2 : 1) (salt).
1-(Isopropylamino)-3-[p-(2-methoxyethyl)phenoxy]-2-propanol (2 : 1) dextro-tartrate salt [56392-17-7].

» Metoprolol Tartrate contains not less than 99.0 percent and not more than 101.0 percent of $(C_{15}H_{25}NO_3)_2 \cdot C_4H_6O_6$, calculated on the dried basis.

Packaging and storage—Preserve in tight, light-resistant containers. Store at 25°, excursions permitted between 15° and 30°.

USP Reference standards ⟨11⟩—*USP Metoprolol Tartrate RS.*
Identification, *Infrared Absorption* ⟨197M⟩.
Specific rotation ⟨781S⟩: between +6.5° and +10.5° (t = 20°).
  Test solution: 20 mg per mL, in water.
pH ⟨791⟩: between 6.0 and 7.0, in a solution (1 in 10).
Loss on drying ⟨731⟩—Dry it in vacuum at 60° for 4 hours: it loses not more than 0.5% of its weight.
Residue on ignition ⟨281⟩: not more than 0.1%.
Heavy metals, *Method I* ⟨231⟩: 0.001%.
Chromatographic purity—
  Standard solution and *Standard dilutions*—Dissolve a suitable quantity of USP Metoprolol Tartrate RS, accurately weighed, in methanol, and dilute quantitatively and stepwise with methanol to obtain solutions having known concentrations of 1.0, 0.5, 0.2, and 0.1 mg per mL, respectively.
  Test solution—Dissolve a quantity of Metoprolol Tartrate in methanol to obtain a solution containing 100 mg per mL.
  Chromatographic chamber—Line a suitable chamber (see *Chromatography* ⟨621⟩) with absorbent paper, and pour into the chamber 250 mL of a mixture of chloroform, methanol, and ammonium hydroxide (80 : 15 : 2). Saturate the chamber for 1.5 hours before using.
  Detecting reagent—Prepare separate solutions of potassium iodide (1 in 100) and soluble starch (prepared by triturating 3 g in 10 mL of cold water and adding the mixture to 90 mL of boiling water with constant stirring). Just prior to use, mix 10 mL of each solution with 3 mL of alcohol.
  Procedure—Apply separately 5-μL portions of the *Test solution* and each of the *Standard dilutions* to a suitable thin-layer chromatographic plate (see *Chromatography* ⟨621⟩) coated with a 0.25-mm layer of chromatographic silica gel mixture. Place the plate in the *Chromatographic chamber,* seal the chamber, and allow the chromatogram to develop until the solvent front has moved about three-fourths of the length of the plate. Remove the plate, and dry in a current of warm air until the odor of ammonia is no longer perceptible (about 45 minutes). Place a beaker containing 0.5 g of potassium permanganate in a chamber. Add 5 mL of 6 N hydrochloric acid to the beaker, and allow to equilibrate for 5 minutes. Place the plate in the chamber for 5 minutes. Remove the plate from the chamber, allow to stand in a current of cool air for 1 hour, and spray with *Detecting reagent.* If spots other than the principal spot are observed in the lane of the *Test solution,* estimate the concentration of each by comparison with the *Standard dilutions:* the spots from the 1.0, 0.5, 0.2, and 0.1 mg per mL *Standard dilutions* correspond to 1.0%, 0.5%, 0.2%, and 0.1% of impurities, respectively; and the sum of any observed impurities in the *Test solution* is not greater than 1.0%.
Organic volatile impurities, *Method I* ⟨467⟩: meets the requirements.

(Official until July 1, 2008)

Assay—Dissolve about 280 mg of Metoprolol Tartrate, accurately weighed, in 20 mL of glacial acetic acid, and titrate with 0.1 N perchloric acid VS, determining the endpoint potentiometrically, using a glass electrode and a calomel electrode containing glacial acetic acid saturated with lithium chloride (see *Titrimetry* ⟨541⟩). Perform a blank determination, and make any necessary correction. Each mL of 0.1 N perchloric acid is equivalent to 34.24 mg of $(C_{15}H_{25}NO_3)_2 \cdot C_4H_6O_6$.

Metoprolol Tartrate Injection

» Metoprolol Tartrate Injection is a sterile solution of Metoprolol Tartrate in Water for Injection. It contains Sodium Chloride as a tonicity-adjusting agent. It contains not less than 90.0 percent and not more than 110.0 percent of the labeled amount of metoprolol tartrate $[(C_{15}H_{25}NO_3)_2 \cdot C_4H_6O_6]$.

Packaging and storage—Preserve in single-dose, light-resistant containers, preferably of Type I or Type II glass.
USP Reference standards ⟨11⟩—*USP Endotoxin RS. USP Metoprolol Tartrate RS. USP Oxprenolol Hydrochloride RS.*
Identification—Place a volume of Injection, equivalent to about 40 mg of metoprolol tartrate, in a separator, add 4 mL of dilute ammonium hydroxide (1 in 3), and extract with 20 mL of chloroform, filtering the chloroform extract through chloroform-pre-rinsed anhydrous sodium sulfate. Evaporate the chloroform to dryness, and place in a freezer to congeal the residue: the IR absorption spectrum of a potassium bromide dispersion of the residue so obtained exhibits maxima only at the same wavelengths as that of a similar preparation of USP Metoprolol Tartrate RS.
Bacterial endotoxins ⟨85⟩—It contains not more than 25.0 USP Endotoxin Units per mg of metoprolol tartrate.
Sterility ⟨71⟩—It meets the requirements when tested as directed for *Membrane Filtration* under *Test for Sterility of the Product to be Examined.*
pH ⟨791⟩: between 5.0 and 8.0.
Other requirements—It meets the requirements under *Injections* ⟨1⟩.
Assay—
  Mobile phase—Prepare a degassed solution by dissolving 961 mg of 1-pentanesulfonic acid sodium salt (monohydrate) and 82 mg of anhydrous sodium acetate in a mixture of 550 mL of methanol and 470 mL of water and adding 0.57 mL of glacial acetic acid.
  Internal standard solution—Dissolve USP Oxprenolol Hydrochloride RS in freshly prepared *Mobile phase* to obtain a solution containing about 720 μg per mL.
  Sodium chloride solution—Dissolve 9.0 g of sodium chloride in water to make 1000 mL.
  Standard preparation—Dissolve an accurately weighed quantity of USP Metoprolol Tartrate RS in *Sodium chloride solution* to obtain a stock solution having a known concentration of about 1000 μg per mL. Mix equal volumes, accurately measured, of this stock solution and of *Internal standard solution.*
  Assay preparation—Dilute an accurately measured volume of Injection, if necessary, quantitatively with *Sodium chloride solution* to obtain a stock solution having a concentration of about 1000 μg per mL. Mix equal volumes, accurately measured, of this stock solution and of *Internal standard solution.*
  Chromatographic system (see *Chromatography* ⟨621⟩)—The liquid chromatograph is equipped with a 254-nm detector and a 3.9-mm × 30-cm column that contains packing L1. The flow rate is about 1 mL per minute. Chromatograph three replicate injections of the *Standard preparation,* and record the peak responses as directed under *Procedure:* the relative standard deviation is not more than 2.0%, and the resolution factor between metoprolol tartrate and oxprenolol hydrochloride is not less than 2.0.
  Procedure—Separately inject equal volumes (about 10 μL) of the *Standard preparation* and the *Assay preparation* into the chromatograph, record the chromatograms, and measure the responses for the

major peaks. The relative retention times are about 0.8 for metoprolol tartrate and 1.0 for oxprenolol hydrochloride. Calculate the quantity, in mg, of metoprolol tartrate [$(C_{15}H_{25}NO_3)_2 \cdot C_4H_6O_6$] in each mL of the Injection taken by the formula:

$$(L / D)(C)(R_U / R_S)$$

in which L is the labeled quantity, in mg, of metoprolol tartrate in the Injection; D is the concentration, in μg per mL, of metoprolol tartrate in the *Assay preparation,* on the basis of the labeled quantity in each mL of Injection taken and the extent of dilution; C is the concentration, in μg per mL, of USP Metoprolol Tartrate RS in the *Standard preparation;* and R_U and R_S are the peak response ratios of metoprolol tartrate to oxprenolol hydrochloride obtained from the *Assay preparation* and the *Standard preparation,* respectively.

Add the following:

▲Metoprolol Tartrate Oral Solution

» Metoprolol Tartrate Oral Solution contains not less than 90.0 percent and not more than 110.0 percent of the labeled amount of metoprolol tartrate [$(C_{15}H_{25}NO_3)_2 \cdot C_4H_6O_6$]. Prepare Metoprolol Tartrate Oral Solution 10 mg per mL as follows (see *Pharmaceutical Compounding—Nonsterile Preparations* ⟨795⟩. See also *Metoprolol Tartrate Oral Suspension*):

Metoprolol Tartrate powder	1 g
Vehicle for Oral Solution (regular or sugar-free), *NF*, a sufficient quantity to make	100 mL

Add Metoprolol Tartrate powder and about 20 mL of Vehicle to a mortar, and mix. Add the Vehicle in small portions almost to volume, and mix thoroughly after each addition. Transfer the contents of the mortar, stepwise and quantitatively, to a calibrated bottle. Add enough Vehicle to bring to final volume, and mix well.

Packaging and storage—Preserve in tight, light-resistant containers. Store at controlled room temperature or in a cold place.
Labeling—Label it to state that it is to be well shaken, and to state the beyond-use date.
USP Reference standards ⟨11⟩—USP Metoprolol Tartrate RS.
pH ⟨791⟩: between 3.6 and 4.6.
Beyond-use date: 60 days after the day on which it was compounded.
Assay—
Mobile phase—Prepare a suitable filtered and degassed solution by dissolving 961 mg of 1-pentanesulfonic acid sodium salt, monohydrate, and 82 mg of anhydrous sodium acetate in a mixture of 550 mL of methanol, 470 mL of water, and 0.57 mL of glacial acetic acid. Make adjustments if necessary (see *System Suitability* under *Chromatography* ⟨621⟩).
Standard preparation—Dissolve USP Metoprolol Tartrate RS in water to obtain a solution having a known concentration of 100 μg per mL.
Assay preparation—Agitate the container of Oral Solution for 30 minutes on a rotating mixer, remove a 5-mL sample, and store in a clear glass vial at −70° until analyzed. At the time of analysis, remove the sample from the freezer, allow it to reach room temperature, and mix on a vortex mixer for 30 seconds. Pipet 1.0 mL of the sample into a 100-mL volumetric flask, and dilute with *Mobile phase* to volume.
Chromatographic system (see *Chromatography* ⟨621⟩)—The liquid chromatograph is equipped with a 254-nm detector and a 4.6-mm × 25-cm analytical column that contains 5-μm packing L1. The flow rate is about 1.0 mL per minute. Chromatograph the *Standard preparation,* and record the peak responses as directed for *Procedure:* the retention time for metoprolol tartrate is about 7.3 minutes; and the relative standard deviation for replicate injections is not more than 1.3%.
Procedure—Separately inject equal volumes (about 20 μL) of the *Standard preparation* and the *Assay preparation* into the chromatograph, record the chromatograms, and measure the responses for the major peaks. Calculate the quantity, in mg, of metoprolol tartrate [$(C_{15}H_{25}NO_3)_2 \cdot C_4H_6O_6$] in the volume of Oral Solution taken by the formula:

$$100(C / V)(r_U / r_S)$$

in which C is the concentration, in μg per mL, of USP Metoprolol Tartrate RS in the *Standard preparation;* V is the volume, in mL, of Oral Solution taken; and r_U and r_S are the peak responses obtained from the *Assay preparation* and the *Standard preparation,* respectively.▲USP31

Add the following:

▲Metoprolol Tartrate Oral Suspension

» Metoprolol Tartrate Oral Suspension contains not less than 90.0 percent and not more than 110.0 percent of the labeled amount of Metoprolol Tartrate [$(C_{15}H_{25}NO_3)_2 \cdot C_4H_6O_6$]. Prepare Metoprolol Tartrate Oral Suspension 10 mg per mL as follows (see *Pharmaceutical Compounding—Nonsterile Preparations* ⟨795⟩. See also *Metoprolol Tartrate Oral Solution*):

Metoprolol Tartrate	1 g
Vehicle: a mixture of Vehicle for Oral Solution, (regular or sugar-free), *NF* and Vehicle for Oral Suspension, *NF* (1 : 1), a sufficient quantity to make	100 mL

If using Tablets, place the Metoprolol Tartrate Tablets in a suitable mortar, and comminute the Tablets, or add Metoprolol Tartrate powder. Add the Vehicle in small portions, and mix well. Transfer the contents of the mortar, stepwise and quantitatively, to a calibrated bottle. Add the Vehicle in portions to rinse the mortar. Add to the preparation to final volume, and mix well.

Packaging and storage—Preserve in tight, light-resistant containers. Store at controlled room temperature, or in a cold place.
Labeling—Label it to state that it is to be well shaken, and to state the beyond-use date.
USP Reference standards ⟨11⟩—USP Metoprolol Tartrate RS.
pH ⟨791⟩: between 3.6 and 4.6.
Beyond-use date: 60 days after the day on which it was compounded.
Assay—
Mobile phase—Prepare a suitable filtered and degassed solution by dissolving 961 mg of 1-pentanesulfonic acid sodium salt, monohydrate, and 82 mg of anhydrous sodium acetate in a mixture of 550 mL of methanol, 470 mL of water, and 0.57 mL of glacial acetic acid. Make adjustments if necessary (see *System Suitability* under *Chromatography* ⟨621⟩).
Standard preparation—Dissolve USP Metoprolol Tartrate RS in water to obtain a solution having a known concentration of 100 μg per mL.

Assay preparation—Agitate the container of Oral Suspension for 30 minutes on a rotating mixer, remove a 5-mL sample, and store in a clear glass vial at −70° until analyzed. At the time of analysis, remove the sample from the freezer, allow it to reach room temperature, and mix with a vortex mixer for 30 seconds. Pipet 1.0 mL of the sample solution into a 100-mL volumetric flask, and dilute with *Mobile phase* to volume.

Chromatographic system (see *Chromatography* ⟨621⟩)—The liquid chromatograph is equipped with a 254-nm detector and a 4.6-mm × 25-cm analytical column that contains 5-μm packing L1. The flow rate is about 1.0 mL per minute. Chromatograph the *Standard preparation*, and record the peak responses as directed for *Procedure:* the retention time for metoprolol tartrate is about 7.3 minutes; and the relative standard deviation for replicate injections is not more than 1.3%.

Procedure—Separately inject equal volumes (about 20 μL) of the *Standard preparation* and the *Assay preparation* into the chromatograph, record the chromatograms, and measure the responses for the major peaks. Calculate the quantity, in mg, of metoprolol tartrate $[(C_{15}H_{25}NO_3)_2 \cdot C_4H_6O_6]$ in the volume of Oral Suspension taken by the formula:

$$100(C/V)(r_U/r_S)$$

in which C is the concentration, in μg per mL, of USP Metoprolol Tartrate RS in the *Standard preparation*; V is the volume, in mL, of Oral Suspension taken; and r_U and r_S are the peak responses obtained from the *Assay preparation* and the *Standard preparation*, respectively.▲USP31

Metoprolol Tartrate Tablets

» Metoprolol Tartrate Tablets contain not less than 90.0 percent and not more than 110.0 percent of the labeled amount of metoprolol tartrate $[(C_{15}H_{25}NO_3)_2 \cdot C_4H_6O_6]$.

Packaging and storage—Preserve in tight, light-resistant containers.

USP Reference standards ⟨11⟩—*USP Metoprolol Tartrate RS. USP Oxprenolol Hydrochloride RS.*

Identification—
A: Place a quantity of finely powdered Tablets, equivalent to about 40 mg of metoprolol tartrate, in a separator, add 25 mL of water and 4 mL of dilute ammonium hydroxide (1 in 3), and extract with 20 mL of chloroform, filtering the chloroform extract through chloroform-prerinsed anhydrous sodium sulfate. Evaporate the chloroform to dryness, and place in a freezer to congeal the residue: the IR absorption spectrum of a potassium bromide dispersion of the residue so obtained exhibits maxima only at the same wavelengths as that of a similar preparation of USP Metoprolol Tartrate RS.

B: Transfer a portion of finely powdered Tablets, equivalent to about 50 mg of metoprolol tartrate, to a 500-mL volumetric flask, dilute with water to volume, and mix. Pass a portion of this solution through a filter of 1 μm or finer porosity: the UV spectrum of the filtrate exhibits maxima and minima at the same wavelengths as that of a solution of USP Metoprolol Tartrate RS in water having a concentration of about 0.1 mg per mL.

C: The retention time of the metoprolol peak in the chromatogram obtained from the *Assay preparation* corresponds to that in the chromatogram of the *Standard preparation* as obtained in the *Assay*.

Dissolution ⟨711⟩—
Medium: simulated gastric fluid TS (without enzyme); 900 mL.
Apparatus 1: 100 rpm.
Time: 30 minutes.
Procedure—Determine the amount of $(C_{15}H_{25}NO_3)_2 \cdot C_4H_6O_6$ dissolved in filtered portions of the solution under test from UV absorbances at the wavelength of maximum absorbance at about 275 nm in comparison with a *Standard* solution having a known concentration of USP Metoprolol Tartrate RS in the same medium.

Tolerances—Not less than 75% (*Q*) of the labeled amount of $(C_{15}H_{25}NO_3)_2 \cdot C_4H_6O_6$ is dissolved in 30 minutes.

Uniformity of dosage units ⟨905⟩: meet the requirements.

Assay—
Solvent mixture—Prepare a mixture of methanol and 0.1 N hydrochloric acid (1 : 1).

Mobile phase—Prepare a suitable and degassed solution by dissolving 961 mg of 1-pentanesulfonic acid sodium salt (monohydrate) and 82 mg of anhydrous sodium acetate in a mixture of 550 mL of methanol and 470 mL of water and adding 0.57 mL of glacial acetic acid.

Standard preparation—Dissolve an accurately weighed quantity of USP Metoprolol Tartrate RS in *Solvent mixture* to obtain a stock solution having a known concentration of about 1000 μg per mL. Transfer 25.0 mL of this solution to a 50-mL volumetric flask, dilute with *Mobile phase* to volume, and mix.

Resolution solution—Prepare a solution of oxprenolol hydrochloride in *Solvent mixture* to obtain a solution containing about 720 μg per mL. Prepare a 1 : 1 mixture of this solution and the stock solution used to prepare the *Standard preparation*.

Assay preparation—Weigh and finely powder not less than 20 Tablets. Transfer an accurately weighed portion of the powder, equivalent to about 50 mg of metoprolol tartrate, to a 50-mL volumetric flask, add 30 mL of *Solvent mixture*, shake by mechanical means for 30 minutes, sonicate for 15 minutes, and heat on a steam bath for 10 minutes. Allow the solution to cool to room temperature, dilute with *Solvent mixture* to volume, and mix. Centrifuge a portion of the solution, and transfer 25.0 mL of the supernatant to a 50-mL volumetric flask, dilute with *Mobile phase* to volume, and mix. Pass a portion of this solution through a filter of 0.5 μm or finer porosity, discarding the first few mL of the filtrate.

Chromatographic system (see *Chromatography* ⟨621⟩)—The liquid chromatograph is equipped with a 254-nm detector and a 3.9-mm × 30-cm column that contains packing L1. The flow rate is about 1 mL per minute. Chromatograph the *Resolution solution*, and record the peak responses as directed under *Procedure*: the relative retention times are about 0.8 for metoprolol and 1.0 for oxprenolol, and the resolution, *R*, between the metoprolol and oxprenolol peaks is not less than 2.0. Chromatograph the *Standard preparation*, and record the peak responses as directed for *Procedure*: the relative standard deviation is not more than 2.0%.

Procedure—Separately inject equal volumes (about 30 μL) of the *Standard preparation* and the *Assay preparation* into the chromatograph, record the chromatograms, and measure the responses for the major peaks. Calculate the quantity, in mg, of metoprolol tartrate $[(C_{15}H_{25}NO_3)_2 \cdot C_4H_6O_6]$ in the portion of Tablets taken by the formula:

$$0.1C(r_U/r_S)$$

in which C is the concentration, in μg per mL, of USP Metoprolol Tartrate RS in the *Standard preparation*; and r_U and r_S are the metoprolol peak responses obtained from the *Assay preparation* and the *Standard preparation*, respectively.

Metoprolol Tartrate and Hydrochlorothiazide Tablets

» Metoprolol Tartrate and Hydrochlorothiazide Tablets contain not less than 90.0 percent and not more than 110.0 percent of the labeled amounts of metoprolol tartrate $[(C_{15}H_{25}NO_3)_2 \cdot C_4H_6O_6]$ and hydrochlorothiazide $(C_7H_8ClN_3O_4S_2)$.

Packaging and storage—Preserve in tight, light-resistant containers.

USP Reference standards ⟨11⟩—*USP Benzothiadiazine Related Compound A RS. USP Hydrochlorothiazide RS. USP Metoprolol Tartrate RS. USP Oxprenolol Hydrochloride RS.*

Identification—

A: Place a quantity of finely powdered Tablets, equivalent to about 100 mg of metoprolol tartrate, in a 50-mL volumetric flask. Add about 30 mL of 0.1 N sodium hydroxide, shake for 20 minutes, dilute with 0.1 N sodium hydroxide to volume, and mix. Filter a portion of this mixture, discarding the first 10 mL of the filtrate. Place 25 mL of the filtrate into a separator, and extract with three 15-mL portions of chloroform, filtering the chloroform extracts through chloroform-prerinsed anhydrous sodium sulfate, and combining the extracts in a suitable container. [NOTE—Retain the aqueous layer remaining after extraction for *Identification* test *B*.] Evaporate the chloroform to dryness, and place in a freezer to congeal the residue: the IR absorption spectrum of a potassium bromide dispersion of the residue so obtained exhibits maxima only at the same wavelengths as that of a similar preparation of USP Metoprolol Tartrate RS.

B: Pass the aqueous layer from *Identification* test *A* through 0.1 N sodium hydroxide-prerinsed cotton. Dilute a portion of the filtrate quantitatively and stepwise with 0.1 N sodium hydroxide to obtain a solution having a concentration of about 0.01 mg of hydrochlorothiazide per mL: the UV absorption spectrum of this solution exhibits maxima and minima at the same wavelengths as a Standard solution prepared as follows. Dissolve 25 mg of USP Hydrochlorothiazide RS in 50 mL of 0.1 N sodium hydroxide in a separator, and extract with three 15-mL portions of chloroform. Discard the chloroform extracts, and pass the aqueous solution through 0.1 N sodium hydroxide-prerinsed cotton. Pipet 2 mL of the filtrate into a 100-mL volumetric flask, dilute with 0.1 N sodium hydroxide to volume, and mix.

Dissolution ⟨711⟩—

Medium: simulated gastric fluid TS (without enzyme); 900 mL.

Apparatus 1: 100 rpm.

Time: 30 minutes.

Determination of dissolved metoprolol tartrate—Remove about 125 mL of the solution under test, allow to cool to room temperature, and filter, discarding the first 25 mL of the filtrate. [NOTE—Retain about 30 mL of the remaining filtrate of the solution under test for the *Determination of dissolved hydrochlorothiazide*.] If necessary, quantitatively dilute a portion of the filtrate with fresh *Dissolution Medium* to obtain a solution having a concentration of about 0.05 mg of metoprolol tartrate per mL. Transfer to separate separators 50.0 mL of the filtrate, 50.0 mL of a Standard solution in *Dissolution Medium* having a known concentration of about 0.05 mg of USP Metoprolol Tartrate RS per mL, and 50.0 mL of *Dissolution Medium* to provide the blank. Add 10 mL of 2.5 N sodium hydroxide to each separator, and extract each with three 15-mL portions of chloroform, filtering the chloroform extracts through pledgets of chloroform-prerinsed glass wool into individual 50-mL volumetric flasks. Dilute the contents of each flask with chloroform to volume, and mix. Determine the absorbances of the solutions from the filtrate and the Standard solution in 2-cm cells at the wavelength of maximum absorbance at about 276 nm, with a suitable spectrophotometer, using the solution from the blank to set the instrument. Calculate the quantity, in mg, of $(C_{15}H_{25}NO_3)_2 \cdot C_4H_6O_6$ dissolved by the formula:

$$900Cf(A_U/A_S)$$

in which C is the concentration, in mg per mL, of USP Metoprolol Tartrate RS in the *Standard solution; f* is the dilution factor for the solution from the filtrate; and A_U and A_S are the absorbances of the solution from the filtrate and of the *Standard solution*, respectively.

Determination of dissolved hydrochlorothiazide—Filter a portion of the filtrate retained from the *Determination of dissolved metoprolol tartrate* through a filter of 0.8 μm or finer porosity, discarding the first 5 mL of the filtrate. If necessary, quantitatively dilute a portion of the filtrate with fresh *Dissolution Medium* to obtain a solution having a concentration of about 0.03 mg of hydrochlorothiazide per mL. Prepare a *Standard solution* in *Dissolution Medium* having a known concentration of about 0.03 mg of USP Hydrochlorothiazide RS per mL. Determine the absorbances of these solutions in 2-cm cells at the wavelength of maximum absorbance at about 316 nm, using *Dissolution Medium* as the blank. Calculate the quantity, in mg, of $C_7H_8ClN_3O_4S_2$ dissolved by the formula:

$$900Cf(A_U/A_S)$$

in which C is the concentration, in mg per mL, of USP Hydrochlorothiazide RS in the *Standard solution; f* is the dilution factor for the solution from the filtrate; and A_U and A_S are the absorbances of the solution from the filtrate and of the *Standard solution*, respectively.

Tolerances—Not less than 80% (*Q*) of the labeled amount of metoprolol tartrate $(C_{15}H_{25}NO_3)_2 \cdot C_4H_6O_6$ and not less than 80% (*Q*) of the labeled amount of hydrochlorothiazide $(C_7H_8ClN_3O_4S_2)$ are dissolved in 30 minutes.

Uniformity of dosage units ⟨905⟩: meet the requirements for *Content Uniformity* with respect to metoprolol tartrate and to hydrochlorothiazide.

Procedure for content uniformity of metoprolol tartrate—Transfer 1 Tablet to a suitable volumetric flask, add 0.1 N hydrochloric acid to about 60% of the nominal volume, sonicate for 15 minutes, and shake by mechanical means for 30 minutes. Dilute with 0.1 N hydrochloric acid to volume to obtain a final solution having a concentration of approximately 1000 μg per mL. Mix, and filter, discarding the first 20 mL of the filtrate. Pipet 10 mL of the filtrate, 10 mL of a Standard solution of USP Metoprolol Tartrate RS in the same medium having a known concentration of about 1000 μg per mL, and 10 mL of 0.1 N hydrochloric acid to provide a blank into individual separators. To each separator add 2.0 mL of 2.5 N sodium hydroxide, and extract with three 25-mL portions of chloroform, passing the chloroform extracts through chloroform-prerinsed glass wool into individual 100-mL volumetric flasks. Dilute with chloroform to volume, and mix. Determine the absorbances of the solutions in 1-cm cells at the wavelength of maximum absorbance at about 276 nm, with a suitable spectrophotometer, using the blank to set the instrument. Calculate the quantity, in mg, of $(C_{15}H_{25}NO_3)_2 \cdot C_4H_6O_6$ in the Tablet by the formula:

$$(T/1000)C(A_U/A_S)$$

in which T is the labeled quantity, in mg, of metoprolol tartrate in the Tablet; C is the concentration, in μg per mL, of USP Metoprolol Tartrate RS in the *Standard solution*; and A_U and A_S are the absorbances of the solution from the Tablet and the *Standard solution*, respectively.

Procedure for content uniformity of hydrochlorothiazide—Transfer 1 Tablet to a 100-mL volumetric flask containing 15 mL of water, and shake by mechanical means for 15 minutes. Add 60 mL of methanol, sonicate for 5 minutes, and shake by mechanical means for 30 minutes. Dilute with methanol to volume, and mix. Centrifuge 40 mL of this suspension. Dilute an accurately measured portion of the supernatant quantitatively with methanol to obtain a solution having a concentration of about 0.05 mg of hydrochlorothiazide per mL. Filter a portion of this solution through a 0.5-μm porosity filter, discarding the first few mL of the filtrate. Use the filtrate as the test solution. Transfer about 25 mg of USP Hydrochlorothiazide RS, accurately weighed, to a 100-mL volumetric flask containing 15 mL of water, dilute with methanol to volume, and mix. Transfer 10.0 mL of this solution to a 50-mL volumetric flask, dilute with methanol to volume, and mix (Standard solution). Concomitantly determine the absorbances of the test solution and the Standard solution at the wavelength of maximum absorbance at about 316 nm, with a suitable spectrophotometer, using methanol as the blank. Calculate the quantity, in mg, of hydrochlorothiazide $(C_7H_8ClN_3O_4S_2)$ in the Tablet taken by the formula:

$$(LC/D)(A_U/A_S)$$

in which L is the labeled quantity, in mg, of hydrochlorothiazide in the Tablet; C is the concentration, in mg per mL, of USP Hydrochlorothiazide RS in the *Standard solution; D* is the concentration, in mg per mL, of hydrochlorothiazide in the test solution based on the labeled quantity in the Tablet and the extent of dilution; and A_U and A_S are the absorbances of the *Test solution* and the *Standard solution*, respectively.

Diazotizable substances—

Standard solution—Weigh accurately 5 mg of USP Benzothiadiazine Related Compound A RS, and dissolve in 2 mL of methanol contained in a 50-mL volumetric flask. Dilute with water to volume, and mix. Pipet 5 mL of the resulting solution into a 100-mL volumetric flask, add 20 mL of methanol, dilute with water to volume, and mix. Each mL of *Standard solution* contains 5 µg of the Reference Standard.

Test solution—Transfer a portion of the powdered Tablets prepared for the *Assay*, accurately weighed and equivalent to 50 mg of hydrochlorothiazide, to a 100-mL volumetric flask containing a mixture of 20 mL of methanol and 20 mL of water. Shake continuously for 5 to 10 minutes, dilute with water to volume, mix, and filter. Use the filtrate as the *Test solution* immediately after preparation.

Procedure—Pipet 5 mL each of the *Standard solution* and the *Test solution* into separate, 50-mL volumetric flasks. Pipet 5 mL of water into a third 50-mL volumetric flask to provide a blank. To each flask add 1 mL of freshly prepared sodium nitrite solution (1 in 100) and 5 mL of dilute hydrochloric acid (1 in 10), and allow to stand for 5 minutes. Add 2 mL of ammonium sulfamate solution (1 in 50), allow to stand for 5 minutes with frequent swirling, then add 2 mL of freshly prepared disodium chromotropate solution (1 in 100) and 10 mL of sodium acetate TS. Dilute with water to volume, and mix. Concomitantly determine the absorbances of the solutions obtained from the *Standard solution* and the *Test solution* at 500 nm, with a suitable spectrophotometer, against the blank. The absorbance of the solution from the *Test solution* does not exceed that of the solution from the *Standard solution*, corresponding to not more than 1.0% of diazotizable substances.

Assay for metoprolol tartrate—

Mobile phase and *Chromatographic system*—Proceed as directed in the *Assay* under *Metoprolol Tartrate Injection*.

Internal standard solution—Dissolve USP Oxprenolol Hydrochloride RS in freshly prepared *Mobile phase* to obtain a solution containing about 360 µg per mL.

Standard preparation—Dissolve an accurately weighed quantity of USP Metoprolol Tartrate RS in 0.1 N hydrochloric acid to obtain a stock solution having a known concentration of about 1000 µg per mL. Transfer 10.0 mL of this stock solution to a suitable separator, add 2.0 mL of 2.5 N sodium hydroxide, and extract with three 25-mL portions of chloroform. Pass the chloroform extracts through chloroform-prerinsed glass wool into a round-bottom flask, and evaporate on a rotary evaporator under vacuum to dryness. Add 20.0 mL of *Internal standard solution* to the flask, sonicate for 3 minutes, and gently swirl to dissolve the residue in the flask.

Assay preparation—Weigh and finely powder not less than 20 Tablets. Transfer an accurately weighed portion of the powder, equivalent to about 100 mg of metoprolol tartrate, to a 100-mL volumetric flask, add 60 mL of 0.1 N hydrochloric acid, heat on a steam bath for 3 minutes, and sonicate for 5 minutes. Shake for 30 minutes. Allow the solution to cool to room temperature, dilute with 0.1 N hydrochloric acid to volume, and mix. Filter a portion of this solution, discarding the first 20 mL of the filtrate. Transfer 10.0 mL of the filtrate to a separator, add 2.0 mL of 2.5 N sodium hydroxide, and extract with three 25-mL portions of chloroform. Pass the chloroform extracts through chloroform-prerinsed glass wool into a round-bottom flask, and evaporate on a rotary evaporator under vacuum to dryness. Add 20.0 mL of *Internal standard solution* to the flask, sonicate for 3 minutes, and gently swirl to dissolve the residue in the flask. Filter a portion of this solution through a filter of 0.5 µm or finer porosity, discarding the first few mL of the filtrate. Use the filtrate as the *Assay preparation*.

Procedure—Proceed as directed for *Procedure* in the *Assay* under *Metoprolol Tartrate Injection*. Calculate the quantity, in mg, of metoprolol tartrate $[(C_{15}H_{25}NO_3)_2 \cdot C_4H_6O_6]$ in the portion of Tablets taken by the formula:

$$0.1C(R_U / R_S)$$

in which C is the concentration, in µg per mL, of USP Metoprolol Tartrate RS in the stock solution used to prepare the *Standard preparation*; and R_U and R_S are the peak response ratios of metoprolol tartrate to oxprenolol hydrochloride obtained from the *Assay preparation* and the *Standard preparation*, respectively.

Assay for hydrochlorothiazide—

Mobile phase—[NOTE—Pass the methanol and water through 0.5-µm porosity filters before use.] Dissolve 1.38 g of monobasic sodium phosphate in 780 mL of water, add 220 mL of methanol, and mix. Degas before use. Make adjustments if necessary (see *System Suitability* under *Chromatography* ⟨621⟩).

Internal standard solution—Dissolve a quantity of sulfanilamide in methanol to obtain a solution containing about 0.4 mg per mL.

System suitability solution—Dissolve a quantity of USP Benzothiadiazine Related Compound A RS in *Internal standard solution* to obtain a solution containing about 1 mg per mL. Mix 1 mL of this solution and 4 mL of methanol.

Standard preparation—Transfer about 50 mg of USP Hydrochlorothiazide RS, accurately weighed, to a 100-mL volumetric flask, add 20.0 mL of *Internal standard solution*, dilute with methanol to volume, and mix.

Assay preparation—Weigh and finely powder not fewer than 20 Tablets. Transfer an accurately weighed portion of the powder, equivalent to about 25 mg of hydrochlorothiazide, to a 50-mL volumetric flask. Add 10.0 mL of *Internal standard solution* and 20 mL of methanol, and sonicate for 5 minutes. Shake by mechanical means for 30 minutes, dilute with methanol to volume, and mix. Centrifuge a portion of this solution, and pass a portion of the supernatant through a 0.5-µm porosity filter, discarding the first few mL of the filtrate. Use the filtrate as the *Assay preparation*.

Chromatographic system (see *Chromatography* ⟨621⟩)—The liquid chromatograph is equipped with a 254-nm detector and a 3.9-mm × 30-cm column that contains packing L1. The flow rate is about 0.6 mL per minute. Chromatograph replicate injections of the *System suitability solution*, and record the peak responses as directed for *Procedure*: the relative retention times are about 0.7 for sulfanilamide and 1.0 for benzothiadiazine related compound A; and the resolution, R, between the peaks is not less than 2.0. Chromatograph the *Standard preparation*, and record the peak responses as directed for *Procedure*: the relative standard deviation for replicate injections is not more than 2.0%.

Procedure—Separately inject equal volumes (about 4 µL) of the *Standard preparation* and the *Assay preparation* into the chromatograph, record the chromatograms, and measure the responses for the major peaks. The relative retention times are about 0.6 for sulfanilamide and 1.0 for hydrochlorothiazide. Calculate the quantity, in mg, of hydrochlorothiazide ($C_7H_8ClN_3O_4S_2$) in the portion of Tablets taken by the formula:

$$50C(R_U / R_S)$$

in which C is the concentration, in mg per mL, of USP Hydrochlorothiazide RS in the *Standard preparation*; and R_U and R_S are the peak response ratios of hydrochlorothiazide to sulfanilamide obtained from the *Assay preparation* and the *Standard preparation*, respectively.

Metrifonate

$C_4H_8Cl_3O_4P$ 257.44
Phosphonic acid, (2,2,2-trichloro-1-hydroxyethyl)-, dimethyl ester.
Dimethyl (2,2,2-trichloro-1-hydroxyethyl)phosphonate   [52-68-6].

» Metrifonate contains not less than 98.0 percent and not more than 100.5 percent of $C_4H_8Cl_3O_4P$, calculated on the anhydrous basis.

Packaging and storage—Preserve in well-closed containers at a temperature not exceeding 25°.
Labeling—Label it to indicate that it is for veterinary use only.
USP Reference standards ⟨11⟩—*USP Metrifonate RS*.
Completeness of solution ⟨641⟩:   meets the requirements, 0.5 g of it being dissolved in methanol.

Color of solution ⟨631⟩—The solution obtained in the test for *Completeness of solution* has no more color than *Matching Fluid F*.
Identification—
  A: *Infrared Absorption* ⟨197K⟩.
  B: *Thin-Layer Chromatographic Identification Test* ⟨201⟩ —
  Test solution: Dissolve 10 mg of Metrifonate in methanol, and dilute with methanol to 10.0 mL.
  Developing solvent sytstem: a mixture of toluene, dioxane, and glacial acetic acid (70 : 25 : 5)
  Procedure—Proceed as directed in the chapter. After allowing the plate to air-dry, spray the plate with a 5% solution of 4-(*p*-nitrobenzyl)pyridine in acetone, and heat at 120 ° for 15 minutes. Before the plate cools, spray it with a 10% solution of tetraethylenepentamine in acetone, and immediately examine the plate: the principal spot in the chromatogram obtained from the *Test solution* corresponds in R_F value, size, and blue color to that in the chromatogram obtained from the Standard solution.
  C: Dissolve 20 mg of Metrifonate in 1 mL of 2 N sodium hydroxide, add 1 mL of pyridine, shake, and heat on a water bath for 2 minutes: a red color develops in the pyridine layer.
  D: To 100 mg of Metrifonate add 0.5 mL of nitric acid, 0.5 mL of a 50% solution of ammonium nitrate, and 0.1 mL of 30 percent hydrogen peroxide, and heat on a water bath for 10 minutes. Heat to boiling, and add 1 mL of ammonium molybdate TS: a yellow color precipitate is formed.
Acidity—Dissolve 2.5 g of it in carbon dioxide-free water, dilute with carbon dioxide-free water to 50 mL, and add 0.1 mL of methyl red TS. Not more than 1.0 mL of 0.1 N sodium hydroxide is required to change the color of the indicator.
Water, *Method I* ⟨921⟩: not more than 0.3%.
Heavy metals ⟨231⟩: 0.001%.
Limit of free chloride—Dissolve 5.0 g of Metrifonate in 30 mL of alcohol, and add a mixture of 100 mL of water and 15 mL of nitric acid. Titrate with 0.1 N silver nitrate VS, determining the endpoint potentiometrically using a silver electrode. Not more than 0.7 mL of 0.1 N silver nitrate is consumed (0.05%).
Chromatographic purity—
  Solution A—Dissolve 1.36 g of monobasic potassium phosphate in water, and dilute with water to 1000 mL. Adjust with phosphoric acid to a pH of 3.0.
  Solution B—Use acetonitrile.
  Mobile phase—Use variable mixtures of *Solution A* and *Solution B* as directed for *Chromatographic system*. Make adjustments if necessary (see *System Suitability* under *Chromatography* ⟨621⟩).
  Diluent—Prepare a mixture of acetonitrile and water (1 : 1).
  Standard preparation—Prepare a solution of USP Metrifonate RS in *Diluent* containing 20 mg per mL.
  Test solution—Transfer 500 mg of Metrifonate, accurately weighed, to a 25-mL volumetric flask, dissolve in and dilute with *Diluent* to volume, and mix.
  Chromatographic system (see *Chromatography* ⟨621⟩)—The liquid chromatograph is equipped with a 210-nm detector and a 4-mm × 25-cm column that contains 5-μm packing L7. The column is maintained at a constant temperature of about 40°. The flow rate is about 1.5 mL per minute. The chromatograph is programmed as follows.

Time (minutes)	Solution A (%)	Solution B (%)	Elution
0	90	10	equilibration (10 minutes)
0–5	90	10	isocratic
5	90→85	10→15	step gradient
5–25	85	15	isocratic
25	85→45	15→55	step gradient
25–end*	45	55	isocratic

*The elution concludes at 3 times the retention time of metrifonate.

  Procedure—Separately inject equal volumes (about 50 μL) of the *Standard solution* and the *Test solution* into the chromatograph, record the chromatograms, and measure the peak areas. Calculate the percentage of each impurity taken by the formula:

$$100F(r_i / r_S)$$

in which F is a response factor, being 0.38 for the desmethylmetrifonate peak, if present at a retention time of 0.5 relative to that of Metrifonate, 0.03 for the dichlorvos peak, if present, at a retention time of 1.9 relative to that of Metrifonate, and 1.0 for any other impurity; r_i is the peak area for the individual impurity obtained from the *Test solution;* and r_S is the peak area for Metrifonate obtained from the *Standard solution:* not more than 1.0% of desmethylmetrifonate, 0.2% of dichlorvos, and 0.5% of any other impurity are found; and a total of not more than 1.0% of impurities other than desmethylmetrifonate and dichlorvos is found.
Assay—Dissolve about 300 mg of Metrifonate, accurately weighed, in 30 mL of alcohol. Add 10 mL of monoethanolamine, and allow to stand for 1 hour at 21 ± 1°. Cool while adding a mixture of 100 mL of water and 15 mL of nitric acid. While maintaining the temperature at 21 ± 1°, titrate with 0.1 N silver nitrate VS, determining the endpoint potentiometrically using a silver electrode. Each mL of 0.1 N silver nitrate is equivalent to 25.74 mg of $C_4H_8Cl_3O_4P$.

Metronidazole

$C_6H_9N_3O_3$ 171.15
1*H*-Imidazole-1-ethanol, 2-methyl-5-nitro-.
2-Methyl-5-nitroimidazole-1-ethanol   [443-48-1].

» Metronidazole contains not less than 99.0 percent and not more than 101.0 percent of $C_6H_9N_3O_3$, calculated on the dried basis.

Packaging and storage—Preserve in well-closed, light-resistant containers. Store at 25°, excursions permitted between 15° and 30°.
USP Reference standards ⟨11⟩—USP Metronidazole RS.
Identification—
  A: *Infrared Absorption* ⟨197K⟩.
  B: *Ultraviolet Absorption* ⟨197U⟩—
  Solution: 20 μg per mL.
  Medium: sulfuric acid in methanol (1 in 350).
Melting range ⟨741⟩: between 159° and 163°.
Loss on drying ⟨731⟩—Dry it at 105° for 2 hours: it loses not more than 0.5% of its weight.
Residue on ignition ⟨281⟩: not more than 0.1%.
Heavy metals, *Method II* ⟨231⟩: 0.005%.
Non-basic substances—A 1-g portion dissolves completely in 10 mL of dilute hydrochloric acid (1 in 2).
Chromatographic purity—Dissolve 100 mg of Metronidazole in 10.0 mL of acetone. Similarly prepare a Standard solution of USP Metronidazole RS in acetone having a concentration of 3.0 mg per mL. Dilute an aliquot of this Standard solution quantitatively and stepwise with acetone to obtain a solution having a concentration of 30 μg per mL (diluted Standard solution). Apply separately 20-μL portions of the test solution, the Standard solution, and the diluted Standard solution to a suitable thin-layer chromatographic plate (see *Chromatography* ⟨621⟩) coated with a 0.25-mm layer of chromatographic silica gel. Allow the spots to dry, and develop the chromatogram in a solvent system consisting of a mixture of chloroform, dehydrated alcohol, diethylamine, and water (80 : 10 : 10 : 1) until the solvent front has moved about three-fourths of the length of the plate. Remove the plate from the developing chamber, mark the solvent front, and allow the solvent to evaporate. Spray the plate with titanium trichloride (20% solution), heat at 110° until the blue-gray color begins to disappear, and cool the plate. *[Caution—Use fast blue B salt spray with adequate ventilation, avoid inhalation of vapors, and avoid contact with the skin]* Spray the plate with fast

blue B salt solution (1 in 100), allow to stand for 3 minutes, and spray with a mixture of alcohol, water, and ammonium hydroxide (50:30:20): the R_F value of the principal spot obtained from the test solution corresponds to that obtained from the Standard solution, and no spot, other than the principal spot, obtained from the test solution is larger or more intense than the principal spot obtained from the diluted Standard solution.

Assay—Dissolve about 100 mg of Metronidazole, accurately weighed, in 20 mL of acetic anhydride, warming slightly to effect solution. Cool, add 1 drop of malachite green TS, and titrate with 0.1 N perchloric acid VS from a 10-mL microburet to a yellow-green endpoint. Perform a blank determination, and make any necessary correction. Each mL of 0.1 N perchloric acid is equivalent to 17.12 mg of $C_6H_9N_3O_3$.

Metronidazole Benzoate

$C_{13}H_{13}N_3O_4$ 275.3
2-(2-Methyl-5-nitroimidazol-1-yl)ethyl benzoate [13182-89-3].

» Metronidazole Benzoate contains not less than 98.5 percent and not more than 101.0 percent of $C_{13}H_{13}N_3O_4$, calculated on the dried basis.

Packaging and storage—Preserve in well-closed, light-resistant containers. Store at 25°, excursions permitted between 15° and 30°.
USP Reference standards ⟨11⟩—*USP Metronidazole RS. USP Metronidazole Benzoate RS. USP Tinidazole Related Compound A RS.*
Identification—
  A: *Infrared Absorption* ⟨197K⟩.
  B: The principal spot in the chromatogram of the *Test solution* corresponds to that in the chromatogram of *Standard solution A*, as obtained in the test for *Related compounds*.
Acidity—Neutralize 40 mL of a mixture of dimethylformamide and water (1:1) with hydrochloric acid or 0.02 M sodium hydroxide, add 0.2 mL of methyl red TS and 2.0 g of Metronidazole Benzoate, mix to dissolve, and titrate with 0.02 M sodium hydroxide: not more than 0.25 mL is required to produce a color change.
Loss on drying ⟨731⟩—Dry it at 80° for 3 hours: it loses not more than 0.5% of its weight.
Residue on ignition ⟨281⟩: not more than 0.1%.
Heavy metals, *Method II* ⟨231⟩: 0.002%.
Related compounds—
  Adsorbent: 0.2-mm layer of chromatographic silica gel mixture.
  Test solution—Transfer about 200 mg of Metronidazole Benzoate, accurately weighed, to a 10-mL volumetric flask, dissolve in and dilute with acetone to volume, and mix.
  Standard solution A—Dissolve an accurately weighed quantity of USP Metronidazole Benzoate RS in acetone, and dilute quantitatively, and stepwise if necessary, with acetone to obtain a solution having a known concentration of about 0.1 mg per mL.
  Standard solution B—Transfer 4.0 mL of *Standard solution A* to a 10-mL volumetric flask, dilute with acetone to volume, and mix.
  Standard solution C—Transfer about 10 mg each of USP Metronidazole RS and USP Tinidazole Related Compound A RS, accurately weighed, to a 50-mL volumetric flask, dissolve in and dilute with acetone to volume, and mix. [NOTE—USP Tinidazole Related Compound A RS is 2-methyl-5-nitroimidazole.]
  Application volume: 10 μL.
  Developing solvent system: ethyl acetate.
  Procedure—Proceed as directed for *Thin-Layer Chromatography* under *Chromatography* ⟨621⟩. Examine the plate under short-wavelength UV light: the test is valid only if the metronidazole and tinidazole related compound A spots obtained from *Standard solution C* are clearly separated: no secondary spot obtained from the *Test solution* is larger or more intense than the principal spot obtained from *Standard solution A* (0.5%); and not more than three spots, excluding the principal spot, obtained from the *Test solution* are larger or more intense than the principal spot obtained from *Standard solution B* (0.2%).
Organic volatile impurities, *Method IV* ⟨467⟩: meets the requirements.
(Official until July 1, 2008)
Assay—Transfer about 250 mg of Metronidazole Benzoate, accurately weighed, to a suitable container, and dissolve with stirring in 50.0 mL of glacial acetic acid. Titrate with 0.1 N perchloric acid, determining the endpoint potentiometrically. Perform a blank determination, and make any necessary correction (see *Titrimetry* ⟨541⟩). Each mL of 0.1 N perchloric acid is equivalent to 27.53 mg of $C_{13}H_{13}N_3O_4$.

Metronidazole Gel

» Metronidazole Gel contains not less than 90.0 percent and not more than 110.0 percent of the labeled amount of metronidazole ($C_6H_9N_3O_3$).

Packaging and storage—Preserve in laminated collapsible tubes at controlled room temperature.
USP Reference standards ⟨11⟩—*USP Metronidazole RS.*
Identification—
  A: *Thin-Layer Chromatographic Identification Test* ⟨201⟩—
  Test solution—Transfer a weighed quantity of the Gel, equivalent to 7.5 mg of metronidazole, to a suitable flask, add 15 mL of water, shake to disperse, and sonicate for about 10 minutes. Elute a portion of this solution through a 10-mm × 15-cm chromatographic column containing a 10-cm length of ion-exchange resin with a pledget of glass wool at the bottom and top of the resin, and collect the eluate in a suitable vial.
  Standard solution: 0.5 mg per mL.
  Application volume: 5 μL.
  Developing solvent system: a mixture of chloroform, methanol, and ammonium hydroxide (6:3:1).
  B: The retention time of the major peak in the chromatogram of the *Assay preparation* corresponds to that in the chromatogram of the *Standard preparation*, as obtained in the *Assay*.
Minimum fill ⟨755⟩: meets the requirements.
pH ⟨791⟩—The apparent pH, determined potentiometrically, is between 4.0 and 6.5.
Assay—
  Mobile phase—Dissolve 1.5 g of monobasic potassium phosphate and 1.3 g of dibasic sodium phosphate in 350 mL of water, add 650 mL of methanol, mix, filter, and degas. Make adjustments if necessary (see *System Suitability* under *Chromatography* ⟨621⟩).
  Standard preparation—Dissolve an accurately weighed quantity of USP Metronidazole RS in *Mobile phase*, and dilute quantitatively, and stepwise if necessary, with *Mobile phase* to obtain a solution having a known concentration of about 0.075 mg per mL.
  Assay preparation—Transfer an accurately weighed quantity of Gel, equivalent to 7.5 mg of metronidazole, to a 100-mL volumetric flask, add 50 mL of *Mobile phase*, and shake by mechanical means for 20 minutes. Dilute with *Mobile phase* to volume, and mix. Centrifuge a portion of this solution until clear, and use the supernatant for injection into the chromatograph.
  Chromatographic system (see *Chromatography* ⟨621⟩)—The liquid chromatograph is equipped with a 254-nm detector and a 4.6-mm × 25-cm column that contains 5-μm packing L7. The flow rate is about 1 mL per minute. Chromatograph the *Standard preparation*, and record the peak heights as directed for *Procedure:* the tailing factor for the metronidazole peak is not more than 2.0; and the relative standard deviation for replicate injections is not more than 2.0%.
  Procedure—Separately inject equal volumes (about 20 μL) of the *Standard preparation* and the *Assay preparation* into the chromatograph, record the chromatograms, and measure the heights of the major peaks. Calculate the quantity, in mg, of metronidazole

($C_6H_9N_3O_3$) in the portion of Gel taken by the formula:

$$100C(r_U / r_S)$$

in which C is the concentration, in mg per mL, of USP Metronidazole RS in the *Standard preparation*; and r_U and r_S are the peak heights of metronidazole obtained from the *Assay preparation* and the *Standard preparation*, respectively.

Metronidazole Injection

» Metronidazole Injection is a sterile, isotonic, buffered solution of Metronidazole in Water for Injection. It contains not less than 90.0 percent and not more than 110.0 percent of the labeled amount of metronidazole ($C_6H_9N_3O_3$).

Packaging and storage—Preserve in single-dose containers of Type I or Type II glass, or in suitable plastic containers, protected from light.

USP Reference standards ⟨11⟩—*USP Endotoxin RS. USP Metronidazole RS.*

Identification—
A: Apply a measured volume of Injection containing 0.025 mg of metronidazole and a measured volume of a solution of USP Metronidazole RS containing 0.025 mg of metronidazole to a suitable thin-layer chromatographic plate (see *Chromatography* ⟨621⟩) coated with a 0.25-mm layer of chromatographic silica gel mixture. Allow the spots to dry, and develop the chromatogram in a solvent system consisting of a mixture of chloroform, methanol, water, and ammonium hydroxide (70 : 28 : 4 : 2) until the solvent front has moved about three-fourths of the length of the plate. Remove the plate from the developing chamber, mark the solvent front, and allow the solvent to evaporate. Locate the spots on the plate by viewing under short-wavelength UV light: the R_F value of the principal spot obtained from the test solution corresponds to that obtained from the Standard solution.
B: The retention time of the major peak obtained from the *Assay preparation* corresponds to that of the *Standard preparation* obtained as directed in the *Assay*.

Bacterial endotoxins ⟨85⟩—It contains not more than 0.35 USP Endotoxin Unit per mg of metronidazole.

pH ⟨791⟩: between 4.5 and 7.0.

Particulate matter ⟨788⟩: meets the requirements under small-volume injections.

Other requirements—It meets the requirements under *Injections* ⟨1⟩.

Assay—
Mobile phase—Prepare a suitable filtered and degassed mixture of monobasic potassium phosphate, prepared by dissolving 0.68 g of monobasic potassium phosphate in 930 mL of water, and methanol (930 : 70), and adjust with 1 M phosphoric acid to a pH of 4.0 ± 0.5.

Standard preparation—Transfer about 25 mg of USP Metronidazole RS, accurately weighed, to a 25-mL volumetric flask, dissolve in methanol, dilute with methanol to volume, and mix. Pipet 2 mL of this solution into a 10-mL volumetric flask containing 2 mL of water, dilute with *Mobile phase* to volume, and mix.

Assay preparation—Transfer an accurately measured volume of Injection, equivalent to about 25 mg of metronidazole, to a 25-mL volumetric flask, dilute with water to volume, and mix. Pipet 2 mL of this solution into a 10-mL volumetric flask containing 2 mL of methanol, dilute with *Mobile phase* to volume, and mix.

Chromatographic system (see *Chromatography* ⟨621⟩)—The liquid chromatograph is equipped with a 320-nm detector and a 4.6-mm × 25-cm column that contains packing L1. The flow rate is about 2.0 mL per minute. Chromatograph five replicate injections of the *Standard preparation*, and record the peak responses as directed under *Procedure*: the relative standard deviation is not more than 2.0%, and the tailing factor is not greater than 2.0.

Procedure—Separately inject equal volumes (about 20 µL) of the *Standard preparation* and the *Assay preparation* into the chromatograph, record the chromatograms, and measure the responses for the major peaks. Calculate the quantity, in mg, of metronidazole ($C_6H_9N_3O_3$) in each mL of the Injection taken by the formula:

$$125C / V(r_U / r_S)$$

in which C is the concentration, in mg per mL, of USP Metronidazole RS in the *Standard preparation*; V is the volume, in mL, of Injection taken; and r_U and r_S are the peak responses for metronidazole obtained from the *Assay preparation* and the *Standard preparation*, respectively.

Metronidazole Tablets

» Metronidazole Tablets contain not less than 90.0 percent and not more than 110.0 percent of the labeled amount of metronidazole ($C_6H_9N_3O_3$).

Packaging and storage—Preserve in well-closed, light-resistant containers.

USP Reference standards ⟨11⟩—*USP Metronidazole RS.*

Identification—
A: To a portion of powdered Tablets, equivalent to about 300 mg of metronidazole, add 20 mL of dilute hydrochloric acid (1 in 100), shake for several minutes, and filter: suitable aliquots of the filtrate respond to *Identification* test B under *Metronidazole*.
B: The retention time of the major peak in the chromatogram of the *Assay preparation* corresponds to that of the *Standard preparation* as obtained in the *Assay*.

Dissolution ⟨711⟩—
Medium: 0.1 N hydrochloric acid; 900 mL.
Apparatus 1: 100 rpm.
Time: 60 minutes.
Procedure—Determine the amount of $C_6H_9N_3O_3$ dissolved from UV absorbances at the wavelength of maximum absorbance at about 278 nm of filtered portions of the solution under test, suitably diluted with 0.1 N hydrochloric acid, in comparison with a Standard solution having a known concentration of USP Metronidazole RS in the same medium.
Tolerances—Not less than 85% (*Q*) of the labeled amount of $C_6H_9N_3O_3$ is dissolved in 60 minutes.

Uniformity of dosage units ⟨905⟩: meet the requirements.
Procedure for content uniformity—Transfer one Tablet to a 250-mL volumetric flask, add about 100 mL of dilute hydrochloric acid (1 in 100), and shake for 30 minutes. Dilute with dilute hydrochloric acid (1 in 100) to volume, and mix. Filter, discarding the first 15 mL of the filtrate. Dilute the filtrate quantitatively with dilute hydrochloric acid (1 in 100), to obtain a solution having a concentration of about 0.2 mg of metronidazole per mL. Pipet 10 mL of this solution into a 100-mL volumetric flask, dilute with dilute hydrochloric acid (1 in 100) to volume, and mix. Concomitantly determine the absorbance of this test solution and that of a similarly prepared Standard solution of USP Metronidazole RS, having a known concentration of about 20 µg per mL, in 1-cm matched cells, at the wavelength of maximum absorbance at about 278 nm, with a suitable spectrophotometer, using dilute hydrochloric acid (1 in 100) as the blank. Calculate the quantity, in mg, of $C_6H_9N_3O_3$ in the Tablet taken by the formula:

$$(TC / D)(A_U / A_S)$$

in which T is the labeled quantity, in mg, of the metronidazole in the Tablet; C is the concentration, in µg per mL, of USP Metronidazole RS in the Standard solution; D is the concentration, in µg per mL, of metronidazole in the test solution, on the basis of the labeled quantity per Tablet and the extent of dilution; and A_U and A_S are the absorbances of the test solution and the Standard solution, respectively.

Assay—

Mobile phase—Prepare a filtered and degassed mixture of water and methanol (80 : 20), making adjustments if necessary (see *System Suitability* under *Chromatography* ⟨621⟩).

Standard preparation—Dissolve an accurately weighed quantity of USP Metronidazole RS in *Mobile phase* to obtain a solution having a known concentration of about 0.5 mg per mL.

Assay preparation—Transfer to a suitable size volumetric flask 10 Tablets, whole or ground, which when diluted with methanol will yield a solution having a concentration of about 10 mg per mL. Add methanol, and shake by mechanical means for 30 minutes or until the Tablets are disintegrated. Dilute with methanol to volume, and allow the solution to stand until the insoluble material has settled. Pipet 5.0 mL of the clear supernatant into a 100-mL volumetric flask, dilute with *Mobile phase* to volume, and mix. Filter the solution.

Chromatographic system (see *Chromatography* ⟨621⟩)—The liquid chromatograph is equipped with a 254-nm detector and a 4.6-mm × 15-cm column that contains packing L7. The flow rate is about 1 mL per minute. Chromatograph the *Standard preparation*, and record the peak response as directed under *Procedure*: the tailing factor is not more than 2, and the relative standard deviation for replicate injections is not more than 2.0%.

Procedure—Separately inject equal volumes (about 10 µL) of the *Standard preparation* and the *Assay preparation* into the chromatograph, record the chromatograms, and measure the peak responses. Calculate the quantity, in mg, of metronidazole ($C_6H_9N_3O_3$) in the portion of Tablets taken by the formula:

$$10(L / D)C(r_U / r_S)$$

in which L is the labeled amount, in mg, of Metronidazole in each Tablet; D is the concentration, in mg per mL, of Metronidazole in the *Assay preparation* based on the labeled quantity per Tablet and the extent of dilution; C is the concentration, in mg per mL, of USP Metronidazole RS in the *Standard preparation;* and r_U and r_S are the metronidazole peak responses obtained from the *Assay preparation* and the *Standard preparation*, respectively.

Metyrapone

$C_{14}H_{14}N_2O$ 226.27
1-Propanone, 2-methyl-1,2-di-3-pyridinyl-.
2-Methyl-1,2-di-3-pyridyl-1-propanone   [54-36-4].

» Metyrapone contains not less than 98.0 percent and not more than 102.0 percent of $C_{14}H_{14}N_2O$, calculated on the dried basis.

Packaging and storage—Preserve in tight containers, protected from heat and light.

USP Reference standards ⟨11⟩—*USP Metyrapone RS.*
Identification—
  A: *Infrared Absorption* ⟨197M⟩.
  B: *Ultraviolet Absorption* ⟨197U⟩—
  Solution: 10 µg per mL.
  Medium: 1 N sulfuric acid.
Loss on drying ⟨731⟩—Dry it in vacuum at room temperature for 6 hours: it loses not more than 0.5% of its weight.
Residue on ignition ⟨281⟩: not more than 0.1%.
Heavy metals, *Method II* ⟨231⟩: 0.001%.
Chromatographic purity—
  Standard solutions—Dissolve USP Metyrapone RS in methanol, and mix to obtain a solution having a known concentration of 0.2 mg per mL. Dilute quantitatively with methanol to obtain *Standard solution A*, containing 40 µg of the Reference Standard per mL, and *Standard solution B*, containing 20 µg of the Reference Standard per mL.

  Test solution—Dissolve an accurately weighed quantity of Metyrapone in methanol to obtain a solution containing 20 mg per mL.

  Procedure—Apply separately 5 µL of the *Test solution* and 5 µL of each *Standard solution* to a suitable thin-layer chromatographic plate (see *Chromatography* ⟨621⟩) coated with a 0.25-mm layer of chromatographic silica gel mixture. Position the plate in a chromatographic chamber, and develop the chromatograms in a solvent system consisting of a mixture of chloroform and methanol (48 : 3) until the solvent front has moved about three-fourths of the length of the plate. Remove the plate from the developing chamber, mark the solvent front, and dry under a current of nitrogen for about 10 minutes. Position the dried plate once again in the same chromatographic chamber, and again develop the chromatograms, until the solvent front has moved about three-fourths of the length of the plate. Remove the plate from the developing chamber, mark the solvent front, and dry under a current of warm air for about 15 minutes. Examine the plate under short-wavelength UV light, and compare the intensities of any secondary spots observed in the chromatogram of the *Test solution* with those of the principal spots in the chromatograms of the *Standard solutions:* no secondary spot from the chromatogram of the *Test solution* is larger or more intense than the principal spot obtained from *Standard solution A* (0.2%), and the sum of the intensities of the secondary spots obtained from the *Test solution* corresponds to not more than 1.0%.
Assay—Transfer about 50 mg of Metyrapone, accurately weighed, to a 100-mL volumetric flask. Dissolve in 1 N sulfuric acid, dilute with the same solvent to volume, and mix. Pipet 2 mL of this solution into a 100-mL volumetric flask, add 1 N sulfuric acid to volume, and mix. Dissolve an accurately weighed quantity of USP Metyrapone RS in 1 N sulfuric acid, and dilute quantitatively and stepwise with 1 N sulfuric acid to obtain a Standard solution having a known concentration of about 10 µg per mL. Concomitantly determine the absorbances of both solutions in 1-cm cells at the wavelength of maximum absorbance at about 260 nm, with a suitable spectrophotometer, using 1 N sulfuric acid as the blank. Calculate the quantity, in mg, of $C_{14}H_{14}N_2O$ in the portion of Metyrapone taken by the formula:

$$5C(A_U / A_S)$$

in which C is the concentration, in µg per mL, of USP Metyrapone RS in the Standard solution, and A_U and A_S are the absorbances of the solution of Metyrapone and the Standard solution, respectively.

Metyrapone Tablets

» Metyrapone Tablets contain not less than 95.0 percent and not more than 105.0 percent of the labeled amount of metyrapone ($C_{14}H_{14}N_2O$).

Packaging and storage—Preserve in tight, light-resistant containers, and avoid exposure to excessive heat.

USP Reference standards ⟨11⟩—*USP Metyrapone RS.*
Identification—
  A: Transfer to a centrifuge tube a quantity of powdered Tablets, equivalent to about 500 mg of metyrapone, add 10 mL of 1 N sodium hydroxide, and mix. Extract with 10 mL of chloroform, centrifuge, and filter: the IR absorption spectrum of this solution, determined in a 0.5-mm cell against chloroform, exhibits maxima only at the same wavelengths as that of a similar solution of USP Metyrapone RS.
  B: Transfer to a centrifuge tube 1 mL of the filtrate obtained in *Identification* test A, add 20 mL of chloroform, and extract with 30 mL of 1 N sulfuric acid, centrifuging and filtering the sulfuric acid layer through a pledget of cotton. Dilute 1 mL of this solution with 1 N sulfuric acid to 100 mL: the UV absorption spectrum of the resulting solution exhibits maxima and minima at the same wavelengths as that of a similar solution of USP Metyrapone RS, concomitantly measured.

Dissolution ⟨711⟩—
Medium: 0.1 N hydrochloric acid; 900 mL.
Apparatus 1: 100 rpm.
Time: 45 minutes.
Procedure—Determine the amount of $C_{14}H_{14}N_2O$ dissolved from UV absorbances at the wavelength of maximum absorbance at about 259 nm of filtered portions of the solution under test, suitably diluted with 0.1 N hydrochloric acid, in comparison with a Standard solution having a known concentration of USP Metyrapone RS in the same medium.
Tolerances—Not less than 60% *(Q)* of the labeled amount of $C_{14}H_{14}N_2O$ is dissolved in 45 minutes.
Uniformity of dosage units ⟨905⟩: meet the requirements.
Assay—
2,4-Dinitrophenylhydrazine in methanol—Shake by mechanical means about 1 g of 2,4-dinitrophenylhydrazine with 75 mL of methanol in a 100-mL flask for about 15 minutes, and filter through paper. Prepare fresh daily.
2,4-Dinitrophenylhydrazine hydrochloride—Mix 2 mL of hydrochloric acid with 23 mL of *2,4-Dinitrophenylhydrazine in methanol*.
Potassium hydroxide in methanol—Dissolve 5 g of potassium hydroxide in 100 mL of methanol, and filter.
Standard preparation—Dissolve an accurately weighed quantity of USP Metyrapone RS in chloroform, and dilute quantitatively and stepwise with chloroform to obtain a solution having a known concentration of about 100 µg per mL.
Assay preparation—Weigh and finely powder not less than 20 Tablets. Transfer an accurately weighed portion of the powder, equivalent to about 25 mg of metyrapone, with the aid of 10 mL of 1 N sodium hydroxide, to a centrifuge tube. Shake gently, and extract with three 15-mL portions of chloroform. Centrifuge each extract, filtering through a pledget of cotton, previously washed with chloroform, into a 50-mL volumetric flask. Add chloroform to volume, and mix. Pipet 5 mL of this solution into a 25-mL volumetric flask, add chloroform to volume, and mix.
Procedure—Pipet 3 mL each of the *Standard preparation*, the *Assay preparation*, and chloroform to provide a blank, into separate 50-mL volumetric flasks. To each flask add 1 mL of *2,4-Dinitrophenylhydrazine hydrochloride*, and shake lightly. Evaporate the solutions on a steam bath to near dryness. Wash down the sides of the flask with 1 mL of chloroform and methanol (1 : 1), and again evaporate the solutions to near dryness. Heat the flasks in an oven maintained at 110° to 120° for 30 minutes. Remove the flasks, pipet 10 mL of *Potassium hydroxide in methanol* into each flask, and heat again in the boiling water bath for 1 minute. Allow to cool to room temperature, insert the stoppers, shake by mechanical means for 5 minutes, add methanol to volume, and mix. Concomitantly determine the absorbances of the solutions in 1-cm cells relative to the blank, at the wavelength of maximum absorbance at about 450 nm, with a suitable spectrophotometer. Calculate the quantity, in mg, of metyrapone ($C_{14}H_{14}N_2O$) in the portion of Tablets taken by the formula:

$$250C(A_U / A_S)$$

in which *C* is the concentration, in mg per mL, of USP Metyrapone RS in the *Standard preparation*, and A_U and A_S are the absorbances of the solutions from the *Assay preparation* and the *Standard preparation*, respectively.

Metyrosine

$C_{10}H_{13}NO_3$ 195.22
L-Tyrosine, α-methyl-, (−)-.
(−)-α-Methyl-L-tyrosine   [672-87-7].

» Metyrosine contains not less than 98.6 percent and not more than 101.0 percent of $C_{10}H_{13}NO_3$, calculated on the dried basis.

Packaging and storage—Preserve in well-closed containers.
USP Reference standards ⟨11⟩—*USP Metyrosine RS.*
Identification—
  A: *Infrared Absorption ⟨197M⟩.*
  B: *Ultraviolet Absorption ⟨197U⟩—*
  Solution: 15 µg per mL.
  Medium: 0.1 N hydrochloric acid.
  Absorptivities at 224 nm, calculated on the dried basis, do not differ by more than 3.0%.
Specific rotation ⟨781S⟩: between +185° and +195° ($t = 30°$; λ = 546 nm; $l = 0.5$ dm).
Test solution: 5 mg per mL, in *Diluent*, with the aid of sonication if necessary. Prepare the *Diluent* as follows.
Solution A—Dissolve 20.0 g of anhydrous sodium acetate in about 150 mL of water in a 250-mL volumetric flask. Add 50.0 mL of glacial acetic acid, dilute with water to volume, and mix.
Solution B—Dissolve 62.5 g of cupric sulfate in water in a 200-mL volumetric flask, dilute with water to volume, and mix.
Diluent—Mix *Solution A* and *Solution B* in a 1000-mL volumetric flask, dilute with water to volume, and mix.
Loss on drying ⟨731⟩—Dry it at a pressure not exceeding 5 mm of mercury at 100° for two hours: it loses not more than 1.0% of its weight.
Residue on ignition ⟨281⟩: not more than 0.1%.
Heavy metals, *Method II* ⟨231⟩:   0.003%.
Organic volatile impurities, *Method IV* ⟨467⟩: meets the requirements.
(Official until July 1, 2008)
Chromatographic purity—
Standard solutions—Dissolve USP Metyrosine RS in a solvent mixture of methanol and ammonium hydroxide (7 : 3) to obtain a solution having a concentration of 10 mg per mL (*Standard solution A*). Pipet 1 mL of *Standard solution A* into a 100-mL volumetric flask, dilute with the same solvent mixture to volume, and mix (*Standard solution B*). Pipet 5 mL of *Standard solution B* into a 10-mL volumetric flask, dilute with the same solvent mixture to volume, and mix (*Standard solution C*). Pipet 5 mL of *Standard solution C* into a 10-mL volumetric flask, dilute with the same solvent mixture to volume, and mix (*Standard solution D*).
Test solution—Dissolve Metyrosine in the solvent mixture of methanol and ammonium hydroxide (7 : 3) to obtain a solution having a concentration of 10 mg per mL.
Procedure—Apply 10-µL portions of *Standard solutions A, B, C,* and *D* and the *Test solution* to a suitable thin-layer chromatographic plate (see *Chromatography ⟨621⟩*) coated with a 0.25-mm layer of chromatographic silica gel mixture and previously washed with methanol. Allow the spots to dry, and develop the chromatogram in a solvent system consisting of a mixture of *n*-propyl alcohol and ammonium hydroxide (7 : 3) until the solvent front has moved about three-fourths of the length of the plate. Remove the plate from the developing chamber, mark the solvent front, and dry the plate. Expose the plate to iodine vapors, and examine under short-wavelength UV light: the chromatogram shows principal spots at about the same R_F value. Estimate the levels of any additional spots observed in the chromatogram of the *Test solution* by comparison with the spots in the chromatograms of *Standard solutions B, C,* and *D:* the sum of the intensities of any spots observed is not greater than that of the principal spot obtained from *Standard solution B,* corresponding to not more than 1%.
Assay—Dissolve about 300 mg of Metyrosine, accurately weighed, in about 100 mL of glacial acetic acid, sonicate for about 5 minutes, and titrate with 0.1 N perchloric acid VS, determining the endpoint potentiometrically, using a platinum ring electrode and a sleeve-type calomel electrode containing 0.1 N lithium perchlorate in glacial acetic acid (see *Titrimetry ⟨541⟩*). Perform a blank determination, and make any necessary correction. Each mL of 0.1 N perchloric acid is equivalent to 19.52 mg of $C_{10}H_{13}NO_3$.

Metyrosine Capsules

» Metyrosine Capsules contain not less than 90.0 percent and not more than 110.0 percent of the labeled amount of metyrosine ($C_{10}H_{13}NO_3$).

Packaging and storage—Preserve in well-closed containers.

USP Reference standards ⟨11⟩—*USP Metyrosine RS*.
Identification—The UV absorption spectrum of a 1 in 10,000 solution of the Capsule contents in dilute hydrochloric acid (1 in 100) exhibits maxima and minima at the same wavelengths as that of a similar solution of USP Metyrosine RS, concomitantly measured.
Dissolution ⟨711⟩—
  Medium: 0.1 N hydrochloric acid; 750 mL.
  Apparatus 1: 100 rpm.
  Time: 60 minutes.
  Procedure—Determine the amount of $C_{10}H_{13}NO_3$ dissolved from UV absorbances at the wavelength of maximum absorbance at about 274 nm of filtered portions of the solution under test, suitably diluted with *Medium*, if necessary, in comparison with a Standard solution having a known concentration of USP Metyrosine RS in the same medium.
  Tolerances—Not less than 75% (*Q*) of the labeled amount of $C_{10}H_{13}NO_3$ is dissolved in 60 minutes.
Uniformity of dosage units ⟨905⟩: meet the requirements.
Assay—
  Standard preparation—Dissolve a suitable quantity of USP Metyrosine RS, accurately weighed, in dilute hydrochloric acid (1 in 100) to obtain a solution having a known concentration of about 100 µg per mL.
  Assay preparation—Combine the contents of not less than 20 Capsules, and transfer an accurately weighed portion of the combined contents, equivalent to about 100 mg of metyrosine, to a 100-mL volumetric flask. Add 50 mL of dilute hydrochloric acid (1 in 100), shake by mechanical means for 45 minutes, dilute with dilute hydrochloric acid (1 in 100) to volume, mix, and filter. Transfer 10.0 mL of the filtrate to a 100-mL volumetric flask, dilute with dilute hydrochloric acid solution (1 in 100) to volume, and mix. Concomitantly determine the absorbances of this solution and the *Standard preparation* at the wavelength of maximum absorbance at about 274 nm, with a suitable spectrophotometer, using dilute hydrochloric acid solution (1 in 100) as the blank. Calculate the quantity, in mg, of metyrosine ($C_{10}H_{13}NO_3$) in the portion of Capsules taken by the formula:

$$C(A_U / A_S)$$

in which *C* is the concentration, in µg per mL, of USP Metyrosine RS in the *Standard preparation*, and A_U and A_S are the absorbances of the solutions obtained from the *Assay preparation* and the *Standard preparation*, respectively.

Mexiletine Hydrochloride

$C_{11}H_{17}NO \cdot HCl$ 215.72
2-Propanamine, 1-(2,6-dimethylphenoxy)-, hydrochloride, (±)-.
(±)-1-Methyl-2-(2,6-xylyloxy)ethylamine hydrochloride   [5370-01-04].

» Mexiletine Hydrochloride contains not less than 98.0 percent and not more than 102.0 percent of $C_{11}H_{17}NO \cdot HCl$, calculated on the dried basis.

Packaging and storage—Preserve in tight containers.
USP Reference standards ⟨11⟩—*USP Mexiletine Hydrochloride RS*.
Identification—
  A: *Infrared Absorption* ⟨197M⟩.
  B: Prepare a test solution by dissolving a suitable quantity of it in methanol to obtain a concentration of about 10 mg per mL. Similarly prepare a Standard solution, using USP Mexiletine Hydrochloride RS. Separately apply 5-µL portions of the test solution and the Standard solution to a suitable thin-layer chromatographic plate (see *Chromatography* ⟨621⟩) coated with a 0.25-mm layer of chromatographic silica gel. Develop the chromatogram in a suitable chromatographic chamber half saturated with solvent vapor, using a solvent system consisting of a mixture of chloroform, methanol, and ammonium hydroxide (425 : 70 : 5) until the solvent front has moved about three-fourths of the length of the plate. Remove the plate from the developing chamber, mark the solvent front, and allow the solvent to evaporate. Spray the plate with a 1 in 500 solution of fast blue BB salt in methanol, and dry the plate at 105° for 15 minutes. Locate the spots on the plate by spraying it with a 1 in 5 solution of potassium hydroxide in methanol: the R_F value of the principal spot obtained from the test solution corresponds to that obtained from the Standard solution.
  C: To 3 mL of a solution (1 in 60) add 1 mL of 6 N ammonium hydroxide, filter, and acidify the filtrate with 2 mL of nitric acid. Then add 1 mL of silver nitrate TS: a curdy, white precipitate is formed, and it is soluble in an excess of 6 N ammonium hydroxide (*presence of chloride*).
pH ⟨791⟩: between 3.5 and 5.5, in a solution (1 in 10).
Loss on drying ⟨731⟩—Dry it at 105° for 2 hours: it loses not more than 0.5% of its weight.
Residue on ignition ⟨281⟩: not more than 0.1%.
Heavy metals, *Method II* ⟨231⟩: 0.001%.
Chromatographic purity—
  Mobile phase, *Standard preparation*, and *Resolution solution*—Prepare as directed in the *Assay*.
  Standard solution—Transfer 10.0 mL of the *Standard preparation* prepared as directed in the *Assay* to a 100-mL volumetric flask, dilute with *Mobile phase* to volume, and mix. This solution contains about 0.2 mg of USP Mexiletine Hydrochloride RS per mL.
  Test solution—Transfer about 100 mg of Mexiletine Hydrochloride, accurately weighed, to a 5-mL volumetric flask, dilute with *Mobile phase* to volume, and mix.
  Chromatographic system (see *Chromatography* ⟨621⟩)—Prepare as directed in the *Assay*, except that the relative standard deviation for replicate injections of the *Standard solution* is not more than 3.0%.
  Procedure—Proceed as directed for *Procedure* in the *Assay*. Calculate the percentage of each impurity observed taken by the formula:

$$500(C / W)(r_U / r_S)$$

in which *C* is the concentration, in mg per mL, of USP Mexiletine Hydrochloride RS in the *Standard solution*, *W* is the weight, in mg, of the Mexiletine Hydrochloride taken to prepare the *Test solution*, r_U is the peak response obtained from an individual impurity observed in the chromatogram of the *Test solution*, and r_S is the mexiletine peak response obtained from the *Standard solution*: not more than 1% of any individual impurity is found, and the total of all observed impurities is not more than 1.5%.
Organic volatile impurities, *Method I* ⟨467⟩: meets the requirements.

(Official until July 1, 2008)

Assay—
  Sodium acetate buffer solution—Dissolve 11.5 g of anhydrous sodium acetate in 500 mL of water, add 3.2 mL of glacial acetic acid, mix, and allow to cool. Adjust with hydrochloric acid to a pH of 4.8 ± 0.1, dilute with water to 1000 mL, and mix.
  Mobile phase—Prepare a suitable filtered and degassed mixture of methanol and *Sodium acetate buffer solution* (600 : 400). Make adjustments if necessary (see *System Suitability* under *Chromatography* ⟨621⟩).

Standard preparation—Dissolve an accurately weighed quantity of USP Mexiletine Hydrochloride RS in *Mobile phase* to obtain a solution having a known concentration of about 2 mg per mL.

Resolution solution—Prepare a solution of 2-phenylethylamine hydrochloride in *Standard preparation* containing about 1 mg per mL.

Assay preparation—Transfer about 100 mg of Mexiletine Hydrochloride, accurately weighed, to a 50-mL volumetric flask, dissolve in and dilute with *Mobile phase* to volume, and mix.

Chromatographic system (see *Chromatography* ⟨621⟩)—The liquid chromatograph is equipped with a 254-nm detector, a guard column containing packing L1, and a 3.9-mm × 30-cm column that contains 10-µm packing L1. The flow rate is about 1 mL per minute. Chromatograph about 20 µL of the *Resolution solution*, and record the peak responses as directed under *Procedure*: the resolution, R, between the 2-phenylethylamine and mexiletine peaks is not less than 3.0. Chromatograph the *Standard preparation*, and record the peak responses as directed under *Procedure*: the relative standard deviation for replicate injections is not more than 2.0%.

Procedure—[NOTE—Use peak areas where peak responses are indicated.] Separately inject equal volumes (about 20 µL) of the *Assay preparation* and the *Standard preparation* into the chromatograph, record the chromatograms, and measure the responses for the major peaks. The relative retention times are about 0.7 for 2-phenylethylamine and 1.0 for mexiletine. Calculate the quantity, in mg, of $C_{11}H_{17}NO \cdot HCl$ in the portion of Mexiletine Hydrochloride taken by the formula:

$$50C(r_U / r_S)$$

in which C is the concentration, in mg per mL, of USP Mexiletine Hydrochloride RS in the *Standard preparation*, and r_U and r_S are the mexiletine peak responses obtained from the *Assay preparation* and the *Standard preparation*, respectively.

Mexiletine Hydrochloride Capsules

» Mexiletine Hydrochloride Capsules contain not less than 90.0 percent and not more than 110.0 percent of the labeled amount of mexiletine hydrochloride ($C_{11}H_{17}NO \cdot HCl$).

Packaging and storage—Preserve in tight containers.

USP Reference standards ⟨11⟩—*USP Mexiletine Hydrochloride RS*.

Identification—

A: Transfer a quantity of Capsule contents, equivalent to about 250 mg of mexiletine hydrochloride, to a suitable test tube, add 10 mL of methanol, and mix on a vortex mixer for 1 minute. Filter the mixture, evaporate the filtrate under a stream of nitrogen to dryness, and dry the residue in vacuum at 60° for 1 hour: the IR absorption spectrum of a mineral oil dispersion of the dried residue so obtained exhibits maxima only at the same wavelengths as that of a similar preparation of USP Mexiletine Hydrochloride RS.

B: The retention time of the major peak in the chromatogram of the *Assay preparation* corresponds to that in the chromatogram of the *Standard preparation*, as obtained in the *Assay*.

Dissolution ⟨711⟩—
Medium: water; 900 mL.
Apparatus 2: 50 rpm.
Time: 30 minutes.
Procedure—Determine the amount of $C_{11}H_{17}NO \cdot HCl$ dissolved from the difference between first derivative values at the wavelengths of maximum and minimum first derivative absorbance in the wavelength range from 230 to 290 nm on filtered portions of the solution under test, suitably diluted with *Dissolution Medium*, if necessary, in comparison with a Standard solution having a known concentration of USP Mexiletine Hydrochloride RS in the same *Medium*.

Tolerances—Not less than 80% (Q) of the labeled amount of $C_{11}H_{17}NO \cdot HCl$ is dissolved in 30 minutes.

Uniformity of dosage units ⟨905⟩: meet the requirements.

Chromatographic purity—

Mobile phase, Standard preparation, and *Resolution solution*—Prepare as directed in the *Assay* under *Mexiletine Hydrochloride*.

Standard solution—Transfer 10.0 mL of the *Standard preparation* prepared as directed in the *Assay* under *Mexiletine Hydrochloride* to a 1000-mL volumetric flask, dilute with *Mobile phase* to volume, and mix. This solution contains about 20 µg of USP Mexiletine Hydrochloride RS per mL.

Test solution—Use the *Assay preparation* prepared as directed in the *Assay*.

Chromatographic system (see *Chromatography* ⟨621⟩)—Prepare as directed in the *Assay* under *Mexiletine Hydrochloride*, except that the relative standard deviation of replicate injections of the *Standard solution* is not more than 3.0%.

Procedure—Separately inject equal volumes (about 20 µL) of the *Standard solution* and the *Test solution* into the chromatograph; record the chromatograms using a high sensitivity setting for the recorder; and measure the areas for the peaks. Calculate the percentage of each impurity observed by the formula:

$$100(C/L)(r_U / r_S)$$

in which C is the concentration, in mg per mL, of USP Mexiletine Hydrochloride RS in the *Standard solution;* L is the quantity, in mg, of mexiletine hydrochloride in each mL of the *Test solution,* based on the labeled amount in the portion of Capsule contents used to prepare the *Assay preparation* and the extent of dilution; r_U is the peak area obtained from an individual impurity observed in the chromatogram of the *Test solution;* and r_S is the mexiletine peak area obtained from the *Standard solution*: not more than 1% of any individual impurity is found; and the total of all observed impurities is not more than 1.5%.

Assay—

Mobile phase, Standard preparation, Resolution solution, and *Chromatographic system*—Prepare as directed in the *Assay* under *Mexiletine Hydrochloride*.

Assay preparation—Weigh the contents of not fewer than 20 Capsules, and calculate the average weight per Capsule. Mix the combined contents of the Capsules, and transfer an accurately weighed portion, equivalent to about 50 mg of mexiletine hydrochloride, to a stoppered, 50-mL centrifuge tube. Add 25.0 mL of *Mobile phase,* insert the stopper, and shake by mechanical means for 15 minutes. Centrifuge, and use the clear supernatant as the *Assay preparation*. [NOTE—Reserve a portion of this solution for use as the *Test solution* in the test for *Chromatographic purity*.]

Procedure—Proceed as directed for *Procedure* in the *Assay* under *Mexiletine Hydrochloride*. Calculate the quantity, in mg, of mexiletine hydrochloride ($C_{11}H_{17}NO \cdot HCl$) in the portion of Capsule contents taken by the formula:

$$25C(r_U / r_S)$$

in which C is the concentration, in mg per mL, of USP Mexiletine Hydrochloride RS in the *Standard preparation;* and r_U and r_S are the mexiletine peak responses obtained from the *Assay preparation* and the *Standard preparation,* respectively.

Mezlocillin Sodium

C₂₁H₂₄NaN₅O₈S₂   561.57
4-Thia-1-azabicyclo[3.2.0]heptane-2-carboxylic acid, 3,3-dimethyl-6-[[[[[3-(methylsulfonyl)-2-oxo-1-imidazolidinyl]carbonyl]amino]phenylacetyl]amino]-7-oxo-, monosodium salt, [2S-[2α,5α,6β(S*)]]-.
Sodium (2S,5R,6R)-3,3-dimethyl-6-[(R)-2-[3-(methylsulfonyl)-2-oxo-1-imidazolidinecarboxamido]-2-phenylacetamido]-7-oxo-4-thia-1-azabicyclo[3.2.0]heptane-2-carboxylate   [59798-30-0].
Monohydrate   579.58

» Mezlocillin Sodium contains the equivalent of not less than 838 μg and not more than 978 μg of mezlocillin ($C_{21}H_{25}N_5O_8S_2$) per mg, calculated on the anhydrous basis.

Packaging and storage—Preserve in tight containers.
Labeling—Where it is intended for use in preparing injectable dosage forms, the label states that it is sterile or must be subjected to further processing during the preparation of injectable dosage forms.
USP Reference standards ⟨11⟩—*USP Mezlocillin Sodium RS. USP Endotoxin RS.*
Identification—
  A: Prepare a test solution containing the equivalent of 4 mg of mezlocillin per mL. Prepare a Standard solution of USP Mezlocillin Sodium RS containing 4 mg per mL. Use within 10 minutes after preparation. Apply separately 5 μL of each solution to a thin-layer chromatographic plate coated with a 0.25-mm layer of chromatographic silica gel mixture (see *Chromatography* ⟨621⟩). Place the plate in a suitable chromatographic chamber, and develop the chromatogram with a solvent system consisting of a mixture of methanol, chloroform, water, and pyridine (90 : 80 : 30 : 10) until the solvent front has moved about three-fourths of the length of the plate. Remove the plate from the chamber, and dry with a current of warm air for 10 minutes. Locate the spots on the plate by exposing it to iodine vapors in a closed chamber for about 30 seconds: the R_F value of the principal spot obtained from the test solution corresponds to that obtained from the Standard solution.
  B: It responds to the tests for *Sodium* ⟨191⟩.
Specific rotation ⟨781S⟩:   between +175° and +195°.
  Test solution: 10 mg per mL, in water.
pH ⟨791⟩:   between 4.5 and 8.0, in a solution (1 in 10).
Water, *Method I* ⟨921⟩:   not more than 6.0%.
Other requirements—Where the label states that Mezlocillin Sodium is sterile, it meets the requirements for *Sterility* and *Bacterial endotoxins* under *Mezlocillin for Injection*. Where the label states that Mezlocillin Sodium must be subjected to further processing during the preparation of injectable dosage forms, it meets the requirements for *Bacterial endotoxins* under *Mezlocillin for Injection*.
Assay—
  Mobile phase—Dissolve 4.9 g of monobasic potassium phosphate and 0.54 g of dibasic potassium phosphate in about 500 mL of water, dilute with water to 1000 mL, and mix. Prepare a suitable mixture of this solution and acetonitrile (855 : 145), and degas. Make adjustments if necessary (see *System Suitability* under *Chromatography* ⟨621⟩).
  Standard preparation—Dissolve a suitable quantity of USP Mezlocillin Sodium RS, accurately weighed, in water to obtain a solution having a known concentration of about 500 μg of mezlocillin ($C_{21}H_{25}N_5O_8S_2$) per mL.
  Assay preparation—Transfer about 110 mg of Mezlocillin Sodium, accurately weighed, to a 200-mL volumetric flask, dissolve in and dilute with water to volume, and mix.
  Chromatographic system (see *Chromatography* ⟨621⟩)—The liquid chromatograph is equipped with a 210-nm detector and a 4-mm × 12.5-cm column containing 5-μm packing L1, and is maintained at 40 ± 1°. The flow rate is about 2 mL per minute. Chromatograph the *Standard preparation*, and record the responses as directed under *Procedure*: the column efficiency is not less than 1500 theoretical plates, the tailing factor is not more than 1.5, and the relative standard deviation for replicate injections is not more than 1.5%.
  Procedure—[NOTE—Use peak areas where peak responses are indicated.] Separately inject equal volumes (about 20 μL) of the *Standard preparation* and the *Assay preparation* into the chromatograph, record the chromatograms, and measure the responses for the major peaks. Calculate the quantity, in μg per mg, of mezlocillin ($C_{21}H_{25}N_5O_8S_2$) in each mg of the Mezlocillin Sodium taken by the formula:

$$200(C/W)(r_U/r_S)$$

in which C is the concentration, in μg per mL, of mezlocillin ($C_{21}H_{25}N_5O_8S_2$) in the *Standard preparation*, W is the weight, in mg, of the portion of Mezlocillin Sodium taken to prepare the *Assay preparation*, and r_U and r_S are the mezlocillin peak responses obtained from the *Assay preparation* and the *Standard preparation*, respectively.

Mezlocillin for Injection

» Mezlocillin for Injection contains an amount of Mezlocillin Sodium equivalent to not less than 90.0 percent and not more than 115.0 percent of the labeled amount of mezlocillin ($C_{21}H_{25}N_5O_8S_2$).

Packaging and storage—Preserve in *Containers for Sterile Solids* as described under *Injections* ⟨1⟩.
USP Reference standards ⟨11⟩—*USP Mezlocillin Sodium RS. USP Endotoxin RS.*
Constituted solution—At the time of use, it meets the requirements for *Constituted Solutions* under *Injections* ⟨1⟩.
Bacterial endotoxins ⟨85⟩—It contains not more than 0.06 USP Endotoxin Unit per mg of mezlocillin.
Sterility ⟨71⟩—It meets the requirements when tested as directed for *Membrane Filtration* under *Test for Sterility of the Product to be Examined*.
Particulate matter ⟨788⟩:   meets the requirements for small-volume injections.
Other requirements—It responds to the *Identification* tests and meets the requirements for *Specific rotation*, *pH*, and *Water* under *Mezlocillin Sodium*. It meets also the requirements for *Uniformity of Dosage Units* ⟨905⟩ and *Labeling* under *Injections* ⟨1⟩.
Assay—
  Mobile phase, Standard preparation, Resolution solution, and *Chromatographic system*—Prepare as directed for the *Assay* under *Mezlocillin Sodium*.
  Assay preparation 1 (where it is represented as being in a single-dose container)—Constitute Mezlocillin for Injection in a volume of water, accurately measured, corresponding to the volume of solvent specified in the labeling. Withdraw all of the withdrawable contents, using a suitable hypodermic needle and syringe, and dilute quantitatively with water to obtain a solution containing about 0.5 mg of mezlocillin per mL.
  Assay preparation 2 (where the label states the quantity of mezlocillin in a given volume of constituted solution)—Constitute Mezlocillin for Injection in a volume of water, accurately measured, corresponding to the volume of solvent specified in the labeling. Dilute an accurately measured portion of the constituted solution quantitatively with water to obtain a solution containing about 0.5 mg of mezlocillin per mL.
  Procedure—[NOTE—Use peak areas where peak responses are indicated.] Separately inject equal volumes (about 20 μL) of the *Standard preparation* and *Assay preparation 1* into the chromatograph, record the chromatograms, and measure the responses for the major

peaks. Calculate the quantity, in mg, of mezlocillin in the container, or in the portion of constituted solution taken by the formula:

$$(L/D)(C/1000)(r_U/r_S)$$

in which L is the labeled quantity, in mg, of mezlocillin in the container, or in the volume of constituted solution taken, D is the concentration, in mg per mL, of mezlocillin in Assay preparation 1 or in Assay preparation 2, on the basis of the labeled quantity in the container, or in the portion of constituted solution taken, respectively, and the extent of dilution, C is the concentration, in µg per mL, of mezlocillin ($C_{21}H_{25}N_5O_8S_2$) in the Standard preparation, and r_U and r_S are the mezlocillin peak responses obtained from the Standard preparation and from Assay preparation 1 or Assay preparation 2, as appropriate.

Mibolerone

$C_{20}H_{30}O_2$ 302.46
Estr-4-en-3-one, 17-hydroxy-7,17-dimethyl-, (7α,17β)-.
17β-Hydroxy-7α,17-dimethylestr-4-en-3-one   [3704-09-4].

» Mibolerone contains not less than 96.0 percent and not more than 106.0 percent of $C_{20}H_{30}O_2$, calculated on the dried basis.

Packaging and storage—Preserve in well-closed containers.
Labeling—Label it to indicate that it is for veterinary use only.

USP Reference standards ⟨11⟩—USP Mibolerone RS.
Identification, Infrared Absorption ⟨197M⟩.
Specific rotation ⟨781S⟩:   between +34° and +40°.
    Test solution: 10 mg per mL, in chloroform.
Loss on drying ⟨731⟩—Dry about 1 g, accurately weighed, in a capillary-stoppered bottle in vacuum at a pressure not exceeding 5 mm of mercury at 60° for 3 hours: it loses not more than 0.5% of its weight.
Residue on ignition ⟨281⟩:   not more than 0.5%.
Assay—
    Mobile phase—Prepare a filtered and degassed mixture of water, tetrahydrofuran, and methanol (60 : 25 : 15). Make adjustments if necessary (see System Suitability under Chromatography ⟨621⟩).
    Internal standard solution—Prepare a solution of progesterone in methanol containing 0.6 mg per mL.
    Standard preparation—Prepare a solution of USP Mibolerone RS in Internal standard solution having a known concentration of about 0.4 mg per mL. Mix, and sonicate if necessary to achieve complete solution.
    Assay preparation—Transfer about 10 mg of Mibolerone, accurately weighed, to a 25-mL volumetric flask, dilute with Internal standard solution to volume, and mix. Sonicate if necessary to achieve complete solution.
    Chromatographic system (see Chromatography ⟨621⟩)—The liquid chromatograph is equipped with a 254-nm detector and a 3.9-mm × 30-cm column that contains packing L1. The flow rate is about 2 mL per minute. Chromatograph the Standard preparation, and record the peak responses as directed for Procedure: the relative retention times are about 0.6 for mibolerone and 1.0 for progesterone; and the relative standard deviation for replicate injections is not more than 2.0%.
    Procedure—Separately inject equal volumes (about 5 µL) of the Standard preparation and the Assay preparation into the chromatograph, record the chromatograms, and measure the responses for the major peaks. Calculate the quantity, in mg, of $C_{20}H_{30}O_2$ in the portion of Mibolerone taken by the formula:

$$25C(R_U/R_S)$$

in which C is the concentration, in mg per mL, of USP Mibolerone RS in the Standard preparation; and R_U and R_S are the ratios of the peak responses of the mibolerone peak and the progesterone peak obtained from the Assay preparation and the Standard preparation, respectively.

Mibolerone Oral Solution

» Mibolerone Oral Solution contains not less than 90.0 percent and not more than 115.0 percent of the labeled amount of mibolerone ($C_{20}H_{30}O_2$).

Packaging and storage—Preserve in tight containers, protected from light.
Labeling—Label it to indicate that it is for veterinary use only.
USP Reference standards ⟨11⟩—USP Mibolerone RS.
Identification—The chromatogram of the Assay preparation exhibits a major peak for mibolerone, the retention time of which corresponds to that in the chromatogram of the Standard preparation, as obtained in the Assay.
Specific gravity ⟨841⟩:   between 1.030 and 1.045.
Assay—
    Internal standard solution—Prepare a solution of 1,3,5-triphenylbenzene in chloroform containing about 0.25 mg per mL.
    Standard preparation—Prepare a solution of USP Mibolerone RS in Internal standard solution having a known concentration of about 0.5 mg per mL.
    Assay preparation—Transfer an accurately weighed portion of Oral Solution, equivalent to about 1000 µg of mibolerone, to a 125-mL separator containing 60 mL of water, and swirl to disperse. Add 30 mL of methylene chloride, shake gently for about 5 minutes, and allow the phases to separate. Drain the lower methylene chloride layer through a pledget of methylene chloride-washed cotton into a 50-mL conical flask. Evaporate to dryness under a current of air. Re-extract the aqueous layer remaining in the separator with an additional 30-mL portion of methylene chloride, draining the filtered methylene chloride extract into the 50-mL conical flask, and evaporating it to dryness. Add 2.0 mL of Internal standard solution, and swirl to dissolve.
    Chromatographic system (see Chromatography ⟨621⟩)—The gas chromatograph is equipped with a flame-ionization detector and a 3-mm × 61-cm column packed with 1% liquid phase G6 on support S1AB. The column is maintained at about 175° and the detector at 195° to 225°. Helium is used as the carrier gas at a flow rate of about 60 mL per minute. Chromatograph the Standard preparation, and record the peak responses as directed for Procedure: the relative retention times are about 0.6 for the internal standard and 1.0 for mibolerone; and the relative standard deviation for replicate injections is not more than 2.0%.
    Procedure—Separately inject equal volumes (about 2 µL) of the Standard preparation and the Assay preparation into the chromatograph, record the chromatograms, and measure the responses for the major peaks. Calculate the quantity, in µg, of mibolerone ($C_{20}H_{30}O_2$) in each mL of the Oral Solution taken by the formula:

$$2000(C/W_U)(D)(R_U/R_S)$$

in which C is the concentration, in mg per mL, of USP Mibolerone RS in the Standard preparation; W_U is the weight, in g, of Oral Solution taken to prepare the Assay preparation; D is the specific gravity of the Oral Solution; and R_U and R_S are the ratios of the peak height response of the mibolerone peak to the internal standard peak obtained from the Assay preparation and the Standard preparation, respectively.

Miconazole

$C_{18}H_{14}Cl_4N_2O$ 416.13

1*H*-Imidazole, 1-2-[(2,4-dichlorophenyl)-2-[(2,4-dichlorophenyl)] methoxy]ethyl]-, (±)-.
(±)-1-[2,4-Dichloro-β-[(2,4-dichlorobenzyl)oxy]phenethyl]imidazole   [22916-47-8].

» Miconazole contains not less than 98.0 percent and not more than 102.0 percent of $C_{18}H_{14}Cl_4N_2O$, calculated on the dried basis.

Packaging and storage—Preserve in well-closed containers, protected from light. Store at 25°, excursions permitted between 15° and 30°.

USP Reference standards ⟨11⟩—*USP Miconazole RS*.
Identification—
  A: *Infrared Absorption* ⟨197K⟩.
  B: Transfer 40 mg to a 100-mL volumetric flask, dissolve in 50 mL of isopropyl alcohol, add 10 mL of 0.1 N hydrochloric acid, dilute with isopropyl alcohol to volume, and mix: the UV absorption spectrum of this solution exhibits maxima and minima at the same wavelengths as that of a similar solution of USP Miconazole RS, concomitantly measured.
Loss on drying ⟨731⟩—Dry it in vacuum at 60° for 4 hours: it loses not more than 0.5% of its weight.
Residue on ignition ⟨281⟩: not more than 0.2%.
Chromatographic purity—Dissolve 30 mg in 3.0 mL of chloroform to obtain the *Test preparation*. Dissolve a suitable quantity of USP Miconazole RS in chloroform to obtain a *Standard solution* having a concentration of 10.0 mg per mL. Quantitatively dilute a portion of this solution with chloroform to obtain a *Diluted standard solution* having a concentration of 100 µg per mL. Apply separate 5-µL portions of the three solutions to the starting line of a suitable thin-layer chromatographic plate (see *Chromatography* ⟨621⟩) coated with a 0.25-mm layer of chromatographic silica gel mixture. Develop the chromatogram in a suitable chamber with a freshly prepared solvent system consisting of a mixture of *n*-hexane, chloroform, methanol, and ammonium hydroxide (60 : 30 : 10 : 1) until the solvent front has moved about three-fourths of the length of the plate. Remove the plate from the chamber, and allow the solvent to evaporate. Expose the plate to iodine vapors in a closed chamber for about 30 minutes, and locate the spots: the R_F value of the principal spot obtained from the *Test solution* corresponds to that obtained from the *Standard solution,* and any other spot obtained from the *Test solution* does not exceed, in size or intensity, the principal spot obtained from the *Diluted standard solution* (1.0%).
Assay—Dissolve about 300 mg of Miconazole, accurately weighed, in 40 mL of glacial acetic acid, add 4 drops of *p*-naphtholbenzein TS, and titrate with 0.1 N perchloric acid VS to a green endpoint. Perform a blank determination, and make any necessary correction. Each mL of 0.1 N perchloric acid is equivalent to 41.61 mg of $C_{18}H_{14}Cl_4N_2O$.

Miconazole Injection

» Miconazole Injection is a sterile solution of Miconazole in Water for Injection. It contains not less than 90.0 percent and not more than 110.0 percent of the labeled amount of miconazole ($C_{18}H_{14}Cl_4N_2O$).

Packaging and storage—Preserve in single-dose containers, preferably of Type I glass, at controlled room temperature.

USP Reference standards ⟨11⟩—*USP Miconazole RS. USP Endotoxin RS*.
Identification—
  Dragendorff's reagent—Dissolve 0.85 g of bismuth subnitrate in a mixture of 40 mL of water and 10 mL of glacial acetic acid (*Solution A*). Dissolve 8 g of potassium iodide in 20 mL of water (*Solution B*). Transfer 5 mL of *Solution A*, 5 mL of *Solution B*, and 20 mL of glacial acetic acid to a 100-mL volumetric flask, dilute with water to volume, and mix.
  Procedure—Transfer a volume of Injection, equivalent to about 50 mg of miconazole, to a 10-mL volumetric flask, dilute with methanol to volume, and mix. Dissolve a suitable quantity of USP Miconazole RS in methanol to obtain a Standard solution having a known concentration of about 5 mg per mL. Apply separate 5-µL portions of the two solutions to the starting line of a suitable thin-layer chromatographic plate (see *Chromatography* ⟨621⟩) coated with a 0.25-mm layer of chromatographic silica gel mixture. Develop the chromatogram in a suitable chamber with a freshly prepared solvent system consisting of a mixture of *n*-hexane, chloroform, methanol, and ammonium hydroxide (60 : 30 : 10 : 1) until the solvent front has moved about three-fourths of the length of the plate. Remove the plate from the chamber, and allow the solvent to evaporate. Locate the spots on the plate by spraying with *Dragendorff's reagent*: the R_F value of one of the principal spots obtained from the test solution corresponds to that obtained from the Standard solution.
Bacterial endotoxins ⟨85⟩—It contains not more than 0.10 USP Endotoxin Unit per mg of miconazole.
pH ⟨791⟩: between 3.7 and 5.7.
Particulate matter ⟨788⟩: meets the requirements under small-volume injections.
Other requirements—It meets the requirements under *Injections* ⟨1⟩.
Assay—
  Mobile phase—Dissolve 5.0 g of ammonium acetate in 200 mL of water, add 300 mL of acetonitrile and 500 mL of methanol, mix, filter, and degas. Make adjustments if necessary (see *System Suitability* under *Chromatography* ⟨621⟩).
  Standard preparation—Dissolve an accurately weighed quantity of USP Miconazole RS in *Mobile phase* and dilute quantitatively, and stepwise if necessary, with *Mobile phase* to obtain a solution having a known concentration of about 0.5 mg per mL. Transfer 10.0 mL of this solution to a 100-mL volumetric flask, dilute with *Mobile phase* to volume, and mix to obtain a *Standard preparation* having a known concentration of about 50 µg per mL.
  Resolution solution—Dissolve suitable quantities of USP Miconazole RS and dibutyl phthalate in *Mobile phase* to obtain a solution containing about 50 µg of each per mL.
  Assay preparation—Transfer an accurately measured volume of Injection, equivalent to about 50 mg of miconazole, to a 100-mL volumetric flask, dilute with *Mobile phase* to volume, and mix. Transfer 10.0 mL of this solution to a 100-mL volumetric flask, dilute with *Mobile phase* to volume, and mix.
  Chromatographic system (see *Chromatography* ⟨621⟩)—The liquid chromatograph is equipped with a 230-nm detector and a 4.6-mm × 30-cm column that contains packing L7. The flow rate is about 2 mL per minute. Chromatograph the *Resolution solution* and the *Standard preparation*, and record the peak responses as directed under *Procedure*: the resolution, *R*, between the dibutyl phthalate and miconazole peaks is not less than 5.0, the tailing factor for the miconazole peak is not more than 1.3, and the relative standard deviation for replicate injections of the *Standard preparation* is not more than 2.0%. The relative retention times are about 0.7 for dibutyl phthalate and 1.0 for miconazole.
  Procedure—[NOTE—Allow the chromatograph to run for at least 16 to 18 minutes between injections to allow for elution of all components associated with the Injection vehicle.] Separately inject equal volumes (about 20 µL) of the *Standard preparation* and the *Assay preparation* into the chromatograph, record the chromatograms, and measure the responses for the major peaks. Calculate the

quantity, in mg, of miconazole ($C_{18}H_{14}Cl_4N_2O$) in each mL of the Injection taken by the formula:

$$(C / V)(r_U / r_S)$$

in which C is the concentration, in µg per mL, of USP Miconazole RS in the *Standard preparation*, V is the volume, in mL, of Injection taken, and r_U and r_S are the peak responses obtained from the *Assay preparation* and the *Standard preparation*, respectively.

Miconazole Nitrate

$C_{18}H_{14}Cl_4N_2O \cdot HNO_3$ 479.14
1*H*-Imidazole, 1-[2-(2,4-dichlorophenyl)-2-[(2,4-dichlorophenyl)methoxy]ethyl]-, mononitrate.
1-[2,4-Dichloro-β-[(2,4-dichlorobenzyl)oxy]phenethyl]imidazole mononitrate   [22832-87-7].

» Miconazole Nitrate contains not less than 98.0 percent and not more than 102.0 percent of $C_{18}H_{14}Cl_4N_2O \cdot HNO_3$, calculated on the dried basis.

Packaging and storage—Preserve in well-closed containers, protected from light.
USP Reference standards ⟨11⟩—*USP Miconazole Nitrate RS. USP Econazole Nitrate RS.*
Identification—
  A: *Infrared Absorption* ⟨197K⟩.
  B: *Ultraviolet Absorption* ⟨197U⟩—
  Solution: 400 µg per mL.
  Medium: 0.1 N hydrochloric acid in isopropyl alcohol (1 in 10).
Loss on drying ⟨731⟩—Dry it at 105° for 2 hours: it loses not more than 0.5% of its weight.
Residue on ignition ⟨281⟩:   not more than 0.2%.
Related compounds—
  Mobile phase—Prepare a filtered and degassed mixture of 0.2 M ammonium acetate, methanol, and acetonitrile (38 : 32 : 30). Make adjustments if necessary (see *System Suitability* under *Chromatography* ⟨621⟩).
  Resolution solution—Dissolve accurately weighed quantities of USP Miconazole Nitrate RS and USP Econazole Nitrate RS in *Mobile phase* to obtain a solution having known concentrations of about 25 µg of each per mL.
  Test solution—Transfer 100 mg of Miconazole Nitrate to a 10-mL volumetric flask, add *Mobile phase* to volume, and mix.
  Diluted test solution—Dilute an accurately measured volume of the *Test solution* quantitatively, and stepwise if necessary, with *Mobile phase* to obtain a solution containing 25 µg of miconazole nitrate per mL.
  Chromatographic system (see *Chromatography* ⟨621⟩)—The liquid chromatograph is equipped with a 235-nm detector and a 4.6-mm × 10-cm column that contains 3-µm packing L1. The flow rate is about 2 mL per minute. Chromatograph the *Resolution solution*, and record the peak responses as directed for *Procedure:* the relative retention times are about 0.5 for econazole and 1.0 for miconazole; the resolution, *R*, between econazole and miconazole is not less than 10; and the relative standard deviation for replicate injections is not more than 2.0%.
  Procedure—Separately inject equal volumes (about 10 µL) of the *Test solution* and *Diluted test solution* into the chromatograph, record the chromatograms for a time that is 1.2 times the retention time of the main peak, and measure the responses of all peaks, excluding the peak representing nitrate ion and any peak producing a response less than 0.2 times the response of the main peak. The response of any individual peak, other than the main peak in the chromatogram of the *Test solution*, is not greater than that of the main peak in the chromatogram of the *Diluted test solution* (0.25%), and the sum of the responses of all peaks, other than the main peak in the chromatogram of the *Test solution*, is not greater than twice the response of the main peak in the chromatogram of the *Diluted test solution* (0.5%).

Assay—Dissolve about 350 mg of Miconazole Nitrate, accurately weighed, in 50 mL of glacial acetic acid, and titrate with 0.1 N perchloric acid VS, determining the endpoint potentiometrically, using a glass-calomel electrode system. Perform a blank determination, and make any necessary correction. Each mL of 0.1 N perchloric acid is equivalent to 47.92 mg of $C_{18}H_{14}Cl_4N_2O \cdot HNO_3$.

Miconazole Nitrate Cream

» Miconazole Nitrate Cream contains not less than 90.0 percent and not more than 110.0 percent of the labeled amount of miconazole nitrate ($C_{18}H_{14}Cl_4N_2O \cdot HNO_3$).

Packaging and storage—Preserve in collapsible tubes or tight containers, and store at controlled room temperature.
Labeling—Cream that is packaged and labeled for use as a vaginal preparation shall be labeled Miconazole Nitrate Vaginal Cream.
USP Reference standards ⟨11⟩—*USP Miconazole Nitrate RS.*
Identification—The retention time of the major peak in the chromatogram of the *Assay preparation* corresponds to that in the chromatogram of the *Standard preparation,* as obtained in the *Assay*.
Minimum fill ⟨755⟩:   meets the requirements.
Assay—
  Buffer solution—Transfer 10 mL of triethylamine to a suitable flask, dilute with 1000 mL of water, adjust with phosphoric acid to a pH of about 2.5, and mix.
  Mobile phase—Prepare a filtered and degassed mixture of *Buffer solution*, methanol, acetonitrile, and tetrahydrofuran (8 : 5 : 4 : 3). Make adjustments if necessary (see *System Suitablility* under *Chromatography* ⟨621⟩).
  Standard preparation—Dissolve an accurately weighed quantity of USP Miconazole Nitrate RS and benzoic acid in *Mobile phase*, and dilute quantitatively, and stepwise if necessary, with *Mobile phase* to obtain a solution having a known concentration of about 0.28 and 0.02 mg per mL for miconazole nitrate and benzoic acid, respectively.
  Assay preparation—Transfer an accurately weighed quantity of Cream, equivalent to about 14 mg of miconazole nitrate, to a 50-mL volumetric flask, dissolve in and dilute with *Mobile phase* to volume, and mix. Sonicate in a water bath at 40° to 45° until the sample is completely dispersed, and mix. Cool the solution to below room temperature, mix, and pass a portion of the solution through a 0.45-µm teflon filter into an HPLC vial.
  Chromatographic system (see *Chromatography* ⟨621⟩)—The liquid chromatograph is equipped with a 225-nm detector and 4.6-mm × 25-cm column that contains packing L11. The flow rate is about 1.0 mL per minute. The column temperature is maintained at 45°. Chromatograph the *Standard preparation*, and record the peak responses as directed for *Procedure:* the column efficiency for miconazole nitrate peak is not less than 7500 theoretical plates; the tailing factor for miconazole nitrate peak is not more than 2.0; and the relative standard deviation for replicate injections of miconazole nitrate is not more than 2.0%. The resolution between miconazole nitrate and benzoic acid is not less than 13.
  Procedure—Separately inject equal volumes (about 10 µL) of the *Standard preparation* and the *Assay preparation* into the chromatograph, record the chromatograms, and measure the responses for the major peaks. Calculate the quantity, in mg, of miconazole nitrate ($C_{18}H_{14}Cl_4N_2O \cdot HNO_3$) in the portion of Cream taken by the formula:

$$50C(r_U / r_S)$$

in which C is the concentration, in mg per mL, of USP Miconazole Nitrate RS in the *Standard preparation;* and r_U and r_S are the peak responses obtained from the *Assay preparation* and the *Standard preparation,* respectively.

Miconazole Nitrate Topical Powder

» Miconazole Nitrate Topical Powder contains not less than 90.0 percent and not more than 110.0 percent of the labeled amount of miconazole nitrate ($C_{18}H_{14}Cl_4N_2O \cdot HNO_3$).

Packaging and storage—Preserve in well-closed containers.

USP Reference standards ⟨11⟩—*USP Miconazole Nitrate RS.*

Identification—Transfer a portion of Topical Powder, equivalent to about 100 mg of miconazole nitrate to a 50-mL beaker, disperse in 40 mL of methanol, and mix for a minimum of 5 minutes. Allow to settle for 5 to 10 minutes, and filter into a 100-mL beaker. Evaporate on a steam bath to dryness. Dry the residue at 105° for 10 minutes: the IR absorption spectrum of a potassium bromide dispersion of the residue so obtained exhibits maxima only at the same wavelengths as that of a similar preparation of USP Miconazole Nitrate RS.

Microbial limits ⟨61⟩—The total count does not exceed 100 microorganisms per g, and tests for *Staphylococcus aureus*, and *Pseudomonas aeruginosa*, are negative.

Minimum fill ⟨755⟩: meets the requirements.

Assay—

Internal standard solution—Dissolve cholestane in chloroform to obtain a solution having a concentration of about 0.5 mg per mL.

Standard preparation—Dissolve an accurately weighed quantity of USP Miconazole Nitrate RS in a mixture of chloroform and methanol (1 : 1) to obtain a solution having a known concentration of about 0.8 mg per mL. Transfer 5.0 mL of this solution to a test tube, add 2.0 mL of *Internal standard solution*, and evaporate at a temperature not higher than 40° with the aid of a current of nitrogen to dryness. Dissolve the residue in 2.0 mL of a mixture of chloroform and methanol (1 : 1), and mix to obtain a *Standard preparation* having a known miconazole nitrate concentration of about 2 mg per mL.

Assay preparation—Transfer an accurately weighed portion of Topical Powder, equivalent to about 20 mg of miconazole nitrate, to a stoppered 50-mL centrifuge tube. Add 25.0 mL of methanol, and shake by mechanical means for 30 minutes to dissolve the miconazole nitrate. Centrifuge to obtain a clear supernatant. Transfer 5.0 mL of this solution to a test tube, add 2.0 mL of *Internal standard solution*, and evaporate at a temperature not higher than 40° with the aid of a current of nitrogen to dryness. Dissolve the residue in 2.0 mL of a mixture of chloroform and methanol (1 : 1).

Chromatographic system (see *Chromatography* ⟨621⟩)—The gas chromatograph is equipped with a flame-ionization detector and a 1.2-m × 2-mm glass column containing 3 percent phase G32 on support S1A. The injection port, detector, and column are maintained at temperatures of about 250°, 300°, and 250°, respectively. Helium is used as the carrier gas, at a flow rate of about 50 mL per minute. Chromatograph the *Standard preparation*, and record the peak responses as directed under *Procedure*: the resolution, *R*, between the cholestane and miconazole nitrate peaks is not less than 2.0, and the relative standard deviation for replicate injections is not more than 3.0%.

Procedure—Separately inject equal volumes (about 5 µL) of the *Standard preparation* and the *Assay preparation* into the chromatograph, record the chromatograms, and measure the responses for the major peaks. The relative retention times for cholestane and miconazole nitrate are about 0.5 and 1.0, respectively. Calculate the quantity, in mg, of miconazole nitrate ($C_{18}H_{14}Cl_4N_2O \cdot HNO_3$) in the portion of Topical Powder taken by the formula:

$$10C(R_U / R_S)$$

in which *C* is the concentration, in mg per mL, of USP Miconazole Nitrate RS in the *Standard preparation*, and R_U and R_S are the peak response ratios of the miconazole nitrate peak to the cholestane peak obtained from the *Assay preparation* and the *Standard preparation*, respectively.

Miconazole Nitrate Vaginal Suppositories

» Miconazole Nitrate Vaginal Suppositories contain not less than 90.0 percent and not more than 110.0 percent of the labeled amount of miconazole nitrate ($C_{18}H_{14}Cl_4N_2O \cdot HNO_3$).

Packaging and storage—Preserve in tight containers, at controlled room temperature.

USP Reference standards ⟨11⟩—*USP Miconazole Nitrate RS.*

Identification—Place a portion of the stock solution, prepared as directed in the *Assay*, containing about 25 mg of miconazole nitrate, in a 50-mL beaker, and evaporate on a steam bath with the aid of a current of filtered air to dryness. Dry the residue at 105° for 10 minutes: the IR absorption spectrum of a potassium bromide dispersion of it so obtained exhibits maxima only at the same wavelengths as that of a similar preparation of USP Miconazole Nitrate RS.

Assay—

Internal standard solution—Dissolve a suitable quantity of cholestane in a mixture of chloroform and methanol (1 : 1) to obtain a solution having a concentration of about 1 mg per mL.

Standard preparation—Dissolve an accurately weighed quantity of USP Miconazole Nitrate RS in methanol to obtain a solution having a known concentration of about 500 µg per mL. Transfer 10.0 mL of this solution to a test tube, and evaporate on a steam bath to dryness with the aid of a current of filtered air. Dissolve the residue in 2.0 mL of *Internal standard solution* to obtain a solution having a concentration of about 2500 µg per mL.

Assay preparation—Transfer 1 Suppository to a stoppered, 50-mL centrifuge tube. Add 30 mL of pentane, and shake by mechanical means for 20 minutes to dissolve the suppository base and to disperse the miconazole nitrate. Centrifuge to obtain a clear supernatant. Aspirate, and discard the clear liquid. Wash the residue with three 20-mL portions of pentane, shaking, centrifuging, and aspirating in the same manner. Discard the pentane washings. Evaporate the residual pentane from the residue with the aid of a current of filtered air. Using small portions of methanol, transfer the residue to a 100-mL volumetric flask. Dissolve in and dilute with methanol to volume, and mix. Transfer an accurately measured volume of this stock solution, equivalent to about 5 mg of miconazole nitrate, to a suitable container, and evaporate to dryness on a steam bath with the aid of a current of filtered air. Dissolve the residue in 2.0 mL of *Internal standard solution*.

Chromatographic system (see *Chromatography* ⟨621⟩)—The gas chromatograph is equipped with a flame-ionization detector and a 2-mm × 1.2-m column packed with 3% phase G32 on support S1A. The carrier gas is helium, flowing at a rate of about 50 mL per minute. The injection port, detector, and column temperatures are maintained at about 250°, 300°, and 250°, respectively. Chromatograph the *Standard preparation*, and record the peak responses as directed for *Procedure*: the relative retention times for cholestane and miconazole nitrate are about 0.44 and 1.0, respectively; the resolution, *R*, between cholestane and miconazole nitrate is not less than 2.0; and the relative standard deviation for replicate injections is not more than 3.0%.

Procedure—Separately inject equal volumes (about 1 µL) of the *Assay preparation* and the *Standard preparation* into the chromatograph, record the chromatograms, and measure the peak responses. Calculate the quantity, in mg, of miconazole nitrate ($C_{18}H_{14}Cl_4N_2O \cdot HNO_3$) in the portion of Suppository taken by the formula:

$$(0.2C/V)(R_U / R_S)$$

in which *C* is the concentration, in µg per mL, of the USP Miconazole Nitrate RS in the *Standard preparation*; *V* is the volume, in mL, of stock solution used to prepare the *Assay preparation*; and R_U and R_S are the ratios of the peak responses of miconazole nitrate to that of cholestane obtained from the *Assay preparation* and *Standard preparation*, respectively.

Milrinone

$C_{12}H_9N_3O$ 211.22
[3,4'-Bipyridine]-5-carbonitrile, 1,6-dihydro-2-methyl-6-oxo-.
1,6-Dihydro-2-methyl-6-oxo[3,4'-bipyridine]-5-carbonitrile
[78415-72-2].

» Milrinone contains not less than 98.5 percent and not more than 101.5 percent of $C_{12}H_9N_3O$, calculated on the anhydrous basis.

Caution—Milrinone is a cardiotonic agent.

Packaging and storage—Preserve in tight containers, and store at controlled room temperature.
USP Reference standards ⟨11⟩—USP Milrinone RS. USP Milrinone Related Compound A RS.
Identification—
   A: *Infrared Absorption* ⟨197K⟩.
   B: The retention time of the major peak in the chromatogram of the *Test solution* corresponds to that in the chromatogram of the *Standard solution*, as obtained in the test for *Chromatographic purity.*
Water, *Method I* ⟨921⟩: not more than 2.0%.
Residue on ignition ⟨281⟩: not more than 0.2%.
Heavy metals, *Method II* ⟨231⟩: 0.002%.
Chromatographic purity—
   pH 7.5 Phosphate buffer—Dissolve 2.7 g of dibasic potassium phosphate in 800 mL of water, add 2.4 mL of triethylamine, adjust with phosphoric acid to a pH of about 7.5, and mix.
   Mobile phase—Prepare a filtered and degassed mixture of *pH 7.5 Phosphate buffer* and acetonitrile (80:20). Make adjustments if necessary (see *System Suitability* under *Chromatography* ⟨621⟩).
   Standard stock solution—Dissolve an accurately weighed quantity of USP Milrinone RS in *Mobile phase* to obtain a solution having a known concentration of about 2 mg per mL, heat in a water bath at approximately 80°, and/or sonicate, if necessary.
   Standard solution—Dilute an appropriate volume of *Standard stock solution* quantitatively, and stepwise if necessary, with *Mobile phase* to obtain a solution having a known concentration of 0.006 mg per mL.
   System suitability solution—Dissolve an accurately weighed quantity of USP Milrinone Related Compound A RS in *Mobile phase* to obtain a solution having a known concentration of about 0.2 mg per mL. Heat in a water bath at approximately 80°, and/or sonicate, if necessary, to dissolve. Transfer 10.0 mL of this solution and 1.0 mL of the *Standard stock solution* to a 100-mL volumetric flask, dilute with *Mobile phase* to volume, and mix.
   Test solution—Transfer about 100 mg of Milrinone, accurately weighed, to a 50-mL volumetric flask, dissolve in and dilute with *Mobile phase* to volume, and mix. Heat in a water bath at approximately 80°, if necessary.
   Chromatographic system (see *Chromatography* ⟨621⟩)—The liquid chromatograph is equipped with a 220-nm detector and a 4.6-mm × 25-cm column that contains packing L7. The flow rate is about 1 mL per minute. Chromatograph the *System suitability solution*, and record the peak responses as directed for *Procedure*: the relative retention times are about 0.6 for milrinone related compound A and 1.0 for milrinone; the resolution, *R*, between milrinone related compound A and milrinone is not less than 4.0; and the relative standard deviation for replicate injections of milrinone is not more than 5.0%.
   Procedure—Separately inject equal volumes (about 20 µL) of the *Test solution* and the *Standard solution* into the chromatograph, record the chromatograms, and measure all the peak responses. Calculate the percentage of each impurity in the portion of Milrinone taken by the formula:

$$5000(C/W)(r_i / r_S)$$

in which *C* is the concentration, in mg per mL, of USP Milrinone RS in the *Standard solution*; *W* is the weight, in mg, of milrinone taken to prepare the *Test solution*; r_i is the peak response for each impurity obtained from the *Test solution*; and r_S is the peak response obtained from the *Standard solution*: not more than 0.3% of any individual impurity is found; and not more than 1.0% of total impurities is found.
Organic volatile impurities, *Method V* ⟨467⟩: meets the requirements.
   Solvent—Use dimethyl sulfoxide.

(Official until July 1, 2008)

Assay—Transfer about 200 mg of Milrinone, accurately weighed, to a 100-mL beaker, and dissolve by stirring in 50 mL of glacial acetic acid. Titrate with 0.1 N perchloric acid VS, determining the endpoint potentiometrically. Perform a blank determination, and make any necessary correction. Each mL of 0.1 N perchloric acid VS is equivalent to 21.12 mg of $C_{12}H_9N_3O$.

Mineral Oil

» Mineral Oil is a mixture of liquid hydrocarbons obtained from petroleum. It may contain a suitable stabilizer.

Packaging and storage—Preserve in tight containers.
Labeling—Label it to indicate the name of any substance added as a stabilizer.
Specific gravity ⟨841⟩: between 0.845 and 0.905.
Viscosity ⟨911⟩—It has a kinematic viscosity of not less than 34.5 centistokes at 40.0°.
Neutrality—Boil 10 mL with an equal volume of alcohol: the alcohol remains neutral to moistened litmus paper.
Readily carbonizable substances—Place 5 mL in a glass-stoppered test tube that previously has been rinsed with chromic acid cleansing mixture (see *Cleaning Glass Apparatus* ⟨1051⟩), then rinsed with water, and dried. Add 5 mL of sulfuric acid containing from 94.5% to 94.9% of H_2SO_4, and heat in a boiling water bath for 10 minutes. After the test tube has been in the bath for 30 seconds, remove it quickly, and, while holding the stopper in place, give three vigorous, vertical shakes over an amplitude of about 5 inches. Repeat every 30 seconds. Do not keep the test tube out of the bath longer than 3 seconds for each shaking period. At the end of 10 minutes from the time when first placed in the water bath, remove the test tube: the Oil may turn hazy, but it remains colorless, or shows a slight pink or yellow color, and the acid does not become darker than the standard color produced by mixing in a similar test tube 3 mL of ferric chloride CS, 1.5 mL of cobaltous chloride CS, and 0.5 mL of cupric sulfate CS, this mixture being overlaid with 5 mL of Oil (see *Readily Carbonizable Substances Test* ⟨271⟩).
Limit of polynuclear compounds—
   Dimethyl sulfoxide—Use spectrophotometric grade dimethyl sulfoxide.
   Standard solution—Dissolve a quantity of naphthalene, accurately weighed, in isooctane, and dilute quantitatively and stepwise with isooctane to obtain a solution having a concentration of 7.0 µg per mL. Determine the absorbance of this solution in a 1-cm cell at the wavelength of maximum absorbance at about 275 nm, using isooctane as the blank.
   Procedure—Transfer 25.0 mL of Mineral Oil and 25 mL of *n*-hexane to a 125-mL separator, and mix. [NOTE—Use only *n*-hexane that previously has been washed by being shaken twice with one-fifth its volume of *Dimethyl sulfoxide*. Use no lubricants other than water on the stopcock, or use a separator equipped with a suitable polymeric stopcock.] Add 5.0 mL of *Dimethyl sulfoxide*, and shake the mixture vigorously for 1 minute. Allow to stand until the lower layer is clear, transfer the lower layer to another 125-mL separator, add 2 mL of *n*-hexane, and shake vigorously. Separate the lower

layer, and determine its absorbance in a 1-cm cell, in the range of 260 nm to 350 nm, using as the blank *Dimethyl sulfoxide* that previously has been shaken vigorously for 1 minute with *n*-hexane in the ratio of 5 mL of *Dimethyl sulfoxide* and 25 mL of *n*-hexane. The absorbance at any wavelength in the specified range is not greater than one-third of the absorbance, at 275 nm, of the *Standard solution*.

Solid paraffin—Fill a tall, cylindrical, standard oil-sample bottle of colorless glass of about 120-mL capacity with Mineral Oil that has been dried previously in a beaker at 105° for 2 hours and cooled to room temperature in a desiccator over silica gel. Insert the stopper, and immerse the bottle in a mixture of ice and water for 4 hours: the test specimen is sufficiently clear that a black line 0.5 mm in width, on a white background, held vertically behind the bottle, is clearly visible.

Mineral Oil Emulsion

» Prepare Mineral Oil Emulsion as follows:

Mineral Oil	500 mL
Acacia, in very fine powder	125 g
Syrup	100 mL
Vanillin	40 mg
Alcohol	60 mL
Purified Water, a sufficient quantity to make	1000 mL

Mix the Mineral Oil with the Powdered Acacia in a dry mortar, add 250 mL of Purified Water all at once, and emulsify the mixture. Then add, in divided portions, triturating after each addition, a mixture of the Syrup, 50 mL of Purified Water, and the Vanillin dissolved in the alcohol. Finally add Purified Water to make the product measure 1000 mL, and mix.

The Vanillin may be replaced by not more than 1 percent of any other official flavoring substance or any mixture of official flavoring substances. Sixty mL of sweet orange peel tincture or 2 g of benzoic acid may be used as a preservative in place of the Alcohol.

For other permissible modifications, see *Emulsions* ⟨1151⟩.

Packaging and storage—Preserve in tight containers.
Alcohol content, *Method I* ⟨611⟩: between 4.0% and 6.0% of C_2H_5OH.

Mineral Oil, Rectal

» Mineral Oil, Rectal, is Mineral Oil that has been suitably packaged.

Packaging and storage—Preserve in tight, single-unit containers.
Specific gravity ⟨841⟩: between 0.845 and 0.905.
Viscosity ⟨911⟩—It has a kinematic viscosity of not less than 34.5 centistokes at 40.0°.
Neutrality—Boil 10 mL with an equal volume of alcohol: the alcohol remains neutral to moistened litmus paper.

Topical Light Mineral Oil

» Topical Light Mineral Oil is Light Mineral Oil that has been suitably packaged.

Packaging and storage—Preserve in tight containers.
Labeling—Label it to indicate the name of any substance added as a stabilizer, and label packages intended for direct use by the public to indicate that it is not intended for internal use.
Specific gravity ⟨841⟩: between 0.818 and 0.880.
Viscosity ⟨911⟩—It has a kinematic viscosity of not more than 33.5 centistokes at 40°.
Neutrality and Solid paraffin—It meets the requirements of the tests for *Neutrality* and *Solid paraffin* under *Mineral Oil*.

Minocycline Hydrochloride

$C_{23}H_{27}N_3O_7 \cdot HCl$ 493.95
2-Naphthacenecarboxamide, 4,7-bis(dimethylamino)-1,4,4a,5,5a,6,11,12a-octahydro-3,10,12,12a-tetrahydroxy-1,11dioxo-, monohydrochloride, [4*S*-(4α,4aα,5aα,12aα)]-.
4,7-Bis(dimethylamino)-1,4,4a,5,5a,6,11,12a-octahydro-3,10,12,12a-tetrahydroxy-1,11-dioxo-2-naphthacenecarboxamide monohydrochloride [*13614-98-7*].

» Minocycline Hydrochloride contains the equivalent of not less than 890 μg and not more than 950 μg of minocycline ($C_{23}H_{27}N_3O_7$) per mg, calculated on the anhydrous basis.

Packaging and storage—Preserve in tight containers, protected from light.
Labeling—Where it is intended for use in preparing injectable dosage forms, the label states that it is sterile or must be subjected to further processing during the preparation of injectable dosage forms.
USP Reference standards ⟨11⟩—*USP Minocycline Hydrochloride RS. USP Endotoxin RS.*
Identification, *Infrared Absorption* ⟨197K⟩: previously dried at 100° for 2 hours.
Crystallinity ⟨695⟩: meets the requirements.
pH ⟨791⟩: between 3.5 and 4.5, in a solution containing the equivalent of 10 mg of minocycline per mL.
Water, *Method I* ⟨921⟩: between 4.3% and 8.0%.
Residue on ignition ⟨281⟩: not more than 0.15%.
Heavy metals, *Method II* ⟨231⟩: 0.005%.
Chromatographic purity—
  Mobile phase, *Resolution solution*, and *Chromatographic system*—Proceed as directed in the *Assay*.
  Test solution 1—Transfer about 25 mg of Minocycline Hydrochloride, accurately weighed, to a 100-mL volumetric flask, dilute with water to volume, and mix. Protect this solution from light, store in a refrigerator, and use within 3 hours.
  Test solution 2—Transfer 1.0 mL of *Test solution 1* to a 50-mL volumetric flask, dilute with water to volume, and mix. Protect this solution from light, store in a refrigerator, and use within 3 hours.
  Test solution 3—Transfer 6.0 mL of *Test solution 2* to a 10-mL volumetric flask, dilute with water to volume, and mix. Protect this solution from light, store in a refrigerator, and use within 3 hours.
  Procedure—Separately inject equal volumes (about 20 μL) of *Test solution 1*, *Test solution 2*, and *Test solution 3* into the chromatograph, record the chromatograms, and measure the areas for all the peaks. [NOTE—Record the chromatogram of *Test solution 1* for

a period of time that is about 2.6 times the retention time of minocycline.] Calculate the percentage of epiminocycline in the portion of Minocycline Hydrochloride taken by the formula:

$$1.2 r_{E1}/r_{M3}$$

in which r_{E1} is the peak response for epiminocycline obtained from *Test solution 1*; and r_{M3} is the peak response for minocycline obtained from *Test solution 3*. Not more than 1.2% is found. Calculate the total percentage of impurities other than epiminocycline in the portion of Minocycline Hydrochloride taken by the formula:

$$2 r_s / r_{M2}$$

in which r_s is the sum of the responses of all impurity peaks other than epiminocycline obtained from *Test solution 1*; and r_{M2} is the peak response for minocycline obtained from *Test solution 2*. Not more than 2.0% of other impurities is found.

Other requirements—Where the label states that Minocycline Hydrochloride is sterile, it meets the requirements for *Sterility Tests* ⟨71⟩ and for *Bacterial endotoxins* under *Minocycline for Injection*. Where the label states that Minocycline Hydrochloride must be subjected to further processing during the preparation of injectable dosage forms, it meets the requirements for *Bacterial endotoxins* under *Minocycline for Injection*.

Assay—
Mobile phase—Prepare a mixture of 0.2 M ammonium oxalate, 0.01 M edetate disodium, dimethylformamide, and tetrahydrofuran (600 : 180 : 120 : 80). Adjust with ammonium hydroxide to a pH of 7.2, and pass through a filter having a 0.5-µm or finer porosity. Make adjustments if necessary (see *System Suitability* under *Chromatography* ⟨621⟩).

Standard preparation—Dissolve an accurately weighed quantity of USP Minocycline Hydrochloride RS in water to obtain a solution having a known concentration of about 500 µg of minocycline ($C_{23}H_{27}N_3O_7$) per mL. Use this solution within 3 hours.

Resolution solution—Transfer 10 mg of USP Minocycline Hydrochloride RS to a 25-mL volumetric flask, add 20 mL of 0.2 M ammonium oxalate, and swirl to dissolve. Heat on a water bath at 60° for 180 minutes, and allow to cool. Dilute with water to volume, and mix.

Assay preparation—Transfer an accurately weighed quantity of Minocycline Hydrochloride, equivalent to about 50 mg of minocycline ($C_{23}H_{27}N_3O_7$), to a 100-mL volumetric flask, add water to volume, and mix.

Chromatographic system (see *Chromatography* ⟨621⟩)—The liquid chromatograph is equipped with a 280-nm detector and a 4.6-mm × 25-cm column that contains 5-µm packing L1, and is maintained at a constant temperature of about 40°. The flow rate is about 1.5 mL per minute. Chromatograph the *Standard preparation*, and record the peak responses as directed for *Procedure*: the capacity factor, k', is not less than 5.0 and not more than 11.5; the tailing factor for the analyte peak is not less than 0.9 and not more than 2.0; and the relative standard deviation for replicate injections is not more than 2.0%. Chromatograph the *Resolution solution* and record the peak responses as directed for *Procedure*: the relative retention times are about 0.7 for epiminocycline and 1.0 for minocycline; and the resolution, *R*, between epiminocycline and minocycline is not less than 4.6.

Procedure—Separately inject equal volumes (about 20 µL) of the *Standard preparation* and the *Assay preparation* into the chromatograph, record the chromatograms, and measure the responses for the major peaks. Calculate the quantity, in µg per mg, of minocycline ($C_{23}H_{27}N_3O_7$), in the portion of Minocycline Hydrochloride taken by the formula:

$$100(C/W)(r_U/r_S)$$

in which *C* is the concentration, in µg per mL, of minocycline ($C_{23}H_{27}N_3O_7$) in the *Standard preparation*; *W* is the weight, in mg, of Minocycline Hydrochloride taken; and r_U and r_S are the peak responses obtained from the *Assay preparation* and the *Standard preparation*, respectively.

Minocycline Hydrochloride Capsules

» Minocycline Hydrochloride Capsules contain the equivalent of not less than 90.0 percent and not more than 115.0 percent of the labeled amount of minocycline ($C_{23}H_{27}N_3O_7$).

Packaging and storage—Preserve in tight, light-resistant containers.

USP Reference standards ⟨11⟩—*USP Minocycline Hydrochloride RS*.

Identification—The retention time of the major peak in the chromatogram of the *Assay preparation* corresponds to that of the *Standard preparation* obtained as directed in the *Assay*.

Dissolution ⟨711⟩—
Medium: water; 900 mL.
Apparatus 2: 50 rpm.
Time: 45 minutes.
Procedure—Determine the amount of $C_{23}H_{27}N_3O_7$ dissolved from UV absorbances at the wavelength of maximum absorbance at about 348 nm of filtered portions of the solution under test, suitably diluted with *Dissolution Medium*, if necessary, in comparison with a Standard solution having a known concentration of USP Minocycline Hydrochloride RS in the same medium.
Tolerances—Not less than 75% (*Q*) of the labeled amount of $C_{23}H_{27}N_3O_7$ is dissolved in 45 minutes.

Uniformity of dosage units ⟨905⟩: meet the requirements.

Water, *Method I* ⟨921⟩: not more than 12.0%.

Assay—
Mobile phase, Standard preparation, Resolution solution, and *Chromatographic system*—Proceed as directed in the *Assay* under *Minocycline Hydrochloride*.

Assay preparation—Weigh the contents of not less than 20 Capsules, and calculate the average weight per Capsule. Mix the combined contents of the Capsules, transfer an accurately weighed portion, equivalent to about 50 mg of minocycline ($C_{23}H_{27}N_3O_7$), to a 100-mL volumetric flask, add about 50 mL of water, and shake to dissolve. Dilute with water to volume, mix, and filter.

Procedure—Proceed as directed for *Procedure* in the *Assay* under *Minocycline Hydrochloride*. Calculate the quantity, in mg, of minocycline ($C_{23}H_{27}N_3O_7$) in the portion of Capsules taken by the formula:

$$0.1C(r_U/r_S).$$

Minocycline for Injection

» Minocycline for Injection is sterile, freeze-dried Minocycline Hydrochloride suitable for parenteral use. It contains the equivalent of not less than 90.0 percent and not more than 120.0 percent of the labeled amount of minocycline ($C_{23}H_{27}N_3O_7$).

Packaging and storage—Preserve in *Containers for Sterile Solids* as described under *Injections* ⟨1⟩, protected from light.

USP Reference standards ⟨11⟩—*USP Minocycline Hydrochloride RS. USP Endotoxin RS*.

Constituted solution—At the time of use, it meets the requirements for *Constituted Solutions* under *Injections* ⟨1⟩.

Identification—The retention time of the major peak in the chromatogram of the *Assay preparation* corresponds to that in the chromatogram of the *Standard preparation*, as obtained in the *Assay*.

Bacterial endotoxins ⟨85⟩—It contains not more than 1.25 USP Endotoxin Units per mg of minocycline.

pH ⟨791⟩: between 2.0 and 3.5, in a solution containing the equivalent of 10 mg of minocycline per mL.

Water, *Method I* ⟨921⟩: not more than 3.0%, the *Test Preparation* being prepared as directed for a hygroscopic specimen.

Particulate matter ⟨788⟩: meets the requirements for small-volume injections.

Limit of epiminocycline—Using the chromatogram of the *Assay preparation* obtained as directed in the *Assay*, calculate the percentage of epiminocycline in the portion of Minocycline for Injection taken by the formula:

$$100 r_e / r_t$$

in which r_e is the area response of any peak in the chromatogram of the *Assay preparation* having a retention time of about 0.86 relative to that of minocycline, and r_t is the total area of the responses of all the peaks in the chromatogram: not more than 6.0% of epiminocycline is found.

Other requirements—It meets the requirements for *Sterility Tests* ⟨71⟩, *Uniformity of Dosage Units* ⟨905⟩, and *Labeling* under *Injections* ⟨1⟩.

Assay—

Mobile phase, *Standard preparation*, *Resolution solution*, and *Chromatographic system*—Proceed as directed in the *Assay* under *Minocycline Hydrochloride*.

Assay preparation 1 (where it is represented as being in a single-dose container)—Constitute Minocycline for Injection in a volume of water, accurately measured, corresponding to the volume of solvent specified in the labeling. Withdraw all of the withdrawable contents, using a hypodermic needle and syringe, and dilute quantitatively with water to obtain a solution containing the equivalent of about 0.5 mg of minocycline ($C_{23}H_{27}N_3O_7$) per mL.

Assay preparation 2 (where the label states the quantity of minocycline in a given volume of constituted solution)—Constitute Minocycline for Injection in a volume of water, accurately measured, corresponding to the volume of solvent specified in the labeling. Dilute an accurately measured portion of the constituted solution quantitatively with water to obtain a solution containing the equivalent of about 0.5 mg of minocycline ($C_{23}H_{27}N_3O_7$) per mL.

Procedure—Proceed as directed for *Procedure* in the *Assay* under *Minocycline Hydrochloride*. Calculate the quantity, in mg, of minocycline ($C_{23}H_{27}N_3O_7$) in the container, or in the portion of constituted solution taken by the formula:

$$0.001 C (L / D)(r_U / r_S)$$

in which L is the labeled quantity, in mg, of minocycline in the container, or in the volume of constituted solution taken; D is the concentration, in mg per mL, of minocycline in *Assay preparation 1* or in *Assay preparation 2*, on the basis of the labeled quantity in the container, or in the portion of constituted solution taken, respectively, and the extent of dilution; and the other terms are as defined therein.

Minocycline Hydrochloride Oral Suspension

» Minocycline Hydrochloride Oral Suspension contains the equivalent of not less than 90.0 percent and not more than 130.0 percent of the labeled amount of minocycline ($C_{23}H_{27}N_3O_7$), and one or more suitable diluents, flavors, preservatives, and wetting agents in an aqueous vehicle.

Packaging and storage—Preserve in tight, light-resistant containers.

USP Reference standards ⟨11⟩—*USP Minocycline Hydrochloride RS*.

Identification—The retention time of the major peak in the chromatogram of the *Assay preparation* corresponds to that of the *Standard preparation* obtained as directed in the *Assay*.

Uniformity of dosage units ⟨905⟩—

FOR SUSPENSION PACKAGED IN SINGLE-UNIT CONTAINERS: meets the requirements.

Deliverable volume ⟨698⟩: meets the requirements.

pH ⟨791⟩: between 7.0 and 9.0.

Assay—

Mobile phase and *Chromatographic system*—Proceed as directed in the *Assay* under *Minocycline Hydrochloride*.

Standard preparation—Dissolve an accurately weighed quantity of USP Minocycline Hydrochloride RS in *Mobile phase* to obtain a solution having a known concentration of about 500 μg of minocycline ($C_{23}H_{27}N_3O_7$) per mL. Use this solution within 1 hour.

Resolution solution—Prepare a solution in water containing 2 mg of USP Minocycline Hydrochloride RS per mL. Transfer 5 mL of this solution to a small beaker, and heat on a steam bath for 60 minutes. Evaporate to dryness, dissolve the residue in about 25 mL of *Mobile phase*, and filter.

Assay preparation—Transfer an accurately measured quantity of Oral Suspension, freshly mixed and free from air bubbles, equivalent to about 50 mg of $C_{23}H_{27}N_3O_7$, to a 100-mL volumetric flask, dilute with *Mobile phase* to volume, mix, and filter. Use this solution within 1 hour.

Procedure—Proceed as directed for *Procedure* in the *Assay* under *Minocycline Hydrochloride*. Calculate the quantity, in mg, of $C_{23}H_{27}N_3O_7$ in each mL of the Oral Suspension taken by the formula:

$$0.1(C/V)(r_U/r_S)$$

in which V is the volume, in mL, of Oral Suspension taken, and the other terms are as defined therein.

Minocycline Hydrochloride Tablets

» Minocycline Hydrochloride Tablets contain the equivalent of not less than 90.0 percent and not more than 115.0 percent of the labeled amount of minocycline ($C_{23}H_{27}N_3O_7$).

Packaging and storage—Preserve in tight, light-resistant containers.

USP Reference standards ⟨11⟩—*USP Minocycline Hydrochloride RS*.

Identification—The retention time of the major peak in the chromatogram of the *Assay preparation* corresponds to that of the *Standard preparation* obtained as directed in the *Assay*.

Dissolution ⟨711⟩—

Medium: water; 900 mL.

Apparatus 2: 50 rpm.

Time: 45 minutes.

Procedure—Determine the amount of $C_{23}H_{27}N_3O_7$ dissolved from UV absorbances at the wavelength of maximum absorbance at about 348 nm of filtered portions of the solution under test, suitably diluted with *Medium*, if necessary, in comparison with a Standard solution having a known concentration of USP Minocycline Hydrochloride RS in the same medium.

Tolerances—Not less than 75% (*Q*) of the labeled amount of $C_{23}H_{27}N_3O_7$ is dissolved in 45 minutes.

Uniformity of dosage units ⟨905⟩: meet the requirements.

Water, *Method I* ⟨921⟩: not more than 12.0%.

Assay—

Mobile phase, *Standard preparation*, *Resolution solution*, and *Chromatographic system*—Proceed as directed in the *Assay* under *Minocycline Hydrochloride*.

Assay preparation—Weigh and finely powder not less than 20 Tablets. Transfer an accurately weighed portion of the powder, equivalent to about 50 mg of minocycline ($C_{23}H_{27}N_3O_7$), to a 100-mL volumetric flask, add about 50 mL of water, and shake for about 1 minute. Dilute with water to volume, mix, and filter.

Procedure—Proceed as directed for *Procedure* in the *Assay* under *Minocycline Hydrochloride*. Calculate the quantity, in mg, of $C_{23}H_{27}N_3O_7$ in the portion of Tablets taken by the formula:

$$0.1C(r_U/r_S).$$

Minoxidil

$C_9H_{15}N_5O$ 209.25
2,4-Pyrimidinediamine, 6-(1-piperidinyl)-, 3-oxide.
2,4-Diamino-6-piperidinopyrimidine 3-oxide   [38304-91-5].

» Minoxidil contains not less than 97.0 percent and not more than 103.0 percent of $C_9H_{15}N_5O$, calculated on the dried basis.

Packaging and storage—Preserve in well-closed containers.
USP Reference standards ⟨11⟩—*USP Minoxidil RS*.
Identification, *Infrared Absorption* ⟨197M⟩—Do not dry specimens.
Loss on drying ⟨731⟩—Dry it at 50° and at a pressure not exceeding 5 mm of mercury for 3 hours: it loses not more than 0.5% of its weight.
Residue on ignition ⟨281⟩:   not more than 0.5%.
Heavy metals, *Method II* ⟨231⟩:   0.002%.
Chromatographic purity—
Mobile phase and *Chromatographic system*—Prepare as directed in the *Assay*.
Test solution—Prepare a solution of Minoxidil in *Mobile phase* having a concentration of about 0.25 mg per mL.
Procedure—Inject about 10 µL of *Test solution* into the chromatograph, record the chromatogram, and measure the peak response for each component. Calculate the total percentage of impurities taken by the formula:

$$100S/(S+A)$$

in which S is the sum of the areas of the minor component peaks detected, and A is the area of the major component. The total of any impurities detected is not more than 1.5%.
Organic volatile impurities, *Method IV* ⟨467⟩: meets the requirements.

(Official until July 1, 2008)

Assay—
Mobile phase—Prepare a solution consisting of a mixture of methanol, water, and glacial acetic acid (700 : 300 : 10), add 3.0 g of docusate sodium per L of solution, and mix. Adjust with perchloric acid to a pH of 3.0, filter, and degas.
Internal standard solution—Prepare a solution of medroxyprogesterone acetate in *Mobile phase* having a concentration of about 0.2 mg per mL.
Standard preparation—Dissolve an accurately weighed quantity of USP Minoxidil RS in *Internal standard solution* to obtain a solution having a known concentration of about 0.25 mg per mL.
Assay preparation—Transfer about 5 mg of Minoxidil, accurately weighed, to a container, add 20.0 mL of *Internal standard solution*, and mix.
Chromatographic system (see *Chromatography* ⟨621⟩)—The liquid chromatograph is equipped with a 254-nm detector and a 4-mm × 25-cm column that contains packing L1. The flow rate is about 1 mL per minute. Chromatograph not less than four replicate injections of the *Standard preparation*, and record the peak responses as directed under *Procedure*: the relative standard deviation is not more than 2.0%, and the resolution, R, between the internal standard and minoxidil is not less than 2.0.

Procedure—Separately inject equal volumes (about 10 µL) of the *Standard preparation* and the *Assay preparation* into the chromatograph, record the chromatograms, and measure the responses for the major peaks. The relative retention times are about 0.8 for the internal standard and 1.0 for minoxidil. Calculate the quantity, in mg, of $C_9H_{15}N_5O$ in the portion of Minoxidil taken by the formula:

$$20C(R_U/R_S)$$

in which C is the concentration, in mg per mL, of USP Minoxidil RS in the *Standard preparation*, and R_U and R_S are the peak response ratios obtained from the *Assay preparation* and the *Standard preparation*, respectively.

Minoxidil Topical Solution

» Minoxidil Topical Solution contains not less than 90.0 percent and not more than 110.0 percent of the labeled amount of minoxidil ($C_9H_{15}N_5O$).

Packaging and storage—Preserve in tight containers.
USP Reference standards ⟨11⟩—*USP Minoxidil RS*.
Identification—
A: *Infrared Absorption* ⟨197M⟩—
Test specimen—Evaporate 1 mL of the Topical Solution under a stream of nitrogen while heating at 50°.
B: The retention time of the major peak for minoxidil in the chromatogram of the *Assay preparation* corresponds to that of the *Standard preparation*, as obtained in the *Assay*.
Assay—
Mobile phase, Internal standard solution, Standard preparation, and *Chromatographic system*—Proceed as directed in the *Assay* under *Minoxidil*.
Assay preparation—Transfer an accurately measured volume of Topical Solution, equivalent to about 100 mg of minoxidil, to a 10-mL volumetric flask, dilute with *Mobile phase* to volume, and mix. Transfer 0.5 mL of this solution to a suitable vial, add 20.0 mL of *Internal standard solution*, and mix.
Procedure—Proceed as directed for *Procedure* in the *Assay* under *Minoxidil*. Calculate the quantity, in mg, of minoxidil ($C_9H_{15}N_5O$) in each mL of the Topical Solution taken by the formula:

$$(400C/V)(R_U/R_S)$$

in which C is the concentration, in mg per mL, of USP Minoxidil RS in the *Standard preparation*, V is the volume, in mL, of the Topical Solution taken for the *Assay preparation*, and R_U and R_S are the ratios of the minoxidil peak to that of the internal standard obtained from the *Assay preparation* and the *Standard preparation*, respectively.

Minoxidil Tablets

» Minoxidil Tablets contain not less than 90.0 percent and not more than 110.0 percent of the labeled amount of minoxidil ($C_9H_{15}N_5O$).

Packaging and storage—Preserve in tight containers.
USP Reference standards ⟨11⟩—*USP Minoxidil RS*.
Identification—Transfer a portion of finely powdered Tablets, equivalent to about 10 mg of minoxidil, to a separator. Add 25 mL of water, and extract with three 15-mL portions of chloroform. Combine the chloroform extracts, and evaporate with the aid of a stream of nitrogen. Wash the inside of the container with about 5 mL of alcohol, add 300 mg of potassium bromide, and evaporate under vacuum at 50° until dry: the IR absorption spectrum of a potassium bromide dispersion prepared from the residue so ob-

tained exhibits maxima at the same wavelengths as that of a similar preparation of USP Minoxidil RS.

Dissolution ⟨711⟩—
Medium: pH 7.2 phosphate buffer (see under *Buffer Solutions* in the section *Reagents, Indicators, and Solutions*); 900 mL.
Apparatus 1: 75 rpm.
Time: 15 minutes.
Procedure—Determine the amount of $C_9H_{15}N_5O$ dissolved from UV absorbances at the wavelength of maximum absorbance of filtered portions of the solution under test, suitably diluted with *Dissolution Medium*, if necessary, in comparison with a *Standard solution* having a known concentration of USP Minoxidil RS in the same medium. For Tablets containing up to 10 mg of minoxidil, measurement is made at about 231 nm; for Tablets containing more than 10 mg, the wavelength used is about 287 nm.
Tolerances—Not less than 75% (*Q*) of the labeled amount of $C_9H_{15}N_5O$ is dissolved in 15 minutes.

Uniformity of dosage units ⟨905⟩: meet the requirements.

Assay—
Mobile phase, Internal standard solution, Standard preparation, and *Chromatographic system*—Proceed as directed in the *Assay* under *Minoxidil*.
Assay preparation—Weigh and finely powder not less than 10 Tablets. To an accurately weighed portion of the powder, equivalent to about 5 mg of minoxidil, add 20.0 mL of *Internal standard solution*, shake for 5 minutes, and centrifuge.
Procedure—Proceed as directed for *Procedure* in the *Assay* under *Minoxidil*. Calculate the quantity, in mg, of minoxidil ($C_9H_{15}N_5O$) in the portion of Tablets taken by the formula:

$$20C(R_U / R_S)$$

in which the terms are as defined therein.

Mirtazapine

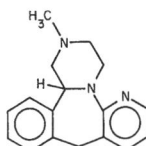

$C_{17}H_{19}N_3$ 265.35
Pyrazino[2,1-*a*]pyrido[2,3-*c*][2]benzazepine,1,2,3,4,10,14b-hexahydro-2-methyl-.
1,2,3,4,10,14b-Hexahydro-2-methylpyrazino[2,1-*a*]pyrido[2,3-*c*][2]-benzazepine   [85650-52-8].

» Mirtazapine contains not less than 98.0 percent and not more than 102.0 percent of $C_{17}H_{19}N_3$, calculated on the anhydrous basis.

Packaging and storage—Preserve in tight containers, and store at controlled room temperature.
Labeling—Label it to indicate whether it is anhydrous or hemihydrate.
USP Reference standards ⟨11⟩—*USP Mirtazapine RS*.
Identification—
  A: *Infrared Absorption* ⟨197K⟩.
  B: The retention time of the major peak in the chromatogram of the *Assay preparation* corresponds to that in the chromatogram of the *Standard preparation*, as obtained in the *Assay*.
Specific rotation ⟨781S⟩: between +2° and −2°.
  Test solution: 10 mg per mL, in denatured alcohol.
Water, *Method I* ⟨921⟩: not more than 1.0% for the anhydrous form and between 1.0% and 3.5% for the hemihydrate form.
Residue on ignition ⟨281⟩: not more than 0.1%.
Heavy metals, *Method II* ⟨231⟩: 0.001%
  Test preparation—Use a weighed quantity, approximately 4.0 g, of Mirtazapine.

Chromatographic purity—
Diluent, Buffer solution, and *Mobile phase*—Proceed as directed in the *Assay*.
Standard solution—Dissolve an accurately weighed quantity of USP Mirtazapine RS in *Diluent,* and dilute quantitatively, and stepwise if necessary, with *Diluent* to obtain a solution having a known concentration of about 15 µg per mL.
Test solution—Transfer about 150 mg of Mirtazapine, accurately weighed, to a 100-mL volumetric flask, dissolve in and dilute with *Diluent* to volume, and mix.
Chromatographic system (see *Chromatography* ⟨621⟩)—The liquid chromatograph is equipped with a 240-nm detector and a 4.6-mm × 25-cm column that contains packing L1. The flow rate is about 1.5 mL per minute. The column temperature is maintained at 40°. Chromatograph the *Standard solution,* and record the peak response as directed for *Procedure:* the tailing factor is not more than 2.0; and the relative standard deviation for replicate injections is not more than 10.0%.
Procedure—Separately inject equal volumes (about 10 µL) of the *Standard solution* and the *Test solution* into the chromatograph, record the chromatograms for about twice the retention time of Mirtazapine, and measure the responses for the major peaks. Calculate the percentage of each impurity in the portion of Mirtazapine taken by the formula:

$$10{,}000F(C/W)\,(r_i / r_S)$$

in which *F* is the relative response factor for the mirtazapine impurities and is equal to 0.24 for 4-methyl-1-(3-methyl-pyridin-2-yl)-2-phenyl-piperazine at a relative retention time of about 1.3, and 1.0 for any other impurity; *C* is the concentration, in mg per mL, of USP Mirtazapine RS in the *Standard solution;* *W* is the weight, in mg, of Mirtazapine taken to prepare the *Test solution;* r_i is the peak response of any impurity obtained from the *Test solution;* and r_S is the mirtazapine peak response obtained from the *Standard solution:* not more than 0.1% of any individual impurity is found, and not more than 0.5% of total impurities is found. [NOTE—Disregard any peak representing less than 0.05% of the main peak and any peak that is due to the *Diluent.*]

Organic volatile impurities, *Method IV* ⟨467⟩: meets the requirements.

(Official until July 1, 2008)

Assay—
Diluent: a mixture of acetonitrile and water (50 : 50).
Buffer solution—Transfer about 36.0 g of tetramethylammonium hydroxide pentahydrate to a 2000-mL volumetric flask, and dissolve in about 1950 mL of water. While stirring, adjust with phosphoric acid to a pH of 7.4, dilute with water to volume, and mix.
Mobile phase—Prepare a filtered and degassed mixture of *Buffer solution,* acetonitrile, methanol, and tetrahydrofuran (65 : 15 : 12.5 : 7.5). Make adjustments if necessary (see *System Suitability* under *Chromatography* ⟨621⟩).
Standard preparation—Dissolve an accurately weighed quantity of USP Mirtazapine RS in *Diluent,* and dilute quantitatively, and stepwise if necessary, with *Diluent* to obtain a solution having a known concentration of about 0.3 mg per mL.
Assay preparation—Transfer about 30 mg of Mirtazapine, accurately weighed, to a 100-mL volumetric flask, dissolve in and dilute with *Diluent* to volume, and mix.
Chromatographic system (see *Chromatography* ⟨621⟩)—The liquid chromatograph is equipped with a 290-nm detector and a 4.6-mm × 25-cm column that contains packing L1. The flow rate is about 1.5 mL per minute. The column temperature is maintained at 40°. Chromatograph the *Standard preparation,* and record the peak response as directed for *Procedure:* the column efficiency is not less than 7000 theoretical plates; the tailing factor is not more than 2.0; and the relative standard deviation for replicate injections is not more than 1.0%.
Procedure—Separately inject equal volumes (about 10 µL) of the *Standard preparation* and the *Assay preparation* into the chromatograph, record the chromatograms, and measure the responses for the

major peaks. Calculate the quantity, in mg, of $C_{17}H_{19}N_3$ in the portion of Mirtazapine taken by the formula:

$$100C(r_U/r_S)$$

in which C is the concentration, in mg per mL, of USP Mirtazapine RS in the *Standard preparation;* and r_U and r_S are the peak responses obtained from the *Assay preparation* and the *Standard preparation,* respectively.

Mirtazapine Tablets

» Mirtazapine Tablets contain not less than 90.0 percent and not more than 110.0 percent of the labeled amount of mirtazapine ($C_{17}H_{19}N_3$).

Packaging and storage—Preserve in tight, light-resistant containers, and store at controlled room temperature.

USP Reference standards ⟨11⟩—USP Mirtazapine RS.
Identification—
  A: *Infrared Absorption* ⟨197K⟩.
  Extraction mixture: a mixture of water and *n*-hexane (1 : 1).
  Test specimen—Transfer a quantity of finely powdered Tablets, equivalent to about 30 mg of mirtazapine, to a suitable centrifuge tube. Add *Extraction mixture* to obtain a solution of about 1 mg of mirtazapine per mL of *n*-hexane. Shake for 5 minutes, and centrifuge. Decant, and evaporate the supernatant.
  Standard specimen—Dissolve an accurately weighed quantity of USP Mirtazapine RS in *Extraction mixture* to obtain a solution having a concentration of about 1 mg of mirtazapine per mL of *n*-hexane. Shake for 5 minutes, and centrifuge. Decant, and evaporate the supernatant.
  B: The retention time of the major peak in the chromatogram of the *Assay preparation* corresponds to that in the chromatogram of the *Standard preparation,* as obtained in the *Assay.*
Dissolution ⟨711⟩—
  Medium: 0.1 N hydrochloric acid; 900 mL.
  Apparatus 2: 50 rpm.
  Time: 15 minutes.
  Procedure—Determine the amount of $C_{17}H_{19}N_3$ dissolved by employing UV absorption at the wavelength of maximum absorbance at about 315 nm on filtered portions of the solution under test, suitably diluted with *Medium,* in comparison with a Standard solution having a known concentration of USP Mirtazapine RS in the same *Medium.*
  Tolerances—Not less than 80% *(Q)* of the labeled amount of $C_{17}H_{19}N_3$ is dissolved in 15 minutes.
Uniformity of dosage units ⟨905⟩: meet the requirements for *Content Uniformity.*
Chromatographic purity—
  Diluent, Buffer solution, and *Mobile phase*—Proceed as directed in the *Assay* under *Mirtazapine.*
  Standard stock solution—Prepare as directed for *Standard preparation* in the *Assay* under *Mirtazapine.*
  Standard solution—Transfer 5.0 mL of the *Standard stock solution* to a 100-mL volumetric flask, dilute with *Diluent* to volume, and mix.
  Test solution—Weigh and finely powder not fewer than 20 Tablets. Transfer an accurately weighed portion of the powder, equivalent to the weight of 1 Tablet, to a suitable conical flask. Add *Diluent* to obtain a solution having a concentration of about 1.5 mg of mirtazapine per mL of *Diluent.* Shake vigorously for 10 minutes, centrifuge an aliquot, and use the clear supernatant.

  Chromatographic system (see *Chromatography* ⟨621⟩)—The liquid chromatograph is equipped with a 240-nm detector and a 4.6-mm × 25-cm column that contains packing L1. The flow rate is about 1.5 mL per minute. The column temperature is maintained at 40°. Chromatograph the *Standard solution,* and record the peak response as directed for *Procedure:* the column efficiency is not less than 7000 theoretical plates; the tailing factor is not more than 2.0; and the relative standard deviation for replicate injections is not more than 10.0%.
  Procedure—Separately inject equal volumes (about 10 µL) of the *Standard solution* and the *Test solution* into the chromatograph, record the chromatograms for about twice the retention time of mirtazapine, and measure the responses for the major peaks. Calculate the percentage of each impurity in the portion of Mirtazapine taken by the formula:

$$5(FV)(C/W)(W_{20}/L)(r_i/r_S)$$

in which F is the relative response factor for the mirtazapine impurities and is equal to 0.24 for 4-methyl-1-(3-methyl-pyridin-2-yl)-2-phenyl-piperazine at a relative retention time of about 1.3, and 1.0 for any other impurity; V is the total volume, in mL, of the *Test solution;* C is the concentration, in mg per mL, of USP Mirtazapine RS in the *Standard solution;* W is the weight, in mg, of the powdered Tablets taken to prepare the *Test solution;* W_{20} is the weight of the 20 Tablets taken; L is the labeled amount, in mg, of mirtazapine in each Tablet; r_i is the peak response of any impurity obtained from the *Test solution;* and r_S is the mirtazapine peak response obtained from the *Standard solution:* not more than 0.2% of any individual impurity is found, and not more than 2.0% of total impurities is found. [NOTE—Disregard any peak representing less than 0.05% of the main peak and any peak that is due to the *Diluent.*]

Assay—

  Diluent, Buffer solution, Mobile phase, and *Standard preparation*—Prepare as directed in the *Assay* under *Mirtazapine.*

  Assay preparation—Weigh and finely powder not fewer than 20 Tablets. Transfer an accurately weighed portion of the powder, equivalent to the weight of 1 Tablet, to a suitable conical flask. Add *Diluent* to obtain a solution having a concentration of about 0.3 mg of mirtazapine per mL of *Diluent.* Shake vigorously for 10 minutes, centrifuge an aliquot, and use the clear supernatant.

  Chromatographic system (see *Chromatography* ⟨621⟩)—The liquid chromatograph is equipped with a 290-nm detector and a 4.6-mm × 25-cm column that contains packing L1. The flow rate is about 1.5 mL per minute. The column temperature is maintained at 40°. Chromatograph the *Standard preparation,* and record the peak response as directed for *Procedure:* the column efficiency is not less than 7000 theoretical plates; the tailing factor is not more than 2.0; and the relative standard deviation for replicate injections is not more than 1.5%.

  Procedure—Separately inject equal volumes (about 10 µL) of the *Standard preparation* and the *Assay preparation* into the chromatograph, record the chromatograms, and measure the responses for the major peaks. Calculate the quantity, in mg, of mirtazapine ($C_{17}H_{19}N_3$) in the portion of Tablets taken by the formula:

$$VC(r_U/r_S)$$

in which V is the volume, in mL, of the *Assay preparation;* C is the concentration, in mg per mL, of USP Mirtazapine RS in the *Standard preparation;* and r_U and r_S are the peak responses obtained from the *Assay preparation* and the *Standard preparation,* respectively.

Mitomycin

$C_{15}H_{18}N_4O_5$ 334.33

Azirino[2′,3′: 3,4]pyrrolo[1,2-a]indole-4,7-dione,6-amino-8-[[(aminocarbonyl)oxy]methyl]-1,1a,2,8,8a,8b-hexahydro-8a-methoxy-5-methyl-, [1aR-(1aα,8β,8aα,8bα)]-.

6-Amino-1,1a,2,8,8a,8b-hexahydro-8-(hydroxymethyl)-8a-methoxy-5-methylazirino[2′,3′: 3,4]-pyrrolo[1,2-a]indole-4,7-dione carbamate (ester).

Mitomycin C   [50-07-7].

» Mitomycin has a potency of not less than 970 µg of $C_{15}H_{18}N_4O_5$ per mg.

Packaging and storage—Preserve in tight, light-resistant containers. Store at 25°, excursion permitted between 15° and 30°.

Labeling—Where it is intended for use in preparing injectable dosage forms, the label states that it is sterile or must be subjected to further processing during the preparation of injectable dosage forms.

USP Reference standards ⟨11⟩—*USP Mitomycin RS.*

Identification—
A: *Infrared Absorption* ⟨197M⟩—Do not dry specimens.
B: *Ultraviolet Absorption* ⟨197U⟩—
 Solution: 5 µg per mL.
 Medium: methanol.
 Absorptivity at 357 nm is not less than 95.0% and not more than 105.0% of USP Mitomycin RS, calculated on the anhydrous basis.

Crystallinity ⟨695⟩: meets the requirements.

pH ⟨791⟩: between 6.0 and 7.5, in an aqueous suspension containing 5 mg per mL.

Water, *Method I* ⟨921⟩: not more than 2.5%.

Other requirements—Where the label states that Mitomycin is sterile, it meets the requirements of the tests for *Sterility* and *Bacterial endotoxins* under *Mitomycin for Injection*. Where the label states that Mitomycin must be subjected to further processing during the preparation of injectable dosage forms, it meets the requirements of the test for *Bacterial endotoxins* under *Mitomycin for Injection*.

Assay—
 Mobile phase—Dissolve 1.54 g of ammonium acetate in 250 mL of methanol, add 5.0 mL of 0.83 N acetic acid and water to make 1000 mL, and mix. Pass through a filter having a 0.5-µm or finer porosity, and degas. Make adjustments if necessary (see *System Suitability* under *Chromatography* ⟨621⟩).
 Standard preparation—Quantitatively dissolve an accurately weighed quantity of USP Mitomycin RS in N,N-dimethylacetamide to obtain a solution having a known concentration of about 0.5 mg per mL.
 Resolution solution—Dissolve suitable quantities of USP Mitomycin RS and 3-ethoxy-4-hydroxybenzaldehyde in N,N-dimethylacetamide to obtain a solution containing about 0.5 mg and 7.5 mg per mL, respectively.
 Assay preparation—Transfer about 25 mg of Mitomycin, accurately weighed, to a 50-mL volumetric flask, add N,N-dimethylacetamide to volume, and mix to dissolve.
 Chromatographic system (see *Chromatography* ⟨621⟩)—The liquid chromatograph is equipped with a 365-nm detector and a 4-mm × 30-cm column that contains packing L11. The flow rate is about 2 mL per minute. Chromatograph the *Resolution solution*, and record the peak responses as directed under *Procedure:* the resolution, R, between the mitomycin and the 3-ethoxy-4-hydroxybenzaldehyde peaks is not less than 1.8. The relative retention times are about 1.0 for mitomycin and 1.4 for 3-ethoxy-4-hydroxybenzaldehyde. Chromatograph the *Standard preparation,* and record the peak responses as directed for *Procedure:* the tailing factor for the mitomycin peak is not more than 1.3; and the relative standard deviation for replicate injections is not more than 2.0%.
 Procedure—Separately inject equal volumes (about 10 µL) of the *Standard preparation* and the *Assay preparation* into the chromatograph, record the chromatograms, and measure the areas for the major peaks. Calculate the quantity, in µg, of $C_{15}H_{18}N_4O_5$ in each mg of the Mitomycin taken by the formula:

$$50(CP/W)(r_U / r_S)$$

in which C is the concentration, in mg per mL, of USP Mitomycin RS in the *Standard preparation;* P is the stated potency, in µg per mg, of the USP Mitomycin RS; W is the weight, in mg, of Mitomycin taken to prepare the *Assay preparation;* and r_U and r_S are the peak areas obtained from the *Assay preparation* and the *Standard preparation,* respectively.

Mitomycin for Injection

» Mitomycin for Injection contains not less than 90.0 percent and not more than 120.0 percent of the labeled amount of mitomycin ($C_{15}H_{18}N_4O_5$).

Packaging and storage—Preserve in *Containers for Sterile Solids* as described under *Injections* ⟨1⟩, protected from light. Store at 25°, excursion permitted between 15° and 30°.

USP Reference standards ⟨11⟩—*USP Endotoxin RS. USP Mitomycin RS.*

Constituted solution—At the time of use, it meets the requirements for *Constituted Solutions* under *Injections* ⟨1⟩.

Identification—Dissolve a quantity in water, and dilute with water to obtain a solution having a concentration of about 1 mg of mitomycin per mL. Apply 2 µL of this solution and 2 µL of a Standard solution of USP Mitomycin RS, similarly prepared to a suitable thin-layer chromatographic plate (see *Chromatography* ⟨621⟩) coated with a 0.25-mm layer of chromatographic silica gel mixture. Allow the spots to dry, and develop the chromatograms in a solvent system consisting of a mixture of butyl alcohol, glacial acetic acid, and water (4 : 2 : 1). Remove the plate from the developing chamber, mark the solvent front, and allow the solvent to evaporate. Spray the plate with a 1 in 100 solution of ninhydrin in alcohol. Heat the plate in an oven at 110° for 15 minutes. Mitomycin appears as a pink spot: the R_F value of the principal spot obtained from the solution under test corresponds to that obtained from the Standard solution.

Bacterial endotoxins ⟨85⟩—It contains not more than 10.0 USP Endotoxin Units per mg of mitomycin.

Sterility ⟨71⟩—It meets the requirements when tested as directed for *Membrane Filtration* under *Test for Sterility of the Product to be Examined.*

pH ⟨791⟩: in the solution constituted as directed in the labeling, between 6.0 and 8.0 where it contains mannitol and between 5.5 and 8.5 where it contains hydroxypropyl betadex.

Water, *Method Ia* ⟨921⟩: not more than 5.0%, the *Test preparation* being prepared as directed for a hygroscopic specimen, using the pooled contents of 5 containers.

Other requirements—It meets the requirements under *Injections* ⟨1⟩ and *Uniformity of Dosage Units* ⟨905⟩.

Assay—
 Mobile phase, Standard preparation, Resolution solution, and *Chromatographic system*—Prepare as directed in the *Assay* under *Mitomycin.*
 Assay preparation—Add an accurately measured volume of N,N-dimethylacetamide to 1 container of Mitomycin for Injection to obtain a solution having a concentration of about 0.5 mg of mitomycin per mL.
 Procedure—Separately inject equal volumes (about 10 µL) of the *Standard preparation* and the *Assay preparation* into the chromatograph, record the chromatograms, and measure the areas for the ma-

jor peaks. Calculate the quantity, in mg, of mitomycin ($C_{15}H_{18}N_4O_5$) in the container of Mitomycin for Injection taken by the formula:

$$(CP/1000)(L/D)(r_U/r_S)$$

in which C is the concentration, in mg per mL, of USP Mitomycin RS in the *Standard preparation*; P is the stated potency, in μg per mg, of USP Mitomycin RS; L is the labeled quantity, in mg, of mitomycin in the container; D is the concentration, in mg per mL, of mitomycin in the *Assay preparation*, on the basis of the labeled quantity and the extent of dilution; and r_U and r_S are the peak areas obtained from the *Assay preparation* and the *Standard preparation*, respectively.

Mitotane

$C_{14}H_{10}Cl_4$ 320.04
Benzene, 1-chloro-2-[2,2-dichloro-1-(4-chlorophenyl)ethyl]-, (±)-.
(±)-1,1-Dichloro-2-(*o*-chlorophenyl)-2-(*p*-chlorophenyl)ethane
[53-19-0].

» Mitotane contains not less than 97.0 percent and not more than 103.0 percent of $C_{14}H_{10}Cl_4$, calculated on the dried basis.

Caution—Handle Mitotane with exceptional care, since it is a highly potent agent.

Packaging and storage—Preserve in tight, light-resistant containers.

USP Reference standards ⟨11⟩—*USP Mitotane RS.*
Identification—
 A: *Infrared Absorption* ⟨197M⟩.
 B: *Ultraviolet Absorption* ⟨197U⟩—
  Solution: 200 μg per mL.
  Medium: methanol.
Melting range ⟨741⟩: between 75° and 81°.
Loss on drying ⟨731⟩—Dry it in vacuum at 60° for 2 hours: it loses not more than 0.5% of its weight.
Residue on ignition ⟨281⟩: not more than 0.5%.
Organic volatile impurities, *Method V* ⟨467⟩: meets the requirements.
 Solvent—Use dimethyl sulfoxide.

(Official until July 1, 2008)

Assay—Dissolve about 0.1 g of Mitotane, accurately weighed, in methanol, and dilute quantitatively and stepwise with methanol to obtain a solution having a concentration of about 200 μg per mL. Similarly prepare a solution in methanol of USP Mitotane RS, diluted quantitatively and stepwise with methanol to yield a Standard solution having a known concentration of about 200 μg per mL. Concomitantly determine the absorbances of both solutions in 1-cm cells at the wavelength of maximum absorbance at about 268 nm, with a suitable spectrophotometer, using methanol as the blank. Calculate the quantity, in mg, of $C_{14}H_{10}Cl_4$ in the portion of Mitotane taken by the formula:

$$0.5C(A_U/A_S)$$

in which C is the concentration, in μg per mL, of USP Mitotane RS in the Standard solution, and A_U and A_S are the absorbances of the solution of Mitotane and the Standard solution, respectively.

Mitotane Tablets

» Mitotane Tablets contain not less than 90.0 percent and not more than 110.0 percent of the labeled amount of mitotane ($C_{14}H_{10}Cl_4$).

Packaging and storage—Preserve in tight, light-resistant containers.

USP Reference standards ⟨11⟩—*USP Mitotane RS.*
Identification—Triturate a quantity of finely powdered Tablets, equivalent to about 500 mg of mitotane, with 10 mL of water, filter on a sintered-glass filter funnel, and wash the residue with two 5-mL portions of water. Transfer the residue to a small beaker, add 4 mL of alcohol, heat to boiling, and filter immediately. Allow the filtrate to cool, filter the crystals of mitotane, wash once with 2 mL of alcohol, and dry in vacuum at 60° for 2 hours: the IR absorption spectrum of a mineral oil dispersion of the mitotane so obtained exhibits maxima only at the same wavelengths as that of a similar preparation of USP Mitotane RS.
Disintegration ⟨701⟩: 15 minutes, the use of disks being omitted.
Uniformity of dosage units ⟨905⟩: meet the requirements.
Assay—
 Standard preparation—Dissolve about 50 mg of USP Mitotane RS, accurately weighed, in methanol, and dilute quantitatively and stepwise with methanol to obtain a solution having a known concentration of about 200 μg per mL.
 Assay preparation—Weigh and finely powder not less than 10 Tablets. Transfer an accurately weighed portion of the powder, equivalent to about 100 mg of mitotane, to a 250-mL volumetric flask, add 100 mL of methanol, and shake occasionally for 5 minutes, then dilute with methanol to volume, and mix. Filter, rejecting the first portion of the filtrate, transfer 25.0 mL of the filtrate to a 50-mL volumetric flask, dilute with methanol to volume, and mix.
 Procedure—Proceed as directed in the *Assay* under *Mitotane*, beginning with "Concomitantly determine the absorbances of both solutions."

Mitoxantrone Hydrochloride

$C_{22}H_{28}N_4O_6 \cdot 2HCl$ 517.40
9,10-Anthracenedione, 1,4-dihydroxy-5,8-bis[[2-[(2-hydroxyethyl)amino]ethyl]amino]-, dihydrochloride.
1,4-Dihydroxy-5,8-bis[[2-[(2-hydroxyethyl)amino]ethyl]amino]anthraquinone dihydrochloride. [70476-82-3].

» Mitoxantrone Hydrochloride contains not less than 97.0 percent and not more than 102.0 percent of $C_{22}H_{28}N_4O_6 \cdot 2HCl$, calculated on the anhydrous basis.

Packaging and storage—Preserve in tight containers.
USP Reference standards ⟨11⟩—*USP Mitoxantrone Hydrochloride RS. USP Mitoxantrone System Suitability Mixture RS.*
Identification, *Infrared Absorption* ⟨197K⟩.
Water, *Method I* ⟨921⟩: not more than 6.0%.
Alcohol—
 Standard solution—Transfer 5.0 mL of dehydrated alcohol to a 250-mL volumetric flask, dilute with water to volume, and mix. Transfer 5.0 mL of this solution to a 500-mL volumetric flask, dilute with water to volume, and mix.
 Internal standard solution—Transfer 5.0 mL of *n*-propyl alcohol to a 250-mL volumetric flask, dilute with water to volume, and mix.

Transfer 5.0 mL of this solution to a 500-mL volumetric flask, dilute with water to volume, and mix.

Standard preparation—Transfer 10.0 mL of the *Standard solution* to a 25-mL volumetric flask, add 10.0 mL of the *Internal standard solution,* dilute with water to volume, and mix. This solution contains 0.063 mg of alcohol (C_2H_5OH) per mL.

Test preparation—Transfer about 100 mg of Mitoxantrone Hydrochloride, accurately weighed, to a 5-mL volumetric flask, add 2.0 mL of the *Internal standard solution,* dilute with water to volume, and mix. Sonicate for 2 minutes and shake for 2 minutes, repeating these actions until the specimen is completely dissolved.

Chromatographic system (see *Chromatography* ⟨621⟩)—The gas chromatograph is equipped with a flame-ionization detector and a 2-mm × 3-m column that contains 20% phase G1 and 0.1% phase G39 on silanized support S1A. Maintain the column at 50° for 5 minutes, then increase the temperature at a rate of 30° per minute. When 140° is reached, maintain that temperature for 20 minutes. Maintain the injection port at 200° and the detection block at 250°. Use helium as the carrier gas at a flow rate of about 15 mL per minute. Make adjustments if necessary (see *System Suitability* under *Chromatography* ⟨621⟩). Chromatograph the *Standard preparation,* and record the peak responses as directed for *Procedure:* the relative retention times are about 0.5 for alcohol and 1.0 for n-propyl alcohol, the resolution, *R,* between the alcohol and the n-propyl alcohol peaks is not less than 6.0, and the tailing factors for the two peaks are not more than 2.0.

Procedure—[NOTE—Use peak areas where peak responses are indicated.] Separately inject equal volumes (about 1 μL) of the *Standard preparation* and the *Test preparation* into the chromatograph, record the chromatograms, and measure the responses for the major peaks. Calculate the percentage of alcohol (C_2H_5OH) in the portion of Mitoxantrone Hydrochloride taken by the formula:

$$500(C/W)(R_U/R_S)$$

in which *C* is the concentration, in mg per mL, of alcohol (C_2H_5OH) in the *Standard preparation;* *W* is the weight, in mg, of Mitoxantrone Hydrochloride taken; and R_U and R_S are the ratios of the response of the alcohol peak to that of the n-propyl alcohol peak obtained from the *Test preparation* and the *Standard preparation,* respectively: not more than 1.5% is found.

Heavy metals ⟨231⟩—Proceed as directed under *Method II,* except in the *Procedure* to filter the final solutions through a suitable acid-resistant membrane filter of 0.22 μm or finer porosity, instead of viewing them over a dark surface: the precipitate on the filter obtained from the *Test Preparation* is not darker than that obtained from the *Standard Preparation.* The limit is 0.002%.

Chromatographic purity—Using the chromatogram of the *Assay preparation* obtained as directed in the *Assay,* calculate the percentage of each impurity in the Mitoxantrone Hydrochloride taken by the formula:

$$100(r_i/r_s)$$

in which r_i is the response of any individual peak, other than the main mitoxantrone peak, and r_s is the sum of the responses of all the peaks in the chromatogram, including that of the main mitoxantrone peak: not more than 1.0% of any individual impurity and not more than 2.0% of total impurities is found.

Assay—

Sodium 1-heptanesulfonate solution—Dissolve 22.0 g of sodium 1-heptanesulfonate in about 150 mL of water, pass through a suitable filter having a 0.5-μm or finer porosity, and transfer the filtrate to a 250-mL volumetric flask. Wash the filter with about 50 mL of water, adding the filtrate to the 250-mL volumetric flask. Add 32.0 mL of glacial acetic acid to the volumetric flask, dilute with water to volume, and mix.

Mobile phase—Prepare a suitable degassed mixture of water, acetonitrile, and *Sodium 1-heptanesulfonate solution* (750 : 250 : 25). Make adjustments if necessary (see *System Suitability* under *Chromatography* ⟨621⟩).

System suitability solution—Prepare a solution of USP Mitoxantrone System Suitability Mixture RS in a suitable volume of *Mobile phase* to obtain a solution containing about 0.2 mg of 8-amino-1,4-dihydroxy-5[[2-[(2-hydroxyethyl)amino]ethyl]amino]-9,10-anthracenedione hydrochloride (mitoxantrone related compound A) and 0.1 mg of mitoxantrone hydrochloride per mL.

Standard preparation—Transfer about 20 mg of USP Mitoxantrone Hydrochloride RS, accurately weighed, to a 50-mL volumetric flask, add 40 mL of *Mobile phase,* and dissolve by sonicating for about 5 minutes. Cool to room temperature, dilute with *Mobile phase* to volume, and mix.

Assay preparation—Transfer about 20 mg of Mitoxantrone Hydrochloride, accurately weighed, to a 50-mL volumetric flask, add 40 mL of *Mobile phase,* and dissolve by sonicating for about 5 minutes. Cool to room temperature, dilute with *Mobile phase* to volume, and mix.

Chromatographic system (see *Chromatography* ⟨621⟩)—The liquid chromatograph is equipped with a 254-nm detector and a 3.9-mm × 30-cm column that contains packing L11. The flow rate is about 3 mL per minute. Chromatograph the *System suitability solution,* and record the peak responses as directed for *Procedure:* the relative retention times are about 0.7 for mitoxantrone and 1.0 for mitoxantrone related compound A; the resolution, *R,* between mitoxantrone and mitoxantrone related compound A is not less than 3.0; and the tailing factor for the mitoxantrone peak is not more than 2.0. Chromatograph the *Standard preparation,* and record the peak responses as directed for *Procedure:* the capacity factor, *k′,* for mitoxantrone is not less than 3.5; and the relative standard deviation for replicate injections is not more than 2.0%.

Procedure—Separately inject equal volumes (about 50 μL) of the *Standard preparation* and the *Assay preparation* into the chromatograph, record the chromatograms, and measure the areas for the major peaks. [NOTE—After use, wash the column with a mixture of acetonitrile and water (50 : 50), and store in this mixture.] Calculate the quantity, in mg, of $C_{22}H_{28}N_4O_6 \cdot 2HCl$ in the portion of Mitoxantrone Hydrochloride taken by the formula:

$$50C(r_U/r_S)$$

in which *C* is the concentration, in mg per mL, of anhydrous mitoxantrone hydrochloride in the *Standard preparation,* as determined from the content of USP Mitoxantrone Hydrochloride RS corrected for the water content determined by a titrimetric water determination; and r_U and r_S are the mitoxantrone peak areas obtained from the *Assay preparation* and the *Standard preparation,* respectively.

Mitoxantrone Injection

» Mitoxantrone Injection is a sterile solution of Mitoxantrone Hydrochloride in Water for Injection. It contains the equivalent of not less than 90.0 percent and not more than 105.0 percent of the labeled amount of mitoxantrone ($C_{22}H_{28}N_4O_6$).

Packaging and storage—Preserve in single-dose or multiple-dose containers, preferably of Type I glass.

Labeling—Label Injection to state both the content of the active moiety and the name of the salt used in formulating the article. Label Mitoxantrone Injection to indicate that it is to be diluted to appropriate strength with water or other suitable fluid prior to administration.

USP Reference standards ⟨11⟩—*USP Mitoxantrone Hydrochloride RS. USP Mitoxantrone System Suitability Mixture RS.*

Identification—Transfer a volume of Injection, equivalent to about 2 mg of mitoxantrone, to a 200-mL volumetric flask, add 100 mL of water and 20 mL of 1 N hydrochloric acid, dilute with water to volume, and mix: the UV absorption spectrum of this solution exhibits maxima and minima at the same wavelengths as that of a similar solution of USP Mitoxantrone Hydrochloride RS.

Bacterial endotoxins ⟨85⟩—It contains not more than 5 Endotoxin Units per mg of mitoxantrone.

Sterility ⟨71⟩—It meets the requirements when tested as directed for *Membrane Filtration* under *Test for Sterility of the Product to be Examined,* the entire contents of each container being used.

Chromatographic purity—Using the chromatogram of the *Assay preparation* obtained as directed in the *Assay*, calculate the percentage of each impurity in the Injection taken by the formula:

$$100(r_i / r_S)$$

in which r_i is the response of any individual peak, other than the main mitoxantrone peak; and r_S is the sum of the responses of all the peaks in the chromatogram, including that of the main mitoxantrone peak: not more than 1.5% of any individual impurity and not more than 3.0% of the total impurities is found.

Other requirements—It meets the requirements under *Injections* ⟨1⟩.

Assay—

Sodium 1-heptanesulfonate solution, Mobile phase, System suitability solution, and *Chromatographic system*—Proceed as directed in the *Assay* under *Mitoxantrone Hydrochloride*.

Standard preparation—Transfer about 23 mg of USP Mitoxantrone Hydrochloride RS, accurately weighed, to a 50-mL volumetric flask, add 40 mL of *Mobile phase*, and dissolve by sonicating for about 5 minutes. Cool to room temperature, dilute with *Mobile phase* to volume, and mix. This solution contains the equivalent of about 0.4 mg of mitoxantrone ($C_{22}H_{28}N_4O_6$) per mL.

Assay preparation—Transfer an accurately measured volume of Injection, equivalent to about 4 mg of mitoxantrone ($C_{22}H_{28}N_4O_6$), to a 10-mL volumetric flask, dilute with *Mobile phase* to volume, and mix.

Procedure—Proceed as directed for *Procedure* in the *Assay* under *Mitoxantrone Hydrochloride*. Calculate the quantity, in mg, of mitoxantrone ($C_{22}H_{28}N_4O_6$) in each mL of the Injection taken by the formula:

$$(444.49 / 517.40)(10C / V)(r_U / r_S)$$

in which 444.49 and 517.40 are the molecular weights of mitoxantrone and mitoxantrone hydrochloride, respectively; V is the volume, in mL, of the portion of Injection taken; and the other terms are as defined therein.

Modafinil

$C_{15}H_{15}NO_2S$ 273.35
Acetamide, 2-[(diphenylmethyl)sulfinyl]-.
2-[(Diphenylmethyl)sulfinyl]-acetamide   [68693-11-8].

» Modafinil contains not less than 98.0 percent and not more than 101.5 percent of $C_{15}H_{15}NO_2S$, calculated on the anhydrous basis.

Packaging and storage—Preserve in well-closed containers. Store at controlled room temperature.

USP Reference standards ⟨11⟩—*USP Modafinil RS. USP Salicylic Acid RS.*

Identification—*Infrared Absorption* ⟨197K⟩.

Water, *Method I* ⟨921⟩: not more than 0.2%.

Residue on ignition ⟨281⟩: not more than 0.1%.

Heavy metals, *Method I* ⟨231⟩—Dissolve the sample in methanol and water solution (60 : 40): not more than 0.002%.

Related compounds—

Buffer, Mobile phase, and *System suitability preparation*—Prepare as directed in the *Assay*.

Test solution—Use the *Assay preparation*.

Chromatographic system (see *Chromatography* ⟨621⟩)—Proceed as directed under *Assay*. Chromatograph the *System suitability preparation,* and record the peak responses as directed for *Procedure:* the relative retention times are listed in the table below; the resolution, *R*, between salicylic acid and modafinil is not less than 1.3; the tailing factor is not more than 1.5; and the relative standard deviation for replicate injections is not more than 2.0% based on the modafinil peak.

Impurity	Relative Retention Time (relative to modafinil)
Salicylic acid*	1.1
Modafinil acid [2-[(diphenylmethyl)sulfinyl] acetic acid]	1.4
Modafinil sulfone [2-[(diphenylmethyl)sulfonyl]acetamide]	1.7
Modafinil ester [2-[(diphenylmethyl)sulfinyl] acetic acid methyl ester]	3.0

*Salicylic acid is used for calculating resolution and is not a potential impurity.

Procedure—Inject a volume (about 20 μL) of the *Test solution* into the chromatograph, record the chromatogram, and measure the peak responses. Calculate the percentage of each related compound in the portion of Modafinil taken by the formula:

$$100(1/F)(r_i / r_s)$$

in which F is the relative response factor for an impurity (F is 0.90 for modafinil sulfone; F is 1 for all other known and unknown impurities); r_i is the individual peak response of each impurity; and r_s is the sum of the responses of all the peaks: not more than 0.5% of any individual known impurity is found, not more than 0.05% of any individual unknown impurity is found, and not more than 1.0% of total impurities is found.

Assay—

Buffer—Dissolve 6.8 g of potassium dihydrogen phosphate in 500 mL of water in a 1000-mL flask. Dilute with water to volume, and mix. Adjust with phosphoric acid to a pH of 2.3.

Mobile phase—Prepare a filtered and degassed mixture of *Buffer* and acetonitrile (65 : 35). Make adjustments if necessary (see *System Suitability* under *Chromatography* ⟨621⟩).

Diluent—Prepare a mixture containing water and acetonitrile (65 : 35), and mix.

System suitability preparation—Dissolve suitable quantities of USP Modafinil RS and USP Salicylic Acid RS in *Diluent* to obtain a solution containing about 0.005 mg per mL and 0.05 mg per mL, respectively.

Standard preparation—Dissolve an accurately weighed quantity of USP Modafinil RS in *Diluent*, and dilute quantitatively, and stepwise if necessary, with *Diluent* to obtain a solution having a known concentration of about 0.1 mg per mL.

Assay preparation—Transfer about 100 mg of Modafinil, accurately weighed, to a 100-mL volumetric flask, dissolve in and dilute with *Diluent* to volume, and mix. Dilute 5.0 mL of this solution with *Diluent* to 50 mL, and mix well.

Chromatographic system (see *Chromatography* ⟨621⟩)—The liquid chromatograph is equipped with a 220-nm detector and a 4.6-mm × 15-cm column that contains 5-μm packing L1. The flow rate is about 1.0 mL per minute. The column temperature is maintained at 40°. Chromatograph the *System suitability preparation,* and record the peak responses as directed for *Procedure:* the relative retention times are about 1.1 for salicylic acid and 1.0 for modafinil; the resolution, *R*, between modafinil and salicylic acid is not less than 1.3; the tailing factor of the modafinil peak is not more than 1.5; and the relative standard deviation for replicate injections is not more than 2.0% based on the modafinil peak.

Procedure—Separately inject equal volumes (about 20 μL) of the *Standard preparation* and the *Assay preparation* into the chromatograph, record the chromatograms, and measure the responses for the modafinil peaks. Calculate the quantity, in mg, of $C_{15}H_{15}NO_2S$ in the portion of Modafinil taken by the formula:

$$1000C(r_U / r_S)$$

in which 1000 is the dilution factor for the *Assay preparation;* C is the concentration, in mg per mL, of USP Modafinil RS in the *Standard preparation;* and r_U and r_S are the peak responses obtained from the *Assay preparation* and the *Standard preparation*, respectively.

Modafinil Tablets

» Modafinil Tablets contain not less than 90.0 percent and not more than 110.0 percent of the labeled amount of modafinil ($C_{15}H_{15}NO_2S$).

Packaging and storage—Preserve in tight containers. Store at controlled room temperature.

USP Reference standards ⟨11⟩—*USP Modafinil RS. USP Salicylic Acid RS.*

Identification, *Infrared Absorption* ⟨197K⟩—Grind 1 Tablet and add 50 mL each of dichloromethane and water. Shake the mixture and allow the layers to separate. Filter a portion of the lower (dichloromethane) layer and evaporate to dryness, using a stream of nitrogen if necessary. Prepare a potassium bromide pellet of the residue. To prepare the Reference Standard potassium bromide dispersion, transfer a quantity (in mg) of USP Modafinil RS, equivalent to the labeled amount of modafinil, to a suitable container, and proceed as directed above beginning with "add 50 mL each of dichloromethane and water."

Dissolution ⟨711⟩—
Medium: 0.1 N hydrochloric acid; 900 mL.
Apparatus 2: 50 rpm.
Time: 30 minutes.
Procedure—Determine the amount of $C_{15}H_{15}NO_2S$ dissolved by employing UV absorption at the wavelength of maximum absorbance at about 222 nm on filtered portions of the solution under test, suitably diluted with *Medium* if necessary, in comparison with a Standard solution having a known concentration of USP Modafinil RS in the same *Medium*.
Tolerances—Not less than 75% (*Q*) of the labeled amount of $C_{15}H_{15}NO_2S$ is dissolved in 30 minutes.

Uniformity of dosage units ⟨905⟩: meet the requirements.

Related compounds—
Buffer, Mobile phase, and *System suitability preparation*—Prepare as directed in the *Assay* under *Modafinil*. Make adjustments if necessary (see *System Suitability* under *Chromatography* ⟨621⟩).
Diluent—Prepare as directed in the *Assay*.
Test solution—Use the *Assay preparation*.
Chromatographic system (see *Chromatography* ⟨621⟩)—Proceed as directed in the *Assay*. Chromatograph the *System suitability preparation*, and record the peak responses as directed for *Procedure*: the relative retention times are presented in the table below; the resolution, *R*, between modafinil and salicylic acid is not less than 1.3; and the relative standard deviation for replicate injections is not more than 2.0% based on the modafinil peak.

Impurity	Relative Retention Time (relative to modafinil)
Salicylic acid*	1.1
Modafinil acid [2-[(diphenylmethyl)sulfinyl] acetic acid]	1.4
Modafinil sulfone [2-[(diphenylmethyl)sulfonyl]acetamide]	1.7

*Salicylic acid is used for calculating resolution and is not a potential impurity.

Procedure—Inject a volume (about 5 µL) of the *Test solution* into the chromatograph, record the chromatogram, and measure all of the peak responses. Calculate the percentage of each impurity in the portion of Tablets taken by the formula:

$$100(1/F)(r_i / r_s)$$

in which *F* is the relative response factor for an impurity (*F* is 0.90 for modafinil sulfone; *F* is 1 for all other known and unknown impurities); r_i is the peak response for each impurity; and r_s is the sum of the responses of all the peaks: not more than 0.5% of any individual impurity is found, not more than 0.1% of any individual unknown impurity is found, and not more than 1.5% of total impurities is found.

Assay—
Buffer, Mobile phase, and *System suitability preparation*—Prepare as directed in the *Assay* under *Modafinil*.
Diluent—Prepare a mixture containing water, acetonitrile, and acetic acid (65 : 35 : 1), and mix.
Standard preparation—Dissolve an accurately weighed quantity of USP Modafinil RS in *Diluent*, and dilute quantitatively, and stepwise if necessary, with *Diluent* to obtain a solution having a known concentration of about 0.4 mg per mL.
Assay preparation—Weigh and finely powder not fewer than 20 Tablets. Transfer an accurately weighed portion of the powder, equivalent to about 100 mg of modafinil, to a 250-mL volumetric flask, add 200 mL of *Diluent*, and sonicate for about 5 minutes with intermittent manual shaking. Dilute with *Diluent* to volume, and mix. Pass a portion of this solution through a filter having a 0.45-µm or finer porosity, and use the filtrate.
Chromatographic system (see *Chromatography* ⟨621⟩)—The liquid chromatograph is equipped with a 220-nm detector and 4.6-mm × 15-cm column that contains 5-µm packing L1. The flow rate is about 1.0 mL per minute. The column temperature is maintained at 40°. Chromatograph the *System suitability preparation*, and record the peak responses as directed for *Procedure*: the relative retention times are about 1.1 for salicylic acid and 1.0 for modafinil; the resolution, *R*, between modafinil and salicylic acid is not less than 1.3; the tailing factor is not more than 1.5; and the relative standard deviation for replicate injections is not more than 2.0% based on the modafinil peak.
Procedure—Separately inject equal volumes (about 5 µL) of the *Standard preparation* and the *Assay preparation* into the chromatograph, record the chromatograms, and measure the responses for the modafinil peaks. Calculate the quantity, in mg, of modafinil ($C_{15}H_{15}NO_2S$) in the portion of Tablets taken by the formula:

$$250C(r_U / r_S)$$

in which *C* is the concentration, in mg per mL, of USP Modafinil RS in the *Standard preparation*; and r_U and r_S are the peak responses obtained from the *Assay preparation* and the *Standard preparation*, respectively.

Molindone Hydrochloride

$C_{16}H_{24}N_2O_2 \cdot HCl$ 312.83

4*H*-Indol-4-one, 3-ethyl-1,5,6,7-tetrahydro-2-methyl-5-(4-morpholinylmethyl)-, monohydrochloride.
3-Ethyl-6,7-dihydro-2-methyl-5-(morpholinomethyl)indol-4(5*H*)-one monohydrochloride [15622-65-8].

» Molindone Hydrochloride contains not less than 98.0 percent and not more than 101.5 percent of $C_{16}H_{24}N_2O_2 \cdot HCl$, calculated on the anhydrous basis.

Packaging and storage—Preserve in tight, light-resistant containers.

USP Reference standards ⟨11⟩—*USP Molindone Hydrochloride RS.*

Identification—
A: *Infrared Absorption* ⟨197K⟩. Do not dry specimens.
B: Prepare a solution in methanol containing 10 mg of molindone hydrochloride per mL. Separately apply 1 µL of this solution and 1 µL of a Standard solution containing 10 mg per mL of USP Molindone Hydrochloride RS in methanol to a thin-layer chromatographic plate (see *Chromatography* ⟨621⟩) coated with a 0.25-mm

layer of chromatographic silica gel mixture, and allow the spots to dry. Protect the chromatogram from light, and develop in a solvent system consisting of a mixture of alcohol, methanol, and 1 N hydrochloric acid (90 : 5 : 5) until the solvent front has moved about three-fourths of the length of the plate. Remove the plate from the developing chamber, mark the solvent front, and allow the solvent to evaporate. Spray the plate with a freshly prepared solution containing 100 mg of potassium ferricyanide dissolved in 20 mL of 10% ferric chloride solution: the principal spot obtained from the test solution corresponds in R_F value and intensity to that obtained from the Standard solution.

C: It responds to the tests for *Chloride* ⟨191⟩.

pH ⟨791⟩: between 4.0 and 5.0, in a solution (1 in 100).

Water, *Method I* ⟨921⟩: not more than 0.5%.

Residue on ignition ⟨281⟩: not more than 0.25%.

Heavy metals, *Method II* ⟨231⟩: not more than 0.003%.

Chromatographic purity—

Mobile phase—Dissolve 1.1 g of sodium octanesulfonate in 600 mL of water, add 400 mL of methanol, 1 mL of glacial acetic acid, and 0.5 mL of triethylamine. Mix, filter through a filter having a porosity of 0.45 µm or less, and degas. Make adjustments if necessary (see *System Suitability* under *Chromatography* ⟨621⟩).

Solvent mixture—Proceed as directed in the *Assay.*

Standard solution—Prepare a solution of USP Molindone Hydrochloride RS in *Solvent mixture* having a known concentration of about 0.01 mg per mL.

Test solution—Transfer about 100 mg of Molindone Hydrochloride, accurately weighed, to a 50-mL volumetric flask, dissolve in and dilute with *Solvent mixture* to volume.

Chromatographic system (see *Chromatography* ⟨621⟩)—The liquid chromatograph is equipped with a 254-nm detector and a 4.6-mm × 25-cm column that contains packing L11. The column temperature is maintained at 35°. The flow rate is about 1.5 mL per minute. Chromatograph the *Standard solution*, and record the peak responses as directed under *Procedure:* the relative standard deviation for replicate injections is not more than 5.0%.

Procedure—Separately inject equal volumes (about 20 µL) of the *Standard solution* and the *Test solution* into the chromatograph, record the chromatograms, and measure the responses of all peaks: no peak from the *Test solution*, other than the molindone peak, is greater than the molindone peak from the *Standard preparation* (0.5%), and the sum of all the impurity peaks is not greater than 2.0%.

Assay—

Mobile phase—Dissolve 1.1 g of sodium octanesulfonate in 480 mL of water, add 520 mL of methanol, 2 mL of glacial acetic acid, and 0.4 mL of triethylamine. Mix, filter through a 0.45-µm filter, and degas. Make adjustments if necessary (see *System Suitability* under *Chromatography* ⟨621⟩).

Solvent mixture—Prepare a mixture of 0.01 N hydrochloric acid and methanol (60 : 40).

Internal standard solution—Dissolve 200 mg of butylparaben in 40 mL of methanol in a 100-mL volumetric flask, dilute with water to volume, and mix.

Standard preparation—Transfer about 25 mg of USP Molindone Hydrochloride RS, accurately weighed, to a 50-mL volumetric flask, add 5.0 mL of *Internal standard solution*, dilute with *Solvent mixture* to volume, and mix.

Assay preparation—Transfer about 50 mg of Molindone Hydrochloride, accurately weighed, to a 100-mL volumetric flask. Add 10.0 mL of *Internal standard solution*, dilute with *Solvent mixture* to volume, and mix.

Chromatographic system (see *Chromatography* ⟨621⟩)—The liquid chromatograph is equipped with a 254-nm detector and a 4.6-mm × 25-cm column that contains packing L11. The column temperature is maintained at 35°. The flow rate is 1.5 mL per minute. Chromatograph the *Standard preparation*, and record the peak responses as directed under *Procedure:* the resolution, *R*, between the molindone and butylparaben peaks is not less than 2, and the relative standard deviation for replicate injections is not more than 2.0%.

Procedure—Separately inject equal volumes (about 10 µL) of the *Standard preparation* and the *Assay preparation* into the chromatograph, record the chromatograms, and measure the responses for the major peaks. The relative retention times are about 0.7 for molindone and 1.0 for butylparaben. Calculate the quantity, in mg, of $C_{16}H_{24}N_2O_2 \cdot HCl$ in the portion of Molindone Hydrochloride taken by the formula:

$$100C(R_U/R_S)$$

in which *C* is the concentration, in mg per mL, of USP Molindone Hydrochloride RS in the *Standard preparation*, and R_U and R_S are the ratios of the peak response of molindone to that of butylparaben obtained from the *Assay preparation* and the *Standard preparation*, respectively.

Molindone Hydrochloride Tablets

» Molindone Hydrochloride Tablets contain not less than 90.0 percent and not more than 110.0 percent of the labeled amount of molindone hydrochloride ($C_{16}H_{24}N_2O_2 \cdot HCl$).

Packaging and storage—Preserve in tight, light-resistant containers.

USP Reference standards ⟨11⟩—*USP Molindone Hydrochloride RS.*

Identification—Dissolve a portion of finely powdered Tablets in methanol to obtain a test solution containing about 2.5 mg of molindone hydrochloride per mL. Separately apply 5 µL of the test solution and 5 µL of a Standard solution of USP Molindone Hydrochloride RS in methanol containing 2.5 mg per mL to a thin-layer chromatographic plate (see *Chromatography* ⟨621⟩) coated with a 0.25-mm layer of chromatographic silica gel mixture. Allow the spots to dry, protect the chromatogram from light, and develop in a solvent system consisting of a mixture of alcohol and 1 N hydrochloric acid (95 : 5). Remove the plate from the developing chamber, mark the solvent front, and allow the solvent to evaporate. Locate the spots on the plate by spraying with Dragendorff's reagent, prepared as directed for *Visualization Technique 3* under *Ordinary Impurities* ⟨466⟩: the R_F value of the principal spot obtained from the test solution corresponds to that obtained from the Standard solution.

Uniformity of dosage units ⟨905⟩: meet the requirements.

Dissolution ⟨711⟩**—**

Medium: 0.1 N hydrochloric acid; 900 mL.

Apparatus 1: 100 rpm.

Time: 30 minutes.

Solvent A—Mix 300 mL of methanol and 700 mL of 0.1 N hydrochloric acid.

Solvent B—Mix 75 mL of methanol and 25 mL of 0.1 N hydrochloric acid.

Standard solution—Transfer about 100 mg of USP Molindone Hydrochloride RS, accurately weighed, to a 250-mL volumetric flask, and dissolve in and dilute with *Solvent A* to volume. Pipet 5.0 mL of this stock solution into a 250-mL volumetric flask, and dilute with *Solvent A* to volume. Pipet 15.0 mL of the diluted stock solution into a 50-mL volumetric flask, and dilute with *Solvent A* to volume.

Test solution—Withdraw a portion of the solution under test, and filter, discarding the first 3 mL of filtrate. Pipet 15.0 mL of this solution into a 25-mL volumetric flask, and dilute with *Solvent B* to volume.

Mobile phase—Dissolve 1.08 g of sodium 1-octanesulfonate in 480 mL of water. Add 520 mL of methanol, 2.0 mL of acetic acid, and 0.4 mL of triethylamine, and mix. Make adjustments if necessary (see *System Suitability* under *Chromatography* ⟨621⟩).

Chromatographic system (see *Chromatography* ⟨621⟩)—The liquid chromatograph is equipped with a 254-nm UV detector and a 4.6-mm × 25-cm column that contains packing L11. The flow rate is about 1.5 mL per minute.

Procedure—Separately inject equal volumes (about 100 µL) of the *Standard solution* and the *Test solution* into the chromatograph, record the chromatograms, and measure the peak heights. Determine the amount of molindone hydrochloride ($C_{16}H_{24}N_2O_2 \cdot HCl$) dissolved.

Tolerances—Not less than 80% *(Q)* of the labeled amount of $C_{16}H_{24}N_2O_2 \cdot HCl$ is dissolved in 30 minutes.

Assay—
Mobile phase, Solvent mixture, Internal standard solution, Standard preparation, and *Chromatographic system*—Proceed as directed in the *Assay* under *Molindone Hydrochloride.*

Assay preparation—Accurately weigh not less than 20 Tablets, grind the Tablets to a homogeneous mixture, and transfer an accurately weighed portion, equivalent to about 50 mg of molindone hydrochloride, to a 250-mL conical flask. Add 10.0 mL of *Internal standard solution* and 90.0 mL of *Solvent mixture,* shake for 30 minutes, and filter.

Procedure—Proceed as directed for *Procedure* in the *Assay* under *Molindone Hydrochloride.* Calculate the quantity, in mg, of molindone hydrochloride ($C_{16}H_{24}N_2O_2 \cdot HCl$) in the portion of Tablets taken by the formula:

$$100C(R_U / R_S)$$

in which *C* is the concentration, in mg per mL, of USP Molindone Hydrochloride RS in the *Standard preparation,* and R_U and R_S are the ratios of the peak response of molindone to that of butylparaben obtained from the *Assay preparation* and the *Standard preparation,* respectively.

Mometasone Furoate

$C_{27}H_{30}Cl_2O_6$ 521.43
Pregna-1,4-diene-3,20-dione, 9,21-dichloro-17-[(2-furanylcarbonyl)oxy]-11-hydroxy-16-methyl-, (11β,16α)-.
9,21-Dichloro-11β,17-dihydroxy-16α-methylpregna-1,4-diene-3,20-dione 17-(2-furoate)   [*83919-23-7*].

» Mometasone Furoate contains not less than 97.0 percent and not more than 102.0 percent of $C_{27}H_{30}Cl_2O_6$, calculated on the dried basis.

Packaging and storage—Preserve in well-closed containers.
USP Reference standards ⟨11⟩—*USP Mometasone Furoate RS.*
Identification—
  A: *Infrared Absorption* ⟨197M⟩.
  B: The retention time of the major peak in the chromatogram of the *Assay preparation* corresponds to that of the *Standard preparation,* both relative to the internal standard, as obtained in the *Assay.*
Specific rotation ⟨781S⟩:   between +56° and +62°.
  Test solution: 5 mg per mL in dioxane.
Loss on drying ⟨731⟩—Dry it at 105° for 3 hours: it loses not more than 0.5% of its weight.
Residue on ignition ⟨281⟩:   not more than 0.1%.
Heavy metals, *Method II* ⟨231⟩:   30 ppm.
Chromatographic purity—
  Standard solutions—Dissolve an accurately weighed quantity of USP Mometasone Furoate RS, and dilute quantitatively with dichloromethane to obtain a solution containing 10 mg per mL. Dilute portions of this solution with dichloromethane to obtain *Standard solutions A, B, C, D,* and *E* containing 0.5 (5%), 0.2 (2%), 0.1 (1%), 0.02 (0.2%), and 0.01 (0.1%) mg per mL, respectively.
  Test solution—Prepare a solution of Mometasone Furoate in dichloromethane containing 10 mg per mL.
  Procedure—Separately apply 40 μL of the *Test solution,* and *Standard solutions A, B, C, D,* and *E* to a thin-layer chromatographic plate (see *Chromatography* ⟨621⟩) coated with a 0.25-mm layer of chromatographic silica gel. Develop the chromatogram in a chamber, previously equilibrated with a solvent system consisting of a mixture of chloroform and ethyl acetate (3 : 1), until the solvent front has moved about three-fourths of the length of the plate. Remove the plate from the developing chamber, mark the solvent front, and air-dry. Examine the plate under short-wavelength UV light. Compare the intensities of any secondary spots observed in the chromatogram of the *Test solution* with those of the principal spots in the chromatogram of the *Standard solutions:* no secondary spot from the chromatogram of the *Test solution* is larger or more intense than the principal spot obtained from *Standard solution C,* and the sum of the intensities of the secondary spots obtained from the *Test solution* is not more than 2.0%.

Assay—
Mobile phase—Prepare a filtered and degassed mixture of methanol and water (65 : 35). Make adjustments if necessary (see *System Suitability* under *Chromatography* ⟨621⟩).

Diluting solution—Prepare a solution consisting of a mixture of methanol, water, and acetic acid (65 : 35 : 0.2).

Internal standard solution—Transfer about 40 mg of beclomethasone dipropionate to a 100-mL volumetric flask, dilute with *Diluting solution* to volume, and mix.

Standard preparation—Dissolve an accurately weighed quantity of USP Mometasone Furoate RS in methanol, and dilute quantitatively, and stepwise if necessary, with *Diluting solution* to obtain a solution having a known concentration of about 0.1 mg per mL. Pipet equal amounts of this solution and the *Internal standard solution,* and dilute quantitatively, and stepwise if necessary, with *Diluting solution* to obtain a solution having a known concentration of about 0.02 mg per mL for mometasone furoate and 0.08 mg per mL for beclomethasone dipropionate.

Assay preparation—Dissolve an accurately weighed quantity of Mometasone Furoate in methanol, and dilute quantitatively, and stepwise if necessary, with *Diluting solution* to obtain a solution having a concentration of about 0.1 mg per mL. Pipet 10.0 mL of this solution and 10.0 mL of the *Internal standard solution* into a 50-mL volumetric flask, dilute with *Diluting solution* to volume, and mix.

Chromatographic system (see *Chromatography* ⟨621⟩)—The liquid chromatograph is equipped with a 254-nm detector and a 4.6-mm × 25-cm column that contains packing L7. The flow rate is about 1.7 mL per minute. Chromatograph the *Standard preparation,* and record the peak responses as directed under *Procedure*: the relative retention times are about 1.6 for beclomethasone dipropionate and 1.0 for mometasone furoate, the resolution, *R,* between the mometasone furoate and beclomethasone dipropionate peaks is not less than 4.0, the tailing factor for the mometasone furoate peak is not more than 1.8, and the relative standard deviation for replicate injections is not more than 2.0%.

Procedure—Separately inject equal volumes (about 20 μL) of the *Standard preparation* and the *Assay preparation* into the chromatograph, record the chromatograms, and measure the responses for the major peaks. Calculate the quantity, in mg, of $C_{27}H_{30}Cl_2O_6$ in the portion of Mometasone Furoate taken by the formula:

$$1000C(R_U / R_S)$$

in which *C* is the concentration, in mg per mL, of USP Mometasone Furoate RS in the *Standard preparation,* and R_U and R_S are the ratios of the mometasone furoate peak to the internal standard peak obtained from the *Assay preparation* and the *Standard preparation,* respectively.

Mometasone Furoate Cream

» Mometasone Furoate Cream is Mometasone Furoate in a suitable cream base. It contains not less than 90.0 percent and not more than 110.0 percent of the labeled amount of mometasone furoate ($C_{27}H_{30}Cl_2O_6$).

Packaging and storage—Preserve in well-closed containers.
USP Reference standards ⟨11⟩—*USP Mometasone Furoate RS.*
Identification—
  A: The retention time of the major peak in the chromatogram of the *Assay preparation* corresponds to that of the *Standard prepa-*

ration, both relative to the internal standard, as obtained in the *Assay*.

B: Prepare a test solution of the Cream in acetonitrile containing 0.2 mg per mL of mometasone furoate. Prepare a Standard solution of USP Mometasone Furoate RS in acetonitrile having the same concentration as the test solution. The test solution so obtained responds to the *Thin-layer Chromatographic Identification Test* ⟨201⟩, a mixture of chloroform and ethyl acetate (3 : 1) being used as the developing solvent.

Microbial limits ⟨61⟩—It meets the requirements of the tests for absence of *Staphylococcus aureus*, *Pseudomonas aeruginosa*, *Escherichia coli*, and *Salmonella* species.

Minimum fill ⟨755⟩: meets the requirements.

Assay—

Mobile phase—Proceed as directed under the *Assay* for *Mometasone Furoate*.

Internal standard solution—Dissolve a suitable quantity of beclomethasone dipropionate in acetonitrile to obtain a solution containing about 0.53 mg per mL.

Standard preparation—Dissolve an accurately weighed quantity of USP Mometasone Furoate RS in acetonitrile, and dilute quantitatively, and stepwise if necessary, with acetonitrile to obtain a solution having a known concentration of about 0.136 mg per mL. Pipet equal amounts of this solution and the *Internal standard solution*, and dilute quantitatively, and stepwise if necessary, with acetonitrile to obtain a solution having known concentrations of about 0.027 mg of mometasone furoate and 0.106 mg of beclomethasone dipropionate per mL.

Assay preparation—Transfer an accurately weighed portion of Cream, equivalent to about 2.0 mg of mometasone furoate, to a 50-mL screw-capped centrifuge tube. Pipet 15.0 mL of *Internal standard solution* and 15.0 mL of acetonitrile into the tube, and attach the cap. Heat in an 85° water bath until the cream completely melts, and shake by hand for 2 minutes. Repeat the heating and shaking. Place the tube in an ice-methanol bath for 10 minutes. Centrifuge to obtain a clear supernatant, and transfer 10.0 mL of the supernatant layer into a 25-mL volumetric flask. Dilute with acetonitrile to volume, and mix.

Chromatographic system (see *Chromatography* ⟨621⟩)—Proceed as directed in the *Assay* under *Mometasone Furoate*.

Procedure—Separately inject equal volumes (about 20 µL) of the *Standard preparation* and the *Assay preparation* into the chromatograph, record the chromatograms, and measure the responses for the major peaks. Calculate the quantity, in mg, of mometasone furoate ($C_{27}H_{30}Cl_2O_6$) in the portion of Cream taken by the formula:

$$75C(R_U / R_S)$$

in which C is the concentration, in mg per mL, of USP Mometasone Furoate RS in the *Standard preparation*, and R_U and R_S are the ratios of the mometasone furoate peak to the internal standard peak obtained from the *Assay preparation* and the *Standard preparation*, respectively.

Mometasone Furoate Ointment

» Mometasone Furoate Ointment is Mometasone Furoate in a suitable ointment base. It contains not less than 90.0 percent and not more than 110.0 percent of the labeled amount of mometasone furoate ($C_{27}H_{30}Cl_2O_6$).

Packaging and storage—Preserve in well-closed containers.

USP Reference standards ⟨11⟩—*USP Mometasone Furoate RS*.

Identification—

A: The retention time of the major peak in the chromatogram of the *Assay preparation* corresponds to that of the *Standard preparation*, both relative to the internal standard, as obtained in the *Assay*.

B: Transfer a quantity of Ointment, equivalent to about 3 mg of mometasone furoate, to a 50-mL screw-capped centrifuge tube. Pipet 5.0 mL of methanol into the tube, and attach the cap. Heat in a steam bath until the ointment completely melts, and shake vigorously until the ointment resolidifies. Place in an ice-water bath for 10 minutes. Centrifuge, and filter a portion of the supernatant. Extract 1 mL of the filtrate with 1 mL of hexane; the lower phase obtained is the test solution. Apply 10 µL of the test solution and 10 µL of a Standard solution of USP Mometasone Furoate RS in methanol containing 0.6 mg per mL to a suitable thin-layer chromatographic plate (see *Chromatography* ⟨621⟩) coated with a 0.25-mm layer of chromatographic silica gel mixture. Allow the spots to dry, and develop the chromatogram in methanol until the solvent front has moved 2 cm from the origin. Remove the plate from the developing chamber and air-dry. Develop the chromatogram in a second solvent system consisting of a mixture of chloroform and ethyl acetate (3 : 1), until the solvent front has moved about three-fourths of the length of the plate. Remove the plate from the developing chamber, mark the solvent front, and allow the spots to air-dry. Examine the plate under short-wavelength UV light: the R_F value of the principal spot obtained from the test solution corresponds to that obtained from the Standard solution.

Microbial limits ⟨61⟩—It meets the requirements of the tests for absence of *Staphylococcus aureus*, *Pseudomonas aeruginosa*, *Escherichia coli*, and *Salmonella* species.

Minimum fill ⟨755⟩: meets the requirements.

Assay—

Mobile phase, Diluting solution, Internal standard solution, Standard preparation, and *Chromatographic system*—Proceed as directed in the *Assay* under *Mometasone Furoate*.

Assay preparation—Transfer an accurately weighed portion of Ointment, equivalent to about 1.0 mg of mometasone furoate, to a 50-mL screw-capped centrifuge tube. Pipet 10.0 mL of *Internal standard solution* and 10.0 mL of *Diluting solution* into the tube, and attach the cap. Heat in an 85° water bath until the ointment completely melts, and shake vigorously by hand until the ointment resolidifies. Repeat heating and shaking two more times. Place the tube in an ice-methanol bath for 10 minutes. Centrifuge to obtain a clear supernatant, and transfer 10.0 mL of the supernatant into a 25-mL volumetric flask. Dilute with *Diluting solution* to volume, and mix.

Procedure—Separately inject equal volumes (about 20 µL) of the *Standard preparation* and the *Assay preparation* into the chromatograph, record the chromatograms, and measure the responses for the major peaks. Calculate the quantity, in mg, of mometasone furoate ($C_{27}H_{30}Cl_2O_6$) in the portion of Ointment taken by the formula:

$$50C(R_U / R_S)$$

in which C is the concentration, in mg per mL, of USP Mometasone Furoate RS in the *Standard preparation,* and R_U and R_S are the ratios of the mometasone furoate peak to the internal standard peak obtained from the *Assay preparation* and the *Standard preparation,* respectively.

Mometasone Furoate Topical Solution

» Mometasone Furoate Topical Solution is Mometasone Furoate in a suitable aqueous vehicle. It contains not less than 90.0 percent and not more than 110.0 percent of the labeled amount of mometasone furoate ($C_{27}H_{30}Cl_2O_6$).

Packaging and storage—Preserve in well-closed containers.

USP Reference standards ⟨11⟩—*USP Mometasone Furoate RS*.

Identification—

A: The retention time of the major peak in the chromatogram of the *Assay preparation* corresponds to that of the *Standard preparation*, both relative to the internal standard, as obtained in the *Assay*.

B: Transfer a quantity of Topical Solution, equivalent to about 2 mg of mometasone furoate, to a 50-mL centrifuge tube. Add 10 mL of water. Extract the aqueous solution with 20 mL of chloroform. Remove the chloroform layer, dry over anhydrous sodium sulfate, and filter through a cotton pledget. Repeat the chloroform extraction and combine the dried extracts. Evaporate the chloroform solution to dryness on a steam bath with a stream of nitrogen. Allow the test specimen to cool to room temperature. Dissolve the residue in a mixture of chloroform and methanol (4 : 1) to obtain a test solution containing 1 mg per mL. Prepare a Standard solution of USP Mometasone Furoate RS having the same concentration as the test solution. The test solution so obtained responds to the *Thin-layer Chromatographic Identification Test* ⟨201⟩, a mixture of chloroform and ethyl acetate (3 : 1) being used as the developing solvent and 20 µL each of test solution and Standard solution being applied to the thin-layer chromatographic plate.

Microbial limits ⟨61⟩—It meets the requirements of the tests for absence of *Staphylococcus aureus*, *Pseudomonas aeruginosa*, *Escherichia coli*, and *Salmonella* species.

pH ⟨791⟩: between 4.0 and 5.0.

Assay—
Mobile phase, *Diluting solution*, *Internal standard solution*, *Standard preparation*, and *Chromatographic system*—Proceed as directed in the *Assay* under *Mometasone Furoate*.

Assay preparation—Transfer an accurately weighed portion of Topical Solution, equivalent to 1.0 mg of mometasone furoate, to a 50-mL volumetric flask. Pipet 10.0 mL of *Internal standard solution* into the flask, dilute with *Diluting solution* to volume, and mix.

Procedure—Separately inject equal volumes (about 20 µL) of the *Standard preparation* and the *Assay preparation* into the chromatograph, record the chromatograms, and measure the responses for the major peaks. Calculate the quantity, in mg, of mometasone furoate ($C_{27}H_{30}Cl_2O_6$) in the portion of Topical Solution taken by the formula:

$$50C(R_U / R_S)$$

in which C is the concentration, in mg per mL, of USP Mometasone Furoate RS in the *Standard preparation*, and R_U and R_S are the ratios of the mometasone furoate peak to the internal standard peak obtained from the *Assay preparation* and the *Standard preparation*, respectively.

Monensin

$C_{36}H_{62}O_{11}$(monensin A) 670.87 $C_{35}H_{60}O_{11}$(monensin B) 656.84 $C_{37}H_{64}O_{11}$(monensin C) 684.90
Monensin.
Stereoisomer of 2-[2-ethyloctahydro-3′-methyl-5′-[tetrahydro-6-hydroxy-6-(hydroxymethyl)-3,5-dimethyl-2*H*-pyran-2-yl][2,2′-bifuran-5-yl]]-9-hydroxy-β-methoxy-α,γ,2,8-tetramethyl-1,6-dioxaspiro[4.5]decan-7-butanoic acid   [*17090-79-8*].

» Monensin is a mixture of antibiotic substances produced by the growth of *Streptomyces cinnamonensis*. It has a potency of not less than 110 µg of monensin per mg.

Packaging and storage—Preserve in well-closed containers. Avoid moisture and excessive heat.

Labeling—Label it to indicate that it is for veterinary use only. Label it also to state that it is for manufacturing, processing, or repackaging.

USP Reference standards ⟨11⟩—*USP Monensin Sodium RS. USP Narasin RS.*

Identification—The chromatogram of the *Assay preparation* obtained as directed in the *Assay* exhibits a major peak for monensin A and a minor peak for monensin B, the retention times of which correspond to those exhibited in the chromatogram of the *Standard preparation*, obtained as directed in the *Assay*.

Loss on drying ⟨731⟩—Dry it in vacuum at 60° for 2 hours: it loses not more than 10% of its weight.

Content of monensin A and B activity—Using the results of the calculations in the *Assay*, calculate the percentage of monensin A activity in the Monensin under test by the formula:

$$100A / P$$

in which A is the potency, in µg per mg, of monensin A in the Monensin under test, as determined in the *Assay*, and P is the potency, in µg of monensin, in each mg of the Monensin under test, as determined in the *Assay*: not less than 90% is found. Calculate the percentage of monensin A activity plus monensin B activity in the Monensin under test by the formula:

$$100(A + B) / P$$

in which B is the potency, in µg per mg, of monensin B in the Monensin under test, as determined in the *Assay*, and the other terms are as defined above: not less than 95% is found.

Assay—
Mobile phase—Prepare a filtered and degassed mixture of methanol, water, and glacial acetic acid (94 : 6 : 0.1). Make adjustments if necessary (see *System Suitability* under *Chromatography* ⟨621⟩).

Neutralized methanol—Add 1 g of sodium bicarbonate to 4 liters of methanol, mix, and filter.

Diluent—Prepare a mixture of methanol and water (9 : 1).

Derivatizing reagent—Dissolve 3 g of vanillin in a mixture of methanol and sulfuric acid (95 : 2). [*Caution—To avoid splattering, add the sulfuric acid carefully and slowly with a pipet; do not pour. Allow the mixture of methanol and sulfuric acid to cool before adding vanillin.*]

Standard preparation—Dissolve an accurately weighed quantity of USP Monensin Sodium RS quantitatively in methanol to obtain a solution containing the equivalent of 1000 µg of monensin per mL. Dilute an accurately measured volume of this stock solution quantitatively with *Diluent* to obtain a solution containing 20.0 µg of monensin per mL.

Assay preparation—Transfer about 500 mg of Monensin, accurately weighed, to a 250-mL flask, add 200.0 mL of *Diluent*, and shake by mechanical means for 1 hour. Allow the solids to settle, and dilute an accurately measured volume of the supernatant quantitatively with *Diluent* to obtain a solution containing about 20 µg of monensin per mL.

Resolution solution—Prepare a solution in *Neutralized methanol* containing about 1 mg of USP Monensin Sodium RS and 3 mg of USP Narasin RS per mL. Transfer 2 mL of this solution to a 200-mL volumetric flask, dilute with *Diluent* to volume, and mix.

Chromatographic system (see *Chromatography* ⟨621⟩)—The liquid chromatograph is equipped with a 4.6-mm × 25-cm column that contains packing L1 and the outlet of which is attached to a tee, the opposing arm of which is attached to a tube from which is pumped the *Derivatizing reagent*, and the outlet of which is connected to a 2-mL postcolumn reaction coil maintained at 98°. The outlet of the reaction coil is connected to a detector set at 520 nm. The *Mobile phase* and the *Derivatizing reagent* flow at the rate of about 0.7 mL per minute. Chromatograph the *Resolution solution*, and record the peak responses as directed under *Procedure*: the relative retention times are about 0.9 for monensin B, 1.0 for monensin A, 1.3 for narasin A, and 1.5 for narasin I, the resolution, R, between the monensin B peak and the monensin A peak is not less than 1.25, and between the monensin A peak and the narasin A peak is not less than 3.5. Chromatograph the *Standard preparation*, and record the peak responses as directed under *Procedure*: the tailing factor is not more than 1.4, and the relative standard deviation for replicate injections is not more than 2.0%. [NOTE—After use, flush the system with methanol.]

Procedure—[NOTE—Use peak areas where peak responses are indicated.] Separately inject equal volumes (about 200 µL) of the *Standard preparation* and the *Assay preparation* into the chromatograph, record the chromatograms, and measure the responses for the major peaks, including a peak for monensin C/D, if present, at a retention time of about 1.1 relative to that of the main monensin A peak in the chromatogram obtained from the *Assay preparation*.

Calculate the quantity, in µg, of monensin A in each mg of the Monensin taken by the formula:

$$(CFD / 100{,}000W)(r_U/r_S)$$

in which C is the concentration, in µg per mL, of monensin activity in the *Standard preparation*, based on the quantity of USP Monensin Sodium RS taken, its designated potency, in µg per mg, and the extent of dilution, F is the designated percentage of monensin A in USP Monensin Sodium RS, D is the dilution factor used in preparing the *Assay preparation*, W is the quantity, in g, of Monensin taken to prepare the *Assay preparation*, and r_U and r_S are the monensin A peak responses obtained from the *Assay preparation* and the *Standard preparation*, respectively. Calculate the quantity, in µg, of monensin B in each mg of the Monensin taken by the same formula, except that r_U is the monensin B peak response obtained from the *Assay preparation* and r_S is the monensin A peak response obtained from the *Standard preparation*. Calculate the quantity, in µg, of monensin C/D in each mg of the Monensin taken by the same formula, except that r_U is the monensin C/D peak response obtained from the *Assay preparation*. Calculate the potency, in µg of monensin, in each mg of the Monensin taken by the formula:

$$A + 0.28B + 1.5C/D$$

in which A is the quantity, in µg, of monensin A in each mg of the Monensin taken, as calculated above, and B is the quantity, in µg, of monensin B in each mg of the Monensin taken, and C/D is the quantity, in µg, of monensin C/D in each mg of Monensin taken, as calculated above.

Monensin Granulated

» Monensin Granulated contains Monensin mixed with suitable diluents, carriers, and inactive ingredients prepared in a granulated form that is free-flowing and free from aggregates. It may contain added Monensin Sodium. It contains not less than 140 mg of monensin per g.

Packaging and storage—Preserve in well-closed containers. Avoid moisture and excessive heat.
Labeling—Label it to indicate that it is for veterinary use only. Label it also to state that it is for manufacturing, processing, or repackaging.
USP Reference standards ⟨11⟩—*USP Monensin Sodium RS. USP Narasin RS.*
Identification—The chromatogram of the *Assay preparation* obtained as directed in the *Assay* exhibits a major peak for monensin A and a minor peak for monensin B, the retention times of which correspond to those exhibited in the chromatogram of the *Standard preparation*, obtained as directed in the *Assay*.
Loss on drying ⟨731⟩—Dry it in vacuum at 60° for 2 hours: it loses not more than 10% of its weight.
Content of monensin A and B activity—Using the results of the calculations in the *Assay*, calculate the percentage of monensin A activity in the Monensin Granulated under test by the formula:

$$100A / P$$

in which A is the potency, in µg per mg, of monensin A in the Monensin Granulated under test, as determined in the *Assay*, and P is the potency, in µg of monensin, in each mg of the Monensin Granulated under test, as determined in the *Assay*: not less than 90% is found. Calculate the percentage of monensin A activity plus monensin B activity in the Monensin Granulated under test by the formula:

$$100(A + B) / P$$

in which B is the potency, in µg per mg, of monensin B in the Monensin Granulated under test, as determined in the *Assay*, and the other terms are as defined above: not less than 95% is found.

Assay—
Mobile phase, Neutralized methanol, Diluent, Derivatizing reagent, Standard preparation, Resolution solution, and *Chromatographic system*—Proceed as directed in the *Assay* under *Monensin*.

Assay preparation—Transfer about 5 g of Monensin Granulated, accurately weighed, to a 250-mL flask, add 200.0 mL of *Diluent*, and shake by mechanical means for 1 hour. Allow the solids to settle, and dilute an accurately measured volume of the supernatant quantitatively with *Diluent* to obtain a solution containing about 20 µg of monensin per mL.

Procedure—Proceed as directed for *Procedure* in the *Assay* under *Monensin*. Calculate the quantity, in mg, of monensin A in each g of the Monensin Granulated taken by the formula:

$$(CFD / 100{,}000W)(r_U/r_S)$$

in which C is the concentration, in µg per mL, of monensin activity in the *Standard preparation*, based on the quantity of USP Monensin Sodium RS taken, its designated potency, in µg per mg, and the extent of dilution, F is the designated percentage of monensin A in USP Monensin Sodium RS, D is the dilution factor used in preparing the *Assay preparation*, W is the quantity, in g, of Monensin Granulated taken to prepare the *Assay preparation*, and r_U and r_S are the monensin A peak responses obtained from the *Assay preparation* and the *Standard preparation*, respectively. Calculate the quantity, in mg, of monensin B in each g of the Monensin Granulated taken by the same formula, except that r_U is the monensin B peak response obtained from the *Assay preparation* and r_S is the monensin A peak response obtained from the *Standard preparation*. Calculate the quantity, in mg, of monensin C/D in each g of the Monensin Granulated taken by the same formula, except that r_U is the monensin C/D peak response obtained from the *Assay preparation*. Calculate the potency, in µg of monensin, in each mg of the Monensin Granulated taken by the formula:

$$A + 0.28B + 1.5C/D$$

in which A is the quantity, in mg, of monensin A in each g of the Monensin Granulated taken, as calculated above, and B is the quantity, in mg, of monensin B in each g of the Monensin Granulated taken, and C/D is the quantity, in mg, of monensin C/D in each g of Monensin Granulated taken, as calculated above.

Monensin Premix

» Monensin Premix contains Monensin Granulated mixed with suitable diluents and inactive ingredients. It contains the equivalent of not less than 85.0 percent and not more than 115.0 percent of the labeled amount of monensin.

Packaging and storage—Preserve in well-closed containers. Avoid moisture and excessive heat.
Labeling—Label it to indicate that it is for veterinary use only. The label bears the statement "Do not feed undiluted."
USP Reference standards ⟨11⟩—*USP Monensin Sodium RS. USP Narasin RS.*
Identification—The chromatogram of the *Assay preparation* obtained as directed in the *Assay* exhibits a major peak for monensin A and a minor peak for monensin B, the retention times of which correspond to those exhibited in the chromatogram of the *Standard preparation* obtained as directed in the *Assay*.
Loss on drying ⟨731⟩—Dry it in vacuum at 60° for 2 hours: it loses not more than 10% of its weight.
Assay—
Mobile phase, Neutralized methanol, Diluent, Derivatizing reagent, Standard preparation, Resolution solution, and *Chromatographic system*—Proceed as directed in the *Assay* under *Monensin*.

Assay preparation—Transfer about 5 g of Premix, accurately weighed, to a 250-mL flask, add 200.0 mL of *Diluent*, and shake by mechanical means for 1 hour. Allow the solids to settle, and dilute an accurately measured volume of the clear supernatant quantitatively with *Diluent* to obtain a solution containing about 20 µg of monensin per mL.

Procedure—Proceed as directed for *Procedure* in the *Assay* under *Monensin*. Calculate the quantity, in mg, of monensin A in each g of the Premix taken by the formula:

$$(CFD / 100{,}000W)(r_U / r_S)$$

in which C is the concentration, in µg per mL, of monensin activity in the *Standard preparation*, based on the quantity of USP Monensin Sodium RS taken, its designated potency, in µg per mg, and the extent of dilution, F is the designated percentage of monensin A in USP Monensin Sodium RS, D is the dilution factor used in preparing the *Assay preparation*, W is the quantity, in g, of Premix taken to prepare the *Assay preparation*, and r_U and r_S are the monensin A peak responses obtained from the *Assay preparation* and the *Standard preparation*, respectively. Calculate the quantity, in mg, of monensin B in each g of the Premix taken by the same formula, except that r_U is the monensin B peak response obtained from the *Assay preparation* and r_S is the monensin A peak response obtained from the *Standard preparation*. Calculate the quantity, in mg, of monensin C/D in each g of the Premix taken by the same formula, except that r_U is the monensin C/D peak response obtained from the *Assay preparation*. Calculate the potency, in mg of monensin, in each g of the Premix taken by the formula:

$$A + 0.28B + 1.5C / D$$

in which A is the quantity, in mg, of monensin A in each g of the Premix taken, as calculated above, and B is the quantity, in mg, of monensin B in each g of the Premix taken, and C/D is the quantity, in mg, of monensin C/D in each g of Premix taken, as calculated above.

Monensin Sodium

$C_{36}H_{61}NaO_{11}$ (monensin A sodium) 692.88 $C_{35}H_{59}NaO_{11}$ (monensin B sodium) 678.85 $C_{37}H_{63}NaO_{11}$ (monensin C sodium) 706.91
Monensin, sodium salt.
Stereoisomer of 2-[2-ethyloctahydro-3′-methyl-5′-[tetrahydro-6-hydroxy-6-(hydroxymethyl)-3,5-dimethyl-2*H*-pyran-2-yl][2,2′-bifuran-5-yl]]-9-hydroxy-β-methoxy-α,γ,2,8-tetramethyl-1,6-dioxaspiro[4.5]decan-7–butanoic acid sodium salt [*22373-78-0*].

» Monensin Sodium has a potency of not less than 800 µg per mg.

Packaging and storage—Preserve in well-closed containers. Avoid moisture and excessive heat.
Labeling—Label it to indicate that it is for veterinary use only. Label it also to state that it is for manufacturing, processing, or repackaging.
USP Reference standards ⟨11⟩—*USP Monensin Sodium RS. USP Narasin RS.*
Identification—The chromatogram of the *Assay preparation* obtained as directed in the *Assay* exhibits a major peak for monensin A and a minor peak for monensin B, the retention times of which correspond to those exhibited in the chromatogram of the *Standard preparation*, as obtained in the *Assay*.
Loss on drying ⟨731⟩—Dry it in vacuum at 60° for 3 hours: it loses not more than 4% of its weight.
Content of monensin A and B activity—Using the results of the calculations in the *Assay*, calculate the percentage of monensin A activity in the Monensin Sodium under test by the formula:

$$100A / P$$

in which A is the potency, in mg per g, of monensin A in the Monensin Sodium under test, as determined in the *Assay*, and P is the potency, in mg of monensin, in each g of the Monensin Sodium under test, as determined in the *Assay*: not less than 90% is found. Calculate the percentage of monensin A activity plus monensin B activity in the Monensin Sodium under test by the formula:

$$100(A + B) / P$$

in which B is the potency, in mg per g, of monensin B in the Monensin Sodium under test, as determined in the *Assay*, and the other terms are as defined above: not less than 95% is found.

Assay—
Mobile phase, Neutralized methanol, Diluent, Derivatizing reagent, Standard preparation, Resolution solution, and *Chromatographic system*—Proceed as directed in the *Assay* under *Monensin*.

Assay preparation—Transfer about 100 mg of Monensin Sodium, accurately weighed, to a 100-mL volumetric flask, dissolve in and dilute with methanol to volume. If necessary, to achieve complete dissolution, sonicate for about 1 minute, and mix. Dilute an accurately measured volume of this solution quantitatively with *Diluent* to obtain a solution containing about 20 µg of monensin per mL.

Procedure—Proceed as directed for *Procedure* in the *Assay* under *Monensin*. Calculate the quantity, in mg, of monensin A in each g of the Monensin Sodium taken by the formula:

$$(CFD / 100{,}000W)(r_U / r_S)$$

in which C is the concentration, in µg per mL, of monensin activity in the *Standard preparation*, based on the quantity of USP Monensin Sodium RS taken, its designated potency, in µg per mg, and the extent of dilution; F is the designated percentage of monensin A in USP Monensin Sodium RS; D is the dilution factor used in preparing the *Assay preparation*; W is the quantity, in g, of Monensin Sodium taken to prepare the *Assay preparation*; and r_U and r_S are the monensin A peak responses obtained from the *Assay preparation* and the *Standard preparation*, respectively. Calculate the quantity, in mg, of monensin B in each g of the Monensin Sodium taken by the same formula, except that r_U is the monensin B peak response obtained from the *Assay preparation*, and r_S is the monensin A peak response obtained from the *Standard preparation*. Calculate the quantity, in mg, of monensin C/D in each g of the Monensin Sodium taken by the same formula, except that r_U is the monensin C/D peak response obtained from the *Assay preparation*. Calculate the potency, in mg of monensin, in each g of the Monensin Sodium taken by the formula:

$$A + 0.28B + 1.5C / D$$

in which A is the quantity, in mg, of monensin A in each g of the Monensin Sodium taken, as calculated above; B is the quantity, in mg, of monensin B in each g of the Monensin Sodium taken; and C/D is the quantity, in mg, of monensin C/D in each g of Monensin Sodium taken, as calculated above.

Monobenzone

$C_{13}H_{12}O_2$ 200.24
Phenol, 4-(phenylmethoxy)-.
p-(Benzyloxy)phenol [*103-16-2*].

» Monobenzone, dried at 105° for 3 hours, contains not less than 98.0 percent and not more than 102.0 percent of $C_{13}H_{12}O_2$.

Packaging and storage—Preserve in tight, light-resistant containers, and avoid exposure to temperatures above 30°.

USP Reference standards ⟨11⟩—USP Monobenzone RS.
Identification—
   A: *Infrared Absorption* ⟨197K⟩.
   B: *Ultraviolet Absorption* ⟨197U⟩—
      Solution: 10 μg per mL.
      Medium: methanol.
   Absorptivities at 292 nm, calculated on the dried basis, do not differ by more than 3.0%.
   C: Transfer about 500 mg of Monobenzone, previously dried, to a 150-mL flask fitted with a reflux condenser, employing a suitable glass joint. Add 5 mL of pyridine and 3 mL of acetic anhydride, reflux for 10 minutes, and cool. Add 100 mL of water and 6 mL of acetone to the flask, and insert a stopper. Cool the contents of the flask in a refrigerator for 1 hour, collect the precipitate in a sintered-glass crucible, and wash the precipitate with water until no odor of pyridine remains. Dry the precipitate for 16 hours in a vacuum desiccator over phosphorus pentoxide. The monobenzone acetate so obtained melts between 110° and 113° when determined as directed for *Class I* (see *Melting Range or Temperature* ⟨741⟩).
Melting range, *Class I* ⟨741⟩: between 117° and 120°.
Loss on drying ⟨731⟩—Dry it at 105° for 3 hours: it loses not more than 1.0% of its weight.
Residue on ignition ⟨281⟩: not more than 0.5%.
Organic volatile impurities, *Method V* ⟨467⟩: meets the requirements.
   Solvent: dimethyl sulfoxide.

(Official until July 1, 2008)

Assay—
   Standard preparation—Dissolve an accurately weighed quantity of USP Monobenzone RS in methanol, and dilute quantitatively, and stepwise if necessary, with methanol to obtain a solution having a known concentration of about 40 μg per mL.
   Assay preparation—Transfer about 100 mg of Monobenzone, accurately weighed, to a 100-mL volumetric flask, dissolve in and dilute with methanol to volume, and mix. Pipet 4 mL of this solution into a 100-mL volumetric flask, dilute with methanol to volume, and mix.
   Procedure—With a suitable spectrophotometer, using methanol as a blank, concomitantly determine the absorbances of the *Standard preparation* and the *Assay preparation* at the wavelength of maximum absorbance at about 292 nm. Calculate the quantity, in mg, of $C_{13}H_{12}O_2$ in the portion of Monobenzone taken by the formula:

$$2500C(A_U / A_S)$$

in which C is the concentration, in mg per mL, of USP Monobenzone RS in the *Standard preparation;* and A_U and A_S are the absorbances obtained from the *Assay preparation* and the *Standard preparation*, respectively.

Monobenzone Cream

» Monobenzone Cream contains not less than 94.0 percent and not more than 106.0 percent of the labeled amount of monobenzone ($C_{13}H_{12}O_2$).

Packaging and storage—Preserve in tight containers, and avoid exposure to temperatures higher than 30°.

USP Reference standards ⟨11⟩—*USP Monobenzone RS.*
Identification—Transfer a quantity of Cream, equivalent to about 500 mg of monobenzone, to a centrifuge bottle, add 100 mL of water, and shake until the cream is completely dispersed. Centrifuge the suspension, decant the supernatant, wash the residue with water, again centrifuge, and decant the water. Transfer the residue to a separator with the aid of water, and adjust the volume to about 100 mL. Extract with four 25-mL portions of chloroform, filtering the extracts through a pledget of cotton into a 150-mL flask. Evaporate the chloroform in a current of warm air, and add 5 mL of pyridine and 3 mL of acetic anhydride to the dry residue. Connect the flask to a reflux condenser, reflux for 10 minutes, cool, and proceed as directed in *Identification* test *C* under *Monobenzone*, beginning with "Add 100 mL of water." It meets the requirements of *Identification* test *C* under *Monobenzone*.

Assay—
   Standard preparation—Prepare as directed in the *Assay* under *Monobenzone*.
   Assay preparation—Transfer an accurately weighed portion of Cream, equivalent to about 200 mg of monobenzone, to a suitable container, add 100 mL of methanol, and shake for about 30 minutes. Transfer the mixture to a 200-mL volumetric flask. Rinse the container with two 25-mL portions of methanol, and add the rinsings to the 200-mL volumetric flask. Dilute with methanol to volume, mix, and filter, discarding the first 20 mL of the filtrate. Pipet 4 mL of this solution into a 100-mL volumetric flask, dilute with methanol to volume, and mix.
   Procedure—Proceed as directed in the *Assay* under *Monobenzone*, but use the *Assay preparation* under *Monobenzone Cream*. Calculate the quantity, in mg, of monobenzone ($C_{13}H_{12}O_2$) in the portion of Cream taken by the formula:

$$5000C(A_U / A_S)$$

in which C is the concentration, in mg per mL, of USP Monobenzone RS in the *Standard preparation* and A_U and A_S are the absorbances obtained from the *Assay preparation* and the *Standard preparation*, respectively.

Morantel Tartrate

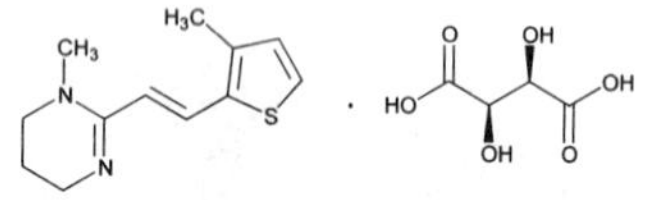

$C_{12}H_{16}N_2S \cdot C_4H_6O_6$ 370.42
Pyrimidine, 1,4,5,6-tetrahydro-1-methyl-2-[2-(3-methyl-2-thienyl)ethenyl]-, (E)-,[R-(R*,R*)]-2,3-dihydroxybutanedioate (1 : 1).
(E)-1,4,5,6-Tetrahydro-1-methyl-2-[2-(3-methyl-2-thienyl)vinyl]pyrimidine tartrate (1 : 1) [26155-31-7].
Morantel [20574-50-9].

Change to read:

» Morantel Tartrate contains not less than ▲96.4▲*USP31* percent and not more than 101.5 percent of $C_{12}H_{16}N_2S \cdot C_4H_6O_6$, calculated on the dried basis.

Packaging and storage—Preserve in well-closed, light-resistant containers. Store at 25°, excursions permitted between 15° and 30°.
Labeling—Label it to indicate it is for veterinary use only.

USP Reference standards ⟨11⟩—*USP Morantel Tartrate RS.*
Clarity and color of solution—Dissolve and dilute 0.25 g to 25.0 mL in carbon dioxide-free water. The solution is clear and yellow to greenish yellow in color.
Identification—
   A: *Infrared Absorption* ⟨197K⟩.
   B: It meets the requirements of the test for *Tartrate* ⟨191⟩.
   C: The retention time of the morantel peak in the chromatogram of the *Test solution* corresponds to that in the chromatogram of *Standard solution 1*, as obtained in the test for *Related compounds*.
Melting temperature ⟨741⟩: 167° to 172°.
pH ⟨791⟩: between 2.8 and 3.9.
   Solution—Dissolve and dilute 0.25 g to 25.0 mL in carbon dioxide-free water.
Loss on drying ⟨731⟩—Dry it at 100° to 105° to constant weight: it loses not more than 1.5% of its weight.

Residue on ignition ⟨281⟩: not more than 0.1%.

Heavy metals, *Method II* ⟨231⟩—not more than 20 ppm.

Change to read:

Related compounds—[NOTE—Conduct this test without exposure to daylight, and with the minimum necessary exposure to artificial light.]

Mobile phase—Mix 3.5 mL of triethylamine and 850 mL of water. Adjust with phosphoric acid to a pH of 2.5. Add 50 mL of tetrahydrofuran and 100 mL of methanol, and mix.

Tartrate solution—Prepare a solution containing about 0.15 mg of tartaric acid per mL in *Mobile phase*.

Standard solution 1—Dissolve an accurately weighed quantity of USP Morantel Tartrate RS in *Mobile phase* to obtain a solution having a known concentration of about 5.0 µg per mL.

Standard solution 2—Dilute 2.0 mL of *Standard solution 1* to 100.0 mL with *Mobile phase*.

System suitability solution—Expose 10 mL of *Standard solution 1* to daylight for 15 minutes before injection.

Test solution—Dissolve an accurately weighed quantity of Morantel Tartrate in *Mobile phase* to obtain a solution having a concentration of about 0.5 mg per mL.

Chromatographic system (see *Chromatography* ⟨621⟩)—The liquid chromatograph is equipped with a 226-nm detector and a 4.6-mm × 25-cm column that contains 5-µm packing L1. The flow rate is about 0.75 mL per minute. Chromatograph the *Tartrate solution, Standard solution 1,* and the *System suitability solution,* and record the peak areas as directed for *Procedure:* using the *System suitability solution,* the resolution, R, between morantel and its preceding peak ((Z)-isomer) is not less than 2. ▲The relative retention times are about 0.8, 1.0, and 1.2 for the morantel (Z)-isomer, morantel, and the morantel 4-methyl isomer (1-methyl-2-[(E)-2-(4-methylthiophen-2-yl)ethenyl]-1,4,5,6 tetrahydropyrimidine), respectively.▲USP31

Procedure—Separately inject equal volumes (about 20 µL) of the *Tartrate solution, Standard solution 1, Standard solution 2,* and the *Test solution* into the chromatograph, record the chromatograms, and measure the areas for the major peaks. Disregarding the tartrate peak and any peak in the chromatogram of the *Test solution* less than the area of the principal peak in the chromatogram of *Standard solution 2*, calculate the area percentage of each impurity, relative to morantel, in the portion of Morantel Tartrate taken by the formula:

$$100(C_S / C_U)(r_i / r_S)$$

in which C_S and C_U are the concentrations of morantel tartrate, in mg per mL, of *Standard solution 1* and the *Test solution,* respectively; and r_i and r_S are the peak areas of each individual impurity and morantel obtained from the *Test solution* and *Standard solution 1,* respectively: ▲not more than 3% of the morantel 4-methyl isomer is found; not more than 0.5% of any other individual impurity is found; and not more than 1% of total other individual impurities is found.▲USP31

Assay—

Dissolve 0.280 g in 40 mL of anhydrous acetic acid. Titrate with 0.1 N perchloric acid VS, determining the endpoint potentiometrically (see *Titrimetry* ⟨541⟩). One mL of 0.1 N perchloric acid is equivalent to 37.04 mg of $C_{12}H_{16}N_2S \cdot C_4H_6O_6$.

Moricizine Hydrochloride

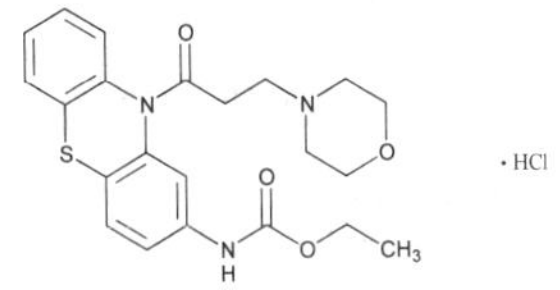

$C_{22}H_{25}N_3O_4S \cdot HCl$

Carbamic acid, [10-[3-(4-morpholinyl)-l-oxopropyl]-10H-phenothiazin-2-yl]-, ethyl ester, hydrochloride.

Ethyl 10-(3-morpholinopropionyl)phenothiazine-2-carbamate, hydrochloride [29560-58-8].

» Moricizine Hydrochloride contains not less than 98.0 percent and not more than 102.0 percent of $C_{22}H_{25}N_3O_4S \cdot HCl$, calculated on the anhydrous and alcohol-free basis.

Packaging and storage—Preserve in tight containers.

USP Reference standards ⟨11⟩—*USP Moricizine Hydrochloride RS.*

Identification—
  A: *Infrared Absorption* ⟨197K⟩.
  B: *Ultraviolet Absorption* ⟨197U⟩—
  Solution: 8 µg per mL.
  Medium: methanol.
  C: Prepare a test solution in methanol containing 20 mg of Moricizine Hydrochloride per mL. Similarly prepare a Standard solution in methanol containing 20 mg of USP Moricizine Hydrochloride RS. Separately apply 5 µL of each solution on a thin-layer chromatographic plate (see *Chromatography* ⟨621⟩) coated with a 0.25-mm layer of chromatographic silica gel mixture. Place the plate in a chromatographic chamber lined with filter paper saturated with a solvent system consisting of a mixture of chloroform, methanol, and diethylamine (91 : 7 : 2). Develop the chromatogram, protected from light, until the solvent front has moved about three-fourths of the length of the plate. Remove the plate from the chamber. Spray the plate with a freshly prepared ferric chloride solution prepared by adding 20 mL of 10% ferric chloride solution to 200 mg of potassium ferricyanide dissolved in 20 mL of water: the R_F value of the blue spot in the chromatogram obtained from the test solution corresponds to that in the chromatogram obtained from the Standard solution.

Clarity of solution—Dissolve 1 g in 30 mL of methanol, sonicating for 5 minutes if necessary. The solution is not less clear than an equal volume of methanol contained in a similar vessel and examined similarly.

Loss on drying ⟨731⟩—Dry it at 105° for 4 hours: it loses not more than 1.0% of its weight.

Water, *Method I* ⟨921⟩: not more than 1.0%.

Residue on ignition ⟨281⟩: not more than 0.1%.

Heavy metals, *Method II* ⟨231⟩: 10 µg per g.

Organic volatile impurities, *Method V* ⟨467⟩: meets the requirements.

(Official until July 1, 2008)

Chromatographic purity—

Mobile phase—Prepare a mixture of water, acetonitrile, and triethylamine (580 : 420 : 1) containing 0.005 M sodium 1-octane sulfonate, and adjust with glacial acetic acid to a pH of 4.2. Make adjustments if necessary (see *System Suitability* under *Chromatography* ⟨621⟩).

Diluent—Prepare a mixture of 0.02 N hydrochloric acid and acetonitrile (58 : 42).

Internal standard solution—Prepare a solution of butamben in *Diluent* containing about 0.1 mg per mL.

Standard solution—Prepare a solution of USP Moricizine Hydrochloride RS in *Diluent* having a known concentration of about 0.10 mg per mL. Transfer 10.0 mL of this solution to a 500-mL volumetric flask, add 25.0 mL of *Internal standard solution,* dilute with *Diluent* to volume, and mix to obtain a solution containing about 0.0020 mg of USP Moricizine Hydrochloride RS per mL. [NOTE—Protect this solution from light.]

Test solution—Transfer about 100 mg of Moricizine Hydrochloride, accurately weighed, to a 100-mL low-actinic volumetric flask, add 5.0 mL of *Internal standard solution*, dilute with *Diluent* to volume, and mix. [NOTE—Protect this solution from light.]

Chromatographic system (see *Chromatography* ⟨621⟩)—The liquid chromatograph is equipped with a 254-nm detector and a 4.6-mm × 25-cm column that contains packing L7 and is maintained at a constant temperature of about 35°. The flow rate is about 2.5 mL per minute. Chromatograph the *Standard solution*, and record the peak responses as directed for *Procedure*: the relative retention times are about 0.6 for moricizine and 1.0 for butamben; the resolution, R, between the moricizine peak and the butamben peak is not less than 2; and the relative standard deviation for replicate injections is not more than 5%.

Procedure—Separately inject equal volumes (about 20 µL) of the *Standard solution* and the *Test solution* into the chromatograph, record the chromatograms for a period of time that is five times the elution time of moricizine, and measure the responses for the peaks, except for the solvent peak. Calculate the percentage of each impurity peak in the portion of Moricizine Hydrochloride taken by the formula:

$$100C(R_i / R_S)$$

in which C is the concentration, in mg per mL, of USP Moricizine Hydrochloride RS in the *Standard solution*, R_i is the ratio of the peak areas of an individual impurity peak to the butamben peak obtained from the *Test solution*, and R_S is the ratio of the peak areas of the moricizine peak to the butamben peak obtained from the *Standard solution*. Any impurity eluting before the moricizine peak is not more than 0.25%, any impurity eluting after the moricizine peak is not more than 0.20%, and the total of all impurities is not more than 1.5%, any impurity of less than 0.1% being disregarded.

Limit of alcohol (C_2H_5OH)—

Standard solution—Transfer 6.0 mL of dehydrated alcohol to a 100-mL volumetric flask, dilute with water to volume, and mix. Transfer 5.0 mL of this solution to a second 100-mL volumetric flask, dilute with water to volume, and mix. Transfer 5.0 mL of this solution to a third 100-mL volumetric flask, dilute with water to volume, and mix. This solution contains 0.1184 mg of C_2H_5OH per mL.

Test solution—Transfer about 1 g of Moricizine Hydrochloride, accurately weighed, to a 50-mL glass-stoppered centrifuge tube, add 19.0 mL of water, and sonicate to dissolve. Transfer 1.0 mL of 3 N ammonium hydroxide to the tube, insert the stopper, and shake the tube by mechanical means for 30 minutes. Centrifuge, draw off a portion of the clear supernatant and filter through a filter having a porosity of 0.5 µm or finer.

Chromatographic system (see *Chromatography* ⟨621⟩)—The gas chromatograph is equipped with a flame-ionization detector and a 4-mm × 1.8-m glass column that contains support S2. The column is maintained at 150°, and the injection port and detector block are maintained at 170°. Helium is used as the carrier gas at a flow rate of about 50 mL per minute. Chromatograph the *Standard solution*, and record the peak responses as directed for *Procedure*: the relative standard deviation for replicate injections is not more than 3%.

Procedure—Separately inject equal volumes (about 5 µL) of the *Standard solution* and the *Test solution* into the chromatograph, record the chromatograms, and measure the peak responses. Calculate the percentage of C_2H_5OH in the portion of Moricizine Hydrochloride taken by the formula:

$$2(C/W)(r_U / r_S)$$

in which C is the concentration, in mg per mL, of C_2H_5OH in the *Standard solution*; W is the weight, in g, of Moricizine Hydrochloride taken to prepare the *Test solution*; and r_U and r_S are the alcohol peak responses obtained from the *Test solution* and the *Standard solution*, respectively. Not more than 0.25% is found.

Content of chloride—Transfer about 400 mg of Moricizine Hydrochloride, accurately weighed, to a conical flask, add 75 mL of methanol, and swirl to dissolve. Add 5 mL of glacial acetic acid, and three drops of eosin Y TS, and titrate with 0.1 N silver nitrate VS to a pink endpoint. Each mL of 0.1 N silver nitrate is equivalent to 3.546 mg of Cl. Not less than 7.49% and not more than 7.80% is found, calculated on the anhydrous and alcohol-free basis.

Assay—

Mobile phase—Prepare a mixture of water, acetonitrile, glacial acetic acid, and triethylamine (580 : 420 : 20 : 1) containing 0.005 M sodium 1-octane sulfonate. Make adjustments if necessary (see *System Suitability* under *Chromatography* ⟨621⟩).

Diluent—Prepare a mixture of 0.02 N hydrochloric acid and acetonitrile (58 : 42).

Internal standard solution—Prepare a solution of butamben in *Diluent* containing about 5 mg per mL.

Standard preparation—Transfer about 25 mg of USP Moricizine Hydrochloride RS, accurately weighed, to a 25-mL low-actinic volumetric flask, add 5.0 mL of *Internal standard solution*, dilute with *Diluent* to volume, and mix. [NOTE—Protect this solution from light.]

Assay preparation—Transfer about 1 mg per mL of Moricizine Hydrochloride, accurately weighed, to a 50-mL low-actinic volumetric flask, add 10.0 mL of *Internal standard solution*, dilute with *Diluent* to volume, and mix. [NOTE—Protect this solution from light.]

Chromatographic system (see *Chromatography* ⟨621⟩)—The liquid chromatograph is equipped with a 254-nm detector and a 4.6-mm × 25-cm column that contains packing L7 and is maintained at a constant temperature of about 35°. The flow rate is about 2.5 mL per minute. Chromatograph the *Standard preparation*, and record the peak responses as directed for *Procedure*: the relative retention times are about 0.6 for moricizine, 1.7 for the reverse Mannich product, 2.0 for the amide hydrolysis product, and 1.0 for butamben; the resolution, R, between the moricizine peak and the butamben peak is not less than 2; and the relative standard deviation for replicate injections is not more than 2%.

Procedure—Separately inject equal volumes (about 10 µL) of the *Standard preparation* and the *Assay preparation* into the chromatograph, record the chromatograms, and measure the responses for the major peaks. Calculate the quantity, in mg, of $C_{22}H_{25}N_3O_4S \cdot HCl$ in the portion of Moricizine Hydrochloride taken by the formula:

$$50C(R_U / R_S)$$

in which C is the concentration, in mg per mL, of USP Moricizine Hydrochloride RS in the *Standard preparation*; and R_U and R_S are the ratios of the peak area responses of moricizine and butamben obtained from the *Assay preparation* and the *Standard preparation*, respectively.

Moricizine Hydrochloride Tablets

» Moricizine Hydrochloride Tablets contain not less than 90.0 percent and not more than 110.0 percent of the labeled amount of moricizine hydrochloride ($C_{22}H_{25}N_3O_4S \cdot HCl$).

Packaging and storage—Preserve in tight containers.

USP Reference standards ⟨11⟩—*USP Moricizine Hydrochloride RS*.

Identification—

A: *Ultraviolet Absorption* ⟨197U⟩—

Test solution—Transfer a portion of finely ground Tablets, equivalent to about 50 mg of moricizine hydrochloride, to a 250-mL volumetric flask, add about 100 mL of 0.1 N hydrochloric acid, shake by mechanical means for 15 minutes, dilute with 0.1 N hydrochloric acid to volume, and mix. Filter a portion of this solution, discarding the first 10 mL of the filtrate. Transfer 10 mL of the filtrate to a 250-mL volumetric flask, dilute with 0.1 N hydrochloric acid to volume, and mix.

Standard solution: 8 µg per mL.

Medium: 0.1 N hydrochloric acid.

B: Shake a Tablet with 10 mL of methanol until it disintegrates, and filter: the filtrate responds to *Identification* test C under *Moricizine Hydrochloride*.

Dissolution ⟨711⟩—
 Medium: 0.1 N hydrochloric acid; 900 mL.
 Apparatus 2: 50 rpm.
 Time: 30 minutes.
 Procedure—Determine the amount of moricizine hydrochloride ($C_{22}H_{25}N_3O_4S \cdot HCl$) dissolved from UV absorbance at about 267 nm of filtered portions of the solution under test, suitably diluted with *Dissolution Medium*, in comparison with a *Standard solution* having a known concentration of USP Moricizine Hydrochloride RS in the same medium.
 Tolerances—Not less than 75% *(Q)* of the labeled amount of moricizine hydrochloride ($C_{22}H_{25}N_3O_4S \cdot HCl$) is dissolved in 30 minutes.

Uniformity of dosage units ⟨905⟩: meet the requirements.

Limit of degradation products—
 Mobile phase—Dissolve 1.08 g of sodium 1-octanesulfonate in 580 mL of water, add 420 mL of acetonitrile, 20 mL of glacial acetic acid, and 1 mL of triethylamine. Adjust with 5 N sodium hydroxide to an apparent pH of 4.5. Mix, and filter through a filter having a porosity of 0.5 µm or finer. Make adjustments if necessary (see *System Suitability* under *Chromatography* ⟨621⟩).
 Diluent—Prepare a mixture of 0.02 N hydrochloric acid and acetonitrile (58 : 42).
 Internal standard solution—Prepare a solution of butamben in *Diluent* containing about 0.2 mg per mL.
 Standard solution—Prepare a solution of USP Moricizine Hydrochloride RS in *Diluent* containing 0.10 mg per mL. Transfer 5.0 mL of this solution to a 50-mL volumetric flask, add 20.0 mL of *Internal standard solution*, dilute with *Diluent* to volume, and mix. [NOTE—Protect this solution from light.]
 Test solution—Transfer 10 Tablets to a 1000-mL flask, add 500.0 mL of *Diluent*, sonicate until the Tablets are disintegrated, and then shake by mechanical means for 30 minutes. Filter this solution, discarding the first 10 mL of the filtrate. Transfer 25.0 mL of the filtrate to a 50-mL volumetric flask, add 20.0 mL of *Internal standard solution*, dilute with *Diluent* to volume, and mix. [NOTE—Protect this solution from light.]
 Chromatographic system (see *Chromatography* ⟨621⟩)—The liquid chromatograph is equipped with a 254-nm detector and a 4.6-mm × 25-cm column that contains packing L7 and is maintained at a constant temperature of about 35°. The flow rate is about 2.5 mL per minute. Chromatograph the *Standard solution*, and record the peak responses as directed under *Procedure*: the relative retention times are about 0.6 for moricizine and 1.0 for butamben, the resolution, *R*, between the moricizine peak and the butamben peak is not less than 2, and the relative standard deviation for replicate injections is not more than 5%.
 Procedure—Separately inject equal volumes (about 20 µL) of the *Standard solution* and the *Test solution* into the chromatograph, record the chromatograms for a period of time that is five times the elution time of moricizine, and measure the responses for the peaks, except for any that elute before moricizine. Calculate the percentage of each impurity peak that elutes after butamben in the portion of Moricizine Hydrochloride taken by the formula:

$$1000(C / L)(R_i / R_S)$$

in which *C* is the concentration, in mg per mL, of USP Moricizine Hydrochloride RS in the *Standard solution*, *L* is the labeled amount, in mg, of moricizine hydrochloride in each Tablet, R_i is the ratio of the peak areas of an individual impurity peak to the butamben peak obtained from the *Test solution*, and R_S is the ratio of the peak areas of the moricizine peak to the butamben peak obtained from the *Standard solution*. The first impurity eluting after the butamben peak is not more than 0.50%, and the second impurity eluting after butamben is not more than 0.25%.

Assay—
 Mobile phase, Diluent, Internal standard solution, Standard preparation, and *Chromatographic system*—Proceed as directed in the *Assay* under *Moricizine Hydrochloride*.
 Assay preparation—Transfer an accurately counted number of Tablets, equivalent to about 4000 mg of moricizine hydrochloride, to a 2000-mL flask, add 1000.0 mL of *Diluent*, and sonicate until the Tablets have disintegrated. Shake by mechanical means for 30 minutes. Filter a portion of this solution, discarding the first 10 mL of the filtrate. Cover the filter funnel with a watch glass to minimize evaporation of the solvent. Transfer 25.0 mL of the filtrate and 20.0 mL of *Internal standard solution* to a 100-mL volumetric flask, dilute with *Diluent* to volume, and mix. [NOTE—Protect this solution from light.]
 Procedure—Proceed as directed for *Procedure* in the *Assay* under *Moricizine Hydrochloride*. Calculate the quantity, in mg, of moricizine hydrochloride ($C_{22}H_{25}N_3O_4S \cdot HCl$) in each Tablet by the formula:

$$4000(C / N)(R_U / R_S)$$

in which *C* is the concentration, in mg per mL, of USP Moricizine Hydrochloride RS in the *Standard preparation*, N is the number of Tablets taken, and R_U and R_S are the ratios of the peak area responses of the moricizine peak to the butamben peak obtained from the *Assay preparation* and the *Standard preparation*, respectively.

Morphine Sulfate

$(C_{17}H_{19}NO_3)_2 \cdot H_2SO_4 \cdot 5H_2O$ 758.83
Morphinan-3,6-diol, 7,8-didehydro-4,5-epoxy-17-methyl, (5α,6α)-, sulfate (2 : 1) (salt), pentahydrate.
7,8-Didehydro-4,5α-epoxy-17-methylmorphinan-3,6α-diol sulfate (2 : 1) (salt) pentahydrate [*6211-15-0*].
Anhydrous   668.77   [*64-31-3*].

» Morphine Sulfate contains not less than 98.0 percent and not more than 102.0 percent of $(C_{17}H_{19}NO_3)_2 \cdot H_2SO_4$, calculated on the anhydrous basis.

Packaging and storage—Preserve in tight, light-resistant containers. Store up to 40° as permitted by the manufacturer.
USP Reference standards ⟨11⟩—*USP Morphine Sulfate RS.*
Identification—
 A: *Infrared Absorption* ⟨197K⟩: dried at 145° for 1 hour.
 B: To 1 mg in a porcelain crucible or small dish add 0.5 mL of sulfuric acid containing, in each mL, 1 drop of formaldehyde TS: an intense purple color is produced at once, and quickly changes to deep blue-violet(*distinction from codeine, which gives at once an intense violet-blue color, and from hydromorphone, which gives at first a yellow to brown color, changing to pink and then to purplish red*).
 C: To a solution of 5 mg in 5 mL of sulfuric acid in a test tube add 1 drop of ferric chloride TS, mix, and heat in boiling water for 2 minutes: a blue color is produced, and when 1 drop of nitric acid is added, it changes to dark red-brown (*codeine and ethylmorphine give the same color reactions, but hydromorphone and papaverine do not produce this color change*).
 D: A solution (1 in 50) responds to the tests for*Sulfate* ⟨191⟩.
Specific rotation ⟨781S⟩: between −107° and −109.5°.
 Test solution: the equivalent of 20 mg per mL, in water.
Acidity—Dissolve 500 mg in 15 mL of water, add 1 drop of methyl red TS, and titrate with 0.020 N sodium hydroxide: not more than 0.50 mL is required to produce a yellow color.
Water, *Method I* ⟨921⟩: between 10.4% and 13.4% is found.
Residue on ignition ⟨281⟩: not more than 0.1%, from 500 mg.
Chloride—To 10 mL of a solution (1 in 100) add 1 mL of 2 N nitric acid and 1 mL of silver nitrate TS: no precipitate or turbidity is produced immediately.
Ammonium salts—Heat 200 mg with 5 mL of 1 N sodium hydroxide on a steam bath for 1 minute: no odor of ammonia is perceptible.
Limit of foreign alkaloids—Dissolve 1.00 g in 10 mL of 1 N sodium hydroxide in a separator, and shake the solution with three successive portions of 15, 10, and 10 mL of chloroform, passing the chloroform solutions through a small filter previously moistened

with chloroform. Shake the combined chloroform solutions with 5 mL of water, separate the chloroform layer, and carefully evaporate on a steam bath to dryness. To the residue add 10.0 mL of 0.020 N sulfuric acid, and heat gently until dissolved. Cool, add 2 drops of methyl red TS, and titrate the excess acid with 0.020 N sodium hydroxide: not less than 7.5 mL is required (1.5%).

Organic volatile impurities, Method I ⟨467⟩: meets the requirements.

(Official until July 1, 2008)

Assay—
*Mobile phase—*Dissolve 0.73 g of sodium 1-heptanesulfonate in 720 mL of water, add 280 mL of methanol and 10 mL of glacial acetic acid, mix, filter, and degas. Make adjustments if necessary (see *System Suitability* under *Chromatography* ⟨621⟩).

*Standard preparation—*Dissolve an accurately weighed quantity of USP Morphine Sulfate RS in *Mobile phase,* and dilute quantitatively, and stepwise if necessary, with *Mobile phase* to obtain a solution having a known concentration of about 0.24 mg per mL. Prepare a fresh solution daily.

*System suitability preparation—*Dissolve suitable quantities of USP Morphine Sulfate RS and phenol in *Mobile phase* to obtain a solution containing about 0.24 and 0.15 mg per mL, respectively.

*Assay preparation—*Transfer about 24 mg of Morphine Sulfate, accurately weighed, to a 100-mL volumetric flask, dissolve in and dilute with *Mobile phase* to volume, and mix.

Chromatographic system (see *Chromatography* ⟨621⟩)—The liquid chromatograph is equipped with a 284-nm detector and a 3.9-mm × 30-cm column that contains packing L1. The flow rate is about 1.5 mL per minute. Chromatograph the *Standard preparation* and the *System suitability preparation,* and record the peak responses as directed for *Procedure:* the relative retention times are about 0.7 for phenol and 1.0 for morphine sulfate; the resolution, R, between phenol and morphine sulfate is not less than 2.0; the tailing factor for the morphine sulfate peak is not more than 2.0; and the relative standard deviation for replicate injections of the *Standard preparation* is not more than 2.0%.

*Procedure—*Separately inject equal volumes (about 25 µL) of the *Standard preparation* and the *Assay preparation* into the chromatograph, record the chromatograms, and measure the responses for the major peaks. Calculate the quantity, in mg, of $(C_{17}H_{19}NO_3)_2 \cdot H_2SO_4$ in the portion of Morphine Sulfate taken by the formula:

$$100C(r_U / r_S)$$

in which C is the concentration, in mg per mL, of anhydrous morphine sulfate in the *Standard preparation,* as determined from the concentration of USP Morphine Sulfate RS corrected for moisture content by a titrimetric water determination; and r_U and r_S are the peak responses obtained from the *Assay preparation* and the *Standard preparation,* respectively.

Morphine Sulfate Extended-Release Capsules

» Morphine Sulfate Extended-Release Capsules contain not less than 90.0 percent and not more than 110.0 percent of the labeled amount of morphine sulfate pentahydrate [$(C_{17}H_{19}NO_3)_2 \cdot H_2SO_4 \cdot 5H_2O$].

Packaging and storage—Preserve in tight, light-resistant containers, and store at controlled room temperature.

USP Reference standards ⟨11⟩—*USP Morphine Sulfate RS.*

Identification—
A: *Infrared Absorption* ⟨197K⟩.
B: The retention time of the major peak in the chromatogram of the *Assay preparation* corresponds to that in the chromatogram of the *Standard preparation,* as obtained in the *Assay.*

Dissolution ⟨711⟩—
*pH 7.5 Phosphate buffer—*Dissolve 6.8 g of monobasic potassium phosphate and 1.6 g of sodium hydroxide in 1 L of water. Adjust with phosphoric acid or 2 N sodium hydroxide to a pH of 7.5.

*Medium—*Proceed as directed for *Procedure* for *Method B* under *Apparatus 1 and Apparatus 2, Delayed-Release Dosage Forms,* observing the following exceptions. Perform *Acid stage* testing, using 500 mL of 0.1 N hydrochloric acid for 1 hour; and perform *Buffer stage* testing, using 500 mL of *pH 7.5 Phosphate buffer* for not less than 8 hours.

Apparatus 1: 100 rpm.
Times: 1, 4, 6, and 9 hours.
Determine the amount of $(C_{17}H_{19}NO_3)_2 \cdot H_2SO_4 \cdot 5H_2O$ dissolved by employing the following method.

*Mobile phase—*Prepare a filtered and degassed mixture of water, methanol, and glacial acetic acid (72 : 28 : 1), containing 0.73 g of sodium 1-heptanesulfonate. Make adjustments if necessary (see *System Suitability* under *Chromatography* ⟨621⟩).

*System suitability solution—*Dissolve suitable quantities of phenol and USP Morphine Sulfate RS in *Mobile phase* to obtain a solution containing about 0.1 mg of each per mL.

*Standard solution—*Dissolve an accurately weighed quantity of USP Morphine Sulfate RS in *pH 7.5 Phosphate buffer,* and dilute quantitatively, and stepwise if necessary, with *pH 7.5 Phosphate buffer* to obtain a solution having a known concentration corresponding to that of the solution under test.

Chromatographic system (see *Chromatography* ⟨621⟩)—The liquid chromatograph is equipped with a 284-nm detector and a 3.9-mm × 30.0-cm column that contains 10-µm packing L1. The flow rate is about 2 mL per minute. Chromatograph the *System suitability solution,* and record the peak responses as directed for *Procedure:* the relative retention times are about 0.8 for phenol and 1.0 for morphine sulfate; the resolution, R, between the phenol and morphine sulfate peaks is not less than 2.0; the tailing factor for the morphine sulfate peak is not more than 2.0; and the relative standard deviation for replicate injections is not more than 2.0%.

*Procedure—*Separately inject equal volumes (about 25 µL) of the *Standard solution* and the filtered portion of the solution under test into the chromatograph, record the chromatograms, and measure the peak responses. Determine the amount of $(C_{17}H_{19}NO_3)_2 \cdot H_2SO_4 \cdot 5H_2O$ dissolved from the measured peak responses.

*Tolerances—*The percentage of the labeled amount of $(C_{17}H_{19}NO_3)_2 \cdot H_2SO_4 \cdot 5H_2O$ dissolved in 1 hour conforms to *Acceptance Table 3.* The percentages of the labeled amount of $(C_{17}H_{19}NO_3)_2 \cdot H_2SO_4 \cdot 5H_2O$ dissolved at the other times specified conform to *Acceptance Table 2.*

Time (hours)	Amount dissolved
1	not more than 10%
4	between 25% and 50%
6	between 50% and 90%
9	not less than 85%

Uniformity of dosage units ⟨905⟩: meet the requirements.

Chromatographic purity—
*Standard solution—*Prepare as directed in the *Assay* for *Standard preparation.*

Diluting solution, Buffer solution, Mobile phase, Resolution solution, and *Chromatographic system—*Proceed as directed in the *Assay.*

*Test solution—*Use the *Assay preparation.*

*Procedure—*Separately inject equal volumes (about 30 µL) of the *Diluting solution* and the *Test solution* into the chromatograph, record the chromatograms, and measure the peak areas, disregarding the peaks corresponding to those obtained in the chromatogram of the *Diluting solution.* Calculate the percentage of each impurity in the portion of Capsules taken by the formula:

$$100(Fr_i / r_M)$$

in which F is the relative response factor equal to 0.25 for any peak with a relative retention time between 2.2 and 2.8 and equal to 1.0 for all other impurity peaks; r_i is the peak response for each impurity obtained from the *Test solution;* and r_M is the peak response for morphine sulfate obtained from the *Test solution:* not more than 1.0% of any individual impurity is found; and not more than 2.0% of total impurities is found.

Assay—

Diluting solution—Use water, and adjust with phosphoric acid to a pH of 3.60.

Buffer solution—Dissolve 13.8 g of monobasic sodium phosphate in 1 L of water.

Mobile phase—Prepare a filtered and degassed mixture of water, *Buffer solution*, acetonitrile, and triethylamine (874.5 : 100 : 25 : 0.5). Make adjustments if necessary (see *System Suitability* under *Chromatography* ⟨621⟩).

Resolution solution—Dissolve an accurately weighed quantity of USP Morphine Sulfate RS in *Diluting solution* to obtain a solution having a known concentration of about 10 mg per mL. Transfer 1.0 mL of this solution to a 10-mL volumetric flask containing 2.0 mL of 30 percent hydrogen peroxide. Heat, with stirring, in a water bath at a temperature of about 80° for about 30 minutes. Cool to room temperature, dilute with *Diluting solution* to volume, and mix.

Standard preparation—Dissolve an accurately weighed quantity of USP Morphine Sulfate RS in *Diluting solution* to obtain a solution having a known concentration of about 1.0 mg per mL.

Assay preparation—Accurately weigh and transfer the contents of 10 Capsules to a suitable volumetric flask to obtain a solution having a final concentration of about 1 mg of morphine sulfate per mL. Add an amount of methanol equivalent to 4.5% of the flask volume. Mix for about 30 minutes, gently swirling every 5 minutes. Add *Diluting solution* up to about half of the flask volume, and sonicate for 5 minutes to dissolve. Rinse the inner wall and neck of the flask with an amount of methanol equivalent to about 0.5% of the flask volume, dilute with *Diluting solution* to volume, and mix. Pass through a suitable filter, and use the clear filtrate.

Chromatographic system (see *Chromatography* ⟨621⟩)—The liquid chromatograph is equipped with a 245-nm detector, a suitable guard column that contains packing L1, and a 3.9-mm × 30.0-cm column that contains 10-μm packing L1. The flow rate is about 2 mL per minute. Chromatograph the *Resolution solution*, and record the peak responses as directed for *Procedure*: the relative retention times are between 1.2 and 1.4 for morphine *N*-oxide and between 2.2 and 2.8 for pseudomorphine; and the resolution, *R*, between the morphine *N*-oxide and morphine sulfate peaks is not less than 2.0. Chromatograph the *Standard preparation*, and record the peak responses as directed for *Procedure*: the relative standard deviation for replicate injections is not more than 2.0%.

Procedure—Separately inject equal volumes (about 30 μL) of the *Standard preparation* and the *Assay preparation* into the chromatograph, record the chromatograms, and measure the peak responses. Calculate the quantity, in mg, of morphine sulfate pentahydrate [(C$_{17}$H$_{19}$NO$_3$)$_2$ · H$_2$SO$_4$ · 5H$_2$O] in the portion of Capsules taken by the formula:

$$CV(r_U / r_S)$$

in which *C* is the concentration, in mg per mL, of USP Morphine Sulfate RS in the *Standard preparation*; *V* is the volume of the volumetric flask used to prepare the *Assay preparation*; and r_U and r_S are the peak responses obtained from the *Assay preparation* and the *Standard preparation*, respectively.

Morphine Sulfate Injection

» Morphine Sulfate Injection is a sterile solution of Morphine Sulfate in Water for Injection. It contains not less than 90.0 percent and not more than 110.0 percent of the labeled amount of morphine sulfate pentahydrate [(C$_{17}$H$_{19}$NO$_3$)$_2$ · H$_2$SO$_4$ · 5H$_2$O]. Injection intended for intramuscular or intravenous administration may contain sodium chloride as a tonicity-adjusting agent, and suitable antioxidants and antimicrobial agents. Injection intended for intrathecal or epidural use may contain sodium chloride as a tonicity-adjusting agent, but contains no other added substances.

Packaging and storage—Preserve in single-dose or in multiple-dose containers, preferably of Type I glass, protected from light. Preserve Injection labeled "Preservative-free" in single-dose containers.

Labeling—It meets the requirements for *Labeling* under *Injections* ⟨1⟩. Label it also to state that the Injection is not to be used if its color is darker than pale yellow, if it is discolored in any other way, or if it contains a precipitate. Injection containing no antioxidant or antimicrobial agents prominently bears on its label the words "Preservative-free," and includes, in its labeling, its routes of administration and the statement that it is not to be heat-sterilized. Injection containing antioxidant or antimicrobial agents includes in its labeling its routes of administration and the statement that it is not for intrathecal or epidural use.

USP Reference standards ⟨11⟩—*USP Morphine Sulfate RS. USP Endotoxin RS.*

Identification—

A: Dilute with methanol, if necessary, a volume of Injection to obtain a solution containing 500 μg per mL. Apply 20 μL of this solution and 20 μL of a solution of USP Morphine Sulfate RS in a mixture of methanol and water (1 : 1) containing 500 μg per mL to a suitable thin-layer chromatographic plate (see *Chromatography* ⟨621⟩) coated with a 250-μm layer of chromatographic silica gel mixture. Allow the spots to dry, and develop the chromatogram in a solvent system consisting of a mixture of acetone, methanol, and ammonium hydroxide (50 : 50 : 1) until the solvent front has moved about three-fourths of the length of the plate. Remove the plate from the developing chamber, mark the solvent front, and allow the solvent to evaporate. Locate the spots on the plate by examination under short-wavelength UV light: the R_F value of the principal spot obtained from the Injection corresponds to that obtained from the Standard solution.

B: It responds to the barium chloride test for *Sulfate* ⟨191⟩.

Bacterial endotoxins ⟨85⟩—It contains not more than 17.0 USP Endotoxin Units per mg of morphine sulfate; if labeled for intrathecal use, it contains not more than 14.29 USP Endotoxin Units per mg of morphine sulfate.

pH ⟨791⟩: between 2.5 and 6.5.

Particulate matter ⟨788⟩—meets the requirements under small-volume Injections.

Other requirements—It meets the requirements under *Injections* ⟨1⟩.

Assay—

Mobile phase, Standard preparation, System suitability preparation, and *Chromatographic system*—Prepare as directed in the *Assay* under *Morphine Sulfate*.

Assay preparation—Transfer an accurately measured volume of Injection, equivalent to about 24 mg of morphine sulfate, to a 100-mL volumetric flask, dilute with *Mobile phase* to volume, and mix.

Procedure—Proceed as directed for *Procedure* in the *Assay* under *Morphine Sulfate*. Calculate the quantity, in mg, of morphine sulfate pentahydrate [(C$_{17}$H$_{19}$NO$_3$)$_2$ · H$_2$SO$_4$ · 5H$_2$O] in each mL of the Injection taken by the formula:

$$(758.85 / 668.77)(100C / V)(r_U / r_S)$$

in which 758.85 and 668.77 are the molecular weights of morphine sulfate pentahydrate and anhydrous morphine sulfate, respectively, *V* is the volume, in mL, of Injection taken, and the other terms are as defined therein.

Morphine Sulfate Suppositories

» Morphine Sulfate Suppositories contain not less than 90.0 percent and not more than 110.0 percent of the labeled amount of morphine sulfate pentahydrate [(C$_{17}$H$_{19}$NO$_3$)$_2$ · H$_2$SO$_4$ · 5H$_2$O].

SUPPOSITORIES COMPOUNDED IN FATTY ACID BASE

Prepare Morphine Sulfate Suppositories in Fatty Acid Base as follows (see *Pharmaceutical Compounding—Nonsterile Preparations* ⟨795⟩):

Morphine Sulfate	50 mg
Silica Gel	25 mg
Fatty Acid Base, a sufficient quantity to make one suppository	

Calibrate the actual molds with the Fatty Acid Base that is used for preparing the Suppositories, and adjust the formula accordingly. Mix thoroughly the Morphine Sulfate and Silica Gel to obtain a uniform powder. Heat the Fatty Acid Base slowly and evenly until melted. Slowly add the powder to the melted base, with stirring. Mix thoroughly, and pour into molds. Cool, trim, and wrap.

Packaging and storage—Preserve in tight containers, and store in a refrigerator.

Labeling—Label Suppositories to state that they are Morphine Sulfate Suppositories in a Fatty Acid Base and to state that they are for rectal use only. Label Suppositories to state that they are to be stored in a refrigerator (2° to 8°). The label also bears a warning that the Suppositories are a specially formulated strength to be used only by the patient for whom they were prescribed, and that wrappers are to be removed prior to use.

USP Reference standards ⟨11⟩—*USP Morphine Sulfate RS*.

Uniformity of dosage units ⟨905⟩: meet the requirements for *Weight Variation*.

Beyond-use date—Ninety days after the day on which they were compounded.

Compliance assay for suppositories compounded in fatty acid base—

Mobile phase—Dissolve 5.5 g of sodium 1-heptanesulfonate in 700 mL of water. Add 300 mL of methanol and 10 mL of glacial acetic acid, mix, filter, and degas. Make adjustments if necessary (see *System Suitability* under *Chromatography* ⟨621⟩).

Standard preparation—Dissolve an accurately weighed quantity of USP Morphine Sulfate RS in *Mobile phase*, and dilute quantitatively, and stepwise if necessary, with *Mobile phase* to obtain a solution having a known concentration of about 0.5 mg per mL. [NOTE—Prepare this solution fresh daily.]

System suitability preparation—Prepare a solution in *Mobile phase* containing, in each mL, about 0.24 mg of USP Morphine Sulfate RS and 0.15 mg of phenol.

Assay preparation—Transfer 1 Suppository to a 60-mL separator containing 20 mL of chloroform and 20 mL of 0.01 N hydrochloric acid, and shake to dissolve the Suppository. Transfer the chloroform layer to a 250-mL separator. Extract the aqueous layer with a second 20-mL portion of chloroform, and combine the chloroform extracts in the 250-mL separator. Wash the chloroform extracts with two additional 20-mL portions of 0.01 N hydrochloric acid, combine the aqueous layers in a 100-mL volumetric flask, dilute with *Mobile phase* to volume, and mix. Pass this solution through a filter having a 0.45-μm or finer porosity, discarding the first 4 mL of the filtrate.

Chromatographic system (see *Chromatography* ⟨621⟩)—The liquid chromatograph is equipped with a 284-nm detector and a 4.6-mm × 25-cm column that contains packing L1. The column temperature is maintained at 30°. The flow rate is about 1.5 mL per minute. Chromatograph the *Standard preparation* and the *System suitability preparation*, and record the peak responses as directed for *Procedure*: the relative retention times are about 0.7 for phenol and 1.0 for morphine; the resolution, R, between phenol and morphine is not less than 2.0; the tailing factor for the morphine peak is not more than 2.0; and the relative standard deviation for replicate injections of the *Standard preparation* is not more than 2.0%.

Procedure—Separately inject equal volumes (about 20 μL) of the *Standard preparation* and the *Assay preparation* into the chromatograph, record the chromatograms, and measure the responses for the major peaks. Calculate the quantity, in mg, of morphine sulfate pentahydrate [$(C_{17}H_{19}NO_3)_2 \cdot H_2SO_4 \cdot 5H_2O$] in the Suppository taken by the formula:

$$(758.83/668.77)(100C)(r_U/r_S)$$

in which 758.83 and 668.77 are the molecular weights of morphine sulfate pentahydrate and anhydrous morphine sulfate, respectively; C is the concentration, in mg per mL, of anhydrous morphine sulfate in the *Standard preparation*, as determined from the concentration of USP Morphine Sulfate RS corrected for moisture content by a titrimetric water determination; and r_U and r_S are the peak responses obtained from the *Assay preparation* and the *Standard preparation*, respectively.

SUPPOSITORIES COMPOUNDED IN POLYETHYLENE GLYCOL BASE

Prepare Morphine Sulfate Suppositories in Polyethylene Glycol Base as follows (see *Pharmaceutical Compounding—Nonsterile Preparations* ⟨795⟩):

Morphine Sulfate	50 mg
Silica Gel	25 mg
Polyethylene Glycol Base, a sufficient quantity to make one suppository	

Calibrate the actual molds with Polyethylene Glycol Base that is used for preparing the Suppositories, and adjust the formula accordingly. Mix thoroughly the Morphine Sulfate and Silica Gel to obtain a uniform powder. Heat the Polyethylene Glycol Base slowly and evenly until melted. Slowly add the powder to the melted base, with stirring. Mix thoroughly, and pour into molds. Cool, trim, and wrap.

Packaging and storage—Preserve in tight containers, and store in a refrigerator. Do not dispense or store polyethylene glycol–base suppositories in polystyrene containers.

Labeling—Label Suppositories to state that they are Morphine Sulfate Suppositories in a Polyethylene Glycol Base and to state that they are for rectal use only. Label Suppositories to state that they are to be stored in a refrigerator (2° to 8°). The label also bears a warning that the Suppositories are a specially formulated strength to be used only by the patient for whom they were prescribed, and that wrappers are to be removed prior to use.

USP Reference standards ⟨11⟩—*USP Morphine Sulfate RS*.

Uniformity of dosage units ⟨905⟩: meet the requirements for *Weight Variation*.

Beyond-use date—Ninety days after the day on which they were compounded.

Compliance assay for suppositories compounded in polyethylene glycol base—

Mobile phase, *Standard preparation*, *System suitability preparation*, and *Chromatographic system*—Proceed as directed in the *Compliance assay for suppositories compounded in fatty acid base*.

Assay preparation—Transfer 1 Suppository to a 100-mL volumetric flask, and add about 70 mL of *Mobile phase*. Sonicate for 15 minutes to dissolve the Suppository, cool, dilute with *Mobile phase* to volume, and mix. Pass a 10-mL portion of the solution through a filter having a 0.45-μm or finer porosity, discarding the first 4 mL of the filtrate.

Procedure—Proceed as directed in the *Compliance assay for suppositories compounded in fatty acid base*. Calculate the quantity, in mg, of morphine sulfate pentahydrate [$(C_{17}H_{19}NO_3)_2 \cdot H_2SO_4 \cdot 5H_2O$] in the Suppository taken by the formula:

$$(758.83/668.77)(100C)(r_U/r_S)$$

in which the terms are as defined therein.

Morrhuate Sodium Injection

» Morrhuate Sodium Injection is a sterile solution of the sodium salts of the fatty acids of Cod Liver Oil. It contains, in each mL, not less than 46.5 mg and not more than 53.5 mg of morrhuate sodium. A suitable antimicrobial agent, not to exceed 0.5 percent, and ethyl alcohol or benzyl alcohol, not to exceed 3.0 percent, may be added.

NOTE—Morrhuate Sodium Injection may show a separation of solid matter on standing. Do not use the material if such solid does not dissolve completely upon warming.

Packaging and storage—Preserve in single-dose or in multiple-dose containers, preferably of Type I glass. It may be packaged in 50-mL multiple-dose containers.

USP Reference standards ⟨11⟩—USP Endotoxin RS.

Identification—Evaporate about 5 mL of the chloroform solution of the fatty acids obtained in the test for *Iodine value of the fatty acids* on a steam bath nearly to dryness, dissolve the residue in 1 mL of chloroform, and add 1 drop of sulfuric acid: a transient red color is produced, and it changes to brown-red.

Bacterial endotoxins ⟨85⟩—It contains not more than 1.4 USP Endotoxin Units per mg of morrhuate sodium.

Acidity and alkalinity—To 5 mL of Injection add 5 mL of alcohol and 2 drops of phenolphthalein TS. If no red color is produced, not more than 0.50 mL of 0.10 N sodium hydroxide is required to impart a distinct red color. If a red color is produced, not more than 0.30 mL of 0.10 N acid is required to discharge it. For concentrations of morrhuate sodium other than 5%, no larger than proportional volumes of alkali and acid are required.

Iodine value of the fatty acids—Transfer to a tared, 125-mL conical flask the solvent hexane solution of the fatty acids obtained in the *Assay*. Evaporate at about 60° to dryness, dry the residue in vacuum over silica gel for 18 hours, and weigh. Dissolve the residue in chloroform to make 100.0 mL of solution, and determine the iodine value (see *Fats and Fixed Oils* ⟨401⟩) on a 25.0-mL aliquot of the solution: the iodine value is not less than 130.

Other requirements—It meets the requirements under *Injections* ⟨1⟩, except that at times it may show a slight turbidity or precipitate.

Assay—Transfer an accurately measured volume of Injection, equivalent to about 500 mg of morrhuate sodium, to a small separator containing 30.0 mL of 0.1 N sulfuric acid VS, add 25 mL of solvent hexane, shake gently, and allow to separate. Withdraw the aqueous layer into a beaker or flask, and wash the solvent hexane layer with two 10-mL portions of water, adding the washings to the main aqueous solution. Retain the hexane solution for the test for *Iodine value of the fatty acids*. Add methyl orange TS, and titrate the excess acid in the aqueous solution with 0.1 N sodium hydroxide VS. Each mL of 0.1 N sulfuric acid is equivalent to 32.4 mg of morrhuate sodium.

Mumps Skin Test Antigen

» Mumps Skin Test Antigen conforms to the regulations of the FDA concerning biologics (see *Biologics* ⟨1041⟩). It is a sterile suspension of formaldehyde-inactivated mumps virus prepared from the extra-embryonic fluids of the mumps virus-infected chicken embryo, concentrated and purified by differential centrifugation, and diluted with isotonic sodium chloride solution. It contains not less than 20 complement-fixing units in each mL. It contains approximately 0.006 M glycine as a stabilizing agent, and it contains a preservative.

Packaging and storage—Preserve at a temperature between 2° and 8°.

Expiration date—The expiration date is not later than 18 months after date of manufacture or date of issue from manufacturer's cold storage (5°, 1 year).

Labeling—Label it to state that it was prepared in embryonated chicken eggs and that a separate syringe and needle are to be used for each individual injection.

Mumps Virus Vaccine Live

» Mumps Virus Vaccine Live conforms to the regulations of the FDA concerning biologics (630.50 to 630.57) (see *Biologics* ⟨1041⟩). It is a bacterially sterile preparation of live virus derived from a strain of mumps virus tested for neurovirulence in monkeys, and for immunogenicity, free from all demonstrable viable microbial agents except unavoidable bacteriophage, and found suitable for human immunization. The strain is grown for the purpose of vaccine production on chicken embryo primary cell tissue cultures derived from pathogen-free flocks, meets the requirements of the specific safety tests in adult and suckling mice; the requirements of the tests in monkey kidney, chicken embryo and human tissue cell cultures and embryonated eggs; and the requirements of the tests for absence of *Mycobacterium tuberculosis* and of avian leucosis, unless the production cultures were derived from certified avian leucosis-free sources and the control fluids were tested for avian leucosis. The strain cultures are treated to remove all intact tissue cells. The Vaccine meets the requirements of the specific tissue culture test for live virus titer, in a single immunizing dose, of not less than the equivalent of 5000 TCID$_{50}$ (quantity of virus estimated to infect 50% of inoculated cultures × 5000) when tested in parallel with the U.S. Reference Mumps Virus, Live. It may contain suitable antimicrobial agents.

Packaging and storage—Preserve in single-dose containers, or in light-resistant, multiple-dose containers, at a temperature between 2° and 8°. Multiple-dose containers for 50 doses are adapted for use only in jet injectors, and those for 10 doses for use by jet or syringe injection.

Expiration date—The expiration date is 1 to 2 years, depending on the manufacturer's data, after date of issue from manufacturer's cold storage (−20°, 1 year).

Labeling—Label the Vaccine in multiple-dose containers to indicate that the contents are intended solely for use by jet injector or for use by either jet or syringe injection, whichever is applicable. Label the Vaccine in single-dose containers, if such containers are not light-resistant, to state that it should be protected from sunlight. Label it also to state that constituted Vaccine should be discarded if not used within 8 hours.

Mupirocin

$C_{26}H_{44}O_9$ 500.62

Nonanoic acid, 9-[[3-methyl-1-oxo-4-[tetrahydro-3,4-dihydroxy-5-[[3-(2-hydroxy-1-methylpropyl)oxiranyl]methyl]-2H-pyran-2-yl]-2-butenyl]oxy]-,[2S-2α(E),3β,4β,5α[2R*, 3R*(1R*,[2R*)]]]-.

(E)-(2S,3R,4R,5S)-5-[(2S,3S,4S,5S)-2,3-Epoxy-5-hydroxy-4-methylhexyl]tetrahydro-3,4-dihydroxy-β-methyl-2H-pyran-2-crotonic acid, ester with 9-hydroxynonanoic acid   [12650-69-0].

» Mupirocin contains not less than 920 µg and not more than 1020 µg of mupirocin ($C_{26}H_{44}O_9$) per mg, calculated on the anhydrous basis.

Packaging and storage—Preserve in tight containers.

USP Reference standards ⟨11⟩—*USP Mupirocin RS. USP Mupirocin Lithium RS.*

Identification—The IR absorption spectrum of a mineral oil dispersion of it exhibits maxima only at the same wavelengths as that of a similar preparation of USP Mupirocin RS.

Crystallinity ⟨695⟩: meets the requirements.

pH ⟨791⟩: between 3.5 and 4.5, in a saturated aqueous solution.

Water, *Method I* ⟨921⟩: not more than 1.0%.

Assay—

pH 6.3 phosphate buffer—Prepare 0.05 M monobasic sodium phosphate, and adjust with 10 N sodium hydroxide to a pH of 6.3 ± 0.2.

Mobile phase—Prepare a suitable mixture of *pH 6.3 phosphate buffer* and acetonitrile (750 : 250), pass through a suitable filter of 0.5 µm or finer porosity, and degas. Make adjustments if necessary (see *System Suitability* under *Chromatography* ⟨621⟩).

Standard preparation—Transfer about 11 mg of USP Mupirocin Lithium RS, accurately weighed, to a 100-mL volumetric flask, add 25 mL of acetonitrile, and swirl to dissolve. Dilute with *pH 6.3 phosphate buffer* to volume, and mix.

Resolution solution—Adjust 10 mL of *Standard preparation* with 6 N hydrochloric acid to a pH of 2.0, allow to stand for 2 hours, and adjust with 5 N sodium hydroxide to a pH of 6.3 ± 0.2.

Assay preparation—Transfer about 11 mg of Mupirocin, accurately weighed, to a 100-mL volumetric flask, add 25 mL of acetonitrile, and swirl to dissolve. Dilute with *pH 6.3 phosphate buffer* to volume, and mix.

Chromatographic system (see *Chromatography* ⟨621⟩)—The liquid chromatograph is equipped with a 229-nm detector and a 4.6-mm × 25-cm column that contains packing L1 based on spherical silica particles. The flow rate is about 2 mL per minute. Chromatograph the *Resolution solution*, and record the peak responses as directed for *Procedure:* the relative retention times are about 0.9 for the mupirocin acid hydrolysis product and 1.0 for mupirocin, and the resolution, *R*, between the mupirocin acid hydrolysis product and mupirocin is not less than 2.0. Chromatograph the *Standard preparation*, and record the peak responses as directed for *Procedure:* the tailing factor is not more than 2, the column efficiency is not less than 1500 theoretical plates when calculated by the formula:

$$5.545(t_r/W_{h/2})^2$$

in which the terms are as defined therein. The relative standard deviation for replicate injections is not more than 2.0%.

Procedure—[NOTE—Use peak areas where peak responses are indicated.] Separately inject equal volumes (about 20 µL) of the *Standard preparation* and the *Assay preparation* into the chromatograph, record the chromatograms, and measure the responses for the major peaks. Calculate the quantity, in µg, of mupirocin ($C_{26}H_{44}O_9$) in each mg of Mupirocin taken by the formula:

$$(M_S E / M_U)(r_U / r_S)$$

in which M_S is the weight, in mg, of USP Mupirocin Lithium RS taken to prepare the *Standard preparation*; *E* is the mupirocin equivalent, in µg per mg, of USP Mupirocin Lithium RS; M_U is the weight, in mg, of mupirocin taken to prepare the *Assay preparation*; and r_U and r_S are the mupirocin peak responses obtained from the *Assay preparation* and the *Standard preparation*, respectively.

Mupirocin Calcium

$C_{52}H_{86}CaO_{18} \cdot 2H_2O$ 1075.34

Nonanoic acid, 9-[[3-Methyl-1-oxo-4-[tetrahydro-3,4-dihydroxy-5-[[3-(2-hydroxy-1-methylpropyl)oxiranyl]methyl]-2H-pyran-2-yl]-2-butenyl]oxy-, calcium salt (2 : 1), dihydrate, [2S-[2α(E),3β,4β,5α[2R*,3R*(1R*,2R*)]]]-.

(αE,2S,3R,4R,5S)-5-[(2S,3S,4S,5S)-2,3-Epoxy-5-hydroxy-4-methylhexyl]tetrahydro-3,4-dihydroxy-β-methyl-2H-pyran-2-crotonic acid, ester with 9-hydroxynonanoic acid, calcium salt (2 : 1), dihydrate   [115074-43-6].

» Mupirocin Calcium contains the equivalent of not less than 865 µg and not more than 936 µg of mupirocin ($C_{26}H_{44}O_9$) per mg.

Packaging and storage—Preserve in tight containers. Store at 25°, excursions permitted between 15° and 30°.

USP Reference standards ⟨11⟩—*USP Mupirocin Calcium RS. USP Mupirocin Lithium RS.*

Identification—

A: *Infrared Absorption* ⟨197M⟩—[NOTE—Do not dry or grind extensively.]

B: *Ultraviolet Absorption* ⟨197U⟩—

Solution: 20 µg per mL.

Medium: methanol.

C: When moistened with hydrochloric acid, it meets the requirements of the flame test for *Calcium* ⟨191⟩.

Specific rotation ⟨781S⟩: between −16° and −20°.

Test solution: 50 mg per mL, in methanol.

Water, *Method I* ⟨921⟩: not less than 3.0% and not more than 4.5%.

Chloride ⟨221⟩—Dissolve 50 mg in a mixture of 1 mL of 2 N nitric acid and 15 mL of methanol. Add 1 mL of silver nitrate TS: the turbidity does not exceed that produced by 0.70 mL of 0.020 N hydrochloric acid (0.5%).

Related compounds—

0.1 M Ammonium acetate—Prepare as directed in the *Assay*.

Mobile phase—Prepare a filtered and degassed mixture of *0.1 M Ammonium acetate* and tetrahydrofuran (70 : 30). Make adjustments if necessary (see *System Suitability* under *Chromatography* ⟨621⟩).

pH 4 Acetate buffer—Transfer about 13.6 g of sodium acetate to a 1000-mL volumetric flask, and dissolve in about 900 mL of water. Adjust with glacial acetic acid to a pH of 4.0, and dilute with water to volume.

Diluent—Prepare a mixture of *pH 4 Acetate buffer* and methanol (1 : 1).

Standard solution—Transfer about 25 mg of USP Mupirocin Lithium RS, accurately weighed, to a 200-mL volumetric flask, dissolve in and dilute with *Diluent* to volume, and mix.

Test solution—Transfer about 50 mg of Mupirocin Calcium, accurately weighed, to a 10-mL volumetric flask, dissolve in and dilute with *Diluent* to volume, and mix.

Resolution solution—Adjust 10 mL of the *Standard solution* with 6 N hydrochloric acid to a pH of 2.0, allow to stand for 20 hours, and adjust with 5 N sodium hydroxide to a pH of 4.0.

Chromatographic system (see *Chromatography* ⟨621⟩)—The liquid chromatograph is equipped with a 240-nm detector and a 4.6-mm × 25-cm column that contains 5-μm packing L7. The flow rate is about 1 mL per minute. Chromatograph the *Resolution solution*, and record the peak responses as directed for *Procedure*: the resolution, R, between the second of two peaks corresponding to hydrolysis products and the peak corresponding to mupirocin is not less than 7.0. Chromatograph the *Standard solution*, and record the peak responses as directed for *Procedure*: the relative retention times are about 0.75 (6 minutes) for pseudomonic acid D and 1.0 (14 minutes) for mupirocin; the column efficiency for the mupirocin peak is not less than 3000 theoretical plates; the tailing factor for the mupirocin peak is not more than 2; and the relative standard deviation of the mupirocin peak for replicate injections is not more than 5%.

Procedure—Separately inject equal volumes (about 20 μL) of the *Standard solution* and the *Test solution* into the chromatograph, and measure the peak area responses for all of the peaks. Calculate the percentage of each related compound in the portion of Mupirocin Calcium taken by the formula:

$$(E/200)(W_S / W_U)(r_i / r_S)$$

in which E is the mupirocin equivalent, in μg per mg, of USP Mupirocin Lithium RS; W_S is the weight, in mg, of USP Mupirocin Lithium RS taken to prepare the *Standard solution*; W_U is the weight, in mg, of Mupirocin Calcium taken to prepare the *Test solution*; r_i is the peak area for any impurity obtained from the *Test solution*; and r_S is the peak area for mupirocin obtained from the *Standard solution*: the area of any peak corresponding to pseudomonic acid D is not greater than 2.5%; the area of any peak, excluding the mupirocin peak and any peak corresponding to pseudomonic acid D, is not greater than 1%; and the sum of the areas of all the peaks, excluding the principal peak, is not greater than 4.5%. Disregard any peak with an area less than 0.05 times the area of the mupirocin peak in the chromatogram obtained from the *Standard solution*.

Assay—

0.1 M Ammonium acetate—Transfer about 7.7 g of ammonium acetate to a 1000-mL volumetric flask, dissolve in about 900 mL of water, adjust with glacial acetic acid to a pH of 5.7, and dilute with water to volume.

Mobile phase—Prepare a filtered and degassed mixture of *0.1 M Ammonium acetate* and tetrahydrofuran (68 : 32). Make adjustments if necessary (see *System Suitability* under *Chromatography* ⟨621⟩).

Standard preparation—Transfer about 25 mg of USP Mupirocin Lithium RS, accurately weighed, to a 200-mL volumetric flask, dissolve in 5 mL of methanol, dilute with *0.1 M Ammonium acetate* to volume, and mix.

Assay preparation—Transfer about 25 mg of Mupirocin Calcium, accurately weighed, to a 200-mL volumetric flask, dissolve in 5 mL of methanol, dilute with *0.1 M Ammonium acetate* to volume, and mix.

Resolution solution—Adjust 10 mL of the *Standard preparation* with 6 N hydrochloric acid to a pH of 2.0, and allow to stand for 20 hours.

Chromatographic system (see *Chromatography* ⟨621⟩)—The liquid chromatograph is equipped with a 230-nm detector and a 4.6-mm × 25-cm column that contains 5-μm packing L7. The flow rate is about 1 mL per minute. Chromatograph the *Resolution solution*, and record the peak responses as directed for *Procedure*: the resolution, R, of the second of the two peaks corresponding to hydrolysis products and the peak corresponding to mupirocin is not less than 7.0. Chromatograph the *Standard preparation*, and record the peak responses as directed for *Procedure*: the relative standard deviation for replicate injections is not more than 1.0%.

Procedure—Separately inject equal volumes (about 20 μL) of the *Standard preparation* and the *Assay preparation* into the chromatograph, and measure the peak area responses for the major peaks.

Calculate the quantity, in μg, of mupirocin ($C_{26}H_{44}O_9$) in each mg of Mupirocin Calcium taken by the formula:

$$E(M_S / M_U)(r_U / r_S)$$

in which E is the designated mupirocin equivalent, in μg, of mupirocin in each mg of USP Mupirocin Lithium RS; M_S is the weight, in mg, of USP Mupirocin Lithium RS taken to prepare the *Standard preparation*; M_U is the weight, in mg, of Mupirocin Calcium taken to prepare the *Assay preparation*; and r_U and r_S are the mupirocin peak area responses obtained from the *Assay preparation* and the *Standard preparation*, respectively.

Mupirocin Cream

» Mupirocin Cream contains a quantity of Mupirocin Calcium equivalent to not less than 90.0 percent and not more than 120.0 percent of the labeled amount of mupirocin ($C_{26}H_{44}O_9$). It may contain one or more suitable buffers, dispersants, and preservatives.

Packaging and storage—Preserve in collapsible tubes or well-closed containers. Store at 25°, excursions permitted between 15° and 30°.

Labeling—Label it to indicate that it contains Mupirocin Calcium and its equivalent content of mupirocin.

USP Reference standards ⟨11⟩—*USP Mupirocin Lithium RS.*

Identification—The retention time of the major peak in the chromatogram of the *Assay preparation* corresponds to that in the chromatogram of the *Standard preparation*, as obtained in the *Assay*.

Minimum fill ⟨755⟩: meets the requirements.

pH ⟨791⟩: between 6.0 and 8.0.

Microbial limits ⟨61⟩—It meets the requirements of the tests for absence of *Staphylococcus aureus* and *Pseudomonas aeruginosa*. The total aerobic microbial count does not exceed 100 cfu per g.

Related compounds—

0.1 M Ammonium acetate, Solution A, Solution B, Mobile phase, pH 6.3 Phosphate buffer, and *Chromatographic system*—Proceed as directed in the *Assay*.

Sodium acetate solution—Add 5.8 mL of glacial acetic acid to 900 mL of water, adjust with sodium hydroxide TS to a pH of 4.0, dilute with water to 1000 mL, and mix.

Tetrahydrofuran solution—Mix 750 mL of tetrahydrofuran and 250 mL of water.

Sodium acetate and tetrahydrofuran solution—Prepare a mixture of *Sodium acetate solution* and *Tetrahydrofuran solution* (50 : 50).

Standard solution—Dissolve an accurately weighed portion of USP Mupirocin Lithium RS in *pH 6.3 Phosphate buffer*. Dilute an accurately measured volume of this solution quantitatively to obtain a solution containing 0.1 mg of mupirocin per mL.

Test stock solution—Transfer an accurately weighed quantity of Cream, equivalent to about 50 mg of mupirocin, to a screw-capped centrifuge tube. Add 5.0 mL of *Tetrahydrofuran solution*, cap, and disperse the Cream by mixing on a vortex mixer and shaking. Add 5.0 mL of *Sodium acetate solution*, cap, and mix. Centrifuge for about 15 minutes. Withdraw the lower layer from the tube, pass it through a filter having a 0.5-μm or finer porosity, and use the filtrate.

Test solution—Transfer 1.0 mL of the *Test stock solution* to a 50-mL volumetric flask, dilute with *Sodium acetate and tetrahydrofuran solution* to volume, mix, and pass through a filter having a 0.5-μm or finer porosity.

pH 4 Acetate buffer—Transfer about 13.6 g of sodium acetate to a 1000-mL volumetric flask, and dissolve in about 900 mL of water. Adjust with glacial acetic acid to a pH of 4.0, and dilute with water to volume.

Chromatographic system (see *Chromatography* ⟨621⟩)—Chromatograph the *Standard solution*, and record the peak responses as directed for *Procedure*: typical retention times are about 16 minutes for pseudomonic acid D and 21 minutes for mupirocin; the relative retention times are 0.36 for pseudomonic acid F, 0.6 for mupirocin degradation product A, 0.63 for mupirocin degradation product B, 0.74 for pseudomonic acid D, 0.9 for pseudomonic acid B, 1.0 for mupirocin, 1.15 for mupirocin related compound A, 1.23 for mupirocin related compound B, 2.03 for pseudomonic acid C, and 2.15 to 2.33 for pseudomonic acid E; the resolution, *R*, between pseudomonic acid D and mupirocin is not less than 3; the column efficiency for the mupirocin peak is not less than 7000 theoretical plates; the tailing factor for the mupirocin peak is not more than 1.75; and the relative standard deviation of the mupirocin peak for replicate injections is not more than 2%.

Procedure—[NOTE—Ensure that buffers, dispersants, or preservatives in the formulation do not interfere with quantification of either impurities or degradation products.] Separately inject equal volumes (about 20 µL) of the *Test stock solution* and the *Test solution* into the chromatograph, and measure the peak responses for all of the peaks that do not correspond to buffers, dispersants, or preservatives. Calculate the percentage of each related compound and degradation product relative to mupirocin in the portion of Cream taken by the formula:

$$2(r_i / r_M)$$

in which r_i is the peak response for each related compound or degradation product obtained from the *Test stock solution;* and r_M is the peak response of the mupirocin peak obtained from the *Test solution:* not more than 3.0% of pseudomonic acid D is found; not more than 8.5% of mupirocin degradation product A is found; not more than 16% of mupirocin degradation product B is found; not more than 1.2% of any other individual impurity or degradation product is found; and not more that 30% of total impurities and degradation products is found.

Assay—

0.1 M Ammonium acetate—Prepare as directed in the *Assay* under *Mupirocin Calcium*.

Solution A—Prepare a filtered and degassed mixture of *0.1 M Ammonium acetate* and tetrahydrofuran (75 : 25).

Solution B—Prepare a filtered and degassed mixture of *0.1 M Ammonium acetate* and tetrahydrofuran (70 : 30).

Mobile phase—Use variable mixtures of *Solution A* and *Solution B* as directed for *Chromatographic system*. Make adjustments if necessary (see *System Suitability* under *Chromatography* ⟨621⟩).

pH 6.3 Phosphate buffer—Dissolve 69 g of monobasic sodium phosphate in 800 mL of water, adjust with sodium hydroxide TS to a pH of 6.3, dilute with water to 1000 mL, and mix.

Standard preparation—Transfer about 21 mg of USP Mupirocin Lithium RS, accurately weighed, to a 200-mL volumetric flask, and dissolve in and dilute with *pH 6.3 Phosphate buffer* to volume.

Assay preparation—Transfer an accurately weighed quantity of Cream, equivalent to about 10 mg of mupirocin, to a 100-mL volumetric flask. Add 50 mL of *pH 6.3 Phosphate buffer* and 25 mL of tetrahydrofuran. Insert the stopper into the flask, mix on a vortex mixer, and shake for 1 to 3 minutes. Dilute with *pH 6.3 Phosphate buffer* to volume. Allow to stand until the oil layer separates out, then dilute the aqueous layer with *pH 6.3 Phosphate buffer* to volume. Repeat 2 to 3 times until as much of the oil layer has separated out as possible. After the final dilution, pass the final solution (bottom layer) through a filter having a 0.5-µm or finer porosity.

Chromatographic system (see *Chromatography* ⟨621⟩)—The liquid chromatograph is equipped with a 240-nm detector and a 4.6-mm × 25-cm column that contains 7-µm packing L7. The flow rate is about 1 mL per minute. Maintain the column at a constant temperature up to 35°. The chromatograph is programmed as follows.

Time (minutes)	Solution A (%)	Solution B (%)	Elution
0	100	0	equilibration
0–6	100	0	isocratic
6–35	100→0	0→100	linear gradient
35–55	0	100	isocratic
55–55.01	0→100	100→0	immediate
55.01–65	100	0	isocratic

Chromatograph the *Standard preparation*, and record the peak responses as directed for *Procedure:* typical retention times are about 16 minutes for pseudomonic acid D and 21 minutes for mupirocin; the resolution, *R*, between pseudomonic acid D and mupirocin is not less than 3; the column efficiency for the mupirocin peak is not less than 7000 theoretical plates; the tailing factor for the mupirocin peak is not more than 1.75; and the relative standard deviation of the mupirocin peak for replicate injections is not more than 2%.

Procedure—Separately inject equal volumes (about 20 µL) of the *Standard preparation* and the *Assay preparation* into the chromatograph, record the chromatograms, and measure the peak area responses for the major peaks. Calculate the weight percent of mupirocin in the portion of Cream taken by the formula:

$$0.05E\,(M_S / M_U)(r_U / r_S)$$

in which M_S is the weight, in mg, of USP Mupirocin Lithium RS taken to prepare the *Standard preparation; E* is the designated mupirocin equivalent, in µg, of mupirocin in each mg of USP Mupirocin Lithium RS; M_U is the weight, in mg, of Cream taken to prepare the *Assay preparation;* and r_U and r_S are the mupirocin peak area responses obtained from the *Assay preparation* and the *Standard preparation,* respectively.

Mupirocin Ointment

» Mupirocin Ointment contains not less than 90.0 percent and not more than 110.0 percent of the labeled amount of mupirocin ($C_{26}H_{44}O_9$).

Packaging and storage—Preserve in collapsible tubes or in well-closed containers.

USP Reference standards ⟨11⟩—*USP Mupirocin Lithium RS.*

Identification—The chromatogram of the *Assay preparation* obtained as directed in the *Assay* exhibits a major peak for mupirocin, the retention time of which corresponds to that exhibited in the chromatogram of the *Standard preparation* obtained as directed in the *Assay*.

Minimum fill ⟨755⟩: meets the requirements.

Assay—

pH 6.3 phosphate buffer, Mobile phase, Standard preparation, Resolution solution, and *Chromatographic system*—Proceed as directed in the *Assay* under *Mupirocin*.

Assay preparation—Dissolve an accurately weighed quantity of Ointment, equivalent to about 10 mg of mupirocin, in 25 mL of acetonitrile. Transfer this solution, with the aid of *pH 6.3 phosphate buffer*, to a 100-mL volumetric flask, dilute with *pH 6.3 phosphate buffer* to volume, and mix.

Procedure—Proceed as directed for *Procedure* in the *Assay* under *Mupirocin*. Calculate the quantity, in mg, of mupirocin ($C_{26}H_{44}O_9$) in the portion of Ointment taken by the formula:

$$(M_S E / 1000)(r_U / r_S)$$

in which the terms are as defined therein.

Myrrh

» Myrrh is the oleo-gum resin obtained from stems and branches of *Commiphora molmol* Engler and other related species of *Commiphora* other than *Commiphora mukul* (Fam. Burseraceae).

Packaging and storage—Preserve in tight containers, and store at controlled room temperature, in a dry place.

Labeling—Label it to indicate the species of *Commiphora* from which the oleo-gum resin was obtained. Label it to indicate that it is intended for topical and oropharyngeal use only.

Botanic characteristics—Myrrh occurs in rounded or irregular tears, or bumps of agglutinated tears, of variable sizes; brownish yellow to reddish brown, covered with some grayish or yellowish dust, externally; rich brown or reddish brown internally, sometimes marked with white spots or lines; thin splinters, translucent or almost transparent; brittle; waxy, granular, conchoidal fracture; characteristic and aromatic odor; aromatic, bitter, and acrid taste.

Identification—

A: Triturate 0.4 g of crushed Myrrh with 1 g of washed sand, shake for a few minutes with 10 mL of ethyl ether, and filter. Evaporate the filtrate to dryness in a porcelain dish, and add a few drops of nitric acid to the residue: a purplish violet color is produced instantly.

B: Transfer 0.1 g of powdered Myrrh to a test tube, and add 1 mL of nitric acid: a red color is produced. Upon addition of a crystal of vanillin, the red color deepens. The red color does not diminish when water is added.

C: *Thin-Layer Chromatographic Identification Test* ⟨201⟩—
Test solution—Transfer 0.5 g of finely powdered Myrrh to a 10-mL centrifuge tube, add 2 mL of alcohol, shake for 1 minute, centrifuge, and filter. Apply 2 µL of the filtrate to the plate.
Standard solution—Dissolve accurately weighed quantities of (E)-anethole, linalool, (–)-bornyl acetate, and (R)-(–)-carvone in toluene, and dilute quantitatively, and stepwise if necessary, with toluene to obtain a solution having known concentrations of about 7 µg per mL of (E)-anethole, 8 µg per mL of linalool, and 10 µg per mL each of (–)-bornyl acetate and (R)-(–)-carvone. Apply 1 µL to the plate.
Developing solvent system: a mixture of toluene and ethyl acetate (93 : 7).
Spray reagent—Dissolve 0.5 mL of *p*-anisaldehyde in 10 mL of glacial acetic acid, add 85 mL of methanol, and mix. Carefully add 5 mL of sulfuric acid, and mix. [NOTE—Prepare fresh immediately before use.]
Procedure—[NOTE—Wash the plate in *Developing solvent system*, and air-dry prior to use.] Proceed as directed in the chapter. Spray the plate with *Spray reagent*, heat in an oven at 100° for 5 minutes, and examine in white light. The chromatogram of the *Standard solution* exhibits four well-resolved spots: an olive-brown spot due to (E)-anethole at an R_F value of about 0.6; an orange-brown spot due to (–)-bornyl acetate at an R_F value of about 0.5; a reddish brown spot due to (R)-(–)-carvone at an R_F value of about 0.4; and a deep gray spot due to linalool at an R_F value of about 0.2. The chromatogram of the *Test solution* exhibits an intense purplish red spot at an R_F value of about 0.7 and two moderately intense purplish red spots at R_F values of about 0.5 and 0.4. The chromatogram of the *Test solution* may exhibit other spots of varying intensities, including a spot at the origin.

D: *Thin-Layer Chromatographic Identification Test* ⟨201⟩—
Test solution—Transfer 0.5 g of finely powdered Myrrh to a test tube containing 5.0 mL of alcohol, and warm the mixture in a water bath for 2 to 3 minutes. Cool, and filter.
Standard solution—Dissolve accurately weighed quantities of (E)-anethole and thymol in alcohol, and dilute quantitatively, and stepwise if necessary, with alcohol to obtain a solution having known concentrations of about 4 µg of (E)-anethole per mL and about 1 mg of thymol per mL.
Developing solvent system: a mixture of toluene and ethyl acetate (98 : 2).
Procedure—Proceed as directed in the chapter. Allow the plate to air-dry, and examine under UV light at 365 nm. The chromatogram of the *Test solution* shows no blue to violet fluorescent zones in the lower third of the chromatogram (*absence of Commiphora mukul*).

Loss on drying ⟨731⟩—Dry 1.0 g of powdered Myrrh between 100° and 105° for 2 hours: it loses not more than 15.0% of its weight.

Foreign organic matter ⟨561⟩: not more than 2%.

Total ash ⟨561⟩: not more than 10.0%.

Acid-insoluble ash ⟨561⟩: not more than 5.0%.

Alcohol-soluble extractives, *Method 2* ⟨561⟩: not less than 40% and not more than 70%.

Water-soluble extractives, *Method 2* ⟨561⟩: not less than 50%.

Volatile oil content ⟨561⟩: not less than 6.0%.

Heavy metals, *Method II* ⟨231⟩: 0.002%.

Myrrh Topical Solution

» Prepare Myrrh Topical Solution as follows:

Myrrh	200 g
A mixture of Alcohol and Water (85 : 15)	900 mL
Alcohol, a sufficient quantity, to make	1000 mL

Macerate about 200 g of coarsely ground Myrrh with an alcohol-water mixture for 48 hours at room temperature in a suitable vessel, which is fitted with a lid and a mechanical stirrer, agitating the mixture with the stirrer. Allow the resulting mixture to stand overnight. Decant the mixture, filter, dilute the filtrate with Alcohol to 1000 mL, and mix.

Labeling—Label it to indicate that it is intended for topical and oropharyngeal use only.

Identification—Using Topical Solution as the *Test solution*, proceed as directed for *Identification* tests *C* and *D* under *Myrrh*.

Alcohol content, *Method II* ⟨611⟩: between 90.0% and 110.0% of the labeled amount of C_2H_5OH.

Other requirements—It meets the requirements for *Packaging and Storage* and *Labeling* for *Tinctures* under *Botanical Extracts* ⟨565⟩.

Nabumetone

$C_{15}H_{16}O_2$ 228.29
2-Butanone, 4-(6-methoxy-2-naphthalenyl)-.
4-(6-Methoxy-2-naphthyl)-2-butanone   [42924-53-8].

» Nabumetone contains not less than 98.0 percent and not more than 101.0 percent of $C_{15}H_{16}O_2$, calculated on the anhydrous basis.

Packaging and storage—Preserve in tight, light-resistant containers.

USP Reference standards ⟨11⟩—*USP Nabumetone RS. USP Nabumetone Related Compound A RS.*

Identification—

A: *Infrared Absorption* ⟨197K⟩.

B: The retention time of the major peak in the chromatogram of the *Assay preparation* corresponds to that in the chromatogram of the *Standard preparation*, as obtained in the *Assay*.

Water, *Method Ic* ⟨921⟩: not more than 0.2%, determined on a 1-g specimen.

Residue on ignition ⟨281⟩: not more than 0.1%.

Heavy metals, *Method II* ⟨231⟩: 0.001%.

Related compounds—
Solution A, Solution B, and *Mobile phase*—Proceed as directed in the *Assay.*

Nabumetone / Official Monographs

System suitability solution—Dissolve accurately weighed quantities of USP Nabumetone RS and USP Nabumetone Related Compound A RS in acetonitrile to obtain a solution having known concentrations of about 1 mg per mL and 1 µg per mL, respectively.

Test solution—Use the *Assay preparation*.

Chromatographic system (see *Chromatography* ⟨621⟩)—Proceed as directed in the *Assay*, except to chromatograph the *System suitability solution*, and record the peak responses as directed for *Procedure*: the relative retention times are about 0.9 for nabumetone related compound A and 1.0 for nabumetone; the resolution, *R*, between nabumetone related compound A and nabumetone is not less than 1.5; the column efficiency is not less than 3600 theoretical plates; the tailing factor determined from the nabumetone peak is between 0.8 and 2.0; and the relative standard deviation for replicate injections is not more than 2.0%.

Procedure—Inject 10 µL of the *Test solution* into the chromatograph, record the chromatogram, and measure all of the peak areas. Calculate the percentage of each impurity in the portion of Nabumetone taken by the formula:

$$100Fr_i/(r_N + \Sigma Fr_i)$$

in which *F* is the relative response factor for each impurity (see the accompanying table for values); r_i is the peak response for each impurity; and r_N is the nabumetone peak response. The limits of impurities are specified in the accompanying table.

Assay—

Solution A—Prepare a filtered and degassed mixture of water and glacial acetic acid (999 : 1).

Solution B—Prepare a filtered and degassed mixture of acetonitrile and tetrahydrofuran (7 : 3).

Mobile phase—Use variable mixtures of *Solution A* and *Solution B* as directed for *Chromatographic system*. Make adjustments if necessary (see *System Suitability* under *Chromatography* ⟨621⟩).

Standard preparation—Dissolve an accurately weighed quantity of USP Nabumetone RS in acetonitrile to obtain a solution having a known concentration of about 1.0 mg per mL.

Assay preparation—Transfer about 100 mg of Nabumetone, accurately weighed, to a 100-mL volumetric flask, dissolve in and dilute with acetonitrile to volume, and mix.

Chromatographic system (see *Chromatography* ⟨621⟩)—The liquid chromatograph is equipped with a 254-nm detector and a 4.6-mm × 15-cm column that contains 4-µm packing L1. The flow rate is about 1.3 mL per minute. The chromatograph is programmed as follows.

Time (minutes)	Solution A (%)	Solution B (%)	Elution
0	60	40	equilibration
0–12	60	40	isocratic
12–28	60→20	40→80	linear gradient
28–29	20→60	80→40	linear gradient
29–30	60	40	isocratic

Chromatograph the *Standard preparation*, and record the peak responses as directed for *Procedure*: the relative standard deviation for replicate injections is not more than 2.0%.

Procedure—Separately inject equal volumes (about 10 µL) of the *Standard preparation* and the *Assay preparation* into the chromatograph, record the chromatograms, and measure the responses for the nabumetone peaks. Calculate the quantity, in mg, of $C_{15}H_{16}O_2$ in the portion of Nabumetone taken by the formula:

$$100C(r_U/r_S)$$

in which *C* is the concentration, in mg per mL, of USP Nabumetone RS in the *Standard preparation*; and r_U and r_S are the peak responses obtained from the *Assay preparation* and the *Standard preparation*, respectively.

Compound	Approximate Relative Retention Time	Relative Response Factor	Limit (w/w, %)
Nabumetone	1.0	—	—
6-Methoxy-2-naphthaldehyde	0.73	0.12	0.1
4-(6'-Methoxy-2'-naphthyl)-butan-2-ol	0.85	0.94	0.1
1-(6'-Methoxy-2'-naphthyl)-but-1-en-3-one (nabumetone related compound A)	0.93	0.25	0.1
5-(6'-Methoxy-2'-naphthyl)-3-methylcyclohex-2-en-1-one	1.2	0.42	0.1
5-(6'-Methoxy-2'-naphthyl)-3-methylcyclohexan-1-one	1.9	1.02	0.1
1,5-Di-(6'-methoxy-2'-naphthyl)-pentan-3-one	2.6	0.91	0.1
6,6-Dimethoxy-2,2'-binaphthyl	2.7	0.10	0.3
Individual unknown impurity	—	—	0.1
Total impurity	—	—	0.8

Nabumetone Tablets

» Nabumetone Tablets contain not less than 95.0 percent and not more than 105.0 percent of the labeled amount of nabumetone ($C_{15}H_{16}O_2$).

Packaging and storage—Preserve in well-closed containers, and store at controlled room temperature.

USP Reference standards ⟨11⟩—*USP Nabumetone RS*.

Identification—The retention time of the major peak in the chromatogram of the *Assay preparation* corresponds to that in the chromatogram of the *Standard preparation*, as obtained in the *Assay*.

Dissolution ⟨711⟩—
Medium: sodium lauryl sulfate solution (2 in 100); 900 mL.
Apparatus 2: 50 rpm.
Time: 45 minutes.
Procedure—Determine the amount of $C_{15}H_{16}O_2$ dissolved from the difference between UV absorbances at the wavelengths of maximum and minimum absorbance at about 270 nm and 296 nm, respectively, on filtered portions of the solution under test, suitably diluted with *Medium*, if necessary, in comparison with a Standard solution having a known concentration of USP Nabumetone RS in the same *Medium*.

Tolerances—Not less than 75% (*Q*) of the labeled amount of $C_{15}H_{16}O_2$ is dissolved in 45 minutes.

Uniformity of dosage units ⟨905⟩: meet the requirements.

Assay—

Mobile phase—Prepare a solution of 6 mL of glacial acetic acid in 350 mL of water. Adjust with 1 N sodium hydroxide to a pH of 3.7, and dilute with water to obtain 400 mL. Prepare a filtered and degassed mixture of acetonitrile and this solution (3 : 2). Make adjustments if necessary (see *System Suitability* under *Chromatography* ⟨621⟩).

Standard preparation—Dissolve an accurately weighed quantity of USP Nabumetone RS in a mixture of methanol and water (9 : 1) to obtain a solution having a known concentration of about 0.5 mg per mL.

Assay preparation—Weigh and finely powder not fewer than 20 Tablets. Transfer an accurately weighed portion of the powder, equivalent to about 500 mg of nabumetone, to a 1000-mL volumetric flask, add about 100 mL of water, and stir with the aid of a magnetic stirrer for 5 minutes. Dilute with methanol to volume, stir for another 15 minutes, and filter.

Chromatographic system (see *Chromatography* ⟨621⟩)—The liquid chromatograph is equipped with a 280-nm detector and an 8-mm × 10-cm column that contains 10-μm packing L1. The flow rate is about 2 mL per minute. Chromatograph the *Standard preparation*, and record the peak responses as directed for *Procedure:* the column efficiency is not less than 1500 theoretical plates; the tailing factor is not more than 1.5; and the relative standard deviation for replicate injections is not more than 2.0%.

Procedure—Separately inject equal volumes (about 20 μL) of the *Standard preparation* and the *Assay preparation* into the chromatograph, record the chromatograms, and measure the responses for the major peaks. Calculate the quantity, in mg, of nabumetone ($C_{15}H_{16}O_2$) in the portion of Tablets taken by the formula:

$$1000C(r_U / r_S)$$

in which C is the concentration, in mg per mL, of USP Nabumetone RS in the *Standard preparation;* and r_U and r_S are the peak responses obtained from the *Assay preparation* and the *Standard preparation*, respectively.

Nadolol

$C_{17}H_{27}NO_4$ 309.40

2,3-Naphthalenediol, 5-[3-[(1,1-dimethylethyl)amino]-2-hydroxypropoxy]-1,2,3,4-tetrahydro-, *cis*-.
1-(*tert*-Butylamino)-3-[(5,6,7,8-tetrahydro-*cis*-6,7-dihydroxy-1-naphthyl)oxy]-2-propanol   [42200-33-9].

» Nadolol contains not less than 98.0 percent and not more than 101.5 percent of $C_{17}H_{27}NO_4$, calculated on the dried basis.

Packaging and storage—Preserve in well-closed containers.
USP Reference standards ⟨11⟩—*USP Nadolol RS.*
Identification, *Infrared Absorption* ⟨197M⟩.
Loss on drying ⟨731⟩—Dry it in vacuum at 60° for 3 hours: it loses not more than 2.0% of its weight.
Residue on ignition ⟨281⟩: not more than 0.1%.
Heavy metals, *Method II* ⟨231⟩: 0.003%.
Racemate composition—Prepare a mineral oil dispersion of Nadolol, previously dried, adjusting the thickness of the mull to give an absorbance reading of 0.6 ± 0.1 at 6.3 μm. Record the spectrum from 6 to 9 μm, using mineral oil in the reference beam. Calculate the percentage of racemate A in the portion of Nadolol taken by the formula:

$$(50 / 0.9)(A_a / A_b)$$

in which 0.9 is the average value of (A_a/A_b) in a mixture of racemates A and B (1 : 1), A_a is the uncorrected absorbance at the wavelength of a maximum absorbance at about 7.90 μm, corresponding to racemate A, and A_b is the uncorrected absorbance at the wavelength of a maximum absorbance at about 8.00 μm, corresponding to racemate B: the content of racemate A is between 40% and 60%.
Chromatographic purity—Prepare the test solution by dissolving about 500 mg of Nadolol in 10.0 mL of a mixture of methanol and chloroform (1 : 1). Prepare a solution of USP Nadolol RS in a mixture of methanol and chloroform (1 : 1) containing about 50 mg per mL. [NOTE—This Standard solution is used only to identify the nadolol zone.] Divide a thin-layer chromatographic plate (see *Chromatography* ⟨621⟩) coated with a 0.25-mm layer of chromatographic silica gel mixture, into four equal sections, the first section to be used for the Standard solution, the next two sections to be used for the test solution, and the last section for the blank. Apply, as streaks, 100 μL of the Standard solution, two 100-μL portions of the test solution, and 100 μL of the mixture of methanol and chloroform (1 : 1) to provide the blank to appropriate sections of the plate, drying each solution as it is applied with a current of cool air. Develop the chromatogram in a solvent system consisting of a mixture of acetone, chloroform, and 2 M ammonium hydroxide (8 : 1 : 1) until the solvent front has moved about three-fourths of the length of the plate. Remove the plate from the developing chamber, air-dry, and locate the bands by viewing under short-wavelength UV light. Identify the nadolol zones by comparison of the chromatograms of the test solution with the chromatogram of the Standard solution. Mark the nadolol zones and the separated impurity zones in the chromatograms of the test solution, and the corresponding zones in the blank section of the plate. Remove the silica gel from the nadolol zone in each chromatogram of the test solution, and transfer to separate 50-mL centrifuge tubes, and similarly transfer the silica gel removed from the corresponding area of the blank chromatogram to a third 50-mL centrifuge tube. Remove the silica gel from the combined impurity zones in each chromatogram of the test solution, and transfer to separate 50-mL centrifuge tubes, and similarly transfer the silica gel removed from the corresponding area of the blank chromatogram to a sixth 50-mL centrifuge tube. Add 30.0 mL of alcohol to each of the 2 tubes containing the mixtures from the nadolol zones and to the third tube containing the corresponding portion of the blank mixture, and add 10.0 mL of alcohol to each of the 2 tubes containing the mixtures from the impurity zones and to the sixth tube containing the corresponding portion of the blank mixture. Shake for 60 minutes, and centrifuge to clarify. Concomitantly determine the absorbances of the supernatants at the wavelength of maximum absorbance at about 278 nm, with a suitable spectrophotometer, using alcohol as the spectrophotometer blank. Calculate the percentage of impurities in the portion of Nadolol taken by the formula:

$$100A_i / (A_i + 3A_U)$$

in which A_i is the average absorbance of the impurity zone eluates corrected for the corresponding blank, and A_U is the average absorbance of the nadolol zone eluates corrected for the corresponding blank: not more than 2.0% is found.
Organic volatile impurities, *Method IV* ⟨467⟩: meets the requirements.

(Official until July 1, 2008)

Assay—
Perchloric acid titrant—Mix 8.5 mL of perchloric acid with 500 mL of glacial acetic acid, cool, dilute with glacial acetic acid to 1000 mL, and mix. Standardize this solution as directed for *Perchloric Acid, Tenth-Normal (0.1 N)* (in *Glacial Acetic Acid*) in the section *Volumetric Solutions* under *Reagents, Indicators, and Solutions.*

Procedure—Transfer about 280 mg of Nadolol, accurately weighed, to a 250-mL conical flask. Add 100 mL of glacial acetic acid, and place in an ultrasonic bath until solution is complete. Add 2 drops of crystal violet TS, and titrate with *Perchloric acid titrant* to an emerald-green endpoint. Perform a blank determination, and make any necessary correction. Each mL of 0.1 N perchloric acid is equivalent to 30.94 mg of $C_{17}H_{27}NO_4$.

Nadolol Tablets

» Nadolol Tablets contain not less than 90.0 percent and not more than 110.0 percent of the labeled amount of nadolol ($C_{17}H_{27}NO_4$).

Packaging and storage—Preserve in tight containers.
USP Reference standards ⟨11⟩—*USP Nadolol RS.*
Identification—Transfer a quantity of powdered Tablets, equivalent to about 50 mg of nadolol, to a conical flask. Add 10 mL of 0.1

N hydrochloric acid, stir for 30 minutes, using a magnetic stirrer, and place in an ultrasonic bath for an additional 30 minutes. Centrifuge, and use the supernatant for the test solution. Apply, as streaks, 100 µL of the test solution and 100 µL of a Standard solution of USP Nadolol RS in 0.1 N hydrochloric acid having a concentration of about 5 mg per mL to a thin-layer chromatographic plate (see *Chromatography* ⟨621⟩) coated with a 0.25-mm layer of chromatographic silica gel mixture. Develop the chromatogram in a solvent system consisting of acetone, chloroform, and 2 N ammonium hydroxide (8 : 1 : 1) until the solvent front has moved about three-fourths of the length of the plate. Remove the plate from the developing chamber, allow the solvent to evaporate, and examine the chromatogram under short-wavelength UV light: the R_F value of the principal spot obtained from the test solution corresponds to that obtained from the Standard solution.

Dissolution ⟨711⟩—
Medium: 0.01 N hydrochloric acid; 900 mL.
Apparatus 1: 100 rpm.
Time: 50 minutes.
Procedure—Determine the amount of $C_{17}H_{27}NO_4$ dissolved, employing the procedure set forth in the *Assay*, except to prepare the *Mobile phase* using 560 mL of methanol and 1440 mL of water instead of 700 mL and 1300 mL, respectively, and adjusting with 0.1 N hydrochloric acid to a pH of 2.5. Use filtered portions of the solution under test, suitably diluted with *Medium*, if necessary, in comparison with a Standard solution having a known concentration of USP Nadolol RS in the same *Medium*.
Tolerances—Not less than 80% (Q) of the labeled amount of $C_{17}H_{27}NO_4$ is dissolved in 50 minutes.

Uniformity of dosage units ⟨905⟩: meet the requirements.

Assay—
Mobile phase—Prepare a filtered and degassed mixture of 700 mL of methanol and 1300 mL of water containing 5.84 g of sodium chloride and 1.0 mL of 0.1 N hydrochloric acid.
Standard preparation—Dissolve an accurately weighed quantity of USP Nadolol RS in *Mobile phase* to obtain a solution having a known concentration of about 0.2 mg per mL.
Assay preparation—Weigh and finely powder not less than 20 Tablets. Weigh accurately a portion of the powder, equivalent to about 20 mg of nadolol, and transfer to a 100-mL volumetric flask. Add about 75 mL of *Mobile phase*, place in an ultrasonic bath for 15 minutes, shaking intermittently, add *Mobile phase* to volume, and mix. Clarify the solution by filtration or centrifugation.
Chromatographic system (see *Chromatography* ⟨621⟩)—The liquid chromatograph is equipped with a 220-nm detector and a 4.6-mm × 25-cm column that contains packing L16. The flow rate is about 1 mL per minute. Chromatograph replicate injections of the *Standard preparation*, and record the peak responses as directed for *Procedure*: the relative standard deviation is not more than 2.0%; and the tailing factor for the nadolol peak is not more than 3.
Procedure—Separately inject equal volumes (about 20 µL) of the *Standard preparation* and the *Assay preparation* into the chromatograph, record the chromatograms, and measure the responses for the major peaks. Calculate the quantity, in mg, of nadolol ($C_{17}H_{27}NO_4$) in the portion of Tablets taken by the formula:

$$100C(r_U / r_S)$$

in which C is the concentration, in mg per mL, of USP Nadolol RS in the *Standard preparation*; and r_U and r_S are the peak responses obtained from the *Assay preparation* and the *Standard preparation*, respectively.

Nadolol and Bendroflumethiazide Tablets

» Nadolol and Bendroflumethiazide Tablets contain not less than 90.0 percent and not more than 110.0 percent of the labeled amounts of nadolol ($C_{17}H_{27}NO_4$) and bendroflumethiazide ($C_{15}H_{14}F_3N_3O_4S_2$).

Packaging and storage—Preserve in tight containers.

USP Reference standards ⟨11⟩—*USP Bendroflumethiazide RS. USP 2,4-Disulfamyl-5-trifluoromethylaniline RS. USP Nadolol RS.*

Identification—The retention times of the major peaks in the chromatogram of the *Assay preparation* correspond to those of the *Standard preparation* obtained as directed in the *Assay*.

Dissolution, *Procedure for a Pooled Sample* ⟨711⟩—[NOTE—Protect solutions from light throughout this test.]
Medium: 0.1 N hydrochloric acid; 900 mL.
Apparatus 2: 50 rpm.
Time: 30 minutes.
Procedure—Determine the amounts of $C_{17}H_{27}NO_4$ and $C_{15}H_{14}F_3N_3O_4S_2$ dissolved, employing the procedure set forth in the *Assay*, using filtered portions of the solution under test, suitably diluted with *Medium*, if necessary, in comparison with a Standard solution having known concentrations of USP Nadolol RS and USP Bendroflumethiazide RS, prepared by dissolving them in the minimal amount of methanol and diluting to the desired concentrations with *Medium*.
Tolerances—Not less than 80% (Q) of the labeled amounts of nadolol ($C_{17}H_{27}NO_4$) and bendroflumethiazide ($C_{15}H_{14}F_3N_3O_4S_2$) are dissolved in 30 minutes.

Uniformity of dosage units ⟨905⟩: meet the requirements for *Content uniformity* with respect to both nadolol and bendroflumethiazide.

Assay—[NOTE—Use low-actinic glassware for the *Assay preparation* and the *Standard preparation*.]
Mobile phase—Dissolve 5.62 g of sodium chloride and 1.97 g of anhydrous sodium acetate in 1000 mL of water in a 2-liter volumetric flask. Add 4.0 mL of glacial acetic acid and 800 mL of methanol, dilute with water to volume, mix, filter, and degas. Make adjustments, if necessary (see *System Suitability* under *Chromatography* ⟨621⟩).
Standard preparation—Dissolve accurately weighed quantities of USP Nadolol RS and USP Bendroflumethiazide RS in methanol and dilute quantitatively, and stepwise if necessary, with methanol to obtain a solution having known concentrations of about 0.4 mg of USP Nadolol RS per mL and about 0.4J mg of USP Bendroflumethiazide RS per mL, J being the ratio of the labeled amount, in mg, of bendroflumethiazide to the labeled amount, in mg, of nadolol per Tablet.
Assay preparation—Weigh and finely powder not less than 20 Tablets. Transfer an accurately weighed portion of the powder, equivalent to about 40 mg of nadolol, to a 100-mL volumetric flask, add methanol and sonicate for 15 minutes with occasional shaking. Dilute with methanol to volume, mix, and centrifuge.
System suitability preparation—Prepare a solution in methanol containing about 0.4 mg each of USP Nadolol RS and USP 2,4-Disulfamyl-5-trifluoromethylaniline RS per mL.
Chromatographic system (see *Chromatography* ⟨621⟩)—The liquid chromatograph is equipped with a 270-nm detector and a 4.6-mm × 30-cm column that contains packing L11. The flow rate is about 1.5 mL per minute. Chromatograph the *System suitability preparation* and the *Standard preparation*, and record the peak responses as directed under *Procedure*: the resolution, R, between the solvent and 2,4-disulfamyl-5-trifluoromethylaniline peaks is not less than 1.4, the resolution, R, between the 2,4-disulfamyl-5-trifluoromethylaniline and nadolol peaks is not less than 1.4, and the resolution, R, between the nadolol and bendroflumethiazide peaks is not less than 1.7. The relative standard deviation for replicate injections of the *Standard preparation* is not more than 3.0%.
Procedure—Separately inject equal volumes (about 20 µL) of the *Standard preparation* and the *Assay preparation* into the chromatograph, record the chromatograms, and measure the responses of the major peaks. The relative retention times are about 0.3 for nadolol and 1.0 for bendroflumethiazide. Calculate the quantity, in mg, of nadolol ($C_{17}H_{27}NO_4$) in the portion of Tablets taken by the formula:

$$100C(r_U / r_S)$$

in which C is the concentration, in mg per mL, of USP Nadolol RS in the *Standard preparation*, and r_U and r_S are the peak responses of nadolol obtained from the *Assay preparation* and the *Standard preparation*, respectively. Calculate the quantity, in mg, of bendroflumethiazide ($C_{15}H_{14}F_3N_3O_4S_2$) in the portion of Tablets taken by the same formula, changing the terms to refer to bendroflumethiazide.

Nafcillin Sodium

$C_{21}H_{21}N_2NaO_5S \cdot H_2O$ 454.48
4-Thia-1-azabicyclo[3.2.0]heptane-2-carboxylic acid, 6-[[(2-ethoxy-1-naphthalenyl)carbonyl]amino]-3,3-dimethyl-7-oxo-, monosodium salt, monohydrate, [2S-(2α,5α,6β)].
Monosodium   (2S,5R,6R)-6-(2-ethoxy-1-naphthamido)-3,3-dimethyl-7-oxo-4-thia-1-azabicyclo[3.2.0]heptane-2-carboxylate monohydrate   [7177-50-6].
Anhydrous   436.47   [985-16-0].

» Nafcillin Sodium has a potency equivalent to not less than 820 μg of nafcillin ($C_{21}H_{22}N_2O_5S$) per mg.

Packaging and storage—Preserve in tight containers.
Labeling—Where it is intended for use in preparing injectable dosage forms, the label states that it is sterile or must be subjected to further processing during the preparation of injectable dosage forms.

USP Reference standards ⟨11⟩—*USP Nafcillin Sodium RS. USP Endotoxin RS.*
Identification—
 A: *Ultraviolet Absorption* ⟨197U⟩—
  Solution: 50 μg per mL.
  Medium: water.
 B: The retention time of the major peak for nafcillin in the chromatogram of the *Assay preparation* corresponds to that in the chromatogram of the *Standard preparation*, as obtained in the *Assay*.
 C: It responds to the tests for *Sodium* ⟨191⟩.
Crystallinity ⟨695⟩: meets the requirements.
pH ⟨791⟩: between 5.0 and 7.0, in a solution containing 30 mg per mL.
Water, *Method I* ⟨921⟩: between 3.5% and 5.3%.
Other requirements—Where the label states that Nafcillin Sodium is sterile, it meets the requirements for *Sterility Tests* ⟨71⟩ and for *Bacterial endotoxins* under *Nafcillin for Injection*. Where the label states that Nafcillin Sodium must be subjected to further processing during the preparation of injectable dosage forms, it meets the requirements for *Bacterial endotoxins* under *Nafcillin for Injection*.
Assay—
 Acetic acid solution—Prepare a 1 in 20 solution of glacial acetic acid and water.
 0.05 M Sodium acetate—Dissolve 6.8 g of sodium acetate in about 800 mL of water, adjust with *Acetic acid solution* to a pH of 7.5, dilute with water to 1000 mL, and mix.
 Mobile phase—Prepare a suitable filtered and degassed mixture of *0.05 M Sodium acetate* and acetonitrile (70 : 30). Make adjustments if necessary (see *System Suitability* under *Chromatography* ⟨621⟩).
 Diluent—Dissolve 6.9 g of sodium citrate in about 800 mL of water, adjust with 1 N hydrochloric acid to a pH of 7.0, dilute with water to 1000 mL, and mix.
 Standard preparation—Dissolve an accurately weighed quantity of USP Nafcillin Sodium RS quantitatively in *Diluent* to obtain a solution having a known concentration of about 400 μg of nafcillin ($C_{21}H_{22}N_2O_5S$) per mL.
 Resolution solution—Prepare a solution of orcinol in water containing about 35 mg per mL. Add 0.5 mL of this solution to 25 mL of *Standard preparation* to obtain a solution containing about 0.7 mg of orcinol and 400 μg of nafcillin per mL.
 Assay preparation—Transfer about 88 mg of Nafcillin Sodium, accurately weighed, to a 200-mL volumetric flask, dilute with *Diluent* to volume, and mix.
 Chromatographic system (see *Chromatography* ⟨621⟩)—The liquid chromatograph is equipped with a 254-nm detector and a 3.9-mm × 30-cm column containing packing L1. The flow rate is about 1 mL per minute. Chromatograph the *Resolution solution*, and record the peak responses as directed for *Procedure:* the relative retention times are about 0.8 for orcinol and 1.0 for nafcillin; and the resolution between the orcinol and nafcillin peaks is not less than 2.0. Chromatograph the *Standard preparation*, and record the responses as directed for *Procedure:* the tailing factor for the analyte peak is not more than 1.5; and the relative standard deviation for replicate injections is not more than 2.0%.
 Procedure—Separately inject equal volumes (about 20 μL) of the *Standard preparation* and the *Assay preparation* into the chromatograph, record the chromatograms, and measure the responses for the major peaks. Calculate the quantity, in μg, of nafcillin ($C_{21}H_{22}N_2O_5S$) in each mg of Nafcillin Sodium taken by the formula:

$$200(C/W)(r_U/r_S)$$

in which C is the concentration, in μg per mL, of nafcillin ($C_{21}H_{22}N_2O_5S$) in the *Standard preparation;* W is the weight, in mg, of the portion of Nafcillin Sodium taken; and r_U and r_S are the nafcillin peak responses obtained from the *Assay preparation* and the *Standard preparation*, respectively.

Nafcillin Sodium Capsules

» Nafcillin Sodium Capsules contain not less than 90.0 percent and not more than 120.0 percent of the labeled amount of nafcillin ($C_{21}H_{22}N_2O_5S$).

Packaging and storage—Preserve in tight containers.
USP Reference standards ⟨11⟩—*USP Nafcillin Sodium RS.*
Dissolution ⟨711⟩—
 Medium: water; 900 mL.
 Apparatus 1: 100 rpm.
 Time: 45 minutes.
 Procedure—Determine the amount of nafcillin ($C_{21}H_{22}N_2O_5S$) by a suitable validated spectrophotometric analysis of a filtered portion of the solution under test, suitably diluted with *Medium*, if necessary, in comparison with a Standard solution having a known concentration of USP Nafcillin Sodium RS in the same medium.
 Tolerances—Not less than 75% (*Q*) of the labeled amount of $C_{21}H_{22}N_2O_5S$ is dissolved in 45 minutes.
Uniformity of dosage units ⟨905⟩: meet the requirements.
Water, *Method I* ⟨921⟩: not more than 5.0%.
Assay—Proceed as directed under *Antibiotics—Microbial Assays* ⟨81⟩, using not less than 5 Capsules blended for 4 ± 1 minutes in a high-speed glass blender jar containing an accurately measured volume of *Buffer No. 1*. Dilute an accurately measured volume of this stock solution quantitatively with *Buffer No. 1* to obtain a *Test Dilution* having a concentration assumed to be equal to the median dose level of the Standard.

Nafcillin Injection

» Nafcillin Injection is a sterile isoosmotic solution of Nafcillin Sodium and one or more buffer substances in Water for Injection. It contains dextrose as a tonicity-adjusting agent. It contains an amount of nafcillin sodium equivalent to not less than 90.0 percent and not more than 120.0 percent of the labeled amount of nafcillin ($C_{21}H_{22}N_2O_5S$). It contains no antimicrobial preservatives.

Packaging and storage—Preserve in *Containers for Injections* as described under *Injections* ⟨1⟩. Maintain in the frozen state.
Labeling—It meets the requirements for *Labeling* under *Injections* ⟨1⟩. The label states that it is to be thawed just prior to use, describes conditions for proper storage of the resultant solution, and directs that the solution is not to be refrozen.
USP Reference standards ⟨11⟩—*USP Endotoxin RS. USP Nafcillin Sodium RS.*
Identification—The retention time of the major peak for nafcillin in the chromatogram of the *Assay preparation* corresponds to that in the chromatogram of the *Standard preparation*, as obtained in the *Assay*.
Bacterial endotoxins ⟨85⟩—It contains not more than 0.13 USP Endotoxin Unit per mg of nafcillin.
Sterility ⟨71⟩—It meets the requirements when tested as directed for *Membrane Filtration* under *Test for Sterility of the Product to be Examined*.
pH ⟨791⟩: between 6.0 and 8.5.
Particulate matter ⟨788⟩: meets the requirements for small-volume injections.
Assay—
 Acetic acid solution, 0.05 M Sodium acetate, Diluent, Mobile phase, Standard preparation, Resolution solution, and Chromatographic system—Proceed as directed in the *Assay* under *Nafcillin Sodium*.
 Assay preparation—Allow one container of Injection to thaw, and mix. Transfer an accurately measured volume of Injection, equivalent to about 40 mg of nafcillin, to a 100-mL volumetric flask, dilute with *Diluent* to volume, and mix.
 Procedure—Proceed as directed for *Procedure* in the *Assay* under *Nafcillin Sodium*. Calculate the quantity, in mg, of nafcillin ($C_{21}H_{22}N_2O_5S$) in each mL of the Injection taken by the formula:

$$0.1(C/V)(r_U/r_S)$$

in which C is the concentration, in µg per mL, of nafcillin in the *Standard preparation*; V is the volume, in mL, of Injection taken to prepare the *Assay preparation*; and r_U and r_S are the nafcillin peak responses obtained from the *Assay preparation* and the *Standard preparation*, respectively.

Nafcillin for Injection

» Nafcillin for Injection contains an amount of Nafcillin Sodium equivalent to not less than 90.0 percent and not more than 120.0 percent of the labeled amount of nafcillin ($C_{21}H_{22}N_2O_5S$).

Packaging and storage—Preserve in *Containers for Sterile Solids* as described under *Injections* ⟨1⟩.
USP Reference standards ⟨11⟩—*USP Endotoxin RS. USP Nafcillin Sodium RS.*
Constituted solution—At the time of use, it meets the requirements for *Constituted Solutions* under *Injections* ⟨1⟩.
Identification—The retention time of the major peak for nafcillin in the chromatogram of the *Assay preparation* corresponds to that in the chromatogram of the *Standard preparation*, as obtained in the *Assay*.
Bacterial endotoxins ⟨85⟩—It contains not more than 0.13 USP Endotoxin Unit per mg of nafcillin.
Sterility ⟨71⟩—It meets the requirements when tested as directed for *Membrane Filtration* under *Test for Sterility of the Product to be Examined*.
pH ⟨791⟩: between 6.0 and 8.5, in the solution constituted as directed in the labeling.
Water, *Method I* ⟨921⟩: between 3.5% and 5.3%.
Particulate matter ⟨788⟩: meets the requirements for small-volume injections.
Other requirements—It meets the requirements for *Uniformity of Dosage Units* ⟨905⟩ and *Labeling* under *Injections* ⟨1⟩.
Assay—
 Acetic acid solution, 0.05 M Sodium acetate, Diluent, Mobile phase, Standard preparation, Resolution solution, and Chromatographic system—Proceed as directed in the *Assay* under *Nafcillin Sodium*.
 Assay preparation 1 (where it is represented as being in a single-dose container)—Constitute Nafcillin for Injection in a volume of water, accurately measured, corresponding to the volume of solvent specified in the labeling. Withdraw all of the withdrawable contents, using a suitable hypodermic needle and syringe, and dilute quantitatively with *Diluent* to obtain a solution having a concentration of about 0.4 mg of nafcillin ($C_{21}H_{22}N_2O_5S$) per mL.
 Assay preparation 2 (where the label states the quantity of nafcillin in a given volume of constituted solution)—Constitute Nafcillin for Injection in a volume of water, accurately measured, corresponding to the volume of solvent specified in the labeling. Dilute an accurately measured volume of the constituted solution quantitatively with *Diluent* to obtain a solution having a concentration of about 0.4 mg of nafcillin ($C_{21}H_{22}N_2O_5S$) per mL.
 Procedure—Proceed as directed for *Procedure* in the *Assay* under *Nafcillin Sodium*. Calculate the quantity, in mg, of nafcillin ($C_{21}H_{22}N_2O_5S$) in the portion of constituted Nafcillin for Injection taken by the formula:

$$(C/1000)(L/D)(r_U/r_S)$$

in which L is the labeled quantity, in mg, of nafcillin in the portion of Nafcillin for Injection taken; D is the concentration, in mg per mL, of nafcillin in *Assay preparation 1* or *Assay preparation 2*, as appropriate, based on the volume of constituted Nafcillin for Injection taken and the extent of dilution; and the other terms are as defined therein.

 Perform the above procedure on 10 containers where it is represented as being in a single-dose container and, if necessary, on 10 containers where the label states the quantity of nafcillin in a given volume of constituted solution. Use the individual results to determine the *Uniformity of dosage units* and the average thereof as the *Assay* value.

Nafcillin Sodium for Oral Solution

» Nafcillin Sodium for Oral Solution contains not less than 90.0 percent and not more than 120.0 percent of the labeled amount of nafcillin ($C_{21}H_{22}N_2O_5S$). It contains one or more suitable buffers, colors, diluents, dispersants, flavors, and preservatives.

Packaging and storage—Preserve in tight containers.
USP Reference standards ⟨11⟩—*USP Nafcillin Sodium RS.*
Uniformity of dosage units ⟨905⟩—
 FOR SOLID PACKAGED IN SINGLE-UNIT CONTAINERS: meets the requirements.
Deliverable volume ⟨698⟩: meets the requirements.
pH ⟨791⟩: between 5.5 and 7.5, in the solution constituted as directed in the labeling.
Water, *Method I* ⟨921⟩: not more than 5.0%.
Assay—Proceed as directed under *Antibiotics—Microbial Assays* ⟨81⟩, using Nafcillin Sodium for Oral Solution constituted as directed in the labeling. Dilute an accurately measured volume of the solution quantitatively with *Buffer No. 1* to obtain a *Test Dilution* having a concentration assumed to be equal to the median dose level of the Standard.

Nafcillin Sodium Tablets

» Nafcillin Sodium Tablets contain not less than 90.0 percent and not more than 120.0 percent of the labeled amount of nafcillin ($C_{21}H_{22}N_2O_5S$).

Packaging and storage—Preserve in tight, light-resistant containers.

USP Reference standards ⟨11⟩—*USP Nafcillin Sodium RS*.
Dissolution ⟨711⟩—
pH 4.0 buffer—Transfer 10.94 g of anhydrous dibasic sodium phosphate and 12.92 g of citric acid monohydrate to a 1-liter volumetric flask, dissolve in water, dilute with water to volume, and mix.
Medium: pH 4.0 buffer; 900 mL.
Apparatus 2: 50 rpm.
Time: 45 minutes.
Procedure—Determine the amount of nafcillin ($C_{21}H_{22}N_2O_5S$) dissolved from UV absorbances, at the wavelength of maximum absorbance at about 280 nm of filtered portions of the solution under test, suitably diluted with *Medium*, if necessary, in comparison with a Standard solution having a known concentration of USP Nafcillin Sodium RS in the same medium.
Tolerances—Not less than 75% (*Q*) of the labeled amount of nafcillin ($C_{21}H_{22}N_2O_5S$) is dissolved in 45 minutes.
Uniformity of dosage units ⟨905⟩: meet the requirements.
Water, *Method I* ⟨921⟩: not more than 5.0%.
Assay—Proceed as directed under *Antibiotics—Microbial Assays* ⟨81⟩, using not less than 5 Tablets blended for 4 ± 1 minutes in a high-speed glass blender jar containing an accurately measured volume of *Buffer No. 1*. Dilute an accurately measured volume of this stock solution quantitatively with *Buffer No. 1* to obtain a *Test Dilution* having a concentration assumed to be equal to the median dose level of the Standard.

Naftifine Hydrochloride

$C_{21}H_{21}N \cdot HCl$ 323.86
1-Naphthalenemethanamine, *N*-methyl-*N*-(3-phenyl-2-propenyl)-, hydrochloride (*E*)-.
(*E*)-*N*-Cinnamyl-*N*-methyl-1-naphthalenemethylamine hydrochloride [65473-14-5].

» Naftifine Hydrochloride contains not less than 99.0 percent and not more than 101.0 percent of $C_{21}H_{21}N \cdot HCl$, calculated on the dried basis.

Packaging and storage—Preserve in tight containers.

USP Reference standards ⟨11⟩—*USP Naftifine Hydrochloride RS*.
Identification, *Infrared Absorption* ⟨197K⟩.
Melting range ⟨741⟩: between 175° and 179°.
Loss on drying ⟨731⟩—Dry over phosphorus pentoxide at 105° for 4 hours: it loses not more than 0.5% of its weight.
Residue on ignition ⟨281⟩: not more than 0.1%.
Heavy metals, *Method II* ⟨231⟩: 0.001%.
Chromatographic purity—
Mobile phase, Standard preparation, and *Chromatographic system*—Proceed as directed in the *Assay*.
Test preparation—Use the *Assay preparation*.
Procedure—Inject a volume (about 15 µL) of the *Test preparation* into the chromatograph, record the chromatogram, and measure the peak responses. Calculate the percentage of each impurity in the portion of Naftifine Hydrochloride taken by the formula:

$$100(r_i / r_S)$$

in which r_i is the peak response for each impurity, and r_S is the sum of the responses of all of the peaks: not more than 0.1% of any individual impurity is found, and the sum of all impurities is not more than 1.0%.
Assay—
Mobile phase—Prepare a filtered and degassed mixture of *n*-hexane, alcohol, dimethylformamide, and formic acid (200 : 60 : 40 : 2), cover tightly with a moisture-proof film, and allow to stand for 12 hours at room temperature. Make adjustments, if necessary (see *System Suitability* under *Chromatography* ⟨621⟩).
Standard preparation—Dissolve an accurately weighed quantity of USP Naftifine Hydrochloride RS in *Mobile phase*, and dilute quantitatively, and stepwise, if necessary, with *Mobile phase* to obtain a solution having a known concentration of about 0.2 mg per mL.
Assay preparation—Transfer about 10 mg of Naftifine Hydrochloride, accurately weighed, to a 50-mL volumetric flask, dissolve in and dilute with *Mobile phase* to volume.
Chromatographic system (see *Chromatography* ⟨621⟩)—The liquid chromatograph is equipped with a 270-nm detector and a 4.6-mm × 25-cm column that contains 5-µm packing L3. The flow rate is about 2.0 mL per minute.
Procedure—Separately inject equal volumes (about 15 µL) of the *Standard preparation* and the *Assay preparation* into the chromatograph, record the chromatograms, and measure the responses for the major peaks. Calculate the quantity, in mg, of $C_{21}H_{21}N \cdot HCl$ in the portion of Naftifine Hydrochloride taken by the formula:

$$50C(r_U / r_S)$$

in which *C* is the concentration, in mg per mL, of USP Naftifine Hydrochloride RS in the *Standard preparation*, and r_U and r_S are the peak responses obtained from the *Assay preparation* and the *Standard preparation*, respectively.

Naftifine Hydrochloride Cream

» Naftifine Hydrochloride Cream contains not less than 90.0 percent and not more than 110.0 percent of Naftifine Hydrochloride ($C_{21}H_{21}N \cdot HCl$) in a water-miscible base.

Packaging and storage—Preserve in tight containers.

USP Reference standards ⟨11⟩—*USP Naftifine Hydrochloride RS*.
Identification—The retention time of the major peak in the chromatogram of the *Assay preparation* corresponds to that of the *Standard preparation* as obtained in the *Assay*.
Microbial limits ⟨61⟩—It meets the requirements of the tests for absence of *Staphylococcus aureus* and *Pseudomonas aeruginosa*.
Minimum fill ⟨755⟩: meets the requirements.
pH ⟨791⟩: between 4.0 and 6.0.
Assay—
Mobile phase, Standard preparation, and *Chromatographic system*—Proceed as directed in the *Assay* under *Naftifine Hydrochloride*.
Assay preparation—Transfer about 1000 mg of Cream, accurately weighed, to a 100-mL volumetric flask, dissolve in 60 mL of methanol, mix vigorously for 2 minutes, and dilute with methanol to volume. Heat at 45° for 5 minutes, and cool to room temperature.
Procedure—Separately inject equal volumes (about 15 µL) of the *Standard preparation* and the *Assay preparation* into the chromatograph, record the chromatograms, and measure the responses for the

major peaks. Calculate the quantity, in mg, of $C_{21}H_{21}N \cdot HCl$ in the portion of Cream taken by the formula:

$$100C(r_U/r_S)$$

in which C is the concentration, in mg per mL, of USP Naftifine Hydrochloride RS in the *Standard preparation,* and r_U and r_S are the peak responses obtained from the *Assay preparation* and the *Standard preparation,* respectively.

Naftifine Hydrochloride Gel

» Naftifine Hydrochloride Gel contains not less than 90.0 percent and not more than 110.0 percent of Naftifine Hydrochloride ($C_{21}H_{21}N \cdot HCl$) in a water-miscible base.

Packaging and storage—Preserve in tight containers.
USP Reference standards ⟨11⟩—*USP Naftifine Hydrochloride RS.*
Identification—The retention time of the major peak in the chromatogram of the *Assay preparation* corresponds to that of the *Standard preparation*as obtained in the *Assay.*
Microbial limits ⟨61⟩—It meets the requirements of the tests for absence of *Staphylococcus aureus* and *Pseudomonas aeruginosa.*
Minimum fill ⟨755⟩: meets the requirements.
pH ⟨791⟩: between 5.5 and 7.5.
Content of alcohol—

Internal standard solution—Transfer 10.0 mL of *n*-propyl alcohol to a 200-mL volumetric flask, dilute with water to volume, and mix.

Standard solution—Prepare a mixture containing an accurately weighed quantity of alcohol in water having a known concentration of about 10.0 mg of alcohol per mL. Transfer 3.0 mL of *Internal standard solution* to a 10-mL volumetric flask, dilute with the alcohol solution, and mix.

Test solution—Transfer about 250 mg of Gel, accurately weighed, to a suitable container. Add 14.0 mL of water and 6.0 mL of *Internal standard solution,* and shake for 15 minutes.

Chromatographic system (see *Chromatography* ⟨621⟩)—The gas chromatograph is equipped with a flame-ionization detector and a 3.2-mm × 1.5-m column packed with 80- to 100-mesh support S3. The column temperature is maintained at 170°, and the injection port and detector are maintained at 200°. Nitrogen is used as the carrier gas, flowing at a rate of 45 mL per minute. Chromatograph the *Standard solution,* and record the peak responses as directed under *Procedure:* the resolution, R, between alcohol and the internal standard is not less than 2.0, the capacity factor, k', is between 2.0 and 3.5 for alcohol and between 6.0 and 8.0 for the internal standard, the tailing factor is not more than 2.5, and the relative standard deviation for replicate injections is not more than 2.5%.

Procedure—Inject equal volumes (about 1 µL) of the *Standard solution* and the *Test solution* into the chromatograph, record the chromatograms, and measure the responses for the major peaks. Calculate the quantity, in mg, of C_2H_5OH in the portion of Gel taken by the formula:

$$5.6C(R_U/R_S)$$

in which C is the concentration, in mg per mL, of C_2H_5OH in the *Standard solution,* and R_U and R_S are the ratios of the peak responses for alcohol to those of the internal standard obtained from the *Test solution* and the *Standard solution,* respectively: the content of C_2H_5OH is between 40% and 45%.

Assay—

Mobile phase, Standard preparation, and *Chromatographic system*—Proceed as directed in the *Assay* under *Naftifine Hydrochloride.*

Assay preparation—Transfer about 1000 mg of Gel, accurately weighed, to a 100-mL volumetric flask, dissolve in 60 mL of methanol, mix vigorously for 2 minutes, and dilute with methanol to volume. Heat at 45° for 5 minutes, and cool to room temperature.

Procedure—Separately inject equal volumes (about 20 µL) of the *Standard preparation* and the *Assay preparation* into the chromatograph, record the chromatograms, and measure the responses for the major peaks. Calculate the quantity, in mg, of $C_{21}H_{21}N \cdot HCl$ in the portion of Gel taken by the formula:

$$100C(r_U/r_S)$$

in which C is the concentration, in mg per mL, of USP Naftifine Hydrochloride RS in the *Standard preparation,* and r_U and r_S are the peak responses obtained from the *Assay preparation* and the *Standard preparation,* respectively.

Nalidixic Acid

$C_{12}H_{12}N_2O_3$ 232.24
1,8-Naphthyridine-3-carboxylic acid, 1-ethyl-1,4-dihydro-7-methyl-4-oxo-.
1-Ethyl-1,4-dihydro-7-methyl-4-oxo-1,8-naphthyridine-3-carboxylic acid [389-08-2].

» Nalidixic Acid contains not less than 99.0 percent and not more than 101.0 percent of $C_{12}H_{12}N_2O_3$, calculated on the dried basis.

Packaging and storage—Preserve in tight containers.
USP Reference standards ⟨11⟩—*USP Nalidixic Acid RS.*
Identification—
 A: *Infrared Absorption* ⟨197K⟩.
 B: *Ultraviolet Absorption* ⟨197U⟩—
  Solution: 5 µg per mL.
  Medium: 0.01 N sodium hydroxide.
  Absorptivities at 258 nm, calculated on the dried basis, do not differ by more than 3.0%.
Melting range ⟨741⟩: between 225° and 231°.
Loss on drying ⟨731⟩—Dry it at 105° for 2 hours: it loses not more than 0.5% of its weight.
Residue on ignition ⟨281⟩: not more than 0.1%.
Heavy metals, *Method II* ⟨231⟩: 0.002%.
Chromatographic purity—

Standard solutions—Prepare a solution of USP Nalidixic Acid RS in chloroform containing 1.0 mg per mL. Dilute quantitatively with chloroform to obtain *Standard solutions* having the following composition:

Standard solution	Dilution	Concentration (mg RS per mL)	Percentage (%, for comparison with test specimen)
A	1 in 10	0.1	0.5
B	1 in 25	0.04	0.2
C	1 in 50	0.02	0.1

Test solution—Dissolve an accurately weighed quantity of Nalidixic Acid in chloroform to obtain a solution containing 20 mg per mL.

Procedure—Apply separately 10 µL of the *Test solution* and 10 µL of each *Standard solution* to a suitable thin-layer chromatographic plate (see *Chromatography* ⟨621⟩) coated with a 0.25-mm layer of chromatographic silica gel mixture. Position the plate in a chromatographic chamber, and develop the chromatograms in a solvent system consisting of a mixture of alcohol, chloroform, and 5 M ammonium hydroxide (70 : 20 : 10) until the solvent front has moved about three-fourths of the length of the plate. Remove the plate from the developing chamber, mark the solvent front, and allow the solvent to evaporate with the aid of warm circulating air. Examine the plate under short-wavelength UV light. Compare the intensities of any secondary spots observed in the chromatogram of the *Test solution* with those of the principal spots in the chromatograms of the *Standard solutions*: no secondary spot is more intense than the principal spot obtained from *Standard solution A* (0.5%), and the sum of the intensities of all secondary spots obtained from the *Test solution* does not exceed 1.0%.

Assay—Dissolve about 250 mg of Nalidixic Acid, accurately weighed, in 30 mL of dimethylformamide that previously has been neutralized to thymolphthalein TS, and titrate with 0.1 N lithium methoxide VS in methanol, using a magnetic stirrer and taking precautions against absorption of atmospheric carbon dioxide. Each mL of 0.1 N lithium methoxide is equivalent to 23.22 mg of $C_{12}H_{12}N_2O_3$.

Nalidixic Acid Oral Suspension

» Nalidixic Acid Oral Suspension contains not less than 95.0 percent and not more than 105.0 percent of the labeled amount of nalidixic acid $C_{12}H_{12}N_2O_3$ in a suitable aqueous vehicle.

Packaging and storage—Preserve in tight containers.

USP Reference standards ⟨11⟩—*USP Nalidixic Acid RS.*

Identification—The retention time of the nalidixic acid peak in the chromatogram of the *Assay preparation* corresponds to that in the chromatogram of the *Standard preparation*, as obtained in the *Assay*.

Uniformity of dosage units ⟨905⟩—
FOR ORAL SUSPENSION PACKAGED IN SINGLE-UNIT CONTAINERS: meets the requirements.

Deliverable volume ⟨698⟩—
FOR ORAL SUSPENSION PACKAGED IN MULTIPLE-UNIT CONTAINERS: meets the requirements.

Assay—
Mobile phase—Prepare a solution of 784 mg of dibasic potassium phosphate in 325 mL of water. To this solution add a solution of 2.62 g of hexadecyltrimethylammonium bromide in 350 mL of methanol. To the combined solution add 325 mL of methanol, mix, filter, and degas. This solution has an apparent pH of about 10. Make adjustments if necessary (see *System Suitability* under *Chromatography* ⟨621⟩).

Internal standard solution—Prepare a solution of sulfanilic acid in *Mobile phase* containing about 0.8 mg per mL.

Standard preparation—Prepare a solution having a known concentration of about 0.18 mg per mL of USP Nalidixic Acid RS in methanol. Transfer 5.0 mL of this solution and 1.0 mL of *Internal standard solution* to a 25-mL volumetric flask, dilute with methanol to volume, and mix.

Assay preparation—Transfer an accurately measured volume of freshly mixed Oral Suspension, equivalent to about 150 mg of nalidixic acid, to a 500-mL volumetric flask, add about 400 mL of methanol, and sonicate for about 30 minutes. Shake by mechanical means for about 30 minutes, sonicate again for about 30 minutes, dilute with methanol to volume, mix, and filter. Transfer 3.0 mL of the clear filtrate and 1.0 mL of *Internal standard solution* to a 25-mL volumetric flask, dilute with methanol to volume, and mix.

Chromatographic system (see *Chromatography* ⟨621⟩)—The liquid chromatograph is equipped with a 254-nm detector and a 3.9-mm × 30-cm column that contains packing L1. The flow rate is about 1.5 mL per minute. Chromatograph the *Standard preparation*, and record the peak responses as directed for *Procedure*: the relative retention times are about 0.7 for sulfanilic acid and 1.0 for nalidixic acid; the resolution, R, between sulfanilic acid and nalidixic acid is not less than 1; and the relative standard deviation for replicate injections is not more than 2.0%.

Procedure—Separately inject equal volumes (about 20 µL) of the *Standard preparation* and the *Assay preparation* into the chromatograph, record the chromatograms, and measure the areas for the major peaks. Calculate the quantity, in mg, of nalidixic acid ($C_{12}H_{12}N_2O_3$) in each mL of the Oral Suspension taken by the formula:

$$(12{,}500/3)(C/V)(R_U/R_S)$$

in which C is the concentration, in mg per mL, of USP Nalidixic Acid RS in the *Standard preparation*; V is the volume, in mL, of Oral Suspension taken to prepare the *Assay preparation*; and R_U and R_S are the ratios of the peak areas for nalidixic acid and sulfanilic acid in the chromatograms obtained from the *Assay preparation* and the *Standard preparation*, respectively.

Nalidixic Acid Tablets

» Nalidixic Acid Tablets contain not less than 93.0 percent and not more than 107.0 percent of the labeled amount of nalidixic acid ($C_{12}H_{12}N_2O_3$).

Packaging and storage—Preserve in tight containers.

USP Reference standards ⟨11⟩—*USP Nalidixic Acid RS.*

Identification—The retention time of the nalidixic acid peak in the chromatogram of the *Assay preparation* corresponds to that in the chromatogram of the *Standard preparation* as obtained in the *Assay*.

Dissolution ⟨711⟩—
Medium: pH 8.60 buffer, prepared by mixing 2.3 volumes of 0.2 M sodium hydroxide with 2.5 volumes of 0.2 M monobasic potassium phosphate and 2.0 volumes of methanol, cooling, mixing with water to obtain 10 volumes of solution, and adjusting, if necessary, by the addition of 1 N sodium hydroxide to a pH of 8.60 ± 0.05. The initial volume for the test is 900 mL.
Apparatus 2: 60 rpm.
Time: 30 minutes.
Procedure—Determine the amount of $C_{12}H_{12}N_2O_3$ dissolved from UV absorbances at the wavelength of maximum absorbance at about 258 nm of filtered portions of the solution under test, suitably diluted with 0.01 N sodium hydroxide, if necessary, in comparison with a Standard solution of known concentration of USP Nalidixic Acid RS in 0.01 N sodium hydroxide, using as the blank a mixture of *Medium* and 0.01 N sodium hydroxide in the same proportions as present in the test solution.
Tolerances—Not less than 80% (*Q*) of the labeled amount of $C_{12}H_{12}N_2O_3$ is dissolved in 30 minutes.

Uniformity of dosage units ⟨905⟩: meet the requirements.

Assay—
Mobile phase, Internal standard solution, Standard preparation, and *Chromatographic system*—Proceed as directed in the *Assay* under *Nalidixic Acid Oral Suspension*.

Assay preparation—Weigh and finely powder not less than 20 Tablets. Transfer an accurately weighed portion of the powder, equivalent to about 150 mg of nalidixic acid, to a 500-mL volumetric flask, add about 400 mL of methanol, and sonicate for about 30 minutes. Shake by mechanical means for about 30 minutes, sonicate again for about 30 minutes, dilute with methanol to volume, mix, and filter. Transfer 3.0 mL of the clear filtrate and 1.0 mL of *Internal standard solution* to a 25-mL volumetric flask, dilute with methanol to volume, and mix.

Procedure—Proceed as directed for *Procedure* in the *Assay* under *Nalidixic Acid Oral Suspension*. Calculate the quantity, in mg, of $C_{12}H_{12}N_2O_3$ in the portion of Tablets taken by the formula:

$$(12{,}500/3)(C)(R_U/R_S)$$

in which the terms are as defined therein.

Nalorphine Hydrochloride

$C_{19}H_{21}NO_3 \cdot HCl$ 347.84
Morphinan-3,6-diol, 7,8-didehydro-4,5-epoxy-17-(2-propenyl)-(5α,6α)-, hydrochloride.
17-Allyl-7,8-didehydro-4,5α-epoxymorphinan-3,6α-diol hydrochloride [57-29-4].

» Nalorphine Hydrochloride contains not less than 97.0 percent and not more than 103.0 percent of $C_{19}H_{21}NO_3 \cdot HCl$, calculated on the dried basis.

Packaging and storage—Preserve in tight, light-resistant containers. Store at 25°, excursions permitted between 15° and 30°.
USP Reference standards ⟨11⟩—*USP Nalorphine Hydrochloride RS*.
Identification—
  A: *Infrared Absorption* ⟨197K⟩.
  B: *Ultraviolet Absorption* ⟨197U⟩—
  Solution: 100 μg per mL.
  Medium: water.
  C: A solution of it responds to the tests for *Chloride* ⟨191⟩.
Specific rotation ⟨781S⟩: between −122° and −125°.
  Test solution: 20 mg per mL, in water.
Loss on drying ⟨731⟩—Dry it in vacuum at 100° for 2 hours: it loses not more than 0.5% of its weight.
Residue on ignition ⟨281⟩: not more than 0.1%.
Assay—Transfer about 25 mg of Nalorphine Hydrochloride, accurately weighed, to a 250-mL volumetric flask, dissolve in and dilute with water to volume, and mix. Concomitantly determine the absorbances of this solution and of a Standard solution of USP Nalorphine Hydrochloride RS in the same medium having a known concentration of about 100 μg per mL in 1-cm cells at the wavelength of maximum absorbance at about 285 nm, with a suitable spectrophotometer, using water as the blank. Calculate the quantity, in mg, of $C_{19}H_{21}NO_3 \cdot HCl$ in the Nalorphine Hydrochloride taken by the formula:

$$0.25C(A_U/A_S)$$

in which *C* is the concentration, in μg per mL, of USP Nalorphine Hydrochloride RS in the Standard solution; and A_U and A_S are the absorbances of the solution of Nalorphine Hydrochloride and the Standard solution, respectively.

Nalorphine Hydrochloride Injection

» Nalorphine Hydrochloride Injection is a suitably buffered, sterile solution of Nalorphine Hydrochloride in Water for Injection. It contains not less than 90.0 percent and not more than 110.0 percent of the labeled amount of nalorphine hydrochloride ($C_{19}H_{21}NO_3 \cdot HCl$).

Packaging and storage—Preserve in single-dose or in multiple-dose containers, preferably of Type I glass.
USP Reference standards ⟨11⟩—*USP Endotoxin RS. USP Nalorphine Hydrochloride RS*.
Identification—Apply 15 μL of Injection and 15 μL of a Standard solution of USP Nalorphine Hydrochloride RS in methanol containing 5 mg per mL to a suitable thin-layer chromatographic plate (see *Chromatography* ⟨621⟩) coated with a 0.25-mm layer of chromatographic silica gel mixture. Allow the applications to dry, and develop the chromatogram in an equilibrated chamber containing methanol until the solvent front has moved about three-fourths of the length of the plate. Remove the plate from the developing chamber, mark the solvent front, and allow the solvent to evaporate. Observe the plate under short- and long-wavelength UV light: the R_F value of the principal spot obtained from the Injection corresponds to that obtained from the Standard solution.
Bacterial endotoxins ⟨85⟩—It contains not more than 11.6 USP Endotoxin Units per mg of nalorphine hydrochloride.
pH ⟨791⟩: between 6.0 and 7.5.
Other requirements—It meets the requirements under *Injections* ⟨1⟩.
Assay—Transfer an accurately measured volume of Injection, equivalent to about 10 mg of nalorphine hydrochloride, to a 25-mL centrifuge separator, add 1 mL of 3 N hydrochloric acid, and dilute with water to about 10 mL. Extract with five 5-mL portions of chloroform, separating the layers by centrifugation before drawing off each chloroform extract, and discard the chloroform extracts. Transfer the aqueous layer to a 100-mL volumetric flask with the aid of water, dilute with water to volume, and mix. Proceed as directed in the *Assay* under *Nalorphine Hydrochloride*, beginning with "Concomitantly determine the absorbances." Calculate the quantity, in mg, of $C_{19}H_{21}NO_3 \cdot HCl$ in each mL of the Injection taken by the formula:

$$(0.1C/V)(A_U/A_S)$$

in which *V* is the volume, in mL, of Injection taken, and *C*, A_U, and A_S are as defined therein.

Naloxone Hydrochloride

$C_{19}H_{21}NO_4 \cdot HCl$ 363.84
Morphinan-6-one, 4,5-epoxy-3,14-dihydroxy-17-(2-propenyl)-, hydrochloride, (5α)-.
17-Allyl-4,5α-epoxy-3,14-dihydroxymorphinan-6-one hydrochloride [357-08-4].
Dihydrate 399.87 [51481-60-8].

» Naloxone Hydrochloride is anhydrous or contains two molecules of water of hydration. It contains not less than 98.0 percent and not more than 100.5 percent of $C_{19}H_{21}NO_4 \cdot HCl$, calculated on the dried basis.

Packaging and storage—Preserve in tight, light-resistant containers. Store at 25°, excursions permitted between 15° and 30°.
USP Reference standards ⟨11⟩—*USP Naloxone RS. USP Noroxymorphone Hydrochloride RS*.
Identification, *Infrared Absorption* ⟨197K⟩—
  Test specimen—Dissolve about 150 mg in 25 mL of water in a small separator, add a few drops of 6 N ammonium hydroxide slowly until no more white precipitate is formed. Extract with three 5-mL portions of chloroform, pass the extracts through a dry filter, collecting the filtrate in a small flask. Evaporate the filtrate on a steam bath to dryness, and dry the residue at 105° for one hour.
Specific rotation ⟨781S⟩: between −170° and −181°.
  Test solution: 25 mg per mL, in water.
Loss on drying ⟨731⟩—Dry it at 105° to constant weight: the anhydrous form loses not more than 0.5% of its weight, and the hydrous form loses not more than 11.0% of its weight.
Noroxymorphone hydrochloride [(−)-4,5α-epoxy-3,14-dihydroxymorphinan-6-one hydrochloride] and other impurities—Transfer about 40 mg, accurately weighed, to a 5-mL volumetric flask, dissolve completely in 2.0 mL of water, add methanol to volume, and mix, to obtain the test solution. Prepare a solution of USP Naloxone RS in chloroform containing about 7.6 mg per mL. Prepare a

solution of USP Noroxymorphone Hydrochloride RS in dilute methanol (3 in 5) containing 0.084 mg per mL. Apply 5 µL each of the test solution and the two Standard solutions to a thin-layer chromatographic plate (see *Chromatography* ⟨621⟩) coated with a 0.25-mm layer of chromatographic silica gel that previously has been activated by heating for 15 minutes at 105°. Immediately place the plate in a suitable chromatographic chamber containing a 1 in 20 solution of methanol in ammoniacal butanol previously prepared by shaking 100 mL of butyl alcohol with 60 mL of ammonium hydroxide solution (1 in 100) and discarding the lower layer. Develop the chromatogram, protected from light, until the solvent front has moved about 10 cm from the point of application. Remove the plate, dry thoroughly, and spray with ferric chloride–potassium ferricyanide reagent prepared, immediately prior to use, by dissolving 100 mg of potassium ferricyanide in 20 mL of ferric chloride solution (1 in 10). Other than the principal spot corresponding in R_F value to that of USP Naloxone RS and the spot at the origin (ammonium chloride), no other spot is more intense than the spot corresponding to that of USP Noroxymorphone Hydrochloride RS (1.0%).

Chloride content—Dissolve about 300 mg, accurately weighed, in 50 mL of methanol contained in a 125-mL conical flask, add 5 mL of glacial acetic acid and 2 drops of eosin Y TS, and titrate with 0.1 N silver nitrate VS to a pink endpoint. Each mL of 0.1 N silver nitrate is equivalent to 3.545 mg of chloride. Not less than 9.54% and not more than 9.94%, calculated on the dried basis, is found.

Assay—Dissolve about 300 mg of Naloxone Hydrochloride, previously dried and accurately weighed, in a mixture of 40 mL of glacial acetic acid and 10 mL of acetic anhydride; add 10 mL of mercuric acetate TS and 1 drop of methyl violet TS; and titrate with 0.1 N perchloric acid VS. Perform a blank determination, and make any necessary correction. Each mL of 0.1 N perchloric acid is equivalent to 36.38 mg of $C_{19}H_{21}NO_4 \cdot HCl$.

Naloxone Hydrochloride Injection

» Naloxone Hydrochloride Injection is a sterile, isotonic solution of Naloxone Hydrochloride in Water for Injection. It contains not less than 90.0 percent and not more than 110.0 percent of the labeled amount of naloxone hydrochloride ($C_{19}H_{21}NO_4 \cdot HCl$). It may contain suitable preservatives.

Packaging and storage—Preserve in single-dose or in multiple-dose containers of Type I glass, protected from light.

USP Reference standards ⟨11⟩—*USP Endotoxin RS. USP Naloxone RS.*

Identification—The retention time of the major peak in the chromatogram of the *Assay preparation* corresponds to that of the *Standard preparation* as obtained in the *Assay*.

Bacterial endotoxins ⟨85⟩—It contains not more than 500 USP Endotoxin Units per mg of Naloxone Hydrochloride.

pH ⟨791⟩: between 3.0 and 6.5.

Limit of 2,2′-bisnaloxone—

Mobile phase, Diluting solvent, System suitability preparation, and Chromatographic system—Prepare as directed in the *Assay*.

Ferric chloride solution—Transfer 4 mL of ferric chloride TS to a 100-mL volumetric flask, dilute with water to volume, and mix.

Identification solution—Dissolve 10 mg of naloxone in 100 mL of 0.1 N hydrochloric acid. Transfer 10.0 mL of this solution to a 100-mL volumetric flask, and add 0.5 mL of *Ferric chloride solution*. Heat on a steam bath for 10 minutes, cool, dilute with water to volume, and mix.

Standard solution—Transfer 2.0 mL of the *Standard preparation* prepared as directed in the *Assay* to a 100-mL volumetric flask, dilute with *Diluting solvent* to volume, and mix.

Test solution—Use the *Assay preparation*.

Procedure—Separately inject equal volumes (about 100 µL) of the *Identification solution*, the *Standard solution*, and the *Test solution* into the chromatograph, record the chromatograms, and measure the areas of the peak responses for naloxone and 2,2′-bisnaloxone. The relative retention times are about 2.8 for the naloxone dimer and 1.0 for naloxone. Calculate the percentage of 2,2′-bisnaloxone in the volume of *Injection* taken by the formula:

$$(100 / L)(363.84 / 327.38)(C / 1.8)(V_b / V)(r_U / r_S)$$

in which L is the labeled quantity, in µg per mL, of naloxone hydrochloride ($C_{19}H_{21}NO_4 \cdot HCl$) in the Injection taken, 363.84 and 327.38 are the molecular weights of anhydrous naloxone hydrochloride and naloxone, respectively, C is the concentration, in µg per mL, of USP Naloxone RS in the *Standard solution*, 1.8 is the ratio of UV absorptivity of 2,2′-bisnaloxone to that of naloxone hydrochloride, V_b is the volume, in mL, of the *Test solution*, V is the volume, in mL, of Injection taken, r_U is the peak response for 2,2′-bisnaloxone obtained from the *Test solution*, and r_S is the peak response for naloxone obtained from the *Standard solution*. Not more than 4.0% is found.

Other requirements—It meets the requirements under *Injections* ⟨1⟩.

Assay—

Mobile phase—Prepare a filtered and degassed mixture of 1.36 g of sodium 1-octanesulfonate, 1.0 g of sodium chloride, 580 mL of water, 420 mL of methanol, and 1.0 mL of phosphoric acid. Make adjustments if necessary (see *System Suitability* under *Chromatography* ⟨621⟩).

Diluting solvent—Transfer 150 mg of edetate disodium to a 2000-mL volumetric flask, and add 0.9 mL of hydrochloric acid. Dilute with water to volume, and mix.

Standard preparation—Dissolve an accurately weighed quantity of USP Naloxone RS in *Diluting solvent*, and dilute quantitatively, and stepwise if necessary, with *Diluting solvent* to obtain a solution having a known concentration of about 10 µg per mL.

Assay preparation 1 (for Injection labeled to contain not more than 100 µg of naloxone hydrochloride per mL)—Transfer an accurately measured volume of Injection, equivalent to about 100 µg of naloxone hydrochloride, to a 10-mL volumetric flask, add *Diluting solvent* to volume, and mix.

Assay preparation 2 (for Injection labeled to contain more than 100 µg of naloxone hydrochloride per mL)—Transfer an accurately measured volume of Injection, equivalent to about 2000 µg of naloxone hydrochloride, to a 200-mL volumetric flask, add *Diluting solvent* to volume, and mix.

System suitability preparation—Prepare a solution in *Diluting solvent* containing about 20 µg of USP Naloxone RS and about 2.5 µg of acetaminophen per mL.

Chromatographic system (see *Chromatography* ⟨621⟩)—The liquid chromatograph is equipped with a 229-nm detector and a 4.6-mm × 25-cm column that contains packing L1. The flow rate is about 1 mL per minute. Chromatograph the *Standard preparation* (about 100 µL) and the *System suitability preparation* (about 20 µL), and record the peak responses as directed under *Procedure*: the resolution, R, between the acetaminophen and naloxone peaks is not less than 8, and the relative standard deviation for replicate injections of the *Standard preparation* is not more than 1.5%.

Procedure—[NOTE—Use peak areas where peak responses are indicated.] Separately inject equal volumes (about 100 µL) of the *Standard preparation* and the appropriate *Assay preparation* into the chromatograph, record the chromatograms, and measure the responses for the major peaks. The relative retention times are about 0.5 for acetaminophen and 1.0 for naloxone. Calculate the quantity, in µg, of $C_{19}H_{21}NO_4 \cdot HCl$ in each mL of the Injection taken by the formula:

$$(363.84 / 327.38)V_a(C / V)(r_U / r_S)$$

in which 363.84 and 327.38 are the molecular weights of anhydrous naloxone hydrochloride and naloxone, respectively; V_a is the volume, in mL, of the *Assay preparation*; C is the concentration, in µg per mL, of USP Naloxone RS in the *Standard preparation*; V is the volume, in mL, of Injection taken; and r_U and r_S are the peak responses obtained from the *Assay preparation* and the *Standard preparation*, respectively.

Naltrexone Hydrochloride

$C_{20}H_{23}NO_4 \cdot HCl$ 377.86

Morphinan-6-one, 17-(cyclopropylmethyl)-4,5-epoxy-3,14-dihydroxy-, hydrochloride, (5α)-.
17-(Cyclopropylmethyl)-4,5α-epoxy-3,14-dihydroxymorphinan-6-one hydrochloride   [16676-29-2].

» Naltrexone Hydrochloride contains not less than 98.0 percent and not more than 102.0 percent of $C_{20}H_{23}NO_4 \cdot HCl$, calculated on the anhydrous, solvent-free basis.

Packaging and storage—Preserve in tight containers.
USP Reference standards ⟨11⟩—*USP Naltrexone RS. USP Naltrexone Related Compound A RS.*
Completeness of solution ⟨641⟩—A 650-mg portion dissolves in 10 mL of water to yield a clear solution.
Identification, *Infrared Absorption* ⟨197K⟩—
 Test specimen—Dissolve about 150 mg in 25 mL of water in a small separator, add a few drops of 6 N ammonium hydroxide slowly until no more white precipitate is formed. Extract with three 5-mL portions of chloroform, filter the extracts through a dry filter, collecting the filtrate in a small flask. Evaporate the filtrate on a steam bath to dryness, and dry the residue at 105° for one hour.
Specific rotation ⟨781S⟩: between −187° and −197°, calculated on the anhydrous, solvent-free basis.
 Test solution: 25 mg per mL, in water.
Water, *Method I* ⟨921⟩—Determine the water content as directed. [NOTE—The result of this test is used in the calculation of *Limit of total solvents*.]
Residue on ignition ⟨281⟩: not more than 0.1%.
Heavy metals, *Method II* ⟨231⟩: not more than 0.002%.
Limit of total solvents—
 Internal standard stock solution—Transfer 6.0 mL of isopropyl alcohol to a 500-mL volumetric flask, dilute with water to volume, and mix. [NOTE—The isopropyl alcohol must be free of alcohol impurities.]
 Internal standard solution—Transfer 5.0 mL of the *Internal standard stock solution* to a 100-mL volumetric flask, dilute with water to volume, and mix.
 Standard solution—Prepare a solution of methanol and alcohol (C_2H_5OH) in water to obtain a solution having a known concentration of about 16 mg of each per mL. Transfer 3.0 mL of this solution and 5.0 mL of *Internal standard stock solution* to a 100-mL volumetric flask, dilute with water to volume, and mix.
 Test solution—Transfer about 75 mg of Naltrexone Hydrochloride, accurately weighed, to a suitable container, add 5.0 mL of *Internal standard solution*, and shake to dissolve.
 Chromatographic system (see *Chromatography* ⟨621⟩)—The gas chromatograph is equipped with a flame-ionization detector and a 4-mm × 1.8-m glass column packed with 80- to 100-mesh support S3. The column temperature is maintained at 150°, and the injection port and detector temperatures are maintained at 170°. Chromatograph the *Standard solution,* and record the peak responses as directed for *Procedure*: the relative retention times are about 0.24 for methanol, 0.53 for alcohol, and 1.0 for isopropyl alcohol.
 Procedure—Separately inject equal volumes (about 5 μL) of the *Standard solution* and the *Test solution* into the gas chromatograph, record the chromatograms, and measure the responses for the major peaks. Calculate the percentages of methanol and alcohol in the portion of Naltrexone Hydrochloride taken by the formula:

$$100(C_S / C_U)(R_U / R_S)$$

in which C_S is the concentration, in mg per mL, of methanol or alcohol (C_2H_5OH) in the *Standard solution*; C_U is the concentration, in mg per mL, of Naltrexone Hydrochloride in the *Test solution*; and R_U and R_S are the peak response ratios of methanol or alcohol to isopropyl alcohol obtained from the *Test solution* and the *Standard solution*, respectively. To the sum of the percentages of methanol and alcohol, add the percentage of water as determined in the test for *Water:* the sum of water and alcoholic solvents is not more than 5.0% for the anhydrous form, and not more than 11.0% for the dihydrate form.
Related compounds—Proceed as directed in the *Assay*. From the chromatogram of the *Assay preparation*, calculate the percentage of each related compound in Naltrexone Hydrochloride taken by the formula:

$$10F(C/W)(r_U / r_S)$$

in which F is the relative response factor for each impurity; C is the concentration, in mg per mL, of USP Naltrexone RS in the *Standard preparation*; W is the weight, in mg, of Naltrexone Hydrochloride taken for the *Assay preparation*; r_U is the peak response of the relevant related compound obtained from the *Assay preparation*; and r_S is the peak response of naltrexone obtained from the *Standard preparation*. [NOTE—The relative response factor is 0.3 for 2,2′-bisnaltrexone and 10-ketonaltrexone, and 1.0 for all other related compound peaks.] Not more than 0.5% of any individual related compound is found; and the total of all related compounds is not more than 1.5%.
Content of chloride—Transfer about 300 mg, accurately weighed, to a 250-mL conical flask, add 50 mL of methanol, 50 mL of water, and 3 mL of nitric acid, and mix to dissolve. Titrate with 0.1 N silver nitrate VS, determining the endpoint potentiometrically. Each mL of 0.1 N silver nitrate is equivalent to 3.545 mg of chloride: between 9.20% and 9.58%, calculated on the anhydrous, solvent-free basis is found.
Assay—
 Solution A—Dissolve about 1.08 g of sodium 1-octanesulfonate and about 23.8 g of sodium acetate in 800 mL of water. Add 1.0 mL of triethylamine and 200 mL of methanol, and mix. Adjust with glacial acetic acid to a pH of 6.5 ± 0.1. Filter and degas prior to use.
 Solution B—Dissolve about 1.08 g sodium 1-octanesulfonate and about 23.8 g sodium acetate in 400 mL of water. Add 1.0 mL triethylamine and 600 mL of methanol, and mix. Adjust with glacial acetic acid to a pH of 6.5 ± 0.1. Filter and degas prior to use.
 Mobile phase—Use variable mixtures of *Solution A* and *Solution B* as directed for *Chromatographic system*.
 Standard preparation—Transfer an accurately weighed quantity of about 22.5 mg of USP Naltrexone RS to a 10-mL volumetric flask. Add 1.5 mL of methanol and 0.6 mL of 0.1 N hydrochloric acid. Dissolve by swirling the flask, and dilute with 0.1 M phosphoric acid to volume.
 Resolution solution—Transfer about 3.0 mg, accurately weighed, of USP Naltrexone Related Compound A RS to a 10-mL volumetric flask. Add 3.0 mL of methanol, and dissolve by swirling. Dilute with 0.1 M phosphoric acid to volume, and mix. Transfer 0.5 mL of this solution to a 10-mL volumetric flask, add 5.0 mL of *Standard preparation*, dilute with 0.1 M phosphoric acid to volume, and mix.
 Assay preparation—Transfer an accurately weighed quantity of about 25 mg of Naltrexone Hydrochloride to a 10-mL volumetric flask. Dissolve in and dilute with 0.1 M phosphoric acid to volume, and mix.
 Chromatographic system (see *Chromatography* ⟨621⟩)—The liquid chromatograph is equipped with a 280-nm detector and a 3.9-mm×15-cm column that contains packing L1 and is programmed to provide, at a flow rate of about 1 mL per minute, a variable mixture of *Solution A* and *Solution B*. At the time the specimen is injected into the chromatograph, the percentage of *Solution A* is 100%; over the next 35 minutes, the proportion of *Solution B* is increased linearly to 100%, and then over the next minute, decreased linearly to 100% of *Solution A*. Allow the system to equilibrate until the late eluting peak has been observed, approximately 17 minutes later. Chromatograph about 20 μL of the *Resolution solution*, and record the peak responses as directed for *Procedure*: the relative retention times are about 0.55 for noroxymorphone, 0.70 for 10-hydroxynaltrexone, 1.0 for naltrexone, 1.26 for naltrexone related compound A, 1.80 for 2,2′-bisnaltrexone, and 1.99 for 10-ketonaltrexone; the resolution, R, between naltrexone and naltrexone related compound A is not less than 2.0; the tailing factor for the naltrexone peak is not greater than 1.4; and the relative standard deviation for replicate injections is not more than 2.0%.

Procedure—Separately inject equal volumes (about 20 µL) of the *Standard preparation* and the *Assay preparation* into the chromatograph, record the chromatograms, and measure the responses for all the peaks. Calculate the quantity, in mg, of $C_{20}H_{23}NO_4 \cdot HCl$ in the portion of Naltrexone Hydrochloride taken by the formula:

$$(377.86/341.41)10C(r_U / r_S)$$

in which 377.86 and 341.41 are the molecular weights of naltrexone hydrochloride and naltrexone, respectively; *C* is the concentration, in mg per mL, of USP Naltrexone RS in the *Standard preparation;* and r_U and r_S are the peak responses of naltrexone obtained from the *Assay preparation* and the *Standard preparation,* respectively.

Naltrexone Hydrochloride Tablets

» Naltrexone Hydrochloride Tablets contain not less than 90.0 percent and not more than 110.0 percent of the labeled amount of naltrexone hydrochloride ($C_{20}H_{23}NO_4 \cdot HCl$).

Packaging and storage—Preserve in tight containers.
USP Reference standards ⟨11⟩—*USP Naltrexone RS. USP Naltrexone Related Compound A RS.*
Identification—The retention time of the major peak for naltrexone in the chromatogram of the *Assay preparation* corresponds to that in the chromatogram of the *Standard preparation,* as obtained in the *Assay.*
Dissolution ⟨711⟩—
 Medium: water; 900 mL.
 Apparatus 2: 50 rpm.
 Time: 60 minutes.
 Determine the amount of $C_{20}H_{23}NO_4 \cdot HCl$ dissolved using the method described below.
 0.05 M Buffer solution—Dissolve 7.0 g of monobasic sodium phosphate in 1 L of water.
 Mobile phase—Prepare a mixture of 600 mL of *0.05 M Buffer solution,* 1.1 g of sodium 1-octane sulfonate monohydrate and 400 mL of methanol. Adjust with dilute sodium hydroxide to a pH of 6.7 ± 0.05, if necessary, filter, and degas. Make adjustments if necessary (see *System Suitability* under *Chromatography* ⟨621⟩).
 Chromatographic system (see *Chromatography* ⟨621⟩)—The liquid chromatograph is equipped with a 280-nm detector and a 3.9-mm × 15-cm column that contains packing L1 and is heated to 45°. The flow rate is about 1 mL per minute. Chromatograph replicate injections of the *Standard solution,* and record the peak responses as directed for *Procedure:* the relative standard deviation is not more than 2.0%.
 Procedure—Inject a volume (about 100 µL) of a filtered portion of the solution under test into the chromatograph, record the chromatogram, and measure the response for the major peak. Calculate the amount of $C_{20}H_{23}NO_4 \cdot HCl$ dissolved in comparison with a Standard solution having a known concentration of USP Naltrexone RS in the same *Medium* and similarly chromatographed.
 Tolerances—Not less than 80% *(Q)* of the labeled amount of $C_{20}H_{23}NO_4 \cdot HCl$ is dissolved in 60 minutes.
Uniformity of dosage units ⟨905⟩: meet the requirements.
Assay—
 Solution A, Solution B, Mobile phase, Resolution solution, Standard preparation, and *Chromatographic system*—Proceed as directed in the *Assay* under *Naltrexone Hydrochloride.*
 Assay preparation—Transfer not fewer than 20 Tablets to a tared container, and determine the average Tablet weight. Grind the Tablets to a homogeneous mixture. Transfer an accurately weighed portion, equivalent to about 250 mg of naltrexone hydrochloride, to a 100-mL volumetric flask. Add about 80 mL of 0.1 M phosphoric acid, and shake or sonicate for at least 30 minutes. Dilute with 0.1 M phosphoric acid to volume, mix, and filter.
 Procedure—Proceed as directed for *Procedure* in the *Assay* under *Naltrexone Hydrochloride.* Calculate the quantity, in mg, of naltrexone hydrochloride ($C_{20}H_{23}NO_4 \cdot HCl$) in the portion of Tablets taken by the formula:

$$(377.86/341.40)100C(r_U / r_S)$$

in which the terms are defined therein.

Nandrolone Decanoate

$C_{28}H_{44}O_3$ 428.65
Estr-4-en-3-one, 17-[(1-oxodecyl)oxy]-, (17β)-.
17β-Hydroxyestr-4-en-3-one decanoate   [*360-70-3*].

» Nandrolone Decanoate contains not less than 97.0 percent and not more than 103.0 percent of $C_{28}H_{44}O_3$, calculated on the dried basis.

Packaging and storage—Preserve in tight, light-resistant containers, and store in a refrigerator.
USP Reference standards ⟨11⟩—*USP Nandrolone RS. USP Nandrolone Decanoate RS.*
Completeness and clarity of solution—A solution in dioxane (1 in 50) is clear.
Identification—
 A: *Infrared Absorption* ⟨197K⟩.
 B: *Ultraviolet Absorption* ⟨197U⟩—
 Solution: 10 µg per mL.
 Medium: alcohol.
 Absorptivities at 239 nm, calculated on the dried basis, do not differ by more than 3.0%.
 C: Prepare a solution in acetone containing 5 mg per mL. Apply 10 µL of this solution and 10 µL of a solution of USP Nandrolone Decanoate RS in acetone containing 5 mg per mL to a suitable thin-layer chromatographic plate (see *Chromatography* ⟨621⟩) coated with a 0.25-mm layer of chromatographic silica gel. Allow the spots to dry, and develop the chromatogram in a solvent system consisting of a mixture of *n*-heptane and acetone (3 : 1) until the solvent front has moved about three-fourths of the length of the plate. Remove the plate from the developing chamber, mark the solvent front, and allow the solvent to evaporate. Locate the spots on the plate by lightly spraying with a solution of sulfuric acid in alcohol (1 in 50) and heating in an oven at 110° for 15 minutes: the R_F value of the principal spot obtained from the test solution corresponds to that obtained from the Standard solution.
Melting range ⟨741⟩: between 33° and 37°.
Specific rotation ⟨781S⟩: between +32° and +36°.
 Test solution: 10 mg per mL, previously dried in dioxane.
Loss on drying ⟨731⟩—Dry it in vacuum over silica gel for 4 hours: it loses not more than 0.5% of its weight.
Organic volatile impurities, *Method V* ⟨467⟩: meets the requirements.
 Solvent: dimethyl sulfoxide.

(Official until July 1, 2008)

Chromatographic purity—
 Mobile phase—Prepare a filtered and degassed mixture of chromatographic *n*-heptane and *n*-propyl alcohol (HPLC grade) (97 : 3). Make adjustments if necessary (see *System suitability* under *Chromatography* ⟨621⟩).
 System suitability solution—Dissolve accurately weighed quantities of USP Nandrolone Decanoate RS, dimethyl phthalate, and USP Nandrolone RS in *Mobile phase,* and dilute quantitatively, and stepwise if necessary, with *Mobile phase* to obtain a solution having known concentrations of about 0.25 mg per mL, 0.25 mg per mL, and 0.16 mg per mL, respectively.

Test solution—Transfer about 13 mg of Nandrolone Decanoate, accurately weighed, to a 50-mL volumetric flask, dissolve in and dilute with *Mobile phase* to volume, and mix.

Chromatographic system (see *Chromatography* ⟨621⟩)—The liquid chromatograph is equipped with a 238-nm detector and a 4.6-mm × 25-cm column that contains packing L10. The flow rate is about 1 mL per minute. Chromatograph the *System suitability solution*, and record the peak responses as directed for *Procedure:* the relative retention times are about 0.67 for dimethyl phthalate and 1.0 for nandrolone decanoate; the resolution, R, between dimethyl phthalate and nandrolone decanoate is not less than 9.0, and the nandrolone peak elutes before 4.5 times the elution time of nandrolone decanoate; the tailing factor is not more than 1.3 for the nandrolone decanoate and dimethyl phthalate peaks; and the relative standard deviation for replicate injections is not more than 2.0%.

Procedure—Inject a volume (about 20 µL) of the *Test solution* into the chromatograph, record the chromatogram, and measure the peak responses. Calculate the percentage of each impurity in the portion of Nandrolone Decanoate taken by the formula:

$$100(r_i / r_s)$$

in which r_i is the peak response for each impurity, and r_s is the sum of the responses of all of the peaks: the sum of all impurities is not more than 3.0%.

Assay—[NOTE—Use low-actinic glassware throughout this procedure.]

Mobile phase—Prepare a filtered and degassed mixture of methanol and water (95 : 5). Make adjustments if necessary (see *System Suitability* under *Chromatography* ⟨621⟩).

Standard preparation—Transfer an accurately weighed quantity of USP Nandrolone Decanoate RS to a suitable volumetric flask, and dilute with methanol to volume to obtain a solution having a known concentration of about 0.2 mg per mL.

Assay preparation—Transfer an accurately weighed quantity of about 20 mg of Nandrolone Decanoate to a 100-mL volumetric flask. Dissolve in and dilute with methanol to volume, and mix.

Chromatographic system (see *Chromatography* ⟨621⟩)—The liquid chromatograph is equipped with a 240-nm detector and an 8-mm × 10-cm analytical column containing packing L1. The flow rate is about 1.0 mL per minute. Chromatograph the *Standard preparation*, and record the peak responses as directed for *Procedure:* the capacity factor, k', is not less than 1.3; the column efficiency is not less than 8000 theoretical plates; the tailing factor is not less than 0.9 and not more than 2.0; and the relative standard deviation for replicate injections is not more than 2.0%.

Procedure—Separately inject equal volumes (about 20 µL) of the *Standard preparation* and the *Assay preparation* into the chromatograph, record the chromatograms, and measure the responses for the major peaks. Calculate the quantity, in mg, of $C_{28}H_{44}O_3$ in the portion of Nandrolone Decanoate taken by the formula:

$$100C(r_U / r_S)$$

in which C is the concentration, in mg per mL, of USP Nandrolone Decanoate RS in the *Standard preparation;* and r_U and r_S are the peak responses obtained from the *Assay preparation* and the *Standard preparation*, respectively.

Nandrolone Decanoate Injection

» Nandrolone Decanoate Injection is a sterile solution of Nandrolone Decanoate in Sesame Oil, with a suitable preservative. It contains not less than 90.0 percent and not more than 110.0 percent of the labeled amount of nandrolone decanoate ($C_{28}H_{44}O_3$).

Packaging and storage—Preserve in single-dose or in multiple-dose containers, preferably of Type I glass, protected from light.

USP Reference standards ⟨11⟩—*USP Nandrolone RS. USP Nandrolone Decanoate RS.*

Identification—Dilute a volume of Injection with acetone to provide a solution containing approximately 5 mg of nandrolone decanoate per mL. This solution responds to *Identification* test C under *Nandrolone Decanoate*, 5-µL portions of the test solution and the Standard solution being used.

Limit of nandrolone—

Standard preparation—Dissolve 25.0 mg of USP Nandrolone RS in 50.0 mL of acetone. Dilute 5.0 mL of this solution with acetone to 50.0 mL, and mix.

Test preparation—Transfer an accurately measured volume of Injection, equivalent to about 50 mg of nandrolone decanoate, to a 10-mL volumetric flask, dilute with acetone to volume, and mix.

Procedure—Apply 10 µL each of the *Standard preparation* and of the *Test preparation* to a suitable thin-layer chromatographic plate (see *Chromatography* ⟨621⟩) coated with a 0.25-mm layer of chromatographic silica gel mixture. Allow the spots to dry, and develop the chromatogram in a solvent system consisting of a mixture of *n*-heptane and acetone (3 : 1) until the solvent front has moved about three-fourths of the length of the plate. Remove the plate from the developing chamber, mark the solvent front, and allow the solvent to evaporate. Return the dry plate to the developing chamber containing the same solvent system, and again develop the chromatogram until the solvent front has moved the same distance from the origin. Remove the plate from the developing chamber, and allow the solvent to evaporate. Locate the spots on the plate by lightly spraying with a 4 in 10 solution of sulfuric acid in methanol and heating at about 100° for 10 minutes. Cool, and examine under long-wavelength UV light: any yellow fluorescent spot from the *Test preparation* at an R_f value of about 0.2 is not greater in size or intensity than that produced by the *Standard preparation* at the same R_f value, corresponding to not more than 1.0% of nandrolone.

Other requirements—It meets the requirements under *Injections* ⟨1⟩.

Assay—

0.02 M Ammonium acetate solution—Transfer about 1.6 g of ammonium acetate to a 1-liter volumetric flask. Dissolve in and dilute with water to volume.

Mobile phase—Prepare a filtered and degassed mixture of alcohol and *0.02 M Ammonium acetate solution* (66 : 34). Make adjustments if necessary (see *System Suitability* under *Chromatography* ⟨621⟩).

Standard preparation—Dissolve an accurately weighed quantity of USP Nandrolone Decanoate RS with tetrahydrofuran, and dilute quantitatively and stepwise if necessary, with tetrahydrofuran to obtain a solution having a known concentration of about 0.2 mg per mL.

Assay preparation—Transfer an accurately measured volume of Injection, equivalent to about 400 mg of nandrolone decanoate to a 200-mL volumetric flask, dilute with tetrahydrofuran to volume, and mix. Transfer 10.0 mL of this solution to a 100-mL volumetric flask, dilute with tetrahydrofuran to volume, and mix.

Chromatographic system (see *Chromatography* ⟨621⟩)—The liquid chromatograph is equipped with a 254-nm detector and a 4.6-mm × 15-cm column containing 5-µm packing L1. The flow rate is about 1.5 mL per minute. The column temperature is maintained at 40°. Chromatograph the *Standard preparation*, and record the peak responses as directed for *Procedure:* the capacity factor, k', for nandrolone decanoate is not less than 5.3; the tailing factor for the Nandrolone Decanoate peak is not more than 1.4; and the relative standard deviation for replicate injections is not more than 2.0%.

Procedure—Separately inject equal volumes (about 10 µL) of the *Standard preparation* and the *Assay preparation* into the chromatograph, record the chromatograms, and measure the responses for the major peaks. Calculate the quantity, in mg, of $C_{28}H_{44}O_3$ in each mL of the Injection taken by the formula:

$$2000(C/V)(r_U / r_S)$$

in which C is the concentration, in mg per mL, of USP Nandrolone Decanoate RS in the *Standard preparation;* V is the volume, in mL, of the injection taken to prepare the *Assay preparation*, and r_U and r_S are the peak responses obtained from the *Assay preparation* and the *Standard preparation*, respectively.

Nandrolone Phenpropionate

$C_{27}H_{34}O_3$ 406.56
Estr-4-en-3-one, 17-(1-oxo-3-phenylpropoxy)-, (17β)-.
17β-Hydroxyestr-4-en-3-one hydrocinnamate [62-90-8].

» Nandrolone Phenpropionate contains not less than 97.0 percent and not more than 103.0 percent of $C_{27}H_{34}O_3$, calculated on the dried basis.

Packaging and storage—Preserve in tight, light-resistant containers.

USP Reference standards ⟨11⟩—*USP Nandrolone Phenpropionate RS.*
Identification—
  A: *Infrared Absorption* ⟨197K⟩.
  B: *Ultraviolet Absorption* ⟨197U⟩—
    Solution: 10 µg per mL.
    Medium: alcohol.
    Absorptivities at 239 nm, calculated on the dried basis, do not differ by more than 3.0%.
  C: Prepare a solution in acetone containing 5 mg per mL. Apply 10 µL of this solution and 10 µL of a solution of USP Nandrolone Phenpropionate RS in acetone containing 5 mg per mL to a suitable thin-layer chromatographic plate (see *Chromatography* ⟨621⟩) coated with a 0.25-mm layer of chromatographic silica gel. Allow the spots to dry, and develop the chromatogram in a solvent system consisting of a mixture of *n*-heptane and acetone (2 : 1) until the solvent front has moved about three-fourths of the length of the plate. Remove the plate from the developing chamber, mark the solvent front, and allow the solvent to evaporate. Locate the spots on the plate by lightly spraying with a 1 in 50 mixture of sulfuric acid in alcohol and heating at 110° for 15 minutes: the R_F value of the principal spot obtained from the test solution corresponds to that obtained from the *Standard solution*.

Melting range ⟨741⟩:   between 95° and 99°.
Specific rotation ⟨781S⟩:   between +48° and +51°.
  Test solution: 20 mg per mL, in dioxane.
Loss on drying ⟨731⟩—Dry it in a suitable vacuum drying tube, using phosphorus pentoxide as the desiccant, at 80° for 3 hours: it loses not more than 0.5% of its weight.
Organic volatile impurities, Method V   ⟨467⟩:   meets the requirements.
  Solvent—Use dimethyl sulfoxide.

(Official until July 1, 2008)

Assay—
  Standard preparation—Prepare as directed under *Single-Steroid Assay* ⟨511⟩, using USP Nandrolone Phenpropionate RS.
  Assay preparation—Weigh accurately about 20 mg of Nandrolone Phenpropionate, previously dried, dissolve it in a sufficient quantity of a mixture of equal volumes of alcohol and chloroform to make 10.0 mL, and mix.
  Procedure—Proceed as directed for *Procedure* under *Single-Steroid Assay* ⟨511⟩, using a solvent system consisting of a mixture of *n*-heptane and acetone (3 : 1), through the fourth sentence of the second paragraph under *Procedure*. Then centrifuge the tubes for 5 minutes, and determine the absorbances of the supernatants in 1-cm cells at the wavelength of maximum absorbance at about 239 nm, with a suitable spectrophotometer, against the blank. Calculate the quantity, in mg, of $C_{27}H_{34}O_3$ in the portion of Nandrolone Phenpropionate taken by the formula:

$$10C(A_U / A_S)$$

in which *C* is the concentration, in mg per mL, of USP Nandrolone Phenpropionate RS in the *Standard preparation*, and A_U and A_S are the absorbances of the solutions from the *Assay preparation* and the *Standard preparation*, respectively.

Nandrolone Phenpropionate Injection

» Nandrolone Phenpropionate Injection is a sterile solution of Nandrolone Phenpropionate in a suitable oil. It contains not less than 90.0 percent and not more than 110.0 percent of the labeled amount of nandrolone phenpropionate ($C_{27}H_{34}O_3$).

Packaging and storage—Preserve in single-dose or in multiple-dose containers, preferably of Type I glass, protected from light.
USP Reference standards ⟨11⟩—*USP Nandrolone RS.*
Identification—Dilute the Injection with acetone to obtain a solution containing 5 mg of nandrolone phenpropionate in each mL. Proceed as directed for *Identification* test *C* under *Nandrolone Phenpropionate*, beginning with "Apply 10 µL of this solution."
Limit of nandrolone—
  Standard preparation—Prepare as directed in the test for *Limit of nandrolone* under *Nandrolone Decanoate Injection*.
  Test preparation—Transfer an accurately measured volume of Injection, equivalent to about 50 mg of nandrolone phenpropionate, to a 10-mL volumetric flask, dilute with acetone to volume, and mix.
  Procedure—Proceed as directed for *Procedure* in the test for *Limit of nandrolone* under *Nandrolone Decanoate Injection*.
Other requirements—It meets the requirements under *Injections* ⟨1⟩.
Assay—
  Isoniazid reagent—Dissolve 500 mg of isoniazid in about 250 mL of methanol, add 0.63 mL of hydrochloric acid, dilute with methanol to 500.0 mL, and mix.
  Standard preparation—Transfer about 25 mg of USP Nandrolone Phenpropionate RS, accurately weighed, to a 100-mL volumetric flask, dissolve in chloroform, dilute with chloroform to volume, and mix. Transfer 5.0 mL of this solution to a 50-mL volumetric flask, dilute with chloroform to volume, and mix.
  Assay preparation—Transfer an accurately measured volume of Injection, equivalent to about 50 mg of nandrolone phenpropionate, to a 200-mL volumetric flask, dilute with chloroform to volume, and mix. Transfer 5.0 mL of this solution to a 50-mL volumetric flask, dilute with chloroform to volume, and mix.
  Procedure—Transfer 5.0 mL each of the *Standard preparation*, of the *Assay preparation*, and of chloroform to provide the blank, to separate 10-mL volumetric flasks, dilute each flask with *Isoniazid reagent* to volume, and mix. Allow the flasks to stand for 1 hour with occasional shaking. Concomitantly determine the absorbances of the solutions in 1-cm cells at the wavelength of maximum absorbance at about 380 nm, with a suitable spectrophotometer, against the blank. Calculate the quantity, in mg, of $C_{27}H_{34}O_3$ in each mL of the Injection taken by the formula:

$$(2C / V)(A_U / A_S)$$

in which *C* is the concentration, in µg per mL, of USP Nandrolone Phenpropionate RS in the *Standard preparation*, *V* is the volume, in mL, of Injection taken, and A_U and A_S are the absorbances of the solutions from the *Assay preparation* and the *Standard preparation*, respectively.

Naphazoline Hydrochloride

$C_{14}H_{14}N_2 \cdot HCl$ 246.74
1*H*-Imidazole,   4,5-dihydro-2-(1-naphthalenylmethyl)-, monohydrochloride.
2-(1-Naphthylmethyl)-2-imidazoline   monohydrochloride [550-99-2].

» Naphazoline Hydrochloride contains not less than 98.0 percent and not more than 102.0 percent of $C_{14}H_{14}N_2 \cdot HCl$, calculated on the dried basis.

Packaging and storage—Preserve in tight, light-resistant containers.

USP Reference standards ⟨11⟩—*USP Naphazoline Hydrochloride RS.*

Identification—

A: *Infrared Absorption* ⟨197K⟩.

B: *Ultraviolet Absorption* ⟨197U⟩—

Solution: 20 µg per mL.

Medium: methanol.

Absorptivities at 280 nm, calculated on the dried basis, do not differ by more than 3.0%.

C: A solution (1 in 100) responds to the tests for *Chloride* ⟨191⟩.

pH ⟨791⟩: between 5.0 and 6.6, in a 1 in 100 solution in carbon dioxide-free water, and the solution is clear and colorless.

Loss on drying ⟨731⟩—Dry it at 105° for 2 hours: it loses not more than 0.5% of its weight.

Residue on ignition ⟨281⟩: not more than 0.2%.

Ordinary impurities ⟨466⟩—

Test solution: methanol.

Standard solution: methanol.

Eluant: a mixture of methanol, glacial acetic acid, and water (8 : 1 : 1).

Visualization: 2.

Assay—

Buffer—In a 1000-mL volumetric flask, dissolve 3.0 g of monobasic potassium phosphate, accurately weighed, in 800 mL of water. Add 3.0 mL of triethylamine, adjust with phosphoric acid to a pH of 3.0, dilute with water to volume, and mix.

Mobile phase—Prepare a filterd and degassed solution of *Buffer* and acetonitrile (80 : 20). Make adjustments if necessary (see *System Suitability* under *Chromatography* ⟨621⟩).

Standard preparation—Dissolve an accurately weighed quantity of USP Naphazoline Hydrochloride RS in water, and dilute quantitatively, and stepwise if necessary, to obtain a concentration of 0.05 mg per mL.

Assay preparation—Transfer about 200 mg of Naphazoline Hydrochloride, accurately weighed, to a 200-mL volumetric flask, and dissolve in and dilute with water to volume. Transfer 5.0 mL of this solution to a 100-mL volumetric flask, dilute with water to volume, and mix.

Chromatographic system (see *Chromatography* ⟨621⟩)—The liquid chromatograph is equipped with a 280-nm detector and a 4.0-mm × 25-cm column that contains packing L1. The flow rate is about 1.5 mL per minute. Chromatograph the *Standard preparation*, and record the peak responses as directed for *Procedure:* the capacity factor, k', is not less than 2.0; the column efficiency is not less than 1500 theoretical plates; the tailing factor is not more than 2.0; and the relative standard deviation for replicate injections of the *Standard preparation* is not more than 2.0%.

Procedure—Separately inject equal volumes (about 20 µL) of the *Standard preparation* and the *Assay preparation* into the chromatograph, record the chromatograms, and measure the responses for the major peaks. Calculate the quantity, in mg, of $C_{14}H_{14}N_2 \cdot HCl$ in the portion of Naphazoline Hydrochloride taken by the formula:

$$4000C(r_U / r_S)$$

in which C is the concentration, in mg per mL, of USP Naphazoline Hydrochloride RS in the *Standard preparation;* and r_U and r_S are the peak responses obtained from the *Assay preparation* and the *Standard preparation,* respectively.

Naphazoline Hydrochloride Nasal Solution

» Naphazoline Hydrochloride Nasal Solution is a solution of Naphazoline Hydrochloride in water adjusted to a suitable pH and tonicity. It contains not less than 90.0 percent and not more than 110.0 percent of the labeled amount of naphazoline hydrochloride ($C_{14}H_{14}N_2 \cdot HCl$).

Packaging and storage—Preserve in tight, light-resistant containers.

USP Reference standards ⟨11⟩—*USP Naphazoline Hydrochloride RS.*

Identification—The retention time of the major peak in the chromatogram of the *Assay preparation* corresponds to that of the *Standard preparation* as obtained in the *Assay*.

Assay—

Mobile phase—Dissolve 1.1 g of sodium 1-heptanesulfonate in about 400 mL of water. Add 250 mL of acetonitrile and 10 mL of glacial acetic acid, dilute with water to 1000 mL, and mix. Sonicate for 10 minutes, filter, and degas to obtain a solution having a pH of about 3.5. Make adjustments if necessary (see *System Suitability* under *Chromatography* ⟨621⟩).

Standard preparation—Dissolve an accurately weighed quantity of USP Naphazoline Hydrochloride RS in water, and dilute quantitatively, and stepwise if necessary, with water to obtain a solution having a known concentration of about 250 µg per mL.

Assay preparation—Pipet a volume of Nasal Solution, equivalent to about 25 mg of naphazoline hydrochloride, into a 100-mL volumetric flask, dilute with water to volume, and mix.

Chromatographic system (see *Chromatography* ⟨621⟩)—The liquid chromatograph is equipped with a 280-nm detector and a 4-mm × 30-cm column that contains packing L11. The flow rate is about 2 mL per minute. Chromatograph the *Standard preparation*, and record the peak responses as directed under *Procedure:* the tailing factor for the naphazoline hydrochloride peak is not more than 2.0, and the relative standard deviation for replicate injections is not more than 1.5%.

Procedure—Separately inject equal volumes (about 15 µL) of the *Standard preparation* and the *Assay preparation* into the chromatograph, record the chromatograms, and measure the responses for the major peaks. Calculate the quantity, in mg, of $C_{14}H_{14}N_2 \cdot HCl$ in each mL of the Nasal Solution taken by the formula:

$$0.1(C / V)(r_U / r_S)$$

in which C is the concentration, in µg per mL, of USP Naphazoline Hydrochloride RS in the *Standard preparation*, V is the volume, in mL, of Nasal Solution taken, and r_U and r_S are the peak responses obtained from the *Assay preparation* and the *Standard preparation,* respectively.

Naphazoline Hydrochloride Ophthalmic Solution

» Naphazoline Hydrochloride Ophthalmic Solution is a sterile, buffered solution of Naphazoline Hydrochloride in water adjusted to a suitable tonicity. It contains not less than 90.0 percent and not more than 115.0 percent of the labeled amount of naphazoline hydrochloride ($C_{14}H_{14}N_2 \cdot HCl$). It contains a suitable preservative.

Packaging and storage—Preserve in tight containers.

USP Reference standards ⟨11⟩—*USP Naphazoline Hydrochloride RS.*

Identification—Place in a separator a volume of Ophthalmic Solution, equivalent to about 25 mg of naphazoline hydrochloride, add 5

mL of 1 N sodium hydroxide, saturate with sodium chloride, and extract with two 25-mL portions of ether. Wash the ether solution with 5 mL of water, pass the ether through a small paper filter, evaporate the filtrate to about 5 mL, transfer the residual solution to a 10- to 15-mL beaker, allow to evaporate spontaneously, and dry the residue at 80° for 1 hour: the naphazoline so obtained melts between 115° and 120° when determined as directed for *Class Ia* under *Melting Range or Temperature* ⟨741⟩.
Sterility ⟨71⟩: meets the requirements.
pH ⟨791⟩: between 5.5 and 7.0.
Assay—
Phosphate buffer—Transfer 3 g of monobasic potassium phosphate to a 1-liter volumetric flask, dissolve in 1000 mL of water and 3 mL of triethylamine, and mix. Adjust with phosphoric acid to a pH of 3, and mix.
Mobile phase—Prepare a filtered and degassed mixture of *Phosphate buffer* and acetonitrile (80 : 20). Make adjustments if necessary (see *System Suitability* under *Chromatography* ⟨621⟩).
Standard preparation—Dissolve an accurately weighed quantity of USP Naphazoline Hydrochloride RS in water, and dilute quantitatively, and stepwise if necessary, with *Mobile phase* to obtain a solution having a known concentration of about 0.05 mg per mL.
Assay preparation—Transfer an accurately measured volume of Ophthalmic Solution, equivalent to about 5.0 mg of naphazoline hydrochloride, to a 100-mL volumetric flask, dissolve in and dilute with *Mobile phase* to volume, and mix.
Chromatographic system (see *Chromatography* ⟨621⟩)—The liquid chromatograph is equipped with a 285-nm detector and a 4.6-mm × 15-cm column that contains packing L11. The flow rate is about 1.5 mL per minute. The column temperature is maintained at 40°. Chromatograph the *Standard preparation*, and record the peak responses as directed under *Procedure:* the column efficiency is not less than 5000 theoretical plates, the tailing factor is not more than 2.0, and the relative standard deviation for replicate injections is not more than 2.0%.
Procedure—Separately inject equal volumes (about 10 µL) of the *Standard preparation* and the *Assay preparation* into the chromatograph, record the chromatograms, and measure the responses for the major peaks. Calculate the quantity, in mg, of $C_{14}H_{14}N_2 \cdot HCl$ in the portion of Ophthalmic Solution taken by the formula:

$$100C(r_U / r_S)$$

in which C is the concentration, in mg per mL, of USP Naphazoline Hydrochloride RS in the *Standard preparation*, and r_U and r_S are the peak responses obtained from the *Assay preparation* and the *Standard preparation*, respectively.

Naphazoline Hydrochloride and Pheniramine Maleate Ophthalmic Solution

» Naphazoline Hydrochloride and Pheniramine Maleate Ophthalmic Solution is a sterile, buffered solution of Naphazoline Hydrochloride and Pheniramine Maleate in water adjusted to a suitable tonicity. It contains not less than 90.0 percent and not more than 110.0 percent of the labeled amount of naphazoline hydrochloride ($C_{14}H_{14}N_2 \cdot HCl$) and pheniramine maleate ($C_{16}H_{20}N_2 \cdot C_4H_4O_4$). It contains a suitable preservative.

Packaging and storage—Preserve in tight containers, and store at a temperature between 20° and 25°, protected from light.
USP Reference standards ⟨11⟩—*USP Naphazoline Hydrochloride RS. USP Pheniramine Maleate RS.*
Identification—
A: Proceed as directed in the following thin-layer chromatographic procedure.

Naphazoline hydrochloride standard solution—Dissolve a quantity of USP Naphazoline Hydrochloride RS in water to obtain a solution containing about 1.5 mg per mL.
Pheniramine maleate standard solution—Dissolve a quantity of USP Pheniramine Maleate RS in water to obtain a solution containing about 6.0 mg per mL.
Test solution—Dilute, if necessary, a volume of Ophthalmic Solution with water to obtain a solution containing about 0.25 mg of naphazoline hydrochloride per mL and 3 mg of pheniramine maleate per mL.
Procedure—Separately apply 5 µL of *Naphazoline hydrochloride standard solution*, 10 µL of *Pheniramine maleate standard solution*, and 30 µL of the *Test solution* to a 20-cm × 20-cm thin-layer chromatographic plate (see *Chromatography* ⟨621⟩) coated with a 0.25-mm layer of silica gel. Allow the spots to dry, then place the plate in a saturated chromatographic chamber, and develop in a solvent system consisting of methanol, water, and acetic acid (8 : 1 : 1) until the solvent front has moved to about 1.5 cm from the top of the plate. Remove the plate from the developing chamber, mark the solvent front, and allow to air-dry. Spray with ninhydrin TS, and place in an oven at 105° to visualize the spots. Both the naphazoline and pheniramine spots are purplish grey in color. The R_F values of the spots obtained from the *Test solution* correspond to those obtained from the *Naphazoline hydrochloride standard solution* and the *Pheniramine maleate standard solution*.
B: The retention times of the major peaks in the chromatogram of the *Assay preparation* correspond to those of the *Standard preparation*, as obtained in the *Assay*.
Sterility ⟨71⟩—It meets the requirements when tested as directed for *Membrane Filtration* under *Test for Sterility of the Product to be Examined*.
pH ⟨791⟩: between 5.7 and 6.3.
Assay—
Buffer solution—Dissolve 14.2 g of anhydrous dibasic sodium phosphate and 20 mL of triethylamine in 1900 mL of water, adjust with phosphoric acid to a pH of 5.6 ± 0.1, dilute with water to make 2000 mL of solution, and mix.
Mobile phase—Prepared a filtered and degassed mixture of *Buffer* and acetonitrile (80 : 20). Make adjustments if necessary (see *System Suitability* under *Chromatography* ⟨621⟩).
Naphazoline hydrochloride stock standard solution—Dissolve an accurately weighed quantity of USP Naphazoline Hydrochloride RS in *Mobile phase* to obtain a solution having a known concentration of about 0.75 mg per mL.
Pheniramine maleate stock standard solution—Dissolve an accurately weighed quantity of USP Pheniramine Maleate RS in *Mobile phase* to obtain a known concentration of about 3.00 mg per mL.
Standard preparation—Transfer 1.0 mL of *Naphazoline hydrochloride stock standard solution* and 3.0 mL of *Pheniramine maleate stock standard solution* to a 25-mL volumetric flask, dilute with *Mobile phase* to volume, and mix to obtain a solution having known concentrations of naphazoline hydrochloride and pheniramine maleate of 0.03 and 0.36 mg per mL, respectively.
Assay preparation—Transfer an accurately measured volume of Ophthalmic Solution, equivalent to about 0.75 mg of naphazoline hydrochloride and 9.0 mg of pheniramine maleate, to a 25-mL volumetric flask, dilute with *Mobile phase* to volume, and mix.
Chromatographic system (see *Chromatography* ⟨621⟩)—The liquid chromatograph is equipped with a 270-nm detector and a 4.6-mm × 15-cm column that contains packing L7. The flow rate is about 1.5 mL per minute. Chromatograph the *Standard preparation*, and record the peak responses as directed for *Procedure:* the resolution, R, between the naphazoline peak and the pheniramine peak is not less than 2; the column efficiency, determined from the naphazoline and pheniramine peaks, is not less than 750 theoretical plates; the tailing factor is not greater than 2.5 for pheniramine; and the relative standard deviation for replicate injections is not more than 2.0%.
Procedure—Separately inject equal volumes (about 25 µL) of the *Standard preparation* and the *Assay preparation* into the chromatograph, record the chromatograms, and measure the responses for the peaks. Calculate the quantity, in mg, of naphazoline hydrochloride

($C_{14}H_{14}N_2 \cdot HCl$) in each mL of the Ophthalmic Solution taken by the formula:

$$25(C/V)(r_U/r_S)$$

in which C is the concentration in mg per mL of USP Naphazoline Hydrochloride RS in the *Standard preparation;* V is the volume, in mL, of Ophthalmic solution taken; and r_U and r_S are the naphazoline peak responses obtained from the *Assay preparation* and the *Standard preparation,* respectively. Calculate the quantity, in mg, of pheniramine maleate ($C_{16}H_{20}N_2 \cdot C_4H_4O_4$) in each mL of the Ophthalmic Solution taken by the same formula, changing the terms to refer to pheniramine maleate.

Naproxen

$C_{14}H_{14}O_3$ 230.26
2-Naphthaleneacetic acid, 6-methoxy-α-methyl-, (S)-.
(+)-(S)-6-Methoxy-α-methyl-2-naphthaleneacetic acid   [22204-53-1].

» Naproxen contains not less than 98.5 percent and not more than 101.5 percent of $C_{14}H_{14}O_3$, calculated on the dried basis.

Packaging and storage—Preserve in tight containers.
USP Reference standards ⟨11⟩—*USP Naproxen RS.*
Identification—
    A: *Infrared Absorption* ⟨197K⟩.
    B: *Ultraviolet Absorption* ⟨197U⟩—
    Solution: 25 µg per mL.
    Medium: methanol.
    Absorptivities at 271 nm, calculated on the dried basis, do not differ by more than 3%.
Specific rotation ⟨781S⟩:   between +83.0° and +89.5°.
    Test solution: 10 mg per mL, in methyl isobutyl ketone.
Loss on drying ⟨731⟩—Dry it at 105° for 3 hours: it loses not more than 0.5% of its weight.
Heavy metals, *Method II* ⟨231⟩:   0.002%.
Chromatographic purity—Dissolve 100 mg of Naproxen in methanol, and dilute with methanol to 5.0 mL to obtain the *Test solution.* Dissolve a suitable quantity of USP Naproxen RS in methanol to obtain a *Standard solution* having a known concentration of about 20 mg per mL. Dilute a portion of this solution quantitatively and stepwise with methanol to obtain three *Comparison solutions* having concentrations of 20, 60, and 100 µg per mL (0.1%, 0.3%, and 0.5% of the *Standard solution*), respectively. Apply separate 10-µL portions of the five solutions to the starting line of a suitable thin-layer chromatographic plate (see *Chromatography* ⟨621⟩) coated with a 0.25-mm layer of chromatographic silica gel mixture. Develop the chromatogram in a solvent system consisting of a mixture of toluene, tetrahydrofuran, and glacial acetic acid (30 : 3 : 1) until the solvent front has moved about three-fourths of the length of the plate. Remove the plate from the chamber, mark the solvent front, air-dry, and view under short-wavelength UV light: the R_F value of the principal spot in the chromatogram of the *Test solution* corresponds to that of the *Standard solution,* and any other spot obtained from the *Test solution* does not exceed, in size or intensity, the principal spot obtained from the 100-µg-per-mL *Comparison solution* (0.5%), and the sum of the intensities of any secondary spots, similarly compared, does not exceed 2.0%.
Organic volatile impurities, *Method V* ⟨467⟩:   meets the requirements.
    Solvent—Use dimethyl sulfoxide.

(Official until July 1, 2008)
Assay—Dissolve about 500 mg of Naproxen, accurately weighed, in a mixture of 75 mL of methanol and 25 mL of water that has been previously neutralized to the phenolphthalein endpoint with 0.1 N sodium hydroxide. Dissolve by gentle warming, if necessary, add phenolphthalein TS, and titrate with 0.1 N sodium hydroxide VS. Each mL of 0.1 N sodium hydroxide is equivalent to 23.03 mg of $C_{14}H_{14}O_3$.

Naproxen Oral Suspension

» Naproxen Oral Suspension contains not less than 90.0 percent and not more than 110.0 percent of the labeled amount of naproxen ($C_{14}H_{14}O_3$).

Packaging and storage—Preserve in tight, light-resistant containers. Store at room temperature.
USP Reference standards ⟨11⟩—*USP Naproxen RS.*
Identification—Prepare a mixture of the *Standard preparation* and the *Assay preparation* (1 : 1), prepared as directed in the *Assay,* and chromatograph as directed in the *Assay:* the chromatogram thus obtained exhibits two main peaks corresponding to naproxen and the internal standard.
Uniformity of dosage units ⟨905⟩—
    FOR ORAL SUSPENSION PACKAGED IN SINGLE-UNIT CONTAINERS: meets the requirements.
Deliverable volume ⟨698⟩—
    FOR ORAL SUSPENSION PACKAGED IN MULTIPLE-UNIT CONTAINERS: meets the requirements.
pH ⟨791⟩:   between 2.2 and 3.7.
Assay—
    Mobile phase—Prepare a mixture of 500 mL of methanol, 500 mL of water, and 2.46 g of anhydrous sodium acetate, and mix until dissolved. Adjust with glacial acetic acid to a pH of 5.8. Make adjustments if necessary (see *System Suitability* under *Chromatography* ⟨621⟩).
    Internal standard solution—Prepare a solution of ethylparaben in methanol containing about 1.1 mg per mL.
    Standard preparation—Transfer about 62.5 mg of USP Naproxen RS, accurately weighed, to a 50-mL volumetric flask, add about 30 mL of methanol, and sonicate to dissolve. Add 5.0 mL of *Internal standard solution,* dilute with methanol to volume, and mix. Transfer 2.0 mL of this solution to a 50-mL volumetric flask, dilute with *Mobile phase* to volume, and mix. This solution contains about 50 µg of USP Naproxen RS and 4.4 µg of ethylparaben per mL.
    Assay preparation—Transfer an accurately measured volume of Oral Suspension, previously well-mixed and free from air bubbles, equivalent to about 125 mg of naproxen, to a 100-mL volumetric flask, using a "to contain" pipet. Rinse the pipet several times with methanol, and add the rinsings to the volumetric flask. Add 10.0 mL of *Internal standard solution,* dilute with methanol to volume, and mix. Transfer 2.0 mL of this solution to a 50-mL volumetric flask, dilute with *Mobile phase* to volume, and mix. Filter, if necessary, to obtain a clear solution.
    Chromatographic system (see *Chromatography* ⟨621⟩)—The liquid chromatograph is equipped with a 254-nm detector and a 3.9-mm × 30-cm column that contains packing L1. The flow rate is about 2 mL per minute. Chromatograph the *Standard preparation,* and record the peak responses as directed for *Procedure:* the relative retention times are about 0.6 for ethylparaben and 1.0 for naproxen; the resolution, R, between ethylparaben and naproxen is not less than 3.0; the tailing factor for the naproxen peak is not more than 2.0; and the relative standard deviation for replicate injections is not more than 1.5%.
    Procedure—Separately inject equal volumes (about 35 µL) of the *Standard preparation* and the *Assay preparation* into the chromatograph, record the chromatograms, and measure the responses for the major peaks. Calculate the quantity, in mg, of naproxen ($C_{14}H_{14}O_3$) in each mL of the Oral Suspension taken by the formula:

$$2.5(C/V)(R_U/R_S)$$

in which C is the concentration, in µg per mL, of USP Naproxen RS in the *Standard preparation;* V is the volume, in mL, of Oral Suspension taken to prepare the *Assay preparation;* and R_U and R_S are the ratios of the response of the naproxen peak to the response of the ethylparaben peak obtained from the *Assay preparation* and the *Standard preparation*, respectively.

Naproxen Tablets

» Naproxen Tablets contain not less than 90.0 percent and not more than 110.0 percent of the labeled amount of naproxen ($C_{14}H_{14}O_3$).

Packaging and storage—Preserve in well-closed containers.

USP Reference standards ⟨11⟩—*USP Naproxen RS*.

Identification—Prepare a mixture of the *Standard preparation* and the *Assay preparation* (1 : 1), prepared as directed in the *Assay*, and chromatograph as directed in the *Assay*: the chromatogram so obtained exhibits two main peaks, corresponding to naproxen and the internal standard.

Dissolution ⟨711⟩—

0.1 M, pH 7.4 phosphate buffer—Dissolve 2.62 g of monobasic sodium phosphate and 11.50 g of anhydrous dibasic sodium phosphate in 1000 mL of water, and mix.

Medium: 0.1 M, pH 7.4 phosphate buffer; 900 mL.

Apparatus 2: 50 rpm.

Time: 45 minutes.

Procedure—Determine the amount of $C_{14}H_{14}O_3$ dissolved from UV absorbances at the wavelength of maximum absorbance at about 332 nm of filtered portions of the solution under test, suitably diluted with *0.1 M, pH 7.4 phosphate buffer*, in comparison with a Standard solution having a known concentration of USP Naproxen RS in the same medium.

Tolerances—Not less than 80% *(Q)* of the labeled amount of $C_{14}H_{14}O_3$ is dissolved in 45 minutes.

Uniformity of dosage units ⟨905⟩: meet the requirements.

Assay—

Mobile phase—Prepare a suitable mixture of acetonitrile, water, and glacial acetic acid (50 : 49 : 1). Make adjustments if necessary (see *System Suitability* under *Chromatography* ⟨621⟩). Increased resolution may be achieved by increasing the proportion of water in the *Mobile phase*.

Solvent mixture—Prepare a suitable mixture of acetonitrile and water (90 : 10).

Internal standard solution—Dilute 5 mL of butyrophenone with acetonitrile to make 100 mL. Dilute 1 mL of the resulting solution with acetonitrile to make 100 mL. Each mL of this solution contains about 0.5 µL of butyrophenone.

Standard preparation—Dissolve an accurately weighed quantity of USP Naproxen RS in *Solvent mixture* to obtain a solution having a known concentration of about 2.5 mg per mL. Transfer 1.0 mL of the resulting solution and 2.0 mL of *Internal standard solution* to a 100-mL volumetric flask, dilute with *Mobile phase* to volume, and mix. This solution contains about 25 µg of USP Naproxen RS per mL.

Assay preparation—Weigh and finely powder not less than 20 Tablets. Transfer an accurately weighed quantity of the powder, equivalent to about 250 mg of naproxen, to a 100-mL volumetric flask. Add 10 mL of water, and sonicate for 10 minutes until the material is completely dispersed. Add about 80 mL of acetonitrile, and sonicate for an additional 5 minutes. Allow the flask to reach room temperature, dilute with acetonitrile to volume, and mix. Allow any insoluble matter to settle, then transfer 1.0 mL of the clear supernatant to a 100-mL volumetric flask, add 2.0 mL of *Internal standard solution*, dilute with *Mobile phase* to volume, and mix.

Chromatographic system (see *Chromatography* ⟨621⟩)—The liquid chromatograph is equipped with a 254-nm detector and a 4.6-mm × 15-cm column that contains 5-µm packing L1. The flow rate is about 1.2 mL per minute. Chromatograph the *Standard preparation*, and record the peak responses as directed under *Procedure*: the column efficiency, determined from the analyte peak, is not less than 4000 theoretical plates when calculated by the formula:

$$5.545(t / W_{h/2})^2$$

the resolution between the analyte and internal standard peaks is not less than 11.5 when calculated by the formula:

$$2(t_2 - t_1) / [1.699(W_{1h/2} + W_{2h/2})]$$

and the relative standard deviation of replicate injections is not more than 1.5%.

Procedure—Separately inject equal volumes (about 20 µL) of the *Standard preparation* and the *Assay preparation* into the chromatograph, record the chromatograms, and measure the responses for the major peaks. The relative retention times are about 0.6 for naproxen and 1.0 for the internal standard. Calculate the quantity, in mg, of $C_{14}H_{14}O_3$ in the portion of Tablets taken by the formula:

$$10C(R_U / R_S)$$

in which C is the concentration, in µg per mL, of USP Naproxen RS in the *Standard preparation*, and R_U and R_S are the ratios of the response of the naproxen peak to the response of the internal standard peak obtained from the *Assay preparation* and the *Standard preparation*, respectively.

Naproxen Delayed-Release Tablets

» Naproxen Delayed-Release Tablets contain not less than 90.0 percent and not more than 110.0 percent of the labeled amount of naproxen ($C_{14}H_{14}O_3$).

Packaging and storage—Preserve in well-closed containers, and store at controlled room temperature.

USP Reference standards ⟨11⟩—*USP Naproxen RS*.

Identification—

A: *Ultraviolet Absorption* ⟨197U⟩—

Test solution—Use the solution under test as obtained in the *Buffer stage* of the *Drug release* test.

Standard solution—Use the Standard solution prepared as directed in the *Buffer stage* of the *Drug release* test.

B: The retention time of the major peak in the chromatogram of the *Assay preparation* corresponds to that in the chromatogram of the *Standard preparation*, as obtained in the *Assay*.

Drug release, Method B ⟨724⟩—

ACID STAGE—

Acid stage medium: 0.1 N hydrochloric acid; 1000 mL.

Apparatus 2: 50 rpm.

Time: 2 hours.

Procedure—Determine the amount of $C_{14}H_{14}O_3$ dissolved by employing UV absorption at the wavelength of maximum absorbance at about 332 nm on filtered portions of the solution under test, suitably diluted with *Acid stage medium*, if necessary, in comparison with a Standard solution having a known concentration of USP Naproxen RS in the same *Acid stage medium*.

Tolerances—Not more than 10% *(Q)* of the labeled amount of $C_{14}H_{14}O_3$ is dissolved in 2 hours.

BUFFER STAGE—

Buffer stage medium: 0.2 M phosphate buffer, pH 6.8; 1000 mL.

Apparatus 2: 50 rpm.

Time: 45 minutes.

Procedure—Determine the amount of $C_{14}H_{14}O_3$ dissolved by employing UV absorption at the wavelength of maximum absorbance at about 332 nm on filtered portions of the solution under test, suitably diluted with *Buffer stage medium*, if necessary, in comparison with a Standard solution having a known concentration of USP Naproxen RS in the same *Buffer stage medium*.

Tolerances—Not less than 80% *(Q)* of the labeled amount of $C_{14}H_{14}O_3$ is dissolved in 45 minutes.

Uniformity of dosage units ⟨905⟩: meet the requirements.

PROCEDURE FOR CONTENT UNIFORMITY—

Mobile phase, Diluent A, Diluent B, and *Chromatographic system*—Proceed as directed in the *Assay.*

Standard solution—Transfer about 12.5 mg of USP Naproxen RS, accurately weighed, to a 50-mL volumetric flask, dilute with *Diluent A* to volume, and mix well. Transfer 10 mL of this solution to a 25-mL volumetric flask, dilute with *Diluent B* to volume, and mix.

Test solution—Transfer 1 Tablet to a 200-mL volumetric flask, and add about 140 mL of *Diluent B.* Shake by mechanical means for 15 minutes, sonicate for 15 minutes, dilute with *Diluent B* to volume, and mix. Pass a portion of this solution through a filter having a porosity of 0.45-μm, pipet 2.0 mL of the filtrate for a 500-mg tablet and 2.5 mL for a 375-mg tablet into a 50-mL volumetric flask, dilute with *Mobile phase* to volume, and mix.

Assay—

Mobile phase—Prepare a filtered and degassed mixture of 1% acetic acid solution and acetonitrile (11 : 9).

Diluent A—Use acetonitrile and water (9 : 1).

Diluent B—Use acetonitrile and water (1 : 1).

Standard stock preparation—Transfer about 12.5 mg of USP Naproxen RS, accurately weighed, to a 25-mL volumetric flask. Dissolve in and dilute with *Diluent A* to volume, and mix.

Standard preparation—Accurately transfer 10.0 mL of the *Standard stock preparation* into a 50-mL volumetric flask, and dilute with *Mobile phase* to volume, and mix.

Assay preparation—Weigh and powder 20 Tablets. Accurately weigh an amount of the powder, equivalent to about 250 mg of naproxen, into a 100-mL volumetric flask, and add about 70 mL of *Diluent B.* Shake by mechanical means for 15 minutes, sonicate for 15 minutes, dilute with *Diluent B* to volume, and mix. Pass this solution through a filter having a porosity of 0.45-μm, transfer 2.0 mL of the filtrate into a 50-mL volumetric flask, dilute with *Mobile phase* to volume, and mix.

Chromatographic system (see *Chromatography* ⟨621⟩)—The liquid chromatograph is equipped with a 254-nm detector and a 4.6-mm × 25-cm column that contains 5-μm packing L1. The flow rate is about 1.0 mL per minute. Chromatograph the *Standard preparation,* and record the peak responses as directed for *Procedure:* the tailing factor of the naproxen peak is not more than 1.5, and the relative standard deviation for replicate injections of the *Standard preparation* is not more than 2.0%.

Procedure—Separately inject equal volumes (about 50 μL) of the *Standard preparation* and the *Assay preparation* into the chromatograph, record the chromatograms, and measure the responses for the naproxen peak. Calculate the quantity, in mg, of naproxen ($C_{14}H_{14}O_3$) in the portion of Tablets taken by the formula:

$$2500C(r_U / r_S)$$

in which *C* is the concentration, in mg per mL, of USP Naproxen RS in the *Standard preparation;* and r_U and r_S are the peak responses obtained from the *Assay preparation* and the *Standard preparation,* respectively.

Naproxen Sodium

$C_{14}H_{13}NaO_3$ 252.24

2-Naphthaleneacetic acid, 6-methoxy-α-methyl-, sodium salt, (*S*)-.
(−)-Sodium   (*S*)-6-methoxy-α-methyl-2-naphthaleneacetate
[26159-34-2].

» Naproxen Sodium contains not less than 98.0 percent and not more than 102.0 percent of $C_{14}H_{13}NaO_3$, calculated on the dried basis.

Packaging and storage—Preserve in tight containers.
USP Reference standards ⟨11⟩—*USP Naproxen Sodium RS.*
Identification—
  A: *Infrared Absorption* ⟨197K⟩.
  B: *Ultraviolet Absorption* ⟨197U⟩—
  Solution: 25 μg per mL.
  Medium: methanol.
Absorptivities at 272 nm, calculated on the dried basis, do not differ by more than 3%.
Specific rotation ⟨781S⟩: between −15.3° and −17.0°.
  Test solution: 50 mg per mL, in 0.1 N sodium hydroxide.
Loss on drying ⟨731⟩—Dry it in vacuum at 105° for 3 hours: it loses not more than 1.0% of its weight.
Heavy metals, *Method I* ⟨231⟩—Dissolve 1.0 g in 20 mL of water in a separator, add 5 mL of 1 N hydrochloric acid, and extract with successive 20-mL, 20-mL, and 10-mL portions of methylene chloride. Discard the methylene chloride extracts, and use the aqueous layer for the test: the limit is 0.002%.
Free naproxen—Dissolve about 5.0 g in 25 mL of water in a separator, and extract the solution with three 15-mL portions of chloroform. Evaporate the combined extracts on a steam bath to dryness. Dissolve the residue in 10 mL of a mixture of methanol and water (3 : 1) previously neutralized with 0.1 N sodium hydroxide to the phenolphthalein endpoint. Add phenolphthalein TS, and titrate with 0.10 N sodium hydroxide: not more than 2.2 mL is consumed (1.0%).
Chromatographic purity—Dissolve 100 mg in 5 mL of methanol. Dissolve a suitable quantity of USP Naproxen Sodium RS in methanol to obtain a *Standard solution* having a known concentration of about 20 mg per mL. Dilute a portion of this solution quantitatively with methanol to obtain three *Comparison solutions* having concentrations of 20, 60, and 100 μg per mL (0.1%, 0.3%, and 0.5% of the *Standard solution*), respectively. Apply separate 10-μL portions of the five solutions on the starting line to a suitable thin-layer chromatographic plate (see *Chromatography* ⟨621⟩) coated with a 0.25-mm layer of chromatographic silica gel mixture. Develop the chromatogram in a solvent system consisting of a mixture of toluene, tetrahydrofuran, and glacial acetic acid (30 : 3 : 1) until the solvent front has moved about three-fourths of the length of the plate. Remove the plate from the chamber, mark the solvent front, air-dry, and view under short-wavelength UV light: the R_F value of the principal spot in the chromatogram of the solution under test corresponds to that of the *Standard solution,* the intensity of any individual secondary spot does not exceed that of the 100-μg-per-mL *Comparison solution* (0.5%), and the sum of the intensities of any secondary spots, similarly compared, does not exceed 2.0%.
Organic volatile impurities, *Method I* ⟨467⟩: meets the requirements.

(Official until July 1, 2008)

Assay—Dissolve about 200 mg of Naproxen Sodium, accurately weighed, in 50 mL of glacial acetic acid containing 2 drops of *p*-naphtholbenzein TS previously neutralized with 0.1 N perchloric acid if necessary. Titrate with 0.1 N perchloric acid VS. Each mL of 0.1 N perchloric acid is equivalent to 25.22 mg of $C_{14}H_{13}NaO_3$.

Naproxen Sodium Tablets

» Naproxen Sodium Tablets contain not less than 90.0 percent and not more than 110.0 percent of the labeled amount of naproxen sodium ($C_{14}H_{13}NaO_3$).

Packaging and storage—Preserve in well-closed containers.
USP Reference standards ⟨11⟩—*USP Naproxen Sodium RS.*
Identification—
  A: Transfer a quantity of finely powdered Tablets, equivalent to about 250 mg of naproxen sodium, to a centrifuge tube, and add 12 mL of water and 1 mL of hydrochloric acid: a dense white precipitate is formed. Centrifuge the mixture: the clear, supernatant responds to the identification test for *Sodium* ⟨191⟩.
  B: Prepare a mixture of the *Standard preparation* and the *Assay preparation* (1 : 1), prepared as directed in the *Assay,* and chro-

matograph as directed in the *Assay:* the chromatogram thus obtained exhibits two main peaks, corresponding to naproxen and the internal standard.

Dissolution ⟨711⟩—

Medium: 0.1 M phosphate buffer (pH 7.4), prepared by dissolving 2.62 g of monobasic sodium phosphate and 11.50 g of anhydrous dibasic sodium phosphate in water to make 1000 mL; 900 mL.

Apparatus 2: 50 rpm.

Time: 45 minutes.

Standard preparation—Dissolve an accurately weighed portion of USP Naproxen Sodium RS in *Medium* to obtain a solution having a known concentration of about 50 µg per mL.

Procedure—Dilute a filtered portion of the solution under test quantitatively with *Medium* as necessary to obtain a solution having a concentration of about 50 µg per mL of $C_{14}H_{13}NaO_3$. Determine the amount of $C_{14}H_{13}NaO_3$ dissolved from UV absorbances at the wavelength of maximum absorbance at about 332 nm of this solution in comparison with the *Standard preparation*.

Tolerances—Not less than 80% *(Q)* of the labeled amount of $C_{14}H_{13}NaO_3$ is dissolved in 45 minutes.

Uniformity of dosage units ⟨905⟩: meet the requirements.

Assay—

Mobile phase, Solvent mixture, Internal standard solution, and *Chromatographic system*—Prepare as directed in the *Assay* under *Naproxen Tablets.*

Standard preparation—Dissolve an accurately weighed quantity of USP Naproxen Sodium RS in *Solvent mixture* to obtain a solution having a concentration of about 2.75 mg per mL. Transfer 1.0 mL of the resulting solution and 2.0 mL of *Internal standard solution* to a 100-mL volumetric flask, dilute with *Mobile phase* to volume, and mix. This solution contains about 27.5 µg of USP Naproxen Sodium RS per mL.

Assay preparation—Weigh and finely powder not less than 20 Tablets. Transfer an accurately weighed quantity of the powder, equivalent to about 275 mg of naproxen sodium, to a 100-mL volumetric flask. Add 10 mL of water, and shake until the material is completely dispersed. Dilute with acetonitrile to volume, and mix. Allow any insoluble matter to settle, then transfer 1.0 mL of the clear supernatant to a 100-mL volumetric flask, add 2.0 mL of *Internal standard solution,* dilute with *Mobile phase* to volume, and mix.

Procedure—Proceed as directed for *Procedure* in the *Assay* under *Naproxen Tablets.* Calculate the quantity, in mg, of $C_{14}H_{13}NaO_3$ in the portion of Tablets taken by the formula:

$$10C(R_U / R_S)$$

in which *C* is the concentration, in µg per mL, of USP Naproxen Sodium RS in the *Standard preparation,* and R_U and R_S are the ratios of the response of the naproxen peak to the response of the internal standard peak obtained from the *Assay preparation* and the *Standard preparation,* respectively.

Narasin Granular

$C_{43}H_{72}O_{11}$ (narasin A)   765.03
$C_{43}H_{70}O_{11}$ (narasin B)   763.01
$C_{44}H_{74}O_{11}$ (narasin D)   779.07
$C_{44}H_{74}O_{11}$ (narasin I)   779.07

Narasin.

2*H*-Pyran-2-acetic acid, α-ethyl-6-[5-[2-(5-ethyltetrahydro-5-hydroxy-6-methyl-2*H*-pyran-2-yl)-15-hydroxy-2,10,12-trimethyl-1,6,8-trioxadispiro[4.1.5.3]pentadec-13-en-9-yl]-2-hydroxy-1,3-dimethyl-4-oxoheptyl]tetrahydro-3,5-dimethyl-.

α-Ethyl-6-[5-[2-(5-ethyltetrahydro-5-hydroxy-6-methyl-2*H*-pyran-2-yl)-15-hydroxy-2,10,12-trimethyl-1,6,8-trioxadispiro[4.1.5.3]pentadec-13-en-9-yl]-2-hydroxy-1,3-dimethyl-4-oxoheptyl]tetrahydro-3,5-dimethyl-2*H*-pyran-2-acetic acid   [55134-13-9].

» Narasin Granular contains narasin mixed with suitable carriers and inactive ingredients prepared in a granular form that is free-flowing and free of aggregates. It contains not less than 100 mg and not more than 160 mg of narasin per g.

Packaging and storage—Preserve in well-closed containers. Avoid moisture and excessive heat.

Labeling—Label it to indicate that it is for animal use only. Label it also to indicate that it is for manufacturing, processing, or repackaging.

USP Reference standards ⟨11⟩—*USP Monensin Sodium RS. USP Narasin RS.*

Identification—The retention time of the major peak for narasin A in the chromatogram of the *Assay preparation* corresponds to that of the *Standard preparation* as obtained in the *Assay.*

Loss on drying ⟨731⟩—Dry it in vacuum at 60° for 3 hours: it loses not more than 10% of its weight.

Powder fineness ⟨811⟩—Not less than 99% passes a No. 30 sieve, and not more than 15% passes a No. 140 sieve.

Content of narasin A—Using the chromatogram of the *Assay preparation* obtained as directed in the *Assay,* calculate the percentage of narasin A by the formula:

$$100A / [A + (D + I)]$$

in which *A* is the narasin A biopotency and *D + I* is the narasin D + *I* biopotency. Not less than 85% of narasin A is found.

Assay—

Diluent—Prepare a mixture of methanol and water (9 : 1).

Mobile phase—Prepare a degassed mixture of methanol, water, and glacial acetic acid (94 : 6 : 0.1). Make adjustments if necessary (see *System Suitability* under *Chromatography* ⟨621⟩).

Neutralized methanol—Add 1 g of sodium bicarbonate to 4 L of methanol, mix, and filter.

Derivatizing reagent—Dissolve 30 g of vanillin in a mixture of methanol and sulfuric acid (950 : 20) in a container protected from light. *[Caution—To avoid splattering, add the sulfuric acid carefully and slowly with a pipet; do not pour. Allow the mixture of methanol and sulfuric acid to cool before adding the vanillin.]* Do not filter.

Resolution solution—Prepare a solution in *Neutralized methanol* containing about 3 mg of USP Narasin RS and 1 mg of USP Monensin Sodium RS per mL. Transfer 2 mL of this solution to a 200-mL volumetric flask, dilute with *Diluent* to volume, and mix.

Standard preparations—Dissolve an accurately weighed quantity of USP Narasin RS in *Neutralized methanol* to obtain a solution having a known concentration of about 1 mg per mL. Transfer 1.0 mL of this stock solution to a 200-mL volumetric flask, and transfer

2.0 mL and 4.0 mL of the stock solution to two separate 100-mL volumetric flasks, dilute each with *Diluent* to volume, and mix. These solutions contain about 5, 20, and 40 µg of USP Narasin RS per mL. Using the designated percentage of narasin A in the USP Narasin RS, calculate the exact narasin A concentration, in µg per mL, in each of the *Standard preparations*.

Assay preparation—Transfer about 5 g of Narasin Granular, accurately weighed, to a suitable container, add 200.0 mL of *Diluent*, and shake by mechanical means for 1 hour. Allow the solids to settle, and quantitatively dilute an accurately measured volume of the supernatant with *Diluent* to obtain a solution containing about 20 µg of narasin per mL. Pass a portion of this solution through a filter having a 0.5-µm or finer porosity, and use the filtrate as the *Assay preparation*.

Chromatographic system (see *Chromatography* ⟨621⟩)—The liquid chromatograph is equipped with a 4.6-mm × 25-cm column that contains packing L1. The column outlet is attached to a tee, the opposing arm is attached to a tube from which is pumped the *Derivatizing reagent*, and the outlet is connected to a 2-mL postcolumn reaction coil maintained at 98°. The outlet of the reaction coil is connected to a detector set at 520 nm. The *Mobile phase* and the *Derivatizing reagent* flow at the rate of about 0.7 mL per minute. Chromatograph the *Resolution solution*, and record the peak responses as directed for *Procedure:* the relative retention times are about 0.7 for monensin B, 0.75 for monensin A, 1.0 for narasin A, and 1.1 for narasin D + I; and the resolution, *R*, between the monensin B peak and the monensin A peak is not less than 1.25, and between the monensin A peak and the narasin A peak not less than 3.5. Chromatograph the *Standard preparations*, and record the peak responses as directed for *Procedure:* the tailing factor for the narasin A peak is not more than 1.4 when calculated by the formula:

$$W_{0.1} / 2f$$

in which $W_{0.1}$ is the width of the peak at 10% of peak height; and f is the distance from the peak maximum to the leading edge of the peak, the distance being measured at a point on the baseline at which 10% peak height is reached. The relative standard deviation for replicate injections is not more than 10%. [NOTE—After use, flush the system with methanol.]

Procedure—Separately inject equal volumes (about 200 µL) of the *Standard preparations* and the *Assay preparation* into the chromatograph, and measure the areas of the peak responses for the narasin A and narasin D + I peaks [NOTE—Narasin D and narasin I will co-elute under this chromatographic system.]

Plot the three narasin peak responses in the chromatograms obtained from the *Standard preparations* versus the concentration, in µg per mL, of narasin A, and draw the straight line best fitting the three plotted points. From the graph so obtained, and the narasin A peak response in the chromatogram obtained from the *Assay preparation*, determine the concentration, C_A, in µg per mL, of narasin A in the *Assay preparation*. From the same graph and the narasin D + I peak response in the chromatogram obtained from the *Assay preparation*, determine the concentration, C_{D+I}, in µg per mL, of narasin D + I in the *Assay preparation*. Calculate the biopotency, in mg per g, in the portion of Narasin Granular taken by the formula:

$$(0.001)(C_A F_A + C_{D+I} F_{D+I})(VE / M)$$

in which F_A is 1.077 representing the biopotency conversion factor for narasin A; F_{D+I} is the biopotency conversion factor for narasin D + I; V is the extraction volume, in mL; E is the dilution factor used in diluting the extract to the final estimated concentration of 20 µg per mL; and M is the weight, in g, of Narasin Granular taken to prepare the *Assay preparation*. Calculate the bioconversion factor, F_{D+I}, for narasin D + I by the formula:

$$(1.510D + 0.012I) / (D + I)$$

in which D and I are the specified percentages of narasin D and narasin I, respectively, in USP Narasin RS; 1.510 is the factor for converting narasin D to narasin D biopotency; and 0.012 is the factor for converting narasin I to narasin I biopotency.

Narasin Premix

» Narasin Premix contains Narasin Granular mixed with suitable diluents and inactive ingredients. It contains not less than 90 percent and not more than 110 percent of the labeled amount of narasin.

Packaging and storage—Preserve in well-closed containers. Avoid moisture and excessive heat.
Labeling—Label it to indicate that it is for animal use only. The label bears the statement, "Do not feed undiluted."

USP Reference standards ⟨11⟩—*USP Monensin Sodium RS. USP Narasin RS.*
Identification—The retention time of the major peak for narasin A in the chromatogram of the *Assay preparation* corresponds to that of the *Standard preparation*, as obtained in the *Assay*.
Loss on drying ⟨731⟩—Dry it in vacuum at 60° for 3 hours: it loses not more than 12% of its weight.
Assay—
Diluent, Mobile phase, Neutralized methanol, Derivatizing reagent, Resolution solution, Standard preparations, and *Chromatographic system*—Proceed as directed in the *Assay* under *Narasin Granular*.

Assay preparation—Transfer about 5 g of Narasin Premix, accurately weighed, to a suitable container, add 200.0 mL of *Diluent*, and shake by mechanical means for 1 hour. Allow the solids to settle, and quantitatively dilute an accurately measured volume of the supernatant with *Diluent* to obtain a solution containing about 20 µg of narasin per mL. Pass a portion of this solution through a filter having a 0.5-µm or finer porosity, and use the filtrate as the *Assay preparation*.

Procedure—Proceed as directed for *Procedure* in the *Assay* under *Narasin Granular*. Calculate the biopotency, in mg per g, in the portion of Narasin Premix taken by the formula:

$$(0.001)(C_A F_A + C_{D+I} F_{D+I})(VE / M)$$

in which M is the weight, in g, of Narasin Premix taken to prepare the *Assay preparation;* and the other terms are as defined therein.

Naratriptan Hydrochloride

$C_{17}H_{25}N_3O_2S \cdot HCl$ 371.93
1*H*-Indole-5-ethanesulfonamide, *N*-methyl-3-(1-methyl-4-piperidinyl)-, monohydrochloride.
N-Methyl-3-(1-methyl-4-piperidyl)indole-5-ethanesulfonamide monohydrochloride [*143388-64-1*].

» Naratriptan Hydrochloride contains not less than 98.0 percent and not more than 101.0 percent of $C_{17}H_{25}N_3O_2S \cdot HCl$, calculated on the anhydrous and solvent free-basis.

Packaging and storage—Preserve in tight containers, and store below 30°.

USP Reference standards ⟨11⟩—*USP Naratriptan Hydrochloride RS. USP Naratriptan Resolution Mixture RS.*
NOTE—When performing assays and tests, store all standard, system suitability, and sample solutions in a cool place, protected from light.

Identification—

A: *Infrared Absorption* ⟨197M⟩.

B: The retention time of the major peak in the chromatogram of the *Assay preparation* corresponds to that in the chromatogram of the *Standard preparation,* as obtained in the *Assay.*

C: It meets the requirements of the test for dry chlorides under *Chloride* ⟨191⟩.

Water, *Method I* ⟨921⟩: not more than 0.5%.

Heavy metals, *Method II* ⟨231⟩: 0.002%.

Chromatographic purity—

0.05 M Ammonium phosphate buffer—Dissolve 5.75 g of monobasic ammonium phosphate in 1000 mL of water, and adjust with phosphoric acid to a pH of 3.00 ± 0.05.

Solution A—Prepare a filtered and degassed mixture of *0.05 M Ammonium phosphate buffer* and acetonitrile (97 : 3).

Solution B—Prepare a filtered and degassed mixture of *0.05 M Ammonium phosphate buffer* and acetonitrile (4 : 1).

Mobile phase—Use variable mixtures of *Solution A* and *Solution B* as directed for *Chromatographic system.* Make adjustments if necessary (see *System Suitability* under *Chromatography* ⟨621⟩).

Resolution solution—Dissolve an accurately weighed quantity of USP Naratriptan Resolution Mixture RS in water to obtain a solution having a known concentration of about 0.11 mg per mL.

Test solution—Dissolve an accurately weighed quantity of Naratriptan Hydrochloride in water to obtain a solution having a known concentration of about 0.11 mg per mL.

Chromatographic system (see *Chromatography* ⟨621⟩)—The liquid chromatograph is equipped with a 225-nm detector and a 4.6-mm × 15-cm column that contains 4-μm packing L1. The column temperature is maintained at 40°. The flow rate is about 1.5 mL per minute. The chromatograph is programmed as follows.

Time (minutes)	Solution A (%)	Solution B (%)	Elution
0–35.0	100→0	0→100	linear gradient
35.0–40.0	0	100	isocratic
40.0–41.0	0→100	100→0	linear gradient
41.0–51.0	100	0	re-equilibration

Chromatograph the *Resolution solution,* and record the peak responses as directed for *Procedure:* the relative retention times are about 1.04 for 2-[3-(1-methyl-1,2,3,6-tetrahydropyridin-4-yl)-1*H*-indol-5-yl]ethanesulfonic acid methylamide (naratriptan related compound B) and 1.0 for naratriptan; and the resolution, *R,* between naratriptan and naratriptan related compound B is not less than 1.5.

Procedure—Inject a volume (about 20 μL) of the *Test solution* into the chromatograph, record the chromatogram, and measure the areas for all of the peaks. Calculate the percentage of each impurity in the portion of Naratriptan Hydrochloride taken by the formula:

$$100(r_i/F)/[r_N+ \Sigma(r_i/F)]$$

in which *F* is the relative response factor (see the accompanying table for values) for each impurity; r_i is the peak response for each impurity; and r_N is the naratriptan peak response (see the accompanying table for limits). In addition to not exceeding the limits listed in the accompanying table, not more than 0.1% of any other individual impurity is found; and not more than 1.5% of total impurities is found.

Organic volatile impurities, *Method IV* ⟨467⟩: meets the requirements.

Solvent—Use dimethyl sulfoxide.

(Official until July 1, 2008)

Assay—

0.01 M Triethylamine phosphate buffer—Dilute 0.6 mL of phosphoric acid with water to 900 mL, and adjust with triethylamine to a pH of 2.5.

Mobile phase—Prepare a filtered and degassed mixture of *0.01 M Triethylamine phosphate buffer* and isopropyl alcohol (9 : 1). Make adjustments if necessary (see *System Suitability* under *Chromatography* ⟨621⟩).

System suitability preparation—Dissolve an accurately weighed quantity of USP Naratriptan Resolution Mixture RS in *Mobile phase* to obtain a solution having a concentration of about 0.7 mg per mL.

Standard preparation—Dissolve an accurately weighed quantity of USP Naratriptan Hydrochloride RS in *Mobile phase,* and dilute quantitatively, and stepwise if necessary, with *Mobile phase* to obtain a solution having a known concentration of about 0.11 mg per mL.

Assay preparation—Transfer about 11 mg of Naratriptan Hydrochloride, accurately weighed, to a 100-mL volumetric flask, dissolve in and dilute with *Mobile phase* to volume, and mix.

Chromatographic system (see *Chromatography* ⟨621⟩)—The liquid chromatograph is equipped with a 282-nm detector and a 4.6-mm × 15-cm column that contains 3-μm packing L11. The column temperature is maintained at 35°. The flow rate is about 1.5 mL per minute. Chromatograph the *System suitability preparation,* and record the peak responses as directed for *Procedure:* the resolution, *R,* between naratriptan related compound A and naraptriptan and between naratriptan related compound B and naratriptan is not less than 1.5. Chromatograph the *Standard preparation,* and record the peak responses as directed for *Procedure:* the relative standard deviation for replicate injections is not more than 1.5%. [NOTE—For identification purposes, the approximate relative retention times are about 0.9 for naratriptan related compound A, 1.0 for naratriptan, and 1.1 for naratriptan related compound B.]

Procedure—Separately inject equal volumes (about 10 μL) of the *Standard preparation* and the *Assay preparation* into the chromatograph, record the chromatograms, and measure the areas for the major peaks. Calculate the quantity, in mg, of $C_{17}H_{25}N_3O_2S \cdot HCl$ in the portion of Naratriptan Hydrochloride taken by the formula:

$$100C(r_U / r_S)$$

in which *C* is the concentration, in mg per mL, of USP Naratriptan Hydrochloride RS in the *Standard preparation;* and r_U and r_S are the peak responses obtained from the *Assay preparation* and the *Standard preparation,* respectively.

Compound Name	Relative Retention Time	Relative Response Factor (*F*)	Limit (%)
3-(1-Methylpiperidin-4-yl)-1*H*-indole	about 0.93	1.0	0.2
2-[3-(1-Methyl-1,2,3,6-tetrahydropyridin-4-yl)-1*H*-indol-5-yl]ethanesulfonic acid methylamide	about 1.04	0.6	0.1
2,2-Bis-[3-(1-methylpiperidin-4-yl)-1*H*-indol-5-yl]ethanesulfonic acid methylamide	about 1.18	0.6	0.2
1-Methyl-4-[5-(2-methylsulfamoyl-ethyl)-1*H*-indol-3-yl]-pyridinium chloride	about 1.25	0.4	0.2
2-[3-(1-Methylpiperidin-4-yl)-5-(2-methylsulfamoyl-ethyl)-indol-1-yl]ethanesulfonic acid methylamide	about 1.36	0.6	0.3
4-[1,5-Bis-(2-methylsulfamoyl-ethyl)-1*H*-indol-3-yl]-1-methylpyridinium chloride	about 1.44	0.5	0.1

Compound Name	Relative Retention Time	Relative Response Factor (F)	Limit (%)
2-[3-(1-Methylpiperidin-4-yl)-1H-indol-5-yl]ethane-sulfonic acid methyl-(2-methylsulfamoyl-ethyl)amide	about 1.48	1.0	0.2
5-Ethyl-3-(1-methylpiperidin-4-yl)-1H-indole	about 1.90	1.00	0.2

Naratriptan Tablets

» Naratriptan Tablets contain an amount of Naratriptan Hydrochloride equivalent to not less than 90.0 percent and not more than 110.0 percent of the labeled amount of naratriptan ($C_{17}H_{25}N_3O_2S$).

Packaging and storage—Preserve in tight containers, and store at controlled room temperature.

USP Reference standards ⟨11⟩—*USP Naratriptan Hydrochloride RS. USP Naratriptan Resolution Mixture RS.*

Identification—
  A: *Thin-Layer Chromatographic Identification Test* ⟨201⟩—
  Diluent—Prepare a mixture of methylene chloride and methanol (1 : 1).
  Adsorbent: high performance thin-layer chromatographic silica gel.
  Test solution—Transfer a number of Tablets, equivalent to 5 mg of naratriptan, to a 25-mL flask, add 1.0 mL of water to wet the Tablets, and gently shake to remove the Tablet film coating. Add 4.5 mL of *Diluent,* and shake for 5 minutes or until the Tablets have dispersed. Centrifuge at 3000 rpm for 10 minutes, and pass through a nylon filter having a 0.45-μm porosity.
  Developing solvent system: a mixture of methylene chloride, alcohol, and triethylamine (10 : 2 : 1).
  B: The retention time of the major peak in the chromatogram of the *Assay preparation* corresponds to that in the chromatogram of the *Standard preparation,* as obtained in the *Assay.*

Dissolution ⟨711⟩—
  Medium: 0.1 N hydrochloric acid; 500 mL, deaerated.
  Apparatus 1: 100 rpm.
  Times: 15 minutes.
  Procedure—Determine the amount of $C_{17}H_{25}N_3O_2S$ dissolved from the difference between first derivative absorbance values at the wavelengths of maximum and minimum in the range from 226 nm to 236 nm on filtered portions of the solution under test, suitably diluted with *Medium,* if necessary, in comparison with a Standard solution having a known concentration of USP Naratriptan Hydrochloride RS in the same *Medium.* [NOTE—Do not sonicate the Standard solution to dissolve. Dissolve the USP Reference Standard with *Medium* at about 37°.]
  Tolerances—Not less than 80% (*Q*) of the labeled amount of $C_{17}H_{25}N_3O_2S$ is dissolved in 15 minutes.

Uniformity of dosage units ⟨905⟩: meet the requirements.

Chromatographic purity—
  0.05 M Ammonium phosphate buffer and *Resolution solution*—Prepare as directed in the test for *Chromatographic purity* under *Naratriptan Hydrochloride.*
  Solution A—Use filtered and degassed *0.05 M Ammonium phosphate buffer.*
  Solution B—Use filtered and degassed acetonitrile.
  Mobile phase—Use variable mixtures of *Solution A* and *Solution B* as directed for *Chromatographic system.* Make adjustments if necessary (see *System Suitability* under *Chromatography* ⟨621⟩).
  Test solution—Transfer 5 Tablets into a suitable amber flask. Add 20.0 mL of 0.1 N sodium hydroxide, and allow to stand for 10 minutes. Sonicate for 10 minutes with regular vigorous swirling of the flask. Add 30.0 mL of *0.05 M Ammonium phosphate buffer,* and mix well. Centrifuge a portion of this solution at 3500 rpm for about 10 minutes, and pass through a suitable filter having a 0.45-μm porosity, discarding the first 3 mL of the filtrate.
  Chromatographic system (see *Chromatography* ⟨621⟩)—The liquid chromatograph is equipped with a 225-nm detector and a 4.6-mm × 15-cm column that contains packing L1. The column temperature is maintained at 40°. The flow rate is about 1.5 mL per minute. The chromatograph is programmed as follows.

Time (minutes)	Solution A (%)	Solution B (%)	Elution
0–35.0	97→80	3→20	linear gradient
35.0–40.0	80	20	isocratic
40.0–41.0	80→97	20→3	linear gradient
41.0–51.0	97	3	re-equilibration

Chromatograph the *Resolution solution,* and record the peak responses as directed for *Procedure:* the relative retention times are about 1.07 for 2-[3-(1-methyl-1,2,3,6-tetrahydropyridin-4-yl)-1H-indol-5-yl]ethanesulfonic acid methylamide (naratriptan related compound B) and 1.0 for naratriptan; and the resolution, *R,* between naratriptan and naratriptan related compound B is not less than 1.5.
  Procedure—Inject a volume (equivalent to about 5 μg of naratriptan hydrochloride) of the *Test solution* into the chromatograph, record the chromatogram, and measure the areas for all of the peaks. Calculate the percentage of each impurity in the portion of Tablets taken by the formula:

$$100(r_i/F)/[r_N + \Sigma(r_i/F)]$$

in which F is the relative response factor (see the accompanying table for values) for each impurity; r_i is the peak response for each impurity; and r_N is the naratriptan peak response (see the accompanying table for limits). In addition to not exceeding the limits listed in the accompanying table, not more than 0.2% of any other individual impurity is found; and not more than 1.5% of total impurities is found.

Assay—
  0.01 M Triethylamine phosphate buffer, Mobile phase, and *Resolution solution*—Prepare as directed in the *Assay* under *Naratriptan Hydrochloride.*
  Standard preparation—Dissolve an accurately weighed quantity of USP Naratriptan Hydrochloride RS in 0.1 N sodium hydroxide to obtain a solution having a known concentration of about 0.2 mg per mL. Dilute an accurately measured volume of this solution in *0.01 M Triethylamine phosphate buffer* to obtain a solution having a known concentration of about 20 μg per mL.
  Assay preparation—Transfer 5 Tablets into an amber 250-mL volumetric flask, add 30 mL of 0.1 N sodium hydroxide, and shake on a wrist-action shaker for at least 30 minutes. Sonicate for 10 minutes with regular vigorous swirling of the flask. Add about 170 mL of *0.01 M Triethylamine phosphate buffer,* and mix well. Allow to cool to room temperature, dilute with *0.01 M Triethylamine phosphate buffer* to volume, and mix. Centrifuge a portion of this solution at 3500 rpm for about 10 minutes, and pass through a suitable filter having a 0.45-μm porosity, discarding the first 3 mL of the filtrate.
  Chromatographic system (see *Chromatography* ⟨621⟩)—The liquid chromatograph is equipped with a 224-nm detector and a 4.6-mm × 15-cm column that contains 5-μm packing L11. The flow rate is about 1.3 mL per minute. Chromatograph the *Resolution solution,* and record the peak responses as directed for *Procedure:* the relative retention times are about 0.9 for 3-(1-methylpiperidin-4-yl)-1H-indole (naratriptan related compound A), 1.0 for naratriptan, and 1.1 for naratriptan related compound B; and the resolution, *R,* between naratriptan related compound A and naratriptan and between naratriptan related compound B and naratriptan is not less than 1.5. Chromatograph the *Standard preparation,* record the chromatogram, and measure the peak response as directed for *Procedure:* the relative standard deviation for replicate injections is not more than 1.5%.
  Procedure—Separately inject equal volumes (equivalent to about 1 μg of naratriptan hydrochloride) of the *Standard preparation* and the *Assay preparation* into the chromatograph, record the chromatograms, and measure the responses for the major peaks. Calculate the

quantity, in mg, of naratriptan ($C_{17}H_{25}N_3O_2S$) in the portion of Tablets taken by the formula:

$$(335.47/371.93)100(C/D)(r_U/r_S)$$

in which 335.47 and 371.93 are the molecular weights of naratriptan and naratriptan hydrochloride, respectively; C is the concentration, in mg per mL, of USP Naratriptan Hydrochloride RS in the *Standard preparation*; D is the concentration, in mg per mL, of naratriptan in the *Assay preparation*, based upon the labeled quantity of naratriptan in the portion of Tablets taken and the extent of dilution; and r_U and r_S are the peak responses obtained from the *Assay preparation* and the *Standard preparation*, respectively.

Compound Name	Relative Retention Time	Relative Response Factor (F)	Limit (%)
2-[3-(1-Methyl-1,2,3,6-tetrahydropyridin-4-yl)-1H-indol-5-yl] ethanesulfonic acid methylamide	about 1.07	0.6	0.2
2,2-Bis-[3-(1-methylpiperidin-4-yl)-1H-indol-5-yl]ethanesulfonic acid methylamide	about 1.26	0.6	0.2
1-Methyl-4-[5-(2-methylsulfamoyl-ethyl)-1H-indol-3-yl]-pyridinium chloride	about 1.33	0.4	0.3
2-[3-(1-methylpiperidin-4-yl)-5-(2-methylsulfamoyl-ethyl)-indol-1-yl]ethanesulfonic acid methylamide	about 1.44	0.6	0.2
4-[1,5-Bis-(2-methylsulfamoyl-ethyl)-1H-indol-3-yl]-1-methylpyridinium chloride	about 1.62	0.5	0.2

Natamycin

$C_{33}H_{47}NO_{13}$ 665.73

Stereoisomer of 22-[(3-amino-3,6-dideoxy-β-D-mannopyranosyl)oxy]-1,3,26-trihydroxy-12-methyl-10-oxo-6,11,28-trioxatricyclo [22.3.1.0^{5,7}]octacosa-8,14,16,18,20-pentaene-25-carboxylic acid   [7681-93-8].

» Natamycin contains not less than 90.0 percent and not more than 102.0 percent of $C_{33}H_{47}NO_{13}$, calculated on the anhydrous basis.

Packaging and storage—Preserve in tight, light-resistant containers.

USP Reference standards ⟨11⟩—USP Natamycin RS.

Identification—Transfer 50 mg, accurately weighed, to a 200-mL volumetric flask, add 5.0 mL of water, and moisten the specimen. Add 100 mL of a 1 in 1000 solution of glacial acetic acid in methanol, and shake by mechanical means in the dark until dissolved. Dilute with the acetic acid-methanol solution to volume, and mix. Transfer 2.0 mL of this solution to a 100-mL volumetric flask, dilute with the acetic acid-methanol solution to volume, and mix: the UV absorption spectrum of the solution so obtained exhibits maxima and minima at the same wavelengths as that of a similar solution of USP Natamycin RS, concomitantly measured.

Crystallinity ⟨695⟩:   meets the requirements.

pH ⟨791⟩:   between 5.0 and 7.5, in an aqueous suspension containing 10 mg per mL.

Water, *Method I* ⟨921⟩:   between 6.0% and 9.0%.

Assay—[NOTE—Throughout the *Assay*, protect from direct light all solutions containing natamycin.]

Mobile phase—Dissolve 3.0 g of ammonium acetate and 1.0 g of ammonium chloride in 760 mL of water, and mix. Add 5.0 mL of tetrahydrofuran and 240 mL of acetonitrile, and mix. Pass this solution through a 0.5 μm or finer porosity filter. Make adjustments if necessary (see *System Suitability* under *Chromatography* ⟨621⟩).

Standard preparation—Transfer about 20 mg of USP Natamycin RS, accurately weighed, to a 100-mL volumetric flask. Add 5.0 mL of tetrahydrofuran, and sonicate for 10 minutes. Add 60 mL of methanol, and swirl to dissolve. Add 25 mL of water, and mix. Allow to cool to room temperature. Dilute with water to volume, and mix. Pass this solution through a suitable membrane filter of 0.5 μm or finer porosity.

Resolution solution—Dissolve 20 mg of Natamycin in a mixture of 99 mL of methanol and 1 mL of 0.1 N hydrochloric acid, and allow to stand for 2 hours. [NOTE—Use this solution within 1 hour.]

Assay preparation—Transfer about 20 mg of Natamycin, accurately weighed, to a 100-mL volumetric flask. Proceed as directed under *Standard preparation*, beginning with "add 5.0 mL of tetrahydrofuran."

Chromatographic system (see *Chromatography* ⟨621⟩)—The liquid chromatograph is equipped with a 303-nm detector and a 4.6-mm × 25-cm analytical column that contains packing L1. [NOTE—A 3.9-mm × 20-mm pre-column may be used to extend the useful life of the analytical column.] The flow rate is about 3 mL per minute. Chromatograph the *Standard preparation*, and record the peak responses as directed for *Procedure* : the column efficiency determined from the analyte peak is not less than 3000 theoretical plates, the tailing factor is not less than 0.8 and not more than 1.3, and the relative standard deviation for replicate injections is not more than 1.0%. Chromatograph the *Resolution solution*, and record the peak responses as directed for *Procedure*: the resolution, R, between natamycin and its methyl ester is not less than 2.5. The relative retention times are about 0.7 for natamycin and 1.0 for its methyl ester.

Procedure—[NOTE—Use peak areas where peak responses are indicated.] Separately inject equal volumes (about 20 μL) of the *Standard preparation* and the *Assay preparation* into the chromatograph, record the chromatograms, and measure the responses for the major peaks. Calculate the percentage of natamycin ($C_{33}H_{47}NO_{13}$) in the portion of Natamycin taken by the formula:

$$0.1(W_S P_S / W_U)(r_U / r_S)$$

in which W_S is the weight, in mg, of USP Natamycin RS taken to prepare the *Standard preparation*; P_S is the stated content, in μg per mg, of USP Natamycin RS; W_U is the weight, in mg, of Natamycin taken to prepare the *Assay preparation*; and r_U and r_S are the peak responses obtained from the *Assay preparation* and the *Standard preparation*, respectively.

Natamycin Ophthalmic Suspension

» Natamycin Ophthalmic Suspension is a sterile suspension of Natamycin in a suitable aqueous vehicle. It contains not less than 90.0 percent and not more than 125.0 percent of the labeled amount of $C_{33}H_{47}NO_{13}$. It contains one or more suitable preservatives.

Packaging and storage—Preserve in tight, light-resistant containers. The containers or individual cartons are sealed and tamper-proof so that sterility is assured at time of first use.

USP Reference standards ⟨11⟩—USP Natamycin RS.
Identification—Transfer a volume of Ophthalmic Suspension, equivalent to about 50 mg of natamycin, to a 200-mL volumetric flask, and add water to make a volume of 5 mL. Proceed as directed in the *Identification* test under *Natamycin*, beginning with "Add 100 mL of a 1 in 1000 solution of glacial acetic acid in methanol:" the specified result is obtained.
Sterility ⟨71⟩—It meets the requirements as directed for *Direct Inoculation of the Culture Medium* under *Test for Sterility of the Product to be Examined,* using 0.25 mL of the Ophthalmic Suspension taken from each container.
pH ⟨791⟩: between 5.0 and 7.5.
Assay—[NOTE—Throughout the *Assay* protect from direct light all solutions containing natamycin.]

Mobile phase, Standard preparation, Resolution solution, and *Chromatographic system*—Proceed as directed in the *Assay* under *Natamycin.*

Assay preparation—Transfer an accurately measured volume of Ophthalmic Suspension, equivalent to about 50 mg of natamycin, to a 250-mL volumetric flask. Add 12.5 mL of tetrahydrofuran, and sonicate for 10 minutes. Add 150 mL of methanol, and swirl to dissolve. Add 60 mL of water, and mix. Allow to cool to room temperature. Dilute with water to volume, and mix. Filter this solution through a suitable membrane filter of 0.5-μm or finer porosity.

Procedure—Proceed as directed in the *Assay* under *Natamycin.* Calculate the quantity, in mg, of $C_{33}H_{47}NO_{13}$ in each mL of the Ophthalmic Suspension taken by the formula:

$$0.25C(P_S/V)(r_U/r_S)$$

in which C is the concentration, in mg per mL, of USP Natamycin RS in the *Standard preparation,* P_S is the stated content, in μg per mg, of USP Natamycin RS, V is the volume, in mL, of Ophthalmic Suspension taken, and r_U and r_S are the peak responses obtained from the *Assay preparation* and the *Standard preparation,* respectively.

Nefazodone Hydrochloride

$C_{25}H_{32}ClN_5O_2 \cdot HCl$ 506.47

3*H*-1,2,4-Triazol-3-one, 2-[3-[4-(3-chlorophenyl)-1-piperazinyl)]propyl]-5-ethyl-2,4-dihydro-4-(2-phenoxyethyl)-, monohydrochloride.
1-[3-[4-(*m*-Chlorophenyl)-1-piperazinyl]propyl]-3-ethyl-4-(2-phenoxyethyl)-Δ²-1,2,4-triazolin-5-one monohydrochloride
[82752-99-6].

» Nefazodone Hydrochloride contains not less than 98.0 percent and not more than 102.0 percent of $C_{25}H_{32}ClN_5O_2 \cdot HCl$, calculated on the dried basis.

Packaging and storage—Preserve in tight containers. Store at a temperature between 15° and 30°.
USP Reference standards ⟨11⟩—USP Nefazodone Hydrochloride RS. USP Nefazodone Related Compound A RS. USP Nefazodone Related Compound B RS.
Completeness of solution ⟨641⟩—A 25 mg per mL solution in methanol meets the requirements.
Identification—
  A: *Infrared Absorption* ⟨197K⟩.
  B: A solution of 10 mg per mL meets the requirements of the test for *Chloride* ⟨191⟩.
Loss on drying ⟨731⟩—Dry it in vacuum at 105° for 3 hours: it loses not more than 0.5% of its weight.
Residue on ignition ⟨281⟩: not more than 0.1%.
Heavy metals, *Method II* ⟨231⟩: 0.001%.
Organic volatile impurities, *Method I* ⟨467⟩: meets the requirements.

(Official until July 1, 2008)

Related compounds—
Diluent—Prepare a solution of water and acetonitrile (50:50).
Solution A—Dissolve 0.77 g of ammonium acetate in about 950 mL of water. Adjust with triethylamine to a pH of 7.10 ± 0.05. Dilute with water to 1 L. Filter and degas.
Solution B—Use filtered and degassed acetonitrile.
Mobile phase—Use variable mixtures of *Solution A* and *Solution B* as directed for *Chromatographic system*. Make adjustments if necessary (see *System Suitability* under *Chromatography* ⟨621⟩).
Standard stock solution—Dissolve an accurately weighed amount of USP Nefazodone Hydrochloride RS in *Diluent* to obtain a solution containing 0.1 mg of nefazodone hydrochloride per mL.
Impurities stock solution—Dissolve accurately weighed quantities of USP Nefazodone Related Compound A RS and USP Nefazodone Related Compound B RS in *Diluent* to obtain a final solution having a known concentration of about 0.1 mg per mL of each compound.
Resolution solution—Dilute a suitable volume of the *Impurities stock solution* with the *Standard stock solution* to obtain a solution having a concentration of about 5 μg per mL each of nefazodone related compounds A and B.
Standard solution—Dilute accurately measured volumes of the *Impurities stock solution* and the *Standard stock solution* quantitatively, and stepwise if necessary, with *Diluent* to obtain a solution having a known concentration of about 1 μg per mL each of nefazodone hydrochloride, nefazodone related compound A, and nefazodone related compound B.
Test solution—Transfer about 100 mg of Nefazodone Hydrochloride, accurately weighed, to a 100-mL volumetric flask, dissolve in and dilute with *Diluent* to volume, and mix.
Chromatographic system (see *Chromatography* ⟨621⟩)—The liquid chromatograph is equipped with a 250-nm detector and a 4.6-mm × 25-cm column that contains 5-μm packing L1. The flow rate is about 1.7 mL per minute. The chromatograph is programmed as follows.

Time (minutes)	Solution A (%)	Solution B (%)	Elution
0	50	50	equilibration
0–10	50→45	50→55	linear gradient
10–16	45→35	55→65	linear gradient
16–25	35	65	isocratic
25–26	35→50	65→50	linear gradient
26–35	50	50	re-equilibration

Chromatograph the *Resolution solution*, and record the peak responses as directed for *Procedure*: the resolution, *R*, between nefazodone related compound A and nefazodone hydrochloride is not less than 4.0 and is not less than 1.5 between nefazodone hydrochloride and nefazodone related compound B. Chromatograph the *Standard solution*, and measure the peak responses as directed for *Procedure*: the relative standard deviation for replicate injections is not more than 5.0% for nefazodone related compound A and nefazodone related compound B. [NOTE—For identification purposes, the relative retention times are about 1.2 for nefazodone related compound A, 1.0 for nefazodone hydrochloride, and 0.94 for nefazodone related compound B.]

Procedure—Inject equal volumes (about 10 μL) of the *Standard solution* and the *Test solution* into the chromatograph, record the chromatograms, and measure the peak responses. Calculate the percentage of each nefazodone related compound in the portion of Nefazodone Hydrochloride taken by the formula:

$$100(C_S/C_T)(r_U/r_S)$$

in which C_S is the concentration, in mg per mL, of the relevant USP Reference Standard in the *Standard solution*; C_T is the concentration of Nefazodone Hydrochloride, in mg per mL, in the *Test solution*; and r_U and r_S are the peak areas of the corresponding nefazodone related compound obtained from the *Test solution* and the *Standard solution*, respectively: not more than 0.2% of nefazodone related compound A is found; not more than 0.2% of nefazodone related compound B is found; not more than 0.1% of any unknown impurity is found; and not more than 0.5% of total impurities is found. [NOTE—Use the peak area for nefazodone hydrochloride in the *Standard solution* as r_S to calculate any unknown impurity.]

Assay—Dissolve about 800 mg of Nefazodone Hydrochloride, accurately weighed, in 50 mL of glacial acetic acid, and add 15 mL of 3% (v/v) mercuric acetate in glacial acetic acid. Titrate with 0.1 N perchloric acid VS, determining the endpoint potentiometrically. Perform a blank determination, and make any necessary correction (see *Titrimetry* ⟨541⟩). Each mL of 0.1 N perchloric acid VS is equivalent to 50.65 mg of $C_{25}H_{32}ClN_5O_2 \cdot HCl$.

Nefazodone Hydrochloride Tablets

» Nefazodone Hydrochloride Tablets contain not less than 90.0 percent and not more than 110.0 percent of the labeled amount of nefazodone hydrochloride ($C_{25}H_{32}ClN_5O_2 \cdot HCl$).

Packaging and storage—Preserve in tight containers. Store at controlled room temperature.

USP Reference standards ⟨11⟩—*USP Nefazodone Hydrochloride RS. USP Nefazodone Related Compound A RS. USP Nefazodone Related Compound B RS.*

Identification—
 A: *Infrared Absorption* ⟨197K⟩.
 B: The retention time of the major peak in the chromatogram of the *Assay preparation* corresponds to that in the chromatogram of the *Standard preparation*, as obtained in the *Assay*.

Dissolution ⟨711⟩—
 Medium: 0.1 N hydrochloric acid; 900 mL, deaerated.
 Apparatus 2: 50 rpm.
 Time: 30 minutes.
 Standard stock solution—Transfer about 70 mg of USP Nefazodone Hydrochloride RS, accurately weighed, to a 50-mL volumetric flask. Add 2.5 mL of methanol, dilute with *Medium* to volume, and mix.
 Standard solution—Dilute the *Standard stock solution* with *Medium* in such a way that the final concentration is similar to the one expected in the *Test solution*.
 Test solution—Use portions of the solution under test passed through a 0.45-μm PVDF filter, discarding the first 5 mL.
 Procedure—Determine the percentage of the labeled amount of nefazodone hydrochloride dissolved by employing UV absorption, using a suitable spectrophotometer, at the wavelength of maximum absorbance at about 246 nm, on the *Test solution* in comparison with the *Standard solution*, using *Medium* as the blank. Calculate the percentage of nefazodone hydrochloride ($C_{25}H_{32}ClN_5O_2 \cdot HCl$) dissolved by the formula:

$$\frac{A_U \times C_S \times 900 \times 100}{A_S \times LC}$$

in which A_U and A_S are the absorbances obtained from the *Test solution* and the *Standard solution*, respectively; C_S is the concentration, in mg per mL, of USP Nefazodone Hydrochloride RS in the *Standard solution*; 900 is the volume, in mL, of *Medium*; 100 is the conversion factor to percentage; and *LC* is the tablet label claim, in mg.
 Tolerances—Not less than 75% (*Q*) of the labeled amount of $C_{25}H_{32}ClN_5O_2 \cdot HCl$ is dissolved in 30 minutes.

Uniformity of dosage units ⟨905⟩: meet the requirements.

Related compounds—
 Dilute acetic acid, Buffer solution, and Mobile phase—Proceed as directed in the *Assay*.

Nefazodone related compound A stock solution—Prepare a solution of USP Nefazodone Related Compound A RS in *Mobile phase* having a known concentration of about 80 μg per mL.
 Nefazodone related compound B stock solution—Prepare a solution of USP Nefazodone Related Compound B RS in *Mobile phase* having a known concentration of about 80 μg per mL.
 System suitability solution—Transfer about 10 mg of USP Nefazodone Hydrochloride RS into a 10-mL volumetric flask. Add 2.0 mL of *Nefazodone related compound A stock solution* and 2.0 mL of *Nefazodone related compound B stock solution*, and mix to dissolve the nefazodone hydrochloride. Dilute with *Mobile phase* to volume, and mix.
 Standard solution—Use the *Standard preparation*, prepared as directed in the *Assay*.
 Test solution—Use the *Assay stock preparation*, prepared as directed in the *Assay*.
 Chromatographic system—Prepare as directed in the *Assay*. Chromatograph the *System suitability solution*, and record the peak responses as directed for *Procedure*. Identify the peaks using the relative retention times given in *Table 1*: the resolution, *R*, between nefazodone related compound A and nefazodone hydrochloride is not less than 2.0; and the resolution, *R*, between nefazodone related compound B and nefazodone hydrochloride is not less than 1.5. [NOTE—Approximate relative retention times are provided in *Table 1* for informational purposes only.]
 Procedure—Inject equal volumes (about 10 μL) of the *Standard solution* and the *Test solution* into the chromatograph, record the chromatograms, and measure the peak responses. Calculate the percentage of individual nefazodone related compounds in the portion of Tablets taken by the formula:

$$100(r_U / r_S)(C_S / C_T)(1/F)$$

in which r_U is the individual peak response for each nefazodone related compound obtained from the *Test solution*; r_S is the response of the corresponding peak in the *Standard solution*, respectively; C_S and C_T are the concentrations, in mg per mL, of nefazodone hydrochloride in the *Standard solution* and the *Test solution*, respectively; and *F* is the relative response factor obtained from *Table 1*. The related compound requirements are listed in *Table 1*.

Table 1

Related Compound	Relative Retention Time	Relative Response Factor (F)	Limit (%)
Nefazodone related compound A	1.4	1.2	0.2
Nefazodone related compound B	0.9	1.0	0.2
Any individual unknown impurity	—	1.0	0.2 each
Total known and unknown	—	—	0.5

Assay—
 Dilute acetic acid—Prepare a mixture of acetic acid and water (1 : 1).
 Buffer solution—Dissolve 0.77 g of ammonium acetate in 1 L of water. Add 1.0 mL of triethylamine, and mix well. Adjust with *Dilute acetic acid* to a pH of 7.10 ± 0.05, and mix.
 Mobile phase—Prepare a filtered and degassed mixture of acetonitrile and *Buffer solution* (58 : 42). Make adjustments if necessary (see *System Suitability* under *Chromatography* ⟨621⟩).
 Standard preparation—Prepare a solution of USP Nefazodone Hydrochloride RS in *Mobile phase* having a known concentration of about 0.1 mg per mL.
 Assay stock preparation—Weigh and finely powder not fewer than 20 Tablets. Transfer an accurately weighed portion of the powder, equivalent to about 250 mg of nefazodone hydrochloride, based on the label claim, to a 250-mL volumetric flask, add about 125 mL of *Mobile phase*, and sonicate for about 10 minutes with occasional shaking. Dilute with *Mobile phase* to volume, and mix to obtain a solution having a concentration of about 1 mg per mL of nefazodone hydrochloride. Pass a portion of this solution through a

filter having a 0.45-μm or finer porosity, and use the filtrate, which has a concentration of about 1 mg per mL of nefazodone hydrochloride.

Assay preparation—Transfer 5.0 mL of *Assay stock preparation* into a 50-mL volumetric flask. Dilute with *Mobile phase* to volume, and mix to obtain a solution having a concentration of 0.1 mg per mL of nefazodone hydrochloride.

Chromatographic system (see *Chromatography* ⟨621⟩)—The liquid chromatograph is equipped with a 250-nm detector and a 4.6-mm × 25-cm column containing 5-μm L1 packing. The flow rate is about 1.0 mL per minute. The column temperature is maintained at 30°. Inject the *Standard preparation,* and record the peak responses as directed for *Procedure:* the tailing factor is not more than 2.0; and the relative standard deviation for replicate injections is not more than 2.0%.

Procedure—Separately inject equal volumes (about 10 μL) of the *Standard preparation* and the *Assay preparation* into the chromatograph, record the chromatograms, and measure the responses for the major peaks. Calculate the quantity, in percent of label claim, of nefazodone hydrochloride ($C_{25}H_{32}ClN_5O_2 \cdot HCl$) in the portion of Tablets taken by the formula:

$$100(C_S / C_U)(r_U / r_S)$$

in which C_S and C_U are the concentrations, in mg per mL, of nefazodone hydrochloride in the *Standard preparation* and the *Assay preparation,* respectively; and r_U and r_S are the peak areas obtained from the *Assay preparation* and the *Standard preparation,* respectively.

Neomycin Sulfate

Neomycin sulfate.
Neomycins sulfate   [1405-10-3].

» Neomycin Sulfate is the sulfate salt of a kind of neomycin, an antibacterial substance produced by the growth of *Streptomyces fradiae* Waksman (Fam. Streptomycetaceae), or a mixture of two or more such salts. It has a potency equivalent to not less than 600 μg of neomycin per mg, calculated on the dried basis.

Packaging and storage—Preserve in tight, light-resistant containers.
Labeling—Where it is intended for use in preparing injectable or other sterile dosage forms, the label states that it is sterile or must be subjected to further processing during the preparation of injectable or other sterile dosage forms.
USP Reference standards ⟨11⟩—*USP Endotoxin RS. USP Neomycin Sulfate RS.*
Identification—
   A: It meets the requirements for neomycin under *Thin-Layer Chromatographic Identification Test* ⟨201BNP⟩.
   B: Dissolve about 10 mg in 1 mL of water, add 5 mL of 15 N sulfuric acid, and heat at 100° for 100 minutes. Allow to cool, add 10 mL of xylene, and shake for 10 minutes. Allow to separate, and decant the xylene layer. To the xylene layer add 10 mL of *p*-bromoaniline TS, and shake: a vivid pink-red color develops upon standing.
   C: A solution (1 in 20) responds to the tests for *Sulfate* ⟨191⟩.
pH ⟨791⟩:   between 5.0 and 7.5, in a solution containing 33 mg of neomycin per mL.
Loss on drying ⟨731⟩—Dry about 100 mg in vacuum at a pressure not exceeding 5 mm of mercury at 60° for 3 hours: it loses not more than 8.0% of its weight.
Other requirements—Where the label states that Neomycin Sulfate is sterile, it meets the requirements for *Sterility* and *Bacterial endotoxins* under *Neomycin for Injection*. Where the label states that Neomycin Sulfate must be subjected to further processing during the preparation of injectable dosage forms, it meets the requirements for *Bacterial endotoxins* under *Neomycin for Injection*. Where it is intended for use in preparing nonparenteral sterile dosage forms, it is exempt from the requirements for *Bacterial endotoxins*.
Assay—Proceed with Neomycin Sulfate as directed under *Antibiotics—Microbial Assays* ⟨81⟩.

Neomycin Boluses

» Neomycin Boluses contain an amount of Neomycin Sulfate equivalent to not less than 90.0 percent and not more than 125.0 percent of the labeled amount of neomycin.

Packaging and storage—Preserve in tight containers.
Labeling—Label Boluses to indicate that they are for veterinary use only.
USP Reference standards ⟨11⟩—*USP Neomycin Sulfate RS.*
Identification—Blend a Bolus with 250 mL of water. Filter a portion of the suspension obtained. If necessary, dilute a portion of the filtrate with water to obtain a test solution containing about 2 mg of neomycin per mL. Dissolve a quantity of USP Neomycin Sulfate RS in water to obtain a Standard solution containing about 2 mg of neomycin per mL. Separately apply 1 μL of each solution to a thin-layer chromatographic plate (see *Chromatography* ⟨621⟩) coated with a 0.25-mm layer of chromatographic silica gel mixture. Develop the chromatogram in a solvent system consisting of a mixture of water, butyl alcohol, glacial acetic acid, and pyridine (35 : 30 : 22 : 6) until the solvent front has moved about three-fourths of the length of the plate. Remove the plate from the developing chamber, mark the solvent front, and dry at about 110° for about 5 minutes. Spray the plate evenly with a solution of ninhydrin (2 mg per mL), and dry the plate at about 100° for about 5 minutes. Locate the spots on the plate: the R_F value of the principal spot in the chromatogram obtained from the test solution corresponds to that of the principal spot in the chromatogram obtained from the Standard solution.
Uniformity of dosage units ⟨905⟩:   meet the requirements for *Weight Variation.*
Disintegration ⟨701⟩:   60 minutes.
Assay—Proceed as directed for the assay of neomycin under *Antibiotics—Microbial Assays* ⟨81⟩, the *Test Dilution* being prepared as follows. Blend an accurately counted number of Boluses (not less than 2) at high speed in a blender jar with a sufficient accurately measured volume of *Buffer No. 3* to obtain a stock solution having a convenient concentration. Dilute this stock solution quantitatively and stepwise with *Buffer No. 3* to obtain a *Test Dilution* having a concentration assumed to be equal to the median dose level of the Standard.

Neomycin Sulfate Cream

» Neomycin Sulfate Cream contains the equivalent of not less than 90.0 percent and not more than 135.0 percent of the labeled amount of neomycin.

Packaging and storage—Preserve in well-closed containers, preferably at controlled room temperature.
USP Reference standards ⟨11⟩—*USP Neomycin Sulfate RS.*
Thin-layer chromatographic identification test ⟨201BNP⟩: meets the requirements.
Minimum fill ⟨755⟩:   meets the requirements.
Assay—Proceed as directed under *Antibiotics—Microbial Assays* ⟨81⟩, using an accurately weighed portion of Cream, equivalent to about 1.75 mg of neomycin, shaken in a separator with about 50 mL of ether, and extracted with four 20-mL portions of *Buffer No. 3.* Combine the aqueous extracts, and dilute with *Buffer No. 3* to an appropriate volume to obtain a stock solution of convenient concentration. Dilute this stock solution quantitatively and stepwise with

Buffer No. 3 to obtain a *Test Dilution* having a concentration assumed to be equal to the median dose level of the Standard.

Neomycin for Injection

» Neomycin for Injection contains an amount of Neomycin Sulfate equivalent to not less than 90.0 percent and not more than 120.0 percent of the labeled amount of neomycin.

Packaging and storage—Preserve in *Containers for Sterile Solids* as described under *Injections* ⟨1⟩.
USP Reference standards ⟨11⟩—*USP Endotoxin RS. USP Neomycin Sulfate RS.*
Thin-layer chromatographic identification test ⟨201BNP⟩: meets the requirements.
Bacterial endotoxins ⟨85⟩—It contains not more than 1.30 USP Endotoxin Units per mg of neomycin.
Sterility ⟨71⟩—It meets the requirements when tested as directed for *Membrane Filtration* under *Test for Sterility of the Product to be Examined*.
Other requirements—It meets the requirements for *pH* and *Loss on drying* under *Neomycin Sulfate* and for *Uniformity of Dosage Units* ⟨905⟩ and *Labeling* under *Injections* ⟨1⟩.
Assay—
Assay preparation 1 (where it is packaged for dispensing)—Constitute Neomycin for Injection as directed in the labeling. Withdraw all of the withdrawable contents, using a suitable hypodermic needle and syringe, and dilute quantitatively with *Buffer No. 3* to obtain a solution having a convenient concentration.
Assay preparation 2 (where it is packaged for dispensing and where the labeling states the quantity of neomycin in a given volume of constituted solution)—Constitute Neomycin for Injection as directed in the labeling. Dilute an accurately measured volume of the constituted solution quantitatively with *Buffer No. 3* to obtain a solution having a convenient concentration.
Procedure—Proceed as directed for neomycin under *Antibiotics—Microbial Assays* ⟨81⟩, using an accurately measured volume of *Assay preparation* diluted quantitatively and stepwise with *Buffer No. 3* to yield a *Test Dilution* having a concentration assumed to be equal to the median dose level of the Standard.

Neomycin Sulfate Ointment

» Neomycin Sulfate Ointment contains the equivalent of not less than 90.0 percent and not more than 135.0 percent of the labeled amount of neomycin.

Packaging and storage—Preserve in well-closed containers, preferably at controlled room temperature.
USP Reference standards ⟨11⟩—*USP Neomycin Sulfate RS.*
Thin-layer chromatographic identification test ⟨201BNP⟩: meets the requirements.
Minimum fill ⟨755⟩: meets the requirements.
Water, *Method I* ⟨921⟩: not more than 1.0%, 20 mL of a mixture of toluene and methanol (7 : 3) being used in place of methanol in the titration vessel.
Assay—Proceed as directed under *Antibiotics—Microbial Assays* ⟨81⟩, using an accurately weighed portion of Ointment, equivalent to about 3.5 mg of neomycin, shaken in a separator with about 50 mL of ether, and extracted with four 20-mL portions of *Buffer No. 3*. Combine the aqueous extracts, and dilute with *Buffer No. 3* to an appropriate volume to obtain a stock solution of convenient concentration. Dilute this stock solution quantitatively and stepwise with *Buffer No. 3* to obtain a *Test Dilution* having a concentration assumed to be equal to the median dose level of the Standard.

Neomycin Sulfate Ophthalmic Ointment

» Neomycin Sulfate Ophthalmic Ointment is a sterile preparation of Neomycin Sulfate in a suitable ointment base. It contains the equivalent of not less than 90.0 percent and not more than 135.0 percent of the labeled amount of neomycin.

Packaging and storage—Preserve in collapsible ophthalmic ointment tubes.
USP Reference standards ⟨11⟩—*USP Neomycin Sulfate RS.*
Thin-layer chromatographic identification test ⟨201BNP⟩: meets the requirements.
Sterility ⟨71⟩: meets the requirements.
Minimum fill ⟨755⟩: meets the requirements.
Water, *Method I* ⟨921⟩: not more than 1.0%, 20 mL of a mixture of toluene and methanol (7 : 3) being used in place of methanol in the titration vessel.
Metal particles—It meets the requirements of the test for *Metal Particles in Ophthalmic Ointments* ⟨751⟩.
Assay—Proceed with Ophthalmic Ointment as directed in the *Assay* under *Neomycin Sulfate Ointment*.

Neomycin Sulfate Oral Solution

» Neomycin Sulfate Oral Solution contains the equivalent of not less than 90.0 percent and not more than 125.0 percent of the labeled amount of neomycin. It may contain one or more suitable colors, flavors, and preservatives.

Packaging and storage—Preserve in tight, light-resistant containers, preferably at controlled room temperature.
USP Reference standards ⟨11⟩—*USP Neomycin Sulfate RS.*
Thin-layer chromatographic identification test ⟨201BNP⟩: meets the requirements.
Uniformity of dosage units ⟨905⟩—
FOR ORAL SOLUTION PACKAGED IN SINGLE-UNIT CONTAINERS: meets the requirements.
Deliverable volume ⟨698⟩—
FOR ORAL SOLUTION PACKAGED IN MULTIPLE-UNIT CONTAINERS: meets the requirements.
pH ⟨791⟩: between 5.0 and 7.5.
Assay—Proceed as directed under *Antibiotics—Microbial Assays* ⟨81⟩, using an accurately measured volume of Oral Solution quantitatively diluted with *Buffer No. 3* to yield a solution having a convenient concentration of neomycin. Quantitatively dilute this stock solution with *Buffer No. 3* to obtain a *Test Dilution* having a concentration assumed to be equal to the median dose level of the Standard.

Neomycin Sulfate Tablets

» Neomycin Sulfate Tablets contain the equivalent of not less than 90.0 percent and not more than 125.0 percent of the labeled amount of neomycin.

Packaging and storage—Preserve in tight containers.
USP Reference standards ⟨11⟩—*USP Neomycin Sulfate RS.*
Thin-layer chromatographic identification test ⟨201BNP⟩—
Test solution—Shake a portion of ground Tablet powder, equivalent to about 70 mg of neomycin (base), with 5 mL of water, and filter. Dilute a portion of this solution with 0.1 N hydrochloric acid

to obtain a solution containing the equivalent of 3.5 mg of neomycin (base) per mL. It meets the requirements.
Disintegration ⟨701⟩: 60 minutes.
Uniformity of dosage units ⟨905⟩: meet the requirements.
Loss on drying ⟨731⟩—Dry about 100 mg of powdered Tablets, accurately weighed, in a capillary-stoppered bottle in vacuum at a pressure not exceeding 5 mm of mercury at 60° for 3 hours: it loses not more than 10.0% of its weight.
Assay—Proceed as directed under *Antibiotics—Microbial Assays* ⟨81⟩, using not less than 5 Tablets blended at high-speed in a blender jar for 3 to 5 minutes with a sufficient accurately measured volume of *Buffer No. 3* to obtain a stock solution having a convenient concentration. Dilute this stock solution quantitatively and stepwise with *Buffer No. 3* to obtain a *Test Dilution* having a concentration assumed to be equal to the median dose level of the Standard.

Neomycin Sulfate and Bacitracin Ointment

» Neomycin Sulfate and Bacitracin Ointment contains the equivalent of not less than 90.0 percent and not more than 130.0 percent of the labeled amounts of neomycin and bacitracin.

Packaging and storage—Preserve in tight, light-resistant containers, preferably at controlled room temperature.

USP Reference standards ⟨11⟩—*USP Bacitracin Zinc RS. USP Neomycin Sulfate RS.*
Thin-layer chromatographic identification test ⟨201BNP⟩: meets the requirements.
Minimum fill ⟨755⟩: meets the requirements.
Water, *Method I* ⟨921⟩: not more than 0.5%, 20 mL of a mixture of toluene and methanol (7 : 3) being used in place of methanol in the titration vessel.
Assay for neomycin—Proceed with Ointment as directed in the *Assay* under *Neomycin Sulfate Ointment.*
Assay for bacitracin—Proceed with Ointment as directed in the *Assay* under *Bacitracin Ointment*

Neomycin Sulfate and Bacitracin Zinc Ointment

» Neomycin Sulfate and Bacitracin Zinc Ointment contains the equivalent of not less than 90.0 percent and not more than 130.0 percent of the labeled amounts of neomycin and bacitracin.

Packaging and storage—Preserve in collapsible tubes or in well-closed containers.

USP Reference standards ⟨11⟩—*USP Bacitracin Zinc RS. USP Neomycin Sulfate RS.*
Thin-layer chromatographic identification test ⟨201BNP⟩: meets the requirements.
Minimum fill ⟨755⟩: meets the requirements.
Water, *Method I* ⟨921⟩: not more than 0.5%, 20 mL of a mixture of toluene and methanol (7 : 3) being used in place of methanol in the titration vessel.
Assay for neomycin and Assay for bacitracin—Proceed with Ointment as directed in the *Assay for neomycin* and in the *Assay for bacitracin* under *Neomycin and Polymyxin B Sulfates and Bacitracin Zinc Ophthalmic Ointment.*

Neomycin Sulfate and Dexamethasone Sodium Phosphate Cream

» Neomycin Sulfate and Dexamethasone Sodium Phosphate Cream contains the equivalent of not less than 90.0 percent and not more than 135.0 percent of the labeled amount of neomycin, and the equivalent of not less than 90.0 percent and not more than 110.0 percent of the labeled amount of dexamethasone phosphate ($C_{22}H_{30}FO_8P$).

Packaging and storage—Preserve in collapsible tubes or in tight containers.

USP Reference standards ⟨11⟩—*USP Dexamethasone RS. USP Dexamethasone Phosphate RS. USP Neomycin Sulfate RS.*
Identification—
  A: It meets the requirements for neomycin under*Thin-Layer Chromatographic Identification Test* ⟨201BNP⟩.
  B: The *Assay preparation*, prepared as directed in the*Assay for dexamethasone phosphate*, meets the requirements for the *Identification* test under *Dexamethasone Sodium Phosphate Cream.*
Minimum fill ⟨755⟩: meets the requirements.
Assay for neomycin—Proceed with Cream as directed in the *Assay* under *Neomycin Sulfate Cream.*
Assay for dexamethasone phosphate—
  Alcohol–aqueous phosphate buffer, 0.05 M Phosphate buffer, Mobile phase, Standard preparation, and *Chromatographic system*—Prepare as directed in the *Assay* under *Dexamethasone Sodium Phosphate Cream.*
  Assay preparation—Using an accurately weighed portion of Cream, prepare as directed in the*Assay* under *Dexamethasone Sodium Phosphate Cream.*
  Procedure—Proceed as directed for *Procedure* in the*Assay* under *Dexamethasone Sodium Phosphate Cream.* Calculate the quantity, in mg, of dexamethasone phosphate ($C_{22}H_{30}FO_8P$) in the portion of Cream taken by the formula:

$$0.1C(r_U / r_S).$$

Neomycin Sulfate and Dexamethasone Sodium Phosphate Ophthalmic Ointment

» Neomycin Sulfate and Dexamethasone Sodium Phosphate Ophthalmic Ointment is a sterile ointment containing Neomycin Sulfate and Dexamethasone Sodium Phosphate. It contains the equivalent of not less than 90.0 percent and not more than 135.0 percent of the labeled amount of neomycin, and the equivalent of not less than 90.0 percent and not more than 110.0 percent of the labeled amount of dexamethasone phosphate ($C_{22}H_{30}FO_8P$).

NOTE—Where Neomycin Sulfate and Dexamethasone Sodium Phosphate Ophthalmic Ointment is prescribed without reference to the quantity of neomycin or dexamethasone phosphate contained therein, a product containing 3.5 mg of neomycin and 0.5 mg of dexamethasone phosphate per g shall be dispensed.

Packaging and storage—Preserve in collapsible ophthalmic ointment tubes.
USP Reference standards ⟨11⟩—*USP Dexamethasone RS. USP Dexamethasone Phosphate RS. USP Neomycin Sulfate RS.*

Identification—

A: It meets the requirements for neomycin under *Thin-Layer Chromatographic Identification Test* ⟨201BNP⟩.

B: The *Assay preparation*, prepared as directed in the *Assay for dexamethasone phosphate*, meets the requirements for the *Identification* test under *Dexamethasone Sodium Phosphate Cream*.

Sterility ⟨71⟩: meets the requirements.

Minimum fill ⟨755⟩: meets the requirements.

Water, *Method I* ⟨921⟩: not more than 1.0%, 20 mL of a mixture of toluene and methanol (7 : 3) being used in place of methanol in the titration vessel.

Metal particles—It meets the requirements of the test for *Metal Particles in Ophthalmic Ointments* ⟨751⟩.

Assay for neomycin—Proceed as directed under *Antibiotics—Microbial Assays* ⟨81⟩, using an accurately weighed portion of Ophthalmic Ointment shaken in a separator with about 50 mL of ether, and extracted with four 20-mL portions of *Buffer No. 3*. Combine the aqueous extracts, and dilute with *Buffer No. 3* to an appropriate volume to obtain a stock solution. Dilute this stock solution quantitatively and stepwise with *Buffer No. 3* to obtain a *Test Dilution* having a concentration assumed to be equal to the median dose level of the Standard.

Assay for dexamethasone phosphate—

Alcohol–aqueous phosphate buffer, *0.05 M Phosphate buffer*, *Mobile phase*, *Standard preparation*, and *Chromatographic system*—Prepare as directed in the *Assay* under *Dexamethasone Sodium Phosphate Cream*.

Assay preparation—Using an accurately weighed portion of Ophthalmic Ointment, prepare as directed in the *Assay* under *Dexamethasone Sodium Phosphate Cream*.

Procedure—Proceed as directed for *Procedure* in the *Assay* under *Dexamethasone Sodium Phosphate Cream*. Calculate the quantity, in mg, of dexamethasone phosphate ($C_{22}H_{30}FO_8P$) in the portion of Ophthalmic Ointment taken by the formula:

$$0.1C(r_U / r_S).$$

Neomycin Sulfate and Dexamethasone Sodium Phosphate Ophthalmic Solution

» Neomycin Sulfate and Dexamethasone Sodium Phosphate Ophthalmic Solution is a sterile, aqueous solution of Neomycin Sulfate and Dexamethasone Sodium Phosphate. It contains the equivalent of not less than 90.0 percent and not more than 130.0 percent of the labeled amount of neomycin, and the equivalent of not less than 90.0 percent and not more than 115.0 percent of the labeled amount of dexamethasone phosphate ($C_{22}H_{30}FO_8P$). It may contain one or more suitable buffers, dispersants, and preservatives.

NOTE—Where Neomycin Sulfate and Dexamethasone Sodium Phosphate Ophthalmic Solution is prescribed, without reference to the amount of neomycin or dexamethasone phosphate contained therein, a product containing 3.5 mg of neomycin and 1.0 mg of dexamethasone phosphate per mL shall be dispensed.

Packaging and storage—Preserve in tight, light-resistant containers, and avoid exposure to excessive heat.

USP Reference standards ⟨11⟩—*USP Dexamethasone RS. USP Dexamethasone Phosphate RS. USP Neomycin Sulfate RS.*

Identification—

A: It meets the requirements for neomycin under *Thin-Layer Chromatographic Identification Test* ⟨201BNP⟩.

B: The *Assay preparation*, prepared as directed in the *Assay for dexamethasone phosphate*, meets the requirements for the *Identification* test under *Dexamethasone Sodium Phosphate Cream*.

Sterility ⟨71⟩: meets the requirements.

pH ⟨791⟩: between 6.0 and 8.0.

Assay for neomycin—Proceed as directed under *Antibiotics—Microbial Assays* ⟨81⟩, using an accurately measured volume of Ophthalmic Solution diluted quantitatively and stepwise with *Buffer No. 3* to yield a *Test Dilution* having a concentration assumed to be equal to the median dose level of the Standard (1.0 µg of neomycin per mL).

Assay for dexamethasone phosphate—

0.002 M Phosphate buffer—Dissolve 0.57 g of dibasic sodium phosphate in water to obtain 2000 mL of solution.

0.10 M Phosphate buffer—Dissolve 13.80 g of monobasic sodium phosphate in water to obtain 1000 mL of solution.

Mobile phase—Prepare a suitable filtered mixture of *0.10 M phosphate buffer* and acetonitrile (690 : 310). Make adjustments if necessary (see *System Suitability* under *Chromatography* ⟨621⟩).

Standard preparation—Dissolve an accurately weighed quantity of USP Dexamethasone Phosphate RS in *0.002 M Phosphate buffer* to obtain a solution having a known concentration of about 125 µg per mL. Transfer 20.0 mL of this solution to a 100-mL volumetric flask, dilute with *0.002 M Phosphate buffer* to volume, mix, and pass through a suitable filter of 1 µm or finer porosity. This solution contains about 25 µg per mL.

Assay preparation—Transfer an accurately measured volume of Ophthalmic Solution, equivalent to about 2.5 mg of dexamethasone phosphate, to a 100-mL volumetric flask, slowly dilute with *0.002 M Phosphate buffer* to volume, mix, and pass through a suitable filter of 1 µm or finer porosity.

Chromatographic system (see *Chromatography* ⟨621⟩)—The liquid chromatograph is equipped with a 254-nm detector and a 4-mm × 30-cm column that contains packing L1. The flow rate is about 1.3 mL per minute. Chromatograph the *Standard preparation*, and measure the peak responses as directed under *Procedure*: the column efficiency is not less than 2000 theoretical plates, the capacity factor, k', for the dexamethasone phosphate peak is not less than 1.05, and the relative standard deviation for replicate injections is not more than 2.0%.

Procedure—[NOTE—Use peak areas where peak responses are indicated.] Separately inject equal volumes (about 50 µL) of the *Standard preparation* and the *Assay preparation* into the chromatograph, record the chromatograms, and measure the areas for the major peaks. Calculate the quantity, in mg, of dexamethasone phosphate ($C_{22}H_{30}FO_8P$), in each mL of the Ophthalmic Solution taken by the formula:

$$0.1(C/V)(r_U / r_S)$$

in which C is the concentration, in µg per mL, of USP Dexamethasone Phosphate RS in the *Standard preparation*; V is the volume, in mL, of Ophthalmic Solution taken; and r_U and r_S are the dexamethasone phosphate peak responses obtained from the *Assay preparation* and the *Standard preparation*, respectively.

Neomycin Sulfate and Fluocinolone Acetonide Cream

» Neomycin Sulfate and Fluocinolone Acetonide Cream contains the equivalent of not less than 90.0 percent and not more than 135.0 percent of the labeled amount of neomycin, and the equivalent of not less than 90.0 percent and not more than 110.0 percent of the labeled amount of fluocinolone acetonide ($C_{24}H_{30}F_2O_6$).

Packaging and storage—Preserve in collapsible tubes or in tight containers.

USP Reference standards ⟨11⟩—*USP Fluocinolone Acetonide RS. USP Neomycin Sulfate RS.*

Identification—
A: It meets the requirements for neomycin under *Thin-Layer Chromatographic Identification Test* ⟨201BNP⟩.
B: It meets the requirements for the *Identification* test under *Fluocinolone Acetonide Cream.*
Minimum fill ⟨755⟩: meets the requirements.
Assay for neomycin—Proceed with Cream as directed in the *Assay* under *Neomycin Sulfate Cream.*
Assay for fluocinolone acetonide—Proceed with Cream as directed in the *Assay* under *Fluocinolone Acetonide Cream.*

Neomycin Sulfate and Fluorometholone Ointment

» Neomycin Sulfate and Fluorometholone Ointment contains the equivalent of not less than 90.0 percent and not more than 135.0 percent of the labeled amount of neomycin, and not less than 90.0 percent and not more than 110.0 percent of the labeled amount of fluorometholone ($C_{22}H_{29}FO_4$).

Packaging and storage—Preserve in collapsible tubes or in well-closed containers.
USP Reference standards ⟨11⟩—*USP Fluorometholone RS. USP Neomycin Sulfate RS.*
Identification—
A: It meets the requirements for neomycin under *Thin-Layer Chromatographic Identification Test* ⟨201BNP⟩.
B: The ratios of the retention time of the main peak to that of the internal standard peak obtained from the *Standard preparation* and the *Assay preparation* as directed in the *Assay for fluorometholone* do not differ by more than 2.0%.
Minimum fill ⟨755⟩: meets the requirements.
Water, *Method I* ⟨921⟩: not more than 1.0%, 20 mL of a mixture of toluene and methanol (7 : 3) being used in place of methanol in the titration vessel.
Assay for neomycin—Proceed with Ointment as directed in the *Assay* under *Neomycin Sulfate Ointment.*
Assay for fluorometholone—
Internal standard solution, Mobile solvent, and *Standard preparation—*Prepare as directed in the *Assay* under *Fluorometholone Cream.*
*Assay preparation—*Transfer an accurately weighed quantity of Ointment, equivalent to about 1 mg of fluorometholone, to a suitable container, add 20.0 mL of *Internal standard solution,* and mix.
*Procedure—*Treat 20.0 mL each of the *Standard preparation* and the *Assay preparation* in the following manner. To each add 10.0 mL of hexane, shake for about 15 minutes, then allow the layers to separate, and centrifuge, if necessary. Using the lower (acetonitrile) layer, proceed as directed for *Procedure* in the *Assay* under *Fluorometholone Cream,* beginning with "Using a suitable microsyringe." Calculate the quantity, in mg, of $C_{22}H_{29}FO_4$ in the portion of Ointment taken by the formula:

$$20C(R_U/R_S)$$

in which the terms are as defined therein.

Neomycin Sulfate and Flurandrenolide Cream

» Neomycin Sulfate and Flurandrenolide Cream contains the equivalent of not less than 90.0 percent and not more than 135.0 percent of the labeled amount of neomycin, and not less than 90.0 percent and not more than 110.0 percent of the labeled amount of flurandrenolide ($C_{24}H_{33}FO_6$).

Packaging and storage—Preserve in collapsible tubes or in tight containers, protected from light.
USP Reference standards ⟨11⟩—*USP Flurandrenolide RS. USP Neomycin Sulfate RS.*
Identification—
A: It meets the requirements for neomycin under *Thin-Layer Chromatographic Identification Test* ⟨201BNP⟩.
B: It meets the requirements for the *Identification* test under *Flurandrenolide Cream.*
Minimum fill ⟨755⟩: meets the requirements.
Assay for neomycin—Proceed with Cream as directed in the *Assay* under *Neomycin Sulfate Ointment.*
Assay for flurandrenolide—Proceed with Cream as directed in the *Assay* under *Flurandrenolide Cream.* Calculate the quantity, in mg, of $C_{24}H_{33}FO_6$ in the portion of Cream taken by the formula:

$$10C(r_U/r_S)$$

in which *C* is the concentration, in mg per mL, of USP Flurandrenolide RS in the *Standard preparation;* and r_U and r_S are the peak responses obtained from the *Assay preparation* and the *Standard preparation,* respectively.

Neomycin Sulfate and Flurandrenolide Lotion

» Neomycin Sulfate and Flurandrenolide Lotion contains the equivalent of not less than 90.0 percent and not more than 130.0 percent of the labeled amount of neomycin, and not less than 90.0 percent and not more than 110.0 percent of the labeled amount of flurandrenolide ($C_{24}H_{33}FO_6$).

Packaging and storage—Preserve in tight containers, protected from light.
USP Reference standards ⟨11⟩—*USP Flurandrenolide RS. USP Neomycin Sulfate RS.*
Identification—
A: It meets the requirements for neomycin under *Thin-Layer Chromatographic Identification Test* ⟨201BNP⟩.
B: It meets the requirements for the *Identification* test under *Flurandrenolide Cream.*
Microbial limits ⟨61⟩—It meets the requirements of the tests for absence of *Staphylococcus aureus* and *Pseudomonas aeruginosa.*
Minimum fill ⟨755⟩: meets the requirements.
Assay for neomycin—Proceed as directed for neomycin under *Antibiotics—Microbial Assays* ⟨81⟩, using an accurately weighed portion of Lotion, equivalent to about 3.5 mg of neomycin, blended for 3 to 5 minutes in a high-speed glass blender jar containing an accurately measured volume of *Buffer No. 3* sufficient to obtain a stock solution having a convenient concentration of neomycin. Dilute an accurately measured volume of this stock solution quantitatively with *Buffer No. 3* to obtain a *Test Dilution* having a concentration of neomycin assumed to be equal to the median dose level of the Standard.
Assay for flurandrenolide—Proceed with Neomycin Sulfate and Flurandrenolide Lotion as directed in the *Assay* under *Flurandrenolide Cream.* Calculate the quantity, in mg, of $C_{24}H_{33}FO_6$ in the portion of Lotion taken by the formula:

$$10C(r_U/r_S)$$

in which *C* is the concentration, in mg per mL, of USP Flurandrenolide RS in the *Standard preparation;* and r_U and r_S are the peak responses obtained from the *Assay preparation* and the *Standard preparation,* respectively.

Neomycin Sulfate and Flurandrenolide Ointment

» Neomycin Sulfate and Flurandrenolide Ointment contains the equivalent of not less than 90.0 percent and not more than 135.0 percent of the labeled amount of neomycin, and not less than 90.0 percent and not more than 110.0 percent of the labeled amount of flurandrenolide ($C_{24}H_{33}FO_6$).

Packaging and storage—Preserve in collapsible tubes or in tight containers, protected from light.
USP Reference standards ⟨11⟩—*USP Flurandrenolide RS. USP Neomycin Sulfate RS.*
Identification—
  A: It meets the requirements for neomycin under*Thin-Layer Chromatographic Identification Test* ⟨201BNP⟩.
  B: It meets the requirements for the *Identification* test under *Flurandrenolide Cream*.
Minimum fill ⟨755⟩: meets the requirements.
Water, *Method I* ⟨921⟩: not more than 1.0%, 20 mL of a mixture of toluene and methanol (7 : 3) being used in place of methanol in the titration vessel.
Assay for neomycin—Proceed with Ointment as directed in the *Assay* under*Neomycin Sulfate Ointment*.
Assay for flurandrenolide—Proceed with Ointment as directed in the *Assay* under*Flurandrenolide Cream*. Calculate the quantity, in mg, of $C_{24}H_{33}FO_6$ in the portion of Ointment taken by the formula:

$$10C(r_U / r_S)$$

in which *C* is the concentration, in mg per mL, of USP Flurandrenolide RS in the *Standard preparation;* and r_U and r_S are the peak responses obtained from the *Assay preparation* and the *Standard preparation*, respectively.

Neomycin Sulfate and Gramicidin Ointment

» Neomycin Sulfate and Gramicidin Ointment contains the equivalent of not less than 90.0 percent and not more than 140.0 percent of the labeled amounts of neomycin and gramicidin.

Packaging and storage—Preserve in collapsible tubes or in well-closed containers.
USP Reference standards ⟨11⟩—*USP Gramicidin RS. USP Neomycin Sulfate RS.*
Thin-Layer Chromatographic Identification Test ⟨201BNP⟩: meets the requirements.
Minimum fill ⟨755⟩: meets the requirements.
Water, *Method I* ⟨921⟩: not more than 1.0%, 20 mL of a mixture of toluene and methanol (7 : 3) being used in place of methanol in the titration vessel.
Assay for neomycin—Proceed with Ointment as directed in the *Assay* under*Neomycin Sulfate Ointment*.
Assay for gramicidin—Proceed as directed for gramicidin under*Antibiotics—Microbial Assays* ⟨81⟩, using an accurately weighed portion of Ointment dissolved in 50 mL of hexanes in a separator, and extracted with four 20-mL portions of 80 percent alcohol. Combine the extracts in a suitable volumetric flask, dilute with alcohol to volume, and mix. Dilute this solution quantitatively and stepwise with alcohol to obtain a*Test Dilution* having a concentration of gramicidin assumed to be equal to the median dose level of the Standard.

Neomycin Sulfate and Hydrocortisone Cream

» Neomycin Sulfate and Hydrocortisone Cream contains the equivalent of not less than 90.0 percent and not more than 135.0 percent of the labeled amount of neomycin, and not less than 90.0 percent and not more than 110.0 percent of the labeled amount of hydrocortisone ($C_{21}H_{30}O_5$).

Packaging and storage—Preserve in collapsible tubes or in well-closed containers.
USP Reference standards ⟨11⟩—*USP Hydrocortisone RS. USP Neomycin Sulfate RS.*
Identification—
  A: It meets the requirements for neomycin under*Thin-Layer Chromatographic Identification Test* ⟨201BNP⟩.
  B: The retention time of the major peaks for hydrocortisone in the chromatogram of the *Assay preparation* corresponds to that in the chromatogram of the *Standard preparation*, as obtained in the *Assay for hydrocortisone*.
Minimum fill ⟨755⟩: meets the requirements.
Assay for neomycin—Proceed with Cream as directed in the *Assay* under*Neomycin Sulfate Ointment*.
Assay for hydrocortisone—Proceed with Cream as directed in the *Assay for hydrocortisone* under *Neomycin and Polymyxin B Sulfates, Bacitracin Zinc, and Hydrocortisone Ophthalmic Ointment*.

Neomycin Sulfate and Hydrocortisone Ointment

» Neomycin Sulfate and Hydrocortisone Ointment contains the equivalent of not less than 90.0 percent and not more than 135.0 percent of the labeled amount of neomycin, and not less than 90.0 percent and not more than 110.0 percent of the labeled amount of hydrocortisone ($C_{21}H_{30}O_5$).

Packaging and storage—Preserve in collapsible tubes or in well-closed containers.
USP Reference standards ⟨11⟩—*USP Hydrocortisone RS. USP Neomycin Sulfate RS.*
Identification—
  A: It meets the requirements for neomycin under*Thin-Layer Chromatographic Identification Test* ⟨201BNP⟩.
  B: The retention time of the major peak for hydrocortisone acetate in the chromatogram of the *Assay preparation* corresponds to that in the chromatogram of the *Standard preparation*, as obtained in the *Assay for hydrocortisone*.
Minimum fill ⟨755⟩: meets the requirements.
Water, *Method I* ⟨921⟩: not more than 1.0%, 20 mL of a mixture of toluene and methanol (7 : 3) being used in place of methanol in the titration vessel.
Assay for neomycin—Proceed with Ointment as directed in the *Assay* under*Neomycin Sulfate Ointment*.
Assay for hydrocortisone—Proceed with Ointment as directed in the *Assay for hydrocortisone* under *Neomycin and Polymyxin B Sulfates, Bacitracin Zinc, and Hydrocortisone Ophthalmic Ointment*.

Neomycin Sulfate and Hydrocortisone Otic Suspension

» Neomycin Sulfate and Hydrocortisone Otic Suspension is a sterile suspension containing not less than 90.0 percent and not more than 130.0 percent of the labeled amount of neomycin, and not less than 90.0 percent and not more than 110.0 percent of the labeled amount of hydrocortisone. It contains Acetic Acid, and may contain one or more suitable buffers, dispersants, and preservatives.

NOTE—Where Neomycin Sulfate and Hydrocortisone Otic Suspension is prescribed, without reference to the quantity of neomycin or hydrocortisone contained therein, a product containing 3.5 mg of neomycin and 10 mg of hydrocortisone per mL shall be dispensed.

Packaging and storage—Preserve in tight, light-resistant containers.

USP Reference standards ⟨11⟩—*USP Hydrocortisone RS. USP Neomycin Sulfate RS.*
Sterility ⟨71⟩: meets the requirements.
pH ⟨791⟩: between 4.5 and 6.0.
Assay for neomycin—Using an accurately measured volume of Otic Suspension, freshly mixed and free from entrapped air, proceed as directed in the *Assay for neomycin* under *Neomycin and Polymyxin B Sulfates and Hydrocortisone Otic Solution.*
Assay for hydrocortisone—
  Mobile phase and *Standard preparation*—Prepare as directed in the *Assay for hydrocortisone content* under *Neomycin and Polymyxin B Sulfates, Bacitracin Zinc, and Hydrocortisone Ophthalmic Ointment.*
  Assay preparation—Transfer 3.0 mL of Otic Suspension, freshly mixed and free from entrapped air, to a 200-mL volumetric flask, dilute with a mixture of methanol and water (1:1) to volume, and mix. Filter the solution, rejecting the first 10 mL of the filtrate.
  Procedure—Proceed as directed for *Procedure* in the *Assay for hydrocortisone content* under *Neomycin and Polymyxin B Sulfates, Bacitracin Zinc, and Hydrocortisone Ophthalmic Ointment.* Calculate the quantity, in mg, of $C_{21}H_{30}O_5$ in each mL of the Otic Suspension taken by the formula:

$$(66.67C)(r_U / r_S)$$

in which C is the concentration, in mg per mL, of USP Hydrocortisone RS in the *Standard preparation*, and r_U and r_S are the peak responses obtained from the *Assay preparation* and the *Standard preparation*, respectively.

Neomycin Sulfate and Hydrocortisone Acetate Cream

» Neomycin Sulfate and Hydrocortisone Acetate Cream contains the equivalent of not less than 90.0 percent and not more than 135.0 percent of the labeled amount of neomycin, and not less than 90.0 percent and not more than 110.0 percent of the labeled amount of hydrocortisone acetate ($C_{23}H_{32}O_6$).

Packaging and storage—Preserve in well-closed containers.
USP Reference standards ⟨11⟩—*USP Hydrocortisone Acetate RS. USP Neomycin Sulfate RS.*

Identification—
  A: It meets the requirements for neomycin under *Thin-Layer Chromatographic Identification Test* ⟨201BNP⟩.
  B: The retention time of the major peak for hydrocortisone acetate in the chromatogram of the *Assay preparation*, corresponds to that in the chromatogram of the *Standard preparation*, as obtained in the *Assay for hydrocortisone acetate*.
Minimum fill ⟨755⟩: meets the requirements.
Assay for neomycin—Proceed with Cream as directed in the *Assay* under *Neomycin Sulfate Ointment.*
Assay for hydrocortisone acetate—Proceed with Cream as directed in the *Assay* under *Hydrocortisone Acetate Lotion.*

Neomycin Sulfate and Hydrocortisone Acetate Lotion

» Neomycin Sulfate and Hydrocortisone Acetate Lotion contains the equivalent of not less than 90.0 percent and not more than 130.0 percent of the labeled amount of neomycin, and not less than 90.0 percent and not more than 110.0 percent of the labeled amount of hydrocortisone acetate ($C_{23}H_{32}O_6$).

Packaging and storage—Preserve in well-closed containers.
USP Reference standards ⟨11⟩—*USP Hydrocortisone Acetate RS. USP Neomycin Sulfate RS.*
Identification—
  A: It meets the requirements for neomycin under *Thin-Layer Chromatographic Identification Test* ⟨201BNP⟩.
  B: The retention time of the major peak for hydrocortisone acetate in the chromatogram of the *Assay preparation* corresponds to that in the chromatogram of the *Standard preparation*, as obtained in the *Assay for hydrocortisone acetate*.
Minimum fill ⟨755⟩: meets the requirements.
Assay for neomycin—Proceed as directed for neomycin under *Antibiotics—Microbial Assays* ⟨81⟩, blending an accurately measured volume of Lotion for 3 to 5 minutes in a high-speed glass blender jar containing an accurately measured volume of *Buffer No. 3*. Dilute an accurately measured volume of the solution so obtained quantitatively and stepwise with *Buffer No. 3* to obtain a *Test Dilution* having a concentration of neomycin assumed to be equal to the median dose level of the *Standard*.
Assay for hydrocortisone acetate—Proceed with Lotion as directed in the *Assay* under *Hydrocortisone Acetate Lotion*.

Neomycin Sulfate and Hydrocortisone Acetate Ointment

» Neomycin Sulfate and Hydrocortisone Acetate Ointment contains the equivalent of not less than 90.0 percent and not more than 135.0 percent of the labeled amount of neomycin, and not less than 90.0 percent and not more than 110.0 percent of the labeled amount of hydrocortisone acetate ($C_{23}H_{32}O_6$).

Packaging and storage—Preserve in collapsible tubes or in well-closed containers.
USP Reference standards ⟨11⟩—*USP Hydrocortisone Acetate RS. USP Neomycin Sulfate RS.*
Identification—
  A: It meets the requirements for neomycin under *Thin-Layer Chromatographic Identification Test* ⟨201BNP⟩.
  B: The retention time of the major peak for hydrocortisone acetate in the chromatogram of the *Assay preparation* corresponds to

that in the chromatogram of the *Standard preparation*, as obtained in the *Assay for hydrocortisone acetate*.
Minimum fill ⟨755⟩: meets the requirements.
Water, *Method I* ⟨921⟩: not more than 1.0%, 20 mL of a mixture of toluene and methanol (7 : 3) being used in place of methanol in the titration vessel.
Assay for neomycin—Proceed with the Ointment as directed in the *Assay* under *Neomycin Sulfate Ointment*.
Assay for hydrocortisone acetate—Proceed with the Ointment as directed in the *Assay* under *Hydrocortisone Acetate Lotion*.

Neomycin Sulfate and Hydrocortisone Acetate Ophthalmic Ointment

» Neomycin Sulfate and Hydrocortisone Acetate Ophthalmic Ointment contains the equivalent of not less than 90.0 percent and not more than 135.0 percent of the labeled amount of neomycin, and not less than 90.0 percent and not more than 110.0 percent of the labeled amount of hydrocortisone acetate ($C_{23}H_{32}O_6$).

Packaging and storage—Preserve in collapsible ophthalmic ointment tubes.
USP Reference standards ⟨11⟩—*USP Hydrocortisone Acetate RS. USP Neomycin Sulfate RS.*
Identification—
  A: It meets the requirements for neomycin under *Thin-Layer Chromatographic Identification Test* ⟨201BNP⟩.
  B: The retention time of the major peak for hydrocortisone acetate in the chromatogram of the *Assay preparation* corresponds to that in the chromatogram of the *Standard preparation*, as obtained in the *Assay for hydrocortisone acetate*.
Sterility ⟨71⟩—It meets the requirements when tested as directed for *Membrane Filtration* under *Test for Sterility of the Product to be Examined*.
Minimum fill ⟨755⟩: meets the requirements.
Water, *Method I* ⟨921⟩: not more than 1.0%, 20 mL of a mixture of toluene and methanol (7 : 3) being used in place of methanol in the titration vessel.
Metal particles—It meets the requirements of the test for *Metal Particles in Ophthalmic Ointments* ⟨751⟩.
Assay for neomycin—Proceed with Ophthalmic Ointment as directed in the *Assay* under *Neomycin Sulfate Ointment*.
Assay for hydrocortisone acetate—Proceed with Ophthalmic Ointment as directed in the *Assay* under *Hydrocortisone Acetate Lotion*.

Neomycin Sulfate and Hydrocortisone Acetate Ophthalmic Suspension

» Neomycin Sulfate and Hydrocortisone Acetate Ophthalmic Suspension is a sterile, aqueous suspension containing the equivalent of not less than 90.0 percent and not more than 130.0 percent of the labeled amount of neomycin, and not less than 90.0 percent and not more than 110.0 percent of the labeled amount of hydrocortisone acetate ($C_{23}H_{32}O_6$).

Packaging and storage—Preserve in tight containers. The containers or individual cartons are sealed and tamper-proof so that sterility is assured at time of first use.
USP Reference standards ⟨11⟩—*USP Hydrocortisone Acetate RS. USP Neomycin Sulfate RS.*

Identification—The chromatogram of the *Assay preparation* obtained as directed in the *Assay for hydrocortisone acetate* exhibits a major peak for hydrocortisone acetate, the retention time of which corresponds with that exhibited in the chromatogram of the *Standard preparation* obtained as directed in the *Assay for hydrocortisone acetate*.
Sterility ⟨71⟩: meets the requirements.
pH ⟨791⟩: between 5.5 and 7.5.
Assay for neomycin—Proceed as directed for neomycin under *Antibiotics—Microbial Assays* ⟨81⟩, using an accurately measured volume of Ophthalmic Suspension, freshly mixed and free from air bubbles, diluted quantitatively and stepwise with *Buffer No. 3* to yield a *Test Dilution* having a concentration assumed to be equal to the median dose level of the Standard.
Assay for hydrocortisone acetate—
  Mobile phase—Prepare a solution containing *n*-butyl chloride, water-saturated *n*-butyl chloride, tetrahydrofuran, methanol, and glacial acetic acid (95 : 95 : 14 : 7 : 6).
  Internal standard solution—Prepare a solution of fluoxymesterone in chloroform containing 0.8 mg per mL.
  Standard preparation—Dissolve about 10 mg of USP Hydrocortisone Acetate RS, accurately weighed, in 10.0 mL of *Internal standard solution*, dilute with about 40 mL of chloroform, and mix.
  Assay preparation—Transfer an accurately measured volume of Ophthalmic Suspension, freshly mixed and free from air bubbles, equivalent to about 10 mg of hydrocortisone acetate, to a suitable container. Add 10.0 mL of *Internal standard solution* and about 40 mL of chloroform, shake vigorously for about 5 minutes, and allow the phases to separate. Use the clear chloroform layer as the *Assay preparation*.
  Chromatographic system (see *Chromatography* ⟨621⟩)—The liquid chromatograph is equipped with a 254-nm detector and a 4-mm × 30-cm column that contains packing L3. The flow rate is about 1 mL per minute. Chromatograph the *Standard preparation*, and record the peak responses as directed for *Procedure:* the resolution, *R*, between the analyte and internal standard peaks is not less than 3.0, and the relative standard deviation for replicate injections is not more than 2.0%.
  Procedure—Separately inject equal volumes (about 15 µL) of the *Standard preparation* and the *Assay preparation* into the chromatograph, record the chromatograms, and measure the responses for the major peaks. The relative retention times are about 0.7 and 1.0 for hydrocortisone acetate and fluoxymesterone, respectively. Calculate the quantity, in mg, of hydrocortisone acetate ($C_{23}H_{32}O_6$) in each mL of the Ophthalmic Suspension taken by the formula:

$$(W / V)(R_U / R_S)$$

in which *W* is the quantity, in mg, of USP Hydrocortisone Acetate RS taken to prepare the *Standard preparation*, *V* is the volume, in mL, of Ophthalmic Suspension taken, and R_U and R_S are the peak response ratios of the hydrocortisone acetate peak to the internal standard peak obtained from the *Assay preparation* and the *Standard preparation*, respectively.

Neomycin Sulfate, Isoflupredone Acetate, and Tetracaine Hydrochloride Ointment

» Neomycin Sulfate, Isoflupredone Acetate, and Tetracaine Hydrochloride Ointment contains the equivalent of not less than 90.0 percent and not more than 120.0 percent of the labeled amount of neomycin, and not less than 92.5 percent and not more than 117.5 percent of the labeled amounts of isoflupredone acetate ($C_{23}H_{29}FO_6$) and tetracaine hydrochloride ($C_{15}H_{24}N_2O_2 \cdot HCl$) in a suitable ointment base.

Packaging and storage—Preserve in collapsible tubes or well-closed containers.
Labeling—Label it to indicate that it is intended for veterinary use only.
USP Reference standards ⟨11⟩—*USP Isoflupredone Acetate RS. USP Neomycin Sulfate RS. USP Tetracaine Hydrochloride RS.*
Identification—
  A: *Thin-Layer Chromatographic Identification Test* ⟨201⟩—
  Test solution—To 2 g of Ointment in a centrifuge tube add 25 mL of chloroform, and heat at 60° for 5 minutes, with occasional shaking. Centrifuge, discard the chloroform layer, add 5 mL of water, shake, and filter. Use the filtrate.
  Standard solution—Prepare a solution containing 2 mg of USP Neomycin Sulfate RS per mL.
  Application volume: 1 µL.
  Developing solvent system: a mixture of water, butyl alcohol, glacial acetic acid, and pyridine (35 : 30 : 22 : 6).
  Spray reagent: a solution of triketohydrindene hydrate in butyl alcohol (2 in 1000).
  Procedure—Proceed as directed in the chapter, except to locate the spots by spraying with *Spray reagent* and heating at 100° for 5 minutes.
  B: The retention time of the major peak for isoflupredone acetate in the chromatogram of the *Assay preparation* corresponds to that in the chromatogram of the *Standard preparation,* as obtained in the *Assay for isoflupredone acetate.*
Minimum fill ⟨755⟩: meets the requirements.
Water, *Method I* ⟨921⟩: not more than 1.0%, a mixture of methanol and chloroform (3 : 2) being used instead of methanol in the titration vessel and the titration vessel being heated to between 45° and 55°.
Assay for neomycin—Proceed as directed under *Antibiotics—Microbial Assays* ⟨81⟩. Place an accurately weighed portion of Ointment in a centrifuge tube with 25 mL of chloroform. Heat at 60° for 3 minutes, shake until the Ointment is dissolved, centrifuge, and remove and discard the chloroform. Add 15 mL of chloroform, shake, centrifuge, and remove and discard the chloroform. Add 5.0 mL of water and 15 mL of chromatographic *n*-heptane, shake, centrifuge, and remove and discard the *n*-heptane layer. Dilute an accurately measured volume of the water layer quantitatively with *Buffer No. 3* to obtain a *Test Dilution* having a concentration of neomycin assumed to be equal to the median dose level of the Standard.
Assay for isoflupredone acetate—
  Mobile phase, Diluent, Internal standard solution, Standard preparation, and *Chromatographic system*—Proceed as directed in the *Assay* under *Isoflupredone Acetate.*
  Assay preparation—Transfer an accurately weighed portion of Ointment, equivalent to about 4 mg of isoflupredone acetate, to a suitable container. Add 8.0 mL of *Internal standard solution,* 32.0 mL of *Diluent,* and about 10 glass beads. Shake for about 15 minutes, centrifuge, and use the clear chloroform portion.
  Procedure—Proceed as directed in the *Assay* under *Isoflupredone Acetate.* Calculate the quantity, in mg, of isoflupredone acetate ($C_{23}H_{29}FO_6$) in the portion of Ointment taken by the formula:

$$W_S(R_U / R_S)$$

in which the terms are as defined therein.
Assay for tetracaine hydrochloride—
  Standard preparation—Prepare a solution in chloroform having a known concentration of about 5.0 µg of USP Tetracaine Hydrochloride RS per mL.
  Assay preparation—Transfer an accurately weighed portion of Ointment, equivalent to about 1.25 mg of tetracaine hydrochloride, to a 250-mL volumetric flask, add about 100 mL of chloroform, and warm on a steam bath for about 3 minutes to dissolve the Ointment. Cool to room temperature, dilute with chloroform to volume, and mix.
  Blank solution—Transfer an accurately weighed portion of the ointment base, equivalent to the weight used in the *Assay preparation,* to a 250-mL volumetric flask. Add 100 mL of chloroform, warm on a steam bath for about 3 minutes to dissolve, and allow to stand until the solution has equilibrated to room temperature. Dilute with chloroform to volume, and mix well.

  Procedure—Concomitantly determine the absorbances of the *Standard preparation,* the *Blank solution,* and the *Assay preparation* with a suitable spectrophotometer at the wavelength of maximum absorbance at about 310 nm, using chloroform to zero the instrument. Calculate the absorbance of the *Blank solution,* A_B, adjusted for weight difference between the *Assay preparation* and the *Blank solution,* by the formula:

$$A(W_T / W_B)$$

in which A is the absorbance of the *Blank solution;* W_T is the weight, in mg, of Ointment taken to prepare the *Assay preparation;* and W_B is the weight, in mg, of the ointment base taken to prepare the *Blank solution.* Calculate the quantity, in mg, of tetracaine hydrochloride ($C_{15}H_{24}N_2O_2 \cdot HCl$) in the portion of Ointment taken by the formula:

$$250C\,[(A_U - A_B)/A_S]$$

in which C is the concentration, in mg per mL, of USP Tetracaine Hydrochloride RS in the *Standard preparation;* A_B is as obtained above; and A_U and A_S are the absorbances of the *Assay preparation* and the *Standard preparation,* respectively.

Neomycin Sulfate, Isoflupredone Acetate, and Tetracaine Hydrochloride Topical Powder

» Neomycin Sulfate, Isoflupredone Acetate, and Tetracaine Hydrochloride Topical Powder contains the equivalent of not less than 90.0 percent and not more than 125.0 percent of the labeled amount of neomycin, and not less than 90.0 percent and not more than 120.0 percent of the labeled amounts of isoflupredone acetate ($C_{23}H_{29}FO_6$) and tetracaine hydrochloride ($C_{15}H_{24}N_2O_2 \cdot HCl$).

Packaging and storage—Preserve in well-closed containers.
Labeling—Label it to indicate that it is intended for veterinary use only.
USP Reference standards ⟨11⟩—*USP Isoflupredone Acetate RS. USP Neomycin Sulfate RS. USP Tetracaine Hydrochloride RS.*
Identification—
  A: *Thin-Layer Chromatographic Identification Test* ⟨201⟩—
  Test solution—Add 20 mL of chloroform to 1 g of Topical Powder, shake for 5 to 10 minutes, and centrifuge. Evaporate a 10-mL portion of the clear solution to dryness, and dissolve the residue in 1 mL of a mixture of chloroform and alcohol (1 : 1).
  Standard solution: 0.5 mg of USP Isoflupredone Acetate RS per mL, in a mixture of chloroform and alcohol (1 : 1).
  Application volume: 30 µL.
  Developing solvent system: a mixture of methylene chloride and methanol (180 : 16), in a paper-lined chromatographic chamber.
  Spray reagent: a solution of sulfuric acid in methanol (70 in 100).
  Procedure—Proceed as directed in the chapter, except to use a plate that has been activated by heating in an oven at 105° for 60 minutes. Allow the plate to cool before using. Locate the spots under short- and long-wavelength UV light. Spray the plate with *Spray reagent,* heat at 90° for 30 minutes, and locate the spots under short- and long-wavelength UV light (*presence of isoflupredone acetate*).
  B: *Thin-Layer Chromatographic Identification Test* ⟨201⟩—
  Test solution—To 1 g of Topical Powder in a centrifuge tube add 5 mL of water, and shake until dissolved. Prepare a suspension of 10 g of cation-exchange resin in 10 mL of water, add 5 mL of a solution of sodium hydroxide (1 in 2), mix, and wash the resin with water until the pH of the wash is about 9. Add 0.3 g of this suspension to the solution of Topical Powder, and shake for 10 seconds.

Centrifuge for 1 minute, and discard the supernatant. Wash the resin in the tube with 10 mL of water, centrifuge, and discard the supernatant. Add 2 mL of 1 M ammonium hydroxide, shake for 10 seconds, and filter. Use the filtrate.

Standard solution, Application volume, Developing solvent system, Spray reagent, and *Procedure*—Proceed as directed in *Identification* test A under *Neomycin Sulfate, Isoflupredone Acetate, and Tetracaine Hydrochloride Ointment* (presence of neomycin).

Minimum fill ⟨755⟩: meets the requirements.

Loss on drying ⟨731⟩—Dry about 2 g in vacuum at a pressure not exceeding 5 mm of mercury at 60° for 3 hours: it loses not more than 8.0% of its weight.

Assay for neomycin—Proceed as directed under *Antibiotics—Microbial Assays* ⟨81⟩, the *Test Dilution* being prepared as follows. Use an accurately weighed quantity of Topical Powder diluted quantitatively with *Buffer No. 3* to obtain a solution having a suitable concentration of neomycin. Dilute this stock solution quantitatively with *Buffer No. 3* to obtain a *Test Dilution* having a concentration assumed to be equal to the median dose level of the Standard.

Assay for isoflupredone acetate—

Mobile phase, Diluent, Internal standard solution, Standard preparation, and *Chromatographic system*—Proceed as directed in the *Assay* under *Isoflupredone Acetate*.

Assay preparation—Transfer an accurately weighed portion of Topical Powder, equivalent to about 4 mg of isoflupredone acetate, to a suitable container. Add 8.0 mL of *Internal standard solution*, 32.0 mL of *Diluent*, and about 10 glass beads. Shake for about 15 minutes, centrifuge, and use the clear chloroform portion.

Procedure—Proceed as directed in the *Assay* under *Isoflupredone Acetate*. Calculate the quantity, in mg, of isoflupredone acetate ($C_{23}H_{29}FO_6$) in the portion of Topical Powder taken by the formula:

$$W_S(R_U/R_S)$$

in which the terms are as defined therein.

Assay for tetracaine hydrochloride—

Standard preparation—Prepare a solution having a known concentration of 5.5 μg of USP Tetracaine Hydrochloride RS per mL.

Assay preparation—Transfer an accurately weighed portion of Topical Powder, equivalent to about 5.5 mg of tetracaine hydrochloride, to a 100-mL volumetric flask, dilute with water to volume, and mix. Pass about 30 mL through a fine, sintered-glass filter. Transfer 10.0 mL of the clear filtrate to a second 100-mL volumetric flask, dilute with water to volume, and mix.

Procedure—Concomitantly determine the absorbances of the *Standard preparation* and the *Assay preparation* at the wavelength of maximum absorbance at about 310 nm, with a suitable spectrophotometer, using water to zero the instrument. Calculate the quantity, in mg, of tetracaine hydrochloride ($C_{15}H_{24}N_2O_2 \cdot HCl$) in the portion of Topical Powder taken by the formula:

$$1000C(A_U/A_S)$$

in which *C* is the concentration, in mg per mL, of USP Tetracaine Hydrochloride RS in the *Standard preparation;* and A_U and A_S are the absorbances of the *Assay preparation* and the *Standard preparation*, respectively.

Neomycin Sulfate and Methylprednisolone Acetate Cream

» Neomycin Sulfate and Methylprednisolone Acetate Cream contains the equivalent of not less than 90.0 percent and not more than 135.0 percent of the labeled amount of neomycin, and not less than 90.0 percent and not more than 110.0 percent of the labeled amount of methylprednisolone acetate ($C_{24}H_{32}O_6$).

Packaging and storage—Preserve in collapsible tubes or in tight containers, protected from light.

USP Reference standards ⟨11⟩—*USP Methylprednisolone Acetate RS. USP Neomycin Sulfate RS.*

Identification—

A: It meets the requirements for neomycin under *Thin-Layer Chromatographic Identification Test* ⟨201BNP⟩.

B: In the thin-layer chromatogram prepared as directed in the *Assay for methylprednisolone acetate*, the R_F value of the principal spot obtained from the *Assay preparation* corresponds to that obtained from the *Standard preparation*, prepared as directed in the *Assay for methylprednisolone acetate*.

Minimum fill ⟨755⟩: meets the requirements.

Assay for neomycin—Proceed with Cream as directed in the *Assay* under *Neomycin Sulfate Ointment*.

Assay for methylprednisolone acetate—Proceed with Cream as directed in the *Assay* under *Methylprednisolone Acetate Cream*.

Neomycin and Polymyxin B Sulfates Cream

» Neomycin and Polymyxin B Sulfates Cream contains the equivalent of not less than 90.0 percent and not more than 130.0 percent of the labeled amounts of neomycin and polymyxin B. It may contain a suitable local anesthetic.

Packaging and storage—Preserve in well-closed containers, preferably at controlled room temperature.

USP Reference standards ⟨11⟩—*USP Neomycin Sulfate RS. USP Polymyxin B Sulfate RS.*

Thin-layer chromatographic identification test ⟨201BNP⟩: meets the requirements.

Minimum fill ⟨755⟩: meets the requirements.

Assay for neomycin—Proceed as directed under *Antibiotics—Microbial Assays* ⟨81⟩, using an accurately weighed portion of Cream, equivalent to about 1.75 mg of neomycin, shaken in a separator with about 50 mL of ether, and extracted with four 20-mL portions of *Buffer No. 3*. Combine the aqueous extracts, and dilute with *Buffer No. 3* to an appropriate volume to obtain a stock solution of convenient concentration. Dilute this stock solution quantitatively and stepwise with *Buffer No. 3* to obtain a *Test Dilution* having a concentration assumed to be equal to the median dose level of the Standard.

Assay for polymyxin B—Proceed as directed under *Antibiotics—Microbial Assays* ⟨81⟩, using an accurately weighed portion of Cream shaken with about 50 mL of ether in a separator, and extracted with four 25-mL portions of *Buffer No. 6*. Combine the aqueous extracts, and dilute with *Buffer No. 6* to an appropriate volume to obtain a stock solution. Dilute this stock solution quantitatively and stepwise with *Buffer No. 6* to obtain a *Test Dilution* having a concentration assumed to be equal to the median dose level of the Standard (10 Polymyxin B Units per mL). Add to each test dilution of the Standard a quantity of USP Neomycin Sulfate RS, dissolved in *Buffer No. 6*, to obtain the same concentration of neomycin present in the *Test Dilution*.

Neomycin and Polymyxin B Sulfates Solution for Irrigation

» Neomycin and Polymyxin B Sulfates Solution for Irrigation is a sterile, aqueous solution containing the equivalent of not less than 90.0 percent and not more than 130.0 percent of the labeled amounts of neomycin and of polymyxin B. It may contain a suitable preservative.

Packaging and storage—Preserve in tight containers.
Labeling—Label it to indicate that it is to be diluted for use in a urinary bladder irrigation and is not intended for injection.
USP Reference standards ⟨11⟩—*USP Neomycin Sulfate RS. USP Polymyxin B Sulfate RS.*
Thin-layer chromatographic identification test ⟨201BNP⟩: meets the requirements.
Sterility ⟨71⟩—It meets the requirements when tested as directed for *Membrane Filtration* under *Test for Sterility of the Product to be Examined.*
pH ⟨791⟩: between 4.5 and 6.0.
Assay for neomycin and Assay for polymyxin B—Proceed with Neomycin and Polymyxin B Sulfates Solution for Irrigation as directed in the *Assay for neomycin* and in the *Assay for polymyxin B* under *Neomycin and Polymyxin B Sulfates and Hydrocortisone Otic Solution.*

Neomycin and Polymyxin B Sulfates Ophthalmic Ointment

» Neomycin and Polymyxin B Sulfates Ophthalmic Ointment is a sterile ointment containing Neomycin Sulfate and Polymyxin B Sulfate. It contains the equivalent of not less than 90.0 percent and not more than 130.0 percent of the labeled amounts of neomycin and polymyxin B.

Packaging and storage—Preserve in collapsible ophthalmic ointment tubes.
USP Reference standards ⟨11⟩—*USP Neomycin Sulfate RS. USP Polymyxin B Sulfate RS.*
Thin-layer chromatographic identification test ⟨201BNP⟩: meets the requirements.
Sterility ⟨71⟩—It meets the requirements when tested as directed for *Membrane Filtration* under *Test for Sterility of the Product to be Examined.*
Minimum fill ⟨755⟩: meets the requirements.
Water, *Method I* ⟨921⟩: not more than 0.5%, 20 mL of a mixture of toluene and methanol (7 : 3) being used in place of methanol in the titration vessel.
Metal particles—It meets the requirements of the test for *Metal Particles in Ophthalmic Ointments* ⟨751⟩.
Assay for neomycin and Assay for polymyxin B—Proceed with Ophthalmic Ointment as directed in the *Assay for neomycin* and in the *Assay for polymyxin B* under *Neomycin and Polymyxin B Sulfates and Bacitracin Zinc Ophthalmic Ointment.*

Neomycin and Polymyxin B Sulfates Ophthalmic Solution

» Neomycin and Polymyxin B Sulfates Ophthalmic Solution contains the equivalent of not less than 90.0 percent and not more than 130.0 percent of the labeled amounts of neomycin and polymyxin B. It may contain one or more suitable buffers, dispersants, irrigants, and preservatives.

Packaging and storage—Preserve in tight containers, and avoid exposure to excessive heat.
USP Reference standards ⟨11⟩—*USP Neomycin Sulfate RS. USP Polymyxin B Sulfate RS.*
Thin-layer chromatographic identification test ⟨201BNP⟩: meets the requirements.
Sterility ⟨71⟩—It meets the requirements when tested as directed for *Membrane Filtration* under *Test for Sterility of the Product to be Examined.*
pH ⟨791⟩: between 5.0 and 7.0.
Assay for neomycin and Assay for polymyxin B—Proceed with Ophthalmic Solution as directed in the *Assay for neomycin* and in the *Assay for polymyxin B* under *Neomycin and Polymyxin B Sulfates and Hydrocortisone Otic Solution.*

Neomycin and Polymyxin B Sulfates and Bacitracin Ointment

» Neomycin and Polymyxin B Sulfates and Bacitracin Ointment contains the equivalent of not less than 90.0 percent and not more than 130.0 percent of the labeled amounts of neomycin, polymyxin B, and bacitracin. It may contain a suitable local anesthetic.

Packaging and storage—Preserve in tight, light-resistant containers, preferably at controlled room temperature.
USP Reference standards ⟨11⟩—*USP Bacitracin Zinc RS. USP Neomycin Sulfate RS. USP Polymyxin B Sulfate RS.*
Thin-layer chromatographic identification test ⟨201BNP⟩: meets the requirements.
Minimum fill ⟨755⟩: meets the requirements.
Water, *Method I* ⟨921⟩: not more than 0.5%, 20 mL of a mixture of toluene and methanol (7 : 3) being used in place of methanol in the titration vessel.
Assay for neomycin and Assay for polymyxin B—Proceed with Ointment as directed in the *Assay for neomycin* and in the *Assay for polymyxin B* under *Neomycin and Polymyxin B Sulfates and Bacitracin Zinc Ophthalmic Ointment.*
Assay for bacitracin—Proceed with Ointment as directed in the *Assay* under *Bacitracin Ointment.*

Neomycin and Polymyxin B Sulfates and Bacitracin Ophthalmic Ointment

» Neomycin and Polymyxin B Sulfates and Bacitracin Ophthalmic Ointment is a sterile ointment containing Neomycin Sulfate, Polymyxin B Sulfate, and Bacitracin. It contains the equivalent of not less than 90.0 percent and not more than 140.0 percent of the labeled amounts of neomycin, polymyxin B, and bacitracin.

Packaging and storage—Preserve in collapsible ophthalmic ointment tubes.
USP Reference standards ⟨11⟩—*USP Bacitracin Zinc RS. USP Neomycin Sulfate RS. USP Polymyxin B Sulfate RS.*
Thin-layer chromatographic identification test ⟨201BNP⟩: meets the requirements.
Sterility ⟨71⟩—It meets the requirements when tested as directed for *Membrane Filtration* under *Test for Sterility of the Product to be Examined.*
Minimum fill ⟨755⟩: meets the requirements.
Water, *Method I* ⟨921⟩: not more than 0.5%, 20 mL of a mixture of toluene and methanol (7 : 3) being used in place of methanol in the titration vessel.
Metal particles—It meets the requirements of the test for *Metal Particles in Ophthalmic Ointments* ⟨751⟩.
Assay for neomycin and Assay for polymyxin B—Proceed with Ophthalmic Ointment as directed in the *Assay for neomycin* and in the *Assay for polymyxin B* under *Neomycin and Polymyxin B Sulfates and Bacitracin Zinc Ophthalmic Ointment.*

Assay for bacitracin—Proceed with Ophthalmic Ointment as directed in the *Assay for bacitracin* under *Bacitracin Ointment*.

Neomycin and Polymyxin B Sulfates, Bacitracin, and Hydrocortisone Acetate Ointment

» Neomycin and Polymyxin B Sulfates, Bacitracin, and Hydrocortisone Acetate Ointment contains the equivalent of not less than 90.0 percent and not more than 130.0 percent of the labeled amounts of neomycin, polymyxin B, and bacitracin, and not less than 90.0 percent and not more than 110.0 percent of the labeled amount of hydrocortisone acetate in a suitable ointment base.

Packaging and storage—Preserve in collapsible tubes or in well-closed containers.
USP Reference standards ⟨11⟩—*USP Bacitracin Zinc RS. USP Hydrocortisone Acetate RS. USP Neomycin Sulfate RS. USP Polymyxin B Sulfate RS.*
Identification—
  A: It meets the requirements under *Thin-Layer Chromatographic Identification Test* ⟨201BNP⟩.
  B: The retention time of the major peak for hydrocortisone acetate in the chromatogram of the *Assay preparation* corresponds to that in the chromatogram of the *Standard preparation*, as obtained in the *Assay for hydrocortisone acetate*.
Minimum fill ⟨755⟩: meets the requirements.
Water, *Method I* ⟨921⟩: not more than 0.5%, 20 mL of a mixture of toluene and methanol (7 : 3) being used in place of methanol in the titration vessel.
Assay for neomycin and Assay for polymyxin B—Proceed with Ointment as directed in the *Assay for neomycin* and in the *Assay for polymyxin B* under *Neomycin and Polymyxin B Sulfates and Bacitracin Zinc Ophthalmic Ointment*.
Assay for bacitracin—Proceed with Ointment as directed in the *Assay* under *Bacitracin Ointment*.
Assay for hydrocortisone acetate—Proceed with Ointment as directed in the *Assay* under *Hydrocortisone Acetate Lotion*.

Neomycin and Polymyxin B Sulfates, Bacitracin, and Hydrocortisone Acetate Ophthalmic Ointment

» Neomycin and Polymyxin B Sulfates, Bacitracin, and Hydrocortisone Acetate Ophthalmic Ointment contains the equivalent of not less than 90.0 percent and not more than 140.0 percent of the labeled amounts of neomycin, polymyxin B, and bacitracin, and not less than 90.0 percent and not more than 110.0 percent of the labeled amount of hydrocortisone acetate, in a suitable ointment base.

Packaging and storage—Preserve in collapsible ophthalmic ointment tubes.
USP Reference standards ⟨11⟩—*USP Bacitracin Zinc RS. USP Hydrocortisone Acetate RS. USP Neomycin Sulfate RS. USP Polymyxin B Sulfate RS.*
Identification—
  A: It meets the requirements under *Thin-Layer Chromatographic Identification Test* ⟨201BNP⟩.
  B: The retention time of the major peak for hydrocortisone acetate in the chromatogram of the *Assay preparation* corresponds to that in the chromatogram of the *Standard preparation*, as obtained in the *Assay for hydrocortisone acetate*.
Sterility ⟨71⟩—It meets the requirements when tested as directed for *Membrane Filtration* under *Test for Sterility of the Product to be Examined*.
Minimum fill ⟨755⟩: meets the requirements.
Water, *Method I* ⟨921⟩: not more than 0.5%, 20 mL of a mixture of toluene and methanol (7 : 3) being used in place of methanol in the titration vessel.
Metal particles—It meets the requirements of the test for *Metal Particles in Ophthalmic Ointments* ⟨751⟩.
Assay for neomycin and Assay for polymyxin B—Proceed with Ophthalmic Ointment as directed in the *Assay for neomycin* and in the *Assay for polymyxin B* under *Neomycin and Polymyxin B Sulfates and Bacitracin Zinc Ophthalmic Ointment*.
Assay for bacitracin—Proceed with Ophthalmic Ointment as directed in the *Assay* under *Bacitracin Ointment*.
Assay for hydrocortisone acetate—Proceed with Ophthalmic Ointment as directed in the *Assay* under *Hydrocortisone Acetate Lotion*.

Neomycin and Polymyxin B Sulfates, Bacitracin, and Lidocaine Ointment

» Neomycin and Polymyxin B Sulfates, Bacitracin, and Lidocaine Ointment contains the equivalent of not less than 90.0 percent and not more than 130.0 percent of the labeled amounts of neomycin, polymyxin B, and bacitracin, and not less than 90.0 percent and not more than 110.0 percent of the labeled amount of lidocaine ($C_{14}H_{22}N_2O$).

Packaging and storage—Preserve in well-closed containers, preferably at controlled room temperature.
USP Reference standards ⟨11⟩—*USP Bacitracin Zinc RS. USP Lidocaine RS. USP Neomycin Sulfate RS. USP Polymyxin B Sulfate RS.*
Identification—
  A: It meets the requirements under *Thin-Layer Chromatographic Identification Test* ⟨201BNP⟩.
  B: The retention time of the major peak for lidocaine in the chromatogram of the *Assay preparation* corresponds to that in the chromatogram of the *Standard preparation*, as obtained in the *Assay for lidocaine*.
Minimum fill ⟨755⟩: meets the requirements.
Water, *Method I* ⟨921⟩: not more than 0.5%, 20 mL of a mixture of toluene and methanol (7 : 3) being used in place of methanol in the titration vessel.
Assay for neomycin and Assay for polymyxin B—Proceed with Ointment as directed in the *Assay for neomycin* and in the *Assay for polymyxin B* under *Neomycin and Polymyxin B Sulfates and Bacitracin Zinc Ophthalmic Ointment*.
Assay for bacitracin—Proceed with Ointment as directed in the *Assay* under *Bacitracin Ointment*.
Assay for lidocaine—
  Mobile phase—Dissolve 4.44 g of docusate sodium in 1000 mL of a mixture of methanol and water (4 : 1), add 1 mL of 0.1 N sulfuric acid, and mix. Make adjustments if necessary (see *System Suitability* under *Chromatography* ⟨621⟩).
  Standard preparation—Dissolve a suitable quantity of USP Lidocaine RS, accurately weighed, in *Mobile phase* to obtain a solution having a known concentration of about 0.4 mg per mL.
  Assay preparation—Transfer an accurately weighed quantity of Ointment, equivalent to about 40 mg of lidocaine, to a separator, add 50 mL of *n*-hexane, and shake until the specimen is in solution. Add 30 mL of *Mobile phase*, shake for 1 minute, and allow the layers to separate. Drain the lower layer into a 100-mL volumetric

flask, and extract the n-hexane layer remaining in the separator with two 30-mL portions of *Mobile phase*, combining the lower layers in the volumetric flask. Dilute the combined extracts in the 100-mL volumetric flask with *Mobile phase* to volume, and mix.

Chromatographic system (see *Chromatography* ⟨621⟩)—The liquid chromatograph is equipped with a 230-nm detector and a 4-mm × 25-cm column that contains packing L1. The flow rate is about 1 mL per minute. Chromatograph the *Standard preparation*, and record the peak response as directed for *Procedure*: the column efficiency determined from the analyte peak is not less than 500 theoretical plates, and the relative standard deviation for replicate injections is not more than 2.0%.

Procedure—Separately inject equal volumes (about 20 µL) of the *Standard preparation* and the *Assay preparation* into the chromatograph, record the chromatograms, and measure the responses for the major peaks. Calculate the quantity, in mg, of lidocaine ($C_{14}H_{22}N_2O$) in the portion of Ointment taken by the formula:

$$100C(r_U / r_S)$$

in which C is the concentration, in mg per mL, of USP Lidocaine RS in the *Standard preparation*, and r_U and r_S are the peak responses obtained from the *Assay preparation* and the *Standard preparation*, respectively.

Neomycin and Polymyxin B Sulfates and Bacitracin Zinc Ointment

» Neomycin and Polymyxin B Sulfates and Bacitracin Zinc Ointment contains the equivalent of not less than 90.0 percent and not more than 130.0 percent of the labeled amounts of neomycin, polymyxin B, and bacitracin. It may contain a suitable local anesthetic.

Packaging and storage—Preserve in well-closed containers, preferably at controlled room temperature.

USP Reference standards ⟨11⟩—*USP Bacitracin Zinc RS. USP Neomycin Sulfate RS. USP Polymyxin B Sulfate RS.*
Thin-layer chromatographic identification test ⟨201BNP⟩: meets the requirements.
Minimum fill ⟨755⟩: meets the requirements.
Water, *Method I* ⟨921⟩: not more than 0.5%, 20 mL of a mixture of toluene and methanol (7 : 3) being used in place of methanol in the titration vessel.
Assay for neomycin, Assay for polymyxin B, and Assay for bacitracin—Proceed with Ointment as directed in the *Assay for neomycin*, in the *Assay for polymyxin B*, and in the *Assay for bacitracin* under *Neomycin and Polymyxin B Sulfates and Bacitracin Zinc Ophthalmic Ointment*.

Neomycin and Polymyxin B Sulfates and Bacitracin Zinc Ophthalmic Ointment

» Neomycin and Polymyxin B Sulfates and Bacitracin Zinc Ophthalmic Ointment contains the equivalent of not less than 90.0 percent and not more than 140.0 percent of the labeled amounts of neomycin, polymyxin B, and bacitracin.

Packaging and storage—Preserve in collapsible ophthalmic ointment tubes.

USP Reference standards ⟨11⟩—*USP Bacitracin Zinc RS. USP Neomycin Sulfate RS. USP Polymyxin B Sulfate RS.*
Thin-layer chromatographic identification test ⟨201BNP⟩: meets the requirements.
Sterility ⟨71⟩: meets the requirements.
Minimum fill ⟨755⟩: meets the requirements.
Water, *Method I* ⟨921⟩: not more than 0.5%, 20 mL of a mixture of toluene and methanol (7 : 3) being used in place of methanol in the titration vessel.
Metal particles—It meets the requirements of the test for *Metal Particles in Ophthalmic Ointments* ⟨751⟩.
Assay for neomycin—Proceed as directed under *Antibiotics—Microbial Assays* ⟨81⟩, using an accurately weighed portion of Ophthalmic Ointment shaken in a separator with about 50 mL of ether, and extracted with four 20-mL portions of *Buffer No. 3*. Combine the aqueous extracts, and dilute with *Buffer No. 3* to an appropriate volume to obtain a stock solution. Dilute this stock solution quantitatively and stepwise with *Buffer No. 3* to obtain a *Test Dilution* having a concentration assumed to be equal to the median dose level of the Standard.
Assay for polymyxin B—Proceed as directed under *Antibiotics—Microbial Assays* ⟨81⟩, using an accurately weighed portion of Ophthalmic Ointment shaken with about 50 mL of ether in a separator, and extracted with four 25-mL portions of *Buffer No. 6*. Combine the aqueous extracts, and dilute with *Buffer No. 6* to an appropriate volume to obtain a stock solution. Dilute this stock solution quantitatively and stepwise with *Buffer No. 6* to obtain a *Test Dilution* having a concentration assumed to be equal to the median dose level of the Standard (10 Polymyxin B Units per mL). Add to each test dilution of the Standard a quantity of Neomycin Standard, dissolved in *Buffer No. 6*, to obtain the same concentration of neomycin present in the *Test Dilution*.
Assay for bacitracin—Proceed as directed under *Antibiotics—Microbial Assays* ⟨81⟩, using an accurately weighed portion of Ophthalmic Ointment shaken with about 50 mL of ether in a separator, and extracted with four 25-mL portions of 0.01 N hydrochloric acid. Combine the acid extracts, and dilute with 0.01 N hydrochloric acid to an appropriate volume to obtain a stock solution. Dilute this stock solution quantitatively and stepwise with *Buffer No. 1* to obtain a *Test Dilution* having a concentration assumed to be equal to the median dose level of the Standard (1.0 Bacitracin Unit per mL). [NOTE—If the stock solution has a concentration of less than 100 Bacitracin Units per mL, add additional hydrochloric acid to each test dilution of the Standard to obtain the same concentration of hydrochloric acid as the *Test Dilution*.]

Neomycin and Polymyxin B Sulfates, Bacitracin Zinc, and Hydrocortisone Ointment

» Neomycin and Polymyxin B Sulfates, Bacitracin Zinc, and Hydrocortisone Ointment contains the equivalent of not less than 90.0 percent and not more than 130.0 percent of the labeled amounts of neomycin, polymyxin B, and bacitracin, and not less than 90.0 percent and not more than 110.0 percent of the labeled amount of hydrocortisone.

Packaging and storage—Preserve in well-closed containers, preferably at controlled room temperature.

USP Reference standards ⟨11⟩—*USP Bacitracin Zinc RS. USP Hydrocortisone RS. USP Neomycin Sulfate RS. USP Polymyxin B Sulfate RS.*
Identification—
A: It meets the requirements under *Thin-Layer Chromatographic Identification Test* ⟨201BNP⟩.
B: The retention time of the major peak for hydrocortisone in the chromatogram of the *Assay preparation* corresponds to that in the chromatogram of the *Standard preparation*, as obtained in the *Assay for hydrocortisone*.

Minimum fill ⟨755⟩: meets the requirements.
Water, *Method I* ⟨921⟩: not more than 0.5%, 20 mL of a mixture of toluene and methanol (7 : 3) being used in place of methanol in the titration vessel.
Assay for neomycin, Assay for polymyxin B, and Assay for bacitracin—Proceed with Ointment as directed in the *Assay for neomycin,* in the *Assay for polymyxin B,* and in the *Assay for bacitracin* under *Neomycin and Polymyxin B Sulfates and Bacitracin Zinc Ophthalmic Ointment.*
Assay for hydrocortisone—Proceed with the Ointment as directed in the *Assay for hydrocortisone* under *Neomycin and Polymyxin B Sulfates, Bacitracin Zinc, and Hydrocortisone Ophthalmic Ointment.*

Neomycin and Polymyxin B Sulfates, Bacitracin Zinc, and Hydrocortisone Ophthalmic Ointment

» Neomycin and Polymyxin B Sulfates, Bacitracin Zinc, and Hydrocortisone Ophthalmic Ointment is a sterile ointment containing Neomycin Sulfate, Polymyxin B Sulfate, Bacitracin Zinc, and Hydrocortisone. It contains the equivalent of not less than 90.0 percent and not more than 140.0 percent of the labeled amounts of neomycin, polymyxin B, and bacitracin, and not less than 90.0 percent and not more than 110.0 percent of the labeled amount of hydrocortisone.

Packaging and storage—Preserve in collapsible ophthalmic ointment tubes.
USP Reference standards ⟨11⟩—*USP Bacitracin Zinc RS. USP Hydrocortisone RS. USP Neomycin Sulfate RS. USP Polymyxin B Sulfate RS.*
Identification—
  A: It meets the requirements under *Thin-Layer Chromatographic Identification Test* ⟨201BNP⟩.
  B: The retention time of the major peak for hydrocortisone in the chromatogram of the *Assay preparation* corresponds to that in the chromatogram of the *Standard preparation,* as obtained in the *Assay for hydrocortisone.*
Sterility ⟨71⟩: meets the requirements.
Minimum fill ⟨755⟩: meets the requirements.
Water, *Method I* ⟨921⟩: not more than 0.5%, 20 mL of a mixture of toluene and methanol (7 : 3) being used in place of methanol in the titration vessel.
Metal particles—It meets the requirements of the test for *Metal Particles in Ophthalmic Ointments* ⟨751⟩.
Assay for neomycin, Assay for polymyxin B, and Assay for bacitracin—Proceed as directed in the *Assay for neomycin,* the *Assay for polymyxin B,* and the *Assay for bacitracin* under *Neomycin and Polymyxin B Sulfates and Bacitracin Zinc Ophthalmic Ointment.*
Assay for hydrocortisone—
  Mobile phase—Prepare a suitable solution of about 500 volumes of methanol, 500 volumes of water, and 1 volume of glacial acetic acid, such that the retention time of hydrocortisone is between 6 and 10 minutes.
  Standard preparation—Dissolve a suitable quantity of USP Hydrocortisone RS, accurately weighed, in methanol and water (1 : 1) to obtain a solution having a known concentration of about 0.15 mg per mL.
  Assay preparation—Transfer to a separator about 1.5 g, accurately weighed, of Ophthalmic Ointment. Add 3 mL of *n*-hexane, and warm gently on a steam bath with mild agitation until dissolved. Add 7 mL of *n*-hexane, mix by swirling, and extract with four 15-mL portions of methanol and water (1 : 1). Collect the extracts in a 100-mL volumetric flask, dilute with methanol and water (1 : 1) to volume, and mix. Filter the solution, rejecting the first 10 mL of the filtrate.

  Chromatographic system (see *Chromatography* ⟨621⟩)—The chromatograph is equipped with a 254-nm detector and a 4-mm × 30-cm column that contains packing L1. The flow rate is about 2 mL per minute. Chromatograph five replicate injections of the *Standard preparation* and record the peak responses as directed under *Procedure:* the relative standard deviation is not more than 2.0%.
  Procedure—Separately inject equal volumes (about 10 µL) of the *Standard preparation* and the *Assay preparation* into the chromatograph by means of a suitable microsyringe or sampling valve, adjusting the specimen size and other operating parameters such that the peak obtained from the *Standard preparation* is about 0.6 full-scale. Record the chromatograms, and measure the responses for the major peaks. Calculate the quantity, in mg per g, of $C_{21}H_{30}O_5$ in the Ophthalmic Ointment taken by the formula:

$$(100C/W)(r_U / r_S)$$

in which *C* is the concentration, in mg per mL, of USP Hydrocortisone RS in the *Standard preparation;* *W* is the weight, in g, of the portion of Ophthalmic Ointment taken; and r_U and r_S are the peak responses obtained from the *Assay preparation* and the *Standard preparation,* respectively.

Neomycin and Polymyxin B Sulfates, Bacitracin Zinc, and Hydrocortisone Acetate Ophthalmic Ointment

» Neomycin and Polymyxin B Sulfates, Bacitracin Zinc, and Hydrocortisone Acetate Ophthalmic Ointment is a sterile ointment containing Neomycin Sulfate, Polymyxin B Sulfate, Bacitracin Zinc, and Hydrocortisone Acetate. It contains the equivalent of not less than 90.0 percent and not more than 140.0 percent of the labeled amounts of neomycin, polymyxin B, and bacitracin, and not less than 90.0 percent and not more than 110.0 percent of the labeled amount of hydrocortisone acetate.

Packaging and storage—Preserve in collapsible ophthalmic ointment tubes.
USP Reference standards ⟨11⟩—*USP Bacitracin Zinc RS. USP Hydrocortisone Acetate RS. USP Neomycin Sulfate RS. USP Polymyxin B Sulfate RS.*
Identification—
  A: It meets the requirements under *Thin-Layer Chromatographic Identification Test* ⟨201BNP⟩.
  B: The retention time of the major peak for hydrocortisone acetate in the chromatogram of the *Assay preparation* corresponds to that in the chromatogram of the *Standard preparation,* as obtained in the *Assay for hydrocortisone acetate.*
Sterility ⟨71⟩—It meets the requirements when tested as directed for *Membrane Filtration* under *Test for Sterility of the Product to be Examined.*
Minimum fill ⟨755⟩: meets the requirements.
Water, *Method I* ⟨921⟩: not more than 0.5%, 20 mL of a mixture of toluene and methanol (7 : 3) being used in place of methanol in the titration vessel.
Metal particles—It meets the requirements of the test for *Metal Particles in Ophthalmic Ointments* ⟨751⟩.
Assay for neomycin, Assay for polymyxin B, and Assay for bacitracin—Proceed with Ophthalmic Ointment as directed in the *Assay for neomycin,* in the *Assay for polymyxin B,* and in the *Assay for bacitracin* under *Neomycin and Polymyxin B Sulfates and Bacitracin Zinc Ophthalmic Ointment.*
Assay for hydrocortisone acetate—Proceed with Ophthalmic Ointment as directed in the *Assay* under *Hydrocortisone Acetate Lotion.*

Neomycin and Polymyxin B Sulfates, Bacitracin Zinc, and Lidocaine Ointment

» Neomycin and Polymyxin B Sulfates, Bacitracin Zinc, and Lidocaine Ointment contains the equivalent of not less than 90.0 percent and not more than 130.0 percent of the labeled amounts of neomycin, polymyxin B, and bacitracin, and not less than 90.0 percent and not more than 110.0 percent of the labeled amount of lidocaine ($C_{14}H_{22}N_2O$).

Packaging and storage—Preserve in well-closed containers, preferably at controlled room temperature.

USP Reference standards ⟨11⟩—*USP Bacitracin Zinc RS. USP Lidocaine RS. USP Neomycin Sulfate RS. USP Polymyxin B Sulfate RS.*

Identification—
A: It meets the requirements under *Thin-Layer Chromatographic Identification Test* ⟨201BNP⟩.
B: The retention time of the major peak for lidocaine in the chromatogram of the *Assay preparation* corresponds to that in the chromatogram of the *Standard preparation*, as obtained in the *Assay for lidocaine*.

Minimum fill ⟨755⟩: meets the requirements.

Water, *Method I* ⟨921⟩: not more than 0.5%, 20 mL of a mixture of toluene and methanol (7 : 3) being used in place of methanol in the titration vessel.

Assay for neomycin—Proceed with Ointment as directed in the *Assay for neomycin* under *Neomycin and Polymyxin B Sulfates and Bacitracin Zinc Ophthalmic Ointment*.

Assay for polymyxin B—Proceed with Ointment as directed in the *Assay for polymyxin B* under *Neomycin and Polymyxin B Sulfates and Bacitracin Zinc Ophthalmic Ointment*.

Assay for bacitracin—Proceed with Ointment as directed in the *Assay for bacitracin* under *Neomycin and Polymyxin B Sulfates and Bacitracin Zinc Ophthalmic Ointment*.

Assay for lidocaine—
Mobile phase, Standard preparation, and *Chromatographic system*—Proceed as directed in the *Assay for lidocaine* under *Neomycin and Polymyxin B Sulfates, Bacitracin, and Lidocaine Ointment*.

Assay preparation—Using the Ointment, proceed as directed for *Assay preparation* in the *Assay for lidocaine* under *Neomycin and Polymyxin B Sulfates, Bacitracin, and Lidocaine Ointment*.

Procedure—Proceed as directed for *Procedure* in the *Assay for lidocaine* under *Neomycin and Polymyxin B Sulfates, Bacitracin, and Lidocaine Ointment*. Calculate the quantity, in mg, of lidocaine ($C_{14}H_{22}N_2O$) in the portion of Ointment taken by the formula:

$$100C(r_U / r_S)$$

in which C is the concentration, in mg per mL, of USP Lidocaine RS in the *Standard preparation*; and r_U and r_S are the lidocaine peak responses obtained from the *Assay preparation* and the *Standard preparation*, respectively.

Neomycin and Polymyxin B Sulfates and Dexamethasone Ophthalmic Ointment

» Neomycin and Polymyxin B Sulfates and Dexamethasone Ophthalmic Ointment contains the equivalent of not less than 90.0 percent and not more than 130.0 percent of the labeled amounts of neomycin and polymyxin B, and not less than 90.0 percent and not more than 110.0 percent of the labeled amount of dexamethasone.

Packaging and storage—Preserve in collapsible ophthalmic ointment tubes.

USP Reference standards ⟨11⟩—*USP Dexamethasone RS. USP Neomycin Sulfate RS. USP Polymyxin B Sulfate RS.*

Identification—
A: It meets the requirements under *Thin-Layer Chromatographic Identification Test* ⟨201BNP⟩.
B: The retention time of the major peak for dexamethasone in the chromatogram of the *Assay preparation* corresponds to that in the chromatogram of the *Standard preparation*, as obtained in the *Assay for dexamethasone*.

Sterility ⟨71⟩—It meets the requirements when tested as directed for *Membrane Filtration* under *Test for Sterility of the Product to be Examined*.

Minimum fill ⟨755⟩: meets the requirements.

Water, *Method Ib* ⟨921⟩: not more than 0.5%, 20 mL of a mixture of toluene and methanol (7 : 3) being used in place of methanol in the titration vessel.

Metal particles—It meets the requirements of the test for *Metal Particles in Ophthalmic Ointments* ⟨751⟩.

Assay for neomycin and Assay for polymyxin B—Proceed with Ophthalmic Ointment as directed in the *Assay for neomycin* and in the *Assay for polymyxin B* under *Neomycin and Polymyxin B Sulfates and Bacitracin Zinc Ophthalmic Ointment*.

Assay for dexamethasone—
Mobile phase—Prepare a suitable aqueous solution of acetonitrile, approximately 1 in 3, such that the retention time of dexamethasone is about 5 minutes.

Standard preparation—Dissolve an accurately weighed quantity of USP Dexamethasone RS in a mixture of acetonitrile and methanol (1 : 1) to obtain a solution having a known concentration of about 60 μg per mL.

Assay preparation—Transfer an accurately weighed portion of Ophthalmic Ointment, equivalent to about 3 mg of dexamethasone, to a suitable test tube, add about 15 mL of cyclohexane, and heat in a water bath at 75 ± 5° for 10 minutes. [NOTE—If the ointment is not fully dissolved, heat on a steam bath for about 30 seconds, place a cap on the test tube, and place on a vortex mixer until all solid material is dissolved.] Filter with suction through a medium-porosity sintered-glass filter. Rinse the test tube twice with 10-mL portions of cyclohexane, filtering the rinsings through the filter, and discard the filtrates. Wash the filter with about 10 mL of a mixture of acetonitrile and methanol (1 : 1), and collect the filtrate in a 50-mL beaker. Wash the test tube and the filter with several 10-mL portions of the same solvent, and combine the washings in the 50-mL beaker. Transfer the contents of the beaker to a 50-mL volumetric flask, with the aid of a mixture of acetonitrile and methanol (1 : 1), dilute with the same solvent to volume, and mix.

Chromatographic system (see *Chromatography* ⟨621⟩)—The liquid chromatograph is equipped with a 254-nm detector and a 4.6-mm × 25-cm column that contains 5- to 10-μm packing L1. The flow rate is about 2 mL per minute. Chromatograph the *Standard preparation*, and record the peak response as directed under *Procedure*: the column efficiency is not less than 4000 theoretical plates, and the relative standard deviation for replicate injections is not more than 1.5%.

Procedure—Separately inject equal volumes (about 10 μL) of the *Standard preparation* and the *Assay preparation* into the chromatograph, record the chromatograms, and measure the responses for the major peaks. Calculate the quantity, in mg, of $C_{22}H_{29}FO_5$ in the portion of Ophthalmic Ointment taken by the formula:

$$50C(r_U / r_S)$$

in which C is the concentration, in μg per mL, of USP Dexamethasone RS in the *Standard preparation*; and r_U and r_S are the peak responses of the *Assay preparation* and the *Standard preparation*, respectively.

Neomycin and Polymyxin B Sulfates and Dexamethasone Ophthalmic Suspension

» Neomycin and Polymyxin B Sulfates and Dexamethasone Ophthalmic Suspension contains the equivalent of not less than 90.0 percent and not more than 130.0 percent of the labeled amounts of neomycin and polymyxin B, and not less than 90.0 percent and not more than 110.0 percent of the labeled amount of dexamethasone. It may contain one or more suitable buffers, stabilizers, preservatives, and suspending agents.

Packaging and storage—Preserve in tight, light-resistant containers in a cool place or at controlled room temperature. The containers or individual cartons are sealed and tamper-proof so that sterility is assured at time of first use.

USP Reference standards ⟨11⟩—*USP Dexamethasone RS. USP Neomycin Sulfate RS. USP Polymyxin B Sulfate RS.*

Identification—Transfer a quantity of Ophthalmic Suspension, equivalent to about 2.5 mg of dexamethasone, to a suitable test tube, add 5 mL of chloroform, mix, and centrifuge. Apply 25 µL of the lower chloroform layer and 25 µL of a Standard solution of USP Dexamethasone RS in chloroform containing 500 µg per mL to a suitable thin-layer chromatographic plate (see *Chromatography* ⟨621⟩) coated with a 0.25-mm layer of chromatographic silica gel. Allow the spots to dry, and develop the chromatogram in a solvent system consisting of a mixture of chloroform and diethylamine (2 : 1) until the solvent front has moved about three-fourths of the length of the plate. Remove the plate from the developing chamber, mark the solvent front, and allow the solvent to evaporate. Locate the spots on the plate by examination under short-wavelength UV light: the R_F value of the principal spot obtained from the test solution corresponds to that obtained from the Standard solution.

Sterility ⟨71⟩—It meets the requirements when tested as directed for *Membrane Filtration* under *Test for Sterility of the Product to be Examined.*

pH ⟨791⟩: between 3.5 and 6.0.

Assay for neomycin—Proceed as directed for neomycin under *Antibiotics—Microbial Assays* ⟨81⟩, using an accurately measured volume of Ophthalmic Suspension, freshly mixed and free from air bubbles, diluted quantitatively and stepwise with *Buffer No. 3* to yield a *Test Dilution* having a concentration assumed to be equal to the median dose level of the Standard.

Assay for polymyxin B—Proceed as directed for polymyxin B under *Antibiotics—Microbial Assays* ⟨81⟩, using an accurately measured volume of Ophthalmic Suspension, freshly mixed and free from air bubbles, diluted quantitatively and stepwise with *Buffer No. 6* to yield a *Test Dilution* having a concentration assumed to be equal to the median dose level of the Standard. Add to each test dilution of the Standard a quantity of USP Neomycin Sulfate RS, dissolved in *Buffer No. 6*, to obtain the same concentration of neomycin as is present in the *Test Dilution.*

Assay for dexamethasone—

Mobile phase and *Chromatographic system*—Proceed as directed in the *Assay for dexamethasone* under *Neomycin and Polymyxin B Sulfates and Dexamethasone Ophthalmic Ointment.*

Standard preparation—Dissolve an accurately weighed quantity of USP Dexamethasone RS in *Mobile phase* to obtain a solution having a known concentration of about 0.12 mg per mL.

Assay preparation—Dilute an accurately measured volume of freshly mixed Ophthalmic Suspension quantitatively with *Mobile phase* to obtain a solution containing about 0.12 mg of dexamethasone per mL.

Procedure—Proceed as directed for *Procedure* in the *Assay for dexamethasone* under *Neomycin and Polymyxin B Sulfates and Dexamethasone Ophthalmic Ointment*. Calculate the quantity, in mg per mL, of $C_{22}H_{29}FO_5$ in the Ophthalmic Suspension taken by the formula:

$$(CL/D)(r_U/r_S)$$

in which L is the labeled quantity, in mg per mL, of dexamethasone in the Ophthalmic Suspension, D is the concentration, in mg per mL, of dexamethasone in the *Assay preparation* based on the labeled quantity in the Ophthalmic Suspension and the extent of dilution, and the other terms are as defined therein.

Neomycin and Polymyxin B Sulfates and Gramicidin Cream

» Neomycin and Polymyxin B Sulfates and Gramicidin Cream contains the equivalent of not less than 90.0 percent and not more than 130.0 percent of the labeled amounts of neomycin, polymyxin B, and gramicidin.

Packaging and storage—Preserve in collapsible tubes or in well-closed containers.

USP Reference standards ⟨11⟩—*USP Gramicidin RS. USP Neomycin Sulfate RS. USP Polymyxin B Sulfate RS.*

Minimum fill ⟨755⟩: meets the requirements.

Assay for neomycin and Assay for polymyxin B—Proceed with Cream as directed in the *Assay for neomycin* and in the *Assay for polymyxin B* under *Neomycin and Polymyxin B Sulfates and Bacitracin Zinc Ophthalmic Ointment.*

Assay for gramicidin—Proceed with Cream as directed in the *Assay for gramicidin* under *Neomycin Sulfate and Gramicidin Ointment.*

Neomycin and Polymyxin B Sulfates and Gramicidin Ophthalmic Solution

» Neomycin and Polymyxin B Sulfates and Gramicidin Ophthalmic Solution is a sterile, isotonic aqueous solution of Neomycin Sulfate, Polymyxin B Sulfate, and Gramicidin. It contains the equivalent of not less than 90.0 percent and not more than 130.0 percent of the labeled amounts of neomycin, polymyxin B, and gramicidin.

Packaging and storage—Preserve in tight containers. The containers or individual cartons are sealed and tamper-proof so that sterility is assured at time of first use.

USP Reference standards ⟨11⟩—*USP Gramicidin RS. USP Neomycin Sulfate RS. USP Polymyxin B Sulfate RS.*

Thin-layer chromatographic identification test ⟨201BNP⟩: meets the requirements.

Sterility ⟨71⟩—It meets the requirements when tested as directed for *Membrane Filtration* under *Test for Sterility of the Product to be Examined.*

pH ⟨791⟩: between 4.7 and 6.0.

Assay for neomycin—Proceed as directed for neomycin under *Antibiotics—Microbial Assays* ⟨81⟩, using an accurately measured volume of Ophthalmic Solution diluted quantitatively and stepwise with *Buffer No. 3* to yield a *Test Dilution* having a concentration assumed to be equal to the median dose level of the Standard.

Assay for polymyxin B—Proceed as directed for polymyxin B under *Antibiotics—Microbial Assays* ⟨81⟩, using an accurately measured volume of Ophthalmic Solution diluted quantitatively and stepwise with *Buffer No. 6* to yield a *Test Dilution* having a concentration assumed to be equal to the median dose level of the Standard. Add to each test dilution of the Standard a quantity of USP

Neomycin Sulfate RS, dissolved in *Buffer No. 6*, to obtain the same concentration of neomycin as is present in the *Test Dilution*.
Assay for gramicidin—Proceed as directed for gramicidin under *Antibiotics—Microbial Assays* ⟨81⟩, using an accurately measured volume of Ophthalmic Solution diluted quantitatively and stepwise with alcohol to yield a *Test Dilution* having a concentration assumed to be equal to the median dose level of the Standard.

Neomycin and Polymyxin B Sulfates, Gramicidin, and Hydrocortisone Acetate Cream

» Neomycin and Polymyxin B Sulfates, Gramicidin, and Hydrocortisone Acetate Cream contains the equivalent of not less than 90.0 percent and not more than 130.0 percent of the labeled amounts of neomycin, polymyxin B, and gramicidin, and not less than 90.0 percent and not more than 110.0 percent of the labeled amount of hydrocortisone acetate ($C_{23}H_{32}O_6$).

Packaging and storage—Preserve in well-closed containers.
USP Reference standards ⟨11⟩—*USP Gramicidin RS. USP Hydrocortisone Acetate RS. USP Neomycin Sulfate RS. USP Polymyxin B Sulfate RS.*
Minimum fill ⟨755⟩: meets the requirements.
Assay for neomycin and Assay for polymyxin B—Proceed with Cream as directed in the *Assay for neomycin* and in the *Assay for polymyxin B* under *Neomycin and Polymyxin B Sulfates and Bacitracin Zinc Ophthalmic Ointment*.
Assay for gramicidin—Proceed with Cream as directed in the *Assay for gramicidin* under *Neomycin Sulfate and Gramicidin Ointment*.
Assay for hydrocortisone acetate—Proceed with Cream as directed in the *Assay* under *Hydrocortisone Acetate Lotion*.

Neomycin and Polymyxin B Sulfates and Hydrocortisone Otic Solution

» Neomycin and Polymyxin B Sulfates and Hydrocortisone Otic Solution is a sterile solution containing the equivalent of not less than 90.0 percent and not more than 130.0 percent of the labeled amounts of neomycin and polymyxin B. It contains not less than 90.0 percent and not more than 110.0 percent of the labeled amount of hydrocortisone. It may contain one or more suitable buffers, dispersants, and solvents.

Packaging and storage—Preserve in tight, light-resistant containers. The containers or individual cartons are sealed and tamper-proof so that sterility is assured at time of first use.
USP Reference standards ⟨11⟩—*USP Hydrocortisone RS. USP Neomycin Sulfate RS. USP Polymyxin B Sulfate RS.*
Sterility ⟨71⟩: meets the requirements.
pH ⟨791⟩: between 2.0 and 4.5.
Assay for neomycin—Proceed as directed under *Antibiotics—Microbial Assays* ⟨81⟩, using an accurately measured volume of Otic Solution diluted quantitatively and stepwise with *Buffer No. 3* to yield a *Test Dilution* having a concentration assumed to be equal to the median dose level of the Standard (1.0 µg of neomycin per mL).
Assay for polymyxin B—Proceed as directed under *Antibiotics—Microbial Assays* ⟨81⟩, using an accurately measured volume of Otic Solution diluted quantitatively and stepwise with *Buffer No. 6* to yield a *Test Dilution* having a concentration assumed to be equal to the median dose level of the Standard (10 Polymyxin B Units per mL). Add to each test dilution of the Standard a quantity of Neomycin Standard, dissolved in *Buffer No. 6*, to obtain the same concentration of neomycin present in the *Test Dilution*.
Assay for hydrocortisone—
Mobile phase, Standard preparation, and *Chromatographic system*—Prepare as directed in the *Assay for hydrocortisone* under *Neomycin and Polymyxin B Sulfates, Bacitracin Zinc and Hydrocortisone Ophthalmic Ointment*.
Assay preparation—Transfer 3.0 mL of Otic Solution to a 200-mL volumetric flask, dilute with a mixture of methanol and water (1:1) to volume, and mix.
Procedure—Proceed as directed for *Procedure* in the *Assay for hydrocortisone* under *Neomycin and Polymyxin B Sulfates, Bacitracin Zinc and Hydrocortisone Ophthalmic Ointment*. Calculate the quantity, in mg, of $C_{21}H_{30}O_5$ in each mL of the Otic Solution taken by the formula:

$$(66.67C)(r_U / r_S)$$

in which C is the concentration, in mg per mL, of USP Hydrocortisone RS in the *Standard preparation,* and r_U and r_S are the peak responses obtained from the *Assay preparation* and the *Standard preparation,* respectively.

Neomycin and Polymyxin B Sulfates and Hydrocortisone Ophthalmic Suspension

» Neomycin and Polymyxin B Sulfates and Hydrocortisone Ophthalmic Suspension is a sterile, aqueous suspension containing the equivalent of not less than 90.0 percent and not more than 130.0 percent of the labeled amounts of neomycin and of polymyxin B. It contains not less than 90.0 percent and not more than 110.0 percent of the labeled amount of hydrocortisone.

Packaging and storage—Preserve in tight containers. The containers or individual cartons are sealed and tamper-proof so that sterility is assured at time of first use.
USP Reference standards ⟨11⟩—*USP Hydrocortisone RS. USP Neomycin Sulfate RS. USP Polymyxin B Sulfate RS.*
Thin-layer chromatographic identification test ⟨201BNP⟩: meets the requirements.
Sterility ⟨71⟩: meets the requirements.
pH ⟨791⟩: between 4.1 and 7.0.
Assay for neomycin—Proceed as directed for neomycin under *Antibiotics—Microbial Assays* ⟨81⟩, using an accurately measured volume of Ophthalmic Suspension, freshly mixed and free from air bubbles, diluted quantitatively and stepwise with *Buffer No. 3* to yield a *Test Dilution* having a concentration assumed to be equal to the median dose level of the Standard.
Assay for polymyxin B—Proceed as directed for polymyxin B under *Antibiotics—Microbial Assays* ⟨81⟩, using an accurately measured volume of Ophthalmic Suspension, freshly mixed and free from air bubbles, diluted quantitatively and stepwise with *Buffer No. 6* to yield a *Test Dilution* having a concentration assumed to be equal to the median dose level of the Standard. Add to each test dilution of the Standard a quantity of Neomycin Sulfate RS, dissolved in *Buffer No. 6*, to yield the same concentration of neomycin as is present in the *Test Dilution*.
Assay for hydrocortisone—
Mobile phase, Standard preparation, and *Chromatographic system*—Prepare as directed in the *Assay for hydrocortisone* under *Neomycin and Polymyxin B Sulfates, Bacitracin Zinc and Hydrocortisone Ophthalmic Ointment*.
Assay preparation—Transfer an accurately measured volume of Ophthalmic Suspension, freshly mixed and free from air bubbles,

equivalent to about 30 mg of hydrocortisone, to a 200-mL volumetric flask, dilute with a mixture of methanol and water (1:1) to volume, and mix. Filter the solution, rejecting the first 10 mL of the filtrate.

Procedure—Proceed as directed for *Procedure* in the *Assay for hydrocortisone* under *Neomycin and Polymyxin B Sulfates, Bacitracin Zinc and Hydrocortisone Ophthalmic Ointment*. Calculate the quantity, in mg, of $C_{21}H_{30}O_5$ in each mL of the Ophthalmic Suspension taken by the formula:

$$200(C/V)(r_U/r_S)$$

in which C is the concentration, in mg per mL, of USP Hydrocortisone RS in the *Standard preparation*; V is the volume, in mL, of Ophthalmic Suspension taken; and r_U and r_S are the peak responses obtained from the *Assay preparation* and the *Standard preparation*, respectively.

Neomycin and Polymyxin B Sulfates and Hydrocortisone Otic Suspension

» Neomycin and Polymyxin B Sulfates and Hydrocortisone Otic Suspension is a sterile suspension containing the equivalent of not less than 90.0 percent and not more than 130.0 percent of the labeled amounts of neomycin and of polymyxin B. It contains not less than 90.0 percent and not more than 110.0 percent of the labeled amount of hydrocortisone. It may contain one or more suitable buffers, dispersants, and preservatives.

Packaging and storage—Preserve in tight, light-resistant containers. The containers or individual cartons are sealed and tamper-proof so that sterility is assured at time of first use.

USP Reference standards ⟨11⟩—*USP Hydrocortisone RS. USP Neomycin Sulfate RS. USP Polymyxin B Sulfate RS.*

Thin-layer chromatographic identification test ⟨201BNP⟩: meets the requirements.

Sterility ⟨71⟩: meets the requirements.

pH ⟨791⟩: between 3.0 and 7.0.

Assay for neomycin and Assay for polymyxin B—Using an accurately measured volume of Otic Suspension, freshly mixed and free from air bubbles, proceed as directed in the *Assay for neomycin* and the *Assay for polymyxin B* under *Neomycin and Polymyxin B Sulfates and Hydrocortisone Otic Solution*.

Assay for hydrocortisone—

Mobile phase, Standard preparation, and *Chromatographic system*—Prepare as directed in the *Assay for hydrocortisone* under *Neomycin and Polymyxin B Sulfates, Bacitracin Zinc and Hydrocortisone Ophthalmic Ointment*.

Assay preparation—Transfer 3.0 mL of Otic Suspension, freshly mixed and free from air bubbles, to a 200-mL volumetric flask, dilute with a mixture of methanol and water (1 : 1) to volume, and mix. Filter the solution, rejecting the first 10 mL of the filtrate.

Procedure—Proceed as directed for *Procedure* in the *Assay for hydrocortisone* under *Neomycin and Polymyxin B Sulfates, Bacitracin Zinc and Hydrocortisone Ophthalmic Ointment*. Calculate the quantity, in mg, of $C_{21}H_{30}O_5$ in each mL of the Otic Suspension taken by the formula:

$$(66.67C)(r_U/r_S)$$

in which C is the concentration, in mg per mL, of USP Hydrocortisone RS in the *Standard preparation*; and r_U and r_S are the peak responses obtained from the *Assay preparation* and the *Standard preparation*, respectively.

Neomycin and Polymyxin B Sulfates and Hydrocortisone Acetate Cream

» Neomycin and Polymyxin B Sulfates and Hydrocortisone Acetate Cream contains the equivalent of not less than 90.0 percent and not more than 130.0 percent of the labeled amounts of neomycin and polymyxin B, and not less than 90.0 percent and not more than 110.0 percent of the labeled amount of hydrocortisone acetate ($C_{23}H_{32}O_6$).

Packaging and storage—Preserve in well-closed containers.

USP Reference standards ⟨11⟩—*USP Hydrocortisone Acetate RS. USP Neomycin Sulfate RS. USP Polymyxin B Sulfate RS.*

Identification—

A: It meets the requirements under *Thin-Layer Chromatographic Identification Test* ⟨201BNP⟩.

B: The retention time of the major peak for hydrocortisone acetate in the chromatogram of the *Assay preparation* corresponds to that in the chromatogram of the *Standard preparation*, as obtained in the *Assay for hydrocortisone acetate*.

Minimum fill ⟨755⟩: meets the requirements.

Assay for neomycin and Assay for polymyxin B—Proceed with Cream as directed in the *Assay for neomycin* and in the *Assay for polymyxin B* under *Neomycin and Polymyxin B Sulfates Cream*.

Assay for hydrocortisone acetate—Proceed with Cream as directed in the *Assay* under *Hydrocortisone Acetate Lotion*.

Neomycin and Polymyxin B Sulfates and Hydrocortisone Acetate Ophthalmic Suspension

» Neomycin and Polymyxin B Sulfates and Hydrocortisone Acetate Ophthalmic Suspension is a sterile suspension of Hydrocortisone Acetate in an aqueous solution of Neomycin Sulfate and Polymyxin B Sulfate. It contains the equivalent of not less than 90.0 percent and not more than 125.0 percent of the labeled amounts of neomycin and polymyxin B, and not less than 90.0 percent and not more than 110.0 percent of the labeled amount of hydrocortisone acetate ($C_{23}H_{32}O_6$). It may contain suitable buffers, preservatives, and suspending agents.

Packaging and storage—Preserve in tight containers. The containers or individual cartons are sealed and tamper-proof so that sterility is assured at time of first use.

USP Reference standards ⟨11⟩—*USP Hydrocortisone Acetate RS. USP Neomycin Sulfate RS. USP Polymyxin B Sulfate RS.*

Sterility ⟨71⟩—It meets the requirements when tested as directed for *Membrane Filtration* under *Test for Sterility of the Product to be Examined*.

pH ⟨791⟩: between 5.0 and 7.0.

Assay for neomycin and Assay for polymyxin B—Proceed with Ophthalmic Suspension as directed in the *Assay for neomycin* and in the *Assay for polymyxin B* under *Neomycin and Polymyxin B Sulfates and Bacitracin Zinc Ophthalmic Ointment*.

Assay for hydrocortisone acetate—Proceed with Ophthalmic Suspension as directed in the *Assay* under *Hydrocortisone Acetate Injectable Suspension*.

Neomycin and Polymyxin B Sulfates and Lidocaine Cream

» Neomycin and Polymyxin B Sulfates and Lidocaine Cream contains the equivalent of not less than 90.0 percent and not more than 130.0 percent of the labeled amounts of neomycin and polymyxin B, and not less than 90.0 percent and not more than 110.0 percent of the labeled amount of lidocaine ($C_{14}H_{22}N_2O$).

Packaging and storage—Preserve in well-closed containers, preferably at controlled room temperature.
USP Reference standards ⟨11⟩—*USP Lidocaine RS. USP Neomycin Sulfate RS. USP Polymyxin B Sulfate RS.*
Identification—
  A: It meets the requirements under *Thin-Layer Chromatographic Identification Test* ⟨201BNP⟩.
  B: The retention time of the major peak for lidocaine in the chromatogram of the *Assay preparation* corresponds to that in the chromatogram of the *Standard preparation*, as obtained in the *Assay for lidocaine*.
Minimum fill ⟨755⟩: meets the requirements.
Assay for neomycin—Proceed with Cream as directed in the *Assay for neomycin* under *Neomycin and Polymyxin B Sulfates Cream.*
Assay for polymyxin B—Proceed with Cream as directed in the *Assay for polymyxin B* under *Neomycin and Polymyxin B Sulfates Cream.*
Assay for lidocaine—
  Mobile phase, Standard preparation, and *Chromatographic system*—Proceed as directed in the *Assay for lidocaine* under *Neomycin and Polymyxin B Sulfates, Bacitracin, and Lidocaine Ointment.*
  Assay preparation—Using Cream, proceed as directed for the *Assay preparation* in the *Assay for lidocaine* under *Neomycin and Polymyxin B Sulfates, Bacitracin, and Lidocaine Ointment.*
  Procedure—Proceed as directed for *Procedure* in the *Assay for lidocaine* under *Neomycin and Polymyxin B Sulfates, Bacitracin, and Lidocaine Ointment*. Calculate the quantity, in mg, of lidocaine ($C_{14}H_{22}N_2O$) in the portion of Cream taken by the formula:

$$100C(r_U / r_S)$$

in which C is the concentration, in mg per mL, of USP Lidocaine RS in the *Standard preparation*; and r_U and r_S are the lidocaine peak responses obtained from the *Assay preparation* and the *Standard preparation*, respectively.

Neomycin and Polymyxin B Sulfates and Pramoxine Hydrochloride Cream

» Neomycin and Polymyxin B Sulfates and Pramoxine Hydrochloride Cream contains the equivalent of not less than 90.0 percent and not more than 130.0 percent of the labeled amounts of neomycin and polymyxin B, and not less than 90.0 percent and not more than 110.0 percent of the labeled amount of pramoxine hydrochloride ($C_{17}H_{27}NO_3 \cdot HCl$).

Packaging and storage—Preserve in well-closed containers, preferably at controlled room temperature.
USP Reference standards ⟨11⟩—*USP Neomycin Sulfate RS. USP Polymyxin B Sulfate RS. USP Pramoxine Hydrochloride RS.*
Identification—
  A: *Thin-Layer Chromatographic Identification Test* ⟨201⟩—
  Test solution—Disperse a quantity of Cream, equivalent to about 25 mg of neomycin, with 20 mL of chloroform in a 60-mL separator. Add 0.2 mL of 2.5 N hydrochloric acid, and shake. Allow the layers to separate for about 30 minutes. Discard the lower chloroform layer, and centrifuge the upper aqueous layer. Use a portion of the centrifuged aqueous layer.
  Standard solution—Dissolve suitable quantities of USP Neomycin Sulfate RS and USP Polymyxin B Sulfate RS in 0.1 N hydrochloric acid to obtain a solution containing the equivalent of about 3.5 mg of neomycin and 10,000 USP Polymyxin B Units per mL.
  Developing solvent system—Dissolve 0.1 g of benzalkonium chloride in a mixture of isopropyl alcohol, water, and ammonium hydroxide (60 : 40 : 10).
  Procedure—Proceed as directed in the chapter. Place the plate in a chromatographic chamber saturated with *Developing solvent system*, and develop the chromatogram. Dry the plate at 105° for about 10 minutes, spray with a solution of ninhydrin in butyl alcohol (1 in 200), and heat the plate at 105° for about 15 minutes. The R_F values of the two principal spots in the chromatogram obtained from the *Test solution* correspond to those of the two principal spots in the chromatogram obtained from the *Standard solution*.
  B: The retention time of the major peak in the chromatogram of the *Assay preparation* corresponds to that in the chromatogram of the *Standard preparation*, as obtained in the *Assay for pramoxine hydrochloride*.
pH ⟨791⟩—Transfer 1 g of Cream to a small beaker, add 10 mL of carbon dioxide-free water, and mix: the pH is between 3.3 and 6.0.
Assay for neomycin—Proceed as directed for neomycin under *Antibiotics—Microbial Assays* ⟨81⟩, using an accurately weighed portion of Cream, equivalent to about 3.5 mg of neomycin, blended for 3 to 5 minutes in a high-speed blender with 249 mL of *Buffer No. 3* and 1 mL of polysorbate 80. Quantitatively dilute an accurately measured volume of this solution with *Buffer No. 3* to obtain a *Test Dilution* having a concentration of neomycin assumed to be equal to the median level of the Standard (1 µg of neomycin per mL).
Assay for polymyxin—Proceed as directed for polymyxin B under *Antibiotics—Microbial Assays* ⟨81⟩, using an accurately weighed portion of Cream, equivalent to about 10,000 USP Polymyxin B Units, blended for 3 to 5 minutes in a high-speed blender with 199 mL of *Buffer No. 6* and 1 mL of polysorbate 80. Quantitatively dilute an accurately measured volume of this solution with *Buffer No. 6* to obtain a *Test Dilution* having a concentration of polymyxin B assumed to be equal to the median dose level of the Standard (10 USP Polymyxin B Units per mL).
Assay for pramoxine hydrochloride—
  Mobile phase—Dissolve 3.5 g of dibasic potassium phosphate in 1000 mL of water. Prepare a mixture of this solution, acetonitrile, and triethylamine (700 : 300 : 2), and adjust with phosphoric acid to a pH of 4.0 ± 0.1. Filter and degas. Make adjustments if necessary (see *System Suitability* under *Chromatography* ⟨621⟩).
  Standard preparation—Prepare a solution of USP Pramoxine Hydrochloride RS in methanol to obtain a solution having a known concentration of about 0.2 mg per mL.
  Assay preparation—Transfer an accurately weighed portion of Cream, equivalent to about 10 mg of pramoxine hydrochloride, to a 50-mL volumetric flask, add about 5 mL of chloroform, and sonicate at about 40° to disperse the Cream. Allow to cool to room temperature, dilute with methanol to volume, and mix. Pass a portion of this solution through a glass fiber filter and a PTFE filter having a 0.45-µm porosity, discarding the first few mL of the filtrate.
  Chromatographic system (see *Chromatography* ⟨621⟩)—The liquid chromatograph is equipped with a 280-nm detector, a guard column that contains packing L7, and a 4.6-mm × 25-cm analytical column that contains packing L7. The column is maintained at a constant temperature of about 40°. The flow rate is about 2 mL per minute. Chromatograph the *Standard preparation*, and record the peak responses as directed for *Procedure*: the relative standard deviation for replicate injections is not more than 2.0%.
  Procedure—Separately inject equal volumes (about 20 µL) of the *Standard preparation* and the *Assay preparation* into the chromatograph, record the chromatograms, and measure the areas for the major peaks. Calculate the quantity, in mg, of pramoxine hydrochloride ($C_{17}H_{27}NO_3 \cdot HCl$) in each g of Cream taken by the formula:

$$50(C/W)(r_U / r_S)$$

in which C is the concentration, in mg per mL, of USP Pramoxine Hydrochloride RS in the *Standard preparation*; W is the weight, in g, of Cream taken to prepare the *Assay preparation;* and r_U and r_S are the peak areas for pramoxine obtained from the *Assay preparation* and the *Standard preparation,* respectively.

Neomycin and Polymyxin B Sulfates and Prednisolone Acetate Ophthalmic Suspension

» Neomycin and Polymyxin B Sulfates and Prednisolone Acetate Ophthalmic Suspension is a sterile suspension of Prednisolone Acetate in an aqueous solution of Neomycin Sulfate and Polymyxin B Sulfate. It contains the equivalent of not less than 90.0 percent and not more than 125.0 percent of the labeled amounts of neomycin and polymyxin B, and not less than 90.0 percent and not more than 110.0 percent of the labeled amount of prednisolone acetate ($C_{23}H_{30}O_6$). It may contain suitable buffers, preservatives, and suspending agents.

Packaging and storage—Preserve in tight containers. The containers or individual cartons are sealed and tamper-proof so that sterility is assured at time of first use.
USP Reference standards ⟨11⟩—*USP Neomycin Sulfate RS. USP Polymyxin B Sulfate RS. USP Prednisolone Acetate RS.*
Identification—The chromatogram of the *Assay preparation* obtained as directed in the *Assay for prednisolone acetate* exhibits a major peak for prednisolone acetate, the retention time of which corresponds to that exhibited in the chromatogram of the *Standard preparation* obtained as directed in the *Assay for prednisolone acetate.*
Sterility ⟨71⟩: meets the requirements.
pH ⟨791⟩: between 5.0 and 7.0.
Assay for neomycin—Proceed as directed for neomycin under *Antibiotics—Microbial Assays* ⟨81⟩, using an accurately measured volume of Ophthalmic Suspension, freshly mixed and free from air bubbles, diluted quantitatively and stepwise with *Buffer No. 3* to yield a *Test Dilution* having a concentration assumed to be equal to the median dose level of the Standard.
Assay for polymyxin B—Proceed as directed for polymyxin B under *Antibiotics—Microbial Assays* ⟨81⟩, using an accurately measured volume of Ophthalmic Suspension, freshly mixed and free from air bubbles, diluted quantitatively and stepwise with *Buffer No. 6* to yield a *Test Dilution* having a concentration assumed to be equal to the median dose level of the Standard. Add to each test dilution of the Standard a quantity of Neomycin Sulfate RS, dissolved in *Buffer No. 6,* to obtain the same concentration of neomycin as is present in the *Test Dilution.*
Assay for prednisolone acetate—
Mobile phase, Internal standard solution, Standard preparation, and *Chromatographic system*—Prepare as directed in the *Assay for prednisolone acetate* under *Neomycin Sulfate and Prednisolone Acetate Ophthalmic Suspension.*
Assay preparation—Transfer an accurately measured volume of Ophthalmic Suspension, freshly mixed and free from air bubbles, equivalent to about 2.5 mg of prednisolone acetate, to a suitable container, add 5.0 mL of *Internal standard solution* and about 100 mL of water-saturated chloroform, and shake by mechanical means for about 15 minutes. Allow to separate for about 15 minutes, and use the clear chloroform layer as the *Assay preparation.*
Procedure—Proceed as directed in the *Assay for prednisolone acetate* under *Neomycin Sulfate and Prednisolone Acetate Ophthalmic Suspension.* Calculate the quantity, in mg, of prednisolone acetate ($C_{23}H_{30}O_6$) in each mL of the Ophthalmic Suspension taken by the formula:

$$0.1(C/V)(R_U/R_S)$$

in which C is the concentration, in μg per mL, of USP Prednisolone Acetate RS in the *Standard preparation,* V is the volume, in mL, of Ophthalmic Suspension taken, and R_U and R_S are the peak response ratios of prednisolone acetate to betamethasone obtained from the *Assay preparation* and the *Standard preparation,* respectively.

Neomycin Sulfate and Prednisolone Acetate Ointment

» Neomycin Sulfate and Prednisolone Acetate Ointment contains the equivalent of not less than 90.0 percent and not more than 135.0 percent of the labeled amount of neomycin, and not less than 90.0 percent and not more than 110.0 percent of the labeled amount of prednisolone acetate ($C_{23}H_{30}O_6$).

Packaging and storage—Preserve in collapsible tubes or in tight containers, protected from light.
USP Reference standards ⟨11⟩—*USP Neomycin Sulfate RS. USP Prednisolone Acetate RS.*
Identification—
A: It meets the requirements for neomycin under *Thin-Layer Chromatographic Identification Test* ⟨201BNP⟩.
B: The retention time of the major peak for prednisolone acetate in the chromatogram of the *Assay preparation* corresponds to that of the *Standard preparation,* as obtained in the *Assay for prednisolone acetate.*
Minimum fill ⟨755⟩: meets the requirements.
Water, *Method I* ⟨921⟩: not more than 1.0%, 20 mL of a mixture of toluene and methanol (7 : 3) being used in place of methanol in the titration vessel.
Assay for neomycin—Proceed with Ointment as directed in the *Assay* under *Neomycin Sulfate Ointment.*
Assay for prednisolone acetate—
Mobile phase, Internal standard solution, Standard preparation, and *Chromatographic system*—Prepare as directed in the *Assay for prednisolone acetate* under *Neomycin Sulfate and Prednisolone Acetate Ophthalmic Suspension.*
Assay preparation—Transfer an accurately weighed portion of Ointment, equivalent to about 1 mg of prednisolone acetate, to a suitable container, add 2.0 mL of *Internal standard solution,* dilute with water-saturated chloroform to about 35 mL, and shake to dissolve the ointment. Transfer about 5 mL of this solution to a suitable container, and evaporate to dryness. Add about 5 mL of water-saturated chloroform, and sonicate for 5 minutes. Filter, and use the clear solution as the *Assay preparation.*
Procedure—Proceed as directed for *Procedure* in the *Assay for prednisolone acetate* under *Neomycin Sulfate and Prednisolone Acetate Ophthalmic Suspension.* Calculate the quantity, in mg, of prednisolone acetate ($C_{23}H_{30}O_6$) in the portion of Ointment taken by the formula:

$$0.04C(R_U/R_S)$$

in which C is the concentration, in μg per mL, of USP Prednisolone Acetate RS in the *Standard preparation,* and R_U and R_S are the peak response ratios of prednisolone acetate to betamethasone obtained from the *Assay preparation* and the *Standard preparation,* respectively.

Neomycin Sulfate and Prednisolone Acetate Ophthalmic Ointment

» Neomycin Sulfate and Prednisolone Acetate Ophthalmic Ointment is a sterile ointment containing Neomycin Sulfate and Prednisolone Acetate. It contains the equivalent of not less than 90.0 percent and not more than 135.0 percent of the labeled amount of neomycin, and not less than 90.0 percent and not more than 110.0 percent of the labeled amount of prednisolone acetate ($C_{23}H_{30}O_6$).

Packaging and storage—Preserve in collapsible ophthalmic ointment tubes.

USP Reference standards ⟨11⟩—*USP Neomycin Sulfate RS. USP Prednisolone Acetate RS.*

Identification—
  A: It meets the requirements for neomycin under *Thin-Layer Chromatographic Identification Test* ⟨201BNP⟩.
  B: The retention time of the major peak for prednisolone acetate in the chromatogram of the *Assay preparation* corresponds to that of the *Standard preparation*, as obtained in the *Assay for prednisolone acetate*.

Sterility ⟨71⟩—It meets the requirements when tested as directed for *Membrane Filtration* under *Test for Sterility of the Product to be Examined*.

Minimum fill ⟨755⟩: meets the requirements.

Water, *Method I* ⟨921⟩: not more than 1.0%, 20 mL of a mixture of toluene and methanol (7 : 3) being used in place of methanol in the titration vessel.

Metal particles—It meets the requirements of the test for *Metal Particles in Ophthalmic Ointments* ⟨751⟩.

Assay for neomycin—Proceed with Ophthalmic Ointment as directed in the *Assay* under *Neomycin Sulfate Ointment*.

Assay for prednisolone acetate—
  Mobile phase, Internal standard solution, Standard preparation, and *Chromatographic system*—Prepare as directed in the *Assay for prednisolone acetate* under *Neomycin Sulfate and Prednisolone Acetate Ophthalmic Suspension*.
  Assay preparation—Using Ophthalmic Ointment, proceed as directed for *Assay preparation* in the *Assay for prednisolone acetate* under *Neomycin Sulfate and Prednisolone Acetate Ointment*.
  Procedure—Proceed as directed for *Procedure* in the *Assay for prednisolone acetate* under *Neomycin Sulfate and Prednisolone Acetate Ophthalmic Suspension*. Calculate the quantity, in mg, of prednisolone acetate ($C_{23}H_{30}O_6$) in the portion of Ophthalmic Ointment taken by the formula:

$$0.04C(R_U / R_S)$$

in which C is the concentration, in μg per mL, of USP Prednisolone Acetate RS in the *Standard preparation*, and R_U and R_S are the peak response ratios of prednisolone acetate to betamethasone obtained from the *Assay preparation* and the *Standard preparation*, respectively.

Neomycin Sulfate and Prednisolone Acetate Ophthalmic Suspension

» Neomycin Sulfate and Prednisolone Acetate Ophthalmic Suspension contains the equivalent of not less than 90.0 percent and not more than 130.0 percent of the labeled amount of neomycin, and not less than 90.0 percent and not more than 110.0 percent of the labeled amount of prednisolone acetate ($C_{23}H_{30}O_6$).

Packaging and storage—Preserve in tight containers. The containers or individual cartons are sealed and tamper-proof so that sterility is assured at time of first use.

USP Reference standards ⟨11⟩—*USP Neomycin Sulfate RS. USP Prednisolone Acetate RS.*

Identification—
  A: Filter a portion of Ophthalmic Suspension, freshly mixed but free from air bubbles, equivalent to about 60 mg of prednisolone acetate, discarding the filtrate. Wash the filter with about 10 mL of water, and dry at 105° for 3 hours: the IR absorption spectrum of a potassium bromide dispersion of the dried residue on the filter so obtained exhibits maxima only at the same wavelengths as that of a similar preparation of USP Prednisolone Acetate RS.
  B: The chromatogram of the *Assay preparation* obtained as directed in the *Assay for prednisolone acetate* exhibits a major peak for prednisolone acetate, the retention time of which corresponds to that exhibited in the chromatogram of the *Standard preparation* obtained as directed in the *Assay for prednisolone acetate*.

Sterility ⟨71⟩—It meets the requirements when tested as directed for *Membrane Filtration* under *Test for Sterility of the Product to be Examined*.

pH ⟨791⟩: between 5.5 and 7.5.

Assay for neomycin—Proceed with Ophthalmic Suspension as directed in the *Assay for neomycin* under *Neomycin and Polymyxin B Sulfates and Prednisolone Acetate Ophthalmic Suspension*.

Assay for prednisolone acetate—
  Mobile phase—Prepare a solution containing *n*-butyl chloride, water-saturated *n*-butyl chloride, tetrahydrofuran, methanol, and glacial acetic acid (95:95:14:7:6).
  Internal standard solution—Prepare a solution of betamethasone in tetrahydrofuran containing 10 mg per mL. Dilute this solution with water-saturated chloroform, and mix to obtain a solution having a concentration of about 1 mg per mL.
  Standard preparation—Dissolve about 5 mg of USP Prednisolone Acetate RS, accurately weighed, in 10.0 mL of *Internal standard solution*. Use sonication, if necessary, dilute with water-saturated chloroform to 200.0 mL, and mix to obtain a solution having a known concentration of about 25 μg per mL.
  Assay preparation—Transfer an accurately measured volume of Ophthalmic Suspension, freshly mixed and free from air bubbles, equivalent to about 2.5 mg of prednisolone acetate, to a suitable container, add 5.0 mL of *Internal standard solution* and about 100 mL of water-saturated chloroform, and shake by mechanical means for about 15 minutes. Allow to separate for about 15 minutes, and use the clear chloroform layer as the *Assay preparation*.
  Chromatographic system (see *Chromatography* ⟨621⟩)—The liquid chromatograph is equipped with a 254-nm detector and a 4-mm × 30-cm column that contains packing L3. The flow rate is about 1 mL per minute. Chromatograph the *Standard preparation*, and record the peak responses as directed for *Procedure:* the resolution, R, between the analyte and internal standard peaks is not less than 3.0, and the relative standard deviation for replicate injections is not more than 2.0%.
  Procedure—Separately inject equal volumes (about 10 μL) of the *Standard preparation* and the *Assay preparation* into the chromatograph, record the chromatograms, and measure the responses for the major peaks. The relative retention times are about 1.6 for betamethasone and 1.0 for prednisolone acetate. Calculate the quantity, in mg, of prednisolone acetate ($C_{23}H_{30}O_6$) in each mL of the Ophthalmic Suspension taken by the formula:

$$0.1(C / V)(R_U / R_S)$$

in which C is the concentration, in μg per mL, of USP Prednisolone Acetate RS in the *Standard preparation*, V is the volume, in mL, of Ophthalmic Suspension taken, and R_U and R_S are the peak response ratios of prednisolone acetate to betamethasone obtained from the *Assay preparation* and the *Standard preparation*, respectively.

Neomycin Sulfate and Prednisolone Sodium Phosphate Ophthalmic Ointment

» Neomycin Sulfate and Prednisolone Sodium Phosphate Ophthalmic Ointment is a sterile ointment containing Neomycin Sulfate and Prednisolone Sodium Phosphate. It contains the equivalent of not less than 90.0 percent and not more than 135.0 percent of the labeled amount of neomycin, and the equivalent of not less than 90.0 percent and not more than 115.0 percent of the labeled amount of prednisolone phosphate ($C_{21}H_{29}O_8P$).

NOTE—Where Neomycin Sulfate and Prednisolone Sodium Phosphate Ophthalmic Ointment is prescribed without reference to the quantity of neomycin or prednisolone phosphate contained therein, a product containing 3.5 mg of neomycin and 2.5 mg of prednisolone phosphate per g shall be dispensed.

Packaging and storage—Preserve in collapsible ophthalmic ointment tubes.

USP Reference standards ⟨11⟩—*USP Neomycin Sulfate RS. USP Prednisolone RS.*
Identification—
   A: It responds to the *Identification* test under *Neomycin Sulfate Cream.*
   B: Shake a quantity of Ophthalmic Ointment, equivalent to about 40 mg of prednisolone phosphate, with 25 mL of sodium chloride solution (1 in 20) and 25 mL of methylene chloride, for 2 minutes. Transfer the methylene chloride layer to a second separator containing 15 mL of sodium chloride (1 in 20). Shake for 1 minute, and discard the methylene chloride layer. Repeat the operation with a second portion of 25 mL of methylene chloride. Combine the aqueous phase from the second separator with the aqueous phase of the first separator. Add 10 mL of *Alkaline phosphatase solution*, prepared as directed in the *Assay for prednisolone phosphate*, and add 50 mL of methylene chloride. Insert the stopper, and allow to stand, with occasional gentle inversion (about once every 15 minutes), for 2 hours. Filter the methylene chloride layer through a dry paper, and evaporate 25 mL of the filtrate to dryness: the residue so obtained responds to *Identification* test A under *Prednisolone.*
Sterility ⟨71⟩: meets the requirements.
Minimum fill ⟨755⟩: meets the requirements.
Water, *Method I* ⟨921⟩: not more than 1.0%, 20 mL of a mixture of toluene and methanol (7:3) being used in place of methanol in the titration vessel.
Metal particles—It meets the requirements of the test for *Metal Particles in Ophthalmic Ointments* ⟨751⟩.
Assay for neomycin—Proceed as directed under *Antibiotics—Microbial Assays* ⟨81⟩, using an accurately weighed portion of Ophthalmic Ointment shaken in a separator with about 50 mL of ether, and extracted with four 20-mL portions of *Buffer No. 3.* Combine the aqueous extracts, and dilute with *Buffer No. 3* to an appropriate volume to obtain a stock solution. Dilute this stock solution quantitatively and stepwise with *Buffer No. 3* to obtain a *Test Dilution* having a concentration assumed to be equal to the median dose level of the Standard.
Assay for prednisolone phosphate—
   pH 9 buffer with magnesium—Prepare as directed in the *Assay* under *Dexamethasone Sodium Phosphate.*
   Alkaline phosphatase solution—Prepare as directed in the *Assay* under *Dexamethasone Sodium Phosphate Injection.*
   Standard preparation—Prepare as directed for *Standard Preparation* under *Assay for Steroids* ⟨351⟩, using USP Prednisolone RS.
   Assay preparation—Transfer an accurately weighed portion of Ophthalmic Ointment, equivalent to about 3 mg of prednisolone phosphate, to a 125-mL separator. Add 25 mL of sodium chloride solution (1 in 20) and 25 mL of methylene chloride, and shake for not less than 2 minutes to disperse the assay specimen. Transfer the methylene chloride layer to a second separator containing 15 mL of sodium chloride solution (1 in 20). Shake for 1 minute, and discard the methylene chloride layer. Repeat the operation with a second portion of 25 mL of methylene chloride. Transfer the aqueous phases from both separators to a 50-mL volumetric flask, rinsing the first separator with the aqueous phase of the second separator. Rinse both separators with the same 5 mL of sodium chloride solution (1 in 20), and add the rinsing to the volumetric flask. Add sodium chloride solution (1 in 20) to volume, and mix.
   Pipet 5 mL of the resulting solution into a 125-mL separator, add 8.0 mL of *Alkaline phosphatase solution*, mix, and allow to stand for 2 hours. Extract the solution with two 25-mL portions of methylene chloride, filtering the extracts through methylene chloride-washed cotton into a small beaker. Evaporate the methylene chloride on a steam bath nearly to dryness, then evaporate with the aid of a current of air to dryness. Dissolve the residue in 25.0 mL of alcohol.
   Prepare a blank by evaporating 50 mL of methylene chloride to dryness and dissolving the residue in 25 mL of alcohol.
   Procedure—Pipet 20 mL each of the *Assay preparation*, the *Standard preparation*, and the blank solution into separate glass-stoppered flasks, and proceed as directed for *Procedure* under *Assay for Steroids* ⟨351⟩, beginning with "add 2.0 mL of a solution prepared by dissolving 50 mg of blue tetrazolium." Calculate the quantity, in mg, of prednisolone phosphate ($C_{21}H_{29}O_8P$) in the portion of Ophthalmic Ointment taken by the formula:

$$0.25C(A_U/A_S)(440.43/360.45)$$

in which C is the concentration, in µg per mL, of USP Prednisolone RS in the *Standard preparation*, A_U and A_S are the absorbances of the solutions from the *Assay preparation* and the *Standard preparation*, respectively, and 440.43 and 360.45 are the molecular weights of prednisolone phosphate and prednisolone, respectively.

Neomycin Sulfate, Sulfacetamide Sodium, and Prednisolone Acetate Ophthalmic Ointment

» Neomycin Sulfate, Sulfacetamide Sodium, and Prednisolone Acetate Ophthalmic Ointment contains the equivalent of not less than 90.0 percent and not more than 135.0 percent of the labeled amount of neomycin, and not less than 90.0 percent and not more than 110.0 percent of the labeled amounts of sulfacetamide sodium ($C_8H_9N_2NaO_3S \cdot H_2O$) and prednisolone acetate ($C_{23}H_{30}O_6$).

Packaging and storage—Preserve in collapsible ophthalmic ointment tubes.
USP Reference standards ⟨11⟩—*USP Neomycin Sulfate RS. USP Prednisolone Acetate RS.*
Identification—
   A: Dissolve a quantity of Ophthalmic Ointment, equivalent to about 1 g of sulfacetamide sodium, in 100 mL of ether in a separator, and extract the mixture with 25 mL of water. Wash the extract with 25 mL of ether, and warm the water extract on a steam bath to remove the last traces of ether. Adjust with 6 N acetic acid to a pH of between 4 and 5, and filter. Wash the precipitate with water, and dry at 105° for 2 hours: the sulfacetamide so obtained melts between 180° and 184°, and responds to *Identification* tests B, D, and E under *Sulfacetamide Sodium.*
   B: To a quantity of Ophthalmic Ointment, equivalent to about 25 mg of prednisolone acetate, add 15 mL of water, extract with two 10-mL portions of peroxide-free ether, discard the ether extracts, and extract with two 10-mL portions of chloroform. Evaporate the combined, clear chloroform extracts, with the aid of a current of air, to dryness: the residue so obtained responds to *Identification* test A under *Prednisolone Acetate.*
Sterility ⟨71⟩—It meets the requirements when tested as directed for *Membrane Filtration* under *Test for Sterility of the Product to be Examined.*
Minimum fill ⟨755⟩: meets the requirements.
Metal particles—It meets the requirements of the test for *Metal Particles in Ophthalmic Ointments* ⟨751⟩.
Assay for neomycin—Proceed with Ophthalmic Ointment as directed in the *Assay* under *Neomycin Sulfate Ointment.*
Assay for sulfacetamide sodium—Weigh accurately a quantity of Ophthalmic Ointment, equivalent to about 500 mg of sulfacetamide sodium, and transfer to a 125-mL separator. Dissolve the ointment in 50 mL of ether, and extract the mixture with six 25-mL portions of water. Warm the combined extracts on a steam bath to remove the last traces of ether, add 20 mL of hydrochloric acid, and proceed

as directed under Nitrite Titration ⟨451⟩, beginning with "cool to 15°." Each mL of 0.1 M sodium nitrite is equivalent to 25.42 mg of $C_8H_9N_2NaO_3S \cdot H_2O$.

Assay for prednisolone acetate—
Standard preparation—Prepare as directed for *Standard Preparation* under *Assay for Steroids* ⟨351⟩, using USP Prednisolone Acetate RS.

Assay preparation—Transfer to a suitable flask an accurately weighed quantity of Ophthalmic Ointment, equivalent to about 10 mg of prednisolone acetate, and add 30 mL of alcohol. Heat on a steam bath to melt the ointment base, and mix. Cool to solidify the ointment base, and filter the alcohol solution into a 100-mL volumetric flask. Repeat the extraction with three 20-mL portions of alcohol, add alcohol to volume, and mix. Pipet 10 mL of this solution into a 100-mL volumetric flask, add alcohol to volume, and mix. Pipet 20 mL of the resulting solution into a glass-stoppered, 50-mL conical flask.

Procedure—Proceed as directed for *Procedure* under *Assay for Steroids* ⟨351⟩. Calculate the quantity, in mg, of $C_{23}H_{30}O_6$ in the portion of Ophthalmic Ointment taken by the formula:

$$C(A_U / A_S).$$

Neomycin Sulfate and Triamcinolone Acetonide Cream

» Neomycin Sulfate and Triamcinolone Acetonide Cream contains the equivalent of not less than 90.0 percent and not more than 135.0 percent of the labeled amount of neomycin, and not less than 90.0 percent and not more than 110.0 percent of the labeled amount of triamcinolone acetonide ($C_{24}H_{34}FO_6$).

Packaging and storage—Preserve in collapsible tubes or in tight containers.

USP Reference standards ⟨11⟩—*USP Neomycin Sulfate RS. USP Triamcinolone Acetonide RS.*
Identification—
  A: It meets the requirements for neomycin under *Thin-Layer Chromatographic Identification Test* ⟨201BNP⟩.
  B: Place 2 g of Cream in a conical flask, add 5.0 mL of chloroform, and shake for 10 minutes. Add 15 mL of alcohol, and shake for an additional 10 minutes. Filter the solution into a centrifuge tube, and evaporate the filtrate to dryness. Dissolve the residue in alcohol to obtain a solution containing about 250 µg of triamcinolone acetonide per mL. Proceed as directed in the *Identification* test under *Triamcinolone Acetonide Cream*, beginning with "Apply 10 µL of this solution": the specified result is observed.
Minimum fill ⟨755⟩: meets the requirements.
Assay for neomycin—Proceed with Cream as directed in the *Assay* under *Neomycin Sulfate Cream*.
Assay for triamcinolone acetonide—Proceed with Cream as directed in the *Assay* under *Triamcinolone Acetonide Cream*.

Neomycin Sulfate and Triamcinolone Acetonide Ophthalmic Ointment

» Neomycin Sulfate and Triamcinolone Acetonide Ophthalmic Ointment contains the equivalent of not less than 90.0 percent and not more than 135.0 percent of the labeled amount of neomycin, and not less than 90.0 percent and not more than 110.0 percent of the labeled amount of triamcinolone acetonide ($C_{24}H_{31}FO_6$).

Packaging and storage—Preserve in collapsible ophthalmic ointment tubes.

USP Reference standards ⟨11⟩—*USP Neomycin Sulfate RS. USP Triamcinolone Acetonide RS.*
Identification—
  A: It meets the requirements for neomycin under *Thin-Layer Chromatographic Identification Test* ⟨201BNP⟩.
  B: Place 2 g of Ophthalmic Ointment in a conical flask, add 5.0 mL of chloroform, and shake for 10 minutes. Add 15 mL of alcohol, and shake for an additional 10 minutes. Filter the solution into a centrifuge tube, and evaporate the filtrate to dryness. Dissolve the residue in alcohol to obtain a solution containing about 250 µg of triamcinolone acetonide per mL. Proceed as directed in the *Identification* test under *Triamcinolone Acetonide Cream*, beginning with "Apply 10 µL of this solution": the specified result is observed.
Sterility ⟨71⟩—It meets the requirements when tested as directed for *Membrane Filtration* under *Test for Sterility of the Product to be Examined*.
Minimum fill ⟨755⟩: meets the requirements.
Water, *Method I* ⟨921⟩: not more than 1.0%, 20 mL of a mixture of toluene and methanol (7 : 3) being used in place of methanol in the titration vessel.
Metal particles—It meets the requirements of the test for *Metal Particles in Ophthalmic Ointments* ⟨751⟩.
Assay for neomycin—Proceed with Ophthalmic Ointment as directed in the *Assay* under *Neomycin Sulfate Ointment*.
Assay for triamcinolone acetonide—Proceed with Ophthalmic Ointment as directed in the *Assay* under *Triamcinolone Acetonide Cream*, except to read "Ophthalmic Ointment" in place of "Cream" throughout.

Neostigmine Bromide

$C_{12}H_{19}BrN_2O_2$ 303.20
Benzenaminium, 3-[[(dimethylamino)carbonyl]oxy]-*N,N,N*-trimethyl-, bromide.
(*m*-Hydroxyphenyl)trimethylammonium bromide dimethylcarbamate [*114-80-7*].

» Neostigmine Bromide contains not less than 98.0 percent and not more than 102.0 percent of $C_{12}H_{19}BrN_2O_2$, calculated on the dried basis.

Packaging and storage—Preserve in tight containers.
USP Reference standards ⟨11⟩—*USP Neostigmine Bromide RS.*
Identification—
  A: *Infrared Absorption* ⟨197K⟩.
  B: A solution (1 in 50) responds to the tests for *Bromide* ⟨191⟩.
Melting range ⟨741⟩: between 171° and 176°, with decomposition.
Loss on drying ⟨731⟩—Dry it at 105° for 3 hours: it loses not more than 2.0% of its weight.
Residue on ignition ⟨281⟩: not more than 0.15%.
Sulfate—Dissolve 250 mg in 10 mL of water, and add 1 mL of 3 N hydrochloric acid and 1 mL of barium chloride TS: no turbidity is produced immediately.
Assay—Dissolve about 750 mg of Neostigmine Bromide, accurately weighed, in a mixture of 70 mL of glacial acetic acid and 20 mL of mercuric acetate TS, add 4 drops of crystal violet TS, and titrate with 0.1 N perchloric acid VS to a blue endpoint. Perform a blank determination, and make any necessary correction. Each mL of 0.1 N perchloric acid is equivalent to 30.32 mg of $C_{12}H_{19}BrN_2O_2$.

Neostigmine Bromide Tablets

» Neostigmine Bromide Tablets contain not less than 93.0 percent and not more than 107.0 percent of the labeled amount of $C_{12}H_{19}BrN_2O_2$.

Packaging and storage—Preserve in tight containers.

USP Reference standards ⟨11⟩—*USP Neostigmine Bromide RS*.

Identification—Extract a quantity of powdered Tablets, equivalent to about 300 mg of neostigmine bromide, with three 10-mL portions of alcohol, filtering after each extraction. Evaporate the combined filtrates under a stream of nitrogen to dryness. Dissolve the residue in 10 mL of water, transfer to a 125-mL separator with the aid of 5 mL of water, extract with 15 mL of ether, and proceed with the following tests.

A: Evaporate 3 mL of the aqueous layer on a steam bath, under a stream of nitrogen, to dryness. Dissolve the residue, warming if necessary, in 1 mL of alcohol. Add 5 mL of chloroform, filter, evaporate the filtrate under a stream of nitrogen to dryness, and dry the residue at 105° for 30 minutes: the IR absorption spectrum of a potassium bromide dispersion of the residue of neostigmine bromide so obtained exhibits maxima only at the same wavelengths as that of a similar preparation of USP Neostigmine Bromide RS.

B: A portion of the aqueous layer responds to the tests for *Bromide* ⟨191⟩.

Dissolution, *Procedure for a Pooled Sample* ⟨711⟩—
  Medium: water; 500 mL.
  Apparatus 2: 50 rpm.
  Time: 45 minutes.
  Procedure—At the specified time interval, withdraw 30 mL of the solution under test, and filter. Pipet 10 mL each of the filtered test solution, a Standard solution having a known concentration of USP Neostigmine Bromide RS, and water to provide a blank, into respective 125-mL separators. Proceed as directed for *Procedure* in the *Assay*, beginning with "Add 15 mL of a solution."
  Tolerances—Not less than 75% (*Q*) of the labeled amount of $C_{12}H_{19}BrN_2O_2$ is dissolved in 45 minutes.

Uniformity of dosage units ⟨905⟩: meet the requirements.

Assay—
  Standard preparation—Dissolve a suitable quantity of USP Neostigmine Bromide RS, accurately weighed, in water, and dilute quantitatively and stepwise with water to obtain a solution having a concentration of about 40 μg per mL.
  Assay preparation—Weigh and finely powder not less than 20 Tablets. Transfer an accurately weighed portion of the powder, equivalent to about 50 mg of neostigmine bromide, to a 100-mL volumetric flask, add about 50 mL of water, shake by mechanical means for about 30 minutes, add water to volume, mix, and filter. Pipet 4 mL of the clear filtrate into a 50-mL volumetric flask, add water to volume, and mix.
  Procedure—Pipet 10 mL each of *Assay preparation* and *Standard preparation* into respective 125-mL separators, and treat each solution as follows. Add 15 mL of a solution prepared by dissolving 25 mg of hexanitrodiphenylamine in methylene chloride to make 250 mL, without grinding the solid or heating the solution. Then add 10 mL of 5 N sodium hydroxide, and shake vigorously for 30 seconds. Collect the methylene chloride layer in a 100-mL volumetric flask, and extract the aqueous layer with three 15-mL portions of methylene chloride, collecting the methylene chloride extracts in each respective flask. Add methylene chloride to volume, and mix. Concomitantly determine the absorbances of both solutions in 1-cm cells at the wavelength of maximum absorbance at about 420 nm, with a suitable spectrophotometer, using methylene chloride as the blank. Calculate the quantity, in mg, of $C_{12}H_{19}BrN_2O_2$ in the portion of Tablets taken by the formula:

$$1.25C(A_U/A_S)$$

in which *C* is the concentration, in μg per mL, of USP Neostigmine Bromide RS in the *Standard preparation*, and A_U and A_S are the absorbances of the solutions from the *Assay preparation* and the *Standard preparation*, respectively.

Neostigmine Methylsulfate

$C_{13}H_{22}N_2O_6S$ 334.39
Benzenaminium, 3-[[(dimethylamino)carbonyl]oxy]-*N*,*N*,*N*-trimethyl-, methyl sulfate.
(*m*-Hydroxyphenyl)trimethylammonium methyl sulfate dimethylcarbamate [*51-60-5*].

» Neostigmine Methylsulfate contains not less than 98.0 percent and not more than 102.0 percent of $C_{13}H_{22}N_2O_6S$, calculated on the dried basis.

Packaging and storage—Preserve in tight containers.

USP Reference standards ⟨11⟩—*USP Neostigmine Methylsulfate RS*.

Identification—
  A: *Infrared Absorption* ⟨197K⟩.
  B: Place about 1 mg in a small porcelain dish, add 2 mL of water and 0.5 mL of sodium hydroxide solution (2 in 5), and evaporate on a steam bath to dryness. Transfer the residue to a small test tube, and quickly heat in a suitable liquid bath to 250°, continuing at that temperature for about 30 seconds. Cool, dissolve the residue in 0.5 mL of water, cool in ice water, and add 1 mL of diazobenzenesulfonic acid TS: a cherry-red color is produced.
  C: Mix about 20 mg with 500 mg of sodium carbonate, and heat the mixture to fusion in a small crucible. Boil the fused mass with 10 mL of water until disintegrated, and filter. Add a few drops of bromine TS to the filtrate, heat to boiling, acidify with hydrochloric acid, and expel the excess bromine by boiling: the resulting solution responds to the tests for *Sulfate* ⟨191⟩.

Melting range ⟨741⟩: between 144° and 149°, determined after drying at 105° for 3 hours.

Loss on drying ⟨731⟩: Dry about 300 mg, accurately weighed, at 105° for 3 hours: it loses not more than 1.0% of its weight.

Residue on ignition ⟨281⟩: not more than 0.1%.

Chloride—To 10 mL of a solution (1 in 50) add 1 mL of 2 N nitric acid and 1 mL of silver nitrate TS: no opalescence is produced immediately.

Sulfate ion—To 10 mL of a solution (1 in 50) add 1 mL of 3 N hydrochloric acid and 1 mL of barium chloride TS: no turbidity is produced immediately.

Assay—Place about 100 mg of Neostigmine Methylsulfate, accurately weighed, in a 500-mL Kjeldahl flask, dissolve in 150 mL of water, and add 40 mL of 2.5 N sodium hydroxide. Connect the flask by means of a distillation trap to a well-cooled condenser that dips into 25 mL of boric acid solution (1 in 25), distill about 150 mL of the contents of the flask, add methyl purple TS to the solution in the receiver, and titrate with 0.02 N sulfuric acid VS. Perform a blank determination, and make any necessary correction. Each mL of 0.02 N sulfuric acid is equivalent to 6.688 mg of $C_{13}H_{22}N_2O_6S$.

Neostigmine Methylsulfate Injection

» Neostigmine Methylsulfate Injection is a sterile solution of Neostigmine Methylsulfate in Water for Injection. It contains not less than 90.0 percent and not more than 110.0 percent of the labeled amount of $C_{13}H_{22}N_2O_6S$.

Packaging and storage—Preserve in single-dose or in multiple-dose containers, protected from light.

USP Reference standards ⟨11⟩—*USP Neostigmine Methylsulfate RS*.

Identification—Transfer a volume of Injection, containing the equivalent of 1 mg of neostigmine methylsulfate, to a small porcelain dish. Evaporate, if necessary, to 2 mL, add 0.5 mL of sodium hydroxide solution (2 in 5), and proceed as directed in *Identification*

test B under *Neostigmine Methylsulfate*, beginning with "evaporate on a steam bath."
pH ⟨791⟩: between 5.0 and 6.5.
Other requirements—It meets the requirements under *Injections* ⟨1⟩.
Assay—
Standard preparation—Dissolve a suitable quantity of USP Neostigmine Methylsulfate RS, accurately weighed, in water, and dilute quantitatively and stepwise with water to obtain a solution having a known concentration of about 40 µg per mL.
Assay preparation—Pipet an accurately measured volume of Injection, equivalent to about 2 mg of neostigmine methylsulfate, into a 50-mL volumetric flask, add water to volume, and mix.
Procedure—Proceed as directed for *Procedure* in the *Assay* under *Neostigmine Bromide Tablets*. Calculate the quantity, in mg, of $C_{13}H_{22}N_2O_6S$ in each mL of the Injection taken by the formula:

$$0.05(C/V)(A_U/A_S)$$

in which C is the concentration, in µg per mL, of USP Neostigmine Methylsulfate RS in the *Standard preparation*, V is the volume, in mL, of Injection taken, and A_U and A_S are the absorbances of the solutions from the *Assay preparation* and the *Standard preparation*, respectively.

Netilmicin Sulfate

$(C_{21}H_{41}N_5O_7)_2 \cdot 5H_2SO_4$ 1441.56

D-Streptamine, O-3-deoxy-4-C-methyl-3-(methylamino)-β-L-arabinopyranosyl-(1→6)-O-[2,6-diamino-2,3,4,6-tetradeoxy-α-D-glycero-hex-4-enopyranosyl-(1→4)]-2-deoxy-N^1-ethyl-, sulfate (2 : 5) (salt).

O-3-Deoxy-4-C-methyl-3-(methylamino)-β-L-arabinopyranosyl-(1→4)-O-[2,6-diamino-2,3,4,6-tetradeoxy-α-D-glycero-hex-4-enopyranosyl-(1→6)]-2-deoxy-N^3-ethyl-L-streptamine sulfate (2 : 5) (salt)   [56391-57-2].

» Netilmicin Sulfate has a potency equivalent to not less than 595 µg of netilmicin ($C_{21}H_{41}N_5O_7$) per mg, calculated on the dried basis. [NOTE—Netilmicin Sulfate is extremely hygroscopic. Protect from exposure to moisture.]

Packaging and storage—Preserve in tight containers.

USP Reference standards ⟨11⟩—*USP Netilmicin Sulfate RS. USP Sisomicin Sulfate RS.*
Identification—
  A: The retention time of the major peak in the chromatogram of the *Assay preparation* corresponds to that in the chromatogram of the *Standard preparation*, as obtained in the *Assay*.
  B: It responds to the tests for *Sulfate* ⟨191⟩.
Specific rotation ⟨781S⟩: between +88° and +96°.
  Test solution: 30 mg per mL, in water.
pH ⟨791⟩: between 3.5 and 5.5, in a solution containing 40 mg of netilmicin per mL.
Loss on drying ⟨731⟩—Dry about 100 mg in vacuum at a pressure not exceeding 5 mm of mercury at 110° for 3 hours: it loses not more than 15.0% of its weight.
Residue on ignition ⟨281⟩: not more than 1.0%, the charred residue being moistened with 2 mL of nitric acid and 5 drops of sulfuric acid.

Chromatographic purity—
Dilute phosphoric acid, Mobile phase, Resolution solution, Assay preparation, and *Chromatographic system*—Proceed as directed in the *Assay*.
Test solution—Use the *Assay preparation*.
Reference solution—Transfer 1.0 mL of the *Test solution* to a 100-mL volumetric flask, dilute with *Mobile phase* to volume, and mix.
Procedure—Separately inject equal volumes (about 20 µL) of the *Test solution* and the *Reference solution* into the chromatograph, and measure the area responses for all the peaks, except those due to the solvent. Calculate the percentage of each impurity in the portion of Netilmicin Sulfate taken by the formula:

$$(r_i/r_S)$$

in which r_i is the peak response of each impurity in the chromatogram obtained from the *Test solution*, and r_S is the netilmicin peak response in the chromatogram obtained from the *Reference solution*: not more than 1% of any individual impurity is found, and not more than 5% of total impurities is found.
Assay—
Dilute phosphoric acid—Dilute 5.0 mL of phosphoric acid with water to 1000 mL, and mix.
Mobile phase—Dissolve 20.22 g of sodium 1-heptanesulfonate in *Dilute phosphoric acid*, dilute with *Dilute phosphoric acid* to 1000 mL, and mix. To 620 mL of this solution add 380 mL of acetonitrile, mix, and pass through a filter having a 0.45-µm porosity. Make adjustments if necessary (see *System Suitability* under *Chromatography* ⟨621⟩).
Resolution solution—Prepare a solution in *Mobile phase* containing about 1 mg of USP Netilmicin Sulfate RS and 1 mg of USP Sisomicin Sulfate RS per mL.
Standard preparation—[NOTE—Use low-actinic glassware.] Dissolve an accurately weighed quantity of USP Netilmicin Sulfate RS in *Mobile phase* to obtain a solution having a known concentration of about 1 mg per mL.
Assay preparation—[NOTE—Use low-actinic glassware.] Transfer about 50 mg of Netilmicin Sulfate, accurately weighed, to a 50-mL volumetric flask. Dissolve in and dilute with *Mobile phase*, to volume, and mix.
Chromatographic system (see *Chromatography* ⟨621⟩)—The chromatograph is equipped with a 205-nm detector and a 4.6-mm × 25-cm column that contains 5-µm packing L1. The flow rate is about 1 mL per minute. Chromatograph the *Resolution solution*, and record the peak responses as directed for *Procedure*: the resolution, R, between sisomicin and netilmicin is not less than 1. Chromatograph the *Standard preparation*, and record the peak responses as directed for *Procedure*: the column efficiency is not less than 3000 theoretical plates; the tailing factor is not more than 2; and the relative standard deviation for replicate injections is not more than 1%.
Procedure—Separately inject equal volumes (about 20 µL) of the *Standard preparation* and the *Assay preparation* into the chromatograph, and measure the area responses for the major peaks. Calculate the quantity, in µg, of netilmicin ($C_{21}H_{41}N_5O_7$) per mg of Netilmicin Sulfate taken by the formula:

$$(W_S P/W_U)(r_U/r_S)$$

in which W_S is the dry weight, in mg, of USP Netilmicin Sulfate RS taken to prepare the *Standard preparation*; P is the designated potency, in µg of netilmicin ($C_{21}H_{41}N_5O_7$) per mg, of USP Netilmicin Sulfate RS; W_U is the dry weight, in mg, of Netilmicin Sulfate taken to prepare the *Assay preparation*; and r_U and r_S are the netilmicin peak responses obtained from the *Assay preparation* and the *Standard preparation*, respectively.

Netilmicin Sulfate Injection

» Netilmicin Sulfate Injection is a sterile solution of Netilmicin Sulfate in Water for Injection. It contains the equivalent of not less than 90.0 percent and not more than 115.0 percent of the labeled amount of netilmicin ($C_{21}H_{41}N_5O_7$). It may contain one or more suitable buffers, chelating agents, and preservatives.

Packaging and storage—Preserve in single-dose or in multiple-dose containers, preferably of Type I glass.
USP Reference standards ⟨11⟩—*USP Endotoxin RS. USP Netilmicin Sulfate RS. USP Sisomicin Sulfate RS.*
Identification—It responds to *Identification* test A under *Netilmicin Sulfate.*
Bacterial endotoxins ⟨85⟩—It contains not more than 1.25 USP Endotoxin Units per mg of netilmicin.
Sterility ⟨71⟩—It meets the requirements when tested as directed for *Membrane Filtration* under *Test for Sterility of the Product to be Examined.*
pH ⟨791⟩: between 3.5 and 6.0.
Particulate matter ⟨788⟩: meets the requirements under small-volume injections.
Other requirements—It meets the requirements under *Injections* ⟨1⟩.
Assay—
Dilute phosphoric acid, Mobile phase, Resolution solution, Standard preparation, and *Chromatographic system*—Proceed as directed in the *Assay* under *Netilmicin Sulfate.*
Assay preparation—Transfer an accurately measured volume of Injection, equivalent to about 100 mg of netilmicin, to a low-actinic, 100-mL volumetric flask. Dilute with *Mobile phase* to volume, and mix.
Procedure—Proceed as directed for *Procedure* in the *Assay* under *Netilmicin Sulfate.* Calculate the quantity, in mg, of netilmicin ($C_{21}H_{41}N_5O_7$) in each mL of Injection taken by the formula:

$$0.1(W_S P/50V)(r_U/r_S)$$

in which V is the volume, in mL, of Injection taken to prepare the *Assay preparation,* and the other terms are as defined therein.

Nevirapine

$C_{15}H_{14}N_4O$ 266.30
6*H*-Dipyrido[3,2-*b*: 2′,3′-*e*][1,4]diazepin-6-one, 11-cyclopropyl-5,11-dihydro-4-methyl-.
11-Cyclopropyl-5,11-dihydro-4-methyl-6*H*-dipyrido[3,2-*b*: 2′,3′-*e*][1,4]diazepin-6-one [*129618-40-2*].
Hemihydrate   275.31

» Nevirapine is anhydrous or contains one-half molecule of water of hydration. It contains not less than 98.0 percent and not more than 102.0 percent of $C_{15}H_{14}N_4O$, calculated on the anhydrous basis.

Packaging and storage—Preserve in tight containers. Store at 25°, excursions permitted between 15° and 30°.
Labeling—Label it to indicate whether it is anhydrous or the hemihydrate.
USP Reference standards ⟨11⟩—*USP Nevirapine Anhydrous RS. USP Nevirapine Hemihydrate RS. USP Nevirapine Related Compound A RS. USP Nevirapine Related Compound B RS.*
Identification—
  A: *Infrared Absorption* ⟨197K⟩—Do not dry the specimens.
  B: The retention time of the major peak in the chromatogram of the *Assay preparation* corresponds to that in the chromatogram of the *Standard preparation,* as obtained in the *Assay.*

Water, *Method I* ⟨921⟩—For Nevirapine anhydrous: not more than 0.2%. For Nevirapine hemihydrate: between 3.1% and 3.9%.
Residue on ignition ⟨281⟩: not more than 0.1%.
Heavy metals, *Method II* ⟨231⟩: 0.001%.
Specified and unspecified impurities—
0.025 M Ammonium phosphate buffer, Mobile phase, Standard stock solution 1, Standard stock solution 2, Standard stock solution 3, and *Resolution solution*—Proceed as directed in the *Assay.*
Standard solution—Transfer 2.0 mL of *Standard stock solution 1* to a 200-mL volumetric flask, dilute with *Mobile phase* to volume, and mix. Transfer 5.0 mL of this solution to a 50-mL volumetric flask, dilute with *Mobile phase* to volume, and mix.
Test solution—Transfer an accurately weighed quantity of Nevirapine, equivalent to about 24 mg of nevirapine anhydrous, to a 100-mL volumetric flask. Add 4 mL of acetonitrile and 80 mL of *Mobile phase,* and sonicate for at least 15 minutes. Allow to cool to room temperature, dilute with *Mobile phase* to volume, and mix.
Chromatographic system—Proceed as directed in the *Assay.* Chromatograph the *Resolution solution* (approximately 25 µL), and record the peak responses as directed for *Procedure:* the relative retention times are about 0.7 for nevirapine related compound B, 1.0 for nevirapine, 1.5 for nevirapine related compound A, and 2.8 for nevirapine impurity C; the resolution, R, between nevirapine related compound B and nevirapine is not less than 5.0; and the resolution between nevirapine and nevirapine related compound A is not less than 7.4. Chromatograph the *Standard solution,* and record the peak responses as directed for *Procedure:* the relative standard deviation for replicate injections is not more than 5.0%.
Procedure—Separately inject equal volumes (about 50 µL) of the *Standard solution* and the *Test solution* into the chromatograph, record the chromatograms for at least 80 minutes, and measure the responses for the major peaks. Calculate the percentage of each impurity in the portion of Nevirapine taken by the formula:

$$10{,}000(1/F)(C/W)(r_i/r_S)$$

in which F is the relative response factor for each impurity, which is equal to 1.3 for nevirapine related compound B and 1.0 for all other impurities; C is the concentration, in mg per mL, of USP Nevirapine Anhydrous RS in the *Standard solution;* W is the weight of Nevirapine, in mg, taken to prepare the *Test solution;* r_i is the peak response for each impurity obtained from the *Test solution;* and r_S is the nevirapine peak response obtained from the *Standard solution:* not more than 0.2% each of nevirapine related compound A, nevirapine related compound B, and nevirapine impurity C is found; not more than 0.1% of any other individual unspecified impurity is found; and not more than 0.6% of total impurities is found.
Organic volatile impurities,   *Method V* ⟨467⟩: meets the requirements.

(Official until July 1, 2008)

Assay—
0.025 M Ammonium phosphate buffer—Transfer 2.88 g of monobasic ammonium phosphate to a 1000-mL volumetric flask, dissolve in 800 mL of water, adjust with 1 N sodium hydroxide to a pH of about 5.0, dilute with water to volume, and mix.
Mobile phase—Prepare a filtered and degassed mixture of *0.025 M Ammonium phosphate buffer* and acetonitrile (4 : 1).
Standard stock solution 1—Transfer an accurately weighed quantity of USP Nevirapine Anhydrous RS to a volumetric flask, add a volume of a mixture of *Mobile phase* and acetonitrile (20 : 1), sonicate for at least 15 minutes, allow to cool to room temperature, dilute with *Mobile phase* to volume, and mix to obtain a solution having a known concentration of about 0.24 mg per mL. [NOTE—Do not use after 78 hours.]
Standard stock solution 2—Transfer an accurately weighed quantity of USP Nevirapine Related Compound A RS to a volumetric flask, add a volume of a mixture of *Mobile phase* and acetonitrile (3 : 1), sonicate for at least 15 minutes, allow to cool to room temperature, dilute with *Mobile phase* to volume, and mix to obtain a solution having a known concentration of about 0.24 mg per mL.
Standard stock solution 3—Transfer an accurately weighed quantity of USP Nevirapine Related Compound B RS to a volumetric flask, add a volume of a mixture of *Mobile phase* and acetonitrile (2.2 : 1), sonicate for at least 30 minutes, allow to cool to room temperature, dilute with *Mobile phase* to volume, and mix to obtain a solution having a known concentration of about 0.06 mg per mL.

Resolution solution—Transfer 3.0 mL of *Standard stock solution 1*, 3.0 mL of *Standard stock solution 2*, and 6.0 mL of *Standard stock solution 3* to a 25-mL volumetric flask, dissolve in and dilute with *Mobile phase* to volume, and mix.

Standard preparation—Transfer 3.0 mL of *Standard stock solution 1* to a 25-mL volumetric flask, dilute with *Mobile phase* to volume, and mix. [NOTE—Do not use after 78 hours.]

Assay preparation—Transfer an accurately weighed quantity of Nevirapine, equivalent to about 24 mg of nevirapine anhydrous, to a 100-mL volumetric flask. Add 4 mL of acetonitrile and 80 mL of *Mobile phase*, sonicate for at least 15 minutes, allow to cool to room temperature, dilute with *Mobile phase* to volume, and mix. Transfer 3.0 mL of this solution to a 25-mL volumetric flask, dilute with *Mobile phase* to volume, and mix.

Chromatographic system (see *Chromatography* ⟨621⟩)—The liquid chromatograph is equipped with a 220-nm detector and a 4.6-mm × 15-cm column that contains 5-µm packing L60 (see *Chromatography* ⟨621⟩). The flow rate is about 1 mL per minute. The column temperature is maintained at 35°. Chromatograph the *Resolution solution* (approximately 25 µL), and record the peak responses as directed for *Procedure*: the relative retention times are about 0.7 for nevirapine related compound B, 1.0 for nevirapine, 1.5 for nevirapine related compound A, and 2.8 for nevirapine impurity C; the resolution, R, between nevirapine related compound B and nevirapine is not less than 5.0; and the resolution between nevirapine and nevirapine related compound A is not less than 7.4. Chromatograph the *Standard preparation*, and record the peak responses as directed for *Procedure*: the relative standard deviation for replicate injections is not more than 2.0%.

Procedure—Separately inject equal volumes (about 25 µL) of the *Standard preparation* and the *Assay preparation* into the chromatograph, record the chromatograms, and measure the responses for the major peaks. Calculate the quantity, in mg, of $C_{15}H_{14}N_4O$ in the portion of Nevirapine taken by the formula:

$$833.33C(r_U / r_S)$$

in which C is the concentration, in mg per mL, of USP Nevirapine Anhydrous RS in the *Standard preparation*; and r_U and r_S are the peak responses obtained from the *Assay preparation* and the *Standard preparation*, respectively.

Nevirapine Oral Suspension

» Nevirapine Oral Suspension contains not less than 90.0 percent and not more than 110.0 percent of the labeled amount of nevirapine ($C_{15}H_{14}N_4O$).

Packaging and storage—Preserve in well-closed containers. Store at 25°, excursions permitted between 15° and 30°.

USP Reference standards ⟨11⟩—*USP Nevirapine Anhydrous RS. USP Nevirapine Related Compound A RS. USP Nevirapine Related Compound B.*

Identification—
 A: *Thin-Layer Chromatographic Identification Test* ⟨201⟩—
 Ferric chloride–potassium ferricyanide reagent—Dissolve 1.35 g of ferric chloride in 25 mL of water. Dissolve 1.64 g of potassium ferricyanide in 25 mL of water. Mix the two solutions immediately before use.

Test solution—Transfer a volume of Oral Suspension, equivalent to about 10 mg of nevirapine, to an 8-mL glass stoppered tube. Pipet 2.0 mL of chloroform into the tube, and shake. Allow the two phases to separate, and then using a disposable glass Pasteur pipet, remove some of the organic layer from the bottom, and transfer to another container.

Standard solution—Dissolve a suitable quantity of USP Nevirapine Anhydrous RS in chloroform to obtain a solution having a known concentration of about 5 mg per mL.

Procedure—Separately apply 5-µL portions of the *Test solution* and the *Standard solution* to a thin-layer chromatographic plate (see *Chromatography* ⟨621⟩) coated with a 0.25-mm layer of chromatographic silica gel 60 F254. Allow the spots to dry, and develop the chromatogram in a chamber saturated with a solvent system consisting of a mixture of ethyl acetate, isopropanol, and concentrated ammonium hydroxide (18 : 2 : 0.1) until the solvent front has moved about 6 to 7 cm from the point of application. Remove the plate from the chamber, mark the solvent front, and dry. Examine the chromatograms under UV light at 254 nm, and outline the spots with a soft pencil. Spray the plate with *Ferric chloride–potassium ferricyanide reagent*: the R_F value (approximately 0.4 to 0.5) of the principal blue spot under UV and after spraying, obtained from the *Test solution*, corresponds to that obtained from the *Standard solution*.

 B: The retention time of the major peak in the chromatogram of the *Assay preparation* corresponds to that in the chromatogram of the *Standard preparation*, as obtained in the *Assay*.

Microbial limits ⟨61⟩—It meets the requirements of the tests for absence of *Escherichia coli*. The total aerobic microbial count does not exceed 100 cfu per mL, and the total combined molds and yeasts count does not exceed 50 cfu per mL.

Dissolution ⟨711⟩—
Medium: 0.1 N hydrochloric acid; 900 mL.
Apparatus 2: 25 rpm.
Time: 45 minutes.
Determine the amount of $C_{15}H_{14}N_4O$ dissolved by employing the following method.

Diluent: a mixture of dehydrated alcohol and water (1 : 1).

Mobile phase—Prepare a filtered and degassed mixture of water and acetonitrile (77 : 23). Make adjustments if necessary (see *System Suitability* under *Chromatography* ⟨621⟩).

System suitability solution—Transfer about 10 mg of USP Nevirapine Anhydrous RS and 15 mg of methylparaben into a 250-mL volumetric flask. Dissolve in approximately 2 mL of *Diluent*, and dilute with *Medium* to volume.

Standard solution—Transfer about 28 mg of USP Nevirapine Anhydrous RS, accurately weighed, into a 500-mL volumetric flask. Add 2 mL of *Diluent*, and sonicate for about 1 minute. Note that the Standard will not be completely dissolved at this point. Dilute with *Medium* to volume, and visually examine the solution to ensure that the Standard is completely dissolved. The final concentration is about 0.056 mg of nevirapine per mL.

Test solution—For sample mixing, gently shake the bottle for approximately 10 seconds by inverting it slowly and rotating it from side to side. The sample should be free of air bubbles. Do not sonicate the sample. Using a 1- to 10-mL suitable positive displacement pipet set at 5 mL, withdraw the equivalent of 50 mg of nevirapine. Remove excess Oral Suspension by wiping the outside of the tip carefully so as not to touch the opening of the tip. Introduce the sample into the dissolution vessel over a 1-to 2-second time period by immersing the tip of the pipet midway between the paddle and the side of the vessel, approximately 1 cm below the meniscus. Similarly dispense the Oral Suspension into the other vessels. At 45 minutes, withdraw 5 mL of the solution under test, and pass through a 0.45-µm nylon filter, discarding the first 2 mL.

Chromatographic system (see *Chromatography* ⟨621⟩)—The chromatograph is equipped with a 214-nm detector, a 3.9-mm × 20-mm guard column that contains packing L1, and a 3.9-mm × 15-cm analytical column that contains 5-µm packing L1. The flow rate is about 1.0 mL per minute. Chromatograph the *System suitability solution*, and record the peak responses as directed for *Procedure*: the resolution, R, between nevirapine and methylparaben is not less than 5.0; and the tailing factor for the nevirapine peak is not more than 1.8. Chromatograph the *Standard solution*, and record the peak responses as directed for *Procedure*: the relative standard deviation for replicate injections is not more than 2.0%.

Procedure—Separately inject equal volumes (about 10 µL) of the *Standard solution* and the *Test solution* into the chromatograph, record the chromatograms for at least 14 minutes, and measure the responses for the nevirapine peaks. Calculate the percentage of $C_{15}H_{14}N_4O$ dissolved by the formula:

$$\frac{r_U \times C_S \times 900 \times 100}{r_S \times V \times LC}$$

in which r_U and r_S are the peak responses obtained from the *Test solution* and the *Standard solution*, respectively; C_S is the concentration, in mg per mL, of USP Nevirapine Anhydrous RS in the *Stan-*

dard solution; 900 is the volume, in mL, of the *Medium;* 100 is the conversion factor to percentage; *V* is the volume, in mL, of Oral Suspension taken; and *LC* is the Oral Suspension label claim, in mg per mL.

Tolerances—Not less than 80% (*Q*) of the labeled amount of $C_{15}H_{14}N_4O$ is dissolved in 45 minutes.

Related compounds—

Potassium phosphate buffer, Solution A, Solution B, Mobile phase, and *Diluent*—Proceed as directed in the *Assay.*

System suitability solution—Proceed as directed in the *Assay.*

Standard stock solution—Use the *Standard stock preparation,* prepared as directed in the *Assay.*

Standard solution—Dilute the *Standard stock solution* quantitatively with *Diluent* to obtain a solution having a known concentration of about 0.3 µg of nevirapine per mL.

Weight determination—Use the weight obtained as directed for *Weight determination* in the *Assay.*

Test solution—Use the *Assay preparation,* prepared as directed in the *Assay.*

Chromatographic system (see *Chromatography* ⟨621⟩)—Proceed as directed in the *Assay:* the relative standard deviation for replicate injections of the *Standard solution* is not more than 10.0%.

Procedure—Separately inject equal volumes (about 20 µL) of the *Standard solution* and the *Test solution* into the chromatograph, record the chromatograms, and measure the peak responses. Calculate the percentage of each unknown impurity in the portion of Oral Suspension taken by the formula:

$$200(C/W_U)(W_A/5)(r_U/r_S)(100/L)$$

in which *C* is the concentration, in mg per mL, of USP Nevirapine Anhydrous RS in the *Standard solution;* W_U is the sample weight, in g, taken to prepare the *Test solution;* W_A is the weight, in g, of 5 mL of Oral Suspension, obtained as directed for *Weight determination;* *L* is the labeled amount, in mg per mL, of nevirapine in the Oral Suspension; r_U is the peak response obtained for each impurity in the *Test solution;* and r_S is the peak response for nevirapine in the *Standard solution.* Not more than 0.1% of any individual unknown impurity is found; and not more than 0.2% of total impurities is found. [NOTE—The excipients and their degradation products should not be included in the determination of impurities.]

Assay—

Diluent—Prepare a mixture of water and methanol (80 : 20).

Potassium phosphate buffer—Dissolve 13.6 g of monobasic potassium phosphate in approximately 1900 mL of water, and adjust with phosphoric acid to a pH of 3.0. Transfer to a 2000-mL volumetric flask, and dilute with water to volume. Mix, filter, and degas.

Solution A: a mixture of *Potassium phosphate buffer* and acetonitrile (97 : 3).

Solution B: a mixture of *Potassium phosphate buffer* and acetonitrile (76 : 24).

Mobile phase—Use variable mixtures of *Solution A* and *Solution B* as directed for *Chromatographic system.* Make adjustments if necessary (see *System Suitability* under *Chromatography* ⟨621⟩).

Standard stock preparation—Transfer about 50 mg of USP Nevirapine Anhydrous RS, accurately weighed, into a 50-mL volumetric flask. Add 20 mL of methanol, and sonicate with intermittent swirling until the sample dissolves. Add water to about 1 cm below the meniscus, cool to room temperature, and dilute with water to volume. The concentration is about 1 mg of nevirapine per mL.

Standard preparation—Dilute the *Standard stock preparation* quantitatively with *Diluent* to obtain a solution having a known concentration of about 0.3 mg of nevirapine per mL.

Stock impurity preparation—Transfer about 3 mg of USP Nevirapine Related Compound A RS and 3 mg of USP Nevirapine Related Compound B RS, accurately weighed, into a 100-mL volumetric flask, add 20 mL of methanol, and sonicate to dissolve. Add water to about 1 cm below the meniscus, cool to room temperature, dilute with water to volume, and mix.

System suitability solution—Transfer 15.0 mL of *Standard stock preparation* and 2.0 mL of *Stock impurity preparation* into a 50-mL volumetric flask, dilute with *Diluent* to volume, and mix.

Weight determination—Using a 1- to 10-mL suitable pipet and a positive displacement tip, withdraw 5.0 mL of the Oral Suspension. The sample should be free of air bubbles. Dispense into a tared vial, and record the weight of the Oral Suspension to ±0.1 mg.

Assay preparation—Using a 1- to 10-mL suitable pipet and a positive displacement tip, withdraw the equivalent of 60 mg of nevirapine. The sample should be free of air bubbles. Remove the excess Oral Suspension by wiping the outside of the tip carefully so as not to touch the opening of the tip, and deliver the sample into a 200-mL tared volumetric flask. Record the sample weight to the nearest ±0.1 mg. Add 40 mL of methanol, and sonicate for about 5 minutes with intermittent swirling. Add water to about 1 cm below the meniscus. Do not shake the flask. Allow the solution to attain room temperature, and dilute with water to volume. Shake the flask gently, and allow to stand for about 5 minutes.

Chromatographic system ⟨621⟩—The liquid chromatograph is equipped with a 254-nm detector, a 4.6-mm × 12.5-mm guard column that contains 5-µm packing L10, and a 4.6-mm × 15-cm analytical column that contains 3.5-µm packing L10. The column temperature is maintained at 35°. The flow rate is about 1.5 mL per minute. The chromatograph is programmed as follows.

Time (minutes)	Solution A (%)	Solution B (%)	Elution
0–1	100	0	isocratic
1–31	100→0	0→100	linear gradient
31–32	0→100	100→0	linear gradient
32–42	100	0	equilibration

Chromatograph the *System suitability solution* (about 20 µL), and record the peak responses as directed for *Procedure:* the resolution, *R,* between nevirapine and nevirapine related compound A is not less than 3.0, and the resolution, *R,* between nevirapine and nevirapine related compound B is not less than 1.7; and the tailing factor for the nevirapine peak is not more than 1.5. Chromatograph the *Standard preparation,* and record the peak responses as directed for *Procedure:* the relative standard deviation for replicate injections is not more than 2.0%.

Procedure—Separately inject equal volumes (about 20 µL) of the *Standard preparation* and the *Assay preparation* into the chromatograph, record the chromatograms, and measure the responses for the nevirapine peak. Calculate the quantity, in mg, of nevirapine ($C_{15}H_{14}N_4O$) in each mL of the Oral Suspension taken by the formula:

$$200(C/W_U)(W_A/5)(r_U/r_S)$$

in which *C* is the concentration, in mg per mL, of USP Nevirapine Anhydrous RS in the *Standard preparation;* W_U is the sample weight, in g, of Oral Suspension taken to prepare the *Assay preparation;* W_A is the weight, in g, of 5 mL of Oral Suspension obtained as directed for *Weight determination;* and r_U and r_S are the peak responses obtained from the *Assay preparation* and the *Standard preparation,* respectively.

Nevirapine Tablets

» Nevirapine Tablets contain not less than 90.0 percent and not more than 110.0 percent of the labeled amount of nevirapine ($C_{15}H_{14}N_4O$).

Packaging and storage—Preserve in well-closed containers. Store at 25°, excursions permitted between 15° and 30°.

USP Reference standards ⟨11⟩—*USP Nevirapine Anhydrous RS. USP Nevirapine Related Compound A RS.*

Identification—

A: *Infrared Absorption* ⟨197K⟩—

Test specimen—Transfer a portion of powdered Tablets equivalent to 25 mg of nevirapine to a 50-mL volumetric flask. Dissolve in 10 mL of methylene chloride. Swirl the solution for about 30 to 60 seconds, and pass through a medium sintered-glass, fritted vacuum funnel. Using a glass syringe, pass the filtrate through a

0.45-μm Teflon filter. Dry the extract at 105° for a minimum of 1 hour.

B: The retention time of the major peak in the chromatogram of the *Assay preparation* corresponds to that in the chromatogram of the *Standard preparation*, as obtained in the *Assay*.

Dissolution ⟨711⟩—

Medium: 0.1 M phosphate buffer, pH 2.0, prepared by transferring 3.9 mL of concentrated phosphoric acid and 5.73 g of monobasic sodium phosphate monohydrate to a 1-L volumetric flask, dissolving in and diluting with water to volume, and if necessary, adjusting with phosphoric acid to a pH of 2.0±0.02; 900 mL.

Apparatus 2: 50 rpm. Use stainless steel paddles only. Do not use paddles coated with polytetrafluoroethylene.

Time: 60 minutes.

Determine the amount of $C_{15}H_{14}N_4O$ dissolved by employing the following method.

Mobile phase, Diluent, and *Chromatographic system*—Proceed as directed in the *Assay*.

Stock standard solution 1—Transfer 27 mg, accurately weighed, of USP Nevirapine Anhydrous RS into a 500-mL volumetric flask. Add 50 mL of alcohol, followed by 250 mL of *Medium*. Sonicate for about 20 minutes to dissolve, allow to cool to room temperature, and dilute with *Medium* to volume.

Stock standard solution 2—Transfer 7 mg, accurately weighed, of USP Nevirapine Related Compound A RS into a 250-mL volumetric flask. Add about 2 mL of *Diluent,* sonicate until completely dissolved, and dilute with *Medium* to volume.

Standard solution—Transfer 25.0 mL of *Stock standard solution 1* into a 100-mL volumetric flask, dilute with *Medium* to volume, and mix well.

Resolution solution—Transfer 25.0 mL of *Stock standard solution 1* into a 50-mL volumetric flask, and dilute with *Medium* to volume. Transfer 25.0 mL of this solution into a 50-mL volumetric flask, dilute with *Stock standard solution 2* to volume, and mix well.

Test solution—Pass 20 mL of the solution under test through a nylon or glass fiber 0.45-μm filter, and dilute with *Medium* to obtain a solution having a final concentration of about 0.0135 mg of nevirapine per mL.

Procedure—Separately inject equal volumes (about 20 μL) of the *Standard solution* and the *Test solution* into the chromatograph, record the chromatograms, and measure the responses for the major peaks. Determine the amount of $C_{15}H_{14}N_4O$ dissolved by the formula:

$$\frac{r_U \times W_S \times D_S \times 900 \times 100}{r_S \times D_U \times LC}$$

in which r_U and r_S are the peak responses obtained from the *Test solution* and the *Standard solution*, respectively; W_S is the amount, in mg, of USP Nevirapine Anhydrous RS taken; D_S is the dilution factor for the *Standard solution;* 900 is the volume, in mL, of *Medium;* 100 is the conversion factor to percentage; D_U is the dilution factor for the *Test solution;* and LC is the Tablet label claim in mg.

Tolerances—Not less than 75% (Q) of the labeled amount of $C_{15}H_{14}N_4O$ is dissolved in 60 minutes.

Uniformity of dosage units ⟨905⟩: meet the requirements.

Chromatographic purity—

Mobile phase, Diluent, Resolution solution, Stock standard solution 1, and *Stock standard solution 2*—Proceed as directed in the *Assay*.

Standard solution—Quantitatively dilute *Stock standard solution 1* with *Diluent* to obtain a solution having a known concentration of about 0.125 μg of nevirapine per mL.

Test solution—Use the *Assay preparation,* as obtained in the *Assay*.

Chromatographic system (see *Chromatography* ⟨621⟩)—Proceed as directed in the *Assay* except that the relative standard deviation for replicate injections of the *Standard solution* is not more than 5.0%.

Procedure—Separately inject equal volumes (about 20 μL) of the *Standard solution* and the *Test solution* into the chromatograph, record the chromatograms for at least 13 minutes, and measure the peak responses. Calculate the percentage of each impurity/degradation product in the portion of Tablets taken by the formula:

$$8000(C/W)(A/L)(r_i / r_S)(100)$$

in which C is the concentration, in mg per mL, of USP Nevirapine Anhydrous RS in the *Standard solution;* W is the weight, in mg, of powdered Tablets taken to prepare the *Test solution;* A is the average weight of each Tablet, in mg; L is the labeled amount, in mg, of nevirapine in each Tablet; r_i is the peak response obtained for each impurity/degradation product in the *Test solution;* and r_S is the peak response for nevirapine in the *Standard solution*. Disregard all peaks due to the solvent or excipients and impurity peaks less than 0.1%. Not more than 0.1% of any individual unknown impurity/degradation product is found; and not more than 0.2% of total unknown impurities/degradation products is found.

Assay—

Mobile phase—Prepare a filtered and degassed mixture of water and acetonitrile (77 : 23). Make adjustments if necessary (see *System Suitability* under *Chromatography* ⟨621⟩).

Diluent—Prepare a mixture of dehydrated alcohol and water (1 : 1).

Stock standard solution 1—Transfer about 25 mg of USP Nevirapine Anhydrous RS, accurately weighed, into a 250-mL volumetric flask, and dissolve in and dilute with *Diluent* to volume.

Stock standard solution 2—Transfer about 5 mg of USP Nevirapine Related Compound A RS, accurately weighed, into a 50-mL volumetric flask, and dissolve in and dilute with *Diluent* to volume.

Standard preparation—Transfer 25.0 mL of *Stock standard solution 1* into a 100-mL volumetric flask, and dilute with *Diluent* to volume. The final concentration is about 0.025 mg of nevirapine per mL.

Resolution solution—Transfer 25.0 mL of *Stock standard solution 1* and 25.0 mL of *Stock standard solution 2* into a 100-mL volumetric flask, dilute with *Diluent* to volume, and mix well.

Assay preparation—Weigh and finely powder not fewer than 20 Tablets. Transfer an accurately weighed portion of the powder, equivalent to 200 mg of nevirapine into a 200-mL volumetric flask, and add about 150 mL of *Diluent*. Sonicate the solution for about 20 minutes, and then shake for about 20 minutes. Cool to room temperature, dilute with *Diluent* to volume, and mix. Centrifuge a portion of the resulting solution at about 1500 rpm for about 5 minutes. Transfer 5.0 mL of the supernatant into a 200-mL volumetric flask, and dilute with *Diluent* to volume. Filter, and discard the first 2 mL of the filtrate.

Chromatographic system (see *Chromatography* ⟨621⟩)—The liquid chromatograph is equipped with a 214-nm detector and a 3.9-mm × 15-cm column containing L1 packing. The column is maintained at ambient temperature. The flow rate is about 1.0 mL per minute. Chromatograph the *Resolution solution* (about 20 μL), and record the peak responses as directed for *Procedure:* the resolution, R, between nevirapine and nevirapine related compound A is not less than 3.0. Chromatograph the *Standard preparation,* and record the peak responses as directed for *Procedure:* the relative standard deviation for replicate injections of the *Standard preparation* is not more than 2.0%.

Procedure—Separately inject equal volumes (about 20 μL) of the *Standard preparation* and the *Assay preparation* into the chromatograph, record the chromatograms, and measure the responses for the nevirapine peak. Calculate the quantity, in mg, of nevirapine ($C_{15}H_{14}N_4O$) in the portion of Tablets taken by the formula:

$$8000C(r_U / r_S)$$

in which C is the concentration, in mg per mL, of USP Nevirapine Anhydrous RS in the *Standard preparation;* and r_U and r_S are the peak responses obtained from the *Assay preparation* and the *Standard preparation,* respectively.

Niacin

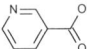

$C_6H_5NO_2$ 123.11
3-Pyridinecarboxylic acid.
Nicotinic acid   [59-67-6].

» Niacin contains not less than 99.0 percent and not more than 101.0 percent of $C_6H_5NO_2$, calculated on the dried basis.

Packaging and storage—Preserve in well-closed containers.
USP Reference standards ⟨11⟩—USP Niacin RS.
Identification—
  A: *Infrared Absorption* ⟨197M⟩.
  B: *Ultraviolet Absorption* ⟨197U⟩—
    Solution: 20 µg per mL.
    Medium: Use the *Buffer solution*, prepared as directed in the *Assay*.
    Ratio: A_{237}/A_{262}, between 0.46 and 0.50.
Loss on drying ⟨731⟩—Dry it at 105° for 1 hour: it loses not more than 1.0% of its weight.
Residue on ignition ⟨281⟩: not more than 0.1%.
Chloride ⟨221⟩—A 0.50-g portion shows no more chloride than corresponds to 0.15 mL of 0.020 N hydrochloric acid (0.02%).
Sulfate ⟨221⟩—A 0.50-g portion shows no more sulfate than corresponds to 0.10 mL of 0.020 N sulfuric acid (0.02%).
Heavy metals, *Method I* ⟨231⟩—Mix 1 g with 4 mL of 1 N acetic acid, dilute with water to 25 mL, heat gently until solution is complete, and cool: the limit is 0.002%.
Ordinary impurities ⟨466⟩—
  Test solution: water.
  Standard solution: water.
  Eluant: a mixture of methanol and 0.1 N hydrochloric acid (9 : 1).
  Visualization: 1.
Organic volatile impurities, *Method IV* ⟨467⟩: meets the requirements.

(Official until July 1, 2008)

Assay—
  Buffer solution—Dissolve 6.8 g of monobasic potassium phosphate in 1 L of water. Adjust with 50% sodium hydroxide solution to a pH of 7.0.
  Assay preparation—Transfer about 200 mg of Niacin, accurately weighed, to a 500-mL volumetric flask; add the *Buffer solution* to dissolve; dilute with the *Buffer solution* to volume; and mix. Transfer 5.0 mL of this solution to a 100-mL volumetric flask, dilute with the *Buffer solution* to volume, and mix.
  Procedure—Concomitantly determine the absorbances of the *Assay preparation* and a solution of USP Niacin RS in the same medium *(Standard preparation)*, at a concentration of about 20 µg per mL, in 1-cm cells at the wavelength of maximum absorbance at about 262 nm, with a suitable spectrophotometer, using the *Buffer solution* as the blank. Calculate the quantity, in mg, of $C_6H_5NO_2$ in the portion of Niacin taken by the formula:

$$10C(A_U/A_S)$$

in which C is the concentration, in µg per mL, of USP Niacin RS in the *Standard preparation*; and A_U and A_S are the absorbances of the solution of the *Assay preparation* and the *Standard preparation*, respectively.

Niacin Injection

» Niacin Injection is a sterile solution of Niacin and niacin sodium in Water for Injection, made with the aid of Sodium Carbonate or Sodium Hydroxide. It contains not less than 95.0 percent and not more than 110.0 percent of the labeled amount of $C_6H_5NO_2$.

Packaging and storage—Preserve in single-dose or in multiple-dose containers, preferably of Type I glass.
USP Reference standards ⟨11⟩—USP Endotoxin RS. USP Niacin RS.
Identification—To a volume of Injection, equivalent to about 100 mg of niacin, add 0.3 mL of 3 N hydrochloric acid, evaporate, if necessary, on a steam bath to about 2 mL, and allow to stand for 1 hour in a cool place. Filter by suction, wash with small volumes of ice-cold water until the last washing does not give a reaction for chloride, and dry at 105° for 1 hour: the niacin so obtained responds to *Identification* tests *A* and *B* under *Niacin*.
Bacterial endotoxins ⟨85⟩—It contains not more than 3.5 USP Endotoxin Units per mg of niacin.
pH ⟨791⟩: between 4.0 and 6.0.
Other requirements—It meets the requirements under *Injections* ⟨1⟩.
Assay—Proceed with Injection as directed for *Chemical Method* under *Niacin or Niacinamide Assay* ⟨441⟩, using *Standard Niacin Preparation* as the *Standard Preparation* in the *Assay Procedure*, and the following as the *Assay Preparation*. Transfer an accurately measured volume of Injection, equivalent to about 50 mg of niacin, to a 500-mL volumetric flask, dilute with water to volume, and mix. Transfer 10.0 mL of this solution to a 200-mL volumetric flask, dilute with water to volume, and mix. Calculate the quantity, in mg, of $C_6H_5NO_2$ in each mL of the Injection taken by the formula:

$$(50/V)(A_U/A_S)$$

in which V is the volume, in mL, of Injection taken.

Niacin Tablets

» Niacin Tablets contain not less than 90.0 percent and not more than 110.0 percent of the labeled amount of $C_6H_5NO_2$.

Packaging and storage—Preserve in well-closed containers.
USP Reference standards ⟨11⟩—USP Niacin RS.
Identification—
  A: Heat a quantity of finely powdered Tablets, equivalent to about 500 mg of niacin, with 25 mL of alcohol on a steam bath for a few minutes, filter, and wash the residue with a few mL of hot alcohol. To the filtrate add 30 mL of water, and evaporate to about 25 mL on the steam bath. Cool, filter if insoluble matter separates, and evaporate the filtrate to about 10 mL. Cool, and place in a refrigerator for 1 hour. Filter the separated niacin with suction, wash it with a few mL of cold alcohol, and dry at 105° for 1 hour: the niacin so obtained responds to *Identification* tests *A* and *B* under *Niacin*.
  B: The retention time of the major peak in the chromatogram of the *Assay preparation* corresponds to that in the chromatogram of the *Standard preparation* obtained as directed in the *Assay*.
Dissolution ⟨711⟩—
  Medium: 0.1 N hydrochloric acid; 900 mL.
  Apparatus 1: 100 rpm.
  Time: 60 minutes.
  Procedure—Determine the amount of $C_6H_5NO_2$ dissolved from UV absorbances at the wavelength of maximum absorbance at about 260 nm of filtered portions of the solution under test, suitably diluted with *Medium*, if necessary, in comparison with a Standard solution having a known concentration of about 0.02 mg of USP Niacin RS per mL in the same medium.
  Tolerances—Not less than 65% (*Q*) of the labeled amount of $C_6H_5NO_2$ is dissolved in 60 minutes.
Uniformity of dosage units ⟨905⟩: meet the requirements.
Assay—
  Mobile phase—Prepare a 0.005 M solution of sodium 1-hexanesulfonate in water. Mix 78 parts of this solution with 14 parts of

methanol, 7 parts of acetonitrile, and 1 part of glacial acetic acid, stir, filter, and degas. Make adjustments if necessary (see *System Suitability* under *Chromatography* ⟨621⟩).

Standard preparation—Transfer an accurately weighed quantity of USP Niacin RS to a suitable volumetric flask, add water, heat on a steam bath, sonicate, shake by mechanical means, cool, and dilute with water to volume to obtain a solution having a known concentration of about 0.5 mg per mL. Transfer 1.0 mL of this solution to a 10-mL volumetric flask, dilute with water to volume, and mix.

Assay preparation—Weigh and finely powder not less than 20 Tablets. Transfer an accurately weighed quantity of the powder equivalent to about 500 mg of Niacin to a 100-mL volumetric flask, add 50 mL of water, and heat on a steam bath for 30 minutes. Sonicate for 2 minutes, shake by mechanical means for 15 minutes, and cool to room temperature. Dilute with water to volume, mix, and filter. Transfer 1.0 mL of this solution to a 100-mL volumetric flask, dilute with water to volume, and mix.

Chromatographic system (see *Chromatography* ⟨621⟩)—The liquid chromatograph is equipped with a 262-nm detector and a 4-mm × 30-cm column that contains packing L1. The flow rate is about 1.3 mL per minute. Chromatograph replicate injections of the *Standard preparation*, and record the peak responses as directed for *Procedure*: the column efficiency determined from the analyte peak is not less than 1000 theoretical plates, the tailing factor for the analyte peak is not more than 2.0, and the relative standard deviation for replicate injections is not more than 2.0%.

Procedure—[NOTE—Use peak areas where peak responses are indicated.] Separately inject equal volumes (about 20 µL) of the *Standard preparation* and the *Assay preparation* into the chromatograph, record the chromatograms, and measure the responses for the major peaks. Calculate the quantity, in mg, of $C_6H_5NO_2$ in the portion of Tablets taken by the formula:

$$10{,}000C(r_U / r_S)$$

in which C is the concentration, in mg per mL, of USP Niacin RS in the *Standard preparation*, and r_U and r_S are the peak responses for niacin obtained from the *Assay preparation* and the *Standard preparation*, respectively.

Niacinamide

$C_6H_6N_2O$ 122.12
3-Pyridinecarboxamide.
Nicotinamide   [98-92-0].

» Niacinamide contains not less than 98.5 percent and not more than 101.5 percent of $C_6H_6N_2O$, calculated on the dried basis.

Packaging and storage—Preserve in tight containers.
USP Reference standards ⟨11⟩—*USP Niacinamide RS*.
Identification—
  A: *Infrared Absorption* ⟨197K⟩.
  B: *Ultraviolet Absorption* ⟨197U⟩—
    Solution: 20 µg per mL.
    Medium: water.
    Ratio: A_{245}/A_{262}, between 0.63 and 0.67.
Melting range ⟨741⟩:   between 128° and 131°.
Loss on drying ⟨731⟩—Dry it over silica gel for 4 hours: it loses not more than 0.5% of its weight.
Residue on ignition ⟨281⟩:   not more than 0.1%.
Heavy metals, *Method II* ⟨231⟩:   0.003%.
Readily carbonizable substances ⟨271⟩—Dissolve 200 mg in 5 mL of sulfuric acid TS: the solution has no more color than *Matching Fluid A*.
Organic volatile impurities, *Method I* ⟨467⟩:   meets the requirements.

(Official until July 1, 2008)

Assay—
Mobile phase—Prepare a filtered and degassed solution containing 0.005 M sodium 1-heptanesulfonate and methanol (70 : 30).

Standard preparation—Transfer about 50 mg of USP Niacinamide RS, accurately weighed, to a 100-mL volumetric flask, dissolve in about 3 mL of water, dilute with *Mobile phase* to volume, and mix. Dilute 4.0 mL of the resulting solution with *Mobile phase* to 50.0 mL, and mix.

Resolution solution—Prepare a solution containing equal volumes of the *Standard preparation* and of a niacin solution similarly prepared and having the same concentration.

Assay preparation—Prepare as directed under *Standard preparation*, using Niacinamide instead of the Reference Standard.

Chromatographic system (see *Chromatography* ⟨621⟩)—The liquid chromatograph is equipped with a 254-nm detector and a 3.9-mm × 30-cm column containing packing L1. The flow rate is about 2 mL per minute. Chromatograph the *Resolution solution*: the resolution, R, between the niacin and niacinamide peaks is not less than 3.0. Chromatograph replicate injections of the *Standard preparation*, and record the peak responses as directed for *Procedure*: the relative standard deviation is not more than 2.0%.

Procedure—Separately inject equal volumes (about 20 µL) of the *Standard preparation* and the *Assay preparation* into the chromatograph, record the chromatograms, and measure the responses for the major peaks. Calculate the quantity, in mg, of $C_6H_6N_2O$ in the portion of Niacinamide taken by the formula:

$$1250C(r_U / r_S)$$

in which C is the concentration, in mg per mL, of USP Niacinamide RS in the *Standard preparation*, and r_U and r_S are the peak responses for the *Assay preparation* and the *Standard preparation*, respectively.

Niacinamide Injection

» Niacinamide Injection is a sterile solution of Niacinamide in Water for Injection. It contains not less than 95.0 percent and not more than 110.0 percent of the labeled amount of $C_6H_6N_2O$.

Packaging and storage—Preserve in single-dose or in multiple-dose containers, preferably of Type I glass.
USP Reference standards ⟨11⟩—*USP Niacinamide RS. USP Endotoxin RS*.
Identification—Dilute a quantity of the Injection, equivalent to about 200 mg of niacinamide, with water to about 10 mL. Add 1 mL of 2.5 N sodium hydroxide, evaporate on a steam bath to dryness, add 5 mL of water, and similarly evaporate to about 1 mL: during the initial evaporation, the odor of ammonia is perceptible. Neutralize to litmus paper with 3 N hydrochloric acid, add 1 mL of the acid in excess, and place the solution in a refrigerator for 2 hours. Then filter, wash the precipitated niacin with small portions of ice-cold water until free from chloride, and dry at 105° for 1 hour: the IR absorption spectrum of a potassium bromide dispersion of the residue so obtained exhibits maxima only at the same wavelengths as that of a similar preparation of USP Niacinamide RS.
Bacterial endotoxins ⟨85⟩—It contains not more than 3.5 USP Endotoxin Units per mg of niacinamide.
pH ⟨791⟩:   between 5.0 and 7.0.
Other requirements—It meets the requirements under *Injections* ⟨1⟩.
Assay—Proceed with Injection as directed for *Chemical Method* under *Niacin or Niacinamide Assay* ⟨441⟩, using *Standard Niacinamide Preparation* as the *Standard Preparation* in the *Assay Procedure*, and the following as the *Assay Preparation*. Dilute an accurately measured volume of Injection, equivalent to about 50 mg of niacinamide, with water to 500 mL in a volumetric flask, and mix. Pipet 10 mL of the solution into a 100-mL volumetric flask,

Niacinamide Tablets

» Niacinamide Tablets contain not less than 90.0 percent and not more than 110.0 percent of the labeled amount of $C_6H_6N_2O$.

Packaging and storage—Preserve in tight containers.
USP Reference standards ⟨11⟩—*USP Niacinamide RS*.
Identification—
 A: Extract a quantity of powdered Tablets, equivalent to about 500 mg of niacinamide, with two 10-mL portions of alcohol, evaporate the filtered alcohol extracts on a steam bath, and dry at 80° for 2 hours: the IR absorption spectrum of a potassium bromide dispersion of the residue so obtained exhibits maxima only at the same wavelengths as that of a similar preparation of USP Niacinamide RS.
 B: From the niacinamide obtained in *Identification* test A, prepare a solution (1 in 50,000), and determine the absorbance of this solution in a 1-cm cell at 245 nm and at 262 nm, with a suitable spectrophotometer, using water as the blank: the ratio A_{245}/A_{262} is between 0.63 and 0.67.

Dissolution, *Procedure for a Pooled Sample* ⟨711⟩—
 Medium: water; 900 mL.
 Apparatus 2: 50 rpm.
 Time: 45 minutes.
 Procedure—Determine the amount of $C_6H_6N_2O$ dissolved, employing the procedure set forth in the *Assay for niacin or niacinamide, pyridoxine hydrochloride, riboflavin, and thiamine* under *Water-soluble Vitamins Tablets*, using filtered portions of the solution under test, suitably diluted with *Dissolution Medium*, if necessary, in comparison with a Standard solution having a known concentration of USP Niacinamide RS in the same medium.
 Tolerances—Not less than 75% (*Q*) of the labeled amount of $C_6H_6N_2O$ is dissolved in 45 minutes.

Uniformity of dosage units ⟨905⟩: meet the requirements.
Assay—Proceed with Tablets as directed for *Chemical Method* under *Niacin or Niacinamide Assay* ⟨441⟩, using *Standard Niacinamide Preparation* as the *Standard Preparation* in the *Assay Procedure*: and the following as the *Assay Preparation*. Weigh and finely powder not less than 10 Tablets. Weigh accurately a quantity of the powder, equivalent to about 25 mg of niacinamide, and transfer with the aid of about 50 mL of water to a 250-mL volumetric flask. Heat, if necessary, until no more dissolves, cool, dilute with water to volume, and mix. Pipet 10 mL of the solution into a 100-mL volumetric flask, dilute with water to volume, and mix. Calculate the quantity, in mg, of $C_6H_6N_2O$ in the portion of Tablets taken by the formula:

$$25(A_U/A_S).$$

Nicotine

$C_{10}H_{14}N_2$ 162.23
3-(1-Methyl-2-pyrrolidinyl)pyridine.
β-Pyridyl-α-*N*-methyl pyrrolidine   [54-11-5].

» Nicotine contains not less than 99.0 percent and not more than 101.0 percent of $C_{10}H_{14}N_2$, calculated on the anhydrous basis.

Packaging and storage—Store under nitrogen in well-closed containers below 25°, protected from light and moisture.
USP Reference standards ⟨11⟩—*USP Nicotine Bitartrate Dihydrate RS*.
Identification, *Ultraviolet Absorption* ⟨197U⟩—
 Solutions—Prepare a solution of Nicotine in water having a concentration of about 1 mg per mL. Transfer 1.0 mL of this solution to a 50-mL volumetric flask, dilute with 0.1 N hydrochloric acid to volume, and mix to obtain the test solution. Transfer an amount of USP Nicotine Bitartrate Dihydrate RS, equivalent to about 50 mg of nicotine, to a 25-mL glass-stoppered tube. Add 5 mL of 6 N ammonium hydroxide, 2 mL of 1 N sodium hydroxide, and 20 mL of *n*-hexane. Shake for 5 minutes, allow the phases to separate, transfer the upper *n*-hexane layer to a vial, and evaporate with a stream of nitrogen gas. [NOTE—Avoid excessive drying to prevent loss of nicotine.] Dissolve the residue of the nicotine so obtained in water to obtain a solution having a concentration of about 1 mg per mL. Dilute 1.0 mL of this solution with 0.1 N hydrochloric acid to 50.0 mL, and mix to obtain the Standard solution.

Specific rotation ⟨781S⟩: between −130° and −143°.
 Test solution: 20 mg per mL, in alcohol.
Water, *Method I* ⟨921⟩: not more than 0.5%.
Heavy metals, *Method II* ⟨231⟩: not more than 0.002%.
Chromatographic purity—
 Test solution—Dissolve about 0.13 g of Nicotine, accurately weighed, in dichloromethane, dilute with dichloromethane to 25.0 mL, and mix.
 Reference solutions—Dilute accurately measured volumes of the *Test solution* quantitatively, and stepwise if necessary, with dichloromethane to obtain *Reference solution A* and *Reference solution B* having concentrations of about 26 µg per mL and 52 µg per mL, respectively.
 Chromatographic system (see *Chromatography* ⟨621⟩)—The gas chromatograph is equipped with a flame-ionization detector maintained at 270° and a 0.53-mm × 30-m fused silica column bonded with a 1.5-µm layer of phase G1. Helium is used as the carrier gas at a flow rate of 20 mL per minute. The column temperature is maintained at 50° for 6 seconds, then programmed to rise from 50° to 250° at 6° per minute, and finally held isothermally at 250° for 3 minutes.
 Procedure—Separately inject equal volumes (about 1 µL) of the *Test solution*, *Reference solution A*, and *Reference solution B* into the chromatograph, and allow the *Test solution* to elute for not less than 2.5 times the retention time of nicotine. Record the chromatograms, and measure all of the peak responses. The sum of the peak responses, excluding that of nicotine, from the *Test solution* is not more than that of the nicotine response from *Reference solution B* (1.0%), and no single peak response is greater than that of the nicotine response from *Reference solution A* (0.5%).

Assay—Dissolve about 60 mg of Nicotine, accurately weighed, in 40 mL of glacial acetic acid, and titrate with 0.1 N perchloric acid VS, determining the endpoint potentiometrically (see *Titrimetry* ⟨541⟩). Perform a blank determination, and make any necessary correction. Each mL of 0.1 N perchloric acid is equivalent to 8.11 mg of $C_{10}H_{14}N_2$.

Nicotine Transdermal System

» Nicotine Transdermal System contains not less than 90.0 percent and not more than 110.0 percent of the labeled amount of nicotine ($C_{10}H_{14}N_2$).

Packaging and storage—Preserve in the hermetic, light-resistant, unit-dose pouch.
Labeling—The labeling indicates the *Drug Release Test* with which the product complies.

---

dilute with water to volume, and mix. Calculate the quantity, in mg, of $C_6H_6N_2O$ in each mL of the Injection taken by the formula:

$$(50/V)(A_U/A_S)$$

in which *V* is the volume, in mL, of Injection taken.

USP Reference standards ⟨11⟩—USP Nicotine Bitartrate Dihydrate RS.

Identification—The retention time of the major peak in the chromatogram of the *Assay preparation* corresponds to that in the chromatogram of the *Standard preparation*, as obtained in the *Assay*.

Drug release ⟨724⟩—

TEST 1—If the product complies with this test, the labeling indicates that it meets USP *Drug Release Test 1*.

Medium: Phosphoric acid solution (1 in 1000); 250 mL, in a tall-form beaker.

Apparatus 7—Proceed as directed in the chapter, using the transdermal system holder–cylinder (see *Figure 4b*). Center the Transdermal System onto a dry, unused 10-cm × 10-cm piece of Cuprophan dialysis membrane with the adhesive side against the membrane, taking care to eliminate air bubbles between the membrane and the release surface. Attach the membrane to the cylinder using two Parker O-rings, such that one of the borders of the transdermal system is aligned to the groove and it is wrapped around the cylinder. The filled beakers are weighed and pre-equilibrated to 32.0 ± 0.3°, prior to immersing the test sample. Reciprocate at a frequency of about 30 cycles per minute with an amplitude of 2.0 ± 0.1 cm. At the end of each time interval, transfer the test sample to a fresh beaker containing the appropriate volume of *Medium*, weighed and pre-equilibrated to 32.0 ± 0.3°. At the end of each release interval, allow the beakers to cool to room temperature, make up for evaporative losses by adding water to obtain the original weight, and mix. This solution is the final *Test solution*.

Times: 2, 12, and 24 hours.

Determine the amount of $C_{10}H_{14}N_2$ released by employing the following method.

Mobile phase—Transfer 0.2 mL of N,N-dimethyloctylamine to a 1-L volumetric flask, add 220 mL of acetonitrile, and mix. Add 300 mL of water, 0.2 mL of glacial acetic acid, 0.20 g of anhydrous sodium acetate, and 0.55 g of sodium 1-dodecanesulfonate, and dilute with water to volume. Mix for 1 hour until clear. Filter and degas. Make adjustments if necessary (see *System Suitability* under *Chromatography* ⟨621⟩). [NOTE—Equilibration of the column may take as long as 3 hours.]

Standard solution—Dissolve an accurately weighed quantity of USP Nicotine Bitartrate Dihydrate RS in *Medium*, and dilute quantitatively, and stepwise if necessary, with *Medium* to obtain a solution having a known concentration of about 0.142 mg of nicotine bitartrate per mL (or 0.046 mg nicotine as free base per mL). [NOTE—About 80 mL of this solution is required in order to prepare the *System suitability solution*.]

System suitability solution—Transfer 8 mg (free base) of nicotine to a 100-mL volumetric flask, and dissolve in 10 mL of acetonitrile. Add 5 mL of 30 percent hydrogen peroxide, and allow 15 minutes to react. Dilute with *Medium* to volume, and mix. Transfer 20 mL of this solution to a 100-mL volumetric flask, dilute with *Standard solution* to volume, and mix.

Chromatographic system (see *Chromatography* ⟨621⟩)—The liquid chromatograph is equipped with a 254-nm detector and a 4.6-mm × 15-cm column that contains packing L1. The flow rate is about 1 mL per minute. Chromatograph the *System suitability solution*, and record the peak responses as directed for *Procedure*: the resolution, R, between nicotine and any degradation peaks is not less than 1.1; the tailing factor is not more than 2.0; and the relative standard deviation for replicate injections is not more than 1.5%.

Procedure—Separately inject equal volumes (about 50 µL) of filtered portions of the *Standard solution* and the solution under test into the chromatograph, record the chromatograms, and measure the responses for the major peaks.

Tolerances—The amount of $C_{10}H_{14}N_2$ released, as a percentage of the labeled amount of the dose absorbed in vivo, at the times specified below, conforms to *Acceptance Table 1*.

Time (hours)	Amount dissolved
0–2	between 31% and 87%
2–12	between 62% and 191%
12–24	between 85% and 261%

TEST 2—If the product complies with this test, the labeling indicates that it meets USP *Drug Release Test 2*.

Phosphate buffer—Dissolve 40.0 g of sodium chloride, 1.0 g of potassium chloride, 8.66 g of dibasic sodium phosphate, and 1.0 g of monobasic potassium phosphate in 5 L of water.

Medium: Phosphate buffer; 500 mL.

Apparatus 6: 50 rpm, double-sided tape being used to attach the Transdermal System to the cylinder.

Times: 6 and 24 hours.

Determine the amount of $C_{10}H_{14}N_2$ released by employing the following method.

Mobile phase—Proceed as directed in the *Assay*.

System suitability solution—Transfer 1.0 mL of the *System suitability solution*, prepared as directed in the *Assay*, to a 100-mL volumetric flask, dilute with *Medium* to volume, and mix.

Standard solution—Pipet 6.0 mL of the *Standard preparation*, prepared as directed in the *Assay*, into a 50-mL volumetric flask, dilute with *Medium* to volume, and mix. Dilute quantitatively and stepwise with *Medium* to obtain an appropriate final concentration.

Test solution—At each of the test times, withdraw a 2-mL aliquot of the solution under test. [NOTE—Replace the aliquots withdrawn for analysis with fresh portions of *Medium*.]

Chromatographic system (see *Chromatography* ⟨621⟩)—The liquid chromatograph is equipped with a 260-nm detector and a 4.6-mm × 12.5-cm column that contains packing L1. The flow rate is about 1 mL per minute. Chromatograph the *Standard solution* used for the 6-hour interval, and record the peak responses as directed for *Procedure*: the resolution, R, between 4,4'-dipyridyl dihydrochloride and nicotine is not less than 5.0; the tailing factor is not more than 2.0; and the relative standard deviation for replicate injections is not more than 2.0%.

Procedure—Separately inject equal volumes (about 100 µL) of the filtered portion of the *Standard solution* and the *Test solution* into the chromatograph, record the chromatograms, and measure the responses for the major peaks.

Tolerances—The amount of $C_{10}H_{14}N_2$ released, as a percentage of the labeled amount of the dose absorbed in vivo, at the times specified, conforms to *Acceptance Table 1*.

Time (hours)	Amount dissolved
6	between 71% and 157%
24	between 156% and 224%

TEST 3—If the product complies with this test, the labeling indicates that it meets USP *Drug Release Test 3*.

Medium: water; 900 mL.

Apparatus 5: 50 rpm, the stainless steel disk assembly being replaced with a 5-cm watch glass for an 11-mg Transdermal System and an 8-cm watch glass for a 22-mg Transdermal System.

Times: 1, 2, and 4 hours.

Standard solution—Prepare a solution of USP Nicotine Bitartrate Dihydrate RS in water having a known concentration of nicotine similar to that of the solution under test.

Procedure—Determine the amount of $C_{10}H_{14}N_2$ released by employing UV absorption at the wavelength of maximum absorbance at about 259 nm, in comparison with the *Standard solution*, using water as the blank.

Tolerances—The amount of $C_{10}H_{14}N_2$ released, as a percentage of the labeled amount of the dose absorbed in vivo, at the times specified, conforms to the following *Acceptance Table*.

Time (hours)	Amount dissolved
1	between 35% and 75%
2	between 55% and 95%
4	not less than 73%

Acceptance Table

Level	Tested	Criteria
L_1	6	No individual value lies outside each of the stated ranges and no individual value is less than the stated amount at the final test time.
L_2	6	The average value of the 12 units ($L_1 + L_2$) lies within each of the stated ranges and is not less than the stated amount at the final test time; none is more than 5% of the labeled content outside each of the stated ranges; and none is more than 5% of the labeled content below the stated amount at the final test time.
L_3	12	The average value of the 24 units ($L_1 + L_2 + L_3$) lies within each of the stated ranges and is not less than the stated amount at the final test time; not more than 2 of the 24 units are more than 5% of labeled content outside each of the stated ranges; not more than 2 of the 24 units are more than 5% of the labeled content below the stated amount at the final test time; and none of the units is more than 10% of the labeled content outside each of the stated ranges or more than 10% of the labeled content below the stated amount at the final test time.

TEST 4—If the product complies with this test, the labeling indicates that it meets USP *Drug Release Test 4*.
Medium: 0.025 N hydrochloric acid; 600 mL.
Apparatus 5: 50 rpm, a convex screen being used to hold the Transdermal System in position during testing.
Times: 4 and 16 hours.
Standard solution and *Procedure*—Proceed as directed under *Test 3*.
Tolerances—The amount of $C_{10}H_{14}N_2$ released, as a percentage of the labeled amount of the dose absorbed in vivo, at the times specified, conforms to *Acceptance Table 1*.

Time (hours)	Amount dissolved
4	between 36% and 66%
16	between 72% and 112%

TEST 5—If the product complies with this test, the labeling indicates that it meets USP *Drug Release Test 5*.
Phosphate buffer, Medium, and *Apparatus*—Proceed as directed under *Test 2*.
Times: 3, 6, and 24 hours.
Mobile phase—Proceed as directed in the *Assay*.
System suitability solution, Standard solution, Test solution, and *Chromatographic system*—Proceed as directed under *Test 2*.
Procedure—Proceed as directed under *Test 2* except to inject about 30 μL.
Tolerances—The amount of $C_{10}H_{14}N_2$ released, as a percentage of the labeled amount of the dose absorbed in vivo, at the times specified, conforms to *Acceptance Table 1*.

Time (hours)	Amount dissolved
3	between 79% and 112%
6	between 108% and 141%
24	between 156% and 202%

Uniformity of dosage units ⟨905⟩: meets the requirements.
Assay—
Mobile phase—Mix 300 mL of acetonitrile, 700 mL of water, and 1 mL of triethylamine, filter, and degas. Make adjustments if necessary (see *System Suitability* under *Chromatography* ⟨621⟩).
Standard preparation—Dissolve an accurately weighed quantity of USP Nicotine Bitartrate Dihydrate RS in water to obtain a stock solution having a known concentration of about 26.87 mg per mL. Quantitatively dilute a volume of the stock solution with methanol to obtain a solution having a known concentration of about 5.37 mg of USP Nicotine Bitartrate Dihydrate RS per mL. [NOTE—This solution contains 1.75 mg of nicotine per mL.]
System suitability solution—Transfer an accurately weighed quantity of about 12.5 mg of 4,4′-dipyridyl dihydrochloride to a 25-mL volumetric flask, add 5.0 mL of the *Standard preparation*, dilute with methanol to volume, and mix.
Assay preparation—Cut an accurately counted number of Transdermal Systems, equivalent to about 175 mg of nicotine, into strips 5 cm² in area. Remove the protective liners, if any, from the strips, and discard. Transfer the strips to a 250-mL flask, and add 100.0 mL of methanol. Insert the stopper into the flask, and shake by mechanical means for about 3 hours. Filter, and use the clear filtrate as the *Assay preparation*.
Chromatographic system (see *Chromatography* ⟨621⟩)—The liquid chromatograph is equipped with a 260-nm detector and a 4.6-mm × 25-cm column containing packing L1. The flow rate is about 1.5 mL per minute. Chromatograph the *System suitability solution*, and record the peak responses as directed for *Procedure*: the resolution, *R*, between nicotine and 4,4′-dipyridyl dihydrochloride is not less than 5.0. Chromatograph the *Standard preparation*, and record the peak responses as directed for *Procedure*: the relative standard deviation for replicate injections is not more than 1.0%.
Procedure—Separately inject equal volumes (about 10 μL) of the *Standard preparation* and the *Assay preparation* into the chromatograph, record the chromatograms, and measure the areas for the major peaks. Calculate the quantity, in mg, of nicotine ($C_{10}H_{14}N_2$) in each Transdermal System taken by the formula:

$$(162.23/462.41)(100C/N)(r_U / r_S)$$

in which 162.23 and 462.41 are the molecular weights of nicotine and anhydrous nicotine bitartrate, respectively; *C* is the concentration, in mg per mL, of USP Nicotine Bitartrate Dihydrate RS in the *Standard preparation*; *N* is the number of Nicotine Transdermal Systems taken for the *Assay preparation*; and r_U and r_S are the nicotine peak responses obtained from the *Assay preparation* and the *Standard preparation*, respectively.

Nicotine Polacrilex

» Nicotine Polacrilex is a weak carboxylic cation-exchange resin prepared from methacrylic acid and divinylbenzene, in complex with nicotine. It contains not less than 95.0 percent and not more than 115.0 percent of the labeled amount of nicotine ($C_{10}H_{14}N_2$), calculated on the anhydrous basis.

Packaging and storage—Preserve in tight containers.
USP Reference standards ⟨11⟩—*USP Nicotine Bitartrate Dihydrate RS. USP Polacrilex Resin RS.*
Identification:
A: *Infrared Absorption* ⟨197K⟩—
Test specimen—Transfer an accurately weighed quantity of Nicotine Polacrilex, equivalent to about 100 mg of nicotine, to a 100-mL glass-stoppered tube. Add 20 mL of 1 M ammonium hydroxide, 5 mL of 10 M sodium hydroxide, and 20 mL of *n*-hexane. Shake for 5

minutes, and allow the phases to separate. Transfer the upper hexane phase to an evaporating dish, and evaporate on a steam bath.

Standard specimen—Use USP Nicotine Bitartrate Dihydrate RS, and proceed as directed for *Test specimen*.

B: *Infrared Absorption* ⟨197K⟩—

Test specimen—Use the residue obtained from the *Assay preparation*. Decant the ammonia solution remaining in each residue, and wash the residue by shaking it with three 10-mL volumes of water, decanting the water phase after each shaking. Wash with 10 mL of 0.1 N hydrochloric acid, decant the liquid, and dry the residue at about 105°.

Standard specimen—Transfer an accurately weighed portion of USP Polacrilex Resin RS, equivalent to the amount of nicotine polacrilex in the *Assay preparation*, to a glass-stoppered tube. Add 10 mL of 1 M ammonium hydroxide. Proceed as directed for *Test specimen*, beginning with "Decant the ammonia".

Nicotine release—Transfer an accurately weighed quantity of Nicotine Polacrilex, equivalent to about 4 mg of nicotine, to a glass-stoppered test tube, add 10.0 mL of sodium chloride solution (0.9 in 100) that has been warmed to 37°, and shake by mechanical means for 10 minutes. Immediately pass the liquid through a dry filter paper, discarding the first mL of the filtrate. Transfer 1.0 mL of the filtrate to a 25-mL volumetric flask, dilute with 0.1 N hydrochloric acid to volume, and mix. Determine the absorbances of the solution in a 1-cm cell at 236 nm and 282 nm and at the wavelength of maximum absorbance at about 259 nm, using 1.0 mL of sodium chloride solution (0.9 in 100) diluted to 25 mL with 0.1 N hydrochloric acid as the blank. Calculate the percentage of nicotine released by the formula:

$$(77400 / CW)(A_{259} - 0.5A_{236} - 0.5A_{282})$$

in which 77400 is a specific absorbance and dilution factor; C is the percentage of nicotine in the Nicotine Polacrilex on the basis of the amount determined in the *Assay*; W is the weight, in mg, of the Nicotine Polacrilex taken; and A_{259}, A_{236}, and A_{282} are the absorbances of the solution under test, corrected for the blank absorbances, at the wavelengths indicated by the subscripts: not less than 70% is released in 10 minutes.

Water, *Method I* ⟨921⟩—Transfer about 1.0 g of Nicotine Polacrilex, accurately weighed, to a 50-mL glass-stoppered test tube, add 20.0 mL of methanol, shake for 30 minutes, and allow to stand for about 30 minutes. Use a 10-mL portion of the methanol layer for the titration: not more than 5.0% is found.

Chromatographic purity—

Mobile phase and *Chromatographic system*—Proceed as directed in the *Assay*.

Standard solution—Transfer 1.0 mL of the *Standard preparation*, prepared as directed in the *Assay*, to a 100-mL volumetric flask, dilute with *Mobile phase* to volume, and mix.

Test solution—Use the *Assay preparation*.

Procedure—[NOTE—Use peak areas where peak responses are indicated.] Separately inject equal volumes (about 20 µL) of the *Standard solution* and the *Test solution* into the chromatograph, and allow the chromatograms to run for not less than two times the retention time of the major peak. Record the chromatograms, and measure the peak responses. Calculate the percentage of each impurity in the portion of Nicotine Polacrilex taken by the formula:

$$(162.23/462.41)(100/3)(100C / W)(r_i / r_S)$$

in which 162.23 and 462.41 are the molecular weights of nicotine and anhydrous nicotine bitartrate, respectively, C is the concentration, in mg per mL, of USP Nicotine Bitartrate Dihydrate RS on the anhydrous basis in the *Standard solution*, W is the weight, in mg, of nicotine in the Nicotine Polacrilex taken, and r_i and r_S are peak responses for the individual impurity and nicotine bitartrate dihydrate obtained from the *Test solution* and the *Standard solution*, respectively: not more than 0.3% of any individual impurity is found, and the sum of all impurities is not more than 1.0%.

Assay—

0.25 M Sodium dodecyl sulfate—Dissolve 18.02 g of sodium dodecyl sulfate in 25 mL of glacial acetic acid and sufficient water to make 250 mL, and mix.

Mobile phase—Mix 640 mL of water, 50 mL of 1 M sodium acetate, and 40 mL of *0.25 M Sodium dodecyl sulfate*, and filter. Add 270 mL of acetonitrile, mix, and degas. Adjust the amount of water if necessary (see *System Suitability* under *Chromatography* ⟨621⟩).

Standard preparation—Dissolve an accurately weighed quantity of USP Nicotine Bitartrate Dihydrate RS in 1 M ammonium hydroxide to obtain a solution having a known concentration of about 6 mg per mL. Transfer 3.0 mL of this solution to a 10-mL volumetric flask, add 3 mL of 1 M acetic acid, dilute with water to volume, and mix.

Assay preparation—Transfer an accurately weighed quantity of Nicotine Polacrilex, equivalent to about 20 mg of nicotine, to a glass-stoppered test tube. Add 10.0 mL of 1 M ammonium hydroxide, shake for 10 minutes, and centrifuge. Transfer 3.0 mL of the clear solution to a 10-mL volumetric flask, add 3 mL of 1 M acetic acid, and dilute with water to volume. [NOTE—Retain the resin residue from centrifugation for use in *Identification* test B.]

Chromatographic system (see *Chromatography* ⟨621⟩)—The liquid chromatograph is equipped with a 254-nm detector and a 3.9-mm × 30-cm column containing packing L1. The flow rate is about 2.0 mL per minute. Chromatograph the *Standard preparation*, and record the peak responses as directed for *Procedure*: the tailing factor is not more than 2.0; and the relative standard deviation for replicate injections is not more than 2.0%.

Procedure—Separately inject equal volumes (about 20 µL) of the *Standard preparation* and the *Assay preparation* into the chromatograph, record the chromatograms, and measure the areas of the major peaks. Calculate the percentage of nicotine ($C_{10}H_{14}N_2$) in the portion of Nicotine Polacrilex taken by the formula:

$$100(162.23 / 462.41)(100C / 3W)(r_U / r_S)$$

in which 162.23 and 462.41 are the molecular weights of nicotine and anhydrous nicotine bitartrate, respectively; C is the concentration, in mg per mL, of USP Nicotine Bitartrate Dihydrate RS on the anhydrous basis in the *Standard preparation;* W is the weight, in mg, of the portion of Nicotine Polacrilex taken; and r_U and r_S are the peak areas obtained from the *Assay preparation* and the *Standard preparation*, respectively.

Nicotine Polacrilex Gum

» Nicotine Polacrilex Gum contains an amount of Nicotine Polacrilex $[(C_4H_6O_2)_x(C_{10}H_{10})_y](C_{10}H_{14}N_2)$ equivalent to not less than 90 percent and not more than 120 percent of the labeled amount of nicotine ($C_{10}H_{14}N_2$).

USP Reference standards ⟨11⟩—*USP Nicotine Bitartrate Dihydrate RS. USP Polacrilex Resin RS.*

Identification—

A: *Developing solvent*—Prepare a mixture of chloroform, acetone, and diethylamine (40 : 5 : 5).

Test solution—Cut several pieces of Gum into small pieces with scissors, and weigh. Transfer a portion of the Gum, equivalent to about 4 mg of nicotine, to a centrifuge tube. Add 5 mL of chloroform, sonicate for about 30 minutes to dissolve the nicotine, and centrifuge for about 10 minutes. Cool to about 15°, and add two 3-mL portions of 0.5 N hydrochloric acid with gentle mixing, and release excess pressure if necessary. Mix the contents of the tube by shaking, and centrifuge the mixture for about 10 minutes. Transfer 5 mL of the upper aqueous layer to a separatory funnel, and adjust with 0.5 N sodium hydroxide solution to a pH greater than 10.0. Add 3 mL of chloroform, and shake gently. Use the chloroform layer as the *Test solution*.

Standard solution—Transfer 10 mg of USP Nicotine Bitartrate Dihydrate RS to a separatory funnel, add 10 mL of water, and mix to dissolve. Adjust with 0.5 N sodium hydroxide to a pH greater than 10.0. Add 3 mL of chloroform, with gentle shaking, and use the chloroform layer as the *Standard solution*.

Procedure—Separately apply 10 µL each of the *Test solution* and the *Standard solution* about 1.5 cm from the lower edge of a thin-layer chromatographic plate (see *Chromatography* ⟨621⟩). Air-dry, place the plate in a chromatographic tank that has been saturated with *Developing solvent*, and develop the chromatogram until the solvent front has moved about 7 cm. Remove the plate from the chamber, and allow to air-dry. Examine the plate under short-wavelength UV light: the R_F value of the principal spot obtained from the *Test solution* corresponds to that obtained from the *Standard solution* (*presence of nicotine*).

B: *Infrared Absorption* ⟨197K⟩—Use USP Polacrilex Resin RS and a test specimen prepared as follows. Cut a piece of Gum into small pieces with scissors. Place the pieces in a 50-mL centrifuge tube, add about 20 mL of *n*-hexane, and place in an ultrasonic bath for about 30 minutes. Centrifuge at about 2500 rpm for about 5 minutes. Decant the hexane phase, and add 10 mL of 2 N hydrochloric acid. Shake the tube carefully, and open the stopper slightly to relieve any excess pressure. Add 10 mL of alcohol, and shake the tube carefully with the stopper slightly open. Centrifuge again as described above, and decant the liquid, taking care to avoid contamination of the precipitate with the gum material. Add 1 mL to 3 mL of water, mix gently to resuspend the precipitate, and filter. Wash the residue on the filter with water and then with alcohol. Dry the filter and residue at about 105° for 1 hour (*presence of polacrilex*).

Uniformity of dosage units ⟨905⟩: meets the requirements.

Assay—

Acetate buffer—Prepare a mixture containing 13.6 g of sodium acetate and 57.2 mL of glacial acetic acid in 1000 mL of water.

Solvent—Prepare a mixture of water, acetonitrile, 0.25 M sodium 1-decanesulfonate, and *Acetate buffer* (785 : 150 : 40 : 25).

Mobile phase—Prepare a mixture containing water, acetonitrile, *Acetate buffer*, and 0.25 M sodium 1-decanesulfonate (685 : 200 : 75 : 40).

Standard preparation—Dissolve an accurately weighed quantity of USP Nicotine Bitartrate Dihydrate RS in *Solvent* to obtain a *Standard stock solution* having a known concentration of about 1.25 mg per mL. Dilute a volume of this solution quantitatively with *Solvent* to obtain a *Standard preparation* having a known concentration of about 125 µg per mL (40 µg of nicotine per mL).

Assay preparation—Place one piece of Gum, accurately weighed, in a stoppered flask, add about 50 mL of *n*-hexane, and transfer 50.0 mL of *Solvent*. Add a stirring bar, insert the stopper in the flask, and stir vigorously for about 30 minutes or until the test specimen has been dispersed. Remove from the stirring mechanism, and allow to stand for about 30 minutes or until the phases have separated. Remove an aliquot of the lower layer, taking care not to remove a large quantity of the insoluble excipients, and filter, discarding the first few mL of the filtrate. Use the clear filtrate as the *Assay preparation*.

Chromatographic system (see *Chromatography* ⟨621⟩)—The liquid chromatograph is equipped with a 254-nm detector and a 4-mm × 30-cm stainless steel column containing packing L1. The flow rate is about 1.5 mL per minute. Chromatograph the *Standard preparation*, record the chromatograms, and measure the peak responses as directed for *Procedure*: the column efficiency is not less than 2500 theoretical plates, the tailing factor is not more than 2.0, and the relative standard deviation for replicate injections is not more than 2.0%.

Procedure—[NOTE—Perform the following procedure on 10 individual pieces of Gum, and use the average of the calculated values as the assay value. Use peak areas where peak responses are indicated.] Separately inject equal volumes (about 50 µL) of the *Standard preparation* and the *Assay preparation* into the chromatograph, record the chromatograms, and measure the peak responses. Calculate the quantity, in mg, of nicotine ($C_{10}H_{14}N_2$) in the Gum taken by the formula:

$$50C(162.23 / 462.41)(r_U / r_S)$$

in which C is the concentration, in mg per mL, of USP Nicotine Bitartrate Dihydrate RS on the anhydrous basis in the *Standard preparation*, 162.23 and 462.41 are the molecular weights of nicotine and anhydrous nicotine bitartrate, respectively, and r_U and r_S are peak responses obtained from the *Assay preparation* and the *Standard preparation*, respectively.

Nifedipine

$C_{17}H_{18}N_2O_6$ 346.33

3,5-Pyridinedicarboxylic acid, 1,4-dihydro-2,6-dimethyl-4-(2-nitrophenyl)-, dimethyl ester.
Dimethyl 1,4-dihydro-2,6-dimethyl-4-(*o*-nitrophenyl)-3,5-pyridinedicarboxylate [21829-25-4].

» Nifedipine contains not less than 98.0 percent and not more than 102.0 percent of $C_{17}H_{18}N_2O_6$, calculated on the dried basis.

Packaging and storage—Preserve in tight, light-resistant containers.

USP Reference standards ⟨11⟩—*USP Nifedipine RS. USP Nifedipine Nitrophenylpyridine Analog RS. USP Nifedipine Nitrosophenylpyridine Analog RS.*

NOTE—Nifedipine, when exposed to daylight and certain wavelengths of artificial light, readily converts to a nitrosophenylpyridine derivative. Exposure to UV light leads to the formation of a nitrophenylpyridine derivative. Perform assays and tests in the dark or under golden fluorescent or other low-actinic light. Use low-actinic glassware.

Identification—

A: *Infrared Absorption* ⟨197K⟩—Do not dry specimens.
B: *Ultraviolet Absorption* ⟨197U⟩—
Spectral range: 450 to 200 nm.
Solution—To a 10-mL volumetric flask containing 14 mg of Nifedipine add 1.0 mL of chloroform, dilute with methanol to volume, and mix. Pipet a 1.0-mL aliquot of the solution into a 100-mL volumetric flask, dilute with methanol to volume, and mix.
Medium: methanol.
C: The retention time of the major peak in the chromatogram of the *Assay preparation* corresponds to that in the chromatogram of the *Standard preparation*, as obtained in the *Assay*.

Melting range, *Class Ia* ⟨741⟩: between 171° and 175°.

Loss on drying ⟨731⟩—Dry it at 105° to constant weight: it loses not more than 0.5% of its weight.

Residue on ignition ⟨281⟩: not more than 0.1%, an ignition temperature of 600° being used.

Heavy metals, *Method II* ⟨231⟩: 0.001%.

Perchloric acid titration—Transfer about 4 g of Nifedipine, accurately weighed, to a 250-mL conical flask, and dissolve in 160 mL of glacial acetic acid with the aid of an ultrasonic bath. Add 3 drops of *p*-naphtholbenzein TS, and titrate to a green endpoint with 0.1 N perchloric acid VS: not more than 0.12 mL of 0.1 N perchloric acid is consumed for each g of Nifedipine.

Chloride and Sulfate—To 5.0 g of Nifedipine in a 140-mL beaker add 4.0 mL of 6 N acetic acid and 46 mL of water. Bring carefully to a boil on a hot plate, cool, and filter through paper free of chloride and sulfate. Use this Nifedipine filtrate for the following tests.

Chloride—Pipet 2.5 mL of the Nifedipine filtrate into a 50-mL color-comparison tube, and add 12.5 mL of water. Into a matched color-comparison tube pipet 10 mL of a Standard solution containing 8.2 µg of sodium chloride per mL corresponding to 5 µg of chloride per mL, add 5.0 mL of water, and mix. To each tube add 0.15 mL of 0.3 M nitric acid and 0.3 mL of silver nitrate TS, and mix: the opalescence exhibited by the Nifedipine filtrate does not exceed that of the Standard solution (0.02%).

Sulfate—Pipet into each of two 50-mL matched color-comparison tubes 1.5 mL of sulfate solution consisting of sufficient potassium sulfate dissolved in water to obtain a sulfate concentration of 10 µg per mL. To each tube add, successively and with continuous shaking, 0.75 mL of alcohol, 0.5 mL of a 6.1% aqueous solution of barium chloride, and 0.25 mL of 6 N acetic acid. Shake for an additional 30 seconds. Pipet into one tube, designated the

Standard tube, 15 mL of the sulfate solution. Pipet into the other tube, designated the Specimen tube, 3 mL of the Nifedipine filtrate and 12 mL of water: the turbidity exhibited by the Specimen tube does not exceed that of the Standard tube (0.05%).

Related compounds—[NOTE—Protect the *Standard nifedipine solution* and the *Test preparation* from actinic light. Conduct this test promptly after preparation of the *Standard nifedipine solution* and the *Test solution*.]

Mobile phase—Prepare as directed in the *Assay*.

Standard nifedipine solution—Dissolve an accurately weighed quantity of USP Nifedipine RS in methanol (about 1 mg per mL), and dilute quantitatively with *Mobile phase* to obtain a solution having a known concentration of about 0.3 mg per mL.

Reference solution 1—Dissolve an accurately weighed quantity of USP Nifedipine Nitrophenylpyridine Analog RS in methanol (about 1 mg per mL), and dilute quantitatively with *Mobile phase* to obtain a solution having a known concentration of about 0.6 µg per mL.

Reference solution 2—Dissolve an accurately weighed quantity of USP Nifedipine Nitrosophenylpyridine Analog RS in methanol (about 1 mg per mL), and dilute quantitatively with *Mobile phase* to obtain a solution having a known concentration of about 0.6 µg per mL.

Standard solution—Transfer 5.0 mL of each of the two *Reference solutions* to a container, add 5.0 mL of *Mobile phase*, and mix.

Test solution—Prepare as directed for the *Assay preparation* in the *Assay*.

System suitability solution—Mix equal volumes of the *Standard nifedipine solution* and of each of the two *Reference solutions*.

Chromatographic system—Prepare as directed in the *Assay*. Chromatograph the *System suitability preparation*, and record the peak responses as directed for *Procedure*: the resolution, R, between the nitrophenylpyridine analog and nitrosophenylpyridine analog peaks is not less than 1.5; the resolution, R, between the nitrosophenylpyridine analog and nifedipine peaks is not less than 1.0; and the relative standard deviation of the response for each analog in replicate injections is not more than 10%. The relative retention times are about 0.8 for the nitrophenylpyridine analog, about 0.9 for the nitrosophenylpyridine analog, and 1.0 for nifedipine.

Procedure—Separately inject equal volumes (about 25 µL) of the *Standard solution* and the *Test solution* into the chromatograph, record the chromatograms, and measure the responses for the major peaks. Calculate the quantity, in mg, of each related compound in the portion of Nifedipine taken by the formula:

$$250C(r_U/r_S)$$

in which C is the concentration, in mg per mL, of the appropriate USP Nifedipine Analog RS, in the *Standard solution*; and r_U and r_S are the peak responses for the corresponding related compound obtained from the *Test solution* and the *Standard solution*, respectively. Not more than 0.2% of each of dimethyl 4-(2-nitrophenyl)-2,6-dimethylpyridine-3,5-dicarboxylate and dimethyl- 4-(2-nitrosophenyl)-2,6-dimethylpyridine-3,5-dicarboxylate, corresponding to Nifedipine Nitrophenylpyridine Analog and Nifedipine Nitrosophenylpyridine Analog, respectively, is found.

Organic volatile impurities, *Method V* ⟨467⟩: meets the requirements.

Solvent: dimethyl sulfoxide.

(Official until July 1, 2008)

Assay—[NOTE—Protect the *Standard preparation* and the *Assay preparation* from actinic light. Conduct the *Assay* promptly after preparation of the *Standard preparation* and the *Assay preparation*.]

Mobile phase—Prepare a suitable mixture of water, acetonitrile, and methanol (50 : 25 : 25), and degas. Make adjustments if necessary (see *System Suitability* under *Chromatography* ⟨621⟩).

Standard preparation—Dissolve an accurately weighed quantity of USP Nifedipine RS in methanol (about 1 mg per mL), and quantitatively dilute with *Mobile phase* to obtain a solution having a known concentration of about 0.1 mg per mL.

Assay preparation—Transfer about 25 mg of Nifedipine, accurately weighed, to a 250-mL volumetric flask. Dissolve in 25 mL of methanol, dilute with *Mobile phase* to volume, and mix to obtain a solution having a concentration of about 0.1 mg per mL.

Chromatographic system (see *Chromatography* ⟨621⟩)—The liquid chromatograph is equipped with a 235-nm detector and a 4.6-mm × 25-cm column that contains 5-µm packing L1. The flow rate is about 1.0 mL per minute. Chromatograph the *Standard preparation*, and record the peak responses as directed for *Procedure*: the column efficiency is not less than 4000 theoretical plates; the tailing factor is not more than 1.5; and the relative standard deviation for replicate injections is not more than 1.0%.

Procedure—Separately inject equal volumes (about 25 µL) of the *Standard preparation* and the *Assay preparation* into the chromatograph, record the chromatograms, and measure the responses for the major peaks. Calculate the quantity, in mg, of $C_{17}H_{18}N_2O_6$ in the portion of Nifedipine taken by the formula:

$$250C(r_U/r_S)$$

in which C is the concentration, in mg per mL, of USP Nifedipine RS in the *Standard preparation*; and r_U and r_S are the peak responses obtained from the *Assay preparation* and the *Standard preparation*, respectively.

Nifedipine Capsules

» Nifedipine Capsules contain not less than 90.0 percent and not more than 110.0 percent of the labeled amount of nifedipine ($C_{17}H_{18}N_2O_6$).

Packaging and storage—Preserve in tight, light-resistant containers at a temperature between 15° and 25°.

USP Reference standards ⟨11⟩—*USP Nifedipine RS. USP Nifedipine Nitrophenylpyridine Analog RS. USP Nifedipine Nitrosophenylpyridine Analog RS.*

NOTE—Nifedipine, when exposed to daylight and certain wavelengths of artificial light, readily converts to a nitrosophenylpyridine derivative. Exposure to UV light leads to the formation of a nitrophenylpyridine derivative. Perform assays and tests in the dark or under golden fluorescent or other low-actinic light. Use low-actinic glassware.

Identification—

A: *Visualizing solution*—In a 100-mL volumetric flask dissolve 3 g of bismuth subnitrate and 30 g of potassium iodide with 10 mL of 3 N hydrochloric acid. Dilute with water to volume, and mix. Prior to use, transfer 10.0 mL of solution to a 100-mL volumetric flask, add 10 mL of 3 N hydrochloric acid, dilute with water to volume, and mix.

Standard solution—Prepare a *Standard solution* of USP Nifedipine RS in methylene chloride containing about 1.2 mg per mL.

Test solution—Using the technique described under *Procedure for content uniformity* in the test for *Uniformity of dosage units*, transfer the contents of 3 Capsules to a centrifuge tube, rinsing the scissors with about 20 mL of 0.1 N sodium hydroxide. Pipet 25 mL of methylene chloride into the tube, insert a stopper, invert several times, and carefully release the pressure in the tube. Insert the stopper again tightly, and shake gently for 1 hour. Centrifuge the tube for 10 minutes at 2000 to 2500 rpm. Remove the supernatant aqueous phase by aspiration with a syringe, and transfer 5.0 mL of the clarified lower layer to a suitable vial.

Procedure—Mix equal portions of the *Standard solution* and the *Test solution*. Apply separately 500 µL each of the *Standard solution*, the *Test solution*, and their mixture to a suitable thin-layer chromatographic plate (see *Chromatography* ⟨621⟩) coated with a 0.5-mm layer of chromatographic silica gel mixture. Allow the spots to dry, and develop the chromatogram, protected from light, in a solvent system consisting of a mixture of ethyl acetate and cyclohexane (1 : 1) until the solvent front has moved about three-fourths of the length of the plate. Remove the plate from the developing chamber, mark the solvent front, and air-dry the plate until no odor is detectable. Immediately view the plate under short-wavelength UV light: each solution exhibits a dark blue major band at the same R_F value of about 0.3. Spray the plate with *Visualizing solution*: each solution exhibits a compact light orange band on a yellow background.

B: The retention time of the major peak in the chromatogram of the *Assay preparation* corresponds to that in the chromatogram of the *Standard preparation,* as obtained in the *Assay.*

Dissolution ⟨711⟩—
Medium: simulated gastric fluid TS (without pepsin); 900 mL.
Apparatus 2: 50 rpm.
Time: 20 minutes.
Standard solution—Dissolve an accurately weighed quantity of USP Nifedipine RS in an amount of methanol not exceeding 2% of the final volume, and dilute quantitatively and stepwise, if necessary, with *Dissolution Medium* to obtain a solution having a known appropriate concentration.
Procedure—Determine the amount of $C_{17}H_{18}N_2O_6$ dissolved by employing UV absorption at the wavelength of maximum absorbance at about 340 nm on filtered portions of the solution under test, suitably diluted with *Dissolution Medium,* if necessary, in comparison with the *Standard solution.* [NOTE—Filters must be checked for absorptive loss of nifedipine.]
Tolerances—Not less than 80% (*Q*) of the labeled amount of $C_{17}H_{18}N_2O_6$ is dissolved in 20 minutes.

Uniformity of dosage units ⟨905⟩: meet the requirements.

Procedure for content uniformity—With the point of a pair of sharp scissors, make a small hole at the end of 1 Capsule. Squeeze most of the contents into a 200-mL volumetric flask, cut the capsule in half, and drop it into the flask. Rinse the scissors with about 20 mL of methanol, quantitatively collecting the rinse in the flask. Dilute with methanol to volume, and mix to obtain the test solution. Dissolve an accurately weighed quantity of USP Nifedipine RS in methanol, and dilute quantitatively and stepwise with methanol to obtain a Standard solution having a known concentration of about 50 µg per mL. Concomitantly determine the absorbances of both solutions in 1-cm cells at the wavelength of maximum absorbance at about 350 nm, with a suitable spectrophotometer, using methanol as the blank. Calculate the quantity, in mg, of nifedipine ($C_{17}H_{18}N_2O_6$) in the Capsule by the formula:

$$(T/D)C(A_U/A_S)$$

in which *T* is the labeled quantity, in mg, of nifedipine in the Capsule; *D* is the concentration, in µg per mL, of nifedipine in the solution from the Capsule, on the basis of the labeled quantity per Capsule and the extent of dilution; *C* is the concentration, in µg per mL, of USP Nifedipine RS in the Standard solution; and A_U and A_S are the absorbances of the solution from the Capsule and the Standard solution, respectively.

Related compounds—[NOTE—Protect the *Standard nifedipine solution* and the *Test solution* from actinic light. Conduct this test promptly after preparation of the *Standard nifedipine solution* and the *Test solution.*]
Mobile phase—Prepare as directed in the *Assay* under *Nifedipine.*
Standard nifedipine solution—Prepare as directed for *Standard nifedipine solution* in the test for *Related compounds* under *Nifedipine.*
Reference solution 1—Prepare as directed for *Reference solution 1* in the test for *Related compounds* under *Nifedipine,* except to make the final known concentration of about 6 µg per mL.
Reference solution 2—Prepare as directed for *Reference solution 2* in the test for *Related compounds* under *Nifedipine,* except to make the final known concentration of about 1.5 µg per mL.
Standard solution—Transfer 5.0 mL of each of the two *Reference solutions* to a container, add 5.0 mL of *Mobile phase,* and mix.
Test solution—Prepare as directed for the *Assay preparation* in the *Assay.*
System suitability solution—Mix equal volumes of the *Standard nifedipine solution* and of each of the two *Reference solutions.*
Chromatographic system—Prepare as directed in the *Assay.* Chromatograph the *System suitability solution,* and record the peak responses as directed for *Procedure:* the resolution, *R,* between the nitrophenylpyridine analog and nitrosophenylpyridine analog peaks is not less than 1.5; the resolution, *R,* between the nitrosophenylpyridine analog and nifedipine peaks is not less than 1.0; and the relative standard deviation determined from the response for each analog in replicate injections is not more than 10%. The relative retention times are about 0.8 for the nitrophenylpyridine analog, about 0.9 for the nitrosophenylpyridine analog, and 1.0 for nifedipine.

Procedure—Separately inject equal volumes (about 25 µL) of the *Standard solution* and the *Test solution* into the chromatograph, record the chromatograms, and measure the responses for the major peaks. Calculate the quantity, in mg, of each related compound in the portion of Capsules taken by the formula:

$$(V/5)C(r_U/r_S)$$

in which *V* is the volume, in mL, of the *Test solution, C* is the concentration, in mg per mL, of the appropriate USP Nifedipine Analog RS in the *Standard solution;* and r_U and r_S are the peak responses of the corresponding related compound obtained from the *Test solution* and the *Standard solution,* respectively: not more than 2.0% of dimethyl 4-(2-nitrophenyl)-2,6-dimethylpyridine-3,5-dicarboxylate, corresponding to nifedipine nitrophenylpyridine analog, and not more than 0.5% of dimethyl 4-(2-nitrosophenyl)-2,6-dimethylpyridine-3,5-dicarboxylate, corresponding to nifedipine nitrosophenylpyridine analog, both relative to the nifedipine content, are found.

Assay—[NOTE—Protect the *Standard preparation* and the *Assay preparation* from actinic light. Conduct the *Assay* promptly after preparation of the *Standard preparation* and the *Assay preparation.*]
Mobile phase and *Standard preparation*—Prepare as directed in the *Assay* under *Nifedipine.*
Assay preparation—Transfer the contents of 5 Capsules with the aid of a small amount of methanol to a volumetric flask, quantitatively dilute with *Mobile phase* to obtain a total volume, *V* mL, of solution having a concentration of about 0.1 mg of nifedipine per mL. Pass through a solvent-resistant filter.
Chromatographic system (see *Chromatography* ⟨621⟩)—The liquid chromatograph is equipped with a 265-nm detector, a 4.6-mm × 25-cm column that contains 5-µm packing L1, and a guard column that contains packing L1. The flow rate is about 1.0 mL per minute. Chromatograph the *Standard preparation,* and record the peak responses as directed for *Procedure:* the column efficiency is not less than 4000 theoretical plates; the tailing factor is not more than 1.5; and the relative standard deviation for replicate injections is not more than 1.0%.
Procedure—Separately inject equal volumes (about 25 µL) of the *Standard preparation* and the *Assay preparation* into the chromatograph, record the chromatograms, and measure the responses for the major peaks. Calculate the quantity, in mg, of nifedipine ($C_{17}H_{18}N_2O_6$) in each Capsule taken by the formula:

$$(V/5)C(r_U/r_S)$$

in which *V* is the volume, in mL, of the *Assay preparation; C* is the concentration, in mg per mL, of USP Nifedipine RS in the *Standard preparation;* and r_U and r_S are the peak responses obtained from the *Assay preparation* and the *Standard preparation,* respectively.

Nifedipine Extended-Release Tablets

» Nifedipine Extended-Release Tablets contain not less than 90.0 percent and not more than 110.0 percent of the labeled amount of nifedipine ($C_{17}H_{18}N_2O_6$).

Packaging and storage—Preserve in tight, light-resistant containers, and store at controlled room temperature.
Labeling—The labeling indicates the *Dissolution Test* with which the product complies.
USP Reference standards ⟨11⟩—*USP Nifedipine RS. USP Nifedipine Nitrophenylpyridine Analog RS. USP Nifedipine Nitrosophenylpyridine Analog RS.*
NOTE—Nifedipine, when exposed to daylight and certain wavelengths of artificial light, readily converts to a nitrosophenylpyridine derivative. Exposure to UV light leads to the formation of a nitrophenylpyridine derivative. Perform assays and tests in the dark or under golden fluorescent or other low-actinic light. Use low-actinic glassware.

Identification—

A: The retention time of the major peak in the chromatogram of the *Assay preparation* corresponds to that in the chromatogram of the *Standard preparation,* as obtained in the *Assay.*

B: *Ultraviolet Absorption* ⟨197U⟩—

Solutions—Prepare a test solution as directed for the *Assay preparation* in the *Assay,* except to dilute further with *Mobile phase* to obtain a solution having a concentration of about 0.02 mg per mL. Prepare the Standard solution as directed for the *Standard preparation* in the *Assay* under *Nifedipine,* except to dilute further with *Mobile phase* to obtain a solution having a known concentration of about 0.02 mg per mL.

Dissolution ⟨711⟩—

TEST 1—If the product complies with this test, the labeling indicates that it meets USP *Dissolution Test 1.*

Medium: water; 50 mL.

Apparatus 7 (see *Drug Release* ⟨724⟩): 15 to 30 cycles per minute. Do not use the reciprocating disk, but use a 25-cm plexiglas rod, the perimeter of the Tablets being affixed to the rod with a water-insoluble glue. The solution containers are 25-mm test tubes, 150 to 200 mm in length, and the water bath is maintained at 37 ± 0.5°. At the end of each specified test interval, the systems are transferred to the next row of new test tubes containing 50 mL of fresh *Medium.*

Times: 4, 8, 12, 16, 20, and 24 hours.

Diluting solution: a mixture of methanol and water (1 : 1).

Standard solutions—Transfer about 50 mg of USP Nifedipine RS, accurately weighed, to a 100-mL volumetric flask, dissolve in 50 mL of methanol, dilute with water to volume, and mix to obtain a Standard stock solution. Quantitatively dilute this Standard stock solution with *Diluting solution* to obtain solutions having suitable known concentrations.

Test solution—Use portions of the solution under test, passed through a 0.4-μm filter, suitably diluted with methanol, and stepwise, if necessary, with *Diluting solution* to obtain a final mixture consisting of equal parts of methanol and water.

Procedure—Determine the amount of $C_{17}H_{18}N_2O_6$ released in the *Test solution* at each 4-hour interval by employing UV absorption at the wavelength of maximum absorbance at about 338 nm, in 0.5-cm cells. [NOTE—For the 4-hour time period, determine the absorbance at 456 nm, and use this determination to correct for excipient interference.]

Tolerances—The cumulative percentages of the labeled amount of nifedipine ($C_{17}H_{18}N_2O_6$), released in vivo and dissolved at the times specified, conform to *Acceptance Table 2.*

Time (hours)	Amount dissolved*
4	between 5% and 17%
8	—
12	between 43% and 80%
16	—
20	—
24	not less than 80%

*The amount dissolved is expressed in terms of the labeled tablet strength rather than in terms of the labeled total contents.

TEST 2—If the product complies with this test, the labeling indicates that it meets USP *Dissolution Test 2.*

Buffer concentrate—Transfer 330.9 g of dibasic sodium phosphate and 38 g of citric acid to a 1-L volumetric flask, add water to dissolve, add 10 mL of phosphoric acid, dilute with water to volume, and mix.

Medium—Mix 125.0 mL of *Buffer concentrate* and 1 L of 10% sodium lauryl sulfate solution, and dilute to 10 L. Adjust if necessary to a pH of 6.8; 900 mL.

Apparatus 2: 50 rpm, with sinkers (see *Figure 1*).

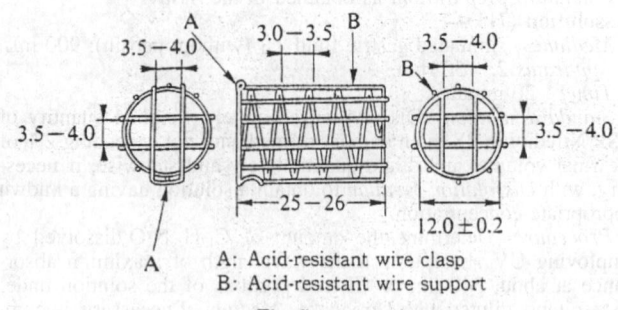

A: Acid-resistant wire clasp
B: Acid-resistant wire support
The figures are in mm.

Figure 1

Times: 3, 6, and 12 hours.

Determine the amount of nifedipine ($C_{17}H_{18}N_2O_6$) dissolved by employing the following method.

Mobile phase—Prepare a filtered and degassed mixture of acetonitrile and water (70 : 30). Make adjustments if necessary (see *System Suitability* under *Chromatography* ⟨621⟩).

Standard solution—Dissolve an accurately weighed quantity of USP Nifedipine RS in methanol to obtain a solution having a known concentration of about 1.11 mg per mL. Dilute quantitatively and stepwise with *Medium* to obtain a solution having a known concentration of 0.1 mg per mL.

Chromatographic system—The liquid chromatograph is equipped with a 350-nm detector and a 4.0-mm × 125-mm column that contains 3-μm packing L1. The flow rate is about 1.5 mL per minute. The column is maintained at about 40°. Chromatograph the *Standard solution,* and record the peak responses as directed for *Procedure:* the column efficiency is not less than 2000 theoretical plates; the tailing factor is not more than 1.5; and the relative standard deviation for replicate injections is not more than 2.0%.

Procedure—Separately inject equal volumes (about 20 μL) of filtered portions of the *Standard solution* and the solution under test into the chromatograph, record the chromatograms, and measure the responses for the major peaks. Determine the amount of nifedipine ($C_{17}H_{18}N_2O_6$) dissolved.

Tolerances—The percentages of the labeled amount of nifedipine ($C_{17}H_{18}N_2O_6$) released in vivo and dissolved at the times specified conform to *Acceptance Table 2.*

Time (hours)	Amount dissolved
3	between 10% and 30%
6	between 40% and 65%
12	not less than 80%

TEST 3—If the product complies with this test, the labeling indicates that it meets USP *Dissolution Test 3.*

FOR TABLETS LABELED TO CONTAIN 30 MG OF NIFEDIPINE—

Phase 1:

Medium: 0.05 M phosphate buffer, pH 7.5; 900 mL.

Apparatus 2: 100 rpm.

Time: 1 hour.

Standard solution—Prepare a solution in *Medium* having an accurately known concentration of about 0.034 mg of USP Nifedipine RS per mL. [NOTE—If necessary, a volume of methanol, not exceeding 10% of the final volume, can be used to help solubilize nifedipine.]

Procedure—[NOTE—After the run, take the Tablet out of the dissolution vessel, adapt a sinker to it, and transfer the Tablet with the sinker to the dissolution vessel containing the *Medium* for Phase 2.] Determine the amount of $C_{17}H_{18}N_2O_6$ released in *Phase 1* from UV absorbances at the wavelength of maximum absorbance at about 238 nm, using filtered portions of the solution under test, in comparison with the *Standard solution,* using the *Medium* as the blank.

Phase 2:

Medium: 0.5% sodium lauryl sulfate in simulated gastric fluid without enzyme, pH 1.2; 900 mL.

Apparatus 2: 100 rpm.

Times: 1, 4, 8, and 12 hours.

Standard solution—Prepare a solution in *Medium* having an accurately known concentration of about 0.034 mg of USP Nifedipine RS per mL. [NOTE—If necessary, a volume of methanol, not exceeding 10% of the final volume, can be used to help solubilize nifedipine.]

Procedure—Determine the amount of $C_{17}H_{18}N_2O_6$ released in *Phase 2* from UV absorbances at the wavelength of maximum absorbance at about 238 nm using filtered portions of the solution under test, in comparison with the *Standard solution*, using *Medium* as the blank.

Tolerances—The cumulative percentages of the labeled amount of nifedipine ($C_{17}H_{18}N_2O_6$), released in vivo and dissolved at the times specified, conform to *Acceptance Table 2*.

Time (hours)	Amount dissolved*
1	not more than 30%
4	between 30% and 55%
8	not less than 60%
12	not less than 80%

*For each dosage unit, add the amount dissolved in phosphate buffer, pH 7.5 from *Phase 1* to the amount dissolved at each time point in *Phase 2*.

FOR TABLETS LABELED TO CONTAIN 60 MG OF NIFEDIPINE—

Phase 1:

Medium: 0.05 M phosphate buffer, pH 7.5; 900 mL.

Procedure—[NOTE—After the run, take the Tablet out of the dissolution vessel, adapt a sinker to it, and transfer the Tablet with the sinker to the dissolution vessel containing the *Medium* for *Phase 2*.] Determine the amount of $C_{17}H_{18}N_2O_6$ released in *Phase 1* from UV absorbances at the wavelength of maximum absorbance at about 238 nm using filtered portions of the solution under test, in comparison with the *Standard solution*, using the *Medium* as the blank.

Apparatus 2: 100 rpm.

Time: 25 minutes.

Standard solution—Prepare a solution in *Medium* having an accurately known concentration of about 0.067 mg of USP Nifedipine RS per mL. If necessary, a volume of methanol, not exceeding 10% of the final volume, can be used to help solubilize nifedipine.

Phase 2:

Medium: 0.5% sodium lauryl sulfate in simulated gastric fluid without enzyme, pH 1.2; 900 mL.

Apparatus 2: 100 rpm.

Times: 1, 4, 8, and 12 hours.

Standard solution—Prepare a solution in *Medium* having an accurately known concentration of about 0.067 mg of USP Nifedipine RS per mL. [NOTE—If necessary, a volume of methanol, not exceeding 10% of the final volume, can be used to help solubilize nifedipine.]

Procedure—Determine the amount of $C_{17}H_{18}N_2O_6$ released in *Phase 2* from UV absorbances at the wavelength of maximum absorbance at about 238 nm, using filtered portions of the solution under test, in comparison with the *Standard solution*, using *Medium* as the blank.

Tolerances—The cumulative percentages of the labeled amount of nifedipine ($C_{17}H_{18}N_2O_6$), released in vivo and dissolved at the times specified, conform to *Acceptance Table 2*.

Time (hours)	Amount dissolved*
1	not more than 30%
4	between 40% and 70%
8	not less than 70%
12	not less than 80%

*For each dosage unit, add the amount dissolved in phosphate buffer, pH 7.5 from *Phase 1* to the amount dissolved at each time point in *Phase 2*.

TEST 4—If the product complies with this test, the labeling indicates that the product meets USP *Dissolution Test 4*.

Medium: 0.5% sodium lauryl sulfate in simulated gastric fluid without enzyme, pH 1.2; 900 mL.

Apparatus 2: 100 rpm.

Times: 1, 4, and 12 hours.

Standard solution—Prepare a solution in *Medium* having an accurately known concentration of about 0.067 mg of USP Nifedipine RS per mL for Tablets labeled to contain 60 mg, and of about 0.034 mg of USP Nifedipine RS per mL for Tablets labeled to contain 30 mg. [NOTE—If necessary, a volume of methanol, not exceeding 10% of the final volume, can be used to help solubilize nifedipine.]

Procedure—Determine the amount of $C_{17}H_{18}N_2O_6$ released from UV absorbances at the wavelength of maximum absorbance at about 238 nm using filtered portions of the solution under test, in comparison with the *Standard solution*, using the *Medium* as the blank.

Tolerances—The cumulative percentages of the labeled amount of nifedipine ($C_{17}H_{18}N_2O_6$), released at the times specified, conform to *Acceptance Table 2*.

FOR TABLETS LABELED TO CONTAIN 30 MG OF NIFEDIPINE

Time (hours)	Amount dissolved
1	between 12% and 35%
4	between 44% and 67%
12	not less than 80%

FOR TABLETS LABELED TO CONTAIN 60 MG OF NIFEDIPINE

Time (hours)	Amount dissolved
1	between 10% and 30%
4	between 40% and 63%
12	not less than 80%

TEST 5—If the product complies with this test, the labeling indicates that the product meets USP *Dissolution Test 5*.

Medium: water; 50 mL.

Apparatus 7 (see *Drug Release* ⟨724⟩)—Use a 25-cm Plexiglas rod, the perimeter of the Tablets being affixed to the rod with a water-insoluble glue; 30 dips per minute. The solution containers are 25-mm test tubes, 150 to 200 mm in length, and the water bath is maintained at 37 ± 0.5°.

Times: 4, 12, and 24 hours.

Diluting solution 1—Prepare a mixture of methanol and acetonitrile (1 : 1).

Diluting solution 2—Prepare a mixture of *Diluting solution 1* and water (1 : 1).

Standard solutions—Transfer about 50 mg of USP Nifedipine RS, accurately weighed, to a 100-mL volumetric flask, dissolve in 50 mL of *Diluting solution 1*, dilute with water to volume, and mix. Quantitatively dilute this solution with *Diluting solution 2* to obtain solutions having known concentrations of 0.01 mg per mL, 0.05 mg per mL, and 0.20 mg per mL that are used at 4, 12, and 24 hours sampling, respectively.

Procedure—[NOTE—For the 4-hour time period, filter the solution under test, and determine the absorbance at 456 nm. Use this absorbance value to correct for excipient interference at the other time points.] Determine the amount of nifedipine released at each interval by employing UV absorption at the wavelength of maximum absorbance at about 338 nm on portions of the solution under test passed through a suitable 0.45-μm filter, suitably diluted, if necessary, with *Diluting solution 1* and water to obtain a final mixture of water, methanol, and acetonitrile (2 : 1 : 1), in comparison with the appropriate *Standard solution*, using 0.5-cm cells, and *Diluting solution 2* as the blank.

Tolerances—The cumulative percentages of the labeled amount of nifedipine, released in vivo and dissolved at the times specified, conform to *Acceptance Table 2*.

Time (hours)	Amount dissolved

2810 Nifedipine / *Official Monographs*

Time (hours)	Amount dissolved
4	not more than 14%
12	between 39% and 75%
24	not less than 75%

Uniformity of dosage units ⟨905⟩: meet the requirements.

Related compounds—[NOTE—Conduct this test promptly after preparation of the *Standard nifedipine solution* and the *Test solution*.]

Mobile phase—Prepare as directed in the *Assay* under *Nifedipine*.

Standard nifedipine solution, Reference solution 1, and *Reference solution 2*—Prepare as directed in the test for *Related compounds* under *Nifedipine*, except to obtain solutions having known concentrations of about 6 µg per mL and 1.5 µg per mL for *Reference solution 1* and *Reference solution 2*, respectively.

System suitability solution—Mix equal volumes of the *Standard nifedipine solution, Reference solution 1,* and *Reference solution 2*.

Standard solution—Transfer 5.0 mL of each *Reference solution* to a container, add 5.0 mL of *Mobile phase*, and mix. Each mL of this solution contains about 2 µg of USP Nifedipine Nitrophenylpyridine Analog RS and 0.5 µg of USP Nifedipine Nitrosophenylpyridine Analog RS.

Test solution—Use a portion of the *Assay preparation*.

Chromatographic system (see *Chromatography* ⟨621⟩)—Prepare as directed in the *Assay*. Chromatograph the *System suitability solution*, and record the peak responses as directed for *Procedure*: the resolution, R, between nitrophenylpyridine analog and nitrosophenylpyridine analog is not less than 1.5; the resolution, R, between nitrosophenylpyridine analog and nifedipine is not less than 1.0; and for each analog, the relative standard deviation for replicate injections is not more than 10%.

Procedure—Separately inject equal volumes (about 25 µL) of the *Standard solution* and the *Test solution* into the chromatograph, record the chromatograms, and measure the responses for the major peaks. Calculate the percentage of each related compound in the portion of Tablets taken by the formula:

$$417(C/W)(r_i/r_S)$$

in which C is the concentration, in µg per mL, of the appropriate analog USP Reference Standard in the *Standard solution*; W is the weight, in mg, of nifedipine in the Tablets taken to prepare the *Test solution*; and r_i and r_S are the peak responses of the corresponding related compound obtained from the *Test solution* and the *Standard solution*, respectively: not more than 2.0% of nifedipine nitrophenylpyridine analog and not more than 0.5% of nifedipine nitrosophenylpyridine analog, both relative to the nifedipine content, are found.

Assay—[NOTE—Conduct the *Assay* promptly after preparation of the *Standard preparation* and the *Assay preparation*.]

Mobile phase and *Standard preparation*—Prepare as directed in the *Assay* under *Nifedipine*.

Assay preparation—Select a number of Tablets, equivalent to about 420 mg of nifedipine. Finely powder the Tablets, and transfer the powder to a 250-mL volumetric flask containing 130 mL of water; or transfer the intact Tablets to a 400-mL, high-speed blender cup containing 130 mL of water, homogenize until a uniform suspension is achieved (about 2 minutes), and transfer the suspension with the aid of a mixture of acetonitrile and methanol (1 : 1) to a 250-mL volumetric flask. Add a mixture of acetonitrile and methanol (1 : 1) to volume, and stir for 30 minutes. Centrifuge the resulting suspension to obtain a clear supernatant stock solution. Transfer 3.0 mL of the stock solution to a 50-mL volumetric flask, dilute with *Mobile phase* to volume, mix, and filter to obtain a solution having a concentration of about 0.1 mg of nifedipine per mL. [NOTE—Reserve a portion of this *Assay preparation* for use as the *Test solution* in the test for *Related compounds*.]

Chromatographic system (see *Chromatography* ⟨621⟩)—The liquid chromatograph is equipped with a 265-nm detector, a 4.6-mm × 25-cm analytical column that contains packing L1, and a 2.1-mm × 3-cm guard column that contains packing L1. The flow rate is about 1 mL per minute. Chromatograph the *Standard preparation*, and record the peak responses as directed for *Procedure*: the column efficiency is not less than 4000 theoretical plates; the tailing factor is not more than 1.5; and the relative standard deviation for replicate injections is not more than 1.0%.

Procedure—Separately inject equal volumes (about 25 µL) of the *Standard preparation* and the *Assay preparation* into the chromatograph, record the chromatograms, and measure the responses for the major peaks. Calculate the quantity, in mg, of nifedipine ($C_{17}H_{18}N_2O_6$) in the Tablets taken by the formula:

$$4167C(r_U/r_S)$$

in which C is the concentration, in mg per mL, of USP Nifedipine RS in the *Standard preparation*; and r_U and r_S are the peak responses obtained from the *Assay preparation* and the *Standard preparation*, respectively.

Nimodipine

$C_{21}H_{26}N_2O_7$ 418.44

3,5-Pyridinedicarboxylic acid, 1,4-dihydro-2,6-dimethyl- 4-(3-nitrophenyl)-, 2-methoxyethyl 1-methylethyl ester.

Isopropyl 2-methoxyethyl 1,4-dihydro-2,6-dimethyl-4-(*m*-nitrophenyl)-3,5-pyridinedicarboxylate [66085-59-4].

» Nimodipine contains not less than 98.5 percent and not more than 101.5 percent of $C_{21}H_{26}N_2O_7$, calculated on the dried basis.

Packaging and storage—Preserve in tight, light-resistant containers, and store at 25°, excursions permitted between 15° and 30°.

USP Reference standards ⟨11⟩—*USP Nimodipine RS. USP Nimodipine Related Compound A RS.*

NOTE—Throughout the following procedures, protect test or assay specimens, the Reference Standards, and solutions containing them by conducting the procedures immediately under subdued light or using low-actinic glassware.

Identification—

A: *Infrared Absorption* ⟨197K⟩.

B: The retention time of the major peak in the chromatogram of the *Test solution* corresponds to that in the chromatogram of *Standard solution 1*, as obtained in the test for *Related compounds*.

Specific rotation ⟨781S⟩: between −10° and +10°.

Test solution: 50 mg per mL, in acetone.

Loss on drying ⟨731⟩—Dry it at 105° for 4 hours: it loses not more than 0.5% of its weight.

Residue on ignition ⟨281⟩: not more than 0.1%.

Related compounds—

Mobile phase—Prepare a filtered and degassed mixture of water, methanol, and tetrahydrofuran (3 : 1 : 1).

Standard solution 1—Transfer an accurately weighed quantity of USP Nimodipine RS to a suitable volumetric flask, dissolve in a volume of tetrahydrofuran equivalent to about 10% of the volume of the volumetric flask, and dilute with *Mobile phase* to volume to obtain a solution containing about 1.6 mg per mL. Dilute an aliquot of this solution with *Mobile phase* to obtain a solution having a known concentration of about 3.2 µg per mL.

Standard solution 2—Transfer accurately weighed quantities of USP Nimodipine RS and USP Nimodipine Related Compound A RS to a suitable volumetric flask, dissolve in a volume of tetrahydrofuran equivalent to about 10% of the volume of the volumetric flask, and dilute with *Mobile phase* to volume to obtain a solution containing 0.8 mg per mL each of USP Nimodipine RS and USP Nimodipine Related Compound A RS. Dilute an aliquot of this solution with *Mobile phase* to obtain a solution having a known concentration of about 1.6 µg per mL each of USP Nimodipine RS and USP Nimodipine Related Compound A RS.

Test solution—Transfer about 40 mg of Nimodipine, accurately weighed, to a 25-mL volumetric flask, dissolve in 2.5 mL of tetrahydrofuran, dilute with *Mobile phase* to volume, and mix.

Chromatographic system (see *Chromatography* ⟨621⟩)—The liquid chromatograph is equipped with a 235-nm detector and a 4.6-mm × 12.5-cm column that contains packing L1. The flow rate is about 2 mL per minute. The column temperature is maintained at 40°. Chromatograph *Standard solution 2*, and record the peak responses as directed for *Procedure:* the resolution, *R*, between nimodipine related compound A and nimodipine is not less than 1.5; and the relative standard deviation for replicate injections is not more than 2.0%. [NOTE—For the purpose of identification, the relative retention times are about 0.9 for nimodipine related compound A and 1.0 for nimodipine.]

Procedure—Separately inject equal volumes (about 20 μL) of *Standard solution 1, Standard solution 2,* and the *Test solution* into the chromatograph, record the chromatograms, and measure the peak responses. [NOTE—Record the chromatogram of the *Test solution* for a period of time equivalent to four times the retention time of nimodipine.] Calculate the percentage of nimodipine related compound A in the portion of Nimodipine taken by the formula:

$$(100/1000)(C_S / C_T)(r_U / r_S)$$

in which C_S is the concentration, in μg per mL, of USP Nimodipine Related Compound A RS in *Standard solution 2*; C_T is the concentration, in mg per mL, of Nimodipine in the *Test solution*; and r_U and r_S are the peak responses of nimodipine related compound A obtained from the *Test solution* and *Standard solution 2*, respectively: not more than 0.1% of nimodipine related compound A is found. Calculate the percentage of any other impurity in the portion of Nimodipine taken by the formula:

$$(100/1000)(C_S / C_T)(r_i / r_S)$$

in which C_S is the concentration, in μg per mL, of USP Nimodipine RS in *Standard solution 1*; C_T is the concentration, in mg per mL, of Nimodipine in the *Test solution*; r_i is the peak response of each impurity obtained from the *Test solution*; and r_S is the peak response of nimodipine obtained from *Standard solution 1*: not more than 0.2% of any other impurity is found; and not more than 0.5% of total impurities is found.

Assay—Transfer about 180 mg of Nimodipine, accurately weighed, to a 100-mL beaker. Dissolve, with gentle heating, by stirring in a mixture of 25 mL of tertiary butyl alcohol and 25 mL of perchloric acid TS. Add 0.1 mL of ferroin TS. Titrate with 0.1 N ceric sulfate VS. Perform a blank determination, and make any necessary correction (see *Titrimetry* ⟨541⟩). Each mL of 0.1 N ceric sulfate is equivalent to 20.92 mg of $C_{21}H_{26}N_2O_7$.

Nitrofurantoin

$C_8H_6N_4O_5$ (anhydrous)   238.16
2,4-Imidazolidinedione, 1-[[(5-nitro-2-furanyl)methylene]amino]-.
1-[(5-Nitrofurfurylidene)amino]hydantoin   [67-20-9].
Monohydrate   256.18   [17140-81-7].

» Nitrofurantoin is anhydrous or contains one molecule of water of hydration. It contains not less than 98.0 percent and not more than 102.0 percent of $C_8H_6N_4O_5$, calculated on the anhydrous basis.

NOTE—Nitrofurantoin and solutions of it are discolored by alkali and by exposure to light, and are decomposed upon contact with metals other than stainless steel and aluminum.

Packaging and storage—Preserve in tight, light-resistant containers.

Labeling—Label it to indicate whether it is anhydrous or hydrous. Nitrofurantoin in the form of macrocrystals is so labeled. The labeling states the specific surface area and which method, specified under *Specific Surface Area* ⟨846⟩, is used.

USP Reference standards ⟨11⟩—*USP Nitrofurantoin RS. USP Nitrofurazone RS. USP Nitrofurfural Diacetate RS.*

Identification—
    A: *Infrared Absorption* ⟨197M⟩: previously dried at 140° for 30 minutes.
    B: The retention time of the major peak in the chromatogram of the *Assay preparation* corresponds to that in the chromatogram of the *Standard preparation*, as obtained in the *Assay*.

Water, *Method III* ⟨921⟩—Dry it at 140° for 30 minutes: the anhydrous form loses not more than 1.0%, and the hydrous form between 6.5% and 7.5%, of its weight.

Specific surface area ⟨846⟩ (where it is labeled as being in the form of macrocrystals)—Outgas a portion of the powder to be placed under test at 150° for 10 minutes at ambient pressure with nitrogen: the limits are between 0.045 m² per g and 0.20 m² per g.

Limit of nitrofurfural diacetate—In a 10-mL volumetric flask dissolve 100 mg of Nitrofurantoin in 1 mL of dimethylformamide, add acetone to volume, and mix. Apply 10 μL of this solution and 10 μL of a Standard solution of USP Nitrofurfural Diacetate RS in a 1 in 10 mixture of dimethylformamide in acetone containing 100 μg per mL to a suitable thin-layer chromatographic plate (see *Chromatography* ⟨621⟩) coated with a 0.25-mm layer of chromatographic silica gel mixture. Allow the spots to dry, and develop the chromatogram in a solvent system consisting of a mixture of chloroform and methanol (9 : 1) until the solvent front has moved about three-fourths of the length of the plate. Remove the plate from the developing chamber, mark the solvent front, allow it to air-dry for 5 minutes, and heat the plate at 105° for 5 minutes. Remove the plate from the oven and, while it is still warm, locate the spots by spraying the plate with a solution prepared by dissolving 0.75 g of phenylhydrazine hydrochloride in 50 mL of water, decolorizing with activated charcoal, adding 25 mL of hydrochloric acid, and mixing with water to produce 200 mL. Any spot produced by the test specimen, at an R_F value of about 0.7, is not greater in size or intensity than that produced by the Standard solution at the same R_F value: not more than 1.0% of nitrofurfural diacetate is found.

Limit of nitrofurazone—
    pH 7.0 Phosphate buffer—Prepare as directed in the *Assay*.
    Mobile phase—Prepare a filtered and degassed mixture of *pH 7.0 Phosphate buffer* and tetrahydrofuran (9 : 1).
    Standard preparation—Prepare a solution of USP Nitrofurazone RS in dimethylformamide containing 5.0 μg per mL. Pipet 2 mL of this solution into a glass-stoppered flask, add 20.0 mL of water, and mix.
    Test preparation—Dissolve 100 mg of Nitrofurantoin in 2.0 mL of dimethylformamide in a glass-stoppered, 25-mL flask. Add 20.0 mL of water, mix, and allow to stand for about 15 minutes to allow precipitate to form. Pass a portion of the solution through a nylon filter having a 0.45-μm porosity, and use the clear filtrate.
    Chromatographic system (see *Chromatography* ⟨621⟩)—The liquid chromatograph is equipped with a 375-nm detector and a 3.9-mm × 30-cm column containing packing L1. The flow rate is about 1.6 mL per minute. Chromatograph the *Standard preparation*, adjusting the operating parameters so that the nitrofurazone peak has a retention time of about 10.5 minutes and its height is about 0.1 full-scale. The relative standard deviation determined from the peak height in replicate injections is not more than 2.0%. Prepare a solution containing about 5.0 μg each of nitrofurazone and nitrofurantoin per mL in dimethylformamide. Dilute this solution 1 : 10 with *Mobile phase*, and inject 60 μL to 100 μL: the resolution, *R*, of the two peaks is not less than 4.0.
    Procedure—Separately inject equal volumes (60 μL to 100 μL) of the *Standard preparation* and the *Test preparation* into the chromatograph, and record the chromatograms. The height of any peak appearing in the chromatogram of the *Test preparation* at a retention time corresponding to that of the main peak from the *Standard preparation* is not greater than the height of the main peak from the *Standard preparation*: not more than 0.01% of nitrofurazone is found.

Assay—

pH 7.0 Phosphate buffer—Dissolve 6.8 g of monobasic potassium phosphate in about 500 mL of water. Add a volume of 1.0 N sodium hydroxide (about 30 mL) sufficient to adjust to a pH of 7.0, dilute with water to 1 liter, and mix.

Mobile phase—Prepare a filtered and degassed mixture of *pH 7.0 Phosphate buffer* and acetonitrile (88 : 12).

Internal standard solution—Prepare a solution containing about 1 mg of acetanilide per mL in water, and mix.

Standard preparation—Dissolve about 50 mg of USP Nitrofurantoin RS, accurately weighed, in 40.0 mL of dimethylformamide in a glass-stoppered flask, add 50.0 mL of *Internal standard solution*, and mix.

Assay preparation—Using about 50 mg of Nitrofurantoin, accurately weighed, proceed as directed for *Standard preparation*.

Chromatographic system (see *Chromatography* ⟨621⟩)—The liquid chromatograph is equipped with a 254-nm detector and a 3.9-mm × 30-cm column that contains packing L1. Chromatograph the *Standard preparation*, adjusting the operating parameters so that the retention time of the nitrofurantoin peak is about 8 minutes and the peak heights are about half full-scale. The resolution, *R*, between acetanilide and nitrofurantoin is not less than 3.0, and the relative standard deviation determined from the ratio of the peak responses in replicate injections is not more than 2.0%.

Procedure—Separately inject equal volumes (5 μL to 10 μL) of the *Standard preparation* and the *Assay preparation* into the chromatograph, record the chromatograms, and measure the responses for the major peaks. Calculate the quantity, in mg, of $C_8H_6N_4O_5$ in the portion of Nitrofurantoin taken by the formula:

$$W(R_U / R_S)$$

in which *W* is the weight, in mg, of USP Nitrofurantoin RS in the *Standard preparation*; and R_U and R_S are the peak response ratios obtained from the *Assay preparation* and the *Standard preparation*, respectively.

Nitrofurantoin Capsules

» Nitrofurantoin Capsules contain not less than 90.0 percent and not more than 110.0 percent of the labeled amount of nitrofurantoin ($C_8H_6N_4O_5$).

Packaging and storage—Preserve in tight, light-resistant containers.

Labeling—Capsules that contain the macrocrystalline form of Nitrofurantoin are so labeled. When more than one *Dissolution* test is given, the labeling states the *Dissolution* test used only if *Test 1* is not used.

USP Reference standards ⟨11⟩—USP Nitrofurantoin RS. USP Nitrofurazone RS.

Identification—

A: Add 10 mL of 6 N acetic acid to a quantity of the contents of Capsules, equivalent to about 100 mg of nitrofurantoin, boil for a few minutes, and filter while hot. Cool to room temperature, collect the precipitate of nitrofurantoin, and dry at 105° for 1 hour: the IR absorption spectrum of a mineral oil dispersion of the precipitate so obtained exhibits maxima only at the same wavelength as that of a similar preparation of USP Nitrofurantoin RS.

B: It responds to *Identification* test B under *Nitrofurantoin*.

Dissolution ⟨711⟩—

TEST 1 (where it is labeled as containing nitrofurantoin macrocrystals)—

Medium: pH 7.2 (±0.05) phosphate buffer; 900 mL.
Apparatus 1: 100 rpm.
Times: 1, 3, and 8 hours.
Procedure—Determine the amount of $C_8H_6N_4O_5$ dissolved by employing UV absorption at the wavelength of maximum absorbance at about 375 nm on filtered portions of the solution under test, suitably diluted with *Medium*, if necessary, in comparison with a *Standard* solution having a known concentration of USP Nitrofurantoin RS in the same *Medium*.

Tolerances—The percentage of the labeled amount of $C_8H_6N_4O_5$ dissolved at the 1-hour point conforms to *Acceptance Table 2*, and the percentages dissolved at the 3- and 8-hour points conform to the criteria for the final test time in *Acceptance Table 2*.

Time (hours)	Amount dissolved
1	between 20% and 60%
3	not less than 45%
8	not less than 60%

TEST 2 (where it is labeled as containing both nitrofurantoin macrocrystalline and monohydrate forms)—If the product complies with this test, the labeling indicates that it meets USP *Dissolution Test 2*.

Acid medium: 0.01 N hydrochloric acid for 1 hour; 900 mL.

pH 7.5 Buffer medium—Prepare a pH 7.5 buffer concentrate by dissolving 62.2 g of potassium hydroxide and 129.3 g of monobasic potassium phosphate in water, dilute with water to 1 L, and mix. After 1 hour change the *Acid medium* to pH 7.5 *Buffer medium* by adding 50 mL of pH 7.5 buffer concentrate, for an additional 6 hours.

Apparatus 2: 100 rpm, with sinkers made of teflon-coated steel wire prepared by forming a coil approximately 22 mm long from a 13-cm length of 20-gauge wire (see *Figure 1*).

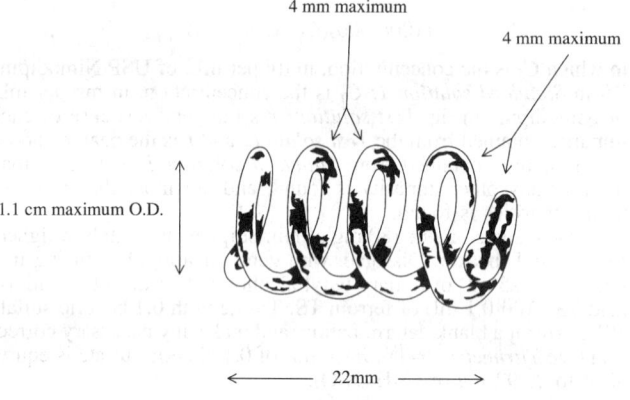

Fig. 1. Sinker.

Times: 1, 3, and 7 hours.

Acid-stage standard solution—Prepare a solution of USP Nitrofurantoin RS in *Acid medium* to obtain a solution having a known concentration of about 0.025 mg per mL.

Buffer-stage standard solution—Prepare a solution of USP Nitrofurantoin RS in *pH 7.5 Buffer medium* to obtain a solution having a known concentration of about 0.075 mg per mL.

Procedure—Determine the amount of $C_8H_6N_4O_5$ dissolved from UV absorbances at the isosbestic wavelength at about 375 nm on filtered portions of each solution under test, suitably diluted, if necessary, with *Acid medium* or *pH 7.5 Buffer medium* when appropriate in comparison with the appropriate *Standard solution*.

Tolerances—The percentages of the labeled amount of $C_8H_6N_4O_5$ dissolved at the specified times conform to the accompanying *Acceptance Table*.

Time (hours)	Amount dissolved (individual)	Amount dissolved (mean)
1	between 2% and 16%	between 5% and 13%
3	between 27% and 69%	between 39% and 56%
7	not less than 68%	not less than 81%

Acceptance Table

Level	Number Tested	Criteria
L_1	12	The mean percentage of dissolved label claim lies within the range for the means at each interval and is not less than the stated amount at the final test time. All individual values lie within the ranges for the individuals at each interval and are not less than the stated amount at the final test time.
L_2	12	The mean percentage of dissolved label claim lies within the range for the means at each interval and is not less than the stated amount at the final test time. Not more than 2 of the 24 individual values lie outside the stated ranges for individuals at each interval, and not more than 2 of 24 are less than the stated amount at the final test time.

TEST 3 (where it is labeled as containing both nitrofurantoin macrocrystalline and monohydrate forms)—If the product complies with this test, the labeling indicates that it meets USP *Dissolution Test 3*.

Acid medium, pH 7.5 Buffer medium, Apparatus 2, Times, Acid-stage standard solution, Buffer stage standard solution, and *Procedure*—Proceed as directed for *Test 2*.

Tolerances—The percentages of the labeled amount of $C_8H_6N_4O_5$ dissolved at the specified times conform to *Acceptance Table 2*.

Time (hours)	Amount dissolved (individual)	Amount dissolved (mean)
1	between 2% and 16%	between 5% and 13%
3	between 50% and 80%	between 55% and 75%
7	not less than 85%	not less than 90%

Uniformity of dosage units ⟨905⟩: meet the requirements.

PROCEDURE FOR CONTENT UNIFORMITY—

Test solution—Transfer the contents of 1 Capsule to a suitable flask, and add a volume of dimethylformamide to obtain a solution having a concentration of about 1.2 mg of nitrofurantoin per mL. Shake the flask for 15 minutes. [NOTE—If necessary, the sample may be homogenized using a disperser.] In the case of a 50- or 100-mg Capsule transfer 40.0 mL of this solution to a suitable flask, and proceed as directed for *Assay preparation* in the *Assay*, beginning with "add 50.0 mL of *Internal standard solution*." In the case of a 25-mg Capsule, transfer 20.0 mL of the solution to a suitable flask, and add 25.0 mL of *Internal standard solution* instead of 50.0 mL.

Procedure—Proceed as directed in the *Assay*, using the following *Test solution* instead of the *Assay preparation*.

Limit of nitrofurazone—

pH 7.0 Phosphate buffer, Mobile phase, Standard preparation, Chromatographic system, and *Procedure*—Proceed as directed in the *Limit of nitrofurazone* test under *Nitrofurantoin*.

Test preparation—Into a glass-stoppered, 25-mL flask weigh a portion of contents of Capsules equivalent to 100 mg of nitrofurantoin. Add 2.0 mL of dimethylformamide, and shake for 5 minutes. Add 20.0 mL of water, mix, and allow to stand for 15 minutes. Pass a portion of the mixture through a 0.45-μm pore size nylon filter.

Assay—

pH 7.0 phosphate buffer, Mobile phase, Internal standard solution, Standard preparation, and *Chromatographic system*—Proceed as directed in the *Assay* under *Nitrofurantoin*.

Assay preparation—Transfer, as completely as possible, the contents of 20 Capsules to a 500-mL flask. Place the emptied capsules in a beaker, add 25 mL of dimethylformamide, and agitate for 1 minute. Decant into the flask containing the Capsule contents. Rinse the emptied capsules with another two 25-mL portions of dimethylformamide, and decant into the flask. Add sufficient dimethylformamide to bring the volume to about 250 mL. Insert the stopper in the flask, and shake by mechanical means for 15 minutes. Dilute with dimethylformamide to volume, and mix. [NOTE—If necessary, the sample may be homogenized using a disperser.] Pass through a medium-porosity, sintered-glass filter into a suitable flask. Transfer an aliquot, equivalent to about 50 mg of nitrofurantoin, to a flask. Add an accurately measured volume of dimethylformamide to bring the volume in the flask to 40.0 mL. To the flask add 50.0 mL of *Internal standard solution*, mix, and cool to room temperature. Pass a portion of the solution through a 0.45-μm pore size nylon filter, discarding the first few mL of the filtrate.

Procedure—Proceed as directed for *Procedure* in the *Assay* under *Nitrofurantoin*. Calculate the quantity, in mg, of nitrofurantoin ($C_8H_6N_4O_5$) in the portion of the powder included in the sample aliquot by the formula:

$$W(R_U / R_S)$$

in which W is the weight, in mg, of USP Nitrofurantoin RS in the *Standard preparation*; and R_U and R_S are the ratios of the peak responses of the nitrofurantoin to the internal standard obtained from the *Assay preparation* and the *Standard preparation*, respectively.

Nitrofurantoin Oral Suspension

» Nitrofurantoin Oral Suspension is a suspension of Nitrofurantoin in a suitable aqueous vehicle. It contains, in each 100 mL, not less than 460 mg and not more than 540 mg of nitrofurantoin ($C_8H_6N_4O_5$).

Packaging and storage—Preserve in tight, light-resistant containers.

USP Reference standards ⟨11⟩—*USP Nitrofurantoin RS. USP Nitrofurantoin Related Compound A RS.*

Identification—

A: To 10 mL of Oral Suspension add 15 mL of acetone, and warm to 50°, with stirring, to coagulate the excipients. Filter, evaporate the acetone with the aid of a warm air blast nearly to dryness, add 10 mL of acetic acid, heat to boiling, and filter while hot. Cool the filtrate to room temperature. Filter the precipitated nitrofurantoin, and dry at 105° for 1 hour: the IR absorption spectrum of a mineral oil dispersion of the precipitate so obtained exhibits maxima only at the same wavelengths as that of a similar preparation of USP Nitrofurantoin RS.

B: It responds to *Identification* test B under *Nitrofurantoin*.

Uniformity of dosage units ⟨905⟩—

FOR ORAL SUSPENSION PACKAGED IN SINGLE-UNIT CONTAINERS: meets the requirements.

Deliverable volume ⟨698⟩—

FOR ORAL SUSPENSION PACKAGED IN MULTIPLE-UNIT CONTAINERS: meets the requirements.

pH ⟨791⟩: between 4.5 and 6.5.

Limit of *N*-(aminocarbonyl)-*N*-[((5-nitro-2-furanyl]methylene)amino]glycine (NF 250) and Assay—

pH 7.0 Phosphate buffer and *Mobile phase*—Prepare as directed in the *Assay* under *Nitrofurantoin*.

Internal standard solution—Dissolve about 13 mg of acetanilide in *Mobile phase,* dilute with *Mobile phase* to 200 mL, and mix.

Standard NF 250 preparation—Prepare a solution of USP Nitrofurantoin Related Compound A RS in *Mobile phase* to contain 125 μg per mL. [NOTE—USP Nitrofurantoin Related Compound A RS is *N*-(aminocarbonyl)-*N*-[((5-nitro-2-furanyl]methylene)amino]glycine.] Dilute 2.0 mL of this solution with *Mobile phase* to 100.0 mL, and mix.

Standard nitrofurantoin preparation—Transfer about 25 mg of USP Nitrofurantoin RS, accurately weighed, to a 100-mL volumetric flask with the aid of about 50 mL of dimethylformamide. Add 20 mL of water, cool to room temperature, and dilute with dimethylformamide to volume to obtain a *Standard solution*. Transfer a 4.0-mL aliquot of this *Standard solution* to a glass-stoppered flask, add 15.0 mL of *Internal standard solution,* and mix.

Assay preparation—Transfer an accurately measured volume of freshly mixed Oral Suspension, equivalent to about 25 mg of nitrofurantoin, to a 100-mL volumetric flask, add 20 mL of water to the flask, and mix. Add about 50 mL of dimethylformamide, and shake the flask for about 20 minutes. Cool to room temperature, and dilute with dimethylformamide to volume. Centrifuge a portion of the solution, and transfer a 4.0-mL aliquot of the supernatant to a glass-stoppered flask. Add 15.0 mL of *Internal standard*, and mix. Filter a portion of the solution through a 5-μm pore size polytef filter, discarding the first few mL of the filtrate.

Test preparation—Transfer an accurately measured volume of the freshly mixed Oral Suspension, equivalent to 5 mg of nitrofurantoin, to a 100-mL volumetric flask. Dilute with *Mobile phase* to volume, and mix. Centrifuge a portion of this solution. Pass a portion of the supernatant through a 5-μm pore size polytef filter, discarding the first few mL of the filtrate.

Chromatographic system (see *Chromatography* ⟨621⟩)—The liquid chromatograph is equipped with both a 254-nm detector and a 375-nm detector and a 3.9-mm × 30-cm column that contains packing L1. For the *Assay*, chromatograph the *Standard nitrofurantoin preparation*, adjusting the operating parameters so that the retention time of the nitrofurantoin peak is about 8 minutes and its peak height is about half full-scale: the relative standard deviation of the ratio of the peak responses in replicate injections is not more than 2.0%, and the resolution, *R*, of the acetanilide and nitrofurantoin peaks is not less than 3.5. The flow rate is about 1.2 mL per minute. For the NF 250 test, adjust the operating parameters so that the NF 250 peak has a retention time of between 3 and 6 minutes and its height is about 0.1 full-scale. The flow rate is about 1.2 mL per minute.

Procedure for limit of N-(aminocarbonyl)-N-[((5-nitro-2-furanyl)methylene)amino]glycine—Inject separately equal volumes (30 μL to 60 μL) of *Standard NF 250 preparation* and the *Test preparation* into the chromatograph, and record the peak responses with the 375-nm detector: the height of any peak appearing in the chromatogram of the *Test preparation* at a retention time corresponding to that of the main peak in the *Standard NF 250 preparation* is not greater than the height of the latter (5.0%).

Procedure for assay—Inject equal volumes (about 15 μL) of *Standard nitrofurantoin preparation* and the *Assay preparation* separately into the chromatograph, and record the peak responses with the 254-nm detector. Calculate the quantity, in mg, of $C_8H_6N_4O_5$ in each mL of the Oral Suspension taken by the formula:

$$0.1(C / V)(R_U / R_S)$$

in which *C* is the concentration, in μg per mL, of USP Nitrofurantoin RS in the *Standard solution*; *V* is the volume, in mL, of Oral Suspension taken; and R_U and R_S are the ratios of the peak responses of the nitrofurantoin to the internal standard obtained from the *Assay preparation* and the *Standard nitrofurantoin preparation*, respectively.

Nitrofurantoin Tablets

» Nitrofurantoin Tablets contain not less than 90.0 percent and not more than 110.0 percent of the labeled amount of nitrofurantoin ($C_8H_6N_4O_5$).

Packaging and storage—Preserve in tight, light-resistant containers.

USP Reference standards ⟨11⟩—*USP Nitrofurantoin RS. USP Nitrofurazone RS.*

Identification—
A: Add 10 mL of 6 N acetic acid to a quantity of powdered Tablets, equivalent to about 100 mg of nitrofurantoin, boil for a few minutes, and filter while hot. Cool to room temperature, collect the precipitate of nitrofurantoin, and dry at 105° for 1 hour: the IR absorption spectrum of a mineral oil dispersion of the precipitate so obtained exhibits maxima only at the same wavelengths as that of a similar preparation of USP Nitrofurantoin RS.

B: It responds to *Identification* test *B* under *Nitrofurantoin*.

Dissolution ⟨711⟩—
Medium: pH 7.2 phosphate buffer (see *Buffer Solutions* in the section *Reagents, Indicators, and Solutions*); 900 mL.
Apparatus 1: 100 rpm.
Times: 60 minutes, 120 minutes.
Standard preparation—Dissolve about 50 mg, accurately weighed, of USP Nitrofurantoin RS in 25 mL of dimethylformamide, dilute with *Dissolution Medium* to 500 mL, mix, and dilute a suitable aliquot of the resulting solution with *Dissolution Medium* to obtain a solution having a known concentration of about 10 μg per mL.
Procedure—Determine the amount of $C_8H_6N_4O_5$ dissolved from absorbances at the wavelength of maximum absorbance at about 375 nm of filtered portions of the solution under test, suitably diluted with *Dissolution Medium*, if necessary, using *Dissolution Medium* as the blank, in comparison with the *Standard preparation*.
Tolerances—Not less than 25% (*Q*) of the labeled amount of $C_8H_6N_4O_5$ is dissolved in 60 minutes, and not less than 85% (*Q*) of the labeled amount of $C_8H_6N_4O_5$ is dissolved in 120 minutes.

Uniformity of dosage units ⟨905⟩: meet the requirements.

Limit of nitrofurazone: meet the requirements of the test for *Nitrofurazone* under *Nitrofurantoin Capsules*, powdered Tablets being used in place of contents of Capsules.

Assay—
pH 7.0 phosphate buffer, Mobile phase, Internal standard solution, Standard preparation, and *Chromatographic system*—Proceed as directed in the *Assay* under *Nitrofurantoin*.

Assay preparation—Weigh and finely powder not less than 20 Tablets. Weigh accurately a portion of the powder, equivalent to about 50 mg of nitrofurantoin, into a glass-stoppered flask. Add 40.0 mL of dimethylformamide, and shake by mechanical means for 15 minutes. Add 50.0 mL of *Internal standard solution*, mix, and cool to room temperature. Pass a portion of the solution through a 0.45-μm pore size nylon filter, discarding the first few mL of the filtrate.

Procedure—Proceed as directed for *Procedure* in the *Assay* under *Nitrofurantoin*. Calculate the quantity, in mg, of $C_8H_6N_4O_5$ in the portion of the powder taken by the formula:

$$W(R_U / R_S)$$

in which *W* is the weight, in mg, of USP Nitrofurantoin RS in the *Standard preparation* and R_U and R_S are the ratios of the peak responses of the nitrofurantoin to the internal standard obtained from the *Assay preparation* and the *Standard preparation*, respectively.

Nitrofurazone

$C_6H_6N_4O_4$ 198.14
Hydrazinecarboxamide, 2-[(5-nitro-2-furanyl)methylene]-.
5-Nitro-2-furaldehyde semicarbazone [59-87-0].

» Nitrofurazone, dried at 105° for 1 hour, contains not less than 98.0 percent and not more than 102.0 percent of $C_6H_6N_4O_4$.

NOTE—Avoid exposing solutions of nitrofurazone at all times to direct sunlight, excessive heat, strong fluorescent lighting, and alkaline materials.

Packaging and storage—Preserve in tight, light-resistant containers, and avoid exposure to direct sunlight and to excessive heat.

USP Reference standards ⟨11⟩—*USP Nitrofurazone RS. USP Nitrofurazone Related Compound A RS.*

Identification—
A: *Infrared Absorption* ⟨197K⟩.
B: *Ultraviolet Absorption* ⟨197U⟩—
Solution: 8 µg per mL, prepared as directed in the *Assay*.
Ratio: A_{306}/A_{375} does not exceed 0.25.
C: Dissolve 400 mg of potassium hydroxide in 10 mL of alcohol. Immediately before use dilute this solution with dimethylformamide to 100 mL. To 10 mL of the prepared solution add a few crystals of Nitrofurazone: a purple solution results.
pH ⟨791⟩—Suspend 1 g in 100 mL of water, shake for 15 minutes, allow the suspension to settle, and filter: the pH of the filtrate is between 5.0 and 7.5.
Loss on drying ⟨731⟩—Dry it at 105° for 1 hour: it loses not more than 0.5% of its weight.
Residue on ignition ⟨281⟩: not more than 0.1%.
Ordinary impurities ⟨466⟩—
Test solution: dimethylformamide.
Standard solution: dimethylformamide.
Application volume: 10 µL.
Eluant: a mixture of chloroform, methanol, and ammonium hydroxide (60 : 24 : 3), in a nonequilibrated chamber.
Visualization: 1.
Limit of 5-nitro-2-furfuraldazine—
Adsorbent: 0.5-mm layer of chromatographic silica gel.
Test solution—Transfer 2.0 g to a 100-mL volumetric flask. Dissolve in 60 mL of dimethylformamide, dilute with acetone to volume, and mix.
Standard solution—Transfer 50.0 mg of USP Nitrofurazone Related Compound A RS to a 100-mL volumetric flask, dissolve in and dilute with dimethylformamide to volume, and mix. [NOTE—USP Nitrofurazone Related Compound A RS is 5-nitro-2-furfuraldazine.] Transfer 5.0 mL of this solution to a 25-mL volumetric flask, add 10 mL of dimethylformamide, dilute with acetone to volume, and mix.
Application volume: 5 µL.
Developing solvent system: a mixture of ethyl acetate and cyclohexane (4 : 1).
Procedure—Proceed as directed for *Thin-Layer Chromatography* under *Chromatography* ⟨621⟩. With a suitable densitometer, equipped with a filter having its maximum transmittance at about 254 nm, locate and scan the spot produced by the *Standard solution* and any spot from the *Test solution* having the same R_F as that produced by the *Standard solution*: the area and intensity of any spot from the *Test solution* are not greater than the area and intensity produced by the spot from the *Standard solution* (0.5%).
Assay—Transfer about 100 mg of Nitrofurazone, previously dried and accurately weighed, to a 250-mL volumetric flask, dissolve in 50 mL of dimethylformamide, dilute with water to volume, and mix. Transfer 5.0 mL of this solution to a 250-mL volumetric flask, dilute with water to volume, and mix. Concomitantly determine the absorbances of this solution and a Standard solution of USP Nitrofurazone RS in the same medium having a known concentration of about 8 µg per mL, in 1-cm cells at the wavelength of maximum absorbance at about 375 nm, with a suitable spectrophotometer, using water as the blank. Calculate the quantity, in mg, of $C_6H_6N_4O_4$ in the Nitrofurazone taken by the formula:

$$12.5C(A_U / A_S)$$

in which C is the concentration, in µg per mL, of USP Nitrofurazone RS in the Standard solution, and A_U and A_S are the absorbances of the solution of Nitrofurazone and the Standard solution, respectively.

Nitrofurazone Ointment

» Nitrofurazone Ointment is Nitrofurazone in a suitable water-miscible base. It contains not less than 90.0 percent and not more than 110.0 percent of the labeled amount of nitrofurazone ($C_6H_6N_4O_4$).

NOTE—Avoid exposure at all times to direct sunlight, excessive heat, strong fluorescent lighting, and alkaline materials.

Packaging and storage—Preserve in tight, light-resistant containers. Avoid exposure to direct sunlight, strong fluorescent lighting, and excessive heat.
USP Reference standards ⟨11⟩—*USP Nitrofurazone RS*.
Completeness of solution—One g dissolves in 9 mL of water to form a clear solution.
Identification—Dissolve 400 mg of potassium hydroxide in a mixture of 9.5 mL of alcohol and 0.5 mL of methanol. Immediately before use, dilute with dimethylformamide to 100 mL. To 10 mL of this solution add a quantity of Ointment, equivalent to about 10 µg of nitrofurazone, and mix: a purple solution results.
Assay—[NOTE—Protect from light all solutions that contain nitrofurazone.]
Triethylamine buffer—Transfer 100 mL of triethylamine to a 1000-mL volumetric flask. Add about 800 mL of water, and cautiously add 80 mL of phosphoric acid. Mix, allow to cool to ambient temperature, dilute with water to volume, mix, and pass through a nylon filter having a 0.5-µm or finer porosity.
Mobile phase—Prepare a filtered and degassed mixture of water, acetonitrile, and *Triethylamine buffer* (790 : 200 : 10). Make any necessary adjustments (see *System Suitability* under *Chromatography* ⟨621⟩).
Standard preparation—Transfer about 50 mg of USP Nitrofurazone RS, accurately weighed, to a 50-mL low-actinic volumetric flask, add 10 mL of dimethylformamide, and swirl to dissolve. Dilute with alcohol to volume, and mix. Transfer 10.0 mL of this solution to a 100-mL low-actinic volumetric flask, dilute with alcohol to volume, and mix. Transfer 10.0 mL of this solution to a 100-mL low-actinic volumetric flask containing 15 mL of alcohol, dilute with water to volume, and mix. This solution contains about 0.01 mg of USP Nitrofurazone RS per mL.
Assay preparation—Transfer an accurately weighed portion of Ointment, equivalent to about 1 mg of nitrofurazone, to a 100-mL low-actinic volumetric flask. Add 0.2 mL of dimethylformamide and about 25 mL of alcohol, and sonicate for about 35 minutes. Dilute with water to volume, mix, and pass through a nylon filter having a 0.5-µm or finer porosity. Use the filtrate.
Chromatographic system (see *Chromatography* ⟨621⟩)—The liquid chromatograph is equipped with a 365-nm detector and a 3.9-mm × 30-cm column that contains packing L1. The flow rate is about 2 mL per minute. Chromatograph the *Standard preparation*, and record the peak responses as directed for *Procedure*: the column efficiency determined from the nitrofurazone peak is not less than 1500 theoretical plates, and the relative standard deviation for replicate injections is not more than 2%.
Procedure—Separately inject equal volumes (about 20 µL) of the *Standard preparation* and the *Assay preparation* into the chromatograph, record the chromatograms, and measure the responses for the major peaks. Calculate the quantity, in mg, of nitrofurazone ($C_6H_6N_4O_4$) in the portion of Ointment taken by the formula:

$$100C(r_U / r_S)$$

in which C is the concentration, in mg per mL, of USP Nitrofurazone RS in the *Standard preparation*; and r_U and r_S are the nitrofurazone peak responses obtained from the *Assay preparation* and the *Standard preparation*, respectively.

Nitrofurazone Topical Solution

» Nitrofurazone Topical Solution contains not less than 95.0 percent and not more than 105.0 percent (w/w) of the labeled amount of $C_6H_6N_4O_4$.

NOTE—Avoid exposure at all times to direct sunlight, excessive heat, and alkaline materials.

Packaging and storage—Preserve in tight, light-resistant containers. Avoid exposure to direct sunlight and excessive heat.

USP Reference standards ⟨11⟩—*USP Nitrofurazone RS*.
Identification—Dissolve 400 mg of potassium hydroxide in a mixture of 9.5 mL of alcohol and 0.5 mL of methanol. Immediately before use dilute with dimethylformamide to 100 mL. To 10 mL of this solution add 1 drop of Topical Solution: a purple solution results.

Assay—[NOTE—Protect from light all solutions that contain nitrofurazone.]
Triethylamine buffer, Mobile phase, Standard preparation, and *Chromatographic system*—Proceed as directed in the *Assay* under *Nitrofurazone Ointment*.
Assay preparation—Transfer an accurately measured portion of Topical Solution, equivalent to about 1 mg of nitrofurazone, to a 100-mL low actinic volumetric flask. Add 0.2 mL of dimethylformamide and about 25 mL of warm (between 40° and 50°) alcohol. Dilute with water to volume, and mix.
Procedure—Proceed as directed in the *Assay* under *Nitrofurazone Ointment*. Calculate the quantity, in mg, of $C_6H_6N_4O_4$ in the portion of Topical Solution taken by the formula:

$$100C(r_U / r_S)$$

in which C is the concentration, in mg per mL, of USP Nitrofurazone RS in the *Standard preparation*, and r_U and r_S are the nitrofurazone peak responses obtained from the *Assay preparation* and the *Standard preparation*, respectively.

Ammonia N 13 Injection

» Ammonia N 13 Injection is a sterile solution of $^{13}NH_3$ in Sodium Chloride Injection, suitable for intravenous administration, in which a portion of the molecules are labeled with radioactive ^{13}N (see *Radiopharmaceuticals for Positron Emission Tomography—Compounding* ⟨823⟩). It contains not less than 90.0 percent and not more than 110.0 percent of the labeled amount of ^{13}N expressed in MBq (or mCi) per mL at the time indicated in the labeling.

Specific activity: no carrier added.
Packaging and storage—Preserve in single-dose or multiple-dose containers that are adequately shielded.
Labeling—Label it to include the following, in addition to the information specified for *Labeling* under *Injections* ⟨1⟩: the time and date of calibration; the amount of ^{13}N as ammonia expressed as total MBq (mCi) per mL, at time of calibration; the expiration time and date; and the statement "Caution—Radioactive Material." The labeling indicates that in making dosage calculations correction is to be made for radioactive decay and also indicates that the radioactive half-life of ^{13}N is 9.96 minutes. The label also includes the statement "Do not use if cloudy or if it contains particulate matter."

USP Reference standards ⟨11⟩—*USP Ammonium Chloride RS*. *USP Endotoxin RS*.
Identification—
A: *Radionuclidic identity*—Its half-life, determined using a suitable detector system (see *Radioactivity* ⟨821⟩ is between 9.5 and 10.5 minutes.
B: *Radiochemical identity*—The retention time of the major peak in the chromatogram of the *Test solution* corresponds to that in the chromatogram of the *Standard solution*, as obtained in the *Radiochemical purity* test.
Bacterial endotoxins ⟨85⟩ (see *Sterilization and Sterility Assurance* under *Radiopharmaceuticals for Positron Emission Tomography—Compounding* ⟨823⟩)—It contains not more than 175/V USP Endotoxin Unit per mL of the Injection, in which V is the maximum administered total dose, in mL, at the expiration time.

pH ⟨791⟩: between 4.5 and 7.5.
Radiochemical purity—
Mobile phase—Add 0.25 mL of concentrated nitric acid to 1000 mL of a mixture of water and methanol (7 : 3), filter, and degas.
Standard solution—Dissolve an accurately weighed quantity of USP Ammonium Chloride RS in water, and dilute quantitatively, and stepwise if necessary, with water to obtain a solution having a known concentration of about 0.1 mg per mL.
Test solution—Use the Injection.
Chromatographic system (see *Chromatography* ⟨621⟩)—The liquid chromatograph is equipped with a 4.1-mm × 25-cm column that contains 10-μm packing L17. It is equipped with a gamma ray detector and a conductivity detector. The flow rate is about 2.0 mL per minute. Chromatograph the *Test solution*, and record the peak responses as directed for *Procedure*: the relative standard deviation for replicate injections is not more than 5%.
Procedure—Prepare a mixture of the *Standard solution* and the *Test solution* (1 : 1), and inject about 20 μL of the mixture into the chromatograph, record the chromatograms, and measure the peak areas. The areas of both the main radioactive and nonradioactive peaks are equal. [NOTE—The volume of Injection may be adjusted to obtain suitable detection system sensitivity.] The radioactivity of the major peak is not less than 95% of the total radioactivity measured. The retention time of the *Test solution* corresponds to the retention time of the *Standard solution*.
Radionuclidic purity—Using a suitable gamma-ray spectrometer (see *Selection of a Counting Assembly* under *Radioactivity* ⟨821⟩), count an appropriate aliquot of the Injection for a period of time sufficient to obtain a gamma spectrum. The resultant gamma spectrum should be analyzed for the presence of identifiable photopeaks which are not characteristic of ^{13}N emissions. Not less than 99.5% of the observed gamma emissions should correspond to the 0.511 MeV, 1.022 MeV, or Compton scatter peaks of ^{13}N.
Chemical purity—This article may be synthesized by different methods and processes and, therefore, contains different impurities. The presence of unlabeled ingredients, reagents, and by-products specific to the process must be controlled, and their potential for physiological or pharmacological effects must be considered.
ALUMINUM (to be determined if Devarda's alloy is used to reduce ^{13}N nitrate/nitrite)—
Aluminum standard solution—Transfer 35.17 mg of aluminum potassium sulfate dodecahydrate, accurately weighed, to a 1000-mL volumetric flask, and dilute with water to volume to obtain a solution having a known concentration of 2 μg of aluminum per mL.
Procedure—Pipet 10 mL of *Aluminum standard solution* into each of two 50-mL volumetric flasks. To each flask add 3 drops of methyl orange TS and 2 drops of 6 N ammonium hydroxide, then add 0.5 N hydrochloric acid, dropwise, until the solution turns red. To one flask add 25 mL of sodium thioglycolate TS, and to the other flask add 1 mL of edetate disodium TS. To each flask add 5 mL of eriochrome cyanine TS and 5 mL of acetate buffer TS, and add water to volume. Immediately determine the absorbance of the solution containing sodium thioglycolate TS at the wavelength of maximum absorbance at about 535 nm, with a suitable spectrophotometer, using the solution containing the edetate disodium TS as a blank. Repeat the procedure using two 1.0-mL aliquots of Injection. Calculate the quantity, in μg per mL, of aluminum in the Injection taken by the formula:

$$20(T_U / T_S)$$

in which T_U and T_S are the absorbances of the solutions from the Injection and the *Aluminum standard solution*, respectively. The concentration of aluminum ion in the Injection is not greater than 10 μg per mL.
Other requirements—It meets the requirements under *Injections* ⟨1⟩, except that the Injection may be distributed or dispensed prior to completion of the test for *Sterility* ⟨71⟩, the latter test being started within 24 hours of final manufacture, and except that it is not subject to the recommendation in *Volume in Container*.
Assay for radioactivity—Using a suitable calibrated system as directed under *Radioactivity* ⟨821⟩, determine the radioactivity, in MBq (or mCi) per mL, of the Injection.

Diluted Nitroglycerin

$C_3H_5N_3O_9$ 227.09
1,2,3-Propanetriol, trinitrate.
Nitroglycerin [55-63-0].

» Diluted Nitroglycerin is a mixture of nitroglycerin ($C_3H_5N_3O_9$) with lactose, dextrose, alcohol, propylene glycol, or other suitable inert excipient to permit safe handling. It contains not less than 90.0 percent and not more than 110.0 percent of the labeled amount of $C_3H_5N_3O_9$. It usually contains not more than 10 percent of nitroglycerin ($C_3H_5N_3O_9$).
Caution—Taking into consideration the concentration and amount of nitroglycerin ($C_3H_5N_3O_9$) in Diluted Nitroglycerin, exercise appropriate precautions when handling this material. Nitroglycerin is a powerful explosive and can be detonated by percussion or excessive heat. Do not isolate nitroglycerin ($C_3H_5N_3O_9$).

Packaging and storage—Preserve in tight, light-resistant containers, and prevent exposure to excessive heat. Store at 25°, excursions permitted between 15° and 30°.
USP Reference standards ⟨11⟩—USP Diluted Nitroglycerin RS.
Identification—
  A: The R_F value of the principal spot in the chromatogram of the *Identification test preparation* corresponds to that in the chromatogram of the *Standard preparation*, as obtained in the test for *Chromatographic purity*.
  B: The retention time of the major peak in the chromatogram of the *Assay preparation* corresponds to that in the chromatogram of the *Standard preparation*, obtained as directed in the *Assay*.
Chromatographic purity—
  Standard solution—Dissolve an accurately weighed quantity of USP Diluted Nitroglycerin RS in methanol, and dilute quantitatively with methanol to obtain a solution having a concentration of 400 µg of nitroglycerin per mL.
  Identification test solution—Prepare a clear solution in methanol containing an amount of Diluted Nitroglycerin equivalent to about 400 µg of nitroglycerin per mL.
  Test solution—Transfer an accurately weighed portion, equivalent to 100 mg of nitroglycerin, to a 5-mL volumetric flask. Dissolve (or suspend) in methanol, dilute with methanol to volume, and mix. Centrifuge a portion, if necessary, to obtain a clear liquid phase.
  Procedure—Apply separately 20 µL of the *Test solution*, 5, 10, 15, and 20 µL of the *Standard solution*, and 20 µL of the *Identification test solution* to a suitable thin-layer chromatographic plate (see *Chromatography* ⟨621⟩) coated with a 0.25-mm layer of chromatographic silica gel mixture. Allow the spots to dry, position the plate in a chromatographic chamber, and develop the chromatograms in a solvent system consisting of a mixture of toluene and ethyl acetate (4 : 1) until the solvent front has moved about three-fourths of the length of the plate. Remove the plate from the developing chamber, mark the solvent front, and allow the solvent to evaporate. Spray the plate with a 1 in 100 solution of diphenylamine in methanol, and irradiate the plate with short- and long-wavelength UV light for about 15 minutes, and examine the chromatogram: any spot obtained from the *Test solution*, other than the principal spot, is not more intense than the spot in the chromatogram from the 20-µL application of the *Standard solution*. Compare the intensities of any secondary spots observed in the chromatogram of the *Test solution* with those of the principal spots in the chromatograms of the *Standard solution* (corresponding to 0.5%, 1.0%, 1.5%, and 2.0%, respectively): the sum of the intensities of the secondary spots obtained in the *Test solution* is not more than 3%. [NOTE—Nitrates of glycerin typically have R_F values of about 0.21, 0.37, and 0.61 for mono-, di-, and tri-substituted glycerins, respectively.]

Assay—
  Mobile phase—Prepare a degassed solution containing equal volumes of methanol and water, making adjustments if necessary (see *System Suitability* under *Chromatography* ⟨621⟩).
  Standard preparation—Dissolve an accurately weighed quantity of USP Diluted Nitroglycerin RS in *Mobile phase* to obtain a solution having a known concentration of about 0.075 mg of nitroglycerin per mL.
  Assay preparation—Transfer an accurately weighed portion of Diluted Nitroglycerin, equivalent to about 7.5 mg of nitroglycerin, to a 100-mL volumetric flask, and dissolve in about 75 mL of *Mobile phase*. If necessary, sonicate for 2 minutes or until the solid is totally dispersed, then shake by mechanical means for 30 minutes. Dilute with *Mobile phase* to volume, mix, and filter.
  Chromatographic system (see *Chromatography* ⟨621⟩)—The liquid chromatograph is equipped with a 220-nm detector and a 4.6-mm × 25-cm column that contains packing L1, and if necessary a short precolumn that contains packing L1. The flow rate is about 1 mL per minute. Chromatograph replicate injections of the *Standard preparation*, and record the peak responses as directed for *Procedure*: the column efficiency is not less than 3000 theoretical plates, the tailing factor for the analyte peak is not more than 2.5, and the relative standard deviation is not more than 3.0%.
  Procedure—Separately inject equal volumes (about 20 µL) of the *Standard preparation* and the *Assay preparation* into the chromatograph by means of a microsyringe or sampling valve, record the chromatograms, and measure the responses for the major peaks. Calculate the quantity, in mg, of $C_3H_5N_3O_9$ in the portion of Diluted Nitroglycerin taken by the formula:

$$100C(r_U / r_S)$$

in which C is the concentration, in mg per mL, of nitroglycerin in the *Standard preparation*, and r_U and r_S are the peak responses of nitroglycerin obtained from the *Assay preparation* and the *Standard preparation*, respectively.

Nitroglycerin Injection

» Nitroglycerin Injection is a sterile solution prepared from Diluted Nitroglycerin; the solvent may contain Alcohol, Propylene Glycol, and Water for Injection. Nitroglycerin Injection contains not less than 90.0 percent and not more than 110.0 percent of the labeled amount of Nitroglycerin ($C_3H_5N_3O_9$).

Packaging and storage—Preserve in single-dose or in multiple-dose containers, preferably of Type I or Type II glass.
Labeling—Where necessary, label it to indicate that it is to be diluted before use.
USP Reference standards ⟨11⟩—USP Diluted Nitroglycerin RS. USP Endotoxin RS.
Identification—The retention time of the major peak in the chromatogram of the *Assay preparation* corresponds to that of the *Standard preparation* obtained as directed in the *Assay*.
Bacterial endotoxins ⟨85⟩—It contains not more than 0.1 USP Endotoxin Unit per µg of nitroglycerin.
pH ⟨791⟩: between 3.0 and 6.5, determined potentiometrically in a solution prepared by adding 5 mL of water and 1 drop of saturated potassium chloride solution to 5 mL of the Injection.
Particulate matter ⟨788⟩: meets the requirements under small-volume injections.
Alcohol content, *Method II* ⟨611⟩: between 90.0% and 110.0% of the labeled amount of C_2H_5OH, isopropyl alcohol being used as the internal standard.
Other requirements—It meets the requirements under *Injections* ⟨1⟩.
Assay—
  Mobile phase, Standard preparation, and *Chromatographic system*—Prepare as directed in the *Assay* under *Diluted Nitroglycerin*.

Assay preparation—Transfer an accurately measured volume of Injection, equivalent to about 7.5 mg of nitroglycerin, to a 100-mL volumetric flask, dissolve in and dilute with *Mobile phase* to volume, and mix.

Procedure—Separately inject equal volumes (about 20 μL) of the *Standard preparation* and the *Assay preparation* into the chromatograph, record the chromatograms, and measure the responses for the major peaks. Calculate the quantity, in mg, of $C_3H_5N_3O_9$ in the portion of Injection taken by the formula:

$$100C(r_U / r_S)$$

in which C is the concentration, in mg per mL, of nitroglycerin in the *Standard preparation*, and r_U and r_S are the peak responses of nitroglycerin obtained from the *Assay preparation* and the *Standard preparation*, respectively.

Nitroglycerin Ointment

» Nitroglycerin Ointment is Diluted Nitroglycerin in a suitable ointment base. It contains not less than 90.0 percent and not more than 115.0 percent of the labeled amount of nitroglycerin ($C_3H_5N_3O_9$).

Packaging and storage—Preserve in tight containers.
Labeling—Label multiple-dose containers with a direction to close tightly, immediately after each use.
USP Reference standards ⟨11⟩—*USP Diluted Nitroglycerin RS*.
Identification—The retention time of the major peak obtained from the *Assay preparation* corresponds to that from the *Standard preparation* as obtained in the *Assay*.
Minimum fill ⟨755⟩: meets the requirements.
Homogeneity—In the case of single-dose containers, perform the *Assay* on specimens from each of 10 containers. In the case of multiple-dose containers, perform the *Assay* on one specimen from the top and one from the bottom of each of 5 containers. Each specimen contains not less than 90.0% and not more than 110.0% of the mean value.
Assay—
Mobile phase, Standard preparation, and *Chromatographic system*—Proceed as directed in the *Assay* under *Diluted Nitroglycerin*.
Assay preparation—Transfer an accurately weighed portion of Ointment, equivalent to about 2.0 mg of nitroglycerin, to a glass-stoppered, 50-mL conical flask, and add 25.0 mL of *Mobile phase*. Immerse for 10 minutes in a water bath maintained at a temperature of 50°, shaking intermittently until the specimen becomes dispersed. Remove from the bath, and shake vigorously for 1 minute to obtain a coagulated solid. Repeat the heating and shaking steps one more time and filter.
Procedure—Separately inject equal volumes of the *Standard preparation* and the *Assay preparation* into the chromatograph, record the chromatograms, and measure the responses for the major peaks. Calculate the quantity, in mg, of $C_3H_5N_3O_9$ in the portion of Ointment taken by the formula:

$$25C(r_U / r_S)$$

in which C is the concentration, in mg per mL, of nitroglycerin in the *Standard preparation*, and r_U and r_S are the peak responses of nitroglycerin obtained from the *Assay preparation* and the *Standard preparation*, respectively.

Nitroglycerin Sublingual Tablets

Former Title: **Nitroglycerin Tablets**

» Nitroglycerin Sublingual Tablets contain not less than 90.0 percent and not more than 115.0 percent of the labeled amount of nitroglycerin ($C_3H_5N_3O_9$).

Packaging and storage—Preserve in tight containers, preferably of glass, and store at controlled room temperature. Each container holds not more than 100 Sublingual Tablets.
Labeling—The labeling indicates that the Sublingual Tablets are for sublingual use, and the label directs that the Sublingual Tablets be dispensed in the original, unopened container, labeled with the following statement directed to the patient. "Warning: To prevent loss of potency, keep these tablets in the original container or in a supplemental nitroglycerin container specifically labeled as being suitable for Nitroglycerin Sublingual Tablets. Close tightly immediately after each use."
USP Reference standards ⟨11⟩—*USP Diluted Nitroglycerin RS*.
Identification—
A: *Thin-Layer Chromatographic Identification Test* ⟨201⟩—
Test solution—Transfer an amount of finely powdered Sublingual Tablets, equivalent to about 1 mg of nitroglycerin, to a glass-stoppered vessel, add 1 mL of acetone, shake by mechanical means for 30 minutes, and filter.
Standard solution: 1 mg per mL, in acetone.
Developing solvent system: a mixture of toluene, ethyl acetate, and glacial acetic acid (16 : 4 : 1).
Procedure—Proceed as directed in the chapter. Spray with a solution of diphenylamine in methanol (1 in 100), and irradiate the plate with short- and long-wavelength UV light for about 10 minutes.
B: The retention time of the major peak in the chromatogram of the *Assay preparation* corresponds to that in the chromatogram of the *Standard preparation,* as obtained in the *Assay*.
Disintegration ⟨701⟩: 2 minutes, determined as set forth for *Sublingual Tablets*.
Uniformity of dosage units ⟨905⟩: meet the requirements.
PROCEDURE FOR CONTENT UNIFORMITY—
Mobile phase, Standard preparation, and *Chromatographic system*—Proceed as directed in the *Assay* under *Diluted Nitroglycerin*.
Test preparation—Transfer 1 Sublingual Tablet to a suitable container, and dissolve in and dilute with *Mobile phase* to obtain a solution containing about 0.075 mg of nitroglycerin per mL.
Procedure—Separately inject equal volumes (about 20 μL) of the *Standard preparation* and the *Test preparation* into the chromatograph, record the chromatograms, and measure the responses for the major peaks. Calculate the quantity, in mg, of nitroglycerin ($C_3H_5N_3O_9$) in the portion of Sublingual Tablets taken by the formula:

$$VC(r_U / r_S)$$

in which V is the volume, in mL, of *Mobile phase* used to prepare the *Test preparation;* C is the concentration, in mg per mL, of USP Diluted Nitroglycerin RS in the *Standard preparation;* and r_U and r_S are the peak responses for nitroglycerin obtained from the *Test preparation* and the *Standard preparation,* respectively. The content of each of the 10 Sublingual Tablets is within the range of 75.0% and 135.0% of the labeled claim. If the content of not more than 1 Sublingual Tablet is outside the range of 75.0% and 135.0% and if the content of none of the Sublingual Tablets is outside the range of 60.0% and 150.0%, test 20 additional units. The requirements are met if the content of each of the additional 20 units falls within the range of 75.0% and 135.0% of the labeled claim.
Assay—
Mobile phase, Standard preparation, and *Chromatographic system*—Prepare as directed in the *Assay* under *Diluted Nitroglycerin*.
Assay preparation—Dissolve not fewer than 20 Sublingual Tablets in *Mobile phase,* and dilute quantitatively, and stepwise if necessary, with *Mobile phase* to obtain a solution containing about 0.075 mg per mL of nitroglycerin.
Procedure—Separately inject equal volumes (about 20 μL) of the *Standard preparation* and the *Assay preparation* into the chromatograph, record the chromatograms, and measure the responses for the major peaks. Calculate the quantity, in mg, of nitroglycerin ($C_3H_5N_3O_9$) per Sublingual Tablet taken by the formula:

$$100 / (TDC)(r_U / r_S)$$

in which T is the number of Sublingual Tablets taken; D is the dilution factor of the *Assay preparation;* C is the concentration, in mg per mL, of USP Diluted Nitroglycerin RS in the *Standard prepara-*

tion; and r_U and r_S are the peak responses for nitroglycerin obtained from the *Assay preparation* and the *Standard preparation,* respectively.

Nitromersol

C₇H₅HgNO₃   351.71
7-Oxa-8-mercurabicyclo[4.2.0]octa-1,3,5-triene, 5-methyl-2-nitro-.
5-Methyl-2-nitro-7-oxa-8-mercurabicyclo[4.2.0]octa-1,3,5-triene [*133-58-4*].

» Nitromersol, dried at 105° for 2 hours, contains not less than 98.0 percent and not more than 100.5 percent of C₇H₅HgNO₃.

Packaging and storage—Preserve in tight, light-resistant containers.
Identification—
   A: A solution (1 in 1000) in 1 N sodium hydroxide possesses a reddish-orange color. The addition of 3 N hydrochloric acid to this solution causes the color to disappear and a yellowish, flocculent precipitate to form.
   B: To a solution prepared by dissolving 250 mg of Nitromersol in 2.5 mL of 1 N sodium hydroxide and diluting with water to 20 mL add about 3 mL of 3 N hydrochloric acid: a yellowish precipitate is formed. Upon filtration, the filtrate is nearly colorless or slightly yellow. Retain the filtrate for the test for *Mercury ions.* Dissolve the precipitate in 20 mL of water to which 2.5 mL of 1 N sodium hydroxide has been added, add 0.5 g of sodium hydrosulfite, and heat to boiling: a heavy deposit of metallic mercury is formed.
Loss on drying ⟨731⟩—Dry it at 105° for 2 hours: it loses not more than 1.0% of its weight.
Residue on ignition ⟨281⟩: not more than 0.1%.
Mercury ions—To the filtrate obtained in *Identification* test *B* add an equal volume of hydrogen sulfide TS: no darkening in color is produced, although a small amount of a flocculent, light yellow precipitate may form.
Alkali-insoluble substances—Add 7 mL of 1 N sodium hydroxide to 1.0 g of Nitromersol, then dilute with water to 20 mL. The resulting solution, upon standing in a glass-stoppered vessel in the dark for 24 hours, shows no more than a slight amount of insoluble material. Collect the insoluble residue, if any, in a tared filter crucible, wash the residue with warm water, and dry at 105° for 1 hour: the weight of the insoluble material does not exceed 1 mg (0.1%).
Uncombined nitrocresol—Shake 500 mg of Nitromersol with 50 mL of benzene, filter, evaporate the filtrate in a tared dish to dryness, and dry the residue at 80° for 2 hours: the weight of the residue does not exceed 5 mg (1%).
Assay—Weigh accurately about 200 mg of Nitromersol, previously ground to a fine powder and dried, and transfer to a 500-mL Kjeldahl flask. Add 15 mL of sulfuric acid, digest cautiously with occasional swirling over a flame until the solution becomes a clear, light yellowish brown, cool, and add, dropwise, enough 30 percent hydrogen peroxide to decolorize the solution. Digest for 2 to 3 minutes, adding more hydrogen peroxide, if necessary, to produce a colorless solution. Cool, dilute with water to about 100 mL, and add potassium permanganate TS until a permanent pink color persists on heating. Then add hydrogen peroxide TS, dropwise, until the color is completely discharged. Cool, and add 5 mL of nitric acid which has been diluted with 10 mL of water. Add 5 mL of ferric ammonium sulfate TS, and titrate with 0.1 N ammonium thiocyanate VS. Each mL of 0.1 N ammonium thiocyanate is equivalent to 17.59 mg of C₇H₅HgNO₃.

Nitromersol Topical Solution

» Nitromersol Topical Solution yields, from each 100 mL, not less than 180.0 mg and not more than 220.0 mg of nitromersol (C₇H₅HgNO₃).

Nitromersol	2 g
Sodium Hydroxide	0.4 g
Sodium Carbonate, monohydrate	4.25 g
Purified Water, a sufficient quantity, to make	1000 mL

Dissolve the Sodium Hydroxide and the monohydrated Sodium Carbonate in 50 mL of Purified Water, add the Nitromersol, and stir until dissolved. Gradually add Purified Water to make 1000 mL.
   NOTE—Prepare dilutions of Nitromersol Topical Solution as needed, since they tend to precipitate upon standing.

Packaging and storage—Preserve in tight, light-resistant containers.
Identification—
   A: To 100 mL add 3 mL of 3 N hydrochloric acid: a yellowish precipitate is formed. Filter, and retain both the filtrate and the precipitate.
   B: Add the precipitate from *Identification* test *A* to 20 mL of water and 2.5 mL of 1 N sodium hydroxide. Add 500 mg of sodium hydrosulfite, and heat to boiling: a heavy deposit of metallic mercury is formed.
Specific gravity ⟨841⟩: between 1.005 and 1.010.
Mercury ions—To the filtrate obtained in *Identification* test *A* add an equal volume of hydrogen sulfide TS: no darkening in color is produced, although a small amount of a flocculent, light yellow precipitate may be formed.
Assay—Transfer 50.0 mL of Topical Solution to a 500-mL Kjeldahl flask, add a few glass beads, and evaporate to about 5 mL. Proceed as directed in the *Assay* under *Nitromersol,* beginning with "Add 15 mL of sulfuric acid."

Nitrous Oxide

N₂O   44.01
Nitrogen oxide (N₂O).
Nitrogen oxide (N₂O)   [*10024-97-2*].

» Nitrous Oxide contains not less than 99.0 percent, by volume, of N₂O.

Packaging and storage—Preserve in cylinders.
   NOTE—The following tests are designed to reflect the quality of Nitrous Oxide in both the vapor and liquid phases that are present in previously unopened cylinders. Reduce the container pressure by means of a regulator. Withdraw the samples for the tests with the least possible release of Nitrous Oxide consistent with proper purging of the sampling apparatus. Measure the gases with a gas volume meter downstream from the detector tubes in order to minimize contamination or change of the specimens. Perform tests in the sequence in which they are listed.
   The various detector tubes called for in the respective tests are listed under *Reagents* in the section *Reagents, Indicators, and Solutions.*
Identification—
   A: With the container temperatures the same and maintained between 15° and 25°, concomitantly read the pressure of the Nitrous Oxide container and of a container of nitrous oxide certified

standard (see under *Reagents* in the section *Reagents, Indicators, and Solutions*). [NOTE—Do not use the nitrous oxide certified standard if it has been depleted to less than half of its full capacity.] The pressure of the Nitrous Oxide container is within 50 psi of that of the nitrous oxide certified standard.

B: Pass 100 ± 5 mL released from the vapor phase of the contents of the Nitrous Oxide container through a carbon dioxide detector tube at the rate specified for the tube: no color change is observed (*distinction from carbon dioxide*).

C: Collect about 100 mL of the gas under test in a 100-mL tube fitted at the top with a stopcock. Open the stopcock, and quickly add a freshly prepared solution of 500 mg of pyrogallol in 2 mL of water and a freshly prepared solution of 12 g of potassium hydroxide in 8 mL of water. Immediately close the stopcock, and mix: the gas is not absorbed, and the solution does not become brown (*distinction from oxygen*).

Water—It meets the requirements of the test for *Water* under *Carbon Dioxide*.

Limit of ammonia—Proceed with Nitrous Oxide as directed in the test for *Carbon monoxide*, except to use an ammonia detector tube: the indicator change corresponds to not more than 0.0025%.

Limit of nitric oxide—Pass 500 ± 50 mL, released from the vapor phase of the contents of the container, through a nitric oxide–nitrogen dioxide detector tube at the rate specified for the tube: the indicator change corresponds to not more than 1 ppm.

Carbon monoxide—Pass 1000 ± 50 mL, released from the vapor phase of the contents of the container, through a carbon monoxide detector tube at the rate specified for the tube: the indicator change corresponds to not more than 0.001%.

Nitrogen dioxide—Arrange a container so that when its valve is opened, a portion of the liquid phase of the contents is released through a piece of tubing of sufficient length to allow all of the liquid to vaporize during passage through it, and to prevent frost from reaching the inlet of the detector tube. Release into the tubing a flow of liquid sufficient to provide 550 mL of the vaporized sample plus any excess necessary to ensure adequate flushing of air from the system. Pass 550 ± 50 mL of this gas through a nitric oxide–nitrogen dioxide detector tube at the rate specified for the tube: the indicator change corresponds to not more than 1 ppm.

Halogens—Pass 1000 ± 50 mL, released from the vapor phase of the contents of the container, through a chlorine detector tube at the rate specified for the tube: the indicator change corresponds to not more than 1 ppm.

Carbon dioxide—Pass 1000 ± 50 mL, released from the vapor phase of the contents of the container, through a carbon dioxide detector tube at the rate specified for the tube: the indicator change corresponds to not more than 0.03%.

Air—Not more than 1.0% of air is present, determined as directed in the *Assay*.

Assay—Introduce a specimen of Nitrous Oxide taken from the liquid phase, as directed in the test for *Nitrogen dioxide*, into a gas chromatograph by means of a gas-sampling valve. Select the operating conditions of the gas chromatograph such that the peak response resulting from the following procedure corresponds to not less than 70% of the full-scale reading. Preferably, use an apparatus corresponding to the general type in which the column is 6 m in length and 4 mm in inside diameter and is packed with porous polymer beads, which permits complete separation of N_2 and O_2 from N_2O, although the N_2 and O_2 may not be separated from each other. Use industrial grade helium (99.99%) as the carrier gas, with a thermal-conductivity detector, and control the column temperature: the peak response produced by the assay specimen exhibits a retention time corresponding to that produced by an air–helium certified standard (see under *Reagents* in the section *Reagents, Indicators, and Solutions*), and is equivalent to not more than 1.0% of air when compared to the peak response of the air-helium certified standard, indicating not less than 99.0%, by volume, of N_2O.

Nizatidine

$C_{12}H_{21}N_5O_2S_2$ 331.46
1,1-Ethenediamine, *N*-[2-[[[2-[(dimethylamino)methyl]-4-thiazolyl]methyl]thio]ethyl]-*N*′-methyl-2-nitro-.
N-[2-[[[2-[(Dimethylamino)methyl]-4-thiazolyl]methyl]thio]ethyl]-*N*′-methyl-2-nitro-1,1-ethenediamine   [76963-41-2].

» Nizatidine contains not less than 98.0 percent and not more than 101.0 percent of $C_{12}H_{21}N_5O_2S_2$, calculated on the dried basis.

Packaging and storage—Preserve in tight, light-resistant containers.

USP Reference standards ⟨11⟩—*USP Nizatidine RS*.
Identification—
 A: *Infrared Absorption* ⟨197K⟩.
 B: The retention time of the major peak in the chromatogram of the *Assay preparation* corresponds to that of the *Standard preparation* as obtained in the *Assay*.
Loss on drying ⟨731⟩—Dry about 2 g, accurately weighed, at 100° for 1 hour: it loses not more than 1.0% of its weight.
Residue on ignition ⟨281⟩: not more than 0.1%.
Heavy metals, *Method II* ⟨231⟩: 0.001%.
Chromatographic purity—
 Solution A—Use *Buffer solution* prepared as directed in the *Assay*.
 Solution B—Use methanol.
 Diluent—Prepare a mixture of *Solution A* and *Solution B* (76 : 24).
 Mobile phase—Use variable mixtures of *Solution A* and *Solution B* as directed for the *Chromatographic system*. Make adjustments if necessary (see *System Suitability* under *Chromatography* ⟨621⟩).
 Standard solutions—Dissolve an accurately weighed quantity of USP Nizatidine RS quantitatively, and stepwise if necessary, in *Diluent*, sonicating if necessary, to obtain a solution having a known concentration of 50 μg per mL (*Standard solution 1*). Quantitatively dilute portions of *Standard solution 1* with *Diluent* to obtain *Standard solution 2* and *Standard solution 3* having known concentrations of 25 μg per mL and 15 μg per mL, respectively.
 Test solution—Prepare a solution of Nizatidine in *Diluent* having a concentration of about 5 mg per mL.
 Chromatographic system (see *Chromatography* ⟨621⟩)—The liquid chromatograph is equipped with a 254-nm detector and a 4.6-mm × 25-cm column that contains 5-μm packing L1. The flow rate is about 1 mL per minute. The chromatograph is programmed as follows.

Time (minutes)	Solution A (%)	Solution B (%)	Elution
0–3	76	24	isocratic
3–20	76→50	24→50	linear gradient
20–45	50	50	isocratic
45–50	50→76	50→24	linear gradient
50–70	76	24	isocratic

Make adjustments to the composition of the *Mobile phase*, if necessary, to obtain a retention time of about 12 minutes for the main nizatidine peak (see *System Suitability* under *Chromatography* ⟨621⟩). Chromatograph *Standard solution 1*, and record the peak areas as directed for *Procedure*: the tailing factor is not more than 2.0.
 Procedure—Separately inject equal volumes (about 50 μL) of *Standard solution 1*, *Standard solution 2*, *Standard solution 3*, and

the *Test solution* into the chromatograph, and allow the *Test solution* to elute for not less than three times the retention time of nizatidine. Record the chromatograms, and measure the areas for all the peaks. The sum of the peak areas, excluding the nizatidine peak area, obtained from the *Test solution* is not more than three times the main peak area obtained from *Standard solution 2*; and no single peak area obtained from the *Test solution* is greater than the main peak area obtained from *Standard solution 3*: not more than 0.3% of any individual impurity is found; and not more than 1.5% of total impurities is found.

Assay—

Buffer solution—Prepare a 0.1 M solution by dissolving 5.9 g of ammonium acetate in 760 mL of water. Add 1 mL of diethylamine, and adjust with acetic acid to a pH of 7.5.

Mobile phase—Prepare a filtered and degassed mixture of *Buffer solution* and methanol (76 : 24). Make adjustments if necessary (see *System Suitability* under *Chromatography* ⟨621⟩).

Standard preparation—Dissolve an accurately weighed quantity of USP Nizatidine RS in *Mobile phase*, sonicating if necessary, to obtain a solution having a known concentration of about 0.3 mg per mL.

Assay preparation—Transfer an accurately weighed quantity of 15 mg of Nizatidine to a 50-mL volumetric flask, dissolve in *Mobile phase*, sonicating if necessary, dilute with *Mobile phase* to volume, and mix.

Chromatographic system (see *Chromatography* ⟨621⟩)—The liquid chromatograph is equipped with a 254-nm detector and a 4.6-mm × 15-cm column that contains 5-μm packing L1. The flow rate is about 1 mL per minute. Chromatograph the *Standard preparation*, and record the peak areas as directed for *Procedure*: the column efficiency is not less than 1500 theoretical plates; the tailing factor is not more than 2.0; and the relative standard deviation for replicate injections is not more than 1.5%.

Procedure—Separately inject equal volumes (about 10 μL) of the *Standard preparation* and the *Assay preparation* into the chromatograph, record the chromatograms, and measure the areas for the major peaks. Calculate the quantity, in mg, of $C_{12}H_{21}N_5O_2S_2$ in the portion of Nizatidine taken by the formula:

$$50C(r_U / r_S)$$

in which C is the concentration, in mg per mL, of USP Nizatidine RS in the *Standard preparation*; and r_U and r_S are the peak areas obtained from the *Assay preparation* and the *Standard preparation*, respectively.

Nizatidine Capsules

» Nizatidine Capsules contain not less than 90.0 percent and not more than 110.0 percent of the labeled amount of nizatidine ($C_{12}H_{21}N_5O_2S_2$).

Packaging and storage—Preserve in tight, light-resistant containers. Store at controlled room temperature.

USP Reference standards ⟨11⟩—USP Nizatidine RS.

Identification—

A: Empty the contents of 2 Capsules into a beaker, add 20 mL of methanol, and swirl for approximately 2 minutes. Filter through a filter paper, and evaporate the methanol solution with a current of cool air to dryness: the IR absorption spectrum of a potassium bromide dispersion of the residue so obtained exhibits maxima only at the same wavelengths as that of a similar preparation of USP Nizatidine RS.

B: The retention time of the major peak in the chromatogram of the *Assay preparation* corresponds to that of the *Standard preparation*, both relative to the internal standard, as obtained in the *Assay*.

Dissolution ⟨711⟩—

Medium: water; 900 mL.
Apparatus 2: 50 rpm.
Time: 30 minutes.

Procedure—Determine the amount of $C_{12}H_{21}N_5O_2S_2$ dissolved from UV absorbances at the wavelength of maximum absorbance at about 314 nm using filtered portions of the solution under test, diluted with water if necessary, in comparison with a Standard solution having a known concentration of USP Nizatidine RS in the same medium.

Tolerances—Not less than 75% (*Q*) of the labeled amount of $C_{12}H_{21}N_5O_2S_2$ is dissolved in 30 minutes.

Uniformity of dosage units ⟨905⟩: meet the requirements.

Chromatographic purity—[NOTE—Use peak areas where peak responses are indicated.]

Buffer solution and *Mobile phase*—Prepare as directed in the *Assay* under *Nizatidine*.

Standard solution—Dissolve an accurately weighed quantity of USP Nizatidine RS in *Mobile phase* and dilute quantitatively, and stepwise if necessary, with *Mobile phase* to obtain a solution having a known concentration of about 40 μg per mL.

Test solution—Remove as completely as possible the contents of not less than 20 Capsules, and mix. Transfer an accurately weighed portion of the powder, equivalent to about 200 mg of nizatidine, to a 100-mL volumetric flask, add 50 mL of *Mobile phase*, and sonicate for about 3 minutes. Dilute with *Mobile phase* to volume, mix, and filter.

System suitability solution—Prepare a solution of nizatidine and phenol in *Mobile phase* containing 40 μg of each per mL.

Chromatographic system (see *Chromatography* ⟨621⟩)—The liquid chromatograph is equipped with a 230-nm detector and a 4.6-mm × 15-cm column that contains 5-μm packing L1. The flow rate is about 1 mL per minute. Chromatograph the *System suitability solution*, and record the peak responses as directed under *Procedure*: the resolution, R, between the nizatidine and phenol peaks is not less than 1.5, the tailing factor for the nizatidine peak is not greater than 1.5, and the relative standard deviation of the nizatidine peak for replicate injections is not more than 2%.

Procedure—Chromatograph about 10 μL of the *Standard solution* and the *Test solution*, and run the chromatograph for twice the elution time of nizatidine. Record the chromatograms, and measure the peak responses. Calculate the percentage of each impurity in the portion of Capsules taken by the formula:

$$2(r_i / r_s)$$

in which r_i is the response of each impurity peak in the *Test solution*, and r_s is the response of the nizatidine peak in the *Standard solution*: not more than 0.5% of any individual impurity and not more than 1.5% of total impurities is found.

Assay—[NOTE—Use peak areas where peak responses are indicated.]

Buffer solution and *Mobile phase*—Prepare as directed in the *Assay* under *Nizatidine*.

Internal standard solution—Prepare a solution of phenol in *Mobile phase* having a concentration of 0.1 mg per mL.

Standard preparation—Dissolve an accurately weighed quantity of USP Nizatidine RS in *Internal standard solution* to obtain a solution having a known concentration of 0.1 mg per mL.

Assay preparation—Weigh accurately not less than 10 Capsules. Remove as completely as possible the contents of the Capsules, and mix the combined contents. Clean and accurately weigh the Capsule shells, and calculate the net weight of the Capsule contents. Transfer an accurately weighed portion of the mixed Capsule contents equivalent to about 500 mg of nizatidine to a 500-mL volumetric flask, add 200 mL of *Internal standard solution*, and sonicate for a few minutes. Cool, dilute with *Internal standard solution* to volume, and mix. Filter a portion of the solution, transfer 1.0 mL of the filtered solution to a 10-mL volumetric flask, dilute with *Internal standard solution* to volume, and mix.

Chromatographic system (see *Chromatography* ⟨621⟩)—The liquid chromatograph is equipped with a 230-nm detector and a 4.6-mm × 15-cm column that contains 5-μm packing L1. The flow rate is about 1 mL per minute. Chromatograph the *Standard preparation*, and record the peak responses as directed for *Procedure*: the resolution, R, between nizatidine and the internal standard phenol, is not less than 3; the tailing factor, T, for the nizatidine peak is not more than 1.6; and the relative standard deviation for replicate injections is not more than 1.5%.

Procedure—Separately inject equal volumes (about 25 μL) of the *Standard preparation* and the *Assay preparation* into the chromatograph, record the chromatograms, and measure the responses for the

major peaks. The relative retention times are about 0.7 for phenol and 1.0 for nizatidine. Calculate the quantity, in mg, of $C_{12}H_{21}N_5O_2S_2$ in the portion of Capsules taken by the formula:

$$5000C(R_U/R_S)$$

in which C is the concentration, in mg per mL, of USP Nizatidine RS in the *Standard preparation*, and R_U and R_S are the ratios of the peak response of the nizatidine to that of the internal standard for the *Assay preparation* and the *Standard preparation*, respectively.

Nonoxynol 9

α-(*p*-Nonylphenyl)-ω-hydroxynona(oxyethylene) [26027-38-3].

» Nonoxynol 9 is an anhydrous liquid mixture consisting chiefly of mononoylphenyl ethers of polyethylene glycols corresponding to the formula:

$$C_9H_{19}C_6H_4(OCH_2CH_2)_nOH$$

in which the average value of *n* is about 9. It contains not less than 90.0 percent and not more than 110.0 percent of nonoxynol 9.

Packaging and storage—Preserve in tight containers.
USP Reference standards ⟨11⟩—*USP Nonoxynol 9 RS*.
Identification—
A: Its IR absorption spectrum, obtained by spreading a capillary film of it between sodium chloride plates, exhibits maxima at 1117 cm^{-1} (strong); at 1512, 1582, and 1610 cm^{-1} (medium, sharp); at 2871, 2928, and 2956 cm^{-1} (strong, unresolved); at 831 cm^{-1} (medium, broad); and at 1250 cm^{-1} (medium, sharp).
B: The retention time of the major peak in the chromatogram of the *Assay preparation* corresponds to that in the chromatogram of the *Standard preparation* as obtained in the *Assay*.
Cloud point—Transfer 1.0 g to a 250-mL beaker, add 99 g of water, and mix to dissolve. Pour about 30 mL of the solution into a 70-mL test tube. Support the test tube in a hot water bath, and stir the contents with a thermometer constantly until the solution becomes cloudy, then remove the test tube from the bath immediately, so that the temperature rises not more than 2° further, and continue stirring. The cloud point is the temperature at which the solution becomes sufficiently clear that the entire thermometer bulb is seen plainly: it is between 52° and 56°.
Acid value ⟨401⟩: not more than 0.2.
Water, *Method I* ⟨921⟩: not more than 0.5%.
Polyethylene glycol—Transfer about 10 g, accurately weighed, to a 250-mL beaker. Add 100 mL of ethyl acetate, and stir on a magnetic stirrer to effect solution. Transfer, with the aid of 100 mL of 5 N sodium chloride, to a pear-shaped, 500-mL separator fitted with a glass stopper. Insert the stopper, and shake vigorously for 1 minute. Remove the stopper carefully to release the pressure. Immerse a thermometer in the mixture, and support the separator so that it is partially immersed in a water bath maintained at 50°. Swirl the separator gently while letting the internal temperature rise to between 40° and 45°, then immediately remove the separator from the bath, dry the outside surface, and drain the salt (lower) layer into another pear-shaped, 500-mL separator. In the same manner, extract the ethyl acetate layer a second time with 100 mL of fresh 5 N sodium chloride, combining the two aqueous extracts. Discard the ethyl acetate layer. Wash the combined aqueous layers with 100 mL of ethyl acetate, using the same technique, and drain the salt (lower) layer into a clean pear-shaped, 500-mL separator. Discard the ethyl acetate layer. Extract the aqueous layer with two successive 100-mL portions of chloroform, draining the chloroform (lower) layers through Whatman folded filter paper 2V, and combining them into a 250-mL beaker. Evaporate on a steam bath to dryness, and continue heating until the odor of chloroform is no longer perceptible. Allow the beaker to cool. Add 25 mL of acetone, and dissolve the residue on a magnetic stirrer. Filter through Whatman folded filter paper 2V into a tared 250-mL beaker, rinsing with two 25-mL portions of acetone. Evaporate on a steam bath to dryness. Dry in vacuum at 60° for 1 hour. Allow the beaker to cool, and weigh: not more than 1.0% of polyethylene glycol is found.

Free ethylene oxide—
Stripped nonoxynol 9—Maintain Nonoxynol 9 at a temperature of 150° with constant stirring in an open vessel until it no longer displays a peak for ethylene oxide when chromatographed as directed below.

Standard solutions—[NOTE—Ethylene oxide is toxic and flammable. Prepare these solutions in a well-ventilated hood, using great care.] Chill all apparatus and reagents used in the preparation of standards in a refrigerator or freezer before use. Fill a chilled pressure bottle with liquid ethylene oxide from a lecture bottle, and store in a freezer when not in use. Use a small piece of polyethylene film to protect the liquid from contact with the rubber gasket. Transfer about 100 mL of chilled isopropyl alcohol to a 500-mL volumetric flask. Using a chilled graduated cylinder, transfer 25 mL of ethylene oxide to the isopropyl alcohol, and swirl gently to mix. Dilute with additional chilled isopropyl alcohol to volume, replace the stopper, and swirl gently to mix. This stock solution contains about 43.6 mg of ethylene oxide per mL. Pipet 25 mL of 0.5 N alcoholic hydrochloric acid, prepared by mixing 45 mL of hydrochloric acid with 1 L of alcohol, into a 500-mL conical flask containing 40 g of magnesium chloride hexahydrate. Shake the mixture to effect saturation. Pipet 10 mL of the ethylene oxide solution into the flask, and add 20 drops of bromocresol green TS. If the solution is not yellow (acid), add an additional volume, accurately measured, of 0.5 N alcoholic hydrochloric acid to give an excess of about 10 mL. Record the total volume of 0.5 N alcoholic hydrochloric acid added. Insert the stopper in the flask, and allow to stand for 30 minutes. Titrate the excess acid with 0.5 N alcoholic potassium hydroxide VS. Perform a blank titration, using 10.0 mL of isopropyl alcohol instead of ethylene oxide solution, adding the same total volume of 0.5 N alcoholic hydrochloric acid, and note the difference in volumes required. Each mL of the difference in volumes of 0.5 N alcoholic potassium hydroxide consumed is equivalent to 22.02 mg of ethylene oxide. Calculate the concentration, in mg per mL, of ethylene oxide in the stock solution. Standardize daily. Store in a refrigerator. Prepare a 1000-ppm standard by pipeting the calculated volume (about 2 mL) of cold stock solution which, on the basis of the standardization, contains 88.6 mg of ethylene oxide, into a container and adding 87.0 g of *Stripped nonoxynol 9*. Prepare 10-, 5-, and 0.5-ppm standards by quantitatively diluting the 1000-ppm standard with additional *Stripped nonoxynol 9*.

Standard preparations—Transfer 5 ± 0.01 g of each *Standard solution* to suitable serum vials equipped with pressure-tight septum closures designed to relieve any excessive pressure, and seal them.

Test preparation—Transfer 5 ± 0.01 g of Nonoxynol 9 to a serum vial of the same kind as the vials used for the *Standard preparations*.

Chromatographic system (see *Chromatography* ⟨621⟩)—Use a gas chromatograph equipped with a flame-ionization detector. Under typical conditions, the instrument contains a 6.4-m × 2.1-mm (ID) nickel column packed with 60-to 80-mesh support S9, the column is maintained at 100°, the injection port is maintained at 160°, the detector is maintained at 200°, and helium is used as the carrier gas at a flow rate of 30 mL per minute. The resolution, *R*, of ethylene oxide and acetaldehyde, upon chromatographing a solution containing 10 μg per mL of each in *Stripped nonoxynol 9*, is not less than 1.5. None of the points used for constructing the straight line *Calibration* curve deviates from the line by more than 10%.

Calibration—Place the vial containing the 10-ppm ethylene oxide *Standard preparation* in an oven, and heat at 90° for 30 minutes. Remove the vial from the oven. Using a gas-tight syringe, immediately inject a 100-μL aliquot of the headspace gas into the gas chromatograph. Obtain the area for the ethylene oxide peak (retention time approximately 8 minutes). Raise the temperature of the column to 200° after ethylene oxide elutes to volatilize heavy components. Re-equilibrate the column at 100°. Repeat the foregoing steps, using the vials containing the 5- and 0.5-ppm *Standard preparation*. Plot area units versus ppm ethylene oxide for the standards on linear graph paper, and draw the best straight line through the points.

Procedure—Place the vial containing the *Test preparation* in an oven, and heat at 90° for 30 minutes. Remove the vial from the oven. Immediately inject a 100-μL aliquot of the headspace gas into the gas chromatograph, and obtain the area for the ethylene oxide peak. Calculate the concentration of ethylene oxide in the test specimen, in ppm, by the formula:

$$r_U S$$

in which r_U is the peak area obtained from the *Test preparation*, and S is the slope of the standard curve, in ppm per area unit. Not more than 1 ppm is found.

Limit of dioxane—

Apparatus—Assemble a closed-system vacuum distillation apparatus, employing glass vacuum stopcocks (*A*, *B*, and *C*), as shown in the accompanying diagram. The concentrator tube (*D*) * is made of borosilicate or quartz (not flint) glass, graduated precisely enough to measure the 0.9 mL or more of distillate collected and marked so that the analyst can dilute accurately to 2.0 mL.

Standard solution—Prepare a solution of dioxane in water having a known concentration of about 100 μg per mL. Use a freshly prepared solution.

Test solution—Transfer 20.0 g to a 50-mL round-bottom flask (*E*) having a 24/40 ground-glass neck joint. Add 1.0 mL of water. Place a small polytef-covered stirring bar in the flask, insert the stopper, and stir to mix. Immerse the flask in an ice bath, and chill for about 1 minute. Wrap heating tape around the tube connecting the concentrator tube (*D*) and the round-bottom flask, and apply about 10 V to the tape. Apply a light coating of high-vacuum silicone grease to the ground-glass joints, and connect the concentrator tube to the 10/30 joint and the round-bottom flask to the 24/40 joint. Immerse the vacuum trap in a Dewar flask filled with liquid nitrogen, close stopcocks *A* and *B*, open stopcock *C*, and begin evacuating the system with a vacuum pump. Prepare a slurry bath from powdered dry ice and methanol, and raise the bath to the neck of the round-bottom flask. After freezing the contents of the flask for about 10 minutes, and when the vacuum system is operating at 0.05-mm pressure or lower, open stopcock *A* for 20 seconds, then close it. Remove the slurry bath, and allow the flask to warm in air for about 1 minute. Immerse the flask in a water bath maintained at a temperature of between 20° and 25°, and after about 5 minutes warm the water bath to between 35° and 40° (sufficient to liquefy most specimens) while stirring slowly but constantly with the magnetic bar. Cool the water in the bath by adding ice, and chill for about 2 minutes. Replace the water bath with the slurry bath, freeze the contents of the round-bottom flask for about 10 minutes, open stopcock *A* for 20 seconds, and then close it. Remove the slurry bath, and repeat the heating steps as before, this time reaching a final temperature of between 45° and 50° or a temperature necessary to melt the specimen completely. If there is any condensation in the tube connecting the round-bottom flask to the concentrator tube, slowly increase the voltage to the heating tape, and heat until condensation disappears.

Stir with the magnetic stirrer throughout the following steps. Very slowly immerse the concentrator tube in a Dewar flask containing liquid nitrogen. *[Caution—When there is liquid distillate in the concentrator tube, immerse the tube in the liquid nitrogen very slowly, or the tube will break.]* Water will begin to distill into the concentrator tube. As ice forms in the concentrator tube, raise the Dewar flask to keep the liquid nitrogen level only slightly below the level of ice in the tube. When water begins to freeze in the neck of the 10/30 joint, or when liquid nitrogen reaches the 2.0-mL graduation mark on the concentrator tube, remove the Dewar flask, and allow the ice to melt without heating. After the ice has melted, check the volume of water that has distilled, and repeat the sequence of chilling and thawing until not less than 0.9 mL of water has been collected. Freeze the tube once again for about 2 minutes, and release the vacuum first by opening stopcock *B*, followed by opening stopcock *A*. Remove the concentrator tube from the apparatus, close it with a greased stopper, and allow the ice to melt without heating. Mix the contents of the concentrator tube by swirling,

---
* A suitable tube is available as Chromaflex concentrator tube, Kontes Glass Co., Vineland, NJ (Catalog No. K42560-0000).

note the volume of distillate, and dilute with water to 2.0 mL, if necessary.

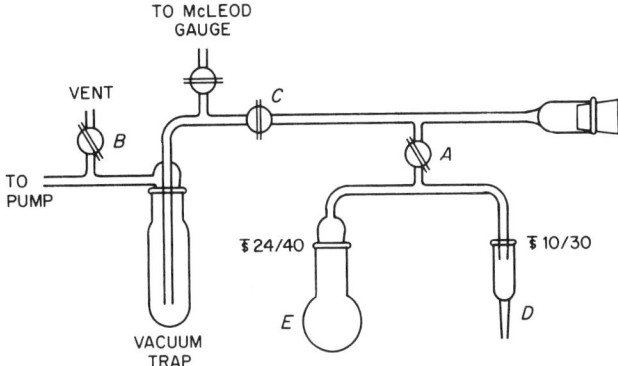

Closed-System Vacuum Distillation Apparatus for Dioxane

Chromatographic system (see *Chromatography* ⟨621⟩)—Use a gas chromatograph equipped with a flame-ionization detector. Under typical conditions, the instrument is equipped with a 2-mm × 1.8-m glass column that contains support S10. The column is maintained at a temperature of about 140°, the injection port at 200°, and the detector at 250°. Nitrogen or helium is the carrier gas, flowing at a rate of about 35 mL per minute. Install an oxygen scrubber between the carrier gas line and the column. Condition the column for about 72 hours at 230° with 30 to 40 mL per minute carrier flow. [NOTE—Support S10 is oxygen-sensitive. Each time a column is installed, flush with carrier gas for 30 to 60 minutes before heating.]

Procedure—Separately inject equal volumes (about 2 to 4 μL) of the *Standard solution* and the *Test solution*. The height of the peak in the chromatogram of the *Test solution* is not greater than that in the chromatogram of the *Standard solution* not more than 10 μg per g is found.

Assay—

Mobile phase—Prepare a degassed solution containing a mixture of methanol and water (80 : 20), making adjustments if necessary (see *System Suitability* under *Chromatography* ⟨621⟩).

Resolution solution—Dissolve octoxynol 9 and USP Nonoxynol 9 RS in *Mobile phase* to obtain a solution containing about 25 mg of each per mL.

Standard preparation—Dissolve an accurately weighed quantity of USP Nonoxynol 9 RS in *Mobile phase* to obtain a solution having a known concentration of about 25 mg per mL.

Assay preparation—Dissolve about 2.5 g of Nonoxynol 9, accurately weighed, in *Mobile phase* in a 100-mL volumetric flask, dilute with *Mobile phase* to volume, and mix.

Chromatographic system—The liquid chromatograph is equipped with a 280-nm detector and a 3.9-mm × 25-cm column that contains 10-μm packing L1. The flow rate is about 1 mL per minute. Chromatograph the *Resolution solution*: the resolution, *R*, is not less than 2.0. Chromatograph replicate injections of the *Standard preparation*: the nonoxynol oligomers elute as a major peak, usually with shoulders and bumps. Include these in the peak response for Nonoxynol 9. The relative standard deviation is not more than 2.0%.

Procedure—Separately inject equal volumes (about 10 μL) of the *Standard preparation* and the *Assay preparation* into the chromatograph, record the chromatograms, and measure the responses for Nonoxynol 9, including any shoulders and bumps. Calculate the quantity, in mg, of Nonoxynol 9 in the portion of specimen taken by the formula:

$$100C(r_U / r_S)$$

in which *C* is the concentration, in mg per mL, of USP Nonoxynol 9 RS in the *Standard preparation*, and r_U and r_S are the peak responses of Nonoxynol 9 obtained from the *Assay* and the *Standard preparation*, respectively.

Norepinephrine Bitartrate

$C_8H_{11}NO_3 \cdot C_4H_6O_6 \cdot H_2O$ 337.28

1,2-Benzenediol, 4-(2-amino-1-hydroxyethyl)-, (R)-,[R-(R*,R*)]-2,3-dihydroxybutanedioate (1 : 1) (salt), monohydrate.
(−)-α-(Aminomethyl)-3,4-dihydroxybenzyl alcohol tartrate (1 : 1) (salt), monohydrate   [69815-49-2].
Anhydrous   319.27   [51-40-1].

» Norepinephrine Bitartrate contains not less than 97.0 percent and not more than 102.0 percent of $C_8H_{11}NO_3 \cdot C_4H_6O_6$, calculated on the anhydrous basis.

Packaging and storage—Preserve in tight, light-resistant containers. Store at 25°, excursions permitted between 15° and 30°.

USP Reference standards ⟨11⟩—*USP Norepinephrine Bitartrate RS.*

Identification—
  A: *Infrared Absorption* ⟨197K⟩.
  B: To a solution of 10 mg in 2 mL of water add 1 drop of ferric chloride TS: an intensely green color develops.
  C: To 10 mL of a solution (1 in 10,000) add 1.0 mL of 0.10 N iodine. Allow to stand for 5 minutes, and add 2.0 mL of 0.10 N sodium thiosulfate: the solution is colorless or has at most a slight pink or slight violet color (*epinephrine* and *isoproterenol* at the same pH, about 3.5, give a strong red-brown or violet color).

Specific rotation ⟨781S⟩:   between −10° and −12°.
  Test solution: 50 mg per mL, in water.

Water, *Method I* ⟨921⟩:   between 4.5% and 5.8%.

Residue on ignition ⟨281⟩:   negligible, from 200 mg.

Limit of arterenone—Its absorptivity (see *Spectrophotometry and Light-scattering* ⟨851⟩) at 310 nm, determined in a solution containing 2 mg per mL, is not more than 0.2.

Assay—Dissolve about 500 mg of Norepinephrine Bitartrate, accurately weighed, in 20 mL of glacial acetic acid, warming slightly if necessary to effect solution. Add 2 drops of crystal violet TS, and titrate with 0.1 N perchloric acid VS. Perform a blank determination, and make any necessary correction. Each mL of 0.1 N perchloric acid is equivalent to 31.93 mg of $C_8H_{11}NO_3 \cdot C_4H_6O_6$.

Norepinephrine Bitartrate Injection

» Norepinephrine Bitartrate Injection is a sterile solution of Norepinephrine Bitartrate in Water for Injection. It contains the equivalent of not less than 90.0 percent and not more than 115.0 percent of the labeled amount of norepinephrine ($C_8H_{11}NO_3$).

Packaging and storage—Preserve in single-dose, light-resistant containers, preferably of Type I glass.

Labeling—Label the Injection in terms of mg of norepinephrine per mL, and, where necessary, label it to indicate that it must be diluted prior to use. The label indicates that the Injection is not to be used if its color is pinkish or darker than slightly yellow or if it contains a precipitate.

USP Reference standards ⟨11⟩— *USP Endotoxin RS. USP Norepinephrine Bitartrate RS.*

Color and clarity—
  Standard solution—Transfer 2.0 mL of 0.100 N iodine VS to a 500-mL volumetric flask, dilute with water to volume, and mix.
  Procedure—Visually examine a portion of the Injection (*Test solution*) in a suitable clear glass test tube against a white background: it is not pinkish and it contains no precipitate. If any yellow color is observed in the *Test solution*, concomitantly determine the absorbances of the *Test solution* and the *Standard solution* in 1-cm cells with a suitable spectrophotometer set at 460 nm: the absorbance of the *Test solution* does not exceed that of the *Standard solution*.

Identification—
  A: It responds to *Identification* test *B* under *Norepinephrine Bitartrate*.
  B: Dilute the Injection with water to a concentration of 1 mg in 5 mL. To 10 mL of the dilution add 2.0 mL of 0.10 N iodine, allow to stand for 5 minutes, then add 3.0 mL of 0.10 N sodium thiosulfate: the solution is colorless or has at most a slight pink or slight violet color (*epinephrine and isoproterenol at the same pH, about 3.5, give a red-brown or violet color*).

Bacterial endotoxins ⟨85⟩—It contains not more than 83.4 USP Endotoxin Units per mg of norepinephrine.

pH ⟨791⟩:   between 3.0 and 4.5.

Particulate matter ⟨788⟩:   meets the requirements for small-volume injections.

Other requirements—It meets the requirements under *Injections* ⟨1⟩.

Assay—
  Mobile phase—Dissolve 1.1 g of sodium 1-heptanesulfonate in 800 mL of water. Add 200 mL of methanol, and adjust with 1 M phosphoric acid to a pH of 3.0 ± 0.1. Pass through a membrane filter. Make adjustments if necessary (see *System Suitability* under *Chromatography* ⟨621⟩).

  Standard preparation—Dissolve an accurately weighed quantity of USP Norepinephrine Bitartrate RS in freshly prepared dilute acetic acid (1 in 25), and dilute quantitatively, and stepwise if necessary, to obtain a solution having a known concentration of about 0.4 mg of norepinephrine bitartrate monohydrate per mL.

  Assay preparation—Transfer an accurately measured volume of Injection, equivalent to about 5 mg of norepinephrine, to a 25-mL volumetric flask, add dilute acetic acid (1 in 25) to volume, and mix.

  System suitability preparation—Dissolve a suitable quantity of isoproterenol hydrochloride in the *Standard preparation* to obtain a solution containing, in each mL, 0.4 mg of USP Norepinephrine Bitartrate RS and 0.4 mg of isoproterenol hydrochloride.

  Chromatographic system (see *Chromatography* ⟨621⟩)—The liquid chromatograph is equipped with a 280-nm detector and a 4.6-mm × 25-cm column that contains packing L1. The flow rate is about 2 mL per minute. Chromatograph the *Standard preparation* and the *System suitability preparation*, and record the peak responses as directed under *Procedure*: the tailing factor for the analyte peak is not more than 2.5, the resolution, *R*, between the norepinephrine and isoproterenol peaks is not less than 4.0, and the relative standard deviation for replicate injections is not more than 2.0%.

  Procedure—Separately inject equal volumes (about 20 μL) of the *Standard preparation* and the *Assay preparation* into the chromatograph, record the chromatograms, and measure the responses for the major peaks. Calculate the quantity, in mg, of norepinephrine ($C_8H_{11}NO_3$) in each mL of the Injection taken by the formula:

$$(169.18 / 337.29)(25C / V)(r_U / r_S)$$

in which 169.18 and 337.29 are the molecular weights of norepinephrine and norepinephrine bitartrate monohydrate, respectively; *C* is the concentration, in mg per mL, of USP Norepinephrine Bitartrate RS in the *Standard preparation*; *V* is the volume, in mL, of Injection taken; and r_U and r_S are the peak responses obtained from the *Assay preparation* and the *Standard preparation*, respectively.

not less than 90.0 percent and not more than 110.0 percent of the labeled amount of mestranol ($C_{21}H_{26}O_2$).

Packaging and storage—Preserve in well-closed containers.

USP Reference standards ⟨11⟩—*USP Mestranol RS. USP Norethindrone RS.*

Identification—Crush 1 Tablet in 1 mL of alcohol in a 15-mL conical centrifuge tube, and centrifuge briefly. Apply 10 μL of this test solution and 10 μL each of solutions containing, respectively, about 1 mg per mL of USP Norethindrone RS in alcohol and about 50 μg per mL of USP Mestranol RS in alcohol at equidistant points along a line about 2.5 cm from the bottom of a thin-layer chromatographic plate (see *Chromatography* ⟨621⟩) coated with a 0.25-mm layer of chromatographic silica gel and previously activated by heating at 105° for 30 minutes. Develop the chromatogram in a mixture of equal volumes of ethyl acetate and cyclohexane in a suitable chamber, previously equilibrated with the solvent mixture, until the solvent front has moved about three-fourths of the length of the plate. Remove the plate, air-dry, and observe under short-wavelength UV light: the principal spot from the test solution appears at the same R_F value as the principal spot from USP Norethindrone RS, at about R_F 0.6. Spray the plate with a sulfuric acid and methanol mixture prepared by cautiously adding and mixing sulfuric acid in small increments to 30 mL of chilled anhydrous methanol in a 100-mL volumetric flask. Adjust to room temperature, dilute with sulfuric acid to volume, and mix. Heat the plate at 105° for 10 minutes: the pink spot from the test solution appears at the same R_F value as the pink spot from USP Mestranol RS (about R_F 0.8).

Dissolution ⟨711⟩—[NOTE—Exercise care in filtering solutions containing mestranol to prevent adsorptive loss of the drug. Centrifugation may be used instead of filtration with nonadsorptive membrane filters. Withdraw dissolution aliquots with glass or polytef pipets or syringes that have been checked for adsorptive loss. Use glass dissolution vessels and polytef-coated or solid polytef paddles.]

Medium: 0.09% sodium lauryl sulfate in 0.1 N hydrochloric acid; 500 mL.
Apparatus 2: 75 rpm.
Time: 60 minutes.

Determine the amounts of norethindrone ($C_{20}H_{26}O_2$) and mestranol ($C_{21}H_{26}O_2$) dissolved, employing the following method.

Mobile phase—Prepare a degassed and filtered mixture of water and acetonitrile (60 : 40). Make adjustments if necessary (see *System Suitability* under *Chromatography* ⟨621⟩).

Chromatographic system (see *Chromatography* ⟨621⟩)—The liquid chromatograph is equipped with a 205-nm detector and a 4.6-mm × 25-cm column that contains packing L10. The flow rate is about 1 mL per minute. Chromatograph replicate injections of a filtered portion of a Standard solution of USP Norethindrone RS and USP Mestranol RS in *Dissolution Medium* having known concentrations similar to those expected in the solution under test, and record the peak responses as directed for *Procedure:* the relative standard deviation is not more than 3.0%. The minimum number of theoretical plates for the norethindrone peak is 4000, and the tailing factors for the norethindrone and mestranol peaks do not exceed 1.5.

Procedure—Separately inject equal volumes (about 200 μL) of the Standard solution and a filtered portion of the solution under test into the chromatograph, record the chromatograms, and measure the responses for the major peaks. The relative retention times are about 0.4 for norethindrone and 1.0 for mestranol. Calculate the quantities of norethindrone and mestranol dissolved by comparison of the corresponding peak responses obtained from the Standard solution and the test solutions.

Tolerances—Not less than 75% (*Q*) of the labeled amount of $C_{20}H_{26}O_2$ and 75% (*Q*) of the labeled amount of $C_{21}H_{26}O_2$ are dissolved in 60 minutes.

Uniformity of dosage units ⟨905⟩: meet the requirements for *Content Uniformity* with respect to norethindrone and to mestranol.

Assay—
Mobile phase—Prepare a filtered and degassed mixture of acetonitrile and water (50 : 50). Make adjustments if necessary (see *System Suitability* under *Chromatography* ⟨621⟩).

Internal standard solution—Transfer about 80 mg of progesterone into a 100-mL volumetric flask, add 50 mL of acetonitrile, dilute with water to volume, and mix.

Mestranol standard stock solution—Dissolve an accurately weighed quantity of USP Mestranol RS in acetonitrile, and dilute quantitatively and stepwise with acetonitrile to obtain a solution having a known concentration of about 0.05 mg per mL.

Norethindrone standard stock solution—Using an accurately weighed quantity of USP Norethindrone RS, prepare a solution in acetonitrile having a known concentration of about 1 mg per mL.

Standard preparation—Transfer 2.0 mL of *Internal standard solution* into a 100-mL volumetric flask. Add accurately measured volumes of *Mestranol standard stock solution* and *Norethindrone standard stock solution* so that the final known concentrations, in mg per mL, of the Reference Standards correspond numerically to about one-fiftieth of the labeled amounts of the corresponding ingredients in the Tablets. Add 50 mL of water, dilute with acetonitrile to volume, and mix.

Assay preparation—Transfer 10 Tablets to a 250-mL volumetric flask, add 50 mL of water, and shake by mechanical means until the Tablets are completely disintegrated. Add 10.0 mL of *Internal standard solution* and 165 mL of acetonitrile, and mix. Sonicate for about 2 minutes. Dilute with acetonitrile to volume, and mix. Allow solid particles to settle, or centrifuge if necessary, to obtain a slightly turbid solution. Transfer 5.0 mL of this solution to a 10-mL volumetric flask, add 1.0 mL of acetonitrile, dilute with water to volume, and mix.

Chromatographic system (see *Chromatography* ⟨621⟩)—The liquid chromatograph is equipped with a 200-nm detector and a 4.6-mm × 15-cm column that contains packing L7. The flow rate is about 1.0 mL per minute. Chromatograph the *Standard preparation*, and record the peak responses as directed for *Procedure:* the column efficiency determined from the mestranol peak is not less than 6000 theoretical plates, the resolution, *R*, between the progesterone and mestranol peaks is not less than 5.0, and the relative standard deviation for six replicate injections is not more than 2.0% (both peaks).

Procedure—Separately inject equal volumes (about 25 μL) of the *Standard preparation* and the *Assay preparation* into the chromatograph, record the chromatograms, and measure the responses for the major peaks. The relative retention times are about 2.5 for mestranol and 1.0 for norethindrone. Calculate the quantities, in mg, of norethindrone ($C_{20}H_{26}O_2$) and mestranol ($C_{21}H_{26}O_2$) in each Tablet taken by the formula:

$$50C(R_U / R_S)$$

in which *C* is the concentration, in mg per mL, of the appropriate USP Reference Standard in the *Standard preparation*, and R_U and R_S are the peak response ratios, at corresponding retention times, obtained from the *Assay preparation* and the *Standard preparation*, respectively.

Norethindrone Acetate

$C_{22}H_{28}O_3$ 340.46
19-Norpregn-4-en-20-yn-3-one, 17-(acetyloxy)-, (17α).9
17-Hydroxy-19-nor-17α-pregn-4-en-20-yn-3-one acetate
[51-98-9].

» Norethindrone Acetate contains not less than 97.0 percent and not more than 103.0 percent of $C_{22}H_{28}O_3$, calculated on the dried basis.

Packaging and storage—Preserve in well-closed containers.
USP Reference standards ⟨11⟩—*USP Norethindrone Acetate RS.*
Completeness of solution—The solution prepared for the determination of *Specific rotation* is clear and free from undissolved solids.
Identification, *Infrared Absorption* ⟨197K⟩.
Specific rotation ⟨781S⟩: between −32° and −38°.
Test solution: 20 mg per mL, in dioxane.
Loss on drying ⟨731⟩—Dry it at 105° for 3 hours: it loses not more than 0.5% of its weight.
Limit of ethynyl group—Proceed as directed in the test for *Ethynyl group* under *Norethindrone*. Not less than 7.13% and not more than 7.57% of ethynyl group is found.

Chromatographic purity—

TEST 1—

Adsorbent: 0.25-mm layer of chromatographic silica gel mixture.

Test solution—Prepare a solution of Norethindrone Acetate in chloroform having a concentration of 10 mg per mL.

Standard stock solution—Prepare a solution of USP Norethindrone Acetate RS in chloroform having a known concentration of 10 mg per mL.

Standard solutions—Dilute accurately measured volumes of the *Standard stock solution* with chloroform to obtain *Standard solutions A, B, C,* and *D* having known concentrations of 150 µg per mL, 50 µg per mL, 30 µg per mL, and 10 µg per mL, respectively.

Application volume: 10 µL, as two 5-µL portions.

Developing solvent system: a mixture of toluene and ethyl acetate (1 : 1).

Procedure—Proceed as directed for *Thin-Layer Chromatography* under *Chromatography* ⟨621⟩, except to apply the solutions along a line 2.5 cm from the edge of the plate. Spray the plate with a mixture of methanol and sulfuric acid (7 : 3), and heat at 100° for 5 minutes. The *Test solution* exhibits a principal spot at the same R_F value as the principal spot of *Standard solution A*. Any individual secondary spot is not more intense than the spot in the chromatogram obtained from *Standard solution B*: not more than 0.5% of any individual impurity is found. The sum of the intensities of all of the secondary spots is not more intense than the spot in the chromatogram obtained from *Standard solution A*: not more than 1.5% of total impurities is found.

TEST 2—

Mobile phase—Prepare a filtered and degassed mixture of acetonitrile and water (6 : 4). Make adjustments if necessary (see *System Suitability* under *Chromatography* ⟨621⟩).

Resolution solution—Dissolve accurately weighed quantities of desoxycorticosterone acetate and USP Norethindrone Acetate RS in *Mobile phase* to obtain a solution having concentrations of about 80 µg of each per mL.

Test solution—Transfer about 62.5 mg of Norethindrone Acetate, accurately weighed, to a 25-mL volumetric flask, dissolve in and dilute with *Mobile phase* to volume, and mix.

Diluted test solution—Transfer 1.0 mL of the *Test solution* to a 100-mL volumetric flask, dilute with *Mobile phase* to volume, and mix.

Chromatographic system (see *Chromatography* ⟨621⟩)—The liquid chromatograph is equipped with a 254-nm detector and a 4.6-mm × 25-cm column that contains packing L1. The flow rate is about 1 mL per minute. Chromatograph the *Resolution solution*, and record the peak responses as directed for *Procedure*: the relative retention times are about 0.83 for desoxycorticosterone acetate and 1.0 for norethindrone acetate; and the resolution, *R*, between desoxycorticosterone acetate and norethindrone acetate is not less than 3.5.

Procedure—Separately inject equal volumes (about 20 µL) of the *Diluted test solution* and the *Test solution* into the chromatograph, record the chromatograms for twice the retention time of norethindrone acetate, and measure all of the peak areas. Calculate the percentage of each impurity in the portion of Norethindrone Acetate taken by the formula:

$$r_i / r_s$$

in which r_i is the peak area for each impurity obtained from the *Test solution;* and r_s is the sum of all the peaks obtained from the *Diluted test solution*. [NOTE—Exclude any peak having a response that is less than 0.025% of the norethindrone acetate peak response obtained from the *Test solution*.] Not more than 0.5% of any individual impurity is found; and not more than 1.0% of total impurities is found.

Organic volatile impurities, *Method IV* ⟨467⟩: meets the requirements.

(Official until July 1, 2008)

Assay—Transfer about 100 mg of Norethindrone Acetate, accurately weighed, to a 200-mL volumetric flask, add alcohol to volume, and mix. Transfer 5.0 mL of this solution to a 250-mL volumetric flask, dilute with alcohol to volume, and mix. Dissolve an accurately weighed quantity of USP Norethindrone Acetate RS in alcohol, and dilute quantitatively and stepwise with alcohol to obtain a Standard solution having a known concentration of about 10 µg per mL. Concomitantly determine the absorbances of both solutions in 1-cm cells at the wavelength of maximum absorbance at about 240 nm, with a suitable spectrophotometer, using alcohol as the blank. Calculate the quantity, in mg, of $C_{22}H_{28}O_3$ in the portion of Norethindrone Acetate taken by the formula:

$$10C(A_U / A_S)$$

in which *C* is the concentration, in µg per mL, of USP Norethindrone Acetate RS in the *Standard solution*, and A_U and A_S are the absorbances of the solution of Norethindrone Acetate and the Standard solution, respectively.

Norethindrone Acetate Tablets

» Norethindrone Acetate Tablets contain not less than 90.0 percent and not more than 110.0 percent of the labeled amount of norethindrone acetate ($C_{22}H_{28}O_3$).

Packaging and storage—Preserve in well-closed containers.

USP Reference standards ⟨11⟩—*USP Norethindrone Acetate RS.*

Identification—It responds to the *Identification* test under *Norethindrone Tablets*, USP Norethindrone Acetate RS being used to prepare the Standard preparation.

Dissolution ⟨711⟩—

Medium: dilute hydrochloric acid (1 in 100) containing 0.02% of sodium lauryl sulfate; 900 mL.

Apparatus 1: 100 rpm.

Time: 60 minutes.

Procedure—Determine the amount of $C_{22}H_{28}O_3$ dissolved from UV absorbances at the wavelength of maximum absorbance at about 248 nm, measured from a baseline drawn from 350 nm through 310 nm and extending beyond the peak maximum, of filtered portions of the solution under test, suitably diluted with *Medium*, in comparison with a Standard solution having a known concentration of USP Norethindrone Acetate RS in the same medium. [NOTE—The Standard solution may be prepared by dissolving the Reference Standard in a volume of methanol, not exceeding 0.5% of the final volume of the solution, and diluting quantitatively with *Dissolution Medium*.]

Tolerances—Not less than 70% (*Q*) of the labeled amount of $C_{22}H_{28}O_3$ is dissolved in 60 minutes.

Uniformity of dosage units ⟨905⟩: meet the requirements.

Procedure for content uniformity—Transfer 1 finely powdered Tablet to a 100-mL volumetric flask with the aid of about 75 mL of alcohol. Heat the alcohol to boiling, and allow the mixture to remain at a temperature just below the boiling point for about 15 minutes, with occasional swirling. Cool to room temperature, dilute with alcohol to volume, mix, and centrifuge a portion of the contents at about 2000 rpm until the solution becomes clear. Dilute a portion of the supernatant quantitatively and stepwise with alcohol to obtain a solution containing approximately 10 µg of norethindrone acetate per mL. Concomitantly determine the absorbances of this solution and of a Standard solution of USP Norethindrone Acetate RS in alcohol having a known concentration of about 10 µg per mL in 1-cm cells at the wavelength of maximum absorbance at about 240 nm, with a suitable spectrophotometer, using alcohol as the blank. Calculate the quantity, in mg, of $C_{22}H_{28}O_3$ in the Tablet taken by the formula:

$$(TC / D)(A_U / A_S)$$

in which *T* is the labeled quantity, in mg, of norethindrone acetate in the Tablet, *C* is the concentration, in µg per mL, of USP Norethindrone Acetate RS in the Standard solution, *D* is the concentration, in µg per mL, of the solution from the Tablet, based upon the labeled quantity per Tablet and the extent of dilution, and A_U and A_S are the absorbances of the solution from the Tablet and the Standard solution, respectively.

Assay—Weigh and finely powder not less than 20 Tablets. Transfer an accurately weighed portion of the powder, equivalent to about 20 mg of norethindrone acetate, to a separator, add 10 mL of water, and extract with three 25-mL portions of chloroform, filtering each extract through chloroform-washed cotton. Evaporate the combined chloroform extracts on a steam bath to dryness, reducing the heat as dryness is approached. Dissolve the residue in alcohol, transfer the solution to a 100-mL volumetric flask, dilute with alcohol to volume, and mix. Transfer a 5.0-mL aliquot to a 100-mL volumetric flask, dilute with alcohol to volume, and mix. Concomitantly determine the absorbances of this solution and a Standard solution of USP Norethindrone Acetate RS in alcohol having a known concentration of about 10 µg per mL in 1-cm cells at the wavelength of maximum absorbance at about 240 nm, with a suitable spectrophotometer, using alcohol as the blank. Calculate the quantity, in mg, of $C_{22}H_{28}O_3$ in the portion of Tablets taken by the formula:

$$2C(A_U / A_S)$$

in which C is the concentration, in µg per mL, of USP Norethindrone Acetate RS in the Standard solution, and A_U and A_S are the absorbances of the solution from the Tablets and the Standard solution, respectively.

Norethindrone Acetate and Ethinyl Estradiol Tablets

» Norethindrone Acetate and Ethinyl Estradiol Tablets contain not less than 90.0 percent and not more than 110.0 percent of the labeled amount of norethindrone acetate ($C_{22}H_{28}O_3$), and not less than 88.0 percent and not more than 112.0 percent of the labeled amount of ethinyl estradiol ($C_{20}H_{24}O_2$).

Packaging and storage—Preserve in well-closed containers.

USP Reference standards ⟨11⟩—*USP Ethinyl Estradiol RS. USP Norethindrone Acetate RS.*

Identification—

A: *Infrared Absorption* ⟨197K⟩—
Test specimen—Wash the isooctane–toluene solution obtained in the *Assay for ethinyl estradiol* with 5 mL of water, filter, and evaporate to dryness.

B: *Thin-Layer Chromatographic Identification Test* ⟨201⟩—
Adsorbent—Use either a 0.1-mm or a 0.25-mm layer of chromatographic silica gel mixture as described in the chapter. Activate the plate at 105° for 60 minutes immediately prior to use.
Test solution—Crush 1 Tablet in 1 mL of alcohol in a 15-mL conical centrifuge tube, and centrifuge briefly.
Standard solution 1: an alcohol solution containing in each mL an amount of USP Norethindrone Acetate RS, accurately weighed, corresponding to the labeled quantity of norethindrone acetate per Tablet.
Standard solution 2: an alcohol solution containing in each mL 50 µg of USP Ethinyl Estradiol RS, accurately weighed.
Application volume: 5 µL.
Developing solvent system: a mixture of chloroform and glacial acetic acid (95 : 5).
Procedure—Proceed as directed in the chapter, except to heat the plate in an oven at 105° for 10 minutes after the solvent evaporates. Remove the plate from the oven, and while it is still hot, spray lightly with dilute sulfuric acid (3 in 4). Observe the plate under long-wavelength UV light: any red fluorescent spot produced by the *Test solution* at an R_F value of about 0.4, and any yellow fluorescent spot produced by the *Test solution* at an R_F value of about 0.2, are not greater in size and intensity than the corresponding spots from *Standard solution 1* and *Standard solution 2*, respectively.

Change to read:
Dissolution ⟨711⟩—
0.025 M Acetate buffer solution—Accurately weigh about 5.22 g of anhydrous sodium acetate and 2.2 g of glacial acetic acid into a 4-L volumetric flask, add 3.5 L of water, and mix. Adjust with 1 N sodium hydroxide to a pH of 5.0 ± 0.2, and dilute with water to volume.

Medium: 0.025 M pH 5.0 acetate buffer with 0.15% sodium lauryl sulfate, prepared by accurately weighing about 6 g of sodium lauryl sulfate into a 4-L volumetric flask, adding 1.5 L of *0.025 M Acetate buffer solution*, mixing, and diluting with *0.025 M Acetate buffer solution* to volume; 600 mL.

Apparatus 2: 75 rpm.
Time: 60 minutes.

Determine the amounts of norethindrone acetate ($C_{22}H_{28}O_3$) and ethinyl estradiol ($C_{20}H_{24}O_2$) dissolved by employing the following method.

Mobile phase—Prepare a filtered and degassed mixture of 0.2% phosphoric acid, acetonitrile, and tetrahydrofuran (540 : 380 : 80). Make adjustments if necessary (see *System Suitability* under *Chromatography* ⟨621⟩).

Standard solution—Dissolve accurately weighed quantities of USP Norethindrone Acetate RS and USP Ethinyl Estradiol RS in a minimum amount of acetonitrile, and dilute quantitatively, and stepwise if necessary, with *Medium* to obtain a solution having known concentrations equivalent to the expected concentrations of the solution under test.

Test solution—Withdraw a 2-mL aliquot using a glass pipet or syringe, and centrifuge at about 2000 rpm for about 5 minutes. Use the supernatant.

Chromatographic system—The liquid chromatograph is equipped with a 242-nm detector and a fluorescent detector with an excitation wavelength set at 210 nm ▲and an emission wavelength set at 310 nm,▲*USP31* a 6-mm × 40-mm column that contains 3-µm packing L1, and a 4-mm × 12.5-mm guard column that contains 5-µm packing L1. The flow rate is about 1 mL per minute. ▲Chromatograph the *Standard solution*, and record the peak responses as directed for *Procedure*: the column efficiency is not less than 500 theoretical plates for ethinyl estradiol and not less than 1400 theoretical plates for norethindrone acetate; the tailing factor for each analyte is not more than 2.0; and the relative standard deviation for each analyte is not more than 2.5%.▲*USP31*

Procedure—Separately inject equal volumes (about 200 µL) of the *Standard solution* and the *Test solution* into the chromatograph, record the chromatograms, and measure the peak responses.

Tolerances—Not less than 80% *(Q)* of the labeled amounts of $C_{22}H_{28}O_3$ and $C_{20}H_{24}O_2$ is dissolved in 60 minutes.

Uniformity of dosage units ⟨905⟩: meet the requirements.

Procedure for content uniformity for ethinyl estradiol—Place 1 Tablet in a 125-mL separator, add 5 mL of water, and shake until the Tablet has disintegrated completely. Add 25.0 mL of a mixture of toluene and isooctane (3 : 2), shake thoroughly, allow to settle, and remove and discard the aqueous phase. Transfer 20.0 mL of the isooctane-toluene solution to a second 125-mL separator, avoiding mechanical transfer of any of the aqueous phase. Transfer 8.0 mL of a solution of USP Ethinyl Estradiol RS in toluene, containing in each mL an amount of ethinyl estradiol equal to one-tenth of the labeled quantity per Tablet, to a third 125-mL separator, and add 12 mL of isooctane. To the second and third separators add 8.0 mL of a 1 in 25 solution of sodium hydroxide in dilute alcohol (1 in 10), shake, allow to settle, and transfer the sodium hydroxide solution from each separator into separate suitable containers. Proceed as directed in the *Assay for ethinyl estradiol*, beginning with "Add, dropwise, 5.0 mL of the sodium hydroxide extract", but determine the absorbances of the final solutions using 5-cm cells. Calculate the quantity, in µg, of $C_{20}H_{24}O_2$ in the Tablet taken by the formula:

$$10C (A_U / A_S)$$

in which C is the concentration, in µg per mL, of the Standard solution in toluene; and A_U and A_S are the absorbances of the test solution and the Standard solution, respectively.

Procedure for content uniformity for norethindrone acetate—Transfer 1 finely powdered Tablet to a 100-mL volumetric flask with the aid of about 75 mL of alcohol, heat to boiling, and allow to remain at a temperature just below the boiling temperature for about 15 minutes, with occasional swirling. Cool to room temperature, dilute with alcohol to volume, and mix. Centrifuge a portion of the contents at about 2000 rpm until the solution becomes clear. If necessary, dilute a portion of the supernatant quantitatively with alcohol to provide a solution containing about 10 µg per mL of norethindrone acetate. Concomitantly determine the absorbances of this solution and of a solution of USP Norethindrone Acetate RS in alcohol having a known concentration of about 10 μg per mL in 1-cm cells at the wavelength of maximum absorbance at about 240 nm, with a suitable spectrophotometer, using alcohol as the blank. Calculate the quantity, in mg, of $C_{22}H_{28}O_3$ in the Tablet taken by the formula:

$$(T/D)C (A_U / A_S)$$

in which T is the labeled quantity, in mg, of norethindrone acetate in the Tablet; D is the concentration, in μg per mL, of norethindrone acetate in the test solution, based on the labeled quantity per Tablet and the extent of dilution; C is the concentration, in μg per mL, of USP Norethindrone Acetate RS in the Standard solution; and A_U and A_S are the absorbances of the solution from the Tablet and the Standard solution, respectively.

Assay for norethindrone acetate—Place 20 Tablets in a 125-mL separator, add 20 mL of water, and shake until the Tablets have disintegrated completely. Extract with three 30-mL portions of chloroform, filtering each extract through chloroform-moistened cotton into a round-bottom, 250-mL flask. Evaporate the combined extracts under vacuum to dryness, with the aid of gentle heat (not more than 40°). Cool, add 5 mL of water and 100.0 mL of a mixture of isooctane and toluene (3 : 2), insert the stopper, and shake for 2 to 3 minutes. Transfer an accurately measured volume of the supernatant isooctane-toluene solution, containing about 1.5 mg of norethindrone acetate, to a round-bottom, 250-mL flask, and similarly evaporate under vacuum to dryness, taking care to assure complete removal of residual toluene. [NOTE—Retain the remaining isooctane-toluene solution for the *Assay for ethinyl estradiol*.] Dissolve the residue in 100.0 mL of alcohol, and mix. Concomitantly determine the absorbances of this solution and a solution of USP Norethindrone Acetate RS in the same medium, having a known concentration of about 15 μg per mL, in 1-cm cells at the wavelength of maximum absorbance at about 240 nm, with a suitable spectrophotometer, using alcohol as the blank. Calculate the quantity, in mg, of norethindrone acetate ($C_{22}H_{28}O_3$) in the accurately measured volume of isooctane-toluene solution of the Tablets taken by the formula:

$$0.1C (A_U / A_S)$$

in which C is the concentration, in μg per mL, of USP Norethindrone Acetate RS in the Standard solution; and A_U and A_S are the absorbances of the solution from the Tablets and the Standard solution, respectively.

Assay for ethinyl estradiol—Transfer 25.0 mL of the isooctane-toluene solution prepared from the Tablets as directed in the *Assay for norethindrone acetate* to a 125-mL separator, avoiding mechanical transfer of any of the aqueous phase. Transfer 10.0 mL of a toluene solution of USP Ethinyl Estradiol RS, containing in each mL a known amount of ethinyl estradiol equal to one-half of the labeled quantity per Tablet, to another 125-mL separator containing 15.0 mL of isooctane. Add 10.0 mL of a 1 in 25 solution of sodium hydroxide in dilute alcohol (1 in 10) to each separator, and shake gently for 3 minutes. Allow to settle, and transfer the sodium hydroxide solution from each separator into separate suitable containers. [NOTE—Retain the isooctane-toluene solution for *Identification* test A.] Add, dropwise, 5.0 mL of the sodium hydroxide extract from the Tablets to 25.0 mL of dilute sulfuric acid (4 in 5) contained in a 150-mL beaker and previously chilled in an ice bath. Stir the acid solution continuously during the addition with the aid of a magnetic stirrer, and keep it in the ice bath. [NOTE—Stir the acid solution rapidly and introduce the alkaline solution near the perimeter of the rapidly swirling acid solution, rather than near the vortex. Add the alkaline solution slowly, dropwise.] Treat 5.0 mL of the sodium hydroxide solution from the Standard in the same manner, and allow the solutions to reach room temperature. Concomitantly determine the absorbances of both solutions in 1-cm cells at the wavelength of maximum absorbance at about 536 nm, with a suitable spectrophotometer, using water as the blank. [NOTE—Use 2-cm cells for Tablets labeled to contain 30 μg or less of ethinyl estra-

diol.] Calculate the quantity, in μg, of ethinyl estradiol ($C_{20}H_{24}O_2$) in the portion of isooctane-toluene solution taken by the formula:

$$10C (A_U / A_S)$$

in which C is the concentration, in μg per mL, of USP Ethinyl Estradiol RS in the Standard solution; and A_U and A_S are the absorbances of the solutions from the Tablets and the Reference Standard, respectively.

Norethynodrel

$C_{20}H_{26}O_2$ 298.42
19-Norpregn-5(10)-en-20-yn-3-one, 17-hydroxy-, (17α)-.
17-Hydroxy-19-nor-17α-pregn-5(10)-en-20-yn-3-one   [68-23-5].

» Norethynodrel contains not less than 97.0 percent and not more than 101.0 percent of $C_{20}H_{26}O_2$.

Packaging and storage—Preserve in well-closed containers.

USP Reference standards ⟨11⟩—USP Norethindrone RS. USP Norethynodrel RS.

Identification, *Infrared Absorption* ⟨197S⟩—
    Solution: 1 in 20.
    Medium: chloroform.

Specific rotation ⟨781S⟩:   between +119° and +125°.
    Test solution: 10 mg per mL, in dioxane.

Limit of ethynyl group—Dissolve 200 mg in about 40 mL of tetrahydrofuran. Add 10 mL of silver nitrate solution (1 in 10), and titrate with 0.1 N sodium hydroxide VS, using either a glass-calomel or a silver-silver chloride electrode system with potassium nitrate filling solution. Each mL of 0.1 N sodium hydroxide is equivalent to 2.503 mg of ethynyl group (–C≡CH). Not less than 8.18% and not more than 8.43% of ethynyl group is found.

Limit of norethindrone—
    Test preparation—Prepare a solution of Norethynodrel in chloroform containing 10 mg per mL.
    Standard solution—Prepare a solution of USP Norethindrone RS in chloroform to contain 1 mg per mL. Dilute 2 mL of the solution with chloroform to 10 mL.
    Procedure—Apply 10-μL volumes of the *Test preparation* and the *Standard solution* (see *Chromatography* ⟨621⟩) to a thin-layer chromatographic plate coated with a 0.25-mm layer of chromatographic silica gel mixture, and allow not more than 5 minutes between spotting the plate and starting development of the chromatogram. Place the plate in a suitable chromatographic chamber previously equilibrated with a mixture of cyclohexane, ethyl acetate, and methanol (60 : 40 : 2), and allow the solvent front to move 15 cm. Spray the plate with dilute sulfuric acid (1 in 2), heat the plate at 105° for 5 minutes, and view under long-wavelength UV light. Locate any norethindrone impurity in the *Test preparation* by comparison with the R_F value from the *Standard solution*. If present, the norethindrone spot from the *Test preparation* is not larger or more intense than the spot from the *Standard solution* (2.0%).

Ordinary impurities ⟨466⟩—
    Test solution: chloroform.
    Standard solution: chloroform.
    Eluant: ether.
    Visualization: 5, followed by viewing under long-wavelength UV light.

Organic volatile impurities, *Method V* ⟨467⟩: meets the requirements.
    Solvent—Use dimethyl sulfoxide.

(Official until July 1, 2008)

Assay—
Standard preparation—Dissolve a suitable quantity of USP Norethynodrel RS, accurately weighed, in methanol, and dilute quantitatively with methanol to obtain a solution having a known concentration of about 1 mg per mL.

Assay preparation—Dissolve about 100 mg of Norethynodrel, accurately weighed, in methanol to make 100.0 mL, and mix.

Procedure—Transfer 10.0 mL each of the *Standard preparation* and the *Assay preparation* to separate 100-mL volumetric flasks. To each flask add 40 mL of methanol, then add 5 mL of a mixture of 3 volumes of hydrochloric acid and 2 volumes of water, mix quickly, and allow to stand at a temperature of about 25° for 1 hour, accurately timed. Prior to the end of the 1-hour period, prepare blanks as follows. Add 1.0 mL each of the *Standard preparation* and the *Assay preparation* to separate 100-mL volumetric flasks, each containing a mixture of 50 mL of methanol and 2 mL of water, dilute each with methanol to volume, and mix. At the end of the 1-hour reaction period, dilute each of the acid-containing solutions with methanol to volume, and mix. Transfer 10.0 mL of each into separate 100-mL volumetric flasks, add 2 mL of water to each, dilute with methanol to volume, and mix. Concomitantly determine the absorbances of the solutions in 1-cm cells at the wavelength of maximum absorbance at about 240 nm, with a suitable spectrophotometer, relative to the corresponding blanks. Calculate the quantity, in mg, of $C_{20}H_{26}O_2$ in the portion of Norethynodrel taken by the formula:

$$100C(A_U / A_S)$$

in which C is the concentration, in mg per mL, of USP Norethynodrel RS in the *Standard preparation*, and A_U and A_S are the absorbances of the solutions from the *Assay preparation* and the *Standard preparation*, respectively.

Norfloxacin

$C_{16}H_{18}FN_3O_3$ 319.33

3-Quinolinecarboxylic acid, 1-ethyl-6-fluoro-1,4-dihydro-4-oxo-7-(1-piperazinyl)-.
1-Ethyl-6-fluoro-1,4-dihydro-4-oxo-7-(1-piperazinyl)-3-quinolinecarboxylic acid   [70458-96-7].

» Norfloxacin contains not less than 99.0 percent and not more than 101.0 percent of $C_{16}H_{18}FN_3O_3$, calculated on the dried basis.

Packaging and storage—Preserve in tight, light-resistant containers.

USP Reference standards ⟨11⟩—*USP Norfloxacin RS*.
Identification—
  A: *Infrared Absorption* ⟨197M⟩.
  B: *Ultraviolet Absorption* ⟨197U⟩—[NOTE—Use low actinic glassware in this procedure.]
    Solution: 5 µg per mL.
    Medium: 0.1 N sodium hydroxide.
    Absorptivities at 273 nm, calculated on the dried basis, do not differ by more than 3.0%.
Loss on drying ⟨731⟩—Dry it in vacuum at a pressure not exceeding 5 mm of mercury at 100° to constant weight: it loses not more than 1.0% of its weight.
Residue on ignition ⟨281⟩:   not more than 0.1%, a platinum crucible being used.
Heavy metals, *Method II* ⟨231⟩:   0.0015%.
Chromatographic purity—Dissolve a quantity of Norfloxacin in a mixture of methanol and methylene chloride (1 : 1) to obtain a test solution containing 8.0 mg per mL. Dissolve 4.0 mg of USP Norfloxacin RS in 1 mL of glacial acetic acid, add 4 mL of methanol, and mix. To 1 mL of this Standard stock solution add 9 mL of the mixture of methanol and methylene chloride (1 : 1) to obtain *Comparison solution A*. Dilute a portion of this solution with an equal volume of the mixture of methanol and methylene chloride (1 : 1) to obtain *Comparison solution B*. Separately apply 5 µL of the test solution, 1, 1.5, and 2 µL of *Comparison solution A*, and 5 µL of *Comparison solution B* to a suitable high-performance thin-layer chromatographic plate (see *Chromatography* ⟨621⟩) coated with a 0.25-mm layer of silica gel mixture, previously washed with methanol and air-dried. The spots of *Comparison solutions A* and *B* are equivalent to 0.2, 0.3, 0.4, and 0.5% of impurities, respectively. Place the plate in a paper-lined chromatographic chamber previously equilibrated with a solvent system consisting of a mixture of chloroform, methanol, toluene, diethylamine, and water (40 : 40 : 20 : 14 : 8). Seal the chamber and allow the chromatogram to develop until the solvent front has moved about nine-tenths of the length of the plate. Remove the plate from the chamber, mark the solvent front, allow the solvent to evaporate, and examine the plate under both short- and long-wavelength UV light. Compare the intensities of any secondary spots observed in the chromatogram of the test solution with those of the principal spots in the chromatograms of *Comparison solutions A* and *B*: the sum of the intensities of secondary spots obtained from the test solution corresponds to not more than 0.5% of impurities.

Assay—Dissolve about 460 mg of Norfloxacin, accurately weighed, in 100 mL of glacial acetic acid. Titrate potentiometrically with 0.1 N perchloric acid VS using a suitable anhydrous electrode system (see *Titrimetry* ⟨541⟩). [NOTE—Remove any aqueous solution in the electrode(s), render anhydrous, and fill with 0.1 N lithium perchlorate in acetic anhydride.] Perform a blank determination, and make any necessary correction. Each mL of 0.1 N perchloric acid is equivalent to 31.93 mg of $C_{16}H_{18}FN_3O_3$.

Norfloxacin Ophthalmic Solution

» Norfloxacin Ophthalmic Solution is a sterile, aqueous solution of Norfloxacin. It contains not less than 90.0 percent and not more than 110.0 percent of the labeled amount of norfloxacin ($C_{16}H_{18}FN_3O_3$).

Packaging and storage—Preserve in tight, light-resistant containers, stored at controlled room temperature.
USP Reference standards ⟨11⟩—*USP Norfloxacin RS*.
Identification—
  A: *Ultraviolet Absorption* ⟨197U⟩—
    Solution: about 0.06 mg of norfloxacin per mL.
    Diluent: 0.1 N hydrochloric acid.
  B: The retention time of the major peak in the chromatogram of the *Assay preparation* corresponds to that in the chromatogram of the *Standard preparation*, as obtained in the *Assay*.
Sterility ⟨71⟩:   meets the requirements.
pH ⟨791⟩:   between 5.0 and 5.4.
Assay—
  Dilute phosphoric acid solution—Prepare a solution of phosphoric acid in water (1 in 1000).
  Mobile phase—Prepare a filtered and degassed mixture of *Dilute phosphoric acid solution* and acetonitrile (850 : 150). Make adjustments if necessary (see *System Suitability* under *Chromatography* ⟨621⟩).
  Standard preparation—Prepare a solution of USP Norfloxacin RS in *Dilute phosphoric acid solution* having a known concentration of about 0.06 mg per mL.
  Resolution solution—Prepare a solution of USP Norfloxacin RS and pipemidic acid in *Dilute phosphoric acid solution* having known concentrations of about 0.06 mg of each per mL.
  Assay preparation—Dilute an accurately measured volume of Ophthalmic Solution quantitatively and stepwise with *Dilute phosphoric acid solution* to obtain a solution having a concentration of about 0.06 mg of norfloxacin per mL.

Chromatographic system (see *Chromatography* ⟨621⟩)—The liquid chromatograph is equipped with a 278-nm detector and a 3.9-mm × 30-cm column that contains packing L1. The column temperature is maintained at 50°. The flow rate is about 0.5 mL per minute. Precondition the column for about 8 hours with 0.01 M monobasic sodium phosphate buffer adjusted with phosphoric acid to a pH of 4.0. Chromatograph the *Resolution solution*, and record the peak responses as directed for *Procedure*: the relative retention times are about 0.8 for pipemidic acid and 1.0 for norfloxacin; and the resolution, R, between the pipemidic acid peak and the norfloxacin peak is not less than 1.2. Chromatograph the *Standard preparation*, and record the peak responses as directed for *Procedure*: the tailing factor for the norfloxacin peak is not more than 2.0; and the relative standard deviation for replicate injections is not more than 2.0%.

Procedure—[NOTE—Use peak areas where peak responses are indicated.] Separately inject equal volumes (about 10 μL) of the *Standard preparation* and the *Assay preparation* into the chromatograph, record the chromatograms, and measure the responses for the major peaks. Calculate the quantity, in mg, of norfloxacin ($C_{16}H_{18}FN_3O_3$) in each mL of the Ophthalmic Solution taken by the formula:

$$(L/D)(C)(r_U/r_S)$$

in which L is the labeled quantity, in mg per mL, of norfloxacin in the Ophthalmic Solution; D is the concentration, in mg per mL, of norfloxacin in the *Assay preparation*, based on the labeled quantity of norfloxacin in each mL of the Ophthalmic Solution and the extent of dilution; C is the concentration, in mg per mL, of USP Norfloxacin RS in the *Standard preparation;* and r_U and r_S are the norfloxacin peak responses obtained from the *Assay preparation* and the *Standard preparation*, respectively.

Norfloxacin Tablets

» Norfloxacin Tablets contain not less than 90.0 percent and not more than 110.0 percent of the labeled amount of norfloxacin ($C_{16}H_{18}FN_3O_3$).

Packaging and storage—Preserve in well-closed containers.

USP Reference standards ⟨11⟩—*USP Norfloxacin RS*.

Identification—
A: The retention time of the major peak in the chromatogram of the *Assay preparation* corresponds to that of the *Standard preparation* obtained as directed in the *Assay*.
B: Shake a quantity of finely powdered Tablets, equivalent to about 75 mg of norfloxacin, with 50 mL of a mixture of acidic methanol (prepared by mixing 1000 mL of methanol and 9 mL of hydrochloric acid) and methylene chloride (1 : 1). Centrifuge a portion of the suspension thus obtained, and use the clear supernatant as the test solution. Apply 50 μL each of the test solution and a standard solution of USP Norfloxacin RS in the same solvent containing 1.5 mg per mL to a suitable thin-layer chromatographic plate (see *Chromatography* ⟨621⟩) coated with a 0.25-mm layer of chromatographic silica gel mixture. Place the plate in a suitable chromatographic chamber that contains and has been equilibrated with a developing system consisting of a mixture of chloroform, methanol, toluene, diethylamine, and water (40 : 40 : 20 : 14 : 8), and develop the chromatogram until the solvent front has moved about three-fourths of the length of the plate. Remove the plate from the chamber, mark the solvent front, and allow the solvent to evaporate. Locate the spots on the plate by examination under short-wavelength UV light: the R_F value of the principal spot obtained from the test solution corresponds to that obtained from the Standard solution.

Dissolution ⟨711⟩—
pH 4.0 buffer—To 900 mL of water in a 1000-mL volumetric flask add 2.86 mL of glacial acetic acid and 1.0 mL of a 50% (w/w) solution of sodium hydroxide, dilute with water to volume, and mix. If necessary, adjust with glacial acetic acid or the sodium hydroxide solution to a pH of 4.0.

Medium: pH 4.0 buffer; 750 mL.
Apparatus 2: 50 rpm.
Time: 30 minutes.

Procedure—Determine the amount of $C_{16}H_{18}FN_3O_3$ dissolved from UV absorbances at the wavelength of maximum absorbance at about 278 nm of filtered portions of the solution under test, suitably diluted with *Medium*, if necessary, in comparison with a Standard solution having a known concentration of USP Norfloxacin RS in the same medium.

Tolerances—Not less than 80% (*Q*) of the labeled amount of $C_{16}H_{18}FN_3O_3$ is dissolved in 30 minutes.

Uniformity of dosage units ⟨905⟩: meet the requirements.

Assay—
Mobile phase—Prepare a filtered and degassed mixture of phosphoric acid solution (1 in 1000) and acetonitrile (850 : 150). Make adjustments if necessary (see *System Suitability* under *Chromatography* ⟨621⟩).

Standard preparation—Dissolve an accurately weighed quantity of USP Norfloxacin RS quantitatively in *Mobile phase*, and dilute quantitatively, and stepwise if necessary, with *Mobile phase* to obtain a solution having a known concentration of about 0.2 mg per mL.

Assay preparation—Weigh and finely powder not less than 20 Tablets. Transfer an accurately weighed portion of the powder, equivalent to about 100 mg of norfloxacin, to a 200-mL volumetric flask. Add 80 mL of *Mobile phase*, sonicate for 10 minutes, dilute with phosphoric acid solution (1 in 1000) to volume, and mix. Transfer 10.0 mL of this solution to a 25-mL volumetric flask, dilute with *Mobile phase* to volume, mix, and filter through a filter having a porosity of 1 μm or less.

Chromatographic system (see *Chromatography* ⟨621⟩)—The liquid chromatograph is equipped with a 275-nm detector and a 3.9-mm × 30-cm column that contains packing L1, and is operated at 40 ± 1.0°. Precondition the column with degassed 0.01 M monobasic sodium phosphate adjusted with phosphoric acid to a pH of 4.0, flowing at a rate of 0.5 mL per minute for 8 hours. For the assay, use a *Mobile phase* flow rate of about 2 mL per minute. Chromatograph the *Standard preparation*, and record the peak responses as directed for *Procedure*: the capacity factor, k', is not less than 2, the column efficiency is not less than 1500 theoretical plates, the tailing factor for the norfloxacin peak is not more than 2.0, and the relative standard deviation for replicate injections is not more than 2.0%.

Procedure—[NOTE—Use peak areas where peak responses are indicated.] Separately inject equal volumes (about 10 μL) of the *Standard preparation* and the *Assay preparation* into the chromatograph, record the chromatograms, and measure the peak responses for the major peaks. Calculate the quantity, in mg, of $C_{16}H_{18}FN_3O_3$ in the portion of Tablets taken by the formula:

$$500C(r_U/r_S)$$

in which C is the concentration, in mg per mL, of USP Norfloxacin RS in the *Standard preparation*, and r_U and r_S are the norfloxacin peak responses obtained from the *Assay preparation* and the *Standard preparation*, respectively.

Norgestimate

$C_{23}H_{31}NO_3$ 369.50
18,19-Dinor-17-pregn-4-en-20-yn-3-one, 17-(acetyloxy)-13-ethyl-, oxime, (17α)-(+)-.
(+)-13-Ethyl-17-hydroxy-18,19-dinor-17α-pregn-4-en-20-yn-3-one oxime acetate (ester)   [35189-28-7].

» Norgestimate is a mixture of *(E)-* and *(Z)-*isomers having a ratio of *(E)-* to *(Z)-*isomer between 1.27 and 1.78 and it contains not less than 98.0 percent and not more than 102.0 percent of $C_{23}H_{31}NO_3$, calculated on the dried basis.

Packaging and storage—Preserve in well-closed containers.
USP Reference standards ⟨11⟩—USP Norgestimate RS. USP Norgestimate Related Compound A RS. USP Deacetylnorgestimate RS.
Identification—
  A: *Infrared Absorption* ⟨197K⟩—
  Test specimen—Use a dispersion in potassium bromide prepared by mixing the specimen with potassium bromide in a 1 to 100 ratio.
  B: The retention time of the major peak in the chromatogram of the *Assay preparation* corresponds to that in the chromatogram of the *Standard preparation,* as obtained in the *Assay.*
Specific rotation ⟨781S⟩: between +40° and +46°.
  Test solution: 10 mg per mL, in chloroform.
Loss on drying ⟨731⟩—Dry it at 105° for 3 hours: it loses not more than 0.5% of its weight.
Residue on ignition ⟨281⟩: not more than 0.3%.
Heavy metals, *Method II* ⟨231⟩: 0.002%.
Limit of residual solvents ⟨467⟩—
  Internal standard solution—Prepare a solution of isobutyl alcohol in dimethylformamide containing 2 µL of isobutyl alcohol per 100 mL of solution.
  Standard solution—Prepare a solution in *Internal standard solution* containing 5 µL each of acetone, alcohol, chloroform, diisopropyl ether, and methanol per 100 mL of solution.
  System suitability solution—Dilute a portion of the *Standard solution* with *Internal standard solution* to obtain a solution containing 0.05 µL each of acetone, alcohol, chloroform, diisopropyl ether, and methanol per 100 mL of solution.
  Test solution—Transfer about 40 mg of Norgestimate and 2 mL of *Internal standard solution* to a 5-mL volumetric flask or a suitable vial, and shake well to dissolve.
  Chromatographic system (see *Chromatography* ⟨621⟩)—The gas chromatograph is equipped with a flame-ionization detector, a 0.53-mm × 30-m fused-silica capillary column bonded with a 1-µm layer of phase G16, and a split injection system. The detector temperature is maintained at about 250°, and the injection port temperature is maintained at about 180°. The chromatograph is programmed as follows. The column temperature is maintained at about 65° for 2.5 minutes, then the temperature is increased at a rate of 35° per minute to 100°, maintained at 100° for 2 minutes, then increased at a rate of 30° per minute to 160°, and maintained at 160° for 2.5 minutes. The carrier gas is helium, flowing at a rate of about 6 mL per minute, and the split flow rate is about 16 mL per minute. Chromatograph the *Internal standard solution,* the *Standard solution,* and the *System suitability solution,* and record the peak responses as directed for *Procedure:* there are no interfering peaks due to dimethylformamide; the retention time of isobutyl alcohol in the chromatogram of the *Internal standard solution* is between 4 and 5 minutes; the signal-to-noise ratio for alcohol obtained from the *System suitability solution* is not less than 2.0; and the relative standard deviation for replicate injections of the *Standard solution,* determined from the peak response ratios of each solvent to the internal standard, is not more than 3.0%.
  Procedure—Separately inject equal volumes (about 1 µL) of the *Standard solution* and the *Test solution* into the chromatograph, record the chromatograms, and measure the responses for the major peaks. Calculate the percentage of each solvent in the portion of Norgestimate taken by the formula:

$$200(CD/W)(R_U/R_S)$$

in which C is the concentration, in mL per mL, of each solvent in the *Standard solution;* D is the density, in mg per mL, of each solvent; W is the weight, in mg, of Norgestimate taken to prepare the *Test solution;* and R_U and R_S are the peak response ratios of the appropriate analyte to the internal standard obtained from the *Test solution* and the *Standard solution,* respectively. *Option 1:* not more than 0.5% each of acetone and alcohol is found, not more than 0.05% of diisopropyl ether is found, not more than 0.006% of chloroform is found, and not more than 0.3% of methanol is found; or *Option 2:* meets the requirements.
Chromatographic purity—
  TEST 1—
  Diluent, Mobile phase, Sensitivity solution, and *Chromatographic system*—Proceed as directed in the *Assay.*
  Standard solution—Use the *Standard preparation,* prepared as directed in the *Assay.*
  Test solution—Use the *Assay preparation.*
  Resolution solution—Dissolve accurately weighed quantities of USP Norgestimate RS, USP Norgestimate Related Compound A RS and USP Deacetylnorgestimate RS in *Diluent* to obtain a solution containing about 0.5 mg of each per mL.
  Chromatographic system (see *Chromatography* ⟨621⟩)—The liquid chromatograph is equipped with a 244-nm detector and a 4.6-mm × 10-cm column that contains 3-µm packing L1. The flow rate is about 1.2 mL per minute. Chromatograph the *Resolution solution,* and record the peak responses as directed for *Procedure:* the relative retention times are about 0.50 for *(Z)-*17-deacetylnorgestimate, about 0.56 for *(E)-*17-deacetylnorgestimate, about 0.72 for norgestimate related compound A, and 1.0 for *(E)-*norgestimate; and the resolution, *R,* between *(Z)-*17-deacetylnorgestimate and *(E)-*17-deacetylnorgestimate is not less than 1.5, and that between *(E)-*17-deacetylnorgestimate and norgestimate related compound A is not less than 1.5.
  Procedure—Separately inject equal volumes (about 25 µL) of the *Standard solution* and the *Test solution* into the chromatograph, record the chromatograms, and measure the peak areas. Calculate the percentage of each impurity in the portion of Norgestimate taken by the formula:

$$5000(CP/W)(r_i/Fr_S)$$

in which C is the concentration, in mg per mL, of USP Norgestimate RS in the *Standard solution;* P is the fraction of *(E)-*norgestimate in USP Norgestimate RS; W is the weight, in mg, of Norgestimate taken to prepare the *Test solution;* r_i is the peak area for each impurity obtained from the *Test solution;* F is the relative response factor for each impurity; and r_S is the peak area of *(E)-*norgestimate, eluting at about 13.5 minutes, obtained from the *Standard solution.* The impurities meet the requirements specified in the table below.

Impurities	Relative Response Time	Relative Response Factor	Limit (not more than)
*(Z)-*17-Deacetylnorgestimate[*]	0.50	0.83	0.3%
*(E)-*Deacetylnorgestimate[*]	0.56	1.13	0.3%
Norgestimate related compound A (levo-norgestrel acetate)	0.72	0.85	0.3%
Any other impurity	—	1.0	0.1%

[*] Provided as a mixture called USP Deacetylnorgestimate RS; their combined limits are not more than 0.3%.

  TEST 2—
  Mobile phase—Prepare a filtered and degassed mixture of cyclohexane and absolute alcohol (50 : 1). Make adjustments if necessary (see *System Suitability* under *Chromatography* ⟨621⟩).
  Standard solution—Dissolve an accurately weighed quantity of USP Norgestimate RS in *Mobile phase,* and dilute quantitatively, and stepwise if necessary, with *Mobile phase* to obtain a solution having a known concentration of about 1.0 mg per mL.
  System suitability solution—Dilute a portion of the *Standard solution* quantitatively, and stepwise if necessary, with *Mobile phase* to obtain a solution having a known concentration of about 0.5 µg per mL.
  Test solution—Transfer about 10 mg of Norgestimate, accurately weighed, to a 10-mL volumetric flask, dissolve in and dilute with *Mobile phase* to volume, and mix.
  Chromatographic system (see *Chromatography* ⟨621⟩)—The liquid chromatograph is equipped with a 210-nm detector and a 4.6-

mm × 25-cm column that contains 5-µm packing L20. The flow rate is about 1 mL per minute. Chromatograph the *System suitability solution,* and record the peak responses as directed for *Procedure:* the signal-to-noise ratio for *(E)*-norgestimate is not less than 3.0. Chromatograph the *Standard solution,* and record the peak areas as directed for *Procedure:* the retention time is about 18.6 minutes for *(E)*-norgestimate; the relative retention times are about 1.0 for *(E)*-norgestimate and 1.1 for *(Z)*-norgestimate; the resolution, *R,* between *(Z)*-norgestimate and *(E)*-norgestimate is not less than 1.5; the tailing factor is not more than 1.5; and the relative standard deviation for replicate injections, determined from the peak area of *(Z)*-norgestimate to *(E)*-norgestimate, is not more than 2.0%.

Procedure—Separately inject equal volumes (about 25 µL) of the *Standard solution* and the *Test solution* into the chromatograph, record the chromatograms, and measure the peak areas. Calculate the percentage of each impurity in the portion of Norgestimate taken by the formula:

$$1000(CP/W)(r_i / Fr_S)$$

in which *C* is the concentration, in mg per mL, of USP Norgestimate RS in the *Standard solution; P* is the fraction of *(E)*-norgestimate in USP Norgestimate RS; *W* is the weight, in mg, of Norgestimate taken to prepare the *Test solution; r_i* is the peak area for each impurity obtained from the *Test solution; F* is the relative response factor and is equal to 1.4 for any peak having a relative retention time of 0.74, 1.5 for any peak having a relative retention time of 0.78, and 1.2 for any peak having a relative retention time of 0.91; and r_S is the peak area of *(E)*-norgestimate obtained from the *Standard solution.* Not more than 0.2% of the impurity having a relative retention time of 0.74 is found; and not more than 0.1% each of the impurities having relative retention times of 0.78 and 0.91 is found. Not more than 1.0% of total impurities is found, the results for *Test 1* and *Test 2* being added.

Organic volatile impurities, Method IV ⟨467⟩: meets the requirements. Chloroform is tested in the *Limit of residual solvents test.*

Solvent—Use dimethyl sulfoxide.

(Official until July 1, 2008)

Assay—

Diluent—Prepare a mixture of methanol and water (4 : 1).

Mobile phase—Prepare a filtered and degassed mixture of water, tetrahydrofuran, and acetonitrile (30 : 11 : 9). Make adjustments if necessary (see System Suitability under *Chromatography* ⟨621⟩).

Standard preparation—Dissolve an accurately weighed quantity of USP Norgestimate RS in *Diluent,* and dilute quantitatively, and stepwise if necessary, with *Diluent* to obtain a solution having a known concentration of about 0.5 mg per mL.

Sensitivity solution—Dilute a portion of *Standard preparation,* quantitatively and stepwise if necessary, with *Diluent* to obtain a solution having a known concentration of about 0.05 µg per mL.

Assay preparation—Transfer about 25 mg of Norgestimate, accurately weighed, to a 50-mL volumetric flask, dissolve in and dilute with *Diluent* to volume, and mix.

Chromatographic system (see *Chromatography* ⟨621⟩)—The liquid chromatograph is equipped with a 244-nm detector and a 4.6-mm × 10-cm column that contains 3-µm packing L1. The flow rate is about 1.2 mL per minute. The column temperature is maintained at about 40°. Chromatograph the *Sensitivity solution,* and record the peak areas as directed for *Procedure:* the signal-to-noise ratio for *(Z)*-norgestimate is not less than 3.0. Chromatograph the *Standard preparation,* and record the peak areas as directed for *Procedure:* the relative retention times are about 0.86 for *(Z)*-norgestimate and 1.0 for *(E)*-norgestimate; the resolution, *R,* between *(Z)*-norgestimate and *(E)*-norgestimate is not less than 1.5; the tailing factor for *(E)*-norgestimate and for *(Z)*-norgestimate is not more than 1.5; and the relative standard deviation for replicate injections, determined from the peak area ratio of *(E)*-norgestimate to *(Z)*-norgestimate, is not more than 2.0%.

Procedure—Separately inject equal volumes (about 25 µL) of the *Standard preparation* and the *Assay preparation* into the chromatograph, record the chromatograms, and measure the areas for the major peaks. Calculate the quantity, in mg, of $C_{23}H_{31}NO_3$ in the portion of Norgestimate taken by the formula:

$$50C(r_U / r_S)$$

in which *C* is the concentration, in mg per mL, of USP Norgestimate RS in the *Standard preparation;* and r_U and r_S are the sums of the peak areas of *(Z)*-norgestimate and *(E)*-norgestimate obtained from the *Assay preparation* and the *Standard preparation,* respectively. Calculate the percentages of the *(Z)*- and *(E)*-isomers, U_Z and U_E, respectively, in the portion of Norgestimate taken by the formula:

$$5000(CP/W)(r_U / r_S)$$

in which *C* is the concentration, in mg per mL, of USP Norgestimate RS in the *Standard preparation; P* is the fraction of *(E)*- or *(Z)*-norgestimate in USP Norgestimate RS; *W* is the weight, in mg, of Norgestimate taken to prepare the *Assay preparation;* and r_U and r_S are the peak responses of the appropriate norgestimate isomer obtained from the *Assay preparation* and the *Standard preparation,* respectively. Calculate the ratio of *(E)*-norgestimate to *(Z)*-norgestimate, that is, the ratio of U_E to U_Z.

Norgestimate and Ethinyl Estradiol Tablets

» Norgestimate and Ethinyl Estradiol Tablets contain not less than 90.0 percent and not more than 110.0 percent of the labeled amounts of norgestimate ($C_{23}H_{31}NO_3$) and ethinyl estradiol ($C_{20}H_{24}O_2$).

Packaging and storage—Preserve in well-closed containers.

USP Reference standards ⟨11⟩—*USP Ethinyl Estradiol RS. USP Norgestimate RS.*

Identification—The retention times of the major peaks in the chromatogram of the *Assay preparation* correspond to those in the chromatogram of the *Standard preparation,* as obtained in the *Assay.*

Disintegration ⟨701⟩: 15 minutes.

Dissolution ⟨711⟩—[NOTE—Exercise care in filtering and handling solutions containing ethinyl estradiol to prevent adsorptive loss of the drug. Centrifugation may be used instead of filtration with nonadsorptive membrane filters. Withdraw dissolution aliquots with glass or polytef pipets or syringes that have been checked for adsorptive loss. Use glass dissolution vessels and polytef-coated or solid polytef paddles.]

Medium: 0.05% polysorbate 20; 600 mL.

Apparatus 2: 75 rpm.

Time: 20 minutes for Tablets labeled as containing 180 µg of $C_{23}H_{31}NO_3$ and 35 µg of $C_{20}H_{24}O_2$; 20 minutes for Tablets labeled as containing 215 µg of $C_{23}H_{31}NO_3$ and 35 µg of $C_{20}H_{24}O_2$; and 30 minutes for Tablets labeled as containing 250 µg of $C_{23}H_{31}NO_3$ and 35 µg of $C_{20}H_{24}O_2$.

Determine the amount of norgestimate ($C_{23}H_{31}NO_3$) and ethinyl estradiol ($C_{20}H_{24}O_2$) dissolved by employing the following method.

Mobile phase—Prepare a degassed mixture of water and isopropyl alcohol (13 : 7). Make adjustments if necessary (see System Suitability under *Chromatography* ⟨621⟩).

Standard solution—Dissolve an accurately weighed quantity of USP Norgestimate RS and USP Ethinyl Estradiol RS in *Medium,* and dilute quantitatively, and stepwise if necessary, with *Medium* to obtain a solution having known concentrations similar to those expected in the *Test solution.* [NOTE—A volume of methanol not exceeding 4% of the total volume of the *Standard solution* may be used to bring the standards into solution prior to dilution with *Medium.*]

Test solution—Use a filtered or centrifuged portion of the solution under test.

Chromatographic system (see *Chromatography* ⟨621⟩)—The liquid chromatograph is equipped with a 254-nm detector (for norgestimate analysis), a spectrofluorometric detector (for ethinyl estradiol analysis) with an excitation wavelength of 234 nm and an emission wavelength of 304 nm, and a 4.6-mm × 25-cm column that contains packing L10. The flow rate is about 1.2 mL per minute. The column temperature is maintained at 40°. Chromatograph the *Standard solution,* and record the peak responses as directed for *Procedure:* the retention times are about 7.5 minutes for ethinyl estradiol and 9.5 minutes for norgestimate; and the relative standard deviation for replicate injections is not more than 3.0% for the ethinyl estradiol and norgestimate peaks.

Procedure—Separately inject equal volumes (about 200 µL) of the *Standard solution* and the *Test solution* into the chromatograph, record the chromatograms, and measure the responses for the major peaks. Calculate the quantity, in mg, of each drug substance dissolved by the formula:

$$600C(r_U / r_S)$$

in which C is the concentration, in mg per mL, of the appropriate analyte in the *Standard solution;* and r_U and r_S are the peak responses obtained from the *Test solution* and the *Standard solution,* respectively.

Tolerances—Not less than 80% *(Q)* of the labeled amounts of $C_{23}H_{31}NO_3$ and $C_{20}H_{24}O_2$ are dissolved in 20 minutes for Tablets labeled as containing 180 µg of $C_{23}H_{31}NO_3$ and 35 µg of $C_{20}H_{24}O_2$, and for Tablets labeled as containing 215 µg of $C_{23}H_{31}NO_3$ and 35 µg of $C_{20}H_{24}O_2$. Not less than 80% *(Q)* of the labeled amounts of $C_{23}H_{31}NO_3$ and $C_{20}H_{24}O_2$ are dissolved in 30 minutes for Tablets labeled as containing 250 µg of $C_{23}H_{31}NO_3$ and 35 µg of $C_{20}H_{24}O_2$.

Uniformity of dosage units ⟨905⟩: meet the requirements.

Chromatographic purity—

Mobile phase—Proceed as directed in the *Assay.*

Standard solution—Use the *Standard preparation,* prepared as directed in the *Assay.*

Test solution—Use the *Assay preparation,* prepared as directed in the *Assay.*

Chromatographic system (see *Chromatography* ⟨621⟩)—The liquid chromatograph is equipped with a detector capable of detecting at 230 nm and 254 nm, simultaneously, and a 4.6-mm × 10-cm column that contains 5-µm packing L1. The flow rate is about 2 mL per minute. Chromatograph the *Standard solution,* and record the peak areas as directed for *Procedure:* the relative retention times are about 0.5 for ethinyl estradiol, 1.0 for *(Z)*-norgestimate, and 1.2 for *(E)*-norgestimate; the resolution, *R,* between *(Z)*-norgestimate and *(E)*-norgestimate is not less than 1.5; and the relative standard deviation for replicate injections of the ethinyl estradiol and norgestimate peaks is not more than 2.0%.

Procedure—Inject a volume (about 50 µL) of the *Test solution* into the chromatograph, record the chromatograms, and measure the areas for the major peaks. Calculate the percentage of the impurity having a relative retention time of about 0.6, relative to the *(Z)*-norgestimate peak, and detected at 230 nm in the portion of Tablets taken by the formula:

$$100(1.31)(r_i / r_s)$$

in which 1.31 is the relative response factor of this impurity; r_i is the peak response for the impurity; and r_s is the sum of the peak responses for *(E)*-norgestimate and *(Z)*-norgestimate: not more than 7.5% is found. Calculate the percentage of any impurity having a relative retention time of about 0.2 or 0.4, relative to the *(Z)*-norgestimate peak, and detected at 254 nm in the portion of Tablets taken by the formula:

$$100(1.54)(C_Z / C_E)(r_i / r_Z)$$

in which 1.54 is the relative response factor of the impurity peaks; C_Z and C_E are the quantities, in mg, of *(Z)*-norgestimate and ethinyl estradiol, respectively, as determined in the *Assay;* r_i is the peak response for each impurity; and r_Z is the peak response for *(Z)*-norgestimate: the sum of the impurities having relative retention times of about 0.2 and 0.4 is not more than 4.0%.

Assay—

Mobile phase—Prepare a degassed mixture of water, tetrahydrofuran, and methanol (13 : 5 : 2). Make adjustments if necessary (see *System Suitability* under *Chromatography* ⟨621⟩).

Internal standard solution—Dissolve an accurately weighed quantity of dibutyl phthalate in methanol to obtain a solution having a concentration of about 0.05 mg per mL.

Standard preparation—Dissolve an accurately weighed quantity of USP Norgestimate RS and USP Ethinyl Estradiol RS in *Internal standard solution,* and dilute quantitatively, and stepwise if necessary, with *Internal standard solution* to obtain a solution having a known concentration of about 7 µg per mL of ethinyl estradiol and a known concentration similar to that expected in the *Assay preparation.* Mix, and pass through a filter having a 0.45-µm porosity.

Assay preparation—Weigh and finely powder not fewer than 20 Tablets. Transfer an accurately weighed portion of the powder, equivalent to about 0.175 mg of ethinyl estradiol, to a 50-mL glass centrifuge tube, and add two glass beads. Add 25.0 mL of *Internal standard solution,* insert the stopper, and mix on a vortex mixer for at least 15 minutes. Sonicate for at least 5 minutes to ensure complete dissolution of the drug substances, mix, and pass through a filter having a 0.45-µm porosity.

Chromatographic system (see *Chromatography* ⟨621⟩)—The liquid chromatograph is equipped with a 230-nm detector and a 4.6-mm × 5-cm column that contains 5-µm packing L1. The flow rate is about 2.1 mL per minute. Chromatograph the *Standard preparation,* and record the peak responses as directed for *Procedure:* the relative retention times are about 0.5 for ethinyl estradiol, 1.0 for *(Z)*-norgestimate, 1.2 for *(E)*-norgestimate and 1.5 for dibutyl phthalate; the resolution, *R,* between *(Z)*-norgestimate and *(E)*-norgestimate is not less than 1.5; and the relative standard deviation of the peak response ratio of ethinyl estradiol, *(Z)*-norgestimate, and *(E)*-norgestimate to dibutyl phthalate from replicate injections is not more than 2.0%.

Procedure—Separately inject equal volumes (about 25 µL) of the *Standard preparation* and the *Assay preparation* into the chromatograph, record the chromatograms, and measure the responses for the major peaks. Calculate the quantity, in mg, of ethinyl estradiol ($C_{20}H_{24}O_2$) in the portion of Tablets taken by the formula:

$$25C(R_U / R_S)$$

in which C is the concentration, in mg per mL, of USP Ethinyl Estradiol RS in the *Standard preparation;* and R_U and R_S are the ratios of the peak responses of ethinyl estradiol to dibutyl phthalate obtained from the *Assay preparation* and the *Standard preparation,* respectively. Calculate the quantity, in mg, of norgestimate ($C_{23}H_{31}NO_3$) in the portion of Tablets taken by the formula:

$$25C[P_A(R_{UA} / R_{SA}) + P_S(R_{US} / R_{SS})]$$

in which C is the concentration, in mg per mL, of USP Norgestimate RS in the *Standard preparation;* P_A and P_S are the corresponding *(E)* and *(Z)* fractions of USP Norgestimate RS; R_{UA} and R_{SA} are the ratios of the peak responses of *(E)*-norgestimate to dibutyl phthalate obtained from the *Assay preparation* and the *Standard preparation,* respectively; and R_{US} and R_{SS} are the ratios of the peak responses of *(Z)*-norgestimate to dibutyl phthalate obtained from the *Assay preparation* and the *Standard preparation,* respectively.

Norgestrel

$C_{21}H_{28}O_2$ 312.45

18,19-Dinorpregn-4-en-20-yn-3-one, 13-ethyl-17-hydroxy-, (17α)-(±)-.

(±)-13-Ethyl-17-hydroxy-18,19-dinor-17α-pregn-4-en-20-yn-3-one   [6533-00-2].

» Norgestrel contains not less than 98.0 percent and not more than 102.0 percent of $C_{21}H_{28}O_2$, calculated on the dried basis.

Packaging and storage—Preserve in well-closed containers.
USP Reference standards ⟨11⟩—*USP Norgestrel RS.*
Identification, *Infrared Absorption* ⟨197K⟩—If differences appear, dissolve portions of both the test specimen and the Reference Standard in ethyl acetate, evaporate the solutions on a steam bath to dryness, and repeat the test.
Melting range, *Class I* ⟨741⟩: between 205° and 212°, but the range between beginning and end of melting does not exceed 4°.
Optical rotation ⟨781A⟩: between −0.1° and +0.1.°
  Test solution: 50 mg, previously dried, per mL, in chloroform.
Loss on drying ⟨731⟩—Dry it at 105° for 3 hours: it loses not more than 0.5% of its weight.
Residue on ignition ⟨281⟩: not more than 0.3%.
Chromatographic purity—
  Phosphomolybdic acid reagent—Add 10 g of phosphomolybdic acid to 100 mL of alcohol, and stir the mixture for not less than 30 minutes. Filter before use.
  Test preparation—Prepare a solution of Norgestrel in chloroform to contain 10.0 mg per mL.
  Standard solution and *Standard dilutions*—Prepare a solution of USP Norgestrel RS in chloroform to contain 10 mg per mL (*Standard solution*). Prepare a series of dilutions of *Standard solution* in chloroform to contain 0.20, 0.10, 0.05, 0.02, and 0.01 mg per mL (*Standard dilutions*).
  Procedure—Apply 10-μL volumes of *Standard solution*, the *Test preparation*, and each of the five *Standard dilutions* at equidistant points along a line 2.5 cm from one edge of a 20- × 20-cm thin-layer chromatographic plate (see *Chromatography* ⟨621⟩) coated with a 0.25-mm layer of chromatographic silica gel mixture and previously activated by heating at 100° for 15 minutes. Place the plate in a suitable developing chamber that contains and has been equilibrated with a mixture of 96 volumes of chloroform and 4 volumes of alcohol, seal the chamber, and allow the chromatogram to develop until the solvent front has moved 15 cm above the line of application. Remove the plate, allow the solvent to evaporate, then spray uniformly with *Phosphomolybdic acid reagent*, and heat it at 105° for 10 to 15 minutes. The lane of the *Test preparation* exhibits its principal spot at the same R_F as the principal spot of *Standard solution*. If spots other than the principal spot are observed in the lane of the *Test preparation*, estimate the concentration of each by comparison with the *Standard dilutions*. The spots from the 0.20-, 0.10-, 0.05-, 0.02-, and 0.01-mg per mL dilutions are equivalent to 2.0, 1.0, 0.5, 0.2, and 0.1% of impurities, respectively. The requirements of the test are met if the sum of the impurities in the *Test preparation* does not exceed 2.0%.
Limit of ethynyl group—Proceed as directed in the test for *Ethynyl group* under *Norethindrone*. Not less than 7.81% and not more than 8.18% of ethynyl group is found.
Assay—Dissolve about 100 mg of Norgestrel, accurately weighed, in alcohol, and dilute quantitatively and stepwise with alcohol to obtain a solution containing about 10 μg per mL. Dissolve an accurately weighed quantity of USP Norgestrel RS in alcohol to obtain a *Standard solution* having a known concentration of about 10 μg per mL. Concomitantly determine the absorbances of both solutions in 1-cm cells at the wavelength of maximum absorbance at about 241 nm, with a suitable spectrophotometer, using alcohol as the blank. Calculate the quantity, in mg, of $C_{21}H_{28}O_2$ in the portion of Norgestrel taken by the formula:

$$10C(A_U / A_S)$$

in which C is the concentration, in μg per mL, of USP Norgestrel RS in the *Standard solution*, and A_U and A_S are the absorbances of the solution of Norgestrel and the *Standard solution*, respectively.

Norgestrel Tablets

» Norgestrel Tablets contain not less than 90.0 percent and not more than 110.0 percent of the labeled amount of norgestrel ($C_{21}H_{28}O_2$).

Packaging and storage—Preserve in well-closed containers.
USP Reference standards ⟨11⟩—*USP Norgestrel RS.*
Identification—Finely powder 20 Tablets, triturate the powder with 5 mL of chloroform, and allow the solids to settle. Apply 60 μL of the extract and 60 μL of a chloroform solution containing about 300 μg of USP Norgestrel RS per mL at points about 3 cm from one edge of a thin-layer chromatographic plate (see *Chromatography* ⟨621⟩) coated with a 0.25-mm layer of chromatographic silica gel mixture. Place the plate in a developing chamber containing a mixture of chloroform and alcohol (96 : 4) to a depth of 2 cm, the chamber having been previously equilibrated with the solvent mixture. Remove the plate when the solvent has moved about 15 cm from the line of application, dry at room temperature, spray with a mixture of 80 volumes of sulfuric acid and 20 volumes of alcohol, and heat at 105° for several minutes: the spot from the solution under test exhibits an R_F value identical to that of the spot from the *Standard* solution, and, when viewed under long-wavelength UV light, exhibits a red fluorescence similar to that from the *Standard* solution.
Disintegration ⟨701⟩: 15 minutes, the use of disks being omitted.
Uniformity of dosage units ⟨905⟩: meet the requirements.
Assay—
  Isoniazid reagent—Dissolve 0.25 g of isoniazid and 0.3 mL of hydrochloric acid in 500 mL of dehydrated alcohol.
  Procedure—Weigh and finely powder not less than 20 Tablets. Transfer an accurately weighed portion of the powder, equivalent to about 75 μg of norgestrel, to a 30-mL separator containing 5 mL of water. Extract with three 5-mL portions of chloroform, shaking for about 1 minute each time, and collecting the chloroform extracts through glass wool, previously moistened with chloroform, into a glass-stoppered test tube. Add 1 mL of dilute hydrochloric acid (1 in 12) to the remaining aqueous phase and extract with a fourth 5-mL portion of chloroform, collecting this chloroform extract as before and combining it with the previous three. To another glass-stoppered test tube transfer 20.0 mL of a solution of USP Norgestrel RS, in chloroform, having a known concentration of about 3.75 μg per mL. Evaporate the contents of both tubes in a water bath with the aid of a current of air to dryness. Add 5.0 mL of *Isoniazid reagent* to each tube, insert the stopper in each tube, and swirl occasionally for 1 hour. Concomitantly determine the absorbances of both solutions in 1-cm cells, at the wavelength of maximum absorbance at about 380 nm, using a suitable spectrophotometer, and using *Isoniazid reagent* as the blank. Calculate the quantity, in μg, of $C_{21}H_{28}O_2$ in the portion of Tablets taken by the formula:

$$20C(A_U / A_S)$$

in which C is the concentration, in μg per mL, of USP Norgestrel RS in the *Standard solution*, and A_U and A_S are the absorbances of the solutions from the Tablets and the *Standard solution*, respectively.

Norgestrel and Ethinyl Estradiol Tablets

» Norgestrel and Ethinyl Estradiol Tablets contain not less than 90.0 percent and not more than 110.0 percent of the labeled amount of norgestrel ($C_{21}H_{28}O_2$) and not less than 90.0 percent and not more than 110.0 percent of the labeled amount of ethinyl estradiol ($C_{20}H_{24}O_2$).

Packaging and storage—Preserve in well-closed containers.

USP Reference standards ⟨11⟩—*USP Ethinyl Estradiol RS. USP Norgestrel RS.*
Identification—The retention times of the major peaks in the chromatogram of the *Assay preparation* correspond to those in the chromatogram of the *Standard preparation,* as obtained in the *Assay.*

Dissolution ⟨711⟩—
Medium: 0.0005% (w/v) polysorbate 80; 500 mL.
Apparatus 2: 75 rpm.
Time: 60 minutes.
Determine the amount of $C_{21}H_{28}O_2$ and $C_{20}H_{24}O_2$ dissolved by employing the following method. [NOTE—Do not use plastics during the preparation of solutions.]
Mobile phase—Prepare a filtered and degassed mixture of water and acetonitrile (3 : 2). Make adjustments if necessary (see *System Suitability* under *Chromatography* ⟨621⟩).
Standard solution[NOTE—A volume of alcohol not exceeding 2% of the final volume of the solution may be used to aid in dissolving the USP Reference Standards.]—Dissolve an accurately weighed quantity of USP Norgestrel RS and USP Ethinyl Estradiol RS in *Medium*, and dilute quantitatively, and stepwise if necessary, with *Medium* to obtain a solution having known concentrations similar to those expected in the *Test solution*.
Test solution—Use a portion of the solution under test filtered through 0.7-μm borosilicate microfiber filter.
Chromatographic system (see *Chromatography* ⟨621⟩)—The liquid chromatograph is equipped with a 247-nm detector (for norgestrel analysis), and a spectrofluorometric detector (for ethinyl estradiol analysis) with an excitation wavelength of about 285 nm and an emission wavelength of 310 nm, and a 4.6-mm × 15-cm column that contains packing L7. The flow rate is about 1 mL per minute. Chromatograph the *Standard solution*, and record the peak responses as directed for *Procedure*: the relative retention times are about 0.7 for ethinyl estradiol and 1.0 for norgestrel; and the relative standard deviation for replicate injections is not more than 3.0% for the ethinyl estradiol and norgestrel peaks.
Procedure—Separately inject equal volumes (about 100 μL) of the *Standard solution* and the *Test solution* into the chromatograph, record the chromatograms, and measure the responses for the major peaks. Calculate the quantities, in mg, of norgestrel ($C_{21}H_{28}O_2$) and ethinyl estradiol ($C_{20}H_{24}O_2$) dissolved by the formula:

$$(500C)(r_U / r_S)$$

in which C is the concentration, in mg per mL, of the appropriate USP Reference Standard in the *Standard solution;* and r_U and r_S are the peak responses obtained from the *Test solution* and the *Standard solution*, respectively.
Tolerances—Not less than 75% (*Q*) of the labeled amount of $C_{21}H_{28}O_2$ and $C_{20}H_{24}O_2$ is dissolved in 60 minutes.

Uniformity of dosage units ⟨905⟩: meet the requirements.

Assay—
Mobile phase—Prepare a degassed mixture of water, acetonitrile, and methanol (45 : 35 : 15). Make adjustments if necessary (see *System Suitability* under *Chromatography* ⟨621⟩).
Standard preparation—Dissolve an accurately weighed quantity of USP Norgestrel RS and USP Ethinyl Estradiol RS in *Mobile phase*, and dilute quantitatively, and stepwise if necessary, with *Mobile phase* to obtain a solution having known concentrations of about 100 μg of norgestrel per mL and 10 μg of ethinyl estradiol per mL.
Assay preparation—Transfer an accurately counted number of Tablets, equivalent to about 10 mg of norgestrel, to a 200-mL volumetric flask. Add 100.0 mL of *Mobile phase*, accurately measured, sonicate for 10 minutes to disintegrate the Tablets, and shake by mechanical means for 20 minutes. Centrifuge the clear portion of the solution at about 2000 rpm for 10 minutes, and filter the clear supernatant.
Chromatographic system (see *Chromatography* ⟨621⟩)—The liquid chromatograph is equipped with a 215-nm detector and a 4.6-mm × 15-cm column that contains 5-μm packing L7. The flow rate is about 1 mL per minute. Chromatograph the *Standard preparation*, and record the peak responses as directed for *Procedure*: the relative retention times are about 1.0 for ethinyl estradiol and 1.5 for norgestrel; the resolution, *R*, between the two major peaks is not less than 2.5; and the relative standard deviation for replicate injections is not more than 2.0%.
Procedure—Separately inject equal volumes (about 50 μL) of the *Standard preparation* and the *Assay preparation* into the chromatograph, record the chromatograms, and measure the responses for the major peaks. Calculate the quantity, in mg, of ethinyl estradiol ($C_{20}H_{24}O_2$) and norgestrel ($C_{21}H_{28}O_2$) in the portion of Tablets taken by the formula:

$$100C(r_U / r_S)$$

in which C is the concentration, in mg per mL, of the relevant USP Reference Standard in the *Standard preparation;* and r_U and r_S are the peak responses for the relevant analyte obtained from the *Assay preparation* and the *Standard preparation*, respectively.

Nortriptyline Hydrochloride

$C_{19}H_{21}N \cdot HCl$ 299.84
1-Propanamine, 3-(10,11-dihydro-5*H*-dibenzo[*a*,*d*]cyclohepten-5-ylidene)-*N*-methyl-, hydrochloride.
10,11-Dihydro-*N*-methyl-5*H*-dibenzo[*a*,*d*]cycloheptene-Δ^5, γ-propylamine hydrochloride   [*894-71-3*].

» Nortriptyline Hydrochloride contains not less than 97.0 percent and not more than 101.5 percent of $C_{19}H_{21}N \cdot HCl$, calculated on the dried basis.

Packaging and storage—Preserve in tight, light-resistant containers.

USP Reference standards ⟨11⟩—*USP Nortriptyline Hydrochloride RS.*

Identification—
A: *Infrared Absorption* ⟨197S⟩—
Solution: 50 mg per mL.
Medium: chloroform.
B: *Ultraviolet Absorption* ⟨197U⟩—
Solution: 10 μg per mL.
Medium: methanol.
Absorptivities at 239 nm, calculated on the dried basis, do not differ by more than 3.0%.
C: It responds to the tests for *Chloride* ⟨191⟩ when tested as specified for alkaloidal hydrochlorides.

Melting range, *Class I* ⟨741⟩: between 215° and 220°, but the range between beginning and end of melting does not exceed 3°.

Loss on drying ⟨731⟩—Dry it at 105° for 3 hours: it loses not more than 0.5% of its weight.

Residue on ignition ⟨281⟩: not more than 0.1%.

Heavy metals, *Method II* ⟨231⟩: 0.001%.

Chromatographic purity—
Adsorbent: chromatographic silica gel mixture.
Test solution—Transfer about 250 mg of Nortriptyline Hydrochloride, accurately weighed, to a 10-mL volumetric flask. Dissolve in and dilute with methanol to volume, and mix.
Standard solutions—Dissolve an accurately weighed quantity of USP Nortriptyline Hydrochloride RS in methanol, and dilute quantitatively, and stepwise if necessary, with methanol to obtain a solution having a known concentration of about 25.0 mg per mL (*Standard solution A*). Dilute appropriate portions of this solution with methanol to obtain *Standard solutions B, C, D, E,* and *F* having known concentrations of 125, 75, 50, 25, and 12.5 μg per mL, respectively. The final concentrations of *Standard solutions B, C, D, E,* and *F* represent 0.5%, 0.3%, 0.2%, 0.1%, and 0.05% of *Standard solution A* concentration, respectively.
Application volume: 5 μL.
Developing solvent system: a mixture of acetonitrile, methanol, and ammonium hydroxide (10 : 1 : 1).
Procedure—Apply equal volumes of the *Test solution* and *Standard solutions A, B, C, D, E,* and *F* as directed in *Ordinary Impurities* ⟨466⟩. Examine the plate under short-wavelength UV light, then spray the plate with Dragendorff's TS, dry the plate with a stream

of nitrogen, and then spray with hydrogen peroxide TS: any secondary spot at an R_F value of 0.78 relative to the nortriptyline spot in the *Test solution* is not greater than the principal spot for *Standard solution D;* any other secondary spot in the *Test solution* is not more than 0.1%; and the sum of all secondary spots is not more than 0.5%.

Organic volatile impurities, Method I ⟨467⟩: meets the requirements.

(Official until July 1, 2008)

Assay—Dissolve about 600 mg of Nortriptyline Hydrochloride, accurately weighed, in 50 mL of glacial acetic acid, add 10 mL of mercuric acetate TS, and titrate with 0.1 N perchloric acid VS, determining the endpoint potentiometrically. Perform a blank determination, and make any necessary correction. Each mL of 0.1 N perchloric acid is equivalent to 29.98 mg of $C_{19}H_{21}N \cdot HCl$.

Nortriptyline Hydrochloride Capsules

» Nortriptyline Hydrochloride Capsules contain nortriptyline hydrochloride equivalent to not less than 90.0 percent and not more than 110.0 percent of the labeled amount of nortriptyline ($C_{19}H_{21}N$).

Packaging and storage—Preserve in tight containers.

USP Reference standards ⟨11⟩—*USP Nortriptyline Hydrochloride RS.*

Identification—
A: Transfer the contents of Capsules, equivalent to about 50 mg of nortriptyline hydrochloride, to a suitable flask. Add 15 mL of chloroform, insert the stopper in the flask, and shake for 15 minutes. Transfer the mixture to a suitable centrifuge tube, and centrifuge at about 2900 rpm for about 5 minutes. Pass through a suitable filter paper containing a small amount of anhydrous sodium sulfate. Evaporate the filtrate to dryness, and dissolve the residue in 0.5 mL of chloroform: the IR absorption spectrum of this solution exhibits maxima only at the same wavelengths as that of a Standard solution prepared by dissolving 50 mg of USP Nortriptyline Hydrochloride RS in 0.5 mL of chloroform.

B: A filtered solution in water of the contents of Capsules, equivalent to nortriptyline hydrochloride solution (1 in 20), responds to the tests for *Chloride* ⟨191⟩, when tested as specified for alkaloidal hydrochlorides.

Dissolution ⟨711⟩—
Medium: water; 500 mL.
Apparatus 1: 100 rpm.
Time: 30 minutes.
Procedure—Determine the amount of $C_{19}H_{21}N$ dissolved, employing the procedure set forth in the *Assay*, making any necessary modifications.
Tolerances—Not less than 80% (*Q*) of the labeled amount of $C_{19}H_{21}N$ is dissolved in 30 minutes.

Uniformity of dosage units ⟨905⟩: meet the requirements.

Assay—
Phosphate buffer—Dissolve 1.63 g of monobasic potassium phosphate in 1 L of water, and adjust with 1 N potassium hydroxide to a pH of 6.7.
Mobile phase—Prepare a filtered and degassed mixture of acetonitrile, methanol, and *Phosphate buffer* (40 : 43 : 17). Make adjustments if necessary (see *System Suitability* under *Chromatography* ⟨621⟩).
Standard preparation—Dissolve an accurately weighed quantity of USP Nortriptyline Hydrochloride RS in methanol, and dilute quantitatively, and stepwise if necessary, with methanol to obtain a solution having a known concentration of about 0.38 mg per mL.
Assay preparation—Weigh, empty, and combine the contents of not less than 20 Capsules. Transfer an accurately weighed portion of the powder, equivalent to about 76 mg of nortriptyline hydrochloride, to a 200-mL volumetric flask, and dissolve in about 150 mL of methanol. Shake by mechanical means for 15 minutes, dilute with methanol to volume, mix, and filter.

Chromatographic system (see *Chromatography* ⟨621⟩)—The liquid chromatograph is equipped with a 239-nm detector and a 4.6-mm × 25-cm column that contains packing L10. The flow rate is about 2.5 mL per minute. Chromatograph the *Standard preparation*, and record the peak responses as directed under *Procedure*: the column efficiency is not less than 500 theoretical plates, the tailing factor is not more than 3.0, and the relative standard deviation for replicate injections is not more than 2.0%.
Procedure—Separately inject equal volumes (about 10 µL) of the *Standard preparation* and the *Assay preparation* into the chromatograph, record the chromatograms, and measure the responses for the major peaks. Calculate the quantity, in mg, of nortriptyline ($C_{19}H_{21}N$) in the portion of Capsules taken by the formula:

$$(263.38 / 299.85)(200C)(r_U / r_S)$$

in which 263.38 and 299.85 are the molecular weights of nortriptyline and nortriptyline hydrochloride, respectively; *C* is the concentration, in mg per mL, of USP Nortriptyline Hydrochloride RS in the *Standard preparation*; and r_U and r_S are the peak responses obtained from the *Assay preparation* and the *Standard preparation*, respectively.

Nortriptyline Hydrochloride Oral Solution

» Nortriptyline Hydrochloride Oral Solution contains nortriptyline hydrochloride equivalent to not less than 90.0 percent and not more than 110.0 percent of the labeled amount of nortriptyline ($C_{19}H_{21}N$).

Packaging and storage—Preserve in tight, light-resistant containers.

USP Reference standards ⟨11⟩—*USP Nortriptyline Hydrochloride RS.*

Identification—
A: Transfer a measured volume of Oral Solution, equivalent to about 50 mg of nortriptyline hydrochloride, to a suitable separator, and render the solution distinctly alkaline (to a pH of 11 or above as indicated by pH indicator paper) by the dropwise addition of 1 N sodium hydroxide. Extract with 15 mL of chloroform, and filter the chloroform extract through about 2 g of anhydrous sodium sulfate that has been previously washed with chloroform. Evaporate the chloroform extract with the aid of heat and a current of air to dryness, and dissolve the residue in 0.5 mL of chloroform: the IR absorption spectrum of this solution exhibits maxima only at the same wavelengths as that of a Standard solution obtained by dissolving 50 mg of USP Nortriptyline Hydrochloride RS in 25 mL of water and proceeding as directed for the test specimen.

B: It responds to the tests for *Chloride* ⟨191⟩, when tested as specified for alkaloidal hydrochlorides.

Uniformity of dosage units ⟨905⟩—
FOR ORAL SOLUTION PACKAGED IN SINGLE-UNIT CONTAINERS: meets the requirements.

Deliverable volume ⟨698⟩—
FOR ORAL SOLUTION PACKAGED IN MULTIPLE-UNIT CONTAINERS: meets the requirements.

pH ⟨791⟩: between 2.5 and 4.0.

Alcohol content, Method II ⟨611⟩: between 3.0% and 5.0% of C_2H_5OH.

Assay—Transfer an accurately measured volume of Oral Solution, equivalent to about 10 mg of nortriptyline, to a 125-mL separator. Add 20 mL of water, mix, and render the solution distinctly alkaline (to a pH of 11 or above as indicated by pH indicator paper) by the dropwise addition of sodium hydroxide solution (1 in 2). Extract the nortriptyline with four 25-mL portions of chloroform, filtering each extract into a 250-mL beaker through about 12 g of anhydrous sodium sulfate previously washed with 25 mL of chloroform. Rinse the sodium sulfate with four 5-mL portions of chloroform, and collect the rinsings in the beaker. Evaporate the combined chloroform solution with the aid of heat and a current of air to about 10 mL.

Transfer the contents of the beaker with the aid of chloroform to a 200-mL volumetric flask. Evaporate the chloroform with the aid of air alone to dryness. *[Caution—Do not use heat.]* Dissolve the residue in 1.7 mL of hydrochloric acid, dilute with water to volume, and mix. Transfer 10.0 mL of the solution to a 50-mL volumetric flask, dilute with water to volume, and mix to obtain the *Assay preparation*. Concomitantly determine the absorbances of the *Assay preparation* and a Standard solution of USP Nortriptyline Hydrochloride RS in water having a known concentration of about 11.4 µg per mL in 1-cm cells at the wavelength of maximum absorbance at about 239 nm, with a suitable spectrophotometer, using water as the blank. Calculate the quantity, in mg, of $C_{19}H_{21}N$ in the portion of Oral Solution taken by the formula:

$$(263.38/299.85)(C)(A_U / A_S)$$

in which 263.38 and 299.85 are the molecular weights of nortriptyline and nortriptyline hydrochloride, respectively; C is the concentration, in µg per mL, of USP Nortriptyline Hydrochloride RS in the Standard solution; and A_U and A_S are the absorbances of the *Assay preparation* and the Standard solution, respectively.

Noscapine

$C_{22}H_{23}NO_7$ 413.42
1(3H)-Isobenzofuranone, 6,7-dimethoxy-3-(5,6,7,8-tetrahydro-4-methoxy-6-methyl-1,3-dioxolo[4,5-g]isoquinolin-5-yl), [S-(R^*,S^*)]-.
Narcotine   [*128-62-1*].

» Noscapine contains not less than 99.0 percent and not more than 100.5 percent of $C_{22}H_{23}NO_7$, calculated on the anhydrous basis.

Packaging and storage—Preserve in well-closed containers.
USP Reference standards ⟨11⟩—*USP Noscapine RS*.
Identification—
  A: *Infrared Absorption* ⟨197K⟩—Do not dry specimens.
  B: *Ultraviolet Absorption* ⟨197U⟩—
    Solution: 60 µg per mL.
    Medium: methanol.
  C: Place about 100 mg in a small porcelain dish, add a few drops of sulfuric acid, and stir: a greenish yellow solution is produced, and on warming it becomes red and then turns violet.
Melting range ⟨741⟩: between 174° and 176°.
Specific rotation ⟨781S⟩: between +42° and +48°.
  Test solution: 20 mg per mL, in 0.1 N hydrochloric acid.
Water, *Method I* ⟨921⟩: not more than 1.0%.
Residue on ignition ⟨281⟩: not more than 0.1%.
Chloride ⟨221⟩—A 700-mg portion shows no more chloride than corresponds to 0.20 mL of 0.020 N hydrochloric acid (0.02%).
Limit of morphine—Dissolve 100 mg in 10 mL of 0.1 N hydrochloric acid. To 1.0 mL of this solution add 5.0 mL of diluted ferricyanide reagent (prepared by dissolving 0.50 g of potassium ferricyanide in 50 mL of water, adding 0.50 mL of ferric chloride TS, and diluting 5.0 mL of the resulting solution to 25.0 mL): no blue or dark green color develops within 1 minute.
Ordinary impurities ⟨466⟩—
  Test solution: chloroform.
  Standard solution: chloroform.
  Eluant: a mixture of ethyl acetate and ether (80 : 20).
  Visualization: 17; then examine the plate immediately.
  Limits—The sum of the intensities of all secondary spots obtained from the *Test solution* corresponds to not more than 1.0%.

Assay—Dissolve about 1.5 g of Noscapine, accurately weighed, in 25 mL of glacial acetic acid. Add 25 mL of dioxane and 5 drops of crystal violet TS, and titrate with 0.1 N perchloric acid VS to a blue endpoint. Perform a blank determination, and make any necessary correction. Each mL of 0.1 N perchloric acid is equivalent to 41.34 mg of $C_{22}H_{23}NO_7$.

Novobiocin Sodium

$C_{31}H_{35}N_2NaO_{11}$ 634.61
Benzamide, *N*-[7-[[3-*O*-(aminocarbonyl)-6-deoxy-5-*C*-methyl-4-*O*-methyl-β-L-*lyxo*-hexopyranosyl]oxy]-4-hydroxy-8-methyl-2-oxo-2*H*-1-benzopyran-3-yl]-4-hydroxy-3-(3-methyl-2-butenyl)-, monosodium salt.
Novobiocin, monosodium salt   [*1476-53-5*].

» Novobiocin Sodium has a potency equivalent to not less than 850 µg of novobiocin ($C_{31}H_{36}N_2O_{11}$) per mg, calculated on the dried basis.

Packaging and storage—Preserve in tight containers.
USP Reference standards ⟨11⟩—*USP Novobiocin RS*.
Identification—
  A: Prepare a test solution by dissolving a quantity of it in methanol to obtain a concentration of about 1 mg of novobiocin per mL. Similarly prepare a Standard solution, using USP Novobiocin RS. Separately apply 1-µL portions of the test solution and the Standard solution to a suitable thin-layer chromatographic plate (see *Chromatography* ⟨621⟩) coated with a 0.25-mm layer of chromatographic silica gel mixture, and allow the spots to dry. Place the plate in a chromatographic chamber equilibrated with a solvent system consisting of a mixture of chloroform, methanol, and ammonium hydroxide (75 : 25 : 1), and develop the chromatogram. When the solvent front has moved about three-fourths of the length of the plate, remove the plate from the chamber, and allow to dry. Locate the spots on the plate by examination under short-wavelength UV light: the R_F value of the principal spot obtained from the test solution corresponds to that obtained from the Standard solution.
  B: The residue obtained by igniting it responds to the tests for *Sodium* ⟨191⟩.
Specific rotation ⟨781S⟩: between −50° and −58°.
  Test solution: 50 mg per mL, in a mixture of methanol and hydrochloric acid (100 : 1).
Crystallinity ⟨695⟩: meets the requirements.
pH ⟨791⟩: between 6.5 and 8.5, in a solution containing 25 mg per mL.
Loss on drying ⟨731⟩—Dry about 100 mg, accurately weighed, in a capillary-stoppered bottle in vacuum at a pressure not exceeding 5 mm of mercury at 60° for 3 hours: it loses not more than 6.0% of its weight.
Residue on ignition ⟨281⟩: between 10.5% and 12.0%, the charred residue being moistened with 2 mL of sulfuric acid and an ignition temperature of 550 ± 50° being used.
Assay—Dissolve a suitable quantity of Novobiocin Sodium, accurately weighed, in an accurately measured volume of *Buffer No. 3* sufficient to obtain a stock solution of convenient concentration. Proceed as directed under *Antibiotics—Microbial Assays* ⟨81⟩, using an accurately measured volume of this stock solution diluted quantitatively and stepwise with *Buffer No. 6* to yield a *Test Dilution* having a concentration assumed to be equal to the median dose level of the Standard.

Novobiocin Sodium Intramammary Infusion

» Novobiocin Sodium Intramammary Infusion is a suspension of Novobiocin Sodium in a suitable vegetable oil vehicle. It contains suitable preservative and suspending agents. It contains the equivalent of not less than 90.0 percent and not more than 125.0 percent of the labeled amount of novobiocin ($C_{31}H_{36}N_2O_{11}$).

Packaging and storage—Preserve in disposable syringes that are well-closed containers.
Labeling—Label it to indicate that it is for veterinary use only.
USP Reference standards ⟨11⟩—*USP Novobiocin RS.*
Water, *Method I* ⟨921⟩: not more than 1.0%, 20 mL of a mixture of toluene and methanol (7 : 3) being used in place of methanol in the titration vessel.
Assay—Proceed as directed for novobiocin under *Antibiotics—Microbial Assays* ⟨81⟩, expelling the contents of a syringe of Intramammary Infusion into a high-speed blender jar containing 1.0 mL of polysorbate 80 and 499.0 mL of *Buffer No. 3*, and blend for 3 to 5 minutes. Allow to stand for 10 minutes, and dilute quantitatively and stepwise with *Buffer No. 6* to obtain a *Test Dilution* having a concentration of novobiocin assumed to be equal to the median dose level of the Standard.

Nystatin

Nystatin.
Nystatin   [*1400-61-9*].

» Nystatin is a substance, or a mixture of two or more substances, produced by the growth of *Streptomyces noursei* Brown et al. (Fam. Streptomycetaceae). It has a potency of not less than 4400 USP Nystatin Units per mg, or, where intended for use in the extemporaneous preparation of oral suspensions, not less than 5000 USP Nystatin Units per mg.

Packaging and storage—Preserve in tight, light-resistant containers.
Labeling—Where packaged for use in the extemporaneous preparation of oral suspensions, the label so states.
USP Reference standards ⟨11⟩—*USP Nystatin RS.*
Identification, *Ultraviolet Absorption* ⟨197U⟩—
 Solution: 10 μg per mL, prepared as follows. Transfer about 50 mg to a glass-stoppered, 100-mL volumetric flask, add 25 mL of methanol and 5 mL of glacial acetic acid to dissolve the specimen, dilute with methanol to volume, and mix. Pipet 2 mL of this solution into a 100-mL volumetric flask, dilute with methanol to volume, and mix.
 Ratio: the ratio ($A_{230}/A_{279(sh)}$) is between 0.90 and 1.25.
Composition—
 Solution A—Prepare a mixture of 0.05 M ammonium acetate and acetonitrile (71 : 29).
 Solution B—Prepare a mixture of acetonitrile and 0.05 M ammonium acetate (60 : 40).
 Mobile phase—Use variable mixtures of *Solution A* and *Solution B* as directed for *Chromatographic system*. Make adjustments if necessary (see *System Suitability* under *Chromatography* ⟨621⟩).
 Standard solution—Quantitatively dissolve an accurately weighed quantity of USP Nystatin RS in dimethyl sulfoxide to obtain a solution having a known concentration of about 0.4 mg per mL. [NOTE—Protect this solution from light and use within 24 hours, if stored in the refrigerator.]
 Test solution—Transfer about 20 mg of Nystatin, accurately weighed, to a low-actinic 50-mL volumetric flask, dissolve in and dilute with dimethyl sulfoxide to volume, and mix. [NOTE—Use this solution within 24 hours, if stored in the refrigerator.]
 System suitability solution—Dissolve about 20 mg of Nystatin in 25 mL of methanol, dilute with water to 50 mL, and mix. To 10.0 mL of this solution add 2.0 mL of diluted hydrochloric acid, and allow to stand at room temperature for 1 hour.
 Chromatographic system (see *Chromatography* ⟨621⟩)—The liquid chromatograph is equipped with a 304-nm detector and a 4.6-mm × 15-cm column that contains base-deactivated end-capped 5-μm packing L1. The column is maintained at a constant temperature of about 30°. The flow rate is about 1 mL per minute. The chromatograph is programmed as follows.

Time (minutes)	Solution A (%)	Solution B (%)	Elution
0–25	100	0	isocratic
25–35	100→0	0→100	gradient
35–40	0	100	isocratic
40–45	0→100	100→0	gradient
45–50	100	0	equilibrium

Chromatograph the *System suitability solution*, and record the peak responses as directed for *Procedure:* the resolution, *R*, between the two major peaks is not less than 3.5. Chromatograph the *Standard solution*, and record the peak responses as directed for *Procedure:* the main nystatin A1 peak elutes at about 14 minutes.
 Procedure—Inject about 20 μL of the *Test solution* into the chromatograph, record the chromatogram, and measure the peak area responses for all of the peaks, disregarding any peaks eluting in less than 2 minutes. Calculate the percentage of each peak by the formula:

$$100 r_i / r_T$$

in which r_i is the response of an individual peak; and r_T is the total of all of the responses, any peaks eluting in less than 2 minutes being disregarded. Not less than 85.0% of nystatin A1 is found; and not more than 4.0% of any other individual component is found.
Suspendibility (where packaged for use in the extemporaneous preparation of oral suspensions)—Transfer about 200 mg, accurately weighed, to a 250-mL beaker containing 200.0 mL of water, and disperse by stirring gently with a stirring rod. Allow to stand for 2 minutes, and observe the suspension: the material is in suspension, and little or no sediment is present on the bottom of the beaker. If there is any sediment, assay the undisturbed suspension as directed for nystatin under *Antibiotics—Microbial Assays* ⟨81⟩, using an accurately measured volume of it blended in a high-speed blender for 3 to 5 minutes with a sufficient accurately measured volume of dimethylformamide to give a concentration of about 400 USP Nystatin Units per mL. Dilute this stock solution quantitatively with *Buffer No. 6* to obtain a *Test Dilution* having a concentration assumed to be equal to the median dose level of the Standard: not less than 90.0% of the expected number of USP Nystatin Units is found, based on the potency obtained in the *Assay*.
Crystallinity (where packaged for use in the extemporaneous preparation of oral suspensions) ⟨695⟩: meets the requirements.
pH ⟨791⟩: between 6.0 and 8.0, in a 3% aqueous suspension.
Loss on drying ⟨731⟩—Dry about 100 mg, accurately weighed, in a capillary-stoppered bottle in vacuum at a pressure not exceeding 5 mm of mercury at 60° for 3 hours: it loses not more than 5.0% of its weight.
Assay—Proceed with Nystatin as directed under *Antibiotics—Microbial Assays* ⟨81⟩.

Nystatin Cream

» Nystatin Cream contains not less than 90.0 percent and not more than 130.0 percent of the labeled amount of USP Nystatin Units.

Packaging and storage—Preserve in collapsible tubes, or in other tight containers, and avoid exposure to excessive heat.
USP Reference standards ⟨11⟩—*USP Nystatin RS.*
Minimum fill ⟨755⟩: meets the requirements.
Assay—Proceed as directed for Nystatin under *Antibiotics—Microbial Assays* ⟨81⟩, blending a suitable accurately weighed portion of Cream in a high-speed blender for 3 to 5 minutes with a sufficient accurately measured volume of dimethylformamide to

give a concentration of about 400 USP Nystatin Units per mL. Dilute this stock solution quantitatively with *Buffer No. 6* to obtain a *Test Dilution* having a concentration assumed to be equal to the median dose level of the Standard.

Nystatin Lotion

» Nystatin Lotion contains not less than 90.0 percent and not more than 140.0 percent of the labeled amount of USP Nystatin Units.

Packaging and storage—Preserve in tight containers, at controlled room temperature.
USP Reference standards ⟨11⟩—*USP Nystatin RS.*
pH ⟨791⟩: between 5.5 and 7.5.
Assay—Proceed with Lotion as directed in the *Assay* under *Nystatin Cream*.

Nystatin Lozenges

» Nystatin Lozenges contain not less than 90.0 percent and not more than 125.0 percent of the labeled amount of USP Nystatin Units.

Packaging and storage—Preserve in tight, light-resistant containers.
USP Reference standards ⟨11⟩—*USP Nystatin RS.*
Disintegration ⟨701⟩: 90 minutes, determined as set forth under *Uncoated Tablets*.
pH ⟨791⟩: between 5.0 and 7.5, in a solution prepared by dissolving 1 Lozenge in 100 mL of water at 37° and allowing the solution to cool to room temperature.
Assay—Proceed as directed for Nystatin under *Antibiotics—Microbial Assays* ⟨81⟩, blending not less than 5 Lozenges for 18 to 20 minutes in a high-speed blender jar containing 100.0 mL of water. Add 400.0 mL of dimethylformamide, and blend for an additional 10 minutes. Dilute an accurately measured volume of this solution quantitatively with a mixture of dimethylformamide and water (4 : 1) to obtain a stock solution containing about 400 USP Nystatin Units per mL. Dilute an accurately measured volume of this stock solution quantitatively with *Buffer No. 6* to obtain a *Test Dilution* having a nystatin concentration assumed to be equal to the median dose level of the Standard. [NOTE—The *Test Dilution* of the specimen and the test dilutions of the Standard contain the same amount of dimethylformamide (about 4%).]

Nystatin Ointment

» Nystatin Ointment contains not less than 90.0 percent and not more than 130.0 percent of the labeled amount of USP Nystatin Units.

Packaging and storage—Preserve in well-closed containers, preferably at controlled room temperature.
USP Reference standards ⟨11⟩—*USP Nystatin RS.*
Minimum fill ⟨755⟩: meets the requirements.
Water, *Method I* ⟨921⟩: not more than 0.5%, 20 mL of a mixture of toluene and methanol (7 : 3) being used in place of methanol in the titration vessel.
Assay—Proceed with Ointment as directed in the *Assay* under *Nystatin Cream*.

Nystatin Topical Powder

» Nystatin Topical Powder is a dry powder composed of Nystatin and Talc. It contains not less than 90.0 percent and not more than 130.0 percent of the labeled amount of USP Nystatin Units.

Packaging and storage—Preserve in well-closed containers.
USP Reference standards ⟨11⟩—*USP Nystatin RS.*
Loss on drying ⟨731⟩—Dry about 100 mg, accurately weighed, in a capillary-stoppered bottle in vacuum at a pressure not exceeding 5 mm of mercury at 60° for 3 hours: it loses not more than 2.0% of its weight.
Assay—Proceed with Topical Powder as directed in the *Assay* under *Nystatin Cream*.

Nystatin Vaginal Suppositories

» Nystatin Vaginal Suppositories contain not less than 90.0 percent and not more than 130.0 percent of the labeled amount of USP Nystatin Units.

Packaging and storage—Preserve in tight, light-resistant containers, at controlled room temperature.
USP Reference standards ⟨11⟩—*USP Nystatin RS.*
Water, *Method I* ⟨921⟩: not more than 1.5%.
Assay—Proceed with Vaginal Suppositories as directed in the *Assay* under *Nystatin Tablets*.

Nystatin Oral Suspension

» Nystatin Oral Suspension contains not less than 90.0 percent and not more than 130.0 percent of the labeled amount of USP Nystatin Units. It contains suitable dispersants, flavors, preservatives, and suspending agents.

Packaging and storage—Preserve in tight, light-resistant containers.
USP Reference standards ⟨11⟩—*USP Nystatin RS.*
Uniformity of dosage units ⟨905⟩—
   FOR SUSPENSION PACKAGED IN SINGLE-UNIT CONTAINERS: meets the requirements, except that under section (*B*)(3) of the *Criteria*, the words "average of the limits" are changed to "upper assay limit."
   Procedure for content uniformity—[NOTE—Use low-actinic glassware. The correction factor, *F*, calculated as directed in section (4) of *Content Uniformity* under *Uniformity of Dosage Units* ⟨905⟩, is invalid if the value obtained by the formula in the second sentence is greater than 25; follow sections (5) and (6), except to substitute 0.750 for 0.900.] Transfer the well-shaken contents of 1 container of Oral Suspension to a 100-mL volumetric flask, dissolve in and dilute with methanol to volume, and mix. Dilute an accurately measured volume of this solution quantitatively, and stepwise if necessary, with methanol to obtain a test solution containing about 25 USP Nystatin Units per mL. Similarly, prepare a Standard solution of USP Nystatin RS in methanol having a known concentration of about 25 USP Nystatin Units per mL. Concomitantly determine the absorbances of the test solution and the Standard solution at the wavelength of maximum absorbance at about 304 nm, with a suitable spectrophotometer, using methanol as the blank. Calculate the

quantity, in USP Nystatin Units, in the container taken by the formula:

$$(CL/D)(A_U/A_S)$$

in which C is the concentration, in USP Nystatin Units per mL, of the Standard solution, L is the labeled quantity, in USP Nystatin Units, in the container, D is the concentration, in USP Nystatin Units, in the test solution, on the basis of the labeled quantity in the container and the extent of dilution, and A_U and A_S are the absorbances of the test solution and the Standard solution, respectively.

Deliverable volume ⟨698⟩: meets the requirements.
pH ⟨791⟩: between 4.5 and 6.0; or if it contains glycerin, between 5.3 and 7.5.
Assay—Proceed as directed for Nystatin under *Antibiotics—Microbial Assays* ⟨81⟩, blending a suitable accurately measured volume of Oral Suspension, freshly mixed and free from air bubbles, for 3 to 5 minutes in a high-speed blender with a sufficient accurately measured volume of dimethylformamide to obtain a solution of convenient concentration. Dilute an accurately measured portion of this solution quantitatively with dimethylformamide to obtain a stock solution containing about 400 USP Nystatin Units per mL. Dilute this stock solution quantitatively with *Buffer No. 6* to obtain a *Test Dilution* having a concentration assumed to be equal to the median dose level of the Standard.

Nystatin for Oral Suspension

» Nystatin for Oral Suspension is a dry mixture of Nystatin with one or more suitable colors, diluents, suspending agents, flavors, and preservatives. It contains the equivalent of not less than 90.0 percent and not more than 140.0 percent of the labeled amount of USP Nystatin Units.

Packaging and storage—Preserve in tight containers.
USP Reference standards ⟨11⟩—*USP Nystatin RS.*
Uniformity of dosage units ⟨905⟩—
 FOR POWDER PACKAGED IN SINGLE-UNIT CONTAINERS: meets the requirements.
Deliverable volume ⟨698⟩—
 FOR POWDER PACKAGED IN MULTIPLE-UNIT CONTAINERS: meets the requirements.
pH ⟨791⟩: between 4.9 and 5.5, in the suspension constituted as directed in the labeling.
Water, *Method I* ⟨921⟩: not more than 7.0%.
Assay—Constitute Nystatin for Oral Suspension as directed in the labeling, and proceed as directed in the *Assay* under *Nystatin Oral Suspension.*

Nystatin Tablets

» Nystatin Tablets contain not less than 90.0 percent and not more than 130.0 percent of the labeled amount of USP Nystatin Units.

Packaging and storage—Preserve in tight, light-resistant containers.
Labeling—Label the Tablets to indicate that they are intended for oral use only (as distinguished from Vaginal Tablets).
USP Reference standards ⟨11⟩—*USP Nystatin RS.*
Disintegration ⟨701⟩: if plain-coated, 120 minutes.
Loss on drying ⟨731⟩—Dry about 100 mg, accurately weighed, of powdered Tablets in a capillary-stoppered bottle in vacuum at a pressure not exceeding 5 mm of mercury at 60° for 3 hours: if plain-coated, it loses not more than 5.0% of its weight; if film-coated, it loses not more than 8.0% of its weight.
Assay—Proceed as directed for Nystatin under *Antibiotics—Microbial Assays* ⟨81⟩, blending not less than 5 Tablets for 3 to 5 minutes in a high-speed blender with a sufficient accurately measured volume of dimethylformamide to obtain a solution of convenient concentration. Dilute an accurately measured portion of this solution quantitatively with dimethylformamide to obtain a stock solution containing about 400 USP Nystatin Units per mL. Dilute this stock solution quantitatively with *Buffer No. 6* to obtain a *Test Dilution* having a concentration assumed to be equal to the median dose level of the Standard.

Nystatin Vaginal Inserts

» Nystatin Vaginal Inserts are composed of Nystatin with suitable binders, diluents, and lubricants. Vaginal Inserts contain not less than 90.0 percent and not more than 140.0 percent of the labeled amount of USP Nystatin Units.

Packaging and storage—Preserve in tight, light-resistant containers and, where so specified in the labeling, in a refrigerator.
USP Reference standards ⟨11⟩—*USP Nystatin RS.*
Disintegration ⟨701⟩: 60 minutes.
Loss on drying ⟨731⟩—Dry about 100 mg, accurately weighed, of powdered Vaginal Inserts in a capillary-stoppered bottle in vacuum at a pressure not exceeding 5 mm of mercury at 60° for 3 hours: it loses not more than 5.0% of its weight.
Assay—Proceed with Vaginal Inserts as directed in the *Assay* under *Nystatin Tablets.*

Nystatin, Neomycin Sulfate, Gramicidin, and Triamcinolone Acetonide Cream

» Nystatin, Neomycin Sulfate, Gramicidin, and Triamcinolone Acetonide Cream contains not less than 90.0 percent and not more than 140.0 percent of the labeled amounts of nystatin, neomycin, and gramicidin, and not less than 90.0 percent and not more than 110.0 percent of the labeled amount of triamcinolone acetonide ($C_{24}H_{31}FO_6$).

Packaging and storage—Preserve in tight containers.
USP Reference standards ⟨11⟩—*USP Gramicidin RS. USP Neomycin Sulfate RS. USP Nystatin RS. USP Triamcinolone Acetonide RS.*
Identification—Place 2 g of Cream in a conical flask, add 5.0 mL of chloroform, and shake for 10 minutes. Add 15 mL of alcohol, and shake for an additional 10 minutes. Filter the solution into a centrifuge tube, and evaporate the filtrate to dryness. Dissolve the residue in alcohol to obtain a solution containing about 250 µg of triamcinolone acetonide per mL. Proceed as directed in the *Identification* test under *Triamcinolone Acetonide Cream*, beginning with "Apply 10 µL of this solution": the specified result is observed.
Minimum fill ⟨755⟩: meets the requirements.
Assay for nystatin—Proceed as directed for nystatin under *Antibiotics—Microbial Assays* ⟨81⟩, blending a suitable, accurately weighed portion of Cream in a high-speed blender for 3 to 5 minutes with a sufficient, accurately measured volume of dimethylformamide to give a convenient concentration. Dilute an accurately measured volume of the solution so obtained quantitatively with dimethylformamide to obtain a stock solution containing about 400

USP Nystatin Units per mL. Dilute an accurately measured volume of this stock solution quantitatively with *Buffer No. 6* to obtain a *Test Dilution* having a concentration of nystatin assumed to be equal to the median dose level of the Standard.

Assay for neomycin—Proceed with Cream as directed in the *Assay* under *Neomycin Sulfate Cream*.

Assay for gramicidin—Proceed as directed for gramicidin under *Antibiotics—Microbial Assays* ⟨81⟩, using an accurately weighed portion of Cream dissolved in 50 mL of hexanes in a separator, and extracted with four 20-mL portions of 80% alcohol. Combine the extracts in a suitable volumetric flask, dilute with alcohol to volume, and mix. Dilute an accurately measured volume of the solution so obtained quantitatively and stepwise with alcohol to obtain a *Test Dilution* having a concentration of gramicidin assumed to be equal to the median dose level of the Standard.

Assay for triamcinolone acetonide—Proceed with Cream as directed in the *Assay* under *Triamcinolone Acetonide Cream*.

Nystatin, Neomycin Sulfate, Gramicidin, and Triamcinolone Acetonide Ointment

» Nystatin, Neomycin Sulfate, Gramicidin, and Triamcinolone Acetonide Ointment contains not less than 90.0 percent and not more than 140.0 percent of the labeled amounts of nystatin, neomycin, and gramicidin, and not less than 90.0 percent and not more than 110.0 percent of the labeled amount of triamcinolone acetonide ($C_{24}H_{31}FO_6$).

Packaging and storage—Preserve in tight containers.

USP Reference standards ⟨11⟩—*USP Gramicidin RS. USP Neomycin Sulfate RS. USP Nystatin RS. USP Triamcinolone Acetonide RS.*

Identification—Place 2 g of Ointment in a conical flask, add 5.0 mL of chloroform, and shake for 10 minutes. Add 15 mL of alcohol, and shake for an additional 10 minutes. Filter the solution into a centrifuge tube, and evaporate the filtrate to dryness. Dissolve the residue in alcohol to obtain a solution containing about 250 µg of triamcinolone acetonide per mL. Proceed as directed in the *Identification* test under *Triamcinolone Acetonide Cream*, beginning with "Apply 10 µL of this solution": the specified result is observed.

Minimum fill ⟨755⟩: meets the requirements.

Water, *Method I* ⟨921⟩: not more than 0.5%, 20 mL of a mixture of toluene and methanol (7 : 3) being used in place of methanol in the titration vessel.

Assay for nystatin—Proceed as directed for nystatin under *Antibiotics—Microbial Assays* ⟨81⟩, blending a suitable, accurately weighed portion of Ointment in a high-speed blender for 3 to 5 minutes with a sufficient, accurately measured volume of dimethylformamide to give a convenient concentration. Dilute an accurately measured volume of the solution so obtained quantitatively with dimethylformamide to obtain a stock solution containing about 400 USP Nystatin Units per mL. Dilute an accurately measured volume of this stock solution quantitatively with *Buffer No. 6* to obtain a *Test Dilution* having a concentration of nystatin assumed to be equal to the median dose level of the Standard.

Assay for neomycin—Proceed with Ointment as directed in the *Assay* under *Neomycin Sulfate Ointment*.

Assay for gramicidin—Proceed as directed for gramicidin under *Antibiotics—Microbial Assays* ⟨81⟩, using an accurately weighed portion of Ointment dissolved in 50 mL of hexanes in a separator, and extracted with four 20-mL portions of 80% alcohol. Combine the extracts in a suitable volumetric flask, dilute with alcohol to volume, and mix. Dilute an accurately measured volume of the solution so obtained quantitatively and stepwise with alcohol to obtain a *Test Dilution* having a concentration of gramicidin assumed to be equal to the median dose level of the Standard.

Assay for triamcinolone acetonide—Proceed with Ointment as directed in the *Assay* under *Triamcinolone Acetonide Cream*, except to read "Ointment" in place of "Cream" throughout.

Nystatin, Neomycin Sulfate, Thiostrepton, and Triamcinolone Acetonide Cream

» Nystatin, Neomycin Sulfate, Thiostrepton, and Triamcinolone Acetonide Cream contains not less than 90.0 percent and not more than 130.0 percent of the labeled amounts of nystatin, neomycin, and thiostrepton, and not less than 90.0 percent and not more than 110.0 percent of the labeled amount of triamcinolone acetonide ($C_{24}H_{31}FO_6$).

Packaging and storage—Preserve in tight containers.

Labeling—Label it to indicate that it is for veterinary use only.

USP Reference standards ⟨11⟩—*USP Nystatin RS. USP Neomycin Sulfate RS. USP Thiostrepton RS. USP Triamcinolone Acetonide RS.*

Identification—Place 2 g of Cream in a conical flask, add 5.0 mL of chloroform, and shake for 10 minutes. Add 15 mL of alcohol, and shake for an additional 10 minutes. Filter the solution into a centrifuge tube, and evaporate the filtrate to dryness. Dissolve the residue in alcohol to obtain a solution containing about 250 µg of triamcinolone acetonide per mL. Proceed as directed in the *Identification* test under *Triamcinolone Acetonide Cream*, beginning with "Apply 10 µL of this solution": the specified result is observed.

Minimum fill ⟨755⟩: meets the requirements.

Assay for nystatin—Proceed as directed for nystatin under *Antibiotics—Microbial Assays* ⟨81⟩, blending a suitable, accurately weighed portion of Cream in a high-speed blender for 3 to 5 minutes with a sufficient, accurately measured volume of dimethylformamide to give a convenient concentration. Dilute an accurately measured volume of the solution so obtained quantitatively with dimethylformamide to obtain a stock solution containing about 400 USP Nystatin Units per mL. Dilute an accurately measured volume of this stock solution quantitatively with *Buffer No. 6* to obtain a *Test Dilution* having a concentration of nystatin assumed to be equal to the median dose level of the Standard.

Assay for neomycin—Proceed as directed for the turbidimetric assay for neomycin under *Antibiotics—Microbial Assays* ⟨81⟩, placing an accurately weighed portion of Cream, equivalent to about 2.5 mg of neomycin, in a 250-mL conical flask, and treating it as follows. Add 50 mL of 0.01 N hydrochloric acid, and shake to disperse the Cream. Transfer the mixture to a 100-mL centrifuge tube. Wash the flask with 40 mL of hexanes, with shaking, and transfer the washing to the centrifuge tube. Stopper the centrifuge tube, shake, and centrifuge for 5 minutes. Draw off the lower aqueous layer, and transfer it to a 250-mL volumetric flask. Repeat the extraction of the hexanes layer remaining in the centrifuge tube with two 50-mL portions of 0.01 N hydrochloric acid, combining the aqueous extracts in the 250-mL volumetric flask. Dilute the contents of the volumetric flask with 0.01 N hydrochloric acid to volume, and mix. Dilute this solution quantitatively and stepwise with *Buffer No. 3* to obtain a *Test Dilution* having a concentration assumed to be equal to the median dose of the Standard.

Assay for thiostrepton—Proceed as directed for thiostrepton under *Antibiotics—Microbial Assays* ⟨81⟩, blending a suitable, accurately weighed portion of Cream in a high-speed blender with a sufficient, accurately measured volume of dimethyl sulfoxide to give a convenient concentration, and filter. Dilute an accurately measured volume of the filtrate so obtained quantitatively with dimethyl sulfoxide to obtain a *Test Dilution* having a concentration of thiostrepton assumed to be equal to the median dose level of the Standard.

Assay for triamcinolone acetonide—Proceed with Cream as directed in the *Assay* under *Triamcinolone Acetonide Cream*.

Nystatin, Neomycin Sulfate, Thiostrepton, and Triamcinolone Acetonide Ointment

» Nystatin, Neomycin Sulfate, Thiostrepton, and Triamcinolone Acetonide Ointment contains not less than 90.0 percent and not more than 130.0 percent of the labeled amounts of nystatin, neomycin, and thiostrepton, and not less than 90.0 percent and not more than 110.0 percent of the labeled amount of triamcinolone acetonide ($C_{24}H_{31}FO_6$).

Packaging and storage—Preserve in tight containers.
Labeling—Label it to indicate that it is for veterinary use only.
USP Reference standards ⟨11⟩—*USP Nystatin RS. USP Neomycin Sulfate RS. USP Thiostrepton RS. USP Triamcinolone Acetonide RS.*
Identification—Place 2 g of Ointment in a conical flask, add 5.0 mL of chloroform, and shake for 10 minutes. Add 15 mL of alcohol, and shake for an additional 10 minutes. Filter the solution into a centrifuge tube, and evaporate the filtrate to dryness. Dissolve the residue in alcohol to obtain a solution containing about 250 μg of triamcinolone acetonide per mL. Proceed as directed in the *Identification* test under *Triamcinolone Acetonide Cream*, beginning with "Apply 10 μL of this solution": the specified result is observed.
Minimum fill ⟨755⟩: meets the requirements.
Assay for nystatin—[NOTE—Protect solutions that contain nystatin from ambient light.]
Ammonium acetate buffer—Dissolve 10.8 ± 1.0 g of ammonium acetate in 2500 mL of water. Adjust with acetic acid to a pH of 6.50 ± 0.05.
Mobile phase—Mix 2500 mL of *Ammonium acetate buffer*, 1000 mL of acetonitrile, and 500 mL of methanol. Pass through a 0.45-μm nylon filter.
BHT solution—Weigh about 1.0 g of butylated hydroxytoluene, and transfer to a 1000-mL volumetric flask. Dilute with methanol to volume, and mix.
Standard preparation—In duplicate, dissolve an accurately weighed quantity of USP Nystatin RS in *BHT solution* to obtain a solution having a known concentration of about 5400 USP Nystatin Units per mL. Store in low-actinic glassware.
System suitability solution—Weigh about 50 mg of USP Nystatin RS, and transfer to a 50-mL low-actinic volumetric flask. Add 0.5 mL of 0.01 N sodium hydroxide, and allow to sit for 1 minute. Add 5 mL of *Ammonium acetate buffer*. Add about 25 mL of methanol, and sonicate to dissolve. Dilute with methanol to volume, and store in low-actinic glassware.
Assay preparation—Thoroughly mix the Ointment prior to sampling. In duplicate, accurately weigh about 1.0 g of Ointment having a known density into a low-actinic sample bottle. Add 20.0 mL of *BHT solution,* and insert a polytef-coated magnetic stir bar having dimensions of about 12.7 × 7.9 mm. Clamp the bottles onto a suitable mixer mill,[1] and mix for a minimum of 5 minutes at about 30 Hz. Centrifuge at about 1350 × g for 5 minutes, or until the supernatant is clear. Transfer the supernatant to low-actinic glassware.
Chromatographic system (see *Chromatography* ⟨621⟩)—The liquid chromatograph is equipped with a 304-nm detector and a 3.9-mm × 15-cm column that contains 4-μm packing L1. The column temperature is maintained at 40°, and the flow rate is about 2.0 mL per minute. [NOTE—Solutions containing nystatin should be stored at 8° until they can be injected into the chromatograph.] Chromatograph the *Standard preparation* and the *System suitability solution*, and record the peak areas as directed for *Procedure:* using the *System suitability solution*, the relative retention times for the nystatin A1 and nystatin A2 peaks are about 1.0 and 1.4, respectively; the column efficiency, using the nystatin A1 peak, is not less than 1200 theoretical plates; the tailing factor is not more than 2.0; and the relative standard deviation for replicate injections is not more than 3.0%. [NOTE—After the conclusion of the run, rinse the column with a mixture of acetonitrile and water (85 : 15) until the baseline is stable, and store in this solution. At the beginning of the next run, rinse with *Mobile phase* until the baseline is stable.]
Procedure—Separately inject equal volumes (about 15 μL) of the duplicate *Standard preparation* and *Assay preparation* into the chromatograph, record the chromatograms, and measure the peak areas for nystatin A1 and nystatin A2. Calculate the quantity, in USP Nystatin Units, of nystatin in the portion of Ointment taken by the formula:

$$20(C_S / W_U)(r_u / r_s)$$

in which C_S is the concentration of USP Nystatin RS, in USP Nystatin Units per mL, of the *Standard preparation*; W_U is the weight, in g, of Ointment taken to prepare the *Assay preparation*; and r_u and r_s are the average peak areas of the sum of nystatin A1 and nystatin A2 obtained from the *Assay preparation* and the *Standard preparation*, respectively.
Assay for neomycin—Proceed as directed for the turbidimetric assay for neomycin under *Antibiotics—Microbial Assays* ⟨81⟩, placing an accurately weighed portion of Ointment, equivalent to about 2.5 mg of neomycin, in a 250-mL conical flask, and treating it as follows. Add 50 mL of hexanes, and shake to disperse the Ointment. Transfer the mixture to a 250-mL separator. Wash the flask with 50 mL of 0.01 N hydrochloric acid, with shaking, and transfer the washing to a separator. Stopper the separator, shake, and allow the layers to separate. Draw off the lower aqueous layer, collecting it in a 250-mL volumetric flask. Repeat the extraction of the hexanes layer remaining in the separator with two or more 50-mL portions of 0.01 N hydrochloric acid, combining the aqueous extracts in the 250-mL volumetric flask. Dilute the contents of the volumetric flask with 0.01 N hydrochloric acid to volume, and mix. Dilute this solution quantitatively and stepwise with *Buffer No. 3* to obtain a *Test Dilution* having a concentration assumed to be equal to the median dose of the Standard.
Assay for thiostrepton—Proceed as directed for thiostrepton under *Antibiotics—Microbial Assays* ⟨81⟩, blending a suitable, accurately weighed portion of Ointment in a high-speed blender with a sufficient, accurately measured volume of dimethyl sulfoxide to give a convenient concentration, and filter. Quantitatively dilute an accurately measured volume of the filtrate so obtained with dimethyl sulfoxide to obtain a *Test Dilution* having a concentration of thiostrepton assumed to be equal to the median dose of the Standard.
Assay for triamcinolone acetonide—Proceed with Ointment as directed in the *Assay* under *Triamcinolone Acetonide Cream*, but read "Ointment" in place of "Cream" throughout.

Nystatin and Triamcinolone Acetonide Cream

» Nystatin and Triamcinolone Acetonide Cream contains not less than 90.0 percent and not more than 140.0 percent of the labeled amount of USP Nystatin Units and not less than 90.0 percent and not more than 110.0 percent of the labeled amount of triamcinolone acetonide ($C_{24}H_{31}FO_6$).

Packaging and storage—Preserve in tight containers.
USP Reference standards ⟨11⟩—*USP Nystatin RS. USP Triamcinolone Acetonide RS.*
Identification—Place 2 g of Cream in a conical flask, add 5.0 mL of chloroform, and shake for 10 minutes. Add 15 mL of alcohol, and shake for an additional 10 minutes. Filter the solution into a centrifuge tube, and evaporate the filtrate to dryness. Dissolve the residue in alcohol to obtain a solution containing about 250 μg of triamcinolone acetonide per mL. Proceed as directed in the *Identification* test under *Triamcinolone Acetonide Cream*, beginning with "Apply 10 μL of this solution": the specified result is observed.

---
[1] A suitable mixer mill can be obtained from Retsch Inc., 74 Walker Lane, Newtown, PA 18940 (www.retsch-us.com; 267-757-0351), product number MM 301.

Minimum fill ⟨755⟩: meets the requirements.
Assay for nystatin—Proceed as directed for nystatin under *Antibiotics—Microbial Assays* ⟨81⟩, blending a suitable, accurately weighed portion of Cream in a high-speed blender for 3 to 5 minutes with a sufficient, accurately measured volume of dimethylformamide to give a convenient concentration. Dilute an accurately measured volume of the solution so obtained quantitatively with dimethylformamide to obtain a stock solution containing about 400 USP Nystatin Units per mL. Dilute an accurately measured volume of this stock solution quantitatively with *Buffer No. 6* to obtain a *Test Dilution* having a concentration of nystatin assumed to be equal to the median dose level of the Standard.
Assay for triamcinolone acetonide—Proceed with Cream as directed in the *Assay* under *Triamcinolone Acetonide Cream*.

Nystatin and Triamcinolone Acetonide Ointment

» Nystatin and Triamcinolone Acetonide Ointment contains not less than 90.0 percent and not more than 140.0 percent of the labeled amount of USP Nystatin Units and not less than 90.0 percent and not more than 110.0 percent of the labeled amount of triamcinolone acetonide ($C_{24}H_{31}FO_6$).

Packaging and storage—Preserve in tight containers.

USP Reference standards ⟨11⟩—*USP Nystatin RS. USP Triamcinolone Acetonide RS.*
Identification—Place 2 g of Ointment in a conical flask, add 5.0 mL of chloroform, and shake for 10 minutes. Add 15 mL of alcohol, and shake for an additional 10 minutes. Filter the solution into a centrifuge tube, and evaporate the filtrate to dryness. Dissolve the residue in alcohol to obtain a solution containing about 250 μg of triamcinolone acetonide per mL. Proceed as directed in the *Identification* test under *Triamcinolone Acetonide Cream*, beginning with "Apply 10 μL of this solution": the specified result is observed.
Minimum fill ⟨755⟩: meets the requirements.
Water, *Method I* ⟨921⟩: not more than 0.5%, 20 mL of a mixture of toluene and methanol (7 : 3) being used in place of methanol in the titration vessel.
Assay for nystatin—Proceed as directed for nystatin under *Antibiotics—Microbial Assays* ⟨81⟩, blending a suitable, accurately weighed portion of Ointment in a high-speed blender for 3 to 5 minutes with a sufficient, accurately measured volume of dimethylformamide to give a convenient concentration. Dilute an accurately measured volume of the solution so obtained quantitatively with dimethylformamide to obtain a stock solution containing about 400 USP Nystatin Units per mL. Dilute an accurately measured volume of this stock solution quantitatively with *Buffer No. 6* to obtain a *Test Dilution* having a concentration of nystatin assumed to be equal to the median dose level of the Standard.
Assay for triamcinolone acetonide—Proceed with Ointment as directed in the *Assay* under *Triamcinolone Acetonide Cream*, except to read "Ointment" in place of "Cream" throughout.

Octinoxate

$C_{18}H_{26}O_3$ 290.40
2-Ethylhexyl 3-(4-methoxyphenyl)-2-propenoate.
2-Propenoic acid, 3-(4-methoxyphenyl)-, 2-ethylhexyl ester.
[5466-77-3].

» Octinoxate contains not less than 95.0 percent and not more than 105.0 percent of $C_{18}H_{26}O_3$, calculated on the as-is basis.

Packaging and storage—Preserve in tight containers, in a cool place.
USP Reference standards ⟨11⟩—*USP Octinoxate RS.*
Identification—
  A: *Infrared Absorption* ⟨197F⟩.
  B: *Ultraviolet Absorption* ⟨197U⟩—
  Solution: 5 μg per mL.
  Medium: alcohol.
Specific gravity ⟨841⟩: between 1.005 and 1.013.
Refractive index ⟨831⟩: between 1.542 and 1.548 at 20°.
Acidity—Transfer 5 mL of Octinoxate to a suitable container, add 50 mL of alcohol, and mix. Add 4 drops of phenolphthalein TS, and titrate with 0.1 N sodium hydroxide: not more than 0.8 mL is consumed.
Chromatographic purity—
  System suitability solution—Prepare a solution of benzyl benzoate and USP Octinoxate RS in acetone containing about 50 mg of each per mL.
  Test solution—Transfer about 5 mL of Octinoxate to a 100-mL volumetric flask, dilute with acetone to volume, and mix.
  Chromatographic system (see *Chromatography* ⟨621⟩)—Proceed as directed in the *Assay*, but chromatograph the *System suitability solution.*
  Procedure—Inject a volume (about 1 μL) of the *Test solution* into the chromatograph, record the chromatogram, and measure the responses for all the peaks. Calculate the percentage of each impurity in the portion of Octinoxate taken by the formula:

$$100(r_i / r_s)$$

in which r_i is the peak response for each impurity; and r_s is the sum of the responses for all the peaks: not more than 0.5% of any individual impurity is found; and not more than 2.0% of total impurities is found.
Assay—
  Internal standard solution—Transfer about 25 mL of benzyl benzoate to a 500-mL volumetric flask, dilute with acetone to volume, and mix.
  Standard preparation—Dilute an accurately measured quantity of USP Octinoxate RS quantitatively, and stepwise if necessary, with *Internal standard solution* to obtain a solution having a known concentration of about 50 mg per mL.
  Assay preparation—Transfer about 5 mL of Octinoxate, accurately measured, to a 100-mL volumetric flask, dilute with *Internal standard solution* to volume, and mix.
  Chromatographic system (see *Chromatography* ⟨621⟩)—The gas chromatograph is equipped with a flame-ionization detector and a 0.32-mm × 25-m column that contains coating G1. The carrier gas is helium, flowing at a rate of about 2 mL per minute. The chromatograph is programmed as follows. Initially the temperature of the column is equilibrated at 80°, then the temperature is increased to 300° over a period of 10 minutes, and maintained at 300° for 10 minutes. The injection port temperature is maintained at 250°, and the detector is maintained at 300°. Chromatograph the *Standard preparation,* and record the peak responses as directed for *Procedure:* the relative retention times are about 0.68 for benzyl benzoate and 1.0 for octinoxate; the resolution, *R,* between benzyl benzoate and octinoxate is not less than 20; the column efficiency is not less than 65,000 theoretical plates; and the relative standard deviation for replicate injections is not more than 2.0%.
  Procedure—Separately inject equal volumes (about 1 μL) of the *Standard preparation* and the *Assay preparation* into the chromatograph, record the chromatograms, and measure the responses for the major peaks. Calculate the quantity, in mg, of $C_{18}H_{26}O_3$ in the portion of Octinoxate taken by the formula:

$$100C(R_U / R_S)$$

in which *C* is the concentration, in mg per mL, of USP Octinoxate RS in the *Standard preparation;* and R_U and R_S are the peak response ratios of octinoxate to benzyl benzoate obtained from the *Assay preparation* and the *Standard preparation,* respectively.

Octisalate

C₁₅H₂₂O₃   250.33
2-Ethylhexyl salicylate.
Benzoic acid, 2-hydroxy-, 2-ethylhexyl ester   [118-60-5].

» Octisalate contains not less than 95.0 percent and not more than 105.0 percent of $C_{15}H_{22}O_3$.

Packaging and storage—Preserve in tight containers.

USP Reference standards ⟨11⟩—*USP Octisalate RS*.

Identification—
  A: *Infrared Absorption* ⟨197F⟩.
  B: *Ultraviolet Absorption* ⟨197U⟩—
    Solution: 5.0 μg per mL.
    Medium: alcohol.
    Absorptivity at 305 nm, calculated on the as-is basis, does not differ by more than 3.0%.

Specific gravity ⟨841⟩: between 1.011 and 1.016.

Refractive index ⟨831⟩: between 1.500 and 1.503 at 20°.

Acidity—Transfer 50 mL of alcohol to a suitable container, add 1 mL of phenol red TS, and add sufficient 0.1 N sodium hydroxide to obtain a persistent pink color. Transfer 50 mL of this solution to a suitable container, add about 5.0 mL of accurately measured Octisalate, mix, and titrate with 0.1 N sodium hydroxide: not more than 0.2 mL of 0.1 N sodium hydroxide per mL of Octisalate is required for neutralization.

Chromatographic purity—
  Test solution—Use the *Assay preparation*.
  Chromatographic system—Proceed as directed in the *Assay*. To evaluate the system suitability requirements, use the *Standard preparation*, as prepared in the *Assay*.
  Procedure—Inject a volume (about 1 μL) of the *Test solution* into the chromatograph, record the chromatogram, and measure all of the peak responses. Calculate the percentage of each impurity in the portion of Octisalate taken by the formula:

$$100(r_i / r_s)$$

in which r_i is the peak response for each impurity, and r_s is the sum of the responses of all the peaks: not more than 0.5% of any individual impurity is found; and not more than 2.0% of total impurities is found.

Assay—
  Standard preparation—Dissolve an accurately weighed quantity of USP Octisalate RS in *tert*-butyl methyl ether, and dilute quantitatively, and stepwise if necessary, with *tert*-butyl methyl ether to obtain a solution having a known concentration of about 20.0 mg per mL.
  Assay preparation—Transfer about 2 g of Octisalate, accurately weighed, to a 100-mL volumetric flask, dilute with *tert*-butyl methyl ether to volume, and mix.
  Chromatographic system (see *Chromatography* ⟨621⟩)—The gas chromatograph is equipped with a flame-ionization detector and a 0.32-mm × 25-m column coated with a 0.1-μm film of phase G1. The carrier gas is helium, flowing at a rate of about 6 mL per minute. The chromatograph is programmed as follows. Initially the temperature of the column is equilibrated at 60°, then the temperature is increased at a rate of 8° per minute to 240°, and is maintained at 240° for 10 minutes. The injection port temperature is maintained at 240°, and the detector temperature is maintained at 260°. Chromatograph the *Standard preparation*, and record the peak responses as directed for *Procedure*: the resolution, *R*, between octisalate and any other peak is not less than 1.0; and the relative standard deviation for replicate injections is not more than 2.0%.
  Procedure—Separately inject equal volumes (about 1 μL) of the *Standard preparation* and the *Assay preparation* into the chromatograph, record the chromatograms, and measure the responses for the major peaks. Calculate the quantity, in mg, of $C_{15}H_{22}O_3$ in the portion of Octisalate taken by the formula:

$$100C(r_U / r_S)$$

in which *C* is the concentration, in mg per mL, of USP Octisalate RS in the *Standard preparation;* and r_U and r_S are the peak responses obtained from the *Assay preparation* and the *Standard preparation*, respectively.

Octocrylene

C₂₄H₂₇NO₂   361.48
2-Propenoic acid, 2-cyano-3,3-diphenyl, 2-ethylhexyl ester.
2-Ethylhexyl 2-cyano-3,3-diphenylacrylate   [6197-30-4].

» Octocrylene contains not less than 95.0 percent and not more than 105.0 percent of $C_{24}H_{27}NO_2$.

Packaging and storage—Preserve in tight containers.

USP Reference standards ⟨11⟩—*USP Octocrylene RS*.

Identification, *Ultraviolet Absorption* ⟨197U⟩—
  Solution: 0.1 mg per mL.
  Medium: methanol.
  Absorptivities, calculated on the as-is basis, do not differ by more than 3.0%.

Specific gravity ⟨841⟩: between 1.045 and 1.055.

Refractive index ⟨831⟩: between 1.561 and 1.571 at 20°.

Acidity—Transfer 60 mL of alcohol to a suitable container, add 1 mL of phenolphthalein TS, and add sufficient 0.1 N sodium hydroxide to obtain a persistent pink color. Transfer 60 mL of this solution to a suitable container, add about 6 g of Octocrylene, accurately weighed, mix, and titrate with 0.1 N sodium hydroxide: not more than 0.18 mL of titrant per g of Octocrylene is necessary to obtain a persistent pink endpoint.

Chromatographic purity—
  Test solution—Use the *Assay preparation*.
  Chromatographic system—Proceed as directed in the *Assay*. To evaluate the system suitability requirements, use the *Standard preparation* prepared as directed in the *Assay*.
  Procedure—Inject a volume (about 1 μL) of the *Test solution* into the chromatograph, record the chromatogram, and measure all of the peak responses. Calculate the percentage of each impurity in the portion of Octocrylene taken by the formula:

$$100(r_i / r_s)$$

in which r_i is the peak response for each impurity; and r_s is the sum of the responses of all the peaks: not more than 0.5% of any individual impurity is found; and not more than 2.0% of total impurities is found.

Assay—
  Standard preparation—Dissolve an accurately weighed quantity of USP Octocrylene RS in acetone, and dilute quantitatively, and stepwise if necessary, with acetone to obtain a solution having a known concentration of about 21.0 mg per mL.
  Assay preparation—Transfer about 2.1 g of Octocrylene, accurately weighed, to a 100-mL volumetric flask, dilute with acetone to volume, and mix.
  Chromatographic system (see *Chromatography* ⟨621⟩)—The gas chromatograph is equipped with a flame-ionization detector and a 0.32-mm × 60-m column coated with a 0.25-μm film of G1. Helium is used as the carrier gas at a flow rate of about 6 mL per minute. The chromatograph is programmed as follows. Initially the temperature of the column is equilibrated at 80°; upon injection, the temperature is increased at a rate of 4° per minute to 280°, and is held at 280° for 10 minutes. The injection port temperature is maintained at 300°, and the detector temperature is maintained at 300°. Chromatograph the *Standard preparation*, and record the peak responses as directed for *Procedure*: the resolution, *R*, between the octocrylene and any other peak is not less than 1.0; and the relative standard deviation for replicate injections is not more than 2.0%.
  Procedure—Separately inject equal volumes (about 1 μL) of the *Standard preparation* and the *Assay preparation* into the chromato-

graph, record the chromatograms, and measure the responses for the major peaks. Calculate the quantity, in mg, of $C_{24}H_{27}NO_2$ in the portion of Octocrylene taken by the formula:

$$100C(r_U/r_S)$$

in which C is the concentration, in mg per mL, of USP Octocrylene RS in the *Standard preparation;* and r_U and r_S are the peak responses obtained from the *Assay preparation* and the *Standard preparation,* respectively.

Ofloxacin

$C_{18}H_{20}FN_3O_4$ 361.38

7*H*-Pyrido[1,2,3-*de*]-1,4-benzoxazine-6-carboxylic acid, 9-fluoro-2,3-dihydro-3-methyl-10-(4-methyl-1-piperazinyl)-7-oxo-, (±)-.
(±)-9-Fluoro-2,3-dihydro-3-methyl-10-(4-methyl-l-piperazinyl)-7-oxo-7*H*-pyrido[1,2,3-*de*]-1,4-benzoxazine-6-carboxylic acid [82419-36-1].

» Ofloxacin contains not less than 98.5 percent and not more than 101.5 percent of $C_{18}H_{20}FN_3O_4$, calculated on the dried basis.

Packaging and storage—Preserve in well-closed containers, protected from light. Store at 25°, excursions permitted between 15° and 30°.

USP Reference standards ⟨11⟩—USP Ofloxacin RS. USP Ofloxacin Related Compound A RS.

Identification—
  A: *Infrared Absorption* ⟨197K⟩.
  B: *Ultraviolet Absorption* ⟨197U⟩—
  Solution: 6.7 µg per mL.
  Medium: 0.1 N hydrochloric acid.

Specific rotation ⟨781S⟩: between +1° and −1°.
  Test solution: 10 mg per mL, in chloroform.

Loss on drying ⟨731⟩—Dry it at 105° for 4 hours: it loses not more than 0.2% of its weight.

Residue on ignition ⟨281⟩: not more than 0.1%.

Arsenic, *Method II* ⟨211⟩: 1 µg per g.

Heavy metals, *Method II* ⟨231⟩: 0.001%.

Related compounds—
  Diluent—Prepare a mixture of water and acetonitrile (6 : 1).
  Mobile phase—Dissolve 4.0 g of ammonium acetate and 7.0 g of sodium perchlorate in 1300 mL of water, adjust with phosphoric acid to a pH of 2.2, and mix. Prepare a filtered and degassed mixture of this solution and 240 mL of acetonitrile. Make adjustments if necessary (see *System Suitability* under *Chromatography* ⟨621⟩).
  System suitability solution—Transfer 10.0 mg of USP Ofloxacin Related Compound A RS and 10.0 mg of USP Ofloxacin RS to a 100-mL volumetric flask, dissolve in and dilute with *Diluent* to volume, and mix. Dilute 10.0 mL of this solution with *Diluent* to 50.0 mL. Dilute 1.0 mL of this solution with *Diluent* to 50.0 mL.
  Standard solution—Quantitatively dissolve an accurately weighed quantity of USP Ofloxacin RS in *Diluent* to obtain a solution that contains 0.0004 mg per mL of ofloxacin.
  Test solution—Quantitatively dissolve an accurately weighed quantity of Ofloxacin in *Diluent* to obtain a solution containing about 0.2 mg per mL.
  Chromatographic system (see *Chromatography* ⟨621⟩)—The liquid chromatograph is equipped with a 294-nm detector and a 4.6-mm × 15-cm column that contains packing L1. The column temperature is maintained at 45°. The flow rate is about 0.5 mL per minute. Chromatograph the *System suitability solution,* and record the peak responses as directed for *Procedure:* the resolution, *R,* between ofloxacin and ofloxacin related compound A is not less than 2.0; and the relative standard deviation for replicate injections is not more than 3.0%.
  Procedure—Inject equal volumes (about 10 µL) of the *Test solution* and the *Standard solution* into the chromatograph, record the chromatograms for a period of time that is about 2.5 times the retention time of the ofloxacin peak, and measure the areas for all of the peaks except the solvent peak. Calculate the percentage of each impurity with an area greater than 0.1 times the average area of the ofloxacin peak obtained from the *Standard solution* by the formula:

$$100(C/C_T)(r_i/r_S)$$

in which C is the concentration, in mg per mL, of USP Ofloxacin RS in the *Standard solution;* C_T is the concentration, in mg per mL, of Ofloxacin in the *Test solution;* r_i is the peak area for an individual impurity; and r_S is the average area of the ofloxacin peak obtained from the *Standard solution:* not more than 0.3% of any individual impurity is found; and the sum of all impurities found is not more than 0.5%.

Limit of methanol and ethanol—
  Internal standard solution—Prepare a solution in sodium hydroxide solution (1 in 100) containing 0.7 µL of *n*-propyl alcohol per mL. Transfer 2.0 mL of this solution to a 250-mL volumetric flask, dilute with the same sodium hydroxide solution (1 in 100) to volume, and mix.
  Standard solution—Prepare a solution in *Internal standard solution* containing 10.0 µg each of methanol and dehydrated alcohol per mL. Transfer 2.0 mL of this solution to a vial fitted with a septum and crimp cap, and seal. Heat the sealed vial at 90° for 2 minutes, and shake for 6 minutes.
  Test solution—Transfer 40 mg of Ofloxacin, accurately weighed, to a vial fitted with a septum and a crimp cap, add 2.0 mL of *Internal standard solution,* and seal the vial. Heat the sealed vial at 90° for 2 minutes, and shake for 6 minutes.
  Blank—Transfer 2.0 mL of the *Internal standard solution* to a vial fitted with a septum and crimp cap, and seal. Heat the sealed vial at 90° for 2 minutes, and shake for 6 minutes.
  Chromatographic system (see *Chromatography* ⟨621⟩)—The gas chromatograph is equipped with a flame-ionization detector, a 0.53-mm × 30-m fused silica column coated with a 3.0-µm film of stationary phase G43, and a fused silica precolumn. Helium is used as the carrier gas at a flow rate of about 7 mL per minute. The injection port and detector temperatures are maintained at about 170° and 250°, respectively. Condition the column with the helium flowing at 200° for 2 hours or until a stable baseline is obtained. For analysis, the column temperature is programmed according to the following steps. It is maintained at 35° for 3 minutes, then increased to 90° at a rate of 20° per minute, then increased further to 200° at a rate of 40° per minute, and then maintained for 2 minutes. Chromatograph the headspace of the *Standard solution,* and record the peak responses as directed for *Procedure:* the relative retention times are about 0.5 for methanol, 0.6 for ethanol, and 1.0 for *n*-propyl alcohol; the resolution, *R,* between the methanol peak and the ethanol peak is not less than 2.0; and the relative standard deviation for replicate injections is not more than 5%.
  Procedure—Use a heated gas tight syringe to make injections of the headspace into the chromatograph. Separately inject equal volumes (about 1 mL) of the headspace of the *Standard solution,* the *Blank,* and the *Test solution* into the chromatograph, record the chromatograms, and measure the peak area responses. Calculate the percentage of methanol and ethanol in the Ofloxacin taken by the formula:

$$(2/W)(R_U - R_B)/(R_S - R_B)$$

in which W is the weight, in mg, of Ofloxacin taken to prepare the *Test solution;* and R_U, R_B, and R_S are the peak response ratios of the relevant alcohol peak to the internal standard peak obtained from the *Test solution,* the *Blank,* and the *Standard solution,* respectively: not more than 0.005% of methanol and not more than 0.05% of ethanol are found.

Assay—Transfer about 100 mg of Ofloxacin, accurately weighed, to a 400-mL beaker, add 275 mL of acetic anhydride, and stir to dissolve. Titrate with 0.1 N perchloric acid VS, determining the endpoint potentiometrically, using a glass-silver chloride electrode system (see *Titrimetry* ⟨541⟩). Use the first of the two inflection points. Perform a blank determination, and make any necessary correction. Each mL of 0.1 N perchloric acid is equivalent to 36.138 mg of $C_{18}H_{20}FN_3O_4$.

Ofloxacin Ophthalmic Solution

» Ofloxacin Ophthalmic Solution is a sterile aqueous solution of Ofloxacin. It contains not less than 90.0 percent and not more than 110.0 percent of the labeled amount of ofloxacin ($C_{18}H_{20}FN_3O_4$).

Packaging and storage—Preserve in tight containers at controlled room temperature.

USP Reference standards ⟨11⟩—USP Ofloxacin RS.
Identification—
  A: *Thin-Layer Chromatographic Identification Test* ⟨201⟩—
  Test solution—Dilute a portion of Ophthalmic Solution with a mixture of chloroform and methanol (1 : 1) to obtain a solution having a concentration of about 0.3 mg of ofloxacin per mL.
  Standard solution—Dissolve an accurately weighed quantity of USP Ofloxacin RS in a mixture of chloroform and methanol (1 : 1) to obtain a solution having a concentration of 3.0 mg per mL. Transfer 5.0 mL of this solution to a 50-mL volumetric flask, add 5 mL of water, dilute with a mixture of chloroform and methanol (1 : 1) to volume, and mix.
  Application volume: 2 µL.
  Developing solvent system: a mixture of chloroform, methanol, and a solution (1 in 30) of ammonium hydroxide (150 : 75 : 15). Saturate a paper-lined chromatographic chamber with this mixture.
  B: The retention time of the ofloxacin peak in the chromatogram of the *Assay preparation* corresponds to that in the chromatogram of the *Standard preparation*, as obtained in the *Assay*.
Sterility ⟨71⟩—It meets the requirements when tested as directed for *Membrane Filtration* under *Test for Sterility of the Product to be Examined*.
pH ⟨791⟩: between 6.0 and 6.8.
Assay—
  Mobile phase—Prepare a filtered and degassed mixture of sodium dodecyl sulfate (0.24% aqueous solution), acetonitrile, and glacial acetic acid (580 : 400 : 20). Make adjustments if necessary (see *System Suitability* under *Chromatography* ⟨621⟩).
  0.05 N Hydrochloric acid—Add 4.0 mL of hydrochloric acid to 500 mL of water, dilute with water to 1000 mL, and mix.
  Resolution solution—Prepare a solution of about 0.1 mg of USP Ofloxacin RS and about 2.4 mg of propylparaben in each mL of acetonitrile.
  Standard preparation—Quantitatively dissolve an accurately weighed quantity of USP Ofloxacin RS in *0.05 N Hydrochloric acid* to obtain a solution having a known concentration of about 0.06 mg per mL.
  Assay preparation—Transfer an accurately measured volume of Ophthalmic Solution, equivalent to about 3 mg of ofloxacin, to a 50-mL volumetric flask, dilute with *0.05 N Hydrochloric acid* to volume, and mix.
  Chromatographic system (see *Chromatography* ⟨621⟩)—The liquid chromatograph is equipped with a 294-nm detector and a 4.6-mm × 25-cm column that contains 5-µm packing L1. The flow rate is about 1.5 mL per minute. The column temperature is maintained at a constant temperature of about 35°. Chromatograph the *Resolution solution*, and record the peak responses as directed for *Procedure:* the resolution, R, between propylparaben and ofloxacin is not less than 2. Chromatograph the *Standard preparation*, and record the peak responses as directed for *Procedure:* the tailing factor is not more than 3; and the relative standard deviation for replicate injections is not more than 2.0%.
  Procedure—Separately inject equal volumes (about 20 µL) of the *Standard preparation* and the *Assay preparation* into the chromatograph, record the chromatograms, and measure the areas for the major peaks. Calculate the quantity, in mg, of ofloxacin ($C_{18}H_{20}FN_3O_4$) in each mL of the Ophthalmic Solution taken by the formula:

$$50(C/V)(r_U/r_S)$$

in which C is the concentration, in mg per mL, of USP Ofloxacin RS in the *Standard preparation*; V is the volume, in mL, of Ophthalmic Solution taken to prepare the *Assay preparation*; and r_U and r_S are the ofloxacin peak areas obtained from the *Assay preparation* and the *Standard preparation*, respectively.

Add the following:

▲Ofloxacin Tablets

» Ofloxacin Tablets contain not less than 90.0 percent and not more than 110.0 percent of the labeled amount of ofloxacin ($C_{18}H_{20}FN_3O_4$).

Packaging and storage—Preserve in well-closed containers, and store at controlled room temperature.
USP Reference standards ⟨11⟩—USP Ofloxacin RS.
Identification—The retention time of the major peak in the chromatogram of the *Assay preparation* corresponds to that in the chromatogram of the *Standard preparation*, as obtained in the *Assay*.
Uniformity of dosage units ⟨905⟩: meet the requirements for *Content Uniformity*.
Related compounds—
  Phosphate buffer—Dissolve 2.72 g of monobasic potassium phosphate in 1000 mL of water. Adjust with diluted phosphoric acid to a pH of 3.3 ± 0.1.
  Solution A—Prepare a filtered and degassed mixture of *Phosphate buffer* and acetonitrile (88 : 12).
  Solution B—Prepare a filtered and degassed mixture of acetonitrile and *Phosphate buffer* (60 : 40).
  Mobile phase—Use variable mixtures of *Solution A* and *Solution B*, as directed for *Chromatographic system*. Make adjustments if necessary (see *System Suitability* under *Chromatography* ⟨621⟩).
  Standard solution—Dissolve an accurately weighed quantity of USP Ofloxacin RS in methanol, and dilute quantitatively, and stepwise if necessary, to obtain a solution having a known concentration of about 4 µg per mL.
  Test solution—Weigh and finely powder not fewer than 20 Tablets. Transfer an accurately weighed portion of the powder, equivalent to about 100 mg of ofloxacin, to a 100-mL volumetric flask, add 70 mL of methanol, and sonicate for about 20 minutes. Dilute with methanol to volume, and mix. Pass a portion of this solution through a filter having a 0.45-µm or finer porosity, discarding the first 5 mL. Use the filtrate.
  Chromatographic system (see *Chromatography* ⟨621⟩)—The liquid chromatograph is equipped with a 294-nm detector and a 4.6-mm × 10-cm column that contains packing L1. The flow rate is about 1.0 mL per minute. The chromatograph is programmed as follows.

Time (minutes)	Solution A (%)	Solution B (%)	Elution
0–8	100	0	isocratic
8–25	100→40	0→60	linear gradient
25–26	40→100	60→0	linear gradient
26–40	100	0	isocratic

Chromatograph the *Standard solution*, and record the peak responses as directed for *Procedure:* the tailing factor is not more than 2.0; and the relative standard deviation for replicate injections is not more than 5.0%.

  Procedure—Separately inject equal volumes (about 10 µL) of the *Standard solution* and the *Test solution* into the chromatograph, record the chromatograms, and measure the responses for the major

[NOTE—Prepare ammonia-saturated dichloromethane as follows. Shake 100 mL of dichloromethane with 30 mL of ammonium hydroxide in a separatory funnel, allow the layers to separate, and use the lower layer.] Remove the plate from the developing chamber, mark the solvent front, allow the solvent to evaporate, and examine the plate under short-wavelength UV light: the chromatograms show principal spots at about the same R_F value. Estimate the intensities of any secondary spots observed in the chromatogram of the *Test solution* by comparison with the spots in the chromatograms of the *Standard solutions*: no secondary spot from the chromatogram of the *Test solution* is larger or more intense than the principal spot obtained from *Standard solution B* (0.3%), and the sum of the intensities of all secondary spots obtained from the *Test solution* is not more intense than the principal spot obtained from *Standard solution A* (1.0%).

METHOD 2—

Diluent—Use *Mobile phase*.

Phosphate buffer, Mobile phase, System suitability solution, and *Chromatographic system*—Proceed as directed in the *Assay*.

Test solution—Dissolve an accurately weighed quantity of Omeprazole in *Diluent* to obtain a solution containing about 0.16 mg per mL. [NOTE—Prepare this solution fresh.]

Procedure—Inject equal volumes (about 40 µL) of the *Test solution* and *Diluent* into the chromatograph, and allow the *Test solution* to elute for not less than two times the retention time of omeprazole. Record the chromatograms, and measure the peak responses. Calculate the percentage of each impurity in the portion of Omeprazole taken by the formula:

$$100(r_i / r_s)$$

in which r_i is the peak response for each impurity, and r_s is the sum of the responses of all of the peaks: not more than 0.3% of any individual impurity is found, and the sum of all impurities is not more than 1.0%.

Assay—

Phosphate buffer—Dissolve 0.725 g of monobasic sodium phosphate and 4.472 g of anhydrous dibasic sodium phosphate in 300 mL of water, dilute with water to 1000 mL, and mix. Dilute 250 mL of this solution with water to 1000 mL. If necessary, adjust the pH with phosphoric acid to 7.6.

Mobile phase—Prepare a filtered and degassed mixture of *Phosphate buffer* and acetonitrile (3 : 1). Make adjustments if necessary (see *System Suitability* under *Chromatography* ⟨621⟩).

Diluent—Prepare a mixture of 0.01 M sodium borate and acetonitrile (3 : 1).

Standard preparation—Dissolve an accurately weighed quantity of USP Omeprazole RS in *Diluent,* and dilute quantitatively, and stepwise if necessary, with *Diluent* to obtain a solution having a known concentration of about 0.2 mg per mL.

Assay preparation—Transfer about 100 mg of Omeprazole, accurately weighed, to a 50-mL volumetric flask, dissolve in and dilute with *Diluent* to volume, and mix. Transfer 5.0 mL of this solution to a 50-mL volumetric flask, dilute with *Diluent* to volume, and mix.

System suitability solution—Dilute a volume of *Standard preparation* with *Diluent* to obtain a solution containing about 0.1 mg of USP Omeprazole RS per mL.

Chromatographic system (see *Chromatography* ⟨621⟩)—The liquid chromatograph is equipped with a 280-nm detector and a 4.6-mm × 15-cm column that contains 5-µm packing L7. The flow rate is about 0.8 mL per minute. Chromatograph the *System suitability solution,* and record the peak responses as directed for *Procedure*: the capacity factor, k', is not less than 6.0; the column efficiency is not less than 3000 theoretical plates; the tailing factor is not more than 1.5; and the relative standard deviation for replicate injections is not more than 1.0%.

Procedure—Separately inject equal volumes (about 20 µL) of the *Standard preparation* and the *Assay preparation* into the chromatograph, record the chromatograms, and measure the responses for the major peaks. Calculate the quantity, in mg, of $C_{17}H_{19}N_3O_3S$ in the portion of Omeprazole taken by the formula:

$$500C(r_U / r_S)$$

in which C is the concentration, in mg per mL, of USP Omeprazole RS in the *Standard preparation;* and r_U and r_S are the peak responses obtained from the *Assay preparation* and the *Standard preparation,* respectively.

Omeprazole Delayed-Release Capsules

» Omeprazole Delayed-Release Capsules contain not less than 90.0 percent and not more than 110.0 percent of the labeled amount of omeprazole ($C_{17}H_{19}N_3O_3S$).

Packaging and storage—Preserve in tight, light-resistant containers. Store between 15° and 30°.

Labeling—When more than one *Dissolution Test* is given, the labeling states the *Dissolution Test* used only if *Test 1* is not used.

USP Reference standards ⟨11⟩—*USP Omeprazole RS.*

Identification—The retention time of the major peak in the chromatogram of the *Assay preparation* corresponds to that in the chromatogram of the *Standard preparation,* as obtained in the *Assay*.

Dissolution ⟨711⟩—

TEST 1—

ACID RESISTANCE STAGE—

Medium: 0.1 N hydrochloric acid; 500 mL.

Apparatus 2: 100 rpm.

Time: 2 hours.

pH 7.6 Phosphate buffer, Mobile phase, and *Chromatographic system*—Proceed as directed for *Buffer stage*.

Standard solution—Transfer about 50 mg of USP Omeprazole RS, accurately weighed, to a 250-mL volumetric flask, dissolve in 50 mL of alcohol, dilute with 0.01 M sodium borate solution to volume, and mix. Transfer 10.0 mL of this solution into a 100-mL volumetric flask, add 20 mL of alcohol, dilute with 0.01 M sodium borate solution to volume, and mix.

Test solution—After 2 hours, filter the *Medium* containing the pellets through a sieve with an aperture of not more than 0.2 mm. Collect the pellets on the sieve, and rinse them with water. Using approximately 60 mL of 0.01 M sodium borate solution, carefully transfer the pellets quantitatively to a 100-mL volumetric flask. Sonicate for about 20 minutes until the pellets are broken up. Add 20 mL of alcohol to the flask, dilute with 0.01 M sodium borate solution to volume, and mix. Dilute an appropriate amount of this solution with 0.01 M sodium borate solution to obtain a solution having a concentration of about 0.02 mg per mL. At level L_1, test 6 units. Test 6 additional units at level L_2, and at level L_3, an additional 12 units are tested. Continue testing through the three levels unless the results conform at either L_1 or L_2.

Procedure—Separately inject equal volumes (about 20 µL) of the *Standard solution* and *Test solution* into the chromatograph, record the chromatograms, and measure the responses for the major peaks. Calculate the quantity, in mg, of omeprazole ($C_{17}H_{19}N_3O_3S$) dissolved in the *Medium* by the formula:

$$T - CD(r_U / r_S)$$

in which T is the labeled quantity, in mg, of omeprazole in the capsule; C is the concentration, in mg per mL, of USP Omeprazole RS in the *Standard solution; D* is the dilution factor used in preparing the *Test solution;* and r_U and r_S are the omeprazole peak responses obtained from the *Test solution* and the *Standard solution,* respectively.

Tolerances—Level L_1: no individual value exceeds 15% of omeprazole dissolved. Level L_2: the average of 12 units is not more than 20% of omeprazole dissolved, and no individual unit is greater than 35% of omeprazole dissolved. Level L_3: the average of 24 units is not more than 20% of omeprazole dissolved, not more than 2 units are greater than 35% of omeprazole dissolved, and no individual unit is greater than 45% of omeprazole dissolved.

BUFFER STAGE—
Medium: pH 6.8 phosphate buffer, 900 mL.
Proceed as directed for *Acid resistance stage* with a new set of capsules from the same batch. After 2 hours, add 400 mL of 0.235 M dibasic sodium phosphate to the 500 mL of 0.1 N hydrochloric acid medium in the vessel. Adjust, if necessary, with 2 N hydrochloric acid or 2 N sodium hydroxide to a pH of 6.8 ± 0.05.
Apparatus 2: 100 rpm.
At the end of 30 minutes, determine the amount of $C_{17}H_{19}N_3O_3S$ dissolved in pH 6.8 phosphate buffer by employing the following method.
pH 10.4, 0.235 M Dibasic sodium phosphate—Dissolve 33.36 g of anhydrous dibasic sodium phosphate in 1000 mL of water, and adjust with 2 N sodium hydroxide to a pH of 10.4 ± 0.1.
pH 6.8 Phosphate buffer—Add 400 mL of 0.1 N hydrochloric acid to 320 mL of *pH 10.4, 0.235 M Dibasic sodium phosphate*, and adjust with 2 N hydrochloric acid or 2 N sodium hydroxide, if necessary, to a pH of 6.8 ± 0.05.
pH 7.6 Phosphate buffer—Dissolve 0.718 g of monobasic sodium phosphate and 4.49 g of dibasic sodium phosphate in 1000 mL of water. Adjust with 2 N hydrochloric acid or 2 N sodium hydroxide, if necessary, to a pH of 7.6 ± 0.1. Dilute 250 mL of this solution with water to 1000 mL.
Mobile phase—Transfer 340 mL of acetonitrile to a 1000-mL volumetric flask, dilute with *pH 7.6 Phosphate buffer* to volume, and pass through a membrane filter having a 0.5-µm or finer porosity. Make adjustments if necessary (see *System Suitability* under *Chromatography* ⟨621⟩).
Standard solution 1 (for Capsules labeled 10 mg)—Dissolve an accurately weighed quantity of USP Omeprazole RS in alcohol to obtain a solution having a known concentration of about 2 mg per mL. Dilute with *pH 6.8 Phosphate buffer* quantitatively, and stepwise if necessary, to obtain a solution having a known concentration of about 0.01 mg per mL. Immediately add 2 mL of 0.25 M sodium hydroxide to 10 mL of this solution, and mix. [NOTE—Do not allow the solution to stand before adding the sodium hydroxide solution.]
Standard solution 2 (for Capsules labeled 20 mg and 40 mg)—Proceed as directed for *Standard solution 1*, except to obtain a solution having a known concentration of about 0.02 mg per mL before mixing with 2 mL of 0.25 M sodium hydroxide.
Test solution 1 (for Capsules containing 10 mg and 20 mg)—Immediately transfer 5.0 mL of the solution under test to a test tube containing 1.0 mL of 0.25 M sodium hydroxide. Mix well, and pass through a membrane filter having a 1.2-µm or finer porosity. Protect from light.
Test solution 2 (for Capsules labeled 40 mg)—Immediately transfer 5.0 mL of the solution under test to a test tube containing 2.0 mL of 0.25 M sodium hydroxide and 5 mL of *pH 6.8 Phosphate buffer*. Mix well, and pass through a membrane filter having a 1.2-µm or finer porosity. Protect from light.
Chromatographic system (see *Chromatography* ⟨621⟩)—The liquid chromatograph is equipped with a 280-nm detector and a 4.0-mm × 12.5-cm analytical column that contains 5-µm packing L7. The flow rate is about 1.0 mL per minute. Chromatograph the appropriate *Standard solution*, and record the peak responses as directed for *Procedure*: the column efficiency is not less than 2000 theoretical plates, and the relative standard deviation for replicate injections is not more than 2.0%.
Procedure—Separately inject equal volumes (about 20 µL) of the appropriate *Standard solution* and the *Test solution* into the chromatograph, record the chromatograms, and measure the responses for the major peaks. Calculate the quantity, in mg, of omeprazole ($C_{17}H_{19}N_3O_3S$) dissolved by the formula:

$$VCD(r_U / r_S)$$

in which V is the volume of *Medium* in each vessel; C is the concentration, in mg per mL, of USP Omeprazole RS in the appropriate *Standard solution*; D is the dilution factor used in preparing the appropriate *Test solution*; and r_U and r_S are the omeprazole peak responses obtained from the appropriate *Test solution* and the *Standard solution*, respectively.
Tolerances—For Capsules labeled 10 and 20 mg, not less than 75% (*Q*) of the labeled amount of $C_{17}H_{19}N_3O_3S$ is dissolved in 30 minutes. For Capsules labeled 40 mg, not less than 70% (*Q*) of the labeled amount of $C_{17}H_{19}N_3O_3S$ is dissolved in 30 minutes. The requirements are met if the quantities dissolved from the product conform to *Acceptance Table 1*.
TEST 2—If the product complies with this test, the labeling indicates that it meets USP *Dissolution Test 2*.
ACID RESISTANCE STAGE—
Medium: 0.1 N hydrochloric acid; 900 mL.
Apparatus 1: 100 rpm.
Time: 2 hours.
Procedure—After 2 hours, remove each sample from the basket, and quantitatively transfer into separate volumetric flasks to obtain a solution having a final concentration of about 0.2 mg per mL. Proceed as directed for the *Assay preparation* in the *Assay*, starting with "Add about 50 mL of *Diluent*". Calculate the quantity, in mg, of omeprazole ($C_{17}H_{19}N_3O_3S$) dissolved in the *Medium* by the formula:

$$T - CD(r_U / r_S)$$

in which T is the assayed quantity, in mg, of omeprazole in the capsule; C is the concentration, in mg per mL, of USP Omeprazole RS in the *Standard solution*; D is the dilution factor used in preparing the *Test solution*; and r_U and r_S are the omeprazole peak responses obtained from *Test solution* and *Standard solution*, respectively.
Tolerances—It complies with the following *Acceptance Table*:

Acceptance Table

Level	Criterion
L_1	the average of the 6 units is not more than 10% of omeprazole dissolved
L_2	the average of the 12 units is not more than 10% of omeprazole dissolved
L_3	the average of the 24 units is not more than 10% of omeprazole dissolved

BUFFER STAGE—
Medium: 0.05 M pH 6.8 phosphate buffer; 900 mL (see *Reagents, Indicators, and Solutions*).
Apparatus 1: 100 rpm.
Time: 45 minutes.
Procedure—Proceed as directed for *Acid resistance stage* with a new set of capsules from the same batch. After 2 hours, replace the acid *Medium* with the buffer *Medium* and continue the test for 45 more minutes. Determine the amount of $C_{17}H_{19}N_3O_3S$ dissolved from UV absorbances at the wavelength of maximum absorbance at about 305 nm on portions of the solutions under test passed through a 0.2-µm nylon filter, in comparison with a Standard solution having a known concentration of USP Omeprazole RS in the same *Medium*.
Tolerances—It complies with *Acceptance Table 1* under *Dissolution* ⟨711⟩. Not less than 75% (*Q*) of the labeled amount of $C_{17}H_{19}N_3O_3S$ is dissolved in 45 minutes.
Uniformity of dosage units ⟨905⟩: meet the requirements.
Chromatographic purity—
Diluent, Solution A, Solution B, Mobile phase, and *Chromatographic system*—Proceed as directed in the *Assay*.
Standard solution—Prepare as directed for the *Standard preparation* in the *Assay*.
Test solution—Use the *Assay preparation*.
Procedure—Separately inject equal volumes (about 10 µL) of the *Standard solution* and the *Test solution* into the chromatograph, record the chromatograms, and measure all of the peak responses. Calculate the percentage of each impurity in the portion of Capsules taken by the formula:

$$10(C/A)(1/F)(r_i / r_S)$$

in which C is the concentration, in µg per mL, of USP Omeprazole RS in the *Standard solution*; A is the quantity, in mg, of omeprazole in the portion of Capsules taken, as determined in the *Assay*; F is the relative response factor (see *Table 1* below for values); r_i is the peak response for each impurity obtained from the *Test solution*; and r_S is the peak response for omeprazole obtained from the *Standard solution*. In addition to not exceeding the limits for each impurity in *Table 1*, not more than 2.0% of total impurities is found.

Table 1

Name	Relative Retention Time	Relative Response Factor (F)	Limit (%)
Thioxopyrido conversion product[1]	0.33	1.6	0.5
5-methoxy-1H-benzimidazole-2-thiol	0.64	3.1	0.5
Any other individual impurity	—	1.0	0.5

[1] Formed in the solution from two isomers: 1,3-dimethyl-8-methoxy-12-thioxopyrido[1′,2′:3,4]imidazo[1,2-a]benzimidazol-2(12H)-one and 1,3-dimethyl-9-methoxy-12-thioxopyrido[1′,2′:3,4]imidazo[1,2-a]benzimidazol-2(12H)-one.

Assay—

Diluent—Dissolve 7.6 g of sodium borate decahydrate in about 800 mL of water. Add 1.0 g of edetate disodium, and adjust with 50% sodium hydroxide solution to a pH of 11.0 ± 0.1. Transfer the solution to a 2000-mL volumetric flask, add 400 mL of dehydrated alcohol, and dilute with water to volume.

Solution A—Prepare a filtered and degassed solution of 6.0 g of glycine in 1500 mL of water. Adjust with 50% sodium hydroxide solution to a pH of 9.0, and dilute with water to 2000 mL.

Solution B—Use a filtered and degassed mixture of acetonitrile and methanol (85 : 15).

Mobile phase—Use variable mixtures of *Solution A* and *Solution B* as directed for *Chromatographic system*. Make adjustments if necessary (see *System Suitability* under *Chromatography* ⟨621⟩).

Standard preparation—Dissolve, by sonicating, an accurately weighed quantity of USP Omeprazole RS in *Diluent*, and dilute quantitatively, and stepwise if necessary, with *Diluent* to obtain a solution having a known concentration of about 0.2 mg per mL.

Assay preparation—Weigh and mix the contents of not fewer than 20 Capsules. Transfer an accurately weighed portion of the mixture, equivalent to about 20 mg of omeprazole, to a 100-mL volumetric flask, add about 50 mL of *Diluent,* and sonicate for 15 minutes. Cool, dilute with *Diluent* to volume, mix, and pass through a membrane filter having 0.45-μm or finer porosity. [NOTE—Bubbles may form just before bringing the solution to volume. Add a few drops of dehydrated alcohol to dissipate the bubbles if they persist for more than a few minutes.]

Chromatographic system (see *Chromatography* ⟨621⟩)—The liquid chromatograph is equipped with a 305-nm detector and a 4.6-mm × 15-cm column that contains 5-μm base-deactivated packing L7. The flow rate is about 1.2 mL per minute. The chromatograph is programmed as follows.

Time (minutes)	Solution A %	Solution B %	Elution
0–20	88→40	12→60	linear gradient
20–21	40→88	60→12	linear gradient
21–25	88	12	isocratic

Chromatograph the *Standard preparation*, and record the peak responses as directed for *Procedure:* the column efficiency is not less than 20,000 theoretical plates; the tailing factor is not less than 0.8 and not more than 2; and the relative standard deviation for replicate injections is not more than 2.0%.

Procedure—Separately inject equal volumes (about 10 μL) of the *Standard preparation* and the *Assay preparation* into the chromatograph, record the chromatograms, and measure the peak responses. Calculate the quantity, in mg, of omeprazole ($C_{17}H_{19}N_3O_3S$) in the portion of Capsules taken by the formula:

$$DC(r_U / r_S)$$

in which D is the dilution factor of the *Assay preparation*; C is the concentration, in mg per mL, of USP Omeprazole RS in the *Standard preparation*; and r_U and r_S are the peak responses obtained from the *Assay preparation* and the *Standard preparation*, respectively.

Ondansetron

$C_{18}H_{19}N_3O$ 293.36

4H-Carbazol-4-one, 1,2,3,9-tetrahydro-9-methyl-3-[(2-methyl-1H-imidazol-1-yl)methyl]-(±)-.
(±)-2,3-Dihydro-9-methyl-3-[(2-methylimidazol-1-yl)methyl]carbazol-4(1H)-one   [99614-02-5].

» Ondansetron contains not less than 98.0 percent and not more than 102.0 percent of $C_{18}H_{19}N_3O$, calculated on the anhydrous basis.

Packaging and storage—Preserve in tight, light-resistant containers at room temperature.

USP Reference standards ⟨11⟩—*USP Ondansetron RS. USP Ondansetron Related Compound C RS. USP Ondansetron Related Compound D RS.*

Identification—
   A: *Infrared Absorption* ⟨197K⟩.
   B: The retention time of the major peak in the chromatogram of the *Assay preparation* corresponds to that in the chromatogram of the *Standard preparation,* as obtained in the *Assay*.

Water, *Method Ia* ⟨921⟩: not more than 3.0%.

Residue on ignition ⟨281⟩: not more than 0.1%.

Chloride ⟨221⟩—To 1 g of the substance under test, add 30 to 40 mL of water, and warm gently, if necessary, until no more dissolves. Mix well, and pass through a filter paper that gives a negative test for chloride. Add 1 mL of nitric acid and 1 mL of silver nitrate TS. Dilute with water to 50 mL. Mix well, and allow to stand for 5 minutes protected from direct sunlight: any turbidity formed is not greater than that produced in a similarly treated control solution containing 0.3 mL of 0.020 N hydrochloric acid (0.02%).

Limit of ondansetron related compound D—

Phosphate buffer—Dissolve about 2.72 g of monobasic potassium phosphate in 900 mL of water. Adjust with 1 N sodium hydroxide or 0.5 N sodium hydroxide to a pH of 5.4, dilute to 1000 mL, and mix.

Mobile phase—Prepare a filtered and degassed mixture of *Phosphate buffer* and acetonitrile (80 : 20). Make adjustments if necessary (see *System Suitability* under *Chromatography* ⟨621⟩).

Standard solution—Dissolve an amount of USP Ondansetron Related Compound D RS in *Mobile phase,* and dilute stepwise with *Mobile phase,* to obtain a solution having a known concentration of about 0.4 μg per mL.

Resolution solution—Prepare a solution of USP Ondansetron Related Compound D RS and USP Ondansetron Related Compound C RS in *Mobile phase* having a known concentration of about 0.6 μg per mL and 1.0 μg per mL, respectively.

Test solution—Transfer about 50 mg of Ondansetron, accurately weighed, to a 100-mL volumetric flask, dissolve in and dilute with *Mobile phase* to volume, and mix.

Chromatographic system (see *Chromatography* ⟨621⟩)—The liquid chromatograph is equipped with a 328-nm detector and a 4.6-mm × 25-cm column that contains packing L10. The column temperature is maintained at 30°. The flow rate is about 1.5 mL per minute. Chromatograph the *Resolution solution,* and record the peak responses as directed for *Procedure:* the relative retention times are about 0.8 for ondansetron related compound C and 1.0 for ondansetron related compound D; and the resolution, R, between ondansetron related compound C and ondansetron related compound D is not less than 1.5. Chromatograph the *Standard solution,* and record the peak responses as directed for *Procedure:* the column efficiency is not less than 8000 theoretical plates; and the relative standard deviation for replicate injections is not more than 2.0%.

Procedure—Separately inject equal volumes (about 20 μL) of the *Standard solution* and the *Test solution* into the chromatograph, record the chromatograms, and measure the responses for the major peaks. Calculate the percentage of ondansetron related compound D in the ondansetron taken by the formula:

$$10(C/W)(r_U/r_S)$$

in which C is the concentration, in μg per mL, of USP Ondansetron Related Compound D RS in the *Standard solution;* W is the weight, in mg, of ondansetron taken to prepare the *Test solution;* and r_U and r_S are the peak responses of ondansetron related compound D obtained from the *Test solution* and the *Standard solution,* respectively: not more than 0.10% is found.

Related compounds—
Phosphate buffer, Mobile phase, Resolution solution, Standard preparation, and *Chromatographic system*—Prepare as directed in the *Assay.*
Test solution—Use the *Assay preparation* prepared as directed in the *Assay.*
Procedure—Inject a volume (about 10 μL) of the *Test solution* into the chromatograph, record the chromatogram, and measure the peak responses. Calculate the percentage of each impurity in the portion of Ondansetron taken by the formula:

$$100(r_i/r_s)$$

in which r_i is the peak area for each impurity; and r_s is the sum of the areas of all the peaks: not more than 0.1% of any individual impurity is found; and not more than 0.5% of total impurities is found, including ondansetron related compound D. [NOTE—Disregard the peak corresponding to ondansetron related compound D at a relative retention time of about 0.4.]

Organic volatile impurities ⟨467⟩: meets the requirements.
(Official until July 1, 2008)

Assay—
Phosphate buffer—Dissolve about 2.72 g of monobasic potassium phosphate in 900 mL of water. Adjust with 1 N sodium hydroxide or 0.5 N sodium hydroxide to a pH of 5.4, dilute to 1000 mL, and mix.
Mobile phase—Prepare a filtered and degassed mixture of *Phosphate buffer* and acetonitrile (52 : 48). Make adjustments if necessary (see *System Suitability* under *Chromatography* ⟨621⟩).
Resolution solution—Prepare a solution of USP Ondansetron RS and USP Ondansetron Related Compound A RS in *Mobile phase* having a known concentration of about 0.09 mg per mL and 0.05 mg per mL, respectively.
Standard preparation—Dissolve an accurately weighed quantity of USP Ondansetron RS in *Mobile phase,* and dilute quantitatively, and stepwise if necessary, with *Mobile phase* to obtain a solution having a known concentration of about 0.090 mg per mL.
Assay preparation—Transfer about 45 mg of Ondansetron, accurately weighed, to a 50-mL volumetric flask, dissolve in and dilute with *Mobile phase* to volume, and mix. Pipet 5.0 mL of this solution into a 50-mL volumetric flask. Dilute with *Mobile phase* to volume, and mix.
Chromatographic system (see *Chromatography* ⟨621⟩)—The liquid chromatograph is equipped with a 216-nm detector and a 4.6-mm 25-cm column that contains packing L10. The flow rate is about 1.5 mL per minute. The column temperature is maintained at 30°. Chromatograph the *Resolution solution,* and record the peak responses as directed for *Procedure:* the relative retention times are about 1.1 for ondansetron related compound A and 1.0 for ondansetron; and the resolution, R, between ondansetron related compound A and ondansetron is not less than 1.5. Chromatograph the *Standard preparation,* and record the peak responses as directed for *Procedure:* the tailing factor is not more than 2.0; and the relative standard deviation for replicate injections is not more than 1.5%.
Procedure—Separately inject equal volumes (about 10 μL) of the *Standard preparation* and the *Assay preparation* into the chromatograph, record the chromatograms, and measure the responses for the ondansetron peaks. Calculate the quantity, in mg, of $C_{18}H_{19}N_3O$ in the portion of Ondansetron taken by the formula:

$$500C(r_U/r_S)$$

in which C is the concentration, in mg per mL, of USP Ondansetron RS in the *Standard preparation;* and r_U and r_S are the peak responses obtained from the *Assay preparation* and the *Standard preparation,* respectively.

Ondansetron Hydrochloride

$C_{18}H_{19}N_3O \cdot HCl \cdot 2H_2O$ 365.86
4*H*-Carbazol-4-one, 1,2,3,9-tetrahydro-9-methyl-3-(2-methyl-1*H*-imidazol-1-yl)methyl-, monohydrochloride, (±)-, dihydrate.
(±)-2,3-Dihydro-9-methyl-3-(2-methylimidazol-1-yl)methyl-carbazol-4(1*H*)-one monohydrochloride dihydrate   [103639-04-9].

» Ondansetron Hydrochloride contains not less than 98.0 percent and not more than 102.0 percent of $C_{18}H_{19}N_3O \cdot HCl$, calculated on the anhydrous basis.

Packaging and storage—Preserve in tight, light-resistant containers. Store at 25°, excursions permitted between 15° and 30°.
USP Reference standards ⟨11⟩—*USP Ondansetron Hydrochloride RS. USP Ondansetron Related Compound A RS. USP Ondansetron Resolution Mixture RS. USP Ondansetron Related Compound C RS. USP Ondansetron Related Compound D RS.*
Identification—
  A: *Infrared Absorption* ⟨197M⟩.
  B: Dissolve 20 mg in 2 mL of water, add 1 mL of 2 M nitric acid, and filter: the filtrate responds to the test for *Chloride* ⟨191⟩.
Water, *Method Ia* ⟨921⟩: between 9.0% and 10.5%.
Residue on ignition ⟨281⟩: not more than 0.1%.
Limit of ondansetron related compound D—
Mobile phase—Prepare a filtered and degassed mixture of 0.02 M monobasic potassium phosphate (previously adjusted with 1 M sodium hydroxide to a pH of 5.4) and acetonitrile (80 : 20). Make adjustments if necessary (see *System Suitability* under *Chromatography* ⟨621⟩).
Standard solution—Dissolve an accurately weighed quantity of USP Ondansetron Related Compound D RS in *Mobile phase,* and dilute quantitatively, and stepwise if necessary, with *Mobile phase* to obtain a solution having a known concentration of about 0.4 μg per mL.
System suitability solution—Dissolve suitable quantities of USP Ondansetron Related Compound D RS and USP Ondansetron Related Compound C RS in *Mobile phase,* and dilute quantitatively, and stepwise if necessary, with *Mobile phase* to obtain a solution having a concentration of about 0.6 μg per mL and 1 μg per mL, respectively.
Test solution—Transfer about 50 mg of Ondansetron Hydrochloride, accurately weighed, to a 100-mL volumetric flask, dissolve in and dilute with *Mobile phase* to volume, and mix.
Chromatographic system (see *Chromatography* ⟨621⟩)—The liquid chromatograph is equipped with a 328-nm detector and a 4.6-mm × 25-cm column that contains packing L10. The flow rate is about 1.5 mL per minute. Chromatograph the *System suitability solution,* and record the peak responses as directed for *Procedure:* the relative retention times are about 0.8 for ondansetron related compound C and 1.0 for ondansetron related compound D; and the resolution, R, between ondansetron related compound C and ondansetron related compound D is not less than 1.5. Chromatograph the *Standard solution,* and record the peak responses as directed for *Procedure:* the column efficiency determined from the analyte peak is not less than 400 theoretical plates; and the relative standard deviation for replicate injections is not more than 2.0%.
Procedure—Separately inject equal volumes (about 20 μL) of the *Standard solution* and the *Test solution* into the chromatograph, record the chromatograms, and measure the responses for the major peaks. Calculate the percentage of ondansetron related compound D in the portion of Ondansetron Hydrochloride taken by the formula:

$$10{,}000(C/W)(r_U/r_S)$$

in which C is the concentration, in mg per mL, of USP Ondansetron Related Compound D RS in the *Standard solution;* W is the weight, in mg, of Ondansetron Hydrochloride taken to prepare the *Test solution;* and r_U and r_S are the peak areas obtained from the *Test solution* and the *Standard solution,* respectively: not more than 0.10% is found.

Chromatographic purity—

METHOD I—

Resolution solution—Dissolve a quantity of USP Ondansetron Resolution Mixture RS in methanol, and dilute quantitatively, and stepwise if necessary, with methanol to obtain a solution having a known concentration of 12.5 mg per mL.

Standard solutions—Dissolve an accurately weighed quantity of USP Ondansetron Hydrochloride RS in methanol, and mix to obtain a solution having a known concentration of about 0.25 mg per mL. Quantitatively dilute this solution with methanol to obtain *Standard solutions,* designated below by letter, having the following compositions:

Standard solution	Dilution	Concentration (µg RS per mL)	Percentage (%, for comparison with test specimen)
A	(1 in 5)	50	0.4
B	(1 in 10)	25	0.2
C	(1 in 20)	12.5	0.1

Test solution—Dissolve an accurately weighed quantity of Ondansetron Hydrochloride in methanol to obtain a solution containing 12.5 mg per mL.

Procedure—Separately apply 20 µL of the *Test solution,* 20 µL of each *Standard solution,* and 20 µL of the *Resolution solution* to a thin-layer chromatographic plate (see *Chromatography* ⟨621⟩) coated with a 0.25-mm layer of chromatographic silica gel mixture. Develop the chromatogram in a solvent system consisting of a mixture of chloroform, ethyl acetate, methanol, and ammonium hydroxide (90 : 50 : 40 : 1) until the solvent front has moved about three-fourths of the length of the plate. Remove the plate from the chamber, mark the solvent front, and allow the solvent to evaporate. Examine the plate under short-wavelength UV light: complete resolution of the three components of the *Resolution solution* spot is found. Compare the intensities of any secondary spots observed in the chromatogram of the *Test solution* with those of the principal spots in the chromatograms of the *Standard solutions:* any secondary spot from the chromatogram of the *Test solution* having an R_F value corresponding to that of the uppermost secondary spot of the *Resolution solution* is not larger or more intense than the principal spot obtained from *Standard solution A* (0.4%); and no other secondary spot from the chromatogram of the *Test solution* is larger or more intense than the principal spot obtained from *Standard solution B* (0.2%).

METHOD II—

Mobile phase and *Chromatographic system*—Proceed as directed in the *Assay.*

Standard solution—Proceed as directed for *Standard preparation* in the *Assay.*

Test solution—Use the *Assay preparation.*

Procedure—Separately inject equal volumes (about 10 µL) of the *Standard solution* and the *Test solution* into the chromatograph, record the chromatograms, and measure the peak responses. Calculate the percentage of each impurity in the portion of Ondansetron Hydrochloride taken by the formula:

$$50{,}000(C/W)(1/F)(r_i / r_S)$$

in which C is the concentration, in mg per mL, of USP Ondansetron Hydrochloride RS in the *Standard solution;* W is the weight, in mg, of Ondansetron Hydrochloride taken to prepare the *Test solution;* F is the relative response factor of the impurities as described in the accompanying table; r_i is the peak area for each impurity in the *Test solution;* and r_S is the peak area of ondansetron obtained from the *Standard solution:* it meets the requirements given in the accompanying table.

Compound Name	Relative Retention Time	Relative Response Factor	Limit (%)
Ondansetron related compound C	about 0.32	1.2	0.2
Ondansetron related compound D*	about 0.34	—	0.1
Imidazole	about 0.49	0.3	0.2
2-methylimidazole	about 0.54	0.4	0.2
Ondansetron	1.0	—	—
Ondansetron related compound A	about 1.10	0.8	0.2
Unknown	—	1.0	0.1
Total	—	—	0.5

*Quantified in the test for *Limit of ondansetron related compound D.*

Assay—

Mobile phase—Prepare a filtered and degassed mixture of 0.02 M monobasic sodium phosphate (previously adjusted with 1 M sodium hydroxide to a pH of 5.4) and acetonitrile (50 : 50). Make adjustments if necessary (see *System Suitability* under *Chromatography* ⟨621⟩).

Standard preparation—Dissolve an accurately weighed quantity of USP Ondansetron Hydrochloride RS in *Mobile phase,* and dilute quantitatively, and stepwise if necessary, with *Mobile phase* to obtain a solution having a known concentration of about 90 µg per mL.

System suitability solution—Dissolve suitable quantities of USP Ondansetron Hydrochloride RS and USP Ondansetron Related Compound A RS in *Mobile phase,* and dilute quantitatively, and stepwise if necessary, with *Mobile phase* to obtain a solution containing about 90 µg per mL and 20 µg per mL, respectively.

Assay preparation—Transfer about 45 mg of Ondansetron Hydrochloride, accurately weighed, to a 50-mL volumetric flask, dissolve in and dilute with *Mobile phase* to volume, and mix. Pipet 5.0 mL of this solution into a 50-mL volumetric flask, dilute with *Mobile phase* to volume, and mix.

Chromatographic system (see *Chromatography* ⟨621⟩)—The liquid chromatograph is equipped with a 216-nm detector and a 4.6-mm × 25-cm column that contains packing L10. The flow rate is about 1.5 mL per minute. Chromatograph the *System suitability solution,* and record the peak responses as directed for *Procedure:* the relative retention times are about 1.0 for ondansetron and 1.1 for ondansetron related compound A; and the resolution, R, between ondansetron related compound A and ondansetron is not less than 1.5. Chromatograph the *Standard preparation,* and record the peak responses as directed for *Procedure:* the tailing factor is not more than 2.0; and the relative standard deviation for replicate injections is not more than 1.5%.

Procedure—Separately inject equal volumes (about 10 µL) of the *Standard preparation* and the *Assay preparation* into the chromatograph, record the chromatograms, and measure the responses for the major peaks. Calculate the quantity, in mg, of $C_{18}H_{19}N_3O \cdot HCl$ in the portion of Ondansetron Hydrochloride taken by the formula:

$$500C(r_U / r_S)$$

in which C is the concentration, in mg per mL, of USP Ondansetron Hydrochloride RS in the *Standard preparation;* and r_U and r_S are the peak areas obtained from the *Assay preparation* and the *Standard preparation,* respectively.

Add the following:

▲Ondansetron Hydrochloride Oral Suspension

» Ondansetron Hydrochloride Oral Suspension is a suspension of Ondansetron Hydrochloride. It contains not less than 90.0 percent and not more than 110.0 percent of the labeled amount of ondansetron ($C_{18}H_{19}N_3O$), calculated on the anhydrous basis. Prepare Ondansetron Hydrochloride Oral Suspension 1.0 mg of Ondansetron Hydrochloride (dihydrate) equivalent to 0.8 mg of Ondansetron per mL as follows (see *Pharmaceutical Compounding—Nonsterile Preparations* ⟨795⟩):

Ondansetron (as Hydrochloride dihydrate)	80 mg
Vehicle: a mixture of Vehicle for Oral Suspension, (regular or sugar-free), *NF*, and Vehicle for Oral Solution, *NF*(1 : 1), a sufficient quantity to make	100 mL

If using Tablets, place the Tablets in a suitable glass mortar, and comminute well, or add Ondansetron Hydrochloride powder. Add 50 mL of the mixed Vehicle in 5-mL portions, and mix well with each addition. Transfer the contents of the mortar, stepwise and quantitatively, to a calibrated bottle. Add sufficient Vehicle to bring the preparation to final volume, and mix well.

Packaging and storage—Preserve in tight, light-resistant containers. Store at controlled room temperature, or in a cold place.
Labeling—Label it to state that it is to be well shaken before use, and to state the beyond-use date. Label content as: Each mL of Ondansetron Hydrochloride Oral Suspension contains 1 mg of Ondansetron Hydrochloride (dihydrate) equivalent to 0.8 mg Ondansetron.
USP Reference standards ⟨11⟩—*USP Ondansetron Hydrochloride RS*.
pH ⟨791⟩: between 3.6 and 4.6.
Beyond-use date: 42 days after the day on which it was compounded.
Assay—
   Mobile phase—Prepare a filtered and degassed solution of 43 mM monobasic potassium phosphate buffer adjusted with a mixture of 1 N sodium hydroxide and acetonitrile (85 : 15) to a pH of 5.4. Make adjustments if necessary (see *System Suitability* under *Chromatography* ⟨621⟩).
   Standard preparation—Dissolve an accurately weighed quantity of USP Ondansetron Hydrochloride RS in *Mobile phase* to obtain a solution having a known concentration of about 4 µg per mL.
   Assay preparation—After each amber plastic vial containing Oral Suspension that is stored at 4° is brought to room temperature, pipet 500 µL of Oral Suspension from each bottle into a 100-mL volumetric flask, and dilute with *Mobile phase* to volume. Pass through a 0.45-µm filter, and keep frozen at −70° until assayed.
   Chromatographic system (see *Chromatography* ⟨621⟩)—The liquid chromatograph is equipped with a 216-nm detector, a 3.9-mm × 20-mm guard column that contains 4-µm packing L10, and a 4.6-mm × 25-cm analytical column that contains 5-µm packing L10. The flow rate is about 1 mL per minute. Chromatograph the *Standard preparation*, and record the peak responses as directed for *Procedure*: the retention time is about 30 minutes for ondansetron hydrochloride; and the relative standard deviation for replicate injections is not more than 1.6%.
   Procedure—Separately inject equal volumes (about 80 µL) of the *Standard preparation* and the *Assay preparation* into the chromatograph, record the chromatograms, and measure the responses for the major peaks. Calculate the quantity, in mg, of ondansetron hydrochloride ($C_{18}H_{19}N_3O \cdot HCl \cdot 2H_2O$) in the volume of Oral Suspension taken by the formula:

$$200(C/V)(r_U/r_S)$$

in which *C* is the concentration, in µg per mL, of USP Ondansetron Hydrochloride RS in the *Standard preparation*; *V* is the volume, in mL, of Oral Suspension taken; and r_U and r_S are the peak responses obtained from the *Assay preparation* and the *Standard preparation*, respectively.
▲*USP31*

Ondansetron Injection

» Ondansetron Injection is a sterile solution of Ondansetron Hydrochloride in Water for Injection or of Ondansetron in Water for Injection prepared with the aid of Hydrochloric Acid. It may contain suitable buffers and/or tonicity adjusting agents. It contains an amount of Ondansetron Hydrochloride equivalent to not less than 95.0 percent and not more than 105.0 percent of the labeled amount of ondansetron ($C_{18}H_{19}N_3O$).

Packaging and storage—Preserve in single-dose or in multiple-dose containers, preferably of Type I glass, at a temperature between 2° and 30°, protected from light.
USP Reference standards ⟨11⟩—*USP Ondansetron Hydrochloride RS. USP Ondansetron Related Compound A RS. USP Ondansetron Related Compound B RS. USP Ondansetron Related Compound C RS. USP Ondansetron Related Compound D RS. USP Endotoxin RS.*
Identification—The retention time of the major peak in the chromatogram of the *Assay preparation* corresponds to that in the chromatogram of the *Standard preparation*, as obtained in the *Assay*.
Bacterial endotoxins ⟨85⟩—It contains not more than 9.9 USP Endotoxin Units per mg of ondansetron hydrochloride.
pH ⟨791⟩: between 3.3 and 4.0.
Particulate matter ⟨788⟩: meets the requirements for small-volume injections.
Limit of ondansetron related compound D—
   Mobile phase, Standard solution, System suitability solution, and *Chromatographic system*—Proceed as directed in the test for *Limit of ondansetron related compound D* under *Ondansetron Hydrochloride*.
   Test solution—Transfer an accurately measured volume of Injection, equivalent to about 10 mg of ondansetron, to a 25-mL volumetric flask, dilute with *Mobile phase* to volume, and mix.
   Procedure—Separately inject equal volumes (about 20 µL) of the *Standard solution* and the *Test solution* into the chromatograph, record the chromatograms, and measure the responses for the major peaks. Calculate the quantity of ondansetron related compound D in the volume of Injection taken by the formula:

$$(2.5/V)(C_S/C_A)(r_U/r_S)$$

in which *V* is the volume, in mL, of Injection taken; C_S is the concentration, in µg per mL, of ondansetron related compound D in the *Standard preparation*; C_A is the concentration, in mg per mL, of ondansetron in the Injection, as determined in the *Assay*; and r_U and r_S are the peak responses obtained from the *Test preparation* and the *Standard preparation*, respectively: not more than 0.12% is found.
Chromatographic purity—
   Mobile phase and *Chromatographic system*—Proceed as directed in the *Assay*.
   System suitability solution—Use the *System suitability solution* prepared as directed in the test for *Limit of ondansetron related compound D* under *Ondansetron Hydrochloride*.
   Test solution—Use the *Assay preparation*.
   Procedure—Inject about 20 µL of the *System suitability solution*, record the chromatogram, and identify the peaks due to ondansetron related compound C and ondansetron related compound D based on their approximate relative retention times of 0.35 and 0.37, respectively. Inject a volume (about 10 µL) of the *Test solution* into the chromatograph, record the chromatogram, and measure the peak responses. [NOTE—Ignore the peak due to ondansetron re-

lated compound D.] Calculate the percentage of each impurity in the volume of Injection taken by the formula:

$$100(r_i / r_s)$$

in which r_i is the peak response for each impurity; and r_s is the sum of the responses of all of the peaks: not more than 0.2% of any individual impurity is found, and the total of all impurities, including the percentage of ondansetron related compound D determined in the test for *Limit of ondansetron related compound D*, is not more than 0.5%.

Other requirements—It meets the requirements under *Injections* ⟨1⟩.

Assay—

Mobile phase—Prepare a filtered and degassed mixture of 0.02 M monobasic potassium phosphate (previously adjusted with 1 M sodium hydroxide to a pH of 5.4), and acetonitrile (50 : 50). Make adjustments if necessary (see *System Suitability* under *Chromatography* ⟨621⟩).

Standard preparation—Dissolve an accurately weighed quantity of USP Ondansetron Hydrochloride RS in *Mobile phase*, and dilute quantitatively, and stepwise if necessary, with *Mobile phase* to obtain a solution having a known concentration of about 0.1 mg per mL.

System suitability solution—Dissolve suitable quantities of USP Ondansetron Hydrochloride RS and USP Ondansetron Related Compound A RS in *Mobile phase*, and dilute quantitatively, and stepwise if necessary, with *Mobile phase* to obtain a solution containing about 0.1 mg per mL and 50 µg per mL, respectively.

Assay preparation—Transfer an accurately measured volume of Injection, equivalent to about 2 mg of ondansetron, to a 25-mL volumetric flask, dilute with *Mobile phase* to volume, and mix.

Chromatographic system (see *Chromatography* ⟨621⟩)—The liquid chromatograph is equipped with a 216-nm detector and a 4.6-mm × 20-cm column that contains packing L10. The flow rate is about 1.5 mL per minute. Chromatograph the *System suitability solution*, and record the peak responses as directed for *Procedure*: the relative retention times are about 1.0 for ondansetron and 1.1 for ondansetron related compound A; and the resolution, R, between ondansetron related compound A and ondansetron is not less than 1.5. Chromatograph the *Standard preparation*, and record the peak responses as directed for *Procedure*: the tailing factor is not more than 2.0; and the relative standard deviation for replicate injections is not more than 1.5%.

Procedure—Separately inject equal volumes (about 10 µL) of the *Standard preparation* and the *Assay preparation* into the chromatograph, record the chromatograms, and measure the responses for the major peaks. Calculate the quantity, in mg, of ondansetron ($C_{18}H_{19}N_3O$) in each mL of the Injection taken by the formula:

$$(293.36 / 329.82)(25C / V)(r_U / r_S)$$

in which 293.36 and 329.82 are the molecular weights of ondansetron and anhydrous ondansetron hydrochloride, respectively; C is the concentration, in mg per mL, on the anhydrous basis, of USP Ondansetron Hydrochloride RS in the *Standard preparation*; V is the volume, in mL, of Injection taken; and r_U and r_S are the peak responses obtained from the *Assay preparation* and the *Standard preparation*, respectively.

Ondansetron Oral Solution

» Ondansetron Oral Solution is a solution of Ondansetron Hydrochloride in a suitable vehicle. It contains not less than 95.0 percent and not more than 105.0 percent of the labeled amount of ondansetron ($C_{18}H_{19}N_3O$).

Packaging and storage—Preserve in well-closed, light-resistant containers.

USP Reference standards ⟨11⟩—*USP Ondansetron Hydrochloride RS. USP Ondansetron Related Compound A RS. USP Ondansetron Related Compound C RS. USP Ondansetron Related Compound D RS.*

Identification—

A: *Thin-Layer Chromatographic Identification Test* ⟨201⟩—

Test solution—Dilute a portion of Oral Solution with a mixture of methanol and water (50 : 50) to obtain a solution containing about 0.2 mg of ondansetron per mL.

Standard solution: 0.25 mg per mL in methanol.

Developing solvent system: chloroform, ethyl acetate, methanol, and ammonium hydroxide (90 : 50 : 40 : 1).

B: The retention time of the major peak in the chromatogram of the *Assay preparation* corresponds to that in the chromatogram of the *Standard preparation*, as obtained in the *Assay*.

Microbial limits ⟨61⟩—It meets the requirements of the tests for absence of *Escherichia coli*. The total aerobic microbial count does not exceed 100 cfu per g, the *Enterobacteriaceae* count does not exceed 10 cfu per g, and the total combined molds and yeasts count does not exceed 50 cfu per g.

Deliverable volume ⟨698⟩: meets the requirements.

pH ⟨791⟩: between 3.3 and 4.0.

Limit of ondansetron related compound D—

Mobile phase—Proceed as directed in the test for *Limit of ondansetron related compound D* under *Ondansetron Hydrochloride*.

System suitability solution—Dissolve suitable quantities of USP Ondansetron Related Compound D RS and USP Ondansetron Related Compound C RS in *Mobile phase*; and dilute quantitatively, and stepwise if necessary, with *Mobile phase* to obtain a solution containing about 0.5 µg per mL and 2 µg per mL, respectively.

Standard solution—Dissolve an accurately weighed quantity of USP Ondansetron Related Compound D RS in *Mobile phase*; and dilute quantitatively, and stepwise if necessary, with *Mobile phase* to obtain a solution having a known concentration of about 0.5 µg per mL.

Test solution—Quantitatively dilute, if necessary, an accurately measured volume of Oral Solution with *Mobile phase* to obtain a solution containing about 0.8 mg of ondansetron per mL.

Chromatographic system (see *Chromatography* ⟨621⟩)—The liquid chromatograph is equipped with a 328-nm detector and a 4.6-mm × 25-cm column that contains packing L10. The flow rate is about 1.5 mL per minute. Chromatograph the *System suitability solution*, and record the peak responses as directed for *Procedure*: the resolution, R, between ondansetron related compound D and ondansetron related compound C is not less than 2.0; the tailing factor for ondansetron related compound D is not more than 2.0; and the relative standard deviation for replicate injections is not more than 4.0%.

Procedure—Separately inject equal volumes (about 20 µL) of the *Standard solution* and the *Test solution* into the chromatograph, record the chromatograms, and measure the responses for the major peaks. Calculate the percentage of ondansetron related compound D in the volume of Oral Solution taken by the formula:

$$100D(C_S / C_A)(r_U / r_S)$$

in which D is the dilution factor for the Oral Solution in the *Test solution*; C_S is the concentration, in µg per mL, of USP Ondansetron Related Compound D RS in the *Standard solution*; C_A is the concentration, in µg per mL, of ondansetron in the Oral Solution, as determined in the *Assay*; and r_U and r_S are the peak responses of ondansetron related compound D obtained from the *Test solution* and the *Standard solution*, respectively: not more than 0.1% is found.

Related compounds—

Mobile phase, System suitability solution, and *Chromatographic system*—Proceed as directed in the *Assay* under *Ondansetron Hydrochloride*.

Standard solution—Prepare as directed for the *Standard preparation*, in the *Assay* under *Ondansetron Hydrochloride*.

Test solution—Use the *Assay preparation*.

Procedure—Separately inject equal volumes (about 10 µL) of *Standard solution* and the *Test solution* into the chromatograph, record the chromatograms, and measure the peak responses. Calculate the percentage of each related compound in the volume of Oral Solution taken by the formula:

$$(293.36/329.82)10{,}000(1/F)(1/V)(C_S/C_A)(r_i/r_S)$$

in which 293.36 and 329.82 are the molecular weights of ondansetron and anhydrous ondansetron hydrochloride, respectively; F is the relative response factor for each known and unknown impurity (the values of relative response factors [RRF] and the limits can be obtained from *Table 1*); V is the volume, in mL, of Oral Solution taken; C_S is the concentration, in mg per mL, on the anhydrous basis, of USP Ondansetron Hydrochloride RS in the *Standard solution*; C_A is the concentration, in mg per mL, of ondansetron in the Oral Solution; r_i is the peak response for any related compound obtained from the *Test solution*; and r_S is the peak response for ondansetron obtained from the *Standard solution*.

Table 1

Related Compound	Approx. RRT	RRF	Limit (%)
Ondansetron related compound D*	0.34	—	0.1
Imidazole	0.40	0.46	0.2
2-Methyl imidazole	0.53	0.54	0.2
Des-*C*-methyl ondansetron hydrochloride	0.62	0.76	0.2
N-Desmethyl ondansetron maleate	0.83	0.73	0.2
Ondansetron related compound A	1.2	0.81	0.2
Unknown	—	1.0	0.2
Total (including ondansetron related compound D)	—	—	0.5

*Quantified from Limit of related compound D test

Assay—

Mobile phase, System suitability solution, Standard preparation, and *Chromatographic system*—Proceed as directed in the *Assay* under *Ondansetron Hydrochloride*.

Assay preparation—Transfer an accurately measured volume of Oral Solution, equivalent to about 9 mg of ondansetron, to a 100-mL volumetric flask; dilute with *Mobile phase* to volume; and mix.

Chromatographic system (see *Chromatography* ⟨621⟩)—The liquid chromatograph is equipped with a 216-nm detector and a 4.6-mm × 25-cm column that contains packing L10. The flow rate is about 1.5 mL per minute. Chromatograph the *System suitability solution*, and record the peak responses as directed for *Procedure*: the relative retention times are about 1.1 for ondansetron related compound A and 1.0 for ondansetron; and the resolution, R, between ondansetron related compound A and ondansetron is not less than 1.5. Chromatograph the *Standard preparation*, and record the peak responses as directed for *Procedure*: the tailing factor is not more than 2.0, and the relative standard deviation for replicate injections is not more than 2.0%.

Procedure—Separately inject equal volumes (about 10 µL) of the *Standard preparation* and the *Assay preparation* into the chromatograph, record the chromatograms, and measure the responses for the major peaks. Calculate the quantity, in mg, of ondansetron ($C_{18}H_{19}N_3O$) in each mL of Oral Solution taken by the formula:

$$(293.36/329.82)100(C/V)(r_U/r_S)$$

in which 293.36 and 329.82 are the molecular weights of ondansetron and anhydrous ondansetron hydrochloride, respectively; C is the concentration, in mg per mL, on the anhydrous basis, of USP Ondansetron Hydrochloride RS in the *Standard preparation*; V is the volume, in mL, of Oral Solution taken; and r_U and r_S are the peak responses obtained from the *Assay preparation* and the *Standard preparation*, respectively.

Ondansetron Orally Disintegrating Tablets

» Ondansetron Orally Disintegrating Tablets contain the equivalent of not less than 90.0 percent and not more than 110.0 percent of the labeled amount of ondansetron ($C_{18}H_{19}N_3O$).

Packaging and storage—Preserve in light-resistant containers. Store at controlled room temperature.

USP Reference standards ⟨11⟩—*USP Ondansetron RS. USP Ondansetron Related Compound A RS. USP Ondansetron Related Compound D RS.*

Identification—The retention time of the major peak in the chromatogram of the *Assay preparation* corresponds to that in the chromatogram of the *Standard preparation*, as obtained in the *Assay*.

Disintegration: not more than 10 seconds.

Dissolution ⟨711⟩—

Medium: 0.1 N hydrochloric acid; 500 mL, deaerated.
Apparatus 2: 50 rpm.
Time: 10 minutes.

Standard solution—Accurately weigh an amount of USP Ondansetron RS, and dilute with *Medium* to obtain a solution having a final concentration of 0.01 mg per mL for Tablets labeled to contain 4 mg, and a final concentration of 0.02 mg per mL for Tablets labeled to contain 8 mg.

Test solution—Pass a portion of the solution under test through a filter.

Procedure—Determine the amount of $C_{18}H_{19}N_3O$ dissolved by UV absorption at the wavelength of maximum absorbance at about 310 nm on portions of the *Test solution* in comparison with the *Standard solution*, using a 1-cm cell. Calculate the amount, in percentage, of ondansetron released by the formula:

$$\frac{A_U \times W_S \times 500 \times P \times 100}{A_S \times D \times L}$$

in which A_U and A_S are the absorbances obtained from the *Test solution* and the *Standard solution*, respectively; W_S is the weight, in mg, of USP Ondansetron RS taken; 500 is the volume, in mL, of *Medium*; 100 is the conversion factor to percentage; D is the dilution factor of the *Standard solution*; and L is the Tablet label claim, in mg.

Tolerances—Not less than 80% (*Q*) of the labeled amount of $C_{18}H_{19}N_3O$ is dissolved in 10 minutes.

Uniformity of dosage units ⟨905⟩: meet the requirements.

Water ⟨921⟩: not more than 4.0%.

Related compounds—

Phosphate buffer—Prepare as directed in the *Assay*.

Mobile phase—Prepare a filtered and degassed mixture of *Phosphate buffer* and acetonitrile (8 : 2). Make adjustments if necessary (see *System Suitability* under *Chromatography* ⟨621⟩).

Ondansetron related compound D solution—Dissolve an amount of USP Ondansetron Related Compound D RS in acetonitrile, and dilute stepwise with *Mobile phase* to obtain a solution having a known concentration of about 0.04 mg per mL.

2-Methylimidazole solution—Dissolve an amount of 2-methylimidazole in acetonitrile, and dilute quantitatively, and stepwise if necessary, with *Mobile phase* to obtain a solution having a known concentration of about 0.04 mg per mL.

Standard stock solution—Dissolve an accurately weighed quantity of USP Ondansetron RS in acetonitrile, and dilute quantitatively, and stepwise if necessary, with *Mobile phase* to obtain a solution having a known concentration of about 0.04 mg per mL.

System suitability solution—Transfer 5.0 mL each of *Standard stock solution*, *2-Methylimidazole solution*, and *Ondansetron related compound D solution* to a 100-mL volumetric flask. Dilute with *Mobile phase* to volume, and mix.

Standard solution—Pipet 5.0 mL of the *Standard stock solution* into a 100-mL volumetric flask, dilute with *Mobile phase* to volume, and mix.

System sensitivity solution—Pipet 10.0 mL of the *Standard solution* into a 100-mL volumetric flask, dilute with *Mobile phase* to volume, and mix.

Test solution—Transfer 10 Tablets to an appropriate volumetric flask so that the final concentration of ondansetron is about 400 µg per mL. Add *Mobile phase* to fill about 60% of the flask capacity. Shake by mechanical means for about 5 minutes, and dilute with *Mobile phase* to volume. Centrifuge a portion of this solution at 3000 rpm for 10 minutes. Use the supernatant.

Chromatographic system (see *Chromatography* ⟨621⟩)—The liquid chromatograph is equipped with a 216-nm detector and a 4.6-mm × 25-cm column that contains packing L10. The flow rate is about 1.5 mL per minute. Chromatograph the *System suitability solution*, and record the peak responses as directed for *Procedure:* the relative retention times are given in *Table 1;* the resolution, *R*, between ondansetron and any adjacent peak is not less than 1.5; the column efficiency is not less than 8000 theoretical plates for ondansetron; and the tailing factor for the ondansetron peak is not more than 2.0. Chromatograph the *System sensitivity solution,* and record the peak responses as directed for *Procedure:* the signal-to-noise ratio for the ondansetron peak is not less than 15. Chromatograph the *Standard solution,* and record the peak responses as directed for *Procedure:* the relative standard deviation for replicate injections is not more than 5.0%.

Procedure—Inject a volume (about 20 µL) of the *Test solution* and the *Standard solution* into the chromatograph, record the chromatograms, and measure the peak responses. Calculate the percentage of each impurity in the portion of Tablets taken by the formula:

$$100(C/F)(V/D)(r_i / r_S)$$

in which *C* is the concentration, in mg per mL, of USP Ondansetron RS in the *Standard solution; F* is the relative response factor for each impurity as specified in *Table 1; V* is the volume, in mL, of the volumetric flask used to prepare the *Test solution; D* is the amount, in mg, of ondansetron in the sample based on the labeled amount and number of Tablets taken; r_i is the peak area of any impurity in the *Test solution;* and r_S is the peak area of ondansetron in the *Standard solution:* it meets the requirements specified in *Table 1.*

Table 1

Compound Name	Relative Retention Time	Relative Response Factor	Limit (%)
2-Methylimidazole	0.16	0.5	0.15
Ondansetron related compound D	0.45	1.2	0.12
Ondansetron	1.0	—	—
Individual unknown impurity	—	1.0	0.1
Total impurities	—	—	0.5

[NOTE—The run time is about 60 minutes.]

Assay—
Diluent: 0.01 N hydrochloric acid.
Phosphate buffer—Dissolve about 2.72 g of monobasic potassium phosphate in 1000 mL of water. Adjust with 1 N sodium hydroxide or 0.5 N sodium hydroxide to a pH of 5.4.
Mobile phase—Prepare a filtered and degassed mixture of *Phosphate buffer* and acetonitrile (52 : 48). Make adjustments if necessary (see *System Suitability* under *Chromatography* ⟨621⟩).
Ondansetron related compound A solution—Dissolve an amount of USP Ondansetron Related Compound A RS in *Diluent,* and dilute stepwise with *Diluent* to obtain a solution having a known concentration of about 0.14 mg per mL.
Concentrated assay preparation—Transfer 10 Tablets to an appropriate volumetric flask so that the final concentration is about 400 µg of ondansetron per mL. Add *Diluent* to fill about 60% of the flask capacity. Shake by mechanical means for about 5 minutes, and dilute with *Diluent* to volume. Filter a portion of this solution through a 0.45-µm polypropylene membrane, discarding the first 5 mL of the filtrate.
System suitability solution—Transfer 8.0 mL of *Ondansetron related compound A solution* and 8.0 mL of the *Standard preparation* to a 50-mL volumetric flask. Dilute with *Diluent* to volume, and mix.
Standard preparation—Dissolve an accurately weighed quantity of USP Ondansetron RS in *Diluent,* and dilute quantitatively, and stepwise if necessary, with *Diluent* to obtain a solution having a known concentration of about 40 µg per mL.
Assay preparation—Transfer 5.0 mL of the *Concentrated assay preparation* to a 50-mL volumetric flask. Dilute with *Diluent* to volume, and mix.
Chromatographic system (see *Chromatography* ⟨621⟩)—The liquid chromatograph is equipped with a 216-nm detector and a 4.6-mm × 25-cm column that contains packing L10. The flow rate is about 1.5 mL per minute. Chromatograph the *System suitability solution,* and record the peak responses as directed for *Procedure:* the relative retention times are about 1.1 for ondansetron related compound A, and 1.0 for ondansetron; the resolution, *R*, between ondansetron related compound A and ondansetron is not less than 1.5; and the tailing factor is not more than 2.0 for the ondansetron peak. Chromatograph the *Standard preparation,* and record the peak responses as directed for *Procedure:* the relative standard deviation for replicate injections is not more than 2.0%.
Procedure—Separately inject equal volumes (about 10 µL) of the *Standard preparation* and the *Assay preparation* into the chromatograph, record the chromatograms, and measure the responses for the ondansetron peaks. Calculate the quantity, in mg, of ondansetron ($C_{18}H_{19}N_3O$) in the portion of Tablets taken by the formula:

$$(10V)C(r_U / r_S)$$

in which *V* is the volume used to prepare the *Concentrated assay preparation; C* is the concentration, in mg per mL, of USP Ondansetron RS in the *Standard preparation;* and r_U and r_S are the peak responses obtained from the *Assay preparation* and the *Standard preparation,* respectively.

Bland Lubricating Ophthalmic Ointment

» Bland Lubricating Ophthalmic Ointment is a sterile ointment of white petrolatum and mineral oil. It may contain Lanolin, Modified Lanolin, or Lanolin Alcohols. It may also contain a suitable antimicrobial preservative.

Packaging and storage—Preserve in suitable collapsible ophthalmic ointment tubes.
Appearance—Transfer a portion of it to a suitable test tube, and examine the sample in front of a light source: the sample should appear translucent.
Color—Examine the extruded ointment for color: it is colorless to light yellow.
Sterility ⟨71⟩—It meets the requirements when tested as directed for *Membrane Filtration* under *Test for Sterility of the Product to be Examined.*
Homogeneity—Transfer about 250 mg of it to a clean microscope slide and examine for separation: no oily or watery substances should be visibly separated from the ointment. Place a cover slip on the ointment and flatten until light readily passes through the sample. Examine for agglomeration: no solid particles are visible.
Acidity or alkalinity—Transfer 20.0 g of it to a 400-mL beaker, add 100 mL of a 1 in 2 mixture of neutralized alcohol and water, agitate thoroughly, and gradually heat to boiling. Boil for 10 minutes. Add 1 mL of phenolphthalein TS and rapidly titrate, with vigorous agitation, with either 0.1 N sodium hydroxide VS (from a colorless alcohol-water layer to a sharp pink endpoint) or 0.1 N hydrochloric acid VS (from a pink alcohol-water layer to a colorless endpoint): not more than 0.40 mL of 0.1 N titrant is required.
Metal particles—It meets the requirements of the test for *Metal Particles in Ophthalmic Ointments* ⟨751⟩.

Opium

» Opium is the air-dried milky exudate obtained by incising the unripe capsules of *Papaver somniferum* Linné or its variety *album* De Candolle (Fam. Papaveraceae). It yields not less than 9.5 percent of anhydrous morphine.

Botanic characteristics—More or less rounded, oval, brick-shaped or elongated, somewhat flattened masses usually about 8 cm to 15 cm in diameter and weighing about 300 g to 2 kg each. Externally, it is pale olive-brown or olive-gray, having a coarse surface and being covered with a thin coating consisting of fragments of poppy leaves and, at times, with fruits of a species of *Rumex* adhering from the packing; it is more or less plastic when fresh, becoming hard or tough on storage. Internally, it is reddish brown and coarsely granular.

Assay—
Chromatographic tubes, Citrate buffer, and *Standard preparation*—Prepare as directed in the *Assay* under *Paregoric.*

Assay preparation—Transfer about 2 g of Opium, accurately weighed, to a 250-mL beaker, add 20 mL of dimethyl sulfoxide, and heat for 20 minutes on a steam bath, intermittently dispersing the substance with a flat-end stirring rod. Allow to stand for 15 minutes to permit undissolved material to settle, and carefully decant the supernatant into a 100-mL volumetric flask. Add another 20 mL of dimethyl sulfoxide to the residue, rinsing the sides of the beaker with dimethyl sulfoxide. Disperse and heat the substance as before, allow to settle, and decant into the volumetric flask. Repeat the dissolution one or two times, until the opium is dissolved (other than for small leaf fragments, sand-like particles, gelatinous materials, etc.). Rinse the beaker, and transfer the residue to the flask with the aid of water. Dilute with water to about 90 mL, and mix. If necessary, add 1 drop of alcohol to dispel any foam. Cool to room temperature, adjust with water to volume, and mix. Pass the resulting solution through a medium-porosity filter paper, discarding the first 20 mL of the filtrate.

Chromatographic columns—Pack a pledget of glass wool at the base of each of the three tubes, and fill with adsorbent using chromatographic siliceous earth as the base of the adsorbent, and tamping it firmly in place. Prepare the tubes as follows. Pack *Column I* in two layers, the lower layer consisting of 3 g of chromatographic siliceous earth mixed with 2 mL of *Citrate buffer* and the upper layer consisting of 3 g of chromatographic siliceous earth mixed with 2.0 mL of the *Assay preparation* and 0.5 mL of *Citrate buffer.* Dry-rinse the beaker in which the components of the two layers have been mixed with 1 g of chromatographic siliceous earth, and add it also to the top of *Column I.* Pack *Column II* with 3 g of chromatographic siliceous earth mixed with 2 mL of dibasic potassium phosphate solution (1 in 5.75). Pack *Column III* with 3 g of chromatographic siliceous earth mixed with 2 mL of sodium hydroxide solution (1 in 50). Place a small pad of glass wool above each column packing.

Procedure—Proceed as directed in the *Assay* under *Paregoric.* Calculate the percentage of anhydrous morphine in the Opium taken by the formula:

$$0.25(C/W)(A_U/A_S)$$

in which C is the concentration, in μg per mL, of anhydrous morphine in the *Standard preparation;* W is the weight, in g, of Opium taken; and A_U and A_S are the corrected absorbances of the solutions from the *Assay preparation* and the *Standard preparation,* respectively.

Powdered Opium

» Powdered Opium is Opium dried at a temperature not exceeding 70°, and reduced to a very fine powder. Powdered Opium yields not less than 10.0 percent and not more than 10.5 percent of anhydrous morphine. It may contain any of the diluents, with the exception of starch, permitted for powdered extracts under *Extracts* ⟨1151⟩.

Packaging and storage—Preserve in well-closed containers.

Botanic characteristics—Consists chiefly of yellowish brown to yellow, more or less irregular and granular fragments of latex, varying from 15 to 150 μm in diameter; a few fragments of strongly lignified, thick-walled, 4- to 5-sided or narrowly elongated, epidermal cells of the poppy capsule; very few fragments of tissues of poppy leaves, poppy capsules, and, occasionally, *Rumex* fruits. In addition, there will be the microscopic characteristics of the diluent if any has been used in the preparation of the powder.

Assay—Proceed with Powdered Opium as directed in the *Assay* under *Opium.*

Opium Tincture

» Opium Tincture contains, in each 100 mL, not less than 0.90 g and not more than 1.10 g of anhydrous morphine.

Opium Tincture may be prepared as follows.

Place 100 g of granulated or sliced Opium in a suitable vessel. [NOTE—Do not use Powdered Opium.] Add 500 mL of boiling water, and allow to stand, with frequent stirring, for 24 hours. Transfer the mixture to a percolator, allow it to drain, percolate with water as the menstruum to complete extraction, and evaporate the percolate to a volume of 400 mL. Boil actively for not less than 15 minutes, and allow to stand overnight. Heat the mixture to 80°, add 50 g of paraffin, and heat until the paraffin is melted. Beat the mixture thoroughly, and cool.

Remove the paraffin, and filter the concentrate, washing the paraffin and the filter with sufficient water to make the filtrate measure 750 mL. Add 188 mL of alcohol to the filtrate, mix, and assay a 10-mL portion of the resulting solution as directed in the *Assay.* Dilute the remaining solution with a mixture of 1 volume of alcohol and 4 volumes of water to obtain a Tincture containing 1 g of anhydrous morphine in each 100 mL. Mix.

Packaging and storage—Preserve in tight, light-resistant containers, and avoid exposure to direct sunlight and to excessive heat.

Alcohol content ⟨611⟩: between 17.0% and 21.0% of C_2H_5OH, determined by the gas-liquid procedure, acetone being used as the internal standard.

Assay—
Chromatographic tubes, Citrate buffer, Standard preparation, and *Chromatographic columns*—Prepare as directed in the *Assay* under *Paregoric.*

Assay preparation—Transfer 10.0 mL of Tincture to a 50-mL volumetric flask containing 10.0 mL of alcohol, add purified water to volume, and mix. Transfer a 2.0-mL aliquot of the solution, equivalent to about 4 mg of Morphine, to a 50-mL beaker, and add 0.5 mL of *Citrate buffer.*

Procedure—Proceed as directed for *Procedure* in the *Assay* under *Paregoric.* Calculate the weight of anhydrous morphine, in g per 100 mL of the Tincture taken by the formula:

$$0.250W(A_U/A_S)$$

in which W is the weight, in mg, of anhydrous morphine in the 50 mL of *Standard preparation,* and A_U and A_S are the corrected ab-

Orphenadrine Citrate

C₁₈H₂₃NO · C₆H₈O₇   461.50
Ethanamine, N,N-dimethyl-2-[(2-methylphenyl)phenylmethoxy]-, (±)-, 2-hydroxy-1,2,3-propanetricarboxylate (1 : 1).
(±)-N,N-Dimethyl-2-[(o-methyl-α-phenylbenzyl)oxy]ethylamine citrate (1 : 1)   [4682-36-4].

» Orphenadrine Citrate contains not less than 98.0 percent and not more than 101.5 percent of C₁₈H₂₃NO · C₆H₈O₇, calculated on the dried basis.

Packaging and storage—Preserve in tight, light-resistant containers.

USP Reference standards ⟨11⟩—*USP Orphenadrine Citrate RS*.

Clarity and color of solution—Mix 1 g of it with 10 mL of a 1 in 28 solution of hydrochloric acid in alcohol: the solution is clear and its absorbance at 436 nm is not greater than 0.050.

Identification—

   A: *Infrared Absorption* ⟨197M⟩.

   B: *Ultraviolet Absorption* ⟨197U⟩—

   Solution: 500 µg per mL.

   Medium: alcohol.

   Absorptivities at 264 nm, calculated on the dried basis, do not differ by more than 3.0%.

Melting range ⟨741⟩: between 134° and 138°.

Loss on drying ⟨731⟩—Dry it at 105° for 3 hours: it loses not more than 0.5% of its weight.

Residue on ignition ⟨281⟩: not more than 0.1%.

Related compounds—

0.05 M Ammonium phosphate buffer, Mobile phase, System sensitivity solution, and *Chromatographic system*—Prepare as directed in the *Assay*.

Standard solution—Use the *Standard preparation*, prepared as directed in the *Assay*.

Test solution—Use the *Assay preparation*, prepared as directed in the *Assay*.

Procedure—Separately inject equal volumes (about 20 µL) of the *Test solution* and the *Standard solution* into the chromatograph, record the chromatogram for at least 2.5 times the retention time of orphenadrine citrate, and measure all of the peak areas. Calculate the percentage of each impurity in the portion of Orphenadrine Citrate taken by the formula:

$$5000F(C/W)(r_i/r_S)$$

in which *C* is the concentration, in mg per mL, of USP Orphenadrine Citrate RS in the *Standard solution*; *W* is the weight, in mg, of the sample taken to prepare the *Test solution*; *F* is the relative response factor described in the table below; r_i is the peak area for each impurity in the *Test solution*; and r_S is the peak area of Orphenadrine Citrate in the *Standard solution*: not more than 0.5% of total impurities is found.

Compound name	Relative Retention Time	Relative Response Factor
Ethyldimethyl [2-(2-methylbenzhydryloxy)ethyl] ammonium chloride	0.25	0.75
2-Methylbenzhydrol	0.51	0.41
Orphenadrine Citrate	1.0	—
N,N-Dimethyl-2-(o-tolyl-o-xyly-loxy)ethylamine	1.54	0.52
Others	—	1.0

Organic volatile impurities, Method I ⟨467⟩: meets the requirements.

(Official until July 1, 2008)

Isomer content—

Solvent—Use carbon tetrachloride.

NMR reference—Use tetramethylsilane.

Test preparation—Place about 1 g of Orphenadrine Citrate and 10 mL of water in a 60-mL separator, slowly add about 20 drops of sodium hydroxide solution (1 in 2), with swirling, to obtain a solution having a pH of about 10, and extract with three 15-mL portions of ether. Combine the ether extracts in a beaker, discarding the aqueous phase, and evaporate to about one-half the volume by warming on a steam bath under a stream of nitrogen. Transfer to a 60-mL separator, wash with three 20-mL portions of water, and dry the ether solution with about 15 g of anhydrous sodium sulfate in a 125-mL conical flask for 1 hour, with intermittent swirling. Decant the dried ether solution through a pledget of glass wool into a small beaker. Rinse the sodium sulfate with two 10-mL portions of ether, and add the rinsings to the beaker. Evaporate most of the ether by warming under a stream of nitrogen, and remove the last traces of ether by drying at a pressure not exceeding 2 mm of mercury at 60°. Transfer 400 mg of the orphenadrine so obtained to a small weighing bottle, add 0.5 mL of carbon tetrachloride and 1 drop of tetramethylsilane, and swirl to dissolve.

Procedure—Proceed as directed for *Relative Method of Quantitation* under *Nuclear Magnetic Resonance* ⟨761⟩, using the calculation formula given therein, in which A_1 is the sum of the average areas of the combined methine peaks associated with the *meta*- and *para*-methylbenzyl isomers, appearing at about 5.23 ppm, and A_2 is the area of the methine peak associated with the *ortho*-methylbenzyl isomer, appearing at about 5.47 ppm, with reference to the tetramethylsilane singlet at 0 ppm, and both n_1 and n_2 are equal to 1: the limit of combined *meta*-and *para*-methylbenzyl isomers is 3.0%.

Assay—

0.05 M Ammonium phosphate buffer—Dissolve 5.8 g of monobasic ammonium phosphate in 1000 mL of water, and adjust with ammonium hydroxide or phosphoric acid to a pH of 7.9 ± 0.05.

Mobile phase—Prepare a filtered and degassed mixture of methanol, *0.05 M Ammonium phosphate buffer*, and acetonitrile (9 : 8 : 3). Make adjustments if necessary (see *System Suitability* under *Chromatography* ⟨621⟩).

Standard preparation—Dissolve an accurately weighed quantity of USP Orphenadrine Citrate RS in *Mobile phase*, and dilute quantitatively, and stepwise if necessary, with *Mobile phase* to obtain a solution having a known concentration of about 0.9 mg per mL.

System sensitivity solution—Dilute a volume of the *Standard preparation* quantitatively, and stepwise if necessary, with *Mobile phase* to obtain a solution having a known concentration of about 0.00045 mg per mL.

Assay preparation—Transfer about 45 mg of Orphenadrine Citrate, accurately weighed, to a 50-mL volumetric flask, dissolve in and dilute with *Mobile phase* to volume, and mix.

Chromatographic system (see *Chromatography* ⟨621⟩)—The liquid chromatograph is equipped with a 220-nm detector and a 4.6-mm × 15-cm column that contains 5-µm packing L1. The flow rate is about 1.5 mL per minute. The column temperature is maintained at 40°. Chromatograph the *Standard preparation*, and record the peak areas as directed for *Procedure*: the column efficiency is not less than 4500 theoretical plates; the tailing factor is not more than 2.0; and the relative standard deviation for replicate injections is not more than 2.0%. Chromatograph the *System sensitivity solution*, and record the peak areas as directed for *Procedure:* the signal-to-noise ratio is not less than 10.

Procedure—Separately inject equal volumes (about 20 µL) of the *Standard preparation* and the *Assay preparation* into the chromatograph, record the chromatograms, and measure the peak areas for orphenadrine citrate. Calculate the quantity, in mg, of $C_{18}H_{23}NO \cdot C_6H_8O_7$ in the portion of Orphenadrine Citrate taken by the formula:

$$50C(r_U/r_S)$$

in which C is the concentration, in mg per mL, of USP Orphenadrine Citrate RS in the *Standard preparation;* and r_U and r_S are the peak responses obtained from the *Assay preparation* and the *Standard preparation,* respectively.

Orphenadrine Citrate Injection

» Orphenadrine Citrate Injection is a sterile solution of Orphenadrine Citrate in Water for Injection, prepared with the aid of Sodium Hydroxide. It contains not less than 93.0 percent and not more than 107.0 percent of the labeled amount of orphenadrine citrate ($C_{18}H_{23}NO \cdot C_6H_8O_7$).

Packaging and storage—Preserve in single-dose or multiple-dose containers, preferably of Type I glass, protected from light.
USP Reference standards ⟨11⟩—USP Endotoxin RS. USP Orphenadrine Citrate RS.
Identification—
A: The retention time of the major peak in the chromatogram of the *Assay preparation* corresponds to that in the chromatogram of the *Standard preparation,* as obtained in the *Assay.*
B: A few drops of Injection respond to the test for *Citrate* ⟨191⟩.
Bacterial endotoxins ⟨85⟩—It contains not more than 5.8 USP Endotoxin Units per mg of orphenadrine citrate.
pH ⟨791⟩: between 5.0 and 6.0.
Related compounds—
0.05 M Ammonium phosphate buffer, Mobile phase, System sensitivity solution, and *Chromatographic system*—Prepare as directed in the *Assay.*
Standard solution—Use the *Standard preparation,* prepared as directed in the *Assay.*
Test solution—Use the *Assay preparation,* prepared as directed in the *Assay.*
Procedure—Separately inject equal volumes (about 20 µL) of the *Test solution* and the *Standard solution* into the chromatograph, record the chromatogram for at least 2.5 times the retention time of orphenadrine citrate, and measure all of the peak areas. Calculate the percentage of each impurity in the portion of Injection taken by the formula:

$$(10{,}000F)(C/V)(1/D)(r_i/r_S)$$

in which F is the relative response factor as found in the table below; C is the concentration, in mg per mL, of USP Orphenadrine Citrate RS in the *Standard solution;* V is the volume, in mL, of Injection taken to prepare the *Test solution;* D is the labeled dose of Injection; r_i is the peak area for each impurity in the *Test solution;* and r_S is the peak area of Orphenadrine Citrate in the *Standard solution:* not more than 4.0% of total impurities is found.

Compound name	Relative Retention Time	Relative Response Factor
Ethyldimethyl [2-(2-methylbenzhydryloxy-)ethyl] ammonium chloride	0.25	0.75
2-Methylbenzhydrol	0.51	0.41

Compound name	Relative Retention Time	Relative Response Factor
Orphenadrine Citrate	1.0	—
N,N-Dimethyl-2-(o-tolyl-o-xylyloxy)ethylamine	1.54	0.52
Others	—	1.0

Other requirements—It meets the requirements under *Injections* ⟨1⟩.
Assay—
0.05 M Ammonium phosphate buffer—Dissolve 5.8 g of monobasic ammonium phosphate in 1000 mL of water, and adjust with ammonium hydroxide or phosphoric acid to a pH of 7.9 ± 0.05.
Mobile phase—Prepare a filtered and degassed mixture of methanol, *0.05 M Ammonium phosphate buffer,* and acetonitrile (9 : 8 : 3). Make adjustments if necessary (see *System Suitability* under *Chromatography* ⟨621⟩).
Standard preparation—Dissolve an accurately weighed quantity of USP Orphenadrine Citrate RS in water, and dilute quantitatively, and stepwise if necessary, with water to obtain a solution having a known concentration of about 0.9 mg per mL.
System sensitivity solution—Dilute a volume of the *Standard preparation* quantitatively, and stepwise if necessary, with water to obtain a solution having a known concentration of about 0.00045 mg per mL.
Assay preparation—Transfer an accurately measured volume of Injection, equivalent to about 90 mg of orphenadrine citrate, to a 100-mL volumetric flask, dilute with water to volume, and mix.
Chromatographic system (see *Chromatography* ⟨621⟩)—The liquid chromatograph is equipped with a 220-nm detector and a 4.6-mm × 15-cm column that contains 5-µm packing L1. The flow rate is about 1.5 mL per minute. The column temperature is maintained at 40°. Chromatograph the *Standard preparation,* and record the peak areas as directed for *Procedure:* the column efficiency is not less than 4500 theoretical plates; the tailing factor is not more than 2.0; and the relative standard deviation for replicate injections is not more than 2.0%. Chromatograph the *System sensitivity solution,* and record the peak areas as directed for *Procedure:* the signal-to-noise ratio is not less than 10.
Procedure—Separately inject equal volumes (about 20 µL) of the *Standard preparation* and the *Assay preparation* into the chromatograph, record the chromatograms, and measure the peak areas for orphenadrine citrate. Calculate the quantity, in mg, of orphenadrine citrate ($C_{18}H_{23}NO \cdot C_6H_8O_7$) in each mL of the Injection taken by the formula:

$$(100C/V)(r_U/r_S)$$

in which C is the concentration, in mg per mL, of USP Orphenadrine Citrate RS in the *Standard preparation;* V is the volume, in mL, of Injection taken; and r_U and r_S are the peak responses obtained from the *Assay preparation* and the *Standard preparation,* respectively.

Oxacillin Sodium

$C_{19}H_{18}N_3NaO_5S \cdot H_2O$ 441.43
4-Thia-1-azabicyclo[3.2.0]heptane-2-carboxylic acid, 3,3-dimethyl-6-[[(5-methyl-3-phenyl-4-isoxazolyl)carbonyl]amino]-7-oxo-, monosodium salt, monohydrate, [2*S*-(2α,5α,6β)]-.
Monosodium (2*S*,5*R*,6*R*)-3,3-dimethyl-6-(5-methyl-3-phenyl-4-isoxazolecarboxamido)-7-oxo-4-thia-1-azabicyclo[3.2.0]heptane-2-carboxylate monohydrate   [7240-38-2].
Anhydrous   423.43   [1173-88-2].

» Oxacillin Sodium contains the equivalent of not less than 815 µg and not more than 950 µg of oxacillin ($C_{19}H_{19}N_3O_5S$) per mg.

Packaging and storage—Preserve in tight containers, at controlled room temperature.
Labeling—Where it is intended for use in preparing injectable dosage forms, the label states that it is sterile or must be subjected to further processing during the preparation of injectable dosage forms.
USP Reference standards ⟨11⟩—*USP Endotoxin RS. USP Oxacillin Sodium RS.*
Identification—
  A: The chromatogram of the *Assay preparation* obtained as directed in the *Assay* exhibits a major peak for oxacillin, the retention time of which corresponds to that exhibited in the chromatogram of the *Standard preparation* obtained as directed in the *Assay.*
  B: It responds to the tests for *Sodium* ⟨191⟩.
Crystallinity ⟨695⟩: meets the requirements.
pH ⟨791⟩: between 4.5 and 7.5, in a solution containing 30 mg per mL.
Water, *Method I* ⟨921⟩: between 3.5% and 5.0%.
Other requirements—Where the label states that Oxacillin Sodium is sterile, it meets the requirements for *Sterility* and *Bacterial endotoxins* under *Oxacillin for Injection*. Where the label states that Oxacillin Sodium must be subjected to further processing during the preparation of injectable dosage forms, it meets the requirements for *Bacterial endotoxins* under *Oxacillin for Injection.*
Assay—
  Mobile phase—Dissolve 1.9 g of monobasic potassium phosphate in 700 mL of water. Add 300 mL of acetonitrile and 100 mL of methanol, and mix. Filter this solution through a 0.5-µm or finer porosity filter, and degas. Make adjustments if necessary (see *System Suitability* under *Chromatography* ⟨621⟩).
  Standard preparation—Dissolve an accurately weighed quantity of USP Oxacillin Sodium RS in water to obtain a solution having a known concentration of about 0.11 mg per mL. [NOTE—Use this *Standard preparation* on the day prepared.]
  Assay preparation—Transfer about 115 mg of Oxacillin Sodium, accurately weighed, to a 200-mL volumetric flask, add water to volume, and mix. Stir with the aid of a magnetic stirrer for 5 minutes to ensure dissolution of the specimen. Transfer 10.0 mL of this solution to a 50-mL volumetric flask, dilute with water to volume, and mix. [NOTE—Use this *Assay preparation* on the day prepared.]
  Chromatographic system (see *Chromatography* ⟨621⟩)—The liquid chromatograph is equipped with a 225-nm detector and a 4-mm × 30-cm column that contains packing L11. The flow rate is about 2 mL per minute. Chromatograph the *Standard preparation*, and record the responses as directed for *Procedure:* the column efficiency is not less than 2000 theoretical plates, the tailing factor is not more than 1.6, and the relative standard deviation for replicate injections is not more than 2.0%.
  Procedure—[NOTE—Use peak areas where peak responses are indicated.] Separately inject equal volumes (about 10 µL) of the *Standard preparation* and the *Assay preparation* into the chromatograph, record the chromatograms, and measure the responses for the major peaks. Calculate the quantity, in µg, of oxacillin ($C_{19}H_{19}N_3O_5S$) in each mg of the Oxacillin Sodium taken by the formula:

$$1000(CE / W)(r_U / r_S)$$

in which C is the concentration, in mg per mL, of USP Oxacillin Sodium RS in the *Standard preparation*; E is the oxacillin equivalent, in µg per mg, of USP Oxacillin Sodium RS; W is the weight, in mg, of the portion of Oxacillin Sodium taken; and r_U and r_S are the oxacillin peak responses obtained from the *Assay preparation* and the *Standard preparation*, respectively.

Oxacillin Sodium Capsules

» Oxacillin Sodium Capsules contain the equivalent of not less than 90.0 percent and not more than 120.0 percent of the labeled amount of oxacillin ($C_{19}H_{19}N_3O_5S$).

Packaging and storage—Preserve in tight containers, at controlled room temperature.
USP Reference standards ⟨11⟩—*USP Oxacillin Sodium RS.*
Identification—The chromatogram of the *Assay preparation* obtained as directed in the *Assay* exhibits a major peak for oxacillin, the retention time of which corresponds to that exhibited in the chromatogram of the *Standard preparation* obtained as directed in the *Assay.*
Dissolution ⟨711⟩—
  Medium: water; 900 mL.
  Apparatus 1: 100 rpm.
  Time: 45 minutes.
  Procedure—Determine the amount of oxacillin ($C_{19}H_{19}N_3O_5S$) by a suitable validated spectrophotometric analysis of a filtered portion of the solution under test, suitably diluted with *Dissolution Medium*, if necessary, in comparison with a Standard solution having a known concentration of USP Oxacillin Sodium RS in the same medium.
  Tolerances—Not less than 75% (Q) of the labeled amount of $C_{19}H_{19}N_3O_5S$ is dissolved in 45 minutes.
Uniformity of dosage units ⟨905⟩: meet the requirements.
Water, *Method I* ⟨921⟩: not more than 6.0%.
Assay—
  Mobile phase, Standard preparation, and *Chromatographic system*—Proceed as directed in the *Assay* under *Oxacillin Sodium.*
  Assay preparation—Remove, as completely as possible, the contents of not less than 10 Capsules, and weigh. Mix, and transfer an accurately weighed portion of the powder, equivalent to about 100 mg of oxacillin ($C_{19}H_{19}N_3O_5S$), to a 200-mL volumetric flask, add water to volume, and mix for 10 minutes with the aid of a magnetic stirrer. Filter about 25 mL of the resulting solution, discarding the first 5 mL of the filtrate. Transfer 10.0 mL of the clear filtrate to a 50-mL volumetric flask, dilute with water to volume, and mix. [NOTE—Use this *Assay preparation* on the day prepared.]
  Procedure—Proceed as directed for *Procedure* in the *Assay* under *Oxacillin Sodium*. Calculate the quantity, in mg, of oxacillin ($C_{19}H_{19}N_3O_5S$) in the portion of Capsule contents taken by the formula:

$$CE(r_U / r_S)$$

in which the terms are as defined therein.

Oxacillin Injection

» Oxacillin Injection is a sterile isoosmotic solution of Oxacillin Sodium in Water for Injection. It contains the equivalent of not less than 90.0 percent and not more than 115.0 percent of the labeled amount of oxacillin ($C_{19}H_{19}N_3O_5S$). It contains dextrose as a tonicity-adjusting agent and one or more suitable buffer substances. It contains no preservatives.

Packaging and storage—Preserve in *Containers for Injections* as described under *Injections* ⟨1⟩. Maintain in the frozen state.
Labeling—It meets the requirements for *Labeling* under *Injections* ⟨1⟩. The label states that it is to be thawed just prior to use, describes conditions for proper storage of the resultant solution, and directs that the solution is not to be refrozen.
USP Reference standards ⟨11⟩—*USP Oxacillin Sodium RS.*
Identification—The chromatogram of the *Assay preparation* obtained as directed in the *Assay* exhibits a major peak for oxacillin, the retention time of which corresponds to that exhibited in the

chromatogram of the *Standard preparation* obtained as directed in the *Assay.*
Pyrogen—It meets the requirements of the *Pyrogen Test* ⟨151⟩, the test dose being a volume of undiluted Injection providing the equivalent of 20 mg of oxacillin per kg.
Sterility ⟨71⟩—It meets the requirements when tested as directed for *Membrane Filtration* under *Test for Sterility of the Product to be Examined.*
pH ⟨791⟩: between 6.0 and 8.5.
Particulate matter ⟨788⟩: meets the requirements for small-volume injections.
Assay—
  Mobile phase, Standard preparation, and *Chromatographic system*—Proceed as directed in the *Assay* under *Oxacillin Sodium.*
  Assay preparation—Allow one container of Injection to thaw, and mix. Transfer an accurately measured volume of Injection, equivalent to about 50 mg of oxacillin, to a 100-mL volumetric flask, dilute with water to volume, and mix. Transfer 10.0 mL of this solution to a 50-mL volumetric flask, dilute with water to volume, and mix. [NOTE—Use this *Assay preparation* on the day prepared.]
  Procedure—Proceed as directed for *Procedure* in the *Assay* under *Oxacillin Sodium.* Calculate the quantity, in mg, of oxacillin ($C_{19}H_{19}N_3O_5S$) in each mL of the Injection taken by the formula:

$$0.5(CE/V)(r_U/r_S)$$

in which *C* is the concentration, in mg per mL, of USP Oxacillin Sodium RS in the *Standard preparation,* *E* is the oxacillin equivalent, in μg per mg, of USP Oxacillin Sodium RS, *V* is the volume, in mL, of Injection taken to prepare the *Assay preparation,* and r_U and r_S are the oxacillin peak responses obtained from the *Assay preparation* and the *Standard preparation,* respectively.

Oxacillin for Injection

» Oxacillin for Injection contains an amount of Oxacillin Sodium equivalent to not less than 90.0 percent and not more than 115.0 percent of the labeled amount of oxacillin ($C_{19}H_{19}N_3O_5S$).

Packaging and storage—Preserve in *Containers for Sterile Solids* as described under *Injections* ⟨1⟩, at controlled room temperature.
USP Reference standards ⟨11⟩—*USP Endotoxin RS. USP Oxacillin Sodium RS.*
Constituted solution—At the time of use, it meets the requirements for *Constituted Solutions* under *Injections* ⟨1⟩.
Identification—The retention time of the oxacillin peak in the chromatogram of the *Assay preparation* corresponds to that in the chromatogram of the *Standard preparation,* as obtained in the *Assay.*
Bacterial endotoxins ⟨85⟩—It contains not more than 0.2 USP Endotoxin Unit per mg of oxacillin.
Sterility ⟨71⟩—It meets the requirements when tested as directed for *Membrane Filtration* under *Test for Sterility of the Product to be Examined.*
Uniformity of dosage units ⟨905⟩: meets the requirements.
  Procedure for content uniformity—Perform the *Assay* on individual containers using *Assay preparation 1* or *Assay preparation 2,* or both, as appropriate.
pH ⟨791⟩: between 6.0 and 8.5, in the solution constituted as directed in the labeling.
Water, *Method I* ⟨921⟩: not more than 6.0%.
Particulate matter ⟨788⟩: meets the requirements for small-volume injections.
Assay—
  Mobile phase, Standard preparation, and *Chromatographic system*—Proceed as directed in the *Assay* under *Oxacillin Sodium.*
  Assay preparation 1 (where it is represented as being in a single-dose container)—Constitute Oxacillin for Injection in a volume of water, accurately measured, corresponding to the volume of solvent specified in the labeling. Withdraw all of the withdrawable contents using a suitable hypodermic needle and syringe, and dilute quantitatively, and stepwise if necessary, with water to obtain a solution containing about 0.1 mg per mL of oxacillin. [NOTE—Use this solution on the day prepared.]
  Assay preparation 2 (where the label states the quantity of oxacillin in a given volume of constituted solution)—Constitute Oxacillin for Injection with a volume of water, accurately measured, corresponding to the volume of solvent specified in the labeling. Dilute an accurately measured volume of the constituted solution quantitatively, and stepwise if necessary, with water to obtain a solution containing about 0.1 mg per mL of oxacillin ($C_{19}H_{19}N_3O_5S$). [NOTE—Use this solution on the day prepared.]
  Procedure—Proceed as directed in the *Assay* under *Oxacillin Sodium.* Calculate the quantity, in mg, of oxacillin ($C_{19}H_{19}N_3O_5S$) in the constituted solution taken by the formula:

$$(L/D)(CE/1000)(r_U/r_S)$$

in which *L* is the labeled quantity, in mg, of oxacillin in the container or in the volume of constituted solution taken; *D* is the concentration, in mg per mL, of oxacillin in *Assay preparation 1* or in *Assay preparation 2,* on the basis of the labeled quantity in the container or in the volume of constituted solution taken, respectively; *C* is the concentration, in mg per mL, of USP Oxacillin Sodium RS in the *Standard preparation; E* is the oxacillin equivalent, in μg per mg, of USP Oxacillin Sodium RS; and r_U and r_S are the oxacillin peak responses obtained from the *Assay preparation* and the *Standard preparation,* respectively. Where the test for *Uniformity of dosage units* has been performed using the *Procedure for content uniformity,* use the average of these determinations as the *Assay* value.

Oxacillin Sodium for Oral Solution

» Oxacillin Sodium for Oral Solution contains the equivalent of not less than 90.0 percent and not more than 120.0 percent of the labeled amount of oxacillin ($C_{19}H_{19}N_3O_5S$). It contains one or more suitable buffers, colors, flavors, preservatives, and stabilizers.

Packaging and storage—Preserve in tight containers at controlled room temperature.
USP Reference standards ⟨11⟩—*USP Oxacillin Sodium RS.*
Identification—The chromatogram of the *Assay preparation* obtained as directed in the *Assay* exhibits a major peak for oxacillin, the retention time of which corresponds to that exhibited in the chromatogram of the *Standard preparation* obtained as directed in the *Assay.*
Uniformity of dosage units ⟨905⟩—
  FOR SOLID PACKAGED IN SINGLE-UNIT CONTAINERS: meets the requirements.
Deliverable volume ⟨698⟩: meets the requirements.
pH ⟨791⟩: between 5.0 and 7.5, in the solution constituted as directed in the labeling.
Water, *Method I* ⟨921⟩: not more than 1.0%.
Assay—
  Mobile phase and *Chromatographic system*—Proceed as directed in the *Assay* under *Oxacillin Sodium.*
  Diluent—Prepare a mixture of water and acetonitrile (700 : 300).
  Standard preparation—Prepare a solution of USP Oxacillin Sodium RS in *Diluent* having a known concentration of about 0.11 mg per mL. [NOTE—Use this solution on the day prepared.]
  Assay preparation—Transfer an accurately measured volume of Oxacillin Sodium for Oral Solution, constituted as directed in the labeling, equivalent to about 250 mg of oxacillin ($C_{19}H_{19}N_3O_5S$), to a 250-mL volumetric flask, dilute with water to volume, and mix. Transfer 5.0 mL of this solution to a 50-mL volumetric flask, dilute with *Diluent* to volume, and mix. Filter about 5 mL of this solution through a 0.5-μm or finer porosity filter, discarding the first 2 mL of the filtrate. Use the clear filtrate as the *Assay preparation.* [NOTE—Use this *Assay preparation* on the day prepared.]

Procedure—Proceed as directed for *Procedure* in the *Assay* under *Oxacillin Sodium*. Calculate the quantity, in mg, of oxacillin ($C_{19}H_{19}N_3O_5S$) in each mL of the constituted Oxacillin Sodium for Oral Solution taken by the formula:

$$2.5(CE / V)(r_U / r_S)$$

in which *V* is the volume, in mL, of the constituted Oxacillin Sodium for Oral Solution taken, and the other terms are as defined therein.

Oxandrolone

$C_{19}H_{30}O_3$ 306.44
2-Oxaandrostan-3-one, 17-hydroxy-17-methyl-, (5α,17β)-.
17β-Hydroxy-17-methyl-2-oxa-5α-androstan-3-one   [53-39-4].

» Oxandrolone contains not less than 98.0 percent and not more than 102.0 percent of $C_{19}H_{30}O_3$, calculated on the dried basis.

Packaging and storage—Preserve in well-closed, light-resistant containers.
USP Reference standards ⟨11⟩—*USP Oxandrolone RS. USP Oxandrolone Related Compound A RS. USP Oxandrolone Related Compound B RS. USP Oxandrolone Related Compound C RS.*
Identification—
  A: *Infrared Absorption* ⟨197K⟩.
  B: The retention time of the major peak in the chromatogram of the *Assay preparation* corresponds to that in the chromatogram of the *Standard preparation*, as obtained in the *Assay*.
Specific rotation ⟨781S⟩: between −18° and −24°.
  Test solution: 10 mg per mL, in chloroform.
Loss on drying ⟨731⟩—Dry it at 105° for 3 hours: it loses not more than 1.0% of its weight.
Residue on ignition ⟨281⟩: not more than 0.2%.
Ordinary impurities ⟨466⟩—
  Test solution: methanol.
  Standard solution: methanol.
  Application volume: 10 µL.
  Eluant: a mixture of toluene and isopropyl alcohol (90 : 10), in a nonequilibrated chamber.
  Visualization: 5.
Organic volatile impurities, *Method V* ⟨467⟩: meets the requirements.
  Solvent—Use dimethyl sulfoxide.

(Official until July 1, 2008)

Assay—
  Mobile phase—Prepare a filtered and degassed mixture of water and acetonitrile (50 : 50). Make adjustments if necessary (see *System Suitability* under *Chromatography* ⟨621⟩).
  System suitability solution—Weigh accurately 30 mg of USP Oxandrolone RS, and place into a 10-mL volumetric flask. Dissolve in and dilute with acetonitrile to volume, and mix.
  Standard preparation—Dissolve an accurately weighed quantity of USP Oxandrolone RS in acetonitrile, and dilute quantitatively, and stepwise if necessary, with acetonitrile to obtain a solution having a known concentration of about 3 mg per mL. [NOTE—Sonicate if necessary to dissolve.]
  Assay preparation—Transfer to a suitable volumetric flask an accurately weighed quantity of Oxandrolone, and dissolve in and dilute with acetonitrile to volume to obtain a solution having a concentration of about 3 mg per mL.
  Chromatographic system (see *Chromatography* ⟨621⟩)—The liquid chromatograph is equipped with a 210-nm detector and a 4.6-mm × 25-cm column that contains packing L1. The flow rate is about 0.8 mL per minute. Chromatograph the *Standard preparation* and the *System suitability solution*, and record the peak responses as directed for *Procedure*: the column efficiency is not less than 2000 theoretical plates; the tailing factor is not more than 2.0; and the relative standard deviation for replicate injections is not more than 2.0%.
  Procedure—Separately inject equal volumes (about 20 µL) of the *Standard preparation* and the *Assay preparation* into the chromatograph, record the chromatograms, and measure the responses for the major peaks. Calculate the quantity, in mg, of $C_{19}H_{30}O_3$ in the portion of Oxandrolone taken by the formula:

$$VC(r_U / r_S)$$

in which *V* is the final volume, in mL, of the *Assay preparation*; *C* is the concentration, in mg per mL, of USP Oxandrolone RS in the *Standard preparation*; and r_U and r_S are the peak responses obtained from the *Assay preparation* and the *Standard preparation*, respectively.

Oxandrolone Tablets

» Oxandrolone Tablets contain not less than 92.0 percent and not more than 108.0 percent of the labeled amount of oxandrolone ($C_{19}H_{30}O_3$).

Packaging and storage—Preserve in tight, light-resistant containers.
Labeling—When more than one *Dissolution Test* is given, the labeling states the *Dissolution Test* used only if *Test 1* is not used.
USP Reference standards ⟨11⟩—*USP Oxandrolone RS.*
Identification—Transfer a portion of finely powdered Tablets, equivalent to about 20 mg of oxandrolone, to a 50-mL stoppered centrifuge tube, add 4 mL of chloroform, shake by mechanical means for 10 minutes, centrifuge for about 15 minutes, and filter a portion of the chloroform layer: the filtrate responds to *Identification test B* under *Oxandrolone*, beginning with "Apply 10 µL each of this solution."

Change to read:
Dissolution ⟨711⟩—
  TEST 1—
  Medium: a solution of water and isopropanol (7 : 3); 500 mL.
  Apparatus 2: 100 rpm.
  Time: 60 minutes.
  Determine the amount of $C_{19}H_{30}O_3$ dissolved by employing the following method.
  Internal standard solution—Dissolve accurately weighed quantities of 17α-methyltestosterone, and dilute quantitatively, and stepwise if necessary, with acetonitrile to obtain a solution having a concentration of about 0.2 mg per mL (for Tablets with a 2.5-mg label claim) and about 0.8 mg per mL (for Tablets with a 10-mg label claim).
  Standard solution—Dissolve an accurately weighed quantity of USP Oxandrolone RS, and dilute quantitatively, and stepwise if necessary, with acetonitrile to obtain a solution having a concentration of about 1 mg per mL.
  Working standard solution—For Tablets labeled to contain 2.5 mg: combine 100 µL of the *Standard solution,* 400 µL of the *Internal standard solution,* and 1500 µL of acetonitrile. For Tablets labeled to contain 10 mg: combine 100 µL of the *Standard solution,* 100 µL of the *Internal standard solution,* and 1800 µL of acetonitrile.
  Test solution—Withdraw 25 mL of the solution under test from the vessel. Pass through a 0.45-µm polytef filter. Transfer 20 mL of the filtrate to a separatory funnel, add 400 µL of the *Internal standard solution,* 40 mL of a 10% potassium chloride solution, and 8 mL of chloroform. In separate separatory funnels, prepare an extraction blank and an internal standard blank in a similar manner using 20 mL of filtered *Medium* in place of the solution under test and excluding the *Internal standard solution* from the extraction

blank. Shake each funnel, and allow the layers to separate. Collect the lower chloroform layer. Repeat the extraction procedure one more time. Evaporate the solvents under a stream of nitrogen at 45° until just dry. Reconstitute the dried residue with 2 mL of acetonitrile (for Tablets with a 2.5-mg label claim) or with 8 mL of acetonitrile (for Tablets with a 10-mg label claim), and sonicate for 10 minutes.

Chromatographic system (see *Chromatography* ⟨621⟩)—The gas chromatograph is equipped with a flame-ionization detector and a 0.53-mm × 30-m column coated with a 0.5-μm phase G27. The carrier gas is helium, flowing at a rate of about 16.8 mL per minute. The injection port and detector temperatures are maintained at 190° and 320°, respectively. The chromatograph is programmed as follows. Upon injection, the column temperature is increased at a rate of 25° per minute to 280°, and maintained at 280° for 3 minutes. Then the column temperature is increased at a rate of 10° per minute to 320°, and maintained at 320° for 3 minutes. Chromatograph the acetonitrile, the extraction blank, and the internal standard blank, and record the peak responses as directed for *Procedure:* the tailing factor is not more than 1.5. Make two injections of the *Working standard solution*, and record the peak responses. The average oxandrolone/Internal standard solution peak area percent comparison is between 98.0% and 102.0%. The resolution, *R*, between the oxandrolone peak and the nearest eluting peak is equal to or greater than 1.5.

Procedure—Separately inject equal volumes (0.5 μL) of the *Working standard solution* and the *Test solution* into the chromatograph, record the chromatograms, and measure the responses for the major peaks. Calculate the percentage of $C_{19}H_{30}O_3$ released by the formula:

$$\frac{C_S \times \text{sample ratio} \times V_{UF} \times 500 \times 100}{\text{Standard ratio} \times V_{UI} \times LC}$$

in which C_S is the concentration, in mg per mL, of oxandrolone in the *Standard solution;* sample ratio is the area ratio of oxandrolone to 17α-methyltestosterone in the sample injection for each *Test solution;* V_{UF} is the final volume, in mL, of the sample after reconstitution of the dry residue; 500 is the volume, in mL, of *Medium;* 100 is the conversion factor to percentage; standard ratio is the mean area ratio of oxandrolone to 17α-methyltestosterone in all injections of the *Standard solution;* V_{UI} is the initial sample volume, in mL, used in the extraction; and *LC* is the tablet label claim, in mg.

Tolerances—Not less than 75% (*Q*) of the labeled amount of oxandrolone ($C_{19}H_{30}O_3$) is dissolved in 60 minutes.

TEST 2—If the product complies with this test, the labeling indicates that it meets USP *Dissolution Test 2*.

Medium: 1% polysorbate 80 in water; 500 mL, deaerated.
Apparatus 2: 100 rpm.
Time: 120 minutes.

Determine the amount of $C_{19}H_{30}O_3$ dissolved by employing the following method.

Mobile phase—Prepare a filtered and degassed mixture of water and acetonitrile (55 : 45). Make adjustments if necessary (see *System Suitability* under *Chromatography* ⟨621⟩).

Standard stock solution—Transfer about 20 mg of USP Oxandrolone RS, accurately weighed, to a 200-mL volumetric flask. Add about 20 mL of acetonitrile, and sonicate to dissolve. Dilute with *Medium* to volume, and mix.

Working standard solution—Quantitatively dilute the *Standard stock solution* with *Medium* to obtain a solution having a final concentration of about 5 μg per mL for Tablets with a label claim of 2.5 mg, or a final concentration of about 20 μg per mL for Tablets with a label claim of 10 mg.

Test solution—Withdraw about 10 mL of the solution under test from the vessel. Centrifuge in a glass tube at 2000 rpm for 10 minutes.

Chromatographic system (see *Chromatography* ⟨621⟩)—The liquid chromatograph is equipped with a refractive index detector and a 4.6-mm × 25-cm column that contains 5-μm packing L1. The column is maintained at 30°, and the detector is maintained at 50°. The flow rate is about 1.5 mL per minute. Chromatograph the *Working standard solution*, and record the peak responses as directed for *Procedure:* the tailing factor is not more than 2.0; the column efficiency is not less than 4000 theoretical plates; and the relative standard deviation for replicate injections is not more than 5.0%.

Procedure—Separately inject equal volumes (about 100 μL) of the *Working standard solution* and the *Test solution* into the chromatograph, record the chromatograms, and measure the responses for the major peaks. Calculate the percentage of $C_{19}H_{30}O_3$ released by the formula:

$$\frac{r_U \times C_S \times D \times 500 \times 100}{r_S \times LC}$$

in which r_U and r_S are the peak responses obtained from the *Test solution* and *Working standard solution*, respectively; C_S is the concentration, in mg per mL, of the *Working standard solution;* *D* is the dilution factor of the *Test solution;* 500 is the volume, in mL, of *Medium;* 100 is the conversion factor to percentage; and *LC* is the tablet label claim, in mg.

Tolerances—Not less than 65% (*Q*) of the labeled amount of $C_{19}H_{30}O_3$ is dissolved in 120 minutes.

TEST 3—If the product complies with this test, the labeling indicates that it meets USP *Dissolution Test 3*.

Medium: 0.1 N hydrochloric acid containing 0.75% of sodium lauryl sulfate; 500 mL, deaerated with helium.
Apparatus 2: 75 rpm.
Time: 90 minutes.

Determine the amount of $C_{19}H_{30}O_3$ released by employing the following method.

Mobile phase—Prepare a filtered and degassed mixture of water and acetonitrile (65 : 35). Make adjustments if necessary (see *System Suitability* under *Chromatography* ⟨621⟩).

Standard stock solution—Transfer about 20 mg, accurately weighed, of USP Oxandrolone RS to a 100-mL volumetric flask. Dissolve in approximately 5 mL of acetonitrile, and sonicate for 10 minutes. Dilute with *Medium* to volume, and mix.

Working standard solution—Transfer 8.0 mL of the *Standard stock solution* to a 200-mL volumetric flask, dilute with *Medium* to volume, and mix.

Test solution—Pass the solution under test through a suitable filter having a porosity of 0.45 μm.

Chromatographic system—The liquid chromatograph is equipped with a refractive index detector and a 4.6-mm × 30-cm column that contains 5-μm packing L1. The flow rate is about 1.0 mL per minute. The temperatures of the detector and the column are both maintained at 35°. Chromatograph the *Working standard solution*, and record the peak responses as directed for *Procedure:* the tailing factor is not more than 2.0; and the relative standard deviation for replicate injections is not more than 5.0%.

Procedure—Separately inject equal volumes (about 200 μL) of the *Working standard solution* and the *Test solution* into the chromatograph, record the chromatograms, and measure the peak responses. Calculate the percentage of $C_{19}H_{30}O_3$ dissolved by the formula:

$$\frac{r_U \times C_S \times 500 \times 100}{r_S \times LC}$$

in which r_U and r_S are the peak responses for the *Test solution* and the *Working standard solution*, respectively; C_S is the concentration, in mg per mL, of oxandrolone in the *Working standard solution;* 500 is the volume, in mL, of *Medium;* 100 is the conversion factor to percentage; and *LC* is the Tablet label claim, in mg.

Tolerances—Not less than 75% (*Q*) of the labeled amount of $C_{19}H_{30}O_3$ is dissolved in 90 minutes.

Uniformity of dosage units ⟨905⟩: meet the requirements.

Assay—
Internal standard solution—Dissolve 100 mg of *n*-octacosane in 200 mL of chloroform.

Standard preparation—Transfer about 50 mg of USP Oxandrolone RS, accurately weighed, to a 100-mL volumetric flask, dissolve in *Internal standard solution*, dilute with *Internal standard solution* to volume, and mix.

Assay preparation—Weigh and finely powder not fewer than 20 Tablets. Transfer an accurately weighed portion of the powder, equivalent to about 5 mg of oxandrolone, to a suitable container, add 10.0 mL of *Internal standard solution,* and shake by mechanical means for 30 minutes. Pass through Whatman No. 2 filter paper, or equivalent, discarding the first 5 mL of the filtrate.

Procedure—Inject separately 2-µL portions of the *Standard preparation* and the *Assay preparation* into a suitable gas chromatograph equipped with a flame-ionization detector (see *Chromatography* ⟨621⟩) and a 4-mm × 2-m glass column, packed with 3% methylsilicone oil on 80- to 100-mesh acid-, base-, and water-washed, flux-calcined, silanized siliceous earth. The column is maintained at about 250°, the injection port is maintained at about 290°, and the detector block is maintained at about 300°; helium is used as the carrier gas at a flow rate of about 60 mL per minute. Calculate the quantity, in mg, of oxandrolone ($C_{19}H_{30}O_3$) in the portion of Tablets taken by the formula:

$$10C(R_U / R_S)$$

in which *C* is the concentration, in mg per mL, of USP Oxandrolone RS in the *Standard preparation;* and R_U and R_S are the ratios of the peak heights of the oxandrolone peak and the internal standard peak from the *Assay preparation* and the *Standard preparation,* respectively.

Oxaprozin

$C_{18}H_{15}NO_3$ 293.32
2-Oxazolepropanoic acid, 4,5-diphenyl-.
4,5-Diphenyl-2-oxazolepropionic acid   [21256-18-8].

» Oxaprozin contains not less than 98.5 percent and not more than 101.5 percent of $C_{18}H_{15}NO_3$, calculated on the dried basis.

NOTE—Because of light sensitivity, protect all oxaprozin samples and Standard solutions from light.

Packaging and storage—Preserve in tight, light-resistant containers, and store at controlled room temperature.
USP Reference standards ⟨11⟩—USP Oxaprozin RS.
Identification—
  A: *Infrared Absorption* ⟨197K⟩: previously dried at 105° for 2 hours.
  B: *Ultraviolet Absorption* ⟨197U⟩: previously dried at 105° for 2 hours. The absorbance of the sample at 285 nm is between 0.455 and 0.495.
  Solution: 10 µg per mL.
  Medium: methanol.
Loss on drying ⟨731⟩—Dry it at 105° for 2 hours: it loses not more than 0.3% of its weight.
Residue on ignition ⟨281⟩: not more than 0.3%.
Arsenic, *Method II* ⟨211⟩: 1 µg per g.
Heavy metals, *Method II* ⟨231⟩: 0.001%.
Chromatographic purity—
  Solution A: 0.1% phosphoric acid adjusted with phosphoric acid to a pH of 2.00 ± 0.1.
  Solution B—Use acetonitrile.
  Mobile phase—Use variable mixtures of *Solution A* and *Solution B* as directed for *Chromatographic system.* Make adjustments if necessary (see *System Suitability* under *Chromatography* ⟨621⟩).
  Diluent A: a mixture of acetonitrile, methylene chloride, and water (48 : 1 : 1).
  Diluent B: a mixture of acetonitrile and water (1 : 1).
  Standard stock solution—Dissolve an accurately weighed quantity of USP Oxaprozin RS in acetonitrile to obtain a solution having a concentration of about 200 µg per mL.

  Standard solution—Transfer 5.0 mL of *Standard stock solution* to a 200-mL volumetric flask, and dilute with *Diluent A* to volume.
  Benzil solution: 200 µg of benzil per mL in acetonitrile.
  Resolution solution—Transfer 5.0 mL of *Benzil solution* and 5.0 mL of *Standard stock solution* to a 100-mL volumetric flask, and dilute with *Diluent A* to volume to obtain a solution having known concentrations of about 10 µg of each per mL.
  Test solution A—[NOTE—*Test solution A* is used to monitor all known and unknown impurities, except imidazolic acid and oximide.] Transfer about 100 mg of Oxaprozin, accurately weighed, to a 100-mL volumetric flask; add 2 mL of methylene chloride, 2 mL of water, and 75 mL of acetonitrile; and sonicate after each solvent is added. Dilute with acetonitrile to volume.
  Test solution B—[NOTE—*Test solution B* is used to monitor only imidazolic acid and oximide.] Transfer about 100 mg of Oxaprozin, accurately weighed, to a 100-mL volumetric flask; add 75 mL of *Diluent B* to dissolve the Oxaprozin; and dilute with *Diluent B* to volume.
  Chromatographic system (see *Chromatography* ⟨621⟩)—The liquid chromatograph is equipped with a 238-nm detector and a 4.6-mm × 15-cm column that contains 5-µm packing L7. The flow rate is 1.0 mL per minute. The chromatograph is programmed as follows.

Time (minutes)	Solution A (%)	Solution B (%)	Elution
0	70	30	equilibration
0–20	70	30	isocratic
21–60	70→0	30→100	linear gradient
60–61	0→70	100→30	linear gradient
61–70	70	30	isocratic

Chromatograph the *Resolution solution,* and record the peak responses as directed for *Procedure:* the relative retention times are about 1.1 for benzil and 1.0 for oxaprozin; and the resolution, *R,* between oxaprozin and benzil is not less than 3.0. Chromatograph the *Standard solution,* and record the peak responses as directed for *Procedure:* the tailing factor is not more than 2.0, and the relative standard deviation for replicate injections is not more than 5.0%.

  Procedure—Inject 20 µL of *Test solution A* and *Test solution B* into the chromatograph, record the chromatogram, and measure the areas for all the peaks. Calculate the percentage of each impurity in the portion of Oxaprozin taken by the formula:

$$100(Fr_i / r_s)$$

in which *F* is the relative response factor and is equal to 1.15 for the imidazolic acid peak with a relative retention time of 0.14, 1.21 for any peak with a relative retention time of 0.42, 0.91 for the oximide peak with a relative retention time of 0.73, 0.85 for any peak with a relative retention time of 0.84, 1.29 for any peak with a relative retention time of 1.08, 1.46 for any peak with a relative retention time of 1.50, and 2.09 for any peak with a relative retention time of 1.57; r_i is the peak response for each impurity; and r_s is the sum of the responses of all the peaks: not more than 0.1% of any individual impurity is found, and not more than 0.5% of total impurities is found. [NOTE—The values of *F* for all known impurities except imidazolic acid and oximide were found using *Test solution A,* and the values of *F* for imidazolic acid and oximide were found using *Test solution B.*]

Organic volatile impurities, *Method V* ⟨467⟩: meets the requirements.
  Solvent—Use dimethyl sulfoxide.

(Official until July 1, 2008)

Assay—Dissolve about 400 mg of Oxaprozin, previously dried at 105° for 2 hours and accurately weighed, in about 100 mL of alcohol in a narrow-mouth container, and titrate with 0.1 N sodium hydroxide VS, determining the endpoint potentiometrically (see *Titrimetry* ⟨541⟩). Each mL of 0.1 N sodium hydroxide is equivalent to 29.332 mg of oxaprozin.

Oxaprozin Tablets

» Oxaprozin Tablets contain not less than 95.0 percent and not more than 105.0 percent of the labeled amount of oxaprozin ($C_{18}H_{15}NO_3$).
NOTE—Because of light sensitivity, protect all oxaprozin samples and Standard solutions from light.

Packaging and storage—Preserve in tight, light-resistant containers, and store at controlled room temperature.
USP Reference standards ⟨11⟩—*USP Oxaprozin RS*.
Identification—
   A: *Thin-Layer Chromatographic Identification Test* ⟨201⟩—
   Test solution: 2 mg per mL of oxaprozin in acetone.
   Developing solvent system: a mixture of ethyl acetate and glacial acetic acid (99 : 1).
   B: The retention time of the major peak in the chromatogram of the *Assay preparation* corresponds to that in the chromatogram of the *Standard preparation*, as obtained in the *Assay*.
Dissolution ⟨711⟩—
   Medium: 0.05 M monobasic potassium phosphate buffer, pH 7.4; 1000 mL.
   Apparatus 2: 75 rpm.
   Time: 45 minutes.
   Procedure—Determine the amount of $C_{18}H_{15}NO_3$ dissolved by employing UV absorption at the wavelength of maximum absorbance at about 286 nm on filtered portions of the solution under test, suitably diluted with *Dissolution Medium*, if necessary, in comparison with a Standard solution having a known concentration of USP Oxaprozin RS in the same *Medium* (an amount of methanol not exceeding 5% of the final volume can be added to help solubilize the USP Reference Standard).
   Tolerances—Not less than 75% (*Q*) of the labeled amount of $C_{18}H_{15}NO_3$ is dissolved in 45 minutes.
Uniformity of dosage units ⟨905⟩: meet the requirements.
Water, *Method Ia* ⟨921⟩: not more than 3.5%.
Assay—
   0.1% Phosphoric acid, pH 2.00 ± 0.10—Add concentrated phosphoric acid, dropwise, to water to obtain a pH of 2.00 ± 0.10.
   Mobile phase—Prepare a filtered and degassed solution of *0.1% Phosphoric acid, pH 2.00 ± 0.10* and acetonitrile (55 : 45).
   Standard preparation—Dissolve an accurately weighed quantity of USP Oxaprozin RS in acetonitrile to obtain a solution having a concentration of about 12 µg of oxaprozin per mL.
   Assay stock preparation—Weigh and finely powder not fewer than 20 Tablets. Transfer an accurately weighed portion of the powder, equivalent to about 60 mg of oxaprozin, to a 100-mL volumetric flask, add about 10 mL of water, and sonicate for 10 minutes. Add about 40 mL of acetonitrile, sonicate for 30 minutes, shake by mechanical means for an additional 30 minutes, add about 30 mL of acetonitrile, and sonicate for 10 minutes. Dilute with acetonitrile to volume.
   Assay preparation—Quantitatively dilute the *Assay stock preparation* with acetonitrile to obtain a solution having a concentration of about 12 µg of oxaprozin per mL.
   Chromatographic system (see *Chromatography* ⟨621⟩)—The liquid chromatograph is equipped with a 285-nm detector and a 4.6-mm × 15-cm column that contains 5-µm packing L7. The flow rate is about 1.0 mL per minute. Chromatograph the *Standard preparation*, and record the peak responses as directed for *Procedure:* the tailing factor is not more than 2.0; and the relative standard deviation for replicate injections is not more than 2.0%.
   Procedure—Separately inject equal volumes (about 20 µL) of the *Standard preparation* and the *Assay preparation* into the chromatograph, record the chromatograms, and measure the responses for the major peaks. Calculate the quantity, in mg, of oxaprozin ($C_{18}H_{15}NO_3$) in the portion of Tablets taken by the formula:

$$100C(r_U / r_S)$$

in which *C* is the concentration in mg per mL of USP Oxaprozin RS in the *Standard preparation*; and r_U and r_S are the peak responses obtained from the *Assay preparation* and the *Standard preparation*, respectively.

Oxazepam

$C_{15}H_{11}ClN_2O_2$ 286.71
2*H*-1,4-Benzodiazepin-2-one, 7-chloro-1,3-dihydro-3-hydroxy-5-phenyl-, (±)-.
(±)-7-Chloro-1,3-dihydro-3-hydroxy-5-phenyl-2*H*-1,4-benzodiazepin-2-one   [604-75-1].

» Oxazepam contains not less than 98.0 percent and not more than 102.0 percent of $C_{15}H_{11}ClN_2O_2$, calculated on the dried basis.

Packaging and storage—Preserve in well-closed containers.
USP Reference standards ⟨11⟩—*USP Oxazepam RS*.
Identification—
   A: *Infrared Absorption* ⟨197K⟩.
   B: *Ultraviolet Absorption* ⟨197U⟩—
   Solution: 4 µg per mL.
   Medium: alcohol.
   Absorptivities at 229 nm, calculated on the dried basis, do not differ by more than 3.0%.
pH ⟨791⟩: between 4.8 and 7.0, in an aqueous suspension (1 in 50).
Loss on drying ⟨731⟩—Dry it at a pressure below 5 mm of mercury at 105° for 3 hours: it loses not more than 2.0% of its weight.
Residue on ignition ⟨281⟩: not more than 0.3%.
Organic volatile impurities, *Method V* ⟨467⟩: meets the requirements.
   Solvent—Use dimethyl sulfoxide.

(Official until July 1, 2008)

Assay—Transfer about 400 mg of Oxazepam, accurately weighed, to a beaker, dissolve in 100 mL of dimethylformamide, and titrate with 0.1 N tetrabutylammonium hydroxide VS, determining the endpoint potentiometrically using a calomel-glass electrode system and taking precautions against absorption of atmospheric carbon dioxide. Perform a blank determination, and make any necessary correction. Each mL of 0.1 N tetrabutylammonium hydroxide is equivalent to 28.67 mg of $C_{15}H_{11}ClN_2O_2$.

Oxazepam Capsules

» Oxazepam Capsules contain not less than 90.0 percent and not more than 110.0 percent of the labeled amount of $C_{15}H_{11}ClN_2O_2$.

Packaging and storage—Preserve in well-closed containers.
USP Reference standards ⟨11⟩—*USP Oxazepam RS*.
Identification—The solution prepared for measurement of absorbance in the *Assay* exhibits a maximum at 229 ± 2 nm.
Dissolution ⟨711⟩—
   Medium: 0.1 N hydrochloric acid; 1000 mL.
   Apparatus 2: 75 rpm.
   Time: 60 minutes.
   Chromatographic system (see *Chromatography* ⟨621⟩)—The liquid chromatograph is fitted with a 232-nm detector and a 4-mm × 15-cm column that contains packing L7. The mobile phase is a degassed mixture of methanol, water, and glacial acetic acid (60 : 40 :

1), and the flow rate is about 2 mL per minute. Chromatograph the Standard solution, and record the peak response as directed for *Procedure:* the tailing factor for the oxazepam peak is not more than 1.5, and the relative standard deviation observed following replicate injections is not more than 3.0%. Make adjustments if necessary (see *System Suitability* under *Chromatography* ⟨621⟩).

Procedure—Inject an accurately measured volume (about 20 µL) of a filtered portion of the solution under test into the chromatograph, record the chromatogram, and measure the response for the major peak. Calculate the quantity of $C_{15}H_{11}ClN_2O_2$ dissolved in comparison with a Standard solution having a known concentration of USP Oxazepam RS in 0.1 N hydrochloric acid [NOTE—a volume of methanol not to exceed 10% of the final total volume may be used to dissolve the Oxazepam reference standard] and similarly chromatographed.

Tolerances—Not less than 75% (Q) of the labeled amount of $C_{15}H_{11}ClN_2O_2$ is dissolved in 60 minutes.

Uniformity of dosage units ⟨905⟩: meet the requirements.

Assay—Remove, as completely as possible, the contents of not less than 20 Capsules, and weigh. Transfer an accurately weighed portion of the mixed powder, equivalent to about 50 mg of oxazepam, to a medium-porosity, sintered-glass funnel that is fitted into a small suction flask. Add 25 mL of alcohol, mix with the aid of a stirring rod, and after about 5 minutes apply gentle suction to remove the extract. Repeat the extraction with four additional 25-mL portions of alcohol, transfer the extracts to a 250-mL volumetric flask, dilute with alcohol to volume, and mix. Transfer 2.0 mL of this solution to a 100-mL volumetric flask, dilute with alcohol to volume, and mix. Concomitantly determine the absorbances of this solution and of a Standard solution of USP Oxazepam RS in the same medium having a known concentration of about 4 µg per mL in 1-cm cells at the wavelength of maximum absorbance at about 229 nm, with a suitable spectrophotometer, using alcohol as the blank. Calculate the quantity, in mg, of $C_{15}H_{11}ClN_2O_2$ in the portion of Capsules taken by the formula:

$$12.5C(A_U/A_S)$$

in which C is the concentration, in µg per mL, of USP Oxazepam RS in the Standard solution, and A_U and A_S are the absorbances of the solution from the Capsules and the Standard solution, respectively.

Oxazepam Tablets

» Oxazepam Tablets contain not less than 90.0 percent and not more than 110.0 percent of the labeled amount of $C_{15}H_{11}ClN_2O_2$.

Packaging and storage—Preserve in well-closed containers.

USP Reference standards ⟨11⟩—*USP Oxazepam RS.*

Identification—The solution prepared for measurement of absorbance in the *Assay* exhibits a maximum at 229 ± 2 nm.

Dissolution ⟨711⟩—
Medium: 0.1 N hydrochloric acid; 1000 mL.
Apparatus 2: 50 rpm.
Time: 60 minutes.
Chromatographic system—The liquid chromatograph is fitted with a 232-nm detector and a 4-mm × 30-cm column that contains packing L7. The mobile phase is a degassed mixture of methanol, water, and glacial acetic acid (60 : 40 : 1), and the flow rate is about 2 mL per minute. In a suitable system, the relative standard deviation observed following replicate injections is not more than 3.0%.
Procedure—Inject an accurately measured volume (about 10 µL) of a filtered portion of the solution under test into the chromatograph by means of a microsyringe or a sampling valve, record the chromatogram, and measure the response for the major peak. Calculate the quantity of $C_{15}H_{11}ClN_2O_2$ dissolved in comparison with a similarly chromatographed Standard solution having a known concentration of USP Oxazepam RS in 0.1 N hydrochloric acid. [NOTE—A volume of alcohol not exceeding 10% of the final total volume of the Standard solution may be used to dissolve the Reference Standard.]

Tolerances—Not less than 80% (Q) of the labeled amount of $C_{15}H_{11}ClN_2O_2$ is dissolved in 60 minutes.

Uniformity of dosage units ⟨905⟩: meet the requirements.

Assay—Weigh and finely powder not less than 20 Tablets. Transfer an accurately weighed portion of the powder, equivalent to about 50 mg of oxazepam, to a medium-porosity, sintered-glass funnel that is fitted into a small suction flask, and proceed as directed in the *Assay* under *Oxazepam Capsules*, beginning with "Add 25 mL of alcohol." Calculate the quantity, in mg, of $C_{15}H_{11}ClN_2O_2$ in the portion of Tablets taken by the formula:

$$12.5C(A_U/A_S)$$

in which C is the concentration, in µg per mL, of USP Oxazepam RS in the Standard solution, and A_U and A_S are the absorbances of the solution from the Tablets and the Standard solution, respectively.

Oxfendazole

$C_{15}H_{13}N_3O_3S$ 315.35
Carbamic acid, 5-(phenylsulfinyl)-1*H*-benzimidazol-2-yl-, methyl ester.
Methyl   5-(phenylsulfinyl)-2-benzimidazolecarbamate [*53716-50-0*].

» Oxfendazole contains not less than 98.0 percent and not more than 100.5 percent of $C_{15}H_{13}N_3O_3S$, calculated on the dried basis.

Packaging and storage—Preserve in well-closed, light-resistant containers.

Labeling—Label it to indicate that it is for veterinary use only.

USP Reference standards ⟨11⟩—*USP Fenbendazole RS. USP Oxfendazole RS.*

Identification—
  A: *Infrared Absorption* ⟨197K⟩.
  B: The appearance of the principal spot in the chromatogram of the *Test solution* corresponds to that in the chromatogram of *Standard solution 1*, as obtained in the test for *Related compounds*.

Loss on drying ⟨731⟩—Dry it in vacuum at a pressure not exceeding 5 mm of mercury at 105° for 2 hours: it loses not more than 1.0% of its weight.

Residue on ignition ⟨281⟩: not more than 0.1%.

Related compounds—
  Diluent—Prepare a mixture of ethyl acetate and glacial acetic acid (4 : 1).
  Standard solution 1—Dissolve a quantity of USP Oxfendazole RS in *Diluent* to obtain a solution having a concentration of 0.1 mg per mL.
  Standard solution 2—Dissolve a quantity of USP Fenbendazole RS in *Diluent* to obtain a solution having a concentration of 0.05 mg per mL.
  Standard solution 3—Prepare a mixture of *Standard solution 1* and *Standard solution 2* (1 : 2).
  Test solution—Dissolve 25 mg of Oxfendazole in *Diluent*, dilute with *Diluent* to 5 mL, and mix.
  Procedure—Separately apply 20 µL portions of *Standard solution 1*, *Standard solution 2*, *Standard solution 3*, and the *Test solution* to a thin-layer chromatographic plate (see *Chromatography* ⟨621⟩) coated with a 0.25-mm layer of chromatographic silica gel mixture. Develop the chromatograms in a solvent system consisting of a mixture of ethyl acetate and glacial acetic acid (95 : 5) until the solvent front has moved about three-fourths of the length of the plate. Remove the plate from the chromatographic chamber, and al-

low to air-dry. Examine the plate under short-wavelength UV light: the chromatogram obtained from *Standard solution 3* shows two clearly separated principal spots. In the chromatogram obtained from the *Test solution*, no spot corresponding to fenbendazole is more intense than the spot in the chromatogram obtained from *Standard solution 2* (1%), and no spot other than the principal spot and no spot corresponding to fenbendazole is more intense than the spot in the chromatogram obtained from *Standard solution 1* (2%).
Assay—Dissolve about 300 mg of Oxfendazole, accurately weighed, in 3 mL of anhydrous formic acid. Add 40 mL of acetic anhydride, and titrate with 0.1 N perchloric acid VS, determining the endpoint potentiometrically. Each mL of 0.1 N perchloric acid is equivalent to 31.54 mg of $C_{15}H_{13}N_3O_3S$.

Oxfendazole Oral Suspension

» Oxfendazole Oral Suspension contains not less than 90.0 percent and not more than 110.0 percent of the labeled amount of oxfendazole ($C_{15}H_{13}N_3O_3S$).

Packaging and storage—Preserve in tight containers, and protect from excessive heat.
Labeling—Label the Suspension to indicate that it is for veterinary use only.
USP Reference standards ⟨11⟩—*USP Oxfendazole RS*.
Identification—The relative retention time of the oxfendazole peak in the chromatogram of the *Assay preparation* corresponds to that in the chromatogram of the *Standard preparation*, as obtained in the *Assay*.
pH ⟨791⟩: between 4.3 and 4.9.
Assay—
  Mobile phase—Prepare a solution of sodium acetate in water containing 2.5 mg per mL, and adjust with glacial acetic acid to a pH of 4.75 ± 0.1. Prepare a mixture of this solution and acetonitrile (800 : 225). Make adjustments if necessary (see *System Suitability* under *Chromatography* ⟨621⟩).
  System suitability solution—Prepare a solution in *Mobile phase* containing in each mL about 1.2 µg of methylparaben, 12 µg of sulfabenzamide, and 72 µg of USP Oxfendazole RS.
  Internal standard solution—Prepare a solution of sulfabenzamide in *Mobile phase* containing about 0.3 mg per mL.
  Standard preparation—Prepare a solution of USP Oxfendazole RS in methanol having a known concentration of about 900 µg per mL. Transfer 20.0 mL of this solution to a 100-mL volumetric flask, add 4.0 mL of *Internal standard solution*, dilute with *Mobile phase* to volume, and mix. This solution contains about 180 µg of USP Oxfendazole RS per mL.
  Assay preparation—Transfer an accurately measured volume of the Suspension, previously well-mixed and free from air bubbles, equivalent to about 450 mg of oxfendazole, to a 500-mL volumetric flask. Add about 30 mL of water, and swirl to disperse. Add about 300 mL of methanol, and dissolve with the aid of sonication. Transfer 20.0 mL of this solution to a 100-mL volumetric flask, add 4.0 mL of *Internal standard solution*, dilute with *Mobile phase* to volume, and mix.
  Chromatographic system (see *Chromatography* ⟨621⟩)—The liquid chromatograph is equipped with a 254-nm detector, a guard column containing packing L2, and a 4.6-mm × 25-cm analytical column that contains packing L1. The flow rate is about 1 mL per minute. Chromatograph the *System suitability solution*, and record the peak responses as directed for *Procedure*: the relative retention times are about 0.7 for sulfabenzamide, 0.8 for methylparaben, and 1.0 for oxfendazole; the resolution, *R*, between the methylparaben peak and the oxfendazole peak is not less than 2.0; the column efficiency determined from the oxfendazole peak is not less than 2000 theoretical plates; and the relative standard deviation of replicate injections is not more than 1.5%. [NOTE—The detector sensitivity may be changed between the peaks to keep the responses on scale.]
  Procedure—Separately inject equal volumes (about 50 µL) of the *Standard preparation* and the *Assay preparation* into the chromatograph, and measure the responses for the major peaks. Calculate the quantity, in mg, of oxfendazole ($C_{15}H_{13}N_3O_3S$) in each mL of the Suspension taken by the formula:

$$2.5(C/V)(R_U/R_S)$$

in which *C* is the concentration, in µg per mL, of USP Oxfendazole RS in the *Standard preparation*; *V* is the volume, in mL, of Suspension taken to prepare the *Assay preparation*; and R_U and R_S are the ratios of the oxfendazole peak response to the sulfabenzamide peak response obtained from the *Assay preparation* and the *Standard preparation*, respectively.

Oxprenolol Hydrochloride

$C_{15}H_{23}NO_3 \cdot HCl$ 301.81
2-Propanol, 1-(*o*-allyloxyphenoxy)-3-isopropylamino-, hydrochloride.
1-(*o*-Allyloxyphenoxy)-3-isopropylamino-2-propanol hydrochloride [6452-73-9].

» Oxprenolol Hydrochloride contains not less than 98.5 percent and not more than 101.0 percent of $C_{15}H_{23}NO_3 \cdot HCl$, calculated on the dried basis.

Packaging and storage—Preserve in well-closed containers.
USP Reference standards ⟨11⟩—*USP Oxprenolol Hydrochloride RS*.
Clarity of solution—Dissolve 1 g in 10 mL of water: solution is clear.
Identification—
  A: *Infrared Absorption* ⟨197K⟩.
  B: A solution of it responds to the tests for *Chloride* ⟨191⟩.
pH ⟨791⟩: between 4.0 and 6.0, in a solution (1 in 10).
Loss on drying ⟨731⟩—Dry about 3 g of it in vacuum at 60° for 6 hours: it loses not more than 0.5% of its weight.
Residue on ignition ⟨281⟩: not more than 0.1%.
Heavy metals, *Method II* ⟨231⟩: 0.001%.
Chromatographic purity—
  Diluting solvent—Prepare a mixture of chloroform and dehydrated alcohol (1 : 1).
  Standard solution A—Prepare a solution of USP Oxprenolol Hydrochloride RS in *Diluting solvent* containing 20 mg per mL.
  Standard solution B—Dilute an accurately measured volume of *Standard solution A* quantitatively, and stepwise if necessary, with *Diluting solvent* to obtain a solution containing 0.08 mg per mL.
  Test solution—Transfer 200 mg of it to a 10-mL volumetric flask, dissolve in *Diluting solvent*, dilute with *Diluting solvent* to volume, and mix.
  Procedure—Apply separate 5-µL portions of the *Test solution* and the *Standard solutions* to the starting line of a suitable thin-layer chromatographic plate (see *Chromatography* ⟨621⟩) coated with a 0.25-mm layer of chromatographic silica gel mixture, previously washed with methanol until the solvent front reaches the top of the plate, dried first in air and then at 100° for 20 minutes, and cooled in a desiccator. Allow the spots to dry. Line a suitable chromatographic chamber with filter paper, saturate the paper with 100 mL of a solvent system consisting of a mixture of ethyl acetate, glacial acetic acid, and water (15 : 5 : 5), and allow to stand for about 30 minutes. Place the plate in the chamber, and develop the chromatogram until the solvent front has moved about three-fourths of the length of the plate. Remove the plate from the chamber and dry at 100° for 15 minutes. Spray the plate uniformly with a detection reagent consisting of a freshly prepared mixture of equal volumes of potassium ferricyanide solution (1 in 100) and ferric chloride solution (1 in 5). Dry the plate in a current of warm air for about 5 minutes or until a spot from *Standard solution B* is visible. Examine the chromatograms in ordinary light: the R_F value of the

ture of this solution and methanol (4 : 1). Make adjustments if necessary (see *System Suitability* under *Chromatography* ⟨621⟩).

System suitability preparation—Dissolve suitable quantities of USP Oxtriphylline RS and theobromine in water to obtain a solution containing about 0.6 mg and 0.3 mg per mL, respectively. Dilute this solution quantitatively, and stepwise if necessary, with water to obtain a solution containing about 60 µg of USP Oxtriphylline RS per mL and about 30 µg of theobromine per mL.

Standard preparation—Dissolve an accurately weighed quantity of USP Oxtriphylline RS in water, and dilute quantitatively, and stepwise if necessary, with water to obtain a solution having a known concentration of about 0.1 mg per mL.

Assay preparation—Place 10 Tablets in a 1000-mL volumetric flask, and add about 700 mL of water. Heat on a steam bath, with occasional shaking, until the Tablets have disintegrated. Cool to room temperature, dilute with water to volume, mix, and filter. Transfer an accurately measured volume of this solution, equivalent to about 20 mg of Oxtriphylline, to a 200-mL volumetric flask, dilute with water to volume, and mix.

Chromatographic system (see *Chromatography* ⟨621⟩)—The liquid chromatograph is equipped with a 275-nm detector and a 3.9-mm × 30-cm column that contains packing L1. The flow rate is about 1 mL per minute. Chromatograph the *System suitability preparation*, and record the peak responses as directed for *Procedure:* the relative retention times are about 0.7 for theobromine and 1.0 for theophylline, and the resolution, *R*, between the theobromine and theophylline peaks is not less than 3.0. Chromatograph the *Standard preparation*, and record the peak responses as directed for *Procedure:* the relative standard deviation for replicate injections is not more than 2.0%.

Procedure—Separately inject equal volumes (about 10 µL) of the *Standard preparation* and the *Assay preparation* into the chromatograph, record the chromatograms, and measure the responses for the major peaks. [NOTE—The major peaks recorded in the chromatograms represent the theophylline moiety of oxtriphylline.] Calculate the quantity, in mg, of $C_7H_8N_4O_2$ in the portion of Tablets taken by the formula:

$$(180.17 / 283.33)(20C / V)(r_U / r_S)$$

in which 180.17 and 283.33 are the molecular weights of anhydrous theophylline and oxtriphylline, respectively; *C* is the concentration, in µg per mL, of USP Oxtriphylline RS in the *Standard preparation*; *V* is the volume, in mL, of solution taken for the *Assay preparation*; and r_U and r_S are the theophylline peak responses obtained from the *Assay preparation* and the *Standard preparation*, respectively.

Oxtriphylline Delayed-Release Tablets

» Oxtriphylline Delayed-Release Tablets contain an amount of oxtriphylline equivalent to not less than 90.0 percent and not more than 110.0 percent of the labeled amount of anhydrous theophylline ($C_7H_8N_4O_2$).

Packaging and storage—Preserve in tight containers.
Labeling—Label the Tablets to state both the content of oxtriphylline and the content of anhydrous theophylline. The label indicates that the Tablets are enteric-coated.
USP Reference standards ⟨11⟩—*USP Oxtriphylline RS.*
Identification—
  A: The retention time exhibited by theophylline in the chromatogram of the *Assay preparation* corresponds to that of theophylline in the chromatogram of the *Standard preparation*, as obtained in the *Assay*.
  B: Transfer a quantity of finely ground Tablets, equivalent to about 100 mg of oxtriphylline, to a suitable test tube, add 10 mL of methanol, shake on a vortex mixer for several minutes, and filter to obtain the test solution. Apply 10 µL of the test solution and 10 µL of a Standard solution of USP Oxtriphylline RS in methanol containing 10 mg per mL to a suitable thin-layer chromatographic plate (see *Chromatography* ⟨621⟩) coated with a 0.25-mm layer of chromatographic silica gel mixture. Allow the applications to dry, and develop the chromatogram in a solvent system consisting of a mixture of chloroform, alcohol, and formic acid (88 : 10 : 2) until the solvent front has moved about three-fourths of the length of the plate. Remove the plate from the developing chamber, mark the solvent front, and allow the solvent to evaporate. Observe the plate under short-wavelength UV light: the principal spot obtained from the test solution corresponds in color, size, and R_F value to that obtained from the Standard solution.

Disintegration ⟨701⟩—Test Tablets as directed for *Enteric-coated Tablets* (see *Disintegration* ⟨701⟩): the tablets do not disintegrate after 30 minutes of agitation in simulated gastric fluid TS; continue agitation in simulated gastric fluid TS for an additional 30 minutes: the tablets may disintegrate during this period; if all of the tablets have not disintegrated, place the basket in simulated intestinal fluid TS, and operate the apparatus: all of the tablets disintegrate within 90 minutes (2.5 hours total disintegration time).

Uniformity of dosage units ⟨905⟩:   meet the requirements.
Assay—
  Mobile phase—Dissolve 6.8 g of monobasic potassium phosphate in water to make 1000 mL, and adjust with 0.1 N potassium hydroxide to a pH of 5.8 ± 0.1. Prepare a filtered and degassed mixture of this solution and methanol (4 : 1). Make adjustments if necessary (see *System Suitability* under *Chromatography* ⟨621⟩).

  Standard preparation—Dissolve an accurately weighed quantity of USP Oxtriphylline RS in water, and dilute quantitatively, and stepwise if necessary, with water to obtain a solution having a known concentration of about 0.1 mg per mL.

  Assay preparation—Place 10 Tablets in a 1000-mL volumetric flask, and add about 700 mL of water. Heat on a steam bath, with occasional shaking, until the Tablets have disintegrated. Cool to room temperature, dilute with water to volume, mix, and filter. Transfer an accurately measured volume of this specimen solution, equivalent to about 20 mg of Oxtriphylline, to a 200-mL volumetric flask, dilute with water to volume, and mix.

  System suitability preparation—Dissolve suitable quantities of USP Oxtriphylline RS and theobromine in water to obtain a solution containing about 0.6 mg and 0.3 mg per mL, respectively. Dilute this solution quantitatively, and stepwise if necessary, with water to obtain a solution containing about 60 µg of USP Oxtriphylline RS per mL and about 30 µg of theobromine per mL.

  Chromatographic system (see *Chromatography* ⟨621⟩)—The liquid chromatograph is equipped with a 275-nm detector and a 3.9-mm × 30-cm column that contains packing L1. The flow rate is about 1 mL per minute. Chromatograph the *Standard preparation* and the *System suitability preparation*, and record the peak responses as directed for *Procedure:* the resolution, *R*, between the theobromine and theophylline peaks is not less than 3.0, and the relative standard deviation for replicate injections of the *Standard preparation* is not more than 2.0%. The relative retention times are about 0.7 for theobromine and 1.0 for theophylline.

  Procedure—Separately inject equal volumes (about 10 µL) of the *Standard preparation* and the *Assay preparation* into the chromatograph, record the chromatograms, and measure the responses for the major peaks. [NOTE—The major peaks recorded in the chromatograms represent the theophylline moiety of oxtriphylline.] Calculate the quantity, in mg, of $C_7H_8N_4O_2$ per Tablet taken by the formula:

$$(180.17 / 283.33)(20C / V)(r_U / r_S)$$

in which 180.17 and 283.33 are the molecular weights of anhydrous theophylline and oxtriphylline, respectively; *C* is the concentration, in µg per mL, of USP Oxtriphylline RS in the *Standard preparation*; *V* is the volume, in mL, of specimen solution taken for the *Assay preparation*; and r_U and r_S are the theophylline peak responses obtained from the *Assay preparation* and the *Standard preparation*, respectively.

Oxtriphylline Extended-Release Tablets

» Oxtriphylline Extended-Release Tablets contain an amount of oxtriphylline equivalent to not less than 90.0

percent and not more than 110.0 percent of the labeled amount of anhydrous theophylline ($C_7H_8N_4O_2$).

Packaging and storage—Preserve in tight containers.

Labeling—Label the Tablets to state both the content of oxtriphylline and the content of anhydrous theophylline. The labeling indicates the *Dissolution Test* with which the product complies.

USP Reference standards ⟨11⟩—*USP Oxtriphylline RS*.

Identification—

A: The retention time exhibited by theophylline in the chromatogram of the *Assay preparation* corresponds to that of theophylline in the chromatogram of the *Standard preparation*, as obtained in the *Assay*.

B: Transfer a quantity of finely ground Tablets, equivalent to about 100 mg of oxtriphylline, to a suitable test tube, and proceed as directed in *Identification* test B under *Oxtriphylline Delayed-Release Tablets*, beginning with "add 10 mL of methanol."

Dissolution ⟨711⟩—

TEST 1 (for products labeled as 400-mg tablets)—If the product complies with this test, the labeling indicates that it meets USP *Dissolution Test 1*. Proceed as directed for *Method B* under *Apparatus 1 and Apparatus 2, Delayed-Release Dosage Forms*, except to use *Acceptance Table 2*.

pH 7.5 Buffer—Transfer 27.22 g of monobasic potassium phosphate to a 4-L volumetric flask, add 1 L of water and 816 mL of 0.2 N sodium hydroxide, and dilute with water to about 3800 mL. Adjust with 0.2 N sodium hydroxide or phosphoric acid to a pH of 7.5, and dilute with water to volume.

Medium: 0.1 N hydrochloric acid for the first hour, then *pH 7.5 Buffer*; 900 mL.

Apparatus 2: 50 rpm.

Procedure—Determine the amount of $C_{12}H_{21}N_5O_3$ dissolved from UV absorbances at the wavelength of maximum absorbance at about 248 nm on filtered portions of the solution under test, diluted with *Medium* if necessary, in comparison with a Standard solution having a known concentration of USP Oxtriphylline RS in the same *Medium*.

Times and Tolerances—

Time (hours)	Amount dissolved
1	between 5% and 30%
3	between 50% and 70%
5	between 65% and 85%
7	not less than 75%

TEST 2 (for products labeled as 600-mg tablets)—If the product complies with this test, the labeling indicates that it meets USP *Dissolution Test 2*. Proceed as directed for *Method B* under *Apparatus 1 and Apparatus 2, Delayed-Release Dosage Forms*, except to use *Acceptance Table 2*.

pH 7.5 Buffer, Apparatus, Medium, and *Procedure*—Proceed as directed for *Test 1*.

Times and Tolerances—

Time (hours)	Amount dissolved
1	between 15% and 40%
3	between 50% and 70%
7	not less than 75%

Uniformity of dosage units ⟨905⟩: meet the requirements.

Assay—Proceed as directed in the *Assay* under *Oxtriphylline Delayed-Release Tablets*, using *Oxtriphylline Extended-Release Tablets*.

Oxybenzone

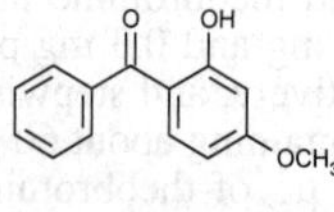

$C_{14}H_{12}O_3$ 228.24
Methanone, (2-hydroxy-4-methoxyphenyl)phenyl-.
2-Hydroxy-4-methoxybenzophenone [131-57-7].

» Oxybenzone contains not less than 97.0 percent and not more than 103.0 percent of $C_{14}H_{12}O_3$, calculated on the dried basis.

Packaging and storage—Preserve in tight, light-resistant containers.

USP Reference standards ⟨11⟩—*USP Oxybenzone RS*.

Identification—
A: *Infrared Absorption* ⟨197K⟩.
B: *Ultraviolet Absorption* ⟨197U⟩—
Solution: 10 µg per mL.
Medium: methanol.
Absorptivities at 287 nm, calculated on the dried basis, do not differ by more than 3.0%.

Congealing temperature ⟨651⟩: not lower than 62.0°.

Loss on drying ⟨731⟩—Dry it in vacuum at 40° for 2 hours: it loses not more than 2.0% of its weight.

Assay—

Standard preparation—Dissolve an accurately weighed quantity of USP Oxybenzone RS in methanol, and quantitatively dilute with methanol, if necessary, to obtain a solution having a known concentration of about 10 µg per mL.

Assay preparation—Dissolve about 100 mg of Oxybenzone, accurately weighed, in methanol in a 100-mL volumetric flask, dilute with methanol to volume, and mix. Agitate gently, if necessary, to hasten solution. Pipet 1 mL of the solution so obtained into a second 100-mL volumetric flask, dilute with methanol to volume, and mix.

Procedure—Concomitantly determine the absorbances of the *Assay preparation* and the *Standard preparation* in 1-cm cells at the wavelength of maximum absorbance at about 287 nm, with a suitable spectrophotometer, using methanol as the blank. Calculate the quantity, in mg, of $C_{14}H_{12}O_3$ in the portion of Oxybenzone taken by the formula:

$$10C(A_U / A_S)$$

in which C is the concentration, in µg per mL, of USP Oxybenzone RS in the *Standard preparation*; and A_U and A_S are the absorbances of the *Assay preparation* and the *Standard preparation*, respectively.

Oxybutynin Chloride

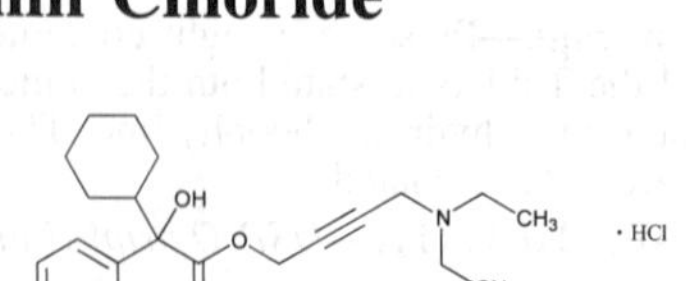

$C_{22}H_{31}NO_3 \cdot HCl$ 393.95
Benzeneacetic acid, α-cyclohexyl-α-hydroxy-, 4-(diethylamino)-2-butynyl ester hydrochloride, (±)-.
4-(Diethylamino)-2-butynyl (±)-α-phenylcyclohexaneglycolate hydrochloride [1508-65-2].

» Oxybutynin Chloride contains not less than 97.0 percent and not more than 101.0 percent of $C_{22}H_{31}NO_3 \cdot HCl$, calculated on the dried basis.

Packaging and storage—Preserve in well-closed containers.

USP Reference standards ⟨11⟩—USP Oxybutynin Chloride RS. USP Oxybutynin Related Compound B RS. USP Oxybutynin Related Compound C RS.

Identification, *Infrared Absorption* ⟨197K⟩.

Melting range ⟨741⟩: between 124° and 129°.

Loss on drying ⟨731⟩: Dry it at 105° for 2 hours: it loses not more than 3% of its weight.

Residue on ignition ⟨281⟩: not more than 0.1%.

Heavy metals, *Method I* ⟨231⟩: 0.002%.

Related compounds—

Phosphate buffer and *Mobile phase*—Prepare as directed in the *Assay*.

System suitability stock solution—Dissolve accurately weighed quantities of USP Oxybutynin Related Compound B RS and USP Oxybutynin Related Compound C RS in *Mobile phase* to obtain a solution having known concentrations of about 100 µg of each USP Reference Standard per mL.

Standard stock solution—Dissolve an accurately weighed quantity of USP Oxybutynin Chloride RS in *Mobile phase* to obtain a solution having a known concentration of about 1.0 mg per mL.

System suitability solution—Transfer 10.0 mL of the *System suitability stock solution* to a 100-mL volumetric flask, add 10.0 mL of the *Standard stock solution,* and dilute with *Mobile phase* to volume.

Standard solution—Transfer 15.0 mL of the *Standard stock solution* to a 100-mL volumetric flask, and dilute with *Mobile phase* to volume. Transfer 5.0 mL of the solution obtained to a separate 100-mL volumetric flask, and dilute with *Mobile phase* to volume. This solution contains about 7.5 µg of USP Oxybutynin Chloride RS per mL.

Test solution—Transfer about 50 mg of Oxybutynin Chloride, accurately weighed, to a 10-mL volumetric flask, dissolve in and dilute with *Mobile phase* to volume, and mix.

Chromatographic system—Prepare as directed in the *Assay*. Chromatograph the *System suitability solution,* and record the peak responses as directed for *Procedure:* the resolution, *R,* between oxybutynin related compound B and oxybutynin related compound C is not less than 1.1; and the relative standard deviation for replicate injections, determined from the oxybutynin peak, is not more than 2.0%.

Procedure—Separately inject equal volumes (about 10 µL) of the *Standard solution* and the *Test solution* into the chromatograph, record the chromatograms for a total time of not less than twice the retention time of the oxybutynin peak, and measure all the peak responses (see *Table 1* for known impurities). Calculate the percentage of each impurity in the portion of Oxybutynin Chloride taken by the formula:

$$(C/W)(1/F)(r_U/r_S)$$

in which *C* is the concentration, in µg per mL, of USP Oxybutynin Chloride RS in the *Standard solution;* *W* is the weight, in mg, of Oxybutynin Chloride taken to prepare the *Test solution;* *F* is the relative response factor for each impurity (see *Table 1* for the values); and r_U and r_S are the peak responses for each impurity obtained from the *Test solution* and for the oxybutynin peak in the *Standard solution,* respectively. [NOTE—For unknown impurities, use the relative response factor of 1.0.]

Table 1

Compound Name	Relative Retention Time	Relative Response Factor (F)	Limit (%)
Oxybutynin related compound A[1]	0.08	1.4	0.5
Diphenyl analog of oxybutynin chloride[2]	0.37	2.7	0.1
Oxybutynin related compound B[3]	0.65	1.3	1.0
Oxybutynin related compound C[4]	0.79	1.0	1.0
Cyclohexenyl analog of oxybutynin chloride[5]	1.8	0.4	1.0
Ethylpropyl analog of oxybutynin chloride[6]	1.9	1.0	0.1

[1] Phenylcyclohexylglycolic acid (cyclohexylmandelic acid, or CHMA)
[2] 4-(Diethylamino)but-2-ynyl 2-hydroxy-2,2-diphenylacetate
[3] Methyl ester of phenylcyclohexylglycolic acid (methyl ester of cyclohexylmandelic acid, or CHMME)
[4] Methylethyl analog of oxybutynin chloride (4-(ethylmethylamino) but-2-ynyl (±)-2-cyclohexyl-2-hydroxy-2-phenylacetate)
[5] 4-(Diethylamino)but-2-ynyl (±)-2-(cyclohex-3-enyl)-2-cyclohexyl-hydroxyacetate
[6] 4-(Ethylpropylamino)but-2-ynyl (±)-2-cyclohexyl-2-hydroxy-2-phenylacetate

In addition to not exceeding the limits for each impurity in *Table 1*, not more than 0.1% of any other single impurity is found; and not more than 1.0% of total impurities is found.

Organic volatile impurities, *Method I* ⟨467⟩: meets the requirements.

(Official until July 1, 2008)

Chloride content—Dissolve about 600 mg of oxybutynin chloride, previously dried and accurately weighed, in 100 mL of water, and add 5 mL of nitric acid. Titrate (see *Titrimetry* ⟨541⟩) with 0.1 N silver nitrate VS, determining the endpoint potentiometrically, using a platinum-silver chloride electrode system. Each mL of 0.1 N silver nitrate is equivalent to 3.545 mg of Cl: the content is between 8% and 10%.

Assay—

Phosphate buffer—Dissolve about 6.67 g of monobasic potassium phosphate and 8.55 g of dibasic potassium phosphate in 1 L of water, and mix.

Mobile phase—Prepare a filtered and degassed mixture of *Phosphate buffer* and acetonitrile (51 : 49). Make adjustments if necessary (see *System Suitability* under *Chromatography* ⟨621⟩).

Standard preparation—Dissolve an accurately weighed quantity of USP Oxybutynin Chloride RS in *Mobile phase*, and dilute quantitatively, and stepwise if necessary, with *Mobile phase* to obtain a solution having a known concentration of about 0.1 mg per mL.

Assay preparation—Transfer about 50 mg of Oxybutynin Chloride, accurately weighed, to a 10-mL volumetric flask, dissolve in and dilute with *Mobile phase* to volume, and mix. Transfer 2.0 mL of this solution to a separate 100-mL volumetric flask, dilute with *Mobile phase* to volume, and mix.

Chromatographic system (see *Chromatography* ⟨621⟩)—The liquid chromatograph is equipped with a 210-nm detector and a 3-µm or 3.5-µm, 4.6-mm × 7.5-cm column that contains packing L7. The column temperature is maintained at 45°. The flow rate is about 1 mL per minute. Chromatograph the *Standard preparation,* and record the peak responses as directed for *Procedure:* the relative standard deviation for replicate injections is not more than 2.0%.

Procedure—Separately inject equal volumes (about 10 µL) of the *Standard preparation* and the *Assay preparation* into the chromatograph, record the chromatograms, and measure the responses for the

major peaks. Calculate the quantity, in mg, of $C_{22}H_{31}NO_3 \cdot HCl$ in the portion of Oxybutynin Chloride taken by the formula:

$$CD(r_U / r_S)$$

in which C is the concentration, in mg per mL, of USP Oxybutynin Chloride RS in the *Standard preparation;* D is the dilution factor for the *Assay preparation;* and r_U and r_S are the peak responses obtained from the *Assay preparation* and the *Standard preparation*, respectively.

Oxybutynin Chloride Oral Solution

» Oxybutynin Chloride Oral Solution contains not less than 90.0 percent and not more than 110.0 percent of the labeled amount of $C_{22}H_{31}NO_3 \cdot HCl$.

Packaging and storage—Preserve in tight, light-resistant containers.

USP Reference standards ⟨11⟩—*USP Oxybutynin Chloride RS.*
Identification—Place a volume of Oral Solution, equivalent to about 50 mg of oxybutynin chloride, in a separator, and extract with 10 mL of chloroform. The extract so obtained responds to the *Thin-Layer Chromatographic Identification Test* ⟨201⟩, methanol being used as the developing solvent, and iodine vapor being used to visualize the spots.
Assay—
pH 4 Phosphate buffer—Place 38 mL of 0.2 M dibasic sodium phosphate in a 100-mL volumetric flask. Dilute with 0.1 M citric acid to volume, and mix. Adjust the pH, if necessary, with either the dibasic sodium phosphate solution or the citric acid solution.
pH 5.6 Phosphate buffer—Place 58 mL of 0.2 M dibasic sodium phosphate in a 100-mL volumetric flask. Dilute with 0.1 M citric acid to volume, and mix. Adjust the pH, if necessary, with either the dibasic sodium phosphate solution or the citric acid solution.
Bromocresol green solution—Transfer 125 mg of bromocresol green to a 25-mL volumetric flask, dissolve in 3.5 mL of 0.05 N sodium hydroxide, dilute with water to volume, and mix.
Standard preparation—Dissolve an accurately weighed quantity of USP Oxybutynin Chloride RS in 0.05 N sulfuric acid to obtain a solution having a known concentration of about 100 µg per mL.
Assay preparation—Transfer an accurately measured volume of Oral Solution, equivalent to about 10 mg of oxybutynin chloride, to a 100-mL volumetric flask, dilute with water to volume, and mix.
Procedure—Separately transfer 10.0 mL of the *Standard preparation* and the *Assay preparation* to separate 125-mL separators. Add 20 mL of *pH 4 Phosphate buffer* to each separator, and extract each solution with a 25-mL portion of chloroform. [NOTE—Allow at least 10 minutes for the layers to separate.] Collect the chloroform extracts in respective 125-mL separators, each containing a mixture of 2 mL of *pH 5.6 Phosphate buffer* and 1 mL of *Bromocresol green solution*. Shake the separators, and filter the chloroform extracts through rayon pledgets, collecting the extracts in respective 100-mL volumetric flasks. Repeat the double extractions with 25-mL portions of chloroform. Wash the rayon pledgets with chloroform, collecting the washings in the respective 100-mL volumetric flasks. Dilute both solutions with chloroform to volume, and mix. Concomitantly determine the absorbances of both solutions at the wavelength of maximum absorbance at about 415 nm, with a suitable spectrophotometer, against a blank prepared using 10 mL of 0.05 N sulfuric acid treated in the same manner as the *Standard preparation* and the *Assay preparation*. Calculate the quantity, in mg, of $C_{22}H_{31}NO_3 \cdot HCl$ in each mL of Oral Solution taken by the formula:

$$(0.1C / V)(A_U / A_S)$$

in which C is the concentration, in µg per mL, of USP Oxybutynin Chloride RS in the *Standard preparation;* V is the volume, in mL, of Oral Solution taken; and A_U and A_S are the absorbances of the solutions from the *Assay preparation* and the *Standard preparation*, respectively.

Oxybutynin Chloride Tablets

» Oxybutynin Chloride Tablets contain not less than 90.0 percent and not more than 110.0 percent of the labeled amount of $C_{22}H_{31}NO_3 \cdot HCl$.

Packaging and storage—Preserve in tight, light-resistant containers.
USP Reference standards ⟨11⟩—*USP Oxybutynin Chloride RS.*
Identification—Add a portion of powdered Tablets, equivalent to about 50 mg of oxybutynin chloride, to 10 mL of chloroform. Mix for two minutes, and centrifuge. The supernatant layer of the solution so obtained responds to the *Thin-Layer Chromatographic Identification Test* ⟨201⟩, methanol being used as the developing solvent and iodine vapor being used to visualize the spots.
Dissolution ⟨711⟩—
Medium: water; 900 mL.
Apparatus 2: 50 rpm.
Time: 30 minutes.
Procedure—Determine the amount of $C_{22}H_{31}NO_3 \cdot HCl$ dissolved using the method set forth in the *Assay*, making any necessary modifications to the concentration of the *Standard preparation* to correspond to that of the solution under test.
Tolerances—Not less than 80% (*Q*) of the labeled amount of $C_{22}H_{31}NO_3 \cdot HCl$ is dissolved in 30 minutes.
Uniformity of dosage units ⟨905⟩: meet the requirements.
Assay—
Solvent A—Add about 0.9 mL of triethylamine to a filtered and deaerated mixture of water and methanol (3200 : 800). Adjust with phosphoric acid to a pH of 3.5 ± 0.05.
Mobile phase—Prepare a degassed and filtered mixture of *Solvent A* and acetonitrile (80 : 20).
Standard preparation—Prepare a solution of USP Oxybutynin Chloride RS in *Mobile phase* having an accurately known concentration of about 0.05 mg per mL.
Assay preparation—Weigh and finely powder not less than 20 Tablets. Transfer an accurately weighed portion of the powder, equivalent to about 50 mg of oxybutynin chloride, to a 1000-mL volumetric flask, add about 400 mL of *Mobile phase*, sonicate for about 10 minutes, shake by mechanical means for about 45 minutes, dilute with *Mobile phase* to volume, and mix.
Chromatographic system—The liquid chromatograph is equipped with a 203-nm detector, and a 4-mm × 30-cm column that contains packing L10. The flow rate is about 2 mL per minute. Chromatograph the *Standard preparation*, and record the chromatogram as directed for *Procedure:* the tailing factor is not more than 2.0, and the relative standard deviation for replicate injections is not more than 2.0%.
Procedure—Separately inject equal volumes (about 20 µL) of the *Standard preparation* and the *Assay preparation* into the chromatograph, record the chromatograms, and measure the responses for the major peaks. Calculate the quantity, in mg, of $C_{22}H_{31}NO_3 \cdot HCl$ in the portion of Tablets taken by the formula:

$$1000C(r_U / r_S)$$

in which C is the concentration, in mg per mL, of USP Oxybutynin Chloride RS in the *Standard preparation*, and r_U and r_S are the oxybutynin peak responses obtained from the *Assay preparation* and the *Standard preparation*, respectively.

Oxybutynin Chloride Extended-Release Tablets

» Oxybutynin Chloride Extended-Release Tablets contain not less than 90.0 percent and not more than 110.0 percent of the labeled amount of oxybutynin chloride ($C_{22}H_{31}NO_3 \cdot HCl$).

Packaging and storage—Preserve in tight containers. Store at controlled room temperature.

USP Reference standards ⟨11⟩—*USP Oxybutynin Chloride RS. USP Oxybutynin Related Compound A RS.*

Identification—

A: *Infrared Absorption* ⟨197⟩—

Test specimen—Add a quantity of finely powdered Tablets, equivalent to about 15 mg of oxybutynin chloride, to 5 mL of water per Tablet. Mix for 1 minute. Adjust with 0.1 N sodium hydroxide to a pH between 7 and 8. Extract the solution twice with 10 mL of ether. Combine the extracts, evaporate the ether, and dry under vacuum over silica gel for at least 30 minutes. Redissolve the dried residue in a small amount of acetone, transfer the solution to an IR salt plate, and evaporate to cast a thin film.

Standard specimen—Dissolve 15 mg of USP Oxybutynin Chloride RS in 5 mL of water. Proceed as directed for the *Test specimen,* beginning with "Adjust with".

B: The retention time of the major peak in the chromatogram of the *Assay preparation* corresponds to that in the chromatogram of the *Standard preparation,* as obtained in the *Assay.*

Drug release ⟨724⟩—

Medium: simulated gastric fluid without enzymes; 50 mL.

Apparatus 7: 30 cycles per minute; 2- to 3-cm amplitude.

Times: 4, 10, and 24 hours.

Determine the amount of $C_{22}H_{31}NO_3 \cdot HCl$ dissolved by employing the following method.

0.035 M Phosphate buffer, pH 2.2—Dissolve about 4.83 g of monobasic sodium phosphate in 1000 mL of water, add 2.3 mL of triethylamine, and adjust with phosphoric acid to a pH of 2.2 ± 0.2.

Acidified water—To 1 L of water add phosphoric acid dropwise to a pH of 3.5, and mix well.

Standard stock solutions—Dissolve accurately weighed quantities of USP Oxybutynin RS in acetonitrile, and dilute quantitatively, and stepwise if necessary, with acetonitrile to obtain solutions having known concentrations of about 250, 300, and 350 µg per mL.

Standard solutions—Prepare a series of dilutions of the *Standard stock solutions* in acidified water having final concentrations similar to those expected in the *Test solution.*

Test solution—Use portions of the solution under test. If the solution is cloudy, centrifuge at 2000 rpm for 10 minutes, and use the supernatant.

Mobile phase—Prepare a suitable filtered and degassed mixture of *0.035 M Phosphate buffer, pH 2.2* and acetonitrile (65 : 35). Make adjustments if necessary (see *System Suitability* under *Chromatography* ⟨621⟩).

System suitability solution—Use a medium range *Standard solution* of USP Oxybutynin Chloride RS.

Chromatographic system (see *Chromatography* ⟨621⟩)—The liquid chromatograph is equipped with a 230-nm detector and a 4.6-mm × 5-cm column that contains packing L11. The flow rate is about 1.5 mL per minute. The column temperature is maintained at about 35°. Chromatograph the *System suitability solution,* and record the peak responses as directed for *Procedure:* the tailing factor is greater than 0.5 and less than 2.5; and the relative standard deviation for replicate injections is not more than 2.0%.

Procedure—Separately inject equal volumes (about 50 µL) of the *Standard solutions* and the *Test solution* into the chromatograph, record the chromatograms, and measure the peak responses. Construct a calibration curve by plotting the peak response versus concentration of the *Standard solutions.* A weighting factor, $1/x$, is applied to the regression line of the calibration curve to enhance the accuracy of the low standard concentrations. Determine the amount of $C_{22}H_{31}NO_3 \cdot HCl$ dissolved in each interval from a linear regression analysis of the calibration curve.

Tolerances—The percentages of the labeled amount of $C_{22}H_{31}NO_3 \cdot HCl$ dissolved at the times specified conform to *Acceptance Table 1.*

FOR TABLETS LABELED TO CONTAIN 5 MG OR 10 MG OF OXYBUTYNIN CHLORIDE:

Time (hours)	Amount dissolved
4	not more than 20%
10	between 34.5% and 59.5%
24	not less than 80%

FOR TABLETS LABELED TO CONTAIN 15 MG OF OXYBUTYNIN CHLORIDE:

Time (hours)	Amount dissolved
4	not more than 20%
10	between 34.5% and 59.5%
24	not less than 75%

Uniformity of dosage units ⟨905⟩: meet the requirements.

Related compounds—

Mobile phase, Diluent, Preparation medium, Impurity stock solution, System suitability solution, and *Chromatographic system*—Proceed as directed in the *Assay.*

Impurity standard solution—Dilute the *Impurity stock solution* with *Diluent* to obtain a solution having a known concentration of about 1 µg of oxybutynin related compound A per mL. [NOTE—Oxybutynin related compound A is phenylcyclohexylglycolic acid.]

Test solution—Use the *Assay preparation.*

Procedure—Separately inject equal volumes (about 50 µL) of the *Impurity standard solution* and the *Test solution* into the chromatograph, record the chromatograms, and measure the peak responses. Calculate the percentage of each impurity in the portion of Tablets taken by the formula:

$$C(r_U / r_S)$$

in which C is the concentration, in µg per mL, of oxybutynin related compound A in the *Impurity standard solution;* and r_U and r_S are the peak responses for each impurity obtained from the *Test solution* and the *Impurity standard solution,* respectively. Disregard any peak less than 0.1%: not more than 1% of oxybutynin related compound A is found, and not more than 2% of total impurities is found.

Assay—

Mobile phase—Prepare a mixture of water, acetonitrile, and triethylamine (65 : 35 : 0.15). Adjust with phosphoric acid to a pH of 3.9, degas, and filter.

Diluent—Use water adjusted with phosphoric acid to a pH of 3.5.

Preparation medium—Prepare a solution of methanol and acetonitrile (1 : 1).

Impurity stock solution—Dissolve an accurately weighed quantity of USP Oxybutynin Related Compound A RS in acetonitrile to obtain a solution having a known concentration of about 0.11 mg per mL.

Standard stock preparation—Dissolve an accurately weighed quantity of USP Oxybutynin Chloride RS in acetonitrile to obtain a solution having a known concentration of about 0.37 mg per mL.

System suitability solution—Transfer 10 mL of the *Standard stock preparation* and 1 mL of the *Impurity stock solution* into a 100-mL volumetric flask, dilute with *Diluent* to volume, and mix.

Standard preparation—Dilute the *Standard stock preparation* with *Diluent* to obtain a solution having a known concentration of about 0.1 mg per mL.

Assay preparation—

FOR TABLETS THAT CONTAIN 5 MG OF OXYBUTYNIN CHLORIDE—Place 10 Tablets in a 500-mL volumetric flask, add 150 mL of *Preparation medium,* and stir for at least 4 hours or until dissolved. Dilute with *Diluent* to volume. Mix thoroughly, centrifuge, and use the clear supernatant.

FOR TABLETS THAT CONTAIN 10 MG OF OXYBUTYNIN CHLORIDE OR MORE—Place 10 Tablets in a 1000-mL volumetric flask, add 300 mL of *Preparation medium,* and stir for at least 4 hours or until dissolved. Dilute with *Diluent* to volume. If necessary, make a further dilution with *Diluent* to obtain a solution having a final concentration equivalent to 0.1 mg per mL of oxybutynin chloride. Mix thoroughly, centrifuge, and use the clear supernatant.

Chromatographic system (see *Chromatography* ⟨621⟩)—The liquid chromatograph is equipped with a 220-nm detector and a 4.6-mm × 15-cm column that contains packing L11. The flow rate is about 1.5 mL per minute. Chromatograph the *System suitability solution,* and record the peak responses as directed for *Procedure:* the relative retention times are about 1.0 for oxybutynin and about 1.6 for oxybutynin related compound A; the resolution, *R*, between oxybutynin and oxybutynin related compound A is not less than 1.5; the tailing factor is greater than 0.75 and not more than 2.5 for each peak; and the relative standard deviation of peak area responses for six replicate injections is not more than 3% for each compound.

Procedure—Separately inject equal volumes (about 50 µL) of the *Standard preparation* and the *Assay preparation* into the chromatograph, record the chromatograms, and measure the area responses for the major peaks. Calculate the quantity, in mg, of oxybutynin chloride ($C_{22}H_{31}NO_3 \cdot HCl$) in the portion of Tablets taken by the formula:

$$CVD(r_U / r_S)$$

in which *C* is the concentration, in mg per mL, of oxybutynin chloride in the *Standard preparation;* *V* is the volume, in mL, of the *Assay preparation;* *D* is the dilution factor; and r_U and r_S are the peak area responses obtained from the *Assay preparation* and the *Standard preparation,* respectively.

Oxycodone Hydrochloride

$C_{18}H_{21}NO_4 \cdot HCl$ 351.82

Morphinan-6-one, 4,5-epoxy-14-hydroxy-3-methoxy-17-methyl-, hydrochloride, (5α)-.

4,5α-Epoxy-14-hydroxy-3-methoxy-17-methylmorphinan-6-one hydrochloride   [124-90-3].

» Oxycodone Hydrochloride contains not less than 97.0 percent and not more than 103.0 percent of $C_{18}H_{21}NO_4 \cdot HCl$, calculated on the anhydrous, solvent-free basis.

Packaging and storage—Preserve in tight containers.

USP Reference standards ⟨11⟩—*USP Oxycodone RS.*

Identification—

A: Dissolve 250 mg in 25 mL of water. Render the solution alkaline with 6 N ammonium hydroxide. Allow the mixture to stand until a precipitate is formed. Filter, wash the precipitate with 50 mL of cold water, and dry for 2 hours at 105°: the precipitate so obtained melts between 218° and 223°, but the range between beginning and end of melting does not exceed 2° (see *Melting Range or Temperature* ⟨741⟩).

B: *Infrared Absorption* ⟨197K⟩: using a portion of the dried precipitate obtained in *Identification* test *A.*

Specific rotation ⟨781S⟩:   between −137° and −149°.

Test solution: 25 mg per mL, in water, calculated on the anhydrous, solvent-free basis.

Water, *Method I* ⟨921⟩:   not more than 7.0%.

Residue on ignition ⟨281⟩:   not more than 0.05%, the use of sulfuric acid being omitted.

Limit of alcohol (C_2H_5OH)—

Internal standard stock solution—Transfer 6.0 mL of isopropyl alcohol to a 500-mL volumetric flask, dilute with water to volume, and mix. [NOTE—The isopropyl alcohol must be free of alcohol impurities.]

Internal standard solution—Transfer 5.0 mL of *Internal standard stock solution* to a 100-mL volumetric flask, dilute with water to volume, and mix.

Standard solution—Prepare a solution of alcohol in water to obtain a solution having a known concentration of about 16 mg of alcohol (C_2H_5OH) per mL. Pipet 3.0 mL of this solution and 5.0 mL of the *Internal standard stock solution* into a 100-mL volumetric flask, dilute with water to volume, and mix.

Test solution—Transfer about 240 mg of Oxycodone Hydrochloride, accurately weighed, to a 15-mL centrifuge tube, add 5.0 mL of *Internal standard solution,* and mix to dissolve.

Chromatographic system (see *Chromatography* ⟨621⟩)—The gas chromatograph is equipped with a flame-ionization detector and a 4-mm × 1.8-m glass column that is packed with 80- to 100-mesh support S3, helium being used as the carrier gas. Prior to use, condition the column overnight at 235° with a slow flow of carrier gas. The column is maintained at 150°, and the injection port and detector temperatures are maintained at 170°. Chromatograph the *Standard solution,* and record the peak responses as directed for *Procedure:* the resolution, *R*, between isopropyl alcohol and alcohol is not less than 2; the tailing factor for alcohol is not more than 1.5; and the relative standard deviation for replicate injections is not more than 2.0%.

Procedure—Separately inject equal volumes (about 5 µL) of the *Standard solution* and the *Test solution* into the chromatograph, record the chromatograms, and measure the responses for the major peaks. Calculate the percentage of C_2H_5OH in the portion of Oxycodone Hydrochloride taken by the formula:

$$100(C_S / C_U)(R_U / R_S)$$

in which C_S is the concentration, in mg per mL, of alcohol (C_2H_5OH) in the *Standard solution;* C_U is the concentration, in mg per mL, of oxycodone hydrochloride in the *Test solution;* and R_U and R_S are the ratios of the alcohol peak to the isopropyl alcohol peak obtained from the *Test solution* and the *Standard solution,* respectively. Not more than 1.0% (w/w) of alcohol (C_2H_5OH) is found.

Chloride content—Dissolve about 300 mg, accurately weighed, in 50 mL of methanol, add 5 mL of glacial acetic acid, and titrate with 0.1 N silver nitrate VS, determining the endpoint potentiometrically. Each mL of 0.1 N silver nitrate is equivalent to 3.545 mg of Cl: the content of Cl is between 9.8% and 10.4%, calculated on the anhydrous, solvent-free basis.

Chromatographic purity—Using the chromatogram of the *Assay preparation* obtained in the *Assay,* calculate the percentage of each impurity in the Oxycodone Hydrochloride taken by the formula:

$$100(r_i / r_s)$$

in which r_i is the peak response for each impurity; and r_s is the sum of the responses of all the peaks: not more than 1.0% of any individual impurity is found; and the sum of all impurities is not more than 2.0%.

Assay—

Mobile phase—Prepare a mixture of 0.005 M sodium 1-hexanesulfonate, methanol, phosphoric acid, and triethylamine (900 : 100 : 5 : 2). Adjust with 50% sodium hydroxide solution to a pH of 2.5 ± 0.1, filter, and degas. Make adjustments if necessary (see *System Suitability* under *Chromatography* ⟨621⟩).

Resolution solution—Prepare a solution in *Mobile phase* containing about 13 µg of codeine phosphate and 9 µg of oxycodone per mL.

Standard preparation—Quantitatively dissolve an accurately weighed quantity of USP Oxycodone RS in *Mobile phase* to obtain a solution having a known concentration of about 0.9 mg per mL.

Assay preparation—Transfer about 100 mg of Oxycodone Hydrochloride, accurately weighed, to a 100-mL volumetric flask, add about 50 mL of *Mobile phase,* and swirl to dissolve. Dilute with *Mobile phase* to volume, and mix. Pass a portion of this solution through a filter having a 0.5-µm or finer porosity, and use the filtrate as the *Assay preparation.*

Chromatographic system (see *Chromatography* ⟨621⟩)—The liquid chromatograph is equipped with a 206-nm detector and a 3.9-mm × 15-cm column that contains 4-µm packing L7 and is maintained at a constant temperature of about 50°. The flow rate is about 1.5 mL per minute. Chromatograph the *Resolution solution,* and record the peak responses as directed for *Procedure:* the relative retention times are about 0.8 for codeine and 1.0 for oxycodone; and the resolution, *R*, between codeine and oxycodone is not less than 3.0. Chromatograph the *Standard preparation,* and record the peak responses as directed for *Procedure:* the tailing factor is between 0.75 and 1.25; and the relative standard deviation for replicate injections is not more than 2.0%.

Procedure—Separately inject equal volumes (about 10 µL) of the *Standard preparation* and the *Assay preparation* into the chromatograph, record the chromatograms for a period of time that is twice the retention time of the main oxycodone peak, and measure the responses for all the peaks. Calculate the quantity, in mg, of $C_{18}H_{21}NO_4 \cdot HCl$ in the portion of Oxycodone Hydrochloride taken by the formula:

$$(351.82/315.37)(100C)(r_U/r_S)$$

in which 351.82 and 315.37 are the molecular weights of oxycodone hydrochloride and oxycodone base, respectively; *C* is the concentration, in mg per mL, of USP Oxycodone RS in the *Standard preparation*; and r_U and r_S are the oxycodone peak area responses obtained from the *Assay preparation* and the *Standard preparation*, respectively.

Oxycodone Hydrochloride Oral Solution

» Oxycodone Hydrochloride Oral Solution contains not less than 90.0 percent and not more than 110.0 percent of the labeled amount of oxycodone hydrochloride ($C_{18}H_{21}NO_4 \cdot HCl$).

Packaging and storage—Preserve in tight, light-resistant containers.

USP Reference standards ⟨11⟩—*USP Oxycodone RS.*
Identification—
　A: Transfer a quantity of Oral Solution, equivalent to about 15 mg of oxycodone, to a separator, add 10 mL of 0.01 N hydrochloric acid, and extract with four 40-mL portions of chloroform, collecting the chloroform extracts in a second separator. Wash the combined chloroform extracts with 5 mL of 0.01 N hydrochloric acid, and discard the chloroform layer. Combine the acidic wash with the aqueous solution remaining in the first separator, and adjust with 6 N ammonium hydroxide to a pH of 9.5 ± 0.5. Extract with one 50-mL and two 20-mL portions of chloroform, and filter the chloroform extracts through chloroform-washed cotton, collecting the filtrate in a 100-mL volumetric flask. Dilute with water-saturated chloroform to volume, and mix (test solution). Similarly prepare a Standard solution using about 12 mg of USP Oxycodone RS and 25 mL of 0.01 N hydrochloric acid, and proceed as directed above beginning with "extract with four 40-mL portions of chloroform." The UV absorption spectrum of the test solution exhibits maxima and minima at the same wavelengths as that of the Standard solution, concomitantly measured.
　B: Separately evaporate 5 mL of the test solution and 5 mL of the Standard solution obtained in *Identification* test *A* just to dryness. Dissolve each residue in 1.0 mL of chloroform. Apply separate 20-µL portions of the solution from the test solution and the solution from the Standard solution to a suitable thin-layer chromatographic plate (see *Chromatography* ⟨621⟩) coated with a 0.25-mm layer of chromatographic silica gel mixture. Allow the spots to dry, and develop the chromatogram in solvent system consisting of a mixture of acetone, toluene, ether, and ammonium hydroxide (6 : 4 : 1 : 0.3) until the solvent front has moved about three-fourths of the length of the plate. Remove the plate from the chamber, mark the solvent front, allow the solvent to evaporate, and spray with iodoplatinate TS: the principal spot obtained from the solution from the test solution corresponds in color, size, and R_F value to that obtained from the solution from the Standard solution, and no other spots are observed.
　C: The retention time of the oxycodone peak in the chromatogram of the *Assay preparation* corresponds to that in the chromatogram of the *Standard preparation* obtained as directed in the *Assay*.
Uniformity of dosage units ⟨905⟩—
　FOR ORAL SOLUTION PACKAGED IN SINGLE-UNIT CONTAINERS: meets the requirements.

Deliverable volume ⟨698⟩—
　FOR ORAL SOLUTION PACKAGED IN MULTIPLE-UNIT CONTAINERS: meets the requirements.
pH ⟨791⟩: between 1.4 and 4.0.
Alcohol content, *Method II* ⟨611⟩ *(if present):* between 85.0% and 115.0% of the labeled amount of C_2H_5OH, determined by the gas-liquid chromatographic method, acetone being used as the internal standard.
Assay—
　Mobile phase, Standard preparation, and *Chromatographic system*—Proceed as directed in the *Assay* under *Oxycodone Hydrochloride Tablets.*
　Assay preparation—Transfer an accurately measured volume of Oral Solution, equivalent to about 5 mg of oxycodone hydrochloride, to a 100-mL volumetric flask, dilute with *Mobile phase* to volume, and mix. Pass a portion of this mixture through a filter having a 0.5-µm or finer porosity, and use the clear filtrate as the *Assay preparation.*
　Procedure—Proceed as directed for *Procedure* in the *Assay* under *Oxycodone Hydrochloride Tablets.* Calculate the quantity, in mg, of oxycodone hydrochloride ($C_{18}H_{21}NO_4 \cdot HCl$) in each mL of the Oral Solution taken by the formula:

$$(351.82/315.37)(100C/V)(r_U/r_S)$$

in which *V* is the volume, in mL, of Oral Solution taken; and the other terms are as defined therein.

Oxycodone Hydrochloride Tablets

» Oxycodone Hydrochloride Tablets contain not less than 90.0 percent and not more than 110.0 percent of the labeled amount of oxycodone hydrochloride ($C_{18}H_{21}NO_4 \cdot HCl$).

Packaging and storage—Preserve in tight, light-resistant containers.

USP Reference standards ⟨11⟩—*USP Oxycodone RS.*
Identification—
　A: The retention time of the oxycodone peak in the chromatogram of the *Assay preparation* corresponds to that in the chromatogram of the *Standard preparation,* as obtained in the *Assay.*
　B: *Thin-Layer Chromatographic Identification Test* ⟨201⟩—
　Test solution—Transfer a portion of powdered Tablets, equivalent to about 5 mg of oxycodone hydrochloride, to a suitable screw-capped tube, add 5 mL of chloroform, sonicate for about 30 seconds, shake for several minutes, and centrifuge. Use the clear supernatant.
　Standard solution: 0.9 mg of USP Oxycodone RS per mL of chloroform.
　Application volume: 20 µL.
　Developing solvent system: a mixture of acetone, toluene, ether, and ammonium hydroxide (6 : 4 : 1 : 0.3).
　Procedure—Proceed as directed in the chapter. Spray with iodoplatinate TS: the R_F value, color, and size of the principal spot obtained from the *Test solution* correspond to those obtained from the *Standard solution;* and no other spot is observed.
Dissolution ⟨711⟩—
　Medium: water; 500 mL.
　Apparatus 2: 50 rpm.
　Time: 45 minutes.
　Procedure—Determine the amount of $C_{18}H_{21}NO_4 \cdot HCl$ dissolved by employing UV absorption at about 225 nm on filtered portions of the solution under test, suitably diluted with *Dissolution Medium,* if necessary, in comparison with a Standard solution having a known concentration of USP Oxycodone RS in 0.1 N hydrochloric acid.
　Tolerances—Not less than 70% *(Q)* of the labeled amount of $C_{18}H_{21}NO_4 \cdot HCl$ is dissolved in 45 minutes.

Uniformity of dosage units ⟨905⟩: meet the requirements.

Assay—

*Mobile phase—*Prepare a suitable mixture of 0.01 M sodium 1-heptanesulfonate, acetonitrile, and glacial acetic acid (74 : 25 : 1). Adjust this mixture with 5 N sodium hydroxide to a pH of 3.5. Make adjustments if necessary (see *System Suitability* under *Chromatography* ⟨621⟩). Filter and degas this solution before use.

*Standard preparation—*Dissolve an accurately weighed quantity of USP Oxycodone RS quantitatively in *Mobile phase* to obtain a solution having a known concentration of about 0.045 mg per mL.

*Assay preparation—*Weigh and finely powder not less than 20 Tablets. Transfer an accurately weighed portion of the powder, equivalent to about 5 mg of oxycodone hydrochloride, to a 100-mL volumetric flask, add about 50 mL of *Mobile phase*, sonicate for about 5 minutes, and shake by mechanical means for about 15 minutes. Dilute with *Mobile phase* to volume, and mix. Filter a portion of this mixture through a filter having a porosity of 0.5 μm or finer, and use the clear filtrate as the *Assay preparation*.

Chromatographic system (see *Chromatography* ⟨621⟩)—The liquid chromatograph is equipped with a 280-nm detector and a 4.6-mm × 15-cm column that contains 5-μm packing L1. The flow rate is about 1.7 mL per minute. Chromatograph the *Standard preparation*, and record the peak responses as directed for *Procedure*: the tailing factor for the oxycodone peak is not more than 2.0, and the relative standard deviation for replicate injections is not more than 2.0%.

*Procedure—*Separately inject equal volumes (about 10 μL) of the *Standard preparation* and the *Assay preparation* into the chromatograph, record the chromatograms, and measure the responses of the oxycodone peaks. Calculate the quantity, in mg, of oxycodone hydrochloride ($C_{18}H_{21}NO_4 \cdot HCl$) in the portion of Tablets taken by the formula:

$$(351.82 / 315.37)(100C)(r_U / r_S)$$

in which 351.82 and 315.37 are the molecular weights of oxycodone hydrochloride and oxycodone base, respectively, C is the concentration, in mg per mL, of USP Oxycodone RS in the *Standard preparation*, and r_U and r_S are the oxycodone peak responses obtained from the *Assay preparation* and the *Standard preparation*, respectively.

Add the following:

▲Oxycodone Hydrochloride Extended-Release Tablets

» Oxycodone Hydrochloride Extended-Release Tablets contain not less than 90.0 percent and not more than 110.0 percent of the labeled amount of oxycodone hydrochloride ($C_{18}H_{21}NO_4 \cdot HCl$).

Packaging and storage—Preserve in tight, light-resistant containers, and store at controlled room temperature.

Labeling—When more than one *Dissolution Test* is given, the labeling states the *Dissolution Test* used only if *Test 1* is not used.

USP Reference standards ⟨11⟩—*USP Oxycodone RS. USP Oxycodone Related Compound A RS.*

Identification—

A: *Thin-Layer Chromatographic Identification Test* ⟨201⟩—

*Test solution—*Transfer a portion of powdered Tablets, equivalent to about 5 mg of oxycodone hydrochloride, to a suitable screw-capped tube, add 5 mL of chloroform, sonicate for about 30 seconds, shake for several minutes, and centrifuge. Use the clear supernatant.

Standard solution: 0.9 mg of USP Oxycodone RS per mL of chloroform.

Application volume: 20 μL.

Developing solvent solution: a mixture of acetone, toluene, ether, and ammonium hydroxide (6 : 4 : 1 : 0.3).

*Procedure—*Proceed as directed in the chapter. Spray with iodoplatinate TS: the R_F value, color, and size of the principal spot obtained from the *Test solution* correspond to those obtained from the *Standard solution*; and no other spot is observed.

B: The retention time of the major peak in the chromatogram of the *Assay preparation* corresponds to that in the chromatogram of the *Standard preparation*, as obtained in the *Assay*.

Dissolution ⟨711⟩—

TEST 1—

Medium: simulated gastric fluid (without enzymes); 900 mL.

Apparatus 1: 100 rpm.

Times: 1, 2, 4, 6, and 8 hours, for Tablets labeled to contain 10 mg, 20 mg, or 40 mg; 1, 2, 4, and 6 hours, for Tablets labeled to contain 80 mg.

Determine the amount of oxycodone ($C_{18}H_{21}NO_4$) dissolved by employing the following method.

*Standard stock solution—*For Tablets labeled to contain 10 mg, transfer about 39.8 mg of USP Oxycodone RS, accurately weighed, into a 100-mL volumetric flask, and dissolve in and dilute with *Medium* to volume. For Tablets labeled to contain 20 mg, 40 mg, or 80 mg, transfer about 39.8 mg of USP Oxycodone RS, accurately weighed, into a 50-mL volumetric flask, and dissolve in and dilute with *Medium* to volume.

*Working standard solution—*Dilute the *Standard stock solution* with *Medium* to obtain solutions containing $L/900$ mg per mL, with L being the oxycodone Tablet label claim, in mg.

*Procedure—*Determine the amount of oxycodone ($C_{18}H_{21}NO_4$) dissolved from UV absorption at a wavelength of about 226 nm (shoulder), using filtered portions of the solution under test, suitably diluted with *Medium*, if necessary, in comparison with the appropriate *Working standard solution*. Use *Medium* as the blank, and a 1.0-cm cell for Tablets labeled to contain 10 mg, 20 mg, or 40 mg; and a 0.5-cm cell for Tablets labeled to contain 80 mg. For Tablets labeled to contain 10 mg, 20 mg, or 40 mg, calculate the amount of oxycodone ($C_{18}H_{21}NO_4$) dissolved by formula (1), in which C is the concentration, in mg per mL, of the appropriate *Working standard solution*; A_U and A_S are the absorbances of the solution under test and of the appropriate *Working standard solution*, respectively; V is the initial volume, in mL, of *Medium* in the vessel; V_S is the volume, in mL, withdrawn from the vessel for previous samplings; C_1 is the concentration, in mg per mL, of oxycodone in the *Medium* determined at 1 hour; C_2 is the concentration, in mg per mL, of oxycodone in the *Medium* determined at 2 hours; C_4 is the concentration, in mg per mL, of oxycodone in the *Medium* determined at 4 hours; C_6 is the concentration, in mg per mL, of oxycodone in the *Medium* determined at 6 hours; C_8 is the concentration, in mg per mL, of oxycodone in the *Medium* determined at 8 hours; 100 is the conversion factor to percentage; and L is the Tablet label claim, in mg.

For Tablets labeled to contain 80 mg, calculate the amount of oxycodone ($C_{18}H_{21}NO_4$) dissolved by formula (2), in which C is the concentration, in mg per mL, of the appropriate *Working standard solution*; A_U and A_S are the absorbances of the solution under test and of the appropriate *Working standard solution*, respectively; V is the initial volume, in mL, of *Medium* in the vessel; V_S is the volume, in mL, withdrawn from the vessel for previous samplings; C_1 is the concentration, in mg per mL, of oxycodone in the *Medium* determined at 1 hour; C_2 is the concentration, in mg per mL, of oxycodone in the *Medium* determined at 2 hours; C_4 is the concentration, in mg per mL, of oxycodone in the *Medium* determined at 4 hours; C_6 is the concentration, in mg per mL, of oxycodone in the *Medium* determined at 6 hours; 100 is the conversion factor to percentage; and L is the Tablet label claim, in mg.

$$\frac{[C \times (A_U / A_S) \times (V - V_S) + (C_1 \times V_S) + (C_2 \times V_S) + (C_4 \times V_S) + (C_6 \times V_S) + (C_8 \times V_S)] \times 100}{L} \quad (1)$$

$$\frac{[C \times (A_U / A_S) \times (V - V_S) + (C_1 \times V_S) + (C_2 \times V_S) + (C_4 \times V_S) + (C_6 \times V_S)] \times 100}{L} \quad (2)$$

Tolerances—The percentages of the labeled amount of oxycodone ($C_{18}H_{21}NO_4$) dissolved at the times specified conform to *Acceptance Table 2*.

FOR TABLETS LABELED TO CONTAIN 10 MG, 20 MG, OR 40 MG:

Time (hours)	Amount dissolved
1	between 20% and 40%
2	between 35% and 55%
4	between 55% and 75%
6	between 70% and 90%
8	not less than 80%

FOR TABLETS LABELED TO CONTAIN 80 MG:

Time (hours)	Amount dissolved
1	between 25% and 45%
2	between 45% and 65%
4	between 65% and 85%
6	not less than 80%

TEST 2—If the product complies with this test, the labeling indicates that the product meets USP *Dissolution Test 2*.
Medium: simulated gastric fluid (without enzymes); 900 mL.
Apparatus 1: 100 rpm.
Times: 1, 4, and 12 hours.
Determine the amount of oxycodone ($C_{18}H_{21}NO_4$) dissolved by employing the following method.
0.85% Phosphoric acid—Dilute 10 mL of phosphoric acid with water to 1 L.
Standard stock solution—Prepare a solution of USP Oxycodone RS in *0.85% Phosphoric acid* containing about 0.9 mg per mL.
Working standard solution—Dilute the *Standard stock solution*, quantitatively and stepwise, with *Medium* to obtain a solution having a concentration of about 40% of the Tablet label claim. [NOTE—This solution is stable for two weeks at room temperature.]
Test solution—Pass the solution under test through a suitable 0.45-µm filter.
Mobile phase—Weigh 23.1 g of monobasic potassium phosphate into a 4-L flask, and dissolve with 3400 mL of water. Add 4 mL of triethylamine, and adjust with *0.85% Phosphoric acid* to a pH of 3.0 ± 0.1. Add 600 mL of methanol and 20 mL of *tert*-butyl methyl ether, and mix well. Filter and degas. Make adjustments if necessary (see *System Suitability* under *Chromatography* ⟨621⟩).
Chromatographic system (see *Chromatography* ⟨621⟩)—The liquid chromatograph is equipped with a 230-nm detector and a 3.9-mm × 30-cm column that contains 10-µm packing L1 and that is maintained at a temperature of 60°. The flow rate is about 1.0 mL per minute. Chromatograph the *Working standard solution*, and record the peak responses as directed for *Procedure*: the tailing factor is not more than 1.5 and not less than 0.75; the capacity factor is not less than 0.5; and the relative standard deviation for replicate injections is not more than 2%.
Procedure—Separately inject equal volumes (about 50 µL) of the *Working standard solution* and the *Test solution* into the chromatograph, record the chromatograms, and measure the peak reponses. Calculate the amount of oxycodone ($C_{18}H_{21}NO_4$) dissolved by formula (3), in which C is the concentration, in mg per mL, of the appropriate *Working standard solution*; r_U and r_S are the peak responses of the solution under test and of the appropriate *Working standard solution*, respectively; V is the initial volume, in mL, of *Medium* in the vessel under test; V_S is the volume, in mL, withdrawn from the vessel for previous samplings; C_1 is the concentration, in mg per mL, of oxycodone in the *Medium* determined at 1 hour; C_4 is the concentration, in mg per mL, of oxycodone in the *Medium* determined at 4 hours; C_{12} is the concentration, in mg per mL, of oxycodone in the *Medium* determined at 12 hours; 100 is the conversion factor to percentage; and L is the Tablet label claim, in mg.

Tolerances—The percentages of the labeled amount of oxycodone ($C_{18}H_{21}NO_4$) dissolved at the times specified conform to *Acceptance Table 2*.

FOR TABLETS LABELED TO CONTAIN 10 MG:

Time (hours)	Amount dissolved
1	between 29% and 49%
4	between 58% and 78%
12	not less than 85%

FOR TABLETS LABELED TO CONTAIN 20 MG:

Time (hours)	Amount dissolved
1	between 33% and 53%
4	between 63% and 83%
12	not less than 85%

FOR TABLETS LABELED TO CONTAIN 40 MG:

Time (hours)	Amount dissolved
1	between 37% and 57%
4	between 68% and 88%
12	not less than 85%

FOR TABLETS LABELED TO CONTAIN 80 MG:

Time (hours)	Amount dissolved
1	between 31% and 51%
4	between 61% and 81%
12	not less than 85%

Uniformity of dosage units ⟨905⟩: meet the requirements.
Assay—
Buffer solution—Dissolve 1.5 g of sodium heptanesulfonate in 740 mL of water. Mix with 10 mL of glacial acetic acid, adjust with 5 N sodium hydroxide solution to a pH of 3.50 ± 0.05, and mix.
Mobile phase—Prepare a filtered and degassed mixture of *Buffer solution* and acetonitrile (75 : 25). Make adjustments if necessary (see *System Suitability* under *Chromatography* ⟨621⟩).
Standard preparation—Dissolve an accurately weighed quantity of USP Oxycodone RS in *Mobile phase*, and dilute quantitatively, and stepwise if necessary, with *Mobile phase* to obtain a solution having a known concentration of about 0.036 mg per mL.
Assay stock preparation—Transfer 10 Tablets into an appropriate volumetric flask, add a volume of a mixture of methanol and acetonitrile (50 : 50) equivalent to 50% of the volumetric flask volume, sonicate for about 10 minutes, and stir for about 20 minutes. Dilute with *Buffer solution* to volume, and mix.
Assay preparation—Transfer a volume of the *Assay stock preparation*, equivalent to 4 mg of oxycodone hydrochloride, into a 100-mL volumetric flask, dilute with *Mobile phase* to volume, and mix. Pass a portion of the solution through a suitable filter, and use the filtrate.

$$\frac{[C \times (r_U / r_S) \times (V - V_S) + (C_1 \times V_S) + (C_4 \times V_S) + (C_{12} \times V_S)] \times 100}{L} \quad (3)$$

Chromatographic system (see *Chromatography* ⟨621⟩)—The liquid chromatograph is equipped with a 280-nm detector and a 4.6-mm × 15-cm column that contains packing L1. The flow rate is about 1.0 mL per minute. Chromatograph the *Standard preparation*, and record the peak responses as directed for *Procedure*: the column efficiency is not less than 4000 theoretical plates; the tailing factor is not more than 2.0; and the relative standard deviation for replicate injections is not more than 2.0%.

Procedure—Separately inject equal volumes (about 20 μL) of the *Standard preparation* and the *Assay preparation* into the chromatograph, record the chromatograms, and measure the responses for the oxycodone peak. Calculate the quantity, in mg, of oxycodone hydrochloride ($C_{18}H_{21}NO_4 \cdot HCl$) in the portion of Tablets taken by the formula:

$$(351.82/315.37)CD(r_U/r_S)$$

in which 351.82 and 315.37 are the molecular weights of oxycodone hydrochloride and oxycodone base, respectively; C is the concentration, in mg per mL, of USP Oxycodone RS in the *Standard preparation*; D is the dilution factor, in mL, for the *Assay preparation*; and r_U and r_S are the peak responses obtained from the *Assay preparation* and the *Standard preparation*, respectively. ▲USP31

Oxycodone and Acetaminophen Capsules

» Oxycodone and Acetaminophen Capsules contain Oxycodone Hydrochloride and Acetaminophen, or Oxycodone Hydrochloride, Oxycodone Terephthalate, and Acetaminophen. Capsules contain not less than 90.0 percent and not more than 110.0 percent of the labeled amounts of oxycodone hydrochloride or oxycodone hydrochloride and oxycodone terephthalate, calculated as total oxycodone ($C_{18}H_{21}NO_4$), and not less than 90.0 percent and not more than 110.0 percent of the labeled amount of acetaminophen ($C_8H_9NO_2$).

Packaging and storage—Preserve in tight, light-resistant containers.

USP Reference standards ⟨11⟩—*USP Acetaminophen RS. USP Oxycodone RS.*

Identification—

A: To a quantity of Capsule contents, equivalent to about 2.5 mg of oxycodone, add 5 mL of a mixture of methanol and water (4 : 1), sonicate for 5 minutes, and shake by mechanical means for 15 minutes. Allow to settle, and use the clear supernatant as the test solution. Prepare a Standard solution of USP Oxycodone RS in the mixture of methanol and water (4 : 1) containing 0.5 mg per mL, and a second Standard solution of USP Acetaminophen RS in the same solvent containing 0.5J mg per mL, J being the ratio of the labeled amount, in mg, of acetaminophen to the labeled amount, in mg, of oxycodone per Capsule. Apply separate 20-μL portions of the test solution and the Standard solutions to a thin-layer chromatographic plate (see *Chromatography* ⟨621⟩) coated with a 0.25-mm layer of silica gel mixture. Allow the spots to dry, and develop the chromatogram in a solvent system consisting of a mixture of butyl alcohol, water, and glacial acetic acid (4 : 2 : 1) until the solvent front has moved about three-fourths of the length of the plate. Remove the plate from the developing chamber, mark the solvent front, and allow the plate to air-dry for about 30 minutes. Expose the plate to iodine vapors in a closed chamber, and locate the spots: the R_F values of the principal spots obtained from the test solution correspond to those obtained from the respective Standard solutions.

B: The retention times of the major peaks in the chromatogram of the *Assay preparation* correspond to those in the chromatogram of the *Standard preparation*, as obtained in the *Assay*.

Dissolution, *Procedure for a Pooled Sample* ⟨711⟩—
Medium: 0.1 N hydrochloric acid; 900 mL.
Apparatus 2: 50 rpm.
Time: 45 minutes.

Procedure—Determine the amounts of oxycodone ($C_{18}H_{21}NO_4$) and acetaminophen ($C_8H_9NO_2$) dissolved, employing the procedure set forth in the *Assay*, making any necessary volumetric adjustments, including adjusting the solution under test to a pH of about 5.5 before injecting.

Tolerances—Not less than 75% (*Q*) of the labeled amounts of $C_{18}H_{21}NO_4$ and $C_8H_9NO_2$ is dissolved in 45 minutes.

Uniformity of dosage units ⟨905⟩: meet the requirements for *Content Uniformity* with respect to oxycodone and for *Weight Variation* with respect to acetaminophen.

Assay—

Solvent mixture—Prepare a suitable mixture of 0.05 M dibasic potassium phosphate and methanol (9 : 1), and adjust with phosphoric acid to a pH of 4.0. Make adjustments if necessary (see *System Suitability* under *Chromatography* ⟨621⟩).

Mobile phase—Add 950 mg of monobasic potassium phosphate to 1000 mL of water. Add 1 mL of phosphoric acid, and stir until dissolved. While stirring, add 1 mL of *n*-nonylamine, and stir until a clear solution is obtained. Adjust with potassium hydroxide TS to a pH of 4.9 ± 0.1. Mix 9 volumes of this solution with 1 volume of methanol. Make adjustments if necessary (see *System Suitability* under *Chromatography* ⟨621⟩).

Oxycodone standard stock solution—Dissolve an accurately weighed quantity of USP Oxycodone RS in *Solvent mixture* to obtain a solution having a known concentration of about 0.075 mg per mL.

Standard preparation—Transfer about 0.75J mg of USP Acetaminophen RS, accurately weighed, J being the ratio of the labeled amount, in mg, of acetaminophen to that of oxycodone equivalent, to a 25-mL volumetric flask, add about 10 mL of *Solvent mixture*, and mix to dissolve. Add 10.0 mL of *Oxycodone standard stock solution*, dilute with *Solvent mixture* to volume, and mix. Transfer 5.0 mL of the solution so obtained to a 50-mL volumetric flask, dilute with *Mobile phase* to volume, and mix. This solution contains about 0.003 mg of USP Oxycodone RS and 0.003J mg of USP Acetaminophen RS per mL.

Assay preparation—Weigh the contents of not fewer than 20 Capsules. Mix the contents, and transfer an accurately weighed portion of the powder, equivalent to about 4.5 mg of oxycodone, to a suitable container. Add 150.0 mL of *Solvent mixture*, and shake by mechanical means for 1 hour. Transfer 5.0 mL of the solution so obtained to a 50-mL volumetric flask, dilute with *Mobile phase* to volume, and mix. Pass the resulting solution through a membrane filter having a 0.5-μm or finer porosity, discarding the first 10 mL of the filtrate. Use the filtrate.

Chromatographic system (see *Chromatography* ⟨621⟩)—The liquid chromatograph is equipped with a 214-nm detector and a 4.6-mm × 25-cm column that contains 5-μm packing L1. The column is maintained at a temperature of 40°. The flow rate is about 2 mL per minute. Chromatograph the *Standard preparation*, and record the peak responses as directed for *Procedure*: the relative retention times are about 0.6 for oxycodone and 1.0 for acetaminophen; the resolution, *R*, between acetaminophen and oxycodone is not less than 2.4; and the relative standard deviation for replicate injections is not more than 2.0%.

Procedure—Separately inject equal volumes (about 20 μL) of the *Standard preparation* and the *Assay preparation* into the chromatograph, record the chromatograms, and measure the responses for the major peaks. Calculate the quantity, in mg, of oxycodone ($C_{18}N_{21}NO_4$) in the portion of Capsules taken by the formula:

$$1500C(r_U/r_S)$$

in which C is the concentration, in mg per mL, of USP Oxycodone RS in the *Standard preparation*; and r_U and r_S are the oxycodone peak responses obtained from the *Assay preparation* and the *Standard preparation*, respectively. Calculate the quantity, in mg, of acetaminophen ($C_8H_9NO_2$) in the portion of Capsules taken by the formula:

$$1500C(r_U / r_S)$$

in which C is the concentration, in mg per mL, of USP Acetaminophen RS in the *Standard preparation;* and r_U and r_S are the acetaminophen peak responses obtained from the *Assay preparation* and the *Standard preparation,* respectively.

Oxycodone and Acetaminophen Tablets

» Oxycodone and Acetaminophen Tablets contain Oxycodone Hydrochloride and Acetaminophen. Tablets contain the equivalent of not less than 90.0 percent and not more than 110.0 percent of the labeled amount of oxycodone ($C_{18}H_{21}NO_4$), and not less than 90.0 percent and not more than 110.0 percent of the labeled amount of acetaminophen ($C_8H_9NO_2$).

Packaging and storage—Preserve in tight, light-resistant containers.

Labeling—The Tablets may be labeled to indicate the content of oxycodone hydrochloride ($C_{18}H_{21}NO_4 \cdot HCl$) equivalent. Each mg of oxycodone is equivalent to 1.116 mg of oxycodone hydrochloride.

USP Reference standards ⟨11⟩—*USP Acetaminophen RS. USP Oxycodone RS.*

Identification—
A: Using a quantity of finely powdered Tablets, equivalent to about 2.5 mg of oxycodone, proceed as directed for *Identification* test A under *Oxycodone and Acetaminophen Capsules:* the specified results are obtained.

B: The retention times of the major peaks in the chromatogram of the *Assay preparation* correspond to those in the chromatogram of the *Standard preparation,* as obtained in the *Assay.*

Dissolution, *Procedure for a Pooled Sample* ⟨711⟩—
Medium: 0.1 N hydrochloric acid; 900 mL.
Apparatus 2: 50 rpm.
Time: 45 minutes.
Procedure—Determine the amounts of oxycodone ($C_{18}H_{21}NO_4$) and acetaminophen ($C_8H_9NO_2$) dissolved, employing the procedure set forth in the *Assay,* making any necessary volumetric adjustments, including adjusting the pH of the solution under test to about 5.5 before injecting.
Tolerances—Not less than 75% (*Q*) of the labeled amounts of $C_{18}H_{21}NO_4$ and $C_8H_9NO_2$ is dissolved in 45 minutes.

Uniformity of dosage units ⟨905⟩: meet the requirements for *Content Uniformity* with respect to oxycodone and for *Weight Variation* with respect to acetaminophen.

Assay—
Solvent mixture, Mobile phase, Oxycodone standard stock solution, Standard preparation, and *Chromatographic system*—Proceed as directed in the *Assay* under *Oxycodone and Acetaminophen Capsules.*

Assay preparation—Weigh and finely powder not fewer than 20 Tablets. Transfer an accurately weighed portion of powder, equivalent to about 4.5 mg of oxycodone ($C_{18}H_{21}NO_4$), to a suitable container. Add 150.0 mL of *Solvent mixture,* and shake by mechanical means for 1 hour. Transfer 5.0 mL of this solution to a 50-mL volumetric flask, dilute with *Mobile phase* to volume, and mix. Pass the resulting solution through a membrane filter having a 0.5-μm or finer porosity, discarding the first 10 mL of the filtrate. Use the filtrate as the *Assay preparation.*

Procedure—Proceed as directed for *Procedure* in the *Assay* under *Oxycodone and Acetaminophen Capsules.* Calculate the quantity, in mg, of oxycodone ($C_{18}N_{21}NO_4$) in the portion of Tablets taken by the formula:

$$1500C(r_U / r_S)$$

in which C is the concentration, in mg per mL, of USP Oxycodone RS in the *Standard preparation;* and r_U and r_S are the peak oxycodone responses obtained from the *Assay preparation* and the *Standard preparation,* respectively. Calculate the quantity, in mg, of acetaminophen ($C_8H_9NO_2$) in the portion of Tablets taken by the formula:

$$1500C(r_U / r_S)$$

in which C is the concentration, in mg per mL, of USP Acetaminophen RS in the *Standard preparation;* and r_U and r_S are the peak acetaminophen responses obtained from the *Assay preparation* and the *Standard preparation,* respectively.

Oxycodone and Aspirin Tablets

» Oxycodone and Aspirin Tablets contain Oxycodone Hydrochloride and Aspirin, or Oxycodone Hydrochloride, Oxycodone Terephthalate, and Aspirin. Tablets contain not less than 93.0 percent and not more than 107.0 percent of the labeled amount of oxycodone ($C_{18}H_{21}NO_4$), and not less than 90.0 percent and not more than 110.0 percent of the labeled amount of aspirin ($C_9H_8O_4$).

Packaging and storage—Preserve in tight, light-resistant containers.

Labeling—Label the Tablets to state both the content of the oxycodone active moiety and the content or contents of the salt or salts of oxycodone used in formulating the article.

USP Reference standards ⟨11⟩—*USP Aspirin RS. USP Oxycodone RS. USP Salicylic Acid RS.*

Identification—The retention times of the oxycodone peak and the aspirin peak in the chromatograms of the respective *Assay preparations* correspond to those of the corresponding analytes of the respective *Standard preparations,* as obtained in the *Assay for oxycodone* and the *Assay for aspirin,* respectively.

Dissolution, *Procedure for a Pooled Sample* ⟨711⟩—
Medium: 0.05 M acetate buffer, prepared by mixing 2.99 g of sodium acetate trihydrate and 1.66 mL of glacial acetic acid with water to obtain 1000 mL of solution having a pH of 4.50 ± 0.05; 500 mL.
Apparatus 1: 50 rpm.
Time: 30 minutes.
Procedure—Determine the amount of $C_{18}H_{21}NO_4$ dissolved using the method for *Assay for oxycodone,* making any necessary volumetric adjustments. Determine the amount of $C_9H_8O_4$ dissolved from UV absorbances at the wavelength of the isobestic point of aspirin and salicylic acid at about 265 nm of filtered portions of the solution under test, suitably diluted with *Medium,* if necessary, in comparison with a Standard solution having a known concentration of USP Aspirin RS in the same medium. [NOTE—Prepare the Standard solution at the time of use. An amount of alcohol not to exceed 1% of the total volume of the Standard solution may be used to bring the Reference Standard into solution prior to dilution with *Medium.*]
Tolerances—Not less than 80% (*Q*) of the labeled amount of $C_{18}H_{21}NO_4$ is dissolved in 30 minutes and not less than 75% (*Q*) of the labeled amount of $C_9H_8O_4$ is dissolved in 30 minutes.

Uniformity of dosage units ⟨905⟩: meet the requirements.

Salicylic acid—
Mobile phase—Dissolve 2 g of sodium 1-heptanesulfonate in a mixture of 850 mL of water and 150 mL of acetonitrile, and adjust with glacial acetic acid to a pH of 3.4. Make adjustments if necessary (see *System Suitability* under *Chromatography* ⟨621⟩).

Diluting solution—Prepare a mixture of acetonitrile and formic acid (99 : 1).

Standard preparation—Dissolve an accurately weighed quantity of USP Salicylic Acid RS in *Diluting solution* to obtain a solution having a known concentration of about 0.008 mg per mL.

Test preparation—Weigh and finely powder not less than 20 Tablets. Transfer an accurately weighed quantity of the powder, equivalent to about 380 mg of aspirin, to a 100-mL volumetric flask, add about 20 mL of *Diluting solution*, and sonicate for about 15 minutes. Dilute with *Diluting solution* to volume, and mix. Centrifuge a portion of this mixture, and use the clear supernatant as the *Test preparation*.

Chromatographic system (see *Chromatography* ⟨621⟩)—The liquid chromatograph is equipped with a 299-nm detector and a 3.9-mm × 30-cm column that contains packing L1. The flow rate is about 2 mL per minute. Chromatograph the *Standard preparation*, and record the responses as directed for *Procedure:* the relative standard deviation for replicate injections is not more than 4.0%.

Procedure—Separately inject equal volumes (about 20 μL) of the *Test preparation* and the *Standard preparation* into the chromatograph, record the chromatograms, and measure the responses for the salicylic acid peaks. Calculate the percentage of salicylic acid in the portion of Tablets taken by the formula:

$$10{,}000(C/a)(r_U/r_S)$$

in which C is the concentration, in mg per mL, of USP Salicylic Acid RS in the *Standard preparation*, a is the quantity, in mg, of aspirin in the portion of Tablets taken, as determined in the *Assay for aspirin*, and r_U and r_S are the salicylic acid peak responses obtained from the *Test preparation* and the *Standard preparation*, respectively: not more than 3.0% is found.

Assay for aspirin—[NOTE—Volumetric flasks should be dried at 105° for not less than 1 hour, and cooled in a desiccator before use.]

Mobile phase—Prepare a mixture of n-heptane and glacial acetic acid (96 : 4), and filter through a filter of 0.5 μm or finer porosity. Make adjustments if necessary (see *System Suitability* under *Chromatography* ⟨621⟩).

Internal standard solution—Prepare solution of 1-naphthol in chloroform containing about 1 mg per mL. [NOTE—Protect this solution from light.]

Standard preparation—Transfer about 163 mg of USP Aspirin RS, accurately weighed, to a 50-mL volumetric flask. Add 2.5 mL of glacial acetic acid, and swirl. Add 25 mL of chloroform, and shake for 10 minutes. Add 5.0 mL of *Internal standard solution*, dilute with chloroform to volume, and mix. [NOTE—Protect this solution from light.]

Assay preparation—Weigh and finely powder not less than 20 Tablets. Transfer an accurately weighed portion of the powder, equivalent to about 325 mg of aspirin, to a 100-mL volumetric flask, add 5 mL of glacial acetic acid, and swirl. Add 50 mL of chloroform, and shake for 10 minutes. Add 10.0 mL of the *Internal standard solution*, dilute with chloroform to volume, mix, and filter. [NOTE—Prepare the *Assay preparation* and the *Standard preparation* concomitantly, and protect from light.]

Chromatographic system (see *Chromatography* ⟨621⟩)—The liquid chromatograph is equipped with a 300-nm detector and a 4.6-mm × 25-cm column containing packing L3. The flow rate is about 4 mL per minute. Chromatograph the *Standard preparation*, and record the peak responses as directed for *Procedure:* the resolution, R, between the 1-naphthol peak and the aspirin peak is not less than 2.0, and the relative standard deviation for replicate injections is not more than 2.0%.

Procedure—[NOTE—Use peak areas where peak responses are indicated.] Separately inject equal volumes (about 20 μL) of the *Standard preparation* and the *Assay preparation* into the chromatograph, record the chromatograms, and measure the responses for the major peaks. The relative retention times are about 0.65 for 1-naphthol and 1.0 for aspirin. Calculate the quantity, in mg, of Aspirin ($C_9H_8O_4$) in the portion of Tablets taken by the formula:

$$100C(R_U/R_S)$$

in which C is the concentration, in mg per mL, of USP Aspirin RS in the *Standard preparation*, and R_U and R_S are the ratios of the aspirin peak response to the 1-naphthol peak response obtained from the *Assay preparation* and the *Standard preparation*, respectively.

Assay for oxycodone—

Mobile phase—Dissolve 2.2 g of sodium 1-octanesulfonate in 740 mL of water, add 260 mL of methanol, 10 mL of glacial acetic acid, and 0.1 mL of triethylamine. Mix, and adjust with 5 N sodium hydroxide to a pH of 6.5 ± 0.1. Filter through a suitable filter of 0.5 μm or finer porosity, and degas. Make adjustments if necessary (see *System Suitability* under *Chromatography* ⟨621⟩).

Diluting solution—Use 0.1 N hydrochloric acid.

Internal standard solution—Transfer about 50 mg of ethylparaben to a 500-mL volumetric flask, add 10 mL of methanol, and swirl to dissolve. Dilute with *Diluting solution* to volume, and mix.

Standard preparation—Dissolve an accurately weighed quantity of USP Oxycodone RS in *Diluting solution*, and dilute quantitatively with *Diluting solution* to obtain a stock solution having a known concentration of about 0.75 mg per mL. Transfer 15.0 mL of this stock solution to a second 100-mL volumetric flask, add 20.0 mL of *Internal standard solution*, dilute with *Diluting solution* to volume, and mix to obtain a *Standard preparation* having a known concentration of about 0.112 mg of USP Oxycodone RS per mL.

Assay preparation—Weigh and finely powder not less than 20 Tablets. Transfer an accurately weighed portion of the powder, equivalent to about 11.2 mg of oxycodone, to a suitable glass-stoppered conical flask, add 50.0 mL of *Diluting solution*, and shake by mechanical means for about 30 minutes. Filter this solution, transfer 25.0 mL of the clear filtrate to a 50-mL volumetric flask, add 10.0 mL of *Internal standard solution*, dilute with *Diluting solution* to volume, and mix. Use this solution as the *Assay preparation*.

Chromatographic system (see *Chromatography* ⟨621⟩)—The liquid chromatograph is equipped with a 280-nm detector and a 3.9-mm × 15-cm column that contains packing L1 and is maintained at a temperature of 50 ± 1.0°. The flow rate is about 1 mL per minute. Chromatograph the *Standard preparation*, and record the responses as directed for *Procedure:* the column efficiency, determined from the oxycodone peak, is not less than 1800 theoretical plates, the resolution, R, between the oxycodone and the ethylparaben peaks is not less than 6, and the relative standard deviation for replicate injections is not more than 2.0%.

Procedure—Separately inject equal volumes (about 30 μL) of the *Standard preparation* and the *Assay preparation* into the chromatograph, record the chromatograms, and measure the responses for the major peaks. The relative retention times are about 0.5 for oxycodone and 1.0 for ethylparaben. Calculate the quantity, in mg, of oxycodone ($C_{18}H_{21}NO_4$) in the portion of Tablets taken by the formula:

$$100C(R_U/R_S)$$

in which C is the concentration, in mg per mL, of USP Oxycodone RS in the *Standard preparation*, and R_U and R_S are the ratios of the responses of the oxycodone peak and the ethylparaben peak obtained from the *Assay preparation* and the *Standard preparation*, respectively.

Oxycodone Terephthalate

$(C_{18}H_{21}NO_4)_2 \cdot C_8H_6O_4$ 796.86

Morphinan-6-one, 4,5-epoxy-14-hydroxy-3-methoxy-17-methyl-, 1,4-benzenedicarboxylate (2 : 1 salt), (5α).

4,5α-Epoxy-14-hydroxy-3-methoxy-17-methylmorphinan-6-one 1,4-benzenedicarboxylate (2 : 1 salt)   [64336-55-6].

» Oxycodone Terephthalate contains not less than 97.0 percent and not more than 103.0 percent of $(C_{18}H_{21}NO_4)_2 \cdot C_8H_6O_4$, calculated on the dried basis.

Packaging and storage—Preserve in tight containers.

USP Reference standards ⟨11⟩—*USP Oxycodone RS.*

Identification—

A: Transfer 50 mL of the filtrate retained from the test for *Terephthalate acid content* to a 125-mL conical flask. Render the solution alkaline with 6 N ammonium hydroxide. Allow the mixture to stand until a precipitate is formed. Filter, wash the precipitate with 50 mL of cold water, and dry for 2 hours at 105°: the precipitate so obtained melts between 218° and 223°, but the range between beginning and end of melting does not exceed 2° (see *Melting Range or Temperature* ⟨741⟩).

B: *Infrared Absorption* ⟨197K⟩: using a portion of the dried precipitate obtained in *Identification* test A, and the USP Oxycodone RS.

C: *Ultraviolet Absorption* ⟨197U⟩—
 Solution: 150 μg per mL.
 Medium: 0.1 N hydrochloric acid.
 Exhibits a maximum at 280 nm.

Loss on drying ⟨731⟩—Dry it at 105° for 4 hours: it loses not more than 1.5% of its weight.

Residue on ignition ⟨281⟩: not more than 1%.

Related compounds—

Solution A—Dissolve 2.2 g of sodium 1-octanesulfonate in 850 mL of water, and add 150 mL of methanol, 20 mL of glacial acetic acid, and 1.0 mL of triethylamine. Mix, pass through a filter having a 0.5-μm or finer porosity, and degas.

Solution B—Dissolve 2.2 g of sodium 1-octanesulfonate in 500 mL of water, and add 500 mL of methanol, 20 mL of glacial acetic acid, and 1.0 mL of triethylamine. Mix, pass through a filter having a 0.5-μm or finer porosity, and degas.

Mobile phase—Use variable mixtures of *Solution A* and *Solution B* as directed for *Chromatographic system*. Make adjustments to either *Solution* as necessary (see *System Suitability* under *Chromatography* ⟨621⟩).

Diluting solution—Use 0.1 N hydrochloric acid.

Standard preparation—Quantitatively dissolve an accurately weighed quantity of USP Oxycodone RS in *Diluting solution* to obtain a stock standard solution having a known concentration of about 0.9 mg per mL. Transfer 10.0 mL of this stock standard solution to a 100-mL volumetric flask, add 20 mL of methanol, dilute with *Diluting solution* to volume, and mix.

Resolution solution—Dissolve a quantity of 4-hydroxybenzoic acid isopropyl ester in methanol to obtain a solution having a concentration of about 0.05 mg per mL. Transfer 20 mL of this solution and 10 mL of the stock standard solution used to prepare the *Standard preparation* to a 100-mL volumetric flask, dilute with *Diluting solution* to volume, and mix.

Test preparation—Transfer about 110 mg of Oxycodone Terephthalate, accurately weighed, to a 10-mL volumetric flask, add 8 mL of methanol, and shake by mechanical means for about 20 minutes to dissolve. Dilute with methanol to volume, and mix.

Chromatographic system (see *Chromatography* ⟨621⟩)—The liquid chromatograph is equipped with a 280-nm detector and a 3.9-mm × 15-cm column that contains packing L1, is maintained at 45 ± 1°, and is programmed to provide variable mixtures of *Mobile phase*. The flow rate is about 1.5 mL per minute. Equilibrate the system with a mobile phase consisting of a mixture of 90% *Solution A* and 10% *Solution B*. After each injection of the *Standard preparation*, *Resolution solution*, and *Test preparation*, the composition of the mobile phase is changed linearly over the next 30 minutes so that at the end of that time it consists of 80% *Solution A* and 20% *Solution B*, and is then changed linearly over the next 20 minutes so that at the end of that time it consists of 100% *Solution B*, which is then maintained for 5 minutes. Chromatograph the *Resolution solution*, and record the peak responses as directed for *Procedure*: the resolution, *R*, between the oxycodone peak and the 4-hydroxybenzoic acid isopropyl ester peak is not less than 8. Chromatograph the *Standard preparation*, and record the peak responses as directed for *Procedure*: the relative standard deviation for replicate injections is not more than 5.0%.

Procedure—Inject about 25 μL of the *Standard preparation* and the *Test preparation* into the chromatograph, record the chromatograms, and measure the peak responses. Calculate the percentage of each impurity in relation to the oxycodone component taken by the formula:

$$1000(398.43/315.37)(C/M)(r_i/r_S)$$

in which 398.43 is one-half of the molecular weight of oxycodone terephthalate; 315.37 is the molecular weight of oxycodone; *C* is the concentration, in mg per mL, of USP Oxycodone RS in the *Standard preparation*; *M* is the quantity, in mg, of Oxycodone Terephthalate taken to prepare the *Test preparation*; r_i is the area of an individual impurity peak obtained from the *Test preparation*; and r_S is the area of the oxycodone peak obtained from the *Standard preparation*. If any impurity is found having a retention time of about 2 in relation to that of the oxycodone peak, divide its apparent percentage by 4.8: no individual impurity exceeds 1.0%, and the sum of all impurities does not exceed 2.0%.

Terephthalic acid content—Transfer about 1 g, accurately weighed, to a 50-mL beaker. Add 25 mL of 0.2 N hydrochloric acid, and heat to boiling with continuous stirring. Cover the beaker with a watch glass, and allow to cool to room temperature. Pass the suspension through a tared, medium-porosity filtering crucible. Transfer any material remaining in the beaker to the crucible with the aid of small portions of cold 0.2 N hydrochloric acid. Wash the material in the crucible with several portions of cold 0.2 N hydrochloric acid. [NOTE—Reserve the combined filtrates for use in *Identification* test A.] Dry the material in the crucible at 105° for 1 hour, allow to cool, and reweigh. The material in the crucible is terephthalic acid. Determine the weight of terephthalic acid, and calculate the percentage of terephthalic acid: between 20.2% and 21.5% of $C_8H_6O_4$ in the Oxycodone Terephthalate, calculated on the dried basis, is found.

Assay—

Mobile phase—Dissolve 2.2 g of sodium 1-octanesulfonate in 740 mL of water, add 260 mL of methanol, 10 mL of glacial acetic acid, and 0.1 mL of triethylamine. Mix, and adjust with 5 N sodium hydroxide to a pH of 6.5 ± 0.1. Pass through a suitable filter having a 0.5-μm or finer porosity, and degas. Make adjustments if necessary (see *System Suitability* under *Chromatography* ⟨621⟩).

Diluting solution—Use 0.1 N hydrochloric acid.

Internal standard solution—Transfer about 50 mg of ethylparaben to a 500-mL volumetric flask, add 10 mL of methanol, and swirl to dissolve. Dilute with *Diluting solution* to volume, and mix.

Standard preparation—Dissolve an accurately weighed quantity of USP Oxycodone RS in *Diluting solution*, and quantitatively dilute with *Diluting solution* to obtain a stock solution having a known concentration of about 0.75 mg per mL. Transfer 15.0 mL of this stock solution to a 100-mL volumetric flask, add 20.0 mL of *Internal standard solution*, dilute with *Diluting solution* to volume, and mix to obtain a *Standard preparation* having a known concentration of about 0.1125 mg of USP Oxycodone RS per mL.

Assay preparation—Transfer about 142 mg of Oxycodone Terephthalate, accurately weighed, to a 200-mL volumetric flask, dilute with *Diluting solution* to volume, and mix. Filter this solution, discarding the first 5 mL of the filtrate. Transfer 10.0 mL of the clear filtrate to a 50-mL volumetric flask, add 10.0 mL of *Internal standard solution*, dilute with *Diluting solution* to volume, and mix. Use this solution as the *Assay preparation*.

Chromatographic system (see *Chromatography* ⟨621⟩)—The liquid chromatograph is equipped with a 280-nm detector and a 3.9-mm × 15-cm column that contains packing L1 and is maintained at a temperature of 50 ± 1.0°. The flow rate is about 1 mL per minute. Chromatograph the *Standard preparation*, and record the responses as directed for *Procedure*: the column efficiency, determined from the oxycodone peak, is not less than 1800 theoretical plates; the resolution, *R*, between oxycodone and ethylparaben is not less than 6; and the relative standard deviation for replicate injections is not more than 2.0%.

Procedure—Separately inject equal volumes (about 30 μL) of the *Standard preparation* and the *Assay preparation* into the chromatograph, record the chromatograms for a period of time that is twice the retention time of the main oxycodone peak, and measure the peak responses for ethylparaben and oxycodone. Calculate the quantity, in mg, of $(C_{18}H_{21}NO_4)_2 \cdot C_8H_6O_4$ in the portion of Oxycodone Terephthalate taken by the formula:

$$(398.43/315.37)(1000C)(R_U/R_S)$$

in which 398.43 is one-half of the molecular weight of oxycodone terephthalate; 315.37 is the molecular weight of oxycodone; C is the concentration, in mg per mL, of USP Oxycodone RS in the *Standard preparation;* and R_U and R_S are the ratios of the peak response of oxycodone to that of ethylparaben obtained from the *Assay preparation* and the *Standard preparation,* respectively.

Oxygen

O_2 32.00
Oxygen.
Oxygen [7782-44-7].

» Oxygen contains not less than 99.0 percent, by volume, of O_2. [NOTE—Oxygen that is produced by the air-liquefaction process is exempt from the requirements of the tests for *Carbon dioxide* and *Carbon monoxide.*]

Packaging and storage—Preserve in cylinders or in a pressurized storage tank. Containers used for Oxygen must not be treated with any toxic, sleep-inducing, or narcosis-producing compounds, and must not be treated with any compound that will be irritating to the respiratory tract when the Oxygen is used.

NOTE—Reduce the container pressure by means of a regulator. Measure the gases with a gas volume meter downstream from the detector tube in order to minimize contamination or change of the specimens.

Labeling—Label it to indicate whether or not it has been produced by the air-liquefaction process. Where it is piped directly from the cylinder or storage tank to the point of use, label each outlet "Oxygen." [NOTE—The various detector tubes called for in the respective tests are listed under *Reagents* in the section *Reagents, Indicators, and Solutions.*]

Identification—
  A: When tested as directed in the *Assay,* not more than 1.0 mL of gas remains.
  B: Pass 100 ± 5 mL released from the vapor phase of the contents of the Oxygen container through a carbon dioxide detector tube at the rate specified for the tube: no color change is observed (*distinction from carbon dioxide*).

Odor—Carefully open the container valve to produce a moderate flow of gas. Do not direct the gas stream toward the face, but deflect a portion of the stream toward the nose: no appreciable odor is discernible.

Carbon dioxide—Pass 1000 ± 50 mL through a carbon dioxide detector tube at the rate specified for the tube: the indicator change corresponds to not more than 0.03%.

Carbon monoxide—Pass 1000 ± 50 mL through a carbon monoxide detector tube at the rate specified for the tube: the indicator change corresponds to not more than 0.001%.

Assay—Place a sufficient quantity of ammonium chloride–ammonium hydroxide solution, prepared by mixing equal volumes of water and ammonium hydroxide and saturating with ammonium chloride at room temperature, in a test apparatus composed of a calibrated 100-mL buret, provided with a two-way stopcock, a gas absorption pipet, and a leveling bulb, both of suitable capacity and all suitably interconnected. Fill the gas absorption pipet with metallic copper in the form of wire coils, wire mesh, or other suitable configuration. Eliminate all gas bubbles from the liquid in the test apparatus. Activate the test solution by performing two or three tests that are not for record purposes. Fill the calibrated buret, all interconnecting tubing, both stopcock openings, and the intake tube with liquid. Draw 100.0 mL of Oxygen into the buret by lowering the leveling bulb. Open the stopcock to the absorption pipet, and force the Oxygen into the absorption pipet by raising the leveling bulb. Agitate the pipet to provide frequent and intimate contact of the liquid, gas, and copper. Continue agitation until no further diminution in volume occurs. Draw the residual gas back into the calibrated buret, and measure its volume: not more than 1.0 mL of gas remains.

Oxygen 93 Percent

» Oxygen 93 Percent is Oxygen produced from air by the molecular sieve process. It contains not less than 90.0 percent and not more than 96.0 percent, by volume, of O_2, the remainder consisting mostly of argon and nitrogen.

Packaging and storage—Preserve in cylinders or in a low pressure collecting tank. Containers used for Oxygen 93 Percent must not be treated with any toxic, sleep-inducing, or narcosis-producing compounds, and must not be treated with any compound that will be irritating to the respiratory tract when the Oxygen 93 Percent is used.

Labeling—Where it is piped directly from the collecting tank to the point of use, label each outlet "Oxygen 93 Percent."

NOTE—The various detector tubes called for in the respective tests are listed under *Reagents* in the section *Reagents, Indicators, and Solutions.*

Where it is preserved in cylinders, reduce the pressure by means of a regulator. Measure the gases with a gas volume meter downstream from the detector tube in order to minimize contamination or change of the specimens.

Identification—
  A: When tested as directed in the *Assay,* not more than 10.0 mL and not less than 4.0 mL of gas remains.
  B: Pass 100 ± 5 mL released from the vapor phase of the contents of the Oxygen 93 Percent container or from the outlet at the point of use through a carbon dioxide detector tube at the rate specified for the tube: no color change is observed (*distinction from carbon dioxide*).

Odor—Carefully open the container valve or system outlet to produce a moderate flow of gas. Do not direct the gas stream toward the face, but deflect a portion of the stream toward the nose: no appreciable odor is discernible.

Carbon dioxide—Pass 1000 ± 50 mL through a carbon dioxide detector tube at the rate specified for the tube: the indicator change corresponds to not more than 0.03%.

Carbon monoxide—Pass 1000 ± 50 mL through a carbon monoxide detector tube at the rate specified for the tube: the indicator change corresponds to not more than 0.001%.

Assay—Place a sufficient quantity of ammonium chloride-ammonium hydroxide solution, prepared by mixing equal volumes of water and ammonium hydroxide and saturating with ammonium chloride at room temperature, in a test apparatus composed of a calibrated 100-mL buret, provided with a two-way stopcock, a gas absorption pipet, and a leveling bulb, both of suitable capacity and all suitably interconnected. Fill the gas absorption pipet with metallic copper in the form of wire coils, wire mesh, or other suitable configuration. Eliminate all gas bubbles from the liquid in the test apparatus. Activate the test solution by performing two or three tests that are not for record purposes. Fill the calibrated buret, all interconnecting tubing, both stopcock openings, and the intake tube with liquid. Draw 100.0 mL of Oxygen 93 Percent into the buret by lowering the leveling bulb. Open the stopcock to the absorption pipet, and force the Oxygen 93 Percent into the absorption pipet by raising the leveling bulb. Agitate the pipet to provide frequent and intimate contact of the liquid, gas, and copper. Continue agitation until no further diminution in volume occurs. Draw the residual gas back into the calibrated buret, and measure its volume: not more than 10.0 mL and not less than 4.0 mL of gas remains.

Water O 15 Injection*

» Water O 15 Injection is a sterile solution of $H_2{}^{15}O$ in Sodium Chloride Injection suitable for intravenous injection, in which a portion of the molecules are labeled with radioactive ^{15}O (see *Radiopharmaceuticals for Positron Emission Tomography—Compounding* ⟨823⟩). It contains not less than 90.0 percent and not more than 110.0 percent of the labeled amount of ^{15}O expressed in MBq (or mCi) per mL at the time indicated in the labeling.

Packaging and storage—Preserve in a single-dose container that is adequately shielded.

Labeling—Label it to include the following, in addition to the information specified for *Labeling* under *Injections* ⟨1⟩: the time and date of calibration; the amount of ^{15}O as water expressed as MBq (mCi) per mL, at time of calibration; total activity at time of calibration; the expiration time and date; and the statement "Caution—Radioactive Material." The labeling indicates that in making dosage calculations, correction is to be made for radioactive decay and also indicates that the radioactive half-life of ^{15}O is 2.03 minutes. The label also includes the statement, "Do not use if cloudy or if it contains particulate matter."

USP Reference standards ⟨11⟩—*USP Endotoxin RS*.

Identification—

A: *Radionuclidic identity*—Its half-life, determined using a suitable detector system (see *Radioactivity* ⟨821⟩), is between 1.83 and 2.08 minutes.

B: *Radiochemical identity*—The retention time of the major peak in the chromatogram of the *Test solution* corresponds to that of the water contained within the product formulation, as obtained in the test for *Radiochemical purity*.

Bacterial endotoxins ⟨85⟩ (see *Sterilization* and *Sterility Assurance* under *Radiopharmaceuticals for Positron Emission Tomography—Compounding* ⟨823⟩)—It contains not more than 175/V Endotoxin Unit per mL of Injection, in which V is the maximum administered total dose, in mL, at the expiration time.

Sterility ⟨71⟩: meets the requirements.

pH ⟨791⟩: between 4.5 and 8.0.

Radiochemical purity—The gas chromatograph (see *Chromatography* ⟨621⟩) is equipped with thermal conductivity and radioactivity detectors and a 0.53-mm × 30-m column coated with a film of G16 stationary phase. The column temperature is maintained at 40°, and the injector and detector temperatures are maintained at 250° and 200°, respectively. The carrier gas is helium, flowing at a rate of about 10 mL per minute. Inject about 50 µL of the Injection into the chromatograph, record the chromatogram, and measure the responses for the major peaks of both the radioactive and the nonradioactive detection systems (the volume of Injection being adjusted, if necessary, to obtain suitable detection system sensitivity): the column efficiency determined from the analyte peak is not less than 10,000 theoretical plates; the tailing factor for the analyte peak is not more than 1.5; and the relative standard deviation for replicate injections is not more than 5%. Not less than 95% of the radioactivity is Water O 15, and the retention time of the Water O 15 corresponds to the retention time of the water contained within the product formulation.

Radionuclidic purity—Using a gamma-ray spectrometer (see *Selection of a Counting Assembly* under *Radioactivity* ⟨821⟩), count an appropriate aliquot of the Injection for a period of time sufficient to obtain a gamma spectrum. The resultant gamma spectrum should be analyzed for the presence of identifiable photopeaks which are not characteristic of ^{15}O emissions. Not less than 99.5% of the observed gamma emissions should correspond to the 0.511 MeV, 1.022 MeV, or Compton scatter peaks of ^{15}O.

Chemical purity—This article can be synthesized by different methods and processes and, therefore, may contain different impurities. The presence of unlabeled ingredients, reagents, and by-products specific to the process must be controlled, and their potential for physiological or pharmacological effects must be considered.

Heavy metals, *Method I* ⟨231⟩: 5 ppm.

Other requirements—It meets the requirements under *Injections* ⟨1⟩, except that the Injection may be distributed or dispensed prior to completion of the test for *Sterility* ⟨71⟩, the latter being started within 24 hours of final manufacture, and except that it is not subject to the recommendation for *Volume in Container*.

Assay for radioactivity—Using a suitable calibrated system as directed under *Radioactivity* ⟨821⟩, determine the radioactivity of the Injection, in MBq (or mCi) per mL.

Oxymetazoline Hydrochloride

$C_{16}H_{24}N_2O \cdot HCl$ 296.84

Phenol, 3-[(4,5-dihydro-1*H*-imidazol-2-yl)methyl]-6-(1,1-dimethylethyl)-2,4-dimethyl-, monohydrochloride.

6-*tert*-Butyl-3-(2-imidazolin-2-ylmethyl)-2,4-dimethylphenol monohydrochloride   [2315-02-8].

» Oxymetazoline Hydrochloride contains not less than 98.5 percent and not more than 101.5 percent of $C_{16}H_{24}N_2O \cdot HCl$, calculated on the dried basis.

Packaging and storage—Preserve in tight containers.

USP Reference standards ⟨11⟩—*USP Oxymetazoline Hydrochloride RS*.

Identification—

A: *Infrared Absorption* ⟨197M⟩.

B: *Ultraviolet Absorption* ⟨197U⟩—

Solution: 100 µg per mL.

Medium: water.

Absorptivities at 279 nm, calculated on the dried basis, do not differ by more than 3.0%.

C: To a solution of about 50 mg in 3 mL of water add 1 mL of 6 N ammonium hydroxide, filter, and acidify the filtrate with nitric acid: the filtrate responds to the tests for *Chloride* ⟨191⟩.

pH ⟨791⟩: between 4.0 and 6.5, in a solution (1 in 20).

Loss on drying ⟨731⟩—Dry it at 105° for 3 hours: it loses not more than 1.0% of its weight.

Residue on ignition ⟨281⟩: not more than 0.1%.

Heavy metals, *Method II* ⟨231⟩: 0.001%.

Assay—

Mobile phase—Prepare a suitable degassed solution of water, methanol, 1 M sodium acetate, and glacial acetic acid (46 : 40 : 10 : 4).

Standard preparation—Prepare a solution in *Mobile phase* of USP Oxymetazoline Hydrochloride RS having a known concentration of about 0.5 mg per mL.

Assay preparation—Transfer about 25 mg of Oxymetazoline Hydrochloride, accurately weighed, to a 50-mL volumetric flask, dissolve in *Mobile phase*, dilute with *Mobile phase* to volume, and mix.

Chromatographic system (see *Chromatography* ⟨621⟩)—The liquid chromatograph is equipped with a 280-nm detector and a 4.6-mm × 0.25-m column that contains packing L9. The flow rate is about 1 mL per minute. Chromatograph five replicate injections of the *Standard preparation*, and record the peak responses as directed for *Procedure:* the tailing factor is not more than 2.0 and the relative standard deviation is not more than 2.0%.

Procedure—Separately inject equal volumes (about 20 µL) of the *Standard preparation* and the *Assay preparation* into the chromatograph, record the chromatograms, and measure the response for the

---

* Assignment of an official United States Adopted Name (USAN) is pending.

major peak. Calculate the quantity, in mg, of $C_{16}H_{24}N_2O \cdot HCl$ in the portion of Oxymetazoline Hydrochloride taken by the formula:

$$50C(r_U/r_S)$$

in which C is the concentration, in mg per mL, of USP Oxymetazoline Hydrochloride RS in the *Standard preparation*, and r_U and r_S are the peak responses obtained from the *Assay preparation* and the *Standard preparation*, respectively.

Oxymetazoline Hydrochloride Nasal Solution

» Oxymetazoline Hydrochloride Nasal Solution is a solution of Oxymetazoline Hydrochloride in water adjusted to a suitable tonicity. It contains not less than 90.0 percent and not more than 110.0 percent of the labeled amount of $C_{16}H_{24}N_2O \cdot HCl$.

Packaging and storage—Preserve in tight containers.

USP Reference standards ⟨11⟩—*USP Oxymetazoline Hydrochloride RS.*

Identification—Place a volume of Nasal Solution, equivalent to about 2.5 mg of oxymetazoline hydrochloride, in a 60-mL separator, and add water to make about 10 mL. Add 2 mL of sodium carbonate solution (1 in 10), extract with 10 mL of chloroform, and transfer the chloroform extract to a second 60-mL separator. Extract the chloroform solution with 10 mL of 0.1 N hydrochloric acid, allow to separate, and discard the chloroform layer. Transfer 8 mL of the acidic aqueous layer to a test tube, neutralize by the dropwise addition of 1 N sodium hydroxide, add 1 drop of 1 N sodium hydroxide in excess, and mix. Add a few drops of sodium nitroferricyanide TS and 2 drops of sodium hydroxide solution (15 in 100), mix, and allow to stand for 10 minutes. Add 0.1 N hydrochloric acid dropwise until the pH is between 8 and 9, and allow to stand for 10 minutes: a violet color develops.

pH ⟨791⟩: between 4.0 and 6.5.

Assay—
Mobile phase—Prepare as directed in the *Assay* under *Oxymetazoline Hydrochloride*.
Standard preparation—Prepare a solution of USP Oxymetazoline Hydrochloride RS in *Mobile phase*, having a known concentration, approximately equal to the labeled concentration of the Nasal Solution.
Assay preparation—Use Nasal Solution.
Chromatographic system and *Procedure*—Proceed as directed in the *Assay* under *Oxymetazoline Hydrochloride*, except to calculate the quantity, in mg, of $C_{16}H_{24}N_2O \cdot HCl$ in each mL of the Nasal Solution taken by the formula:

$$C(r_U/r_S)$$

in which the terms are as defined therein.

Oxymetazoline Hydrochloride Ophthalmic Solution

» Oxymetazoline Hydrochloride Ophthalmic Solution is a sterile, buffered solution of Oxymetazoline Hydrochloride in water adjusted to a suitable tonicity. It contains not less than 90.0 percent and not more than 110.0 percent of the labeled amount of $C_{16}H_{24}N_2O \cdot HCl$. It contains a suitable preservative.

Packaging and storage—Preserve in tight containers.
USP Reference standards ⟨11⟩—*USP Oxymetazoline Hydrochloride RS.*
Identification—A volume of Ophthalmic Solution, equivalent to about 2.5 mg of oxymetazoline hydrochloride, responds to the *Identification* test under *Oxymetazoline Hydrochloride Nasal Solution*.
Sterility ⟨71⟩: meets the requirements.
pH ⟨791⟩: between 5.8 and 6.8.
Assay—
Mobile phase—Prepare as directed in the *Assay* under *Oxymetazoline Hydrochloride*.
Standard preparation—Prepare a solution of USP Oxymetazoline Hydrochloride RS in *Mobile phase*, having a known concentration approximately equal to the labeled concentration of the Ophthalmic Solution.
Assay preparation—Use Ophthalmic Solution.
Chromatographic system and *Procedure*—Proceed as directed in the *Assay* under *Oxymetazoline Hydrochloride*, except to calculate the quantity, in mg, of $C_{16}H_{24}N_2O \cdot HCl$ in each mL of the Ophthalmic Solution taken by the formula:

$$C(r_U/r_S)$$

in which the terms are as defined therein.

Oxymetholone

$C_{21}H_{32}O_3$ 332.48

Androstan-3-one, 17-hydroxy-2-(hydroxymethylene)-17-methyl-, (5α,17β)-.
17β-Hydroxy-2-(hydroxymethylene)-17-methyl-5α-androstan-3-one   [434-07-1].

» Oxymetholone contains not less than 97.0 percent and not more than 103.0 percent of $C_{21}H_{32}O_3$, calculated on the dried basis.

Packaging and storage—Preserve in well-closed containers.
USP Reference standards ⟨11⟩—*USP Oxymetholone RS.*
Completeness of solution—Dissolve 100 mg in 5 mL of dioxane: the solution is clear and free from undissolved solid.
Identification—
A: *Infrared Absorption* ⟨197K⟩.
B: *Ultraviolet Absorption* ⟨197U⟩—
Solution: 10 μg per mL.
Medium: 0.01 N methanolic sodium hydroxide.
Melting range ⟨741⟩: between 172° and 180°.
Specific rotation ⟨781S⟩: between +34° and +38°.
Test solution: 20 mg per mL, in dioxane.
Loss on drying ⟨731⟩—Dry it in vacuum over phosphorus pentoxide for 4 hours: it loses not more than 1.0% of its weight.
Organic volatile impurities, *Method V* ⟨467⟩: meets the requirements.
Solvent—Use dimethyl sulfoxide.
(Official until July 1, 2008)
Assay—
Standard preparation—Prepare as directed under *Single-steroid Assay* ⟨511⟩, using USP Oxymetholone RS.
Assay preparation—Weigh accurately about 20 mg of Oxymetholone, previously dried, dissolve in a sufficient quantity of a mixture of equal volumes of alcohol and chloroform to make 10.0 mL, and mix.
Procedure—Proceed as directed for *Procedure* under *Single-steroid Assay* ⟨511⟩, using a solvent system consisting of a mixture of benzene and alcohol (98 : 2), through the fourth sentence of the second paragraph under *Procedure*. Then centrifuge the tubes for 5

minutes, and determine the absorbances of the supernatants in 1-cm cells at the wavelength of maximum absorbance at about 315 nm, with a suitable spectrophotometer, against the blank. [NOTE—Use 0.01 N alcoholic sodium hydroxide, rather than alcohol, to elute the silica gel bands.] Calculate the quantity, in mg, of $C_{21}H_{32}O_3$ in the portion of Oxymetholone taken by the formula:

$$10C(A_U / A_S)$$

in which C is the concentration, in mg per mL, of USP Oxymetholone RS in the *Standard preparation*, and A_U and A_S are the absorbances of the solutions from the *Assay preparation* and the *Standard preparation*, respectively.

Oxymetholone Tablets

» Oxymetholone Tablets contain not less than 90.0 percent and not more than 110.0 percent of the labeled amount of $C_{21}H_{32}O_3$.

Packaging and storage—Preserve in well-closed containers.

USP Reference standards ⟨11⟩—*USP Oxymetholone RS*.

Identification—Mix an amount of powdered Tablets, equivalent to about 50 mg of oxymetholone, with 15 mL of solvent hexane, and stir occasionally for 15 minutes. Centrifuge the mixture, and decant and discard the solvent hexane. Extract the residue with two 10-mL portions of solvent hexane, centrifuging and decanting as before, and discard the solvent hexane. Add 25 mL of chloroform to the residue, mix by shaking for 1 to 2 minutes, and filter. Evaporate the filtrate to about 3 mL, add a few mL of solvent hexane to induce crystallization, and evaporate to dryness: the IR absorption spectrum of a potassium bromide dispersion prepared from the oxymetholone so obtained, and previously dried, exhibits maxima only at the same wavelengths as that of a similar preparation of USP Oxymetholone RS, crystallized from the same solvent mixture.

Dissolution ⟨711⟩—

Medium: 0.05 M pH 8.5 alkaline borate buffer (see under *Solutions* in the section *Reagents, Indicators, and Solutions*); 900 mL.

Apparatus 1: 100 rpm.

Time: 45 minutes.

Procedure—Determine the amount of $C_{21}H_{32}O_3$ dissolved from UV absorbances at the wavelength of maximum absorbance at about 313 nm of filtered portions of the solution under test, suitably diluted with *Dissolution Medium* if necessary, in comparison with a Standard solution having a known concentration of USP Oxymetholone RS in the same medium. [NOTE—An amount of acetonitrile not to exceed 5% of the total volume of the Standard solution may be used to bring the Reference Standard into solution prior to dilution with *Dissolution Medium*.]

Tolerances—Not less than 75% (Q) of the labeled amount of $C_{21}H_{32}O_3$ is dissolved in 45 minutes.

Uniformity of dosage units ⟨905⟩: meet the requirements.

Procedure for content uniformity—Transfer 1 finely powdered Tablet to a 100-mL volumetric flask with the aid of about 75 mL of methanol. Heat the methanol to boiling, and allow to remain at a temperature just below the boiling point for 15 minutes with occasional swirling. Cool to room temperature, dilute with methanol to volume, and mix. Centrifuge a portion of the mixture at about 2000 rpm until the solution becomes clear. Transfer a portion of the supernatant, equivalent to about 1 mg of oxymetholone, to a 100-mL volumetric flask. Add 10 mL of a 1 in 250 solution of sodium hydroxide in methanol, and dilute with methanol to volume. Without delay, concomitantly determine the absorbances of this solution and a freshly prepared Standard solution of USP Oxymetholone RS in the same medium having a known concentration of about 10 μg per mL in 1-cm cells at the wavelength of maximum absorbance at about 315 nm, with a suitable spectrophotometer, using a 1 in 2500 solution of sodium hydroxide in methanol as the blank. Calculate the quantity, in mg, of $C_{21}H_{32}O_3$ in the Tablet taken by the formula:

$$(TC / D)(A_U / A_S)$$

in which T is the labeled quantity, in mg, of oxymetholone in the Tablet, C is the concentration, in μg per mL, of USP Oxymetholone RS in the Standard solution, D is the concentration, in μg per mL, of oxymetholone in the solution from the Tablet, based upon the labeled quantity per Tablet and the extent of dilution, and A_U and A_S are the absorbances of the solution from the Tablet and the Standard solution, respectively.

Assay—Weigh and finely powder not less than 20 Tablets. Transfer an accurately weighed portion of the powder, equivalent to about 20 mg of oxymetholone, to a separator, add 10 mL of water, and extract with three 25-mL portions of chloroform, filtering each extract through chloroform-washed cotton. Evaporate the combined chloroform extracts on a steam bath to dryness, reducing the application of heat as dryness is approached. Dissolve the residue in methanol, transfer to a 100-mL volumetric flask, dilute with methanol to volume, and mix. Transfer 5.0 mL of the solution to a 100-mL volumetric flask, add 10 mL of a 1 in 250 solution of sodium hydroxide in methanol, dilute with methanol to volume, and mix. Without delay, concomitantly determine the absorbances of this solution and a freshly prepared Standard solution of USP Oxymetholone RS in the same medium having a known concentration of about 10 μg per mL in 1-cm cells at the wavelength of maximum absorbance at about 315 nm, with a suitable spectrophotometer, using a 1 in 2500 solution of sodium hydroxide in methanol as the blank. Calculate the quantity, in mg, of $C_{21}H_{32}O_3$ in the portion of Tablets taken by the formula:

$$2C(A_U / A_S)$$

in which C is the concentration, in μg per mL, of USP Oxymetholone RS in the Standard solution, and A_U and A_S are the absorbances of the solution from the Tablets and the Standard solution, respectively.

Oxymorphone Hydrochloride

$C_{17}H_{19}NO_4 \cdot HCl$ 337.80

Morphinan-6-one, 4,5-epoxy-3,14-dihydroxy-17-methyl-, hydrochloride, (5α)-.

4,5α-Epoxy-3,14-dihydroxy-17-methylmorphinan-6-one hydrochloride [*357-07-3*].

» Oxymorphone Hydrochloride contains not less than 97.0 percent and not more than 102.0 percent of $C_{17}H_{19}NO_4 \cdot HCl$, calculated on the dried basis.

Packaging and storage—Preserve in tight, light-resistant containers. Store at 25°, excursions permitted between 15° and 30°.

USP Reference standards ⟨11⟩—*USP Oxymorphone RS*.

Identification—

A: Dissolve about 250 mg in 25 mL of water, and render the solution alkaline with a saturated solution of sodium bicarbonate. Extract the liberated oxymorphone with two 15-mL portions of chloroform. Reserve the chloroform extracts, combined in a second separator, for *Identification* test *B*: the aqueous phase, acidified with 2 N nitric acid, responds to the tests for *Chloride* ⟨191⟩.

B: Wash the combined chloroform extracts from *Identification* test *A* with 5 mL of water, and filter. Evaporate the chloroform solution on a steam bath nearly to dryness, then add a few mL of ether, and continue the evaporation with stirring until the solvent is removed: the IR absorption spectrum of a 1 in 50 solution in alcohol-free chloroform of the oxymorphone so obtained, determined in a 0.5-mm cell, exhibits maxima only at the same wavelengths as that of a similar solution of USP Oxymorphone RS.

C: The UV absorption spectrum of a 1 in 6500 solution in 0.1 N hydrochloric acid exhibits maxima and minima at the same wavelengths as that of a solution of USP Oxymorphone RS, prepared by dissolving about 20 mg of the Reference Standard in 10 mL of 1 N hydrochloric acid and diluting with water to 100.0 mL. The ratio A_{281}/A_{264} is 1.75 ± 0.2.

D: Dissolve 10 mg in 1 mL of water, and add a few drops of ferric chloride TS: a blue color is produced immediately.

Specific rotation ⟨781S⟩: between $-145°$ and $-155°$.
 Test solution: 100 mg per mL, in water.

Acidity—Dissolve 300 mg in 10 mL of water, add 1 drop of methyl red TS, and titrate with 0.020 N sodium hydroxide: not more than 0.30 mL is required to produce a yellow color.

Loss on drying ⟨731⟩—Dry it at 105° for 18 hours: it loses not more than 8.0% of its weight.

Residue on ignition ⟨281⟩: not more than 0.3%.

Limit of nonphenolic substances—Dissolve 1 g in 15 mL of water, add 5 mL of sodium hydroxide solution (2 in 25), and extract with three 10-mL portions of chloroform. Filter the combined extracts through a small chloroform-moistened filter paper, and wash the filtrate with 5 mL of water. Filter the chloroform layer through chloroform-moistened filter paper into a tared, 50-mL beaker, and evaporate on a steam bath with the aid of a gentle current of filtered air to dryness. Dry the beaker and residue at 105° for 1 hour, and weigh: the residue so obtained does not exceed 15 mg.

Ordinary impurities ⟨466⟩—
 Test solution: methanol.
 Standard solution: methanol.
 Eluant: a mixture of dehydrated alcohol, cyclohexane, and ammonium hydroxide (10 : 5 : 1).
 Visualization: 1.

Chloride content—Dissolve about 300 mg, accurately weighed, in 50 mL of methanol in a glass-stoppered flask, add 5 mL of glacial acetic acid and 3 drops of eosin Y TS, and titrate with 0.1 N silver nitrate VS. Each mL of 0.1 N silver nitrate is equivalent to 3.545 mg of Cl: the content is between 10.2% and 10.8%, calculated on the dried basis.

Assay—Transfer about 700 mg of Oxymorphone Hydrochloride, accurately weighed, to a glass-stoppered flask containing 50 mL of glacial acetic acid and 10 mL of mercuric acetate TS. Add 3 mL of acetic anhydride and 1 drop of methyl violet TS, and titrate with 0.1 N perchloric acid VS to a clear blue color. Perform a blank determination, and make any necessary correction. Each mL of 0.1 N perchloric acid is equivalent to 33.78 mg of $C_{17}H_{19}NO_4 \cdot HCl$.

Oxymorphone Hydrochloride Injection

» Oxymorphone Hydrochloride Injection is a sterile solution of Oxymorphone Hydrochloride in Water for Injection. It contains not less than 93.0 percent and not more than 107.0 percent of the labeled amount of $C_{17}H_{19}NO_4 \cdot HCl$.

Packaging and storage—Preserve in single-dose or in multiple-dose containers of Type I glass, protected from light.

USP Reference standards ⟨11⟩—*USP Oxymorphone RS. USP Endotoxin RS.*

Identification—The solution prepared for measurement of absorbance in the *Assay* exhibits maxima and minima at the same wavelengths as the *Standard preparation* prepared as directed in the *Assay.*

Bacterial endotoxins ⟨85⟩—It contains not more than 238.1 USP Endotoxin Units per mg of oxymorphone hydrochloride.

pH ⟨791⟩: between 2.7 and 4.5.

Other requirements—It meets the requirements under *Injections* ⟨1⟩.

Assay—
 Standard preparation—Transfer about 45 mg of USP Oxymorphone RS, accurately weighed, to a 50-mL volumetric flask, dissolve in about 10 mL of chloroform, dilute with chloroform to volume, and mix. Transfer 15.0 mL of this solution to a 100-mL volumetric flask, dilute with chloroform to volume, and mix. The concentration of USP Oxymorphone RS in the *Standard preparation* is about 135 μg per mL.

 Assay preparation—Transfer an accurately measured volume of Injection, equivalent to about 15 mg of oxymorphone hydrochloride, to a 125-mL separator, and add water, if necessary, to bring the volume to 15 mL. Adjust by the addition of hydrochloric acid to a pH of less than 2, extract with five 15-mL portions of chloroform, and discard the chloroform extracts. Adjust the aqueous phase with ammonium hydroxide to a pH of 9.5, and extract with four 20-mL portions of chloroform. Filter the chloroform extracts through a chloroform-moistened pledget of cotton into a 100-mL volumetric flask, dilute with chloroform to volume, and mix.

 Procedure—Concomitantly determine the absorbances of the solutions in 1-cm cells at the wavelength of maximum absorbance at about 282 nm, with a suitable spectrophotometer, using chloroform as the blank. Calculate the quantity, in mg, of $C_{17}H_{19}NO_4 \cdot HCl$ in each mL of the Injection taken by the formula:

$$(337.80 / 301.34)(0.1C / V)(A_U / A_S)$$

in which 337.80 and 301.34 are the molecular weights of oxymorphone hydrochloride and oxymorphone, respectively; C is the concentration, in μg per mL, of USP Oxymorphone RS in the *Standard preparation*; V is the volume, in mL, of Injection taken; and A_U and A_S are the absorbances of the *Assay preparation* and the *Standard preparation*, respectively.

Oxymorphone Hydrochloride Suppositories

» Oxymorphone Hydrochloride Suppositories contain not less than 93.0 percent and not more than 107.0 percent of the labeled amount of $C_{17}H_{19}NO_4 \cdot HCl$.

Packaging and storage—Preserve in well-closed containers, and store in a refrigerator.

USP Reference standards ⟨11⟩—*USP Oxymorphone RS.*

Identification—Place a number of Suppositories, equivalent to 5 mg of oxymorphone hydrochloride, in a 125-mL separator. Add 25 mL of 0.1 N hydrochloric acid, and shake without heating until the specimen is dissolved. Wash the solution with five 25-mL portions of chloroform, shaking the separator gently to avoid forming emulsions, and discard the chloroform washings. Adjust with 6 N ammonium hydroxide to a pH of about 9.5, using short-range pH indicator paper, and extract with three 25-mL portions of chloroform, filtering the extracts through chloroform-moistened glass wool into a 200-mL round-bottom flask. Evaporate the combined extracts to dryness, using a rotary evaporator. Add 25 mL of 0.1 N hydrochloric acid, insert the stopper, and swirl to dissolve the residue: the UV absorption spectrum of the solution so obtained exhibits maxima and minima at the same wavelengths as that of a similar solution of USP Oxymorphone RS, concomitantly measured.

Assay—
 Mobile phase—0.05 M sodium borate adjusted to a pH of about 9.1.

 Internal standard solution—Prepare a solution of procaine hydrochloride in 0.01 N hydrochloric acid having a concentration of about 3 mg per mL.

 Standard preparation—Using an accurately weighed quantity of USP Oxymorphone RS, prepare a solution in 0.01 N hydrochloric acid having a known concentration of about 4.5 mg per mL, sonicating, if necessary, to effect solution. Transfer 10.0 mL of this solution, 10.0 mL of the *Internal standard solution*, and 5.0 mL of 0.01 N hydrochloric acid to a 125-mL separator. Extract with four 25-mL portions of chloroform, discarding the chloroform layer each time. Transfer the aqueous layer to a suitable flask, and bubble filtered air through the solution for 10 minutes to remove final traces of chloroform. The concentration of USP Oxymorphone RS in the *Standard preparation* is about 1.8 mg per mL.

Assay preparation—Transfer a number of Suppositories, accurately counted and equivalent to about 50 mg of oxymorphone hydrochloride, to a 125-mL separator. Add 15.0 mL of 0.01 N hydrochloric acid, 10.0 mL of *Internal standard solution*, and 25 mL of chloroform. Shake until the suppositories dissolve. Discard the chloroform layer. Extract the aqueous layer with three 25-mL portions of chloroform, discarding the chloroform each time. Transfer the aqueous layer to a suitable flask and bubble filtered air through the solution for 10 minutes to remove final traces of chloroform.

Chromatographic system (see *Chromatography* ⟨621⟩)—The liquid chromatograph is equipped with a 254-nm detector and a 2.1-mm × 100-cm column that contains packing L12. The flow rate is about 1 mL per minute. Chromatograph five replicate injections of the *Standard preparation*, and record the peak responses as directed for *Procedure*: the relative standard deviation is not more than 2.0%, and the resolution factor between oxymorphone hydrochloride and procaine hydrochloride is not less than 1.5.

Procedure—Separately inject equal volumes (about 15 μL) of the *Standard preparation* and the *Assay preparation* into the chromatograph by means of a suitable microsyringe or sampling valve, record the chromatograms, and measure the responses for the major peaks. The retention times are about 5 and 7.5 minutes for oxymorphone hydrochloride and procaine hydrochloride, respectively. Calculate the quantity, in mg, of $C_{17}H_{19}NO_4 \cdot HCl$ in each Suppository taken by the formula:

$$(337.80 / 301.34)(25C/N)(R_U / R_S)$$

in which 337.80 and 301.34 are the molecular weights of oxymorphone hydrochloride and oxymorphone, respectively; *C* is the concentration, in mg per mL, of USP Oxymorphone RS in the *Standard preparation*; *N* is the number of Suppositories taken; and R_U and R_S are the ratios of the peak responses of oxymorphone hydrochloride and procaine hydrochloride obtained from the *Assay preparation* and the *Standard preparation*, respectively.

Oxytetracycline

$C_{22}H_{24}N_2O_9 \cdot 2H_2O$ 496.47

2-Naphthacenecarboxamide, 4-(dimethylamino)-1,4,4a,5,5a,6,11,12a-octahydro-3,5,6,10,12,12a-hexahydroxy-6-methyl-1,11-dioxo-, [4S-(4α,4aα,5α,5aα,6β,12aα)]-, dihydrate.

4-(Dimethylamino)-1,4,4a,5,5a,6,11,12a-octahydro-3,5,6,10,12,12a-hexahydroxy-6-methyl-1,11-dioxo-2-naphthacene-carboxamide dihydrate [*6153-64-6*].

Anhydrous   460.44   [*79-57-2*].

» Oxytetracycline has a potency equivalent to not less than 832 μg of $C_{22}H_{24}N_2O_9$ per mg.

Packaging and storage—Preserve in tight, light-resistant containers.

Labeling—Where it is intended for use in preparing injectable dosage forms, the label states that it is sterile or must be subjected to further processing during the preparation of injectable dosage forms.

USP Reference standards ⟨11⟩—*USP Endotoxin RS. USP Oxytetracycline RS.*

Identification—
A: *Ultraviolet Absorption* ⟨197U⟩—
Solution: 20 μg per mL.
Medium: 0.1 N hydrochloric acid.
Absorptivity at 353 nm, calculated on the anhydrous basis, is between 96.0% and 104.0% of that of USP Oxytetracycline RS, the potency of the Reference Standard being taken into account.
B: To 1 mg add 2 mL of sulfuric acid: a light red color is produced.

Crystallinity ⟨695⟩: meets the requirements.

pH ⟨791⟩: between 4.5 and 7.0, in an aqueous suspension containing 10 mg per mL.

Water, *Method I* ⟨921⟩: between 6.0% and 9.0%.

Other requirements—Where the label states that Oxytetracycline is sterile, it meets the requirements for *Sterility* and *Bacterial endotoxins* under *Oxytetracycline for Injection*. Where the label states that Oxytetracycline must be subjected to further processing during the preparation of injectable dosage forms, it meets the requirements for *Bacterial endotoxins* under *Oxytetracycline for Injection*.

Assay—

Tetrabutylammonium hydrogen sulfate solution—Dissolve 1 g of tetrabutylammonium hydrogen sulfate in 100 mL of water. Adjust with 1 N sodium hydroxide to a pH of 7.5.

Edetate disodium solution—Dissolve 0.04 g of edetate disodium in 100 mL of water. Adjust with 1 N sodium hydroxide to a pH of 7.5.

pH 7.5 Phosphate buffer—Prepare a mixture of 0.33 M dibasic potassium phosphate and 0.33 M monobasic sodium phosphate (85 : 15). Adjust, if necessary, by adding more of the appropriate component to a pH of 7.5.

Mobile phase—Transfer, with the aid of 200 mL of water, 50 g of tertiary butyl alcohol to a 1000-mL volumetric flask. Add 60 mL of *pH 7.5 Phosphate buffer*, 50 mL of *Tetrabutylammonium hydrogen sulfate solution*, and 10 mL of *Edetate disodium solution*, and dilute with water to volume. Degas before use. Make adjustments if necessary (see *System Suitability* under *Chromatography* ⟨621⟩).

Standard preparation—Dissolve an accurately weighed quantity of USP Oxytetracycline RS in 0.01 N hydrochloric acid to obtain a solution having a known concentration of about 0.22 mg per mL.

System suitability solution—Prepare a solution of tetracycline hydrochloride in 0.01 N hydrochloric acid containing about 0.2 mg per mL. Mix 3 mL of this solution and 1.5 mL of the *Standard preparation*, and dilute with water to 25 mL.

Assay preparation—Transfer about 44 mg of Oxytetracycline to a 200-mL volumetric flask, add about 25 mL of 0.01 N hydrochloric acid, swirl to dissolve, dilute with 0.01 N hydrochloric acid to volume, and mix.

Chromatographic system (see *Chromatography* ⟨621⟩)—The liquid chromatograph is equipped with a 254-nm detector and a 4.6-mm × 25-cm column that contains packing L21 and is maintained at 60 ± 2°. The flow rate is about 1 mL per minute. Chromatograph the *System suitability solution*, and record the peak responses as directed for *Procedure*: the relative retention times are about 0.6 for oxytetracycline and 1.0 for tetracycline; and the resolution, *R*, between the oxytetracycline peak and the tetracycline peak is not less than 5. Chromatograph the *Standard preparation*, and record the peak responses as directed for *Procedure*: the tailing factor is not more than 1.25; and the relative standard deviation for replicate injections is not more than 1.0%.

Procedure—[NOTE—Use peak areas where peak responses are indicated.] Separately inject equal volumes (about 20 μL) of the *Standard preparation* and the *Assay preparation* into the chromatograph, record the chromatograms, and measure the responses for the major peaks. Calculate the quantity, in μg, of $C_{22}H_{24}N_2O_9$ in each mg of the Oxytetracycline taken by the formula:

$$200(CP / W)(r_U / r_S)$$

in which *C* is the concentration, in mg per mL, of USP Oxytetracycline RS in the *Standard preparation*; *P* is the assigned potency, in μg per mg, of USP Oxytetracycline RS; *W* is the weight, in mg, of the Oxytetracycline taken to prepare the *Assay preparation*; and r_U and r_S are the oxytetracycline peak responses obtained from the *Assay preparation* and the *Standard preparation*, respectively.

Oxytetracycline Injection

» Oxytetracycline Injection is a sterile solution of Oxytetracycline with or without one or more suitable anesthetics, antioxidants, buffers, complexing agents, preservatives, and solvents. It contains the equivalent of not less than 90.0 percent and not more than 120.0 percent of the labeled amount of Oxytetracycline ($C_{22}H_{24}N_2O_9$).

Packaging and storage—Preserve in single-dose or multiple-dose containers, protected from light.
USP Reference standards ⟨11⟩—*USP Endotoxin RS. USP Oxytetracycline RS.*
Identification—To an accurately measured volume of Injection, equivalent to about 50 mg of oxytetracycline, add 50 mL of methanol, and shake. Using the clear solution so obtained as the *Test Solution*, proceed as directed for *Method II* under *Identification—Tetracyclines* ⟨193⟩.
Bacterial endotoxins ⟨85⟩—It contains not more than 0.4 USP Endotoxin Unit per mg of oxytetracycline.
Sterility ⟨71⟩—It meets the requirements when tested as directed for *Membrane Filtration* under *Test for Sterility of the Product to be Examined*.
pH ⟨791⟩: between 8.0 and 9.0.
Assay—
Tetrabutylammonium hydrogen sulfate solution, Edetate disodium solution, pH 7.5 Phosphate buffer, Mobile phase, Standard preparation, System suitability solution, and *Chromatographic system*—Proceed as directed in the *Assay* under *Oxytetracycline*.
Assay preparation—Transfer an accurately measured volume of Injection, equivalent to about 100 mg of oxytetracycline, to a 500-mL volumetric flask, dilute with 0.01 N hydrochloric acid to volume, and mix.
Procedure—Proceed as directed for *Procedure* in the *Assay* under *Oxytetracycline*. Calculate the quantity, in mg, of $C_{22}H_{24}N_2O_9$ in each mL of the Injection taken by the formula:

$$0.5(CP/V)(r_U/r_S)$$

in which C is the concentration, in mg per mL, of USP Oxytetracycline RS in the *Standard preparation*; V is the volume, in mL, of Injection taken to prepare the *Assay preparation*; and the other terms are as defined therein.

Oxytetracycline Tablets

» Oxytetracycline Tablets contain the equivalent of not less than 90.0 percent and not more than 120.0 percent of the labeled amount of $C_{22}H_{24}N_2O_9$.

Packaging and storage—Preserve in tight, light-resistant containers.
USP Reference standards ⟨11⟩—*USP Oxytetracycline RS.*
Identification—Shake a suitable quantity of finely powdered Tablets with methanol to obtain a solution containing about 1 mg of oxytetracycline per mL, and filter. Using the filtrate as the *Test Solution*, proceed as directed for *Method II* under *Identification—Tetracyclines* ⟨193⟩.
Dissolution ⟨711⟩—
Medium: 0.1 N hydrochloric acid; 900 mL.
Apparatus 1: 100 rpm.
Time: 45 minutes.
Procedure—Determine the amount of $C_{22}H_{24}N_2O_9$ dissolved from UV absorbances at the wavelength of maximum absorbance at about 353 nm of filtered portions of the solution under test, suitably diluted with *Dissolution Medium*, if necessary, in comparison with a Standard solution having a known concentration of USP Oxytetracycline RS in the same medium.
Tolerances—Not less than 75% (*Q*) of the labeled amount of $C_{22}H_{24}N_2O_9$ is dissolved in 45 minutes.
Uniformity of dosage units ⟨905⟩: meet the requirements.
Water, *Method I* ⟨921⟩: not more than 7.5%.
Assay—
Tetrabutylammonium hydrogen sulfate solution, Edetate disodium solution, pH 7.5 Phosphate buffer, Mobile phase, Standard preparation, Resolution solution, and *Chromatographic system*—Proceed as directed in the *Assay* under *Oxytetracycline*.
Assay preparation—Weigh and finely powder not less than 20 Tablets. Transfer an accurately weighed portion of the powder, equivalent to about 100 mg of oxytetracycline, to a 500-mL volumetric flask, add about 25 mL of 0.01 N hydrochloric acid, and mix. Dilute with 0.01 N hydrochloric acid to volume, and mix. Filter a portion of this solution through a 0.5-µm or finer porosity filter, and use the filtrate as the *Assay preparation*.
Procedure—Proceed as directed for *Procedure* in the *Assay* under *Oxytetracycline*. Calculate the quantity, in mg, of $C_{22}H_{24}N_2O_9$ in the portion of Tablets taken by the formula:

$$0.5(CP)(r_U/r_S)$$

in which C is the concentration, in mg per mL, of USP Oxytetracycline RS in the *Standard preparation*, and the other terms are as defined therein.

Oxytetracycline and Nystatin Capsules

» Oxytetracycline and Nystatin Capsules contain not less than 90.0 percent and not more than 120.0 percent of the labeled amount of oxytetracycline ($C_{22}H_{24}N_2O_9$), and not less than 90.0 percent and not more than 135.0 percent of the labeled amount of USP Nystatin Units.

Packaging and storage—Preserve in tight, light-resistant containers.
USP Reference standards ⟨11⟩—*USP Oxytetracycline RS. USP Nystatin RS*
Identification—Shake a suitable quantity of Capsule contents with methanol to obtain a solution containing about 1 mg of oxytetracycline per mL, and filter. Using the filtrate as the *Test Solution*, proceed as directed for *Method II* under *Identification—Tetracyclines* ⟨193⟩.
Dissolution ⟨711⟩—
Medium: 0.1 N hydrochloric acid; 900 mL.
Apparatus 1: 100 rpm.
Time: 45 minutes.
Procedure—Determine the amount of oxytetracycline ($C_{22}H_{24}N_2O_9$) dissolved from UV absorbances at the wavelength of maximum absorbance at about 353 nm of filtered portions of the solution under test, suitably diluted with *Dissolution Medium*, if necessary, in comparison with a Standard solution having a known concentration of USP Oxytetracycline RS in the same medium.
Tolerances—Not less than 75% (*Q*) of the labeled amount of $C_{22}H_{24}N_2O_9$ is dissolved in 45 minutes.
Uniformity of dosage units ⟨905⟩: meet the requirements for *Weight Variation* with respect to oxytetracycline.
Water, *Method I* ⟨921⟩: not more than 7.5%.
Assay for oxytetracycline—Place not less than 5 Capsules in a high-speed glass blender jar containing an accurately measured volume of 0.1 N hydrochloric acid, and blend for 3 to 5 minutes, so that the stock solution so obtained contains not less than 150 µg of oxytetracycline ($C_{22}H_{24}N_2O_9$) per mL. Proceed as directed under *Antibiotics—Microbial Assays* ⟨81⟩, using an accurately measured volume of this stock solution diluted quantitatively and stepwise with water to yield a *Test Dilution* having a concentration of oxytetracycline assumed to be equal to the median dose level of the Standard.
Assay for nystatin—Proceed as directed for Nystatin under *Antibiotics—Microbial Assays* ⟨81⟩, blending not less than 5 Capsules for 3 to 5 minutes in a high-speed blender with a sufficient accurately

measured volume of dimethylformamide to obtain a solution of convenient concentration. Dilute an accurately measured portion of this solution quantitatively with dimethylformamide to obtain a stock solution containing about 400 USP Nystatin Units per mL. Dilute this stock solution quantitatively with *Buffer No. 6* to obtain a *Test Dilution* having a concentration of nystatin assumed to be equal to the median dose level of the Standard.

Oxytetracycline and Nystatin for Oral Suspension

» Oxytetracycline and Nystatin for Oral Suspension is a dry mixture of Oxytetracycline and Nystatin with one or more suitable buffers, colors, diluents, flavors, suspending agents, and preservatives. When constituted as directed in the labeling, it contains not less than 90.0 percent and not more than 120.0 percent of the labeled amount of oxytetracycline ($C_{22}H_{24}N_2O_9$), and not less than 90.0 percent and not more than 135.0 percent of the labeled amount of USP Nystatin Units.

Packaging and storage—Preserve in tight, light-resistant containers, at controlled room temperature.

USP Reference standards ⟨11⟩—*USP Oxytetracycline RS. USP Nystatin RS*

Identification—To a quantity of Oxytetracycline and Nystatin for Oral Suspension (powder), equivalent to about 50 mg of oxytetracycline, add 50 mL of methanol, shake, and allow the mixture to settle. Using the clear supernatant as the *Test Solution*, proceed as directed for *Method II* under *Identification—Tetracyclines* ⟨193⟩.

Uniformity of dosage units ⟨905⟩—

FOR SOLID PACKAGED IN SINGLE-UNIT CONTAINERS: meets the requirements for *Content Uniformity* with respect to oxytetracycline and nystatin.

Deliverable volume ⟨698⟩: meets the requirements.

pH ⟨791⟩: between 4.5 and 7.5, in the suspension constituted as directed in the labeling.

Water, *Method I* ⟨921⟩: not more than 2.0%.

Assay for oxytetracycline—Constitute Oxytetracycline and Nystatin for Oral Suspension as directed in the labeling. Transfer an accurately measured volume of the suspension so obtained, freshly mixed and free from air bubbles, to a suitable volumetric flask, dilute with 0.1 N hydrochloric acid to volume so that the stock solution so obtained contains not less than 150 μg of oxytetracycline per mL, and mix. Proceed as directed for oxytetracycline under *Antibiotics—Microbial Assays* ⟨81⟩, using an accurately measured volume of the stock solution diluted quantitatively and stepwise with water to yield a *Test Dilution* having a concentration assumed to be equal to the median dose level of the Standard.

Assay for nystatin—Constitute Oxytetracycline and Nystatin for Oral Suspension as directed in the labeling. Transfer an accurately measured volume of the suspension so obtained, freshly mixed and free from air bubbles, to a blender jar containing a sufficient, accurately measured volume of dimethylformamide to yield a solution of convenient concentration, and blend at high speed for 3 to 5 minutes. Dilute an accurately measured volume of this solution quantitatively with dimethylformamide to obtain a stock solution containing about 400 USP Nystatin Units per mL. Proceed as directed for nystatin under *Antibiotics—Microbial Assays* ⟨81⟩, using an accurately measured volume of this solution diluted quantitatively with *Buffer No. 6* to yield a *Test Dilution* having a concentration of nystatin assumed to be equal to the median dose level of the Standard.

Oxytetracycline Calcium

$C_{44}H_{46}CaN_4O_{18}$ 958.93

2-Naphthacenecarboxamide, 4-(dimethylamino)-1,4,4a,5,5a,6,11,12a-octahydro-3,5,6,10,12,12a-hexahydroxy-6-methyl-1,11-dioxo-, calcium salt, [4S-(4α,4aα,5α,5aα,6β,12aα)]-.

4-(Dimethylamino)-1,4,4a,5,5a,6,11,12a-octahydro-3,5,6,10,12,12a-hexahydroxy-6-methyl-1,11-dioxo 2-naphthacenecarboxamide calcium salt [*15251-48-6*].

» Oxytetracycline Calcium has a potency equivalent to not less than 865 μg of oxytetracycline ($C_{22}H_{24}N_2O_9$) per mg, calculated on the anhydrous basis.

Packaging and storage—Preserve in tight, light-resistant containers, and store in a cool place.

USP Reference standards ⟨11⟩—*USP Oxytetracycline RS*.

Identification—Dissolve a suitable quantity in methanol to obtain a *Test Solution* containing 1 mg of oxytetracycline per mL, and proceed as directed for *Method II* under *Identification—Tetracyclines* ⟨193⟩.

Crystallinity ⟨695⟩: meets the requirements.

pH ⟨791⟩: between 6.0 and 8.0, in an aqueous suspension containing 25 mg per mL.

Water, *Method I* ⟨921⟩: between 8.0% and 14.0%.

Calcium content—Proceed as directed under *Residue on Ignition* ⟨281⟩, except to ignite at 550 ± 50° instead of at 800 ± 25°: the weight of residue so obtained, multiplied by 0.2944, gives the equivalent of calcium in the Oxytetracycline Calcium taken. The calcium content is between 3.85% and 4.35%, calculated on the anhydrous basis.

Assay—Dissolve an accurately weighed quantity of Oxytetracycline Calcium in an accurately measured volume of 0.1 N hydrochloric acid to obtain a stock solution having a concentration of about 1000 μg of oxytetracycline per mL. Proceed as directed for oxytetracycline under *Antibiotics—Microbial* ⟨81⟩, using an accurately measured volume of the stock solution diluted quantitatively and stepwise with water to yield a *Test Dilution* having a concentration assumed to be equal to the median dose level of the Standard.

Oxytetracycline Calcium Oral Suspension

» Oxytetracycline Calcium Oral Suspension contains the equivalent of not less than 90.0 percent and not more than 120.0 percent of the labeled amount of oxytetracycline ($C_{22}H_{24}N_2O_9$). It contains one or more suitable buffers, colors, flavors, preservatives, stabilizers, and suspending agents. In addition, it may contain N-acetylglucosamine.

Packaging and storage—Preserve in tight, light-resistant containers.

USP Reference standards ⟨11⟩—*USP Oxytetracycline RS*.

Identification—Shake a suitable quantity of Oral Suspension with methanol to obtain a solution containing 1 mg of oxytetracycline per mL, and filter. Using the filtrate as the *Test Solution*, proceed as directed for *Method II* under *Identification—Tetracyclines* ⟨193⟩.

Uniformity of dosage units ⟨905⟩—

FOR SOLID PACKAGED IN SINGLE-UNIT CONTAINERS: meets the requirements.

Deliverable volume ⟨698⟩: meets the requirements.

pH ⟨791⟩: between 5.0 and 8.0.

Assay—Transfer an accurately measured quantity of Oral Suspension, freshly mixed and free from air bubbles, equivalent to about 150 mg of oxytetracycline, to a 1000-mL volumetric flask, dilute with 0.1 N hydrochloric acid to volume, and mix. Proceed as directed for oxytetracycline under *Antibiotics—Microbial Assays* ⟨81⟩, using an accurately measured volume of this stock solution diluted quantitatively and stepwise with water to yield a *Test Dilution* having a concentration assumed to be equal to the median dose level of the Standard.

Oxytetracycline Hydrochloride

$C_{22}H_{24}N_2O_9 \cdot HCl$ 496.90
2-Naphthacenecarboxamide, 4-(dimethylamino)-1,4,4a,5,5a,6,11,12a-octahydro-3,5,6,10,12,12a-hexahydroxy-6-methyl-1,11-dioxo-, monohydrochloride, [4S-(4α,4aα,5α,5aα,6β,12aα)]-.
4-(Dimethylamino)-1,4,4a,5,5a,6,11,12a-octahydro-3,5,6,10,12,12a-hexahydroxy-6-methyl-1,11-dioxo-2-naphthacenecarboxamide monohydrochloride [2058-46-0].

» Oxytetracycline Hydrochloride has a potency equivalent to not less than 835 µg of oxytetracycline ($C_{22}H_{24}N_2O_9$) per mg, calculated on the dried basis.

Packaging and storage—Preserve in tight, light-resistant containers.
Labeling—Where it is intended for use in preparing injectable or ophthalmic dosage forms, the label states that it is sterile or must be subjected to further processing during the preparation of injectable or ophthalmic dosage forms.
USP Reference standards ⟨11⟩—*USP Endotoxin RS. USP Oxytetracycline RS.*
Identification—
 A: *Ultraviolet Absorption* ⟨197U⟩—
  Solution: 20 µg per mL.
  Medium: 0.1 N hydrochloric acid.
  Absorptivity, calculated on the dried basis, at 353 nm is between 88.2% and 96.8% of that of USP Oxytetracycline RS, the potency of the Reference Standard being taken into account.
 B: To 1 mg add 2 mL of sulfuric acid: a light red color is produced.
Crystallinity ⟨695⟩: meets the requirements.
pH ⟨791⟩: between 2.0 and 3.0, in a solution containing 10 mg per mL.
Loss on drying ⟨731⟩—Dry about 100 mg, accurately weighed, in a capillary-stoppered bottle in vacuum at a pressure not exceeding 5 mm of mercury at 60° for 3 hours: it loses not more than 2.0% of its weight.
Other requirements—Where the label states that Oxytetracycline Hydrochloride is sterile, it meets the requirements for *Sterility* and *Bacterial endotoxins* under *Oxytetracycline for Injection*. Where the label states that Oxytetracycline Hydrochloride must be subjected to further processing during the preparation of injectable dosage forms, it meets the requirements for *Bacterial endotoxins* under *Oxytetracycline for Injection*. Where it is intended for use in preparing ophthalmic dosage forms, it is exempt from the requirements for *Bacterial endotoxins*.
Assay—
 Tetrabutylammonium hydrogen sulfate solution, Edetate disodium solution, pH 7.5 Phosphate buffer, Mobile phase, Standard preparation, System suitability solution, and *Chromatographic system*—Proceed as directed in the *Assay* under *Oxytetracycline*.
 Assay preparation—Transfer about 44 mg of Oxytetracycline Hydrochloride to a 200-mL volumetric flask, add about 25 mL of 0.01 N hydrochloric acid, swirl to dissolve, dilute with 0.01 N hydrochloric acid to volume, and mix.
 Procedure—Proceed as directed in the *Assay* under *Oxytetracycline*. Calculate the quantity, in µg, of oxytetracycline ($C_{22}H_{24}N_2O_9$) in each mg of Oxytetracycline Hydrochloride taken by the formula:

$$200(CP/W)(r_U/r_S)$$

in which the terms are as defined therein.

Oxytetracycline Hydrochloride Capsules

» Oxytetracycline Hydrochloride Capsules contain the equivalent of not less than 90.0 percent and not more than 120.0 percent of the labeled amount of oxytetracycline ($C_{22}H_{24}N_2O_9$).

Packaging and storage—Preserve in tight, light-resistant containers.
USP Reference standards ⟨11⟩—*USP Oxytetracycline RS.*
Identification—Shake a suitable quantity of Capsule contents with methanol to obtain a solution containing 1 mg of oxytetracycline per mL, and filter. Using the filtrate as the *Test Solution*, proceed as directed for *Method II* under *Identification—Tetracyclines* ⟨193⟩.
Dissolution ⟨711⟩—
 Medium: water; 900 mL.
 Apparatus 2: 75 rpm.
 Time: 60 minutes.
 Procedure—Determine the amount of $C_{22}H_{24}N_2O_9$ dissolved from UV absorbances at the wavelength of maximum absorbance at about 273 nm of filtered portions of the solution under test, suitably diluted with water, in comparison with a Standard solution having a known concentration of USP Oxytetracycline RS in the same medium, using 5 mL of 0.1 N hydrochloric acid to dissolve the Standard.
 Tolerances—Not less than 80% (*Q*) of the labeled amount of $C_{22}H_{24}N_2O_9$ is dissolved in 60 minutes.
Uniformity of dosage units ⟨905⟩: meet the requirements.
Loss on drying ⟨731⟩—Dry about 100 mg of Capsule contents, accurately weighed, in a capillary-stoppered bottle in vacuum at a pressure not exceeding 5 mm of mercury at 60° for 3 hours: it loses not more than 5.0% of its weight.
Assay—
 Tetrabutylammonium hydrogen sulfate solution, Edetate disodium solution, pH 7.5 Phosphate buffer, Mobile phase, Standard preparation, Resolution solution, and *Chromatographic system*—Proceed as directed in the *Assay* under *Oxytetracycline*.
 Assay preparation—Remove, as completely as possible, the contents of not less than 20 Capsules, and mix. Transfer an accurately weighed portion of the powder, equivalent to about 100 mg of oxytetracycline, to a 500-mL volumetric flask, add about 50 mL of 0.01 N hydrochloric acid, and swirl to dissolve. Dilute with 0.01 N hydrochloric acid to volume, mix, and filter a portion of the solution through a 0.5-µm or finer porosity filter. Use the filtrate as the *Assay preparation*.
 Procedure—Proceed as directed for *Procedure* in the *Assay* under *Oxytetracycline*. Calculate the quantity, in mg, of oxytetracycline ($C_{22}H_{24}N_2O_9$) in the portion of Capsules taken by the formula:

$$0.5(CP)(r_U/r_S)$$

in which the terms are as defined therein.

Oxytetracycline for Injection

» Oxytetracycline for Injection contains an amount of Oxytetracycline Hydrochloride equivalent to not less than 90.0 percent and not more than 115.0 percent of the labeled amount of oxytetracycline ($C_{22}H_{24}N_2O_9$).

Packaging and storage—Preserve in *Containers for Sterile Solids* as described under *Injections* ⟨1⟩, protected from light.
USP Reference standards ⟨11⟩—*USP Oxytetracycline RS. USP Endotoxin RS.*
Constituted solution—At the time of use, it meets the requirements for *Constituted Solutions* under *Injections* ⟨1⟩.

Bacterial endotoxins ⟨85⟩—It contains not more than 0.4 USP Endotoxin Unit per mg of oxytetracycline.
Sterility ⟨71⟩—It meets the requirements when tested as directed for *Membrane Filtration* under *Test for Sterility of the Product to be Examined*, *Fluid D* being used instead of *Fluid A*.
pH ⟨791⟩: between 1.8 and 2.8, in a solution containing 25 mg per mL.
Loss on drying ⟨731⟩—Dry about 100 mg, accurately weighed, in a capillary-stoppered bottle in vacuum at a pressure not exceeding 5 mm of mercury at 60° for 3 hours: it loses not more than 3.0% of its weight.
Particulate matter ⟨788⟩: meets the requirements for small-volume injections.
Other requirements—It responds to *Identification* test *B* under *Oxytetracycline Hydrochloride*. It also meets the requirements for *Uniformity of Dosage Units* ⟨905⟩ and *Labeling* under *Injections* ⟨1⟩.
Assay—
Tetrabutylammonium hydrogen sulfate solution, Edetate disodium solution, pH 7.5 Phosphate buffer, Mobile phase, Standard preparation, System suitability solution, and *Chromatographic system*—Proceed as directed in the *Assay* under *Oxytetracycline*.
Assay preparation 1 (where it is represented as being in a single-dose container)—Constitute Oxytetracycline for Injection in a volume of water, accurately measured, corresponding to the volume of solvent specified in the labeling. Withdraw all of the withdrawable contents, using a suitable hypodermic needle and syringe, and dilute quantitatively with 0.01 N hydrochloric acid to obtain a solution having a concentration of about 0.2 mg of oxytetracycline per mL.
Assay preparation 2 (where the label states the quantity of oxytetracycline in a given volume of constituted solution)—Constitute Oxytetracycline for Injection in a volume of water, accurately measured, corresponding to the volume of solvent specified in the labeling. Dilute an accurately measured volume of the constituted solution quantitatively with 0.01 N hydrochloric acid to obtain a solution having a concentration of about 0.2 mg of oxytetracycline per mL.
Procedure—Proceed as directed for *Procedure* in the *Assay* under *Oxytetracycline*. Calculate the quantity, in mg, of oxytetracycline ($C_{22}H_{24}N_2O_9$) withdrawn from the container or in the portion of constituted solution taken by the formula:

$$(L/D)(CP)(r_U/r_S)$$

in which L is the labeled quantity, in mg, of oxytetracycline ($C_{22}H_{24}N_2O_9$) in the container or in the portion of constituted solution taken; D is the concentration, in mg per mL, of oxytetracycline in *Assay preparation 1* or in *Assay preparation 2*, based on the labeled quantity in the container or in the portion of constituted solution taken, respectively, and the extent of dilution; and the other terms are as defined therein.

Oxytetracycline Hydrochloride Soluble Powder

» Oxytetracycline Hydrochloride Soluble Powder is a dry mixture of Oxytetracycline Hydrochloride and one or more suitable excipients. It contains not less than 90.0 percent and not more than 110.0 percent of the labeled amount of oxytetracycline hydrochloride ($C_{22}H_{24}N_2O_9 \cdot HCl$).

Packaging and storage—Preserve in well-closed containers.
Labeling—Label it to indicate that it is for oral veterinary use only.
USP Reference standards ⟨11⟩—*USP Oxytetracycline RS*.
Identification—
A: Shake a quantity of Soluble Powder with methanol to obtain a solution containing about 1 mg of oxytetracycline hydrochloride per mL. Filter if necessary to obtain a clear solution. Using the filtrate as the *Test solution*, proceed as directed for *Method II* under *Identification—Tetracyclines* ⟨193⟩.
B: The retention time of the major peak in the chromatogram of the *Assay preparation* corresponds to that in the chromatogram of the *Standard preparation*, as obtained in the *Assay*.
pH ⟨791⟩: between 1.5 and 3.0, in the solution obtained as directed in the labeling.
Loss on drying ⟨731⟩—Dry about 100 mg, accurately weighed, in a capillary-stoppered bottle in vacuum at a pressure not exceeding 5 mm of mercury at 60° for 3 hours: it loses not more than 3.0% of its weight.
Minimum fill ⟨755⟩: meets the requirements.
Assay—
Tetrabutylammonium hydrogen sulfate solution, Edetate disodium solution, pH 7.5 Phosphate buffer, Mobile phase, Standard preparation, System suitability solution, and *Chromatographic system*—Proceed as directed in the *Assay* under *Oxytetracycline*.
Assay preparation—Transfer an accurately weighed portion of the Soluble Powder, equivalent to about 100 mg of oxytetracycline hydrochloride, to a 500-mL volumetric flask, dilute with 0.01 N hydrochloric acid to volume, and mix. Pass a portion of this solution through a filter having a 0.5-μm or finer porosity. Use the filtrate as the *Assay preparation*.
Procedure—Proceed as directed for *Procedure* in the *Assay* under *Oxytetracycline*. Calculate the quantity, in g, of oxytetracycline hydrochloride ($C_{22}H_{24}N_2O_9 \cdot HCl$) in each g of Soluble Powder taken by the formula:

$$0.5(496.90/460.44)(CP/W)(r_U/r_S)$$

in which 496.90 and 460.44 are the molecular weights of oxytetracycline hydrochloride and oxytetracycline, respectively; C is the concentration, in mg per mL, of USP Oxytetracycline RS in the *Standard preparation*; P is the assigned potency, in μg of oxytetracycline per mg, of USP Oxytetracycline RS; W is the weight, in g, of Soluble Powder taken to prepare the *Assay preparation*; and r_U and r_S are the oxytetracycline peak responses obtained from the *Assay preparation* and the *Standard preparation*, respectively.

Oxytetracycline Hydrochloride and Hydrocortisone Acetate Ophthalmic Suspension

» Oxytetracycline Hydrochloride and Hydrocortisone Acetate Ophthalmic Suspension is a sterile suspension of Oxytetracycline Hydrochloride and Hydrocortisone Acetate in a suitable oil vehicle with one or more suitable suspending agents. It contains the equivalent of not less than 90.0 percent and not more than 115.0 percent of the labeled amount of oxytetracycline ($C_{22}H_{24}N_2O_9$) and not less than 90.0 percent and not more than 110.0 percent of the labeled amount of hydrocortisone acetate ($C_{23}H_{32}O_6$).

Packaging and storage—Preserve in tight, light-resistant containers. The containers are sealed and tamper-proof so that sterility is assured at time of first use.
USP Reference standards ⟨11⟩—*USP Oxytetracycline RS. USP Hydrocortisone Acetate RS*.
Sterility ⟨71⟩—It meets the requirements when tested as directed for *Direct Inoculation of the Culture Medium* under *Test for Sterility of the Product to be Examined* using 0.25 mL of specimen.
Water, *Method I* ⟨921⟩: not more than 1.0%, 60 mL of a mixture of methanol and chloroform (2 : 1) being used instead of methanol in the titration vessel.
Assay for oxytetracycline—Transfer an accurately measured volume of Ophthalmic Suspension to a separator, add 50 mL of ether, and shake. Add 25 mL of 0.1 N hydrochloric acid, shake, and allow to separate. Collect the acid layer, and repeat the extraction with

three additional 25-mL portions of 0.1 N hydrochloric acid. Combine the acid extracts in a 200-mL volumetric flask, dilute with 0.1 N hydrochloric acid to volume, and mix. Proceed as directed for oxytetracycline under *Antibiotics—Microbial Assays* ⟨81⟩, using an accurately measured volume of this solution diluted quantitatively and stepwise with water to obtain a *Test Dilution* having a concentration assumed to be equal to the median dose level of the *Standard*.

Assay for hydrocortisone acetate—

Mobile phase—Prepare a degassed and filtered mixture of water and methanol (50 : 50).

Standard preparation—Dissolve an accurately weighed quantity of USP Hydrocortisone Acetate RS in a mixture of *Mobile phase* and alcohol (80 : 20) to obtain a solution having a known concentration of about 0.06 mg per mL.

Assay preparation—Transfer an accurately measured volume of Ophthalmic Suspension, equivalent to about 30 mg of hydrocortisone acetate, to a separator containing 25 mL of pH 9.0 alkaline borate buffer (see under *Buffer Solutions* in the section *Reagents, Indicators, and Solutions*). Extract with four 25-mL portions of chloroform, filtering each chloroform extract through a thin layer of chloroform-washed anhydrous sodium sulfate into a 250-mL volumetric flask. Rinse the sodium sulfate with chloroform, collecting the filtrate in the volumetric flask, dilute with chloroform to volume, and mix. Transfer 25.0 mL of the resulting solution to a 50-mL conical flask, and evaporate slowly with the aid of mild heat until about 5 mL remains. Add about 15 mL of alcohol, and evaporate slowly until about 5 mL remains. Transfer this solution to a 50-mL volumetric flask, dilute with a mixture of *Mobile phase* and alcohol (80 : 20) to volume, and mix.

Chromatographic system (see *Chromatography* ⟨621⟩)—The liquid chromatograph is equipped with a 254-nm detector and a 3.9-mm × 30-cm column that contains packing L1. The flow rate is about 1 mL per minute. Chromatograph the *Standard preparation*, and record the peak responses as directed for *Procedure:* the column efficiency determined from the analyte peak is not less than 235 theoretical plates, the tailing factor for the analyte peak is not more than 1.7, and the relative standard deviation of replicate injections is not more than 2.0%.

Procedure—Separately inject equal volumes (about 25 µL) of the *Standard preparation* and the *Assay preparation* into the chromatograph, record the chromatograms, and measure the responses for the major peaks. Calculate the quantity, in mg, of $C_{23}H_{32}O_6$ in each mL of the Ophthalmic Suspension taken by the formula:

$$500(C / V)(r_U / r_S)$$

in which C is the concentration, in mg per mL, of USP Hydrocortisone Acetate RS in the *Standard preparation*; V is the volume, in mL, of Ophthalmic Suspension taken; and r_U and r_S are the peak responses obtained from the *Assay preparation* and the *Standard preparation*, respectively.

Oxytetracycline Hydrochloride and Hydrocortisone Ointment

» Oxytetracycline Hydrochloride and Hydrocortisone Ointment contains the equivalent of not less than 90.0 percent and not more than 115.0 percent of the labeled amount of oxytetracycline ($C_{22}H_{24}N_2O_9$), and not less than 90.0 percent and not more than 110.0 percent of the labeled amount of hydrocortisone.

Packaging and storage—Preserve in collapsible tubes or in well-closed, light-resistant containers.

USP Reference standards ⟨11⟩—USP Oxytetracycline RS. USP Hydrocortisone RS.

Minimum fill ⟨755⟩: meets the requirements.

Water, *Method I* ⟨921⟩: not more than 1.0%, 20 mL of a mixture of toluene and methanol (7 : 3) being used in place of methanol in the titration vessel.

Assay for oxytetracycline—Transfer a suitable, accurately weighed quantity of Ointment to a separator, add 50 mL of ether, and shake. Add 20 mL of 0.1 N hydrochloric acid, shake, and allow to separate. Collect the acid layer, and repeat the extraction with three additional 20-mL portions of 0.1 N hydrochloric acid. Combine the acid extracts in a 100-mL volumetric flask, dilute with 0.1 N hydrochloric acid to volume, and mix. Quantitatively dilute a portion of this solution with 0.1 N hydrochloric acid so that the solution so obtained contains not less than 150 µg of oxytetracycline per mL. Proceed as directed for oxytetracycline under *Antibiotics—Microbial Assays* ⟨81⟩, using an accurately measured volume of this solution diluted quantitatively and stepwise with water to yield a *Test Dilution* having a concentration assumed to be equal to the median dose level of the *Standard*.

Assay for hydrocortisone—Proceed with Ointment as directed in the *Assay for hydrocortisone* under *Neomycin and Polymyxin B Sulfate, Bacitracin Zinc, and Hydrocortisone Ophthalmic Ointment.*

Oxytetracycline Hydrochloride and Polymyxin B Sulfate Ointment

» Oxytetracycline Hydrochloride and Polymyxin B Sulfate Ointment contains the equivalent of not less than 90.0 percent and not more than 120.0 percent of the labeled amount of oxytetracycline ($C_{22}H_{24}N_2O_9$), and not less than 90.0 percent and not more than 125.0 percent of the labeled amount of polymyxin B.

Packaging and storage—Preserve in collapsible tubes, or in well-closed, light-resistant containers.

USP Reference standards ⟨11⟩—USP Oxytetracycline RS. USP Polymyxin B Sulfate RS.

Minimum fill ⟨755⟩: meets the requirements.

Water, *Method I* ⟨921⟩: not more than 1.0%, 10 mL of a mixture of toluene and methanol (7 : 3) being used in place of methanol in the titration vessel.

Assay for oxytetracycline—Proceed with Ointment as directed in the *Assay for oxytetracycline* under *Oxytetracycline Hydrochloride and Hydrocortisone Ointment.*

Assay for polymyxin B—Transfer an accurately weighed quantity of Ointment, equivalent to about 10,000 USP Polymyxin B Units, to a 15-mL centrifuge tube, add 10 mL of ether, stir, and centrifuge for 10 minutes. Decant and discard the clear ether. Wash the residue with 10 mL of ether, centrifuge for 10 minutes, decanting and discarding the clear ether. Wash the residue with several 10-mL portions of acetone, centrifuging, decanting, and discarding each washing until the yellow color is removed from the residue. [NOTE—Take care not to remove any of the residue with the washings.] Add 0.2 mL of polysorbate 80 to the residue, and mix. Transfer the mixture to a 100-mL volumetric flask with the aid of *Buffer No. 6*, dilute with the same solvent to volume, and mix. Proceed as directed for polymyxin B under *Antibiotics—Microbial Assays* ⟨81⟩, using an accurately measured volume of this solution diluted quantitatively with *Buffer No. 6* to yield a *Test Dilution* having a concentration of polymyxin B assumed to be equal to the median dose level of the *Standard*.

Oxytetracycline Hydrochloride and Polymyxin B Sulfate Ophthalmic Ointment

» Oxytetracycline Hydrochloride and Polymyxin B Sulfate Ophthalmic Ointment is a sterile ointment containing Oxytetracycline Hydrochloride and Polymyxin B Sulfate. It contains the equivalent of not less than 90.0 percent and not more than 120.0 percent of the labeled amount of oxytetracycline, and not less than 90.0 percent and not more than 125.0 percent of the labeled amount of polymyxin B.

Packaging and storage—Preserve in collapsible ophthalmic ointment tubes.
USP Reference standards ⟨11⟩—*USP Oxytetracycline RS. USP Polymyxin B Sulfate RS.*
Sterility ⟨71⟩: meets the requirements.
Minimum fill ⟨755⟩: meets the requirements.
Water, *Method I* ⟨921⟩: not more than 1.0%, 20 mL of a mixture of toluene and methanol (7 : 3) being used in place of methanol in the titration vessel.
Metal particles—It meets the requirements of the test for *Metal Particles in Ophthalmic Ointments* ⟨751⟩.
Assay for oxytetracycline—Proceed with Ophthalmic Ointment as directed in the *Assay for oxytetracycline* under *Oxytetracycline Hydrochloride and Hydrocortisone Ointment*.
Assay for polymyxin B—Proceed with Ophthalmic Ointment as directed in the *Assay for polymyxin B* under *Oxytetracycline Hydrochloride and Polymyxin B Sulfate Ointment*.

Oxytetracycline Hydrochloride and Polymyxin B Sulfate Topical Powder

» Oxytetracycline Hydrochloride and Polymyxin B Sulfate Topical Powder contains the equivalent of not less than 90.0 percent and not more than 120.0 percent of the labeled amounts of oxytetracycline ($C_{22}H_{24}N_2O_9$) and polymyxin B in a suitable, fine powder base.

Packaging and storage—Preserve in well-closed containers.
USP Reference standards ⟨11⟩—*USP Oxytetracycline RS. USP Polymyxin B Sulfate RS.*
Minimum fill ⟨755⟩: meets the requirements.
Loss on drying ⟨731⟩—Dry about 100 mg, accurately weighed, in a capillary-stoppered bottle in vacuum at a pressure not exceeding 5 mm of mercury at 60° for 3 hours: it loses not more than 2.0% of its weight.
Assay for oxytetracycline—Transfer a suitable, accurately weighed quantity of Topical Powder to a glass blender jar containing a sufficient, accurately measured volume of 0.1 N hydrochloric acid to yield a stock solution containing not less than 150 µg of oxytetracycline per mL, and blend at high speed for 3 to 5 minutes. Proceed as directed for oxytetracycline under *Antibiotics—Microbial Assays* ⟨81⟩, using an accurately measured volume of this solution diluted quantitatively and stepwise with water to obtain a *Test Dilution* having a concentration of oxytetracycline assumed to be equal to the median dose level of the Standard.
Assay for polymyxin B—Transfer an accurately weighed quantity of Topical Powder, equivalent to about 10,000 USP Polymyxin B Units, to a 50-mL centrifuge tube, add 15 mL of acetone and 0.05 mL of hydrochloric acid, and stir. Add 20 mL of acetone, and centrifuge for 10 minutes. Decant and discard the clear liquid. Add 15 mL of acetone and 0.05 mL of hydrochloric acid to the residue, stir, add 20 mL of acetone, and centrifuge for 10 minutes, decanting and discarding the clear liquid. [NOTE—Take care not to discard any of the residue with the clear liquid.] Add 5 mL of *Buffer No. 6* to the residue, and mix. Transfer the mixture to a 100-mL volumetric flask with the aid of *Buffer No. 6*, dilute with the same solvent to volume, and mix. Proceed as directed for polymyxin B under *Antibiotics—Microbial Assays* ⟨81⟩, using an accurately measured volume of this stock solution diluted quantitatively with *Buffer No. 6* to obtain a *Test Dilution* having a concentration of polymyxin B assumed to be equal to the median dose level of the Standard.

Oxytetracycline Hydrochloride and Polymyxin B Sulfate Vaginal Inserts

» Oxytetracycline Hydrochloride and Polymyxin B Sulfate Vaginal Inserts contain the equivalent of not less than 90.0 percent and not more than 120.0 percent of the labeled amounts of oxytetracycline ($C_{22}H_{24}N_2O_9$) and polymyxin B.

Packaging and storage—Preserve in well-closed containers.
USP Reference standards ⟨11⟩—*USP Oxytetracycline RS. USP Polymyxin B Sulfate RS.*
Loss on drying ⟨731⟩—Dry about 100 mg, accurately weighed, of powdered Vaginal Inserts in a capillary-stoppered bottle in vacuum at a pressure not exceeding 5 mm of mercury at 60° for 3 hours: it loses not more than 3.0% of its weight.
Assay for oxytetracycline—Place not fewer than 5 Vaginal Inserts in a high-speed blender jar containing an accurately measured volume of 0.1 N hydrochloric acid, so that the stock solution obtained after blending for 3 to 5 minutes contains not less than 150 µg of oxytetracycline per mL. Proceed as directed for oxytetracycline under *Antibiotics—Microbial Assays* ⟨81⟩, using an accurately measured volume of this solution diluted quantitatively and stepwise with water to obtain a *Test Dilution* having a concentration of oxytetracycline assumed to be equal to the median dose level of the Standard.
Assay for polymyxin B—Weigh and finely powder not fewer than 5 Vaginal Inserts. Transfer an accurately weighed portion of the powder, equivalent to about 100,000 USP Polymyxin B Units, to a filter funnel equipped with a solvent-resistant membrane filter (1-µm or finer porosity). Wash the powder with five 20-mL portions of acetone, applying vacuum, and discarding the accumulated filtrate. [NOTE—If necessary, wash the powder with additional portions of acetone to remove any yellow color.] Carefully transfer the filter and the washed powder to a beaker containing about 400 mL of *Buffer No. 6* (see *Antibiotics—Microbial Assays* ⟨81⟩), and stir. Transfer the contents of the beaker to a 500-mL volumetric flask with the aid of *Buffer No. 6*, dilute with the same solvent to volume, and mix. Proceed as directed for polymyxin B under *Antibiotics—Microbial Assays* ⟨81⟩, using an accurately measured volume of this solution diluted quantitatively and stepwise with *Buffer No. 6* to yield a *Test Dilution* having a concentration of polymyxin B assumed to be equal to the median dose level of the Standard.

Oxytocin

CYIQNCPLG

$C_{43}H_{66}N_{12}O_{12}S_2$ 1007.19
Oxytocin.
Oxytocin   [50-56-6].

» Oxytocin is a nonapeptide hormone having the property of causing the contraction of uterine smooth muscle and of the myoepithelial cells within the mammary gland. It is prepared by synthesis or obtained from the posterior lobe of the pituitary of healthy domestic animals used for food by man. Its oxytocic activity is not less than 400 USP Oxytocin Units per mg.

Packaging and storage—Preserve in tight containers, preferably of Type I glass, in a refrigerator.

USP Reference standards ⟨11⟩—*USP Oxytocin RS. USP Vasopressin RS.*

Microbial limits ⟨61⟩—The total bacterial count does not exceed 200 cfu per g. For products of animal origin, it meets also the requirements of the tests for absence of *Salmonella* species and *Escherichia coli*.

Identification—
  A: The retention time of the oxytocin peak in the chromatogram of the *Assay preparation* corresponds to that in the chromatogram of the *Standard preparation* as obtained in the *Assay*.
  B: Obtain the uterus from a 120- to 200-g rat in diestrus. Suspend one horn of the uterus in a bath at 32° containing, in each L of water, 9.0 g of sodium chloride, 0.42 g of potassium chloride, 0.16 g of calcium chloride, 0.50 g of sodium bicarbonate, 0.25 g of dextrose, and 0.0053 g of magnesium chloride. Oxygenate the bath solution with a mixture of 95% oxygen and 5% carbon dioxide. Record the contractions of the muscle on a recorder, using an isotonic and linear transducer. Add to the bath two appropriate dilutions of USP Oxytocin RS, and record the contraction of the muscle following each dilution. The appropriate dilutions are determined to give clearly distinctive submaximal contractions. Replace the solution in the bath with a fresh solution, and wait until the muscle is relaxed. Dissolve or dilute the preparation to be tested in a suitable diluent to obtain responses on the addition of two doses similar to the one used with the Standard solution. The magnitude of the contractions obtained with the Standard solution is comparable to the contractions obtained with the test solution.

Vasopressor activity (for product labeled of animal origin)—Proceed as directed in the *Assay* under *Vasopressin*, except to prepare a dilution of the Standard solution of USP Vasopressin RS containing 0.1 USP Vasopressin Unit per mL. The vasopressic activity of the test preparation is not more than 0.1 USP Vasopressin Unit per mL.

Ordinary impurities—The sum of the responses of impurities in the chromatogram of the *Assay preparation* obtained in the *Assay* is not more than 5% of the area of the oxytocin peak.

Assay—
  Mobile phase A—Prepare a buffer solution of 0.1 M monobasic sodium phosphate.
  Mobile phase B—Prepare a filtered and degassed mixture of acetonitrile in water (1 : 1). Make adjustments if necessary (see *System Suitability* under *Chromatography* ⟨621⟩).
  Diluent—Dissolve 5.0 g of chlorobutanol in 5.0 mL of glacial acetic acid, add 5.0 g of alcohol, 1.1 g of sodium acetate, and 1000 mL of water, and mix.
  Standard preparation—Dissolve the entire contents of a vial of USP Oxytocin RS in a known volume of *Diluent*. [NOTE—The solution may be diluted as necessary to a working concentration range for the assay.]
  Assay preparation—Dissolve an accurately weighed quantity of Oxytocin in *Diluent* to obtain a solution containing about 10 USP Oxytocin Units per mL.
  Chromatographic system (see *Chromatography* ⟨621⟩)—The liquid chromatograph is equipped with a variable wavelength detector set at 220 nm and a 12.0-cm × 4.6-mm column that contains 5-μm packing L1, and is programmed to provide variable mixtures of *Mobile phase A* and *Mobile phase B*. The column is maintained at room temperature, and the flow rate is about 1.5 mL per minute. The system is equilibrated with a mixture of 70% *Mobile phase A* and 30% *Mobile phase B*. After each injection of the *Standard preparation* and the *Assay preparation*, the composition of the mobile phase is changed linearly over the next 20 minutes so that it consists of a mixture of 50% *Mobile phase A* and 50% *Mobile phase B*. Chromatograph the *Standard preparation*, and record the chromatograms as directed for *Procedure*. Adjust the flow rate or the composition of the *Mobile phase* such that the retention time of oxytocin is approximately 10 minutes and between 15 and 17 minutes for chlorobutanol. The resolution, *R*, between oxytocin and the nearest adjacent peak is not less than 1.5, and the relative standard deviation for replicate injections is not more than 2.0% for oxytocin.
  Procedure—Separately inject three equal volumes (about 100 μL) of the *Assay preparation* and the *Standard preparation* into the chromatograph, and record the chromatograms as described under *Chromatographic system*. Identify the peaks, and determine the area of the oxytocin peak. Calculate the potency of oxytocin in USP Oxytocin Units per mg by the formula:

$$C(r_U/r_S)(V/W)$$

in which *C* is the concentration, in USP Oxytocin Units per mL, of the *Standard preparation*; and r_U and r_S are the mean peak responses obtained from the *Assay preparation* and the *Standard preparation*, respectively; *V* is the volume of sample solution in which the sample was dissolved; and *W* is the amount, in mg, of oxytocin dissolved in the sample solution.

Oxytocin Injection

» Oxytocin Injection is a sterile solution of Oxytocin in a suitable diluent. Each mL of Oxytocin Injection possesses an oxytocic activity of not less than 90.0 percent and not more than 110.0 percent of that stated on the label in USP Oxytocin Units.

Change to read:

Packaging and storage—Preserve in single-dose or multiple-dose containers, preferably of Type I glass ▲or in suitable plastic containers.▲*USP31*

Labeling—Label it to indicate its oxytocic activity in USP Oxytocin Units per mL. Label it also to state the animal source if naturally derived, or to state that it is synthetic.

USP Reference standards ⟨11⟩—*USP Endotoxin RS. USP Oxytocin RS.*

Bacterial endotoxins ⟨85⟩—It contains not more than 35.7 Endotoxin Units per USP Oxytocin Unit.

pH ⟨791⟩: between 3.0 and 5.0.

Particulate matter ⟨788⟩: meets the requirements for small-volume injections.

Other requirements—It meets the requirements under *Injections* ⟨1⟩.

Assay—Proceed as directed for *Oxytocin* except to use undiluted Injection as the *Assay preparation* and to allow not less than 25 minutes between injections. Calculate the potency, in USP Oxytocin Units per mL, by the formula:

$$C(r_U/r_S)$$

in which *C* is the concentration, in USP Oxytocin Units per mL, of the *Standard preparation*; and r_U and r_S are the mean values of the peak responses obtained from the *Assay preparation* and the *Standard preparation*, respectively.

Oxytocin Nasal Solution

» Oxytocin Nasal Solution is a solution of Oxytocin in a suitable diluent. It contains suitable preservatives, and is packaged in a form suitable for nasal administration. Each mL of Oxytocin Nasal Solution possesses an oxytocic activity of not less than 85.0 percent and not more than 120.0 percent of that stated on the label in USP Oxytocin Units.

Packaging and storage—Preserve in containers suitable for administering the contents by spraying into the nasal cavities with the patient in the upright position, or for instillation in drop form.
Labeling—Label it to indicate that it is for intranasal administration only. Label it to state the origin (animal or synthetic), and the animal source of the product if of animal origin.
USP Reference standards ⟨11⟩—*USP Oxytocin RS. USP Vasopressin RS.*
pH ⟨791⟩: between 3.7 and 4.3.
Vasopressor activity (for product labeled of animal origin)—Proceed as directed in the *Assay* under *Vasopressin*, except to use a Standard solution of USP Vasopressin RS containing 0.1 USP Vasopressin Unit per mL and to use a test solution prepared by diluting a volume of Nasal Solution to a concentration of 10 USP Oxytocin Units per mL. The vasopressic activity of the test solution is not more than 0.1 USP Oxytocin Unit per mL.
Assay—
Mobile phase A, Mobile phase B, Diluent, Standard preparation, and *Chromatographic system*—Proceed as directed in the *Assay* under *Oxytocin.*
Assay preparation—Quantitatively dilute an accurately measured volume of Nasal Solution in *Diluent* to obtain a solution containing about 10 USP Oxytocin Units per mL.
Procedure—Separately inject three equal volumes (about 100 µL) of the *Assay preparation* and the *Standard preparation* into the chromatograph, record the chromatograms, and measure the responses for the major peaks. Calculate the potency, in USP Oxytocin Units per mL, in the portion of Nasal Solution taken by the formula:

$$C(r_U / r_S)$$

in which C is the concentration, in USP Oxytocin Units per mL, of USP Oxytocin RS in the *Standard preparation;* and r_U and r_S are the mean peak responses obtained for oxytocin from the *Assay preparation* and the *Standard preparation,* respectively.

Paclitaxel

$C_{47}H_{51}NO_{14}$ 853.91
Benzenepropanoic acid, β-(benzoylamino)-α-hydroxy-, 6,12b-bis(acetyloxy)-12-(benzoyloxy)-2a,3,4,4a,5,6,9,10,11,12,12a,12b-dodecahydro-4,11-dihydroxy-4a,8,13,13-tetramethyl-5-oxo-7,11-methano-1*H*-cyclodeca[3,4]benz[1,2-*b*]oxet-9-yl ester, [2a*R*-[2aα,4β,4aβ,6β,9α(α*R**,β–*S**),11α,12α,12aα,12bα]]-.
(2a*R*,4*S*,4a*S*,6*R*,9*S*,11*S*,12*S*,12a*R*,12b*S*)-1,2a,3,4,4a,6,9,10,11,12,12a,12b-Dodecahydro-4,6,9,11,12,12b-hexahydroxy-4a,8,13,13-tetramethyl-7,11-methano-5*H*-cyclodeca[3,4]-benz[1,2-*b*]oxet-5-one 6,12b-diacetate, 12-benzoate, 9-ester with (2*R*,3*S*)-*N*-benzoyl-3-phenylisoserine [33069-62-4].

» Paclitaxel contains not less than 97.0 percent and not more than 102.0 percent of $C_{47}H_{51}NO_{14}$, calculated on the anhydrous, solvent-free basis.

Caution—Paclitaxel is cytotoxic. Great care should be taken to prevent inhaling particles of Paclitaxel and exposing the skin to it.

Packaging and storage—Preserve in tight, light-resistant containers, and store at controlled room temperature.

Labeling—The labeling indicates the type of process used to produce the material and the *Related compounds* test with which the material complies.
USP Reference standards ⟨11⟩—*USP Endotoxin RS. USP Paclitaxel RS. USP Paclitaxel Related Compound A RS. USP Paclitaxel Related Compound B RS.*
Identification—
  A: *Infrared Absorption* ⟨197K⟩.
  B: The retention time of the major peak in the chromatogram of the *Assay preparation* corresponds to that in the chromatogram of the *Standard preparation,* as obtained in the *Assay.*
Specific rotation ⟨781S⟩: between –49.0° and –55.0° at 20°, calculated on the anhydrous, solvent-free basis.
  Test solution: 10 mg per mL, in methanol.
Microbial limits ⟨61⟩—The total aerobic microbial count does not exceed 100 cfu per g. It meets the requirements of the tests for the absence of *Staphylococcus aureus, Pseudomonas aeruginosa, Salmonella* species, and *Escherichia coli.*
Bacterial endotoxins ⟨85⟩—It contains not more than 0.4 USP Endotoxin Unit per mg of paclitaxel.
Water, *Method Ic* ⟨921⟩: not more than 4.0%.
Residue on ignition ⟨281⟩: not more than 0.2%.
Heavy metals, *Method II* ⟨231⟩: 0.002%.
Related compounds—
  TEST 1 *(for material labeled as isolated from natural sources)*—If the material complies with this test, the labeling indicates that it meets *USP Related compounds Test 1.*
  Diluent—Prepare as directed in the *Assay.*
  Solution A—Prepare filtered and degassed acetonitrile.
  Solution B—Prepare filtered and degassed water.
  Mobile phase—Use variable mixtures of *Solution A* and *Solution B* as directed for *Chromatographic system.* Make adjustments if necessary (see *System Suitability* under *Chromatography* ⟨621⟩).
  System suitability solution—Dissolve accurately weighed quantities of USP Paclitaxel Related Compound A RS and USP Paclitaxel Related Compound B RS in methanol to obtain a solution having known concentrations of about 10 µg of each per mL. Transfer 5.0 mL of this solution to a 50-mL volumetric flask, dilute with *Diluent* to volume, and mix.
  Standard solution—Dissolve, with the aid of sonication, an accurately weighed quantity of USP Paclitaxel RS in *Diluent,* and dilute quantitatively, and stepwise if necessary, with *Diluent* to obtain a solution having a known concentration of about 5 µg per mL.
  Test solution—Use the *Assay preparation.*
  Chromatographic system (see *Chromatography* ⟨621⟩)—The liquid chromatograph is equipped with a 227-nm detector and a 4.6-mm × 25-cm column that contains 5-µm packing L43. The flow rate is about 2.6 mL per minute. The column temperature is maintained at 30°. The chromatograph is programmed as follows.

Time (minutes)	Solution A (%)	Solution B (%)	Elution
0–35	35	65	isocratic
35–60	35→80	65→20	linear gradient
60–70	80→35	20→65	linear gradient
70–80	35	65	isocratic

Chromatograph the *System suitability solution,* and record the peak responses as directed for *Procedure:* the relative retention times are about 0.78 for paclitaxel related compound A and 0.86 for paclitaxel related compound B (relative to the retention time for paclitaxel obtained from the *Test solution*); and the resolution, *R,* between paclitaxel related compound A and paclitaxel related compound B is not less than 1.0. Chromatograph the *Standard solution,* and record the peak responses as directed for *Procedure:* the relative standard deviation for replicate injections is not more than 2.0%.
  Procedure—Inject a volume (about 15 µL) of the *Test solution* into the chromatograph, record the chromatogram, and measure the

areas for the major peaks. Calculate the percentage of each impurity in the portion of Paclitaxel taken by the formula:

$$100(Fr_i / r_U)$$

in which F is the relative response factor for each impurity peak (see *Table 1* for values); r_i is the peak area for each individual impurity; and r_U is the peak area for paclitaxel.

Table 1

Relative Retention Time	Relative Response Factor (F)	Name	Limit (%)
0.24	1.29	Baccatin III	0.2
0.53	1.00	10-Deacetylpaclitaxel	0.5
0.57	1.00	7-Xylosylpaclitaxel	0.2
0.78	1.26	Cephalomannine (paclitaxel related compound A)	a_1[1]
0.78	1.26	2″,3″-Dihydrocephalomannine	a_2[1]
0.86	1.00	10-Deacetyl-7-epipaclitaxel (paclitaxel related compound B)	0.5
1.10	1.00	Benzyl analog[3]	b_1[2]
1.10	1.00	3″,4″-Dehydropaclitaxel C	b_2[2]
1.40	1.00	7-Epicephalomannine	0.3
1.85	1.00	7-Epipaclitaxel	0.5

[1] Resolution may be incomplete for these peaks, depending upon the relative amounts present; the sum of a_1 and a_2 is not more than 0.5%.
[2] Resolution may be incomplete for these peaks depending upon the relative amounts present; the sum of b_1 and b_2 is not more than 0.5%.
[3] The following chemical name is assigned to the related compound, benzyl analog: Baccatin III 13-ester with (2R,3S)-2-hydroxy-3-phenyl-3-(2-phenylacetylamino)propanoic acid.

In addition to not exceeding the limits for paclitaxel related impurities in *Table 1*, not more than 0.1% of any other single impurity is found; and not more than 2.0% of total impurities is found.

TEST 2 *(for material labeled as produced by a semisynthetic process)*—If the material complies with this test, the labeling indicates that it meets *USP Related compounds Test 2*.

Diluent—Use acetonitrile.

Solution A—Use a filtered and degassed mixture of water and acetonitrile (3 : 2).

Solution B—Use filtered and degassed acetonitrile.

Mobile phase—Use variable mixtures of *Solution A* and *Solution B* as directed for *Chromatographic system*. Make adjustments if necessary (see *System Suitability* under *Chromatography* ⟨621⟩).

System suitability solution—Dissolve accurately weighed quantities of USP Paclitaxel RS and USP Paclitaxel Related Compound B RS in *Diluent*, using shaking and sonication if necessary, to obtain a solution having known concentrations of about 0.96 mg and 0.008 mg per mL, respectively.

Test solution—Transfer about 10 mg of Paclitaxel, accurately weighed, to a 10-mL volumetric flask; dissolve in and dilute with *Diluent* to volume, using shaking and sonication if necessary; and mix.

Chromatographic system (see *Chromatography* ⟨621⟩)—The liquid chromatograph is equipped with a 227-nm detector and a 4.6-mm × 15-cm column that contains 3-µm packing L1. The flow rate is about 1.2 mL per minute. The column temperature is maintained at 35°. The chromatograph is programmed as follows.

Time (minutes)	Solution A (%)	Solution B (%)	Elution
0–20	100	0	isocratic
20–60	100→10	0→90	linear gradient
60–62	10→100	90→0	linear gradient
62–70	100	0	isocratic

Chromatograph the *System suitability solution,* and record the peak responses as directed for *Procedure*: the relative retention times are about 0.94 for paclitaxel related compound B and 1.0 for paclitaxel; the resolution, R, between paclitaxel related compound B and paclitaxel is not less than 1.2; and the relative standard deviation for replicate injections is not more than 2.0%.

Procedure—Separately inject equal volumes (about 15 µL) of the *Diluent* and the *Test solution* into the chromatograph, record the chromatograms, and measure the areas for all the peaks. Disregard any peaks due to the *Diluent*. Calculate the percentage of each impurity in the portion of Paclitaxel taken by the formula:

$$100(Fr_i / r_s)$$

in which F is the relative response factor for each impurity (see *Table 2* for values); r_i is the peak area for each impurity obtained from the *Test solution;* and r_s is the sum of the areas of all the peaks obtained from the *Test solution*.

Table 2

Relative Retention Time	Relative Response factor (F)	Name	Limit (%)
0.11	1.24	10-Deacetylbaccatin III	0.1
0.20	1.29	Baccatin III	0.2
0.42	1.39	Photodegradant[2]	0.1
0.47	1.00	10-Deacetylpaclitaxel	0.5
0.80	1.00	2-Debenzoylpaclitaxel-2-pentenoate	0.7
0.92[1]	1.00	Oxetane ring opened, acetyl and benzoyl[2]	x_1
0.92[1]	1.00	10-Acetoacetylpaclitaxel	x_2
0.94[1]	1.00	10-Deacetyl-7-epipaclitaxel (paclitaxel related compound B)	x_3
1.37	1.00	7-Epipaclitaxel	0.4
1.45	1.00	10,13-Bis-sidechainpaclitaxel[2]	0.5
1.54	1.00	7-Acetylpaclitaxel	0.6
1.80	1.75	13-Tes-baccatin III	0.1
2.14	1.00	7-Tes-paclitaxel	0.3

[1] Resolution may be incomplete for these peaks depending upon the relative amounts present; the sum of x_1, x_2, and x_3 is not more than 0.4%.
[2] The following chemical names are assigned to the related compounds Photodegradant, Oxetane ring opened, acetyl and benzoyl, and 10,13-Bissidechainpaclitaxel:
Photodegradant
(1R,2R,4S,5S,7R,10S,11R,12S,13S,15S,16S)-2,10-diacetyloxy-5,13-dihydroxy-4,16,17,17-tetramethyl-8-oxa-3-oxo-12-phenylcarbonyloxypentacyclo[11.3.1.0^{1,11}.0^{4,11}.0^{7,10}]heptadec-15-yl
(2R,3S)-2-hydroxy-3-phenyl-3-(phenylcarbonylamino)propanoate
Oxetane ring opened, acetyl and benzoyl migrated
(1S,2S,3R,4S,5S,7S,8S,10R,13S)-5,10-diacetyloxy-1,2,4,7-tetrahydroxy-8,12,15,15-tetramethyl-9-oxo-4-(phenylcarbonyloxymethyl)tricyclo[9.3.1.0^{3,8}]pentadec-11-en-13-yl
(2R,3S)-2-hydroxy-3-phenyl-3-(phenylcarbonylamino)propanoate
10,13-Bissidechainpaclitaxel
Baccatin III 13-ester with (2R,3S)-2-hydroxy-3-phenyl-3-(phenylcarbonylamino)propanoic acid, 10-ester with (2S,3S)-2-hydroxy-3-phenyl-3-(phenylcarbonylamino)propanoic acid

In addition to not exceeding the limits for paclitaxel related impurities in *Table 2*, not more than 0.1% of any other single impurity is found; and not more than 2.0% of total impurities is found.

Organic volatile impurities, *Method IV* ⟨467⟩: meets the requirements.

(Official until July 1, 2008)

Assay—

Diluent—Prepare a mixture of methanol and acetic acid (200 : 1).

Mobile phase—Prepare a filtered and degassed mixture of water and acetonitrile (11 : 9). Make adjustments if necessary (see *System Suitability* under *Chromatography* ⟨621⟩).

Standard preparation—Dissolve, using sonication if necessary, an accurately weighed quantity of USP Paclitaxel RS in *Diluent*, and dilute quantitatively, and stepwise if necessary, with *Diluent* to obtain a solution having a known concentration of about 1 mg per mL.

Assay preparation—Transfer about 10 mg of Paclitaxel, accurately weighed, to a 10-mL volumetric flask. Dissolve in *Diluent*, using sonication if necessary, dilute with *Diluent* to volume, and mix.

Chromatographic system (see *Chromatography* ⟨621⟩)—The liquid chromatograph is equipped with a 227-nm detector and a 4.6-mm × 25-cm column that contains 5-μm packing L43. The flow rate is about 1.5 mL per minute. Chromatograph the *Standard preparation*, and record the peak responses as directed for *Procedure*: the tailing factor is between 0.7 and 1.3; and the relative standard deviation for replicate injections is not more than 1.5%.

Procedure—Separately inject equal volumes (about 10 μL) of the *Standard preparation* and the *Assay preparation* into the chromatograph, record the chromatograms, and measure the areas for the major peaks. Calculate the quantity, in mg, of $C_{47}H_{51}NO_{14}$ in the portion of Paclitaxel taken by the formula:

$$10C(r_U / r_S)$$

in which C is the concentration, in mg per mL, of USP Paclitaxel RS in the *Standard preparation;* and r_U and r_S are the peak responses for paclitaxel obtained from the *Assay preparation* and the *Standard preparation*, respectively.

Paclitaxel Injection

» Paclitaxel Injection is a sterile, stabilized solution of Paclitaxel, suitable for dilution for intravenous administration. It contains not less than 90.0 percent and not more than 110.0 percent of the labeled amount of paclitaxel ($C_{47}H_{51}NO_{14}$).

Packaging and storage—Preserve in single-dose or multiple-dose containers, preferably of Type I glass, at controlled room temperature.

Labeling—Label it to indicate that it is to be diluted with a suitable parenteral vehicle prior to intravenous infusion.

USP Reference standards ⟨11⟩—*USP Endotoxin RS. USP Paclitaxel RS. USP Paclitaxel Related Compound B RS.*

Identification—

A: The retention time of the major peak in the chromatogram of the *Test solution* corresponds to that in the chromatogram of the *Standard solution*, as obtained in the test for *Limit of degradation products*.

B: The retention time of the major peak in the chromatogram of the *Assay preparation* corresponds to that in the chromatogram of the *Standard preparation*, as obtained in the *Assay*.

Bacterial endotoxins ⟨85⟩—It contains not more than 0.67 USP Endotoxin Unit per mg of paclitaxel.

pH ⟨791⟩: between 3.0 and 7.0, in a solution (1 in 10).

Limit of degradation products—

Solution A—Prepare a filtered and degassed mixture of water and acetonitrile (3 : 2).

Solution B—Use filtered and degassed acetonitrile.

Mobile phase—Use variable mixtures of *Solution A* and *Solution B* as directed for *Chromatographic system*. Make adjustments if necessary (see *System Suitability* under *Chromatography* ⟨621⟩).

Standard solution—Dissolve accurately weighed quantities of USP Paclitaxel RS and USP Paclitaxel Related Compound B RS in acetonitrile, and dilute quantitatively, and stepwise if necessary, to obtain solutions having known concentrations of about 1.2 mg per mL and 0.006 mg per mL, respectively.

Test solution—Quantitatively dilute an accurately measured volume of Injection with acetonitrile to obtain a solution containing about 1.2 mg of paclitaxel per mL, and mix.

Chromatographic system (see *Chromatography* ⟨621⟩)—The liquid chromatograph is equipped with a 227-nm detector and a 4.6-mm × 15-cm column that contains 3-μm packing L1. The flow rate is about 1.2 mL per minute. The column temperature is maintained at 35°. The chromatograph is programmed as follows.

Time (minutes)	Solution A (%)	Solution B (%)	Elution
0–26	100	0	isocratic
26–66	100→17	0→83	linear gradient
66–67	17→100	83→0	linear gradient
67–75	100	0	isocratic

Chromatograph the *Standard solution*, and record the peak responses as directed for *Procedure*: the resolution, R, between paclitaxel related compound B and paclitaxel is not less than 1.2; and the relative standard deviation for replicate injections is not more than 2.0%.

Procedure—Separately inject equal volumes (about 10 μL) of the *Standard solution* and the *Test solution* into the chromatograph, record the chromatograms, and measure the areas of the analyte peaks. Calculate the percentage of each degradation product in the volume of Injection taken by the formula:

$$100(C_S / C_U)(r_i / r_S)$$

in which C_S is the concentration, in mg per mL, of USP Paclitaxel Related Compound B RS in the *Standard solution;* C_U is the concentration, in mg per mL, of paclitaxel in the *Test solution*, based on the labeled amount of paclitaxel per mL of Injection; r_i is the peak area for each degradation product obtained from the *Test solution;* and r_S is the peak area for paclitaxel related compound B obtained from the *Standard solution*. In addition to not exceeding the limits stated in *Table 1*, not more than 0.1% of any other paclitaxel degradation product is found; and not more than 2.0% of total paclitaxel degradation products is found.

Table 1.

Relative Retention Time	Name	Limit (%)
0.19	Baccatin III	0.8
0.21	Ethyl ester side chain	0.4
0.50	10-Deacetylpaclitaxel	0.8
0.95	10-Deacetyl-7-epipaclitaxel (paclitaxel related compound B)	0.5
1.40	7-Epipaclitaxel	0.6

Other requirements—It meets the requirements under *Injections* ⟨1⟩.

Assay—

Diluent—Transfer 200 μL of glacial acetic acid to a 1-liter volumetric flask containing about 500 mL of methanol, mix, and dilute with methanol to volume.

Mobile phase—Prepare a filtered and degassed mixture of water and acetonitrile (11 : 9). Make adjustments if necessary (see *System Suitability* under *Chromatography* ⟨621⟩).

Standard preparation—Dissolve an accurately weighed quantity of USP Paclitaxel RS in *Diluent* to obtain a solution having a known concentration of about 0.6 mg per mL.

Assay preparation—Quantitatively dilute an accurately measured volume of Injection with *Diluent* to obtain a solution containing about 0.6 mg of paclitaxel per mL.

Chromatographic system (see *Chromatography* ⟨621⟩)—The liquid chromatograph is equipped with a 227-nm detector and a 4.0-mm × 25-cm column that contains 5-μm packing L43. The flow rate is about 1.5 mL per minute. Chromatograph the *Standard preparation*, and record the peak responses as directed for *Procedure*: the retention time of the paclitaxel peak is between 6.0 and 10.0 minutes; and the relative standard deviation for replicate injections is not more than 1.5%.

Procedure—Separately inject equal volumes (about 10 µL) of the *Standard preparation* and the *Assay preparation* into the chromatograph, record the chromatograms, and measure the responses for the paclitaxel peaks. Calculate the quantity, in mg, of paclitaxel ($C_{47}H_{51}NO_{14}$) in each mL of the Injection taken by the formula:

$$(L/D)C(r_U / r_S)$$

in which L is the labeled quantity, in mg, of paclitaxel in each mL of Injection; D is the concentration, in mg per mL, of paclitaxel in the *Assay preparation*, based on the labeled quantity; C is the concentration, in mg per mL, of USP Paclitaxel RS in the *Standard preparation*; and r_U and r_S are the peak responses obtained from the *Assay preparation* and the *Standard preparation*, respectively.

Padimate O

$C_{17}H_{27}NO_2$ 277.40
Benzoic acid, 4-(dimethylamino)-, 2-ethylhexyl ester.
2-Ethylhexyl *p*-(dimethylamino)benzoate [*21245-02-3*].

» Padimate O contains not less than 97.0 percent and not more than 103.8 percent of $C_{17}H_{27}NO_2$.

Packaging and storage—Preserve in tight, light-resistant containers.
USP Reference standards ⟨11⟩—*USP Padimate O RS*.
Identification—
 A: *Infrared Absorption* ⟨197F⟩.
 B: *Ultraviolet Absorption* ⟨197U⟩—
  Solution: 5 µg per mL.
  Medium: alcohol.
  Absorptivities at 312 nm do not differ by more than 4.0%.
Specific gravity ⟨841⟩: between 0.990 and 1.000.
Refractive index ⟨831⟩: between 1.5390 and 1.5430.
Acid value ⟨401⟩: not more than 1.0.
Saponification value ⟨401⟩: between 195 and 215, reflux temperature being maintained for 4 hours.
Chromatographic purity—
 Chromatographic system (see *Chromatography* ⟨621⟩)—The gas chromatograph is equipped with a flame-ionization detector and a 3-mm × 1.8-m stainless steel column packed with 10 percent liquid phase G9 on support S1A. The column temperature is programmed at a rate of 10° per minute from 150° to 250°, then maintained at 250° for 10 minutes, and helium is used as the carrier gas.
 Procedure—Chromatograph 2 µL of a 1 in 100 solution of Padimate O in chloroform: the response due to padimate O is not less than 98.0% of the sum of the responses on the chromatogram, exclusive of the chloroform peak.
Assay—Dissolve about 500 mg of Padimate O, accurately weighed, in 75 mL of acetic anhydride, and titrate with 0.1 N perchloric acid VS, determining the endpoint potentiometrically. Each mL of 0.1 N perchloric acid is equivalent to 27.74 mg of $C_{17}H_{27}NO_2$.

Padimate O Lotion

» Padimate O Lotion contains not less than 90.0 percent and not more than 110.0 percent of the labeled amount of $C_{17}H_{27}NO_2$.

Packaging and storage—Preserve in tight, light-resistant containers.
USP Reference standards ⟨11⟩—*USP Padimate O RS*.
Identification—The retention time of the major peak in the chromatogram of the *Assay preparation* corresponds to that in the chromatogram of the *Standard preparation*, as obtained in the *Assay*.
Assay—
 Mobile phase—Prepare a suitable filtered and degassed solution containing methanol, water, and glacial acetic acid (85 : 15 : 0.5).
 Standard preparation—Dissolve an accurately weighed quantity of USP Padimate O RS in isopropyl alcohol and dilute quantitatively, and stepwise if necessary, with isopropyl alcohol to obtain a solution having a known concentration of about 100 µg per mL.
 Assay preparation—Transfer an accurately weighed quantity of Lotion, equivalent to about 100 mg of Padimate O, to a 100-mL volumetric flask, and add about 75 mL of isopropyl alcohol. Heat gently with swirling until the specimen is dispersed. Cool to room temperature, dilute with isopropyl alcohol to volume, and mix. Pipet 10.0 mL of this solution into a 100-mL volumetric flask, dilute with isopropyl alcohol to volume, and mix.
 Chromatographic system (see *Chromatography* ⟨621⟩)—The liquid chromatograph is equipped with a 308-nm detector and a 4.6-mm × 25-cm column that contains 5-µm *base-deactivated* packing L1. The flow rate is about 1.5 mL per minute. Chromatograph the *Standard preparation*, and record the peak responses as directed under *Procedure*: the tailing factor is not more than 2.5 and the relative standard deviation for replicate injections is not more than 2.0%.
 Procedure—Separately inject equal volumes (about 10 µL) of the *Standard preparation* and the *Assay preparation* into the chromatograph, record the chromatograms, and measure the responses for the major peaks. Calculate the quantity, in mg, of $C_{17}H_{27}NO_2$ in the portion of Lotion taken by the formula:

$$C(r_U / r_S)$$

in which C is the concentration, in µg per mL, of USP Padimate O RS in the *Standard preparation*, and r_U and r_S are the peak responses for padimate O obtained from the *Assay preparation* and the *Standard preparation*, respectively.

Pamabrom

$C_{11}H_{18}BrN_5O_3$ 348.20
8-Bromo-3,7-dihydro-1,3-dimethyl-1-*H*-purine-2,6-dione compound with 2-amino-2-methyl-1-propanol (1 : 1).
8-Bromotheophylline compound with 2-amino-2-methyl-1-propanol (1 : 1) [*606-04-02*].

» Pamabrom contains not less than 72.2 percent and not more than 76.6 percent of 8-bromotheophylline ($C_7H_7BrN_4O_2$), calculated on the anhydrous basis; and not less than 24.6 percent and not more than 26.6 percent of 2-amino-2-methyl-1-propanol ($C_4H_{11}NO$), calculated on the anhydrous basis.

Packaging and storage—Preserve in well-closed containers.
USP Reference standards ⟨11⟩—*USP 8-Bromotheophylline RS. USP Theophylline RS*.
Identification—It responds to the *Thin-layer Chromatographic Identification Test* ⟨201⟩, using a solvent system consisting of a mixture of xylene, methanol, and glacial acetic acid (11 : 2 : 1) and a *Standard solution* and a *Test solution* prepared as directed below: the R_F value of the principal spot, which appears as a dark spot against a green background, from the *Test solution* corresponds to that obtained from the *Standard solution*.
 Standard solution—Transfer an accurately weighed quantity of about 20 mg of USP 8-Bromotheophylline RS to a 100-mL volu-

metric flask, add 25 mL of water, 50 mL of methanol, and a small amount of dilute ammonium hydroxide. Swirl the flask to effect solution. Dilute the contents of the flask with methanol to volume, and mix.

Test solution—Transfer an accurately weighed quantity of about 25 mg of Pamabrom to a 100-mL volumetric flask, add 25 mL of water, and swirl to dissolve. Dilute the contents of the flask with methanol to volume, and mix.

Water, *Method I* ⟨921⟩: not more than 3%.
Heavy metals, *Method II* ⟨231⟩: 20 µg per g.
Limit of theophylline—
Diluting solution, Mobile phase, and *Chromatographic system*—Proceed as directed in the *Assay for 8-bromotheophylline*.

Standard solution—Dissolve an accurately weighed quantity of USP Theophylline RS in *Diluting solution*, add a few drops of ammonium hydroxide, sonicating if necessary, to obtain a solution having a known concentration of about 1 mg of USP Theophylline RS per mL. Dilute a volume of this solution quantitatively, and stepwise if necessary, with *Diluting solution* to obtain a solution having a known concentration of about 5 µg per mL.

Test solution—Transfer an accurately weighed quantity of about 200 mg of Pamabrom to a 200-mL volumetric flask. Add about 50 mL of *Diluting solution*, and sonicate for 5 minutes. Cool to room temperature, dilute with *Diluting solution* to volume, and mix.

Procedure—Separately inject equal volumes (about 20 µL) of the *Standard solution* and the *Test solution* into the chromatograph, record the chromatograms, and measure the responses for the major peaks. Calculate the percentage of theophylline in the portion of Pamabrom taken by the formula:

$$20(C/W)(r_U/r_S)$$

in which C is the concentration, in µg per mL, of USP Theophylline RS in the *Standard solution*, W is the weight, in mg, of Pamabrom taken, and r_U and r_S are the peak responses of theophylline obtained from the *Test solution* and the *Standard solution*, respectively: not more than 0.5% is found.

Assay for 8-bromotheophylline—
Diluting solution—Prepare a mixture of water and methanol (70 : 30).

Mobile phase—Prepare a filtered and degassed mixture of water, methanol, and glacial acetic acid (69 : 30 : 1), filter, and degas. Make adjustments if necessary (see *System Suitability* under *Chromatography* ⟨621⟩).

Internal standard solution—Dissolve an accurately weighed quantity of caffeine in *Diluting solution*, and dilute quantitatively, and stepwise if necessary, to obtain a solution having a concentration of about 125 µg of caffeine per mL.

Standard preparation—Dissolve an accurately weighed quantity of USP 8-Bromotheophylline RS in *Diluting solution*, add a few drops of ammonium hydroxide, sonicating if necessary, to obtain a solution having a known concentration of about 0.75 mg of USP 8-Bromotheophylline RS per mL. Transfer 5.0 mL of this solution to a 100-mL volumetric flask, add 10.0 mL of *Internal standard solution*, dilute with *Mobile phase* to volume, mix, and filter.

Assay preparation—Transfer an accurately weighed quantity of about 200 mg of Pamabrom to a 200-mL volumetric flask, add about 50 mL of *Diluting solution* and two drops of ammonium hydroxide, and sonicate for 5 minutes. [NOTE—If a hazy solution is present after 5 minutes of sonication, add 1 additional drop of ammonium hydroxide.] Cool, dilute with *Diluting solution* to volume, and mix. Transfer 5.0 mL of this solution to a 100-mL volumetric flask, add 10.0 mL of *Internal standard solution*, dilute with *Mobile phase* to volume, mix, and filter.

Chromatographic system (see *Chromatography* ⟨621⟩)—The liquid chromatograph is equipped with a 280-nm detector and a 4.6-mm × 15-cm column that contains packing L1. The flow rate is about 1.5 mL per minute. Chromatograph 20 µL of the *Standard preparation*, and record the peak responses as directed under *Procedure*: the relative retention times are about 0.6 for caffeine and 1.0 for 8-bromotheophylline, the resolution, R, between caffeine and 8-bromotheophylline is not less than 2.0, and the relative standard deviation for replicate injections is not more than 2.0%.

Procedure—Separately inject equal volumes (about 20 µL) of the *Standard preparation* and the *Assay preparation* into the chromatograph, record the chromatograms, and measure the responses for the major peaks. Calculate the quantity, in mg, of 8-bromotheophylline ($C_7H_7BrN_4O_2$) in the portion of Pamabrom taken by the formula:

$$4000C(R_U/R_S)$$

in which C is the concentration, in mg per mL, of USP 8-Bromotheophylline RS in the *Standard preparation*, and R_U and R_S are the peak response ratios of the 8-bromotheophylline peak and the internal standard peak obtained from the *Assay preparation* and the *Standard preparation*, respectively.

Assay for 2-amino-2-methyl-1-propanol—Dissolve about 1 g of Pamabrom, accurately weighed, in 10 mL of water by warming gently on a steam bath until the solution is clear. Cool, add methyl orange TS, and titrate with 0.5 N hydrochloric acid VS. Perform a blank determination, and make any necessary correction (see *Titrimetry* ⟨541⟩). Each mL of 0.5 N hydrochloric acid is equivalent to 44.57 mg of $C_4H_{11}NO$.

Pamidronate Disodium

$C_3H_9NNa_2O_7P_2 \cdot 5H_2O$ 369.11
Phosphonic acid, (3-amino-1-hydroxypropylidene)bis-, disodium salt, pentahydrate.
Disodium dihydrogen (3-amino-1-hydroxypropylidene)diphosphonate, pentahydrate   [*109552-15-0*].
Anhydrous   279.06   [*57248-88-1*].

» Pamidronate Disodium contains not less than 98.0 percent and not more than 102.0 percent of $C_3H_9NNa_2O_7P_2$, calculated on the anhydrous basis.

Packaging and storage—Preserve in tight containers. Store at a temperature not exceeding 30°.
USP Reference standards ⟨11⟩—USP Beta Alanine RS. USP Pamidronate Disodium RS.
Clarity and color of solution—
Test preparation 1—Dissolve 1.0 g in 50 mL of water with gentle warming. Cool to room temperature.

Test preparation 2—Dissolve 1.0 g in 25 mL of 2 N sodium hydroxide solution with gentle warming. Cool to room temperature.

Procedure—Examine *Test preparation 1* and *Test preparation 2*: the solutions are clear. Separately measure the absorbance of each of these solutions at 420 nm in 4-cm cells, using water as the blank for *Test preparation 1* and using 2 N sodium hydroxide solution as the blank for *Test preparation 2*: the absorbance of each solution is not more than 0.10.
Identification—
A: *Infrared Absorption* ⟨197K⟩.
B: The retention time of the major peak in the chromatogram of the *Assay preparation* corresponds to that in the chromatogram of the *Standard preparation*, as obtained in the *Assay*.
C: It meets the requirements of the pyroantimonate precipitate test for *Sodium* ⟨191⟩.
Microbial limits ⟨61⟩—The total aerobic microbial count does not exceed 1000 cfu per g, and the total combined yeasts and molds count does not exceed 100 cfu per g.
pH ⟨791⟩: between 7.8 and 8.8, in a solution (1 in 100).
Water, *Method I* ⟨921⟩: between 23.0% and 25.5%.
Heavy metals, *Method II* ⟨231⟩: 20 µg per g.
Related compounds—
TEST 1—
Adsorbent: 0.25-mm layer of chromatographic silica gel mixture.

Test solution—Transfer 30 mg of Pamidronate Disodium to a 10-mL volumetric flask, dissolve in and dilute with water to volume, and mix.

Standard solution—Dissolve an accurately weighed quantity of USP Beta Alanine RS in water, and dilute quantitatively, and stepwise if necessary, with water to obtain a solution containing 0.006 mg of beta alanine per mL.

Application volume: 10 µL.

Developing solvent system: a mixture of methanol, diisopropyl ether, and 25% ammonia (9 : 8 : 4).

Spray reagent—Dissolve 0.2 g of ninhydrin in 100 mL of a mixture of butyl alcohol and 2 N acetic acid (95 : 5).

Procedure—Proceed as directed for *Thin-Layer Chromatography* under *Chromatography* ⟨621⟩. Dry the plate between 100° and 105° until the ammonia disappears completely. Spray with *Spray reagent*, and heat between 100° and 105° for about 15 minutes. Examine the plate under white light. The spot obtained from the *Test solution* having an R_F value of about 0.5 is not greater in size or intensity than the corresponding spot obtained from the *Standard solution*: not more than 0.2% of beta alanine is found. Evaluate any other additional spot in the chromatogram of the *Test solution*, and determine the percentage of total other impurities (excluding beta alanine).

TEST 2—

Mobile phase—Proceed as directed in the *Assay*.

Impurity stock solution 1—Transfer about 300 mg of ortho-phosphoric acid, accurately weighed, to a 1000-mL volumetric flask, dissolve in and dilute with water to volume, and mix.

Impurity stock solution 2—Transfer about 250 mg of phosphorous acid, accurately weighed, to a 1000-mL volumetric flask, dissolve in and dilute with water to volume, and mix.

Impurity standard solution—Transfer 2.0 mL each of *Impurity stock solution 1* and *Impurity stock solution 2* to a 50-mL volumetric flask, dilute with water to volume, and mix.

Test solution—Prepare as directed for the *Assay preparation*.

Chromatographic system (see *Chromatography* ⟨621⟩)—Proceed as directed in the *Assay*. Chromatograph the *Impurity standard solution*, and record the peak responses as directed for *Procedure*: the elution order is a phosphate peak followed by the phosphite peak; the resolution, R, between the two peaks is not less than 2.5; the relative standard deviation for replicate injections, determined from the phosphate peak, is not more than 10%; and the relative standard deviation for replicate injections, determined from the phosphite peak, is not more than 20%.

Procedure—Separately inject equal volumes (about 100 µL) of the *Impurity standard solution* and the *Test solution* into the chromatograph, record the chromatograms, and measure the responses for the major peaks. Calculate the percentage of phosphates as ortho-phosphoric acid in the portion of Pamidronate Disodium taken by the formula:

$$0.2(W_1/W)(r_U/r_S)$$

in which W_1 is the weight, in mg, of ortho-phosphoric acid taken to prepare the *Impurity stock solution 1*; W is the weight, in mg, of Pamidronate Disodium taken to prepare the *Test solution*; and r_U and r_S are the phosphate peak responses obtained from the *Test solution* and the *Impurity standard solution*, respectively: not more than 0.5% of phosphate, determined as ortho-phosphoric acid, is found.

Calculate the percentages of phosphites as phosphorous acid in the portion of Pamidronate Disodium taken by the formula:

$$0.2(W_2/W)(r_U/r_S)$$

in which W_2 is the weight, in mg, of phosphorous acid taken to prepare the *Impurity stock solution 2*; W is as defined above; and r_U and r_S are the phosphite peak responses obtained from the *Test solution* and the *Impurity standard solution*, respectively: not more than 0.5% of phosphite, determined as phosphorous acid, is found; and not more than 0.5% of total phosphate and phosphite combined is found.

Calculate the percentage of any other impurity in the portion of Pamidronate Disodium taken by the formula:

$$0.2(W_1/W)(r_i/r_S)$$

in which W_1 and W are as defined above; r_i is the peak response of any other impurity in the *Test solution*; and r_S is the response of the phosphate peak obtained from the *Impurity standard solution*: not more than 0.5% of total other impurities (excluding beta alanine, phosphate as ortho-phosphoric acid, and phosphite as phosphorous acid) is found, the results for *Test 1* and *Test 2* being added.

Alcohol content, Method II ⟨611⟩: not more than 0.3% is found.

Assay—

Mobile phase—To 2500 mL of water, add 0.47 mL of anhydrous formic acid, adjust with 2 N sodium hydroxide solution to a pH of 3.5, filter, and degas. Make adjustments if necessary (see *System Suitability* under *Chromatography* ⟨621⟩). [NOTE—The small amounts of formic acid have a strong influence on the retention times.]

Standard preparation—Dissolve an accurately weighed quantity of USP Pamidronate Disodium RS in water, and dilute quantitatively, and stepwise if necessary, with water to obtain a solution having a known concentration of about 2 mg per mL.

Assay preparation—Transfer about 100 mg of Pamidronate Disodium, accurately weighed, to a 50-mL volumetric flask, dissolve in and dilute with water to volume, and mix.

Chromatographic system (see *Chromatography* ⟨621⟩)—The liquid chromatograph is equipped with a refractive index detector and a 4.6-mm × 10-cm column that contains packing L23. The flow rate is about 1.0 mL per minute. The column temperature is maintained at 35°. Chromatograph the *Standard preparation*, and record the peak responses as directed for *Procedure*: the tailing factor is not less than 0.3 and not more than 1.2; and the relative standard deviation for replicate injections is not more than 2.0%.

Procedure—Separately inject equal volumes (about 100 µL) of the *Standard preparation* and the *Assay preparation* into the chromatograph, record the chromatograms, and measure the responses for the major peaks. Calculate the quantity, in mg, of $C_3H_9NNa_2O_7P_2$ in the portion of Pamidronate Disodium taken by the formula:

$$50C(r_U/r_S)$$

in which C is the concentration, in mg per mL, of USP Pamidronate Disodium RS in the *Standard preparation*; and r_U and r_S are the peak responses obtained from the *Assay preparation* and the *Standard preparation*, respectively.

Pamidronate Disodium for Injection

Change to read:

» Pamidronate Disodium for Injection is a sterile, freeze-dried mixture of Pamidronate Disodium and suitable excipients. It contains not less than •93.0 percent•₃ and not more than 108.0 percent of the labeled amount of pamidronate disodium ($C_3H_9NNa_2O_7P_2$).

Packaging and storage—Preserve in *Containers for Sterile Solids*, as described under *Injections* ⟨1⟩. Store at controlled room temperature.

USP Reference standards ⟨11⟩—*USP Beta Alanine RS. USP Endotoxin RS. USP Pamidronate Disodium RS.*

Constituted solution—At the time of use, it meets the requirements for *Constituted Solutions* under *Injections* ⟨1⟩.

Identification—The retention time of the major peak in the chromatogram of the *Assay preparation* corresponds to that in the chromatogram of the *Standard preparation*, as obtained in the *Assay*.

Bacterial endotoxins ⟨85⟩—It contains not more than 3.88 USP Endotoxin Units per mg of anhydrous pamidronate disodium.

Uniformity of dosage units ⟨905⟩: meets the requirements for *Weight Variation*.

pH ⟨791⟩: between 6.0 and 7.0, determined in a solution constituted as directed in the labeling.

Particulate matter ⟨788⟩: meets the requirements for small-volume injections.

Water, *Method Ia* ⟨921⟩: not more than 5%.

Limit of beta alanine—

Adsorbent, Application volume, Developing solvent system, and *Spray reagent*—Proceed as directed for *Related compounds, Test 1* under *Pamidronate Disodium.*

Standard solution—Dissolve an accurately weighed quantity of USP Beta Alanine RS in water, and dilute quantitatively, and stepwise if necessary, with water to obtain a solution containing 0.0075 mg of beta alanine per mL.

Test solution—Reconstitute the vial with the appropriate amount of water to obtain a solution having a concentration of 3 mg of anhydrous pamidronate disodium per mL, based on the label claim.

Procedure—Proceed as directed for *Thin-Layer Chromatography* under *Chromatography* ⟨621⟩. Dry the plate between 100° and 105° until the ammonia disappears completely. Spray with *Spray reagent,* and heat between 100° and 105° for about 15 minutes. Examine the plate under white light. The spot having an R_F value of about 0.5 obtained from the *Test solution* is not greater in size or intensity than the corresponding spot obtained from the *Standard solution:* not more than 0.25% of beta alanine is found.

Other requirements—It meets the requirements under *Sterility Tests* ⟨71⟩ and for *Labeling* under *Injections* ⟨1⟩.

Assay—

Mobile phase and *Chromatographic system*—Proceed as directed in the *Assay* under *Pamidronate Disodium.*

Standard preparation—Dissolve an accurately weighed quantity of USP Pamidronate Disodium RS in water, and dilute quantitatively, and stepwise if necessary, with water to obtain a solution having a known concentration of about 2.5 mg per mL. Calculate the concentration, C_S, of anhydrous pamidronate disodium, the molecular weights of anhydrous and pentahydrate pamidronate disodium being 279.06 and 369.11, respectively.

Assay preparation—Constitute a suitable number of vials of Pamidronate Disodium for Injection with the appropriate amount of water to obtain a solution having a known concentration of about 2 mg of anhydrous pamidronate disodium per mL, based on the label claim.

Procedure—Separately inject equal volumes (about 100 μL) of the *Standard preparation* and the *Assay preparation* into the chromatograph, record the chromatograms, and measure the responses for the major peaks. Calculate the percentage of $C_3H_9NNa_2O_7P_2$ in the portion of Pamidronate Disodium for Injection taken by the formula:

$$100(C_S / C_U)(r_U / r_S)$$

in which C_S is as defined under the *Standard preparation;* C_U is the concentration, in mg per mL, of anhydrous pamidronate disodium in the *Assay preparation;* and r_U and r_S are the peak responses obtained from the *Assay preparation* and the *Standard preparation,* respectively.

Pancreatin

Pancreatin.
Pancreatin [8049-47-6].

» Pancreatin is a substance containing enzymes, principally amylase, lipase, and protease, obtained from the pancreas of the hog, *Sus scrofa* Linné var. *domesticus* Gray (Fam. Suidae) or of the ox, *Bos taurus* Linné (Fam. Bovidae). Pancreatin contains, in each mg, not less than 25 USP Units of amylase activity, not less than 2.0 USP Units of lipase activity, and not less than 25 USP Units of protease activity. Pancreatin of a higher digestive power may be labeled as a whole-number multiple of the three minimum activities or may be diluted by admixture with lactose, or with sucrose containing not more than 3.25 percent of starch, or with pancreatin of lower digestive power.

NOTE—One USP Unit of amylase activity is contained in the amount of pancreatin that decomposes starch at an initial rate such that 0.16 μEq of glycosidic linkage is hydrolyzed per minute under the conditions of the *Assay for amylase activity.*

One USP Unit of lipase activity is contained in the amount of pancreatin that liberates 1.0 μEq of acid per minute at a pH of 9.0 and 37° under the conditions of the *Assay for lipase activity.*

One USP Unit of protease activity is contained in the amount of pancreatin that under the conditions of the *Assay for protease activity* hydrolyzes casein at an initial rate such that there is liberated per minute an amount of peptides not precipitated by trichloroacetic acid that gives the same absorbance at 280 nm as 15 nmol of tyrosine.

Packaging and storage—Preserve in tight containers, at a temperature not exceeding 30°.

USP Reference standards ⟨11⟩—*USP Bile Salts RS. USP Pancreatin Amylase and Protease RS. USP Pancreatin Lipase RS.*

Microbial limits ⟨61⟩—It meets the requirements of the test for absence of *Salmonella* species and *Escherichia coli.*

Loss on drying ⟨731⟩—Dry it in vacuum at 60° for 4 hours: it loses not more than 5.0% of its weight.

Fat—Place 2.0 g of Pancreatin in a flask of about 50-mL capacity, add 20 mL of ether, insert the stopper, and set it aside for 2 hours, mixing by rotating at frequent intervals. Decant the supernatant ether by means of a guiding rod into a plain filter about 7 cm in diameter, previously moistened with ether, and collect the filtrate in a tared beaker. Repeat the extraction with a 10-mL portion of ether, proceeding as directed before, then with another 10-mL portion of ether, and transfer the ether and the remainder of the Pancreatin to the filter. Allow to drain, evaporate the ether spontaneously, and dry the residue at 105° for 2 hours: the residue of fat obtained from Pancreatin possessing three or more times the three minimum activities weighs not more than 120 mg (6.0%); that obtained from Pancreatin possessing less than three times the three minimum activities weighs not more than 60 mg (3.0%).

Assay for amylase activity (*Starch digestive power*)—

pH 6.8 phosphate buffer—On the day of use, dissolve 13.6 g of monobasic potassium phosphate in water to make 500 mL of solution. Dissolve 14.2 g of anhydrous dibasic sodium phosphate in water to make 500 mL of solution. Mix 51 mL of the monobasic potassium phosphate solution with 49 mL of the dibasic sodium phosphate solution. If necessary, adjust by the dropwise addition of the appropriate solution to a pH of 6.8.

Substrate solution—On the day of use, stir a portion of purified soluble starch equivalent to 2.0 g of dried substance with 10 mL of water, and add this mixture to 160 mL of boiling water. Rinse the beaker with 10 mL of water, add it to the hot solution, and heat to boiling, with continuous mixing. Cool to room temperature, and add water to make 200 mL.

Standard preparation—Weigh accurately about 20 mg of USP Pancreatin Amylase and Protease RS into a suitable mortar. Add about 30 mL of *pH 6.8 phosphate buffer,* and triturate for 5 to 10 minutes. Transfer the mixture with the aid of *pH 6.8 phosphate buffer* to a 50-mL volumetric flask, dilute with *pH 6.8 phosphate buffer* to volume, and mix. Calculate the activity, in USP Units of amylase activity per mL, of the resulting solution from the declared potency on the label of the USP Reference Standard.

Assay preparation—For Pancreatin having about the same amylase activity as the USP Pancreatin Amylase and Protease RS, weigh accurately about 40 mg of Pancreatin into a suitable mortar. [NOTE—For Pancreatin having a different amylase activity, weigh accurately the amount necessary to obtain an *Assay preparation* having amylase activity per mL corresponding approximately to that of the *Standard preparation.*] Add about 3 mL of *pH 6.8 phosphate buffer,* and triturate for 5 to 10 minutes. Transfer the mixture with the aid of *pH 6.8 phosphate buffer* to a 100-mL volumetric flask, dilute with *pH 6.8 phosphate buffer* to volume, and mix.

Procedure—Prepare four stoppered, 250-mL conical flasks, and mark them *S*, *U*, *BS*, and *BU*. Pipet into each flask 25 mL of *Substrate solution*, 10 mL of *pH 6.8 phosphate buffer*, and 1 mL of sodium chloride solution (11.7 in 1000), insert the stoppers, and mix. Place the flasks in a water bath maintained at 25 ± 0.1°, and allow them to equilibrate. To flasks *BU* and *BS* add 2 mL of 1 N hydrochloric acid, mix, and return the flasks to the water bath. To flasks *U* and *BU* add 1.0-mL portions of the *Assay preparation*, and to flasks *S* and *BS* add 1.0 mL of the *Standard preparation*. Mix each, and return the flasks to the water bath. After 10 minutes, accurately timed from the addition of the enzyme, add 2-mL portions of 1 N hydrochloric acid to flasks *S* and *U*, and mix. To each flask, with continuous stirring, add 10.0 mL of 0.1 N iodine VS, and immediately add 45 mL of 0.1 N sodium hydroxide. Place the flasks in the dark at a temperature between 15° and 25° for 15 minutes. To each flask add 4 mL of 2 N sulfuric acid, and titrate with 0.1 N sodium thiosulfate VS to the disappearance of the blue color. Calculate the amylase activity, in USP Units per mg, of the Pancreatin taken by the formula:

$$100(C_S / W_U)(V_{BU} - V_U) / (V_{BS} - V_S)$$

in which C_S is the amylase activity of the *Standard preparation*, in USP Units per mL, W_U is the amount, in mg, of Pancreatin taken, and V_U, V_S, V_{BU}, and V_{BS} are the volumes, in mL, of 0.1 N sodium thiosulfate consumed in the titration of the solutions in flasks *U*, *S*, *BU*, and *BS*, respectively.

Assay for lipase activity (Fat digestive power)—

Acacia solution—Centrifuge a solution of acacia (1 in 10) until clear. Use only the clear solution.

Olive oil substrate—Combine 165 mL of *Acacia solution*, 20 mL of olive oil, and 15 g of crushed ice in the cup of an electric blender. Cool the mixture in an ice bath to 5°, and homogenize at high speed for 15 minutes, intermittently cooling in an ice bath to prevent the temperature from exceeding 30°.

Test for suitability of mixing as follows. Place a drop of the homogenate on a microscope slide, and gently press a cover slide in place to spread the liquid. Examine the entire field under high power (43× objective lens and 5× ocular), using an eyepiece equipped with a calibrated micrometer. The substrate is satisfactory if 90% of the particles do not exceed 2 μm in diameter and none exceeds 10 μm in diameter.

Buffer solution—Dissolve 60 mg of tris(hydroxymethyl)aminomethane and 234 mg of sodium chloride in water to make 100 mL.

Bile salts solution—Prepare a solution to contain 80.0 mg of USP Bile Salts RS in each mL.

Standard test dilution—Suspend about 200 mg of USP Pancreatin Lipase RS, accurately weighed, in about 3 mL of cold water in a mortar, triturate for 10 minutes, and add cold water to a volume necessary to produce a concentration of 8 to 16 USP Units of lipase activity per mL, based upon the declared potency on the label of the USP Reference Standard. Maintain the suspension at 4°, and mix before using. For each determination withdraw 5 to 10 mL of the cold suspension, and allow the temperature to rise to 20° before pipeting the exact volume.

Assay test dilution—Suspend about 200 mg of Pancreatin, accurately weighed, in about 3 mL of cold water in a mortar, triturate for 10 minutes, and add cold water to a volume necessary to produce a concentration of 8 to 16 USP Units of lipase activity per mL, based upon the estimated potency of the test material. Maintain the suspension at 4°, and mix before using. For each determination withdraw 5 to 10 mL of the cold suspension, and allow the temperature to rise to 20° before pipeting the exact volume.

Procedure—Mix 10.0 mL of *Olive oil substrate*, 8.0 mL of *Buffer solution*, 2.0 mL of *Bile salts solution*, and 9.0 mL of water in a jacketed glass vessel of about 50-mL capacity, the outer chamber of which is connected to a thermostatically controlled water bath. Cover the mixture, and stir continuously with a mechanical stirring device. With the mixture maintained at a temperature of 37 ± 0.1°, add 0.1 N sodium hydroxide VS, from a microburet inserted through an opening in the cover, and adjust to a pH of 9.20 potentiometrically using a calomel-glass electrode system. Add 1.0 mL of the *Assay test dilution*, and then continue adding the 0.1 N sodium hydroxide VS for 5 minutes to maintain the pH at 9.0. Determine the volume of 0.1 N sodium hydroxide VS added after each minute.

In the same manner, titrate 1.0 mL of *Standard test dilution*.

Calculation of potency—Plot the volume of 0.1 N sodium hydroxide VS titrated against time. Using only the points which fall on the straight-line segment of the curve, calculate the mean acidity released per minute by the test specimen and the Standard. Taking into consideration the dilution factors, calculate the lipase activity, in USP Units, of the Pancreatin taken by comparison to the activity of the Standard, using the lipase activity stated on the label of USP Pancreatin Lipase RS.

Assay for protease activity (Casein digestive power)—

Casein substrate—Place 1.25 g of finely powdered casein in a 100-mL conical flask containing 5 mL of water, shake to form a suspension, add 10 mL of 0.1 N sodium hydroxide, shake for 1 minute, add 50 mL of water, and shake for about 1 hour to dissolve the casein. The resulting solution should have a pH of about 8. If necessary, adjust the pH to about 8, using 1 N sodium hydroxide or 1 N hydrochloric acid. Transfer the solution to a 100-mL volumetric flask, dilute with water to volume, and mix. Use this substrate on the day it is prepared.

Buffer solution—Dissolve 6.8 g of monobasic potassium phosphate and 1.8 g of sodium hydroxide in 950 mL of water in a 1000-mL volumetric flask, adjust to a pH of 7.5 ± 0.2, using 0.2 N sodium hydroxide, dilute with water to volume, and mix. Store this solution in a refrigerator.

Trichloroacetic acid solution—Dissolve 50 g of trichloroacetic acid in 1000 mL of water. Store this solution at room temperature.

Filter paper—Determine the suitability of the filter paper by filtering a 5-mL portion of *Trichloroacetic acid solution* through the paper and measuring the absorbance of the filtrate at 280 nm, using an unfiltered portion of the same *Trichloroacetic acid solution* as the blank: the absorbance is not more than 0.04. If the absorbance is more than 0.04, the filter paper may be washed repeatedly with *Trichloroacetic acid solution* until the absorbance of the filtrate, determined as above, is not more than 0.04.

Standard test dilution—Add about 100 mg of USP Pancreatin Amylase and Protease RS, accurately weighed, to 100.0 mL of *Buffer solution*, and mix by shaking intermittently at room temperature for about 25 minutes. Dilute quantitatively with *Buffer solution* to obtain a concentration of about 2.5 USP Units of protease activity per mL, based on the potency declared on the label of the Reference Standard.

Assay test dilution—Weigh accurately about 100 mg of Pancreatin into a mortar. Add about 3 mL of *Buffer solution*, and triturate for 5 to 10 minutes. Transfer the mixture with the aid of *Buffer solution* to a 100-mL volumetric flask, dilute with *Buffer solution* to volume, and mix. Dilute quantitatively with *Buffer solution* to obtain a dilution that corresponds in activity to that of the *Standard test dilution*.

Procedure—Label test tubes in duplicate S_1, S_2, and S_3 for the standard series, and *U* for the sample. Pipet into tubes S_1 2.0 mL, into S_2 and *U* 1.5 mL, and into S_3 1.0 mL of *Buffer solution*. Pipet into tubes S_1 1.0 mL, into S_2 1.5 mL, and into S_3 2.0 mL of the *Standard test dilution*. Pipet into tubes *U* 1.5 mL of the *Assay test dilution*. Pipet into one tube each of S_1, S_2, S_3, and *U* 5.0 mL of *Trichloroacetic acid solution*, and mix. Designate these tubes as S_{1B}, S_{2B}, S_{3B}, and U_B, respectively. Prepare a blank by mixing 3 mL of *Buffer solution* and 5 mL of *Trichloroacetic acid solution* in a separate test tube marked *B*. Place all the tubes in a 40° water bath, insert a glass stirring rod into each tube, and allow for temperature equilibration. At zero time, add to each tube, at timed intervals, 2.0 mL of the *Casein substrate*, preheated to the bath temperature, and mix. Sixty minutes, accurately timed, after the addition of the *Casein substrate* stop the reaction in tubes S_1, S_2, S_3, and *U* by adding 5.0 mL of *Trichloroacetic acid solution* at the corresponding time intervals, stir, and remove all the tubes from the bath. Allow to stand for 10 minutes at room temperature for complete protein precipitation, and filter. The filtrates must be free from haze. Determine the absorbances of the filtrates, in 1-cm cells, at 280 nm, with a suitable spectrophotometer, using the filtrate from the blank (tube *B*) to set the instrument.

Calculation of potency—Correct the absorbance values for the filtrates from tubes S_1, S_2, and S_3 by subtracting the absorbance values for the filtrates from tubes S_{1B}, S_{2B}, and S_{3B}, respectively, and plot the corrected absorbance values against the corresponding volumes of the *Standard test dilution* used. From the curve, using the corrected absorbance value ($U - U_B$) for the Pancreatin taken, and taking into consideration the dilution factors, calculate the protease activity, in USP Units, of the Pancreatin taken by comparison with that of the Standard, using the protease activity stated on the label of USP Pancreatin Amylase and Protease RS.

Pancreatin Tablets

» Pancreatin Tablets contain not less than 90.0 percent of the labeled amount of pancreatin.

Packaging and storage—Preserve in tight containers, preferably at a temperature not exceeding 30°.
Labeling—Label the Tablets to indicate minimum pancreatin fat digestive power; i.e., single strength, double strength, triple strength.
USP Reference standards ⟨11⟩—*USP Bile Salts RS. USP Pancreatin Amylase and Protease RS. USP Pancreatin Lipase RS.*
Microbial limits ⟨61⟩—Tablets meet the requirements of the test for absence of *Salmonella* species and *Escherichia coli*.
Disintegration ⟨701⟩: 60 minutes.
Assay for amylase activity (*Starch digestive power*)—Weigh and finely powder not fewer than 20 Tablets, avoiding the production of heat during the process. Proceed as directed in the *Assay for amylase activity* under *Pancreatin*, using as the assay preparation an accurately weighed portion of the powder, equivalent to 40 mg of pancreatin. (Use an inversely proportionate amount of the powder if the Tablets are labeled to contain a whole-number multiple of the minimum requirement for pancreatin digestive activity.)
Assay for lipase activity (*Fat digestive power*)—
  Acacia solution, Olive oil substrate, Buffer solution, Bile salts solution, and *Standard test dilution*—Prepare as directed in the *Assay for lipase activity* under *Pancreatin*.
  Assay test dilution—Proceed as directed for *Assay test dilution* in the *Assay for lipase activity* under *Pancreatin*, using as the assay preparation an accurately weighed portion of the powder, prepared as directed in the *Assay for amylase activity*, equivalent to about 200 mg of pancreatin.
  Procedure and *Calculation of potency*—Proceed as directed in the *Assay for lipase activity* under *Pancreatin*.
Assay for protease activity (*Casein digestive power*)—
  Casein substrate, Buffer solution, Trichloroacetic acid solution, Filter paper and *Standard test dilution*—Prepare as directed in the *Assay for protease activity* under *Pancreatin*.
  Assay test dilution—Add an accurately weighed portion of the powder, prepared as directed in the *Assay for amylase activity*, equivalent to about 100 mg of pancreatin, to 100.0 mL of *Buffer solution*, and mix by shaking intermittently at room temperature for 25 minutes. Dilute quantitatively with *Buffer solution* to obtain a dilution that corresponds in activity to the *Standard test dilution*.
  Procedure and *Calculation of potency*—Proceed as directed in the *Assay for protease activity* under *Pancreatin*.

Pancrelipase

» Pancrelipase is a substance containing enzymes, principally lipase, with amylase and protease, obtained from the pancreas of the hog, *Sus scrofa* Linné var. *domesticus* Gray (Fam. Suidae). It contains, in each mg, not less than 24 USP Units of lipase activity, not less than 100 USP Units of amylase activity, and not less than 100 USP Units of protease activity.

NOTE—One USP Unit of amylase activity is contained in the amount of pancrelipase that decomposes starch at an initial rate such that 0.16 µEq of glycosidic linkage is hydrolyzed per minute under the conditions of the *Assay for amylase activity*.
One USP Unit of lipase activity is contained in the amount of pancrelipase that liberates 1.0 µEq of acid per minute at pH 9.0 and 37° under the conditions of the *Assay for lipase activity*.
One USP Unit of protease activity is contained in the amount of pancrelipase that under the conditions of the *Assay for protease activity*, hydrolyzes casein at an initial rate such that there is liberated per minute an amount of peptides not precipitated by trichloroacetic acid that gives the same absorbance at 280 nm as 15 nmol of tyrosine.

Packaging and storage—Preserve in tight containers, preferably at a temperature not exceeding 25°.
Labeling—Label it to indicate lipase activity in USP Units.
USP Reference standards ⟨11⟩—*USP Bile Salts RS. USP Pancreatin Amylase and Protease RS. USP Pancreatin Lipase RS.*
Microbial limits ⟨61⟩—It meets the requirements of the tests for absence of *Salmonella* species and *Escherichia coli*.
Loss on drying ⟨731⟩—Dry it in vacuum at 60° for 4 hours: it loses not more than 5.0% of its weight.
Fat—Place 2.0 g of Pancrelipase in a flask of about 50-mL capacity, add 20 mL of ether, insert the stopper, and set aside for 2 hours, mixing by rotating at frequent intervals. Decant the supernatant ether by means of a guiding rod into a plain filter about 7 cm in diameter, previously moistened with ether, and collect the filtrate in a tared beaker. Repeat the extraction with a 10-mL portion of ether, then with another 10-mL portion of ether, transfer the ether and the remainder of the Pancrelipase to the filter. Allow to drain, evaporate the ether spontaneously, and dry the residue at 105° for 2 hours: the residue of fat weighs not more than 100 mg (5.0%).
Assay for amylase activity (*Starch digestive power*)—
  pH 6.8 Phosphate buffer—On the day of use, dissolve 13.6 g of monobasic potassium phosphate in water to make 500 mL of solution. Dissolve 14.2 g of anhydrous dibasic sodium phosphate in water to make 500 mL of solution. Mix 51 mL of the monobasic potassium phosphate solution with 49 mL of the dibasic sodium phosphate solution. If necessary, adjust by the dropwise addition of the appropriate solution to a pH of 6.8.
  Substrate solution—On the day of use, stir a portion of purified soluble starch equivalent to 2.0 g of dried substance with 10 mL of water, and add this mixture to 160 mL of boiling water. Rinse the beaker with 10 mL of water, add it to the hot solution, and heat to boiling, with continuous mixing. Cool to room temperature, and add water to make 200 mL.
  Standard preparation—Weigh accurately about 20 mg of USP Pancreatin Amylase and Protease RS into a suitable mortar. Add about 30 mL of *pH 6.8 Phosphate buffer*, and triturate for 5 to 10 minutes. Transfer the mixture with the aid of *pH 6.8 Phosphate buffer* to a 50-mL volumetric flask, dilute with *pH 6.8 phosphate buffer* to volume, and mix. Calculate the activity, in USP Units of amylase activity per mL, of the resulting solution from the declared potency on the label of the Reference Standard.
  Assay preparation—For Pancrelipase having about 4 times the amylase activity of the USP Pancreatin Amylase and Protease RS, weigh accurately about 10 mg of Pancrelipase into a suitable mortar. [NOTE—For Pancrelipase having a different amylase activity, weigh accurately the amount necessary to obtain an *Assay preparation* having amylase activity per mL corresponding approximately to that of the *Standard preparation*.] Add about 3 mL of *pH 6.8 Phosphate buffer*, and triturate for 5 to 10 minutes. Transfer the mixture with the aid of *pH 6.8 Phosphate buffer* to a 100-mL volumetric flask, dilute with *pH 6.8 Phosphate buffer* to volume, and mix.
  Procedure—Prepare four stoppered, 250-mL conical flasks, and mark them *S, U, BS,* and *BU*. Pipet into each flask 25 mL of *Substrate solution*, 10 mL of *pH 6.8 Phosphate buffer*, and 1 mL of sodium chloride solution (11.7 in 1000), insert the stoppers, and mix. Place the flasks in a water bath maintained at 25 ± 0.1°, and allow them to equilibrate. To flasks *BU* and *BS* add 2 mL of 1 N

hydrochloric acid, mix, and return the flasks to the water bath. To flasks *U* and *BU* add 1.0-mL portions of *Assay preparation*, and to flasks *S* and *BS* add 1.0 mL of *Standard preparation*. Mix each, and return the flasks to the water bath. After 10 minutes, accurately timed from the addition of the enzyme, add 2-mL portions of 1 N hydrochloric acid to flasks *S* and *U*, and mix. To each flask, with continuous stirring, add 10.0 mL of 0.1 N iodine VS, and immediately add 45 mL of 0.1 N sodium hydroxide. Place the flasks in the dark at a temperature between 15° and 25° for 15 minutes. To each flask add 4 mL of 2 N sulfuric acid, and titrate with 0.1 N sodium thiosulfate VS to the disappearance of the blue color. Calculate the amylase activity, in USP Units per mg, of the Pancrelipase taken by the formula:

$$100(C_S / W_U)(V_{BU} - V_U) / (V_{BS} - V_S)$$

in which C_S is the amylase activity of the *Standard preparation*, in USP Units per mL, W_U is the amount, in mg, of Pancrelipase taken, and V_U, V_S, V_{BU}, and V_{BS} are the volumes, in mL, of 0.1 N sodium thiosulfate consumed in the titration of the solutions in flasks *U*, *S*, *BU*, and *BS*, respectively.

Assay for lipase activity (*Fat digestive power*)—

Acacia solution—Centrifuge a solution of acacia (1 in 10) until clear. Use only the clear solution.

Olive oil substrate—Combine 165 mL of *Acacia solution*, 20 mL of olive oil, and 15 g of crushed ice in the cup of an electric blender. Cool the mixture in an ice bath to 5°, and homogenize at high speed for 15 minutes, intermittently cooling in an ice bath to prevent the temperature from exceeding 30°.

Test for suitability of mixing as follows. Place a drop of the homogenate on a microscope slide, and gently press a cover slide in place to spread the liquid. Examine the entire field under high power (43× objective lens and 5× ocular), using an eyepiece equipped with a calibrated micrometer. The substrate is satisfactory if 90% of the particles do not exceed 2 µm in diameter and none exceeds 10 µm in diameter.

Buffer solution—Dissolve 60 mg of tris(hydroxymethyl)aminomethane and 234 mg of sodium chloride in water to make 100 mL.

Bile salts solution—Prepare a solution to contain 80.0 mg of USP Bile Salts RS in each mL.

Standard test dilution—Suspend about 200 mg of USP Pancreatin Lipase RS, accurately weighed, in about 3 mL of cold water in a mortar, triturate for 10 minutes, and add cold water to a volume necessary to produce a concentration of 8 to 16 USP Units of lipase activity per mL, based upon the declared potency on the label of the Reference Standard. Maintain the suspension at 4°, and mix before using. For each determination withdraw 5 to 10 mL of the cold suspension, and allow the temperature to rise to 20° before pipeting the exact volume.

Assay test dilution—Suspend about 200 mg of Pancrelipase, accurately weighed, in about 3 mL of cold water in a mortar, triturate for 10 minutes, and add cold water to a volume necessary to produce a concentration of 8 to 16 USP Units of lipase activity per mL, based upon the estimated potency of the test material. Maintain the suspension at 4°, and mix before using. For each determination withdraw 5 to 10 mL of the cold suspension, and allow the temperature to rise to 20° before pipeting the exact volume.

Procedure—Mix 10.0 mL of *Olive oil substrate*, 8.0 mL of *Buffer solution*, 2.0 mL of *Bile salts solution*, and 9.0 mL of water in a jacketed glass vessel of about 50-mL capacity, the outer chamber of which is connected to a thermostatically controlled water bath. Cover the mixture, and stir continuously with a mechanical stirring device. With the mixture maintained at a temperature of 37 ± 0.1°, add 0.1 N sodium hydroxide VS, from a microburet inserted through an opening in the cover, to adjust the pH to 9.20 potentiometrically using a calomel-glass electrode system. Add 1.0 mL of *Assay test dilution*, and then continue adding the 0.1 N sodium hydroxide VS for 5 minutes to maintain the pH at 9.0. Determine the volume of 0.1 N sodium hydroxide VS added after each minute.

In the same manner titrate 1.0 mL of *Standard test dilution*.

Calculation of potency—Plot the volume of 0.1 N sodium hydroxide VS titrated against time. Using only the points which fall on the straight-line segment of the curve, calculate the mean acidity released per minute by the test specimen and the Standard. Taking into consideration the dilution factors, calculate the lipase activity, in USP Units, of the Pancrelipase taken by comparison to the activity of the Reference Standard, using the lipase activity stated on the label of USP Pancreatin Lipase RS.

Assay for protease activity (*Casein digestive power*)—

Casein substrate—Place 1.25 g of finely powdered casein in a 100-mL conical flask containing 5 mL of water, shake to form a suspension, add 10 mL of 0.1 N sodium hydroxide, shake for 1 minute, add 50 mL of water, and shake for about 1 hour to dissolve the casein. If necessary, adjust to a pH of about 8, using 1 N sodium hydroxide or 1 N hydrochloric acid. Transfer the solution quantitatively to a 100-mL volumetric flask, dilute with water to volume, and mix. Use this substrate on the day it is prepared.

Buffer solution—Dissolve 6.8 g of monobasic potassium phosphate and 1.8 g of sodium hydroxide in 950 mL of water in a 1000-mL volumetric flask, adjust to a pH of 7.5 ± 0.2, using 0.2 N sodium hydroxide, dilute with water to volume, and mix. Store this solution in a refrigerator.

Trichloroacetic acid solution—Dissolve 50 g of trichloroacetic acid in 1000 mL of water. This solution may be stored at room temperature.

Filter paper—Determine the suitability of the filter paper by filtering a 5-mL portion of *Trichloroacetic acid solution* through the paper and measuring the absorbance of the filtrate at 280 nm, using an unfiltered portion of the same *Trichloroacetic acid solution* as the blank: the absorbance is not more than 0.04. If the absorbance is more than 0.04, wash the filter paper repeatedly with *Trichloroacetic acid solution* until the absorbance of the filtrate, determined as above, is not more than 0.04.

Standard test dilution—Add about 100 mg of USP Pancreatin Amylase and Protease RS, accurately weighed, to 100.0 mL of *Buffer solution*, and mix by shaking intermittently at room temperature for about 25 minutes. Dilute quantitatively with *Buffer solution* to produce a concentration of about 2.5 USP Units of protease activity per mL, based upon the declared potency on the label of the Reference Standard.

Assay test dilution—Weigh accurately about 100 mg of Pancrelipase into a suitable mortar. Add about 3 mL of *Buffer solution*, and triturate for 5 to 10 minutes. Transfer the mixture with the aid of *Buffer solution* to a 100-mL volumetric flask, dilute with *Buffer solution* to volume, and mix. Dilute quantitatively with *Buffer solution* to obtain a dilution that corresponds in activity to the *Standard test dilution*.

Procedure—Label test tubes in duplicate S_1, S_2, and S_3 for the standard series, and *U* for the sample. Pipet into tubes S_1 2.0 mL, into S_2 and *U* 1.5 mL, and into S_3 1.0 mL of *Buffer solution*. Pipet into tubes S_1 1.0 mL, into S_2 1.5 mL, and into S_3 2.0 mL of the *Standard test dilution*. Pipet into tubes *U* 1.5 mL of the *Assay test dilution*. Pipet into one tube each of S_1, S_2, S_3, and *U* 5.0 mL of *Trichloroacetic acid solution*, and mix. Designate these tubes as S_{1B}, S_{2B}, S_{3B}, and U_B, respectively. Prepare a blank by mixing 3 mL of *Buffer solution* and 5 mL of *Trichloroacetic acid solution* in a separate test tube marked *B*. Place all the tubes in a 40° water bath, insert a glass stirring rod into each tube, and allow for temperature equilibration. At zero time, add to each tube, at timed intervals, 2.0 mL of the *Casein substrate*, preheated to the bath temperature, and mix. Sixty minutes, accurately timed, after the addition of the *Casein substrate* stop the reaction in tubes S_1, S_2, S_3, and *U* by adding 5.0 mL of *Trichloroacetic acid solution* at the corresponding time intervals, stir, and remove all the tubes from the bath. Allow to stand at room temperature for 10 minutes for complete protein precipitation, and filter. The filtrates must be free from haze. Determine the absorbances of the filtrates, in 1-cm cells, at 280 nm, with a suitable spectrophotometer, using the filtrate from the blank (tube *B*) to set the instrument.

Calculation of potency—Correct the absorbance values for the filtrates from tubes S_1, S_2, and S_3 by subtracting the absorbance values for the filtrates from tubes S_{1B}, S_{2B}, and S_{3B}, respectively, and plot the corrected absorbance values against the corresponding volumes of the *Standard test dilution* used. From the curve, using the corrected absorbance value ($U - U_B$) for the Pancrelipase taken, and taking into consideration the dilution factors, calculate the protease activity, in USP Units, of the Pancrelipase taken by comparison with that of the Standard, using the protease activity stated on the label of USP Pancreatin Amylase and Protease RS.

Pancrelipase Capsules

» Pancrelipase Capsules contain an amount of Pancrelipase equivalent to not less than 90.0 percent and not more than 150.0 percent of the labeled lipase activity expressed in USP Units, the labeled activity being not less than 8000 USP Units per Capsule. They contain, in each Capsule, the pancrelipase equivalent of not less than 30,000 USP Units of amylase activity, and not less than 30,000 USP Units of protease activity.

Packaging and storage—Preserve in tight containers, preferably with a desiccant, at a temperature not exceeding 25°.
Labeling—Label the Capsules to indicate lipase activity in USP Units.
USP Reference standards ⟨11⟩—*USP Bile Salts RS. USP Pancreatin Amylase and Protease RS. USP Pancreatin Lipase RS.*
Microbial limits ⟨61⟩—Capsules meet the requirements of the tests for absence of *Salmonella* species and *Escherichia coli*.
Loss on drying ⟨731⟩—Dry the contents of 10 Capsules in vacuum at 60° for 4 hours: it loses not more than 5.0% of its weight.
Assay—Weigh the contents of not less than 10 Capsules, and determine the average weight per capsule. Mix the combined contents, and proceed as directed for *Assay for amylase activity*, *Assay for lipase activity*, and *Assay for protease activity* under *Pancrelipase*.

Pancrelipase Delayed-Release Capsules

» Pancrelipase Delayed-Release Capsules contain an amount of Pancrelipase equivalent to not less than 90.0 percent and not more than 165.0 percent of the labeled lipase. It contains not less than 90.0 percent of the labeled activities of amylase and protease expressed in the respective USP Units.

Packaging and storage—Preserve in tight containers at controlled room temperature.
Labeling—Label the Capsules to indicate lipase, amylase, and protease activities in USP Units. The label also indicates that the Capsule contents are enteric-coated.
USP Reference standards ⟨11⟩—*USP Bile Salts RS. USP Pancreatin Amylase and Protease RS. USP Pancreatin Lipase RS.*
Microbial limits ⟨61⟩—Capsules meet the requirements of the tests for absence of *Salmonella* species and *Escherichia coli*.
Dissolution ⟨711⟩—
  PART 1—
  Medium: simulated gastric fluid TS, without enzyme; 800 mL.
  Apparatus 1: 100 rpm.
  Time: 60 minutes.
  PART 2—
  pH 6.0 phosphate buffer—Dissolve 8 g of sodium chloride and 36.8 g of monobasic potassium phosphate in 4000 mL of water. Adjust with 2 N sodium hydroxide to a pH of 6.0 ± 0.1.
  Medium: pH 6.0 phosphate buffer; 800 mL.
  Apparatus 2: 100 rpm.
  Time: 30 minutes.
  Standard solution—Proceed as directed under *Standard test dilution* in the *Assay for lipase activity* under *Pancrelipase*, except to use the *Dissolution Medium* in place of cold water.
  Test solution—Empty the contents of 10 Capsules, and transfer an accurately weighed portion of the contents, equivalent to the concentration of USP Units of lipase activity per mL in the *Standard solution* (between 8 and 16 Units per mL), to *Apparatus 1*.
  Procedure—Proceed according to the conditions for *Part 1*. After 1 hour, remove the baskets, and allow the excess *Dissolution Medium* to drain. Transfer the contents of each basket to the dissolution vessels in *Part 2* with the aid of a few mL of *Dissolution Medium*. Proceed according to the conditions for *Part 2*. After 30 minutes, remove a 10-mL portion of the solution under test, transfer to a test tube, and cool to 4°. Proceed as directed in the *Assay for lipase activity* under *Pancrelipase*.
  Tolerances—Not less than 75% (Q) of the labeled USP Units of lipase activity per Capsule is dissolved.
Loss on drying ⟨731⟩—Dry the contents of 10 Capsules in vacuum at 60° for 4 hours: the test specimen loses not more than 5.0% of its weight.
Assay—Weigh the contents of not less than 10 Capsules, and determine the average weight per Capsule. Grind the contents, mix the combined contents, and proceed as directed in the *Assay for lipase activity*, the *Assay for amylase activity*, and the *Assay for protease activity* under *Pancrelipase*.

Pancrelipase Tablets

» Pancrelipase Tablets contain an amount of Pancrelipase equivalent to not less than 90.0 percent and not more than 150.0 percent of the labeled lipase activity expressed in USP Units, the labeled activity being not less than 8000 USP Units per Tablet. They contain, in each Tablet, the pancrelipase equivalent of not less than 30,000 USP Units of amylase activity, and not less than 30,000 USP Units of protease activity.

Packaging and storage—Preserve in tight containers, preferably with a desiccant, at a temperature not exceeding 25°.
Labeling—Label the Tablets to indicate the lipase activity in USP Units.
USP Reference standards ⟨11⟩—*USP Bile Salts RS. USP Pancreatin Amylase and Protease RS. USP Pancreatin Lipase RS.*
Microbial limits ⟨61⟩—Tablets meet the requirements of the test for absence of *Salmonella* species and *Escherichia coli*.
Disintegration ⟨701⟩: 75 minutes.
Loss on drying ⟨731⟩—Dry about 5 g, accurately weighed, of finely ground Tablets in vacuum at 60° for 4 hours: it loses not more than 5.0% of its weight.
Assay—Weigh and finely powder not less than 20 Tablets, avoiding the production of heat during the process, and proceed as directed for *Assay for amylase activity*, *Assay for lipase activity*, and *Assay for protease activity* under *Pancrelipase*.

Pancuronium Bromide

$C_{35}H_{60}Br_2N_2O_4$ 732.67
Piperidinium, 1,1'-[(2β,3α,5α,16β,17β)-3,17-bis(acetyloxy)androstane-2,16-diyl]bis[1-methyl]-, dibromide.
1,1'-(3α,17β-Dihydroxy-5α-androstan-2β,16β-ylene)bis[1-methylpiperidinium]dibromide diacetate.
2β,16β-Dipiperidino-5α-androstane-3α,17β-diol diacetate dimethobromide [15500-66-0].

» Pancuronium Bromide contains not less than 98.0 percent and not more than 102.0 percent of $C_{35}H_{60}Br_2N_2O_4$, calculated on the anhydrous basis.

Packaging and storage—Preserve in tight containers, protected from light and moisture. Store between 15° and 25°.

USP Reference standards ⟨11⟩—*USP Pancuronium Bromide RS. USP Vecuronium Bromide RS.*

Identification—
  A: *Infrared Absorption* ⟨197K⟩.
  B: The R_F value of the principal spot in the chromatogram of the *Test solution* corresponds to that of the chromatogram of *Standard solution 2,* as obtained in the test for *Related compounds.*
  C: A solution (1 in 10) meets the requirements of the tests for *Bromide* ⟨191⟩.

Clarity of solution—
  Hydrazine sulfate solution—Transfer 1.0 g of hydrazine sulfate to a 100-mL volumetric flask, dissolve in and dilute with water to volume, and mix. Allow to stand for 4 to 6 hours before use.
  Methenamine solution—Transfer 2.5 g of methenamine to a 100-mL glass-stoppered flask, add 25 mL of water, insert the glass stopper, and mix to dissolve.
  Primary opalescent suspension—[NOTE—This suspension is stable for 2 months, provided it is stored in a glass container free from surface defects. The suspension must not adhere to the glass and must be well mixed before use.] Transfer 25.0 mL of *Hydrazine sulfate solution* to the *Methenamine solution* in the 100-mL glass-stoppered flask. Mix, and allow to stand for 24 hours.
  Opalescence standard—[NOTE—This suspension should not be used beyond 24 hours after preparation.] Transfer 15.0 mL of the *Primary opalescent suspension* to a 1000-mL volumetric flask, dilute with water to volume, and mix.
  Reference suspensions—Transfer 5.0 mL of the *Opalescence standard* to a 100-mL volumetric flask, dilute with water to volume, and mix to obtain *Reference suspension A.* Transfer 10.0 mL of the *Opalescence standard* to a second 100-mL volumetric flask, dilute with water to volume, and mix to obtain *Reference suspension B.*
  Test solution—Dissolve 50 mg of Pancuronium Bromide in about 20 mL of water, dilute with water to 25 mL, and mix.
  Procedure—Transfer a sufficient portion of the *Test solution* to a test tube of colorless, transparent, neutral glass with a flat base and an internal diameter of 15 to 25 mm to obtain a depth of 40 mm. Similarly transfer portions of *Reference suspension A, Reference suspension B,* and water to separate matching test tubes. Compare the *Test solution, Reference suspension A, Reference suspension B,* and water in diffused daylight, viewing vertically against a black background (see *Visual Comparison* under *Spectrophotometry and Light-Scattering* ⟨851⟩). [NOTE—The diffusion of light must be such that *Reference suspension A* can readily be distinguished from water, and *Reference suspension B* can readily be distinguished from *Reference suspension A.*] The *Test solution* shows the same or more clarity than *Reference suspension A.*

Color of solution—
  Standard stock solution—Prepare a solution of ferric chloride CS, cobaltous chloride CS, cupric sulfate CS, and a 10 g per L hydrochloric acid solution (3 : 3 : 2.4 : 1.6).
  Standard solution—[NOTE—Prepare this solution just before use.] Transfer 1 mL of *Standard stock solution* to a 100-mL volumetric flask, dilute with hydrochloric acid (10 g per L) solution to volume, and mix.
  Test solution—Use the *Test solution* prepared as directed in the test for *Clarity of solution.*
  Procedure—Transfer a sufficient portion of the *Test solution* to a test tube of colorless, transparent, neutral glass with a flat base and an external diameter of 15 to 25 mm to obtain a depth of 40 mm. Similarly transfer a portion of the *Standard solution* and water to separate matching test tubes. Compare the *Test solution* (see *Visual Comparison* under *Spectrophotometry and Light-Scattering* ⟨851⟩): the *Test solution* is not more intensely colored than the *Standard solution* or water.

Specific rotation ⟨781S⟩: between +39° and +43°.
  Test solution: 30 mg per mL, in water.

Water, *Method I* ⟨921⟩: not more than 8.0%.

Residue on ignition ⟨281⟩: not more than 0.1%.

Related compounds—
  Adsorbent: 0.2-mm layer of chromatographic silica gel mixture.

  Test solution—Prepare a solution of Pancuronium Bromide in methylene chloride containing 10 mg per mL.
  Diluted test solution—Dilute 1.0 mL of the *Test solution* with methylene chloride to 50 mL, and mix. Dilute 1.0 mL of the resulting solution with methylene chloride to 20 mL, and mix.
  Standard solution 1—Prepare a solution in methylene chloride containing 0.1 mg of USP Vecuronium Bromide RS and 10 mg of USP Pancuronium Bromide RS per mL.
  Standard solution 2—Prepare a solution of USP Pancuronium Bromide RS in methylene chloride containing 10 mg per mL.
  Developing solvent system: a mixture of isopropyl alcohol, acetonitrile, and a 400 g per L solution of sodium iodide (85 : 10 : 5).
  Procedure—Apply separately 5-μL portions of the *Test solution, Diluted test solution, Standard solution 1,* and *Standard solution 2* to a suitable thin-layer chromatographic plate (see *Thin-Layer Chromatography* under *Chromatography* ⟨621⟩). Develop in an unlined and unsaturated tank over a path of 8 cm. Spray the plate with a 20 g per L solution of sodium nitrite, and allow to dry for 5 minutes. Spray the plate with Dragendorff's TS, and cover the plate with a transparent glass cover. Any spot in the chromatogram obtained from the *Test solution* due to vecuronium bromide is not more intense than the corresponding spot in the chromatogram obtained from *Standard solution 1:* equivalent to not more than 1.0% of vecuronium bromide. Any other spot in the chromatogram obtained from the *Test solution,* except for the principal spot and any spot due to vecuronium bromide, is not more intense than the spot in the chromatogram obtained from the *Diluted test solution:* equivalent to not more than 0.1% of any individual impurity. In a valid test, the chromatogram obtained from *Standard solution 1* shows two clearly separated spots. The R_F values for pancuronium bromide and vecuronium bromide are about 0.5 and 0.64, respectively.

Assay—Transfer about 200 mg of Pancuronium Bromide, accurately weighed, to a 100-mL beaker, and dissolve by stirring in 50 mL of acetic anhydride. Titrate with 0.1 N perchloric acid VS, determining the endpoint potentiometrically. Perform a blank determination, and make any necessary correction (see *Titrimetry* ⟨541⟩). Each mL of 0.1 N perchloric acid is equivalent to 36.63 mg of $C_{35}H_{60}Br_2N_2O_4$.

Panthenol

$C_9H_{19}NO_4$ 205.25
Butanamide, 2,4-dihydroxy-*N*-(3-hydroxypropyl)-3,3-dimethyl-, (±)-.
(±)-2,4-Dihydroxy-*N*-(3-hydroxypropyl)-3,3-dimethylbutyramide.
(±)-Pantothenyl alcohol   [16485-10-2].

» Panthenol is a racemic mixture of the dextrorotatory and levorotatory isomers of panthenol. It contains not less than 99.0 percent and not more than 102.0 percent of $C_9H_{19}NO_4$, calculated on the dried basis.

Packaging and storage—Preserve in tight containers.

USP Reference standards ⟨11⟩—*USP Racemic Panthenol RS.*

Identification—
  A: *Infrared Absorption* ⟨197M⟩.
  B: To 1 mL of a solution (1 in 10) add 5 mL of 1 N sodium hydroxide and 1 drop of cupric sulfate TS, and shake vigorously: a deep blue color develops.
  C: To 1 mL of a solution (1 in 100) add 1 mL of 1 N hydrochloric acid, and heat on a steam bath for about 30 minutes. Cool, add 100 mg of hydroxylamine hydrochloride, mix, and add 5 mL of 1 N sodium hydroxide. Allow to stand for 5 minutes, then adjust with 1 N hydrochloric acid to a pH of between 2.5 and 3.0, and add 1 drop of ferric chloride TS: a purplish-red color develops.

Melting range, *Class I* ⟨741⟩: between 64.5° and 68.5°.
Specific rotation ⟨781S⟩: between −0.05° and +0.05°.
Test solution: 50 mg per mL, in water.
Loss on drying ⟨731⟩—Dry it in vacuum over phosphorus pentoxide at 56° for 4 hours: it loses not more than 0.5% of its weight.
Residue on ignition ⟨281⟩: not more than 0.1%.
Limit of aminopropanol—Transfer about 10 g, accurately weighed, to a 50-mL flask, and dissolve in 25 mL of water. Add bromothymol blue TS, and titrate with 0.01 N sulfuric acid VS to a yellow endpoint. Each mL of 0.01 N sulfuric acid is equivalent to 750 µg of aminopropanol. Not more than 0.10% is found.
Organic volatile impurities, *Method I* ⟨467⟩: meets the requirements.

(Official until July 1, 2008)

Assay—
Potassium biphthalate solution—Dissolve 20.42 g of potassium biphthalate in glacial acetic acid contained in a 1000-mL volumetric flask. If necessary, warm the mixture on a steam bath to achieve complete solution, observing precautions against absorption of moisture. Cool to room temperature, dilute with glacial acetic acid to volume, and mix.
Procedure—Transfer about 400 mg of Panthenol, accurately weighed, to a 300-mL flask fitted to a reflux condenser by means of a standard-taper glass joint, add 50.0 mL of 0.1 N perchloric acid VS, and reflux for 5 hours. Cool, observing precautions to prevent atmospheric moisture from entering the condenser, and rinse the condenser with glacial acetic acid, collecting the rinsings in the flask. Add 5 drops of crystal violet TS, and titrate with *Potassium biphthalate solution* to a blue-green endpoint. Perform a blank determination, and note the difference in volumes required. Each mL of the difference in volumes of 0.1 N perchloric acid consumed is equivalent to 20.53 mg of $C_9H_{19}NO_4$.

Papain

Papain.
Papain [9001-73-4].

» Papain is a purified proteolytic substance derived from *Carica papaya* Linné (Fam. Caricaceae). Papain, when assayed as directed herein, contains not less than 6000 Units per mg. Papain of a higher digestive power may be reduced to the official standard by admixture with papain of lower activity, lactose, or other suitable diluents.

One USP Unit of Papain activity is the activity that releases the equivalent of 1 µg of tyrosine from a specified casein substrate under the conditions of the *Assay*, using the enzyme concentration that liberates 40 µg of tyrosine per mL of test solution.

Packaging and storage—Preserve in tight, light-resistant containers, in a cool place.
USP Reference standards ⟨11⟩—*USP Papain RS*.
pH ⟨791⟩: between 4.8 and 6.2, in a solution (1 in 50).
Loss on drying ⟨731⟩—Dry it in a vacuum oven at 60° for 4 hours: it loses not more than 7.0% of its weight.
Assay (*Casein digestive power*)—
Dibasic sodium phosphate, 0.05 M—Dissolve 7.1 g of anhydrous dibasic sodium phosphate in water to make 1000 mL. Add 1 drop of toluene as a preservative.
Citric acid, 0.05 M—Dissolve 10.5 g of citric acid monohydrate in water to make 1000 mL. Add 1 drop of toluene as a preservative.
Casein substrate—Disperse 1 g of Hammersten-type casein in 50 mL of *0.05 M Dibasic sodium phosphate*. Place in a boiling water bath for 30 minutes with occasional stirring. Cool to room temperature, and add *0.05 M Citric acid* to adjust to a pH of 6.0 ± 0.1. Stir the solution rapidly and continuously during the addition of the *0.05 M Citric acid* to prevent precipitation of the casein. Dilute with water to 100 mL. Prepare fresh daily.

Buffer solution (Phosphate-Cysteine Disodium ethylenediaminetetraacetate Buffer)—Dissolve 3.55 g of anhydrous dibasic sodium phosphate in 400 mL of water in a 500-mL volumetric flask. Add 7.0 g of disodium edetate and 3.05 g of cysteine hydrochloride monohydrate. Adjust with 1 N hydrochloric acid or 1 N sodium hydroxide to a pH of 6.0 ± 0.1, dilute with water to volume, and mix. Prepare fresh daily.
Trichloroacetic acid solution—Dissolve 30 g of reagent grade trichloroacetic acid in water, and dilute with water to 100 mL. This solution may be stored at room temperature.
Standard preparation—Weigh accurately 100 mg of USP Papain RS in a 100-mL volumetric flask, and add *Buffer solution* to dissolve. Dilute with *Buffer solution* to volume, and mix. Transfer 2.0 mL of this solution to a 50-mL volumetric flask, dilute with *Buffer solution* to volume, and mix. Use within 30 minutes after preparation.
Assay preparation—Transfer an accurately weighed amount of Papain, equivalent to about 100 mg of USP Papain RS, to a 100-mL volumetric flask, dilute with *Buffer solution* to volume, and mix. Transfer 2.0 mL of this solution to a 50-mL volumetric flask, dilute with *Buffer solution* to volume, and mix.
Procedure—Into each of 12 test tubes (18- × 150-mm) pipet 5.0 mL of *Casein substrate*. Place in a water bath at 40°, and allow 10 minutes to reach bath temperature. Into each of two of the tubes (the tests are run in duplicate except for the blanks) labeled S_1, pipet 1.0 mL of the *Standard preparation* and 1.0 mL of the *Buffer solution*, mix by swirling, note zero time, insert the stopper, and replace in the bath. Into each of 2 other tubes, labeled S_2, pipet 1.5 mL of *Standard preparation* and 0.5 mL of *Buffer solution*, and proceed as before. Repeat this procedure for 2 tubes, labeled S_3, to which 2.0 mL of *Standard preparation* is added, and for 2 tubes, labeled U_2, to which 1.5 mL of *Assay preparation* and 0.5 mL of *Buffer solution* are added. After 60 minutes, accurately timed, add to all 12 tubes 3.0 mL of *Trichloroacetic acid solution*, and shake vigorously. With the 4 tubes to which no *Standard preparation* or *Assay preparation* were added, prepare blanks by pipeting, respectively, 1.0 mL of *Standard preparation* and 1.0 mL of *Buffer solution*; 1.5 mL of *Standard preparation* and 0.5 mL of *Buffer solution*; 2.0 mL of *Standard preparation*; and 1.5 mL of *Assay preparation* and 0.5 mL of *Buffer solution*. Replace all tubes in the 40° water bath, for 30 to 40 minutes, to allow to coagulate fully the precipitated protein. Filter through medium-porosity filter paper, discarding the first 3 mL of the filtrate (filtrates used are clear). Read the absorbances, at 280 nm, of the filtrates of all solutions against their respective blanks. Plot the absorbance readings for S_1, S_2, and S_3 against the enzyme concentration of each corresponding level. By interpolation from this curve, taking into consideration dilution factors, calculate the potency in Units, in the weight of Papain taken by the formula:

$$(50{,}000\,/\,3)CA$$

in which 50,000/3 is a factor derived by the expression 100(50/2)(10/1.5), C is the concentration, in mg per mL, obtained from the standard curve, and A is the activity of the Reference Standard in Units per mg.

Papain Tablets for Topical Solution

» Papain Tablets for Topical Solution contain not less than 100.0 percent of the labeled potency.

Packaging and storage—Preserve in tight, light-resistant containers in a cool place.
USP Reference standards ⟨11⟩—*USP Papain RS*.
Completeness of solution ⟨641⟩—Prepare a solution of 50 Tablets in 500.0 mL of water, allow to stand for 4 hours, filter through 2 superimposed, matched-weight, 47-mm diameter, 0.8-µm porosity membrane filters, and wash the residue by rinsing the flask at the sides of the holder with water. Dry both filters in a desiccator under vacuum, over phosphorus pentoxide, for 6 to 18 hours, weigh the filters separately, and subtract the weight of the lower filter from

that of the upper filter: the difference in the weights is not more than 50 mg (1 mg per Tablet).
Microbial limits ⟨61⟩—It meets the requirements of the tests for absence of *Staphylococcus aureus* and *Pseudomonas aeruginosa*.
Disintegration ⟨701⟩: not more than 15 minutes at 23 ± 2°.
pH ⟨791⟩: between 6.9 and 8.0, determined in a solution of 1 Tablet in 10 mL.
Assay—
Dibasic sodium phosphate, 0.05 M; Citric acid, 0.05 M; Casein substrate; Buffer solution; Trichloroacetic acid solution; and *Standard preparation*—Prepare as directed in the *Assay* under *Papain*.
Assay preparation—Place a counted number of Papain Tablets for Topical Solution, equivalent to about 600,000 USP Units of Papain, in a 100-mL volumetric flask, dissolve in *Buffer solution*, dilute with *Buffer solution* to volume, and mix. Transfer 2.0 mL of this solution to a 50-mL volumetric flask, dilute with *Buffer solution* to volume, and mix.
Procedure—Proceed as directed for *Procedure* in the *Assay* under *Papain*. By interpolation from the standard curve, calculate the potency, in Units, in the number of Tablets taken by the formula:

$$(50,000 / 3)CA$$

in which the factors are as defined therein.

Papaverine Hydrochloride

$C_{20}H_{21}NO_4 \cdot HCl$ 375.85
Isoquinoline, 1-[(3,4-dimethoxyphenyl)methyl]-6,7-dimethoxy-, hydrochloride.
6,7-Dimethoxy-1-veratrylisoquinoline hydrochloride [61-25-6].

» Papaverine Hydrochloride contains not less than 98.5 percent and not more than 100.5 percent of $C_{20}H_{21}NO_4 \cdot HCl$, calculated on the dried basis.

Packaging and storage—Preserve in tight, light-resistant containers. Store at 25°, excursions permitted between 15° and 30°.
USP Reference standards ⟨11⟩—*USP Papaverine Hydrochloride RS*.
Completeness of solution—A 1 in 15 solution in chloroform is clear and free from undissolved solid.
Identification—
 A: *Infrared Absorption* ⟨197K⟩.
 B: *Ultraviolet Absorption* ⟨197U⟩—
 Solution: 2.5 μg per mL.
 Medium: 0.1 N hydrochloric acid.
 Absorptivities at 251 nm, calculated on the dried basis, do not differ by more than 3.0%.
 C: A solution (1 in 50) responds to the tests for *Chloride* ⟨191⟩.
pH ⟨791⟩: between 3.0 and 4.5, in a solution (1 in 50).
Loss on drying ⟨731⟩—Dry it at 105° for 2 hours: it loses not more than 0.5% of its weight.
Residue on ignition ⟨281⟩: not more than 0.1%.
Limit of cryptopine, thebaine, or other organic impurities—Dissolve 50 mg in 2 mL of sulfuric acid in a small test tube: the resulting solution is not more yellow-brown in color than *Matching Fluid S* (see *Readily Carbonizable Substances Test* ⟨271⟩), and it is not more pink than a standard prepared, in equal volume, by diluting 3.0 mL of 0.1 N potassium permanganate with water to 1000 mL.
Organic volatile impurities, *Method IV* ⟨467⟩: meets the requirements.

(Official until July 1, 2008)
Assay—Dissolve about 700 mg of Papaverine Hydrochloride, accurately weighed, in 80 mL of glacial acetic acid; add 10 mL of mercuric acetate TS and 1 drop of crystal violet TS; and titrate with 0.1 N perchloric acid VS to a blue-green endpoint. Perform a blank determination, and make any necessary correction. Each mL of 0.1 N perchloric acid is equivalent to 37.59 mg of $C_{20}H_{21}NO_4 \cdot HCl$.

Papaverine Hydrochloride Injection

» Papaverine Hydrochloride Injection is a sterile solution of Papaverine Hydrochloride in Water for Injection. It contains not less than 95.0 percent and not more than 105.0 percent of the labeled amount of $C_{20}H_{21}NO_4 \cdot HCl$.

Packaging and storage—Preserve in single-dose or multiple-dose containers, preferably of Type I glass.
USP Reference standards ⟨11⟩—*USP Endotoxin RS. USP Papaverine Hydrochloride RS*.
Identification—
 A: Add 2 mL of alcohol to 1 mL of Injection, and evaporate on a steam bath, with the aid of a stream of nitrogen, to dryness. Dry the residue at 105° for 2 hours: it responds to *Identification* test *A* under *Papaverine Hydrochloride*.
 B: It responds to *Identification* test *C* under *Papaverine Hydrochloride*.
Bacterial endotoxins ⟨85⟩—It contains not more than 2.9 USP Endotoxin Units per mg of papaverine hydrochloride.
pH ⟨791⟩: not less than 3.0.
Other requirements—It meets the requirements under *Injections* ⟨1⟩.
Assay—Transfer 1.0 mL of Injection to a 200-mL volumetric flask, and dilute with water to volume. Pipet 3 mL of this solution into a separator, add 10 mL of water, and render alkaline with 6 N ammonium hydroxide. Extract the alkaloid with successive 5-mL portions of chloroform, and evaporate the extracts to dryness. Dissolve the residue in 0.1 N hydrochloric acid, and dilute with the same medium to 100.0 mL. Concomitantly determine the absorbances of this solution and of a Standard solution of USP Papaverine Hydrochloride RS in 0.1 N hydrochloric acid having a known concentration of about 4.5 μg per mL in 1-cm cells at the wavelength of maximum absorbance at about 251 nm, with a suitable spectrophotometer, using 0.1 N hydrochloric acid as the blank. Calculate the quantity, in mg, of $C_{20}H_{21}NO_4 \cdot HCl$ in the portion of Injection taken by the formula:

$$6.67C(A_U / A_S)$$

in which C is the concentration, in μg per mL, of USP Papaverine Hydrochloride RS in the Standard solution, and A_U and A_S are the absorbances of the solution from the Injection and the Standard solution, respectively.

Papaverine Hydrochloride Tablets

» Papaverine Hydrochloride Tablets contain not less than 93.0 percent and not more than 107.0 percent of the labeled amount of $C_{20}H_{21}NO_4 \cdot HCl$.

Packaging and storage—Preserve in tight containers.
USP Reference standards ⟨11⟩—*USP Papaverine Hydrochloride RS*.
Identification—Add a portion of powdered Tablets, equivalent to about 30 mg of papaverine hydrochloride, to 10 mL of 0.1 N hydrochloric acid in a separator. Extract the mixture with 10 mL of chloroform, filter the chloroform phase through paper, evaporate the solvent on a steam bath, and dry the residue at 105° for 2 hours: it responds to *Identification* test *A* under *Papaverine Hydrochloride*.

Dissolution ⟨711⟩—
Medium: water; 900 mL.
Apparatus 1: 100 rpm.
Time: 30 minutes.
Procedure—Determine the amount of $C_{20}H_{21}NO_4 \cdot HCl$ dissolved from UV absorbances at the wavelength of maximum absorbance at about 250 nm on filtered portions of the solution under test, suitably diluted with 0.1 N hydrochloric acid, in comparison with a Standard solution having a known concentration of USP Papaverine Hydrochloride RS in the same *Medium*.
Tolerances—Not less than 80% (*Q*) of the labeled amount of $C_{20}H_{21}NO_4 \cdot HCl$ is dissolved in 30 minutes.

Uniformity of dosage units ⟨905⟩: meet the requirements.
Procedure for content uniformity—Transfer 1 finely powdered Tablet to a 250-mL volumetric flask, add 50 mL of water and 3 mL of hydrochloric acid, mix, and allow to stand for 15 minutes with occasional agitation. Dilute with water to volume, mix, and filter, discarding the first 20 mL of the filtrate. Dilute a portion of the subsequent filtrate quantitatively and stepwise, if necessary, with water to provide a solution containing approximately 2.4 µg of papaverine hydrochloride per mL. Concomitantly determine the absorbances of this solution and a solution of USP Papaverine Hydrochloride RS, in the same medium at a concentration of about 2.4 µg per mL, in 1-cm cells, at the wavelength of maximum absorbance at about 250 nm, with a suitable spectrophotometer, using water as the blank. Calculate the quantity, in mg, of $C_{20}H_{21}NO_4 \cdot HCl$ in the Tablet by the formula:

$$(TC/D)(A_U/A_S)$$

in which *T* is the labeled quantity, in mg, of papaverine hydrochloride in the Tablet; *C* is the concentration, in µg per mL, of USP Papaverine Hydrochloride RS in the Standard solution; *D* is the concentration, in µg per mL, of the solution from the Tablet based upon the labeled quantity per Tablet and the extent of dilution; and A_U and A_S are the absorbances of the solution from the Tablet and the Standard solution, respectively.

Assay—Weigh and finely powder not less than 20 Tablets. Transfer an accurately weighed portion of the powder, equivalent to about 30 mg of papaverine hydrochloride, to a glass-stoppered conical flask, add about 100 mL of 0.1 N hydrochloric acid, and shake by mechanical means for 15 minutes. Filter the mixture into a 200-mL volumetric flask, and add 0.1 N hydrochloric acid to volume. Proceed as directed in the *Assay* under *Papaverine Hydrochloride Injection*, beginning with "Pipet 3 mL of this solution into a separator." Calculate the quantity, in mg, of $C_{20}H_{21}NO_4 \cdot HCl$ in the portion of Tablets taken by the formula:

$$6.67C(A_U/A_S)$$

in which *C* is the concentration, in µg per mL, of USP Papaverine Hydrochloride RS in the Standard solution, and A_U and A_S are the absorbances of the solution from the Tablets and the Standard solution, respectively.

Parachlorophenol

C_6H_5ClO 128.56
Phenol, 4-chloro-.
p-Chlorophenol   [*106-48-9*].

» Parachlorophenol contains not less than 99.0 percent and not more than 100.5 percent of C_6H_5ClO.

Packaging and storage—Preserve in tight, light-resistant containers.
Clarity and reaction of solution—A 1 in 100 solution is clear and is acid to litmus.

Identification—
A: To a 1 in 100 solution of it add bromine TS dropwise: a white precipitate is formed, and at first it redissolves, but then it becomes permanent as an excess of the reagent is added.
B: Add 1 drop of ferric chloride TS to 10 mL of a 1 in 100 solution of it: the solution acquires a violet-blue color.
C: Heat a few crystals, held on a copper wire, in the edge of a nonluminous flame: a green color is imparted to the flame.
D: To a mixture of 1 g of it and 5 mL of sodium hydroxide solution (1 in 3) add 1.5 g of monochloroacetic acid. Shake, and heat on a steam bath for 1 hour. Cool, dilute with 15 mL of water, and acidify with hydrochloric acid. Extract with 50 mL of ether, wash the ether solution with 10 mL of cold water, then extract the ether solution with 25 mL of sodium carbonate solution (1 in 20). Acidify the solution with hydrochloric acid, collect the resulting precipitate on a filter, and recrystallize it from hot water: the resulting parachlorophenoxyacetic acid melts between 154° and 158°.

Congealing temperature ⟨651⟩: between 42° and 44°.
Limit of nonvolatile residue—Heat about 1 g, accurately weighed, in a tared container on a steam bath until it is volatilized, and dry at 105° for 1 hour: not more than 0.1% of residue remains.
Chloride—Acidify 10 mL of a 1 in 100 solution with 2 N nitric acid, and add a few drops of silver nitrate TS: no turbidity or opalescence is produced.
Assay—Transfer about 1 g of Parachlorophenol, accurately weighed, to a 500-mL volumetric flask, dissolve in and dilute with water to volume, and mix. Transfer a 25.0-mL portion of the solution to an iodine flask, cool in an ice bath to about 4°, and add 20.0 mL of 0.1 N bromine VS. Add 5 mL of hydrochloric acid, and immediately insert the stopper. Maintain the flask at a temperature of 4° for 30 minutes, shaking at frequent intervals. Allow it to stand for 15 minutes, remove the stopper just sufficiently to introduce quickly 5 mL of potassium iodide solution (1 in 5), taking care that no bromine vapor escapes, and at once insert the stopper in the flask. Shake thoroughly, remove the stopper, and rinse it and the neck of the flask with a small portion of water, allowing the washings to flow into the flask. Shake the mixture, and titrate the liberated iodine with 0.1 N sodium thiosulfate VS, using 3 mL of starch TS as the indicator. Perform a blank determination (see *Residual Titrations* under *Titrimetry* ⟨541⟩). Each mL of 0.1 N bromine is equivalent to 3.214 mg of C_6H_5ClO.

Camphorated Parachlorophenol

» Camphorated Parachlorophenol is a triturated mixture that contains not less than 33.0 percent and not more than 37.0 percent of parachlorophenol (C_6H_5ClO) and not less than 63.0 percent and not more than 67.0 percent of camphor ($C_{10}H_{16}O$). The sum of the percentages of parachlorophenol and camphor is not less than 97.0 and not more than 103.0.

Packaging and storage—Preserve in tight, light-resistant containers.
Assay for parachlorophenol—Transfer about 1 g of Camphorated Parachlorophenol, accurately weighed, to a wide-mouth conical flask, and add a few glass beads, 6 mL of sodium hydroxide solution (1 in 2), and 130 mL of water. Heat the solution to boiling, add 70 mL of potassium permanganate solution (3 in 50), and continue to boil for 20 minutes. To the hot solution add 40 mL of 0.1 N silver nitrate. Add 50 mL of 18 N sulfuric acid, and sodium sulfite crystals, in divided portions and with swirling until the permanganate color is discharged and no manganese dioxide remains. Boil until the vapors are no longer acid to litmus, keeping the volume nearly constant by the addition of water. Add 5 mL of nitric acid, and continue to boil for 5 minutes. Cool, and collect the precipitate on a tared filtering crucible, wash well with water, then with 10 mL of alcohol, dry at 105° for 1 hour, cool, and weigh. Each 1.000 g of the silver chloride so obtained is equivalent to 897.0 mg of C_6H_5ClO.

Assay for camphor—Transfer about 300 mg of Camphorated Parachlorophenol, accurately weighed, to a 200-mL pressure bottle containing 50 mL of freshly prepared dinitrophenylhydrazine TS. Close the pressure bottle, immerse it in a water bath, and maintain it at about 75° for 4 hours. Cool to room temperature, then transfer the contents to a beaker with the aid of 100 mL of 3 N sulfuric acid and allow it to stand overnight. Collect the precipitate on a tared filtering crucible, wash with 100 mL of 3 N sulfuric acid and then with 75 mL of cold water, in divided portions, to remove the acid. Dry at 80° for 2 hours, cool, and weigh. The weight of the precipitate so obtained, multiplied by 0.4581, represents the weight of $C_{10}H_{16}O$ in the sample taken.

Paraldehyde

$C_6H_{12}O_3$ 132.16
1,3,5-Trioxane, 2,4,6-trimethyl-.
2,4,6-Trimethyl-s-trioxane   [123-63-7].

» NOTE—Paraldehyde is subject to oxidation to form acetic acid. It may contain a suitable stabilizer.

Packaging and storage—Preserve in well-filled, tight, light-resistant containers, preferably of Type I or Type II glass, holding not more than 30 mL, at a temperature not exceeding 25°. Paraldehyde may be shipped in bulk containers holding a minimum of 22.5 kg (50 lb) to commercial drug repackagers only.

Labeling—The label of all containers of Paraldehyde, including those dispensed by the pharmacist, includes a statement directing the user to discard the unused contents of any container that has been opened for more than 24 hours.

NOTE—The label of bulk containers of Paraldehyde directs the commercial drug repackager to demonstrate compliance with the USP purity tests for Paraldehyde immediately prior to repackaging, and not to repackage from a container that has been opened longer than 24 hours.

Identification—Heat it with a small quantity of 2 N sulfuric acid: acetaldehyde, recognizable by its pungent odor, is produced.

Congealing temperature ⟨651⟩: not lower than 11°.

Distilling range, Method I ⟨721⟩—It distills completely between 120° and 126°, a correction factor of 0.050° per mm being applied as necessary.

Acidity—To a solution of 6.0 mL in 100 mL of water add 5 drops of phenolphthalein TS, and titrate with 1.0 N sodium hydroxide: not more than 0.50 mL is required to produce a pink color (0.5% as acetic acid).

Chloride—To 5 mL of a solution (1 in 10) add 1 drop of nitric acid and 3 drops of silver nitrate TS: no opalescence is produced immediately.

Sulfate—To 5 mL of a solution (1 in 10) add 1 drop of hydrochloric acid and 3 drops of barium chloride TS: no turbidity is produced.

Limit of nonvolatile residue—Heat 5.0 mL in a small, tared evaporating dish on a steam bath: no disagreeable odor is noticeable as the last portions evaporate, and, when dried at 105° for 1 hour, not more than 3 mg of residue remains (0.06%).

Limit of acetaldehyde—Place 100 mL of water in a 250-mL conical flask, add 5.0 mL of Paraldehyde, and shake the mixture gently until solution is complete. Add 5 mL of hydroxylamine hydrochloride solution (3.5 in 100). Shake the mixture gently for 30 seconds, add methyl orange TS, and titrate immediately with 0.50 N sodium hydroxide. Perform a blank titration: the difference between the titers does not exceed 1 mL of 0.50 N sodium hydroxide (0.4%).

Paramethasone Acetate

$C_{24}H_{31}FO_6$ 434.50
Pregna-1,4-diene-3,20-dione, 21-(acetyloxy)-6-fluoro-11,17-dihydroxy-16-methyl-, (6α,11β,16α)-.
6α-Fluoro-11β,17,21-trihydroxy-16α-methylpregna-1,4-diene-3,20-dione 21-acetate   [1597-82-6].

» Paramethasone Acetate contains not less than 95.0 percent and not more than 101.0 percent of $C_{24}H_{31}FO_6$, calculated on the dried basis.

Packaging and storage—Preserve in tight containers.
USP Reference standards ⟨11⟩—USP Paramethasone Acetate RS.
Identification—
 A: Infrared Absorption ⟨197K⟩.
 B: Ultraviolet Absorption ⟨197U⟩—
  Solution: 20 µg per mL.
  Medium: methanol.
 Absorptivities at 242 nm, calculated on the dried basis, do not differ by more than 4.0%.
 C: Prepare a solution of Paramethasone Acetate in a mixture of chloroform and methanol (1 : 1) containing 2 mg per mL. Apply 10 µL each of this solution and a chloroform-methanol (1 : 1) solution of USP Paramethasone Acetate RS containing 2 mg per mL to a suitable thin-layer chromatographic plate (see Chromatography ⟨621⟩) coated with a 0.25-mm layer of chromatographic silica gel mixture. Allow the spots to dry, and develop the chromatogram in a solvent system consisting of a mixture of methylene chloride, nitromethane, and glacial acetic acid (60 : 40 : 1) until the solvent front has moved about three-fourths of the length of the plate. Remove the plate from the developing chamber, and allow to dry in air for 15 minutes. Return the plate to the developing chamber, and develop again, in the same solvent system, until the solvent front has moved about three-fourths of the length of the plate. Remove the plate from the developing chamber, mark the solvent front, and allow the solvent to evaporate. Locate the spots on the plate by examination under short-wavelength UV light: the R_F value of the principal spot obtained from the test solution corresponds to that obtained from the Standard solution.

Specific rotation ⟨781S⟩: between +67° and +77°.
 Test solution: 10 mg per mL, in chloroform.

X-ray diffraction ⟨941⟩—The X-ray diffraction pattern of Paramethasone Acetate conforms to either one or a mixture of the patterns described by the data in the accompanying table.

Form A		Form B	
d	I/I_1	d	I/I_1
12.09	10	11.62	20
8.42	20	7.80	8
7.78	10	7.13	10
6.41	100	6.50	60
5.65	100	5.98	100
5.50	10	5.63	70
5.18	2	5.30	100
4.59	30	4.85	60
4.41	20	4.65	60
4.24	40	4.43	8
3.93	20	4.30	2
3.64	30b	3.93	60
3.48	15	3.72	6

Form A		Form B	
d	I/I_1	d	I/I_1
3.27	20	3.58	4
3.12	30	3.45	4
3.03	8	3.26	10
2.90	2	3.09	10
2.82	8	2.96	10
2.70	10	2.88	10
2.61	8	2.81	6b
2.51	10	2.66	8b
2.35	2	2.55	6
2.29	8	2.48	6b
2.24	6	2.38	10
2.11	4	2.30	6
2.08	2	2.26	8
2.04	4	2.19	6
2.00	4	2.11	10
1.95	1	2.04	8
1.92	4	1.99	10
1.87	2		
1.84	2		
1.82	1		

Loss on drying ⟨731⟩—Dry it in vacuum at 105° for 4 hours: it loses not more than 1.0% of its weight.

Assay—

Standard preparation—Prepare as directed under *Single-Steroid Assay* ⟨511⟩, using USP Paramethasone Acetate RS to prepare a solution containing approximately 10 mg per mL.

Assay preparation—Weigh accurately about 50 mg of Paramethasone Acetate, previously dried, dissolve it in a sufficient quantity of a mixture of equal volumes of alcohol and chloroform to make 5.0 mL, and mix.

Procedure—Proceed as directed for *Procedure* under *Single-steroid Assay* ⟨511⟩, applying 10 µL each of the *Assay preparation* and the *Standard preparation* to the chromatographic plate, and using a solvent system consisting of methylene chloride, nitromethane, and glacial acetic acid (60 : 40 : 1), through the fourth sentence of the second paragraph under *Procedure*. Then centrifuge the tubes for 5 minutes, and determine the absorbances of the supernatants in 1-cm cells at the wavelength of maximum absorbance at about 242 nm, against the blank. Calculate the quantity, in mg, of $C_{24}H_{31}FO_6$ in the portion of Paramethasone Acetate taken by the formula:

$$5C(A_U/A_S)$$

in which C is the concentration, in mg per mL, of USP Paramethasone Acetate RS in the *Standard preparation*, and A_U and A_S are the absorbances of the solutions from the *Assay preparation* and the *Standard preparation*, respectively.

Paramethasone Acetate Tablets

» Paramethasone Acetate Tablets contain not less than 85.0 percent and not more than 115.0 percent of the labeled amount of $C_{24}H_{31}FO_6$.

Packaging and storage—Preserve in well-closed containers.

USP Reference standards ⟨11⟩—*USP Paramethasone Acetate RS.*

Identification—The IR absorption spectrum of the *Assay preparation*, prepared as directed in the *Assay*, exhibits maxima only at the same wavelengths as that of the *Standard preparation*, prepared as directed in the *Assay*.

Disintegration ⟨701⟩: 15 minutes, the use of disks being omitted.

Uniformity of dosage units ⟨905⟩: meet the requirements.

Procedure for content uniformity—Transfer 1 finely powdered Tablet to a 50-mL volumetric flask, add 25 mL of chloroform, and shake by mechanical means for 15 minutes. Dilute with chloroform to volume, mix, and filter, discarding the first 20 mL of the filtrate. Dilute a portion of the subsequent filtrate quantitatively and stepwise, if necessary, with chloroform to obtain a solution containing approximately 20 µg of paramethasone acetate per mL. Transfer 10.0 mL each of this solution and of a solution of USP Paramethasone Acetate RS in the same medium having a known concentration of about 20 µg per mL to separate 25-mL volumetric flasks, and transfer 10 mL of chloroform to a third flask to provide the blank. To each flask add 3.0 mL of a 1 in 4000 solution of blue tetrazolium in alcohol and 5.0 mL of a 1 in 20 solution of tetramethylammonium hydroxide TS in alcohol, mixing after each addition. Fifteen minutes, accurately timed, after the addition of the last reagent, add 1 mL of glacial acetic acid to each flask, dilute with chloroform to volume, and mix. Concomitantly determine the absorbances of the solutions in 1-cm cells at the wavelength of maximum absorbance at about 525 nm, with a suitable spectrophotometer, against the blank. Calculate the quantity, in mg, of $C_{24}H_{31}FO_6$ in the Tablet taken by the formula:

$$(TC/D)(A_U/A_S)$$

in which T is the labeled quantity, in mg, of paramethasone acetate in the Tablet, C is the concentration, in µg per mL, of USP Paramethasone Acetate RS in the *Standard solution*, D is the concentration, in µg per mL, of the solution from the Tablet, based upon the labeled quantity per Tablet and the extent of dilution, and A_U and A_S are the absorbances of the solution from the Tablet and the Standard solution, respectively.

Assay—

Standard preparation—Transfer about 6 mg of USP Paramethasone Acetate RS, accurately weighed, to a separator containing 15 mL of water, and proceed as directed under *Assay preparation*, beginning with "add 3 drops of hydrochloric acid."

Assay preparation—Weigh and finely powder not less than 20 Tablets. Transfer an accurately weighed portion of the powder, equivalent to about 6 mg of paramethasone acetate, to a separator containing 15 mL of water, add 3 drops of hydrochloric acid, and heat on a steam bath for 5 minutes, mixing frequently. Cool the separator to room temperature, add 4 drops of sodium hydroxide solution (1 in 2), and immediately extract with four 25-mL portions of chloroform. Filter the extracts through anhydrous sodium sulfate, collecting the extracts in a beaker. [*Caution—Do not allow the filter paper to extend above the top of the funnel.*] Rinse the filter with several small portions of chloroform, add the rinsings to the beaker, and evaporate the chloroform on a steam bath with the aid of a current of air until about 3 mL remains. Transfer the residual liquid, with the aid of several small portions of chloroform, to a glass-stoppered, 10-mL conical flask, and evaporate on a steam bath with the aid of a current of air to dryness. Add 2.0 mL of chloroform to the flask, insert the stopper, and mix to dissolve the residue.

Procedure—Concomitantly determine the absorbances of the solutions in 1-mm cells at the wavelength of maximum absorbance at 6.04 µm, with a suitable IR spectrophotometer, using chloroform as the blank. Calculate the quantity, in mg, of $C_{24}H_{31}FO_6$ in the portion of Tablets taken by the formula:

$$W(A_U/A_S)$$

in which W is the weight, in mg, of USP Paramethasone Acetate RS used in preparing the *Standard preparation*, and A_U and A_S are the absorbances of the *Assay preparation* and the *Standard preparation*, respectively.

Paregoric

» Paregoric yields, from each 100 mL, not less than 35 mg and not more than 45 mg of anhydrous morphine. Paregoric may be prepared as follows:

Powdered Opium	4.3 g
Suitable essential oil(s)	—
Benzoic Acid	3.8 g
Diluted Alcohol	900 mL
Glycerin	38 mL
To make about	950 mL

Macerate for 5 days the Powdered Opium, Benzoic Acid, and essential oil(s), with occasional agitation, in a mixture of 900 mL of Diluted Alcohol and 38 mL of Glycerin. Then filter, and pass enough Diluted Alcohol through the filter to obtain 950 mL of total filtrate. Assay a portion of this filtrate as directed herein, and dilute the remainder with a sufficient quantity of Diluted Alcohol containing, in each 100 mL, 400 mg of Benzoic Acid, 4 mL of Glycerin, and sufficient essential oil(s) to yield a solution containing, in each 100 mL, 40 mg of anhydrous morphine.

NOTE—Paregoric may be prepared also by using Opium or Opium Tincture instead of Powdered Opium, the anhydrous morphine content being adjusted to 40 mg in each 100 mL and the alcohol content being adjusted to 45 percent.

Packaging and storage—Preserve in tight, light-resistant containers, and avoid exposure to direct sunlight and to excessive heat.
Alcohol content ⟨611⟩: between 43.0% and 47.0% of C_2H_5OH, determined by the gas-liquid procedure, acetone being used as the internal standard.
Assay—
Chromatographic tubes—Prepare three similar tubes, each about 260 mm long and consisting of about 200 mm of 25-mm tubing and about 6 cm of 6-mm tubing. In each of the tubes, place a pledget of glass wool at a point where the 6-mm tubing is constricted slightly, about 2 cm from the junction.
Citrate buffer—Mix equal volumes of 0.1 M sodium citrate and 0.1 M citric acid.
Standard preparation—Prepare a solution by dissolving an accurately weighed quantity of USP Morphine Sulfate RS, equivalent to about 40 mg of anhydrous morphine, in 0.5 mL of triethylamine contained in a 100-mL volumetric flask, and add methanol to volume. Pipet 10 mL of this solution into a 50-mL volumetric flask, add 1 mL each of triethylamine and hydrochloric acid, and add water-saturated chloroform to volume.
Assay preparation—Evaporate 10.0 mL of Paregoric (equivalent to about 4 mg of morphine) on a steam bath under a stream of air to about 2 mL, and cool. [NOTE—Avoid reducing the volume to less than 2 mL.] Add 0.5 mL of *Citrate buffer*.
Chromatographic columns—Fill the three tubes with adsorbent prepared as follows, using chromatographic siliceous earth as the base of the adsorbent, and tamp it firmly in place. Pack *Column I* in two layers, the lower layer consisting of 3 g of chromatographic siliceous earth mixed with 2 mL of *Citrate buffer* and the upper layer of 3 g of chromatographic siliceous earth mixed with the *Assay preparation*. Dry-rinse the beaker in which the components of the two layers have been mixed with 1 g of chromatographic siliceous earth, and add it also to the top of *Column I*. Pack *Column II* with 3 g of chromatographic siliceous earth mixed with 2 mL of dibasic potassium phosphate solution (1 in 5.75). Pack *Column III* with 3 g of chromatographic siliceous earth mixed with 2 mL of sodium hydroxide solution (1 in 50). Place a small pad of glass wool above each column packing.
Procedure—[NOTES—(1) Use water-saturated solvents throughout this procedure; (2) prepare eluants fresh daily; and (3) avoid bringing the solutions into contact with metal.] Wash *Column I* with 100 mL of ether, followed by 100 mL of chloroform, rinse the tip of the column with chloroform, and discard the solvents. In the following operations, rinse each column tip before discarding the column or changing receivers. Mount the three columns vertically so that the effluent from *Column I* flows into *Column II*, and the effluent from the latter flows into *Column III*. Pass through the three columns 5 mL of a 1 in 5 solution of triethylamine in chloroform, followed by four 10-mL portions of a 1 in 100 solution of triethylamine in chloroform, allowing each portion to pass through completely before subsequent additions. Discard *Column I*. Pass three 5-mL portions of the 1 in 100 solution of triethylamine in chloroform through the two remaining columns. Discard *Column II*. Wash *Column III* successively with 10 mL of the 1 in 100 solution of triethylamine in chloroform, 50 mL of chloroform, 2 mL of a 1 in 10 solution of glacial acetic acid in chloroform, and 50 mL of a 1 in 100 solution of glacial acetic acid in chloroform. Discard all washings. Arrange to collect eluate from *Column III* in a 50-mL volumetric flask containing 10 mL of methanol and 1 mL of hydrochloric acid. Elute the column with 5 mL of a 1 in 5 solution of triethylamine in chloroform, followed by 33 mL of a 1 in 100 solution of triethylamine in chloroform. Dilute with chloroform to volume, and mix. Concomitantly record the spectra of this solution and the *Standard preparation* in 1-cm cells, with a suitable spectrophotometer, from 255 nm to 360 nm, using chloroform as the blank, and plot the corresponding wavelength-absorbance curves. Correct the absorbance of each solution, at the wavelength of maximum absorbance at about 285 nm, by extrapolating the portion of the baseline curve between 340 nm and 310 nm to this wavelength. Calculate the weight of anhydrous morphine, in mg per 100 mL of Paregoric, taken by the formula:

$$10W(A_U / A_S)$$

in which W is the weight, in mg, of anhydrous morphine in the 50 mL of *Standard preparation*, and A_U and A_S are the corrected absorbances of the solution from the *Assay* and the *Standard preparation*, respectively.

Paricalcitol

$C_{27}H_{44}O_3$ 416.64
19-Nor-1-α,25-dihydroxyvitamin D_2.
(1α,3β,7E,22E)-19-Nor-9,10-secoergosta-5,7,22-triene-1,3,25-triol.
(7E,22E)-19-Nor-9,10-secoergosta-5,7,22-triene-1α,3β,25-triol
[*131918-61-1*].

» Paricalcitol contains not less than 97.0 percent and not more than 103.0 percent of $C_{27}H_{44}O_3$, calculated on the dried basis.

Caution—Handle Paricalcitol with exceptional care because it is very potent. Care should be taken to prevent inhaling particles of Paricalcitol and exposing the skin to it.

Packaging and storage—Preserve in tight, light-resistant containers, and store under argon in a freezer.
USP Reference standards ⟨11⟩—USP Paricalcitol RS. USP Paricalcitol Solution RS.
Identification—
A: *Infrared Absorption* ⟨197K⟩.
B: The retention time of the major peak in the chromatogram of the *Assay preparation* corresponds to that in the chromatogram of the *Standard preparation*, as obtained in the *Assay*.
Loss on drying (see *Thermal Analysis* ⟨891⟩)—Determine the percentage of volatile substances by thermogravimetric analysis on an appropriately calibrated instrument, using about 8 mg of Paricalcitol, accurately weighed. Heat at a rate of 5° per minute between ambient temperature and 150° in an atmosphere of nitrogen

at a flow rate of 40 mL per minute. From the thermogram determine the accumulated loss in weight: it loses not more than 2.0% of its weight.

Chromatographic purity—[NOTE—Use low-actinic glassware to prepare solutions of Paricalcitol.]

Diluent—Prepare a mixture of water and dehydrated alcohol (1 : 1).

Butylparaben solution—Transfer about 25 mg of butylparaben to a 100-mL volumetric flask, dilute with *Diluent* to volume, and mix.

Solution A—Use filtered and degassed water.

Solution B—Use filtered and degassed acetonitrile.

Mobile phase—Use variable mixtures of *Solution A* and *Solution B*, as directed for *Chromatographic system*. Make adjustments if necessary (see *System Suitability* under *Chromatography* ⟨621⟩).

Standard solution—Dilute USP Paricalcitol Solution RS in *Diluent* to a known concentration of about 0.1 µg of paricalcitol per mL.

Control standard solution—Transfer 3.0 mL of the *Standard solution* to a 10.0-mL volumetric flask, dilute with *Diluent* to volume, and mix.

Test stock solution—Prepare a solution of Paricalcitol in dehydrated alcohol, having a known concentration of about 200 µg per mL.

Resolution solution—Transfer 1 mL of the *Butylparaben solution* and 1 mL of the *Test stock solution* to a 100-mL volumetric flask, dilute with *Diluent* to volume, and mix. Transfer 1 mL of this solution to a 10-mL volumetric flask, dilute with *Diluent* to volume, and mix.

Test solution—Prepare a mixture of the *Test stock solution* and water (1 : 1).

Chromatographic system (see *Chromatography* ⟨621⟩)—The liquid chromatograph is equipped with a 252-nm detector and a 4.6-mm × 25-cm column that contains 5-µm packing L1. The flow rate is about 2 mL per minute. The chromatograph is programmed as follows.

Time (minutes)	Solution A (%)	Solution B (%)	Elution
0–10	95	5	isocratic
10–30	95→45	5→55	linear gradient
30–40	45	55	isocratic
40–45	45→0	55→100	linear gradient
45–50	0	100	isocratic

Chromatograph the *Resolution solution*, and record the peak responses as directed for *Procedure:* the resolution, R, between paricalcitol and butylparaben is not less than 12.0. Chromatograph the *Standard solution* and the *Control standard solution*, and record the peak responses as directed for *Procedure:* the area ratio for the paricalcitol peak from the *Standard solution* to that from the *Control standard solution* is between 1.8 and 4.0; and the relative standard deviation for replicate injections of the *Standard solution* is not more than 10.0%.

Procedure—Separately inject equal volumes (about 100 µL) of the *Diluent*, the *Standard solution*, and the *Test solution* into the chromatograph, record the chromatograms, and measure the peak responses, disregarding any peaks corresponding to those obtained from the *Diluent*. Calculate the percentage of each impurity in the portion of Paricalcitol taken by the formula:

$$100(C_S / C_U)(r_i / r_S)$$

in which C_S and C_U are the concentrations, in µg per mL, of paricalcitol in the *Standard solution* and the *Test solution*, respectively; r_i is the peak response for each impurity obtained from the *Test solution*; and r_S is the paricalcitol peak response obtained from the *Standard solution*: not more than 0.1% of any individual impurity is found; and not more than 0.5% of total impurities is found.

Assay—[NOTE—Use low-actinic glassware to prepare solutions of paricalcitol.]

Mobile phase—Prepare a filtered and degassed mixture of methanol and water (4 : 1). Make adjustments if necessary (see *System Suitability* under *Chromatography* ⟨621⟩).

Diluent—Prepare a mixture of methanol and water (1 : 1).

Standard preparation—Transfer an accurately weighed amount of USP Paricalcitol RS to a suitable volumetric flask, dissolve in a minimum amount of dehydrated alcohol, and dilute with *Diluent* to volume. Further dilute this solution quantitatively, and stepwise if necessary, with *Diluent* to obtain a solution having a known concentration of about 5.0 µg per mL.

Assay preparation—Transfer an accurately weighed amount of Paricalcitol to a suitable volumetric flask, dissolve in a minimum amount of dehydrated alcohol, and dilute with *Diluent* to volume. Further dilute this solution quantitatively, and stepwise if necessary, with *Diluent* to obtain a solution having a known concentration of about 5.0 µg per mL.

Chromatographic system (see *Chromatography* ⟨621⟩)—The liquid chromatograph is equipped with a 252-nm detector and a 4.6-mm × 25-cm column that contains 5-µm packing L1. The flow rate is about 2 mL per minute. Chromatograph the *Standard preparation*, and record the peak responses as directed for *Procedure*: the tailing factor is not more than 2.0; and the relative standard deviation for replicate injections is not more than 2.0%.

Procedure—Separately inject equal volumes (about 100 µL) of the *Standard preparation* and the *Assay preparation* into the chromatograph, record the chromatograms, and measure the responses for the major peaks. Calculate the percentage of $C_{27}H_{44}O_3$ in the portion of Paricalcitol taken by the formula:

$$100(C_S / C_U)(r_U / r_S)$$

in which C_U and C_S are the concentrations, in µg per mL, of paricalcitol in the *Assay preparation* and the *Standard preparation*, respectively; and r_U and r_S are the paricalcitol peak responses obtained from the *Assay preparation* and the *Standard preparation*, respectively.

Paricalcitol Injection

» Paricalcitol Injection is a sterile solution of Paricalcitol in a mixture of Water for Injection, Propylene Glycol, and Alcohol. It contains not less than 90.0 percent and not more than 110.0 percent of the labeled amount of paricalcitol ($C_{27}H_{44}O_3$). It contains no antimicrobial agents.

Packaging and storage—Preserve in single-dose containers, preferably of Type I glass. Store at controlled room temperature.

USP Reference standards ⟨11⟩—*USP Endotoxin RS. USP Paricalcitol Solution RS.*

Identification—The retention time of the major peak in the chromatogram of the *Assay preparation* corresponds to that in the chromatogram of the *Standard preparation*, as obtained in the *Assay*.

Bacterial endotoxins ⟨85⟩—It contains not more than 10 USP Endotoxin Units per µg of paricalcitol.

Particulate matter ⟨788⟩: meets the requirements for small-volume injections.

Limit of aluminum ⟨206⟩—

Nitric acid diluent—Dilute 4 mL of nitric acid to 2000 mL with water.

Matrix modifier solution—Dissolve 1.5 g of magnesium nitrate in 1000 mL of water.

Standard stock solution—Proceed as directed in the chapter under *Standard Preparations*, beginning with "Treat some aluminum wire" and ending with "Cool, and transfer the solution, with the aid of water, to a 100-mL volumetric flask, dilute with water to volume, and mix." Transfer 2 mL of this solution to a second 100-mL volumetric flask, dilute with water to volume, and mix. Transfer 2 mL of this solution to a third 100-mL volumetric flask, dilute with water to volume, and mix. This solution contains about 0.4 µg of aluminum per mL.

Standard solutions—Dilute accurately measured portions of the *Standard stock solution* with *Nitric acid diluent* to obtain solutions having known concentrations of about 2.5, 5.0, 10, 20, and 50 ng of aluminum per mL.

Test solution—Dilute 4.0 mL of Injection with 6.0 mL of *Nitric acid diluent* or use an appropriate dilution to obtain a solution having a concentration not greater than 0.02 µg of aluminum per mL.

System suitability solution—Dilute 9.5 mL of the *Test solution* with 0.5 mL of the *Standard stock solution*. If the resulting solution contains more than 0.04 µg of aluminum per mL, prepare an alternate dilution having a concentration between about 0.02 and 0.04 µg of aluminum per mL.

Procedure—Concomitantly determine the absorbances of the *Standard solutions*, the *System suitability solution*, and the *Test solution* at the aluminum emission line at 309.3 nm with a suitable atomic absorption spectrophotometer (see *Spectrophotometry and Light-Scattering* ⟨851⟩) equipped with an aluminum hollow-cathode lamp and a flameless electrically heated furnace. Under typical conditions, the sample volume is 20 µL, the volume of the *Matrix modifier solution* is 5 µL, the injection temperature is 100°, and the oven conditions are as follows [NOTE—These conditions may be optimized for each instrument]:

Step	Temperature
Drying 1	110°
Drying 2	130°
Drying 3	200°
Pyrrolysis	1100°
Read	2300°
Clean Out	2450°

Plot the absorbances of the *Standard solutions* versus the content of aluminum, in ng per mL, drawing a straight line best fitting the five points: the correlation coefficient is not less than 0.995; the recovery for the *System suitability solution* is between 80% and 120%; and the duplicate injections must agree within 0.0024 µg per mL. From the graph so obtained, determine the quantity of aluminum, C, in µg, found in each mL of the *Test solution*. Calculate the quantity, in µg, of aluminum in each mL of the Injection taken by the formula:

$$CD,$$

in which C is as defined above; and D is the dilution factor used to prepare the *Test solution*: not more than 0.5 µg per mL is found.

Related compounds—

Diluent—Prepare a mixture of water and acetonitrile (1 : 1).

Solution A—Prepare a filtered and degassed mixture of water and acetonitrile (85 : 15).

Solution B—Use filtered and degassed acetonitrile.

Mobile phase—Use variable mixtures of *Solution A* and *Solution B* as directed for *Chromatographic system*. Make adjustments if necessary (see *System Suitability* under *Chromatography* ⟨621⟩).

Standard solution—Prepare a solution of USP Paricalcitol Solution RS in *Diluent* having a known concentration of paricalcitol equal to about 0.5% of the labeled concentration of the Injection.

Control standard solution—Transfer 5.0 mL of the *Standard solution* to a 25.0-mL volumetric flask, dilute with *Diluent* to volume, and mix.

Degradation stock solution—Accurately dilute about 1 mL of USP Paricalcitol Solution RS with *Diluent* to 5 mL.

Degradation solution 1—Transfer about 1 mL of the *Degradation stock solution* and 0.1 mL of 30 percent hydrogen peroxide into a 10-mL container, and allow to stand at room temperature for 1 hour. Dilute with *Diluent* to 10 mL, and mix.

Degradation solution 2—Place about 1 mL of the *Degradation stock solution* and 1 mL of 0.1 N hydrochloric acid in a 10-mL container. Mix, and heat at 70° for 1 hour. Cool to room temperature, dilute with *Diluent* to 10 mL, and mix.

Test solution—Use the Injection.

Chromatographic system (see *Chromatography* ⟨621⟩)—The liquid chromatograph is equipped with a 252-nm detector, a 4.6-mm × 7.5-cm guard column that contains packing L1, and a 4.6-mm × 25-cm column that contains 5-µm packing L1. The flow rate is about 1 mL per minute. The chromatograph is programmed as follows.

Time (minutes)	Solution A (%)	Solution B (%)	Elution
0–25	65→5	35→95	linear gradient
25–45	5	95	isocratic

Chromatograph the *Standard solution* and the *Control standard solution*, and record the peak responses as directed for *Procedure*: the area ratio for the paricalcitol peak from the *Standard solution* to that from the *Control standard solution* is between 4.0 and 6.0; and the relative standard deviation for replicate injections of the *Standard solution* is not more than 5.0%.

Procedure—Chromatograph the *Degradation solution 1*, and identify the paricalcitol peak and the peaks due to the related compounds listed in *Table 1*.

Table 1

Relative Retention Time	Name	Limit in the Test solution, (%)
0.63	Related compound A	1.0
0.79	Related compound B	1.0

Chromatograph the *Degradation solution 2*, and identify the paricalcitol peak and the peaks due to the related compounds listed in *Table 2*. The resolution, R, between the paricalcitol peak and the related compound D peak is not less than 1.0.

Table 2

Relative Retention Time	Name	Limit in the Test solution, (%)
0.89	Related compound C	1.0
0.95	Related compound D	1.0
1.32	Related compound E[*]	1.0
1.57	Related compound F	1.0
1.66	Related compound G	1.0
1.74	Related compound H	1.0
1.79	Related compound I	1.0

[*] NOTE—This peak is very small (approximately 3 to 5 times the signal-to-noise ratio).

Separately inject equal volumes (about 100 to 200 µL) of the *Diluent* and the *Test solution*, in duplicate, into the chromatograph, record the chromatograms, and measure the peak responses, disregarding any peaks corresponding to those obtained from the *Diluent*. Calculate the percentage of each impurity in the portion of Injection taken by the formula:

$$100(C/L)(r_i / r_S)$$

in which C is the concentration, in µg per mL, of paricalcitol in the *Standard solution*, calculated on the basis of the content of paricalcitol in the USP Paricalcitol Solution RS; L is the labeled amount, in µg per mL, of paricalcitol in the Injection; r_i is the peak response for each impurity obtained from the *Test solution*; and r_S is the paricalcitol peak response obtained from the *Standard solution*: in addition to not exceeding the limits for impurities in *Tables 1* and *2*, not more than 2.0% of total impurities is found.

Content of propylene glycol and alcohol—

Mobile phase—Prepare a filtered and degassed 0.01 N sulfuric acid solution.

Alcohol standard solution—Transfer 2.0 mL of dehydrated alcohol to a 10-mL volumetric flask, dilute with water to volume, and mix.

Propylene glycol standard solution—Transfer 3.0 mL of propylene glycol to a 10-mL volumetric flask, dilute with water to volume, and mix.

Standard solution—Transfer 5.0 mL each of *Alcohol standard solution* and *Propylene glycol standard solution* to a 50-mL volumetric flask, dilute with water to volume, and mix.

Test solution—Transfer 5.0 mL of the Injection to a 50-mL volumetric flask, dilute with water to volume, and mix.

Procedure—Separately inject equal volumes (about 20 µL) of a portion of the solution under test, previously passed through a suitable 0.45-µm membrane filter, and the *Standard solution* into the chromatograph, record the chromatograms, and measure the responses for the major peaks. Calculate the quantity of $C_{19}H_{20}FNO_3$ dissolved based on the peak responses obtained from the solution under test and the *Standard solution*.

Tolerances—Not less than 80% (*Q*) of the labeled amount of $C_{19}H_{20}FNO_3$ is dissolved in 60 minutes.

Uniformity of dosage units ⟨905⟩: meet the requirements.

PROCEDURE FOR CONTENT UNIFORMITY—

Buffer solution, Mobile phase, and *Chromatographic system*—Proceed as directed in the *Assay*.

Standard solution—Use the *Standard preparation,* prepared as directed in the *Assay*.

Test solution—Place 1 Tablet in a suitable volumetric flask, and add a volume of a hydrochloric acid solution (7 in 1000), equivalent to about 25% of the flask volume. Allow the Tablet to disintegrate, dilute with methanol to volume, and mix to obtain a solution containing about 0.1 mg of paroxetine per mL. Centrifuge a portion of the solution.

Procedure—Proceed as directed in the *Assay*. Calculate the quantity, in mg, of $C_{19}H_{20}FNO_3$ in the Tablet taken by the formula:

$$VC(329.37/365.83)(r_U / r_S)$$

in which *V* is the volume of the flask used; r_U and r_S are the peak responses obtained from the *Test solution* and the *Standard solution,* respectively; and the other terms are as defined therein.

Assay—

Buffer solution—Prepare a mixture of water, phosphoric acid, and triethylamine (100 : 0.6 : 0.3).

Mobile phase—Prepare a filtered and degassed mixture of *Buffer solution* and acetonitrile (7 : 3). Make adjustments if necessary (see *System Suitability* under *Chromatography* ⟨621⟩).

Standard preparation—Dissolve an accurately weighed quantity of USP Paroxetine Hydrochloride RS in methanol, and dilute quantitatively, and stepwise if necessary, with methanol to obtain a solution having a known concentration of about 0.1 mg per mL.

Assay preparation—Weigh and finely powder not fewer than 20 Tablets. Transfer an accurately weighed portion of the powder, equivalent to about 100 mg of paroxetine, to a 200-mL volumetric flask, dissolve in and dilute with methanol to volume, and mix. Centrifuge a portion of this solution for 6 minutes. Transfer 20 mL of the supernatant to a 100-mL volumetric flask, dilute with methanol to volume, and mix.

Chromatographic system (see *Chromatography* ⟨621⟩)—The liquid chromatograph is equipped with a 295-nm detector and a 4.6-mm × 3.3-cm column that contains 3-µm packing L7. The flow rate is about 2.0 mL per minute. Chromatograph the *Standard preparation,* and record the peak responses as directed for *Procedure*: the column efficiency is not less than 750 theoretical plates; the tailing factor is not more than 4; and the relative standard deviation for replicate injections is not more than 2.0%.

Procedure—Separately inject equal volumes (about 5 µL) of the *Standard preparation* and the *Assay preparation* into the chromatograph, record the chromatograms, and measure the responses for the major peaks. Calculate the quantity, in mg, of paroxetine ($C_{19}H_{20}FNO_3$) in the portion of Tablets taken by the formula:

$$1000C(329.37/365.83)(r_U / r_S)$$

in which *C* is the concentration, in mg per mL, of USP Paroxetine Hydrochloride RS in the *Standard preparation;* 329.37 and 365.83 are the molecular weights for paroxetine and paroxetine hydrochloride, respectively; and r_U and r_S are the peak responses obtained from the *Assay preparation* and the *Standard preparation,* respectively.

Pectin

Pectin.
Pectin [9000-69-5].

» Pectin is a purified carbohydrate product obtained from the dilute acid extract of the inner portion of the rind of citrus fruits or from apple pomace. It consists chiefly of partially methoxylated polygalacturonic acids.

Pectin yields not less than 6.7 percent of methoxy groups (–OCH₃) and not less than 74.0 percent of galacturonic acid ($C_6H_{10}O_7$), calculated on the dried basis.

NOTE—Commercial pectin for the production of jellied food products is standardized to the convenient "150 jelly grade" by addition of dextrose or other sugars, and sometimes contains sodium citrate or other buffer salts. This monograph refers to the pure pectin to which no such additions have been made.

Packaging and storage—Preserve in tight containers.

Labeling—Label it to indicate whether it is of apple or of citrus origin.

Identification—

A: Heat 1 g with 9 mL of water on a steam bath until a solution is formed, replacing water lost by evaporation: it forms a stiff gel on cooling.

B: To a solution (1 in 100) add an equal volume of alcohol: a translucent, gelatinous precipitate is formed (*distinction from most gums*).

C: To 5 mL of a solution (1 in 100) add 1 mL of 2 N sodium hydroxide, and allow to stand at room temperature for 15 minutes: a gel or semigel forms (*distinction from tragacanth*).

D: Acidify the gel from the preceding test with 3 N hydrochloric acid, and shake: a voluminous, colorless, gelatinous precipitate forms, which upon boiling becomes white and flocculent (*pectic acid*).

Microbial limits ⟨61⟩—It meets the requirements of the test for absence of *Salmonella* species.

Loss on drying ⟨731⟩—Dry it at 105° for 3 hours: it loses not more than 10.0% of its weight.

Arsenic, *Method II* ⟨211⟩: 3 ppm.

Lead—Add 2.0 g of Pectin to 20 mL of nitric acid in a 250-mL conical flask, mix, and heat the contents carefully until the Pectin is dissolved. Continue the heating until the volume is reduced to about 7 mL. Cool rapidly to room temperature, transfer to a 100-mL volumetric flask, and dilute with water to volume. A 50.0-mL portion of this solution contains not more than 5 µg of lead (corresponding to not more than 0.0005% of Pb) when tested according to the limit test for *Lead* ⟨251⟩, 15 mL of ammonium citrate solution, 3 mL of potassium cyanide solution, and 500 µL of hydroxylamine hydrochloride solution being used. After the first dithizone extractions, wash the combined chloroform layers with 5 mL of water, discarding the water layer and continuing in the usual manner by extracting with 20 mL of dilute nitric acid (1 in 100).

Sugars and organic acids—Place 1 g in a 500-mL flask, moisten it with 3 to 5 mL of alcohol, pour in rapidly 100 mL of water, shake, and allow to stand until solution is complete. To this solution add 100 mL of alcohol containing 0.3 mL of hydrochloric acid, mix, and filter rapidly. Measure 25 mL of the filtrate into a tared dish, evaporate the liquid on a steam bath and dry the residue in a vacuum oven at 50° for 2 hours: the weight of the residue does not exceed 20 mg.

Organic volatile impurities, *Method IV* ⟨467⟩: meets the requirements.

(Official until July 1, 2008)

Assay for methoxy groups—Transfer 5.00 g of Pectin to a suitable beaker, and stir for 10 minutes with a mixture of 5 mL of hydrochloric acid and 100 mL of 60 percent alcohol. Transfer to a sintered-glass filter (30- to 60-mL crucible or Büchner type, coarse), and wash with six 15-mL portions of the hydrochloric acid—60 percent alcohol mixture, followed by 60 percent alcohol until the filtrate is free from chlorides. Finally wash with 20 mL of alcohol, dry for 1 hour at 105°, cool, and weigh. Transfer exactly one-tenth of the total net weight of the dried sample (representing 500 mg of the original unwashed sample) to a 250-mL conical flask, and moisten with 2 mL of alcohol. Add 100 mL of carbon dioxide-free water, insert the stopper, and swirl occasionally until the Pectin is completely dissolved. Add 5 drops of phenolphthalein TS, titrate with 0.5 N sodium hydroxide VS, and record the results as the *initial titer*. Add 20.0 mL of 0.5 N sodium hydroxide VS, insert the stopper, shake vigorously, and allow to stand for 15 minutes. Add 20.0 mL of 0.5 N hydrochloric acid VS, and shake until the pink color disappears. Add phenolphthalein TS, and titrate with 0.5 N sodium hydroxide VS to a faint pink color that persists after vigorous shaking: record this value as the *saponification titer*. Each mL of 0.5 N sodium hydroxide used in the *saponification titer* is equivalent to 15.52 mg of –OCH₃.

Assay for galacturonic acid—Each mL of 0.5 N sodium hydroxide used in the total titration (the *initial titer* added to the *saponification titer*) in the *Assay for methoxy groups* is equivalent to 97.07 mg of $C_6H_{10}O_7$.

Penbutolol Sulfate

$(C_{18}H_{29}NO_2)_2 \cdot H_2SO_4$ 680.94
2-Propanol, 1-(2-cyclopentylphenoxy)-3-[(1,1-dimethylethyl)amino]-, (*S*)-, sulfate (2 : 1) (salt).
(*S*)-1-(*tert*-Butylamino)-3-(*o*-cyclopentylphenoxy)-2-propanol sulfate (2 : 1) (salt)   [38363-32-5].

» Penbutolol Sulfate contains not less than 98.0 percent and not more than 102.0 percent of $(C_{18}H_{29}NO_2)_2 \cdot H_2SO_4$, calculated on the anhydrous basis.

Packaging and storage—Preserve in tight, light-resistant containers.

USP Reference standards ⟨11⟩—USP Penbutolol Sulfate RS.
Identification—
  A: *Infrared Absorption* ⟨197M⟩.
  B: A solution (10 mg per mL) responds to the tests for *Sulfate* ⟨191⟩.
Loss on drying ⟨731⟩—Dry it at 105° for 3 hours: it loses not more than 1.0% of its weight.
Residue on ignition ⟨281⟩:   not more than 0.2%.
Specific rotation ⟨781S⟩:   between −22° and −26°, determined at 20°.
  Test solution: 10 mg per mL, in methanol.
Chromatographic purity—
  *Organic phase—*Prepare a mixture of methanol and acetonitrile (610 : 390). Make adjustments if necessary (see *System Suitability* under *Chromatography* ⟨621⟩).
  *Aqueous phase—*Dissolve 11 g of sodium 1-heptanesulfonate in 1000 mL of water, add 5.0 mL of triethylamine, adjust with phosphoric acid to a pH of 2.70 ± 0.05, and filter through a filter having a porosity of 0.5 μm or finer. Make adjustments if necessary (see *System Suitability* under *Chromatography* ⟨621⟩).
  *Solvent mixture—*Prepare a mixture of *Organic phase* and *Aqueous phase* (600 : 400).
  *Test solution—*Transfer about 50 mg of Penbutolol Sulfate to a 25-mL volumetric flask, dissolve in and dilute with *Solvent mixture* to volume, and mix.
  *Diluted test solution—*Transfer 1.0 mL of the *Test solution* to a 100-mL volumetric flask, dilute with *Solvent mixture* to volume, and mix.
  Chromatographic system (see *Chromatography* ⟨621⟩)—The liquid chromatograph is equipped with a 271-nm detector, a preinjection guard column that contains packing L4, and a 4.6-mm × 25-cm analytical column that contains packing L1 and is maintained at a constant temperature between ambient and 40°, and is programmed to provide variable mixtures of *Organic phase* and *Aqueous phase*.

Before each injection, the system is equilibrated with a mobile phase consisting of a mixture of 60% *Organic phase* and 40% *Aqueous phase*. After each injection, this composition of the mobile phase is maintained for 15 minutes, then the proportion of *Organic phase* is increased linearly over the next 20 minutes so that the mobile phase consists of 80% *Organic phase* and 20% *Aqueous phase*. The proportion of *Organic phase* is then decreased to 60% over 1 minute. The flow rate is about 1 mL per minute. Chromatograph the *Diluted test solution*, and record the peak responses as directed for *Procedure*: the resolution, *R*, between the penbutolol peak and any impurity peak is not less than 1.5, and the tailing factor is not more than 2, when calculated by the formula:

$$W_{0.1} / 2f$$

in which $W_{0.1}$ is the width of the peak at 10% of peak height.
  Procedure—[NOTE—Use peak areas where peak responses are indicated.] Separately inject equal volumes (about 20 μL) of the *Solvent mixture*, the *Test solution*, and the *Diluted test solution* into the chromatograph, and measure the peak responses for all the peaks. Calculate the percentage of each individual impurity in the Penbutolol Sulfate taken by the formula:

$$r_i / r_D$$

in which r_i is the peak response for an individual impurity in the chromatogram of the *Test solution*, and r_D is the penbutolol peak response obtained from the *Diluted test solution*: not more than 1.2% of any impurity is found.
Assay—
  *Organic phase—*Prepare a mixture of methanol and acetonitrile (610 : 390). Make adjustments if necessary (see *System Suitability* under *Chromatography* ⟨621⟩).
  *Aqueous phase—*Dissolve 11 g of sodium 1-heptanesulfonate in 1000 mL of water, add 5.0 mL of triethylamine, adjust with phosphoric acid to a pH of 2.70 ± 0.05, and filter through a filter having a porosity of 0.5 μm or finer. Make adjustments if necessary (see *System Suitability* under *Chromatography* ⟨621⟩).
  *Mobile phase—*Prepare a mixture of *Organic phase* and *Aqueous phase* (650 : 350). Make adjustments if necessary (see *System Suitability* under *Chromatography* ⟨621⟩).
  *Internal standard solution—*Prepare a solution of 3,4-dimethylbenzophenone in *Mobile phase* containing about 0.01 mg per mL.
  *Standard preparation—*Transfer about 24 mg of USP Penbutolol Sulfate RS, accurately weighed, to a 100-mL volumetric flask, dissolve in and dilute with *Internal standard solution* to volume, and mix.
  *Assay preparation—*Transfer about 24 mg of Penbutolol Sulfate, accurately weighed, to a 100-mL volumetric flask, dissolve in and dilute with *Internal standard solution* to volume, and mix.
  Chromatographic system (see *Chromatography* ⟨621⟩)—The liquid chromatograph is equipped with a 271-nm detector and a 4.6-mm × 25-cm column that contains packing L1. The flow rate is about 1 mL per minute. Chromatograph the *Standard preparation*, and record the peak responses as directed for *Procedure*: the relative retention times are about 0.9 for penbutolol and 1.0 for 3,4-dimethylbenzophenone, and the resolution, *R*, between the penbutolol peak and the 3,4-dimethylbenzophenone peak is not less than 1.5, and the relative standard deviation for replicate injections is not more than 2.0%.
  *Procedure—*Separately inject equal volumes (about 20 μL) of the *Standard preparation* and the *Assay preparation* into the chromatograph, record the chromatograms, and measure the areas of the responses for the major peaks. Calculate the quantity, in mg, of $(C_{18}H_{29}NO_2)_2 \cdot H_2SO_4$ in the portion of Penbutolol Sulfate taken by the formula:

$$100C(R_U / R_S)$$

in which *C* is the concentration, in mg per mL, of USP Penbutolol Sulfate RS in the *Standard preparation*, and R_U and R_S are the ratios of the penbutolol peak response to the internal standard peak response obtained from the *Assay preparation* and the *Standard preparation*, respectively.

Penbutolol Sulfate Tablets

» Penbutolol Sulfate Tablets contain not less than 90.0 percent and not more than 110.0 percent of the labeled amount of $(C_{18}H_{29}NO_2)_2 \cdot H_2SO_4$.

Packaging and storage—Preserve in well-closed, light-resistant containers.

USP Reference standards ⟨11⟩—*USP Penbutolol Sulfate RS.*
Identification, *Ultraviolet Absorption* ⟨197U⟩—
  Solution: Sonicate a weighed portion of ground Tablets in sufficient methanol to obtain a solution containing about 0.4 mg of penbutolol sulfate per mL. Filter this solution, and dilute a portion of the filtrate with methanol to obtain a solution containing about 0.06 mg of penbutolol sulfate per mL.
Dissolution ⟨711⟩—
  Medium: water; 900 mL.
  Apparatus 2: 50 rpm.
  Time: 30 minutes.
  Mobile phase—Dissolve 2 g of ammonium acetate in 250 mL of water, add 750 mL of acetonitrile, mix, and adjust with glacial acetic acid to a pH of 6.0. Filter and degas. Make adjustments if necessary (see *System Suitability* under *Chromatography* ⟨621⟩).
  Standard solution—Dissolve an accurately weighed quantity of USP Penbutolol Sulfate RS quantitatively in water to obtain a stock solution having a known concentration of about 0.018 mg per mL. Mix 10.0 mL of this solution and 10.0 mL of acetonitrile, and filter through a filter having a 0.5-μm or finer porosity.
  Test solution—Filter about 30 mL of the solution under test. Mix 10.0 mL of the filtrate and 10.0 mL of acetonitrile, and filter through a filter having a 0.5-μm or finer porosity.
  Chromatographic system (see *Chromatography* ⟨621⟩)—The liquid chromatograph is equipped with a 272-nm detector, a 4.6-mm × 15-cm column that contains 5-μm diameter packing L10. The flow rate is about 2.5 mL per minute. Chromatograph the *Standard solution*, and record the peak responses as directed for *Procedure:* the relative standard deviation for replicate injections is not more than 2.5%.
  Procedure—Separately inject equal volumes (about 50 μL) of the *Standard solution* and the *Test solution* into the chromatograph, and measure the areas of the responses for the penbutolol peaks. Calculate the quantity, in mg, of $(C_{18}H_{29}NO_2)_2 \cdot H_2SO_4$ dissolved by the formula:

$$1800C(r_U / r_S)$$

in which C is the concentration, in mg per mL, of USP Penbutolol Sulfate RS in the *Standard solution*, and r_U and r_S are the penbutolol peak responses obtained from the *Test solution* and the *Standard solution*, respectively.
  Tolerances—Not less than 75% (Q) of the labeled amount of $(C_{18}H_{29}NO_2)_2 \cdot H_2SO_4$ is dissolved in 30 minutes.
Chromatographic purity—Examine the chromatogram of the *Assay preparation* obtained in the *Assay*. If an impurity peak is observed at a retention time of 0.8 relative to that of penbutolol, calculate the percentage of that impurity by the formula:

$$100r_i / r_s$$

in which r_i is the response of the impurity peak, and r_s is the sum of the responses of all of the peaks. If the percentage exceeds 1.2%, perform the following test.
  Organic phase, Aqueous phase, Solvent mixture, and *Chromatographic system*—Proceed as directed in the test for *Chromatographic purity* under *Penbutolol Sulfate.*
  Test solution—Transfer an accurately weighed portion of powdered Tablets, equivalent to about 100 mg of penbutolol sulfate, to a 50-mL volumetric flask, dilute with *Solvent mixture* to volume, mix, and filter.
  Diluted test solution—Transfer 1.0 mL of the *Test solution* to a 100-mL volumetric flask, dilute with *Solvent mixture* to volume, and mix.
  Procedure—Proceed as directed for *Procedure* in the test for *Chromatographic purity* under *Penbutolol Sulfate.* Calculate the percentage of each individual impurity in the portion of Tablets taken by the formula:

$$r_i / r_D$$

in which the terms are as defined therein: not more than 1.2% of any impurity is found.
Assay—
  Organic phase, Aqueous phase, and *Mobile phase*—Proceed as directed in the *Assay* under *Penbutolol Sulfate.*
  Standard preparation—Dissolve an accurately weighed quantity of USP Penbutolol Sulfate RS quantitatively in *Mobile phase* to obtain a solution having a known concentration of about 0.2 mg per mL.
  Resolution solution—Prepare a solution of 3,4-dimethylbenzophenone in *Standard preparation* containing about 0.01 mg of 3,4-dimethylbenzophenone per mL.
  Assay preparation—Weigh and finely powder not less than 20 Tablets. Transfer an accurately weighed portion of the powder, equivalent to about 20 mg of penbutolol sulfate, to a 100-mL volumetric flask, dilute with *Mobile phase* to volume, and mix. Sonicate for about 10 minutes, and filter a portion through a filter having a 0.5-μm or finer porosity, discarding the first 5 mL of the filtrate. Use the clear filtrate as the *Assay preparation.*
  Chromatographic system (see *Chromatography* ⟨621⟩)—The liquid chromatograph is equipped with a 270-nm detector and a 4.6-mm × 15-cm column that contains 5-μm diameter packing L1. The flow rate is about 1 mL per minute. Chromatograph the *Resolution solution*, and record the peak responses as directed for *Procedure:* the relative retention times are about 0.7 for penbutolol and 1.0 for 3,4-dimethylbenzophenone, and the tailing factor is not more than 1.4, when calculated by the formula:

$$W_{0.1} / 2f$$

in which $W_{0.1}$ is the width of the peak at 10% of peak height, the resolution, R, between the penbutolol peak and the 3,4-dimethylbenzophenone peak is not less than 5, and the relative standard deviation for replicate injections is not more than 2.0%.
  Procedure—[NOTE—Use peak areas where peak responses are indicated.] Separately inject equal volumes (about 20 μL) of the *Standard preparation* and the *Assay preparation* into the chromatograph, record the chromatograms, and measure the responses for the major peaks. Calculate the quantity, in mg, of $(C_{18}H_{29}NO_2)_2 \cdot H_2SO_4$ in the portion of Tablets taken by the formula:

$$100C(r_U / r_S)$$

in which C is the concentration, in mg per mL, of USP Penbutolol Sulfate RS in the *Standard preparation*, and r_U and r_S are the penbutolol peak responses obtained from the *Assay preparation* and the *Standard preparation*, respectively.

Penicillamine

$C_5H_{11}NO_2S$ 149.21
D-Valine, 3-mercapto-.
D-3-Mercaptovaline   [52-67-5].

» Penicillamine contains not less than 97.0 percent and not more than 102.0 percent of $C_5H_{11}NO_2S$, calculated on the dried basis.

Packaging and storage—Preserve in tight containers.

USP Reference standards ⟨11⟩—*USP Penicillamine RS. USP Penicillin G Potassium RS. USP Penicillamine Disulfide RS.*

Penicillamine / Official Monographs

Identification—
A: *Infrared Absorption* ⟨197M⟩(50 mg in 300 mg).
B: Dissolve 10 mg in 5 mL of water, and add 1 drop of 5 N sodium hydroxide and 20 mg of ninhydrin: a blue or violet-blue color is produced immediately.
C: Dissolve 20 mg in 4 mL of water, add 2 mL of phosphotungstic acid solution (1 in 10), and heat nearly to boiling: a deep blue color is produced immediately.
Specific rotation ⟨781S⟩: between −60.5° and −64.5°.
Test solution: 50 mg per mL, in 1.0 N sodium hydroxide.
pH ⟨791⟩: between 4.5 and 5.5, in a solution (1 in 100).
Loss on drying ⟨731⟩—Dry about 100 mg, accurately weighed, in a capillary-stoppered bottle in vacuum at a pressure not exceeding 5 mm of mercury at 60° for 3 hours: it loses not more than 0.5% of its weight.
Residue on ignition ⟨281⟩: not more than 0.1%, the charred residue being moistened with 2 mL of nitric acid and 5 drops of sulfuric acid.
Heavy metals, *Method II* ⟨231⟩: not more than 0.002%.
Limit of penicillin activity—
pH 2.5 Buffer—Dissolve 100 g of monobasic potassium phosphate in water, add 0.2 mL of hydrochloric acid, dilute with water to 1000 mL, and mix. Adjust, if necessary, with phosphoric acid or with 10 N potassium hydroxide to a pH of 2.5.
Standard preparation—Prepare as directed for Penicillin G in Table 2 under *Antibiotics—Microbial Assays* ⟨81⟩, except to prepare a final stock solution containing 100 Penicillin G Units per mL and six test dilutions ranging from 0.005 Penicillin G Unit per mL to 0.2 Penicillin G Unit per mL, and to use a median dose of the Standard of 0.050 Penicillin G Unit per mL.
Test preparation—Dissolve 1.0 g in water to make 18.0 mL, transfer 9.0 mL of this solution to a separator, add 20 mL of amyl acetate and 1 mL of *pH 2.5 Buffer*, and shake. Allow the layers to separate, and draw off the aqueous layer into a second separator, retaining the amyl acetate extract in the first separator. Check the pH of the aqueous layer, and if it is greater than 3.0 adjust it with hydrochloric acid to a pH of 2.5, and extract with 20 mL of amyl acetate. Discard the aqueous layer, and add the amyl acetate extract to the first separator. Wash the combined amyl acetate extracts with 10 mL of diluted *pH 2.5 Buffer* (1 in 10), and discard the aqueous layer. Extract the amyl acetate with 10.0 mL of *Buffer No. 1* (see *Phosphate Buffers and Other Solutions* in the section *Media and Diluents* under *Antibiotics—Microbial Assays* ⟨81⟩). Use a portion of the buffer extract as *Test solution A*. To a 5-mL portion of the extract add 0.1 mL of penicillinase solution, and incubate at 36° to 37.5° for 60 minutes (*Test solution B*).
Preparation of inoculum—Prepare as directed under *Antibiotics—Microbial Assays* ⟨81⟩, using *Micrococcus luteus* (ATCC 9341) as the test organism, and an inoculum that gives clear sharp zones of inhibition 17 mm to 21 mm in diameter with the median dose level of the Standard.
Procedure—Proceed as directed for the *Cylinder-Plate Method* under *Antibiotics—Microbial Assays* ⟨81⟩, using 10 mL of Medium 1 for the base layer and 4 mL of inoculated Medium 4 for the seed layer, and incubating the plates at 29° to 31°, except on each test plate to fill 2 cylinders with *Test solution A*, 2 cylinders with *Test solution B*, and 2 cylinders with the median dose of the Standard. If *Test solution A* yields no zone of inhibition, the test is negative for penicillin. If *Test solution A* yields a zone of inhibition and *Test solution B* does not, penicillin is present. Determine its level from the standard curve: not more than 0.01 Penicillin G Unit is found in each mL of *Test solution A* (0.2 Penicillin G Unit per g).
Mercury—
NOTE—Mercuric dithizonate is light-sensitive. Perform this test in subdued light.
Dithizone stock solution—Dissolve 40 mg of dithizone in 1000 mL of chloroform.
Dithizone titrant—Dilute 30.0 mL of *Dithizone stock solution* with chloroform to 100.0 mL. This solution contains approximately 12 mg of dithizone per L.
Standard solution—Transfer 135.4 mg of mercuric chloride to a 100-mL volumetric flask, add 0.25 N sulfuric acid to volume, and mix. This solution contains the equivalent of 100 mg of Hg in 100 mL.

Diluted standard solution—Pipet 2 mL of *Standard solution* into a 100-mL volumetric flask, add 0.25 N sulfuric acid to volume, and mix. Each mL of this solution contains the equivalent of 20 µg of Hg.
Standardization—Pipet 1 mL of *Diluted standard solution* into a 250-mL separator, and add 100 mL of 0.25 N sulfuric acid, 90 mL of water, and 10 mL of hydroxylamine hydrochloride solution (1 in 5). Then add 1 mL of edetate disodium solution (1 in 50), 1 mL of glacial acetic acid, and 5 mL of chloroform, shake for 1 minute, allow to separate, and discard the chloroform layer. To the solution add *Dithizone titrant*, in portions of 0.3 mL to 0.5 mL, from a 10-mL buret. After each addition, shake the mixture 20 times, and allow the chloroform layer to separate and discard it. Continue until an addition of *Dithizone titrant* remains green after the shaking. Calculate the quantity, in µg, of mercury equivalent to 1 mL of *Dithizone titrant* by dividing 20 by the number of mL of *Dithizone titrant* added.
Procedure—Transfer 500 mg of Penicillamine to a 650-mL Kjeldahl flask containing a few glass beads, incline the flask at an angle of about 45°, and add 2.5 mL of nitric acid through a small funnel placed in the mouth of the flask. Allow the mixture to stand at room temperature until nitrous oxide fumes are evolved and vigorous reaction subsides (5 to 30 minutes). Add 2.5 mL of sulfuric acid through the funnel, and heat, gently at first and then to the production of fumes of sulfur trioxide, then cool. Cautiously add 2.5 mL of nitric acid, again heat to the production of sulfur trioxide fumes, and cool. Repeat the treatment with nitric acid and heat, then cool, and cautiously add 50 mL of water, rinsing the funnel and collecting the rinsings in the flask. Remove the funnel, boil the solution down to approximately half its volume (about 25 mL), and cool to room temperature. Transfer to a 250-mL separator with the aid of water, and add water to make about 50 mL. Add 1 mL of edetate disodium solution (1 in 50) and 1 mL of glacial acetic acid, and extract with small portions of chloroform until the last chloroform extract remains colorless. Discard the chloroform extract, and add 50 mL of 0.25 N sulfuric acid, 90 mL of water, and 10 mL of hydroxylamine hydrochloride solution (1 in 5). Add *Dithizone titrant*, in portions of 0.3 mL to 0.5 mL, from a 10-mL buret. After each addition, shake the mixture 20 times, and allow the chloroform layer to separate and discard it. Continue until an addition of *Dithizone titrant* remains green after the shaking. Calculate the amount of mercury present: the limit is 10 µg (0.002%).
Limit of penicillamine disulfide—
Diluent, Mobile phase, and *Resolution solution*—Prepare as directed in the *Assay.*
Standard preparation—Dissolve an accurately weighed quantity of USP Penicillamine Disulfide RS in *Diluent* to obtain a solution having a known concentration of about 0.025 mg per mL.
Test preparation—Use the *Assay preparation*.
Chromatographic system—Proceed as directed in the *Assay*. Chromatograph the *Standard preparation*, and record the penicillamine disulfide peak responses as directed for *Procedure:* the relative standard deviation for replicate injections is not more than 2.0%.
Procedure—[NOTE—Use peak areas where peak responses are indicated.] Separately inject equal volumes (about 20 µL) of the *Standard preparation* and the *Test preparation* into the chromatograph, record the chromatograms, and measure the responses for the penicillamine disulfide peaks. Calculate the percentage of penicillamine disulfide ($C_{10}H_{20}N_2O_4S_2$) in the Penicillamine taken by the formula:

$$100C(r_U / r_S)$$

in which C is the concentration, in mg per mL, of USP Penicillamine Disulfide RS in the *Standard preparation*, and r_U and r_S are the penicillamine disulfide peak responses obtained from the *Test preparation* and the *Standard preparation*, respectively: not more than 1.0% of penicillamine disulfide is found.
Assay—
Diluent—Dissolve 1.0 g of edetate disodium in water to make 1000 mL of solution.
Mobile phase—Dissolve 6.9 g of monobasic sodium phosphate and 0.20 g of sodium 1-hexanesulfonate in water to make 1000 mL of solution. Adjust with phosphoric acid to a pH of 3.0 ± 0.1, and filter through a suitable filter of 1 µm or finer porosity. Make adjustments if necessary (see *System Suitability* under *Chromatography* ⟨621⟩).

Resolution solution—Prepare a solution in *Diluent* containing about 1 mg of USP Penicillamine RS and 0.1 mg of USP Penicillamine Disulfide RS per mL.

Standard preparation—Dissolve an accurately weighed quantity of USP Penicillamine RS in *Diluent* to obtain a solution having a concentration of about 1.25 mg per mL.

Assay preparation—Transfer about 125 mg of Penicillamine, accurately weighed, to a 100-mL volumetric flask, dissolve in and dilute with *Diluent* to volume, and mix.

Chromatographic system (see *Chromatography* ⟨621⟩)—The liquid chromatograph is equipped with a 210-nm detector and a 3.9-mm × 30-cm column containing packing L1. The flow rate is about 1.6 mL per minute. Chromatograph the *Resolution solution*, and record the responses as directed for *Procedure*: the relative retention times are about 0.7 for penicillamine and 1.0 for penicillamine disulfide, and the resolution, *R*, between the penicillamine peak and the penicillamine disulfide peak is not less than 3.0. Chromatograph the *Standard preparation*, and record the responses as directed for *Procedure*: the relative standard deviation for replicate injections is not more than 1.0%.

Procedure—[NOTE—Use peak areas where peak responses are indicated.] Separately inject equal volumes (about 20 µL) of the *Standard preparation* and the *Assay preparation* into the chromatograph, record the chromatograms, and measure the responses for the major peaks. Calculate the quantity, in mg, of penicillamine ($C_5H_{11}NO_2S$) in the portion of Penicillamine taken by the formula:

$$100C(r_U / r_S)$$

in which *C* is the concentration, in mg per mL, of USP Penicillamine RS in the *Standard preparation*, and r_U and r_S are the penicillamine peak responses obtained from the *Assay preparation* and the *Standard preparation*, respectively.

Penicillamine Capsules

» Penicillamine Capsules contain not less than 90.0 percent and not more than 110.0 percent of the labeled amount of $C_5H_{11}NO_2S$.

Packaging and storage—Preserve in tight containers.

USP Reference standards ⟨11⟩—USP Penicillamine RS. USP Penicillamine Disulfide RS.

Identification—The contents of the Capsules respond to *Identification* test A under *Penicillamine Tablets* and to *Identification* test C under *Penicillamine*.

Dissolution ⟨711⟩—
  Medium: 0.1 N hydrochloric acid; 900 mL.
  Apparatus 1: 100 rpm.
  Time: 30 minutes.
  PROCEDURE FOR A POOLED SAMPLE—
  Dilute hydrochloric acid—Dilute 37 mL of hydrochloric acid with water to 1 L.
  Ammonium sulfamate reagent—Dissolve 250 mg of ammonium sulfamate in 100 mL of *Dilute hydrochloric acid*.
  N-(1-Naphthyl)ethylenediamine dihydrochloride reagent—Dissolve 100 mg of N-(1-naphthyl)ethylenediamine dihydrochloride in 100 mL of *Dilute hydrochloric acid*.
  Sulfanilamide–mercuric chloride reagent—Dissolve 100 mg of sulfanilamide and 100 mg of mercuric chloride in 100 mL of *Dilute hydrochloric acid*.
  Sodium nitrite reagent—Dissolve 200 mg of sodium nitrite in 100 mL of dilute sulfuric acid (1 in 50). Prepare fresh.
  Standard solution—Dissolve an accurately weighed quantity of USP Penicillamine RS in 0.1 N hydrochloric acid to obtain a solution having a known concentration of about 250 µg per mL.
  Procedure—Pipet an aliquot of the filtered test solution, estimated to contain about 278 µg of penicillamine, into a 100-mL volumetric flask. Into a similar flask pipet an equivalent volume of 0.1 N hydrochloric acid to provide a reagent blank, and into a third 100-mL volumetric flask pipet 1 mL of *Standard solution*. Treat each flask as follows. Add by pipet 3 mL of *Sodium nitrite reagent*, and mix by swirling occasionally. After 5 minutes, add 10 mL of *Ammonium sulfamate reagent*, swirl, and allow to stand for an additional 5 minutes. Add 5 mL of *Sulfanilamide–mercuric chloride reagent*, swirl, and immediately add 10 mL of *N-(1-Naphthyl)ethylenediamine dihydrochloride reagent*. Dilute with water to volume, and mix. Determine the absorbances of both solutions in 1-cm cells at the wavelength of maximum absorbance at about 540 nm, with a suitable spectrophotometer, against the reagent blank. Calculate the percentage dissolution of the Capsule taken by the formula:

$$90(C/WV)(A_U / A_S)$$

in which *C* is the concentration, in µg per mL, of USP Penicillamine RS in the *Standard solution*; *W* is the labeled quantity, in mg, of penicillamine in the Capsule; *V* is the volume, in mL, of the aliquot of test solution used; and A_U and A_S are the absorbances of the solutions from the test solution and the *Standard solution*, respectively.

Tolerances—Not less than 80% (*Q*) of the labeled amount of $C_5H_{11}NO_2S$ is dissolved in 30 minutes.

PROCEDURE FOR A UNIT SAMPLE —
  Buffer solution—Prepare a 50-mM solution of monobasic potassium phosphate buffer, pH 3.0.
  Mobile phase—Prepare a filtered and degassed mixture of *Buffer solution* and methanol (97 : 3). Make adjustments if necessary (see *System Suitability* under *Chromatography* ⟨621⟩).
  Standard solution—Prepare a solution of USP Penicillamine RS in 0.1 N hydrochloric acid having a known concentration corresponding to the content of 1 Capsule dissolved in 900 mL of *Medium*.
  Resolution solution—Prepare a solution of USP Penicillamine Disulfide RS in 0.1 N hydrochloric acid having a known concentration of about 0.002 mg per mL.
  Test solution—Proceed as directed for *Procedure for Capsules, Uncoated Tablets, and Plain Coated Tablets* under *Dissolution* ⟨711⟩. After 30 minutes, withdraw about 10 mL of solution from each vessel, and immediately pass each aliquot through a 0.45-µm polyvinylidene difluoride filter paper. Discard the first 2 mL of filtered solution, and chromatograph the remaining filtrate.
  Chromatographic system (see *Chromatography* ⟨621⟩)—The liquid chromatograph is equipped with a 210-nm detector and a 4.6-mm × 15-cm column that contains 5-µm packing L1. The flow rate is about 1.0 mL per minute. Chromatograph the *Standard solution*, and record the peak responses as directed for *Procedure*: the tailing factor is not more than 2.0, and the relative standard deviation for replicate injections is not more than 2.0%. Chromatograph the *Resolution solution*, and record the peak responses as directed for *Procedure*: the resolution, *R*, between penicillamine and penicillamine disulfide is not less than 2.0.
  Procedure—Separately inject equal volumes (about 30 µL) of the *Standard solution* and the *Test solution* into the chromatograph, record the chromatograms, and measure the responses for the major peaks. Calculate the amount, in percentage, of $C_5H_{11}NO_2S$ released by the formula:

$$\frac{r_U \times C_S \times 900 \times 100}{r_S \times LC}$$

in which r_U and r_S are the peak areas obtained from the *Test solution* and the *Standard solution*, respectively; C_S is the concentration, in mg per mL, of the *Standard solution*; 900 is the volume, in mL, of *Medium*; 100 is the conversion factor to percentage; and *LC* is the label claim, in mg, for each Capsule.

Tolerances—Not less than 80% (*Q*) of the labeled amount of $C_5H_{11}NO_2S$ is dissolved in 30 minutes.

Uniformity of dosage units ⟨905⟩:   meet the requirements.

Loss on drying ⟨731⟩—Dry about 100 mg of Capsule contents, accurately weighed, in a capillary-stoppered bottle in vacuum at a pressure not exceeding 5 mm of mercury at 60° for 3 hours: it loses not more than 1.0% of its weight.

Limit of penicillamine disulfide—
  Diluent, Mobile phase, and *Resolution solution*—Proceed as directed in the *Assay* under *Penicillamine*

Standard preparation—Dissolve an accurately weighed quantity of USP Penicillamine Disulfide RS in *Diluent* to obtain a solution having a known concentration of about 0.025 mg per mL.

Test preparation—Use the *Assay preparation*.

Chromatographic system—Proceed as directed in the *Assay* under *Penicillamine*. Chromatograph the *Standard preparation*, and record the penicillamine disulfide peak responses as directed for *Procedure*: the relative standard deviation for replicate injections is not more than 2.0%.

Procedure—[NOTE—Use peak areas where peak responses are indicated.] Separately inject equal volumes (about 20 µL) of the *Standard preparation* and the *Test preparation* into the chromatograph, record the chromatograms, and measure the responses for the penicillamine disulfide peaks. Calculate the percentage of penicillamine disulfide ($C_{10}H_{20}N_2O_4S_2$) in the Capsules taken by the formula:

$$100(C/L)(V/N)(r_U / r_S)$$

in which C is the concentration, in mg per mL, of USP Penicillamine Disulfide RS in the *Standard preparation*; L is the quantity, in mg, of penicillamine in each Capsule based on the labeled amount; V is the volume, in mL, of the volumetric flask used to prepare the *Assay preparation* in the *Assay*; N is the number of Capsules used to prepare the *Assay preparation* in the *Assay*; and r_U and r_S are the penicillamine disulfide peak responses obtained from the *Test preparation* and the *Standard preparation*, respectively: not more than 2.0% of penicillamine disulfide is found.

Assay—

Diluent, Mobile phase, Resolution solution, Standard preparation, and *Chromatographic system*—Proceed as directed in the *Assay* under *Penicillamine*.

Assay preparation—Carefully open and transfer the contents of not fewer than 10 Capsules, accurately counted, to a suitable volumetric flask of such volume that when treated as described below, a solution is obtained that contains about 1.25 mg of penicillamine per mL. Add the empty Capsule shells to the flask, and add sufficient *Diluent* to the flask to fill it to about three-fourths of its capacity. Shake for 1 minute, and allow the mixture to stand for 90 minutes. Dilute with *Diluent* to volume, and mix. Filter a portion of this solution through a suitable filter of 1 µm or finer porosity, and use the clear filtrate as the *Assay preparation*.

Procedure—Proceed as directed for *Procedure* in the *Assay* under *Penicillamine*. Calculate the quantity, in mg, of penicillamine ($C_5H_{11}NO_2S$) in each Capsule taken by the formula:

$$C(V/N)(r_U / r_S)$$

in which C is the concentration, in mg per mL, of USP Penicillamine RS in the *Standard preparation*; V is the volume, in mL, of the volumetric flask used to prepare the *Assay preparation*; N is the number of Capsules used to prepare the *Assay preparation*; and r_U and r_S are the penicillamine peak responses obtained from the *Assay preparation* and the *Standard preparation*, respectively.

Penicillamine Tablets

» Penicillamine Tablets contain not less than 90.0 percent and not more than 110.0 percent of the labeled amount of $C_5H_{11}NO_2S$.

Packaging and storage—Preserve in tight containers.

USP Reference standards 〈11〉—USP Penicillamine RS. USP Penicillamine Disulfide RS.

Identification—

A: Transfer a portion of finely powdered Tablets, equivalent to about 100 mg of penicillamine, to a 10-mL volumetric flask, dilute with methanol to volume, add 2 drops of 3 N hydrochloric acid, mix, and filter. Use the filtrate as the test solution. Prepare a Standard solution by dissolving 100 mg of USP Penicillamine RS in 10 mL of methanol, adding 2 drops of 3 N hydrochloric acid, and mixing. Separately apply 10-µL portions of the test solution and the Standard solution to a suitable thin-layer chromatographic plate (see *Chromatography* 〈621〉) coated with a 0.25-mm layer of chromatographic silica gel mixture, heated at 105° for 30 minutes, and allowed to cool before use. Allow the spots to dry, and develop the chromatogram in a solvent system consisting of a mixture of butyl alcohol, glacial acetic acid, and water (8:2:2) until the solvent front has moved about three-fourths of the length of the plate. Remove the plate, mark the solvent front, allow the solvent to evaporate, and place the plate in an atmosphere of iodine vapors. After a few minutes, spray the plate with a 1 in 300 solution of ninhydrin in dehydrated alcohol, heat it at 105° for about 10 minutes, allow it to cool, and examine it: the R_F values, colors, and intensities of the principal spots obtained from the test solution correspond to those obtained from the Standard solution.

B: A portion of powdered Tablets responds to *Identification* test C under *Penicillamine*.

Dissolution 〈711〉—

Medium: 0.5% edetate disodium and 0.05% sodium lauryl sulfate solution; 900 mL.

Apparatus 1: 100 rpm.

Time: 60 minutes.

Mobile phase—Prepare a filtered and degassed solution of 0.01 M dibasic sodium phosphate and 0.01 M monobasic potassium phosphate (60:40). If necessary, adjust the solution by the addition of 0.01 M dibasic sodium phosphate or 0.01 M monobasic potassium phosphate to a pH of 7.0 ± 0.1.

Standard solution—Prepare a solution of USP Penicillamine RS in 0.5% edetate disodium and 0.05% sodium lauryl sulfate solution having an accurately known concentration of about 0.28 mg per mL.

Chromatographic system (see *Chromatography* 〈621〉)—The liquid chromatograph is equipped with a 254-nm detector and a 3.9-mm × 30-cm column that contains packing L1. The flow rate is about 1 mL per minute. Chromatograph replicate injections of the *Standard solution*, and record the peak responses as directed for *Procedure*: the relative standard deviation is not more than 2.0%, and the resolution factor between the solvent peak and penicillamine is not less than 1.5.

Procedure—Separately inject equal volumes (about 80 µL) of the *Standard solution* and a filtered portion of the solution under test into the chromatograph, record the chromatograms, measure the responses for the major peaks, and calculate the amount of $C_5H_{11}NO_2S$ dissolved per Tablet.

Tolerances—Not less than 80% (*Q*) of the labeled amount of $C_5H_{11}NO_2S$ is dissolved in 60 minutes.

Uniformity of dosage units 〈905〉: meet the requirements.

Loss on drying 〈731〉—Dry about 100 mg of finely ground Tablets, accurately weighed, in a capillary-stoppered bottle in vacuum at a pressure not exceeding 5 mm of mercury at 60° for 3 hours: it loses not more than 3.0% of its weight.

Penicillamine disulfide—

Diluent—Prepare as directed in the *Assay*.

Mobile phase, Resolution solution, and *Chromatographic system*—Proceed as directed in the *Assay* under *Penicillamine*.

Standard preparation—Dissolve an accurately weighed quantity of USP Penicillamine Disulfide RS in *Diluent* to obtain a solution having a known concentration of about 0.025 mg per mL.

Test preparation—Use the *Assay preparation*.

Chromatographic system—Proceed as directed in the *Assay* under *Penicillamine*. Chromatograph the *Standard preparation*, and record the penicillamine disulfide peak responses as directed for *Procedure*: the relative standard deviation for replicate injections is not more than 2.0%.

Procedure—[NOTE—Use peak areas where peak responses are indicated.] Separately inject equal volumes (about 20 µL) of the *Standard preparation* and the *Test preparation* into the chromatograph, record the chromatograms, and measure the responses for the penicillamine disulfide peaks. Calculate the percentage of penicillamine disulfide ($C_{10}H_{20}N_2O_4S_2$) in the portion of Tablets taken by the formula:

$$20{,}000(C / L)(r_U / r_S)$$

in which C is the concentration, in mg per mL, of USP Penicillamine Disulfide RS in the *Standard preparation*, L is the quantity, in mg, of penicillamine in each Tablet based on the labeled amount, and r_U and r_S are the penicillamine disulfide peak responses obtained from the *Test preparation* and the *Standard preparation*, respectively: not more than 3.0% of penicillamine disulfide is found.

Assay—

Diluent—Dissolve 5.0 g of edetate disodium in water to make 1000 mL of solution.

Mobile phase, Resolution solution, and *Chromatographic system*—Proceed as directed in the *Assay* under *Penicillamine*.

Standard preparation—Dissolve an accurately weighed quantity of USP Penicillamine RS in *Diluent* to obtain a solution having a known concentration of about 1.25 mg per mL.

Assay preparation—Weigh and finely powder not less than 20 Tablets. Transfer an accurately weighed portion of the powder, equivalent to about 250 mg of penicillamine, to a 200-mL volumetric flask, add about 150 mL of *Diluent*, shake for 5 minutes, and allow the mixture to stand for 90 minutes. Dilute with *Diluent* to volume, and mix. Filter a portion of this solution through a suitable filter of 1 µm or finer porosity, and use the clear filtrate as the *Assay preparation*.

Procedure—Proceed as directed for *Procedure* in the *Assay* under *Penicillamine*. Calculate the quantity, in mg, of penicillamine ($C_5H_{11}NO_2S$) in the portion of Tablets taken by the formula:

$$200C(r_U/r_S)$$

in which C is the concentration, in mg per mL, of USP Penicillamine RS in the *Standard preparation*, and r_U and r_S are the penicillamine peak responses obtained from the *Assay preparation* and the *Standard preparation*, respectively.

Penicillin G, Neomycin, Polymyxin B, Hydrocortisone Acetate, and Hydrocortisone Sodium Succinate Topical Suspension

» Penicillin G, Neomycin, Polymyxin B, Hydrocortisone Acetate, and Hydrocortisone Sodium Succinate Topical Suspension is a suspension of Penicillin G Procaine, Neomycin Sulfate, Polymyxin B Sulfate, Hydrocortisone Acetate, and Hydrocortisone Sodium Succinate in a suitable vehicle. It contains not less than 90.0 percent and not more than 140.0 percent of the labeled amounts of neomycin, penicillin G, and polymyxin B, and not less than 90.0 percent and not more than 110.0 percent of the labeled amounts of hydrocortisone acetate ($C_{23}H_{32}O_6$) and hydrocortisone sodium succinate ($C_{25}H_{33}NaO_8$).

Packaging and storage—Preserve in well-closed containers.

Labeling—Label Topical Suspension to indicate that it is for veterinary use only.

USP Reference standards ⟨11⟩—*USP Neomycin Sulfate RS. USP Penicillin G Potassium RS. USP Polymyxin B Sulfate RS. USP Hydrocortisone Acetate RS. USP Hydrocortisone Hemisuccinate RS.*

Identification—

A: Using a similar portion of Topical Suspension, proceed as directed in *Identification* test *B* under *Neomycin and Polymyxin B Sulfates Cream:* the indicated result is obtained.

B: It responds to the *Identification* test under *Penicillin G Procaine Intramammary Infusion*.

C: The chromatogram of the *Assay preparation* obtained as directed in the *Assay for hydrocortisone acetate and hydrocortisone sodium succinate* exhibits major peaks for hydrocortisone acetate and hydrocortisone sodium succinate, the retention times of which, relative to that of the internal standard, correspond to those for hydrocortisone acetate and hydrocortisone hemisuccinate exhibited in the chromatogram of the *Standard preparation* obtained as directed in the *Assay for hydrocortisone acetate and hydrocortisone sodium succinate*.

Water, *Method I* ⟨921⟩: not more than 1.0%, 20 mL of a mixture of toluene and methanol (7 : 3) being used in place of methanol in the titration vessel.

Assay for penicillin G—Proceed with the Topical Suspension as directed in the *Assay for penicillin G* under *Penicillin G Procaine, Neomycin and Polymyxin B Sulfates, and Hydrocortisone Acetate Topical Suspension*.

Assay for neomycin—Proceed with the Topical Suspension as directed in the *Assay for neomycin* under *Penicillin G Procaine, Neomycin and Polymyxin B Sulfates, and Hydrocortisone Acetate Topical Suspension*.

Assay for polymyxin B—Proceed with the Topical Suspension as directed in the *Assay for polymyxin B* under *Penicillin G Procaine, Neomycin and Polymyxin B Sulfates, and Hydrocortisone Acetate Topical Suspension*.

Assay for hydrocortisone acetate and hydrocortisone sodium succinate—

Mobile phase—Prepare a filtered and degassed mixture of butyl chloride, water-saturated butyl chloride, tetrahydrofuran, methanol, and glacial acetic acid (544 : 544 : 58 : 29 : 25). Make adjustments if necessary (see *System Suitability* under *Chromatography* ⟨621⟩).

Extraction solution—Prepare a mixture of chloroform and glacial acetic acid (1000 : 30).

Internal standard solution—Prepare a solution in tetrahydrofuran containing about 1.4 mg of methylprednisolone per mL.

Standard preparation—Transfer about 7.5 mg of USP Hydrocortisone Acetate RS, accurately weighed, and 7.5J mg of USP Hydrocortisone Hemisuccinate RS, accurately weighed, to a conical flask, *J* being the ratio of the labeled amount, in mg, of hydrocortisone sodium succinate to the labeled amount, in mg, of hydrocortisone acetate in the Topical Suspension. Add 5.0 mL of *Internal standard solution* and about 95 mL of *Extraction solution*, and mix.

Resolution solution—Dissolve about 3.7 mg of penicillin G procaine in 10 mL of *Standard preparation*.

Assay preparation—Transfer an accurately measured portion of well-mixed Topical Suspension, equivalent to about 7.5 mg of hydrocortisone acetate, to a conical flask. Add 5.0 mL of *Internal standard solution* and about 95 mL of *Extraction solution*, and shake by mechanical means for about 15 minutes. Centrifuge a portion of this mixture, and use the clear supernatant as the *Assay preparation*.

Chromatographic system (see *Chromatography* ⟨621⟩)—The liquid chromatograph is equipped with a 254-nm detector, a guard column containing packing L3, and a 3.9-mm × 30-cm analytical column that contains packing L3. The flow rate is about 1 mL per minute. Chromatograph the *Resolution solution*, and measure the peak responses as directed for *Procedure:* the relative retention times for penicillin G procaine, hydrocortisone acetate, hydrocortisone hemisuccinate, and methylprednisone are about 0.3, 0.4, 0.7, and 1.0, respectively, and the resolution, *R*, between penicillin G procaine and hydrocortisone acetate is not less than 1.5. Chromatograph the *Standard preparation*, and record the peak responses as directed for *Procedure:* the relative standard deviation of the ratios of the hydrocortisone acetate peak to the internal standard peak and the hydrocortisone sodium succinate peak to the internal standard peak is not more than 2%.

Procedure—Separately inject equal volumes (about 20 µL) of the *Standard preparation* and the *Assay preparation* into the chromatograph, record the chromatograms, and measure the responses for the major peaks. Calculate the quantity, in mg, of hydrocortisone acetate in the portion of Topical Suspension taken by the formula:

$$W(R_U/R_S)$$

in which *W* is the quantity, in mg, of USP Hydrocortisone Acetate RS taken to prepare the *Standard preparation*, and R_U and R_S are the ratios of the hydrocortisone acetate peak response to the internal standard peak response obtained from the *Assay preparation* and the *Standard preparation*, respectively. Calculate the quantity, in mg, of hydrocortisone sodium succinate in the portion of Topical Suspension taken by the formula:

$$(484.52 / 462.54)(W)(R_U / R_S)$$

in which 484.52 and 462.54 are the molecular weights of hydrocortisone sodium succinate and anhydrous hydrocortisone hemisuccinate, respectively, W is the quantity, in mg, of USP Hydrocortisone Hemisuccinate RS taken to prepare the *Standard preparation*, and R_U and R_S are the ratios of the hydrocortisone hemisuccinate peak response to the internal standard peak response obtained from the *Assay preparation* and the *Standard preparation*, respectively.

Penicillin G Benzathine

$(C_{16}H_{18}N_2O_4S)_2 \cdot C_{16}H_{20}N_2 \cdot 4H_2O$ 981.19
4-Thia-1-azabicyclo[3.2.0]heptane-2-carboxylic acid, 3,3-dimethyl-7-oxo-6-[(phenylacetyl)amino-], 2[S-(2α,5α,6β)]-, compd. with N,N'-bis(phenylmethyl)-1,2-ethanediamine (2 : 1), tetrahydrate.
(2S,5R,6R)-3,3-Dimethyl-7-oxo-6-(2-phenylacetamido)-4-thia-1-azabicyclo[3.2.0]heptane-2-carboxylic acid compound with N,N'-dibenzylethylenediamine (2 : 1), tetrahydrate   [41372-02-5].
Anhydrous   909.15   [1538-09-6].

» Penicillin G Benzathine has a potency of not less than 1090 Penicillin G Units and not more than 1272 Penicillin G Units per mg.

Packaging and storage—Preserve in tight containers.
Labeling—Where it is intended for use in preparing injectable dosage forms, the label states that it is sterile or must be subjected to further processing during the preparation of injectable dosage forms.
USP Reference standards ⟨11⟩—*USP Endotoxin RS. USP Penicillin G Benzathine RS. USP Penicillin G Potassium RS.*
Identification, *Ultraviolet Absorption* ⟨197U⟩—
    Solution: 500 µg per mL.
    Medium: methanol.
    Absorptivity at 263 nm is between 85.0% and 110.0% of that of USP Penicillin G Benzathine RS.
Crystallinity ⟨695⟩: meets the requirements.
Bacterial endotoxins ⟨85⟩—Where the label states that Penicillin G Benzathine is sterile or that it must be subjected to further processing during the preparation of injectable dosage forms it contains not more than 0.01 USP Endotoxin Unit per 100 Penicillin G Units.
Sterility ⟨71⟩—Where the label states that Penicillin G Benzathine is sterile it meets the requirements when tested as directed in the section *Direct Inoculation of the Culture Medium* under *Test for Sterility of the Product to be Examined*, except to use Fluid Thioglycollate Medium and Soybean–Casein Digest Medium containing polysorbate 80 solution (1 in 200) and an amount of sterile penicillinase sufficient to inactivate the penicillin G in each tube, and to shake the vessels once daily.
pH ⟨791⟩: between 4.0 and 6.5, in a solution prepared by dissolving 50 mg in 50 mL of dehydrated alcohol, adding 50 mL of water, and mixing.
Water, *Method I* ⟨921⟩: between 5.0% and 8.0%.
Benzathine content—To about 1 g of Penicillin G Benzathine, accurately weighed, add 30 mL of a saturated solution of sodium chloride and 10 mL of 5 N sodium hydroxide, and extract with four 50-mL portions of ether. Wash the combined ether extracts with three 10-mL portions of water. Extract the combined water washings with 25 mL of ether, and add the ether extract to the water-washed combined ether extracts. Evaporate this combined ether solution to a volume of about 5 mL, add 2 mL of dehydrated alcohol, and evaporate to dryness. Dissolve the residue in 50 mL of glacial acetic acid, add 1 mL of *p*-naphtholbenzein TS, and titrate with 0.1 N perchloric acid VS to a green endpoint. Perform a blank determination, and make any necessary correction. Each mL of 0.1 N perchloric acid is equivalent to 12.02 mg of benzathine ($C_{16}H_{20}N_2$): between 24.0% and 27.0% of benzathine in Penicillin G Benzathine, calculated on the anhydrous basis, is found.
Assay—
    0.05 M phosphate buffer, pH 6.0—Dissolve 6.8 g of monobasic potassium phosphate in 900 mL of water, adjust with 1 N sodium hydroxide to a pH of 6.0, dilute with water to 1000 mL, and mix.
    Mobile phase—Prepare a mixture of *0.05 M phosphate buffer, pH 6.0* and acetonitrile (4 : 1), pass through a membrane filter having a 5-µm or finer porosity, and degas. Make adjustments if necessary (see *System Suitability* under *Chromatography* ⟨621⟩).
    Standard preparation—Transfer about 40 mg of USP Penicillin G Potassium RS, accurately weighed, to a 50-mL volumetric flask, add 10 mL of acetonitrile and 5 mL of methanol, and swirl to dissolve. Without delay, dilute with *0.05 M phosphate buffer, pH 6.0* to volume, and mix.
    System suitability preparation—Prepare a solution of penicillin V potassium in *Mobile phase* containing about 1 mg per mL. Mix equal volumes of this solution and the *Standard preparation*.
    Assay preparation—Transfer about 53 mg of Penicillin G Benzathine, accurately weighed, to a 50-mL volumetric flask, add 10 mL of acetonitrile and 5 mL of methanol, and swirl to dissolve. Without delay, dilute with *0.05 M phosphate buffer, pH 6.0* to volume, and mix.
    Chromatographic system (see *Chromatography* ⟨621⟩)—The liquid chromatograph is equipped with a 225-nm detector and a 4-mm × 30-cm column that contains packing L1. The flow rate is about 2 mL per minute. Chromatograph the *Standard preparation* and the *System suitability preparation*, and record the peak responses as directed for *Procedure*: the relative retention times are about 0.7 for penicillin G and 1.0 for penicillin V; the resolution, R, between penicillin G and penicillin V is not less than 2.0; the column efficiency determined from the analyte peak is not less than 600 theoretical plates; and the relative standard deviation for replicate injections of the *Standard preparation* is not more than 1.0%.
    Procedure—Separately inject equal volumes (about 10 µL) of the *Standard preparation* and the *Assay preparation* into the chromatograph, record the chromatograms, and measure the responses for the major peaks. Calculate the potency, in Penicillin G Units per mg, of the Penicillin G Benzathine taken by the formula:

$$50(CP / W)(r_U / r_S)$$

in which C is the concentration, in mg per mL, of USP Penicillin G Potassium RS in the *Standard preparation*; P is the stated potency, in Penicillin G Units per mg, of USP Penicillin G Potassium RS; W is the quantity, in mg, of Penicillin G Benzathine taken to prepare the *Assay preparation*; and r_U and r_S are the penicillin G peak responses obtained from the *Assay preparation* and the *Standard preparation*, respectively.

Penicillin G Benzathine Injectable Suspension

» Penicillin G Benzathine Injectable Suspension is a sterile suspension of Penicillin G Benzathine in Water for Injection with one or more suitable buffers, dispersants, preservatives, and suspending agents. It contains not less than 90.0 percent and not more than 115.0 percent of the labeled amount of penicillin.

Packaging and storage—Preserve in single-dose or multiple-dose containers, preferably of Type I or Type II glass, in a refrigerator.
USP Reference standards ⟨11⟩—*USP Endotoxin RS. USP Penicillin G Benzathine RS. USP Penicillin G Potassium RS.*
Identification—It responds to the *Identification* test under *Penicillin G Benzathine Oral Suspension.*

Bacterial endotoxins ⟨85⟩—It contains not more than 0.01 Endotoxin Unit per 100 Penicillin G Units.
Sterility ⟨71⟩—It meets the requirements when tested as directed for *Direct Inoculation of the Culture Medium* under *Test for Sterility of the Product to be Examined*, except to use Fluid Thioglycollate Medium and Soybean–Casein Digest Medium containing polysorbate 80 solution (1 in 200) and an amount of sterile penicillinase sufficient to inactivate the penicillin G in each vessel, and to shake the vessels once daily.
pH ⟨791⟩: between 5.0 and 7.5.
Other requirements—It meets the requirements under *Injections* ⟨1⟩.
Assay—
  Standard preparation—Using USP Penicillin G Potassium RS, prepare as directed for *Standard preparation* under *Iodometric Assay—Antibiotics* ⟨425⟩.
  Assay preparation—Using a suitable hypodermic needle and syringe, withdraw an accurately measured volume of Injectable Suspension, equivalent to about 300,000 Penicillin G Units, and dilute quantitatively with 1.0 N sodium hydroxide to obtain an *Assay preparation* containing about 2000 Penicillin G Units per mL. Pipet 2.0 mL of this solution into a glass-stoppered, 125-mL conical flask.
  Blank preparation—Using a suitable hypodermic needle and syringe, withdraw an accurately measured volume of Injectable Suspension, equivalent to about 300,000 Penicillin G Units, and quantitatively dilute with *Buffer No. 1* to obtain a suspension containing about 2000 Penicillin G Units per mL. Pipet 2 mL of this solution into a glass-stoppered, 125-mL conical flask.
  Procedure—Proceed as directed for *Procedure* under *Iodometric Assay—Antibiotics* ⟨425⟩, except in performing the *Inactivation and Titration* to omit the addition of 1.0 N sodium hydroxide to the *Assay preparation*, and in performing the *Blank Determination* to use the *Blank preparation* in place of the *Assay preparation*. Calculate the quantity, in Penicillin G Units, in each mL of the Injectable Suspension taken by the formula:

$$(L/2D)(F)(B-I)$$

in which L is the labeled quantity, in Penicillin G Units per mL, in the Injectable Suspension taken, and D is the concentration, in Penicillin G Units per mL, in the *Assay preparation* on the basis of the labeled quantity in the Injectable Suspension and the extent of dilution, and the other terms are as defined therein.

Penicillin G Benzathine Oral Suspension

» Penicillin G Benzathine Oral Suspension contains not less than 90.0 percent and not more than 120.0 percent of the labeled amount of penicillin G. It contains one or more suitable buffers, colors, dispersants, flavors, and preservatives.

Packaging and storage—Preserve in tight containers.
USP Reference standards ⟨11⟩—*USP Penicillin G Benzathine RS. USP Penicillin G Potassium RS.*
Identification—Mix a portion of it with methanol to obtain a solution containing about 3000 Penicillin G Units per mL. Apply 20 µL of this test solution and 20 µL of a Standard solution of USP Penicillin G Benzathine RS in methanol containing 2.5 mg per mL to a suitable thin-layer chromatographic plate (see *Chromatography* ⟨621⟩) coated with a 0.25-mm layer of chromatographic silica gel, and allow the spots to dry. Using an unlined developing chamber, develop the chromatogram in a solvent system consisting of a mixture of methanol, acetonitrile, and ammonium hydroxide (70 : 30 : 3) until the solvent front has moved about three-fourths of the length of the plate. Remove the plate from the developing chamber, and allow to air-dry. Spray the plate uniformly with a spray reagent prepared as follows. Dissolve 20 g of tartaric acid and 1.7 g of bismuth subnitrate in 80 mL of water. Add 2.5 mL of this solution, 2.5 mL of potassium iodide solution (4 in 10), and 10 g of tartaric acid to 50 mL of water, and mix. Examine the chromatograms: the principal spot obtained from the test solution corresponds in R_F value to that obtained from the Standard solution.
Uniformity of dosage units ⟨905⟩—
  FOR SUSPENSION PACKAGED IN SINGLE-UNIT CONTAINERS: meets the requirements.
Deliverable volume ⟨698⟩: meets the requirements.
pH ⟨791⟩: between 6.0 and 7.0.
Assay—
  Standard preparation—Using Penicillin G Potassium RS, prepare as directed for *Standard preparation* under *Iodometric Assay—Antibiotics* ⟨425⟩.
  Assay preparation—Dilute an accurately measured volume of Oral Suspension, freshly mixed and free from air bubbles, quantitatively with 1.0 N sodium hydroxide to obtain a solution having a concentration of about 2000 Penicillin G Units per mL. Pipet 2 mL of this solution into a glass-stoppered, 125-mL conical flask.
  Blank preparation—Dilute an accurately measured volume of Oral Suspension, freshly mixed and free from air bubbles, quantitatively with *Buffer No. 1* to obtain a suspension containing about 2000 Penicillin G Units per mL. Pipet 2 mL of this solution into a glass-stoppered, 125-mL conical flask.
  Procedure—Proceed as directed for *Procedure* under *Iodometric Assay—Antibiotics* ⟨425⟩, except in performing the *Inactivation and titration* to omit the addition of 1.0 N sodium hydroxide to the *Assay preparation*, and in performing the *Blank determination* to use the *Blank preparation* in place of the *Assay preparation*. Calculate the quantity, in Penicillin G Units, in each mL of the Oral Suspension taken by the formula:

$$(L/2D)(F)(B-I)$$

in which L is the labeled quantity, in Penicillin G Units per mL, in the Oral Suspension taken, and D is the concentration, in Penicillin G Units per mL, of the *Assay preparation* on the basis of the labeled quantity in the Oral Suspension and the extent of dilution.

Penicillin G Benzathine Tablets

» Penicillin G Benzathine Tablets contain not less than 90.0 percent and not more than 120.0 percent of the labeled amount of penicillin G.

Packaging and storage—Preserve in tight containers.
USP Reference standards ⟨11⟩—*USP Penicillin G Potassium RS. USP Penicillin G Benzathine RS.*
Identification—Shake a suitable quantity of finely powdered Tablets with methanol to obtain a solution containing about 3000 Penicillin G Units per mL, and filter: the filtrate so obtained responds to the *Identification* test under *Penicillin G Benzathine Oral Suspension*.
Disintegration ⟨701⟩: 60 minutes, simulated gastric fluid TS being used in place of water as the test medium.
Uniformity of dosage units ⟨905⟩: meet the requirements.
Water, *Method I* ⟨921⟩: not more than 8.0%.
Assay—
  Standard preparation—Using Penicillin G Potassium RS, prepare as directed for *Standard preparation* under *Iodometric Assay—Antibiotics* ⟨425⟩.
  Assay preparation—Weigh and finely powder not less than 20 Tablets. Transfer a portion of the powder, accurately weighed, equivalent to about 200,000 Penicillin G Units, to a 100-mL volumetric flask, add 10 mL of 1.0 N sodium hydroxide, and mix. Allow to stand for 15 minutes, add 10 mL of 1.2 N hydrochloric acid, dilute with water to volume, and mix. Pipet 2 mL of this solution into a glass-stoppered, 125-mL conical flask.
  Blank preparation—Transfer an accurately weighed portion of the powdered Tablets remaining from the preparation of the *Assay preparation*, equivalent to about 200,000 Penicillin G Units, to a 100-mL volumetric flask, dilute with *Buffer No. 1* to volume, and

mix. Pipet 2 mL of this solution into a glass-stoppered, 125-mL conical flask.

Procedure—Proceed as directed for *Procedure* under *Iodometric Assay—Antibiotics* ⟨425⟩, except in performing the *Inactivation and titration* to omit the addition of 1.0 N sodium hydroxide and 1.2 N hydrochloric acid, and in the *Blank determination* to use the *Blank preparation* in place of the *Assay preparation*. Calculate the quantity, in Penicillin G Units, in the portion of Tablets taken by the formula:

$$(T/2D)(F)(B - I)$$

in which T is the labeled quantity, in Penicillin G Units, in each Tablet, and D is the concentration, in Penicillin G Units per mL, of the *Assay preparation* on the basis of the labeled quantity in each Tablet and the extent of dilution.

Penicillin G Benzathine and Penicillin G Procaine Injectable Suspension

» Penicillin G Benzathine and Penicillin G Procaine Injectable Suspension is a sterile suspension of Penicillin G Benzathine and Penicillin G Procaine or, when labeled for veterinary use only, of Penicillin G Benzathine and penicillin G procaine, in Water for Injection. It may contain one or more suitable buffers, preservatives, and suspending agents. It contains not less than 90.0 percent and not more than 115.0 percent of the labeled amounts of penicillin G benzathine and penicillin G procaine.

Packaging and storage—Preserve in single-dose or multiple-dose containers, preferably of Type I or Type III glass.
Labeling—Where it is intended for veterinary use only, it is so labeled.

USP Reference standards ⟨11⟩—*USP Penicillin G Benzathine RS. USP Penicillin G Potassium RS. USP Procaine Hydrochloride RS. USP Endotoxin RS.*
Identification—
A: It responds to the *Identification* test under *Penicillin G Benzathine Oral Suspension*: the spot obtained from the test solution, corresponding in R_F value to that obtained from the Standard solution, is completely resolved from a second spot, produced by penicillin G procaine.
B: It responds to the *Identification* test under *Penicillin G Procaine*.
Crystallinity ⟨695⟩ (where it is prepared from penicillin G procaine and is labeled as intended for veterinary use only)—Dilute a portion of the Injectable Suspension, equivalent to about 300,000 Penicillin G Units, with water to obtain a volume of 10 mL, and centrifuge. Remove and discard the supernatant fluid. Resuspend the residue in 10 mL of water, and centrifuge. Remove and discard the supernatant fluid. Dry the residue in a vacuum desiccator. The dried residue meets the requirements.
pH ⟨791⟩: between 5.0 and 7.5.
Limit of soluble penicillin G and procaine (where it is prepared from penicillin G procaine and is labeled for veterinary use only)—
Mobile phase—Dissolve 4 g of sodium 1-hexanesulfonate and 5.44 g of monobasic potassium phosphate in 760 mL of water, adjust with phosphoric acid to a pH of 2.5, dilute with acetonitrile to 1000 mL, and mix. Pass through a filter having a 0.5-µm or finer porosity, and degas. Make adjustments if necessary (see *System Suitability* under *Chromatography* ⟨621⟩).
pH 6.0 Phosphate buffer—Dissolve 16 g of monobasic potassium phosphate and 4 g of dibasic sodium phosphate in water, dilute with water to 200 mL, adjust with phosphoric acid or 1 N sodium hydroxide to a pH of 6.0.

Diluent—Transfer 60 mL of butyl alcohol, 100 mL of acetonitrile, and 10 mL of *pH 6.0 Phosphate buffer* to a 500-mL volumetric flask, dilute with water to volume, and mix.
Standard solution—Transfer about 24 mg of USP Penicillin G Potassium RS, accurately weighed, and about 8 mg of USP Procaine Hydrochloride RS, accurately weighed, to a 100-mL volumetric flask, add 12 mL of butyl alcohol and 20 mL of acetonitrile, and shake to dissolve. Add 2 mL of *pH 6.0 Phosphate buffer* to volume, and mix.
Test solution—Centrifuge about 20 mL of the Suspension. Remove the supernatant fluid, and pass it through a filter having a 5-µm or finer porosity. Transfer 5.0 mL of the clear filtrate to a 50-mL volumetric flask, dilute with *Diluent* to volume, and mix.
Chromatographic system (see *Chromatography* ⟨621⟩)—The liquid chromatograph is equipped with a 204-nm detector and a 4-mm × 15-cm column that contains 5-µm packing L1. The flow rate is about 1 mL per minute. Chromatograph the *Standard solution*, and record the peak responses as directed for *Procedure*: the relative standard deviation for replicate injections is not more than 0.3%.
Procedure—Separately inject equal volumes (about 5 µL) of the *Standard solution* and the *Test solution* into the chromatograph, record the chromatograms, and measure the responses for the major peaks. Calculate the percentage of penicillin G ($C_{16}H_{18}N_2O_4S$) in the *Test solution* by the formula:

$$(334.40 / 372.48)(C)(r_U/r_S)$$

in which 334.40 and 372.48 are the molecular weights of penicillin G and penicillin G potassium respectively; C is the concentration, in mg per mL, of USP Penicillin G Potassium RS in the *Standard solution*; and r_U and r_S are the responses of the penicillin G peaks in the chromatograms of the *Test solution* and the *Standard solution*, respectively: not more than 1% is found. Calculate the percentage of procaine ($C_{13}H_{20}N_2O_2$) in the *Test solution* by the formula:

$$(236.32 / 272.78)(C)(r_U/r_S)$$

in which 236.32 and 272.78 are the molecular weights of procaine and procaine hydrochloride, respectively; C is the concentration, in mg per mL, of USP Procaine Hydrochloride RS in the *Standard solution*; and r_U and r_S are the responses of the procaine peaks in the chromatograms of the *Test solution* and the *Standard solution*, respectively: not more than 1% is found.
Other requirements—It meets the requirements for *Bacterial endotoxins* and *Sterility* under *Penicillin G Procaine Injectable Suspension*. It meets also the requirements under *Injections* ⟨1⟩.
Assay for penicillin G procaine—
Standard preparations—Transfer about $14k$ mg of USP Procaine Hydrochloride RS, accurately weighed, to a 500-mL volumetric flask, and dissolve in 2 mL of 0.5 N sodium hydroxide, k being the ratio of the labeled number of Penicillin G Procaine Units to the labeled number of Penicillin G Benzathine Units in the Injectable Suspension. After 15 minutes, add 1 mL of 1.2 N hydrochloric acid, dilute with water to volume, and mix. This stock solution contains about $28k$ µg of USP Procaine Hydrochloride RS per mL. Transfer 1.0, 2.0, 3.0, 4.0, and 5.0 mL, respectively, of this stock solution to each of five 25-mL volumetric flasks. Transfer 4.0, 3.0, 2.0, and 1.0 mL of water to the first four flasks, respectively.
Assay preparation—Where the Injectable Suspension is represented as being in a single-dose container, withdraw all of the withdrawable contents, using a suitable hypodermic needle and syringe. Where the label states the quantities of penicillin G benzathine and penicillin G procaine in a given volume of Injectable Suspension, remove an accurately measured volume of the Injectable Suspension. For each 300,000 Penicillin G Benzathine Units in the specimen of Injectable Suspension taken, add 20 mL of 0.5 N sodium hydroxide, and mix. After 15 minutes, add 0.5 mL of 1.2 N hydrochloric acid for each mL of 0.5 N sodium hydroxide used, and dilute quantitatively with water to obtain a solution containing 36 Penicillin G Procaine Units per mL. Transfer 5.0 mL of this solution to a 50-mL volumetric flask.
Procedure—To each of the flasks containing the *Standard preparations* and the *Assay preparation*, and to a seventh 50-mL volumetric flask containing 5.0 mL of water to provide the blank, add 0.5 mL of 4 N hydrochloric acid, 1.0 mL of sodium nitrite solution (1 in 1000), 1.0 mL of ammonium sulfamate solution (1 in 200),

and 1.0 mL of N-(1-naphthyl)ethylenediamine dihydrochloride solution (1 in 1000), mixing and allowing 2 minutes to elapse after each addition. Dilute the contents of each flask with water to volume, and mix. Concomitantly determine the absorbances of the solutions from the *Standard preparations* and the *Assay preparation* at the wavelength of maximum absorbance at about 550 nm, with a suitable spectrophotometer, using the blank to set the instrument at zero. Plot the absorbance values of solutions from the *Standard preparations* versus concentration, in mg per mL, of procaine hydrochloride in the solutions from the *Standard preparations*, and draw the straight line best fitting the five plotted points. From the graph so obtained, determine the concentration (*C*), in mg per mL, of procaine hydrochloride in the solution from the *Assay preparation*. Calculate the quantity, in Penicillin G Procaine Units in each container or in each mL of the Injectable Suspension taken by the formula:

$$(588.73 / 272.78)(1009.1)(CL/D)$$

in which 588.73 and 272.78 are the molecular weights of penicillin G procaine monohydrate and procaine hydrochloride, respectively; 1009.1 is the theoretical potency, in Penicillin G Units, in each mg of penicillin G procaine; *L* is the labeled amount, in Penicillin G Procaine Units in each container or in each mL of Injectable Suspension taken; and *D* is the concentration, in Penicillin G Procaine Units per mL, of the solution from the *Assay preparation*, on the basis of the labeled amount in each container or in each mL of Injectable Suspension taken and the extent of dilution.

Assay for penicillin G benzathine—

Standard preparation—Using USP Penicillin G Potassium RS, prepare as directed for *Standard preparation* under *Iodometric Assay—Antibiotics* ⟨425⟩.

Assay preparation—Where the Injectable Suspension is represented as being in a single-dose container, withdraw all of the withdrawable contents, using a suitable hypodermic needle and syringe. Where the label states the quantities of penicillin G benzathine and penicillin G procaine in a given volume of Injectable Suspension, remove an accurately measured volume of Injectable Suspension, freshly mixed but free from air bubbles. Dilute the specimen of Injectable Suspension taken quantitatively with 1 N sodium hydroxide to obtain a solution containing about 2000 Penicillin G Units per mL. Pipet 2 mL of this solution into each of two glass-stoppered, 125-mL conical flasks.

Blank preparation—Prepare as directed for *Assay preparation*, except to use *Buffer No. 1* instead of 1.0 N sodium hydroxide.

Procedure—Proceed as directed for *Procedure* under *Iodometric Assay—Antibiotics* ⟨425⟩, except in performing the *Inactivation and Titration* to omit the addition of 1.0 N sodium hydroxide to the *Assay preparation*, and in performing the *Blank Determination* to use the *Blank preparation* in place of the *Assay preparation*. Calculate the total quantity, *T*, in Penicillin G Units, in each mL of the Injectable Suspension taken by the formula:

$$(L/2D)(F)(B - I)$$

in which *L* is the labeled quantity, in Penicillin G Units in each container, or per mL, in the Injectable Suspension taken; and *D* is the concentration, in Penicillin G Units per mL, in the *Assay preparation* on the basis of the labeled quantity in the Injectable Suspension and the extent of dilution. Calculate the quantity, in Penicillin G Benzathine Units, in each container, or in each mL, of the Injectable Suspension taken by the formula:

$$T - P$$

in which *P* is the quantity, in Penicillin G Procaine Units, in each container, or in each mL, of Injectable Suspension taken, as determined in the *Assay for penicillin G procaine*.

Penicillin G Potassium

$C_{16}H_{17}KN_2O_4S$ 372.48

4-Thia-1-azabicyclo[3.2.0]heptane-2-carboxylic acid, 3,3-dimethyl-7-oxo-6-[(phenylacetyl)amino-], monopotassium salt, [2S-(2α,5α,6β)]-.

Monopotassium   (2S,5R,6R)-3,3-dimethyl-7-oxo-6-(2-phenylacetamido)-4-thia-1-azabicyclo[3.2.0]heptane-2-carboxylate [*113-98-4*].

» Penicillin G Potassium has a potency of not less than 1440 Penicillin G Units and not more than 1680 Penicillin G Units per mg.

Packaging and storage—Preserve in tight containers.

Labeling—Where it is intended for use in preparing injectable dosage forms, the label states that it is sterile or must be subjected to further processing during the preparation of injectable dosage forms.

USP Reference standards ⟨11⟩**—***USP Penicillin G Potassium RS*.

Identification—

A: *Infrared Absorption* ⟨197K⟩.

B: It responds to the flame test for *Potassium* ⟨191⟩.

Crystallinity ⟨695⟩: meets the requirements.

pH ⟨791⟩: between 5.0 and 7.5, in a solution containing 60 mg per mL.

Loss on drying ⟨731⟩**—**Dry about 100 mg, accurately weighed, in a capillary-stoppered bottle in vacuum at 60° for 3 hours: it loses not more than 1.5% of its weight.

Other requirements—Where the label states that Penicillin G Potassium is sterile, it meets the requirements for *Sterility* and *Bacterial endotoxins* under *Penicillin G Potassium for Injection*. Where the label states that Penicillin G Potassium must be subjected to further processing during the preparation of injectable dosage forms, it meets the requirements for *Bacterial endotoxins* under *Penicillin G Potassium for Injection*.

Assay—

Mobile phase—Prepare a mixture of 0.01 M monobasic potassium phosphate and methanol (60 : 40). Make adjustments if necessary (see *System Suitability* under *Chromatography* ⟨621⟩).

Resolution solution—Prepare a solution in water containing about 0.1 mg each of USP Penicillin G Potassium RS and 2-phenylacetamide per mL.

Standard preparation—Transfer about 5 mg of USP Penicillin G Potassium RS, accurately weighed, to a 50-mL volumetric flask, add about 45 mL of water, and shake to dissolve. Dilute with water to volume, and mix. This solution contains the equivalent of about 160 Penicillin G Units per mL.

Assay preparation—Transfer about 5 mg of Penicillin G Potassium, accurately weighed, to a 50-mL volumetric flask, add about 45 mL of water, and shake to dissolve. Dilute with water to volume, and mix.

Chromatographic system (see *Chromatography* ⟨621⟩)—The liquid chromatograph is equipped with a 220-nm detector and a 4.6-mm × 10-cm column that contains 5-μm packing L1. The flow rate is about 1 mL per minute. Chromatograph the *Resolution solution*, and record the peak responses as directed for *Procedure*: the relative retention times are about 0.8 for 2-phenylacetamide and 1.0 for penicillin G; and the resolution, *R*, between 2-phenylacetamide and penicillin G is not less than 2.0. Chromatograph the *Standard preparation*, and record the peak responses as directed for *Procedure*: the column efficiency is not less than 1000 theoretical plates; the tailing factor is not more than 2.0; and the relative standard deviation for replicate injections is not more than 2.0%.

Procedure—Separately inject equal volumes (about 10 μL) of the *Standard preparation* and the *Assay preparation* into the chromatograph, record the chromatograms, and measure the responses for the

major peaks. Calculate the potency, in Penicillin G Units per mg, of the Penicillin G Potassium taken by the formula:

$$(PW_S/W_U)(r_U/r_S)$$

in which P is the specified potency, in Penicillin G Units per mg, of USP Penicillin G Potassium RS; W_S and W_U are the weights, in mg, of USP Penicillin G Potassium RS and the Penicillin G Potassium taken to prepare the Standard preparation and the Assay preparation, respectively; and r_U and r_S are the penicillin G peak responses obtained from the Assay preparation and the Standard preparation, respectively.

Penicillin G Potassium Injection

» Penicillin G Potassium Injection is a sterile isoosmotic solution of Penicillin G Potassium in Water for Injection. It contains one or more suitable buffers and a tonicity-adjusting agent. It contains not less than 90.0 percent and not more than 115.0 percent of the labeled number of Penicillin G Units.

Packaging and storage—Preserve in single-dose containers, as described under Injections ⟨1⟩. Maintain in the frozen state.
Labeling—It meets the requirements for Labeling under Injections ⟨1⟩. The label states that it is to be thawed just prior to use, describes conditions for proper storage of the resultant solution, and directs that the solution is not to be refrozen.
USP Reference standards ⟨11⟩—USP Endotoxin RS. USP Penicillin G Potassium RS.
Identification—The chromatogram of the Assay preparation obtained as directed in the Assay exhibits a major peak for penicillin G, the retention time of which corresponds to that exhibited in the chromatogram of the Standard preparation having a concentration of 200 Penicillin G Units per mL, obtained as directed in the Assay.
Bacterial endotoxins ⟨85⟩—It contains not more than 0.01 USP Endotoxin Unit per 100 Penicillin G Units.
Sterility ⟨71⟩—It meets the requirements when tested as directed for Membrane Filtration under Test for Sterility of the Product to be Examined.
pH ⟨791⟩: between 5.5 and 8.0.
Particulate matter ⟨788⟩: meets the requirements under small-volume injections.
Assay—
  Sodium citrate buffer—Dissolve 0.8 g of sodium citrate (dihydrate) in about 150 mL of water, adjust with 0.1 N hydrochloric acid to a pH of 6.8, dilute with water to 200 mL, and mix.
  Potassium phosphate buffer—Dissolve 10 g of monobasic potassium phosphate in 900 mL of water, adjust with phosphoric acid to a pH of 4.15, dilute with water to 1000 mL, and mix.
  Mobile phase—Prepare a suitable mixture of Potassium phosphate buffer and methanol (550 : 450), filter through a filter of 0.5 μm or finer porosity, and degas. Make adjustments if necessary (see System Suitability under Chromatography ⟨621⟩).
  Standard preparations—Prepare a standard stock solution of USP Penicillin G Potassium RS in Sodium citrate buffer containing a known concentration of about 2000 Penicillin G Units per mL. To three separate 100-mL volumetric flasks transfer 5.0, 10.0, and 15.0 mL of the standard stock solution, dilute with water to volume, and mix. These solutions contain about 100, 200, and 300 Penicillin G Units per mL, respectively.
  Assay preparation 1 (where it is represented as being in a single-dose container)—Allow 1 container of Injection to thaw, and mix. Withdraw all of the withdrawable contents, using a suitable hypodermic needle and syringe, and dilute quantitatively with water to obtain a solution containing about 200 Penicillin G Units per mL.
  Assay preparation 2 (where the label states the quantity of penicillin G in a given volume of Injection)—Allow 1 container of Injection to thaw, and mix. Dilute an accurately measured volume of the Injection quantitatively with water to obtain a solution containing about 200 Penicillin G Units per mL.

Chromatographic system (see Chromatography ⟨621⟩)—The liquid chromatograph is equipped with a 225-nm detector and a 4.6-mm × 10-cm column containing 5-μm packing L1. The flow rate is about 1 mL per minute. Chromatograph the Standard preparation having a concentration of about 200 Penicillin G Units per mL, and record the peak responses as directed for Procedure: the tailing factor for the penicillin G peak is not more than 2, and the relative standard deviation for replicate injections is not more than 2%.
Procedure—Separately inject equal volumes (about 10 μL) of the Standard preparations and the appropriate Assay preparation into the chromatograph, record the chromatograms, and measure the responses for the major peaks. Plot the peak responses obtained from the Standard preparations versus concentration, in Penicillin G Units per mL, and draw the straight line best fitting the three plotted points. From the graph so obtained, determine the number, N, of Penicillin G Units in each mL of the appropriate Assay preparation. Calculate the number of Penicillin G Units in the container, or in each mL of the Injection taken by the formula:

$$(NL/D)$$

in which L is the labeled number of Penicillin G Units in the container, or in each mL of Injection taken, and D is the number of Penicillin G Units in each mL of Assay preparation 1, or of Assay preparation 2, as appropriate, on the basis of the labeled number of Penicillin G Units in the container, or in each mL of the Injection taken, and the extent of dilution.

Penicillin G Potassium for Injection

» Penicillin G Potassium for Injection is sterile Penicillin G Potassium or a sterile, dry mixture of Penicillin G Potassium with not less than 4.0 percent and not more than 5.0 percent of Sodium Citrate, of which not more than 0.15 percent may be replaced by Citric Acid. It has a potency of not less than 90.0 percent and not more than 120.0 percent of the labeled number of Penicillin G Units. In addition, where it contains Sodium Citrate it has a potency of not less than 1335 and not more than 1595 Penicillin G Units per mg.

Packaging and storage—Preserve in Containers for Sterile Solids as described under Injections ⟨1⟩.
USP Reference standards ⟨11⟩—USP Endotoxin RS. USP Penicillin G Potassium RS.
Constituted solution—At the time of use, it meets the requirements for Constituted Solutions under Injections ⟨1⟩.
Identification—Prepare a solution of it containing about 12,000 Penicillin G Units per mL in a solvent mixture consisting of acetone, 0.1 M citric acid, and 0.1 M sodium citrate (2 : 1 : 1). Prepare a Standard solution of USP Penicillin G Potassium RS containing about 12,000 Penicillin G Units per mL in the same solvent mixture. Apply separately 20 μL of each solution to a thin-layer chromatographic plate (see Chromatography ⟨621⟩) coated with a 0.25-mm layer of chromatographic silica gel mixture. Place the plate in a suitable chromatographic chamber, and develop the chromatogram in a solvent system consisting of a mixture of toluene, dioxane, and glacial acetic acid (90 : 25 : 4) until the solvent front has moved about three-fourths of the length of the plate. Remove the plate from the chamber, mark the solvent front, and allow to air-dry. Spray the plate with starch TS followed by dilute iodine TS (1 in 10). Penicillin G appears as a white spot on a purple background: the R_F value of the penicillin G spot obtained from the test solution corresponds to that obtained from the Standard solution.
Crystallinity ⟨695⟩: meets the requirements.
Bacterial endotoxins ⟨85⟩—It contains not more than 0.01 USP Endotoxin Unit per 100 Penicillin G Units.
Sterility ⟨71⟩—It meets the requirements when tested as directed for Membrane Filtration under Test for Sterility of the Product to be Examined.

pH ⟨791⟩: between 5.0 and 7.5, in a solution containing 60 mg per mL, or, where packaged for dispensing, in the solution constituted as directed in the labeling, except where it is labeled as containing sodium citrate it is between 6.0 and 8.5.

Loss on drying ⟨731⟩—Dry about 100 mg, accurately weighed, in a capillary-stoppered bottle in vacuum at 60° for 3 hours: it loses not more than 1.5% of its weight.

Particulate matter ⟨788⟩: meets the requirements for small-volume injections.

Other requirements—It meets the requirements for *Uniformity of Dosage Units* ⟨905⟩, and *Labeling* under *Injections* ⟨1⟩.

Assay—

Mobile phase, Standard preparation, Resolution solution, and *Chromatographic system*—Proceed as directed in the *Assay* under *Penicillin G Potassium*.

Assay preparation 1 (where it is represented as being in a single-dose container)—Constitute Penicillin G Potassium for Injection as directed in the labeling. Withdraw all of the withdrawable contents, using a hypodermic needle and syringe, and quantitatively dilute with water to obtain a solution containing about 160 Penicillin G Units per mL.

Assay preparation 2 (where the label states the quantity of penicillin G in a given volume of constituted solution)—Constitute Penicillin G Potassium for Injection as directed in the labeling. Quantitatively dilute an accurately measured volume of the constituted solution with water to obtain a solution containing about 160 Penicillin G Units per mL.

Assay preparation 3 (where it contains Sodium Citrate)—Transfer about 50 mg of the Penicillin G Potassium for Injection, accurately weighed, to a 500-mL volumetric flask, add about 400 mL of water, and shake to dissolve. Dilute with water to volume, and mix.

Procedure—Proceed as directed for *Procedure* in the *Assay* under *Penicillin G Potassium*. Calculate the number of Penicillin G Units in the container or in the portion of constituted solution taken by the formula:

$$(L/D)(PW_S/50)(r_U/r_S)$$

in which L is the labeled quantity of Penicillin G Units in the container or in the volume of constituted solution taken; D is the concentration, in Penicillin G Units per mL, of *Assay preparation 1* or *Assay preparation 2*, on the basis of the labeled quantity in the container or in the portion of constituted solution taken and the extent of dilution; P is the specified potency, in Penicillin G Units per mg, of USP Penicillin G Potassium RS; W_S is the weight, in mg, of USP Penicillin G Potassium RS taken to prepare the *Standard preparation;* and r_U and r_S are the penicillin G peak responses obtained from the *Assay preparation* and the *Standard preparation,* respectively. Calculate the potency, in Penicillin G Units per mg, of the Penicillin G Potassium for Injection taken by the formula:

$$10(W_S/W_U)(P)(r_U/r_S)$$

in which W_S and W_U are the weights, in mg, of USP Penicillin G Potassium RS and Penicillin G Potassium for Injection taken to prepare the *Standard preparation* and *Assay preparation 3*, respectively, and the other terms are as defined above. Perform the above procedure on 10 containers (where it is represented as being in a single-dose container) and, if necessary, on 10 containers (where the label states the quantity of penicillin G in a given volume of constituted solution). Use the individual results to determine the *Uniformity of dosage units* and the average thereof as the *Assay* value.

Penicillin G Potassium for Oral Solution

» Penicillin G Potassium for Oral Solution is a dry mixture of Penicillin G Potassium and one or more suitable buffers, colors, diluents, flavors, and preservatives. It contains not less than 90.0 percent and not more than 130.0 percent of the labeled number of Penicillin G Units when constituted as directed in the labeling.

Packaging and storage—Preserve in tight containers.

USP Reference standards ⟨11⟩—*USP Penicillin G Potassium RS.*

Identification—Shake a portion of it, equivalent to about 100,000 Penicillin G Units, with 8 mL of a solvent mixture consisting of acetone, 0.1 M citric acid, and 0.1 M sodium citrate (2 : 1 : 1): the solution so obtained responds to the *Identification* test under *Penicillin G Potassium for Injection*.

Uniformity of dosage units ⟨905⟩—

FOR SOLID PACKAGED IN SINGLE-UNIT CONTAINERS: meets the requirements.

Deliverable volume ⟨698⟩: meets the requirements.

pH ⟨791⟩: between 5.5 and 7.5, in the solution constituted as directed in the labeling.

Water, *Method I* ⟨921⟩: not more than 1.0%.

Assay—

Standard preparation—Prepare as directed for *Standard preparation* under *Iodometric Assay—Antibiotics* ⟨425⟩, using USP Penicillin G Potassium RS.

Assay preparation—Dilute an accurately measured volume of solution of Penicillin G Potassium for Oral Solution, constituted as directed in the labeling, quantitatively and stepwise with *Buffer No. 1* (see *Media and Diluents* under *Antibiotics—Microbial Assay* ⟨81⟩) to obtain a solution containing about 2000 Penicillin G Units per mL. Pipet 2 mL of this solution into each of two glass-stoppered, 125-mL conical flasks.

Procedure—Proceed as directed for *Procedure* under *Iodometric Assay—Antibiotics* ⟨425⟩. Calculate the quantity, in Penicillin G Units, in each mL of the constituted solution of Penicillin G Potassium for Oral Solution taken by the formula:

$$(L/2D)(F)(B - I)$$

in which L is the labeled quantity, in Penicillin G Units per mL in the constituted solution of Penicillin G Potassium for Oral Solution, and D is the concentration, in Units per mL, of Penicillin G in the *Assay preparation* on the basis of the labeled quantity in the constituted solution of Penicillin G Potassium for Oral Solution and the extent of dilution.

Penicillin G Potassium Tablets

» Penicillin G Potassium Tablets contain not less than 90.0 percent and not more than 120.0 percent of the labeled number of Penicillin G Units.

Packaging and storage—Preserve in tight containers.

USP Reference standards ⟨11⟩—*USP Penicillin G Potassium RS.*

Identification—Shake a quantity of ground Tablet powder, equivalent to about 100,000 Penicillin G Units, with 8 mL of a solvent mixture consisting of acetone, 0.1 M citric acid, and 0.1 M sodium citrate (2 : 1 : 1), and filter: the filtrate so obtained responds to the *Identification* test under *Penicillin G Potassium for Injection*.

Dissolution ⟨711⟩—

Medium: pH 6.0 phosphate buffer (see *Buffer Solutions* in the section *Reagents, Indicators, and Solutions*); 900 mL.

Apparatus 2: 75 rpm.

Time: 60 minutes.

Standard preparation—Dissolve an accurately weighed quantity of USP Penicillin G Potassium RS in *Dissolution Medium*, and dilute quantitatively with the same solvent to obtain a solution having a known concentration of about 400 Penicillin G Units per mL.

Procedure—Filter the solution under test, dilute with *Dissolution Medium*, if necessary, and proceed as directed for *Procedure* in the section *Antibiotics—Hydroxylamine Assay*, under *Automated Meth-*

ods of Analysis ⟨16⟩. Calculate the number of Penicillin G Units in each mL of the solution taken by the formula:

$$C(A_U / A_S)$$

in which C is the concentration, in Penicillin G Units per mL, of the *Standard preparation*.

Tolerances—Not less than 70% *(Q)* of the labeled amount of Penicillin G Units is dissolved in 60 minutes.

Uniformity of dosage units ⟨905⟩: meet the requirements.

Loss on drying ⟨731⟩—Dry about 100 mg, accurately weighed, of powdered Tablets in a capillary-stoppered bottle in vacuum at 60° for 3 hours: it loses not more than 1.0% of its weight.

Assay—

Standard preparation—Prepare as directed for *Standard preparation* under *Iodometric Assay—Antibiotics* ⟨425⟩, using USP Penicillin G Potassium RS.

Assay preparation—Place not less than 5 Tablets in a high-speed glass blender jar containing an accurately measured volume of *Buffer No. 1*, and blend for 4 ± 1 minutes. Dilute an accurately measured volume of this stock solution quantitatively with *Buffer No. 1* to obtain an *Assay preparation* containing about 2000 Penicillin G Units per mL. Pipet 2 mL of this solution into each of two glass-stoppered, 125-mL conical flasks.

Procedure—Proceed as directed for *Procedure* under *Iodometric Assay—Antibiotics* ⟨425⟩. Calculate the quantity, in Penicillin G Units in each Tablet taken by the formula:

$$(L / 2D)(F)(B - I)$$

in which L is the labeled quantity, in Penicillin G Units, in each Tablet, and D is the concentration, in Units per mL, of Penicillin G in the *Assay preparation* on the basis of the labeled quantity in each Tablet and the extent of dilution.

Penicillin G Procaine

$C_{16}H_{18}N_2O_4S \cdot C_{13}H_{20}N_2O_2 \cdot H_2O$ 588.72

4-Thia-1-azabicyclo[3.2.0]heptane-2-carboxylic acid, 3,3-dimethyl-7-oxo-6-[(phenylacetyl)amino-], 2S-(2α,5α,6β)-, compd. with 2-(diethylamino)ethyl 4-aminobenzoate (1 : 1) monohydrate.

(2S,5R,6R)-3,3-Dimethyl-7-oxo-6-(2-phenylacetamido)-4-thia-1-azabicyclo[3.2.0]heptane-2-carboxylic acid compound with 2-(diethylamino)ethyl *p*-aminobenzoate (1 : 1) monohydrate [6130-64-9].

Anhydrous   570.71   [54-35-3].

» Penicillin G Procaine has a potency of not less than 900 Penicillin G Units and not more than 1050 Penicillin G Units per mg.

Packaging and storage—Preserve in *Containers for Sterile Solids* as described under *Injections* ⟨1⟩.

Labeling—Where it is intended for use in preparing injectable dosage forms, the label states that it is sterile or must be subjected to further processing during the preparation of injectable dosage forms.

USP Reference standards ⟨11⟩—*USP Penicillin G Potassium RS. USP Procaine Hydrochloride RS. USP Endotoxin RS.*

Identification—Prepare a solution of it containing about 12,000 Penicillin G Units per mL in a solvent mixture consisting of acetone, 0.1 M citric acid, and 0.1 M sodium citrate (2 : 1 : 1). Prepare a Standard solution of USP Penicillin G Potassium RS containing about 12,000 Penicillin G Units per mL in the same solvent mixture (*Standard solution A*). Prepare a Standard solution of USP Procaine Hydrochloride RS containing about 5 mg per mL in the same solvent system (*Standard solution B*). Apply separately 20 μL of each solution to a thin-layer chromatographic plate (see *Chromatography* ⟨621⟩) coated with a 0.25-mm layer of chromatographic silica gel mixture. Place the plate in a suitable chromatographic chamber, and develop the chromatogram in a solvent system consisting of a mixture of toluene, dioxane, and glacial acetic acid (90 : 25 : 4) until the solvent front has moved about three-fourths of the length of the plate. Remove the plate from the chamber, mark the solvent front, and allow to air-dry. Examine the plate under short- and long-wavelength UV light, noting the positions of the spots. Spray the plate with starch TS followed by dilute iodine TS (1 in 10). Penicillin G appears as a white spot on a purple background: the R_F value of the penicillin G spot obtained from the test solution corresponds to that obtained from *Standard solution A*. Spray the location of the spots visualized with UV light with a 1 in 20 solution of *p*-dimethylaminobenzaldehyde in methanol. Procaine appears as a bright yellow spot: the R_F value of the procaine spot obtained from the test solution corresponds to that obtained from *Standard solution B*.

Crystallinity ⟨695⟩: meets the requirements.

Bacterial endotoxins ⟨85⟩—Where the label states that Penicillin G Procaine is sterile or that it must be subjected to further processing during the preparation of injectable dosage forms it contains not more than 0.01 USP Endotoxin Unit per 100 Penicillin G Units.

Sterility ⟨71⟩—Where the label states that Penicillin G Procaine is sterile it meets the requirements when tested as directed for *Membrane Filtration* under *Test for Sterility of the Product to be Examined*, except to use *Fluid A* to which has been added sufficient sterile penicillinase to inactivate the penicillin G and to swirl the vessel until solution is complete before filtering.

pH ⟨791⟩: between 5.0 and 7.5, in a (saturated) solution containing about 300 mg per mL.

Water, *Method I* ⟨921⟩: between 2.8% and 4.2%.

Content of Penicillin G and procaine—

Mobile phase—Dissolve 14 g of monobasic potassium phosphate and 6.5 g of tetrabutylammonium hydroxide solution (4 in 10) in about 700 mL of water, adjust with 1 N potassium hydroxide to a pH of 7.0, dilute with water to 1000 mL, and mix. Mix 500 mL of this solution, 250 mL of acetonitrile, and 250 mL of water. Adjust with 1 N potassium hydroxide or dilute phosphoric acid (1 in 10) to a pH of 7.5 ± 0.05, filter through a membrane filter of 5 μm or finer porosity, and degas. Make adjustments if necessary (see *System Suitability* under *Chromatography* ⟨621⟩).

Standard preparation—Using accurately weighed quantities of USP Penicillin G Potassium RS and USP Procaine Hydrochloride RS, prepare a solution in *Mobile phase* having known concentrations of about 0.8 mg per mL and 0.54 mg per mL, respectively.

Test preparation—Transfer about 70 mg of Penicillin G Procaine, accurately weighed, to a 50-mL volumetric flask, add about 30 mL of *Mobile phase*, sonicate to dissolve, dilute with *Mobile phase* to volume, and mix.

Resolution solution—Prepare a solution of penicillin V potassium in *Mobile phase* containing 2.4 mg per mL. Mix 1 volume of this solution and 3 volumes of *Standard preparation*.

Chromatographic system (see *Chromatography* ⟨621⟩)—The liquid chromatograph is equipped with a 235-nm detector and a 4-mm × 30-cm column that contains 10-μm packing L1. The flow rate is about 1 mL per minute. Chromatograph the *Standard preparation*, and record the peak responses as directed for *Procedure*: the relative standard deviation for replicate injections is not more than 3.0%. Chromatograph about 10 μL of the *Resolution solution*, and record the peak responses as directed for *Procedure*: the resolution, *R*, between penicillin G and penicillin V is not less than 2.0.

Procedure—Separately inject equal volumes (about 10 μL) of the *Standard preparation* and the *Test preparation* into the chromatograph, record the chromatograms, and measure the responses for the major peaks. The relative retention times are 1.0 for procaine and about 2.2 for penicillin G. Calculate the percentage of penicillin G ($C_{16}H_{18}N_2O_4S$) in the specimen under test by the formula:

$$50C(G_S / W_U)(r_U / r_S)$$

in which C is the concentration, in mg per mL, of USP Penicillin G Potassium RS in the *Standard preparation*, G_S is the designated penicillin G content, in percentage, of USP Penicillin G Potassium RS, W_U is the amount, in mg, of Penicillin G Procaine taken, and r_U and r_S are the responses of the penicillin G peaks obtained from the *Test preparation* and the *Standard preparation*, respectively: between 51.0% and 59.6% of $C_{16}H_{18}N_2O_4S$ is found. Calculate the percentage of procaine ($C_{13}H_{20}N_2O_2$) in the specimen under test by the formula:

$$(236.32 / 272.78)(5000C / W_U)(r_U / r_S)$$

in which 236.32 and 272.78 are the molecular weights of procaine and procaine hydrochloride, respectively, C is the concentration, in mg per mL, of USP Procaine Hydrochloride RS in the *Standard preparation*, W_U is the amount, in mg, of Penicillin G Procaine taken, and r_U and r_S are the responses of the procaine peaks obtained from the *Test preparation* and the *Standard preparation*, respectively: between 37.5% and 43.0% is found.

Assay—
  Standard preparation—Using USP Penicillin G Potassium RS, prepare as directed for *Standard preparation* under *Iodometric Assay—Antibiotics* ⟨425⟩.
  Assay preparation—Prepare as directed for *Assay Preparation* under *Iodometric Assay—Antibiotics* ⟨425⟩, except to dissolve about 100 mg of Penicillin G Procaine, accurately weighed, in 2.0 mL of methanol, and to dilute quantitatively with *Buffer No. 1* to obtain a solution containing about 2000 Penicillin G Units per mL.
  Procedure—Proceed as directed for *Procedure* under *Iodometric Assay—Antibiotics* ⟨425⟩. Calculate the potency, in Penicillin G Units per mg, of the Penicillin G Procaine taken by the formula:

$$F(B - I) / (2D)$$

in which D is the concentration, in mg per mL, of the *Assay preparation*, on the basis of the weight of Penicillin G Procaine taken and the extent of dilution, and the other terms are as defined therein.

Penicillin G Procaine Intramammary Infusion

» Penicillin G Procaine Intramammary Infusion is a suspension of Penicillin G Procaine in a suitable vegetable oil vehicle. It may contain one or more buffers, dispersants, preservatives, and thickening agents. It contains not less than 90.0 percent and not more than 115.0 percent of the labeled amount of penicillin G.

Packaging and storage—Preserve in well-closed disposable syringes.
Labeling—Label it to indicate that it is for veterinary use only.
USP Reference standards ⟨11⟩—*USP Penicillin G Potassium RS. USP Penicillin G Procaine RS.*
Identification—Transfer a portion of it, equivalent to about 100,000 Penicillin G Units, to a test tube, add 25 mL of methanol, and shake. Allow to separate, and use the methanol layer as the test solution. Prepare a Standard solution of USP Penicillin G Procaine RS in methanol containing about 4.5 mg per mL. Apply separately 10 µL of each solution to a thin-layer chromatographic plate (see *Chromatography* ⟨621⟩) coated with a 0.25-mm layer of chromatographic silica gel mixture. Allow the spots to dry, and develop the chromatogram in a solvent system consisting of a mixture of butanol, isopropyl alcohol, acetone, and water (4 : 4 : 2 : 2) until the solvent front has moved about three-fourths of the length of the plate. Remove the plate from the developing chamber, mark the solvent front, and allow the solvent to evaporate. Expose the plate to iodine vapors in a closed chamber for about 15 minutes, and locate the spots: the R_F values and colors of the two principal spots obtained from the test solution correspond to those obtained from the Standard solution.
Water, *Method I* ⟨921⟩: not more than 1.4%, 20 mL of a mixture of toluene and methanol (7 : 3) being used in place of methanol in the titration vessel.
Assay—Proceed as directed under *Antibiotics—Microbial Assays* ⟨81⟩, expelling the contents of 1 syringe of Intramammary Infusion into a high-speed glass blender jar containing 499.0 mL of *Buffer No. 1* and 1.0 mL of polysorbate 80, and blending for 3 to 5 minutes. Allow to stand for about 10 minutes, and dilute an accurately measured volume of the aqueous phase quantitatively and stepwise with *Buffer No. 1* to obtain a *Test Dilution* having a concentration assumed to be equal to the median dose level of the Standard.

Penicillin G Procaine Injectable Suspension

» Penicillin G Procaine Injectable Suspension is a sterile suspension of Penicillin G, Procaine or, where labeled for veterinary use only of sterile penicillin G procaine, in Water for Injection and contains one or more suitable buffers dispersants, or suspending agents, and a suitable preservative. It may contain procaine hydrochloride in a concentration not exceeding 2.0 percent, and may contain one or more suitable stabilizers. It contains not less than 90.0 percent and not more than 115.0 percent of the labeled amount of penicillin G, the labeled amount being not less than 300,000 Penicillin G Units per mL or per container.

Packaging and storage—Preserve in single-dose or multiple-dose containers, preferably of Type I or Type III glass, in a refrigerator.
Labeling—Where it is intended for veterinary use only, the label so states.
USP Reference standards ⟨11⟩—*USP Endotoxin RS. USP Penicillin G Potassium RS. USP Procaine Hydrochloride RS.*
Identification—It responds to the *Identification* test under *Penicillin G Procaine*.
Crystallinity ⟨695⟩ (where it is prepared from penicillin G procaine and is labeled for veterinary use only): meets the requirements, the dried residue prepared as directed in the test for *Pencillin G and procaine contents* being used.
Bacterial endotoxins ⟨85⟩—It contains not more than 0.01 USP Endotoxin Unit per 100 Penicillin G Units.
Sterility ⟨71⟩—It meets the requirements when tested as directed for *Membrane Filtration* under *Test for Sterility of the Product to be Examined*, except to use a portion of specimen from each container equivalent to 300,000 Penicillin G Units, instead of the minimum volume specified in the *Table 2, Minimum Quantity to be Used for Each Medium*, and to use Fluid A to which has been added sufficient sterile penicillinase to inactivate the penicillin G and to swirl the vessel until solution is complete before filtering. If the Injectable Suspension contains lecithin, use *Fluid D*. If it contains carboxymethylcellulose sodium, add sufficient sterile carboxymethylcellulase to *Fluid A* or *Fluid D* to dissolve the carboxymethylcellulose sodium before filtering. If it does not dissolve completely, proceed as directed for *Direct Inoculation of the Culture Medium* under *Test for Sterility of the Product to be Examined*, except to use Fluid Thioglycollate Medium and Soybean–Casein Digest Medium containing an amount of sterile penicillinase sufficient to inactivate the penicillin G in each vessel.
pH ⟨791⟩: between 5.0 and 7.5.
Penicillin G and procaine contents (where it is prepared from penicillin G procaine and is labeled for veterinary use only)—Dilute a portion of it, equivalent to about 300,000 Penicillin G Units, with water to obtain a volume of 10 mL, centrifuge, and remove and discard the supernatant. Resuspend the sediment in 10 mL of water, centrifuge, and remove and discard the supernatant. Dry the sediment in a vacuum desiccator containing silica gel for 18 hours at a temperature not exceeding 25°. The dried material meets the requirements of the test for *Penicillin G and procaine contents* under *Penicillin G Procaine*. [NOTE—Reserve a portion of the dried material for the test for *Crystallinity*.]
Other requirements—It meets the requirements under *Injections* ⟨1⟩.

Assay—

Standard preparation—Using USP Penicillin G Potassium RS, prepare as directed for *Standard preparation* under *Iodometric Assay—Antibiotics* ⟨425⟩.

Assay preparation 1 (where it is represented as being in a single-dose container)—Withdraw all of the withdrawable contents of the Injectable Suspension, using a suitable hypodermic needle and syringe, and dilute quantitatively with *Buffer No. 1* to obtain a solution containing about 2000 Penicillin G Units per mL. Pipet 2 mL of this solution into each of two glass-stoppered, 125-mL conical flasks.

Assay preparation 2 (where the label states the quantity of penicillin G procaine in a given volume of Injectable Suspension)—Dilute an accurately measured volume of Injectable Suspension quantitatively with *Buffer No. 1* to obtain a solution containing about 2000 Penicillin G Units per mL. Pipet 2.0 mL of this solution into each of two glass-stoppered, 125-mL conical flasks.

Procedure—Proceed as directed for *Procedure* under *Iodometric Assay—Antibiotics* ⟨425⟩. Calculate the quantity, in Penicillin G Units, in the container, or in the portion of Injectable Suspension taken, by the formula:

$$(L/2D)(F)(B - I)$$

in which L is the labeled quantity in Penicillin G Units, in the container, or in the volume of Injectable Suspension taken; and D is the concentration, in Penicillin G Units per mL, of *Assay preparation 1*, or of *Assay preparation 2*, on the basis of the labeled quantity in the container, or in the portion of Injectable Suspension taken, respectively, and the extent of dilution.

Penicillin G Procaine for Injectable Suspension

» Penicillin G Procaine for Injectable Suspension is a sterile mixture of Penicillin G Procaine and one or more suitable buffers, dispersants, or suspending agents, and preservatives. It contains not less than 90.0 percent and not more than 115.0 percent of the labeled amount of penicillin G, the labeled amount being not less than 300,000 Penicillin G Units per container or per mL of constituted Suspension.

Packaging and storage—Preserve in single-dose or multiple-dose containers, preferably of Type I or Type III glass.

USP Reference standards ⟨11⟩—*USP Endotoxin RS. USP Penicillin G Potassium RS. USP Procaine Hydrochloride RS.*

Identification—It responds to the *Identification* test under *Penicillin G Procaine.*

pH ⟨791⟩: between 5.0 and 7.5, when constituted as directed in the labeling.

Water, *Method I* ⟨921⟩: between 2.8% and 4.2%.

Other requirements—It meets the requirements for *Bacterial endotoxins* and *Sterility* under *Penicillin G Procaine Injectable Suspension*. It meets also the requirements under *Injections* ⟨1⟩ and *Uniformity of Dosage Units* ⟨905⟩.

Assay—

Standard preparation—Using USP Penicillin G Potassium RS, prepare as directed for *Standard preparation* under *Iodometric Assay—Antibiotics* ⟨425⟩.

Assay preparation 1 (where it is represented as being in a single-dose container)—Constitute Penicillin G Procaine for Injectable Suspension as directed in the labeling. Withdraw all of the withdrawable contents, using a suitable hypodermic needle and syringe, and dilute quantitatively with *Buffer No. 1* to obtain a solution containing about 2000 Penicillin G Units per mL. Pipet 2 mL of this solution into each of two glass-stoppered, 125-mL conical flasks.

Assay preparation 2 (where the label states the quantity of penicillin G procaine in a given volume of constituted suspension)—Constitute Penicillin G Procaine for Injectable Suspension as directed in the labeling. Dilute an accurately measured volume of the constituted injectable suspension quantitatively with *Buffer No. 1* to obtain a solution containing about 2000 Penicillin G Units per mL. Pipet 2 mL of this solution into each of two glass-stoppered, 125-mL conical flasks.

Procedure—Proceed as directed for *Procedure* under *Iodometric Assay—Antibiotics* ⟨425⟩. Calculate the quantity, in Penicillin G Units, in the container, or in the portion of constituted injectable suspension taken by the formula:

$$(L/2D)(F)(B-I)$$

in which L is the labeled quantity, in Penicillin G Units, in the container, or in the volume of constituted injectable suspension taken, and D is the concentration, in Penicillin G Units per mL, of *Assay preparation 1* or of *Assay preparation 2* on the basis of the labeled quantity in the container or in the portion of constituted injectable suspension taken, respectively, and the extent of dilution.

Penicillin G Procaine and Dihydrostreptomycin Sulfate Intramammary Infusion

» Penicillin G Procaine and Dihydrostreptomycin Sulfate Intramammary Infusion is a suspension of Penicillin G Procaine and Dihydrostreptomycin Sulfate in a suitable vegetable oil vehicle. It may contain suitable gelling and thickening agents. It contains not less than 90.0 percent and not more than 120.0 percent of the labeled amounts of Penicillin G Units and of dihydrostreptomycin ($C_{21}H_{41}N_7O_{12}$).

Packaging and storage—Preserve in well-closed, disposable syringes.

Labeling—Label it to indicate that it is intended for veterinary use only.

USP Reference standards ⟨11⟩—*USP Dihydrostreptomycin Sulfate RS. USP Penicillin G Potassium RS. USP Penicillin G Procaine RS.*

Identification—

A: It responds to the *Identification* test under *Penicillin G Procaine Intramammary Infusion.*

B: Place a portion of it, equivalent to about 100 mg of dihydrostreptomycin, in a separator, add 20 mL of chloroform and 20 mL of water, and shake by mechanical means for 15 minutes. Allow to separate, and discard the lower chloroform layer. Repeat the extraction with a 20-mL portion of chloroform, discarding the chloroform layer. Use the aqueous layer as the test solution. Prepare a Standard solution of USP Dihydrostreptomycin Sulfate RS in water containing 6.5 mg per mL. Apply separately 30 µL of each solution to a thin-layer chromatographic plate (see *Chromatography* ⟨621⟩) coated with a 0.25-mm layer of chromatographic silica gel mixture. Allow the spots to dry, and develop the chromatogram in a solvent system consisting of a mixture of *n*-propyl alcohol, water, pyridine, and glacial acetic acid (15 : 12 : 10 : 2) until the solvent front has moved about three-fourths of the length of the plate. Remove the plate from the developing chamber, mark the solvent front, and allow the solvent to evaporate. Spray the plate with a reagent prepared by dissolving 2 g of ninhydrin in 100 mL of alcohol and adding 20 mL of glacial acetic acid, heat the plate at 110° for 10 minutes, and examine the chromatograms: the R_F value and color of the principal spot obtained from the test solution correspond to those obtained from the Standard solution.

Water, *Method I* ⟨921⟩: not more than 1.4%, 20 mL of a mixture of toluene and methanol (7 : 3) being used in the titration vessel in place of methanol.

Assay for penicillin G—Proceed as directed for penicillin G under *Antibiotics—Microbial Assays* ⟨81⟩, expelling the contents of 1 syringe of Intramammary Infusion into a high-speed glass blender jar containing 499.0 mL of *Buffer No. 1* and 1.0 mL of polysorbate 80, and blending for 3 to 5 minutes. Allow to stand for about 10 minutes, and dilute an accurately measured volume of the aqueous phase quantitatively and stepwise with *Buffer No. 1* to obtain a *Test Dilution* having a concentration of penicillin G assumed to be equal to the median dose level of the Standard.

Assay for dihydrostreptomycin—Proceed as directed for the cylinder-plate assay for dihydrostreptomycin under *Antibiotics—Microbial Assays* ⟨81⟩, expelling the contents of 1 syringe of Intramammary Infusion into a high-speed glass blender jar containing 499.0 mL of *Buffer No. 3* and 1.0 mL of polysorbate 80, and blending for 3 to 5 minutes. Allow to stand for about 10 minutes, and to an accurately measured volume of the aqueous phase add an accurately measured volume of penicillinase sufficient to inactivate the penicillin G contained therein. Dilute this solution quantitatively with *Buffer No. 3* to obtain a *Test Dilution* having a concentration of dihydrostreptomycin assumed to be equal to the median dose level of the Standard, and store at 37° for 30 minutes before filling the cylinders.

Penicillin G Procaine and Dihydrostreptomycin Sulfate Injectable Suspension

» Penicillin G Procaine and Dihydrostreptomycin Sulfate Injectable Suspension is a sterile suspension of Penicillin G Procaine in a solution of Dihydrostreptomycin Sulfate in Water for Injection, and contains one or more suitable buffers, preservatives, and dispersing or suspending agents. It may contain Procaine Hydrochloride in a concentration not exceeding 2.0 percent, and it may contain one or more suitable stabilizers. It contains not less than 90.0 percent and not more than 115.0 percent of the labeled amounts of Penicillin G Units and of dihydrostreptomycin ($C_{21}H_{41}N_7O_{12}$).

Packaging and storage—Preserve in single-dose or multiple-dose, tight containers.
Labeling—Label it to indicate that it is intended for veterinary use only.
USP Reference standards ⟨11⟩—*USP Dihydrostreptomycin Sulfate RS. USP Endotoxin RS. USP Penicillin G Potassium RS.*
Identification—It responds to *Identification* tests A and B under *Penicillin G Procaine, Dihydrostreptomycin Sulfate, Chlorpheniramine Maleate, and Dexamethasone Suspension.*
Bacterial endotoxins ⟨85⟩—It contains not more than 0.01 USP Endotoxin Unit per 100 Penicillin G Units.
Sterility ⟨71⟩—It meets the requirements when tested as directed for *Membrane Filtration* under *Test for Sterility of the Product to be Examined*, except to use a portion of specimen from each container equivalent to 300,000 Penicillin G Units, instead of the minimum volume specified in the *Table 2, Minimum Quantity to be Used for Each Medium* and to use *Fluid A* to which has been added sufficient sterile penicillinase to inactivate the penicillin G and to swirl the vessel until solution is complete before filtering. If the Injectable Suspension contains lecithin, use *Fluid D* to which has been added sufficient penicillinase to inactivate the penicillin G and to swirl the vessel until solution is complete before filtering. If it contains carboxymethylcellulose sodium, add also sufficient sterile carboxymethylcellulase to *Fluid A* or *Fluid D* to dissolve the carboxymethylcellulose sodium before filtering. If it does not dissolve completely, proceed as directed for *Direct Inoculation of the Culture Medium* under *Test for Sterility of the Product to be Examined*, except to use Fluid Thioglycollate Medium containing an amount of sterile penicillinase sufficient to inactivate the penicillin G in each vessel.

pH ⟨791⟩: between 5.0 and 8.0.
Assay for penicillin G—
Standard preparation—Using USP Penicillin G Potassium RS, prepare as directed for *Standard preparation* under *Iodometric Assay—Antibiotics* ⟨425⟩.
Assay preparation—Dilute an accurately measured volume of Injectable Suspension quantitatively with *Buffer No. 1* to obtain a solution containing about 2000 Penicillin G Units per mL. Pipet 2 mL of this solution into each of two glass-stoppered, 125-mL conical flasks.
Procedure—Proceed as directed for *Procedure* under *Iodometric Assay—Antibiotics* ⟨425⟩, except in the *Blank Determination* to add 0.1 mL of 1.2 N hydrochloric acid immediately before the 10.0 mL of 0.01 N iodine VS. Calculate the quantity, in Penicillin G Units, in the portion of Injectable Suspension taken by the formula:

$$(L/2D)(F)(B - I)$$

in which L is the labeled quantity, in Penicillin G Units, in the volume of Injectable Suspension taken, and D is the concentration, in Penicillin G Units per mL, of the *Assay preparation*, on the basis of the labeled quantity in the portion of Injectable Suspension taken and the extent of dilution, and the other terms are as defined therein.
Assay for dihydrostreptomycin—Proceed as directed for the turbidimetric assay for dihydrostreptomycin under *Antibiotics—Microbial Assays* ⟨81⟩, using an accurately measured volume of Injectable Suspension diluted quantitatively with water to yield a *Test Dilution* having a concentration assumed to be equal to the median dose level of the Standard.

Penicillin G Procaine, Dihydrostreptomycin Sulfate, Chlorpheniramine Maleate, and Dexamethasone Injectable Suspension

» Penicillin G Procaine, Dihydrostreptomycin Sulfate, Chlorpheniramine Maleate, and Dexamethasone Injectable Suspension is a sterile suspension of Penicillin G Procaine and Dexamethasone in a solution of Sterile Dihydrostreptomycin Sulfate and Chlorpheniramine Maleate in Water for Injection. It contains one or more suitable buffers, preservatives, and dispersing or suspending agents. It may contain Procaine Hydrochloride in a concentration not exceeding 2.0 percent, and it may contain one or more suitable stabilizers. It contains not less than 90.0 percent and not more than 115.0 percent of the labeled amounts of Penicillin G Units and of dihydrostreptomycin ($C_{21}H_{41}N_7O_{12}$), and not less than 90.0 percent and not more than 110.0 percent of the labeled amounts of chlorpheniramine maleate ($C_{16}H_{19}ClN_2 \cdot C_4H_4O_4$) and of dexamethasone ($C_{22}H_{29}FO_5$).

Packaging and storage—Preserve in single-dose or multiple-dose, tight containers, in a cool place.
Labeling—Label it to indicate that it is intended for veterinary use only.
USP Reference standards ⟨11⟩—*USP Penicillin G Potassium RS. USP Penicillin G Procaine RS. USP Dihydrostreptomycin Sulfate RS. USP Chlorpheniramine Maleate RS. USP Dexamethasone RS. USP Endotoxin RS.*
Identification—
A: Transfer, with the aid of water, a portion of the Injectable Suspension, freshly mixed and free from air bubbles, equivalent to about 400,000 Penicillin G Units, to a separator, add 50 mL of chloroform, and shake by mechanical means for 15 minutes. Allow to

separate, and filter the lower chloroform layer through about 4 g of anhydrous sodium sulfate supported on a pledget of glass wool, collecting the filtrate in a 100-mL volumetric flask. Repeat the extraction with two 25-mL portions of chloroform, combining the filtrates in the 100-mL volumetric flask. Dilute with chloroform to volume, and mix. [NOTE—Retain the aqueous phase for *Identification* test *B*.] Prepare a Standard solution of USP Penicillin G Procaine RS in chloroform containing about 4.5 mg per mL. Apply separately 10 μL of each solution to a thin-layer chromatographic plate (see *Chromatography* ⟨621⟩) coated with a 0.25-mm layer of chromatographic silica gel mixture. Allow the spots to dry, and develop the chromatogram in a solvent system consisting of a mixture of butanol, isopropyl alcohol, acetone, and water (4 : 4 : 2 : 2) until the solvent front has moved about three-fourths of the length of the plate. Remove the plate from the developing chamber, mark the solvent front, and allow the solvent to evaporate. Expose the plate to iodine vapors in a closed chamber for about 15 minutes, and locate the spots: the R_F values and colors of the two principal spots obtained from the test solution correspond to those obtained from the Standard solution.

B: Dilute the aqueous phase retained from *Identification* test *A* with water to obtain a test solution containing about 5 mg of dihydrostreptomycin per mL. Prepare a Standard solution of USP Dihydrostreptomycin Sulfate RS in water containing 6.5 mg per mL. Apply separately 30 μL of each solution to a thin-layer chromatographic plate (see *Chromatography* ⟨621⟩) coated with a 0.25-mm layer of chromatographic silica gel mixture. Allow the spots to dry, and develop the chromatogram in a solvent system consisting of a mixture of *n*-propyl alcohol, water, pyridine, and glacial acetic acid (15 : 12 : 10 : 2) until the solvent front has moved about three-fourths of the length of the plate. Remove the plate from the developing chamber, mark the solvent front, and allow the solvent to evaporate. Spray the plate with a reagent prepared by dissolving 2 g of ninhydrin in 100 mL of alcohol and adding 20 mL of glacial acetic acid, heat the plate at 110° for 10 minutes, and examine the chromatograms: the R_F value and color of the principal spot obtained from the test solution correspond to those obtained from the Standard solution.

C: The chromatogram of the *Assay preparation* obtained as directed in the *Assay for chlorpheniramine maleate* exhibits a major peak for chlorpheniramine, the retention time of which corresponds to that exhibited in the chromatogram of the *Standard preparation* similarly determined, both relative to the internal standard.

D: The chromatogram of the *Assay preparation* obtained as directed in the *Assay for dexamethasone* exhibits a major peak for dexamethasone, the retention time of which corresponds to that exhibited in the chromatogram of the *Standard preparation* similarly determined, both relative to the internal standard.

Bacterial endotoxins ⟨85⟩—It contains not more than 0.01 Endotoxin Unit per 100 Penicillin G Units.

pH ⟨791⟩: between 5.0 and 6.0.

Other requirements—It meets the requirements of the test for *Sterility* under *Penicillin G Procaine and Dihydrostreptomycin Sulfate Injectable Suspension*, and the requirements under *Injections* ⟨1⟩.

Assay for penicillin G—
Standard preparation—Using USP Penicillin G Potassium RS, prepare as directed for *Standard preparation* under *Iodometric Assay—Antibiotics* ⟨425⟩.

Assay preparation—Dilute an accurately measured volume of Injectable Suspension, freshly mixed and free from air bubbles, quantitatively with *Buffer No. 1* to yield a solution containing about 2000 Penicillin G Units per mL. Pipet 2 mL of this solution into each of two glass-stoppered, 125-mL conical flasks.

Procedure—Proceed as directed for *Procedure* under *Iodometric Assay—Antibiotics* ⟨425⟩, except in the *Blank Determination* to add 0.1 mL of 1.2 N hydrochloric acid immediately before the 10.0 mL of 0.01 N iodine VS. Calculate the quantity, in Penicillin G Units, in the portion of Injectable Suspension taken by the formula:

$$(L / 2D)(F)(B - I)$$

in which *L* is the labeled quantity, in Penicillin G Units, in the volume of Injectable Suspension taken, and *D* is the concentration, in Penicillin G Units per mL, of the *Assay preparation*, on the basis of the labeled quantity in the portion of Injectable Suspension taken and the extent of dilution, and the other terms are as defined therein.

Assay for dihydrostreptomycin—Proceed as directed for the turbidimetric assay for dihydrostreptomycin under *Antibiotics—Microbial Assays* ⟨81⟩, using an accurately measured volume of Injectable Suspension, freshly mixed and free from air bubbles, diluted quantitatively with water to yield a *Test Dilution* having a concentration of dihydrostreptomycin assumed to be equal to the median dose level of the Standard.

Assay for chlorpheniramine maleate—
Internal standard solution—Prepare a solution of brompheniramine maleate in water having a concentration of about 7 mg per mL.

Standard preparation—Dissolve an accurately weighed quantity of USP Chlorpheniramine Maleate RS in water to obtain a stock solution having a known concentration of about 6 mg per mL. Transfer 5.0 mL of this solution to a 50-mL centrifuge tube. Add 5.0 mL of *Internal standard solution*, and adjust with sodium hydroxide solution (1 in 2) to a pH of about 10. Add 25.0 mL of hexanes, place the cap on the tube, shake for about 2 minutes, and centrifuge. Use the upper hexanes layer as the *Standard preparation*.

Assay preparation—Transfer an accurately measured volume of Injectable Suspension, freshly mixed and free from air bubbles, equivalent to about 30 mg of chlorpheniramine maleate, to a 50-mL centrifuge tube. Proceed as directed under *Standard preparation*, beginning with "Add 5.0 mL of *Internal standard solution*." Use the upper hexanes layer as the *Assay preparation*.

Chromatographic system (see *Chromatography* ⟨621⟩)—The gas chromatograph is equipped with a flame-ionization detector, and contains a 4-mm × 1.8-m glass column packed with 1.2% liquid phase G16 and 0.5% potassium hydroxide on 100- to 120-mesh support S1A. The column is maintained isothermally at about 180°, and the injection port and the detector block are maintained at about 200°. Dry nitrogen is used as the carrier gas at a flow rate of about 50 mL per minute. Chromatograph the *Standard preparation*, and record the peak responses as directed for *Procedure*: the resolution, *R*, between the analyte and internal standard peaks is not less than 2.0, and the relative standard deviation for replicate injections is not more than 2.0%.

Procedure—Separately inject equal volumes (about 1.5 μL) of the *Standard preparation* and the *Assay preparation* into the chromatograph, record the chromatograms, and measure the responses for the major peaks. The relative retention times are about 0.75 for chlorpheniramine and 1.0 for brompheniramine. Calculate the quantity, in mg, of chlorpheniramine maleate ($C_{16}H_{19}ClN_2 \cdot C_4H_4O_4$) in each mL of the Injectable Suspension taken by the formula:

$$5(C / V)(R_U / R_S)$$

in which *C* is the concentration of USP Chlorpheniramine Maleate RS in the stock solution used to prepare the *Standard preparation*, *V* is the volume, in mL, of Injectable Suspension taken, and R_U and R_S are the peak response ratios of the chlorpheniramine maleate peak to the internal standard peak obtained from the *Assay preparation* and the *Standard preparation*, respectively.

Assay for dexamethasone—
Mobile phase—Prepare a suitable filtered mixture of water and acetonitrile (2 : 1). Make adjustments if necessary (see *System Suitability* under *Chromatography* ⟨621⟩).

Internal standard solution—Dissolve about 30 mg of beclomethasone in 2 mL of methanol in a 50-mL volumetric flask, dilute with methylene chloride to volume, and mix.

Standard preparation—Transfer about 25 mg of USP Dexamethasone RS, accurately weighed, to a 50-mL volumetric flask. Add about 1 mL of methanol, swirl to dissolve, dilute with methylene chloride to volume, and mix. Transfer 5.0 mL of this solution to a suitable flask, and add 5.0 mL of *Internal standard solution*. Heat the flask on a steam bath, and evaporate under a stream of nitrogen just to dryness. Add 10.0 mL of methanol to the flask, and swirl to dissolve the residue. This *Standard preparation* contains about 0.25 mg of USP Dexamethasone RS and 0.3 mg of beclomethasone per mL.

Assay preparation—Transfer an accurately measured volume of Injectable Suspension, freshly mixed and free from air bubbles, equivalent to about 2.5 mg of dexamethasone, to a separator containing 50 mL of 0.1 N hydrochloric acid, add 5.0 mL of *Internal* standard solution, and extract with four 25-mL portions of methylene chloride, combining the extracts in a second separator. Wash the combined extracts with 50 mL of sodium bicarbonate solution (1 in 20), filtering the lower methylene chloride layer through about 4 g of anhydrous sodium sulfate supported on a cotton pledget previously washed with methylene chloride, and collecting the filtrate in a suitable flask. Wash the aqueous layer with 25 mL of methylene chloride, and filter the lower methylene chloride layer through the same filter, collecting the filtrate in the same flask. Heat the flask on a steam bath, and evaporate under a stream of nitrogen just to dryness. Add 10.0 mL of methanol, and swirl to dissolve the residue.

Chromatographic system (see *Chromatography* ⟨621⟩)—The liquid chromatograph is equipped with a 254-nm detector and a 4-mm × 30-cm column that contains packing L1. The flow rate is about 1.2 mL per minute. Chromatograph the *Standard preparation*, and record the peak responses as directed for *Procedure:* the resolution, *R*, of the analyte and the internal standard peaks is not less than 2.0, and the relative standard deviation for replicate injections is not more than 2.0%.

Procedure—Separately inject equal volumes (about 10 μL) of the *Standard preparation* and the *Assay preparation* into the chromatograph, record the chromatograms, and measure the responses for the major peaks. The relative retention times are about 0.8 for dexamethasone and 1.0 for beclomethasone. Calculate the quantity, in mg, of dexamethasone ($C_{22}H_{29}FO_5$) in each mL of the Injectable Suspension taken by the formula:

$$10(C/V)(R_U/R_S)$$

in which *C* is the concentration, in mg per mL, of USP Dexamethasone RS in the *Standard preparation*, *V* is the volume, in mL, of Injectable Suspension taken, and R_U and R_S are the peak response ratios of the dexamethasone peak to the internal standard peak obtained from the *Assay preparation* and the *Standard preparation*, respectively.

Penicillin G Procaine, Dihydrostreptomycin Sulfate, and Prednisolone Injectable Suspension

» Penicillin G Procaine, Dihydrostreptomycin Sulfate, and Prednisolone Injectable Suspension is a sterile suspension of Penicillin G Procaine and Prednisolone in a solution of Dihydrostreptomycin Sulfate in Water for Injection. It contains one or more suitable buffers, dispersants, preservatives, and suspending agents. It may contain not more than 2.0 percent of procaine hydrochloride, and one or more suitable stabilizing agents. It contains not less than 90.0 percent and not more than 115.0 percent of the labeled number of Penicillin G Units, not less than 90.0 percent and not more than 115.0 percent of the labeled amount of dihydrostreptomycin ($C_{21}H_{41}N_7O_{12}$), and not less than 90.0 percent and not more than 110.0 percent of the labeled amount of prednisolone ($C_{21}H_{28}O_5$).

Packaging and storage—Preserve in single-dose or multiple-dose, tight containers.
Labeling—Label it to indicate that it is intended for veterinary use only, and is not to be used in animals to be slaughtered for human consumption.
USP Reference standards ⟨11⟩—*USP Penicillin G Potassium RS. USP Dihydrostreptomycin Sulfate RS. USP Prednisolone RS. USP Endotoxin RS.*
Identification—It responds to *Identification* tests A and B under *Penicillin G Procaine, Dihydrostreptomycin Sulfate, Chlorpheniramine Maleate, and Dexamethasone Injectable Suspension.*
Bacterial endotoxins ⟨85⟩—It contains not more than 0.01 Endotoxin Unit per 100 Penicillin G Units.
Other requirements—It meets the requirements of the test for *Sterility*, and for *pH* under *Penicillin G Procaine and Dihydrostreptomycin Sulfate Injectable Suspension.*
Assay for penicillin G—
Standard preparation—Using USP Penicillin G Potassium RS, prepare as directed for *Standard preparation* under *Iodometric Assay—Antibiotics* ⟨425⟩.
Assay preparation—Dilute an accurately measured volume of Injectable Suspension quantitatively with *Buffer No. 1* to obtain a solution containing about 2000 Penicillin G Units per mL. Pipet 2 mL of this solution into each of two glass-stoppered, 125-mL conical flasks.
Procedure—Proceed as directed for *Procedure* under *Iodometric Assay—Antibiotics* ⟨425⟩, except in the *Blank Determination* to add 0.1 mL of 1.2 N hydrochloric acid immediately before the 10.0 mL of 0.01 N iodine VS. Calculate the quantity, in Penicillin G Units, in the portion of Injectable Suspension taken by the formula:

$$(L/2D)(F)(B-I)$$

in which *L* is the labeled quantity, in Penicillin G Units, in the volume of Injectable Suspension taken, *D* is the concentration, in Penicillin G Units per mL, of the *Assay preparation*, on the basis of the labeled quantity in the portion of Injectable Suspension taken and the extent of dilution, and the other terms are as defined therein.
Assay for dihydrostreptomycin—Proceed as directed for the turbidimetric assay for dihydrostreptomycin as directed under *Antibiotics—Microbial Assays* ⟨81⟩, using an accurately measured volume of Injectable Suspension diluted quantitatively with water to yield a *Test Dilution* having a concentration assumed to be equal to the median dose level of the Standard.
Assay for prednisolone—
Standard preparation—Prepare as directed for *Standard Preparation* under *Single-steroid Assay* ⟨511⟩, using USP Prednisolone RS.
Assay preparation—Transfer to a separator an accurately measured volume of Injectable Suspension, and add 15 mL of water. Extract with three 25-mL portions and finally with one 20-mL portion of chloroform, filtering each portion through chloroform-washed cotton into a 100-mL volumetric flask. Add chloroform to volume, and mix. Pipet 20 mL of this solution into a suitable glass-stoppered flask or tube, evaporate the chloroform on a steam bath just to dryness, cool, and dissolve the residue in 2.0 mL, accurately measured, of a mixture of equal volumes of chloroform and alcohol.
Procedure—Proceed as directed for *Single-Steroid Assay* ⟨511⟩, using *Solvent A* to develop the chromatogram. Calculate the quantity, in mg, of prednisolone ($C_{21}H_{28}O_5$) in each mL of the Injectable Suspension taken by the formula:

$$0.01(C/V)(A_U/A_S)$$

in which the terms are as defined therein.

Penicillin G Procaine, Neomycin and Polymyxin B Sulfates, and Hydrocortisone Acetate Topical Suspension

» Penicillin G Procaine, Neomycin and Polymyxin B Sulfates, and Hydrocortisone Acetate Topical Suspension is a suspension of Penicillin G Procaine, Neomycin Sulfate, Polymyxin B Sulfate and Hydrocortisone Acetate in Peanut Oil or Sesame Oil. It may contain one or more suitable dispersing and suspending agents. It contains not less than 90.0 percent and not more than 140.0 percent of the labeled amounts of Penicillin G Units, of neomycin, and of polymyxin B Units, and not less than 90.0 percent and not more than 110.0 percent of the labeled amount of hydrocortisone acetate ($C_{23}H_{32}O_6$).

Packaging and storage—Preserve in well-closed containers.
Labeling—Label it to indicate that it is intended for veterinary use only.
USP Reference standards ⟨11⟩—*USP Penicillin G Potassium RS. USP Neomycin Sulfate RS. USP Polymyxin B Sulfate RS. USP Hydrocortisone Acetate RS.*
Water, *Method I* ⟨921⟩: not more than 1.0%, 20 mL of a mixture of toluene and methanol (7:3) being used in place of methanol in the titration vessel.
Assay for penicillin G—Proceed as directed for penicillin G under *Antibiotics—Microbial Assays* ⟨81⟩, using an accurately measured volume of Topical Suspension blended for 2 minutes in a high-speed glass blender jar with 499.0 mL of *Buffer No. 1* and 1.0 mL of polysorbate 80. Allow to stand for 10 minutes, and dilute an accurately measured volume of the aqueous phase quantitatively and stepwise with *Buffer No. 1* to obtain a *Test Dilution* having a concentration of penicillin G assumed to be equal to the median dose level of the *Standard*.
Assay for neomycin—Proceed as directed for neomycin under *Antibiotics—Microbial Assays* ⟨81⟩, using an accurately measured volume of Topical Suspension shaken in a separator with about 50 mL of ether, and extracted with four 20-mL portions of *Buffer No. 3*. Combine the aqueous extracts, and dilute with *Buffer No. 3* to an appropriate volume to obtain a stock solution. To an accurately measured volume of this stock solution add an accurately measured volume of penicillinase sufficient to inactivate the penicillin G therein, heat at 37° for 30 minutes, and dilute quantitatively and stepwise with *Buffer No. 3* to obtain a *Test Dilution* having a concentration of neomycin assumed to be equal to the median dose level of the *Standard*.
Assay for polymyxin B—Proceed as directed for polymyxin B under *Antibiotics—Microbial Assays* ⟨81⟩, using an accurately measured volume of Topical Suspension blended for 2 minutes in a high-speed glass blender jar containing 499.0 mL of *Buffer No. 6* and 1.0 mL of polysorbate 80. Allow to stand for 10 minutes, and to an accurately measured volume of the aqueous phase add an accurately measured volume of penicillinase sufficient to inactivate the penicillin G therein. Heat the solution at 37° for 30 minutes, and dilute quantitatively and stepwise with *Buffer No. 6* to obtain a *Test Dilution* having a concentration of polymyxin assumed to be equal to the median dose level of the *Standard*. Add to each test dilution of the *Standard* a quantity of USP Neomycin Sulfate RS dissolved in *Buffer No. 6* to obtain the same concentration of neomycin present in the *Test Dilution*.
Assay for hydrocortisone acetate—Using an accurately measured volume of Topical Suspension, proceed as directed in the *Assay* under *Hydrocortisone Acetate Lotion*.

Penicillin G Procaine and Novobiocin Sodium Intramammary Infusion

» Penicillin G Procaine and Novobiocin Sodium Intramammary Infusion is a suspension of Penicillin G Procaine and Novobiocin Sodium in a suitable vegetable oil vehicle. It contains a suitable preservative and suspending agent. It contains not less than 90.0 percent and not more than 125.0 percent of the labeled amounts of Penicillin G Units and novobiocin ($C_{31}H_{36}N_2O_{11}$).

Packaging and storage—Preserve in disposable syringes that are well-closed containers.
Labeling—Label it to indicate that it is for veterinary use only.
USP Reference standards ⟨11⟩—*USP Novobiocin RS. USP Penicillin G Potassium RS.*
Water, *Method I* ⟨921⟩: not more than 1.0%, 20 mL of a mixture of toluene and methanol (7:3) being used in place of methanol in the titration vessel.
Assay for penicillin G—Proceed as directed for penicillin G under *Antibiotics—Microbial Assays* ⟨81⟩, except to use *Staphylococcus aureus* ATCC No. 12692 as the test organism. Prepare the inoculum by growing the organism at 32° to 35° for 24 hours on Medium 1 to which has been added a solution of novobiocin sodium, containing the equivalent of 2.5 mg of novobiocin per mL that has been filtered through a membrane filter having a 0.2-µm porosity, so that the medium contains the equivalent of 10 µg of novobiocin per mL. Use an inoculum composition of about 5 mL of stock suspension in each 100 mL of Medium 1. Expel the contents of a syringe of Intramammary Infusion into a high-speed glass blender jar containing 1.0 mL of polysorbate 80 and 499.0 mL of *Buffer No. 1*, and blend for 3 to 5 minutes. Allow to stand for 10 minutes, and dilute an accurately measured volume of the aqueous phase quantitatively and stepwise with *Buffer No. 1* to obtain a *Test Dilution* having a concentration of penicillin G assumed to be equal to the median dose level of the *Standard*.
Assay for novobiocin—Proceed as directed for novobiocin under *Antibiotics—Microbial Assays* ⟨81⟩, expelling the contents of a syringe of Intramammary Infusion into a high-speed blender jar containing 1.0 mL of polysorbate 80 and 499.0 mL of *Buffer No. 3*, and blend for 3 to 5 minutes. Allow to stand for 10 minutes. To an accurately measured volume of the aqueous phase add sufficient penicillinase to inactivate the penicillin G therein, and dilute quantitatively and stepwise with *Buffer No. 6* to obtain a *Test Dilution* having a concentration of novobiocin assumed to be equal to the median dose level of the *Standard*. [NOTE—Store this *Test Dilution* at 37° for 30 minutes and allow to cool before using it to fill the cylinders on the plates.]

Penicillin G Sodium

$C_{16}H_{17}N_2NaO_4S$ 356.37

4-Thia-1-azabicyclo[3.2.0]heptane-2-carboxylic acid, 3,3-dimethyl-7-oxo-6-[(phenylacetyl)amino-], 2S-(2α,5α,6β-, monosodium salt.
Monosodium   (2S,5R,6R)-3,3-dimethyl-7-oxo-6-(2-phenylacetamido)-4-thia-1-azabicyclo[3.2.0]heptane-2-carboxylate [69-57-8].

» Penicillin G Sodium has a potency of not less than 1500 Penicillin G Units and not more than 1750 Penicillin G Units per mg.

Packaging and storage—Preserve in tight containers.
Labeling—Where it is intended for use in preparing injectable dosage forms, the label states that it is sterile or must be subjected to further processing during the preparation of injectable dosage forms.
USP Reference standards ⟨11⟩—*USP Endotoxin RS. USP Penicillin G Potassium RS. USP Penicillin G Sodium RS.*
Identification—
A: *Infrared Absorption* ⟨197K⟩.
B: It responds to the tests for *Sodium* ⟨191⟩.
Crystallinity ⟨695⟩: meets the requirements.
pH ⟨791⟩: between 5.0 and 7.5, in a solution containing 60 mg per mL.
Loss on drying ⟨731⟩—Dry about 100 mg, accurately weighed, in a capillary-stoppered bottle in vacuum at a pressure not exceeding 5 mm of mercury at 60° for 3 hours: it loses not more than 1.5% of its weight.
Other requirements—Where the label states that Penicillin G Sodium is sterile, it meets the requirements for *Sterility* and *Bacterial*

endotoxins under *Penicillin G Sodium for Injection*. Where the label states that Penicillin G Sodium must be subjected to further processing during the preparation of injectable dosage forms, it meets the requirements for *Bacterial endotoxins* under *Penicillin G Sodium for Injection*.

Assay—
Mobile phase, Resolution solution, Standard preparation, and *Chromatographic system*—Proceed as directed in the *Assay* under *Penicillin G Potassium*.

Assay preparation—Transfer about 5 mg of Penicillin G Sodium, accurately weighed, to a 50-mL volumetric flask, add about 45 mL of water, and shake to dissolve. Dilute with water to volume, and mix.

Procedure—Proceed as directed in the *Assay* under *Penicillin G Potassium*. Calculate the potency, in Penicillin G Units per mg, of Penicillin G Sodium taken by the formula:

$$(PW_S / W_U)(r_U / r_S)$$

in which W_U is the weight of Penicillin G Sodium taken to prepare the *Assay preparation*, and the other terms are as defined therein.

Penicillin G Sodium for Injection

» Penicillin G Sodium for Injection is sterile Penicillin G Sodium or a sterile mixture of Penicillin G Sodium and not less than 4.0 percent and not more than 5.0 percent of Sodium Citrate, of which not more than 0.15 percent may be replaced by Citric Acid. It contains not less than 90.0 percent and not more than 120.0 percent of the labeled amount of penicillin G. In addition, where it contains Sodium Citrate it has a potency of not less than 1420 and not more than 1667 Penicillin G Units per mg.

Packaging and storage—Preserve in *Containers for Sterile Solids* as described under *Injections* ⟨1⟩.
USP Reference standards ⟨11⟩—*USP Endotoxin RS. USP Penicillin G Potassium RS.*
Constituted solution—At the time of use, it meets the requirements for *Constituted Solutions* under *Injections* ⟨1⟩.
Identification—It responds to the *Identification* test under *Penicillin G Potassium for Injection*.
Crystallinity ⟨695⟩: meets the requirements.
Sterility ⟨71⟩—It meets the requirements when tested as directed for *Membrane Filtration* under *Test for Sterility of the Product to be Examined*.
Bacterial endotoxins ⟨85⟩—It contains not more than 0.01 USP Endotoxin Unit per 100 Penicillin G Units.
pH ⟨791⟩: between 5.0 and 7.5, in a solution containing 60 mg per mL, except where it is labeled as containing sodium citrate it is between 6.0 and 7.5.
Loss on drying ⟨731⟩—Dry about 100 mg, accurately weighed, in a capillary-stoppered bottle in vacuum at a pressure not exceeding 5 mm of mercury at 60° for 3 hours: it loses not more than 1.5% of its weight.
Particulate matter ⟨788⟩: meets the requirements for small-volume injections.
Other requirements—It meets the requirements for *Uniformity of Dosage Units* ⟨905⟩ and *Labeling* under *Injections* ⟨1⟩.
Assay—
Mobile phase, Standard preparation, Resolution solution, and *Chromatographic system*—Proceed as directed in the *Assay* under *Penicillin G Sodium*.

Assay preparation 1 (where it is represented as being in a single-dose container)—Constitute Penicillin G Sodium for Injection as directed in the labeling. Withdraw all of the withdrawable contents, using a hypodermic needle and syringe, and quantitatively dilute with water to obtain a solution containing about 160 Penicillin G Units per mL.

Assay preparation 2 (where the label states the quantity of penicillin G in a given volume of constituted solution)—Constitute Penicillin G Sodium for Injection as directed in the labeling. Quantitatively dilute an accurately measured volume of the constituted solution with water to obtain a solution containing about 160 Penicillin G Units per mL.

Assay preparation 3 (where it contains Sodium Citrate)—Transfer about 50 mg of the Penicillin G Sodium for Injection, accurately weighed, to a 500-mL volumetric flask, add about 400 mL of water, and shake to dissolve. Dilute with water to volume, and mix.

Procedure—Proceed as directed for *Procedure* in the *Assay* under *Penicillin G Sodium*. Calculate the number of Penicillin G Units in the container or in the portion of constituted solution taken by the formula:

$$(L/D)(PW_S / 50)(r_U / r_S)$$

in which L is the labeled quantity of Penicillin G Units in the container or in the volume of constituted solution taken; D is the concentration, in Penicillin G Units per mL, of *Assay preparation 1* or *Assay preparation 2*, on the basis of the labeled quantity in the container or in the portion of constituted solution taken and the extent of dilution; P is the specified potency, in Penicillin G Units per mg, of USP Penicillin G Potassium RS; W_S is the weight, in mg, of USP Penicillin G Potassium RS taken to prepare the *Standard preparation;* and r_U and r_S are the penicillin G peak responses obtained from the *Assay preparation* and the *Standard preparation,* respectively. Calculate the potency, in Penicillin G Units per mg, of the Penicillin G Sodium for Injection taken by the formula:

$$10(W_S / W_U)(P)(r_U / r_S)$$

in which W_S and W_U are the weights, in mg, of USP Penicillin G Potassium RS and Penicillin G Sodium for Injection taken to prepare the *Standard preparation* and *Assay preparation 3*, respectively; and the other terms are as defined above. Perform the above procedure on 10 containers (where it is represented as being in a single-dose container) and, if necessary, on 10 containers (where the label states the quantity of penicillin G in a given volume of constituted solution). Use the individual results to determine the *Uniformity of dosage units* and the average thereof as the *Assay* value.

Penicillin V

$C_{16}H_{18}N_2O_5S$ 350.39
4-Thia-1-azabicyclo[3.2.0]heptane-2-carboxylic acid, 3,3-dimethyl-7-oxo-6-(phenoxyacetyl)amino-, 2S-(2α,5α,6β)-.
(2S,5R,6R)-3,3-Dimethyl-7-oxo-6-(2-phenoxyacetamido)-4-thia-1-azabicyclo[3.2.0]heptane-2-carboxylic acid   [87-08-1].

» Penicillin V has a potency of not less than 1525 and not more than 1780 Penicillin V Units per mg.

Packaging and storage—Preserve in tight containers.
Labeling—Label it to indicate that it is to be used in the manufacture of nonparenteral drugs only.
USP Reference standards ⟨11⟩—*USP Penicillin V Potassium RS. USP Penicillin V RS.*
Identification, *Infrared Absorption* ⟨197K⟩—Do not dry specimens.
Crystallinity ⟨695⟩: meets the requirements.
pH ⟨791⟩: between 2.5 and 4.0, in a suspension containing 30 mg per mL.
Water, *Method I* ⟨921⟩: not more than 2.0%.
Phenoxyacetic acid—
Diluent—Use pH 6.6 phosphate buffer (see *Buffer Solutions* in the section *Reagents, Indicators, and Solutions*).

Mobile phase—Prepare a mixture of water, acetonitrile, and glacial acetic acid (65 : 35 : 1). Make adjustments if necessary (see *System Suitability* under *Chromatography* ⟨621⟩).

Standard solution—Dissolve an accurately weighed quantity of phenoxyacetic acid quantitatively in *Diluent* to obtain a solution having a known concentration of about 0.1 mg per mL.

Test solution—Dissolve an accurately weighed quantity of Penicillin V quantitatively in *Diluent* to obtain a solution containing 20.0 mg per mL. [NOTE—Use this solution on the day prepared.]

Chromatographic system (see *Chromatography* ⟨621⟩)—The liquid chromatograph is equipped with a 254-nm detector and a 4.6-mm × 25-cm column containing 5-µm packing L1. The flow rate is about 1 mL per minute. Chromatograph the *Standard solution*, and record the responses as directed for *Procedure*: the tailing factor is not more than 1.5, and the relative standard deviation for replicate injections is not more than 2.0%.

Procedure—[NOTE—Use peak areas where peak responses are indicated.] Separately inject equal volumes (about 20 µL) of the *Standard solution* and the *Test solution* into the chromatograph, record the chromatograms, and measure the responses for the phenoxyacetic acid peaks. Calculate the percentage of phenoxyacetic acid in the portion of Penicillin V taken by the formula:

$$5C(r_U / r_S)$$

in which C is the concentration, in mg per mL, of phenoxyacetic acid in the *Standard solution*, and r_U and r_S are the phenoxyacetic acid peak responses obtained from the *Test solution* and the *Standard solution*, respectively. Not more than 0.5% is found.

Limit of *p*-hydroxypenicillin V—Using the chromatogram of the *Assay preparation* obtained as directed in the *Assay*, calculate the percentage of *p*-hydroxypenicillin V in the portion of Penicillin V taken by the formula:

$$100 r_p / r_s$$

in which r_p is the *p*-hydroxypenicillin V peak response; and r_s is the sum of the *p*-hydroxypenicillin V and penicillin V peak responses: not more than 5.0% is found.

Assay—

Mobile phase—Prepare a suitable filtered and degassed mixture of water, acetonitrile, and glacial acetic acid (650 : 350 : 5.75). Make adjustments if necessary (see *System Suitability* under *Chromatography* ⟨621⟩).

Standard preparation—Dissolve an accurately weighed quantity of USP Penicillin V Potassium RS in *Mobile phase* to obtain a solution having a known concentration of about 2.5 mg per mL.

Assay preparation—Transfer about 125 mg of Penicillin V, accurately weighed, to a 50-mL volumetric flask, dilute with *Mobile phase* to volume, and mix.

Resolution solution—Prepare a solution in *Mobile phase* containing about 2.5 mg of penicillin G potassium and 2.5 mg of penicillin V potassium per mL.

Chromatographic system (see *Chromatography* ⟨621⟩)—The liquid chromatograph is equipped with a 254-nm detector and a 4-mm × 30-cm column that contains packing L1. The flow rate is about 1 mL per minute. Chromatograph the *Resolution solution*, and record the peak responses as directed for *Procedure*: the relative retention times are about 0.8 for penicillin G and 1.0 for penicillin V, the column efficiency determined from the penicillin V peak is not less than 1800 theoretical plates, and the resolution, R, between penicillin G and penicillin V is not less than 3.0. Chromatograph the *Standard preparation*, and record the peak responses as directed for *Procedure*: the relative standard deviation for replicate injections is not more than 1.0%.

Procedure—Separately inject equal volumes (about 10 µL) of the *Standard preparation* and the *Assay preparation* into the chromatograph, record the chromatograms, and measure the responses for the major penicillin V peaks and any *p*-hydroxypenicillin V peaks with a retention time of about 0.4 relative to that of the main penicillin V peak. Calculate the quantity, in USP Penicillin V Units, in each mg of the Penicillin V taken by the formula:

$$50(CP / W_U)(r_U / r_S)$$

in which C is the concentration, in mg per mL, of USP Penicillin V Potassium RS in the *Standard preparation*, P is the designated potency, in USP Penicillin V Units per mg, of USP Penicillin V Potassium RS, W_U is the weight, in mg, of Penicillin V taken to prepare the *Assay preparation*, and r_U and r_S are the sums of the *p*-hydroxypenicillin V and penicillin V peak responses obtained from the *Assay preparation* and the *Standard preparation*, respectively.

Penicillin V for Oral Suspension

» Penicillin V for Oral Suspension is a dry mixture of Penicillin V with or without one or more suitable buffers, colors, flavors, and suspending agents. It contains not less than 90.0 percent and not more than 120.0 percent of the labeled number of Penicillin V Units when constituted as directed.

Packaging and storage—Preserve in tight containers.
Labeling—It may be labeled in terms of the weight of penicillin V contained therein, in addition to or instead of Units, on the basis that 1600 Penicillin V Units are equivalent to 1 mg of penicillin V.
USP Reference standards ⟨11⟩—*USP Penicillin V Potassium RS. USP Penicillin V RS.*
Identification—The retention time of the penicillin V peak in the chromatogram of the *Assay preparation* corresponds to that in the chromatogram of the *Standard preparation*, as obtained in the *Assay*.
Uniformity of dosage units ⟨905⟩—
FOR SOLID PACKAGED IN SINGLE-UNIT CONTAINERS: meets the requirements.
Deliverable volume ⟨698⟩: meets the requirements.
pH ⟨791⟩: between 2.0 and 4.0, in the suspension constituted as directed in the labeling.
Water, *Method I* ⟨921⟩: not more than 1.0%.
Assay—

Mobile phase, Standard preparation, Resolution solution, and *Chromatographic system*—Proceed as directed in the *Assay* under *Penicillin V*.

Assay preparation—Transfer an accurately measured volume of Penicillin V for Oral Suspension, freshly mixed and free from air bubbles, constituted as directed in the labeling, equivalent to about 400,000 USP Penicillin V Units, to a 100-mL volumetric flask, dilute with *Mobile phase* to volume, and mix. Filter a portion of this solution through a suitable filter having a 0.5-µm or finer porosity, and use the filtrate as the *Assay preparation*.

Procedure—Proceed as directed for *Procedure* in the *Assay* under *Penicillin V*. Calculate the number of USP Penicillin V Units in each mL of the constituted Penicillin V for Oral Suspension taken by the formula:

$$100(CP / V)(r_U / r_S)$$

in which V is the volume, in mL, of constituted Penicillin V for Oral Suspension taken, and the other terms are as defined therein.

Penicillin V Tablets

» Penicillin V Tablets contain not less than 90.0 percent and not more than 120.0 percent of the labeled number of Penicillin V Units.

Packaging and storage—Preserve in tight containers.
Labeling—The Tablets may be labeled in terms of the weight of penicillin V contained therein, in addition to or instead of Units, on the basis that 1600 Penicillin V Units are equivalent to 1 mg of penicillin V.

USP Reference standards ⟨11⟩—*USP Penicillin V Potassium RS. USP Penicillin V RS.*

Identification—The retention time of the penicillin V peak in the chromatogram of the *Assay preparation* corresponds to that in the chromatogram of the *Standard preparation,* as obtained in the *Assay.*

Dissolution ⟨711⟩—
  Medium: water; 900 mL.
  Apparatus 2: 50 rpm.
  Time: 45 minutes.
  Procedure—Determine the amount of penicillin V ($C_{16}H_{18}N_2O_5S$) by a suitable validated spectrophotometric analysis of a filtered portion of the solution under test, suitably diluted with *Dissolution Medium,* if necessary, in comparison with a Standard solution having a known concentration of USP Penicillin V Potassium RS in the same medium.
  Tolerances—Not less than 75% (*Q*) of the labeled amount of $C_{16}H_{18}N_2O_5S$ is dissolved in 45 minutes.

Uniformity of dosage units ⟨905⟩: meet the requirements.

Water, *Method I* ⟨921⟩: not more than 3.0%.

Assay—
  Mobile phase, Standard preparation, Resolution solution, and *Chromatographic system*—Proceed as directed in the *Assay* under *Penicillin V.*
  Assay preparation—Weigh and finely powder not less than 20 Tablets. Transfer an accurately weighed portion of the powder, equivalent to about 400,000 USP Penicillin V Units, to a 100-mL volumetric flask, dilute with *Mobile phase* to volume, and shake for about 5 minutes. Filter a portion of this solution through a suitable filter of 0.5 µm or finer porosity, and use the filtrate as the *Assay preparation.*
  Procedure—Proceed as directed for *Procedure* in the *Assay* under *Penicillin V.* Calculate the number of USP Penicillin V Units in the portion of Tablets taken by the formula:

$$100CP(r_U / r_S)$$

in which the terms are as defined therein.

Penicillin V Benzathine

($C_{16}H_{18}N_2O_5S)_2 \cdot C_{16}H_{20}N_2$ 941.12
4-Thia-1-azabicyclo[3.2.0]heptane-2-carboxylic acid, 3,3-dimethyl-7-oxo-6-[(2-phenoxyacetyl)amino-], [2*S*-(2α,5α,6β)]-, compd. with *N,N'*-bis(phenylmethyl)-1,2-ethanediamine (2 : 1).
(2*S*,5*R*,6*R*)-3,3-Dimethyl-7-oxo-6-(2-phenoxyacetamido)-4-thia-1-azabicyclo[3.2.0]heptane-2-carboxylic acid compound with *N,N'*-dibenzylethylenediamine (2 : 1) [5928-84-7].
Tetrahydrate 1013.21 [63690-57-3].

» Penicillin V Benzathine has a potency of not less than 1060 and not more than 1240 Penicillin V Units per mg.

Packaging and storage—Preserve in tight containers.

USP Reference standards ⟨11⟩—*USP Penicillin V Potassium RS.*

Crystallinity ⟨695⟩: meets the requirements.

pH ⟨791⟩: between 4.0 and 6.5, in a suspension containing about 30 mg per mL.

Water, *Method I* ⟨921⟩: between 5.0% and 8.0%.

Penicillin V content—Transfer about 40 mg, accurately weighed, to a 100-mL volumetric flask, add methanol to volume, and mix. Concomitantly determine the absorbances of this solution and of a similarly prepared Standard solution prepared with about 30 mg of USP Penicillin V Potassium RS at the wavelength of maximum absorbance at about 276 nm. Determine the percentage of penicillin V taken by the formula:

$$P(a_U / a_S)$$

in which *P* is the percentage content of penicillin V in the USP Penicillin V Potassium RS, and a_U and a_S are the absorptivities of the solution of the specimen and the Standard solution, respectively: between 62.3% and 72.5% is found.

Assay—
  Standard preparation—Prepare as directed for *Standard preparation* under *Iodometric Assay—Antibiotics* ⟨425⟩, using USP Penicillin V Potassium RS.
  Assay preparations—Dissolve a quantity of Penicillin V Benzathine in 1.0 N sodium hydroxide to obtain a solution containing 2000 Penicillin V Units per mL. Pipet 2 mL of this solution into a glass-stoppered, 125-mL conical flask, and use as the *Assay preparation* for *Inactivation and titration.* Dilute a quantity of Penicillin V Benzathine quantitatively with water to obtain a suspension containing 2000 Penicillin V Units per mL. Pipet 2 mL of this suspension into a glass-stoppered, 125-mL conical flask, and use as the *Assay preparation* for the *Blank determination.*
  Procedure—Proceed as directed for *Procedure* under *Iodometric Assay—Antibiotics* ⟨425⟩, except in the *Inactivation and titration* of the specimen to omit the addition of 2.0 mL of 1.0 N sodium hydroxide. Calculate the potency, in Penicillin V Units per mg, in the Penicillin V Benzathine taken by the formula:

$$(F)(B - I) / (2D)$$

in which *D* is the concentration, in mg per mL, of the *Assay preparation* for *Inactivation and titration* on the basis of the weight of Penicillin V Benzathine taken and the extent of dilution.

Penicillin V Benzathine Oral Suspension

» Penicillin V Benzathine Oral Suspension contains not less than 90.0 percent and not more than 120.0 percent of the labeled number of Penicillin V Units per mL. It contains one or more suitable buffers, colors, dispersants, flavors, and preservatives.

Packaging and storage—Preserve in tight containers, and store in a refrigerator.

Labeling—It may be labeled in terms of the weight of penicillin V contained therein, in addition to or instead of Units, on the basis that 1600 Penicillin V Units are equivalent to 1 mg of penicillin V.

USP Reference standards ⟨11⟩—*USP Penicillin V Potassium RS.*

Uniformity of dosage units ⟨905⟩—
  FOR SUSPENSION PACKAGED IN SINGLE-UNIT CONTAINERS: meets the requirements.

Deliverable volume ⟨698⟩: meets the requirements.

pH ⟨791⟩: between 6.0 and 7.0.

Assay—
  Standard preparation—Prepare as directed for *Standard preparation* under *Iodometric Assay—Antibiotics* ⟨425⟩, using USP Penicillin V Potassium RS.
  Assay preparations—Dilute an accurately measured volume of Oral Suspension, freshly mixed and free from air bubbles, quantitatively with 1.0 N sodium hydroxide to obtain a solution containing 2000 Penicillin V Units per mL. Pipet 2 mL of this solution into a glass-stoppered, 125-mL conical flask, and use as the *Assay preparation* for *Inactivation and titration.* Dilute an accurately measured volume of Oral Suspension quantitatively with water to obtain a suspension containing 2000 Penicillin V Units per mL. Pipet 2 mL of this suspension into a glass-stoppered, 125-mL conical flask, and use as the *Assay preparation* for the *Blank determination.*
  Procedure—Proceed as directed for *Procedure* under *Iodometric Assay—Antibiotics* ⟨425⟩, except in the *Inactivation and titration* to omit the addition of 2.0 mL of 1.0 N sodium hydroxide. Calculate

the quantity, in Penicillin V Units, in each mL of the Oral Suspension taken by the formula:

$$(T/2D)F(B - I)$$

in which T is the labeled quantity, in Penicillin V Units per mL, in the Oral Suspension, and D is the concentration, in Penicillin V Units per mL, in the *Assay preparation* for *Inactivation and titration* on the basis of the volume of Oral Suspension taken and the extent of dilution.

Penicillin V Potassium

$C_{16}H_{17}KN_2O_5S$ 388.48

4-Thia-1-azabicyclo[3.2.0]heptane-2-carboxylic acid, 3,3-dimethyl-7-oxo-[6-(phenoxyacetyl)amino]-, monopotassium salt, [2S-(2α,5α,6β)]-.
Monopotassium   (2S,5R,6R)-3,3-dimethyl-7-oxo-6-(2-phenoxyacetamido)-4-thia-1-azabicyclo[3.2.0]heptane-2-carboxylate [*132-98-9*].

» Penicillin V Potassium has a potency of not less than 1380 and not more than 1610 Penicillin V Units per mg.

Packaging and storage—Preserve in tight containers.
Labeling—Label it to indicate that it is to be used in the manufacture of nonparenteral drugs only.
USP Reference standards ⟨11⟩—*USP Penicillin V Potassium RS*.
Identification—
  A: *Infrared Absorption* ⟨197K⟩.
  B: It responds to the flame test for *Potassium* ⟨191⟩.
Specific rotation ⟨781S⟩:   between +220° and +235°.
  Test solution: 10 mg per mL, in carbon dioxide-free water.
Crystallinity ⟨695⟩:   meets the requirements.
pH ⟨791⟩:   between 4.0 and 7.5, in a solution containing 30 mg per mL.
Loss on drying ⟨731⟩—Dry about 100 mg in a capillary-stoppered bottle in vacuum at 60° for 3 hours: it loses not more than 1.5% of its weight.
Phenoxyacetic acid—
  Diluent, Mobile phase, Standard solution, and *Chromatographic system*—Proceed as directed in the test for *Phenoxyacetic acid* under *Penicillin V*.
  Test solution—Dissolve an accurately weighed quantity of Penicillin V Potassium quantitatively in *Diluent* to obtain a solution containing 20.0 mg per mL. [NOTE—Use this solution on the day prepared.]
  Procedure—Proceed as directed for *Procedure* in the test for *Phenoxyacetic acid* under *Penicillin V*. Calculate the percentage of phenoxyacetic acid in the portion of Penicillin V Potassium taken by the formula:

$$5C(r_U/r_S)$$

in which C is the concentration, in mg per mL, of phenoxyacetic acid in the *Standard solution*, and r_U and r_S are the phenoxyacetic acid peak responses obtained from the *Test solution* and the *Standard solution*, respectively. Not more than 0.5% is found.
Limit of *p*-hydroxypenicillin V—Using the chromatogram of the *Assay preparation* obtained as directed in the *Assay*, calculate the percentage of *p*-hydroxypenicillin V in the portion of Penicillin V Potassium taken by the formula:

$$100r_p/r_U$$

in which r_p is the *p*-hydroxypenicillin V peak response, and r_U is the sum of the *p*-hydroxypenicillin V and penicillin V peak responses: not more than 5.0% is found.
Assay—
  Mobile phase, Standard preparation, Resolution solution, and *Chromatographic system*—Proceed as directed in the *Assay* under *Penicillin V*.
  Assay preparation—Transfer about 125 mg of Penicillin V Potassium, accurately weighed, to a 50-mL volumetric flask, dilute with *Mobile phase* to volume, and mix.
  Procedure—Proceed as directed for *Procedure* in the *Assay* under *Penicillin V*. Calculate the quantity, in USP Penicillin V Units, in each mg of the Penicillin V Potassium taken by the formula:

$$50(CP/W_U)(r_U/r_S)$$

in which W_U is the weight, in mg, of Penicillin V Potassium taken to prepare the *Assay preparation*, and the other terms are as defined therein.

Penicillin V Potassium for Oral Solution

» Penicillin V Potassium for Oral Solution is a dry mixture of Penicillin V Potassium with or without one or more suitable buffers, colors, flavors, preservatives, and suspending agents. It contains not less than 90.0 percent and not more than 135.0 percent of the labeled number of Penicillin V Units when constituted as directed.

Packaging and storage—Preserve in tight containers.
Labeling—It may be labeled in terms of the weight of penicillin V contained therein, in addition to or instead of Units, on the basis that 1600 Penicillin V Units are equivalent to 1 mg of penicillin V.
USP Reference standards ⟨11⟩—*USP Penicillin V Potassium RS*.
Identification—The retention time of the penicillin V peak in the chromatogram of the *Assay preparation* corresponds to that in the chromatogram of the *Standard preparation,* as obtained in the *Assay*.
Uniformity of dosage units ⟨905⟩—
  FOR SOLID PACKAGED IN SINGLE-UNIT CONTAINERS: meets the requirements.
Deliverable volume ⟨698⟩:   meets the requirements.
pH ⟨791⟩:   between 5.0 and 7.5, when constituted as directed in the labeling.
Water, *Method I* ⟨921⟩:   not more than 1.0%.
Assay—
  Mobile phase, Standard preparation, Resolution solution, and *Chromatographic system*—Proceed as directed in the *Assay* under *Penicillin V*.
  Assay preparation—Transfer an accurately measured volume of Penicillin V Potassium for Oral Solution, constituted as directed in the labeling, equivalent to about 400,000 USP Penicillin V Units, to a 100-mL volumetric flask, dilute with *Mobile phase* to volume, and mix. Filter a portion of this solution through a suitable filter having a 0.5-μm or finer porosity, and use the filtrate as the *Assay preparation*.
  Procedure—Proceed as directed for *Procedure* in the *Assay* under *Penicillin V*. Calculate the number of USP Penicillin V Units

in each mL of the constituted Penicillin V Potassium for Oral Solution taken by the formula:

$$100(CP/V)(r_U/r_S)$$

in which V is the volume, in mL, of constituted Penicillin V Potassium for Oral Suspension taken, and the other terms are as defined therein.

Penicillin V Potassium Tablets

» Penicillin V Potassium Tablets contain not less than 90.0 percent and not more than 120.0 percent of the labeled number of Penicillin V Units.

Packaging and storage—Preserve in tight containers.
Labeling—Label the chewable Tablets to indicate that they are to be chewed before swallowing. The Tablets may be labeled in terms of the weight of penicillin V contained therein, in addition to or instead of Units, on the basis that 1600 Penicillin V Units are equivalent to 1 mg of penicillin V.

USP Reference standards ⟨11⟩—*USP Penicillin V Potassium RS*.
Identification—The retention time of the penicillin V peak in the chromatogram of the *Assay preparation* corresponds to that in the chromatogram of the *Standard preparation*, as obtained in the *Assay*.

Dissolution ⟨711⟩—
Medium: pH 6.0 phosphate buffer (see *Buffer Solutions* in the section *Reagents, Indicators, and Solutions*); 900 mL.
Apparatus 2: 50 rpm.
Time: 45 minutes.
Procedure—Determine the amount of Penicillin V Units by a suitable validated spectrophotometric analysis of a filtered portion of the solution under test, suitably diluted with *Dissolution Medium*, if necessary, in comparison with a Standard solution of USP Penicillin V Potassium RS in the same medium having a known concentration of Penicillin V Units.
Tolerances—Not less than 75% (*Q*) of the labeled amount of Penicillin V Units is dissolved in 45 minutes.

Uniformity of dosage units ⟨905⟩: meet the requirements.
Loss on drying ⟨731⟩—Dry about 100 mg in a capillary-stoppered bottle in vacuum at 60° for 3 hours: it loses not more than 1.5% of its weight.

Assay—
Mobile phase, Standard preparation, Resolution solution, and *Chromatographic system*—Proceed as directed in the *Assay* under *Penicillin V*.
Assay preparation—Weigh and finely powder not less than 20 Tablets. Transfer an accurately weighed portion of the powder, equivalent to about 400,000 USP Penicillin V Units, to a 100-mL volumetric flask, dilute with *Mobile phase* to volume, and shake for about 5 minutes. Filter a portion of this solution through a suitable filter having a 0.5-μm or finer porosity, and use the filtrate as the *Assay preparation*.
Procedure—Proceed as directed for *Procedure* in the *Assay* under *Penicillin V*. Calculate the number of USP Penicillin V Units in the portion of Tablets taken by the formula:

$$100CP(r_U/r_S)$$

in which the terms are as defined therein.

Pentazocine

$C_{19}H_{27}NO$ 285.43
2,6-Methano-3-benzazocin-8-ol, 1,2,3,4,5,6-hexahydro-6,11-dimethyl-3-(3-methyl-2-butenyl)-, (2α,6α,11*R**)-.
(2*R**,6*R**,11*R**)-1,2,3,4,5,6-Hexahydro-6,11-dimethyl-3-(3-methyl-2-butenyl)-2,6-methano-3-benzazocin-8-ol   [359-83-1].

» Pentazocine contains not less than 98.0 percent and not more than 101.5 percent of $C_{19}H_{27}NO$, calculated on the dried basis.

Packaging and storage—Preserve in tight, light-resistant containers.
USP Reference standards ⟨11⟩—*USP Pentazocine RS*.
Identification—
  A: *Infrared Absorption* ⟨197K⟩.
  B: *Ultraviolet Absorption* ⟨197U⟩—
    Solution: 80 μg per mL.
    Medium: 0.01 N hydrochloric acid.
    Absorptivities at 278 nm, calculated on the dried basis, do not differ by more than 3.0%.
Melting range ⟨741⟩: between 147° and 158°, with slight darkening.
Loss on drying ⟨731⟩—Dry it at a pressure not exceeding 5 mm of mercury at 60° to constant weight: it loses not more than 1.0% of its weight.
Residue on ignition ⟨281⟩: not more than 0.2%.
Ordinary impurities ⟨466⟩—
  Test solution: methanol.
  Standard solution: methanol.
  Eluant: a mixture of chloroform, methanol, and isopropylamine (94 : 3 : 3).
  Visualization—Heat the plate in an oven at 105° for 15 minutes, cool, follow with visualization technique 17, and view under short-wavelength UV light.
Assay—Dissolve about 500 mg of Pentazocine, accurately weighed, in 50 mL of glacial acetic acid, add 1 drop of crystal violet TS, and titrate with 0.1 N perchloric acid VS to a green endpoint. Perform a blank determination, and make any necessary correction. Each mL of 0.1 N perchloric acid is equivalent to 28.54 mg of $C_{19}H_{27}NO$.

Pentazocine Hydrochloride

$C_{19}H_{27}NO \cdot HCl$ 321.88
2,6-Methano-3-benzazocin-8-ol, 1,2,3,4,5,6-hexahydro-6,11-dimethyl-3-(3-methyl-2-butenyl)-, hydrochloride, (2α,6α,11*R**)-.
(2*R**,6*R**,11*R**)-1,2,3,4,5,6-Hexahydro-6,11-dimethyl-3-(3-methyl-2-butenyl)-2,6-methano-3-benzazocin-8-ol hydrochloride [64024-15-3].

» Pentazocine Hydrochloride contains not less than 98.0 percent and not more than 102.0 percent of $C_{19}H_{27}NO \cdot HCl$, calculated on the dried basis.

Packaging and storage—Preserve in tight, light-resistant containers.

USP Reference standards ⟨11⟩—*USP Pentazocine RS.*
Identification—
  A: *Ultraviolet Absorption* ⟨197U⟩—
    Solution: 80 μg per mL of pentazocine.
    Medium: 0.01 N hydrochloric acid.
    Absorptivities at 278 nm, calculated on the dried basis, do not differ by more than 3.0%. [NOTE—The molecular weight of pentazocine ($C_{19}H_{27}NO$) is 285.43.]
  B: Dissolve 50 mg of USP Pentazocine RS in 25 mL of 0.01 N hydrochloric acid in a separator, and use this in place of the Standard solution specified under *Identification—Organic Nitrogenous Bases* ⟨181⟩: Pentazocine Hydrochloride meets the requirements of the test.
  C: A solution (1 in 100) responds to the tests for *Chloride* ⟨191⟩.
Loss on drying ⟨731⟩—Dry it at a pressure not exceeding 5 mm of mercury at 100° to constant weight: it loses not more than 1.0% of its weight.
Residue on ignition ⟨281⟩: not more than 0.2%.
Ordinary impurities ⟨466⟩—
  Test solution: methanol.
  Standard solution: methanol, USP Pentazocine RS being used.
  Eluant: a mixture of chloroform, methanol, and isopropylamine (94 : 3 : 3).
  Visualization—Heat the plate in an oven at 105° for 15 minutes, cool, follow with visualization technique 17, and view under short-wavelength UV light.
  Limits—The total of any ordinary impurities observed does not exceed 1.0%.
Assay—Dissolve about 650 mg of Pentazocine Hydrochloride, accurately weighed, in 50 mL of glacial acetic acid, and add 10 mL of mercuric acetate TS. Add 1 drop of crystal violet TS, and titrate with 0.1 N perchloric acid VS to a green endpoint. Perform a blank determination, and make any necessary correction. Each mL of 0.1 N perchloric acid is equivalent to 32.19 mg of $C_{19}H_{27}NO \cdot HCl$.

Pentazocine and Acetaminophen Tablets

(Monograph under this title—to become official February 1, 2009)

» Pentazocine and Acetaminophen Tablets contain an amount of Pentazocine Hydrochloride equivalent to not less than 90.0 percent and not more than 110.0 percent of the labeled amount of pentazocine ($C_{19}H_{27}NO$) and not less than 90.0 percent and not more than 110.0 percent of the labeled amount of acetaminophen ($C_8H_9NO_2$).

Packaging and storage—Preserve in tight, light-resistant containers.
USP Reference standards ⟨11⟩—*USP Acetaminophen RS. USP Pentazocine RS.*
Thin-layer chromatographic identification test ⟨201⟩—
  Test solution—Transfer a quantity of finely powdered Tablets, equivalent to about 5 mg of pentazocine and 130 mg of acetaminophen, to a suitable flask, and add 5 mL of a mixture of chloroform and methanol (1 : 1), shake, and allow the solids to settle. Use the supernatant.
  Standard solutions—Prepare a solution of USP Pentazocine RS in a mixture of chloroform and methanol (1 : 1) containing 1 mg per mL (*Standard solution A*). Using the same solvent, prepare a solution of USP Acetaminophen RS containing 26 mg per mL (*Standard solution B*).
  Developing solvent system: a mixture of ethyl acetate, methanol, and formic acid (90 : 5 : 5).
  Procedure—Evaporate the solvents in cool, circulating air. After developing and examining the spots, spray the plate with iodoplatinate reagent prepared by dissolving 300 mg of platinic chloride in 100 mL of water and adding 100 mL of potassium iodide solution (6 in 100): the chromatogram obtained with the *Test solution* shows two principal spots that correspond in R_F values, size, and intensity of color with the spots obtained from *Standard solutions A* and *B*.
Uniformity of dosage units ⟨905⟩: meet the requirements.
  PROCEDURE FOR CONTENT UNIFORMITY OF PENTAZOCINE AND ACETAMINOPHEN—
  Solvent—Prepare a mixture of acetonitrile and 0.035 N sulfuric acid (6 : 4).
  Mobile phase—Prepare a mixture of 0.005 M monobasic sodium phosphate, tetrahydrofuran, and phosphoric acid (950 : 50 : 1). Make adjustments if necessary (see *System Suitability* under *Chromatography* ⟨621⟩).
  Pentazocine standard stock solution—Dissolve an accurately weighed quantity of USP Pentazocine RS in *Solvent*, and dilute quantitatively with *Solvent* to obtain a solution having a known concentration of about 0.25 mg per mL.
  Standard solution—Transfer an accurately weighed quantity of USP Acetaminophen RS to a suitable volumetric flask, add a sufficient volume of *Pentazocine standard stock solution*, and mix to dissolve the acetaminophen. Dilute with *Mobile phase* to volume, and mix to obtain known concentrations of about 0.0125 mg and 0.325 mg of pentazocine and acetaminophen per mL, respectively.
  Test solution—Transfer 1 Tablet to a 100-mL volumetric flask, add 50 mL of *Solvent,* and sonicate for about 30 minutes. Dilute with *Solvent* to volume, and mix. Pass a portion of this solution through a paper filter, covering the funnel with a watch glass, and discarding the first few mL of the filtrate. Dilute 5.0 mL of the filtrate with *Mobile phase* to 100 mL, and pass this solution through a membrane filter having a 0.5-μm or finer porosity.
  System suitability solution—Transfer about 32.5 mg of USP Acetaminophen RS to a 100-mL volumetric flask, dissolve in and dilute with *Solvent* to volume, and mix. Transfer 1.0 mL of this solution to a 100-mL volumetric flask, add 5.0 mL of *Pentazocine standard stock solution,* dilute with *Mobile phase* to volume, and mix.
  Chromatographic system (see *Chromatography* ⟨621⟩)—The liquid chromatograph is equipped with a 220-nm detector and a 9.4-mm × 10-cm column that contains 5-μm packing L1. The flow rate is about 1.5 mL per minute. Chromatograph the *System suitability solution*, and record the peak responses as directed for *Procedure*: the relative retention times are about 0.2 for acetaminophen and 1.0 for pentazocine; the resolution, *R*, between pentazocine and acetaminophen is not less than 7; and the relative standard deviation for replicate injections is not more than 2.0% for the pentazocine and acetaminophen peaks.
  Procedure—Separately inject equal volumes (about 10 μL) of the *Standard solution* and the *Test solution* into the liquid chromatograph, and measure the responses for the pentazocine and the acetaminophen peaks. Calculate the quantity, in mg, of pentazocine ($C_{19}H_{27}NO$) and acetaminophen ($C_8H_9NO_2$) in the portion of Tablets taken by the formula:

$$2000C(r_U / r_S)$$

in which *C* is the concentration, in mg per mL, of the appropriate USP Reference Standard in the *Standard solution;* and r_U and r_S are the peak responses for the corresponding analyte obtained from the *Test solution* and the *Standard solution*, respectively.
Assay for pentazocine—
  Mobile phase—Prepare a mixture of chloroform, methanol, and isopropylamine (96 : 4 : 0.2).
  Diluent—Prepare a mixture of methanol and 0.035 N sulfuric acid (1 : 1).
  Standard preparation—Dissolve an accurately weighed quantity of USP Pentazocine RS in *Diluent*, and dilute quantitatively with the same solvent to obtain a stock solution having a known concentration of about 0.5 mg per mL. Transfer 10.0 mL of this stock solution to a 125-mL separator. Add 30 mL of water and 5 mL of sodium carbonate solution (1 : 10), and mix. Extract with 60 mL of chloroform, pass the chloroform layer through filter paper, collecting the filtrate in a 100-mL volumetric flask, dilute with chloroform to volume, and mix.
  Assay preparation—Weigh and finely powder not fewer than 20 Tablets. Transfer an accurately weighed portion of the powder, equivalent to about 25 mg of pentazocine to a 50-mL glass-stop-

pered cylinder, add 50.0 mL of *Diluent,* and shake intermittently for about 15 minutes. Sonicate for about 2 minutes, allow the solids to settle, and transfer 10.0 mL of the supernatant to a 125-mL separator. [NOTE—Save the remainder of the supernatant for use in the *Assay for acetaminophen.*] Add 30 mL of water and 5 mL of sodium carbonate solution (1 : 10) to the separator, and mix. Extract with 60 mL of chloroform, pass the chloroform layer through filter paper, collecting the filtrate in a 100-mL volumetric flask, dilute with chloroform to volume, and mix.

Chromatographic system (see *Chromatography* ⟨621⟩)—The liquid chromatograph is equipped with a 280-nm detector and a 4.6-mm × 25-cm column that contains 10-μm packing L3. The flow rate is about 1.2 mL per minute. Chromatograph the *Standard preparation,* and record the peak responses as directed for *Procedure:* the column efficiency is not less than 1000 theoretical plates; the tailing factor is not more than 3.0; and the relative standard deviation for replicate injections is not more than 2.0%.

Procedure—Separately inject equal volumes (about 20 μL) of the *Standard preparation* and the *Assay preparation* into the liquid chromatograph, record the chromatograms, and measure the responses for the pentazocine peaks. Calculate the quantity, in mg, of pentazocine ($C_{19}H_{27}NO$) in the portion of Tablets taken by the formula:

$$50C(r_U / r_S)$$

in which C is the concentration, in mg per mL, of USP Pentazocine RS in the stock solution used to prepare the *Standard preparation;* and r_U and r_S are the peak responses obtained from the *Assay preparation* and the *Standard preparation,* respectively.

Assay for acetaminophen—

Mobile phase and *Diluent*—Proceed as directed in the *Assay for pentazocine.*

Standard preparation—Transfer about 130 mg of USP Acetaminophen RS, accurately weighed, to a 10-mL volumetric flask, dissolve in and dilute with *Diluent* to volume, and mix. Transfer 2.0 mL of this solution to a 200-mL volumetric flask, and dilute with ethyl acetate to volume, and mix.

Assay preparation—Transfer 2.0 mL of the supernatant reserved from the *Assay for pentazocine* to a 200-mL volumetric flask, dilute with ethyl acetate to volume, and mix.

Chromatographic system (see *Chromatography* ⟨621⟩)—The liquid chromatograph is equipped with a 254-nm detector and a 4.6-mm × 25-cm column that contains 10-μm packing L3. The flow rate is about 1.4 mL per minute. Chromatograph the *Standard preparation,* and record the peak responses as directed for *Procedure:* the column efficiency is not less than 1000 theoretical plates; the tailing factor is not more than 3.0; and the relative standard deviation for replicate injections is not more than 2.0%.

Procedure—Separately inject equal volumes (about 10 μL) of the *Standard preparation* and the *Assay preparation* into the chromatograph, record the chromatograms, and measure the responses for the acetaminophen peak. Calculate the quantity, in mg, of acetaminophen ($C_8H_9NO_2$) in the portion of Tablets taken by the formula:

$$100C(r_U / r_S)$$

in which C is the concentration, in mg per mL, of USP Acetaminophen RS in the *Standard preparation;* and r_U and r_S are the peak responses obtained from the *Assay preparation* and the *Standard preparation,* respectively.

Pentazocine and Aspirin Tablets

» Pentazocine and Aspirin Tablets contain an amount of Pentazocine Hydrochloride equivalent to not less than 90.0 percent and not more than 110.0 percent of the labeled amount of pentazocine ($C_{19}H_{27}NO$) and not less than 90.0 percent and not more than 110.0 percent of the labeled amount of aspirin ($C_9H_8O_4$).

Packaging and storage—Preserve in tight, light-resistant containers.

USP Reference standards ⟨11⟩—*USP Aspirin RS. USP Pentazocine RS. USP Salicylic Acid RS.*

Thin-layer chromatographic identification test ⟨201⟩—

Test solution—Shake a quantity of finely powdered Tablets, equivalent to about 25 mg of pentazocine and 650 mg of aspirin, with 10 mL of a mixture of chloroform and methanol (1 : 1) in an ultrasonic bath for 2 minutes. Allow the solids to settle.

Standard solutions—Prepare a solution of USP Pentazocine RS in a mixture of chloroform and methanol (1 : 1) containing 2.5 mg per mL. Using the same solvent, prepare a solution of USP Aspirin RS containing 65 mg per mL.

Developing solvent system: ethyl acetate, methanol, and formic acid (90 : 5 : 5).

Procedure—Evaporate the solvents from the spots in warm circulating air. Place the plate in the developing chamber, and after developing the plate, remove it, and mark the solvent front. Evaporate the solvents thoroughly in warm circulating air, and examine the plate under short-wavelength UV light. Expose the plate to iodine vapor for about 5 minutes, and observe. Then spray the plate with an iodoplatinate spray reagent prepared by dissolving 300 mg of platinic chloride in 100 mL of water and adding 100 mL of potassium iodide solution (6 in 100): the chromatogram obtained with the *Test solution* shows two principal spots which correspond in R_F values, size, and intensity of color with the spots obtained with the *Standard solutions.*

Nonaspirin salicylates—

Ferric chloride–urea reagent—To a mixture of 8 mL of ferric chloride solution (6 in 10) and 42 mL of 0.05 N hydrochloric acid add 60 g of urea. Dissolve the urea by swirling and without the aid of heat, and adjust the resulting solution, if necessary, with 6 N hydrochloric acid to a pH of 3.2. Prepare on the day of use.

Procedure—Insert a small pledget of glass wool above the stem constriction of a 20- × 2.5-cm chromatographic tube, and uniformly pack with a mixture of about 1 g of chromatographic siliceous earth and 0.5 mL of 5 M phosphoric acid. Directly above this layer, pack a similar mixture of about 3 g of chromatographic siliceous earth and 2 mL of *Ferric chloride–urea reagent.* To an accurately weighed quantity of finely powdered Tablets, equivalent to about 50 mg of aspirin, add 10 mL of chloroform, stir for 3 minutes, and transfer to the chromatographic adsorption column with the aid of 5 mL of chloroform. Pass 50 mL of chloroform in several portions through the column, rinse the tip of the chromatographic tube with chloroform, and discard the eluate. If the purple zone reaches the bottom of the tube, discard the column, and repeat the test with a smaller quantity of powdered Tablets.

Elute the adsorbed salicylic acid into a 100-mL volumetric flask containing 20 mL of methanol and 4 drops of hydrochloric acid by passing two 10-mL portions of a 1 in 10 solution of glacial acetic acid in water-saturated ether, and then 30 mL of chloroform, through the column, and dilute the eluate with chloroform to volume. Dissolve a suitable, accurately weighed quantity of salicylic acid in chloroform to obtain a Standard solution containing 150 μg of salicylic acid per mL. Pipet 5 mL of this solution into a 50-mL volumetric flask containing 10 mL of methanol, 2 drops of hydrochloric acid, and 10 mL of a 1 in 10 solution of glacial acetic acid in ether. Add chloroform to volume, and mix. Concomitantly determine the absorbances of both solutions in 1-cm cells at the wavelength of maximum absorbance at about 306 nm, using as the blank a suitable mixture of the same composition as that of the Standard solution: the absorbance of the solution from the Tablets does not exceed that of the Standard solution, any necessary adjustment being made for having used a smaller sample (3.0%).

Dissolution ⟨711⟩—

Medium: water; 900 mL.

Apparatus 1: 80 rpm.

Time: 30 minutes.

Strongly basic, anion-exchange resin—Mix a suitable quantity of anion-exchange resin with 10 volumes of dilute glacial acetic acid (1 in 50) and shake for 20 minutes. Allow the resin to settle, and decant the supernatant. Repeat the acetic acid washing four more times. Wash with water until 5.0 mL of the water wash gives a negligible response when substituted for 5.0 mL of the *Test solu-*

tion, and carried through the *Determination of dissolved pentazocine* below.

Test solution—To a suitable 50-mL flask, add 0.4 g of *Strongly basic anion-exchange resin*, and 25 mL of the solution under test. Shake by mechanical means for 15 minutes. Allow to settle, and use the clear supernatant in the following determinations.

Determination of dissolved pentazocine—
STANDARD SOLUTION—Prepare a solution in dilute glacial acetic acid (1 in 50) containing 13 µg of USP Pentazocine RS per mL.
PROCEDURE—Transfer 5.0 mL portions of the *Test solution*, the *Standard solution*, and water to serve as the reagent blank, into three separate 125-mL separators. To each separator add 10 mL of a filtered 1 in 4000 solution of bromocresol purple in dilute glacial acetic acid (1 in 50) and 20.0 mL of chloroform. Insert the stopper, and shake gently for 1 minute, accurately timed. Allow the layers to separate, and determine the absorbances of the clear chloroform layers from the *Standard solution* and the *Test solution* in 1-cm cells at the wavelength of maximum absorbance at about 408 nm with a suitable spectrophotometer against the chloroform layer from the reagent blank. Determine the amount of pentazocine ($C_{19}H_{27}NO$) in the *Test solution* by comparison with the *Standard solution*.

Determination of dissolved aspirin—
STANDARD SOLUTION—Prepare a solution containing 15 µg of USP Salicylic Acid RS per mL of 0.1 N sodium hydroxide.
PROCEDURE—Transfer 1.0 mL of the *Test solution* to a 25-mL volumetric flask containing 1.0 mL of sodium hydroxide solution (1 in 10), and swirl. Allow to stand for 10 minutes. Dilute with water to volume, and mix. Concomitantly determine the absorbances of the *Test solution* and of the *Standard solution* in 1-cm cells at the wavelength of maximum absorbance at about 296 nm with a suitable spectrophotometer, using 0.1 N sodium hydroxide as the blank. Calculate the quantity, in mg, of aspirin ($C_9H_8O_4$) in the *Test solution* by comparison with the *Standard solution*, using the quantity (180.16/138.12), the ratio of the molecular weight of aspirin to that of salicylic acid, to convert the amount of salicylic acid measured to the amount of aspirin in the *Test solution*.

Tolerances—Not less than 80% *(Q)* of the labeled amount of $C_{19}H_{27}NO$ and not less than 70% *(Q)* of the labeled amount of $C_9H_8O_4$ are dissolved in 30 minutes.

Uniformity of dosage units ⟨905⟩: meet the requirements.

Assay—
Chromatographic column—Use a 200-mm tube consisting of about a 90-mm length of 22-mm tubing fused to about a 100-mm length of 5-mm tubing having a stopcock at the bottom of this section. Place a pledget of glass wool at the bottom of the 5-mm portion just above the stopcock. Transfer a suitable quantity of sulfonic acid cation-exchange resin to a beaker and wash three times with water, discarding the water wash each time by decantation. Cover the resin with a mixture of methanol and 6 N hydrochloric acid (1 : 1), and allow to stand for 1 hour. Decant the acid wash; if it is colored yellow or orange, repeat this step until the wash is almost colorless. Then wash the resin by repeated 15-minute soakings in a mixture of methanol and water (1 : 1) followed by decantation until the wash is neutral to wide-range indicator paper. Fill the tube to a height of 100 mm with slurry of the washed resin in a mixture of methanol and water (1 : 1). Wash the column with 25 mL of methanol and water (1 : 1).

Test solutions—Weigh and finely powder not fewer than 20 Tablets. Transfer a portion of the freshly powdered Tablets, equivalent to about 25 mg of pentazocine and 650 mg of aspirin, accurately weighed, to a tared 250-mL flask. Add 100.0 mL of a mixture of methanol and water (1 : 1), and shake by mechanical means for 20 minutes. Centrifuge a suitable quantity for 5 minutes. Transfer 25.0 mL of the clear supernatant to the prepared *Chromatographic column*, followed by five 10-mL portions of the mixture of methanol and water (1 : 1), collecting the eluate in a 250-mL volumetric flask containing 10.0 mL of 2.5 N sodium hydroxide. Dilute with water to volume, and mix. Reserve this as *Test solution 1* for the *Determination of aspirin*. Next pass through the column five 5-mL portions of a mixture of methanol and 6 N hydrochloric acid (1 : 1) followed by 10 mL of water. Collect the eluate in a 100-mL volumetric flask, dilute with water to volume, and use this as *Test solution 2* for the *Determination of pentazocine*.

Determination of aspirin—
STANDARD SOLUTION—Prepare a solution of USP Salicylic Acid RS in 0.1 N sodium hydroxide having a known concentration of about 18 µg per mL.
PROCEDURE—Pipet 4 mL of *Test solution 1* into a 100-mL volumetric flask, dilute with 0.1 N sodium hydroxide to volume, and mix (*Diluted test solution*). Concomitantly determine the absorbances of the *Diluted test solution* and the *Standard solution* in 1-cm cells at the wavelength of maximum absorbance at about 296 nm with a suitable spectrophotometer, using 0.1 N sodium hydroxide as the blank. Calculate the quantity, in mg, of aspirin ($C_9H_8O_4$), in the portion of Tablets taken by the formula:

$$25C(180.16/138.12)(A_U/A_S)$$

in which C is the concentration, in µg per mL, of USP Salicylic Acid RS in the *Standard solution*; (180.16/138.12) is the ratio of the molecular weight of aspirin to that of salicylic acid; and A_U and A_S are the absorbances of *Diluted test solution* and the *Standard solution*, respectively.

Determination of pentazocine—
STANDARD SOLUTION—Prepare a solution of USP Pentazocine RS in a mixture of water, methanol, and 6 N hydrochloric acid (6 : 1 : 1) having a known concentration of about 62.5 µg per mL.
PROCEDURE—Concomitantly determine the absorbances of *Test solution 2* and the *Standard solution*, in 1-cm cells at the wavelength of maximum absorbance at about 278 nm, with a suitable spectrophotometer, using the solvent for the *Standard solution* as the blank. Calculate the quantity, in mg, of pentazocine ($C_{19}H_{27}NO$) in the portion of Tablets taken by the formula:

$$0.4C(A_U/A_S)$$

in which C is the concentration, in µg per mL, of USP Pentazocine RS in the *Standard solution*; and A_U and A_S are the absorbances of *Test solution 2* and the *Standard solution*, respectively.

Pentazocine and Naloxone Tablets

» Pentazocine and Naloxone Tablets contain amounts of Pentazocine Hydrochloride and Naloxone Hydrochloride equivalent to not less than 90.0 percent and not more than 110.0 percent of the labeled amounts of pentazocine ($C_{19}H_{27}NO$) and naloxone ($C_{19}H_{21}NO_4$).

Packaging and storage—Preserve in tight, light-resistant containers.

USP Reference standards ⟨11⟩—*USP Naloxone RS. USP Pentazocine RS.*

Identification—Crush 1 Tablet in 10 mL of a mixture of chloroform and methanol (1 : 1), and mix. Sonicate for about 2 minutes, and filter (*Solution A*). Evaporate 5 mL of *Solution A* to dryness on a steam bath under a stream of nitrogen. Dissolve the residue in 0.2 mL of the mixture of chloroform and methanol (1 : 1) (*Solution B*). Apply 10 µL of *Solution A*, 5 µL of *Solution B*, 10 µL of a Standard solution of USP Pentazocine RS in the 1 : 1 mixture of chloroform and methanol containing 5.0 mg per mL, and 5 µL of a Standard solution of USP Naloxone RS in the 1 : 1 mixture of chloroform and methanol containing 1.3 mg per mL to a suitable thin-layer chromatographic plate (see *Chromatography* ⟨621⟩) coated with a 0.25-mm layer of chromatographic silica gel mixture. Develop the chromatograms in a solvent system consisting of a mixture of 1-butanol, water, and glacial acetic acid (70 : 20 : 10) until the solvent front has moved about three-fourths of the length of the plate. Remove the plate from the developing chamber, mark the solvent front, and dry under a current of warm air. Spray the plate with Folin-Ciocalteu Phenol TS followed by sodium hydroxide solution (1 in 10). Tests *Solution A* and *Solution B* exhibit spots having the same R_F values and approximately the same size and shape as their respective Standard solutions.

Dissolution ⟨711⟩—
Medium: water; 900 mL.
Apparatus 2: 50 rpm.
Time: 45 minutes.
Procedure—Determine the amount of $C_{19}H_{27}NO$ dissolved from UV absorption at the wavelength of maximum absorbance at about 279 nm (corrected for absorbance at 305 nm) on filtered portions of the solution under test, suitably diluted with *Dissolution Medium*, if necessary, in comparison with a Standard solution having a known concentration of USP Pentazocine RS prepared by dissolving the standard in a minimum volume of 0.1 N hydrochloric acid (about 4 mL per 100 mg) and diluting quantitatively and stepwise with water.
Tolerances—Not less than 75% (*Q*) of the labeled amount of pentazocine ($C_{19}H_{27}NO$) is dissolved in 45 minutes.

Uniformity of dosage units ⟨905⟩: meet the requirements.
PROCEDURE FOR CONTENT UNIFORMITY FOR PENTAZOCINE AND NALOXONE—
Solvent mixture—Use a mixture containing methanol, water, and phosphoric acid (500 : 500 : 1).
Mobile phase—Prepare a filtered and degassed mixture by dissolving 675 mg of sodium 1-octanesulfonate and 426 mg of anhydrous dibasic sodium phosphate in 625 mL of water, and mix. Add 475 mL of methanol and 10 mL of phosphoric acid. Make adjustments if necessary (see *System Suitability* under *Chromatography* ⟨621⟩).
Strong anion-exchange resin—Transfer about 30 g of strong anion-exchange resin to a 250-mL beaker. Wash the resin with two 200-mL portions of water, decanting the water after each wash. Wash with two 200-mL portions of dilute glacial acetic acid (1 in 20), decanting the first wash, and filter with the aid of suction.
Standard stock solution—Transfer about 20 mg of USP Naloxone RS, accurately weighed, to a 100-mL volumetric flask. Dissolve in and dilute with *Solvent mixture* to volume, and mix.
Standard solution—Transfer about 100 mg of USP Pentazocine RS, accurately weighed, to a 50-mL volumetric flask. Dissolve in about 30 mL of *Solvent mixture*. Add 5.0 mL of the *Standard stock solution*, dilute with *Solvent mixture* to volume, and mix.
Test solution—Transfer 1 Tablet to a 25-mL glass-stoppered cylinder. Add 25.0 mL of *Solvent mixture*. Sonicate for 10 minutes, and shake intermittently for 15 minutes. Filter into a glass-stoppered conical flask. Add about 125 mg of *Strong anion-exchange resin*, and shake for 30 minutes.
Chromatographic system (see *Chromatography* ⟨621⟩)—The liquid chromatograph is equipped with a 229-nm detector and a 4.6-mm × 25-cm column that contains packing L1. The flow rate is about 1.5 mL per minute. Chromatograph the *Standard solution*, and record the peak responses as directed for *Procedure*: the relative retention times are about 0.3 for naloxone and 1.0 for pentazocine; the resolution, *R*, between pentazocine and naloxone is not less than 6; and the relative standard deviation for replicate injections is not more than 2.0%.
Procedure—Separately inject equal volumes (about 20 µL) of the *Standard solution* and the *Test solution* into the chromatograph, adjusting the operating parameters such that satisfactory chromatography and peak responses are obtained with the *Standard solution*. Record the chromatograms, and measure the areas for the major peaks. Calculate the quantities, in mg, of pentazocine ($C_{19}H_{27}NO$) and naloxone ($C_{19}H_{21}NO_4$) in the Tablet taken by the same formula:

$$25C(r_U / r_S)$$

in which *C* is the concentration, in mg per mL, of the appropriate USP Reference Standard in the *Standard solution;* and r_U and r_S are the peak responses for the corresponding analyte obtained from the *Test solution* and the *Standard solution*, respectively.

Assay for pentazocine and naloxone—Proceed as directed for *Procedure for content uniformity for pentazocine and naloxone*, except to use the following *Assay preparation* in place of the *Test solution*, and to prepare the *Standard preparation* as directed for the *Standard solution*.
Assay preparation—Weigh and finely powder not fewer than 20 Tablets. Transfer an accurately weighed portion of the powder, equivalent to about 100 mg of pentazocine, to a 100-mL volumetric flask, and add 50.0 mL of the *Solvent mixture*. Sonicate for 5 minutes, and shake intermittently for 15 minutes. Filter into a glass-stoppered conical flask. Add about 250 mg of *Strong anion-exchange resin*, and shake for 30 minutes.
Procedure—Proceed as directed for *Procedure* under *Uniformity of dosage units*. Calculate the quantities, in mg, of pentazocine ($C_{19}H_{27}NO$) and naloxone ($C_{19}H_{21}NO_4$), in the portion of the finely powdered Tablets taken by the same formula:

$$50C(r_U / r_S)$$

in which *C* is the concentration, in mg per mL, of the appropriate USP Reference Standard in the *Standard preparation;* and r_U and r_S are the peak responses of the corresponding analyte obtained from the *Assay preparation* and the *Standard preparation*, respectively.

Pentazocine Injection

$C_{19}H_{27}NO \cdot C_3H_6O_3$ 375.50
2,6-Methano-3-benzazocin-8-ol, 1,2,3,4,5,6-hexahydro-6,11-dimethyl-3-(3-methyl-2-butenyl)-, (2α,6α,11*R**)-, compd. with 2-hydroxypropanoic acid (1 : 1).
(2*R**,6*R**,11*R**)-1,2,3,4,5,6-Hexahydro-6,11-dimethyl-3-(3-methyl-2-butenyl)-2,6-methano-3-benzazocin-8-ol lactate (salt) [*17146-95-1*].

» Pentazocine Injection is a sterile solution of Pentazocine in Water for Injection, prepared with the aid of Lactic Acid. It contains not less than 95.0 percent and not more than 105.0 percent of the labeled amount of pentazocine ($C_{19}H_{27}NO$).

Packaging and storage—Preserve in single-dose or multiple-dose containers, preferably of Type I glass.

USP Reference standards ⟨11⟩—*USP Endotoxin RS. USP Pentazocine RS.*

Identification—
A: Transfer a volume of Injection, equivalent to about 15 mg of lactic acid, to a 50-mL conical flask, add 1 mL of 2 N sulfuric acid, and mix. Add, dropwise, potassium permanganate solution (3.2 in 100), until a slight excess has been added, as evidenced by a violet color. [NOTE—The addition of a large excess of potassium permanganate may result in a false negative test for lactate.] Moisten a piece of filter paper with a color-indicating solution (previously prepared by dissolving 250 mg of sodium nitroferricyanide in water to make 9 mL of solution, adding 1 mL of morpholine, and mixing). Place the moistened filter paper over the conical flask opening, and heat the solution moderately: the acetaldehyde fumes produced turn the moistened filter paper blue.
B: Dissolve 50 mg of USP Pentazocine RS in 25 mL of 0.01 N hydrochloric acid in a separator, and use this in place of the Standard solution specified under *Identification—Organic Nitrogenous Bases* ⟨181⟩: a volume of Injection, equivalent to about 50 mg of pentazocine, meets the requirements of the test.

Bacterial endotoxins ⟨85⟩—It contains not more than 5.8 USP Endotoxin Units per mg of pentazocine.

pH ⟨791⟩: between 4.0 and 5.0.

Other requirements—It meets the requirements under *Injections* ⟨1⟩.

Assay—
Ion-exchange column—Place a pledget of glass wool in the base of a 6-mm (ID) tube equipped with a stopcock, and fill the tube to a height of about 25 mm with a styrene-divinylbenzene cation-exchange resin that has been previously soaked in 3 N hydrochloric acid for not less than 2 hours. Pass 10 mL of methanol through the column followed by 50 mL of 3 N hydrochloric acid, then wash the column with water until the eluate is neutral. *[Caution—Do not permit the column to become dry at anytime.]*
Standard preparation—Transfer about 60 mg of USP Pentazocine RS, accurately weighed, to a 50-mL volumetric flask, dilute with a mixture of equal volumes of methanol and 6 N hydrochloric acid to volume, and mix. Transfer 10.0 mL of this solution to a 100-mL volumetric flask, dilute with the mixture of methanol and 6 N hydrochloric acid to volume, and mix. The concentration of USP

Pentazocine RS in the *Standard preparation* is about 120 μg per mL.

Assay preparation—Dilute an accurately measured volume of Injection, equivalent to about 60 mg of pentazocine, with water to 10.0 mL, and mix. Transfer 2.0 mL of this solution to the column, then pass 100 mL of water through the column at a rate of about 2 mL per minute, and discard the eluate. Place a 100-mL volumetric flask under the column, and pass through the column a mixture of equal volumes of methanol and 6 N hydrochloric acid until approximately 95 mL of eluate has been collected. Remove the flask, dilute with the mixture of methanol and 6 N hydrochloric acid to volume, and mix.

Procedure—Concomitantly determine the absorbances of the *Assay preparation* and the *Standard preparation* in 1-cm cells at the wavelength of maximum absorbance at about 278 nm, with a suitable spectrophotometer, using a mixture of equal volumes of methanol and 6 N hydrochloric acid as the blank. Calculate the quantity, in mg, of pentazocine ($C_{19}H_{27}NO$) in each mL of the Injection taken by the formula:

$$(0.5C/V)(A_U/A_S)$$

in which C is the concentration, in μg per mL, of USP Pentazocine RS in the *Standard preparation*; V is the volume, in mL, of Injection taken; and A_U and A_S are the absorbances of the *Assay preparation* and the *Standard preparation*, respectively.

Pentetic Acid

$C_{14}H_{23}N_3O_{10}$ 393.35
Glycine, *N,N*-bis[2-[bis(carboxymethyl)amino]ethyl].
Diethylenetriaminepentaacetic acid [67-43-6].

» Pentetic Acid contains not less than 98.0 percent and not more than 100.5 percent of $C_{14}H_{23}N_3O_{10}$.

Packaging and storage—Preserve in well-closed containers.
USP Reference standards ⟨11⟩—*USP Pentetic Acid RS*.
Identification, *Infrared Absorption* ⟨197K⟩.
Residue on ignition ⟨281⟩: not more than 0.2%.
Heavy metals, *Method II* ⟨231⟩: 0.005%.
Limit of nitrilotriacetic acid—
 Cupric acetate solution—Dissolve 20 g of cupric acetate in a mixture of 800 mL of water and 10 mL of glacial acetic acid. Adjust with 1 N sodium hydroxide to a pH of 4.2, dilute with water to obtain 1000 mL of solution, and filter.
 Mobile phase—Prepare a mixture of 1600 mL of water, 40 mL of glacial acetic acid, 30.4 mL of 0.5 M dodecyltriethylammonium phosphate, and 20 mL of *Cupric acetate solution*. Adjust with 1 N sodium hydroxide to a pH of 4.0, dilute with water to obtain 2000 mL of solution, filter through a filter having a 0.5-μm or finer porosity, and degas. Make adjustments if necessary (see *System Suitability* under *Chromatography* ⟨621⟩).
 Stock standard solution—Transfer about 50 mg of nitrilotriacetic acid, accurately weighed, to a 100-mL volumetric flask, dilute with *Cupric acetate solution* to volume, and mix.
 Standard solution—Transfer 1.0 mL of the *Stock standard solution* to a 25-mL volumetric flask, dilute with *Cupric acetate solution* to volume, and mix. This solution contains about 0.02 mg of nitrilotriacetic acid per mL.
 Test solution—Transfer about 2 g of Pentetic Acid, accurately weighed, to a 100-mL volumetric flask. Add about 70 mL of *Cupric acetate solution*, and swirl to dissolve. Sonicate, if necessary, to dissolve. Dilute with *Cupric acetate solution* to volume, and mix.
 Resolution solution—Transfer 1.0 mL of the *Stock standard solution* to a 25-mL volumetric flask, dilute with *Test solution* to volume, and mix.
 Chromatographic system (see *Chromatography* ⟨621⟩)—The liquid chromatograph is equipped with a 290-nm detector and a 4.6-mm × 25-cm column that contains 5-μm packing L1 that has been highly deactivated (carbon loading of about 30%). The flow rate is about 1 mL per minute. Equilibrate the column by passing, in sequence, water, methanol, and water for about 15 minutes each, and then *Mobile phase* for about 45 minutes. Chromatograph the *Resolution solution*, and record the peak responses as directed for *Procedure*: the resolution, R, between pentetic acid and nitrilotriacetic acid is not less than 2.0, and the relative retention times are about 0.6 for pentetic acid and 1.0 for nitrilotriacetic acid. Chromatograph the *Standard solution*, and record the peak responses as directed for *Procedure*: the relative standard deviation for replicate injections is not more than 5.0%.
 Procedure—Separately inject equal volumes (about 20 μL) of the *Standard solution* and the *Test solution* into the chromatograph, and measure the responses for the major peaks. Calculate the percentage of nitrilotriacetic acid in the portion of Pentetic Acid taken by the formula:

$$10,000(C/W)(r_U/r_S)$$

of which C is the concentration, in mg per mL, of nitrilotriacetic acid in the *Standard solution*, W is the weight, in mg, of Pentetic Acid taken to prepare the *Test solution*, and r_U and r_S are the nitrilotriacetic acid peak responses obtained from the *Test solution* and the *Standard solution*, respectively. The limit is 0.1%.

Iron—Using 1.5 g of specimen, proceed as directed in the test for *Iron* under *Edetic Acid*. The color of the test solution is not deeper than that of the solution containing the standard iron solution (0.01%).
Assay—Transfer about 200 mg of Pentetic Acid, accurately weighed, to a 125-mL conical flask, add 50 mL of water and 1.5 mL of 1 N sodium hydroxide, and swirl to dissolve the specimen. Add 10 mL of 0.1 N ammonium thiocyanate, and mix. Add about 40 mL of methyl ethyl ketone, mix, and allow the layers to separate. Titrate with 0.05 N ferric ammonium sulfate VS, stirring continuously. As the titration proceeds, the aqueous phase turns from colorless to yellow, and the organic phase remains colorless. As the endpoint is approached, stop the titration, mix, and allow the layers to separate. Add 0.1-mL increments of 0.05 N ferric ammonium sulfate VS, mixing and allowing the layers to separate after each addition, until the organic layer turns from colorless to pink. Each mL of 0.05 N ferric ammonium sulfate consumed is equivalent to 19.668 mg of $C_{14}H_{23}N_3O_{10}$.

Pentobarbital

$C_{11}H_{18}N_2O_3$ 226.27
2,4,6(1*H*,3*H*,5*H*)-Pyrimidinetrione, 5-ethyl-5-(1-methylbutyl)-, (±)-.
(±)-5-Ethyl-5-(1-methylbutyl)barbituric acid [76-74-4].

» Pentobarbital contains not less than 98.0 percent and not more than 102.0 percent of $C_{11}H_{18}N_2O_3$, calculated on the dried basis. Where the material is labeled as intended solely for veterinary use, Pentobarbital contains not less than 97.0 percent and not more than 102.0 percent of $C_{11}H_{18}N_2O_3$, calculated on the dried basis.

Packaging and storage—Preserve in tight containers.

USP Reference standards ⟨11⟩—*USP Pentobarbital RS*.
Identification—
  A: *Infrared Absorption* ⟨197S⟩—
  Solution: 7 in 100.
  Medium: chloroform.
  B: *Ultraviolet Absorption* ⟨197U⟩—
  Solution: 16 μg per mL.
  Medium: 0.1 N sodium hydroxide.
  C: The retention time of the major peak in the chromatogram of the *Assay preparation* corresponds to that in the chromatogram of the *Standard preparation,* as obtained in the *Assay.*
Melting range, *Class I* ⟨741⟩: between 127° and 133°.
Loss on drying ⟨731⟩—Dry it at 105° for 2 hours: it loses not more than 1.0% of its weight.
Residue on ignition ⟨281⟩: not more than 0.1%.
Heavy metals, *Method II* ⟨231⟩: 0.002%.
Organic volatile impurities, *Method V* ⟨467⟩: meets the requirements.
  Solvent—Use dimethyl sulfoxide.

(Official until July 1, 2008)

Related compounds—
  Mobile phase—Prepare as directed in the *Assay.*
  Standard solution—Dissolve an accurately weighed quantity of USP Pentobarbital RS in *Mobile phase,* and dilute quantitatively, and stepwise if necessary, with *Mobile phase* to obtain a solution having a known concentration of about 0.001 mg per mL.
  Test solution—Transfer about 100 mg of Pentobarbital, accurately weighed, to a 100-mL volumetric flask, add about 80 mL of *Mobile phase,* and sonicate until dissolved. Dilute with *Mobile phase* to volume, and mix.
  Chromatographic system (see *Chromatography* ⟨621⟩)—The liquid chromatograph is equipped with a 214-nm detector and a 4.6-mm × 25-cm column that contains 5-μm packing L1. The flow rate is about 1.0 mL per minute. Chromatograph the *Standard solution,* and record the peak responses as directed for *Procedure:* the capacity factor, k', is not less than 2.5; the column efficiency is not less than 15,000 theoretical plates; the tailing factor is not more than 1.5; and the relative standard deviation for replicate injections is not more than 15.0%.
  Procedure—Separately inject equal volumes (about 10 μL) of the *Standard solution* and *Test solution* into the chromatograph, record the chromatograms, and measure the areas for the major peaks. Calculate the percentage of any impurity in the portion of Pentobarbital taken by the formula:

$$(10{,}000/F)(C/W)(r_i/r_S)$$

in which C is the concentration, in mg per mL, of USP Pentobarbital RS in the *Standard solution;* F is the relative response factor of the impurity according to the table below; W is the weight, in mg, of pentobarbital, on the dried basis, used to prepare the *Test solution;* r_i is the peak area for any impurity in the *Test solution;* and r_S is the peak area for pentobarbital in the *Standard solution:* the impurities meet the requirements given in the table below:

Compound Name	Relative Retention Time	Relative Response Factor	Limit (%)
6-Imino-5-ethyl-5-(1-methylbutyl) barbituric acid	about 0.39	1.5	0.2
5-Ethyl-5-(1-ethyl-propyl) barbituric acid*	about 0.93	1.0	0.1
Pentobarbital	1.0	—	—
5-Ethyl-5-(1,3-dimethylbutyl) barbituric acid	about 1.5	0.9	0.3

*Where the material is labeled as intended solely for veterinary use, the limit of 5-ethyl-5-(1-ethylpropyl) barbituric acid is 3.0%.

Compound Name	Relative Retention Time	Relative Response Factor	Limit (%)
Unknown impurities	—	1.0	0.1
Total	—	—	0.5

*Where the material is labeled as intended solely for veterinary use, the limit of 5-ethyl-5-(1-ethylpropyl) barbituric acid is 3.0%.

Assay—
  Mobile phase—Prepare a filtered and degassed pH 3.5 mixture of 0.01 M monobasic potassium phosphate and acetonitrile (65 : 35). Make adjustments if necessary (see *System Suitability* under *Chromatography* ⟨621⟩).
  Standard preparation—Dissolve an accurately weighed quantity of USP Pentobarbital RS in *Mobile phase,* and dilute quantitatively, and stepwise if necessary, with *Mobile phase* to obtain a solution having a known concentration of about 0.1 mg per mL.
  Assay preparation—Transfer about 100 mg of Pentobarbital, accurately weighed, to a 100-mL volumetric flask, add about 80 mL of *Mobile phase,* and sonicate until dissolved. Dilute with *Mobile phase* to volume, and mix. Transfer 10.0 mL of this solution to a 100-mL volumetric flask. Dilute with *Mobile phase* to volume, and mix.
  Chromatographic system (see *Chromatography* ⟨621⟩)—The liquid chromatograph is equipped with a 214-nm detector and a 4.6-mm × 25-cm column that contains 5-μm packing L1. The flow rate is about 1.0 mL per minute. Chromatograph the *Standard preparation,* and record the peak responses as directed for *Procedure:* the capacity factor, k', is not less than 2.5; the column efficiency is not less than 15,000 theoretical plates; the tailing factor is not more than 1.5; and the relative standard deviation for replicate injections is not more than 2.0%.
  Procedure—Separately inject equal volumes (about 10 μL) of the *Standard preparation* and the *Assay preparation* into the chromatograph, record the chromatograms, and measure the responses for the major peaks. Calculate the quantity, in mg, of $C_{11}H_{18}N_2O_3$ in the portion of Pentobarbital taken by the formula:

$$1000C(r_U/r_S)$$

in which C is the concentration, in mg per mL, of USP Pentobarbital RS in the *Standard preparation;* and r_U and r_S are the peak areas obtained from the *Assay preparation* and the *Standard preparation,* respectively.

Pentobarbital Oral Solution

» Pentobarbital Oral Solution contains not less than 92.5 percent and not more than 107.5 percent of the labeled amount of pentobarbital ($C_{11}H_{18}N_2O_3$).

Packaging and storage—Preserve in tight containers.

USP Reference standards ⟨11⟩—*USP Pentobarbital RS*.
Identification—Dilute a volume of Oral Solution with alcohol to obtain a concentration of about 1 mg of pentobarbital per mL. Apply 50 μL of this solution and 50 μL of a Standard solution of USP Pentobarbital RS in alcohol containing 1 mg per mL as streaks about 1 cm in length along the spotting line to a suitable thin layer chromatographic plate (see *Chromatography* ⟨621⟩) coated with a 0.25-mm layer of chromatographic silica gel mixture. Allow the streaks to dry, and develop the chromatogram in a solvent system consisting of a mixture of isopropyl alcohol, ammonium hydroxide, chloroform, and acetone (9 : 4 : 2 : 2) until the solvent front has moved about three-fourths of the length of the plate. Remove the plate from the developing chamber, mark the solvent front, and allow the solvent to evaporate. Locate the spots by viewing the plate under short-wavelength light: the R_F value of the principal spot obtained from the test solution corresponds to that obtained from the Standard solution.

Alcohol content, *Method I* ⟨611⟩: between 16.0% and 20.0% of C_2H_5OH.

Assay—
Internal standard solution—Dissolve an accurately weighed quantity of *n*-tricosane in chloroform, and quantitatively dilute with chloroform to obtain a solution having a known concentration of about 0.6 mg per mL.

Standard preparation—Dissolve accurately weighed quantities of USP Pentobarbital RS and *n*-tricosane in chloroform, and quantitatively dilute with chloroform to obtain a solution that contains, in each mL, known amounts of about 1 mg of USP Pentobarbital RS and about 0.4 mg of *n*-tricosane.

Assay preparation—Transfer an accurately measured volume of Oral Solution, equivalent to about 20 mg of pentobarbital, to a separator, add 1 mL of dilute hydrochloric acid (1 in 5), and extract with four 10-mL portions of chloroform. Filter the extracts through about 15 g of anhydrous sodium sulfate that is supported on a funnel by a small pledget of glass wool. Collect the combined filtrate in a 50-mL volumetric flask, wash the sodium sulfate with 5 mL of chloroform, dilute with chloroform to volume, and mix. Combine 4.0 mL of this solution with 1.0 mL of *Internal standard solution* in a suitable container, and reduce the volume to about 1.5 mL by evaporation, with the aid of a stream of dry nitrogen, at room temperature.

Chromatographic system and *System suitability*—Proceed as directed for *Chromatographic System* and *System Suitability* under *Barbiturate Assay* ⟨361⟩, the resolution, *R*, between pentobarbital and *n*-tricosane being not less than 2.3. [NOTE—Relative retention times are, approximately, 0.5 for *n*-tricosane and 1.0 for pentobarbital.]

Procedure—Proceed as directed for *Procedure* under *Barbiturate Assay* ⟨361⟩. Calculate the quantity, in mg, of pentobarbital ($C_{11}H_{18}N_2O_3$) in each mL of the Oral Solution taken by the formula:

$$12.5(R_U)(Q_S)(C_i) / V(R_S)$$

in which *V* is the volume, in mL, of Oral Solution taken; and the other terms are as defined therein.

Pentobarbital Sodium

$C_{11}H_{17}N_2NaO_3$ 248.25
2,4,6(1*H*,3*H*,5*H*)-Pyrimidinetrione, 5-ethyl-5-(1-methylbutyl)-, monosodium salt.
Sodium 5-ethyl-5-(1-methylbutyl)barbiturate   [57-33-0].

» Pentobarbital Sodium contains not less than 98.0 percent and not more than 102.0 percent of $C_{11}H_{17}N_2NaO_3$, calculated on the dried basis. Where the material is labeled as intended solely for veterinary use, Pentobarbital Sodium contains not less than 97.0 percent and not more than 102.0 percent of $C_{11}H_{17}N_2NaO_3$, calculated on the dried basis.

Packaging and storage—Preserve in tight containers.
USP Reference standards ⟨11⟩—USP Pentobarbital RS.
Completeness of solution—Mix 1.0 g with 10 mL of carbon dioxide-free water: after 1 minute, the solution is clear and free from undissolved solid.
Identification—
  A: *Ultraviolet Absorption* ⟨197U⟩—
    Solution: 10 μg per mL.
    Medium: dilute ammonium hydroxide (1 in 200).
  B: The retention time of the major peak in the chromatogram of the *Assay preparation* corresponds to that in the chromatogram of the *Standard preparation,* as obtained in the *Assay.*
  C: Ignite about 200 mg: the residue effervesces with acids, and meets the requirements of the tests for *Sodium* ⟨191⟩.
pH ⟨791⟩: between 9.8 and 11.0, in the solution prepared in the test for *Completeness of solution.*
Loss on drying ⟨731⟩—Dry it at 105° for 6 hours: it loses not more than 3.5% of its weight.

Heavy metals, *Method II* ⟨231⟩: 0.003%.
Related compounds—
Mobile phase—Prepare as directed in the *Assay.*
Standard solution—Dissolve an accurately weighed quantity of USP Pentobarbital RS in *Mobile phase,* and dilute quantitatively, and stepwise if necessary, with *Mobile phase* to obtain a solution having a known concentration of about 0.001 mg per mL.

Test solution—Transfer about 110 mg of Pentobarbital Sodium, accurately weighed, to a 100-mL volumetric flask, add about 80 mL of *Mobile phase,* and sonicate until dissolved. Dilute with *Mobile phase* to volume, and mix.

Chromatographic system (see *Chromatography* ⟨621⟩)—The liquid chromatograph is equipped with a 214-nm detector and a 4.6-mm × 25-cm column that contains 5-μm packing L1. The flow rate is about 1.0 mL per minute. Chromatograph the *Standard solution,* and record the peak responses as directed for *Procedure:* the capacity factor, *k'*, is not less than 2.5; the column efficiency is not less than 15,000 theoretical plates; the tailing factor is not more than 1.5; and the relative standard deviation for replicate injections is not more than 15.0%.

Procedure—Separately inject equal volumes (about 10 μL) of the *Standard solution* and *Test solution* into the chromatograph, record the chromatograms, and measure the areas for the major peaks. Calculate the percentage of any impurity in the portion of Pentobarbital Sodium taken by the formula:

$$(248.25/226.27)(10{,}000/F)(C/W)(r_i/r_S)$$

in which 248.25 and 226.27 are the molecular weights of pentobarbital sodium and pentobarbital, respectively; *F* is the relative response factor of the impurity according to the table below; *C* is the concentration, in mg per mL, of USP Pentobarbital RS in the *Standard solution;* *W* is the weight, in mg, of Pentobarbital Sodium, on the dried basis, used to prepare the *Test solution;* r_i is the peak area for any impurity in the *Test solution;* and r_S is the peak area for pentobarbital in the *Standard solution:* the impurities meet the requirements given in the table below:

Compound Name	Relative Retention Time	Relative Response Factor	Limit (%)
6-Imino-5-ethyl-5-(1-methylbutyl)barbituric acid	about 0.39	1.5	0.2
5-Ethyl-5-(1-ethylpropyl)barbituric acid*	about 0.93	1.0	0.1
Pentobarbital	1.0	—	—
5-Ethyl-5-(1,3-dimethylbutyl)barbituric acid	about 1.5	0.9	0.3
Unknown impurities	—	1.0	0.1
Total	—	—	0.5

*Where the material is labeled as intended solely for veterinary use, the limit of 5-ethyl-5-(1-ethylpropyl) barbituric acid is 3.0%.

Organic volatile impurities, *Method I* ⟨467⟩: meets the requirements.

(Official until July 1, 2008)

Assay—[NOTE—Use the value for *Loss on drying* obtained at the same time as the preparation of the *Test solution* in the test for *Related compounds* and the *Assay preparation* in the *Assay.*]

Mobile phase, Standard preparation, and *Chromatographic system*—Proceed as described in the *Assay* under *Pentobarbital.*

Assay preparation—Transfer about 110 mg of Pentobarbital Sodium, accurately weighed, to a 100-mL volumetric flask, add about 80 mL of *Mobile phase,* and sonicate until dissolved. Dilute with *Mobile phase* to volume, and mix. Transfer 10.0 mL of this solution to a 100-mL volumetric flask. Dilute with *Mobile phase* to volume, and mix.

Procedure—Separately inject equal volumes (about 10 µL) of the *Standard preparation* and the *Assay preparation* into the chromatograph, record the chromatograms, and measure the responses for the major peaks. Calculate the quantity, in mg, of $C_{11}H_{17}N_2NaO_3$ in the portion of Pentobarbital Sodium taken by the formula:

$$(248.25/226.27)1000C(r_U/r_S)$$

in which 248.25 and 226.27 are the molecular weights of pentobarbital sodium and pentobarbital, respectively; C is the concentration, in mg per mL, of USP Pentobarbital RS in the *Standard preparation;* and r_U and r_S are the peak areas obtained from the *Assay preparation* and the *Standard preparation*, respectively.

Pentobarbital Sodium Capsules

» Pentobarbital Sodium Capsules contain not less than 92.5 percent and not more than 107.5 percent of the labeled amount of $C_{11}H_{17}N_2NaO_3$.

Packaging and storage—Preserve in tight containers.

USP Reference standards⟨11⟩—*USP Pentobarbital RS.*

Identification—Mix a quantity of the contents of Capsules, equivalent to about 100 mg of pentobarbital sodium, with 15 mL of water in a separator. Filter, if necessary, and saturate the solution with sodium chloride. To the solution add 2 mL of hydrochloric acid, shake, and extract the liberated pentobarbital with five 25-mL portions of chloroform. Filter each extract through a pledget of chloroform-washed cotton, or other suitable filter, into a beaker, and finally wash the separator and the filter with several small portions of chloroform. Evaporate the combined filtrate and washings on a steam bath with the aid of a current of air, add 10 mL of ether, again evaporate, recrystallize the residue from hot alcohol, and dry the recrystallized residue at 105° for 30 minutes: the residue so obtained responds to *Identification* test A under *Pentobarbital Sodium.*

Dissolution ⟨711⟩—
Medium: water; 900 mL.
Apparatus 1: 100 rpm.
Time: 45 minutes.
Standard preparation—Dissolve an accurately weighed quantity of USP Pentobarbital RS in freshly prepared dilute ammonium hydroxide (1 in 20) to obtain a solution having a known concentration of about 10 µg of pentobarbital per mL. The concentration of pentobarbital, multiplied by 1.097, represents the equivalent amount of pentobarbital sodium.
Procedure—Determine the amount of $C_{11}H_{17}N_2NaO_3$ dissolved from UV absorbances at the wavelength of maximum absorbance at about 240 nm on filtered portions of the solution under test, suitably diluted with freshly prepared dilute ammonium hydroxide (1 in 20), in comparison with the *Standard preparation.*
Tolerances—Not less than 75% (*Q*) of the labeled amount of $C_{11}H_{17}N_2NaO_3$ is dissolved in 45 minutes.

Uniformity of dosage units ⟨905⟩: meet the requirements.

Procedure for content uniformity—Transfer the contents of 1 Capsule to a 250-mL volumetric flask, with the aid of about 5 mL of alcohol. Add 10 mL of freshly prepared dilute ammonium hydroxide (1 in 200), and without delay dilute with the same solution to volume. Mix, filter if necessary, and discard the first 20 mL of the filtrate. Dilute a portion of the clear solution with dilute ammonium hydroxide (1 in 200) to obtain a solution having a concentration of about 10 µg of pentobarbital sodium per mL. Dissolve a suitable quantity of USP Pentobarbital RS in dilute ammonium hydroxide (1 in 200) to obtain a Standard solution having a known concentration of about 10 µg per mL. Concomitantly determine the absorbances of both solutions in 1-cm cells at the wavelength of maximum absorbance at about 240 nm, with a suitable spectrophotometer, using dilute ammonium hydroxide (1 in 200) as the blank.

Calculate the quantity, in mg, of $C_{11}H_{17}N_2NaO_3$ in the Capsule taken by the formula:

$$1.097(T/C_U)C_S(A_U/A_S)$$

in which T is the labeled quantity, in mg, of pentobarbital sodium in the Capsule, C_U is the concentration, in µg per mL, of pentobarbital sodium in the solution from the Capsule contents, on the basis of the labeled quantity per Capsule and the extent of dilution, C_S is the concentration, in µg per mL, of USP Pentobarbital RS in the Standard solution, and A_U and A_S are the absorbances of the solution from the Capsule contents and the Standard solution, respectively.

Assay—
Internal standard—*n*-Tricosane.
Internal standard solution—Dissolve an accurately weighed quantity of *n*-tricosane in chloroform, and quantitatively dilute with chloroform to obtain a solution having a known concentration of about 0.4 mg per mL.
Standard preparation—Dissolve accurately weighed quantities of USP Pentobarbital RS and *n*-tricosane in chloroform, and quantitatively dilute with chloroform to obtain a solution that contains, in each mL, known amounts of about 0.9 mg of USP Pentobarbital RS and about 0.4 mg of *n*-tricosane.
Assay preparation—Weigh not less than 20 Capsules, and transfer the contents as completely as possible to a suitable container. Remove any residual powder from the empty capsules with the aid of a current of air, and weigh the capsule shells, determining the weight of the contents by difference. Mix the contents of the Capsules, transfer an accurately weighed portion of the powder, equivalent to about 50 mg of pentobarbital sodium, to a separator. Add 15 mL of water and 1 mL of hydrochloric acid, and extract with five 25-mL portions of chloroform. Filter the extracts through about 15 g of anhydrous sodium sulfate that is supported on a funnel by a small pledget of glass wool. Collect the combined filtrate in a 100-mL volumetric flask, wash the sodium sulfate with 15 mL of chloroform, collecting the washing with the filtrate, dilute with chloroform to volume, and mix. Combine 2.0 mL of this solution with 1.0 mL of *Internal standard solution* in a suitable container, and reduce the volume to about 1 mL by evaporation, with the aid of a stream of dry nitrogen, at room temperature.
Chromatographic system and *System suitability*—Proceed as directed for *Chromatographic System* and *System Suitability* under *Barbiturate Assay* ⟨361⟩, the resolution, *R*, between pentobarbital and *n*-tricosane being not less than 2.3. [NOTE—Relative retention times are, approximately, 0.5 for *n*-tricosane barbital and 1.0 for pentobarbital.]
Procedure—Proceed as directed for *Procedure* under *Barbiturate Assay* ⟨361⟩. Calculate the quantity, in mg, of $C_{11}H_{17}N_2NaO_3$ in the portion of Capsules taken by the formula:

$$(248.25/226.27)(50)(R_U)(Q_S)(C_i/R_S)$$

in which 248.25 and 226.27 are the molecular weights of pentobarbital sodium and pentobarbital, respectively.

Pentobarbital Sodium Injection

» Pentobarbital Sodium Injection is a sterile solution of Pentobarbital Sodium in a suitable solvent. Pentobarbital may be substituted for the equivalent amount of Pentobarbital Sodium, for adjustment of the pH. The Injection contains the equivalent of not less than 92.0 percent and not more than 108.0 percent of the labeled amount of $C_{11}H_{17}N_2NaO_3$.

Packaging and storage—Preserve in single-dose or multiple-dose containers, preferably of Type I glass. The Injection may be packaged in 50-mL containers.

Labeling—The label indicates that the Injection is not to be used if it contains a precipitate.

USP Reference standards ⟨11⟩—*USP Endotoxin RS. USP Pentobarbital RS.*

Identification—The retention time of the major peak in the chromatogram of the *Assay preparation* corresponds to that in the chromatogram of the *Standard preparation*, as obtained in the *Assay*.

Bacterial endotoxins ⟨85⟩—It contains not more than 0.8 USP Endotoxin Unit per mg of pentobarbital sodium.

pH ⟨791⟩: between 9.0 and 10.5.

Other requirements—It meets the requirements under *Injections* ⟨1⟩.

Assay—

Mobile phase—Prepare a filtered and degassed pH 3.5 mixture of 0.01 M monobasic potassium phosphate and acetonitrile (65 : 35). Make adjustments if necessary (see *System Suitability* under *Chromatography* ⟨621⟩).

Standard preparation—Dissolve an accurately weighed quantity of USP Pentobarbital RS in *Mobile phase*, and dilute quantitatively, and stepwise if necessary, with *Mobile phase* to obtain a solution having a known concentration of about 0.1 mg per mL.

Assay preparation—Quantitatively dilute a suitable volume of Injection with *Mobile phase* to obtain a solution having a known concentration of about 0.1 mg per mL.

Chromatographic system (see *Chromatography* ⟨621⟩)—The liquid chromatograph is equipped with a 214-nm detector and a 4.6-mm × 25-cm column that contains 5-μm packing L1. The flow rate is about 1.0 mL per minute. Chromatograph the *Standard preparation*, and record the peak responses as directed for *Procedure*: the capacity factor, k', is not less than 2.5; the column efficiency is not less than 15,000 theoretical plates; the tailing factor is not more than 1.5; and the relative standard deviation for replicate injections is not more than 2.0%.

Procedure—Separately inject equal volumes (about 10 μL) of the *Standard preparation* and the *Assay preparation* into the chromatograph, record the chromatograms, and measure the responses for the major peaks. Calculate the percentage of $C_{11}H_{17}N_2NaO_3$ in the portion of Injection taken by the formula:

$$100(248.25/226.27)(C_S / C_U)(r_U / r_S)$$

in which 248.25 and 226.27 are the molecular weights of pentobarbital sodium and pentobarbital, respectively; C_S is the concentration, in mg per mL, of USP Pentobarbital RS in the *Standard preparation*; C_U is the final concentration, in mg per mL, of the *Assay preparation*; and r_U and r_S are the peak areas obtained from the *Assay preparation* and the *Standard preparation*, respectively.

Pentoxifylline

$C_{13}H_{18}N_4O_3$ 278.31

1*H*-Purine-2,6-dione, 3,7-dihydro-3,7-dimethyl-1-(5-oxohexyl)-.
1-(5-Oxohexyl)theobromine   [6493-05-6].

» Pentoxifylline contains not less than 98.0 percent and not more than 102.0 percent of $C_{13}H_{18}N_4O_3$.

Packaging and storage—Preserve in well-closed containers.

USP Reference standards ⟨11⟩—*USP Pentoxifylline RS*.

Completeness of solution ⟨641⟩—Solution in carbon dioxide-free water (1 in 50) meets the requirements.

Identification—

A: *Infrared Absorption* ⟨197K⟩.

B: *Ultraviolet Absorption* ⟨197U⟩—

Solution: 0.01 mg per mL.

Medium: water.

Absorptivities at 274 nm, calculated on the dried basis, do not differ by more than 3.0%.

Melting range, *Class I* ⟨741⟩: between 104° and 107°.

Acidity—Dissolve about 1 g in 50 mL of carbon dioxide-free water, and add 1 drop of bromothymol blue TS: not more than 0.2 mL of 0.01 N sodium hydroxide is required in order to produce a color change.

Loss on drying ⟨731⟩—Dry it in vacuum at 60° for 3 hours: it loses not more than 0.5% of its weight.

Residue on ignition ⟨281⟩:   not more than 0.1%.

Chloride ⟨221⟩—A 2.0-g portion shows no more chloride than corresponds to 0.31 mL of 0.020 N hydrochloric acid (0.011%).

Sulfate ⟨221⟩—A 1.0-g portion shows no more sulfate than corresponds to 0.20 mL of 0.020 N sulfuric acid (0.02%).

Heavy metals, *Method II* ⟨231⟩:   0.001%.

Chromatographic purity—

Perchloric acid solution and *Mobile phase*—Prepare as directed in the *Assay*.

System suitability solution—Dissolve accurately weighed quantities of caffeine and USP Pentoxifylline RS in *Mobile phase* to obtain a solution containing about 0.0007 mg per mL and 0.35 mg per mL, respectively.

Standard solution—Dissolve an accurately weighed quantity of USP Pentoxifylline RS in *Mobile phase* to obtain a solution having a known concentration of about 0.0007 mg per mL.

Test solution—Dissolve an accurately weighed quantity of Pentoxifylline in *Mobile phase* to obtain a solution having a concentration of about 0.35 mg per mL.

Chromatographic system (see *Chromatography* ⟨621⟩)—Proceed as directed in the *Assay*. Chromatograph the *System suitability solution*, and record the peak responses as directed for *Procedure*: the resolution, R, between caffeine and pentoxifylline is not less than 10.0. Chromatograph the *Standard solution*, and record the peak responses for pentoxifylline as directed for *Procedure*: the relative standard deviation for replicate injections is not more than 5.0%.

Procedure—Separately inject equal volumes (about 20 μL) of the *Standard solution* and the *Test solution* into the chromatograph, and allow the chromatogram to run five times longer than the retention time for the pentoxifylline. Measure the areas of all the peaks in the *Test solution*, except that for pentoxifylline. Calculate the percentage of each impurity in the portion of Pentoxifylline taken by the formula:

$$286C(r_i / r_S)$$

in which C is the concentration, in mg per mL, of USP Pentoxifylline RS in the *Standard solution*; r_i is the peak area response for each impurity obtained from the *Test solution*; and r_S is the peak area response for pentoxifylline obtained from the *Standard solution*: not more than 0.2% of any individual impurity is found, and not more than 0.5% of total impurities is found.

Organic volatile impurities, *Method V* ⟨467⟩:   meets the requirements.

(Official until July 1, 2008)

Assay—

Perchloric acid solution—Dissolve 1.0 g of perchloric acid in 1000 mL of water, and mix.

Mobile phase—Prepare a filtered and degassed mixture of *Perchloric acid solution*, acetonitrile, tetrahydrofuran, and methanol (80 : 15 : 2.5 : 2). Make adjustments if necessary (see *System Suitability* under *Chromatography* ⟨621⟩).

System suitability solution—Dissolve suitable quantities of caffeine and USP Pentoxifylline RS in *Mobile phase* to obtain a solution containing 0.024 mg per mL and 0.048 mg per mL, respectively.

Standard preparation—Dissolve an accurately weighed quantity of USP Pentoxifylline RS in *Mobile phase*, and dilute quantitatively, and stepwise if necessary, with *Mobile phase* to obtain a solution having a known concentration of about 0.05 mg per mL.

Assay preparation—Transfer about 25 mg of Pentoxifylline, accurately weighed, to a 100-mL volumetric flask, dissolve in and dilute with *Mobile phase* to volume, and mix. Pipet 5.0 mL of the solution so obtained to a 25-mL volumetric flask, dilute with *Mobile phase* to volume, and mix.

Chromatographic system (see *Chromatography* ⟨621⟩)—The liquid chromatograph is equipped with a 273-nm detector and a 4.6-mm × 25-cm column that contains 5-μm packing L1. The flow rate is about 0.7 mL per minute. Chromatograph the *System suitability solution*, and record the peak responses as directed for *Procedure*: the resolution, R, between caffeine and pentoxifylline is not less than 10.0. Chromatograph the *Standard preparation*, and record the peak responses as directed for *Procedure:* the relative standard deviation for replicate injections is not more than 2.0%.

Procedure—Separately inject equal volumes (about 10 µL) of the *Standard preparation* and the *Assay preparation* into the chromatograph, record the chromatograms, and measure the responses for the major pentoxifylline peaks. Calculate the quantity, in mg, of $C_{13}H_{18}N_4O_3$ in the portion of Pentoxifylline taken by the formula:

$$500C(r_U / r_S)$$

in which C is the concentration, in mg per mL, of USP Pentoxifylline RS in the *Standard preparation;* and r_U and r_S are the peak responses obtained from the *Assay preparation* and the *Standard preparation,* respectively.

Pentoxifylline Extended-Release Tablets

» Pentoxifylline Extended-Release Tablets contain not less than 95.0 percent and not more than 105.0 percent of the labeled amount of pentoxifylline ($C_{13}H_{18}N_4O_3$).

Packaging and storage—Preserve in well-closed containers. Protect from light, and store between 15° and 30°.
Labeling—The labeling indicates the *Dissolution Test* with which the product complies.
USP Reference standards ⟨11⟩—*USP Pentoxifylline RS.*
Identification—
A: *Infrared Absorption* ⟨197K⟩—
Test specimen—Finely powder not fewer than 5 Tablets. (A coarse screen may be used to separate the powder from the tablet film-coating if necessary.) Transfer an accurately weighed portion of the powder, equivalent to about 200 mg of pentoxifylline, to a 15-mL centrifuge tube, add about 10 mL of methanol, cap the tube, and shake vigorously for about 5 minutes. Centrifuge for about 5 minutes to allow undissolved material to settle. Decant the supernatant into a suitable beaker, and evaporate the solution with the aid of a current of air to dryness at about 35°. Dissolve the residue in about 15 mL of methylene chloride, transfer to a separatory funnel, add about 10 mL of water, and shake. Allow the layers to separate, transfer the methylene chloride layer, and pass through a funnel partially filled with anhydrous sodium sulfate, collecting the filtrate in a small beaker. Evaporate the solution with the aid of a current of air to dryness at about 35°. Dissolve the residue so obtained in 8 to 10 mL of ether, and then chill in an ice bath, if necessary, to induce crystallization. Collect the crystals on filter paper, wash with about 2 mL of cold ether, and allow to air-dry. Prepare a mixture of about 1.5% (w/w) of the crystals in potassium bromide.
B: The retention time of the major peak in the chromatogram of the *Assay preparation* corresponds to that in the chromatogram of the *Standard preparation,* as obtained in the *Assay.*
Dissolution ⟨711⟩—
TEST 1—If the product complies with this test, the labeling indicates that it meets USP *Dissolution Test 1.*
Medium: water; 900 mL or 1000 mL.
Apparatus 2: 100 rpm.
Times: 1, 4, 8, and 12 hours.
Procedure—Determine the amount of $C_{13}H_{18}N_4O_3$ dissolved by employing UV absorption at the wavelength of maximum absorbance at about 274 nm on filtered portions of the solution under test, suitably diluted with *Medium,* if necessary, in comparison with a Standard solution having a known concentration of USP Pentoxifylline RS in the same *Medium.*
Tolerances—The percentages of the labeled amount of $C_{13}H_{18}N_4O_3$ dissolved at the times specified conform to *Acceptance Table 2.*

Time (hours)	Amount dissolved
1	not more than 30%
4	between 30% and 55%
8	not less than 60%
12	not less than 80%

TEST 2—If the product complies with this test, the labeling indicates that it meets USP *Dissolution Test 2.*
Medium: water; 900 mL.
Apparatus 2: 75 rpm.
Times: 1, 6, 10, and 20 hours.
Procedure—Proceed as directed for *Test 1.*
Tolerances—The percentages of the labeled amount of $C_{13}H_{18}N_4O_3$ dissolved at the times specified conform to the following table.

Time (hours)	Amount dissolved
1	between 8% and 30%
6	between 35% and 60%
10	between 53% and 78%
20	not less than 80%

TEST 3—If the product complies with this test, the labeling indicates that it meets USP *Dissolution Test 3.*
Medium: water; 900 mL.
Apparatus 1: 100 rpm.
Times: 2, 8, 12, and 20 hours.
Procedure—Proceed as directed for *Test 1.*
Tolerances—The percentages of the labeled amount of $C_{13}H_{18}N_4O_3$ dissolved at the times specified conform to the following table.

Time (hours)	Amount dissolved
2	between 15% and 35%
8	between 55% and 75%
12	between 75% and 95%
20	not less than 85%

TEST 4—If the product complies with this test, the labeling indicates that it meets USP *Dissolution Test 4.*
Medium: water; 900 mL.
Apparatus 2: 50 rpm.
Times: 1, 8, and 24 hours.
Procedure—Proceed as directed for *Test 1.*
Tolerances—The percentages of the labeled amount of $C_{13}H_{18}N_4O_3$ dissolved at the times specified conform to the following table.

Time (hours)	Amount dissolved
1	between 0% and 20%
8	between 35% and 60%
24	not less than 80%

TEST 5—If the product complies with this test, the labeling indicates that it meets USP *Dissolution Test 5.*
Medium: water; 900 mL.
Apparatus 2: 75 rpm.
Times: 1, 2, 4, 6, and 20 hours.
Procedure—Proceed as directed for *Test 1,* except to use the wavelength of maximum absorbance at about 264 nm instead of 274 nm.
Tolerances—The percentages of the labeled amount of $C_{13}H_{18}N_4O_3$ dissolved at the times specified conform to the following table.

Time (hours)	Amount dissolved
1	between 5% and 25%
2	between 10% and 35%
4	between 20% and 50%
6	between 30% and 60%
20	not less than 80%

TEST 6—If the product complies with this test, the labeling indicates that it meets USP *Dissolution Test 6*.
Medium: simulated gastric fluid (without enzymes); 900 mL.
Apparatus 2: 50 rpm.
Times: 2, 8, 12, and 24 hours.
Procedure—Proceed as directed for *Test 1*.
Tolerances—The percentages of the labeled amount of $C_{13}H_{18}N_4O_3$ dissolved at the times specified conform to the following table.

Time (hours)	Amount dissolved
2	between 10% and 30%
8	between 40% and 60%
12	between 55% and 75%
24	not less than 85%

TEST 7—If the product complies with this test, the labeling indicates that it meets USP *Dissolution Test 7*.
Medium: water; 900 mL.
Apparatus 2: 50 rpm.
Times: 1, 3, 8, and 18 hours.
Procedure—Proceed as directed for *Test 1*.
Tolerances—The percentages of the labeled amount of $C_{13}H_{18}N_4O_3$ dissolved at the times specified conform to the following table.

Time (hours)	Amount dissolved
1	not more than 25%
3	between 25% and 45%
8	between 55% and 75%
18	not less than 80%

TEST 8—If the product complies with this test, the labeling indicates that it meets USP *Dissolution Test 8*.
Medium: water; 900 mL.
Apparatus 2: 75 rpm.
Times: 1, 2, 4, 10, and 16 hours.
Procedure—Proceed as directed for *Test 1*.
Tolerances—The percentages of the labeled amount of $C_{13}H_{18}N_4O_3$ dissolved at the times specified conform to the following table.

Time (hours)	Amount dissolved
1	between 10% and 20%
2	between 15% and 35%
4	between 25% and 45%
10	between 55% and 75%
16	not less than 80%

TEST 9—If the product complies with this test, the labeling indicates that it meets USP *Dissolution Test 9*.
Medium: water; 900 mL.
Apparatus 2: 50 rpm.
Times: 1, 3, 6, 12, and 18 hours.
Procedure—Proceed as directed for *Test 1*, except to use the wavelength of maximum absorbance at about 230 nm instead of 274 nm.
Tolerances—The percentages of the labeled amount of $C_{13}H_{18}N_4O_3$ dissolved at the times specified conform to the following table.

Time (hours)	Amount dissolved
1	between 0% and 20%
3	between 20% and 40%
6	between 30% and 60%
12	between 50% and 80%
18	not less than 80%

TEST 10—If the product complies with this test, the labeling indicates that it meets USP *Dissolution Test 10*.
Medium: water; 900 mL.
Apparatus 2: 75 rpm.
Times: 1, 6, 12, and 20 hours.
Procedure—Proceed as directed for *Test 1*.
Tolerances—The percentages of the labeled amount of $C_{13}H_{18}N_4O_3$ dissolved at the times specified conform to the following table.

Time (hours)	Amount dissolved
1	not more than 20%
6	between 35% and 65%
12	between 60% and 90%
20	not less than 80%

Uniformity of dosage units ⟨905⟩: meet the requirements.
Chromatographic purity—
Perchloric acid solution, Mobile phase, Extracting solution, and *System suitability solution*—Prepare as directed in the *Assay*.
Standard solution—Dissolve an accurately weighed quantity of USP Pentoxifylline RS in *Extracting solution* containing an amount of methanol equal to 0.8% of the total volume to be used, and dilute quantitatively, and stepwise if necessary, with *Extracting solution* to obtain a solution having a known concentration of about 0.96 µg per mL.
Test solution—Transfer 10.0 mL of the first dilution filtrate from the *Assay preparation* to a 25-mL volumetric flask, dilute with *Extracting solution* to volume, and mix. The final concentration of pentoxifylline in this solution is about 0.32 mg per mL.
Chromatographic system (see *Chromatography* ⟨621⟩)—Proceed as directed in the *Assay*. Chromatograph the *Standard solution,* and record the peak responses for pentoxifylline as directed for *Procedure*: the relative standard deviation for replicate injections is not more than 5.0%.
Procedure—Separately inject equal volumes (about 10 µL) of the *Standard solution* and the *Test solution* into the chromatograph, and allow the chromatogram to run five times longer than the retention time of the pentoxifylline peak. Record the chromatograms, and measure all the peak responses from the *Test solution,* except that for pentoxifylline. Calculate the percentage of each impurity in the portion of Tablets taken by the formula:

$$312C(r_i / r_S)$$

in which C is the concentration, in mg per mL, of USP Pentoxifylline RS in the *Standard solution*; r_i is the peak response for each impurity obtained from the *Test solution*; and r_S is the peak response for pentoxifylline obtained from the *Standard solution*: not more than 0.3% of any individual impurity is found; and not more than 1.0% of total impurities is found.
Assay—
Perchloric acid solution—Dissolve 1.0 g of perchloric acid in 1000 mL of water, and mix.
Mobile phase—Prepare a filtered and degassed mixture of *Perchloric acid solution,* acetonitrile, tetrahydrofuran, and methanol (80 : 15 : 2.5 : 2). Make adjustments if necessary (see *System Suitability* under *Chromatography* ⟨621⟩).
Extracting solution—Prepare a mixture of water and alcohol (7 : 3).
System suitability solution—Transfer about 20 mg of USP Pentoxifylline RS and about 10 mg of caffeine, each accurately weighed, to a 25-mL volumetric flask. Add 0.2 mL of methanol, and swirl the flask to distribute the methanol. Dilute with *Extracting solution* to volume, and mix. Pipet 3.0 mL of the resulting solution into a 50-mL volumetric flask, dilute with *Extracting solution* to volume, and mix.
Standard preparation—Dissolve an accurately weighed quantity of USP Pentoxifylline RS in *Extracting solution* containing an amount of methanol equal to 0.8% of the total volume to be used, and dilute quantitatively, and stepwise if necessary, with *Extracting solution* to obtain a solution having a known concentration of about 0.048 mg per mL.
Assay preparation—Weigh and finely powder not fewer than 20 Tablets. Transfer an accurately weighed portion of the powder, equivalent to about 40 mg of pentoxifylline, to a 50-mL volumetric flask. Pipet 0.4 mL of methanol into the flask, and swirl for at least

1 minute. Add about 30 mL of *Extracting solution,* and sonicate for 60 minutes with occasional swirling of the flask. Add an additional 15 mL of *Extracting solution,* allow to cool to room temperature, dilute with *Extracting solution* to volume, and mix. Centrifuge or pass through a suitable filter. Reserve a portion of this first dilution for preparation of the *Test solution* in the *Chromatographic purity* test. Pipet 3.0 mL of the clear solution into a 50-mL volumetric flask, dilute with *Extracting solution* to volume, and mix.

Chromatographic system (see *Chromatography* ⟨621⟩)—The liquid chromatograph is equipped with a 273-nm detector and a 4.6-mm × 25-cm column that contains packing L1. The flow rate is about 0.7 mL per minute. Chromatograph the *System suitability solution,* and record the peak responses as directed for *Procedure:* the resolution, *R,* between caffeine and pentoxifylline is not less than 10.0. Chromatograph the *Standard preparation,* and record the peak responses for pentoxifylline as directed for *Procedure:* the relative standard deviation for replicate injections is not more than 2.0%.

Procedure—Separately inject equal volumes (about 10 µL) of the *Standard preparation* and the *Assay preparation* into the chromatograph, record the chromatograms, and measure the responses for the major peaks. Calculate the quantity, in mg, of pentoxifylline ($C_{13}H_{18}N_4O_3$) in the portion of Tablets taken by the formula:

$$833C(r_U/r_S)$$

in which *C* is the concentration, in mg per mL, of USP Pentoxifylline RS in the *Standard preparation;* and r_U and r_S are the peak responses obtained from the *Assay preparation* and the *Standard preparation,* respectively.

Peppermint Spirit

» Peppermint Spirit contains, in each 100 mL, not less than 9.0 mL and not more than 11.0 mL of peppermint oil.

Peppermint Oil................	100 mL
Peppermint, in coarse powder......	10 g
Alcohol, a sufficient quantity, to make	1000 mL

Macerate the peppermint leaves, freed as much as possible from stems and coarsely powdered, for 1 hour in 500 mL of purified water, and then strongly express them. Add the moist, macerated leaves to 900 mL of alcohol, and allow the mixture to stand for 6 hours with frequent agitation. Filter, and to the filtrate add the oil and add alcohol to make the product measure 1000 mL.

Packaging and storage—Preserve in tight containers, protected from light.

Alcohol content, *Method II* ⟨611⟩: between 79.0% and 85.0% of C_2H_5OH.

Assay—Transfer 5.0 mL of Spirit to a Babcock bottle, graduated to 8%, add 1.0 mL of kerosene, and mix. Add saturated calcium chloride solution, acidified with hydrochloric acid, almost to fill the bulb of the bottle. Rotate the bottle vigorously to ensure mixing, and then add a sufficient quantity of the calcium chloride solution to bring the separated oil into the neck of the bottle. Centrifuge at about 1500 rpm for 5 minutes, and read the volume of oil in the stem. Subtract five divisions for the kerosene added, and multiply the remaining number of divisions by 4.2 to obtain the volume, in mL, of peppermint oil in 100 mL of the Spirit.

Perflubron

C_8BrF_{17} 498.96
Octane, 1-bromo-1,1,2,2,3,3,4,4,5,5,6,6,7,7,8,8,8-heptadecafluoro-.
1-Bromoheptadecafluorooctane.
Perfluorooctyl bromide   [423-55-2].

» Perflubron contains not less than 98.0 and not more than 100.0 percent of C_8BrF_{17}.

Packaging and storage—Preserve in tight, light-resistant containers.
USP Reference standards ⟨11⟩—*USP Perflubron RS.*
Identification—
  A: Record the IR absorption spectrum, using a gas cell. The spectrum so obtained exhibits maxima only at the same wavelengths as that of a similar preparation of USP Perflubron RS.
  B: The retention time of the major peak in the chromatogram of the test specimen, obtained as directed in the *Assay,* corresponds to that of USP Perflubron RS, similarly chromatographed.
Specific gravity ⟨841⟩:   between 1.922 and 1.925.
Chromatographic purity—
  Chromatographic system (see *Chromatography* ⟨621⟩)—The gas chromatograph is equipped with a split injection port with a split ratio, range of 1 : 45 to 1 : 100, a flame-ionization detector, and a 0.25-mm × 60-m column coated with a 1-µm film of phase G2. Hydrogen is used as the carrier gas. The chromatograph is programmed to maintain the column temperature at 35° for 7 minutes, then to increase the temperature at a rate of 20° per minute to 185°, and held at this temperature for 4.5 minutes. The injection port is maintained between 200° and 220° and the detector at a temperature above 200°.
  Procedure—Inject a volume (about 0.2 µL) of Perflubron into the chromatograph, record the chromatogram, and measure the areas of the peak responses. Calculate the percentage of each individual impurity in the portion of Perflubron taken by the formula:

$$100(r_i/r_s)$$

in which r_i is the peak response of the individual impurity, and r_s is the sum of the responses of all the peaks: not more than 0.20% of any individual impurity is found.
Nonvolatile residue—Transfer 75 g of Perflubron to a tared evaporating dish, evaporate to dryness, and dry the residue at 105° for 1 hour: the weight of the residue so obtained does not exceed 1.5 mg (0.002%).
Assay—
  Chromatographic system—Proceed as directed in the test for *Chromatographic purity.*
  Procedure—Inject about 0.2 µL of Perflubron into the chromatograph, record the chromatograms, and measure the areas of the peak responses. Calculate the percentage of C_8BrF_{17} in the portion of Perflubron taken by the formula:

$$100(r_U/r_s)$$

in which r_U is the peak response for perflubron obtained from the test specimen, and r_s is the sum of the responses of all of the peaks.

Perflutren Protein-Type A Microspheres Injectable Suspension

» Perflutren Protein-Type A Microspheres Injectable Suspension is a sterile, nonpyrogenic suspension of microspheres produced by dispersing perflutren (octafluoropropane) gas in an aqueous solution of diluted sterile Albumin Human. It contains not less than 0.8 percent and not more than 1.2 percent protein. It may contain stabilizers, but contains no preservatives.

Packaging and storage—Preserve in single-dose, tight containers that contain perflutren gas in the headspace, and store in a refrigerator.

Labeling—Label it to indicate that perflutren gas is contained within the microspheres. The labeling also provides the following warnings: "Do not use if lower layer is cloudy or turbid, contains visible foreign matter, or if the contents do not appear as a homogeneous, opaque, milky-white suspension after mixing. Do not use if the upper white layer of product is absent. Do not inject air into the vial. Invert the vial, and gently rotate to resuspend the microspheres. Do not use if, after resuspension, the solution appears to be clear rather than opaque milky-white."

USP Reference standards ⟨11⟩—*USP Endotoxin RS*.

Bacterial endotoxins ⟨85⟩—It contains not more than 0.5 USP Endotoxin Unit per mL of Perflutren Protein-Type A Microspheres Injectable Suspension.

Safety—It meets the requirements for biologics as set forth for *Safety Tests—Biologicals* under *Biological Reactivity Tests, In Vivo* ⟨88⟩.

Sterility ⟨71⟩: meets the requirements.

pH ⟨791⟩: between 6.4 and 7.4.

Microsphere size and concentration—

Electrolyte solution—Use filtered and buffered saline electrolyte solution.[1]

Diluent—Prepare a solution that contains, in each L of water, 1.5 g of sodium lauryl sulfate and 0.1 g of thimerosal. Prior to use, pass the solution through a 0.2-µm nylon filter. [NOTE—The *Diluent* is to be used exclusively to prepare the *Reference stock solution* described below; it must not be used to prepare the *Test solution*.]

Reference stock solution—Transfer a quantity of NIST traceable microspheres suspension containing about 0.5 g of microspheres directly into a tared centrifuge tube equipped with a cap, and weigh.[2] Using the density and concentration of the microspheres obtained from the Certificate of Analysis, calculate the volume occupied by the microspheres and the number of microspheres in the portion taken. Calculate the target total volume, in mL, by dividing the number of microspheres in the portion taken by the target concentration of 2.0×10^8 microspheres per mL. Calculate the target *Diluent* volume by subtracting the volume occupied by the microspheres from the target total volume. Transfer the target volume of *Diluent* to the centrifuge tube containing the portion of microspheres taken, and mix the tube vigorously for 1 hour. The prepared *Reference stock solution*, which contains a suspension of microspheres with a target mean particle diameter of 5.2 µm and a concentration of 2.0×10^8 microspheres per mL, is divided into smaller containers and stored at 5°.

Reference solution—Equilibrate the *Reference stock solution* to room temperature, and mix thoroughly. Immediately transfer 20 µL of the *Reference stock solution* to a beaker containing 200 mL of *Electrolyte solution*, mix, and analyze immediately.

Blank solution—Use 200 mL of *Electrolyte solution*.

Test solution—Allow the Injectable Suspension to equilibrate to room temperature. Invert the vial, and gently rotate to resuspend the microspheres. [NOTE—After resuspension, the contents should appear as a homogeneous, opaque, milky-white suspension.] Immediately withdraw a 20-µL aliquot, transfer to a beaker containing 200 mL of *Electrolyte solution*, mix, and analyze immediately.

Test apparatus—Use a multichannel particle analyzer that operates on the electrical zone-sensing principle.[3] The analyzer is fitted and calibrated with an aperture tube having a 50-µm orifice. The multichannel particle analyzer is equipped with software capable of data-smoothing, data extrapolation, distribution graphing, and data conversion. Analyze the *Blank solution*, the *Reference solution*, and the *Test solution* as directed for *Procedure:* the total count in the *Blank solution* is not more than 500; the mean particle diameter of microspheres in the *Reference solution* is within 5% of the mean particle diameter of microspheres in the *Reference stock solution*; the concentration of the *Reference solution* is within 10% of the concentration of the *Reference stock solution*; and the coincidence effect in the analysis of the *Test solution* is not more than 5%.

Procedure—Rinse the orifice of the aperture tube with *Electrolyte solution* before and after analyzing each preparation. Place the *Blank solution* in the apparatus, and adjust the vacuum on the sample stand so that the counting begins about 12 seconds after the analyzer is set to the counting position. Set the data acquisition to stop when one of the following conditions is met: preset length of time, preset volume, preset number of counts in any channel, or total counts. Collect the count versus the channel data for the *Blank solution*, and analyze using the data-smoothing, data extrapolation, distribution graphing, and data conversion features of the system software. In the same manner, analyze the *Reference solution* and the *Test solution*. The *Test solution* data are normalized and expressed as the number of microspheres per mL: the concentration of microspheres is between 5.0×10^8 and 8.0×10^8 per mL. Calculate the percentage of microspheres less than 10 µm in size in the portion of Injectable Suspension taken by the formula:

$$100(P_A / P_B)$$

in which P_A is the number of microspheres in the 1- to 10-µm size range, and P_B is the number of microsphere particles in the 1- to 32-µm size range. Not fewer than 93% of microsphere particles is smaller than 10 µm.

Container headspace content—

Reference solutions—Use 99% perflutren reference standard[4] (electronic grade perflutren gas of at least 99 molar % purity) and 60% perflutren reference standard[4] (an electronic grade gas in air mixture containing 60 molar % perflutren gas).

Blank solution—Use ambient air.

Test solution—Use gas from the container headspace.

Chromatographic system (see *Chromatography* ⟨621⟩)—The gas chromatograph is equipped with a thermal conductivity detector and a 0.53-mm × 25-m fused-silica (porous layer open tubular) column coated with Al_2O_3 / KCl (aluminum oxide deactivated with potassium chloride).[5] The carrier gas is helium with a flow rate adjusted to obtain a retention time of about 1.5 to 1.8 minutes for perflutren. The column temperature is maintained at about 65°, the injection port temperature is maintained at about 130°, and the detector temperature is maintained at about 180°. Chromatograph the *Reference solutions* as directed for *Procedure:* the resolution, R, between perflutren and air is not less than 2; and the relative standard deviation for replicate injections is not more than 5%. The measured value for the 99% perflutren reference standard is within 5% of the nominal value.

Procedure—Using a gas-tight syringe, separately inject 10 µL of the *Blank solution*, the *Reference solutions*, and the *Test solution* into the chromatograph. Record the chromatograms, and measure the responses for the major peaks. The percentages of perflutren in the 99% perflutren reference standard and in the *Test solution* are calculated by comparing the peak areas in each with the peak areas obtained from the 60% perflutren reference standard. The container headspace of Injectable Suspension contains not less than 60% of perflutren gas.

Microsphere perflutren content—

Reference stock solutions—The 97% decafluorobutane reference standard is decafluorobutane gas of at least 97 molar % purity.[6] The 5% decafluorobutane–5% perflutren reference standard is a mixture containing 5 molar % decafluorobutane gas and 5 molar % perflutren gas in air.[7] The 99% perflutren reference standard is electronic grade perflutren gas of at least 99 molar % purity.[4]

Analysis vial—Transfer 100 µL of 97% decafluorobutane reference standard gas and 100 µL of glacial acetic acid to a 2-mL vial equipped with a septum cap.

---

[1] Filtered and buffered saline electrolyte solution is available as ISOTON® II from Beckman Coulter, Inc., Fullerton, CA.
[2] Microspheres with a mean particle diameter of 5 µm are available as NIST traceable Dynospheres from Bangs Laboratories, Inc., Fishers, IN.
[3] A suitable multichannel particle analyzer is available as the Multisizer Model IIe from Beckman Coulter, Inc., Fullerton, CA.
[4] A suitable grade of perflutren (octafluoropropane) is available from Air Products and Chemicals, Inc., Allentown, PA.
[5] The column is available from Varian U.S.A. Chrompack, Walnut Creek, CA, catalog number CP7517, as an Al_2O_3/KCl PLOT column (0.53-mm ID, 25-m length).
[6] The gas is available under product code 03047567SR-LD from Scott Medical Products, Plumsteadville, PA.
[7] The mixture of the two gases in air is available under product code 03047566SR-LD from Scott Medical Products, Plumsteadville, PA.

Reference solution—Transfer 100 µL of 99% perflutren reference standard and 0.75 mL of 1% Albumin Human to an *Analysis vial*, and incubate by mixing for at least 3 hours.

Test solution—Allow a vial of the Injectable Suspension to equilibrate to room temperature. Invert the vial, and gently rotate to resuspend the microspheres. [NOTE—After resuspension, the contents of the vial should appear as a homogeneous, opaque, milky-white suspension.] Withdraw 0.75 mL of Injectable Suspension, and transfer to another *Analysis vial*. Incubate the *Test solution* by mixing for at least 3 hours.

Chromatographic system (see *Chromatography* ⟨621⟩)—Prepare as directed for *Container headspace content*. The carrier gas is helium with a flow rate adjusted to obtain the following retention times: 1.0 to 1.1 minutes for air, 1.3 to 1.5 minutes for perflutren, and 1.5 to 2.5 minutes for decafluorobutane. The column temperature is maintained at about 85°, and then after elution of the perflutren the temperature is increased at a rate of 50° per minute to 120°, and maintained at 120° for 2 minutes. The injection port temperature is maintained at about 130°, and the detector temperature is maintained at about 180°. Chromatograph the 5% decafluorobutane–5% perflutren reference standard and the *Reference solution* as directed for *Procedure*: the resolution, *R*, between air and perflutren is not less than 2; the resolution, *R*, between perflutren and decafluorobutane is not less than 5; the relative standard deviation determined from the perflutren peak response for the *Reference solution* is not more than 5%; and the relative standard deviation determined from the response ratios for replicate injections of the 5% decafluorobutane–5% perflutren reference standard is not more than 5%.

Procedure—Inject 20 µL of the headspace gas from the vials containing the *Reference solution* and the *Test solution* into the gas chromatograph. Record the chromatograms, and measure the areas for the major peaks. Calculate the quantity, in mg per mL, of perflutren in the portion of Injectable Suspension taken by the formula:

$$0.188(M/V)(R_S/R_U)$$

in which *M* is the number of µmols of decafluorobutane in an *Analysis vial* after addition of the Injectable Suspension; *V* is the volume, in mL, of Injectable Suspension added to the *Analysis vial*; and R_S and R_U are the peak area ratios of decafluorobutane to perflutren obtained from the *Reference solution* and the *Test solution*, respectively. The quantity of perflutren in the Injectable Suspension is between 0.11 mg per mL and 0.33 mg per mL.

Other requirements—It meets the requirements under *Injections* ⟨1⟩, except that it is not subject to the requirement for *Particulate Matter* under *Constituted Solutions*.

Assay for protein—

Diluted antifoam reagent—Transfer 100 µL of antifoam reagent[8] to a suitable container, and dilute with water to 10 mL.

Blank preparation—Transfer 500 µL of Sodium Chloride Injection to a culture tube. Dilute the contents of the tube with water to 2 mL, and add 10 µL of *Diluted antifoam reagent*.

Standard preparations—Transfer 25-, 50-, 62.5-, 75-, and 100-µL aliquots of protein standard solution[9] containing 8 g per dL into separate tubes. Dilute the contents of each tube with water to 2.00 mL, and add 10 µL of *Diluted antifoam reagent* to each tube. During the *Procedure*, the addition of 3.0 mL of biuret reagent TS to each of the tubes produces *Standard preparations* with protein concentrations of 0.4, 0.8, 1.0, 1.2, and 1.6 mg per mL.

Assay preparation—Equilibrate each container of Injectable Suspension to room temperature, and mix each for at least 5 minutes to ensure a homogeneous suspension. Vent the container, and transfer 500-µL aliquots into separate tubes. Dilute the contents of each tube with water to 2 mL, and add 10 µL of *Diluted antifoam reagent*.

Procedure—To each of the tubes containing the *Blank preparation*, *Standard preparations*, and *Assay preparation*, add 3.0 mL of biuret reagent TS, mix, and allow to stand for 30 minutes, accurately timed, for maximum color development. The *Blank preparation*, *Standard preparations*, and *Assay preparation* are treated

---
[8] Available as Antifoam Reagent, catalog number 2210, from Dow Corning Corporation, Midland, MI.
[9] Available as Bovine Serum Albumin, SRM 927c, Standard Reference Materials, National Institute of Standards and Technology, Gaithersburg, MD.

---

identically. Using the *Blank preparation*, set the absorbance equal to zero. Determine the absorbance of each of the *Standard preparations* and the *Assay preparation* in 1-cm cells with a suitable spectrophotometer at a wavelength of 540 nm. Using linear regression, analyze the data obtained for each of the *Standard preparations*. Calculate the correlation coefficient, slope, and *y*-intercept values: the correlation coefficient is not less than 0.995. Calculate the quantity, in mg, of protein in each mL of the Injectable Suspension by the formula:

$$10[(A_U - y\text{-intercept})/\text{slope}]$$

in which 10 is the dilution factor; and A_U is the absorbance of the *Assay preparation*: the calculated quantity of protein in the Injectable Suspension is between 8 and 12 mg per mL.

Pergolide Mesylate

$C_{19}H_{26}N_2S \cdot CH_4O_3S$ 410.60

Ergoline, 8-[(methylthio)methyl]-6-propyl-, monomethanesulfonate, (8β)-.
8β-[(Methylthio)methyl]-6-propylergoline monomethanesulfonate   [66104-23-2].

» Pergolide Mesylate contains not less than 97.5 percent and not more than 102.0 percent of $C_{19}H_{26}N_2S \cdot CH_4O_3S$, calculated on the dried basis.

Packaging and storage—Preserve in tight, light-resistant containers.

USP Reference standards ⟨11⟩—*USP Pergolide Mesylate RS*. *USP Pergolide Sulfoxide RS*.
Identification, *Infrared Absorption* ⟨197K⟩.
Specific rotation ⟨781S⟩: between −17° and −23° at 20°.
Test solution: 10 mg per mL, in dimethylformamide.
Loss on drying ⟨731⟩—Dry it in vacuum at 105° for 1 hour: it loses not more than 0.5% of its weight.
Residue on ignition ⟨281⟩: not more than 0.1%.
Heavy metals, *Method II* ⟨231⟩: 0.001%.
Chromatographic purity—

Solution A—Prepare a filtered and degassed mixture of 5.0 mL of morpholine with 995 mL of water, and adjust with phosphoric acid to a pH of 7.0.

Solution B—Prepare a filtered and degassed mixture of methanol, acetonitrile, and tetrahydrofuran (1 : 1 : 1). Make adjustments if necessary (see *System Suitability* under *Chromatography* ⟨621⟩).

Mobile phase—Use variable mixtures of *Solution A* and *Solution B* as directed for *Chromatographic system* (see *System Suitability* under *Chromatography* ⟨621⟩).

Standard solution 1—Dissolve an accurately weighed quantity of USP Pergolide Mesylate RS in methanol, and dilute quantitatively, and stepwise if necessary, with methanol to obtain a solution having a known concentration of about 30 µg per mL.

Standard solution 2—Dilute 10.0 mL of *Standard solution 1* to 50 mL with methanol.

Test solution—Transfer about 60 mg of Pergolide Mesylate, accurately weighed, to a 10-mL volumetric flask, dissolve in and dilute with methanol to volume, and mix.

Chromatographic system (see *Chromatography* ⟨621⟩)—The liquid chromatograph is equipped with a 280-nm detector and a 4.6-mm × 25-cm column that contains base-deactivated packing L1. The flow rate is about 1 mL per minute. The column temperature is maintained at 40°. The chromatograph is programmed as follows.

Time (minutes)	Solution A (%)	Solution B (%)	Elution
0	70	30	equilibration
0–35	70→0	30→100	linear gradient

Chromatograph *Standard solution 1*, and record the peak responses as directed for*Procedure*: the column efficiency is not less than 10,000 theoretical plates; the tailing factor is not more than 1.5; and the relative standard deviation for replicate injections is not more than 2.0%.

Procedure—Separately inject equal volumes (about 10 µL) of *Standard solution 1*, *Standard solution 2*, the *Test solution*, and a methanol blank into the chromatograph, record the chromatograms, and measure all of the peak responses. Disregard the contributions due to any peaks found in the methanol blank. The sum of the peak responses, excluding that of pergolide, from the *Test solution* is not more than the pergolide peak response obtained from *Standard solution 1* (0.5%), and no single peak response is more than the pergolide peak response obtained from *Standard solution 2* (0.1%).

Organic volatile impurities, Method IV ⟨467⟩: meets the requirements.
Solvent: dimethylformamide. [NOTE—Do not add sodium sulfate.]

(Official until July 1, 2008)

Assay—
Diluent—Dissolve 5 mg of methionine in 500 mL of 0.01 N hydrochloric acid. Add 500 mL of methanol, and mix.

Mobile phase—Prepare a solution of 0.009 M sodium 1-octanesulfonate containing 1.0 mL of glacial acetic acid per L. Prepare a filtered and degassed mixture of this solution, methanol, and acetonitrile (2 : 1 : 1). Make adjustments if necessary (see *System Suitability* under *Chromatography* ⟨621⟩).

Resolution solution—Dissolve about 4 mg of USP Pergolide Sulfoxide RS and 8 mg of USP Pergolide Mesylate RS in 50 mL of *Diluent*.

Standard preparation—Dissolve an accurately weighed quantity of USP Pergolide Mesylate RS in*Diluent*, and dilute quantitatively, and stepwise if necessary, with *Diluent* to obtain a solution having a known concentration of about 0.13 mg per mL.

Assay preparation—Transfer about 6.5 mg of Pergolide Mesylate, accurately weighed, to a 50-mL volumetric flask, dissolve in and dilute with *Diluent* to volume, and mix.

Chromatographic system (see *Chromatography* ⟨621⟩)—The liquid chromatograph is equipped with a 280-nm detector and a 4.6-mm × 25-cm column that contains base-deactivated packing L7. The flow rate is about 1 mL per minute. The column temperature is maintained at 40°. Chromatograph the *Resolution solution*, and record the peak responses as directed for *Procedure*: the resolution, R, between pergolide sulfoxide and pergolide is not less than 12.0. Chromatograph the *Standard preparation*, and record the peak responses as directed for *Procedure*: the tailing factor is not more than 1.5; and the relative standard deviation for replicate injections is not more than 2.0%.

Procedure—Separately inject equal volumes (about 10 µL) of the *Standard preparation* and the *Assay preparation* into the chromatograph, record the chromatograms, and measure the responses for the pergolide peaks. Calculate the quantity, in mg, of $C_{19}H_{26}N_2S \cdot CH_4O_3S$ in the portion of Pergolide Mesylate taken by the formula:

$$50C(r_U / r_S)$$

in which C is the concentration, in mg per mL, of USP Pergolide Mesylate RS in the *Standard preparation*; and r_U and r_S are the peak responses obtained from the *Assay preparation* and the*Standard preparation*, respectively.

Pergolide Tablets

» Pergolide Tablets contain an amount of Pergolide Mesylate equivalent to not less than 90.0 percent and not more than 110.0 percent of the labeled amount of pergolide ($C_{19}H_{26}N_2S$).

Packaging and storage—Preserve in tight, light-resistant containers.

USP Reference standards ⟨11⟩—*USP Pergolide Mesylate RS. USP Pergolide Sulfoxide RS.*

Thin-layer chromatographic identification test ⟨201⟩—
Adsorbent: 0.25-mm layer of binder-free silica gel.

Test solution—Transfer a number of Tablets, equivalent to 1 mg of pergolide, to a separator containing 20 mL of methylene chloride and 10 mL of 0.1 N sodium hydroxide. Shake until the Tablets have disintegrated, allow the layers to separate, and drain the methylene chloride layer through a small funnel containing about 1 g of anhydrous sodium sulfate, collecting the filtrate in a suitable stoppered vessel. Wash the sodium sulfate with a few mL of methylene chloride, adding these washes to the filtrate, and evaporate to dryness under a stream of nitrogen. Redissolve the residue in 2 mL of a mixture of methylene chloride and methanol (1 : 1).

Standard solution: 0.65 mg per mL, in a mixture of methylene chloride and methanol (1 : 1).

Application volume: 20 µL.

Developing solvent system: a mixture of chloroform, methanol, and ethyl acetate (8 : 1 : 1). Allow the plate to equilibrate for about 10 minutes in the developing chamber prior to development.

Procedure—Proceed as directed in the chapter. Place the plate in a chamber containing iodine vapors, and locate the spots.

Dissolution ⟨711⟩—
Medium: simulated gastric fluid TS (without enzymes) containing 20 µg of L-cysteine per mL; 500 mL.

Apparatus 2: 50 rpm.

Time: 30 minutes.

Determine the amount of $C_{19}H_{26}N_2S$ dissolved by employing the following method.

Mobile phase—Prepare a filtered and degassed mixture of acetonitrile, water, and triethylamine, (21 : 19 : 0.08). Adjust with phosphoric acid to a pH of 5.0. Make adjustments if necessary (see *System Suitability* under*Chromatography* ⟨621⟩).

Triethylamine phosphate suspension—Add 1.0 mL of triethylamine to 500 mL of acetonitrile, mix, and adjust with phosphoric acid to a pH of 5.0. A white precipitate will form. Stir continuously during use.

Resolution solution—Prepare a solution of USP Pergolide Mesylate RS and USP Pergolide Sulfoxide RS containing a known amount of each equivalent to the labeled amount of pergolide in each 500 mL of *Medium*.

Standard solution—Transfer about 16 mg of USP Pergolide Mesylate RS, accurately weighed, to a 250-mL volumetric flask, dissolve in 10.0 mL of methanol, dilute with *Medium* to volume, and mix. Dilute this solution quantitatively and stepwise with *Medium* to obtain a solution having a known concentration equivalent to the labeled amount of pergolide in each 500 mL.

Chromatographic system (see *Chromatography* ⟨621⟩)—The liquid chromatograph is equipped with a fluorometer set to an excitation wavelength of 224 nm and an emission wavelength of 350 nm and with a 4.6-mm × 15-cm column that contains base-deactivated packing L10. The flow rate is about 2 mL per minute. Chromatograph the*Resolution solution*, and record the peak responses as directed for *Procedure*: the resolution, R, between pergolide sulfoxide and pergolide is not less than 1.0. Chromatograph the *Standard solution*, and record the peak responses as directed for *Procedure*: the relative standard deviation for replicate injections, determined from the pergolide peak, is not more than 2.0%.

Procedure—Immediately before injection, pipet 2.0 mL of *Triethylamine phosphate suspension*, continuously stirred, into a suitable container containing 5.0 mL of the solution for injection, and mix to obtain a clear solution. Separately inject equal volumes (about 200 µL) of the *Standard solution* and filtered portions of the solutions under test into the chromatograph, record the chromatograms, and measure the areas for the major peaks. Calculate the amount, in mg, of pergolide ($C_{19}H_{26}N_2S$) dissolved by the formula:

$$500C(314.50/410.60)(r_U/r_S)$$

in which C is the concentration, in µg per mL, of USP Pergolide Mesylate RS in the *Standard solution;* 314.50 and 410.60 are the molecular weights of pergolide and pergolide mesylate, respectively; and r_U and r_S are the peak areas obtained from the solution under test and the *Standard solution*, respectively.

Tolerances—Not less than 75% *(Q)* of the labeled amount of $C_{19}H_{26}N_2S$ is dissolved in 30 minutes.

Uniformity of dosage units ⟨905⟩: meet the requirements.

Chromatographic purity—

Mobile phase, System suitability solution, Standard preparation, and *Chromatographic system*—Proceed as directed in the *Assay*.

Diluted standard preparation—Transfer 3.0 mL of the *Standard preparation* to a 50-mL volumetric flask. Dilute with *Mobile phase* to volume, and mix.

Test preparation—Use the *Assay preparation*.

Procedure—Separately inject equal volumes (about 100 µL) of the *Diluted standard preparation* and the *Test preparation* into the chromatograph, and measure all of the peak responses. Calculate the percentage of each impurity in the Tablets by the formula:

$$20C(314.50/410.60)(r_i/r_S)$$

in which C is the concentration, in µg per mL, of USP Pergolide Mesylate RS in the *Diluted standard preparation;* 314.50 and 410.60 are the molecular weights of pergolide and pergolide mesylate, respectively; r_i is the peak response of the individual impurity obtained from the *Test preparation;* and r_S is the peak response of pergolide obtained from the *Diluted standard preparation:* not more than 6.0% of pergolide sulfoxide is found; not more than 0.5% of any individual impurity, excluding pergolide sulfoxide, is found; and not more than 1.0% of total impurities, excluding pergolide sulfoxide, is found.

Assay—

Mobile phase—Prepare a solution of 0.038 M sodium 1-octanesulfonate containing 0.0077 mg of methionine per mL and 2.45 mL of glacial acetic acid per L. Adjust with 5 N sodium hydroxide to a pH of 4.1. Prepare a filtered and degassed mixture of this solution and acetonitrile (65 : 35). Make adjustments if necessary (see *System Suitability* under *Chromatography* ⟨621⟩).

System suitability solution—Prepare a solution of USP Pergolide Mesylate RS and USP Pergolide Sulfoxide RS in *Mobile phase* having a known concentration of about 6.5 µg per mL of pergolide mesylate and 0.1 µg per mL of pergolide sulfoxide.

Standard preparation—Dissolve an accurately weighed quantity of USP Pergolide Mesylate RS in *Mobile phase*, and dilute quantitatively and stepwise with *Mobile phase* to obtain a solution having a known concentration of about 6.5 µg per mL.

Assay preparation—Place 20 whole Tablets into a suitable stoppered container, add *Mobile phase*, shake and sonicate until the Tablets have dissolved, and quantitatively dilute to obtain a solution containing about 5 µg per mL of pergolide.

Chromatographic system (see *Chromatography* ⟨621⟩)—The liquid chromatograph is equipped with a fluorometer set to an excitation wavelength of 280 nm and an emission wavelength of 335 nm and with a 4.6-mm × 7.5-cm column that contains base-deactivated packing L7. The flow rate is about 1.5 mL per minute. The column temperature is maintained at 35°. Chromatograph the *System suitability solution*, and record the peak responses as directed for *Procedure:* the resolution, *R*, between pergolide sulfoxide and pergolide is not less than 12.0; and the relative standard deviation for replicate injections is not more than 2.0%.

Procedure—Separately inject equal volumes (about 100 µL) of the *Standard preparation* and the *Assay preparation* into the chromatograph, and measure the responses for the major peaks. Calculate the quantity, in mg, of pergolide ($C_{19}H_{26}N_2S$) in the portion of Tablets taken by the formula:

$$0.001C(314.50/410.60)(r_U/r_S)$$

in which C is the concentration, in µg per mL, of USP Pergolide Mesylate RS in the *Standard preparation;* 314.50 and 410.60 are the molecular weights of pergolide and pergolide mesylate, respectively; and r_U and r_S are the peak responses obtained from the *Assay preparation* and the *Standard preparation*, respectively.

Perphenazine

$C_{21}H_{26}ClN_3OS$ 403.97

1-Piperazineethanol, 4-[3-(2-chloro-10*H*-phenothiazin-10-yl)-propyl-].

4-[3-(2-Chlorophenothiazin-10-yl)propyl]-1-piperazineethanol [*58-39-9*].

» Perphenazine contains not less than 98.0 percent and not more than 102.0 percent of $C_{21}H_{26}ClN_3OS$, calculated on the dried basis.

Packaging and storage—Preserve in tight, light-resistant containers.

USP Reference standards ⟨11⟩—USP Perphenazine RS. USP Perphenazine Sulfoxide RS.

Clarity and color of solution—Dissolve 500 mg in 25 mL of methanol: the solution is clear and not more than light yellow.

NOTE—Throughout the following procedures, protect test or assay specimens, the USP Reference Standard, and solutions containing them, by conducting the procedures without delay, under subdued light, or using low-actinic glassware.

Identification—

A: *Infrared Absorption* ⟨197M⟩.

B: *Ultraviolet Absorption* ⟨197U⟩—

Solution: 10 µg per mL.

Medium: methanol.

Absorptivities at 257 nm, calculated on the dried basis, do not differ by more than 2.5%.

Melting range, *Class I* ⟨741⟩: between 94° and 100°.

Loss on drying ⟨731⟩—Dry it in vacuum at 65° for 3 hours: it loses not more than 0.5% of its weight.

Residue on ignition ⟨281⟩: not more than 0.1%.

Ordinary impurities ⟨466⟩—

Test solution: a mixture of acetone and methanol (3 : 1).

Standard solution: solutions of USP Perphenazine Sulfoxide RS in a mixture of acetone and methanol (3 : 1) except that the solution having a concentration of 0.01 mg per mL is replaced with a solution having a concentration of 0.02 mg per mL.

Eluant: a mixture of acetone and ammonium hydroxide (95 : 5).

Visualization: 1.

Organic volatile impurities, *Method V* ⟨467⟩: meets the requirements.

Solvent—Use dimethyl sulfoxide.

(Official until July 1, 2008)

Assay—Dissolve about 400 mg of Perphenazine, previously dried and accurately weighed, in 50 mL of glacial acetic acid, warming slightly to effect solution. Cool to room temperature, add 10 mL of acetic anhydride, and allow to stand for 5 minutes. Add 1 drop of crystal violet TS, and titrate with 0.1 N perchloric acid VS to a green endpoint. Perform a blank determination, and make any necessary correction. Each mL of 0.1 N perchloric acid is equivalent to 20.20 mg of $C_{21}H_{26}ClN_3OS$.

Perphenazine Injection

» Perphenazine Injection is a sterile solution of Perphenazine in Water for Injection, prepared with the aid of Citric Acid. It contains not less than 90.0 percent and not more than 110.0 percent of the labeled amount of $C_{21}H_{26}ClN_3OS$, as the citrate.

Packaging and storage—Preserve in single-dose or multiple-dose containers, preferably of Type I glass, protected from light.

USP Reference standards ⟨11⟩—*USP Endotoxin RS. USP Perphenazine RS.*

NOTE—Throughout the following procedures, protect test or assay specimens, the USP Reference Standard, and solutions containing them, by conducting the procedures without delay, under subdued light, or using low-actinic glassware.

Identification—Dilute 1 mL with methanol to 5 mL. Apply 5 µL each of this solution and a solution of USP Perphenazine RS in methanol containing 1 mg per mL to a suitable thin-layer chromatographic plate, coated with a 0.25-mm layer of chromatographic silica gel. Develop the chromatogram in a solvent system consisting of a mixture of acetone and ammonium hydroxide (200 : 1) until the solvent front has moved about 15 cm. Air-dry the plate, and spray lightly with a solution of iodoplatinic acid prepared by dissolving 100 mg of chloroplatinic acid in 1 mL of 1 N hydrochloric acid, adding 25 mL of potassium iodide solution (4 in 100), diluting with water to 100 mL, and adding 0.50 mL of formic acid: the R_F value of the principal spot obtained from the Injection corresponds to that obtained from the Standard solution.

Bacterial endotoxins ⟨85⟩—It contains not more than 35.7 USP Endotoxin Units per mg of perphenazine.

pH ⟨791⟩: between 4.2 and 5.6.

Other requirements—It meets the requirements under *Injections* ⟨1⟩.

Assay—

Acid-alcohol solution—Transfer 10 mL of hydrochloric acid to a 1000-mL flask containing 500 mL of alcohol and 300 mL of water. Dilute with water to volume.

Palladium chloride solution—Dissolve 100 mg of palladium chloride in a mixture of 1 mL of hydrochloric acid and 50 mL of water in a 100-mL volumetric flask, heating on a steam bath to effect solution. Cool, dilute with water to volume, and mix. Store in an amber bottle and use within 30 days. On the day of use, transfer 50 mL to a 500-mL volumetric flask, add 4 mL of hydrochloric acid and 4.1 g of anhydrous sodium acetate, dilute with water to volume, and mix.

Standard preparation—Dissolve an accurately weighed quantity of USP Perphenazine RS in *Acid-alcohol solution* to obtain a solution having a known concentration of about 150 µg per mL.

Assay preparation—Dilute 3.0 mL of Injection with *Acid-alcohol solution* to 100 mL in a volumetric flask.

Procedure—Mix 10.0 mL each of the *Assay preparation* and the *Standard preparation* with 15.0 mL of *Palladium chloride solution*, filter, if necessary, and concomitantly determine the absorbances of these solutions, against a reagent blank, in 1-cm cells at the wavelength of maximum absorbance at about 480 nm, with a suitable spectrophotometer. Calculate the quantity, in mg, of $C_{21}H_{26}ClN_3OS$ in the volume of Injection taken by the formula:

$$0.1C(A_U/A_S)$$

in which C is the concentration, in µg per mL, of USP Perphenazine RS in the *Standard preparation*, and A_U and A_S are the absorbances of the solutions from the *Assay preparation* and the *Standard preparation*, respectively.

Perphenazine Oral Solution

» Perphenazine Oral Solution contains not less than 90.0 percent and not more than 110.0 percent of the labeled amount of perphenazine ($C_{21}H_{26}ClN_3OS$).

Packaging and storage—Preserve in well-closed, light-resistant containers.

USP Reference standards ⟨11⟩—*USP Perphenazine RS.*

NOTE—Throughout the following procedures, protect test or assay specimens, the USP Reference Standard, and solutions containing them, by conducting the procedures without delay, under subdued light, or using low-actinic glassware.

Identification—It meets the requirements for the *Identification* test under *Perphenazine Injection*.

Uniformity of dosage units ⟨905⟩—

FOR ORAL SOLUTION PACKAGED IN SINGLE-UNIT CONTAINERS: meets the requirements.

Deliverable volume ⟨698⟩—

FOR ORAL SOLUTION PACKAGED IN MULTIPLE-UNIT CONTAINERS: meets the requirements.

Limit of perphenazine sulfoxide—

Mobile phase, Resolution solution, Standard preparation, and *Chromatographic system*—Proceed as directed in the *Assay*.

Test preparation—Transfer an accurately measured portion of Oral Solution, equivalent to about 16 mg of perphenazine, to a 200-mL volumetric flask, dissolve in and dilute with methanol to volume, mix, and filter.

Procedure—Inject a volume (about 10 µL) of the *Test preparation* into the chromatograph, record the chromatogram, and measure the peak responses. Calculate the percentage of perphenazine sulfoxide in the portion of Oral Solution taken by the formula:

$$100(r_i/r_s)$$

in which r_i is the peak response of perphenazine sulfoxide (relative retention time of about 0.72); and r_s is the sum of the responses of all the peaks: not more than 5.0% of perphenazine sulfoxide is found.

Assay—

Mobile phase—Prepare a filtered and degassed mixture of 0.01 M ammonium acetate, acetonitrile, and methanol (48 : 39 : 13). Adjust with glacial acetic acid to a pH of 4.5. Make adjustments if necessary (see *System Suitability* under *Chromatography* ⟨621⟩).

Resolution solution—Dissolve suitable quantities of brompheniramine maleate and USP Perphenazine RS in methanol to obtain a solution having known concentrations of about 40 µg per mL and 8 µg per mL, respectively.

Standard preparation—Dissolve an accurately weighed quantity of USP Perphenazine RS in methanol, dilute quantitatively, and stepwise if necessary, with methanol to obtain a solution having a known concentration of about 8.0 µg per mL, and filter.

Assay preparation—Transfer an accurately measured portion of Oral Solution, equivalent to about 16 mg of perphenazine, to a 200-mL volumetric flask, dissolve in and dilute with methanol to volume, and mix. Dilute quantitatively, and stepwise if necessary, with methanol to obtain a solution having a concentration of about 8.0 µg per mL, and filter.

Chromatographic system (see *Chromatography* ⟨621⟩)—The liquid chromatograph is equipped with a 254-nm detector and a 3.9-mm × 30-cm column that contains packing L11. The flow rate is about 1.5 mL per minute. Chromatograph the *Resolution solution*, and record the peak responses as directed for *Procedure*: the relative retention times are about 0.6 for brompheniramine and 1.0 for perphenazine; and the resolution, R, between brompheniramine and perphenazine is not less than 3.0. Chromatograph the *Standard preparation*, and record the peak responses as directed for *Procedure*: the tailing factor is not more than 3.0; and the relative standard deviation for replicate injections is not more than 2.0%.

Procedure—Separately inject equal volumes (about 10 µL) of the *Standard preparation* and the *Assay preparation* into the chromatograph, record the chromatograms, and measure the responses for the major peaks. Calculate the quantity, in mg, of perphenazine

($C_{21}H_{26}ClN_3OS$) in the portion of Oral Solution taken by the formula:

$$2000C(r_U / r_S)$$

in which C is the concentration, in mg per mL, of USP Perphenazine RS in the *Standard preparation*; and r_U and r_S are the peak responses obtained from the *Assay preparation* and the *Standard preparation*, respectively.

Perphenazine Syrup

» Perphenazine Syrup contains not less than 90.0 percent and not more than 110.0 percent of the labeled amount of perphenazine ($C_{21}H_{26}ClN_3OS$).

Packaging and storage—Preserve in well-closed, light-resistant containers.

USP Reference standards ⟨11⟩—*USP Perphenazine RS*.

NOTE—Throughout the following procedures, protect test or assay specimens, the USP Reference Standard, and solutions containing them, by conducting the procedures without delay, under subdued light, or using low-actinic glassware.

Identification—Add 10 mL of water to a volume of Syrup, equivalent to about 4 mg of perphenazine, render alkaline by dropwise addition of sodium hydroxide to a pH of 11 to 12, and extract with four 5-mL portions of chloroform, combining the extracts through a bed of anhydrous sodium sulfate in a funnel into a beaker. Evaporate the extracts on a steam bath nearly to dryness, and dissolve the residue in 4 mL of methanol: the solution so obtained responds to the *Identification* test under *Perphenazine Injection*.

Uniformity of dosage units ⟨905⟩—
FOR SYRUP PACKAGED IN SINGLE-UNIT CONTAINERS: meets the requirements.

Deliverable volume ⟨698⟩—
FOR SYRUP PACKAGED IN MULTIPLE-UNIT CONTAINERS: meets the requirements.

Assay—

Acid-alcohol solution and *Palladium chloride solution*—Prepare as directed in the *Assay* under *Perphenazine Injection*.

Standard preparation—Dissolve an accurately weighed quantity of USP Perphenazine RS in *Acid-alcohol solution* to obtain a solution having a known concentration of about 160 µg per mL.

Assay preparation—Transfer an accurately measured volume of Syrup, equivalent to about 6 mg of perphenazine, to a 25-mL volumetric flask, dilute with water to volume, and mix. Transfer 10 mL to a 125-mL separator, add 25 mL of water, adjust with ammonium hydroxide to a pH of 10 to 11, and extract with four 20-mL portions of chloroform, filtering the extracts through anhydrous sodium sulfate. Evaporate the combined extracts on a steam bath with the aid of a stream of nitrogen to about 5 mL. Complete the evaporation without application of heat, and dissolve the residue in 15.0 mL of *Acid-alcohol solution*, filtering if necessary.

Procedure—Mix 10.0 mL each of the *Assay preparation* and the *Standard preparation* with 15.0 mL of *Palladium chloride solution*, filter if necessary, and concomitantly determine the absorbances of these solutions, against a reagent blank, in 1-cm cells at the wavelength of maximum absorbance at about 480 nm, with a suitable spectrophotometer. Calculate the quantity, in mg, of perphenazine ($C_{21}H_{26}ClN_3OS$) in each mL of the Syrup taken by the formula:

$$0.0375(C/V)(A_U / A_S)$$

in which C is the concentration, in µg per mL, of USP Perphenazine RS in the *Standard preparation*; V is the volume, in mL, of Syrup taken; and A_U and A_S are the absorbances of the solutions from the *Assay preparation* and the *Standard preparation*, respectively.

Perphenazine Tablets

» Perphenazine Tablets contain not less than 90.0 percent and not more than 110.0 percent of the labeled amount of $C_{21}H_{26}ClN_3OS$.

Packaging and storage—Preserve in tight, light-resistant containers.

USP Reference standards ⟨11⟩—*USP Perphenazine RS*.

NOTE—Throughout the following procedures, protect test or assay specimens, the USP Reference Standard, and solutions containing them, by conducting the procedures without delay, under subdued light, or using low-actinic glassware.

Identification—Shake a portion of finely powdered Tablets, equivalent to about 5 mg of perphenazine, with about 10 mL of chloroform, filter, evaporate the filtrate on a steam bath nearly to dryness, and dissolve the residue in 5 mL of methanol: the solution so obtained responds to the *Identification* test under *Perphenazine Injection*.

Dissolution ⟨711⟩—
Medium: 0.1 N hydrochloric acid; 900 mL.
Apparatus 2: 50 rpm.
Time: 45 minutes.
Procedure—Determine the amount of $C_{21}H_{26}ClN_3OS$ dissolved from UV absorbances at the wavelength of maximum absorbance at about 257 nm of filtered portions of the solution under test, suitably diluted with *Dissolution Medium*, if necessary, in comparison with a Standard solution having a known concentration of USP Perphenazine RS in the same medium.

Tolerances—Not less than 75% (*Q*) of the labeled amount of $C_{21}H_{26}ClN_3OS$ is dissolved in 45 minutes.

Uniformity of dosage units ⟨905⟩: meet the requirements.

Assay—

Acid-alcohol solution and *Palladium chloride solution*—Prepare as directed in the *Assay* under *Perphenazine Injection*.

Standard preparation—Prepare as directed in the *Assay* under *Perphenazine Syrup*.

Assay preparation—Weigh and finely powder not less than 20 Tablets. Transfer a portion of the powder, equivalent to about 4 mg of perphenazine, to a glass-stoppered conical flask, pipet into the flask 25 mL of *Acid-alcohol solution*, shake by mechanical means for 30 minutes, and centrifuge a portion of the mixture. The clear supernatant fluid is the *Assay preparation*.

Procedure—Proceed as directed for *Procedure* in the *Assay* under *Perphenazine Injection*. Calculate the quantity, in mg, of $C_{21}H_{26}ClN_3OS$ in the portion of Tablets taken by the formula:

$$0.025C(A_U / A_S)$$

in which C is the concentration, in µg per mL, of USP Perphenazine RS in the *Standard preparation*, and A_U and A_S are the absorbances of the solutions from the *Assay preparation* and the *Standard preparation*, respectively.

Perphenazine and Amitriptyline Hydrochloride Tablets

» Perphenazine and Amitriptyline Hydrochloride Tablets contain not less than 90.0 percent and not more than 110.0 percent of the labeled amounts of perphenazine ($C_{21}H_{26}ClN_3OS$) and amitriptyline hydrochloride ($C_{20}H_{23}N \cdot HCl$).

Packaging and storage—Preserve in well-closed containers.

USP Reference standards ⟨11⟩—*USP Amitriptyline Hydrochloride RS. USP Perphenazine RS*.

NOTE—Throughout the following procedures, protect test or assay specimens, the USP Reference Standard, and solutions containing them, by conducting the procedures without delay, under subdued light, or using low-actinic glassware.

Identification—Transfer a portion of powdered Tablets, equivalent to about 40 mg of perphenazine, to a 100-mL volumetric flask containing about 50 mL of alcohol. Agitate for 20 minutes, add alcohol to volume, mix, and filter or centrifuge. Separately prepare two Standard solutions containing 0.4 mg per mL of USP Perphenazine RS and USP Amitriptyline Hydrochloride RS, respectively, in alcohol. Separately apply 5 μL of the test solution and 5 μL of each Standard solution to a thin-layer chromatographic plate (see *Chromatography* ⟨621⟩) coated with a 0.25-mm layer of chromatographic silica gel mixture. Develop the chromatogram using a solvent system consisting of a mixture of cyclohexane, ethyl acetate, and diethylamine (85 : 25 : 5) until the solvent front has moved about 15 cm. Remove the plate from the developing chamber, air-dry for 20 minutes, and examine the plate under short-wavelength UV light: the R_F values of the principal spots obtained from the test solution correspond to those obtained from the Standard solutions.

Dissolution ⟨711⟩—
  Medium: 0.1 N hydrochloric acid; 900 mL.
  Apparatus 2: 50 rpm.
  Time: 60 minutes.
  Procedure—[NOTE—Due to potential decrease in the recovery of perphenazine when multiple injections are made from a vial, no more than two withdrawals should be made from any single vial.] Determine the amounts of perphenazine and amitriptyline hydrochloride in solution in filtered portions of the solution under test, in comparison with a Standard solution having known concentrations of USP Perphenazine RS and USP Amitriptyline Hydrochloride RS in the same medium, as directed for *Procedure* in the Assay.
  Tolerances—Not less than 75% (*Q*) of the labeled amounts of perphenazine ($C_{21}H_{26}ClN_3OS$) and amitriptyline hydrochloride ($C_{20}H_{23}N \cdot HCl$) is dissolved in 60 minutes.

Uniformity of dosage units ⟨905⟩: meet the requirements for *Content uniformity* with respect to perphenazine and to amitriptyline hydrochloride.

Assay—
  Mobile phase—Prepare a filtered and degassed mixture of water, acetonitrile, methanol, and methanesulfonic acid (490 : 310 : 200 : 2). Make adjustments if necessary (see *System Suitability* under *Chromatography* ⟨621⟩).
  Standard preparation—Dissolve an accurately weighed quantity of USP Perphenazine RS in methanol, and dilute quantitatively with methanol to obtain a solution having a known concentration of about 0.8 mg per mL (*Solution P*). Transfer 4*J* mg of USP Amitriptyline Hydrochloride RS to a 50-mL volumetric flask, *J* being the ratio of the labeled amount, in mg, of amitriptyline hydrochloride to the labeled amount, in mg, of perphenazine per Tablet. Add 5.0 mL of *Solution P* and 20 mL of 0.2 N acetic acid, shake, and sonicate to dissolve the USP Reference Standards. Dilute with methanol to volume, and mix. Pipet 25 mL of this solution into a 100-mL volumetric flask, dilute with a mixture of methanol and 0.04 N acetic acid (3 : 2) to volume, and mix to obtain a *Standard preparation* having known concentrations of about 20 μg of USP Perphenazine RS per mL and about 20*J* μg of USP Amitriptyline Hydrochloride RS per mL.
  Assay preparation—Transfer 10 Tablets to a 250-mL volumetric flask, add 100 mL of 0.2 N acetic acid, and shake the mixture until the Tablets have disintegrated. Add methanol to volume, mix, and filter. Dilute an accurately measured volume (V_F mL) of the clear filtrate quantitatively with a mixture of methanol and 0.04 N acetic acid (3 : 2) to obtain a solution (V_A mL) containing about 20 μg of perphenazine per mL, and filter through a membrane filter.
  Chromatographic system (see *Chromatography* ⟨621⟩)—The liquid chromatograph is equipped with a 254-nm detector and a 3.9-mm × 30-cm column that contains packing L1. The flow rate is about 1 mL per minute, and is adjusted until the relative retention times for perphenazine and amitriptyline are about 1 and 1.5, respectively. Chromatograph the *Standard preparation*, and record the peak responses as directed for *Procedure:* the relative standard deviation is not more than 2.0% for replicate injections, and the resolution, *R*, between perphenazine and amitriptyline is not less than 4.
  Procedure—Separately inject equal volumes (about 20 μL) of the *Standard preparation* and the *Assay preparation* into the chromatograph, record the chromatograms, and measure the responses for the major peaks. Calculate the quantity, in mg, of perphenazine ($C_{21}H_{26}ClN_3OS$) in each Tablet taken by the formula:

$$0.25(C/10)(V_A/V_F)(r_U/r_S)$$

in which *C* is the concentration, in μg per mL, of USP Perphenazine RS in the *Standard preparation*, V_A is the volume, in mL, of the *Assay preparation*, V_F is the volume, in mL, of the filtrate taken for the *Assay preparation*, and r_U and r_S are the responses of the perphenazine peaks obtained from the *Assay preparation* and the *Standard preparation*, respectively. Calculate the quantity, in mg, of amitriptyline hydrochloride ($C_{20}H_{23}N \cdot HCl$) taken by the same formula, reading amitriptyline hydrochloride instead of perphenazine.

Pertussis Immune Globulin

» Pertussis Immune Globulin conforms to the regulations of the FDA concerning biologics (see *Biologics* ⟨1041⟩). It is a sterile, nonpyrogenic solution of globulins derived from the blood plasma of adult human donors who have been immunized with pertussis vaccine such that each 1.25 mL contains not less than the amount of immune globulin to be equivalent to 25 mL of human hyperimmune serum. It may contain 0.3 M glycine as a stabilizing agent, and it contains a suitable preservative.

Packaging and storage—Preserve at a temperature between 2° and 8°.

Expiration date—The expiration date is not later than 3 years after date of issue from manufacturer's cold storage (5°, 3 years).

Labeling—Label it to state that it is not intended for intravenous injection.

Petrolatum

» Petrolatum is a purified mixture of semisolid hydrocarbons obtained from petroleum. It may contain a suitable stabilizer.

Packaging and storage—Preserve in well-closed containers.

Labeling—Label it to indicate the name and proportion of any added stabilizer.

Color—Melt about 10 g on a steam bath, and pour about 5 mL of the liquid into a clear-glass 15- × 150-mm test tube, keeping the petrolatum melted. The petrolatum is not darker than a solution made by mixing 3.8 mL of ferric chloride CS and 1.2 mL of cobaltous chloride CS in a similar tube, the comparison of the two being made in reflected light against a white background, the petrolatum tube being held directly against the background at such an angle that there is no fluorescence.

Specific gravity ⟨841⟩: between 0.815 and 0.880 at 60°.

Melting range, *Class III* ⟨741⟩: between 38° and 60°.

Consistency—
  Apparatus—Determine the consistency of Petrolatum by means of a penetrometer fitted with a polished cone-shaped metal plunger weighing 150 g, having a detachable steel tip of the following dimensions: the tip of the cone has an angle of 30°, the point being truncated to a diameter of 0.381 ± 0.025 mm, the base of the tip is 8.38 ± 0.05 mm in diameter, and the length of the tip is 14.94 ± 0.05 mm. The remaining portion of the cone has an angle of 90°, is about 28 mm in height, and has a maximum diameter at the base of about 65 mm. The containers for the test are flat-bottom metal cylinders that are 100 ± 6 mm in diameter and not less than 65 mm in

height. They are constructed of at least 1.6-mm (16-gauge) metal, and are provided with well-fitting, water-tight covers.

Procedure—Place the required number of containers in an oven, and bring them and a quantity of Petrolatum to a temperature of 82 ± 2.5°, pour the Petrolatum into one or more of the containers, filling to within 6 mm of the rim. Cool to 25 ± 2.5° over a period of not less than 16 hours, protected from drafts. Two hours before the test, place the containers in a water bath at 25 ± 0.5°. If the room temperature is below 23.5° or above 26.5°, adjust the temperature of the cone to 25 ± 0.5° by placing it in the water bath.

Without disturbing the surface of the substance under test, place the container on the penetrometer table, and lower the cone until the tip just touches the top surface of the test substance at a spot 25 mm to 38 mm from the edge of the container. Adjust the zero setting and quickly release the plunger, then hold it free for 5 seconds. Secure the plunger, and read the total penetration from the scale. Make three or more trials, each so spaced that there is no overlapping of the areas of penetration. Where the penetration exceeds 20 mm, use a separate container of the test substance for each trial. Read the penetration to the nearest 0.1 mm. Calculate the average of the three or more readings, and conduct further trials to a total of 10 if the individual results differ from the average by more than ±3%: the final average of the trials is not less than 10.0 mm and not more than 30.0 mm, indicating a consistency value between 100 and 300.

Acidity—If the addition of phenolphthalein TS in the test for *Alkalinity* produces no pink color, add 0.1 mL of methyl orange TS: no red or pink color is produced.

Alkalinity—Introduce 35 g into a suitable beaker, add 100 mL of boiling water, cover, and place on a stirring hot-plate maintained at the boiling point of water. After 5 minutes, allow the phases to separate. Draw off the separated water into a casserole, wash the petrolatum further with two 50-mL portions of boiling water, and add the washings to the casserole. To the pooled washings add 1 drop of phenolphthalein TS, and boil: the solution does not acquire a pink color.

Residue on ignition ⟨281⟩—Heat 2 g in an open porcelain or platinum dish over a Bunsen flame: it volatilizes without emitting an acrid odor and on ignition yields not more than 0.1% of residue.

Organic acids—Weigh 20.0 g, add 100 mL of a 1 in 2 mixture of neutralized alcohol and water, agitate thoroughly, and heat to boiling. Add 1 mL of phenolphthalein TS, and titrate rapidly with 0.1 N sodium hydroxide VS, with vigorous agitation to the production of a sharp pink endpoint, noting the color change in the alcohol-water layer: not more than 400 µL of 0.100 N sodium hydroxide is required.

Fixed oils, fats, and rosin—Digest 10 g with 50 mL of 5 N sodium hydroxide at 100° for 30 minutes. Separate the water layer, and acidify it with 5 N sulfuric acid: no oily or solid matter separates.

Hydrophilic Petrolatum

» Prepare Hydrophilic Petrolatum as follows:

Cholesterol	30 g
Stearyl Alcohol	30 g
White Wax	80 g
White Petrolatum	860 g
To make	1000 g

Melt the Stearyl Alcohol and White Wax together on a steam bath, then add the Cholesterol, and stir until completely dissolved. Add the White Petrolatum, and mix. Remove from the bath, and stir until the mixture congeals.

White Petrolatum

» White Petrolatum is a purified mixture of semisolid hydrocarbons obtained from petroleum, and wholly or nearly decolorized. It may contain a suitable stabilizer.

Color—Melt about 10 g on a steam bath, and pour 5 mL of the liquid into a clear-glass, 16-× 150-mm bacteriological test tube: the warm, melted liquid is not darker than a solution made by mixing 1.6 mL of ferric chloride CS and 3.4 mL of water in a similar tube, the comparison of the two being made in reflected light against a white background, the tubes being held directly against the background at such an angle that there is no fluorescence.

Residue on ignition ⟨281⟩—Heat 2 g in an open porcelain or platinum dish over a flame: it volatilizes without emitting an acrid odor and on ignition yields not more than 0.05% of residue.

Other requirements—It meets the requirements for *Packaging and storage*, *Labeling*, *Specific gravity*, *Melting range*, *Consistency*, *Alkalinity*, *Acidity*, *Organic acids*, and *Fixed oils, fats, and rosin* under *Petrolatum*.

Phenazopyridine Hydrochloride

$C_{11}H_{11}N_5 \cdot HCl$ 249.70
2,6-Pyridinediamine, 3-(phenylazo)-, monohydrochloride.
2,6-Diamino-3-(phenylazo)pyridine monohydrochloride   [136-40-3].

» Phenazopyridine Hydrochloride contains not less than 99.0 percent and not more than 101.0 percent of $C_{11}H_{11}N_5 \cdot HCl$, calculated on the dried basis.

Packaging and storage—Preserve in tight containers.

USP Reference standards ⟨11⟩—*USP Phenazopyridine Hydrochloride RS*.

Identification—
  A: *Infrared Absorption* ⟨197K⟩.
  B: *Ultraviolet Absorption* ⟨197U⟩—
  Solution: 5 µg per mL.
  Medium: sulfuric acid in alcohol (1 in 360).
  C: Prepare a solution of it in alcohol containing about 0.2 mg per mL. Transfer 10 mL of this solution to a glass-stoppered, 100-mL graduated cylinder, add chloroform to volume, and mix. Apply 10 µL of the solution so obtained to a suitable thin-layer chromatographic plate (see *Chromatography* ⟨621⟩) coated with a 0.25-mm layer of chromatographic silica gel. Apply to the same plate 10 µL of a Standard solution of USP Phenazopyridine Hydrochloride RS in the same medium having a known concentration of about 0.02 mg per mL. Develop the chromatogram in a solvent system consisting of a mixture of chloroform, ethyl acetate, and methanol (85 : 10 : 5) until the solvent front has moved about three-fourths of the length of the plate. Remove the plate from the chamber and allow it to dry. Locate the spots by spraying the plate lightly with 2 N hydrochloric acid: the R_F of the principal spot in the chromatogram of the test solution corresponds to that obtained from the Standard solution.

Loss on drying ⟨731⟩—Dry it at 105° for 4 hours: it loses not more than 1.0% of its weight.

Residue on ignition ⟨281⟩: not more than 0.2%.

Water-insoluble substances—Dissolve about 2 g, accurately weighed, in 200 mL of water, heat to boiling, then heat in a covered container on a steam bath for 1 hour. Filter through a tared, fine-porosity, sintered-glass crucible, wash thoroughly with water, and dry at 105° to constant weight: the weight of the residue does not

exceed 0.1% of the weight of Phenazopyridine Hydrochloride taken.
Heavy metals, *Method II* ⟨231⟩: 0.002%.
Ordinary impurities ⟨466⟩—
Test solution—Prepare a solution of it in alcohol having a concentration of 2.0 mg per mL.
Standard solutions—Prepare solutions of USP Phenazopyridine Hydrochloride RS in alcohol containing 0.04, 0.02, and 0.01 mg per mL, respectively.
Eluant: a mixture of chloroform, ethyl acetate, and methanol (85 : 10 : 5).
Visualization—Spray the plate with 5 N hydrochloric acid.
Assay—Transfer about 100 mg of Phenazopyridine Hydrochloride, accurately weighed, to a 200-mL volumetric flask. Add about 100 mL of a mixture of sulfuric acid and alcohol (1 in 360), heat gently on a steam bath for 10 minutes, shake by mechanical means to dissolve, cool to room temperature, dilute with the alcoholic sulfuric acid to volume, and mix. Transfer 10.0 mL of this solution to a 100-mL volumetric flask, dilute with the alcoholic sulfuric acid to volume, and mix. Transfer 5.0 mL of the resulting solution to a 50-mL volumetric flask, dilute with the alcoholic sulfuric acid to volume, and mix. Concomitantly determine the absorbances of this solution and a Standard solution of USP Phenazopyridine Hydrochloride RS in the same medium having a known concentration of about 5 μg per mL, in 1-cm cells at the wavelength of maximum absorbance at about 390 nm, with a suitable spectrophotometer, using dilute alcoholic sulfuric acid (1 in 360) as the blank. Calculate the quantity, in mg, of $C_{11}H_{11}N_5 \cdot HCl$ in the Phenazopyridine Hydrochloride taken by the formula:

$$20C(A_U/A_S)$$

in which C is the concentration, in μg per mL, of USP Phenazopyridine Hydrochloride RS in the Standard solution, and A_U and A_S are the absorbances of the solution of Phenazopyridine Hydrochloride and the Standard solution, respectively.

Phenazopyridine Hydrochloride Tablets

» Phenazopyridine Hydrochloride Tablets contain not less than 90.0 percent and not more than 110.0 percent of the labeled amount of phenazopyridine hydrochloride ($C_{11}H_{11}N_5 \cdot HCl$).

Packaging and storage—Preserve in tight containers.

USP Reference standards ⟨11⟩—*USP Phenazopyridine Hydrochloride RS*.
Identification—Transfer a quantity of finely ground Tablets, equivalent to about 50 mg of phenazopyridine hydrochloride, to a 125-mL separator, add 50 mL of water, 1 mL of 1 N hydrochloric acid, and 5 mL of a saturated sodium chloride solution, and shake to dissolve. Extract with two 25-mL portions of chloroform, and discard the chloroform. Add 5 mL of 1 N sodium hydroxide to the aqueous solution, and extract with one 50-mL portion of chloroform. Transfer the chloroform layer to a second 125-mL separator, and wash with one 50-mL portion of 0.1 N sodium hydroxide. Filter the chloroform layer through a pledget of cotton previously washed with chloroform. Add 5 drops of hydrochloric acid to the filtrate, and evaporate under a current of air on a steam bath to dryness. Add 5 mL of alcohol, and evaporate. Dry the residue at 105° for 4 hours: the IR absorption spectrum of a potassium bromide dispersion of the dried residue so obtained exhibits maxima only at the same wavelengths as that of a similar preparation of USP Phenazopyridine Hydrochloride RS.
Dissolution ⟨711⟩—
Medium: water; 900 mL.
Apparatus 2: 50 rpm.
Time: 45 minutes.
Procedure—Determine the amount of $C_{11}H_{11}N_5 \cdot HCl$ dissolved from UV absorbances at the wavelength of maximum absorbance at about 422 nm on filtered portions of the solution under test, suitably diluted with *Dissolution Medium* in comparison with a Standard solution having a known concentration of USP Phenazopyridine Hydrochloride RS in the same *Medium*.
Tolerances—Not less than 75% (*Q*) of the labeled amount of $C_{11}H_{11}N_5 \cdot HCl$ is dissolved in 45 minutes.
Uniformity of dosage units ⟨905⟩: meet the requirements.
Assay—
Phosphate buffer—Dissolve 2.64 g of dibasic ammonium phosphate in about 900 mL of water. Adjust with phosphoric acid to a pH of 3.0, dilute with water to 1000 mL, and mix.
Mobile phase—Prepare a mixture of *Phosphate buffer* and methanol (50 : 50). Make adjustments if necessary (see *System Suitability* under *Chromatography* ⟨621⟩).
Standard preparation—Transfer about 50 mg of USP Phenazopyridine Hydrochloride RS, accurately weighed, to a 100-mL volumetric flask. Add 50 mL of methanol, and swirl to dissolve. Dilute with *Phosphate buffer* to volume, mix, and pass through a filter having a 0.5-μm or finer porosity.
Assay preparation—Weigh and finely powder not fewer than 20 Tablets. Transfer an accurately weighed portion of the powder, equivalent to about 100 mg of phenazopyridine hydrochloride, to a 200-mL volumetric flask. Add 100 mL of methanol, and sonicate for 10 minutes. Add about 75 mL of *Phosphate buffer*, and sonicate for an additional 10 minutes, with occasional mixing. Dilute with *Phosphate buffer* to volume, and mix. Pass this solution through a filter having a 0.5-μm or finer porosity.
Chromatographic system (see *Chromatography* ⟨621⟩)—The liquid chromatograph is equipped with a 220-nm detector and a 3.9-mm × 30-cm column that contains packing L1. The flow rate is about 1.5 mL per minute. Chromatograph the *Standard preparation*, and record the responses as directed for *Procedure:* the column efficiency is not less than 1400 theoretical plates; the tailing factor for the analyte peak is not more than 2.0; and the relative standard deviation for replicate injections is not more than 2.0%.
Procedure—Separately inject equal volumes (about 10 μL) of the *Standard preparation* and the *Assay preparation* into the chromatograph, record the chromatograms, and measure the responses for the major peaks. Calculate the quantity, in mg, of $C_{11}H_{11}N_5 \cdot HCl$ in the portion of Tablets taken by the formula:

$$200C(r_U/r_S)$$

in which C is the concentration, in mg per mL, of USP Phenazopyridine Hydrochloride RS in the *Standard preparation;* and r_U and r_S are the phenazopyridine peak responses obtained from the *Assay preparation* and the *Standard preparation*, respectively.

Phendimetrazine Tartrate

$C_{12}H_{17}NO \cdot C_4H_6O_6$ 341.36
Morpholine, 3,4-dimethyl-2-phenyl-, (2*S-trans*)-, [*R*-(*R**,*R**)]-2,3-dihydroxybutanedioate (1 : 1).
(2*S*,3*S*)-3,4-Dimethyl-2-phenylmorpholine L-(+)-tartrate (1 : 1) [50-58-8].

» Phendimetrazine Tartrate contains not less than 98.0 percent and not more than 102.0 percent of $C_{12}H_{17}NO \cdot C_4H_6O_6$, calculated on the dried basis.

Packaging and storage—Preserve in tight containers.

USP Reference standards ⟨11⟩—*USP Phendimetrazine Tartrate RS*.

Identification—

A: *Infrared Absorption* ⟨197K⟩.

B: *Ultraviolet Absorption* ⟨197U⟩—

Solution: 1 mg per mL.

Medium: methanol.

C: It responds to the test for *Tartrate* ⟨191⟩.

Melting range ⟨741⟩: between 182° and 188°, with decomposition, but the range between beginning and end of melting does not exceed 3°.

Specific rotation ⟨781S⟩: between +32° and +36°.

Test solution: 100 mg per mL, in water.

pH ⟨791⟩: between 3.0 and 4.0, in a solution (1 in 40).

Loss on drying ⟨731⟩—Dry it to constant weight at 105°: it loses not more than 0.5% of its weight.

Residue on ignition ⟨281⟩: not more than 0.1%.

Chloride ⟨221⟩—A 1.0-g portion shows no more chloride than corresponds to 0.50 mL of 0.020 N hydrochloric acid (0.035%).

Sulfate ⟨221⟩—A 1.0-g portion shows no more sulfate than corresponds to 0.10 mL of 0.020 N sulfuric acid (0.01%).

Heavy metals ⟨231⟩: 0.001%.

Chromatographic purity—Dissolve 500 mg in water, dilute with water to 5.0 mL, and mix. Apply 10 μL of this preparation and 10 μL of an aqueous solution of USP Phendimetrazine Tartrate RS containing about 100 mg per mL to the starting line to a suitable thin-layer chromatographic plate (see *Chromatography* ⟨621⟩) coated with a 0.25-mm layer of chromatographic silica gel mixture. Develop the chromatogram in a suitable chamber with a solvent system consisting of a mixture of acetone, methanol, and ammonium hydroxide (50 : 50 : 1) until the solvent front has moved about three-fourths of the length of the plate. Remove the plate from the chamber, air-dry, view under short-wavelength UV light, and observe the location of the spots. Expose the plate to iodine vapors in a closed chamber: yellow spots appear at the same locations as the spots observed under UV light, and the R_F value of the spot obtained from the test preparation corresponds to that obtained from the Standard solution, and no other spot is obtained.

Organic volatile impurities, Method I ⟨467⟩: meets the requirements.

(Official until July 1, 2008)

L-*erythro* isomer—Dissolve 3.0 g of Phendimetrazine Tartrate in 25 mL of sodium hydroxide solution (1 in 20) in a suitable separator. Add 25 mL of sodium hydroxide solution (1 in 2), swirl, and allow the phendimetrazine base to separate. Discard the lower, alkaline layer, and collect the upper layer, centrifuging, if necessary, to obtain a clear liquid. Inject 1.0 μL of this liquid into a suitable gas chromatograph equipped with a flame-ionization detector, a 100 : 1 specimen splitter, and a 25-m × 0.25-mm capillary column, the inside wall of which is coated with a 0.4-μm film of liquid phase G1. The temperatures of the injection port, column, and detector block are 250°, 140°, and 280°, respectively. The carrier gas is helium. Preferably using an electronic integrator, determine the areas of all peaks in the chromatogram. The retention times are about 8.5 minutes for the D-*threo* isomer and 9 minutes for the L-*erythro* isomer. Calculate the percentage of L-*erythro*isomer in the test specimen taken by the formula:

$$100(r_U / r_S)$$

in which r_U is the peak area response of the L-*erythro*isomer peak and r_S is the sum of the areas of the L-*erythro*isomer peak and the D-*threo* isomer peak: the limit is 0.1%.

Assay—Transfer to a beaker about 500 mg of Phendimetrazine Tartrate, accurately weighed, and dissolve in 50 mL of glacial acetic acid. Add 1 drop of crystal violet TS, and titrate with 0.1 N perchloric acid VS to a green endpoint. Perform a blank determination, and make any necessary correction. Each mL of 0.1 N perchloric acid is equivalent to 34.14 mg of $C_{12}H_{17}NO \cdot C_4H_6O_6$.

Phendimetrazine Tartrate Capsules

» Phendimetrazine Tartrate Capsules contain not less than 95.0 percent and not more than 105.0 percent of the labeled amount of $C_{12}H_{17}NO \cdot C_4H_6O_6$.

Packaging and storage—Preserve in tight containers.

USP Reference standards ⟨11⟩—*USP Phendimetrazine Tartrate RS*.

Identification—

A: Shake a quantity of Capsule contents, equivalent to about 300 mg of phendimetrazine tartrate, with about 50 mL of water, filter, and transfer the filtrate to a 200-mL separator. Add 3 mL of 12.5 N sodium hydroxide, and extract with two 50-mL portions of chloroform. Extract the combined chloroform extracts in a 250-mL separator with two 15-mL portions of 0.5 N hydrochloric acid, and evaporate the combined aqueous extracts on a steam bath to dryness. Dissolve the residue in 5 mL of acetone, and add 50 mL of anhydrous ether to the solution. On standing, phendimetrazine hydrochloride crystallizes out. Filter the precipitate, wash with anhydrous ether, and dry at 105°: the crystals so obtained melt between 189° and 193°, but the range between beginning and end of melting does not exceed 2°.

B: A portion of Capsule contents responds to the test for *Tartrate* ⟨191⟩.

Dissolution ⟨711⟩—

Medium: water; 900 mL.

Apparatus 1: 100 rpm.

Time: 60 minutes.

pH 7.5 Phosphate buffer—Prepare a solution of 0.025 M monobasic potassium phosphate, and adjust with 1 N potassium hydroxide to a pH of 7.5.

Mobile phase—Prepare a suitable degassed and filtered mixture of acetonitrile and *pH 7.5 Phosphate buffer* (65 : 35).

Chromatographic system (see *Chromatography* ⟨621⟩)—The liquid chromatograph is equipped with a 210-nm detector and a 4-mm × 15-cm column that contains packing L15. The flow rate is about 1 mL per minute. Chromatograph three replicate injections of the Standard solution, and record the peak responses as directed for *Procedure:* the relative standard deviation is not more than 3.0%.

Procedure—Separately inject equal volumes (about 50 μL) of the Standard solution and a filtered aliquot of the solution under test into the chromatograph, record the chromatograms, and measure the responses for the major peaks. Calculate the percentage of $C_{12}H_{17}NO \cdot C_4H_6O_6$ dissolved in comparison with a Standard solution of USP Phendimetrazine Tartrate RS, similarly prepared and chromatographed.

Tolerances—Not less than 70% (*Q*) of the labeled amount of $C_{12}H_{17}NO \cdot C_4H_6O_6$ is dissolved in 60 minutes.

Uniformity of dosage units ⟨905⟩: meet the requirements.

Assay—

Mobile phase—Dissolve 1.1 g of sodium 1-heptanesulfonate in 575 mL of water, add 400 mL of methanol, 25 mL of dilute acetic acid (14 in 100), and mix. Adjust with glacial acetic acid to a pH of 3.0 ± 0.1, if necessary. Filter through a 0.45-μm membrane filter, and degas. Make adjustments if necessary (see *System Suitability* under *Chromatography* ⟨621⟩).

Diluent—Prepare a mixture of water, methanol, and dilute acetic acid (14 in 100) (57.5 : 40 : 2.5).

Internal standard solution—Prepare a solution of salicylamide in *Diluent* having a concentration of about 0.1 mg per mL.

Standard preparation—Dissolve an accurately weighed quantity of USP Phendimetrazine Tartrate RS in *Internal standard solution*, and dilute quantitatively with *Internal standard solution* to obtain a solution having a known concentration of about 0.7 mg of USP Phendimetrazine Tartrate RS per mL.

Assay preparation—Remove, as completely as possible, the contents of not fewer than 20 Capsules, and weigh accurately. Mix the combined contents, and transfer an accurately weighed quantity of the powder, equivalent to about 35 mg of phendimetrazine tartrate, to a 50-mL volumetric flask, add 25 mL of *Internal standard solution*, and sonicate for about 15 minutes. Cool the solution to room temperature, dilute with *Internal standard solution* to volume, mix, and filter through a 0.45-µm membrane filter.

Chromatographic system (see *Chromatography* ⟨621⟩)—The liquid chromatograph is equipped with a 256-nm detector and a 3.9-mm × 30-cm column that contains packing L1. The flow rate is about 1 mL per minute. Chromatograph the *Standard preparation*, and record the peak responses as directed for *Procedure*: the resolution, R, between the analyte and internal standard peaks is not less than 3.0, and the relative standard deviation for replicate injections is not more than 1.0%.

Procedure—Separately inject equal volumes (about 20 µL) of the *Standard preparation* and the *Assay preparation* into the chromatograph, record the chromatograms, and measure the responses for the major peaks. The relative retention times are about 0.5 for salicylamide and 1.0 for phendimetrazine tartrate. Calculate the quantity, in mg, of $C_{12}H_{17}NO \cdot C_4H_6O_6$ in the portion of Capsules taken by the formula:

$$50C(R_U / R_S)$$

in which C is the concentration, in mg per mL, of USP Phendimetrazine Tartrate RS in the *Standard preparation*, and R_U and R_S are the peak response ratios obtained from the *Assay preparation* and the *Standard preparation*, respectively.

Phendimetrazine Tartrate Tablets

» Phendimetrazine Tartrate Tablets contain not less than 90.0 percent and not more than 110.0 percent of the labeled amount of $C_{12}H_{17}NO \cdot C_4H_6O_6$.

Packaging and storage—Preserve in well-closed containers.

USP Reference standards ⟨11⟩—*USP Phendimetrazine Tartrate RS*.

Identification—A quantity of finely powdered Tablets, equivalent to about 300 mg of phendimetrazine tartrate, responds to the *Identification* tests under *Phendimetrazine Tartrate Capsules*.

Dissolution ⟨711⟩—
 Medium: water; 900 mL.
 Apparatus 1: 100 rpm.
 Time: 60 minutes.
 pH 7.5 Phosphate buffer—Prepare a solution of 0.025 M monobasic potassium phosphate, and adjust to a pH of 7.5 by the addition of 1 N potassium hydroxide.
 Mobile phase—Prepare a suitable degassed and filtered mixture of acetonitrile and *pH 7.5 Phosphate buffer* (65 : 35).
 Chromatographic system (see *Chromatography* ⟨621⟩)—The liquid chromatograph is equipped with a 210-nm detector and a 4-mm × 15-cm column that contains packing L15. The flow rate is about 1.0 mL per minute. Chromatograph three replicate injections of the Standard solution, and record the peak responses as directed for *Procedure*: the relative standard deviation is not more than 3.0%.
 Procedure—Separately inject equal volumes (about 50 µL) of the Standard solution and a filtered aliquot of the solution under test into the chromatograph, record the chromatograms, and measure the responses for the major peaks. Calculate the percentage of $C_{12}H_{17}NO \cdot C_4H_6O_6$ dissolved in comparison with a Standard solution of USP Phendimetrazine Tartrate RS, similarly prepared and chromatographed.
 Tolerances—Not less than 70% (Q) of the labeled amount of $C_{12}H_{17}NO \cdot C_4H_6O_6$ is dissolved in 60 minutes.

Uniformity of dosage units ⟨905⟩: meet the requirements.

Assay—
 Mobile phase, Diluent, Internal standard solution, Standard preparation, and *Chromatographic system*—Prepare as directed in the *Assay* under *Phendimetrazine Tartrate Capsules*.
 Assay preparation—Weigh and finely powder not fewer than 20 Tablets. Transfer an accurately weighed portion of the powder, equivalent to about 35 mg of phendimetrazine tartrate, to a 50-mL volumetric flask, add 25 mL of *Internal standard solution*, and sonicate for about 15 minutes. Cool the solution to room temperature, dilute with *Internal standard solution* to volume, mix, and filter through a 0.45-µm membrane filter.

Procedure—Proceed as directed for *Procedure* in the *Assay* under *Phendimetrazine Tartrate Capsules*. Calculate the quantity, in mg, of $C_{12}H_{17}NO \cdot C_4H_6O_6$ in the portion of Tablets taken by the formula:

$$50C(R_U / R_S)$$

in which C is the concentration, in mg per mL, of USP Phendimetrazine Tartrate RS in the *Standard preparation*, and R_U and R_S are the peak response ratios obtained from the *Assay preparation* and the *Standard preparation*, respectively.

Phenelzine Sulfate

$C_8H_{12}N_2 \cdot H_2SO_4$ 234.27
Hydrazine, (2-phenylethyl)-, sulfate (1 : 1).
Phenethylhydrazine sulfate (1 : 1).   [156-51-4].

» Phenelzine Sulfate contains not less than 98.0 percent and not more than 102.0 percent of $C_8H_{12}N_2 \cdot H_2SO_4$, calculated on the dried basis.

Packaging and storage—Preserve in tight containers, protected from heat and light.

USP Reference standards ⟨11⟩—*USP Phenelzine Sulfate RS*.

Identification—
 A: *Infrared Absorption* ⟨197K⟩.
 B: Dissolve 100 mg in 5 mL of water, render the solution alkaline with 1 N sodium hydroxide, and add 1 mL of alkaline cupric tartrate TS: a red to yellow-red precipitate is formed.
 C: A solution (1 in 10) meets the requirements of the tests for *Sulfate* ⟨191⟩.

Melting range ⟨741⟩: between 164° and 168°.

pH ⟨791⟩: between 1.4 and 1.9, in a solution (1 in 100).

Loss on drying ⟨731⟩—Dry it at a pressure not exceeding 5 mm of mercury over silica gel at 80° for 2 hours: it loses not more than 1.0% of its weight.

Heavy metals, *Method I* ⟨231⟩: 0.002%.

Limit of hydrazine—
 Mobile phase—Prepare a filtered and degassed mixture of methanol and 1% monobasic ammonium phosphate solution (75 : 25). Make adjustments if necessary (see *System Suitability* under *Chromatography* ⟨621⟩).
 Standard solution—Transfer an accurately weighed quantity of about 42.0 mg of hydrazine sulfate, equivalent to about 10 mg of hydrazine, to a 100-mL volumetric flask. Dissolve in water, sonicate for about 5 minutes, dilute with methanol to volume, and mix. Dilute an accurately measured volume of this solution quantitatively and stepwise with methanol to obtain a solution having a known concentration of 5.0 µg of hydrazine per mL. Transfer 5.0 mL of this solution to a 200-mL volumetric flask, add 50 mL of methanol and 0.7 mL of ammonium hydroxide, and shake to mix. Add 0.5 mL of salicylaldehyde, shake by mechanical means for about 5 minutes, dilute with methanol to volume, sonicate for about 2 minutes, and mix.
 Test solution—Transfer about 25.8 mg of Phenelzine Sulfate, accurately weighed, to a 200-mL volumetric flask, dissolve in about 50 mL of methanol, and sonicate. Add 0.7 mL of ammonium hydroxide, shake to mix, add 0.5 mL of salicylaldehyde, shake by mechanical means for about 5 minutes, dilute with methanol to volume, sonicate for about 2 minutes, and mix.
 Chromatographic system (see *Chromatography* ⟨621⟩)—The liquid chromatograph is equipped with a 340-nm detector and a 4.6-mm × 25-cm column that contains 5-µm packing L1. Chromatograph the *Standard solution*, and record the peak areas as directed for *Procedure*: the relative retention times for salicylaldehyde, phen-

elzine sulfate derivative, and hydrazine sulfate derivative are about 0.21, 0.47, and 1.0, respectively; the column efficiency determined from the analyte peak is not less than 4500 theoretical plates; the resolution, R, between phenelzine and salazine (derivatized hydrazine) is not less than 1.25; and the relative standard deviation for replicate injections is not more than 7%.

Procedure—Separately inject equal volumes (about 50 µL) of the *Standard solution* and the *Test solution* into the chromatograph, record the chromatograms, and measure the peak areas for salazine (derivatized hydrazine). Calculate the percentage of hydrazine in the portion of Phenelzine Sulfate taken by the formula:

$$20(C/W)(r_U/r_S)$$

in which C is the concentration, in µg per mL, of hydrazine base in the *Standard solution*; W is the weight, in mg, of Phenelzine Sulfate taken to prepare the *Test solution*; and r_U and r_S are the salazine peak areas obtained from the *Test solution* and the *Standard solution*, respectively: not more than 0.1% is found.

Ordinary impurities ⟨466⟩—
 Test solution: a mixture of methanol and water (1 : 1).
 Standard solution: a mixture of methanol and water (1 : 1).
 Eluant: acetone. [NOTE—Prewash the plate with *Eluant*, and dry.]
 Visualization: 1.

Organic volatile impurities, *Method I* ⟨467⟩: meets the requirements.

(Official until July 1, 2008)

Assay—
 Ion-pair solution, Mobile phase, Standard preparation, and *Chromatographic system*—Proceed as directed in the *Assay* under *Phenelzine Sulfate Tablets*.
 Assay preparation—Transfer about 26 mg of Phenelzine Sulfate, accurately weighed, to a 100-mL volumetric flask, dissolve in and dilute with *Mobile phase* to volume, and mix.
 Procedure—Separately inject equal volumes (about 20 µL) of the *Standard preparation* and the *Assay preparation* into the chromatograph, record the chromatograms, and measure the peak responses. Calculate the quantity, in mg, of $C_8H_{12}N_2 \cdot H_2SO_4$ in the portion of Phenelzine Sulfate taken by the formula:

$$100C(r_U/r_S)$$

in which C is the concentration, in mg per mL, of USP Phenelzine Sulfate RS in the *Standard preparation;* and r_U and r_S are the peak responses obtained from the *Assay preparation* and the *Standard preparation,* respectively.

Phenelzine Sulfate Tablets

» Phenelzine Sulfate Tablets contain an amount of phenelzine sulfate ($C_8H_{12}N_2 \cdot H_2SO_4$) equivalent to not less than 90.0 percent and not more than 110.0 percent of the labeled amount of phenelzine ($C_8H_{12}N_2$).

Packaging and storage—Preserve in tight containers, protected from heat and light.

USP Reference standards ⟨11⟩—*USP Phenelzine Sulfate RS.*

Identification—Extract a portion of powdered Tablets, equivalent to about 30 mg of phenelzine, with 10 mL of water, and filter: the filtrate responds to *Identification* tests B and C under *Phenelzine Sulfate.*

Disintegration ⟨701⟩—Place 1 tablet in each of the 6 tubes of the basket and, if the tablets have a soluble external coating, immerse the basket in water at room temperature for 5 minutes. Then add a disk to each tube, and operate the apparatus, using simulated gastric fluid TS maintained at 37 ± 2° as the immersion fluid. After 30 minutes of operation in simulated gastric fluid TS, lift the basket from the fluid, and observe the tablets. If the tablets have not disintegrated completely, substitute simulated intestinal fluid TS maintained at 37 ± 2° as the immersion fluid. Continue the test for a total period of time, including previous exposure to water and simulated gastric fluid TS, of 1 hour and 30 minutes. Lift the basket from the fluid, and observe the tablets: all of the tablets have disintegrated completely. If 1 or 2 tablets fail to disintegrate completely, repeat the test on 12 additional tablets: not less than 16 of the total 18 tablets tested disintegrate completely.

Uniformity of dosage units ⟨905⟩: meet the requirements.

Assay—
 Ion-pair solution—Dissolve about 6.8 g of monobasic potassium phosphate and about 2.16 g of sodium 1-octanesulfonate in 1000 mL of water, and mix. Adjust with phosphoric acid to a pH of 3.0, and filter.
 Mobile phase—Prepare a filtered and degassed mixture of *Ion-pair solution* and methanol (60 : 40). Make adjustments if necessary (see *System Suitability* under *Chromatography* ⟨621⟩).
 Standard preparation—Dissolve an accurately weighed quantity of USP Phenelzine Sulfate RS in *Mobile phase*, and dilute quantitatively, and stepwise if necessary, with *Mobile phase* to obtain a solution having a known concentration of about 258 µg per mL.
 Assay preparation—Transfer not less than 20 Tablets to a suitable container, add about 300 mL of *Mobile phase*, and homogenize until dissolved. Transfer this solution to a 500-mL volumetric flask, dilute with *Mobile phase* to volume, mix, centrifuge, and filter, discarding the first 5 mL of the filtrate. Transfer a portion of the filtrate, equivalent to about 12.9 mg of phenelzine sulfate, to a 50-mL volumetric flask, dilute with *Mobile phase* to volume, and mix.
 Chromatographic system (see *Chromatography* ⟨621⟩)—The liquid chromatograph is equipped with a 210-nm detector and a 3.9-mm × 15-cm column that contains packing L1. The flow rate is about 1.0 mL per minute. Chromatograph the *Standard preparation*, and record the peak responses as directed for *Procedure*: the column efficiency is not less than 3000 theoretical plates, the tailing factor is not more than 2.0, and the relative standard deviation for replicate injections is not more than 2.0%.
 Procedure—Separately inject equal volumes (about 20 µL) of the *Standard preparation* and the *Assay preparation* into the chromatograph, record the chromatograms, and measure the responses for the major peaks. Calculate the quantity, in µg, of phenelzine ($C_8H_{12}N_2$) in the *Assay preparation* by the formula:

$$(136.20 / 234.27)(50C)(r_U/r_S)$$

in which 136.20 and 234.27 are the molecular weights of phenelzine and phenelzine sulfate, respectively, C is the concentration, in µg per mL, of USP Phenelzine Sulfate RS in the *Standard preparation*, and r_U and r_S are the peak responses obtained from the *Assay preparation* and the *Standard preparation*, respectively.

Pheniramine Maleate

$C_{16}H_{20}N_2 \cdot C_4H_4O_4$ 356.42

2-[α-[2-Dimethylaminoethyl]benzyl]pyridine bimaleate.
N,N-Dimethyl-3-phenyl-3-(2-pyridyl)propylamine hydrogen maleate   [132-20-7].

» Pheniramine Maleate contains not less than 98.0 percent and not more than 102.0 percent of $C_{16}H_{20}N_2 \cdot C_4H_4O_4$, calculated on the dried basis.

Packaging and storage—Preserve in well-closed containers.

USP Reference standards ⟨11⟩—*USP Pheniramine Maleate RS.*
Identification, *Infrared Absorption* ⟨197K⟩.
Melting range, *Class I* ⟨741⟩: between 104° and 109°.
pH ⟨791⟩: between 4.5 and 5.5, in a solution (10 mg per mL).
Loss on drying ⟨731⟩—Dry it in vacuum at 65° for 6 hours: it loses not more than 0.5% of its weight.

Residue on ignition ⟨281⟩: not more than 0.5%.
Heavy metals, *Method I* ⟨231⟩: 0.002%.
Chromatographic purity—

0.005 M Octane sulfonic acid—Transfer 1.08 g of sodium 1-octane sulfonate to a 1-liter volumetric flask. Dilute with 1.5% (v/v) acetic acid solution to volume, add 5.0 mL of triethylamine, mix, and filter.

Mobile phase—Prepare a filtered and degassed mixture of *0.005 M Octane sulfonic acid* and acetonitrile (39 : 11). Make adjustments if necessary (see *System Suitability* under *Chromatography* ⟨621⟩).

System suitability solution—Dissolve suitable quantities of phenylethyl alcohol and USP Pheniramine Maleate RS in water to obtain a solution containing about 3.6 and 0.24 mg per mL, respectively.

Test solution—Transfer about 24 mg of Pheniramine Maleate, accurately weighed, to a 100-mL volumetric flask, dissolve in and dilute with water to volume, and mix.

Chromatographic system (see *Chromatography* ⟨621⟩)—The liquid chromatograph is equipped with a 265-nm detector and a 3.9-mm × 30-cm column that contains packing L1. The flow rate is about 2 mL per minute. Chromatograph the *System suitability solution,* and record the peak responses as directed for *Procedure:* the relative retention times are about 0.5 phenylethyl alcohol and 1.0 for pheniramine maleate, and the resolution, *R,* between phenylethyl alcohol and pheniramine maleate is not less than 2.0, the tailing factor is not more than 2.5, and the relative standard deviation for replicate injections is not more than 2.0%.

Procedure—Inject a volume (about 10 µL) of the *Test solution* into the chromatograph, record the chromatogram, and measure the peak responses. Calculate the percentage of each impurity (not including the solvent peak and maleic acid, if observed) in the portion of Pheniramine Maleate taken by the formula:

$$100(r_i / r_s)$$

in which r_i is the peak response for each impurity, and r_s is the sum of the responses of all of the peaks: not more than 0.5% of any individual impurity is found, and not more than 2.0% of total impurities is found.

Organic volatile impurities, *Method IV* ⟨467⟩: meets the requirements.

(Official until July 1, 2008)

Assay—Dissolve about 500 mg of Pheniramine Maleate, accurately weighed, in 25 mL of glacial acetic acid. Add 2 drops of crystal violet TS, and titrate with 0.1 N perchloric acid VS. Perform a blank determination, and make any necessary corrections. Each mL of 0.1 N perchloric acid is equivalent to 17.82 mg of $C_{16}H_{20}N_2 \cdot C_4H_4O_4$.

Phenmetrazine Hydrochloride

$C_{11}H_{15}NO \cdot HCl$ 213.70
Morpholine, 3-methyl-2-phenyl-, hydrochloride.
3-Methyl-2-phenylmorpholine hydrochloride   [1707-14-8].

» Phenmetrazine Hydrochloride, dried at 105° for 2 hours, contains not less than 98.0 percent and not more than 102.0 percent of $C_{11}H_{15}NO \cdot HCl$.

Packaging and storage—Preserve in tight containers.

USP Reference standards ⟨11⟩—*USP Phenmetrazine Hydrochloride RS.*

Identification—
  A: *Infrared Absorption* ⟨197S⟩—
  Solution: 1 in 20.
  Medium: chloroform.
  B: *Ultraviolet Absorption* ⟨197U⟩—
  Solution: 500 µg per mL.
  Medium: 0.5 N hydrochloric acid.
Melting range, *Class Ia* ⟨741⟩: between 172° and 182°, but the range between beginning and end of melting does not exceed 3°.
pH ⟨791⟩: between 4.5 and 5.5, in a solution (1 in 40).
Loss on drying ⟨731⟩—Dry it at 105° for 2 hours: it loses not more than 0.5% of its weight.
Residue on ignition ⟨281⟩: not more than 0.1%.
Sulfate ⟨221⟩—A 2.0-g portion shows no more sulfate than corresponds to 0.20 mL of 0.020 N sulfuric acid (0.01%).
Chloride content—Transfer about 350 mg, previously dried and accurately weighed, to a 250-mL beaker. Add about 125 mL of water and 10 drops of sulfuric acid, and stir for 15 minutes with a magnetic stirrer. Titrate the solution potentiometrically with 0.1 N silver nitrate VS, using a silver-mercurous sulfate electrode system with a saturated salt bridge of potassium sulfate. Each mL of 0.1 N silver nitrate is equivalent to 3.545 mg of Cl: the content is between 16.3% and 17.0%.
Heavy metals, *Method II* ⟨231⟩: 0.001%.
Ordinary impurities ⟨466⟩—
  Test solution: methanol.
  Standard solution: methanol.
  Eluant: a mixture of chloroform, absolute alcohol, and ammonium hydroxide (80 : 20 : 1).
  Visualization: 1.
Organic volatile impurities, *Method I* ⟨467⟩: meets the requirements.

(Official until July 1, 2008)

Assay—Transfer to a 200-mL volumetric flask about 100 mg of Phenmetrazine Hydrochloride, previously dried and accurately weighed. Dissolve in 0.5 N hydrochloric acid, dilute with 0.5 N hydrochloric acid to volume, and mix to obtain the *Assay preparation.* Concomitantly determine the absorbances of the *Assay preparation* and of a Standard solution of USP Phenmetrazine Hydrochloride RS, in the same medium having a known concentration of about 500 µg per mL, in 1-cm cells, at the wavelength of maximum absorbance at about 256 nm, with a suitable spectrophotometer, using 0.5 N hydrochloric acid as the blank. Calculate the quantity, in mg, of $C_{11}H_{15}NO \cdot HCl$ in the Phenmetrazine Hydrochloride taken by the formula:

$$0.2C(A_U / A_S)$$

in which *C* is the concentration, in µg per mL, of USP Phenmetrazine Hydrochloride RS in the Standard solution, and A_U and A_S are the absorbances from the *Assay preparation* and the Standard solution, respectively.

Phenmetrazine Hydrochloride Tablets

» Phenmetrazine Hydrochloride Tablets contain not less than 93.0 percent and not more than 107.0 percent of the labeled amount of $C_{11}H_{15}NO \cdot HCl$.

Packaging and storage—Preserve in tight containers.

USP Reference standards ⟨11⟩—*USP Phenmetrazine Hydrochloride RS.*

Identification—Dissolve 5 Tablets in 40 mL of water in a 250-mL separator. Add 3 mL of sodium hydroxide solution (1 in 2), and extract with two 50-mL portions of chloroform. Extract the combined chloroform extracts in a 250-mL separator with two 15-mL portions of 0.5 N hydrochloric acid, and evaporate the combined aqueous extracts on a steam bath to dryness. Dissolve the residue in 5 mL of acetone, and add 50 mL of anhydrous ether to the solution. On standing, phenmetrazine hydrochloride will crystallize out. Filter the precipitate, wash with anhydrous ether, and dry at 105°: the crystals so obtained melt within a range of 3° between 172° and 182° (see *Melting Range or Temperature* ⟨741⟩).

Dissolution ⟨711⟩—
  Medium: water; 900 mL.
  Apparatus 2: 50 rpm.
  Time: 45 minutes.
  Procedure—Determine the amount of $C_{11}H_{15}NO \cdot HCl$ dissolved from UV absorbances at the wavelength of maximum absorbance at about 256 nm on filtered portions of the solution under test, suitably diluted with *Dissolution Medium*, if necessary, in comparison with a Standard solution having a known concentration of USP Phenmetrazine Hydrochloride RS in the same *Medium*.
  Tolerances—Not less than 75% (*Q*) of the labeled amount of $C_{11}H_{15}NO \cdot HCl$ is dissolved in 45 minutes.

Uniformity of dosage units ⟨905⟩: meet the requirements.

Assay—Weigh and finely powder not fewer than 20 Tablets. Transfer an accurately weighed portion of the powder, equivalent to about 250 mg of phenmetrazine hydrochloride, to a 250-mL volumetric flask, add about 125 mL of 0.5 N hydrochloric acid, shake by mechanical means for 1 hour, dilute with 0.5 N hydrochloric acid to volume, and mix. Transfer 50.0 mL of the solution to a 250-mL separator, add 5 mL of sodium hydroxide solution (1 in 2), and extract with four 50-mL portions of chloroform, collecting the chloroform extracts in a second 250-mL separator. Extract the combined chloroform extracts with six 15-mL portions of 0.5 N hydrochloric acid, collecting the aqueous extracts in a 100-mL volumetric flask, and dilute with 0.5 N hydrochloric acid to volume to obtain the *Assay preparation*. Concomitantly determine the absorbances of the *Assay preparation* and of a Standard solution of USP Phenmetrazine Hydrochloride RS in the same medium, having a known concentration of about 500 µg per mL, in 1-cm cells, at the wavelength of maximum absorbance at about 256 nm, with a suitable spectrophotometer, using 0.5 N hydrochloric acid as the blank. Calculate the quantity, in mg, of $C_{11}H_{15}NO \cdot HCl$ in the portion of Tablets taken by the formula:

$$0.5C(A_U/A_S)$$

in which *C* is the concentration, in µg per mL, of USP Phenmetrazine Hydrochloride RS in the Standard solution, and A_U and A_S are the absorbances from the *Assay preparation* and the Standard solution, respectively.

Phenobarbital

$C_{12}H_{12}N_2O_3$ 232.24
2,4,6(1*H*,3*H*,5*H*)-Pyrimidinetrione, 5-ethyl-5-phenyl-.
5-Ethyl-5-phenylbarbituric acid [50-06-6].

» Phenobarbital contains not less than 98.0 percent and not more than 101.0 percent of $C_{12}H_{12}N_2O_3$, calculated on the dried basis.

Packaging and storage—Preserve in well-closed containers.

USP Reference standards ⟨11⟩—*USP Phenobarbital RS.*

Identification—
  A: The IR absorption spectrum of a potassium bromide dispersion of it exhibits maxima only at the same wavelengths as that of a similar preparation of USP Phenobarbital RS. If a difference appears, dissolve portions of both the test specimen and the USP Reference Standard in a suitable solvent, evaporate the solutions to dryness, and repeat the test on the residues.
  B: The retention time of the major peak in the chromatogram of the *Assay preparation* corresponds to that of the *Standard preparation*, both relative to the internal standard, as obtained in the *Assay*.

Melting range ⟨741⟩: between 174° and 178°, but the range between beginning and end of melting does not exceed 2°.

Loss on drying ⟨731⟩—Dry it at 105° for 2 hours: it loses not more than 1.0% of its weight.

Residue on ignition ⟨281⟩: not more than 0.15%.

Organic volatile impurities, Method V ⟨467⟩: meets the requirements.
  Solvent—Use dimethyl sulfoxide.
  (Official until July 1, 2008)

Assay—
  pH 4.5 Buffer solution—Dissolve about 6.6 g of sodium acetate trihydrate and 3.0 mL of glacial acetic acid in 1000 mL of water, and adjust, if necessary, with glacial acetic acid to a pH of 4.5 ± 0.1.
  Mobile phase—Prepare a filtered and degassed mixture of *pH 4.5 Buffer solution* and methanol (3 : 2), making adjustments if necessary (see *System Suitability* under *Chromatography* ⟨621⟩).
  Internal standard solution—Dissolve a sufficient quantity of caffeine in a mixture of methanol and *pH 4.5 Buffer solution* (1 : 1) to obtain a solution having a concentration of about 125 µg per mL.
  Standard preparation—Dissolve about 20 mg of USP Phenobarbital RS, accurately weighed, in 15.0 mL of *Internal standard solution*. Sonicate if necessary.
  Assay preparation—Transfer about 20 mg of Phenobarbital, accurately weighed, to a conical flask, add 15.0 mL of *Internal standard solution*, mix, and sonicate for 15 minutes. Filter through a membrane filter (0.5 µm or finer porosity) before use.
  Chromatographic system (see *Chromatography* ⟨621⟩)—The liquid chromatograph is equipped with a 254-nm detector and a 4-mm × 25-cm column that contains packing L1. The flow rate is about 2 mL per minute. Chromatograph the *Standard preparation*, and record the peak responses as directed for *Procedure:* the resolution, *R*, between the analyte and the internal standard peaks is not less than 1.2, the tailing factor for the analyte and the internal standard peaks is not greater than 2.0, and the relative standard deviation for replicate injections is not more than 2.0%.
  Procedure—Separately inject equal volumes (about 10 µL) of the *Standard preparation* and the *Assay preparation* into the chromatograph, record the chromatograms, and measure the responses for the major peaks. The relative retention times are about 0.6 for caffeine and 1.0 for phenobarbital. Calculate the quantity, in mg, of $C_{12}H_{12}N_2O_3$ in the portion of Phenobarbital taken by the formula:

$$W(R_U/R_S)$$

in which *W* is the weight, in mg, of USP Phenobarbital RS taken for the *Standard preparation*, and R_U and R_S are the peak response ratios obtained from the *Assay preparation* and the *Standard preparation*, respectively.

Phenobarbital Oral Solution

» Phenobarbital Oral Solution contains not less than 90.0 percent and not more than 110.0 percent of the labeled amount of phenobarbital ($C_{12}H_{12}N_2O_3$).

Packaging and storage—Preserve in tight, light-resistant containers.

USP Reference standards ⟨11⟩—*USP Phenobarbital RS.*

Identification—
  A: Place 10 mL of Oral Solution in a separator containing 20 mL of water, add 5 mL of 1 N sodium hydroxide, and extract with two 10-mL portions of chloroform, discarding the chloroform extracts. Add 5 mL of 3 N hydrochloric acid, and extract with two 25-mL portions of chloroform, filtering the extracts through paper into a beaker. Remove the chloroform by evaporation on a steam bath, and dry the residue at 105° for 2 hours: the residue so obtained meets the requirements for *Identification* test A under *Phenobarbital*.
  B: The retention time of the major peak in the chromatogram of the *Assay preparation* corresponds to that in the chromatogram of

the *Standard preparation*, both relative to the internal standard, as obtained in the *Assay*.

Alcohol content, *Method II* ⟨611⟩: between 12.0% and 15.0% of C_2H_5OH.

Assay—
pH 4.5 Buffer solution, Mobile phase, and *Chromatographic system*—Prepare as directed in the *Assay* under *Phenobarbital*.

Diluent—Prepare a mixture of methanol and *pH 4.5 Buffer solution* (2 : 1).

Internal standard solution—Dissolve a sufficient quantity of caffeine in *Diluent* to obtain a solution having a concentration of about 1.7 mg per mL.

Standard preparation—Transfer about 33 mg of USP Phenobarbital RS, accurately weighed, to a 25-mL volumetric flask containing 2.0 mL of *Internal standard solution*. Dilute with *Diluent* to volume, and mix.

Assay preparation—Transfer a quantity of Oral Solution, equivalent to about 33 mg of phenobarbital, to a 25-mL volumetric flask containing 2.0 mL of *Internal standard solution*. Dilute with *Diluent* to volume, and mix.

Procedure—Proceed as directed for *Procedure* in the *Assay* under *Phenobarbital*. Calculate the quantity, in mg, of phenobarbital ($C_{12}H_{12}N_2O_3$) in the portion of the Oral Solution taken by the formula:

$$W(R_U / R_S)$$

in which the terms are as defined therein.

Phenobarbital Tablets

» Phenobarbital Tablets contain not less than 90.0 percent and not more than 110.0 percent of the labeled amount of $C_{12}H_{12}N_2O_3$.

Packaging and storage—Preserve in well-closed containers.

USP Reference standards ⟨11⟩—*USP Phenobarbital RS*.
Identification—
A: Triturate a quantity of finely powdered Tablets, equivalent to about 60 mg of phenobarbital, with 50 mL of chloroform, and filter. Evaporate the clear filtrate to dryness, and dry at 105° for 2 hours: the residue so obtained responds to *Identification* test A under *Phenobarbital*.
B: The retention time of the major peak in the chromatogram of the *Assay preparation* corresponds to that of the *Standard preparation*, both relative to the internal standard, as obtained in the *Assay*.

Dissolution ⟨711⟩—
Medium: water; 900 mL.
Apparatus 2: 50 rpm.
Time: 45 minutes.
Procedure—Determine the amount of $C_{12}H_{12}N_2O_3$ dissolved from UV absorbances at the wavelength of maximum absorbance at about 240 nm on filtered portions of the solution under test, suitably diluted with pH 9.6 alkaline borate buffer (see *Buffer Solutions* in the section *Reagents, Indicators, and Solutions*), in comparison with a Standard solution having a known concentration of USP Phenobarbital RS in the same *Medium*.
Tolerances—Not less than 75% (*Q*) of the labeled amount of $C_{12}H_{12}N_2O_3$ is dissolved in 45 minutes.

Uniformity of dosage units ⟨905⟩: meet the requirements.

Assay—
pH 4.5 Buffer solution, Mobile phase, Internal standard solution, Standard preparation, and *Chromatographic system*—Prepare as directed in the *Assay* under *Phenobarbital*.

Assay preparation—Weigh and finely powder not fewer than 20 Tablets. Weigh accurately a portion of the powder, equivalent to about 20 mg of phenobarbital, add 15.0 mL of *Internal standard solution*, mix, and sonicate for 15 minutes. Filter through a membrane filter having a 0.5-μm or finer porosity before use.

Procedure—Proceed as directed for *Procedure* in the *Assay* under *Phenobarbital*. Calculate the quantity, in mg, of $C_{12}H_{12}N_2O_3$ in the portion of Tablets taken by the formula:

$$(W)(R_U / R_S)$$

in which the terms are as defined therein.

Phenobarbital Sodium

$C_{12}H_{11}N_2NaO_3$ 254.22
2,4,6(1*H*,3*H*,5*H*)-Pyrimidinetrione, 5-ethyl-5-phenyl-, monosodium salt.
Sodium 5-ethyl-5-phenylbarbiturate   [57-30-7].

» Phenobarbital Sodium contains not less than 98.5 percent and not more than 101.0 percent of $C_{12}H_{11}N_2NaO_3$, calculated on the dried basis.

Packaging and storage—Preserve in tight containers.
Labeling—Where it is intended for use in preparing injectable dosage forms, the label states that it is sterile or must be subjected to further processing during the preparation of injectable dosage forms.

USP Reference standards ⟨11⟩—*USP Phenobarbital RS. USP Endotoxin RS*.
Completeness of solution—Mix 1.0 g with 10 mL of carbon dioxide-free water: after 1 minute, the solution is clear and free from undissolved solid.
Identification—
A: Dissolve about 50 mg of Phenobarbital Sodium in 15 mL of water in a separator, add 2 mL of hydrochloric acid, shake, and extract the liberated phenobarbital with four 25-mL portions of chloroform. Filter the combined extracts through a pledget of cotton or other suitable filter into a beaker, and wash the separator and the filter with several small portions of chloroform. Evaporate a 50-mL portion of the chloroform solution of phenobarbital on a steam bath with the aid of a current of air. Add 10 mL of ether, again evaporate, and dry the residue at 105° for 2 hours: the IR absorption spectrum of a potassium bromide dispersion of the residue so obtained exhibits maxima only at the same wavelengths as that of a similar preparation of USP Phenobarbital RS.
B: Ignite about 200 mg: the residue effervesces with acids, and responds to the tests for *Sodium* ⟨191⟩.
C: The relative retention time of the major peak in the chromatogram of the *Assay preparation* corresponds to that in the chromatogram of the *Standard preparation*, as obtained in the *Assay*.

pH ⟨791⟩: between 9.2 and 10.2, in the solution prepared in the test for *Completeness of solution*.
Loss on drying ⟨731⟩—Dry it at 150° for 4 hours: it loses not more than 7.0% of its weight.
Heavy metals ⟨231⟩—Dissolve 2.0 g in 52 mL of water. Add slowly, with vigorous stirring, 8 mL of 1 N hydrochloric acid, and filter, discarding the first 5 mL of the filtrate. Dilute 20 mL of the subsequent filtrate with water to 25 mL: the limit is 0.003%.
Organic volatile impurities, *Method I* ⟨467⟩: meets the requirements.

(Official until July 1, 2008)

Other requirements—Where the label states that Phenobarbital Sodium is sterile, it meets the requirements for *Sterility Tests* ⟨71⟩ and for *Bacterial endotoxins* under *Phenobarbital Sodium for Injection*. Where the label states that Phenobarbital Sodium must be subjected to further processing during the preparation of injectable dosage forms, it meets the requirements for *Bacterial endotoxins* under *Phenobarbital Sodium for Injection*.

Assay—
pH 4.5 Buffer solution, Mobile phase, Internal standard solution, Standard preparation, and *Chromatographic system*—Prepare as directed in the *Assay* under *Phenobarbital*.

Assay preparation—Transfer about 22 mg of Phenobarbital Sodium, accurately weighed, to a conical flask, add 15.0 mL of *Internal standard solution*, mix, and sonicate for 15 minutes. Pass through a membrane filter having a 0.5-μm or finer porosity before use.

Procedure—Proceed as directed for *Procedure* in the *Assay* under *Phenobarbital*. Calculate the quantity, in mg, of $C_{12}H_{11}N_2NaO_3$ in the portion of Phenobarbital Sodium taken by the formula:

$$(254.22 / 232.24)(W)(R_U / R_S)$$

in which 254.22 and 232.24 are the molecular weights of phenobarbital sodium and phenobarbital, respectively; and the other terms are as defined therein.

Phenobarbital Sodium Injection

» Phenobarbital Sodium Injection is a sterile solution of Phenobarbital Sodium in a suitable solvent. Phenobarbital may be substituted for the equivalent amount of Phenobarbital Sodium, for adjustment of the pH. The Injection contains the equivalent of not less than 90.0 percent and not more than 105.0 percent of the labeled amount of $C_{12}H_{11}N_2NaO_3$.

Packaging and storage—Preserve in single-dose or multiple-dose containers, preferably of Type I glass.
Labeling—The label indicates that the Injection is not to be used if it contains a precipitate.
USP Reference standards ⟨11⟩—*USP Phenobarbital RS. USP Endotoxin RS.*
Identification—
  A: Transfer to a separator a volume of Injection, equivalent to about 50 mg of phenobarbital sodium, add 15 mL of water, add 2 mL of hydrochloric acid, shake, and extract the liberated phenobarbital with four 25-mL portions of chloroform. Filter the combined extracts through a pledget of cotton or other suitable filter into a beaker, and wash the separator and the filter with several small portions of chloroform. Evaporate a 50-mL portion of the chloroform solution of phenobarbital on a steam bath with the aid of a current of air. Add 10 mL of ether, again evaporate, and dry the residue at 105° for 2 hours: the IR absorption spectrum of a potassium bromide dispersion of the residue so obtained exhibits maxima only at the same wavelengths as that of a similar preparation of USP Phenobarbital RS.
  B: The retention time of the major peak in the chromatogram of the *Assay preparation* corresponds to that of the *Standard preparation*, both relative to the internal standard, as obtained in the *Assay*.
Bacterial endotoxins ⟨85⟩—It contains not more than 0.3 USP Endotoxin Unit per mg of phenobarbital sodium.
pH ⟨791⟩: between 9.2 and 10.2.
Other requirements—It meets the requirements under *Injections* ⟨1⟩.
Assay—
  pH 4.5 Buffer solution, Mobile phase, Internal standard solution, and *Chromatographic system*—Prepare as directed in the *Assay* under *Phenobarbital*.
  Standard preparation—Transfer about 15 mg of USP Phenobarbital RS, accurately weighed, to a 50-mL volumetric flask, add 25 mL of *Mobile phase*, and sonicate if necessary to dissolve. Add 15.0 mL of *Internal standard solution*, dilute with *Mobile phase* to volume, and mix to obtain a solution having a known concentration of about 0.3 mg of USP Phenobarbital RS per mL.
  Assay preparation—Transfer an accurately measured volume of Injection, equivalent to about 65 mg of phenobarbital sodium, to a 100-mL volumetric flask, dilute with *Mobile phase* to volume, and mix. Transfer 25.0 mL of this solution to a 50-mL volumetric flask, add 15.0 mL of *Internal standard solution*, dilute with *Mobile phase* to volume, and mix.

Procedure—Proceed as directed for *Procedure* in the *Assay* under *Phenobarbital*. Calculate the quantity, in mg, of $C_{12}H_{11}N_2NaO_3$ in each mL of the Injection taken by the formula:

$$(254.22 / 232.24)(4W / V)(R_U / R_S)$$

in which 254.22 and 232.24 are the molecular weights of phenobarbital sodium and phenobarbital, respectively, V is the volume, in mL, of Injection taken, and the other terms are as defined therein.

Phenobarbital Sodium for Injection

» Phenobarbital Sodium for Injection is Phenobarbital Sodium suitable for parenteral use.

Packaging and storage—Preserve in *Containers for Sterile Solids* as described under *Injections* ⟨1⟩.
USP Reference standards ⟨11⟩—*USP Phenobarbital RS. USP Endotoxin RS.*
Constituted solution—At the time of use, it meets the requirements for *Constituted Solutions* under *Injections* ⟨1⟩.
Bacterial endotoxins ⟨85⟩—It contains not more than 0.8 USP Endotoxin Unit per mg of phenobarbital sodium.
Other requirements—It conforms to the Definition, responds to the *Identification* tests, and meets the requirements for *Completeness of solution, pH, Loss on drying, Heavy metals*, and *Assay* under *Phenobarbital Sodium*. It meets also the requirements for *Sterility Tests* ⟨71⟩, *Uniformity of Dosage Units* ⟨905⟩, and *Labeling* under *Injections* ⟨1⟩.

Phenol

C_6H_6O 94.11
Phenol.
Phenol [108-95-2].

» Phenol contains not less than 99.0 percent and not more than 100.5 percent of C_6H_6O, calculated on the anhydrous basis. It may contain a suitable stabilizer.
Caution—Avoid contact with skin, since serious burns may result.

Packaging and storage—Preserve in tight, light-resistant containers.
Labeling—Label it to indicate the name and amount of any substance added as a stabilizer.
Clarity of solution and reaction—A solution (1 in 15) is clear, and is neutral or acid to litmus paper.
Identification—
  A: To a solution add bromine TS: a white precipitate is formed, and it dissolves at first but becomes permanent as more of the reagent is added.
  B: To 10 mL of a solution (1 in 100) add 1 drop of ferric chloride TS: a violet color is produced.
Congealing temperature ⟨651⟩: not lower than 39°.
Water, *Method I* ⟨921⟩: not more than 0.5%.
Limit of nonvolatile residue—Heat about 5 g, accurately weighed, in a tared porcelain dish on a steam bath until it has evaporated, and dry the residue at 105° for 1 hour: not more than 0.05% of residue remains.
Organic volatile impurities, *Method I* ⟨467⟩: meets the requirements.

(Official until July 1, 2008)

Assay—Place about 2 g of Phenol, accurately weighed, in a 1000-mL volumetric flask, dilute with water to volume, and mix. Pipet 20 mL of the solution into an iodine flask, add 30.0 mL of 0.1 N bromine VS, then add 5 mL of hydrochloric acid, and immediately insert the stopper. Shake the flask repeatedly during 30 minutes, allow it to stand for 15 minutes, add quickly 5 mL of potassium iodide solution (1 in 5), taking precautions against the escape of bromine vapor, and at once insert the stopper in the flask. Shake thoroughly, remove the stopper, and rinse it and the neck of the flask with a small quantity of water, so that the washing flows into the flask. Add 1 mL of chloroform, shake the mixture, and titrate the liberated iodine with 0.1 N sodium thiosulfate VS, adding 3 mL of starch TS as the endpoint is approached. Perform a blank determination (see *Residual Titrations* under *Titrimetry* ⟨541⟩). Each mL of 0.1 N bromine is equivalent to 1.569 mg of C_6H_6O.

Camphorated Phenol Topical Gel

» Camphorated Phenol Topical Gel is a mixture of camphor and phenol in a suitable gel vehicle. It contains not less than 90.0 percent and not more than 110.0 percent of the labeled amount of camphor ($C_{10}H_{16}O$) and phenol (C_6H_6O).

Packaging and storage—Preserve in tight containers. Store at room temperature, avoid excessive heat, and close cover after each use.

USP Reference standards ⟨11⟩—*USP Camphor RS. USP Phenol RS.*

Identification—The retention times of the camphor and phenol peaks in the chromatograms of the *Assay preparation* correspond to those in the chromatograms of the *Standard preparation*, as obtained in the *Assay* for camphor and phenol.

Assay—

Internal standard solution—Transfer 250 mg, accurately weighed, of *n*-dodecane to a 25-mL volumetric flask, dilute with chloroform to volume, and mix.

Standard preparation—Transfer about 96 mg of USP Phenol RS, accurately weighed, to a 10-mL volumetric flask. Add about 224 mg of USP Camphor RS, accurately weighed, to the flask. Dilute with chloroform to volume, and mix. Combine 5.0 mL of this solution with 5.0 mL of *Internal standard solution* in a 50-mL volumetric flask, dilute with chloroform to volume, and mix.

Assay preparation—Transfer about 1 g of Topical Gel, accurately weighed, to a 50-mL flask. Add 5.0 mL of *Internal standard solution*, dilute with chloroform to volume, and mix.

Chromatographic system (see *Chromatography* ⟨621⟩)—The gas chromatograph is equipped with a flame-ionization detector (200°) and a 2-mm × 1.8-m glass column packed with 100- to 120-mesh S1A, coated with 15% G44. The carrier gas is helium. Adjust the column temperature to about 140° so that the relative retention times are 0.3 for phenol, 0.8 for camphor, and 1.0 for the internal standard. Chromatograph the *Standard preparation*, and record the peak responses as directed for *Procedure*: the resolution, *R*, between the camphor peak and the internal standard peak is not less than 2.0 and between the phenol peak and the camphor peak is not less than 5.0; and the relative standard deviation of the peak response ratio of the camphor peak and phenol peak to the internal standard peak for five consecutive injections of the *Standard preparation* is not more than 2.0%.

Procedure—Inject 1 to 2 μL of the *Assay preparation* and the *Standard preparation* into the gas chromatograph, record the chromatograms, and determine the peak response ratios. Calculate the percentage of camphor (w/w) and the percentage of phenol (w/w) in the sample according to the formula:

$$(50W_R / W)(r_U / r_S)$$

in which W_R is the weight, in mg, of the appropriate USP Reference Standard in the *Standard preparation*; *W* is the weight of Topical Gel, in mg, taken to prepare the *Assay preparation*; and r_U and r_S are the response ratios of the corresponding analyte peaks in the *Assay preparation* and the *Standard preparation*, respectively.

Camphorated Phenol Topical Solution

» Camphorated Phenol Topical Solution is a solution of Camphor and Phenol in Eucalyptus Oil and Light Mineral Oil. It contains not less than 90.0 percent and not more than 110.0 percent of the labeled amount of camphor ($C_{10}H_{16}O$) and phenol (C_6H_6O).

Packaging and storage—Preserve in tight containers. Store at room temperature, avoid excessive heat, and close cover after each use.

USP Reference standards ⟨11⟩—*USP Camphor RS. USP Phenol RS.*

Identification—The retention times of the camphor and phenol peaks in the chromatograms of the *Assay preparation* correspond to those in the chromatograms of the *Standard preparation*, as obtained in the *Assay*.

Specific gravity ⟨841⟩: between 0.840 and 0.865.

Assay—

Internal standard solution—Transfer 250 mg, accurately weighed, of *n*-dodecane to a 25-mL volumetric flask, dilute with chloroform to volume, and mix.

Standard preparation—Transfer about 96 mg of USP Phenol RS, accurately weighed, to a 10-mL volumetric flask. Add about 224 mg of USP Camphor RS, accurately weighed, to the flask. Dilute with chloroform to volume, and mix. Combine 5.0 mL of this solution with 5.0 mL of *Internal standard solution* in a 50-mL volumetric flask, dilute with chloroform to volume, and mix.

Assay preparation—Transfer about 1 g of Topical Solution, accurately weighed, to a 50-mL volumetric flask. Add 5.0 mL of *Internal standard solution*, dilute with chloroform to volume, and mix.

Chromatographic system (see *Chromatography* ⟨621⟩)—The gas chromatograph is equipped with a flame-ionization detector, maintained at a temperature of 200°, and a 2-mm × 1.8-m glass column packed with 100- to 120-mesh S1A, coated with 15% G44. The carrier gas is helium. Adjust the column temperature to about 140° so that the relative retention times are 0.3 for phenol, 0.8 for camphor, and 1.0 for the internal standard. Chromatograph the *Standard preparation*, and record the peak responses as directed for *Procedure*: the resolution, *R*, between camphor and the internal standard is not less than 2.0, and between phenol and camphor is not less than 5.0; and the relative standard deviation of the peak response ratio of camphor and phenol to the internal standard for five consecutive injections of the *Standard preparation* is not more than 2.0%.

Procedure—Separately inject 1 to 2 μL of the *Assay preparation* and the *Standard preparation* into the gas chromatograph, record the chromatograms, and determine the peak response ratios. Calculate the percentage of camphor (w/w) and the percentage of phenol (w/w) in the portion of Topical Solution taken by the formula:

$$(50W_R / W)(R_U / R_S)$$

in which W_R is the weight, in mg, of the appropriate USP Reference Standard in the *Standard preparation*; *W* is the weight of Topical Solution, in mg, taken to prepare the *Assay preparation*; and R_U and R_S are the response ratios of the corresponding analyte peaks in the *Assay preparation* and the *Standard preparation*, respectively.

Liquefied Phenol

» Liquefied Phenol is Phenol maintained in a liquid condition by the presence of about 10 percent of water. It contains not less than 89.0 percent by weight of C_6H_6O. It may contain a suitable stabilizer.

Caution—Avoid contact with skin because serious burns may result.

NOTE—When phenol is to be mixed with a fixed oil, mineral oil, or white petrolatum, use crystalline Phenol, not Liquefied Phenol.

Packaging and storage—Preserve in tight, light-resistant glass containers.
Labeling—Label it to indicate the name and amount of any substance added as a stabilizer.
Distilling range, *Method I* ⟨721⟩:   not higher than 182.5°, an air-cooled condenser being used.
Organic volatile impurities, *Method I*   ⟨467⟩:   meets the requirements.

(Official until July 1, 2008)

Other requirements—It responds to the *Identification* tests, and meets the requirements of the tests for *Clarity of solution and reaction* and *Nonvolatile residue,* under *Phenol.*
Assay—Proceed with Liquefied Phenol as directed in the *Assay* under *Phenol.*

Phenoxybenzamine Hydrochloride

$C_{18}H_{22}ClNO \cdot HCl$ 340.29
Benzenemethanamine, *N*-(2-chloroethyl)-*N*-(1-methyl-2-phenoxy-ethyl)-, hydrochloride.
N-(2-Chloroethyl)-*N*-(1-methyl-2-phenoxyethyl)benzylamine hydrochloride [*63-92-3*].

» Phenoxybenzamine Hydrochloride contains not less than 98.0 percent and not more than 101.0 percent of $C_{18}H_{22}ClNO \cdot HCl$, calculated on the dried basis.

Packaging and storage—Preserve in well-closed containers.
USP Reference standards ⟨11⟩—*USP Phenoxybenzamine Hydrochloride RS.*
Identification—
  A: *Infrared Absorption* ⟨197K⟩.
  B: *Ultraviolet Absorption* ⟨197U⟩—
    Solution: 1 mg per mL.
    Medium: methanol.
    Absorptivities at 275 nm, calculated on the dried basis, do not differ by more than 3.0%.
Melting range, *Class I* ⟨741⟩:   between 136° and 141°.
Loss on drying ⟨731⟩—Dry it in vacuum at 60° for 2 hours: it loses not more than 0.5% of its weight.
Ordinary impurities ⟨466⟩—
  Test solution: methanol.
  Standard solution: methanol.
  Eluant: a mixture of toluene and acetone (1 : 1).
  Visualization: 1.
Organic volatile impurities, *Method V*   ⟨467⟩:   meets the requirements.
  Solvent—Use dimethyl sulfoxide.

(Official until July 1, 2008)

Assay—Dissolve about 500 mg of Phenoxybenzamine Hydrochloride, accurately weighed, in 50 mL of glacial acetic acid, add 15 mL of mercuric acetate TS, and titrate with 0.1 N perchloric acid VS, determining the endpoint potentiometrically. Perform a blank determination, and make any necessary correction. Each mL of 0.1 N perchloric acid is equivalent to 34.03 mg of $C_{18}H_{22}ClNO \cdot HCl$.

Phenoxybenzamine Hydrochloride Capsules

» Phenoxybenzamine Hydrochloride Capsules contain not less than 90.0 percent and not more than 110.0 percent of the labeled amount of $C_{18}H_{22}ClNO \cdot HCl$.

Packaging and storage—Preserve in well-closed containers.
USP Reference standards ⟨11⟩—*USP Phenoxybenzamine Hydrochloride RS.*
Identification—The UV absorption spectrum of the solution employed for measurement of absorbance in the *Assay* exhibits maxima and minima at the same wavelengths as that of a similar solution of USP Phenoxybenzamine Hydrochloride RS, concomitantly measured. The ratio A_{268}/A_{272} of the maximum at 268 ± 2 nm and the minimum at 272 ± 2 nm is between 1.75 and 1.95.
Dissolution ⟨711⟩—
  Medium: 0.1 N hydrochloric acid; 500 mL.
  Apparatus 1: 100 rpm.
  Time: 45 minutes.
  Procedure—Determine the amount of $C_{18}H_{22}ClNO \cdot HCl$ dissolved from UV absorbances at the wavelength of maximum absorbance at about 267 nm on filtered portions of the solution under test, suitably diluted with *Dissolution Medium,* if necessary, in comparison with a Standard solution having a known concentration of USP Phenoxybenzamine Hydrochloride RS in the same *Medium.*
  Tolerances—Not less than 75% (*Q*) of the labeled amount of $C_{18}H_{22}ClNO \cdot HCl$ is dissolved in 45 minutes.

Change to read:
Uniformity of dosage units ⟨905⟩:   meet the requirements.
  ▲PROCEDURE FOR CONTENT UNIFORMITY—
    Buffer solution, Mobile phase, and *Chromatographic system*—Proceed as directed in the *Assay.*
    Standard solution—Proceed as directed for *Standard preparation* in the *Assay.*
    Test solution—Carefully open 10 Capsules and transfer each immediately into separate volumetric flasks, including the capsule shells. Add acetonitrile, approximately about 60% of the volume of the flask, and sonicate for 15 minutes with occasional stirring. Cool the flask and dilute with acetonitrile to volume to prepare a solution having a known concentration of 0.2 mg per mL. [NOTE—The capsule shell does not dissolve.] Cool, dilute with acetonitrile to volume, mix, and pass through a 0.45-μm nylon membrane filter, discarding the first few mL of the filtrate. Use the subsequent filtrate as the *Test solution.*
    Procedure—Separately inject equal volumes (about 10 μL) of the *Standard solution* and the *Test solution* into the chromatograph, record the chromatograms, and measure the responses for the major peaks. Calculate the quantity, in mg, of phenoxybenzamine hydrochloride in the Capsules taken by the formula:

$$T \, (C_S / C_U)(r_U / r_S)$$

in which *T* is the labeled quantity, in mg, of phenoxybenzamine hydrochloride in the Capsules taken; C_S is the concentration, in mg per mL, of USP Phenoxybenzamine Hydrochloride RS in the *Standard solution;* C_U is the concentration, in mg per mL, of phenoxybenzamine hydrochloride in the *Test solution,* based on the labeled quantity per Capsule and the extent of dilution; and r_U and r_S are the peak responses obtained from the *Test solution* and the *Standard solution,* respectively.▲USP31

Add the following:
▲**Related compounds**—
  Buffer solution, Mobile phase, System suitability solution, and *Chromatographic system*—Proceed as directed in the *Assay.*
  Standard solution—Proceed as directed for *Standard preparation* in the *Assay.*

Test solution—Use the *Assay preparation*.
Procedure—Proceed as directed in the *Assay*. Calculate the percentage of each individual impurity by the formula:

$$(100 / F)(r_i / r_s)$$

in which F is the relative response factor, which is 1.1 for the known degradant phenoxybenzamine tertiary amine and 1 for all other individual impurities; r_i is the peak response for the individual impurity obtained from the *Test solution*; and r_s is the sum of all the peak responses obtained from the *Test solution*. Not more than 0.5% of phenoxybenzamine tertiary amine is found; not more than 0.1% of any other specified or unspecified individual impurity (degradant) is found; and not more than 0.5% total of all the specified and unspecified impurities is found.▲USP31

Change to read:
Assay—
▲*Buffer solution*—Dissolve 1.1 g of anhydrous monobasic sodium phosphate in 500 mL of water. Adjust with concentrated phosphoric acid to a pH of 3.0.

Mobile phase—Prepare a filtered and degassed mixture of *Buffer solution* and acetonitrile (45 : 55).

Standard preparation—Prepare a solution of USP Phenoxybenzamine Hydrochloride RS in acetonitrile having a known concentration of 0.2 mg per mL. Sonicate for 5 minutes to mix well.

System suitability solution—Prepare a solution of 0.5 mL of 0.1 N sodium hydroxide and 10 mL of the *Standard preparation* taken in a vial. [NOTE—Basic solutions of phenoxybenzamine hydrochloride will produce the known degradant tertiary amine phenoxybenzamine (the second major peak that elutes before the phenoxybenzamine peak and has a relative retention time of about approximately 0.3 minutes) and an unknown related substance. Severe degradation of the drug substance will be observed if the solution is allowed to stand for more than 1 hour.]

Assay preparation—Remove, as completely as possible, the contents of not fewer than 20 Capsules, and weigh. Transfer an accurately weighed portion of the mixed powder, equivalent to about 10 mg of phenoxybenzamine hydrochloride, to a 50-mL volumetric flask. Add about 40 mL of acetonitrile, and sonicate for 15 minutes with occasional swirling. Cool, and dilute with acetonitrile to volume to obtain a solution having a phenoxybenzamine hydrochloride concentration of 0.2 mg per mL, based on the label claim. Allow the sample to stand undisturbed for 30 minutes such that the undissolved material settles to the bottom. Transfer the top clear solution into HPLC vials, and use as the *Assay preparation*.

Chromatographic system—The liquid chromatograph is equipped with a 268-nm detector and a 4.6-mm × 150-cm column that contains packing L7. The flow rate is about 1.0 mL per minute. The column is maintained at ambient temperatures. Chromatograph the *System suitability solution*, and record the peak responses as directed for *Procedure*: the resolution R, between the phenoxybenzamine hydrochloride and the unknown peak that elutes after the phenoxybenzamine peak (approximately at about 9.4 minutes) is not less than 4. Chromatograph the *Standard preparation*, and record the peak responses as directed for *Procedure*: the relative standard deviation for an average of five injections determined from the phenoxybenzamine hydrochloride peak is not more than 2%.

Procedure—Separately inject equal volumes (about 10 μL) of the *Standard preparation* and the *Assay preparation* into the chromatograph, record the chromatograms, and measure the responses for the major peaks. Calculate the quantity, in percentage of label claim, of phenoxybenzamine hydrochloride ($C_{18}H_{22}ClNO \cdot HCl$) in the portion of Capsules taken by the formula:

$$(100(C_S / C_U)(r_U / r_S)$$

in which C_S is the concentration, in mg per mL, of USP Phenoxybenzamine Hydrochloride RS in the *Standard preparation*; C_U is the concentration, in mg per mL, of phenoxybenzamine hydrochloride in the *Assay preparation*; and r_U and r_S are the peak responses obtained from the *Assay preparation* and the *Standard preparation*, respectively.▲USP31

Phensuximide

$C_{11}H_{11}NO_2$ 189.21
2,5-Pyrrolidinedione, 1-methyl-3-phenyl-, (±)-.
(±)-N-Methyl-2-phenylsuccinimide   [86-34-0].

» Phensuximide contains not less than 97.0 percent and not more than 103.0 percent of $C_{11}H_{11}NO_2$, calculated on the anhydrous basis.

Packaging and storage—Preserve in tight containers.
USP Reference standards ⟨11⟩—*USP Phensuximide RS*.
Identification—
   A: *Infrared Absorption* ⟨197K⟩.
   B: *Ultraviolet Absorption* ⟨197U⟩—
   Solution: 400 μg per mL.
   Medium: alcohol.
Melting range, *Class I* ⟨741⟩: between 68° and 74°.
Water, *Method I* ⟨921⟩: not more than 1.0%.
Residue on ignition ⟨281⟩: not more than 0.5%.
Limit of cyanide—Dissolve 1.0 g in 10 mL of warm alcohol, and add 3 drops of ferrous sulfate TS, 1 mL of 1 N sodium hydroxide, and a few drops of ferric chloride TS. Warm gently, and finally acidify with 2 N sulfuric acid: no blue precipitate or blue color is formed within 15 minutes.
Ordinary impurities ⟨466⟩—
   Test solution: 200 mg of phensuximide per mL in methylene chloride.
   Standard solutions: 1.0, 2.0, and 4.0 mg per mL in methylene chloride.
   Application volume: 5 μL.
   Eluant: a mixture of ethyl acetate and hexanes (1 : 1).
   Visualization: 6.
Organic volatile impurities, *Method V* ⟨467⟩: meets the requirements.
   Solvent—Use dimethyl sulfoxide.

(Official until July 1, 2008)
Assay—Transfer about 200 mg of Phensuximide, accurately weighed, to a 50-mL volumetric flask. Dissolve in 40 mL of alcohol, dilute with alcohol to volume, and mix. Transfer 5.0 mL of this solution to a 50-mL volumetric flask, dilute with alcohol to volume, and mix. Concomitantly determine the absorbances of this solution and of a Standard solution of USP Phensuximide RS, in the same medium having a known concentration of about 400 μg per mL, in 1-cm cells at the wavelength of maximum absorbance at about 258 nm, with a suitable spectrophotometer, using alcohol as the blank. Calculate the quantity, in mg, of $C_{11}H_{11}NO_2$ in the Phensuximide taken by the formula:

$$0.5C(A_U / A_S)$$

in which C is the concentration, in μg per mL, of USP Phensuximide RS in the Standard solution, and A_U and A_S are the absorbances of the solution from Phensuximide and the Standard solution, respectively.

Phensuximide Capsules

» Phensuximide Capsules contain not less than 93.0 percent and not more than 107.0 percent of the labeled amount of $C_{11}H_{11}NO_2$.

Packaging and storage—Preserve in tight containers.
USP Reference standards ⟨11⟩—*USP Phensuximide RS.*
Identification—
  A: The contents of Capsules respond to *Identification* test A under *Phensuximide.*
  B: The retention time exhibited by phensuximide in the chromatogram of the *Assay preparation* corresponds to that of phensuximide in the chromatogram of the *Standard preparation,* as obtained in the *Assay.*
Dissolution ⟨711⟩—
  Medium: water; 900 mL.
  Apparatus 1: 100 rpm.
  Time: 120 minutes.
  Procedure—Determine the amount of $C_{11}H_{11}NO_2$ dissolved, employing the procedure set forth in the *Assay,* making any necessary modifications.
  Tolerances—Not less than 75% (*Q*) of the labeled amount of $C_{11}H_{11}NO_2$ is dissolved in 120 minutes.
Uniformity of dosage units ⟨905⟩: meet the requirements.
Assay—
  Mobile phase—Prepare a filtered and degassed mixture of water and acetonitrile (55 : 45). Make adjustments if necessary (see *System Suitability* under *Chromatography* ⟨621⟩).
  Standard preparation—Dissolve an accurately weighed quantity of USP Phensuximide RS in *Mobile phase* to obtain a solution having a known concentration of about 1 mg per mL.
  Assay preparation—Place 10 Capsules in a 500-mL volumetric flask, and add 280 mL of water. Sonicate in a water bath at 40° to 50°, with occasional shaking, until the Capsules have broken, and cool to room temperature. Dilute with acetonitrile to volume, mix, and filter. Transfer an accurately measured volume of this specimen solution, equivalent to about 50 mg of Phensuximide, to a 50-mL volumetric flask, dilute with *Mobile phase* to volume, and mix.
  Chromatographic system (see *Chromatography* ⟨621⟩)—The liquid chromatograph is equipped with a 254-nm detector and a 3.9-mm × 30-cm column that contains packing L1. The flow rate is about 1 mL per minute. Chromatograph the *Standard preparation,* and record the peak responses as directed for *Procedure:* the column efficiency determined from the analyte peak is not less than 2100 theoretical plates, and the relative standard deviation for replicate injections is not more than 1.5%.
  Procedure—Separately inject equal volumes (about 20 µL) of the *Standard preparation* and the *Assay preparation* into the chromatograph, record the chromatograms, and measure the responses for the major peaks. Calculate the quantity, in mg, of $C_{11}H_{11}NO_2$ per Capsule taken by the formula:

$$2500(C/V)(r_U/r_S)$$

in which *C* is the concentration, in mg per mL, of USP Phensuximide RS in the *Standard preparation,* *V* is the volume, in mL, of specimen solution taken for the *Assay preparation,* and r_U and r_S are the phensuximide peak responses obtained from the *Assay preparation* and the *Standard preparation,* respectively.

Phentermine Hydrochloride

$C_{10}H_{15}N \cdot HCl$ 185.69
Benzeneethanamine, α,α-dimethyl-, hydrochloride.
α,α-Dimethylphenethylamine hydrochloride   [*1197-21-3*].

» Phentermine Hydrochloride contains not less than 98.0 percent and not more than 101.0 percent of $C_{10}H_{15}N \cdot HCl$, calculated on the dried basis.

Packaging and storage—Preserve in tight containers.
USP Reference standards ⟨11⟩—*USP Phentermine Hydrochloride RS.*

Identification—
  A: *Infrared Absorption* ⟨197K⟩.
  B: *Ultraviolet Absorption* ⟨197U⟩—
    Solution: 600 µg per mL.
    Medium: 0.1 N hydrochloric acid.
    Absorptivities at 256 nm, calculated on the dried basis, do not differ by more than 2.0%.
  C: It responds to the tests for *Chloride* ⟨191⟩.
Melting range ⟨741⟩: between 202° and 205°.
pH ⟨791⟩: between 5.0 and 6.0, in a solution (1 in 50).
Loss on drying ⟨731⟩—Dry it at 105° for 3 hours: it loses not more than 2.0% of its weight.
Residue on ignition ⟨281⟩: not more than 0.1%.
Chromatographic purity—
  Standard preparations—Dissolve an accurately weighed quantity of USP Phentermine Hydrochloride RS in chloroform to obtain *Standard preparation A* having a known concentration of 2 mg per mL. Dilute this solution quantitatively with chloroform to obtain *Standard preparations,* designated below by letter, having the following compositions:

Standard preparation	Dilution	Concentration (mg RS per mL)	Percentage (%, for comparison with test specimen)
A	(undiluted)	2.0	1.0
B	(1 in 2)	1.0	0.5
C	(1 in 5)	0.4	0.2
D	(1 in 10)	0.2	0.1

  Test preparation—Dissolve an accurately weighed quantity of Phentermine Hydrochloride in chloroform to obtain a solution containing 200 mg per mL.
  Procedure—Apply separately 10 µL of the *Test preparation* and 10 µL of each *Standard preparation* to a suitable thin-layer chromatographic plate (see *Chromatography* ⟨621⟩) coated with a 0.25-mm layer of chromatographic silica gel mixture. Position the plate in a chromatographic chamber, and develop the chromatograms in a solvent system consisting of a mixture of chloroform, cyclohexane, and diethylamine (50 : 40 : 10) until the solvent front has moved about three-fourths of the length of the plate. Remove the plate from the developing chamber, mark the solvent front, and allow the solvent to evaporate in air. Examine the plate under short-wavelength UV light. Compare the intensities of any secondary spots observed in the chromatogram of the *Test preparation* with those of the principal spots in the chromatograms of the *Standard preparations:* the sum of the intensities of secondary spots obtained from the *Test preparation* corresponds to not more than 1.0% of related compounds, with no single impurity corresponding to more than 0.5%.
Organic volatile impurities, *Method I* ⟨467⟩: meets the requirements.

(Official until July 1, 2008)
Assay—Dissolve about 400 mg of Phentermine Hydrochloride, accurately weighed, in 40 mL of glacial acetic acid, and add 10 mL of mercuric acetate TS, warming slightly to effect solution. Cool to room temperature, and titrate with 0.1 N perchloric acid VS, determining the endpoint potentiometrically. Perform a blank determination, and make any necessary correction. Each mL of 0.1 N perchloric acid is equivalent to 18.57 mg of $C_{10}H_{15}N \cdot HCl$.

Phentermine Hydrochloride Capsules

» Phentermine Hydrochloride Capsules contain not less than 90.0 percent and not more than 110.0 percent of the labeled amount of $C_{10}H_{15}N \cdot HCl$.

Packaging and storage—Preserve in tight containers.
USP Reference standards ⟨11⟩—*USP Phentermine Hydrochloride RS.*

Identification—
A: Stir a portion of the Capsule contents in acetone to prepare a solution containing about 1 mg of phentermine hydrochloride per mL, and filter using an acetone resistant filter. Transfer 1 mL of the clear filtrate to a mortar containing about 200 mg of potassium bromide, triturate with a pestle, and air-dry to allow the acetone to evaporate. Place in an oven at 125° for 30 minutes to dry the mixture: the IR absorption spectrum of a potassium bromide dispersion prepared from the residue exhibits maxima only at the same wavelengths as that of a similar preparation of USP Phentermine Hydrochloride RS.

B: The retention time of the major peak in the chromatogram of the *Assay preparation* corresponds to that in the chromatogram of the *Standard preparation*, as obtained in the *Assay*.

Dissolution, *Procedure for a Pooled Sample* ⟨711⟩—
Medium: water; 900 mL. Use 500 mL for Capsules containing 15 mg of phentermine hydrochloride or less.
Apparatus 2: 50 rpm.
Time: 45 minutes.
Procedure—Determine the amount of $C_{10}H_{15}N \cdot HCl$ dissolved, employing the procedure set forth in the *Assay*, making any necessary modifications including concentration of the analyte in the volume of test solution taken.
Tolerances—Not less than 75% (*Q*) of the labeled amount of $C_{10}H_{15}N \cdot HCl$ is dissolved in 45 minutes.

Uniformity of dosage units ⟨905⟩: meet the requirements.

Assay—
Mobile phase—Dissolve 1.1 g of sodium 1-heptanesulfonate in 575 mL of water. Add 25 mL of dilute glacial acetic acid (14 in 100) and 400 mL of methanol. Adjust dropwise, if necessary, with glacial acetic acid to a pH of 3.3 ± 0.1. Filter through a 0.5-µm membrane filter. The volume of methanol may be adjusted to provide a suitable retention time for phentermine hydrochloride (about 8 minutes).

Standard preparation—Using an accurately weighed quantity of USP Phentermine Hydrochloride RS, prepare a solution in 0.04 M phosphoric acid having a known concentration of about 0.4 mg per mL.

Assay preparation—Remove, as completely as possible, the contents of not fewer than 20 Capsules, and weigh. Transfer an accurately weighed portion of the mixed powder, equivalent to about 20 mg of phentermine hydrochloride, to a 50-mL volumetric flask. Add 40 mL of 0.04 M phosphoric acid, and sonicate for 15 minutes. Dilute with 0.04 M phosphoric acid to volume, and mix. Filter through a 0.5-µm membrane filter, discarding the first few mL of the filtrate.

Chromatographic system (see *Chromatography* ⟨621⟩)—The liquid chromatograph is equipped with a 254-nm detector and a 3.9-mm × 30-cm column that contains packing L1. The flow rate is about 2 mL per minute. Chromatograph three replicate injections of the *Standard preparation*, and record the peak response as directed for *Procedure:* the relative standard deviation is not more than 2.0%.

Procedure—Separately inject equal volumes (about 50 µL) of the *Standard preparation* and the *Assay preparation* into the chromatograph by means of a suitable sampling valve, record the chromatograms, and measure the responses for the major peaks. Calculate the quantity, in mg, of $C_{10}H_{15}N \cdot HCl$ in the portion of Capsules taken by the formula:

$$50C(r_U / r_S)$$

in which *C* is the concentration, in mg per mL, of USP Phentermine Hydrochloride RS in the *Standard preparation*, and r_U and r_S are the peak responses obtained from the *Assay preparation* and the *Standard preparation*, respectively.

Phentermine Hydrochloride Tablets

» Phentermine Hydrochloride Tablets contain not less than 90.0 percent and not more than 110.0 percent of the labeled amount of phentermine hydrochloride ($C_{10}H_{15}N \cdot HCl$).

Packaging and storage—Preserve in tight containers.

USP Reference standards ⟨11⟩—*USP Phentermine Hydrochloride RS*.

Identification—
A: A portion of finely powdered Tablets meets the requirements for *Identification* test A under *Phentermine Hydrochloride Capsules*.

B: The retention time of the major peak in the chromatogram of the *Assay preparation* corresponds to that in the chromatogram of the *Standard preparation*, as obtained in the *Assay*.

Dissolution, *Procedure for a Pooled Sample* ⟨711⟩—
Medium: water; 900 mL. Use 500 mL for Tablets containing 15 mg of phentermine hydrochloride or less.
Apparatus 2: 50 rpm.
Time: 45 minutes.
Determine the amount of $C_{10}H_{15}N \cdot HCl$ dissolved by employing the following method.

Ion-pair solution—Dissolve 1.1 g of sodium 1-heptanesulfonate in 1 L of water. Add 3.5 mL of glacial acetic acid, and mix.

Mobile phase—Prepare a filtered and degassed mixture of methanol and *Ion-pair solution* (21 : 19). Adjust with phosphoric acid to a pH of 2.5. Make adjustments if necessary (see *System Suitability* under *Chromatography* ⟨621⟩).

Standard solution—Dissolve an accurately weighed quantity of USP Phentermine Hydrochloride RS in water, and dilute quantitatively, and stepwise if necessary, with water to obtain a solution having a known concentration approximately equivalent to the *Test solution*.

Test solution—Use a filtered portion of the pooled sample under test.

Chromatographic system (see *Chromatography* ⟨621⟩)—The liquid chromatograph is equipped with a 208-nm detector and a 4.6-mm × 25-cm column that contains packing L1. The flow rate is about 1 mL per minute. Chromatograph the *Standard solution*, and record the peak responses as directed for *Procedure:* the tailing factor is not more than 2.0; and the relative standard deviation for replicate injections is not more than 2.0%.

Procedure—Separately inject equal volumes (about 25 µL) of the *Standard solution* and the *Test solution* into the chromatograph, record the chromatograms, and measure the peak responses. Determine the amount, in mg, of phentermine hydrochloride ($C_{10}H_{15}N \cdot HCl$) dissolved by the formula:

$$VC(r_U / r_S)$$

in which *V* is the volume of dissolution media used per vessel; *C* is the concentration, in mg per mL, of USP Phentermine Hydrochloride RS in the *Standard solution;* and r_U and r_S are the peak responses obtained from the *Test solution* and the *Standard solution*, respectively.

Tolerances—Not less than 75% (*Q*) of the labeled amount of $C_{10}H_{15}N \cdot HCl$ is dissolved in 45 minutes.

Uniformity of dosage units ⟨905⟩: meet the requirements.

Procedure for content uniformity—Proceed as directed in the *Assay*, except to prepare the *Test preparations* as follows. Transfer 1 Tablet to each of 10 suitable containers, add 1 mL of water and 10 mL of *Internal standard solution* to each, mix, sonicate for about 10 minutes after each Tablet has disintegrated, and filter.

Assay—
Mobile phase—Prepare a suitably degassed solution containing 0.03% diethylamine in methanol. Make adjustments if necessary (see *System Suitability* under *Chromatography* ⟨621⟩).

Internal standard solution—Prepare a solution of caffeine in *Mobile phase* having a final concentration of about 0.02 mg per mL.

Standard preparation—Transfer an accurately weighed amount of USP Phentermine Hydrochloride RS, equivalent to about 7.5 mg of phentermine hydrochloride, to a 10-mL volumetric flask. Add *Internal standard solution* to volume, and mix.

Assay preparation—Weigh and finely powder not fewer than 20 Tablets. Transfer an accurately weighed portion of the powder, equivalent to about 7.5 mg, to a suitable flask. Pipet 10.0 mL of *Internal standard solution* into the flask. Insert the stopper, mix, and sonicate for about 10 minutes. Pass through a filter having a 0.5-µm porosity.

Chromatographic system (see *Chromatography* ⟨621⟩)—The liquid chromatograph is equipped with a 254-nm detector and a 4.6-mm × 25-cm column that contains packing L1. The flow rate is about 1.5 mL per minute. Chromatograph the *Standard preparation*, and record the peak responses as directed for *Procedure*: the relative retention times are about 0.5 for caffeine and 1.0 for phentermine; the resolution, *R*, between caffeine and phentermine is not less than 4; the column efficiency determined from the analyte peak is not less than 2000 theoretical plates; and the relative standard deviation for replicate injections is not more than 2.0%.

Procedure—Separately inject equal volumes (about 10 µL) of the *Standard preparation* and the *Assay preparation* into the chromatograph, record the chromatograms, and measure the responses for the major peaks. Calculate the quantity, in mg, of phentermine hydrochloride ($C_{10}H_{15}N \cdot HCl$) in the portion of Tablets taken by the formula:

$$10C(R_U / R_S)$$

in which *C* is the concentration, in mg per mL, of USP Phentermine Hydrochloride RS in the *Standard preparation*; and R_U and R_S are the peak response ratios of phentermine to the internal standard obtained from the *Assay preparation* and the *Standard preparation*, respectively.

Phentolamine Mesylate

$C_{17}H_{19}N_3O \cdot CH_4O_3S$ 377.46

Phenol, 3-[[(4,5-dihydro-1*H*-imidazol-2-yl)methyl](4-methylphenyl)amino]-, monomethanesulfonate (salt).

m-[*N*-(2-Imidazolin-2-ylmethyl)-*p*-toluidino]phenol monomethanesulfonate (salt)   [65-28-1].

» Phentolamine Mesylate contains not less than 98.0 percent and not more than 102.0 percent of $C_{17}H_{19}N_3O \cdot CH_4O_3S$, calculated on the dried basis.

Packaging and storage—Preserve in tight, light-resistant containers. Store at 25°, excursions permitted between 15° and 30°.

USP Reference standards ⟨11⟩—*USP Phentolamine Mesylate RS.*

Identification—

A: *Infrared Absorption* ⟨197M⟩.

B: *Ultraviolet Absorption* ⟨197U⟩—

Solution: 20 µg per mL.

Medium: water.

C: The R_F value of the principal spot in the chromatogram of the *Identification preparation* corresponds to that of *Standard preparation A* as obtained in the test for *Chromatographic purity*.

Loss on drying ⟨731⟩—Dry it in vacuum at 60° for 4 hours: it loses not more than 0.5% of its weight.

Residue on ignition ⟨281⟩: not more than 0.1%.

Sulfate ⟨221⟩—A 0.10-g portion shows no more sulfate than corresponds to 0.20 mL of 0.020 N sulfuric acid (0.2%).

Chromatographic purity—

Standard preparations—Dissolve USP Phentolamine Mesylate RS in methanol, and mix to obtain *Standard preparation A* having a known concentration of 50 µg per mL. Quantitatively dilute with methanol to obtain *Standard preparations*, designated below by letter, having the following compositions:

Standard preparation	Dilution	Concentration (µg RS per mL)	Percentage (%, for comparison with test specimen)
A	(undiluted)	50	0.5
B	(3 in 5)	30	0.3
C	(1 in 5)	10	0.1

Test preparation—Dissolve an accurately weighed quantity of Phentolamine Mesylate in methanol to obtain a solution containing 10 mg per mL.

Identification preparation—Dilute a portion of the *Test preparation* quantitatively with methanol to obtain a solution containing 50 µg per mL.

Detection reagent—Prepare (1) a solution of 1 g of potassium ferricyanide in 20 mL of water, and (2) a solution of 1.9 g of ferric chloride in 20 mL of water. Just prior to use, mix equal volumes of the solutions.

Procedure— Apply separately 5 µL of the *Test preparation*, 5 µL of the *Identification preparation*, and 5 µL of each *Standard preparation* to a suitable thin-layer chromatographic plate (see *Chromatography* ⟨621⟩) coated with a 0.25-mm layer of chromatographic silica gel, and allow to dry. Position the plate in a chromatographic chamber, and develop the chromatograms in a solvent system consisting of a mixture of chloroform, diethylamine, and methanol (15 : 3 : 2) until the solvent front has moved about three-fourths of the length of the plate. Remove the plate from the developing chamber, mark the solvent front, and dry the plate at 100° for 1 hour. Spray the plate with *Detection reagent*. Within 15 minutes after spraying, compare the intensities of any secondary spots observed in the chromatogram of the *Test preparation* with those of the principal spots in the chromatograms of the *Standard preparations*: no secondary spot from the chromatogram of the *Test preparation* is larger or more intense than the principal spot obtained from *Standard preparation A* (0.5%), and the sum of the intensities of all secondary spots obtained from the *Test preparation* corresponds to not more than 1.0%.

Assay—

0.1 N Tetrabutylammonium hydroxide in isopropyl alcohol—Dilute with dehydrated isopropyl alcohol a commercially available 25% solution of tetrabutylammonium hydroxide in methanol, and standardize as directed under *Tetrabutylammonium Hydroxide, Tenth-Normal (0.1 N)* (see *Volumetric Solutions* in the section *Reagents, Indicators, and Solutions*), using dehydrated isopropyl alcohol instead of dimethylformamide.

Procedure—Dissolve with the aid of sonication, if necessary, about 300 mg of Phentolamine Mesylate, accurately weighed, in 100 mL of dehydrated isopropyl alcohol. Titrate in an atmosphere of nitrogen with *0.1 N Tetrabutylammonium hydroxide in isopropyl alcohol*, determining the endpoint potentiometrically, using a glass electrode and a calomel electrode containing a saturated solution of tetramethylammonium chloride in dehydrated isopropyl alcohol (see *Titrimetry* ⟨541⟩). Perform a blank determination, and make any necessary correction. Each mL of 0.1 N tetrabutylammonium hydroxide is equivalent to 37.75 mg of $C_{17}H_{19}N_3O \cdot CH_4O_3S$.

Phentolamine Mesylate for Injection

» Phentolamine Mesylate for Injection is sterile Phentolamine Mesylate or a sterile mixture of Phentolamine Mesylate with a suitable buffer or suitable diluents. It contains not less than 90.0 percent and not more than 110.0 percent of the labeled amount of $C_{17}H_{19}N_3O \cdot CH_4O_3S$.

Packaging and storage—Preserve in *Containers for Sterile Solids* as described under *Injections* ⟨1⟩.

USP Reference standards ⟨11⟩—USP Phentolamine Mesylate RS. USP Endotoxin RS.

Constituted solution—At the time of use, it meets the requirements for *Constituted Solutions* under *Injections* ⟨1⟩.

Identification—Mix a portion of it, equivalent to about 40 mg of phentolamine mesylate, with about 15 mL of chloroform. Filter into a beaker, and evaporate to dryness, taking precautions against introducing moisture: the residue so obtained responds to *Identification* test A under *Phentolamine Mesylate*.

Bacterial endotoxins ⟨85⟩—It contains not more than 5.8 USP Endotoxin Units per mg of phentolamine mesylate.

Uniformity of dosage units ⟨905⟩: meets the requirements.

Procedure for content uniformity—Dissolve the contents of 1 container in water to provide a solution containing about 20 µg of phentolamine mesylate per mL. Concomitantly determine the absorbances of this solution and of a solution of USP Phentolamine Mesylate RS, in the same medium, at a concentration of about 20 µg per mL, in 1-cm cells at the wavelength of maximum absorbance at about 278 nm, with a suitable spectrophotometer, using water as the blank. Calculate the quantity, in mg, of $C_{17}H_{19}N_3O \cdot CH_4O_3S$ in the Phentolamine Mesylate for Injection taken by the formula:

$$(T/D)C(A_U/A_S)$$

in which T is the labeled quantity, in mg, of phentolamine mesylate in the Phentolamine Mesylate for Injection, D is the concentration, in µg per mL, of phentolamine mesylate in the solution from the Phentolamine Mesylate for Injection, based on the labeled quantity per container and the extent of dilution, C is the concentration, in µg per mL, of USP Phentolamine Mesylate RS in the Standard solution, and A_U and A_S are the absorbances of the solution from the Phentolamine Mesylate for Injection and the Standard solution, respectively.

pH ⟨791⟩: between 4.5 and 6.5, in a freshly prepared solution having a concentration of about 1 in 100.

Other requirements—It meets the requirements for *Sterility Tests* ⟨71⟩ and *Labeling* under *Injections* ⟨1⟩.

Assay—

Standard preparation—Transfer about 25 mg of USP Phentolamine Mesylate RS, accurately weighed, to a 50-mL volumetric flask, add water to volume, and mix.

Assay preparation—Dissolve the contents of 10 containers of Phentolamine Mesylate for Injection in a volume of water corresponding to the volume of solvent specified in the labeling. Transfer an aliquot, equivalent to about 25 mg of phentolamine mesylate, to a 50-mL volumetric flask, add water to volume, and mix.

Procedure—Pipet 5-mL portions, respectively, of the *Standard preparation*, *Assay preparation*, and water to provide a blank, into separate 125-mL separators. Into each separator pipet 5-mL portions of 0.1 N hydrochloric acid and saturated picric acid solution. Extract with three 25-mL portions of chloroform, filtering each portion through chloroform-washed cotton into a 100-mL volumetric flask. Dilute with chloroform to volume, and mix. Concomitantly determine the absorbances of the solutions from the *Assay preparation* and the *Standard preparation* in 1-cm cells at the wavelength of maximum absorbance at about 410 nm, with a suitable spectrophotometer, against the blank. Calculate the quantity, in mg, of $C_{17}H_{19}N_3O \cdot CH_4O_3S$ in the aliquot of Phentolamine Mesylate for Injection taken by the formula:

$$50C(A_U/A_S)$$

in which C is the concentration, in mg per mL, of USP Phentolamine Mesylate RS in the *Standard preparation*, and A_U and A_S are the absorbances of the solutions from the *Assay preparation* and the *Standard preparation*, respectively.

Phenylalanine

$C_9H_{11}NO_2$ 165.19
L-Phenylalanine.
L-Phenylalanine [63-91-2].

» Phenylalanine contains not less than 98.5 percent and not more than 101.5 percent of $C_9H_{11}NO_2$, as L-phenylalanine, calculated on the dried basis.

Packaging and storage—Preserve in well-closed containers.

USP Reference standards ⟨11⟩—USP L-*Phenylalanine RS.* USP L-*Tyrosine RS.*

Identification, *Infrared Absorption* ⟨197K⟩.

Specific rotation ⟨781S⟩: between −32.7° and −34.7°.

Test solution: 20 mg per mL, in water.

pH ⟨791⟩: between 5.4 and 6.0, in a solution (1 in 100).

Loss on drying ⟨731⟩—Dry it at 105° for 3 hours: it loses not more than 0.3% of its weight.

Residue on ignition ⟨281⟩: not more than 0.4%.

Chloride ⟨221⟩—A 0.73-g portion shows no more chloride than corresponds to 0.50 mL of 0.020 N hydrochloric acid (0.05%).

Sulfate ⟨221⟩—A 0.33-g portion shows no more sulfate than corresponds to 0.10 mL of 0.020 N sulfuric acid (0.03%).

Iron ⟨241⟩: 0.003%.

Heavy metals, *Method II* ⟨231⟩: 0.0015%.

Chromatographic purity—

Adsorbent: 0.25-mm layer of chromatographic silica gel mixture.

Diluent—Prepare a mixture of glacial acetic acid and water (50 : 50).

Test solution—Dissolve an accurately weighed quantity of Phenylalanine in *Diluent* to obtain a solution having a concentration of 10 mg per mL. Apply 5 µL.

Standard solution—Dissolve an accurately weighed quantity of USP L-Phenylalanine RS in *Diluent* to obtain a solution having a known concentration of about 0.05 mg per mL. Apply 5 µL. [NOTE—This solution has a concentration equivalent to about 0.5% of that of the *Test solution*.]

System suitability solution—Prepare a solution in *Diluent* containing 0.4 mg each of USP L-Phenylalanine RS and USP L-Tyrosine RS per mL. Apply 5 µL.

Spray reagent—Dissolve 0.2 g of ninhydrin in 100 mL of a mixture of butyl alcohol and 2 N acetic acid (95 : 5).

Developing solvent system—Prepare a mixture of butyl alcohol, glacial acetic acid, and water (60 : 20 : 20).

Procedure—Proceed as directed for *Thin-Layer Chromatography* under *Chromatography* ⟨621⟩. After air-drying the plate, spray with *Spray reagent*, and heat between 100° and 105° for about 15 minutes. Examine the plate under white light. The chromatogram obtained from the *System suitability solution* exhibits two clearly separated spots. Any secondary spot in the chromatogram obtained from the *Test solution* is not larger or more intense than the principal spot in the chromatogram obtained from the *Standard solution*: not more than 0.5% of any individual impurity is found; and not more than 2.0% of total impurities is found.

Organic volatile impurities, *Method I* ⟨467⟩: meets the requirements.

(Official until July 1, 2008)

Assay—Transfer about 160 mg of Phenylalanine, accurately weighed, to a 125-mL flask, dissolve in a mixture of 3 mL of formic acid and 50 mL of glacial acetic acid, and titrate with 0.1 N perchloric acid VS, determining the endpoint potentiometrically. Perform a blank determination, and make any necessary correction. Each mL of 0.1 N perchloric acid is equivalent to 16.52 mg of $C_9H_{11}NO_2$.

Phenylbutazone

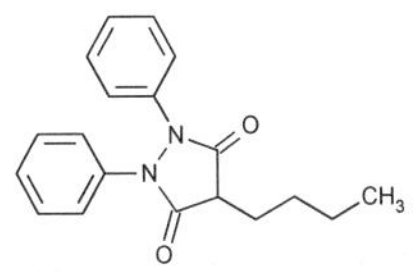

$C_{19}H_{20}N_2O_2$ 308.37
3,5-Pyrazolidinedione, 4-butyl-1,2-diphenyl-.
4-Butyl-1,2-diphenyl-3,5-pyrazolidinedione [50-33-9].

» Phenylbutazone contains not less than 98.0 percent and not more than 102.0 percent of $C_{19}H_{20}N_2O_2$, calculated on the dried basis.

Packaging and storage—Preserve in tight containers.
USP Reference standards 〈11〉—*USP Phenylbutazone RS.*
Identification—
  A: *Infrared Absorption* 〈197K〉.
  B: *Ultraviolet Absorption* 〈197U〉—
  Solution: 10 µg per mL.
  Medium: sodium hydroxide solution (1 in 2500).
  Absorptivities at 264 nm, calculated on the dried basis, do not differ by more than 2.0%.
Melting range 〈741〉: between 104° and 107°.
Loss on drying 〈731〉—Dry it in vacuum at a pressure of 30 ± 10 mm of mercury at 80° for 4 hours: it loses not more than 0.5% of its weight.
Residue on ignition 〈281〉: not more than 0.1%, 2.0 g being used for the test.
Chloride 〈221〉—Boil 2.0 g with 60 mL of water for 5 minutes, cool, and filter. To a 30-mL portion of the filtrate add 1 mL of 2 N nitric acid and 1 mL of silver nitrate TS: the filtrate shows no more chloride than corresponds to 0.10 mL of 0.020 N hydrochloric acid (0.007%).
Sulfate 〈221〉—To a 30-mL portion of the filtrate obtained in the test for *Chloride* add 2 mL of barium chloride TS: the mixture shows no more sulfate than corresponds to 0.10 mL of 0.020 N sulfuric acid (0.01%).
Heavy metals, *Method II* 〈231〉: 0.001%.
Organic volatile impurities, *Method V* 〈467〉: meets the requirements.
  Solvent—Use dimethyl sulfoxide.

(Official until July 1, 2008)

Assay—
  Acetate buffer—Transfer 2.72 g of sodium acetate to a 1000-mL beaker, and dissolve in about 700 mL of water. Adjust with glacial acetic acid to a pH of 4.1. Filter through a 0.5-µm filter, dilute with filtered water to 1000 mL, and mix.
  Mobile phase—Prepare a filtered and degassed mixture of acetonitrile with 560 mL of *Acetate buffer* (440 : 560). Make adjustments if necessary (see *System Suitability* under *Chromatography* 〈621〉).
  Internal standard solution—Dissolve 300 mg of desoxycorticosterone acetate in 200 mL of acetonitrile, and mix.
  Standard preparation—Dissolve an accurately weighed quantity of USP Phenylbutazone RS in acetonitrile, with the aid of sonication, and dilute quantitatively with acetonitrile to obtain a solution having a concentration of about 1.4 mg per mL. Pipet 10 mL of this solution into a 50-mL volumetric flask, add 10.0 mL of *Internal standard solution*, dilute with acetonitrile to volume, and mix. [NOTE—Use this solution within 8 hours of its preparation.]
  Assay preparation—Transfer about 140 mg of Phenylbutazone, accurately weighed, to a 100-mL volumetric flask, add 75 mL of acetonitrile, and sonicate to dissolve. Dilute with acetonitrile to volume, and mix. Pipet 10 mL of this solution into a 50-mL volumetric flask, add 10.0 mL of *Internal standard solution*, dilute with acetonitrile to volume, and mix. [NOTE—Use this solution within 8 hours of its preparation.]
  Chromatographic system (see *Chromatography* 〈621〉)—The liquid chromatograph is equipped with a 254-nm detector and a 4.6-mm × 25-cm column that contains packing L7, preceded by a precolumn that contains packing L2. The flow rate is about 2.4 mL per minute. Chromatograph the *Standard preparation,* and record the peak responses as directed for *Procedure:* the resolution, *R*, of phenylbutazone and the internal standard is not less than 3.5, and the relative standard deviation of the ratio of their peak responses in replicate injections is not more than 2.0%.
  Procedure—Separately inject equal volumes (about 25 µL) of the *Standard preparation* and the *Assay preparation* into the chromatograph, record the chromatograms, and measure the responses for the major peaks. The relative retention times are about 1.0 for the internal standard and 0.7 for phenylbutazone. Calculate the quantity, in mg, of $C_{19}H_{20}N_2O_2$ in the portion of Phenylbutazone taken by the formula:

$$500C(R_U / R_S)$$

in which *C* is the concentration, in mg per mL, of USP Phenylbutazone RS in the *Standard preparation;* and R_U and R_S are the ratios of the peak response of the phenylbutazone to that of the internal standard for the *Assay preparation* and the *Standard preparation,* respectively.

Phenylbutazone Boluses

Change to read:

» Phenylbutazone Boluses contain not less than 90.0 percent and not more than 110.0 percent of the labeled amount of phenylbutazone ($C_{19}H_{20}N_2O_2$) ▲and nominally not less than 1 g of phenylbutazone per bolus.▲USP31

Packaging and storage—Preserve in well-closed containers.
Labeling—Label Boluses to indicate that they are for veterinary use only.
USP Reference standards 〈11〉—*USP Phenylbutazone RS.*
Identification—
  A: Transfer a portion of powdered Boluses, equivalent to about 500 mg of phenylbutazone, to a 250-mL conical flask, add 100 mL of solvent hexane, and heat the mixture under reflux for 15 minutes. Filter the hot mixture, and allow the filtrate to cool. Separate the crystals thus formed by filtration, and dry in vacuum at 80° for 30 minutes: the phenylbutazone so obtained responds to *Identification* test A under *Phenylbutazone.*
  B: The retention time of the phenylbutazone peak in the chromatogram of the *Assay preparation* corresponds to that in the chromatogram of the *Standard preparation,* as obtained in the *Assay.*
Disintegration 〈701〉: 45 minutes with disks, determined as directed for *Uncoated Tablets,* simulated gastric fluid being used as the immersion fluid.
Uniformity of dosage units 〈905〉—meet the requirements for *Weight Variation.*
Assay—
  Acetate buffer, Mobile phase, Internal standard solution, Standard preparation, and *Chromatographic system*—Proceed as directed in the *Assay* under *Phenylbutazone.*
  Assay preparation—Weigh and finely powder a Phenylbutazone Bolus. Transfer an accurately weighed portion of the powder, equivalent to about 500 mg of phenylbutazone, to a 250-mL volumetric flask. Transfer 10.0 mL of water to the flask, and shake by mechanical means for 15 minutes. Add about 120 mL of acetonitrile, and sonicate until insoluble material is dispersed into fine particles. Shake by mechanical means for 20 minutes, dilute with acetonitrile to volume, and mix. Transfer 7.0 mL of this solution to a 50-mL volumetric flask, add 10.0 mL of *Internal standard solution,* dilute with acetonitrile to volume, and mix. Pass a portion of this solution through a filter having a porosity of 0.5 µm or finer, discarding the first few mL of the filtrate. Use the clear filtrate as the *Assay preparation.* [NOTE—Use this solution within 8 hours of its preparation.]

Procedure—Proceed as directed for *Procedure* in the *Assay* under *Phenylbutazone*. Calculate the quantity, in mg, of $C_{19}H_{20}N_2O_2$ in the portion of the Bolus taken by the formula:

$$1786C\,(R_U/R_S)$$

in which C is the concentration, in mg per mL, of USP Phenylbutazone RS in the *Standard preparation*, and R_U and R_S are the ratios of the peak responses of phenylbutazone to that of the internal standard obtained from the *Assay preparation* and the *Standard preparation*, respectively.

Phenylbutazone Injection

» Phenylbutazone Injection is a sterile solution of Phenylbutazone in Sterile Water for Injection. It contains not less than 90.0 percent and not more than 110.0 percent of the labeled amount of $C_{19}H_{20}N_2O_2$.

Packaging and storage—Preserve in single-dose or multiple-dose containers, preferably of Type I glass. Protect from light, and store in a refrigerator.
Labeling—Label Injection to indicate that it is for veterinary use only.
USP Reference standards ⟨11⟩—*USP Phenylbutazone RS*.
Clarity of solution—The Injection is essentially free from particles of foreign matter that can be observed on visual inspection.
Identification—
  A: Transfer a volume of Injection, equivalent to about 500 mg of phenylbutazone, to a 250-mL conical flask, add 100 mL of solvent hexane, and heat the mixture under reflux for 15 minutes. Filter the hot mixture, and allow the filtrate to cool. Separate the crystals thus formed by filtration, and dry in vacuum at 80° for 30 minutes: the phenylbutazone so obtained responds to *Identification* test A under *Phenylbutazone*.
  B: The retention time of the phenylbutazone peak in the chromatogram of the *Assay preparation* corresponds to that in the chromatogram of the *Standard preparation* as obtained in the *Assay*.
Sterility ⟨71⟩—It meets the requirements when tested as directed for *Membrane Filtration* under *Test for Sterility of the Product to be Examined*.
Bacterial endotoxins ⟨85⟩—It contains not more than 1.1 USP Endotoxin Units per mg of phenylbutazone.
pH ⟨791⟩: between 9.5 and 10.0.
Other requirements—It meets the requirements under *Injections* ⟨1⟩.
Assay—
  Acetate buffer, Mobile phase, Internal standard solution, Standard preparation, and *Chromatographic system*—Proceed as directed in the *Assay* under *Phenylbutazone*.
  Assay preparation—Transfer an accurately measured volume of Injection, equivalent to about 200 mg of phenylbutazone, to a 100-mL volumetric flask. Dilute with acetonitrile to volume, and mix. Transfer 7.0 mL of this solution to a 50-mL volumetric flask, add 10.0 mL of *Internal standard solution*, dilute with acetonitrile to volume, and mix. [NOTE—Use this solution within 8 hours of its preparation.]
  Procedure—Proceed as directed for *Procedure* in the *Assay* under *Phenylbutazone*. Calculate the quantity, in mg, of $C_{19}H_{20}N_2O_2$ in each mL of the Injection taken by the formula:

$$350(C/V)(R_U/R_S)$$

in which C is the concentration, in mg per mL, of USP Phenylbutazone RS in the *Standard preparation*, V is the volume, in mL, of Injection taken to prepare the *Assay preparation*, and R_U and R_S are the ratios of the peak responses of phenylbutazone to that of the internal standard obtained from the *Assay preparation* and the *Standard preparation*, respectively.

Phenylbutazone Tablets

Change to read:
» Phenylbutazone Tablets contain not less than 93.0 percent and not more than 107.0 percent of the labeled amount of phenylbutazone ($C_{19}H_{20}N_2O_2$) ▲and nominally not more than 200 mg of phenylbutazone per Tablet.▲USP31

Packaging and storage—Preserve in tight containers.

Add the following:
▲**Labeling**—Label Tablets to indicate that they are for veterinary use only.▲USP31
USP Reference standards ⟨11⟩—*USP Phenylbutazone RS*.
Identification—Transfer to a 250-mL conical flask a portion of powdered Tablets, equivalent to about 500 mg of phenylbutazone, add 100 mL of solvent hexane, and heat the mixture under reflux for 15 minutes. Filter the hot mixture, and allow the filtrate to cool. Separate the crystals thus formed by filtration, and dry in vacuum at 80° for 30 minutes: the phenylbutazone so obtained responds to *Identification* test A under *Phenylbutazone*.
Dissolution ⟨711⟩—
  Medium: pH 7.5 simulated intestinal fluid TS (without the enzyme); 900 mL.
  Apparatus 1: 100 rpm.
  Time: 30 minutes.
  Procedure—Determine the amount of $C_{19}H_{20}N_2O_2$ dissolved by employing UV absorption at the wavelength of maximum absorbance at about 264 nm on filtered portions of the solution under test, suitably diluted, if necessary, with *Medium,* using a suitable spectrophotometer, 1-cm cells, and *Medium* as the blank, in comparison with a solution of known concentration of USP Phenylbutazone RS in the same *Medium*.
  Tolerances—Not less than 70% (*Q*) is dissolved in 30 minutes.
Uniformity of dosage units ⟨905⟩: meet the requirements.
  Procedure for content uniformity—Transfer 1 Tablet to a 100-mL volumetric flask, add 60 mL of methanol, and shake by mechanical means for about 20 minutes or until the tablet is completely disintegrated. Dilute with methanol to volume, and mix. Filter a portion of mixture, discarding the first 10 mL of the filtrate. Dilute an accurately measured portion of the filtrate with sodium hydroxide solution (1 in 2500) to obtain a solution containing about 10 µg per mL. Prepare a solution of USP Phenylbutazone RS in methanol having a known concentration of about 1 mg per mL. Quantitatively dilute a portion of this solution with sodium hydroxide solution (1 in 2500) to obtain a Standard solution having a final known concentration of about 10 µg per mL. Concomitantly determine the absorbances of the solution from the Tablet and the Standard solution at the wavelength of maximum absorbance at about 264 nm with a suitable spectrophotometer, using sodium hydroxide solution (1 in 2500) as the blank. Calculate the quantity, in mg, of $C_{19}H_{20}N_2O_2$ in the Tablet by the formula:

$$(TC/D)(A_U/A_S)$$

in which T is the labeled quantity, in mg, of phenylbutazone in the Tablet; C is the concentration, in µg per mL, of USP Phenylbutazone RS in the Standard solution; D is the concentration, in µg per mL, of phenylbutazone in the solution from the Tablet based on the labeled quantity per Tablet and the extent of dilution; and A_U and A_S are the absorbances of the solution from the Tablet and the Standard solution, respectively.
Assay—
  Acetate buffer, Mobile phase, Internal standard solution, Standard preparation, and *Chromatographic system*—Proceed as directed in the *Assay* under *Phenylbutazone*.
  Assay preparation—Weigh and finely powder not fewer than 20 Tablets. Accurately weigh a portion of the powder, equivalent to about 500 mg of phenylbutazone, and transfer to a 250-mL volumetric flask. Pipet 50 mL of water into the flask, and shake by

mechanical means for 15 minutes. Add about 120 mL of acetonitrile, and sonicate until insoluble material is dispersed into fine particles. Shake by mechanical means for 20 minutes, dilute with acetonitrile to volume, and mix. Centrifuge a portion of this solution. Pipet 7 mL of the solution into a 50-mL volumetric flask, add 10.0 mL of *Internal standard solution,* dilute with acetonitrile to volume, and mix. Pass a portion through a 0.5-µm filter, discarding the first few mL of the filtrate. [NOTE—Use this solution within 8 hours of its preparation.]

Procedure—Proceed as directed for *Procedure* in the *Assay* under *Phenylbutazone.* Calculate the quantity, in mg, of phenylbutazone ($C_{19}H_{20}N_2O_2$) in the portion of Tablets taken by the formula:

$$1786C (R_U / R_S)$$

in which C is the concentration, in mg per mL, of USP Phenylbutazone RS in the *Standard preparation;* and R_U and R_S are the ratios of the peak response of phenylbutazone to that of the internal standard for the *Assay preparation* and the *Standard preparation,* respectively.

Phenylephrine Bitartrate

$C_9H_{13}NO_2 \cdot C_4H_6O_6$ 317.3

R-2-(Methylamino)-1-(3-hydroxyphenyl)ethanol-, (2R,3R)-2,3-dihydroxybutanedioate (1 : 1) (salt).
(–)-1-(3-Hydroxyphenyl)-2-methylaminoethanol, hydrogen tartrate.
(–)-3 Hydroxy-α-[(methylamino)methyl]benzenemethanol, hydrogen tartrate.
1-m-Hydroxy-α-[(methylamino)methyl]benzyl alcohol, hydrogen tartrate   [*17162-39-9*].

» Phenylephrine Bitartrate contains not less than 99.0 percent and not more than 100.5 percent of $C_9H_{13}NO_2 \cdot C_4H_6O_6$, calculated on the dried basis.

Packaging and storage—Preserve in tight, light-resistant containers. Store at controlled room temperature.
USP Reference standards ⟨11⟩—*USP Norphenylephrine Hydrochloride RS. USP Phenylephrine Hydrochloride RS.*
Identification—
  A: *Infrared Absorption* ⟨197K⟩.
  B: The alkaline filtrate from the test for *Specific rotation* responds positively to the test for *Tartrate* ⟨191⟩.
Specific rotation ⟨781S⟩: between –53° and –57° for the prepared sample.
  Test solution—Prepare a sample solution of about 240 mg per mL in water. Make the solution slightly alkaline by adding concentrated ammonium hydroxide dropwise. Rub the wall of the vessel with a glass rod so that the base precipitates out. Filter the base under suction, wash with a little water and acetone, and dry at 105° for 2 hours. Prepare and measure a 50 mg per mL solution of base precipitate in 1 M hydrochloric acid.
pH ⟨791⟩: between 3.0 and 4.0 in 10% w/v aqueous solution.
Loss on drying ⟨731⟩—Dry at 105° to a constant weight: it loses not more than 0.5% of its weight.
Residue on ignition ⟨281⟩: not more than 0.1%.
Chromatographic purity—
  Buffer solution—Dissolve 3.25 g of 1-octanesulfonic acid sodium salt monohydrate in 1 L of water. Adjust slowly with 3 M phosphoric acid to a pH of 2.8.
  Solution A—Prepare a filtered and degassed mixture of *Buffer solution* and acetonitrile (9 : 1).
  Solution B—Prepare a filtered and degassed mixture of acetonitrile and *Buffer solution* (9 : 1).
  Diluent—Prepare a mixture of *Solution A* and *Solution B* (8 : 2).
  System suitability solution—Dissolve accurately weighed quantities of USP Phenylephrine Hydrochloride RS and USP Norphenylephrine Hydrochloride RS in *Diluent,* and dilute quantitatively, and stepwise if necessary, to obtain a solution having known concentrations of about 1.0 mg per mL and 0.9 µg per mL, respectively.
  Blank solution—Prepare a solution containing 0.8 mg per mL L(+)-tartaric acid in *Diluent.*

  Test solution—Transfer 78 mg of Phenylephrine Bitartrate, accurately weighed, to a 50-mL volumetric flask. Dissolve in and dilute with *Diluent* to volume, and mix.
  Chromatographic system (see *Chromatography* ⟨621⟩)—The liquid chromatograph is equipped with a 215-nm detector and a 4-mm × 5.5-cm column that contains packing L1. The column and injection port temperatures are maintained at 45 ± 2°. The flow rate is about 1.5 mL per minute. The chromatograph is programmed as follows.

Time (minutes)	Solution A (%)	Solution B (%)	Elution
0	93	7	equilibration
0–10	93→70	7→30	linear gradient
10–10.1	70→93	30→7	linear gradient
10.1–18	93	7	equilibration

Chromatograph the *System suitability solution,* and record the peak responses as directed for *Procedure:* the resolution, R, between norphenylephrine and (–)-phenylephrine is not less than 1.5; the tailing factor of (–)-phenylephrine is less than 1.8; and the relative standard deviation for replicate injections is not more than 5%.
  Procedure—Separately inject equal volumes (about 4 µL) of the *Blank solution* and the *Test solution* into the chromatograph, record the chromatograms, and measure all of the peak responses. Calculate the percentage of each impurity in the portion of Phenylephrine Bitartrate taken by the formula:

$$100(r_i / r_s)$$

in which r_i is the peak response for each impurity, and r_s is the sum of the responses of all the peaks. [NOTE—Examine the chromatogram of the *Blank solution* for peaks and disregard any corresponding peaks observed in the chromatogram of the *Test solution.*] The limits of impurities are specified in the accompanying table.

Compound	Approximate Relative Retention Time	Limit (%)
Phenylephrine	1.0	—
Norphenylephrine	0.9	0.2
Phenylephrone	1.2	0.1
Benzylphenylephrine	2.9	0.2
Benzylphenylephrone	3.1	0.1
Individual unknown impurity	—	0.1
Total impurity	—	0.5

Assay—Transfer about 280 mg of Phenylephrine Bitartrate, accurately weighed, to a 100-mL beaker, and dissolve by stirring in 60 mL of glacial acetic acid. Titrate with 0.1 N perchloric acid, determining the endpoint potentiometrically. Perform a blank determination (see *Titrimetry* ⟨541⟩), and make the necessary correction. Each mL of 0.1 N perchloric acid is equivalent to 31.73 mg of $C_9H_{13}NO_2 \cdot C_4H_6O_6$.

Phenylephrine Hydrochloride

$C_9H_{13}NO_2 \cdot HCl$ 203.67
Benzenemethanol, 3-hydroxy-α-[(methylamino)methyl]-, hydrochloride (R)-.
(–)-*m*-Hydroxy-α-[(methylamino)methyl]benzyl alcohol hydrochloride   [*61-76-7*].

» Phenylephrine Hydrochloride contains not less than 97.5 percent and not more than 102.5 percent of $C_9H_{13}NO_2 \cdot HCl$, calculated on the dried basis.

Packaging and storage—Preserve in tight, light-resistant containers. Store at 25°, excursions permitted between 15° and 30°.
USP Reference standards ⟨11⟩—*USP Phenylephrine Hydrochloride RS.*
Identification—
 A: *Infrared Absorption* ⟨197K⟩.
 B: A solution (1 in 100) responds to the tests for *Chloride* ⟨191⟩.
Melting range ⟨741⟩: between 140° and 145°.
Specific rotation ⟨781S⟩: between −42° and −47.5°.
 Test solution: 50 mg per mL, in water.
Loss on drying ⟨731⟩—Dry it at 105° for 2 hours: it loses not more than 1.0% of its weight.
Residue on ignition ⟨281⟩: not more than 0.2%.
Sulfate ⟨221⟩—A solution of 50 mg in 25 mL of water shows no more turbidity than corresponds to 0.10 mL of 0.020 N sulfuric acid (0.20%).
Limit of ketones—Dissolve 200 mg in 1 mL of water, add 2 drops of sodium nitroferricyanide TS, then add 1 mL of 1 N sodium hydroxide, followed by 0.6 mL of glacial acetic acid: the color of the final solution is not deeper than that obtained in a control solution prepared with 1 mL of dilute acetone (1 in 2000).
Chromatographic purity—
 Standard preparations—Dissolve an accurately weighed quantity of USP Phenylephrine Hydrochloride RS in methanol to obtain a solution having a known concentration of 1 mg per mL. Quantitatively dilute with methanol to obtain *Standard preparations* having the following compositions:

Standard Preparation	Dilution	Concentration (μg RS per mL)	Percentage (%, for comparison with test specimen)
A	(1 in 2)	500	1.0
B	(1 in 4)	250	0.5
C	(1 in 10)	100	0.2
D	(1 in 20)	50	0.1

 Test preparation—Dissolve an accurately weighed quantity of Phenylephrine Hydrochloride in methanol to obtain a solution containing 50 mg per mL.
 Procedure—Apply separately 5 μL of the *Test preparation* and 5 μL of each *Standard preparation* to a suitable thin-layer chromatographic plate (see *Chromatography* ⟨621⟩) coated with a 0.25-mm layer of chromatographic silica gel mixture. Position the plate in a chromatographic chamber and develop the chromatograms in a solvent system consisting of a mixture of *n*-butyl alcohol, water, and formic acid (7 : 2 : 1) until the solvent front has moved about three-fourths of the length of the plate. Remove the plate from the developing chamber, mark the solvent front, and allow the solvent to evaporate in warm, circulating air. Examine the plate under short-wavelength UV light. Then spray the plate with a saturated solution of *p*-nitrobenzenediazonium tetrafluoroborate followed by sodium carbonate solution (1 in 10). Compare the intensities of any secondary spots observed in the chromatogram of the *Test preparation* with those of the principal spots in the chromatograms of the *Standard preparations*: the sum of the intensities of secondary spots obtained from the *Test preparation* corresponds to not more than 1.0% of related compounds, with no single impurity corresponding to more than 0.5%.
Chloride content—Dissolve about 300 mg, accurately weighed, in 5 mL of water. Add 5 mL of glacial acetic acid and 50 mL of methanol, then add eosin Y TS, and titrate with 0.1 N silver nitrate VS. Each mL of 0.1 N silver nitrate is equivalent to 3.545 mg of Cl. Not less than 17.0% and not more than 17.7% of Cl is found, calculated on the dried basis.

Assay—Dissolve about 100 mg of Phenylephrine Hydrochloride, accurately weighed, in 20 mL of water contained in an iodine flask, add 50.0 mL of 0.1 N bromine VS, then add 5 mL of hydrochloric acid, and immediately insert the stopper. Shake the flask, and allow to stand for 15 minutes. Introduce quickly 10 mL of potassium iodide solution (1 in 10), allow to stand for 5 minutes, shake thoroughly, remove the stopper, and rinse it and the neck of the flask with a small quantity of water into the flask. Titrate the liberated iodine with 0.1 N sodium thiosulfate VS, adding 3 mL of starch TS as the endpoint is approached. Perform a blank determination (see *Residual Titrations* under *Titrimetry* ⟨541⟩). Each mL of 0.1 N bromine is equivalent to 3.395 mg of $C_9H_{13}NO_2 \cdot HCl$.

Phenylephrine Hydrochloride Injection

» Phenylephrine Hydrochloride Injection is a sterile solution of Phenylephrine Hydrochloride in Water for Injection. It contains not less than 90.0 percent and not more than 115.0 percent of the labeled amount of $C_9H_{13}NO_2 \cdot HCl$.

Packaging and storage—Preserve in single-dose or multiple-dose containers, preferably of Type I glass, protected from light.
USP Reference standards ⟨11⟩—*USP Phenylephrine Hydrochloride RS. USP Endotoxin RS.*
Identification—Concentrate or dilute, if necessary, a suitable volume of Injection to a concentration of about 10 mg per mL. Apply 2 μL of this solution and of a Standard solution of USP Phenylephrine Hydrochloride RS, containing about 10 mg per mL, at points about 2.5 cm from the bottom edge of a suitable thin-layer chromatographic plate (see *Chromatography* ⟨621⟩) coated with a 0.25-mm layer of chromatographic silica gel. Dry the spots in a current of warm air, and develop the chromatogram in a suitable chromatographic chamber with a mixture of methanol, water, and ammonium hydroxide (72 : 25 : 3) until the solvent front has moved about 12 cm. Dry the plate in warm air, and spray it with alcoholic potassium hydroxide TS. Dry at 60° for 15 minutes, and spray the plate with *p*-nitroaniline TS: the reddish orange spot obtained from the test solution corresponds in color, size, and intensity to that obtained from the Standard solution.
Bacterial endotoxins ⟨85⟩—It contains not more than 25.0 USP Endotoxin Units per mg of phenylephrine hydrochloride.
pH ⟨791⟩: between 3.0 and 6.5.
Other requirements—It meets the requirements under *Injections* ⟨1⟩.
Assay—
 Mobile phase—Prepare and filter a mixture of methanol and water (1 : 1) containing 1.1 g of sodium 1-octanesulfonate per liter, adjusted with 3 M phosphoric acid to a pH of 3.0. Make adjustments if necessary (see *System Suitability* under *Chromatography* ⟨621⟩).
 Dilution solvent—Prepare a mixture of methanol and water (1 : 1), adjusted with 3 M phosphoric acid to a pH of 3.0.
 System suitability solution—Dissolve about 50 mg each of USP Phenylephrine Hydrochloride RS and USP Epinephrine Bitartrate RS in 5 mL of water, dilute with *Dilution solvent* to 25.0 mL, and mix. Further dilute 5.0 mL of the resulting solution with *Dilution solvent* to 25.0 mL, and mix to obtain a solution having a concentration of about 0.4 mg of phenylephrine hydrochloride and 0.4 mg of epinephrine bitartrate per mL.
 Standard preparation—Dissolve about 50 mg of USP Phenylephrine Hydrochloride RS, accurately weighed, in 10 mL of water, dilute with *Dilution solvent* to 25.0 mL, and mix. Further dilute 5.0 mL of the resulting solution with *Dilution solvent* to 25.0 mL, and mix to obtain a solution having a known concentration of about 0.4 mg per mL.
 Assay preparation—Transfer an accurately measured volume of Injection, equivalent to about 10 mg of phenylephrine hydrochloride, to a 25-mL volumetric flask. Dilute with *Dilution solvent* to volume, and mix.
 Chromatographic system (see *Chromatography* ⟨621⟩)—The liquid chromatograph is equipped with a 280-nm detector and a 4.6-

mm × 25-cm column that contains packing L1. The flow rate is about 1 mL per minute. Chromatograph the *System suitability solution*, and record the responses for the major peaks: the resolution, *R*, between epinephrine and phenylephrine is not less than 1.0. Chromatograph replicate injections of the *Standard preparation*, and record the peak responses as directed for *Procedure:* the relative standard deviation is not more than 2.0%.

Procedure—Separately inject equal volumes (about 20 μL) of the *Standard preparation* and the *Assay preparation* into the chromatograph, record the chromatograms, and measure the responses for the major peaks. Calculate the quantity, in mg, of $C_9H_{13}NO_2 \cdot HCl$ in each mL of the Injection taken by the formula:

$$(25C / V)(r_U / r_S)$$

in which *C* is the concentration, in mg per mL, of USP Phenylephrine Hydrochloride RS in the *Standard preparation*, *V* is the volume, in mL, of Injection taken, and r_U and r_S are the peak responses obtained from the *Assay preparation* and the *Standard preparation*, respectively.

Phenylephrine Hydrochloride Nasal Jelly

» Phenylephrine Hydrochloride Nasal Jelly contains not less than 90.0 percent and not more than 110.0 percent of the labeled amount of $C_9H_{13}NO_2 \cdot HCl$.

Packaging and storage—Preserve in tight containers.

USP Reference standards ⟨11⟩—*USP Phenylephrine Hydrochloride RS.*
Identification—Dissolve a suitable quantity in water to obtain a solution having a concentration of about 60 μg per mL, and centrifuge, if necessary: the UV absorption spectrum of the solution so obtained exhibits maxima and minima at the same wavelengths as that of a similar solution of USP Phenylephrine Hydrochloride RS, concomitantly measured.
Minimum fill ⟨755⟩: meets the requirements.
Assay—
Mobile phase—Prepare a mixture of methanol and water (1 : 1) containing 1.1 g of sodium 1-octanesulfonate per liter, adjust with phosphoric acid to a pH of 3.0, filter, and degas. Make adjustments to the methanol and water ratio, if necessary (see *System Suitability* under *Chromatography* ⟨621⟩).
Dilution solvent—Prepare a mixture of methanol and water (1 : 1), and adjust with phosphoric acid to a pH of 3.0.
Standard preparation—Dissolve an accurately weighed quantity of USP Phenylephrine Hydrochloride RS in *Dilution solvent* to obtain a Stock standard solution having a known concentration of about 2 mg per mL. Dilute an accurately measured volume of this solution with *Dilution solvent* to obtain the *Standard preparation* having a known concentration of about 0.1 mg per mL.
Assay preparation—Transfer an accurately weighed amount of Nasal Jelly, equivalent to about 10 mg of phenylephrine hydrochloride, to a 100-mL volumetric flask. Dilute with *Dilution solvent* to volume, and mix.
Resolution solution—Transfer 5.0 mL of Stock standard solution to a 100-mL volumetric flask, add 10 mg of USP Epinephrine Bitartrate RS, dilute with *Dilution solvent* to volume, and mix.
Chromatographic system (see *Chromatography* ⟨621⟩)—The liquid chromatograph is equipped with a 280-nm detector and a 4.6-mm × 25-cm column that contains packing L1. The flow rate is about 1 mL per minute. Chromatograph the *Resolution solution*: the resolution, *R*, is not less than 1.5, and the tailing factor for the phenylephrine peak is not more than 2.0. Chromatograph replicate injections of the *Standard preparation*: the relative standard deviation is not more than 2.0%.
Procedure—Separately inject equal volumes (about 20 μL) of the *Standard preparation* and the *Assay preparation* into the chromatograph, record the chromatograms, and measure the responses for the major peaks. Calculate the quantity, in mg, of $C_9H_{13}NO_2 \cdot HCl$ in the portion of Nasal Jelly taken by the formula:

$$100C(r_U / r_S)$$

in which *C* is the concentration, in mg per mL, of USP Phenylephrine Hydrochloride RS in the *Standard preparation*, and r_U and r_S are the peak responses obtained from the *Assay preparation* and the *Standard preparation*, respectively.

Phenylephrine Hydrochloride Nasal Solution

» Phenylephrine Hydrochloride Nasal Solution contains not less than 90.0 percent and not more than 115.0 percent of the labeled amount of $C_9H_{13}NO_2 \cdot HCl$.

Packaging and storage—Preserve in tight, light-resistant containers.

USP Reference standards ⟨11⟩—*USP Phenylephrine Hydrochloride RS.*
Identification—It responds to the *Identification* test under *Phenylephrine Hydrochloride Injection*.
Assay—
Mobile phase, Dilution solvent, Standard preparation, Resolution solution, and *Chromatographic system*—Prepare as directed in the *Assay* under *Phenylephrine Hydrochloride Nasal Jelly*.
Assay preparation—Transfer an accurately measured volume of Nasal Solution, equivalent to about 10 mg of phenylephrine hydrochloride, to a 100-mL volumetric flask. Dilute with *Dilution solvent* to volume, and mix.
Procedure—Separately inject equal volumes (about 20 μL) of the *Standard preparation* and the *Assay preparation* into the chromatograph, record the chromatograms, and measure the responses for the major peaks. Calculate the quantity, in mg, of $C_9H_{13}NO_2 \cdot HCl$ in each mL of the Nasal Solution taken by the formula:

$$100(C / V)(r_U / r_S)$$

in which *C* is the concentration, in mg per mL, of USP Phenylephrine Hydrochloride RS in the *Standard preparation*, *V* is the volume, in mL, of Nasal Solution taken, and r_U and r_S are the peak responses obtained from the *Assay preparation* and the *Standard preparation*, respectively.

Phenylephrine Hydrochloride Ophthalmic Solution

» Phenylephrine Hydrochloride Ophthalmic Solution is a sterile, aqueous solution of Phenylephrine Hydrochloride. It contains not less than 90.0 percent and not more than 115.0 percent of the labeled amount of $C_9H_{13}NO_2 \cdot HCl$. It may contain a suitable antimicrobial agent and buffer and may contain suitable antioxidants.

Packaging and storage—Preserve in tight, light-resistant containers of not more than 15-mL size.

USP Reference standards ⟨11⟩—*USP Phenylephrine Hydrochloride RS.*
Identification—It responds to the *Identification* test under *Phenylephrine Hydrochloride Injection*.
Sterility ⟨71⟩: meets the requirements.
pH ⟨791⟩: between 4.0 and 7.5 for buffered Ophthalmic Solution; between 3.0 and 4.5 for unbuffered Ophthalmic Solution.

Assay—
Mobile phase, Dilution solvent, Standard preparation, Resolution solution, and Chromatographic system—Prepare as directed in the Assay under Phenylephrine Hydrochloride Nasal Jelly.

Assay preparation—Transfer an accurately measured volume of Ophthalmic Solution, equivalent to about 10 mg of phenylephrine hydrochloride, to a 100-mL volumetric flask. Dilute with Dilution solvent to volume, and mix.

Procedure—Separately inject equal volumes (about 20 µL) of the Standard preparation and the Assay preparation into the chromatograph, record the chromatograms, and measure the responses for the major peaks. Calculate the quantity, in mg, of $C_9H_{13}NO_2 \cdot HCl$ in each mL of Ophthalmic Solution taken by the formula:

$$100(C/V)(r_U/r_S)$$

in which C is the concentration, in mg per mL, of USP Phenylephrine Hydrochloride RS in the Standard preparation, V is the volume, in mL, of Ophthalmic Solution taken, and r_U and r_S are the peak responses obtained from the Assay preparation and the Standard preparation, respectively.

Phenylethyl Alcohol

$C_8H_{10}O$ 122.17
Benzeneethanol.
Phenethyl alcohol   [60-12-8].

Packaging and storage—Preserve in tight, light-resistant containers, and store in a cool, dry place.
USP Reference standards ⟨11⟩—USP Phenylethyl Alcohol RS.
Identification, Infrared Absorption ⟨197F⟩.
Specific gravity ⟨841⟩: between 1.017 and 1.020.
Refractive index ⟨831⟩: between 1.531 and 1.534 at 20°.
Residue on ignition ⟨281⟩—Evaporate 10 mL in a suitable crucible, and ignite to constant weight: the limit is 0.005%.
Chlorinated compounds—Wind a 1.5- × 5-cm strip of 20-mesh copper gauze around the end of a copper wire. Heat the gauze in the nonluminous flame of a Bunsen burner until it glows without coloring the flame green. Permit the gauze to cool, and heat several times until a good coat of oxide has formed. Apply with a medicine dropper 2 drops of Phenylethyl Alcohol to the cooled gauze, ignite, and permit it to burn freely in the air. Again cool the gauze, add 2 more drops of Phenylethyl Alcohol, and burn as before. Continue this process until a total of 6 drops has been added and ignited, and then hold the gauze in the outer edge of the Bunsen flame, adjusted to a height of about 4 cm: no transient green color or other color is imparted to the flame.
Aldehyde—Shake 5 mL with 5 mL of 1 N sodium hydroxide, and allow to stand for 1 hour: no yellow color appears in the organic (top) layer.
Organic volatile impurities, Method IV ⟨467⟩: meets the requirements.

(Official until July 1, 2008)

Phenylpropanolamine Bitartrate

$C_9H_{13}NO \cdot C_4H_6O_6$ 301.30
(R^*,S^*)-($\pm$)-α-(1-Aminoethyl)benzenemethanol bitartrate   [67244-90-0].

» Phenylpropanolamine Bitartrate contains not less than 98.0 percent and not more than 101.0 percent of $C_9H_{13}NO \cdot C_4H_6O_6$, calculated on the dried basis.

Packaging and storage—Preserve in tight, light-resistant containers.
USP Reference standards ⟨11⟩—USP Cathinone Hydrochloride RS. USP Dextroamphetamine Sulfate RS. USP Phenylpropanediol RS. USP Phenylpropanolamine Bitartrate RS. USP Phenylpropanolamine Hydrochloride RS.
Identification—
  A: Infrared Absorption ⟨197K⟩.
  B: It responds to the test for Tartrate ⟨191⟩.
Melting range, Class I ⟨741⟩: between 150° and 164°.
pH ⟨791⟩: between 3.1 and 3.7, in a solution (3 in 100).
Loss on drying ⟨731⟩—Dry it at 65° for 3 hours: it loses not more than 1.0% of its weight.
Residue on ignition ⟨281⟩: not more than 0.1%.
Heavy metals, Method I ⟨231⟩—Dissolve 1 g in 5 mL of water, add 1 mL of 1 N acetic acid, and dilute with water to 25 mL: the limit is 0.002%.
Limit of cathinone hydrochloride—Proceed as directed for Limit of cathinone hydrochloride under Phenylpropanolamine Hydrochloride.
Limit of amphetamine hydrochloride and phenylpropanediol—
  Mobile phase—Prepare a mixture of 20 mL of 10% tetramethylammonium hydroxide and 5 mL of phosphoric acid, dilute with water to a volume of 1000 mL, and mix. To 896 mL of the resulting solution add 100 mL of methanol, 4 mL of tetrahydrofuran, and mix. Filter and degas the mixture. Make adjustments if necessary (see System Suitability under Chromatography ⟨621⟩).
  Standard solution A—Dissolve accurately weighed quantities of USP Phenylpropanolamine Hydrochloride RS and USP Dextroamphetamine Sulfate RS in water to obtain a solution having known concentrations of about 100 mg of USP Phenylpropanolamine Hydrochloride RS per mL and 1 µg of USP Dextroamphetamine Sulfate RS per mL.
  Standard solution B—Dissolve an accurately weighed quantity of USP Phenylpropanediol RS in water, and dilute quantitatively, and stepwise if necessary, with water to obtain a solution having a known concentration of about 0.1 mg per mL.
  Resolution solution—Dissolve accurately weighed quantities of USP Phenylpropanolamine Hydrochloride RS and USP Dextroamphetamine Sulfate RS in water to obtain a solution containing about 5 µg of each per mL.
  Test solution—Transfer about 1000 mg of Phenylpropanolamine Bitartrate, accurately weighed, to a 10-mL volumetric flask, dilute with water to volume, and mix.
  Chromatographic system (see Chromatography ⟨621⟩)—The liquid chromatograph is equipped with a 215-nm detector and a 4.6-mm × 15-cm column that contains spherical 5-µm packing L1. The flow rate is about 2.0 mL per minute. Separately chromatograph the Resolution solution and each Standard solution, and record the peak responses as directed for Procedure: the relative retention times are about 1.0 for phenylpropanolamine, between 1.9 and 2.1 for dextroamphetamine, and between 2.3 and 2.7 for phenylpropanediol; the resolution, R, between phenylpropanolamine and dextroamphetamine in the chromatogram of the Resolution solution is not less than 5.0; and the relative standard deviation for replicate injections of the Standard solutions is not more than 3.0%.
  Procedure—Separately inject equal volumes (about 20 µL) of Standard solution A, Standard solution B, and the Test solution into the chromatograph, record the chromatograms, and measure the responses for the major peaks. Calculate the percentage of phenylpropanediol in the portion of Phenylpropanolamine Bitartrate taken by the formula:

$$1000C/W(r_U/r_S)$$

in which C is the concentration, in mg per mL, of USP Phenylpropanediol RS in Standard solution B; W is the weight, in mg, of Phenylpropanolamine Bitartrate taken to prepare the Test solution; and r_U and r_S are the peak responses obtained from the Test solution and the Standard solution B, respectively. The limit of phenylpropanediol is not more than 0.2%.

Calculate the percentage of amphetamine hydrochloride in the portion of Phenylpropanolamine Bitartrate taken by the formula:

$$(343.34 / 368.49)(C / W)(r_U / r_S)$$

in which 343.34 is twice the molecular weight of amphetamine hydrochloride; 368.49 is the molecular weight of dextroamphetamine sulfate; C is the concentration, in µg per mL, of USP Dextroamphetamine Sulfate RS in *Standard solution A*; W is the weight, in mg, of Phenylpropanolamine Bitartrate taken to prepare the *Test solution*; and r_U and r_S are the amphetamine peak responses obtained from the *Test solution* and *Standard solution A*, respectively. The limit of amphetamine hydrochloride is not more than 0.001%.

Organic volatile impurities, *Method I* ⟨467⟩: meets the requirements.

(Official until July 1, 2008)

Assay—Dissolve about 500 mg of Phenylpropanolamine Bitartrate, previously dried and accurately weighed, in 50 mL of glacial acetic acid. Add 10 mL of mercuric acetate TS and 2 drops of crystal violet TS, and titrate with 0.1 N perchloric acid VS to a green endpoint. Perform a blank determination, and make any necessary correction. Each mL of 0.1 N perchloric acid is equivalent to 30.13 mg of $C_9H_{13}NO \cdot C_4H_6O_6$.

Phenylpropanolamine Hydrochloride

$C_9H_{13}NO \cdot HCl$ 187.67
Benzenemethanol, α-(1-aminoethyl)-, hydrochloride, (R^*,S^*)-, (±).
(±)-Norephedrine hydrochloride [154-41-6].

» Phenylpropanolamine Hydrochloride contains not less than 98.0 percent and not more than 101.0 percent of $C_9H_{13}NO \cdot HCl$, calculated on the dried basis.

Packaging and storage—Preserve in tight, light-resistant containers.

USP Reference standards ⟨11⟩—*USP Cathinone Hydrochloride RS. USP Dextroamphetamine Sulfate RS. USP Phenylpropanolamine Hydrochloride RS.*

Identification—
  A: *Infrared Absorption* ⟨197K⟩.
  B: *Ultraviolet Absorption* ⟨197U⟩—
    Solution: 500 µg per mL.
    Medium: water.
    Absorptivities at 256 nm, calculated on the dried basis, do not differ by more than 3.0%.
  C: Dissolve 1 g in 10 mL of water, add 10 mL of saturated sodium carbonate solution, and mix. Separate the precipitate by vacuum filtration, using a medium-porosity, sintered-glass filter, and wash with three 5-mL portions of ice-cold water. Dry the crystals at 80° for 1 hour: the phenylpropanolamine so obtained melts between 101° and 104° (see *Melting Range or Temperature* ⟨741⟩).

Melting range, *Class I* ⟨741⟩: between 191° and 196°.

pH ⟨791⟩: between 4.2 and 5.5, in a solution (3 in 100).

Loss on drying ⟨731⟩—Dry it at 105° for 2 hours: it loses not more than 0.5% of its weight.

Residue on ignition ⟨281⟩: not more than 0.1%.

Heavy metals, *Method I* ⟨231⟩—Dissolve 1 g in 5 mL of water, add 1 mL of 1 N acetic acid, and dilute with water to 25 mL: the limit is 0.002%.

Limit of cathinone hydrochloride—Transfer 2.5 g to a 25-mL volumetric flask, add dilute hydrochloric acid (1 in 120) to volume, and mix. Concomitantly determine the absorbances of this solution and a Standard solution of USP Cathinone Hydrochloride RS in the same medium having a known concentration of 100 µg per mL in 1-cm cells at the wavelength of maximum absorbance at about 285 nm, using dilute hydrochloric acid (1 in 120) as the blank: the absorbance of the test solution is not greater than that of the Standard solution. Not more than 0.10% is found.

Limit of amphetamine hydrochloride—

Mobile phase—Prepare a filtered and degassed mixture of water, acetonitrile, phosphoric acid, and triethylamine (950 : 50 : 8 : 5). Make adjustments if necessary (see *System suitability* under *Chromatography* ⟨621⟩).

System suitability solution—Dissolve suitable quantities of USP Phenylpropanolamine Hydrochloride RS and USP Dextroamphetamine Sulfate RS in water to obtain a solution containing about 5 µg of each per mL.

Amphetamine stock solution—Dissolve an accurately weighed quantity of USP Dextroamphetamine Sulfate RS in water, and dilute quantitatively, and stepwise if necessary, with water to obtain a solution having a known concentration of about 2.5 µg per mL.

Phenylpropanolamine stock solution—Transfer about 2.5 g of Phenylpropanolamine Hydrochloride, accurately weighed, to a 10-mL volumetric flask, dilute with water to volume, and dissolve, using sonication if necessary.

Standard solution—Transfer 4.0 mL of *Phenylpropanolamine stock solution*, accurately measured, to a 10-mL volumetric flask, add 4.0 mL of *Amphetamine stock solution*, dilute with water to volume, and mix to obtain a solution having known concentrations of about 100 mg per mL and 1 µg per mL, respectively.

Test solution—Transfer about 4.0 mL of *Phenylpropanolamine stock solution*, accurately measured, to a 10-mL volumetric flask, dilute with water to volume, and mix.

Chromatographic system (see *Chromatography* ⟨621⟩)—The liquid chromatograph is equipped with a 206-nm detector and a 4.6-mm × 25-cm column that contains 5-µm, base-deactivated packing L1. The flow rate is about 1 mL per minute. Chromatograph the *System suitability solution*, and record the peak responses as directed for *Procedure:* the relative retention times are 1.0 for phenylpropanolamine and 2.1 for amphetamine; the resolution, R, between phenylpropanolamine and amphetamine is not less than 15; and the column efficiency is not less than 10,000 theoretical plates. Chromatograph the *Standard solution*, and record the peak responses as directed for *Procedure:* the relative standard deviation of the amphetamine peak for replicate injections is not more than 3.0%.

Procedure—Separately inject equal volumes (about 5 µL) of the *Standard solution* and the *Test solution* into the chromatograph, record the chromatograms, and measure the responses at the locus of the amphetamine peak. Calculate the percentage of amphetamine hydrochloride in the portion of Phenylpropanolamine Hydrochloride taken by the formula:

$$0.2(171.67/368.49)(C_S / C_U)[r_U /(r_S - r_U)]$$

in which 171.67 and 368.49 are the molecular weights of amphetamine hydrochloride and amphetamine sulfate, respectively; C_S is the concentration, in µg per mL, of USP Dextroamphetamine Sulfate RS in the *Standard solution*; C_U is the concentration, in mg per mL, of Phenylpropanolamine Hydrochloride in the *Test solution*; and r_U and r_S are the peak responses of amphetamine obtained from the *Test solution* and the *Standard solution*, respectively: not more than 0.001% is found.

Organic volatile impurities, *Method I* ⟨467⟩: meets the requirements.

(Official until July 1, 2008)

Assay—Dissolve about 500 mg of Phenylpropanolamine Hydrochloride, accurately weighed, in 50 mL of glacial acetic acid. Add 10 mL of mercuric acetate TS and 2 drops of crystal violet TS, and titrate with 0.1 N perchloric acid VS to a green endpoint. Perform a blank determination, and make any necessary correction. Each mL of 0.1 N perchloric acid is equivalent to 18.77 mg of $C_9H_{13}NO \cdot HCl$.

Phenylpropanolamine Hydrochloride Capsules

» Phenylpropanolamine Hydrochloride Capsules contain not less than 90.0 percent and not more than 110.0 percent of the labeled amount of phenylpropanolamine hydrochloride ($C_9H_{13}NO \cdot HCl$).

Packaging and storage—Preserve in tight, light-resistant containers.

USP Reference standards ⟨11⟩—*USP Phenylpropanolamine Hydrochloride RS.*

Identification—The retention time of the major peak in the chromatogram of the *Assay preparation* corresponds to that in the chromatogram of the *Standard preparation*, as obtained in the *Assay*.

Dissolution, *Procedure for a pooled sample* ⟨711⟩—
 Medium: water; 900 mL.
 Apparatus 1: 100 rpm.
 Time: 45 minutes.
 Procedure—Determine the amount of phenylpropanolamine hydrochloride dissolved, employing the procedure set forth in the *Assay*, making any necessary volumetric adjustments.
 Tolerances—Not less than 75% (*Q*) of the labeled amount of $C_9H_{13}NO \cdot HCl$ is dissolved in 45 minutes.

Uniformity of dosage units ⟨905⟩: meet the requirements.

Assay—
 Mobile phase—[NOTE—Prepare the *Mobile phase* one day prior to use.] Prepare a filtered and degassed mixture of water, methanol, tetramethylammonium hydroxide solution (1 in 10), and phosphoric acid (700 : 300 : 14 : 3.5). Make adjustments if necessary (see *System Suitability* under *Chromatography* ⟨621⟩).
 Internal standard solution—Prepare a solution of theophylline in methanol containing 0.1 mg per mL.
 Standard preparation—Dissolve an accurately weighed quantity of USP Phenylpropanolamine Hydrochloride RS in *Internal standard solution* to obtain a solution having a known concentration of about 3 mg per mL.
 Assay preparation—Remove as completely as possible the contents of not fewer than 20 Capsules, weigh, and mix. Transfer an accurately weighed portion of the combined contents, equivalent to about 750 mg of phenylpropanolamine hydrochloride, to a suitable container. Add 250.0 mL of *Internal standard solution*, mix, sonicate for 30 minutes, allow to stand overnight, and filter.
 Chromatographic system (see *Chromatography* ⟨621⟩)—The liquid chromatograph is equipped with a 254-nm detector and a 4-mm × 30-cm column that contains packing L11. The flow rate is about 1.5 mL per minute. Chromatograph the *Standard preparation*, and record the peak responses as directed for *Procedure*: the relative retention times are about 0.6 for phenylpropanolamine and 1.0 for theophylline; the resolution, *R*, between phenylpropanolamine and theophylline is not less than 5.0; and the relative standard deviation for replicate injections is not more than 2.0%.
 Procedure—Separately inject equal volumes (about 5 µL) of the *Standard preparation* and the *Assay preparation* into the chromatograph, record the chromatograms, and measure the responses for the major peaks. Calculate the quantity, in mg, of phenylpropanolamine hydrochloride ($C_9H_{13}NO \cdot HCl$) in the portion of Capsules taken by the formula:

$$(250C)(R_U / R_S)$$

in which *C* is the concentration, in mg per mL, of USP Phenylpropanolamine Hydrochloride RS in the *Standard preparation*; and R_U and R_S are the peak response ratios of phenylpropanolamine and theophylline obtained from the *Assay preparation* and the *Standard preparation*, respectively.

Phenylpropanolamine Hydrochloride Extended-Release Capsules

» Phenylpropanolamine Hydrochloride Extended-Release Capsules contain not less than 90.0 percent and not more than 110.0 percent of the labeled amount of phenylpropanolamine hydrochloride ($C_9H_{13}NO \cdot HCl$).

Packaging and storage—Preserve in tight, light-resistant containers.

Labeling—The labeling indicates the USP *Dissolution Test* with which the product complies.

USP Reference standards ⟨11⟩—*USP Phenylpropanolamine Hydrochloride RS.*

Identification—The retention time of the phenylpropanolamine peak in the chromatogram of the *Assay preparation* corresponds to that in the chromatogram of the *Standard preparation*, both relative to the internal standard, as obtained in the *Assay*.

Dissolution ⟨711⟩—
 TEST 1—If the product complies with this test, the labeling indicates that it meets USP *Dissolution Test 1*.
 Medium: water; 1000 mL.
 Apparatus 1: 100 rpm.
 Times: 3, 6, and 12 hours.
 Determine the amount of $C_9H_{13}NO \cdot HCl$ dissolved by employing the following method.
 Solvent A—Dissolve 1.9 g of sodium 1-hexanesulfonate in 700 mL of water, add 50 mL of 1 M monobasic sodium phosphate and 20 mL of 0.25 N triethylammonium phosphate (prepared by mixing 500 mL of a solution containing 25.3 g of triethylamine and 500 mL of a solution containing 9.6 g of phosphoric acid), and mix. Dilute with water to 1 L, and mix.
 Mobile phase—Prepare a filtered and degassed mixture of *Solvent A* and methanol (100 : 82). Make adjustments if necessary (see *System Suitablity* under *Chromatography* ⟨621⟩).
 Chromatographic system (see *Chromatography* ⟨621⟩)—The liquid chromatograph is equipped with a 210-nm detector and a 4.6-mm × 25-cm column that contains packing L1. The flow rate is about 1.5 mL per minute. Chromatograph replicate injections of a *Standard solution*, and record the peak responses as directed for *Procedure*: the tailing factor for the analyte peak is not more than 1.5, and the relative standard deviation for replicate injections is not more than 2%.
 Procedure—Inject an accurately measured volume (about 50 µL) of a filtered portion of the solution under test into the chromatograph, record the chromatogram, and measure the response for the major peak. Calculate the quantity of $C_9H_{13}NO \cdot HCl$ dissolved by comparison with a Standard solution having a known concentration of USP Phenylpropanolamine Hydrochloride RS in the same *Medium* and similarly chromatographed.
 Tolerances—The percentages of the labeled amount of $C_9H_{13}NO \cdot HCl$ dissolved at the times specified conform to *Acceptance Table 2*

Time (hours)	Amount dissolved
3	between 15% and 45%
6	between 40% and 70%
12	not less than 70%

Uniformity of dosage units ⟨905⟩: meet the requirements.

Assay—
 Mobile phase—[NOTE—Prepare the *Mobile phase* one day prior to use.] Prepare a filtered and degassed mixture of water, methanol, 10% tetramethylammonium hydroxide, and phosphoric acid (700 : 300 : 14 : 3.5). Make adjustments if necessary (see *Chromatography* ⟨621⟩).
 Internal standard solution—Prepare a solution of Theophylline in methanol having a final concentration of about 0.1 mg per mL.
 Standard preparation—Prepare a solution of USP Phenylpropanolamine Hydrochloride RS in *Internal standard solution* having an accurately known concentration of 3 mg per mL.

Assay preparation—Transfer the accurately weighed contents of a counted number of Capsules, equivalent to about 750 mg of phenylpropanolamine hydrochloride, to a container. Add 250.0 mL of *Internal standard solution*, mix, sonicate for 30 minutes, allow to stand overnight, and filter.

Chromatographic system (see *Chromatography* ⟨621⟩)—The liquid chromatograph is equipped with a 254-nm detector and a 4-mm × 30-cm column that contains packing L11. The flow rate is about 1.5 mL per minute. Chromatograph replicate injections of the *Standard preparation*, and record the peak responses as directed for *Procedure*: the relative standard deviation is not more than 2.0%, and the resolution, *R*, between phenylpropanolamine and theophylline is not less than 5.0.

Procedure—Separately inject equal volumes (about 5 µL) of the *Standard preparation* and the *Assay preparation* into the chromatograph, record the chromatograms, and measure the responses for the major peaks. The relative retention times are about 0.6 for phenylpropanolamine and 1.0 for theophylline. Calculate the quantity, in mg, of phenylpropanolamine hydrochloride ($C_9H_{13}NO \cdot HCl$) in each of the Capsules taken by the formula:

$$(250C/N)(R_U/R_S)$$

in which *C* is the concentration, in mg per mL, of USP Phenylpropanolamine Hydrochloride RS in the *Standard preparation*; *N* is the number of Capsules taken; and R_U and R_S are the peak response ratios obtained from the *Assay preparation* and the *Standard preparation*, respectively.

Phenylpropanolamine Hydrochloride Oral Solution

» Phenylpropanolamine Hydrochloride Oral Solution contains not less than 90.0 percent and not more than 110.0 percent of the labeled amount of phenylpropanolamine hydrochloride ($C_9H_{13}NO \cdot HCl$).

Packaging and storage—Preserve in tight containers.

USP Reference standards ⟨11⟩—*USP Phenylpropanolamine Hydrochloride RS*.

Identification—The retention time of the major peak in the chromatogram of the *Assay preparation* corresponds to that of the *Standard preparation*, as obtained in the *Assay*.

Uniformity of dosage units ⟨905⟩—
FOR ORAL SOLUTION PACKAGED IN SINGLE-UNIT CONTAINERS: meets the requirements.

Deliverable volume ⟨698⟩—
FOR ORAL SOLUTION PACKAGED IN MULTIPLE-UNIT CONTAINERS: meets the requirements.

Alcohol content (*if present*) ⟨611⟩: between 90.0% and 110.0% of the labeled amount of C_2H_5OH.

Assay—

Solvent A, Mobile phase, Standard preparation, and *Chromatographic system*—Proceed as directed in the *Assay* under *Phenylpropanolamine Hydrochloride Tablets*.

Assay preparation—Transfer an accurately measured volume of Oral Solution, equivalent to about 750 mg of phenylpropanolamine hydrochloride, to a 200-mL volumetric flask, dilute with methanol to volume, and mix. Transfer 1.0 mL of this solution to a 10-mL volumetric flask, dilute with methanol to volume, and mix.

Procedure—Proceed as directed for *Procedure* in the *Assay* under *Phenylpropanolamine Hydrochloride Tablets*. Calculate the quantity, in mg per mL, of phenylpropanolamine hydrochloride ($C_9H_{13}NO \cdot HCl$) in the portion of Oral Solution taken by the formula:

$$2(C/V)(r_U/r_S)$$

in which *C* is the concentration, in µg per mL, of USP Phenylpropanolamine Hydrochloride RS in the *Standard preparation*; *V* is the volume, in mL, of Oral Solution taken; and r_U and r_S are the peak responses obtained from the *Assay preparation* and the *Standard preparation*, respectively.

Phenylpropanolamine Hydrochloride Tablets

» Phenylpropanolamine Hydrochloride Tablets contain not less than 90.0 percent and not more than 110.0 percent of the labeled amount of phenylpropanolamine hydrochloride ($C_9H_{13}NO \cdot HCl$).

Packaging and storage—Preserve in tight, light-resistant containers.

USP Reference standards ⟨11⟩—*USP Phenylpropanolamine Hydrochloride RS*.

Identification—The retention time of the major peak in the chromatogram of the *Assay preparation* corresponds to that in the chromatogram of the *Standard preparation*, as obtained in the *Assay*.

Dissolution, *Procedure for a pooled sample* ⟨711⟩—
Medium: water; 900 mL.
Apparatus 2: 50 rpm.
Time: 45 minutes.
Procedure—Determine the amount of phenylpropanolamine hydrochloride dissolved, employing the procedure set forth in the *Assay*, making any necessary volumetric adjustments.
Tolerances—Not less than 75% (*Q*) of the labeled amount of $C_9H_{13}NO \cdot HCl$ is dissolved in 45 minutes.

Uniformity of dosage units ⟨905⟩: meet the requirements.

Assay—

Solvent A—Dissolve 1.9 g of sodium 1-hexanesulfonate in 700 mL of water, add 50 mL of 1 M monobasic sodium phosphate and 20 mL of 0.25 N triethylammonium phosphate (prepared by mixing 500 mL of a solution containing 25.3 g of triethylamine and 500 mL of a solution containing 9.6 g of phosphoric acid), and mix. Dilute with water to 1 liter, and mix.

Mobile phase—Prepare a filtered and degassed mixture of *Solvent A* and methanol (100 : 82). Make adjustments if necessary (see *Chromatography* ⟨621⟩).

Standard preparation—Dissolve an accurately weighed quantity of USP Phenylpropanolamine Hydrochloride RS in methanol, and dilute quantitatively with methanol to obtain a solution having a known concentration of about 375 µg per mL.

Assay preparation—Weigh and finely powder not fewer than 20 Tablets. Transfer an accurately weighed portion of the powder, equivalent to about 750 mg of phenylpropanolamine hydrochloride, to a 200-mL volumetric flask. Add about 150 mL of methanol, and sonicate for about 10 minutes. Dilute with methanol to volume, and mix. Transfer 10.0 mL of this solution to a 100-mL volumetric flask, dilute with methanol to volume, mix, and filter.

Chromatographic system (see *Chromatography* ⟨621⟩)—The liquid chromatograph is equipped with a 254-nm detector and a 3.9-mm × 30-cm column that contains packing L1. The flow rate is about 1.5 mL per minute. Chromatograph the *Standard preparation*, and record the peak responses as directed for *Procedure*: the tailing factor for the analyte peak is not more than 2.5; and the relative standard deviation for replicate injections is not more than 2.0%.

Procedure—Separately inject equal volumes (about 70 µL) of the *Standard preparation* and the *Assay preparation* into the chromatograph, record the chromatograms, and measure the responses for the major peaks. Calculate the quantity, in mg, of $C_9H_{13}NO \cdot HCl$ in the portion of Tablets taken by the formula:

$$2C(r_U/r_S)$$

in which *C* is the concentration, in µg per mL, of USP Phenylpropanolamine Hydrochloride RS in the *Standard preparation*; and r_U and r_S are the peak responses obtained from the *Assay preparation* and the *Standard preparation*, respectively.

Phenylpropanolamine Hydrochloride Extended-Release Tablets

» Phenylpropanolamine Hydrochloride Extended-Release Tablets contain not less than 90.0 percent and not more than 110.0 percent of the labeled amount of phenylpropanolamine hydrochloride ($C_9H_{13}NO \cdot HCl$).

Packaging and storage—Preserve in tight, light-resistant containers.
Labeling—The labeling states the in vitro *Dissolution* test conditions of *Times* and *Tolerances,* as directed under *Dissolution.*
USP Reference standards ⟨11⟩—*USP Phenylpropanolamine Hydrochloride RS.*
Identification—The retention time of the phenylpropanolamine peak in the chromatogram of the *Assay preparation* corresponds to that in the chromatogram of the *Standard preparation,* both relative to the internal standard, as obtained in the *Assay.*
Dissolution ⟨711⟩—
  Medium: water; 1000 mL.
  Apparatus 1: 100 rpm.
  Times and *Tolerances:* as specified in the *Labeling;* use *Acceptance Table 2.*
  Determine the amount of $C_9H_{13}NO \cdot HCl$ dissolved, employing the following method.
  Solvent A, Mobile phase, Chromatographic system, and *Procedure*—Proceed as directed in *Test 1* for *Dissolution* under *Phenylpropanolamine Hydrochloride Extended-Release Capsules.*
Uniformity of dosage units ⟨905⟩: meet the requirements.
Assay—
  Solvent A—Dissolve 1.9 g of sodium 1-hexanesulfonate in 700 mL of water, add 50 mL of 1 M monobasic sodium phosphate and 20 mL of 0.25 N triethylammonium phosphate (prepared by mixing 500 mL of a solution containing 25.3 g of triethylamine and 500 mL of a solution containing 9.6 g of phosphoric acid), and mix. Dilute with water to 1 L, and mix.
  Mobile phase—Prepare a filtered and degassed mixture of *Solvent A* and methanol (100 : 82). Make adjustments if necessary (see *Chromatography* ⟨621⟩).
  Standard preparation—Dissolve an accurately weighed quantity of USP Phenylpropanolamine Hydrochloride RS in methanol, and quantitatively dilute with methanol to obtain a solution having a known concentration of about 375 µg per mL.
  Assay preparation—Weigh and finely powder not fewer than 20 Tablets. Transfer an accurately weighed portion of the powder, equivalent to about 750 mg of phenylpropanolamine hydrochloride, to a 200-mL volumetric flask. Add about 150 mL of methanol and sonicate for about 10 minutes. Dilute with methanol to volume, and mix. Transfer 10.0 mL of this solution to a 100-mL volumetric flask, dilute with methanol to volume, and mix. Use a filtered portion of the solution.
  Chromatographic system (see *Chromatography* ⟨621⟩)—The liquid chromatograph is equipped with a 254-nm detector and a 3.9-mm × 30-cm column that contains packing L1. The flow rate is about 1.5 mL per minute. Chromatograph the *Standard preparation,* and record the peak responses as directed for *Procedure:* the tailing factor for the analyte peak is not more than 2.5, and the relative standard deviation for replicate injections is not more than 2.0%.
  Procedure—Inject an accurately measured volume (about 70 µL) of the *Standard preparation* and the *Assay preparation* into the chromatograph, record the chromatograms, and measure the responses for the major peaks. Calculate the quantity, in mg, of phenylpropanolamine hydrochloride ($C_9H_{13}NO \cdot HCl$) in the portion of Tablets taken by the formula:

$$2C(r_U / r_S)$$

in which C is the concentration, in µg per mL, of USP Phenylpropanolamine Hydrochloride RS; and r_U and r_S are the peak responses obtained from the *Assay preparation* and the *Standard preparation,* respectively.

Phenyltoloxamine Citrate

$C_{17}H_{21}NO \cdot C_6H_8O_7$ 447.47
N,N-Dimethyl-2-(α-phenyl-*o*-tolyloxy)ethylamine, citrate (1 : 1) salt.
2-(2-Dimethylaminoethoxy)diphenylmethane, citrate (1 : 1) salt
Phenyltoloxamine dihydrogen citrate   [1176-08-5].

» Phenyltoloxamine Citrate contains not less than 99.0 percent and not more than 101.0 percent of $C_{17}H_{21}NO \cdot C_6H_8O_7$, calculated on the dried basis.

Packaging and storage—Preserve in well-closed containers. Store at room temperature.
USP Reference standards ⟨11⟩—*USP Phenyltoloxamine Citrate RS. USP Phenyltoloxamine Related Compound A RS.*
Identification, *Infrared Absorption* ⟨197K⟩.
Melting range, *Class Ia* ⟨741⟩: between 137° and 143°.
pH ⟨791⟩: between 3.2 and 4.2, in a solution (1 in 100).
Loss on drying ⟨731⟩—Dry it in vacuum at 80° for 3 hours: it loses not more than 0.5% of its weight.
Residue on ignition ⟨281⟩: not more than 0.1%.
Heavy metals, *Method I* ⟨231⟩: 20 µg per g.
Related compounds—
  Resolution solution—In a separatory funnel dissolve about 10 mg each of USP Phenyltoloxamine Citrate RS and USP Phenyltoloxamine Related Compound A RS, accurately weighed, in 50 mL of water. Add 5 mL of ammonium hydroxide, and extract with three 10-mL portions of methylene chloride. Combine the extracts, dry the solution over anhydrous sodium sulfate, and gently evaporate to dryness. Dissolve the residue in 20 mL of methylene chloride.
  Test solution—In a separatory funnel dissolve about 400 mg of Phenyltoloxamine Citrate, accurately weighed, in 50 mL of water. Proceed as directed for *Resolution solution,* beginning with "Add 5 mL of ammonium hydroxide."
  Chromatographic system (see *Chromatography* ⟨621⟩)—The gas chromatograph is equipped with a split injection system, a flame-ionization detector, and a 0.32-mm × 25-m column coated with a 0.45-µm film of phase G27. The carrier gas is helium, flowing at a rate of about 29 cm per second, with a split flow rate of about 25 mL per minute. The column temperature is programmed as follows. Initially the temperature of the column is equilibrated at 190° for 3 minutes, then the temperature is increased at a rate of 4° per minute to 240°, and maintained at 240° for 8 minutes. The injection port and the detector temperatures are maintained at 280°. Chromatograph the *Resolution solution,* and record the peak responses as directed for *Procedure:* the resolution, R, between phenyltoloxamine and phenyltoloxamine related compound A is not less than 1.5.
  Procedure—Inject a volume (about 1 µL) of the *Test solution* into the chromatograph, record the chromatograms, and measure the peak responses. Calculate the percentage of each impurity in the portion of Phenyltoloxamine Citrate taken by the formula:

$$100(r_i / r_s)$$

in which r_i is the peak response of each impurity; and r_s is the sum of the responses of all the peaks, excluding the solvent peaks: not more than 0.2% of phenyltoloxamine related compound A; not more than 0.1% of any other individual impurity; and not more than 1.0% of total impurities is found.
Organic volatile impurities, *Method I* ⟨467⟩: meets the requirements.

(Official until July 1, 2008)
Assay—Dissolve about 0.5 g of Phenyltoloxamine Citrate, accurately weighed, in 80 mL of glacial acetic acid, and titrate with 0.1 N perchloric acid VS, determining the endpoint potentiometrically. Perform a blank determination, and make any necessary cor-

rection (see Titrimetry ⟨541⟩). Each mL of 0.1 N perchloric acid is equivalent to 44.75 mg of $C_{17}H_{21}NO \cdot C_6H_8O_7$.

Phenytoin

$C_{15}H_{12}N_2O_2$ 252.27
2,4-Imidazolidinedione, 5,5-diphenyl-.
5,5-Diphenylhydantoin   [57-41-0].

» Phenytoin contains not less than 98.0 percent and not more than 102.0 percent of $C_{15}H_{12}N_2O_2$, calculated on the dried basis.

Packaging and storage—Preserve in tight containers.
USP Reference standards ⟨11⟩—USP Phenytoin RS.
Clarity and color of solution—Dissolve 1 g in a mixture of 5 mL of 1 N sodium hydroxide and 20 mL of water: the solution is clear and not darker than pale yellow.
Identification, Infrared Absorption ⟨197K⟩.
Loss on drying ⟨731⟩—Dry it at 105° for 4 hours: it loses not more than 1.0% of its weight.
Heavy metals, Method II ⟨231⟩: 0.002%.
Chromatographic purity—
  Mobile phase—Prepare as directed in the Assay.
  Standard solution—Dissolve an accurately weighed quantity of USP Phenytoin RS in methanol, and dilute quantitatively, and stepwise if necessary, with methanol to obtain a solution having a known concentration of about 10 µg per mL.
  Test solution—Use Assay preparation A, prepared as directed in the Assay.
  Resolution solution—Prepare a solution of benzoin in methanol having a concentration of about 10 µg per mL. Dissolve 10 mg of USP Phenytoin RS in 10.0 mL of the benzoin solution.
  Chromatographic system (see Chromatography ⟨621⟩)—The liquid chromatograph is equipped with a 220-nm detector and a 4.6-mm × 25-cm column that contains 5-µm packing L1. The flow rate is about 1.5 mL per minute. Chromatograph the Resolution solution, and record the peak responses as directed for Procedure: the relative retention times are about 0.75 for phenytoin and 1.0 for benzoin; and the resolution, R, is not less than 1.5.
  Procedure—[NOTE—Use peak areas where peak responses are indicated.] Separately inject equal volumes (about 20 µL) of the Standard solution and the Test solution into the chromatograph, record the chromatograms, and measure the responses for all of the peaks. Calculate the percentage of each impurity peak in the Test solution taken by the formula:

$$100(C/D)(r_i/r_S)$$

in which C is the concentration, in µg per mL, of USP Phenytoin RS in the Standard solution; D is the concentration, in µg per mL, of phenytoin in the Test solution; r_i is the peak response for each impurity; and r_S is the peak response for phenytoin in the Standard solution: not more than 0.9% total impurities is found, excluding benzophenone.
Limit of benzophenone—
  Mobile phase and *Test solution*—Prepare as directed in the test for Chromatographic purity.
  Standard solution—Dissolve an accurately weighed quantity of benzophenone in methanol, and dilute quantitatively, and stepwise if necessary, with methanol to obtain a solution having a known concentration of about 1.0 µg per mL.
  Chromatographic system (see Chromatography ⟨621⟩)—Use the same system as directed in the test for Chromatographic purity except to chromatograph three injections of the Standard solution, and record the peak responses as directed for Procedure: the relative standard deviation is not more than 5.0%.
  Procedure—[NOTE—Use peak areas where peak responses are indicated.] Separately inject equal volumes (about 20 µL) of the Standard solution and the Test solution into the chromatograph, record the chromatograms, and measure the responses for all of the peaks. The relative retention times are about 0.25 for phenytoin and 1.0 for benzophenone. Calculate the percentage of benzophenone in the portion of Phenytoin taken by the formula:

$$100(C/D)(r_U/r_S)$$

in which C is the concentration, in µg per mL, of benzophenone in the Standard solution; D is the concentration, in µg per mL, of phenytoin in the Test solution; and r_U and r_S are the benzophenone peak responses obtained from the Test solution and the Standard solution, respectively: not more than 0.1% of benzophenone is found.
Organic volatile impurities, Method V ⟨467⟩: meets the requirements.
  Solvent—Use dimethyl sulfoxide.

(Official until July 1, 2008)

Assay—
  Mobile phase—Prepare a filtered and degassed mixture of methanol and water (55 : 45). Make adjustments if necessary (see System Suitability under Chromatography ⟨621⟩).
  Standard preparation—Dissolve, with the aid of sonication if necessary, an accurately weighed quantity of USP Phenytoin RS in Mobile phase, and dilute quantitatively, and stepwise if necessary, with Mobile phase to obtain a solution having a known concentration of about 100 µg per mL.
  Assay preparation—Transfer about 100 mg of Phenytoin, accurately weighed, to a 100-mL volumetric flask, dissolve in and dilute with methanol to volume, and mix (Assay preparation A). Transfer 10.0 mL of this solution to a second 100-mL volumetric flask, dilute with Mobile phase to volume, and mix (Assay preparation B).
  Resolution solution—Prepare a solution of benzoin in Mobile phase having a concentration of about 1.5 mg per mL. Mix 1.0 mL of this solution and 9.0 mL of the Standard preparation.
  Chromatographic system (see Chromatography ⟨621⟩)—The liquid chromatograph is equipped with a 220-nm detector and a 4.6-mm × 25-cm column that contains 5-µm packing L1. The flow rate is about 1.5 mL per minute. Chromatograph the Standard preparation, and record the peak responses as directed for Procedure: the relative standard deviation is not more than 1.0%. Chromatograph the Resolution solution. The relative retention times are about 0.75 for phenytoin and 1.0 for benzoin; the resolution, R, is not less than 1.5; and the tailing factor for the phenytoin peak is not more than 1.5.
  Procedure—Separately inject equal volumes (about 20 µL) of the Standard preparation and Assay preparation B into the chromatograph, record the chromatograms, and measure the responses for the major peaks. Calculate the quantity, in mg, of $C_{15}H_{12}N_2O_2$ in the portion of Phenytoin taken by the formula:

$$(1000C)(r_U/r_S)$$

in which C is the concentration, in mg per mL, of USP Phenytoin RS in the Standard preparation; and r_U and r_S are the peak responses obtained from the Assay preparation and the Standard preparation, respectively.

Phenytoin Oral Suspension

» Phenytoin Oral Suspension is Phenytoin suspended in a suitable medium. It contains not less than 95.0 percent and not more than 105.0 percent of the labeled amount of phenytoin ($C_{15}H_{12}N_2O_2$).

Packaging and storage—Preserve in tight containers. Avoid freezing.
Labeling—The label bears a statement that the patient must use an accurately calibrated measuring device with multiple-dose containers.

USP Reference standards ⟨11⟩—USP Phenytoin RS.
Identification—
  A: Shake a volume of Oral Suspension, equivalent to about 100 mg of phenytoin, with 50 mL of a mixture of ether and chloroform (1 in 2) in a separator, evaporate the extract to dryness, and dry in vacuum at 105° for 4 hours: the phenytoin so obtained melts between 292° and 299° with some decomposition, the procedure for *Class I* being used (see *Melting Range or Temperature* ⟨741⟩).
  B: Dissolve 50 mg of the residue obtained in *Identification* test A in 50 mL of chloroform, with slight warming if necessary. To 5 mL of this solution add 0.2 mL of a freshly prepared solution of cobaltous acetate in methanol (1 in 100) and 1 mL of a freshly prepared solution of isopropylamine in methanol (1 in 20), and mix: a violet to red-violet color is produced.

Dissolution ⟨711⟩—
  0.05 M Tris buffer—Dissolve 36.3 g of tris(hydroxymethyl)aminomethane and 60 g of sodium lauryl sulfate in 6 L of water, adjust with hydrochloric acid to a pH of 7.5 ± 0.05, and degas.
  Medium: 0.05 M Tris buffer; 900 mL.
  Apparatus 2: 35 rpm.
  Time: 60 minutes.
  Dissolution procedure—Shake the sample suspension well, about 100 shakes. Using a 5-mL syringe, collect approximately 5 mL of suspension, and record the weight. With the paddles lowered, gently empty the contents of each syringe into the bottom of each vessel containing the *Medium*. Start rotating the paddles. Reweigh each syringe, and determine the amount of suspension delivered into each vessel. At the end of 60 minutes, remove 4 mL from each vessel, and pass through a 0.45-μm nylon filter presaturated with *Medium*.
  Determine the amount of $C_{15}H_{12}N_2O_2$ dissolved by employing the following method.
  0.02 M Sodium phosphate buffer—Dissolve 2.76 g of monobasic sodium phosphate in 1 L of water.
  Mobile phase—Prepare a filtered and degassed mixture of *0.02 M Sodium phosphate buffer*, methanol, and acetonitrile (50 : 27 : 23), and mix. Adjust with phosphoric acid to a pH of 3.0. Make adjustments if necessary (see *System Suitability* under *Chromatography* ⟨621⟩).
  Standard solution—Transfer about 70 mg of USP Phenytoin RS, accurately weighed, to a 500-mL volumetric flask. Dissolve in 15 mL of methanol, dilute with *Medium* to volume, and mix.
  Chromatographic system (see *Chromatography* ⟨621⟩)—The liquid chromatograph is equipped with a 240-nm detector and a 4.6-mm × 15-cm column that contains packing L1. The flow rate is about 1 mL per minute. Chromatograph the *Standard solution*, and record the responses as directed for *Procedure*: the column efficiency is not less than 5400 theoretical plates; the tailing factor is not more than 2.0; and the relative standard deviation for replicate injections is not more than 2.0%.
  Procedure—Separately inject equal volumes (about 10 μL) of the *Standard solution* and the solution under test into the chromatograph, record the chromatograms, and measure the responses for the major peaks. Calculate the quantity, in mg, of $C_{15}H_{12}N_2O_2$ dissolved. [NOTE—The density of Oral Suspension must be determined and used in calculating the quantity, in mg, of phenytoin dissolved.]
  Tolerances—Not less than 80% (Q) of the labeled amount of $C_{15}H_{12}N_2O_2$ is dissolved in 60 minutes.

Uniformity of dosage units ⟨905⟩—
  FOR ORAL SUSPENSION PACKAGED IN SINGLE-UNIT CONTAINERS: meets the requirements.

Deliverable volume ⟨698⟩—
  FOR ORAL SUSPENSION PACKAGED IN MULTIPLE-UNIT CONTAINERS: meets the requirements.

Assay—
  Mobile phase—Prepare a filtered and degassed mixture of water, methanol, acetonitrile, 0.5% triethylamine in water, and 1.74 N acetic acid (191 : 100 : 40 : 1.3 : 1). Make adjustments if necessary.
  Standard preparation—Dissolve an accurately weighed quantity of USP Phenytoin RS in methanol, and dilute quantitatively, and stepwise if necessary, with *Mobile phase* to obtain a solution having a known concentration of about 0.625 mg per mL.
  Assay preparation—Transfer a quantity of Oral Suspension, equivalent to about 125 mg of phenytoin, into a 200-mL volumetric flask, rinse the pipet with 40 mL of methanol, and add the rinsings to the flask. Add about 50 mL of *Mobile phase*, dilute with methanol to volume, mix, sonicate, and filter.
  Chromatographic system (see *Chromatography* ⟨621⟩)—The liquid chromatograph is equipped with a 229-nm detector and a 4.6-mm × 25-cm column that contains packing L1. The flow rate is about 1.5 mL per minute. Chromatograph the *Standard preparation*, and record the peak responses as directed for *Procedure*: the tailing factor is not more than 1.5; and the relative standard deviation for replicate injections is not more than 2.0%.
  Procedure—Separately inject equal volumes (about 10 μL) of the *Standard preparation* and the *Assay preparation* into the chromatograph, record the chromatograms, and measure the responses for the major peaks. Calculate the quantity, in mg, of phenytoin ($C_{15}H_{12}N_2O_2$) in the portion of Oral Suspension taken by the formula:

$$200C(r_U / r_S)$$

in which *C* is the concentration, in mg per mL, of USP Phenytoin RS in the *Standard preparation*; and r_U and r_S are the peak responses obtained from the *Assay preparation* and the *Standard preparation*, respectively.

Phenytoin Tablets

(Current title—not to change until February 1, 2010)
Monograph title change—to become official February 1, 2010
See **Phenytoin Chewable Tablets**

» Phenytoin Tablets contain not less than 95.0 percent and not more than 105.0 percent of the labeled amount of $C_{15}H_{12}N_2O_2$.

Packaging and storage—Preserve in well-closed containers.
Labeling—Label the Tablets to indicate that they are to be chewed.

USP Reference standards ⟨11⟩—USP Phenytoin RS.
Identification—The retention time of the major peak in the chromatogram of the *Assay preparation* corresponds to that in the chromatogram of the *Standard preparation*, as obtained in the *Assay*.

Dissolution ⟨711⟩—
  0.05 M Tris buffer—Dissolve 60.5 g of tris(hydroxymethyl)aminomethane in 6 liters of water. Dilute with water to 10 liters, and adjust with phosphoric acid to a pH of 9.0 ± 0.05. Dissolve 100 g of sodium lauryl sulfate in about 6 liters of the prepared buffer, transfer this solution to the remaining buffer solution, and mix.
  Medium: 0.05 M Tris buffer; 900 mL.
  Apparatus 2: 100 rpm.
  Time: 120 minutes.
  Determine the amount of $C_{15}H_{12}N_2O_2$ dissolved by employing the following method.
  Triethylamine solution, Mobile phase, and *Chromatographic system*—Proceed as directed in the *Assay*.
  Standard solution—Dissolve an accurately weighed quantity of USP Phenytoin RS in methanol to obtain a solution having a known concentration of 3.0 mg per mL. Transfer a portion of this solution to a suitable container, and dilute quantitatively, and stepwise if necessary, with *Dissolution Medium* to obtain a concentration of 0.06 mg per mL. Transfer 10.0 mL of this solution to a 50-mL volumetric flask, dilute with *Mobile phase* to volume, and mix.
  Test solution—Withdraw a portion of the solution under test, and filter, discarding the first 3 mL of the filtrate. Pipet 10.0 mL of this solution into a 50-mL volumetric flask, dilute with *Mobile phase* to volume, and mix.
  Procedure—Separately inject equal volumes (about 25 μL) of the *Standard solution* and the *Test solution* into the chromatograph, record the chromatograms, and measure the areas of the peak responses. Determine the amount of $C_{15}H_{12}N_2O_2$ dissolved by comparison of the peak responses obtained from the *Standard solution* and the *Test solution*.
  Tolerances—Not less than 70% (Q) of the labeled amount of $C_{15}H_{12}N_2O_2$ is dissolved in 120 minutes.

Uniformity of dosage units ⟨905⟩: meet the requirements.

Assay—

*Triethylamine solution—*Transfer 1 mL of triethylamine to a 100-mL volumetric flask, dilute with water to volume, and mix.

*Mobile phase—*Prepare a filtered and degassed mixture of water, methanol, acetonitrile, *Triethylamine solution,* and acetic acid (500 : 270 : 230 : 5 : 1). Make adjustments if necessary (see *System Suitability* under *Chromatography* ⟨621⟩).

*Standard preparation—*Dissolve an accurately weighed quantity of USP Phenytoin RS in *Mobile phase,* and dilute quantitatively, and stepwise if necessary, with *Mobile phase* to obtain a solution having a known concentration of about 0.5 mg per mL.

*Assay preparation—*Weigh and finely powder not fewer than 20 Tablets. Transfer an accurately weighed portion of the powder, equivalent to about 250 mg of phenytoin, to a 500-mL volumetric flask, dissolve in and dilute with *Mobile phase* to volume, and mix.

Chromatographic system (see *Chromatography* ⟨621⟩)—The liquid chromatograph is equipped with a 254-nm detector and a 4.6-mm × 25-cm column that contains packing L1. The flow rate is about 1.5 mL per minute. Chromatograph the *Standard preparation,* and record the peak responses as directed for *Procedure:* the column efficiency is not less than 6500 theoretical plates, the tailing factor is not more than 1.5, and the relative standard deviation for replicate injections is not more than 2.0%.

*Procedure—*Separately inject equal volumes (about 25 μL) of the *Standard preparation* and the *Assay preparation* into the chromatograph, record the chromatograms, and measure the responses for the major peaks. Calculate the quantity, in mg, of $C_{15}H_{12}N_2O_2$ in the portion of Tablets taken by the formula:

$$500C(r_U / r_S)$$

in which *C* is the concentration, in mg per mL, of USP Phenytoin RS in the *Standard preparation,* and r_U and r_S are the peak responses obtained from the *Assay preparation* and the *Standard preparation,* respectively.

Phenytoin Chewable Tablets

(Monograph under this new title—to become official February 1, 2010)
(Current monograph title is Phenytoin Tablets)

» Phenytoin Chewable Tablets contain not less than 95.0 percent and not more than 105.0 percent of the labeled amount of $C_{15}H_{12}N_2O_2$.

Packaging and storage—Preserve in well-closed containers.

Labeling—Label the Chewable Tablets to indicate that they are to be chewed.

USP Reference standards ⟨11⟩—*USP Phenytoin RS.*

Identification—The retention time of the major peak in the chromatogram of the *Assay preparation* corresponds to that of the major peak in the chromatogram of the *Standard preparation,* as obtained in the *Assay.*

Dissolution ⟨711⟩—

*0.05 M Tris buffer—*Dissolve 60.5 g of tris(hydroxymethyl)aminomethane in 6 L of water. Dilute with water to 10 L, and adjust with phosphoric acid to a pH of 9.0 ± 0.05. Dissolve 100 g of sodium dodecyl sulfate in about 6 L of the prepared buffer, transfer this solution to the remaining buffer solution, and mix.

Medium: 0.05 M Tris buffer; 900 mL.
Apparatus 2: 100 rpm.
Time: 120 minutes.

Determine the amount of $C_{15}H_{12}N_2O_2$ dissolved by employing the following method.

Triethylamine solution, Mobile phase, and *Chromatographic system—*Proceed as directed in the *Assay.*

*Standard solution—*Dissolve an accurately weighed quantity of USP Phenytoin RS in methanol to obtain a solution having a known concentration of 3.0 mg per mL. Transfer a portion of this solution to a suitable container, and dilute quantitatively, and stepwise if necessary, with *Medium* to obtain a concentration of 0.06 mg per mL. Transfer 10.0 mL of this solution to a 50-mL volumetric flask, dilute with *Mobile phase* to volume, and mix.

*Test solution—*Withdraw a portion of the solution under test, and filter, discarding the first 3 mL of the filtrate. Pipet 10.0 mL of this solution into a 50-mL volumetric flask, dilute with *Mobile phase* to volume, and mix.

*Procedure—*Separately inject equal volumes (about 25 μL) of the *Standard solution* and the *Test solution* into the chromatograph, record the chromatograms, and measure the areas of the peak responses. Determine the amount of $C_{15}H_{12}N_2O_2$ dissolved by comparison of the peak responses obtained from the *Standard solution* and the *Test solution.*

*Tolerances—*Not less than 70% *(Q)* of the labeled amount of $C_{15}H_{12}N_2O_2$ is dissolved in 120 minutes.

Uniformity of dosage units ⟨905⟩: meet the requirements.

Assay—

*Triethylamine solution—*Transfer 1 mL of triethylamine to a 100-mL volumetric flask, dilute with water to volume, and mix.

*Mobile phase—*Prepare a filtered and degassed mixture of water, methanol, acetonitrile, *Triethylamine solution,* and acetic acid (500 : 270 : 230 : 5 : 1). Make adjustments if necessary (see *System Suitability* under *Chromatography* ⟨621⟩).

*Standard preparation—*Dissolve an accurately weighed quantity of USP Phenytoin RS in *Mobile phase,* and dilute quantitatively, and stepwise if necessary, with *Mobile phase* to obtain a solution having a known concentration of about 0.5 mg per mL.

*Assay preparation—*Weigh and finely powder not fewer than 20 Chewable Tablets. Transfer an accurately weighed portion of the powder, equivalent to about 250 mg of phenytoin, to a 500-mL volumetric flask, dissolve in and dilute with *Mobile phase* to volume, and mix.

Chromatographic system (see *Chromatography* ⟨621⟩)—The liquid chromatograph is equipped with a 254-nm detector and a 4.6-mm × 25-cm column that contains packing L1. The flow rate is about 1.5 mL per minute. Chromatograph the *Standard preparation,* and record the peak responses as directed for *Procedure:* the column efficiency is not less than 6500 theoretical plates; the tailing factor is not more than 1.5; and the relative standard deviation for replicate injections is not more than 2.0%.

*Procedure—*Separately inject equal volumes (about 25 μL) of the *Standard preparation* and the *Assay preparation* into the chromatograph, record the chromatograms, and measure the responses for the major peaks. Calculate the quantity, in mg, of $C_{15}H_{12}N_2O_2$ in the portion of Chewable Tablets taken by the formula:

$$500C(r_U / r_S)$$

in which *C* is the concentration, in mg per mL, of USP Phenytoin RS in the *Standard preparation;* and r_U and r_S are the peak responses obtained from the *Assay preparation* and the *Standard preparation,* respectively.

(Official February 1, 2010)

Phenytoin Sodium

$C_{15}H_{11}N_2NaO_2$ 274.25
2,4-Imidazolidinedione, 5,5-diphenyl-, monosodium salt.
5,5-Diphenylhydantoin sodium salt   [630-93-3].

» Phenytoin Sodium contains not less than 98.0 percent and not more than 102.0 percent of $C_{15}H_{11}N_2NaO_2$, calculated on the dried basis.

Packaging and storage—Preserve in tight containers.

USP Reference standards ⟨11⟩—*USP Phenytoin RS. USP Phenytoin Related Compound A RS. USP Phenytoin Related Compound B RS.*

Clarity and color of solution—Dissolve 1.0 g in 20 mL of carbon dioxide-free water, and add 0.10 N sodium hydroxide until the hydrolyzed phenytoin is dissolved: not more than 4.0 mL of the 0.10 N sodium hydroxide is required to produce a clear, colorless solution.

Identification—
A: Dissolve about 300 mg of Phenytoin Sodium, accurately weighed, in about 50 mL of water in a separator. Add 10 mL of 3 N hydrochloric acid, and extract with three successive portions, measuring 100, 60, and 30 mL, respectively, of a 1 in 2 mixture of ether and chloroform. Evaporate the combined extracts, and dry the residue of phenytoin at 105° for 4 hours: the IR absorption spectrum of a potassium bromide dispersion of the residue so obtained exhibits maxima only at the same wavelengths as that of a similar preparation of USP Phenytoin RS.
B: It responds to the flame test for *Sodium* ⟨191⟩.
Loss on drying ⟨731⟩—Dry it at 105° for 4 hours: it loses not more than 2.5% of its weight.
Heavy metals, *Method II* ⟨231⟩: 0.002%.
Related compounds—
Mobile phase, Standard stock preparation, System suitability stock solution, and *System suitability solution*—Prepare as directed in the *Assay.*
Standard solution—Dissolve accurately weighed quantities of benzophenone, USP Phenytoin RS, USP Phenytoin Related Compound A RS, and USP Phenytoin Related Compound B RS in *Mobile phase,* and dilute quantitatively, and stepwise if necessary, with *Mobile phase* to obtain a solution having known concentrations of 0.5 μg per mL, 1 μg per mL, 9 μg per mL, and 9 μg per mL, respectively.
Test solution—Use the *Assay stock preparation.*
Chromatographic system—Proceed as directed in the *Assay,* except to inject the *Standard solution* instead of the *Standard preparation:* the relative standard deviation for replicate injections is not more than 5.0% for each compound.
Procedure—Separately inject equal volumes (about 20 μL) of the *Standard solution* and the *Test solution* into the chromatograph, record the chromatograms, and measure the peak responses. Calculate the percentage of phenytoin related compound A, phenytoin related compound B, and benzophenone in the portion of Phenytoin Sodium taken by the formula:

$$100(C/D)(r_i / r_S)$$

in which C is the concentration, in μg per mL, of the respective analyte in the *Standard solution;* D is the concentration, in μg per mL, of Phenytoin Sodium in the *Test solution;* and r_i and r_S are the peak responses for phenytoin related compound A, phenytoin related compound B, or benzophenone obtained from the *Test solution* and the *Standard solution,* respectively: not more than 0.9% each of phenytoin related compound A and phenytoin related compound B is found, and not more than 0.1% of benzophenone is found. Calculate the percentage of every other impurity in the portion of Phenytoin Sodium taken by the formula:

$$100(274.25/252.27)(C/D)(r_i / r_S)$$

in which C is the concentration, in μg per mL, of USP Phenytoin RS in the *Standard solution;* 274.25 and 252.27 are the molecular weights of phenytoin sodium and phenytoin, respectively; r_i and r_S are the peak responses of each impurity obtained from the *Test solution* and the *Standard solution,* respectively; and the other term is as defined above. Not more than 0.9% of total impurities is found, excluding benzophenone.
Organic volatile impurities, *Method V* ⟨467⟩: meets the requirements.
Solvent—Use dimethyl sulfoxide.

(Official until July 1, 2008)

Assay—
Mobile phase—Prepare a filtered and degassed mixture of 0.05 M monobasic ammonium phosphate buffer, adjusted to a pH of 2.5 with phosphoric acid, acetonitrile, and methanol (45 : 35 : 20). Make adjustments if necessary (see *System Suitability* under *Chromatography* ⟨621⟩).
Standard stock preparation—Transfer about 100 mg of USP Phenytoin RS, accurately weighed, to a 100-mL volumetric flask, dissolve in *Mobile phase,* and sonicate, if necessary, to dissolve.
System suitability stock solution—Transfer 5.0 mL of the *Standard stock preparation* to a 50-mL volumetric flask, and dilute with *Mobile phase* to volume to obtain a solution having a known concentration of about 100 μg per mL.
System suitability solution—Transfer about 75.0 mg of benzoin to a 50-mL volumetric flask, dissolve in 10 mL of methanol, and dilute with a mixture of 0.05 M monobasic ammonium phosphate buffer, previously adjusted with phosphoric acid to a pH of 2.5 and acetonitrile (45 : 35), to volume. Transfer 1.0 mL of the solution so obtained to a 10-mL volumetric flask, and dilute with the *System suitability stock solution* to volume.
Standard preparation—Transfer 5 mL of the *Standard stock preparation* to a 100-mL volumetric flask, and dilute with *Mobile phase* to volume.
Assay stock preparation—Transfer about 100 mg of Phenytoin Sodium, accurately weighed, to a 100-mL volumetric flask, dissolve in and dilute with *Mobile phase* to volume, and mix.
Assay preparation—Transfer 5.0 mL of the *Assay stock preparation* to a 100-mL volumetric flask, dilute with *Mobile phase* to volume, and mix.
Chromatographic system—The liquid chromatograph is equipped with a 220-nm detector and a 4.6-mm × 25-cm column that contains 5-μm packing L1. The flow rate is about 1.5 mL per minute. Chromatograph the *Standard preparation,* and record the responses as directed for *Procedure:* the relative standard deviation for replicate injections is not more than 1.0%. Chromatograph the *System suitability solution,* and record the peak responses as directed for *Procedure:* the relative retention times are 1.0 for phenytoin and about 1.3 for benzoin; the column efficiency is not less than 9400 theoretical plates for the phenytoin peak; the tailing factor is not more than 1.5; and the resolution, R, between phenytoin and benzoin is not less than 1.5.
Procedure—Separately inject equal volumes (about 20 μL) of the *Standard preparation* and the *Assay preparation* into the chromatograph, record the chromatograms, and measure the peak responses for the major peaks. Calculate the quantity, in mg, of $C_{15}H_{11}N_2NaO_2$ in the portion of Phenytoin Sodium taken by the formula:

$$2000C(274.25/252.27)(r_U / r_S)$$

in which C is the concentration, in mg per mL, of USP Phenytoin RS in the *Standard preparation;* 274.25 and 252.27 are the molecular weights of phenytoin sodium and phenytoin, respectively; and r_U and r_S are the peak responses obtained from the *Assay preparation* and the *Standard preparation,* respectively.

Extended Phenytoin Sodium Capsules

» Extended Phenytoin Sodium Capsules contain not less than 95.0 percent and not more than 105.0 percent of the labeled amount of phenytoin sodium ($C_{15}H_{11}N_2NaO_2$).

Packaging and storage—Preserve in tight, light-resistant containers. Protect from moisture. Store at controlled room temperature.
Labeling—When more than one *Dissolution* test is given, the labeling states the *Dissolution* test used only if *Test 1* is not used.
USP Reference standards ⟨11⟩—*USP Phenytoin RS. USP Phenytoin Related Compound A RS. USP Phenytoin Related Compound B RS.*
Identification—
A: The contents of Capsules meet the requirements of *Identification* test A under *Phenytoin Sodium.*
B: The contents of Capsules meet the requirements of the flame test for *Sodium* ⟨191⟩.
Dissolution ⟨711⟩—
Test 1:
Medium: water; 900 mL.
Apparatus 1: 50 rpm.
Times: 30, 60, and 120 minutes.
Determine the amount of $C_{15}H_{11}N_2NaO_2$ dissolved by employing the following method.

Mobile phase—Prepare a filtered and degassed mixture of methanol and water (7 : 3). Make adjustments if necessary (see *System Suitability* under *Chromatography* ⟨621⟩).

Standard solution—Prepare a solution of USP Phenytoin RS in methanol, and dilute with water to obtain a solution having a concentration similar to that of the solution under test.

Chromatographic system (see *Chromatography* ⟨621⟩)—The liquid chromatograph is equipped with a 229-nm detector and a 4.6-mm × 25-cm column that contains packing L1. The flow rate is about 1 mL per minute. Chromatograph the *Standard solution*, and record the peak responses as directed for *Procedure:* the column efficiency is not less than 3200 theoretical plates; the tailing factor is not more than 2.0; and the relative standard deviation for replicate injections is not more than 2.0%.

Procedure—Separately inject equal volumes (about 10 μL) of the *Standard solution* and the solution under test into the chromatograph, record the chromatograms, and measure the responses for the major peaks. Calculate the quantity, in mg, of phenytoin sodium ($C_{15}H_{11}N_2NaO_2$) dissolved by the formula:

$$(274.25/252.27)900C(r_U/r_S)$$

in which 274.25 and 252.27 are the molecular weights of phenytoin sodium and phenytoin, respectively; C is the concentration, in mg per mL, of USP Phenytoin RS in the *Standard solution;* and r_U and r_S are the peak responses obtained from the solution under test and the *Standard solution*, respectively.

Tolerances (for products labeled as 30-mg capsules)—The percentage of the labeled amount of $C_{15}H_{11}N_2NaO_2$ dissolved is not more than 40% *(Q)* in 30 minutes, is 56% *(Q′)* in 60 minutes, and is not less than 65% *(Q″)* in 120 minutes. The requirements are met if the quantities dissolved from the Capsules tested conform to the accompanying *Acceptance Table*.

Acceptance Table

Stage	Number Tested	Acceptance Criteria
S_1	6	Each unit is within the range between $Q - 15\%$ and $Q - 5\%$, is within the range $Q′ \pm 10\%$, and is not less than $Q″ + 5\%$ at the stated *Times*.
S_2	6	Average of 12 units ($S_1 + S_2$) is within the range between $Q - 10\%$ and Q, is within the range $Q′ \pm 8\%$, and is not less than $Q″$; no unit is outside the range between $Q - 20\%$ and $Q + 10\%$, no unit is outside the range $Q′ \pm 18\%$, and no unit is less than $Q″ - 10\%$ at the stated *Times*.
S_3	12	Average of 24 units ($S_1 + S_2 + S_3$) is within the range between $Q - 10\%$ and Q, is within the range $Q′ \pm 8\%$ and is not less than $Q″$; not more than 2 units are outside the range between $Q - 20\%$ and $Q + 10\%$, and no unit is outside the range $Q - 30\%$ and $Q + 20\%$; not more than 2 units are outside the range $Q′ \pm 18\%$, and no unit is outside the range $Q′ \pm 25\%$; not more than 2 units are less than $Q″ - 10\%$, and no unit is less than $Q″ - 20\%$ at the stated *Times*.

Tolerances (for products labeled as 100-mg capsules)—The percentage of the labeled amount of $C_{15}H_{11}N_2NaO_2$ dissolved is not more than 45% *(Q)* in 30 minutes, is 60% *(Q′)* in 60 minutes, and is not less than 70% *(Q″)* in 120 minutes. The requirements are met if the quantities dissolved from the Capsules tested conform to the accompanying *Acceptance Table*.

Acceptance Table

Stage	Number Tested	Acceptance Criteria
S_1	6	Each unit is within the range between $Q - 25\%$ and $Q - 5\%$, is equal to $Q′ \pm 20\%$, and is not less than $Q″ + 5\%$ at the stated *Times*.
S_2	6	Average of 12 units ($S_1 + S_2$) is within the range between $Q - 20\%$ and Q, is within the range $Q′ \pm 15\%$, and is not less than $Q″$; no unit is outside the range between $Q - 30\%$ and $Q + 10\%$, no unit is outside the range $Q′ \pm 25\%$, and no unit is less than $Q″ - 10\%$ at the stated *Times*.
S_3	12	Average of 24 units ($S_1 + S_2 + S_3$) is within the range between $Q - 20\%$ and Q, is within the range $Q′ \pm 15\%$ and is not less than $Q″$; not more than 2 units are outside the range between $Q - 30\%$ and $Q + 10\%$, and no unit is outside the range between $Q - 40\%$ and $Q + 20\%$; not more than 2 units are outside the range $Q′ \pm 25\%$, and no unit is outside the range $Q′ \pm 35\%$; not more than 2 units are less than $Q″ - 10\%$, and no unit is less than $Q″ - 20\%$ at the stated *Times*.

Test 2: If the product complies with this test, the labeling indicates that it meets USP *Dissolution Test 2*. Proceed as directed in *Test 1*, except for using *Apparatus 1* at 75 rpm and the following *Tolerances*.

Tolerances (for products labeled as 100-mg capsules)—The percentage of the labeled amount of $C_{15}H_{11}N_2NaO_2$ dissolved is not more than 45% *(Q)* in 30 minutes, is 65% *(Q′)* in 60 minutes, and is not less than 70% *(Q″)* in 120 minutes. The requirements are met if the quantities dissolved from the Capsules tested conform to the accompanying *Acceptance Table*.

Acceptance Table

Stage	Number Tested	Acceptance Criteria
S_1	6	Each unit is within the range between $Q - 25\%$ and $Q - 5\%$, is equal to $Q' \pm 20\%$, and is not less than $Q'' + 5\%$ at the stated *Times*.
S_2	6	Average of 12 units ($S_1 + S_2$) is within the range between $Q - 25\%$ and $Q - 5\%$, is within the range of $Q' - 20\%$ and $Q' + 10\%$, and is not less than Q''; no unit is outside the range between $Q - 30\%$ and $Q + 5\%$, no unit is outside the range $Q' - 25\%$ and $Q' + 20\%$, and no unit is less than $Q'' - 10\%$ at the stated *Times*.
S_3	12	Average of 24 units ($S_1 + S_2 + S_3$) is within the range between $Q - 25\%$ and $Q - 5\%$, is within the range of $Q' - 20\%$ and $Q' + 10\%$, and is not less than Q''; not more than 2 units are outside the range between $Q - 30\%$ and $Q + 5\%$; and no unit is outside the range of $Q - 40\%$ and $Q + 15\%$; not more than 2 units are outside the range $Q' - 25\%$ and $Q' + 20\%$, and no unit is outside the range $Q' - 35\%$ and $Q' + 25\%$; not more than 2 units are less than $Q'' - 10\%$; and no unit is less than $Q'' - 20\%$ at the stated *Times*.

Test 3: If the product complies with this test, the labeling indicates that it meets USP*Dissolution Test 3*.
Medium: water; 900 mL.
Apparatus 1: 75 rpm.
Times: 30, 60, and 120 minutes.
Determine the amount of $C_{15}H_{11}N_2NaO_2$ dissolved by employing the method described under *Test 1*.
Tolerances (for products labeled as 200-mg and 300-mg capsules)—The percentage of the labeled amount of $C_{15}H_{11}N_2NaO_2$ dissolved is not more than 30% *(Q)* in 30 minutes, is 50% *(Q')* in 60 minutes, and is not less than 60% *(Q'')* in 120 minutes. The requirements are met if the quantities dissolved from the Capsules tested conform to the accompanying *Acceptance Table*.

Acceptance Table

Stage	Number Tested	Acceptance Criteria
S_1	6	Each unit is within the range between $Q - 20\%$ and $Q + 5\%$, is equal to $Q' - 20\%$ and $Q' + 25\%$, and is not less than $Q'' + 5\%$ at the stated *Times*.
S_2	6	Average of 12 units ($S_1 + S_2$) is within the range between $Q - 20\%$ and Q, is within the range of $Q' \pm 20\%$, and is not less than Q''; no unit is outside the range between $Q - 25\%$ and $Q + 10\%$, no unit is outside the range $Q' \pm 25\%$, and no unit is less than $Q'' - 10\%$ at the stated *Times*.
S_3	12	Average of 24 units ($S_1 + S_2 + S_3$) is within the range between $Q - 20\%$ and Q, is within the range of $Q' \pm 20\%$, and is not less than Q''; not more than 2 units are outside the range between $Q - 25\%$ and $Q + 10\%$, and no unit is outside the range $Q - 25\%$ and $Q + 15\%$; not more than 2 units are outside the range $Q' \pm 25\%$; and no unit is outside the range $Q' \pm 30\%$; not more than 2 units are less than $Q'' - 10\%$; and no unit is less than $Q'' - 20\%$ at the stated *Times*.

Uniformity of dosage units ⟨905⟩: meet the requirements.
PROCEDURE FOR CONTENT UNIFORMITY—
Phosphate buffer and *Mobile phase*—Proceed as directed in the *Assay*.
Standard solution—Dissolve an accurately weighed quantity of USP Phenytoin RS in methanol, and dilute quantitatively, and stepwise if necessary, with *Mobile phase* to obtain a solution having a known concentration of about 0.5 mg per mL.
Test solution—Place one intact Capsule or one opened capsule with its contents in a suitable container, add approximately 15 mL of methanol, and place in a shaking water bath at 37° for 30 minutes. Sonicate for 60 minutes with occasional shaking. Dilute with methanol to volume, and mix. Dilute with *Mobile phase*, if necessary, to obtain a final concentration of about 0.5 mg per mL.
Chromatographic system (see *Chromatography* ⟨621⟩)—Proceed as directed in the *Assay*, except to chromatograph the *Standard solution* instead of the *Standard preparation*.
Procedure—Proceed as directed in the *Assay*, except to inject the *Standard solution* and the *Test solution* instead of the *Standard preparation* and the *Assay preparation*.

Related compounds—
Phosphate buffer and *Mobile phase*—Proceed as directed in the *Assay*.
Standard solution—Dissolve accurately weighed quantities of USP Phenytoin RS, USP Phenytoin Related Compound A RS, and USP Phenytoin Related Compound B RS in methanol, and dilute quantitatively, and stepwise if necessary, with methanol to obtain a solution having known concentrations of about 600, 3, and 3 µg per mL, respectively.
Test solution—Use the *Assay preparation*.
Chromatographic system (see *Chromatography* ⟨621⟩)—Prepare as directed in the *Assay*. Chromatograph the *Standard solution*, and record the peak responses as directed for *Procedure:* the relative retention times are about 0.38 for phenytoin related compound A, 0.45 for phenytoin related compound B, and 1.0 for phenytoin; the resolution, *R*, between phenytoin related compound B and phenytoin is not less than 8, and the resolution, *R*, between phenytoin related compound A and phenytoin related compound B is not less than 1.5; the tailing factor for the phenytoin peak is not more than 2.0; and the relative standard deviation for replicate injections is not more than 2.0% determined from phenytoin, and not more than 5.0% determined from phenytoin related compound A or phenytoin related compound B.

Procedure—Separately inject equal volumes (about 10 µL) of the *Standard solution* and the *Test solution* into the chromatograph, record the chromatograms, and measure the responses for the major peaks. Calculate the quantity, in µg, of each phenytoin related compound in the portion of Capsules taken by the formula:

$$100C(r_U / r_S)$$

in which *C* is the concentration, in µg per mL, of the appropriate USP Reference Standard in the *Standard solution;* and r_U and r_S are the peak responses for the corresponding phenytoin related compound obtained from the *Test solution* and the *Standard solution*, respectively: not more than 0.5% of phenytoin related compound A is found; and not more than 1.0% of phenytoin related compound B is found.

Assay—
Phosphate buffer—Prepare a solution of 0.05 M monobasic potassium phosphate in water, adjust with phosphoric acid to a pH of 3.5, and mix.
Mobile phase—Prepare a filtered and degassed mixture of methanol and *Phosphate buffer* (11 : 9). Make adjustments if necessary (see *System Suitability* under *Chromatography* ⟨621⟩).
Standard preparation—Dissolve an accurately weighed quantity of USP Phenytoin RS in methanol, and dilute quantitatively, and stepwise if necessary, with *Mobile phase* to obtain a solution having a known concentration of about 0.6 mg per mL.
Assay preparation—Transfer the contents of 10 Capsules to a 250-mL volumetric flask. Add about 150 mL of methanol, and sonicate for 20 minutes. Cool to room temperature, dilute with methanol to volume, mix, and filter. Transfer an accurately measured portion of the filtered solution, equivalent to about 60 mg of phenytoin, to a 100-mL volumetric flask, dilute with *Mobile phase* to volume, and mix.
Chromatographic system (see *Chromatography* ⟨621⟩)—The liquid chromatograph is equipped with a 229-nm detector and a 4.6-mm × 25-cm column that contains packing L1. The flow rate is about 1 mL per minute. Chromatograph the *Standard preparation*, and record the peak responses as directed for *Procedure*: the column efficiency is not less than 3000 theoretical plates; the tailing factor is not more than 2.0; and the relative standard deviation for replicate injections is not more than 2.0%.
Procedure—Separately inject equal volumes (about 10 µL) of the *Standard preparation* and the *Assay preparation* into the chromatograph, record the chromatograms, and measure the responses for the major peaks. Calculate the quantity, in mg, of phenytoin sodium ($C_{15}H_{11}N_2NaO_2$) in the portion of Capsules taken by the formula:

$$(274.25/252.27)100C(r_U / r_S)$$

in which 274.25 and 252.27 are the molecular weights of phenytoin sodium and phenytoin, respectively; *C* is the concentration, in mg per mL, of USP Phenytoin RS in the *Standard preparation;* and r_U and r_S are the peak responses obtained from the *Assay preparation* and the *Standard preparation*, respectively.

Prompt Phenytoin Sodium Capsules

» Prompt Phenytoin Sodium Capsules contain not less than 95.0 percent and not more than 105.0 percent of the labeled amount of $C_{15}H_{11}N_2NaO_2$.

Packaging and storage—Preserve in tight containers.
Labeling—Label the Capsules with the statement "Not for once-a-day dosing," printed immediately under the official name, in a bold and contrasting color and/or enclosed within a box.
USP Reference standards ⟨11⟩—USP Phenytoin RS. USP Phenytoin Sodium RS.
Identification—
A: The contents of Capsules respond to *Identification* test A under *Phenytoin Sodium*.
B: The contents of Capsules respond to the flame test for *Sodium* ⟨191⟩.

Dissolution ⟨711⟩—
Medium: water; 900 mL.
Apparatus 1: 50 rpm.
Time: 30 minutes.
Procedure—Determine the amount of $C_{15}H_{11}N_2NaO_2$ dissolved by measuring the UV absorbance at 258 nm on filtered portions of the solution under test, suitably diluted with *Dissolution Medium* if necessary, in comparison with a Standard solution having a known concentration of USP Phenytoin Sodium RS in the same *Medium*.
Tolerances—Not less than 85% *(Q)* of the labeled amount of $C_{15}H_{11}N_2NaO_2$ is dissolved in 30 minutes.
Uniformity of dosage units ⟨905⟩: meet the requirements.
Procedure for content uniformity—Proceed as directed in the test for *Uniformity of dosage units* under *Extended Phenytoin Sodium Capsules*.
Assay—Proceed with Capsules as directed in the *Assay* under *Extended Phenytoin Sodium Capsules*.

Phenytoin Sodium Injection

» Phenytoin Sodium Injection is a sterile solution of Phenytoin Sodium with Propylene Glycol and Alcohol in Water for Injection. It contains not less than 95.0 percent and not more than 105.0 percent of the labeled amount of $C_{15}H_{11}N_2NaO_2$.

NOTE—Do not use the Injection if it is hazy or contains a precipitate.

Packaging and storage—Preserve in single-dose or multiple-dose containers, preferably of Type I glass, at controlled room temperature.
USP Reference standards ⟨11⟩—USP Phenytoin RS. USP Endotoxin RS.
Identification—
A: Transfer a volume of Injection, equivalent to about 250 mg of phenytoin sodium, to a separator containing 25 mL of water. Extract, in the order listed, with 50-, 30-, and 30-mL portions of ethyl acetate. Wash each extract with two 20-mL portions of sodium acetate solution (1 in 100). Evaporate the combined ethyl acetate extracts, and dry the residue of phenytoin at 105° to constant weight: the IR absorption spectrum of a potassium bromide dispersion of the residue so obtained exhibits maxima only at the same wavelengths as that of a potassium bromide dispersion of USP Phenytoin RS.
B: It responds to the flame test for *Sodium* ⟨191⟩.
Bacterial endotoxins ⟨85⟩—It contains not more than 0.3 USP Endotoxin Unit per mg of phenytoin sodium.
pH ⟨791⟩: between 10.0 and 12.3.
Alcohol and propylene glycol content—
Internal standard solution—Pipet 8 mL of methanol and 20 mL of ethylene glycol into a 100-mL volumetric flask, dilute with water to volume, and mix.
Alcohol solution—Pipet 6 mL of dehydrated alcohol into a 100-mL volumetric flask, dilute with water to volume, and mix.
Propylene glycol solution—Pipet 20 mL of propylene glycol into a 100-mL volumetric flask, dilute with water to volume, and mix.
Standard preparation—Pipet 10 mL each of *Internal standard solution*, *Alcohol solution*, and *Propylene glycol solution* into a 100-mL volumetric flask, dilute with water to volume, and mix.
Test preparation—Pipet 5 mL of Injection and 10 mL of *Internal standard solution* into a 100-mL volumetric flask, dilute with water to volume, and mix.
Chromatographic system (see *Chromatography* ⟨621⟩)—The gas chromatograph is equipped with a flame-ionization detector and a 1.8-m × 2.0-mm (ID) glass column packed with 50- to 80-mesh silanized packing S3. The column is maintained at a temperature of 140° for 3 minutes, programmed at a rate of 6° per minute to a temperature of 190°, and maintained at 190° for 6 minutes, helium being used as the carrier gas at a flow rate of about 40 mL per minute. The injection port and detector are maintained at a temperature

of 200°. Chromatograph five replicate injections of the *Standard preparation*, and record the chromatograms: the resolution, R, between methanol and alcohol is not less than 2.0, the resolution, R, between ethylene glycol and propylene glycol is not less than 3.0, and the relative standard deviation is not more than 2.0%.

Procedure—Separately inject equal volumes (about 2 μL) of the *Standard preparation* and the *Test preparation* into the chromatograph, record the chromatograms, and measure the responses for the major peaks. The order of elution is methanol, alcohol, ethylene glycol, and propylene glycol in order of increasing retention time: the relative retentions are about 1.0 for methanol and 2.2 for alcohol with respect to methanol and alcohol peaks, and about 1.0 for ethylene glycol and 1.4 for propylene glycol with respect to the ethylene glycol and propylene glycol peaks. Calculate the relative response ratio for the alcohol peak with respect to the methanol peak and for the propylene glycol peak with respect to the ethylene glycol peak. Calculate the alcohol content, in percentage, taken by the formula:

$$12(R_U / R_S)$$

in which R_U and R_S are the relative response ratios for the methanol and alcohol peaks obtained from the *Test preparation* and the *Standard preparation*, respectively. Calculate the propylene glycol content, in percentage, taken by the formula:

$$40(R'_U / R'_S)$$

in which R'_U and R'_S are the relative response ratios for the ethylene glycol and propylene glycol peaks obtained from the *Test preparation* and the *Standard preparation*, respectively. The alcohol content is not less than 9.0% and not more than 11.0%, and the propylene glycol content is not less than 37.0% and not more than 43.0%.

Particulate matter ⟨788⟩: meets the requirements under small-volume Injections.

Other requirements—It meets the requirements under *Injections* ⟨1⟩.

Assay—

Mobile phase—Prepare a suitable degassed and filtered mixture of methanol and water (55 : 45).

Standard preparation—Dissolve an accurately weighed portion of USP Phenytoin RS in *Mobile phase* to obtain a solution having a known concentration of about 230 μg per mL.

Assay preparation—Transfer an accurately measured volume of Injection, equivalent to 250 mg of phenytoin sodium, to a volumetric flask and dilute quantitatively and stepwise with *Mobile phase* to obtain a solution having a concentration of about 250 μg of phenytoin sodium per mL.

Chromatographic system (see *Chromatography* ⟨621⟩)—The liquid chromatograph is equipped with a 254-nm detector and a 3.9-mm × 25-cm column that contains packing L1. The flow rate is about 1.5 mL per minute. Chromatograph replicate injections of the *Standard preparation*, and record the peak responses as directed for *Procedure*: the relative standard deviation is not more than 2.0%, and the tailing factor is not more than 2.0.

Procedure—Separately inject equal volumes (about 20 μL) of the *Standard preparation* and the *Assay preparation* into the chromatograph, record the chromatograms, and measure the response for the major peak. Calculate the quantity, in mg, of $C_{15}H_{11}N_2NaO_2$ in each mL of the Injection taken by the formula:

$$(274.25 / 252.27)(C / V)(r_U / r_S)$$

in which 274.25 and 252.27 are the molecular weights of phenytoin sodium and phenytoin, respectively, C is the concentration, in μg per mL, of USP Phenytoin RS in the *Standard preparation*, V is the volume, in mL, of Injection taken, and r_U and r_S are the peak responses obtained from the *Assay preparation* and the *Standard preparation*, respectively.

Chromic Phosphate P 32 Suspension

» Chromic Phosphate P 32 Suspension is a sterile, aqueous suspension of radioactive chromic phosphate P 32 in a 30 percent Dextrose solution suitable for intraperitoneal, intrapleural, or interstitial administration. It contains not less than 90.0 percent and not more than 110.0 percent of the labeled amount of ^{32}P as chromic phosphate expressed in megabecquerels (millicuries) per mL at the time indicated in the labeling. It may contain a preservative or a stabilizer. Other chemical forms of radioactivity do not exceed 5.0 percent of the total radioactivity.

Packaging and storage—Preserve in single-dose or multiple-dose containers.

Labeling—Label it to include the following, in addition to the information specified for *Labeling* under *Injections* ⟨1⟩: the time and date of calibration; the amount of ^{32}P as labeled chromic phosphate expressed as total megabecquerels (millicuries) and concentration as megabecquerels (millicuries) per mL at the time of calibration; the expiration date; and the statements, "Caution—Radioactive Material," and "For intracavitary use only." The labeling indicates that in making dosage calculations, correction is to be made for radioactive decay, and also indicates that the radioactive half-life of ^{32}P is 14.3 days.

USP Reference standards ⟨11⟩—*USP Endotoxin RS.*

Radionuclide identification—

A: The beta radiation of the Suspension, measured according to the procedure set forth under *Radioactivity* ⟨821⟩, shows a mass absorption coefficient within ±5% of the value found for a specimen of a known standard of the same radionuclide when determined under identical counting conditions and geometry.

B: Its beta-ray spectrum is identical to that of a specimen of ^{32}P of known purity showing no distinct photopeaks and no energies greater than 1.710 MeV.

Bacterial endotoxins ⟨85⟩—It contains not more than 175/V USP Endotoxin Unit per mL of the Injection, when compared with the USP Endotoxin RS, in which V is the maximum recommended total dose, in mL, at the expiration date or time.

pH ⟨791⟩: between 3.0 and 5.0.

Radiochemical purity—Place a measured volume of Suspension, to provide a count rate of about 20,000 counts per minute, about 2.5 cm from one end of a 25-mm × 300-mm strip of chromatographic paper (see *Chromatography* ⟨621⟩), and allow to dry. Develop the chromatogram by ascending chromatography, using water as the solvent, and air-dry: the radioactivity in the chromic phosphate is not less than 95.0% of the total radioactivity when measured at the origin.

Other requirements—It meets the requirements under *Injections* ⟨1⟩, except that the Suspension may be distributed or dispensed prior to the completion of the test for *Sterility*, the latter test being started on the day of final manufacture, and except that it is not subject to the recommendations on *Volume in Container*.

Assay for dextrose—

Periodic acid reagent solution—Dissolve 8.5 g of sodium metaperiodate in 80 mL of 1 N sulfuric acid, dilute with water to 100 mL, and mix.

Assay preparation—Decant the supernatant from sterile Suspension into a disposable centrifuge tube, and centrifuge. Pipet 1.0 mL of the clear supernatant into a 25-mL volumetric flask, dilute with water to volume, and mix.

Procedure—Pipet 50 mL of *Periodic acid reagent solution* into a 250-mL conical flask, add 3.0 mL of the *Assay preparation*, swirl, cover the flask, and allow to stand at room temperature for 2 hours. Add, in the order named and with rapid stirring, 50 mL of a saturated solution of sodium bicarbonate, 50.0 mL of 0.1 N potassium arsenite VS, 4 mL of potassium iodide solution (1 in 5), and 20 g of sodium bicarbonate. Stir the solution at room temperature for 15 minutes. Titrate with 0.1 N iodine VS, using 3 mL of starch TS as the indicator. Perform a blank determination, and make any necessary correction. Each mL of 0.1 N iodine is equivalent to 1.802 mg of dextrose ($C_6H_{12}O_6$). Not less than 27.0% and not more than 33.0% is found.

Assay for radioactivity—Using a suitable counting assembly (see *Assay, Beta-emitting* under *Radioactivity* ⟨821⟩), determine the ra-

Sodium Phosphate P 32 Solution

Phosphoric-^{32}P acid, disodium salt.
Dibasic sodium phosphate-^{32}P [7635-46-3].

» Sodium Phosphate P 32 Solution is a solution suitable for either oral or intravenous administration, containing radioactive phosphorus (^{32}P) processed in the form of Dibasic Sodium Phosphate from the neutron bombardment of elemental sulfur. Nonradioactive Dibasic Sodium Phosphate may be added during the processing. Sodium Phosphate P 32 Solution contains not less than 90.0 percent and not more than 110.0 percent of the labeled amount of ^{32}P as phosphate expressed in megabecquerels (microcuries or millicuries) per mL at the time indicated in the labeling. Other chemical forms of radioactivity are absent.

Packaging and storage—Preserve in single-dose or multiple-dose containers that previously have been treated to prevent adsorption.
Labeling—Label it to include the following: the time and date of calibration; the amount of ^{32}P as phosphate expressed in total megabecquerels (microcuries or millicuries) and in megabecquerels (microcuries or in millicuries) per mL at the time of calibration; the name and quantity of any added preservative or stabilizer; a statement of the intended use, whether oral or intravenous; a statement of whether the contents are intended for diagnostic or therapeutic use; the expiration date; and the statements "Caution—Radioactive Material," and "Not for intracavitary use." The labeling indicates that in making dosage calculations, correction is to be made for radioactive decay, and also indicates that the radioactive half-life of ^{32}P is 14.3 days.
USP Reference standards ⟨11⟩—*USP Endotoxin RS*.
Radionuclide identification—
  A: The beta radiation of the Solution, measured according to the procedure set forth under *Radioactivity* ⟨821⟩, shows a mass absorption coefficient within ±5% of the value found for a specimen of a known standard of the same radionuclide when determined under identical counting conditions and geometry.
  B: Its beta-ray and/or bremsstrahlung spectrum is identical to that of a specimen of ^{32}P of known purity showing no distinct photopeaks and no energies greater than 1.710 MeV.
Bacterial endotoxins ⟨85⟩—It contains not more than 175/*V* USP Endotoxin Unit per mL of the Injection, when compared with the USP Endotoxin RS, in which *V* is the maximum recommended total dose, in mL, at the expiration date or time.
pH ⟨791⟩: between 5.0 and 6.0.
Radiochemical purity—Place a measured volume, appropriately diluted with phosphoric acid solution (1 in 20) such that it provides a count rate of about 20,000 counts per minute, about 45 mm from the end of a 25- × 300-mm strip of chromatographic paper (see *Chromatography* ⟨621⟩), and allow to dry. Develop the chromatogram by descending chromatography, using a mixture of tertiary butyl alcohol, water, and formic acid (40 : 20 : 5). Allow to dry, and determine the position of the phosphoric acid by spraying the paper with a solution prepared by dissolving 5 g of ammonium molybdate in 100 mL of water and pouring, with constant stirring, into a mixture of 12 mL of nitric acid and 24 mL of water. Determine the position of the radioactivity distribution by scanning with a collimated radiation detector. The radioactivity appears in one band only, corresponding in R_F value to the phosphoric acid.
Other requirements—Solution intended for intravenous use meets the requirements under *Injections* ⟨1⟩, except that the Solution may be distributed or dispensed prior to completion of the test for *Sterility*, the latter test being started on the day of final manufacture, and except that it is not subject to the recommendation on *Volume in Container*.
Assay for radioactivity—Using a suitable counting assembly (see *Assay, Beta-emitting* under *Radioactivity* ⟨821⟩), determine the radioactivity, in MBq (mCi) per mL, of Solution by use of a calibrated system as directed under *Radioactivity* ⟨821⟩).

Physostigmine

$C_{15}H_{21}N_3O_2$ 275.35
Pyrrolo[2,3-*b*]indol-5-ol, 1,2,3,3a,8,8a-hexahydro-1,3a,8-trimethyl-, methylcarbamate (ester), (3a*S-cis*).
Physostigmine.
1,2,3,3aβ,8,8aβ-Hexahydro-1,3a,8-trimethylpyrrolo[2,3-*b*]indol-5-yl methylcarbamate   [57-47-6].

» Physostigmine is an alkaloid usually obtained from the dried ripe seed of *Physostigma venenosum* Balfour (Fam. Leguminosae). It contains not less than 97.0 percent and not more than 102.0 percent of $C_{15}H_{21}N_3O_2$, calculated on the dried basis.

Packaging and storage—Preserve in tight, light-resistant containers.
USP Reference standards ⟨11⟩—*USP Physostigmine Salicylate RS*.
Identification—It meets the requirements of the test for *Identification—Organic Nitrogenous Bases* ⟨181⟩, USP Physostigmine Salicylate RS being used, and 1 g of sodium bicarbonate being used in place of the 2 mL of 1 N sodium hydroxide specified.
Specific rotation ⟨781S⟩: between −236° and −246° (λ= 365 nm).
  Test solution: 10 mg per mL, in methanol.
Loss on drying ⟨731⟩—Dry it over silica gel for 24 hours: it loses not more than 1.0% of its weight.
Residue on ignition ⟨281⟩: negligible, from 100 mg.
Readily carbonizable substances ⟨271⟩—Dissolve 100 mg in 5 mL of sulfuric acid TS: at the end of 5 minutes the solution has no more color than *Matching Fluid I*.
Assay—Dissolve about 175 mg of Physostigmine, accurately weighed, in 25 mL of chloroform. Add 25 mL of glacial acetic acid, and titrate with 0.02 N perchloric acid in dioxane VS, determining the endpoint potentiometrically. Perform a blank determination, and make any necessary correction. Each mL of 0.02 N perchloric acid is equivalent to 5.507 mg of $C_{15}H_{21}N_3O_2$.

Physostigmine Salicylate

$C_{15}H_{21}N_3O_2 \cdot C_7H_6O_3$ 413.47
Pyrrolo[2,3-*b*]indol-5-ol, 1,2,3,3a,8,8a-hexahydro-1,3a,8-trimethyl-, methylcarbamate (ester), (3a*S-cis*)-, mono-(2-hydroxybenzoate).
Physostigmine monosalicylate   [57-64-7].

» Physostigmine Salicylate contains not less than 97.0 percent and not more than 102.0 percent of $C_{15}H_{21}N_3O_2 \cdot C_7H_6O_3$, calculated on the dried basis.

Packaging and storage—Preserve in tight, light-resistant containers. Store at 25°, excursions permitted between 15° and 30°.

USP Reference standards ⟨11⟩—*USP Physostigmine Salicylate RS*.

Identification—
A: It responds to the *Identification* test under *Physostigmine*.
B: It responds to the tests for *Salicylate* ⟨191⟩.
Specific rotation ⟨781S⟩: between −91° and −94°.
Test solution: 10 mg per mL, in water.
Loss on drying ⟨731⟩—Dry it over silica gel for 24 hours: it loses not more than 1.0% of its weight.
Residue on ignition ⟨281⟩: negligible, from 100 mg.
Sulfate—Precipitate the salicylic acid from 10 mL of a cold, saturated solution of Physostigmine Salicylate with a slight excess of 3 N hydrochloric acid, filter, and to the filtrate add 5 drops of barium chloride TS: no turbidity is produced immediately.
Readily carbonizable substances ⟨271⟩—Dissolve 100 mg in 5 mL of sulfuric acid TS: at the end of 5 minutes the solution has no more color than *Matching Fluid I*.
Assay—Dissolve about 250 mg of Physostigmine Salicylate, accurately weighed, in 25 mL of chloroform. Add 25 mL of glacial acetic acid, and titrate with 0.02 N perchloric acid in dioxane VS, determining the endpoint potentiometrically. Perform a blank determination, and make any necessary correction. Each mL of 0.02 N perchloric acid is equivalent to 8.270 mg of $C_{15}H_{21}N_3O_2 \cdot C_7H_6O_3$.

Physostigmine Salicylate Injection

» Physostigmine Salicylate Injection is a sterile solution of Physostigmine Salicylate in Water for Injection. It contains not less than 90.0 percent and not more than 110.0 percent of the labeled amount of physostigmine salicylate ($C_{15}H_{21}N_3O_2 \cdot C_7H_6O_3$). It may contain an antimicrobial agent and an antioxidant.

NOTE—Do not use the Injection if it is more than slightly discolored.

Packaging and storage—Preserve in single-dose containers, preferably of Type I glass, protected from light.
USP Reference standards ⟨11⟩—*USP Benzyl Alcohol RS. USP Endotoxin RS. USP Physostigmine Salicylate RS.*
Identification—
A: It responds to the *Identification* test under *Physostigmine*.
B: It responds to the tests for *Salicylate* ⟨191⟩.
Bacterial endotoxins ⟨85⟩—It contains not more than 83.4 USP Endotoxin Units per mg of physostigmine salicylate.
pH ⟨791⟩: between 3.5 and 5.0.
Other requirements—It meets the requirements under *Injections* ⟨1⟩.
Assay—
*0.05 M Ammonium acetate—*Dissolve 3.85 g of ammonium acetate in 1 L of water, and adjust, if necessary, with glacial acetic acid or ammonium hydroxide to a pH of 6 ± 0.1.
*Mobile phase—*Prepare a filtered and degassed mixture of equal volumes of acetonitrile and *0.05 M Ammonium acetate*. Make adjustments if necessary (see *System Suitability* under *Chromatography* ⟨621⟩).
*Benzyl alcohol–benzaldehyde solution—*Prepare a mixture of 100 µL of USP Benzyl Alcohol RS and 1 µL of benzaldehyde in 400 mL of acetonitrile.
*Standard preparation—*Dissolve an accurately weighed quantity of USP Physostigmine Salicylate RS in *Benzyl alcohol–benzaldehyde solution,* and dilute quantitatively, and stepwise if necessary, with *Benzyl alcohol–benzaldehyde solution* to obtain a solution having a known concentration of about 30 µg per mL.
*Assay preparation—*Transfer an accurately measured volume of Injection, equivalent to about 3 mg of physostigmine salicylate, to a 100-mL volumetric flask, dilute with acetonitrile to volume, and mix.
Chromatographic system (see *Chromatography* ⟨621⟩)—The liquid chromatograph is equipped with a 254-nm detector and a 3.9-mm × 30-cm column that contains packing L1. The flow rate is about 2 mL per minute. Separately chromatograph 10-µL portions of the *Benzyl alcohol–benzaldehyde solution* and the *Standard preparation,* and record the peak responses as directed for *Procedure* [NOTE—If the components of the *Benzyl alcohol–benzaldehyde solution* co-elute, the *Standard preparation* will exhibit only two peaks instead of three]: in a suitable system, benzyl alcohol and benzaldehyde elute before physostigmine; the resolution, *R*, between the physostigmine peak and the adjacent peak (benzyl alcohol or benzaldehyde or the combination of these) is not less than 2.0; the column efficiency determined from the analyte peak is not less than 1200 theoretical plates; and the relative standard deviation for replicate injections is not more than 2.0%.
*Procedure—*Separately inject equal volumes (about 10 µL) of the *Standard preparation* and the *Assay preparation* into the chromatograph, record the chromatograms, and measure the responses for the major peaks. Calculate the quantity, in mg, of physostigmine salicylate ($C_{15}H_{21}N_3O_2 \cdot C_7H_6O_3$) in each mL of the Injection taken by the formula:

$$0.1(C/V)(r_U/r_S)$$

in which *C* is the concentration, in µg per mL, of USP Physostigmine Salicylate RS in the *Standard preparation; V* is the volume, in mL, of Injection taken; and r_U and r_S are the peak responses obtained from the *Assay preparation* and the *Standard preparation,* respectively.

Physostigmine Salicylate Ophthalmic Solution

» Physostigmine Salicylate Ophthalmic Solution is a sterile, aqueous solution of Physostigmine Salicylate. It contains not less than 90.0 percent and not more than 110.0 percent of the labeled amount of $C_{15}H_{21}N_3O_2 \cdot C_7H_6O_3$. It may contain suitable antimicrobial agents, buffers, and stabilizers, and suitable additives to increase its viscosity.

Packaging and storage—Preserve in tight, light-resistant containers.
USP Reference standards ⟨11⟩—*USP Physostigmine Salicylate RS.*
Identification—It responds to the *Identification* tests under *Physostigmine Salicylate*.
Sterility ⟨71⟩: meets the requirements.
pH ⟨791⟩: between 2.0 and 4.0.
Assay—
0.05 M Ammonium acetate and *Mobile phase—*Prepare as directed in the *Assay* under *Physostigmine Salicylate Injection*.
*Standard preparation—*Dissolve an accurately weighed quantity of USP Physostigmine Salicylate RS in acetonitrile, and dilute quantitatively, and stepwise if necessary, with acetonitrile, to obtain a solution having a known concentration of about 30 µg per mL.
*Assay preparation—*Transfer an accurately measured volume of Ophthalmic Solution, equivalent to about 3 mg of physostigmine salicylate, to a 100-mL volumetric flask, dilute with acetonitrile to volume, and mix.
Chromatographic system (see *Chromatography* ⟨621⟩)—The liquid chromatograph is equipped with a 254-nm detector and a 3.9-mm × 30-cm column that contains packing L1. The flow rate is about 2 mL per minute. Chromatograph the *Standard preparation* and record the peak responses as directed for *Procedure:* the column efficiency determined from the analyte peak is not less than 1200 theoretical plates, and the relative standard deviation for replicate injections is not more than 2.0%.
*Procedure—*Proceed as directed for *Procedure* in the *Assay* under *Physostigmine Salicylate Injection*. Calculate the quantity, in

mg, of $C_{15}H_{21}N_3O_2 \cdot C_7H_6O_3$ in each mL of the Ophthalmic Solution taken by the formula:

$$0.1(C/V)(r_U/r_S)$$

in which the terms are as defined therein.

Physostigmine Sulfate

$(C_{15}H_{21}N_3O_2)_2 \cdot H_2SO_4$ 648.77
Pyrrolo[2,3-*b*]indol-5-ol, 1,2,3,3a,8,8a-hexahydro-1,3a,8-trimethyl-, methylcarbamate (ester), (3a*S-cis*)-, sulfate (2 : 1).
Physostigmine sulfate (2 : 1)   [64-47-1].

» Physostigmine Sulfate contains not less than 97.0 percent and not more than 102.0 percent of $(C_{15}H_{21}N_3O_2)_2 \cdot H_2SO_4$, calculated on the dried basis.

Packaging and storage—Preserve in tight, light-resistant containers.
USP Reference standards ⟨11⟩—*USP Physostigmine Salicylate RS.*
Identification—
  A: It responds to the *Identification* test under *Physostigmine.*
  B: A solution (1 in 100) responds to the tests for *Sulfate* ⟨191⟩.
Specific rotation ⟨781S⟩: between −116° and −120°.
  Test solution: 10 mg per mL, in water.
Loss on drying ⟨731⟩—Dry it at 105° to constant weight: it loses not more than 1.0% of its weight.
Residue on ignition ⟨281⟩: negligible, from 100 mg.
Readily carbonizable substances—It meets the requirements of the test for *Readily carbonizable substances* under *Physostigmine.*
Assay—Dissolve about 200 mg of Physostigmine Sulfate, accurately weighed, in 25 mL of water. Render the solution alkaline by the addition of about 1 g of sodium bicarbonate, and extract with one 25-mL and five 10-mL portions of chloroform, each time shaking vigorously for 1 minute. Filter each extract through glass wool. Add 15 mL of glacial acetic acid and 10 mL of acetic acid anhydride to the combined chloroform extracts, and titrate with 0.02 N perchloric acid VS, determining the endpoint potentiometrically. Perform a blank determination, and make any necessary correction. Each mL of 0.02 N perchloric acid is equivalent to 6.488 mg of $(C_{15}H_{21}N_3O_2)_2 \cdot H_2SO_4$.

Physostigmine Sulfate Ophthalmic Ointment

» Physostigmine Sulfate Ophthalmic Ointment contains not less than 90.0 percent and not more than 110.0 percent of the labeled amount of $(C_{15}H_{21}N_3O_2)_2 \cdot H_2SO_4$. It is sterile.

Packaging and storage—Preserve in collapsible ophthalmic ointment tubes.
USP Reference standards ⟨11⟩—*USP Physostigmine Salicylate RS.*
Identification—
  A: Place about 20 g of Ophthalmic Ointment in a beaker, add about 25 mL of water, and heat gently on a steam bath, with continuous stirring, until the ointment base has melted. Cool to congeal the ointment base, and decant the aqueous solution through a filter into a separator. Draw off a 2-mL portion, and reserve for *Identification test B:* the solution in the separator meets the requirements of the test for *Identification—Organic Nitrogenous Bases* ⟨181⟩, USP Physostigmine Salicylate RS being used, and 1 g of sodium bicarbonate being used in place of the 2 mL of 1 N sodium hydroxide specified.
  B: A 2-mL portion of the aqueous solution obtained in *Identification test A* responds to the tests for *Sulfate* ⟨191⟩.
Sterility ⟨71⟩: meets the requirements.
Metal particles—It meets the requirements of the test for *Metal Particles in Ophthalmic Ointments* ⟨751⟩.
Assay—
  0.05 M Ammonium acetate and *Mobile phase*—Prepare as directed in the *Assay* under *Physostigmine Salicylate Injection.*
  Standard preparation—Dissolve an accurately weighed quantity of USP Physostigmine Salicylate RS in acetonitrile, and dilute quantitatively, and stepwise if necessary, with acetonitrile, to obtain a solution having a known concentration of about 40 μg per mL.
  Assay preparation—Transfer an accurately weighed quantity of Ophthalmic Ointment, equivalent to about 3 mg of physostigmine sulfate, to a 60-mL separator. Add 20 mL of spectrophotometric grade *n*-hexane, and extract with four 20-mL portions of acetonitrile. Collect the acetonitrile extracts in a 100-mL volumetric flask, dilute with acetonitrile to volume, and mix.
  Chromatographic system (see *Chromatography* ⟨621⟩)—Proceed as directed for *Chromatographic system* in the *Assay* under *Physostigmine Salicylate Ophthalmic Solution.*
  Procedure—Proceed as directed for *Procedure* in the *Assay* under *Physostigmine Salicylate Injection.* Calculate the quantity, in mg, of $(C_{15}H_{21}N_3O_2)_2 \cdot H_2SO_4$ in the portion of the Ophthalmic Ointment taken by the formula:

$$(648.77/413.47)(0.05C)(r_U/r_S)$$

in which 648.77 and 413.47 are the molecular weights of physostigmine sulfate and physostigmine salicylate, respectively, *C* is the concentration, in μg per mL, of USP Physostigmine Salicylate RS in the *Standard preparation.*

Phytonadione

E component

$C_{31}H_{46}O_2$ 450.70
1,4-Naphthalenedione, 2-methyl-3-(3,7,11,15-tetramethyl-2-hexadecenyl)-, [*R*-[*R*,R*-(E)*]]-.
Phylloquinone   [84-80-0].

» Phytonadione is a mixture of *E* and *Z* isomers containing not less than 97.0 percent and not more than 103.0 percent of $C_{31}H_{46}O_2$. It contains not more than 21.0 percent of the *Z* isomer.

Packaging and storage—Preserve in tight, light-resistant containers.
USP Reference standards ⟨11⟩—*USP Phytonadione RS.*
Identification—
  A: *Infrared Absorption* ⟨197F⟩.
  B: *Ultraviolet Absorption* ⟨197U⟩—
    Solution: 10 μg per mL.
    Medium: *n*-hexane.
  Absorptivities at 248 nm do not differ by more than 3.0%.
Refractive index ⟨831⟩: between 1.523 and 1.526.
Reaction—A 1 in 20 solution of it in dehydrated alcohol is neutral to litmus.
Limit of menadione—Mix about 20 mg with 0.5 mL of a mixture of equal volumes of 6 N ammonium hydroxide and alcohol, then add 1 drop of ethyl cyanoacetate, and shake gently: no purple or blue color is produced.
Z isomer content—[NOTE—Protect solutions containing Phytonadione from exposure to light.]
  Mobile phase, Internal standard solution, Assay preparation, Chromatographic system, and *Procedure*—Proceed as directed in

the *Assay*, except to calculate the percentage of Z isomer taken by the formula:

$$100r_Z / (r_Z + r_E)$$

in which r_Z is the peak area of the (Z)-phytonadione isomer peak and r_E is the peak area of the (E)-phytonadione isomer peak obtained from the *Assay preparation*.

Assay—[NOTE—Protect solutions containing Phytonadione from exposure to light.]

Mobile phase—Prepare a filtered and degassed solution of *n*-hexane and *n*-amyl alcohol (2000 : 1.5).

Internal standard solution—Dissolve cholesteryl benzoate in *Mobile phase* to obtain a solution having a concentration of 2.5 mg per mL.

Standard preparation—Transfer about 60 mg of USP Phytonadione RS, accurately weighed, to a 50-mL volumetric flask, add 20 mL of *Mobile phase*, mix, dilute with *Mobile phase* to volume, and again mix. Pipet 4 mL of the resulting solution into a 50-mL volumetric flask, dilute with *Mobile phase* to volume, and mix. Pipet 10 mL of this solution and 7 mL of *Internal standard solution* into a 25-mL volumetric flask, dilute with *Mobile phase* to volume, and mix.

Assay preparation—Prepare as directed under *Standard preparation*, using Phytonadione instead of the Reference Standard.

Chromatographic system (see *Chromatography* ⟨621⟩)—The liquid chromatographic is equipped with a 254-nm detector and a 4.6-mm × 25-cm column that contains packing L3. The flow rate is about 1 mL per minute. Chromatograph replicate injections of the *Standard preparation*, and record the peak responses as directed for *Procedure*: the relative standard deviation is not more than 2.0%, and the resolution, R, between (Z)-phytonadione and (E)-phytonadione is not less than 1.5.

Procedure—Separately inject equal volumes (about 50 µL) of the *Standard preparation* and the *Assay preparation* into the chromatograph, record the chromatograms, and measure the responses for the major peaks. The relative retention times are about 0.7 for the internal standard, 0.9 for (Z)-phytonadione, and 1.0 for (E)-phytonadione. Calculate the quantity, in mg, of $C_{31}H_{46}O_2$ in the portion of Phytonadione taken by the formula:

$$1.56C(R_U / R_S)$$

in which C is the concentration, in µg per mL, of USP Phytonadione RS in the *Standard preparation*, and R_U and R_S are the relative peak response ratios for the *Assay preparation* and the *Standard preparation*, respectively. Calculate R_U and R_S by the formula:

(response for the (Z)-phytonadione peak + response for the (E)-phytonadione peak) / response for the internal standard peak.

Phytonadione Injectable Emulsion

» Phytonadione Injectable Emulsion is a sterile, aqueous dispersion of Phytonadione. It contains not less than 90.0 percent and not more than 110.0 percent of the labeled amount of $C_{31}H_{46}O_2$. It contains suitable solubilizing and/or dispersing agents.

Packaging and storage—Preserve in single-dose or multiple-dose containers, preferably of Type I glass, protected from light.

USP Reference standards ⟨11⟩—*USP Phytonadione RS. USP Endotoxin RS.*

Identification—The retention time of the major peak in the chromatogram of the *Assay preparation* corresponds to that in the chromatogram of the *Standard preparation*, as obtained in the *Assay*.

Bacterial endotoxins ⟨85⟩—It contains not more than 14.0 USP Endotoxin Units per mg of phytonadione.

pH ⟨791⟩: between 3.5 and 7.0.

Other requirements—It meets the requirements under *Injections* ⟨1⟩.

Assay—[NOTE—Use low-actinic glassware throughout this assay, and otherwise protect the solutions from exposure to light.]

Mobile phase—Prepare a suitable degassed mixture of dehydrated alcohol and water (95 : 5).

Standard preparation—Dissolve an accurately weighed quantity of USP Phytonadione RS in *Mobile phase* to obtain a solution having a known concentration of about 1 mg per mL. Pipet 1 mL of this solution into a 10-mL volumetric flask, dilute with *Mobile phase* to volume, and mix to obtain a *Standard preparation* having a known concentration of about 0.1 mg per mL.

Assay preparation 1 (containing 10 mg or more of phytonadione per mL)—Pipet a volume of Injectable Emulsion, equivalent to 10 mg of phytonadione, into a 10-mL volumetric flask, dilute with *Mobile phase* to volume, and mix. Pipet 1 mL of this solution into a 10-mL volumetric flask, dilute with *Mobile phase* to volume, and mix.

Assay preparation 2 (containing less than 10 mg of phytonadione per mL)—Pipet a volume of Injectable Emulsion, equivalent to 1 mg of phytonadione, into a 10-mL volumetric flask, dilute with *Mobile phase* to volume, and mix.

Chromatographic system (see *Chromatography* ⟨621⟩)—The liquid chromatograph is equipped with a 254-nm detector and a 4-mm × 25-cm column that contains packing L1. The flow rate is about 0.7 mL per minute. Chromatograph five replicate injections of the *Standard preparation*, and record the peak responses as directed for *Procedure*: the relative standard deviation is not more than 1.5%.

Procedure—Separately inject equal volumes (about 10 µL) of the *Standard preparation* and the appropriate *Assay preparation* into the chromatograph, record the chromatograms, and measure the peak response for the major peak. Calculate the quantity, in mg, of $C_{31}H_{46}O_2$ in each mL of the Injectable Emulsion taken by the formula:

$$D(C/V)(r_U / r_S)$$

in which D is 100 if the Injectable Emulsion contains 10 mg or more of phytonadione per mL, or 10 if the Injectable Emulsion contains less than 10 mg of phytonadione per mL; C is the concentration, in mg per mL, of USP Phytonadione RS in the *Standard preparation*; V is the volume, in mL, of Injectable Emulsion taken; and r_U and r_S are the peak responses of phytonadione obtained from the appropriate *Assay preparation* and the *Standard preparation*, respectively.

Phytonadione Tablets

» Phytonadione Tablets contain not less than 90.0 percent and not more than 110.0 percent of the labeled amount of $C_{31}H_{46}O_2$.

Packaging and storage—Preserve in well-closed, light-resistant containers.

USP Reference standards ⟨11⟩—*USP Phytonadione RS.*

Identification—

A: Transfer a portion of finely powdered Tablets, equivalent to about 10 mg of phytonadione, to a 1000-mL volumetric flask, add 750 mL of dehydrated alcohol, and shake vigorously. Dilute with dehydrated alcohol to volume, mix, and filter: the UV absorption spectrum of the filtrate exhibits maxima and minima at the same wavelengths as that of a 1 in 100,000 solution of USP Phytonadione RS in dehydrated alcohol concomitantly measured.

B: The retention time of the major peak in the chromatogram of the *Assay preparation* corresponds to that in the chromatogram of the *Standard preparation*, as obtained in the *Assay*.

Disintegration ⟨701⟩: 30 minutes.

Uniformity of dosage units ⟨905⟩: meet the requirements.

Assay—[NOTE—Use low-actinic glassware throughout the *Assay*, and otherwise protect the solutions from light.]

Mobile phase—Prepare a suitable filtered and degassed mixture of dehydrated alcohol and water (95 : 5).

Standard preparation—Prepare a solution of USP Phytonadione RS in dehydrated alcohol having a known concentration of about 0.10 mg per mL.

Assay preparation—Weigh and finely powder not less than 20 Tablets. Transfer a portion of the powdered Tablets, equivalent to about 5 mg of phytonadione, to a 50-mL volumetric flask, add 20 mL of dehydrated alcohol, and shake by mechanical means for 15 minutes. Dilute with dehydrated alcohol to volume, mix, and filter.

Chromatographic system (see *Chromatography* ⟨621⟩)—The liquid chromatograph is equipped with a 254-nm detector and a 4-mm × 30-cm column that contains packing L1. The flow rate is about 1.5 mL per minute. Chromatograph three replicate injections of the *Standard preparation*, and record the peak responses as directed for *Procedure*: the column efficiency determined from the analyte peak is not less than 915 theoretical plates, the relative standard deviation is not more than 2.0%, and the tailing factor is not more than 2.0.

Procedure—Separately inject equal volumes (about 10 µL) of the *Standard preparation* and the *Assay preparation* into the chromatograph, record the chromatograms, and measure the response for the major peak. Calculate the quantity, in mg, of $C_{31}H_{46}O_2$, in the portion of Tablets taken by the formula:

$$50C(r_U / r_S)$$

in which C is the concentration, in mg per mL, of USP Phytonadione RS in the *Standard preparation*, and r_U and r_S are the peak responses obtained from the *Assay preparation* and the *Standard preparation*, respectively.

Pilocarpine

$C_{11}H_{16}N_2O_2$ 208.26
2(3H)-Furanone, 3-ethyldihydro-4-[(1-methyl-1H-imidazol-5-yl)methyl]-, (3S-cis)-.
Pilocarpine [92-13-7].

» Pilocarpine contains not less than 95.0 percent and not more than 100.5 percent of pilocarpine ($C_{11}H_{16}N_2O_2$), calculated on the anhydrous basis.

Packaging and storage—Preserve in tight, light-resistant containers, in a cold place.
USP Reference standards ⟨11⟩—USP Pilocarpine RS. USP Pilocarpine Nitrate RS.
Identification—
  A: *Infrared Absorption* ⟨197F⟩.
  B: *Ultraviolet Absorption* ⟨197U⟩—
  Solution: 20 µg per mL.
  Medium: water.
Specific rotation ⟨781S⟩: between +102° and +107°.
  Test solution: 20 mg per mL, in pH 6.0 phosphate buffer.
Refractive index ⟨831⟩: between 1.5170 and 1.5210 at 25°, determined in a liquid specimen. If crystals are present, first warm to about 40°.
Water, *Method I* ⟨921⟩: not more than 0.5%.
Chloride—
  Standard chloride solution—Transfer 165 mg of sodium chloride to a 100-mL volumetric flask, and dissolve in and dilute with water to volume. Transfer 25.0 mL of this solution to a 1000-mL volumetric flask, and dilute with water to volume. This solution contains 25 µg of chloride per mL.
  Test solution—Transfer about 1.0 g of Pilocarpine, accurately weighed, to a 100-mL volumetric flask, dissolve in and dilute with water to volume.
  Procedure—Transfer 5.0 mL of the *Test solution* to a test tube, add 0.6 mL of diluted nitric acid and 0.3 mL of silver nitrate TS: any opalescence produced is not greater than that produced by an identically treated solution containing 5.0 mL of the *Standard chloride solution* (0.25%).
Sulfate—
  Standard sulfate solution—Dissolve 148 mg of anhydrous sodium sulfate in water, and dilute with water to 100 mL. Dilute 10.0 mL of this solution with water to 1000 mL. This solution contains 10 µg of sulfate per mL.
  Procedure—To about 1 g of Pilocarpine in a test tube add 1 mL of 6 N hydrochloric acid and 4 mL of water, and mix. For the control, transfer 4.0 mL of *Standard sulfate solution* to a test tube, add 1 mL of 6 N hydrochloric acid, and mix. Adjust both solutions with pH indicator paper by the dropwise addition of 3 N hydrochloric acid or 6 N ammonium hydroxide, if necessary, to a pH of between 2 and 3. Add water to maintain the same volume in the control and test specimen tubes. To each tube add 1 mL of barium chloride TS, and mix: any turbidity produced in the specimen tube after 10 minutes' standing is not greater than that produced in the control (0.004%).
Limit of nitrate—
  Standard preparation—Prepare a solution of USP Pilocarpine Nitrate RS to contain 43 µg per mL. This solution contains the equivalent of 10 µg of nitrate ion per mL.
  Test preparation—Prepare a solution of Pilocarpine to contain 200 mg per mL.
  Procedure—Transfer 0.5-mL portions of the *Test preparation* and of the *Standard preparation*, respectively, to separate test tubes, and to each tube add 1 drop of a 1 in 100 solution of sulfanilic acid in 5 N acetic acid and 1 drop of a 3 in 1000 solution of N-(1-naphthyl)ethylenediamine dihydrochloride in 5 N acetic acid. Adjust the *Standard preparation* and the *Test preparation* with pH indicator paper by the dropwise addition of 3 N hydrochloric acid or 1 N ammonium hydroxide, if necessary to a pH of between 2 and 3. To each solution add a few granules of acid-washed, nitrate-free zinc. Heat the test tubes in a water bath at a temperature of about 32°. Allow 5 minutes for the development of a pink color: any pink color observed in the *Test preparation* is not greater than that observed in the *Standard preparation* (0.005%).
Related compounds—
  Buffer solution, Mobile phase, System suitability preparation, and *Chromatographic system*—Proceed as directed in the *Assay*.
  Standard solution—Prepare a solution in water of isopilocarpine nitrate to contain 1.5 µg per mL.
  Test preparation—Prepare as directed for *Assay preparation* in the *Assay*.
  Procedure—Separately inject equal volumes (about 40 µL) of the *Standard solution* and the *Test preparation* into the chromatograph, record the chromatograms, and measure the responses for all the peaks. Calculate the percentage of isopilocarpine in the portion of Pilocarpine taken by the formula:

$$(208.26 / 271.27)50(C / W)(r_U / r_S)$$

in which 208.26 and 271.27 are the molecular weights of pilocarpine and isopilocarpine nitrate, respectively, C is the concentration, in µg per mL, of isopilocarpine nitrate in the *Standard solution*, W is the weight, in mg, of Pilocarpine taken, and r_U and r_S are the peak responses due to isopilocarpine in the *Test preparation* and the *Standard solution*, respectively: not more than 2% of isopilocarpine is found. Calculate the percentage of all other impurities from the chromatogram of the *Test preparation* taken by the formula:

$$(208.26 / 271.27)50(C / W)(r_i / r_s)$$

in which r_i is the peak response due to the impurity: no one impurity corresponding to one of the four peaks in the *System suitability preparation* exceeds 3%; no other individual impurity exceeds 0.5%. The sum total of all impurities, including isopilocarpine, is not more than 5.0%.
Assay—
  Buffer solution—Transfer 13.5 mL of phosphoric acid to a 1-liter beaker containing 700 mL of water. Add 3 mL of triethylamine, and dilute with water to 1000 mL. Adjust with 20% sodium hydroxide to a pH of 3.0.
  Mobile phase—Prepare a filtered and degassed mixture of *Buffer solution* and methanol (98 : 2). Make adjustments if necessary (see

System Suitability under *Chromatography* ⟨621⟩). [NOTE—Do not store this *Mobile phase* for more than 2 days.]

Standard preparation—Prepare a solution in water having an accurately known concentration of about 40 μg of USP Pilocarpine Nitrate RS per mL. [NOTE—Use this solution within 24 hours of its preparation.]

Assay preparation—Transfer an accurately weighed quantity of about 15 mg of Pilocarpine to a 500-mL volumetric flask. Dilute with water to volume, and mix. [NOTE—Use this solution within 24 hours of its preparation.]

System suitability preparation—Transfer accurately weighed quantities of about 30 mg each of pilocarpine hydrochloride and isopilocarpine nitrate to a 50-mL volumetric flask, and dilute with water to volume. Transfer 25 mL of this solution to a suitable flask, add 5 mL of 1 N sodium hydroxide, and reflux for 1 hour. Cool, and adjust the solution with 0.25 M phosphoric acid to a pH of 7.0. Quantitatively transfer this solution to a 50-mL volumetric flask, dilute with water to volume, and mix. Dilute the remaining original solution with water to volume, and mix. Add 1 mL each of the refluxed and unrefluxed solutions to a 10-mL volumetric flask, dilute with water to volume, and mix.

Chromatographic system (see *Chromatography* ⟨621⟩)—The liquid chromatograph is equipped with a 215-nm detector and a 4.6-mm × 12.5-cm column that contains 3-μm packing L1. The flow rate is about 1.0 mL per minute. Chromatograph replicate injections of the *Standard preparation*, and record the peak responses as directed for *Procedure*: the relative standard deviation is not more than 2.0%. Chromatograph the *System suitability preparation*, and record the peak responses as directed for *Procedure*: four peaks are observed; the resolution, R, between two adjacent peaks is not less than 1.2, the column efficiency determined for the pilocarpine peak is not less than 1500 theoretical plates, and the tailing factor, T, for the pilocarpine peak is not greater than 1.5. The relative retention times for the major peaks are about 0.67 for isopilocarpine, 0.76 for pilocarpine, 0.85 for pilocarpic acid, and 1.0 for isopilocarpic acid.

Procedure—Separately inject equal volumes (about 40 μL) of the *Standard preparation* and the *Assay preparation* into the chromatograph, record the chromatograms, and measure the responses for all the peaks. Calculate the quantity, in mg, of pilocarpine ($C_{11}H_{16}N_2O_2$) in the portion of Pilocarpine taken by the formula:

$$(208.26 / 271.27)500C(r_U / r_S)$$

in which 208.26 and 271.27 are the molecular weights of pilocarpine and pilocarpine nitrate, respectively, C is the concentration, in mg per mL, of USP Pilocarpine Nitrate RS in the *Standard preparation*, and r_U and r_S are the peak responses for pilocarpine obtained from the *Assay preparation* and the *Standard preparation*, respectively.

Pilocarpine Ocular System

» Pilocarpine Ocular System contains not less than 85.0 percent and not more than 115.0 percent of the labeled amount of pilocarpine ($C_{11}H_{16}N_2O_2$). It is sterile.

Packaging and storage—Preserve in single-dose containers in a cold place.

USP Reference standards ⟨11⟩—*USP Pilocarpine RS. USP Pilocarpine Hydrochloride RS. USP Pilocarpine Nitrate RS.*

Identification—Cut around the inside margin of the Ocular System, then discard the ring encircling the Ocular System, extract the remaining portion with 0.5 mL of methanol in a small capped vial, shaking vigorously for 1 to 2 minutes. Evaporate the methanol extract on a sodium chloride plate forming a thin film: the IR absorption spectrum of the film exhibits maxima only at the same wavelengths as that of a similar preparation of USP Pilocarpine RS.

Sterility ⟨71⟩: meets the requirements.

Uniformity of dosage units ⟨905⟩: meets the requirements for capsules.

Drug release pattern—Place each of the Ocular Systems in suitable porous holders made of an inert material, and suspend each from a nickel wire. To the upper end of the wire attach a tag identifying the specimen. Put each assembly into a test tube containing 27.0 mL of saline TS so that the system lies at the bottom of the tube and the identifying tag extends from the open top of the tube. Put the tubes into a horizontally reciprocating shaker in which the temperature is maintained at 37 ± 0.5°. Agitate the tubes with a horizontal amplitude of about 4 cm and a frequency of about 35 cycles per minute. At 7, 24, 48, 72, 96, and 168 hours, remove the assemblies from their tubes, and each time replace them in similar tubes containing 27.0 mL of fresh saline TS. Determine the amount of pilocarpine in solution in each tube, after adjusting the volume to 27.0 mL to make up for any evaporative losses, by measuring the UV absorbance in 1-cm cells at the wavelength of maximum absorbance at about 215 nm, with a suitable spectrophotometer, against saline TS as the blank. Concomitantly measure the absorbance of a *Standard solution* of USP Pilocarpine Hydrochloride RS having a known concentration of about 20 μg in each mL of saline TS. Calculate the quantity, in μg, of $C_{11}H_{16}N_2O_2$ in each solution taken by the formula:

$$(208.26 / 244.72)(A_U / A_S)27C$$

in which 208.26 and 244.72 are the molecular weights of pilocarpine and pilocarpine hydrochloride, respectively; A_U and A_S are the absorbances of the test solution and the Standard solution, respectively; and C is the concentration, in μg per mL, of USP Pilocarpine Hydrochloride RS in the Standard solution. Calculate the amount of pilocarpine released in 168 hours by adding the pilocarpine content of each set of tubes collected over 168 hours.

Tolerances—The amount of $C_{11}H_{16}N_2O_2$ from each Ocular System released during the total 0 to 168 hours tested conforms to *Acceptance Table 1* under *Drug Release* ⟨724⟩. The drug release range for this time period is not less than 80.0% and not more than 120.0% of the labeled release pattern.

Assay—

Buffer solution, Mobile phase, Standard preparation, System suitability preparation, and *Chromatographic system*—Proceed as directed in the *Assay* under *Pilocarpine*.

Assay preparation—Select not fewer than 10 Ocular Systems. Cut each System into 4 pieces, transfer quantitatively to a 500-mL volumetric flask, and rinse all cutting utensils with 20 to 30 mL of methanol into the flask. Make additional rinses of the utensils with about 250 mL of *Mobile phase*, and collect all the rinses in the flasks. Allow the flasks to stand for 30 minutes, sonicate for about 15 minutes, dilute with water to volume, and mix. Transfer an aliquot of the supernatant, equivalent to 6 mg of pilocarpine to a 200-mL volumetric flask, dilute with water to volume, mix, and filter.

Procedure—Proceed as directed for *Procedure* in the *Assay* under *Pilocarpine*. Calculate the quantity, in mg, of pilocarpine in each Ocular System taken by the formula:

$$(208.26 / 271.27)(10 / V)(C / N)(r_U / r_S)$$

in which 208.26 and 271.27 are the molecular weights of pilocarpine and pilocarpine nitrate, respectively; V is the volume, in mL, of the supernatant taken (see *Assay preparation*); C is the concentration, in μg per mL, of USP Pilocarpine Nitrate RS in the *Standard preparation*; N is the number of Ocular Systems taken; and r_U and r_S are the peak responses for pilocarpine obtained from the *Assay preparation* and the *Standard preparation*, respectively.

Pilocarpine Hydrochloride

$C_{11}H_{16}N_2O_2 \cdot HCl$ 244.72

2(3H)-Furanone, 3-ethyldihydro-4-[(1-methyl-1H-imidazol-5-yl)methyl]-, monohydrochloride, (3S-cis)-.
Pilocarpine monohydrochloride   [54-71-7].

» Pilocarpine Hydrochloride contains not less than 98.5 percent and not more than 101.0 percent of $C_{11}H_{16}N_2O_2 \cdot HCl$, calculated on the dried basis.

Packaging and storage—Preserve in tight, light-resistant containers.

USP Reference standards ⟨11⟩—*USP Pilocarpine Hydrochloride RS.*
Identification—
  A: *Infrared Absorption* ⟨197M⟩.
  B: A solution (1 in 20) responds to the tests for *Chloride* ⟨191⟩.
Melting range ⟨741⟩: between 199° and 205°, but the range between beginning and end of melting does not exceed 3°.
Specific rotation ⟨781S⟩: between +88.5° and +91.5°.
  Test solution: 20 mg per mL, in water.
Loss on drying ⟨731⟩—Dry it at 105° for 2 hours: it loses not more than 3.0% of its weight.
Readily carbonizable substances ⟨271⟩—Dissolve 250 mg in 5 mL of sulfuric acid TS: the solution has no more color than *Matching Fluid B*.
Ordinary impurities ⟨466⟩—
  Test solution: dehydrated alcohol.
  Standard solution: dehydrated alcohol.
  Eluant: a mixture of hexanes, dehydrated alcohol, and ammonium hydroxide (70 : 30 : 1).
  Visualization: 17.
  Limits: not more than 1%.
Other alkaloids—Dissolve 200 mg in 20 mL of water, and divide the solution into two portions. To one portion add a few drops of 6 N ammonium hydroxide, and to the other add a few drops of potassium dichromate TS: no turbidity is produced in either solution.
Assay—Dissolve about 500 mg of Pilocarpine Hydrochloride, accurately weighed, in a mixture of 20 mL of glacial acetic acid and 10 mL of mercuric acetate TS, warming slightly to effect solution. Cool the solution to room temperature, add 2 drops of crystal violet TS, and titrate with 0.1 N perchloric acid VS. Perform a blank determination, and make any necessary correction. Each mL of 0.1 N perchloric acid is equivalent to 24.47 mg of $C_{11}H_{16}N_2O_2 \cdot HCl$.

Pilocarpine Hydrochloride Ophthalmic Solution

» Pilocarpine Hydrochloride Ophthalmic Solution is a sterile, buffered, aqueous solution of Pilocarpine Hydrochloride. It contains not less than 90.0 percent and not more than 110.0 percent of the labeled amount of $C_{11}H_{16}N_2O_2 \cdot HCl$. It may contain suitable antimicrobial agents and stabilizers, and suitable additives to increase its viscosity.

Packaging and storage—Preserve in tight containers.

USP Reference standards ⟨11⟩—*USP Pilocarpine Hydrochloride RS.*
Identification—The retention time of the major peak in the chromatogram of the *Assay preparation* corresponds to that in the chromatogram of the *Standard preparation,* as obtained in the *Assay.*
Sterility ⟨71⟩: meets the requirements.
pH ⟨791⟩: between 3.5 and 5.5.
Assay—
  Mobile phase—Mix 300 mL of a 1 in 50 solution of ammonium hydroxide in isopropyl alcohol and 700 mL of *n*-hexane. Filter through a 0.5-μm filter before using.
  Standard preparation—Using an accurately weighed quantity of USP Pilocarpine Hydrochloride RS, prepare a solution having a known concentration of about 1.6 mg per mL.
  Assay preparation—Transfer an accurately measured volume of Ophthalmic Solution, equivalent to about 80 mg of pilocarpine hydrochloride, to a 50-mL volumetric flask. Dilute with methanol to volume, and mix.
  Chromatographic system (see *Chromatography* ⟨621⟩)—The liquid chromatograph is equipped with a 220-nm detector and a 4.6-mm × 25-cm column that contains packing L3. The flow rate is about 2 mL per minute. Chromatograph three replicate injections of the *Standard preparation,* and record the peak responses as directed for *Procedure:* the relative standard deviation is not more than 2.0%.
  Procedure—Separately inject equal volumes (about 10 μL) of the *Standard preparation* and the *Assay preparation* into the chromatograph by means of a suitable microsyringe or sampling valve, record the chromatograms, and measure the responses for the major peaks. The retention time is about 16 minutes for pilocarpine hydrochloride. Calculate the quantity, in mg, of $C_{11}H_{16}N_2O_2 \cdot HCl$ in each mL of the Ophthalmic Solution taken by the formula:

$$50(C / V)(r_U / r_S)$$

in which *C* is the concentration, in mg per mL, of USP Pilocarpine Hydrochloride RS in the *Standard preparation,* *V* is the volume, in mL, of Ophthalmic Solution taken, and r_U and r_S are the peak responses obtained from the *Assay preparation* and the *Standard preparation,* respectively.

Pilocarpine Nitrate

$C_{11}H_{16}N_2O_2 \cdot HNO_3$ 271.27
2(3*H*)-Furanone, 3-ethyldihydro-4-[(1-methyl-1*H*-imidazol-5-yl)methyl]-, (3*S-cis*)-, mononitrate.
Pilocarpine mononitrate [148-72-1].

» Pilocarpine Nitrate contains not less than 98.5 percent and not more than 101.0 percent of $C_{11}H_{16}N_2O_2 \cdot NO_3$, calculated on the dried basis.

Packaging and storage—Preserve in tight, light-resistant containers.
USP Reference standards ⟨11⟩—*USP Pilocarpine Nitrate RS.*
Identification—
  A: *Infrared Absorption* ⟨197K⟩.
  B: Mix a solution (1 in 10) with an equal volume of ferrous sulfate TS, and superimpose the mixture upon 5 mL of sulfuric acid contained in a test tube: the zone of contact becomes brown.
Melting range ⟨741⟩: between 171° and 176°, with decomposition, but the range between beginning and end of melting does not exceed 3°.
Specific rotation ⟨781S⟩: between +79.5° and +82.5°.
  Test solution: 20 mg per mL, in water.
Loss on drying ⟨731⟩—Dry it at 105° for 2 hours: it loses not more than 2.0% of its weight.
Readily carbonizable substances ⟨271⟩—Dissolve 100 mg in 5 mL of sulfuric acid TS: the solution has no more color than *Matching Fluid A*.
Chloride—To 5 mL of a solution (1 in 50), acidified with nitric acid, add a few drops of silver nitrate TS: no opalescence is produced immediately.
Other alkaloids—Dissolve 200 mg in 20 mL of water, and divide the solution into two portions. To one portion add a few drops of 6 N ammonium hydroxide and to the other add a few drops of potassium dichromate TS: no turbidity is produced in either solution.
Assay—Dissolve about 600 mg of Pilocarpine Nitrate, accurately weighed, in 30 mL of glacial acetic acid, warming slightly to effect solution. Cool to room temperature, and titrate with 0.1 N perchloric acid VS, determining the endpoint potentiometrically. Perform a blank determination, and make any necessary correction. Each mL of 0.1 N perchloric acid is equivalent to 27.13 mg of $C_{11}H_{16}N_2O_2 \cdot NO_3$.

Pilocarpine Nitrate Ophthalmic Solution

» Pilocarpine Nitrate Ophthalmic Solution is a sterile, buffered, aqueous solution of Pilocarpine Nitrate. It contains not less than 90.0 percent and not more than

110.0 percent of the labeled amount of $C_{11}H_{16}N_2O_2 \cdot HNO_3$. It may contain suitable antimicrobial agents and stabilizers, and suitable additives to increase its viscosity.

Packaging and storage—Preserve in tight, light-resistant containers.

USP Reference standards ⟨11⟩—*USP Pilocarpine Nitrate RS.*

Identification—
  A: The retention time of the major peak in the chromatogram of the *Assay preparation* corresponds to that in the chromatogram of the *Standard preparation* obtained as directed in the *Assay*.
  B: It responds to *Identification* test B under *Pilocarpine Nitrate*.

Sterility ⟨71⟩: meets the requirements.

pH ⟨791⟩: between 4.0 and 5.5.

Assay—Proceed with Ophthalmic Solution as directed in the *Assay* under *Pilocarpine Hydrochloride Ophthalmic Solution*, except to read pilocarpine nitrate instead of pilocarpine hydrochloride throughout and to calculate the quantity, in mg, of $C_{11}H_{16}N_2O_2 \cdot HNO_3$ in each mL of the Ophthalmic Solution taken by the formula given therein.

Pimozide

$C_{28}H_{29}F_2N_3O$ 461.55

2*H*-Benzimidazol-2-one, 1-[1-[4,4-bis(4-fluorophenyl)butyl]-4-piperidinyl]-1,3-dihydro-.
1-[1-[4,4-Bis(*p*-fluorophenyl)butyl]-4-piperidyl]-2-benzimidazolinone [2062-78-4].

» Pimozide contains not less than 98.0 percent and not more than 102.0 percent of $C_{28}H_{29}F_2N_3O$, calculated on the dried basis.

Packaging and storage—Preserve in tight, light-resistant containers.

USP Reference standards ⟨11⟩—*USP Pimozide RS.*

Identification—
  A: *Infrared Absorption* ⟨197K⟩.
  B: *Ultraviolet Absorption* ⟨197U⟩—
    Solution: 35 μg per mL.
    Medium: 0.1 N hydrochloric acid in methanol (1 in 10).

Melting range, *Class I* ⟨741⟩: between 216° and 220°.

Loss on drying ⟨731⟩—Dry it in vacuum at 80° for 4 hours: it loses not more than 0.5% of its weight.

Residue on ignition ⟨281⟩: not more than 0.2%, a 2-g portion and a platinum crucible being used for the test.

Heavy metals, *Method II* ⟨231⟩: 0.002%.

Ordinary impurities ⟨466⟩—
  Test solution: chloroform.
  Standard solution: chloroform.
  Eluant: a mixture of cyclohexane and acetone (1 : 1).
  Visualization: 1, then 17.
  Limit—The total of any ordinary impurities observed does not exceed 1.0%.

Organic volatile impurities, *Method V* ⟨467⟩: meets the requirements.
  Solvent—Use dimethyl sulfoxide.

(Official until July 1, 2008)

Assay—Dissolve about 320 mg of Pimozide, accurately weighed, in 40 mL of glacial acetic acid. Titrate with 0.1 N perchloric acid VS, determining the endpoint potentiometrically. Perform a blank determination, and make any necessary correction. Each mL of 0.1 N perchloric acid is equivalent to 46.16 mg of $C_{28}H_{29}F_2N_3O$.

Pimozide Tablets

» Pimozide Tablets contain not less than 90.0 percent and not more than 110.0 percent of the labeled amount of $C_{28}H_{29}F_2N_3O$.

Packaging and storage—Preserve in tight, light-resistant containers.

USP Reference standards ⟨11⟩—*USP Pimozide RS.*

Identification—The retention time of the major peak in the chromatogram of the *Assay preparation* corresponds to that of the *Standard preparation*, both relative to the internal standard, as obtained in the *Assay*.

Dissolution, *Procedure for a Pooled Sample* ⟨711⟩—
  Medium: 0.01 N hydrochloric acid; 900 mL.
  Apparatus 2: 50 rpm.
  Time: 30 minutes.
  Standard preparation—Transfer about 27 mg of USP Pimozide RS, accurately weighed, to a 250-mL volumetric flask containing 1 mL of lactic acid. Heat on a steam bath to dissolve, add about 80 mL of hot water, and shake. Cool, dilute with water to volume, and mix. Dilute the solution quantitatively with 0.01 N hydrochloric acid to obtain a solution having a known concentration approximately the same as that of the solution under test (assuming complete dissolution).
  Procedure—Transfer a portion of the solution under test to a suitable container, and centrifuge until clear. Pipet a volume of the supernatant, estimated to contain about 110 μg of pimozide (assuming complete dissolution), into a suitable container. Pipet an equal volume of the *Standard preparation* into a second container. To each container add 20 mL of 1 N sodium hydroxide and 20.0 mL of chloroform. Shake each mixture by mechanical means for 15 minutes, and centrifuge. Aspirate and discard the aqueous layers, and transfer the chloroform layers to separate clean beakers. Determine the amount of $C_{28}H_{29}F_2N_3O$ dissolved from absorbances of the chloroform layers obtained from the solution under test and the *Standard preparation*, in 5-cm cells at the wavelength of maximum absorbance at about 277 nm.
  Tolerances—Not less than 80% *(Q)* of the labeled amount of $C_{28}H_{29}F_2N_3O$ is dissolved in 30 minutes.

Uniformity of dosage units ⟨905⟩: meet the requirements.
  Procedure for content uniformity—Place 1 tablet in a 50-mL flask, add 5.0 mL of 0.1 N hydrochloric acid, and shake by mechanical means for 30 minutes. Add 20.0 mL of methanol, and shake by mechanical means for 20 minutes. Dilute, if necessary, quantitatively with methanol to obtain a solution having a concentration of about 40 μg of pimozide per mL, mix, and centrifuge. Concomitantly determine the absorbance of the supernatant and of a solution of USP Pimozide RS in the same medium having a known concentration of about 40 μg per mL in 1-cm cells at the wavelength of maximum absorbance at about 277 nm, with a suitable spectrophotometer, using a mixture of 0.1 N hydrochloric acid and methanol (1 in 10) as the blank. Calculate the quantity, in mg, of $C_{28}H_{29}F_2N_3O$ in the Tablet taken by the formula:

$$(TC/D)(A_U/A_S)$$

in which *T* is the labeled quantity, in mg, of pimozide in the Tablet, *C* is the concentration, in μg per mL, of USP Pimozide RS in the *Standard solution*, *D* is the concentration, in μg per mL, of pimozide in the solution from the Tablet based upon the labeled quantity per Tablet and the extent of dilution, and A_U and A_S are the absorbances of the solution from the Tablet and the Standard solution, respectively.

Assay—[NOTE—Protect all pimozide solutions from light.]
  Ammonium acetate solution—Dissolve 500 mg of ammonium acetate in 100 mL of water, and mix.

Mobile phase—Prepare a filtered and degassed mixture of acetonitrile and *Ammonium acetate solution* (65 : 35), making adjustments if necessary (see *System Suitability* under *Chromatography* ⟨621⟩).

Internal standard solution—Dissolve 3,4-dimethylbenzophenone in a mixture of methanol and tetrahydrofuran (1 : 1) to obtain a solution having a concentration of about 1 mg per mL.

Standard preparation—Transfer about 25 mg of USP Pimozide RS, accurately weighed, to a 50-mL volumetric flask, add 10 mL of *Internal standard solution*, dilute with a mixture of methanol and tetrahydrofuran (1 : 1) to volume, and mix.

Assay preparation—Weigh and finely powder not less than 20 Tablets. Transfer an accurately weighed portion of the powder, equivalent to about 25 mg of pimozide, to a 50-mL volumetric flask. Add 10 mL of *Internal standard solution* and 20 mL of a mixture of methanol and tetrahydrofuran (1 : 1), and shake by mechanical means for 30 minutes. Dilute with a mixture of methanol and tetrahydrofuran (1 : 1) to volume, and centrifuge. Use the clear supernatant as the *Assay preparation*.

Chromatographic system (see *Chromatography* ⟨621⟩)—The liquid chromatograph is equipped with a 280-nm detector and a 4.6-mm × 25-cm column that contains 5-μm packing L1. The flow rate is about 2 mL per minute. Chromatograph replicate injections of the *Standard preparation*, and record the peak responses as directed for *Procedure*: the relative standard deviation is not more than 2.0%, and the resolution, R, between the analyte and the internal standard peaks is not less than 1.3.

Procedure—Separately inject equal volumes (about 10 μL) of the *Standard preparation* and the *Assay preparation* into the chromatograph, record the chromatograms, and measure the responses for the major peaks. The relative retention times are about 0.7 for pimozide and 1.0 for the internal standard. Calculate the quantity, in mg, of $C_{28}H_{29}F_2N_3O$ in the portion of Tablets taken by the formula:

$$50C(R_U / R_S)$$

in which C is the concentration, in mg per mL, of USP Pimozide RS in the *Standard preparation*, and R_U and R_S are the ratios of the pimozide peak response to the internal standard peak response obtained from the *Assay preparation* and the *Standard preparation*, respectively.

Pindolol

$C_{14}H_{20}N_2O_2$ 248.32

2-Propanol,1-(1*H*-indol-4-yloxy)-3-(1-methylethyl)amino-.
1-(Indol-4-yloxy)-3-(isopropylamino)-2-propanol   [*13523-86-9*].

» Pindolol contains not less than 98.5 percent and not more than 101.0 percent of $C_{14}H_{20}N_2O_2$, calculated on the dried basis.

Packaging and storage—Preserve in well-closed containers, protected from light.

USP Reference standards ⟨11⟩—*USP Pindolol RS.*

Identification—
  A: *Infrared Absorption* ⟨197K⟩.
  B: *Ultraviolet Absorption* ⟨197U⟩—
  Solution: 20 μg per mL.
  Medium: hydrochloric acid in methanol (1 in 1200).
  C: The retention time of the major peak in the chromatogram of the *Assay preparation* corresponds to that in the chromatogram of the *Standard preparation*, as obtained in the *Assay*.

Melting range ⟨741⟩:   between 169° and 173°, but the range between beginning and end of melting does not exceed 3°.

Loss on drying ⟨731⟩—Dry it at 105° for 4 hours: it loses not more than 0.5% of its weight.

Residue on ignition ⟨281⟩:   not more than 0.1%.
Heavy metals, *Method II* ⟨231⟩:   0.002%.
Chromatographic purity—

Mobile phase—Prepare a mixture of 0.05 M sodium acetate, previously adjusted with glacial acetic acid to a pH of 5.0, and acetonitrile (65 : 35), and filter through a filter having a 0.5-μm or finer porosity. Make adjustments if necessary (see *System Suitability* under *Chromatography* ⟨621⟩). Decreasing the acetonitrile concentration results in less resolution between pindolol and impurities that elute on the tail of the pindolol peak; increasing the acetonitrile concentration results in less resolution between impurities with longer retention times.

Resolution solution—Prepare as directed for *Resolution solution* in the *Assay*.

Test solution—Use the stock solution used to prepare the *Assay preparation* in the *Assay*.

Chromatographic system (see *Chromatography* ⟨621⟩)—Proceed as directed in the *Chromatographic system* under the *Assay*.

Procedure—[NOTE—Use peak areas where peak responses are indicated.] Separately inject equal volumes (about 10 μL) of the *Resolution solution* and the *Test solution* into the chromatograph, record the chromatograms, and measure the responses for all of the peaks. Calculate the percentage of each impurity in the portion of Pindolol taken by the formula:

$$10,000(C / W)(r_U / r_S)$$

in which C is the concentration, in mg per mL, of USP Pindolol RS in the *Resolution solution*, W is the weight, in mg, of the portion of Pindolol taken to prepare the *Test solution*, r_U is the peak response of an individual impurity, and r_S is the pindolol peak response obtained from the *Resolution solution*. Not more than 0.5% of any individual impurity is found, and the total of all impurities does not exceed 2.0%.

Organic volatile impurities, *Method V* ⟨467⟩:   meets the requirements.

Solvent—Use dimethyl sulfoxide.

(Official until July 1, 2008)

Assay—

Mobile phase—Prepare a mixture of 0.05 *M* sodium acetate, previously adjusted with glacial acetic acid to a pH of 5.0, and acetonitrile (65 : 35), and filter through a filter having a 0.5-μm or finer porosity. Make adjustments if necessary (see *System Suitability* under *Chromatography* ⟨621⟩).

Resolution solution—Prepare a solution in *Mobile phase* having known concentrations of about 0.005 mg of USP Pindolol RS per mL and about 0.005 mg of indole per mL.

Standard preparation—Transfer about 100 mg of USP Pindolol RS, accurately weighed, to a 100-mL volumetric flask, add about 90 mL of *Mobile phase*, and dissolve by sonicating for about 5 minutes. Cool, dilute with *Mobile phase* to volume, and mix. Transfer 5.0 mL of this solution to a 50-mL volumetric flask, dilute with *Mobile phase* to volume, and mix.

Assay preparation—Transfer about 100 mg of Pindolol, accurately weighed, to a 100-mL volumetric flask, add about 90 mL of *Mobile phase*, and dissolve by sonicating for about 5 minutes. Cool, dilute with *Mobile phase* to volume, and mix. Transfer 5.0 mL of this stock solution to a 50-mL volumetric flask, dilute with *Mobile phase* to volume, and mix.

Chromatographic system (see *Chromatography* ⟨621⟩)—The liquid chromatograph is equipped with a 219-nm detector and a 4.6-mm × 15-cm column containing 3-μm packing L10. The flow rate is about 1 mL per minute. Chromatograph the *Resolution solution*, and record the responses as directed for *Procedure*: the relative retention times are about 0.5 for indole and 1.0 for pindolol, the resolution, R, between the indole and pindolol is not less than 7, the column efficiency determined from the pindolol peak is not less than 3000 theoretical plates, and the relative standard deviation of the pindolol peak response for replicate injections is not more than 2%.

Procedure—[NOTE—Use peak areas where peak responses are indicated.] Separately inject equal volumes (about 10 μL) of the *Standard preparation* and the *Assay preparation* into the chromatograph, record the chromatograms, and measure the responses for the major peaks. Calculate the quantity, in mg, of $C_{14}H_{20}N_2O_2$ in the portion of Pindolol taken by the formula:

$$1000C(r_U/r_S)$$

in which C is the concentration, in mg per mL, of USP Pindolol RS in the *Standard preparation*, and r_U and r_S are the pindolol peak responses obtained from the *Assay preparation* and the *Standard preparation*, respectively.

Pindolol Tablets

» Pindolol Tablets contain not less than 90.0 percent and not more than 110.0 percent of the labeled amount of pindolol ($C_{14}H_{20}N_2O_2$).

Packaging and storage—Preserve in well-closed containers, protected from light.

USP Reference standards ⟨11⟩—*USP Pindolol RS.*
Identification—
A: Examine the chromatograms obtained in the test for *Chromatographic purity:* the principal spot obtained from the *Test solution* is similar in R_F value, color, and intensity to that obtained from the *Standard stock solution*.
B: The retention time exhibited by pindolol in the chromatogram of the *Assay preparation* corresponds to that of pindolol in the chromatogram of the *Standard preparation*, as obtained in the *Assay*.

Dissolution, *Procedure for a Pooled Sample* ⟨711⟩—
Medium: 0.1 N hydrochloric acid; 500 mL.
Apparatus 2: 50 rpm.
Time: 15 minutes.
Mobile phase and *Chromatographic system*—Proceed as directed in the *Assay*.
Standard solution—Dissolve an accurately weighed quantity of USP Pindolol RS in *Dissolution Medium* to obtain a solution having a known concentration of about $0.002J$ mg per mL, J being the labeled quantity, in mg, of pindolol in each Tablet. Mix equal volumes of this solution and of *Mobile phase* to obtain the *Standard solution*.
Resolution solution—Dissolve a quantity of nortriptyline hydrochloride in *Standard solution* to obtain a solution having a concentration of about 0.005 mg of nortriptyline hydrochloride per mL.
Test solution—Filter a portion of the solution under test. Mix equal volumes of the filtrate and of *Mobile phase* to obtain the *Test solution*.
Procedure—Proceed as directed for *Procedure* under the *Assay*. Calculate the quantity of $C_{14}H_{20}N_2O_2$ dissolved by the formula:

$$500C(r_U/r_S)$$

in which C is the concentration, in mg per mL, of USP Pindolol RS in the *Standard solution;* and r_U and r_S are the pindolol peak responses obtained from the *Test solution* and the *Standard solution*, respectively.
Tolerances—Not less than 80% (Q) of the labeled amount of $C_{14}H_{20}N_2O_2$ is dissolved in 15 minutes.

Uniformity of dosage units ⟨905⟩: meet the requirements.
Chromatographic purity—[NOTE—Protect solutions and chromatographic plate (after application of solutions) from light.]
p-Dimethylaminobenzaldehyde spray—Dissolve 1 g of *p*-dimethylaminobenzaldehyde in a mixture of 50 mL of hydrochloric acid and 50 mL of alcohol, and mix. [NOTE—Store this solution in a tightly closed, light-resistant container, and discard after 4 weeks.]
Solvent mixture—Prepare a solution of methanol and glacial acetic acid (99 : 1).
Standard stock solution—Dissolve an accurately weighed quantity of USP Pindolol RS in *Solvent mixture* to obtain a solution containing 5.0 mg per mL.
Standard solution 1—Dilute an accurately measured volume of *Standard stock solution* quantitatively and stepwise with *Solvent mixture* to obtain a solution containing 0.025 mg per mL.
Standard solution 2—Dilute 6.0 mL of *Standard solution 1* with *Solvent mixture* to 10.0 mL, and mix.
Standard solution 3—Dilute 4.0 mL of *Standard solution 1* with *Solvent mixture* to 10.0 mL, and mix.
Standard solution 4—Dilute 2.0 mL of *Standard solution 1* with *Solvent mixture* to 10.0 mL, and mix.
Test solution—[NOTE—Prepare this solution immediately before use, and apply last.] Transfer a portion of powdered Tablets, equivalent to 50 mg of pindolol, to a 50-mL flask, add 10.0 mL of *Solvent mixture*, insert the stopper in the flask, and shake by mechanical means for 15 minutes. Centrifuge a portion of the resultant suspension, and promptly test the clear supernatant.
Procedure—Prepare a lined chromatographic chamber (see *Chromatography* ⟨621⟩) with a developing solvent consisting of a mixture of methylene chloride, methanol, and formic acid (75 : 23.5 : 1.5), and equilibrate for 30 minutes. Separately apply 2-µL portions of the *Standard stock solution*, each of the *Standard solutions*, and the *Test solution* to a thin-layer chromatographic plate coated with a 0.25-mm layer of chromatographic silica gel. Place the plate in the chromatographic chamber, and allow the solvent front to move about two-thirds of the length of the plate. Remove the plate from the chamber, immediately spray with the *p-Dimethylaminobenzaldehyde spray*, heat the plate at 60° for 15 minutes, and promptly examine the chromatogram: no individual secondary spot observed in the chromatogram of the *Test solution* is greater in size or intensity than the principal spot observed in the chromatogram of *Standard solution 1*, corresponding to 0.5%, and the total of any such spots observed does not exceed 3.0%. [NOTE—In a valid determination, spots from all solutions must be visible.]

Assay—
Ammonium carbonate solution—Dissolve 300 mg of ammonium carbonate in 50 mL of water, and mix.
Mobile phase—Prepare a filtered and degassed mixture of acetonitrile, methanol, and *Ammonium carbonate solution* (475 : 475 : 50), making adjustments, if necessary (see *System Suitability* under *Chromatography* ⟨621⟩).
Standard preparation—Prepare a solution of USP Pindolol RS in *Mobile phase* to obtain a solution having a known concentration of about 0.2 mg per mL.
Resolution solution—Dissolve a quantity of nortriptyline hydrochloride in *Standard preparation* to obtain a solution having a concentration of about 0.2 mg of nortriptyline hydrochloride per mL.
Assay preparation—Weigh and finely powder not less than 20 Tablets. Transfer an accurately weighed portion of the powder, equivalent to about 20 mg of pindolol, to a 100-mL volumetric flask. Add 4 mL of water, and sonicate for 2 minutes, with occasional shaking to disperse the powder. Add 30 mL of *Mobile phase*, sonicate for 15 minutes, and allow to cool. Dilute with *Mobile phase* to volume, mix, and filter. Use the clear filtrate as the *Assay preparation*.
Chromatographic system (see *Chromatography* ⟨621⟩)—The liquid chromatograph is equipped with a 254-nm detector and a 4.6-mm × 25-cm column that contains packing L16. The flow rate is about 3 mL per minute. Chromatograph the *Resolution solution*, and record the peak responses as directed for *Procedure*: the resolution between pindolol and nortriptyline is not less than 1.5. Chromatograph the *Standard preparation*, and record the peak responses as directed for *Procedure*: the relative standard deviation for replicate injections is not more than 2.0%.
Procedure—Separately inject equal volumes (about 10 µL) of the *Standard preparation* and the *Assay preparation* into the chromatograph, record the chromatograms, and measure the responses for the major peaks. The relative retention times are about 0.6 for pindolol and 1.0 for nortriptyline. Calculate the quantity, in mg, of pindolol ($C_{14}H_{20}N_2O_2$) in the portion of Tablets taken by the formula:

$$100C(r_U/r_S)$$

in which C is the concentration, in mg per mL, of USP Pindolol RS in the *Standard preparation;* and r_U and r_S are the pindolol peak responses obtained from the *Assay preparation* and the *Standard preparation*, respectively.

Piperacillin

$C_{23}H_{27}N_5O_7S \cdot H_2O$ 535.57

4-Thia-1-azabicyclo[3.2.0]heptane-2-carboxylic acid, 6-[[[[(4-ethyl-2,3-dioxo-1-piperazinyl)carbonyl]amino]phenylacetyl]amino]-3,3-dimethyl-7-oxo-, monohydrate, [2S-2α,5α,6β(S*)]].
(2S,5R,6R)-6-[(R)-2-(4-ethyl-2,3-dioxo-1-piperazinecarboxamido)-2-phenylacetamido]-3,3-dimethyl-7-oxo-4-thia-1-azabicyclo[3.2.0]heptaic acid monohydrate   [66258-76-2].
Anhydrous   517.56   [61477-96-1].

» Piperacillin contains not less than 960 µg and not more than 1030 µg of piperacillin ($C_{23}H_{27}N_5O_7S$) per mg, calculated on the anhydrous basis.

Packaging and storage—Preserve in well-closed containers.
Labeling—Where it is intended for use in preparing injectable dosage forms, the label states that it is sterile or must be subjected to further processing during the preparation of injectable dosage forms.
USP Reference standards ⟨11⟩—USP Piperacillin RS. USP Ampicillin RS. USP Endotoxin RS.
Identification, *Infrared Absorption* ⟨197K⟩.
Water, *Method I* ⟨921⟩:   between 2.0% and 4.0%.
Heavy metals, *Method II* ⟨231⟩:   0.002%.
Specific rotation ⟨781S⟩:   between +155° and +175°.
 Test solution: 40 mg per mL, in methanol.
Related compounds—
 TEST 1—
 Mobile phase and *Chromatographic system*—Prepare as directed in the *Assay*.
 Standard piperacillin solution—Transfer about 40 mg of USP Piperacillin RS, accurately weighed, to a 100-mL volumetric flask, add a few drops of methanol to dissolve it, dilute with *Mobile phase* to volume, and mix. Transfer 5.0 mL of this solution to a 50-mL volumetric flask, dilute with *Mobile phase* to volume, and mix. [NOTE—Use these solutions within 1 hour.]
 Standard ampicillin solution—Prepare a solution of USP Ampicillin RS in *Mobile phase* having a known concentration of about 0.08 mg per mL.
 Test solution—Use the *Assay preparation*.
 Procedure—Separately inject equal volumes (about 10 µL) of the *Test solution,* the *Standard ampicillin solution,* and the *Standard piperacillin solution,* and proceed as directed in the *Assay*. Calculate the percentage of ampicillin in the portion of Piperacillin taken by the formula:

$$10C(P/W)(r_U/r_{Sa})$$

in which C is the concentration, in mg per mL, of USP Ampicillin RS in the *Standard ampicillin solution;* P is the designated potency, in µg of ampicillin per mg, of USP Ampicillin RS; W is the weight, in mg, of Piperacillin taken to prepare the *Test solution;* and r_U and r_{Sa} are the peak responses of ampicillin obtained from the *Test solution* and the *Standard ampicillin solution,* respectively: not more than 0.2% of ampicillin is found.
 Calculate the percentage of piperacillin related compound A (4-carboxy-α-[2-(4-ethyl-2,3-dioxo-1-piperazinecarboxamido-2-phenylacetamido]-5,5-dimethyl-2-thiazolidinacetic acid), piperacillin related compound B (1-ethyl-2,3-piperazinedione), and piperacillin related compound C (2-(3-acetyl-4-carboxy-5,5-dimethyl-2-thiazolidinyl)-N-[N-[(4-ethyl-2,3-dioxo-1-piperazinyl)-carbonyl]-2-phenylglycyl]glycine) in the portion of Piperacillin taken by the formula:

$$10C(P/W)(RRF_i)(r_i/r_{Sp})$$

in which C is the concentration, in mg per mL, of USP Piperacillin RS in the *Standard piperacillin solution; P* is the designated potency, in µg of piperacillin per mg, of USP Piperacillin RS; W is the weight, in mg, of Piperacillin taken to prepare the *Test solution;* RRF_i is the response factor of an individual piperacillin related compound relative to the response of piperacillin, specifically 1.4 for piperacillin related compound A, 0.41 for piperacillin related compound B, and 0.93 for piperacillin related compound C; r_i is the response of each impurity peak obtained from the *Test solution;* and r_{Sp} is the peak response of piperacillin obtained from the *Standard piperacillin solution:* not more than 1.0% of piperacillin related compound A, not more than 0.2% of piperacillin related compound B, and not more than 0.4% of piperacillin related compound C is found.
 TEST 2—
 Mobile phase—Prepare a mixture of methanol, water, 0.2 M monobasic sodium phosphate, and 0.4 M tetrabutylammonium hydroxide (615 : 282 : 100 : 3). Adjust with phosphoric acid to a pH of 5.50 ± 0.02, and degas. Make adjustments if necessary (see *System Suitability* under *Chromatography* ⟨621⟩).
 Standard stock solution—Transfer about 20 mg of USP Piperacillin RS, accurately weighed, to a 50-mL volumetric flask, add a few drops of methanol to dissolve it, dilute with *Mobile phase* to volume, and mix. [NOTE—Use this solution within 1 hour.]
 Standard solution—Transfer 5.0 mL of the *Standard stock solution* to a 50-mL volumetric flask, dilute with *Mobile phase* to volume, and mix. [NOTE—Use this solution within 1 hour.]
 Test solution—Transfer about 40 mg of Piperacillin, accurately weighed, to a 100-mL volumetric flask, add a few drops of methanol to dissolve it, dilute with *Mobile phase* to volume, and mix. [NOTE—Use this solution within 1 hour.]
 Chromatographic system (see *Chromatography* ⟨621⟩)—The liquid chromatograph is equipped with a 220-nm detector and a 4.6-mm × 25-cm column that contains packing L1. The flow rate is about 1 mL per minute. Chromatograph the *Standard solution,* and record the peak responses as directed for *Procedure*: the relative retention times are about 1.0 for piperacillin and 2.55 for 6-[2-[6-[2-(4-ethyl-2,3-dioxo-1-piperazinecarboxamido)-2-phenylacetamido]-3,3-dimethyl-7-oxo-4-thia-1-azabicyclo[3.2.0]heptane-2-carboxamido]-2-phenylacetamido]-3,3-dimethyl-7-oxo-4-thia-1-azabicyclo[3.2.0]heptane-2-carboxylic acid (piperacillin related compound D); and the relative standard deviation for replicate injections is not more than 2%.
 Procedure—Separately inject equal volumes (about 10 µL) of the *Standard solution* and the *Test solution* into the chromatograph, record the chromatograms, and measure the peak responses for piperacillin and piperacillin related compound D. Calculate the percentage of piperacillin related compound D in the portion of Piperacillin taken by the formula:

$$10C(1.47)(P/W)(r_i/r_S)$$

in which C is the concentration, in mg per mL, of USP Piperacillin RS in the *Standard solution;* 1.47 is the relative response factor for piperacillin related compound D; P is the designated potency, in µg of piperacillin per mg, of USP Piperacillin RS; W is the weight, in mg, of Piperacillin taken to prepare the *Test solution;* r_i is the impurity peak response obtained from the *Test solution;* and r_S is the peak response of piperacillin obtained from the *Standard solution:* not more than 2.0% of piperacillin related compound D is found. The sum of all impurities found in *Test 1* and *Test 2* is not more than 3.8%.
Other requirements—Where the label states that Piperacillin is sterile, it meets the requirements for *Sterility* and *Bacterial endotoxins* under *Piperacillin for Injection.* Where the label states that Piperacillin must be subjected to further processing during the preparation of injectable dosage forms, it meets the requirements for *Bacterial endotoxins* under *Piperacillin for Injection.*
Assay—
 Mobile phase—Prepare a mixture of methanol, water, 0.2 M monobasic sodium phosphate, and 0.4 M tetrabutylammonium hy-

droxide (450 : 447 : 100 : 3). Adjust with phosphoric acid to a pH of 5.50 ± 0.02. Make adjustments if necessary (see *System Suitability* under *Chromatography* ⟨621⟩).

Standard preparation—Transfer about 40 mg of USP Piperacillin RS, accurately weighed, to a 100-mL volumetric flask, add a few drops of methanol to dissolve it, dilute with *Mobile phase* to volume, and mix. [NOTE—Use this solution within 1 hour.]

Resolution solution—Prepare a solution in *Mobile phase* containing in each mL about 0.1 mg of USP Ampicillin RS and 0.2 mg of USP Piperacillin RS.

Assay preparation—Transfer about 40 mg of Piperacillin, accurately weighed, to a 100-mL volumetric flask, add a few drops of methanol to dissolve it, dilute with *Mobile phase* to volume, and mix. [NOTE—Use this solution within 1 hour.]

Chromatographic system (see *Chromatography* ⟨621⟩)—The liquid chromatograph is equipped with a 220-nm detector and a 4.6-mm × 25-cm column that contains packing L1. The flow rate is about 1 mL per minute. Chromatograph the *Resolution solution*, and record the peak responses as directed for *Procedure*: the relative retention times are about 0.24 for piperacillin related compound B, 0.31 for ampicillin, 0.37 for piperacillin related compound C, 0.62 for related compound A, and 1.0 for piperacillin, the resolution, R, between ampicillin and piperacillin is not less than 16, and the tailing factor for the piperacillin peak is not more than 1.2. Chromatograph the *Standard preparation*, and record the peak responses as directed for *Procedure*: the relative standard deviation for replicate injections is not more than 2%.

Procedure—Separately inject equal volumes (about 10 µL) of the *Standard preparation* and the *Assay preparation* into the chromatograph, record the chromatograms, and measure the responses for the major peaks. Calculate the potency, in µg of piperacillin ($C_{23}H_{27}N_5O_7S$) per mg, of the portion of Piperacillin taken by the formula:

$$100(CP/W)(r_U/r_S)$$

in which C is the concentration, in mg per mL, of USP Piperacillin RS in the *Standard preparation*; P is the designated potency, in µg of piperacillin per mg, of USP Piperacillin RS; W is the weight, in mg, of Piperacillin taken to prepare the *Assay preparation*; and r_U and r_S are the piperacillin peak responses obtained from the *Assay preparation* and the *Standard preparation*, respectively.

Piperacillin Sodium

$C_{23}H_{26}N_5NaO_7S$ 539.54

4-Thia-1-azabicyclo[3.2.0]heptane-2-carboxylic acid, 6-[[[[(4-ethyl-2,3-dioxo-1-piperazinyl)carbonyl]amino]phenylacetyl]amino]-3,3-dimethyl-7-oxo-, monosodium salt, [2S-[2α,5α,6β(S*)]].

Sodium (2S,5R,6[R])-6-[(R)-2-(4-ethyl-2,3-dioxo-1-piperazine-carboxamido)-2-phenylacetamido]-3,3-dimethyl-7-oxo-4-thia-1-azabicyclo[3.2.0]heptane-2-carboxylate   [59703-84-3].

» Piperacillin Sodium has a potency equivalent to not less than 863 µg and not more than 1007 µg of piperacillin ($C_{23}H_{27}N_5O_7S$) per mg, calculated on the anhydrous basis.

Packaging and storage—Preserve in tight containers.

Labeling—Where it is intended for use in preparing injectable dosage forms, the label states that it is sterile or must be subjected to further processing during the preparation of injectable dosage forms.

USP Reference standards ⟨11⟩—*USP Piperacillin RS. USP Ampicillin RS. USP Endotoxin RS.*

Identification—

A: The chromatogram obtained from the *Assay preparation* in the *Assay* exhibits a major peak for piperacillin, the retention time of which corresponds to that exhibited by the *Standard preparation*, and the chromatogram compares qualitatively to that obtained from the *Standard preparation*.

B: It responds to the tests for *Sodium* ⟨191⟩.

pH ⟨791⟩: between 5.5 and 7.5, in a solution containing 400 mg per mL.

Water, *Method I* ⟨921⟩: not more than 1.0%, the method of *Test preparation* described for hygroscopic substances being used.

Related compounds—

Mobile phase and *Chromatographic system*—Proceed as directed in the *Assay* under *Piperacillin*.

Standard piperacillin solution—Proceed as directed in the *Related compounds, Test 1* under *Piperacillin*.

Test solution—Use the *Assay preparation*.

Procedure—Separately inject equal volumes (about 10 µL) of the *Test solution* and the *Standard piperacillin* and proceed as directed in the *Assay*. Calculate the percentage of piperacillin related compound A and piperacillin related compound C in the portion of Piperacillin taken by the formula:

$$10C(P/W)(RRF_i)(r_i/r_{Sp})$$

in which C is the concentration, in mg per mL, of USP Piperacillin RS in the *Standard piperacillin solution*, P is the designated potency, in µg of piperacillin per mg, of USP Piperacillin RS, W is the weight, in mg, of Piperacillin Sodium taken to prepare the *Test solution*, RRF_i is the response factor of an individual piperacillin related compound relative to the response of piperacillin, specifically 1.4 for piperacillin related compound A and 0.93 for piperacillin related compound C, r_i is the response of the impurity peak, if any, observed in the chromatogram of the *Test solution* at a retention time corresponding to piperacillin related compound A or piperacillin related compound C, and r_{Sp} is the peak response of the piperacillin peak in the chromatogram of the *Standard piperacillin solution*: not more than 3.5% of piperacillin related compound A and not more than 1.0% of piperacillin related compound C is found.

Other requirements—Where the label states that Piperacillin Sodium is sterile, it meets the requirements for *Sterility* and *Bacterial endotoxins* under *Piperacillin for Injection*. Where the label states that Piperacillin Sodium must be subjected to further processing during the preparation of injectable dosage forms, it meets the requirements for *Bacterial endotoxins* under *Piperacillin for Injection*.

Assay—

Mobile phase, Standard preparation, Resolution solution, and *Chromatographic system*—Proceed as directed in the *Assay* under *Piperacillin*.

Assay preparation—Transfer about 20 mg of Piperacillin Sodium, accurately weighed, to a 50-mL volumetric flask. Add about 35 mL of *Mobile phase*, and shake to dissolve. Dilute with *Mobile phase* to volume, and mix.

Procedure—Separately inject equal volumes (about 10 µL) of the *Standard preparation* and the *Assay preparation* into the chromatograph, record the chromatograms, and measure the responses for the major peaks. Calculate the potency, in µg of piperacillin ($C_{23}H_{27}N_5O_7S$) per mg, of the portion of Piperacillin taken by the formula:

$$(50CP/W)(r_U/r_S)$$

in which C is the concentration, in mg per mL, of USP Piperacillin RS in the *Standard preparation*, P is the designated potency, in µg of piperacillin per mg, of USP Piperacillin RS, W is the weight, in mg, of Piperacillin Sodium taken to prepare the *Assay preparation*, and r_U and r_S are the piperacillin peak responses obtained from the *Assay preparation* and the *Standard preparation*, respectively.

Piperacillin for Injection

» Piperacillin for Injection contains an amount of piperacillin sodium equivalent to not less than 90.0 percent and not more than 120.0 percent of the labeled amount of piperacillin ($C_{23}H_{27}N_5O_7S$).

Packaging and storage—Preserve in *Containers for Sterile Solids* as described under *Injections* ⟨1⟩.

USP Reference standards ⟨11⟩—*USP Piperacillin RS. USP Ampicillin RS. USP Endotoxin RS.*
Constituted solution—At the time of use, it meets the requirements for *Constituted Solutions* under *Injections* ⟨1⟩.
Bacterial endotoxins ⟨85⟩—It contains not more than 0.07 USP Endotoxin Unit per mg of piperacillin.
Sterility ⟨71⟩—It meets the requirements when tested as directed for *Membrane Filtration* under *Test for Sterility of the Product to be Examined.*
pH ⟨791⟩: between 4.8 and 6.8, in a solution containing 200 mg of piperacillin per mL.
Water, *Method I* ⟨921⟩: not more than 0.9%.
Particulate matter ⟨788⟩: meets the requirements for small volume injections.
Related compounds—
  Mobile phase and *Chromatographic system*—Proceed as directed in the *Assay* under *Piperacillin.*
  Standard piperacillin solution—Proceed as directed in the *Related compounds, Test 1* under *Piperacillin.*
  Test solution 1 and *Test solution 2*—Use *Assay preparation 1* and *Assay preparation 2*, respectively, and proceed as directed under the *Assay.*
  Procedure—Separately inject equal volumes (about 10 µL) of the *Test solutions* and the *Standard piperacillin solution*, and proceed as directed in the *Assay*. Calculate the percentage of piperacillin related compound A and piperacillin related compound C in the portion of Piperacillin for Injection taken by the formula:

$$0.1C(P/A)(RRF_i)(r_i/r_{Sp})$$

in which C is the concentration, in mg per mL, of USP Piperacillin RS in the *Standard piperacillin solution*, P is the designated potency, in µg of piperacillin per mg, of USP Piperacillin RS, A is the quantity, in mg, of piperacillin in each mL of *Test solution 1* or *Test solution 2*, RRF_i is the response factor of an individual piperacillin related compound relative to the response of piperacillin, specifically 1.4 for piperacillin related compound A and 0.93 for piperacillin related compound C, r_i is the response of each impurity peak, if any, observed in the chromatogram of the *Test solution* at a retention time corresponding to piperacillin related compound A or piperacillin related compound C, and r_{Sp} is the peak response of the piperacillin peak in the chromatogram of the *Standard piperacillin solution*: not more than 3.5% of piperacillin related compound A and not more than 1.0% of piperacillin related compound C is found.
Other requirements—It responds to the *Identification* test under *Piperacillin* and meets the requirements for *Uniformity of Dosage Units* ⟨905⟩ and *Labeling* under *Injections* ⟨1⟩.
Assay—
  Mobile phase, Standard preparation, Resolution solution, and *Chromatographic system*—Proceed as directed in the *Assay* under *Piperacillin.*
  Assay preparation 1 (where it is labeled for use as a single-dose container)—Constitute Piperacillin for Injection in a volume of water, accurately measured, corresponding to the volume of solvent specified in the labeling. Withdraw all of the withdrawable contents, using a suitable hypodermic needle and syringe, and dilute quantitatively with *Mobile phase* to obtain a solution containing about 0.4 mg of piperacillin per mL.
  Assay preparation 2 (where the label states the quantity of piperacillin in a given volume of the constituted solution)—Constitute Piperacillin for Injection in a volume of water, accurately measured, corresponding to the volume of solvent specified in the labeling. Dilute an accurately measured volume of the constituted solution quantitatively with *Mobile phase* to obtain a solution containing about 0.4 mg of piperacillin per mL.
  Procedure—Separately inject equal volumes (about 10 µL) of the *Standard preparation* and the *Assay preparations* into the chromatograph, record the chromatograms, and measure the responses for the major peaks. Calculate the quantity, in mg of piperacillin ($C_{23}H_{27}N_5O_7S$) in the container, or in the portion of constituted solution taken by the formula:

$$(L/D)(CP/1000)(r_U/r_S)$$

in which L is the labeled quantity, in mg, of piperacillin in the container or in the volume of constituted solution taken, D is the concentration, in mg of piperacillin per mL, of *Assay preparation 1* or *Assay preparation 2*, based on the labeled quantity in the container or in the portion of constituted solution taken, respectively, and the extent of dilution, C is the concentration, in mg per mL, of USP Piperacillin RS in the *Standard preparation*, P is the designated potency, in µg of piperacillin per mg, of USP Piperacillin RS, and r_U and r_S are the piperacillin peak responses obtained from the *Assay preparation* and the *Standard preparation*, respectively.

Piperazine

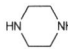

$C_4H_{10}N_2$ 86.14
Piperazine.
Piperazine   [110-85-0].

» Piperazine contains not less than 98.0 percent and not more than 101.0 percent of $C_4H_{10}N_2$, calculated on the anhydrous basis.

Packaging and storage—Preserve in tight containers, protected from light.
Color of solution—Dissolve 10.0 g in water, and dilute with water to 50.0 mL: the solution has no more color than a standard solution prepared by adding 2.0 mL of ferric chloride CS to water and diluting with water to 50.0 mL, when compared in matched color-comparison tubes.
Identification—It responds to *Identification* test A under *Piperazine Citrate.*
Melting range ⟨741⟩: between 109° and 113°.
Water, *Method I* ⟨921⟩: not more than 2.0%.
Primary amines and ammonia—Dissolve 200 mg in 10 mL of water, add 1 mL of acetone and 0.5 mL of freshly prepared sodium nitroferricyanide solution (1 in 10), mix, and allow to stand for 10 minutes, accurately timed. Determine the absorbance of this solution at 520 nm and at 600 nm, using a reagent blank as the reference solution. The ratio A_{600}/A_{520} is not more than 0.5 (equivalent to about 0.7% of primary amines and ammonia).
Assay—Weigh accurately about 150 mg of Piperazine, and dissolve in 75 mL of glacial acetic acid. Titrate potentiometrically with 0.1 N perchloric acid VS, using a silver-glass electrode system. As the endpoint is approached, warm the solution to 60° to 70°, then complete the titration. Perform a blank determination, and make any necessary correction. Each mL of 0.1 N perchloric acid is equivalent to 4.307 mg of $C_4H_{10}N_2$.

Piperazine Citrate

$(C_4H_{10}N_2)_3 \cdot 2C_6H_8O_7 \cdot xH_2O$ (anhydrous)   642.65
Piperazine, 2-hydroxy-1,2,3-propanetricarboxylate (3 : 2), hydrate.
Piperazine citrate (3 : 2) hydrate   [41372-10-5].
Anhydrous   642.66   [144-29-6].

» Piperazine Citrate contains not less than 98.0 percent and not more than 100.5 percent of $(C_4H_{10}N_2)_3 \cdot 2C_6H_8O_7$, calculated on the anhydrous basis.

Packaging and storage—Preserve in well-closed containers.
Identification—
   A: Dissolve about 200 mg in 5 mL of 3 N hydrochloric acid, and add, with stirring, 1 mL of sodium nitrite solution (1 in 2). Chill in an ice bath for 15 minutes, stirring if necessary, to induce crystallization, filter the precipitate on a sintered-glass funnel, wash with 10 mL of cold water, and dry at 105°: the N,N'-dinitrosopiperazine so obtained melts between 156° and 160°.
   B: It responds to the tests for *Citrate* ⟨191⟩.
Water, *Method I* ⟨921⟩:   not more than 12.0%.
Primary amines and ammonia—Dissolve 500 mg in 10 mL of water. Add 1 mL of 2.5 N sodium hydroxide, 1 mL of acetone, and 1 mL of sodium nitroferricyanide TS. Mix, and allow to stand for 10 minutes, accurately timed. Determine the absorbance of this solution at 520 nm and at 600 nm, using a blank consisting of the same quantities of the same reagents, but substituting water for the sodium hydroxide solution. The ratio A_{600}/A_{520} is not more than 0.50 (equivalent to about 0.7% of primary amines and ammonia).
Assay—Dissolve about 200 mg of Piperazine Citrate, accurately weighed, in 100 mL of glacial acetic acid TS, warming slightly if necessary to effect solution. Add crystal violet TS, and titrate with 0.1 N perchloric acid VS. Perform a blank determination, and make any necessary correction. Each mL of 0.1 N perchloric acid is equivalent to 10.71 mg of $(C_4H_{10}N_2)_3 \cdot 2C_6H_8O_7$.

Piperazine Citrate Syrup

» Piperazine Citrate Syrup is prepared from Piperazine Citrate or from Piperazine to which an equivalent amount of Citric Acid is added. It contains an amount of piperazine citrate equivalent to not less than 93.0 percent and not more than 107.0 percent of the labeled amount of piperazine hexahydrate ($C_4H_{10}N_2 \cdot 6H_2O$).

Packaging and storage—Preserve in tight containers.
Identification—
   A: To 2 mL of Syrup add 5 mL of 3 N hydrochloric acid, then add, with stirring, 1 mL of sodium nitrite solution (1 in 2). Chill in an ice bath for 15 minutes, stirring if necessary, to induce crystallization, filter the precipitate on a sintered-glass funnel, wash with 10 mL of cold water, and dry at 105°: the N,N'-dinitrosopiperazine so obtained melts between 156° and 160°.
   B: It responds to the tests for *Citrate* ⟨191⟩.
Assay—Determine the specific gravity of Syrup, and transfer an accurately weighed portion of the Syrup, equivalent to about 200 mg of piperazine citrate, to a 250-mL beaker. Add 10 mL of water and 75 mL of trinitrophenol TS, stir well, and allow to stand in a refrigerator for not less than 2 hours. Collect the precipitate in a tared filtering crucible, wash with five 10-mL portions of dehydrated alcohol, and dry at 105° to constant weight. [*Caution—Picrates may explode.*] The weight of the dipicrate, multiplied by 0.3568, gives the equivalent of $C_4H_{10}N_2 \cdot 6H_2O$ in the portion of Syrup taken.

Piperazine Citrate Tablets

» Piperazine Citrate Tablets contain an amount of piperazine citrate equivalent to not less than 93.0 percent and not more than 107.0 percent of the labeled amount of piperazine hexahydrate ($C_4H_{10}N_2 \cdot 6H_2O$).

Packaging and storage—Preserve in tight containers.
Identification—
   A: Finely powder a number of Tablets, equivalent to about 200 mg of piperazine citrate, mix with 5 mL of 3 N hydrochloric acid, and filter. To the filtrate add, with stirring, 1 mL of sodium nitrite solution (1 in 2). Chill in an ice bath for 15 minutes, stirring if necessary, to induce crystallization, filter the precipitate on a sintered-glass funnel, wash with 10 mL of cold water, and dry at 105°: the N,N'-dinitrosopiperazine so obtained melts between 156° and 160°.
   B: To a quantity of powdered Tablets, equivalent to about 500 mg of piperazine citrate, add 10 mL of water, shake, and filter: the filtrate responds to the tests for *Citrate* ⟨191⟩.
Dissolution, *Procedure for a Pooled Sample* ⟨711⟩—
   Medium: water; 900 mL.
   Apparatus 2: 50 rpm.
   Time: 45 minutes.
   Procedure—Determine the amount of piperazine hexahydrate ($C_4H_{10}N_2 \cdot 6H_2O$) dissolved, employing the procedure set forth in the *Assay*, making any necessary modifications.
   Tolerances—Not less than 75% (*Q*) of the labeled amount of $C_4H_{10}N_2 \cdot 6H_2O$ is dissolved in 45 minutes.
Uniformity of dosage units ⟨905⟩:   meet the requirements.
Assay—Weigh and finely powder not less than 20 Tablets. Shake an accurately weighed portion of the powder, equivalent to about 200 mg of piperazine citrate, for 1 hour with 10 mL of a mixture of 1 part of 3 N hydrochloric acid and 3 parts of water, filter, and wash the residue with two 10-mL portions of water. To the combined extract and washings add 75 mL of trinitrophenol TS, and proceed as directed in the *Assay* under *Piperazine Citrate Syrup*, beginning with "stir well."

Piroxicam

$C_{15}H_{13}N_3O_4S$ 331.35
2*H*-1,2-Benzothiazine-3-carboxamide, 4-hydroxy-2-methyl-*N*-2-pyridinyl-, 1,1-dioxide.
4-Hydroxy-2-methyl-*N*-2-pyridyl-2*H*-1,2-benzothiazine-3-carboxamide 1,1-dioxide   [36322-90-4].

» Piroxicam contains not less than 97.0 percent and not more than 103.0 percent of $C_{15}H_{13}N_3O_4S$.

Packaging and storage—Preserve in tight, light-resistant containers.
USP Reference standards ⟨11⟩—*USP Piroxicam RS*.
Identification—
   A: *Infrared Absorption* ⟨197M⟩—Do not dry specimens.
   B: *Ultraviolet Absorption* ⟨197U⟩—
      Solution: 10 μg per mL.
      Medium: hydrochloric acid in methanol (1 in 1200).
   C: Prepare a test solution of it in a mixture of chloroform and methanol (1 : 1) containing 1 mg per mL. Similarly prepare a Standard solution, using USP Piroxicam RS. Separately apply 20-μL portions of the test solution and the Standard solution to a suitable thin-layer chromatographic plate (see *Chromatography* ⟨621⟩) coated with a 0.25-mm layer of chromatographic silica gel. Allow

Foreign organic matter ⟨561⟩: not more than 0.50%.

Plasma Protein Fraction

» Plasma Protein Fraction conforms to the regulations of the federal Food and Drug Administration concerning biologics (640.90 to 640.96) (see *Biologics* ⟨1041⟩). It is a sterile preparation of serum albumin and globulin obtained by fractionating material (source blood, plasma, or serum) from healthy human donors, the source material being tested for the absence of hepatitis B surface antigen. It is made by a process that yields a product having protein components of approved composition and sedimentation coefficient content. Not less than 83 percent of its total protein is albumin and not more than 17 percent of its total protein consists of alpha and beta globulins. Not more than 1 percent of its total protein has the electrophoretic properties of gamma globulin. It is a solution containing, in each 100 mL, 5 g of protein, and it contains not less than 94 percent and not more than 106 percent of the labeled amount. It contains no added antimicrobial agent, but it contains sodium acetyltryptophanate with or without sodium caprylate as a stabilizing agent. It has a sodium content of not less than 130 mEq per L and not more than 160 mEq per L and a potassium content of not more than 2 mEq per L. It has a pH between 6.7 and 7.3, measured in a solution diluted to contain 1 percent of protein with 0.15 M sodium chloride. It meets the requirements of the test for heat stability.

Packaging and storage—Preserve at the temperature indicated on the label.

Expiration date—The minimum expiration date is not later than 5 years after issue from manufacturer's cold storage (5°, 1 year) if labeling recommends storage between 2° and 10°; not later than 3 years after issue from manufacturer's cold storage (5°, 1 year) if labeling recommends storage at temperatures not higher than 30°.

Labeling—Label it to state that it is not to be used if it is turbid and that it is to be used within 4 hours after the container is entered. Label it also to state the osmotic equivalent in terms of plasma and the sodium content.

Platelet Concentrate

» Platelet Concentrate conforms to the regulations of the federal Food and Drug Administration concerning biologics (640.20 to 640.27) (see *Biologics* ⟨1041⟩). It contains the platelets taken from plasma obtained by whole blood collection, by plasma pheresis, or by platelet pheresis, from a single suitable human donor of whole blood; or from a plasma pheresis donor; or from a platelet pheresis donor who meets the criteria described in the product license application (in which case the collection procedure is as described therein), except where a licensed physician has determined that the recipient is to be transfused with the platelets from a specific donor (in which case the platelet pheresis procedure is performed under the supervision of a licensed physician who is aware of the health status of the donor and has certified that the donor's health permits such procedure). In all cases, the collection of source material is made by a single, uninterrupted venipuncture with minimal damage to and manipulation of the donor's tissue. Concentrate consists of such platelets suspended in a specified volume of the original plasma, the separation of plasma and resuspension of the platelets being done in a closed system, within 4 hours of collection of the whole blood or plasma. The separation of platelets is by a procedure shown to yield an unclumped product without visible hemolysis, with a content of not less than 5.5×10^{10} platelets per unit in not less than 75 percent of the units tested, and the volume of original plasma used for resuspension of the separated platelets is such that the product has a pH of not less than 6 during the storage period when kept at the selected storage temperature, the selected storage temperature and corresponding volume of resuspension plasma being either 30 mL to 50 mL of plasma for storage at 20° to 24°, or 20 mL to 30 mL of plasma for storage at 1° to 6°. It meets the aforementioned requirements for platelet count, pH, and actual plasma volume, when tested 72 hours after preparation.

Packaging and storage—Preserve in hermetic containers of colorless, transparent, sterile, pyrogen-free Type I or Type II glass, or of a suitable plastic material (see *Transfusion and Infusion Assemblies* ⟨161⟩). Preserve at the temperature relevant to the volume of resuspension plasma, either between 20° and 24° or between 1° and 6°, the latter except during shipment, when the temperature may be between 1° and 10°.

Expiration time—The expiration time is not more than 72 hours from the time of collection of the source material.

Labeling—In addition to the labeling requirements of Whole Blood applicable to this product, label it to state the volume of original plasma present, the kind and volume of anticoagulant solution present in the original plasma, the blood group designation of the source blood, and the hour of expiration on the stated expiration date. Where labeled for storage at 20° to 24°, label it also to state that a continuous gentle agitation shall be maintained, or where labeled for storage at 1° to 6°, to state that such agitation is optional. Label it also with the type and result of a serologic test for syphilis, or to indicate that it was nonreactive in such test; with the type and result of a test for hepatitis B surface antigen, or to indicate that it was nonreactive in such test; with a warning that it is to be used as soon as possible but not more than 4 hours after entering the container; to state that a filter is to be used in the administration equipment; and to state that the instruction circular provided is to be consulted for directions for use.

Plicamycin

$C_{52}H_{76}O_{24}$ 1085.15
Plicamycin.
Plicamycin.
[2S-[2α,3β(1R*,3R*,4S*)]]-6-[[2,6-Dideoxy-3-O-(2,6-dideoxy-β-D-arabino-hexopyranosyl)-β-D-arabino-hexopyranosyl]oxy]-2-[(O-2,6-dideoxy-3-C-methyl-β-D-ribo-hexopyranosyl-(1→4)-O-2,6-dideoxy-α-D-lyxo-hexopyranosyl-(1→3)-2,6-dideoxy-β-D-arabino-hexopyranosyl)oxy]-3-(3,4-dihydroxy-1-methyl-2-oxopentyl)-3,4-dihydro-8,9-dihydroxy-7-methyl-1(2H)-anthracenone   [18378-89-7].

» Plicamycin has a potency of not less than 900 μg of $C_{52}H_{76}O_{24}$ per mg, calculated on the dried basis.

Packaging and storage—Preserve in tight, light-resistant containers, at a temperature between 2° and 8°.
USP Reference standards ⟨11⟩—*USP Plicamycin RS.*
Identification—
  A: *Infrared Absorption* ⟨197K⟩.
  B: The chromatogram obtained from the *Assay preparation* in the *Assay* exhibits a major peak for plicamycin the retention time of which corresponds to that exhibited by the *Standard preparation*, and the chromatogram compares qualitatively to that obtained from the *Standard preparation*.
Crystallinity ⟨695⟩: meets the requirements.
pH ⟨791⟩: between 4.5 and 5.5, in a solution containing 0.5 mg per mL.
Loss on drying ⟨731⟩—Dry about 100 mg, accurately weighed, in vacuum at a pressure not exceeding 5 mm of mercury at 25° for 4 hours: it loses not more than 8.0% of its weight.
Assay—[NOTE—Prepare solutions of plicamycin in low-actinic glassware.]
  Mobile phase—Prepare a suitable filtered and degassed mixture of 650 mL of 0.01 M phosphoric acid and 350 mL of acetonitrile.
  Standard preparations—Dissolve an accurately weighed quantity of USP Plicamycin RS in *Mobile phase* to obtain a solution having a concentration of 500 μg of plicamycin per mL. Dilute this solution with *Mobile phase* to obtain solutions containing 50, 100, and 150 μg of plicamycin per mL.
  Assay preparation—Transfer about 5 mg of Plicamycin, accurately weighed, to a 50-mL volumetric flask. Dissolve in *Mobile phase*, dilute with *Mobile phase* to volume, and mix.
  Chromatographic system (see *Chromatography* ⟨621⟩)—The liquid chromatograph is equipped with a 278-nm detector and a 4.6-mm × 25-cm column that contains packing L1. The flow rate is about 1.3 mL per minute. Chromatograph replicate injections of the *Standard preparation*, and record the peak responses as directed for *Procedure:* the relative standard deviation is not more than 2.0%.
  Procedure—Separately inject equal volumes (about 10 μL) of the *Standard preparations* and the *Assay preparation* into the chromatograph by means of a suitable microsyringe or sampling valve, record the chromatograms, and measure the responses for the major peaks. The retention time is about 13 minutes for plicamycin. Plot the peak responses of the *Standard preparations* versus concentration, in μg per mL, of plicamycin, and draw the straight line best fitting the three plotted points. From the graph so obtained, determine the concentration, in μg per mL, of plicamycin in the *Assay preparation*. Calculate the potency, in μg of $C_{52}H_{76}O_{24}$ per mg, taken by the formula:

$$(50C / W)$$

in which *C* is the concentration, in μg per mL, of plicamycin in the *Assay preparation*, and *W* is the weight, in mg, of Plicamycin taken.

Plicamycin for Injection

» Plicamycin for Injection is a sterile, dry mixture of Plicamycin and Mannitol. It may contain a suitable buffer. It contains not less than 90.0 percent and not more than 110.0 percent of the labeled amount of plicamycin ($C_{52}H_{76}O_{24}$).

Packaging and storage—Preserve in light-resistant *Containers for Sterile Solids* as described under *Injections* ⟨1⟩, at a temperature between 2° and 8°.
Labeling—Label it with the mandatory instruction to consult the professional information for dosage and warnings, and with the warning that it is intended for hospital use only, under the direct supervision of a physician.
USP Reference standards ⟨11⟩—*USP Plicamycin RS. USP Endotoxin RS.*
Constituted solution—At the time of use, it meets the requirements for *Constituted Solutions* under *Injections* ⟨1⟩.
Identification—Transfer a suitable quantity to a centrifuge tube, add methanol to obtain a solution having a concentration of about 0.5 mg of plicamycin per mL, mix, and centrifuge to obtain a clear solution. Apply 100 μL of this solution and 100 μL of a Standard solution of USP Plicamycin RS, similarly prepared to a suitable thin-layer chromatographic plate (see *Chromatography* ⟨621⟩) coated with a 0.25-mm layer of chromatographic silica gel mixture. Allow the spots to dry, and develop the chromatograms in a solvent system consisting of a mixture chloroform and methanol (1 : 1) for about 60 minutes. Remove the plate from the developing chamber, mark the solvent front, and allow the solvent to evaporate. Spray the plate with a (1 : 1) mixture of ferric chloride solution (1 in 100) and potassium ferricyanide solution (1 in 100). Observe the blue spots under a long-wavelength UV light: the R_F value of the principal spot obtained from the test solution corresponds to that obtained from the Standard solution (R_F about 0.7). Spots of trace components at R_F values of about 0.4 and 0.5 are not more intense than similar spots obtained from the Standard solution.
Bacterial endotoxins ⟨85⟩—It contains not more than 100.0 USP Endotoxin Units per mg of plicamycin.
Sterility ⟨71⟩—It meets the requirements when tested as directed for *Membrane Filtration* under *Test for Sterility of the Product to be Examined.*
pH ⟨791⟩: between 5.0 and 7.5, in the solution constituted as directed in the labeling.
Water, *Method I* ⟨921⟩: not more than 2.0%.
Assay—[NOTE—Prepare solutions of plicamycin in low-actinic glassware.]
  Mobile phase, Standard preparation, and *Chromatographic system*—Proceed as directed in the *Assay* under *Plicamycin.*
  Assay preparation—Dilute the contents of 1 container of Plicamycin for Injection quantitatively with *Mobile phase* to obtain a solution containing about 100 μg of plicamycin per mL.
  Procedure—Proceed as directed for *Procedure* in the *Assay* under *Plicamycin.* Calculate the quantity, in mg, of plicamycin ($C_{52}H_{76}O_{24}$) in the container by the formula:

$$C(L / D)$$

in which *C* is the concentration, in μg per mL, of plicamycin in the *Assay preparation;* *L* is the labeled quantity, in mg, of plicamycin in the container; and *D* is the concentration, in μg per mL, of plicamycin in the *Assay preparation* on the basis of the labeled quantity in the container and the extent of dilution.

Podophyllum

» Podophyllum consists of the dried rhizomes and roots of *Podophyllum peltatum* Linné (Fam. Berberidaceae). It yields not less than 5.0 percent of podophyllum resin.

Botanic characteristics—
Podophyllum—Consists of nearly cylindrical rhizomes, jointed, compressed or flattened somewhat on upper and lower surfaces, and sometimes branched. It occurs as pieces of rhizome up to 20 cm in length, with internodes from 2 mm to 9 mm in diameter, some of the nodes being somewhat thickened. The rhizome is dusky red to light yellowish brown, longitudinally wrinkled or nearly smooth, with irregular, somewhat V-shaped scars of scale leaves; some of the nodes are annulate, the upper portion having large, circular, depressed stem-scars and buds or stem-bases. On the lower portion there are numerous root-scars or roots, the latter from 2 cm to 7 cm in length and about 2 mm in thickness. The fracture is short and weak, the fractured surface being yellowish orange to pale yellow or grayish white.
Histology—The rhizome shows an outer portion consisting of a brown epidermis, often necrosed, and 1 to 3 layers of brown to olive-brown suberized cells; a cortex about 20 cells in width, consisting chiefly of nearly isodiametric cells, the cells containing single or compound starch grains and resin masses and, in scattered cells of the nodes, rosette aggregates of calcium oxalate; a circle of from 16 to 34 open collateral vascular bundles, separated by rather wide medullary rays, each bundle containing a few lignified vessels, a more or less distinct cambium, and a rather large phloem. The pith is large, the cells being more or less rounded and containing starch grains and reddish brown resin masses. The roots show an epidermal layer of brownish suberized cells and a single row of hypodermal cells; a broad cortex of thin-walled nearly isodiametric cells; a distinct endodermis of tangentially elongated cells having uniformly thickened walls; and a 4- to 7-rayed vascular bundle.
Powdered Podophyllum—It is pale brown to weak yellow and has a slight odor. It contains numerous starch grains, simple or 2- to 6-compound, the individual grains being spheroidal, plano- to angular-convex, or polygonal, up to 20 μm in diameter; occasional rosette aggregates of calcium oxalate, up to 80 μm in diameter; vessels with simple pits or reticulate thickenings; fragments of starch- and resin-bearing parenchyma and reddish brown to yellow cork cells.
Indian podophyllum—*Podophyllum peltatum* is differentiated from *Podophyllum hexandrum* Royle (Indian podophyllum) by the reaction described in the test for *Distinction from resin of Indian podophyllum* under *Podophyllum Resin*.
Acid-insoluble ash ⟨561⟩: not more than 2.0%.
Organic volatile impurities, *Method IV* ⟨467⟩: meets the requirements.

(Official until July 1, 2008)
Foreign organic matter ⟨561⟩: not more than 2.0%.
Assay—Place 10 g of Podophyllum, in fine powder, in a 125-mL conical flask, add 35 mL of alcohol, and reflux on a steam bath for 3 hours. Transfer the mixture to a small percolator, and percolate slowly with warm alcohol until the percolate measures 95 mL. Cool, add sufficient alcohol to the percolate to make it measure 100.0 mL, and mix. Transfer 10.0 mL of this percolate to a separator, and add 10 mL of chloroform and 10 mL of dilute hydrochloric acid (7 in 500). Shake the mixture, allow it to separate, draw off the alcohol-chloroform layer into a second separator, and wash the acid layer with three 15-mL portions of a mixture of chloroform and alcohol (2 : 1), adding the washings to the second separator. Add 10 mL of dilute hydrochloric acid (7 in 500) to the combined extract and washings, again shake the mixture, allow it to separate, and draw off the alcohol-chloroform layer into a tared vessel. Wash the acid layer three times with 15-mL portions of the alcohol-chloroform mixture, adding the washings to the tared vessel. Evaporate the combined extracts on a steam bath to approximately 1 mL, add 5 mL of dehydrated alcohol, again evaporate to dryness, and dry the residue at 80° for 4 hours: the weight of this residue is the weight of resin in 1 g of the Podophyllum taken.

Podophyllum Resin

» Podophyllum Resin is the powdered mixture of resins extracted from Podophyllum by percolation with Alcohol and subsequent precipitation from the concentrated percolate upon addition to acidified water. It contains not less than 40.0 percent and not more than 50.0 percent of hexane-insoluble matter. [*Caution—Podophyllum Resin is highly irritating to the eye and to mucous membranes in general.*]

Packaging and storage—Preserve in tight, light-resistant containers.
Identification—
 A: It is soluble in 1 N potassium hydroxide or in 1 N sodium hydroxide, forming a yellow liquid, which gradually becomes darker on standing and from which the resin is precipitated by hydrochloric acid.
 B: A hot solution of it deposits most of its solids on cooling, and if the cooled liquid is filtered, the filtrate turns brown upon the addition of a few drops of ferric chloride TS.
Residue on ignition ⟨281⟩: not more than 1.5%.
Distinction from resin of Indian podophyllum—Add 400 mg to 3 mL of 60 percent alcohol, then add 0.5 mL of 1 N potassium hydroxide, shake the mixture gently, and allow to stand for 2 hours: it does not gelatinize.
Hexane-insoluble matter—Transfer about 1 g of Podophyllum Resin, accurately weighed, to a glass-stoppered, 100-mL conical flask, add 30.0 mL of chloroform, insert the stopper tightly, and shake for 30 minutes, using a mechanical wrist-action shaker, or equivalent. Filter with suction through a medium- or fine-porosity, sintered-glass filter, into a small filter flask. Wash the conical flask and the filter with two 5-mL portions of chloroform, adding the washings to the filtrate. Transfer the filtrate with the aid of chloroform to a 50-mL volumetric flask, add chloroform to volume, and mix. Pipet 20 mL of the resulting solution into a 250-mL conical flask containing 160 mL of solvent hexane. Gently swirl, allow to stand for 10 minutes, and transfer the resulting precipitate to a tared, fine-porosity, sintered-glass filter, wash the flask and the precipitate with two 20-mL portions of solvent hexane, dry the precipitate at 70° for 1 hour, and weigh the *Hexane-insoluble matter* so obtained. Multiply by 2.5 to find the amount present in the quantity of Podophyllum Resin taken.

Podophyllum Resin Topical Solution

» Podophyllum Resin Topical Solution is a solution in Alcohol consisting of Podophyllum Resin and an alcoholic extract of Benzoin. It contains, in each 100 mL, not less than 10 g and not more than 13 g of hexane-insoluble matter.[*Caution—Podophyllum Resin Topical Solution is highly irritating to the eye and to mucous membranes in general.*]

Packaging and storage—Preserve in tight, light-resistant containers.
Identification—
 A: A 1 in 5 solution in chloroform is levorotatory.
 B: The precipitate obtained as directed in the test for *Hexane-insoluble matter* responds to *Identification* test A under *Podophyllum Resin*.
Alcohol content ⟨611⟩: between 69.0% and 72.0% of C_2H_5OH.
Hexane-insoluble matter—Using a 10.0-mL quantity of the Topical Solution, proceed as directed for *Hexane-insoluble matter* under *Podophyllum Resin*. Multiply the weight of hexane-insoluble matter found by 2.5 to find the amount present in the 10.0 mL taken.

Poliovirus Vaccine Inactivated

» Poliovirus Vaccine Inactivated conforms to the regulations of the federal Food and Drug Administration concerning biologics (630.1 to 630.6) (see *Biologics* ⟨1041⟩). It is a sterile aqueous suspension of inactivated poliomyelitis virus of Types 1, 2, and 3. The virus strains are grown separately in primary cell cultures of monkey kidney tissue, and from a virus suspension with a virus titer of not less than $10^{6.5}$ TCID$_{50}$ measured in comparison with the U. S. Reference Poliovirus of the corresponding type, are inactivated so as to reduce the virus titer by a factor of 10^{-8}, and after inactivation are combined in suitable proportions.

No extraneous protein, capable of producing allergenic effects upon injection into human subjects, is added to the final virus production medium. If animal serum is used at any stage, its calculated concentration in the final medium does not exceed 1 part per million. Suitable antimicrobial agents may be used during the production. The single strain harvests or virus pools prior to inactivation meet the requirements of the specific mouse, guinea pig, and rabbit tests for absence of B virus and *Mycobacterium tuberculosis*, and the tissue culture test for absence of SV-40 virus. The single strain or trivalent virus pools after inactivation meet the requirements of the specific tissue culture and monkey tests for absence of active poliovirus, the mouse test for absence of lymphocytic choriomeningitis virus, and the tissue culture safety test for absence of SV-40 virus or other active viruses. The Vaccine meets the requirements of the specific monkey potency test by virus neutralizing antibody production, based on the U. S. Reference Poliovirus Antiserum, such that the ratio of the geometric mean titer of the group of monkey serums representing the vaccine to the mean titer value of the reference serum is not less than 1.29 for Type 1, 1.13 for Type 2, and 0.72 for Type 3.

Packaging and storage—Preserve at a temperature between 2° and 8°.

Expiration date—The expiration date is not later than 1 year after date of issue from manufacturer's cold storage (5°, 1 year).

Labeling—Label it to state that it is to be well shaken before use. Label it also to state that it was prepared in monkey tissue cultures.

Poloxalene

Oxirane, methyl-, polymer with oxirane.
Polyethylene-polypropylene glycol   [9003-11-6].

» Poloxalene is a synthetic block copolymer of ethylene oxide and propylene oxide. It contains not less than 98.0 percent and not more than 103.0 percent of poloxalene.

Packaging and storage—Preserve in tight containers, protected from light. Store in a cool place.

USP Reference standards ⟨11⟩—*USP Poloxalene RS*.

Labeling—Label it to indicate that it is for veterinary use only.

Identification—
Color reagent—Dissolve 12.7 g of ammonium thiocyanate and 2.0 g of cobalt nitrate in 100 mL of water.
Procedure—Add 10 mL of ethylene chloride to 0.5 g of Poloxalene, and shake for 1 minute. Add 1 mL of *Color reagent*, and shake for 1 minute: a blue color is produced in the lower layer.

Average molecular weight—
Phthalic anhydride-pyridine solution—Prepare as directed in the test for *Average molecular weight* under *Poloxamer*.
Procedure—Using about 12 g of Poloxalene, accurately weighed, proceed as directed for *Procedure* in the test for *Average molecular weight* under *Poloxamer*: the average molecular weight is between 2850 and 3150.

pH ⟨791⟩:   between 5.0 and 7.5, in a solution (1 in 40).

Water, *Method Ia* ⟨921⟩:   not more than 0.4%.

Hydroxyl value ⟨401⟩—
Esterification reagent—Dissolve 166 g of phthalic anhydride and 28 g of imidazole in 1000 mL of pyridine, and allow to stand for 2 hours before using. Store in a light-resistant bottle.
Procedure—Transfer a quantity of Poloxalene, determined by dividing 420 by the expected hydroxyl value and accurately weighed, to a glass-stoppered, 250-mL conical flask, and add 25.0 mL of *Esterification reagent*. Transfer 25.0 mL of *Esterification reagent* to a second glass-stoppered, 250-mL conical flask to provide the reagent blank. Add glass beads to the flasks, swirl to dissolve the Poloxalene, and fit both flasks with glass-jointed reflux condensers previously rinsed with 10 mL of pyridine, and heat on a steam bath for 15 minutes. Add 10 mL of pyridine through each condenser, insert the stoppers, and cool under running water for 1 minute. After removing the condensers, add 10 mL of water and 1 mL of phenolphthalein TS, and titrate with 0.5 N sodium hydroxide VS to a light pink endpoint that persists for at least 15 seconds. Calculate the hydroxyl value by the formula:

$$(56.11 N / W)(B - U)$$

in which N is the normality of the 0.5 N sodium hydroxide titrant; W is the weight, in g, of the Poloxalene taken; B and U are the volumes, in mL, of 0.5 N sodium hydroxide consumed by the reagent blank and the solution of Poloxalene, respectively. [NOTE—If B minus U is greater than 10 mL, repeat the test using a smaller sample.] The hydroxyl value is between 36.0 and 40.0.

Cloud point—Add 10 g of Poloxalene to 190.0 mL of water in a 250-mL beaker. Add a magnetic stirring bar, place on a stirrer and hot plate, and stir until dissolution is complete. Place a probe from an electronic thermometer with an accuracy of 0.2° in the solution within 3 mm of the stirring bar. Continue stirring at a rate that minimizes the formation of bubbles. Adjust the hot plate so that the temperature of the solution increases at a rate of about 1° per minute. Continue to view the solution, and record the temperature when the probe can no longer be seen. This occurs between 42.5° and 46.5°.

Assay—
Standard preparation—Dissolve an accurately weighed quantity of USP Poloxalene RS in ethylene dichloride to obtain a solution having a known concentration of about 0.1575 mg per mL.
Assay preparation—Transfer about 105 mg of Poloxalene, accurately weighed, to a 100-mL volumetric flask, add about 85 mL of ethylene dichloride, and swirl to dissolve. Dilute with ethylene dichloride to volume, and mix. Transfer 15.0 mL of this solution to a second 100-mL volumetric flask, dilute with ethylene dichloride to volume, and mix.
Procedure—Transfer 10.0 mL of the *Standard preparation*, the *Assay preparation*, and ethylene dichloride (to serve as a blank) to glass-stoppered tubes, add 4.0 mL of the *Color reagent* specified in the *Identification* test, shake vigorously for 3 minutes, and then centrifuge for 5 minutes. Carefully remove the lower ethylene dichloride layers from the three tubes, and using the ethylene dichloride layer from the tube containing the blank to zero the spectrophotometer, determine the UV absorbance at 630 nm of the solutions from the *Standard preparation* and the *Assay preparation*. Calculate the

percentage of poloxalene in the portion of Poloxalene taken by the formula:

$$100(A_U / A_S)(C_S / C_U)$$

in which A_U and A_S are the absorbances of the solutions from the *Assay preparation* and the *Standard preparation*, respectively; and C_S and C_U are the concentrations, in mg per mL, of the *Standard preparation* and the *Assay preparation*, respectively.

Polycarbophil

Polycarbophil.
Polycarbophil   [9003-97-8].

» Polycarbophil is polyacrylic acid cross-linked with divinyl glycol.

Packaging and storage—Preserve in tight containers.
Identification—
  A: A dispersion (1 in 100) is orange with thymol blue TS and yellow with cresol red TS.
  B: Adjust a dispersion (1 in 100) with 1 M sodium hydroxide to a pH of about 7.5. A very viscous gel is produced.
pH ⟨791⟩—To 1.0 g add 100 mL of water, and shake by mechanical means for 1 hour: the pH of the mixture is not more than 4.0.
Loss on drying ⟨731⟩—Dry it in vacuum at 45° for 4 hours: it loses not more than 1.5% of its weight.
Residue on ignition ⟨281⟩: not more than 4.0%.
Absorbing power—Transfer about 50 mg, accurately weighed, to an accurately tared 50-mL centrifuge tube fitted with a tight closure. Add 35 mL of sodium bicarbonate solution (1.5 in 100), and shake manually, venting as necessary to release liberated carbon dioxide. Shake and vent at least 3 times. Close the tube tightly, and shake vigorously by mechanical means for 60 minutes. Centrifuge at 2000 rpm for 1 hour. By means of a 50-mL syringe fitted with a 13-gauge needle, draw off the supernatant taking care that the solid material is not disturbed. Repeat the process of the addition of 35 mL of sodium bicarbonate solution, of the shaking, and of the withdrawing of supernatant. Accurately weigh the tube with its contents, and calculate the weight of the absorbed solution by subtracting the weight of Polycarbophil taken and the tare weight of the tube. The absorbed weight is not less than 62 g per g of Polycarbophil on the dried basis.
Limit of acrylic acid—
  pH 3.0 phosphate buffer—Prepare 0.01 M monobasic potassium phosphate, and adjust with phosphoric acid to a pH of 3.0 ± 0.5.
  Mobile phase—Prepare a degassed solution consisting of *pH 3.0 phosphate buffer* and methanol (8 : 2).
  Standard solution—Dissolve an accurately weighed quantity of acrylic acid in water to obtain a solution containing 1.0 mg per mL. Dilute quantitatively, and stepwise if necessary, with a 2.5% alum solution to obtain a solution having a known concentration of about 30 µg per mL.
  Test solution—Transfer about 0.1 g of Polycarbophil into a vial. Add 20 mL of a 2.5% alum solution and mix. Heat at 50° for 20 minutes, then shake for 1 hour, centrifuge, and filter.
  Chromatographic system (see *Chromatography* ⟨621⟩)—The liquid chromatograph is equipped with a 210-nm detector and a 3.9-mm × 30-cm column that contains packing L1. The flow rate is about 2.0 mL per minute. Chromatograph the *Standard solution*, and record peak responses as directed for *Procedure:* the relative standard deviation for replicate injections of the *Standard solution* is not more than 5.0%, and the tailing factor is not more than 2.5.
  Procedure—Separately inject equal volumes (about 20 µL) of the *Standard solution* and the *Test solution* into the chromatograph, record the chromatograms, and measure the response for the acrylic acid peak. Calculate the percentage of acrylic acid in the portion of Polycarbophil taken by the formula:

$$(0.002C / W)(r_U / r_S)$$

in which *C* is the concentration, in µg per mL, of acrylic acid, *W* is the weight, in g, of Polycarbophil taken, and r_U and r_S are the acrylic acid peak responses obtained from the *Test solution* and the *Standard solution*, respectively: not more than 0.3% acrylic acid is found.
Limit of ethyl acetate—
  Internal standard solution—Dissolve an accurately weighed quantity of methyl ethyl ketone in methanol, and dilute quantitatively, and stepwise if necessary, to obtain a solution having a known concentration of about 0.075 mg per mL.
  Standard solution—Dissolve 0.225 mg, accurately weighed, of ethyl acetate into a 10-mL volumetric flask. Add 2.0 mL of the *Internal standard solution*, dilute with methanol to volume, and mix.
  Test solution—Transfer about 50 mg of Polycarbophil into a 10-mL volumetric flask. Add 2.0 mL of the *Internal standard solution*, dilute with methanol to volume, and mix.
  Chromatographic system (see *Chromatography* ⟨621⟩)—The gas chromatograph is equipped with a flame-ionization detector and a 10-ft. × 2-mm column that contains 1% liquid phase G25 on support S12. The column is maintained at about 160°, and the injection port and detector block are maintained at about 250°. The carrier gas is dry helium flowing at a rate of about 30 mL per minute. Chromatograph the *Standard solution*, and record the chromatogram as directed for *Procedure:* the relative retention times are about 1.3 for ethyl acetate, and 1.0 for methyl ethyl ketone, and the relative standard deviation for replicate injections of the ethyl acetate peak is not more than 2%.
  Procedure—Separately inject equal volumes (about 2 µL) of the *Test solution* and the *Standard solution* into the chromatograph, record the chromatograms, and measure the responses for the major peaks. Calculate the percentage of ethyl acetate in the portion of Polycarbophil taken by the formula:

$$(0.001C / W)(R_U / R_S)$$

in which *C* is the concentration of ethyl acetate, in µg per mL, *W* is the weight of Polycarbophil, in g, and R_U and R_S are the ratios of the responses of the ethyl acetate peak to the methyl ethyl ketone peak obtained from the *Test solution* and the *Standard solution*, respectively: not more than 0.45% is found.
Organic volatile impurities, Method IV ⟨467⟩: meets the requirements.

(Official until July 1, 2008)

Polyethylene Glycol 3350 and Electrolytes for Oral Solution

(Title for this monograph—to become official August 1, 2012). (Prior to August 1, 2012, the current practice of labeling the article of commerce with the name PEG 3350 and Electrolytes for Oral Solution may be continued. Use of the name Polyethylene Glycol 3350 and Electrolytes for Oral Solution will be permitted as of August 1, 2007, but the use of this name will not be mandatory until August 12, 2012. The 60-month extension will provide the time needed by the manufacturers and users to make necessary changes.)

» Polyethylene Glycol 3350 and Electrolytes for Oral Solution is a mixture of Polyethylene Glycol 3350, Sodium Bicarbonate, Sodium Chloride, Sodium Sulfate (anhydrous), and Potassium Chloride. When constituted as directed in the labeling it contains not less than 90.0 percent and not more than 110.0 percent of the labeled amounts of polyethylene glycol 3350, potassium (K^+), sodium (Na^+), bicarbonate (HCO_3^-), chloride (Cl^-), and sulfate ($SO_4^=$), the labeled amounts per L being 10 mmol (10 mEq) of potassium, 125 mmol (125 mEq) of sodium, 20 mmol (20 mEq) of bicarbonate, 35 mmol (35 mEq) of chloride, and 40 mmol (80 mEq) of sulfate.

Packaging and storage—Preserve in tight containers.
Completeness of solution ⟨641⟩: meets the requirements.
Identification—
  A: The IR absorption spectrum of a mineral oil dispersion of it in a calcium fluoride cell exhibits maxima only at the same wavelengths as that of a similar preparation of polyethylene glycol 3350.
  B: A solution (1 in 20) responds to the tests for *Sodium* ⟨191⟩, *Potassium* ⟨191⟩, *Bicarbonate* ⟨191⟩, *Sulfate* ⟨191⟩, and *Chloride* ⟨191⟩.
pH ⟨791⟩: between 7.5 and 9.5, in the solution prepared as directed in the labeling.
Uniformity of dosage units ⟨905⟩: meets the requirements.
Osmolarity ⟨785⟩: between 235 and 304 mOsmol, in the solution prepared as directed in the labeling.
Assay for potassium and sodium—

Mobile phase—Dilute 0.5 mL of nitric acid with water to obtain 4000 mL of solution. Degas, and place the solution in a suitable plastic container. Make adjustments if necessary (see *System Suitability* under *Chromatography* ⟨621⟩).

Internal standard solution—Dissolve a suitable quantity of ammonium bromide in water to obtain a solution having a concentration of about 2 mg per mL.

Standard preparation—To a 100-mL volumetric flask transfer about 90 mg of potassium chloride, previously dried at 105° for 2 hours and accurately weighed, and about 880 mg of sodium chloride, previously dried at 105° for 2 hours and accurately weighed, dilute with water to volume, and mix. Transfer 5.0 mL of this solution to a 500-mL volumetric flask, add 10.0 mL of *Internal standard solution*, dilute with water to volume, and mix. Pass this solution through a filter having a 0.5-μm or finer porosity, and store the filtrate in a suitable plastic container. This *Standard preparation* contains about 9 μg (0.00012 mEq) of potassium chloride and about 88 μg (0.0015 mEq) of sodium chloride per mL.

Assay preparation—Constitute the contents of a container of Polyethylene Glycol 3350 and Electrolytes for Oral Solution with an accurately measured volume of water, as specified in the labeling. Transfer 6.0 mL of this stock solution, equivalent to about 0.06 mEq of potassium, to a 500-mL volumetric flask, add 10 mL of *Internal standard solution*, dilute with water to volume, and mix. This solution contains about 0.00012 mEq of potassium and 0.0015 mEq of sodium per mL. [NOTE—Reserve the remaining portion of the stock solution for the *Assay for bicarbonate*, and reserve the remaining portion of the *Assay preparation* for the *Assay for chloride and sulfate* and the *Assay for polyethylene glycol 3350*.]

Chromatographic system (see *Chromatography* ⟨621⟩)—The liquid chromatograph is equipped with a conductivity detector, a 4-mm × 5-cm guard column containing packing L22, and a 4-mm × 30-cm analytical column maintained at 35 ± 1° containing packing L22. The flow rate is about 0.9 mL per minute. Chromatograph the *Standard preparation* as directed for *Procedure*: the relative retention times are about 0.6 for sodium, 0.8 for ammonium, and 1.0 for potassium; the resolution, *R*, between the sodium and ammonium peaks is not less than 1.1, and between the ammonium and potassium peaks is not less than 0.9. [NOTE—Maintain column backpressure at less than 1000 pounds per square inch. Backpressure may be reduced by changing the in-line filters and frits in the columns. Column efficiency may be improved by backflushing the analytical column with 30 mL of 0.1 N nitric acid or by injecting four successive 100-μL portions of 0.1 N nitric acid into the chromatograph.]

Procedure—[NOTE—Use peak heights where peak responses are indicated.] Separately inject equal volumes (about 10 μL) of the *Standard preparation* and the *Assay preparation* into the chromatograph, record the chromatograms, and measure the responses for the major peaks. Calculate the mEq of potassium per L of constituted Oral Solution taken by the formula:

$$(500/74.55)(C/6)(R_U/R_S)$$

in which 74.55 is the molecular weight of potassium chloride; *C* is the concentration, in μg per mL, of potassium chloride in the *Standard preparation*; and R_U and R_S are the peak response ratios of potassium to ammonium obtained from the *Assay preparation* and the *Standard preparation*, respectively. Calculate the mEq of sodium per L of constituted Oral Solution taken by the formula:

$$(500/58.44)(C/6)(R_U/R_S)$$

in which 58.44 is the molecular weight of sodium chloride; *C* is the concentration, in μg per mL, of sodium chloride in the *Standard preparation*; and R_U and R_S are the peak response ratios of sodium to ammonium obtained from the *Assay preparation* and the *Standard preparation*, respectively.

Assay for bicarbonate—Transfer 400.0 mL of the stock solution remaining from the *Assay for potassium and sodium*, equivalent to about 672 mg of sodium bicarbonate (8 mEq), to a suitable container, add methyl red TS, and titrate with 1 N sulfuric acid VS. Calculate the mEq of bicarbonate (HCO_3^-) per L of constituted Oral Solution taken by the formula:

$$2.5V_A$$

in which V_A is the volume, in mL, of 1 N sulfuric acid consumed.

Assay for chloride and sulfate—

Mobile phase—Transfer 34 g of boric acid, 8.6 g of lithium hydroxide, 23.5 mL of gluconic acid solution (1 : 1), and 125 mL of glycerin to a 1000-mL volumetric flask, dissolve in water, dilute with water to volume, and mix. Add 15 mL of this buffer solution to 865 mL of water, mix, and degas. Add 120 mL of acetonitrile, mix, and degas. [NOTE—Protect the *Mobile phase* from air to prevent absorption of carbon dioxide.] Make adjustments if necessary (see *System Suitability* under *Chromatography* ⟨621⟩). Increasing the proportion of buffer solution decreases the retention times of the analytes.

Internal standard solution—Dissolve a suitable quantity of ammonium bromide in water to obtain a solution having a concentration of about 2.2 mg per mL.

Standard preparation—To a 100-mL volumetric flask transfer about 246 mg of sodium chloride (4.2 mEq), previously dried at 105° for 2 hours and accurately weighed, and about 682 mg of anhydrous sodium sulfate (9.6 mEq), previously dried at 105° for 2 hours and accurately weighed, dilute with water to volume, and mix. Transfer 5.0 mL of this solution to a 500-mL volumetric flask, add 10.0 mL of *Internal standard solution*, dilute with water to volume, and mix. Filter this solution through a 0.5-μm or finer porosity filter, and store the filtrate in a suitable glass container. This *Standard preparation* contains about 24.6 μg of sodium chloride (0.00042 mEq of chloride) and about 68.2 μg of sodium sulfate (0.00096 mEq of sulfate) per mL.

Assay preparation—Use the *Assay preparation* prepared as directed in the *Assay for potassium and sodium*. This solution contains about 0.042 mEq of chloride and 0.096 mEq of sulfate per mL.

Chromatographic system (see *Chromatography* ⟨621⟩)—The liquid chromatograph is equipped with a conductivity detector, a 4-mm × 5-cm guard column containing packing L23, and a 4-mm × 30-cm analytical column maintained at 35 ± 1° containing packing L23. The flow rate is about 0.9 mL per minute. Chromatograph the *Standard preparation* as directed for *Procedure*: the relative retention times are about 0.25 for chloride, 0.4 for bromide, and 1.0 for sulfate, the resolution, *R*, between the chloride and bromide peaks is not less than 1.5 and between the bromide and sulfate peaks is not less than 4.5. [NOTE—Maintain column backpressure at less than 1000 pounds per square inch. Backpressure may be reduced by changing the in-line filters and frits in the columns. Column efficiency may be improved by backflushing the analytical column with 50 mL of the buffer solution used to prepare the *Mobile phase*.]

Procedure—[NOTE—Use peak heights where peak responses are indicated.] Separately inject equal volumes (about 10 μL) of the *Standard preparation* and the *Assay preparation* into the chromatograph, record the chromatograms, and measure the responses for the major peaks. Calculate the mEq of chloride per L of constituted Oral Solution taken by the formula:

$$(500/58.44)(C/6)(R_U/R_S)$$

in which 58.44 is the molecular weight of sodium chloride, *C* is the concentration, in μg per mL, of sodium chloride in the *Standard preparation*, and R_U and R_S are the peak response ratios of chloride to bromide obtained from the *Assay preparation* and the *Standard preparation*, respectively. Calculate the mEq of sulfate per L of constituted Oral Solution taken by the formula:

$$(500 / 71.02)(C / 6)(R_U / R_S)$$

in which 71.02 is one-half of the molecular weight of sodium sulfate, C is the concentration, in µg per mL, of anhydrous sodium sulfate in the *Standard preparation*, and R_U and R_S are the peak response ratios of sulfate to bromide obtained from the *Assay preparation* and the *Standard preparation*, respectively.

Assay for polyethylene glycol 3350—
Salt solution—Prepare a solution in water containing 0.35 mg of sodium chloride, 0.18 mg of potassium chloride, 0.40 mg of sodium bicarbonate, 1.37 mg of anhydrous sodium sulfate, and 0.88 mg of ammonium bromide per mL.
Mobile phase—Dilute 40.0 mL of *Salt solution* with water to 1000 mL. Make adjustments if necessary (see *System Suitability* under *Chromatography* ⟨621⟩).
Standard preparation—Transfer about 360 mg of polyethylene glycol 3350, accurately weighed, to a 500-mL volumetric flask, add 20.0 mL of *Salt solution* and about 250 mL of water, dissolve by swirling, dilute with water to volume, and mix. This *Standard preparation* contains about 0.72 mg of polyethylene glycol 3350 per mL.
Assay preparation—Use the *Assay preparation* prepared as directed in the *Assay for potassium and sodium*. This solution contains about 0.72 mg of polyethylene glycol 3350 per mL.
Chromatographic system (see *Chromatography* ⟨621⟩)—[NOTE—Use peak heights where peak responses are indicated.] The liquid chromatograph is equipped with a refractive index detector maintained at 34 ± 0.5°, a 7.8-mm × 4.5-cm guard column containing packing L25, and a 7.8-mm × 30-cm analytical column containing packing L25 and maintained at ambient temperature. The flow rate is about 1 mL per minute. Chromatograph the *Standard preparation* as directed for *Procedure*: the relative standard deviation for replicate injections is not more than 1.5%. [NOTE—Maintain column backpressure at less than 1000 pounds per square inch. Backpressure may be reduced by cleaning the frits in the guard column or by replacing the guard column. Baseline drift may be reduced by maintaining strict control of ambient temperature, by insulating the lines, the *Mobile phase* reservoir, and the columns, and by increasing the time of equilibration.]
Procedure—Separately inject equal volumes (about 20 µL) of the *Standard preparation* and the *Assay preparation* into the chromatograph, record the chromatograms, and measure the responses for the major peaks. Calculate the content, in g, of polyethylene glycol 3350 per L of constituted Oral Solution taken by the formula:

$$500(C / 6)(r_U / r_S)$$

in which C is the concentration, in mg per mL, of polyethylene glycol 3350 in the *Standard preparation*, and r_U and r_S are the polyethylene glycol 3350 peak responses obtained from the *Assay preparation* and the *Standard preparation*, respectively.

Polymyxin B Sulfate

Polymyxin B, sulfate.
Polymyxin B sulfate   [1405-20-5].

» Polymyxin B Sulfate is the sulfate salt of a kind of polymyxin, a substance produced by the growth of *Bacillus polymyxa* (Prazmowski) Migula (Fam. Bacillaceae), or a mixture of two or more such salts. It has a potency of not less than 6000 Polymyxin B Units per mg, calculated on the dried basis.

Packaging and storage—Preserve in tight, light-resistant containers.
Labeling—Where packaged for prescription compounding, the label states the number of Polymyxin B Units in the container and per milligram, that it is not intended for manufacturing use, that it is not sterile, and that its potency cannot be assured for longer than 60 days after opening. Where it is intended for use in preparing injectable or other sterile dosage forms, the label states that it is sterile or must be subjected to further processing during the preparation of injectable or other sterile dosage forms.

USP Reference standards ⟨11⟩—*USP Polymyxin B Sulfate RS.*
Identification—
A: *Liquid Chromatographic Identification Test—*
Mobile phase—Prepare a mixture of 0.1 M tribasic sodium phosphate and acetonitrile (77 : 23), and adjust with phosphoric acid to a pH of 3.0. Make adjustments if necessary (see *System Suitability* under *Chromatography* ⟨621⟩).
Standard solution—Prepare a solution of USP Polymyxin B Sulfate RS in *Mobile phase* having a concentration of about 3.5 mg per mL. Protect this solution from light.
Test solution—Prepare a solution of Polymyxin B Sulfate in *Mobile phase* having a concentration of about 3.5 mg per mL. Protect this solution from light.
Chromatographic system (see *Chromatography* ⟨621⟩)—The liquid chromatograph is equipped with a 212-nm detector and a 4.6-mm × 25-cm column that contains 5-µm packing L1. The flow rate is about 1 mL per minute.
Procedure—Separately inject equal volumes (about 10 µL) of the *Standard solution* and the *Test solution* into the chromatograph, and record the chromatograms. The chromatogram obtained from the *Test solution* corresponds qualitatively to that obtained from the *Standard solution*, exhibiting a major peak corresponding to polymyxin B1 and peaks at relative retention times of about 0.5 (polymyxin B2) and 0.6 (polymyxin B3).
B: Dissolve 2 mg in 5 mL of water, add 5 mL of 2.5 N sodium hydroxide, mix, and add 5 drops of cupric sulfate solution (1 in 100), shaking after the addition of each drop: a reddish violet color is produced.
C: A solution (1 in 20) meets the requirements of the tests for *Sulfate* ⟨191⟩.
pH ⟨791⟩:   between 5.0 and 7.5, in a solution containing 5 mg per mL.
Loss on drying ⟨731⟩—Dry about 100 mg, accurately weighed, in a capillary-stoppered bottle in vacuum at 60° for 3 hours: it loses not more than 7.0% of its weight.
Content of phenylalanine—Transfer about 0.375 g of Polymyxin B Sulfate, accurately weighed, to a 100-mL volumetric flask, dissolve in and dilute with 0.1 N hydrochloric acid to volume, and mix. Measure the absorbances of this solution at the maxima at about 264 nm (A_{264}), 258 nm (A_{258}), and 252 nm (A_{252}), and the absorbances at 280 nm (A_{280}) and 300 nm (A_{300}). Calculate the percentage of phenylalanine in the portion of Polymyxin B Sulfate taken by the formula:

$$(9.4787/W)(A_{258} - 0.5A_{252} + 0.5A_{264} - 1.84A_{280} + 0.8A_{300})$$

in which W is the weight, in g, of Polymyxin B Sulfate taken: it contains between 9% and 12% of phenylalanine, calculated on the dried basis.
Other requirements—If for prescription compounding, it meets the requirements for *Residue on ignition* under *Polymyxin B for Injection*. Where the label states that Polymyxin B Sulfate is sterile, it meets the requirements for *Sterility Tests* ⟨71⟩ and, where intended for injectable dosage forms, for *Pyrogen* under *Polymyxin B for Injection*. Where the label states that Polymyxin B Sulfate must be subjected to further processing during the preparation of injectable dosage forms, it meets the requirements for *Pyrogen* under *Polymyxin B for Injection*.
Assay—Proceed with Polymyxin B Sulfate as directed under *Antibiotics—Microbial Assays* ⟨81⟩.

Polymyxin B for Injection

» Polymyxin B for Injection contains an amount of Polymyxin B Sulfate equivalent to not less than 90.0

percent and not more than 120.0 percent of the labeled amount of polymyxin B.

Packaging and storage—Preserve in *Containers for Sterile Solids* as described under *Injections* ⟨1⟩, protected from light.
Labeling—Label it to indicate that where it is administered intramuscularly and/or intrathecally, it is to be given only to patients hospitalized so as to provide constant supervision by a physician.
USP Reference standards ⟨11⟩—*USP Polymyxin B Sulfate RS*.
Constituted solution—At the time of use, it meets the requirements for *Constituted Solutions* under *Injections* ⟨1⟩.
Thin-layer chromatographic identification test ⟨201BNP⟩: meets the requirements.
Pyrogen—It meets the requirements of the *Pyrogen Test* ⟨151⟩, the test dose being 1.0 mL per kg of a solution in pyrogen-free saline TS containing 20,000 Polymyxin B Units per mL.
Sterility ⟨71⟩—It meets the requirements when tested as directed for *Membrane Filtration* under *Test for Sterility of the Product to be Examined*.
Particulate matter ⟨788⟩: meets the requirements for small-volume injections.
Residue on ignition ⟨281⟩: not more than 5.0%, the charred residue being moistened with 2 mL of nitric acid and 5 drops of sulfuric acid.
Heavy metals, *Method II* ⟨231⟩: not more than 0.01%.
Other requirements—It meets the requirements for *pH* and *Loss on drying* under *Polymyxin B Sulfate*. It also meets the requirements for *Uniformity of Dosage Units* ⟨905⟩ and for *Labeling* under *Injections* ⟨1⟩.
Assay—
  Assay preparation 1 (where it is represented as being in a single-dose container)—Constitute Polymyxin B for Injection in a volume of water, accurately measured, corresponding to the volume of solvent specified in the labeling. Withdraw all of the withdrawable contents, using a suitable hypodermic needle and syringe, and dilute quantitatively with *Buffer No. 6* to obtain a solution containing a convenient number of Polymyxin B Units per mL.
  Assay preparation 2 (where the label states the quantity of polymyxin B in a given volume of constituted solution)—Constitute 1 container of Polymyxin B for Injection in a volume of water, accurately measured, corresponding to the volume of solvent specified in the labeling. Dilute an accurately measured volume of the constituted solution quantitatively with *Buffer No. 6* to obtain a solution containing a convenient number of Polymyxin B Units per mL.
  Procedure—Proceed as directed under *Antibiotics—Microbial Assays* ⟨81⟩, using an accurately measured volume of *Assay preparation* diluted quantitatively with *Buffer No. 6* to yield a *Test Dilution* having a concentration assumed to be equal to the median dose level of the Standard.

Polymyxin B Sulfate and Bacitracin Zinc Topical Aerosol

» Polymyxin B Sulfate and Bacitracin Zinc Topical Aerosol contains the equivalent of not less than 90.0 percent and not more than 130.0 percent of the labeled amounts of polymyxin B and bacitracin.

Packaging and storage—Preserve in pressurized containers, and avoid exposure to excessive heat.
USP Reference standards ⟨11⟩—*USP Polymyxin B Sulfate RS*. *USP Bacitracin Zinc RS*.
Identification—Collect in a suitable container the expelled contents of 1 Aerosol container, shake with a volume of 0.1 N hydrochloric acid sufficient to obtain a solution containing about 500 USP Bacitracin Units per mL, centrifuge, and use the clear supernatant as the test solution. Proceed as directed under *Thin-Layer Chromatographic Identification Test* ⟨201BNP⟩. The specified result is observed.
Microbial limits—Collect aseptically in a suitable container half the contents expelled from 5 containers, dissolve in 500 mL of *Fluid A* containing 0.25 g of sodium thioglycollate and adjusted with sodium hydroxide to a pH of 6.6 ± 0.6, pass through a membrane filter as directed for *Membrane Filtration* under *Test for Sterility of the Product to be Examined* under *Sterility Tests* ⟨71⟩, except to place the filter on the surface of Soybean–Casein Digest Agar Medium in a Petri dish, incubate for 7 days at 30° to 35°, and count the number of colonies on the filter. Similarly prepare a second specimen, except to incubate at 20° to 25°. Not more than 20 colonies are observed from the two specimens. It meets also the requirements of the tests for absence of *Staphylococcus aureus* and *Pseudomonas aeruginosa* under *Microbial Limit Tests* ⟨61⟩.
Water, *Method I* ⟨921⟩—Store 1 container of Topical Aerosol in a freezer for not less than 2 hours, open the container, and transfer 10.0 mL of the freshly mixed specimen to a titration vessel containing 20 mL of a mixture of toluene and methanol (7 : 3) instead of methanol. In titrating the specimen, determine the endpoint at a temperature of 10° or higher: not more than 0.5% of water is found.
Other requirements—It meets the requirements for *Pressure Test*, *Minimum Fill*, and *Leakage Test* under *Aerosols, Metered-Dose Inhalers, and Dry Powder Inhalers* ⟨601⟩.
Assay for polymyxin B—Proceed as directed for polymyxin B under *Antibiotics—Microbial Assays* ⟨81⟩, expelling the entire contents of 1 container of Topical Aerosol, according to the directions in the labeling, into a 2000-mL conical flask held in a horizontal position. Add 500.0 mL of 0.01 N hydrochloric acid, and shake to dissolve. Immediately dilute an accurately measured volume of this acidic solution quantitatively and stepwise with *Buffer No. 6* to obtain a *Test Dilution* having a concentration of polymyxin B assumed to be equal to the median dose level of the Standard.
Assay for bacitracin—Proceed as directed for bacitracin under *Antibiotics—Microbial Assays* ⟨81⟩, using an accurately measured volume of the acidic solution obtained in the *Assay for polymyxin B* immediately diluted quantitatively and stepwise with *Buffer No. 1* to yield a *Test Dilution* having a bacitracin concentration assumed to be equal to the median dose level of the Standard. [NOTE—Add additional hydrochloric acid to each test dilution of the Standard to obtain the same concentration of hydrochloric acid as in the *Test Dilution*.]

Polymyxin B Sulfate and Bacitracin Zinc Topical Powder

» Polymyxin B Sulfate and Bacitracin Zinc Topical Powder contains not less than 90.0 percent and not more than 130.0 percent of the labeled amounts of polymyxin B and bacitracin.

Packaging and storage—Preserve in well-closed containers.
USP Reference standards ⟨11⟩—*USP Polymyxin B Sulfate RS*. *USP Bacitracin Zinc RS*.
Microbial limits—Collect aseptically in a suitable container about 1 g from not less than 5 containers, dissolve in 500 mL of *Fluid A*, filter through a membrane filter as directed for *Membrane Filtration* under *Test for Sterility of the Product to be Examined* under *Sterility Tests* ⟨71⟩, except to place the filter on the surface of Soybean–Casein Digest Agar Medium in a Petri dish, incubate for 7 days at 30° to 35°, and count the number of colonies on the filter. Similarly prepare a second specimen, except to incubate at 20° to 25°. Not more than 20 colonies are observed from the two specimens. It meets also the requirements of the tests for absence of *Staphylococcus aureus* and *Pseudomonas aeruginosa* under *Microbial Limit Tests* ⟨61⟩.
Water, *Method I* ⟨921⟩: not more than 7.0%.
Assay for polymyxin B—Proceed as directed for polymyxin B under *Antibiotics—Microbial Assays* ⟨81⟩, using an accurately weighed portion of Topical Powder, equivalent to about 5000 USP Polymyxin B Units, shaken with 20 mL of water in a suitable volumetric flask. Dilute with *Buffer No. 6* to volume, and mix. Dilute an

accurately measured volume of the solution so obtained quantitatively with *Buffer No. 6* to obtain a *Test Dilution* having a concentration of polymyxin B assumed to be equal to the median dose level of the Standard.

Assay for bacitracin—Proceed as directed for bacitracin under *Antibiotics—Microbial Assays* ⟨81⟩, using an accurately weighed portion of Topical Powder, equivalent to about 800 USP Bacitracin Units, added to a 100-mL volumetric flask, dilute with 0.01 N hydrochloric acid to volume, and mix. Dilute this solution quantitatively with *Buffer No. 1* to obtain a *Test Dilution* having a concentration assumed to be equal to the median dose level of the Standard. In preparing each test dilution of the Standard, add additional hydrochloric acid to each to obtain the same concentration of hydrochloric acid as in the *Test Dilution*.

Polymyxin B Sulfate and Hydrocortisone Otic Solution

» Polymyxin B Sulfate and Hydrocortisone Otic Solution is a sterile solution containing not less than 90.0 percent and not more than 130.0 percent of the labeled amount of polymyxin B, and not less than 90.0 percent and not more than 110.0 percent of the labeled amount of hydrocortisone ($C_{21}H_{30}O_5$). It may contain one or more suitable buffers and preservatives.

NOTE—Where Polymyxin B Sulfate and Hydrocortisone Otic Solution is prescribed without reference to the quantity of polymyxin B or hydrocortisone contained therein, a product containing 10,000 Polymyxin B Units and 5 mg of hydrocortisone per mL shall be dispensed.

Packaging and storage—Preserve in tight, light-resistant containers.
USP Reference standards ⟨11⟩—*USP Polymyxin B Sulfate RS. USP Hydrocortisone RS.*
Sterility ⟨71⟩: meets the requirements.
pH ⟨791⟩: between 3.0 and 5.0.
Assay for polymyxin B—Proceed with Otic Solution as directed under *Antibiotics—Microbial Assays* ⟨81⟩, using an accurately measured volume of Otic Solution diluted quantitatively with *Buffer No. 6* to yield a *Test Dilution* having a concentration assumed to be equal to the median dose level of the Standard.
Assay for hydrocortisone—
Mobile phase—Prepare a suitable solution of about 500 volumes of methanol, 500 volumes of water, and 1 volume of glacial acetic acid, such that the retention time of hydrocortisone is between 6 and 10 minutes.
Standard preparation—Dissolve a suitable quantity of USP Hydrocortisone RS, accurately weighed, in a mixture of methanol and water (1 : 1) to obtain a solution having a known concentration of about 0.15 mg per mL.
Assay preparation—Transfer an accurately measured volume of Otic Solution, equivalent to about 15 mg of hydrocortisone, to a 100-mL volumetric flask, dilute with a mixture of methanol and water (1 : 1) to volume, and mix.
Chromatographic system (see *Chromatography* ⟨621⟩)—The chromatograph is equipped with a 254-nm detector and a 4-mm × 30-cm column that contains packing L1. The flow rate is about 2 mL per minute. Chromatograph five replicate injections of the *Standard preparation*, and record the peak responses as directed for *Procedure*: the relative standard deviation is not more than 2.0%.
Procedure—Separately inject equal volumes (about 10 µL) of the *Standard preparation* and the *Assay preparation* into the chromatograph by means of a suitable microsyringe or sampling valve, adjusting the specimen size and other operating parameters such that the peak obtained from the *Standard preparation* is about 0.6 full-scale. Record the chromatograms, and measure the responses for the major peaks. Calculate the quantity, in mg, of $C_{21}H_{30}O_5$ in each mL of the Otic Solution taken by the formula:

$$(100C / V)(H_U / H_S)$$

in which *C* is the concentration, in mg per mL, of USP Hydrocortisone RS in the *Standard preparation*, *V* is the volume, in mL, of the portion of Otic Solution taken, and H_U and H_S are the peak responses obtained from the *Assay preparation* and the *Standard preparation*, respectively.

Polymyxin B Sulfate and Trimethoprim Ophthalmic Solution

» Polymyxin B Sulfate and Trimethoprim Ophthalmic Solution is a sterile, isotonic, aqueous solution of Polymyxin B Sulfate and Trimethoprim Sulfate or of Polymyxin B Sulfate and Trimethoprim that has been solubilized with Sulfuric Acid. It contains not less than 90.0 percent and not more than 130.0 percent of the labeled amount of polymyxin B and the equivalent of not less than 90.0 percent and not more than 110.0 percent of the labeled amount of trimethoprim ($C_{14}H_{18}N_4O_3$). It contains one or more preservatives.

Packaging and storage—Preserve in tight, light-resistant containers, and store at controlled room temperature.
Labeling—Label it to indicate that it is to be stored at 15° to 25°, protected from light.
USP Reference standards ⟨11⟩—*USP Polymyxin B Sulfate RS. USP Trimethoprim RS.*
Identification—
  A: It meets the requirements for polymyxin B under *Thin-Layer Chromatographic Identification Test* ⟨201BNP⟩.
  B: The retention time of the trimethoprim peak in the chromatogram of the *Assay preparation* corresponds to that in the chromatogram of the *Standard preparation*, as obtained in the *Assay for trimethoprim*.
Sterility ⟨71⟩—It meets the requirements when tested as directed for *Membrane Filtration* under *Test for Sterility of the Product to be Examined*.
pH ⟨791⟩: between 4.0 and 6.2.
Assay for polymyxin B—Proceed as directed for polymyxin B under *Antibiotics—Microbial Assays* ⟨81⟩, using an accurately measured volume of Ophthalmic Solution, diluted quantitatively and stepwise with *Buffer No. 6*, to obtain a *Test Dilution* having a concentration of polymyxin B assumed to be equal to the median dose level of the Standard.
Assay for trimethoprim—
Diluent—Prepare a mixture of 0.01 N hydrochloric acid and acetonitrile (870 : 130).
Mobile phase—Dissolve 1.65 g of ethanesulfonic acid in 1000 mL of a mixture of water and acetonitrile (870 : 130). Adjust with 10 N sodium hydroxide or 0.1 N hydrochloric acid to a pH of 3.5. Pass this solution through a filter having a 0.5-µm or finer porosity, and degas. Make adjustments if necessary (see *System Suitability* under *Chromatography* ⟨621⟩).
Standard preparation—Dissolve an accurately weighed quantity of USP Trimethoprim RS in *Diluent* to obtain a solution having a known concentration of about 0.04 mg per mL.
Assay preparation—Transfer an accurately measured volume of Ophthalmic Solution, equivalent to about 1 mg of trimethoprim, to a 25-mL volumetric flask, dilute with *Diluent* to volume, and mix.
Chromatographic system (see *Chromatography* ⟨621⟩)—The liquid chromatograph is equipped with a 254-nm detector and a 3.9-mm × 30-cm column that contains packing L11. The flow rate is about 1.5 mL per minute. Chromatograph the *Standard preparation*, and record the peak responses as directed for *Procedure*: the tailing factor is not more than 1.5, when calculated at 10% height of

the peak; and the relative standard deviation for replicate injections is not more than 2.0%.

Procedure—Separately inject equal volumes (about 10 µL) of the *Standard preparation* and the *Assay preparation* into the chromatograph, record the chromatograms, and measure the responses for the major peaks. Calculate the quantity, in mg, of trimethoprim ($C_{14}H_{18}N_4O_3$) in each mL of the Ophthalmic Solution taken by the formula:

$$25(C/V)(r_U / r_S)$$

in which C is the concentration, in mg per mL, of USP Trimethoprim RS in the *Standard preparation*; V is the volume, in mL, of Ophthalmic Solution taken to prepare the *Assay preparation*; and r_U and r_S are the trimethoprim peak area responses obtained from the *Assay preparation* and the *Standard preparation*, respectively.

Polyvinyl Alcohol

(C_2H_4O)$_n$
Ethenol, homopolymer.
Vinyl alcohol polymer   [9002-89-5].

» Polyvinyl Alcohol is a water-soluble synthetic resin, represented by the formula:

$$(C_2H_4O)_n$$

in which the average value of n lies between 500 and 5000. It is prepared by 85 percent to 89 percent hydrolysis of polyvinyl acetate. The apparent viscosity, in centipoises, at 20°, of a solution containing 4 g of Polyvinyl Alcohol in each 100 g is not less than 85.0 percent and not more than 115.0 percent of that stated on the label.

Packaging and storage—Preserve in well-closed containers.
Viscosity—After determining the *Loss on drying*, weigh a quantity of undried Polyvinyl Alcohol, equivalent to 6.00 g on the dried basis. Over a period of seconds, transfer the test specimen with continuous slow stirring to about 140 mL of water contained in a suitable tared flask. When the specimen is well-wetted, increase the rate of stirring, avoiding mixing in excess air. Heat the mixture to 90°, and maintain the temperature at 90° for about 5 minutes. Discontinue heating, and continue stirring for 1 hour. Add water to make the mixture weigh 150 g. Resume stirring to obtain a homogenous solution. Filter the solution through a tared 100-mesh screen into a 250-mL conical flask, cool to about 15°, mix, and proceed as directed under *Viscosity* ⟨911⟩.
pH ⟨791⟩: between 5.0 and 8.0, in a solution (1 in 25).
Loss on drying ⟨731⟩—Dry it at 110° to constant weight: it loses not more than 5.0% of its weight.
Residue on ignition ⟨281⟩: not more than 2.0%.
Water-insoluble substances—Wash the tared 100-mesh screen used in the test for *Viscosity* with two 25-mL portions of water, and dry at 110° for 1 hour: not more than 6.4 mg of water-insoluble substances is found (0.1%).
Organic volatile impurities, *Method I* ⟨467⟩: meets the requirements.

(Official until July 1, 2008)
Degree of hydrolysis—
Procedure—Transfer about 1 g of Polyvinyl Alcohol, previously dried at 110° to constant weight and accurately weighed, to a wide-mouth, 250-mL conical flask fitted by means of a suitable glass joint to a reflux condenser. Add 35 mL of dilute methanol (3 in 5), and mix gently to assure complete wetting of the solid. Add 3 drops of phenolphthalein TS, and add 0.2 N hydrochloric acid or 0.2 N sodium hydroxide, if necessary, to neutralize. Add 25.0 mL of 0.2 N sodium hydroxide VS, and reflux gently on a hot plate for 1 hour. Wash the condenser with 10 mL of water, collecting the washings in the flask, cool, and titrate with 0.2 N hydrochloric acid VS. Concomitantly perform a blank determination in the same manner, using the same quantity of 0.2 N sodium hydroxide VS.

Calculation of saponification value—Calculate the saponification value by the formula:

$$[(B - A)N56.11] / W$$

in which B and A are the volumes, in mL, of 0.2 N hydrochloric acid VS consumed in the titration of the blank and the test preparation, respectively, N is the exact normality of the hydrochloric acid solution, W is the weight, in g, of the portion of Polyvinyl Alcohol taken, and 56.11 is the molecular weight of potassium hydroxide.

Calculation of degree of hydrolysis—Calculate the degree of hydrolysis, expressed as percentage of hydrolysis of polyvinyl acetate, by the formula:

$$100 - [7.84S / (100 - 0.075S)]$$

in which S is the saponification value of the Polyvinyl Alcohol taken: between 85% and 89% is found.

Sulfurated Potash

Thiosulfuric acid, dipotassium salt, mixture with potassium sulfide (K_2S_x).
Dipotassium thiosulfate mixture with potassium sulfide (K_2S_x) [39365-88-3].

» Sulfurated Potash is a mixture composed chiefly of potassium polysulfides and potassium thiosulfate. It contains not less than 12.8 percent of sulfur (S) in combination as sulfide.

Packaging and storage—Preserve in tight containers. Containers from which it is to be taken for immediate use in compounding prescriptions contain not more than 120 g.
Identification—
A: To a 1 in 10 solution add an excess of 6 N acetic acid: hydrogen sulfide is evolved, and sulfur is precipitated.
B: Filter the mixture from *Identification* test A, and add to the filtrate an excess of sodium bitartrate TS: an abundant, white, crystalline precipitate is formed within 15 minutes.
Organic volatile impurities, *Method IV* ⟨467⟩: meets the requirements.

(Official until July 1, 2008)
Assay for sulfides—Transfer 10 to 15 pieces of Sulfurated Potash to a mortar, and reduce to a fine powder. Transfer about 1 g of the powder, accurately weighed, to a 250-mL beaker, and dissolve in 50 mL of water. Filter, if necessary, and wash or dilute with water to 75 mL. Add, with constant stirring, 50 mL of cupric sulfate solution (1 in 20), and allow the mixture to stand, with occasional stirring, for 10 minutes. Filter through a retentive filter, and wash the precipitate with 200 mL of 0.25 N hydrochloric acid, taking care to avoid breaking up the cake. (If the filtrate is not blue in color, discard the assay specimen, and start over, using a larger volume of cupric sulfate solution.) Ignite the precipitate in a tared dish at 1000° for 1 hour, cool in a desiccator, and weigh: the weight of the cupric oxide so obtained, multiplied by 0.4030, represents the weight of S in the specimen under assay.

Potassium Acetate

$C_2H_3KO_2$ 98.14
Acetic acid, potassium salt.
Potassium acetate   [127-08-2].

» Potassium Acetate contains not less than 99.0 percent and not more than 100.5 percent of $C_2H_3KO_2$, calculated on the dried basis.

Packaging and storage—Preserve in tight containers.
Identification—A solution (1 in 10) responds to the tests for *Potassium* ⟨191⟩ and for *Acetate* ⟨191⟩.
pH ⟨791⟩: between 7.5 and 8.5, in a solution (1 in 20).
Loss on drying ⟨731⟩—Dry it at 150° for 2 hours: it loses not more than 1.0% of its weight.
Heavy metals, *Method I* ⟨231⟩—Prepare the *Test Preparation* as follows. Dissolve 1 g in 10 mL of water, add 3.0 mL of glacial acetic acid, dilute with water to 25 mL, and adjust with glacial acetic acid to a pH between 3.8 and 4.0, measured with a pH meter. Prepare the *Monitor Preparation* as directed for *Test Preparation*, 2.0 mL of *Standard Lead Solution* being added: the limit is 0.002%.
Limit of sodium—
  Potassium chloride solution—Dissolve 100 g of potassium chloride in water to make 1000 mL.
  Standard solutions—Transfer 127.1 mg of sodium chloride, previously dried at 105° for 2 hours and accurately weighed, to a 500-mL volumetric flask, add water to volume, and mix. Transfer 10.0 mL of this solution to a 100-mL volumetric flask, dilute with water to volume, and mix. Transfer 2.0, 5.0, and 10.0 mL of this solution to separate 100-mL volumetric flasks, add 10.0 mL of *Potassium chloride solution* to each flask, dilute with water to volume, and mix. These *Standard solutions* contain 0.2, 0.5, and 1.0 µg of sodium per mL, respectively. [NOTE—Concentrations of sodium in the *Standard solutions* may be modified to fit the linear or working range of the atomic absorption spectrophotometer.]
  Test solution—Transfer about 0.2 g of Potassium Acetate, accurately weighed, to a 100-mL volumetric flask containing about 50 mL of water, and swirl to dissolve. Add 10.0 mL of *Potassium chloride solution*, dilute with water to volume, and mix. [NOTE—The concentration of Potassium Acetate in the *Test solution* may be modified by using a different quantity or by further dilution to bring the absorption response within the range of responses obtained from the *Standard solutions*.]
  Blank solution—Transfer 10.0 mL of *Potassium chloride solution* to a 100-mL volumetric flask, dilute with water to volume, and mix.
  Procedure—Concomitantly determine the absorbances of the *Standard solutions* and the *Test solution* at the sodium emission line of 589 nm, with a suitable atomic absorption spectrophotometer (see *Spectrophotometry and Light-Scattering* ⟨851⟩) equipped with a sodium hollow-cathode lamp and an oxidizing air–acetylene flame, using the *Blank solution* to zero the instrument. Plot the absorbances of the *Standard solutions* versus concentration, in µg per mL, of sodium, and draw the straight line best fitting the plotted points. From the graph so obtained, determine the concentration C, in µg per mL, of sodium in the *Test solution*. Calculate the percentage of sodium in the portion of Potassium Acetate taken by the formula:

$$CD/10,000W$$

in which W is the quantity, in g, of Potassium Acetate taken to prepare the *Test solution*; and D is the extent of dilution of the *Test solution*: not more than 0.03% of sodium is found.
Assay—Dissolve about 200 mg of Potassium Acetate, previously dried and accurately weighed, in 25 mL of glacial acetic acid, add 2 drops of crystal violet TS, and titrate with 0.1 N perchloric acid VS to a green endpoint. Perform a blank determination, and make any necessary correction. Each mL of 0.1 N perchloric acid is equivalent to 9.814 mg of $C_2H_3KO_2$.

Potassium Acetate Injection

» Potassium Acetate Injection is a sterile solution of Potassium Acetate in Water for Injection. It contains not less than 95.0 percent and not more than 105.0 percent of the labeled amount of $C_2H_3KO_2$.

Packaging and storage—Preserve in single-dose or in multiple-dose containers, preferably of Type I or Type II glass.
Labeling—The label states the potassium acetate content in terms of weight and of milliequivalents in a given volume. Label the Injection to indicate that it is to be diluted to appropriate strength with water or other suitable fluid prior to administration. The label states also the total osmolar concentration in mOsmol per L. Where the contents are less than 100 mL, or where the label states that the Injection is not for direct injection but is to be diluted before use, the label alternatively may state the total osmolar concentration in mOsmol per mL.
USP Reference standards ⟨11⟩—*USP Endotoxin RS*.
Identification—It responds to the tests for *Potassium* ⟨191⟩ and for *Acetate* ⟨191⟩.
Bacterial endotoxins ⟨85⟩—It contains not more than 8.80 USP Endotoxin Units per mEq.
pH ⟨791⟩: between 5.5 and 8.0, when diluted with water to 1.0% of potassium acetate.
Particulate matter ⟨788⟩: meets the requirements under small-volume injections.
Other requirements—It meets the requirements under *Injections* ⟨1⟩.
Assay—
  Potassium stock solution—Dissolve 190.7 mg of potassium chloride, previously dried at 105° for 2 hours, in water. Transfer to a 1000-mL volumetric flask, dilute with water to volume, and mix. Transfer 100.0 mL of this solution to a 1000-mL volumetric flask, dilute with water to volume, and mix. This solution contains 10 µg of potassium (equivalent to 19.07 µg of potassium chloride) per mL.
  Standard preparations—To separate 100-mL volumetric flasks transfer 10.0, 15.0, and 20.0 mL, respectively, of *Potassium stock solution*. To each flask add 2.0 mL of sodium chloride solution (1 in 5) and 1.0 mL of hydrochloric acid, dilute with water to volume, and mix. The *Standard preparations* contain, respectively, 1.0, 1.5, and 2.0 µg of potassium per mL.
  Assay preparation—Transfer an accurately measured volume of Injection, equivalent to about 2 g of potassium acetate, to a 500-mL volumetric flask, dilute with water to volume, and mix. Transfer 5.0 mL of the solution to a 250-mL volumetric flask, dilute with water to volume, and mix. Transfer 5.0 mL of the resulting solution to a 100-mL volumetric flask, add 2.0 mL of sodium chloride solution (1 in 5) and 1.0 mL of hydrochloric acid, dilute with water to volume, and mix.
  Procedure—Concomitantly determine the absorbances of the *Standard preparations* and the *Assay preparation* at the potassium emission line of 766.5 nm, with a suitable atomic absorption spectrophotometer (see *Spectrophotometry and Light-scattering* ⟨851⟩) equipped with a potassium hollow-cathode lamp and an air–acetylene flame, using water as the blank. Plot the absorbance of the *Standard preparation* versus concentration, in µg per mL, of potassium, and draw the straight line best fitting the three plotted points. From the graph so obtained, determine the concentration, in µg per mL, of potassium in the *Assay preparation*. Calculate the quantity, in mg, of $C_2H_3KO_2$ in the portion of Injection taken by the formula:

$$500C(2.510)$$

in which C is the concentration, in µg per mL, of potassium in the *Assay preparation*, and 2.510 is the ratio of the molecular weight of potassium acetate to the atomic weight of potassium.

Potassium Bicarbonate

$KHCO_3$ 100.12
Carbonic acid, monopotassium salt.
Monopotassium carbonate   [298-14-6].

» Potassium Bicarbonate contains not less than 99.5 percent and not more than 101.5 percent of $KHCO_3$, calculated on the dried basis.

Packaging and storage—Preserve in well-closed containers.
Identification—A solution (1 in 10) responds to the tests for *Potassium* ⟨191⟩ and for *Bicarbonate* ⟨191⟩.
Loss on drying ⟨731⟩—Dry it over silica gel for 4 hours: it loses not more than 0.3% of its weight.
Normal carbonate—Grind 3.0 g of Potassium Bicarbonate with 25 mL of alcohol and 5 mL of water in a porcelain mortar. Add 3 drops of phenolphthalein TS, and titrate slowly with barium chloride solution, prepared by dissolving 12.216 g of barium chloride in 300 mL of water and diluting with alcohol to obtain 1000 mL of solution, until the suspension becomes colorless. Continue the grinding for 2 minutes, and if the color turns pink, continue the titration with the barium chloride solution to a colorless end-point. Repeat the grinding for 2 minutes and the addition of the barium chloride solution, if necessary, until the suspension is colorless after 2 minutes of grinding. Each mL of the barium chloride solution is equivalent to 6.911 mg of K_2CO_3: not more than 2.5% is found.
Heavy metals, *Method I* ⟨231⟩—To 2 g add 5 mL of water and 8 mL of 3 N hydrochloric acid, heat to boiling, and maintain that temperature for 1 minute. Add 1 drop of phenolphthalein TS and sufficient 6 N ammonium hydroxide, dropwise, to give the solution a faint pink color. Cool, add 2 mL of 1 N acetic acid, and then dilute with water to 25 mL: the limit is 0.001%.
Organic volatile impurities, *Method IV* ⟨467⟩: meets the requirements.

(Official until July 1, 2008)

Assay—Dissolve about 4 g of Potassium Bicarbonate, accurately weighed, in 100 mL of water, add methyl red TS, and titrate with 1 N hydrochloric acid VS. Add the acid slowly, with constant stirring, until the solution becomes faintly pink. Heat the solution to boiling, cool, and continue the titration until the pink color no longer fades after boiling. Each mL of 1 N hydrochloric acid is equivalent to 100.1 mg of $KHCO_3$.

Potassium Bicarbonate Effervescent Tablets for Oral Solution

» Potassium Bicarbonate Effervescent Tablets for Oral Solution contain not less than 90.0 percent and not more than 110.0 percent of the labeled amount of K.

Packaging and storage—Preserve in tight containers, protected from excessive heat.
Labeling—The label states the potassium content in terms of weight and in terms of milliequivalents. Where the Tablets are packaged in individual pouches, the label instructs the user not to open until the time of use.
Identification—One Tablet dissolves in 100 mL of water with effervescence. The collected gas responds to the test for *Bicarbonate* ⟨191⟩, and the resulting solution responds to the test for *Potassium* ⟨191⟩.
Uniformity of dosage units ⟨905⟩: meet the requirements.
Assay—
Potassium stock solution and *Standard preparations*—Prepare as directed in the *Assay* under *Potassium Chloride Oral Solution*.
Assay preparation—Transfer 10 Tablets to a 2000-mL volumetric flask, dissolve in 200 mL of water, swirl until effervescence ceases, dilute with water to volume, and mix. Filter, and quantitatively dilute an accurately measured volume of the filtrate with water to obtain a solution containing 30 μg of potassium per mL. Transfer 5.0 mL of the resulting solution to a 100-mL volumetric flask, add 2.0 mL of sodium chloride solution (1 in 5) and 1.0 mL of hydrochloric acid, dilute with water to volume, and mix.
Procedure—Proceed as directed for *Procedure* in the *Assay* under *Potassium Chloride Oral Solution*. Calculate the quantity, in mg, of K in each Tablet taken by the formula:

$$L(C/D)$$

in which L is the labeled quantity, in mg, of potassium in each Tablet, C is the concentration, in μg per mL, of potassium in the *Assay preparation*, and D is the concentration, in μg per mL, of potassium in the *Assay preparation* on the basis of the labeled quantity in each Tablet and the extent of dilution.

Potassium Bicarbonate and Potassium Chloride for Effervescent Oral Solution

» Potassium Bicarbonate and Potassium Chloride for Effervescent Oral Solution contains not less than 90.0 percent and not more than 110.0 percent of the labeled amounts of K and Cl.

Packaging and storage—Preserve in tight containers, protected from excessive heat.
Labeling—The label states the potassium and chloride contents in terms of weight and in terms of milliequivalents. Where packaged in individual pouches, the label instructs the user not to open until the time of use.
Identification—A 3-g portion dissolves in 100 mL of water with effervescence. The collected gas so obtained responds to the test for *Bicarbonate* ⟨191⟩, and the resulting solution responds to the tests for *Potassium* ⟨191⟩ and for *Chloride* ⟨191⟩.
Minimum fill ⟨755⟩—
FOR SOLID PACKAGED IN MULTIPLE-UNIT CONTAINERS: meets the requirements.
Uniformity of dosage units ⟨905⟩—
FOR SOLID PACKAGED IN SINGLE-UNIT CONTAINERS: meets the requirements.
Assay for potassium—
Potassium stock solution and *Standard preparations*—Prepare as directed in the *Assay* under *Potassium Chloride Oral Solution*.
Assay preparation—Weigh and mix the contents of not less than 20 containers of Potassium Bicarbonate and Potassium Chloride for Effervescent Oral Solution. Transfer an accurately weighed portion of the powder, equivalent to about 6 g of potassium, to a 1000-mL volumetric flask, dissolve in about 200 mL of water, dilute with water to volume, and mix. Transfer 5.0 mL of this solution to a second 1000-mL volumetric flask, dilute with water to volume, and mix. Transfer 5.0 mL of the resulting solution to a 100-mL volumetric flask, add 2.0 mL of sodium chloride solution (1 in 5) and 1.0 mL of hydrochloric acid, dilute with water to volume, and mix.
Procedure—Proceed as directed for *Procedure* in the *Assay* under *Potassium Chloride Oral Solution*. Calculate the quantity, in mg, of K in the portion of Potassium Bicarbonate and Potassium Chloride for Effervescent Oral Solution taken by the formula:

$$400C$$

in which C is the concentration, in μg per mL, of potassium in the *Assay preparation*.
Assay for chloride—Weigh and mix the contents of not less than 20 containers of Potassium Bicarbonate and Potassium Chloride for Effervescent Oral Solution. Transfer a portion of the powder, equivalent to about 900 mg of chloride, to a 2000-mL volumetric flask. Add about 200 mL of water, swirl until effervescence ceases, dilute with water to volume, and mix. Transfer 25.0 mL of this solution to a 250-mL conical flask, add 50.0 mL of 0.1 N silver nitrate VS and 15 mL of nitric acid, and boil, with constant swirling, until the solution is colorless. Cool to room temperature, add water to make about 150 mL, then add 5 mL of ferric ammonium sulfate TS, and titrate the excess silver nitrate with 0.1 N ammonium thiocyanate VS to a permanent faint brown endpoint. Each mL of 0.1 N silver nitrate is equivalent to 3.545 mg of Cl.

Potassium Bicarbonate and Potassium Chloride Effervescent Tablets for Oral Solution

» Potassium Bicarbonate and Potassium Chloride Effervescent Tablets for Oral Solution contain not less than 90.0 percent and not more than 110.0 percent of the labeled amounts of K and Cl.

Packaging and storage—Preserve in tight containers, protected from excessive heat.
Labeling—The label states the potassium and chloride contents in terms of weight and in terms of milliequivalents. Where the Tablets are packaged in individual pouches, the label instructs the user not to open until the time of use.
Identification—One Tablet dissolves in 100 mL of water with effervescence. The collected gas responds to the test for *Bicarbonate* ⟨191⟩, and the resulting solution responds to the tests for *Potassium* ⟨191⟩ and for *Chloride* ⟨191⟩.
Uniformity of dosage units ⟨905⟩: meet the requirements.
Assay for potassium—
 Potassium stock solution and *Standard preparations*—Prepare as directed in the *Assay* under *Potassium Chloride Oral Solution*.
 Assay preparation—Transfer 10 Tablets to a 2000-mL volumetric flask, dissolve in 200 mL of water, swirl until effervescence ceases, dilute with water to volume, and mix. Filter, and quantitatively dilute an accurately measured volume of the filtrate with water to obtain a solution containing 30 µg of potassium per mL. Transfer 5.0 mL of the resulting solution to a 100-mL volumetric flask, add 2.0 mL of sodium chloride solution (1 in 5) and 1.0 mL of hydrochloric acid, dilute with water to volume, and mix.
 Procedure—Proceed as directed for *Procedure* in the *Assay* under *Potassium Chloride Oral Solution*. Calculate the quantity, in mg, of K in each Tablet taken by the formula:

$$L(C/D)$$

in which L is the labeled quantity, in mg, of potassium in each Tablet; C is the concentration, in µg per mL, of potassium in the *Assay preparation*, and D is the concentration, in µg per mL, of potassium in the *Assay preparation* on the basis of the labeled quantity in each Tablet and the extent of dilution.

Assay for chloride—Transfer a number of Tablets, equivalent to about 900 mg of chloride, to a 2000-mL volumetric flask. Add about 200 mL of water, swirl until effervescence ceases, dilute with water to volume, and mix. Transfer 25.0 mL of this solution to a 250-mL conical flask, add 50.0 mL of 0.1 N silver nitrate VS and 15 mL of nitric acid, and boil, with constant swirling, until the supernatant is colorless. Cool to room temperature, add sufficient water to make a volume of about 150 mL, add 5 mL of ferric ammonium sulfate TS, and titrate the excess silver nitrate with 0.1 N ammonium thiocyanate VS to a permanent faint brown endpoint. Each mL of 0.1 N silver nitrate is equivalent to 3.545 mg of Cl. Calculate the quantity, in mg, of chloride (Cl) in each Tablet by dividing the total amount of chloride in the Tablets taken by the number of Tablets taken.

Potassium and Sodium Bicarbonates and Citric Acid Effervescent Tablets for Oral Solution

» Potassium and Sodium Bicarbonates and Citric Acid Effervescent Tablets for Oral Solution contain not less than 90.0 percent and not more than 110.0 percent of the labeled amounts of potassium bicarbonate ($KHCO_3$), sodium bicarbonate ($NaHCO_3$), and anhydrous citric acid ($C_6H_8O_7$).

Packaging and storage—Preserve in tight containers.
Labeling—Label it to state the sodium content. The label states also that the Tablets are to be dissolved in water before being taken.
USP Reference standards ⟨11⟩—*USP Citric Acid RS*.
(Official January 1, 2009)
Identification—One Tablet dissolves in 100 mL of water with effervescence. The collected gas responds to the test for *Bicarbonate* ⟨191⟩, and the resulting solution responds to the tests for *Potassium* ⟨191⟩ and for *Sodium* ⟨191⟩. The resulting solution responds also to the test for *Citrate* ⟨191⟩, 3 to 5 drops of it and 20 mL of the mixture of pyridine and acetic anhydride being used.
Acid-neutralizing capacity ⟨301⟩—The acid consumed by the minimum single dose recommended in the labeling is not less than 5 mEq.
Assay for potassium bicarbonate and sodium bicarbonate—
 Potassium chloride stock solution—Prepare a solution of potassium chloride, previously dried at 125° for 30 minutes and accurately weighed, in water to obtain a solution having a known concentration of about 7.5 mg per mL.
 Sodium chloride stock solution—Prepare a solution of sodium chloride, previously dried at 125° for 30 minutes and accurately weighed, in water to obtain a solution having a known concentration of about 7 mg per mL.
 Lithium diluent solution—Transfer 1.04 g of lithium nitrate to a 1000-mL volumetric flask, add a suitable nonionic surfactant, then add water to volume, and mix.
 Standard preparation—Transfer 5.0 mL of *Potassium chloride stock solution* and 5.0 mL of *Sodium chloride stock solution* to a 50-mL volumetric flask, dilute with water to volume, and mix. Each mL of this intermediate solution contains about 0.75 mg of potassium chloride and 0.7 mg of sodium chloride. Transfer 5.0 mL of this solution to a 100-mL volumetric flask, dilute with *Lithium diluent solution* to volume, and mix.
 Assay preparation 1—Weigh and finely powder not fewer than 20 Tablets. [NOTE—Tablets and powder are hygroscopic. After removal from the container, grind the Tablets promptly in an atmosphere of low relative humidity, and weigh the powder promptly.] Transfer an accurately weighed portion of the powder, equivalent to about 3000 mg of potassium bicarbonate, to a 1000-mL volumetric flask, dissolve in 500 mL of water, swirl until effervescence ceases, dilute with water to volume, and mix. Dilute an accurately measured volume of this stock solution quantitatively with water to obtain a test solution containing about 1 mg of potassium bicarbonate per mL, on the basis of the labeled quantity. Transfer 5.0 mL of this solution to a 100-mL volumetric flask, dilute with *Lithium diluent solution* to volume, and mix.
 Assay preparation 2—Dilute an accurately measured volume of the stock solution used to prepare *Assay preparation 1* quantitatively with water to obtain a test solution containing about 1 mg of sodium bicarbonate per mL, on the basis of the labeled quantity. Transfer 5.0 mL of this solution to a 100-mL volumetric flask, dilute with *Lithium diluent solution* to volume, and mix.
 Procedure—Using a suitable flame photometer, adjusted to read zero with *Lithium diluent solution*, concomitantly determine the potassium flame emission readings for the *Standard preparation* and *Assay preparation 1* at the wavelength of maximum emission at about 766 nm. Calculate the quantity, in mg, of potassium bicarbonate ($KHCO_3$) in each Tablet taken by the formula:

$$(100.12/74.55)(LC/D)(R_{U,K}/R_{S,K})$$

in which 100.12 and 74.55 are the molecular weights of potassium bicarbonate and potassium chloride, respectively; L is the labeled quantity, in mg, of potassium bicarbonate in each Tablet; C is the concentration, in mg per mL, of potassium chloride in the intermediate solution used to prepare the *Standard preparation*; D is the concentration, in mg per mL, of potassium bicarbonate in the test solution used to prepare *Assay preparation 1*, on the basis of the labeled quantity of potassium bicarbonate in each Tablet and the extent of dilution; and $R_{U,K}$ and $R_{S,K}$ are the potassium emission readings obtained from *Assay preparation 1* and the *Standard preparation*, respectively. Similarly determine the sodium flame emission readings for the *Standard preparation* and *Assay preparation 2* at the wavelength of maximum emission at about 589 nm. Calculate the quantity, in mg, of sodium bicarbonate (NaHCO₃) in each Tablet taken by the formula:

$$(84.01/58.44)(LC/D)(R_{U,Na}/R_{S,Na})$$

in which 84.01 and 58.44 are the molecular weights of sodium bicarbonate and sodium chloride, respectively; *L* is the labeled quantity, in mg, of sodium bicarbonate in each Tablet; *C* is the concentration, in mg per mL, of sodium chloride in the intermediate solution used to prepare the *Standard preparation*; *D* is the concentration, in mg per mL, of sodium bicarbonate in the test solution used to prepare *Assay preparation 2*, on the basis of the number of Tablets taken, the labeled quantity of sodium bicarbonate in each Tablet, and the extent of dilution; and $R_{U,Na}$ and $R_{S,Na}$ are the sodium emission readings obtained from *Assay preparation 2* and the *Standard preparation*, respectively.

Assay for anhydrous citric acid—

Cation-exchange column—Mix 10 g of styrenedivinylbenzene cation-exchange resin with 50 mL of water in a suitable beaker. Allow the resin to settle, and decant the supernatant until a slurry of resin remains. Pour the slurry into a 14-mm × 30-cm glass chromatographic tube (having a sealed-in, coarse-porosity porous glass disk and fitted with a stopcock), and allow to settle as a homogeneous bed. Wash the resin bed with about 100 mL of water, closing the stopcock when the water level is about 2 mm above the resin bed.

Procedure—Transfer an accurately measured volume of the stock solution used to prepare *Assay preparation 1* in the *Assay for potassium bicarbonate and sodium bicarbonate*, equivalent to about 40 mg of anhydrous citric acid, carefully onto the top of the resin bed in the *Cation-exchange column*. Place a 250-mL conical flask below the column, open the stopcock, and allow to flow until the solution has entered the resin bed. Elute the column with 60 mL of water at a flow rate of about 5 mL per minute, collecting about 65 mL of the eluate in a suitable flask. Boil the eluate for 1 minute, cool, add 5 drops of phenolphthalein TS, swirl the flask, and titrate with 0.02 N sodium hydroxide VS to a pink endpoint. Each mL of 0.02 N sodium hydroxide is equivalent to 1.281 mg of anhydrous citric acid (C₆H₈O₇).

(Official until January 1, 2009)

Assay for anhydrous citric acid—

Mobile Phase, Standard Preparation 1, and *Chromatographic System*—Proceed as directed under *Assay for Citric Acid/Citrate and Phosphate* ⟨345⟩.

Assay preparation—Transfer an accurately measured volume of the stock solution used to prepare *Assay preparation 1* in the *Assay for potassium bicarbonate and sodium bicarbonate*, equivalent to about 40 mg of anhydrous citric acid, into a suitable volumetric flask, and proceed as directed for *Assay Preparation for Citric Acid/Citrate Assay* under *Assay for Citric Acid/Citrate and Phosphate* ⟨345⟩.

Procedure—Proceed as directed for *Procedure* under ⟨345⟩, and calculate the quantity, in mg, of anhydrous citric acid (C₆H₈O₇) in the portion of Tablets taken by the formula:

$$0.001(192.12/189.10)C_S\,D(r_U/r_S)$$

in which 192.12 is the molecular weight of anhydrous citric acid; 189.10 is the molecular weight of citrate (C₆H₅O₇); C_S is the concentration, in μg per mL, of citrate in *Standard Preparation 1*; *D* is the dilution factor; and r_U and r_S are the citrate peak areas obtained from the *Assay preparation* and *Standard Preparation 1*, respectively.

(Official January 1, 2009)

Potassium Bitartrate

C₄H₅KO₆ 188.18
Butanedioic acid 2,3-dihydroxy-, [R-(R*,R*)]-, monopotassium salt.
Potassium hydrogen tartrate [868-14-4].

» Potassium Bitartrate, dried at 105° for 3 hours, contains not less than 99.0 percent and not more than 101.0 percent of C₄H₅KO₆.

Packaging and storage—Preserve in tight containers.
Identification—
A: Ignite it: it leaves a residue that imparts a reddish purple color to a nonluminous flame.
B: A saturated solution of it yields a yellowish orange precipitate with sodium cobaltinitrite TS.
C: A solution (1 in 10) responds to the tests for *Tartrate* ⟨191⟩.
Insoluble matter—Mix 500 mg of it with 3 mL of 6 N ammonium hydroxide: no undissolved residue remains.
Limit of ammonia—

Sodium hypochlorite solution—Use a commercially available solution that contains between 4.0% and 6.0% of sodium hypochlorite.

Oxidizing solution—[NOTE—Prepare on the day of use.] Prepare a mixture of alkaline sodium citrate TS and *Sodium hypochlorite solution* (4 : 1).

Diluted sodium nitroferricyanide solution—Prepare a mixture of water and sodium nitroferricyanide TS (10 : 1).

Standard solution—Transfer 300 mg of ammonium chloride, previously dried over silica gel for 4 hours, to a 1-L volumetric flask, and dilute with water to volume. This solution contains 100 μg of ammonia per mL. Dilute this solution quantitatively, and stepwise if necessary, with water to obtain a solution having a concentration of 0.25 μg of ammonia per mL.

Test solution—Transfer 250 mg of Potassium Bitartrate to a 100-mL volumetric flask, and dissolve in and dilute with water to volume. Heat gently to facilitate the dissolution.

Procedure—[NOTE—Carefully follow the order of addition stated below.] Separately transfer 6.0 mL each of the *Standard solution* and the *Test solution* to two color-comparison tubes. To each tube add 0.4 mL of phenol TS, 0.4 mL of *Diluted sodium nitroferricyanide solution*, and 1.0 mL of *Oxidizing solution*. Dilute with water to 10 mL, mix, and allow to stand for 1 hour: the color of the *Test solution* is not darker than the color of the *Standard solution* (0.01%).

Heavy metals, *Method I* ⟨231⟩—Mix 2 g of it with 15 mL of water, and add 6 N ammonium hydroxide dropwise until solution is complete. Add 1 drop of phenolphthalein TS, and add just sufficient 1 N acetic acid dropwise to discharge the pink color. Add 2 mL of 1 N acetic acid, and dilute with water to 25 mL: the limit is 0.002%.

Assay—Dry about 6 g of Potassium Bitartrate at 105° for 3 hours, allow to cool, and weigh accurately. Dissolve in 100 mL of boiling water, add a few drops of phenolphthalein TS, and titrate with 1 N sodium hydroxide VS to a pink endpoint. Perform a blank determination, and make any necessary correction. Each mL of 1 N sodium hydroxide is equivalent to 188.2 mg of C₄H₅KO₆.

Potassium Bromide

KBr 119.0
Potassium bromide.
Potassium bromide [7758-02-3].

» Potassium Bromide contains not less than 98.0 percent and not more than 100.5 percent of KBr, calculated on the dried basis. It contains no added substances.

Packaging and storage—Preserve in well-closed containers, and store at room temperature.
Appearance of solution: clear and colorless.
Test solution—Dissolve 10.0 g in carbon dioxide-free water, and dilute with the same solvent to 100 mL.
Identification—
A: A solution containing 4.5 mg of potassium bromide responds to the test for *Bromide* ⟨191⟩.
B: Responds to the test for *Potassium* ⟨191⟩.
Acidity or alkalinity—To 10 mL of the solution prepared for the test for *Appearance of solution,* add 0.1 mL of bromothymol blue TS: not more than 0.5 mL of 0.01 N hydrochloric acid or 0.01 N sodium hydroxide is required to change the color of this solution.
Loss on drying ⟨731⟩—Dry it at 100° to 105° for 3 hours: it loses not more than 1.0% of its weight.
Bromates—
Starch–mercuric iodide solution—Triturate 1.0 g of soluble starch with 5 mL of water and pour the mixture into 100 mL of boiling water, containing 10 mg of mercuric iodide.
Procedure—To 10 mL of the solution prepared for the test for *Appearance of solution* add 1 mL of *Starch–mercuric iodide solution,* 0.1 mL of a 100 g per L solution of potassium iodide, and 0.25 mL of 0.5 M sulfuric acid. Allow to stand protected from light for 5 minutes: no blue or violet color develops.
Limit of chlorine: not more than 0.6%.
Nitric acid solution and *Ferric ammonium sulfate solution*—Proceed as directed in the *Assay*.
Procedure—Dissolve 1.000 g of Potassium Bromide in 20 mL of *Nitric acid solution* in a conical flask, add and mix 5 mL of 30 percent hydrogen peroxide, and heat in a water bath until the solution is colorless. Rinse the sides of the flask with a small quantity of water, and heat in a water bath for 15 minutes. Allow to cool, dilute with water to 50 mL, and add 5.0 mL of silver nitrate VS and 1 mL of dibutyl phthalate. Mix, and back titrate the excess silver nitrate with ammonium thiocyanate VS (see *Titrimetry* ⟨541⟩), using 5 mL of *Ferric ammonium sulfate solution* as the indicator. Perform a blank titration. Not more than 1.7 mL of silver nitrate VS is used.
Iodides—To 5 mL of the solution prepared for the test for *Appearance of solution* add 0.15 mL of a 10.5 g per 100 mL ferric chloride solution, and 2 mL of dichloromethane. Shake, and allow to separate. The lower layer is colorless.
Sulfates ⟨221⟩—A 2.0-g portion shows no more sulfate than corresponds to 0.2 mL of 0.020 N sulfuric acid (0.01%).
Limit of iron: not more than 20 ppm.
Citric acid solution—Prepare a 200 g citric acid per mL solution.
Iron standard solution—Transfer 0.863 g of ferric ammonium sulfate to a 500-mL volumetric flask, and dissolve in 25 mL of dilute sulfuric acid. Dilute with water to volume. Transfer 1.0 mL of the resulting solution to a 10-mL volumetric flask, and dilute with water to volume. Transfer 2.5 mL of this resulting solution to a 50-mL volumetric flask, and dilute with water to volume. [NOTE—Prepare immediately before use.]
Test solution—Transfer 5 mL of the solution prepared for the test for *Appearance of solution* to a 10-mL volumetric flask, and dilute with water to volume.
Procedure—To 10 mL each of the *Iron standard solution* and the *Test solution* add 2.0 mL of the *Citric acid solution* and 0.1 mL of thioglycolic acid. Make alkaline to litmus with ammonia water, and dilute with water to 20 mL. After 5 minutes, any pink color in the *Test solution* is not more intense than that in the *Iron standard solution*.
Magnesium and alkaline-earth metals—To 200 mL of water add 0.1 g of hydroxylamine hydrochloride, 10 mL of pH 10.0 ammonia–ammonium chloride buffer (prepared by dissolving 5.4 g of ammonium chloride in 20 mL of water, adding 20 mL of ammonium hydroxide and diluting to 100 mL), 1 mL of 0.1 M zinc sulfate, and about 0.2 g of eriochrome black T trituration. Heat to about 40°. Titrate this solution (see *Titrimetry* ⟨541⟩) with 0.01 M edetate disodium VS until the violet color changes to deep blue. To this solution add 10.0 g of Potassium Bromide dissolved in 100 mL of water. If the color changes to violet, titrate the solution with 0.01 M edetate disodium VS to a deep blue endpoint. The volume of 0.01 M edetate disodium consumed in the second titration does not exceed 5.0 mL (0.02%, calculated as Ca).
Heavy metals, *Method I* ⟨231⟩: not more than 10 ppm.
Assay—
Nitric acid solution—Dilute 14 mL of nitric acid with water to 100 mL.
Ferric ammonium sulfate solution—Transfer 10 g of ferric ammonium sulfate to a 100-mL volumetric flask. Dissolve in and dilute with water to volume.
Procedure—Dissolve 2.000 g of Potassium Bromide in water, and dilute with water to 100.0 mL. To 10.0 mL of the solution add 50 mL of water, 5 mL of *Nitric acid solution,* 25.0 mL of silver nitrate VS, and 2 mL of dibutyl phthalate. Mix, and back titrate the excess silver nitrate with ammonium thiocyanate VS (see *Titrimetry* ⟨541⟩), using 2 mL of *Ferric ammonium sulfate solution* as the indicator, shaking vigorously towards the endpoint. Each mL of 0.1 M silver nitrate is equivalent to 11.90 mg of KBr. Calculate the percent content of Potassium Bromide, corrected for the chloride content, by the formula:

$$a - 3.357b$$

in which *a* is the percent content of KBr and KCl obtained, calculated as KBr; and *b* is the percent content of chlorides.

Potassium Carbonate

K$_2$CO$_3$ (anhydrous)   138.21
Carbonic acid, dipotassium salt.
Dipotassium carbonate   [584-08-7].
Sesquihydrate   165.23

» Potassium Carbonate contains not less than 99.5 percent and not more than 100.5 percent of K$_2$CO$_3$, calculated on the dried basis.

Packaging and storage—Preserve in well-closed containers.
Identification— It responds to the tests for *Potassium* ⟨191⟩ and for *Carbonate* ⟨191⟩.
Loss on drying ⟨731⟩—Dry it at 180° for 4 hours: it loses not more than 0.5% of its weight.
Insoluble substances—Dissolve 1 g in 20 mL of water: the solution is complete, clear, and colorless.
Heavy metals ⟨231⟩—Dissolve 4.0 g in 10 mL of water, add 15 mL of 3 N hydrochloric acid, and heat to boiling. Add 1 drop of phenolphthalein TS, and neutralize with 1 N sodium hydroxide until the solution is faintly pink in color. Cool, and dilute with water to 25 mL: the limit is 0.0005%.
Organic volatile impurities, *Method I* ⟨467⟩: meets the requirements.
(Official until July 1, 2008)
Assay—Transfer the dried potassium carbonate obtained in the test for *Loss on drying* to a flask with the aid of 150 mL of water, add 4 drops of methyl orange TS, and titrate with 1 N hydrochloric acid VS. Each mL of 1 N hydrochloric acid is equivalent to 69.11 mg of K$_2$CO$_3$.

Potassium Chloride

KCl   74.55
Potassium chloride.
Potassium chloride   [7447-40-7].

» Potassium Chloride contains not less than 99.0 percent and not more than 100.5 percent of KCl, calculated on the dried basis.

Packaging and storage—Preserve in well-closed containers.
Labeling—Where Potassium Chloride is intended for use in hemodialysis, it is so labeled.

Identification—A solution (1 in 20) responds to the tests for *Potassium* ⟨191⟩ and for *Chloride* ⟨191⟩.

Acidity or alkalinity—To a solution of 5.0 g in 50 mL of carbon dioxide–free water add 3 drops of phenolphthalein TS: no pink color is produced. Then add 0.30 mL of 0.020 N sodium hydroxide: a pink color is produced.

Loss on drying ⟨731⟩—Dry it at 105° for 2 hours: it loses not more than 1.0% of its weight.

Iodide or bromide—

IODIDE—

Standard stock solution—Transfer an accurately weighed quantity, about 41 mg, of potassium iodide to a 25-mL volumetric flask. Dissolve in and dilute with water to volume, and mix.

Standard solution—Dilute 1.0 mL of *Standard stock solution* with water to 25 mL, and mix. Dilute 2.0 mL of this solution with water to 8 mL, and proceed as directed for *Test solution* beginning with "Add 1 mL each of chloroform".

Test solution—Dissolve 2 g of Potassium Chloride in 8 mL of water. Add 1 mL each of chloroform and diluted hydrochloric acid, then add 2 drops of a chloramine T solution (0.1 in 100), and shake gently. The violet color of the chloroform layer is not darker than that of a concomitantly prepared *Standard solution*: the limit is 0.005%.

BROMIDE—

Standard solution—Transfer an accurately weighed quantity, about 32 mg, of sodium bromide to a 25-mL volumetric flask. Dissolve in and dilute with water to volume, and mix. Dilute 2.0 mL of this solution with water to 8 mL, and proceed as directed for *Test solution* beginning with "Add 1 mL each of chloroform".

Test solution—Dissolve 2 g of Potassium Chloride in 8 mL of water. Add 1 mL each of chloroform and diluted hydrochloric acid, then add 5 drops of a chloramine T solution (1 in 100), and shake gently. The brown color of the chloroform layer is not darker than that of a concomitantly prepared *Standard solution*: the limit is 0.1%.

Aluminum ⟨206⟩ (where it is labeled as intended for use in hemodialysis)—Proceed as directed using 2.0 g of Potassium Chloride to prepare the *Test Preparation*: the limit is 1 µg per g.

Calcium and magnesium—To 20 mL of a solution (1 in 100) add 2 mL each of 6 N ammonium hydroxide, ammonium oxalate TS, and dibasic sodium phosphate TS: no turbidity is produced within 5 minutes.

Sodium—A solution (1 in 20), tested on a platinum wire, does not impart a pronounced yellow color to a nonluminous flame.

Heavy metals ⟨231⟩—Dissolve 2.0 g in 25 mL of water: the limit is 0.001%.

Organic volatile impurities, *Method I* ⟨467⟩: meets the requirements.

(Official until July 1, 2008)

Assay—Dissolve about 200 mg of Potassium Chloride, accurately weighed, in 10 mL of water. Add 10 mL of glacial acetic acid, 75 mL of methanol, and 3 drops of eosin Y TS. Titrate, with shaking, with 0.1 N silver nitrate VS to a pink endpoint. Each mL of 0.1 N silver nitrate is equivalent to 7.455 mg of KCl.

Potassium Chloride Extended-Release Capsules

» Potassium Chloride Extended-Release Capsules contain not less than 90.0 percent and not more than 110.0 percent of the labeled amount of KCl.

Packaging and storage—Preserve in tight containers at a temperature not exceeding 30°.

Identification—A portion of the filtrate obtained as directed under *Assay* in the *Assay* responds to the tests for *Potassium* ⟨191⟩ and for *Chloride* ⟨191⟩.

Dissolution ⟨711⟩—

Medium: water; 900 mL.

Apparatus 1: 100 rpm.

Time: 2 hours.

Potassium stock solution and *Standard preparations*—Prepare as directed in the *Assay* under *Potassium Chloride Oral Solution*.

Procedure—Filter the solution under test, and dilute quantitatively with *Dissolution Medium* to obtain a test solution containing about 60 µg of potassium chloride per mL. Add 5.0 mL of the test solution to a 100-mL volumetric flask, add 2.0 mL of sodium chloride solution (1 in 5) and 1.0 mL of hydrochloric acid, dilute with water to volume, mix, and proceed as directed for *Procedure* in the *Assay* under *Potassium Chloride Oral Solution*. Calculate the quantity, in mg, of KCl dissolved by the formula:

$$(900F)(1.907C)$$

in which F is the extent of dilution of the solution under test, and the other terms are as defined therein.

Tolerances—Not more than 35% (Q) of the labeled amount of KCl is dissolved in 2 hours. The requirements are met if the quantities dissolved from the Capsules tested conform to the accompanying acceptance table instead of the table shown under *Dissolution* ⟨711⟩.

Acceptance Table

Stage	Number Tested	Acceptance Criteria
S_1	6	Each unit is within the range $Q \pm 30\%$.
S_2	6	Average of 12 units ($S_1 + S_2$) is within the range between $Q - 30\%$ and $Q + 35\%$, and no unit is outside the range $Q \pm 40\%$.
S_3	12	Average of 24 units ($S_1 + S_2 + S_3$) is within the range between $Q - 30\%$ and $Q + 35\%$, and not more than 2 units are outside the range $Q \pm 40\%$.

Uniformity of dosage units ⟨905⟩: meet the requirements.

Assay—

Potassium stock solution and *Standard preparations*—Prepare as directed in the *Assay* under *Potassium Chloride Oral Solution*.

Assay preparation—Place not less than 20 Capsules in a suitable container with 400 mL of water, heat to boiling, and boil for 20 minutes. Allow to cool, transfer the solution to a 1000-mL volumetric flask, dilute with water to volume, and mix. Filter, discarding the first 20 mL of the filtrate. Transfer an accurately measured volume of the subsequent filtrate, equivalent to about 60 mg of potassium chloride, to a 1000-mL volumetric flask, dilute with water to volume, and mix. (Retain a portion of the filtrate for use in the *Identification* test.) Transfer 5.0 mL of the resulting solution to a 100-mL volumetric flask, add 2.0 mL of sodium chloride solution (1 in 5) and 1.0 mL of hydrochloric acid, dilute with water to volume, and mix.

Procedure—Proceed as directed for *Procedure* in the *Assay* under *Potassium Chloride Oral Solution*. Calculate the quantity, in mg, of KCl in each Capsule taken by the formula:

$$(TC/D)(1.907)$$

in which T is the labeled quantity, in mg, of potassium chloride in each Capsule, D is the concentration, in µg per mL, of potassium chloride in the *Assay preparation*, based on the labeled quantity per Capsule and the extent of dilution, and the other terms are as defined therein.

Potassium Chloride for Injection Concentrate

» Potassium Chloride for Injection Concentrate is a sterile solution of Potassium Chloride in Water for Injection. It contains not less than 95.0 percent and not more than 105.0 percent of the labeled amount of KCl.

Packaging and storage—Preserve in single-dose or in multiple-dose containers, preferably of Type I or Type II glass.

Labeling—The label states the potassium chloride content in terms of weight and of milliequivalents in a given volume. Label the Concentrate to indicate that it is to be diluted to appropriate strength with water or other suitable fluid prior to administration. Immediately following the name, the label bears the boxed warning:

> **Concentrate Must be Diluted Before Use**

This warning is not required when the liquid preparation is in a *Pharmacy bulk package* and the label thereon states prominently "Pharmacy Bulk Package—Not for direct infusion."

The cap of the container and the overseal of the cap must be black, and both bear the words: "Must Be Diluted" in readily legible type, in a color that stands out from its background OR the overseal may be of a clear plastic material through which the black cap is visible and the printing is readily legible.

When the nature of the container-closure system prevents compliance, the design shall follow the intent of this requirement as closely as possible, the black color being used beneath the words "Must be Diluted," which are so placed that words are readily visible as the contents of the container are being removed. Ampuls shall be identified by a black band or a series of black bands above the constriction. The label states also the total osmolar concentration in mOsmol per L. Where the contents are less than 100 mL, the label alternatively may state the total osmolar concentration in mOsmol per mL.

USP Reference standards ⟨11⟩—*USP Endotoxin RS*.

Identification—It responds to the tests for *Potassium* ⟨191⟩ and for *Chloride* ⟨191⟩.

Bacterial endotoxins ⟨85⟩: It contains not more than 8.80 USP Endotoxin Units per mEq.

pH ⟨791⟩: between 4.0 and 8.0.

Particulate matter ⟨788⟩: meets the requirements under small-volume injections.

Other requirements—It meets the requirements under *Injections* ⟨1⟩.

Assay—

Potassium stock solution and *Standard preparations*—Prepare as directed in the *Assay* under *Potassium Chloride Oral Solution*.

Assay preparation—Transfer an accurately measured volume of Concentrate, equivalent to about 600 mg of potassium chloride, to a 500-mL volumetric flask, dilute with water to volume, and mix. Proceed as directed for *Assay preparation* in the *Assay* under *Potassium Chloride Oral Solution*, beginning with "Transfer 5.0 mL of the solution to a 100-mL volumetric flask."

Procedure—Proceed as directed for *Procedure* in the *Assay* under *Potassium Chloride Oral Solution*. Calculate the quantity, in mg, of KCl in the portion of Concentrate taken by the formula:

$$200C(1.907)$$

in which the terms are as defined therein.

Potassium Chloride Oral Solution

» Potassium Chloride Oral Solution contains not less than 95.0 percent and not more than 105.0 percent of the labeled amount of KCl. It may contain alcohol.

Packaging and storage—Preserve in tight containers.

Identification—Carefully evaporate about 5 mL to dryness, and ignite the residue at dull-red heat to remove all organic matter. Cool, dissolve the residue in 10 mL of water, and filter: the filtrate responds to the tests for *Potassium* ⟨191⟩ and for *Chloride* ⟨191⟩.

Alcohol content (*if present*) ⟨611⟩: not less than 90.0% and not more than 115.0% of the labeled amount, the labeled amount being not more than 7.5% of C_2H_5OH, determined by the gas-liquid chromatographic procedure, acetone being used as the internal standard.

Assay—

Potassium stock solution—Dissolve 190.7 mg of potassium chloride, previously dried at 105° for 2 hours, in water. Transfer to a 1000-mL volumetric flask, dilute with water to volume, and mix. Transfer 100.0 mL of this solution to a 1000-mL volumetric flask, dilute with water to volume, and mix. This solution contains 10 μg of potassium (equivalent to 19.07 μg of potassium chloride) per mL.

Standard preparations—To separate 100-mL volumetric flasks transfer 10.0, 15.0, and 20.0 mL, respectively, of *Potassium stock solution*. To each flask add 2.0 mL of sodium chloride solution (1 in 5) and 1.0 mL of hydrochloric acid, dilute with water to volume, and mix. The *Standard preparations* contain, respectively, 1.0, 1.5, and 2.0 μg of potassium per mL.

Assay preparation—Transfer an accurately measured volume of Oral Solution, equivalent to about 600 mg of potassium chloride, to a 500-mL volumetric flask, dilute with water to volume, and mix. Transfer 5.0 mL of the solution to a 100-mL volumetric flask, dilute with water to volume, and mix. Transfer 5.0 mL of the resulting solution to a 100-mL volumetric flask, add 2.0 mL of sodium chloride solution (1 in 5) and 1.0 mL of hydrochloric acid, dilute with water to volume, and mix.

Procedure—Concomitantly determine the absorbances of the *Standard preparations* and the *Assay preparation* at the potassium emission line of 766.5 nm, with a suitable atomic absorption spectrophotometer (see *Spectrophotometry and Light-scattering* ⟨851⟩) equipped with a potassium hollow-cathode lamp and an air–acetylene flame, using water as the blank. Plot the absorbance of the *Standard preparation* versus concentration, in μg per mL, of potassium, and draw the straight line best fitting the three plotted points. From the graph so obtained, determine the concentration, in μg per mL, of potassium in the *Assay preparation*. Calculate the quantity, in mg, of KCl in the portion of Oral Solution taken by the formula:

$$200C(1.907)$$

in which C is the concentration, in μg per mL, of potassium in the *Assay preparation*, and 1.907 is the ratio of the molecular weight of potassium chloride to the atomic weight of potassium.

Potassium Chloride for Oral Solution

» Potassium Chloride for Oral Solution is a dry mixture of Potassium Chloride and one or more suitable colors, diluents, and flavors. It contains not less than 90.0 percent and not more than 110.0 percent of the labeled amount of KCl.

Packaging and storage—Preserve in tight containers.

Labeling—The label states the Potassium Chloride (KCl) content in terms of weight and in terms of milliequivalents.

Identification—Ignite about 200 mg at a temperature not above 600°, in order to remove all organic matter, cool, dissolve the residue in 10 mL of water, and filter: the filtrate responds to the tests for *Potassium* ⟨191⟩ and for *Chloride* ⟨191⟩.

Minimum fill ⟨755⟩—

FOR SOLID PACKAGED IN MULTIPLE-UNIT CONTAINERS: meets the requirements.

Uniformity of dosage units ⟨905⟩—

FOR SOLID PACKAGED IN SINGLE-UNIT CONTAINERS: meets the requirements.

Assay—
Potassium stock solution and *Standard preparations*—Prepare as directed in the *Assay* under *Potassium Chloride Oral Solution*.

Assay preparation 1 (where it is packaged in unit-dose containers)—Weigh and mix the contents of not less than 20 containers of Potassium Chloride for Oral Solution. Transfer an accurately weighed portion of the powder, equivalent to about 1.5 g of potassium chloride, to a 500-mL volumetric flask, dissolve in water, dilute with water to volume, and mix. Transfer 5.0 mL of the solution to a 250-mL volumetric flask, dilute with water to volume, and mix. Transfer 5.0 mL of the resulting solution to a 100-mL volumetric flask, add 2.0 mL of sodium chloride solution (1 in 5) and 1.0 mL of hydrochloric acid, dilute with water to volume, and mix.

Assay preparation 2 (where it is packaged in multiple-unit containers)—Transfer an accurately weighed portion of Potassium Chloride for Oral Solution, equivalent to about 1.5 g of potassium chloride, to a 500-mL volumetric flask, dissolve in water, dilute with water to volume, and mix. Proceed as directed for *Assay preparation 1*, beginning with "Transfer 5.0 mL of the solution."

Procedure—Proceed as directed for *Procedure* in the *Assay* under *Potassium Chloride Oral Solution*. Calculate the quantity of KCl, in mg, in the portion of Potassium Chloride for Oral Solution taken by the formula:

$$500C(1.907)$$

in which *C* is as defined therein.

Potassium Chloride Extended-Release Tablets

» Potassium Chloride Extended-Release Tablets contain not less than 90.0 percent and not more than 110.0 percent of the labeled amount of potassium chloride (KCl).

Packaging and storage—Preserve in tight containers at a temperature not exceeding 30°.
Labeling—The labeling states with which *Assay preparation* the product complies only if *Assay preparation 1* is not used.
Identification—A portion of the filtrate obtained as directed for the designated *Assay preparation* in the *Assay* meets the requirements of the tests for *Potassium* ⟨191⟩ and for *Chloride* ⟨191⟩.
Dissolution ⟨711⟩—
  Medium: water; 900 mL.
  Apparatus 2: 50 rpm.
  Time: 2 hours.
  Potassium stock solution—Prepare as directed in the *Assay* under *Potassium Chloride Oral Solution*.
  Standard solutions—Prepare as directed for *Standard preparations* in the *Assay* under *Potassium Chloride Oral Solution*.
  Procedure—Filter the solution under test, and dilute quantitatively with *Dissolution Medium* to obtain a test solution containing about 60 μg of potassium chloride per mL. Place 5.0 mL of the test solution in a 100-mL volumetric flask, add 2.0 mL of sodium chloride solution (1 in 5) and 1.0 mL of hydrochloric acid, dilute with water to volume, mix, and proceed as directed for *Procedure* in the *Assay* under *Potassium Chloride Oral Solution*. Calculate the quantity, in mg, of KCl dissolved by the formula:

$$(900F)(1.907C)$$

in which *F* is the extent of dilution of the solution under test, and the other terms are as defined therein.
  Tolerances—Not more than 35% (*Q*) of the labeled amount of KCl is dissolved in 2 hours. The requirements are met if the quantities dissolved from the Tablets tested conform to the accompanying acceptance table instead of the table shown under *Dissolution* ⟨711⟩.

Acceptance Table

Stage	Number Tested	Acceptance Criteria
S_1	6	Each unit is within the range $Q \pm 30\%$.
S_2	6	Average of 12 units ($S_1 + S_2$) is within the range between $Q - 30\%$ and $Q + 35\%$, and no unit is outside the range $Q \pm 40\%$.
S_3	12	Average of 24 units ($S_1 + S_2 + S_3$) is within the range between $Q - 30\%$ and $Q + 35\%$, and not more than 2 units outside the range $Q \pm 40\%$.

Uniformity of dosage units ⟨905⟩: meet the requirements.
Assay—[NOTES—If necessary, first score nonsugar-coated tablets. Retain a portion of the filtrate of either *Assay preparation 1* or *Assay preparation 2* for use in the test for *Identification*.]

Potassium stock solution and *Standard preparations*—Prepare as directed in the *Assay* under *Potassium Chloride Oral Solution*.

Assay preparation 1—Place not fewer than 20 Tablets in a suitable container with 400 mL of water, heat to boiling, and boil for 20 minutes. Allow to cool, transfer the solution to a 1000-mL volumetric flask, dilute with water to volume, and mix. Filter, discarding the first 20 mL of the filtrate. Transfer an accurately measured volume of the subsequent filtrate, equivalent to about 60 mg of potassium chloride, to a 1000-mL volumetric flask, dilute with water to volume, and mix.

Assay preparation 2 (For formulations containing crystals coated with hydrophobic polymers)—Place not fewer than 20 Tablets in a 2000-mL volumetric flask. Add 1200 mL of a mixture of acetonitrile and water (1 : 1), and shake by mechanical means, or stir using a magnetic bar for 90 minutes. Dilute with the mixture of acetonitrile and water (1 : 1) to volume. Allow to stand for 90 minutes. Pass through a filter having a 0.2-μm porosity. Transfer an accurately measured volume of the filtrate, quantitatively dilute with water to obtain a solution having a concentration of about 0.06 mg per mL, and mix. [NOTE—Retain a portion of the filtrate for use in the test for *Identification*.]. Transfer 5.0 mL of the resulting solution to a 100-mL volumetric flask, add 2.0 mL of sodium chloride solution (1 in 5) and 1.0 mL of hydrochloride acid, dilute with water to volume, and mix.

Procedure—Proceed as directed in the *Assay* under *Potassium Chloride Oral Solution*. Calculate the quantity, in mg, of potassium chloride (KCl) in each Tablet taken by the formula:

$$1.907(TC/D)$$

in which *T* is the labeled quantity, in mg, of potassium chloride in each Tablet; *D* is the concentration, in μg per mL, of potassium chloride in the designated *Assay preparation*, based on the labeled quantity per Tablet and the extent of dilution; and the other terms are as defined therein.

Potassium Chloride in Dextrose Injection

» Potassium Chloride in Dextrose Injection is a sterile solution of Potassium Chloride and Dextrose in Water for Injection. It contains not less than 95.0 percent and not more than 110.0 percent of the labeled amount of Potassium Chloride (KCl) and not less than 95.0 percent and not more than 105.0 percent of the labeled amount of dextrose ($C_6H_{12}O_6 \cdot H_2O$). It contains no antimicrobial agents.

Packaging and storage—Preserve in single-dose glass or plastic containers. Glass containers are preferably of Type I or Type II glass.

Labeling—The label states the total osmolar concentration in mOsmol per L. Where the contents are less than 100 mL, or where the label states that the Injection is not for direct injection but is to be diluted before use, the label alternatively may state the total osmolar concentration in mOsmol per mL. The content of potassium, in milliequivalents, is prominently displayed on the label.

USP Reference standards ⟨11⟩—*USP Endotoxin RS.*

Identification—It responds to the *Identification* test under *Dextrose*, to the flame test for *Potassium* ⟨191⟩, and to the tests for *Chloride* ⟨191⟩.

Bacterial endotoxins ⟨85⟩—It contains not more than 0.5 USP Endotoxin Unit per mL.

pH ⟨791⟩: between 3.5 and 6.5, determined on a portion diluted with water, if necessary, to a concentration of not more than 5% of dextrose.

Limit of 5-hydroxymethylfurfural and related substances—Dilute an accurately measured volume of Injection, equivalent to 1.0 g of $C_6H_{12}O_6 \cdot H_2O$, with water to 500.0 mL. Determine the absorbance of this solution in a 1-cm cell at 284 nm, with a suitable spectrophotometer, using water as the blank: the absorbance is not more than 0.25.

Other requirements—It meets the requirements of the test for *Heavy metals* under *Dextrose Injection*, and meets the requirements under *Injections* ⟨1⟩.

Assay for dextrose—Transfer an accurately measured volume of Injection, containing between 2 and 5 g of dextrose, to a 100-mL volumetric flask. Add 0.2 mL of 6 N ammonium hydroxide, dilute with water to volume, and mix. Determine the angular rotation in a suitable polarimeter tube (see *Optical Rotation* ⟨781⟩). Calculate the percentage (g per 100 mL) of dextrose ($C_6H_{12}O_6 \cdot H_2O$) in the portion of Injection taken by the formula:

$$(100/52.9)(198.17/180.16)AR$$

in which 100 is the percentage; 52.9 is the midpoint of the specific rotation range for anhydrous dextrose, in degrees; 198.17 and 180.16 are the molecular weights for dextrose monohydrate and anhydrous dextrose, respectively; A is 100 mm divided by the length of the polarimeter tube, in mm; and R is the observed rotation, in degrees.

Assay for potassium chloride—Transfer an accurately measured volume of Injection, equivalent to between 75 and 150 mg of potassium chloride, to a conical flask, add water, if necessary, to bring the volume to about 10 mL, and add 10 mL of glacial acetic acid, 75 mL of methanol, and 3 drops of eosin Y TS. Titrate, with shaking, with 0.1 N silver nitrate VS to a pink endpoint. Each mL of 0.1 N silver nitrate is equivalent to 7.455 mg of KCl.

Potassium Chloride in Dextrose and Sodium Chloride Injection

» Potassium Chloride in Dextrose and Sodium Chloride Injection is a sterile solution of Potassium Chloride, Dextrose, and Sodium Chloride in Water for Injection. It contains not less than 95.0 percent and not more than 110.0 percent of the labeled amounts of potassium (K) and chloride (Cl) and not less than 95.0 percent and not more than 105.0 percent of the labeled amounts of dextrose ($C_6H_{12}O_6 \cdot H_2O$) and sodium (Na). It contains no antimicrobial agents.

Packaging and storage—Preserve in single-dose containers, preferably of Type I or Type II glass, or of a suitable plastic.

Labeling—The label states the potassium, sodium, and chloride contents in terms of milliequivalents in a given volume. The label states also the total osmolar concentration in mOsmol per L. Where the contents are less than 100 mL, the label alternatively may state the total osmolar concentration in mOsmol per mL.

USP Reference standards ⟨11⟩—*USP Endotoxin RS.*

Identification—

A: It responds to the flame test for *Sodium* ⟨191⟩.

B: To 2 mL of Injection add 5 mL of sodium cobaltinitrite TS: a yellow precipitate is formed immediately. If necessary, centrifuge the solution and examine the precipitate (*presence of potassium*).

C: It responds to the tests for *Chloride* ⟨191⟩.

D: It responds to the *Identification* test under *Dextrose*.

Bacterial endotoxins ⟨85⟩—It contains not more than 0.5 USP Endotoxin Unit per mL.

pH ⟨791⟩: between 3.5 and 6.5.

Heavy metals ⟨231⟩—Transfer to a suitable vessel a volume, in mL, of Injection, calculated to two significant figures by the formula:

$$0.2/[(G_K L_K) + (G_D L_D) + (G_S L_S)]$$

in which G_K, G_D, and G_S are the labeled amounts, in g, of potassium chloride, dextrose, and sodium chloride, respectively, in each 100 mL of Injection, and L_K, L_D, and L_S are the limits, in percentage, for *Heavy metals* specified under *Potassium Chloride*, *Dextrose*, and *Sodium Chloride*, respectively. Adjust the volume by evaporation or addition of water to 25 mL, as necessary: it passes the test.

5-hydroxymethylfurfural and related substances—Dilute an accurately measured volume of Injection, equivalent to 1.0 g of $C_6H_{12}O_6 \cdot H_2O$, with water to 500.0 mL. Determine the absorbance of this solution in a 1-cm cell at 284 nm, with a suitable spectrophotometer, using water as the blank: the absorbance is not more than 0.25.

Other requirements—It meets the requirements under *Injections* ⟨1⟩.

Assay for potassium and sodium—

Internal standard solution, Potassium stock solution, Sodium stock solution, Stock standard preparation, and *Standard preparation*—Prepare as directed in the *Assay for potassium and sodium* under *Potassium Chloride in Sodium Chloride Injection*.

Assay preparation—Transfer 5.0 mL of Potassium Chloride in Dextrose and Sodium Chloride Injection to a 500-mL volumetric flask, dilute with *Internal standard solution* to volume, and mix.

Procedure—Proceed as directed for *Procedure* in the *Assay for potassium and sodium* under *Potassium Chloride in Sodium Chloride Injection*.

Assay for chloride—Transfer an accurately measured volume of Injection, equivalent to about 55 mg of chloride, to a conical flask, and add 10 mL of glacial acetic acid, 75 mL of methanol, and 3 drops of eosin Y TS. Titrate, with shaking, with 0.1 N silver nitrate VS to a pink endpoint. Each mL of 0.1 N silver nitrate is equivalent to 3.545 mg of Cl. Each mg of chloride is equivalent to 0.0282 mEq of Cl.

Assay for dextrose—Transfer an accurately measured volume of Injection, containing between 2 g and 5 g of dextrose, to a 100-mL volumetric flask. Add 0.2 mL of 6 N ammonium hydroxide, dilute with water to volume, and mix. Determine the angular rotation in a suitable polarimeter tube (see *Optical Rotation* ⟨781⟩). Calculate the percentage (g per 100 mL) of dextrose ($C_6H_{12}O_6 \cdot H_2O$) in the portion of Injection taken by the formula:

$$(100/52.9)(198.17/180.16)AR$$

in which 100 is the percentage; 52.9 is the midpoint of the specific rotation range for anhydrous dextrose, in degrees; 198.17 and 180.16 are the molecular weights for dextrose monohydrate and anhydrous dextrose, respectively; A is 100 mm divided by the length of the polarimeter tube, in mm; and R is the observed rotation, in degrees.

Potassium Chloride, Potassium Bicarbonate, and Potassium Citrate Effervescent Tablets for Oral Solution

» Potassium Chloride, Potassium Bicarbonate, and Potassium Citrate Effervescent Tablets for Oral Solution contain not less than 90.0 percent and not more than 110.0 percent of the labeled amounts of K and Cl.

Packaging and storage—Preserve in tight containers, protected from excessive heat.
Labeling—The label states the potassium and chloride contents in terms of weight and in terms of milliequivalents. Where Tablets are packaged in individual pouches, the label instructs the user not to open until the time of use.
Identification—One Tablet dissolves in 100 mL of water with effervescence. The collected gas responds to the test for *Bicarbonate* ⟨191⟩, and the resulting solution responds to the tests for *Potassium* ⟨191⟩, for *Chloride* ⟨191⟩, and for *Citrate* ⟨191⟩.
Uniformity of dosage units ⟨905⟩: meet the requirements for *Weight Variation*.
Assay for potassium—
Potassium stock solution and *Standard preparations*—Prepare as directed in the *Assay* under *Potassium Chloride Oral Solution*.
Assay preparation—Transfer 10 Potassium Chloride, Potassium Bicarbonate, and Potassium Citrate Effervescent Tablets for Oral Solution to a 2000-mL volumetric flask, dissolve in 200 mL of water, swirl until effervescence ceases, dilute with water to volume, and mix. Filter, and quantitatively dilute an accurately measured volume of the filtrate with water to obtain a solution containing 30 µg of potassium per mL. Transfer 5.0 mL of the resulting solution to a 100-mL volumetric flask, add 2.0 mL of sodium chloride solution (1 in 5) and 1.0 mL of hydrochloric acid, dilute with water to volume, and mix.
Procedure—Proceed as directed for *Procedure* in the *Assay* under *Potassium Chloride Oral Solution*. Calculate the quantity, in mg, of potassium (K) in each Tablet taken by the formula:

$$L(C/D)$$

in which L is the labeled quantity, in mg, of potassium in each Tablet, C is the concentration, in µg per mL, of potassium in the *Assay preparation*, and D is the concentration, in µg per mL, of potassium in the *Assay preparation* on the basis of the labeled quantity in each Tablet and the extent of dilution.
Assay for chloride—Transfer a number of Potassium Chloride, Potassium Bicarbonate, and Potassium Citrate Effervescent Tablets for Oral Solution, equivalent to about 900 mg of chloride, to a 2000-mL volumetric flask. Add about 200 mL of water, swirl until effervescence ceases, dilute with water to volume, and mix. Transfer 25.0 mL of this solution to a 250-mL conical flask, add 50.0 mL of 0.1 N silver nitrate VS and 15 mL of nitric acid, and boil, with constant swirling, until the supernatant is colorless. Cool to room temperature, add sufficient water to make a volume of about 150 mL, add 5 mL of ferric ammonium sulfate TS, and titrate the excess silver nitrate with 0.1 N ammonium thiocyanate VS to a permanent faint brown endpoint. Each mL of 0.1 N silver nitrate is equivalent to 3.545 mg of Cl. Calculate the quantity, in mg, of chloride (Cl) in each Tablet by dividing the total amount of chloride in the Tablets taken by the number of Tablets taken.

Potassium Chloride in Lactated Ringer's and Dextrose Injection

» Potassium Chloride in Lactated Ringer's and Dextrose Injection is a sterile solution of Calcium Chloride, Potassium Chloride, Sodium Chloride, and Sodium Lactate in Water for Injection. It contains, in each 100 mL, not less than 285.0 mg and not more than 315.0 mg of sodium (as NaCl and $C_3H_5NaO_3$), not less than 4.90 mg and not more than 6.00 mg of calcium (Ca, equivalent to not less than 18.0 mg and not more than 22.0 mg of $CaCl_2 \cdot 2H_2O$), and not less than 231.0 mg and not more than 261.0 mg of lactate ($C_3H_5O_3$, equivalent to not less than 290.0 mg and not more than 330.0 mg of $C_3H_5NaO_3$). It contains not less than 95.0 percent and not more than 105.0 percent of the labeled amount of Potassium Chloride (KCl), not less than 90.0 percent and not more than 105.0 percent of the labeled amount of dextrose ($C_6H_{12}O_6 \cdot H_2O$), and not less than 90.0 percent and not more than 110.0 percent of the labeled amount of chloride (Cl, as NaCl, KCl, and $CaCl_2 \cdot 2H_2O$). It contains no antimicrobial agents.

Packaging and storage—Preserve in single-dose glass or plastic containers. Glass containers are preferably of Type I or Type II glass.
Labeling—The label states the total osmolar concentration in mOsmol per L. Where the contents are less than 100 mL, the label alternatively may state the total osmolar concentration in mOsmol per mL. The label includes also the warning: "Not for use in the treatment of lactic acidosis."
USP Reference standards ⟨11⟩—*USP Sodium Lactate RS. USP Endotoxin RS.*
Identification—
A: It responds to the *Identification* test under *Dextrose Injection*.
B: It responds to the flame tests for *Sodium* ⟨191⟩ and for *Potassium* ⟨191⟩, to the test for *Chloride* ⟨191⟩, and to the ammonium oxalate test for *Calcium* ⟨191⟩.
C: The retention time of the lactate peak in the chromatogram of the *Assay preparation* corresponds to that of the *Standard preparation* as obtained in the *Assay for lactate*.
Bacterial endotoxins ⟨85⟩—It contains not more than 0.5 USP Endotoxin Unit per mL.
pH ⟨791⟩: between 3.5 and 6.5.
Heavy metals ⟨231⟩—Transfer to a suitable vessel a volume, in mL, of Injection, calculated to two significant figures by the formula:

$$0.2 / [(G_S L_S) + (G_K L_K) + (G_C L_C) + (G_L L_L) + (G_D L_D)]$$

in which G_S, G_K, G_C, G_L, and G_D are the labeled amounts, in g, of sodium chloride, potassium chloride, calcium chloride, sodium lactate, and dextrose, respectively, in each 100 mL of Injection, and L_S, L_K, L_C, L_L, and L_D are the limits, in percentage, for *Heavy metals* specified under *Sodium Chloride*, *Potassium Chloride*, *Calcium Chloride*, *Sodium Lactate*, and *Dextrose*, respectively. Adjust the volume by evaporation or addition of water to 25 mL, as necessary: it meets the requirements of the test.
Limit of 5-hydroxymethylfurfural and related substances—Dilute an accurately measured volume of Injection, equivalent to 1.0 g of $C_6H_{12}O_6 \cdot H_2O$, with water to 500.0 mL. Determine the absorbance of this solution in a 1-cm cell at 284 nm, with a suitable spectrophotometer, using water as the blank: the absorbance is not more than 0.25.
Other requirements—It meets the requirements under *Injections* ⟨1⟩.
Assay for calcium—[NOTE—Concentrations of the *Standard preparations* and the *Assay preparation* may be modified to fit the linear or working range of the atomic absorption spectrophotometer.]
Lanthanum chloride solution and *Blank solution*—Prepare as directed in the *Assay for calcium* under *Ringer's Injection*.
Calcium stock solution and *Standard preparations*—Prepare as directed in the *Assay for calcium* under *Ringer's Injection*.
Assay preparation—Transfer 30.0 mL of Injection (equivalent to about 1.6 mg of calcium), to a 100-mL volumetric flask containing 5.0 mL of *Lanthanum chloride solution*. Dilute the contents of the flask with water to volume, and mix.

Procedure—Proceed as directed in the *Assay for calcium* under *Ringer's Injection*. Calculate the quantity, in mg, of calcium in each 100 mL of the Injection taken by the formula:

$$C/3$$

in which C is the concentration, in µg per mL, of calcium in the *Assay preparation*, as determined from the graph.

Assay for potassium—Proceed with Injection as directed in the *Assay for potassium* under *Ringer's Injection*.

Assay for sodium—Proceed with Injection as directed in the *Assay for sodium* under *Ringer's Injection*.

Assay for chloride—Proceed with Injection as directed in the *Assay for chloride* under *Ringer's Injection*.

Assay for lactate—

Mobile phase, Resolution solution, Standard preparation, Chromatographic system, and *Procedure*—Proceed as directed in the *Assay for lactate* under *Lactated Ringer's Injection*.

Assay preparation—Use undiluted Injection.

Procedure—Proceed as directed in the *Assay for lactate* under *Lactated Ringer's Injection*. Calculate the concentration, in mg per mL, of lactate ($C_3H_5O_3$) in the *Assay preparation* taken by the formula:

$$C(89.07/112.06)(r_U/r_S)$$

in which the terms are as defined therein.

Assay for dextrose—Proceed with Injection as directed in the *Assay for dextrose* under *Ringer's and Dextrose Injection*.

Potassium Chloride in Sodium Chloride Injection

» Potassium Chloride in Sodium Chloride Injection is a sterile solution of Potassium Chloride and Sodium Chloride in Water for Injection. It contains not less than 95.0 percent and not more than 110.0 percent of the labeled amounts of potassium (K) and chloride (Cl) and not less than 95.0 percent and not more than 105.0 percent of the labeled amount of sodium (Na). It contains no antimicrobial agents.

Packaging and storage—Preserve in single-dose containers, preferably of Type I or Type II glass, or of a suitable plastic.

Labeling—The label states the potassium, sodium, and chloride contents in terms of milliequivalents in a given volume. The label states also the total osmolar concentration in mOsmol per L. Where the contents are less than 100 mL, the label alternatively may state the total osmolar concentration in mOsmol per mL.

USP Reference standards ⟨11⟩—*USP Endotoxin RS.*

Identification—

A: It responds to the flame test for *Sodium* ⟨191⟩.

B: To 2 mL of Injection add 5 mL of sodium cobaltinitrite TS: a yellow precipitate is formed immediately. If necessary, centrifuge the solution and examine the precipitate (*presence of potassium*).

C: It responds to the tests for *Chloride* ⟨191⟩.

Bacterial endotoxins ⟨85⟩—It contains not more than 0.5 USP Endotoxin Unit per mL.

pH ⟨791⟩: between 3.5 and 6.5.

Heavy metals ⟨231⟩—Transfer to a suitable vessel a volume, in mL, of Injection, calculated to two significant figures by the formula:

$$0.2/[(G_K L_K) + (G_S L_S)]$$

in which G_K and G_S are the labeled amounts, in g, of potassium chloride and sodium chloride, respectively, in each 100 mL of Injection, and L_K and L_S are the limits, in percentage, for *Heavy metals* specified under *Potassium Chloride* and *Sodium Chloride*, respectively. Adjust the volume by evaporation or addition of water to 25 mL, as necessary: it passes the test.

Other requirements—It meets the requirements under *Injections* ⟨1⟩.

Assay for potassium and sodium—

Internal standard solution—Transfer 1.04 g of lithium nitrate to a 1000-mL volumetric flask, add a suitable nonionic surfactant, then add water to volume, and mix.

Potassium stock solution—Transfer 18.64 g of potassium chloride, previously dried at 105° for 2 hours and accurately weighed, to a 250-mL volumetric flask, add water to volume, and mix. Each mL of this stock solution contains 39.10 mg (1 mEq) of potassium.

Sodium stock solution—Transfer 14.61 g of sodium chloride, previously dried at 105° for 2 hours and accurately weighed, to a 250-mL volumetric flask, add water to volume, and mix.

Stock standard preparation—Transfer 0.1J mL of *Potassium stock solution* and 0.1J' mL of *Sodium stock solution* to a 100-mL volumetric flask, J and J' being the labeled amounts, in mEq per liter, of potassium and sodium, respectively, in the Injection. Dilute with water to volume, and mix. Each mL of this solution contains 0.0391J mg of potassium (K) and 0.02299J' mg of sodium (Na).

Standard preparation—Transfer 5.0 mL of *Stock standard preparation* to a 500-mL volumetric flask, dilute with *Internal standard solution* to volume, and mix.

Assay preparation—Transfer 5.0 mL of Injection to a 500-mL volumetric flask, dilute with *Internal standard solution* to volume, and mix.

Procedure—Using a suitable flame photometer, adjusted to read zero with *Internal standard solution*, concomitantly determine the flame emission readings for the *Standard preparation* and the *Assay preparation* at the wavelengths of maximum emission for potassium, sodium, and lithium (766 nm, 589 nm, and 671 nm, respectively). Calculate the quantity, in mg, of K in each mL of the Injection taken by the formula:

$$C(R_{U,766}/R_{U,671})(R_{S,671}/R_{S,766})$$

in which C is the concentration, in mg per mL, of potassium in the *Stock standard preparation*, $R_{U,766}$ and $R_{U,671}$ are the emission readings at the wavelengths identified by the subscript numbers obtained from the *Assay preparation*, and $R_{S,671}$ and $R_{S,766}$ are the emission readings at the wavelengths identified by the subscript numbers obtained from the *Standard preparation*. Each mg of potassium is equivalent to 0.02558 mEq of potassium. Calculate the quantity, in mg, of Na in each mL of the Injection taken by the formula:

$$C(R_{U,589}/R_{U,671})(R_{S,671}/R_{S,589})$$

in which C is the concentration, in mg per mL, of sodium in the *Stock standard preparation*, $R_{U,589}$ and $R_{U,671}$ are the emission readings at the wavelengths identified by the subscript numbers obtained for the *Assay preparation*, and $R_{S,671}$ and $R_{S,589}$ are the emission readings at the wavelengths identified by the subscript numbers obtained from the *Standard preparation*. Each mg of sodium is equivalent to 0.04350 mEq of sodium.

Assay for chloride—Transfer an accurately measured volume of Injection, equivalent to about 55 mg of chloride, to a conical flask, and add 10 mL of glacial acetic acid, 75 mL of methanol, and 3 drops of eosin Y TS. Titrate, with shaking, with 0.1 N silver nitrate VS to a pink endpoint. Each mL of 0.1 N silver nitrate is equivalent to 3.545 mg of Cl. Each mg of chloride is equivalent to 0.0282 mEq of Cl.

Potassium Citrate

$C_6H_5K_3O_7 \cdot H_2O$ 324.41
1,2,3-Propanetricarboxylic acid, 2-hydroxy-, tripotassium salt, monohydrate.
Tripotassium citrate monohydrate   [6100-05-6].
Anhydrous   306.40   [866-84-2].

» Potassium Citrate contains not less than 99.0 percent and not more than 100.5 percent of $C_6H_5K_3O_7$, calculated on the dried basis.

Packaging and storage—Preserve in tight containers.
Identification—A solution (1 in 10) responds to the tests for *Potassium* ⟨191⟩ and for *Citrate* ⟨191⟩.
Alkalinity—A solution of 1.0 g in 20 mL of water is alkaline to litmus, but after the addition of 0.20 mL of 0.10 N sulfuric acid, no pink color is produced by the addition of 1 drop of phenolphthalein TS.
Loss on drying ⟨731⟩—Dry it at 180° for 4 hours: it loses between 3.0% and 6.0% of its weight.
Tartrate—To a solution of 1 g in 1.5 mL of water in a test tube add 1 mL of 6 N acetic acid, and scratch the walls of the test tube with a glass rod: no crystalline precipitate is formed.
Heavy metals, *Method I* ⟨231⟩—Dissolve 2 g in 25 mL of water, and proceed as directed for *Test Preparation*, except to use glacial acetic acid to adjust the pH: the limit is 0.001%.
Organic volatile impurities, *Method I* ⟨467⟩: meets the requirements.

(Official until July 1, 2008)

Assay—Dissolve about 200 mg of Potassium Citrate, accurately weighed, in 25 mL of glacial acetic acid. Add 2 drops of crystal violet TS, and titrate with 0.1 N perchloric acid VS to a green endpoint. Perform a blank determination, and make any necessary correction. Each mL of 0.1 N perchloric acid is equivalent to 10.21 mg of $C_6H_5K_3O_7$.

Potassium Citrate Extended-Release Tablets

» Potassium Citrate Extended-Release Tablets contain not less than 90.0 percent and not more than 110.0 percent of the labeled amount of potassium citrate ($C_6H_5K_3O_7$).

Packaging and storage—Preserve in tight containers.
USP Reference standards ⟨11⟩—*USP Citric Acid RS*.

(Official January 1, 2009)

Identification—
   A: Powder 5 Tablets, mix with 20 mL of water, and filter: the filtrate responds to the tests for *Potassium* ⟨191⟩.
   B: A portion of powdered Tablets containing about 50 mg of potassium citrate responds to the test for *Citrate* ⟨191⟩, 20 mL of the mixture of pyridine and acetic anhydride being used.
Dissolution ⟨711⟩—
   Medium: water; 900 mL.
   Apparatus 2: 50 rpm.
   Times: 30 minutes, 1 hour, and 3 hours.
   Potassium stock solution and *Standard preparation*—Prepare as directed in the *Assay* under *Potassium Chloride Oral Solution*.
   Procedure—Filter the solution under test, and dilute quantitatively with *Medium* to obtain a test solution containing about 60 µg of potassium citrate per mL. Transfer 5.0 mL of the test solution to a 100-mL volumetric flask, add 2.0 mL of sodium chloride solution (1 in 5) and 1.0 mL of hydrochloric acid, dilute with water to volume, mix, and proceed as directed for *Procedure* in the *Assay* under *Potassium Chloride Oral Solution*. Calculate the quantity, in mg, of $C_6H_5K_3O_7$ dissolved by the formula:

$$900F(2.612C)$$

in which F is the extent of dilution of the solution under test; 2.612 is the ratio of the molecular weight of anhydrous potassium citrate to three times the atomic weight of potassium; and C is the concentration, in µg per mL, of potassium in the test solution.
   Tolerances—The percentages of the labeled amount of $C_6H_5K_3O_7$ dissolved from the Tablets are not more than 45% (Q) in 30 minutes, not more than 60% (Q') in 1 hour, and not less than 80% (Q'') in 3 hours. The requirements are met if the quantities dissolved from the Tablets tested conform to the accompanying table instead of the table shown under *Dissolution* ⟨711⟩.

Acceptance Table

Stage	Number Tested	Acceptance Criteria
S_1	6	Each unit is within the range between $Q \pm 10\%$ and $Q' \pm 10\%$, and is not less than $Q'' + 5\%$ at the stated *Times*.
S_2	6	Average of 12 units ($S_1 + S_2$) is within the range between $Q \pm 10\%$ and $Q' \pm 10\%$ and is not less than Q''; no unit is outside the range between $Q \pm 15\%$ and $Q' \pm 15\%$, and no unit is less than $Q'' - 5\%$ at the stated *Times*.
S_3	12	Average of 24 units ($S_1 + S_2 + S_3$) is within the range between $Q \pm 10\%$ and $Q' \pm 10\%$ and is not less than Q''; not more than 1 unit is outside the range between $Q \pm 15\%$, not more than 1 unit is outside the range between $Q' \pm 15\%$, and not more than 1 unit is less than $Q'' - 5\%$ at the stated *Times*.

Uniformity of dosage units ⟨905⟩: meet the requirements.
Potassium content—
   Potassium stock solution and *Standard preparations*—Prepare as directed in the *Assay* under *Potassium Chloride Oral Solution*.
   Assay preparation—Transfer 3.0 mL of the clear filtrate, reserved from the *Assay*, to a 100-mL volumetric flask, add 2.0 mL of sodium chloride solution (1 in 5) and 1.0 mL of hydrochloric acid, dilute with water to volume, and mix.
   Procedure—Proceed as directed for *Procedure* in the *Assay* under *Potassium Chloride Oral Solution*. Calculate the quantity, in mg, of potassium (K) in the portion of Tablets taken by the formula:

$$(100C/3)$$

in which C is as defined therein: the quantity, in mg, of potassium found in the portion of Tablets taken is not less than 36.4% and not more than 40.2% of the quantity, in mg, of potassium citrate in the portion of Tablets taken, as determined in the *Assay*.
Assay—
   Standard preparation—Dissolve a suitable quantity of citric acid, previously dried at 90° for 3 hours and accurately weighed, in water to obtain a solution having a known concentration of about 1.0 mg of anhydrous citric acid per mL.
   Assay preparation—Weigh and finely powder not fewer than 20 Tablets. Transfer an accurately weighed portion of the powder, equivalent to about 200 mg of potassium citrate, to a 1000-mL volumetric flask, add about 300 mL of hot water, and shake by mechanical means for 15 minutes. Allow to cool, dilute with water to volume, and mix. Filter, discarding the first 30 mL of the filtrate.

Transfer 20.0 mL of the clear filtrate to a 25-mL volumetric flask, dilute with water to volume, and mix. [NOTE—Reserve the remaining filtrate for the test for *Potassium content.*]

Standard curve—Pipet aliquots of 8, 9, 10, 11, and 12 mL, respectively, of the *Standard preparation* into separate 100-mL volumetric flasks, dilute with water to volume, and mix. These solutions contain about 0.08, 0.09, 0.10, 0.11, and 0.12 mg of anhydrous citric acid per mL, respectively. Continue as directed for *Procedure.* Plot the resultant absorbances versus the respective concentrations, in mg per mL, of the standard solutions.

Procedure—Pipet 1 mL of the *Assay preparation* into a suitable test tube. To a second test tube add 1.0 mL of water to serve as a reference blank. To each tube add 1.3 mL of pyridine, and mix by swirling. To one tube at a time add 5.7 mL of acetic anhydride, and mix, using a rotary vortex stirrer. Immediately place in a water bath maintained at 31 ± 1.0°, and allow the color to develop for 33 ± 1 minutes. Determine the absorbance against the reference blank in 2.5-cm cells at 425 nm, taking care to measure the absorbance of each solution at the same elapsed time from mixing. Calculate the quantity, in mg, of potassium citrate ($C_6H_5K_3O_7$) in the portion of Tablets taken by the formula:

$$(306.40/192.13)(1250C)$$

in which 306.40 and 192.13 are the molecular weights of anhydrous potassium citrate and anhydrous citric acid, respectively; and C is the concentration, in mg per mL, of anhydrous citric acid read from the *Standard curve.*

(Official until January 1, 2009)

Assay—
Mobile phase, Standard Preparation 1, and *Chromatographic System*—Proceed as directed under *Assay for Citric Acid/Citrate and Phosphate* ⟨345⟩.

Assay preparation—Weigh and finely powder not fewer than 20 Tablets. Transfer an accurately weighed portion of the powder, equivalent to about 200 mg of potassium citrate, to a 1000-mL volumetric flask, add about 300 mL of hot water, and shake by mechanical means for 15 minutes. Allow to cool, dilute with water to volume, and mix. Filter, discarding the first 30 mL of the filtrate. Transfer an aliquot of the clear filtrate into a suitable volumetric flask, and dilute with water and freshly prepared sodium hydroxide solution to obtain a solution containing about 20 μg per mL of citrate in 1 mM sodium hydroxide. [NOTE—Reserve the remaining filtrate for the test for *Potassium content.*]

Procedure—Proceed as directed for *Procedure* under ⟨345⟩, and calculate the quantity, in mg, of potassium citrate ($C_6H_5K_3O_7$) in the portion of Tablets taken by the formula:

$$0.001(306.39/189.10)C_S D(r_U / r_S)$$

in which 306.39 is the molecular weight of potassium citrate; 189.10 is the molecular weight of citrate ($C_6H_5O_7$); C_S is the concentration, in μg per mL, of citrate in *Standard Preparation 1; D* is the dilution factor; and r_U and r_S are the citrate peak areas obtained from the *Assay preparation* and *Standard Preparation 1,* respectively.

(Official January 1, 2009)

Potassium Citrate and Citric Acid Oral Solution

» Potassium Citrate and Citric Acid Oral Solution is a solution of Potassium Citrate and Citric Acid in a suitable aqueous medium. It contains, in each 100 mL, not less than 7.55 g and not more than 8.35 g of potassium (K), and not less than 12.18 g and not more than 13.46 g of citrate ($C_6H_5O_7$), equivalent to not less than 20.9 g and not more than 23.1 g of potassium citrate monohydrate ($C_6H_5K_3O_7 \cdot H_2O$); and not less than 6.34 g and not more than 7.02 g of citric acid monohydrate ($C_6H_8O_7 \cdot H_2O$).

NOTE—The potassium ion content of Potassium Citrate and Citric Acid Oral Solution is approximately 2 mEq per mL.

Packaging and storage—Preserve in tight containers.
USP Reference standards ⟨11⟩—*USP Citric Acid RS.*
(Official January 1, 2009)
Identification—
A: To 2 mL of a dilution of Oral Solution (1 in 40) add 5 mL of sodium cobaltinitrite TS: a yellow precipitate is formed immediately (*presence of potassium*).
B: To a mixture of 1 mL of Oral Solution with 1 mL of hydrochloric acid add 10 mL of cobalt-uranyl acetate TS, and stir with a glass rod: no precipitate or turbidity forms after 15 minutes, and the solution remains clear (*absence of sodium*).
C: It responds to the test for *Citrate* ⟨191⟩, 3 to 5 drops of Oral Solution and 20 mL of the mixture of pyridine and acetic anhydride being used.
pH ⟨791⟩: between 4.9 and 5.4.
Assay for potassium—
Potassium stock solution, Sodium stock solution, Lithium diluent solution, and *Standard preparation*—Prepare as directed in the *Assay for sodium and potassium* under *Tricitrates Oral Solution.*

Assay preparation—Transfer an accurately measured volume of Oral Solution, equivalent to about 2 g of potassium citrate monohydrate, to a 200-mL volumetric flask, dilute with water to volume, and mix. Transfer 50 μL of this solution to a 10-mL volumetric flask, dilute with *Lithium diluent solution* to volume, and mix.

Procedure—Using a suitable flame photometer, adjusted to read zero with *Lithium diluent solution,* concomitantly determine the potassium flame emission readings for the *Standard preparation* and the *Assay preparation* at the wavelength of maximum emission at about 766 nm. Calculate the quantity, in g, of K in the portion of Oral Solution taken by the formula:

$$(18.64/12.5)(39.10/74.55)(R_{U,K} / R_{S,K})$$

in which 18.64 is the weight, in g, of potassium chloride in the *Potassium stock solution;* 39.10 is the atomic weight of potassium; 74.55 is the molecular weight of potassium chloride; and $R_{U,K}$ and $R_{S,K}$ are the potassium emission readings obtained for the *Assay preparation* and the *Standard preparation,* respectively.
Assay for citrate—
Cation-exchange column—Mix 10 g of styrene-divinylbenzene cation-exchange resin with 50 mL of water in a suitable beaker. Allow the resin to settle, and decant the supernatant until a slurry of resin remains. Pour the slurry into a 15-mm × 30-cm glass chromatographic tube (having a sealed-in, coarse-porosity fritted disk and fitted with a stopcock), and allow to settle as a homogeneous bed. Wash the resin bed with about 100 mL of water, closing the stopcock when the water level is about 2 mm above the resin bed.

Procedure—Pipet 15 mL of Oral Solution into a 250-mL volumetric flask, dilute with water to volume, and mix. Pipet 5 mL of this solution carefully onto the top of the resin bed in the *Cation-exchange column.* Place a 250-mL conical flask below the column, open the stopcock, and allow to flow until the solution has entered the resin bed. Elute the column with 60 mL of water at a flow rate of about 5 mL per minute, collecting about 65 mL of the eluate. Add 5 drops of phenolphthalein TS to the eluate, swirl the flask, and titrate with 0.02 N sodium hydroxide VS. Record the buret reading, and calculate the volume *(B)* of 0.02 N sodium hydroxide consumed. Each mL of the difference between the volume *(B)* and the volume *(A)* of 0.02 N sodium hydroxide consumed in the *Assay for citric acid* is equivalent to 1.261 mg of $C_6H_5O_7$.

(Official until January 1, 2009)
Assay for citrate—
Mobile Phase, Standard Preparation 1, and *Chromatographic System*—Proceed as directed under *Assay for Citric Acid/Citrate and Phosphate* ⟨345⟩.

Assay preparation—Pipet 15 mL of Oral Solution into a suitable volumetric flask, and proceed as directed for *Assay Preparation for Citric Acid/Citrate Assay* under *Assay for Citric Acid/Citrate and Phosphate* ⟨345⟩.

Procedure—Proceed as directed for *Procedure* under ⟨345⟩, and calculate the concentration, in mg per mL, of citrate ($C_6H_5O_7$) in the Oral Solution taken by the formula:

$$0.001 C_S (D/V)(r_U/r_S) - A(189.10/210.14)$$

in which C_S is the concentration, in µg per mL, of citrate in *Standard preparation 1*; D is the dilution factor; V is the volume of Oral Solution used in the preparation of the *Assay preparation*; r_U and r_S are the citrate peak areas obtained from the *Assay preparation* and *Standard Preparation 1*, respectively; 189.10 is the molecular weight of citrate ($C_6H_5O_7$); 210.14 is the molecular weight of citric acid monohydrate ($C_6H_8O_7 \cdot H_2O$); and A is the concentration of citric acid monohydrate, in mg per mL, determined in the *Assay for citric acid*.

(Official January 1, 2009)

Assay for citric acid—Transfer 15 mL of Oral Solution, accurately measured, to a 250-mL volumetric flask, dilute with water to volume, and mix. Pipet 5 mL of this solution into a suitable flask, add 25 mL of water and 5 drops of phenolphthalein TS, and titrate with 0.02 N sodium hydroxide VS to a pink endpoint. Record the buret reading, and calculate the volume (A) of 0.02 N sodium hydroxide consumed. Each mL of 0.02 N sodium hydroxide is equivalent to 1.401 mg of $C_6H_8O_7 \cdot H_2O$.

Potassium Gluconate

$C_6H_{11}KO_7$ (anhydrous)   234.25
D-Gluconic acid, monopotassium salt.
Monopotassium D-gluconate   [*299-27-4*].
Monohydrate   252.26   [*35398-15-3*].

» Potassium Gluconate is anhydrous or contains one molecule of water of hydration. It contains not less than 97.0 percent and not more than 103.0 percent of $C_6H_{11}KO_7$, calculated on the dried basis.

Packaging and storage—Preserve in tight containers.
Labeling—Label it to indicate whether it is anhydrous or the monohydrate.
USP Reference standards ⟨11⟩—*USP Potassium Gluconate RS.*
Identification—
  A: *Infrared Absorption* ⟨197M⟩.
  B: It responds to the flame test for *Potassium* ⟨191⟩.
  C: It responds to *Identification* test B under *Calcium Gluconate*.
Loss on drying ⟨731⟩—Dry it in vacuum at 105° for 4 hours: the anhydrous form loses not more than 3.0% of its weight, and the monohydrate loses between 6.0% and 7.5% of its weight.
Heavy metals, *Method I* ⟨231⟩—Dissolve 1 g in 10 mL of water, add 6 mL of 3 N hydrochloric acid, and dilute with water to 25 mL: the limit is 0.002%.
Reducing substances—Transfer 1.0 g to a 250-mL conical flask, dissolve in 10 mL of water, and add 25 mL of alkaline cupric citrate TS. Cover the flask, boil gently for 5 minutes, accurately timed, and cool rapidly to room temperature. Add 25 mL of 0.6 N acetic acid, 10.0 mL of 0.1 N iodine VS, and 10 mL of 3 N hydrochloric acid, and titrate with 0.1 N sodium thiosulfate VS, adding 3 mL of starch TS as the endpoint is approached. Perform a blank determination, omitting the specimen, and note the difference in volumes required. Each mL of the difference in volume of 0.1 N sodium thiosulfate consumed is equivalent to 2.7 mg of reducing substances (as dextrose): the limit is 1.0%.
Organic volatile impurities, *Method I* ⟨467⟩: meets the requirements.

(Official until July 1, 2008)

Assay—
Potassium stock solution—Dissolve 190.7 mg of potassium chloride, previously dried at 105° for 2 hours, in water. Transfer to a 1000-mL volumetric flask, dilute with water to volume, and mix. Transfer 100.0 mL of this solution to a 1000-mL volumetric flask, dilute with water to volume, and mix. This solution contains 10 µg of potassium (equivalent to 19.07 µg of potassium chloride) per mL.

Standard preparations—To separate 100-mL volumetric flasks transfer 10.0, 15.0, and 20.0 mL, respectively, of *Potassium stock solution*. To each flask add 2.0 mL of sodium chloride solution (1 in 5) and 1.0 mL of hydrochloric acid, dilute with water to volume, and mix. The *Standard preparations* contain, respectively, 1.0, 1.5, and 2.0 µg of potassium per mL.

Assay preparation—Transfer about 180 mg of Potassium Gluconate, accurately weighed, to a 1000-mL volumetric flask, add water to volume, and mix. Filter a portion of the solution. Transfer 5.0 mL of the filtrate to a 100-mL volumetric flask, add 2.0 mL of sodium chloride solution (1 in 5) and 1.0 mL of hydrochloric acid, dilute with water to volume, and mix.

Procedure—Concomitantly determine the absorbances of the *Standard preparations* and the *Assay preparation* at the potassium emission line of 766.5 nm, with a suitable atomic absorption spectrophotometer (see *Spectrophotometry and Light-scattering* ⟨851⟩) equipped with a potassium hollow-cathode lamp and an air–acetylene flame, using water as the blank. Plot the absorbance of the *Standard preparation* versus concentration, in µg per mL, of potassium, and draw the straight line best fitting the three plotted points. From the graph so obtained, determine the concentration, in µg per mL, of potassium in the *Assay preparation*. Calculate the weight, in mg, of $C_6H_{11}KO_7$ in the Potassium Gluconate taken by the formula:

$$20C(234.25/39.10)$$

in which C is the concentration, in µg per mL, of potassium in the *Assay preparation*, 234.25 is the molecular weight of potassium gluconate, and 39.10 is the atomic weight of potassium.

Potassium Gluconate Oral Solution

» Potassium Gluconate Oral Solution contains not less than 95.0 percent and not more than 105.0 percent of the labeled amount of potassium gluconate ($C_6H_{11}KO_7$).

Packaging and storage—Preserve in tight, light-resistant containers.
Identification—
  A: It meets the requirements of the flame test for *Potassium* ⟨191⟩.
  B: Evaporate 5 mL on a steam bath to dryness: a mineral oil dispersion of the residue exhibits an IR absorption maximum in the spectral region between 6.2 and 6.25 µm (*carboxylic acid salt*).
Alcohol content, *Method II* ⟨611⟩: between 4.5% and 5.5% of C_2H_5OH.
Assay—
Potassium stock solution and *Standard preparations*—Prepare as directed in the *Assay* under *Potassium Gluconate*.

Assay preparation—Transfer an accurately measured volume of Oral Solution, equivalent to about 1.8 g of potassium gluconate, to a 1000-mL volumetric flask, dilute with water to volume, and mix. Transfer 10.0 mL of the solution to a 100-mL volumetric flask, dilute with water to volume, and mix. Transfer 5.0 mL of the resulting solution to a 100-mL volumetric flask, add 2.0 mL of sodium chloride solution (1 in 5) and 1.0 mL of hydrochloric acid, dilute with water to volume, and mix.

Procedure—Proceed as directed for *Procedure* in the *Assay* under *Potassium Gluconate*. Calculate the quantity, in mg, of potassium gluconate (C₆H₁₁KO₇) in each mL of the Oral Solution taken by the formula:

$$(200C / V)(234.25 / 39.10)$$

in which V is the volume of Oral Solution taken; 234.25 is the molecular weight of potassium gluconate; and 39.10 is the atomic weight of potassium.

Potassium Gluconate Tablets

» Potassium Gluconate Tablets contain not less than 95.0 percent and not more than 105.0 percent of the labeled amount of C₆H₁₁KO₇.

Packaging and storage—Preserve in tight containers.
USP Reference standards ⟨11⟩—*USP Potassium Gluconate RS.*
Identification—
  A: The IR absorption spectrum of a mineral oil dispersion prepared from finely powdered Tablets exhibits maxima only at the same wavelengths as that of a similar preparation of USP Potassium Gluconate RS.
  B: Triturate a portion of powdered Tablets with a few mL of water, and filter: the filtrate responds to the flame test for *Potassium* ⟨191⟩.
Dissolution ⟨711⟩—
  Medium: water; 900 mL.
  Apparatus 2: 100 rpm.
  Time: 45 minutes.
  Procedure—Determine the amount of C₆H₁₁KO₇ dissolved, employing the procedure set forth in the *Assay*, making any necessary modifications.
  Tolerances—Not less than 75% (*Q*) of the labeled amount of C₆H₁₁KO₇ is dissolved in 45 minutes.
Uniformity of dosage units ⟨905⟩: meet the requirements.
Assay—
  Potassium stock solution and *Standard preparations*—Prepare as directed in the *Assay* under *Potassium Gluconate*.
  Assay preparation—Weigh and finely powder not less than 20 Tablets. Transfer an accurately weighed portion of the powder, equivalent to about 1.8 g of potassium gluconate, to a 1000-mL volumetric flask, add water to volume, and mix to dissolve. Filter a portion of the solution, transfer 10.0 mL of the filtrate to a 100-mL volumetric flask, dilute with water to volume, and mix. Transfer 5.0 mL of the resulting solution to a 100-mL volumetric flask, add 2.0 mL of sodium chloride solution (1 in 5) and 1.0 mL of hydrochloric acid, dilute with water to volume, and mix.
  Procedure—Proceed as directed for *Procedure* in the *Assay* under *Potassium Gluconate*. Calculate the quantity, in mg, of C₆H₁₁KO₇ in the portion of Tablets taken by the formula:

$$200C(234.25 / 39.10)$$

in which 234.25 is the molecular weight of potassium gluconate and 39.10 is the atomic weight of potassium.

Potassium Gluconate and Potassium Chloride Oral Solution

» Potassium Gluconate and Potassium Chloride Oral Solution is a solution of Potassium Gluconate and Potassium Chloride in a suitable aqueous medium. It contains not less than 90.0 percent and not more than 110.0 percent of the labeled amounts of potassium (K) and chloride (Cl).

Packaging and storage—Preserve in tight containers.
Labeling—Label it to state the potassium and chloride contents in terms of milliequivalents of each in a given volume of Oral Solution.
Identification—
  A: To 2 mL of a dilution of Oral Solution (1 in 40) add 5 mL of sodium cobaltinitrite TS: a yellow precipitate is formed immediately (*presence of potassium*).
  B: Evaporate 5 mL on a steam bath to dryness: a mineral oil dispersion of the residue so obtained exhibits an IR absorption maximum in the spectral region between 6.2 and 6.25 μm (*carboxylic acid salt*).
  C: It responds to the tests for *Chloride* ⟨191⟩.
Assay for potassium—
  Potassium stock solution—Dissolve in water 0.9535 g of potassium chloride, previously dried at 105° for 2 hours. Transfer to a 500-mL volumetric flask, dilute with water to volume, and mix. This solution contains 1000 μg of potassium per mL.
  Standard preparations—To separate 200-mL volumetric flasks transfer 19.0 mL and 25.0 mL, respectively, of *Potassium stock solution*, dilute with water to volume, and mix. The *Standard preparations* contain 95.0 μg and 125.0 μg of potassium per mL, respectively.
  Assay preparation—Transfer an accurately measured volume of Oral Solution, equivalent to about 782 mg (20 mEq) of potassium, to a 100-mL volumetric flask, dilute with water to volume, and mix. Transfer 7.0 mL of the resulting solution to a 500-mL volumetric flask, dilute with water to volume, and mix.
  Procedure—Concomitantly determine the absorbances of the *Standard preparations* and the *Assay preparation* at the resonance line of 766.5 nm, with a suitable atomic absorption spectrophotometer (see *Spectrophotometry and Light-scattering* ⟨851⟩) equipped with a potassium hollow-cathode lamp and an air–acetylene flame, using water as the blank. Plot the absorbances of the *Standard preparations* versus concentration, in μg per mL, of potassium. From the graph so obtained, determine the concentration, C, in μg per mL, of potassium in the *Assay preparation*. Calculate the quantity, in mg, of potassium in each mL of the Oral Solution taken by the formula:

$$(50 / 7)(C / V)$$

in which V is the volume, in mL, of Oral Solution taken. Each mg of potassium is equivalent to 0.02558 mEq.
Assay for chloride—
  Ionic strength adjusting solution—Use 5 M sodium nitrate.
  Procedure—Transfer an accurately measured volume of Oral Solution, equivalent to about 100 mg (2.8 mEq) of chloride, to a suitable beaker. Add 2.0 mL of *Ionic strength adjusting solution* and water to make about 100 mL, and titrate with 0.1 N silver nitrate VS, determining the endpoint potentiometrically, using a silver-sulfide specific ion-selective electrode and a double-junction reference electrode containing potassium nitrate solution (1 in 10). Perform a blank determination, and make any necessary correction. Each mL of 0.1 N silver nitrate is equivalent to 3.545 mg of chloride (Cl). Each mg of chloride is equivalent to 0.0282 mEq of Cl.

Potassium Gluconate and Potassium Chloride for Oral Solution

» Potassium Gluconate and Potassium Chloride for Oral Solution is a dry mixture of Potassium Gluconate and Potassium Chloride and one or more suitable colors, diluents, and flavors. It contains not less than 90.0 percent and not more than 110.0 percent of the labeled amounts of potassium (K) and chloride (Cl).

Packaging and storage—Preserve in tight containers.
Labeling—Label it to state the potassium and chloride contents in terms of milliequivalents. Where packaged in unit-dose pouches, the label instructs the user not to open until the time of use.

Identification—

A: Ignite about 200 mg at a temperature not above 600°, in order to remove all organic matter, cool, dissolve the residue in 10 mL of water, and filter: the filtrate responds to the tests for *Potassium* ⟨191⟩ and for *Chloride* ⟨191⟩.

B: A mineral oil dispersion of it exhibits an IR absorption maximum in the spectral region between 6.2 and 6.25 μm (*carboxylic acid salt*).

Minimum fill ⟨755⟩: meets the requirements.

Assay for potassium—

Potassium stock solution—Dissolve in water 0.9535 g of potassium chloride, previously dried at 105° for 2 hours. Transfer to a 500-mL volumetric flask, dilute with water to volume, and mix. This solution contains 1000 μg of potassium per mL.

Standard preparations—To separate 200-mL volumetric flasks transfer 19.0 mL and 25.0 mL, respectively, of the *Potassium stock solution*, dilute with water to volume, and mix. The *Standard preparations* contain 95.0 μg and 125.0 μg of potassium per mL, respectively.

Assay preparation 1 (where it is packaged in unit-dose containers)—Weigh and mix the contents of not less than 20 containers of Potassium Gluconate and Potassium Chloride for Oral Solution. Transfer an accurately weighed portion of the powder, equivalent to about 782 mg (20 mEq) of potassium, to a 100-mL volumetric flask, dilute with water to volume, and mix. Transfer 7.0 mL of this stock solution to a 500-mL volumetric flask, dilute with water to volume, and mix.

Assay preparation 2 (where it is packaged in multiple-unit containers)—Transfer an accurately weighed portion of Potassium Gluconate and Potassium Chloride for Oral Solution, equivalent to about 780 mg (20 mEq) of potassium, to a 100-mL volumetric flask, dissolve in water, dilute with water to volume, and mix. Transfer 7.0 mL of this stock solution to a 500-mL volumetric flask, dilute with water to volume, and mix.

Procedure—Concomitantly determine the absorbances of the *Standard preparations* and the *Assay preparation* at the resonance line of 766.5 nm, with a suitable atomic absorption spectrophotometer (see *Spectrophotometry and Light-scattering* ⟨851⟩) equipped with a potassium hollow-cathode lamp and an air–acetylene flame, using water as the blank. Plot the absorbances of the *Standard preparations* versus concentration, in μg per mL, of potassium. From the graph so obtained, determine the concentration, C, in μg per mL, of potassium in the *Assay preparation*. Calculate the quantity, in mg, of potassium in the portion of Potassium Gluconate and Potassium Chloride for Oral Solution taken by the formula:

$$50C / 7.$$

Each mg of potassium is equivalent to 0.02558 mEq.

Assay for chloride—

Ionic strength adjusting solution—Use 5 M sodium nitrate.

Assay preparation 1 (where it is packaged in unit-dose containers)—Weigh and mix the contents of not less than 20 containers of Potassium Gluconate and Potassium Chloride for Oral Solution. Transfer an accurately weighed portion of the powder, equivalent to about 100 mg (2.8 mEq) of chloride, to a suitable beaker.

Assay preparation 2 (where it is packaged in multiple-unit containers)—Transfer an accurately weighed portion of Potassium Gluconate and Potassium Chloride for Oral Solution, equivalent to about 100 mg (2.8 mEq) of chloride, to a suitable beaker.

Procedure—Add 2.0 mL of *Ionic strength adjusting solution* to *Assay preparation 1* or *Assay preparation 2*, add water to make about 100 mL, and titrate with 0.1 N silver nitrate VS, determining the endpoint potentiometrically, using a silver-sulfide specific ion-selective electrode and a double-junction reference electrode containing potassium nitrate solution (1 in 10). Perform a blank determination, and make any necessary correction. Each mL of 0.1 N silver nitrate is equivalent to 3.545 mg of chloride (Cl). Each mg of chloride is equivalent to 0.0282 mEq of Cl.

Potassium Gluconate and Potassium Citrate Oral Solution

» Potassium Gluconate and Potassium Citrate Oral Solution is a solution of Potassium Gluconate and Potassium Citrate in a suitable aqueous medium. It contains not less than 90.0 percent and not more than 110.0 percent of the labeled amount of potassium (K).

Packaging and storage—Preserve in tight containers.

Labeling—Label it to state the potassium content in terms of milliequivalents in a given volume of Oral Solution.

Identification—

A: To 2 mL of a dilution of Oral Solution (1 in 40) add 5 mL of sodium cobaltinitrite TS: a yellow precipitate is formed immediately (*presence of potassium*).

B: It responds to the test for *Citrate* ⟨191⟩, 3 to 5 drops of Oral Solution and 20 mL of the mixture of pyridine and acetic anhydride being used.

Assay for potassium—

Potassium stock solution—Dissolve in water 0.9535 g of potassium chloride, previously dried at 105° for 2 hours. Transfer to a 500-mL volumetric flask, dilute with water to volume, and mix. This solution contains 1000 μg of potassium per mL.

Standard preparations—To separate 200-mL volumetric flasks transfer 19.0 mL and 25.0 mL, respectively, of *Potassium stock solution*, dilute with water to volume, and mix. The *Standard preparations* contain 95.0 μg and 125.0 μg of potassium per mL, respectively.

Assay preparation—Transfer an accurately measured volume of Oral Solution, equivalent to about 782 mg (20 mEq) of potassium, to a 100-mL volumetric flask, dilute with water to volume, and mix. Transfer 7.0 mL of this solution to a 500-mL volumetric flask, dilute with water to volume, and mix.

Procedure—Concomitantly determine the absorbances of the *Standard preparations* and the *Assay preparation* at the resonance line of 766.5 nm, with a suitable atomic absorption spectrophotometer (see *Spectrophotometry and Light-scattering* ⟨851⟩) equipped with a potassium hollow-cathode lamp and an air–acetylene flame, using water as the blank. Plot the absorbances of the *Standard preparations* versus concentration, in μg per mL, of potassium. From the graph so obtained, determine the concentration, C, in μg per mL, of potassium in the *Assay preparation*. Calculate the quantity, in mg, of potassium in each mL of the Oral Solution taken by the formula:

$$(50 / 7)(C / V)$$

in which V is the volume, in mL, of Oral Solution taken. Each mg of potassium is equivalent to 0.02558 mEq.

Potassium Gluconate, Potassium Citrate, and Ammonium Chloride Oral Solution

» Potassium Gluconate, Potassium Citrate, and Ammonium Chloride Oral Solution is a solution of Potassium Gluconate, Potassium Citrate, and Ammonium Chloride in a suitable aqueous medium. It contains not less than 90.0 percent and not more than 110.0 percent of the labeled amounts of potassium (K) and chloride (Cl).

Packaging and storage—Preserve in tight containers.

Labeling—Label it to state the potassium and chloride contents in terms of milliequivalents of each in a given volume of Oral Solution.

Identification—

A: To 2 mL of a dilution of Oral Solution (1 in 40) add 5 mL of sodium cobaltinitrite TS: a yellow precipitate is formed immediately (*presence of potassium*).

B: It responds to the test for *Citrate* ⟨191⟩, 3 to 5 drops of Oral Solution and 20 mL of the mixture of pyridine and acetic anhydride being used.

C: It responds to the tests for *Ammonium* ⟨191⟩ and for *Chloride* ⟨191⟩.

Assay for potassium—

Potassium stock solution—Dissolve in water 0.9535 g of potassium chloride, previously dried at 105° for 2 hours. Transfer to a 500-mL volumetric flask, dilute with water to volume, and mix. This solution contains 1000 µg of potassium per mL.

Standard preparations—To separate 200-mL volumetric flasks transfer 19.0 mL and 25.0 mL, respectively, of the *Potassium stock solution*, dilute with water to volume, and mix. The *Standard preparations* contain 95.0 µg and 125.0 µg of potassium per mL, respectively.

Assay preparation—Transfer an accurately measured volume of Oral Solution, equivalent to about 782 mg (20 mEq) of potassium, to a 100-mL volumetric flask, dilute with water to volume, and mix. Transfer 7.0 mL of this solution to a 500-mL volumetric flask, dilute with water to volume, and mix.

Procedure—Concomitantly determine the absorbances of the *Standard preparations* and the *Assay preparation* at the resonance line of 766.5 nm, with a suitable atomic absorption spectrophotometer (see *Spectrometry and Light-scattering* ⟨851⟩) equipped with a potassium hollow-cathode lamp and an air–acetylene flame, using water as the blank. Plot the absorbances of the *Standard preparations* versus concentration, in µg per mL, of potassium. From the graph so obtained, determine the concentration, *C*, in µg per mL, of potassium in the *Assay preparation*. Calculate the quantity, in mg, of potassium in each mL of the Oral Solution taken by the formula:

$$(50/7)(C/V)$$

in which *V* is the volume, in mL, of Oral Solution taken. Each mg of potassium is equivalent to 0.02558 mEq.

Assay for chloride—

Ionic strength adjusting solution—Use 5 M sodium nitrate.

Procedure—Transfer an accurately measured volume of Oral Solution, equivalent to about 100 mg (2.8 mEq) of chloride, to a suitable beaker. Add 2.0 mL of *Ionic strength adjusting solution* and water to make about 100 mL, and titrate with 0.1 N silver nitrate VS, determining the endpoint potentiometrically, using a silver-sulfide specific ion-selective electrode and a double-junction reference electrode containing potassium nitrate solution (1 in 10). Perform a blank determination, and make any necessary correction. Each mL of 0.1 N silver nitrate is equivalent to 3.545 mg of chloride (Cl). Each mg of chloride is equivalent to 0.0282 mEq of Cl.

Potassium Guaiacolsulfonate

$C_7H_7KO_5S \cdot \frac{1}{2}H_2O$ 251.30

Benzenesulfonic acid, hydroxymethoxy-, monopotassium salt, hemihydrate.
Potassium hydroxymethoxybenzenesulfonate hemihydrate [78247-49-1].
Anhydrous   242.30

» Potassium Guaiacolsulfonate contains not less than 98.0 percent and not more than 102.0 percent of $C_7H_7KO_5S$, calculated on the anhydrous basis.

Packaging and storage—Preserve in well-closed, light-resistant containers.

USP Reference standards ⟨11⟩—*USP Potassium Guaiacolsulfonate RS*.

Identification—

A: *Infrared Absorption* ⟨197M⟩: between 7 µm and 13 µm, previously dried at 105° for 18 hours.

B: *Ultraviolet Absorption* ⟨197U⟩—
Solution: 50 µg per mL, prepared as directed in the *Assay*.

C: A solution (1 in 10) responds to the tests for *Potassium* ⟨191⟩.

Water, *Method I* ⟨921⟩:   between 3.0% and 6.0%.

Selenium ⟨291⟩:   0.003%.

Sulfate—To 10 mL of a solution (1 in 20) add 5 drops of barium chloride TS, and acidify with hydrochloric acid: no turbidity is produced in 1 minute.

Heavy metals ⟨231⟩—Dissolve 1.0 g in 1 mL of 1 N acetic acid, and dilute with water to 25 mL. The limit is 0.002%.

Assay—Transfer about 250 mg of Potassium Guaiacolsulfonate, accurately weighed, to a 500-mL volumetric flask, dissolve in 400 mL of water, dilute with water to volume, and mix. Dilute 10.0 mL of this solution with pH 7.0 phosphate buffer to 100.0 mL, and mix. Concomitantly determine the absorbances of this solution and a Standard solution of USP Potassium Guaiacolsulfonate RS in the same medium, having a known concentration of about 50 µg per mL, in 1-cm cells at the wavelength of maximum absorbance at about 279 nm, with a suitable spectrophotometer, using a 1 in 10 mixture of water and pH 7.0 phosphate buffer as the blank. Calculate the quantity, in mg, of $C_7H_7KO_5S$ in the Potassium Guaiacolsulfonate taken by the formula:

$$5C(A_U/A_S)$$

in which *C* is the concentration, in µg per mL, calculated on the anhydrous basis, of USP Potassium Guaiacolsulfonate RS in the Standard solution, and A_U and A_S are the absorbances of the preparation under assay and the Standard solution, respectively.

Potassium Iodide

KI   166.00
Potassium iodide.
Potassium iodide   [7681-11-0].

» Potassium Iodide contains not less than 99.0 percent and not more than 101.5 percent of KI, calculated on the dried basis.

Packaging and storage—Preserve in well-closed containers.

Identification—A solution of it meets the requirements of the tests for *Potassium* ⟨191⟩ and for *Iodide* ⟨191⟩.

Alkalinity—Dissolve 1.0 g in 10 mL of water, and add 0.1 mL of 0.1 N sulfuric acid and 1 drop of phenolphthalein TS: no color is produced.

Loss on drying ⟨731⟩—Dry it at 105° for 4 hours: it loses not more than 1.0% of its weight.

Iodate—Dissolve 1.1 g in sufficient ammonia- and carbon dioxide-free water to obtain 10 mL of solution, and transfer to a color-comparison tube. Add 1 mL of starch TS and 0.25 mL of 1.0 N sulfuric acid, mix, and compare the color with that of a control containing, in a similar volume, 100 mg of Potassium Iodide, 1 mL of standard iodate solution [prepare by diluting 1 mL of potassium iodate solution (1 in 2500) with water to 100 mL], 1 mL of starch TS, and 0.25 mL of 1.0 N sulfuric acid. Any color produced in the solution of the test specimen does not exceed that in the control: not more than 4 µg per g is found.

Limit of nitrate, nitrite, and ammonia—To a solution of 1 g in 5 mL of water contained in a test tube of about 40-mL capacity add 5 mL of 1 N sodium hydroxide and about 200 mg of aluminum wire. Insert a pledget of purified cotton in the upper portion of the test tube, and place a piece of moistened red litmus paper over the mouth of the tube. Heat the test tube and its contents in a steam bath for 15 minutes: no blue coloration of the paper is discernible.

Thiosulfate and barium—Dissolve 0.5 g in 10 mL of ammonia- and carbon dioxide-free water, and add 2 drops of 2 N sulfuric acid: no turbidity develops within 1 minute.
Heavy metals ⟨231⟩—Dissolve 2.0 g in 25 mL of water: the limit is 0.001%.
Organic volatile impurities, *Method I* ⟨467⟩: meets the requirements.

(Official until July 1, 2008)
Assay—Dissolve about 500 mg of Potassium Iodide, accurately weighed, in about 10 mL of water, and add 35 mL of hydrochloric acid. Titrate with 0.05 M potassium iodate VS until the dark brown solution which is produced becomes pale brown. Add 2 to 3 drops of amaranth TS, and continue the titration slowly until the red color just changes to yellow. Each mL of 0.05 M potassium iodate is equivalent to 16.60 mg of KI.

Potassium Iodide Oral Solution

» Potassium Iodide Oral Solution contains not less than 94.0 percent and not more than 106.0 percent of the labeled amount of KI.

NOTE—If Potassium Iodide Oral Solution is not to be used within a short time, add 0.5 mg of sodium thiosulfate for each g of KI. Products that have data to demonstrate acceptable stability without the addition of thiosulfate are exempt from this requirement. Crystals of potassium iodide may form in Potassium Iodide Oral Solution under normal conditions of storage, especially if refrigerated.

Packaging and storage—Preserve in tight, light-resistant containers.
Identification—It responds to the tests for *Potassium* ⟨191⟩ and for *Iodide* ⟨191⟩.
Uniformity of dosage units ⟨905⟩—
FOR ORAL SOLUTION PACKAGED IN SINGLE-UNIT CONTAINERS: meets the requirements.
Deliverable volume ⟨698⟩—
FOR ORAL SOLUTION PACKAGED IN MULTIPLE-UNIT CONTAINERS: meets the requirements.
Assay—Dilute an accurately measured volume of Oral Solution with water to obtain a solution containing about 50 mg of potassium iodide per mL. To 10.0 mL of this solution, in a 150-mL beaker, add about 40 mL of water, 25 mL of alcohol, and 1.0 mL of 1 N nitric acid. Titrate with 0.1 N silver nitrate VS, determining the endpoint potentiometrically, using silver-calomel electrodes and a salt bridge containing 4 percent agar in a saturated potassium nitrate solution. Perform a blank determination, and make any necessary correction. Each mL of 0.1 N silver nitrate is equivalent to 16.60 mg of KI.

Potassium Iodide Tablets

» Potassium Iodide Tablets contain not less than 94.0 percent and not more than 106.0 percent of the labeled amount of KI for Tablets of 300 mg or more, and not less than 92.5 percent and not more than 107.5 percent for Tablets of less than 300 mg.

Packaging and storage—Preserve in tight containers.
Identification—A filtered solution of powdered Tablets responds to the tests for *Potassium* ⟨191⟩ and for *Iodide* ⟨191⟩.

Dissolution ⟨711⟩—
FOR UNCOATED TABLETS—
Medium: water; 900 mL.
Apparatus 2: 50 rpm.
Time: 15 minutes.
Procedure—Determine the amount of KI dissolved from UV absorbances at the wavelength of maximum absorbance at about 227 nm of filtered portions of the solutions under test, suitably diluted with *Dissolution Medium*, if necessary, in comparison with a Standard solution having a known concentration of potassium iodide in the same medium.
Tolerances—Not less than 75% (*Q*) of the labeled amount of KI is dissolved in 15 minutes.
Uniformity of dosage units ⟨905⟩: meet the requirements.
Assay—Weigh and finely powder not less than 20 Tablets. Transfer a portion of the powder, equivalent to about 1.2 g of potassium iodide, to a 250-mL volumetric flask, add 100 mL of water, shake for 20 minutes, dilute with water to volume, and mix. Filter through paper, discarding the first 20 mL of the filtrate. Transfer 100.0 mL of the filtrate, 25 mL of alcohol, and 1.0 mL of 1 N nitric acid to a 200-mL beaker. Titrate with 0.1 N silver nitrate VS, determining the endpoint potentiometrically, using silver-calomel electrodes and a salt bridge containing 4 percent agar in a saturated potassium nitrate solution. Perform a blank determination, and make any necessary correction. Each mL of 0.1 N silver nitrate is equivalent to 16.60 mg of KI.

Potassium Iodide Delayed-Release Tablets

» Potassium Iodide Delayed-Release Tablets contain not less than 94.0 percent and not more than 106.0 percent of the labeled amount of KI for Tablets of 300 mg or more, and not less than 92.5 percent and not more than 107.5 percent for Tablets of less than 300 mg.

Packaging and storage—Preserve in tight containers.
Disintegration ⟨701⟩—Proceed as directed for *Delayed-Release (enteric coated) Tablets:* the Tablets do not disintegrate after 1 hour of agitation in simulated gastric fluid TS, but they disintegrate within 90 minutes in simulated intestinal fluid TS.
Other requirements—Tablets respond to the *Identification* test and meet the requirements for *Uniformity of dosage units* and *Assay* under *Potassium Iodide Tablets*.

Potassium Nitrate

KNO_3 101.10
Potassium nitrate.
Potassium nitrate [7757-79-1].

» Potassium Nitrate contains not less than 99.0 percent and not more than 100.5 percent of KNO_3.

Packaging and storage—Preserve in tight containers.
Identification—A solution of it responds to the tests for *Potassium* ⟨191⟩ and for *Nitrate* ⟨191⟩.
Chloride ⟨221⟩—A 500-mg portion of it shows no more chloride than corresponds to 0.21 mL of 0.020 N hydrochloric acid (0.03%).
Sulfate ⟨221⟩—Dissolve 100 mg of Potassium Nitrate in 10 mL of water, add 15 mL of 6 N hydrochloric acid, and evaporate to dryness on a steam bath. To the residue so obtained add 7 mL of 6 N hydrochloric acid, and evaporate to dryness on a steam bath. Dissolve the residue so obtained in about 35 mL of water and, if necessary, neutralize with hydrochloric acid using litmus paper indicator. Filter, if necessary, to obtain a clear test solution. This test solution shows no more sulfate than corresponds to 0.10 mL of 0.020 N sulfuric acid (0.1%).

Arsenic, *Method I* ⟨211⟩: 3 ppm.
Lead—A solution of 0.5 g of it in 20 mL of water contains not more than 5 µg of lead (corresponding to not more than 0.001% of Pb) when tested as directed under *Lead* ⟨251⟩.
Heavy metals, *Method I* ⟨231⟩: 0.002%.
Iron ⟨241⟩: not more than 0.001%.
Limit of sodium—
  Stock test solution—Transfer 1.0 g of Potassium Nitrate to a 500-mL volumetric flask, add water to dissolve it, dilute with water to volume, and mix. [NOTE—The concentration of potassium nitrate in this solution may be modified by using a different quantity or by further dilution to bring the absorption response within the working range of the atomic absorption spectrophotometer.]
  Stock standard solution—Transfer 127.1 mg of sodium chloride, previously dried at 105° for 2 hours and accurately weighed, to a 500-mL volumetric flask, add water to volume, and mix. Transfer 5.0 mL of this solution to a second 500-mL volumetric flask, dilute with water to volume, and mix. This solution contains 1.0 µg of sodium per mL.
  Procedure—Transfer 5.0 mL of *Stock test solution* to each of three 25-mL volumetric flasks. To these flasks, respectively, add 0.0, 5.0, and 10.0 mL of *Stock standard solution*, dilute with water to volume, and mix. These flasks contain 0.0, 0.20, and 0.40 µg of added sodium per mL, respectively. [NOTE—Concentrations of sodium in these solutions may be modified to fit the linear or working range of the atomic absorption spectrophotometer.] Concomitantly determine the absorbances of these solutions at the sodium emission line of 589 nm with an atomic absorption spectrophotometer (see *Spectrophotometry and Light-scattering* ⟨851⟩) equipped with a sodium hollow-cathode lamp and an oxidizing flame, using water to zero the instrument. Plot the absorbances of the three solutions versus concentration, in µg of added sodium per mL, draw the straight line best fitting the plotted points, and extrapolate the line until it intercepts the concentration axis. From the graph so obtained determine the concentration, C, in µg of sodium per mL, of the solution containing 0.0 mL of the *Stock standard solution*. Calculate the percentage of sodium in the portion of Potassium Nitrate taken by multiplying C by 0.25: the limit is 0.1%.
Limit of nitrite—
  Sulfanilic acid solution—Prepare a solution containing 1 mg of sulfanilic acid per mL.
  N-(1-Naphthyl)ethylenediamine dihydrochloride solution—Prepare a solution containing 1 mg of *N*-(1-naphthyl)ethylenediamine dihydrochloride per mL. [NOTE—When stored in a low-actinic glass bottle, this solution may be used for 1 week.]
  Standard solutions—Transfer 150.0 mg of sodium nitrite to a 100-mL volumetric flask, dilute with water to volume, and mix. Transfer 10.0 mL of this solution to a 1000-mL volumetric flask, dilute with water to volume, and mix. This solution contains 15 µg of sodium nitrite (10 µg of nitrite) per mL. Transfer 1.0 mL and 2.0 mL of this solution to separate 50-mL beakers, and add 19 and 18 mL of water to the respective beakers.
  Test solution—Transfer 4.0 g of Potassium Nitrate to a 50-mL beaker, add 20 mL of water, and swirl to dissolve.
  Procedure—To the beakers containing the *Standard solutions* and the *Test solution* add 5.0 mL of *Sulfanilic acid solution* and 5.0 mL of diluted hydrochloric acid, and allow to stand for 3 minutes. Add 5.0 mL of *N-(1-Naphthyl)ethylenediamine dihydrochloride solution* to each beaker, mix, and allow to stand for 15 minutes. Concomitantly determine the absorbances of the solutions at 550 nm. The absorbance of the solution from the *Test solution* does not exceed that of the solution from the *Standard solution* containing 20 µg of nitrite (5 µg per g).
Assay—[NOTE—Use water that is carbon dioxide- and ammonia-free.]
  Cation-exchange column—Transfer strongly acidic styrene-divinylbenzene cation-exchange resin (16-to 50-mesh) to a 2-cm diameter chromatographic column to a depth of about 20 cm.
  Procedure—Dissolve about 400 mg of Potassium Nitrate, accurately weighed, in 100 mL of water. Pass this solution through the *Cation-exchange column* at a rate of about 5 mL per minute, and collect the eluate in a 500-mL conical flask. Wash the resin in the column with water at a rate of about 10 mL per minute, collecting the eluate in the conical flask. Add 0.15 mL of phenolphthalein TS to the flask, and after 5 minutes titrate with 0.1 N sodium hydroxide VS to a pink endpoint. Continue collecting the wash from the column, and continue titrating, if necessary, until a 50-mL increment of eluate requires no further addition of sodium hydroxide. Each mL of 0.1 N sodium hydroxide is equivalent to 10.11 mg of KNO₃.

Potassium Nitrate Solution

» Potassium Nitrate Solution contains not less than 98.0 percent and not more than 102.0 percent of the labeled amount of KNO₃.

Packaging and storage—Preserve in tight containers.
Identification—It responds to the tests for *Potassium* ⟨191⟩ and for *Nitrate* ⟨191⟩.
Chloride ⟨221⟩—An accurately measured portion of Solution, equivalent to 500 mg of potassium nitrate, shows no more chloride than corresponds to 0.21 mL of 0.020 N hydrochloric acid (0.03%, based on the potassium nitrate content of the Solution).
Sulfate ⟨221⟩—Dilute an accurately measured portion of Solution, equivalent to 100 mg of potassium nitrate, with water to obtain 10 mL of solution, add 15 mL of 6 N hydrochloric acid, and evaporate to dryness on a steam bath. To the residue so obtained add 7 mL of 6 N hydrochloric acid, and evaporate to dryness on a steam bath. Dissolve the residue so obtained in about 35 mL of water and, if necessary, neutralize with hydrochloric acid using litmus paper indicator. Filter, if necessary, to obtain a clear test solution. This test solution shows no more sulfate than corresponds to 0.10 mL of 0.020 N sulfuric acid (0.1%, based on the potassium nitrate content of the Solution).
Arsenic, *Method I* ⟨211⟩: 3 ppm, based on the potassium nitrate content of the Solution, an accurately measured portion of Solution, equivalent to 1.0 g of potassium nitrate, being tested.
Lead—Dilute an accurately measured portion of Solution, equivalent to 500 mg of potassium nitrate, with water to obtain 20 mL of test solution. This test solution contains not more than 5 µg of lead (corresponding to not more than 0.001% of Pb, based on the potassium nitrate content of the Solution) when tested as directed under *Lead* ⟨251⟩.
Heavy metals, *Method I* ⟨231⟩: 0.002%, based on the potassium nitrate content of the Solution.
Iron ⟨241⟩: not more than 0.001%, based on the potassium nitrate content of the Solution, an accurately measured portion of Solution, equivalent to 1.0 g of potassium nitrate, being tested.
Limit of sodium—
  Stock test solution—Transfer an accurately measured portion of Solution, equivalent to 1.0 g of potassium nitrate, to a 500-mL volumetric flask, add water to volume, and mix. [NOTE—The concentration of potassium nitrate in this solution may be modified by using a different quantity or by further dilution to bring the absorption response within the working range of the atomic absorption spectrophotometer.]
  Stock standard solution—Proceed as directed in the *Limit of sodium* test under *Potassium Nitrate*.
  Procedure—Proceed as directed in the *Limit of sodium* test under *Potassium Nitrate*. Calculate the percentage of sodium in the portion of Solution taken by multiplying C by 0.25: the limit is 0.1%, based on the potassium nitrate content of the Solution.
Limit of nitrite—
  Sulfanilic acid solution, N-(1-Naphthyl)ethylenediamine dihydrochloride solution, and *Standard solutions*—Proceed as directed in the *Limit of nitrite* test under *Potassium Nitrate*.
  Test solution—Transfer an accurately measured portion of the Solution, equivalent to 4.0 g of potassium nitrate, to a 50-mL beaker, add sufficient water to obtain 20 mL of solution, and mix.
  Procedure—Proceed as directed in the *Limit of nitrite* test under *Potassium Nitrate*. The absorbance of the solution from the *Test solution* does not exceed that of the solution from the *Standard solution* containing 20 µg of nitrite (5 µg per g, based on the potassium nitrate content of the Solution).

Assay—[NOTE—Use water that is carbon dioxide- and ammonia-free.]

Cation-exchange column—Transfer strongly acidic styrene-divinylbenzene cation-exchange resin (16- to 50-mesh) to a 2-cm diameter chromatographic column to a depth of about 20 cm.

Procedure—Transfer an accurately measured portion of Solution, equivalent to about 400 mg of potassium nitrate, to a beaker and add sufficient water to obtain 100 mL of solution. Proceed as directed in the *Assay* under *Potassium Nitrate* beginning with "Pass this solution through . . . ." Each mL of 0.1 N sodium hydroxide is equivalent to 10.11 mg of KNO₃.

Potassium Perchlorate

» Potassium Perchlorate contains not less than 99.0 percent and not more than 100.5 percent of KClO₄, calculated on the dried basis.

Caution: Great care should be taken in handling Potassium Perchlorate in solution or in the dry state, as explosions may occur if it is brought into contact with organic or other readily oxidizable substances.

Packaging and storage—Preserve in well-closed containers.
Identification—
  A: Ignite a small portion of a solution (1 in 10) on a platinum wire in a nonluminous flame: a transient violet color is imparted to the flame.
  B: Add a few drops of methylene blue solution (1 in 1000) to the solution (1 in 10): a violet-colored precipitate is formed.
pH ⟨791⟩: between 5.0 and 6.5, in a 0.1 M solution.
Loss on drying ⟨731⟩—Dry it over silica gel for 12 hours: it loses not more than 0.5% of its weight.
Insoluble substances—Dissolve 20 g in 150 mL of warm water, pass through a tared medium-porosity filtering crucible, and wash with three 50-mL portions of warm water. Dry the residue at 105° for 3 hours: the weight of the residue does not exceed 1 mg (0.005%).
Chloride ⟨221⟩—A 5.0-g portion shows no more chloride than corresponds to 0.20 mL of 0.020 N hydrochloric acid (0.003%).
Heavy metals, *Method I* ⟨231⟩: 0.001%.
Limit of sodium—Ignite a small portion of a solution (1 in 10) on a platinum wire in a nonluminous flame: no pronounced yellow color is imparted to the flame.
Organic volatile impurities, *Method I* ⟨467⟩: meets the requirements.

(Official until July 1, 2008)

Assay—
Mobile phase—Transfer 16.6 g of phthalic acid to a 100-mL volumetric flask, dissolve in and dilute with methanol to volume, and mix. Transfer 10.0 mL of this solution to a 1000-mL flask, dilute with water to volume, and mix. Adjust with about 450 mg of lithium hydroxide to a pH of 4.5, filter, and degas.
Standard preparation—Transfer about 50 mg of potassium perchlorate, accurately weighed, to a 50-mL volumetric flask, dilute with water to volume, and mix. Transfer 10.0 mL of this solution to a 100-mL volumetric flask, dilute with water to volume, and mix to obtain a solution having a known concentration of about 0.1 mg per mL.
Assay preparation—Using about 50 mg of Potassium Perchlorate, accurately weighed, proceed as directed for the *Standard preparation*.
Chromatographic system (see *Chromatography* ⟨621⟩)—The liquid chromatograph is equipped with a conductivity detector and a 4.6-mm × 7.5-cm column that contains 6-µm packing L23. The flow rate is about 1.2 mL per minute. Chromatograph the *Standard preparation*, and record the peak responses as directed for *Procedure*: the tailing factor is not more than 1.5; and the relative standard deviation for replicate injections is not more than 2.0%.
Procedure—Separately inject equal volumes (about 50 µL) of the *Standard preparation* and the *Assay preparation* into the chromatograph, record the chromatograms, and measure the responses for the major peaks. Calculate the quantity, in mg, of KClO₄ in the portion of Potassium Perchlorate taken by the formula:

$$500C(r_U / r_S)$$

in which C is the concentration, in mg per mL, of potassium perchlorate in the *Standard preparation*; and r_U and r_S are the peak responses obtained from the *Assay preparation* and the *Standard preparation*, respectively.

Potassium Perchlorate Capsules

» Potassium Perchlorate Capsules contain not less than 90.0 percent and not more than 110.0 percent of the labeled amount of potassium perchlorate (KClO₄).

Packaging and storage—Preserve in tight, light-resistant containers.
USP Reference standards ⟨11⟩—*USP Potassium Perchlorate RS*.
Identification—
  A: Dissolve the contents of 5 Capsules in 20 mL of water, and filter: the filtrate responds to the tests for *Potassium* ⟨191⟩.
  B: Add a few drops of methylene blue solution (1 in 1000) to the filtrate obtained in *Identification* test A: a violet-colored precipitate is obtained.
Disintegration ⟨701⟩: 30 minutes, 1 N hydrochloric acid maintained at 37 ± 2° being used as the immersion fluid.
Uniformity of dosage units ⟨905⟩: meet the requirements for *Content Uniformity*.
Assay—
Mobile phase, Standard preparation, and *Chromatographic system*—Proceed as directed in the *Assay* under *Potassium Perchlorate*.
Assay preparation—Mix the contents of not less than 10 Capsules, and transfer an accurately weighed portion of the mixed powder, equivalent to about 200 mg of potassium perchlorate, to a 200-mL volumetric flask, dilute with water to volume, and mix. Pass through a filter having 0.22-µm pore size, transfer 10.0 mL of the clear filtrate to a 100-mL volumetric flask, dilute with water to volume, and mix.
Procedure—Proceed as directed in the *Assay* under *Potassium Perchlorate*. Calculate the quantity, in mg, of potassium perchlorate (KClO₄) in the portion of Capsules taken by the formula:

$$2000C(r_U / r_S)$$

in which the terms are as defined therein.

Potassium Permanganate

KMnO₄   158.03
Permanganic acid (HMnO₄), potassium salt.
Potassium permanganate (KMnO₄)   [7722-64-7].

» Potassium Permanganate contains not less than 99.0 percent and not more than 100.5 percent of KMnO₄, calculated on the dried basis.

Caution: Observe great care in handling Potassium Permanganate, as dangerous explosions may occur if it is brought into contact with organic or other readily oxidizable substances, either in solution or in the dry state.

Packaging and storage—Preserve in well-closed containers.
Identification—A solution of it is deep violet-red when concentrated and pink when highly diluted, and responds to the tests for *Permanganate* ⟨191⟩.

Loss on drying ⟨731⟩—Dry it over silica gel for 18 hours: it loses not more than 0.5% of its weight.
Insoluble substances—Dissolve 2.0 g in 150 mL of water that previously has been warmed to steam-bath temperature, and filter immediately through a tared, medium-porosity filtering crucible. Wash the filter with three 50-mL portions of the warm water, and dry the filtering crucible and the residue at 105° for 3 hours: not more than 4 mg of residue is obtained (0.2%).
Assay—Transfer about 1000 mg of Potassium Permanganate, accurately weighed, and for each mg of Potassium Permanganate taken, 2.13 mg of sodium oxalate, previously dried at 110° to constant weight and accurately weighed, to a 500-mL conical flask. Add 150 mL of water and 20 mL of 7 N sulfuric acid, heat to about 80°, and titrate the excess oxalic acid with 0.03 N potassium permanganate VS. Calculate the quantity, in mg, of KMnO$_4$ in the portion of Potassium Permanganate taken by the formula:

$$0.4718W_S - 0.9482V$$

in which 0.4718 is the KMnO$_4$ equivalent, in mg, of each mg of sodium oxalate, W_S is the weight, in mg, of sodium oxalate taken, 0.9482 is the quantity of KMnO$_4$, in mg, in each mL of 0.03 N potassium permanganate, and V is the volume, in mL, of 0.03 N potassium permanganate consumed.

Dibasic Potassium Phosphate

K$_2$HPO$_4$ 174.18
Phosphoric acid, dipotassium salt.
Dipotassium hydrogen phosphate   [7758-11-4].

» Dibasic Potassium Phosphate contains not less than 98.0 percent and not more than 100.5 percent of K$_2$HPO$_4$, calculated on the dried basis.

Packaging and storage—Preserve in well-closed containers.
Identification—A solution (1 in 20) responds to the tests for *Potassium* ⟨191⟩ and for *Phosphate* ⟨191⟩.
pH ⟨791⟩: between 8.5 and 9.6, in a solution (1 in 20).
Loss on drying ⟨731⟩—Dry it at 105° to constant weight: it loses not more than 1.0% of its weight.
Insoluble substances—Dissolve 10 g in 100 mL of hot water, filter through a tared filtering crucible, wash the insoluble residue with hot water, and dry at 105° for 2 hours: the weight of the residue so obtained does not exceed 20 mg (0.2%).
Carbonate—To 1 g add 3 mL of water and 2 mL of 3 N hydrochloric acid: not more than a few bubbles are evolved.
Chloride ⟨221⟩—A 1.0-g portion shows no more chloride than corresponds to 0.40 mL of 0.020 N hydrochloric acid (0.03%).
Sulfate ⟨221⟩—A 0.20-g portion shows no more sulfate than corresponds to 0.20 mL of 0.020 N sulfuric acid (0.1%).
Arsenic, *Method I* ⟨211⟩: 3 ppm.
Iron—Dissolve 0.33 g in 10 mL of water, add 6 mL of hydroxylamine hydrochloride solution (1 in 10) and 4 mL of orthophenanthroline solution prepared by dissolving 1 g of orthophenanthroline in 1000 mL of water containing 1 mL of 3 N hydrochloric acid, and dilute with water to 25 mL: any red color produced within 1 hour is not darker than that of a control prepared from 1 mL of *Standard Iron Solution* (see *Iron* ⟨241⟩): the limit is 0.003%.
Sodium ⟨191⟩—A solution (1 in 10) tested on a platinum wire imparts no pronounced yellow color to a nonluminous flame.
Heavy metals, *Method I* ⟨231⟩: Dissolve a portion equivalent to 4.2 g of K$_2$HPO$_4$ in enough water to make 50 mL of stock solution. Transfer 12 mL of this stock solution to a 50-mL color-comparison tube (*Test Preparation*). Transfer 11 mL of the stock solution to a second color-comparison tube containing 1.0 mL of *Standard Lead Solution* (*Monitor Preparation*). Transfer 1.0 mL of *Standard Lead Solution* and 11 mL of water to a third color-comparison tube (*Standard Preparation*). Proceed as directed for *Procedure*, omitting the dilution to 50 mL: the limit is 0.001%.

Limit of fluoride—Proceed as directed in the test for *Fluoride* under *Dibasic Calcium Phosphate*. The limit is 0.001%.
Limit of monobasic or tribasic salt—Dissolve 3 g in 30 mL of water, cool to 20°, and add 3 drops of thymol blue TS: a blue color is produced, which is changed to yellow (with a greenish tinge) by the addition of not more than 0.4 mL of 1 N hydrochloric acid.
Assay—Transfer 40.0 mL of 1 N hydrochloric acid to a 250-mL beaker, add 50 mL of water, and titrate potentiometrically with 1 N sodium hydroxide VS to the endpoint. Record the volume of 1 N sodium hydroxide VS consumed as the blank. Transfer about 5.2 g of Dibasic Potassium Phosphate, accurately weighed, to a 250-mL beaker, add 50 mL of water and 40.0 mL of 1 N hydrochloric acid VS, stir until dissolved, and proceed as directed in the *Assay* under *Dibasic Sodium Phosphate*, beginning with "Titrate the excess acid." Where A is equal to or less than B, each mL of the volume A of 1 N sodium hydroxide is equivalent to 174.2 mg of K$_2$HPO$_4$. Where A is greater than B, each mL of the volume $2B - A$ of 1 N sodium hydroxide is equivalent to 174.2 mg of K$_2$HPO$_4$.

Potassium Phosphates Injection

» Potassium Phosphates Injection is a sterile solution of Monobasic Potassium Phosphate and Dibasic Potassium Phosphate in Water for Injection. It contains not less than 95.0 percent and not more than 105.0 percent of the labeled amounts of monobasic potassium phosphate (KH$_2$PO$_4$) and dibasic potassium phosphate (K$_2$HPO$_4$). It contains no bacteriostat or other preservative.

Packaging and storage—Preserve in single-dose containers, preferably of Type I glass.
Labeling—The label states the potassium content in terms of milliequivalents in a given volume, and states also the elemental phosphorus content in terms of millimoles in a given volume. Label the Injection to indicate that it is to be diluted to appropriate strength with water or other suitable fluid prior to administration, and that once opened any unused portion is to be discarded. The label states also the total osmolar concentration in mOsmol per L. Where the contents are less than 100 mL, or where the label states that the Injection is not for direct injection but is to be diluted before use, the label alternatively may state the total osmolar concentration in mOsmol per mL.
USP Reference standards ⟨11⟩—*USP Endotoxin RS*.
Identification—It responds to the tests for *Potassium* ⟨191⟩ and for *Phosphate* ⟨191⟩.
Bacterial endotoxins ⟨85⟩—It contains not more than 1.10 USP Endotoxin Units per mg of potassium phosphates.
Particulate matter ⟨788⟩: meets the requirements for small-volume Injections.
Other requirements—It meets the requirements under *Injections* ⟨1⟩.
Assay for monobasic potassium phosphate—Transfer an accurately measured volume of Injection, equivalent to about 300 mg of monobasic potassium phosphate, to a 100-mL beaker, and dilute with water to about 50 mL. Place the electrodes of a suitable pH meter in the solution, and titrate with 0.1 N sodium hydroxide VS to the inflection point to a pH of about 9.1. Each mL of 0.1 N sodium hydroxide is equivalent to 13.61 mg of KH$_2$PO$_4$.
Assay for dibasic potassium phosphate—Transfer an accurately measured volume of Injection, equivalent to about 300 mg of dibasic potassium phosphate, to a 100-mL beaker, and dilute with water to about 50 mL. Place the electrodes of a suitable pH meter in the solution, and titrate with 0.1 N hydrochloric acid VS to the inflection point to a pH of about 4.2. Each mL of 0.1 N hydrochloric acid is equivalent to 17.42 mg of K$_2$HPO$_4$.

Potassium Sodium Tartrate

$C_4H_4KNaO_6 \cdot 4H_2O$ 282.22
Butanedioic acid, 2,3-dihydroxy-, [R-(R*,R*)]-, monopotassium monosodium salt, tetrahydrate.
Monopotassium monosodium tartrate tetrahydrate [6100-16-9; 6381-59-5].
Anhydrous   210.16   [304-59-6].

» Potassium Sodium Tartrate contains not less than 99.0 percent and not more than 102.0 percent of $C_4H_4KNaO_6$, calculated on the anhydrous basis.

Packaging and storage—Preserve in tight containers.
Identification—
  A: Ignite it: it emits the odor of burning sugar and leaves a residue that is alkaline to litmus and that effervesces with acids.
  B: To 10 mL of a solution (1 in 20) add 10 mL of 6 N acetic acid: a white, crystalline precipitate is formed within 15 minutes.
  C: A solution (1 in 10) responds to the tests for *Tartrate* ⟨191⟩.
Alkalinity—A solution of 1.0 g in 20 mL of water is alkaline to litmus, but after the addition of 0.20 mL of 0.10 N sulfuric acid no pink color is produced by the addition of 1 drop of phenolphthalein TS.
Water, *Method I* ⟨921⟩:   between 21.0% and 27.0%.
Limit of ammonia—
  Sodium hypochlorite solution—Use a commercially available solution that contains between 4.0% and 6.0% of sodium hypochlorite.
  Oxidizing solution—[NOTE—Prepare on the day of use.] Prepare a mixture of alkaline sodium citrate TS and *Sodium hypochlorite solution* (4 : 1).
  Diluted sodium nitroferricyanide solution—Prepare a mixture of water and sodium nitroferricyanide TS (10 : 1).
  Standard solution—Transfer 300 mg of ammonium chloride, previously dried over silica gel for 4 hours, to a 1-L volumetric flask, and dilute with water to volume. This solution contains 100 µg of ammonia per mL. Dilute this solution quantitatively, and stepwise if necessary, with water to obtain a solution having a concentration of 1.0 µg of ammonia per mL.
  Test solution—Transfer 5.0 g of Potassium Sodium Tartrate to a 100-mL volumetric flask, and dissolve in and dilute with water to volume.
  Procedure—[NOTE—Carefully follow the order of addition stated below.] Separately transfer 4.0 mL of each of the *Standard solution* and the *Test solution* to two color-comparison tubes. To each tube add 0.4 mL of phenol TS, 0.4 mL of *Diluted sodium nitroferricyanide solution,* and 1.0 mL of *Oxidizing solution*. Dilute with water to 10 mL, mix, and allow to stand for 1 hour: the color of the *Test solution* is not darker than the color of the *Standard solution* (0.002%).
Heavy metals, *Method II* ⟨231⟩:   0.001%.
Assay—Weigh accurately about 2 g of Potassium Sodium Tartrate in a tared porcelain crucible, and ignite, gently at first, until the salt is thoroughly carbonized, protecting the carbonized salt from the flame at all times. Cool the crucible, place it in a glass beaker, and break up the carbonized mass with a glass rod. Without removing the glass rod or the crucible, add 50 mL of water and 50.0 mL of 0.5 N sulfuric acid VS, cover the beaker, and boil the solution for 30 minutes. Filter, and wash with hot water until the last washing is neutral to litmus. Cool the combined filtrate and washings, add methyl red-methylene blue TS, and titrate the excess acid with 0.5 N sodium hydroxide VS. Perform a blank determination (see *Residual Titrations* under *Titrimetry* ⟨541⟩). Each mL of 0.5 N sulfuric acid is equivalent to 52.54 mg of $C_4H_4KNaO_6$.

Povidone

$(C_6H_9NO)_n$
2-Pyrrolidinone, 1-ethenyl-, homopolymer.
1-Vinyl-2-pyrrolidinone polymer   [9003-39-8].

» Povidone is a synthetic polymer consisting essentially of linear 1-vinyl-2-pyrrolidinone groups, the degree of polymerization of which results in polymers of various molecular weights. The different types of Povidone are characterized by their viscosity in aqueous solution, relative to that of water, expressed as a K-value. (See the section on *K-value* below.) The K-value of Povidone having a stated (nominal) K-value of 15 or less is not less than 85.0 percent and not more than 115.0 percent of the stated values. The K-value of Povidone having a stated K-value or a stated K-value range with an average of more than 15 is not less than 90.0 percent and not more than 108.0 percent of the stated value or of the average of the stated range.

Packaging and storage—Preserve in tight containers.
Labeling—Label it to state, as part of the official title, the K-value or K-value range of the Povidone.
Identification—
  A: To 10 mL of a solution (1 in 50) add 20 mL of 1 N hydrochloric acid and 5 mL of potassium dichromate TS: an orange-yellow precipitate is formed.
  B: Dissolve 75 mg of cobalt nitrate and 300 mg of ammonium thiocyanate in 2 mL of water. To this solution add 5 mL of a solution of Povidone (1 in 50), and render the resulting solution acid by the addition of 3 N hydrochloric acid: a pale blue precipitate is formed.
  C: To 5 mL of a solution (1 in 200) add a few drops of iodine TS: a deep red color is produced.
pH ⟨791⟩:   between 3.0 and 7.0, in a solution (1 in 20).
Water, *Method I* ⟨921⟩:   not more than 5.0%.
Residue on ignition ⟨281⟩:   not more than 0.1%.
Lead ⟨251⟩—Dissolve 1.0 g in 25 mL of water: the limit is 10 ppm.
Limit of aldehydes—
  Phosphate buffer—Transfer 8.3 g of potassium pyrophosphate to a 500-mL volumetric flask, and dissolve in 400 mL of water. Adjust, if necessary, with 1 N hydrochloric acid to a pH of 9.0, dilute with water to volume, and mix.
  Aldehyde dehydrogenase solution—Transfer a quantity of lyophilized aldehyde dehydrogenase equivalent to 70 units to a glass vial, dissolve in 10.0 mL of water, and mix. [NOTE—This solution is stable for 8 hours at 4°.]
  NAD solution—Transfer 40 mg of nicotinamide adenine dinucleotide to a glass vial, dissolve in 10.0 mL of *Phosphate buffer,* and mix. [NOTE—This solution is stable for 4 weeks at 4°.]
  Standard preparation—Add about 2 mL of water to a glass weighing bottle, and weigh accurately. Add about 100 mg (about 0.13 mL) of freshly distilled acetaldehyde, and weigh accurately. Transfer this solution to a 100-mL volumetric flask. Rinse the weighing bottle with several portions of water, transferring each rinsing to the 100-mL volumetric flask. Dilute the solution in the 100-mL volumetric flask with water to volume, and mix. Store at 4° for about 20 hours. Pipet 1 mL of this solution into a 100-mL volumetric flask, dilute with water to volume, and mix.
  Test preparation—Transfer about 2 g of Povidone, accurately weighed, to a 100-mL volumetric flask, dissolve in 50 mL of *Phosphate buffer,* dilute with *Phosphate buffer* to volume, and mix. Insert a stopper into the flask, heat at 60° for 1 hour, and cool to room temperature.

Procedure—Pipet 0.5 mL each of the *Standard preparation,* the *Test preparation,* and water to provide the reagent blank into separate 1-cm cells. Add 2.5 mL of *Phosphate buffer* and 0.2 mL of *NAD solution* to each cell. Cover the cells to exclude oxygen. Mix by inversion, and allow to stand for 2 to 3 minutes at 22 ± 2°. Determine the absorbances of the solutions at a wavelength of 340 nm, using water as the reference. Add 0.05 mL of *Aldehyde dehydrogenase solution* to each cell. Cover the cells to exclude oxygen. Mix by inversion, and allow to stand for 5 minutes at 22 ± 2°. Determine the absorbances of the solutions at a wavelength of 340 nm, using water as the reference. Calculate the percentage of aldehydes, expressed as acetaldehyde, in the Povidone taken by the formula:

$$10(C/W)\left[\frac{(A_{U2} - A_{U1}) - (A_{B2} - A_{B1})}{(A_{S2} - A_{S1}) - (A_{B2} - A_{B1})}\right],$$

in which C is the concentration, in mg per mL, of acetaldehyde in the *Standard preparation;* W is the weight, in g, of Povidone taken; A_{U1}, A_{S1}, and A_{B1} are the absorbances of the solutions obtained from the *Test preparation,* *Standard preparation,* and water reagent blank, respectively, before addition of the *Aldehyde dehydrogenase solution;* and A_{U2}, A_{S2}, and A_{B2} are the absorbances of the solutions obtained from the *Test preparation,* *Standard preparation,* and water reagent blank, respectively, after addition of the *Aldehyde dehydrogenase solution:* not more than 0.05% is found.

Limit of hydrazine—Transfer 2.5 g to a 50-mL centrifuge tube, add 25 mL of water, and mix to dissolve. Add 500 µL of a 1 in 20 solution of salicylaldehyde in methanol, swirl, and heat in a water bath at 60° for 15 minutes. Allow to cool, add 2.0 mL of toluene, insert a stopper in the tube, shake vigorously for 2 minutes, and centrifuge. Apply 10 µL of the clear upper toluene layer in the centrifuge tube and 10 µL of a Standard solution of salicylaldazine in toluene containing 9.38 µg per mL to a suitable thin-layer chromatographic plate (see *Chromatography* ⟨621⟩) coated with a 0.25-mm layer of dimethylsilanized chromatographic silica gel mixture. Allow the spots to dry, and develop the chromatogram in a solvent system consisting of a mixture of methanol and water (2 : 1) until the solvent front has moved about three-fourths of the length of the plate. Remove the plate from the developing chamber, mark the solvent front, and allow the solvent to evaporate. Locate the spots on the plate by examination under UV light at a wavelength of 365 nm: salicylaldazine appears as a fluorescent spot having an R_F value of about 0.3, and the fluorescence of any salicylaldazine spot from the test specimen is not more intense than that produced by the spot obtained from the Standard solution (1 ppm of hydrazine).

Vinylpyrrolidinone—

Mobile phase—Prepare a mixture of water and methanol (80 : 20).

Resolution solution—Transfer 10 mg of vinylpyrrolidinone and 500 mg of vinyl acetate, accurately weighed, to a 100-mL volumetric flask, and dissolve in and dilute with methanol to volume. Transfer 1.0 mL of this solution to a 100-mL volumetric flask, dilute with *Mobile phase* to volume, and mix.

Standard solution—Transfer an accurately weighed quantity of 50 mg of vinylpyrrolidinone to a 100-mL volumetric flask, dilute with methanol to volume, and mix. Transfer 1.0-mL of this solution to a 100-mL volumetric flask, dilute with methanol to volume, and mix. Transfer 5.0 mL of this solution to a 100-mL volumetric flask, dilute with *Mobile phase* to volume, and mix.

Test solution—Transfer an accurately weighed quantity of about 250 mg of Povidone to a 10-mL volumetric flask, dilute with *Mobile phase* to volume, and mix.

Chromatographic system (see *Chromatography* ⟨621⟩)—The liquid chromatograph is equipped with a 235-nm detector, a 4.0-mm × 2.5-cm guard column containing packing L7, and a 4.0-mm × 25-cm analytical column containing 5-µm packing L7. [NOTE—The analysis can also be performed with a 4.0-mm × 30-mm or a 4.6-mm × 30-mm guard column containing packing L7 and with a 4.6-mm × 25-cm analytical column containing 5-µm packing L7.] The column temperature is maintained at about 40°. Adjust the flow rate so that the retention time of vinylpyrrolidinone is about 10 minutes. Chromatograph the *Resolution solution,* and record the peak responses as directed for *Procedure:* the resolution, R, between vinylpyrrolidinone and vinyl acetate is not less than 2.0. Chromatograph the *Standard solution,* and record the peak responses as directed for *Procedure:* the relative standard deviation for replicate injections is not more than 2.0%.

Procedure—Separately inject equal volumes (about 50 µL) each of the *Standard solution* and the *Test solution* into the chromatograph, record the chromatograms, and measure the responses for the vinylpyrrolidinone peak. [NOTE—If necessary, after each injection of the *Test solution,* wash the polymeric material of Povidone from the guard column by passing the *Mobile phase* through the column backwards for about 30 minutes at the same flow rate.] Calculate the percentage of vinylpyrrolidinone in the sample taken by the formula:

$$1000(C/W)(r_U / r_S)$$

in which C is the concentration, in mg per mL, of vinylpyrrolidinone in the *Standard solution;* W is the weight, in mg, of Povidone taken to prepare the *Test solution;* and r_U and r_S are the peak responses for vinylpyrrolidinone obtained from the *Test solution* and *Standard solution,* respectively: not more than 0.001% is found.

K-value—Accurately weigh a quantity of undried Povidone equivalent on the anhydrous basis to the amount specified in the following table:

Nominal K-value	g
≤18	5.00
>18 to ≤95	1.00
>95	0.10

Dissolve it in about 50 mL of water in a 100-mL volumetric flask, dilute with water to volume, and mix. Allow to stand for 1 hour. Determine the viscosity, using a capillary-tube viscosimeter (see *Viscosity* ⟨911⟩), of this solution at 25 ± 0.2°. Calculate the K-value of Povidone by the formula:

$$[\sqrt{300c \log z + (c + 1.5c \log z)^2} + 1.5c \log z - c]/(0.15c + 0.003c^2),$$

in which c is the weight, in g, on the anhydrous basis, of the specimen tested in each 100.0 mL of solution; and z is the viscosity of the test solution relative to that of water.

Nitrogen content—Proceed as directed under *Nitrogen Determination, Method II* ⟨461⟩, using about 0.1 g of Povidone, accurately weighed. In the procedure, omit the use of hydrogen peroxide, use 5 g of a powdered mixture of potassium sulfate, cupric sulfate, and titanium dioxide (33 : 1 : 1), instead of potassium sulfate and cupric sulfate (10 : 1), and heat until a clear, light-green solution is obtained, then heat for a further 45 minutes: the nitrogen content, on the anhydrous basis, is not less than 11.5% and not more than 12.8%.

Povidone-Iodine

$(C_6H_9NO)_n \cdot xI$

2-Pyrrolidinone, 1-ethenyl-, homopolymer, compd. with iodine.
1-Vinyl-2-pyrrolidinone polymer, compound with iodine [25655-41-8].

» Povidone-Iodine is a complex of Iodine with Povidone. It contains not less than 9.0 percent and not more than 12.0 percent of available iodine (I), calculated on the dried basis.

Packaging and storage—Preserve in tight containers.
Identification—
   A: Add 1 drop of a solution (1 in 10) to a mixture of 1 mL of starch TS and 9 mL of water: a deep blue color is produced.
   B: Spread 1 mL of a solution (1 in 10) over an area of about 20 cm × 20 cm on a glass plate, and allow to air-dry at room temperature in an atmosphere of low humidity overnight: a brown, dry, non-smearing film is formed, and it dissolves readily in water.
Loss on drying ⟨731⟩—Dry 5.0 g of it at 105° until the difference between two successive weighings at 1-hour intervals is not greater than 5.0 mg: it loses not more than 8.0% of its weight.
Residue on ignition ⟨281⟩: not more than 0.025%, from 2 g.
Iodide ion—
   Determination of total iodine—Dissolve about 500 mg of Povidone-Iodine, accurately weighed, in 100 mL of water in a 250-mL conical flask. Add sodium bisulfite TS until the color of iodine has disappeared. Add 25.0 mL of 0.1 N silver nitrate VS and 10 mL of nitric acid, and mix. Titrate the excess silver nitrate with 0.1 N ammonium thiocyanate VS, using ferric ammonium sulfate TS as the indicator. Perform a blank determination (see *Residual Titrations* under *Titrimetry* ⟨541⟩). Each mL of 0.1 N silver nitrate is equivalent to 12.69 mg of I. From the percentage of total iodine, calculated on the dried basis, subtract the percentage of available iodine (see *Assay for available iodine*), to obtain the percentage of iodide ion. Not more than 6.6%, calculated on the dried basis, is found.
Heavy metals, *Method II* ⟨231⟩:   0.002%.
Nitrogen content ⟨461⟩—Not less than 9.5% and not more than 11.5% of N is found, calculated on the dried basis.
Assay for available iodine—Place about 5 g of Povidone-Iodine, accurately weighed, in a 400-mL beaker, and add 200 mL of water. Cover the beaker, and stir by mechanical means at room temperature for not more than 1 hour to dissolve as completely as possible. Titrate immediately with 0.1 N sodium thiosulfate VS, adding 3 mL of starch TS as the endpoint is approached. Perform a blank determination, and make any necessary correction. Each mL of 0.1 N sodium thiosulfate is equivalent to 12.69 mg of I.

Povidone-Iodine Topical Aerosol

» Povidone-Iodine Topical Aerosol is a solution of Povidone-Iodine under nitrogen in a pressurized container. It contains not less than 85.0 percent and not more than 120.0 percent of the labeled amount of iodine (I).

Packaging and storage—Preserve in pressurized containers, and avoid exposure to excessive heat.
Identification—Spray Topical Aerosol into a beaker or flask until about 50 mL has been collected, and allow to stand for 5 minutes to allow the entrapped propellant to escape. (Retain portions of the solution so obtained for the *pH* and *Assay* procedures.) The solution meets the requirements of the following tests.
   A: Add 1 mL of a dilution containing about 0.05% of iodine to a mixture of 1 mL of starch TS and 9 mL of water: a deep blue color is produced.
   B: Transfer 10 mL to a 50-mL conical flask, avoiding contact with the neck of the flask. Cover the mouth of the flask with a small disk of filter paper, and wet it with 1 drop of starch TS: no blue color appears within 60 seconds.
pH ⟨791⟩—The pH of the solution prepared for the *Identification* tests is not more than 6.0.
Other requirements—It meets the requirements for *Pressure Test, Minimum Fill,* and *Leakage Test* under *Aerosols, Nasal Sprays, Metered-Dose Inhalers, and Dry Powder Inhalers* ⟨601⟩.
Assay—Transfer an accurately measured volume of the solution of Topical Aerosol prepared for the *Identification* tests, equivalent to about 50 mg of iodine, to a 100-mL beaker, and dilute with water to a total volume of not less than 30 mL. Titrate immediately with 0.02 N sodium thiosulfate VS, determining the endpoint potentiometrically, using a platinum-calomel electrode system. Perform a blank determination, and make any necessary correction. Each mL of 0.02 N sodium thiosulfate is equivalent to 2.538 mg of iodine (I).

Povidone-Iodine Ointment

» Povidone-Iodine Ointment is an emulsion, solution, or suspension of Povidone-Iodine in a suitable water-soluble ointment base. It contains not less than 85.0 percent and not more than 120.0 percent of the labeled amount of iodine (I).

Packaging and storage—Preserve in tight containers.
Identification—
   A: Add 1 mL of an alcohol dilution of it containing about 0.05% of iodine to a mixture of 1 mL of starch TS and 9 mL of water: a deep blue color is produced.
   B: Place 10 g in a 50-mL beaker, avoiding contact with the walls of the beaker. Cover the mouth of the beaker with a disk of filter paper, and wet it with 1 drop of starch TS: no blue color appears within 60 seconds.
Minimum fill ⟨755⟩: meets the requirements.
pH ⟨791⟩: between 1.5 and 6.5, determined in a solution (1 in 20).
Assay—Transfer an accurately weighed quantity of Ointment, equivalent to about 50 mg of iodine, to a 100-mL beaker, add water to make a total volume of not less than 30 mL, and stir until the ointment is dissolved. Titrate immediately with 0.02 N sodium thiosulfate VS, determining the endpoint potentiometrically, using a platinum-calomel electrode system. Perform a blank determination, and make any necessary correction. Each mL of 0.02 N sodium thiosulfate is equivalent to 2.538 mg of I.

Povidone-Iodine Cleansing Solution

» Povidone-Iodine Cleansing Solution is a solution of Povidone-Iodine with one or more suitable surface-active agents. It contains not less than 85.0 percent and not more than 120.0 percent of the labeled amount of iodine (I). It may contain a small amount of alcohol.

Packaging and storage—Preserve in tight containers.
Identification—
   A: It responds to *Identification* tests A and B under *Povidone-Iodine Topical Aerosol*.
   B: To 2 mL of it in a glass-stoppered test tube add 1 mL of peanut oil and 4 mL of water, and shake vigorously for 10 seconds. Allow to stand for 3 minutes: a stable emulsion is formed.
pH ⟨791⟩: between 1.5 and 6.5.
Alcohol content (*if present*) ⟨611⟩:   between 90.0% and 110.0% of the labeled amount of C_2H_5OH.
Assay—Transfer to a 100-mL beaker an accurately measured volume of Solution, equivalent to about 50 mg of iodine, and add water to make a total volume of not less than 30 mL. Titrate immediately with 0.02 N sodium thiosulfate VS, determining the endpoint potentiometrically, using a platinum-calomel electrode system. Perform a blank determination, and make any necessary correction. Each mL of 0.02 N sodium thiosulfate is equivalent to 2.538 mg of I.

Povidone-Iodine Topical Solution

» Povidone-Iodine Topical Solution is a solution of Povidone-Iodine. It contains not less than 85.0 percent and not more than 120.0 percent of the labeled amount of iodine (I). It may contain a small amount of alcohol.

Packaging and storage—Preserve in tight containers.
Identification—It responds to *Identification* tests *A* and *B* under *Povidone-Iodine Topical Aerosol*.
pH ⟨791⟩: between 1.5 and 6.5.
Alcohol content (*if present*) ⟨611⟩: between 90.0% and 110.0% of the labeled amount of C_2H_5OH.
Assay—Transfer to a 100-mL beaker an accurately measured volume of *Topical Solution*, equivalent to about 50 mg of iodine, and add water to make a total volume of not less than 30 mL. Titrate immediately with 0.02 N sodium thiosulfate VS, determining the endpoint potentiometrically, using a platinum-calomel electrode system. Perform a blank determination, and make any necessary correction. Each mL of 0.02 N sodium thiosulfate is equivalent to 2.538 mg of I.

Pralidoxime Chloride

$C_7H_9ClN_2O$ 172.61
Pyridinium, 2-(hydroxyimino)methyl-1-methyl-, chloride.
2-Formyl-1-methylpyridinium chloride oxime   [51-15-0].

» Pralidoxime Chloride contains not less than 97.0 percent and not more than 102.0 percent of $C_7H_9ClN_2O$, calculated on the dried basis.

Packaging and storage—Preserve in well-closed containers.
Labeling—Where it is intended for use in preparing injectable dosage forms, the label states that it is sterile or must be subjected to further processing during the preparation of injectable dosage forms.
USP Reference standards ⟨11⟩—*USP Pralidoxime Chloride RS*. *USP Endotoxin RS*.
Identification—
  A: *Infrared Absorption* ⟨197M⟩.
  B: A solution (1 in 10) responds to the tests for *Chloride* ⟨191⟩.
  C: The retention time of the major peak in the chromatogram of the *Assay preparation* corresponds to that in the chromatogram of the *Standard preparation*, as obtained in the *Assay*.
Melting range ⟨741⟩: between 215° and 225°, with decomposition.
Loss on drying ⟨731⟩—Dry it at 105° for 3 hours: it loses not more than 2.0% of its weight.
Residue on ignition ⟨281⟩: not more than 0.5%.
Heavy metals, *Method I* ⟨231⟩: 0.002%.
Chloride content—Dissolve about 300 mg, accurately weighed, in 150 mL of water, add 20 mL of glacial acetic acid and 10 drops of (*p-tert*-octylphenoxy)nonaethoxyethanol, and titrate with 0.1 N silver nitrate VS, determining the endpoint potentiometrically. Perform a blank determination, and make any necessary correction. Each mL of 0.1 N silver nitrate is equivalent to 3.545 mg of Cl. Not less than 20.2% and not more than 20.8%, calculated on the dried basis, is found.
Other requirements—Where the label states that Pralidoxime Chloride is sterile, it meets the requirements for *Sterility Tests* ⟨71⟩ and for *Bacterial endotoxins* under *Pralidoxime Chloride for Injection*. Where the label states that Pralidoxime Chloride must be subjected to further processing during the preparation of injectable dosage forms, it meets the requirements for *Bacterial endotoxins* under *Pralidoxime Chloride for Injection*.
Assay—
  Dilute phosphoric acid solution—Transfer 10 mL of phosphoric acid to a 100-mL volumetric flask containing 50 mL of water, and mix. Dilute with water to volume, and mix.

  Tetraethylammonium chloride solution—Transfer about 170 mg of tetraethylammonium chloride to a 1-liter volumetric flask, add 3.4 mL of *Dilute phosphoric acid solution*, and add water to dissolve the mixture. Dilute with water to volume, and mix.
  Mobile phase—Prepare a filtered and degassed mixture of acetonitrile and *Tetraethylammonium chloride solution* (52 : 48). Make adjustments if necessary (see *System Suitability* under *Chromatography* ⟨621⟩).
  Standard preparation—Dissolve a suitable quantity of USP Pralidoxime Chloride RS, accurately weighed, in water to obtain a *Standard solution* having a known concentration of about 1.25 mg per mL. (Reserve a portion of the *Standard solution* for the *System suitability preparation*.) Pipet 2.0 mL of this solution into a 100-mL volumetric flask, dilute with *Mobile phase* to volume, and mix.
  Assay preparation—Transfer about 62.5 mg of Pralidoxime Chloride, accurately weighed, to a 50-mL volumetric flask, dissolve in water, dilute with water to volume, mix, and filter. Pipet 2.0 mL of this solution into a 100-mL volumetric flask, dilute with *Mobile phase* to volume, and mix.
  System suitability preparation—Prepare a solution of pyridine-2-aldoxime in water having a concentration of 0.65 mg per mL. Transfer 2.0 mL of this solution to a 100-mL volumetric flask, add 2.0 mL of the *Standard solution*, dilute with *Mobile phase* to volume, and mix.
  Chromatographic system (see *Chromatography* ⟨621⟩)—The liquid chromatograph is equipped with a 270-nm detector and a 3- to 5-mm × 25-cm column containing 5-µm packing L1. The flow rate is about 1.2 mL per minute. Chromatograph the *Standard preparation* and the *System suitability preparation* by injecting about 15 µL of these preparations, and record the peak responses as directed for *Procedure*: the resolution, *R*, between the pyridine-2-aldoxime and pralidoxime chloride peaks is not less than 4.0; the column efficiency determined from the analyte peak is not less than 4000 theoretical plates; the tailing factor for the analyte peak is not more than 2.5; and the relative standard deviation for replicate injections is not more than 2.0%.
  Procedure—Separately inject equal volumes (about 15 µL) of the *Standard preparation* and the *Assay preparation* into the chromatograph, record the chromatograms, and measure the responses for the major peaks. The relative retention times are about 0.6 for pyridine-2-aldoxime and 1.0 for pralidoxime chloride. Calculate the quantity, in mg, of $C_7H_9ClN_2O$ in the portion of Pralidoxime Chloride taken by the formula:

$$2.5C(r_U / r_S)$$

in which *C* is the concentration, in µg per mL, of USP Pralidoxime Chloride RS in the *Standard preparation*; and r_U and r_S are the peak responses obtained from the *Assay preparation* and the *Standard preparation*, respectively.

Pralidoxime Chloride for Injection

» Pralidoxime Chloride for Injection contains not less than 90.0 percent and not more than 110.0 percent of the labeled amount of pralidoxime chloride ($C_7H_9ClN_2O$).

Packaging and storage—Preserve in *Containers for Sterile Solids* as described under *Injections* ⟨1⟩.
USP Reference standards ⟨11⟩—*USP Pralidoxime Chloride RS*. *USP Endotoxin RS*.
Completeness of solution ⟨641⟩—The contents of 1 container dissolve in 10 mL of water to yield a clear solution.
Constituted solution—At the time of use, it meets the requirements for *Constituted Solutions* under *Injections* ⟨1⟩.
Bacterial endotoxins ⟨85⟩—It contains not more than 0.10 USP Endotoxin Unit per mg of pralidoxime chloride.
pH ⟨791⟩: between 3.5 and 4.5, in a solution (1 in 20).
Other requirements—It conforms to the Definition, responds to the *Identification* tests, and meets the requirements for *Loss on drying* and *Heavy metals* under *Pralidoxime Chloride*. It meets also the

requirements for *Sterility Tests* ⟨71⟩, *Uniformity of Dosage Units* ⟨905⟩, and *Labeling* under *Injections* ⟨1⟩.

Assay—
Dilute phosphoric acid solution, Tetraethylammonium chloride solution, Mobile phase, Standard preparation, System suitability preparation, and *Chromatographic system—*Proceed as directed in the *Assay* under *Pralidoxime Chloride.*

*Assay preparation—*Select an accurately counted number of containers of Pralidoxime Chloride for Injection, the combined contents of which are equivalent to about 10 g of pralidoxime chloride. Dissolve the contents of each container in water, and combine all of the solutions in a 1000-mL volumetric flask. Rinse each container with water, and add the rinsings to the volumetric flask. Dilute with water to volume, and mix. Transfer 25.0 mL of the resulting solution to a 200-mL volumetric flask, dilute with water to volume, and mix. Transfer 2.0 mL of this solution to a 100-mL volumetric flask, dilute with *Mobile phase* to volume, and mix.

*Procedure—*Proceed as directed for *Procedure* in the *Assay* under *Pralidoxime Chloride.* Calculate the quantity, in mg, of pralidoxime chloride ($C_7H_9ClN_2O$) in each container of Pralidoxime Chloride for Injection taken by the formula:

$$400(C/N)(r_U/r_S)$$

in which N is the number of containers selected for the *Assay preparation,* and the other terms are as defined therein.

Pramoxine Hydrochloride

$C_{17}H_{27}NO_3 \cdot HCl$ 329.86
Morpholine, 4-[3-(4-butoxyphenoxy)propyl]-, hydrochloride.
4-[3-(*p*-Butoxyphenoxy)propyl]morpholine hydrochloride [637-58-1].

» Pramoxine Hydrochloride contains not less than 98.0 percent and not more than 102.0 percent of $C_{17}H_{27}NO_3 \cdot HCl$, calculated on the dried basis.

Packaging and storage—Preserve in tight containers.
USP Reference standards ⟨11⟩—*USP Pramoxine Hydrochloride RS.*
Identification—
   A: *Infrared Absorption* ⟨197K⟩.
   B: The retention time of the major peak in the chromatogram of the *Assay preparation* corresponds to that in the chromatogram of the *Standard preparation,* as obtained in the *Assay.*
   C: It meets the requirements of the tests for *Chloride* ⟨191⟩.
Melting range ⟨741⟩: between 170° and 174°.
Loss on drying ⟨731⟩—Dry it at 105° for 1 hour: it loses not more than 1.0% of its weight.
Residue on ignition ⟨281⟩: not more than 0.1%.
Assay—
   *pH 7.5 Phosphate buffer—*Dissolve 8.71 g of dibasic potassium phosphate in about 800 mL of water, adjust with dilute phosphoric acid (1 in 10) to a pH of 7.5 ± 0.1, add water to make 1000 mL, and mix.
   *Mobile phase—*Prepare a filtered and degassed mixture of acetonitrile and *pH 7.5 Phosphate buffer* (55 : 45). Make adjustments if necessary (see *System Suitability* under *Chromatography* ⟨621⟩).
   *Standard preparation—*Dissolve an accurately weighed quantity of USP Pramoxine Hydrochloride RS in *Mobile phase* to obtain a solution having a known concentration of about 0.5 mg per mL.
   *Assay preparation—*Transfer about 50 mg of Pramoxine Hydrochloride, accurately weighed, to a 100-mL volumetric flask, dissolve in and dilute with *Mobile phase* to volume, and mix.
   Chromatographic system (see *Chromatography* ⟨621⟩)—The liquid chromatograph is equipped with a 224-nm detector and a 4.6-mm × 25-cm column that contains packing L1. The column temperature is maintained at 40°, and the flow rate is about 2 mL per minute. Chromatograph the *Standard preparation,* and record the peak responses as directed for *Procedure:* the column efficiency is not less than 1500 theoretical plates; the tailing factor is not more than 1.5; and the relative standard deviation for replicate injections is not more than 1.5%.
   *Procedure—*Separately inject equal volumes (about 20 µL) of the *Standard preparation* and the *Assay preparation* into the chromatograph, record the chromatograms, and measure the responses for the major peaks. Calculate the quantity, in mg, of $C_{17}H_{27}NO_3 \cdot HCl$ in the portion of Pramoxine Hydrochloride taken by the formula:

$$100C(r_U/r_S)$$

in which C is the concentration, in mg per mL, of USP Pramoxine Hydrochloride RS in the *Standard preparation;* and r_U and r_S are the peak responses obtained from the *Assay preparation* and the *Standard preparation,* respectively.

Pramoxine Hydrochloride Cream

» Pramoxine Hydrochloride Cream contains not less than 90.0 percent and not more than 110.0 percent of the labeled amount of $C_{17}H_{27}NO_3 \cdot HCl$ in a suitable water-miscible base.

Packaging and storage—Preserve in tight containers.
USP Reference standards ⟨11⟩—*USP Pramoxine Hydrochloride RS.*
Identification—
   A: Dissolve a quantity of Cream, equivalent to about 50 mg of pramoxine hydrochloride, in a mixture of 25 mL of methanol and 75 mL of ether, and extract with three 25-mL portions of a mixture of equal volumes of 3 N hydrochloric acid and water. Discard the methanol-ether solution, render the combined extracts alkaline with 25 mL of 5 N sodium hydroxide, and extract the pramoxine with 50 mL of chloroform. Evaporate the clear chloroform extract with the aid of a current of air to dryness: the UV absorption spectrum of a 1 in 100,000 solution of the residue so obtained, in 0.1 N hydrochloric acid, exhibits maxima and minima at the same wavelengths as that of a similar solution of the residue similarly obtained from USP Pramoxine Hydrochloride RS, concomitantly measured.
   B: To a 5-mg portion of the pramoxine obtained in *Identification* test *A* add 1 drop of nitric acid. To the yellow solution cautiously add 5 drops of ammonium hydroxide: a red-brown precipitate is formed.
Microbial limits ⟨61⟩—It meets the requirements of the tests for absence of *Staphylococcus aureus* and *Pseudomonas aeruginosa.*
Minimum fill ⟨755⟩: meets the requirements.
Assay—
   *pH 7.5 phosphate buffer—*Dissolve 3.5 g of dibasic potassium phosphate in 100 mL of water, and adjust the solution by the addition of phosphoric acid solution (1 : 1) to a pH of 7.5 ± 0.1.
   *Mobile phase—*Prepare a suitable degassed and filtered mixture of acetonitrile, water, and *pH 7.5 phosphate buffer* (22 : 17 : 1).
   *Internal standard solution—*Prepare a solution of dibutyl phthalate in methanol having a final concentration of about 4 µL per mL.
   *Standard preparation—*Prepare a solution of USP Pramoxine Hydrochloride RS in methanol having a known concentration of about 2 mg per mL. Pipet 10 mL of this solution and 5 mL of *Internal standard solution* into a 100-mL volumetric flask, dilute with methanol to volume, mix, and filter.
   *Assay preparation—*Transfer an accurately weighed portion of Cream, equivalent to about 18 mg of pramoxine hydrochloride, to a glass-stoppered, 250-mL conical flask. Add 15.0 mL of isopropyl alcohol and 40.0 mL of methanol, heat on a steam bath, with swirling, to dissolve the Cream, add 40.0 mL of methanol and 5.0 mL of *Internal standard solution,* and mix. Cool the flask to a temperature of 10° or less to precipitate the waxes, and filter the solution.
   Chromatographic system (see *Chromatography* ⟨621⟩)—The liquid chromatograph is equipped with a 224-nm detector, a 4.6-mm × 3-cm guard column that contains packing L1, and a 4-mm × 30-cm

analytical column that contains packing L1. The flow rate is about 2 mL per minute. Chromatograph three replicate injections of the *Standard preparation*, and record the peak responses as directed for *Procedure:* the relative standard deviation is not more than 2.0%, and the resolution factor between pramoxine hydrochloride and dibutyl phthalate is not less than 2.4.

Procedure—Separately inject equal volumes (about 20 µL) of the *Standard preparation* and the *Assay preparation* into the chromatograph, record the chromatograms, and measure the responses for the major peaks. The relative retention times are about 0.8 for pramoxine hydrochloride and 1.0 for dibutyl phthalate. Calculate the quantity, in mg, of pramoxine hydrochloride in the portion of Cream taken by the formula:

$$100C(R_U / R_S)$$

in which C is the concentration, in mg per mL, of USP Pramoxine Hydrochloride RS in the *Standard preparation*, and R_U and R_S are the peak response ratios of pramoxine hydrochloride and internal standard obtained from the *Assay preparation* and the *Standard preparation*, respectively.

Pramoxine Hydrochloride Jelly

» Pramoxine Hydrochloride Jelly contains not less than 94.0 percent and not more than 106.0 percent of the labeled amount of $C_{17}H_{27}NO_3 \cdot HCl$.

Packaging and storage—Preserve in tight containers, preferably in collapsible tubes.

USP Reference standards ⟨11⟩—*USP Pramoxine Hydrochloride RS.*

Identification—Place a quantity of Jelly, equivalent to about 5 mg of pramoxine hydrochloride, in a glass-stoppered conical flask, add 25 mL of chloroform, and shake for 15 minutes. Filter into a small porcelain evaporating dish, and evaporate in a current of air on a steam bath. Add 1 drop of nitric acid to the residue, and to the resulting yellow solution cautiously add 5 drops of ammonium hydroxide: a red-brown precipitate is formed.

Microbial limits ⟨61⟩—It meets the requirements of the tests for absence of *Staphylococcus aureus* and *Pseudomonas aeruginosa*.

Assay—

Standard preparation—Dissolve a suitable quantity of USP Pramoxine Hydrochloride RS, accurately weighed, in 0.5 N sulfuric acid, and dilute quantitatively with the same solvent to obtain a solution having a known concentration of about 150 µg per mL.

Assay preparation—[NOTE—If emulsions form, 2 to 5 mL of alcohol may be added to separate the phases.] Transfer an accurately weighed quantity of Jelly, equivalent to about 15 mg of pramoxine hydrochloride, to a small beaker, and dissolve the Jelly in 0.1 N sulfuric acid, using four 5-mL portions, warming each portion on a steam bath, and transferring to a 125-mL separator. Shake the separator vigorously after each transfer to complete dissolution of the Jelly. To the cooled solution in the separator add 20 mL of ether, shake carefully, and proceed as directed for *Assay Preparation* under *Salts of Organic Nitrogenous Bases* ⟨501⟩, beginning with "filter the acid phase into a second 125-mL separator," except to combine the final 0.5 N sulfuric acid extracts in a 100-mL volumetric flask, dilute with the acid to volume, and mix.

Procedure—Proceed as directed under *Salts of Organic Nitrogenous Bases* ⟨501⟩, diluting 20.0 mL each of the *Standard preparation* and the *Assay preparation* with 0.5 N sulfuric acid to 50.0 mL, and determining the absorbances at the wavelength of maximum absorbance at about 286 nm. Calculate the quantity, in mg, of $C_{17}H_{27}NO_3 \cdot HCl$ in the portion of Jelly taken by the formula:

$$0.1C(A_U / A_S)$$

in which C is the concentration, in µg per mL, of USP Pramoxine Hydrochloride RS in the *Standard preparation*.

Pravastatin Sodium

$C_{23}H_{35}NaO_7$ 446.51

1-Naphthaleneheptanoic acid, 1,2,6,7,8,8a-hexahydro-β,δ,6-trihydroxy-2-methyl-8-(2-methyl-1-oxobutoxy)-, monosodium salt, [1S-[1α($\beta S^*,\delta S^*$),2α,6α,8$\beta(R^*)$,8aα]]-.

Sodium (+)-($\beta R,\delta R$,1S, 2S,6S,8S,8aR)-1,2,6,7,8,8a-hexahydro-β,δ,6,8-tetrahydroxy-2-methyl-1-naphthaleneheptanoate, 8-[(2S)-2-methylbutyrate]   [81131-70-6].

» Pravastatin Sodium contains not less than 97.5 percent and not more than 102.0 percent of $C_{23}H_{35}NaO_7$, calculated on the anhydrous and solvent-free basis.

Packaging and storage—Preserve in tight containers. Store as per labeling instructions. Possible storage conditions could include the following, in the presence of stability data supporting the condition: Store under nitrogen in a cold place. Store at room temperature.

USP Reference standards ⟨11⟩—*USP Pravastatin 1,1,3,3-Tetramethylbutylamine RS. USP Pravastatin Sodium RS. USP Pravastatin Related Compound A RS.*

Identification—

A: *Infrared Absorption* ⟨197K⟩.

B: It meets the requirements of the pyroantimonate precipitation test for *Sodium* ⟨191⟩.

Specific rotation ⟨781⟩:   between +150° and +160° (at 20°), calculated on the anhydrous and solvent-free basis.

Test solution: 5 mg per mL in water.

pH ⟨791⟩:   between 7.2 and 9.0, in a solution (1 in 20).

Water, *Method I* ⟨921⟩:   not more than 4.0%.

Heavy metals, *Method II* ⟨231⟩:   0.002%.

Limit of alcohol *(if present)*—

Test solution—Transfer about 0.2 g of Pravastatin Sodium, accurately weighed, to a 20-mL volumetric flask, dilute with water to volume, and mix. Pipet 5 mL of this solution into a vial fitted with a septum and a crimp cap, add 1 mL of water, seal the vial, and mix. Heat the sealed vial at 80° for 60 minutes.

Standard solution—Pipet 2 mL of dehydrated alcohol into a 100-mL volumetric flask, dilute with water to volume, and mix. Pipet 10 mL of this solution into a 100-mL volumetric flask, dilute with water to volume, and mix. Pipet 1 mL of this solution into a vial fitted with a septum and a crimp cap, and calculate the amount of alcohol, W_A, added, in g, the specific gravity of dehydrated alcohol being 0.79 g per mL. Add 5 mL of the *Test solution* to the same vial, seal the vial, and mix. Heat the sealed vial at 80° for 60 minutes.

Blank solution—Pipet 6 mL of water into a vial fitted with a septum and a crimp cap, and seal the vial. Heat the sealed vial at 80° for 60 minutes.

Chromatographic system (see *Chromatography* ⟨621⟩)—The gas chromatograph is equipped with a flame-ionization detector and a 0.53-mm × 30-m fused silica capillary column coated with a 3-µm film of stationary phase G43. The carrier gas is helium, with a split ratio of 1 : 5, and flowing with a linear velocity of about 35 cm per second. The chromatograph is programmed as follows. The column temperature is maintained at 40° for 20 minutes, then the temperature is increased at a rate of 10° per minute to 240°, and maintained at 240° for 20 minutes. The transfer line temperature is maintained at 85°, the injection port temperature is maintained at 140°, and the detector is maintained at 250°. Chromatograph the *Blank solution*, and record the peak responses as directed for *Procedure:* no interfering peaks are observed.

Procedure—Separately inject equal volumes (about 1 mL) of headspace gas of the *Standard solution* and the *Test solution* into the chromatograph, record the chromatograms, and measure the area responses for the major peaks. Calculate the percentage (w/w) of alcohol in the portion of Pravastatin Sodium taken by the formula:

$$100(W_A/W)(V/5)[r_U/(r_S-r_U)]$$

in which W_A is as defined above; W is the weight, in g, of Pravastatin Sodium taken to prepare the *Test solution*; V is the volume, in mL, of the *Test solution*; 5 is the volume, in mL, of the *Test solution* taken; and r_U and r_S are the peak area responses of alcohol obtained from the *Test solution* and the *Standard solution*, respectively: not more than 3.0% is found.

Chromatographic purity—[NOTE—The *Standard solution* and the *Test solution* are maintained at 15° until injected into the chromatograph.]

Diluent—Prepare a mixture of methanol and water (1 : 1).

Buffer pH 7.0—Prepare a 0.08 M phosphoric acid solution, adjust with triethylamine to a pH of 7.0, and mix.

Solution A—Prepare a filtered and degassed mixture of water, *Buffer pH 7.0*, and acetonitrile (52 : 30 : 18).

Solution B—Prepare a filtered and degassed mixture of acetonitrile, *Buffer pH 7.0*, and water (60 : 30 : 10).

Mobile phase—Use variable mixtures of *Solution A* and *Solution B* as directed for *Chromatographic system*. Make adjustments if necessary (see *System Suitability* under *Chromatography* ⟨621⟩).

Standard solution—Dissolve an accurately weighed quantity of USP Pravastatin 1,1,3,3-Tetramethylbutylamine RS in *Diluent*, and dilute quantitatively, and stepwise if necessary, with *Diluent* to obtain a solution having a known concentration of about 1.25 μg of pravastatin 1,1,3,3-tetramethylbutylamine per mL.

System suitability solution—Dissolve accurately weighed quantities of USP Pravastatin 1,1,3,3-Tetramethylbutylamine RS and USP Pravastatin Related Compound A RS in *Diluent* to obtain a solution containing about 0.6 mg of USP Pravastatin 1,1,3,3-tetramethylbutylamine RS and 0.001 mg of USP Pravastatin Related Compound A RS per mL. [NOTE—USP Pravastatin Related Compound A RS is a sodium salt of 3α-hydroxyisocompactin acid.]

Test solution—Transfer about 50 mg of Pravastatin Sodium, accurately weighed, to a 100-mL volumetric flask, dissolve in and dilute with *Diluent* to volume, and mix.

Chromatographic system (see *Chromatography* ⟨621⟩—The liquid chromatograph is equipped with a 238-nm detector and a 4.6-mm × 7.5-cm column that contains 3.5-μm packing L1. Alternatively, a 4.0-mm × 10-cm column that contains 3-μm packing L1 can be used. The flow rate is about 1 mL per minute. The chromatograph is programmed as follows.

Time (minutes)	Solution A (%)	Solution B (%)	Elution
0–3.0	100	0	isocratic
3.0–26.5	100→0	0→100	linear gradient
26.5–26.6	0→100	100→0	linear gradient
26.6–30.0	100	0	re-equilibration

Chromatograph the *System suitability solution*, and record the peak responses as directed for *Procedure*: the relative retention times are about 1.0 for pravastatin and 1.1 for pravastatin related compound A; and the resolution, R, between pravastatin and pravastatin related compound A is not less than 2.0. Chromatograph the *Standard solution*, and record the peak responses as directed for *Procedure*: the relative standard deviation for replicate injections is not more than 10.0%.

Procedure—Separately inject equal volumes (about 10 μL) of the *Standard solution* and the *Test solution* into the chromatograph, record the chromatograms, identify the impurities listed in *Table 1*, and measure the peak responses. Calculate the percentage of each impurity in the portion of Pravastatin Sodium taken by the formula:

$$100 \times (446.51/553.78)C(V/W)(r_i/r_S)$$

in which 446.51 and 553.78 are the molecular weights of pravastatin sodium and pravastatin 1,1,3,3-tetramethylbutylamine, respectively; C is the concentration, in mg per mL, of pravastatin 1,1,3,3-tetramethylbutylamine in the *Standard solution*; V is the volume, in mL, of the *Test solution*; W is the weight, in mg, of Pravastatin Sodium taken to prepare the *Test solution*; r_i is the peak response for each impurity obtained from the *Test solution*; and r_S is the pravastatin peak response obtained from the *Standard solution*. In addition to not exceeding the limits for each impurity specified in *Table 1*, not more than 0.1% of any other individual impurity is found, and not more than 0.6% of total impurities is found.

Table 1

Name	Relative Retention Time	Limit (%)
3″-Hydroxypravastatin	0.33	0.2
6′-Epipravastatin	0.92	0.3
3α-Hydroxyisocompactin[1]	1.1	0.2
Pentanoyl impurity[2]	1.2	0.2
Pravastatin lactone	1.8	0.2
Compactin	3.1	0.2

[1] Sodium (3R,5R)-3,5-dihydroxy-7-[(1S,2S,3S,8S,8aR)-3-hydroxy-2-methyl-8-[[(2S)-2-methylbutanoyl]oxy]-1,2,3,7,8,8a-hexahydronaphthalen-1-yl]heptanoate (pravastatin related compound A).

[2] (3R,5R)-3,5-dihydroxy-7-[(1S,2S,6S,8S,8aR)-6-hydroxy-2-methyl-8-[[(2S)-2-methylpentanoyl]oxy]-1,2,6,7,8,8a-hexahydronaphthalen-1-yl]heptanoic acid.

Assay—

Solution A—Prepare a 0.08 M phosphoric acid solution, adjust with a 25% sodium hydroxide solution to a pH of 5.0, mix, filter, and degas.

Solution B—Use acetonitrile.

Mobile phase—Use variable mixtures of *Solution A* and *Solution B* as directed for *Chromatographic system*. Make adjustments if necessary (see *System Suitability* under *Chromatography* ⟨621⟩).

Standard preparation—Dissolve an accurately weighed quantity of USP Pravastatin 1,1,3,3-Tetramethylbutylamine RS in methanol, and dilute quantitatively, and stepwise if necessary, with methanol to obtain a solution having a known concentration of about 0.25 mg of pravastatin 1,1,3,3-tetramethylbutylamine per mL.

System suitability preparation—Dissolve accurately weighed quantities of USP Pravastatin 1,1,3,3-Tetramethylbutylamine RS and USP Pravastatin Related Compound A RS in methanol to obtain a solution containing about 0.25 mg of USP Pravastatin 1,1,3,3-Tetramethylbutylamine RS and 0.001 mg of USP Pravastatin Related Compound A RS per mL.

Assay preparation—Transfer about 20 mg of Pravastatin Sodium, accurately weighed, to a 100-mL volumetric flask, dissolve in and dilute with methanol to volume, and mix.

Chromatographic system (see *Chromatography* ⟨621⟩—The liquid chromatograph is equipped with a 238-nm detector and a 4.0-mm × 10-cm column that contains 3-μm packing L1. The flow rate is about 1 mL per minute. The chromatograph is programmed as follows.

Time (minutes)	Solution A (%)	Solution B (%)	Elution
0–7.0	80→72	20→28	linear gradient
7.0–10.0	72→50	28→50	linear gradient
10.0–17.0	50	50	isocratic
17.0–17.1	50→80	50→20	linear gradient
17.1–20.0	80	20	re-equilibration

Chromatograph the *System suitability preparation*, and record the peak responses as directed for *Procedure*: the relative retention times are about 1.0 for pravastatin and 1.2 for pravastatin related compound A; the resolution, R, between pravastatin and pravastatin related compound A is not less than 1.2; and the relative standard deviation for replicate injections for the pravastatin peak is not more than 2.0%.

Procedure—Separately inject equal volumes (about 10 μL) of the *Standard preparation* and the *Assay preparation* into the chromatograph, record the chromatograms, and measure the responses for the

pravastatin peaks. Calculate the quantity, in mg, of $C_{23}H_{35}NaO_7$ in the portion of Pravastatin Sodium taken by the formula:

$$(446.51/553.78)VC(r_U/r_S)$$

in which 446.51 and 553.78 are the molecular weights of pravastatin sodium and pravastatin 1,1,3,3-tetramethylbutylamine, respectively; V is the volume, in mL, of the *Assay preparation;* C is the concentration, in mg per mL, of pravastatin 1,1,3,3-tetramethylbutylamine in the *Standard preparation;* and r_U and r_S are the responses of the pravastatin peak obtained from the *Assay preparation* and the *Standard preparation,* respectively.

Pravastatin Sodium Tablets

» Pravastatin Sodium contains not less than 90.0 percent and not more than 110.0 percent of the labeled amount of pravastatin sodium ($C_{23}H_{35}NaO_7$).

Packaging and storage—Preserve in tight containers. Protect from moisture and light. Store at controlled room temperature.

USP Reference standards ⟨11⟩—*USP Pravastatin Related Compound B RS. USP Pravastatin Sodium RS. USP Pravastatin 1,1,3,3-Tetramethylbutylamine RS.*

Identification—
  A: The retention time of the major peak in the chromatogram of the *Assay preparation* corresponds to that in the chromatogram of the *Standard preparation,* as obtained in the *Assay.*
  B: *Ultraviolet Absorption* ⟨197U⟩—Finely powder a number of Tablets, and extract with water a portion equivalent to about 10 mg of pravastatin sodium. The UV absorption spectrum of a solution of pravastatin sodium in water containing about 10 μg per mL exhibits maxima at the same wavelength as that of a similar solution of USP Pravastatin Sodium RS, concomitantly measured between 220 and 340 nm.

Dissolution ⟨711⟩—
  Medium: water; 900 mL.
  Apparatus 2: 50 rpm.
  Time: 30 minutes.
  *Procedure—*Determine the amount of $C_{23}H_{35}NaO_7$ dissolved by employing UV absorption at the wavelength of maximum absorbance at about 238 nm on filtered portions of the solution under test, suitably diluted with *Medium,* if necessary, in comparison with a Standard solution having a known concentration of USP Pravastatin 1,1,3,3-Tetramethylbutylamine RS in the same *Medium.* [NOTE—To express the concentration of the Standard solution as pravastatin sodium, use the conversion factor of (446.51/553.78), in which 446.51 and 553.78 are the molecular weights of pravastatin sodium and pravastatin 1,1,3,3-tetramethylbutylamine, respectively.]
  *Tolerances—*Not less than 80% (*Q*) of the labeled amount of $C_{23}H_{35}NaO_7$ is dissolved in 30 minutes.

Uniformity of dosage units ⟨905⟩: meet the requirements.

Related compounds—
  Mobile phase and *Chromatographic system—*Proceed as directed in the *Assay.*
  *Test solution—*Use the *Assay preparation,* prepared as directed in the *Assay.* [NOTE—Use this solution within 24 hours of preparation.]
  *Procedure—*Inject a volume (about 20 μL) of the *Test solution* into the chromatograph, record the chromatograms for up to 4 times the retention time of the pravastatin peak, identify the impurities listed in *Table 1,* and measure the peak responses. Calculate the percentage of each impurity in the portion of Tablets taken by the formula:

$$100(r_i/r_s)$$

in which r_i is the peak response of the individual impurity, and r_s is the sum of the responses of all the peaks obtained from the *Test solution.* In addition to not exceeding the limits of each impurity in *Table 1,* not more than 0.2% of any unspecified individual impurity is found, and not more than 3% of total impurities is found. Disregard the peak due to pravastatin related compound B that elutes at the relative retention time of about 0.7 and the peak due to 3″-hydroxypravastatin at the relative retention time of about 0.3, as these impurities are controlled in the drug substance monograph. Disregard any impurity that is less than 0.05%.

Table 1

Name	Relative Retention Time	Limit (%)
Oxidation impurity[1]	0.5	1
Pravastatin sodium	1.0	n/a
Specified unknown impurity 1	1.6	0.2
Specified unknown impurity 2	1.8	0.2
Pravastatin lactone	2.1	2
Specified unknown impurity 3	2.8	0.2
Specified unknown impurity 4	3.2	0.2
Specified unknown impurity 5	3.8	0.2

[1] Sodium (3R,5R)-3,5-dihydroxy-7-((1S,2S)-6-hydroxy-2-methyl-1,2-dihydronaphthalen-1-yl)heptanoate.

Assay—[NOTE—The *Standard preparation, Assay stock preparation,* and *Assay preparation* can be stored for up to 7 days at room temperature.]

*Mobile phase—*Prepare a filtered and degassed mixture of methanol, water, glacial acetic acid, and triethylamine (500 : 500 : 1 : 1). Make adjustments if necessary (see *System Suitability* under *Chromatography* ⟨621⟩).

*Diluent 1—*Transfer 16.4 g of anhydrous sodium acetate into a 2000-mL volumetric flask. Add 1600 mL of water, adjust with glacial acetic acid to a pH of 5.6, dilute with water to volume, and mix.

*Diluent 2—*Prepare a mixture of *Diluent 1* and methanol (80 : 20).

*Standard preparation—*Transfer an accurately weighed quantity of USP Pravastatin 1,1,3,3-Tetramethylbutylamine RS to a suitable volumetric flask, and dissolve in *Diluent 1* using sonication to obtain a solution having a known concentration of about 0.6 mg of pravastatin 1,1,3,3-tetramethylbutylamine per mL. Dilute 5.0 mL of this solution with *Diluent 2* to 25.0 mL, and mix.

*Assay stock preparation—*Transfer not fewer than 5 Tablets to a suitable volumetric flask with at least a ($NL\times2$)-mL capacity, N being the number of Tablets transferred, and L being the label claim per Tablet, filled to at least 80% capacity with *Diluent 1.* [NOTE—It is necessary to fill the flask to 80% capacity to maintain the correct pH throughout the preparation.] Shake for at least 1 hour, and sonicate for at least 15 minutes with periodic shaking of the flask by hand, until the Tablets have completely disintegrated. Allow to cool, and dilute with *Diluent 1* to volume. Centrifuge a portion of the solution for 15 minutes at 2000 rpm, or filter.

*Assay preparation—*Dilute approximately 5 mL of the *Assay stock preparation* with *Diluent 2* to obtain a solution having an expected concentration of about 0.1 mg per mL, based on the label claim.

*Resolution solution—*Transfer about 2 mg of USP Pravastatin Related Compound B RS to a 10-mL volumetric flask. Dissolve in and dilute with methanol to volume. Transfer 0.1 mL of this solution and 1.0 mL of the *Standard preparation* to a small tube, and mix. [NOTE—Pravastatin related compound B is the 6′-epipravastatin sodium.]

Chromatographic system (see *Chromatography* ⟨621⟩)—The liquid chromatograph is equipped with a 238-nm detector and a 4.6-mm × 5-cm column than contains endcapped packing L1. Alternatively, a 3.9-mm × 7.5-cm column containing endcapped packing L1 can be used. The flow rate is about 1.0 mL per minute. Chromatograph the *Resolution solution,* and record the peak responses as directed for *Procedure:* the relative retention times are about 0.7 for pravastatin related compound B and 1.0 for pravastatin; the reso-

3056 **Pravastatin** / *Official Monographs*

lution, R, between the pravastatin related compound B and the pravastatin peaks is not less than 3.0. Chromatograph the *Standard preparation*, and record the peak responses as directed for *Procedure*: the relative standard deviation for replicate injections is not more than 2.0%.

Procedure—Separately inject equal volumes (about 20 µL) of the *Standard preparation* and the *Assay preparation* into the chromatograph, record the chromatograms, and measure the peak response for pravastatin. Calculate the percentage of pravastatin sodium ($C_{23}H_{35}NaO_7$) in the portion of Tablets taken by the formula:

$$100(446.51/553.78)(CVD/NL)(r_U / r_S)$$

in which 100 is the conversion factor to percentage; 446.51 and 553.78 are the molecular weights of pravastatin sodium and pravastatin 1,1,3,3-tetramethylbutylamine, respectively; C is the concentration, in mg per mL, of pravastatin 1,1,3,3-tetramethylbutylamine in the *Standard preparation*; V is the volume, in mL, of the *Assay stock preparation*; D is the dilution factor of the *Assay preparation*; N is the number of Tablets taken to prepare the *Assay stock preparation*; L is the label claim, in mg of pravastatin sodium per Tablet; and r_U and r_S are the pravastatin peak responses obtained from the *Assay preparation* and the *Standard preparation*, respectively.

Praziquantel

$C_{19}H_{24}N_2O_2$ 312.41
4*H*-Pyrazino[2,1-*a*]isoquinolin-4-one, 2-(cyclohexylcarbonyl)-1,2,3,6,7,11b-hexahydro-.
2-(Cyclohexylcarbonyl)-1,2,3,6,7,11b-hexahydro-4*H*-pyrazino-[2,1-*a*]isoquinolin-4-one   [55268-74-1].

» Praziquantel contains not less than 98.5 percent and not more than 101.0 percent of $C_{19}H_{24}N_2O_2$, calculated on the dried basis.

Packaging and storage—Preserve in well-closed, light-resistant containers.
USP Reference standards ⟨11⟩—*USP Praziquantel RS. USP Praziquantel Related Compound A RS. USP Praziquantel Related Compound B RS. USP Praziquantel Related Compound C RS.*
Identification, *Infrared Absorption* ⟨197K⟩.
Melting range ⟨741⟩: between 136° and 142°.
Loss on drying ⟨731⟩—Dry it in vacuum at a pressure not exceeding 5 mm of mercury at 50° over phosphorus pentoxide for 2 hours: it loses not more than 0.5% of its weight.
Residue on ignition ⟨281⟩: not more than 0.1%.
Phosphate—
Cupric sulfate solution—Dissolve 250 mg of cupric sulfate and 4.5 g of ammonium acetate in sufficient 2 N acetic acid to obtain 100 mL of solution.
4-Amino-3-hydroxy-1-naphthalenesulfonic acid solution—Grind in a mortar 5 g of sodium sulfite, 94.3 g of sodium metabisulfite, and 700 mg of 4-amino-3-hydroxy-1-naphthalenesulfonic acid. Dissolve 1.5 g of this mixture in 10 mL of water, heating gently if necessary. Use this solution only when freshly prepared.
Standard solution—Dissolve 143.3 mg of dried monobasic potassium phosphate in water to make 1000 mL of solution. Transfer 5.0 mL of this solution to a 100-mL volumetric flask, dilute with water to volume, and mix. This solution contains the equivalent of 5 µg of phosphate (PO_4) in each mL.
Test solution—Add 30 mL of water to 500 mg of specimen, and heat to boiling. Allow to cool, and filter, collecting the filtrate in a 50-mL volumetric flask. Wash the filter with water, collecting the washings in the volumetric flask, dilute with water to volume, and mix.

Procedure—Treat 10 mL of *Test solution* and 10 mL of *Standard solution* as follows. To each add 5 mL of *Cupric sulfate solution*, 2 mL of ammonium molybdate solution (3 in 100), 1 mL of *4-Amino-3-hydroxy-1-naphthalenesulfonic acid solution*, and 1 mL of perchloric acid solution (3 in 100), mix, and allow to stand for 15 minutes: the *Test solution* does not have a blue color that is darker than that of the *Standard solution* (0.05%).
Heavy metals, *Method II* ⟨231⟩: 0.002%.
Related compounds—
Mobile phase and *Chromatographic system*—Prepare as directed in the *Assay*.
Standard preparation—Dissolve accurately weighed quantities of USP Praziquantel Related Compound A RS, USP Praziquantel Related Compound B RS, and USP Praziquantel Related Compound C RS in *Mobile phase* to obtain a single solution having known concentrations of about 0.04 mg of each per mL.
Test preparation—Transfer about 200 mg of Praziquantel, accurately weighed, to a 10-mL volumetric flask, dissolve in and dilute with *Mobile phase* to volume, and mix.
Procedure—Separately inject equal volumes (about 10 µL) of the *Standard preparation* and the *Test preparation* into the chromatograph, record the chromatograms, and measure the responses for the peaks. The relative retention times are about 0.8 for praziquantel related compound A, 1.0 for praziquantel, 1.8 for praziquantel related compound B, and 2.1 for praziquantel related compound C. Calculate, in turn, the percentages of 2-benzoyl-1,2,3,6,7,11b-hexahydro-4*H*-pyrazino[2,1-*a*]isoquinolin-4-one (praziquantel related compound A), 2-(cyclohexylcarbonyl)-2,3,6,7-tetrahydro-4*H*-pyrazino[2,1-*a*]isoquinolin-4-one (praziquantel related compound B), and 2-(N-formylhexahydrohippuroyl)-1,2,3,4-tetrahydroisoquinolin-1-one (praziquantel related compound C) in the portion of Praziquantel taken by the formula:

$$1000(C/W)(r_U / r_S)$$

in which C is the concentration, in mg per mL, of the respective USP Reference Standard taken to prepare the *Standard preparation*; W is the weight, in mg, of Praziquantel taken to prepare the *Test preparation*; and r_U and r_S are the peak responses at corresponding retention times, obtained from the *Test preparation* and the *Standard preparation*, respectively. Not more than 0.2% of each is found.
Assay—
Mobile phase—Prepare a suitable degassed mixture of acetonitrile and water (60 : 40). Make adjustments if necessary (see *System Suitability* under *Chromatography* ⟨621⟩).
Standard preparation—Dissolve an accurately weighed quantity of USP Praziquantel RS in *Mobile phase*, and dilute quantitatively, and stepwise if necessary, with *Mobile phase* to obtain a solution having a known concentration of about 0.18 mg per mL.
Assay preparation—Transfer about 36 mg of Praziquantel, accurately weighed, to a 20-mL volumetric flask, dissolve in and dilute with *Mobile phase* to volume, and mix. Transfer 5.0 mL of the solution so obtained to a 50-mL volumetric flask, dilute with *Mobile phase* to volume, and mix.
Chromatographic system (see *Chromatography* ⟨621⟩)—The liquid chromatograph is equipped with a 210-nm detector and a 4-mm × 25-cm column that contains 10-µm packing L1. The flow rate is about 1.5 mL per minute. Chromatograph the *Standard preparation*, and record the peak responses as directed for *Procedure*: the tailing factor is not more than 1.5; and the relative standard deviation for replicate injections is not more than 1.0%.
Procedure—Separately inject equal volumes (about 10 µL) of the *Standard preparation* and the *Assay preparation* into the chromatograph, record the chromatograms, and measure the responses for the major peaks. Calculate the quantity, in mg, of $C_{19}H_{24}N_2O_2$ in the portion of Praziquantel taken by the formula:

$$200C(r_U / r_S)$$

in which C is the concentration, in mg per mL, of USP Praziquantel RS in the *Standard preparation*; and r_U and r_S are the peak responses obtained from the *Assay preparation* and the *Standard preparation*, respectively.

Praziquantel Tablets

» Praziquantel Tablets contain not less than 90.0 percent and not more than 110.0 percent of the labeled amount of $C_{19}H_{24}N_2O_2$.

Packaging and storage—Preserve in tight containers.

USP Reference standards ⟨11⟩—*USP Praziquantel RS*.

Identification—Transfer a quantity of powdered Tablets, equivalent to about 30 mg of Praziquantel, to a centrifuge tube, add 5 mL of methanol, agitate for 5 minutes, and centrifuge. Use the clear supernatant as the test solution. Apply separately, as 1-cm wide bands, 10 µL each of the test solution and a Standard solution of USP Praziquantel RS in methanol containing 6 mg per mL to a thin-layer chromatographic plate (see *Chromatography* ⟨621⟩) coated with a 0.25-mm layer of chromatographic silica gel mixture. Develop the chromatogram in an unsaturated chamber, using ethyl acetate as the developing solvent, until the solvent front has moved about 8 cm. Remove the plate from the chamber, air-dry, and examine under short-wavelength UV light: the R_F value of the principal band in the chromatogram of the test solution corresponds to that obtained for the Standard solution.

Dissolution ⟨711⟩—

Medium: 0.1 N hydrochloric acid containing 2.0 mg of sodium lauryl sulfate per mL; 900 mL.

Apparatus 2: 50 rpm.

Time: 60 minutes.

Standard preparation—Dissolve an accurately weighed quantity of USP Praziquantel RS in methanol to obtain a solution having a known concentration of about *L*/90 mg per mL, *L* being the labeled quantity, in mg, of praziquantel in each Tablet. Transfer 5.0 mL of this solution to a 50-mL volumetric flask, dilute with *Dissolution Medium* to volume, and mix.

Procedure—Determine the amount of $C_{19}H_{24}N_2O_2$ dissolved from UV absorbances at the wavelength of maximum absorbance at about 263 nm of filtered portions of the solution under test in comparison with the *Standard preparation*.

Tolerances—Not less than 75% (*Q*) of the labeled amount of $C_{19}H_{24}N_2O_2$ is dissolved in 60 minutes.

Uniformity of dosage units ⟨905⟩: meet the requirements.

Assay—

Mobile phase and *Chromatographic system*—Proceed as directed in the *Assay* under *Praziquantel*.

Standard preparation—Dissolve an accurately weighed quantity of USP Praziquantel RS in *Mobile phase*, and dilute quantitatively, and stepwise if necessary, with *Mobile phase* to obtain a solution having a known concentration of about 0.18 mg per mL.

Assay preparation—Weigh and finely powder not less than 20 Tablets. Transfer an accurately weighed portion of the powder, equivalent to about 150 mg of praziquantel, to a 100-mL volumetric flask, add 70 mL of *Mobile phase*, sonicate for 5 minutes, dilute with *Mobile phase* to volume, mix, and filter. Transfer 3.0 mL of the filtrate to a 25-mL volumetric flask, dilute with *Mobile phase* to volume, and mix.

Procedure—Proceed as directed for *Procedure* in the *Assay* under *Praziquantel*. Calculate the quantity, in mg, of $C_{19}H_{24}N_2O_2$ in the portion of Tablets taken by the formula:

$$2500(C/3)(r_U/r_S)$$

in which *C* is the concentration, in mg per mL, of USP Praziquantel RS in the *Standard preparation*, and r_U and r_S are the peak responses obtained from the *Assay preparation* and the *Standard preparation*, respectively.

Prazosin Hydrochloride

$C_{19}H_{21}N_5O_4 \cdot HCl$ 419.86

Piperazine, 1-(4-amino-6,7-dimethoxy-2-quinazolinyl)-4-(2-furanylcarbonyl)-, monohydrochloride.

1-(4-Amino-6,7-dimethoxy-2-quinazolinyl)-4-(2-furoyl)piperazine monohydrochloride [19237-84-4].

» Prazosin Hydrochloride contains not less than 97.0 percent and not more than 103.0 percent of $C_{19}H_{21}N_5O_4 \cdot HCl$, calculated on the anhydrous basis.

Caution—Care should be taken to prevent inhaling particles of Prazosin Hydrochloride and to prevent its contacting any part of the body.

Packaging and storage—Preserve in tight, light-resistant containers.

Labeling—Label it to indicate whether it is anhydrous or is the polyhydrate.

USP Reference standards ⟨11⟩—*USP Prazosin Hydrochloride RS*.

Identification—

A: *Infrared Absorption* ⟨197K⟩—Obtain the test specimen as follows. Dissolve about 20 mg of it in 20 mL of methanol, with the aid of gentle heat, and evaporate to dryness. Dry the residue in vacuum at 130° for 3 hours. Proceed as directed with the residue so obtained and a similar preparation of USP Prazosin Hydrochloride RS.

B: *Ultraviolet Absorption* ⟨197U⟩—

Solution: 7 µg per mL.

Medium: methanolic 0.01 N hydrochloric acid.

Absorptivities at 329 nm and 246 nm, calculated on the anhydrous basis, do not differ by more than 4.0%.

C: Prepare a test solution of it in a mixture of chloroform, methanol, and diethylamine (10 : 10 : 1) containing 5 mg per mL, and proceed as directed under *Thin-layer Chromatographic Identification Test* ⟨201⟩, using a solvent system consisting of a mixture of ethyl acetate and diethylamine (19 : 1).

D: It responds to the tests for *Chloride* ⟨191⟩.

Water, *Method I* ⟨921⟩: not more than 2.0% for the anhydrous form; between 8.0% and 15.0% for the polyhydrate form.

Residue on ignition ⟨281⟩: not more than 0.4%, determined on a 1-g portion, accurately weighed.

Heavy metals, *Method II* ⟨231⟩: 0.005%.

Iron—

Standard preparation—Dissolve 100 mg of iron wire, accurately weighed, in 10 mL of hydrochloric acid, with boiling. Cool, transfer to a 1000-mL volumetric flask, dilute with water to volume, and mix. Dilute quantitatively and stepwise with 0.2 N nitric acid to obtain a solution containing 4.0 µg of iron per mL.

Test preparation—Dissolve the residue obtained in the test for *Residue on ignition* in 20 mL of 2 N nitric acid. Slowly evaporate this solution to approximately 5 mL, transfer to a 25-mL volumetric flask, using 0.2 N nitric acid as a wash solvent, dilute with 0.2 N nitric acid to volume, and mix.

Procedure—Concomitantly determine the absorbances of the *Standard preparation* and the *Test preparation* at the wavelength of maximum absorbance at about 248 nm, with a suitable atomic absorption spectrophotometer (see *Apparatus* under *Spectrophotometry and Light-scattering* ⟨851⟩) equipped with an iron hollow-cathode lamp and an air–acetylene flame, using water as the blank: the absorbance of the *Test preparation* is not more than that of the *Standard preparation* (0.010%).

Nickel—

Standard preparation—Dissolve 100 mg of nickel, accurately weighed, in 10 mL of nitric acid with the aid of boiling. Cool, transfer to a 1000-mL volumetric flask, dilute with water to volume, and mix. Dilute quantitatively and stepwise with 0.2 N nitric acid to obtain a solution containing 4.0 µg of nickel per mL.

Test preparation—Use the *Test preparation* prepared as directed in the test for *Iron*.

Procedure—Concomitantly determine the absorbances of the *Standard preparation* and the *Test preparation* at the wavelength of maximum absorbance at about 232 nm, with a suitable atomic absorption spectrophotometer (see *Apparatus* under *Spectrophotometry and Light-scattering* ⟨851⟩) equipped with a nickel hollow-cathode lamp and an air–acetylene flame, using water as the blank: the absorbance of the *Test preparation* is not more than that of the *Standard preparation* (0.010%).

Ordinary impurities ⟨466⟩—
  Test solution: a mixture of chloroform, methanol, and diethylamine (10 : 10 : 1).
  Standard solution: a mixture of chloroform, methanol, and diethylamine (10 : 10 : 1).
  Eluant: a mixture of ethyl acetate and diethylamine (19 : 1).
  Visualization: 1.

Organic volatile impurities, *Method IV* ⟨467⟩: meets the requirements.

(Official until July 1, 2008)

Assay—
  Mobile phase—Mix 700 mL of methanol, 300 mL of water, and 10 mL of glacial acetic acid. Add diethylamine in sufficient quantity (about 0.2 mL) such that the retention time of prazosin hydrochloride is between 6 and 10 minutes. Degas the solution.

  Standard preparation—Transfer about 100 mg of USP Prazosin Hydrochloride RS, accurately weighed, to a 100-mL volumetric flask, dissolve in and dilute with methanol to volume, and mix. Dilute this solution quantitatively with a mixture of methanol and water (7 : 3) to obtain a solution having a known concentration of about 30 µg per mL.

  Assay preparation—Transfer about 100 mg of Prazosin Hydrochloride, accurately weighed, to a 100-mL volumetric flask, dissolve in and dilute with methanol to volume, and mix. Pipet 3 mL of this solution into a 100-mL volumetric flask, dilute with a mixture of methanol and water (7 : 3) to volume, and mix.

  Chromatographic system (see *Chromatography* ⟨621⟩)—The liquid chromatograph is equipped with a 254-nm detector and a 4.6-mm × 25-cm column that contains packing L3. The flow rate is adjusted to obtain a retention time of between 6 and 10 minutes for prazosin hydrochloride. Chromatograph the *Standard preparation*, and record the peak responses as directed for *Procedure*: the relative standard deviation for replicate injections is not more than 2.0%.

  Procedure—Inject equal volumes (about 5 µL) of the *Standard preparation* and the *Assay preparation* into the chromatograph, using a suitable microsyringe or sampling valve, and measure the peak responses at identical retention times. Calculate the quantity, in mg, of $C_{19}H_{21}N_5O_4 \cdot HCl$ in the Prazosin Hydrochloride taken by the formula:

$$(C / 0.3)(r_U / r_S)$$

in which C is the concentration, in µg per mL, of USP Prazosin Hydrochloride RS, calculated on the anhydrous basis, in the *Standard preparation*, and r_U and r_S are the peak responses obtained from the *Assay preparation* and the *Standard preparation*, respectively.

Prazosin Hydrochloride Capsules

» Prazosin Hydrochloride Capsules contain an amount of $C_{19}H_{21}N_5O_4 \cdot HCl$ equivalent to not less than 90.0 percent and not more than 110.0 percent of the labeled amount of prazosin ($C_{19}H_{21}N_5O_4$).

Caution—Care should be taken to prevent inhaling particles of Prazosin Hydrochloride and to prevent its contacting any part of the body.

Packaging and storage—Preserve in well-closed, light-resistant containers.

USP Reference standards ⟨11⟩—*USP Prazosin Hydrochloride RS.*

Identification—To a portion of the contents of Capsules, equivalent to about 10 mg of prazosin, add 20 mL of a mixture of chloroform and methanol (1 : 1), shake by mechanical means for 10 minutes, and centrifuge. Apply as separate 7.5-cm streaks 100 µL of this solution and 100 µL of a Standard solution of USP Prazosin Hydrochloride RS in a mixture of chloroform and methanol (1 : 1) containing about 0.5 mg per mL to a suitable thin-layer chromatographic plate (see *Chromatography* ⟨621⟩) coated with a 0.25-mm layer of chromatographic silica gel mixture. Allow the streaks to dry, and develop the chromatogram in a solvent system consisting of a mixture of ethyl acetate and diethylamine (19 : 1) until the solvent front has moved about three-fourths of the length of the plate. Remove the plate from the developing chamber, mark the solvent front, allow the solvent to evaporate, and view under short-wavelength UV light: prazosin appears as a dark blue band on a yellow-green fluorescent background, and the R_F value of the prazosin band obtained from the solution from the Capsule contents corresponds to that obtained from the Standard solution. Spray the plate evenly with a 1 in 50 solution of hydrochloric acid in potassium iodoplatinate TS: the R_F value of the principal band obtained from the solution from the Capsule contents corresponds to that obtained from the Standard solution.

Dissolution ⟨711⟩—
  Medium: 0.1 N hydrochloric acid containing 3% sodium lauryl sulfate; 900 mL.
  Apparatus 1: 100 rpm.
  Time: 60 minutes.
  Procedure—Determine the amount of $C_{19}H_{21}N_5O_4$ dissolved, employing the procedure set forth in the *Assay*, using a filtered portion of the solution under test as the *Assay preparation* in comparison with a Standard solution having a known concentration of USP Prazosin Hydrochloride RS in the same *Medium*.
  Tolerances—Not less than 75% (*Q*) of the labeled amount of $C_{19}H_{21}N_5O_4$ is dissolved in 60 minutes.

Uniformity of dosage units ⟨905⟩: meet the requirements.

  Procedure for content uniformity—Transfer the contents of a Capsule to a 100-mL volumetric flask, add 50 mL of 0.01 N methanolic hydrochloric acid containing 30% water, shake by mechanical means for 15 minutes, adjust with the same solvent to volume, and mix. Filter through a membrane filter having a porosity of 1.2 µm and dilute, if necessary, a portion of the filtrate with the same solvent to a concentration of about 10 µg of prazosin per mL. Prepare a Standard solution of USP Prazosin Hydrochloride RS in the same solvent having a known concentration of about 11 µg per mL. Concomitantly determine the absorbances of the solution from the Capsule contents and the Standard solution in 1-cm cells at the wavelength of maximum absorbance at about 330 nm, with a suitable spectrophotometer, using the solvent as the blank. Calculate the quantity, in mg, of prazosin ($C_{19}H_{21}N_5O_4$) in the Capsule taken by the formula:

$$(383.40/419.86)(0.001DC)(A_U / A_S)$$

in which 383.40 and 419.86 are the molecular weights of prazosin and prazosin hydrochloride, respectively; D is the dilution factor for the Capsule contents; C is the concentration, in µg per mL, of USP Prazosin Hydrochloride RS, calculated on the anhydrous basis, in the Standard solution; and A_U and A_S are the absorbances of the solution from the Capsule contents and the Standard solution, respectively.

Assay—
  Mobile phase, Chromatographic system, and *Procedure*—Proceed as directed in the *Assay* under *Prazosin Hydrochloride*.
  Acid–methanol solution—To 300 mL of water in a 1000-mL volumetric flask, add 0.85 mL of hydrochloric acid, dilute with methanol to volume, and mix. Transfer 300 mL of this solution to a 500-mL volumetric flask, dilute with methanol to volume, and mix.
  Standard preparation—Prepare a solution of USP Prazosin Hydrochloride RS in *Acid–methanol solution* having a known concentration of about 0.2 mg per mL. Pipet 5 mL of this solution into a 100-mL volumetric flask, add 45.0 mL of *Acid–methanol solution*, dilute with methanol to volume, and mix.

Assay preparation—Remove, as completely as possible, the contents of not less than 20 Capsules, and weigh. Transfer a quantity of the contents, accurately weighed, equivalent to about 1 mg of prazosin hydrochloride, to a glass-stoppered flask containing 50.0 mL of *Acid–methanol solution*, and shake by mechanical means for 30 minutes. Place the flask in an ultrasonic bath for 30 minutes, cool to room temperature, and filter the contents through a membrane filter (5 μm or finer porosity). Transfer 25.0 mL of the filtrate to a 50-mL volumetric flask, dilute with methanol to volume, and mix.

Procedure—Proceed as directed for *Procedure* in the *Assay* under *Prazosin Hydrochloride*. Calculate the quantity, in mg, of prazosin ($C_{19}H_{21}N_5O_4$) in the portion of the contents of Capsules taken by the formula:

$$(383.40/419.86)(0.1C)(r_U/r_S)$$

in which 383.40 and 419.86 are the molecular weights of prazosin and prazosin hydrochloride, respectively; *C* is the concentration, in μg per mL, of USP Prazosin Hydrochloride RS, calculated on the anhydrous basis, in the *Standard preparation*; and r_U and r_S are the peak responses obtained from the *Assay preparation* and the *Standard preparation*, respectively.

Prednicarbate

$C_{27}H_{36}O_8$ 488.57

(1) Pregna-1,4-diene-3,20-dione, 17-[(ethoxycarbonyl)oxy]-11-hydroxy-21-(1-oxopropoxy)-, (11β)-.
(2) 11β,17,21-Trihydroxypregna-1,4-diene-3,20-dione 17-(ethyl carbonate) 21-propionate   [73771-04-7].

» Prednicarbate contains not less than 97.0 percent and not more than 102.0 percent of $C_{27}H_{36}O_8$, calculated on the dried basis.

Packaging and storage—Preserve in well-closed, light-resistant containers.

USP Reference standards ⟨11⟩—*USP Prednicarbate RS. USP Prednicarbate Related Compound A RS.*

Identification—
  A: *Infrared Absorption* ⟨197K⟩.
  B: The retention time of the major peak in the chromatogram of the *Assay preparation* corresponds to that in the chromatogram of the *Standard preparation*, as obtained in the *Assay*.

Specific rotation ⟨781S⟩:   between +60° and +66°.
  Test solution: 10 mg per mL, in alcohol.

Loss on drying ⟨731⟩—Dry it at 105° for 6 hours: it loses not more than 0.5% of its weight.

Chromatographic purity—
  Mobile phase, Resolution solution, and *Chromatographic system*—Prepare as directed in the *Assay*.
  Test solution—Use the *Assay preparation*.
  Diluted test solution—Transfer 1 mL of the *Test solution* to a 200-mL volumetric flask, dissolve in and dilute with *Mobile phase* to volume, and mix.
  Procedure—Separately inject equal volumes (about 20 μL) of the *Test solution* and the *Diluted test solution* into the chromatograph, record the chromatograms, and measure the response for the prednicarbate peak obtained from the *Diluted test solution*. Obtain from the *Test solution* the peak responses for prednicarbate related compound A and for all peaks other than prednicarbate. Continue the chromatography for twice the retention time of prednicarbate. Calculate the percentage of the related compound and all the impurities in the portion of Prednicarbate taken by the formula:

$$0.5(r_T/r_{DT})$$

in which r_T is the peak response for each individual impurity peak obtained from the *Test solution*; and r_{DT} is the peak response of the main peak in the chromatogram of the *Diluted test solution*: not more than 1.0% of prednicarbate related compound A is found; not more than 0.5% of any other individual impurity is found, with the exception of the main peak and the peak corresponding to prednicarbate related compound A; and not more than 2.0% of total impurities is found. Disregard any peak (0.0125%) with an area less than 0.025 times the area of the main peak in the chromatogram obtained from the *Diluted test solution*.

Assay—
  Mobile phase—Prepare a filtered and degassed mixture of water and acetonitrile (60 : 50). Make adjustments if necessary (see *System Suitability* under *Chromatography* ⟨621⟩).
  Resolution solution—Dissolve suitable quantities of USP Prednicarbate Related Compound A RS and Prednicarbate in *Mobile phase* to obtain a solution containing about 3 μg of each per mL. [NOTE—Prepare all solutions just prior to use.]
  Standard preparation—Dissolve an accurately weighed quantity of USP Prednicarbate RS in *Mobile phase,* and dilute quantitatively, and stepwise if necessary, with *Mobile phase* to obtain a solution having a known concentration of about 0.6 mg per mL.
  Assay preparation—Transfer about 30 mg of Prednicarbate, accurately weighed, to a 50-mL volumetric flask, dissolve in and dilute with *Mobile phase* to volume, and mix.
  Chromatographic system (see *Chromatography* ⟨621⟩)—The liquid chromatograph is equipped with a 243-nm detector and a 4-mm × 12.5-cm column that contains packing L1. The flow rate is about 0.7 mL per minute. Chromatograph the *Resolution solution,* and record the peak responses as directed for *Procedure:* the relative retention times are about 1.1 for prednicarbate related compound A and 1.0 for prednicarbate; and the resolution, *R*, between prednicarbate and prednicarbate related compound A is not less than 3.0.
  Procedure—Separately inject equal volumes (about 20 μL) of the *Standard preparation* and the *Assay preparation* into the chromatograph, record the chromatograms, and measure the responses for the prednicarbate peaks. Continue the chromatography for twice the retention time of prednicarbate. Calculate the quantity, in mg, of $C_{27}H_{36}O_8$ in the portion of Prednicarbate taken by the formula:

$$50C(r_U/r_S)$$

in which *C* is the concentration, in mg per mL, of USP Prednicarbate RS in the *Standard preparation*; and r_U and r_S are the peak responses obtained from the *Assay preparation* and the *Standard preparation*, respectively.

Prednicarbate Cream

» Prednicarbate Cream contains not less than 90.0 percent and not more than 110.0 percent of the labeled amount of prednicarbate ($C_{27}H_{36}O_8$). It may contain a suitable preservative.

Packaging and storage—Preserve in tight, light-resistant containers, and store at controlled room temperature.

USP Reference standards ⟨11⟩—*USP Prednicarbate RS. USP Prednicarbate Related Compound A RS. USP Prednicarbate Related Compound B RS. USP Prednicarbate Related Compound C RS.*

Identification—The retention time of the prednicarbate peak in the chromatogram of the *Assay preparation* corresponds to that in the chromatogram of the *Standard preparation*, as obtained in the *Assay*.

Consistency—At room temperature, a string of Cream having a length of 2 cm retains its shape on a glass plate for at least 10 minutes. It can be spread easily and has no visible lumps.

Microbial limits ⟨61⟩—It meets the requirements of the tests for absence of *Staphylococcus aureus* and *Pseudomonas aeruginosa*. The total aerobic bacterial count does not exceed 100 cfu per g.

Minimum fill ⟨755⟩: meets the requirements.

pH ⟨791⟩: between 3.5 and 5.0, in a solution prepared in the following manner. Add 15 mL of boiling water to 3.5 g of Cream in a 50-mL centrifuge tube, and shake vigorously until an emulsion is formed. Loosen the cap, and place in a steam bath for 5 minutes. Centrifuge the hot solution. After cooling to room temperature, collect the lower aqueous solution in a glass tube, and determine the pH.

Related compounds—

Solution A, Solution B, Mobile phase, Solution 1, Solution 2, and Resolution solution—Prepare as directed in the *Assay*.

Standard stock solution—Prepare as directed for *Standard stock preparation* in the *Assay*.

Standard solution—Prepare as directed for *Standard preparation* in the *Assay*.

System sensitivity solution—Dilute 1.0 mL of the *Standard solution* with dehydrated alcohol to 50.0 mL. Dilute 1.0 mL of the solution thus obtained with *Solution A* to 20.0 mL.

Test solution—Prepare as directed for the *Assay preparation*.

Chromatographic system—Proceed as directed in the *Assay*. Chromatograph the *System sensitivity solution*: the signal-to-noise ratio is not less than 3. Chromatograph the *Resolution solution*, and record the peak responses as directed for *Procedure*: the relative retention times are about 0.57 for prednicarbate related compound B, 0.64 for prednicarbate related compound C, 1.0 for prednicarbate, and 1.04 for prednicarbate related compound A.

Procedure—Inject a volume (about 60 µL) of the *Test solution* into the chromatograph, record the chromatogram, and measure the peak responses. Calculate the percentage of each related compound and unknown impurity in the portion of Cream taken by the formula:

$$100(r_i / r_s)$$

in which r_i is the peak response for each individual impurity obtained from the *Test solution*, and r_s is the sum of the peak responses obtained from the *Test solution*: not more than 2.0% of prednicarbate related compound B and not more than 2.0% of prednicarbate related compound C is found; not more than 0.5% of any individual related compound is found; and not more than 5.0% of total related compounds is found.

Assay—

Solution A—Prepare a 0.01 M solution of monobasic potassium phosphate in water.

Solution B—Prepare a mixture of acetonitrile and dehydrated alcohol (2 : 1).

Mobile phase—Use variable mixtures of *Solution A* and *Solution B* as directed for *Chromatographic system*. Make adjustments if necessary (see *System Suitability* under *Chromatography* ⟨621⟩).

Standard stock preparation—Dissolve an accurately weighed quantity of USP Prednicarbate RS in dehydrated alcohol, and dilute quantitatively, and stepwise if necessary, with dehydrated alcohol to obtain a solution having a known concentration of 0.3 mg per mL.

Standard preparation—Transfer 10.0 mL of the *Standard stock preparation* to a 100-mL volumetric flask, add 15 mL of tetrahydrofuran and 30 mL of *Solution B*, and dilute with *Solution A* to volume.

Assay preparation—Transfer an accurately weighed quantity of Cream, equivalent to about 3.0 mg of prednicarbate, to a 100-mL volumetric flask. Add 15 mL of tetrahydrofuran, shake vigorously, and allow to stand in an ultrasonic bath until the sample has dissolved. Add 20 mL of dehydrated alcohol, and shake vigorously. Add 20 mL of acetonitrile, and shake vigorously. Immediately dilute with *Solution A* to volume, and shake vigorously. Allow to stand in an ice bath for at least 15 minutes. Shake the samples vigorously, and pass through a folded paper filter. Pass the filtrate through a membrane filter of 0.45-µm porosity.

Solution 1—Prepare a solution containing 0.3 mg per mL each of USP Prednicarbate Related Compound B RS and USP Prednicarbate Related Compound C RS in dehydrated alcohol.

Solution 2—Transfer about 15 mg of USP Prednicarbate Related Compound A RS, accurately weighed, to a 50-mL volumetric flask; add 1.0 mL of *Solution 1*, and dilute with dehydrated alcohol to volume.

Resolution solution—Transfer 10.0 mL of the *Standard preparation* to a volumetric flask; add 1.0 mL of *Solution 2*, 1 mL of tetrahydrofuran, and 2 mL of acetonitrile; and dilute with *Solution A* to 20.0 mL.

Chromatographic system (see *Chromatography* ⟨621⟩)—The liquid chromatograph is equipped with a 243-nm detector and a 4.0-mm × 25-cm column that contains 5-µm packing L1. The column temperature is maintained at 40°. The flow rate is about 1 mL per minute. The chromatograph is programmed as follows.

Time (minutes)	Solution A (%)	Solution B (%)	Elution
0–5	67	33	equilibration
5–45	67→40	33→60	linear gradient
45–50	40	60	isocratic
50–55	40→20	60→80	linear gradient
55–70	20	80	isocratic
70–75	20→67	80→33	linear gradient
75–85	67	33	isocratic

Chromatograph the *Resolution solution*, and record the peak responses as directed for *Procedure*: the resolution, *R*, between prednicarbate and prednicarbate related compound A is not less than 1.5. Chromatograph the *Standard preparation*, and record the peak responses as directed for *Procedure*: the tailing factor for the prednicarbate peak is between 0.7 and 1.5; and the relative standard deviation for replicate injections is not more than 2.0%.

Procedure—Separately inject equal volumes (about 60 µL) of the *Standard preparation* and the *Assay preparation* into the chromatograph, record the chromatograms, and measure the peak responses. Calculate the quantity, in mg, of prednicarbate ($C_{27}H_{36}O_8$) in each g of Cream taken by the formula:

$$100(C/W)(r_U / r_S)$$

in which *C* is the concentration, in mg per mL, of USP Prednicarbate RS in the *Standard preparation*; *W* is the weight, in g, of Cream taken; and r_U and r_S are the prednicarbate peak responses obtained from the *Assay preparation* and the *Standard preparation*, respectively.

Prednicarbate Ointment

» Prednicarbate Ointment contains not less than 90.0 percent and not more than 110.0 percent of the labeled amount of prednicarbate ($C_{27}H_{36}O_8$), in a suitable ointment base.

Packaging and storage—Preserve in tight, light-resistant containers, and store at controlled room temperature.

USP Reference standards ⟨11⟩—USP Prednicarbate RS. USP Prednicarbate Related Compound A RS. USP Prednicarbate Related Compound B RS. USP Prednicarbate Related Compound C RS.

Identification—It meets the requirements of the *Identification* test under *Prednicarbate Cream*.

Consistency—At room temperature, a string of Ointment having a length of 2 cm retains its shape on a glass plate for at least 10 minutes. It can be spread easily and has no visible lumps.

Microbial limits ⟨61⟩—It meets the requirements of the tests for absence of *Staphylococcus aureus* and *Pseudomonas aeruginosa*. The total aerobic bacterial count does not exceed 100 cfu per g.

Minimum fill ⟨755⟩: meets the requirements.

Related compounds—

Solution A, Solution B, Mobile phase, Solution 1, Solution 2, and Resolution solution—Prepare as directed for the *Assay* under *Prednicarbate Cream*.

Standard stock solution—Prepare as directed for the *Standard stock preparation* in the *Assay* under *Prednicarbate Cream*.

System sensitivity solution—Prepare as directed in the test for *Related compounds* under *Prednicarbate Cream*.

Test solution—Prepare as directed for the *Assay preparation* under *Prednicarbate Cream*.

Chromatographic system—Prepare as directed for the *Assay* under *Prednicarbate Cream*. Chromatograph the *System sensitivity solution*, and record the peak responses as directed for *Procedure*: the signal-to-noise ratio is not less than 3. Chromatograph the *Resolution solution*, and record the responses as directed for *Procedure*: the relative retention times are about 0.57 for prednicarbate related compound B, 0.64 for prednicarbate related compound C, 1.0 for prednicarbate, and 1.04 for prednicarbate related compound A.

Procedure—Inject a volume (about 60 μL) of the *Test solution* into the chromatograph, record the chromatogram, and measure the peak responses. Calculate the percentage of each related compound and unknown impurity in the portion of Ointment taken by the formula:

$$100(r_i / r_s)$$

in which r_i is the peak response for each impurity obtained from the *Test solution*, and r_s is the sum of all the peak responses obtained from the *Test solution*: not more than 2.0% of prednicarbate related compound B and not more than 2.0% of prednicarbate related compound C is found; not more than 0.5% of any individual related compound is found; and not more than 5.0% of total related compounds is found.

Assay—

Solution A, Solution B, Mobile phase, Standard stock preparation, Standard preparation, Assay preparation, Solution 1, Solution 2, and *Resolution solution*—Prepare as directed in the *Assay* under *Prednicarbate Cream*.

Chromatographic system (see *Chromatography* ⟨621⟩)—The liquid chromatograph is equipped with a 243-nm detector and a 4.0-mm × 25-cm column that contains 5-μm packing L1. The column temperature is maintained at 40°. The flow rate is about 1 mL per minute. The chromatograph is programmed as follows.

Time (minutes)	Solution A (%)	Solution B (%)	Elution
0–5	67	33	equilibration
5–45	67→40	33→60	linear gradient
45–50	40	60	isocratic
50–55	40→20	60→80	linear gradient
55–70	20	80	isocratic
70–75	20→67	80→33	linear gradient
75–85	67	33	isocratic

Chromatograph the *Resolution solution*, and record the peak responses as directed for *Procedure*: the resolution, *R*, between prednicarbate and prednicarbate related compound A is not less than 1.5. Chromatograph the *Standard preparation*, and record the peak responses as directed for *Procedure*: the tailing factor for the prednicarbate peak is between 0.7 and 1.5; and the relative standard deviation for replicate injections is not more than 2.0%.

Procedure—Separately inject equal volumes (about 60 μL) of the *Standard preparation* and the *Assay preparation* into the chromatograph, record the chromatograms, and measure the peak responses. Calculate the quantity, in mg, of prednicarbate ($C_{27}H_{36}O_8$) in each g of Ointment taken by the formula:

$$100(C/W)(r_U / r_S)$$

in which *C* is the concentration, in mg per mL, of USP Prednicarbate RS in the *Standard preparation*; *W* is the weight, in g, of Ointment taken; and r_U and r_S are the prednicarbate peak responses obtained from the *Assay preparation* and the *Standard preparation*, respectively.

Prednisolone

$C_{21}H_{28}O_5$ (anhydrous) 360.45
Pregna-1,4-diene-3,20-dione, 11,17,21-trihydroxy-, (11β)-.
11β,17,21-Trihydroxypregna-1,4-diene-3,20-dione (anhydrous) [50-24-8].
Sesquihydrate 387.48 [52438-85-4].

» Prednisolone is anhydrous or contains one and one-half molecules of water of hydration. It contains not less than 97.0 percent and not more than 102.0 percent of $C_{21}H_{28}O_5$, calculated on the dried basis.

Packaging and storage—Preserve in well-closed containers.
Labeling—Label it to indicate whether it is anhydrous or hydrous.
USP Reference standards ⟨11⟩—*USP Prednisolone RS.*
Identification—
 A: *Infrared Absorption* ⟨197K⟩.
 B: *Ultraviolet Absorption* ⟨197U⟩—
 Solution: 10 μg per mL.
 Medium: methanol.
 Absorptivities at 242 nm, calculated on the dried basis, do not differ by more than 2.5%. If a difference appears, dissolve portions of both the test specimen and the Reference Standard in ethyl acetate, evaporate the solutions to dryness, and repeat the test on the residues.
Specific rotation ⟨781S⟩: between +97° and +103°.
 Test solution: 10 mg per mL, in dioxane.
Loss on drying ⟨731⟩—Dry it in vacuum at 105° for 3 hours: anhydrous Prednisolone loses not more than 1.0%, and hydrous Prednisolone not more than 7.0%, of its weight.
Residue on ignition ⟨281⟩: negligible, from 100 mg.
Selenium ⟨291⟩: 0.003%, a 200-mg test specimen being used.
Chromatographic purity—
 Solution A—Prepare a filtered and degassed mixture of water and acetonitrile (77 : 23).
 Solution B—Prepare a filtered and degassed mixture of water and acetonitrile (60 : 40).
 Mobile phase—Use variable mixtures of *Solution A* and *Solution B* as directed for *Chromatographic system*. Make adjustments if necessary (see *System Suitability* under *Chromatography* ⟨621⟩).
 Diluent: a mixture of water and acetonitrile (1 : 1).
 Standard solution—Dissolve an accurately weighed quantity of USP Prednisolone RS in *Diluent*, and dilute quantitatively, and stepwise if necessary, with *Diluent* to obtain a solution having a known concentration of about 0.01 mg per mL.
 System suitability solution—Dissolve an accurately weighed quantity of USP Prednisolone RS and hydrocortisone in *Diluent* to obtain a solution having a known concentration of about 1 mg per mL and 0.06 mg per mL, respectively.
 Test solution—Transfer about 25 mg of Prednisolone, accurately weighed, to a 25-mL volumetric flask, dissolve in and dilute with *Diluent* to volume, and mix.
 Chromatographic system (see *Chromatography* ⟨621⟩)—The liquid chromatograph is equipped with a 254-nm detector and a 4.6-mm × 30-cm column that contains 5-μm packing L1. The flow rate is about 1.5 mL per minute. The column temperature is maintained at 40°. The chromatograph is programmed as follows.

Time (minutes)	Solution A (%)	Solution B (%)	Elution
0	100	0	equilibration
0–25	100	0	isocratic
25–45	100→0	0→100	linear gradient

Time (minutes)	Solution A (%)	Solution B (%)	Elution
45–60	0	100	isocratic
60–61	0→100	100→0	linear gradient
61–100	100	0	re-equilibration

Chromatograph the *System suitability solution,* and record the peak responses as directed for *Procedure:* the relative retention times for prednisolone and hydrocortisone are about 1.0 and 1.06, respectively; and the height of the smallest peak is not less than 2 times the height of the valley between the prednisolone and hydrocortisone peaks. Chromatograph the *Standard solution,* and record the peak responses as directed for *Procedure:* the relative standard deviation for replicate injections is not more than 5.0% for the prednisolone peak.

Procedure—Separately inject equal volumes (about 20 μL) of the *Standard solution* and *Test solution* into the chromatograph, record the chromatograms, and measure the responses for the major peaks. Calculate the percentage of each impurity in the portion of Prednisolone taken by the formula:

$$2500(C/W)(r_i/r_S)$$

in which C is the concentration, in mg per mL, of USP Prednisolone RS in the *Standard solution;* W is the weight, in mg, of prednisolone used to prepare the *Test solution;* r_i is the peak response for each impurity in the *Test solution;* and r_S is the peak response obtained from the *Standard solution:* no impurity greater than 1.0% and only one peak greater than 0.5% is found; and not more than 2.0% of total impurities is found.

Assay—

Mobile phase—Prepare a solution containing a mixture of butyl chloride, water-saturated butyl chloride, tetrahydrofuran, methanol, and glacial acetic acid (95 : 95 : 14 : 7 : 6). Make adjustments if necessary (see *System Suitability* under *Chromatography* ⟨621⟩).

Internal standard solution—Prepare a solution of betamethasone in tetrahydrofuran containing 5 mg per mL. Dilute this solution with water-saturated chloroform, and mix to obtain a solution having a final concentration of 0.5 mg per mL.

Standard preparation—Transfer about 10 mg of USP Prednisolone RS, accurately weighed, to a 100-mL volumetric flask, and dissolve in 5.0 mL of methanol. Add 20.0 mL of *Internal standard solution,* and mix. Dilute with water-saturated chloroform to 100.0 mL, and mix.

Assay preparation—Transfer about 10 mg of Prednisolone, accurately weighed, to a 100-mL volumetric flask, and dissolve in 5.0 mL of methanol. Add 20.0 mL of *Internal standard solution,* and mix. Dilute with water-saturated chloroform to 100.0 mL, and mix.

Chromatographic system (see *Chromatography* ⟨621⟩)—The liquid chromatograph is equipped with a 254-nm detector and a 4-mm × 30-cm column that contains packing L3. The flow rate is about 1 mL per minute. Chromatograph four replicate injections of the *Standard preparation,* and record the peak responses as directed for *Procedure:* the relative retention times are about 0.7 for betamethasone and 1.0 for prednisolone; the resolution, R, between prednisolone and betamethasone is not less than 3.5; and the relative standard deviation for replicate injections is not more than 2.0%.

Procedure—Separately inject equal volumes (about 10 μL) of the *Standard preparation* and the *Assay preparation* into the chromatograph, record the chromatograms, and measure the responses for the major peaks. Calculate the quantity, in mg, of $C_{21}H_{28}O_5$ in the portion of Prednisolone taken by the formula:

$$0.1C(R_U/R_S)$$

in which C is the concentration, in μg per mL, of USP Prednisolone RS in the *Standard preparation;* and R_U and R_S are the peak response ratios of prednisolone to the internal standard obtained from the *Assay preparation* and the *Standard preparation,* respectively.

Prednisolone Cream

» Prednisolone Cream contains not less than 90.0 percent and not more than 110.0 percent of the labeled amount of $C_{21}H_{28}O_5$, in a suitable cream base.

Packaging and storage—Preserve in collapsible tubes or in tight containers.

USP Reference standards ⟨11⟩—*USP Prednisolone RS.*

Identification—Evaporate in a test tube to dryness about 5 mL of the dilute solution obtained in the *Assay.* Add 2 to 3 mL of warm perchloric acid, mix, and warm on a steam bath for about 2 minutes: a blood-red color develops. Add 5 mL of water: the color is not discharged.

Minimum fill ⟨755⟩: meets the requirements.

Assay—

Sulfuric acid reagent—Prepare a solution of sulfuric acid, dehydrated alcohol, and water solution (4 : 3 : 3).

Modified phenylhydrazine-sulfuric acid TS—Dissolve 65 mg of phenylhydrazine hydrochloride in 100 mL of *Sulfuric acid reagent.*

Standard preparation—Dissolve in dehydrated alcohol a suitable quantity, accurately weighed, of USP Prednisolone RS, and dilute quantitatively and stepwise with dehydrated alcohol to obtain a solution having a known concentration of about 0.1 mg per mL.

Assay preparation—To an accurately weighed portion of Cream, equivalent to about 20 mg of prednisolone, add 25 mL of dehydrated alcohol. Warm on a steam bath to disperse the assay specimen, then chill to congeal it. Filter through paper, previously washed with dehydrated alcohol, into a 200-mL volumetric flask. Repeat twice more, starting with "add 25 mL of dehydrated alcohol." Dilute with dehydrated alcohol to volume. (Retain about 5 mL of this dilution for the *Identification* test.)

Procedure—Pipet 2 mL of *Assay preparation* into each of two 50-mL conical flasks (identify as *Assay preparation* and *Assay preparation blank*). Pipet 2 mL of *Standard preparation* into each of two 50-mL conical flasks (identify as *Standard preparation* and *Standard preparation blank*). Pipet 2 mL of dehydrated alcohol into a 50-mL conical flask (identify as *Reagent blank*). Add 20.0 mL of *Sulfuric acid reagent* to the *Assay preparation blank* and to the *Standard preparation blank.* Add 20.0 mL of *Modified phenylhydrazine-sulfuric acid* to the *Assay preparation,* to the *Standard preparation,* and to the *Reagent blank,* respectively. Maintain the flasks in a water bath at 60° for about 45 minutes, then chill in a water-ice bath. Filter each through a fine-porosity, sintered-glass funnel, and identify the filtrate flasks correspondingly. Concomitantly determine the absorbances of the solutions at the wavelength of maximum absorbance at about 410 nm, with a suitable spectrophotometer, against dehydrated alcohol. Calculate the quantity, in mg, of $C_{21}H_{28}O_5$ in the portion of Cream taken by the formula:

$$200C[(A_U - A_{UB} - A_R)/(A_S - A_{SB} - A_R)]$$

in which C is the concentration, in mg per mL, of USP Prednisolone RS in the *Standard preparation,* A_U and A_S are the absorbances of the solutions from the *Assay preparation* and the *Standard preparation,* respectively, A_{UB} and A_{SB} are the absorbances of the solutions from the *Assay preparation blank* and the *Standard preparation blank,* respectively, and A_R is the absorbance of the *Reagent blank.*

Prednisolone Oral Solution

» Prednisolone Oral Solution contains not less than 90.0 percent and not more than 110.0 percent of the labeled amount of prednisolone ($C_{21}H_{28}O_5$). It may contain alcohol.

Packaging and storage—Preserve in tight, light-resistant containers.

USP Reference standards ⟨11⟩—USP Prednisolone RS.
Identification—The retention time of the major peak in the chromatogram of the *Assay preparation* corresponds to that in the chromatogram of the *Standard preparation,* as obtained in the *Assay.*
pH ⟨791⟩: between 3.0 and 4.5.
Alcohol content, *Method II* ⟨611⟩(*if present*): not less than 90.0% and not more than 115.0% of the labeled amount.
Assay—
Citrate buffer—Prepare a 0.0033 M solution of citric acid in water, adjust with 1 N sodium hydroxide to a pH of 6.2, and mix.
Diluting solution: a mixture of methanol and water (1 : 1).
Mobile phase—Prepare a filtered and degassed mixture of *Citrate buffer* and methanol (31 : 19). Make adjustments if necessary (see *System Suitability* under *Chromatography* ⟨621⟩).
System suitability solution—Dissolve suitable quantities of prednisolone and hydrocortisone in a mixture of methanol and water (1 : 1) to obtain a solution containing about 100 µg per mL and 90 µg per mL, respectively.
Standard preparation—Dissolve an accurately weighed quantity of USP Prednisolone RS in *Diluting solution,* and dilute quantitatively, and stepwise if necessary, with *Diluting solution* to obtain a solution having a known concentration of about 0.1 mg per mL.
Assay preparation—Transfer an accurately measured volume of Oral Solution, equivalent to about 5.0 mg of prednisolone, to a 50-mL volumetric flask, dissolve in *Diluting solution,* shake by mechanical means for 15 minutes, dilute with *Diluting solution* to volume, and mix.
Chromatographic system (see *Chromatography* ⟨621⟩)—The liquid chromatograph is equipped with a 254-nm detector and a 4.6-mm × 15-cm column that contains packing L10. The flow rate is about 1 mL per minute. Chromatograph the *System suitability solution,* and record the peak responses as directed for *Procedure*: the relative retention times are about 0.8 for hydrocortisone and 1.0 for prednisolone; the resolution, *R*, between hydrocortisone and prednisolone is not less than 2.5; and the relative standard deviation for replicate injections is not more than 2.0%.
Procedure—Separately inject equal volumes (about 10 µL) of the *Standard preparation* and the *Assay preparation* into the chromatograph, record the chromatograms, and measure the responses for the major peaks. Calculate the quantity, in mg, of prednisolone ($C_{21}H_{28}O_5$) in the volume of Oral Solution taken by the formula:

$$50C(r_U / r_S)$$

in which *C* is the concentration, in mg per mL, of USP Prednisolone RS in the *Standard preparation;* and r_U and r_S are the peak responses obtained from the *Assay preparation* and the *Standard preparation,* respectively.

Prednisolone Tablets

» Prednisolone Tablets contain not less than 90.0 percent and not more than 110.0 percent of the labeled amount of $C_{21}H_{28}O_5$.

Packaging and storage—Preserve in well-closed containers.
USP Reference standards ⟨11⟩—USP Prednisolone RS.
Identification—Pulverize a number of Tablets, equivalent to about 50 mg of prednisolone, and digest with 25 mL of chloroform for 15 minutes. Filter the mixture, and evaporate the filtrate on a steam bath to dryness. Wash the residue with two 10-mL portions of hot solvent hexane, decanting the supernatant each time and discarding it. Digest the residue with 25 mL of dehydrated alcohol, warming slightly, for 15 minutes. Filter the warm solution, and evaporate the filtrate to a volume of 2 to 3 mL. Add solvent hexane until the mixture just becomes turbid, chill it to effect crystallization, collect the crystals, and dry them at 60° for 1 hour: the crystals of prednisolone so obtained respond to *Identification* test A under *Prednisolone.*

Dissolution ⟨711⟩—
Medium: water; 900 mL.
Apparatus 2: 50 rpm.
Time: 30 minutes.
Procedure—Determine the amount in solution on filtered portions of the *Dissolution Medium,* suitably diluted at the wavelength of maximum absorbance at about 246 nm, with a suitable spectrophotometer in comparison with a Standard solution having a known concentration of USP Prednisolone RS. An amount of alcohol not to exceed 5% of the total volume of the Standard solution may be used to bring the prednisolone standard into solution prior to dilution with water.
Tolerances—Not less than 70% (*Q*) of the labeled amount of $C_{21}H_{28}O_5$ is dissolved in 30 minutes.
Uniformity of dosage units ⟨905⟩: meet the requirements.
Procedure for content uniformity—
Mobile phase, Internal standard solution, Standard preparation, and *Chromatographic system*—Prepare as directed in the *Assay* under *Prednisolone.*
Test preparation—Place 1 tablet in a suitable container. Place 0.5 mL of water directly on the tablet, and allow to stand until disintegrated (about 30 minutes). Gently agitate the container to ensure that the tablet is completely disintegrated. Add 2.0 mL of *Internal standard solution* for each mg of labeled tablet strength, and sonicate for about 10 minutes. Dilute with a quantity of water-saturated chloroform approximately four times the volume of added *Internal standard solution.* Add a few glass beads, close the container, and shake vigorously for about 30 minutes. Centrifuge, or allow to stand until a clear solution is obtained. Analyze the clear solution as directed under *Procedure.*
Procedure—Proceed as directed for *Procedure* in the *Assay* under *Prednisolone.* Calculate the quantity, in mg, of $C_{21}H_{28}O_5$ in the Tablet taken by the formula:

$$(FW_S)(R_U / R_S)$$

in which *F* is the ratio of the volume of the *Internal standard solution,* in mL, in the *Test preparation* to the volume, in mL, of the *Internal standard solution* in the *Standard preparation,* W_S is the weight, in mg, of USP Prednisolone RS taken for the *Standard preparation,* and the other terms are as defined therein.
Assay—
Mobile phase, Internal standard solution, Standard preparation, and *Chromatographic system*—Prepare as directed in the *Assay* under *Prednisolone.*
Assay preparation—Weigh and finely powder not less than 10 Tablets. Transfer an accurately weighed portion of the powder, equivalent to about 10 mg of prednisolone, to a 100-mL volumetric flask. Add 20.0 mL of *Internal standard solution,* and sonicate for 10 minutes. Dilute with water-saturated chloroform to volume, and shake for 30 minutes. Centrifuge this mixture, and use the clear supernatant.
Procedure—Proceed as directed for *Procedure* in the *Assay* under *Prednisolone.* Calculate the quantity, in mg, of $C_{21}H_{28}O_5$ in the portion of Tablets taken by the formula:

$$0.1C(R_U / R_S)$$

in which the terms are as defined therein.

Prednisolone Acetate

$C_{23}H_{30}O_6$ 402.49
Pregna-1,4-diene-3,20-dione, 21-(acetyloxy)-11,17-dihydroxy-, (11β)-.
11β,17,21-Trihydroxypregna-1,4-diene-3,20-dione 21-acetate [52-21-1].

» Prednisolone Acetate contains not less than 97.0 percent and not more than 102.0 percent of $C_{23}H_{30}O_6$, calculated on the dried basis.

Packaging and storage—Preserve in well-closed containers. Store at 25°, excursions permitted between 15° and 30°.

USP Reference standards ⟨11⟩—*USP Prednisolone Acetate RS.*
Identification—
  A: *Infrared Absorption* ⟨197K⟩.
  B: *Ultraviolet Absorption* ⟨197U⟩—
    Solution: 10 μg per mL.
    Medium: methanol.
    Absorptivities at 242 nm, calculated on the dried basis, do not differ by more than 2.5%.
Specific rotation ⟨781S⟩: between +112° and +119°.
    Test solution: 10 mg per mL, in dioxane.
Loss on drying ⟨731⟩—Dry it at 105° for 3 hours: it loses not more than 1.0% of its weight.
Chromatographic purity—
  Mobile phase—Prepare a filtered and degassed mixture of isooctane, butyl chloride and methanol (49 : 49 : 2). Make adjustments if necessary (see *System Suitability* under *Chromatography* ⟨621⟩).
  Test solution—Transfer about 10 mg of Prednisolone Acetate, accurately weighed, to a suitable container, dissolve in 10 mL of chloroform, and mix.
  Chromatographic system (see *Chromatography* ⟨621⟩)—The liquid chromatograph is equipped with a 254-nm detector and a 6.0-mm × 4.0-cm column that contains packing L3. The flow rate is about 3 mL per minute. Chromatograph the *Test solution,* and record the peak responses as directed for *Procedure:* the column efficiency is not less than 800 theoretical plates; and the relative standard deviation for replicate injections is not more than 2.0%.
  Procedure—Inject a volume (about 10 μL) of the *Test solution* into the chromatograph, record the chromatogram, and measure all the peak responses. Calculate the percentage of each impurity in the portion of Prednisolone Acetate taken by the formula:

$$100(r_i / r_s)$$

in which r_i is the peak response for each impurity; and r_s is the sum of the responses for all the peaks: not more than 1.0% of any individual impurity is found; and not more than 2.0% of total impurities is found.
Assay—
  Mobile phase—Prepare a solution containing a mixture of *n*-butyl chloride, water-saturated *n*-butyl chloride, tetrahydrofuran, methanol, and glacial acetic acid (95 : 95 : 14 : 7 : 6). Make adjustments if necessary (see *System Suitability* under *Chromatography* ⟨621⟩).
  Internal standard solution—Prepare a solution of betamethasone in tetrahydrofuran containing 10 mg per mL. Dilute this solution with water-saturated chloroform, and mix to obtain a solution having a final concentration of about 1 mg of betamethasone per mL.
  Standard preparation—Transfer about 10 mg of USP Prednisolone Acetate RS, accurately weighed, to a 100-mL volumetric flask; add 20.0 mL of *Internal standard solution;* and dissolve, using sonication if necessary. Dilute with water-saturated chloroform to volume, and mix. Dilute 5.0 mL of the solution so obtained with water-saturated chloroform to 20.0 mL to obtain a solution having a known concentration of about 25 μg of USP Prednisolone Acetate RS per mL.
  Assay preparation—Transfer about 10 mg of Prednisolone Acetate, accurately weighed, to a 100-mL volumetric flask; add 20.0 mL of *Internal standard solution;* and dissolve, using sonication if necessary. Dilute with water-saturated chloroform to volume, and mix. Dilute 5.0 mL of the solution so obtained with water-saturated chloroform to 20.0 mL.
  Chromatographic system (see *Chromatography* ⟨621⟩)—The liquid chromatograph is equipped with a 254-nm detector and a 4-mm × 30-cm column that contains packing L3. The flow rate is about 1 mL per minute. Chromatograph the *Standard preparation,* and record the peak responses as directed for *Procedure:* the relative retention times are about 1.6 for betamethasone and 1.0 for prednisolone acetate; the resolution, *R*, between prednisolone acetate and betamethasone is not less than 3.0; and the relative standard deviation for replicate injections is not more than 2.0%.
  Procedure—Separately inject equal volumes (about 10 μL) of the *Standard preparation* and the *Assay preparation* into the chromatograph, record the chromatograms, and measure the responses for the major peaks. Calculate the quantity, in mg, of $C_{23}H_{30}O_6$ in the portion of Prednisolone Acetate taken by the formula:

$$0.4C(R_U / R_S)$$

in which *C* is the concentration, in μg per mL, of USP Prednisolone Acetate RS in the *Standard preparation;* and R_U and R_S are the peak response ratios obtained from the *Assay preparation* and the *Standard preparation,* respectively.

Prednisolone Acetate Injectable Suspension

» Prednisolone Acetate Injectable Suspension is a sterile suspension of Prednisolone Acetate in a suitable aqueous medium. It contains not less than 90.0 percent and not more than 110.0 percent of the labeled amount of $C_{23}H_{30}O_6$.

Packaging and storage—Preserve in single-dose or in multiple-dose containers, preferably of Type I glass.
USP Reference standards ⟨11⟩—*USP Prednisolone Acetate RS.*
Identification—Allow a volume of Injectable Suspension, equivalent to about 50 mg of prednisolone acetate, to settle. Decant and discard the supernatant. Dissolve the residue in 6 mL of alcohol. Evaporate the solution, with the aid of a current of air, to half its volume, when crystallization occurs. Chill, if necessary, to aid crystallization. Filter the crystals, and allow to dry with the aid of a current of air: the crystals so obtained respond to *Identification* test A under *Prednisolone Acetate*.
pH ⟨791⟩: between 5.0 and 7.5.
Other requirements—It meets the requirements under *Injections* ⟨1⟩.
Assay—
  Mobile phase—Prepare a filtered and degassed mixture of water and acetonitrile (60 : 40). Make adjustments if necessary (see *System Suitability* under *Chromatography* ⟨621⟩).
  Methanol-acetonitrile solution—Prepare a solution by mixing equal volumes of methanol and acetonitrile.
  Standard preparation—Dissolve an accurately weighed quantity of USP Prednisolone Acetate RS in *Methanol-acetonitrile solution,* and dilute quantitatively, and stepwise if necessary, with *Methanol-acetonitrile solution* to obtain a solution having a known concentration of about 0.1 mg per mL.
  Assay preparation—Transfer an accurately measured volume of Injectable Suspension, equivalent to about 50 mg of prednisolone acetate, to a 50-mL volumetric flask, add *Methanol-acetonitrile solution* to volume, and mix. Pipet 5 mL of this solution into a second 50-mL volumetric flask, dilute with *Methanol-acetonitrile solution* to volume, and mix.
  Chromatographic system (see *Chromatography* ⟨621⟩)—The liquid chromatograph is equipped with a 254-nm detector and a 4.6-mm × 25-cm column that contains packing L1. The flow rate is about 1 mL per minute. Chromatograph the *Standard preparation,* and record the peak response as directed for *Procedure:* the capacity factor, *k′*, is not less than 3.0, and the relative standard deviation for replicate injections is not more than 3.0%.
  Procedure—Separately inject equal volumes (about 10 μL) of the *Standard preparation* and the *Assay preparation* into the chromatograph, record the chromatograms, and measure the responses for the major peaks. Calculate the quantity, in mg, of $C_{23}H_{30}O_6$ in each mL of the Injectable Suspension taken by the formula:

$$500(C / V)(r_U / r_S)$$

in which *C* is the concentration, in mg per mL, of USP Prednisolone Acetate RS in the *Standard preparation, V* is the volume, in mL, of Injectable Suspension taken, and r_U and r_S are the peak responses for prednisolone acetate obtained from the *Assay preparation* and the *Standard preparation,* respectively.

Prednisolone Acetate Ophthalmic Suspension

» Prednisolone Acetate Ophthalmic Suspension is a sterile, aqueous suspension of prednisolone acetate containing a suitable antimicrobial preservative. It may contain suitable buffers, stabilizers, and suspending and viscosity agents. It contains not less than 90.0 percent and not more than 115.0 percent of the labeled amount of $C_{23}H_{30}O_6$.

Packaging and storage—Preserve in tight containers.

USP Reference standards ⟨11⟩—*USP Prednisolone Acetate RS.*

Identification—Transfer a volume of Ophthalmic Suspension, equivalent to about 7.5 mg of Prednisolone Acetate, to a test tube, add 5 mL of chloroform, and shake. Centrifuge, and apply 20 µL of the chloroform layer and 20 µL of a Standard solution of USP Prednisolone Acetate RS in chloroform containing 1.5 mg per mL on a thin-layer chromatographic plate (see *Chromatography* ⟨621⟩) coated with a 0.25-mm layer of chromatographic silica gel mixture. Develop the chromatogram in a mixture of chloroform and acetone (4 : 1) until the solvent front has moved about three-fourths the length of the plate. Mark the solvent front, and locate the spots on the plate by examining under UV light: the R_F value of the principal spot obtained from the solution under test corresponds to that obtained from the Standard solution.

Sterility ⟨71⟩: meets the requirements.

pH ⟨791⟩: between 5.0 and 6.0.

Assay—

Mobile phase—Prepare a suitably filtered and degassed solution of water and acetonitrile (3 : 2). Make adjustments if necessary (see *System Suitability* under *Chromatography* ⟨621⟩).

Standard preparation—Dissolve an accurately weighed quantity of USP Prednisolone Acetate RS in a mixture of acetonitrile and water (1 : 1) to obtain a solution having a known concentration of about 0.1 mg per mL.

System suitability preparation—Prepare a solution of prednisolone in a mixture of acetonitrile and methanol (1 : 1) having a concentration of about 0.1 mg per mL. Mix equal volumes of this solution and the *Standard preparation*.

Assay preparation—Transfer an accurately measured volume of Ophthalmic Suspension, equivalent to about 5 mg of prednisolone acetate, to a 50-mL volumetric flask. Dilute with a mixture of acetonitrile and water (1 : 1) to volume, and mix.

Chromatographic system (see *Chromatography* ⟨621⟩)—The liquid chromatograph is equipped with a 254-nm detector and a column that contains packing L1. The flow rate is about 2 mL per minute. Chromatograph the *Standard preparation* and the *System suitability preparation*, and record the peak responses as directed for *Procedure:* the relative retention times are 0.5 for prednisolone and 1.0 for prednisolone acetate, the column efficiency is not less than 7000 theoretical plates, the tailing factor is not more than 2.0, and the resolution, *R*, between prednisolone and prednisolone acetate is not less than 2.0.

Procedure—Separately inject equal volumes (about 10 µL) of the *Standard preparation* and the *Assay preparation* into the chromatograph, record the chromatograms, and measure the responses for the major peaks. Calculate the quantity, in mg, of $C_{23}H_{30}O_6$ in each mL of the Ophthalmic Suspension taken by the formula:

$$50(C / V)(r_U / r_S)$$

in which *C* is the concentration, in mg per mL, of USP Prednisolone Acetate RS in the *Standard preparation*, *V* is the volume, in mL, of Ophthalmic Suspension taken, and r_U and r_S are the peak responses obtained from the *Assay preparation* and the *Standard preparation*, respectively.

Prednisolone Hemisuccinate

$C_{25}H_{32}O_8$ 460.52

Pregna-1,4-diene-3,20-dione, 21-(3-carboxy-1-oxopropoxy)-11,17-dihydroxy-, (11β)-.

11β,17,21-Trihydroxypregna-1,4-diene-3,20-dione 21-(hydrogen succinate)   [*2920-86-7*].

» Prednisolone Hemisuccinate contains not less than 98.0 percent and not more than 102.0 percent of $C_{25}H_{32}O_8$, calculated on the dried basis.

Packaging and storage—Preserve in tight containers.

USP Reference standards ⟨11⟩—*USP Prednisolone Hemisuccinate RS.*

Identification—
  A: *Infrared Absorption* ⟨197K⟩.
  B: *Ultraviolet Absorption* ⟨197U⟩—
  Solution: 20 µg per mL.
  Medium: methanol.
  Absorptivities at 243 nm, calculated on the dried basis, do not differ by more than 3.0%.

Specific rotation ⟨781S⟩: between +99° and +104°.
  Test solution: 6.7 mg per mL, in dioxane.

Loss on drying ⟨731⟩—Dry it in vacuum at 65° for 3 hours: it loses not more than 0.5% of its weight.

Residue on ignition ⟨281⟩: negligible, from 100 mg.

Assay—

Standard preparation—Dissolve an accurately weighed quantity of USP Prednisolone Hemisuccinate RS in a mixture of equal volumes of alcohol and chloroform to obtain a solution having a known concentration of about 8 mg per mL.

Assay preparation—Weigh accurately about 80 mg of Prednisolone Hemisuccinate, previously dried, dissolve in a mixture of equal volumes of alcohol and chloroform to make 10.0 mL, and mix.

Procedure—Use a 20- × 20-cm chromatographic plate coated with a 0.25-mm layer of chromatographic silica gel mixture, which has been activated by heating at 105° for 1 hour. Using a solvent system consisting of a mixture of 5 parts of butyl alcohol, 4 parts of acetic acid, and 1 part of water, proceed as directed for *Procedure* under *Single-steroid Assay* ⟨511⟩, ending with "Centrifuge the tubes for 5 minutes," except to apply 50 µL in place of 200 µL of the solutions to the plate. Concomitantly determine the absorbances of the solutions in 1-cm cells at the wavelength of maximum absorbance at about 243 nm, with a suitable spectrophotometer, against the blank. Calculate the quantity, in mg, of $C_{25}H_{32}O_8$ in the portion of Prednisolone Hemisuccinate taken by the formula:

$$10C(A_U / A_S)$$

in which *C* is the concentration, in mg per mL, of USP Prednisolone Hemisuccinate RS in the *Standard preparation*, and A_U and A_S are the absorbances of the solutions from the *Assay preparation* and the *Standard preparation*, respectively.

Prednisolone Sodium Phosphate

$C_{21}H_{27}Na_2O_8P$ 484.39

Pregna-1,4-diene-3,20-dione, 11,17-dihydroxy-21-(phosphonooxy)-, disodium salt, (11β)-.

11β,17,21-Trihydroxypregna-1,4-diene-3,20-dione 21-(disodium phosphate)   [*125-02-0*].

» Prednisolone Sodium Phosphate contains not less than 96.0 percent and not more than 102.0 percent of $C_{21}H_{27}Na_2O_8P$, calculated on the dried basis.

Packaging and storage—Preserve in tight containers.
USP Reference standards ⟨11⟩—*USP Prednisolone RS. USP Prednisolone Sodium Phosphate RS.*
Identification—
A: *Infrared Absorption* ⟨197K⟩.
B: The residue from the ignition of about 20 mg of it meets the requirements of the tests for *Sodium* ⟨191⟩ and for *Phosphate* ⟨191⟩.
Specific rotation ⟨781S⟩: between +95° and +102°.
Test solution: 10 mg per mL, in a mixture of pH 7.0 phosphate buffer and carbon dioxide-free water (9 : 1).
pH ⟨791⟩: between 7.5 and 10.5, in a solution (1 in 100).
Water, *Method I* ⟨921⟩: not more than 6.5%.
Phosphate ions—
Standard phosphate solution—Dissolve 143.3 mg of dried monobasic potassium phosphate, KH_2PO_4, in water to make 1000.0 mL. This solution contains the equivalent of 0.10 mg of phosphate (PO_4) in each mL.
Phosphate reagent A—Dissolve 5 g of ammonium molybdate in 1 N sulfuric acid to make 100 mL.
Phosphate reagent B—Dissolve 350 mg of *p*-methylaminophenol sulfate in 50 mL of water, add 20 g of sodium bisulfite, mix to dissolve, and dilute with water to 100 mL.
Procedure—Dissolve about 50 mg of Prednisolone Sodium Phosphate, accurately weighed, in a mixture of 10 mL of water and 5 mL of 2 N sulfuric acid contained in a 25-mL volumetric flask, by warming if necessary. Add 1 mL each of *Phosphate reagent A* and *Phosphate reagent B*, dilute with water to 25 mL, mix, and allow to stand at room temperature for 30 minutes. Similarly and concomitantly, prepare a standard solution, using 5.0 mL of *Standard phosphate solution* instead of the 50 mg of the substance under test. Concomitantly determine the absorbances of both solutions in 1-cm cells at 730 nm, with a suitable spectrophotometer, using water as the blank. The absorbance of the test solution is not more than that of the standard solution. The limit is 1.0% of phosphate (PO_4).
Selenium ⟨291⟩: 0.003%, a 200-mg test specimen being used.
Free prednisolone—Dissolve 50.0 mg of Prednisolone Sodium Phosphate, accurately weighed, in water to make 25.0 mL. Pipet 5 mL of the solution into a glass-stoppered, 50-mL tube, add 25.0 mL of methylene chloride, insert the stopper, mix by gentle shaking, and allow to stand until the methylene chloride layer is clear (about 20 minutes). Determine the absorbance of the methylene chloride solution in a 1-cm cell at 241 nm, with a suitable spectrophotometer, using methylene chloride as the blank. Calculate the quantity, in mg, of free prednisolone in the portion of Prednisolone Sodium Phosphate weighed by comparison with the absorbance of the untreated methylene chloride solution of USP Prednisolone RS obtained as directed in the *Assay*: not more than 0.5 mg is found (1.0%).
Assay—
pH 9 buffer with magnesium—Mix 3.1 g of boric acid and 500 mL of water in a 1-liter volumetric flask, add 21 mL of 1 N sodium hydroxide and 10 mL of 0.1 M magnesium chloride, dilute with water to volume, and mix.
Alkaline phosphatase solution—Transfer 250 mg of alkaline phosphate enzyme to a 25-mL volumetric flask, dissolve by adding *pH 9 buffer with magnesium* to volume, and mix. Prepare this solution fresh daily.
Standard preparation—Dissolve a suitable, accurately weighed quantity of USP Prednisolone RS in methylene chloride, and dilute quantitatively and stepwise with methylene chloride to obtain a solution having a known concentration of about 16 μg per mL. Pipet 100 mL of the solution into a glass-stoppered, 100-mL cylinder, and add 1.0 mL of *Alkaline phosphatase solution* and 1.0 mL of water. Allow to stand, with occasional gentle inversion, for 2 hours.
Assay preparation—Dissolve about 100 mg of Prednisolone Sodium Phosphate, accurately weighed, in water that has been saturated with methylene chloride, to make 50.0 mL, and mix. Pipet 10 mL of this solution into a 125-mL separator, and shake with two 25-mL portions of water-washed methylene chloride, discarding the methylene chloride layers.

Procedure—Pipet 1 mL of the *Assay preparation* into a glass-stoppered, 100-mL cylinder, add 1.0 mL of *Alkaline phosphatase solution* and about 50 mL of methylene chloride, insert the stopper, and allow to stand, with occasional gentle inversion (about once every 15 minutes), for 2 hours. Add methylene chloride to volume, mix, and allow to stand until the methylene chloride layer is clear (about 20 minutes). Concomitantly and without delay, determine the absorbances of the methylene chloride solution obtained from the *Assay preparation* and the *Standard preparation* at 241 nm, with a suitable spectrophotometer, using methylene chloride as the blank. Calculate the quantity, in mg, of $C_{21}H_{27}Na_2O_8P$ in the portion of Prednisolone Sodium Phosphate taken by the formula:

$$1.344[5C(A_U/A_S)]$$

in which 1.344 is the ratio of the molecular weight of prednisolone sodium phosphate to that of prednisolone, *C* is the concentration, in μg per mL, of USP Prednisolone RS in the *Standard preparation*, and A_U and A_S are the absorbances of the solution from the *Assay preparation* and the *Standard preparation*, respectively.

Prednisolone Sodium Phosphate Injection

» Prednisolone Sodium Phosphate Injection is a sterile solution of Prednisolone Sodium Phosphate in Water for Injection. It contains not less than 90.0 percent and not more than 110.0 percent of the labeled amount of prednisolone phosphate ($C_{21}H_{29}O_8P$), present as the disodium salt.

Packaging and storage—Preserve in single-dose or in multiple-dose containers, preferably of Type I glass, protected from light.
USP Reference standards ⟨11⟩—*USP Prednisolone RS. USP Endotoxin RS.*
Identification—
A: Dissolve 65 mg of phenylhydrazine hydrochloride in 100 mL of dilute sulfuric acid (3 in 5), add 5 mL of isopropyl alcohol, and mix. Heat 5 mL of this solution with 1 mL of *Assay preparation* (obtained as directed in the *Assay*) at 70° for 2 hours: a yellow color develops.
B: It responds to *Identification* test A under *Prednisolone Sodium Phosphate*.
Bacterial endotoxins ⟨85⟩—It contains not more than 5.0 USP Endotoxin Units per mg of prednisolone phosphate.
pH ⟨791⟩: between 7.0 and 8.0.
Particulate matter ⟨788⟩: meets the requirements under small-volume injections.
Other requirements—It meets the requirements under *Injections* ⟨1⟩.
Assay—
pH 9 buffer with magnesium—Prepare as directed in the *Assay* under *Prednisolone Sodium Phosphate*.
Alkaline phosphatase solution—Prepare as directed in the *Assay* under *Prednisolone Sodium Phosphate*.
Standard preparation—Prepare as directed in the *Assay* under *Prednisolone Sodium Phosphate*.
Assay preparation—Pipet a volume of Injection, equivalent to about 100 mg of prednisolone phosphate, into a separator containing 20 mL of water. Wash the solution with two 10-mL portions of methylene chloride, and discard the washings. Transfer the aqueous layer to a 50-mL volumetric flask, dilute with water to volume, and mix.
Procedure—Proceed as directed for *Procedure* in the *Assay* under *Prednisolone Sodium Phosphate*. Calculate the quantity, in mg, of $C_{21}H_{29}O_8P$ in each mL of the Injection taken by the formula:

$$6.11(C/V)(A_U/A_S)$$

in which *C* is the concentration, in μg per mL, of USP Prednisolone RS in the *Standard preparation*, *V* is the volume, in mL, of Injection taken, and A_U and A_S are the absorbances of the solution from the *Assay preparation* and the *Standard preparation*, respectively.

Prednisolone Sodium Phosphate Ophthalmic Solution

» Prednisolone Sodium Phosphate Ophthalmic Solution is a sterile solution of Prednisolone Sodium Phosphate in a buffered, aqueous medium. It contains not less than 90.0 percent and not more than 115.0 percent of the labeled amount of prednisolone phosphate ($C_{21}H_{29}O_8P$), present as the disodium salt.

Packaging and storage—Preserve in tight, light-resistant containers.

USP Reference standards ⟨11⟩—*USP Prednisolone RS.*
Identification—It responds to *Identification* test A under *Prednisolone Sodium Phosphate* and to *Identification* test A under *Prednisolone Sodium Phosphate Injection.*
Sterility ⟨71⟩: meets the requirements.
pH ⟨791⟩: between 6.2 and 8.2.
Assay—Proceed with Ophthalmic Solution as directed in the *Assay* under *Prednisolone Sodium Phosphate Injection.*

Prednisolone Sodium Succinate for Injection

$C_{25}H_{31}NaO_8$ 482.50
Pregna-1,4-diene-3,20-dione, 21-(3-carboxy-1-oxopropoxy)-11,17-dihydroxy-, monosodium salt, (11β)-.
11β,17,21-Trihydroxypregna-1,4-diene-3,20-dione 21-(sodium succinate)   [1715-33-9].

» Prednisolone Sodium Succinate for Injection is sterile prednisolone sodium succinate prepared from Prednisolone Hemisuccinate with the aid of Sodium Hydroxide or Sodium Carbonate. It contains the equivalent of not less than 90.0 percent and not more than 110.0 percent of the labeled amount of prednisolone ($C_{21}H_{28}O_5$). It contains suitable buffers.

Packaging and storage—Preserve in *Containers for Sterile Solids* as described under *Injections* ⟨1⟩.
USP Reference standards ⟨11⟩—*USP Prednisolone Hemisuccinate RS. USP Endotoxin RS.*
Constituted solution—At the time of use, it meets the requirements for *Constituted Solutions* under *Injections* ⟨1⟩.
Identification—Place about 50 mg in a separator, add 20 mL of water and 2 mL of 3 N hydrochloric acid, and extract with 25 mL of chloroform. Filter the extract into a suitable beaker, evaporate on a steam bath to dryness, and dry the residue at 60° for 1 hour: the residue so obtained responds to *Identification* test A under *Prednisolone Hemisuccinate.*
Bacterial endotoxins ⟨85⟩—It contains not more than 5.8 USP Endotoxin Units per mg of prednisolone.
pH ⟨791⟩: between 6.7 and 8.0, determined in the solution constituted as directed in the labeling.

Loss on drying ⟨731⟩—Dry it at 105° for 3 hours: it loses not more than 2.0% of its weight.
Particulate matter ⟨788⟩: meets the requirements under small-volume injections.
Other requirements—It meets the requirements for *Sterility Tests* ⟨71⟩, *Uniformity of Dosage Units* ⟨905⟩ and *Labeling* under *Injections* ⟨1⟩.
Assay—
Standard preparation—Dissolve about 64 mg of USP Prednisolone Hemisuccinate RS, accurately weighed, in about 100 mL of alcohol, add 5.0 mL of water, dilute with alcohol to 200.0 mL, and mix. Dilute 4.0 mL of this solution with alcohol to 100.0 mL, and mix. Pipet 20 mL of the resulting solution into a glass-stoppered, 50-mL conical flask.
Assay preparation—Transfer an accurately weighed portion of Prednisolone Sodium Succinate for Injection, equivalent to about 50 mg of prednisolone, to a 200-mL volumetric flask, dissolve in 5.0 mL of water, add alcohol to volume, and mix. Dilute 4.0 mL of this mixture with alcohol to 100.0 mL, and mix. Pipet 20 mL of the resulting solution into a glass-stoppered, 50-mL conical flask.
Procedure—Proceed as directed under *Assay for Steroids* ⟨351⟩. Calculate the quantity, in mg, of $C_{21}H_{28}O_5$ in the portion of Prednisolone Sodium Succinate for Injection taken by the formula:

$$5C(0.7827)(A_U / A_S)$$

in which C is the concentration, in μg per mL, of USP Prednisolone Hemisuccinate RS in the *Standard preparation*, 0.7827 is the ratio of the molecular weight of prednisolone to that of prednisolone hemisuccinate, and A_U and A_S are the absorbances of the solutions from the *Assay preparation* and the *Standard preparation*, respectively.

Prednisolone Tebutate

$C_{27}H_{38}O_6$(monohydrate)   476.60
Pregna-1,4-diene-3,20-dione, 11,17-dihydroxy-21-(3,3-dimethyl-1-oxobutyl)oxy-, (11β)-.
11β,17,21-Trihydroxypregna-1,4-diene-3,20-dione 21-(3,3-dimethylbutyrate)   [7681-14-3].

» Prednisolone Tebutate contains not less than 97.0 percent and not more than 103.0 percent of $C_{27}H_{38}O_6$, calculated on the dried basis.

Packaging and storage—Preserve in tight containers sealed under sterile nitrogen, in a cold place.
USP Reference standards ⟨11⟩—*USP Prednisolone Tebutate RS.*
Identification—
A: Dissolve a portion of it in acetone, and evaporate to dryness: the IR absorption spectrum of a mineral oil dispersion of the residue so obtained, previously dried at a pressure not exceeding 5 mm of mercury at 105° for 4 hours, exhibits maxima only at the same wavelengths as that of a similar preparation of USP Prednisolone Tebutate RS.
B: *Ultraviolet Absorption* ⟨197U⟩—
Solution: 20 μg per mL.
Medium: methanol.
Absorptivities at 242 nm, calculated on the dried basis, do not differ by more than 3.0%.
Specific rotation ⟨781S⟩: between +100° and +115°.
Test solution: 10 mg per mL, in chloroform.
Loss on drying ⟨731⟩—Dry it at a pressure not exceeding 5 mm of mercury at 105° for 4 hours: it loses not more than 5.0% of its weight.

Residue on ignition ⟨281⟩: not more than 0.1%.
Selenium ⟨291⟩: 0.003%, a 200-mg specimen being used.
Assay—
  Mobile solvent—Prepare a mixture of isooctane, tetrahydrofuran, and alcohol (89 : 10 : 1).
  Standard preparation—Dissolve a suitable quantity of USP Prednisolone Tebutate RS, accurately weighed, in a mixture of tetrahydrofuran and isooctane (1 : 1) to obtain a solution having a known concentration of about 1 mg per mL.
  Assay preparation—Weigh accurately about 50 mg of Prednisolone Tebutate, transfer to a 50-mL volumetric flask, dilute with tetrahydrofuran and isooctane (1 : 1) to volume, and mix.
  Procedure—Inject separately 25-µL volumes of the *Standard preparation* and the *Assay preparation* into a suitable high-pressure liquid chromatograph equipped with a constant flow pump and a 30-cm × 3.9-mm column that contains packing L3, is operated at 25°, and is equipped with an UV detector capable of monitoring absorption at 254 nm. The flow rate is about 1.0 mL per minute. The retention time for Prednisolone Tebutate is about 30 minutes, but the chromatogram is run for about 45 minutes. Five replicate injections of the *Standard preparation* show a relative standard deviation of not more than 1.5%. Calculate the quantity, in mg, of $C_{27}H_{38}O_6$ in the portion of Prednisolone Tebutate taken by the formula:

$$50C(R_U / R_S)$$

in which C is the concentration, in mg per mL, of USP Prednisolone Tebutate RS in the *Standard preparation*, and R_U and R_S are the peak areas obtained from the *Assay preparation* and the *Standard preparation*, respectively.

Prednisolone Tebutate Injectable Suspension

» Prednisolone Tebutate Injectable Suspension is a sterile suspension of Prednisolone Tebutate in a suitable aqueous medium. It contains not less than 90.0 percent and not more than 110.0 percent of the labeled amount of $C_{27}H_{38}O_6$.

Packaging and storage—Preserve in single-dose or in multiple-dose containers, preferably of Type I glass.
USP Reference standards ⟨11⟩—*USP Prednisolone Tebutate RS. USP Endotoxin RS.*
Identification, *Ultraviolet Absorption* ⟨197U⟩—
  Solution: Dilute a portion of the Injectable Suspension with methanol to obtain a solution having a concentration of about 20 µg per mL.
Bacterial endotoxins ⟨85⟩—It contains not more than 8.8 USP Endotoxin Units per mg of prednisolone tebutate.
pH ⟨791⟩: between 6.0 and 8.0.
Other requirements—It meets the requirements under *Injections* ⟨1⟩.
Assay—
  Mobile solvent—Prepare a mixture of isooctane, tetrahydrofuran, and alcohol (89 : 10 : 8).
  Standard preparation—Dissolve an accurately weighed quantity of USP Prednisolone Tebutate RS in a mixture of tetrahydrofuran and isooctane (1 : 1) to obtain a solution having a known concentration of about 1 mg per mL.
  Assay preparation—Transfer to a separator an accurately measured volume, freshly mixed, of Injectable Suspension, equivalent to about 100 mg of prednisolone tebutate, and dilute with about 10 mL of water. Extract with three 25-mL portions of methylene chloride, filtering each portion through methylene chloride-washed cotton into a 100-mL volumetric flask. Add methylene chloride to volume, and mix. Pipet 10 mL of this solution into a 50-mL centrifuge tube, evaporate the methylene chloride on a steam bath just to dryness, cool, and dissolve the residue in 10.0 mL of tetrahydrofuran and isooctane (1 : 1). Filter through a 1-µm membrane filter.
  Procedure—Introduce equal volumes, about 10 µL, of the *Assay preparation* and the *Standard preparation* into a high-pressure liquid chromatograph (see *Chromatography* ⟨621⟩), operated at room temperature, by means of a suitable microsyringe or sampling valve, adjusting the sample size and other operating parameters such that the peak obtained with the *Standard preparation* is about 0.6 full-scale. Typically, the apparatus is fitted with a 3.9-mm × 30-cm column containing packing L3 and is equipped with an UV detector capable of monitoring absorption at 254 nm and a suitable recorder. In a suitable chromatogram, the coefficient of variation for five replicate injections of a single specimen is not more than 3.0%. Measure the height of the peaks, at identical retention times, obtained with the *Assay preparation* and the *Standard preparation*. Calculate the quantity, in mg, of $C_{27}H_{38}O_6$, in the volume of Injectable Suspension taken by the formula:

$$100C(r_U / r_S)$$

in which C is the concentration, in mg per mL, of USP Prednisolone Tebutate RS in the *Standard preparation*, and r_U and r_S are the peak heights obtained from the *Assay preparation* and the *Standard preparation*, respectively.

Prednisone

$C_{21}H_{26}O_5 \cdot H_2O$ 376.46
Pregna-1,4-diene-3,11,20-trione monohydrate, 17,21-dihydroxy-.
17,21-Dihydroxypregna-1,4-diene-3,11,20-trione monohydrate.
Anhydrous 358.44 [53-03-2].

» Prednisone contains one molecule of water of hydration or is anhydrous. It contains not less than 97.0 percent and not more than 102.0 percent of $C_{21}H_{26}O_5$, calculated on the anhydrous basis.

Packaging and storage—Preserve in well-closed containers.
Labeling—Label to indicate whether it is hydrous or anhydrous.
USP Reference standards ⟨11⟩—*USP Prednisone RS.*
Identification—
  A: *Infrared Absorption* ⟨197K⟩—If a difference appears, dissolve portions of both the test specimen and the Reference Standard in methanol, evaporate the solutions to dryness, and repeat the tests.
  B: Dissolve about 6 mg in 2 mL of sulfuric acid, and allow to stand for 5 minutes: an orange color is produced. Pour the solution into 10 mL of water: the color changes first to yellow and then, gradually, to bluish green.
Specific rotation ⟨781S⟩: between +167° and +175°.
  Test solution: 5 mg per mL, in dioxane.
Water, *Method I:* not more than 5.0% is found for Prednisone monohydrate, and not more than 1.0% is found for anhydrous Prednisone.
Residue on ignition ⟨281⟩: negligible, from 100 mg.
Chromatographic purity—
  Mobile phase—Prepare a filtered and degassed mixture of chloroform and methanol (98 : 2). Make adjustments if necessary (see *System Suitability* under *Chromatography* ⟨621⟩).
  Test solution—Transfer about 25 mg of Prednisone, accurately weighed, to a suitable container, dissolve in 20 mL of *Mobile phase*, and mix.
  Chromatographic system (see *Chromatography* ⟨621⟩)—The liquid chromatograph is equipped with a 254-nm detector and a 6.0-mm × 4.0-cm column that contains packing L3. The flow rate is about 1 mL per minute. Chromatograph the *Test solution*, and record the peak responses as directed for *Procedure*: the column efficiency is not less than 2,500 theoretical plates; and the relative standard deviation for replicate injections is not more than 2.0%.

Procedure—Inject a volume (about 5 μL) of the *Test solution* into the chromatograph, record the chromatogram, and measure the peak responses. Calculate the percentage of each impurity in the portion of Prednisone taken by the formula:

$$100(r_i / r_s)$$

in which r_i is the peak response for each impurity; and r_s is the sum of the responses of all peaks: not more than 1.5% of any individual impurity is found, and not more than 2.0% of total impurities is found.

Assay—
Mobile phase—Prepare a suitable filtered mixture of water, peroxide-free tetrahydrofuran, and methanol (688 : 250 : 62) such that at a flow rate of 1.0 mL per minute, the retention times of prednisone and acetanilide are about 8 and 6 minutes, respectively.

Internal standard solution—Prepare a solution of acetanilide in dilute methanol (1 in 2) having a concentration of about 110 μg per mL.

Standard preparation—Using an accurately weighed quantity of USP Prednisone RS, prepare a solution in dilute methanol (1 in 2) having a known concentration of about 0.2 mg per mL. Transfer 5.0 mL of this solution and 5.0 mL of the *Internal standard solution* to a 50-mL volumetric flask. Add dilute methanol (1 in 2) to volume, and mix to obtain a *Standard preparation* having a known concentration of about 20 μg of USP Prednisone RS per mL. Prepare this solution fresh.

Assay preparation—Using about 50 mg of Prednisone, accurately weighed, proceed as directed for *Standard preparation*, beginning with "prepare a solution in dilute methanol (1 in 2)."

Chromatographic system (see *Chromatography* ⟨621⟩)—The liquid chromatograph is equipped with a 254-nm detector and a 4-mm × 25-cm column that contains packing L1. Chromatograph five replicate injections of the *Standard preparation*, and record the peak responses as directed for *Procedure*: the relative standard deviation is not more than 2.0%; and the resolution factor between prednisone and the internal standard is not less than 3. Adjust the operating parameters so that the peak obtained from the *Standard preparation* is about one-half full-scale.

Procedure—Separately inject equal volumes (about 10 μL) of the *Standard preparation* and the *Assay preparation* into the chromatograph by means of a suitable microsyringe or sampling valve, record the chromatograms, and measure the responses at equivalent retention times. Calculate the quantity, in mg, of $C_{21}H_{26}O_5$ in the portion of Prednisone taken by the formula:

$$2.5C(R_U / R_S)$$

in which C is the concentration, in μg per mL, of USP Prednisone RS in the *Standard preparation*; and R_U and R_S are the peak response ratios of the prednisone peak to the internal standard peak obtained from the *Assay preparation* and the *Standard preparation*, respectively.

Prednisone Oral Solution

» Prednisone Oral Solution contains not less than 90.0 percent and not more than 110.0 percent of the labeled amount of prednisone ($C_{21}H_{26}O_5$).

Packaging and storage—Preserve in tight containers.
USP Reference standards ⟨11⟩—*USP Prednisone RS*.
Identification—Shake 50 mL of Oral Solution with 25 mL of chloroform for 5 minutes. Filter the chloroform extract through a pledget of cotton and a layer of anhydrous sodium sulfate, and evaporate on a warm water bath with the aid of a current of air to about 3 mL. Continue the evaporation to dryness at room temperature. Wash the residue with two 10-mL portions of hot solvent hexane, decanting the solvent and discarding it each time. Digest the residue with 25 mL of warm dehydrated alcohol for 15 minutes. Filter the mixture, and evaporate the filtrate to about 3 mL. Add solvent hexane until the mixture becomes slightly cloudy, and chill in a freezer to promote the formation of crystals. Collect the crystals, and dry at 60° for 1 hour: the crystals meet the requirements for *Identification* test A under *Prednisone*.

Uniformity of dosage units ⟨905⟩—
FOR ORAL SOLUTION PACKAGED IN SINGLE-UNIT CONTAINERS: meets the requirements.

Deliverable volume ⟨698⟩—
FOR ORAL SOLUTION PACKAGED IN MULTIPLE-UNIT CONTAINERS: meets the requirements.

pH ⟨791⟩: between 2.6 and 4.5.
Alcohol content, *Method II* ⟨611⟩: between 2.0% and 6.0% is found.

Assay—
Mobile phase—Dissolve 1.36 g of monobasic potassium phosphate in 600 mL of water, add 400 mL of methanol, pass through a 0.2-μm membrane filter, and degas. Make adjustments if necessary (see *System Suitability* under *Chromatography* ⟨621⟩).

Standard preparation—Using an accurately weighed quantity of USP Prednisone RS, prepare a solution in alcohol containing 1 mg per mL. Dilute 4 volumes of this solution quantitatively with 96 volumes of water to obtain a *Standard preparation* having a known concentration of about 40 μg per mL.

Assay preparation—Transfer an accurately measured volume of Oral Solution, equivalent to about 10 mg of prednisone, to a 250-mL volumetric flask. Dilute with water to volume, and mix.

Chromatographic system (see *Chromatography* ⟨621⟩)—The liquid chromatograph is equipped with a 254-nm detector and a 3.9-mm × 30-cm column that contains packing L1. The flow rate is about 1.5 mL per minute. Chromatograph the *Standard preparation*, and record the peak responses as directed for *Procedure*: the tailing factor for the analyte peak is not more than 2.0; and the relative standard deviation for replicate injections is not more than 2.0%.

Procedure—Separately inject equal volumes (about 10 μL) of the *Standard preparation* and the *Assay preparation* into the chromatograph by means of a sampling valve, record the chromatograms, and measure the responses for the major peaks. Calculate the quantity, in mg, of prednisone ($C_{21}H_{26}O_5$) in each mL of the Oral Solution taken by the formula:

$$(0.25C/V)(r_U / r_S)$$

in which C is the concentration, in μg per mL, of USP Prednisone RS in the *Standard preparation*; V is the volume, in mL, of Oral Solution taken; and r_U and r_S are the peak responses obtained from the *Assay preparation* and the *Standard preparation*, respectively.

Prednisone Injectable Suspension

» Prednisone Injectable Suspension is a sterile suspension of Prednisone in a suitable aqueous medium. It contains not less than 90.0 percent and not more than 110.0 percent of the labeled amount of $C_{21}H_{26}O_5$.

Packaging and storage—Preserve in multiple-dose containers, preferably of Type I glass.
Labeling—Label it to indicate that it is for veterinary use only. Label it to indicate that it is for intramuscular administration only.
USP Reference standards ⟨11⟩—*USP Prednisone RS. USP Endotoxin RS*.
Identification—The retention time of the major peak in the chromatogram of the *Assay preparation* corresponds to that of the *Standard preparation*, both relative to the internal standard, as obtained in the *Assay*.
pH ⟨791⟩: between 3.0 and 7.0.
Sterility ⟨71⟩—It meets the requirements when tested as directed for *Direct Inoculation of the Culture Medium* under *Test for Sterility of the Product to be Examined*.
Bacterial endotoxins ⟨85⟩—It contains not more than 2.27 Endotoxin Units per mg of prednisone.
Other requirements—It meets the requirements under *Injections* ⟨1⟩.

Assay—

Mobile phase—Prepare a filtered and degassed mixture of methanol and 0.05 M monobasic potassium phosphate (350 : 300). Make adjustments if necessary (see *System Suitability* under *Chromatography* ⟨621⟩).

Internal standard solution—Dissolve a quantity of betamethasone in methanol to obtain a solution containing about 0.4 mg per mL.

Standard preparation—Dissolve an accurately weighed quantity of USP Prednisone RS in methanol, and dilute quantitatively, and stepwise if necessary, with methanol to obtain a solution having a known concentration of about 0.25 mg per mL. Transfer 10.0 mL of this solution to a 50-mL volumetric flask. Add 10.0 mL of *Internal standard solution*, dilute with methanol to volume, and mix.

Assay preparation—Transfer an accurately measured volume of well-mixed Suspension, equivalent to about 80 mg of prednisone, to a 100-mL volumetric flask. Dilute with methanol to volume, and mix. Transfer 3.0 mL of this solution to a 50-mL volumetric flask. Add 10.0 mL of *Internal standard solution*, dilute with methanol to volume, and mix.

Chromatographic system (see *Chromatography* ⟨621⟩)—The liquid chromatograph is equipped with a 254-nm detector and a 4-mm × 30-cm column that contains packing L1. The flow rate is about 1 mL per minute. Chromatograph the *Standard preparation*, and record the peak responses as directed for *Procedure:* the relative retention times are about 1.9 for betamethasone and 1.0 for prednisone, the resolution, *R*, between the prednisone peak and the betamethasone peak is not less than 3.5, and the relative standard deviation for replicate injections is not more than 2.0%.

Procedure—Separately inject equal volumes (about 10 µL) of the *Standard preparation* and the *Assay preparation* into the chromatograph, record the chromatograms, and measure the responses for the analyte peaks. Calculate the quantity, in mg, of prednisone in each mL of the Suspension taken by the formula:

$$5000(C / 3V)(R_U / R_S)$$

in which *C* is the concentration, in mg per mL, of USP Prednisone RS in the *Standard preparation*, *V* is the volume, in mL, of the Suspension taken to prepare the *Assay preparation*, and R_U and R_S are the ratios of the prednisone peak to the internal standard peak obtained from the *Assay preparation* and the *Standard preparation*, respectively.

Prednisone Tablets

» Prednisone Tablets contain not less than 90.0 percent and not more than 110.0 percent of the labeled amount of $C_{21}H_{26}O_5$.

Packaging and storage—Preserve in well-closed containers.

USP Reference standards ⟨11⟩—*USP Prednisone RS*.

Identification—Into a 50-mL beaker containing a portion of pulverized Tablets, equivalent to about 10 mg of prednisone, add 10 mL of water, and mix to form a slurry. Transfer the slurry to a 3-cm × 13-cm column packed with diatomaceous earth, and allow to be absorbed for a period of 10 minutes. Elute the column with 60 mL of water-washed ether, evaporate the eluate on a steam bath to dryness, wash the residue with three 20-mL portions of *n*-heptane, and filter. Dry the residue at 105° for 30 minutes: the crystals respond to *Identification* tests *A* and *B* under *Prednisone*.

Dissolution ⟨711⟩—

Medium: water; use 500 mL of the *Dissolution Medium* for Tablets labeled to contain 10 mg of prednisone or less, and 900 mL for Tablets labeled to contain more than 10 mg of prednisone.

Apparatus 2: 50 rpm.

Time: 30 minutes.

Procedure—Determine the amount of $C_{21}H_{26}O_5$ dissolved from UV absorbances at the wavelength of maximum absorbance at about 242 nm of filtered portions of the solution under test, suitably diluted with *Dissolution Medium*, if necessary, in comparison with a Standard solution having a known concentration of USP Prednisone RS in the same medium. An amount of alcohol not to exceed 5% of the total volume of the Standard solution may be used to bring the prednisone standard into solution prior to dilution with water.

Tolerances—Not less than 80% *(Q)* of the labeled amount of $C_{21}H_{26}O_5$ is dissolved in 30 minutes.

Uniformity of dosage units ⟨905⟩: meet the requirements.

Procedure for content uniformity—

Mobile phase, Internal standard solution, Standard preparation, and *Chromatographic system*—Proceed as directed in the *Assay* under *Prednisone*.

Test preparation—Place 1 Tablet in a volumetric flask of such size that when the contents are diluted to volume the resulting solution has a concentration of about 0.2 mg of prednisone per mL. Add 5 mL of water, swirl, sonicate for 1 minute, add a volume of methanol equal to one-half the volume of the volumetric flask, and sonicate again for 1 minute. Dilute with water to volume, and mix. Transfer 5.0 mL of this solution and 5.0 mL of the *Internal standard solution* to a 50-mL volumetric flask, add dilute methanol (1 in 2) to volume, and mix. Filter through a 5-µm filter, discarding the first 20 mL of the filtrate.

Procedure—Proceed as directed for *Procedure* in the *Assay* under *Prednisone*, except to calculate the quantity, in mg, of $C_{21}H_{26}O_5$ in the Tablet taken by the formula:

$$DC(R_U / R_S)$$

in which *D* is the dilution factor for the *Test preparation* and the other terms are as defined therein.

Assay—

Mobile phase, Internal standard solution, Standard preparation, and *Chromatographic system*—Proceed as directed in the *Assay* under *Prednisone*.

Assay preparation—Weigh and finely powder not less than 20 Tablets. Transfer an accurately weighed portion of the powder, equivalent to about 20 mg of prednisone, to a 100-mL volumetric flask. Add 5 mL of water, sonicate for 1 minute, add 50 mL of methanol, and sonicate again for 1 minute. Dilute with water to volume, and mix. Transfer 5.0 mL of this solution and 5.0 mL of the *Internal standard solution* to a 50-mL volumetric flask, add dilute methanol (1 in 2) to volume, and mix. Filter through a 5-µm filter, discarding the first 20 mL of the filtrate.

Procedure—Proceed as directed for *Procedure* in the *Assay* under *Prednisone*, except to calculate the quantity, in mg, of $C_{21}H_{26}O_5$ in the portion of Tablets taken by the formula:

$$C(R_U / R_S)$$

in which the terms are as defined therein.

Prilocaine

$C_{13}H_{20}N_2O$ 220.31

Propranamide, *N*-(2-methylphenyl)-2-(propylamino)-.

2-(Propylamino)-*o*-propionotoluidide.

(*RS*)-*N*-(2-methylphenyl)-2-(propylamino)propanamide   [721-50-6].

» Prilocaine contains not less than 99.0 percent and not more than 101.0 percent of $C_{13}H_{20}N_2O$, calculated on the anhydrous basis.

Packaging and storage—Preserve in well-closed containers, and store below 25°.

USP Reference standards ⟨11⟩—*USP Prilocaine RS. USP Prilocaine Related Compound A RS. USP Prilocaine Related Compound B RS.*

Identification, *Infrared Absorption* ⟨197K⟩—Because of the low melting point of prilocaine, the mortar, pestle, and potassium bromide must be at ambient temperature. Record the IR spectrum using the diffuse reflectance technique.

Melting range, *Class 1a* ⟨741⟩: between 36° and 39°, without previous drying.

Water, *Method Ia* ⟨921⟩: not more than 0.5%, determined on 1.00 g of sample.

Residue on ignition ⟨281⟩: not more than 0.1%.

Limit of prilocaine related compound A—

Mobile phase—Prepare as directed under *Related compounds*.

Standard solution—Dissolve an accurately weighed quantity of USP Prilocaine Related Compound A RS in *Mobile phase*, and dilute quantitatively, and stepwise if necessary, with *Mobile phase* to obtain a solution having a known concentration of about 1.3 µg per mL.

Test solution—Transfer about 100 mg of Prilocaine, accurately weighed, to a 10-mL volumetric flask, dissolve and dilute with *Mobile phase* to volume, and mix.

Chromatographic system (see *Chromatography* ⟨621⟩)—Use the system as described under *Related compounds*. Chromatograph the *Standard solution,* and record the peak responses as directed for *Procedure*: the signal-to-noise ratio of the major peak should be greater than 10.

Procedure—Separately inject equal volumes (about 20 µL) of the *Standard solution* and the *Test solution* into the chromatograph, record the chromatograms, and measure the responses for the major peaks: any peak corresponding to prilocaine related compound A (*o*-toluidine) in the *Test solution* is not greater than the response of the major peak in the *Standard solution* (0.01%).

Related compounds—

Buffer—Dilute 1.3 mL of a 1 M monobasic sodium phosphate solution (1.38 g diluted with water to 10 mL) and 32.5 mL of a 0.5 M anhydrous disodium hydrogen phosphate solution (7.1 g diluted with water to 100 mL) with water to 1 L. The pH of this solution is 8.0. Make adjustments as needed.

Mobile phase—Prepare a degassed mixture of *Buffer* and acetonitrile (73 : 27). Make adjustments if necessary (see *System Suitability* under *Chromatography* ⟨621⟩).

System suitability solution—Dissolve accurately weighed quantities of USP Prilocaine RS and USP Prilocaine Related Compound B RS in *Mobile phase,* and dilute quantitatively, and stepwise if necessary, with *Mobile phase* to obtain a solution having known concentrations of about 2.5 µg per mL and 3.0 µg per mL, respectively.

Test solution—Transfer about 25 mg of Prilocaine, accurately weighed, to a 10-mL volumetric flask, dilute with *Mobile phase* to volume, and mix.

Chromatographic system (see *Chromatography* ⟨621⟩)—The liquid chromatograph is equipped with a 240-nm detector and a 4.6-mm × 15-cm column that contains 5-µm packing L1. The flow rate is about 1 mL per minute. Chromatograph the *System suitability solution,* and record the peak responses as directed for *Procedure:* the relative retention times are about 1.19 for prilocaine related compound B and 1.0 for prilocaine; the resolution, *R*, between prilocaine and prilocaine related compound B is not less than 3.0; and the signal-to-noise ratio for the prilocaine peak is not less than 10.

Procedure—Inject a volume (about 20 µL) of the *Test solution* into the chromatograph, record the chromatograms, and measure the peak responses. Run the chromatograms for at least 1.5 times the retention of prilocaine. Check the stability of the baseline by injecting *Mobile phase*. Calculate the percentage of each impurity in the portion of Prilocaine taken by the formula:

$$100(r_i / r_s)$$

in which r_i is the individual peak response of each impurity; and r_s is the sum of the responses of all the peaks: not more than 0.2% of any individual impurity is found; not more than one impurity exceeds 0.1%, and not more than 0.5% of total impurities is found.

Assay—Dissolve 400 mg of Prilocaine, accurately weighed, in 50 mL of glacial acetic acid. Titrate with 0.1 N perchloric acid VS, determining the endpoint potentiometrically. Perform a blank determination, and make any necessary correction (see *Titrimetry* ⟨541⟩). Each mL of 0.1 N perchloric acid is equivalent to 22.03 mg of $C_{13}H_{20}N_2O$.

Prilocaine Hydrochloride

$C_{13}H_{20}N_2O \cdot HCl$ 256.77

Propanamide, *N*-(2-methylphenyl)-2-(propylamino)-, monohydrochloride.

2-(Propylamino)-*o*-propionotoluidide monohydrochloride [1786-81-8].

» Prilocaine Hydrochloride contains not less than 99.0 percent and not more than 101.0 percent of $C_{13}H_{20}N_2O \cdot HCl$, calculated on the dried basis.

Packaging and storage—Preserve in well-closed containers.

USP Reference standards ⟨11⟩—*USP Prilocaine Hydrochloride RS.*

Identification—

A: *Infrared Absorption* ⟨197K⟩.

B: Dissolve about 300 mg in 5 mL of water, add 4 mL of 6 N ammonium hydroxide, and extract with 50 mL of chloroform. Filter the extract, and evaporate the filtrate on a steam bath with the aid of a current of air. Dissolve about 100 mg of the prilocaine so obtained in 1 mL of alcohol, add 10 drops of cobaltous chloride TS, and shake for 2 minutes: a bright green color develops, and a precipitate is formed.

C: Dissolve about 100 mg in 3 mL of water, render the solution alkaline with 6 N ammonium hydroxide, and filter: the filtrate responds to the tests for *Chloride* ⟨191⟩.

Melting range, *Class I* ⟨741⟩: between 166° and 169°.

Loss on drying ⟨731⟩—Dry it at 105° for 4 hours: it loses not more than 0.3% of its weight.

Residue on ignition ⟨281⟩: not more than 0.1%.

Heavy metals, *Method I* ⟨231⟩: 0.002%.

Assay—Dissolve about 500 mg of Prilocaine Hydrochloride, accurately weighed, in 50 mL of glacial acetic acid, add 10 mL of mercuric acetate TS and 2 drops of crystal violet TS, and titrate with 0.1 N perchloric acid VS to a blue-green endpoint. Perform a blank determination, and make any necessary correction. Each mL of 0.1 N perchloric acid is equivalent to 25.68 mg of $C_{13}H_{20}N_2O \cdot HCl$.

Prilocaine Hydrochloride Injection

» Prilocaine Hydrochloride Injection is a sterile solution of Prilocaine Hydrochloride in Water for Injection. It contains not less than 95.0 percent and not more than 105.0 percent of the labeled amount of $C_{13}H_{20}N_2O \cdot HCl$.

Packaging and storage—Preserve in single-dose or in multiple-dose containers, preferably of Type I glass.

USP Reference standards ⟨11⟩—*USP Prilocaine Hydrochloride RS. USP Endotoxin RS.*

Identification—

A: It meets the requirements under *Identification—Organic Nitrogenous Bases* ⟨181⟩.

B: It responds to *Identification* test B under *Prilocaine Hydrochloride*.

Bacterial endotoxins ⟨85⟩—It contains not more than 0.9 USP Endotoxin Unit per mg of prilocaine hydrochloride.

pH ⟨791⟩: between 6.0 and 7.0.

Other requirements—It meets the requirements under *Injections* ⟨1⟩.

Assay—
Mobile phase—Mix 50 mL of glacial acetic acid and 930 mL of water, and adjust with 1 N sodium hydroxide to a pH of 3.40. Mix about 4 volumes of this solution with 1 volume of acetonitrile, such that the retention time of prilocaine is about 4 to 6 minutes. Filter through a membrane filter (1 μm or finer porosity), and degas. Make adjustments if necessary (see *System Suitability* under *Chromatography* ⟨621⟩).

Standard preparation—Dissolve an accurately weighed quantity of USP Prilocaine Hydrochloride RS quantitatively in *Mobile phase* to obtain a solution having a known concentration of about 4 mg per mL.

Assay preparation—Transfer an accurately measured volume of Injection, equivalent to about 200 mg of prilocaine hydrochloride, to a 50-mL volumetric flask, dilute with *Mobile phase* to volume, and mix.

Resolution preparation—Prepare a solution of procainamide hydrochloride in *Mobile phase* containing about 900 μg per mL. Mix 2 mL of this solution and 20 mL of *Standard preparation*.

Chromatographic system (see *Chromatography* ⟨621⟩)—The liquid chromatograph is equipped with a 254-nm detector and a 3.9-mm × 30-cm column that contains packing L1, and is operated at a temperature between 20° and 25° maintained at ±1.0° of the selected temperature. The flow rate is about 1.5 mL per minute. Chromatograph the *Standard preparation*, and record the peak responses as directed for *Procedure:* the relative standard deviation for replicate injections is not more than 1.5%. Chromatograph about 10 μL of the *Resolution preparation*, and record the peak responses as directed for *Procedure:* the resolution, R, between the prilocaine and procainamide peaks is not less than 2.0.

Procedure—[NOTE—Use peak areas where peak responses are indicated.] Separately inject equal volumes (about 10 μL) of the *Standard preparation* and the *Assay preparation* into the liquid chromatograph, record the chromatograms, and measure the responses for the major peaks. Calculate the quantity, in mg, of $C_{13}H_{20}N_2O \cdot HCl$ in each mL of the Injection taken by the formula:

$$(50)(C/V)(r_U/r_S)$$

in which C is the concentration, in mg per mL, of USP Prilocaine Hydrochloride RS in the *Standard preparation*, V is the volume, in mL, of Injection taken, and r_U and r_S are the peak responses obtained from the *Assay preparation* and the *Standard preparation*, respectively.

Prilocaine and Epinephrine Injection

» Prilocaine and Epinephrine Injection is a sterile solution prepared from Prilocaine Hydrochloride and Epinephrine with the aid of Hydrochloric Acid in Water for Injection, or a sterile solution of Prilocaine Hydrochloride and Epinephrine Bitartrate in Water for Injection. The content of epinephrine does not exceed 0.002 percent (1 in 50,000). Prilocaine and Epinephrine Injection contains the equivalent of not less than 95.0 percent and not more than 105.0 percent of the labeled amount of prilocaine hydrochloride ($C_{13}H_{20}N_2O \cdot HCl$) and the equivalent of not less than 90.0 percent and not more than 115.0 percent of the labeled amount of epinephrine ($C_9H_{13}NO_3$).

Packaging and storage—Preserve in single-dose or in multiple-dose, light-resistant containers, preferably of Type I glass.

Labeling—The label indicates that the Injection is not to be used if its color is pinkish or darker than slightly yellow or if it contains a precipitate.

USP Reference standards ⟨11⟩—*USP Prilocaine Hydrochloride RS. USP Epinephrine Bitartrate RS. USP Endotoxin RS.*

Color and clarity—Using the Injection as the *Test solution*, proceed as directed for *Color and clarity* under *Epinephrine Injection*.

Identification—
A: It responds to *Identification* test B under *Prilocaine Hydrochloride*.

B: The chromatogram of the *Assay preparation* obtained as directed in the *Assay for prilocaine hydrochloride* exhibits a major peak for prilocaine, the retention time of which corresponds to that exhibited in the chromatogram of the *Standard preparation* obtained as directed in the *Assay for prilocaine hydrochloride*.

C: The chromatogram of the *Assay preparation* obtained as directed in the *Assay for epinephrine* exhibits a major peak for epinephrine, the retention time of which corresponds to that exhibited in the chromatogram of the *Standard preparation* obtained as directed in the *Assay for epinephrine*.

Bacterial endotoxins ⟨85⟩—It contains not more than 0.9 USP Endotoxin Unit per mg of prilocaine hydrochloride.

pH ⟨791⟩: between 3.3 and 5.5.

Other requirements—It meets the requirements under *Injections* ⟨1⟩.

Assay for prilocaine hydrochloride—
Mobile phase, Standard preparation, Resolution preparation, and *Chromatographic system*—Proceed as directed in the *Assay* under *Prilocaine Hydrochloride Injection*.

Assay preparation—Transfer an accurately measured volume of Injection, equivalent to about 200 mg of prilocaine hydrochloride, to a 50-mL volumetric flask, dilute with *Mobile phase* to volume, and mix.

Procedure—[NOTE—Use peak areas where peak responses are indicated.] Separately inject equal volumes (about 10 μL) of the *Assay preparation* and the *Standard preparation* into the chromatograph, record the chromatograms, and measure the responses for the major peaks. Calculate the quantity, in mg, of prilocaine hydrochloride ($C_{13}H_{20}N_2O \cdot HCl$) in each mL of the Injection taken by the formula:

$$50(C/V)(r_U/r_S)$$

in which C is the concentration, in mg per mL, of USP Prilocaine Hydrochloride RS in the *Standard preparation*, V is the volume, in mL, of Injection taken, and r_U and r_S are the prilocaine peak responses obtained from the *Assay preparation* and the *Standard preparation*, respectively.

Assay for epinephrine—
Mobile phase—Mix 50 mL of glacial acetic acid and 930 mL of water, and adjust with 1 N sodium hydroxide to a pH of 3.40. Dissolve 1.1 g of sodium 1-heptanesulfonate in this solution, add 1.0 mL of 0.1 M disodium ethylenediaminetetraacetate, and mix. Mix about 9 volumes of this solution with 1 volume of methanol. Filter through a membrane filter (1 μm or finer porosity), and degas. Make adjustments if necessary (see *System Suitability* under *Chromatography* ⟨621⟩).

Standard preparation—Dissolve an accurately weighed quantity of USP Epinephrine Bitartrate RS in *Mobile phase* to obtain a solution having a known concentration of about 9 μg of epinephrine bitartrate per mL. Pipet 10 mL of this solution into a 50-mL volumetric flask, dilute with *Mobile phase* to volume, and mix to obtain a *Standard preparation* having a known concentration of about 1.8 μg of epinephrine bitartrate per mL.

Assay preparation—Transfer an accurately measured volume of Injection, equivalent to about 50 μg of epinephrine, to a 50-mL volumetric flask, dilute with *Mobile phase* to volume, and mix.

Chromatographic system (see *Chromatography* ⟨621⟩)—The liquid chromatograph is fitted with a 30-cm × 3.9-mm stainless steel column packed with packing L1, and is equipped with an electrochemical detector held at a potential of +650 mV, a controller capable of regulating the background current, and a suitable recorder, and it is operated at a temperature between 20° and 25° maintained at ±1.0° of the selected temperature. The flow rate is about 1 mL per minute. Chromatograph the *Standard preparation* as directed for *Procedure:* the relative standard deviation of the peak responses of successive injections of the *Standard preparation* is not more than 1.5%.

Procedure—Separately inject equal volumes (about 20 μL) of the *Assay preparation* and the *Standard preparation* into the chromatograph, record the chromatograms, and measure the responses for the major peaks. Calculate the quantity, in µg, of epinephrine ($C_9H_{13}NO_3$) in each mL of the Injection taken by the formula:

$$(183.21 / 333.30)50(C / V)(r_U / r_S)$$

in which 183.21 and 333.30 are the molecular weights of epinephrine and epinephrine bitartrate, respectively, C is the concentration, in µg per mL, of USP Epinephrine Bitartrate RS in the *Standard preparation*, V is the volume, in mL, of Injection taken, and r_U and r_S are the peak responses obtained from the *Assay preparation* and the *Standard preparation*, respectively.

Primaquine Phosphate

$C_{15}H_{21}N_3O \cdot 2H_3PO_4$ 455.34
1,4-Pentanediamine, N^4-(6-methoxy-8-quinolinyl)-, (±)-, phosphate (1 : 2).
(±)-8-[(4-Amino-1-methylbutyl)amino]-6-methoxyquinoline phosphate (1 : 2) [*63-45-6*].

» Primaquine Phosphate contains not less than 98.0 percent and not more than 102.0 percent of $C_{15}H_{21}N_3O \cdot 2H_3PO_4$, calculated on the dried basis.

Packaging and storage—Preserve in well-closed, light-resistant containers.

USP Reference standards ⟨11⟩—*USP Primaquine Phosphate RS.*
Identification—
 A: *Infrared Absorption* ⟨197K⟩.
 B: The residue obtained by ignition responds to the test for pyrophosphate as described under *Phosphate* ⟨191⟩.
Loss on drying ⟨731⟩—Dry it at 105° for 2 hours: it loses not more than 1.0% of its weight.
Organic volatile impurities, *Method I* ⟨467⟩: meets the requirements.
(Official until July 1, 2008)
Assay—Dissolve about 700 mg of Primaquine Phosphate, accurately weighed, in about 75 mL of water in a beaker, add 10 mL of hydrochloric acid, and proceed as directed under *Nitrite Titration* ⟨451⟩, beginning with "cool to about 15°." Each mL of 0.1 M sodium nitrite is equivalent to 45.53 mg of $C_{15}H_{21}N_3O \cdot 2H_3PO_4$.

Primaquine Phosphate Tablets

» Primaquine Phosphate Tablets contain not less than 93.0 percent and not more than 107.0 percent of the labeled amount of $C_{15}H_{21}N_3O \cdot 2H_3PO_4$.

Packaging and storage—Preserve in well-closed, light-resistant containers.

USP Reference standards ⟨11⟩—*USP Primaquine Phosphate RS.*
Identification—Digest a quantity of finely powdered Tablets, equivalent to about 25 mg of primaquine phosphate, with 10 mL of water for 15 minutes, and filter.
 A: Dilute 0.1 mL of the filtrate with 1 mL of water, and add 1 drop of gold chloride TS: a violet-blue color is produced at once.
 B: To the remainder of the filtrate add 5 mL of trinitrophenol TS: a yellow precipitate is formed. Wash the precipitate with cold water, and dry at 105° for 2 hours: the picrate melts between 208° and 215°. [*Caution—Picrates may explode.*]

Dissolution ⟨711⟩—
 Medium: 0.01 N hydrochloric acid; 900 mL.
 Apparatus 2: 50 rpm.
 Time: 60 minutes.
 Determine the amount of $C_{15}H_{21}N_3O \cdot 2H_3PO_4$ dissolved by employing the following method.
 1-Pentanesulfonate sodium solution—Add about 961 mg of sodium 1-pentanesulfonate and 1 mL of glacial acetic acid to 400 mL of water, and mix.
 Mobile phase—Prepare a filtered and degassed mixture of methanol and *1-Pentanesulfonate sodium solution* (60 : 40). Make adjustments if necessary (see *System Suitability* under *Chromatography* ⟨621⟩).
 Chromatographic system (see *Chromatography* ⟨621⟩)—The liquid chromatograph is equipped with a 254-nm detector and a 3.9-mm × 30-cm column that contains packing L1. The flow rate is about 2 mL per minute. Chromatograph replicate injections of the Standard solution and record the peak responses as directed for *Procedure:* the relative standard deviation is not more than 3.0%.
 Procedure—Separately inject into the chromatograph equal volumes (about 20 µL) of the solution under test and a Standard solution having a known concentration of USP Primaquine Phosphate RS in the same *Medium*, and record the chromatograms. Measure the responses for the major peaks, and calculate the amount of $C_{15}H_{21}N_3O \cdot 2H_3PO_4$ dissolved.
 Tolerances—Not less than 80% (*Q*) of the labeled amount of $C_{15}H_{21}N_3O \cdot 2H_3PO_4$ is dissolved in 60 minutes.
Uniformity of dosage units ⟨905⟩: meet the requirements.
 Procedure for content uniformity—Transfer 1 Tablet, previously crushed or finely powdered, to a beaker, add 5 mL of hydrochloric acid and about 25 g of crushed ice, then add water to bring the total volume to about 50 mL. Proceed as directed under *Nitrite Titration* ⟨451⟩, beginning with "slowly titrate," and using as the titrant 0.01 M sodium nitrite VS, freshly prepared from 0.1 M sodium nitrite. Concomitantly perform a blank titration, and make any necessary correction. Each mL of 0.01 M sodium nitrite is equivalent to 4.553 mg of $C_{15}H_{21}N_3O \cdot 2H_3PO_4$.
Assay—Weigh and finely powder not less than 30 Tablets. Weigh accurately a portion of the powder, equivalent to about 700 mg of primaquine phosphate, and transfer to a beaker. Add 50 mL of water and sufficient hydrochloric acid to provide about 5 mL in excess, and proceed as directed under *Nitrite Titration* ⟨451⟩, beginning with "cool to about 15°." Each mL of 0.1 M sodium nitrite is equivalent to 45.53 mg of $C_{15}H_{21}N_3O \cdot 2H_3PO_4$.

Primidone

$C_{12}H_{14}N_2O_2$ 218.25
4,6(1*H*,5*H*)-Pyrimidinedione, 5-ethyldihydro-5-phenyl-.
5-Ethyldihydro-5-phenyl-4,6(1*H*,5*H*)-pyrimidinedione [*125-33-7*].

» Primidone contains not less than 98.0 percent and not more than 102.0 percent of $C_{12}H_{14}N_2O_2$, calculated on the dried basis.

Packaging and storage—Preserve in well-closed containers.

USP Reference standards ⟨11⟩—*USP Primidone RS.*
Identification—
 A: *Infrared Absorption* ⟨197K⟩—If a difference appears, dissolve portions of both the tests specimen and the Reference Standard in alcohol, evaporate the solutions to dryness, and repeat the tests.

B: *Ultraviolet Absorption* ⟨197U⟩—
Solution: 400 μg per mL.
Medium: alcohol.
Absorptivities at 257 nm, calculated on the dried basis, do not differ by more than 3.0%.
C: Fuse 0.20 g with 0.20 g of anhydrous sodium carbonate: ammonia is evolved.
Melting range ⟨741⟩: between 279° and 284°.
Loss on drying ⟨731⟩—Dry it at 105° for 2 hours: it loses not more than 0.5% of its weight.
Residue on ignition ⟨281⟩: not more than 0.2%.
Ordinary impurities ⟨466⟩—
Test solution—Prepare a solution in methanol having a known concentration of 2 mg per mL.
Standard solutions—Prepare solutions in methanol having known concentrations of 2, 10, 20, and 40 μg per mL.
Eluant: a mixture of butyl alcohol, glacial acetic acid, and water (5 : 3 : 2).
Visualization—Expose the plate to chlorine gas for about 15 minutes, air-dry until the chlorine has dissipated (about 15 minutes), and follow with visualization technique 20.
Organic volatile impurities, *Method V* ⟨467⟩: meets the requirements.
Solvent—Use dimethyl sulfoxide.

(Official until July 1, 2008)
Assay—Transfer about 40 mg of Primidone, accurately weighed, to a 100-mL volumetric flask. Add 70 mL of alcohol, and boil gently to dissolve. Cool, and add alcohol to volume. Determine the absorbances in a 2-cm cell, with a suitable spectrophotometer, using alcohol as the blank, at the minima that occur at about 254 nm and 261 nm and at the maximum that occurs at about 257 nm. Concomitantly determine the absorbances of a Standard solution in alcohol of USP Primidone RS, similarly prepared to have a known concentration of about 400 μg per mL. Calculate the quantity, in mg, of $C_{12}H_{14}N_2O_2$ in the Primidone taken by the formula:

$$0.1C(2A_{257} - A_{254} - A_{261})_U / (2A_{257} - A_{254} - A_{261})_S$$

in which C is the concentration, in μg per mL, of USP Primidone RS in the Standard solution, and the parenthetic expressions are the differences in the absorbances of the two solutions at the wavelengths indicated by the subscripts for the solution of Primidone (U) and the Standard solution (S), respectively.

Primidone Oral Suspension

» Primidone Oral Suspension is a suspension of Primidone in a suitable aqueous vehicle. It contains, in each 100 mL, not less than 4.5 g and not more than 5.5 g of primidone ($C_{12}H_{14}N_2O_2$).

Packaging and storage—Preserve in tight, light-resistant containers.
USP Reference standards ⟨11⟩—*USP Primidone RS.*
Identification—The retention time of the major peak in the chromatogram of the *Assay preparation* corresponds to that in the chromatogram of the *Standard preparation*, both relative to the internal standard, as obtained in the *Assay*.
Uniformity of dosage units ⟨905⟩—
FOR ORAL SUSPENSION PACKAGED IN SINGLE-UNIT CONTAINERS: meets the requirements.
Deliverable volume ⟨698⟩—
FOR ORAL SUSPENSION PACKAGED IN MULTIPLE-UNIT CONTAINERS: meets the requirements.
pH ⟨791⟩: between 5.5 and 8.5.
Assay—
Internal standard solution—Dissolve a suitable quantity of androsterone in alcohol to obtain a solution having a final concentration of about 10 mg per mL.
Standard preparation—Transfer about 100 mg of USP Primidone RS, accurately weighed, to a 100-mL volumetric flask, add 65 mL of alcohol, and boil for 1 hour. Allow to cool to ambient temperature, add 10.0 mL of *Internal standard solution*, dilute with alcohol to volume, mix, and filter.
Assay preparation—Transfer an accurately weighed quantity of well-mixed Oral Suspension, equivalent to about 50 mg of primidone, to a 50-mL volumetric flask; add 35 mL of alcohol; and boil for 1 hour. Allow to cool to ambient temperature, add 5.0 mL of *Internal standard solution*, dilute with alcohol to volume, mix, and filter.
Chromatographic system (see *Chromatography* ⟨621⟩)—The gas chromatograph is equipped with a flame-ionization detector and a 4.0-mm × 120-cm column packed with 10% liquid phase G3 on support S1AB. Helium is used as the carrier gas at a flow rate of about 40 mL per minute. The detector and injection port temperatures are maintained at about 310°, and the column temperature is maintained at about 260°. Chromatograph three replicate injections of the *Standard preparation*, and record the peak responses as directed for *Procedure*: the relative standard deviation is not more than 2.0%; and the resolution factor between primidone and androsterone is not less than 1.5.
Procedure—Separately inject equal volumes (about 3 μL) of the *Standard preparation* and the *Assay preparation* into the chromatograph, record the chromatograms, and measure the responses for the major peaks. The relative retention times are about 0.8 for primidone and 1.0 for androsterone. Calculate the quantity, in mg, of primidone ($C_{12}H_{14}N_2O_2$) in each mL of the Oral Suspension taken by the formula:

$$0.5D(W_S / W_U)(R_U / R_S)$$

in which D is the density, in g per mL, of the Oral Suspension; W_S is the weight, in mg, of the Standard used; W_U is the weight, in mg, of Oral Suspension taken; and R_U and R_S are the relative response factors obtained from the *Assay preparation* and the *Standard preparation*, respectively.

Primidone Tablets

» Primidone Tablets contain not less than 95.0 percent and not more than 105.0 percent of the labeled amount of $C_{12}H_{14}N_2O_2$.

Packaging and storage—Preserve in well-closed containers.
Labeling—Tablets intended solely for veterinary use are so labeled.
USP Reference standards ⟨11⟩—*USP Primidone RS.*
Identification—The retention time of the major peak in the chromatogram of the *Assay preparation* corresponds to that of the *Standard preparation*, both relative to the internal standard, obtained as directed in the *Assay*.
Dissolution ⟨711⟩—
Medium: water; 900 mL.
Apparatus 2: 50 rpm.
Time: 60 minutes.
Procedure—[NOTE—Perform baseline corrections, if necessary, in determining the absorbance by extrapolating the baseline through the absorbance minima at about 300 and 280 nm and beyond 257 nm.] Determine the amount of $C_{12}H_{14}N_2O_2$ dissolved from UV absorbances at the wavelength of maximum absorbance at about 257 nm of filtered portions of the solution under test, suitably diluted with *Dissolution Medium*, if necessary, in comparison with a *Standard solution* having a known concentration of USP Primidone RS in the same medium.
Tolerances—Not less than 75% (*Q*) of the labeled amount of $C_{12}H_{14}N_2O_2$ is dissolved in 60 minutes.
Uniformity of dosage units ⟨905⟩: meet the requirements.
Assay—
Internal standard solution—Dissolve a suitable quantity of androsterone in alcohol to obtain a solution having a final concentration of about 10 mg per mL.
Standard preparation—Transfer about 100 mg of USP Primidone RS, accurately weighed, to a 100-mL volumetric flask, add 65 mL of alcohol, and boil for 1 hour. Allow to cool to ambient tempera-

ture, add 10.0 mL of *Internal standard solution*, dilute with alcohol to volume, mix, and filter.

Assay preparation—Weigh and finely powder not less than 20 Tablets. Transfer an accurately weighed portion of the powder, equivalent to about 50 mg of primidone, to a 50-mL volumetric flask, add 35 mL of alcohol, and boil for 1 hour. Allow to cool to ambient temperature, add 5.0 mL of *Internal standard solution*, dilute with alcohol to volume, mix, and filter.

Chromatographic system (see *Chromatography* ⟨621⟩)—The gas chromatograph is equipped with a flame-ionization detector and a 4.0-mm × 120-cm column packed with 10% liquid phase G3 on support S1AB. Helium is used as the carrier gas at a flow rate of about 40 mL per minute. The detector and injector temperatures are maintained at about 310° and the column temperature is maintained at about 260°. Chromatograph three replicate injections of the *Standard preparation*, and record the peak responses as directed for *Procedure:* the relative standard deviation is not more than 2.0%, and the resolution factor between primidone and androsterone is not less than 1.5.

Procedure—Separately inject equal volumes (about 3 μL) of the *Standard preparation* and the *Assay preparation* into the chromatograph, record the chromatograms, and measure the responses for the major peaks. The relative retention times are about 0.8 for primidone and 1.0 for androsterone. Calculate the quantity, in mg, of $C_{12}H_{14}N_2O_2$ in the portion of Tablets taken by the formula:

$$50C(R_U / R_S)$$

in which C is the concentration, in mg per mL, of USP Primidone RS in the *Standard preparation*, and R_U and R_S are the relative response factors obtained from the *Assay preparation* and the *Standard preparation*, respectively.

Probenecid

$C_{13}H_{19}NO_4S$ 285.36
Benzoic acid, 4-[(dipropylamino)sulfonyl]-.
p-(Dipropylsulfamoyl)benzoic acid   [57-66-9].

» Probenecid contains not less than 98.0 percent and not more than 101.0 percent of $C_{13}H_{19}NO_4S$, calculated on the dried basis.

Packaging and storage—Preserve in well-closed containers.

USP Reference standards ⟨11⟩—*USP Probenecid RS*.
Identification—
  A: *Infrared Absorption* ⟨197K⟩.
  B: *Ultraviolet Absorption* ⟨197U⟩—
  Solution: 20 μg per mL.
  Medium: alcohol.
  Absorptivities at 248 nm, calculated on the dried basis, do not differ by more than 3.0%.
Melting range ⟨741⟩: between 198° and 200°.
Acidity—To 2.0 g add 100 mL of water, heat on a steam bath for 30 minutes, cool, filter, and dilute with water to 100.0 mL. To 25.0 mL of this solution add 1 drop of phenolphthalein TS, and titrate with 0.10 N sodium hydroxide: not more than 0.50 mL is required to produce a pink color.
Loss on drying ⟨731⟩—Dry it at 105° for 4 hours: it loses not more than 0.5% of its weight.
Residue on ignition ⟨281⟩: not more than 0.1%.
Selenium ⟨291⟩: not more than 0.003%, a 100-mg test specimen, mixed with 100 mg of magnesium oxide, being used.

Heavy metals, *Method II* ⟨231⟩: not more than 0.002%.
Chromatographic purity—
  Mobile phase, Assay preparation, and *Chromatographic system*—Proceed as directed in the *Assay*.
  Test preparation—Use the *Assay preparation*.
  Procedure—Inject about 20 μL of the *Test preparation* into the chromatograph, record the chromatograms, and measure the responses for all of the peaks. Calculate the percentages of each peak, other than the solvent peak and the probenecid peak, in the portion of Probenecid taken by the formula:

$$100(r_I / r_T)$$

in which r_I is the response of each peak and r_T is the sum of the responses of all of the peaks, excluding that of the solvent peak: not more than 0.5% of any individual impurity and not more than 2.0% of total impurities is found.
Organic volatile impurities, *Method V* ⟨467⟩: meets the requirements.
  Solvent—Use dimethyl sulfoxide.

(Official until July 1, 2008)

Assay—
  Sodium phosphate solution—Prepare in glacial acetic acid solution (1 in 100) a 0.05 M solution of monobasic sodium phosphate, and adjust with phosphoric acid to a pH of 3.0.
  Mobile phase—Prepare a degassed and filtered mixture (50:50) of *Sodium phosphate solution* and a 1 in 100 solution of glacial acetic acid in acetonitrile. Make adjustments if necessary (see *System Suitability* under *Chromatography* ⟨621⟩).
  Standard preparation—Dissolve an accurately weighed quantity of USP Probenecid RS in *Mobile phase* to obtain a solution having a known concentration of about 0.50 mg per mL.
  Assay preparation—Transfer about 50 mg of Probenecid, accurately weighed, to a 100-mL volumetric flask, dissolve in and dilute with *Mobile phase* to volume, and mix.
  Chromatographic system (see *Chromatography* ⟨621⟩)—The liquid chromatograph is equipped with a 254-nm detector and a 3.9-mm × 30-cm column that contains packing L11. The flow rate is about 1 mL per minute. Chromatograph the *Standard preparation*, and record the peak responses as directed for *Procedure:* the tailing factor is not more than 2.3, the number of theoretical plates is not less than 3900, and the relative standard deviation for replicate injections is not more than 1.5%.
  Procedure—Separately inject equal volumes (about 20 μL) of the *Standard preparation* and the *Assay preparation* into the chromatograph, record the chromatograms, and measure the responses for the major peaks. Calculate the quantity, in mg, of $C_{13}H_{19}NO_4S$ in the portion of Probenecid taken by the formula:

$$100C(r_U / r_S)$$

in which C is the concentration, in mg per mL, of USP Probenecid RS in the *Standard preparation*, and r_U and r_S are the peak responses obtained from the *Assay preparation* and the *Standard preparation*, respectively.

Probenecid Tablets

» Probenecid Tablets contain not less than 93.0 percent and not more than 107.0 percent of the labeled amount of $C_{13}H_{19}NO_4S$.

Packaging and storage—Preserve in well-closed containers.
USP Reference standards ⟨11⟩—*USP Probenecid RS*.
Identification—
  A: *Ultraviolet Absorption* ⟨197U⟩—
  Solution: Assay preparation.
  B: Finely powder a quantity of Tablets, equivalent to about 500 mg of probenecid, triturate the powder with alcohol, and filter. Evaporate the filtrate to about 20 mL, cool, acidify with hydrochloric acid until acid to litmus, remove the crystals by filtration, and recrystallize from diluted alcohol: the probenecid so obtained melts between 196° and 200°, as determined by the method for

Class Ia under *Melting Range or Temperature* ⟨741⟩, and responds to *Identification* test A under *Probenecid*.

Dissolution ⟨711⟩—
 Medium: simulated intestinal fluid TS, prepared without pancreatin, pH 7.5 ± 0.1; 900 mL.
 Apparatus 2: 75 rpm.
 Time: 30 minutes.
 Procedure—Determine the amount of $C_{13}H_{19}NO_4S$ dissolved by employing UV absorption at the wavelength of maximum absorbance at about 244 nm on filtered portions of the solution under test, suitably diluted with 0.1 N sodium hydroxide, if necessary, in comparison with a Standard solution having a known concentration of USP Probenecid RS.
 Tolerances—Not less than 80% *(Q)* of the labeled amount of $C_{13}H_{19}NO_4S$ is dissolved in 30 minutes.

Uniformity of dosage units ⟨905⟩: meet the requirements.

Assay—Weigh and finely powder not less than 20 Tablets. Weigh accurately a portion of the powder, equivalent to about 100 mg of probenecid, and transfer to a 250-mL volumetric flask. Add chloroform to volume, and mix. Filter a portion of the chloroform solution, discarding the first 20 to 25 mL of the filtrate, and pipet 5 mL of the filtrate into a 125-mL separator containing 10 mL of chloroform. Extract the chloroform layer with four 15-mL portions of sodium carbonate solution (1 in 100). Render the combined extracts distinctly acid with 5 N hydrochloric acid, and extract with four 20-mL portions of chloroform, filtering each extract through a small pledget of cotton into a 100-mL volumetric flask. Wash the cotton filter with 10 mL of chloroform, add chloroform to volume, and mix. Dissolve an accurately weighed quantity of USP Probenecid RS in chloroform, and dilute quantitatively and stepwise with chloroform to obtain a Standard solution having a known concentration of about 20 µg per mL. Concomitantly determine the absorbances of both solutions in 1-cm cells at the wavelength of maximum absorbance at about 257 nm, with a suitable spectrophotometer, using chloroform as the blank. Calculate the quantity, in mg, of $C_{13}H_{19}NO_4S$ in the portion of Tablets taken by the formula:

$$5C(A_U / A_S)$$

in which *C* is the concentration, in µg per mL, of USP Probenecid RS in the Standard solution; and A_U and A_S are the absorbances of the solution from the Tablets and the Standard solution, respectively.

Probenecid and Colchicine Tablets

» Probenecid and Colchicine Tablets contain not less than 90.0 percent and not more than 115.0 percent of the labeled amount of colchicine ($C_{22}H_{25}NO_6$) and not less than 90.0 percent and not more than 110.0 percent of the labeled amount of probenecid ($C_{13}H_{19}NO_4S$).

Packaging and storage—Preserve in well-closed, light-resistant containers.

USP Reference standards ⟨11⟩—*USP Colchicine RS. USP Probenecid RS.*

Identification—
 Probenecid standard solution—Prepare a solution of USP Probenecid RS in chloroform having a concentration of about 1 mg per mL.
 Colchicine standard solution—Prepare a solution of USP Colchicine RS in chloroform having a concentration of about 1 mg per mL.
 Probenecid test solution—Using a portion of finely powdered Tablets, prepare a filtered solution in chloroform having a concentration of about 1 mg of probenecid per mL.
 Colchicine test solution—Transfer a quantity of finely powdered Tablets, equivalent to about 0.5 mg of colchicine, to a container, add 15 mL of water, mix, and filter, collecting the filtrate. Extract the filtrate with 25 mL of chloroform, and evaporate the chloroform extract to a volume of about 1 mL.
 Procedure (see *Chromatography* ⟨621⟩)—Apply separately 5-µL portions of the *Probenecid test solution* and the *Probenecid standard solution*, a 7-µL portion of the *Colchicine test solution*, and a 3.5-µL portion of the *Colchicine standard solution* to a thin-layer chromatographic plate, coated with a 0.25-mm layer of chromatographic silica gel mixture. Allow the spots to dry, and develop the chromatogram in a solvent system consisting of a mixture of methanol and ammonium hydroxide (100 : 1.5) until the solvent front has moved about three-fourths of the length of the plate. Remove the plate from the developing chamber, allow the solvent to evaporate, and view the plate under short-wavelength UV light: the R_F value of the principal spot in the chromatogram obtained from the *Probenecid test solution* corresponds to that obtained from the *Probenecid standard solution*. The R_F value of the principal spot in the chromatogram obtained from the *Colchicine test solution* corresponds to that obtained from the *Colchicine standard solution*.

Dissolution ⟨711⟩—
 Medium: pH 6.8 phosphate buffer (see under *Buffer Solutions* in the section *Reagents, Indicators, and Solutions*); 900 mL.
 Apparatus 2: 50 rpm.
 Time: 30 minutes.
 Procedure for probenecid—Determine the amount of $C_{13}H_{19}NO_4S$ dissolved from UV absorbances at the wavelength of maximum absorbance at about 244 nm of filtered portions of the solution under test, suitably diluted with 0.1 N sodium hydroxide, if necessary, in comparison with a Standard solution having a known concentration of USP Probenecid RS.
 Procedure for colchicine—Extract a filtered 200-mL portion of the solution under test with two 25-mL portions of chloroform, collecting the chloroform extracts in a suitable flask. Evaporate the combined extracts to a small volume, and transfer to a 10-mL volumetric flask. Rinse the flask with small portions of chloroform, and add the rinsings to the 10-mL volumetric flask. Dilute with chloroform to volume, and mix. Determine the amount of $C_{22}H_{25}NO_6$ dissolved from absorbances, at the wavelength of maximum absorbance at about 350 nm, of this solution, using chloroform as the blank, in comparison with a Standard solution in chloroform having a known concentration of USP Colchicine RS.
 Tolerances—Not less than 80% *(Q)* of the labeled amounts of $C_{22}H_{25}NO_6$ and $C_{13}H_{19}NO_4S$ are dissolved in 30 minutes.

Uniformity of dosage units ⟨905⟩: meet the requirements.

Assay for probenecid—
 Standard preparation—Dissolve an accurately weighed quantity of USP Probenecid RS on 0.1 N sodium hydroxide, and dilute quantitatively and stepwise with 0.1 N sodium hydroxide to obtain a solution having a known concentration of about 10 µg per mL.
 Assay preparation—Weigh and finely powder not less than 20 Tablets. Weigh accurately a portion of the powder, equivalent to about 250 mg of probenecid, and transfer to a 250-mL volumetric flask. Add 0.1 N sodium hydroxide to volume, and mix. Filter a portion of the solution, discarding the first 20 mL of the filtrate, pipet 2 mL of the filtrate into a 200-mL volumetric flask, dilute with 0.1 N sodium hydroxide to volume, and mix.
 Procedure—Concomitantly determine the absorbances of the *Assay preparation* and the *Standard preparation* at the wavelength of maximum absorbance at about 244 nm, with a suitable spectrophotometer, using 0.1 N sodium hydroxide as the blank. Calculate the quantity, in mg, of $C_{13}H_{19}NO_4S$ in the portion of Tablets taken by the formula:

$$25C(A_U / A_S)$$

in which *C* is the concentration, in µg per mL, of USP Probenecid RS in the *Standard preparation*, and A_U and A_S are the absorbances of the *Assay preparation* and the *Standard preparation*, respectively.

Assay for colchicine—[NOTE—Conduct this procedure without delay, under subdued light, using low-actinic glassware.]
 Alcoholic sodium carbonate solution—Dissolve 5.0 g of anhydrous sodium carbonate in 900 mL of water, add 100 mL of isopropyl alcohol, and mix.
 Standard preparation—Dissolve an accurately weighed quantity of USP Colchicine RS in *Alcoholic sodium carbonate solution*, and dilute quantitatively and stepwise with *Alcoholic sodium carbonate solution* to obtain a solution having a known concentration of about 10 µg per mL.

Assay preparation—Weigh and finely powder not less than 20 Probenecid and Colchicine Tablets. Weigh accurately a portion of the powder, equivalent to about 1 mg of colchicine, and transfer to a 100-mL volumetric flask. Add 75 mL of *Alcoholic sodium carbonate solution*, shake for 30 minutes, dilute with *Alcoholic sodium carbonate solution* to volume, mix, and filter, discarding the first 20 mL of the filtrate.

Procedure—Concomitantly determine the absorbances of the *Assay preparation* and the *Standard preparation* at the wavelength of maximum absorbance at about 350 nm, with a suitable spectrophotometer, using *Alcoholic sodium carbonate solution* as the blank. Calculate the quantity, in mg, of $C_{22}H_{25}NO_6$ in the portion of Tablets taken by the formula:

$$0.1C(A_U / A_S)$$

in which C is the concentration, in μg per mL, of USP Colchicine RS in the *Standard preparation*, and A_U and A_S are the absorbances of the *Assay preparation* and the *Standard preparation*, respectively.

Probucol

$C_{31}H_{48}O_2S_2$ 516.84
Phenol, 4,4′-[(1-methylethylidene)bis(thio)]bis[2,6-bis(1,1-dimethylethyl)-.
Acetone bis(3,5-di-*tert*-butyl-4-hydroxyphenyl) mercaptole [23288-49-5].

» Probucol contains not less than 98.0 percent and not more than 102.0 percent of $C_{31}H_{48}O_2S_2$, calculated on the dried basis.

Packaging and storage—Preserve in well-closed, light-resistant containers.
USP Reference standards ⟨11⟩—*USP Probucol RS. USP Probucol Related Compound A RS. USP Probucol Related Compound B RS. USP Probucol Related Compound C RS.*
Identification, *Infrared Absorption* ⟨197K⟩.
Melting range, *Class I* ⟨741⟩: between 124° and 127°, a dried specimen being used.
Loss on drying ⟨731⟩—Dry it in vacuum at 80° for 1 hour: it loses not more than 1.0% of its weight.
Residue on ignition ⟨281⟩: 0.1%.
Heavy metals, *Method II* ⟨231⟩: 0.002%.
Related compounds—
Mobile phase—Prepare a mixture of *n*-hexane and dehydrated alcohol (4000 : 1). Make adjustments, if necessary (see *System Suitability* under *Chromatography* ⟨621⟩).
Reference solution 1—Dissolve an accurately weighed quantity of USP Probucol Related Compound A RS in *n*-hexane, and dilute quantitatively and stepwise with *n*-hexane to obtain a solution having a known concentration of about 10 μg per mL.
Reference solution 2—Dissolve an accurately weighed quantity of USP Probucol Related Compound B RS in *n*-hexane, and dilute quantitatively with *n*-hexane to obtain a solution having a known concentration of about 0.1 mg per mL.
Reference solution 3—Dissolve an accurately weighed quantity of USP Probucol Related Compound C RS in *n*-hexane, and dilute quantitatively with *n*-hexane to obtain a solution having a known concentration of about 1 mg per mL.
Standard solution—Transfer about 10 mg of USP Probucol RS, accurately weighed, to a 50-mL volumetric flask. Add 1 mL of *Reference solution 1*, 4 mL of *Reference solution 2*, and 10 mL of *Reference solution 3*, and dilute with *n*-hexane to volume.

Test solution—Transfer about 1 g of Probucol, accurately weighed, to a 25-mL volumetric flask, dissolve in and dilute with *n*-hexane to volume, and mix.
System suitability solution—Pipet 1 mL of *Reference solution 2* and 1 mL of the *Test solution* into a 200-mL volumetric flask, dilute with *n*-hexane to volume, and mix.
Chromatographic system (see *Chromatography* ⟨621⟩)—The liquid chromatograph is equipped with 254-nm and 420-nm detectors, connected in series, and a 4.6-mm × 25-cm column that contains packing L3. The flow rate is about 1 mL per minute. Chromatograph the *System suitability solution*, and record the peak responses detected at 254 nm, for related compound B and probucol. Related compound B elutes first; the resolution, R, of the peaks is not less than 2.5; and the relative standard deviation for replicate injections, determined from the probucol peak, is not more than 2%.
Procedure—Separately inject equal volumes (about 20 μL) of the *Standard solution* and the *Test solution* into the chromatograph, record the chromatograms, and measure the peak areas. The order of elution is compound C, compound B, compound A, and finally probucol. Compound A is detected at 420 nm, and the others are detected at 254 nm. Calculate the percentage of each related compound in the portion of Probucol taken by the formula:

$$2500(C / W)(r_U / r_S)$$

in which C is the concentration, in mg per mL, of the respective probucol related compound in the *Standard solution;* W is the weight, in mg, of Probucol taken; and r_U and r_S are the peak areas obtained from the *Test solution;* and the *Standard solution*, respectively: not more than 0.0005% of compound A; not more than 0.02% of compound B; and not more than 0.5% of compound C are found.
Organic volatile impurities, *Method V* ⟨467⟩: meets the requirements.
Solvent—Use dimethyl sulfoxide.

(Official until July 1, 2008)

Assay—
Mobile phase—Prepare a degassed and filtered mixture of acetonitrile and water (85 : 15). Make adjustments, if necessary (see *System Suitability* under *Chromatography* ⟨621⟩).
System suitability preparation—To about 56 mg of Probucol add 10 mL of *n*-propyl alcohol, and dissolve the Probucol. Add 1.0 mL of 70% *tert*-butyl hydroperoxide, and mix. Cover loosely, and heat on a steam bath at about 90° for 30 minutes. Allow to cool to room temperature, dilute with a mixture of *n*-propyl alcohol and water (17 : 14) to 200 mL, and mix. Dilute 25 mL of this solution with *Mobile phase* to 100 mL.
Standard preparation—Dissolve an accurately weighed quantity of USP Probucol RS in *Mobile phase*, and dilute quantitatively and stepwise with *Mobile phase* to obtain a solution having a known concentration of about 63 μg per mL.
Assay preparation—Transfer about 63 mg of Probucol, accurately weighed, to a 50-mL volumetric flask. Dissolve in and dilute with *Mobile phase* to volume, and mix. Pipet 5 mL of this solution into a 100-mL volumetric flask, dilute with *Mobile phase* to volume, and mix.
Chromatographic system (see *Chromatography* ⟨621⟩)—The liquid chromatograph is equipped with a 242-nm detector and a 4.6-mm × 25-cm column that contains packing L7. The flow rate is about 2.0 mL per minute. Chromatograph the *System suitability preparation*, and record the peaks for the degradation product and probucol at relative retention times of approximately 0.8 and 1.0, respectively. The resolution, R, of the peaks is not less than 2.0. Chromatograph the *Standard preparation*: the relative standard deviation for replicate injections is not more than 1.0%.
Procedure—Separately inject equal volumes (about 50 μL) of the *Standard preparation* and the *Assay preparation* into the chromatograph, record the chromatograms, and measure the areas for the major peaks. Calculate the quantity, in mg, of $C_{31}H_{48}O_2S_2$ in the portion of Probucol taken by the formula:

$$C(r_U / r_S)$$

in which C is the concentration, in μg per mL, of USP Probucol RS in the *Standard preparation;* and r_U and r_S are the peak areas obtained from the *Assay preparation* and the *Standard preparation*, respectively.

Probucol Tablets

» Probucol Tablets contain not less than 90.0 percent and not more than 110.0 percent of the labeled amount of $C_{31}H_{48}O_2S_2$.

Packaging and storage—Preserve in well-closed, light-resistant containers.

USP Reference standards ⟨11⟩—*USP Probucol RS*.

Identification—

   A: Place an amount of powdered Tablets, equivalent to 15 to 20 mg of probucol, in the depression of a spot plate, and add two drops of sulfuric acid: an intense yellow color is produced immediately. The color corresponds to that obtained from a similar preparation of USP Probucol RS.

   B: Transfer a quantity of finely ground Tablets, equivalent to about 1000 mg of probucol, to a copper centrifuge tube. Add 5 mL of methylene chloride, cap the tube, and mix for about 30 seconds on a vortex mixer. Centrifuge at about 7000 rpm for 10 minutes. Decant the supernatant, and place about 1 mL of this solution on each side of a potassium bromide plate, holding the plate at an angle so that a thin film is formed on the plate: the IR absorption spectrum of the clear film so obtained exhibits maxima only at the same wavelengths as that of a similar preparation of USP Probucol RS.

Uniformity of dosage units ⟨905⟩: meet the requirement for *Weight Variation*.

Assay—

   Mobile phase, System suitability preparation, and *Chromatographic system*—Proceed as directed in the *Assay* under *Probucol*.

   Standard preparation—Dissolve an accurately weighed quantity of USP Probucol RS in *Mobile phase*, and dilute quantitatively and stepwise with *Mobile phase* to obtain a solution having a known concentration of about 50 µg per mL.

   Assay preparation—Weigh and finely powder not less than 20 Tablets. Transfer an accurately weighed quantity of the powder, equivalent to about 500 mg of probucol, to a 100-mL volumetric flask, add 80 mL of *Mobile phase*, and stir the mixture vigorously for about 1 hour. Dilute with *Mobile phase* to volume, and mix. Transfer 1.0 mL of this solution to a 100-mL volumetric flask, dilute with *Mobile phase* to volume, mix, and filter.

   Procedure—Separately inject equal volumes (about 50 µL) of the *Standard preparation* and the *Assay preparation* into the chromatograph, record the chromatograms, and measure the responses for the major peaks. Calculate the quantity, in mg, of $C_{31}H_{48}O_2S_2$ in the portion of Tablets taken by the formula:

$$10C(r_U/r_S)$$

in which *C* is the concentration, in µg per mL, of USP Probucol RS in the *Standard preparation*, and r_U and r_S are the peak responses obtained from the *Assay preparation* and the *Standard preparation*, respectively.

Procainamide Hydrochloride

$C_{13}H_{21}N_3O \cdot HCl$ 271.79
Benzamide, 4-amino-*N*-[2-(diethylamino)ethyl]-, monohydrochloride.
p-Amino-*N*-[2-(diethylamino)ethyl]benzamide monohydrochloride   [614-39-1].

» Procainamide Hydrochloride contains not less than 98.0 percent and not more than 102.0 percent of $C_{13}H_{21}N_3O \cdot HCl$, calculated on the dried basis.

Packaging and storage—Preserve in tight containers. Store at 25°, excursions permitted between 15° and 30°.

USP Reference standards ⟨11⟩—*USP Aminobenzoic Acid RS. USP Procainamide Hydrochloride RS*.

Identification—

   A: *Infrared Absorption* ⟨197K⟩.

   B: *Standard solution*—Use the *Standard solution* containing 0.2 mg of USP Procainamide Hydrochloride RS per mL, prepared as directed under *Ordinary impurities*.

   Test solution—Dilute the *Test solution*, prepared as directed under *Ordinary impurities*, with methanol to obtain a solution containing about 0.2 mg of procainamide hydrochloride per mL.

   Adsorbent, Eluant, and *Visualization*—Prepare as directed in *Ordinary impurities*.

   Procedure—Proceed as directed for *Procedure* under *Ordinary impurities* ⟨466⟩: the R_F value of the principal spot obtained from the *Test solution* corresponds to that obtained from the *Standard solution*.

Melting range ⟨741⟩: between 165° and 169°.

Loss on drying ⟨731⟩—Dry it at 105° for 4 hours: it loses not more than 0.3% of its weight.

Residue on ignition ⟨281⟩: not more than 0.1%.

Heavy metals, *Method II* ⟨231⟩: 0.002%.

Ordinary impurities ⟨466⟩—

   Test solution: methanol.
   Standard solution: methanol.
   Adsorbent: chromatographic silica gel.
   Eluant: a mixture of chloroform, methanol, and ammonium hydroxide (70 : 30 : 0.7).
   Visualization: 1, followed by spraying with a 1 in 2000 solution of fluorescamine in acetone and viewing with UV light at 366 nm.

Organic volatile impurities, *Method I* ⟨467⟩: meets the requirements.

(Official until July 1, 2008)

Limit of free *p*-aminobenzoic acid—

   Mobile phase and *Resolution solution*—Proceed as directed in the *Assay*.

   Standard solution—Quantitatively dissolve an accurately weighed quantity of USP Aminobenzoic Acid RS in *Mobile phase* to obtain a solution having a known concentration of about 0.25 µg per mL.

   Test solution—Transfer 25.0 mL of the stock solution used to prepare the *Assay preparation* to a 50-mL volumetric flask, dilute with *Mobile phase* to volume, and mix. This solution contains about 0.25 mg of procainamide hydrochloride per mL.

   Chromatographic system—Proceed as directed for *Chromatographic system* in the *Assay*. In addition, the tailing factor for the *p*-aminobenzoic acid peak in the chromatogram obtained from the *Resolution solution* is not more than 2.0; and the relative standard deviation for replicate injections of the *Standard solution* is not more than 3.0%.

   Procedure—Separately inject equal volumes (about 20 µL) of the *Standard solution* and the *Test solution* into the chromatograph, record the chromatograms, and measure the responses for the *p*-aminobenzoic acid peaks. Calculate the percentage of *p*-aminobenzoic acid in the portion of Procainamide Hydrochloride taken by the formula:

$$20(C/W)(r_U/r_S)$$

in which C is the concentration, in µg per mL, of USP Aminobenzoic Acid RS in the *Standard solution;* W is the weight, in mg, of Procainamide Hydrochloride taken to prepare the stock solution for the *Assay preparation;* and r_U and r_S are the p-aminobenzoic acid peak responses obtained from the *Test solution* and the *Standard solution,* respectively. The limit is 0.1%.

Assay—
Mobile phase—Prepare a suitable mixture of water, methanol, and triethylamine (140 : 60 : 1); adjust with phosphoric acid to a pH of 7.5 ± 0.1; filter; and degas. Make adjustments if necessary (see *System Suitability* under *Chromatography* ⟨621⟩).

Standard preparation—Quantitatively dissolve an accurately weighed quantity of USP Procainamide Hydrochloride RS in *Mobile phase* to obtain a solution having a known concentration of about 0.5 mg per mL. Quantitatively dilute an accurately measured volume of this stock solution with *Mobile phase* to obtain a *Standard preparation* having a known concentration of about 0.05 mg per mL.

Resolution solution—Dissolve a quantity of p-aminobenzoic acid in *Mobile phase* to obtain a solution containing about 0.1 mg per mL. Pipet 10 mL of this solution and 10 mL of the stock solution used to prepare the *Standard preparation* to a 100-mL volumetric flask, dilute with *Mobile phase* to volume, and mix.

Assay preparation—Transfer about 50 mg of Procainamide Hydrochloride, accurately weighed, to a 100-mL volumetric flask; dissolve in and dilute with *Mobile phase* to volume and mix. Transfer 10.0 mL of this stock solution to a second 100-mL volumetric flask, dilute with *Mobile phase* to volume, and mix.

Chromatographic system (see *Chromatography* ⟨621⟩)—The liquid chromatograph is equipped with a 280-nm detector and a 3.9-mm × 30-cm column that contains 10-µm packing L1. The flow rate is about 1 mL per minute. Chromatograph the *Resolution solution,* and record the peak responses as directed for *Procedure:* the resolution, R, between the p-aminobenzoic acid and procainamide peaks is not less than 5.0. The relative retention times are about 0.5 for p-aminobenzoic acid and 1.0 for procainamide hydrochloride. Chromatograph the *Standard preparation,* and record the peak responses as directed for *Procedure:* the relative standard deviation for replicate injections is not more than 2.0%.

Procedure—Separately inject equal volumes (about 20 µL) of the *Standard preparation* and the *Assay preparation* into the chromatograph, record the chromatograms, and measure the responses for the major peaks. Calculate the quantity, in mg, of $C_{13}H_{21}N_3O \cdot HCl$ in the portion of Procainamide Hydrochloride taken by the formula:

$$1000C(r_U/r_S)$$

in which C is the concentration, in mg per mL, of USP Procainamide Hydrochloride RS in the *Standard preparation;* and r_U and r_S are the peak responses obtained from the *Assay preparation* and the *Standard preparation,* respectively.

Procainamide Hydrochloride Capsules

» Procainamide Hydrochloride Capsules contain not less than 95.0 percent and not more than 105.0 percent of the labeled amount of $C_{13}H_{21}N_3O \cdot HCl$.

Packaging and storage—Preserve in tight containers.
USP Reference standards ⟨11⟩—*USP Procainamide Hydrochloride RS.*
Identification—Capsules respond to the *Thin-Layer Chromatographic Identification Test* ⟨201⟩, 5 µL of the clear supernatant used to prepare the *Assay preparation* in the *Assay* and 5 µL of the stock solution used to prepare the *Standard preparation* in the *Assay* being applied to the plate, and a solvent system consisting of a mixture of ethyl acetate, methanol, and ammonium hydroxide (22 : 2 : 1) being used to develop the chromatogram.

Dissolution ⟨711⟩—
Medium: 0.01 N hydrochloric acid; 900 mL.
Apparatus 2: 50 rpm.
Time: 90 minutes.
Procedure—Determine the amount of $C_{13}H_{21}N_3O \cdot HCl$ dissolved by employing UV absorption at the wavelength of maximum absorbance at about 275 nm on filtered portions of the solution under test, suitably diluted with an amount of 0.01 N sodium hydroxide that is not less than twice the volume of the portion of test solution taken, in comparison with a Standard solution having a known concentration of USP Procainamide Hydrochloride RS in the same media.
Tolerances—Not less than 75% (*Q*) of the labeled amount of $C_{13}H_{21}N_3O \cdot HCl$ is dissolved in 90 minutes.
Uniformity of dosage units ⟨905⟩: meet the requirements.
Assay—
Mobile phase, Standard preparation, Resolution solution, and *Chromatographic system*—Prepare as directed in the *Assay* under *Procainamide Hydrochloride.*

Assay preparation—Accurately weigh and mix the contents of 20 Capsules. Transfer an accurately weighed portion of the mixture, equivalent to about 500 mg of procainamide hydrochloride, to a 500-mL volumetric flask. Add about 350 mL of methanol to the flask, and sonicate for 10 minutes in a 40° water bath. Allow the flask to cool to room temperature, dilute with methanol to volume, and mix. Centrifuge a portion of the suspension, transfer 5.0 mL of the clear supernatant obtained to a 100-mL volumetric flask, dilute with *Mobile phase* to volume, and mix. [NOTE—Reserve the remainder of the clear supernatant for the *Identification* test.]

Procedure—Proceed as directed for *Procedure* in the *Assay* under *Procainamide Hydrochloride.* Calculate the quantity, in mg, of $C_{13}H_{21}N_3O \cdot HCl$ in the portion of Capsule contents taken by the formula:

$$10,000C(r_U/r_S)$$

in which C is the concentration, in mg per mL, of USP Procainamide Hydrochloride RS in the *Standard preparation,* and r_U and r_S are the peak responses obtained from the *Assay preparation* and the *Standard preparation,* respectively.

Procainamide Hydrochloride Injection

» Procainamide Hydrochloride Injection is a sterile solution of Procainamide Hydrochloride in Water for Injection. It contains not less than 95.0 percent and not more than 105.0 percent of the labeled amount of $C_{13}H_{21}N_3O \cdot HCl$.

Packaging and storage—Preserve in single-dose or in multiple-dose containers, preferably of Type I glass.
Labeling—Label it to indicate that the Injection is not to be used if it is darker than slightly yellow, or is discolored in any other way.

USP Reference standards ⟨11⟩—*USP Procainamide Hydrochloride RS. USP Endotoxin RS.*
Identification—It responds to the *Thin-Layer Chromatographic Identification Test* ⟨201⟩, 5 µL of the clear supernatant being used to prepare the *Assay preparation* in the *Assay* and 5 µL of the stock solution being used to prepare the *Standard preparation* in the *Assay* being applied to the plate, and a solvent system consisting of a mixture of ethyl acetate, methanol, and ammonium hydroxide (22 : 2 : 1) being used to develop the chromatogram.
Bacterial endotoxins ⟨85⟩—It contains not more than 0.35 USP Endotoxin Unit per mg of procainamide hydrochloride.
pH ⟨791⟩: between 4.0 and 6.0.
Particulate matter ⟨788⟩: meets the requirements under Small-volume injections.
Other requirements—It meets the requirements under *Injections* ⟨1⟩.

Assay—
Mobile phase, Standard preparation, Resolution solution, and *Chromatographic system*—Prepare as directed in the *Assay* under *Procainamide Hydrochloride*.

Assay preparation—Transfer an accurately measured volume of Injection, equivalent to about 500 mg of procainamide hydrochloride, to a 500-mL volumetric flask, dilute with methanol to volume, and mix. Transfer 5.0 mL of this stock solution to a 100-mL volumetric flask, reserving the remainder of the stock solution for the *Identification* test. Dilute with *Mobile phase* to volume, and mix.

Procedure—Proceed as directed for *Procedure* in the *Assay* under *Procainamide Hydrochloride*. Calculate the quantity, in mg, of $C_{13}H_{21}N_3O \cdot HCl$ in each mL of the Injection taken by the formula:

$$10{,}000(C / V)(r_U / r_S)$$

in which C is the concentration, in mg per mL, of USP Procainamide Hydrochloride RS in the *Standard preparation*, V is the volume, in mL, of Injection taken, and r_U and r_S are the peak responses obtained from the *Assay preparation* and the *Standard preparation*, respectively.

Procainamide Hydrochloride Tablets

» Procainamide Hydrochloride Tablets contain not less than 95.0 percent and not more than 105.0 percent of the labeled amount of $C_{13}H_{21}N_3O \cdot HCl$.

Packaging and storage—Preserve in tight containers.

USP Reference standards ⟨11⟩—*USP Procainamide Hydrochloride RS.*

Identification—Tablets respond to the *Thin-Layer Chromatographic Identification Test* ⟨201⟩, 5 μL of the clear supernatant used to prepare the *Assay preparation* in the *Assay* and 5 μL of the stock solution used to prepare the *Standard preparation* in the *Assay* being applied to the plate, and a solvent system consisting of a mixture of ethyl acetate, methanol, and ammonium hydroxide (22 : 2 : 1) being used to develop the chromatogram.

Dissolution ⟨711⟩—
Medium: 0.1 N hydrochloric acid; 900 mL.
Apparatus 2: 50 rpm.
Time: 60 minutes.
Procedure—Determine the amount of $C_{13}H_{21}N_3O \cdot HCl$ dissolved by employing UV absorption at the wavelength of maximum absorbance at about 275 nm on filtered portions of the solution under test, suitably diluted with an amount of 0.01 N sodium hydroxide that is not less than twice the volume of the portion of test solution taken, in comparison with a Standard solution having a known concentration of USP Procainamide Hydrochloride RS in the same media.
Tolerances—Not less than 80% (*Q*) of the labeled amount of $C_{13}H_{21}N_3O \cdot HCl$ is dissolved in 60 minutes.

Uniformity of dosage units ⟨905⟩: meet the requirements.

Assay—
Mobile phase, Standard preparation, Resolution solution, and *Chromatographic system*—Proceed as directed in the *Assay* under *Procainamide Hydrochloride*.

Assay preparation—Weigh and finely powder not less than 20 Procainamide Hydrochloride Tablets. Transfer an accurately weighed portion of the powder, equivalent to about 500 mg of procainamide hydrochloride, to a 500-mL volumetric flask, add about 350 mL of methanol, and sonicate for 10 minutes in a 40° water bath. Allow the flask to cool to room temperature, dilute with methanol to volume, and mix. Centrifuge a portion of the suspension, transfer 5.0 mL of the clear supernatant obtained to a 100-mL volumetric flask, reserving the remainder of the clear supernatant for the *Identification* test. Dilute with *Mobile phase* to volume, and mix.

Procedure—Proceed as directed for *Procedure* in the *Assay* under *Procainamide Hydrochloride*. Calculate the quantity of $C_{13}H_{21}N_3O \cdot HCl$ in the portion of Tablets taken by the formula:

$$10{,}000C(r_U / r_S)$$

in which C is the concentration, in mg per mL, of USP Procainamide Hydrochloride RS in the *Standard preparation*, and r_U and r_S are the procainamide peak responses obtained from the *Assay preparation* and the *Standard preparation*, respectively.

Procainamide Hydrochloride Extended-Release Tablets

» Procainamide Hydrochloride Extended-Release Tablets contain not less than 93.0 percent and not more than 107.0 percent of the labeled amount of procainamide hydrochloride ($C_{13}H_{21}N_3O \cdot HCl$).

Packaging and storage—Preserve in tight containers.
Labeling—The labeling indicates the *Dissolution Test* with which the product complies.

USP Reference standards ⟨11⟩—*USP Procainamide Hydrochloride RS.*

Identification—It responds to the *Thin-Layer Chromatographic Identification Test* ⟨201⟩, 5 μL of the stock solution prepared as directed for *Assay preparation* in the *Assay* and 5 μL of the *Stock standard solution* being applied to the plate, and a solvent system consisting of a mixture of ether, methanol, and ammonium hydroxide (25 : 5 : 1) being used to develop the chromatogram.

Dissolution ⟨711⟩—
TEST 1—If the product complies with this test, the labeling indicates that the product meets USP *Dissolution Test 1*.
Medium: 0.1 N hydrochloric acid; 900 mL.
Apparatus 2: 50 rpm.
Times: 1, 4, and 6 hours.
Procedure—Determine the amount of $C_{13}H_{21}N_3O \cdot HCl$ dissolved from UV absorbances at the wavelength of maximum absorbance at about 224 nm, using filtered portions of the solution under test, diluted with *Medium*, if necessary, in comparison with a Standard solution having a known concentration of USP Procainamide Hydrochloride RS in the same *Medium*.
Tolerances—The percentage of the labeled amount of $C_{13}H_{21}N_3O \cdot HCl$ dissolved at the times specified conforms to *Acceptance Table 2*.

Time (hours)	Amount dissolved
1	between 30% and 60%
4	between 60% and 90%
6	not less than 75%

TEST 2—If the product complies with this test, the labeling indicates that the product meets USP *Dissolution Test 2*.
Medium—Proceed as directed for *Method B* under *Delayed-Release Dosage Forms*.
ACID STAGE: 0.1 N hydrochloric acid; 900 mL for 1 hour.
BUFFER STAGE: 0.05 M phosphate buffer, pH 7.5; 900 mL (see *Buffer Solutions* under *Reagents, Indicators, and Solutions*) for not less than 8 hours.
Apparatus 2: 50 rpm, with sinkers.
Times: 1, 4, and 8 hours.
Procedure—Proceed as directed for *Procedure* in *Test 1*.
Tolerances—The percentages of the labeled amount of $C_{13}H_{21}N_3O \cdot HCl$ dissolved at the times specified conform to *Acceptance Table 2*.

Time (hours)	Amount dissolved
1	between 30% and 60%
4	between 60% and 90%
8	not less than 80%

TEST 3—If the product complies with this test, the labeling indicates that the product meets USP *Dissolution Test 3*.
Medium—Proceed as directed under *Test 2*.
Apparatus 2: 50 rpm, with sinkers.
Times: 1, 3, 6, and 8 hours.
Procedure—Proceed as directed for *Procedure* in *Test 1*.
Tolerances—The percentages of the labeled amount of $C_{13}H_{21}N_3O \cdot HCl$ dissolved at the times specified conform to *Acceptance Table 2*.

Time (hours)	Amount dissolved
1	between 25% and 50%
3	between 40% and 75%
6	between 65% and 90%
8	not less than 80%

TEST 4—If the product complies with this test, the labeling indicates that the product meets USP *Dissolution Test 4*.
Medium: 0.1 N hydrochloric acid; 900 mL.
Apparatus 1: 50 rpm.
Times: 1, 2, 4, 8, and 14 hours.
Procedure—Proceed as directed for *Procedure* in *Test 1*.
Tolerances—The percentages of the labeled amount of $C_{13}H_{21}N_3O \cdot HCl$ dissolved at the times specified conform to *Acceptance Table 2*.

Time (hours)	Amount dissolved
1	not more than 30%
2	between 25% and 45%
4	between 45% and 75%
8	between 70% and 90%
14	not less than 80%

TEST 5—If the product complies with this test the labeling indicates that the product meets USP *Dissolution Test 5*.
Medium—Proceed as directed for *Method B* under *Delayed-Release Dosage Forms*.
ACID STAGE: 0.1 N hydrochloric acid; 1000 mL for 1 hour.
BUFFER STAGE: 0.05 M phosphate buffer, pH 7.5; 1000 mL (see *Buffer Solutions* under *Reagents, Indicators, and Solutions*) for not less than 8 hours.
Apparatus 2: 50 rpm, with sinkers.
Times: 1, 4, 6, and 8 hours.
Procedure—Proceed as directed for *Procedure* in *Test 1*.
Tolerances—Proceed as directed for *Tolerances* in *Test 2*.
FOR 500 MG TABLETS—

Time (hours)	Amount dissolved
1	between 30% and 45%
4	between 55% and 75%
6	not less than 65%
8	not less than 75%

FOR 750 AND 1000 MG TABLETS—

Time (hours)	Amount dissolved
1	between 30% and 50%
4	between 60% and 80%
6	between 70% and 90%
8	not less than 75%

TEST 6—If the product complies with this test, the labeling indicates that the product meets USP *Dissolution Test 6*.
Medium—Proceed as directed for *Test 2*.
Apparatus 2: 50 rpm.
Times: 1, 4, and 8 hours.
Procedure—Proceed as directed for *Procedure* in *Test 1*.
Tolerances—Proceed as directed for *Tolerances* in *Test 2*.
FOR 250 MG TABLETS—

Time (hours)	Amount dissolved
1	between 30% and 60%
4	between 60% and 90%
8	not less than 80%

FOR 500 MG TABLETS—

Time (hours)	Amount dissolved
1	between 30% and 50%
4	between 60% and 80%
8	not less than 85%

FOR 750 MG TABLETS—

Time (hours)	Amount dissolved
1	between 30% and 50%
4	between 60% and 80%
8	not less than 80%

TEST 8—If the product complies with this test, the labeling indicates that the product meets USP *Dissolution Test 8*.
Medium—Proceed as directed for *Method B* under *Delayed-Release Dosage Forms*.
ACID STAGE: 0.1 N hydrochloric acid; 900 mL for 1 hour.
BUFFER STAGE: 0.05 M phosphate buffer, pH 7.5; 900 mL (see *Buffer Solutions* under *Reagents, Indicators, and Solutions*) for not less than 8 hours.
Apparatus 2: 50 rpm, with sinkers.
Times: 1, 4, 6, and 8 hours.
Procedure—Proceed as directed for *Procedure* in *Test 1*.
Tolerances—Proceed as directed for *Tolerances* in *Test 2*.

Time (hours)	Amount dissolved
1	between 33% and 50%
4	between 70% and 85%
6	not less than 80%
8	not less than 85%

Uniformity of dosage units ⟨905⟩: meet the requirements.
Assay—
Mobile phase—Prepare a suitable mixture of water, methanol, and triethylamine (140 : 60 : 1), adjust with phosphoric acid to a pH of 7.5, filter, and degas. Make adjustments if necessary (see *System Suitability* under *Chromatography* ⟨621⟩).
Standard preparation—Dissolve an accurately weighed quantity of USP Procainamide Hydrochloride RS in *Mobile phase* to obtain a solution having a known concentration of about 0.5 mg per mL (*Stock standard solution*). Quantitatively dilute an accurately measured volume of this solution with *Mobile phase* to obtain a solution having a known concentration of about 0.05 mg per mL (*Standard preparation*).
Assay preparation—Transfer not fewer than 10 Tablets, accurately counted, to a 1000-mL volumetric flask, and add 100 mL of a mixture of methanol and methylene chloride (1 : 1). Place the flask in a 40° sonicator bath, and sonicate, with occasional shaking, until the Tablets have disintegrated completely. Add about 700 mL of methanol, and sonicate for 10 minutes, with occasional shaking. Allow to cool, dilute with methanol to volume, and mix. Filter a portion of this solution, discarding the first 10 mL of the filtrate. Quantitatively dilute an accurately measured volume of the filtrate with *Mobile phase* to obtain a solution having a concentration of about 0.5 mg of procainamide hydrochloride per mL. Use a portion of this stock solution for the *Identification* test. Quantitatively dilute another accurately measured volume of the stock solution with *Mo-*

bile phase to obtain a solution having a concentration of about 0.05 mg per mL (*Assay preparation*).

Resolution solution—Prepare a solution of *p*-aminobenzoic acid in *Mobile phase* containing 0.1 mg per mL. Pipet 10 mL of this solution and 10 mL of the *Stock standard* into a 100-mL volumetric flask, dilute with *Mobile phase* to volume, and mix.

Chromatographic system (see *Chromatography* ⟨621⟩)—The liquid chromatograph is equipped with a 280-nm detector and a 3.9-mm × 30-cm column that contains 10-μm packing L1. The flow rate is about 1 mL per minute. Chromatograph the *Resolution solution*: the resolution, *R*, is not less than 2.0. Chromatograph replicate injections of the *Standard preparation*: the relative standard deviation is not more than 2.0%.

Procedure—Separately inject equal volumes (about 20 μL) of the *Standard preparation* and the *Assay preparation* into the chromatograph, record the chromatograms, and measure the responses for the major peaks. The relative retention times are about 0.5 for *p*-aminobenzoic acid and 1.0 for procainamide. Calculate the quantity, in mg, of procainamide hydrochloride ($C_{13}H_{21}N_3O \cdot HCl$) per Tablet taken by the formula:

$$(L / D)(C)(r_U / r_S)$$

in which *L* is the labeled quantity, in mg, of procainamide hydrochloride in each Tablet; *D* is the concentration, in mg per mL, of procainamide hydrochloride in the *Assay preparation*, based on the number of Tablets taken, the labeled quantity per Tablet, and the extent of dilution; *C* is the concentration, in mg per mL, of USP Procainamide Hydrochloride RS in the *Standard preparation*; and r_U and r_S are the peak responses obtained from the *Assay preparation* and the *Standard preparation*, respectively.

Procaine Hydrochloride

$C_{13}H_{20}N_2O_2 \cdot HCl$ 272.78

Benzoic acid, 4-amino-, 2-(diethylamino)ethyl ester, monohydrochloride.
2-(Diethylamino)ethyl *p*-aminobenzoate monohydrochloride [51-05-8].

» Procaine Hydrochloride contains not less than 99.0 percent and not more than 101.0 percent of $C_{13}H_{20}N_2O_2 \cdot HCl$, calculated on the dried basis.

Packaging and storage—Preserve in well-closed containers.
Labeling—Where it is intended for use in preparing injectable dosage forms, the label states that it is sterile or must be subjected to further processing during the preparation of injectable dosage forms.

USP Reference standards ⟨11⟩—*USP Endotoxin RS. USP Procaine Hydrochloride RS*.
Identification—
  A: *Infrared Absorption* ⟨197K⟩.
  B: Dissolve 10 mg in 1 mL of water, add 1 drop each of hydrochloric acid and sodium nitrite solution (1 in 10), then add 1 mL of a solution prepared by dissolving 0.2 g of 2-naphthol in 10 mL of sodium hydroxide solution (1 in 10), and shake: a scarlet-red precipitate is formed.
  C: It responds to the tests for *Chloride* ⟨191⟩.
Melting range ⟨741⟩: between 153° and 158°.
Bacterial endotoxins ⟨85⟩—Where the label states that Procaine Hydrochloride is sterile or must be subjected to further processing during the preparation of injectable dosage forms, it contains not more than 0.6 USP Endotoxin Unit per mg of procaine hydrochloride.

Sterility ⟨71⟩—It meets the requirements when tested as directed for *Membrane Filtration* under *Test for Sterility of the Product to be Examined*.
Acidity—To a solution of 1.0 g in 25 mL of water add 1 drop of methyl red TS, and titrate with 0.020 N sodium hydroxide: not more than 0.50 mL is required for neutralization.
Loss on drying ⟨731⟩—Dry it over silica gel for 18 hours: it loses not more than 1.0% of its weight.
Residue on ignition ⟨281⟩: not more than 0.15%.
Heavy metals ⟨231⟩: 0.002%.
Chromatographic purity—
  Solvent—Prepare a mixture of methanol and trichloroethane (7 : 3).
  Standard preparations—Prepare a solution of USP Procaine Hydrochloride RS in *Solvent* containing 1.6 mg per mL. Dilute quantitatively with *Solvent* to obtain Standard preparations having the following compositions:

Standard preparation	Dilution	Concentration (mg RS per mL)	Percentage (%, for comparison with test specimen)
A	2.5 in 10	0.4	0.5
B	2.0 in 10	0.32	0.4
C	1.0 in 10	0.16	0.2
D	0.5 in 10	0.08	0.1

Test preparation—Transfer 1.6 g of Procaine Hydrochloride, accurately weighed, to a suitable capped container, add 20 mL of *Solvent*, close the container, and sonicate for 2 minutes. Use this solution as the *Test preparation*.

Procedure—Apply separately 10 μL of the *Test preparation* and 10 μL of each *Standard preparation* to a suitable thin-layer chromatographic plate (see *Chromatography* ⟨621⟩) coated with a 0.25-mm layer of chromatographic silica gel mixture, prewashed with methanol and allowed to dry. Use a double-trough chromatographic chamber. Fill one trough with ammonium hydroxide, and allow the chamber to equilibrate for 1 hour. Position the plate in the other trough, and develop the chromatogram in a solvent system consisting of a mixture of methylene chloride and methanol (95 : 6) until the solvent front has moved about three-fourths of the length of the plate. Remove the plate from the developing chamber, mark the solvent front, and allow the solvent to evaporate. Examine the plate under short-wavelength UV light. Compare the intensities of any secondary spots observed in the chromatogram of the *Test preparation* with those of the principal spots in the chromatograms of the *Standard preparations*: no secondary spot is more intense than the principal spot obtained from *Standard* (0.5%), and the sum of the intensities of all secondary spots obtained from the *Test preparation* does not exceed 1.0%.

Assay—Transfer about 0.5 g of Procaine Hydrochloride, accurately weighed, to a beaker, add 100 mL of cold water, 5 mL of hydrochloric acid, and 100 mg of potassium bromide, and stir until dissolved. Proceed as directed under *Nitrite Titration* ⟨451⟩, beginning with "cool to about 15°." Perform a blank determination, and make any necessary correction. Each mL of 0.1 M sodium nitrite is equivalent to 27.28 mg of $C_{13}H_{20}N_2O_2 \cdot HCl$.

Procaine Hydrochloride Injection

» Procaine Hydrochloride Injection is a sterile solution of Procaine Hydrochloride in Water for Injection. It contains not less than 95.0 percent and not more than 105.0 percent of the labeled amount of $C_{13}H_{20}N_2O_2 \cdot HCl$.

Packaging and storage—Preserve in single-dose or in multiple-dose containers, preferably of Type I or Type II glass. The Injection may be packaged in 100-mL multiple-dose containers.

USP Reference standards ⟨11⟩—*USP Procaine Hydrochloride RS. USP Endotoxin RS.*
Identification—Evaporate a portion of Injection, equivalent to about 20 mg of procaine hydrochloride, on a steam bath just to dryness, and dry over silica gel for 18 hours: the residue responds to *Identification* tests A and B under *Procaine Hydrochloride*.
Bacterial endotoxins ⟨85⟩—It contains not more than 0.6 USP Endotoxin Unit per mg of procaine hydrochloride.
pH ⟨791⟩: between 3.0 and 5.5.
Particulate matter ⟨788⟩: meets the requirements under Small-volume injections.
Other requirements—It meets the requirements under *Injections* ⟨1⟩.
Assay—
Standard preparation—Transfer to a 125-mL separator about 50 mg, accurately weighed, of USP Procaine Hydrochloride RS, and dilute with water to 20 mL.
Assay preparation—Transfer to a 125-mL separator an accurately measured volume of Injection, equivalent to about 50 mg of procaine hydrochloride, and dilute with water to 20 mL.
Procedure—To the *Standard preparation* and also to the *Assay preparation* add 5 mL of 6 N ammonium hydroxide, then treat each as follows. Extract with five 25-mL portions of chloroform, and filter the combined extracts through about 1 g of anhydrous sodium sulfate supported on a pledget of glass wool. Receive the filtrate in a 200-mL volumetric flask, add chloroform to volume, and mix. Transfer 3.0 mL of this solution to a 100-mL volumetric flask, add chloroform to volume, and mix. Concomitantly determine the absorbances of both solutions at the wavelength of maximum absorbance at about 280 nm, with a suitable spectrophotometer, using chloroform as the blank. Calculate the quantity, in mg, of $C_{13}H_{20}N_2O_2 \cdot HCl$ in each mL of the Injection taken by the formula:

$$(W/V)(A_U/A_S)$$

in which W is the weight, in mg, of USP Procaine Hydrochloride RS used, V is the volume, in mL, of Injection taken, and A_U and A_S are the absorbances of the solutions from the *Assay preparation* and the *Standard preparation*, respectively.

Procaine Hydrochloride and Epinephrine Injection

» Procaine Hydrochloride and Epinephrine Injection is a sterile solution of Procaine Hydrochloride and Epinephrine Hydrochloride in Water for Injection. The content of epinephrine does not exceed 0.002 percent (1 in 50,000). It contains not less than 95.0 percent and not more than 105.0 percent of the labeled amount of procaine hydrochloride ($C_{13}H_{20}N_2O_2 \cdot HCl$), and not less than 90.0 percent and not more than 115.0 percent of the labeled amount of epinephrine ($C_9H_{13}NO_3$).

Packaging and storage—Preserve in single-dose or in multiple-dose, light-resistant containers, preferably of Type I or Type II glass.
Labeling—The label indicates that the Injection is not to be used if its color is pinkish or darker than slightly yellow or if it contains a precipitate.
USP Reference standards ⟨11⟩—*USP Procaine Hydrochloride RS. USP Epinephrine Bitartrate RS. USP Endotoxin RS.*
Color and clarity—Using the Injection as the *Test solution*, proceed as directed for *Color and clarity* under *Epinephrine Injection*.
Identification—Evaporate a portion of Injection, equivalent to about 20 mg of procaine hydrochloride, on a steam bath just to dryness, and dry over silica gel for 18 hours, protected from light: the residue responds to *Identification* tests A and B under *Procaine Hydrochloride*.
Bacterial endotoxins ⟨85⟩—It contains not more than 0.6 USP Endotoxin Unit per mg of procaine hydrochloride.

pH ⟨791⟩: between 3.0 and 5.5.
Content of epinephrine—
Alkaline ascorbate reagent—Mix 100 mL of alcohol, 80 mL of sodium hydroxide solution (1 in 5), and 8 mL of ascorbic acid solution (1 in 50). Prepare fresh on the day of use.
Standard preparation—Place about 18 mg of USP Epinephrine Bitartrate RS, accurately weighed, in a 100-mL volumetric flask, add sodium bisulfite solution (1 in 1000) to volume, and mix. Dilute this solution quantitatively with water to obtain a solution having a known concentration of about 10 µg of epinephrine per mL.
Procedure—Pipet a volume of Injection, equivalent to about 10 µg of epinephrine, into a 50-mL beaker. Into another 50-mL beaker pipet 1 mL of *Standard preparation*. Treat the contents of each beaker as follows. Add 10 mL of dilute hydrochloric acid (1 in 120), and heat gently to reduce the volume of solution to about 5 mL. Allow to cool to room temperature, then add 5 mL of sodium acetate solution (1 in 5), followed by 0.5 mL of potassium ferricyanide solution (1 in 400), and mix. At 2 minutes, accurately timed, after the last addition, add 20 mL of *Alkaline ascorbate reagent*, transfer the contents to a corresponding 50-mL volumetric flask with the aid of water, add water to volume, and mix. At 15 to 20 minutes after the addition of the *Alkaline ascorbate reagent*, determine the fluorescences of each solution and of a reagent blank, with a suitable fluorometer, with an excitation wavelength setting of 420 nm and a fluorescence wavelength setting of 520 nm. Calculate the quantity, in µg, of $C_9H_{13}NO_3$ in each mL of Injection taken by the formula:

$$(C/V)[(I_U - B)/(I_S - B)]$$

in which C is the concentration of epinephrine, in µg per mL, of USP Epinephrine Bitartrate RS in the *Standard preparation*, V is the volume, in mL, of Injection taken, and I_U, I_S, and B are the fluorescence readings of the solutions from the Injection, the *Standard preparation*, and the reagent blank, respectively.
Other requirements—It meets the requirements under *Injections* ⟨1⟩.
Assay—
Standard preparation—Transfer to a 125-mL separator about 50 mg, accurately weighed, of USP Procaine Hydrochloride RS, and dilute with water to 20 mL.
Assay preparation—Transfer to a 125-mL separator an accurately measured volume of Injection, equivalent to about 50 mg of procaine hydrochloride, and dilute with water to 20 mL.
Procedure—To the *Standard preparation* and also to the *Assay preparation* add 5 mL of 6 N ammonium hydroxide, then treat each as follows. Extract with five 25-mL portions of chloroform, and filter the combined extracts through about 1 g of anhydrous sodium sulfate supported on a pledget of glass wool. Receive the filtrate in a 200-mL volumetric flask, add chloroform to volume, and mix. Transfer 3.0 mL of this solution to a 100-mL volumetric flask, add chloroform to volume, and mix. Concomitantly determine the absorbances of both solutions at the wavelength of maximum absorbance at about 280 nm, with a suitable spectrophotometer, using chloroform as the blank. Calculate the quantity, in mg, of $C_{13}H_{20}N_2O_2 \cdot HCl$ in each mL of the Injection taken by the formula:

$$(W/V)(A_U/A_S)$$

in which W is the weight, in mg, of USP Procaine Hydrochloride RS used, V is the volume, in mL, of Injection taken, and A_U and A_S are the absorbances of the solutions obtained from the *Assay preparation* and the *Standard preparation*, respectively.

Procaine and Tetracaine Hydrochlorides and Levonordefrin Injection

» Procaine and Tetracaine Hydrochlorides and Levonordefrin Injection is a sterile solution of Procaine Hydrochloride, Tetracaine Hydrochloride, and

Levonordefrin in Water for Injection. It contains not less than 95.0 percent and not more than 105.0 percent of the labeled amount of procaine hydrochloride ($C_{13}H_{20}N_2O_2 \cdot HCl$), not less than 95.0 percent and not more than 105.0 percent of the labeled amount of tetracaine hydrochloride ($C_{15}H_{24}N_2O_2 \cdot HCl$), and not less than 90.0 percent and not more than 110.0 percent of the labeled amount of levonordefrin ($C_9H_{13}NO_3$).

Packaging and storage—Preserve in single-dose or in multiple-dose containers, preferably of Type I glass.
Labeling—The label indicates that the Injection is not to be used if its color is pinkish or darker than slightly yellow or if it contains a precipitate.
USP Reference standards ⟨11⟩—*USP Epinephrine Bitartrate RS. USP Endotoxin RS.*
Color and clarity—Using the Injection as the *Test solution*, proceed as directed for *Color and clarity* under *Mepivacaine Hydrochloride and Levonordefrin Injection*.
Identification—
  A: Mix 10 mL of Injection with 10 mL of 3 N hydrochloric acid, cool to 0° in an ice bath, add 5 mL of sodium nitrite solution (1 in 5), stirring gently, add 2 mL of a solution of 0.1 g of 2-naphthol in 5 mL of 1 N sodium hydroxide, and observe immediately: a bright orange-red precipitate is formed (*presence of a primary aminophenyl group*).
  B: It responds to the tests for *Chloride* ⟨191⟩.
  C: To about 25 mL of Injection add 1 drop of ferric chloride TS: the solution immediately turns a light green and changes to a light blue within 1 minute. Add 2 drops of 3 N hydrochloric acid: the color reverts to light green (*presence of levonordefrin*).
Bacterial endotoxins ⟨85⟩—It contains not more than 0.6 USP Endotoxin Unit per mg of procaine hydrochloride.
pH ⟨791⟩: between 3.5 and 5.0.
Other requirements—It meets the requirements under *Injections* ⟨1⟩.
Assay for procaine hydrochloride—Transfer 25.0 mL of Injection to a 250-mL beaker, add 10 mL of dilute hydrochloric acid (1 in 2), 15 mL of water, and 1.0 mL of formaldehyde solution, and allow to stand for 3 minutes. Titrate with 0.1 M sodium nitrite VS, using starch iodide paper as an external indicator. Perform a blank determination, and make any necessary correction. Calculate the quantity, in mg, of $C_{13}H_{20}N_2O_2 \cdot HCl$ in each mL of the Injection taken by the formula:

$$(272.78 / 25)(V_2M_2 - 0.5V_1M_1)$$

in which V_2 is the volume, in mL, and M_2 is the exact molarity of the 0.1 M sodium nitrite solution used in the titration, V_1 and M_1 are as defined under *Assay for tetracaine hydrochloride*, and 272.78 is the molecular weight of procaine hydrochloride.
Assay for tetracaine hydrochloride—Transfer 50.0 mL of Injection to a 100-mL beaker, add 5 g of sodium acetate and 5 mL of isopropyl alcohol, and stir until the sodium acetate is dissolved. Add 1.5 mL of potassium thiocyanate solution (75 in 100), and stir while cooling in an ice bath. Keep in the ice bath for 1 hour, stirring about four times during the period. Do not stir excessively. Prepare a filtering crucible with double suitable filter paper, connect to a suction flask, and moisten the paper with a few drops of the clear supernatant. Remove the excess liquid by suction. Filter the mixture, and dry by suction. Transfer the entire contents of the crucible to the original beaker, and rinse the crucible with 10 mL of dilute hydrochloric acid (1 in 2), followed by 30 mL of water. Transfer the rinsings to the beaker. Cool in ice, and titrate with 0.02 M sodium nitrite VS, using starch iodide paper as an external indicator. Perform a blank determination, using 10 mL of dilute hydrochloric acid (1 in 2) and 30 mL of water, and make any necessary correction. Calculate the quantity, in mg, of $C_{15}H_{24}N_2O_2 \cdot HCl$ in each mL of the Injection taken by the formula:

$$(300.83 / 50)(V_1M_1)$$

in which V_1 is the volume, in mL, and M_1 is the exact molarity of the 0.02 M sodium nitrite used in the titration, and 300.83 is the molecular weight of tetracaine hydrochloride.

Assay for levonordefrin—
Ferro-citrate solution, Buffer solution, and *Standard preparation*—Prepare as directed under *Epinephrine Assay* ⟨391⟩.
Assay preparation—Proceed with Injection as directed for *Assay Preparation* under *Epinephrine Assay* ⟨391⟩, except to read "levonordefrin" where "epinephrine" is specified.
Procedure—Proceed as directed for *Procedure* under *Epinephrine Assay* ⟨391⟩. Calculate the quantity, in mg, of levonordefrin ($C_9H_{13}NO_3$) in each mL of the Injection taken by the formula:

$$(183.21 / 333.30)(0.05C / V)(A_U / A_S)$$

in which 183.21 and 333.30 are the molecular weights of levonordefrin and epinephrine bitartrate, respectively, C is the concentration, in μg per mL, of USP Epinephrine Bitartrate RS in the *Standard preparation,* and V is the volume, in mL, of Injection taken.

Procarbazine Hydrochloride

$C_{12}H_{19}N_3O \cdot HCl$ 257.76
Benzamide, *N*-(1-methylethyl)-4-[(2-methylhydrazino)methyl]-, monohydrochloride.
N-Isopropyl-α-(2-methylhydrazino)-*p*-toluamide   monohydrochloride   [366-70-1].

» Procarbazine Hydrochloride contains not less than 98.5 percent and not more than 100.5 percent of $C_{12}H_{19}N_3O \cdot HCl$.
Caution: Handle Procarbazine Hydrochloride with exceptional care, since it is a highly potent agent

Packaging and storage—Preserve in tight, light-resistant containers.
USP Reference standards ⟨11⟩—*USP Procarbazine Hydrochloride RS.*
Identification—
  A: *Infrared Absorption* ⟨197M⟩.
  B: *Ultraviolet Absorption* ⟨197U⟩—[NOTE—Use low-actinic glassware throughout this test.]
  Solution: 10 μg per mL.
  Medium: 0.1 N hydrochloric acid.
  Absorptivities at 232 nm do not differ by more than 3.0%.
Residue on ignition ⟨281⟩:   not more than 0.1%.
Heavy metals, *Method II* ⟨231⟩:   0.002%.
Organic volatile impurities, *Method I* ⟨467⟩:   meets the requirements.
(Official until July 1, 2008)
Assay—Dissolve about 0.75 g of Procarbazine Hydrochloride, accurately weighed, in 100 mL of water. Titrate with 0.1 N sodium hydroxide VS, determining the endpoint potentiometrically, using a calomel-glass electrode system. Each mL of 0.1 N sodium hydroxide is equivalent to 25.78 mg of $C_{12}H_{19}N_3O \cdot HCl$.

Procarbazine Hydrochloride Capsules

» Procarbazine Hydrochloride Capsules contain not less than 90.0 percent and not more than 110.0 percent of the labeled amount of procarbazine ($C_{12}H_{19}N_3O$).

Packaging and storage—Preserve in tight, light-resistant containers.

USP Reference standards ⟨11⟩—USP Procarbazine Hydrochloride RS.
Identification—The polarogram of the solution employed for measurement in the *Assay* exhibits a half-wave potential ($E_{1/2}$) within ±0.03 volt of that of USP Procarbazine Hydrochloride RS, similarly measured ($E_{1/2}$ is about −0.16 volt against a saturated calomel electrode).
Dissolution ⟨711⟩—
  Medium: water; 900 mL.
  Apparatus 2: 50 rpm.
  Time: 45 minutes.
  Procedure—Determine the amount of procarbazine ($C_{12}H_{19}N_3O$) dissolved from UV absorbances at the wavelength of maximum absorbance at about 233 nm of filtered portions of the solution under test, suitably diluted with water, in comparison with a Standard solution having a known concentration of USP Procarbazine Hydrochloride RS in the same medium.
  Tolerances—Not less than 75% (*Q*) of the labeled amount of $C_{12}H_{19}N_3O$ is dissolved in 45 minutes.
Uniformity of dosage units ⟨905⟩: meet the requirements.
Assay—
  pH 12 buffer—Dissolve 5.43 mL of phosphoric acid, 4.60 mL of glacial acetic acid, and 4.95 g of boric acid in water to make 2000 mL. To 100 mL of this solution add 100 mL of 0.2 N sodium hydroxide. Prior to use, deaerate this solution by bubbling with scrubbed nitrogen.
  Procedure—[NOTE—Use low-actinic glassware throughout this procedure.] Weigh the contents of not less than 20 Capsules, and determine the average weight per capsule. Mix the combined contents to obtain a homogeneous sample. Transfer an accurately weighed portion of this powder, equivalent to about 60 mg of procarbazine hydrochloride, to a 100-mL volumetric flask that previously has been flushed with nitrogen. Dissolve in *pH 12 buffer*, dilute with *pH 12 buffer* to volume, and centrifuge a portion of this solution at about 1500 rpm for about 3 minutes. Transfer 10 mL to 15 mL of the solution to a polarographic cell that is regulated at 25 ± 0.1°. Deaerate by bubbling scrubbed nitrogen through the solution for 5 minutes. Insert the dropping mercury electrode of a suitable polarograph, which is capable of measuring a current of 10 microamperes, using an average capillary, a mercury column height of 56 cm, and a drop rate of approximately 4 per second. Record the polarogram from −0.75 volt to +0.25 volt, using a saturated calomel electrode as the reference electrode. Determine the height of the current at a point 200 mV anodic of the half-wave potential. Calculate the quantity, in mg, of $C_{12}H_{19}N_3O$ in the portion of Capsule contents taken by the formula:

$$100(0.8585C)[i_U / i_S]$$

in which 0.8585 is the ratio of the molecular weight of procarbazine to that of procarbazine hydrochloride, i_U is the observed current of the solution from the Capsule contents and i_S is that determined similarly in a solution of USP Procarbazine Hydrochloride RS, the concentration of which is *C* mg per mL (about 600 μg per mL).

Prochlorperazine

$C_{20}H_{24}ClN_3S$ 373.94
10*H*-Phenothiazine, 2-chloro-10-[3-(4-methyl-1-piperazinyl)propyl]-.
2-Chloro-10-[3-(4-methyl-1-piperazinyl)propyl]phenothiazine [*58-38-8*].

» Prochlorperazine contains not less than 98.0 percent and not more than 101.0 percent of $C_{20}H_{24}ClN_3S$.

Packaging and storage—Preserve in tight, light-resistant containers.
USP Reference standards ⟨11⟩—USP Prochlorperazine Maleate RS.
  NOTE—Throughout the following procedures, protect test or assay specimens, the Reference Standard, and solutions containing them, by conducting the procedures without delay, under subdued light, or using low-actinic glassware.
Identification—It meets the requirements under *Identification—Organic Nitrogenous Bases* ⟨181⟩, USP Prochlorperazine Maleate RS being used as the standard for comparison.
Residue on ignition ⟨281⟩: not more than 0.1%.
Ordinary impurities ⟨466⟩—
  Test solution: methanol.
  Standard solution: methanol.
  Eluant: a mixture of methanol and ammonium hydroxide (100 : 1).
  Visualization: 1.
Assay—Transfer about 400 mg of Prochlorperazine, accurately weighed, to a 125-mL conical flask, add 30 mL of glacial acetic acid, and warm on a steam bath to dissolve. Add 2 drops of crystal violet TS, and titrate with 0.1 N perchloric acid VS to a blue endpoint. Perform a blank determination, and make any necessary correction. Each mL of 0.1 N perchloric acid is equivalent to 18.70 mg of $C_{20}H_{24}ClN_3S$.

Prochlorperazine Oral Solution

» Prochlorperazine Oral Solution contains an amount of prochlorperazine edisylate equivalent to not less than 92.0 percent and not more than 108.0 percent of the labeled amount of prochlorperazine ($C_{20}H_{24}ClN_3S$).

Packaging and storage—Preserve in tight, light-resistant containers.
USP Reference standards ⟨11⟩—USP Prochlorperazine Maleate RS.
  NOTE—Throughout the following procedures, protect test or assay specimens, the USP Reference Standard, and solutions containing them, by conducting the procedures without delay, under subdued light, or using low-actinic glassware.
Identification—
  A: To 2 mL of Oral Solution add 3 mL of water and 3 or 4 drops of ferric chloride TS: a stable red color is produced.
  B: To 1 mL of Oral Solution add 10 mL of bromine TS, previously warmed to room temperature: essentially no color change occurs (distinction from *chlorpromazine hydrochloride*, which immediately produces a green color).
Uniformity of dosage units ⟨905⟩—
  FOR ORAL SOLUTION PACKAGED IN SINGLE-UNIT CONTAINERS: meets the requirements.
Deliverable volume ⟨698⟩—
  FOR ORAL SOLUTION PACKAGED IN MULTIPLE-UNIT CONTAINERS: meets the requirements.
Assay—
  Ion-pairing solution—Transfer 4.33 g of sodium 1-octanesulfonate, accurately weighed, to a 1-L volumetric flask. Dissolve in 500 mL of water, add 4.0 mL of glacial acetic acid, dilute with water to volume, and mix.
  Mobile phase—Prepare a filtered and degassed mixture of *Ion-pairing solution*, acetonitrile, and methanol (50 : 40 : 10). Make adjustments if necessary (see *System Suitability* under *Chromatography* ⟨621⟩).
  Diluting solution—Prepare a mixture containing 1000 mL of distilled water, 8.6 mL of concentrated hydrochloric acid, and 1000 mL of methanol.
  Standard stock solution—Dissolve an accurately weighed quantity of USP Prochlorperazine Maleate RS in *Diluting solution;* and dilute quantitatively, and stepwise if necessary, with *Diluting solution* to obtain a solution having a known concentration of about 1.0 mg per mL.

Internal standard solution—Prepare a solution of trifluoperazine hydrochloride in *Diluting solution* containing about 0.9 mg per mL.

Standard preparation—Pipet 10.0 mL of the *Standard stock solution* and 10.0 mL of the *Internal standard solution* into a 100-mL volumetric flask. Dilute with *Diluting solution* to volume, and mix.

Assay preparation—Transfer a quantity of Oral Solution, equivalent to about 10.0 mg of prochlorperazine, to a 100-mL volumetric flask; add 10.0 mL of *Internal standard solution*; dilute with *Diluting solution* to volume; and mix.

Chromatographic system (see *Chromatography* ⟨621⟩)—The liquid chromatograph is equipped with a 254-nm detector and a 3.9-mm × 15-cm column that contains 10-μm packing L1. The flow rate is about 1.5 mL per minute. Chromatograph the *Standard preparation*, and record the peak responses as directed for *Procedure*: the relative retention times are about 1.3 for trifluoperazine and 1.0 for prochlorperazine; the resolution, R, between prochlorperazine and the internal standard is not less than 2.0; the tailing factor is not more than 2.0; and the relative standard deviation for replicate injections is not more than 2.0%.

Procedure—Separately inject equal volumes (about 10 μL) of the *Standard preparation* and the *Assay preparation* into the chromatograph, record the chromatograms, and measure the responses for the major peaks. Calculate the quantity, in mg, of prochlorperazine ($C_{20}H_{24}ClN_3S$) in the portion of Oral Solution taken by the formula:

$$(373.94/606.09)(100C)(R_U/R_S)$$

in which 373.94 and 606.09 are the molecular weights of prochlorperazine and prochlorperazine maleate, respectively; C is the concentration, in mg per mL, of USP Prochlorperazine Maleate RS in the *Standard preparation*; and R_U and R_S are the ratios of the prochlorperazine peak to the internal standard peak obtained from the *Assay preparation* and the *Standard preparation*, respectively.

Prochlorperazine Suppositories

» Prochlorperazine Suppositories contain not less than 90.0 percent and not more than 110.0 percent of the labeled amount of $C_{20}H_{24}ClN_3S$.

Packaging and storage—Preserve in tight containers at a temperature below 37°. Do not expose the unwrapped Suppositories to sunlight.

USP Reference standards ⟨11⟩—*USP Prochlorperazine Maleate RS*.

NOTE—Throughout the following procedures, protect test or assay specimens, the Reference Standard, and solutions containing them, by conducting the procedures without delay, under subdued light, or using low-actinic glassware.

Identification—

A: Place a quantity of Suppositories, equivalent to about 5 mg of prochlorperazine, in a test tube, add 4 mL of dilute hydrochloric acid (1 in 2), warm on a steam bath to melt the solid, and swirl to mix: a pink color develops in the aqueous layer.

B: To the solution from *Identification* test *A* add 10 mL of bromine TS, and mix: essentially no color change occurs (distinction from *chlorpromazine*, which immediately produces a green color).

Assay—

Standard preparation—Transfer about 40 mg of USP Prochlorperazine Maleate RS, accurately weighed, to a 250-mL separator containing 75 mL of ether. Add 0.5 mL of 6 N ammonium hydroxide, and proceed as directed for *Assay preparation*, beginning with "Extract with four 65-mL portions of dilute hydrochloric acid (1 in 100)."

Assay preparation—Weigh, mash, and then mix not less than 15 Suppositories. Transfer an accurately weighed quantity of the mass, equivalent to about 25 mg of prochlorperazine, to a 100-mL beaker. Dissolve in 50 mL of ether, and transfer to a 250-mL separator with the aid of three 25-mL portions of ether. Extract with four 65-mL portions of dilute hydrochloric acid (1 in 100), collecting the aqueous extracts in a 500-mL volumetric flask. Aerate the combined extracts for 15 to 20 minutes to remove dissolved ether. Add dilute hydrochloric acid (1 in 100) to volume, and mix. Filter a portion of the solution through filter paper, discarding the first 25 mL of the filtrate. To 25.0 mL of the subsequent filtrate add dilute hydrochloric acid (1 in 100) to make 200.0 mL, and mix.

Procedure—Concomitantly determine the absorbances of the *Standard preparation* and the *Assay preparation* in 1-cm cells at 254 nm and at 278 nm, with a suitable spectrophotometer, using dilute hydrochloric acid (1 in 100) as the blank. Calculate the quantity, in mg, of $C_{20}H_{24}ClN_3S$ in the portion of Suppositories taken by the formula:

$$0.617W(A_{254} - A_{278})_U / (A_{254} - A_{278})_S$$

in which 0.617 is the ratio of the molecular weight of prochlorperazine to that of prochlorperazine maleate, W is the weight, in mg, of USP Prochlorperazine Maleate RS in the *Standard preparation*, and the parenthetic expressions are the differences in the absorbances of the two solutions at the wavelengths indicated by the subscripts, for the *Assay preparation* (U) and the *Standard preparation* (S), respectively.

Prochlorperazine Edisylate

$C_{20}H_{24}ClN_3S \cdot C_2H_6O_6S_2$ 564.14
10*H*-Phenothiazine, 2-chloro-10-[3-(4-methyl-1-piperazinyl)propyl]-,1,2-ethanedisulfonate (1 : 1).
2-Chloro-10-[3-(4-methyl-1-piperazinyl)propyl]phenothiazine 1,2-ethanedisulfonate (1 : 1)   [*1257-78-9*].

» Prochlorperazine Edisylate contains not less than 98.0 percent and not more than 101.5 percent of $C_{20}H_{24}ClN_3S \cdot C_2H_6O_6S_2$, calculated on the dried basis.

Packaging and storage—Preserve in tight, light-resistant containers.

USP Reference standards ⟨11⟩—*USP Prochlorperazine Maleate RS*.

NOTE—Throughout the following procedures, protect test or assay specimens, the Reference Standard, and solutions containing them, by conducting the procedures without delay, under subdued light, or using low-actinic glassware.

Identification—

A: It meets the requirements under *Identification—Organic Nitrogenous Bases* ⟨181⟩, USP Prochlorperazine Maleate RS being used as the standard for comparison.

B: Fuse about 100 mg with a few pellets of sodium hydroxide: the cooled melt responds to the test for *Sulfite* ⟨191⟩.

Loss on drying ⟨731⟩—Dry it in vacuum at 100° for 3 hours: it loses not more than 0.5% of its weight.

Residue on ignition ⟨281⟩: not more than 0.1%.

Selenium ⟨291⟩: 0.003%, a 100-mg test specimen, mixed with 100 mg of magnesium oxide, being used.

Ordinary impurities ⟨466⟩—

Test solution: a mixture of methanol and ammonium hydroxide (9 : 1).

Standard solution: a mixture of methanol and ammonium hydroxide (9 : 1).

Eluant: a mixture of chloroform, toluene, alcohol, and ammonium hydroxide (50 : 50 : 50 : 0.5).

Spray reagent—Mix 2 mL of chloroplatinic acid solution (1 in 10) and 50 mL of potassium iodide solution (4 in 100). Dilute with water to 100 mL, and acidify with 1 N hydrochloric acid.

Visualization: 1, followed by *Spray reagent.*
Organic volatile impurities, *Method I* ⟨467⟩: meets the requirements.

(Official until July 1, 2008)
Assay—Transfer about 750 mg of Prochlorperazine Edisylate, accurately weighed, to a separator containing 40 mL of water, and shake to effect solution. Render the solution alkaline with ammonium hydroxide, and extract with three 25-mL portions of ether. Wash the combined ether extracts once with about 25 mL of water, discard the washing, and evaporate the ether solution on a steam bath to dryness. Dissolve the residue in 60 mL of glacial acetic acid, add crystal violet TS, and titrate with 0.1 N perchloric acid VS. Perform a blank determination, and make any necessary correction. Each mL of 0.1 N perchloric acid is equivalent to 28.21 mg of $C_{20}H_{24}ClN_3S \cdot C_2H_6O_6S_2$.

Prochlorperazine Edisylate Injection

» Prochlorperazine Edisylate Injection is a sterile solution of Prochlorperazine Edisylate in Water for Injection. It contains an amount of prochlorperazine edisylate equivalent to not less than 90.0 percent and not more than 110.0 percent of the labeled amount of prochlorperazine ($C_{20}H_{24}ClN_3S$).

Packaging and storage—Preserve in single-dose or in multiple-dose containers, preferably of Type I glass, protected from light.
USP Reference standards ⟨11⟩—*USP Prochlorperazine Maleate RS. USP Endotoxin RS.*
NOTE—Throughout the following procedures, protect test or assay specimens, the Reference Standard, and solutions containing them, by conducting the procedures without delay, under subdued light, or using low-actinic glassware.
Identification—It meets the requirements under *Identification—Organic Nitrogenous Bases* ⟨181⟩, USP Prochlorperazine Maleate RS being used as the standard for comparison.
Bacterial endotoxins ⟨85⟩—It contains not more than 17.9 USP Endotoxin Units per mg of prochlorperazine.
pH ⟨791⟩: between 4.2 and 6.2.
Other requirements—It meets the requirements under *Injections* ⟨1⟩.
Assay—
Phosphate buffer—Transfer about 2.68 grams of dibasic sodium phosphate, heptahydrate to a 1-L volumetric flask, add 950 mL of water, and adjust to a pH of 3.0 with phosphoric acid, dilute to volume, and mix.
Mobile phase—Prepare a filtered and degassed mixture of acetonitrile and *Phosphate buffer* (7 : 3). Make adjustments if necessary (see *System Suitability* under *Chromatography* ⟨621⟩).
Standard preparation—Dissolve an accurately weighed quantity of USP Prochlorperazine Maleate RS in *Mobile phase*, and dilute quantitatively, and stepwise if necessary, with *Mobile phase* to obtain a solution having a known concentration of prochlorperazine of about 0.1 mg per mL.
Assay preparation—Transfer an accurately measured portion of Injection, equivalent to about 10 mg of prochlorperazine, to a 100-mL volumetric flask, dissolve in *Mobile phase*, and dilute with *Mobile phase* to volume.
Chromatographic system (see *Chromatography* ⟨621⟩)—The liquid chromatograph is equipped with a 254-nm detector and a 3.9-mm × 30-cm column that contains packing L1. The flow rate is about 1.5 mL per minute. The column temperature is maintained at 40°. Chromatograph the *Standard preparation*, and record the peak responses as directed for *Procedure:* the column efficiency is not less than 3000 theoretical plates, the tailing factor is not more than 2.5, and the relative standard deviation for replicate injections is not more than 2.0%.
Procedure—Separately inject equal volumes (about 10 μL) of the *Standard preparation* and the *Assay preparation* into the chromatograph, record the chromatograms, and measure the responses for the major peaks. Calculate the quantity, in mg, of prochlorperazine ($C_{20}H_{24}ClN_3S$) in the portion of Injection taken by the formula:

$$100(373.94 / 606.09)C(r_U / r_S)$$

in which 373.94 and 606.09 are the molecular weights of prochlorperazine and prochlorperazine maleate, respectively, C is the concentration, in mg per mL, of USP Prochlorperazine Maleate RS in the *Standard preparation*, and r_U and r_S are the peak responses obtained from the *Assay preparation* and the *Standard preparation*, respectively.

Prochlorperazine Maleate

$C_{20}H_{24}ClN_3S \cdot 2C_4H_4O_4$ 606.09
10*H*-Phenothiazine, 2-chloro-10-[3-(4-methyl-1-piperazinyl)-propyl]-, (Z)-2-butenedioate (1 : 2).
2-Chloro-10-[3-(4-methyl-1-piperazinyl)propyl]phenothiazine maleate (1 : 2)   [84-02-6].

» Prochlorperazine Maleate contains not less than 98.0 percent and not more than 101.5 percent of $C_{20}H_{24}ClN_3S \cdot 2C_4H_4O_4$, calculated on the dried basis.

Packaging and storage—Preserve in tight, light-resistant containers.
USP Reference standard ⟨11⟩—*USP Prochlorperazine Maleate RS.*
NOTE—Throughout the following procedures, protect test or assay specimens, the Reference Standard, and solutions containing them, by conducting the procedures without delay, under subdued light, or using low-actinic glassware.
Identification, *Infrared Absorption* ⟨197K⟩.
Loss on drying ⟨731⟩—Dry it in vacuum at 60° for 2 hours: it loses not more than 0.5% of its weight.
Residue on ignition ⟨281⟩: not more than 0.1%.
Ordinary impurities ⟨466⟩—
Test solution: a mixture of methanol and 1 N sodium hydroxide (9 : 1).
Standard solution: a mixture of methanol and 1 N sodium hydroxide (9 : 1).
Eluant: a mixture of methanol and ammonium hydroxide (100 : 1).
Visualization: 1.
Organic volatile impurities, *Method V* ⟨467⟩: meets the requirements.
Solvent—Use dimethyl sulfoxide.

(Official until July 1, 2008)
Assay—Transfer to a beaker about 400 mg of Prochlorperazine Maleate, accurately weighed, and dissolve in 30 mL of chloroform, warming on a steam bath to effect solution. Add 100 mL of glacial acetic acid, cool to room temperature, and titrate with 0.05 N perchloric acid VS, determining the endpoint potentiometrically. Perform a blank determination, and make any necessary correction. Each mL of 0.05 N perchloric acid is equivalent to 15.15 mg of $C_{20}H_{24}ClN_3S \cdot 2C_4H_4O_4$.

Prochlorperazine Maleate Tablets

» Prochlorperazine Maleate Tablets contain an amount of prochlorperazine maleate equivalent to not less than 95.0 percent and not more than 105.0 percent of the labeled amount of prochlorperazine ($C_{20}H_{24}ClN_3S$).

Packaging and storage—Preserve in well-closed containers, protected from light.
USP Reference standards ⟨11⟩—*USP Prochlorperazine Maleate RS.*

NOTE—Throughout the following procedures, protect test or assay specimens, the Reference Standard, and solutions containing them, by conducting the procedures without delay, under subdued light, or using low-actinic glassware.

Identification—The retention time of the major peak in the chromatogram of the *Assay preparation* corresponds to that in the chromatogram of the *Standard preparation*, as obtained in the *Assay*.

Dissolution 〈711〉—
  Medium: 0.1 N hydrochloric acid; 500 mL.
  Apparatus 2: 75 rpm.
  Time: 60 minutes.
  Procedure—Determine the amount of prochlorperazine ($C_{20}H_{24}ClN_3S$) dissolved from UV absorbances at the wavelength of maximum absorbance at about 254 nm of filtered portions of the solution under test, suitably diluted with *Dissolution Medium*, if necessary, in comparison with a Standard solution having a known concentration of USP Prochlorperazine Maleate RS in the same *Medium*.
  Tolerances—Not less than 75% (*Q*) of the labeled amount of $C_{20}H_{24}ClN_3S$ is dissolved in 60 minutes.

Uniformity of dosage units 〈905〉: meet the requirements.

Assay—
  Ion-pairing solution—Transfer 4.33 g of sodium 1-octanesulfonate, accurately weighed, to a 1-liter volumetric flask. Dissolve in 500 mL of water, add 4.0 mL of glacial acetic acid, dilute with water to volume, and mix.
  Mobile phase—Prepare a suitable filtered and degassed mixture of *Ion-pairing solution*, acetonitrile, and methanol (45 : 40 : 15).
  Standard preparation—Dissolve an accurately weighed quantity of USP Prochlorperazine Maleate RS in *Mobile phase* to obtain a solution having a known concentration of about 0.2 mg per mL.
  Assay preparation—Weigh and finely powder not less than 20 Tablets. Transfer an accurately weighed portion of the powder, equivalent to about 20 mg of prochlorperazine maleate, to a 100-mL volumetric flask. Add 60 mL of *Mobile phase*, sonicate for 3 minutes, and shake by mechanical means for 30 minutes. Dilute with *Mobile phase* to volume, mix, and filter, discarding the first 10 mL of filtrate.
  Chromatographic system (see *Chromatography* 〈621〉)—The liquid chromatograph is equipped with a 254-nm detector and a 3.9-mm × 30-cm column that contains packing L1. The flow rate is about 2 mL per minute. Chromatograph the *Standard preparation*, and record the peak responses as directed for *Procedure*: the tailing factor for the analyte peak is not more than 2.0; and the relative standard deviation for replicate injections is not more than 2.0%.
  Procedure—Separately inject equal volumes (about 10 µL) of the *Standard preparation* and the *Assay preparation* into the chromatograph, record the chromatograms, and measure the responses for the major peaks. Calculate the quantity, in mg, of prochlorperazine ($C_{20}H_{24}ClN_3S$) in the portion of Tablets taken by the formula:

$$(373.94 / 606.09)(100C)(r_U / r_S)$$

in which 373.94 and 606.09 are the molecular weights of prochlorperazine and prochlorperazine maleate, respectively; *C* is the concentration, in mg per mL, of USP Prochlorperazine Maleate RS in the *Standard preparation*; and r_U and r_S are the peak responses obtained from the *Assay preparation* and the *Standard preparation*, respectively.

Procyclidine Hydrochloride

$C_{19}H_{29}NO \cdot HCl$ 323.90
1-Pyrrolidinepropanol, α-cyclohexyl-α-phenyl-, hydrochloride.
α-Cyclohexyl-α-phenyl-1-pyrrolidinepropanol hydrochloride [1508-76-5].

» Procyclidine Hydrochloride contains not less than 99.0 percent and not more than 101.0 percent of $C_{19}H_{29}NO \cdot HCl$, calculated on the dried basis.

Packaging and storage—Preserve in tight, light-resistant containers, and store in a dry place.

USP Reference standards 〈11〉—*USP Procyclidine Hydrochloride RS*.

Identification—
  A: *Infrared Absorption* 〈197K〉.
  B: Dissolve about 250 mg in 10 mL of water in a separator, render alkaline with 6 N ammonium hydroxide, and extract with three 10-mL portions of ether. Filter the ether extracts slowly through a layer of about 2 g of anhydrous granular sodium sulfate supported on glass wool, evaporate the ether with a current of warm air, and scratch the surface of the container to induce crystallization of the residue: the procyclidine so obtained melts between 83° and 87°, the procedure for *Class I* being used (see *Melting Range or Temperature* 〈741〉).
  C: A solution (1 in 100) responds to the tests for *Chloride* 〈191〉.

pH 〈791〉: between 5.0 and 6.5, in a solution (1 in 100).

Loss on drying 〈731〉—Dry it in vacuum at 105° for 4 hours: it loses not more than 0.5% of its weight.

Residue on ignition 〈281〉: not more than 0.1%.

Related compounds—Dissolve approximately 200 mg of Procyclidine Hydrochloride in 20 mL of water, and render the solution alkaline by adding 1.5 mL of 6 N ammonium hydroxide. Extract with three 15-mL portions of chloroform, wash the combined extracts with 20 mL of water, discard the water washing, and filter the chloroform solution through a layer of 3 to 4 g of anhydrous granular sodium sulfate supported on glass wool. Reduce the volume to 5 mL by evaporating with the aid of gentle heat and a current of air. Inject 2 µL of this solution into a suitable gas chromatograph (see *Chromatography* 〈621〉) equipped with a flame-ionization detector, and record the chromatogram to 2.5 relative to the retention time of the principal (procyclidine) peak. Under typical conditions, the instrument contains a 1-m × 2-mm glass column packed with 10% polyethylene glycol 20,000 and 2% potassium hydroxide on packing S1A. The column is maintained at a temperature of 180°, the injection port is maintained at 210°, the detector block is maintained at about 220°, and dry helium is used as the carrier gas at a flow rate of about 60 mL per minute. From the total area under the curve, excluding the solvent peak, calculate the percentage of total impurities by area normalization: not more than 4.0% is found.

Organic volatile impurities, *Method V* 〈467〉: meets the requirements.

(Official until July 1, 2008)

Assay—Dissolve about 700 mg of Procyclidine Hydrochloride, accurately weighed, in 75 mL of glacial acetic acid in a 250-mL beaker, warming, if necessary, to effect solution. Cool, add 10 mL of mercuric acetate TS, and titrate with 0.1 N perchloric acid VS, determining the endpoint potentiometrically. Perform a blank determination, and make any necessary correction. Each mL of 0.1 N perchloric acid is equivalent to 32.39 mg of $C_{19}H_{29}NO \cdot HCl$.

Procyclidine Hydrochloride Tablets

» Procyclidine Hydrochloride Tablets contain not less than 93.0 percent and not more than 107.0 percent of the labeled amount of $C_{19}H_{29}NO \cdot HCl$.

Packaging and storage—Preserve in tight containers, and store in a dry place.

USP Reference standards 〈11〉—*USP Procyclidine Hydrochloride RS*.

Identification—
  A: Triturate a portion of finely powdered Tablets, equivalent to about 10 mg of procyclidine hydrochloride, with 20 mL of chloroform, filter, evaporate the filtrate on a steam bath to dryness, and dry the residue at 105° for 1 hour: the IR absorption spectrum of a

potassium bromide dispersion of the procyclidine hydrochloride so obtained exhibits maxima only at the same wavelengths as that of a similar preparation of USP Procyclidine Hydrochloride RS.

B: A portion of finely powdered Tablets, equivalent to about 50 mg of procyclidine hydrochloride, responds to *Identification test B* under *Procyclidine Hydrochloride*.

Dissolution, *Procedure for a Pooled Sample* ⟨711⟩—
  Medium: water; 900 mL.
  Apparatus 2: 50 rpm.
  Time: 45 minutes.
  Procedure—Determine the amount of $C_{19}H_{29}NO \cdot HCl$ dissolved, employing the procedure set forth in the *Assay*, making any necessary modifications.
  Tolerances—Not less than 75% (Q) of the labeled amount of $C_{19}H_{29}NO \cdot HCl$ is dissolved in 45 minutes.

Uniformity of dosage units ⟨905⟩: meet the requirements.

Related compounds—Using a portion of powdered Tablets, equivalent to 200 mg of procyclidine hydrochloride, proceed as directed in the test for *Related compounds* under *Procyclidine Hydrochloride*.

Assay—
  Bromocresol purple solution—Dissolve 250 mg of bromocresol purple in dilute glacial acetic acid (1 in 50) to make 1000 mL.
  Standard preparation—Transfer about 25 mg of USP Procyclidine Hydrochloride RS, accurately weighed, to a 100-mL volumetric flask, add water to volume, and mix. Transfer 10.0 mL of this solution to a second 100-mL volumetric flask, dilute with *Bromocresol purple solution* to volume, and mix. The concentration of the *Standard preparation* is about 25 µg per mL.
  Assay preparation—Weigh and finely powder not less than 20 Tablets. Transfer an accurately weighed portion of the powder, equivalent to about 2.5 mg of procyclidine hydrochloride, to a 100-mL volumetric flask, add 10.0 mL of water, and mix. Dilute with *Bromocresol purple solution* to volume, mix, and allow the undissolved particles to settle. Use the supernatant as directed in the *Procedure*.
  Procedure—Transfer 5.0 mL each of the *Standard preparation* and the *Assay preparation* to individual 60-mL separators. Transfer 0.5 mL of water and 4.5 mL of *Bromocresol purple solution* to a third separator to provide the blank. Extract each solution with 20.0 mL of chloroform, and filter each extract, discarding the first 5 mL of the filtrate. Concomitantly determine the absorbance of each subsequent filtrate in a 1-cm cell at the wavelength of maximum absorbance at about 405 nm, with a suitable spectrophotometer, against the blank. Calculate the quantity, in mg, of $C_{19}H_{29}NO \cdot HCl$ in the portion of Tablets taken by the formula:

$$0.1C(A_U / A_S)$$

in which C is the concentration, in µg per mL, of USP Procyclidine Hydrochloride RS in the *Standard preparation*, and A_U and A_S are the absorbances of the solutions from the *Assay preparation* and the *Standard preparation*, respectively.

Progesterone

$C_{21}H_{30}O_2$ 314.47
Pregn-4-ene-3,20-dione.
Progesterone [57-83-0].

» Progesterone contains not less than 97.0 percent and not more than 103.0 percent of $C_{21}H_{30}O_2$, calculated on the dried basis.

Packaging and storage—Preserve in tight, light-resistant containers. Store at 25°, excursions permitted between 15° and 30°.

USP Reference standards ⟨11⟩—*USP Progesterone RS*.

Identification—
  A: *Infrared Absorption* ⟨197K⟩.
  B: *Ultraviolet Absorption* ⟨197U⟩—
    Solution: 10 µg per mL.
    Medium: methanol.

Melting range ⟨741⟩: between 126° and 131°. It may exist also in a polymorphic modification, melting at about 121°.

Specific rotation ⟨781S⟩: between +175° and +183°.
  Test solution: 20 mg per mL, in dioxane.

Loss on drying ⟨731⟩—Dry it in vacuum over silica gel for 4 hours: it loses not more than 0.5% of its weight.

Assay—
  Mobile phase—Prepare a filtered and degassed mixture of water and isopropyl alcohol (72 : 28). Make adjustments if necessary (see *System Suitability* under *Chromatography* ⟨621⟩).
  Internal standard solution—Transfer about 66 mg of methyltestosterone to a 10-mL volumetric flask, add dilute alcohol (85 in 100) to volume, and mix.
  Standard preparation—Dissolve an accurately weighed quantity of USP Progesterone RS in dilute alcohol (85 in 100) to obtain a solution having a known concentration of about 2.5 mg per mL. Transfer 4.0 mL of this solution to a 10-mL volumetric flask, add 1.0 mL of *Internal standard solution,* then add dilute alcohol (85 in 100) to volume, and mix to obtain a solution having a known concentration of about 1 mg of USP Progesterone RS per mL.
  Assay preparation—Transfer about 10 mg of Progesterone, accurately weighed, to a 10-mL volumetric flask, add 1.0 mL of *Internal standard solution,* then add dilute alcohol (85 in 100) to volume, and mix.
  Chromatographic system (see *Chromatography* ⟨621⟩)—The liquid chromatograph is equipped with a 254-nm detector and a 4-mm × 30-cm column that contains 10-µm packing L1. The flow rate is about 1.5 mL per minute. Chromatograph the *Standard preparation*, and record the peak responses as directed for *Procedure:* the resolution, R, between the analyte and internal standard peaks is not less than 3.5; and the relative standard deviation for replicate injections is not more than 1.5%.
  Procedure—Separately inject equal volumes (5 µL) of the *Standard preparation* and the *Assay preparation* into the chromatograph, record the chromatograms, and measure the responses for the major peaks. The relative retention times are about 2.0 for progesterone and 1.0 for methyltestosterone. Calculate the quantity, in mg, of $C_{21}H_{30}O_2$ in the portion of Progesterone taken by the formula:

$$10C(R_U / R_S)$$

in which C is the concentration, in mg per mL, of USP Progesterone RS in the *Standard preparation;* and R_U and R_S are the peak response ratios obtained from the *Assay preparation* and the *Standard preparation*, respectively.

Progesterone Injection

» Progesterone Injection is a sterile solution of Progesterone in a suitable solvent. It contains not less than 90.0 percent and not more than 110.0 percent of the labeled amount of $C_{21}H_{30}O_2$.

Packaging and storage—Preserve in single-dose or in multiple-dose containers, preferably of Type I or Type III glass.

USP Reference standards ⟨11⟩—*USP Progesterone RS*.

Identification—Insert a pledget of fine glass wool into the base of a chromatographic tube of about 200 × 25 mm. Mix 8.0 mL of nitromethane with 7.0 g of purified siliceous earth in a 150-mL beaker until uniform, and transfer to the chromatographic tube, packing lightly with a suitable tamping rod. Pack a pledget of glass wool on the top of the column. Dilute 1 mL of the Injection with *n*-heptane to obtain a solution having a concentration of about 1 mg of progesterone per mL. Transfer 4.0 mL of this solution to the prepared column. Pass 300 mL of *n*-heptane through the column, discarding the first 120 mL of the eluate. Collect the subsequent eluate in a 250-mL beaker. Evaporate the solution under a stream of nitrogen on a steam bath to about 50 mL, transfer to a 100-mL beaker, and evaporate to dryness. Remove the last traces of *n*-heptane by adding 1 mL of methanol and again drying. Dry the specimen over silica gel for 4 hours: the IR absorption spectrum of a potassium bromide dispersion of the residue so obtained exhibits maxima only at the same wavelengths as that of a similar preparation of USP Progesterone RS.

Other requirements—It meets the requirements under *Injections* $\langle 1 \rangle$.

Assay—

Mobile phase—Prepare a degassed mixture of alcohol and water (11 : 9). Make adjustments if necessary (see *System Suitability* under *Chromatography* $\langle 621 \rangle$).

Standard preparation—Dissolve an accurately weighed quantity of USP Progesterone RS in 20 mL of tetrahydrofuran, and dilute quantitatively, and stepwise if necessary, with alcohol to obtain a solution having a known concentration of about 0.08 mg per mL.

Assay preparation—Transfer an accurately measured volume of Injection, equivalent to about 100 mg of progesterone, to a 100-mL volumetric flask, add 20 mL of tetrahydrofuran to dissolve, and dilute with alcohol to volume. Transfer 8 mL of this solution to a 100-mL volumetric flask, dilute with alcohol to volume, and mix.

Chromatographic system (see *Chromatography* $\langle 621 \rangle$)—The liquid chromatograph is equipped with a 254-nm detector and a 4.6-mm × 25-cm column that contains 5-μm packing L1. The flow rate is about 1 mL per minute. The column temperature is maintained at about 40°. Chromatograph a sample of dimethyl sulfoxide, and identify the retention time, t_α, of this nonretarded compound to calculate the capacity factor, k'. Chromatograph the *Standard preparation*, and record the peak responses as directed for *Procedure*: the capacity factor, k', for progesterone is not less than 2.0; the tailing factor is not more than 2.0; and the relative standard deviation for replicate injections is not more than 2.0%.

Procedure—Separately inject equal volumes (about 10 μL) of the *Standard preparation* and the *Assay preparation* into the chromatograph, record the chromatograms, and measure the responses for the major peaks. [NOTE—The run time for the *Assay preparation* must be at least twice that of the *Standard preparation*.] Calculate the quantity, in mg, of progesterone ($C_{21}H_{30}O_2$) in each mL of Injection taken by the formula:

$$1250(C/V)(r_U / r_S)$$

in which C is the concentration, in mg per mL, of USP Progesterone RS in the *Standard preparation*; V is the volume, in mL, of Injection taken; and r_U and r_S are the peak responses for progesterone obtained from the *Assay preparation* and the *Standard preparation*, respectively.

Progesterone Intrauterine Contraceptive System

» Progesterone Intrauterine Contraceptive System contains not less than 90.0 percent and not more than 110.0 percent of the labeled amount of $C_{21}H_{30}O_2$. It is sterile.

Packaging and storage—Preserve in sealed, single-unit containers.

USP Reference standards $\langle 11 \rangle$—*USP Progesterone RS*.

Identification—Cut off and discard the sealed ends of the drug-containing cores of 2 Systems, and force the contents of the tubes into a small centrifuge tube. Add 3 mL of methanol, insert the stopper in the tube, mix, centrifuge, and transfer the clear, supernatant to a small beaker. Evaporate the methanol to dryness, wash the residue with two 4-mL portions of cyclohexane, and discard the washings. Dry the residue in vacuum at 50° to constant weight: the IR absorption spectrum of a mineral oil dispersion of the dried residue so obtained exhibits maxima only at the same wavelengths as that of a similar preparation of USP Progesterone RS.

Sterility $\langle 71 \rangle$: meets the requirements.
Uniformity of dosage units $\langle 905 \rangle$: meets the requirements.
Chromatographic purity—

Test solution—Remove the drug-containing core from 1 System, as directed in the *Assay*, transferring it to a small flask with 25 mL of methanol. Shake vigorously for several minutes, and allow the insoluble portion to settle. The resulting supernatant is the *Test solution*.

Procedure—Divide a 20- × 20-cm thin-layer chromatographic plate, coated with a 0.25-mm layer of chromatographic silica gel mixture, into sections 2 cm apart. In successive sections of the plate, on a line 2 cm from the lower edge of the plate and parallel to it, apply 1 μL, 2 μL, 3 μL, and 100 μL of the *Test solution*. Develop the plate in a suitable pre-equilibrated chromatographic chamber with a solvent system consisting of a mixture of chloroform and ethyl acetate (2 : 1) until the solvent front has moved 10 cm above the point of application of the spots. Remove the plate, and allow to air-dry. Observe the dried plate under short-wavelength UV light (254 nm). If spots other than the principal spot are observed in the lane of the 100-μL specimen, estimate the concentration of each by comparison with the 1-μL (1%), 2-μL (2%), and 3-μL (3%) spots. The requirement is met if the sum of impurities in the 100-μL specimen does not exceed 3%.

Drug release pattern—Remove the attached sutures from 10 Systems, and secure each system to a corrosion-resistant wire of sufficient length such that the systems are completely immersed during the shaking operation but do not touch the bottoms of the flasks. Suspend each system by the attached wire from the arm of a mechanical shaker designed to travel 2.5 cm in each direction in a vertically reciprocating cycle, at a speed of 2.5 cycles per second, so that each system is immersed in a separate 250-mL volumetric flask containing 230 mL of water, pre-equilibrated to 60 ± 0.1°. Immerse the volumetric flasks in an insulated constant-temperature water bath, maintained at 60 ± 0.1° and having a suitable means of maintaining the water level, so that the water level of the bath is above the water level in the flasks. Employ a rack or other suitable means of support for the flasks in the water bath.

Operate the shaker under the conditions described above for 23.5 hours, then remove the flasks and the systems from the bath. Remove the systems from the flasks, and immerse each system in a different flask containing 230 mL of water, pre-equilibrated to 60 ± 0.1°, and immerse these flasks in the water bath. Repeat this shaking operation daily for 12 days, using different flasks each day.

Determine the quantity of progesterone in the solutions from each of the 12 days of testing as follows. Immediately add 15 mL of methanol to each solution, allow to cool to room temperature, dilute with water to volume, and mix. Concomitantly determine the UV absorbances of each test solution and of a solution of USP Progesterone RS in the same medium, having a known concentration of about 7 μg per mL, in 2-cm cells at the wavelength of maximum absorbance at about 248 nm, with a suitable spectrophotometer, against a blank of water and methanol (47 : 3). Calculate the progesterone release rate, in mg per day, in the solutions taken by the formula:

$$(A_U / A_S)(24 / 23.5)0.25C$$

in which A_U and A_S are the absorbances of the test solution and the Standard solution, respectively; and C is the concentration, in μg per mL, of USP Progesterone RS in the Standard solution. For the time points specified, the drug-release pattern conforms to *Acceptance Table 1* under *Drug Release* $\langle 724 \rangle$.

Day	Release Rate (mg per day)
6	1.05–1.45
9	0.95–1.35
12	0.90–1.30

Assay—Cut off the lower sealed end of the drug-containing core of a number of Progesterone Intrauterine Contraceptive Systems, sufficient to provide about 400 mg of progesterone, forcing the viscous liquid core into a 1000-mL volumetric flask. Cut the core sections in half lengthwise, using a sharp blade, taking precautions not to contaminate either the core material or the outside of the membranes. Transfer all of these sections of the systems to the flask containing the core material. Add about 500 mL of methanol to the flask, shake vigorously for 5 to 10 minutes, dilute with methanol to volume, and centrifuge a portion of the solution. Dilute 10.0 mL of the clear, supernatant with methanol to 250 mL, and mix. Concomitantly determine the absorbances of this solution and of a Standard solution of USP Progesterone RS, previously dried and accurately weighed, in methanol having a known concentration of about 16 µg of progesterone per mL, in 1-cm cells at the wavelength of maximum absorbance at about 241 nm, with a suitable spectrophotometer, using methanol as the blank. Calculate the quantity, in mg, of $C_{21}H_{30}O_2$ in each System taken by the formula:

$$25(C / N)(A_U / A_S)$$

which C is the concentration, in µg per mL, of USP Progesterone RS in the Standard solution; N is the number of Systems taken; and A_U and A_S are the absorbances of the test solution and the Standard solution, respectively.

Progesterone Injectable Suspension

» Progesterone Injectable Suspension is a sterile suspension of Progesterone in Water for Injection. It contains not less than 93.0 percent and not more than 107.0 percent of the labeled amount of $C_{21}H_{30}O_2$.

Packaging and storage—Preserve in single-dose or in multiple-dose containers, preferably of Type I glass.
USP Reference standards ⟨11⟩—*USP Progesterone RS. USP Methyltestosterone RS.*
Identification—Filter a volume of well-shaken Injectable Suspension, equivalent to not less than 100 mg of progesterone, through a medium-porosity, sintered-glass crucible, filtering again through the same crucible if the fluid is not clear. Wash with several 5-mL portions of water until 2 mL of the last washing, evaporated on a steam bath, leaves no weighable residue: the washed solid, dried at 105° to constant weight, melts between 126° and 131°, and responds to *Identification* test A under *Progesterone*.
pH ⟨791⟩: between 4.0 and 7.5.
Other requirements—It meets the requirements under *Injections* ⟨1⟩.
Assay—
  Mobile phase—Prepare a filtered and degassed mixture of water and isopropyl alcohol (72 : 28). Make adjustments if necessary (see *System Suitability* under *Chromatography* ⟨621⟩.)
  Diluent—Prepare a mixture of alcohol and water (85 in 100).
  Internal standard solution—Dissolve an accurately weighed quantity of USP Methyltestosterone RS in *Diluent* to obtain a solution containing about 6.6 mg per mL.
  Standard preparation—Dissolve an accurately weighed quantity of USP Progesterone RS in *Diluent*, and dilute quantitatively, and stepwise if necessary, with *Diluent* to obtain a solution having a known concentration of about 2.5 mg per mL.
  Standard curve—To four separate polytef-lined, screw-capped centrifuge tubes, pipet 3-, 4-, 5-, and 6-mL portions, respectively, of the *Standard preparation*. Add *Diluent* to each tube to make about 8 mL of solution. Transfer 1.0 mL of *Internal standard solution* to each tube, and mix.
  Assay preparation—Transfer an accurately measured volume of Injectable Suspension, equivalent to about 25 mg progesterone, to a polytef-lined, screw-capped, 25 mL test tube. Add 16 mL of *Diluent*, and shake until clear. Add 2.0 mL of *Internal standard solution*, and mix.
  Chromatographic system (see *Chromatography* ⟨621⟩)—The liquid chromatograph is equipped with a 254-nm detector and a 2.1-mm × 1-m column that contains packing L2. The chromatographic conditions are such that retention times of the internal standard and progesterone are between 3 and 6 minutes and 7 and 11 minutes, respectively. Chromatograph any solution of the *Standard curve*, and record the peak areas as directed for *Procedure*: the resolution, R, between progesterone and methyltestosterone is not less than 3.5;

and the relative standard deviation for replicate injections is not more than 1.5%.
  Procedure—Separately inject equal volumes (5.0 µL) of each solution of the *Standard curve* and the *Assay preparation* into the chromatograph, record the chromatograms, and measure the peak areas. Plot the progesterone to methyltestosterone peak ratio versus the concentration, in mg per mL, of progesterone in the *Standard curve* solutions. Extrapolate the progesterone to methyltestosterone peak ratio of the *Assay preparation* in the *Standard curve* so obtained, and determine the progesterone concentration, C, in mg per mL, in the *Assay preparation*. Calculate the amount, in mg, of progesterone ($C_{21}H_{30}O_2$) in each mL of the Injectable Suspension taken by the formula:

$$V/A(C)$$

in which V is the total volume of the *Assay preparation*; A is the volume in mL of Injectable Suspension taken; and C is the concentration of progesterone in the *Assay preparation* calculated above.

Progesterone Vaginal Suppositories

Change to read:
» Progesterone Vaginal Suppositories contain not less than 90.0 percent and not more than 110.0 percent of the labeled amount of progesterone ($C_{21}H_{30}O_2$).
SUPPOSITORIES COMPOUNDED IN FATTY ACID BASE
Prepare Progesterone Vaginal Suppositories in fatty acid base as follows (see *Pharmaceutical Compounding—Nonsterile Preparations* ⟨795⟩):

Progesterone (micronized)
▲▲USP31 . . . . 25 mg to 600 mg
Fatty acid base, a sufficient
  quantity to make one suppository

Calibrate the actual molds with the fatty acid base that is used for preparing the suppositories, and adjust the formula accordingly. ▲▲USP31 Heat the fatty acid base slowly and evenly until melted. Slowly add the ▲Progesterone▲USP31 powder to the melted base, with stirring. Mix thoroughly, and pour into molds. Cool in a refrigerator until solidified, trim, and wrap.

Packaging and storage—Preserve in well-closed, light-resistant containers. Store in a refrigerator.
Labeling—Label Suppositories to state that they are Progesterone Vaginal Suppositories in a Fatty Acid Base and to state the content, in mg, of progesterone per suppository. Label Suppositories to state that they are to be stored in a refrigerator (2° to 8°). Label them to state that they are to be used only as directed, and that wrappers are to be removed prior to use.
USP Reference standards ⟨11⟩—*USP Methyltestosterone RS. USP Progesterone RS.*
Uniformity of dosage units ⟨905⟩: meet the requirements for *Weight Variation*.
Beyond-use date—Ninety days after the day on which they were compounded.
Assay for suppositories compounded in fatty acid base—
  Alcohol mixture—Prepare a mixture of dehydrated alcohol, isopropyl alcohol, and methanol (90 : 5 : 5).
  Mobile phase—Prepare a filtered and degassed mixture of *Alcohol mixture* and water (55 : 45). Make adjustments if necessary (see *System Suitability* under *Chromatography* ⟨621⟩).

Diluted alcohol mixture—Prepare a mixture of *Alcohol mixture* and water (7 : 3).

Resolution solution—Dissolve an accurately weighed quantity of USP Methyltestosterone RS in *Mobile phase*, and dilute quantitatively, and stepwise if necessary, with *Mobile phase* to obtain a solution having a known concentration of about 0.4 mg per mL. Separately and similarly prepare a solution in *Mobile phase* having a known concentration of about 0.4 mg of USP Progesterone RS per mL. Transfer 2.0 mL of each solution to a 10-mL volumetric flask, dilute with *Mobile phase* to volume, and mix.

Standard preparation 1—Dissolve an accurately weighed quantity of USP Progesterone RS in *n*-propyl alcohol, and dilute quantitatively, and stepwise if necessary, with *n*-propyl alcohol to obtain a solution having a known concentration of about 0.25 mg per mL. Mix 5.0 mL of this solution with 10.0 mL of *Diluted alcohol mixture*.

Standard preparation 2—Dissolve an accurately weighed quantity of USP Progesterone RS in *n*-propyl alcohol, and dilute quantitatively, and stepwise if necessary, with *n*-propyl alcohol to obtain a solution having a known concentration of about 3 mg per mL. Transfer 3.0 mL of this solution to a 100-mL volumetric flask, dilute with *Diluted alcohol mixture* to volume, and mix.

Assay preparation 1—Transfer 1 Suppository, containing not more than 100 mg of progesterone, to a 100-mL volumetric flask, dissolve in about 90 mL of *n*-propyl alcohol, heat at 45° for 4 minutes, sonicate for 10 minutes, cool, dilute with *n*-propyl alcohol to volume, and mix. Dilute quantitatively, and stepwise if necessary, with *n*-propyl alcohol, sonicating if necessary, to obtain a solution containing about 0.25 mg of progesterone per mL. Transfer 5.0 mL of this solution to a 50-mL centrifuge tube, add 10.0 mL of *Diluted alcohol mixture*, mix, sonicate for 1 minute, and centrifuge for 10 minutes at 2000 rpm. Pass the supernatant through a filter having a 0.45-μm or finer porosity, discarding the first 4 mL of the filtrate.

Assay preparation 2—Transfer 1 Suppository, containing more than 100 mg of progesterone, to a 200-mL volumetric flask, dissolve in about 180 mL of *n*-propyl alcohol, heat at 45° for 8 minutes, sonicate for 5 minutes, cool, dilute with *n*-propyl alcohol to volume, and mix. Dilute quantitatively, and stepwise if necessary, sonicating each dilution for 1 minute, to obtain a solution containing about 0.09 mg of progesterone per mL. Transfer about 15 mL of this solution to a 50-mL centrifuge tube, and centrifuge for 10 minutes at 2000 rpm. Pass the supernatant through a filter having a 0.45-μm or finer porosity, discarding the first 4 mL of the filtrate.

Chromatographic system (see *Chromatography* ⟨621⟩)—The liquid chromatograph is equipped with a 245-nm detector and a 3.9-mm × 30-cm column that contains packing L1. The column temperature is maintained at 40°. The flow rate is about 1.0 mL per minute. Chromatograph the *Resolution solution*, and record the peak responses as directed for *Procedure*: the relative retention times are about 0.8 for methyltestosterone and 1.0 for progesterone; the resolution, *R*, between methyltestosterone and progesterone is not less than 2.0; the tailing factor is not more than 2.0 for the progesterone peak; and the relative standard deviation for replicate injections is not more than 2.0% for progesterone.

Procedure—Separately inject equal volumes (about 10 μL) of *Standard preparation 1* and *Assay preparation 1*, or of *Standard preparation 2* and *Assay preparation 2*, into the chromatograph, record the chromatograms, and measure the areas for the major peaks. Calculate the quantity, in mg, of progesterone ($C_{21}H_{30}O_2$) in the Suppository taken by the formula:

$$300CD(r_U / r_S)$$

in which *C* is the concentration, in mg per mL, of USP Progesterone RS in the *Standard preparation*; *D* is the dilution factor for obtaining the *Assay preparation*; and r_U and r_S are the peak responses obtained from the *Assay preparation* and the *Standard preparation*, respectively.

Change to read:
SUPPOSITORIES COMPOUNDED IN POLYETHYLENE GLYCOL BASE
Prepare Progesterone Vaginal Suppositories in polyethylene glycol base as follows (see *Pharmaceutical Compounding—Nonsterile Preparations* ⟨795⟩):

Progesterone (micronized)   25 mg to 600 mg
▲USP31   ▲USP31
Polyethylene glycol base, a sufficient quantity to make one suppository

Calibrate the actual molds with polyethylene glycol base that is used for preparing the Suppositories, and adjust the formula accordingly. ▲USP31 Heat the polyethylene glycol base slowly and evenly until melted. Slowly add the ▲Progesterone▲USP31 powder to the melted base, with stirring. Mix thoroughly, and pour into molds. Cool, trim, and wrap.

Packaging and storage—Preserve in tight, light-resistant containers. Do not dispense or store polyethylene glycol–base suppositories in polystyrene containers. Store in a refrigerator.

Labeling—Label Suppositories to state that they are Progesterone Vaginal Suppositories in a Polyethylene Glycol Base and to state the content, in mg, of progesterone per suppository. Label Suppositories to state that they are to be stored in a refrigerator (2° to 8°). Label them to state that they are to be used only as directed, that wrappers are to be removed prior to use, and that, if necessary, they may be moistened prior to insertion.

USP Reference standards ⟨11⟩—*USP Methyltestosterone RS. USP Progesterone RS.*

Uniformity of dosage units ⟨905⟩: meet the requirements for *Weight Variation*.

Beyond-use date—Ninety days after the day on which they were compounded.

Assay for suppositories compounded in polyethylene glycol base—

Alcohol mixture, Mobile phase, Resolution solution, and *Chromatographic system*—Proceed as directed in the compliance *Assay for suppositories compounded in fatty acid base*.

Standard preparation—Dissolve an accurately weighed quantity of USP Progesterone RS in *Mobile phase*, and dilute quantitatively, and stepwise if necessary, with *Mobile phase*, to obtain a solution having a known concentration of about 0.1 mg per mL.

Assay preparation—Dissolve 1 Suppository in 200 mL of *Mobile phase*, and dilute quantitatively, and stepwise if necessary, with *Mobile phase* to obtain a solution containing about 0.1 mg of progesterone per mL. Pass a 10-mL portion of the mixture through a filter having a 0.45-μm or finer porosity, discarding the first 4 mL of the filtrate.

Procedure—Separately inject equal volumes (about 10 μL) of the *Standard preparation* and the *Assay preparation* into the chromatograph, record the chromatograms, and measure the areas for the major peaks. Calculate the quantity, in mg, of progesterone ($C_{21}H_{30}O_2$) in the Suppository taken by the formula:

$$200CD(r_U / r_S)$$

in which *C* is the concentration, in mg per mL, of USP Progesterone RS in the *Standard preparation*; *D* is the dilution factor for obtaining the *Assay preparation*; and r_U and r_S are the peak responses obtained from the *Assay preparation* and the *Standard preparation*, respectively.

Proline

$C_5H_9NO_2$ 115.13
L-Proline.
L-Proline. [*147-85-3*].

» Proline contains not less than 98.5 percent and not more than 101.5 percent of $C_5H_9NO_2$, as L-proline, calculated on the dried basis.

Packaging and storage—Preserve in well-closed containers.
USP Reference standards ⟨11⟩—*USP L-Proline RS. USP L-Threonine RS.*
Identification, *Infrared Absorption* ⟨197K⟩.
Specific rotation ⟨781S⟩: between −84.3° and −86.3°.
   Test solution: 40 mg per mL, in water.
Loss on drying ⟨731⟩—Dry it at 105° for 3 hours: it loses not more than 0.4% of its weight.
Residue on ignition ⟨281⟩:   not more than 0.4%.
Chloride ⟨221⟩—A 0.73-g portion shows no more chloride than corresponds to 0.50 mL of 0.020 N hydrochloric acid (0.05%).
Sulfate ⟨221⟩—A 0.33-g portion shows no more sulfate than corresponds to 0.10 mL of 0.020 N sulfuric acid (0.03%).
Iron ⟨241⟩:   0.003%.
Heavy metals, *Method I* ⟨231⟩:   0.0015%.
Chromatographic purity—
   Adsorbent: 0.25-mm layer of chromatographic silica gel mixture.
   Test solution—Dissolve an accurately weighed quantity of Proline in 0.1 N hydrochloric acid to obtain a solution having a concentration of 10 mg per mL. Apply 5 µL.
   Standard solution—Dissolve an accurately weighed quantity of USP L-Proline RS in 0.1 N hydrochloric acid to obtain a solution having a known concentration of about 0.05 mg per mL. Apply 5 µL. [NOTE—This solution has a concentration equivalent to about 0.5% of that of the *Test solution.*]
   System suitability solution—Prepare a solution in 0.1 N hydrochloric acid containing 0.4 mg each of USP L-Proline RS and USP L-Threonine RS per mL. Apply 5 µL.
   Spray reagent—Dissolve 0.2 g of ninhydrin in 100 mL of a mixture of butyl alcohol and 2 N acetic acid (95 : 5).
   Developing solvent system—Prepare a mixture of butyl alcohol, glacial acetic acid, and water (60 : 20 : 20).
   Procedure—Proceed as directed for *Thin-Layer Chromatography* under *Chromatography* ⟨621⟩. After air-drying the plate, spray with *Spray reagent,* and heat between 100° and 105° for about 15 minutes. Examine the plate under white light. The chromatogram obtained from the *System suitability solution* exhibits two clearly separated spots. Any secondary spot in the chromatogram obtained from the *Test solution* is not larger or more intense than the principal spot in the chromatogram obtained from the *Standard solution:* not more than 0.5% of any individual impurity is found; and not more than 2.0% of total impurities is found.
Organic volatile impurities, *Method I* ⟨467⟩:   meets the requirements.

(Official until July 1, 2008)

Assay—Transfer about 100 mg of Proline, accurately weighed, to a 125-mL flask, dissolve in a mixture of 3 mL of formic acid and 50 mL of glacial acetic acid, and titrate with 0.1 N perchloric acid VS, determining the endpoint potentiometrically. Perform a blank determination, and make any necessary correction. Each mL of 0.1 N perchloric acid is equivalent to 11.51 mg of $C_5H_9NO_2$.

Promazine Hydrochloride

$C_{17}H_{20}N_2S \cdot HCl$ 320.88
10*H*-Phenothiazine-10-propanamine,   *N,N*-dimethyl-, monohydrochloride.
10-3-(Dimethylamino)propylphenothiazine monohydrochloride [*53-60-1*].

» Promazine Hydrochloride, dried at 105° for 2 hours, contains not less than 98.0 percent and not more than 102.0 percent of $C_{17}H_{20}N_2S \cdot HCl$.

Packaging and storage—Preserve in tight, light-resistant containers.
USP Reference standards ⟨11⟩—*USP Promazine Hydrochloride RS.*
Completeness and clarity of solution—A solution of it (1 in 10) and a 1 in 10 solution of it in chloroform are practically clear and show not more than a light yellow color.
   NOTE—Throughout the following procedures, protect test or assay specimens, the Reference Standard, and solutions containing them, by conducting the procedures without delay, under subdued light, or using low-actinic glassware.
Identification—
   A: *Infrared Absorption* ⟨197K⟩.
   B: Determine the absorbance of the assay solution employed for measurement of absorbance in the *Assay* at 301 nm, using 0.1 N hydrochloric acid as the blank. Similarly determine the absorbance of a 1 in 10 dilution of this solution, prepared with the same acid, at the wavelength of maximum absorbance at about 252 nm: the ratio $10(A_{252}/A_{301})$ is between 7.1 and 7.9.
   C: It responds to the tests for *Chloride* ⟨191⟩.
Melting range, *Class I* ⟨741⟩:   between 172° and 182°, but the range between beginning and end of melting does not exceed 3°.
pH ⟨791⟩:   between 4.2 and 5.2, in a solution (1 in 20).
Loss on drying ⟨731⟩—Dry it at 105° for 2 hours: it loses not more than 0.5% of its weight.
Residue on ignition ⟨281⟩:   not more than 0.1%.
Selenium ⟨291⟩—The absorbance of the solution from the *Test Solution,* prepared with 100 mg of Promazine Hydrochloride and 200 mg of magnesium oxide, is not greater than one-half that from the *Standard Solution* (0.003%).
Heavy metals, *Method II* ⟨231⟩:   0.005%.
Chromatographic purity—[NOTE—Perform this test under conditions of subdued light and with no unnecessary delays between the preparation of the solutions and the development of the chromatographic plate.]
   Developing solvent—Mix 95 volumes of toluene with 15 volumes of alcohol and 1 volume of ammonium hydroxide.
   Standard preparations—Dissolve an accurately weighed quantity of USP Promazine Hydrochloride RS in methanol to obtain *Standard preparation A* having a known concentration of 0.4 mg per mL. Dilute quantitatively with methanol to obtain *Standard preparations* having the following compositions:

Standard preparation	Dilution	Concentration (µg RS per mL)	Percentage (%, for comparison with test specimens)
A	(undiluted)	400	2.0
B	(1 in 2)	200	1.0
C	(3 in 10)	120	0.6
D	(1 in 10)	40	0.2

   Test preparation—Dissolve an accurately weighed quantity of Promazine Hydrochloride in methanol to obtain a solution containing 20 mg per mL.
   Procedure—Apply separately 10 µL of the *Test preparation* and 10 µL of each *Standard preparation* to a suitable thin-layer chromatographic plate (see *Chromatography* ⟨621⟩) coated with a 0.25-mm layer of chromatographic silica gel mixture, and allow to dry. Position the plate in a chromatographic chamber and develop the chromatograms in the *Developing solvent* until the solvent front has moved about three-fourths of the length of the plate. Remove the plate from the developing chamber, mark the solvent front, and allow the solvent to evaporate by air drying for 15 minutes. Examine the plate under short-wavelength UV light. Compare the intensities of any secondary spots observed in the chromatogram of the *Test preparation* with those of the principal spots in the chromatograms of the *Standard preparations:* the sum of the intensities of secondary spots obtained from the *Test preparation* corresponds to not more than 2.0% of related compounds, with no single impurity corresponding to more than 1.0%.
Organic volatile impurities, *Method I* ⟨467⟩:   meets the requirements.

(Official until July 1, 2008)

Assay—[NOTE—Use low-actinic glassware.] Transfer about 50 mg of Promazine Hydrochloride, previously dried and accurately weighed, to a 1000-mL volumetric flask, add 0.1 N hydrochloric acid to volume, and mix. Without delay, concomitantly determine the absorbances of this solution and of a Standard solution of USP Promazine Hydrochloride RS in the same medium having a known concentration of about 50 µg per mL in 1-cm cells at the wavelength of maximum absorbance at about 301 nm, with a suitable spectrophotometer, using 0.1 N hydrochloric acid as the blank. Calculate the quantity, in mg, of $C_{17}H_{20}N_2S \cdot HCl$ in the portion of Promazine Hydrochloride taken by the formula:

$$C(A_U / A_S)$$

which C is the concentration, in µg per mL, of USP Promazine Hydrochloride RS in the Standard solution, and A_U and A_S are the absorbances of the solution of Promazine Hydrochloride and the Standard solution, respectively.

Promazine Hydrochloride Injection

» Promazine Hydrochloride Injection is a sterile solution of Promazine Hydrochloride in Water for Injection. It contains not less than 95.0 percent and not more than 110.0 percent of the labeled amount of $C_{17}H_{20}N_2S \cdot HCl$.

Packaging and storage—Preserve in single-dose or in multiple-dose containers, preferably of Type I glass, protected from light.

USP Reference standards ⟨11⟩—*USP Promazine Hydrochloride RS. USP Endotoxin RS.*
  NOTE—Throughout the following procedures, protect test or assay specimens, the Reference Standard, and solutions containing them, by conducting the procedures without delay, under subdued light, or using low-actinic glassware.
Identification—
  A: It meets the requirements under *Identification—Organic Nitrogenous Bases* ⟨181⟩.
  B: It responds to *Identification* test B under *Promazine Hydrochloride.*
Bacterial endotoxins ⟨85⟩—It contains not more than 1.8 USP Endotoxin Units per mg of promazine hydrochloride.
pH ⟨791⟩: between 4.0 and 5.5.
Other requirements—It meets the requirements under *Injections* ⟨1⟩.
Assay—[NOTE—Use low-actinic glassware.] Transfer a volume of Injection, equivalent to about 50 mg of promazine hydrochloride, to a 100-mL volumetric flask, dilute with 0.1 N hydrochloric acid to volume, and mix. Transfer 10.0 mL of the solution to a 250-mL separator, add 20 mL of water, render alkaline with ammonium hydroxide, and extract with four 25-mL portions of ether. Extract the combined ether extracts with five 15-mL portions of 0.1 N hydrochloric acid, collecting the aqueous extracts in a 100-mL volumetric flask. Aerate to remove residual ether, dilute with 0.1 N hydrochloric acid to volume, and mix. Without delay, concomitantly determine the absorbances of this solution and of a Standard solution of USP Promazine Hydrochloride RS in the same medium having a known concentration of about 50 µg per mL in 1-cm cells at the wavelength of maximum absorbance at about 301 nm, with a suitable spectrophotometer, using 0.1 N hydrochloric acid as the blank. Calculate the quantity, in mg, of $C_{17}H_{20}N_2S \cdot HCl$ in each mL of the Injection taken by the formula:

$$(C / V)(A_U / A_S)$$

in which C is the concentration, in µg per mL, of USP Promazine Hydrochloride RS in the Standard solution, V is the volume, in mL, of Injection taken, and A_U and A_S are the absorbances of the solution from the Injection and the Standard solution, respectively.

Promazine Hydrochloride Oral Solution

» Promazine Hydrochloride Oral Solution contains not less than 95.0 percent and not more than 110.0 percent of the labeled amount of $C_{17}H_{20}N_2S \cdot HCl$.

Packaging and storage—Preserve in tight, light-resistant containers.
USP Reference standards ⟨11⟩—*USP Promazine Hydrochloride RS.*
  NOTE—Throughout the following procedures, protect test or assay specimens, the Reference Standard, and solutions containing them, by conducting the procedures without delay, under subdued light, or using low-actinic glassware.
Identification—
  A: Dilute a volume of Oral Solution, equivalent to about 50 mg of promazine hydrochloride, with 0.01 N hydrochloric acid to 25 mL, and proceed as directed under *Identification—Organic Nitrogenous Bases* ⟨181⟩, beginning with "Transfer the liquid to a separator": the Oral Solution meets the requirements of the test.
  B: It responds to *Identification* test B under *Promazine Hydrochloride.*
pH ⟨791⟩: between 5.0 and 5.5.
Assay—[NOTE—Use low-actinic glassware.] Transfer an accurately measured volume of Oral Solution, or a quantitative dilution of it in water, equivalent to about 10 mg of promazine hydrochloride, to a 250-mL separator. Add water to adjust the volume to about 45 mL, add 3 mL of sodium hydroxide solution (1 in 10), mix, and extract the promazine with five 25-mL portions of ether. Wash the combined ether extracts with 25 mL of water, and discard the aqueous washings. Extract the combined ether extract with one 50-mL and four 25-mL portions of 0.1 N hydrochloric acid. Filter the acid extracts through a pledget of cotton washed with 0.1 N hydrochloric acid into a 250-mL volumetric flask, dilute with the same acid to volume, and mix. Without delay, concomitantly determine the absorbances of this solution and of a Standard solution of USP Promazine Hydrochloride RS in the same medium having a known concentration of about 40 µg per mL in 1-cm cells at the wavelength of maximum absorbance at about 301 nm, with a suitable spectrophotometer, using 0.1 N hydrochloric acid as the blank. Calculate the quantity, in mg, of $C_{17}H_{20}N_2S \cdot HCl$ in each mL of the Oral Solution taken by the formula:

$$(0.25C / V)(A_U / A_S)$$

in which C is the concentration, in µg per mL, of USP Promazine Hydrochloride RS in the Standard solution, V is the volume, in mL, of Oral Solution taken, and A_U and A_S are the absorbances from the assay solution and the Standard solution, respectively.

Promazine Hydrochloride Syrup

» Promazine Hydrochloride Syrup contains not less than 95.0 percent and not more than 110.0 percent of the labeled amount of $C_{17}H_{20}N_2S \cdot HCl$.

Packaging and storage—Preserve in tight, light-resistant containers.
USP Reference standards ⟨11⟩—*USP Promazine Hydrochloride RS.*
  NOTE—Throughout the following procedures, protect test or assay specimens, the Reference Standard, and solutions containing them, by conducting the procedures without delay, under subdued light, or using low-actinic glassware.
Identification—It responds to *Identification* test B under *Promazine Hydrochloride.*
Assay—[NOTE—Use low-actinic glassware.] Transfer a volume of Syrup, equivalent to about 10 mg of promazine hydrochloride, to a 250-mL separator. Proceed as directed in the *Assay* under *Promazine Hydrochloride Oral Solution*, beginning with "Add water to

adjust the volume to about 45 mL." Calculate the quantity, in mg, of $C_{17}H_{20}N_2S \cdot HCl$ in each mL of the Syrup taken by the formula:

$$(0.25C/V)(A_U/A_S)$$

in which C is the concentration, in µg per mL, of USP Promazine Hydrochloride RS in the Standard solution, V is the volume, in mL, of Syrup taken, and A_U and A_S are the absorbances of the solution from the Syrup and the Standard solution, respectively.

Promazine Hydrochloride Tablets

» Promazine Hydrochloride Tablets contain not less than 95.0 percent and not more than 110.0 percent of the labeled amount of $C_{17}H_{20}N_2S \cdot HCl$.

Packaging and storage—Preserve in tight, light-resistant containers.

USP Reference standards ⟨11⟩—*USP Promazine Hydrochloride RS.*
NOTE—Throughout the following procedures, protect test or assay specimens, the Reference Standard, and solutions containing them, by conducting the procedures without delay, under subdued light, or using low-actinic glassware.

Identification—
A: Shake a portion of powdered Tablets, equivalent to about 50 mg of promazine hydrochloride, with 25 mL of 0.01 N hydrochloric acid for 5 minutes, and filter: the solution meets the requirements under *Identification—Organic Nitrogenous Bases* ⟨181⟩.
B: It responds to *Identification* test *B* under *Promazine Hydrochloride*.

Disintegration ⟨701⟩: 30 minutes, with disks.
Uniformity of dosage units ⟨905⟩: meet the requirements.
Assay—[NOTE—Use low-actinic glassware.] Weigh and finely powder not less than 20 Tablets. Transfer an accurately weighed portion of the powder, equivalent to about 50 mg of promazine hydrochloride, to a 100-mL volumetric flask. Add 50 mL of 0.1 N hydrochloric acid, and shake by mechanical means for about 1 hour. Dilute with 0.1 N hydrochloric acid to volume, mix, and centrifuge a portion of the mixture. Transfer 10.0 mL of the clear, supernatant to a 250-mL separator, and proceed as directed in the *Assay* under *Promazine Hydrochloride Injection*, beginning with "add 20 mL of water." Calculate the quantity, in mg, of $C_{17}H_{20}N_2S \cdot HCl$ in the portion of Tablets taken by the formula:

$$C(A_U/A_S)$$

in which C is the concentration, in µg per mL, of USP Promazine Hydrochloride RS in the Standard solution, and A_U and A_S are the absorbances of the solution from the Tablets and the Standard solution, respectively.

Promethazine Hydrochloride

$C_{17}H_{20}N_2S \cdot HCl$ 320.88
10*H*-Phenothiazine-10-ethanamine, *N,N,*α-trimethyl-, monohydrochloride, (±)-.
(±)-10-[2-(Dimethylamino)propyl]phenothiazine monohydrochloride [58-33-3].

» Promethazine Hydrochloride contains not less than 97.0 percent and not more than 101.5 percent of $C_{17}H_{20}N_2S \cdot HCl$, calculated on the dried basis.

Packaging and storage—Preserve in tight, light-resistant containers.

USP Reference standards ⟨11⟩—*USP Promethazine Hydrochloride RS.*

Completeness and clarity of solution—Separately prepare a 1 in 10 solution of it in water and 1 in 10 solution of it in chloroform: each solution is practically clear and shows not more than a light yellow color.
NOTE—Throughout the following procedures, protect test or assay specimens, the Reference Standard, and solutions containing them, by conducting the procedures without delay, under subdued light, or using low-actinic glassware.

Identification—
A: *Infrared Absorption* ⟨197K⟩.
B: It responds to the tests for *Chloride* ⟨191⟩.

pH ⟨791⟩: between 4.0 and 5.0, in a solution (1 in 20).
Loss on drying ⟨731⟩—Dry it at 105° for 4 hours: it loses not more than 0.5% of its weight.
Residue on ignition ⟨281⟩: not more than 0.1%.
Related substances—
Standard preparation and *Standard dilutions*—Dissolve an accurately weighed quantity of USP Promethazine Hydrochloride RS in methylene chloride to obtain a solution containing 10.0 mg per mL (*Standard preparation*). Prepare a series of quantitative dilutions of the *Standard preparation* in methylene chloride to contain 0.2, 0.1, 0.05, and 0.025 mg per mL (*Standard dilutions*) corresponding to 2.0%, 1.0%, 0.5%, and 0.25% of impurities, respectively.
Test solution—Dissolve 100 mg, accurately weighed, of Promethazine Hydrochloride in 10.0 mL of methylene chloride.
Procedure—Using a 20- × 20-cm thin-layer chromatographic plate (see *Chromatography* ⟨621⟩) coated with a 0.25-mm layer of silica gel mixture, apply 10-µL portions of the *Test preparation*, the *Standard preparation*, and each of the *Standard dilutions* 2.5 cm from the lower edge of the plate. Develop the plate in an unsaturated tank containing a mixture of ethyl acetate, acetone, alcohol, and ammonium hydroxide (90 : 45 : 2 : 1). After the solvent has moved not less than 10 cm, air-dry the plate, and view under short-wavelength UV light: the R_F value of the principal spot obtained from the *Test preparation* corresponds to that from the *Standard preparation*. Estimate the concentration of any other spots observed in the lane for the *Test preparation* by comparison with the *Standard dilutions*: the sum of the impurities is not greater than 2.0%, and no single impurity is greater than 1.0%.
Assay—Dissolve about 700 mg of Promethazine Hydrochloride, accurately weighed, in a mixture of 75 mL of glacial acetic acid and 10 mL of mercuric acetate TS. Add 1 drop of crystal violet TS, and titrate with 0.1 N perchloric acid VS to a blue endpoint. Perform a blank determination, and make any necessary correction. Each mL of 0.1 N perchloric acid is equivalent to 32.09 mg of $C_{17}H_{20}N_2S \cdot HCl$.

Promethazine Hydrochloride Injection

» Promethazine Hydrochloride Injection is a sterile solution of Promethazine Hydrochloride in Water for Injection. It contains not less than 95.0 percent and not more than 110.0 percent of the labeled amount of $C_{17}H_{20}N_2S \cdot HCl$.

Packaging and storage—Preserve in single-dose or in multiple-dose containers, preferably of Type I glass, protected from light.

USP Reference standards ⟨11⟩—*USP Promethazine Hydrochloride RS. USP Endotoxin RS.*
NOTE—Throughout the following procedures, protect test or assay specimens, the Reference Standard, and solutions containing

them, by conducting the procedures without delay, under subdued light, or using low-actinic glassware.

Identification—Add a volume of Injection, equivalent to about 50 mg of promethazine hydrochloride, to 20 mL of dilute hydrochloric acid (1 in 1000) contained in a separator. Wash the solution with a 20-mL portion of methylene chloride, discarding the washing. Add 2 mL of 1 N sodium hydroxide and 20 mL of methylene chloride, and shake for 2 minutes. Evaporate the methylene chloride extract on a steam bath with the aid of a stream of nitrogen to dryness. Dissolve the residue in 4 mL of carbon disulfide, filter through paper, if necessary, and determine the IR absorption spectrum as directed under *Identification—Organic Nitrogenous Bases* ⟨181⟩, obtaining the spectrum of USP Promethazine Hydrochloride RS as directed: the Injection meets the requirements of the test.

Bacterial endotoxins ⟨85⟩—It contains not more than 5.0 USP Endotoxin Units per mg of promethazine hydrochloride.

pH ⟨791⟩: between 4.0 and 5.5.

Other requirements—It meets the requirements under *Injections* ⟨1⟩.

Assay—

Mobile phase—Dissolve 1 g of sodium 1-pentanesulfonate in 500 mL of water, add 500 mL of acetonitrile and 5 mL of glacial acetic acid, filter, and degas. Make adjustments if necessary (see *System Suitability* under *Chromatography* ⟨621⟩).

Standard preparation—Dissolve an accurately weighed quantity of USP Promethazine Hydrochloride RS in *Mobile phase*, and dilute quantitatively, and stepwise if necessary, with the same solvent to obtain a solution having a known concentration of about 0.1 mg per mL.

Assay preparation—Transfer an accurately measured volume of Injection, equivalent to about 50 mg of promethazine hydrochloride, to a 50-mL volumetric flask, dilute with *Mobile phase* to volume, and mix. Transfer 10.0 mL of the resulting solution to a 100-mL volumetric flask, dilute with *Mobile phase* to volume, and mix.

System suitability preparation—Dissolve a suitable quantity of phenothiazine in *Standard preparation* to obtain a solution containing about 10 µg of phenothiazine per mL.

Chromatographic system (see *Chromatography* ⟨621⟩)—The liquid chromatograph is equipped with a 254-nm detector and a 4.6-mm × 30-cm column that contains packing L11. The flow rate is about 1.5 mL per minute. Chromatograph the *System suitability preparation*, and record the peak responses as directed for *Procedure*: the resolution, R, between the promethazine and phenothiazine peaks is not less than 3.0, and the relative standard deviation for replicate injections is not more than 2.0%.

Procedure—Separately inject equal volumes (about 30 µL) of the *Standard preparation* and the *Assay preparation* into the chromatograph, record the chromatograms, and measure the responses for the major peaks. The relative retention times are 1.0 for promethazine and about 1.6 for phenothiazine. Calculate the quantity, in mg, of $C_{17}H_{20}N_2S \cdot HCl$ in each mL of the Injection taken by the formula:

$$500(C/V)(r_U/r_S)$$

in which C is the concentration, in mg per mL, of USP Promethazine Hydrochloride RS in the *Standard preparation*, V is the volume, in mL, of Injection taken, and r_U and r_S are the peak responses obtained from the *Assay preparation* and the *Standard preparation*, respectively.

Promethazine Hydrochloride Oral Solution

» Promethazine Hydrochloride Oral Solution contains not less than 90.0 percent and not more than 110.0 percent of the labeled amount of promethazine hydrochloride ($C_{17}H_{20}N_2S \cdot HCl$).

Packaging and storage—Preserve in tight, light-resistant containers.

USP Reference standards ⟨11⟩—*USP Promethazine Hydrochloride RS.*

NOTE—Throughout the following procedures, protect test or assay specimens, the Reference Standard, and solutions containing them, by conducting the procedures without delay, under subdued light, or using low-actinic glassware.

Identification—Treat 25 mL of Oral Solution as directed in the *Assay*, ending with "using a current of air only." Dissolve the residue in 2.5 mL of carbon disulfide, filter through paper if necessary, and determine the IR absorption spectrum as directed under *Identification—Organic Nitrogenous Bases* ⟨181⟩, obtaining the spectrum of USP Promethazine Hydrochloride RS as directed: the Oral Solution meets the requirements of the test.

Assay—[NOTE—Use low-actinic glassware in this assay.] Transfer an accurately measured volume of Oral Solution, equivalent to about 25 mg of promethazine hydrochloride, to a 250-mL separator. Add 10 mL of ammonium hydroxide, and extract the promethazine base with six 40-mL portions of chloroform. Wash the combined chloroform extracts with 25 mL of dilute hydrochloric acid (1 in 9). Wash the acid solution with 25 mL of chloroform, and add the washings to the main chloroform extract. Evaporate the chloroform extract on a steam bath, with the aid of a current of air, to a volume of 5 to 10 mL, and finally evaporate, using only a current of air, to dryness. Dissolve the residue, with slight warming, in dilute sulfuric acid (1 in 100), and transfer to a 500-mL volumetric flask with the aid of additional acid. Cool, add dilute sulfuric acid (1 in 100) to volume, mix, and filter, rejecting the first half of the filtrate. Dissolve an accurately weighed quantity of USP Promethazine Hydrochloride RS in dilute sulfuric acid (1 in 100), and dilute quantitatively and stepwise with the dilute acid to obtain a Standard solution having a known concentration of about 50 µg per mL. Concomitantly determine the absorbances of both solutions in 1-cm cells at the wavelength of maximum absorbance at about 298 nm, with a suitable spectrophotometer, using dilute sulfuric acid (1 in 100) as the blank. Calculate the quantity, in mg, of promethazine hydrochloride ($C_{17}H_{20}N_2S \cdot HCl$) in each mL of the Oral Solution taken by the formula:

$$500(C/V)(A_U/A_S)$$

in which C is the concentration, in mg per mL, of USP Promethazine Hydrochloride RS in the Standard solution; V is the volume, in mL, of Oral Solution taken; and A_U and A_S are the absorbances of the solution from the Oral Solution and the Standard solution, respectively.

Promethazine Hydrochloride Suppositories

» Promethazine Hydrochloride Suppositories contain not less than 95.0 percent and not more than 110.0 percent of the labeled amount of $C_{17}H_{20}N_2S \cdot HCl$.

Packaging and storage—Preserve in tight, light-resistant containers, and store in a cold place.

USP Reference standards ⟨11⟩—*USP Promethazine Hydrochloride RS.*

NOTE—Throughout the following procedures, protect test or assay specimens, the Reference Standard, and solutions containing them, by conducting the procedures without delay, under subdued light, or using low-actinic glassware.

Identification—Transfer a number of Suppositories, equivalent to about 50 mg of promethazine hydrochloride, to a 250-mL separator. Add 75 mL of solvent hexane and 25 mL of 0.01 N hydrochloric acid; shake to dissolve the solids. Using the aqueous phase, filtered through paper if necessary, proceed as directed under *Identification—Organic Nitrogenous Bases* ⟨181⟩, beginning with "Transfer the liquid to a separator."

Assay—

Palladium chloride solution—Add 5 mL of hydrochloric acid to a beaker containing 500 mg of palladium chloride. Warm on a steam bath to obtain a complete solution. Slowly add 200 mL of hot water. (If necessary, continue warming and add additional hydrochloric acid to maintain complete solution.) Transfer the solution to a 500-mL volumetric flask, and dilute with water to volume. To 50 mL of this solution add 250 mL of 2 M sodium acetate, and adjust with hydrochloric acid to a pH of 4.0. Transfer the solution to a 500-mL volumetric flask, dilute with water to volume, and mix.

Standard preparation—Using an accurately weighed quantity of USP Promethazine Hydrochloride RS, prepare a solution in 0.05 N hydrochloric acid containing about 0.1 mg in each mL. Protect the solution from light.

Assay preparation—Weigh 10 Suppositories and calculate the average. Carefully melt them, avoiding the use of excessive heat, and mix. Add 30 mL of hexanes to an accurately weighed portion, equivalent to about 50 mg of promethazine hydrochloride. Warm gently to dissolve, and transfer to a low-actinic separator. Rinse the transfer container with several small portions of the hexanes and 0.05 N hydrochloric acid, and add the rinsings to the separator. Extract with five 20-mL portions of 0.05 N hydrochloric acid shaking gently to avoid emulsions. Drain through glass wool prewashed with 0.05 N hydrochloric acid. Collect in a 500-mL low-actinic volumetric flask. Rinse the glass wool with additional 0.05 N hydrochloric acid, dilute the combined filtrate with 0.05 N hydrochloric acid to volume, and mix.

Procedure—Pipet 2.0 mL of the *Standard preparation*, *Assay preparation*, and 0.05 N hydrochloric acid into separate test tubes. Add 3.0 mL of *Palladium chloride solution* to each, and mix. Concomitantly determine the absorbances of the *Standard preparation* and the *Assay preparation* in 1-cm cells at the wavelength of maximum absorbance at about 450 nm, with a suitable spectrophotometer, using the hydrochloric acid-palladium chloride solution as the reagent blank in the reference cell. Calculate the quantity, in mg, of $C_{17}H_{20}N_2S \cdot HCl$ in the portion of Suppositories taken by the formula:

$$500C(A_U / A_S)$$

in which C is the concentration, in mg per mL, of USP Promethazine Hydrochloride RS in the *Standard preparation*, and A_U and A_S are the absorbances of the solutions from the *Assay preparation* and the *Standard preparation*, respectively.

Promethazine Hydrochloride Tablets

» Promethazine Hydrochloride Tablets contain not less than 95.0 percent and not more than 110.0 percent of the labeled amount of promethazine hydrochloride ($C_{17}H_{20}N_2S \cdot HCl$).

Packaging and storage—Preserve in tight, light-resistant containers.

USP Reference standards ⟨11⟩—*USP Promethazine Hydrochloride RS.*

NOTE—Throughout the following procedures, protect test or assay specimens, the Reference Standard, and solutions containing them, by conducting the procedures without delay, under subdued light, or using low-actinic glassware.

Identification—Shake a quantity of powdered Tablets, equivalent to about 50 mg of promethazine hydrochloride, with 30 mL of chloroform, and filter into a beaker. Evaporate the chloroform, dissolve the residue in 40 mL of dilute hydrochloric acid (1 in 1000), and transfer the liquid to a separator. In a second separator, dissolve 50 mg of USP Promethazine Hydrochloride RS in 40 mL of dilute hydrochloric acid (1 in 1000). Treat each solution as follows. Add 2 mL of 1 N sodium hydroxide and 15 mL of carbon disulfide, and shake for 2 minutes. Centrifuge if necessary to clarify the lower phase, and pass through a dry filter, collecting the filtrate in a small flask provided with a glass stopper. Reduce the volume of the carbon disulfide extracts to 4 to 5 mL, and proceed as directed under *Identification—Organic Nitrogenous Bases* ⟨181⟩, beginning with "Determine the absorption spectra."

Dissolution ⟨711⟩—
Medium: 0.01 N hydrochloric acid; 900 mL.
Apparatus 1: 100 rpm.
Time: 45 minutes.
Procedure—Determine the amount of $C_{17}H_{20}N_2S \cdot HCl$ dissolved by employing UV absorption at the wavelength of maximum absorbance at about 249 nm on filtered portions of the solution under test, suitably diluted with *Dissolution Medium*, in comparison with a Standard solution having a known concentration of USP Promethazine Hydrochloride RS in the same *Medium*.
Tolerances—Not less than 75% (*Q*) of the labeled amount of $C_{17}H_{20}N_2S \cdot HCl$ is dissolved in 45 minutes.

Uniformity of dosage units ⟨905⟩: meet the requirements.
Procedure for content uniformity—Transfer 1 finely powdered Tablet to a 100-mL volumetric flask, add 50 mL of citric acid solution (1 in 100), and shake by mechanical means for 15 minutes. Dilute with citric acid solution (1 in 100) to volume, and centrifuge about 50 mL of the mixture. Dilute an accurately measured portion of the clear solution, equivalent to 5 mg of promethazine hydrochloride, quantitatively with citric acid solution (1 in 100) to 100 mL. Concomitantly determine the absorbance of this solution and a Standard solution of USP Promethazine Hydrochloride RS in the same medium, having a known concentration of about 50 µg per mL, in 1-cm cells at the wavelength of maximum absorbance at about 298 nm, with a suitable spectrophotometer, using citric acid solution (1 in 100) as the blank. Calculate the quantity, in mg, of $C_{17}H_{20}N_2S \cdot HCl$ in the Tablet by the formula:

$$(TC / D)(A_U / A_S)$$

in which T is the labeled quantity, in mg, of promethazine hydrochloride in the Tablet; D is the concentration, in µg per mL, of promethazine hydrochloride in the test solution based on the labeled quantity per Tablet and the extent of dilution; C is the concentration, in µg per mL, of USP Promethazine Hydrochloride RS in the Standard solution; and A_U and A_S are the absorbances of the solution from the Tablet and the Standard solution, respectively.

Assay—
Buffered palladium chloride solution—Transfer 500 mg of palladium chloride to a 250-mL beaker, add 5 mL of hydrochloric acid, and warm on a steam bath. Add 200 mL of hot water in small quantities while stirring until solution is complete. Cool, dilute with water to 500 mL, and mix. Transfer 25 mL of this solution to a 500-mL volumetric flask. Add 50 mL of 1 N sodium acetate and 48 mL of 1 N hydrochloric acid, dilute with water to volume, and mix.

Standard preparation—Transfer about 31 mg of USP Promethazine Hydrochloride RS, accurately weighed, to a low-actinic 250-mL volumetric flask. Dissolve in 0.1 N hydrochloric acid, dilute with 0.1 N hydrochloric acid to volume, and mix.

Assay preparation—Weigh and finely powder not fewer than 20 Tablets. Transfer an accurately weighed portion of the powder, equivalent to about 6.25 mg of promethazine hydrochloride, to a low-actinic 125-mL separator. Add 20 mL of saturated potassium chloride solution, 10 mL of 1 N sodium hydroxide, and 10 mL of methanol, and extract the promethazine with three 20-mL portions of *n*-heptane. Filter the heptane extracts through anhydrous sodium sulfate and collect them in a low-actinic 125-mL separator. Extract the promethazine from the *n*-heptane solution with three 15-mL portions of 0.1 N hydrochloric acid, collect the acid extracts in a low-actinic 50-mL volumetric flask, dilute with 0.1 N hydrochloric acid to volume, and mix.

Procedure—Into separate test tubes, pipet 2-mL portions of the *Standard preparation*, the *Assay preparation*, and 0.1 N hydrochloric acid to provide a blank. Add 3.0 mL of *Buffered palladium chloride solution* to each tube, and mix. Concomitantly determine the absorbances of the solutions at the wavelength of maximum absorbance at about 470 nm, using a suitable spectrophotometer, and using the blank in the reference cell. Calculate the quantity, in mg, of promethazine hydrochloride ($C_{17}H_{20}N_2S \cdot HCl$) in the portion of Tablets taken by the formula:

$$50C(A_U / A_S)$$

in which C is the concentration, in mg per mL, of USP Promethazine Hydrochloride RS in the *Standard preparation*; and A_U and A_S

3098 Promethazine / *Official Monographs*

are the absorbances of the solutions from the *Assay preparation* and the *Standard preparation*, respectively.

Propafenone Hydrochloride

$C_{21}H_{27}NO_3 \cdot HCl$ 377.90
1-Propanone, 1-[2-[2-hydroxy-3-(propylamino)propoxy]phenyl]-3-phenyl-, hydrochloride.
2′-[2-Hydroxy-3-(propylamino)propoxy]-3-phenylpropiophenone hydrochloride   [34183-22-7].

» Propafenone Hydrochloride contains not less than 98.0 percent and not more than 102.0 percent of $C_{21}H_{27}NO_3 \cdot HCl$, calculated on the dried basis.

Packaging and storage—Preserve in tight, light-resistant containers, and store at a temperature between 15° and 30°.
USP Reference standards ⟨11⟩—*USP Propafenone Hydrochloride RS*.
Clarity of solution—Dissolve 1.0 g in 30 mL of hot water, and observe without delay: the solution initially is clear.
Identification—
  A: *Infrared Absorption* ⟨197K⟩.
  B: Dissolve 0.5 g of propafenone hydrochloride in 50 mL of water with heating. Adjust with 0.1 N sodium hydroxide to a pH of 9.5 to 10.0: a precipitate is formed. Cool the mixture, and filter. Add 1 mL of 6 N nitric acid and 2 to 3 drops of 0.1 N silver nitrate to the filtrate: a precipitate is formed, which dissolves upon the addition of a few drops of ammonium hydroxide.
Melting range ⟨741⟩:   between 171° and 175°.
pH ⟨791⟩:   between 5.0 and 6.2 in a solution (1 in 200).
Loss on drying ⟨731⟩—Dry it at 105° to constant weight; it loses not more than 0.5% of its weight.
Residue on ignition ⟨281⟩:   not more than 0.1%.
Heavy metals, *Method II* ⟨231⟩:   20 ppm.
Limit of methanol and acetone—
  Standard solution—Prepare a solution, in dimethyl sulfoxide, containing 2.0 μg of methanol and 20.0 μg of acetone.
  Test solution—Dissolve an accurately weighed portion of the material to be tested in dimethyl sulfoxide to obtain a final solution having a known concentration of about 20 mg of the test material per mL.
  Chromatographic system (see *Chromatography* ⟨621⟩)—The gas chromatograph is equipped with a flame-ionization detector, a 0.53-mm × 30-m fused silica analytical column coated with a 3.0-μm G43 stationary phase, and a 0.53-mm × 5-m silica guard column deactivated with phenylmethyl siloxane. The carrier gas is helium with a linear velocity of about 35 cm per second. The injection port and detector temperatures are maintained at 140° and 260°, respectively. The column temperature is programmed according to the following steps. It is maintained at 40° for 20 minutes, then increased rapidly to 240°, and maintained at 240° for 20 minutes. Inject the *Standard solution*, and record the peak responses as directed for *Procedure*: the relative standard deviation of the individual peak responses from replicate injections is not more than 15%.
  Procedure—Separately inject equal volumes (about 1 μL) of the *Standard solution* and the *Test solution* into the chromatograph, record the chromatograms, and measure the peak responses. Identify, based on retention time, any peaks present in the chromatogram of the *Test solution*, and calculate the amounts of methanol and acetone present. Not more than 100 ppm of methanol and 1000 ppm of acetone are found.
Chromatographic purity—
  Mobile phase—Prepare a filtered and degassed mixture of 2.5 mM tetrabutylammonium hydrogen sulfate and acetonitrile (16 : 9).

Make adjustments if necessary (see *System Suitability* under *Chromatography* ⟨621⟩).
  Diluent—Prepare a mixture of acetonitrile and water (9 : 1).
  Standard solution—Dissolve an accurately weighed quantity of USP Propafenone Hydrochloride RS in *Diluent*, and dilute quantitatively, and stepwise if necessary, with *Diluent* to obtain a solution having a known concentration of about 5 μg per mL.
  Test solution—Transfer about 50 mg of Propafenone Hydrochloride, accurately weighed, to a 50-mL volumetric flask, dissolve in 5 mL of *Diluent*, dilute with *Mobile phase* to volume, and mix.
  Chromatographic system (see *Chromatography* ⟨621⟩)—The liquid chromatograph is equipped with a 222-nm detector and a 3.9-mm × 15-cm column that contains packing L10. The flow rate is about 1.0 mL per minute. Chromatograph the *Standard solution*, and record the peak responses as directed for *Procedure*: the column efficiency is not less than 2000 theoretical plates; and the relative standard deviation for replicate injections is not more than 15%.
  Procedure—Separately inject a volume (about 10 μL) of the *Standard solution* and the *Test solution* into the chromatograph, and allow the *Test solution* to elute for not less than eight times the retention time of propafenone. Record the chromatogram, and measure the peak responses for all the peaks: the sum of the peak responses, other than that of propafenone, in the chromatogram of the *Test solution* is not more than two times the propafenone response obtained from the *Standard solution* (1.0%); and no other peak response, other than that of propafenone, in the chromatogram of the *Test solution* is greater than the propafenone response obtained from the *Standard solution* (0.5%).
Assay—Transfer about 250 mg of Propafenone Hydrochloride, accurately weighed, to a 125-mL flask. Dissolve in 30 mL of methanol, add 15 mL of mercuric acetate TS, and titrate with 0.1 N perchloric acid VS, determining the endpoint potentiometrically. Perform a blank determination, and make any necessary correction. Each mL of 0.1 N perchloric acid is equivalent to 37.79 mg of $C_{21}H_{27}NO_3 \cdot HCl$.

Propantheline Bromide

$C_{23}H_{30}BrNO_3$ 448.39
2-Propanaminium, *N*-methyl-*N*-(1-methylethyl)-*N*-[2-[(9*H*-xanthen-9-ylcarbonyl)oxy]ethyl]-, bromide.
(2-Hydroxyethyl)diisopropylmethylammonium bromide xanthene-9-carboxylate   [50-34-0].

» Propantheline Bromide contains not less than 98.0 percent and not more than 102.0 percent of $C_{23}H_{30}BrNO_3$, calculated on the dried basis.

Packaging and storage—Preserve in well-closed containers.
USP Reference standards ⟨11⟩—*USP Xanthanoic Acid RS. USP Xanthone RS. USP Propantheline Bromide RS. USP Propantheline Bromide Related Compound A RS*.
Identification—
  A: Prepare 3 mL of a solution in chloroform having a concentration of about 6 mg per mL, and reserve a 1-mL portion for *Identification test B*. In a well-ventilated hood, apply 2 mL of this solution dropwise to a salt plate while continuously evaporating the solvent with the aid of an IR heat lamp and a current of dry air. Heat the residue at 105° for 15 minutes: the IR absorption spectrum of the residue on the single salt plate exhibits maxima only at the same wavelengths as that of a similar preparation of USP Propantheline Bromide RS, treated in the same manner.
  B: Apply 5 μL of the chloroform solution retained from *Identification test A* and 5 μL of a Standard solution of USP Propantheline Bromide RS in chloroform containing 6 mg per mL to a suit-

able thin-layer chromatographic plate (see *Chromatography* ⟨621⟩) coated with a 0.25-mm layer of chromatographic silica gel. Develop the chromatogram in a solvent system consisting of a mixture of 1 N hydrochloric acid and acetone (1 : 1) until the solvent front has moved about three-fourths of the length of the plate. Remove the plate from the developing chamber, mark the solvent front, and dry at 105° for 5 minutes. Spray the plate with potassium-bismuth iodide TS, and heat at 105° for 5 minutes: the R_F value of the principal spot obtained from the test solution corresponds to that obtained from the Standard solution.

C: To 5 mL of a solution (1 in 100) add 2 mL of 2 N nitric acid: this solution responds to the tests for *Bromide* ⟨191⟩, except that in the test that liberates bromine, the chloroform layer may be yellow.

Loss on drying ⟨731⟩—Dry it at 105° for 4 hours: it loses not more than 0.5% of its weight.

Residue on ignition ⟨281⟩: not more than 0.1%.

Related compounds—

pH 3.5 buffer solution—Dissolve 17.3 g of sodium dodecyl sulfate in 1000 mL of water containing 10 mL of phosphoric acid in a 2000-mL volumetric flask. Add 250 mL of 0.5 M sodium hydroxide and, while stirring, adjust with 0.5 M sodium hydroxide or dilute phosphoric acid (1 in 10) to a pH of 3.5 ± 0.05, dilute with water to volume, and mix.

Mobile phase—Prepare a filtered and degassed mixture of acetonitrile and *pH 3.5 buffer solution* (55 : 45). Make adjustments if necessary (see *System Suitability* under *Chromatography* ⟨621⟩).

Standard solution—Dissolve accurately weighed quantities of USP Propantheline Bromide Related Compound A RS, USP Xanthanoic Acid RS, and USP Xanthone RS in *Mobile phase*, and dilute quantitatively, and stepwise if necessary, with *Mobile phase* to obtain a solution having a known concentration of about 6.0 µg of propantheline bromide related compound A per mL, and about 1.5 µg each of xanthanoic acid and xanthone per mL.

Test solution—Transfer about 60 mg of Propantheline Bromide, accurately weighed, to a 200-mL volumetric flask, dissolve in *Mobile phase*, dilute with *Mobile phase* to volume, and mix.

Chromatographic system (see *Chromatography* ⟨621⟩)—The liquid chromatograph is equipped with a 254-nm detector and a 4.6-mm × 25-cm column that contains packing L7. The flow rate is about 2.0 mL per minute. Chromatograph the *Standard solution*, and record peak responses as directed for *Procedure*: the resolution, *R*, between the least resolved peaks is not less than 1.2; and the relative standard deviation for replicate injections of the *Standard solution* is not more than 6.0% for each component.

Procedure—Separately inject equal volumes (about 50 µL) of the *Standard solution* and the *Test solution* into the chromatograph, record the chromatograms for a total time of not less than 1.5 times the retention time of the propantheline bromide peak, and measure the response for each peak, except the peaks at or before the void volume. Calculate the percentage of xanthanoic acid, xanthone, and propantheline bromide related compound A greater than or equal to 0.1% in the portion of Propantheline Bromide taken by the formula:

$$20C/W(r_U / r_S)$$

in which *C* is the concentration, in µg, of xanthanoic acid, xanthone, or propantheline bromide related compound A per mL of the *Standard solution*; *W* is the weight, in mg, of Propantheline Bromide taken; and r_U and r_S are the related compound peak responses obtained from the *Test solution* and the *Standard solution*, respectively: not more than 2.0% of propantheline bromide related compound A and 0.5% each of xanthone and xanthanoic acid is found. Calculate the percentage of all unknown impurities greater than or equal to 0.1% by the formula:

$$100r_i / r_t$$

in which r_i is the response of the unknown impurity peak; and r_t is the sum of the responses of all the measured peaks observed in the chromatogram: the sum total of all known and unknown impurities is not more than 3.0%.

Organic volatile impurities, *Method I* ⟨467⟩: meets the requirements.

(Official until July 1, 2008)

Bromide content—Weigh accurately about 500 mg, and dissolve in 40 mL of water. Add 10 mL of glacial acetic acid and 40 mL of methanol, then add eosin Y TS, and titrate with 0.1 N silver nitrate VS. Each mL of 0.1 N silver nitrate is equivalent to 7.990 mg of Br. Not less than 17.5% and not more than 18.2% of Br, calculated on the dried basis, is found.

Assay—Dissolve about 600 mg of Propantheline Bromide, accurately weighed, in a mixture of 20 mL of glacial acetic acid and 15 mL of mercuric acetate TS, warming slightly if necessary to effect solution. Cool to room temperature, and titrate with 0.1 N perchloric acid VS, determining the endpoint potentiometrically. Perform a blank determination, and make any necessary correction. Each mL of 0.1 N perchloric acid is equivalent to 44.84 mg of $C_{23}H_{30}BrNO_3$.

Propantheline Bromide Tablets

» Propantheline Bromide Tablets contain not less than 90.0 percent and not more than 110.0 percent of the labeled amount of $C_{23}H_{30}BrNO_3$.

Packaging and storage—Preserve in well-closed containers.

USP Reference standards ⟨11⟩—*USP Xanthanoic Acid RS. USP Xanthone RS. USP Propantheline Bromide RS. USP Propantheline Bromide Related Compound A RS.*

Identification—

A: Finely powder a number of Tablets, equivalent to about 90 mg of propantheline bromide, and triturate the powder with 10 mL of chloroform. Filter, and wash the filter with 10 mL of chloroform, collecting the filtrate and washing in a separator. Add 10 mL of water, shake, and discard the chloroform layer. Wash the aqueous layer with two 10-mL portions of ether, and discard the ether washings. Filter the aqueous solution, and evaporate on a steam bath with the aid of a current of dry air to dryness. Dissolve the residue in 5 mL of chloroform, mix, and proceed as directed in *Identification* test A under *Propantheline Bromide*, beginning with "In a well-ventilated hood": the specified result is observed.

B: The chromatogram of the *Assay preparation* obtained as directed in the *Assay* exhibits a major peak for propantheline bromide, the retention time of which corresponds to that exhibited in the chromatogram of the *Standard preparation*.

Dissolution, *Procedure for a Pooled Sample* ⟨711⟩—

Medium: pH 4.5 (±0.05) Acetate buffer prepared by mixing 1.64 g of anhydrous sodium acetate and 1.25 mL of glacial acetic acid with 500 mL of water, and diluting with water to obtain 1000 mL of solution having a pH of 4.50 ± 0.05; 500 mL.

Apparatus 2: 50 rpm.

Time: 45 minutes.

Determine the amount of propantheline bromide dissolved using the following method.

pH 3.5 buffer solution, Mobile phase, and *Chromatographic system*—Prepare as directed under *Assay*.

Procedure—Inject a volume (about 50 µL) of a filtered portion of the solution under test into the chromatograph, record the chromatogram, and measure the response for the major peak. Calculate the quantity of $C_{23}H_{30}BrNO_3$ dissolved in comparison with a Standard solution having a known concentration of USP Propantheline Bromide RS in the same medium and similarly chromatographed.

Tolerances—Not less than 75% (*Q*) of the labeled amount of $C_{23}H_{30}BrNO_3$ is dissolved in 45 minutes.

Uniformity of dosage units ⟨905⟩: meet the requirements.

Related compounds—

pH 3.5 buffer solution and *Mobile phase*—Prepare as directed for *Related compounds* under *Propantheline Bromide*.

Standard solution—Dissolve accurately weighed quantities of USP Propantheline Bromide Related Compound A RS, USP Xanthanoic Acid RS, and USP Xanthone RS in *Mobile phase*, and dilute quantitatively and stepwise if necessary, with *Mobile phase* to obtain a solution having known concentrations of about 12.0 µg of propantheline bromide related compound A per mL, and about 3.0 µg each of xanthanoic acid and xanthone per mL.

Test solution—Use the *Assay preparation* prepared as directed under *Assay*.

Chromatographic system (see *Chromatography* ⟨621⟩)—The liquid chromatograph is equipped with a 254-nm detector and a 4.6-mm × 25-cm column that contains packing L7. The flow rate is about 2.0 mL per minute. Chromatograph the *Standard solution*, and record the peak responses as directed for *Procedure:* the resolution, R, between the least resolved peaks is not less than 1.2; and the relative standard deviation for replicate injections of the *Standard solution* is not more than 6.0% for each component or, if the *Assay* is performed concomitantly, the relative standard deviation for the propantheline bromide peak in the replicate injections of the *Standard solution* is not more than 2.0%.

Procedure—Separately inject equal volumes (about 50 μL) of the *Standard solution* and the *Test solution* into the chromatograph, record the chromatograms, and measure the responses for the major peaks. Calculate the percentage of xanthanoic acid, xanthone, and propantheline bromide related compound A greater than or equal to 0.1% in the portion of Tablets taken by the formula:

$$100C/C_X(r_U/r_S)$$

in which C is the concentration, in μg, of xanthanoic acid, xanthone, or propantheline bromide related compound A per mL of the *Standard solution*; C_X is the theoretical concentration, in μg per mL, of Propantheline Bromide in the *Test solution*; and r_U and r_S are the related compound peak responses obtained from the *Test solution* and the *Standard solution*, respectively: not more than 4.0% of propantheline bromide related compound A and 1.0% each of xanthone and xanthanoic acid are found.

Assay—

pH 3.5 buffer solution and *Mobile phase*—Prepare as directed for *Related compounds* under *Propantheline Bromide*.

Standard preparation—Dissolve an accurately weighed quantity of USP Propantheline Bromide RS in *Mobile phase* to obtain a solution having a known concentration of about 0.3 mg per mL.

Assay preparation—Weigh and finely powder not less than 20 Tablets. Transfer an accurately weighed portion of the powder, equivalent to 15 mg of propantheline bromide, to a 50-mL volumetric flask, dissolve in *Mobile phase*, dilute with *Mobile phase* to volume, mix, and filter.

Chromatographic system (see *Chromatography* ⟨621⟩)—The liquid chromatograph is equipped with a 254-nm detector and a 4.6-mm × 25-cm column that contains packing L7. The flow rate is about 2.0 mL per minute. Chromatograph the *Standard preparation*, and record peak responses as directed for *Procedure:* the relative standard deviation for replicate injections is not more than 2.0%.

Procedure—Separately inject equal volumes (about 50 μL) of the *Standard preparation* and the *Assay preparation* into the chromatograph, record the chromatograms, and measure the peak responses. Calculate the quantity, in mg, of $C_{23}H_{30}BrNO_3$ in the portion of Tablets taken by the formula:

$$50C(r_U/r_S)$$

in which C is the concentration, in mg per mL, of USP Propantheline Bromide RS in the *Standard preparation*; and r_U and r_S are the peak responses due to Propantheline Bromide obtained from the *Assay preparation* and the *Standard preparation*, respectively.

Proparacaine Hydrochloride

$C_{16}H_{26}N_2O_3 \cdot HCl$ 330.85

Benzoic acid, 3-amino-4-propoxy-, 2-(diethylamino)ethyl ester, monohydrochloride.

2-(Diethylamino)ethyl 3-amino-4-propoxybenzoate monohydrochloride   [5875-06-9].

» Proparacaine Hydrochloride contains not less than 97.0 percent and not more than 103.0 percent of $C_{16}H_{26}N_2O_3 \cdot HCl$, calculated on the dried basis.

Packaging and storage—Preserve in well-closed containers.

USP Reference standard ⟨11⟩—*USP Proparacaine Hydrochloride RS*.

Identification—

A: It meets the requirements under *Identification—Organic Nitrogenous Bases* ⟨181⟩.

B: Dissolve 50 mg, accurately weighed, in water to make 250.0 mL, and mix. Pipet 10 mL of this solution into a 100-mL volumetric flask, add 2 mL of 10 percent, pH 6.0 phosphate buffer (see *Buffer Solutions* in the section *Reagents, Indicators, and Solutions*), add water to volume, and mix: the UV absorption spectrum of the solution exhibits maxima and minima at the same wavelengths as that of a similar solution of USP Proparacaine Hydrochloride RS, concomitantly measured, and the respective absorptivities, calculated on the dried basis, at the wavelength of maximum absorbance at about 310 nm do not differ by more than 3.0%.

C: A solution (1 in 50) responds to the tests for *Chloride* ⟨191⟩, the procedure for alkaloidal hydrochlorides being used.

Melting range ⟨741⟩: between 178° and 185°, but the range between beginning and end of melting does not exceed 2°.

Loss on drying ⟨731⟩—Dry it at 105° for 3 hours: it loses not more than 0.5% of its weight.

Residue on ignition ⟨281⟩: not more than 0.15%.

Ordinary impurities ⟨466⟩—

Test solution: methanol.

Standard solution: methanol.

Eluant: a mixture of butyl alcohol, water, and glacial acetic acid (5 : 3 : 1).

Visualization: 1; 17.

Assay—Place 250 mg of Proparacaine Hydrochloride, accurately weighed, in a 250-mL conical flask, add 80 mL of a 1 in 20 solution of acetic anhydride in glacial acetic acid, and heat on a steam bath for 10 minutes. Cool to room temperature, add 10 mL of mercuric acetate TS and 1 or 2 drops of crystal violet TS, and titrate with 0.1 N perchloric acid VS to a blue-green endpoint. Perform a blank determination, and make any necessary correction. Each mL of 0.1 N perchloric acid is equivalent to 33.09 mg of $C_{16}H_{26}N_2O_3 \cdot HCl$.

Proparacaine Hydrochloride Ophthalmic Solution

» Proparacaine Hydrochloride Ophthalmic Solution is a sterile, aqueous solution of Proparacaine Hydrochloride. It contains not less than 95.0 percent and not more than 110.0 percent of the labeled amount of $C_{16}H_{26}N_2O_3 \cdot HCl$.

Packaging and storage—Preserve in tight, light-resistant containers.

Labeling—Label it to indicate that it is to be stored in a refrigerator after the container is opened.

USP Reference standards ⟨11⟩—*USP Proparacaine Hydrochloride RS*.

Identification—To 1 mL of Ophthalmic Solution in a test tube add 5 mL of dilute hydrochloric acid (1 in 100), mix, and cool in an ice bath for 2 minutes. Add 2 drops of sodium nitrite solution (1 in 10), stir, and cool again for 2 minutes. Add 1 mL of a solution prepared by dissolving 200 mg of 2-naphthol in 10 mL of 1 N sodium hydroxide: a scarlet-red precipitate is formed. Add 5 mL of acetone: the precipitate does not dissolve.

Sterility ⟨71⟩: meets the requirements.

pH ⟨791⟩: between 3.5 and 6.0.

Assay—

pH 7.5 buffer—Dissolve 6.8 g of monobasic potassium phosphate in 1000 mL of water, add 5 mL of triethylamine, and adjust with 5

N potassium hydroxide to a pH of 7.5. Filter through a filter having a porosity of 0.5 µm or finer, and degas.

Mobile phase—Prepare a mixture of *pH 7.5 buffer* and acetonitrile (60 : 40). Make adjustments if necessary (see *System Suitability* under *Chromatography* ⟨621⟩).

Standard preparation—Transfer about 25 mg of USP Proparacaine Hydrochloride RS, accurately weighed, to a 25-mL volumetric flask, dissolve in and dilute with water to volume, and mix. Transfer 5.0 mL of this stock solution to a 50-mL volumetric flask, dilute with *Mobile phase* to volume, and mix. [NOTE—Use this solution within 6 hours.]

Assay preparation—Transfer an accurately measured volume of Ophthalmic Solution, equivalent to about 10 mg of proparacaine hydrochloride, to a 100-mL volumetric flask, dilute with *Mobile phase* to volume, and mix. [NOTE—Use this solution within 6 hours.]

Chromatographic system (see *Chromatography* ⟨621⟩)—The liquid chromatograph is equipped with a 270-nm detector and a 4.6-mm × 15-cm column that contains 5-µm spherical packing L10. The flow rate is about 1.5 mL per minute. Chromatograph the *Standard preparation*, and record the peak responses as directed for *Procedure*: the tailing factor is not more than 1.5, the column efficiency is not less than 3000 theoretical plates, and the relative standard deviation for replicate injections is not more than 2.0%.

Procedure—[NOTE—Use peak areas where peak responses are indicated.] Separately inject equal volumes (about 10 µL) of the *Standard preparation* and the *Assay preparation* into the chromatograph, record the chromatograms, and measure the responses for the major peaks. Calculate the quantity, in mg, of $C_{16}H_{26}N_2O_3 \cdot HCl$ in each mL of the Ophthalmic Solution taken by the formula:

$$100(C / V)(r_U / r_S)$$

in which C is the concentration, in mg per mL, of USP Proparacaine Hydrochloride RS in the *Standard preparation*, V is the volume, in mL, of Ophthalmic Solution taken, and r_U and r_S are the proparacaine peak responses obtained from the *Assay preparation* and the *Standard preparation*, respectively.

Propofol

$C_{12}H_{18}O$ 178.27
Phenol, 2,6-bis(1-methylethyl).
2,6-Diisopropylphenol   [2078-54-8].

» Propofol contains not less than 98.0 percent and not more than 102.0 percent of $C_{12}H_{18}O$.

Packaging and storage—Preserve in tight containers under an atmosphere of inert gas, and protect from light. Store at room temperature.

Labeling—The labeling indicates the *Related compounds* test with which the article complies if a test other than *Test 1* is used.

USP Reference standards ⟨11⟩—*USP Propofol RS. USP Propofol Related Compound A RS. USP Propofol Related Compound B RS. USP Propofol Related Compound C RS. USP Propofol Resolution Mixture RS.*

Identification, *Infrared Absorption* ⟨197F⟩.

Refractive index ⟨831⟩:   between 1.5125 and 1.5145 at 20°.

Related compounds—[NOTE—On the basis of knowledge of the manufacturing process, either (1) *Related compounds Test 1* is performed in conjunction with the *Limit of propofol related compound A*, *Limit of propofol related compound B Test 1*, and *Assay Test 1* procedures; or (2) *Related compounds Test 2* is performed in conjunction with the *Limit of propofol related compound B Test 2* and the *Assay Test 2* procedures.]

TEST 1—

Resolution solution—Dissolve an accurately weighed quantity of USP Propofol Resolution Mixture RS in methanol, and dilute quantitatively, and stepwise if necessary, with methanol to obtain a solution having a concentration of about 100 mg per mL.

Standard solution—Dissolve an accurately weighed quantity of USP Propofol RS in methanol, and dilute quantitatively, and stepwise if necessary, with methanol to obtain a solution having a concentration of about 0.1 mg per mL.

Test solution—Transfer about 1000 mg of Propofol, accurately weighed, to a 10-mL volumetric flask, dissolve in and dilute with methanol to volume, and mix.

Chromatographic system (see *Chromatography* ⟨621⟩)—Proceed as directed under *Assay Test 1*, except to chromatograph the *Standard solution* six times and chromatograph the *Resolution solution*: the relative retention time is about 0.18 for 2,6-diisopropylphenyl-isopropyl ether, 1.0 for propofol, and about 1.1 for 2-isopropyl-6-*n*-propylphenol; the resolution, *R*, between propofol and 2-isopropyl-6-*n*-propylphenol is not less than 2. Chromatograph the *Standard solution* six times, and record the peak responses as directed for *Procedure*: the column efficiency determined from the propofol peak is not less than 5000 theoretical plates; and the relative standard deviation for replicate injections is not more than 3.5%.

Procedure—Separately inject equal volumes (about 1.0 µL) of the *Resolution solution,* the *Standard solution,* and the *Test solution* into the chromatograph, record the chromatograms, and measure all the peak responses. Calculate the percentage of each impurity in the portion of Propofol taken by the formula:

$$0.1(r_i / r_S)$$

in which r_i is the peak response for each impurity obtained from the *Test solution;* and r_S is the peak response for propofol obtained from the *Standard solution:* not more than 0.1% of 2,6-diisopropylphenyl-isopropyl ether is found; not more than 0.1% of each other individual impurity is found; and not more than 0.3% of total impurities is found.

TEST 2—

Mobile phase—Prepare as directed in *Assay Test 2*.

System suitability solution 1—Transfer 5 µL of USP Propofol RS and 15 µL of USP Propofol Related Compound B RS to a 50-mL volumetric flask, dissolve in and dilute with hexane to volume, and mix.

System suitability solution 2—Dissolve an accurately weighed quantity of USP Propofol Related Compound A RS and accurate volumes of the propofol that is under test and USP Propofol Related Compound C RS in hexane, and dilute quantitatively, and stepwise if necessary, with hexane to obtain a solution having known concentrations of 0.25 mg of propofol related compound A per mL, 100 µL of propofol per mL, and 5 µL of propofol related compound C per mL.

Test solution—Transfer about 1000 mg of Propofol, accurately weighed, to a 10-mL volumetric flask, dissolve in and dilute with hexane to volume, and mix.

Reference solution—Dilute 1 mL of the *Test solution* with hexane to 100 mL, and mix. Dilute 1 mL of this solution with hexane to 10 mL, and mix.

Chromatographic system (see *Chromatography* ⟨621⟩)—Proceed as directed in *Assay Test 2*. Chromatograph *System suitability solution 1* and *System suitability solution 2*, and record the peak responses as directed for *Procedure:* the relative retention times are about 0.8 for propofol related compound B from *System suitability solution 1*, 0.5 for 2,6-diisopropylphenylisopropyl ether, 1.0 for propofol, and 5.0 for propofol related compound A from *System suitability solution 2;* and the resolution, *R*, between propofol related compound B and propofol is at least 4.0.

Procedure—Separately inject a volume (about 10 µL) of the *Test solution* and the *Reference solution* into the chromatograph, record the chromatogram, and measure all peak responses. Calculate the percentage of each impurity in the portion of Propofol taken by the formula:

$$0.1(r_i / r_S)(1/F)$$

in which r_i is the peak response for each impurity obtained from the *Test solution;* r_S is the peak response for propofol obtained from the

Reference solution; and *F* is the response factor. *F* is 0.2 for 2,6-diisopropylphenylisopropyl ether and 4.0 for propofol related compound A: not more than 0.2% of 2,6-diisopropylphenylisopropyl ether is found; not more than 0.01% of propofol related compound A is found; not more than 0.05% of each of the other individual impurities is found; and not more than 0.3% of total impurities is found.

Limit of propofol related compound A—[NOTE—This test is to be performed in conjunction with *Related compounds Test 1.*]

Mobile phase—Prepare a filtered and degassed mixture of acetonitrile, water, and methanol (50 : 40 : 10).

Standard solution—Prepare a solution in methanol containing 20 µg per mL of USP Propofol Related Compound A RS.

Test solution—Transfer about 500 mg of Propofol, accurately weighed, to a 25-mL volumetric flask, dissolve in and dilute with methanol to volume, and mix.

Chromatographic system (see *Chromatography* ⟨621⟩)—The liquid chromatograph is equipped with a 270-nm detector and a 4.6-mm × 15-cm column that contains packing L1. The flow rate is about 1.5 mL per minute. Chromatograph the *Standard solution* six times, and record the peak responses as directed for *Procedure:* the column efficiency, based on the propofol related compound A peak, is not less than 6000 theoretical plates; and the relative standard deviation for replicate injections for propofol related compound A peaks is not more than 15%.

Procedure—Separately inject equal volumes (about 20 µL) of the *Standard solution* and the *Test solution* into the chromatograph, record the chromatograms, and measure the peak responses for propofol related compound A. Calculate the percentage of propofol related compound A in the portion of Propofol taken by the formula:

$$0.01(r_U / r_S)$$

in which r_U and r_S are the peak responses for propofol related compound A obtained from the *Test solution* and the *Standard solution*, respectively: not more than 0.1% of propofol related compound A is found.

Limit of propofol related compound B—

TEST 1—[NOTE—This is to be performed in conjunction with *Related compounds Test 1.*]

Sample solution: neat.

Procedure—Examine the portion of Propofol taken at 330 nm using air as the blank (see *Ultraviolet Absorption* ⟨197U⟩. The absorbance of the *Sample solution* is not more than 0.4 absorbance units (0.1%).

TEST 2—[NOTE—This is to be performed in conjunction with *Related compounds Test 2.*]

Mobile phase—Prepare as directed under *Assay Test 2*.

Standard stock solution—Dissolve about 5 mg of USP Propofol Related Compound B RS in hexane, and dilute with hexane to 50 mL.

Standard solution—Dilute 5 mL of the *Standard stock solution* with hexane to 100 mL.

Test solution—Dissolve about 0.5 g of Propofol in hexane, and dilute with hexane to 10 mL.

Chromatographic system (see *Chromatography* ⟨621⟩)—Prepare as directed under *Assay Test 2* except that the liquid chromatograph is equipped with a detector at 254 nm. Chromatograph the *Standard solution* and the *Test solution*, and record the peak responses as directed for *Procedure:* the relative retention time for propofol related compound B is about 0.8 and 1.0 for propofol.

Procedure—Separately inject equal volumes (about 20 µL) of the *Standard solution* and the *Test solution* into the chromatograph, record the chromatograms, and measure the peak responses. Calculate the percentage of propofol related compound B in the portion of Propofol taken by the formula:

$$100(C_S / C_U)(r_U / r_S)$$

in which C_S is the concentration, in mg per mL, of the *Standard solution;* C_U is the concentration, in mg per mL, of propofol in the *Test solution;* and r_U and r_S are the peak responses obtained from the *Test solution* and the *Standard solution*, respectively: not more than 0.05% of propofol related compound B is found.

Assay—

TEST 1—[NOTE—This is to be performed in conjunction with *Related compounds Test 1.*]

Standard preparation—Dissolve an accurately weighed quantity of USP Propofol RS in methanol, and dilute quantitatively, and stepwise if necessary, with methanol to obtain a solution having a concentration of about 10 mg per mL.

Assay preparation—Transfer about 250 mg of Propofol, accurately weighed, to a 25-mL volumetric flask, and dissolve in and dilute with methanol to volume.

Chromatographic system (see *Chromatography* ⟨621⟩)—The gas chromatograph is equipped with a flame-ionization detector and a 0.53-mm × 30-m column coated with a 1.2-µm phase G16. The carrier gas is helium, flowing at a rate of about 8 mL per minute. The injection port and the detector temperatures are maintained at 250° and 300°, respectively. The chromatograph is programmed as follows. Upon injection, the column temperature is maintained at 145° for 20 minutes; the temperature is increased at a rate of 5° per minute to 200° and maintained at 200° for 5 minutes. Chromatograph the *Standard preparation* five times, and record the peak responses as directed for *Procedure:* the column efficiency determined from the propofol peak is not less than 5000 theoretical plates; the tailing factor is not more than 2.5; and the relative standard deviation for replicate injections is not more than 1.5%.

Procedure—Separately inject equal volumes (about 1.0 µL) of the *Standard preparation* and the *Assay preparation* into the chromatograph, record the chromatograms, and measure the responses for the major peaks. Calculate the percentage of $C_{12}H_{18}O$ in the portion of Propofol taken by the formula:

$$100(C_S / C_U)(r_U / r_S)$$

in which C_S is the concentration, in mg per mL, of USP Propofol RS in the *Standard preparation;* C_U is the concentration, in mg per mL, of Propofol in the *Assay preparation;* and r_U and r_S are the peak responses obtained from the *Assay preparation* and the *Standard preparation*, respectively.

TEST 2—[NOTE—This is to be performed in conjunction with *Related compounds Test 2.*]

Mobile phase—Prepare a filtered and degassed mixture of hexane, acetonitrile, and alcohol (990 : 7.5 : 1). Make adjustments if necessary (see *System Suitability* under *Chromatography* ⟨621⟩).

Standard preparation—Dissolve an accurately weighed quantity of USP Propofol RS in hexane, and dilute quantitatively, and stepwise if necessary, with hexane to obtain a solution having a concentration of about 2.4 mg per mL.

Assay preparation—Transfer about 240 mg of Propofol, accurately weighed, to a 100-mL volumetric flask, dissolve in and dilute with hexane to volume, and mix.

Chromatographic system (see *Chromatography* ⟨621⟩)—The liquid chromatograph is equipped with a 275-nm detector and 4.6-mm × 20-cm column that contains 5-µm packing L3. The flow rate is about 2 mL per minute. Chromatograph the *Standard preparation*, and record the peak responses as directed for *Procedure:* the tailing factor is not more than 1.5; and the relative standard deviation for replicate injections is not more than 2.0%.

Procedure—Separately inject equal volumes (about 10 µL) of the *Standard preparation* and the *Assay preparation* into the chromatograph, record the chromatograms, and measure the responses for the propofol peaks. Calculate the quantity, in mg, of $C_{12}H_{18}O$ in the portion of Propofol taken by formula:

$$100(C_S / C_U)(r_U / r_S)$$

in which C_S is the concentration, in mg per mL, of USP Propofol RS in the *Standard preparation;* C_U is the concentration, in mg per mL, of Propofol in the *Assay preparation;* and r_U and r_S are the peak responses obtained from the *Assay preparation* and the *Standard preparation*, respectively.

Propoxycaine Hydrochloride

$C_{16}H_{26}N_2O_3 \cdot HCl$ 330.85

Benzoic acid, 4-amino-2-propoxy-, 2-(diethylamino)ethyl ester, monohydrochloride.
2-(Diethylamino)ethyl 4-amino-2-propoxybenzoate monohydrochloride [550-83-4].

» Propoxycaine Hydrochloride, dried at 105° for 3 hours, contains not less than 98.0 percent and not more than 102.0 percent of $C_{16}H_{26}N_2O_3 \cdot HCl$.

Packaging and storage—Preserve in well-closed, light-resistant containers.
USP Reference standards ⟨11⟩—*USP Propoxycaine Hydrochloride RS.*
Identification—
  A: *Infrared Absorption* ⟨197K⟩.
  B: *Ultraviolet Absorption* ⟨197U⟩—
  Solution: 10 μg per mL.
  Medium: water.
  Absorptivities at 303 nm, calculated on the dried basis, do not differ by more than 3.0%.
  C: A solution (1 in 100) responds to the tests for *Chloride* ⟨191⟩.
Melting range, *Class I* ⟨741⟩: between 146° and 151°.
Loss on drying ⟨731⟩—Dry it at 105° for 3 hours: it loses not more than 0.5% of its weight.
Residue on ignition ⟨281⟩: not more than 0.2%.
Chromatographic purity—
  Solvent—Prepare a mixture of chloroform and methanol (9 : 1).
  Standard preparations—Dissolve a quantity of USP Propoxycaine Hydrochloride RS in *Solvent*, and dilute quantitatively, and stepwise if necessary, with *Solvent* to obtain a solution containing 0.5 mg per mL. Dilute quantitatively with *Solvent* to obtain Standard preparations having the following compositions:

Standard preparation	Dilution	Concentration (mg RS per mL)	Percentage (%, for comparison with test specimen)
A	1 in 2	0.25	0.5
B	1 in 5	0.10	0.2
C	1 in 10	0.05	0.1

Test preparation—Dissolve an accurately weighed quantity of Propoxycaine Hydrochloride in *Solvent* to obtain a solution containing 50 mg per mL.
  Procedure—Apply separately 5 μL of the *Test preparation* and 5 μL of each *Standard preparation* to a suitable thin-layer chromatographic plate (see *Chromatography* ⟨621⟩) coated with a 0.25-mm layer of chromatographic silica gel mixture. Position the plate in a chromatographic chamber, and develop the chromatograms in a solvent system consisting of a mixture of chloroform, methanol, and isopropylamine (96 : 2 : 2) until the solvent front has moved about three-fourths of the length of the plate. Remove the plate from the developing chamber, mark the solvent front, and allow the solvent to evaporate, with the aid of warm circulating air. Examine the plate under short-wavelength UV light, and again after exposing the plate to iodine vapors for a few minutes and spraying it with 7 N sulfuric acid. In each instance, compare the intensities of any secondary spots observed in the chromatogram of the *Test preparation* with those of the principal spots in the chromatograms of the *Standard preparations*: no secondary spot is more intense than the principal spot obtained from *Standard preparation A* (0.5%), and the sum of the intensities of all secondary spots obtained from the *Test preparation* does not exceed 1.0%.
Assay—Dissolve about 500 mg of Propoxycaine Hydrochloride, previously dried and accurately weighed, in 200 mL of ice-cold water containing 1 g of potassium bromide and 2.5 mL of hydrochloric acid, and titrate with 0.1 M sodium nitrite VS, using starch iodide paper as an external indicator. Perform a blank determination, and make any necessary correction. Each mL of 0.1 M sodium nitrite is equivalent to 33.09 mg of $C_{16}H_{26}N_2O_3 \cdot HCl$.

Propoxycaine and Procaine Hydrochlorides and Levonordefrin Injection

» Propoxycaine and Procaine Hydrochlorides and Levonordefrin Injection is a sterile solution of Propoxycaine Hydrochloride, Procaine Hydrochloride, and Levonordefrin in Water for Injection. It contains not less than 95.0 percent and not more than 105.0 percent of the labeled amount of propoxycaine hydrochloride ($C_{16}H_{26}N_2O_3 \cdot HCl$), not less than 95.0 percent and not more than 105.0 percent of the labeled amount of procaine hydrochloride ($C_{13}H_{20}N_2O_2 \cdot HCl$), and not less than 90.0 percent and not more than 110.0 percent of the labeled amount of levonordefrin ($C_9H_{13}NO_3$).

Packaging and storage—Preserve in single-dose containers, preferably of Type I glass.
Labeling—The label indicates that the Injection is not to be used if its color is pinkish or darker than slightly yellow or if it contains a precipitate.
USP Reference standards ⟨11⟩—*USP Propoxycaine Hydrochloride RS. USP Procaine Hydrochloride RS. USP Epinephrine Bitartrate RS. USP Endotoxin RS.*
Color and clarity—Using the Injection as the *Test solution*, proceed as directed for *Color and clarity* under *Mepivacaine Hydrochloride and Levonordefrin Injection*.
Identification—
  A: Cool a mixture of 10 mL of Injection and 10 mL of 3 N hydrochloric acid in an ice bath to 0°, add 5 mL of sodium nitrite solution (1 in 5), stirring gently, and 2 mL of a solution of 0.1 g of 2-naphthol in 5 mL of 1 N sodium hydroxide, and observe immediately: a bright orange-red precipitate is formed (*presence of a primary aminophenyl group*).
  B: It responds to the tests for *Chloride* ⟨191⟩.
  C: To about 25 mL of Injection add 1 drop of ferric chloride TS: the solution immediately turns a light green and changes to a light blue within 1 minute. Add 2 drops of 3 N hydrochloric acid: the color reverts to light green (*presence of levonordefrin*).
Bacterial endotoxins ⟨85⟩—It contains not more than 0.8 USP Endotoxin Unit per mg of propoxycaine hydrochloride.
pH ⟨791⟩: between 3.5 and 5.0.
Other requirements—It meets the requirements under *Injections* ⟨1⟩.
Assay for propoxycaine and procaine hydrochlorides—
  Standard propoxycaine hydrochloride preparation—Prepare, by quantitative and stepwise dilution, a solution in dilute hydrochloric acid (1 in 6) containing about 50 μg of USP Propoxycaine Hydrochloride RS, accurately weighed, in each mL.
  Standard procaine hydrochloride preparation—Prepare, by quantitative and stepwise dilution, a solution in dilute hydrochloric acid (1 in 6) containing about 200 μg of USP Procaine Hydrochloride RS, accurately weighed, in each mL.
  Assay preparation—Transfer an accurately measured volume of Injection, equivalent to about 100 mg of procaine hydrochloride, to a 125-mL separator containing 25 mL of chloroform and 10 mL of water. Add 5 mL of sodium carbonate TS, shake vigorously, allow the layers to separate, and transfer the chloroform layer to a second

separator. Extract the aqueous layer with two 10-mL portions of chloroform, adding the extracts to the second separator. Extract the combined chloroform extracts with 35 mL of dilute hydrochloric acid (1 in 6), transfer the chloroform to a third separator, and transfer the acid extract to a 100-mL volumetric flask. Extract the chloroform with two 10-mL portions of dilute hydrochloric acid (1 in 6), add the acid extracts to the volumetric flask, add dilute hydrochloric acid (1 in 6) to volume, and mix. Transfer 15.0 mL of this solution to a second 100-mL volumetric flask, add dilute hydrochloric acid (1 in 6) to volume, and mix.

Procedure—Concomitantly determine the absorbances of the *Standard preparations* and the *Assay preparation* in 1-cm cells at 296 and 272 nm, with a suitable spectrophotometer, using water as the blank. Calculate the quantity, in mg, of propoxycaine hydrochloride ($C_{16}H_{26}N_2O_3 \cdot HCl$) in each mL of the Injection taken by the formula:

$$(0.667C/V)(A_{296}A_4 - A_{272}A_3)/(A_1A_4 - A_2A_3)$$

in which C is the concentration, in μg per mL, of USP Propoxycaine Hydrochloride RS in the *Standard propoxycaine hydrochloride preparation*.

Calculate the quantity, in mg, of procaine hydrochloride ($C_{13}H_{20}N_2O_2 \cdot HCl$) in each mL of the Injection taken by the formula:

$$(0.667C/V)(A_{272}A_1 - A_{296}A_2)/(A_1A_4 - A_2A_3)$$

in which C is the concentration, in μg per mL, of USP Procaine Hydrochloride RS in the *Standard procaine hydrochloride preparation*, V is the volume, in mL, of Injection taken, A_1 and A_2 are the absorbances of the *Standard propoxycaine hydrochloride preparation* at 296 and 272 nm, respectively, A_3 and A_4 are the absorbances of the *Standard procaine hydrochloride preparation* at 296 and 272 nm, respectively, and A_{296} and A_{272} are the absorbances of the *Assay preparation* at 296 and 272 nm, respectively.

Assay for levonordefrin—

Ferro-citrate solution, *Buffer solution*, and *Standard preparation*—Prepare as directed under *Epinephrine Assay* ⟨391⟩.

Assay preparation—Proceed with Injection as directed for *Assay Preparation* under *Epinephrine Assay* ⟨391⟩, except to read "levonordefrin" where "epinephrine" is specified.

Procedure—Proceed as directed for *Procedure* under *Epinephrine Assay* ⟨391⟩. Calculate the quantity, in mg, of levonordefrin ($C_9H_{13}NO_3$) in each mL of the Injection taken by the formula:

$$(183.21/333.30)(0.05C/V)(A_U/A_S)$$

in which 183.21 and 333.30 are the molecular weights of levonordefrin and epinephrine bitartrate, respectively, C is the concentration, in μg per mL, of USP Epinephrine Bitartrate RS in the *Standard preparation*, and V is the volume, in mL, of Injection taken.

Propoxycaine and Procaine Hydrochlorides and Norepinephrine Bitartrate Injection

» Propoxycaine and Procaine Hydrochlorides and Norepinephrine Bitartrate Injection is a sterile solution of Propoxycaine Hydrochloride, Procaine Hydrochloride, and Norepinephrine Bitartrate in Water for Injection. It contains not less than 95.0 percent and not more than 105.0 percent of the labeled amount of propoxycaine hydrochloride ($C_{16}H_{26}N_2O_3 \cdot HCl$), not less than 95.0 percent and not more than 105.0 percent of the labeled amount of procaine hydrochloride ($C_{13}H_{20}N_2O_2 \cdot HCl$), and an amount of norepinephrine bitartrate ($C_8H_{11}NO_3 \cdot C_4H_6O_6 \cdot H_2O$) equivalent to not less than 90.0 percent and not more than 110.0 percent of the labeled amount of norepinephrine ($C_8H_{11}NO_3$).

Packaging and storage—Preserve in single-dose or in multiple-dose containers, preferably of Type I glass.

Labeling—The label indicates that the Injection is not to be used if its color is pinkish or darker than slightly yellow or if it contains a precipitate.

USP Reference standards ⟨11⟩—*USP Propoxycaine Hydrochloride RS. USP Procaine Hydrochloride RS. USP Norepinephrine Bitartrate RS. USP Endotoxin RS.*

Color and clarity—Using the Injection as the *Test solution*, proceed as directed for *Color and clarity* under *Norepinephrine Bitartrate Injection*.

Identification—

A: Cool a mixture of 10 mL of Injection and 10 mL of 3 N hydrochloric acid in an ice bath to 0°, add 5 mL of sodium nitrite solution (1 in 5), stirring gently, and 2 mL of a solution of 0.1 g of 2-naphthol in 5 mL of 1 N sodium hydroxide, and observe immediately: a bright orange-red precipitate is formed (*presence of a primary aminophenyl group*).

B: It responds to the tests for *Chloride* ⟨191⟩.

C: To about 5 mL of Injection add 1 drop of ferric chloride TS: a green color develops (*presence of norepinephrine bitartrate*).

Bacterial endotoxins ⟨85⟩—It contains not more than 0.8 USP Endotoxin Unit per mg of propoxycaine hydrochloride.

pH ⟨791⟩: between 3.5 and 5.0.

Other requirements—It meets the requirements under *Injections* ⟨1⟩.

Assay for propoxycaine and procaine hydrochlorides—

Standard propoxycaine hydrochloride preparation—Prepare, by quantitative and stepwise dilution, a solution in 2 N hydrochloric acid containing about 50 μg of USP Propoxycaine Hydrochloride RS, accurately weighed, in each mL.

Standard procaine hydrochloride preparation—Prepare, by quantitative and stepwise dilution, a solution in 2 N hydrochloric acid containing about 200 μg of USP Procaine Hydrochloride RS, accurately weighed, in each mL.

Assay preparation—Transfer an accurately measured volume of Injection, equivalent to about 100 mg of procaine hydrochloride, to a 125-mL separator containing 25 mL of chloroform and 10 mL of water. Add 5 mL of sodium carbonate TS, shake vigorously, allow the layers to separate, and transfer the chloroform layer to a second separator. Extract the aqueous layer with two 10-mL portions of chloroform, adding the extracts to the second separator. Extract the combined chloroform extracts with 35 mL of 2 N hydrochloric acid, transfer the chloroform to a third separator, and transfer the acid extract to a 100-mL volumetric flask. Extract the chloroform with two 10-mL portions of 2 N hydrochloric acid, add the acid extracts to the volumetric flask, dilute with 2 N hydrochloric acid to volume, and mix. Transfer 15.0 mL of this solution to a second 100-mL volumetric flask, dilute with 2 N hydrochloric acid to volume, and mix.

Procedure—Concomitantly determine the absorbances of the *Standard preparations* and the *Assay preparation*, in 1-cm cells, at 296 nm and 272 nm, with a suitable spectrophotometer, using water as the blank.

Calculate the quantity, in mg, of propoxycaine hydrochloride ($C_{16}H_{26}N_2O_3 \cdot HCl$) in each mL of the Injection taken by the formula:

$$(0.667C/V)(A_{296}A_4 - A_{272}A_3)/(A_1A_4 - A_2A_3)$$

in which C is the concentration, in μg per mL, of USP Propoxycaine Hydrochloride RS in the *Standard propoxycaine hydrochloride preparation*, V is the volume, in mL, of Injection taken, A_1 and A_2 are the absorbances of the *Standard propoxycaine hydrochloride preparation* at 296 nm and 272 nm, respectively, A_3 and A_4 are the absorbances of the *Standard procaine hydrochloride preparation* at 296 nm and 272 nm, respectively, and A_{296} and A_{272} are the absorbances of the *Assay preparation* at 296 nm and 272 nm, respectively.

Calculate the quantity, in mg, of procaine hydrochloride ($C_{13}H_{20}N_2O_2 \cdot HCl$) in each mL of the Injection taken by the formula:

$$(0.667C/V)(A_{272}A_1 - A_{296}A_2)/(A_1A_4 - A_2A_3)$$

in which C is the concentration, in µg per mL, of USP Procaine Hydrochloride RS in the *Standard procaine hydrochloride preparation*, and V is the volume, in mL, of Injection taken.

Assay for norepinephrine—
Ferro-citrate solution, Buffer solution, and *Standard preparation*—Prepare as directed under *Epinephrine Assay* ⟨391⟩, except to read "USP Norepinephrine Bitartrate RS" for "USP Epinephrine Bitartrate RS" throughout.

Assay preparation—Prepare as directed for *Assay Preparation* under *Epinephrine Assay* ⟨391⟩ except to read "norepinephrine" where "epinephrine" is specified.

Procedure—Proceed as directed for *Procedure* under *Epinephrine Assay* ⟨391⟩. Calculate the quantity, in mg, of norepinephrine ($C_8H_{11}NO_3$) in each mL of the Injection taken by the formula:

$$(169.18/319.27)(0.05C/V)(A_U/A_S)$$

in which 169.18 and 319.27 are the molecular weights of norepinephrine and norepinephrine bitartrate, respectively, C is the concentration, in µg per mL, calculated on the anhydrous basis, of USP Norepinephrine Bitartrate RS in the *Standard preparation*, and V is the volume, in mL, of Injection taken.

Propoxyphene Hydrochloride

$C_{22}H_{29}NO_2 \cdot HCl$ 375.93

Benzeneethanol, α-[2-(dimethylamino)-1-methylethyl]-α-phenyl-, propanoate (ester), hydrochloride, [S-(R*,S*)]-.
(2S,3R)-(+)-4-(Dimethylamino)-3-methyl-1,2-diphenyl-2-butanol propionate (ester) hydrochloride   [1639-60-7].

» Propoxyphene Hydrochloride contains not less than 98.0 percent and not more than 101.0 percent of $C_{22}H_{29}NO_2 \cdot HCl$, calculated on the dried basis.

Packaging and storage—Preserve in tight containers.

USP Reference standards ⟨11⟩—*USP Propoxyphene Hydrochloride RS. USP Propoxyphene Related Compound A RS. USP Propoxyphene Related Compound B RS.*

Identification—
A: *Infrared Absorption* ⟨197S⟩—
Solution: 1 in 20.
Medium: chloroform.
B: Dissolve 0.25 g of Propoxyphene Hydrochloride in 15 mL of Purified Water, and treat 3 mL of this solution with 1 mL of 6 N ammonium hydroxide to precipitate the propoxyphene base. Filter to remove the precipitate, acidify the filtrate with 2 mL of nitric acid, and add 1 mL of silver nitrate TS: a white, curdy precipitate that is soluble in an excess of 6 N ammonium hydroxide confirms the presence of silver chloride.

Melting range ⟨741⟩: between 163.5° and 168.5°, but the range between beginning and end of melting does not exceed 3°.

Specific rotation ⟨781S⟩: between +52° and +57°.
Test solution: 10 mg per mL, in water, freshly prepared.

Loss on drying ⟨731⟩—Dry it at 105° for 3 hours: it loses not more than 1.0% of its weight.

Related compounds—
Mobile phase and *Chromatographic system*—Proceed as directed in the *Assay*.
Standard stock solution—Accurately weigh about 10 mg each of USP Propoxyphene Related Compound A RS and USP Propoxyphene Related Compound B RS into a 50-mL volumetric flask, dissolve using 2 mL of methanol, dilute with *Mobile phase* to volume, and mix.

Standard solution—Transfer 5.0 mL of the *Standard stock solution* to a 50-mL volumetric flask, dilute with *Mobile phase* to volume, and mix.

Test solution—Use the *Assay preparation*.

System suitability solution—Dissolve an accurately weighed quantity of USP Propoxyphene Hydrochloride RS in *Standard solution*, and dilute quantitatively, and stepwise if necessary, to obtain a solution having known concentrations of about 4.5 mg per mL of USP Propoxyphene Hydrochloride RS, about 0.02 mg per mL of USP Propoxyphene Related Compound A RS, and about 0.02 mg per mL of USP Propoxyphene Related Compound B RS.

Chromatographic system—Chromatograph the *System suitability solution*, and record the peak responses as directed for *Procedure:* the relative retention times are about 0.63 for propoxyphene related compound A, 0.78 for propoxyphene related compound B, and 1.0 for propoxyphene hydrochloride; the resolution, R, between propoxyphene related compound B and propoxyphene related compound A is not less than 2.0; and the relative standard deviation for replicate injections is not more than 2.0%.

Procedure—Separately inject equal volumes (about 50 µL) of the *Test solution* and the *Standard solution* into the chromatograph, record the chromatograms, and measure the peak responses. Calculate the quantity, in mg, of propoxyphene related compound A in the portion of Propoxyphene Hydrochloride taken by the formula:

$$50C(r_U/r_S)$$

in which C is the concentration, in mg per mL, of USP Propoxyphene Related Compound A RS in the *Standard solution;* and r_U and r_S are the propoxyphene related compound A peak responses obtained from the *Test solution* and *Standard solution,* respectively. Not more than 0.5% of propoxyphene related compound A is found. Calculate the quantity, in mg, of propoxyphene related compound B as the hydrochloride in the portion of Propoxyphene Hydrochloride taken by the formula:

$$50C(361.93/325.45)(r_U/r_S)$$

in which C is the concentration, in mg per mL, of USP Propoxyphene Related Compound B RS in the *Standard solution;* 361.93 and 325.45 are the molecular weights of propoxyphene related compound B as the hydrochloride and propoxyphene related compound B, respectively; and r_U and r_S are the propoxyphene related compound B peak responses obtained from the *Test solution* and *Standard solution*, respectively. Not more than 0.6% of propoxyphene related compound B as the hydrochloride is found.

Organic volatile impurities, *Method I* ⟨467⟩: meets the requirements.

(Official until July 1, 2008)

Assay—
0.1 M Monobasic ammonium phosphate buffer, pH 6.3—Dissolve 11.5 g of monobasic ammonium phosphate and 1.0 mL of triethylamine in 1000 mL of water, adjust with 10% sodium hydroxide to a pH of 6.3 ± 0.05, and mix.

Mobile phase—Prepare a filtered and degassed mixture of methanol and *0.1 M Monobasic ammonium phosphate buffer, pH 6.3* (67 : 33). Make adjustments if necessary (see *System Suitability* under *Chromatography* ⟨621⟩).

Standard preparation—Dissolve an accurately weighed quantity of USP Propoxyphene Hydrochloride RS in *Mobile phase* to obtain a solution having a known concentration of about 5.0 mg per mL.

Assay preparation—Transfer about 250 mg of Propoxyphene Hydrochloride, accurately weighed, to a 50-mL volumetric flask, dissolve in and dilute with *Mobile phase* to volume, and mix.

Chromatographic system (see *Chromatography* ⟨621⟩)—The liquid chromatograph is equipped with a 254-nm detector and a 3.9-mm × 30-cm column that contains packing L1. The flow rate is about 1.5 mL per minute. Chromatograph the *Standard preparation*, and record the peak responses as directed for *Procedure:* the retention time of propoxyphene hydrochloride is about 9 minutes; the tailing factor for the propoxyphene hydrochloride peak is not more than 3.5; and the relative standard deviation for replicate injections is not more than 2.0%.

Procedure—Separately inject equal volumes (about 50 µL) of the *Standard preparation* and the *Assay preparation* into the chromatograph, record the chromatograms, and measure the responses for the major peaks. Calculate the quantity, in mg, of $C_{22}H_{29}NO_2 \cdot HCl$ in the portion of Propoxyphene Hydrochloride taken by the formula:

$$50C(r_U / r_S)$$

in which C is the concentration, in mg per mL, of USP Propoxyphene Hydrochloride RS in the *Standard preparation;* and r_U and r_S are the peak responses obtained from the *Assay preparation* and the *Standard preparation*, respectively.

Propoxyphene Hydrochloride Capsules

» Propoxyphene Hydrochloride Capsules contain not less than 92.5 percent and not more than 107.5 percent of the labeled amount of $C_{22}H_{29}NO_2 \cdot HCl$.

Packaging and storage—Preserve in tight containers.
USP Reference standards ⟨11⟩—*USP Propoxyphene Hydrochloride RS.*
Identification—Transfer an accurately weighed quantity of Capsule contents remaining from the preparation of the *Assay preparation* in the *Assay*, equivalent to about 320 mg of propoxyphene hydrochloride, to a 100-mL volumetric flask. Add 20 mL of acetone, and sonicate for about 1 minute. Dilute the solution with water to volume, and mix. Allow to stand until the excipients have settled, usually about 15 to 20 minutes. Transfer 40.0 mL of this solution to a 125-mL separator containing 20 mL of sodium carbonate solution (1 in 10), and swirl the mixture for 3 minutes. Add 25.0 mL of chloroform, insert the stopper, and shake the mixture by mechanical means for 1 hour. Filter the chloroform extract through a layer of anhydrous sodium sulfate into a suitable beaker. Prepare a Standard solution as follows. Transfer about 125 mg of USP Propoxyphene Hydrochloride RS, accurately weighed, to a 125-mL separator containing 8 mL of acetone, 32 mL of water, and 20 mL of sodium carbonate solution (1 in 10), and swirl the mixture for 3 minutes. Proceed as directed for the test solution, beginning with "Add 25.0 mL of chloroform." Use the chloroform solutions obtained from the Capsule contents and from the USP Propoxyphene Hydrochloride RS for the following tests.
  A: The IR absorption spectrum of the chloroform solution of the contents of Capsules, concentrated if necessary by evaporating a portion on a steam bath with the aid of a current of air to about one-fifth of its volume, exhibits maxima only at the same wavelengths as that of a similar preparation of USP Propoxyphene Hydrochloride RS.
  B: Transfer 20.0 mL of the test solution and 20.0 mL of the Standard solution to separate beakers, and evaporate on a steam bath with the aid of a current of air to about 5 mL. Remove the beakers from the steam bath, and continue evaporation with the aid of a current of air until the chloroform is completely evaporated. Add 5.0 mL of 0.1 N hydrochloric acid to each, and dissolve the residue. Using the solution obtained from the test solution, determine the specific rotation (see *Optical Rotation* ⟨781⟩), in which c, the concentration of propoxyphene hydrochloride per 100 mL of solution, is calculated as follows:

$$0.0064(W_U / W_T)A$$

in which W_U is the weight, in mg, of the portion of Capsule contents taken, W_T is the average weight, in mg, of the contents of each Capsule, and A is the quantity, in mg, of propoxyphene hydrochloride per Capsule, as obtained in the *Assay*. Using the solution obtained from the Standard solution, determine the specific rotation, c, being calculated by multiplying the weight, in mg, of USP Propoxyphene Hydrochloride RS taken by 0.016. The specific rotation obtained from the solution from the test solution is not less than 95.0% of that obtained from the solution from the Standard solution.
  C: The chromatogram of the *Assay preparation* obtained as directed in the *Assay* exhibits a major peak for propoxyphene hydrochloride, the retention time of which corresponds to that exhibited in the chromatogram of the *Standard preparation* obtained as directed in the *Assay*.

Dissolution ⟨711⟩—
  Medium: pH 4.5 acetate buffer, prepared as directed in the test for *Dissolution* under *Propoxyphene Hydrochloride, Aspirin, and Caffeine Capsules;* 500 mL.
  Apparatus 1: 100 rpm.
  Time: 60 minutes.
  Procedure—Proceed as directed in the *Assay* using a filtered portion of the solution under test diluted with *Diluent*, and a Standard solution having an accurately known concentration of USP Propoxyphene Hydrochloride RS in *Diluent*. Calculate the amount of propoxyphene hydrochloride dissolved.
  Tolerances—Not less than 85% *(Q)* of the labeled amount of $C_{22}H_{29}NO_2 \cdot HCl$ is dissolved in 60 minutes.
Uniformity of dosage units ⟨905⟩: meet the requirements.
Assay—
  Phosphate buffer—Dissolve 6.8 g of monobasic potassium phosphate in about 900 mL of water. Add 2.0 mL of triethylamine, mix, and adjust by the addition of phosphoric acid to a pH of 3.0 ± 0.1. Dilute with water to 1 liter, and mix.
  Diluent—Prepare a mixture of water and acetonitrile (3 : 2).
  Mobile phase—Prepare a filtered and degassed mixture of *Phosphate buffer* and acetonitrile (3 : 2). Make adjustments if necessary (see *System Suitability* under *Chromatography* ⟨621⟩).
  Standard preparation—Dissolve an accurately weighed quantity of USP Propoxyphene Hydrochloride RS in *Diluent* with the aid of sonication to obtain a solution having a known concentration of about 325 µg per mL. Transfer 2.0 mL of this solution to a 100-mL volumetric flask, dilute with *Diluent* to volume, and mix to obtain a *Standard preparation* having a known concentration of about 6.5 µg per mL.
  Assay preparation—Remove, as completely as possible, the contents of not less than 20 Capsules. Weigh the contents, and determine the average weight per capsule. Mix the combined contents, and transfer an accurately weighed quantity of the powder, equivalent to about 65 mg of propoxyphene hydrochloride, to a 200-mL volumetric flask. Add about 50 mL of *Diluent*, sonicate for 5 minutes, and shake by mechanical means for 15 minutes. Dilute with *Diluent* to volume, mix, and filter, discarding the first 20 mL of the filtrate. Transfer 2.0 mL of the filtrate to a 100-mL volumetric flask, dilute with *Diluent* to volume, and mix.
  Chromatographic system (see *Chromatography* ⟨621⟩)—The liquid chromatograph is equipped with a 220-nm detector and a 4.6-mm × 3.3-cm column that contains 3-µm packing L1 that is base-deactivated. Precondition the column for at least 30 minutes with *Mobile phase*. The flow rate is about 1 mL per minute. Chromatograph the *Standard preparation*, and record the peak responses as directed for *Procedure:* the tailing factor for the propoxyphene hydrochloride peak is not more than 2, and the relative standard deviation for replicate injections is not more than 2.0%.
  Procedure—Separately inject equal volumes (about 10 µL) of the *Standard preparation* and the *Assay preparation* into the chromatograph, record the chromatograms, and measure the peak responses for the major peaks. Calculate the quantity, in mg, of $C_{22}H_{29}NO_2 \cdot HCl$ in the portion of Capsules taken by the formula:

$$10C(r_U / r_S)$$

in which C is the concentration, in µg per mL, of USP Propoxyphene Hydrochloride RS in the *Standard preparation*, and r_U and r_S are the propoxyphene hydrochloride peak responses obtained from the *Assay preparation* and the *Standard preparation*, respectively.

Propoxyphene Hydrochloride and Acetaminophen Tablets

» Propoxyphene Hydrochloride and Acetaminophen Tablets contain not less than 90.0 percent and not more than 110.0 percent of the labeled amounts of propoxyphene hydrochloride ($C_{22}H_{29}NO_2 \cdot HCl$) and acetaminophen ($C_8H_9NO_2$).

Packaging and storage—Preserve in tight containers.
USP Reference standards ⟨11⟩—*USP Acetaminophen RS. USP Propoxyphene Hydrochloride RS.*
Identification—Transfer 1 finely ground Tablet to a test tube. If the Tablets are coated, first immerse the Tablet in acetone for 1½ minutes, remove the shell, and grind. Add 5 mL of methanol, shake for 5 minutes, and centrifuge. Use the clear supernatant as the *Test solution.* Prepare a *Standard solution* in methanol containing, in each mL, 130 mg of USP Acetaminophen RS and 13 mg of USP Propoxyphene Hydrochloride RS. Apply 5 μL of the *Test solution* on a line parallel to and about 2 cm from the bottom edge of a 20- × 5-cm thin-layer chromatographic plate (see *Chromatography* ⟨621⟩) coated with chromatographic silica gel mixture, and apply 5 μL of the *Standard solution* separately on the starting line. Place the plate in a developing chamber containing a mixture of butyl acetate, chloroform, and formic acid (60 : 40 : 20), and develop the chromatogram until the solvent front has moved about 15 cm above the line of application. Remove the plate, allow to dry in a hood, and view under short-wavelength UV light: the R_F value of the principal spot from the *Test solution* corresponds to that from the *Standard solution.* Spray the plate with iodoplatinate TS: the R_F value of the orange-brown spot from the *Test solution* corresponds to that from the *Standard solution.*

Dissolution, *Procedure for a Pooled Sample* ⟨711⟩—
 Medium: pH 4.5 acetate buffer, prepared as directed in the test for *Dissolution* under *Propoxyphene Hydrochloride, Aspirin and Caffeine Capsules*; 700 mL.
 Apparatus 2: 50 rpm.
 Time: 30 minutes.
 Procedure—Proceed as directed in the *Assay*, using a filtered portion of the solution under test, diluted with *Mobile phase*, and a *Standard solution* having accurately known concentrations of USP Propoxyphene Hydrochloride RS and USP Acetaminophen RS in *Mobile phase.* Calculate the amounts of propoxyphene hydrochloride ($C_{22}H_{29}NO_2 \cdot HCl$) and acetaminophen ($C_8H_9NO_2$) dissolved.
 Tolerances—Not less than 80% *(Q)* of the labeled amount of $C_{22}H_{29}NO_2 \cdot HCl$ and not less than 80% *(Q)* of the labeled amount of $C_8H_9NO_2$ are dissolved in 30 minutes.

Uniformity of dosage units ⟨905⟩: meet the requirements for *Content Uniformity* with respect to propoxyphene hydrochloride.

Assay—
 Mobile phase—Mix 0.15% diethylamine in water, adjusted with phosphoric acid to a pH of 3.2 ± 0.2, and acetonitrile (4 : 1). Sonicate for 15 minutes, and filter through a filter having a porosity of 0.5 μm or finer. Make adjustments if necessary (see *System Suitability* under *Chromatography* ⟨621⟩).
 Standard preparation 1—Transfer about 2*J* mg of USP Acetaminophen RS, accurately weighed, to a 10-mL volumetric flask, *J* being the ratio of the labeled amount, in mg, of acetaminophen to the labeled amount, in mg, of propoxyphene hydrochloride in each Tablet. Transfer about 2 mg of USP Propoxyphene Hydrochloride RS, accurately weighed, to the same flask. Add about 5 mL of *Mobile phase*, swirl to dissolve, dilute with *Mobile phase* to volume, and mix. This solution contains about 0.2 mg of USP Propoxyphene Hydrochloride RS and 0.2*J* mg of USP Acetaminophen RS per mL.
 Standard preparation 2—Transfer 5.0 mL of *Standard preparation 1* to a 100-mL volumetric flask, dilute with *Mobile phase* to volume, and mix. This solution contains about 0.01*J* mg of USP Acetaminophen RS per mL.
 Assay preparation 1—Weigh and finely powder not less than 20 Tablets. Transfer an accurately weighed portion of the powder, equivalent to about 40 mg of propoxyphene hydrochloride, to a 200-mL volumetric flask, add about 150 mL of *Mobile phase*, shake by mechanical means for 30 minutes, sonicate for 5 minutes, dilute with *Mobile phase* to volume, mix, and filter, discarding the first 20 mL of the filtrate. Use the clear filtrate as *Assay preparation 1*.
 Assay preparation 2—Transfer 5.0 mL of *Assay preparation 1* to a 100-mL volumetric flask, dilute with *Mobile phase* to volume, and mix.
 Chromatographic system (see *Chromatography* ⟨621⟩)—The liquid chromatograph is equipped with a 210-nm detector and a 254-nm detector and a 3.9-mm × 30-cm column that contains packing L1. The flow rate is about 1 mL per minute. Chromatograph *Standard preparation 1*, and record the responses as directed for *Procedure:* the tailing factor for the propoxyphene peak is not more than 2.0, and the relative standard deviation for replicate injections is not more than 2.0%. Chromatograph *Standard preparation 2*, and record the responses as directed for *Procedure:* the tailing factor for the acetaminophen peak is not more than 1.5, and the relative standard deviation for replicate injections is not more than 2.0%.
 Procedure—[NOTE—Use peak areas where peak responses are indicated.] Separately inject equal volumes (about 20 μL) of *Standard preparation 1*, *Standard preparation 2*, *Assay preparation 1*, and *Assay preparation 2* into the chromatograph, record the chromatograms using both the 210-nm and the 254-nm detectors, and measure the responses for the propoxyphene hydrochloride peaks obtained using the 210-nm detector and for the acetaminophen peaks obtained using the 254-nm detector. Calculate the quantity, in mg, of propoxyphene hydrochloride ($C_{22}H_{29}NO_2 \cdot HCl$) in the portion of Tablets taken by the formula:

$$200C(r_U / r_S)$$

in which C is the concentration, in μg per mL, of USP Propoxyphene Hydrochloride RS in *Standard preparation 1*, and r_U and r_S are the propoxyphene hydrochloride peak responses obtained from *Assay preparation 1* and *Standard preparation 1*, respectively. Calculate the quantity, in mg, of acetaminophen ($C_8H_9NO_2$) in the portion of Tablets taken by the formula:

$$4000C(r_U / r_S)$$

in which C is the concentration, in mg per mL, of USP Acetaminophen RS in *Standard preparation 2*, and r_U and r_S are the acetaminophen peak responses obtained from *Assay preparation 2* and *Standard preparation 2*, respectively.

Propoxyphene Hydrochloride, Aspirin, and Caffeine Capsules

» Propoxyphene Hydrochloride, Aspirin, and Caffeine Capsules contain not less than 90.0 percent and not more than 110.0 percent of the labeled amounts of propoxyphene hydrochloride ($C_{22}H_{29}NO_2 \cdot HCl$), aspirin ($C_9H_8O_4$), and caffeine ($C_8H_{10}N_4O_2$).

NOTE—Where Propoxyphene Hydrochloride, Aspirin, and Caffeine Capsules are prescribed, the quantity of propoxyphene hydrochloride is to be specified. Where the Capsules are prescribed without reference to the quantity of aspirin or caffeine contained therein, a product containing 389 mg of aspirin and 32.4 mg of caffeine shall be dispensed.

Packaging and storage—Preserve in tight containers at controlled room temperature.
USP Reference standards ⟨11⟩—*USP Aspirin RS. USP Caffeine RS. USP Propoxyphene Hydrochloride RS. USP Salicylic Acid RS.*
Identification—
 A: Place an amount of the finely powdered contents of Capsules, equivalent to about 65 mg of propoxyphene hydrochloride, in a test tube, add 5 mL of methanol, shake for 5 minutes, and centrifuge. The clear supernatant is the test solution. Dissolve weighed amounts of USP Propoxyphene Hydrochloride RS, USP Aspirin RS, and USP Caffeine RS corresponding, proportionately, to the amounts of propoxyphene hydrochloride, aspirin, and caffeine in the Capsules to obtain a Standard solution having a known concentration of about 13 mg of propoxyphene hydrochloride per mL. Apply 10 μL each of the test solution and the Standard solution to a suitable thin-layer chromatographic plate (see *Chromatography* ⟨621⟩) coated with a 0.25-mm layer of chromatographic silica gel mixture. Develop the chromatograms in a solvent system consisting

of a mixture of chloroform, butyl acetate, and formic acid (30 : 20 : 10) until the solvent front has moved about three-fourths of the length of the plate. Remove the plate from the developing chamber, mark the solvent front, allow it to dry in a fume hood, and examine the plate under short-wavelength UV light: the chromatogram of the test solution exhibits 3 principal spots that correspond in R_F value and intensity with those obtained from the Standard solution.

B: The *Assay preparation* prepared as directed in the *Assay for propoxyphene hydrochloride and caffeine* is dextrorotatory.

Dissolution ⟨711⟩—
Medium: pH 4.5 acetate buffer; 500 mL.
Apparatus 1: 100 rpm.
Time: 60 minutes.
pH 4.5 acetate buffer—Dissolve 2.99 g of sodium acetate trihydrate in 200 mL of water, add 1.66 mL of glacial acetic acid, dilute with water to 1000 mL, and mix.
Determination of dissolved aspirin—Transfer 5.0 mL of a filtered portion of the solution under test to a 25-mL volumetric flask. Concurrently pipet 5 mL of a standard solution, prepared by dissolving 35 mg of accurately weighed USP Aspirin RS in 50.0 mL of *pH 4.5 acetate buffer*, into a second 25-mL volumetric flask. Proceed as directed for *Procedure* in the *Assay for aspirin*, beginning with "Into each flask pipet 5 mL of *Sodium hydroxide reagent*." Concomitantly determine the absorbances of both solutions against a similarly treated blank of 5.0 mL of *pH 4.5 acetate buffer*. Determine the amount of aspirin ($C_9H_8O_4$) in solution by comparison with the Standard solution.
Determination of dissolved propoxyphene hydrochloride—
INTERNAL STANDARD SOLUTION—Dissolve *n*-tricosane in chloroform to obtain a solution containing about 0.06 mg per mL.
STANDARD PREPARATION—Dissolve an accurately weighed quantity of USP Propoxyphene Hydrochloride RS in *pH 4.5 acetate buffer* to obtain a solution having a known concentration (between 0.06 and 0.13 mg per mL) that corresponds to the concentration of propoxyphene hydrochloride that is estimated for the solution under test, based on the labeled content of the Capsules and the extent of dissolution.
PROCEDURE—Transfer equal, accurately measured, volumes (between 5.0 and 10.0 mL) of filtered portions of the solution under test and the *Standard preparation* into separate, screw-capped centrifuge tubes. To each tube add 5.0 mL of sodium carbonate solution (1 in 5), and shake. Extract with one 5.0-mL portion of *Internal standard solution*, and one 5.0-mL portion of chloroform, and shake each extract for 5 minutes. Pass the organic layers through phase-separating paper. Evaporate to about 1 mL, and inject a 10-μL portion into a suitable gas chromatograph equipped with a flame-ionization detector. Proceed as directed for *Procedure* in the *Assay for propoxyphene hydrochloride and caffeine*, beginning with "The column is typically 60 cm × 4 mm." Determine the amount of propoxyphene hydrochloride ($C_{22}H_{29}NO_2 \cdot HCl$) in solution by comparison with the *Standard preparation*.
Tolerances—Not less than 75% (*Q*) of the labeled amount of $C_9H_8O_4$ is dissolved in 60 minutes, and not less than 85% (*Q*) of the labeled amount of $C_{22}H_{29}NO_2 \cdot HCl$ is dissolved in 60 minutes.

Uniformity of dosage units ⟨905⟩: meet the requirements for *Content Uniformity* with respect to propoxyphene hydrochloride and to caffeine.

Free salicylic acid—
Ferric chloride-urea reagent—Dissolve by swirling, without the aid of heat, 60 g of urea in a mixture of 8 mL of ferric chloride solution (6 in 10) and 42 mL of 0.05 N hydrochloric acid. Adjust this solution, if necessary, with 6 N hydrochloric acid to a pH of 3.2.
Standard preparation—Transfer 15.0 mg of USP Salicylic Acid RS, accurately weighed, to a 100-mL volumetric flask, add chloroform to volume, and mix. Transfer 10.0 mL of this solution to a 100-mL volumetric flask containing 20 mL of methanol, 4 drops of hydrochloric acid, and 20 mL of a 1 in 10 solution of glacial acetic acid in ether, dilute with chloroform to volume, and mix.
Test preparation—Pack a pledget of glass wool in the base of a 25- × 200-mm chromatographic tube. In a beaker, prepare a mixture of 6 g of chromatographic siliceous earth, 2 mL of freshly prepared *Ferric chloride-urea reagent*, and 40 mL of chloroform. Transfer the mixture to the chromatographic tube. Rinse the beaker with 15 mL of chloroform, transfer to the column, and pack tightly. Place a small amount of glass wool at the top of the column. Weigh accurately a quantity of the finely powdered contents of Capsules, equivalent to about 50 mg of aspirin, mix with 10 mL of chloroform by stirring for 3 minutes, and transfer to the chromatographic column with the aid of 10 mL of chloroform. Pass 40 mL of chloroform through the column, rinse the tip of the chromatographic tube with chloroform, and discard the eluate. Prepare as a receiver a 100-mL volumetric flask containing 20 mL of methanol and 4 drops of hydrochloric acid, and elute any salicylic acid from the column with 20 mL of a 1 in 10 solution of glacial acetic acid in ether that recently has been saturated with water, followed by 30 mL of chloroform. Dilute the eluate with chloroform to volume, and mix.
Procedure—Concomitantly determine the absorbances of the *Standard preparation* and the *Test preparation* in 1-cm cells at the wavelength of maximum absorbance at about 306 nm, with a suitable spectrophotometer, using as the blank a solvent mixture of the same composition as that used for the *Standard preparation*: the absorbance of the *Test preparation* does not exceed that of the *Standard preparation* (3.0%, calculated on the basis of the labeled content of aspirin).

Assay for propoxyphene hydrochloride and caffeine—
Internal standard solution—Dissolve *n*-tricosane in chloroform to obtain a solution having a concentration of about 0.6 mg per mL.
Standard preparation—Transfer to a 50-mL volumetric flask accurately weighed quantities of about 32 mg of USP Propoxyphene Hydrochloride RS, about 32*J* mg of USP Aspirin RS, and about 32*J'* mg of USP Caffeine RS, where *J* is the ratio of the labeled amount, in mg, of aspirin to the labeled amount, in mg, of propoxyphene hydrochloride per Capsule, and *J'* is the ratio of the labeled amount, in mg, of caffeine to the labeled amount, in mg, of propoxyphene hydrochloride per Capsule. Add 10 mL of acetone, and swirl to dissolve the reference standards completely. Dilute with water to volume, and mix.
Assay preparation—Remove as completely as possible the contents of 20 Capsules, and transfer an accurately weighed portion of the powder, equivalent to 65 mg of propoxyphene hydrochloride, to a 100-mL volumetric flask containing 20 mL of acetone. If the Capsules contain a pellet (propoxyphene hydrochloride) as well as a powder, finely grind the pellets, then mix with the powder before proceeding. Sonicate for about 1 minute. Dilute the milky solution with water to volume, and mix. Filter, discarding the first 20 mL of the filtrate.
Procedure for propoxyphene hydrochloride and *caffeine*—Transfer 5.0-mL aliquots of the *Assay preparation* and the *Standard preparation* to separate 60-mL separators. To each add 5.0 mL of sodium carbonate solution (1 in 5) and 5.0 mL of *Internal standard solution*. Shake vigorously for 5 minutes, and allow the layers to separate. Drain the chloroform layer through phase-separating paper, suitably supported in a funnel, into a screw-capped test tube. Extract with one 5-mL portion of chloroform, and drain the chloroform layer through phase-separating paper. Evaporate the combined chloroform extracts, using a stream of dry nitrogen, to a final volume of about 2 mL. Inject separately a suitable volume, equivalent to about 6.4 μg of propoxyphene, of the chloroform extracts from the *Assay preparation* and the *Standard preparation* into a suitable gas chromatograph equipped with a flame-ionization detector. The column is typically 60 cm × 3 mm and is packed with 3% methyl phenyl silicone, liquid phase on 80- to 100-mesh chromatographic siliceous earth. The temperature of the injection port is 200°, the column temperature is 175°, and the carrier gas, nitrogen, has a flow rate of about 60 mL per minute. Relative retention times are about 0.65 for caffeine, 1.0 for the internal standard, and 1.7 for propoxyphene. In a suitable chromatogram, the resolution factor is not less than 1.0 between any two peaks, the relative standard deviation for five replicate injections of the *Standard preparation* is not more than 2.0, and the tailing factor for caffeine is not greater than 1.5. Calculate the quantities, in mg, of propoxyphene hydrochloride ($C_{22}H_{29}NO_2 \cdot HCl$) and caffeine ($C_8H_{10}N_4O_2$), respectively, in the portion taken for the *Assay preparation* by the same formula:

$$100C(R_U / R_S)$$

in which *C* is the concentration, in mg per mL, of the appropriate USP Reference Standard in the *Standard preparation*, and R_U and R_S are the ratios of the peak areas of the corresponding analyte to those of the internal standard obtained from the *Assay preparation* and the *Standard preparation*, respectively.

Assay for aspirin—

Sodium hydroxide reagent—Dissolve 1 g of polyoxyethylene (23) lauryl ether in about 100 mL of hot water contained in a 1000-mL volumetric flask. Dilute with water to about 600 mL, and dissolve 10 g of sodium hydroxide in this solution. Dilute with water to volume, and mix.

Ferric nitrate reagent—Mix 70 mL of nitric acid with about 600 mL of water contained in a 1000-mL volumetric flask. Dissolve 40 g of ferric nitrate [Fe(NO$_3$)$_3$ · 9H$_2$O] in this solution, dilute with water to volume, and mix.

Standard preparation and *Assay preparation*—Prepare as directed in the *Assay for propoxyphene hydrochloride and caffeine* to obtain solutions having concentrations of about 4 mg of aspirin per mL.

Procedure—Into separate 25-mL volumetric flasks pipet 2 mL each of the *Standard preparation* and the *Assay preparation*, and 2 mL of dilute acetone (1 in 5) to provide the blank. Into each flask pipet 5 mL of *Sodium hydroxide reagent*, mix by gentle swirling, and allow to stand at room temperature for 8 minutes. Dilute with *Ferric nitrate reagent* to volume, and mix. Concomitantly determine the absorbances of both solutions against the blank in 1-cm cells at the wavelength of maximum absorbance at about 530 nm, taking care to allow the solutions to reach an equilibrium temperature in the cell compartment. The color intensity is temperature-dependent. Calculate the quantity, in mg, of aspirin (C$_9$H$_8$O$_4$) in the portion taken for the *Assay preparation* by the formula:

$$100C(A_U / A_S)$$

in which C is the concentration, in mg per mL, of USP Aspirin RS in the *Standard preparation*, and A_U and A_S are the absorbances of the solutions from the *Assay preparation* and the *Standard preparation*, respectively.

Propoxyphene Napsylate

C$_{22}$H$_{29}$NO$_2$ · C$_{10}$H$_8$O$_3$S · H$_2$O   565.72
Benzeneethanol, α-[2-(dimethylamino)-1-methylethyl]-α-phenyl-, propanoate (ester), [S-(R*,S*)]-, compd. with 2-naphthalenesulfonic acid (1 : 1), monohydrate.
(αS,1R)-α-[2-(Dimethylamino)-1-methylethyl]-α-phenylphenethyl propionate compound with 2-naphthalenesulfonic acid (1 : 1) monohydrate   [*26570-10-5*].
Anhydrous   547.72   [*17140-78-2*].

» Propoxyphene Napsylate contains not less than 97.0 percent and not more than 103.0 percent of C$_{22}$H$_{29}$NO$_2$ · C$_{10}$H$_8$O$_3$S, calculated on the anhydrous basis.

Packaging and storage—Preserve in tight containers.

USP Reference standards ⟨11⟩—*USP Propoxyphene Napsylate RS. USP Propoxyphene Related Compound A RS. USP Propoxyphene Related Compound B RS.*

Identification—

A: *Infrared Absorption* ⟨197K⟩: previously dried at 105° for 3 hours.

B: *Ultraviolet Absorption* ⟨197U⟩—

Solution: 40 µg per mL.

Medium: methanol.

Absorptivities at 275 nm, calculated on the anhydrous basis, do not differ by more than 3.0%.

Melting range, *Class I* ⟨741⟩: between 158° and 165°, but the range between beginning and end of melting does not exceed 4°, determined after drying at 105° for 3 hours.

Specific rotation ⟨781S⟩: between +35° and +43°.
Test solution: 10 mg per mL, in chloroform.
Water, *Method I* ⟨921⟩: between 2.5% and 5.0%.
Residue on ignition ⟨281⟩: not more than 0.5%.
Heavy metals, *Method II* ⟨231⟩: 0.003%.
Related compounds—

Mobile phase and *Chromatographic system*—Proceed as directed in the *Assay*.

Standard stock solution—Accurately weigh about 10 mg each of USP Propoxyphene Related Compound A RS and USP Propoxyphene Related Compound B RS into a 50-mL volumetric flask, dissolve using 2 mL of methanol, dilute with *Mobile phase* to volume, and mix.

Standard solution—Transfer 5.0 mL of the *Standard stock solution* to a 50-mL volumetric flask, dilute with *Mobile phase* to volume, and mix.

System suitability solution—Dissolve an accurately weighed quantity of USP Propoxyphene Napsylate RS in *Standard solution*, and dilute quantitatively, and stepwise if necessary, to obtain a solution having known concentrations of about 4.5 mg per mL of USP Propoxyphene Napsylate RS, about 0.02 mg per mL of USP Propoxyphene Related Compound A RS, and about 0.02 mg per mL of USP Propoxyphene Related Compound B RS.

Test solution—Use the *Assay preparation*.

Chromatographic system—Chromatograph the *System suitability solution*, and record the peak responses as directed for *Procedure*: the relative retention times are about 0.63 for propoxyphene related compound A, 0.78 for propoxyphene related compound B, and 1.0 for propoxyphene napsylate; the resolution, R, between propoxyphene related compound B and propoxyphene related compound A is not less than 2.0; and the relative standard deviation for replicate injections is not more than 2.0%.

Procedure—Separately inject equal volumes (about 50 µL) of the *Standard solution* and the *Test solution* into the chromatograph, record the chromatograms, and measure the peak responses. Calculate the quantity, in mg, of propoxyphene related compound A in the portion of Propoxyphene Napsylate taken by the formula:

$$50C(491.67/319.88)(r_U / r_S)$$

in which C is the concentration, in mg per mL, of USP Propoxyphene Related Compound A RS in the *Standard solution*; 491.67 and 319.88 are the molecular weights of propoxyphene related compound A napsylate and propoxyphene related compound A, respectively; and r_U and r_S are the propoxyphene related compound A peak responses obtained from the *Test solution* and the *Standard solution*, respectively: not more than 0.5% of propoxyphene related compound A napsylate is found. Calculate the quantity, in mg, of propoxyphene related compound B napsylate in the portion of Propoxyphene Napsylate taken by the formula:

$$50C(533.71/325.45)(r_U / r_S)$$

in which C is the concentration, in mg per mL, of USP Propoxyphene Related Compound B RS in the *Standard solution*; 533.71 and 325.45 are the molecular weights of propoxyphene related compound B napsylate and propoxyphene related compound B, respectively; and r_U and r_S are the propoxyphene related compound B peak responses obtained from the *Test solution* and the *Standard solution*, respectively. Not more than 0.6% of propoxyphene related compound B napsylate is found.

Organic volatile impurities, *Method V* ⟨467⟩: meets the requirements.

Solvent—Use dimethyl sulfoxide.

(Official until July 1, 2008)

Assay—

0.1 M Monobasic ammonium phosphate buffer, pH 6.3—Dissolve 11.5 g of monobasic ammonium phosphate and 1.0 mL of triethylamine in 1000 mL of water, adjust with 10% sodium hydroxide to a pH of 6.3 ± 0.05, and mix.

Mobile phase—Prepare a filtered and degassed mixture of methanol and *0.1 M Monobasic ammonium phosphate buffer, pH 6.3* (67 : 33). Make adjustments if necessary (see *System Suitability* under *Chromatography* ⟨621⟩).

Standard preparation—Dissolve an accurately weighed quantity of USP Propoxyphene Napsylate RS in *Mobile phase* to obtain a solution having a known concentration of about 5.0 mg per mL.

Assay preparation—Transfer about 250 mg of Propoxyphene Napsylate, accurately weighed, to a 50-mL volumetric flask, dissolve in and dilute with *Mobile phase* to volume, and mix.

Chromatographic system (see *Chromatography* ⟨621⟩)—The liquid chromatograph is equipped with a 254-nm detector and a 3.9-mm × 30-cm column that contains packing L1. The flow rate is about 1.5 mL per minute. Chromatograph the *Standard preparation*, and record the peak responses as directed for *Procedure:* the retention time of propoxyphene napsylate is about 9 minutes; the tailing factor for the propoxyphene napsylate peak is not more than 3.5; and the relative standard deviation for replicate injections is not more than 2.0%.

Procedure—Separately inject equal volumes (about 50 µL) of the *Standard preparation* and the *Assay preparation* into the chromatograph, record the chromatograms, and measure the responses for the major peaks. Calculate the quantity, in mg, of $C_{22}H_{29}NO_2 \cdot C_{10}H_8O_3S$ in the portion of Propoxyphene Napsylate taken by the formula:

$$50C(r_U / r_S)$$

in which C is the concentration, in mg per mL, of USP Propoxyphene Napsylate RS in the *Standard preparation;* and r_U and r_S are the peak responses obtained from the *Assay preparation* and the *Standard preparation,* respectively.

Propoxyphene Napsylate Oral Suspension

» Propoxyphene Napsylate Oral Suspension contains not less than 90.0 percent and not more than 110.0 percent of the labeled amount of propoxyphene napsylate ($C_{22}H_{29}NO_2 \cdot C_{10}H_8O_3S \cdot H_2O$).

Packaging and storage—Preserve in tight containers, protected from light. Avoid freezing.

USP Reference standards ⟨11⟩—USP Propoxyphene Napsylate RS.

Identification—Transfer a volume of Oral Suspension, equivalent to about 100 mg of propoxyphene napsylate, to a small flask, mix with 10 mL of chloroform, and filter: the chloroform solution is dextrorotatory (see *Optical Rotation* ⟨781⟩).

Uniformity of dosage units ⟨905⟩—
FOR ORAL SUSPENSION PACKAGED IN SINGLE-UNIT CONTAINERS: meets the requirements.

Deliverable volume ⟨698⟩—
FOR ORAL SUSPENSION PACKAGED IN MULTIPLE-UNIT CONTAINERS: meets the requirements.

Alcohol content, *Method II* ⟨611⟩: between 0.5% and 1.5% of C_2H_5OH.

Assay—
Diethylamine phosphate buffer, Diluent, Mobile phase, Standard preparation, and *Chromatographic system*—Proceed as directed in the *Assay* under *Propoxyphene Napsylate Tablets.*

Assay preparation—Transfer an accurately weighed quantity of the well-mixed Oral Suspension, equivalent to about 50 mg of propoxyphene napsylate monohydrate, to a 100-mL volumetric flask. Dissolve in and dilute with a solution of acetonitrile in water (2 in 5) to volume, and mix. Further dilute 10.0 mL of the resulting solution to 50 mL with the solution of acetonitrile in water (2 in 5).

Procedure—Separately inject equal volumes (about 20 µL) of the *Standard preparation* and the *Assay preparation* into the chromatograph, record the chromatograms, and measure the areas for the propoxyphene peaks. Calculate the quantity, in mg, of propoxyphene napsylate ($C_{22}H_{29}NO_2 \cdot C_{10}H_8O_3S \cdot H_2O$) in each mL of the Oral Suspension taken by the formula:

$$(565.72/547.72)500C(D/W_U)(r_U / r_S)$$

in which 565.72 and 547.72 are the molecular weights of propoxyphene napsylate and anhydrous propoxyphene napsylate, respectively; C is the concentration, in mg per mL, of anhydrous USP Propoxyphene Napsylate RS in the *Standard preparation;* D is the density, in g per mL, of the Oral Suspension; W_U is the weight, in g, of the Oral Suspension taken; and r_U and r_S are the peak responses obtained from the *Assay preparation* and the *Standard preparation,* respectively.

Propoxyphene Napsylate Tablets

» Propoxyphene Napsylate Tablets contain not less than 90.0 percent and not more than 110.0 percent of the labeled amount of $C_{22}H_{29}NO_2 \cdot C_{10}H_8O_3S \cdot H_2O$.

Packaging and storage—Preserve in tight containers.

USP Reference standards ⟨11⟩—USP Propoxyphene Napsylate RS.

Identification—Transfer a portion of finely powdered Tablets, equivalent to about 100 mg of propoxyphene napsylate, to a small flask, and mix with 10 mL of chloroform. Add 10 mL of *pH 12.5 borate buffer* (prepared as directed in the *Assay* under *Propoxyphene Napsylate*), shake for 3 minutes, allow to stand until most of the emulsion has broken, and filter the chloroform solution: the chloroform solution is dextrorotatory (see *Optical Rotation* ⟨781⟩).

Dissolution ⟨711⟩—
Medium: pH 4.5 *acetate buffer*, prepared as directed in the *Dissolution* test under *Propoxyphene Hydrochloride, Aspirin, and Caffeine Capsules;* 500 mL.
Apparatus 1: 100 rpm.
Time: 60 minutes.
Determine the amount of $C_{22}H_{29}NO_2 \cdot C_{10}H_8O_3S \cdot H_2O$ dissolved by employing the following method.

Diethylamine phosphate buffer, Mobile phase, and *Chromatographic system*—Proceed as directed in the *Assay*.

Standard solution—Dissolve an accurately weighed quantity of USP Propoxyphene Napsylate RS in *Dissolution Medium* to obtain a solution having a known concentration of about 0.1 mg per mL.

Test solution—Quantitatively dilute a filtered portion of the solution under test with *Dissolution Medium* to obtain a solution having a concentration of about 0.1 mg of propoxyphene napsylate per mL.

Procedure—Separately inject equal volumes (about 20 µL) of the *Standard solution* and the *Test solution* into the chromatograph, record the chromatograms, and measure the areas for the propoxyphene peaks. Calculate the quantity, in mg, of $C_{22}H_{29}NO_2 \cdot C_{10}H_8O_3S \cdot H_2O$ dissolved by the formula:

$$(565.72 / 547.72)500CD(r_U / r_S)$$

in which 565.72 and 547.72 are the molecular weights of propoxyphene napsylate and anhydrous propoxyphene napsylate, respectively; C is the concentration, in mg per mL, of USP Propoxyphene Napsylate RS in the *Standard solution;* D is the dilution factor used to prepare the *Test solution;* and r_U and r_S are the peak responses obtained from the *Test solution* and the *Standard solution,* respectively.

Tolerances—Not less than 75% (*Q*) of the labeled amount of $C_{22}H_{29}NO_2 \cdot C_{10}H_8O_3S \cdot H_2O$ is dissolved in 60 minutes.

Uniformity of dosage units ⟨905⟩: meet the requirements.

Assay—
Diethylamine phosphate buffer—Mix 5.0 mL of diethylamine with 995 mL of water, and adjust with phosphoric acid to a pH of 3.2.

Diluent—Prepare a mixture of *Diethylamine phosphate buffer* and acetonitrile (4 : 1).

Mobile phase—Prepare a mixture of *Diethylamine phosphate buffer* and acetonitrile (3 : 2). Sonicate for 15 minutes, and pass through a filter having a 0.5-µm or finer porosity. Make adjustments if necessary (see *System Suitability* under *Chromatography* ⟨621⟩).

Standard preparation—Dissolve an accurately weighed quantity of USP Propoxyphene Napsylate RS in *Diluent* to obtain a solution having a known concentration of about 0.1 mg per mL.

Assay preparation—Weigh and finely powder not fewer than 20 Tablets. Transfer an accurately weighed portion of the powder, equivalent to about 5 Tablets, to a 1000-mL volumetric flask. Dissolve in and dilute with *Diluent* to volume, and mix. Further dilute 10.0 mL of the resulting solution with *Diluent*, mix, and filter or centrifuge to obtain a clear solution having a concentration of about 0.1 mg per mL.

Chromatographic system (see *Chromatography* ⟨621⟩)—The liquid chromatograph is equipped with a 217-nm detector and a 3.9-mm × 30-cm column containing packing L1. The flow rate is about 1 mL per minute. Chromatograph the *Standard preparation*, and record the responses as directed for *Procedure*: the tailing factor is not more than 1.5; and the relative standard deviation for replicate injections is not more than 2.0%.

Procedure—Separately inject equal volumes (about 20 µL) of the *Standard preparation* and the *Assay preparation* into the chromatograph, record the chromatograms, and measure the areas for the propoxyphene peaks. Calculate the quantity, in mg, of propoxyphene napsylate ($C_{22}H_{29}NO_2 \cdot C_{10}H_8O_3S \cdot H_2O$) in the portion of the Tablets taken by the formula:

$$(565.72 / 547.72)1000CD(r_U / r_S)$$

in which 565.72 and 547.72 are the molecular weights of propoxyphene napsylate monohydrate and anhydrous propoxyphene napsylate, respectively; C is the concentration, in mg per mL, of USP Propoxyphene Napsylate RS in the *Standard preparation*; D is the dilution factor used to prepare the *Assay preparation*; and r_U and r_S are the responses obtained from the *Assay preparation* and the *Standard preparation*, respectively.

Propoxyphene Napsylate and Acetaminophen Tablets

» Propoxyphene Napsylate and Acetaminophen Tablets contain not less than 90.0 percent and not more than 110.0 percent of the labeled amounts of propoxyphene napsylate ($C_{22}H_{29}NO_2 \cdot C_{10}H_8O_3S \cdot H_2O$) and acetaminophen ($C_8H_9NO_2$).

Packaging and storage—Preserve in tight containers, at controlled room temperature.

USP Reference standards ⟨11⟩—*USP Acetaminophen RS. USP Propoxyphene Napsylate RS.*

Identification—

A: Transfer the finely ground contents of 1 Tablet to a test tube, add 5 mL of methanol, shake for 5 minutes, and centrifuge. Use the clear supernatant as the test solution. Prepare a Standard solution in methanol containing, in each mL, about 20 mg of USP Propoxyphene Napsylate RS and 130 mg of USP Acetaminophen RS. Apply 10 µL of the test solution on a line parallel to and about 2 cm from the bottom edge of a 20- × 5-cm thin-layer chromatographic plate (see *Chromatography* ⟨621⟩) coated with chromatographic silica gel mixture, and apply 10 µL of the Standard solution separately on the starting line. Place the plate in a developing chamber containing a mixture of chloroform, butyl acetate, and formic acid (50 : 50 : 20), and develop the chromatogram until the solvent front has moved about 15 cm above the line of application. Remove the plate, allow to dry in a hood, and view under short-wavelength UV light: the solution under test exhibits two principal spots having intensities and R_F values identical to those of the two principal spots obtained from the Standard solution.

B: The retention time of the major peak for propoxyphene in the chromatogram of the *Assay preparation* corresponds to that in the chromatogram of the *Standard preparation*, as obtained in the *Assay for propoxyphene napsylate*.

C: The retention time of the major peak for acetaminophen in the chromatogram of the *Assay preparation* corresponds to that in the chromatogram of the *Standard preparation*, as obtained in the *Assay for acetaminophen*.

Dissolution ⟨711⟩—

Medium: pH 4.5 acetate buffer, prepared as directed in the test for *Dissolution* under *Propoxyphene Hydrochloride, Aspirin, and Caffeine Capsules*; 500 mL.

Apparatus 1: 100 rpm.

Time: 60 minutes.

Determine the amount of propoxyphene napsylate monohydrate ($C_{22}H_{29}NO_2 \cdot C_{10}H_8O_3S \cdot H_2O$) dissolved by employing the following method.

Diethylamine phosphate buffer, Mobile phase, and *Chromatographic system*—Proceed as directed in the *Assay* under *Propoxyphene Napsylate Tablets*.

Standard solution—Transfer about 10 mg of USP Propoxyphene Napsylate RS and about 10J mg of USP Acetaminophen RS, both accurately weighed, to a 100-mL volumetric flask, J being the ratio of the labeled amount, in mg, of acetaminophen to the labeled amount, in mg, of propoxyphene napsylate in each Tablet. Dissolve in and dilute with *Dissolution Medium* to volume, and mix. This solution contains about 0.1 mg of USP Propoxyphene Napsylate RS and 0.1J mg of USP Acetaminophen RS per mL. [NOTE—Retain a portion of this solution for use in preparing the *Standard solution* when determining the amount of acetaminophen dissolved.]

Test solution and *Procedure*—Proceed as directed in the *Dissolution* test under *Propoxyphene Napsylate Tablets*.

Determine the amount of acetaminophen ($C_8H_9NO_2$) dissolved by employing the following method.

Diethylamine phosphate buffer—Prepare as directed in the *Assay* under *Propoxyphene Napsylate Tablets*.

Mobile phase, Chromatographic system, and *Procedure*—Proceed as directed in the *Assay for acetaminophen*.

Standard solution A—Transfer 10.0 mL of the *Standard solution* to a 100-mL volumetric flask, dilute with *Dissolution Medium* to volume, and mix. This solution contains about 0.01J mg of USP Acetaminophen RS per mL.

Test solution A—Quantitatively dilute a filtered portion of the solution under test with *Dissolution Medium* to obtain a solution having a concentration of about 0.01J mg of acetaminophen per mL.

Tolerances—Not less than 75% (*Q*) of the labeled amounts of $C_{22}H_{29}NO_2 \cdot C_{10}H_8O_3S \cdot H_2O$ and $C_8H_9NO_2$ is dissolved in 60 minutes.

Uniformity of dosage units ⟨905⟩: meet the requirements for *Content Uniformity* with respect to propoxyphene napsylate and acetaminophen.

Assay for propoxyphene napsylate—

Diethylamine phosphate buffer, Diluent, Mobile phase, and *Chromatographic system*—Proceed as directed in the *Assay* under *Propoxyphene Napsylate Tablets*.

Standard preparation—Transfer about 10 mg of USP Propoxyphene Napsylate RS and about 10J mg of USP Acetaminophen RS, both accurately weighed, to a 100-mL volumetric flask, J being the ratio of the labeled amount, in mg, of acetaminophen to the labeled amount, in mg, of propoxyphene napsylate in each Tablet. Dissolve in and dilute with *Diluent* to volume, and mix. This solution contains about 0.1 mg of USP Propoxyphene Napsylate RS and 0.1J mg of USP Acetaminophen RS per mL. [NOTE—Retain a portion of the *Standard preparation* for use in the *Assay for acetaminophen*.]

Assay preparation and *Procedure*—Proceed as directed in the *Assay* under *Propoxyphene Napsylate Tablets*. [NOTE—Retain a portion of the *Assay preparation* for use in the *Assay for acetaminophen*.]

Assay for acetaminophen—

Diethylamine phosphate buffer—Prepare as directed in the *Assay* under *Propoxyphene Napsylate Tablets*.

Mobile phase—Prepare a mixture of *Diethylamine phosphate buffer* and acetonitrile (4 : 1). Sonicate for 15 minutes, and pass through a filter having a 0.5-µm or finer porosity. Make adjustments if necessary (see *System Suitability* under *Chromatography* ⟨621⟩).

Standard preparation—Transfer 10.0 mL of the *Standard preparation* prepared as directed in the *Assay for propoxyphene napsylate* to a 100-mL volumetric flask, dilute with *Mobile phase* to volume, and mix. This solution contains about 0.01*J* mg of USP Acetaminophen RS per mL.

Assay preparation—Transfer 10.0 mL of the *Assay preparation* prepared as directed in the *Assay for propoxyphene napsylate* to a 100-mL volumetric flask, dilute with *Mobile phase* to volume, and mix.

Chromatographic system (see *Chromatography* ⟨621⟩)—The liquid chromatograph is equipped with a 245-nm detector and a 3.9-mm × 30-cm column containing packing L1. The flow rate is about 1 mL per minute. Chromatograph the *Standard preparation*, and record the responses as directed for *Procedure*: the tailing factor is not more than 1.5; and the relative standard deviation for replicate injections is not more than 2.0%.

Procedure—Separately inject equal volumes (about 20 µL) of the *Standard preparation* and the *Assay preparation* into the chromatograph, record the chromatograms, and measure the areas for the acetaminophen peaks. Calculate the quantity, in mg, of acetaminophen ($C_8H_9NO_2$) in the portion of Tablets taken by the formula:

$$5000CD(r_U/r_S)$$

in which *C* is the concentration, in mg per mL, of USP Acetaminophen RS in the *Standard preparation*; *D* is the dilution factor used to prepare the *Assay preparation* in the *Assay for propoxyphene napsylate*; and r_U and r_S are the peak responses obtained from the *Assay preparation* and the *Standard preparation*, respectively.

Propoxyphene Napsylate and Aspirin Tablets

» Propoxyphene Napsylate and Aspirin Tablets contain not less than 90.0 percent and not more than 110.0 percent of the labeled amounts of propoxyphene napsylate ($C_{22}H_{29}NO_2 \cdot C_{10}H_8O_3S \cdot H_2O$) and aspirin ($C_9H_8O_4$).

Packaging and storage—Preserve in tight containers, at controlled room temperature.
USP Reference standards ⟨11⟩—*USP Propoxyphene Napsylate RS. USP Aspirin RS. USP Salicylic Acid RS.*
Identification—
A: Transfer the finely ground contents of 1 Tablet to a test tube, add 5 mL of methanol, shake for 5 minutes, and centrifuge. Use the clear supernatant as the *Test solution*. Prepare a *Standard solution* in methanol containing, in each mL, about 65 mg of USP Aspirin RS and 20 mg of USP Propoxyphene Napsylate RS. Apply 10 µL of the *Test solution* on a line parallel to and about 2 cm from the bottom edge of a 20- × 5-cm thin-layer chromatographic plate (see *Chromatography* ⟨621⟩) coated with chromatographic silica gel mixture, and apply 10 µL of the *Standard solution* separately on the starting line. Place the plate in a developing chamber containing a mixture of chloroform, butyl acetate, and formic acid (60 : 40 : 20), and develop the chromatogram until the solvent front has moved about 15 cm above the line of application. Remove the plate, allow to dry in a hood, and view under short-wavelength UV light: the solution under test exhibits two principal spots having intensities and R_F values identical to those of the two principal spots obtained from the *Standard solution*.
B: The *Assay preparation* prepared as directed in the *Assay* is dextrorotatory.
Dissolution ⟨711⟩—
Medium: pH 4.5 acetate buffer, prepared as directed in the test for *Dissolution* under *Propoxyphene Hydrochloride, Aspirin, and Caffeine Capsules*; 500 mL.
Apparatus 1: 100 rpm.
Time: 60 minutes.
Determination of dissolved propoxyphene napsylate—
Internal standard solution and *pH 9.0 buffer*—Prepare as directed in the test for *Dissolution* under *Propoxyphene Hydrochloride, Aspirin, and Caffeine Capsules*.

Standard preparation and *Procedure*—Proceed as directed in the test for *Dissolution* under *Propoxyphene Napsylate Tablets*.
Determination of dissolved aspirin—Proceed as directed for *Determination of dissolved aspirin* in the test for *Dissolution* under *Propoxyphene Hydrochloride, Aspirin, and Caffeine Capsules*.
Tolerances—Not less than 75% (*Q*) of the labeled amount of $C_{22}H_{29}NO_2 \cdot C_{10}H_8O_3S \cdot H_2O$ and not less than 75% (*Q*) of the labeled amount of $C_9H_8O_4$ are dissolved in 60 minutes.
Uniformity of dosage units ⟨905⟩: meet the requirements for *Content Uniformity* with respect to propoxyphene napsylate.
Free salicylic acid—
Ferric chloride-urea reagent—Dissolve by swirling, without the aid of heat, 60 g of urea in a mixture of 8 mL of ferric chloride solution (6 in 10) and 42 mL of 0.05 N hydrochloric acid. Adjust this solution by the addition of 6 N hydrochloric acid to a pH of 3.2, if necessary.
Standard preparation—Transfer 15.0 mg of USP Salicylic Acid RS, accurately weighed, to a 100-mL volumetric flask, add chloroform to volume, and mix. Transfer 10.0 mL of this solution to a 100-mL volumetric flask containing 20 mL of methanol, 4 drops of hydrochloric acid, and 20 mL of a 1 in 10 solution of glacial acetic acid in ether, dilute with chloroform to volume, and mix.
Test preparation—Pack a pledget of glass wool in the base of a 25- × 200-mm chromatographic tube. In a beaker, prepare a mixture of 6 g of chromatographic siliceous earth, 2 mL of freshly prepared *Ferric chloride-urea reagent*, and 40 mL of chloroform. Transfer the mixture to the chromatographic tube. Rinse the beaker with 15 mL of chloroform, transfer to the column, and pack tightly. Place a small amount of glass wool at the top of the column. Weigh accurately a quantity of the finely powdered contents of Tablets, equivalent to about 50 mg of aspirin, mix with 10 mL of chloroform by stirring for 3 minutes, and transfer with the aid of 10 mL of chloroform to the chromatographic column. Pass 40 mL of chloroform through the column, rinse the tip of the chromatographic tube with chloroform, and discard the eluate. Prepare as a receiver a 100-mL volumetric flask containing 20 mL of methanol and 4 drops of hydrochloric acid, and elute any salicylic acid from the column by passing 20 mL of a 1 in 10 solution of glacial acetic acid in ether that recently has been saturated with water, followed by 30 mL of chloroform. Dilute the eluate with chloroform to volume, and mix.
Procedure—Concomitantly determine the absorbances of the *Standard preparation* and the *Test preparation* in 1-cm cells at the wavelength of maximum absorbance at about 306 nm, with a suitable spectrophotometer, using as the blank a solvent mixture of the same composition as that used for the *Standard preparation*: the absorbance of the *Test preparation* does not exceed that of the *Standard preparation* (3.0%, calculated on the basis of the labeled content of aspirin).
Assay for propoxyphene napsylate—
Internal standard solution—Dissolve *n*-tricosane in chloroform to obtain a solution containing about 0.6 mg per mL.
Standard preparation—Transfer 50 mg of USP Propoxyphene Napsylate RS and 163 mg of USP Aspirin RS, all accurately weighed, to a 50-mL volumetric flask. Add 10 mL of acetone, and swirl to dissolve the Reference Standards completely. Dilute with water to volume, and mix.
Assay preparation—Weigh and finely powder not fewer than 20 Tablets. Transfer an accurately weighed portion of the powder, equivalent to about 100 mg of propoxyphene napsylate, to a 100-mL volumetric flask containing 20 mL of acetone, and sonicate for about 1 minute. Dilute the milky solution with water to volume, mix, and filter, discarding the first 20 mL of the filtrate.
Procedure—Transfer 5.0-mL aliquots of the *Assay preparation* and the *Standard preparation* to separate 60-mL containers. To each add 5.0 mL of sodium carbonate solution (1 in 5) and 5.0 mL of *Internal standard solution*. Shake vigorously for 5 minutes, and allow the layers to separate. Drain the chloroform layer through phase-separating paper, suitably supported in a funnel, into a screw-capped test tube. Extract with one 5-mL portion of chloroform, and drain the chloroform layer through phase-separating paper. Evaporate the combined chloroform extracts, using a stream of dry nitrogen, to a final volume of about 2 mL. Inject separately a suitable volume, equivalent to about 6.4 µg of propoxyphene, of the chloroform extracts from the *Assay preparation* and the *Standard preparation* into a suitable gas chromatograph equipped with a flame-ion-

ization detector. The column is typically 120 cm × 3 mm and is packed with 3% phase G3 on support S1A. The temperature of the injection port is 200°, the column temperature is 175°, and the carrier gas is nitrogen flowing at the rate of about 60 mL per minute. Relative retention times are 1.0 for the internal standard, and 1.7 for propoxyphene. In a suitable chromatogram, the resolution factor is not less than 1.0 and the relative standard deviation for five replicate injections of the *Standard preparation* is not more than 2.0. Calculate the quantity, in mg, of $C_{22}H_{29}NO_2 \cdot C_{10}H_8O_3S \cdot H_2O$ in the portion of Tablets taken by the formula:

$$(565.72 / 547.72)(100C)(R_U / R_S)$$

in which 565.72 and 547.72 are the molecular weights of propoxyphene napsylate monohydrate and anhydrous propoxyphene napsylate, respectively, C is the concentration, in mg per mL, of anhydrous propoxyphene napsylate in the *Standard preparation*, as determined from the concentration of USP Propoxyphene Napsylate RS corrected for moisture content by a titrimetric water determination, and R_U and R_S are the peak response ratios obtained from the *Assay preparation* and the *Standard preparation*, respectively.

Assay for aspirin—

Sodium hydroxide reagent—Dissolve 1 g of polyoxyethylene (23) lauryl ether in about 100 mL of hot water contained in a 1000-mL volumetric flask. Dilute with water to about 600 mL, and dissolve 10 g of sodium hydroxide in this solution. Dilute with water to volume, and mix.

Ferric nitrate reagent—Mix 70 mL of nitric acid with about 600 mL of water contained in a 1000-mL volumetric flask. Dissolve 40 g of ferric nitrate [$Fe(NO_3)_3 \cdot 9H_2O$] in this solution, dilute with water to volume, and mix.

Standard preparation and *Assay preparation*—Prepare as directed in the *Assay for propoxyphene napsylate.*

Procedure—Into separate 25-mL volumetric flasks pipet 2 mL each of the *Standard preparation* and the *Assay preparation*, and 2 mL of dilute acetone (2 in 10) to provide the blank. Into each flask pipet 5 mL of *Sodium hydroxide reagent*, mix by gentle swirling, and allow to stand at room temperature for 8 minutes. Dilute with *Ferric nitrate reagent* to volume, and mix. Concomitantly determine the absorbances of both solutions against the blank in 1-cm cells at the wavelength of maximum absorbance at about 530 nm, taking care to allow the solutions to reach an equilibrium temperature in the cell compartment. The color intensity is temperature-dependent. Calculate the quantity, in mg, of $C_9H_8O_4$ in the portion taken for the *Assay preparation* by the formula:

$$100C(A_U / A_S)$$

in which C is the concentration, in mg per mL, of USP Aspirin RS in the *Standard preparation*, and A_U and A_S are the absorbances of the solutions from the *Assay preparation* and *Standard preparation*, respectively.

Propranolol Hydrochloride

$C_{16}H_{21}NO_2 \cdot HCl$ 295.80

2-Propanol, 1-[(1-methylethyl)amino]-3-(1-naphthalenyloxy)-, hydrochloride, (±)-.

(±)-1-(Isopropylamino)-3-(1-naphthyloxy)-2-propanol hydrochloride [*318-98-9*].

» Propranolol Hydrochloride contains not less than 98.0 percent and not more than 101.5 percent of $C_{16}H_{21}NO_2 \cdot HCl$, calculated on the dried basis.

Packaging and storage—Preserve in well-closed containers. Store at 25°, excursions permitted between 15° and 30°.

USP Reference standards ⟨11⟩—*USP Propranolol Hydrochloride RS.*

Identification—

A: *Infrared Absorption* ⟨197M⟩.

B: The retention time of the major peak for propranolol in the chromatogram of the *Assay preparation* corresponds to that in the chromatogram of the *Standard preparation,* as obtained in the *Assay.*

C: It responds to the tests for *Chloride* ⟨191⟩.

Melting range, *Class Ia* ⟨741⟩: between 162° and 165°.

Specific rotation ⟨781S⟩: between −1.0° and +1.0°.

Test solution: 40 mg per mL, in water.

Loss on drying ⟨731⟩—Dry it at 105° for 4 hours: it loses not more than 0.5% of its weight.

Residue on ignition ⟨281⟩: not more than 0.1%.

Organic volatile impurities, *Method I* ⟨467⟩: meets the requirements.

(Official until July 1, 2008)

Assay—

Mobile phase—Dissolve 0.5 g of sodium dodecyl sulfate in 18 mL of 0.15 M phosphoric acid, add 90 mL of acetonitrile and 90 mL of methanol, dilute with water to make 250 mL, mix, and pass through a filter having a 0.5-μm or finer porosity. Make adjustments if necessary (see *System Suitability* under *Chromatography* ⟨621⟩).

Standard preparation—Quantitatively dissolve an accurately weighed quantity of USP Propranolol Hydrochloride RS in methanol to obtain a stock solution having a known concentration of about 1 mg per mL. Transfer 5.0 mL of this solution to a 25-mL volumetric flask, dilute with methanol to volume, mix, and pass through a filter having a 0.7-μm or finer porosity. This solution contains about 0.2 mg of USP Propranolol Hydrochloride RS per mL.

Resolution solution—Prepare a solution of procainamide hydrochloride in methanol containing about 0.25 mg per mL. Transfer 5 mL of this solution and 5 mL of the stock solution used to prepare the *Standard preparation* to a 25-mL volumetric flask, dilute with methanol to volume, and mix.

Assay preparation—Transfer about 50 mg of Propranolol Hydrochloride, accurately weighed, to a 50-mL volumetric flask, add 45 mL of methanol, shake, and sonicate for 5 minutes. Dilute with methanol to volume, mix, and pass through a filter having a 0.7-μm or finer porosity. Transfer 5.0 mL of this solution to a 25-mL volumetric flask, dilute with methanol to volume, and mix.

Chromatographic system (see *Chromatography* ⟨621⟩)—The liquid chromatograph is equipped with a 290-nm detector and a 4.6-mm × 25-cm column that contains 5-μm packing L7. The flow rate is about 1.5 mL per minute. Chromatograph the *Resolution solution,* and record the peak responses as directed for *Procedure:* the relative retention times are about 0.6 for procainamide and 1.0 for propranolol; and the resolution, *R,* between the procainamide and the propranolol peaks is not less than 2.0. Chromatograph the *Standard preparation,* and record the peak responses as directed for *Procedure:* the tailing factor for the propranolol peak is not more than 3.0; and the relative standard deviation for replicate injections is not more than 2.0%.

Procedure—Separately inject equal volumes (about 20 μL) of the *Standard preparation* and the *Assay preparation* into the chromatograph, record the chromatograms, and measure the responses for the major peaks. Calculate the quantity, in mg, of $C_{16}H_{21}NO_2 \cdot HCl$ in the portion of Propranolol Hydrochloride taken by the formula:

$$250C(r_U / r_S)$$

in which C is the concentration, in mg per mL, of USP Propranolol Hydrochloride RS in the *Standard preparation;* and r_U and r_S are the propranolol peak responses obtained from the *Assay preparation* and the *Standard preparation,* respectively.

Propranolol Hydrochloride Extended-Release Capsules

» Propranolol Hydrochloride Extended-Release Capsules contain not less than 90.0 percent and not more than 110.0 percent of the labeled amount of propranolol hydrochloride ($C_{16}H_{21}NO_2 \cdot HCl$).

Packaging and storage—Preserve in well-closed containers.
Labeling—The labeling states the *Dissolution Test* with which the product complies.
USP Reference standards ⟨11⟩—*USP Propranolol Hydrochloride RS.*
Identification—Transfer the contents of a number of Capsules, equivalent to about 160 mg of propranolol hydrochloride, to a glass mortar. Add about 5 mL of water, and triturate the mixture with a glass pestle. Transfer the suspension to a centrifuge tube with the aid of about 10 mL of water. Add 1 mL of 1 N sodium hydroxide, and mix. Add 15 mL of ether, and shake by mechanical means for about 5 minutes. Centrifuge the mixture, and transfer as much of the ether layer as possible to a second centrifuge tube. Add 0.1 mL of hydrochloric acid to the ether extract, and shake. Centrifuge, and discard the ether layer. Add 15 mL of ether to the precipitate, and shake by mechanical means for about 5 minutes. Centrifuge, and discard the ether layer. Dry the precipitate in vacuum at about 45° for 30 minutes. Transfer a small amount of the dried precipitate to a mortar, and grind to a fine powder: the IR absorption spectrum of a mineral oil dispersion of the powder so obtained exhibits maxima only at the same wavelengths as that of a similar preparation of USP Propranolol Hydrochloride RS.

Dissolution ⟨711⟩—
TEST 1—If the product complies with this test, the labeling indicates that it meets USP *Dissolution Test 1*.
pH 1.2 Buffer solution—Dissolve 2.0 g of sodium chloride in water, add 7.0 mL of hydrochloric acid, dilute with water to 1 L, and mix.
pH 6.8 Buffer solution—Dissolve 21.72 g of anhydrous dibasic sodium phosphate and 4.94 g of citric acid monohydrate in water, dilute with water to 1 L, and mix.
Media—Proceed as directed under *Method B* for *Delayed-Release Dosage Forms*, using 900 mL of *pH 1.2 Buffer solution* during the *Acid stage*, run for 1.5 hours, and use the acceptance criteria given under *Acceptance Table 3*. For the *Buffer stage*, use 900 mL of *pH 6.8 Buffer solution*, run for the time specified, and use the acceptance criteria given under *Tolerances*.
Apparatus 1: 100 rpm.
Times: 1.5, 4, 8, 14, and 24 hours.
Procedure—Using filtered portions of the solution under test, diluted if necessary, determine the amount of $C_{16}H_{21}NO_2 \cdot HCl$ dissolved, using UV absorbances at the wavelength of maximum absorbance at about 320 nm, with respect to a baseline drawn from 355 nm through 340 nm, by comparison with a *Standard solution* in water having a known concentration of USP Propranolol Hydrochloride RS.
Tolerances—The percentages of the labeled amount of $C_{16}H_{21}NO_2 \cdot HCl$ dissolved at the times specified conform to *Acceptance Table 2*.

Time (hours)	Amount dissolved
1.5	not more than 30%
4	between 35% and 60%
8	between 55% and 80%
14	between 70% and 95%
24	between 81% and 110%

TEST 2—If the product complies with this test, the labeling indicates that it meets USP *Dissolution Test 2*.
pH 1.2 Buffer solution—Dissolve 2.0 g of sodium chloride in water, add 7.0 mL of hydrochloric acid, dilute with water to 1 L, and mix.
pH 7.5 Buffer solution—Dissolve 6.8 g of monobasic potassium phosphate and 1.6 g of sodium hydroxide in 900 mL of water, adjust with 1 N sodium hydroxide to a pH of 7.5, dilute with water to 1 L, and mix.
Media—Proceed as directed under *Method B* for *Delayed-Release Dosage Forms*, using 900 mL of *pH 1.2 Buffer solution* during the *Acid stage*, run for 1 hour, and use the acceptance criteria given under *Acceptance Table 3*. For the *Buffer stage*, use 900 mL of *pH 7.5 Buffer solution*, run for the time specified, and use the acceptance criteria given under *Tolerances*.
Apparatus 1: 50 rpm.
Times: 1, 3, 6, and 12 hours.
Procedure—Using filtered portions of the solution under test, diluted if necessary, determine the amount of $C_{16}H_{21}NO_2 \cdot HCl$ dissolved, using UV absorbances at the wavelength of maximum absorbance at about 320 nm, with respect to a baseline drawn from 355 nm through 340 nm, by comparison with a *Standard solution* in water having a known concentration of USP Propranolol Hydrochloride RS.
Tolerances—The percentages of the labeled amount of $C_{16}H_{21}NO_2 \cdot HCl$ dissolved at the times specified conform to *Acceptance Table 2*.

Time (hours)	Amount dissolved
1	not more than 20%
3	between 20% and 45%
6	between 45% and 80%
12	not less than 80%

Uniformity of dosage units ⟨905⟩: meet the requirements.
Procedure for content uniformity—Transfer the contents of 1 Capsule to a 100-mL volumetric flask, add about 70 mL of methanol, swirl occasionally for 30 minutes, and sonicate for about 1 minute, and then swirl occasionally for an additional 30 minutes. Dilute with methanol to volume, mix, and centrifuge a portion of the solution. Quantitatively dilute an accurately measured volume of the clear solution with methanol to obtain a solution containing about 40 µg of propranolol hydrochloride per mL. Concomitantly determine the absorbances of this solution and a *Standard solution* of USP Propranolol Hydrochloride RS in methanol having a known concentration of about 40 µg per mL, in 1-cm cells at the wavelength of maximum absorbance at about 290 nm, with a suitable spectrophotometer, using methanol as the blank. Calculate the quantity, in mg, of $C_{16}H_{21}NO_2 \cdot HCl$ in the Capsule taken by the formula:

$$(LC / D)(A_U / A_S)$$

in which *L* is the labeled quantity, in mg, of propranolol hydrochloride in the Capsule; *C* is the concentration, in µg per mL, of USP Propranolol Hydrochloride RS in the *Standard solution*; *D* is the concentration, in µg per mL, of the solution from the Capsule, based on the labeled quantity per Capsule and the extent of dilution; and A_U and A_S are the absorbances of the solution from the Capsule and the *Standard solution*, respectively.

Assay—
Phosphate buffer—Dissolve 13.6 g of monobasic potassium phosphate in 2 L of water, and mix. Pass the solution through a filter having a 0.5-µm or finer porosity before use.
Mobile phase—Prepare a suitable degassed mixture of *Phosphate buffer* and acetonitrile (650 : 350). Make adjustments if necessary (see *System Suitability* under *Chromatography* ⟨621⟩).
Diluting solvent—Mix 650 mL of water with 350 mL of acetonitrile.
Standard preparation—Dissolve an accurately weighed quantity of USP Propranolol Hydrochloride RS in methanol, and dilute quantitatively and stepwise with methanol to obtain a solution having a known concentration of about 200 µg per mL. Transfer 5.0 mL of this solution to a 50.0-mL volumetric flask, add *Diluting solvent* to volume, and mix.
Assay preparation—Transfer the contents of 10 Capsules, accurately counted, to a 500-mL volumetric flask. Add 300 mL of methanol, and swirl by mechanical means for 2 hours. Allow to stand for about 16 hours, then sonicate for one-half hour, and swirl for one-half hour. Quantitatively dilute with methanol to volume,

mix, and centrifuge a portion of the solution. Dilute an accurately measured volume of the clear solution with *Diluting solvent* to obtain a solution having a concentration of about 20 µg of propranolol hydrochloride per mL.

Chromatographic system (see *Chromatography* ⟨621⟩)—The liquid chromatograph is equipped with a 220-nm detector and a 4-mm × 15-cm column that contains 5-µm packing L1. The flow rate is about 2 mL per minute. Chromatograph the *Standard preparation*, and record the peak responses as directed for *Procedure*: the retention time of propranolol is about 5 to 9 minutes; the column efficiency determined from the analyte peak is not less than 1000 theoretical plates; the tailing factor for the analyte peak is not more than 3; and the relative standard deviation for replicate injections is not more than 2%.

Procedure—Separately inject equal volumes (about 20 µL) of the *Standard preparation* and the *Assay preparation* into the chromatograph, record the chromatograms, and measure the responses for the major peaks. Calculate the quantity, in mg, of propranolol hydrochloride ($C_{16}H_{21}NO_2 \cdot HCl$) in each Capsule taken by the formula:

$$(LC / D)(r_U / r_S)$$

in which L is the labeled quantity, in mg, of propranolol hydrochloride in each Capsule; C is the concentration, in µg per mL, of USP Propranolol Hydrochloride RS in the *Standard preparation*; D is the concentration, in µg of propranolol hydrochloride per mL, of the *Assay preparation*, based on the labeled quantity per Capsule, the number of Capsules taken, and the extent of dilution; and r_U and r_S are the peak responses obtained from the *Assay preparation* and the *Standard preparation*, respectively.

Propranolol Hydrochloride Injection

» Propranolol Hydrochloride Injection is a sterile solution of Propranolol Hydrochloride in Water for Injection. It contains not less than 90.0 percent and not more than 110.0 percent of the labeled amount of $C_{16}H_{21}NO_2 \cdot HCl$.

Packaging and storage—Preserve in single-dose, light-resistant containers, preferably of Type I glass.

USP Reference standards ⟨11⟩—*USP Propranolol Hydrochloride RS. USP Endotoxin RS.*
Identification—The chromatogram of the *Assay preparation* obtained as directed in the *Assay* exhibits a major peak for propranolol, the retention time of which corresponds to that exhibited in the chromatogram of the *Standard preparation* obtained as directed in the *Assay*.
Bacterial endotoxins ⟨85⟩—It contains not more than 55.6 USP Endotoxin Units per mg of propranolol hydrochloride.
pH ⟨791⟩: between 2.8 and 4.0.
Other requirements—It meets the requirements under *Injections* ⟨1⟩.
Assay—
Mobile phase, Standard preparation, Resolution solution, and *Chromatographic system*—Prepare as directed in the *Assay* under *Propranolol Hydrochloride*.
Assay preparation—Transfer an accurately measured volume of Injection, equivalent to about 5 mg of propranolol hydrochloride, to a 25-mL volumetric flask, dilute with methanol to volume, and mix.
Procedure—Proceed as directed for *Procedure* in the *Assay* under *Propranolol Hydrochloride*. Calculate the quantity, in mg, of $C_{16}H_{21}NO_2 \cdot HCl$ in each mL of the Injection taken by the formula:

$$25(C / V)(r_U / r_S)$$

in which C is the concentration, in mg per mL, of USP Propranolol Hydrochloride in the *Standard preparation*, V is the volume, in mL, of Injection taken, and r_U and r_S are the propranolol peak responses obtained from the *Assay preparation* and the *Standard preparation*, respectively.

Propranolol Hydrochloride Tablets

» Propranolol Hydrochloride Tablets contain not less than 90.0 percent and not more than 110.0 percent of the labeled amount of $C_{16}H_{21}NO_2 \cdot HCl$.

Packaging and storage—Preserve in well-closed, light-resistant containers.

USP Reference standards ⟨11⟩—*USP Propranolol Hydrochloride RS.*
Identification—The chromatogram of the *Assay preparation* obtained as directed in the *Assay* exhibits a major peak for propranolol, the retention time of which corresponds to that exhibited in the chromatogram of the *Standard preparation* obtained as directed in the *Assay*.
Dissolution ⟨711⟩—
Medium: dilute hydrochloric acid (1 in 100); 1000 mL.
Apparatus 1: 100 rpm.
Time: 30 minutes.
Procedure—Determine the amount of $C_{16}H_{21}NO_2 \cdot HCl$ dissolved from UV absorbances at the wavelength of maximum absorbance at about 289 nm of filtered portions of the solution under test, suitably diluted with *Medium*, if necessary, in comparison with a Standard solution having a known concentration of USP Propranolol Hydrochloride RS in the same medium.
Tolerances—Not less than 75% (*Q*) of the labeled amount of $C_{16}H_{21}NO_2 \cdot HCl$ is dissolved in 30 minutes.
Uniformity of dosage units ⟨905⟩: meet the requirements.
Procedure for content uniformity—Transfer 1 Tablet to a 100-mL volumetric flask, add 5 mL of dilute hydrochloric acid (1 in 100), and let stand, swirling occasionally, until it is disintegrated. Add about 70 mL of methanol, and sonicate for about 1 minute. Dilute with methanol to volume, mix, and centrifuge a portion of the solution. Dilute an aliquot of the clear solution quantitatively with methanol to provide a solution containing about 40 µg of propranolol hydrochloride per mL. Concomitantly determine the absorbances of this solution and of a solution of USP Propranolol Hydrochloride RS in methanol, at a known concentration of about 40 µg per mL, in 1-cm cells at the wavelength of maximum absorbance at about 290 nm, with a suitable spectrophotometer, using methanol as the blank. Calculate the quantity, in mg, of $C_{16}H_{21}NO_2 \cdot HCl$ in the Tablet by the formula:

$$(T / D)C(A_U / A_S)$$

in which T is the labeled quantity, in mg, of propranolol hydrochloride in the Tablet, D is the concentration, in µg per mL, of the solution from the Tablet, based on the labeled quantity per Tablet and the extent of dilution, C is the concentration, in µg per mL, of USP Propranolol Hydrochloride RS in the Standard solution, and A_U and A_S are the absorbances of the solution from the Tablet and the Standard solution, respectively.
Assay—
Mobile phase, Standard preparation, Resolution solution, and *Chromatographic system*—Prepare as directed in the *Assay* under *Propranolol Hydrochloride*.
Assay preparation—Weigh and finely powder not less than 20 Tablets. Transfer an accurately weighed portion of the powder, equivalent to about 50 mg of propranolol hydrochloride, to a 50-mL volumetric flask, add 40 mL of methanol, shake, and sonicate for 5 minutes. Dilute with methanol to volume, mix, and filter through a 0.7-µm or finer porosity filter. Transfer 5.0 mL of this solution to a 25-mL volumetric flask, dilute with methanol to volume, and mix.
Procedure—Proceed as directed for *Procedure* in the *Assay* under *Propranolol Hydrochloride*. Calculate the quantity, in mg, of $C_{16}H_{21}NO_2 \cdot HCl$ in the portion of Tablets taken by the formula:

$$250C(r_U / r_S)$$

in which C is the concentration, in mg per mL, of USP Propranolol Hydrochloride in the *Standard preparation*, and r_U and r_S are the propranolol peak responses obtained from the *Assay preparation* and the *Standard preparation*, respectively.

Propranolol Hydrochloride and Hydrochlorothiazide Extended-Release Capsules

» Propranolol Hydrochloride and Hydrochlorothiazide Extended-Release Capsules contain not less than 90.0 percent and not more than 110.0 percent of the labeled amounts of propranolol hydrochloride ($C_{16}H_{21}NO_2 \cdot HCl$) and hydrochlorothiazide ($C_7H_8ClN_3O_4S_2$).

Packaging and storage—Preserve in well-closed containers.
USP Reference standards ⟨11⟩—*USP Benzothiadiazine Related Compound A RS. USP Hydrochlorothiazide RS. USP Propranolol Hydrochloride RS.*
Identification—
A: Transfer the contents of a number of Capsules, equivalent to about 100 mg of hydrochlorothiazide, to a 20-mesh sieve. Break up any large lumps with the aid of a spatula, and collect the powder that passes through the sieve. [NOTE—Retain the material on the screen for *Identification* test *B*.] Transfer the powder that passed through the sieve to a screw-capped, 35-mL centrifuge tube, add 5 mL of solvent hexane, and shake for 5 minutes. Centrifuge, and discard the solvent. To the residue in the centrifuge tube add 10 mL of 1 N sodium hydroxide, shake, and filter, collecting the filtrate in a separator. Wash the filter with 5 mL of water, and collect the washing in the separator. Add 50 mL of ether to the separator, shake for 2 minutes, and allow the phases to separate. Drain the aqueous layer into a beaker, adjust with 6 N hydrochloric acid to a pH of about 2, induce crystallization by scratching the inner surface of the beaker with a glass rod, and allow to stand until crystallization is complete. Collect the crystals on a filter, and dry at 105° for 30 minutes. Grind the crystals to a fine powder: the IR absorption spectrum of a mineral oil dispersion of the powder so obtained exhibits maxima only at the same wavelengths as that of a similar preparation of USP Hydrochlorothiazide RS.
B: Wash the material retained on the screen from *Identification* test *A* with a small amount of water, discarding the washings. Transfer the particles remaining on the screen to a glass mortar, add about 5 mL of water, and triturate the mixture with a glass pestle. Transfer the suspension, with the aid of about 10 mL of water, to a 35-mL screw-capped centrifuge tube, add about 1 mL of 1 N sodium hydroxide, and mix. Add about 15 mL of ether, and shake by mechanical means for 5 minutes. Centrifuge the mixture, and transfer as much of the ether layer as possible to a second centrifuge tube. Add 0.1 mL of hydrochloric acid to the ether extract, and shake. Centrifuge, and discard the ether. Add about 15 mL of ether to the residue, and shake by mechanical means for 5 minutes. Centrifuge, and discard the ether layer. Dry the residue in vacuum at 45° for 30 minutes. Grind the crystals to a fine powder: the IR absorption spectrum of a mineral oil dispersion of the powder so obtained exhibits maxima only at the same wavelengths as that of a similar preparation of USP Propranolol Hydrochloride RS.
C: The retention times of the major peaks for propanolol hydrochloride and hydrochlorothiazide in the chromatogram of the *Assay preparation* correspond to those exhibited in the chromatogram of the *Standard preparation*, as obtained in the *Assay.*
Dissolution ⟨711⟩—
pH 1.5 Buffer solution, pH 6.8 Buffer solution, Media, and *Apparatus*—Proceed as directed in the test for *Dissolution* under *Propranolol Hydrochloride Extended-Release Capsules.*
Analytical method—Determine the amounts of hydrochlorothiazide ($C_7H_8ClN_3O_4S_2$) and propranolol hydrochloride ($C_{16}H_{21}NO_2 \cdot HCl$) dissolved, using the following method.
Standard stock solution A—Prepare a solution of USP Propranolol Hydrochloride RS in dilute hydrochloric acid (1 in 100) having a known concentration of about 0.4 mg per mL.
Standard stock solution B—Dissolve an accurately weighed quantity of USP Hydrochlorothiazide RS in 0.25 N sodium hydroxide to obtain a solution having a concentration of about 25 mg per mL. Quantitatively dilute this solution with water to obtain a solution having a known concentration of about 0.5 mg per mL.
Standard solution—Prepare, by combining aliquots of *Standard stock solutions A* and *B*, and diluting with dilute hydrochloric acid (1 in 100), solutions bracketing the expected concentration of the samples at the various time points.
Times: 30 minutes; 1.5, 4, 8, 14, and 24 hours.
Procedure—Use an automatic analyzer consisting of a liquid sampler, a proportioning pump, two UV spectrophotometers, and a manifold consisting of the components illustrated in the diagram under *Automated Methods of Analysis* ⟨16⟩. Start the sampler and conduct determinations at a rate of 30 per hour, using a ratio of about 1:1 for the sample to wash time. Calculate the amounts of $C_7H_8ClN_3O_4S_2$ and $C_{16}H_{21}NO_2 \cdot HCl$ dissolved by comparison with the *Standard solution.*
Tolerances (hydrochlorothiazide)—Use *Acceptance Table 1*. Not less than 80% (*Q*) of the labeled amount of $C_7H_8ClN_3O_4S_2$ is dissolved in 30 minutes.
Tolerances (propranolol hydrochloride)—The percentages of the labeled amount of $C_{16}H_{21}NO_2 \cdot HCl$ dissolved at the times specified conform to *Acceptance Table 2*.

Time (hours)	Amount dissolved (%)
1.5	not more than 30%
4	between 35% and 60%
8	between 55% and 80%
14	between 70% and 95%
24	between 83% and 108%

Uniformity of dosage units ⟨905⟩: meet the requirements for *Content Uniformity* with respect to propranolol hydrochloride and to hydrochlorothiazide.
Procedure for content uniformity—
Apparatus—Use an automatic analyzer consisting of (1) a 20-channel peristaltic pump; (2) an UV spectrophotometer equipped with a 10-mm flow cell and a 293-nm detector; (3) an UV spectrophotometer equipped with a 10-mm flow cell and a 273-nm detector; (4) recording devices for each of the two aforementioned detectors; and (5) a manifold consisting of components illustrated in the pertinent diagram in the chapter *Automated Methods of Analysis* ⟨16⟩.
Standard hydrochlorothiazide stock solution—Dissolve an accurately weighed quantity of USP Hydrochlorothiazide RS in methanol to obtain a solution having a known concentration of about 5 mg per mL.
Standard propranolol hydrochloride stock solution—Dissolve an accurately weighed quantity of USP Propranolol Hydrochloride RS in methanol to obtain a solution having a known concentration of about 5*J* mg per mL, *J* being the ratio of the labeled amount, in mg, of propranolol hydrochloride to the labeled amount, in mg, of hydrochlorothiazide per Capsule.
Standard preparation—Transfer 10.0 mL of the *Standard hydrochlorothiazide stock solution*, 10.0 mL of the *Standard propranolol hydrochloride stock solution*, and 10.0 mL of methanol to a 100-mL volumetric flask, dilute with 0.12 N hydrochloric acid to volume, and mix.
Test preparations—Transfer the contents of an appropriate number of individual Capsules to separate 100-mL volumetric flasks, rinsing each empty Capsule shell with 2 mL of methanol, and adding the rinsings to the respective volumetric flasks. Add 28 mL of methanol to each flask, and mix by mechanical means for 30 minutes. Dilute the contents of each flask with 0.12 N hydrochloric acid to volume, and mix.
Procedure—With the sampler in the standby position, pump all reagents through the system until a stable baseline is achieved. Activate the sampler, and allow one cycle to pass without introducing the *Standard preparation* or the *Test preparations*, then introduce a 5-mL portion of the *Standard preparation* into the sampler for the next two cycles and for every sixth cycle thereafter. Disregard the first value for the *Standard preparation*. Add the *Test preparations* to the sampler at the rate of 30 per hour, using a ratio of about 1:1 for the sample to wash time, to follow the second 5-mL portion of the *Standard preparation*. Record the absorbance values, and calculate each peak value by the difference between peak height and

baseline. Calculate the quantity, in mg, of hydrochlorothiazide ($C_7H_8ClN_3O_4S_2$) per Capsule taken by the formula:

$$100C(A_U/A_S)$$

in which C is the concentration, in mg per mL, of USP Hydrochlorothiazide RS in the *Standard preparation;* A_U is the absorbance at 273 nm of the individual *Test preparation;* and A_S is the averaged absorbance at 273 nm of the *Standard preparations.* Make any necessary correction of the results obtained as follows.
(1) Calculate the correction, F', by the formula:

$$F' = A/P'$$

in which A is the weight of active ingredient equivalent to 1 average dosage unit obtained by the *Assay* procedure; and P' is the weight of active ingredient equivalent to 1 average dosage unit calculated as the mean of the dosage units tested by the *Content Uniformity* procedure.
(2) If F' is between 0.970 and 1.030, no correction is required.
(3) If F' is not between 0.970 and 1.030, calculate the weight of active ingredient in each dosage unit by multiplying each of the weights found using the special procedure by F'.

Calculate the quantity, in mg, of propranolol hydrochloride ($C_{16}H_{21}NO_2 \cdot HCl$) per Capsule by the same formula, in which C is the concentration, in mg per mL, of USP Propranolol Hydrochloride RS in the *Standard preparation;* A_U is the absorbance at 293 nm of the individual *Test preparation;* and A_S is the averaged absorbance at 293 nm of the *Standard preparations.* Make any necessary correction of the results obtained as directed above.

Related compounds—

Tetrabutylammonium hydroxide solution, Buffer, Mobile phase, Standard preparation, and *Chromatographic system*—Prepare as directed in the *Assay.*

Standard solution—Transfer about 25 mg of USP Benzothiadiazine Related Compound A RS, accurately weighed, to a 200-mL volumetric flask, add 30 mL of methanol, and swirl to dissolve. Dilute with *Buffer* to volume, and mix. Dilute an accurately measured volume of this solution quantitatively, and stepwise if necessary, with *Mobile phase* to obtain a solution having a known concentration of about 0.5 μg per mL.

Test solution—Use the *Assay preparation* prepared as directed in the *Assay.*

Procedure—Proceed as directed for *Procedure* in the *Assay,* except to inject equal volumes (about 50 μL) of the *Standard solution* and the *Test solution.* Calculate the percentage of benzothiadiazine related compound A in the Capsules taken by the formula:

$$1000(C/NL)(r_U/r_S)$$

in which C is the concentration, in μg per mL, of USP Benzothiadiazine Related Compound A RS in the *Standard solution;* N is the number of Capsules taken to prepare the *Test solution;* L is the labeled amount, in mg, of hydrochlorothiazide in each Capsule taken; and r_U and r_S are the peak responses of benzothiadiazine related compound A obtained from the *Test solution* and the *Standard solution,* respectively: not more than 1.0% is present.

Assay—

Tetrabutylammonium hydroxide solution—Use a suitable aqueous or methanolic solution having a known concentration of tetrabutylammonium hydroxide.

Buffer—Dissolve 31.25 g of monobasic potassium phosphate in 500 mL of water in a 1000-mL volumetric flask. Add 18.75 mL of phosphoric acid, mix, and add a volume of *Tetrabutylammonium hydroxide solution* equivalent to about 13 g of tetrabutylammonium hydroxide. Dilute with water to volume, and mix. Dilute 100 mL of this solution with water to obtain 1000 mL of solution, adjusting, if necessary, with phosphoric acid or 10 N potassium hydroxide to a pH of 2.4 ± 0.1.

Mobile phase—Prepare a suitable mixture of *Buffer* and methanol (850 : 150). Make adjustments if necessary (see *System Suitability* under *Chromatography* ⟨621⟩).

Standard hydrochlorothiazide stock solution—Transfer about 25 mg of USP Hydrochlorothiazide RS, accurately weighed, to a 100-mL volumetric flask, add 15 mL of methanol, and sonicate for 5 minutes, adding ice to the bath, if necessary, to maintain the temperature at not more than 20°. Dilute with *Buffer* to volume, and mix. Use this solution within 3 days.

Standard propranolol hydrochloride stock solution—Dissolve an accurately weighed quantity of USP Propranolol Hydrochloride RS in *Mobile phase* to obtain a solution having a known concentration of about 0.25J mg per mL, J being the ratio of the labeled quantity, in mg, of propranolol hydrochloride to the labeled quantity, in mg, of hydrochlorothiazide per Capsule.

Standard preparation—Transfer 5.0 mL of *Standard hydrochlorothiazide stock solution* and 5.0 mL of *Standard propranolol hydrochloride stock solution* to a 25-mL volumetric flask, dilute with *Mobile phase* to volume, and mix. This solution contains about 50 μg of hydrochlorothiazide and 50Jμg of propranolol hydrochloride per mL. Use this solution within 3 days.

Assay preparation—Carefully open an accurately counted number of Capsules, equivalent to about 500 mg of hydrochlorothiazide, and transfer the contents and the Capsule shells to a 500-mL volumetric flask. Add 5.0 mL of water to the flask, and allow to stand for 5 minutes. Dilute with methanol to volume, mix, and sonicate for 10 minutes, adding ice to the bath, if necessary, to maintain the temperature at not more than 20°. Remove the flask from the bath, and shake it occasionally for 1 hour. Centrifuge a portion of the contents of the flask, if necessary, to obtain a clear solution. Transfer 5.0 mL of the clear solution to a 100-mL volumetric flask, add 10.0 mL of methanol, dilute with *Buffer* to volume, and mix.

Chromatographic system (see *Chromatography* ⟨621⟩)—The liquid chromatograph is equipped with a 220-nm detector and a 4-mm × 15-cm column that contains packing L1. The flow rate is about 1.5 mL per minute. Chromatograph the *Standard preparation,* and record the peak responses as directed for *Procedure:* the column efficiency determined from the propranolol peak is not less than 2500 theoretical plates when calculated by the formula:

$$5.545(t/W_{h/2})^2$$

the tailing factor for the hydrochlorothiazide and propranolol peaks is not more than 1.5; and the relative standard deviation for replicate injections is not more than 2.0%.

Procedure—Separately inject equal volumes (about 50 μL) of the *Standard preparation* and the *Assay preparation* into the chromatograph, record the chromatograms, and measure the areas for the major peaks. The retention time for propranolol is between 12 and 25 minutes; and the relative retention times are about 0.25 for benzothiadiazine related compound A, 0.4 for hydrochlorothiazide, and 1.0 for propranolol. Calculate the quantities, in mg, of hydrochlorothiazide ($C_7H_8ClN_3O_4S_2$) and propranolol hydrochloride ($C_{16}H_{21}NO_2 \cdot HCl$) in each Capsule taken by the same formula:

$$10(C/N)(r_U/r_S)$$

in which C is the concentration, in μg per mL, of USP Propranolol Hydrochloride RS or USP Hydrochlorothiazide RS in the *Standard preparation;* N is the number of Capsules taken to prepare the *Assay preparation;* and r_U and r_S are the peak responses of the corresponding analyte obtained from the *Assay preparation* and the *Standard preparation,* respectively.

Propranolol Hydrochloride and Hydrochlorothiazide Tablets

» Propranolol Hydrochloride and Hydrochlorothiazide Tablets contain not less than 90.0 percent and not more than 110.0 percent of the labeled amounts of propranolol hydrochloride ($C_{16}H_{21}NO_2 \cdot HCl$) and hydrochlorothiazide ($C_7H_8ClN_3O_4S_2$).

Packaging and storage—Preserve in well-closed containers.

USP Reference standards ⟨11⟩—*USP Benzothiadiazine Related Compound A RS. USP Hydrochlorothiazide RS. USP Propranolol Hydrochloride RS.*

Identification—

A: Infrared Absorption ⟨197M⟩—

Test specimen—Transfer a quantity of finely powdered Tablets, equivalent to about 100 mg of propranolol hydrochloride, to a 50-mL centrifuge tube, add 15 mL of water and 1 mL of 1 N sodium hydroxide, and mix. Add 20 mL of ether, cap the tube, and shake by mechanical means for 5 minutes. Centrifuge the mixture, and transfer as much of the ether layer as possible to a second centrifuge tube. Add 0.05 mL of hydrochloric acid to the ether extract, and shake. Centrifuge, and discard the ether layer. Add 20 mL of ether to the residue in the tube, and shake by mechanical means for 5 minutes. Centrifuge, and discard the ether layer. Dry the residue in the tube in vacuum at about 50° for 30 minutes. Transfer a small amount of the dried residue to a mortar, and grind to fine powder.

Standard specimen: a similar preparation of USP Propranolol Hydrochloride RS.

B: Infrared Absorption ⟨197M⟩—

Test specimen—Transfer a quantity of finely powdered Tablets, equivalent to about 100 mg of hydrochlorothiazide, to a 35-mL centrifuge tube, add 30 mL of acetone, mix, and allow to stand for 30 minutes, with occasional shaking. Centrifuge, and decant the acetone extract into a beaker, discarding the residue in the centrifuge tube. Evaporate the acetone extract on a steam bath to dryness, add 10 mL of 0.1 N sodium hydroxide, and mix, using a spatula to dislodge any residue from the beaker. Transfer the suspension to a 125-mL separator, and wash the beaker with about 5 mL of water, adding the washing to the separator. Add 50 mL of ether to the separator, shake for 2 minutes, and allow the phases to separate. Draw off the clear lower layer, filtering it into a beaker. Add 1 N hydrochloric acid dropwise with stirring until a pH of about 2 is reached. [NOTE—Precipitation occurs during the addition of the acid.] When precipitation is complete, decant the supernatant, and wash the precipitate with 5 mL of water. Dry the precipitate at 105° for 30 minutes.

Standard specimen: a similar preparation of USP Hydrochlorothiazide RS.

Dissolution ⟨711⟩—

Medium: 0.01 N hydrochloric acid; 900 mL.
Apparatus 1: 100 rpm.
Time: 30 minutes.

Procedure—Filter a portion of the solution under test, transfer 10.0 mL of the filtrate to a suitable capped bottle, and add 5.0 mL of water, 1.0 mL of 5 N sodium hydroxide, and 25.0 mL of n-heptane. Cap the bottle, shake by mechanical means for 5 minutes, and allow the layers to separate, centrifuging if necessary, to obtain clear upper (n-heptane) and lower (aqueous) extracts. Determine the quantity, in μg, of propranolol hydrochloride ($C_{16}H_{21}NO_2 \cdot HCl$) in each mL of the n-heptane extract by employing UV absorption at the wavelength of maximum absorbance at about 293 nm, in comparison with an n-heptane Standard solution obtained by similarly treating and extracting a mixture of 5.0 mL of an aqueous solution having a known concentration of USP Propranolol Hydrochloride RS and 5.0 mL of a 0.005 N sodium hydroxide solution having a known concentration of USP Hydrochlorothiazide RS, using a blank consisting of the n-heptane extract obtained by similarly treating and extracting 10.0 mL of water. Determine the quantity, in μg, of hydrochlorothiazide ($C_7H_8ClN_3O_4S_2$) in each mL of the aqueous extract by employing UV absorption at the wavelength of maximum absorbance at about 273 nm, in comparison with the aqueous extract remaining from the preparation of the n-heptane Standard solution, using as a blank the aqueous extract remaining from the preparation of the n-heptane blank extract. Calculate the quantity, in mg, of $C_{16}H_{21}NO_2 \cdot HCl$ dissolved by multiplying the quantity, in μg, of propranolol hydrochloride in each mL of the n-heptane extract from the solution under test by 2.25. Calculate the quantity, in mg, of $C_7H_8ClN_3O_4S_2$ dissolved by multiplying the quantity, in μg, of hydrochlorothiazide in each mL of the aqueous extract from the solution under test by 1.44.

Tolerances—Not less than 80% *(Q)* of the labeled amount of $C_{16}H_{21}NO_2 \cdot HCl$ and not less than 80% *(Q)* of the labeled amount of $C_7H_8ClN_3O_4S_2$ is dissolved in 30 minutes.

Uniformity of dosage units ⟨905⟩: meet the requirements for *Content Uniformity* with respect to propranolol hydrochloride and hydrochlorothiazide.

Procedure for content uniformity—Transfer a Tablet to a suitable container, and add 500.0 mL of 0.1 N hydrochloric acid. Shake until the Tablet has disintegrated, sonicate for 30 seconds, shake by mechanical means for 30 minutes, and then repeat the sonication and shaking. Centrifuge a portion of the solution, and transfer 6.0 mL of the clear supernatant and 15.0 mL of water to a suitable capped bottle. Add 1.0 mL of 5 N sodium hydroxide and 25.0 mL of n-heptane, cap the bottle, shake by mechanical means for 5 minutes, and allow the layers to separate, centrifuging, if necessary, to obtain clear upper (n-heptane) and lower (aqueous) layers (test solutions). Prepare a similar Standard solution by mixing 6.0 mL of 0.1 N hydrochloric acid, 3.0 mL of water, 6.0 mL of an aqueous solution having a known concentration of USP Propranolol Hydrochloride RS, and 6.0 mL of a 0.04 N sodium hydroxide solution having a known concentration of USP Hydrochlorothiazide RS, and proceeding as directed for the test solutions, beginning with "Add 1.0 mL of 5 N sodium hydroxide." Prepare similar blank n-heptane and aqueous extracts by adding 6.0 mL of 0.1 N hydrochloric acid to 15.0 mL of water, and proceeding as directed for the test solutions, beginning with "Add 1.0 mL of 5 N sodium hydroxide". Concomitantly determine the absorbances of the n-heptane test solution and the n-heptane Standard solution at the wavelength of maximum absorbance at about 293 nm, using the n-heptane blank extract to set the instrument. Calculate the quantity, in mg, of propranolol hydrochloride ($C_{16}H_{21}NO_2 \cdot HCl$) in the Tablet taken by the formula:

$$(12.5 / 6)(C)(A_U / A_S)$$

in which *C* is the concentration, in μg per mL, of USP Propranolol Hydrochloride RS in the n-heptane Standard solution; and A_U and A_S are the absorbances at 293 nm of the n-heptane test solution and the n-heptane Standard solution, respectively. Concomitantly determine the absorbances of the aqueous test solution and the aqueous Standard solution at the wavelength of maximum absorbance at about 273 nm, using the aqueous blank extract to set the instrument. Calculate the quantity, in mg, of hydrochlorothiazide ($C_7H_8ClN_3O_4S_2$) in the Tablet taken by the formula:

$$(11 / 6)(C)(A_U / A_S)$$

in which *C* is the concentration, in μg per mL, of USP Hydrochlorothiazide RS in the aqueous Standard solution; and A_U and A_S are the absorbances at 273 nm of the aqueous test solution and the aqueous Standard solution, respectively.

Related compounds—

Tetrabutylammonium hydroxide solution, Buffer, Mobile phase, and *Chromatographic system*—Proceed as directed under *Assay*.

Standard solution—Dissolve an accurately weighed quantity of USP Benzothiadiazine Related Compound A RS in methanol to obtain a solution having a known concentration of about 0.5 mg per mL. Transfer an accurately measured volume of this solution, and dilute quantitatively, and stepwise if necessary, with *Mobile phase* to obtain a solution having a known concentration of about 0.5 μg per mL.

Test solution—Use the *Assay preparation* prepared as directed in the *Assay*.

Chromatographic system—Proceed as directed under *Assay*, except to chromatograph the *Standard solution*: the relative standard deviation for replicate injections is not more than 5.0%.

Procedure—Separately inject equal volumes (about 50 μL) of the *Standard solution* and *Test solution* into the chromatograph, record the chromatograms, and measure the peak areas. Calculate the percentage of benzothiadiazine related compound A in the portion of Tablets taken by the formula:

$$50(C/L)(r_U / r_S)$$

in which *C* is the concentration in μg per mL, of USP Benzothiadiazine Related Compound A RS in the *Standard solution;* *L* is the amount, in mg, of hydrochlorothiazide in the portion of Tablets taken, based on the labeled amount; and r_U and r_S are the peak areas of benzothiadiazine related compound A obtained from the *Test solution* and *Standard solution,* respectively: not more than 1.0% is found.

Assay—

Tetrabutylammonium hydroxide solution—Use a suitable aqueous or methanolic solution having a known concentration of tetrabutylammonium hydroxide.

Buffer—Dissolve 6.8 g of monobasic potassium phosphate in 1000 mL of water in a 2000-mL volumetric flask. Add 3.4 mL of phosphoric acid and a volume of *Tetrabutylammonium hydroxide solution* equivalent to about 2.6 g of tetrabutylammonium hydroxide, dilute with water to volume, and mix. Adjust, if necessary, with phosphoric acid or 10 N potassium hydroxide to a pH of 2.5 ± 0.1, and pass through a filter having a 0.5-μm or finer porosity.

Mobile phase—Prepare a suitable mixture of *Buffer* and methanol (850 : 150). Make adjustments if necessary (see *System Suitability* under *Chromatography* ⟨621⟩) so that the retention time of propranolol is between 12 and 25 minutes.

Standard hydrochlorothiazide stock solution—Transfer about 25 mg of USP Hydrochlorothiazide RS, accurately weighed, to a 100-mL volumetric flask, add 15 mL of methanol, and mix to dissolve. Dilute with *Buffer* to volume, and mix.

Standard propranolol hydrochloride stock solution—Dissolve an accurately weighed quantity of USP Propranolol Hydrochloride RS in *Mobile phase* to obtain a solution having a known concentration of about 0.25*J* mg per mL, *J* being the ratio of the labeled quantity, in mg, of propranolol hydrochloride to the labeled quantity, in mg, of hydrochlorothiazide per Tablet.

Standard preparation—Transfer 5.0 mL of *Standard hydrochlorothiazide stock solution* and 5.0 mL of *Standard propranolol hydrochloride stock solution* to a 25-mL volumetric flask, dilute with *Mobile phase* to volume, and mix. This solution contains about 50 μg of hydrochlorothiazide and 50*J*μg of propranolol hydrochloride per mL.

Assay preparation—Weigh and finely powder not fewer than 20 Tablets. Transfer an accurately weighed portion of the powder, equivalent to about 25 mg of hydrochlorothiazide, to a 500-mL volumetric flask. Add 5 mL of water, mix, and allow to stand for 5 minutes, with occasional swirling. Add 75 mL of methanol, mix, and sonicate for 10 minutes, with occasional swirling, adding ice to the bath, if necessary, to maintain the temperature at not more than 20°. Add about 350 mL of *Buffer* to the flask, and sonicate for 10 minutes, with occasional swirling, maintaining the temperature of the bath at not more than 20°. Dilute with *Buffer* to volume, and mix. Centrifuge a portion of this solution, if necessary, to obtain a clear solution (*Assay preparation*).

Chromatographic system (see *Chromatography* ⟨621⟩)—The liquid chromatograph is equipped with a 270-nm detector and a 4-mm × 15-cm column that contains 5-μm packing L1. The flow rate is about 1.5 mL per minute. Chromatograph the *Standard preparation*, and record the peak responses as directed for *Procedure*: the column efficiency determined from the propranolol peak is not less than 2500 theoretical plates; the tailing factor for the propranolol and hydrochlorothiazide peaks is not more than 1.5; and the relative standard deviation for replicate injections is not more than 2.0%. [NOTE—The relative retention times are about 0.25 for benzothiadiazine related compound A, 0.4 for hydrochlorothiazide, and 1.0 for propranolol.]

Procedure—Separately inject equal volumes (about 50 μL) of the *Standard preparation* and the *Assay preparation* into the chromatograph, record the chromatograms, and measure the areas for the major peaks. Calculate the quantities, in mg, of propranolol hydrochloride ($C_{16}H_{21}NO_2 \cdot HCl$) and hydrochlorothiazide ($C_7H_8ClN_3O_4S_2$) in the portion of Tablets taken by the same formula:

$$0.5C(r_U / r_S)$$

in which *C* is the concentration, in μg per mL, of the appropriate Reference Standard in the *Standard preparation;* and r_U and r_S are the peak responses of the corresponding analyte obtained from the *Assay preparation* and the *Standard preparation*, respectively.

Propylene Glycol

$C_3H_8O_2$ 76.09
1,2-Propanediol.
1,2-Propanediol   [*57-55-6*].

» Propylene Glycol contains not less than 99.5 percent of $C_3H_8O_2$.

Packaging and storage—Preserve in tight containers.

USP Reference standards ⟨11⟩—USP Propylene Glycol RS.
Identification, *Infrared Absorption* ⟨197F⟩ on undried specimen.
Specific gravity ⟨841⟩:   between 1.035 and 1.037.
Acidity—Add 1 mL of phenolphthalein TS to 50 mL of water, then add 0.1 N sodium hydroxide until the solution remains pink for 30 seconds. Then add 10 mL of Propylene Glycol, accurately measured, and titrate with 0.10 N sodium hydroxide until the original pink color returns and remains for 30 seconds: not more than 0.20 mL of 0.10 N sodium hydroxide is required.
Water, *Method I* ⟨921⟩:   not more than 0.2%.
Residue on ignition—Heat 50 g in a tared 100-mL shallow dish until it ignites, and allow it to burn without further application of heat in a place free from drafts. Cool, moisten the residue with 0.5 mL of sulfuric acid, and ignite to constant weight: the weight of the residue does not exceed 3.5 mg.
Chloride ⟨221⟩—A 1-mL portion shows no more chloride than corresponds to 0.10 mL of 0.020 N hydrochloric acid (0.007%).
Sulfate ⟨221⟩—A 5.0-mL portion shows no more sulfate than corresponds to 0.30 mL of 0.020 N sulfuric acid (0.006%).
Heavy metals ⟨231⟩—Mix 4.0 mL with water to make 25 mL: the limit is 5 ppm.
Organic volatile impurities, *Method IV* ⟨467⟩: meets the requirements.

(Official until July 1, 2008)

Assay—

Chromatographic system (see *Chromatography* ⟨621⟩)—The gas chromatograph is equipped with a thermal conductivity detector, and contains a 1-m × 4-mm column packed with 5% G16 on support S5. The injection port temperature is 240°, the detector temperature is 250°, and the column temperature is programmed at a rate of 5° per minute from 120° to 200°, and helium is used as the carrier gas. The approximate retention time for propylene glycol is 5.7 minutes, and the approximate retention times for the 3 isomers of dipropylene glycol, when present, are 8.2, 9.0, and 10.2 minutes, respectively.

Procedure—Inject a suitable volume, typically about 10 μL, of Propylene Glycol into a suitable gas chromatograph, and record the chromatogram. Calculate the percentage of $C_3H_8O_2$ in the Propylene Glycol by dividing the area under the propylene glycol peak by the sum of the areas under all of the peaks, excluding those due to air and water, and multiplying by 100.

Propylhexedrine

$C_{10}H_{21}N$ 155.28
Cyclohexaneethanamine, *N*,α-dimethyl-, (±)-.
(±)-*N*,α-Dimethylcyclohexaneethylamine   [*101-40-6*].

» Propylhexedrine contains not less than 98.0 percent and not more than 101.0 percent of $C_{10}H_{21}N$.

Packaging and storage—Preserve in tight containers.

Identification—

A: To 3 mL of water contained in a small flask add about 0.1 mL of it and 0.5 mL of 1 N hydrochloric acid, and agitate the mixture until clear. Add 20 mL of trinitrophenol TS, insert the stopper in the flask, shake vigorously for a few minutes, and allow to stand for 2 hours. Filter, wash the precipitate with about 20 mL of cold water, and dry in vacuum at 60° for 4 hours: the picrate so obtained melts between 108° and 110° (see *Melting Range or Temperature* ⟨741⟩). *[Caution: Picrates may explode.]*

B: A solution, prepared as directed in *Identification* test A, yields a brown precipitate with iodine TS and a white precipitate with mercuric-potassium iodide TS.

Specific gravity ⟨841⟩: between 0.848 and 0.852.

Assay—Tare a glass-stoppered conical flask containing about 15 mL of water, add quickly about 0.5 mL of Propylhexedrine, and again weigh. Add to the contents of the flask 30 mL of neutralized alcohol, then add methyl red TS, and titrate with 0.1 N sulfuric acid VS. Perform a blank determination, and make any necessary correction. Each mL of 0.1 N sulfuric acid is equivalent to 15.53 mg of $C_{10}H_{21}N$.

Propylhexedrine Inhalant

» Propylhexedrine Inhalant consists of cylindrical rolls of suitable fibrous material impregnated with Propylhexedrine, usually aromatized, and contained in a suitable inhaler. The inhaler contains not less than 90.0 percent and not more than 125.0 percent of the labeled amount of $C_{10}H_{21}N$.

Packaging and storage—Preserve in tight containers (inhalers), and avoid exposure to excessive heat.

Identification—Place the contents of 1 inhaler in a glass-stoppered flask, add 50 mL of methanol, and allow to stand for 1 hour with frequent agitation. Filter, pressing out the roll on the filter. Add to the filtrate 1 N hydrochloric acid until it is slightly acid to moistened litmus paper, then add 30 mL of water, and evaporate to about 20 mL. Cool, transfer to a small separator, and shake with 10 mL of ether. Withdraw the water layer, warm it on a steam bath to expel any ether, and dilute to about 25 mL. From 10 mL of the solution, precipitate the propylhexedrine with trinitrophenol TS as directed in *Identification* test A under *Propylhexedrine*: the propylhexedrine picrate so obtained melts between 108° and 110° (see *Melting Range or Temperature* ⟨741⟩). *[Caution—Picrates may explode.]*

Assay—Place the contents of 2 inhalers of Inhalant in the thimble of a continuous-extraction apparatus, and quickly assemble the apparatus. Rinse each of the emptied inhalers with about 20 mL of methanol, pouring the rinsings through the condenser into the extraction flask. Add through the condenser 20 mL to 30 mL of methanol, and extract for 15 to 20 cycles. Cool the extract, transfer it completely with the aid of small portions of methanol to a 100-mL volumetric flask, dilute with methanol to volume, and mix. To 50.0 mL of the solution add 25.0 mL of 0.1 N sulfuric acid VS, and evaporate to about 40 mL. Cool, add methyl red TS, and titrate the excess acid with 0.1 N sodium hydroxide VS. Each mL of 0.1 N sulfuric acid is equivalent to 15.53 mg of $C_{10}H_{21}N$.

Propyliodone

$C_{10}H_{11}I_2NO_3$ 447.01
1(4*H*)-Pyridineacetic acid, 3,5-diiodo-4-oxo-, propyl ester.
Propyl 3,5-diiodo-4-oxo-1(4*H*)pyridineacetate   [587-61-1].

» Propyliodone contains not less than 99.0 percent and not more than 101.0 percent of $C_{10}H_{11}I_2NO_3$, calculated on the dried basis.

Packaging and storage—Preserve in tight, light-resistant containers. Store at 25°, excursions permitted between 15° and 30°.

Identification—

A: Heat 100 mg with a few drops of sulfuric acid: violet vapors are evolved.

B: Reflux 1 g with 10 mL of 1 N sodium hydroxide for 30 minutes, add 10 mL of water, and acidify to litmus paper with hydrochloric acid: the precipitate of 3,5-diiodo-4-oxo-1(4*H*)-pyridineacetic acid, after being washed with water and dried at 105°, melts at about 245°.

Melting range ⟨741⟩: between 187° and 190°.

Acidity—Dissolve 1.0 g in 40 mL of hot *n*-propyl alcohol previously neutralized to phenolphthalein TS, cool, and allow to stand in an ice bath for 15 minutes with frequent shaking. Filter, wash the residue with neutralized *n*-propyl alcohol, combine the filtrate and washings, add phenolphthalein TS, and titrate with 0.050 N sodium hydroxide to a pink color that persists for 15 seconds: not more than 0.15 mL of 0.050 N sodium hydroxide is required for neutralization.

Loss on drying ⟨731⟩—Dry it at 105° to constant weight: it loses not more than 0.5% of its weight.

Residue on ignition ⟨281⟩: not more than 0.1%.

Iodine and iodide—Shake 2.4 g with 30 mL of water for 15 minutes, filter, and to 10 mL of filtrate add 1 mL of 2 N nitric acid, 1 mL of sodium nitrite solution (1 in 500), and 2 mL of chloroform. Shake, and centrifuge: any purple color in the chloroform layer is not darker than that obtained with a mixture of 6 mL of water and 4 mL of potassium iodide solution (2.6 in 100,000) treated in the same manner (0.01% of I).

Heavy metals, *Method II* ⟨231⟩: 0.002%.

Assay—Using about 15 mg of Propyliodone, accurately weighed, proceed as directed in the *Assay* under *Iodoquinol*. Each mL of 0.02 N sodium thiosulfate is equivalent to 0.7450 mg of $C_{10}H_{11}I_2NO_3$.

Propyliodone Injectable Oil Suspension

» Propyliodone Injectable Oil Suspension is a sterile suspension of Propyliodone in Peanut Oil. It contains not less than 57.0 percent and not more than 63.0 percent of $C_{10}H_{11}I_2NO_3$.

Packaging and storage—Preserve in single-dose, light-resistant containers.

Identification—Mix 1 g of Injectable Oil Suspension with 20 mL of solvent hexane, filter the diluted suspension through a fine-porosity, sintered-glass crucible, and wash the residue free from peanut oil with the solvent hexane: the residue responds to the *Identification* tests under *Propyliodone*, and, after being dried at 105° to constant weight, melts between 187° and 190°.

Weight per mL—Transfer 60 to 70 mL of well-shaken Injectable Oil Suspension to a 250-mL beaker, place in a vacuum desiccator, and cautiously apply vacuum. When vigorous frothing has ceased, apply a pressure of about 10 mm of mercury for 15 minutes. Remove the specimen, mix gently with a spatula without stirring in any air bubbles, adjust its temperature to about 20°, and fill a clean, dry, tared 50-mL pycnometer with it. Adjust the temperature of the filled pycnometer to 25°, remove any excess of the specimen, weigh, and calculate the net weight. The weight per mL is between 1.236 g and 1.276 g.

Iodine and iodide—Disperse 3.3 mL in 125 mL of alcohol-free chloroform, add 25 mL of sodium hydroxide solution (1 in 2500), and shake. Separate the aqueous layer, shake it with 125 mL of alcohol-free chloroform, and discard the chloroform. Proceed with 10 mL of the aqueous layer as directed in the test for *Iodine and iodide* under *Propyliodone*, beginning with "add 1 mL of 2 N nitric acid."
Other requirements—It meets the requirements under *Injections* ⟨1⟩.

Assay—Open 1 container of Injectable Oil Suspension, stir the contents with a glass rod until mixed, replace the closure, and shake. Quickly transfer about 30 mg of Injectable Oil Suspension to a tared combustion capsule, and weigh accurately. Using this as the assay specimen, proceed as directed in the *Assay* under *Iodoquinol*. Each mL of 0.02 N sodium thiosulfate is equivalent to 0.7450 mg of $C_{10}H_{11}I_2NO_3$. From the weight of Injectable Oil Suspension taken and the observed *Weight per mL*, calculate the weight of propyliodone in each mL of Injectable Oil Suspension.

Propylthiouracil

$C_7H_{10}N_2OS$ 170.23
4(1*H*)-Pyrimidinone, 2,3-dihydro-6-propyl-2-thioxo-.
6-Propyl-2-thiouracil   [51-52-5].

» Propylthiouracil contains not less than 98.0 percent and not more than 100.5 percent of $C_7H_{10}N_2OS$, calculated on the dried basis.

Packaging and storage—Preserve in well-closed, light-resistant containers.
USP Reference standards ⟨11⟩—*USP Propylthiouracil RS*.
Identification, *Infrared Absorption* ⟨197K⟩.
Melting range ⟨741⟩:   between 218° and 221°.
Loss on drying ⟨731⟩—Dry it at 105° for 2 hours: it loses not more than 0.5% of its weight.
Residue on ignition ⟨281⟩:   not more than 0.1%.
Selenium ⟨291⟩:   0.003%, a 200-mg specimen being used.
Heavy metals, *Method II* ⟨231⟩:   0.002%.
Ordinary impurities ⟨466⟩—
  Test solution: methanol.
  Standard solution: methanol.
  Application volume: 10 µL.
  Eluant: a mixture of toluene, ethyl acetate, and formic acid (50 : 45 : 5), in a nonequilibrated chamber.
  Visualization: 1.
Organic volatile impurities, *Method V* ⟨467⟩:   meets the requirements.
  Solvent—Use dimethyl sulfoxide.

(Official until July 1, 2008)
Assay—Weigh accurately about 300 mg of Propylthiouracil, transfer to a 500-mL conical flask, and add 30 mL of water. Add from a buret about 30 mL of 0.1 N sodium hydroxide VS, heat to boiling, and agitate until solution is complete. Wash down any particles on the wall of the flask with a few mL of water, then add about 50 mL of 0.1 N silver nitrate while mixing, and boil gently for 7 minutes. Cool to room temperature, and continue to titrate with 0.1 N sodium hydroxide VS, determining the endpoint potentiometrically, using a glass-calomel electrode system. Each mL of 0.1 N sodium hydroxide is equivalent to 8.512 mg of $C_7H_{10}N_2OS$.

Propylthiouracil Tablets

» Propylthiouracil Tablets contain not less than 93.0 percent and not more than 107.0 percent of the labeled amount of $C_7H_{10}N_2OS$.

Packaging and storage—Preserve in well-closed containers.
USP Reference standards ⟨11⟩—*USP Propylthiouracil RS*.
Identification—
  A: Boil a quantity of finely powdered Tablets, equivalent to about 100 mg of propylthiouracil, with 10 mL of alcohol under a reflux condenser for 20 minutes. Filter while hot, and evaporate the filtrate on a steam bath to dryness: a portion of the residue responds to the *Identification* tests under *Propylthiouracil*.
  B: The chromatogram of the *Assay preparation* obtained as directed in the *Assay* exhibits a major peak, the retention time of which corresponds to that exhibited in the chromatogram of the *Standard preparation*.
Dissolution ⟨711⟩—
  Medium: water; 900 mL.
  Apparatus 1:   100 rpm.
  Time: 30 minutes.
  Procedure—Determine the amount of $C_7H_{10}N_2OS$ dissolved from UV absorbances at the wavelength of maximum absorbance at about 274 nm of filtered portions of the solution under test, suitably diluted with *Dissolution Medium*, in comparison with a Standard solution having a known concentration of USP Propylthiouracil RS in the same medium.
  Tolerances—Not less than 85% (*Q*) of the labeled amount of $C_7H_{10}N_2OS$ is dissolved in 30 minutes.
Uniformity of dosage units ⟨905⟩:   meet the requirements.
Assay—
  0.025 M Phosphate buffer—Transfer an accurately weighed quantity of 3.40 g of monobasic potassium phosphate to a 1000-mL beaker. Add 500 mL of water, and stir until dissolved. Adjust the resulting solution with phosphoric acid or 0.1 N sodium hydroxide to a pH of 4.6. Add 500 mL of water to this solution, and mix.
  Mobile phase—Prepare a filtered and degassed mixture of *0.025 M Phosphate buffer* and acetonitrile (80 : 20). Make adjustments if necessary (see *System Suitability* under *Chromatography* ⟨621⟩).
  Standard preparation—Transfer an accurately weighed quantity of about 25 mg of USP Propylthiouracil RS to a 50-mL volumetric flask, add 5 mL of methanol, and sonicate for 5 minutes. Add 25 mL of water, and shake by mechanical means for 15 minutes. Dilute with water to volume, and mix. Transfer 10.0 mL of this solution to a 100-mL volumetric flask, dilute with water to volume, and mix to obtain a solution having a known concentration of about 50 µg per mL.
  Assay preparation—Weigh and finely powder not fewer than 20 Tablets. Transfer an accurately weighed portion of the powder equivalent to about 50 mg of propylthiouracil to a 100-mL volumetric flask, add 10 mL of methanol, and sonicate for 5 minutes. Add 50 mL of water, and shake by mechanical means for 20 minutes. Dilute with water to volume, mix, and filter. Transfer 10.0 mL of this solution to a 100-mL volumetric flask, dilute with water to volume, and mix.
  Chromatographic system (see *Chromatography* ⟨621⟩)—The liquid chromatograph is equipped with a 272-nm detector and a 4.6-mm × 10-cm column that contains 5-µm packing L1. The flow rate is about 1 mL per minute. Chromatograph the *Standard preparation*, and record the peak responses as described for *Procedure*: the column efficiency, determined from the analyte peak, is not less than 3500 theoretical plates, the tailing factor, *T*, for the propylthiouracil peak is not more than 2.0, and the relative standard deviation for replicate injections is not more than 2.0%.
  Procedure—Separately inject equal volumes (about 20 µL) of the *Standard preparation* and the *Assay preparation* into the chromatograph, record the chromatograms, and measure the peak area re-

sponses for the major peaks. Calculate the quantity, in mg, of $C_7H_{10}N_2OS$ in the portion of Tablets taken by the formula:

$$1000C(r_U / r_S)$$

in which C is the concentration, in mg per mL, of USP Propylthiouracil RS in the *Standard preparation*, and r_U and r_S are the peak area responses of propylthiouracil obtained from the *Assay preparation* and the *Standard preparation*, respectively.

Protamine Sulfate

» Protamine Sulfate is a purified mixture of simple protein principles obtained from the sperm or testes of suitable species of fish, which has the property of neutralizing heparin. Each mg of Protamine Sulfate, calculated on the dried basis, neutralizes not less than 100 USP Heparin Units.

Packaging and storage—Preserve in tight containers, in a refrigerator.
USP Reference standards ⟨11⟩—*USP Heparin Sodium RS*.
Loss on drying ⟨731⟩—Dry it at 105° for 3 hours: it loses not more than 5% of its weight.
Ultraviolet absorbance—The difference in absorbance of a 1.0% solution in water between 260 nm and 280 nm against a water blank, is not greater than 0.1 (see *Spectrophotometry and Light-Scattering* ⟨851⟩).
Sulfate—Dissolve about 150 mg, accurately weighed, in 75 mL of water, add 5 mL of 3 N hydrochloric acid, heat to boiling, and while maintaining at the boiling point, slowly add 10 mL of barium chloride TS. Cover the vessel, and allow the mixture to stand on a steam bath for 1 hour. Filter, wash the precipitate with several portions of hot water, dry, and ignite to constant weight. The weight of the barium sulfate, multiplied by 0.4117, represents the weight of sulfate in the portion of Protamine Sulfate taken. Not less than 16% and not more than 22%, calculated on the dried basis, is found.
Nitrogen content—Determine the nitrogen content as directed under *Method II* (see *Nitrogen Determination* ⟨461⟩). Not less than 22.5% and not more than 25.5% of N, calculated on the dried basis, is found.
Assay—
 Assay preparation—Dissolve a suitable quantity of Protamine Sulfate, accurately weighed, in Water for Injection to obtain a solution having a concentration of 1 mg per mL, calculated on the dried basis.
 Plasma—Prepare as directed for *Preparation of plasma* in the *Assay* under *Heparin Sodium*.
 Heparin preparation—On the day of the assay, prepare a solution of USP Heparin Sodium RS in saline TS to give a final concentration of 115 USP Heparin Units per mL.
 Calcium-thromboplastin solution—Dissolve in calcium chloride solution (1 in 50) a quantity of thromboplastin that is sufficient, as determined by preliminary trial if necessary, to produce clotting in about 35 seconds in a mixture consisting of equal volumes of plasma and a mixture of 4 volumes of saline TS and 1 volume of the prepared calcium-thromboplastin solution.
 Procedure—Into each of 10 meticulously cleansed, 13- × 100-mm test tubes pipet 2.5 mL of *Plasma*. Place the tubes in a water bath at 37 ± 0.2°, and to each of nine of them add 0.5 mL of *Assay preparation*. Into the tenth tube, to provide the control, pipet 2 mL of saline TS and 0.5 mL of *Calcium-thromboplastin solution*, noting the time, to the nearest second, of adding the latter. While mixing with a wire loop, note the time of the first appearance of fibrin fibers, and record it to the nearest second. The elapsed time is the normal clotting time of the plasma. Pipet into the nine remaining tubes the following volumes, in mL, of *Heparin preparation*: 0.43, 0.45, 0.47, 0.49, 0.50, 0.51, 0.53, 0.55, and 0.57, respectively. To each tube add saline TS to make 4.5 mL. Taking the tubes in random order, add 0.5 mL of *Calcium-thromboplastin solution*, and note the clotting time in each tube in the same manner as for the control tube.
 Calculation—Calculate the number of USP Heparin Units neutralized per mg taken by the formula:

$$N_S / W_U$$

in which N_S is the number of USP Heparin Units, and W_U is the number of mg of Protamine Sulfate in the last tube prior to the first one in which the clotting time is not less than 2 seconds longer than that in the control tube.

Protamine Sulfate Injection

» Protamine Sulfate Injection is a sterile, isotonic solution of Protamine Sulfate. It contains not less than 90.0 percent and not more than 120.0 percent of the labeled amount of protamine sulfate.

Packaging and storage—Preserve in single-dose containers, preferably of Type I glass. Store at controlled room temperature.
Labeling—Label it to indicate the approximate neutralization capacity in USP Heparin Units.
USP Reference standards ⟨11⟩—*USP Endotoxin RS. USP Heparin Sodium RS*.
Identification—It responds to the tests for *Sulfate* ⟨191⟩.
Bacterial endotoxins ⟨85⟩—It contains not more than 7.0 USP Endotoxin Units per mg of protamine sulfate.
Other requirements—It meets the requirements under *Injections* ⟨1⟩.
Assay—Using as the *Assay preparation* a solution prepared by diluting with Water for Injection an accurately measured volume of Injection to give an estimated final concentration of protamine sulfate of 1 mg per mL, proceed as directed in the *Assay* under *Protamine Sulfate*. The potency, in mg of protamine sulfate in each mL of the Injection, is given by the formula:

$$v / V$$

in which v and V are the volumes, in mL, respectively, of the *Heparin preparation* and of the Injection present in the last tube prior to the first one in which the clotting time is not less than 2 seconds longer than that in the control tube.

Protamine Sulfate for Injection

» Protamine Sulfate for Injection is a sterile mixture of Protamine Sulfate with one or more suitable, dry diluents. It contains not less than 90.0 percent and not more than 120.0 percent of the labeled amount of protamine sulfate.

Packaging and storage—Preserve in *Containers for Sterile Solids* as described under *Injections* ⟨1⟩. Preserve the accompanying solvent in single-dose or in multiple-dose containers, preferably of Type I glass.
Labeling—Label it to indicate the approximate neutralization capacity in USP Heparin Units.
USP Reference standards ⟨11⟩—*USP Endotoxin RS. USP Heparin Sodium RS*.
Constituted solution—At the time of use, it meets the requirements for *Constituted Solutions* under *Injections* ⟨1⟩.
Bacterial endotoxins ⟨85⟩—It contains not more than 7.0 USP Endotoxin Units per mg of protamine sulfate.
pH and clarity of solution—Dissolve it in the solvent recommended in the labeling: the pH of the solution is between 6.5 and 7.5, and the solution is clear.

Other requirements—Both it and the accompanying solvent meet the requirements for *Sterility Tests* ⟨71⟩ and *Labeling* under *Injections* ⟨1⟩. It meets also the requirements for *Uniformity of Dosage Units* ⟨905⟩.

Assay—Using as the *Assay preparation* a solution prepared by dissolving the contents of 1 container of Protamine Sulfate for Injection in Water for Injection to give a final concentration of about 1 mg of protamine sulfate per mL, proceed as directed in the *Assay* under *Protamine Sulfate*. Calculate the potency, in mg, of protamine sulfate in each mL of the *Assay preparation* taken by the formula:

$$v/V$$

in which v and V are the volumes, in mL, respectively, of the *Heparin preparation* and the *Assay preparation* present in the last tube prior to the first one in which the clotting time is not less than 2 seconds longer than in the control tube.

Protein Hydrolysate Injection

» Protein Hydrolysate Injection is a sterile solution of amino acids and short-chain peptides, which represent the approximate nutritive equivalent of the casein, lactalbumin, plasma, fibrin, or other suitable protein from which it is derived by acid, enzymatic, or other methods of hydrolysis. It may be modified by partial removal and restoration or addition of one or more amino acids. It may contain alcohol, dextrose, or other carbohydrate suitable for intravenous infusion. Not less than 50.0 percent of the total nitrogen present is in the form of α-amino nitrogen.

Packaging and storage—Preserve in single-dose containers, preferably of Type I or Type II glass, and avoid excessive heat.

Labeling—The label of the immediate container bears in a subtitle the name of the protein from which the hydrolysate has been derived and the word "modified" if one or more of the "essential" amino acids has been partially removed, restored, or added. The label bears a statement of the pH range; the name and percentage of any added other nutritive ingredient; the method of hydrolysis; the nature of the modification, if any, in amino acid content after hydrolysis; the percentage of each essential amino acid or its equivalent; the approximate protein equivalent, in g per liter; the approximate number of calories per liter; the percentage of the total nitrogen in the form of α-amino nitrogen; and the quantity of the sodium and of the potassium ions present in each 100 mL of the Injection. Injection that contains not more than 30 mg of sodium per 100 mL may be labeled "Protein Hydrolysate Injection, Low Sodium," or by a similar title the approximate equivalent thereof.

The label states the total osmolar concentration in mOsmol per L. Where the contents are less than 100 mL, or where the label states that the Injection is not for direct injection but is to be diluted before use, the label alternatively may state the total osmolar concentration in mOsmol per mL.

USP Reference standards ⟨11⟩—*USP Endotoxin RS*.

Non-antigenicity—

Sensitizing solution—Select a suitable quantity of the protein identical in nature and quality with that from which the hydrolysate was manufactured, and subject it to the same hydrolytic process used in manufacturing the hydrolysate but reduce the time of hydrolysis to one-third. For purposes of preservation add, if desired, 0.5% of chlorobutanol, and package the sensitizing solution in 100-mL multiple-dose containers. Store in a cold place.

Preparation of animals—Select healthy guinea pigs each weighing between 420 and 480 g. Inject each animal intraperitoneally with 6 mL of the sensitizing solution on the second, fourth, and sixth days of each of two successive weeks. Use the sensitized animals not less than 30 days and not more than 37 days after the last sensitizing dose. Re-sensitize any animals not used during the 7-day period by injecting intraperitoneally a booster dose of 6 mL of the sensitizing solution, and use re-sensitized animals not less than 9 days and not more than 16 days after the injection of the booster dose.

Procedure—Inject, intravenously, 3 mL of Injection, at the rate of 2 mL per minute, using a 5-mL syringe fitted with a 27-gauge needle, into each of five guinea pigs prepared as described above. During the injection and during the 15 minutes following, observe the animals for any of the following symptoms: (1) licking the nose or rubbing the nose with forefeet; (2) ruffling of the fur; (3) labored breathing; (4) sneezing or coughing (three or more times); (5) retching. The requirements of the test are met if none of the injected animals show more than two of the listed symptoms and none show rales, convulsions, or prostration, or die. If none of the listed symptoms are observed, test the sensitivity of the animals by injecting into one of them 3 mL of the sensitizing solution intravenously at the rate of 2 mL per minute: the animal shows positive signs of anaphylaxis such as rales, convulsions, prostration, and/or death in addition to one or more of the lesser reaction symptoms.

Bacterial endotoxins ⟨85⟩—It contains not more than 0.5 USP Endotoxin Unit per mg of protein hydrolysate.

Biological adequacy—It meets the requirements under *Protein—Biological Adequacy Test* ⟨141⟩.

pH ⟨791⟩: between 4.0 and 7.0, determined potentiometrically, but the variation from the pH range stated on the label is not greater than ±0.5 pH unit.

Content of α-amino nitrogen—Dilute 5.0 mL of a 5% Injection, or an appropriate volume of any other concentration, to 25 mL. Adjust to a pH of 7, potentiometrically, by the addition of 0.1 N sodium hydroxide or 0.1 N hydrochloric acid. Add 10 mL of formaldehyde TS, previously adjusted to a pH of 9.0, potentiometrically, then while stirring the solution, preferably with a mechanical stirrer, and with a suitable glass electrode in the system, add 0.1 N sodium hydroxide VS slowly toward the end, until a pH of 9.0 is reached. Continue stirring for 2 minutes, check the pH, and adjust if necessary. Record the volume of 0.1 N sodium hydroxide VS added in the titration. Each mL of 0.10 N sodium hydroxide corresponds to 1.4 mg of α-amino nitrogen.

Nitrogen content—Using 0.1 mL of Injection, determine the nitrogen content as directed under *Method II* (see *Nitrogen Determination* ⟨461⟩).

Potassium content—

Standard solutions—Prepare four standard solutions (numbered 1, 2, 3, and 4) each containing a suitable wetting agent and 25.0 mEq of sodium (1.46 g of sodium chloride) per liter, and to the solutions add, respectively, 0-, 2.0-, 3.0-, and 4.0-mg supplements of potassium, in the form of the chloride, per L. If necessary, because of changes in the sensitivity of the instrument mentioned below, vary the levels of concentration of the potassium, keeping the ratios between solutions approximately as given.

Standard graph—Set a suitable flame photometer to a wavelength of 766 nm. Adjust the instrument to zero transmittance with solution 1. Then adjust the instrument to 100% transmittance with solution 4. Read the percent transmittance of solutions 2 and 3. Plot the observed transmittance of solutions 2, 3, and 4 as the ordinate and the concentration as the abscissa on arithmetic coordinate paper.

Procedure—Pipet a portion of the Injection containing approximately 300 μg of potassium, or a quantity corresponding to the concentration of the *Standard solutions*, into a 100-mL volumetric flask. Add a small amount of wetting agent, and dilute to volume with a sodium solution of such strength that the final sodium concentration is 25.0 mEq per L. Adjust the instrument to zero transmittance with solution 1 and to 100% transmittance with solution 4. Read the percent transmittance of the test solution and, by reference to the standard potassium graph, calculate the potassium content of the Injection in mg of potassium per mL.

Sodium content—Proceed as directed under *Potassium content*, with the following modifications: (1) prepare the *Standard solutions* to contain 6.00 mEq of potassium (447 mg of potassium chloride), and substitute sodium for the stated quantities of potassium; (2) prepare the *Standard graph* with the flame photometer set at 589 nm instead of 766 nm; and (3) under *Procedure* read "sodium" for "potassium" throughout, but in the second sentence read "a potassium solution of such strength that the final potassium concentra-

Protriptyline Hydrochloride

$C_{19}H_{21}N \cdot HCl$ 299.84
5*H*-Dibenzo[*a,d*]cycloheptene-5-propanamine, *N*-methyl-, hydrochloride.
N-Methyl-5*H*-dibenzo[*a,d*]cycloheptene-5-propylamine hydrochloride   [1225-55-4].

» Protriptyline Hydrochloride contains not less than 99.0 percent and not more than 101.0 percent of $C_{19}H_{21}N \cdot HCl$, calculated on the dried basis.

Packaging and storage—Preserve in well-closed containers.
USP Reference standards ⟨11⟩—*USP Protriptyline Hydrochloride RS.*
Identification—
  A: *Infrared Absorption* ⟨197M⟩.
  B: *Ultraviolet Absorption* ⟨197U⟩—
  Solution: 10 µg per mL.
  Medium: 0.1 N methanolic hydrochloric acid.
  Absorptivities at 292 nm, calculated on the dried basis, do not differ by more than 3.0%.
  C: It responds to the test for *Chloride* ⟨191⟩, when tested as specified for alkaloidal hydrochlorides.
  D: Its X-ray diffraction pattern (see *X-ray Diffraction* ⟨941⟩) conforms to that of USP Protriptyline Hydrochloride RS.
pH ⟨791⟩: between 5.0 and 6.5, in a solution (1 in 100).
Loss on drying ⟨731⟩—Dry it at a pressure below 5 mm of mercury at 60° to constant weight: it loses not more than 0.3% of its weight.
Residue on ignition ⟨281⟩: not more than 0.1%.
Heavy metals, *Method II* ⟨231⟩: 0.001%.
Organic volatile impurities, *Method I* ⟨467⟩: meets the requirements.
(Official until July 1, 2008)
Assay—Transfer about 700 mg of Protriptyline Hydrochloride, accurately weighed, to a 125-mL conical flask, and dissolve in 30 mL of glacial acetic acid. Add crystal violet TS and 10 mL of mercuric acetate TS, and titrate with 0.1 N perchloric acid VS to a green endpoint. Perform a blank determination, and make any necessary correction. Each mL of 0.1 N perchloric acid is equivalent to 29.98 mg of $C_{19}H_{21}N \cdot HCl$.

Protriptyline Hydrochloride Tablets

» Protriptyline Hydrochloride Tablets contain not less than 90.0 percent and not more than 110.0 percent of the labeled amount of $C_{19}H_{21}N \cdot HCl$.

Packaging and storage—Preserve in tight containers.
USP Reference standards ⟨11⟩—*USP Protriptyline Hydrochloride RS.*
Identification—
  A: The retention time of the major peak in the chromatogram of the *Assay preparation* corresponds to that in the chromatogram of the *Standard preparation*, as obtained in the *Assay*.
  B: A filtered solution of finely powdered Tablets, equivalent to protriptyline hydrochloride solution (1 in 20), meets the requirements of the tests for *Chloride* ⟨191⟩, when tested as specified for alkaloidal hydrochlorides.
Dissolution ⟨711⟩—
  Medium: water; 900 mL.
  Apparatus 1: 100 rpm.
  Time: 45 minutes.
  Procedure—Determine the amount of $C_{19}H_{21}N \cdot HCl$ dissolved from UV absorbances at the wavelength of maximum absorbance at about 290 nm of filtered portions of the solution under test, suitably diluted with *Dissolution Medium*, if necessary, in comparison with a Standard solution having a known concentration of USP Protriptyline Hydrochloride RS in the same medium.
  Tolerances—Not less than 75% *(Q)* of the labeled amount of $C_{19}H_{21}N \cdot HCl$ is dissolved in 45 minutes.
Uniformity of dosage units ⟨905⟩: meet the requirements.
  PROCEDURE FOR CONTENT UNIFORMITY—
  Solution A, Solution B, Mobile phase, Diluent, Standard preparation, and *Chromatographic system*—Proceed as directed in the *Assay*.
  Test preparation—Transfer 1 finely powdered Tablet to a 50-mL volumetric flask, add about 1 mL of 2.5 N hydrochloric acid and 5 mL of water for each 5 mg of protriptyline hydrochloride, and shake by mechanical means for 20 minutes or until the Tablet is fully disintegrated. Add 5 mL of alcohol for each 5 mg of protriptyline hydrochloride, and shake for an additional 10 minutes. Dilute with water to volume, mix, and pass through a 0.45-µm membrane filter, discarding the first 1.5 mL of the filtrate. Use the subsequent filtrate as the *Test preparation*.
  Procedure—Proceed as directed in the *Assay*. Calculate the quantity, in mg, of protriptyline hydrochloride ($C_{19}H_{21}N \cdot HCl$) in the Tablet taken by the formula:

$$(TC/D)(r_U/r_S)$$

in which *T* is the labeled quantity, in mg, of protriptyline hydrochloride in the Tablet; *C* is the concentration, in µg per mL, of USP Protriptyline Hydrochloride RS in the *Standard preparation*; *D* is the concentration, in µg per mL, of protriptyline hydrochloride in the *Test preparation*, based on the labeled quantity per Tablet and the extent of dilution; and r_U and r_S are the peak responses obtained from the *Test preparation* and the *Standard preparation*, respectively.
Assay—
  Solution A—Prepare a filtered and degassed solution of 22.0 g of monobasic sodium phosphate and 3.78 g of sodium 1-hexanesulfonate in 1900 mL of water. Adjust with phosphoric acid to a pH of 2.90, and dilute with water to volume in a 2000-mL volumetric flask. Make adjustments if necessary (see *System Suitability* under *Chromatography* ⟨621⟩).
  Solution B—Use filtered and degassed acetonitrile. Make adjustments if necessary (see *System Suitability* under *Chromatography* ⟨621⟩).
  Mobile phase—Use variable mixtures of *Solution A* and *Solution B* as directed for *Chromatographic system*.
  Diluent—Add 200 mL of alcohol to a 1000-mL volumetric flask. Add 40 mL of 2.5 N hydrochloric acid, dilute with water to volume, and mix.
  Standard preparation—Dissolve an accurately weighed quantity of USP Protriptyline Hydrochloride RS in *Diluent*, and dilute quantitatively, and stepwise if necessary, with *Diluent* to obtain a solution having a known concentration of about 0.20 µg per mL.
  Assay preparation—Weigh and finely powder not fewer than 20 Tablets. Transfer an accurately weighed portion of the powder, equivalent to about 40 mg of protriptyline hydrochloride, to a 200-mL volumetric flask, add 40 mL of alcohol, and shake by mechanical means for 5 minutes. Add 40 mL of water and 8 mL of 2.5 N hydrochloric acid, and shake for an additional 10 minutes. Dilute with water to volume, and mix. Pass through a 0.45-µm membrane filter, discarding the first 5 mL of the filtrate. Use the subsequent filtrate as the *Assay preparation*.
  Chromatographic system (see *Chromatography* ⟨621⟩)—The liquid chromatograph is equipped with a 280-nm detector and a 4.6-mm × 15-cm column containing 5-µm base-deactivated packing L7.

The flow rate is about 1.5 mL per minute. The chromatograph is programmed as follows.

Time (minutes)	Solution A (%)	Solution B (%)	Elution
0	83	17	equilibration
0–15	83→50	17→50	linear gradient
15–20	50	50	isocratic
20–25	50→83	50→17	linear gradient
25–30	83	17	re-equilibration

Chromatograph the *Standard preparation* and record the peak responses as directed for *Procedure:* the column efficiency is not less than 25,000 theoretical plates; the tailing factor is not more than 2.5; and the relative standard deviation is not more than 2.0%.

Procedure—Separately inject equal volumes (about 20 µL) of the *Assay preparation* and the *Standard preparation* into the chromatograph, record the chromatograms, and measure the responses for the major peaks. Calculate the quantity, in mg, of protriptyline hydrochloride ($C_{19}H_{21}N \cdot HCl$) in the portion of Tablets taken by the formula:

$$200C(r_U/r_S)$$

in which C is the concentration, in mg per mL, of USP Protriptyline Hydrochloride RS in the *Standard preparation;* and r_U and r_S are the peak responses obtained from the *Assay preparation* and the *Standard preparation*, respectively.

Pseudoephedrine Hydrochloride

$C_{10}H_{15}NO \cdot HCl$ 201.69

Benzenemethanol, α-[1-(methylamino)ethyl]-, [S-(R*,R*)]-, hydrochloride.
(+)-Pseudoephedrine hydrochloride   [345-78-8].

» Pseudoephedrine Hydrochloride contains not less than 98.0 percent and not more than 100.5 percent of $C_{10}H_{15}NO \cdot HCl$, calculated on the dried basis.

Packaging and storage—Preserve in tight, light-resistant containers.

USP Reference standards ⟨11⟩—*USP Pseudoephedrine Hydrochloride RS.*
Identification—
   A: *Infrared Absorption* ⟨197K⟩.
   B: A solution responds to the tests for *Chloride* ⟨191⟩.
Melting range, *Class I* ⟨741⟩: between 182° and 186°, but the range between beginning and end of melting does not exceed 2°.
Specific rotation ⟨781S⟩: between +61.0° and +62.5°.
   Test solution: 50 mg per mL, in water.
pH ⟨791⟩: between 4.6 and 6.0, in a solution (1 in 20).
Loss on drying ⟨731⟩—Dry it at 105° for 3 hours: it loses not more than 0.5% of its weight.
Residue on ignition ⟨281⟩: not more than 0.1%.
Ordinary impurities ⟨466⟩—
   Test solution: alcohol.
   Standard solution: alcohol.
   Eluant: a mixture of alcohol, glacial acetic acid, and water (10 : 3 : 1).
   Visualization—Dry the plate overnight in a hood or for 2 hours with a current from a hot air dryer. In a pre-equilibrated closed chamber, on the bottom of which there are iodine crystals, expose the plate to iodine vapors for not less than 30 minutes.

Organic volatile impurities, *Method V* ⟨467⟩: meets the requirements, except to maintain the injection port temperature at 70°, instead of at 140°.
(Official until July 1, 2008)
Assay—Dissolve about 400 mg of Pseudoephedrine Hydrochloride, accurately weighed, in a mixture of 50 mL of glacial acetic acid and 10 mL of mercuric acetate TS, add 1 drop of crystal violet TS, and titrate with 0.1 N perchloric acid VS to a blue-green endpoint. Perform a blank determination, and make any necessary correction. Each mL of 0.1 N perchloric acid is equivalent to 20.17 mg of $C_{10}H_{15}NO \cdot HCl$.

Pseudoephedrine Hydrochloride Extended-Release Capsules

» Pseudoephedrine Hydrochloride Extended-Release Capsules contain not less than 90.0 percent and not more than 110.0 percent of the labeled amount of pseudoephedrine hydrochloride ($C_{10}H_{15}NO \cdot HCl$).

Packaging and storage—Preserve in tight containers.
USP Reference standards ⟨11⟩—*USP Pseudoephedrine Hydrochloride RS.*
Identification—
   A: A portion of Capsule contents, equivalent to about 180 mg of pseudoephedrine hydrochloride, meets the requirements of *Identification* test A under *Pseudoephedrine Hydrochloride Extended-Release Tablets.*
   B: The retention time of the major peak in the chromatogram of the *Assay preparation* corresponds to that in the chromatogram of the *Standard preparation,* as obtained in the *Assay.*
Dissolution ⟨711⟩—
   Medium: water; 900 mL.
   Apparatus 2: 50 rpm.
   Times: 3, 6, and 12 hours.
   Procedure—Determine the amount of $C_{10}H_{15}NO \cdot HCl$ dissolved, employing the procedure set forth in the *Assay,* using a filtered portion of the solution under test as the *Assay preparation* in comparison with a *Standard* solution having a known concentration of USP Pseudoephedrine Hydrochloride RS in the same *Medium.*
   Tolerances—The percentages of the labeled amount of $C_{10}H_{15}NO \cdot HCl$ dissolved at the times specified conform to *Acceptance Table 2.*

Time (hours)	Amount dissolved
3	between 20% and 50%
6	between 45% and 75%
12	not less than 75%

Uniformity of dosage units ⟨905⟩: meet the requirements.
Assay—
   Mobile phase, Standard preparation, and *Chromatographic system*—Proceed as directed in the *Assay* under *Pseudoephedrine Hydrochloride Extended-Release Tablets.*
   Assay preparation—Remove, as completely as possible, the contents of not fewer than 20 Capsules, weigh, and mix. Transfer an accurately weighed portion of the combined contents, equivalent to about 120 mg of pseudoephedrine hydrochloride, to a 100-mL volumetric flask, add 10 mL of 0.01 N hydrochloric acid, and sonicate for 10 minutes. Cool to room temperature. Dilute with 0.01 N hydrochloric acid to volume, mix, and filter.
   Procedure—Proceed as directed in the *Assay* under *Pseudoephedrine Hydrochloride Extended-Release Tablets.* Calculate the quantity, in mg, of pseudoephedrine hydrochloride ($C_{10}H_{15}NO \cdot HCl$) in the portion of Capsules taken by the formula:

$$100C(r_U/r_S)$$

in which C is the concentration, in mg per mL, of USP Pseudoephedrine Hydrochloride RS in the *Standard preparation;* and r_U

and r_S are the peak responses obtained from the *Assay preparation* and the *Standard preparation*, respectively.

Pseudoephedrine Hydrochloride Oral Solution

» Pseudoephedrine Hydrochloride Oral Solution contains not less than 90.0 percent and not more than 110.0 percent of the labeled amount of pseudoephedrine hydrochloride ($C_{10}H_{15}NO \cdot HCl$).

Packaging and storage—Preserve in tight, light-resistant containers.

USP Reference standards ⟨11⟩—*USP Pseudoephedrine Hydrochloride RS*.

Identification—Extract a volume of Oral Solution, equivalent to about 120 mg of pseudoephedrine hydrochloride, with two 30-mL portions of ether, discard the extracts, and add 4 mL of 1 N sodium hydroxide. Extract with 30 mL of chloroform, and evaporate the chloroform on a steam bath, avoiding overheating: the pseudoephedrine so obtained melts at about 118°, the procedure for *Class I* being used (see *Melting Range or Temperature* ⟨741⟩), and when 50 mg is dissolved in 10 mL of 0.1 N hydrochloric acid, the resulting solution is dextrorotatory.

Reaction—It is acid to litmus.

Uniformity of dosage units ⟨905⟩—
FOR ORAL SOLUTION PACKAGED IN SINGLE-UNIT CONTAINERS: meets the requirements.

Deliverable volume ⟨698⟩—
FOR ORAL SOLUTION PACKAGED IN MULTIPLE-UNIT CONTAINERS: meets the requirements.

Assay—
Mobile phase—Prepare a filtered and degassed mixture of alcohol and 0.40% ammonium acetate solution (17 : 3). Make adjustments if necessary (see *System Suitability* under *Chromatography* ⟨621⟩).

Standard preparation—Dissolve an accurately weighed quantity of USP Pseudoephedrine Hydrochloride RS in 0.01 N hydrochloric acid to obtain a solution having a known concentration of about 1.2 mg per mL.

Assay preparation—Transfer an accurately measured volume of Oral Solution, equivalent to about 60 mg of pseudoephedrine hydrochloride, to a 50-mL volumetric flask, dilute with 0.01 N hydrochloric acid to volume, mix, and filter.

Chromatographic system (see *Chromatography* ⟨621⟩)—The liquid chromatograph is equipped with a 254-nm detector and a 4.6-mm × 25-cm column that contains packing L3. The flow rate is about 1.5 mL per minute. Chromatograph five replicate injections of the *Standard preparation*, and record the peak responses as directed for *Procedure:* the tailing factor is not more than 2.0; and the relative standard deviation for replicate injections is not more than 2.0%.

Procedure—Separately inject equal volumes (about 10 μL) of the *Standard preparation* and the *Assay preparation* into the chromatograph, record the chromatograms, and measure the responses for the major peaks. Calculate the quantity, in mg, of pseudoephedrine hydrochloride ($C_{10}H_{15}NO \cdot HCl$) in each mL of the Oral Solution taken by the formula:

$$50(C/V)(r_U/r_S)$$

in which C is the concentration, in mg per mL, of USP Pseudoephedrine Hydrochloride RS in the *Standard preparation*; V is the volume, in mL, of Oral Solution taken; and r_U and r_S are the peak responses obtained from the *Assay preparation* and the *Standard preparation*, respectively.

Pseudoephedrine Hydrochloride Tablets

» Pseudoephedrine Hydrochloride Tablets contain not less than 90.0 percent and not more than 110.0 percent of the labeled amount of pseudoephedrine hydrochloride ($C_{10}H_{15}NO \cdot HCl$).

Packaging and storage—Preserve in tight containers.

USP Reference standards ⟨11⟩—*USP Pseudoephedrine Hydrochloride RS*.

Identification—
A: *Thin-Layer Chromatographic Identification Test* ⟨201⟩—
Test solution—Transfer 1 tablet to a glass-stoppered tube, add 10 mL of water, and shake or mix until the tablet completely disintegrates. Sonicate for 5 minutes, centrifuge for 5 minutes, and pass through a nylon filter.
Standard solution—Dissolve an accurately weighed quantity of USP Pseudoephedrine Hydrochloride RS in water to obtain a solution having a known concentration of about 3 mg per mL.
Developing solvent system—Prepare a mixture of butyl alcohol, glacial acetic acid, and water (8 : 2 : 2).
Procedure—Proceed as directed in the chapter. The R_F value and appearance of the principal spot obtained from the *Test solution* correspond to that obtained from the *Standard solution*.
B: The retention time of the major peak in the chromatogram of the *Assay preparation* corresponds to that in the chromatogram of the *Standard solution,* as obtained in the *Assay*.

Dissolution, *Procedure for a Pooled Sample* ⟨711⟩—
Medium: water; 900 mL.
Apparatus 2: 50 rpm.
Time: 45 minutes.
Determine the amount of $C_{10}H_{15}NO \cdot HCl$ dissolved by employing the following method.
Mobile phase—Proceed as directed in the *Assay*.
Chromatographic system (see *Chromatography* ⟨621⟩)—The liquid chromatograph is equipped with a 214-nm detector and a 4.6-mm × 25-cm column that contains packing L3. The flow rate is about 1.5 mL per minute. Chromatograph the Standard solution, and record the peak responses as directed for *Procedure:* the tailing factor is not more than 2.0; and the relative standard deviation for replicate injections is not more than 2.0%.
Procedure—Inject a volume of a filtered portion of the solution under test into the chromatograph, record the chromatograms, and measure the responses for the major peaks. Calculate the quantity of $C_{10}H_{15}NO \cdot HCl$ dissolved in comparison with a Standard solution having a known concentration of USP Pseudoephedrine Hydrochloride RS in the same medium and similarly chromatographed.
Tolerances—Not less than 75% *(Q)* of the labeled amount of $C_{10}H_{15}NO \cdot HCl$ is dissolved in 45 minutes.

Uniformity of dosage units ⟨905⟩: meet the requirements, the following method being employed for chewable tablets.
PROCEDURE FOR CONTENT UNIFORMITY—
Mobile phase and *Chromatographic system*—Proceed as directed in the *Assay* under *Pseudoephedrine Hydrochloride Oral Solution*.
Standard preparation—Dissolve an accurately weighed quantity of USP Pseudoephedrine Hydrochloride RS in a mixture of 0.01 N hydrochloric acid and methanol (4 : 1) to obtain a solution having a known concentration of about 0.15 mg per mL.
Test preparation—Transfer 1 Tablet, accurately weighed, into a 100-mL volumetric flask, add 20 mL of methanol, and shake for 30 minutes. Add about 25 mL of 0.01 N hydrochloric acid, and sonicate to dissolve. Cool to room temperature, dilute with 0.01 N hydrochloric acid to volume, mix, and filter.
Procedure—Proceed as directed in the *Assay*.

Assay—
Mobile phase, Standard preparation, and *Chromatographic system*—Proceed as directed in the *Assay* under *Pseudoephedrine Hydrochloride Oral Solution*.
Assay preparation—Weigh and finely powder not fewer than 20 Tablets. Transfer an accurately weighed portion of the powder, equivalent to about 120 mg of pseudoephedrine hydrochloride, to a 100-mL volumetric flask, add 0.01 N hydrochloric acid, and soni-

cate to dissolve. Cool to room temperature. Dilute with 0.01 N hydrochloric acid to volume, mix, and filter.

Procedure—Separately inject equal volumes (about 10 µL) of the *Standard preparation* and the *Assay preparation* into the chromatograph, record the chromatograms, and measure the responses for the major peaks. Calculate the quantity, in mg, of pseudoephedrine hydrochloride ($C_{10}H_{15}NO \cdot HCl$) in the portion of Tablets taken by the formula:

$$100C(r_U / r_S)$$

in which C is the concentration, in mg per mL, of USP Pseudoephedrine Hydrochloride RS in the *Standard preparation*; and r_U and r_S are the peak responses obtained from the *Assay preparation* and the *Standard preparation*, respectively.

Pseudoephedrine Hydrochloride Extended-Release Tablets

» Pseudoephedrine Hydrochloride Extended-Release Tablets contain not less than 90.0 percent and not more than 110.0 percent of the labeled amount of pseudoephedrine hydrochloride ($C_{10}H_{15}NO \cdot HCl$).

Packaging and storage—Preserve in tight containers.
Labeling—When more than one *Dissolution Test* is given, the labeling states the *Dissolution Test* used only if *Test 1* is not used.
USP Reference standards ⟨11⟩—*USP Pseudoephedrine Hydrochloride RS.*
Identification—
A: *Infrared Absorption* ⟨197K⟩—
Test specimen—Triturate a number of Tablets, equivalent to about 180 mg of pseudoephedrine hydrochloride, and filter with about 10 mL of chloroform collected using vacuum filtration. Maintain the vacuum until no further filtrate can be collected, and evaporate the chloroform on a steam bath, taking care to avoid overheating. Recrystallize the residue from a small amount of dehydrated alcohol.
B: The retention time of the major peak in the chromatogram of the *Assay preparation* corresponds to that in the chromatogram of the *Standard preparation,* as obtained in the *Assay.*
Dissolution ⟨711⟩—
FOR PRODUCTS LABELED FOR DOSING EVERY 12 HOURS—
TEST 1—
Medium: water; 900 mL.
Apparatus 2: 50 rpm.
Times: 1, 3, and 6 hours.
Standard solution—Dissolve an accurately weighed quantity of USP Pseudoephedrine Hydrochloride RS in water, and dilute quantitatively, and stepwise if necessary, with water to obtain a solution having a known concentration of about 0.13 mg per mL.
Procedure—Determine the amount of $C_{10}H_{15}NO \cdot HCl$ dissolved by employing the procedure set forth in the *Assay*. Separately inject equal volumes (about 50 µL) of the *Standard solution* and the filtered solution under test. Calculate the amount of $C_{10}H_{15}NO \cdot HCl$ dissolved per Tablet.
Times and Tolerances—The percentage of the labeled amount of $C_{10}H_{15}NO \cdot HCl$ dissolved at the times given conforms to *Acceptance Table 2*.

Time (hours)	Amount dissolved
1	between 25% and 45%
3	between 50% and 75%
6	not less than 75%

TEST 3—If the product complies with this test, the labeling indicates that it meets USP *Dissolution Test 3*.
Medium, Apparatus, and *Times*—Proceed as directed for *Test 1*.
Procedure—Determine the amount of $C_{10}H_{15}NO \cdot HCl$ dissolved by employing UV absorption at the wavelength of maximum absorbance at about 214 nm on portions of the solution under test, filtered through a 0.45-µm filter and suitably diluted with *Medium,* if necessary, in comparison with a Standard solution having a known concentration of USP Pseudoephedrine Hydrochloride RS in the same *Medium.*
Times and Tolerances—The percentage of the labeled amount of $C_{10}H_{15}NO \cdot HCl$ dissolved at the times given conforms to *Acceptance Table 2*.

Time (hours)	Amount dissolved
1	between 25% and 45%
3	between 60% and 80%
6	not less than 80%

FOR PRODUCTS LABELED FOR DOSING EVERY 24 HOURS—
TEST 2—If the product complies with this test, the labeling indicates that it meets USP *Dissolution Test 2*.
Medium: 0.9% sodium chloride in water; 50 mL.
Apparatus 7 (see *Drug Release* ⟨724⟩): 30 cycles per minute; 2–3 cm amplitude. To prepare the sample, see *Figure 1* below that illustrates the following steps:
1. Place one Tablet on a 5- × 5-cm nylon netting.
2. Fold netting over the Tablet. Continue folding until the Tablet is enclosed in netting.
3. Fold netting so that the two open ends meet. The Tablet should be enveloped in the center of the netting.
4. Insert rod (see *Figure 4c* under *Drug Release* ⟨724⟩) through netting to secure the Tablet.
5. Secure netting with HPLC plastic ferrules or other appropriate device. Trim the excess netting. Attach each sample holder to the vertically reciprocating sample holder.

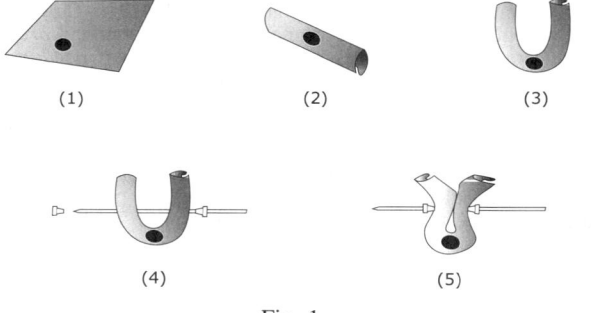

Fig. 1

Times: 2, 8, 14, and 24 hours.
Determine the amount of $C_{10}H_{15}NO \cdot HCl$ dissolved by employing the following method.
0.05 M Phosphate buffer, pH 6.8—Transfer 200 mL of water to a 1000-mL volumetric flask. Add 3.4 mL of phosphoric acid and 5 mL of triethylamine. Add water to almost 900 mL. Adjust with 1 N sodium hydroxide to a pH of about 6.8, dilute with water to volume, and mix.
Mobile phase—Prepare a filtered and degassed mixture of *0.05 M Phosphate buffer, pH 6.8* and methanol (9 : 1).
System suitability solution—Dissolve an accurately weighed quantity of USP Pseudoephedrine Hydrochloride RS in water, and dilute quantitatively, and stepwise if necessary, with water to obtain a solution having a known concentration of about 0.4 mg per mL.
Standard solutions—Prepare solutions in water having accurately known concentrations of USP Pseudoephedrine Hydrochloride RS in a range around the expected concentration of the solution under test at each time interval.
Chromatographic system (see *Chromatography* ⟨621⟩)—The liquid chromatograph is equipped with a 254-nm detector and a 4.6-mm × 5-cm column that contains packing L1. The flow rate is about 1.5 mL per minute. Chromatograph the *System suitability solution,* and record the peak responses as directed for *Procedure:* the tailing factor for the analyte peak is not more than 2; and the relative standard deviation for replicate injections is not more than 2.0%.
Procedure—Separately inject equal volumes (about 10 µL) of the *Standard solutions* and the solution under test into the chromato-

graph, record the chromatograms, and measure the responses for the major peak. Construct a calibration curve by plotting the peak response versus concentration of the *Standard solutions*. Determine the amount of $C_{10}H_{15}NO \cdot HCl$ dissolved at each time interval from a linear regression analysis of the calibration curve.

Times and *Tolerances*—The percentage of the labeled amount of $C_{10}H_{15}NO \cdot HCl$ dissolved at the times given conforms to *Acceptance Table 2*.

Time (hours)	Amount dissolved
2	between 20% and 35%
8	between 40% and 65%
14	between 60% and 90%
24	not less than 85%

Uniformity of dosage units ⟨905⟩: meet the requirements.

Assay—

Mobile phase—Prepare a filtered and degassed mixture of alcohol and ammonium acetate solution (1 in 250) (17 : 3).

Standard preparation—Dissolve an accurately weighed quantity of USP Pseudoephedrine Hydrochloride RS in alcohol to obtain a solution having a known concentration of about 1.2 mg per mL.

Assay preparation—Transfer not fewer than 20 Tablets to a suitable container, add 500 mL of alcohol, and homogenize until the Tablets are dispersed. Quantitatively transfer the contents of the container to a 1000-mL volumetric flask, dilute with alcohol to volume, mix, and allow to stand for the solids to settle. Transfer 25.0 mL of the supernatant into a 50-mL volumetric flask, dilute with alcohol to volume, and mix. Pass a portion of this solution through a 0.45-μm filter before injection.

Chromatographic system (see *Chromatography* ⟨621⟩)—The liquid chromatograph is equipped with a 254-nm detector and a 4.6-mm × 15-cm column that contains packing L3. The flow rate is about 0.7 mL per minute. Chromatograph the *Standard preparation*, and record the peak responses as directed for *Procedure*: the tailing factor is not more than 2.5; and the relative standard deviation for replicate injections is not more than 2.0%.

Procedure—Separately inject equal volumes (about 10 μL) of the *Standard preparation* and the *Assay preparation* into the chromatograph, record the chromatograms, and measure the responses for the major peaks. Calculate the quantity, in mg, of pseudoephedrine hydrochloride ($C_{10}H_{15}NO \cdot HCl$) in the portion of Tablets taken by the formula:

$$100C(r_U / r_S)$$

in which C is the concentration, in mg per mL, of USP Pseudoephedrine Hydrochloride RS in the *Standard preparation*; and r_U and r_S are the peak responses obtained from the *Assay preparation* and the *Standard preparation*, respectively.

Pseudoephedrine Hydrochloride, Carbinoxamine Maleate, and Dextromethorphan Hydrobromide Oral Solution

» Pseudoephedrine Hydrochloride, Carbinoxamine Maleate, and Dextromethorphan Hydrobromide Oral Solution contains not less than 90.0 percent and not more than 110.0 percent of the labeled amounts of carbinoxamine maleate ($C_{16}H_{19}ClN_2O \cdot C_4H_4O_4$), dextromethorphan hydrobromide ($C_{18}H_{25}NO \cdot HBr$), and pseudoephedrine hydrochloride ($C_{10}H_{15}NO \cdot HCl$).

Packaging and storage—Preserve in tight, light-resistant containers, and store at controlled room temperature.

USP Reference standards ⟨11⟩—*USP Carbinoxamine Maleate RS. USP Dextromethorphan Hydrobromide RS. USP Pseudoephedrine Hydrochloride RS.*

Identification

A: The retention times of the carbinoxamine maleate and dextromethorphan hydrobromide peaks in the chromatogram of the *Assay preparation* correspond to those in the chromatogram of the *Standard preparation*, as obtained in the *Assay for carbinoxamine maleate and dextromethorphan hydrobromide*.

B: The retention time of the pseudoephedrine hydrochloride peak in the chromatogram of the *Assay preparation* corresponds to that in the chromatogram of the *Standard preparation*, as obtained in the *Assay for pseudoephedrine hydrochloride*.

Microbial limits ⟨61⟩—The total aerobic microbial count does not exceed 100 per g, the total combined molds and yeasts count does not exceed 10 per g, and it meets the requirements of the tests for absence of *Salmonella* species and *Escherichia coli*.

Uniformity of dosage units ⟨905⟩—

FOR ORAL SOLUTION PACKAGED IN SINGLE-UNIT CONTAINERS: meets the requirements.

Deliverable volume ⟨698⟩—

FOR ORAL SOLUTION PACKAGED IN MULTIPLE-UNIT CONTAINERS: meets the requirements.

pH ⟨791⟩: between 3.0 and 5.0.

Alcohol content, *Method II* ⟨611⟩ *(if present)*: between 90.0% and 110.0% of the labeled amount of C_2H_5OH is found.

Assay for carbinoxamine maleate and dextromethorphan hydrobromide—

pH 5.5 buffer—Dissolve about 4.4 g of dibasic potassium phosphate in 1000 mL of water. Adjust with phosphoric acid to a pH of 5.5.

Mobile phase—Prepare a filtered and degassed mixture of methanol and *pH 5.5 buffer* (60 : 40). Make adjustments if necessary (see *System Suitability* under *Chromatography* ⟨621⟩).

Standard preparation—Dissolve accurately weighed quantities of USP Carbinoxamine Maleate RS and USP Dextromethorphan Hydrobromide RS in water, and dilute quantitatively, and stepwise if necessary, with water to obtain a solution having known concentrations of about 0.1 mg per mL of carbinoxamine maleate and 0.3 mg per mL of dextromethorphan hydrobromide.

Assay preparation—Transfer an accurately measured volume of Oral Solution to a volumetric flask, and dilute with water to volume to obtain a solution having concentrations of about 0.1 mg per mL of carbinoxamine maleate and 0.3 mg per mL of dextromethorphan hydrobromide, and mix.

Chromatographic system (see *Chromatography* ⟨621⟩)—The liquid chromatograph is equipped with a 225-nm detector and a 4.6-mm × 25-cm column that contains packing L9. The flow rate is about 1.5 mL per minute. Chromatograph the *Standard preparation*, and record the peak responses as directed for *Procedure*: the relative retention times are about 0.8 for dextromethorphan and 1.0 for carbinoxamine; the resolution, R, between carbinoxamine and dextromethorphan is not less than 3.0; the tailing factor for the dextromethorphan peak is not more than 2.0; and the relative standard deviation for replicate injections is not more than 2.0%.

Procedure—Separately inject equal volumes (about 20 μL) of the *Standard preparation* and the *Assay preparation* into the chromatograph, record the chromatograms, and measure the responses for the analyte peaks. Calculate the quantities, in mg, of carbinoxamine maleate ($C_{16}H_{19}ClN_2O \cdot C_4H_4O_4$) and dextromethorphan hydrobromide ($C_{18}H_{25}NO \cdot HBr$) in each mL in the volume of Oral Solution taken by the formula:

$$C(VD)(r_U / r_S)$$

in which C is the concentration, in mg per mL, of the appropriate Reference Standard in the *Standard preparation*; V is the volume of Oral Solution taken; D is the dilution factor used for the *Assay preparation*; and r_U and r_S are the peak responses for the appropriate analyte obtained from the *Assay preparation* and the *Standard preparation*, respectively.

Assay for pseudoephedrine hydrochloride—

pH 5.5 buffer and *Mobile phase*—Proceed as directed in the *Assay for carbinoxamine maleate and dextromethorphan hydrobromide*.

Standard preparation—Dissolve an accurately weighed quantity of USP Pseudoephedrine Hydrochloride RS in water, and dilute quantitatively, and stepwise if necessary, with water to obtain a solution having a known concentration of about of 1.2 mg per mL of pseudoephedrine hydrochloride.

Assay preparation—Transfer an accurately measured volume of Oral Solution to a volumetric flask, dilute with water to volume to obtain a solution having a concentration of about 1.2 mg per mL of pseudoephedrine hydrochloride, and mix.

Chromatographic system (see *Chromatography* ⟨621⟩)—The liquid chromatograph is equipped with a 257-nm detector and a 4.6-mm × 25-cm column that contains packing L9. The flow rate is about 1.5 mL per minute. Chromatograph the *Standard preparation*, and record the peak responses as directed for *Procedure*: the column efficiency is not less than 1000 theoretical plates; and the relative standard deviation for replicate injections is not more than 2.0%.

Procedure—Separately inject equal volumes (about 20 μL) of the *Standard preparation* and the *Assay preparation* into the chromatograph, record the chromatograms, and measure the responses for the analyte peaks. Calculate the quantity, in mg, of pseudoephedrine hydrochloride ($C_{10}H_{15}NO \cdot HCl$) in each mL in the volume of Oral Solution taken by the formula:

$$C(VD)(r_U / r_S)$$

in which C is the concentration, in mg per mL, of USP Pseudoephedrine Hydrochloride RS in the *Standard preparation*; V is the volume of Oral Solution taken; D is the dilution factor used for the *Assay preparation*; and r_U and r_S are the peak responses for pseudoephedrine hydrochloride obtained from the *Assay preparation* and the *Standard preparation*, respectively.

Pseudoephedrine Sulfate

$(C_{10}H_{15}NO)_2 \cdot H_2SO_4$ 428.54
Benzenemethanol, α-[1-(methylamino)ethyl]-, [S-(R*,R*)]-, sulfate (2 : 1) (salt).
(+)-Pseudoephedrine sulfate (2 : 1) (salt)   [7460-12-0].

» Pseudoephedrine Sulfate contains not less than 98.0 percent and not more than 100.5 percent of $(C_{10}H_{15}NO)_2 \cdot H_2SO_4$, calculated on the dried basis.

Packaging and storage—Preserve in tight, light-resistant containers.
USP Reference standards ⟨11⟩—*USP Pseudoephedrine Sulfate RS.*
Identification—
  A: *Infrared Absorption* ⟨197K⟩.
  B: *Ultraviolet Absorption* ⟨197U⟩—
  Solution: 500 μg per mL.
  Medium: water.
Absorptivities at 257 nm, calculated on the dried basis, do not differ by more than 3.0%.
  C: A solution of it responds to the test for *Sulfate* ⟨191⟩.
Melting range, *Class I* ⟨741⟩: between 174° and 179°, but the range between beginning and end of melting does not exceed 2°.
Specific rotation ⟨781S⟩: between +56.0° and +59.0°.
  Test solution: 50 mg per mL, in water.
pH ⟨791⟩: between 5.0 and 6.5 in a solution (1 in 20).
Loss on drying ⟨731⟩—Dry it at 105° for 2 hours: it loses not more than 2.0% of its weight.
Residue on ignition ⟨281⟩: not more than 0.1%.
Chloride ⟨221⟩—A 200-mg portion shows no more chloride than corresponds to 0.4 mL of 0.02 N hydrochloric acid (0.14%).
Heavy metals—Treat a solution of 1.0 g in 20 mL of dilute alcohol (1 in 2) with 5 mL of sodium hydroxide solution (1 in 20) and 5 drops of sodium sulfide TS: the color developed is not darker than that of a blank determination performed simultaneously, containing 10 ppm of standard lead solution (see *Heavy Metals* ⟨231⟩).

Ordinary impurities ⟨466⟩—
  Test solution: alcohol.
  Standard solution: alcohol.
  Eluant: a mixture of alcohol, glacial acetic acid, and water (10 : 3 : 1).
  Visualization: Expose the plate for 24 hours to iodine vapors in a pre-equilibrated closed chamber, on the bottom of which there are iodine crystals.
Assay—Dissolve about 150 mg of Pseudoephedrine Sulfate, accurately weighed, in 50 mL of glacial acetic acid. Titrate with 0.1 N perchloric acid VS, determining the endpoint potentiometrically. Perform a blank determination, and make any necessary correction. Each mL of 0.1 N perchloric acid is equivalent to 42.85 mg of $(C_{10}H_{15}NO)_2 \cdot H_2SO_4$.

Psyllium Hemicellulose

» Psyllium Hemicellulose is the alkali soluble fraction of the husk from *Plantago ovata* Forssk. It consists of a combination of highly substituted arabinoxylan polysaccharides. These polysaccharides are linear chains of xylose units (β-(1→4)-xylan) to which are attached single units of arabinose and additional xylose. Rhamnose, galactose, glucose, and rhamnosyluronic acid residues are also present as minor constituents. It contains not less than 75.0 percent of dietary soluble fiber, calculated on the dried basis.

Packaging and storage—Preserve in tight containers. Store at 25°, excursions permitted between 15° and 30°.
Identification—
  A: The powdered mucilage stains red with ruthenium red TS and lead acetate TS.
  B: It meets the requirements of the test for *Swell volume*.
Total acidity—To a beaker, transfer 40 mL of the supernatant as obtained below in the test for *Swell volume* without disturbing the gel. Add 1 mL of phenolphthalein TS, and titrate with 0.03 N sodium hydroxide. Not more than 1.8 mL is consumed.
Microbial limits ⟨61⟩—The total aerobic microbial count does not exceed 1000 cfu per g and the total combined molds and yeasts count does not exceed 100 cfu per g. It meets the requirements of the tests for absence of *Salmonella* species and *Escherichia coli*.
Loss on drying ⟨731⟩—Dry at 105° for 3 hours: it loses not more than 12.0% of its weight.
Total ash ⟨561⟩: not more than 5.0%.
Acid-insoluble ash ⟨561⟩: not more than 1.0%.
Limit of alcohol—
  Internal standard solution—Transfer 5.0 mL of *n*-propyl alcohol into a 500-mL volumetric flask containing approximately 450 mL of water. Dilute with water to volume, insert the stopper into the flask, and mix well.
  Standard stock solution—Transfer 5.0 mL of absolute alcohol at 20 ± 2° into a 500-mL volumetric flask containing approximately 450 mL of water. Dilute with water to volume, insert the stopper into the flask, and mix well.
  Standard solution—Transfer 10.0 mL of the *Standard stock solution* and 10.0 mL of *Internal standard solution* into a 100-mL volumetric flask. Dilute with water to volume, insert the stopper into the flask, and mix well.
  Test solution—Transfer 0.5 g of Psyllium Hemicellulose, accurately weighed, into a 150-mL conical flask. Add about 90 mL of water, insert the stopper into the flask, and stir rapidly for 3 hours using a magnetic stirrer. Add 10.0 mL of the *Internal standard solution*, and mix well. Pass the sample through a filter having a 0.45-μm porosity.
  Chromatographic system (see *Chromatography* ⟨621⟩)—The gas chromatograph is equipped with a flame-ionization detector and a 0.53-mm × 30-m fused silica analytical column coated with 3.0-μm G43 stationary phase. A 0.53-mm × 2-m fused silica guard column may be used. The chromatograph is programmed as follows. Ini-

tially, the column temperature is equilibrated at 40° for 5 minutes. The temperature is then increased at a rate of 10° per minute to 230°, and is maintained at 230° for 3 minutes. The injection port temperature is maintained at 250°, and the detector is maintained at 300°. The carrier gas is helium. The split flow ratio is about 10 : 1, and the flow rate is maintained at about 4.0 mL per minute. Inject the *Standard solution,* and record the peak responses as directed for *Procedure:* the relative standard deviation for replicate injections is not more than 2%.

Procedure—Separately inject equal volumes (about 0.5 µL) of the *Standard solution* and the *Test solution* into the chromatograph, record the chromatograms, and measure the responses for all the peaks. Calculate the percentage of alcohol in the portion of Psyllium Hemicellulose taken by the formula:

$$1000(C/W)(R_U / R_S)$$

in which C is the concentration, in mg per mL, of alcohol in the *Standard stock solution;* W is the weight, in mg, of Psyllium Hemicellulose taken; and R_U and R_S are the ratios of the peak responses of alcohol to those of *n*-propyl alcohol from the *Test solution* and the *Standard solution,* respectively: not more than 12.0% (w/w) is found.

Organic volatile impurities, Method IV ⟨467⟩: meets the requirements.

(Official until July 1, 2008)

Heavy metals, Method II ⟨231⟩: 10 µg per g.

Swell volume—Add 0.50 g of Psyllium Hemicellulose to a glass-stoppered, 100-mL graduated mixing cylinder. To avoid material clumping, hold the cylinder at a 45° angle, and gently rotate it while using a wash bottle to forcefully add about 30 mL of water. Add water to bring the total volume to 100 mL, and cap the cylinder. Invert the cylinder several times until a uniform suspension is achieved, and allow to stand. Gently invert the cylinder several times again at 4 hours and 8 hours after the initial sample preparation, and allow to stand. Allow the gel to settle for 16 hours. Determine the volume of the gel: not less than 80 mL per g of Psyllium Hemicellulose is found.

Content of soluble dietary fiber—

Alcohol solution—Transfer 82.0 mL of alcohol to a 100-mL volumetric flask, dilute with water to volume, and mix.

Buffer solution—Dissolve 1.95 g of 2-(*N*-morpholino)-ethanesulfonic acid and 1.22 g of tris(hydroxymethyl)aminomethane in 170 mL of water. Adjust with 6 N sodium hydroxide to a pH of 8.2, dilute with water to 200 mL, and mix. [NOTE—It is important to adjust the pH to 8.2 at 24°. If the *Buffer solution* temperature is 20°, adjust the pH to 8.3; if the temperature is 28°, adjust the pH to 8.1. For deviations between 20° and 28°, adjust by interpolation.]

Acid solution—Prepare 0.561 N hydrochloric acid by dissolving 9.35 mL of 6 N hydrochloric acid in 70 mL of water. Dilute with water to 100.0 mL, and mix.

Phosphate buffer—Prepare a pH 6.0 phosphate buffer (see *Buffer Solutions* under *Reagents, Indicators, and Solutions*).

Protease solution—Dissolve 5 mg of protease in 0.1 mL of *Phosphate buffer.*

Enzyme purity—To ensure the absence of undesirable enzymatic activities and the presence of desirable enzymatic activities, proceed as directed for *Test preparations* and *Procedure* using the substrates listed in the following table in place of Psyllium Hemicellulose.

Substrate	Weight in g	Activity Tested
Pectin	0.2	Pectinase
Arabinogalactan	0.2	Hemicellulase
β-Glucan	0.2	β-Glucanase
Wheat starch	1.0	α-Amylase and amyloglucosidase
Corn starch	1.0	α-Amylase and amyloglucosidase
Casein	0.3	Protease

The enzyme preparation is suitable if more than 90% of the original weight of pectin, arabinogalactan, and β-glucan is recovered; not more than 2% of the original weight of casein and corn starch is recovered; and not more than 1% of the original weight of wheat starch is recovered. [NOTE—Test the enzyme purity of every new lot of enzyme and at 6-month intervals thereafter.]

Blank preparations—Using two 400-mL tall-form beakers, appropriately labeled, proceed as directed for *Procedure* without Psyllium Hemicellulose.

Test preparations—Weigh accurately, in duplicate, approximately 0.2 g of Psyllium Hemicellulose, previously milled to very fine powder. [NOTE—Duplicates should differ by less than 1 mg in weight.] Transfer duplicate samples to appropriately labeled 400-mL, tall-form beakers, and proceed as directed for *Procedure*.

Procedure—Treat each preparation in the following manner. Add 40 mL of *Buffer solution* to the beaker. [NOTE—For the *Test preparation,* stir until Psyllium Hemicellulose is completely dispersed.] Add 125 µL of heat-stable α-amylase solution, and stir to ensure uniform mixing. Cover the beaker with aluminum foil, and incubate over a water bath maintained at 95° to 100° for 15 minutes, with continuous agitation. [NOTE—Start timing once the water bath temperature reaches 95°; a total time of 35 minutes is usually sufficient.] Remove the beaker from the water bath, and cool to 60°. Remove the aluminum foil, scrape any ring from inside the beaker, and disperse any gels in the bottom of the beaker with a spatula. Rinse the walls of the beaker and the spatula with 10 mL of water, collecting the rinsings in the beaker. Add 500 µL of *Protease solution.* Cover with aluminum foil, and incubate over a water bath maintained at 60 ± 3° for 30 minutes with continuous agitation. [NOTE—Start timing when the bath temperature reaches 60°.] Remove the foil, and transfer 5 mL of *Acid solution* while stirring. Adjust, if necessary, with 1 N sodium hydroxide or 1 N hydrochloric acid to a pH of 4.28 ± 0.07 at 60°. [NOTE—It is important to adjust the pH to 4.28 while the solution in the beaker is maintained at 60°, otherwise the pH will increase at lower temperatures.] Add 150 µL of amyloglucosidase solution while stirring. Cover with aluminum foil, and incubate over a water bath maintained at 60 ± 3° for 30 minutes with constant agitation. [NOTE—Start timing once the water bath reaches 60°.] Transfer approximately 40 mL of the beaker contents to a 50-mL centrifuge tube, and sonicate the tube contents for 3 minutes.* Centrifuge at 10,000–14,000 rpm for 10 minutes. Carefully pour the supernatant into an appropriately labeled 600-mL tared beaker. Do not disturb any pellet in the bottom of the centrifuge tube. Add the remaining sample from the original 400-mL beaker into the centrifuge tube still containing the pellet. Rinse the 400-mL beaker with 15–20 mL of water, and add the rinsing to the 50-mL centrifuge tube. Centrifuge the sample at 10,000–14,000 rpm for 10 minutes. Carefully pour the supernatant into the 600-mL beaker containing the first supernatant. Add 390 mL (measured before heating) of alcohol at 60° to the 600-mL beaker. Cover the beaker, and allow to stand for at least 1 hour to form a precipitate.

Place 3 g of chromatographic siliceous earth into a clean air-dried crucible with a fritted disk. Heat the crucible containing chromatographic siliceous earth at 525° in a muffle furnace for at least 4 hours. Cool. Pass deionized water through the crucible while applying constant suction. Rinse with acetone, and allow to air-dry. Store the crucible in a convection oven at approximately 130° for at least 2 hours before use. Weigh the prepared crucible to 0.1 mg before use. Wet the chromatographic siliceous earth in the crucible using a stream of *Alcohol solution* from a washing bottle, and apply suction to evenly distribute the chromatographic siliceous earth over the fritted disk. Maintaining the suction, transfer the supernatant and precipitate from the beaker to the crucible, and filter. Transfer any solid residue in the beaker with the aid of *Alcohol solution.* [NOTE—In some cases, gums may form during filtration, trapping liquid in the residue. If so, break the surface film with a spatula to improve filtration.] Wash the residue in the crucible sequentially with 30 mL of *Alcohol solution,* 20 mL of alcohol, and 20 mL of acetone. Dry the crucible containing the residue at 100° in a convection oven for at least 4 hours, cool to room temperature in a desiccator. Determine the weight of the residue *(R).*

Use one of the duplicate residues from the *Test preparations* and one of the blank residues from the *Blank preparations* to determine

---

*A suitable sonicator is Sonifier 250 (or equivalent), equipped with a 12-mm tip, from Branson Ultrasonic Corp., Danbury, CT, in which an output control value of 3 and a cycle time of 75% generates a power output of 43 W.

the protein content, in mg, by placing the residue in a 500-mL Kjeldahl flask, and proceeding as directed for *Method I* under *Nitrogen Determination* ⟨461⟩. The protein content is determined by multiplying the content of nitrogen found by 6.25. Incinerate the residue from the remaining duplicate of the *Test preparation* and the *Blank preparation* as directed for *Total Ash* under *Articles of Botanical Origin* ⟨561⟩ at a reduced temperature of 525°, and determine the ash content as directed. Calculate the corrected average weight of the blank, in mg, B, by the formula:

$$R_B - P_B - A_B$$

in which R_B is the weight, in mg, of the average blank residue for duplicate blank determinations; P_B is the content, in mg, of protein found in the blank; and A_B is the content, in mg, of ash found in the blank. Calculate the content of soluble dietary fiber, in percentage, by the formula:

$$100(R_U - P_U - A_U - B)/W_U$$

in which R_U is the weight, in mg, of average residue for the duplicate *Test preparations*; P_U is the content of protein, in mg, found in the Psyllium Hemicellulose; A_U is the content of ash, in mg, found in the Psyllium Hemicellulose; B is the average weight of the blank as calculated above; and W_U is the average weight, in mg, of the Psyllium Hemicellulose taken.

Psyllium Husk

» Psyllium Husk is the cleaned, dried seed coat (epidermis) separated by winnowing and thrashing from the seeds of *Plantago ovata* Forssk., known in commerce as Blond Psyllium or Indian Psyllium or Ispaghula, or from *Plantago arenaria* Waldst. & Kit. (*Plantago psyllium* L.) known in commerce as Spanish or French Psyllium (Fam. Plantaginaceae), in whole or in powdered form.

Packaging and storage—Preserve in well-closed containers, secured against insect attack (see *Preservation* under *Vegetable and Animal Drugs* in the *General Notices*).

Botanic characteristics—

Histology—Husk—The epidermis is composed of large cells having transparent walls filled with mucilage, and the cells swell rapidly in aqueous mounts and appear polygonal to slightly rounded in a surface view, when viewed from above (from below they appear elongated to rectangular). The swelling takes place mainly in the radial direction. The mucilage of the epidermal cells stains red with ruthenium red and lead acetate TS. The very occasional starch granules that are present in some of the epidermal cells, and that may be found embedded in the mucilage, are small and simple or compounded with four or more components.

Powdered Psyllium Seed Husk—It is a pale to medium buff-colored powder, having a slight pinkish tinge and a weak characteristic odor. Occasional single and 2- to 4-compound starch granules, the individual grains being spheroidal plano to angular convex from 2 to 10 µm in diameter, are found embedded in the mucilage. Entire or broken epidermal cells are filled with mucilage. In surface view, the epidermal cells appear polygonal to slightly rounded. Mucilage stains red with ruthenium red TS and lead acetate TS. Some of the elongated and rectangular cells representing the lower part of epidermis and also radially swollen epidermal cells can be found.

Identification—

A: *Mounted in cresol*—Cells, viewed microscopically, are composed of polygonal prismatic cells having 4 to 6 straight or slightly wavy walls.

B: *Mounted in alcohol and irrigated with water*—Viewed microscopically, the mucilage in the outer part of the epidermal cells swells rapidly and goes into solution.

Microbial limits ⟨61⟩—The total combined molds and yeasts count does not exceed 1000 cfu per g, and it meets the requirements of the test for absence of *Salmonella* species and *Escherichia coli*.

Total ash ⟨561⟩: not more than 4.0%.

Acid-insoluble ash ⟨561⟩: not more than 1.0%.

Water, *Method II* ⟨921⟩: not more than 12.0%.

Light extraneous matter—[NOTE—Perform this test in a well-ventilated hood.] Transfer 99 to 101 g of Psyllium Husk, weighed to 0.1 g accuracy, to a 1000-mL tall-form beaker. Add about 800 mL of trichloroethylene, previously adjusted to a temperature of 24° to 26°, and maintain this temperature throughout the test. Stir the husk for about 5 seconds, and allow it to settle while protecting the surface from drafts in the hood. Remove the floating material with a spoon made of 50-mesh screen, and transfer the material to a piece of filter paper in a dish. Stir the husk mixture again, allow it to settle, remove the floating material again, and combine it with the material on the paper. Repeat this procedure until no more material appears on the surface. Dry the removed material with the paper in a hood and then in an oven at 40° for 3 hours. Cool to room temperature. Weigh the filter paper with the material. Brush the material off the paper, weigh the paper, and then calculate the percentage of light extraneous matter: no more than 5% is found.

Insect infestation—Transfer 25 g to a 250-mL beaker, add sufficient solvent hexane to saturate, add an additional 75 to 100 mL of solvent hexane, and allow to stand for 10 minutes, stirring occasionally with a stirring rod. Wet a sheet of filter paper with alcohol, and filter the mixture with the aid of vacuum. Discard the filtrate. Transfer the residue to the original beaker with the aid of alcohol. Add alcohol to bring the volume to 150 mL above the level of the transferred residue. Boil for 10 minutes. Filter through alcohol-wetted paper as above. Prepare a trap flask, consisting of a 2000-mL graduated, narrow-mouth conical flask into which is inserted a rubber disk supported on a stiff metal rod about 4 mm in diameter and longer than the height of the flask, the rod being threaded at the lower end and furnished with nuts and washers to hold the disk in place, and the disk being of the proper shape and size to prevent liquid in the body of the flask from spilling when it is pressed up against the neck from the inside. Transfer the residue to the trap flask, completing the transfer with the aid of hot water. Add sufficient hot water to bring the volume to 1000 mL. Add 20 mL of hydrochloric acid. Raise the rod, and support it so that the rubber disk is held above the liquid level. Rinse the rubber disk with hot water. Spray the inside of the neck of the flask with an antifoam spray. Boil for 30 minutes, and cool to room temperature. Add 40 mL of solvent hexane, and agitate for 1 minute by tilting the flask and moving the rod vertically with wrist action. Allow to stand for 5 minutes. Add water to bring the level of liquid to the neck of the flask, and allow to stand for 20 minutes. Simultaneously rotate the disk to free it from settled material, and raise it as far as possible into the neck of the flask. Prepare a sheet of ruled filter paper, with lines approximately 5 mm apart for filtration by moistening it with water and placing it on a vacuum funnel. Transfer the material trapped in the neck of the flask to the filter with the aid of water. If necessary, wash the paper with alcohol to remove traces of hexane. Place the paper on a 100-mm petri dish that has been wetted with a solution containing equal volumes of glycerin and alcohol. Add 35 mL of solvent hexane to the flask, and gently stir with the trapping rod. Add water to bring the liquid level into the neck of the flask. Allow to stand for 15 minutes. Using the same technique as before, transfer the trapped material onto a separate paper. Examine the papers at 30× magnification: in the case of powdered Psyllium Husk, not more than 400 insect fragments, including mites and psocids, can be seen; in the case of whole Psyllium Husk, not more than 100 insect fragments, including mites and psocids, can be seen.

Swell volume—Transfer 250 mL of simulated intestinal fluid TS without enzymes to a glass-stoppered, 500-mL graduated cylinder. Gradually, with shaking, add 3.5 g of the Psyllium Husk until a uniform, smooth suspension is obtained. Dilute with the same fluid to 500 mL. Shake the cylinder for about 1 minute every 30 minutes for 8 hours. Allow the gel to settle for 16 hours (total time 24 hours). Determine the volume of the gel: it is not less than 40 mL per g for powdered Psyllium Husk, and not less than 35 mL per g for whole Psyllium Husk.

Psyllium Hydrophilic Mucilloid for Oral Suspension

» Psyllium Hydrophilic Mucilloid for Oral Suspension is a dry mixture of Psyllium Husk with suitable additives.

Packaging and storage—Preserve in tight containers.

Identification—Microscopically, it shows the presence of fragmented Psyllium Husk, as described for *Histology—Husk* in the section, *Botanic characteristics*, under *Psyllium Husk*.

Microbial limits ⟨61⟩—It meets the requirements of the tests for absence of *Salmonella* species and of *Escherichia coli*.

Swell volume—Transfer 250 mL of simulated intestinal fluid TS without enzymes to a glass-stoppered, 500-mL graduated cylinder. Gradually, with shaking, add an amount of Psyllium Hydrophilic Mucilloid for Oral Suspension, equivalent to 3.5 g of psyllium husk, and shake until a uniform, smooth suspension is obtained. Dilute with the same fluid to 500 mL. Shake the cylinder for about 1 minute every 30 minutes for 8 hours. Allow the gel to settle for 16 hours (total time 24 hours). Determine the volume of the gel: it is not less than 110 mL.

Pumice

» Pumice is a substance of volcanic origin, consisting chiefly of complex silicates of aluminum, potassium, and sodium.

Packaging and storage—Preserve in well-closed containers.

Labeling—Label powdered Pumice to indicate, in descriptive terms, the fineness of the powder.

Powdered Pumice meets the following requirements:

"Pumice Flour" or "Superfine Pumice": not less than 97.0% of pumice flour or superfine pumice passes through a No. 200 standard mesh sieve.

"Fine Pumice": not less than 95.0% of fine pumice passes through a No. 150 standard mesh sieve and not more than 75.0% passes through a No. 200 standard mesh sieve.

"Coarse Pumice": not less than 95.0% of coarse pumice passes through a No. 60 standard mesh sieve and not more than 5.0% passes through a No. 200 standard mesh sieve.

Water-soluble substances—Boil 10 g with 50 mL of water for 30 minutes, adding water from time to time to maintain approximately the original volume, and then filter: the filtrate is neutral to litmus, and one-half of this filtrate, when evaporated and dried at 105° for 1 hour, yields not more than 10 mg of residue (0.20%).

Acid-soluble substances—Boil 1 g of Pumice with 25 mL of 3 N hydrochloric acid for 30 minutes, adding water from time to time to maintain approximately the original volume, then filter the liquid. Add 5 drops of sulfuric acid to the filtrate, evaporate to dryness, ignite, and weigh the residue: not more than 60 mg of residue is obtained (6.0%).

Iron—Acidify the remaining half of the filtrate from the test for *Water-soluble substances* with hydrochloric acid, and add a few drops of potassium ferrocyanide TS: no blue color is produced.

Pyrantel Pamoate

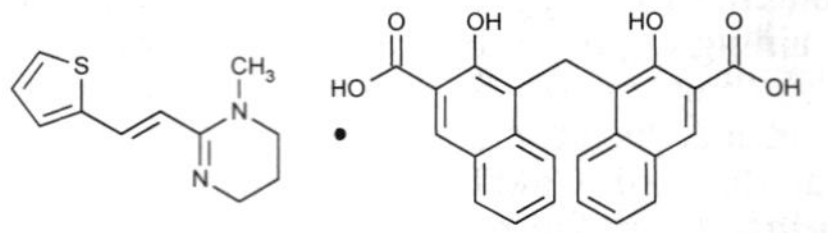

$C_{11}H_{14}N_2S \cdot C_{23}H_{16}O_6$ 594.68

Pyrimidine, 1,4,5,6-tetrahydro-1-methyl-2-[2-(2-thienyl)ethenyl]-, (*E*)-, compd. with 4,4′-methylenebis[3-hydroxy-2-naphthalenecarboxylic acid] (1 : 1).

(*E*)-1,4,5,6-Tetrahydro-1-methyl-2-[2-(2-thienyl)vinyl]pyrimidine 4,4′-methylenebis[3-hydroxy-2-naphthoate](1 : 1)   [22204-24-6]

» Pyrantel Pamoate contains not less than 97.0 percent and not more than 103.0 percent of $C_{34}H_{30}N_2O_6S$, calculated on the dried basis.

Packaging and storage—Preserve in well-closed, light-resistant containers.

USP Reference standards ⟨11⟩—*USP Pamoic Acid RS. USP Pyrantel Pamoate RS.*

Identification—
A: *Infrared Absorption* ⟨197K⟩.
B: *Ultraviolet Absorption* ⟨197U⟩—
Solution: 16 µg per mL.
Medium: methanol.
C: The chromatogram of the *Assay preparation* obtained as directed in the *Assay* exhibits major peaks due to pyrantel base and pamoic acid, the retention times of which correspond to those exhibited in the chromatogram of the *Standard preparation* obtained as directed in the *Assay*.

Loss on drying ⟨731⟩—Dry it in vacuum at 60° for 3 hours: it loses not more than 2.0% of its weight.

Residue on ignition ⟨281⟩:   not more than 0.5%, from 1.33 g.

Heavy metals, *Method II* ⟨231⟩:   0.005%.

Limit of iron ⟨241⟩—To the residue obtained in the test for *Residue on ignition* add 3 mL of hydrochloric acid and 2 mL of nitric acid, and evaporate on a steam bath to dryness. Dissolve the residue in 2 mL of hydrochloric acid with the aid of gentle heat. Add 18 mL of hydrochloric acid, dilute with water to 50 mL, and mix. Dilute 5 mL of this solution with water to 47 mL: the limit is 0.0075%.

Related compounds—
TEST 1—
Chromatographic sheet—Impregnate 18- × 56-cm filter paper (Whatman No. 1 or equivalent) with a freshly prepared 7 : 3 mixture of acetone and glycine–sodium chloride–hydrochloric acid buffer solution (prepared by mixing 3 volumes of a solution that is 0.3 M with respect to both glycine and sodium chloride with 7 volumes of 0.3 M hydrochloric acid). Press the impregnated paper uniformly between white, nonfluorescent blotters to remove the excess solvent.
Test solutions: 0.2 and 20 mg per mL, in a mixture of chloroform, methanol, and ammonium hydroxide (10 : 10 : 1).
Standard solutions: 0.2 and 20 mg per mL, in a mixture of chloroform, methanol, and ammonium hydroxide (10 : 10 : 1).
Application volume: 20 µL.
Developing solvent system: a mixture of ethyl acetate, butyl alcohol, and water (10 : 1 : 1).
Procedure—Proceed as directed for *Descending Chromatography* under *Chromatography* ⟨621⟩. Develop for 16 to 20 hours. Remove the sheet from the chamber, air-dry for 10 minutes, transfer to an air-circulating oven, and dry at 60° for 30 minutes. Examine the chromatogram on a 254-nm UV scanner screen: the R_F value of the principal spot from the *Test solution* corresponds to that obtained from the appropriate *Standard solution;* and no spot in the chromatogram of the more concentrated *Test solution*, other than the principal spot, is larger or more intense than the principal spot from the less concentrated *Test solution*.

TEST 2—

Adsorbent: 0.25-mm layer of chromatographic silica gel mixture.

Test stock solution—Transfer about 100 mg of Pyrantel Pamoate, accurately weighed, to a 10-mL volumetric flask, dissolve in and dilute with dimethylformamide to volume, and mix.

Test solution—Transfer 1.0 mL of the *Test stock solution* to a 100-mL volumetric flask, dilute with dimethylformamide to volume, and mix.

Standard solution—Transfer about 50 mg of USP Pyrantel Pamoate RS to a 5-mL volumetric flask, dilute with dimethylformamide to volume, and mix.

Developing solvent system: a mixture of ethyl acetate, water, and glacial acetic acid (3 : 1 : 1).

Procedure—Proceed as directed for *Thin-Layer Chromatography* under *Chromatography* ⟨621⟩, except to line the developing chamber with filter paper, and allow to equilibrate. Apply 5-µL portions of the *Test stock solution*, the *Test solution*, and the *Standard solution* to the plate, and allow to dry. Develop the chromatogram until the solvent front has moved about 10 cm. Remove the plate from the developing chamber, and allow to air-dry for about 10 minutes. Examine the plate under short-wavelength UV light. The chromatograms obtained from the *Test stock solution* and the *Test solution* exhibit spots for pyrantel and the pamoate moiety at relative positions corresponding to those obtained from the chromatogram of the *Standard solution*: the R_F value of pyrantel is about 0.3, and the R_F value of the pamoate moiety is about 0.8. No spot obtained from the *Test stock solution*, other than that of pyrantel and the pamoate moiety, is more intense than the pyrantel spot obtained from the *Test solution*.

Content of pamoic acid—

Mobile phase and *Chromatographic system*—Prepare as directed in the *Assay*.

Standard solution—Dissolve an accurately weighed quantity of USP Pamoic Acid RS in *Mobile phase* to obtain a solution having a known concentration of about 0.52 mg per mL. Transfer 1.0 mL of this solution to a 10-mL volumetric flask, dilute with *Mobile phase* to volume, and mix.

Test solution—Use the *Assay preparation*.

Procedure—Inject equal volumes (about 20 µL) of the *Standard solution* and the *Test solution* into the chromatograph, record the chromatograms, and record the peak responses as directed in the *Assay*. Calculate the quantity, in mg, of $C_{23}H_{16}O_6$ in the portion of Pyrantel Pamoate taken by the formula:

$$1000C(r_U / r_S)$$

in which C is the concentration, in mg per mL, of USP Pamoic Acid RS in the *Standard solution* and r_U and r_S are the peak responses for pamoic acid obtained from the *Test solution* and the *Standard solution*, respectively: the content of pamoic acid is between 63.4% and 67.3%, calculated on the dried basis.

Assay—[NOTE—Use low-actinic glassware in preparing solutions of pyrantel pamoate, and otherwise protect the solutions from unnecessary exposure to bright light. Complete the *Assay* without prolonged interruption.]

Mobile phase—Prepare a mixture of acetonitrile, acetic acid, water, and diethylamine (92.8 : 3 : 3 : 1.2), filter, and degas. Make adjustments if necessary (see *System Suitability* under *Chromatography* ⟨621⟩). [NOTE—Increasing the amount of acetonitrile in *Mobile phase* increases retention times. Increasing the amount of acetic acid, water, and diethylamine decreases retention times. Should the *Mobile phase* need to be adjusted, maintain the ratios among acetic acid, water, and diethylamine (1 : 1 : 0.4).]

Standard preparation—Prepare a solution in *Mobile phase* having an accurately known concentration of about 80 µg of USP Pyrantel Pamoate RS per mL.

Assay preparation—Transfer about 80 mg of Pyrantel Pamoate, accurately weighed, to a 100-mL volumetric flask, dissolve in and dilute with *Mobile phase* to volume, and mix. Dilute 1.0 mL of this solution with *Mobile phase* to 10.0 mL, and mix.

Chromatographic system (see *Chromatography* ⟨621⟩)—The liquid chromatograph is equipped with a 288-nm detector and 4.6-mm × 25-cm column that contains packing L3. The flow rate is about 1.0 mL per minute. Chromatograph the *Standard preparation,* and record the peak responses as directed for *Procedure:* the resolution, R, between pyrantel and pamoic acid is not less than 10.0; the number of theoretical plates for the pyrantel peak is not less than 8000; the tailing factor for the pyrantel peak is not greater than 1.3; and the relative standard deviation for replicate injections is not more than 1.0%.

Procedure—Separately inject equal volumes (about 20 µL) of the *Standard preparation* and the *Assay preparation* into the chromatograph, record the chromatograms obtained for a period of not less than 2.5 times the retention times of pyrantel, and measure the responses for the major peaks. The relative retention times for pamoic acid and pyrantel are about 0.6 and 1.0, respectively. Calculate the quantity, in mg, of $C_{34}H_{30}N_2O_6S$ in the portion of Pyrantel Pamoate taken by the formula:

$$1000C(r_U / r_S)$$

in which C is the concentration, in mg, of USP Pyrantel Pamoate RS in the *Standard preparation,* and r_U and r_S are the peak responses for pyrantel obtained from the *Assay preparation* and the *Standard preparation,* respectively.

Pyrantel Pamoate Oral Suspension

» Pyrantel Pamoate Oral Suspension is a suspension of Pyrantel Pamoate in a suitable aqueous vehicle. It contains not less than 90.0 percent and not more than 110.0 percent of the labeled amount of pyrantel ($C_{11}H_{14}N_2S$).

Packaging and storage—Preserve in tight, light-resistant containers.

USP Reference standards ⟨11⟩—*USP Pyrantel Pamoate RS.*

Identification—[See *Note* in the *Assay*.]

A: Dilute a suitable volume of Oral Suspension with 0.05 N methanolic ammonium hydroxide to obtain a solution having a concentration of about 8 mg of pyrantel pamoate per mL. Similarly prepare a Standard solution of USP Pyrantel Pamoate RS. Shake both solutions by mechanical means, and centrifuge to obtain clear solutions. Apply a 100-µL portion of each solution to a 20- × 20-cm thin-layer chromatographic plate (see *Chromatography* ⟨621⟩) coated with a 0.50-mm layer of silica gel mixture. Develop the plate in a suitable chromatographic chamber containing the upper phase obtained by shaking together methyl isobutyl ketone, formic acid, and water (2 : 1 : 1). Develop the plate until the solvent front is about 2 cm from the top edge of the plate. Remove the plate, allow the solvent to evaporate, and examine the plate under UV light at about 365 nm: the R_F value of the principal spot from the test solution corresponds to that obtained from the Standard solution.

B: [NOTE—Prepare 0.05 N methanolic ammonium hydroxide by transferring 0.8 mL of ammonium hydroxide to a 250-mL volumetric flask containing 100 mL of methanol, diluting with methanol to volume, and mixing.] Dilute a suitable volume of Oral Suspension with 0.05 N methanolic ammonium hydroxide to obtain a solution having a concentration of about 16 mg of pyrantel pamoate per mL. Similarly prepare a Standard solution of USP Pyrantel Pamoate RS. Shake both solutions by mechanical means, and centrifuge to obtain clear solutions. Apply a 20-µL portion of each solution to an 18- × 24-cm sheet of chromatographic paper (Whatman No. 1 or equivalent) that previously has been prepared as follows. Impregnate the paper with a freshly prepared solution obtained by mixing 7 volumes of acetone and 3 volumes of glycine-sodium chloride-hydrochloric acid buffer solution (prepared by mixing 3 volumes of a solution that is 0.3 M with respect to both glycine and sodium chloride with 7 volumes of 0.3 M hydrochloric acid). Press the impregnated paper uniformly between white, nonfluorescent blotters to remove the excess solvent. Place the spotted chromatographic paper in a suitable chromatographic chamber, and develop by descending chromatography (see *Chromatography* ⟨621⟩), using as the solvent system the upper phase obtained by mixing ethyl acetate, butanol, and water (10 : 1 : 1). After developing for 20 hours, remove the paper from the chamber, air-dry for 10 minutes, transfer to an air-circulating oven, and dry at 60° for 30 minutes: the R_F

value of the principal spot from the solution under test corresponds to that obtained from the Standard solution.

C: The retention times of the major peaks due to pyrantel base and pamoic acid in the chromatogram of the *Assay preparation* correspond to those in the chromatogram of the *Standard preparation,* as obtained in the *Assay.*

Uniformity of dosage units ⟨905⟩—
FOR ORAL SUSPENSION PACKAGED IN SINGLE-UNIT CONTAINERS: meets the requirements.

Deliverable volume ⟨698⟩—
FOR ORAL SUSPENSION PACKAGED IN MULTIPLE-UNIT CONTAINERS: meets the requirements.

pH ⟨791⟩: between 4.5 and 6.0.

Assay—[NOTE—Use low-actinic glassware in preparing solutions of pyrantel pamoate, and otherwise protect the solutions from unnecessary exposure to bright light. Complete the assay without prolonged interruption.]

Mobile phase, Standard preparation, and *Chromatographic system*—Proceed as directed in the *Assay* under *Pyrantel Pamoate.*

Assay preparation—Transfer by means of a pipet an accurately measured volume of Oral Suspension, equivalent to about 200 mg of pyrantel pamoate, into a 100-mL volumetric flask, disperse, and dilute with water to volume. While stirring the dispersion with a magnetic stirrer, transfer 1.0 mL of the aliquot to a 25-mL volumetric flask, dissolve in and dilute with *Mobile phase* to volume, mix, and filter.

Procedure—Separately inject equal volumes (about 20 µL) of the *Standard preparation* and the *Assay preparation* into the chromatograph, record the chromatograms obtained for a period of not less than 2.5 times the retention times of pyrantel base, and measure the responses for the major peaks. The relative retention times for pamoic acid and pyrantel base are about 0.6 and 1.0, respectively. Calculate the quantity, in mg, of pyrantel ($C_{11}H_{14}N_2S$) in each mL of the Oral Suspension taken by the formula:

$$2500(0.347)(C/V)(r_U/r_S)$$

in which 0.347 is the ratio of the molecular weight of pyrantel to that of pyrantel pamoate; C is the concentration, in mg per mL, of USP Pyrantel Pamoate RS in the *Standard preparation;* V is the volume, in mL, of Oral Suspension taken; and r_U and r_S are the peak responses for pyrantel base obtained from the *Assay preparation* and the *Standard preparation,* respectively.

Pyrazinamide

$C_5H_5N_3O$ 123.11
Pyrazinecarboxamide.
Pyrazinecarboxamide   [98-96-4].

» Pyrazinamide contains not less than 99.0 percent and not more than 101.0 percent of $C_5H_5N_3O$, calculated on the anhydrous basis.

Packaging and storage—Preserve in well-closed containers.

USP Reference standards ⟨11⟩—*USP Pyrazinamide RS.*

Identification—
A: *Infrared Absorption* ⟨197M⟩.
B: *Ultraviolet Absorption* ⟨197U⟩—
Solution: 10 µg per mL.
Medium: water.
Absorptivities at 268 nm, calculated on the dried basis, do not differ by more than 3.0%.
C: Boil 20 mg with 5 mL of 5 N sodium hydroxide: the odor of ammonia is perceptible.

Melting range ⟨741⟩: between 188° and 191°.
Water, *Method I* ⟨921⟩: not more than 0.5%.
Residue on ignition ⟨281⟩: not more than 0.1%.
Heavy metals, *Method II* ⟨231⟩: 0.001%.
Organic volatile impurities, *Method I* ⟨467⟩: meets the requirements.

(Official until July 1, 2008)

Assay—Place about 300 mg of Pyrazinamide, accurately weighed, in a 500-mL Kjeldahl flask, dissolve in 100 mL of water, and add 75 mL of 5 N sodium hydroxide. Connect the flask by means of a distillation trap to a well-cooled condenser, the delivery tube of which dips into 20 mL of boric acid solution (1 in 25) contained in a suitable receiver. Boil gently for 20 minutes, avoiding insofar as possible distilling any of the liquid, then boil vigorously to complete the distillation of the ammonia. Cool the liquid in the receiver if necessary, add methyl purple TS, and titrate with 0.1 N hydrochloric acid VS. Perform a blank determination, and make any necessary correction. Each mL of 0.1 N hydrochloric acid is equivalent to 12.31 mg of $C_5H_5N_3O$.

Pyrazinamide Tablets

» Pyrazinamide Tablets contain not less than 93.0 percent and not more than 107.0 percent of the labeled amount of pyrazinamide ($C_5H_5N_3O$).

Packaging and storage—Preserve in well-closed containers.

USP Reference standards ⟨11⟩—*USP Pyrazinamide RS.*

Identification—
A: To a quantity of powdered Tablets, equivalent to about 1 g of pyrazinamide, add about 75 mL of isopropyl alcohol, heat on a steam bath, and filter while hot. Allow to cool, filter the crystals that form, and dry at 105° for 1 hour: the IR absorption spectrum of a mineral oil dispersion of the dried crystals so obtained exhibits maxima only at the same wavelengths as that of a similar preparation of USP Pyrazinamide RS. If a difference appears, dissolve portions of both the dried crystals and the Reference Standard in acetone, evaporate the solutions to dryness, and repeat the test on the residues.
B: The dried crystals obtained in *Identification* test *A* meet the requirements for *Identification* test *B* under *Pyrazinamide.*
C: To 20 mg of the dried crystals obtained in *Identification* test *A* add 5 mL of 5 N sodium hydroxide, and heat gently over an open flame: the odor of ammonia is perceptible.

Dissolution ⟨711⟩—
Medium: water; 900 mL.
Apparatus 2: 50 rpm.
Time: 45 minutes.
Procedure—Determine the amount of $C_5H_5N_3O$ dissolved by employing UV absorption at the wavelength of maximum absorbance at about 268 nm on filtered portions of the solution under test, suitably diluted with *Dissolution Medium,* if necessary, in comparison with a Standard solution having a known concentration of USP Pyrazinamide RS in the same *Medium.*
Tolerances—Not less than 75% (*Q*) of the labeled amount of $C_5H_5N_3O$ is dissolved in 45 minutes.

Uniformity of dosage units ⟨905⟩: meet the requirements.

Assay—
Mobile phase—Prepare pH 8.0 phosphate buffer (see *Buffer Solutions* in the section *Reagents, Indicators, and Solutions*), and adjust with phosphoric acid to a pH of 3.0. Mix 10 mL of acetonitrile with 1 L of this solution, filter, and degas. Make adjustments if necessary (see *System Suitability* under *Chromatography* ⟨621⟩).

Standard preparation—Transfer an accurately weighed quantity of USP Pyrazinamide RS to a suitable volumetric flask, dissolve in water, sonicating to dissolve, dilute with water to volume, and mix to obtain a solution having a known concentration of about 0.1 mg per mL. Transfer 20.0 mL of the solution to a 50-mL volumetric flask, dilute with water to volume, and mix.

System suitability solution—Transfer 1 mL of hydrochloric acid to a 5-mL volumetric flask, dilute with *Standard preparation* to volume, and mix. Keep this solution on a boiling water bath for 5 minutes, and cool.

Assay preparation—Accurately weigh not fewer than 20 Tablets, and grind to a fine powder. Transfer an accurately weighed quantity of the powder, equivalent to about 100 mg of pyrazinamide, to a 500-mL volumetric flask, add 300 mL of water, and sonicate for 10 minutes. Dilute with water to volume, and mix. Filter a portion of this solution, discarding the first few mL of the filtrate. Transfer 20.0 mL of this filtrate to a 100-mL volumetric flask, dilute with water to volume, and mix.

Chromatographic system (see *Chromatography* ⟨621⟩)—The liquid chromatograph is equipped with a 270-nm detector and a 3.9-mm × 15-cm column that contains packing L1. The flow rate is about 1 mL per minute. Chromatograph the *Standard preparation*, and record the peak responses as directed for *Procedure*: the column efficiency is not less than 2500 theoretical plates; and the tailing factor for the pyrazinamide peak is not more than 1.3. Chromatograph the *System suitability solution*, and record the peak responses as directed for *Procedure*: the relative retention times are about 0.45 for pyrazinoic acid and 1.0 for pyrazinamide; and the resolution, *R*, between pyrazinamide and pyrazinoic acid is not less than 6.0.

Procedure—Separately inject equal volumes (about 20 µL) of the *Standard preparation* and the *Assay preparation* into the chromatograph, record the chromatograms, and measure the responses for the major peaks. Calculate the quantity, in mg, of pyrazinamide ($C_5H_5N_3O$) in the portion of Tablets taken by the formula:

$$2.5C(r_U / r_S)$$

in which *C* is the concentration, in µg, of USP Pyrazinamide RS in the *Standard preparation*; and r_U and r_S are the peak responses obtained from the *Assay preparation* and the *Standard preparation*, respectively.

Pyrethrum Extract

» Pyrethrum Extract is a mixture of three naturally occurring, closely related insecticidal esters of chrysanthemic acid (Pyrethrins I: jasmolin I, cinerin I, and pyrethrin I) and three closely related esters of pyrethric acid (Pyrethrins II: jasmolin II, cinerin II, and pyrethrin II). It contains not less than 90.0 percent and not more than 110.0 percent of the labeled amount of pyrethrins (sum of Pyrethrins I and Pyrethrins II). The ratio of Pyrethrins I to Pyrethrins II in the Extract is not less than 0.8 and not more than 2.8. It may contain pigments characteristic of chrysanthemum species, triglyceride oils, terpenoids, and carotenoid. It may also contain suitable solvents and antioxidants. It contains no other added substances.

Packaging and storage—Preserve in tight, light-resistant containers.

USP Reference standards ⟨11⟩—*USP Pyrethrum Extract RS*.

Identification—The retention times of the major peaks in the chromatogram of the *Assay preparation* correspond to those in the chromatogram of the *Standard preparation*, as obtained in the *Assay*.

Assay—

Mobile phase—Prepare a filtered and degassed mixture of hexanes and tetrahydrofuran (97.75 : 2.25). Make adjustments if necessary (see *System Suitability* under *Chromatography* ⟨621⟩).

Standard preparation—Dissolve an accurately weighed quantity of USP Pyrethrum Extract RS in hexanes, and dilute stepwise with hexanes to obtain a solution having a known concentration of about 0.5 mg of pyrethrins per mL.

Assay preparation—Transfer an accurately weighed quantity of Extract, equivalent to about 50 mg of pyrethrins, to a 100-mL volumetric flask, dilute with hexanes to volume, and mix.

Chromatographic system (see *Chromatography* ⟨621⟩)—The liquid chromatograph is equipped with a 240-nm detector and a 4.6-mm × 25-cm column that contains 5-µm packing L10. The flow rate is about 1.5 mL per minute. Chromatograph the *Standard preparation*, and record the peak responses as directed for *Procedure*: the resolution, *R*, between the individual pyrethrin peaks is not less than 2.0; and the relative standard deviation for replicate injections is not more than 1.0%.

Procedure—Separately inject equal volumes (about 10 µL) of the *Standard preparation* and the *Assay preparation* into the chromatograph, record the chromatograms, and measure the responses for the six major peaks. The relative retention times are about 0.78 to 0.80 for jasmolin I; 0.86 to 0.87 for cinerin I; 1.0 for pyrethrin I; 1.95 to 2.15 for jasmolin II; 2.15 to 2.4 for cinerin II; and 2.55 to 2.88 for pyrethrin II. Calculate the quantity, in mg, of pyrethrins in the portion of Extract taken by the formula:

$$100\Sigma[C_{Si}(r_{Ui}/r_{Si})]$$

in which C_{Si} is the concentration, in mg per mL, of the individual pyrethrin of interest in the *Standard preparation*; and r_{Ui} and r_{Si} are the peak responses obtained from the *Assay preparation* and the *Standard preparation*, respectively. Calculate the ratio of Pyrethrins I to Pyrethrins II in the portion of the Extract taken by the formula:

$$A/B$$

in which *A* and *B* are the sums of the quantities of Pyrethrins I and Pyrethrins II, respectively.

Pyridostigmine Bromide

$C_9H_{13}BrN_2O_2$ 261.12

Pyridinium, 3-[[(dimethylamino)carbonyl]oxy]-1-methyl-, bromide. 3-Hydroxy-1-methylpyridinium bromide dimethylcarbamate [*101-26-8*].

» Pyridostigmine Bromide contains not less than 98.5 percent and not more than 100.5 percent of $C_9H_{13}BrN_2O_2$, calculated on the dried basis.

Packaging and storage—Preserve in tight containers.

USP Reference standards ⟨11⟩—*USP Pyridostigmine Bromide RS*.

Identification—

A: *Infrared Absorption* ⟨197K⟩.

B: *Ultraviolet Absorption* ⟨197U⟩—

Solution: 35 µg per mL.

Medium: 0.1 N hydrochloric acid.

Absorptivities at 269 nm, calculated on the dried basis, do not differ by more than 3.0%.

C: To about 100 mg in a test tube add 0.6 mL of 1 N sodium hydroxide: an orange color develops. When the mixture is heated, the color changes to yellow, and a strip of moistened red litmus paper held over the top of the test tube turns blue.

D: A solution (1 in 50) responds to tests for *Bromide* ⟨191⟩.

Melting range ⟨741⟩: between 154° and 157°, the test specimen having been previously dried.

Loss on drying ⟨731⟩—Dry it in a suitable vacuum drying tube, using phosphorus pentoxide as the desiccant, at 100° for 4 hours: it loses not more than 2.0% of its weight.

Residue on ignition ⟨281⟩: not more than 0.1%.

Ordinary impurities ⟨466⟩—

Test solution: methanol.

Standard solution: methanol.

Eluant: a mixture of methanol and water (1 : 1); the thin-layer chromatographic plate coating material is cellulose with a fluorescent indicator.

Visualization: 1.
Organic volatile impurities, *Method I* ⟨467⟩: meets the requirements.

(Official until July 1, 2008)
Assay—Dissolve about 850 mg of Pyridostigmine Bromide, accurately weighed, in 80 mL of glacial acetic acid. Add 25 mL of mercuric acetate TS and 2 drops of quinaldine red TS, and titrate with 0.1 N perchloric acid in dioxane VS to a colorless endpoint. Perform a blank determination, and make any necessary correction. Each mL of 0.1 N perchloric acid is equivalent to 26.11 mg of $C_9H_{13}BrN_2O_2$.

Pyridostigmine Bromide Injection

» Pyridostigmine Bromide Injection is a sterile solution of Pyridostigmine Bromide in a suitable medium. It contains not less than 90.0 percent and not more than 110.0 percent of the labeled amount of $C_9H_{13}BrN_2O_2$.

Packaging and storage—Preserve in single-dose containers, preferably of Type I glass, protected from light.

USP Reference standards ⟨11⟩—*USP Pyridostigmine Bromide RS. USP Endotoxin RS.*
Identification—
    A: The solution prepared for measurement of absorbance in the *Assay* exhibits maxima and minima at the same wavelengths as that of a similar solution of USP Pyridostigmine Bromide RS, concomitantly measured.
    B: To 2 mL of Injection add 1 mL of 2 N nitric acid: the solution so obtained responds to the tests for *Bromide* ⟨191⟩.
Bacterial endotoxins ⟨85⟩—It contains not more than 17.0 USP Endotoxin Units per mg of pyridostigmine bromide.
pH ⟨791⟩: between 4.5 and 5.5.
Other requirements—It meets the requirements under *Injections* ⟨1⟩.
Assay—Transfer to a suitable separator an accurately measured volume of Injection, equivalent to about 20 mg of pyridostigmine bromide. Add 10 mL of 1 N hydrochloric acid, and mix. Extract with four 20-mL portions and one 15-mL portion of ethyl ether, and discard the extracts. Transfer the aqueous layer to a 100-mL volumetric flask, using about 25 mL of water to aid the transfer. Place the flask on a steam bath and warm, with the aid of a stream of nitrogen, to evaporate any residual ether, then cool the flask to room temperature, dilute with water to volume, and mix. Dilute 20.0 mL of the resulting solution with 0.1 N hydrochloric acid to 100.0 mL, and mix. Dissolve an accurately weighed quantity of USP Pyridostigmine Bromide RS in 0.1 N hydrochloric acid to obtain a Standard solution having a known concentration of about 40 μg per mL. Concomitantly determine the absorbances of both solutions in 1-cm cells at the wavelength of maximum absorbance at about 269 nm, with a suitable spectrophotometer, using 0.1 N hydrochloric acid as the blank. Calculate the quantity, in mg, of $C_9H_{13}BrN_2O_2$ in each mL of the Injection taken by the formula:

$$(0.5C/V)(A_U/A_S)$$

in which C is the concentration, in μg per mL, of USP Pyridostigmine Bromide RS in the Standard solution, V is the volume, in mL, of Injection taken, and A_U and A_S are the absorbances of the solution from the Injection and the Standard solution, respectively.

Pyridostigmine Bromide Oral Solution

» Pyridostigmine Bromide Oral Solution contains, in each 100 mL, not less than 1.08 g and not more than 1.32 g of pyridostigmine bromide ($C_9H_{13}BrN_2O_2$).

Packaging and storage—Preserve in tight, light-resistant containers.
USP Reference standards ⟨11⟩—*USP Pyridostigmine Bromide RS.*
Identification—To 5 mL of Oral Solution in a separator add 100 mL of 2.5 N hydrochloric acid, and mix. Extract with five 20-mL portions of chloroform, place 2 mL of the aqueous solution in a 50-mL volumetric flask, and add water to volume: the UV absorption spectrum of this solution exhibits maxima and minima at the same wavelengths as that of a similar solution of USP Pyridostigmine Bromide RS, concomitantly measured.
Assay—
    Phosphate solution—Dissolve 38 g of monobasic sodium phosphate and 2 g of anhydrous dibasic sodium phosphate in water to make 1000 mL. Adjust the pH, if necessary, by slight variation of the ratio of the two ingredients, to 5.3 ± 0.1.
    Bromocresol green solution—Dissolve 250 mg of bromocresol green sodium salt in 250 mL of *Phosphate solution*.
    Standard preparation—Dissolve a suitable quantity of USP Pyridostigmine Bromide RS, accurately weighed, in water, to obtain a solution having a known concentration of about 1.2 mg per mL.
    Assay preparation—Transfer an accurately measured volume of Oral Solution, equivalent to about 120 mg of pyridostigmine bromide, to a 100-mL volumetric flask, add water to volume, and mix.
    Procedure—Transfer 10 mL each, accurately measured, of the *Assay preparation* and the *Standard preparation* to separate 125-mL separators. Into each separator pipet 10 mL of water, 20 mL of *Phosphate solution*, and 5 mL of *Bromocresol green solution*. Extract each solution with six 15-mL portions of chloroform, collecting the chloroform extracts in respective 100-mL volumetric flasks, then add chloroform to volume in each flask, and mix. Concomitantly determine the absorbances of both solutions in 1-cm cells at the wavelength of maximum absorbance at about 415 nm, with a suitable spectrophotometer, using chloroform as the blank. Calculate the quantity, in mg, of pyridostigmine bromide ($C_9H_{13}BrN_2O_2$) in the portion of Oral Solution taken by the formula:

$$100C(A_U/A_S)$$

in which C is the concentration, in mg per mL, of USP Pyridostigmine Bromide RS in the *Standard preparation;* and A_U and A_S are the absorbances of the solutions obtained from the *Assay preparation* and the *Standard preparation*, respectively.

Pyridostigmine Bromide Tablets

» Pyridostigmine Bromide Tablets contain not less than 95.0 percent and not more than 105.0 percent of the labeled amount of $C_9H_{13}BrN_2O_2$.

Packaging and storage—Preserve in tight containers.
USP Reference standards ⟨11⟩—*USP Pyridostigmine Bromide RS.*
Identification—
    A: The retention time of the major peak in the chromatogram of the *Assay preparation* corresponds to that of the *Standard preparation* as obtained in the *Assay*.
    B: Shake a quantity of finely powdered Tablets, equivalent to about 100 mg of pyridostigmine bromide, with 20 mL of water for 5 minutes, and filter the mixture: the filtrate responds to the tests for *Bromide* ⟨191⟩.
Dissolution ⟨711⟩—
    Medium: water; 900 mL.
    Apparatus 2: 50 rpm.
    Time: 60 minutes.
    Procedure—Determine the amount of $C_9H_{13}BrN_2O_2$ dissolved from UV absorbances at the wavelength of maximum absorbance at about 270 nm of filtered portions of the solution under test, suitably diluted with water, in comparison with a Standard solution having a known concentration of USP Pyridostigmine Bromide RS in the same medium.
    Tolerances—Not less than 80% (*Q*) of the labeled amount of $C_9H_{13}BrN_2O_2$ is dissolved in 60 minutes.

Uniformity of dosage units ⟨905⟩: meet the requirements.

Assay—

*Buffer solution—*Mix 11.2 g of phosphoric acid with 500 mL of water, and adjust with a 50% solution of sodium hydroxide in water to a pH of 7.0. Dilute with water to 1000 mL.

*Mobile phase—*Dissolve 1 g of sodium 1-heptanesulfonate in 500 mL of water in a 1000-mL volumetric flask, and add 5.0 mL of triethylamine and 100 mL of acetonitrile. Dilute with water to volume, and mix. Adjust with phosphoric acid to a pH of 3.0. Make adjustments if necessary (see *System Suitability* under *Chromatography* ⟨621⟩).

*Standard preparation—*Dissolve an accurately weighed quantity of USP Pyridostigmine Bromide RS in *Buffer solution*, and dilute quantitatively, and stepwise if necessary, to obtain a solution having a known concentration of 0.25 mg per mL.

*Assay preparation—*Weigh and finely powder not less than 20 Tablets. Transfer an accurately weighed portion of the powder, equivalent to about 50 mg of pyridostigmine bromide, to a 200-mL volumetric flask, add 100 mL of *Buffer solution*, and shake for 30 minutes. Dilute with *Buffer solution* to volume, mix, and centrifuge. Use a portion of the supernatant as the *Assay preparation*.

Chromatographic system (see *Chromatography* ⟨621⟩)—The liquid chromatograph is equipped with a 270-nm detector and a 4-mm × 30-cm column that contains packing L1. The flow rate is about 2 mL per minute. Chromatograph the *Standard preparation*, and record the peak responses as directed for *Procedure*: the tailing factor is not more than 1.5, and the relative standard deviation for replicate injections is not more than 1.0%.

*Procedure—*Separately inject equal volumes (about 20 μL) of the *Standard preparation* and the *Assay preparation* into the chromatograph, record the chromatograms, and measure the responses for the major peaks. Calculate the quantity, in mg, of $C_9H_{13}BrN_2O_2$ in the portion of Tablets taken by the formula:

$$200C(r_U / r_S)$$

in which C is the concentration, in mg per mL, of USP Pyridostigmine Bromide RS in the *Standard preparation*, and r_U and r_S are the peak responses obtained from the *Assay preparation* and the *Standard preparation*, respectively.

Pyridoxine Hydrochloride

$C_8H_{11}NO_3 \cdot HCl$ 205.64
3,4-Pyridinedimethanol, 5-hydroxy-6-methyl-, hydrochloride.
Pyridoxol hydrochloride   [58-56-0].

» Pyridoxine Hydrochloride contains not less than 98.0 percent and not more than 102.0 percent of $C_8H_{11}NO_3 \cdot HCl$, calculated on the dried basis.

Packaging and storage—Preserve in tight, light-resistant containers.

USP Reference standards ⟨11⟩—*USP Pyridoxine Hydrochloride RS.*

Identification—

    A: *Infrared Absorption* ⟨197M⟩.
    B: It responds to the tests for *Chloride* ⟨191⟩.

Loss on drying ⟨731⟩—Dry it in vacuum over silica gel for 4 hours: it loses not more than 0.5% of its weight.

Residue on ignition ⟨281⟩: not more than 0.1%.

Heavy metals, *Method II* ⟨231⟩:   0.003%.

Organic volatile impurities, *Method I* ⟨467⟩: meets the requirements.

(Official until July 1, 2008)

Chloride content—Dissolve about 500 mg, accurately weighed, in 50 mL of methanol in a glass-stoppered flask. Add 5 mL of glacial acetic acid and 2 to 3 drops of eosin Y TS, and titrate with 0.1 N silver nitrate VS. Each mL of 0.1 N silver nitrate is equivalent to 3.545 mg of Cl. Not less than 16.9% and not more than 17.6% of Cl, calculated on the dried basis, is found.

Assay—

*Mobile phase—*Mix 20 mL of glacial acetic acid, 1.2 g of sodium 1-hexanesulfonate, and about 1400 mL of water in a 2000-mL volumetric flask. Adjust with glacial acetic acid or 1 N sodium hydroxide to a pH of 3.0. Add 470 mL of methanol, dilute with water to volume, mix, and filter through a 0.5-μm filter. Make adjustments if necessary (see *System Suitability* under *Chromatography* ⟨621⟩).

*Internal standard solution—*Dissolve p-hydroxybenzoic acid in *Mobile phase* to obtain a solution having a concentration of 5 mg per mL.

*Standard preparation—*Dissolve about 50 mg of USP Pyridoxine Hydrochloride RS, accurately weighed, in *Mobile phase* in a 100-mL volumetric flask, dilute with *Mobile phase* to volume, and mix. Transfer 10.0 mL of the resulting solution to a 100-mL volumetric flask, add 1.0 mL of *Internal standard solution*, dilute with *Mobile phase* to volume, and mix to obtain a solution having a known concentration of about 0.05 mg per mL.

*Assay preparation—*Dissolve about 50 mg of Pyridoxine Hydrochloride, accurately weighed, in *Mobile phase* in a 100-mL volumetric flask, dilute with *Mobile phase* to volume, and mix. Transfer 10.0 mL of the resulting solution to a 100-mL volumetric flask, add 1.0 mL of *Internal standard solution*, dilute with *Mobile phase* to volume, and mix.

Chromatographic system (see *Chromatography* ⟨621⟩)—The liquid chromatograph is equipped with a 280-nm detector and a 4.6-mm × 25-cm column that contains packing L1. The flow rate is about 1.5 mL per minute. Chromatograph the *Standard preparation*, and record the peak responses as directed for *Procedure*: the resolution, R, of the pyridoxine and p-hydroxybenzoic acid peaks is not less than 2.5, and the relative standard deviation for replicate injections is not more than 3.0%.

*Procedure—*Separately inject equal volumes (about 20 μL) of the *Standard preparation* and the *Assay preparation* into the chromatograph, record the chromatograms, and measure the responses for the major peaks. The relative retention times are about 0.7 for pyridoxine and 1.0 for p-hydroxybenzoic acid. Calculate the quantity, in mg, of $C_8H_{11}NO_3 \cdot HCl$ in the portion of Pyridoxine Hydrochloride taken by the formula:

$$1000C(R_U / R_S)$$

in which C is the concentration, in mg per mL, of USP Pyridoxine Hydrochloride RS in the *Standard preparation*, and R_U and R_S are the ratios of the peak responses of pyridoxine to internal standard obtained from the *Assay preparation* and the *Standard preparation*, respectively.

Pyridoxine Hydrochloride Injection

» Pyridoxine Hydrochloride Injection is a sterile solution of Pyridoxine Hydrochloride in Water for Injection. It contains not less than 95.0 percent and not more than 115.0 percent of the labeled amount of Pyridoxine Hydrochloride ($C_8H_{11}NO_3 \cdot HCl$).

Packaging and storage—Preserve in single-dose or in multiple-dose containers, preferably of Type I glass, protected from light.

USP Reference standards ⟨11⟩—*USP Endotoxin RS. USP Pyridoxine Hydrochloride RS.*

Identification—Evaporate a volume of Injection, equivalent to about 50 mg of pyridoxine hydrochloride, on a steam bath to dryness. Add 5 mL of dehydrated alcohol, and again evaporate to dryness. Dry the residue at 105° for 3 hours: the residue so obtained responds to *Identification* tests *A* and *B* under *Pyridoxine Hydrochloride*.

Bacterial endotoxins ⟨85⟩—It contains not more than 0.4 USP Endotoxin Unit per mg of pyridoxine hydrochloride.

pH ⟨791⟩: between 2.0 and 3.8.
Other requirements—It meets the requirements under *Injections* ⟨1⟩.
Assay—
Ammonium chloride–ammonium hydroxide buffer—Dissolve 16 g of ammonium chloride in 70 mL of water, add 16 mL of ammonium hydroxide, dilute with water to 100 mL, mix, and filter.
Chlorimide solution—Dissolve 40 mg of 2,6-dichloroquinonechlorimide in 100 mL of isopropyl alcohol. Store the solution in a refrigerator, and use within 1 month. Do not use the solution if it has become pink.
Standard stock solution—Dissolve a suitable quantity of USP Pyridoxine Hydrochloride RS, accurately weighed, in 0.1 N hydrochloric acid, quantitatively dilute with the same solvent to obtain a solution having a known concentration of about 0.1 mg per mL, and mix. Keep the solution in an amber bottle, in a cool place.
Standard preparation—In a 100-mL volumetric flask dilute 10.0 mL of the *Standard stock solution* with water to volume, and mix. Prepare this solution daily as needed.
Assay preparation—Dilute an accurately measured volume of Injection, equivalent to about 100 mg of pyridoxine hydrochloride, quantitatively and stepwise with water to a concentration of about 10 μg of pyridoxine hydrochloride per mL.
Procedure—
(a) Pipet 5 mL of the clear *Assay preparation* into a flask, add 25.0 mL of isopropyl alcohol, and mix. Pipet 5 mL of the isopropyl alcohol dilution into a glass-stoppered, 25-mL graduated cylinder or test tube; and add in succession, mixing after each addition, 1.0 mL of *Ammonium chloride–ammonium hydroxide buffer*, 1.0 mL of sodium acetate solution (1 in 5), and 1.0 mL of water. Cool to about 25°, then add 1.0 mL of *Chlorimide solution*, and shake vigorously for 10 seconds, accurately timed. Ninety seconds, accurately timed, after the addition of the *Chlorimide solution*, determine the absorbance at the wavelength of maximum absorbance at about 650 nm, with a suitable spectrophotometer, using water as the blank. [NOTE—Make the reading promptly to avoid errors due to fading of the color.] Designate the absorbance as A_U.
(b) Repeat procedure (a), but substitute 1.0 mL of boric acid solution (1 in 20) for the 1.0 mL of water. Designate the absorbance as A_U'.
(c) Repeat procedure (a), but substitute 5.0 mL of the *Standard preparation* for the 5.0 mL of the *Assay preparation*. Designate the absorbance as A_S.
(d) Repeat procedure (c), but substitute 1.0 mL of boric acid solution (1 in 20) for the 1.0 mL of water. Designate the absorbance as A_S'.
Calculate the quantity, in mg, of pyridoxine hydrochloride ($C_8H_{11}NO_3 \cdot HCl$) in each mL of the Injection taken by the formula:

$$10(C/V)(A_U - A_U') / (A_S - A_S')$$

in which C is the concentration, in μg per mL, of USP Pyridoxine Hydrochloride RS in the *Standard preparation*; V is the volume, in mL, of Injection taken; and the other terms are as defined above.

Pyridoxine Hydrochloride Tablets

» Pyridoxine Hydrochloride Tablets contain not less than 95.0 percent and not more than 115.0 percent of the labeled amount of $C_8H_{11}NO_3 \cdot HCl$.

Packaging and storage—Preserve in well-closed containers, protected from light.

USP Reference standards ⟨11⟩—*USP Pyridoxine Hydrochloride RS*.
Identification—To a quantity of powdered Tablets, equivalent to about 100 mg of pyridoxine hydrochloride, add about 5 mL of water. Shake the mixture, filter into a test tube, and add 2 or 3 drops of ferric chloride TS: an orange to deep red color is produced.

Dissolution, *Procedure for a Pooled Sample* ⟨711⟩—
Medium: water; 900 mL.
Apparatus 2: 50 rpm.
Time: 45 minutes.
Procedure—Determine the amount of $C_8H_{11}NO_3 \cdot HCl$ dissolved employing the procedure set forth in the *Assay for niacin or niacinamide, pyridoxine hydrochloride, riboflavin, and thiamine* under *Water-Soluble Vitamins Tablets* by using filtered portions of the solution under test suitably diluted with *Dissolution Medium*, if necessary, in comparison with a Standard solution having a known concentration of USP Pyridoxine Hydrochloride RS in the same medium.
Tolerances—Not less than 75% (*Q*) of the labeled amount of $C_8H_{11}NO_3 \cdot HCl$ is dissolved in 45 minutes.
Uniformity of dosage units ⟨905⟩: meet the requirements.
Procedure for content uniformity—Transfer 1 Tablet, previously finely powdered, to a 500-mL volumetric flask containing about 300 mL of water, shake for about 30 minutes, and dilute with water to volume. Filter a portion of the mixture, discarding the first 25 mL of the filtrate. Dilute a suitable aliquot of the subsequent filtrate quantitatively and stepwise with dilute hydrochloric acid (1 in 100) so that the concentration of pyridoxine hydrochloride is about 10 μg per mL. Dissolve an accurately weighed quantity of USP Pyridoxine Hydrochloride RS in dilute hydrochloric acid (1 in 100), and dilute quantitatively and stepwise with the same solvent to obtain a Standard solution having a known concentration of about 10 μg per mL. Concomitantly determine the absorbances of both solutions in 1-cm cells at the wavelength of maximum absorbance at about 290 nm, with a suitable spectrophotometer, using dilute hydrochloric acid (1 in 100) as the blank. Calculate the quantity, in mg, of $C_8H_{11}NO_3 \cdot HCl$ in the Tablet taken by the formula:

$$(T/D)C(A_U/A_S)$$

in which T is the labeled quantity, in mg, of pyridoxine hydrochloride in the Tablet, D is the dilution factor, C is the concentration, in μg per mL, of USP Pyridoxine Hydrochloride RS in the Standard solution, and A_U and A_S are the absorbances of the solution from the Tablet and the Standard solution, respectively.

Assay—Weigh and finely powder not less than 20 Tablets. Weigh accurately a portion of the powder, equivalent to about 10 mg of pyridoxine hydrochloride, and transfer, with the aid of water, to a conical flask. Add 5 mL of hydrochloric acid, then dilute with water to about 250 mL, and heat on a steam bath until disintegration is complete. Cool, transfer to a 1000-mL volumetric flask, dilute with water to volume, mix, and centrifuge a portion of the mixture. Using the clear supernatant as the *Assay preparation*, proceed as directed in the *Assay* under *Pyridoxine Hydrochloride Injection*, calculating the quantity, in mg, of $C_8H_{11}NO_3 \cdot HCl$ in the portion of Tablets taken by the formula:

$$C(A_U - A_U') / (A_S - A_S')$$

in which C is the concentration, in μg per mL, of USP Pyridoxine Hydrochloride RS in the *Standard preparation*, and the other terms are as defined therein.

Pyrilamine Maleate

$C_{17}H_{23}N_3O \cdot C_4H_4O_4$ 401.47
1,2-Ethanediamine, *N*-[(4-methoxyphenyl)methyl]-*N'*,*N'*-dimethyl-*N*-2-pyridinyl-, (*Z*)-2-butenedioate (1 : 1).
2-[[2-(Dimethylamino)ethyl](*p*-methoxybenzyl)amino]pyridine maleate (1 : 1)   [59-33-6].

» Pyrilamine Maleate, dried in vacuum over phosphorus pentoxide for 5 hours, contains not less than 98.0 percent and not more than 100.5 percent of $C_{17}H_{23}N_3O \cdot C_4H_4O_4$.

Packaging and storage—Preserve in tight, light-resistant containers.

USP Reference standards⟨11⟩—*USP Pyrilamine Maleate RS*.

Identification—
  A: *Infrared Absorption* ⟨197K⟩.
  B: *Ultraviolet Absorption* ⟨197U⟩—
  Solution: 10 µg per mL.
  Medium: 0.5 N sulfuric acid.
  Absorptivities at 236 nm and 312 nm, calculated on the dried basis, do not differ by more than 3.0%.

Melting range, *Class I* ⟨741⟩: between 99° and 103°.

Loss on drying ⟨731⟩—Dry it in vacuum over phosphorus pentoxide for 5 hours: it loses not more than 0.5% of its weight.

Residue on ignition ⟨281⟩: not more than 0.1%.

Related compounds—
  TEST 1—
  Standard solution—Dissolve an accurately weighed quantity of USP Pyrilamine Maleate RS in a mixture of methanol and ammonium hydroxide (200 : 1) to obtain a solution having a known concentration of about 0.4 mg per mL. Quantitatively dilute this solution with the mixture of methanol and ammonium hydroxide (200 : 1) to obtain *Standard solutions A, B,* and *C* having the following compositions:

Standard solution	Dilution	Concentration (mg of RS per mL)	Percentage (%, for comparison with test specimen)
A	(1 in 4)	0.1	0.5
B	(3 in 20)	0.06	0.3
C	(1 in 20)	0.02	0.1

Test solution—Dissolve an accurately weighed quantity of Pyrilamine Maleate in a mixture of methanol and ammonium hydroxide (200 : 1) to obtain a solution having a known concentration of about 20 mg per mL.

Eluant: ethyl acetate, diethylamine, *n*-hexane, and methanol (93 : 7 : 1 : 1).

Procedure—Apply separately 10 µL of the *Test solution* and 10 µL of each of the three *Standard solutions* to a suitable thin-layer chromatographic plate (see *Chromatography* ⟨621⟩) coated with a 0.25-mm layer of chromatographic silica gel mixture. [NOTE—The plate has been prewashed for 2 hours with *Eluant* and dried.] Allow the spots on the plate to dry. Place the plate in a chromatographic chamber and develop the chromatograms in *Eluant* until the solvent front has moved about three-fourths of the length of the plate. Remove the plate from the developing chamber, mark the solvent front, and air-dry the plate. View the plate under short-wavelength UV light and compare the intensities of any secondary spots from the chromatogram of the *Test solution* with those of the principal spots from the chromatograms of the *Standard solutions*. No secondary spot from the chromatogram of the *Test solution* is larger or more intense than the principal spot from *Standard solution A* (0.5%), and the sum of the intensities of all secondary spots from the *Test solution* corresponds to not more than 1.0%.

TEST 2—
Mobile phase—Prepare a filtered and degassed mixture of 0.01 M ammonium acetate, methanol, and triethylamine (40 : 60 : 0.1). Make adjustments, if necessary (see *System Suitability* under *Chromatography* ⟨621⟩).

Standard solution—Dissolve an accurately weighed quantity of USP Pyrilamine Maleate RS in *Mobile phase* to obtain a solution having a known concentration of about 0.5 µg per mL.

Test solution—Transfer about 50 mg of Pyrilamine Maleate, accurately weighed, to a 100-mL volumetric flask, dissolve in and dilute with *Mobile phase* to volume, and mix.

Chromatographic system (see *Chromatography* ⟨621⟩)—The liquid chromatograph is equipped with a 254-nm detector and a 4.0-mm × 30-cm column that contains packing L11. The flow rate is about 1.0 mL per minute. Chromatograph the *Standard solution*, and record the peak responses as directed for *Procedure:* the relative standard deviation for replicate injections is not more than 5.0%.

Procedure—Inject a volume (about 20 µL) of the *Test solution* into the chromatograph, run the chromatograph for 25 minutes, record the chromatograms, and measure the peak area responses, but do not measure the maleate peak area response, which elutes near the void volume. Calculate the percentage of each impurity in the portion of pyrilamine taken by the formula:

$$10{,}000(C / W)(r_i / r_S)$$

in which C is the concentration, in mg per mL, of USP Pyrilamine Maleate RS in the *Standard solution;* W is the weight, in mg, of the Pyrilamine Maleate taken to prepare the *Test solution;* r_i is the peak area response for each impurity; and r_S is the response of the *Standard solution:* not more than 0.3% of any individual impurity is found, and not more than 1.0% of total impurities is found.

Organic volatile impurities, *Method I* ⟨467⟩: meets the requirements.

(Official until July 1, 2008)

Assay—Dissolve about 400 mg of Pyrilamine Maleate, previously dried and accurately weighed, in 50 mL of glacial acetic acid. Add 1 drop of crystal violet TS, and titrate with 0.1 N perchloric acid VS to a blue-green endpoint. Perform a blank determination, and make any necessary correction. Each mL of 0.1 N perchloric acid is equivalent to 20.07 mg of $C_{17}H_{23}N_3O \cdot C_4H_4O_4$.

Pyrilamine Maleate Tablets

» Pyrilamine Maleate Tablets contain not less than 93.0 percent and not more than 107.0 percent of the labeled amount of $C_{17}H_{23}N_3O \cdot C_4H_4O_4$.

Packaging and storage—Preserve in well-closed containers.

USP Reference standards ⟨11⟩—*USP Pyrilamine Maleate RS*.

Identification—Tablets meet the requirements under *Identification—Organic Nitrogenous Bases* ⟨181⟩.

Dissolution, *Procedure for a Pooled Sample* ⟨711⟩—
  Medium: water; 900 mL.
  Apparatus 2: 50 rpm.
  Time: 45 minutes.
  Procedure—Determine the amount of $C_{17}H_{23}N_3O \cdot C_4H_4O_4$ dissolved, employing the procedure set forth in the *Assay*, making any necessary modifications.
  Tolerances—Not less than 75% (*Q*) of the labeled amount of $C_{17}H_{23}N_3O \cdot C_4H_4O_4$ is dissolved in 45 minutes.

Uniformity of dosage units ⟨905⟩: meet the requirements.

Assay—Proceed with Tablets as directed under *Salts of Organic Nitrogenous Bases* ⟨501⟩, determining the absorbance at the wavelength of maximum absorbance at about 312 nm. Calculate the quantity, in mg, of $C_{17}H_{23}N_3O \cdot C_4H_4O_4$ in the portion of Tablets taken by the formula:

$$0.05C(A_U / A_S)$$

in which C is the concentration, in µg per mL, calculated on the dried basis, of USP Pyrilamine Maleate RS in the *Standard Preparation*.

Pyrimethamine

$C_{12}H_{13}ClN_4$ 248.71
2,4-Pyrimidinediamine, 5-(4-chlorophenyl)-6-ethyl-.
2,4-Diamino-5-(p-chlorophenyl)-6-ethylpyrimidine   [58-14-0].

» Pyrimethamine contains not less than 99.0 percent and not more than 101.0 percent of $C_{12}H_{13}ClN_4$, calculated on the dried basis.

Packaging and storage—Preserve in tight, light-resistant containers.
USP Reference standards ⟨11⟩—*USP Pyrimethamine RS.*
Identification—
  A: *Infrared Absorption* ⟨197K⟩.
  B: Mix about 100 mg with 500 mg of anhydrous sodium carbonate, and ignite the mixture. Cool, add 5 mL of hot water, heat for 5 minutes on a steam bath, filter, and neutralize the filtrate with nitric acid: the solution responds to the test for *Chloride* ⟨191⟩.
Melting range ⟨741⟩: between 238° and 242°.
Loss on drying ⟨731⟩—Dry it at 105° for 4 hours: it loses not more than 0.5% of its weight.
Residue on ignition ⟨281⟩: not more than 0.1%.
Ordinary impurities ⟨466⟩—
  Test solution: a mixture of methanol and chloroform (1 : 1).
  Standard solution: a mixture of methanol and chloroform (1 : 1).
  Eluant: a mixture of n-propyl alcohol, glacial acetic acid, and water (8 : 1 : 1).
  Visualization: 2.
Organic volatile impurities, *Method V* ⟨467⟩: meets the requirements.
  Solvent—Use dimethyl sulfoxide.
  (Official until July 1, 2008)
Assay—Dissolve about 200 mg of Pyrimethamine, accurately weighed, in 25 mL of glacial acetic acid, warming slightly to effect solution. Cool the solution to room temperature, add 4 drops of quinaldine red TS, and titrate with 0.1 N perchloric acid VS. Perform a blank determination, and make any necessary correction. Each mL of 0.1 N perchloric acid is equivalent to 24.87 mg of $C_{12}H_{13}ClN_4$.

Pyrimethamine Tablets

» Pyrimethamine Tablets contain not less than 93.0 percent and not more than 107.0 percent of the labeled amount of pyrimethamine ($C_{12}H_{13}ClN_4$).

Packaging and storage—Preserve in tight, light-resistant containers.
USP Reference standards ⟨11⟩—*USP Pyrimethamine RS.*
Identification—
  A: The UV absorption spectrum of the *Assay Preparation* exhibits maxima at the same wavelengths as that of a similar solution of USP Pyrimethamine RS.
  B: To a quantity of powdered Tablets, equivalent to about 250 mg of pyrimethamine, add 25 mL of acetone, boil for 2 minutes, and filter through a sintered-glass crucible. Repeat this treatment three times with 25-mL portions of acetone. Evaporate the combined filtrates carefully on a steam bath with the aid of a current of air to dryness: the residue responds to *Identification* test *A* under *Pyrimethamine,* and melts between 237° and 242° (see *Melting Range or Temperature* ⟨741⟩).

Dissolution ⟨711⟩—
  Medium: 0.1 N hydrochloric acid; 900 mL.
  Apparatus 2: 50 rpm.
  Time: 45 minutes.
  Procedure—Determine the amount of $C_{12}H_{13}ClN_4$ dissolved by employing UV absorption at the wavelength of maximum absorbance at about 273 nm on filtered portions of the solution under test, suitably diluted with *Dissolution Medium,* if necessary, in comparison with a Standard solution having a known concentration of USP Pyrimethamine RS in the same *Medium.*
  Tolerances—Not less than 75% (*Q*) of the labeled amount of $C_{12}H_{13}ClN_4$ is dissolved in 45 minutes.
Uniformity of dosage units ⟨905⟩: meet the requirements.
  Procedure for content uniformity—Transfer 1 Tablet to a 100-mL volumetric flask, add 25 mL of 0.1 N hydrochloric acid, warm the flask on a steam bath for 5 minutes, cool, dilute with 0.1 N hydrochloric acid to volume, mix, and filter, rejecting the first few mL of the filtrate. Pipet a portion of the clear filtrate, equivalent to about 2.5 mg of pyrimethamine, into a 250-mL volumetric flask, dilute with 0.1 N hydrochloric acid to volume, and mix. Dissolve an accurately weighed quantity of USP Pyrimethamine RS in 0.1 N hydrochloric acid, and dilute quantitatively and stepwise with 0.1 N hydrochloric acid to obtain a Standard solution having a known concentration of about 10 µg per mL. Concomitantly determine the absorbances of both solutions in 1-cm cells at the wavelength of maximum absorbance at about 273 nm, with a suitable spectrophotometer, using 0.1 N hydrochloric acid as the blank. Calculate the quantity, in mg, of $C_{12}H_{13}ClN_4$ in the Tablet taken by the formula:

$$(T/D)C(A_U/A_S)$$

in which *T* is the labeled quantity, in mg, of pyrimethamine in the Tablet; *D* is the concentration, in µg per mL, of pyrimethamine in the solution from the Tablet, on the basis of the labeled quantity per Tablet and the extent of dilution; *C* is the concentration, in µg per mL, of USP Pyrimethamine RS in the Standard solution; and A_U and A_S are the absorbances of the solution from the Tablet and the Standard solution, respectively.
Assay—Proceed with Tablets as directed under *Salts of Organic Nitrogenous Bases* ⟨501⟩, diluting 5.0 mL each of the *Standard Preparation* and the *Assay Preparation,* respectively, with 0.5 N sulfuric acid to 200.0 mL and determining the absorbances of both solutions in 1-cm cells at the wavelength of maximum absorbance at about 273 nm. Calculate the quantity, in mg, of pyrimethamine ($C_{12}H_{13}ClN_4$) in the portion of Tablets taken by the formula:

$$50C(A_U/A_S)$$

in which *C* is the concentration, in mg per mL, of USP Pyrimethamine RS in the *Standard Preparation;* and A_U and A_S are as defined in the chapter.

Pyroxylin

Cellulose, nitrate.
Pyroxylin   [9004-70-0].

» Pyroxylin is a product obtained by the action of a mixture of nitric and sulfuric acids on cotton and consists chiefly of cellulose tetranitrate $(C_{12}H_{16}N_4O_{18})_n$.

  NOTE—Dry Pyroxylin is a light yellow, matted mass of filaments, resembling raw cotton in appearance, but harsh to the touch. *It is exceedingly flammable,* burning, when unconfined, very rapidly and with a luminous flame. When kept in well-closed bottles and exposed to light, it is decomposed with the evolution of nitrous vapors, leaving a carbonaceous residue.
  Pyroxylin available commercially is moistened with about 30 percent of alcohol or other suitable solvent. The alcohol or other solvent must be allowed to evaporate from the Pyroxylin to yield the dried substance de-

scribed in this Pharmacopeia. Pyroxylin moistened with alcohol or other solvent may be used in the tests set forth in this monograph, provided the weight of test specimen taken corresponds to the specified amount of dry Pyroxylin.

Packaging and storage—Preserve loosely packed in cartons, protected from light.
Labeling—The label bears a caution statement to the effect that Pyroxylin is highly flammable.
Viscosity ⟨911⟩—Dissolve 48.8 g in a mixture of 88 g of alcohol and 193.2 g of toluene, and when solution is complete, add 70 g of ethyl acetate, and mix. Transfer the solution to the cup of a rotational type of viscosimeter, adjust the temperature to 25°, and determine the viscosity, making certain that the apparent viscosity reaches equilibrium before taking the final reading: the viscosity is between 110 and 147 poises.
Residue on ignition ⟨281⟩—Saturate about 500 mg, accurately weighed, with alcohol in a dish placed in cold water, and ignite the Pyroxylin at the top. When combustion is complete, heat the dish to redness, and cool: not more than 0.3% of residue remains.
Acidity and water-soluble substances—Stir 1.0 g with 20 mL of water for 10 minutes, and filter: the filtrate does not have an acid reaction to litmus. Evaporate 10 mL of the filtrate on a steam bath to dryness, and dry the residue at 105° for 1 hour: not more than 1.5 mg of residue remains.
Organic volatile impurities, *Method V* ⟨467⟩: meets the requirements.
  Solvent—Use dimethyl sulfoxide as the solvent.

(Official until July 1, 2008)

Pyrvinium Pamoate

$C_{75}H_{70}N_6O_6$ 1151.40
Quinolinium, 6-(dimethylamino)-2-[2-(2,5-dimethyl-1-phenyl]-1*H*-pyrrol-[3-yl]ethenyl]-1-methyl-, salt with 4,4′-methylenebis[3-hydroxy-[2-naphthalenecarboxylic acid] (2 : 1).
6-(Dimethylamino)-2-[2-(2,5-dimethyl-1-phenylpyrrol-3-yl)vinyl]-1-methylquinolinium 4,4′-methylenebis[3-hydroxy-2-naphthoate] (2 : 1)   [3546-41-6].

» Pyrvinium Pamoate contains not less than 96.0 percent and not more than 104.0 percent of $C_{75}H_{70}N_6O_6$, calculated on the anhydrous basis.

Packaging and storage—Preserve in tight, light-resistant containers.
USP Reference standards ⟨11⟩—*USP Pyrvinium Pamoate RS*.
Identification—
  A: *Infrared Absorption* ⟨197K⟩.
  B: A solution of it in a 1 in 200 solution of glacial acetic acid in methanol, prepared as directed in the *Assay*, exhibits absorbance maxima at about 358 nm and at about 505 nm, and the ratio A_{505}/A_{358} is between 1.93 and 2.07.
Water, *Method I* ⟨921⟩: not more than 6.0%, a 200-mg specimen being used for the test, and a mixture of 10 mL of methanol and 10 mL of chloroform being used as the solvent.
Residue on ignition ⟨281⟩: not more than 0.5%.
Assay—[NOTE—Use low-actinic flasks in preparing the solutions, and otherwise protect the solutions from unnecessary exposure to bright light. Complete the assay without prolonged interruption.] Dissolve about 250 mg of Pyrvinium Pamoate, accurately weighed, in 125 mL of glacial acetic acid in a 250-mL volumetric flask, dilute with methanol to volume, and mix. Transfer 5 mL of this solution to a 500-mL volumetric flask, dilute with methanol to volume, and mix. Similarly dissolve an accurately weighed quantity of USP Pyrvinium Pamoate RS in glacial acetic acid, using 1 mL for each 2 mg taken, and dilute quantitatively and stepwise with methanol to obtain a Standard solution having a known concentration of about 10 μg per mL. Concomitantly determine the absorbances of both solutions in 1-cm cells at the wavelength of maximum absorbance at about 505 nm, with a suitable spectrophotometer, using methanol as the blank. Calculate the quantity, in mg, of $C_{75}H_{70}N_6O_6$ in the portion of Pyrvinium Pamoate taken by the formula:

$$25C(A_U/A_S)$$

in which C is the concentration, in μg per mL, of USP Pyrvinium Pamoate RS in the Standard solution, calculated on the anhydrous basis, and A_U and A_S are the absorbances of the solution of Pyrvinium Pamoate and the Standard solution, respectively.

Pyrvinium Pamoate Oral Suspension

» Pyrvinium Pamoate Oral Suspension contains, in each 100 mL, an amount of pyrvinium pamoate equivalent to not less than 0.90 g and not more than 1.10 g of pyrvinium ($C_{26}H_{28}N_3^+$).

Packaging and storage—Preserve in tight, light-resistant containers.
USP Reference standards ⟨11⟩—*USP Pyrvinium Pamoate RS*.
Identification—The absorption spectrum, between 300 nm and 600 nm, of the solution employed for measurement of absorbance in the *Assay* exhibits maxima and minima at the same wavelengths as that of a similar solution of USP Pyrvinium Pamoate RS, concomitantly measured.
Uniformity of dosage units ⟨905⟩—
  FOR ORAL SUSPENSION PACKAGED IN SINGLE-UNIT CONTAINERS: meets the requirements.
Deliverable volume ⟨698⟩—
  FOR ORAL SUSPENSION PACKAGED IN MULTIPLE-UNIT CONTAINERS: meets the requirements.
pH ⟨791⟩: between 6.0 and 8.0, determined potentiometrically.
Assay—[NOTE—Use low-actinic flasks in preparing the solutions, and otherwise protect the solutions from unnecessary exposure to bright light. Complete the assay without prolonged interruption.] Using a pipet calibrated "to contain," transfer 5 mL of Oral Suspension, freshly mixed and free from air bubbles, to a 250-mL volumetric flask. Complete the transfer by rinsing the pipet with 10 mL of methanol. Add 100 mL of glacial acetic acid, and mix to dissolve the pyrvinium pamoate. Dilute this solution with methanol to volume, and mix. Transfer 3 mL of the resulting solution to a 100-mL volumetric flask, dilute with methanol to volume, and mix. Dissolve an accurately weighed quantity of USP Pyrvinium Pamoate RS in glacial acetic acid, using 4 mL for each 3 mg taken, and dilute quantitatively and stepwise with methanol to obtain a Standard solution having a known concentration of about 9 μg per mL. Concomitantly determine the absorbances of both solutions in 1-cm cells at the wavelength of maximum absorbance at about 505 nm, with a suitable spectrophotometer, using methanol as the blank. Calculate the quantity, in g per 100 mL, of pyrvinium ($C_{26}H_{28}N_3^+$) in the Oral Suspension taken by the formula:

$$0.1667C(0.6644A_U/A_S)$$

in which C is the concentration, in μg per mL, of USP Pyrvinium Pamoate RS in the Standard solution, calculated on the anhydrous basis; 0.6644 is the ratio of the molecular weight of pyrvinium to one-half the molecular weight of pyrvinium pamoate; and A_U and A_S are the absorbances of the solution prepared from the Oral Suspension and the Standard solution, respectively.

Pyrvinium Pamoate Tablets

» Pyrvinium Pamoate Tablets contain an amount of pyrvinium pamoate equivalent to not less than 92.0 percent and not more than 108.0 percent of the labeled amount of pyrvinium ($C_{26}H_{28}N_3^+$).

Packaging and storage—Preserve in tight, light-resistant containers.

USP Reference standards ⟨11⟩—*USP Pyrvinium Pamoate RS.*
Identification—Tablets respond to the *Identification* test under *Pyrvinium Pamoate Oral Suspension.*
Disintegration ⟨701⟩: 30 minutes.
Uniformity of dosage units ⟨905⟩: meet the requirements.
Assay—[NOTE—Use low-actinic flasks in preparing the solutions, and otherwise protect the solutions from unnecessary exposure to bright light. Complete the assay without prolonged interruption.] Place a number of Tablets, equivalent to 500 mg of pyrvinium, in a 500-mL volumetric flask, and add 25 mL of water and 25 mL of acetone. Completely disintegrate the tablets by heating on the steam bath for 10 minutes with frequent mixing, allowing part of the acetone to boil off slowly. To the hot mixture add 250 mL of glacial acetic acid, and mix occasionally for 5 minutes without further heating, to dissolve the pyrvinium pamoate. Dilute with methanol to volume at room temperature, and mix. Centrifuge a portion of the mixture until a clear solution is obtained. Transfer 3 mL of the clear supernatant to a 500-mL volumetric flask, dilute with methanol to volume, and mix. Dissolve an accurately weighed quantity of USP Pyrvinium Pamoate RS in glacial acetic acid, using 1 mL for each 3 mg taken, and dilute quantitatively and stepwise with methanol to obtain a Standard solution having a known concentration of about 9 µg per mL. Concomitantly determine the absorbances of both solutions in 1-cm cells at the wavelength of maximum absorbance at about 505 nm, with a suitable spectrophotometer, using methanol as the blank. Calculate the quantity, in mg, of pyrvinium ($C_{26}H_{28}N_3^+$) in the portion of Tablets taken by the formula:

$$83.3C(0.6644A_U/A_S)$$

in which C is the concentration, in µg per mL, of USP Pyrvinium Pamoate RS in the Standard solution, calculated on the anhydrous basis, 0.6644 is the ratio of the molecular weight of pyrvinium to one-half the molecular weight of pyrvinium pamoate, and A_U and A_S are the absorbances of the solution from the Tablets and the Standard solution, respectively.

Quazepam

$C_{17}H_{11}ClF_4N_2S$ 386.80
2*H*-1,4-Benzodiazepine-2-thione, 7-chloro-5-(2-fluorophenyl)-1,3-dihydro-1-(2,2,2-trifluoroethyl)-.
7-Chloro-5-(*o*-fluorophenyl)-1,3-dihydro-1-(2,2,2-trifluoroethyl)-2*H*-1,4-benzodiazepine-2-thione   [36735-22-5].

» Quazepam contains not less than 98.5 percent and not more than 101.5 percent of $C_{17}H_{11}ClF_4N_2S$, calculated on the dried basis.

Packaging and storage—Preserve in well-closed containers.
USP Reference standards ⟨11⟩—*USP Quazepam RS. USP Quazepam Related Compound A RS.*
Identification—
  A: *Infrared Absorption* ⟨197M⟩.
  B: The R_F value of the principal spot in the chromatogram of the *Test solution* obtained in the test for *Related compounds* corresponds to that in the chromatogram of *Standard solution A*.
Melting range ⟨741⟩: between 146° and 151°, but the range between beginning and end of melting does not exceed 2°.
Loss on drying ⟨731⟩—Dry it at 105° for 4 hours: it loses not more than 0.5% of its weight.
Residue on ignition ⟨281⟩: not more than 0.2%.
Heavy metals, *Method II* ⟨231⟩: not more than 20 µg per g.
Related compounds—
  Test solution—Prepare a solution of Quazepam in methylene chloride containing 20 mg per mL.
  Standard solution A—Dissolve an accurately weighed quantity of USP Quazepam RS in methylene chloride to obtain a solution having a known concentration of about 20 mg per mL.
  Standard solution B—Dissolve an accurately weighed quantity of USP Quazepam RS in methylene chloride to obtain a solution having a known concentration of about 0.04 mg per mL (0.2%).
  Standard solution C—Dissolve an accurately weighed quantity of USP Quazepam Related Compound A RS in methylene chloride to obtain a solution having a known concentration of about 0.2 mg per mL (1%).
  Procedure—Separately apply 5 µL of the *Test solution* and 5 µL of each of the *Standard solutions* to a thin-layer chromatographic plate (see *Chromatography* ⟨621⟩) coated with a 0.25-mm layer of chromatographic silica gel. Allow the spots to dry, and develop the chromatogram in a solvent system consisting of a mixture of cyclohexane, ethyl acetate, and ether (170 : 40 : 25) in a paper-lined tank until the solvent front has moved about three-fourths of the length of the plate. Remove the plate from the developing chamber, mark the solvent front, allow to air-dry, and examine the plate under short-wavelength UV light. Compare the intensity of the secondary spot in the chromatogram of the *Test solution* having the same R_F value as that of the primary spot of *Standard solution C*: the spot is not larger or more intense than the principal spot in the chromatogram of *Standard solution C*. Compare the intensities of any additional secondary spots observed in the chromatogram of the *Test solution* with that of the principal spot in the chromatogram of *Standard solution B*: the sum of the intensities of the additional secondary spots obtained from the *Test solution* corresponds to not more than 0.2%.
Assay—Dissolve about 500 mg of Quazepam, accurately weighed, in 150 mL of acetic anhydride. Titrate with 0.1 N perchloric acid VS, determining the endpoint potentiometrically, using a glass-calomel electrode system. Perform a blank determination, and make any necessary correction. Each mL of 0.1 N perchloric acid is equivalent to 38.68 mg of $C_{17}H_{11}ClF_4N_2S$.

Quazepam Tablets

» Quazepam Tablets contain not less than 90 percent and not more than 110.0 percent of quazepam ($C_{17}H_{11}ClF_4N_2S$).

Packaging and storage—Preserve in a well-closed container.
USP Reference standards ⟨11⟩—*USP Ethylparaben RS. USP Quazepam RS. USP Quazepam Related Compound A RS.*
Identification—
  A: The retention time of the major peak in the chromatogram of the *Assay preparation* corresponds to that in the chromatogram of the *Standard preparation*, both relative to the internal standard as obtained in the *Assay*.
  B: The R_F value of the principal spot in the chromatogram of the *Test solution* obtained in the test for *Related compounds* corresponds to that in the chromatogram of *Standard solution A*.

Dissolution ⟨711⟩—
Medium: 1% sodium lauryl sulfate; 900 mL.
Apparatus 2: 50 rpm.
Time: 30 minutes.
*Procedure—*Determine the amount of $C_{17}H_{11}ClF_4N_2S$ dissolved from UV absorbances at the wavelength of maximum absorbance at about 287 nm on filtered portions of the solution under test in comparison with a Standard solution having a known concentration of USP Quazepam RS dissolved in a small volume of methanol and diluted with *Dissolution Medium*.
*Tolerances—*Not less than 80% (*Q*) of the labeled amount of $C_{17}H_{11}ClF_4N_2S$ is dissolved in 30 minutes.

Uniformity of dosage units ⟨905⟩: meet the requirements.

Related compounds—
*Test solution—*Grind 10 Tablets to a fine powder. Dissolve an accurately weighed portion of the powder in methylene chloride to obtain a solution having a concentration of 10 mg of quazepam per mL. Mix for 30 minutes, and centrifuge.
*Standard solution A—*Dissolve an accurately weighed quantity of USP Quazepam RS in methylene chloride to obtain a solution having a known concentration of about 10 mg per mL.
*Standard solution B—*Dissolve an accurately weighed quantity of USP Quazepam RS in methylene chloride to obtain a solution having a known concentration of about 0.04 mg per mL (0.2%).
*Standard solution C—*Dissolve an accurately weighed quantity of USP Quazepam Related Compound A RS in methylene chloride to obtain a solution having a known concentration of about 0.3 mg per mL (1.5%).
*Procedure—*Separately apply 10 µL each of the *Test Solution* and *Standard solution A* and 5 µL each of *Standard solutions B* and *C* to a thin-layer chromatographic plate (see *Chromatography* ⟨621⟩) coated with a 0.25-mm layer of chromatographic silica gel. Allow the spots to dry, and develop the chromatogram in a solvent system consisting of a mixture of cyclohexane, ethyl acetate, and ether (170 : 40 : 25) in a paper-lined tank until the solvent front has moved about three-fourths of the length of the plate. Remove the plate from the developing chamber, mark the solvent front, allow to air-dry, and examine the plate under short-wavelength UV light. Compare the intensity of the secondary spot in the chromatogram of the *Test solution* having the same R_F value as the principal spot in the chromatogram of *Standard solution C*. The spot is not larger or more intense than the principal spot obtained from *Standard solution C*. Compare the intensities of any additional secondary spots observed in the chromatogram of the *Test solution* with that of the principal spot in the chromatogram of *Standard solution B:* no additional secondary spot from the chromatogram of the *Test solution* is larger or more intense than the principal spot obtained from *Standard solution B,* and the sum of the intensities of the additional secondary spots obtained from the *Test solution* is not more than 0.6%.

Assay—
*Mobile phase—*Prepare a filtered and degassed mixture of methanol and water (7 : 3). Make adjustments, if necessary (see *System Suitability* under *Chromatography* ⟨621⟩).
*Internal standard solution—*Dissolve an accurately weighed quantity of USP Ethylparaben RS in methanol, and dilute quantitatively, and stepwise if necessary, with methanol to obtain a solution containing about 0.19 mg per mL.
*Standard preparation—*Dissolve an accurately weighed quantity of USP Quazepam RS in *Internal standard solution,* and dilute quantitatively, and stepwise if necessary, with *Internal standard solution* to obtain a solution having a known concentration of about 1.5 mg of quazepam per mL.
*Assay preparation—*Weigh and finely powder not fewer than 10 Tablets. Transfer an accurately weighed portion of powder, equivalent to about 15 mg of quazepam, to a 50-mL screw-capped centrifuge tube. Add 10.0 mL of *Internal standard solution,* and centrifuge for 30 minutes.
Chromatographic system (see *Chromatography* ⟨621⟩)—The liquid chromatograph is equipped with a 254-nm detector and a 4.6-mm × 25-cm column that contains packing L7. The flow rate is about 1.5 mL per minute. Chromatograph the *Standard preparation,* and record the peak responses as directed for *Procedure:* the resolution, *R,* between ethylparaben and quazepam is not less than 5.5; and the relative standard deviation for replicate injections is not more than 2.0%. [NOTE—For identification purposes, the relative retention times are about 0.4 for ethylparaben and 1.0 for quazepam.]
*Procedure—*Separately inject equal volumes (about 5 µL) of the *Standard preparation* and the *Assay preparation* into the chromatograph, record the chromatograms, and measure the responses for the major peaks. Calculate the quantity, in mg, of quazepam ($C_{17}H_{11}ClF_4N_2S$) in the portion of Tablets taken by the formula:

$$10C(R_U / R_S)$$

in which *C* is the concentration, in mg per mL, of USP Quazepam RS in the *Standard preparation;* and R_U and R_S are the ratios of the peak response of quazepam to that of ethylparaben obtained from the *Assay preparation* and the *Standard preparation,* respectively.

Quinapril Hydrochloride

$C_{25}H_{30}N_2O_5 \cdot HCl$ 474.98

3-Isoquinolinecarboxylic acid, 2-[2-[[1-(ethoxycarbonyl)-3-phenylpropyl]amino]-1-oxopropyl]-1,2,3,4-tetrahydro-, monohydrochloride, [3S-[2[R*(R*)],3R*]].
(S)-2-[(S)-N-[(S)-1-Carboxy-3-phenylpropyl]alanyl]-1,2,3,4-tetrahydro-3-isoquinolinecarboxylic acid, 1-ethyl ester, monohydrochloride [82586-55-8].

» Quinapril Hydrochloride contains not less than 98.5 percent and not more than 101.5 percent of $C_{25}H_{30}N_2O_5 \cdot HCl$, calculated on the anhydrous basis.

Packaging and storage—Preserve in well-closed containers, and store at controlled room temperature.

USP Reference standards ⟨11⟩—*USP Quinapril Hydrochloride RS. USP Quinapril Related Compound A RS. USP Quinapril Related Compound B RS.*

Identification—
A: *Infrared Absorption* ⟨197K⟩.
B: The retention time of the major peak in the chromatogram of the *Assay preparation* corresponds to that in the chromatogram of the *Standard preparation,* as obtained in the *Assay.*

Specific rotation ⟨781S⟩: between +14.4° and +15.4°.
Test solution: 20 mg per mL, in methanol.

Water, *Method I* ⟨921⟩: not more than 1.0%.

Residue on ignition ⟨281⟩: not more than 0.1%.

Heavy metals, *Method II* ⟨231⟩: 0.002%.

Limit of residual solvents—
*Standard stock solution—*Transfer about 50 mL of dimethylformamide to a 200-mL volumetric flask. Add about 75 mg each of acetone and acetonitrile and 30 mg each of methylene chloride and toluene, each accurately weighed by difference, and mix. Dilute with dimethylformamide to volume, and mix.
*System suitability solution 1—*Transfer about 25 mL of dimethylformamide to a 50-mL volumetric flask. Add 35 µL of dehydrated alcohol and 25 mL of methylene chloride. Dilute with dimethylformamide to volume, and mix. Transfer 1.0 mL of this solution to a 50-mL volumetric flask, dilute with dimethylformamide to volume, and mix.
*System suitability solution 2—*Transfer 2.0 mL of the *Standard stock solution* to a 50-mL volumetric flask, dilute with dimethylformamide to volume, and mix.
*Standard solution—*Transfer 4.0 mL of the *Standard stock solution* to a 50-mL volumetric flask, dilute with dimethylformamide to volume, and mix.
*Test solution—*Transfer about 60 mg of Quinapril Hydrochloride, accurately weighed, to a suitable headspace vial, add 5.0 mL of dimethylformamide, seal, and shake to dissolve.

Chromatographic system (see *Chromatography* ⟨621⟩)—The gas chromatograph is equipped with a flame-ionization detector, a headspace sampler, a 0.53-mm × 30-m fused-silica column coated with a 1.0-μm film of phase G16, and a split injection system. The carrier gas is helium, flowing at a rate of 6 mL per minute. The split flow rate is about 100 mL per minute, with a back pressure of 3.5 psi. The oven temperature of the headspace sampler is maintained at 60°, and the vial pressure is maintained at 6.1 psi. The temperature of the headspace loop and transfer lines is maintained at 65°. The vials are equilibrated for 10 minutes prior to injection, and injection occurs every 36 minutes. The chromatograph is programmed as follows. Initially the column temperature is maintained at 35° for 10 minutes, then the temperature is increased at a rate of 7° per minute to 150°, and maintained at 150° for 4 minutes. The injection port temperature is maintained at 180°, and the detector is maintained at 240°. Chromatograph *System suitability solution 1*, and record the peak responses as directed for *Procedure*: the relative retention times are about 0.94 for methylene chloride and 1.0 for alcohol; the resolution, R, between methylene chloride and alcohol is not less than 1.2; the column efficiency, determined from the methylene chloride peak, is not less than 4900 theoretical plates; and the tailing factor for the methylene chloride peak is not more than 1.7. Chromatograph *System suitability solution 2*, and record the peak responses as directed for *Procedure*: the relative standard deviation for replicate injections is not more than 15.0%.

Procedure—Separately inject equal volumes (about 1 mL) of the gaseous headspace of the *Standard solution* and the *Test solution* into the chromatograph, record the chromatograms, and measure the areas for the major peaks. Separately calculate the percentages, by weight, of acetone, acetonitrile, methylene chloride, and toluene in the portion of Quinapril Hydrochloride taken by the formula:

$$0.2(W_S / W_Q)(r_U / r_S)$$

in which W_S is the weight, in mg, of the appropriate solvent taken to prepare the *Standard solution*; W_Q is the weight, in mg, of Quinapril Hydrochloride taken to prepare the *Test solution*; and r_U and r_S are the peak responses of the relevant solvent obtained from the *Test solution* and the *Standard solution*, respectively: not more than 0.25% each of acetone and acetonitrile is found; and not more than 0.1% each of methylene chloride and toluene is found.

Related compounds—
Diluent, Mobile phase, and *Chromatographic system*—Prepare as directed in the *Assay*.

System suitability solution—Prepare as directed for the *System suitability preparation* in the *Assay*.

Standard solution—Dissolve accurately weighed quantities of USP Quinapril Related Compound A RS and USP Quinapril Related Compound B RS in *Diluent* to obtain a solution having known concentrations of about 0.5 mg of each per mL. Transfer 1.0 mL of this solution to a 100-mL volumetric flask, dilute with *Diluent* to volume, and mix.

Test solution—Use the *Assay preparation*.

Procedure—Separately inject equal volumes (about 10 μL) of the *Standard solution* and the *Test solution* into the chromatograph, record the chromatograms, and measure the areas for the major peaks. Calculate the percentage of each quinapril related compound in the portion of Quinapril Hydrochloride taken by the formula:

$$100(V_U / W_U)C_S(r_U / r_S)$$

in which V_U is the volume, in mL, of the *Test solution*; W_U is the weight, in mg, of Quinapril Hydrochloride taken to prepare the *Test solution*; C_S is the concentration, in mg per mL, of the relevant USP Reference Standard in the *Standard solution*; and r_U and r_S are the peak areas of the corresponding quinapril related compound obtained from the *Test solution* and the *Standard solution*, respectively: not more than 0.5% each of quinapril related compound A and quinapril related compound B is found. Calculate the percentage of each impurity in the portion of Quinapril Hydrochloride taken by the formula:

$$100(r_i / r_s)$$

in which r_i is the peak response for each impurity obtained from the *Test solution*; and r_s is the sum of the responses of all the peaks obtained from the *Test solution*: not more than 0.2% of any individual impurity, other than quinapril related compound A and quinapril related compound B, is found; and not more than 2.0% of total impurities is found.

Content of chloride—Transfer about 100 mg of Quinapril Hydrochloride, accurately weighed, to a 100-mL beaker. Dissolve in 50 mL of water and 10 mL of alcohol. Acidify with nitric acid. Titrate with 0.01 N silver nitrate VS, and determine the endpoint potentiometrically, using suitable electrodes (see *Titrimetry* ⟨541⟩). Perform a blank determination, and make any necessary correction. Each mL of 0.01 N silver nitrate is equivalent to 0.3545 mg of chloride: not less than 7.2% and not more than 7.6% of chloride is found.

Assay—
Diluent—Prepare a mixture of pH 6.5, 0.025 M monobasic ammonium phosphate solution and acetonitrile (3 : 2).

Mobile phase—Prepare a filtered and degassed mixture of water, acetonitrile, and methanesulfonic acid (72 : 28 : 0.1). Make adjustments if necessary (see *System Suitability* under *Chromatography* ⟨621⟩).

System suitability preparation—Dissolve accurately weighed quantities of USP Quinapril Hydrochloride RS, USP Quinapril Related Compound A RS, and USP Quinapril Related Compound B RS in *Diluent* to obtain a solution having known concentrations of about 2 mg of USP Quinapril Hydrochloride RS per mL and 0.005 mg each of USP Quinapril Related Compound A RS and USP Quinapril Related Compound B RS per mL.

Standard preparation—Dissolve an accurately weighed quantity of USP Quinapril Hydrochloride RS in *Diluent* to obtain a solution having a known concentration of about 2 mg per mL.

Assay preparation—Transfer about 100 mg of Quinapril Hydrochloride, accurately weighed, to a 50-mL volumetric flask, dissolve in and dilute with *Diluent* to volume, and mix.

Chromatographic system (see *Chromatography* ⟨621⟩)—The liquid chromatograph is equipped with a 214-nm detector, a 4.6-mm × 3-cm guard column that contains 5-μm packing L10, and a 4.6-mm × 25-cm column that contains 5-μm packing L10. The flow rate is about 1.5 mL per minute. Chromatograph the *System suitability preparation*, and record the peak responses as directed for *Procedure*: the resolution between quinapril and quinapril related compound A is not less than 1.75; the resolution between quinapril and quinapril related compound B is not less than 3.5; the column efficiency is not less than 550 theoretical plates; and the relative standard deviation for replicate injections is not more than 2.0%.

Procedure—Separately inject equal volumes (about 10 μL) of the *Standard preparation* and the *Assay preparation* into the chromatograph, record the chromatograms, and measure the areas for the quinapril hydrochloride peaks. Calculate the quantity, in mg, of $C_{25}H_{30}N_2O_5 \cdot HCl$ in the portion of Quinapril Hydrochloride taken by the formula:

$$50C(r_U / r_S)$$

in which C is the concentration, in mg per mL, of USP Quinapril Hydrochloride RS in the *Standard preparation*; and r_U and r_S are the peak responses obtained from the *Assay preparation* and the *Standard preparation*, respectively.

Quinapril Tablets

» Quinapril Tablets contain an amount of Quinapril Hydrochloride equivalent to not less than 90.0 percent and not more than 110.0 percent of the labeled amount of quinapril ($C_{25}H_{30}N_2O_5$).

Packaging and storage—Preserve in well-closed containers. Store at controlled room temperature.

USP Reference standards ⟨11⟩—*USP Quinapril Hydrochloride RS. USP Quinapril Related Compound A RS. USP Quinapril Related Compound B RS.*

Identification—
A: *Thin-Layer Chromatographic Identification Test* ⟨201⟩—
Test solution—Transfer a quantity of finely powdered Tablets, equivalent to about 10.0 mg of quinapril, to a 15-mL centrifuge tube; add 5 mL of methanol; mix; and centrifuge for 10 minutes.
Standard solution—Transfer about 10.8 mg of USP Quinapril Hydrochloride RS to a 15-mL centrifuge tube, add 5 mL of methanol, mix, and centrifuge for 10 minutes.
Application volume: 25 μL.
Developing solvent system: a mixture of methanol and ethyl acetate (1 : 1).
Procedure—Proceed as directed in the chapter, except to wash the plate in methanol and air-dry it prior to use.
B: The retention time of the major peak in the chromatogram of the *Assay preparation* corresponds to that in the chromatogram of the *Standard preparation*, as obtained in the *Assay*.

Dissolution ⟨711⟩—
Medium: water; 900 mL.
Apparatus 1: 100 rpm.
Time: 30 minutes.
Procedure—Determine the amount of $C_{25}H_{30}N_2O_5$ dissolved by employing the procedure set forth in the *Assay*, using a filtered portion of the solution under test as the *Assay preparation*, using methanol to prepare the *Standard preparation*, and making any necessary volumetric adjustments with water.
Tolerances—Not less than 80% (*Q*) of the labeled amount of $C_{25}H_{30}N_2O_5$ is dissolved in 30 minutes.

Uniformity of dosage units ⟨905⟩: meet the requirements.
PROCEDURE FOR CONTENT UNIFORMITY—
Solvent, Buffered solvent, Mobile phase, and *Chromatographic system*—Prepare as directed in the *Assay*.
Standard solution—Prepare as directed for *Standard preparation* in the *Assay*.
Test solution—Transfer 1 Tablet to a volumetric flask. Add a volume of *Solvent*, equivalent to about one-half the flask volume; sonicate for 5 minutes; and shake by mechanical means for about 15 minutes. Dilute with *Solvent* to volume, mix, and pass through a suitable filter, discarding the first portion of the filtrate. Dilute a portion of the filtrate quantitatively, and stepwise if necessary, with *Solvent* to obtain a solution containing about 0.108 mg of quinapril hydrochloride per mL.
Procedure—Separately inject equal volumes (about 20 μL) of the *Standard solution* and the *Test solution* into the chromatograph, record the chromatograms, and measure the areas of the major peaks. Calculate the quantity, in mg, of quinapril ($C_{25}H_{30}N_2O_5$) in each Tablet taken by the formula:

$$(438.52/474.98)C(L/D)(r_U / r_S)$$

in which 438.52 and 474.98 are the molecular weights of quinapril and quinapril hydrochloride, respectively; *C* is the concentration, in mg per mL, of USP Quinapril Hydrochloride RS in the *Standard solution*; *L* is the labeled quantity, in mg, of quinapril in each Tablet; *D* is the concentration, in mg per mL, of quinapril hydrochloride in the *Test solution*; and r_U and r_S are the quinapril peak areas obtained from the *Test solution* and the *Standard solution*, respectively.

Related compounds—
Solvent, Buffered solvent, and *Mobile phase*—Prepare as directed in the *Assay*.
Resolution solution—Dissolve accurately weighed quantities of USP Quinapril Hydrochloride RS, USP Quinapril Related Compound A RS, and USP Quinapril Related Compound B RS in *Solvent* to obtain a solution having known concentrations of about 0.1 mg of USP Quinapril Hydrochloride RS and 0.005 mg each of USP Quinapril Related Compound A RS and USP Quinapril Related Compound B RS per mL.
Standard solution—Dissolve accurately weighed quantities of USP Quinapril Related Compound A RS and USP Quinapril Related Compound B RS in *Solvent*, and dilute quantitatively, and stepwise if necessary, to obtain a solution having known concentrations of about 0.5 μg each of USP Quinapril Related Compound A RS and USP Quinapril Related Compound B RS per mL.
Test solution—Use the *Assay preparation*.
Chromatographic system—Prepare as directed in the *Assay*. Chromatograph the *Resolution solution*, and record the peak areas as directed for *Procedure:* the relative retention times are about 0.6 for quinapril related compound B, 1.0 for quinapril, and 2.0 for quinapril related compound A; and the resolution, *R,* between quinapril and quinapril related compound A and between quinapril and quinapril related compound B is not less than 2.0. Chromatograph the *Standard solution,* and record the peak areas as directed for *Procedure:* the column efficiency is not less than 600 theoretical plates; the tailing factor for the quinapril and quinapril related compound A peaks is less than 1.5 and that for the quinapril related compound B peak is less than 2.0; and the relative standard deviation for replicate injections is not more than 2.0% for quinapril and not more than 3.0% for each quinapril related compound.
Procedure—Separately inject equal volumes (about 20 μL) of the *Standard solution* and the *Test solution* into the chromatograph, record the chromatograms, and measure the areas of the major peaks. Calculate the quantity, in mg, of each quinapril related compound in the portion of Tablets taken by the formula:

$$500CD(r_U / r_S)$$

in which *C* is the concentration, in mg per mL, of the appropriate USP Reference Standard in the *Standard solution; D* is the dilution factor used to prepare the *Test solution;* and r_U and r_S are the peak areas of the corresponding quinapril related compound obtained from the *Test solution* and the *Standard solution,* respectively: not more than 1.0% of quinapril related compound A is found; not more than 3.0% of quinapril related compound B is found; and not more than 3.6% of total impurities is found.

Assay—
Solvent—Prepare a mixture of water and acetonitrile (65 : 35).
Buffered solvent—Prepare a mixture of pH 6.5, 0.05 M dibasic potassium phosphate and acetonitrile (65 : 35).
Mobile phase—Prepare a filtered and degassed mixture of water, acetonitrile, and methanesulfonic acid (65 : 35 : 0.2). Make adjustments if necessary (see *System Suitability* under *Chromatography* ⟨621⟩).
Standard preparation—Dissolve an accurately weighed quantity of USP Quinapril Hydrochloride RS in *Solvent* to obtain a solution having a known concentration of about 1.08 mg per mL. Quantitatively dilute with *Buffered solvent* to obtain a solution having a known concentration of about 0.108 mg per mL.
Assay preparation—Transfer 10 Tablets to a 500-mL volumetric flask, add about 300 mL of *Solvent,* and sonicate until the Tablets have disintegrated. Shake by mechanical means for about 15 minutes, dilute with *Solvent* to volume, mix, and centrifuge. Dilute quantitatively, and stepwise if necessary, with *Solvent* to obtain a solution having a concentration of about 0.1 mg of quinapril per mL; and pass through a suitable filter, discarding the first portion of the filtrate.
Chromatographic system (see *Chromatography* ⟨621⟩)—The liquid chromatograph is equipped with a 214-nm detector and a 6.0-mm × 4-cm column that contains 3-μm packing L10. The flow rate is about 1.2 mL per minute. Chromatograph the *Standard preparation,* and record the peak areas as directed for *Procedure:* the column efficiency is not less than 600 theoretical plates; the tailing factor is not more than 1.5; and the relative standard deviation for replicate injections is not more than 2.0%.
Procedure—Separately inject equal volumes (about 20 μL) of the *Standard preparation* and the *Assay preparation* into the chromatograph, record the chromatograms, and measure the areas for the major peaks. Calculate the quantity, in mg, of quinapril ($C_{25}H_{30}N_2O_5$) in the portion of Tablets taken by the formula:

$$500CD(438.52/474.98)(r_U / r_S)$$

in which *C* is the concentration, in mg per mL, of USP Quinapril Hydrochloride RS in the *Standard preparation; D* is the dilution factor used to prepare the *Assay preparation;* 438.52 and 474.98 are the molecular weights of quinapril and quinapril hydrochloride, respectively; and r_U and r_S are the peak areas obtained from the *Assay preparation* and the *Standard preparation,* respectively.

Quinidine Gluconate

$C_{20}H_{24}N_2O_2 \cdot C_6H_{12}O_7$ 520.57
Cinchonan-9-ol, 6'-methoxy-, (9S)-, mono-D-gluconate (salt)
Quinidine mono-D-gluconate (salt)   [7054-25-3].

» Quinidine Gluconate is the gluconate of an alkaloid that may be obtained from various species of *Cinchona* and their hybrids, or from *Remijia pedunculata* Flückiger (Fam. Rubiaceae), or prepared from quinine. Quinidine Gluconate contains not less than 99.0 percent and not more than 100.5 percent of total alkaloid salt, calculated as $C_{20}H_{24}N_2O_2 \cdot C_6H_{12}O_7$, on the dried basis.

Packaging and storage—Preserve in well-closed, light-resistant containers. Store at 25°, excursions permitted between 15° and 30°.

USP Reference standards ⟨11⟩—*USP Quinidine Gluconate RS. USP Quininone RS.*

Identification—
  A: A 1 in 2000 solution in dilute sulfuric acid (1 in 350) exhibits a vivid blue fluorescence. On the addition of a few drops of hydrochloric acid, the fluorescence disappears.
  B: In the test for *Chromatographic purity*, the R_F value of the principal spot obtained from the *Test preparation* corresponds to that from the *Standard preparation*.
  C: A solution (1 in 50) is dextrorotatory.
  D: Dissolve 700 mg in 5 mL of water with the aid of heat, and add 1 mL of glacial acetic acid and 200 mg of phenylhydrazine hydrochloride. Heat in a water bath for 15 minutes, cool, and scratch the inner surface of the tube with a glass rod: orange crystals are formed.

Loss on drying ⟨731⟩—Dry it at 105° for 1 hour: it loses not more than 0.5% of its weight.

Residue on ignition ⟨281⟩:   not more than 0.15%.

Heavy metals, *Method II* ⟨231⟩:   0.001%.

Limit of dihydroquinidine gluconate—
  Methanesulfonic acid solution—Add 35.0 mL of methanesulfonic acid to 20.0 mL of glacial acetic acid, dilute with water to 500 mL, and mix.
  Diethylamine solution—Dissolve 10.0 mL of diethylamine in water to obtain 100 mL of solution.
  Mobile phase—Prepare a filtered and degassed mixture of water, acetonitrile, *Methanesulfonic acid solution,* and *Diethylamine solution* (860 : 100 : 20 : 20). Adjust with *Diethylamine solution* to a pH of 2.6.
  System suitability solution—Transfer about 10 mg each of quinidine gluconate and dihydroquinidine hydrochloride to a 50-mL volumetric flask. Dissolve in about 5 mL of methanol, dilute with *Mobile phase* to volume, and mix.
  Test solution—Transfer about 26 mg of Quinidine Gluconate to a 100-mL volumetric flask, dissolve in and dilute with *Mobile phase* to volume, and mix.
  Chromatographic system (see *Chromatography* ⟨621⟩)—The liquid chromatograph is equipped with a 235-nm detector and a 3.9-mm × 30-cm column that contains packing L1. Chromatograph the *System suitability solution,* and proceed as directed for *Procedure:* the relative retention times for quinidine and dihydroquinidine are 1 and 1.5, respectively; the resolution, *R*, between the quinidine and dihydroquinidine is not less than 2.5; and the relative standard deviation for the peak response is not more than 2.0%.
  Procedure—Inject about 50 µL of the *Test solution* into the chromatograph, record the chromatogram, and measure the peak responses. The response of the dihydroquinidine peak is not greater than 0.25 that of the quinidine peak (20.0%).

Chromatographic purity—
  Standard preparation—Prepare a solution of USP Quinidine Gluconate RS in diluted alcohol to contain 6 mg per mL.
  Diluted standard preparation—Dilute a portion of the *Standard preparation* with diluted alcohol to a concentration of 0.06 mg per mL.
  Related substances preparation—Prepare a solution in diluted alcohol containing in each mL 0.04 mg of USP Quininone RS (corresponding to 0.06 mg of the gluconate), and 0.08 mg of cinchonine (corresponding to 0.12 mg of the gluconate).
  Test preparation—Prepare a solution of Quinidine Gluconate in diluted alcohol to contain 6 mg per mL.
  Procedure—Apply 10-µL portions of the *Test preparation,* the *Standard preparation,* the *Diluted standard preparation,* and the *Related substances preparation* to a suitable thin-layer chromatographic plate (see *Chromatography* ⟨621⟩) coated with a 0.25-mm layer of chromatographic silica gel. Allow to dry, and develop the chromatogram in a solvent system consisting of a mixture of chloroform, acetone, and diethylamine (5 : 4 : 1), the solvent chamber being used without previous equilibration. When the solvent front has moved about 15 cm, remove the plate from the chamber, mark the solvent front, and allow the solvent to evaporate. Spray the chromatogram with glacial acetic acid. Locate the spots on the plate by examination under long-wavelength UV light. Any spot produced by the *Test preparation* at the R_F value of a spot produced by the *Related substances preparation* is not greater in size or intensity than that corresponding spot. Apart from these spots and from the spots appearing at the R_F value of Quinidine Gluconate and dihydroquinidine gluconate (the two spots most evident from the *Standard preparation*), any additional fluorescent spot is not greater in size or intensity than the principal spot of the *Diluted standard preparation*. Spray the plate with potassium iodoplatinate TS. Any spot produced by the *Test preparation* is not greater in size or intensity than a corresponding spot from the *Related substances preparation*.

Organic volatile impurities, *Method I* ⟨467⟩:   meets the requirements.

(Official until July 1, 2008)

Assay—Dissolve about 150 mg of Quinidine Gluconate, accurately weighed, in 10 mL of glacial acetic acid, heating gently if necessary. Cool the solution, add 20 mL of acetic anhydride and 4 drops of *p*-naphtholbenzein TS, and titrate with 0.1 N perchloric acid VS from a 10-mL microburet to a green endpoint. Perform a blank determination, and make any necessary correction. Each mL of 0.1 N perchloric acid is equivalent to 26.03 mg of total alkaloid salt, calculated as $C_{20}H_{24}N_2O_2 \cdot C_6H_{12}O_7$.

Quinidine Gluconate Injection

» Quinidine Gluconate Injection is a sterile solution of Quinidine Gluconate in Water for Injection. It contains, in each mL, amounts of quinidine gluconate and dihydroquinidine gluconate totaling not less than 76 mg and not more than 84 mg of quinidine gluconate, calculated as $C_{20}H_{24}N_2O_2 \cdot C_6H_{12}O_7$.

Packaging and storage—Preserve in single-dose or in multiple-dose containers, preferably of Type I glass.

USP Reference standards ⟨11⟩—*USP Quinidine Gluconate RS. USP Quininone RS. USP Endotoxin RS.*

Identification—
  A: A 1 in 150 solution of Injection in dilute sulfuric acid (1 in 350) exhibits a vivid blue fluorescence. On the addition of a few drops of hydrochloric acid, the fluorescence disappears.
  B: A solution of Injection (1 in 4) is dextrorotatory.
  C: In the test for *Chromatographic purity*, the R_F value of the principal spot obtained from the *Test preparation* corresponds to that from the *Standard preparation*.

Bacterial endotoxins ⟨85⟩—It contains not more than 0.6 USP Endotoxin Unit per mg of quinidine gluconate.

Chromatographic purity—Mix an accurately measured volume of Injection, equivalent to 80 mg of quinidine gluconate, with 25 mL of water, add 2 drops of 2 N sulfuric acid, and extract with 50 mL of ether, discarding the ether extract. To the aqueous solution add 2 mL of 1 N sodium hydroxide, extract with 50 mL of ether, wash the extract with 25 mL of water, and discard the aqueous solutions. Evaporate the ether extract just to dryness, and dissolve the residue in 10 mL of alcohol. Using this as the test solution, proceed as directed in the test for *Chromatographic purity* under *Quinidine Gluconate*, beginning with "Apply 10-μL portions of the *Test preparation*."

Other requirements—It meets the requirements under *Injections* ⟨1⟩.

Assay—

Methanesulfonic acid solution, Diethylamine solution, Mobile phase, System suitability solution, and *Chromatographic system*— Proceed as directed in the test for *Limit of dihydroquinidine gluconate* under *Quinidine Gluconate*.

Standard preparation—Transfer about 26 mg of USP Quinidine Gluconate RS, accurately weighed, to a 100-mL volumetric flask, dissolve in and dilute with *Mobile phase* to volume, and mix.

Assay preparation—Transfer an accurately measured volume of Injection, equivalent to about 400 mg of quinidine gluconate, to a 50-mL volumetric flask, add methanol to volume, and mix. Transfer 3.0 mL of this solution to a 100-mL volumetric flask, dilute with *Mobile phase* to volume, and mix.

Procedure—Separately inject equal volumes (about 50 μL) of the *Standard preparation* and the *Assay preparation* into the chromatograph. Calculate the quantity, in mg, of the sum of quinidine gluconate and dihydroquinidine gluconate in each mL of the Injection taken by the formula:

$$(5000/3)(C/V)(r_{b,U} + r_{d,U}) / (r_{b,S} + r_{d,S})$$

in which C is the concentration, in mg per mL, of USP Quinidine Gluconate RS in the *Standard preparation*; V is the volume, in mL, of Injection taken; $r_{b,U}$ and $r_{b,S}$ are the peak responses of quinidine obtained from the *Assay preparation* and the *Standard preparation*, respectively; and $r_{d,U}$ and $r_{d,S}$ are the peak responses of dihydroquinidine obtained from the *Assay preparation* and the *Standard preparation*, respectively.

Quinidine Gluconate Extended-Release Tablets

» Quinidine Gluconate Extended-Release Tablets contain amounts of quinidine gluconate and dihydroquinidine gluconate totaling not less than 90.0 percent and not more than 110.0 percent of the labeled amount of quinidine gluconate, calculated as quinidine gluconate ($C_{20}H_{24}N_2O_2 \cdot C_6H_{12}O_7$).

Packaging and storage—Preserve in well-closed, light-resistant containers.

Labeling—The labeling indicates the *Dissolution Test* with which the product complies.

USP Reference standards ⟨11⟩—USP Quinidine Gluconate RS. USP Quininone RS.

Identification—

A: Shake a quantity of powdered Tablets, equivalent to about 50 mg of quinidine gluconate, with 100 mL of dilute sulfuric acid (1 in 350), and filter: the filtrate so obtained exhibits a vivid blue fluorescence when viewed under long-wavelength UV light. On the addition of hydrochloric acid, the fluorescence disappears.

B: The retention time of the major peak in the chromatogram of the *Assay preparation* corresponds to that in the chromatogram of the *Standard preparation*, as obtained in the *Assay*.

C: In the test for *Chromatographic purity*, the R_F value of the principal spot obtained from the *Test solution* corresponds to that obtained from the *Standard solution*.

Dissolution ⟨711⟩—

TEST 1—If the product complies with this test, the labeling indicates that it meets USP *Dissolution Test 1*.

Medium: pH 5.4, 0.1 M acetate buffer prepared as follows. Add 6.9 g of anhydrous sodium acetate and 0.525 mL of glacial acetic acid to 1 L of water, and mix. Adjust with 0.1 N hydrochloric acid or 0.1 N sodium hydroxide to a pH of 5.4; 900 mL.

Apparatus 2: 75 rpm.

Times: 1, 2, 4, and 8 hours.

Procedure—Determine the amount of $C_{20}H_{24}N_2O_2 \cdot C_6H_{12}O_7$ dissolved from UV absorbances at the wavelength of maximum absorbance at about 235 nm, using filtered aliquots of the solution under test, diluted with *Medium* if necessary, in comparison with a Standard solution having a known concentration of USP Quinidine Gluconate RS in the same *Medium*.

Tolerances—The percentages of the labeled amount of quinidine gluconate dissolved at the times specified conform to *Acceptance Table 2*.

Time (hours)	Amount dissolved
1	between 30% and 50%
2	between 45% and 65%
4	between 60% and 85%
8	not less than 85%

TEST 4—If the product complies with this test, the labeling indicates that it meets USP *Dissolution Test 4*.

Medium: 0.1 N hydrochloric acid; 600 mL.

Apparatus 2: 75 rpm.

Times and *Procedure*—Proceed as directed for *Test 1*.

Tolerances—The percentages of the labeled amount of quinidine gluconate dissolved at the times specified conform to *Acceptance Table 2*.

Time (hours)	Amount dissolved
1	between 30% and 45%
2	between 45% and 60%
4	between 60% and 80%
8	not less than 85%

TEST 5—If the product complies with this test, the labeling indicates that it meets USP *Dissolution Test 5*.

Medium, Apparatus, and *Procedure*—Proceed as directed for *Test 1*, using 8-mesh sinker baskets.[*]

Times: 1, 2, and 4 hours.

Tolerances—The percentages of the labeled amount of quinidine gluconate dissolved at the times specified conform to *Acceptance Table 2*.

Time (hours)	Amount dissolved
1	between 20% and 50%
2	between 40% and 70%
4	not less than 75%

Uniformity of dosage units ⟨905⟩: meet the requirements.

Procedure for content uniformity—Quantitatively transfer 1 intact or powdered Tablet to a 250-mL volumetric flask, and add about 125 mL of 0.1 N hydrochloric acid. Heat the sample with frequent agitation just to boiling, and cool to room temperature. Dilute with 0.1 N hydrochloric acid to volume, mix, and filter, discarding the first 20 mL of the filtrate. Concomitantly determine the absorbance of this solution, quantitatively diluted with 0.1 N hydrochloric acid, if necessary, and a Standard solution of USP Quinidine Gluconate RS in 0.1 N hydrochloric acid having a known concentration of about 0.0525 mg per mL, in 1-cm cells, at the wavelength of maximum absorbance at about 347 nm, with a suitable spectrophotometer, using 0.1 N hydrochloric acid as the blank. Calculate the quantity, in mg, of active ingredients, calculated as quinidine

---

[*] A suitable sinker is available from VanKel, www.varianinc.com, catalog number 12-3062.

gluconate ($C_{20}H_{24}N_2O_2 \cdot C_6H_{12}O_7$), in the Tablet taken by the formula:

$$(TC/D)(A_U/A_S)$$

in which T is the labeled quantity, in mg, of quinidine gluconate in the Tablet; D is the concentration, in mg per mL, of quinidine gluconate in the solution from the Tablet, based on the labeled quantity per Tablet and the extent of dilution; C is the concentration, in mg per mL, of USP Quinidine Gluconate RS in the Standard solution; and A_U and A_S are the absorbances of the solution from the Tablet and the Standard solution, respectively.

Chromatographic purity—
Standard solution—Prepare a solution of USP Quinidine Gluconate RS in diluted alcohol to contain 6 mg per mL.
Diluted standard solution—Dilute a portion of the *Standard solution* with diluted alcohol to a concentration of 0.06 mg per mL.
Quininone solution—Prepare a solution in diluted alcohol containing in each mL 0.04 mg of USP Quininone RS (corresponding to 0.06 mg of the gluconate).
Test solution—Shake a quantity of powdered Tablets, equivalent to about 150 mg of quinidine gluconate, with 25 mL of diluted alcohol for 10 minutes, and filter.
Procedure—Apply 10-µL portions of the *Test solution*, the *Standard solution*, the *Diluted standard solution*, and the *Quininone solution* to a suitable thin-layer chromatographic plate (see *Chromatography* ⟨621⟩) coated with a 0.25-mm layer of chromatographic silica gel. Allow to dry, and develop the chromatogram in a solvent system consisting of a mixture of chloroform, acetone, and diethylamine (5 : 4 : 1), the solvent chamber being used without previous equilibration. When the solvent front has moved about 15 cm, remove the plate from the chamber, mark the solvent front, and allow the solvent to evaporate. Spray the chromatogram with glacial acetic acid. Locate the spots on the plate by examination under long-wavelength UV light. Any spot produced by the *Test solution* at the R_F value of a spot produced by the *Quininone solution* is not greater in size or intensity than that corresponding spot. Apart from these spots and from the spots appearing at the R_F value of quinidine gluconate and dihydroquinidine gluconate (the two spots most evident from the *Standard solution*), any additional fluorescent spot is not greater in size or intensity than the principal spot obtained from the *Diluted standard solution*.

Assay—
Methanesulfonic acid solution—Add 35.0 mL of methanesulfonic acid to 20.0 mL of glacial acetic acid, dilute with water to 500 mL, and mix.
Diethylamine solution—Dissolve 10.0 mL of diethylamine in water to obtain 100 mL of solution.
Mobile phase—Prepare a suitable filtered and degassed mixture of water, acetonitrile, *Methanesulfonic acid solution*, and *Diethylamine solution* (860 : 100 : 20 : 20). Adjust with *Diethylamine solution* to a pH of 2.6 if found to be lower.
System suitability preparation—Transfer about 10 mg each of quinidine gluconate and dihydroquinidine chloride to a 50-mL volumetric flask. Dissolve in about 5 mL of methanol, dilute with *Mobile phase* to volume, and mix.
Standard preparation—Transfer about 20 mg of USP Quinidine Gluconate RS, accurately weighed, to a 100-mL volumetric flask, dissolve in and dilute with *Mobile phase* to volume, and mix.
Assay preparation—Weigh and finely powder not fewer than 20 Tablets. Transfer an accurately weighed portion of the powder, equivalent to about 160 mg of quinidine gluconate, to a 100-mL volumetric flask, add about 80 mL of a mixture of methanol and water (1 : 1), and sonicate until evenly dispersed. Cool to room temperature, dilute with a mixture of methanol and water (1 : 1) to volume, mix, and filter, discarding the first 20 mL of the filtrate. Transfer 3.0 mL of the filtrate to a 25-mL volumetric flask, dilute with *Mobile phase* to volume, and mix.
Chromatographic system (see *Chromatography* ⟨621⟩)—The liquid chromatograph is equipped with a 235-nm detector and a 3- to 5-mm × 25- to 30-cm column that contains packing L1. The flow rate is about 1.5 mL per minute. Chromatograph the *System suitability preparation*, and record the peak responses as directed for *Procedure*: the typical relative retention times for quinidine and dihydroquinidine are 1 and 1.5, respectively; and the resolution, R, between quinidine and dihydroquinidine is not less than 1.2. Chromatograph the *Standard preparation*, and record the peak responses as directed for *Procedure*: the relative standard deviation for replicate injections is not more than 2.0%.
Procedure—Separately inject equal volumes (about 20 µL) of the *Standard preparation* and the *Assay preparation* into the chromatograph, record the chromatograms, and measure the responses for the quinidine and dihydroquinidine peaks. Calculate the quantity, in mg, of the sum of quinidine gluconate and dihydroquinidine gluconate in the portion of Tablets taken by the formula:

$$(2500/3)C(r_{b,U} + r_{d,U}) / (r_{b,S} + r_{d,S})$$

in which C is the concentration, in mg per mL, of USP Quinidine Gluconate RS in the *Standard preparation*; $r_{b,U}$ and $r_{b,S}$ are the peak responses of quinidine obtained from the *Assay preparation* and the *Standard preparation*, respectively; and $r_{d,U}$ and $r_{d,S}$ are the peak responses of dihydroquinidine obtained from the *Assay preparation* and the *Standard preparation*, respectively.

Quinidine Sulfate

($C_{20}H_{24}N_2O_2$)$_2 \cdot H_2SO_4 \cdot 2H_2O$ 782.94
Cinchonan-9-ol, 6′-methoxy-, (9S)-, sulfate (2 : 1) (salt), dihydrate.
Quinidine sulfate (2 : 1) (salt) dihydrate   [6591-63-5].
Anhydrous   746.93   [50-54-4].

» Quinidine Sulfate is the sulfate of an alkaloid obtained from various species of *Cinchona* and their hybrids and from *Remijia pedunculata* Flückiger (Fam. Rubiaceae), or prepared from quinine. It contains not less than 99.0 percent and not more than 101.0 percent of total alkaloid salt, calculated as ($C_{20}H_{24}N_2O_2$)$_2 \cdot H_2SO_4$, on the anhydrous basis.

Packaging and storage—Preserve in well-closed, light-resistant containers.
USP Reference standards ⟨11⟩—*USP Quinidine Sulfate RS. USP Quininone RS.*
Identification—
   A: A 1 in 2000 solution in dilute sulfuric acid (1 in 350) exhibits a vivid blue fluorescence. On the addition of a few drops of hydrochloric acid, the fluorescence disappears.
   B: In the test for *Chromatographic purity*, the R_F value of the principal spot obtained from the *Test preparation* corresponds to that from the *Standard preparation*.
   C: A 1 in 50 solution made with the aid of a few drops of hydrochloric acid responds to the tests for *Sulfate* ⟨191⟩.
Specific rotation ⟨781⟩: between +275° and +288°, calculated on the anhydrous basis, determined in a solution in 0.1 N hydrochloric acid containing 200 mg in each 10 mL.
Water, *Method I* ⟨921⟩: between 4.0% and 5.5%.
Residue on ignition ⟨281⟩: not more than 0.1%.
Chloroform-alcohol-insoluble substances—Warm 2 g with 15 mL of a mixture of chloroform and dehydrated alcohol (2 : 1) at about 50° for 10 minutes. Filter through a tared, sintered-glass filter, using gentle suction. Wash the filter with five 10-mL portions of the chloroform-alcohol mixture, dry at 105° for 1 hour, and weigh: the weight of the residue does not exceed 2 mg (0.1%).
Heavy metals, *Method II* ⟨231⟩: 0.001%.
Limit of dihydroquinidine sulfate—
Methanesulfonic acid solution—Add 35.0 mL of methanesulfonic acid to 20.0 mL of glacial acetic acid, dilute with water to 500 mL, and mix.
Diethylamine solution—Dissolve 10.0 mL of diethylamine in water to obtain 100 mL of solution.

Mobile phase—Prepare a filtered and degassed mixture of water, acetonitrile, *Methanesulfonic acid solution*, and *Diethylamine solution* (860 : 100 : 20 : 20). Adjust with *Diethylamine* to a pH of 2.6.

System suitability solution—Transfer about 10 mg each of quinidine sulfate and dihydroquinidine hydrochloride to a 50-mL volumetric flask. Dissolve in about 5 mL of methanol, dilute with *Mobile phase* to volume, and mix.

Test solution—Transfer about 20 mg of Quinidine Sulfate to a 100-mL volumetric flask, dissolve in and dilute with *Mobile phase* to volume, and mix.

Chromatographic system (see *Chromatography* ⟨621⟩)—The liquid chromatograph is equipped with a 235-nm detector and a 3.9-mm × 30-cm column that contains packing L1. Chromatograph the *System suitability solution*, and proceed as directed for *Procedure:* the relative retention times for quinidine and dihydroquinidine are 1 and 1.5, respectively, the resolution, *R*, between the quinidine and dihydroquinidine is not less than 2.5, and the relative standard deviation for the peak response is not more than 2.0%.

Procedure—Inject about 50 μL of the *Test solution* into the chromatograph, record the chromatogram, and measure the peak responses. The response of the dihydroquinidine peak is not greater than 0.25 that of the quinidine peak (20.0%).

Chromatographic purity—

Standard preparation—Prepare a solution of USP Quinidine Sulfate RS in diluted alcohol to contain 6 mg per mL.

Diluted standard preparation—Dilute a portion of the *Standard preparation* with diluted alcohol to a concentration of 0.06 mg per mL.

Related substances preparation—Prepare a solution in diluted alcohol containing in each mL 0.05 mg of USP Quininone RS (corresponding to 0.06 mg of the sulfate), and 0.10 mg of cinchonine (corresponding to 0.12 mg of the sulfate).

Test preparation—Prepare a solution of Quinidine Sulfate in diluted alcohol to contain 6 mg per mL.

Procedure—Apply 10-μL portions of the *Test preparation*, the *Standard preparation*, the *Diluted standard preparation*, and the *Related substances preparation* to a suitable thin-layer chromatographic plate (see *Chromatography* ⟨621⟩) coated with a 0.25-mm layer of chromatographic silica gel. Allow to dry, and develop the chromatogram in a solvent system consisting of a mixture of chloroform, acetone, and diethylamine (5 : 4 : 1), the solvent chamber being used without previous equilibration. When the solvent front has moved about 15 cm, remove the plate from the chamber, mark the solvent front, and allow the solvent to evaporate. Spray the chromatogram with glacial acetic acid. Locate the spots on the plate by examination under long-wavelength UV light. Any spot produced by the *Test preparation* at the R_F value of a spot produced by the *Related substances preparation* is not greater in size or intensity than that corresponding spot. Apart from these spots and from the spots appearing at the R_F value of Quinidine Sulfate and dihydroquinidine sulfate (the two spots most evident from the *Standard preparation*), any additional fluorescent spot is not greater in size or intensity than the principal spot of the *Diluted standard preparation*. Spray the plate with potassium iodoplatinate TS. Any spot produced by the *Test preparation* is not greater in size or intensity than a corresponding spot from the *Related substances preparation*.

Organic volatile impurities, *Method I* ⟨467⟩: meets the requirements.

(Official until July 1, 2008)

Assay—Dissolve about 200 mg of Quinidine Sulfate, accurately weighed, in 20 mL of acetic anhydride, and proceed as directed in the *Assay* under *Quinidine Gluconate*, beginning with [add] "4 drops of *p*-naphtholbenzein TS." Each mL of 0.1 N perchloric acid is equivalent to 24.90 mg of total alkaloid salt, calculated as $(C_{20}H_{24}N_2O_2)_2 \cdot H_2SO_4$.

Quinidine Sulfate Capsules

» Quinidine Sulfate Capsules contain amounts of quinidine sulfate and dihydroquinidine sulfate totaling not less than 90.0 percent and not more than 110.0 percent of the labeled amount of quinidine sulfate, calculated as $(C_{20}H_{24}N_2O_2)_2 \cdot H_2SO_4 \cdot 2H_2O$.

Packaging and storage—Preserve in tight, light-resistant containers.

USP Reference standards ⟨11⟩—*USP Quinidine Sulfate RS. USP Quininone RS.*

Identification—

A: Shake a quantity of the contents of Capsules, equivalent to about 100 mg of quinidine sulfate, with 10 mL of dilute sulfuric acid (1 in 350), and filter: an appropriate dilution of the filtrate exhibits a vivid blue fluorescence. On the addition of a few drops of hydrochloric acid the fluorescence disappears.

B: In the test for *Chromatographic purity*, the R_F value of the principal spot obtained from the *Test preparation* corresponds to that from the *Standard preparation*.

C: Shake a quantity of the contents of Capsules, equivalent to about 100 mg of quinidine sulfate, with 10 mL of dilute hydrochloric acid (1 in 100), and filter: the filtrate responds to the tests for *Sulfate* ⟨191⟩.

Dissolution ⟨711⟩—

Medium: 0.01 N hydrochloric acid; 900 mL.
Apparatus 1: 100 rpm.
Time: 30 minutes.

Procedure—Determine the amount of $(C_{20}H_{24}N_2O_2)_2 \cdot H_2SO_4 \cdot 2H_2O$ dissolved by employing UV absorption at the wavelength of maximum absorbance at about 248 nm on filtered portions of the solution under test, suitably diluted with *Dissolution Medium*, in comparison with a Standard solution having a known concentration of USP Quinidine Sulfate RS in the same *Medium*.

Tolerances—Not less than 85% (*Q*) of the labeled amount of $(C_{20}H_{24}N_2O_2)_2 \cdot H_2SO_4 \cdot 2H_2O$ is dissolved in 30 minutes.

Uniformity of dosage units ⟨905⟩: meet the requirements.

Procedure for content uniformity—Transfer the contents of 1 Capsule to a 250-mL volumetric flask, add about 175 mL of dilute hydrochloric acid (1 in 100), and shake by mechanical means for 30 minutes. Add dilute hydrochloric acid (1 in 100) to volume, and mix. Filter a portion of the mixture, discarding the first 20 mL of the filtrate. Concomitantly determine the absorbances of this solution, quantitatively diluted, if necessary, and a Standard solution of USP Quinidine Sulfate RS in dilute hydrochloric acid (1 in 100) having a known concentration of about 40 μg per mL, in 1-cm cells, at the wavelength of maximum absorbance at about 345 nm, with a suitable spectrophotometer, using water as the blank. Calculate the quantity, in mg, of active ingredients, calculated as quinidine sulfate $[(C_{20}H_{24}N_2O_2)_2 \cdot H_2SO_4 \cdot 2H_2O]$, in the Capsule taken by the formula:

$$(TC/D)(A_U/A_S)$$

in which *T* is the labeled quantity, in mg, of quinidine sulfate in the Capsule, *D* is the concentration, in μg per mL, of quinidine sulfate in the solution from the Capsule, based on the labeled quantity per Capsule and the extent of dilution, *C* is the concentration, in μg per mL, of USP Quinidine Sulfate RS in the Standard solution, and A_U and A_S are the absorbances of the solution from the Capsule and the Standard solution, respectively.

Chromatographic purity—Shake a quantity of the contents of Capsules, equivalent to about 150 mg of quinidine sulfate, with 25 mL of diluted alcohol for 10 minutes, and filter. Using this as the *Test preparation,* proceed as directed in the test for *Chromatographic purity* under *Quinidine Sulfate*.

Assay—

Methanesulfonic acid solution, Diethylamine solution, Mobile phase, System suitability solution, and *Chromatographic system*—Proceed as directed for *Limit of dihydroquinidine sulfate* under *Quinidine Sulfate*.

Standard preparation—Transfer about 20 mg of USP Quinidine Sulfate RS, accurately weighed, to a 100-mL volumetric flask, dissolve in and dilute with *Mobile phase* to volume, and mix.

Assay preparation—Transfer the contents of not fewer than 20 Capsules to a container, and mix. Transfer an accurately weighed portion of the powder, equivalent to about 160 mg of quinidine sulfate, to a 100-mL volumetric flask, add 80 mL of methanol, and shake the flask by mechanical means for 30 minutes. Dilute with methanol to volume, mix, and filter, discarding the first 10 mL of the filtrate. Transfer 3.0 mL of the filtrate to a 25-mL volumetric flask, dilute with *Mobile phase* to volume, and mix.

Procedure—Separately inject equal volumes (about 50 µL) of the *Standard preparation* and the *Assay preparation* into a chromatograph. Calculate the quantity, in mg, of the sum of quinidine sulfate and dihydroquinidine sulfate in the portion of Capsules taken by the formula:

$$(2500/3)C(r_{b,U} + r_{d,U})/(r_{b,S} + r_{d,S})$$

in which C is the concentration, in mg per mL, of USP Quinidine Sulfate RS in the *Standard preparation*; $r_{b,U}$ and $r_{b,S}$ are the peak responses of quinidine obtained from the *Assay preparation* and the *Standard preparation*, respectively; and $r_{d,U}$ and $r_{d,S}$ are the peak responses of dihydroquinidine obtained from the *Assay preparation* and the *Standard preparation*, respectively.

Add the following:

▲Quinidine Sulfate Oral Suspension

» Quinidine Sulfate Oral Suspension contains not less than 90.0 percent and not more than 110.0 percent of the labeled amount of quinidine sulfate [$(C_{20}H_{24}N_2O_2)_2 \cdot H_2SO_4 \cdot 2H_2O$]. Prepare Quinidine Sulfate Oral Suspension 10 mg per mL as follows (see *Pharmaceutical Compounding—Nonsterile Preparations* ⟨795⟩):

Quinidine Sulfate	1 g
Vehicle: a mixture of Vehicle for Oral Solution (regular or sugar-free), *NF*, and Vehicle for Oral Suspension, *NF* (1 : 1), a sufficient quantity to make	100 mL

If using Quinidine Sulfate Tablets, place in a suitable mortar, and comminute into a fine powder, or add Quinidine Sulfate powder to the mortar. Add about 15 mL of the Vehicle, and mix to a uniform paste. Add the Vehicle in small portions almost to volume, and mix thoroughly after each addition. Transfer the contents of the mortar, stepwise and quantitatively, to the calibrated bottle. Add sufficient Vehicle to volume, and mix well.

Packaging and storage—Preserve in tight, light-resistant containers. Store at room temperature, or in a cold place.
Labeling—Label it to state that it is to be well shaken before use, and to state the beyond-use date.
USP Reference standards ⟨11⟩—*USP Quinidine Sulfate RS*.
pH ⟨791⟩: between 3.4 and 4.4.
Beyond-use date: 60 days after the day on which it was compounded.
Assay—
Methanesulfonic acid solution—Add 35.0 mL of methanesulfonic acid to 20.0 mL of glacial acetic acid, dilute with water to 500 mL, and mix.
Diethylamine solution—Dissolve 10.0 mL of diethylamine in water to obtain 100 mL of solution.
Mobile phase—Prepare a suitable filtered and degassed solution of water, acetonitrile, *Methanesulfonic acid solution,* and *Diethylamine solution* (80 : 20 : 2 : 2). Make adjustments if necessary (see *System Suitability* under *Chromatography* ⟨621⟩).

Standard preparation—Dissolve USP Quinidine Sulfate RS in *Mobile phase* to obtain a solution having a known concentration of about 100 µg per mL.

Assay preparation—Agitate the container of Oral Suspension for 30 minutes on a rotating mixer, remove a 5-mL sample, and store in a clear glass vial at –70° until analyzed. At the time of analysis, remove the sample from the freezer, allow it to reach room temperature, and mix on a vortex mixer for 30 seconds. Pipet 1.0 mL of the sample solution into a 100-mL volumetric flask, and dilute with *Mobile phase* to volume.

Chromatographic system (see *Chromatography* ⟨621⟩)—The liquid chromatograph is equipped with a 235-nm detector and a 4.6-mm × 25-cm analytical column that contains 5-µm packing L1. The flow rate is about 1.0 mL per minute. Chromatograph the 100 µg per mL *Standard preparation,* and record the peak responses as directed for *Procedure:* the retention time for quinidine sulfate is about 8.5 minutes, and the relative standard deviation for replicate injections is not more than 1.0%.

Procedure—Separately inject equal volumes (about 20 µL) of the *Standard preparation* and the *Assay preparation* into the chromatograph, record the chromatograms, and measure the responses for the major peaks. Calculate the quantity, in mg, of quinidine sulfate [$(C_{20}H_{24}N_2O_2)_2 \cdot H_2SO_4 \cdot 2H_2O$] in the volume of Oral Suspension taken by the formula:

$$100(C/V)(r_U/r_S)$$

in which C is the concentration, in µg per mL, of USP Quinidine Sulfate RS in the *Standard preparation;* V is the volume, in mL, of Oral Suspension taken; and r_U and r_S are the peak responses obtained from the *Assay preparation* and the *Standard preparation,* respectively.
▲USP31

Quinidine Sulfate Tablets

» Quinidine Sulfate Tablets contain amounts of quinidine sulfate and dihydroquinidine sulfate totaling not less than 90.0 percent and not more than 110.0 percent of the labeled amount of quinidine sulfate, calculated as $(C_{20}H_{24}N_2O_2)_2 \cdot H_2SO_4 \cdot 2H_2O$.

Packaging and storage—Preserve in well-closed, light-resistant containers.
USP Reference standards ⟨11⟩—*USP Quinidine Sulfate RS. USP Quininone RS*.
Identification—The Tablets meet the requirements of the tests for *Identification* under *Quinidine Sulfate Capsules*, powdered Tablets being used in place of the contents of Capsules.
Dissolution ⟨711⟩—
Medium: 0.01 N hydrochloric acid; 900 mL.
Apparatus 1: 100 rpm.
Time: 30 minutes.
Procedure—Determine the amount of $(C_{20}H_{24}N_2O_2)_2 \cdot H_2SO_4 \cdot 2H_2O$ dissolved by employing UV absorption at the wavelength of maximum absorbance at about 248 nm on filtered portions of the solution under test, suitably diluted with *Dissolution Medium*, in comparison with a Standard solution having a known concentration of USP Quinidine Sulfate RS in the same *Medium*.
Tolerances—Not less than 85% (*Q*) of the labeled amount of $(C_{20}H_{24}N_2O_2)_2 \cdot H_2SO_4 \cdot 2H_2O$ is dissolved in 30 minutes.
Uniformity of dosage units ⟨905⟩: meet the requirements.
Procedure for content uniformity—Proceed as directed for *Procedure for content uniformity* in the test for *Uniformity of dosage units* under *Quinidine Sulfate Capsules*, using 1 powdered Tablet instead of the contents of 1 Capsule.
Chromatographic purity—Shake a quantity of powdered Tablets, equivalent to about 150 mg of quinidine sulfate, with 25 mL of diluted alcohol for 10 minutes, and filter. Using the filtrate as the *Test preparation,* proceed as directed in the test for *Chromatographic purity* under *Quinidine Sulfate*.

Assay—Proceed as directed in the *Assay* under *Quinidine Sulfate Capsules*, using powdered Tablets.

Quinidine Sulfate Extended-Release Tablets

» Quinidine Sulfate Extended-Release Tablets contain amounts of quinidine sulfate and dihydroquinidine sulfate totaling not less than 90.0 percent and not more than 110.0 percent of the labeled amount of quinidine sulfate, calculated as $(C_{20}H_{24}N_2O_2)_2 \cdot H_2SO_4 \cdot 2H_2O$.

Packaging and storage—Preserve in well-closed, light-resistant containers.

Labeling—The labeling indicates the *Dissolution Test* with which the product complies.

USP Reference standards ⟨11⟩—*USP Quinidine Sulfate RS. USP Quininone RS.*

Identification—
  A: Shake a quantity of powdered Tablets, equivalent to about 50 mg of quinidine sulfate, with 100 mL of dilute sulfuric acid (1 in 350), and filter: the filtrate so obtained exhibits a vivid blue fluorescence. On the addition of a few drops of hydrochloric acid, the fluorescence disappears.
  B: In the test for *Chromatographic purity*, the R_F value of the principal spot obtained from the *Test preparation* corresponds to that from the *Standard preparation*.
  C: Shake a quantity of the powdered Tablets, equivalent to about 100 mg of quinidine sulfate, with 10 mL of dilute hydrochloric acid (1 in 100), and filter: the filtrate so obtained meets the requirements of the tests for *Sulfate* ⟨191⟩.

Dissolution ⟨711⟩—
  TEST 1—If the product complies with this test, the labeling indicates that it meets USP *Dissolution Test 1*.
  Medium: 0.1 N hydrochloric acid; 900 mL.
  Apparatus 1: 100 rpm.
  Times: 1, 4, and 12 hours.
  Procedure—Using filtered portions of the solution under test, diluted with 0.1 N hydrochloric acid if necessary, determine the amount of $(C_{20}H_{24}N_2O_2)_2 \cdot H_2SO_4 \cdot 2H_2O$ dissolved from UV absorbances at the wavelength of maximum absorbance at about 248 nm by comparison with a Standard solution having a known concentration of USP Quinidine Sulfate RS in the same *Medium*.
  Tolerances—The percentages of the labeled amount of $(C_{20}H_{24}N_2O_2)_2 \cdot H_2SO_4 \cdot 2H_2O$ dissolved at the times specified conform to *Acceptance Table 2*.

Time (hours)	Amount dissolved
1	between 20% and 50%
4	between 43% and 73%
12	not less than 70%

  TEST 2—If the product complies with this test, the labeling indicates that it meets USP *Dissolution Test 2*.
  Medium: 0.1 N hydrochloric acid; 900 mL.
  Apparatus 1: 100 rpm.
  Times: 1, 4, and 12 hours.
  Procedure—Proceed as directed for *Test 1*.
  Tolerances—The percentages of the labeled amount of $(C_{20}H_{24}N_2O_2)_2 \cdot H_2SO_4 \cdot 2H_2O$ dissolved at the times specified conform to *Acceptance Table 2*.

Time (hours)	Amount dissolved
1	between 10% and 35%
4	between 30% and 55%
12	not less than 75%

Uniformity of dosage units ⟨905⟩: meet the requirements.
  Procedure for content uniformity—Proceed as directed for *Procedure for content uniformity* in the test for *Uniformity of dosage units* under *Quinidine Sulfate Capsules*, using 1 powdered Tablet instead of the contents of 1 Capsule.

Chromatographic purity—Shake a quantity of powdered Tablets, equivalent to about 150 mg of quinidine sulfate, with 25 mL of diluted alcohol for 10 minutes, and filter. Using the filtrate as the *Test preparation*, proceed as directed in the test for *Chromatographic purity* under *Quinidine Sulfate*.

Assay—Proceed as directed in the *Assay* under *Quinidine Sulfate Capsules*, using powdered Tablets.

Quinine Sulfate

$(C_{20}H_{24}N_2O_2)_2 \cdot H_2SO_4 \cdot 2H_2O$ 782.94
Cinchonan-9-ol, 6'-methoxy-, (8α,9R)-, sulfate (2:1) (salt), dihydrate.
Quinine sulfate (2:1) (salt) dihydrate   [6119-70-6].
Anhydrous   746.93   [804-63-7].

» Quinine Sulfate is the sulfate of an alkaloid obtained from the bark of species of *Cinchona*. It contains not less than 99.0 percent and not more than 101.0 percent of total alkaloid salt, calculated as $(C_{20}H_{24}N_2O_2)_2 \cdot H_2SO_4$, on the anhydrous basis.

Packaging and storage—Preserve in well-closed, light-resistant containers.

USP Reference standards ⟨11⟩—*USP Quinine Sulfate RS. USP Quininone RS.*

Identification—
  A: A 1 in 2000 solution in dilute sulfuric acid (1 in 350) exhibits a vivid blue fluorescence. On the addition of a few drops of hydrochloric acid, the fluorescence disappears.
  B: In the test for *Chromatographic purity*, the R_F value of the principal spot obtained from the *Test preparation* corresponds to that from the *Standard preparation*.
  C: A solution (1 in 50) made with the aid of a few drops of hydrochloric acid responds to the tests for *Sulfate* ⟨191⟩.

Specific rotation ⟨781S⟩: between −235° and −245°.
  Test solution: 20 mg per mL, in 0.1 N hydrochloric acid.

Water, *Method I* ⟨921⟩: between 4.0% and 5.5%.

Residue on ignition ⟨281⟩: not more than 0.1%.

Heavy metals, *Method II* ⟨231⟩: 0.001%.

Chloroform-alcohol-insoluble substances—Warm 2 g with 15 mL of a mixture of chloroform and dehydrated alcohol (2:1) at about 50° for 10 minutes. Filter through a tared, sintered-glass filter, using gentle suction. Wash the filter with five 10-mL portions of the chloroform-alcohol mixture, dry at 105° for 1 hour, and weigh: the weight of the residue does not exceed 2 mg (0.1%).

Chromatographic purity—
  Standard preparation—Prepare a solution of USP Quinine Sulfate RS in diluted alcohol to contain 6 mg per mL.
  Diluted standard preparation—Dilute a portion of the *Standard preparation* with diluted alcohol to a concentration of 0.06 mg per mL.
  Related substances preparation—Prepare a solution in diluted alcohol containing in each mL 0.05 mg each of USP Quininone RS (corresponding to 0.06 mg of the sulfate), and 0.10 mg of cinchonidine (corresponding to 0.12 mg of the sulfate).
  Test preparation—Prepare a solution of Quinine Sulfate in diluted alcohol to contain 6 mg per mL.

Procedure—Apply 10-μL portions of the *Test preparation*, the *Standard preparation*, the *Diluted standard preparation*, and the *Related substances preparation* to a suitable thin-layer chromatographic plate (see *Chromatography* ⟨621⟩) coated with a 0.25-mm layer of chromatographic silica gel. Allow to dry, and develop the chromatogram in a solvent system consisting of a mixture of chloroform, acetone, and diethylamine (5 : 4 : 1), the solvent chamber being used without previous equilibration. When the solvent front has moved about 15 cm, remove the plate from the chamber, mark the solvent front, and allow the solvent to evaporate. Spray the chromatogram with glacial acetic acid. Locate the spots on the plate by examination under long-wavelength UV light. Any spot produced by the *Test preparation* at the R_F value of a spot produced by the *Related substances preparation* is not greater in size or intensity than that corresponding spot. Apart from these spots and from the spot appearing at the R_F value of Quinine Sulfate, any additional fluorescent spot is not greater in size or intensity than the spot of the *Diluted standard preparation*. Spray the plate with potassium iodoplatinate TS. Any spot produced by the *Test preparation* is not greater in size or intensity than a corresponding spot from the *Related substances preparation*.

Limit of dihydroquinine sulfate—
Methanesulfonic acid solution—Add 35.0 mL of methanesulfonic acid to 20.0 mL of glacial acetic acid, dilute with water to 500 mL, and mix.
Diethylamine solution—Dissolve 10.0 mL of diethylamine in water to obtain 100 mL of solution.
Mobile phase—Prepare a suitable filtered and degassed mixture of water, acetonitrile, *Methanesulfonic acid solution*, and *Diethylamine solution* (860 : 100 : 20 : 20). Adjust with *Diethylamine solution* to a pH of 2.6 if found to be lower.
System suitability preparation—Transfer about 10 mg each of quinine sulfate and dihydroquinine to a 50-mL volumetric flask. Dissolve in about 5 mL of methanol, dilute with *Mobile phase* to volume, and mix.
System suitability test—Chromatograph injections of the *System suitability preparation* as directed for *Procedure*: the relative retention times for quinine and dihydroquinine are about 1 and 1.5, respectively. The resolution between the quinine and dihydroquinine peaks is not less than 1.2. The relative standard deviation for the peak response of quinine is not more than 2.0%.
Test preparation—Transfer about 20 mg of Quinine Sulfate to a 100-mL volumetric flask, dissolve in and dilute with *Mobile phase* to volume, and mix.
Procedure (see *Chromatography* ⟨621⟩)—Inject about 50 μL of the *Test preparation* into a chromatograph equipped with a 235-nm detector and a 3.9-mm × 30-cm column that contains packing L1. The response of the dihydroquinine peak is not greater than one-ninth that of the quinine peak (10.0%).

Organic volatile impurities, *Method IV* ⟨467⟩: meets the requirements.

(Official until July 1, 2008)

Assay—Dissolve about 200 mg of Quinine Sulfate, accurately weighed, in 20 mL of acetic anhydride, add 4 drops of *p*-naphtholbenzein TS, and titrate with 0.1 N perchloric acid VS from a 10-mL microburet to a green endpoint. Perform a blank determination, and make any necessary correction. Each mL of 0.1 N perchloric acid is equivalent to 24.90 mg of total alkaloid salt, calculated as $(C_{20}H_{24}N_2O_2)_2 \cdot H_2SO_4$.

Quinine Sulfate Capsules

» Quinine Sulfate Capsules contain amounts of quinine sulfate and dihydroquinine sulfate totaling not less than 90.0 percent and not more than 110.0 percent of the labeled amount of quinine sulfate, calculated as $(C_{20}H_{24}N_2O_2)_2 \cdot H_2SO_4 \cdot 2H_2O$.

Packaging and storage—Preserve in tight containers.
USP Reference standards ⟨11⟩—*USP Quinine Sulfate RS. USP Quininone RS.*

Identification—
A: Shake well a quantity of the contents of Capsules, equivalent to about 100 mg of quinine sulfate, with 100 mL of dilute sulfuric acid (1 in 350), and filter. An appropriate dilution of the filtrate exhibits a vivid blue fluorescence. On the addition of a few drops of hydrochloric acid the fluorescence disappears.
B: In the test for *Chromatographic purity*, the R_F value of the principal spot obtained from the *Test preparation* corresponds to that from the *Standard preparation*.
C: Shake a quantity of the contents of Capsules, equivalent to about 20 mg of quinine sulfate, with 10 mL of dilute hydrochloric acid (1 in 100), and filter: the filtrate responds to the tests for *Sulfate* ⟨191⟩.
D: The retention time of the major peak in the chromatogram of the *Assay preparation* corresponds to that in the chromatogram of the *Standard preparation*, obtained as directed in the *Assay*.

Dissolution ⟨711⟩—
Medium: 0.1 N hydrochloric acid; 900 mL.
Apparatus 1: 100 rpm.
Time: 45 minutes.
Procedure—Determine the amount of $(C_{20}H_{24}N_2O_2)_2 \cdot H_2SO_4 \cdot 2H_2O$ dissolved by employing UV absorption at the wavelength of maximum absorbance at about 248 nm on filtered portions of the solution under test, suitably diluted with *Dissolution Medium*, in comparison with a Standard solution having a known concentration of USP Quinine Sulfate RS in the same *Medium*.
Tolerances—Not less than 75% *(Q)* of the labeled amount of $(C_{20}H_{24}N_2O_2)_2 \cdot H_2SO_4 \cdot 2H_2O$ is dissolved in 45 minutes.

Uniformity of dosage units ⟨905⟩: meet the requirements.
Procedure for content uniformity—Transfer the contents of 1 Capsule to a 250-mL volumetric flask, add about 175 mL of dilute hydrochloric acid (1 in 100), and shake by mechanical means for 30 minutes. Add dilute hydrochloric acid (1 in 100) to volume, and mix. Filter a portion of the mixture, discarding the first 20 mL of the filtrate. Concomitantly determine the absorbances of this solution, quantitatively diluted, if necessary, and a Standard solution of USP Quinine Sulfate RS in dilute hydrochloric acid (1 in 100) having a known concentration of about 40 μg per mL, in 1-cm cells, at the wavelength of maximum absorbance at about 345 nm, with a suitable spectrophotometer, using water as the blank. Calculate the quantity, in mg, of active ingredients, calculated as quinine sulfate $[(C_{20}H_{24}N_2O_2)_2 \cdot H_2SO_4 \cdot 2H_2O]$, in the Capsule taken by the formula:

$$(TC/D)(A_U/A_S)$$

in which *T* is the labeled quantity, in mg, of quinine sulfate in the Capsule, *D* is the concentration, in μg per mL, of quinine sulfate in the solution from the Capsule, based on the labeled quantity per Capsule and the extent of dilution, *C* is the concentration, in μg per mL, of USP Quinine Sulfate in the Standard solution, and A_U and A_S are the absorbances of the solution from the Capsule and the Standard solution, respectively.

Chromatographic purity—Shake a quantity of the contents of Capsules, equivalent to about 150 mg of quinine sulfate, with 25 mL of diluted alcohol for 10 minutes, and filter. Using this as the test solution, proceed as directed in the test for *Chromatographic purity* under *Quinine Sulfate*.

Assay—
Methanesulfonic acid solution, Diethylamine solution, Mobile phase, System suitability preparation, and *System suitability test*—Proceed as directed in the test for *Limit of dihydroquinine sulfate* under *Quinine Sulfate*.
Standard preparation—Transfer about 20 mg of USP Quinine Sulfate RS, accurately weighed, to a 100-mL volumetric flask, dissolve in and dilute with *Mobile phase* to volume, and mix.
Assay preparation—Transfer the contents of not less than 20 Capsules to a container, and mix. Transfer an accurately weighed portion of the powder, equivalent to about 160 mg of quinine sulfate, to a 100-mL volumetric flask, add 80 mL of methanol, and shake the flask by mechanical means for 30 minutes. Dilute with methanol to volume, and filter, discarding the first 10 mL of the filtrate. Transfer 3.0 mL of the filtrate to a 25-mL volumetric flask, dilute with *Mobile phase* to volume, and mix.
Procedure (see *Chromatography* ⟨621⟩)—Inject equal volumes (about 50 μL) of the *Standard preparation* and the *Assay prepara-*

tion into a chromatograph equipped with a 235-nm detector and a 3.9-mm × 30-cm column that contains packing L1. Calculate the quantity, in mg, of the sum of quinine sulfate and dihydroquinine sulfate in the portion of Capsules taken by the formula:

$$(2500/3)C(r_{b,U} + r_{d,U})/(r_{b,S} + r_{d,S})$$

in which C is the concentration, in mg per mL, of USP Quinine Sulfate RS in the *Standard preparation*, $r_{b,U}$ and $r_{b,S}$ are the peak area responses of quinine obtained from the *Assay preparation* and the *Standard preparation*, respectively, and $r_{d,U}$ and $r_{d,S}$ are the peak area responses of dihydroquinine obtained from the *Assay preparation* and the *Standard preparation*, respectively.

Quinine Sulfate Tablets

» Quinine Sulfate Tablets contain amounts of quinine sulfate and dihydroquinine sulfate totaling not less than 90.0 percent and not more than 110.0 percent of the labeled amount of quinine sulfate, calculated as $(C_{20}H_{24}N_2O_2)_2 \cdot H_2SO_4 \cdot 2H_2O$.

Packaging and storage—Preserve in well-closed containers.

USP Reference standards ⟨11⟩—*USP Quinine Sulfate RS. USP Quininone RS.*
Identification—
   A: Shake well a quantity of powdered Tablets, equivalent to about 100 mg of quinine sulfate, with 100 mL of dilute sulfuric acid (1 in 350), and filter. An appropriate dilution of the filtrate exhibits a vivid blue fluorescence. On the addition of a few drops of hydrochloric acid the fluorescence disappears.
   B: In the test for *Chromatographic purity*, the R_F value of the principal spot obtained from the *Test preparation* corresponds to that from the *Standard preparation*.
   C: Shake a quantity of powdered Tablets, equivalent to about 20 mg of quinine sulfate, with 10 mL of dilute hydrochloric acid (1 in 100), and filter: the filtrate responds to the tests for *Sulfate* ⟨191⟩.
   D: The retention time of the major peak in the chromatogram of the *Assay preparation* corresponds to that in the chromatogram of the *Standard preparation*, obtained as directed in the *Assay*.
Dissolution ⟨711⟩—
   Medium: 0.01 N hydrochloric acid; 900 mL.
   Apparatus 1: 100 rpm.
   Time: 45 minutes.
   Procedure—Determine the amount of $(C_{20}H_{24}N_2O_2)_2 \cdot H_2SO_4 \cdot 2H_2O$ dissolved by employing UV absorption at the wavelength of maximum absorbance at about 248 nm on filtered portions of the solution under test, suitably diluted with *Dissolution Medium*, in comparison with a Standard solution having a known concentration of USP Quinine Sulfate RS in the same *Medium*.
   Tolerances—Not less than 75% (*Q*) of the labeled amount of $(C_{20}H_{24}N_2O_2)_2 \cdot H_2SO_4 \cdot 2H_2O$ is dissolved in 45 minutes.
Uniformity of dosage units ⟨905⟩: meet the requirements.
   Procedure for content uniformity—Proceed as directed for *Procedure for content uniformity* under *Uniformity of dosage units* under *Quinine Sulfate Capsules*, using 1 powdered Tablet instead of the contents of 1 Capsule.
Chromatographic purity—Shake a quantity of powdered Tablets, equivalent to about 150 mg of quinine sulfate, with 25 mL of diluted alcohol for 10 minutes, and filter. Using this as the test solution, proceed as directed in the test for *Chromatographic purity* under *Quinine Sulfate*.
Assay—
   Methanesulfonic acid solution, Diethylamine solution, Mobile phase, System suitability preparation, and *System suitability test*—Proceed as directed in the test for *Limit of dihydroquinine sulfate* under *Quinine Sulfate*.

   Standard preparation—Transfer about 20 mg of USP Quinine Sulfate RS, accurately weighed, to a 100-mL volumetric flask, dissolve in and dilute with *Mobile phase* to volume, and mix.
   Assay preparation—Weigh and finely powder not less than 20 Tablets. Transfer an accurately weighed portion of the powder, equivalent to about 160 mg of quinine sulfate, to a 100-mL volumetric flask, add 80 mL of methanol, and shake the flask by mechanical means for 30 minutes. Dilute with methanol to volume, and filter, discarding the first 10 mL of the filtrate. Transfer 3.0 mL of the filtrate to a 25-mL volumetric flask, dilute with *Mobile phase* to volume, and mix.
   Procedure (see *Chromatography* ⟨621⟩)—Inject equal volumes (about 50 µL) of the *Standard preparation* and the *Assay preparation* into a chromatograph equipped with a 235-nm detector and a 3.9-mm × 30-cm column that contains packing L1. Calculate the quantity, in mg, of the sum of quinine sulfate and dihydroquinine sulfate in the portion of Tablets taken by the formula:

$$(2500/3)C(r_{b,U} + r_{d,U})/(r_{b,S} + r_{d,S})$$

in which C is the concentration, in mg per mL, of USP Quinine Sulfate RS in the *Standard preparation*, $r_{b,U}$ and $r_{b,S}$ are the peak area responses of quinine obtained from the *Assay preparation* and the *Standard preparation*, respectively, and $r_{d,U}$ and $r_{d,S}$ are the peak area responses of dihydroquinine obtained from the *Assay preparation* and the *Standard preparation*, respectively.

Rabies Immune Globulin

» Rabies Immune Globulin conforms to the regulations of the FDA concerning biologics (see *Biologics* ⟨1041⟩). It is a sterile, nonpyrogenic, slightly opalescent solution consisting of globulins derived from blood plasma or serum that has been tested for the absence of hepatitis B surface antigen, derived from selected adult human donors who have been immunized with rabies vaccine and have developed high titers of rabies antibody. It has a potency such that when labeled as 150 International Units (IU) per mL, it has a geometric mean lower limit (95% confidence) potency value of not less than 110 IU per mL, and proportionate lower limit potency values for other labeled potencies, based on the U.S. Standard Rabies Immune Globulin and using the CVS Virus challenge, by neutralization test in mice or tissue culture. It contains not less than 10 g and not more than 18 g of protein per 100 mL, of which not less than 80 percent is monomeric immunoglobulin G, having a sedimentation coefficient in the range of 6.0 to 7.5S, with no fragments having a sedimentation coefficient less than 6S and no aggregates having a sedimentation coefficient greater than 12S. It contains 0.3 M glycine as a stabilizing agent, and it contains a suitable preservative. It has a pH between 6.4 and 7.2, measured in a solution diluted to contain 1 percent of protein with 0.15 M sodium chloride. It meets the requirements of the test for heat stability.

Packaging and storage—Preserve at a temperature between 2° and 8°.

Expiration date—The expiration date is not later than 1 year after date of issue from manufacturer's cold storage (5°, 1 year).

Labeling—Label it to state that it is not for intravenous injection.

Rabies Vaccine

» Rabies Vaccine conforms to the regulations of the FDA concerning biologics (see *Biologics* ⟨1041⟩). It is a sterile preparation, in dried or liquid form, of inactivated rabies virus harvested from inoculated diploid cell cultures. The cell cultures are shown to consist of diploid cells by tests of karyology, to be non-tumorigenic by tests in hamsters treated with anti-lymphocytic serum (ALS) and to be free from extraneous agents by tests in animals or cell-culture systems. The harvested virus meets the requirements for identity by serological tests, for absence of infectivity by tests in mice or cell-culture systems, and for absence of extraneous agents by tests in animals or cell-culture systems. The Vaccine meets the requirements for absence of live virus by tests using a suitable virus amplification system involving inoculation and incubation of sensitive cell cultures for not less than 14 days followed by inoculation of the cell-culture fluid thereafter into not less than 20 adult mice. It has a potency of rabies antigen equivalent to not less than 2.5 International Units for Rabies Vaccine, per dose, determined with the specific mouse protection test using the U.S. Standard Rabies Vaccine. It meets the requirements for general safety (see *Safety Tests—Biologicals* under *Biological Reactivity Tests, in Vivo* ⟨88⟩).

Packaging and storage—Preserve at a temperature between 2° and 8°.

Expiration date—The expiration date is not later than 2 years after date of issue from manufacturer's cold storage (5°, 1 year).

Labeling—Label it to state that it contains rabies antigen equivalent to not less than 2.5 IU per dose and that it is intended for intramuscular injection only.

Racepinephrine

$C_9H_{13}NO_3$ 183.20

1,2-Benzenediol, 4-[1-hydroxy-2-(methylamino)ethyl]-, (±)-.
(±)-3,4-Dihydroxy-α-[(methylamino)methyl]benzyl alcohol   [329-65-7].

» Racepinephrine is a racemic mixture of the enantiomorphs of epinephrine. It contains not less than 97.0 percent and not more than 102.0 percent of $C_9H_{13}NO_3$, calculated on the dried basis.

Packaging and storage—Preserve in tight, light-resistant containers.

USP Reference standards ⟨11⟩—*USP Epinephrine Bitartrate RS. USP Norepinephrine Bitartrate RS.*

Identification—To 5 mL of pH 4.0 acid phthalate buffer (see *Buffer Solutions* in the section *Reagents, Indicators, and Solutions*) add 0.5 mL of a solution of Racepinephrine (1 in 1000) and 1.0 mL of 0.1 N iodine. Mix, and allow to stand for 5 minutes. Add 2 mL of sodium thiosulfate solution (1 in 40): a deep red color is produced.

Specific rotation ⟨781S⟩:   between −1° and +1°.

Test solution: 10 mg per mL, in 0.6 N hydrochloric acid.

Loss on drying ⟨731⟩—Dry it in vacuum over silica gel for 18 hours: it loses not more than 2.0% of its weight.

Residue on ignition ⟨281⟩:   not more than 0.5%.

Limit of adrenalone—Its absorptivity (see *Spectrophotometry and Light-scattering* ⟨851⟩) at 310 nm, determined in a solution in dilute hydrochloric acid (1 in 200) containing 2 mg per mL, is not more than 0.2.

Limit of norepinephrine—

Epinephrine standard solution—Dilute with methanol an accurately measured volume of a solution of USP Epinephrine Bitartrate RS in formic acid containing about 364 mg per mL to obtain a solution having a concentration of about 20 mg per mL.

Norepinephrine standard solution—Dilute with methanol an accurately measured volume of a solution of USP Norepinephrine Bitartrate RS in formic acid containing 16 mg per mL to obtain a solution having a known concentration of 1.6 mg per mL.

Test solution—Dissolve 200 mg of Racepinephrine in 1.0 mL of formic acid, dilute with methanol to 10.0 mL, and mix.

Procedure—Apply 5-μL portions of *Epinephrine standard solution*, *Norepinephrine standard solution*, and *Test solution* to a suitable thin-layer chromatographic plate (see *Chromatography* ⟨621⟩) coated with a 0.25-mm layer of chromatographic silica gel mixture. Allow to dry, and develop the chromatogram in an unsaturated tank using a solvent system consisting of a mixture of *n*-butanol, water, and formic acid (7 : 2 : 1) until the solvent front has moved about three-fourths of the length of the plate. Remove the plate from the developing chamber, mark the solvent front, and allow the solvent to evaporate in warm circulating air. Spray with Folin-Ciocalteu Phenol TS, followed by sodium carbonate solution (1 in 10): the R_F value of the principal spot obtained from the *Test solution* corresponds to that obtained from the *Epinephrine standard solution*. Any spot obtained from the *Test solution* is not larger nor more intense than the spot with the same R_F value obtained from the *Norepinephrine standard solution*, corresponding to not more than 4.0% of norepinephrine.

Organic volatile impurities, Method V ⟨467⟩:   meets the requirements.

Solvent—Use dimethyl sulfoxide.

(Official until July 1, 2008)

Assay—

Ferro-citrate solution, *Buffer solution*, and *Standard preparation*—Prepare as directed under *Epinephrine Assay* ⟨391⟩.

Assay preparation—Transfer about 10 mg of Racepinephrine, accurately weighed, to a 1-liter volumetric flask. Dilute with sodium bisulfite solution (1 in 500) to volume, and mix.

Procedure—Proceed as directed for *Procedure* under *Epinephrine Assay* ⟨391⟩. Calculate the quantity, in mg, of $C_9H_{13}NO_3$ in the portion of Racepinephrine taken by the formula:

$$(183.20 / 333.29)C(A_U / A_S)$$

in which 183.20 and 333.29 are the molecular weights of racepinephrine and epinephrine bitartrate, respectively, C is the concentration, in μg per mL, of USP Epinephrine Bitartrate RS in the *Standard preparation*, and A_U and A_S are the absorbances of the solutions from the *Assay preparation* and the *Standard preparation*, respectively.

Racepinephrine Inhalation Solution

» Racepinephrine Inhalation Solution is a sterile solution of Racepinephrine in Purified Water prepared with the aid of Hydrochloric Acid or of Racepinephrine Hydrochloride in Purified Water. It contains not less than 90.0 percent and not more than 110.0 percent of the labeled amount of racepinephrine ($C_9H_{13}NO_3$).

Packaging and storage—Preserve in tight, light-resistant containers. Do not freeze.

Labeling—The label indicates that the Inhalation Solution is not to be used if its color is pinkish or darker than slightly yellow or if it contains a precipitate.

USP Reference standards ⟨11⟩—*USP Epinephrine Bitartrate RS*.

Color and clarity—

Standard solution—Transfer 2.0 mL of 0.100 N iodine VS to a 500-mL volumetric flask, dilute with water to volume, and mix.

Procedure—Visually examine a portion of the Inhalation Solution (*Test solution*) in a suitable clear glass test tube against a white background: it is not pinkish and it contains no precipitate. If any yellow color is observed in the *Test solution*, concomitantly determine the absorbances of the *Test solution* and the *Standard solution* in 1-cm cells with a suitable spectrophotometer set at 460 nm: the absorbance of the *Test solution* does not exceed that of the *Standard solution*.

Identification—To 5 mL of pH 4.0 acid phthalate buffer (see *Buffer Solutions* in the section *Reagents, Indicators, and Solutions*) add 0.5 mL of Inhalation Solution and 1.0 mL of 0.1 N iodine. Mix, and allow to stand for 5 minutes. Add 2 mL of sodium thiosulfate solution (1 in 40): a deep red color is produced.

Sterility ⟨71⟩: meets the requirements.

pH ⟨791⟩: between 2.0 and 3.5.

Assay—

Mobile phase—Prepare a filtered and degassed mixture of 0.05 M monobasic sodium phosphate and methanol (85 : 15). Dissolve a suitable quantity of sodium 1-octanesulfonate in this mixture to obtain a solution that is 0.005 M with respect to sodium 1-octanesulfonate. Make adjustments if necessary (see *System Suitability* under *Chromatography* ⟨621⟩).

Standard preparation—Dissolve an accurately weighed quantity of USP Epinephrine Bitartrate RS in a mixture of 0.05 M monobasic sodium phosphate and methanol (85 : 15), and dilute quantitatively, and stepwise if necessary, with the same solvent mixture to obtain a solution having a known concentration of about 0.1 mg per mL.

Assay preparation—Transfer an accurately measured volume of Inhalation Solution, equivalent to about 11 mg of racepinephrine, to a 200-mL volumetric flask, dilute with a mixture of 0.05 M monobasic sodium phosphate and methanol (85 : 15) to volume, and mix.

System suitability preparation—Dissolve a suitable quantity of dopamine hydrochloride in a mixture of 0.05 M monobasic sodium phosphate and methanol (85 : 15) to obtain a solution containing about 0.1 mg per mL. Transfer 20.0 mL of this solution to a 50-mL volumetric flask. Add 5.0 mL of the *Standard preparation,* dilute with a mixture of 0.05 M monobasic sodium phosphate and methanol (85 : 15) to volume, and mix.

Chromatographic system (see *Chromatography* ⟨621⟩)—The liquid chromatograph is equipped with a 280-nm detector and a 4.6-mm × 25-cm column that contains 5-μm packing L1. The flow rate is about 1 mL per minute. Chromatograph the *Standard preparation* and the *System suitability preparation*, and record the peak responses as directed for *Procedure:* the tailing factor for the analyte peak is not more than 1.2, the resolution, *R,* between the dopamine and analyte peak is not less than 5.0, and the relative standard deviation for replicate injections is not more than 2.0%.

Procedure—Separately inject equal volumes (about 10 μL) of the *Standard preparation* and the *Assay preparation* into the chromatograph, record the chromatograms, and measure the responses for the major peaks. Calculate the quantity, in mg, of $C_9H_{13}NO_3$ in each mL of the Inhalation Solution taken by the formula:

$$(183.20 / 333.29)(200)(C / V)(r_U / r_S)$$

in which 183.20 and 333.29 are the molecular weights of racepinephrine and epinephrine bitartrate, respectively; *C* is the concentration, in mg per mL, of USP Epinephrine Bitartrate RS in the *Standard preparation;* *V* is the volume, in mL, of Inhalation Solution taken; and r_U and r_S are the peak responses obtained from the *Assay preparation* and the *Standard preparation,* respectively.

Racepinephrine Hydrochloride

$C_9H_{13}NO_3 \cdot HCl$ 219.67

» Racepinephrine Hydrochloride is a racemic mixture of the hydrochlorides of the enantiomorphs of epinephrine. It contains not less than 97.0 percent and not more than 102.0 percent of $C_9H_{13}NO_3 \cdot HCl$, calculated on the anhydrous basis.

Packaging and storage—Preserve in tight, light-resistant containers.

USP Reference standards ⟨11⟩—*USP Epinephrine Bitartrate RS*. *USP Norepinephrine Bitartrate RS*.

Change to read:

Identification—

A: ▲*Ultraviolet Absorption* ⟨197U⟩—

Solution: 50 μg per mL. [NOTE—Use USP Epinephrine Bitartrate RS in the preparation of the *Standard solution*.]

Medium: water.▲*USP31*

B: ▲A solution (1 in 100) meets the requirements of the tests for *Chloride* ⟨191⟩.▲*USP31*

Specific rotation ⟨781S⟩: between −1° and +1°.

Test solution: 10 mg per mL, in 0.12 N hydrochloric acid.

Water, *Method I* ⟨921⟩: not more than 0.5%.

Residue on ignition ⟨281⟩: not more than 0.5%.

Organic volatile impurities, *Method I* ⟨467⟩: meets the requirements.

(Official until July 1, 2008)

Other requirements—It meets the requirements for *Limit of adrenalone* and *Limit of norepinephrine* under *Racepinephrine*.

Assay—

Mobile phase—Prepare a filtered and degassed solution of 0.17 N acetic acid. Make adjustments if necessary (see *System Suitability* under *Chromatography* ⟨621⟩).

Standard preparation—Dissolve an accurately weighed quantity of USP Epinephrine Bitartrate RS in *Mobile phase* to obtain a solution having a known concentration of about 150 μg per mL.

Assay preparation—Transfer about 25 mg of Racepinephrine Hydrochloride, accurately weighed, to a 100-mL volumetric flask. Dissolve in and dilute with *Mobile phase* to volume, and mix. Transfer 4.0 mL of this solution to a 10-mL volumetric flask, dilute with *Mobile phase* to volume, and mix to obtain a solution containing about 100 μg per mL.

Chromatographic system (see *Chromatography* ⟨621⟩)—The liquid chromatograph is equipped with a 278-nm detector and a 4.6-mm × 15-cm column that contains packing L1. The flow rate is about 2.0 mL per minute. Chromatograph the *Standard preparation*, and record the peak responses as directed for *Procedure:* the relative standard deviation for replicate injections is not more than 2.0%.

Procedure—Separately inject equal volumes (about 25 μL) of the *Standard preparation* and the *Assay preparation* into the chromatograph, record the chromatograms, and measure the responses for the major peaks. Calculate the quantity, in mg, of $C_9H_{13}NO_3 \cdot HCl$ in the portion of Racepinephrine Hydrochloride taken by the formula:

$$0.25C(219.67 / 333.30)(r_U / r_S)$$

in which *C* is the concentration, in μg per mL, of USP Epinephrine Bitartrate RS in the *Standard preparation:* 219.67 and 333.30 are the molecular weights of racepinephrine hydrochloride and epinephrine bitartrate, respectively; and r_U and r_S are the peak responses obtained from the *Assay preparation* and the *Standard preparation,* respectively.

Ramipril

$C_{23}H_{32}N_2O_5$ 416.51

Cyclopenta[b]pyrrole-2-carboxylic acid, 1-[2-[[1-(ethoxycarbonyl)-3-phenylpropyl]amino]-1-oxopropyl]octahydro-, [2S-[1[R*(R*)],2α,3aβ,6aβ]]-.

(2S,3aS,6aS)-1-[(S)-N-[(S)-1-Carboxy-3-phenylpropyl]alanyl] octahydrocyclopenta[b]pyrrole-2-carboxylic acid, 1-ethyl ester [87333-19-5].

» Ramipril contains not less than 98.0 percent and not more than 102.0 percent of $C_{23}H_{32}N_2O_5$, calculated on the dried basis.

Packaging and storage—Preserve in tight containers.

USP Reference standards ⟨11⟩—*USP Ramipril RS. USP Ramipril Related Compound A RS. USP Ramipril Related Compound B RS. USP Ramipril Related Compound C RS. USP Ramipril Related Compound D RS.*

Identification, *Infrared Absorption* ⟨197K⟩.

Melting range ⟨741⟩: between 105° and 112°.

Specific rotation ⟨781S⟩: between +32.0° and +38.0°, determined at 20°.

Test solution: 10 mg per mL, in 0.1 M methanolic hydrochloric acid.

Loss on drying ⟨731⟩—Dry it in vacuum at a pressure not exceeding 5 mm of mercury at 60° for 6 hours: it loses not more than 0.2% of its weight.

Residue on ignition ⟨281⟩: not more than 0.1%.

Limit of palladium—

Diluent—Prepare a mixture of water and nitric acid (997 : 3).

Standard stock solution—Transfer about 50 mg of palladium metal, accurately weighed, to a 100-mL volumetric flask, dissolve in 9 mL of hydrochloric acid, and dilute with water to volume.

Standard solutions—Dilute the *Standard stock solution* quantitatively, and stepwise if necessary, with *Diluent* to obtain solutions containing 0.02, 0.03, and 0.05 μg of palladium per mL.

Test solution—Transfer about 200 mg of Ramipril, accurately weighed, to a 100-mL volumetric flask, and dissolve in and dilute with *Diluent* to volume.

Blank solution—Transfer about 150 mg of magnesium nitrate to a 100-mL volumetric flask, and dissolve in and dilute with *Diluent* to volume.

Procedure—Concomitantly determine the absorbances of equal volumes of the *Standard solutions* and the *Test solution* (about 20 μL), at the palladium emission line at 247.6 nm, with a suitable atomic absorption spectrophotometer (see *Spectrophotometry and Light-Scattering* ⟨851⟩) equipped with a palladium hollow-cathode lamp, using a 10-μL injection of *Blank solution* as the blank. Plot the absorbances of the *Standard solutions* versus concentration, in μg per mL, of palladium, and draw the straight line best fitting the three plotted points. From the graph so obtained, determine the concentration, C_P, in μg per mL, of palladium in the *Test solution*. Calculate the percentage of palladium in the portion of Ramipril taken by the formula:

$$0.1 C_P / C_R$$

in which C_R is the concentration, in mg per mL, of Ramipril taken to prepare the *Test solution*. The limit is 0.002%.

Related compounds—

Solution A—Dissolve 2.0 g of sodium perchlorate in a mixture of 800 mL of water and 0.5 mL of triethylamine, adjust with phosphoric acid to a pH of about 3.6 ± 0.1, add 200 mL of acetonitrile, and mix.

Solution B—Dissolve 2.0 g of sodium perchlorate in a mixture of 300 mL of water and 0.5 mL of triethylamine, adjust with phosphoric acid to a pH of about 2.6 ± 0.1, add 700 mL of acetonitrile, and mix.

Mobile phase—Use variable filtered and degassed mixtures of *Solution A* and *Solution B* as directed for *Chromatographic system*. Make adjustments if necessary (see *System Suitability* under *Chromatography* ⟨621⟩).

Test solution—Transfer about 25 mg of Ramipril, accurately weighed, to a 25-mL volumetric flask, dissolve in and dilute with *Solution A* to volume, and mix. [NOTE—Keep the *Test solution* cold until injected.]

Resolution solution—Dissolve a quantity of USP Ramipril RS, USP Ramipril Related Compound A RS, USP Ramipril Related Compound B RS, USP Ramipril Related Compound C RS, and USP Ramipril Related Compound D RS in *Solution B* to obtain a solution with a concentration of about 0.5 mg of each per mL.

Standard solution—Dissolve an accurately weighed quantity of USP Ramipril RS in *Solution B*, and dilute quantitatively, and stepwise if necessary, with *Solution B* to obtain a solution having a known concentration of about 0.005 mg per mL.

Chromatographic system (see *Chromatography* ⟨621⟩)—The liquid chromatograph is equipped with a 210-nm detector and a 4.0-mm × 25-cm column that contains 3-μm packing L1, and is maintained at a temperature of 65°. The flow rate is about 1 mL per minute. The chromatograph is programmed as follows.

Time (minutes)	Solution A (%)	Solution B (%)	Elution
0–6	90	10	isocratic
6–7	90→75	10→25	linear gradient
7–20	75→65	25→35	linear gradient
20–30	65→25	35→75	linear gradient
30–40	25	75	isocratic
40–45	25→90	75→10	linear gradient
45–55	90	10	isocratic

NOTE—Make adjustments at the 75 : 25 ratio stage, if necessary, to achieve elution of ramipril between 16 and 19 minutes after injection of the *Standard solution*. Chromatograph the *Resolution solution*, and record the peak responses as directed for *Procedure*: the resolution, *R*, between ramipril related compound A and ramipril is not less than 3.0. Similarly chromatograph the *Test solution*, and record the peak responses as directed for *Procedure*: the retention time for ramipril is between 16 and 19 minutes; and the tailing factor for the ramipril peak is between 0.8 and 2.0. Chromatograph the *Standard solution*, and record the peak responses as directed for *Procedure*: the relative standard deviation for replicate injections is not more than 5.0%. [NOTE—The relative retention times are about 0.8 for ramipril related compound A, 1.0 for ramipril, 1.3 for ramipril related compound B, 1.5 for ramipril related compound C, and 1.6 for ramipril related compound D.]

Procedure—Separately inject equal volumes (about 10 μL) of the *Test solution* and the *Standard solution* into the chromatograph, record the chromatograms, and measure the peak response for ramipril obtained from the *Standard solution* and the responses of all the peaks, other than the ramipril peak, obtained from the *Test solution*. Calculate the percentage of each related compound and unknown impurity in the portion of Ramipril taken by the formula:

$$100 F (C_S / C_T)(r_i / r_S)$$

in which *F* is the relative response factor for the related compound, which is 2.4 for ramipril related compound C, and 1.0 for all other individual impurities; C_S is the concentration, in mg per mL, of USP Ramipril RS in the *Standard solution*; C_T is the concentration, in mg per mL, of ramipril in the *Test solution*; r_i is the peak response for each individual peak obtained from the *Test solution*; and r_S is the ramipril peak response obtained from the *Standard solution*: not more than 0.5% of ramipril related compound A, ramipril related compound B, ramipril related compound C, or ramipril related compound D is found; not more than 0.1% of any other individual impurity is found; and not more than 1.0% of total impurities is found.

Assay—
Sodium dodecyl sulfate solution—Prepare a 0.1% solution of sodium dodecyl sulfate. Adjust with phosphoric acid to a pH of 2.4 ± 0.1, filter, and degas.
Mobile phase—Prepare a mixture of *Sodium dodecyl sulfate solution* and acetonitrile (55 : 45). Adjust with phosphoric acid to a pH of 2.75 ± 0.1, filter, and degas. Make adjustments if necessary (see *System Suitability* under *Chromatography* ⟨621⟩).
System suitability preparation—Dissolve accurately weighed quantities of USP Ramipril RS and USP Ramipril Related Compound A RS in *Mobile phase* to obtain a solution having known concentrations of about 0.2 mg per mL and 0.01 mg per mL, respectively.
Standard preparation—Dissolve an accurately weighed quantity of USP Ramipril RS in *Mobile phase* to obtain a solution having a known concentration of about 0.2 mg per mL.
Assay preparation—Transfer about 100 mg of Ramipril, accurately weighed, to a 100-mL volumetric flask, dissolve in about 10 mL of acetonitrile, dilute with *Mobile phase* to volume, and mix. Pipet about 10 mL of this stock solution to a 50-mL volumetric flask, dilute with *Mobile phase* to volume, and mix.
Chromatographic system (see *Chromatography* ⟨621⟩)—The liquid chromatograph is equipped with a 210-nm detector and a 4.6-mm × 15-cm column that contains packing L1. The flow rate is about 1.8 mL per minute. Chromatograph the *System suitability preparation*, and record the peak responses as directed for *Procedure*: the resolution, *R*, between ramipril and ramipril related compound A is not less than 2.0; the column efficiency determined from the ramipril peak is not less than 4000 theoretical plates; and the relative standard deviation for replicate injections determined from the ramipril peak is not more than 1.0%.
Procedure—Separately inject equal volumes (about 20 μL) of the *Standard preparation* and the *Assay preparation* into the chromatograph, record the chromatograms, and measure the responses for all of the peaks. Calculate the quantity, in mg, of $C_{23}H_{32}N_2O_5$ in the portion of Ramipril taken by the formula:

$$500C(r_U / r_S)$$

in which *C* is the concentration, in mg per mL, of USP Ramipril RS in the *Standard preparation*; and r_U and r_S are the peak responses obtained from the *Assay preparation* and the *Standard preparation*, respectively.

Ranitidine Hydrochloride

$C_{13}H_{22}N_4O_3S \cdot HCl$ 350.87
1,1-Ethenediamine, *N*-[2-[[[5-[(dimethylamino)methyl]-2-furanyl]-methyl]thio]ethyl]-*N'*-methyl-2-nitro-, monohydrochloride.
N-[2-[[[5-[(Dimethylamino)methyl]-2-furanyl]methyl]thio]ethyl]-*N'*-methyl-2-nitro-1,1-ethenediamine, hydrochloride   [66357-59-3].

» Ranitidine Hydrochloride contains not less than 97.5 percent and not more than 102.0 percent of $C_{13}H_{22}N_4O_3S \cdot HCl$, calculated on the dried basis.

Packaging and storage—Preserve in tight, light-resistant containers.

USP Reference standards ⟨11⟩—*USP Ranitidine Hydrochloride RS. USP Ranitidine Resolution Mixture RS.*
Identification—
   A: *Infrared Absorption* ⟨197M⟩.
   B: *Ultraviolet Absorption* ⟨197U⟩—
   Solution: 10 μg per mL.
   Medium: water.
      Absorptivities at 229 nm and 315 nm, calculated on the dried basis, do not differ by more than 3.0%.

   C: A solution of it meets the requirements of the tests for *Chloride* ⟨191⟩.
pH ⟨791⟩:   between 4.5 and 6.0, in a solution (1 in 100).
Loss on drying ⟨731⟩—Dry it in vacuum at 60° for 3 hours: it loses not more than 0.75% of its weight.
Residue on ignition ⟨281⟩:   not more than 0.1%.

Change to read:
Chromatographic purity—
   Diluent, Mobile phase, Resolution solution, and *Chromatographic system*—Proceed as directed in the *Assay*.
   Standard solution—Prepare as directed for *Standard preparation* in the *Assay*.
   Test solution—Prepare as directed for *Assay preparation* in the *Assay*.
   Procedure—Separately inject equal volumes (about 10 μL) of the *Standard solution* and the *Test solution* into the chromatograph, record the chromatograms, and identify the ranitidine peak and the peaks due to impurities and degradation products listed in the table below.

Name	Relative Retention Time
Ranitidine simple nitroacetamide▲1▲USP31	0.14
Ranitidine oxime▲2▲USP31	0.21
Ranitidine amino alcohol▲3▲USP31	0.45
Ranitidine diamine▲4▲USP31	0.57
Ranitidine *S*-oxide ▲5▲USP31	0.64
Ranitidine *N*-oxide▲6▲USP31	0.72
Ranitidine complex nitroacetamide▲7▲USP31	0.84
Ranitidine formaldehyde adduct▲8▲USP31	1.36
Ranitidine *bis*-compound▲9▲USP31	1.75

[1]▲*N*-Methyl-2-nitroacetamide.▲USP31
[2]▲3-(Methylamino)-5,6-dihydro-2*H*-1,4-thiazin-2-one oxime.▲USP31
[3]▲{5-[(Dimethylamino)methyl]furan-2-yl}methanol.▲USP31
[4]▲5-{[(2-Aminoethyl)thio]methyl}-*N,N*-dimethyl-2-furanmethanamine (Ranitidine related compound A).▲USP31
[5]▲ *N*-{2-[({5-[(Dimethylamino)methyl]-2-furanyl}methyl)sulfinyl]ethyl}-*N'*-methyl-2-nitro-1,1-ethenediamine (Ranitidine related compound C).▲USP31
[6]▲ *N,N*-Dimethyl(5-{[(2-{[1-(methylamino)-2-nitroethenyl]amino}ethyl)sulphanyl]methyl}furan-2-yl)methanamine *N*-oxide.▲USP31
[7]▲ *N*-{2-[({5-[(Dimethylamino)methyl]furan-2-yl}methyl)sulphanyl]ethyl}-2-nitroacetamide.▲USP31
[8]▲2,2'-Methylenebis(*N*-{2-[({5-[(dimethylamino)methyl]furan-2-yl}methyl)sulphanyl]ethyl}-*N'*-methyl-2-nitroethene-1,1-diamine).▲USP31
[9]▲*N,N'*-bis{2-[({5-[(Dimethylamino)methyl]-2-furanyl}methyl)thio]ethyl}-2-nitro-1,1-ethenediamine (Ranitidine related compound B).▲USP31

Measure the responses for the major peaks, and calculate the percentage of each impurity in the portion of Ranitidine Hydrochloride taken by the formula:

$$▲100CV/W(r_i / r_S)▲USP31$$

in which *C* is the concentration, in mg per mL, of ranitidine hydrochloride in the *Standard solution*; ▲*V* is the volume, in mL, of the *Test solution*;▲USP31 *W* is the weight, in mg, of Ranitidine Hydrochloride taken to prepare the *Test solution*; r_i is the peak response for each impurity obtained from the *Test solution*; and r_S is the ranitidine peak response obtained from the *Standard solution*: not more than 0.3% of ranitidine bis-compound is found, not more than 0.1% of any other single impurity is found, and not more than 0.5% of total impurities is found.
Organic volatile impurities, *Method IV* ⟨467⟩: meets the requirements.

(Official until July 1, 2008)

Change to read:
Assay—
Phosphate buffer—Place approximately 1900 mL of water in a 2.0-L volumetric flask, accurately add 6.8 mL of phosphoric acid, and mix. Accurately add 8.6 mL of 50% sodium hydroxide solution, and dilute with water to volume. If necessary, adjust with 50%

sodium hydroxide solution or phosphoric acid to a pH of 7.1, and filter.

Solution A—Prepare a mixture of *Phosphate buffer* and acetonitrile (98 : 2).

Solution B—Prepare a mixture of *Phosphate buffer* and acetonitrile (78 : 22).

Mobile phase—Use variable mixtures of *Solution A* and *Solution B* as directed for *Chromatographic system*. Make adjustments if necessary (see *System Suitability* under *Chromatography* ⟨621⟩).

Diluent—Use *Solution A*.

Standard preparation—Dissolve an accurately weighed quantity of USP Ranitidine Hydrochloride RS in *Diluent* to obtain a solution having a known concentration of about 0.125 mg of ranitidine hydrochloride per mL.

Resolution solution—Transfer about 1.3 mg of USP Ranitidine Resolution Mixture RS to a 10-mL volumetric flask, and dissolve in and dilute with *Diluent* to volume. [NOTE—USP Ranitidine Resolution Mixture RS contains ranitidine hydrochloride and four related impurities: ranitidine amino alcohol hemifumarate, ranitidine diamine hemifumarate, ranitidine N-oxide, and ranitidine complex nitroacetamide.]

Assay preparation—Transfer about 25 mg of Ranitidine Hydrochloride, accurately weighed, to a 200-mL volumetric flask. Dissolve in and dilute with *Diluent* to volume, and mix.

Chromatographic system (see *Chromatography* ⟨621⟩)—The liquid chromatograph is equipped with a 230-nm detector and a 4.6-mm × 10-cm column containing 3.5-µm packing L1 that is stable from pH 1 to 12. The flow rate is about 1.5 mL per minute. The column temperature is maintained at 35°. The chromatograph is programmed as follows.

Time (minutes)	Solution A (%)	Solution B (%)	Elution
0–10	100→0	0→100	linear gradient
10–15	0	100	isocratic
15–16	0→100	100→0	linear gradient
16–20	100	0	re-equilibration

Chromatograph the *Resolution solution*, and identify the peaks using the table of impurities and degradation products (found above): the resolution, *R*, between the peaks for ranitidine N-oxide and ranitidine complex nitroacetamide is not less than 1.5. Chromatograph the *Standard preparation*, and record the peak responses as directed for *Procedure*: the relative standard deviation for replicate injections is not more than 1.0%.

Procedure—Separately inject equal volumes (about 10 µL) of the *Standard preparation* and the *Assay preparation* into the chromatograph, record the chromatograms, and measure the areas for the major peaks. Calculate the ▲percentage▲USP31 of $C_{13}H_{22}N_4O_3S \cdot HCl$ in the portion of Ranitidine Hydrochloride taken by the formula:

$$▲100(C_S/C_U)(r_U/r_S)▲USP31$$

in which ▲ C_S and C_U are the concentrations, in mg per mL, of ranitidine hydrochloride in the *Standard preparation* and the *Assay preparation*, respectively;▲USP31 and r_U and r_S are the peak responses obtained from the *Assay preparation* and the *Standard preparation*, respectively.

Ranitidine Injection

» Ranitidine Injection is a sterile solution of Ranitidine Hydrochloride in Water for Injection. It contains the equivalent of not less than 90.0 percent and not more than 110.0 percent of the labeled amount of ranitidine ($C_{13}H_{22}N_4O_3S$).

Packaging and storage—Preserve in single-dose or in multiple-dose containers of Type I glass, protected from light. Store below 30°. Do not freeze.

Labeling—Label Injection to state both the content of the active moiety and the content of the salt used in formulating the article.

USP Reference standards ⟨11⟩—*USP Ranitidine Hydrochloride RS. USP Ranitidine Related Compound A RS. USP Ranitidine Related Compound C RS.*

Identification—

A: The R_F value of the principal spot observed in the chromatogram of the *Test preparation* obtained as directed in the *Chromatographic purity* test corresponds to that obtained from the *Standard preparation*.

B: The retention time of the major peak in the chromatogram of the *Assay preparation* corresponds to that in the chromatogram of the *Standard preparation*, as obtained in the *Assay*.

Bacterial endotoxins ⟨85⟩—It contains not more than 7.00 USP Endotoxin Units per mg of ranitidine.

pH ⟨791⟩: between 6.7 and 7.3.

Particulate matter ⟨788⟩: meets the requirements under small-volume injections.

Chromatographic purity—

Test preparation—Dilute Injection quantitatively with water, if necessary, to obtain a solution containing 25 mg of ranitidine per mL. [NOTE—Use Injection of lower concentration without dilution as directed under *Procedure*.]

Standard preparation—Dissolve USP Ranitidine Hydrochloride RS in water to obtain a solution having a known concentration of 560 µg per mL. Dilute portions of this *Standard preparation* quantitatively with water to obtain solutions having concentrations of 280 µg per mL (*Diluted standard preparation A*), 140 µg per mL (*Diluted standard preparation B*), 84 µg per mL (*Diluted standard preparation C*), 28 µg per mL (*Diluted standard preparation D*), and 14 µg per mL (*Diluted standard preparation E*), respectively.

Resolution preparation—Dissolve USP Ranitidine Related Compound A RS in methanol to obtain a solution having a known concentration of 1.27 mg per mL.

Procedure—Apply separately 10 µL of the *Standard preparation*, *Diluted standard preparations A, B, C, D* and *E*, and the required volume of the *Test preparation*, equivalent to 250 µg of ranitidine, to a suitable thin-layer chromatographic plate (see *Chromatography* ⟨621⟩) coated with a 0.25-mm layer of chromatographic silica gel mixture. In addition, apply separately a further loading of the same volume of the *Test preparation* to the same plate, and on top of this application, apply 10 µL of the *Resolution preparation*. Allow the spots to dry, and develop the chromatograms in a solvent system consisting of a mixture of ethyl acetate, isopropyl alcohol, ammonium hydroxide, and water (25 : 15 : 5 : 1) until the solvent front has moved not less than 15 cm from the origin. Remove the plate from the developing chamber, mark the solvent front, and allow to air-dry. Expose the plate to iodine vapors in a closed chamber until the chromatogram is fully revealed. Examine the plate and compare the intensities of any secondary spots observed in the chromatogram of the *Test preparation* with those of the principal spots in the chromatograms of the *Standard preparation* and *Diluted standard preparations (A, B, C, D,* and *E*): the system suitability requirements are met when there is complete resolution between the primary spots of the *Test preparation*, and the *Resolution preparation* and if a spot is observed in the chromatogram of *Diluted standard preparation E*. The major secondary spot is not greater in size or intensity than the principal spot produced by the *Standard preparation* (2.0%), and no other secondary spot is greater in size or intensity than the principal spot produced by *Diluted standard preparation A* (1.0%). The sum of the intensities of all secondary spots obtained from the *Test preparation*, corresponds to not more than 5.0%.

Other requirements—It meets the requirements under *Injections* ⟨1⟩.

Assay—

Mobile phase—Prepare a filtered and degassed mixture of methanol and 0.1 M aqueous ammonium acetate (85 : 15). Make adjustments if necessary (see *System Suitability* under *Chromatography* ⟨621⟩).

Standard preparation—Dissolve an accurately weighed quantity of USP Ranitidine Hydrochloride RS in *Mobile phase* to obtain a solution having a known concentration of about 0.112 mg (equivalent to 0.100 mg of ranitidine base) per mL.

System suitability solution—Dissolve accurately weighed quantities of USP Ranitidine Hydrochloride RS and USP Ranitidine Related Compound C RS in *Mobile phase* to obtain a solution having known concentrations of about 0.112 mg per mL and 0.01 mg per mL, respectively.

Assay preparation—Dilute an accurately measured volume of Injection, quantitatively and stepwise if necessary, with *Mobile phase* to obtain a solution having a concentration of 0.1 mg of ranitidine per mL.

Chromatographic system (see *Chromatography* ⟨621⟩)—The liquid chromatograph is equipped with a 322-nm detector and a 4.6-mm × 20- to 30-cm column that contains packing L1. The flow rate is about 2 mL per minute. Chromatograph the *System suitability solution*, and record the peak responses as directed for *Procedure*: the resolution, R, between ranitidine hydrochloride and N-[2-[[[5-[(dimethylamino)methyl]-2-furanyl]methyl]sulfinyl]ethyl]-N'-methyl-2-nitro-1,1-ethenediamine (ranitidine related compound C) is not less than 1.5. Chromatograph the *Standard preparation*, and record the peak responses as directed for *Procedure*: the tailing factor for the ranitidine hydrochloride peak is not more than 2.0; the column efficiency determined from the ranitidine hydrochloride peak is not less than 700 theoretical plates; and the relative standard deviation for replicate injections is not more than 2%.

Procedure—Separately inject equal volumes (about 10 µL) of the *Standard preparation* and the *Assay preparation* into the chromatograph, record the chromatograms, and measure the area responses for the major peaks. Calculate the quantity, in mg, of $C_{13}H_{22}N_4O_3S$ in the portion of Injection taken by the formula:

$$(314.40 / 350.87)(L / D)(C)(r_U / r_S)$$

in which 314.40 and 350.87 are the molecular weights of ranitidine and ranitidine hydrochloride, respectively; L is the labeled quantity of ranitidine in the Injection taken; D is the concentration, in mg per mL, of ranitidine in the *Assay preparation* on the basis of the labeled quantity and the extent of dilution; C is the concentration, in mg per mL, of USP Ranitidine Hydrochloride RS in the *Standard preparation*; and r_U and r_S are the peak area responses obtained from the *Assay preparation* and the *Standard preparation*, respectively.

Ranitidine Oral Solution

» Ranitidine Oral Solution is a solution of Ranitidine Hydrochloride in water. It contains the equivalent of not less than 90.0 percent and not more than 110.0 percent of the labeled amount of ranitidine ($C_{13}H_{22}N_4O_3S$).

Packaging and storage—Preserve in tight, light-resistant containers. Store below 25°. Do not freeze.

USP Reference standards ⟨11⟩—*USP Ranitidine Hydrochloride RS. USP Ranitidine Related Compound A RS. USP Ranitidine Related Compound C RS.*

Identification—
A: The R_F value of the principal spot observed in the chromatogram of the *Test preparation* obtained as directed in the *Chromatographic purity* test corresponds to that obtained from the *Standard preparation*.
B: The retention time of the major peak in the chromatogram of the *Assay preparation* corresponds to that in the chromatogram of the *Standard preparation*, as obtained in the *Assay*.

Microbial limits ⟨61⟩—It meets the requirements of the tests for absence of *Salmonella* species and *Escherichia coli;* and the total aerobic microbial count does not exceed 100 cfu per mL.

pH ⟨791⟩: between 6.7 and 7.5.

Chromatographic purity—
Test preparation—[NOTE—Apply a quantity of extractives from Oral Solution to the chromatographic plate so as to achieve a nominal loading of 200 µg of ranitidine.] Transfer a weighed quantity of Oral Solution, equivalent to 10 mg of ranitidine, to a suitable syringe. Attach the tip of the syringe to the top of a cartridge (11 mm × 12 mm) of volume 0.5 mL containing 0.4 g of an L1 packing for high-pressure liquid chromatography that has been previously prepared by passage of 10 mL of methanol followed by passage of 20 mL of 0.5 M ammonia solution. Add 2.0 mL of 0.5 M ammonia solution to the syringe and force the mixture slowly through the cartridge. Repeat with 2 further 3-mL portions of 0.5 M ammonia solution. Discard all the liquid that has traversed the cartridge. Pass 5 mL of a mixture of 0.1 M hydrochloric acid and methanol (3 : 1) through the cartridge, and collect the eluant in a clean round-bottom, 25-mL flask. Repeat this with another 5-mL portion of the same eluting mixture and collect the eluant in the same flask. Evaporate the contents of the flask to dryness at a temperature not exceeding 30°. Redissolve the residue in 1.0 mL of a mixture of methanol and water (50 : 50).

Standard preparation—Dissolve USP Ranitidine Hydrochloride RS in a mixture of methanol and water (50 : 50) to obtain a solution having a known concentration of 448 µg (equivalent to 400 µg of ranitidine) per mL. Dilute portions of this *Standard preparation* quantitatively with the mixture of methanol and water (50 : 50) to obtain solutions having concentrations of 224 µg per mL *(Diluted standard preparation A)*, 112 µg per mL *(Diluted standard preparation B)*, 56 µg per mL *(Diluted standard preparation C)*, 22 µg per mL *(Diluted standard preparation D)*, and 11 µg per mL *(Diluted standard preparation E)*, respectively.

Resolution preparation—Dissolve USP Ranitidine Related Compound A RS in methanol to obtain a solution having a known concentration of 1.27 mg per mL.

Procedure—Apply separately 10 µL of the *Standard preparation*, the *Diluted standard preparations (A, B, C, D, and E)*, and 20 µL (superposition of 2 × 10 µL) of the *Test preparation* to a suitable thin-layer chromatographic plate (see *Chromatography* ⟨621⟩) coated with a 0.25-mm layer of chromatographic silica gel mixture. In addition, apply separately a further loading of 10 µL of the *Test preparation* to the same plate, and on top of this application, apply 10 µL of the *Resolution preparation*. Allow the spots to dry, and develop the chromatograms in a solvent system consisting of a mixture of ethyl acetate, isopropyl alcohol, ammonium hydroxide, and water (25 : 15 : 5 : 1) until the solvent front has moved not less than 15 cm from the origin. Remove the plate from the developing chamber, mark the solvent front, and allow to air-dry. Expose the plate to iodine vapors in a closed chamber until the chromatogram is fully revealed. Examine the plate and compare the intensities of any secondary spots observed in the chromatogram of the *Test preparation* with those of the principal spots in the chromatograms of the *Standard preparation* and *Diluted standard preparations (A, B, C, D, and E)*: the system suitability requirements are met when there is complete resolution between the primary spots of the *Test preparation* and the *Resolution preparation* and if a spot is observed in the chromatogram of *Diluted standard preparation E*. The major secondary spot is not greater in size or intensity than the principal spot produced by the *Standard preparation* (2.0%), and no other secondary spot is greater in size or intensity than the principal spot produced by *Diluted standard preparation A* (1.0%). The sum of the intensities of all secondary spots obtained from the *Test preparation* corresponds to not more than 5.0%. [NOTE—Spots established as arising from other components in the formulation are to be ignored.]

Assay—
Mobile phase, Standard preparation, System suitability solution, and Chromatographic system—Prepare as directed in the *Assay* under *Ranitidine Injection*, the chromatographic column being fitted with a suitable pre-column also containing packing L1.

Assay preparation—Dilute an accurately measured quantity of Oral Solution, quantitatively, and stepwise if necessary, with *Mobile phase* to obtain a solution having a concentration of 0.1 mg of ranitidine per mL.

Procedure—Separately inject an equal quantity (about 10 µL) of the *Standard preparation* and the *Assay preparation* into the chromatograph, record the chromatograms, and measure the area responses for the major peaks. Calculate the quantity, in mg, of ranitidine ($C_{13}H_{22}N_4O_3S$) in the portion of Oral Solution taken by the formula:

$$(314.40 / 350.87)(L / D)(C)(r_U / r_S)$$

in which 314.40 and 350.87 are the molecular weights of ranitidine and ranitidine hydrochloride respectively; L is the labeled quantity of ranitidine in the Oral Solution taken; D is the concentration, in mg per mL, of ranitidine in the *Assay preparation*, on the basis of the labeled quantity and the extent of dilution; C is the concentration, in mg per mL, of USP Ranitidine Hydrochloride RS in the *Standard preparation*; and r_U and r_S are the peak area responses obtained from the *Assay preparation* and the *Standard preparation*, respectively.

Ranitidine Tablets

» Ranitidine Tablets contain an amount of ranitidine hydrochloride ($C_{13}H_{22}N_4O_3S \cdot HCl$) equivalent to not less than 90.0 percent and not more than 110.0 percent of the labeled amount of ranitidine ($C_{13}H_{22}N_4O_3S$).

Packaging and storage—Preserve in tight, light-resistant containers.

USP Reference standards ⟨11⟩—*USP Ranitidine Hydrochloride RS. USP Ranitidine Related Compound A RS. USP Ranitidine Related Compound C RS.*

Identification—
  A: The R_F value of the principal spot observed in the chromatogram of the *Test preparation* obtained as directed in the *Chromatographic purity* test corresponds to that obtained from the *Standard preparation*.
  B: The retention time of the major peak in the chromatogram of the *Assay preparation* corresponds to that of the major peak in the chromatogram of the *Standard preparation* as obtained in the *Assay*.
  C: Shake a quantity of crushed Tablets, equivalent to about 100 mg of ranitidine, with 2 mL of water, and filter: the filtrate responds to the tests for *Chloride* ⟨191⟩.

Dissolution ⟨711⟩—
  Medium: water; 900 mL.
  Apparatus 2: 50 rpm.
  Time: 45 minutes.
  Procedure—Determine the amount of $C_{13}H_{22}N_4O_3S$ dissolved from UV absorbances at the wavelength of maximum absorbance at about 314 nm using filtered portions of the solution under test, suitably diluted with water, if necessary, in comparison with a Standard solution having a known concentration of USP Ranitidine Hydrochloride RS in the same medium.
  Tolerances—Not less than 80% *(Q)* of the labeled amount of $C_{13}H_{22}N_4O_3S$ is dissolved in 45 minutes.

Uniformity of dosage units ⟨905⟩: meet the requirements.

Chromatographic purity—
  Test preparation—Prepare a filtered solution in methanol containing 20 mg of ranitidine per mL (equivalent to 22.4 mg of ranitidine hydrochloride per mL) by shaking an appropriate number of Tablets in a suitable volume of methanol until the tablets have disintegrated completely.
  Standard preparations—Dissolve USP Ranitidine Hydrochloride RS in methanol to obtain a solution having a known concentration of 0.22 mg per mL. Dilute portions of this *Standard preparation* quantitatively with methanol to obtain solutions having concentrations of 110 µg per mL (*Diluted standard preparation A*), 66 µg per mL (*Diluted standard preparation B*), 22 µg per mL (*Diluted standard preparation C*), and 11 µg per mL (*Diluted standard preparation D*), respectively.
  Resolution preparation—Dissolve USP Ranitidine Related Compound A RS, 5-[[(2-aminoethyl)thio]methyl]-*N,N*-dimethyl-2-furanmethanamine, hemifumarate salt, in methanol to obtain a solution having a known concentration of 1.27 mg per mL.
  Procedure—Apply separately 10 µL of the *Test preparation*, the *Standard preparation*, and *Diluted standard preparations A, B, C,* and *D* to a suitable thin-layer chromatographic plate (see *Chromatography* ⟨621⟩) coated with a 0.25-mm layer of chromatographic silica gel mixture. In addition, apply separately 10 µL of the *Test preparation* to the same plate, and on top of this application, apply 10 µL of the *Resolution preparation*. Allow the spots to dry, and develop the chromatograms in a solvent system consisting of a mixture of ethyl acetate, isopropyl alcohol, ammonium hydroxide, and water (25 : 15 : 5 : 1) until the solvent front has moved not less than 15 cm from the origin. Remove the plate from the developing chamber, mark the solvent front, and air-dry. Expose the plate to iodine vapor in a closed chamber until the chromatogram is fully revealed. Examine the plate, and compare the intensities of any secondary spots observed in the chromatogram of the *Test preparation* with those of the principal spots in the chromatograms of the *Standard preparation* and *Diluted standard preparations A, B, C,* and *D:* the system suitability requirements are met if there is complete resolution between the primary spots in the chromatogram of the combined *Test preparation* and the *Resolution preparation*, and if a spot is observed in the chromatogram of *Diluted standard preparation D*. No single secondary spot exhibits an intensity greater than that of *Diluted standard preparation A* (0.5%), and no other secondary spot exhibits an intensity greater than that of *Diluted standard preparation B* (0.3%). The sum of the intensities of all secondary spots obtained from the *Test preparation* correspond to not more than 2.0%.

Assay—
  Mobile phase, Standard preparation, System suitability solution, and *Chromatographic system*—Prepare as directed in the *Assay* under *Ranitidine Injection*.
  Assay preparation—Transfer 10 Tablets to a minimum of 250 mL of *Mobile phase*, accurately measured. Shake the mixture until the Tablets have disintegrated completely, and filter. Dilute the filtrate quantitatively, and stepwise if necessary, with *Mobile phase* to obtain a solution having a concentration of ranitidine similar to that of the *Standard preparation*.
  Procedure—Separately inject equal volumes (about 10 µL) of the *Standard preparation* and the *Assay preparation* into the chromatograph, record the chromatograms, and measure the area responses for the major peaks. Calculate the quantity, in mg, of $C_{13}H_{22}N_4O_3S$ in the portion of Tablets taken by the formula:

$$(314.40 / 350.87)(L / D)(C)(r_U / r_S)$$

in which 314.40 and 350.87 are the molecular weights of ranitidine and ranitidine hydrochloride, respectively; L is the labeled amount, in mg, of ranitidine in each tablet; D is the concentration, in mg per mL, of ranitidine in the *Assay preparation*, based on the labeled quantity per Tablet and the extent of dilution; C is the concentration, in mg per mL, of USP Ranitidine Hydrochloride RS in the *Standard preparation*; and r_U and r_S are the peak area responses obtained from the *Assay preparation* and the *Standard preparation*, respectively.

Ranitidine in Sodium Chloride Injection

» Ranitidine in Sodium Chloride Injection is a sterile solution of Ranitidine Hydrochloride and Sodium Chloride in Water for Injection. It contains not less than 90.0 percent and not more than 110.0 percent of the labeled amounts of both ranitidine ($C_{13}H_{22}N_4O_3S$) and sodium chloride.

Packaging and storage—Preserve in glass containers, preferably of Type I or Type II glass, or in containers of suitable plastic, protected from light. Store at a temperature between 2° and 25°. Do not freeze.

USP Reference standards ⟨11⟩—*USP Ranitidine Hydrochloride RS. USP Ranitidine Related Compound A RS. USP Ranitidine Related Compound C RS.*

Identification—
  A: The R_F value of the principal spot observed in the chromatogram of the *Test preparation* obtained as directed in the *Chromatographic purity* test corresponds to that obtained from the *Standard preparation*.

B: The retention time of the major peak in the chromatogram of the *Assay preparation* corresponds to that in the chromatogram of the *Standard preparation* as obtained in the *Assay*.

C: Meets the requirements of the tests for *Sodium* ⟨191⟩ and for *Chloride* ⟨191⟩.

Bacterial endotoxins ⟨85⟩—It contains not more than 7.0 USP Endotoxin Units per mg of ranitidine.

pH ⟨791⟩: between 6.7 and 7.3.

Chromatographic purity—

Test preparation—[NOTE—Apply a quantity of extractives from Injection to the chromatographic plate to achieve a nominal loading of 200 µg of ranitidine.] Transfer an accurately measured volume of Injection, equivalent to 10 mg of ranitidine, to a suitable flask, add about 5 times this volume of alcohol, and evaporate to dryness at a temperature not exceeding 30°. Redissolve the residue in 1.0 mL of a mixture of methanol and water (50 : 50).

Standard preparation—Dissolve USP Ranitidine Hydrochloride RS in a mixture of methanol and water (50 : 50) to obtain a *Standard preparation* having a known concentration of 672 µg (equivalent to 600 µg of ranitidine base) per mL. Dilute portions of this *Standard preparation* quantitatively, and stepwise if necessary, with the mixture of methanol and water (50 : 50) to obtain solutions having concentrations of 448 µg per mL (*Diluted standard preparation A*), 224 µg per mL (*Diluted standard preparation B*), 112 µg per mL (*Diluted standard preparation C*), 56 µg per mL (*Diluted standard preparation D*), and 11 µg per mL (*Diluted standard preparation E*), respectively.

Resolution preparation—Dissolve USP Ranitidine Related Compound A RS in methanol to obtain a solution having a known concentration of 1.27 mg per mL.

Procedure—Apply separately 10 µL of the *Standard preparation*, the *Diluted standard preparations* (*A, B, C, D,* and *E*) and 20 µL (superposition of 2 × 10 µL) of the *Test preparation* to a suitable thin-layer chromatographic plate (see *Chromatography* ⟨621⟩) coated with a 0.25-mm layer of chromatographic silica gel mixture. In addition, apply separately a further loading of 10 µL of the *Test preparation* to the same plate, and on top of this application, apply 10 µL of the *Resolution preparation*. Allow the spots to dry, and develop the chromatograms in a solvent system consisting of a mixture of ethyl acetate, isopropyl alcohol, ammonium hydroxide, and water (25 : 15 : 5 : 1) until the solvent front has moved not less than 15 cm from the origin. Remove the plate from the developing chamber, mark the solvent front, and allow to air-dry. Expose the plate to iodine vapors in a closed chamber until the chromatogram is fully revealed. Examine the plate and compare the intensities of any secondary spots observed in the chromatogram of the *Test preparation* with those of the principal spots in the chromatograms of the *Standard preparation* and *Diluted standard preparations* (*A, B, C, D,* and *E*): the system suitability requirements are met when there is complete resolution between the primary spots of the *Test preparation* and the *Resolution preparation* and if a spot is observed in the chromatogram of *Diluted standard preparation E*. The major secondary spot is not greater in size or in intensity than the principal spot produced by the *Standard preparation* (3.0%), and no other secondary spot is greater in size or intensity than the principal spot produced by *Diluted standard preparation A* (2.0%). The sum of the intensities of all secondary spots obtained from the *Test preparation* corresponds to not more than 6.0%.

Other requirements—It meets the requirements under *Injections* ⟨1⟩.

Assay for ranitidine—

Mobile phase, Standard preparation, System suitability solution, and *Chromatographic system*—Prepare as directed in the *Assay* under *Ranitidine Injection*.

Assay preparation—Dilute an accurately measured volume of Injection, quantitatively and stepwise if necessary, with *Mobile phase* to obtain a solution having a concentration of 0.1 mg of ranitidine per mL.

Procedure—Separately inject equal volumes (about 10 µL) of the *Standard preparation* and the *Assay preparation* into the chromatograph, record the chromatograms, and measure the area responses for the major peaks. Calculate the quantity, in mg, of $C_{13}H_{22}N_4O_3S$ in the portion of Injection taken by the formula:

$$(314.40 / 350.87)(L/D)(C)(r_U / r_S)$$

in which 314.40 and 350.87 are the molecular weights of ranitidine and ranitidine hydrochloride, respectively; L is the labeled quantity of ranitidine in the Injection taken; D is the concentration, in mg per mL, of ranitidine in the *Assay preparation*, on the basis of the labeled quantity and the extent of dilution; C is the concentration, in mg per mL, of USP Ranitidine Hydrochloride RS in the *Standard preparation*; and r_U and r_S are the peak area responses obtained from the *Assay preparation* and the *Standard preparation*, respectively.

Assay for sodium chloride—Dilute an accurately measured volume of Injection, quantitatively and stepwise if necessary, with water to obtain a suitable volume of a solution having a concentration of about 0.5 mg of sodium chloride per mL. Titrate with 0.1 N silver nitrate VS using a silver-silver chloride electrode. Each mL of 0.1 N silver nitrate is equivalent to 3.545 mg of chloride. From the determined concentration per mL, subtract the quantity $(35.453/314.40)W$ so as to correct for the chloride present as ranitidine hydrochloride where W is the quantity, in mg per mL, of ranitidine as determined in the *Assay for ranitidine*. Multiplication of the answer by 1.648 gives the amount of sodium chloride per mL.

Rauwolfia Serpentina

» Rauwolfia Serpentina is the dried root of *Rauwolfia* (Linné) Bentham ex Kurz (Fam. Apocynaceae), sometimes having fragments of rhizome and aerial stem bases attached. It contains not less than 0.15 percent of reserpine-rescinnamine group alkaloids, calculated as reserpine.

Packaging and storage—Preserve in well-closed containers, and store at controlled room temperature, in a dry place, secure against insect attack (see *Preservation* under *Vegetable and Animal Drugs* in the *General Notices*).

USP Reference standards ⟨11⟩—*USP Rauwolfia Serpentina RS. USP Reserpine RS.*

Botanic characteristics—

Unground Rauwolfia Serpentina root—This occurs as segments usually from 5 to 15 cm in length (pieces sometimes shorter) and from 3 to 20 mm in diameter. The pieces are subcylindrical to tapering, rather tortuous or curved, rarely branched, but bearing occasional twisted rootlets, which are larger, more abundant, and more rigid and woody on the thicker parts of the roots. Externally, light brown to grayish yellow to grayish brown, dull, rough or slightly wrinkled longitudinally yet peculiarly smooth to the touch, occasionally showing small circular rootlet scars in the larger pieces, with some exfoliation of the bark in small areas to reveal the paler wood beneath. When scraped, the bark separates readily from the wood. Fracture short, but irregular, the longer pieces readily breaking with a snap, slightly fibrous marginally. The freshly fractured surfaces show a rather thin layer of grayish yellow bark, with the pale yellowish white wood constituting about 80% of the radius. The smoothed transverse surface of larger pieces shows a finely radiate stele with three or more clearly marked growth rings; a small knob-like protuberance is frequently noticeable at the center. The wood is hard and of relatively low density. The odor is indistinct, earthy, reminiscent of stored white potatoes.

Histology—A transverse section of Rauwolfia Serpentina root shows externally two to eight alternating strata of cork cells, the strata with larger cells alternating with strata made up of markedly smaller cells (*distinction from R. canescens*). Each stratum composed of smaller cells includes from three to five tangentially arranged cell layers, while each stratum made up of larger cells includes from one to six tangential layers. In a cross-sectional view, the largest central cells of the larger cell group measure 40 to 90 µm radially and up to 75 µm tangentially (although usually smaller), while the cells of the smaller cell groups measure about 5 to 20 µm radially and up to 75 μm tangentially. The walls are thin and suberized. The secondary cortex consists of several rows of tangentially elongated to isodiametric parenchyma cells, most being densely filled with starch grains; others (the short latex cells) occur singly or in short series and contain brown resin masses. The secondary phloem is relatively narrow and is made up of phloem parenchyma (bearing starch grains and less commonly tabular to angular calcium oxalate crystals up to 20 μm in length; also, occasionally, with some brown resin masses in outer cells and phloem rays) interlaid with scattered sieve tissue and traversed by phloem rays two to four cells in width. Sclerenchyma cells (stone cells and fibers) are absent in root (*distinction from other species of Rauwolfia*). Cambium is indistinct, narrow, dark, and wavering. The secondary xylem represents the large bulk of the root and shows one or more prominent annual rings with a denser core of wood about 500 μm across at the center. The xylem is composed of many wood wedges separated by xylem rays, and on closer examination reveals vessels in interrupted radial rows, much xylem parenchyma, many large-celled xylem rays, few wood fibers, and tracheids, all lignified-walled. The xylem fibers occur in both tangential and radial rows. The xylem rays are 1 to 12, occasionally up to 16, cells in width.

Rauwolfia Serpentina rhizome—Histology—This is similar to that of root except for the presence of a prominent cortex, pericycle fibers, bicollateral vascular bundles, and a small central pith. The pericycle fibers occur singly or in groups of two to five, have thick, nonlignified walls, tapering, often lobed ends, with subterminal enlargements having thin walls and broad lumina. Vessel elements up to 485 μm are found. The xylem rays are one to four cells in width, with lignified and pitted walls. Internal phloem strands occur embedded in the outer region of the pith. The xylem fibers are somewhat less wavy than those of the root. The pith consists of starch parenchyma cells, among which are scattered short latex cells with yellowish contents stained brown with iodine TS.

Ground Rauwolfia Serpentina root—This is brownish to reddish gray in color. Present are very numerous starch grains (mostly simple, two- to three-compound, occasionally four-compound); simple grains spheroid, ovate, muller-shaped, plano-to angular-convex, or irregular; hilum simple, Y-shaped, stellate, or irregularly cleft; unaltered grains 6 to 34 μm (average 20 μm) in diameter, mostly in the lower range (maximum sizes larger than in *R. canescens* and *R. micrantha*); altered grains up to about 50 μm in diameter; large unaltered grains show polarization cross clearly; calcium oxalate prisms and cluster crystals scattered, about 10 to 15 μm in size; brown resin masses and yellowish granular secretion masses occur occasionally; isolated cork cells elongated, up to 90 μm in length; phelloderm and phloem parenchyma cells similar in appearance; vessels subcylindrical, up to 360 μm in length and from about 20 μm up to 57 μm in diameter (narrower than in *R. canescens*) (the wall markings generally consist of simple pits, with bordered pits adjacent to xylem ray cells), the vessel end walls oblique to transverse, generally with openings in the end walls, some vessels showing tyloses; tracheids pitted, with moderately thick, tapering, beaded walls, with relatively broad lumina, polygonal in cross-section; xylem parenchyma cells with moderately thick walls with simple circular pits, cells polygonal in cross-section, bearing considerable starch; phloem and xylem-ray cells with pitted walls bearing much starch, sometimes with brown resin masses, xylem fibers with thick heavily lignified walls showing small transverse and oblique linear pits and pointed simple to bifurcate ends, measuring from 200 to 750 μm in length (shorter than in *R. micrantha* and *R. canescens*). No phloem fibers or sclereids are present in root (colorless nonlignified pericycle or primary phloem fibers, single or in small groups, may be present from rhizome or stem tissues).

Microbial limits ⟨61⟩—Rauwolfia Serpentina (as the ground root) meets the requirements of the test for absence of *Salmonella* species.

Loss on drying ⟨731⟩—Dry it at 100° to constant weight: it loses not more than 12.0% of its weight.

Acid-insoluble ash ⟨561⟩: not more than 2.0%.

Stems and other foreign organic matter ⟨561⟩—It contains not more than 2.0% of stems and not more than 3.0% of other foreign organic matter.

Chemical identification—[NOTE—In this procedure, use formamide treated as directed in the specifications for Formamide (see under *Reagents* in the section *Reagents, Indicators, and Solutions*) if it has an ammoniacal odor.]

Immobile solvent—Dilute 30 mL of formamide with acetone to 100 mL.

Mobile solvent A—Mix 90 mL of isooctane, 60 mL of carbon tetrachloride, 4 mL of piperidine, and 2 mL of tertiary butyl alcohol.

Mobile solvent B—Mix 75 mL of chloroform, 75 mL of isooctane, and 2 mL of tertiary butyl alcohol.

Spray solution—Dissolve 25 g of trichloroacetic acid in 100 mL of methanol.

Standard solution—Warm a 1-g portion of USP Rauwolfia Serpentina RS with 5 mL of alcohol at 55° to 65° for 30 minutes, with occasional mixing. Cool, and filter.

Test preparation—Reduce 10 g of Rauwolfia Serpentina root to a fine powder. Treat a 1-g portion as in the preparation of the *Standard solution*.

Procedure A—Line the sides of a chromatographic chamber suitable for ascending chromatography (see *Chromatography* ⟨621⟩) with blotting paper. Transfer *Mobile solvent A* to the bottom of the container, and cover the chamber. Immerse a 20- × 20-cm sheet of filter paper (Whatman No. 1 or equivalent) in the *Immobile solvent*, and blot between paper toweling. Allow the acetone solvent to evaporate completely. Apply about 1-μL portions of the *Test preparation* and of the *Standard solution* to a line 2.5 cm from the bottom of the filter paper. Allow to dry. Apply a 2-μL portion of the *Immobile solvent* to each spot, allow to dry, and suspend the paper so that it dips into the *Mobile solvent*. Cover the chamber, and after about 1 hour, when the *Mobile solvent* has risen approximately seven-eighths of the height of the paper, remove the chromatogram, and dry at 90° in a current of air. Spray the paper lightly and evenly with the *Spray solution*, and dry at 90° for 10 minutes.

Procedure B—Use the apparatus described in *Procedure A*, but containing a glass trough with about 2 mL of ammonium hydroxide to saturate the atmosphere of the tank with NH_3. Transfer *Mobile solvent B* to the bottom of the tank outside the trough. Complete the test as described in *Procedure A*, omitting the trichloroacetic acid spray. Examine both chromatograms under UV light, and note the fluorescent spots. In both chromatograms the *Test preparation* yields spots corresponding in position and color to those of the *Standard solution*.

Organic volatile impurities, Method IV ⟨467⟩: meets the requirements.

(Official until July 1, 2008)

Assay—

Apparatus—A medium-sized continuous-extraction apparatus provided with a 250-mL flask and a 35- × 80-mm thimble is convenient, although a smaller apparatus may be used.

Solvents: alcohol, chloroform, and 1,1,1-trichloroethane. Use 1,1,1-trichloroethane having a boiling range between 73° and 76°.

Standard solution—Dissolve 20.0 mg of USP Reserpine RS in 25 mL of hot alcohol, cool, dilute with alcohol to 50.0 mL, and mix. When stored in a tightly-stoppered, light-resistant bottle in the dark, this solution is chromogenically stable for several weeks. Dilute 5.0 mL with alcohol to 100.0 mL, and mix before using.

Procedure—Extract about 2.5 g of finely powdered Rauwolfia Serpentina, accurately weighed, in a continuous-extraction apparatus for 4 hours. Use about 100 mL of vigorously boiling alcohol as solvent, and a few boiling chips to prevent bumping. Protect the flask and thimble and all solutions of Rauwolfia Serpentina alkaloids from direct or strong light. Wash the extract into a 100-mL volumetric flask with alcohol, cool, dilute with alcohol to volume, and mix. Transfer 20.0 mL to a separator containing 200 mL of 0.5 N sulfuric acid, mix, and extract with three 25-mL portions of 1,1,1-trichloroethane. Lubricate stopcocks only with lubricants insoluble in trichloroethane or chloroform (polytef stopcocks are satisfactory). Drain the lower phase as completely as possible. Wash each of the 1,1,1-trichloroethane extracts in a second separator containing 50 mL of 0.5 N sulfuric acid, and discard the trichloroethane extracts. Extract the weakly basic alkaloids from the first acid solution with 25-, 15-, 15-, 10-, 10-, and 10-mL portions of chloroform. Wash each chloroform extract with the acid in the second separator, then with two 10-mL portions of sodium bicarbonate solution (1 in 50) in two additional separators. Filter the chloroform extracts through chloroform-washed cotton into a 100-mL volumetric flask containing 10 mL of alcohol. Dilute with alcohol to volume, and mix. Transfer duplicate 10.0-mL aliquots to glass-stoppered, 25-mL conical flasks, and mix with 4 mL of alcohol. Evaporate with gentle heating almost to dryness, place in a vacuum desiccator, and evaporate to dryness. Dissolve the residues by agitating with 5.0 mL of alcohol. Transfer duplicate 5.0-mL aliquots of the *Standard solution* to flasks. Add 2.0 mL of 0.5 N sulfuric acid to one of the test specimen flasks and to one of the standard flasks (the blanks). Add to the other flasks 1.0 mL of 0.5 N sulfuric acid and 1.0 mL of sodium nitrite solution (3 in 1000). Mix the contents of each flask, and warm in a water bath at 50° to 60° for 20 minutes. Cool, add to each flask 500 µL of sulfamic acid solution (1 in 20), and mix. After stabilization of the solution colors, determine their absorbances in 1-cm cells at 390 nm, relative to a blank consisting of a mixture of alcohol and water (2 : 1). The quantity, in mg, of reserpine-rescinnamine group alkaloids in the specimen taken is given by the formula:

$$5(A - A_0) / (S - S_0)$$

in which A and A_0 are the absorbances of the nitrite-treated specimen and specimen blank, respectively, and S and S_0 are the corresponding absorbances for the solutions from the respective *Standard solution* aliquots.

Powdered Rauwolfia Serpentina

» Powdered Rauwolfia Serpentina is Rauwolfia Serpentina reduced to a fine or a very fine powder, and adjusted, if necessary, to conform to the requirements for reserpine-rescinnamine group alkaloids by admixture with lactose or starch or with a powdered rauwolfia serpentina containing a higher or lower content of these alkaloids. It contains not less than 0.15 percent and not more than 0.20 percent of reserpine-rescinnamine group alkaloids, calculated as reserpine.

Packaging and storage—Preserve in well-closed containers, and store at controlled room temperature, in a dry place, secure against insect attack (see *Preservation* under *Vegetable and Animal Drugs*, and the *General Notices*).
USP Reference standards ⟨11⟩—USP Rauwolfia Serpentina RS. USP Reserpine RS.
Identification—It conforms to the requirements for *Ground Rauwolfia Serpentina* root under *Botanic characteristics* and meets the requirements of the test for *Chemical identification* under *Rauwolfia Serpentina*.
Microbial limit ⟨61⟩—It meets the requirements of the test for absence of *Salmonella* species.
Acid-insoluble ash ⟨561⟩: not more than 2.0%.
Assay—Proceed with Powdered Rauwolfia Serpentina as directed in the *Assay* under *Rauwolfia Serpentina*.

Rauwolfia Serpentina Tablets

» Rauwolfia Serpentina Tablets contain an amount of reserpine-rescinnamine group alkaloids, calculated as reserpine, equivalent to not less than 0.15 percent and not more than 0.20 percent of the labeled amount of powdered rauwolfia serpentina.

Packaging and storage—Preserve in tight, light-resistant containers.
USP Reference standards ⟨11⟩—USP Rauwolfia Serpentina RS. USP Reserpine RS.
Identification—The powdered rauwolfia serpentina in the Tablets conforms to the requirements for *Ground Rauwolfia Serpentina* root under *Botanic characteristics* and meets the requirements of the test for *Chemical identification* under *Rauwolfia Serpentina*.
Microbial limits ⟨61⟩—Tablets meet the requirements of the test for absence of *Salmonella* species.
Disintegration ⟨701⟩: 1 hour, with disks using simulated gastric fluid TS, without enzyme.
Uniformity of dosage units ⟨905⟩: meet the requirements.
Assay—Weigh and finely powder not less than 20 Tablets. Weigh accurately a portion of this powder, equivalent to 2.5 g of powdered rauwolfia serpentina, and proceed as directed for *Procedure* in the *Assay* under *Rauwolfia Serpentina*.

Purified Rayon

» Purified Rayon is a fibrous form of bleached, regenerated cellulose.

Alkalinity or acidity—Immerse about 10 g in 100 mL of recently boiled and cooled water, and decant 25-mL portions of the water, with the aid of a glass rod, into each of two dishes. To one portion add 3 drops of phenolphthalein TS, and to the other portion add 1 drop of methyl orange TS: neither portion appears pink when viewed against a white background.
Residue on ignition ⟨281⟩: not more than 1.50%, determined on a 5.0-g test specimen.
Acid-insoluble ash—To the residue obtained in the test for *Residue on ignition*, add 25 mL of 3 N hydrochloric acid, and boil for 5 minutes. Collect the insoluble matter on a tared filtering crucible, wash with hot water, ignite, and weigh: the residue weighs not more than 63.0 mg (1.25%).
Water-soluble substances—Proceed as directed in the test for *Water-soluble substances* under *Purified Cotton*: the residue weighs not more than 100 mg (1.0%).
Fiber length and absorbency—Remove it from its wrappings, and condition it for not less than 4 hours in a standard atmosphere of 65 ± 2% relative humidity at 21 ± 1.1°. Determine the *Fiber length* and *Absorbency* as follows.
   Fiber length—Determine the fiber length of Purified Rayon as directed for *Fiber Length* under *Cotton* ⟨691⟩: not less than 70.0%, by weight, of the fibers are 19 mm or greater in length, and not more than 5.0%, by weight, of the fibers are 6.3 mm or less in length.
   Absorbency—Proceed as directed for the *Absorbency Test* under *Cotton* ⟨691⟩: submersion is complete in 5 seconds, and the rayon retains not less than 16 times its weight of water.
Other requirements—It meets the requirements of the tests for *Dyes* and *Other foreign matter* under *Purified Cotton*.

Oral Rehydration Salts

» Oral Rehydration Salts is a dry mixture of Sodium Chloride, Potassium Chloride, Sodium Bicarbonate, and Dextrose (anhydrous). Alternatively, it may contain Sodium Citrate (anhydrous or dihydrate) instead of Sodium Bicarbonate. It may contain Dextrose (monohydrate) instead of Dextrose (anhydrous), provided that the Sodium Bicarbonate or Sodium Citrate is packaged in a separate, accompanying container. It contains the equivalent of not less than 90.0 percent and not more than 110.0 percent of the amounts of sodium (Na^+), potassium (K^+), chloride (Cl^-), and bicarbonate (HCO_3^-) or citrate ($C_6H_5O_7^{-3}$), calculated from the labeled amounts of Sodium Chloride, Potassium Chloride, and Sodium Bicarbonate [or Sodium Citrate (anhydrous or dihydrate)]. It contains not less than 90.0

percent and not more than 110.0 percent of the labeled amounts of anhydrous dextrose ($C_6H_{12}O_6$), or dextrose monohydrate ($C_6H_{12}O_6 \cdot H_2O$). It may contain suitable flavors.

Packaging and storage—Preserve in tight containers, and avoid exposure to temperatures in excess of 30°. The Sodium Bicarbonate or Sodium Citrate component may be omitted from the mixture and packaged in a separate, accompanying container.

Labeling—The label indicates prominently whether Sodium Bicarbonate or Sodium Citrate is a component by the placement of the word "Bicarbonate" or "Citrate," as appropriate, in juxtaposition to the official title. The label states the name and quantity, in g, of each component in each unit-dose container, or in a stated quantity, in g, of Salts in a multiple-unit container. The label states the net weight in each container and provides directions for constitution. Where packaged in individual unit-dose pouches, the label instructs the user not to open until the time of use. The label states also that any solution that remains unused 24 hours after constitution is to be discarded.

USP Reference standards ⟨11⟩—*USP Citric Acid RS*.
(Official January 1, 2009)

Identification—
A: It meets the requirements of the flame tests for *Sodium* ⟨191⟩ and for *Potassium* ⟨191⟩.
B: It meets the requirements of the tests for *Chloride* ⟨191⟩.
C: Where it contains Sodium Bicarbonate, it dissolves with effervescence, and the collected gas so obtained meets the requirements of the tests for *Bicarbonate* ⟨191⟩.
D: Where it contains Sodium Citrate, it meets the requirements of the test for *Citrate* ⟨191⟩, 3 to 5 drops of the solution constituted as directed in the labeling and 20 mL of the mixture of pyridine and acetic anhydride being used.
E: Where it contains Dextrose, add a few drops of the solution constituted as directed in the labeling to 5 mL of hot alkaline cupric tartrate TS: a copious red precipitate of cuprous oxide is formed (*presence of dextrose*).

Loss on drying ⟨731⟩—Dry it at 50° to constant weight: it loses not more than 1.0% of its weight.

Minimum fill ⟨755⟩—Proceed as directed, except to change the requirements following "The average net weight of the contents of the 10 containers is not less than the labeled amount, and the net weight of the contents of any single container is not less than" to read "95% and not more than 105% of the labeled amount. If the contents of not more than 1 container are less than 95% but not less than 90% of the labeled amount or more than 105% but not more than 110% of the labeled amount, determine the net weight of the contents of 20 additional containers. The average net weight of the contents of 30 containers is not less than the labeled amount, and the net weight of the contents of not more than 1 of the 30 containers is less than 95% but not less than 90% of the labeled amount or more than 105% but not more than 110% of the labeled amount."

NOTE—In performing the *Assay for sodium and potassium,* the *Assay for chloride,* the *Assay for bicarbonate,* and the *Assay for citrate,* calculate from the labeled amounts of sodium chloride, potassium chloride, and sodium bicarbonate or sodium citrate the total equivalent amounts of sodium (Na^+), potassium (K^+), chloride (Cl^-), and bicarbonate (HCO_3^-), [or citrate ($C_6H_5O_7^{-3}$)] contained therein. (See accompanying table.)

pH ⟨791⟩: between 7.0 and 8.8, in the solution constituted as directed in the labeling.

Assay for dextrose—Transfer the contents of 1 or more unit-dose containers of Oral Rehydration Salts, or an accurately weighed portion of the contents of 1 multiple-unit container, equivalent to about 20 g of dextrose, to a 100-mL volumetric flask, dilute with water to volume, and mix. Transfer 50.0 mL of this stock solution to a 100-mL volumetric flask. Add 0.2 mL of 6 N ammonium hydroxide, dilute with water to volume, and mix. [NOTE—Reserve the remaining stock solution for the *Assay for sodium and potassium,* the *Assay for chloride,* the *Assay for bicarbonate,* and the *Assay for citrate.*] Determine the angular rotation in a suitable polarimeter tube (see *Optical Rotation* ⟨781⟩). Where the Oral Rehydration Salts is labeled to contain anhydrous dextrose, calculate the percentage (g per 100 mL) of $C_6H_{12}O_6$ in the portion of Oral Rehydration Salts taken by the formula:

$$(100/52.9)AR$$

in which 100 is the percentage; 52.9 is the midpoint of the specific rotation range for anhydrous dextrose, in degrees; A is 100 mm divided by the length of the polarimeter tube, in mm; and R is the observed rotation, in degrees. Where the Oral Rehydration Salts is labeled to contain dextrose monohydrate, calculate the percentage (g per 100 mL) of $C_6H_{12}O_6 \cdot H_2O$ in the portion of Oral Rehydration Salts taken by the formula:

$$(100/52.9)(198.17/180.16)AR$$

in which 100 is the percentage; 52.9 is the midpoint of the specific rotation range for anhydrous dextrose, in degrees; 198.17 and 180.16 are the molecular weights for dextrose monohydrate and anhydrous dextrose, respectively; A is 100 mm divided by the length of the polarimeter tube, in mm; and R is the observed rotation, in degrees.

Assay for sodium and potassium—
Sodium stock solution—Transfer 14.61 g of sodium chloride, previously dried at 105° for 2 hours and accurately weighed, to a 250-mL volumetric flask, add water to volume, and mix.

Potassium stock solution—Transfer 18.64 g of potassium chloride, previously dried at 105° for 2 hours and accurately weighed, to a 250-mL volumetric flask, add water to volume, and mix.

Lithium diluent solution—Transfer 1.04 g of lithium nitrate to a 1000-mL volumetric flask, add a suitable nonionic surfactant, then add water to volume, and mix.

Standard preparation—Transfer 5.0 mL of *Sodium stock solution* and 5.0 mL of *Potassium stock solution* to a 500-mL volumetric flask, dilute with water to volume, and mix. Transfer 5.0 mL of the resulting solution to a 100-mL volumetric flask, dilute with *Lithium diluent solution* to volume, and mix. Each mL of this solution contains 0.01150 mg of sodium (Na^+) and 0.01955 mg of potassium (K^+).

Assay preparation 1—Dilute an accurately measured volume of the stock solution remaining from the *Assay for dextrose* quantitatively, and stepwise if necessary, with water to obtain a solution containing about 0.23 mg of sodium (Na^+) per mL. Transfer 5.0 mL of the resulting solution to a 100-mL volumetric flask, dilute with *Lithium diluent solution* to volume, and mix.

Assay preparation 2—Dilute an accurately measured volume of the stock solution remaining from the *Assay for dextrose* quantitatively, and stepwise if necessary, with water to obtain a solution containing about 0.39 mg of potassium per mL. Transfer 5.0 mL of the resulting solution to a 100-mL volumetric flask, dilute with *Lithium diluent solution* to volume, and mix.

Procedure—Using a suitable flame photometer, adjusted to read zero with *Lithium diluent solution,* concomitantly determine the sodium flame emission readings for the *Standard preparation* and *Assay preparation 1* at the wavelength of maximum emission at about 589 nm. Calculate the quantity, in mg, of Na^+ in the unit-dose container or containers taken or in the portion of powder taken from the multiple-unit container by the formula:

$$0.23(L_{Na}/D_{Na})(R_{U,Na}/R_{S,Na})$$

in which L_{Na} is the quantity, in mg, of sodium (Na^+) in the unit-dose container or containers taken or in the portion of powder taken from the multiple-unit container, calculated from the labeled quantities of sodium chloride and sodium bicarbonate (or sodium citrate); D_{Na} is the concentration, in mg per mL, of sodium in *Assay preparation 1,* based on the volume taken of the stock solution remaining from the *Assay for dextrose* and the extent of dilution; and $R_{U,Na}$ and $R_{S,Na}$ are the sodium emission readings obtained from *Assay preparation 1* and the *Standard preparation,* respectively. Similarly determine the potassium flame emission readings from the *Standard preparation* and *Assay preparation 2* at the wavelength of maximum emission at about 766 nm. Calculate the quantity, in mg, of K^+ in the unit-dose container or containers taken or in the portion of powder taken from the multiple-unit container by the formula:

$$0.391(L_K / D_K)(R_{U,K} / R_{S,K})$$

in which L_K is the quantity, in mg, of potassium in the unit-dose container or containers taken or in the portion of powder taken from the multiple-unit container, calculated from the labeled quantity of potassium chloride; D_K is the concentration, in mg per mL, of potassium in *Assay preparation 2*, based on the volume taken of the stock solution remaining from the *Assay for dextrose* and the extent of dilution; and $R_{U,K}$ and $R_{S,K}$ are the potassium emission readings obtained from *Assay preparation 2* and the *Standard preparation*, respectively.

Assay for chloride—Transfer an accurately measured volume of the stock solution remaining from the *Assay for dextrose*, equivalent to about 55 mg of chloride (Cl^-), to a suitable container, and titrate with 0.1 N silver nitrate VS until the silver chloride flocculates and the mixture acquires a faint pink color using potassium chromate TS as the indicator. Calculate the quantity, in mg, of Cl^- in the unit-dose container or containers taken or in the portion of powder taken from the multiple-unit container by the formula:

$$354.5 T / v$$

in which T is the volume, in mL, of 0.1 N silver nitrate consumed; and v is the volume, in mL, of stock solution taken.

Assay for bicarbonate *(if present)*—Transfer an accurately measured volume of the stock solution remaining from the *Assay for dextrose*, equivalent to about 100 mg of bicarbonate (HCO_3^-), to a suitable beaker, add 25 mL of water and 3 drops of methyl orange TS, and titrate with 0.1 N hydrochloric acid VS. Calculate the quantity, in mg, of HCO_3^- in the unit-dose container or containers taken or in the portion of powder taken from the multiple-unit container, by the formula:

$$610.2 T / v$$

in which T is the volume, in mL, of 0.1 N hydrochloric acid consumed; and v is the volume, in mL, of the stock solution taken.

Assay for citrate *(if present)*—

Mobile phase—Dissolve 20 g of ammonium sulfate in a mixture of water and acetonitrile (980 : 20). Make adjustments if necessary (see *System Suitability* under *Chromatography* ⟨621⟩).

Standard preparation—Dissolve an accurately weighed quantity of sodium citrate, previously dried at 180° for 18 hours, in water to obtain a solution having a known concentration of about 2.5 mg of anhydrous sodium citrate per mL.

Assay preparation—Transfer an accurately measured volume of the stock solution remaining from the *Assay for dextrose*, equivalent to about 180 mg of citrate ($C_6H_5O_7^{-3}$), to a 100-mL volumetric flask, dilute with water to volume, and mix.

Chromatographic system (see *Chromatography* ⟨621⟩)—The liquid chromatograph is equipped with a 220-nm detector and a 4.8-mm × 20-cm column that contains packing L8. The flow rate is about 2 mL per minute. Chromatograph the *Standard preparation*, and record the peak response as directed for *Procedure*: the retention time for the citrate peak is about 3 minutes, the column efficiency is not less than 1000 theoretical plates, the tailing factor is not more than 2.0, and the relative standard deviation for replicate injections is not more than 2.0%. [NOTE—The column may be equilibrated before use by making a series of injections of the *Standard preparation* over a period of several hours. If the tailing factor is greater than 2, the equilibration may be facilitated by adding 1 g of sodium citrate to each 1000 mL of the *Mobile phase* and pumping this solution through the column at about 0.5 mL per minute for several hours. The column must then be washed with *Mobile phase* for a few minutes before use.]

Procedure—Separately inject equal volumes (about 20 µL) of the *Standard preparation* and the *Assay preparation* into the chromatograph, record the chromatograms, and measure the responses for the major peaks. Calculate the quantity, in mg, of $C_6H_5O_7^{-3}$ in the unit-dose container or containers taken or in the portion of powder taken from the multiple-unit container by the following formula:

$$(189.12 / 258.07)(10{,}000\,C / v)(r_U / r_S)$$

in which 189.12 and 258.07 are the molecular weights of citrate ($C_6H_5O_7^{-3}$) and anhydrous sodium citrate, respectively, C is the concentration, in mg per mL, of anhydrous sodium citrate in the *Standard preparation*, v is the volume, in mL, of the stock solution taken to prepare the *Standard preparation*, and r_U and r_S are the citrate peak responses obtained from the *Assay preparation* and the *Standard preparation*, respectively.

(Official until January 1, 2009)

Assay for citrate *(if present)*—

Mobile phase, Standard Preparation 1, and *Chromatographic System*—Proceed as directed under *Assay for Citric Acid/Citrate and Phosphate* ⟨345⟩.

Assay preparation—Transfer an accurately measured volume of the stock solution remaining from the *Assay for dextrose*, equivalent to about 180 mg of citrate ($C_6H_5O_7^{-3}$), to a suitable volumetric flask, and proceed as directed for *Assay Preparation for Citric Acid/Citrate Assay* under *Assay for Citric Acid/Citrate and Phosphate* ⟨345⟩.

Procedure—Proceed as directed for *Procedure* under ⟨345⟩. Calculate the quantity, in mg, of citrate ($C_6H_5O_7^{-3}$) in the portion of Oral Rehydration Salts taken by the formula:

$$0.001\,C_S\,D(r_U / r_S)$$

in which C_S is the concentration, in µg per mL, of citrate in *Standard Preparation 1*; D is the dilution factor; and r_U and r_S are the citrate peak areas obtained from the *Assay preparation* and *Standard Preparation 1*, respectively.

	mg equivalent of each g of component				
Component	Na^+	K^+	Cl^-	HCO_3^-	$C_6H_5O_7^{-3}$
Sodium Chloride	393.4		606.6		
Potassium Chloride		524.4	475.6		
Sodium Bicarbonate	273.6			726.4	
Anhydrous Sodium Citrate	267.2				732.8
Sodium Citrate Dihydrate	234.5				643.0

(Official January 1, 2009)

Repaglinide

C₂₇H₃₆N₂O₄   452.59

(S)-2-Ethyoxy-4-[2-[[methyl-1-[2-[(1-piperidinyl)phenyl]butyl]
amino]-2-oxoethyl]-benzoic acid.
(+)-2-Ethoxy-α-[[(S)-α-isobutyl-o-piperidinobenzyl]carbamoyl]-p-toluic acid   [135062-02-1].

» Repaglinide contains not less than 98.0 percent and not more than 101.0 percent of $C_{27}H_{36}N_2O_4$, calculated on the dried basis.

Packaging and storage—Preserve in tight containers.
USP Reference standards ⟨11⟩—USP Repaglinide RS. USP Repaglinide Related Compound A RS. USP Repaglinide Related Compound B RS. USP Repaglinide Related Compound C RS.
Identification—
  A: *Infrared Absorption* ⟨197K⟩.
  B: *Ultraviolet Absorption* ⟨197U⟩—
  Solution: 25 μg per mL.
  Medium: methanol.
Specific rotation ⟨781S⟩: between +6.3° and +7.3°, at 20°.
  Test solution: 50 mg per mL, in methanol.
Loss on drying (see *Thermal Analysis* ⟨891⟩)—Determine the percentage of volatile substances by thermogravimetric analysis on an appropriately calibrated instrument, using about 30 mg of Repaglinide, accurately weighed. Heat the specimen at the rate of 10° per minute between 30° and 210° in an atmosphere of nitrogen at a flow rate of 200 mL per minute. From the thermogram, determine the accumulated loss in weight between 30° and 200°: it loses not more than 0.7% of its weight.
Residue on ignition ⟨281⟩: not more than 0.1%, an ignition temperature of 600 ± 25° being used.
Heavy metals, *Method II* ⟨231⟩: 0.001%.
Chromatographic purity—
  Solution A—Prepare a filtered and degassed monobasic potassium phosphate solution (3 in 1000). Adjust with 1 N sodium hydroxide to a pH of 7.0.
  Solution B—Use filtered and degassed methanol.
  Mobile phase—Use variable mixtures of *Solution A* and *Solution B* as directed for *Chromatographic system*. Make adjustments if necessary (see *System Suitability* under *Chromatography* ⟨621⟩).
  System suitability solution—Dissolve accurately weighed quantities of USP Repaglinide RS, USP Repaglinide Related Compound A RS, USP Repaglinide Related Compound B RS, and USP Repaglinide Related Compound C RS in methanol to obtain a solution having known concentrations of about 10 mg of USP Repaglinide RS per mL and 100 μg each of the related compound Reference Standards per mL.
  Test solution—Transfer about 100 mg of Repaglinide, accurately weighed, to a 10-mL volumetric flask, dissolve in and dilute with methanol to volume, and mix.
  Standard solution—Transfer 0.1 mL of the *Test solution* to a 10-mL volumetric flask, dilute with methanol to volume, and mix.
  Chromatographic system (see *Chromatography* ⟨621⟩)—Prepare as directed in the *Assay*, except to program the chromatograph as follows.

Time (minutes)	Solution A (%)	Solution B (%)	Elution
0	50	50	equilibration
0–2	50→30	50→70	linear gradient
2–8	30	70	isocratic
8–12	30→5	70→95	linear gradient
12–15	5	95	isocratic

Chromatograph the *System suitability solution*, and record the peak areas as directed for *Procedure:* the relative retention times are about 0.3 for repaglinide related compound B, 0.9 for repaglinide related compound C, 1.0 for repaglinide, and 1.6 for repaglinide related compound A. Chromatograph the *Standard solution*, and record the peak areas as directed for *Procedure:* the relative standard deviation for replicate injections is not more than 10%.
  Procedure—Separately inject equal volumes (about 3 μL) of the *Test solution* and the *Standard solution* into the chromatograph, record the chromatograms, and measure the peak areas. Calculate the percentage of each impurity, other than repaglinide related compound A, in the portion of Repaglinide taken by the formula:

$$r_i / r_S$$

in which r_i is the peak response for each impurity obtained from the *Test solution;* and r_S is the peak response of repaglinide obtained from the *Standard solution*. For repaglinide related compound A, use the same formula, but multiply the result by a response factor equal to 2.0: not more than 0.1% of any individual impurity is found, and not more than 0.5% of total impurities is found.

Assay—
  Buffer solution—Prepare a monobasic potassium phosphate solution (1 in 1000), and adjust with phosphoric acid to a pH of 2.5.
  Mobile phase—Prepare a filtered and degassed mixture of methanol and *Buffer solution* (80 : 20).
  System suitability preparation—Dissolve accurately weighed quantities of USP Repaglinide RS and USP Repaglinide Related Compound B RS in methanol to obtain a solution having known concentrations of about 500 μg per mL and 40 μg per mL, respectively.
  Standard preparation—Dissolve an accurately weighed quantity of USP Repaglinide RS in methanol, and dilute quantitatively, and stepwise if necessary, with methanol to obtain a solution having a known concentration of about 500 μg per mL.
  Assay preparation—Transfer about 25 mg of Repaglinide, accurately weighed, to a 50-mL volumetric flask, dissolve in and dilute with methanol to volume, and mix.
  Chromatographic system (see *Chromatography* ⟨621⟩)—The liquid chromatograph is equipped with a 240-nm detector and a 4.6-mm × 12.5-cm column that contains 5-μm packing L1. The flow rate is about 1.0 mL per minute. The column temperature is maintained at 45°. Chromatograph the *System suitability preparation*, and record the peak areas as directed for *Procedure:* the relative retention times are about 1.0 for repaglinide and 0.4 for repaglinide related compound B. Chromatograph the *Standard preparation*, and record the peak areas as directed for *Procedure:* the relative standard deviation for replicate injections is not more than 2.0%.
  Procedure—Separately inject equal volumes (about 10 μL) of the *Standard preparation* and the *Assay preparation* into the chromatograph, record the chromatograms, and measure the areas for the major peaks. Calculate the quantity, in mg, of $C_{27}H_{36}N_2O_4$ in the portion of Repaglinide taken by the formula:

$$50C(r_U / r_S)$$

in which C is the concentration, in mg per mL, of USP Repaglinide RS in the *Standard preparation;* and r_U and r_S are the peak responses obtained from the *Assay preparation* and the *Standard preparation*, respectively.

Repaglinide Tablets

» Repaglinide Tablets contain not less than 95.0 percent and not more than 105.0 percent of the labeled amount of repaglinide ($C_{27}H_{36}N_2O_4$).

Packaging and storage—Preserve in tight containers.

USP Reference standards ⟨11⟩—USP Repaglinide RS. USP Repaglinide Related Compound A RS.

Identification—

A: *Thin-Layer Chromatographic Identification Test ⟨201⟩*—

Test solution—Transfer an accurately weighed quantity of powdered Tablets, equivalent to about 10 mg of repaglinide, to a suitable container, add 10 mL of a mixture of methanol and methylene chloride (1 : 1), shake for 15 minutes, and centrifuge.

Developing solvent system: a mixture of toluene, methylene chloride, and methanol (2 : 2 : 1).

B: The retention time and UV spectrum of the major peak in the chromatogram of the *Assay preparation* correspond to those in the chromatogram of the *Standard preparation,* as obtained in the *Assay.*

Dissolution ⟨711⟩—

Medium: pH 5.0 buffer, prepared by mixing 10.2 g of citric acid monohydrate and 18.16 g of dibasic sodium phosphate dihydrate with 1 L of water; 900 mL.

Apparatus 2: 75 rpm.

Time: 30 minutes.

Determine the amount of $C_{27}H_{36}N_2O_4$ dissolved by employing the following method.

Buffer solution—Prepare a monobasic potassium phosphate solution (1.5 in 1000), and adjust with phosphoric acid to a pH of 2.3.

Mobile phase—Prepare a filtered and degassed mixture of acetonitrile, *Buffer solution*, and methanol (49 : 40 : 11).

Standard solution—Transfer about 22 mg of USP Repaglinide RS, accurately weighed, to a 100-mL volumetric flask, dissolve in and dilute with methanol to volume, and mix. Transfer 5.0 mL of this solution to a 100-mL volumetric flask, and dilute with methanol to volume. Transfer 5.0 mL of the resulting solution to a 100-mL volumetric flask, add 25 mL of methanol, dilute with *Medium* to volume, and mix.

Chromatographic system (see *Chromatography ⟨621⟩*)—The liquid chromatograph is equipped with a fluorometric detector, set at an excitation wavelength of 244 nm and an emission wavelength of 348 nm, and a 4.0-mm × 12.5-cm column that contains 10-μm packing L1. The column temperature is maintained at 40°. The flow rate is about 1.0 mL per minute. Chromatograph the *Standard solution*, and record the peak responses as directed for *Procedure:* the capacity factor, k', is about 1.8; the tailing factor is between 0.5 and 2.0; and the relative standard deviation for replicate injections is not more than 2.0%.

Procedure—Separately inject equal volumes (about 20 μL) of the *Standard solution* and a filtered portion of the solution under test into the chromatograph, record the chromatograms, and measure the areas for the major peaks. Calculate the quantity of $C_{27}H_{36}N_2O_4$ dissolved by comparing the measured peak responses of the *Standard solution* and the solution under test.

Tolerances—Not less than 70% (*Q*) of the labeled amount of $C_{27}H_{36}N_2O_4$ is dissolved in 30 minutes.

Uniformity of dosage units ⟨905⟩: meet the requirements.

Loss on drying ⟨731⟩—Dry about 2 g of finely ground Tablets, accurately weighed, at 105° for 3 hours: it loses not more than 6.0% of its weight.

Chromatographic purity—

pH 4.0 Phosphate buffer, *pH 2.5 Phosphate buffer*, *Diluent*, and *Mobile phase*—Proceed as directed in the *Assay.*

Standard solution 1, Standard solution 2, and *System suitability solution*—Proceed as directed in the *Assay* for *Standard preparation 1, Standard preparation 2,* and *System suitability preparation,* respectively.

Standard solution 3—Transfer 2.5 mL of *Standard solution 2* to a 1-liter volumetric flask, dilute with *Diluent* to volume, and mix.

Test solution—Use the *Assay preparation.*

Chromatographic system (see *Chromatography ⟨621⟩*)—The liquid chromatograph is equipped with a 210-nm diode array detector and a 4.0-mm × 6-cm column that contains 5-μm packing L1. The column temperature is maintained at 40°. The flow rate is about 1.0 mL per minute. Chromatograph the *System suitability solution,* and record the peak responses as directed for *Procedure:* the capacity factors, k', for repaglinide and repaglinide related compound A are about 4.9 and 1.2, respectively; the resolution, *R,* between the two peaks is not less than 7.0; and the tailing factor is between 0.8 and 2.0. Chromatograph *Standard solution 3*, and record the peak responses as directed for *Procedure:* the relative standard deviation for replicate injections is not more than 10%.

Procedure—Separately inject equal volumes (about 20 μL) of *Standard solution 2* and the *Test solution* into the chromatograph, record the chromatograms, and measure all of the peak responses. Calculate the percentage of each impurity in the portion of Tablets taken by the formula:

$$100(r_i / r_S)$$

in which r_i is the peak response for each impurity in the *Test solution;* and r_S is the repaglinide peak response obtained from *Standard solution 2:* not more than 0.5% of total impurities is found.

Assay—

pH 4.0 Phosphate buffer—Prepare a monobasic ammonium phosphate solution (2 in 1000), and adjust with phosphoric acid to a pH of 4.0.

pH 2.5 Phosphate buffer—Prepare a monobasic ammonium phosphate solution (2 in 1000), and adjust with phosphoric acid to a pH of 2.5.

Diluent—Prepare a mixture of methanol and *pH 4.0 Phosphate buffer* (7 : 3).

Mobile phase—Prepare a filtered and degassed mixture of methanol and *pH 2.5 Phosphate buffer* (7 : 3).

Standard preparation 1—Dissolve an accurately weighed quantity of USP Repaglinide RS in methanol to obtain a solution having a known concentration of about 800 μg per mL.

Standard preparation 2—Transfer 5.0 mL of *Standard preparation 1* to a 50-mL volumetric flask, dilute with *Diluent* to volume, and mix.

System suitability preparation—Dissolve an accurately weighed quantity of USP Repaglinide Related Compound A RS in methanol to obtain a solution having a known concentration of about 80 μg per mL. Transfer 1.0 mL of this solution to a 50-mL volumetric flask, add 5.0 mL of *Standard preparation 1*, dilute with *Diluent* to volume, and mix.

Assay preparation—Transfer 8 whole Tablets to a suitable volumetric flask, and dissolve in and dilute with *Diluent* to volume to obtain a solution having a concentration of about 80 μg per mL. Stir for 20 minutes with the aid of a magnetic stirrer, and filter a portion of the solution.

Chromatographic system (see *Chromatography ⟨621⟩*)—The liquid chromatograph is equipped with a 245-nm diode array detector and a 4.0-mm × 6-cm column that contains 5-μm packing L1. The column temperature is maintained at 40°. The flow rate is about 1.0 mL per minute. Chromatograph the *System suitability preparation,* and record the peak responses as directed for *Procedure:* the capacity factors, k', for repaglinide and repaglinide related compound A are about 4.9 and 1.2, respectively; the resolution, *R,* between the two peaks is not less than 7.0; and the tailing factor is between 0.8 and 2.0. Chromatograph *Standard preparation 2*, and record the peak responses as directed for *Procedure:* the relative standard deviation for replicate injections is not more than 2.0%.

Procedure—Separately inject equal volumes (about 20 μL) of *Standard preparation 2* and the *Assay preparation* into the chromatograph, record the chromatograms, and measure the areas for the major peaks. Calculate the quantity, in mg, of repaglinide ($C_{27}H_{36}N_2O_4$) in each of the Tablets taken by the formula:

$$(VC/8)(r_U / r_S)$$

in which *V* is the volume, in mL, of *Diluent* used in the *Assay preparation;* *C* is the concentration, in mg per mL, of USP Repaglinide RS in *Standard preparation 2;* and r_U and r_S are the peak responses obtained from the *Assay preparation* and *Standard preparation 2,* respectively.

Reserpine

$C_{33}H_{40}N_2O_9$ 608.68
Yohimban-16-carboxylic acid, 11,17-dimethoxy-18-[(3,4,5-trimethoxybenzoyl)oxy]-, methyl ester, $(3\beta,16\beta,17\alpha,18\beta,20\alpha)$-.
Methyl 18β-hydroxy-11,17α-dimethoxy-3β,20α-yohimban-16β-carboxylate 3,4,5-trimethoxybenzoate (ester)   [50-55-5].

» Reserpine contains not less than 97.0 percent and not more than 101.0 percent of $C_{33}H_{40}N_2O_9$, calculated on the dried basis.

Packaging and storage—Preserve in tight, light-resistant containers. Store at 25°, excursions permitted between 15° and 30°.

USP Reference standards ⟨11⟩—*USP Reserpine RS.*

Identification—

  A: *Infrared Absorption* ⟨197K⟩.

  B: [NOTE—Conduct this test promptly, with a minimum exposure to light.] Dissolve 25.0 mg of it, previously dried, in 0.25 mL of chloroform; mix with about 30 mL of methanol previously warmed to 50°; transfer the mixture with the aid of warm methanol to a 250-mL volumetric flask; cool the solution to room temperature; dilute with methanol to volume; and mix. Pipet 10 mL of this solution into a 50-mL volumetric flask, add 36 mL of chloroform, dilute with methanol to volume, and mix: the UV absorption spectrum of a 1 in 50,000 solution so obtained exhibits the same maxima in the range of 255 nm to 350 nm as that of a similar solution of USP Reserpine RS, concomitantly measured; and the respective absorptivities, determined with reference to a mixture of 36 volumes of chloroform and 14 volumes of methanol as the blank, at the wavelength of maximum absorbance at about 268 nm, do not differ by more than 3.0%.

Loss on drying ⟨731⟩—Dry it at 60° for 3 hours: it loses not more than 0.5% of its weight.

Residue on ignition ⟨281⟩: not more than 0.1%.

Assay—

  Mobile phase—Prepare a filtered and degassed 1 : 1 mixture of acetonitrile and ammonium chloride solution (1 in 100). Make adjustments if necessary (see *System Suitability* under *Chromatography* ⟨621⟩). The pH is about 5.6.

  Standard preparation—Dissolve an accurately weighed quantity of USP Reserpine RS in *Mobile phase*, and dilute quantitatively, and stepwise if necessary, with *Mobile phase* to obtain a solution having a known concentration of about 10 μg per mL.

  Assay preparation—Transfer about 10 mg of Reserpine, accurately weighed, to a 100-mL volumetric flask. Dilute with *Mobile phase* to volume, and mix. Dilute 1.0 mL of this solution with 9.0 mL of *Mobile phase*, and mix.

  Chromatographic system (see *Chromatography* ⟨621⟩)—The liquid chromatograph is equipped with a 268-nm detector and a 4.6-mm × 25-cm column that contains packing L1. The flow rate is about 1.5 mL per minute. Chromatograph the *Standard preparation*, and record the peak responses as directed for *Procedure*: the column efficiency determined from the analyte peak is not less than 1500 theoretical plates; the tailing factor for the analyte peak is not more than 1.5; and the relative standard deviation for replicate injections is not more than 2.0%.

  Procedure—Separately inject equal volumes (about 20 μL) of the *Standard preparation* and the *Assay preparation* into the chromatograph, record the chromatograms, and measure the responses for the major peaks. Calculate the quantity, in mg, of $C_{33}H_{40}N_2O_9$ in the portion of Reserpine taken by the formula:

$$C(r_U/r_S)$$

in which C is the concentration, in μg per mL, of USP Reserpine RS in the *Standard preparation;* and r_U and r_S are the peak responses obtained from the *Assay preparation* and the *Standard preparation,* respectively.

Reserpine Injection

» Reserpine Injection is a sterile solution of Reserpine in Water for Injection, prepared with the aid of a suitable acid. It contains not less than 90.0 percent and not more than 110.0 percent of the labeled amount of $C_{33}H_{40}N_2O_9$. It contains suitable antioxidants.

Packaging and storage—Preserve in single-dose (or, if stabilizers are present, in multiple-dose), light-resistant containers, preferably of Type I glass.

USP Reference standards ⟨11⟩—*USP Reserpine RS. USP Endotoxin RS.*

Identification—It responds to the *Identification* test under *Reserpine Oral Solution*.

Bacterial endotoxins ⟨85⟩—It contains not more than 71.5 USP Endotoxin Units per mg of reserpine.

pH ⟨791⟩: between 3.0 and 4.0.

Other alkaloids—[NOTE—Conduct this test promptly after preparation of the test and standard solutions.] Pipet 10 mL each of the citric acid solution of the Injection, and of *Solution 1* used in preparing the *Standard preparation,* respectively, obtained as directed in the *Assay,* into two separators. To the Injection solution add 100 mL of saturated sodium bicarbonate solution, and to *Solution 1* add 10 mL of water, 10 drops of saturated sodium bicarbonate solution, and 90 mL of water, and extract both of the resulting solutions with 50 mL of ether. Transfer the aqueous phase to another separator, extract with a second 50-mL portion of ether, and discard the aqueous layers. Wash the ether layers in succession with two 25-mL portions of water, and discard the washings. Extract the combined ether layers with three 15-mL portions of 2 N sulfuric acid, collect the extracts in a 50-mL volumetric flask, add 2 N sulfuric acid to volume, and mix. The absorption spectrum of the solution from the Injection, in the range of 255 to 350 nm, measured in a 1-cm cell, 2 N sulfuric acid being used as the blank, exhibits maxima and minima only at the same wavelengths as that of the solution from the *Standard preparation,* concomitantly measured. Calculate the quantity, in mg, of total alkaloids in each mL of the Injection taken by the formula:

$$10(I/SV)$$

in which I is the absorbance of the solution from the Injection at the wavelength of maximum absorbance at about 268 nm; S is that of the solution from the *Standard preparation*; and V is the volume, in mL, of Injection taken. The content of total alkaloids is not more than 114.0% of the labeled amount of $C_{33}H_{40}N_2O_9$, and does not differ by more than 10.0% from the amount of $C_{33}H_{40}N_2O_9$ determined in the *Assay.*

Other requirements—It meets the requirements under *Injections* ⟨1⟩.

Assay—

  Standard preparation—Dissolve 25.0 mg of USP Reserpine RS, accurately weighed, in 0.25 mL of chloroform, mix with about 30 mL of methanol previously warmed to 50°, transfer the mixture to a 250-mL volumetric flask with the aid of warm methanol, cool the solution to room temperature, dilute with methanol to volume, and mix (*Solution 1*). Protect the solution from light. Just prior to use in the *Assay,* pipet 10 mL of *Solution 1* into a 50-mL volumetric flask, add 36 mL of chloroform, and dilute with methanol to volume (*Standard preparation*).

Assay preparation—Transfer to a 100-mL volumetric flask an accurately measured volume of Injection, equivalent to about 10 mg of reserpine, and dilute with citric acid solution (1 in 50) to volume.

Procedure—Pipet 10 mL of the *Assay preparation* into a separator, or a suitably stoppered, 50-mL centrifuge tube, add 10 mL of chloroform, and shake for 2 minutes. Separate and withdraw the chloroform. Wash the citric acid solution with two 10-mL portions of chloroform, adding the washings to the main chloroform solution. To the combined chloroform solutions add 10 mL of sodium bicarbonate solution (1 in 100), shake for 2 minutes, and separate. Withdraw the chloroform, filtering it through a pledget of cotton, into a 50-mL volumetric flask containing 14.0 mL of methanol. Extract the aqueous bicarbonate layer in the extraction vessel with two 2-mL portions of chloroform, passing each portion successively through the filter into the volumetric flask. Add chloroform to volume, and mix.

Pipet duplicate 5-mL aliquots of the chloroform-methanol solution and of the *Standard preparation* into separate, 10-mL volumetric flasks. Add 2.0 mL of a 1 in 10 solution of hydrochloric acid in methanol to each flask. To one flask of each pair of duplicates (representing the *Standard preparation* and the extracted *Assay preparation*) add 1.0 mL of a 3 in 1000 solution of sodium nitrite in dilute methanol (1 in 2). To the second flask of each pair (constituting the blanks) add 1 mL of dilute methanol (1 in 2). Mix, and allow to stand for 30 minutes. Add 0.5 mL of ammonium sulfamate solution (1 in 20) to each flask, add methanol to volume, mix, and allow to stand for 10 minutes. Determine the absorbance of each solution in a 1-cm cell at the wavelength of maximum absorbance at about 390 nm, with a suitable spectrophotometer, using a mixture of methanol, chloroform, and water (5.4 : 3.6 : 1) as the blank. Calculate the quantity, in mg, of $C_{33}H_{40}N_2O_9$ in each mL of the Injection taken by the formula:

$$10(A - A_0)_U / V(A - A_0)_S$$

in which V is the volume, in mL, of Injection taken, and the parenthetic expressions are the differences in absorbances of the nitrite-treated and blank solutions, respectively, from the *Assay preparation* (U) and the *Standard preparation* (S).

Reserpine Oral Solution

» Reserpine Oral Solution contains not less than 90.0 percent and not more than 110.0 percent of the labeled amount of reserpine ($C_{33}H_{40}N_2O_9$).

Packaging and storage—Preserve in tight, light-resistant containers.

USP Reference standards ⟨11⟩—*USP Reserpine RS*.

Identification—Evaporate about 2 mL of the chloroform-methanol solution obtained from the *Assay preparation* as directed for *Procedure* in the *Assay*, in a test tube to dryness, add to the residue 0.5 mL of glacial acetic acid, swirl for 1 to 2 minutes, and add 1 mL of a 1 in 50 solution of vanillin in hydrochloric acid: a pink color is produced, and it becomes deep violet-red within a few minutes or as a result of warming the solution for 10 to 20 seconds.

Alcohol content ⟨611⟩: between 11.0% and 13.0% of C_2H_5OH.

Assay—

Standard preparation—Dissolve 25.0 mg of USP Reserpine RS, accurately weighed, in 0.25 mL of chloroform, mix with about 30 mL of methanol previously warmed to 50°, transfer the mixture to a 250-mL volumetric flask with the aid of warm methanol, cool the solution to room temperature, dilute with methanol to volume, and mix (*Solution 1*). Protect the solution from light. Just prior to use in the *Assay*, pipet 10 mL of *Solution 1* into a 50-mL volumetric flask, add 36 mL of chloroform, and dilute with methanol to volume (*Standard preparation*).

Procedure—Transfer an accurately measured volume of Oral Solution, equivalent to about 1 mg of reserpine, into a separator or a suitably stoppered, 50-mL centrifuge tube, add 5 mL of citric acid solution (1 in 50) and 10 mL of chloroform, and shake for 2 minutes. Separate and withdraw the chloroform. Wash the citric acid solution with two 10-mL portions of chloroform, adding the washings to the main chloroform solution. To the combined chloroform solutions add 10 mL of sodium bicarbonate solution (1 in 100), shake for 2 minutes, and separate. Withdraw the chloroform, filtering it through a pledget of cotton, into a 50-mL volumetric flask containing 14.0 mL of methanol. Extract the aqueous bicarbonate layer in the extraction vessel with two 2-mL portions of chloroform, passing each portion successively through the filter into the volumetric flask. Add chloroform to volume, and mix (*Assay preparation*).

Pipet duplicate 5-mL aliquots of the chloroform-methanol solution and of the *Standard preparation* into separate, 10-mL volumetric flasks. Add 2.0 mL of a 1 in 10 solution of hydrochloric acid in methanol to each flask. To one flask of each pair of duplicates (representing the *Standard preparation* and the extracted *Assay preparation*) add 1.0 mL of a 3 in 1000 solution of sodium nitrite in dilute methanol (1 in 2). To the second flask of each pair (constituting the blanks) add 1 mL of dilute methanol (1 in 2). Mix, and allow to stand for 30 minutes. Add 0.5 mL of ammonium sulfamate solution (1 in 20) to each flask, add methanol to volume, mix, and allow to stand for 10 minutes. Determine the absorbance of each solution in a 1-cm cell at the wavelength of maximum absorbance at about 390 nm, with a suitable spectrophotometer, using a mixture of methanol, chloroform, and water (5.4 : 3.6 : 1) as the blank. Calculate the quantity, in mg, of reserpine ($C_{33}H_{40}N_2O_9$) in each mL of the Oral Solution taken by the formula:

$$(A - A_0)_U / V(A - A_0)_S$$

in which V is the volume, in mL, of Oral Solution taken; and the parenthetic expressions are the differences in absorbances of the nitrite-treated and blank solutions, respectively, from the *Assay preparation* (U) and the *Standard preparation* (S).

Reserpine Tablets

» Reserpine Tablets contain not less than 90.0 percent and not more than 110.0 percent of the labeled amount of reserpine ($C_{33}H_{40}N_2O_9$).

Packaging and storage—Preserve in tight, light-resistant containers.

USP Reference standards ⟨11⟩—*USP Reserpine RS*.

Identification—Evaporate about 2 mL of the *Test solution*, obtained from the test for *Other alkaloids*, in a test tube to dryness, add to the residue 0.5 mL of the glacial acetic acid, swirl for 1 to 2 minutes, and add 1 mL of a 1 in 50 solution of vanillin in hydrochloric acid: a pink color is produced, and it becomes deep violet-red within a few minutes or as a result of warming the solution for 10 to 20 seconds.

Dissolution ⟨711⟩—[NOTE—Do not substitute membrane filters for filter paper where the filtration of reserpine-containing solutions is indicated. Reserpine has been shown to be adsorbed onto membranes.]

Medium: 0.1 N acetic acid; 500 mL.
Apparatus 1: 100 rpm.
Time: 45 minutes.

p-Toluenesulfonic acid solution—Dissolve 1 g of *p*-toluenesulfonic acid in 100 mL of glacial acetic acid.

Standard solution—Dissolve an accurately weighed quantity of USP Reserpine RS in glacial acetic acid, and dilute quantitatively, and stepwise if necessary, with glacial acetic acid to obtain a solution having a known concentration of about 0.1 µg per mL.

Test solution—Pipet an aliquot of the filtered solution under test, containing about 11 µg of reserpine, into a 125-mL separatory funnel. Extract with three 10-mL portions of chloroform, collecting the extracts in a 100-mL volumetric flask, dilute with glacial acetic acid to volume, and mix.

Procedure—Into three individual 50-mL test tubes, pipet 10 mL each of the *Standard solution*, the *Test solution*, and glacial acetic acid to provide the blank. Treat each as follows. Add 10 mL of *p-Toluenesulfonic acid solution*, insert a stopper, and mix gently.

Place in a steam bath for 10 minutes. Remove from the steam bath, and cool. Determine the amount of $C_{33}H_{40}N_2O_9$ dissolved from the fluorescences of the *Test solution* and the *Standard solution* using a suitable spectrophotometer arranged to deliver activation radiation at 390 nm and to measure the resultant fluorescence at the emission wavelength of about 480 nm.

Tolerances—Not less than 75% *(Q)* of the labeled amount of $C_{33}H_{40}N_2O_9$ is dissolved in 45 minutes.

Uniformity of dosage units ⟨905⟩: meet the requirements.

Procedure for content uniformity—

Phosphoric acid-methanol solution—Dilute 20 mL of phosphoric acid with 200 mL of methanol, then dilute with water to 1000 mL, and mix.

Vanadium pentoxide reagent—Prepare a saturated solution of vanadium pentoxide in phosphoric acid by shaking by mechanical means for 1 hour 100 mg of vanadium pentoxide with 100 mL of phosphoric acid. Allow undissolved solids to settle overnight, and filter the supernatant through a medium-porosity, sintered-glass funnel.

Standard solution—Using an accurately weighed quantity of USP Reserpine RS, prepare a solution in *Phosphoric acid-methanol solution* having a known concentration of about 0.002 mg per mL.

Test preparation—Place 1 Tablet in a suitable container, and add an accurately measured volume of *Phosphoric acid-methanol solution* so that the concentration of the final solution is about 0.002 mg of reserpine per mL. Shake by mechanical means until the tablet is completely disintegrated. Filter before using.

Procedure—With the *Apparatus* set as described for *Automated Dissolution Test for Reserpine Tablets* under *Automated Methods of Analysis* ⟨16⟩, conduct determinations of one Standard per five Tablets. Calculate the quantity, in mg, of reserpine ($C_{33}H_{40}N_2O_9$) in the Tablet taken by the formula:

$$CD(I_U / I_S)$$

in which *C* is the concentration, in mg per mL, of USP Reserpine RS in the *Standard solution*; *D* is the dilution factor for the *Test preparation*; and I_U and I_S are the fluorescence intensities obtained from the *Test preparation* and the *Standard solution*, respectively.

Other alkaloids—

Adsorbent—Use acid-washed chromatographic siliceous earth.

Chromatographic tube—Select a chromatographic tube about 200 mm long and about 22 mm in internal diameter that is constricted to an outlet at the lower end. Insert at the constriction a small pledget of glass wool, previously washed with chloroform and air-dried.

Chromatographic column—Mix 1 g of *Adsorbent* with 0.5 mL of freshly prepared sodium bicarbonate solution (1 in 50) in a 100-mL beaker until the mixture appears fluffy and uniformly moistened, transfer to the *Chromatographic tube*, and tamp lightly with a packing rod to a thickness of about 7 to 9 mm. Mix uniformly 1 g of *Adsorbent* with 0.5 mL of freshly prepared citric acid solution (1 in 200), transfer to the *Chromatographic tube*, and tamp lightly with a packing rod. Mix uniformly 1 g of *Adsorbent* with 0.5 mL of water, transfer to the *Chromatographic tube*, and tamp lightly with a packing rod.

Blank mixture—Combine 1 mL of dimethyl sulfoxide and 2 g of *Adsorbent* in a suitable container, and stir thoroughly until the mass is uniformly wetted and free from lumps.

Blank solution—Transfer the *Blank mixture* through a powder funnel to a prepared *Chromatographic column*. Scrub the beaker with about 1 g of *Adsorbent*, and add it through the funnel to the tube. Wipe the spatula, beaker, and funnel with a tuft of glass wool, previously washed with chloroform and air-dried. Place the glass wool in the tube, and press it down on the column with the packing rod, so that the overall height of the column is between 55 mm and 65 mm. Rinse the spatula, beaker, and funnel with the first portion of the chloroform used to elute the specimen. Elute the reserpine with 45 mL of chloroform. [NOTE—A properly packed column elutes in 4 to 8 minutes.] Collect the eluate in a 50-mL volumetric flask containing 14 mL of methanol. Rinse the tip of the column with chloroform, add chloroform to volume, and mix.

Standard solution—[NOTE—Use actinic glassware for this solution.] Dissolve 25.0 mg of USP Reserpine RS, accurately weighed, in 0.25 mL of chloroform, and mix with about 30 mL of methanol previously warmed to 50°. Transfer the mixture to a 250-mL volumetric flask with the aid of warm methanol, cool the solution to room temperature, dilute with methanol to volume, and mix. Just before use, pipet 10 mL of this solution into a 50-mL volumetric flask, add 36 mL of chloroform, dilute with methanol to volume, and mix.

Test mixture—Weigh and finely powder, to pass a 60-mesh sieve, not fewer than 20 Tablets. Weigh accurately a portion of the powder, equivalent to about 1 mg of reserpine, but not more than 1 g of the powder, and transfer to a 150-mL beaker. Dry-mix the powder with about 500 mg of *Adsorbent*, then mix with 1 mL of dimethyl sulfoxide (immobile solvent). Stir thoroughly until the mass is uniformly wetted and free from lumps, and allow the mixture to stand for 5 minutes. Add another 500 mg of *Adsorbent*, and thoroughly work it into the mass. Again add an amount of *Adsorbent* so that the total amount added is 2 g, and disperse it completely in the mass.

Test solution—Transfer the *Test mixture* through a powder funnel to a prepared *Chromatographic column*. Proceed as directed for *Blank solution* beginning with "Scrub the beaker with about 1 g of *Adsorbent*."

Procedure—Determine the UV absorption spectrum of the *Test solution*, between 255 and 350 nm, using the *Blank solution* in the reference cell. Similarly, determine the UV absorption spectrum of the *Standard solution*, using a solution of 3.6 volumes of chloroform and 1.4 volumes of methanol as the blank. The two spectra are similar, and the ratio, A_{268}/A_{295}, for the *Test solution* does not differ by more than 4.0% from the corresponding ratio for the *Standard solution*. Calculate the quantity, in mg, of reserpine ($C_{33}H_{40}N_2O_9$) in the portion of Tablets taken by the formula:

$$A_U / A_S$$

in which A_U and A_S are the absorbances of the *Test solution* and the *Standard solution*, respectively, at the absorption maximum at about 268 nm. The result so obtained does not differ more than 6.0% from that obtained in the *Assay*.

Assay—

Mobile phase, Standard preparation, and *Chromatographic system*—Proceed as directed in the *Assay* under *Reserpine*.

Assay preparation—Weigh and finely powder not fewer than 20 Tablets. Transfer an accurately weighed quantity of the powder, equivalent to about 1 mg of reserpine, to a 100-mL volumetric flask. Add *Mobile phase* to volume, and mix. Filter a portion through a 0.8-μm or finer membrane disk.

Procedure—Proceed as directed for *Procedure* in the *Assay* under *Reserpine*, and calculate the quantity, in mg, of reserpine ($C_{33}H_{40}N_2O_9$) in the portion of Tablets taken by the formula:

$$0.1C(r_U / r_S)$$

in which the terms are as defined therein.

Reserpine and Chlorothiazide Tablets

» Reserpine and Chlorothiazide Tablets contain not less than 90.0 percent and not more than 110.0 percent of the labeled amount of reserpine ($C_{33}H_{40}N_2O_9$) and not less than 93.0 percent and not more than 107.0 percent of the labeled amount of chlorothiazide ($C_7H_6ClN_3O_4S_2$).

Packaging and storage—Preserve in tight, light-resistant containers.

USP Reference standards ⟨11⟩—*USP Reserpine RS. USP Chlorothiazide RS.*

Identification—

A: Transfer a quantity of powdered Tablets, equivalent to about 1 mg of reserpine, to a stoppered, 50-mL centrifuge tube. Add 20 mL of citric acid solution (1 in 50), and shake until the powder is suspended. Extract the mixture with two 20-mL portions of chloroform, centrifuge, and withdraw the chloroform, filtering each extract through a pledget of cotton into a 50-mL volumetric flask. Dilute with chloroform to volume, and mix: the UV absorption spectrum of the solution so obtained exhibits maxima and minima at the same wavelengths as that of a similar solution of USP Reserpine RS, concomitantly measured (*presence of reserpine*).

B: Transfer a quantity of powdered Tablets, equivalent to about 50 mg of chlorothiazide, to a test tube containing 10 mL of acetone, agitate for 5 minutes, and centrifuge. Use the clear supernatant as the Test solution. Separately apply 10 µL each of the Test solution and a Standard solution of USP Chlorothiazide RS in acetone containing 5 mg per mL to a thin-layer chromatographic plate (see *Chromatography* ⟨621⟩) coated with a 0.25-mm layer of chromatographic silica gel mixture and previously washed with methanol. Develop the chromatogram in a solvent system consisting of a mixture of ethyl acetate and isopropyl alcohol (17 : 3) until the solvent front has moved about three-fourths of the length of the plate. Remove the plate from the chamber, air-dry, and examine under short-wavelength UV light: the R_F value of the principal spot in the chromatogram of the Test solution corresponds to that obtained from the Standard solution (*presence of chlorothiazide*).

Dissolution ⟨711⟩—

Medium: mixture of pH 8.0 phosphate buffer (see *Buffer Solutions* in the section *Reagents, Indicators, and Solutions*) and *n*-propyl alcohol (3 : 2); 900 mL.

Apparatus 2: 75 rpm.

Time: 60 minutes.

Determination of dissolved reserpine—

STANDARD PREPARATION—Dissolve about 34 mg of USP Reserpine RS, accurately weighed, in a 50-mL volumetric flask containing 5 mL of chloroform, dilute with *n*-propyl alcohol to volume (*Solution 1*), and mix. Pipet 1 mL of *Solution 1* into a 50-mL volumetric flask, dilute with *n*-propyl alcohol to volume (*Solution 2*), and mix. Pipet 1 mL of *Solution 2* into a 100-mL volumetric flask, dilute with *Dissolution Medium* to volume, and mix to obtain the *Standard preparation*.

PROCEDURE—Filter a portion of the solution under test through paper, and transfer 5.0 mL of the clear filtrate to a 25-mL volumetric flask. Pipet 5 mL of the *Standard preparation* into a separate 25-mL volumetric flask. Treat each flask as follows: Add 5 drops of hydrochloric acid and 5 mL of a mixture of water, alcohol, and sulfuric acid (29 : 20 : 1), and mix. Add by pipet 5 mL of sodium nitrite solution (3 in 1000), dilute with alcohol to volume, mix, and allow to stand for 30 minutes. Concomitantly determine the fluorescences of the solution under test and the *Standard preparation* in a suitable spectrophotometer arranged to deliver activation radiation at 405 nm and to measure the resultant fluorescence at the emission wavelength of about 500 nm. Calculate the amount of reserpine ($C_{33}H_{40}N_2O_9$) dissolved.

Determination of dissolved chlorothiazide—

STANDARD PREPARATION—Transfer about 27 mg of USP Chlorothiazide RS, accurately weighed, to a 50-mL volumetric flask containing 5 mL of methanol, swirl to dissolve, dilute with *Dissolution Medium* to volume, and mix. Pipet 2 mL of this solution into a 100-mL volumetric flask, dilute with *Dissolution Medium* to volume, and mix.

PROCEDURE—Determine the amount of chlorothiazide ($C_7H_6ClN_3O_4S_2$) dissolved from UV absorbances at the wavelength of maximum absorbance at about 292 nm of filtered portions of the solution under test, suitably diluted with *Dissolution Medium*, in comparison with the *Standard preparation*.

Tolerances—Not less than 75% (*Q*) of the labeled amount of $C_{33}H_{40}N_2O_9$ is dissolved in 60 minutes, and not less than 75% (*Q*) of the labeled amount of $C_7H_6ClN_3O_4S_2$ is dissolved in 60 minutes.

Uniformity of dosage units ⟨905⟩: meet the requirements with respect to chlorothiazide and to reserpine.

Procedure for content uniformity for reserpine—

Standard preparation—Prepare as directed for *Standard preparation* in the *Assay for reserpine*.

Test preparation—Weigh 1 Tablet, grind to a fine powder, and transfer to a stoppered, 50-mL centrifuge tube. Add 25.0 mL of chloroform and methanol solution (1 : 1), shake by mechanical means for 15 minutes, and centrifuge. Pipet 4 mL of the clear supernatant into a 100-mL volumetric flask, dilute with the chloroform and methanol solution to volume, and mix.

Procedure—Proceed as directed for *Procedure* in the *Assay for reserpine*. Calculate the quantity, in mg, of $C_{33}H_{40}N_2O_9$, in the Tablet taken by the formula:

$$(W_t / W_U)(TC / D)(I_U / I_S)$$

in which W_t is the weight, in mg, of the Tablet, W_U is the weight, in mg, of the portion of Tablet taken, T is the labeled quantity, in mg, of reserpine in the Tablet, C is the concentration, in µg per mL, of USP Reserpine RS in the *Standard preparation*, D is the concentration, in µg per mL, of reserpine in the *Test preparation*, based upon the labeled quantity per Tablet and the extent of dilution, and I_U and I_S are the fluorescence intensities of the solutions from the *Test preparation* and the *Standard preparation*, respectively.

Procedure for content uniformity for chlorothiazide—

Standard preparation—Prepare as directed for *Standard preparation* under *Assay for chlorothiazide*.

Test preparation—Transfer 1 Tablet to a 500-mL volumetric flask, add 300 mL of 0.1 N sodium hydroxide, and sonicate, swirling the flask intermittently, until the Tablet is dissolved. Dilute with 0.1 N sodium hydroxide to volume, mix, and filter, discarding the first 15 mL of the filtrate. Dilute a portion of the clear filtrate quantitatively with 0.1 N sodium hydroxide to obtain a solution having a concentration of about 10 µg of chlorothiazide per mL.

Procedure—Proceed as directed for *Procedure* in the *Assay for chlorothiazide*. Calculate the quantity, in mg, of $C_7H_6ClN_3O_4S_2$, in the Tablet taken by the formula:

$$(TC / D)(A_U / A_S)$$

in which T is the labeled quantity, in mg, of chlorothiazide in the Tablet, C is the concentration, in µg per mL, of USP Chlorothiazide RS in the *Standard preparation*, D is the concentration, in µg per mL, of chlorothiazide in the *Test preparation*, based upon the labeled quantity per Tablet and the extent of dilution, and A_U and A_S are the absorbances of the solutions from the *Test preparation* and the *Standard preparation*, respectively.

Assay for reserpine—

Standard preparation—Dissolve about 25 mg of USP Reserpine RS, accurately weighed, in 1 mL of chloroform contained in a 50-mL volumetric flask, dilute with methanol to volume, and mix. Dilute a portion of this solution quantitatively and stepwise with chloroform and methanol solution (1 : 1) to obtain a solution having a known concentration of about 0.2 µg of reserpine per mL.

Assay preparation—Weigh and finely powder not less than 20 Tablets. Transfer an accurately weighed portion of the powder, equivalent to about 1 mg of reserpine, to a stoppered, 50-mL centrifuge tube, add 25.0 mL of chloroform and methanol solution (1 : 1), shake by mechanical means for 15 minutes, and centrifuge. Dilute a portion of the clear supernatant quantitatively and stepwise with chloroform and methanol solution (1 : 1) to obtain a solution having a concentration of about 0.2 µg of reserpine per mL.

Procedure—Separately transfer 5.0 mL of the *Assay preparation*, 5.0 mL of the *Standard preparation*, and 5.0 mL of chloroform and methanol solution (1 : 1) to provide the reagent blank, respectively, to three 25-mL volumetric flasks. To each flask add 0.5 mL of hydrochloric acid, 1.0 mL of a 3 in 1000 solution of sodium nitrite in dilute methanol (1 in 2), mix, and allow to stand for 30 minutes. Add 1 mL of ammonium sulfamate solution (1 in 20) to each flask, add chloroform and methanol solution (1 : 1) to volume, mix, and allow to stand for 10 minutes. Concomitantly determine the fluorescence intensities of the solutions in a suitable spectrophotometer arranged to deliver activation radiation at 405 nm and to measure the resultant fluorescence at the emission wavelength of about 500 nm. Calculate the quantity, in mg, of $C_{33}H_{40}N_2O_9$ in the portion of Tablets taken by the formula:

$$5C(I_U / I_S)$$

in which C is the concentration, in µg per mL, of USP Reserpine RS in the *Standard preparation*, and I_U and I_S are the fluorescence intensities of the solutions from the *Assay preparation* and the *Standard preparation*, respectively.

Assay for chlorothiazide—

Standard preparation—Dissolve an accurately weighed quantity of USP Chlorothiazide RS in 0.1 N sodium hydroxide, and dilute quantitatively and stepwise with 0.1 N sodium hydroxide to obtain a solution having a known concentration of about 10 µg per mL. Use a freshly prepared solution.

Assay preparation—Weigh and finely powder not less than 20 Tablets. Transfer an accurately weighed portion of the powder, equivalent to about 250 mg of chlorothiazide, to a 500-mL volumetric flask, add about 300 mL of 0.1 N sodium hydroxide, and shake by mechanical means for 15 minutes. Dilute with 0.1 N sodium hydroxide to volume, and mix. Filter through paper, discarding the first 15 mL of the filtrate. Pipet 2 mL of the clear filtrate into a 100-mL volumetric flask, dilute with 0.1 N sodium hydroxide to volume, and mix.

Procedure—Concomitantly determine the absorbances of the *Standard preparation* and the *Assay preparation* in 1-cm cells at the wavelength of maximum absorbance at about 292 nm, with a suitable spectrophotometer, using 0.1 N sodium hydroxide as the blank. Calculate the quantity, in mg, of $C_7H_6ClN_3O_4S_2$, in the portion of Tablets taken by the formula:

$$25C(A_U / A_S)$$

in which C is the concentration, in µg per mL, of USP Chlorothiazide RS in the *Standard preparation*, and A_U and A_S are the absorbances of the *Assay preparation* and the *Standard preparation*, respectively.

Reserpine, Hydralazine Hydrochloride, and Hydrochlorothiazide Tablets

» Reserpine, Hydralazine Hydrochloride, and Hydrochlorothiazide Tablets contain not less than 90.0 percent and not more than 110.0 percent of the labeled amount of reserpine ($C_{33}H_{40}N_2O_9$), and not less than 93.0 percent and not more than 107.0 percent of the labeled amounts of hydralazine hydrochloride ($C_8H_8N_4 \cdot HCl$) and hydrochlorothiazide ($C_7H_8ClN_3O_4S_2$).

NOTE—Where Reserpine, Hydralazine Hydrochloride, and Hydrochlorothiazide Tablets are prescribed, without reference to the quantity of reserpine, hydralazine hydrochloride, or hydrochlorothiazide contained therein, a product containing 0.1 mg of reserpine, 25 mg of hydralazine hydrochloride, and 15 mg of hydrochlorothiazide shall be dispensed.

Packaging and storage—Preserve in tight, light-resistant containers.

USP Reference standards ⟨11⟩—*USP Reserpine RS. USP Hydralazine Hydrochloride RS. USP Hydrochlorothiazide RS. USP Benzothiadiazine Related Compound A RS.*

Identification—

A: Transfer a quantity of finely powdered Tablets, equivalent to about 100 mg of hydralazine hydrochloride, to a glass-stoppered flask. Add 40 mL of dilute hydrochloric acid (1 in 12), shake by mechanical means for 5 minutes, and filter, discarding the first few mL of the filtrate. Transfer 20 mL of the filtrate to a separator. Extract with a 10-mL portion of methylene chloride, and discard the methylene chloride. To the aqueous phase add 2 mL of sodium nitrite solution (14 in 1000) and 10 mL of methylene chloride, and shake by mechanical means for 5 minutes. Allow the layers to separate, and drain the methylene chloride through sodium sulfate that has been pre-washed with methylene chloride, into a 50-mL beaker. Evaporate over gentle heat with the aid of nitrogen to dryness: the IR absorption spectrum of a potassium bromide dispersion of the residue so obtained exhibits maxima only at the same wavelengths as that of a similar preparation of USP Hydralazine Hydrochloride RS, similarly treated (*presence of hydralazine hydrochloride*).

B: Transfer a quantity of finely powdered Tablets, equivalent to about 1 mg of reserpine, to a 50-mL centrifuge tube. Add 20 mL of cyclohexane, shake by mechanical means for 15 minutes, centrifuge, and discard the cyclohexane. Repeat the extraction with two additional 20-mL portions of cyclohexane, shaking by mechanical means for 2 minutes each time. To the residue add 10 mL of chloroform, shake for 2 minutes, and filter through a medium-porosity, sintered-glass funnel into another 50-mL centrifuge tube. Extract the chloroform with 10 mL of 1.0 N hydrochloric acid, discarding the aqueous acid layer. Extract the chloroform with 10 mL of 0.5 N sodium hydroxide. Centrifuge for 5 minutes, and withdraw the chloroform with a syringe, passing the chloroform through cotton into a 50-mL volumetric flask containing 40 mL of methanol. Dilute with chloroform to volume, and mix: the UV absorption spectrum of the solution so obtained exhibits maxima and minima at the same wavelengths as that of a similar solution of USP Reserpine RS, concomitantly measured (*presence of reserpine*).

C: The UV absorption spectrum of the solution from the *Assay preparation*, obtained as directed for *Procedure* in the Assay for hydrochlorothiazide, exhibits maxima and minima at the same wavelengths as that of the solution from the *Standard preparation*, prepared as directed in the *Assay for hydrochlorothiazide*, similarly measured (*presence of hydrochlorothiazide*).

Disintegration ⟨701⟩: 30 minutes.

Uniformity of dosage units ⟨905⟩: meet the requirements for *Content Uniformity* with respect to reserpine, to hydralazine hydrochloride, and to hydrochlorothiazide.

Procedure for content uniformity—

Apparatus—Use an automatic analyzer consisting of (1) a solid sampler with 100-mL dissolution capability; (2) a 20-channel peristaltic pump; (3) a continuous filtering device; (4) a colorimeter equipped with a 2-mm flow cell and analysis capability at 530 nm; (5) a UV spectrophotometer equipped with a 10-mm flow cell and analysis capability at 271 nm; (6) a spectrofluorometer equipped with a 2-mm flow cell and analysis capability of 365 nm activation energy and 495 nm fluorescence; (7) recording devices for each of the three aforementioned detectors; and (8) a manifold consisting of components illustrated in the pertinent diagram in the chapter *Automated Methods of Analysis* ⟨16⟩. Prepare the ion-exchange column listed in the manifold as follows. Wash sulfonic acid cation-exchange resin (40- to 60-mesh) with isopropyl alcohol until the alcohol shows no appreciable UV absorption at 271 nm, then add sufficient 1 N hydrochloric acid to cover the resin. Drain off the acid, and wash the resin with an equivalent volume of 1 N sodium hydroxide and then again with 1 N hydrochloric acid. Finally wash the resin with water until the effluent is neutral to litmus. Draw the resin into a 10-mm length of "solvaflex" tubing (1 mm ID) by vacuum, and plug each end with glass wool.

Saturated vanadium pentoxide (V_2O_5)—Stir for about 6 hours or shake by mechanical means for 2 hours about 100 mg of vanadium pentoxide powder with 100 mL of phosphoric acid. Filter through a medium-porosity, sintered-glass funnel. This solution is stable for 1 month.

0.3% Hydrogen peroxide (H_2O_2)—Dilute 1 mL of 30 percent hydrogen peroxide with water to 100 mL. Prepare fresh daily.

Blue tetrazolium reagent (B.T.)—Dissolve 760 mg of blue tetrazolium in 3.8 liters of a mixture of dehydrated alcohol and methanol (19 : 1).

Tetramethylammonium hydroxide (T.M.A.H.)—Dilute 38 mL of tetramethylammonium hydroxide solution (1 in 10) with dehydrated alcohol and methanol (19 : 1) to 3.8 liters.

Solvent, *wash*, and *diluent*—Prepare by mixing equal volumes of methanol and water. Add 1 mL of phosphoric acid to each 3.8 liters.

Standard preparation—Accurately weigh about 42.0 mg of USP Reserpine RS into a 200-mL volumetric flask, dissolve in methanol, and dilute with methanol to volume. Pipet 10 mL of this solution into a 100-mL volumetric flask containing about 315.0 mg of USP Hydrochlorothiazide RS and about 525.0 mg of USP Hydralazine Hydrochloride RS, accurately weighed. Dissolve in *Solvent*, and dilute with *Solvent* to volume. (A 5-mL aliquot represents 1 standard Tablet.)

Procedure—With the sampler in the standby position, pump all reagents through the system until a stable baseline is achieved. Activate the sampler, and allow one cycle to pass without introducing the Tablets or the *Standard preparation*, then pipet a 5-mL aliquot of the *Standard preparation* into the hopper at the solvent addition portion for the next two cycles and for every sixth cycle thereafter. Disregard the first value for the *Standard preparation*. Add the Tablets to the sampler at the rate of 20 per hour to follow the second 5-mL aliquot of the *Standard preparation*. Record the absorbance and fluorescence values, and calculate each peak value by the difference between peak height and baseline. Calculate the quantity, in mg per Tablet, taken by the formula:

$$(0.005 / 1.05)C(A_U / A_S)$$

in which C is the concentration, in µg per mL, of the appropriate Reference Standard in the *Standard preparation*, A_U is the absorbance of the Tablet, and A_S is the averaged absorbance of the *Standard preparations*.

Diazotizable substances—

Standard solution—Weigh accurately 25 mg of USP Benzothiadiazine Related Compound A RS, dissolve in 5 mL of methanol contained in a 50-mL volumetric flask, dilute with water to volume, and mix. Pipet 4 mL of this solution into a 100-mL volumetric flask, dilute with water to volume, and mix.

Test solution—Transfer a portion of the powdered Tablets prepared for the *Assay for hydrochlorothiazide*, accurately weighed and equivalent to about 100 mg of hydrochlorothiazide, to a 100-mL volumetric flask, and add a mixture of 20 mL of methanol and 20 mL of water. Shake continuously for 5 to 10 minutes, dilute with water to volume, mix, and filter. Use the filtrate as the *Test solution*.

Procedure—Pipet 5 mL each of the *Standard solution* and the *Test solution* into separate, 50-mL volumetric flasks. Pipet 5 mL of water into a third 50-mL volumetric flask to provide the blank. To each flask add 1 mL of freshly prepared sodium nitrite solution (1 in 100) and 5 mL of dilute hydrochloric acid (1 in 12), and allow to stand for 5 minutes. Add 2 mL of ammonium sulfamate solution (1 in 50), allow to stand for 5 minutes with frequent swirling, then add 2 mL of freshly prepared disodium chromotropate solution (1 in 100) and 10 mL of sodium acetate TS. Dilute with water to volume, and mix. Concomitantly determine the absorbances of the solutions from the *Standard solution* and the *Test solution* in 1-cm cells at the wavelength of maximum absorbance at about 500 nm, with a suitable spectrophotometer, against the blank. The absorbance of the solution from the *Test solution* does not exceed that of the solution from the *Standard solution*, corresponding to not more than 2.0% of diazotizable substances.

Assay for reserpine—

Standard preparation—Dissolve about 25 mg of USP Reserpine RS, accurately weighed, in chloroform in a 50-mL volumetric flask, and dilute with chloroform to volume (*Solution 1*). Pipet 10 mL of *Solution 1* into a 50-mL volumetric flask, and dilute with chloroform to volume. Protect the solution from light.

Assay preparation—Weigh and finely powder not less than 20 Tablets. Transfer an accurately weighed portion of the powder, equivalent to about 1 mg of reserpine, to a separator or a stoppered, 50-mL centrifuge tube containing 10 mL of citric acid solution (1 in 50). Shake vigorously until the powder is completely suspended. Add 10 mL of chloroform, and proceed as directed for *Procedure*, beginning with "shake thoroughly for 2 minutes."

Procedure—[NOTE—Conduct the entire procedure quickly, without exposure to direct sunlight. Perform the extractions in a suitable separator or in a suitably stoppered, 50-mL centrifuge tube, and separate by centrifuging, withdrawing the portion to be retained into a hypodermic syringe fitted with a square-tipped, 14-gauge, 15-cm needle.] Pipet 10 mL of the *Standard preparation* into the extraction vessel, add 10 mL of citric acid solution (1 in 50), and shake thoroughly for 2 minutes. Separate and withdraw the chloroform. Wash the citric acid solution with two 10-mL portions of chloroform, adding the washings to the main chloroform solution. To the combined chloroform solutions add 10 mL of citric acid solution (1 in 50), shake for 2 minutes, and separate and withdraw the chloroform. To the combined chloroform solutions add 10 mL of sodium bicarbonate solution (1 in 100), shake for 2 minutes, and separate. Withdraw the chloroform, filtering it through a pledget of cotton, into a 50-mL volumetric flask containing 14.0 mL of methanol. Extract the aqueous bicarbonate layer in the extraction vessel with two 2-mL portions of chloroform, passing each portion successively through the filter into the volumetric flask. Add chloroform to volume, and mix. Pipet duplicate 5-mL aliquots of the chloroform-methanol solutions into separate, 10-mL volumetric flasks. Add 2.0 mL of a 1 in 10 solution of hydrochloric acid in methanol to each flask. To one flask of each pair of duplicates (representing the extracted *Standard preparation* and the extracted *Assay preparation*) add 1.0 mL of a 3 in 1000 solution of sodium nitrite in dilute methanol (1 in 2). To the second flask of each pair (constituting the blanks) add 1 mL of dilute methanol (1 in 2). Mix, and allow to stand for 30 minutes. Add 0.5 mL of ammonium sulfamate solution (1 in 20) to each flask, add methanol to volume, mix, and allow to stand for 10 minutes. Determine the absorbance of each solution in a 1-cm cell at the wavelength of maximum absorbance at about 390 nm, with a suitable spectrophotometer, relative to the absorbance of a mixture of methanol, chloroform, and water (5.4 : 3.6 : 1). Calculate the quantity, in mg, of $C_{33}H_{40}N_2O_9$ in the portion of Tablets taken by the formula:

$$0.01C(A - A_0)_U / (A - A_0)_S$$

in which C is the concentration, in µg per mL, of USP Reserpine RS in the *Standard preparation*, and the parenthetic expressions are the differences in absorbances of the nitrite-treated and blank solutions, respectively, from the *Assay preparation* (U) and the *Standard preparation* (S).

Assay for hydralazine hydrochloride—

Sodium acetate solution—Dissolve 27.2 g of sodium acetate trihydrate in 50 mL of water, bring to room temperature, and dilute with water to 100 mL.

Ferric ammonium sulfate solution—Dissolve 1.8 g of ferric ammonium sulfate in 4 mL of dilute hydrochloric acid (1 in 12), and dilute with water to 100 mL. Filter, and use the clear filtrate. Prepare fresh.

1,10-Phenanthroline solution—Shake 300 mg of 1,10-phenanthroline with 100 mL of water for 1 hour. Filter, and use the clear filtrate. Prepare fresh.

Standard preparation—Dissolve about 50 mg of USP Hydralazine Hydrochloride RS, accurately weighed, in water in a 100-mL volumetric flask, and dilute with water to volume. Pipet 10 mL of this solution into a 100-mL volumetric flask, dilute with water to volume, and mix.

Assay preparation—Weigh and finely powder not less than 20 Tablets. Transfer to a 200-mL volumetric flask an accurately weighed portion of the powder, equivalent to about 100 mg of hydralazine hydrochloride, add 100 mL of water, and shake by mechanical means for 30 minutes. Dilute with water to volume, mix, and filter through paper, discarding the first 15 mL of the filtrate. Pipet 10 mL of the clear filtrate into a 100-mL volumetric flask, and dilute with water to volume.

Procedure—Pipet 10 mL each of the *Assay preparation*, the *Standard preparation*, and water to provide the blank, into separate, 200-mL volumetric flasks. To each flask add 5 mL of acetic acid solution (12 in 100), 5 mL of *Sodium acetate solution*, 2 mL of *1,10-Phenanthroline solution*, and 1 mL of *Ferric ammonium sulfate solution*, mix, and allow to stand in the dark for 30 minutes. Dilute with water to volume, and mix. Concomitantly determine the absorbances of both solutions in 1-cm cells at the wavelength of maximum absorbance at about 510 nm, with a suitable spectrophotometer, against the blank. Calculate the quantity, in mg, of $C_8H_8N_4 \cdot HCl$ in the portion of Tablets taken by the formula:

$$2C(A_U / A_S)$$

in which C is the concentration, in µg per mL, of USP Hydralazine Hydrochloride RS in the *Standard preparation*, and A_U and A_S are the absorbances of the solutions from the *Assay preparation* and the *Standard preparation*, respectively.

Assay for hydrochlorothiazide—

Methanolic sodium hydroxide solution—Dissolve 40 g of sodium hydroxide in 125 mL of water, cool, and dilute with methanol to 500 mL. Filter before use.

Column preparation—Weigh about 10 g of sulfonic acid cation exchange resin into a 250-mL beaker. Add 75 mL of methanol, and stir the mixture with a magnetic stirrer for 30 minutes. Place a glass wool plug at the lower end of a glass chromatographic column (15 mm × 45-cm long), equipped with a stopcock to regulate the eluant flow. Transfer and pack the slurry in portions into the prepared column to a height of 10 cm. If air is trapped, remove by tapping, stirring, or back-flushing the column. Place a glass wool plug on top of the resin bed after packing. Wash the resin with consecutive 100-mL portions of a 1 in 5 solution of hydrochloric acid in methanol, and of methanol, then of *Methanolic sodium hydroxide solution* and of methanol, respectively, using a flow rate of approximately 4 mL per minute. Wash the sodium form of the resin with 150 mL of a 1 in 5 solution of hydrochloric acid in methanol, followed by not less than 100 mL of methanol. The UV spectrum of the last few mL of the methanol washing conforms to that of the methanol.

Standard preparation—Mix about 40 mg of USP Hydrochlorothiazide RS, accurately weighed, with 4 mL of water in a 200-mL volumetric flask. Add 150 mL of methanol, warm gently on a steam bath for a few minutes, and shake by mechanical means for 20 minutes. Dilute with methanol to volume, and mix.

Assay preparation—Weigh and finely powder not less than 20 Tablets. Transfer an accurately weighed portion of the powder, equivalent to about 20 mg of hydrochlorothiazide, to a 100-mL volumetric flask. Add 2 mL of water, mix, and add 75 mL of methanol. Warm gently on a steam bath for a few minutes, and shake by mechanical means for 20 minutes. Dilute with methanol to volume, and mix. Centrifuge a portion of the mixture, and use the clear solution as the *Assay preparation*.

Procedure—Keeping the column stopcocks closed, pipet 4 mL of the clear *Assay preparation* on the top of the resin bed of 1 column, and pipet 4 mL of the *Standard preparation* on the top of the second column. Place a 100-mL volumetric flask beneath each of the columns, and collect the eluate. Adjust the flow rate to approximately 2 mL per minute, and allow the solution to flow until it just disappears into the upper glass wool plug. Close the stopcock, carefully add 25 mL of methanol, and further elute each column with the same flow rate as before. Repeat with two additional 25-mL portions of methanol. Dilute the contents of each flask with methanol to volume. Concomitantly determine the absorbances of both solutions at the wavelength of maximum absorbance at about 271 nm, with a suitable spectrophotometer, using methanol as the blank. Calculate the quantity, in mg, of $C_7H_8ClN_3O_4S_2$ in the portion of Tablets taken by the formula:

$$0.1C(A_U/A_S)$$

in which C is the concentration, in µg per mL, of USP Hydrochlorothiazide RS in the *Standard preparation,* and A_U and A_S are the absorbances of the solution from the *Assay preparation* and the *Standard preparation,* respectively.

Reserpine and Hydrochlorothiazide Tablets

» Reserpine and Hydrochlorothiazide Tablets contain not less than 90.0 percent and not more than 110.0 percent of the labeled amount of reserpine ($C_{33}H_{40}N_2O_9$), and not less than 93.0 percent and not more than 107.0 percent of the labeled amount of hydrochlorothiazide ($C_7H_8ClN_3O_4S_2$).

Packaging and storage—Preserve in tight, light-resistant containers.

USP Reference standards ⟨11⟩—*USP Reserpine RS. USP Hydrochlorothiazide RS. USP Benzothiadiazine Related Compound A RS.*

Identification—

A: Transfer a quantity of powdered Tablets, equivalent to 1 mg of reserpine, to a stoppered, 50-mL centrifuge tube. Add 20 mL of citric acid solution (1 in 50), and shake until the powder is suspended. Extract the mixture with two 20-mL portions of chloroform, centrifuge, and withdraw the chloroform, filtering each extract through a pledget of cotton into a 50-mL volumetric flask. Dilute with chloroform to volume, and mix: the UV absorption spectrum of the solution exhibits maxima and minima at the same wavelengths as that of a similar solution of USP Reserpine RS, concomitantly measured (*presence of reserpine*).

B: Transfer a quantity of powdered Tablets, equivalent to about 50 mg of hydrochlorothiazide, to a test tube containing 10 mL of acetone, agitate for 5 minutes, and centrifuge. Use the clear supernatant as the Test solution. Separately apply 10 µL each of the Test solution and a Standard solution of USP Hydrochlorothiazide RS in acetone containing 5 mg per mL to a thin-layer chromatographic plate (see *Chromatography* ⟨621⟩) coated with a 0.25-mm layer of chromatographic silica gel mixture and previously washed with methanol. Develop the chromatogram in a solvent system consisting of a mixture of ethyl acetate and isopropyl alcohol (17 : 3) until the solvent front has moved about three-fourths of the length of the plate. Remove the plate from the chamber, air-dry, and examine under short-wavelength UV light: the R_F value of the principal spot in the chromatogram of the Test solution corresponds to that obtained from the Standard solution (*presence of hydrochlorothiazide*).

Dissolution ⟨711⟩—

Medium: mixture of 0.1 N hydrochloric acid and *n*-propyl alcohol (3 : 2); 900 mL.

Apparatus 2: 50 rpm.

Times: 45 minutes, 60 minutes.

Determination of dissolved reserpine—

PHOSPHATE BUFFER—Dissolve 6.8 g of monobasic potassium phosphate in 1 L of water, mix thoroughly, and adjust with phosphoric acid to a pH of 3.0 ± 0.05.

MOBILE PHASE—Prepare a filtered and degassed mixture of *Phosphate buffer* and acetonitrile (65 : 35). Make adjustments if necessary (see *System Suitability* under *Chromatography* ⟨621⟩).

STANDARD STOCK PREPARATION—Dissolve an accurately weighed quantity of USP Reserpine RS in *Medium*, and dilute quantitatively and stepwise if necessary, with *Medium* to obtain a solution having a known concentration of about 0.14 µg per mL.

STANDARD PREPARATION—Transfer 8.0 mL of *Standard stock preparation* to a 25-mL volumetric flask. Dilute with *Mobile phase* to volume, and mix to obtain a solution having a known concentration of about 0.044 µg per mL.

TEST PREPARATION—Filter a portion of the solution under test, and transfer 8.0 mL to a 25-mL volumetric flask. Dilute with *Mobile phase* to volume, and mix.

CHROMATOGRAPHIC SYSTEM (see *Chromatography* ⟨621⟩)—The liquid chromatograph is equipped with a fluorescence detector (excitation at 270 nm and detection at 360 nm) and a 4.6-mm × 15-cm column that contains packing L11. The flow rate is about 2.0 mL per minute. Chromatograph the *Standard preparation,* and record the peak responses as directed for *Procedure*: the capacity factor, k', is not less than 2.0; the column efficiency is not less than 3000 theoretical plates; the tailing factor is not more than 2.0; and the relative standard deviation for replicate injections is not more than 2.0%.

PROCEDURE—Separately inject equal volumes (about 100 µL) of the *Standard preparation* and the *Assay preparation* into the chromatograph, record the chromatograms, and measure the responses for the reserpine peak. Calculate the quantity, in mg, of reserpine ($C_{33}H_{40}N_2O_9$) dissolved by the formula:

$$2813C(r_U/r_S)$$

in which C is the concentration, in mg per mL, of USP Reserpine RS in the *Standard preparation;* and r_U and r_S are the peak responses obtained from the *Test preparation* and the *Standard preparation,* respectively.

Determination of dissolved hydrochlorothiazide—

STANDARD PREPARATION—Dissolve about 27 mg of USP Hydrochlorothiazide RS, accurately weighed, in a 50-mL volumetric flask containing 5 mL of methanol, dilute with *Dissolution Medium* to volume, and mix. Pipet 2 mL of this solution into a 100-mL volumetric flask, dilute with *Dissolution Medium* to volume, and mix.

PROCEDURE—Determine the amount of hydrochlorothiazide ($C_7H_8ClN_3O_4S_2$) dissolved from UV absorption, at the wavelength of maximum absorbance at about 271 nm, on filtered portions of the solution under test, suitably diluted with *Dissolution Medium*, in comparison with the *Standard preparation.*

Tolerances—Not less than 80% (*Q*) of the labeled amount of $C_{33}H_{40}N_2O_9$ is dissolved in 45 minutes and not less than 80% (*Q*) of the labeled amount of $C_7H_8ClN_3O_4S_2$ is dissolved in 60 minutes.

Uniformity of dosage units ⟨905⟩: meet the requirements with respect to reserpine and to hydrochlorothiazide.

Procedure for content uniformity for reserpine—

STANDARD PREPARATION—Prepare as directed for *Standard preparation* under *Assay for reserpine*.

TEST SOLUTION—Weigh 1 Tablet, grind to a fine powder, and transfer to a stoppered, 50-mL centrifuge tube. Add 25.0 mL of a mixture of chloroform and methanol solution (1 : 1), shake by mechanical means for 15 minutes, and centrifuge. Pipet 4 mL of the clear supernatant into a 100-mL volumetric flask, dilute with the chloroform-methanol solution to volume, and mix.

PROCEDURE—Proceed as directed for *Procedure* under *Assay for reserpine*. Calculate the quantity, in mg, of $C_{33}H_{40}N_2O_9$, in the Tablet taken by the formula:

$$(W_t / W_U)(TC/D)(I_U / I_S)$$

in which W_t is the weight, in mg, of the Tablet; W_U is the weight, in mg, in the portion of Tablet taken; T is the labeled quantity, in mg, of reserpine in the Tablet; C is the concentration, in µg per mL, of USP Reserpine RS in the *Standard preparation*; D is the concentration, in µg per mL, of reserpine in the *Test solution*, based upon the labeled quantity per Tablet and the extent of dilution; and I_U and I_S are the fluorescence intensities of the solutions from the *Test solution* and the *Standard preparation*, respectively.

Procedure for content uniformity for hydrochlorothiazide—

STANDARD PREPARATION—Prepare as directed for *Standard preparation* under *Assay for hydrochlorothiazide*.

TEST SOLUTION—Transfer 1 Tablet to a 250-mL volumetric flask, add 150 mL of 0.1 N sodium hydroxide, and sonicate, swirling the flask intermittently, until the tablet is dissolved. Dilute with 0.1 N sodium hydroxide to volume, mix, and filter, discarding the first 15 mL of the filtrate. Dilute a portion of the clear filtrate quantitatively and stepwise with 0.1 N sodium hydroxide to obtain a solution having a concentration of about 10 µg of hydrochlorothiazide per mL.

PROCEDURE—Proceed as directed for *Procedure* under *Assay for hydrochlorothiazide*. Calculate the quantity, in mg, of $C_7H_8ClN_3O_4S_2$, in the Tablet taken by the formula:

$$(TC/D)(A_U / A_S)$$

in which T is the labeled quantity, in mg, of hydrochlorothiazide in the Tablet; C is the concentration, in µg per mL, of USP Hydrochlorothiazide RS in the *Standard preparation*; D is the concentration, in µg per mL, of hydrochlorothiazide in the *Test solution*, based upon the labeled quantity per Tablet and the extent of dilution; and A_U and A_S are the absorbances of the solutions from the *Test solution* and the *Standard preparation*, respectively.

Diazotizable substances—

*Standard solution—*Accurately weigh 25 mg of USP Benzothiadiazine Related Compound A RS, dissolve in 5 mL of methanol contained in a 100-mL volumetric flask, dilute with water to volume, and mix. Pipet 4 mL of this solution into a 100-mL volumetric flask, dilute with water to volume, and mix.

*Test solution—*Transfer a portion of finely powdered Tablets, accurately weighed and equivalent to about 100 mg of hydrochlorothiazide, to a 100-mL volumetric flask, and add 20 mL of methanol and 20 mL of water. Shake continuously for 5 to 10 minutes, dilute with water to volume, mix, and filter. Use the filtrate as the *Test solution*.

*Procedure—*Pipet 5 mL each of the *Standard solution* and the *Test solution* into separate, 50-mL volumetric flasks. Pipet 5 mL of water into a third 50-mL volumetric flask to provide the blank. To each flask add 1 mL of freshly prepared sodium nitrite solution (1 in 100) and 5 mL of dilute hydrochloric acid (1 in 12), and allow to stand for 5 minutes. Add 2 mL of ammonium sulfamate solution (1 in 50), shake vigorously, allow to stand for 5 minutes, then add 2 mL of freshly prepared disodium chromotropate solution (1 in 100) and 10 mL of sodium acetate TS. Dilute with water to volume, and mix. Concomitantly determine the absorbances of the solutions from the *Standard solution* and the *Test solution* in 1-cm cells at the wavelength of maximum absorbance at about 500 nm, with a suitable spectrophotometer, against the blank. The absorbance of the solution from the *Test solution* does not exceed that of the solution from the *Standard solution*, corresponding to not more than 1.0% of diazotizable substances.

Assay for reserpine—

*Standard preparation—*Dissolve about 25 mg of USP Reserpine RS, accurately weighed, in 1 mL of chloroform contained in a 50-mL volumetric flask, dilute with methanol to volume, and mix. Dilute a portion of this solution quantitatively and stepwise with chloroform and methanol solution (1 : 1) to obtain a solution having a known concentration of about 0.2 µg of reserpine per mL.

*Assay preparation—*Weigh and finely powder not fewer than 20 Tablets. Transfer to a stoppered, 50-mL centrifuge tube an accurately weighed portion of the powder, equivalent to about 1 mg of reserpine, add 25.0 mL of a mixture of chloroform and methanol solution (1 : 1), shake by mechanical means for 15 minutes, and centrifuge. Dilute a portion of the clear supernatant quantitatively and stepwise with a mixture of chloroform and methanol solution (1 : 1) to obtain a solution having a concentration of about 0.2 µg of reserpine per mL.

*Procedure—*Separately transfer 5.0 mL of the *Assay preparation*, 5.0 mL of the *Standard preparation*, and 5.0 mL of a mixture of chloroform and methanol solution (1 : 1) to provide the reagent blank, respectively, to three 25-mL volumetric flasks. To each flask add 0.5 mL of hydrochloric acid, 1.0 mL of a 3 in 1000 solution of sodium nitrite in dilute methanol (1 in 2), mix, and allow to stand for 30 minutes. Add 1 mL of ammonium sulfamate solution (1 in 20) to each flask, add chloroform and methanol solution (1 : 1) to volume, mix, and allow to stand for 10 minutes. Concomitantly determine the fluorescence intensities of the solutions in a suitable spectrophotometer arranged to deliver activation radiation at 405 nm and to measure the resultant fluorescence at the emission wavelength of about 500 nm. Calculate the quantity, in mg, of $C_{33}H_{40}N_2O_9$ in the portion of Tablets taken by the formula:

$$5C(I_U / I_S)$$

in which C is the concentration, in µg per mL, of USP Reserpine RS in the *Standard preparation*, and I_U and I_S are the fluorescence intensities of the solutions from the *Assay preparation* and the *Standard preparation*, respectively.

Assay for hydrochlorothiazide—

*Standard preparation—*Dissolve an accurately weighed quantity of USP Hydrochlorothiazide RS in 0.1 N sodium hydroxide, and dilute quantitatively and stepwise with 0.1 N sodium hydroxide to obtain a solution having a known concentration of about 10 µg of hydrochlorothiazide per mL. Use a freshly prepared solution.

*Assay preparation—*Weigh and finely powder not fewer than 20 Tablets. Weigh accurately a portion of the powder, equivalent to about 50 mg of hydrochlorothiazide, and transfer to a 500-mL volumetric flask. Add 200 mL of 0.1 N sodium hydroxide, shake by mechanical means for 15 minutes, dilute with the same solvent to volume, and mix. Filter a portion of the solution through paper, discarding the first 15 mL of the filtrate, and transfer 10.0 mL of the clear filtrate to a 100-mL volumetric flask. Dilute with 0.1 N sodium hydroxide to volume, and mix.

*Procedure—*Concomitantly determine the absorbances of the *Standard preparation* and the *Assay preparation* in 1-cm cells at the wavelength of maximum absorbance, at about 274 nm, with a suitable spectrophotometer, using 0.1 N sodium hydroxide as the blank. Calculate the quantity, in mg, of $C_7H_8ClN_3O_4S_2$ in the portion of Tablets taken by the formula:

$$5C(A_U / A_S)$$

in which C is the concentration, in µg per mL, of USP Hydrochlorothiazide RS in the *Standard preparation*, and A_U and A_S are the absorbances of the solutions from the *Assay preparation* and the *Standard preparation*, respectively.

Resorcinol

$C_6H_6O_2$ 110.11
1,3-Benzenediol
Resorcinol [108-46-3].

» Resorcinol contains not less than 99.0 percent and not more than 100.5 percent of $C_6H_6O_2$, calculated on the dried basis.

Packaging and storage—Preserve in well-closed, light-resistant containers.
USP Reference standards ⟨11⟩—*USP Resorcinol RS*.
Identification—
  A: *Infrared Absorption* ⟨197K⟩—[NOTE—If necessary to recrystallize, dissolve in dehydrated alcohol.]
  B: Dissolve 100 mg in 2 mL of 1 N sodium hydroxide, add 1 drop of chloroform, and heat the mixture: an intense crimson color is produced. Then add a slight excess of hydrochloric acid: the color changes to pale yellow.
  C: To 10 mL of a solution (1 in 100) add 1 drop of ferric chloride TS: a blue-violet color is produced, and it fades slowly.
Melting range ⟨741⟩: between 109° and 111°.
Loss on drying ⟨731⟩—Dry it over silica gel for 4 hours: it loses not more than 1.0% of its weight.
Residue on ignition ⟨281⟩: not more than 0.05%.
Phenol—Heat gently a solution (1 in 20): the odor of phenol is not perceptible.
Catechol—To 10 mL of a solution (1 in 20) previously mixed with 2 drops of 1 N acetic acid add 0.5 mL of lead acetate TS: no turbidity is produced.
Ordinary impurities ⟨466⟩—
  Test solution: methanol.
  Standard solution: methanol.
  Eluant: a mixture of hexanes and ethyl acetate (70 : 30).
  Visualization: 17 and then 1.
  Application volume: 10 μL.
  Limits: not more than 1.0%.
Organic volatile impurities, *Method IV* ⟨467⟩: meets the requirements.

(Official until July 1, 2008)
Assay—Dissolve about 1.5 g of Resorcinol, accurately weighed, in water to make 500.0 mL. Transfer to an iodine flask 25.0 mL of the resulting solution, add 50.0 mL of 0.1 N bromine VS, dilute with 50 mL of water, add 5 mL of hydrochloric acid, and at once insert the stopper in the flask. Shake for 1 minute, allow to stand for 2 minutes, and add 10 mL of potassium iodide TS while slightly loosening the stopper. Shake thoroughly, allow to stand for 5 minutes, remove the stopper, and rinse it and the neck of the flask with 20 mL of water into the flask. Titrate the liberated iodine with 0.1 N sodium thiosulfate VS, adding starch TS as the endpoint is approached. Perform a blank determination. From the volume of 0.1 N sodium thiosulfate VS used, calculate the volume, in mL, of 0.1 N bromine VS consumed by the resorcinol. Each mL of 0.1 N bromine is equivalent to 1.835 mg of $C_6H_6O_2$.

Compound Resorcinol Ointment

» Prepare Compound Resorcinol Ointment as follows:

Resorcinol	60 g
Zinc Oxide	60 g
Bismuth Subnitrate	60 g
Juniper Tar	20 g
Yellow Wax	100 g
Petrolatum	290 g
Lanolin	280 g
Glycerin	130 g
To make	1000 g

Melt the Yellow Wax and the Lanolin in a dish on a steam bath. Triturate the Zinc Oxide and the Bismuth Subnitrate with the Petrolatum until smooth, and add it to the melted mixture. Dissolve the Resorcinol in the Glycerin, incorporate the solution with the warm mixture just prepared, then add the Juniper Tar, and stir the Ointment until it congeals.

Packaging and storage—Preserve in tight containers, and avoid prolonged exposure to temperatures exceeding 30°.

Resorcinol and Sulfur Topical Suspension

Former monograph title: Resorcinol and Sulfur Lotion

» Resorcinol and Sulfur Topical Suspension is Resorcinol and Sulfur in a suitable hydroalcoholic vehicle. It contains not less than 90.0 percent and not more than 110.0 percent of the labeled amount of resorcinol ($C_6H_6O_2$) and not less than 95.0 percent and not more than 110.0 percent of the labeled amount of sulfur (S).

Packaging and storage—Preserve in tight containers.
USP Reference standards ⟨11⟩—*USP Resorcinol RS*.
Identification—
  A: Transfer a quantity of Topical Suspension, equivalent to about 20 mg of resorcinol, to a 15-mL centrifuge tube, add 5 mL of 5 N sodium hydroxide, mix, and centrifuge the mixture for 5 minutes. Decant the supernatant into a test tube, and retain the residue for *Identification* test B. Add 0.5 mL of chloroform, mix, and heat on a steam bath: an intense crimson color is produced. Add a slight excess of hydrochloric acid: the color changes to pale yellow *(presence of resorcinol)*.
  B: Place a small portion of the residue from the centrifuge tube in *Identification* test A on the tip of a spatula, and burn it: sulfur dioxide, which turns moistened starch-iodate paper blue, is formed *(presence of sulfur)*.
Alcohol content ⟨611⟩—Determine by the gas-liquid chromatographic method, acetone being used as the internal standard: it contains between 90.0% and 110.0% of the labeled amount of C_2H_5OH.
Assay for resorcinol—
  Mobile phase—Prepare a suitable degassed solution of water, acetonitrile, and methanol (about 55 : 7 : 6) such that the retention times of resorcinol and caffeine are about 3 minutes and 4 minutes, respectively.
  Internal standard solution—Dissolve about 140 mg of caffeine in 2 mL of chloroform, add methanol to make 100 mL, and mix.
  Standard preparation—Transfer 50 mg of USP Resorcinol RS, accurately weighed, to a 25-mL volumetric flask, dilute with methanol to volume, and mix. Transfer 10.0 mL of this solution and 5.0 mL of *Internal standard solution* to a 100-mL volumetric flask, dilute with methanol to volume, and mix.
  Assay preparation—Transfer an accurately weighed portion of Topical Suspension, equivalent to about 20 mg of resorcinol, to a 150-mL beaker. Add 40 mL of methanol and 5.0 mL of *Internal standard solution*, and heat on a steam bath for 5 minutes. Cool the mixture to room temperature, and decant the liquid into a 100-mL volumetric flask. Wash the residue in the beaker by adding 20 mL of methanol to the beaker. Heat on a steam bath for 5 minutes, cool

the mixture to room temperature, and decant the liquid into the volumetric flask. Repeat the washing, heating, cooling, and decanting. Dilute the contents of the volumetric flask with methanol to volume, and mix.

Procedure—Introduce equal volumes (about 10 µL) of the *Assay preparation* and the *Standard preparation* into a high-pressure liquid chromatograph (see *Chromatography* ⟨621⟩), operated at room temperature, by means of a suitable microsyringe or sampling valve, adjusting the specimen size and other operating parameters such that the peak obtained from the *Standard preparation* is about 0.6 full scale. Typically, the apparatus is fitted with a 4-mm × 30-cm column containing packing L1 and is equipped with an UV detector capable of monitoring absorption at 280 nm, and a suitable recorder. In a suitable chromatogram the coefficient of variation for five replicate injections of the *Standard preparation* is not more than 3.0%. Measure the peak responses at equivalent retention times, obtained from the *Assay preparation* and the *Standard preparation,* and calculate the quantity, in mg, of resorcinol ($C_6H_6O_2$) in the portion of Topical Suspension taken by the formula:

$$(100C)(R_U/R_S)$$

in which *C* is the concentration, in mg per mL, of USP Resorcinol RS in the *Standard preparation;* and R_U and R_S are the ratios of the responses of the resorcinol and caffeine peaks obtained from the *Assay preparation* and the *Standard preparation,* respectively.

Assay for sulfur—Transfer an accurately weighed portion of Topical Suspension, equivalent to about 85 mg of sulfur, to a suitable flask, add 40 mL of sodium sulfite solution (1 in 20), a few drops of antifoam, and a few boiling chips, and boil under a reflux condenser for 1 hour. Cool to room temperature, add 10 mL of formaldehyde solution and 6 mL of 6 N acetic acid, and dilute with water to 150 mL. Add 3 mL of starch TS, and titrate with 0.1 N iodine VS until a permanent blue color is produced. Each mL of 0.1 N iodine is equivalent to 3.206 mg of sulfur (S).

Resorcinol Monoacetate

$C_8H_8O_3$ 152.15
1,3-Benzenediol, monoacetate.
Resorcinol monoacetate   [*102-29-4*].

Packaging and storage—Preserve in tight, light-resistant containers.

Identification—

A: Fuse 3 drops with about 300 mg of phthalic anhydride and about 50 mg of zinc chloride: a small portion of the fused mixture when dissolved in 10 mL of 1 N sodium hydroxide produces an intense yellow-green fluorescence typical of fluorescein.

B: Dissolve 0.5 mL in 3 mL of alcohol, add 3 drops of sulfuric acid, and boil: ethyl acetate, recognizable by its odor, is evolved.

Specific gravity ⟨841⟩:   between 1.203 and 1.207.

Acidity—A solution of 10 mL of Resorcinol Monoacetate in 20 mL of benzene, when shaken with 100 mL of water, requires not more than 0.50 mL of 0.10 N sodium hydroxide for neutralization, methyl orange TS being used as the indicator.

Loss on drying ⟨731⟩—Dry it on a steam bath for 1 hour: it loses not more than 2.5% of its weight.

Residue on ignition ⟨281⟩:   not more than 0.1%.

Organic volatile impurities, *Method I* ⟨467⟩: meets the requirements.

(Official until July 1, 2008)

Ribavirin

$C_8H_{12}N_4O_5$ 244.20
1*H*-1,2,4-Triazole-3-carboxamide, 1-*β*-D-ribofuranosyl-.
1-*β*-D-Ribofuranosyl-1*H*-1,2,4-triazole-3-carboxamide   [*36791-04-5*].

» Ribavirin contains not less than 98.9 percent and not more than 101.5 percent of $C_8H_{12}N_4O_5$, calculated on the dried basis.

Packaging and storage—Preserve in tight containers.
USP Reference standards ⟨11⟩—*USP Ribavirin RS.*
Identification—
  A: *Infrared Absorption* ⟨197K⟩.
  B: *Thin-Layer Chromatographic Identification Test* ⟨201⟩—
  Test solution: 10 mg per mL.
  Developing solvent system: a mixture of acetonitrile and 0.1 M ammonium chloride (9 : 2).
  Spray reagent—Mix 0.5 mL of anisaldehyde, 0.5 mL of sulfuric acid, 0.1 mL of glacial acetic acid, and 9 mL of alcohol.
  Procedure—Proceed as directed in the chapter. Allow the plate to air-dry for about 15 minutes, spray with *Spray reagent*, heat the plate at 110° for 30 minutes, and locate the spots on the plate by examining the plate in daylight.
Specific rotation ⟨781S⟩:   between −33.5° and −37.0° (*t* = 20°).
  Test solution: 10 mg per mL, in water.
pH ⟨791⟩:   between 4.0 and 6.5, in a solution (1 in 50), to each 50 mL of which has been added 0.2 mL of a saturated potassium chloride solution.
Loss on drying ⟨731⟩:   Dry it at 105° for 5 hours: it loses not more than 0.5% of its weight.
Residue on ignition ⟨281⟩:   not more than 0.25%.
Heavy metals, *Method II* ⟨231⟩:   0.001%.
Chromatographic purity—
  Mobile phase, Standard preparation, Test solution, and *Chromatographic system*—Prepare as directed in the *Assay*.
  Procedure—Inject about 10 µL of the *Test solution* into the chromatograph, record the chromatogram, and measure the responses of all the peaks, except that of the solvent peak. Calculate the percentage of each peak, other than that of the solvent peak and the main ribavirin peak, by the formula:

$$100r_i/r_t$$

in which r_i is the response of the individual peak, and r_t is the sum of the responses of all the peaks in the chromatogram: not more than 0.25% of any individual peak is found, and the sum of all such peaks does not exceed 1.0%.
Assay—
  Mobile phase—Adjust water with sulfuric acid to a pH of 2.5 ± 0.1. Filter through a suitable filter of 0.5-µm or finer porosity, and degas. Make adjustments if necessary (see *System Suitability* under *Chromatography* ⟨621⟩).
  Standard preparation—Dissolve an accurately weighed quantity of USP Ribavirin RS quantitatively in *Mobile phase* to obtain a solution having a known concentration of about 0.025 mg per mL.
  Test solution—Transfer about 50 mg of Ribavirin, accurately weighed, to a 100-mL volumetric flask, add about 50 mL of *Mobile phase*, swirl to dissolve, dilute with *Mobile phase* to volume, and mix.
  Assay preparation—Transfer 5.0 mL of the *Test solution* to a 100-mL volumetric flask, dilute with *Mobile phase* to volume, and mix.
  Chromatographic system (see *Chromatography* ⟨621⟩)—The liquid chromatograph is equipped with a 207-nm detector and a 7.8-

mm × 10-cm column that contains packing L17 and is operated at 65 ± 0.5°. The flow rate is about 1 mL per minute. Chromatograph the *Standard preparation,* and record the peak responses as directed for *Procedure*: the tailing factor for the ribavirin peak is not less than 0.7 and not more than 1.5, and the relative standard deviation for replicate injections is not more than 0.5%.

Procedure—Separately inject equal volumes (about 10 µL) of the *Standard preparation* and the *Assay preparation* into the chromatograph, record the chromatograms, and measure the peak area responses for the major peaks. Calculate the quantity, in mg, of $C_8H_{12}N_4O_5$ in the portion of Ribavirin taken by the formula:

$$2000C(r_U / r_S)$$

in which C is the concentration, in mg per mL, of USP Ribavirin RS in the *Standard preparation,* and r_U and r_S are the ribavirin peak area responses obtained from the *Assay preparation* and the *Standard preparation,* respectively.

Ribavirin for Inhalation Solution

» Ribavirin for Inhalation Solution is a sterile, freeze-dried form of ribavirin. When constituted as directed in the labeling, the inhalation solution so obtained contains not less than 95.0 percent and not more than 105.0 percent of the labeled amount of ribavirin ($C_8H_{12}N_4O_5$).

Packaging and storage—Preserve in tight containers, in a dry place at controlled room temperature.
Labeling—The labeling indicates that Ribavirin for Inhalation Solution must be constituted with a measured volume of Sterile Water for Injection or with Sterile Water for Inhalation containing no preservatives, and that the constituted solution is to be administered only by a small-particle aerosol generator.
USP Reference standards ⟨11⟩—*USP Ribavirin RS.*
Identification—It responds to the *Identification* tests under *Ribavirin.*
Sterility ⟨71⟩—It meets the requirements when tested as directed for *Membrane Filtration* under *Test for Sterility of the Product to be Examined.*
pH ⟨791⟩: between 4.0 and 6.5, in the solution constituted as directed in the labeling, to each 50 mL of which has been added 0.2 mL of a saturated potassium chloride solution.
Chromatographic purity—
 Mobile phase, Standard preparation, Test solution, and *Chromatographic system*—Prepare as directed in the *Assay.*
 Procedure—Inject about 10 µL of the *Test solution* into the chromatograph, record the chromatogram, and measure the responses of all the peaks, except that of the solvent peak. Calculate the percentage of each peak, other than that of the ribavirin peak, in the chromatogram of the *Test solution* by the formula:

$$100 r_i / r_t$$

in which r_i is the response of the individual peak, and r_t is the sum of the responses of all the peaks in the chromatogram: not more than 0.25% of any individual peak is found, and the sum of all such peaks does not exceed 1.0%.
Other requirements—It meets the requirements for *Specific rotation, Loss on drying, Residue on ignition,* and *Heavy metals* under *Ribavirin.*
Assay—
 Mobile phase, Standard preparation, and *Chromatographic system*—Prepare as directed in the *Assay* under *Ribavirin.*
 Test solution—Constitute Ribavirin for Inhalation Solution as directed in the labeling, using an accurately measured volume of diluent. Transfer an accurately measured volume of the constituted inhalation solution, equivalent to about 100 mg of ribavirin, to a 200-mL volumetric flask, dilute with *Mobile phase* to volume, and mix.
 Assay preparation—Transfer 5.0 mL of the *Test solution* to a 100-mL volumetric flask, dilute with *Mobile phase* to volume, and mix.

Procedure—Proceed as directed for *Procedure* in the *Assay* under *Ribavirin.* Calculate the quantity, in mg, of ribavirin ($C_8H_{12}N_4O_5$) in each mL of the constituted Inhalation Solution taken by the formula:

$$4000(C / V)(r_U / r_S)$$

in which V is the volume, in mL, of constituted Inhalation Solution taken, and the other terms are as defined therein.

Riboflavin

$C_{17}H_{20}N_4O_6$ 376.36
Riboflavine.
Riboflavine   [83-88-5].

» Riboflavin contains not less than 98.0 percent and not more than 102.0 percent of $C_{17}H_{20}N_4O_6$, calculated on the dried basis.

Packaging and storage—Preserve in tight, light-resistant containers.
USP Reference standards ⟨11⟩—*USP Riboflavin RS.*
Identification—A solution of 1 mg in 100 mL of water is pale greenish yellow by transmitted light, and has an intense yellowish-green fluorescence that disappears upon the addition of mineral acids or alkalies.
Specific rotation ⟨781S⟩: between −115° and −135°.
 Test solution: 5 mg per mL, in 0.05 M sodium hydroxide free from carbonate. Measure the specific rotation within 30 minutes of preparation.
Loss on drying ⟨731⟩—Dry about 500 mg at 105° for 2 hours: it loses not more than 1.5% of its weight.
Residue on ignition ⟨281⟩: not more than 0.3%.
Limit of lumiflavin—Prepare alcohol-free chloroform just prior to use, as follows. Shake 20 mL of chloroform gently but thoroughly with 20 mL of water for 3 minutes, draw off the chloroform layer, and wash twice more with 20-mL portions of water. Finally, filter the chloroform through a dry filter paper, shake it for 5 minutes with 5 g of powdered anhydrous sodium sulfate, allow the mixture to stand for 2 hours, and decant or filter the clear chloroform. Shake 25 mg of Riboflavin with 10 mL of the alcohol-free chloroform for 5 minutes, and filter: the absorbance of the filtrate, determined in 1-cm cells at a wavelength of 440 nm, with a suitable spectrophotometer, alcohol-free chloroform being used as the blank, does not exceed 0.025.
Organic volatile impurities, Method IV ⟨467⟩: meets the requirements.

(Official until July 1, 2008)
Assay—[NOTE—Conduct the entire procedure without exposure to direct sunlight.] Place about 50 mg of Riboflavin, accurately weighed, in a 1000-mL volumetric flask containing about 50 mL of water. Add 5 mL of 6 N acetic acid and sufficient water to make about 800 mL. Heat on a steam bath, protected from light, with frequent agitation until dissolved. Cool to about 25°, dilute with water to volume, and mix. Dilute this solution quantitatively and stepwise with water to bring it within the operating sensitivity of the fluorometer used. In the same manner, prepare a Standard solution to contain, in each mL, an accurately weighed quantity, of USP Riboflavin RS, equivalent to that of the Riboflavin solution prepared as directed above, and measure the intensity of its fluorescence in a fluorometer at about 530 nm. (An excitation wavelength of about 444 nm is preferable.) Immediately after the reading, add to the solution about 10 mg of sodium hydrosulfite, stirring with a glass

rod until dissolved, and at once measure the fluorescence again. The difference between the two readings represents the intensity of the fluorescence due to the Standard. Similarly, measure the intensity of the fluorescence of the final solution of the Riboflavin being assayed at about 530 nm, before and after the addition of sodium hydrosulfite. Calculate the quantity, in µg per mL, of $C_{17}H_{20}N_4O_6$ in the final solution of Riboflavin taken by the formula:

$$C(I_U / I_S)$$

in which C is the concentration, in µg per mL, of USP Riboflavin RS in the final solution of the Standard, and I_U and I_S are the corrected fluorescence values observed for the solutions of the Riboflavin and Standard, respectively.

Riboflavin Injection

» Riboflavin Injection is a sterile solution of Riboflavin in Water for Injection. It contains not less than 95.0 percent and not more than 120.0 percent of the labeled amount of $C_{17}H_{20}N_4O_6$. It may contain niacinamide or other suitable solubilizers.

Packaging and storage—Preserve in light-resistant, in single-dose or in multiple-dose containers, preferably of Type I glass.
USP Reference standards ⟨11⟩—*USP Riboflavin RS. USP Endotoxin RS.*
Identification—It responds to the *Identification* test under *Riboflavin*.
Bacterial endotoxins ⟨85⟩—It contains not more than 7.1 USP Endotoxin Units per mg of riboflavin.
pH ⟨791⟩: between 4.5 and 7.0.
Other requirements—It meets the requirements under *Injections* ⟨1⟩.
Assay—Dilute an accurately measured volume of not less than 1 mL of Injection to make a solution containing approximately 0.1 µg of riboflavin per mL. Using this as the *Assay Preparation*, proceed as directed under *Riboflavin Assay* ⟨481⟩. Calculate the quantity, in mg, of $C_{17}H_{20}N_4O_6$ in each mL of the Injection taken by the formula:

$$C(A / B)$$

in which C is the concentration, in mg per mL, of $C_{17}H_{20}N_4O_6$ obtained for the *Assay Preparation*, A is the test specimen dilution volume, in mL, and B is the volume, in mL, of Injection taken.

Riboflavin Tablets

» Riboflavin Tablets contain not less than 95.0 percent and not more than 115.0 percent of the labeled amount of $C_{17}H_{20}N_4O_6$.

Packaging and storage—Preserve in tight, light-resistant containers.
USP Reference standards ⟨11⟩—*USP Riboflavin RS.*
Dissolution ⟨711⟩—
 Medium: water; 900 mL.
 Apparatus 2: 50 rpm.
 Time: 45 minutes.
 Procedure—Determine the amount of $C_{17}H_{20}N_4O_6$ dissolved, employing the procedure set forth in the *Assay for niacin or niacinamide, pyridoxine hydrochloride, riboflavin, and thiamine* under *Water-soluble Vitamins Tablets* using filtered portions of the solution under test, suitably diluted with *Dissolution Medium* if necessary, in comparison with a Standard solution having a known concentration of USP Riboflavin RS in the same medium.
 Tolerances—Not less than 75% (*Q*) of the labeled amount of $C_{17}H_{20}N_4O_6$ is dissolved in 45 minutes.

Uniformity of dosage units ⟨905⟩: meet the requirements.
Assay—Weigh and finely powder not fewer than 20 Tablets. Weigh accurately a portion of the powder, equivalent to about 20 mg of riboflavin, transfer to a 250-mL flask, and add 150 mL of 0.1 N hydrochloric acid. Shake vigorously, and wash down the sides of the flask with sufficient 0.1 N hydrochloric acid to ensure that the pH remains below 1.5 during the subsequent period of heating. Heat the mixture on a steam bath, with frequent agitation, until the riboflavin has dissolved, or in an autoclave at 121° for 30 minutes. Cool, adjust the mixture, with vigorous agitation, to a pH of 5 to 6 with 1 N sodium hydroxide, transfer to a 1000-mL volumetric flask, dilute with water to volume, and mix. If the solution is not clear, filter through paper known not to adsorb riboflavin. Dilute an aliquot of the clear solution quantitatively and stepwise with water to make a final measured volume that contains approximately 0.1 µg of riboflavin per mL. Using this as the *Assay Preparation*, proceed as directed under *Riboflavin Assay* ⟨481⟩. Calculate the quantity, in mg, of $C_{17}H_{20}N_4O_6$ in the portion of powdered Tablets taken by the formula:

$$200,000C / W$$

in which C is the concentration, in mg per mL, of $C_{17}H_{20}N_4O_6$ obtained for the *Assay Preparation*, and W is the weight, in mg, of powdered Tablets. Calculate the quantity, in mg, of $C_{17}H_{20}N_4O_6$ in each Tablet.

Riboflavin 5′-Phosphate Sodium

$C_{17}H_{20}N_4NaO_9P \cdot 2H_2O$ 514.36
Riboflavin 5′-(dihydrogen phosphate), monosodium salt, dihydrate.
Riboflavine 5′-(sodium hydrogen phosphate), dihydrate
Anhydrous   478.33   [130-40-5].

» Riboflavin 5′-Phosphate Sodium contains not less than the equivalent of 73.0 percent and not more than the equivalent of 79.0 percent of riboflavin ($C_{17}H_{20}N_4O_6$), calculated on the dried basis.

Packaging and storage—Preserve in tight, light-resistant containers.
USP Reference standards ⟨11⟩—*USP Riboflavin RS. USP Phosphated Riboflavin RS.*
Identification—
 A: Dissolve 1 mg in 100 mL of water: the solution is pale greenish yellow by transmitted light, and it exhibits an intense yellowish green fluorescence under long-wavelength UV light that disappears upon the addition of mineral acids or alkalies.
 B: To 0.5 g add 10 mL of nitric acid, evaporate the mixture on a water bath to dryness, ignite the residue until the carbon is removed, dissolve the residue in 5 mL of water, and filter: the filtrate so obtained responds to the tests for *Sodium* ⟨191⟩ and for *Phosphate* ⟨191⟩.
 Specific rotation ⟨781S⟩: between +37.0° and +42.0°, determined within 15 minutes.
  Test solution: 15 mg per mL, in 5 N hydrochloric acid.
pH ⟨791⟩: between 5.0 and 6.5, in a solution (1 in 100).
Loss on drying ⟨731⟩—Dry it in vacuum over phosphorus pentoxide at 100° for 5 hours: it loses not more than 7.5% of its weight.
Residue on ignition ⟨281⟩: not more than 25.0%.
Free phosphate—
 Acid molybdate solution—Dilute 25 mL of ammonium molybdate solution (7 in 100) with water to 200 mL. To this dilution add slowly 25 mL of 7.5 N sulfuric acid, and mix.

Ferrous sulfate solution—Just prior to use, prepare a 1 in 10 solution of ferrous sulfate in 0.15 N sulfuric acid.

Standard preparation—Prepare a solution in water containing 44.0 µg of monobasic potassium phosphate in each mL.

Test preparation—Transfer 300 mg of Riboflavin 5′-Phosphate Sodium to a 100-mL volumetric flask, dissolve in and dilute with water to volume, and mix.

Procedure—Transfer 10.0 mL each of the *Standard preparation* and the *Test preparation* to separate 50-mL conical flasks, add 10.0 mL of *Acid molybdate solution* and 5.0 mL of *Ferrous sulfate solution* to each flask, and mix. Concomitantly determine the absorbances of the solutions, in 1-cm cells, at the wavelength of maximum absorbance at about 700 nm, with a suitable spectrophotometer, using as the blank a mixture of 10.0 mL of water, 10.0 mL of *Acid molybdate solution*, and 5.0 mL of *Ferrous sulfate solution*: the absorbance of the solution from the *Test preparation* is not greater than that from the *Standard preparation* (1% as PO_4).

Free riboflavin and riboflavin diphosphates—[NOTE—Conduct this test so that all solutions are protected from actinic light at all stages, preferably by using low-actinic glassware.]

Mobile phase—Mix 850 mL of 0.054 M monobasic potassium phosphate with 150 mL of methanol, filter, and degas the solution. Make adjustments if necessary (see *System Suitability* under *Chromatography* ⟨621⟩).

Standard preparation—Transfer 60 mg of USP Riboflavin RS, accurately weighed, to a 250-mL volumetric flask, dissolve carefully in 1 mL of hydrochloric acid, dilute with water to volume, and mix. Pipet a 4-mL aliquot into a 100-mL volumetric flask, dilute with *Mobile phase* to volume, and mix.

Test preparation—Transfer 100.0 mg of Riboflavin 5′-Phosphate Sodium to a 100-mL volumetric flask, dissolve in 50 mL of water, dilute with *Mobile phase* to volume, and mix. Pipet 8 mL of this solution into a 50-mL volumetric flask, dilute with *Mobile phase* to volume, and mix.

System suitability preparation—Dissolve USP Phosphated Riboflavin RS in water to obtain a solution containing 2 mg per mL. Add an equal volume of *Mobile phase*, and mix. Dilute 8 mL of this solution with *Mobile phase* to 50 mL, and mix.

Chromatographic system (see *Chromatography* ⟨621⟩)—The liquid chromatograph is equipped with a fluorometric detector set at 440-nm excitation wavelength and provided with a 470-nm emission filter or set at about 530 nm for a fluorescence detector that uses a monochromator for emission wavelength selection, and a 3.9-mm × 30-cm column that contains packing L1. The flow rate is about 2.0 mL per minute. Chromatograph the *System suitability preparation*, and record the peak responses. The retention time for riboflavin 5′-monophosphate is about 20 to 25 minutes, and the approximate relative retention times for the components are as follows:

Riboflavin 3′4′-diphosphate:	0.23
Riboflavin 3′5′-diphosphate:	0.39
Riboflavin 4′5′-diphosphate:	0.58
Riboflavin 3′-monophosphate:	0.70
Riboflavin 4′-monophosphate:	0.87
Riboflavin 5′-monophosphate:	1.00
Riboflavin:	1.63

The resolution, R, between the peaks for riboflavin 4′-monophosphate and riboflavin 5′-monophosphate is not less than 1.0, and the relative standard deviation of the response for riboflavin 5′-monophosphate in replicate injections is not more than 1.5%.

Procedure—Separately inject equal volumes (about 100 µL) of the *Standard preparation*, the *Test preparation*, and the *System suitability preparation* into the chromatograph. Measure the peak responses obtained from the *Standard preparation* and the *Test preparation*, identifying the peaks to be measured in the chromatogram of the *Test preparation* by comparison of retention times with those of the peaks in the chromatogram of the *System suitability preparation*. Calculate the percentage of free riboflavin taken by the formula:

$$625C(r_F / r_S)$$

and calculate the percentage of riboflavin in the form of riboflavin diphosphates taken by the formula:

$$625C(r_D / r_S)$$

in which C is the concentration, in mg per mL, of USP Riboflavin RS in the *Standard preparation*, r_F is the riboflavin peak response, if any, obtained from the *Test preparation*, r_D is the sum of the responses for any of the 3 riboflavin diphosphate peaks obtained from the *Test preparation*, and r_S is the riboflavin peak response obtained from the *Standard preparation*. Not more than 6.0% of free riboflavin and not more than 6.0% of riboflavin diphosphates, as riboflavin, calculated on the dried basis, are found.

Limit of lumiflavin—Prepare alcohol-free chloroform just prior to use, as follows. Shake 20 mL of chloroform gently but thoroughly with 20 mL of water for 3 minutes, draw off the chloroform layer, and wash twice more with 20-mL portions of water. Finally filter the chloroform through a dry filter paper, shake it for 5 minutes with 5 g of powdered anhydrous sodium sulfate, allow the mixture to stand for 2 hours, and decant or filter the clear chloroform. Shake 35 mg of Riboflavin 5′-Phosphate Sodium with 10 mL of the alcohol-free chloroform for 5 minutes, and filter: the absorbance of the filtrate so obtained, determined in 1-cm cells at a wavelength of 440 nm, with a suitable spectrophotometer, alcohol-free chloroform being used as the blank, does not exceed 0.025.

Organic volatile impurities, *Method IV* ⟨467⟩: meets the requirements.

(Official until July 1, 2008)

Assay—[NOTE—Conduct the assay so that all solutions are protected from actinic light at all stages, preferably by using low-actinic glassware.]

Standard preparation—Transfer about 35 mg of USP Riboflavin RS, accurately weighed, to a 250-mL conical flask, add 20 mL of pyridine and 75 mL of water, and dissolve the riboflavin by frequent shaking. Transfer the solution to a 1000-mL volumetric flask, dilute with water to volume, and mix. Transfer 10.0 mL of this solution to a second 1000-mL volumetric flask, add sufficient 0.1 N sulfuric acid (about 4 mL) so that the final pH of the solution is between 5.9 and 6.1, dilute with water to volume, and mix. The *Standard preparation* so obtained contains about 0.35 µg of riboflavin per mL.

Assay preparation—Transfer about 50 mg of Riboflavin 5′-Phosphate Sodium, accurately weighed, to a 250-mL conical flask, add 20 mL of pyridine and 75 mL of water, and dissolve by frequent shaking. Transfer the solution to a 1000-mL volumetric flask, dilute with water to volume, and mix. Transfer 10.0 mL of this solution to a second 1000-mL volumetric flask, add sufficient 0.1 N sulfuric acid (about 4 mL) so that the final pH of the solution is between 5.9 and 6.1, dilute with water to volume, and mix.

Procedure—With a suitable fluorometer, determine the maximum fluorescence intensities, I_S and I_U, of the *Standard preparation* and the *Assay preparation*, respectively, at about 530 nm, using an excitation wavelength of about 440 nm. Calculate the quantity, in mg, of $C_{17}H_{20}N_4O_6$ in the portion of Riboflavin 5′-Phosphate Sodium taken by the formula:

$$100C(I_U / I_S)$$

in which C is the concentration, in µg per mL, of USP Riboflavin RS in the *Standard preparation*.

Rifabutin

$C_{46}H_{62}N_4O_{11}$ 847.00

(9S,12E,14S,15R,16S,17R,18R,19R,20S,21S,22E,24Z)-6,16,18,20-Tetrahydroxy-1′-isobutyl-14-methoxy-7,9,15,17,19,21,25-heptamethylspiro[9,4-(epoxypentadeca[1,11,13]trienimino)-2H-furo[2′,3′: 7,8]naphth[1,2-d]imidazole-2,4′-piperidine]-5,10,26-(3H,9H)-trione-16-acetate   [72559-06-9].

» Rifabutin contains not less than 950 µg and not more than 1020 µg of $C_{46}H_{62}N_4O_{11}$ per mg, calculated on the anhydrous basis.

Packaging and storage—Preserve in well-closed containers, protected from light and from excessive heat.

USP Reference standards ⟨11⟩—*USP Rifabutin RS*.
Identification—
  A: *Infrared Absorption* ⟨197K⟩.
  B: The retention time of the major peak in the chromatogram of the *Assay preparation* corresponds to that in the chromatogram of the *Standard preparation* obtained as directed in the *Assay*.
Water, *Method I* ⟨921⟩:   not more than 2.5%.
Limit of N-isobutylpiperidone—Prepare a test solution of Rifabutin in a mixture of chloroform and methanol (1 : 1) containing 10 mg per mL. Prepare a series of *Standard* solutions of N-isobutylpiperidone in a mixture of chloroform and methanol (1 : 1) containing 0.005, 0.01, 0.02, 0.05, and 0.1 mg per mL, respectively. Separately apply 10-µL spots of the test solution and the Standard solutions to the starting line of a thin-layer chromatographic plate (see *Chromatography* ⟨621⟩) coated with a 0.25-mm layer of chromatographic silica gel mixture, and allow to dry. Develop the chromatograms in a solvent system consisting of a mixture of hexanes and acetone (100 : 30) in an equilibrated unlined chromatographic chamber until the solvent front has moved about three-fourths of the length of the plate. Remove the plate from the chromatographic chamber, allow the plate to air-dry, and place it in an iodine vapor chamber until the spots are visible (about 5 minutes). Remove the plate from the chamber, spray the plate with starch TS, and examine the plate: no spot in the chromatogram of the test solution at an R_F value corresponding to that of N-isobutylpiperidone is more intense than that of the principal spot observed in the chromatogram obtained from the Standard solution containing 0.05 mg of N-isobutylpiperidone per mL (0.5%).
Chromatographic purity—Using the chromatogram of the *Assay preparation* obtained as directed in the *Assay*, calculate the percentage of impurities by the formula:

$$100(r_i/r_S)$$

in which r_i is the response of an individual impurity and r_S is the sum of the responses of all peaks: any impurity peak detected at a retention time of about 0.5, 0.6, 0.8, or 1.4 relative to the retention time of the rifabutin peak does not exceed 1.0%, not more than 0.5% of any other impurity is detected, and the total of all impurity peaks is not more than 3.0%.
Assay—
  0.1 M Monobasic potassium phosphate—Prepare a solution containing 13.6 g of monobasic potassium phosphate per L.
  Mobile phase—Prepare a mixture of acetonitrile and *0.1 M Monobasic potassium phosphate* (50 : 50). Adjust by dropwise addition of 2 N sodium hydroxide to a pH of 6.5 ± 0.1. Filter through a 0.5-µm or finer porosity filter, and degas. Make adjustments if necessary (see *System Suitability* under *Chromatography* ⟨621⟩).
  Standard preparation—Transfer about 25 mg of USP Rifabutin RS, accurately weighed, to a 50-mL volumetric flask. Add 5 mL of acetonitrile, dilute with *Mobile phase* to volume, and mix.
  Assay preparation—Transfer about 25 mg of Rifabutin, accurately weighed, to a 50-mL volumetric flask. Add 5 mL of acetonitrile, dilute with *Mobile phase* to volume, and mix.
  Resolution solution—Dissolve about 10 mg of Rifabutin and 2 mL of methanol, add 1 mL of 2 N sodium hydroxide, and allow to stand for about 4 minutes. Add 1 mL of 2 N hydrochloric acid, and dilute with *Mobile phase* to 50 mL. [NOTE—Portions of this solution may be stored in the frozen state for future use.]
  Chromatographic system (see *Chromatography* ⟨621⟩)—The liquid chromatograph is equipped with a 254-nm detector and a 4.6-mm × 12.5-cm column that contains 5-µm diameter packing L7. The flow rate is about 1 mL per minute. Chromatograph the *Resolution solution*, and record the peak responses as directed for *Procedure*: the chromatogram exhibits a major peak for a degradant, two minor peaks for degradants, and a major peak for rifabutin at relative retention times of about 0.5, 0.6, 0.8, and 1.0, respectively. The resolution, R, between the rifabutin peak and the degradant peak eluting at a relative retention time of about 0.8 is not less than 1.3. Chromatograph the *Standard preparation*, and record the peak responses as directed for *Procedure*: the column efficiency is not less than 2000 theoretical plates, and the relative standard deviation for replicate injections is not more than 2.0%.
  Procedure—Separately inject equal volumes (about 10 µL) of the *Standard preparation* and the *Assay preparation* into the chromatograph, record the chromatograms for a period of time that is twice the retention time of the major rifabutin peak, and measure the area responses for the major peaks. Calculate the quantity, in µg, of $C_{46}H_{62}N_4O_{11}$ in each mg of Rifabutin taken by the formula:

$$50(CP/W)(r_U/r_S)$$

in which C is the concentration, in mg per mL, of USP Rifabutin RS in the *Standard preparation*, P is the designated potency, in µg per mg, of USP Rifabutin RS, W is the weight, in mg, of Rifabutin taken to prepare the *Assay preparation*, and r_U and r_S are the rifabutin peak area responses obtained from the *Assay preparation* and the *Standard preparation*, respectively.

Rifabutin Capsules

» Rifabutin Capsules contain not less than 90.0 percent and not more than 110.0 percent of the labeled amount of $C_{46}H_{62}N_4O_{11}$.

Packaging and storage—Preserve in well-closed containers, protected from light and from excessive heat.

USP Reference standards ⟨11⟩—*USP Rifabutin RS*.
Identification—
  A: *Ultraviolet Absorption* ⟨197U⟩—
  Solution—Prepare the test solution as follows. Suspend a quantity of Capsule contents, equivalent to about 200 mg of rifabutin, in 20 mL of methanol, sonicate for about 5 minutes, and filter through a 0.5-µm or finer porosity filter. Dilute a portion of the filtrate quantitatively, and stepwise if necessary, with methanol to obtain a solution having a concentration of about 20 µg per mL. Prepare a Standard solution by dissolving a quantity of USP Rifabutin RS in methanol, with the aid of sonication, to obtain a solution having a concentration of about 20 µg per mL, and filter through a 0.5-µm or finer porosity filter.
  Medium: methanol.
  B: The retention time of the major peak in the chromatogram of the *Assay preparation* corresponds to that in the chromatogram of the *Standard preparation* obtained as directed in the *Assay*.

Dissolution—
Medium: 0.01 N hydrochloric acid; 900 mL.
Apparatus 1: 100 rpm.
Time: 45 minutes.
*Procedure—*Determine the amount of $C_{46}H_{62}N_4O_{11}$ dissolved from UV absorbances at the wavelength of maximum absorbance at about 280 nm of filtered portions of the solution under test, suitably diluted with *Dissolution Medium*, in comparison with a Standard solution having a known concentration of USP Rifabutin RS in the same medium, taking into account its designated potency.
*Tolerances—*Not less than 75% *(Q)* of the labeled amount of $C_{46}H_{62}N_4O_{11}$ is dissolved in 45 minutes.

Chromatographic purity—Using the chromatogram of the *Assay preparation* obtained as directed in the *Assay*, calculate the percentage of impurities by the formula:

$$100(r_i / r_S)$$

in which r_i is the response of an individual impurity and r_S is the sum of the responses of all peaks: any impurity peak detected at a retention time of about 0.5, 0.6, 0.8, or 1.4 relative to the retention time of the rifabutin peak does not exceed 1.0%, not more than 0.5% of any other impurity is detected, and the total of all impurity peaks is not more than 4.5%.

Assay—
0.1 M Monobasic potassium phosphate, Mobile phase, Standard preparation, Resolution solution, and *Chromatographic system—*Proceed as directed in the *Assay* under *Rifabutin*.

*Assay preparation—*Remove as completely as possible the contents of not less than 20 Capsules, weigh accurately, and determine the average weight of the Capsule contents. Transfer an accurately weighed portion of the powder, equivalent to about 25 mg of rifabutin, to a 50-mL volumetric flask. Add 5 mL of acetonitrile, dilute with *Mobile phase* to volume, and mix. Filter through a 0.5-μm or finer porosity filter, and use the filtrate as the *Assay preparation*.

*Procedure—*Proceed as directed for *Procedure* in the *Assay* under *Rifabutin*. Calculate the quantity, in mg, of $C_{46}H_{62}N_4O_{11}$ in the portion of Capsules taken by the formula:

$$0.05CP(r_U / r_S)$$

in which the terms are as defined therein.

Rifampin

$C_{43}H_{58}N_4O_{12}$ 822.94
Rifamycin, 3-[[[(4-methyl-1-piperazinyl)imino]methyl]-.
5,6,9,17,19,21-Hexahydroxy-23-methoxy-2,4,12,16,18,20,22-
  heptamethyl-8-[N-(4-methyl-1-piperazinyl)formimidoyl]-2,7-
  (epoxypentadeca[1,11,13]trienimino)naphtho[2,1-b]furan-1,11-
  (2H)-dione 21-acetate   [13292-46-1].

» Rifampin contains not less than 95.0 percent and not more than 103.0 percent of $C_{43}H_{58}N_4O_{12}$, calculated on the dried basis.

Packaging and storage—Preserve in tight, light-resistant containers, protected from excessive heat.

USP Reference standards ⟨11⟩—USP Rifampin RS. USP Rifampin Quinone RS.

Identification, *Infrared Absorption* ⟨197M⟩.
Crystallinity ⟨695⟩: meets the requirements.
pH ⟨791⟩: between 4.5 and 6.5, in a suspension (1 in 100).
Loss on drying ⟨731⟩—Dry about 100 mg in a capillary-stoppered bottle in vacuum at 60° for 4 hours: it loses not more than 2.0% of its weight.

Related substances—
Phosphate buffer, Mobile phase, Solvent mixture, Resolution solution, and *Chromatographic system—*Proceed as directed in the *Assay*.

*Stock test preparation—*Transfer about 200 mg of Rifampin to a 100-mL volumetric flask, dissolve in and dilute with acetonitrile to volume, and mix. Sonicate for about 30 seconds, if necessary, to ensure dissolution. [NOTE—Use this solution within 2 hours.]

*Test preparation—*Transfer 5.0 mL of *Stock test* to a 50-mL volumetric flask, dilute with *Solvent* to volume, and mix. [NOTE—Prepare this solution immediately prior to injection into the chromatograph.]

*Dilute test preparation—*Transfer 10.0 mL of *Stock test preparation* to a 100-mL volumetric flask, dilute with acetonitrile to volume, and mix. Transfer 5.0 mL of the resulting solution to a 50-mL volumetric flask, dilute with acetonitrile to volume, and mix. Transfer 5.0 mL of this solution to another 50-mL volumetric flask, dilute with *Solvent mixture* to volume, and mix. [NOTE—Prepare this final dilution immediately prior to injection into the chromatograph.]

*Procedure—*Separately inject equal volumes (about 50 μL) of the *Test preparation* and the *Dilute test preparation* into the chromatograph, record the chromatograms, and measure the responses for all of the peaks. Calculate the percentage of each related substance by the formula:

$$r_{Ti} / (r_D + 0.01 \Sigma r_{Ti})$$

in which r_{Ti} is the area of the peak of the individual related substance in the chromatogram obtained from the *Test preparation*, r_D is the area of the rifampin peak in the chromatogram obtained from the *Dilute test preparation*, and Σr_{Ti} is the sum of the areas of all of the peaks of the related substances obtained in the chromatogram of the *Test preparation*: not more than 1.5% of rifampin quinone is found, not more than 1.0% of any other individual related substance is found, and a total of not more than 3.5% of all individual related substances, other than rifampin quinone, having retention times of up to 3 in relation to the retention time of rifampin is found.

Assay—
*Phosphate buffer—*Dissolve 136.1 g of monobasic potassium phosphate in about 500 mL of water, add 6.3 mL of phosphoric acid, dilute with water to 1000 mL, and mix.

*Mobile phase—*Prepare a suitable mixture of water, acetonitrile, *Phosphate buffer*, 1.0 M citric acid, and 0.5 M sodium perchlorate (510 : 350 : 100 : 20 : 20), filter through a suitable filter of 0.7 μm or finer porosity, and degas. Make adjustments if necessary (see *System Suitability* under *Chromatography* ⟨621⟩).

*Solvent mixture—*Prepare a mixture of water, acetonitrile, 1.0 M dibasic potassium phosphate, 1.0 M monobasic potassium phosphate, and 1.0 M citric acid (640 : 250 : 77 : 23 : 10).

*Standard preparation—*Transfer about 40 mg of USP Rifampin RS, accurately weighed, to a 200-mL volumetric flask. Dissolve in and dilute with acetonitrile to volume, and mix. Sonicate for about 30 seconds, if necessary, to ensure dissolution. [NOTE—Use this solution within 5 hours.] Transfer 10.0 mL of this solution to a 100-mL volumetric flask, dilute with *Solvent mixture* to volume, and mix. [NOTE—Prepare this final dilution immediately prior to injection into the chromatograph.]

*Assay preparation—*Using Rifampin, proceed as directed for *Standard preparation*.

*Resolution solution—*Dissolve suitable quantities of USP Rifampin RS and USP Rifampin Quinone RS in acetonitrile to obtain a solution containing about 0.1 mg of each per mL. Transfer 1.0 mL of this solution to a 10-mL volumetric flask, dilute with *Solvent mixture* to volume, and mix.

Chromatographic system (see *Chromatography* ⟨621⟩)—The liquid chromatograph is equipped with a 254-nm detector and a 4.6-mm × 10-cm column that contains 5-μm packing L7. The flow rate is about 1.5 mL per minute. Chromatograph the *Resolution solution*, and record the peak responses as directed for *Procedure:* the resolution, *R*, between the rifampin quinone and rifampin peaks is not less than 4.0. Chromatograph the *Standard preparation*, and record the peak responses as directed for *Procedure*: the column efficiency determined from the rifampin peak is not less than 1000 theoretical plates, and the relative standard deviation for replicate injections is not more than 1.0%.

Procedure—Separately inject equal volumes (about 50 µL) of the *Standard preparation* and the *Assay preparation* into the chromatograph, record the chromatograms, and measure the area responses for the major peaks. The relative retention times are about 0.6 for rifampin quinone and 1.0 for rifampin. Calculate the quantity, in mg, of rifampin ($C_{43}H_{58}N_4O_{12}$) in the portion of Rifampin taken to prepare the *Assay preparation* by the formula:

$$2000C(r_U / r_S)$$

in which C is the concentration, in mg per mL, calculated on the dried basis, of USP Rifampin RS in the *Standard preparation*, and r_U and r_S are the area responses of the rifampin peaks obtained from the *Assay preparation* and the *Standard preparation*, respectively.

Rifampin Capsules

» Rifampin Capsules contain not less than 90.0 percent and not more than 110.0 percent of the labeled amount of $C_{43}H_{58}N_4O_{12}$.

Packaging and storage—Preserve in tight, light-resistant containers, protected from excessive heat.

USP Reference standards ⟨11⟩—USP Rifampin RS. USP Rifampin Quinone RS.

Identification—
A: Triturate a quantity of Capsule contents, equivalent to about 50 mg of rifampin, with 5 mL of chloroform, and filter. Apply 3 µL each of the filtrate (test solution) and of a solution of USP Rifampin RS in chloroform containing 10 mg per mL to a suitable thin-layer chromatographic plate (see *Chromatography* ⟨621⟩) coated with a 0.25-mm layer of chromatographic silica gel mixture. Allow the spots to dry, and develop the chromatogram in an equilibrated chromatographic chamber containing a solvent system consisting of a mixture of chloroform and methanol (90 : 10) until the solvent front has moved about one-half of the length of the plate. Remove the plate from the developing chamber, mark the solvent front, and allow the solvent to evaporate. Locate the red spots on the plate: the R_F value of the principal spot obtained from the test solution corresponds to that obtained from the Standard solution.
B: The chromatogram of the *Assay preparation* exhibits a major peak for rifampin, the retention time of which corresponds to that exhibited in the chromatogram of the *Standard preparation*, as obtained in the *Assay*.

Dissolution ⟨711⟩—
Medium: 0.1 N hydrochloric acid; 900 mL.
Apparatus 1: 100 rpm.
Time: 45 minutes.
Procedure—Determine the amount of $C_{43}H_{58}N_4O_{12}$ dissolved from absorbances at the wavelength of maximum absorbance at about 475 nm on filtered portions of the solution under test, suitably diluted, if necessary, with *Dissolution Medium*, in comparison with a Standard solution having a known concentration of USP Rifampin RS, calculated on the dried basis, in the same *Medium*, prepared concomitantly and held in the water bath for the *Time* specified.
Tolerances—Not less than 75% (*Q*) of the labeled amount of $C_{43}H_{58}N_4O_{12}$ is dissolved in 45 minutes.

Uniformity of dosage units ⟨905⟩: meet the requirements.

Procedure for content uniformity—
Phosphate buffer, *Mobile phase*, *Solvent mixture*, *Diluent*, *Standard preparation*, *Resolution solution*, and *Chromatographic system*—Proceed as directed in the *Assay*.
Test preparation—Transfer the contents of 1 Capsule to a suitable volumetric flask so that when diluted to volume as directed below, each mL of solution contains about 1.5 mg of rifampin. Rinse the Capsule shell with a small quantity of *Solvent mixture*, and add the washing to the volumetric flask. Add *Solvent mixture* until the flask is about four-fifths full. Proceed as directed for *Assay preparation* in the *Assay*, beginning with "Sonicate for about 5 minutes."
Procedure—Proceed as directed for *Procedure* in the *Assay*. Calculate the quantity, in mg, of $C_{43}H_{58}N_4O_{12}$ in the Capsule content by the formula:

$$(LC / D)(r_U / r_S)$$

in which L is the labeled quantity, in mg, of rifampin in the Capsule, C is the concentration, in mg per mL, of USP Rifampin RS, calculated on the dried basis, in the *Standard preparation*, D is the concentration, in mg per mL, of rifampin in the *Test preparation*, based on the labeled quantity per Capsule and the extent of dilution, and r_U and r_S are the rifampin peak responses obtained from the *Test preparation* and the *Standard preparation*, respectively.

Loss on drying ⟨731⟩—Dry about 100 mg of Capsule contents in a capillary-stoppered bottle in vacuum at 60° for 3 hours: it loses not more than 3.0% of its weight.

Assay—
Phosphate buffer—Dissolve 136.1 g of monobasic potassium phosphate in about 500 mL of water, add 6.3 mL of phosphoric acid, dilute with water to 1000 mL, and mix (pH 3.1 ± 0.1).
Mobile phase—Prepare a suitable mixture of water, acetonitrile, *Phosphate buffer*, 1.0 M citric acid, and 0.5 M sodium perchlorate (510 : 350 : 100 : 20 : 20), filter through a suitable filter of 0.7 µm or finer porosity, and degas. Make adjustments if necessary (see *System Suitability* under *Chromatography* ⟨621⟩).
Solvent mixture—Prepare a mixture of acetonitrile and methanol (1 : 1).
Diluent—Prepare a suitable mixture of water, acetonitrile, 1.0 M dibasic sodium phosphate, 1.0 M monobasic potassium phosphate, and 1.0 M citric acid (640 : 250 : 77 : 23 : 10).
Standard preparation—Dissolve an accurately weighed quantity of USP Rifampin RS in *Solvent mixture* to obtain a solution having a known concentration of about 1.5 mg per mL, sonicating for about 30 seconds, if necessary, to ensure dissolution. Transfer 10.0 mL of this solution to a 50-mL volumetric flask, dilute with acetonitrile to volume, and mix. [NOTE—Use this working solution within 5 hours.] Transfer 5.0 mL of the working solution to a 50-mL volumetric flask, dilute with *Diluent* to volume, and mix. Each mL of this solution contains about 0.03 mg of USP Rifampin RS. [NOTE—Inject this *Standard preparation* into the chromatograph within 30 to 60 seconds after preparation.]
Assay preparation—Remove, as completely as possible, the contents of not less than 20 Capsules, and weigh accurately. Mix the Capsule contents, and transfer an accurately weighed portion of the powder, equivalent to about 300 mg of rifampin, to a 200-mL volumetric flask, and add about 180 mL of *Solvent mixture*. Sonicate for about 5 minutes, allow to equilibrate to room temperature, dilute with *Solvent mixture* to volume, and mix. Transfer 10.0 mL of the resulting solution to a 50-mL volumetric flask, dilute with acetonitrile to volume, and mix. [NOTE—Use this solution within 5 hours.] Transfer 5.0 mL of this solution to a 50-mL volumetric flask, dilute with *Diluent* to volume, and mix. [NOTE—Inject this *Assay preparation* into the chromatograph within 30 to 60 seconds after preparation.]
Resolution solution—Dissolve USP Rifampin Quinone RS in *Solvent mixture* to obtain a solution containing about 0.1 mg per mL. Transfer 1.5 mL of this solution and 5.0 mL of the working solution used to prepare the *Standard preparation* to a 50-mL volumetric flask, dilute with *Diluent* to volume, and mix.
Chromatographic system (see *Chromatography* ⟨621⟩)—The liquid chromatograph is equipped with a 254-nm detector and a 4.6-mm × 10-cm column that contains 5-µm packing L7. The flow rate is about 1.5 mL per minute. Chromatograph the *Resolution solution*, and record the peak responses as directed for *Procedure*: the relative retention times are about 0.6 for rifampin quinone and 1.0 for rifampin, and the resolution, *R*, between the rifampin quinone and rifampin peaks is not less than 4.0. Chromatograph the *Standard preparation*, and record the peak responses as directed for *Procedure*: the relative standard deviation for replicate injections is not more than 1.0%.
Procedure—Separately inject equal volumes (about 50 µL) of the *Standard preparation* and the *Assay preparation* into the chromatograph, record the chromatograms, and measure the area responses

for the major peaks. Calculate the quantity, in mg, of $C_{43}H_{58}N_4O_{12}$ in the portion of Capsules taken by the formula:

$$10,000C(r_U / r_S)$$

in which C is the concentration, in mg per mL, of USP Rifampin RS, calculated on the dried basis, in the *Standard preparation*, and r_U and r_S are the rifampin peak area responses obtained from the *Assay preparation* and the *Standard preparation*, respectively.

Rifampin for Injection

» Rifampin for Injection contains not less than 90.0 percent and not more than 115.0 percent of the labeled amount of rifampin ($C_{43}H_{58}N_4O_{12}$).

Packaging and storage—Preserve in *Containers for Sterile Solids* as described under *Injections* ⟨1⟩.
USP Reference standards ⟨11⟩—*USP Rifampin RS. USP Rifampin Quinone RS. USP Endotoxin RS.*
Identification—
  A: It responds to *Identification* test A under *Rifampin Capsules*, the test solution being prepared by dissolving the contents of a container in chloroform to obtain a solution containing about 10 mg of rifampin per mL.
  B: The retention time of the rifampin peak in the chromatogram of the *Assay preparation* corresponds to that in the chromatogram of the *Standard preparation* as obtained in the *Assay*.
Bacterial endotoxins ⟨85⟩—Dissolve Rifampin for Injection in endotoxin-free water to obtain a stock solution containing 10 mg of rifampin per mL. Dilute the stock solution quantitatively, and stepwise if necessary, with endotoxin-free water to obtain a solution containing 0.12 mg of rifampin per mL: it contains not more than 0.5 USP Endotoxin Unit per mg of rifampin.
Sterility ⟨71⟩—It meets the requirements when tested as directed for *Membrane Filtration* under *Test for Sterility of the Product to be Examined*.
pH ⟨791⟩: between 7.8 and 8.8, in a solution containing 60 mg of rifampin per mL.
Water, *Method I* ⟨921⟩: not more than 1.0%.
Particulate matter ⟨788⟩: meets the requirements for small-volume injections.
Assay—
  Phosphate buffer, Mobile phase, Solvent mixture, Standard preparation, Resolution solution, and *Chromatographic system*—Prepare as directed in the *Assay* under *Rifampin*.
  Assay preparation 1 (where it is represented as being in a single-dose container)—Constitute a container of Rifampin for Injection in a volume of water, accurately measured, corresponding to the volume of diluent specified in the labeling. [NOTE—Use this solution within 2 hours.] Withdraw all of the withdrawable contents, using a suitable hypodermic needle and syringe, and transfer to a suitable volumetric flask of such capacity that when diluted with acetonitrile to volume, a solution is obtained containing about 6 mg of rifampin ($C_{43}H_{58}N_4O_{12}$) per mL. [NOTE—Use this stock solution within 5 hours.] Dilute an accurately measured volume of this stock solution quantitatively and stepwise with *Solvent mixture* to obtain a solution having a concentration of about 0.02 mg of rifampin per mL. [NOTE—Prepare this final dilution immediately prior to injection into the chromatograph.]
  Assay preparation 2 (where the label states the quantity of rifampin in a given volume of constituted solution)—Constitute a container of Rifampin for Injection in a volume of water, accurately measured, equivalent to the volume of diluent specified in the labeling. [NOTE—Use this solution within 2 hours.] Dilute an accurately measured volume of the constituted solution quantitatively and stepwise with acetonitrile to obtain a solution having a concentration of about 0.2 mg of rifampin ($C_{43}H_{58}N_4O_{12}$) per mL. [NOTE—Use this stock solution within 5 hours.] Transfer 10.0 mL of this solution to a 100-mL volumetric flask, dilute with *Solvent mixture* to volume, and mix. [NOTE—Prepare this final dilution immediately prior to the injection into the chromatogram.]

  Procedure—Proceed as directed for *Procedure* in the *Assay* under *Rifampin*. Calculate the quantity, in mg, of rifampin ($C_{43}H_{58}N_4O_{12}$) withdrawn from the container of constituted Rifampin for Injection, or in the volume of constituted Rifampin for Injection taken by the formula:

$$(L / D)(C)(r_U / r_S)$$

in which L is the labeled quantity, in mg, of rifampin in the container, or in the volume of constituted solution taken, D is the concentration, in mg per mL, of rifampin in *Assay preparation 1* or in *Assay preparation 2*, on the basis of the labeled quantity in the container, or in the volume of constituted solution taken, and the extent of dilution, C is the concentration, in mg per mL, calculated on the dried basis, of USP Rifampin RS in the *Standard preparation*, and r_U and r_S are the rifampin peak responses obtained from *Assay preparation 1*, or *Assay preparation 2*, and the *Standard preparation*, respectively.

Rifampin Oral Suspension

» Rifampin Oral Suspension contains not less than 90.0 percent and not more than 110.0 percent of the labeled amount of rifampin ($C_{43}H_{58}N_4O_{12}$). Use Rifampin or the number of Rifampin Capsules that contain the designated amount of Rifampin, and prepare Rifampin Oral Suspension as follows (see *Pharmaceutical Compounding—Nonsterile Preparations* ⟨795⟩):

Rifampin	1.20 g
Syrup, a sufficient quantity to make ...	120 mL

Transfer 1.20 g of Rifampin, or the contents of Rifampin Capsules, into a mortar. [NOTE—If necessary, gently crush the Capsule contents with a pestle to produce a fine powder.] Add about 2 mL of Syrup to the mortar, and triturate until a smooth paste is formed. Add about 10 mL of Syrup, and triturate to form a suspension. Continue to add Syrup, until about 80 mL has been added. Transfer this suspension to a 120-mL pre-calibrated light-resistant glass or plastic prescription bottle. Rinse the mortar and pestle with successive small portions of Syrup, and add the rinses to the bottle. Shake vigorously. If necessary, add Citric Acid or Sodium Citrate to adjust to a pH of 5.0. Add a suitable flavor if desired. Add sufficient Syrup to make the product measure 120 mL, and shake vigorously to produce the Oral Suspension.

Packaging and storage—Preserve in a tight, light-resistant glass or plastic prescription bottle, with a child-resistant closure. Store at controlled room temperature.
Labeling—Label it to state that the Suspension is to be well shaken. Label it to state that it contains 50 mg of rifampin in 5 mL of Oral Suspension.
USP Reference standards ⟨11⟩—*USP Rifampin RS. USP Rifampin Quinone RS.*
pH ⟨791⟩: between 4.5 and 5.5.
Beyond-use date—Thirty days after the day on which it was compounded.
Assay—
  Phosphate buffer, Solvent mixture, and *Resolution solution*—Prepare as directed in the *Assay* under *Rifampin*.
  Mobile phase—Prepare a suitable mixture of water, acetonitrile, *Phosphate buffer*, 1.0 M citric acid, and 0.5 M sodium perchlorate (500 : 360 : 100 : 20 : 20), pass through a suitable filter having a

0.7-μm or finer porosity, and degas. Make adjustments if necessary (see *System Suitability* under *Chromatography* ⟨621⟩).

Diluent—Prepare a mixture of acetonitrile and water (1 : 1).

Standard preparation—Dissolve an accurately weighed quantity of USP Rifampin RS in *Diluent* to obtain a solution having a known concentration of about 0.5 mg per mL, sonicating for about 30 seconds, if necessary, to dissolve. Transfer 5.0 mL of this solution to a 50-mL, low-actinic volumetric flask, dilute with *Diluent* to volume, and mix. [NOTE—Use this preparation within 1 hour.]

Assay preparation—Transfer 5.0 mL of Oral Suspension, freshly mixed and free from air bubbles, to a 100-mL, low-actinic volumetric flask, dissolve in and dilute with *Diluent* to volume, and mix. Transfer 5.0 mL of the resulting solution to a 50-mL, low-actinic volumetric flask, dilute with *Diluent* to volume, and mix.

Chromatographic system (see *Chromatography* ⟨621⟩)—The liquid chromatograph is equipped with a 254-nm detector and a 4.6-mm × 10-cm column that contains 5-μm packing L7. Chromatograph the *Resolution solution*, and record the peak responses as directed for *Procedure*: the relative retention times are about 0.6 for rifampin quinone and 1.0 for rifampin; and the resolution, *R*, between the rifampin quinone and rifampin is not less than 4.0. Chromatograph the *Standard preparation*, and record the peak responses as directed for *Procedure*: the relative standard deviation for replicate injections is not more than 1.0%.

Procedure—Separately inject equal volumes (about 20 μL) of the *Standard preparation* and the *Assay preparation* into the chromatograph, record the chromatograms, and measure the areas for the major peaks. Calculate the quantity, in mg, of rifampin ($C_{43}H_{58}N_4O_{12}$) in the portion of Oral Suspension taken by the formula:

$$1000C(r_U / r_S)$$

in which *C* is the concentration, in mg per mL, of USP Rifampin RS, calculated on the dried basis, in the *Standard preparation*; and r_U and r_S are the rifampin peak responses obtained from the *Assay preparation* and the *Standard preparation*, respectively.

Rifampin and Isoniazid Capsules

» Rifampin and Isoniazid Capsules contain not less than 90.0 percent and not more than 130.0 percent of the labeled amount of rifampin ($C_{43}H_{58}N_4O_{12}$) and not less than 90.0 percent and not more than 110.0 percent of the labeled amount of isoniazid ($C_6H_7N_3O$).

NOTE—Where Rifampin and Isoniazid Capsules are prescribed without reference to the quantity of rifampin or isoniazid contained therein, a product containing 300 mg of rifampin and 150 mg of isoniazid shall be dispensed.

Packaging and storage—Preserve in tight, light-resistant containers, and avoid exposure to excessive heat.

USP Reference standards ⟨11⟩—*USP Rifampin RS. USP Isoniazid RS*.

Identification—

A: *Thin-Layer Chromatographic Identification Test* ⟨201⟩—

Test solution—Transfer a portion of Capsule contents, equivalent to about 120 mg of rifampin, to a suitable flask, add 20 mL of methanol, and shake for several minutes. Pass this suspension through a filter having a 1-μm or finer porosity, discarding the first few mL of the filtrate. Dilute a volume of the filtrate with an equal volume of acetone, and mix.

Standard solutions—Dissolve a quantity of USP Rifampin RS in methanol to obtain a solution containing 6 mg per mL. Add an equal volume of acetone, and mix. Dissolve a quantity of USP Isoniazid RS in methanol to obtain a solution containing 2.5 mg per mL. Add an equal volume of acetone, and mix.

Application volume: 2 μL.

Developing solvent solution: a mixture of acetone and glacial acetic acid (100 : 1).

B: The retention times of the rifampin and isoniazid peaks in the chromatogram of the *Assay preparation* correspond to those of rifampin and isoniazid in the chromatogram of the *Standard preparation*, as obtained in the *Assay for rifampin and isoniazid*.

Dissolution ⟨711⟩—

Medium: 0.1 N hydrochloric acid; 900 mL.

Apparatus 1: 100 rpm.

Time: 45 minutes.

Determine the amount of rifampin ($C_{43}H_{58}N_4O_{12}$) dissolved by employing the following method.

Phosphate buffer solution—Dissolve 15.3 g of dibasic potassium phosphate and 80.0 g of monobasic potassium phosphate into a 1-L volumetric flask, mix, dilute with water to volume, and mix.

Isoniazid standard solution—Accurately weigh about 66 mg of USP Isoniazid RS into a 100-mL volumetric flask. Dissolve in and dilute with 0.1 N hydrochloric acid to volume, and mix.

Standard stock solution—Accurately weigh about 66 mg of USP Rifampin RS into a 200-mL volumetric flask, dissolve in 10 mL of 0.1 N hydrochloric acid, and mix. Add 50.0 mL of *Isoniazid standard solution*, dilute with 0.1 N hydrochloric acid to volume, and mix. [NOTE—Prepare this solution immediately before the test is performed, and place in the dissolution bath at the start of the test.]

Standard solution—At the end of the test run, transfer a 5.0-mL aliquot of the *Standard stock solution* and 10.0 mL of *Phosphate buffer solution* to a 50-mL volumetric flask. Dilute with water to volume, and mix. [NOTE—Analyze the solution immediately, if possible, and if not, within 3 hours after final dilution.]

Test solution—At the end of the test run, withdraw a 25-mL aliquot, and filter, discarding the first 10 mL of the filtrate. Allow to cool for about 10 minutes, and transfer 5.0 mL of the filtrate and 10.0 mL of the *Phosphate buffer solution* to a 50-mL volumetric flask. Dilute with water to volume, and mix. [NOTE—Analyze the solution immediately, if possible, and if not, within 3 hours after final dilution.]

Determine the amount of rifampin ($C_{43}H_{58}N_4O_{12}$) dissolved from absorbances at the wavelength of maximum absorbance at about 475 nm of the *Standard solution* and the *Test solution*.

Determine the amount of isoniazid ($C_6H_7N_3O$) dissolved by employing the following method.

Mobile phase—Prepare a filtered and degassed mixture of water, *Phosphate buffer solution*, and methanol (850 : 100 : 50). Make adjustments if necessary (see *System Suitability* under *Chromatography* ⟨621⟩).

Chromatographic system (see *Chromatography* ⟨621⟩)—The liquid chromatograph is equipped with a 254-nm detector and a 4.0-mm × 30-cm column that contains 10-μm packing L1. The flow rate is about 1.5 mL per minute.

Procedure—Separately inject equal volumes (about 50 μL) of the *Standard solution* and the *Test solution* into the chromatograph, record the chromatograms, and measure the responses for the isoniazid peaks.

Tolerances—Not less than 75% (*Q*) of the labeled amount of $C_{43}H_{58}N_4O_{12}$ and not less than 80% (*Q*) of the labeled amount of $C_6H_7N_3O$ are dissolved in 45 minutes.

Loss on drying ⟨731⟩—Dry about 100 mg of Capsule contents in a capillary-stoppered bottle in vacuum at 60° for 3 hours: it loses not more than 3.0% of its weight.

Assay for rifampin and isoniazid—

Buffer solution—Dissolve 1.4 g of dibasic sodium phosphate in 1 L of water, and adjust with phosphoric acid to a pH of 6.8.

Solution A—Prepare a filtered and degassed mixture of *Buffer solution* and acetonitrile (96 : 4).

Solution B—Prepare a filtered and degassed mixture of acetonitrile and *Buffer solution* (55 : 45).

Mobile phase—Use variable mixtures of *Solution A* and *Solution B* as directed for *Chromatographic system*. Make adjustments if necessary (see *System Suitability* under *Chromatography* ⟨621⟩).

Standard preparation—Dissolve accurately weighed quantities of USP Rifampin RS and USP Isoniazid RS in a mixture of *Buffer solution* and methanol (96 : 4) to obtain a solution having known concentrations of about 0.16 mg per mL and 0.08 mg per mL, respectively. [NOTE—Use this solution within 10 minutes.]

Assay preparation—Weigh the contents of not fewer than 10 Capsules, mix, and transfer an accurately weighed portion of the powder, equivalent to about 8 mg of isoniazid, to a 100-mL volumetric flask, and add about 90 mL of *Buffer solution*. Sonicate for about 10 minutes, allow to equilibrate to room temperature, dilute with *Buffer solution* to volume, and mix. [NOTE—Use this solution within 2 hours.]

Chromatographic system (see *Chromatography* ⟨621⟩)—The liquid chromatograph is equipped with a 238-nm detector and a 4.6-mm × 25-cm column that contains 5-μm base-deactivated packing L1. The flow rate is about 1.5 mL per minute. The chromatograph is programmed as follows.

Time (minutes)	Solution A (%)	Solution B (%)	Elution
0	100	0	equilibration
0–5	100	0	isocratic
5–6	100→0	0→100	linear gradient
6–15	0	100	isocratic

Chromatograph the *Standard preparation*, and record the peak responses as directed for *Procedure*: the relative retention times are about 2.6 and 1.0 for rifampin and isoniazid, respectively; the column efficiency is not less than 50,000 and not less than 6,000 theoretical plates for rifampin and isoniazid, respectively; the tailing factors are not more than 2.0; and the relative standard deviation for replicate injections is not more than 2.0%.

Procedure—Separately inject equal volumes (about 20 μL) of the *Standard preparation* and the *Assay preparation* into the chromatograph, record the chromatograms, and measure the peak responses. Calculate the quantity, in mg, of rifampin ($C_{43}H_{58}N_4O_{12}$) and isoniazid ($C_6H_7N_3O$) in the portion of Capsules taken by the formula:

$$100C(r_U/r_S)$$

in which C is the concentration, in mg per mL, of USP Rifampin RS, calculated on the dried basis, or of USP Isoniazid RS, as appropriate, in the *Standard preparation*; and r_U and r_S are the peak responses obtained from the corresponding analytes obtained from the *Assay preparation* and the *Standard preparation*, respectively.

Rifampin, Isoniazid, and Pyrazinamide Tablets

» Rifampin, Isoniazid, and Pyrazinamide Tablets contain not less than 90.0 percent and not more than 110.0 percent of the labeled amounts of rifampin ($C_{43}H_{58}N_4O_{12}$), isoniazid ($C_6H_7N_3O$), and pyrazinamide ($C_5H_5N_3O$).

Packaging and storage—Preserve in tight, light-resistant containers at controlled room temperature.

USP Reference standards ⟨11⟩—*USP Isoniazid RS. USP Pyrazinamide RS. USP Rifampin RS.*

Identification—

A: *Thin-Layer Chromatographic Identification Test* ⟨201⟩—

Test solution—Transfer an accurately weighed portion of ground Tablets, equivalent to about 120 mg of rifampin, to a suitable flask, add 20 mL of methanol, and shake for several minutes. Pass this suspension through a filter having a 1-μm or finer porosity, discarding the first few mL of the filtrate. Dilute a volume of the filtrate with an equal volume of acetone, and mix.

Standard solutions—Dissolve a quantity of USP Rifampin RS in methanol to obtain a solution containing 6 mg per mL. Add an equal volume of acetone, and mix. Dissolve a quantity of USP Isoniazid RS in methanol to obtain a solution containing 2.5 mg per mL. Add an equal volume of acetone, and mix. Dissolve a quantity of USP Pyrazinamide RS in methanol to obtain a solution containing 15 mg per mL. Add an equal volume of acetone, and mix.

Application volume: 2 μL.

Developing solvent system: a mixture of acetone and glacial acetic acid (100 : 1).

B: The retention times of the rifampin, isoniazid, and pyrazinamide peaks in the chromatogram of the *Assay preparation* correspond to those of rifampin, isoniazid, and pyrazinamide in the chromatogram of the *Standard preparation*, as obtained in the *Assay for rifampin, isoniazid, and pyrazinamide*.

Dissolution ⟨711⟩—

Medium: simulated gastric fluid TS, without pepsin; 900 mL.

Apparatus 1: 100 rpm.

Time: 30 minutes.

Standard stock solution—Prepare a solution in *Medium* having known concentrations of about 0.22 mg of USP Isoniazid RS and 1.3 mg of USP Pyrazinamide RS per mL. Use this solution on the day prepared.

Intermediate standard solution—Transfer about 27 mg of USP Rifampin RS, accurately weighed, to a 200-mL volumetric flask, add 50.0 mL of the *Standard stock solution*, and swirl to dissolve. Dilute with *Medium* to volume, and mix. Place this flask into the dissolution bath immediately prior to starting the tablet dissolution. Withdraw the flask from the dissolution bath at the same time that the solutions under test are withdrawn.

Determine the amount of $C_{43}H_{58}N_4O_{12}$ dissolved by employing the following method.

Standard solution—Transfer 10.0 mL of the *Intermediate standard solution* to a 50-mL volumetric flask, dilute with *Medium* to volume, and mix.

Procedure—Transfer 10.0 mL of the filtered solution under test to a separate 50-mL volumetric flask, dilute with *Medium* to volume, and mix. Concomitantly determine the UV absorbances at 475 nm of the solution obtained and the *Standard solution*, using the *Medium* as the blank. Calculate the quantity, in mg, of rifampin ($C_{43}H_{58}N_4O_{12}$) dissolved by the formula:

$$4500C(A_U/A_S)$$

in which C is the concentration, in mg per mL, of USP Rifampin RS in the *Standard solution*; and A_U and A_S are the absorbances of the solution under test and the *Standard solution*, respectively.

Tolerances—Not less than 80% (*Q*) of the labeled amount of rifampin ($C_{43}H_{58}N_4O_{12}$) is dissolved in 30 minutes.

Determine the amount of $C_6H_7N_3O$ and $C_5H_5N_3O$ dissolved by employing the following method.

Mobile phase—Prepare a filtered and degassed mixture of water, 1 M monobasic potassium phosphate, and acetonitrile (860 : 100 : 40). Make adjustments if necessary (see *System Suitability* under *Chromatography* ⟨621⟩).

System suitability solution—Prepare a solution of isonicotinic acid in *Medium* containing about 0.125 mg per mL. Transfer 10 mL of this solution and 4 mL of the *Standard stock solution* to a 100-mL volumetric flask containing 15 mL of 1 M dibasic potassium phosphate and 30 mL of *Mobile phase*. Dilute with *Mobile phase* to volume, and mix.

Standard solution—Transfer 15.0 mL of the *Intermediate standard solution* to a 100-mL volumetric flask containing 15 mL of 1 M dibasic potassium phosphate and 30 mL of *Mobile phase*. Dilute with *Mobile phase* to volume, and mix. This solution may be used for 20 hours.

Test solution—Withdraw 60 mL of the solution under test, and filter, discarding the first 20 mL of the filtrate. Centrifuge the filtrate for 5 minutes. Transfer 15.0 mL of this solution to a 100-mL volumetric flask containing 15 mL of 1 M dibasic potassium phosphate and 30 mL of *Mobile phase*. Dilute with *Mobile phase* to volume, and mix. This solution may be used for 20 hours.

Chromatographic system (see *Chromatography* ⟨621⟩)—The liquid chromatograph is equipped with a 254-nm detector and a 4.6-mm × 30-cm column that contains packing L44. The flow rate is about 1 mL per minute. Chromatograph the *System suitability solution*, and record the peak responses as directed for *Procedure*: the relative retention times are about 0.7 for isonicotinic acid, 1.0 for pyrazinamide, and 1.8 for isoniazid; and the resolution, *R*, between isonicotinic acid and pyrazinamide is not less than 2.5 and between pyrazinamide and isoniazid not less than 4.0. Chromatograph the *Standard solution*, and record the peak responses as directed for *Procedure*: the relative standard deviations determined from the pyrazinamide and isoniazid responses for replicate injections are not more than 1.5%.

Procedure—Separately inject equal volumes (about 50 μL) of the *Standard solution* and the *Test solution* into the chromatograph, record the chromatograms, and measure the areas for the major peaks. Calculate the quantity, in mg, of isoniazid ($C_6H_7N_3O$) dissolved by the formula:

$$6000C(r_U / r_S)$$

in which C is the concentration, in mg per mL, of USP Isoniazid RS in the *Standard solution*; and r_U and r_S are the isoniazid peak areas obtained from the *Test solution* and the *Standard solution*, respectively. Calculate the quantity, in mg, of pyrazinamide ($C_5H_5N_3O$) dissolved by the same formula, except to read "USP Pyrazinamide RS" where "USP Isoniazid RS" is specified, and "pyrazinamide" where "isoniazid" is specified.

Tolerances—Not less than 80% *(Q)* of the labeled amount of isoniazid ($C_6H_7N_3O$) and not less than 75% of the labeled amount of pyrazinamide ($C_5H_5N_3O$) are dissolved in 30 minutes.

Uniformity of dosage units ⟨905⟩: meet the requirements.

Loss on drying—Dry about 100 mg of powdered Tablets, accurately weighed, in a capillary-stoppered bottle in vacuum at 60° for 3 hours: it loses not more than 3.0% of its weight.

Assay for rifampin, isoniazid, and pyrazinamide—

Buffer solution—Dissolve 1.4 g of dibasic sodium phosphate in 1 L of water, and adjust with phosphoric acid to a pH of 6.8.

Solution A—Prepare a filtered and degassed mixture of *Buffer solution* and acetonitrile (96 : 4).

Solution B—Prepare a filtered and degassed mixture of acetonitrile and *Buffer solution* (55 : 45).

Mobile phase—Use variable mixtures of *Solution A* and *Solution B* as directed for *Chromatographic system*. Make adjustments if necessary (see *System Suitability* under *Chromatography* ⟨621⟩).

Standard preparation—Dissolve accurately weighed quantities of USP Rifampin RS, USP Isoniazid RS, and USP Pyrazinamide RS in a mixture of *Buffer solution* and methanol (96 : 4) to obtain a solution having known concentrations of about 0.16 mg per mL, 0.08 mg per mL, and 0.43 mg per mL, respectively. [NOTE—Use this solution within 10 minutes.]

Assay preparation—Weigh and finely powder not fewer than 20 Tablets. Transfer an accurately weighed quantity of the powder, equivalent to about 8 mg of isoniazid, to a 100-mL volumetric flask, and add about 90 mL of *Buffer solution*. Sonicate for about 10 minutes, allow to equilibrate to room temperature, dilute with *Buffer solution* to volume, and mix. [NOTE—Use this solution within 2 hours.]

Chromatographic system (see *Chromatography* ⟨621⟩)—The liquid chromatograph is equipped with a 238-nm detector and a 4.6-mm × 25-cm column that contains 5-μm base-deactivated packing L1. The flow rate is about 1.5 mL per minute. The chromatograph is programmed as follows.

Time (minutes)	Solution A (%)	Solution B (%)	Elution
0	100	0	equilibration
0–5	100	0	isocratic
5–6	100→0	0→100	linear gradient
6–15	0	100	isocratic

Chromatograph the *Standard preparation*, and record the peak responses as directed for *Procedure*: the relative retention times are about 1.8, 0.7, and 1.0 for rifampin, isoniazid, and pyrazinamide, respectively; the resolution, *R*, between isoniazid and pyrazinamide is not less than 4; the column efficiency is not less than 50,000, not less than 6,000, and not less than 10,000 theoretical plates for rifampin, isoniazid, and pyrazinamide, respectively; the tailing factor is not more than 2.0; and the relative standard deviation for replicate injections is not more than 2.0%.

Procedure—Separately inject equal volumes (about 20 μL) of the *Standard preparation* and the *Assay preparation* into the chromatograph, record the chromatograms, and measure the peak responses. Calculate the quantities, in mg, of rifampin ($C_{43}H_{58}N_4O_{12}$), isoniazid ($C_6H_7N_3O$), and pyrazinamide ($C_5H_5N_3O$) in the portion of Tablets taken by the formula:

$$100C(r_U / r_S)$$

in which C is the concentration, in mg per mL, of USP Rifampin RS, calculated on the dried basis, or of USP Isoniazid RS or of USP Pyrazinamide RS, as appropriate, in the *Standard preparation;* and r_U and r_S are the peak responses obtained from the corresponding analytes obtained from the *Assay preparation* and the *Standard preparation*, respectively.

Rifampin, Isoniazid, Pyrazinamide, and Ethambutol Hydrochloride Tablets

» Rifampin, Isoniazid, Pyrazinamide, and Ethambutol Hydrochloride Tablets contain not less than 90.0 percent and not more than 110.0 percent of the labeled amounts of rifampin ($C_{43}H_{58}N_4O_{12}$), isoniazid ($C_6H_7N_3O$), pyrazinamide ($C_5H_5N_3O$), and ethambutol hydrochloride ($C_{10}H_{24}N_2O_2 \cdot 2HCl$).

Packaging and storage—Preserve in tight, light-resistant containers, and store at controlled room temperature.

USP Reference standards ⟨11⟩—*USP Ethambutol Hydrochloride RS. USP Isoniazid RS. USP Pyrazinamide RS. USP Rifampin RS.*

Identification—

A: The retention times of the rifampin, isoniazid, and pyrazinamide peaks in the chromatogram of the *Assay preparation* correspond to those in the chromatogram of the *Standard preparation*, as obtained in the *Assay for rifampin, isoniazid, and pyrazinamide.*

B: The retention time of the ethambutol peak in the chromatogram of the *Assay preparation* corresponds to that in the chromatogram of the *Standard preparation*, as obtained in the *Assay for ethambutol hydrochloride.*

Dissolution ⟨711⟩—

Medium: 10 mM pH 6.8 sodium phosphate buffer, prepared by dissolving 7 g of anhydrous dibasic sodium phosphate in 5 L of water, and adjusting with phosphoric acid to a pH of 6.8; 900 mL.

Apparatus 2: 100 rpm.

Time: 45 minutes.

Procedure—Determine the amounts of rifampin ($C_{43}H_{58}N_4O_{12}$), isoniazid ($C_6H_7N_3O$), pyrazinamide ($C_5H_5N_3O$), and ethambutol hydrochloride ($C_{10}H_{24}N_2O_2 \cdot 2HCl$) dissolved using filtered portions of the solution under test and by employing the procedures set forth in the *Assay for rifampin, isoniazid, and pyrazinamide* and the *Assay for ethambutol hydrochloride.*

Tolerances—Not less than 75% *(Q)* of the labeled amounts of $C_{43}H_{58}N_4O_{12}$, $C_6H_7N_3O$, $C_5H_5N_3O$, and $C_{10}H_{24}N_2O_2 \cdot 2HCl$ is dissolved in 45 minutes.

Loss on drying—Dry about 100 mg of powdered Tablets in a capillary-stoppered bottle in vacuum at 60° for 3 hours: it loses not more than 3.0% of its weight.

Assay for rifampin, isoniazid, and pyrazinamide—

Buffer solution—Dissolve 1.4 g of anhydrous dibasic sodium phosphate in 1 L of water, and adjust with phosphoric acid to a pH of 6.8.

Solution A—Prepare a filtered and degassed mixture of *Buffer solution* and acetonitrile (96 : 4).

Solution B—Prepare a filtered and degassed mixture of acetonitrile and *Buffer solution* (55 : 45).

Mobile phase—Use variable mixtures of *Solution A* and *Solution B* as directed for *Chromatographic system*. Make adjustments if necessary (see *System Suitability* under *Chromatography* ⟨621⟩).

Standard preparation—Dissolve accurately weighed quantities of USP Rifampin RS, USP Isoniazid RS, and USP Pyrazinamide RS in a mixture of *Buffer solution* and methanol (96 : 4) to obtain a solution having known concentrations of about 0.16 mg per mL, 0.08 mg per mL, and 0.43 mg per mL, respectively. [NOTE—Use this solution within 10 minutes.]

Assay preparation—Weigh and finely powder not fewer than 20 Tablets. Transfer an accurately weighed quantity of the powder, equivalent to about 8 mg of isoniazid, to a 100-mL volumetric flask, and add about 90 mL of *Buffer solution*. Sonicate for about 10 minutes, allow to equilibrate to room temperature, dilute with *Buffer solution* to volume, and mix. [NOTE—Use this solution within 2 hours.]

Chromatographic system (see *Chromatography* ⟨621⟩)—The liquid chromatograph is equipped with a 238-nm detector and a 4.6-mm × 25-cm column that contains a 5-μm base-deactivated packing L1. The flow rate is about 1.5 mL per minute. The chromatograph is programmed as follows.

Time (minutes)	Solution A (%)	Solution B (%)	Elution
0	100	0	equilibration
0–5	100	0	isocratic
5–6	100→0	0→100	linear gradient
6–15	0	100	isocratic

Chromatograph the *Standard preparation,* and record the peak responses as directed for *Procedure:* the relative retention times for rifampin, isoniazid, and pyrazinamide are about 1.8, 0.7, and 1.0, respectively; the resolution, *R*, between isoniazid and pyrazinamide is not less than 4; the column efficiencies, determined from the rifampin, isoniazid, and pyrazinamide peaks are not less than 50,000 theoretical plates, 6000 theoretical plates, and 10,000 theoretical plates, respectively; the tailing factor is not more than 2.0; and the relative standard deviation for replicate injections is not more than 2.0%.

Procedure—Separately inject equal volumes (about 20 μL) of the *Standard preparation* and the *Assay preparation* into the chromatograph, record the chromatograms, and measure the peak responses. Calculate the quantities, in mg, of rifampin ($C_{43}H_{58}N_4O_{12}$), isoniazid ($C_6H_7N_3O$), and pyrazinamide ($C_5H_5N_3O$) in the portion of Tablets taken by the formula:

$$100C(r_U/r_S)$$

in which *C* is the concentration, in mg per mL, of the appropriate USP Reference Standard in the *Standard preparation;* and r_U and r_S are the peak responses of the corresponding analyte obtained from the *Standard preparation* and the *Assay preparation,* respectively.

Assay for ethambutol hydrochloride—

Diluent—Dissolve 1.4 g of anhydrous dibasic sodium phosphate in 1 L of water, and adjust with phosphoric acid to a pH of 6.8.

Buffer solution—Mix 1.0 mL of triethylamine and 1 L of water, and adjust with phosphoric acid to a pH of 7.0.

Mobile phase—Prepare a filtered and degassed mixture of acetonitrile and *Buffer solution* (50 : 50). Make adjustments if necessary (see *System Suitability* under *Chromatography* ⟨621⟩).

Standard preparation—Dissolve an accurately weighed quantity of USP Ethambutol Hydrochloride RS in *Diluent* to obtain a solution having a known concentration of about 0.3 mg per mL.

Assay preparation—Weigh and finely powder not fewer than 20 Tablets. Transfer an accurately weighed quantity of the powder, equivalent to about 30 mg of ethambutol hydrochloride, to a 100-mL volumetric flask, and add about 90 mL of *Diluent*. Sonicate for about 10 minutes, allow to equilibrate to room temperature, dilute with *Diluent* to volume, and mix. Pass a portion of this solution through a filter, discarding the first 10 mL of the filtrate.

Chromatographic system (see *Chromatography* ⟨621⟩)—The liquid chromatograph is equipped with a 200-nm detector and a 4.6-mm × 15-cm column that contains a 5-μm base-deactivated packing L10. The flow rate is about 1.0 mL per minute. Chromatograph the *Standard preparation,* and record the peak responses as directed for *Procedure:* the tailing factor is not more than 3; and the relative standard deviation for replicate injections is not more than 2.0%.

Procedure—Separately inject equal volumes (about 100 μL) of the *Standard preparation* and the *Assay preparation* into the chromatograph, record the chromatograms, and measure the peak responses. Calculate the quantity, in mg, of ethambutol hydrochloride ($C_{10}H_{24}N_2O_2 \cdot 2HCl$) in the portion of Tablets taken by the formula:

$$100C(r_U/r_S)$$

in which *C* is the concentration, in mg per mL, of USP Ethambutol Hydrochloride RS in the *Standard preparation;* and r_U and r_S are the ethambutol peak responses obtained from the *Assay preparation* and the *Standard preparation,* respectively.

Rimantadine Hydrochloride

$C_{12}H_{21}N \cdot HCl$ 215.77

Tricyclo[3.3.1.1^{3,7}]-decane-1-methanamine, α-methyl-, hydrochloride.

α-Methyl-1-adamantanemethylamine hydrochloride   [1501-84-4].

» Rimantadine Hydrochloride contains not less than 98.0 percent and not more than 102.0 percent of $C_{12}H_{21}N \cdot HCl$, calculated on the dried basis.

Packaging and storage—Preserve in well-closed containers, and store between 15° to 30°.

USP Reference standards ⟨11⟩—*USP Rimantadine Hydrochloride RS.*

Identification—
 A: *Infrared Absorption* ⟨197K⟩.
 B: The retention time of the rimantadine peak in the chromatogram of the *Assay preparation* corresponds to that in the chromatogram of the *Standard preparation,* as obtained in the *Assay.*

X-ray diffraction ⟨941⟩—The X-ray diffraction pattern conforms to that of USP Rimantadine Hydrochloride RS, similarly determined.

Loss on drying ⟨731⟩—Dry it at 105° for 3 hours: it loses not more than 0.5% of its weight.

Residue on ignition ⟨281⟩:   not more than 0.2%.

Heavy metals, *Method II* ⟨231⟩:   20 μg per g.

Ordinary impurities ⟨466⟩—

Test solution—Transfer 100 mg of Rimantadine Hydrochloride to a 10-mL centrifuge tube, add 2 mL of 1 N sodium hydroxide, and mix. Add 2 mL of chloroform, and mix on a vortex mixer for 1 minute. Allow the layers to separate, and apply 10 μL of the organic layer.

Standard solution—Proceed as directed for the *Test solution,* using USP Rimantadine Hydrochloride RS in place of the test specimen.

Eluant: a mixture of ethyl acetate, methanol, and ammonium hydroxide (80 : 10 : 4).

Procedure—Use a low-actinic glass tank. Dry the plate in a stream of hot air, then heat in an oven at 105° for 30 minutes. Allow the plate to cool to room temperature.

Visualization—Place the plate in an atmosphere of chlorine, prepared by mixing 1.5% potassium permanganate solution and diluted hydrochloric acid (1 : 1), for about 90 minutes. Allow to air-dry for 60 minutes, and follow with visualization technique 20.

Limit of toluene—

Standard solution—Transfer 10 μL of toluene to a 100-mL volumetric flask, dilute with chloroform to volume, and mix.

Test solution—Transfer about 750 mg of Rimantadine Hydrochloride, accurately weighed, to a 10-mL volumetric flask, dilute with chloroform to volume, and mix.

Chromatographic system (see *Chromatography* ⟨621⟩)—The gas chromatograph is equipped with a flame-ionization detector and a 2-mm × 2-m column that contains 80- to 100-mesh support S1A. The column temperature is maintained at about 200°, and nitrogen is used as the carrier gas. The injection port and detector temperatures are maintained at about 250°. Chromatograph the *Standard solution,* and record the peak responses as directed for *Procedure:* the tailing factor is not more than 1.5 for toluene; and the relative standard deviation for replicate injections is not more than 2.0%.

Procedure—Separately inject equal volumes (about 5 µL) of the *Standard solution* and the *Test solution* into the chromatograph, record the chromatograms for 9 minutes, and measure the responses for the toluene peaks. Calculate the percentage of toluene in the portion of Rimantadine Hydrochloride taken by the formula:

$$0.867(100/W_U)(r_U / r_S)$$

in which 0.867 is the specific gravity of toluene; W_U is the weight, in mg, of Rimantadine Hydrochloride taken to prepare the *Test solution;* and r_U and r_S are the toluene peak responses obtained from the *Test solution* and the *Standard solution,* respectively: not more than 0.1% is found.

Assay—

Internal standard solution—Transfer about 400 mg of *n*-eicosane to a 250-mL volumetric flask, dilute with hexane to volume, and mix.

Standard preparation—Transfer about 40 mg of USP Rimantadine Hydrochloride RS, accurately weighed, to a 50-mL centrifuge tube, add 15 mL of 1 N sodium hydroxide, and mix. Add 25.0 mL of *Internal standard solution,* and shake by mechanical means for about 15 minutes. Allow the layers to separate, and filter a portion of the top hexane layer through anhydrous sodium sulfate. Use the clear filtrate.

Assay preparation—Using about 40 mg of Rimantadine Hydrochloride, accurately weighed, proceed as directed for *Standard preparation.*

Chromatographic system (see *Chromatography* ⟨621⟩)—The gas chromatograph is equipped with a flame-ionization detector and a 4-mm × 1.8-m glass column that is packed with 3% phase G19 on 100- to 200-mesh support S1A. The column temperature is maintained at about 160°, and the injection port and detector temperatures are maintained at about 250°. Nitrogen is used as the carrier gas. Adjust the carrier flow rate and temperature so that the *n*-eicosane elutes at about 8 minutes. Chromatograph the *Standard preparation,* and record the peak responses as directed for *Procedure:* the tailing factor is not more than 2.0 for rimantadine; and the relative standard deviation for replicate injections is not more than 2.0%.

Procedure—Separately inject equal volumes (about 2 µL) of the *Standard preparation* and the *Assay preparation* into the chromatograph, record the chromatograms, and measure the responses for the major peaks. Calculate the quantity, in mg, of $C_{12}H_{21}N \cdot HCl$ in the portion of Rimantadine Hydrochloride taken by the formula:

$$25C(R_U / R_S)$$

in which C is the concentration, in mg per mL, of USP Rimantadine Hydrochloride in the *Standard preparation;* and R_U and R_S are the ratios of the rimantadine peak response to the *n*-eicosane peak response obtained from the *Assay preparation* and the *Standard preparation,* respectively.

Rimantadine Hydrochloride Tablets

» Rimantadine Hydrochloride Tablets contain not less than 90.0 percent and not more than 110.0 percent of the labeled amount of rimantadine hydrochloride ($C_{12}H_{21}N \cdot HCl$).

Packaging and storage—Preserve in tight, light-resistant containers, and store between 15° to 30°.

USP Reference standards ⟨11⟩—*USP Rimantadine Hydrochloride RS.*

Identification—

A: The retention time of the rimantadine peak in the chromatogram of the *Assay preparation* corresponds to that in the chromatogram of the *Standard preparation,* as obtained in the *Assay.*

B: [*Caution—Avoid contact with o-tolidine when performing this test, and conduct the test in a well-ventilated hood.*] Weigh and finely powder not fewer than 5 Tablets. Transfer a portion of the powder, equivalent to 100 mg of rimantadine hydrochloride, to a 10-mL centrifuge tube, add 2 mL of 1 N sodium hydroxide, and mix. Add 2 mL of chloroform, and mix on a vortex mixer for 1 minute. Allow the layers to separate, and use the organic layer as the test solution. Separately apply 10 µL of the test solution and 10 µL of a Standard solution of USP Rimantadine Hydrochloride RS, similarly prepared, to a suitable thin-layer chromatographic plate (see *Chromatography* ⟨621⟩) coated with a 0.25-mm layer of chromatographic silica gel. Place the plate in a low-actinic glass chromatographic chamber, and develop the chromatogram in a solvent system consisting of a mixture of ethyl acetate, methanol, and ammonium hydroxide (80 : 10 : 4) until the solvent front has moved about three-fourths of the length of the plate. Remove the plate from the chamber, dry it in a stream of hot air, and then heat in an oven at 105° for 30 minutes. Allow the plate to cool to room temperature. Place the dried plate in an atmosphere of chlorine, prepared from a mixture of 1.5% potassium permanganate solution and 3 N hydrochloric acid (1 : 1), for about 90 minutes. Remove the plate, and allow it to air-dry for 60 minutes. Prepare a spray reagent as follows. Dissolve 160 mg of *o*-tolidine in 30 mL of glacial acetic acid, dilute with water to 500 mL, add 1 g of potassium iodide, and mix until the potassium iodide is dissolved. Locate the spots on the plate by spraying with the spray reagent: the R_F value of the principal spot in the chromatogram of the test solution corresponds to that of the principal spot obtained from the Standard solution.

Uniformity of dosage units ⟨905⟩: meet the requirements.

Dissolution ⟨711⟩—

Medium: water; 900 mL.

Apparatus 2: 50 rpm.

Time: 30 minutes.

Procedure—Determine the amount of $C_{12}H_{21}N \cdot HCl$ dissolved, employing the procedure set forth in the *Assay.*

Tolerances—Not less than 80% (*Q*) of the labeled amount of $C_{12}H_{21}N \cdot HCl$ is dissolved in 30 minutes.

Assay—

Internal standard solution, Standard preparation, and *Chromatographic system*—Proceed as directed in the *Assay* under *Rimantadine Hydrochloride.*

Assay preparation—Weigh and finely powder not fewer than 20 Tablets. Transfer an accurately weighed portion of the powder, equivalent to about 40 mg of rimantadine hydrochloride, to a 50-mL centrifuge tube, add 15 mL of 1 N sodium hydroxide, and mix. Add 25.0 mL of *Internal standard solution,* and shake by mechanical means for about 15 minutes. Allow the layers to separate, and filter a portion of the top hexane layer through anhydrous sodium sulfate. Use the clear filtrate as the *Assay preparation.*

Procedure—Separately inject equal volumes (about 2 µL) of the *Standard preparation* and the *Assay preparation* into the chromatograph, record the chromatograms, and measure the responses for the major peaks. Calculate the quantity, in mg, of rimantadine hydrochloride ($C_{12}H_{21}N \cdot HCl$) in the portion of Tablets taken by the formula:

$$25C(R_U / R_S)$$

in which C is the concentration, in mg per mL, of USP Rimantadine Hydrochloride RS in the *Standard preparation;* and R_U and R_S are the ratios of the rimantadine peak response to the *n*-eicosane peak response obtained from the *Assay preparation* and the *Standard preparation,* respectively.

Rimexolone

C₂₄H₃₄O₃   370.52

Androsta-1,4-diene-3-one, 11-hydroxy-16,17-dimethyl-17-(1-oxopropyl)-, (11β, 16α, 17β)-.

11β-Hydroxy-16α,17α-dimethyl-17-propionylandrosta-1,4-diene-3-one   [49697-38-3].

» Rimexolone contains not less than 97.0 percent and not more than 102.0 percent of $C_{24}H_{34}O_3$, calculated on the dried basis.

Packaging and storage—Preserve in well-closed containers.

USP Reference standards ⟨11⟩—*USP Rimexolone RS.*

Identification—
    A: *Infrared Absorption* ⟨197K⟩.
    B: Prepare a test solution in chloroform containing 10 mg per mL. Separately apply 5 μL of this solution and 5 μL of a Standard solution of USP Rimexolone RS in chloroform containing 10 mg per mL to a thin-layer chromatographic plate (see *Chromatography* ⟨621⟩) coated with a 0.25-mm layer of chromatographic silica gel mixture. Allow the spots to dry, and develop the chromatogram in a solvent system consisting of a mixture of chloroform and methanol (19 : 1) until the solvent front has moved about three-fourths of the length of the plate. Remove the plate from the developing chamber, mark the solvent front, and allow the solvent to evaporate. Observe the plate under short-wavelength UV light: the R_F value of the principal spot obtained from the test solution corresponds to that of the principal spot obtained from the Standard solution.

Specific rotation ⟨781S⟩: between +47° and +54°.
    Test solution: 20 mg per mL, in chloroform.

Loss on drying ⟨731⟩—Dry it in vacuum at 105° for 3 hours: it loses not more than 1.0% of its weight.

Residue on ignition ⟨281⟩: not more than 0.1%.

Heavy metals, *Method II* ⟨231⟩: 0.002%.

Chromatographic purity—
    Mobile phase and *Chromatographic system*—Proceed as directed in the *Assay.*
    Test solution—Proceed as directed for *Assay preparation* in the *Assay.*
    Procedure—Inject a volume (about 20 μL) of the *Test solution* into the chromatograph, record the chromatogram, and measure the peak responses. Calculate the percentage of each impurity in the portion of Rimexolone taken by the formula:

$$100(r_i / r_s)$$

in which r_i is the peak response for each impurity, and r_s is the sum of the responses of all of the peaks: not more than 1.0% of any individual impurity is found, and the sum of all impurities is not more than 2.0%.

Organic volatile impurities, *Method V* ⟨467⟩: meets the requirements.

(Official until July 1, 2008)

Assay—
    Mobile phase—Prepare a filtered and degassed mixture of acetonitrile and water (6 : 4). Make adjustments if necessary (see *System Suitability* under *Chromatography* ⟨621⟩).
    Standard preparation—Dissolve an accurately weighed quantity of USP Rimexolone RS in methanol, and dilute quantitatively, and stepwise if necessary, with *Mobile phase* to obtain a solution having a known concentration of about 0.2 mg per mL.
    Assay preparation—Transfer about 25 mg of Rimexolone, accurately weighed, to a 25-mL volumetric flask, dissolve in and dilute with methanol to volume. Transfer 5.0 mL of this solution to a 25 mL-volumetric flask, dilute with *Mobile phase* to volume, and mix.
    Chromatographic system (see *Chromatography* ⟨621⟩)—The liquid chromatograph is equipped with a 242-nm detector and a 4.6-mm × 25-cm column that contains packing L1. The flow rate is about 1 mL per minute. Chromatograph the *Standard preparation*, and record the peak responses as directed for *Procedure:* the capacity factor, k', is not less than 1.5, the column efficiency is not less than 3000 theoretical plates, the tailing factor is not more than 2.0, and the relative standard deviation for replicate injections is not more than 2.0%.
    Procedure—Separately inject equal volumes (about 20 μL) of the *Standard preparation* and the *Assay preparation* into the chromatograph, record the chromatograms, and measure the responses for the major peaks. Calculate the quantity, in mg, of $C_{24}H_{34}O_3$ in the portion of Rimexolone taken by the formula:

$$125C(r_U / r_S)$$

in which C is the concentration, in mg per mL, of USP Rimexolone RS in the *Standard preparation*, and r_U and r_S are the peak responses obtained from the *Assay preparation* and the *Standard preparation*, respectively.

Rimexolone Ophthalmic Suspension

» Rimexolone Ophthalmic Suspension is a sterile suspension of Rimexolone in a suitable aqueous medium. It contains not less than 90.0 percent and not more than 110.0 percent of the labeled amount of rimexolone ($C_{24}H_{34}O_3$). It may contain suitable stabilizers, buffers, and antimicrobial agents.

Packaging and storage—Preserve in well-closed containers.

USP Reference standards ⟨11⟩—*USP Rimexolone RS.*

Identification—The retention time of the major peak in the chromatogram of the *Assay preparation* corresponds to that in the chromatogram of the *Standard preparation*, as obtained in the *Assay.*

Viscosity ⟨911⟩: between 50 and 350 centipoises.

Sterility ⟨71⟩: meets the requirements.

pH ⟨791⟩: between 6.0 and 8.0.

Assay—
    Mobile phase, Standard preparation, Chromatographic system—Proceed as directed in the *Assay* under *Rimexolone.*
    Assay preparation—Transfer an accurately weighed portion of Ophthalmic Suspension, equivalent to about 25 mg of Rimexolone, to a 25-mL volumetric flask, dilute with methanol to volume, and sonicate for 2 minutes. Transfer 5.0 mL of this suspension to a 25-mL volumetric flask, dilute with *Mobile phase* to volume, mix, and filter.
    Procedure—Separately inject equal volumes (about 20 μL) of the *Standard preparation* and the *Assay preparation* into the chromatograph, record the chromatograms, and measure the responses for the major peaks. Calculate the quantity, in mg, of rimexolone ($C_{24}H_{34}O_3$) in the portion of Ophthalmic Suspension taken by the formula:

$$125C(r_U / r_S)$$

in which C is the concentration, in mg per mL, of USP Rimexolone RS in the *Standard preparation*, and r_U and r_S are the peak responses obtained from the *Assay preparation* and the *Standard preparation*, respectively.

Ringer's Injection

» Ringer's Injection is a sterile solution of Sodium Chloride, Potassium Chloride, and Calcium Chloride in Water for Injection. It contains, in each 100 mL, not less than 323.0 mg and not more than 354.0 mg of sodium (Na, equivalent to not less than 820.0 mg and not more than 900.0 mg of NaCl); not less than 14.9 mg and not more than 16.5 mg of potassium (K, equivalent to not less than 28.5 mg and not more than 31.5 mg of KCl); not less than 8.20 mg and not more than 9.80 mg of calcium (Ca, equivalent to not less than 30.0 mg and not more than 36.0 mg of $CaCl_2 \cdot 2H_2O$); and not less than 523.0 mg and not more than 580.0 mg of chloride (Cl, as NaCl, KCl, and $CaCl_2 \cdot 2H_2O$). Ringer's Injection contains no antimicrobial agents.

NOTE—The calcium, chloride, potassium, and sodium ion contents of Ringer's Injection are approximately 4.5, 156, 4, and 147.5 milliequivalents per liter, respectively.

Sodium Chloride	8.6 g
Potassium Chloride	0.3 g
Calcium Chloride	0.33 g
Water for Injection, a sufficient quantity to make	1000 mL

Dissolve the three salts in the Water for Injection, filter until clear, place in suitable containers, and sterilize.

Packaging and storage—Preserve in single-dose glass or plastic containers. Glass containers are preferably of Type I or Type II glass.

Labeling—The label states the total osmolar concentration in mOsmol per L. Where the contents are less than 100 mL, the label alternatively may state the total osmolar concentration in mOsmol per mL.

USP Reference standards ⟨11⟩—*USP Endotoxin RS*.

Identification—It responds to the flame tests for *Sodium* ⟨191⟩ and *Potassium* ⟨191⟩, to the ammonium oxalate test for *Calcium* ⟨191⟩, and to the tests for *Chloride* ⟨191⟩.

Bacterial endotoxins ⟨85⟩—It contains not more than 0.5 USP Endotoxin Unit per mL.

pH ⟨791⟩: between 5.0 and 7.5.

Heavy metals ⟨231⟩—Evaporate 67 mL to a volume of about 20 mL, add 2 mL of 1 N acetic acid, and dilute with water to 25 mL: the limit is 0.3 ppm.

Other requirements—It meets the requirements under *Injections* ⟨1⟩.

Assay for calcium—[NOTE—Concentrations of the *Standard preparations* and the *Assay preparation* may be modified to fit the linear or working range of the atomic absorption spectrophotometer.]

Lanthanum chloride solution—Transfer 17.69 g of lanthanum chloride to a 200-mL volumetric flask, add 100 mL of water, and carefully add 50 mL of hydrochloric acid. Mix, and allow to cool. Dilute with water to volume, and mix.

Blank solution—Transfer 5.0 mL of *Lanthanum chloride solution* to a 100-mL volumetric flask, dilute with water to volume, and mix.

Calcium stock solution—Transfer 499.5 mg of primary standard calcium carbonate to a 200-mL volumetric flask, and add 10 mL of water. Carefully add 5 mL of diluted hydrochloric acid, and swirl to dissolve the calcium carbonate. Dilute with water to volume, and mix. This solution contains 1000 μg of calcium (Ca) per mL.

Standard preparations—To three separate 100-mL volumetric flasks, each containing 5.0 mL of *Lanthanum chloride solution*, add 1.0, 1.5, and 2.0 mL, respectively, of *Calcium stock solution*. Dilute the contents of each flask with water to volume, and mix. These three solutions contain, 10.0, 15.0, and 20.0 μg, respectively, of calcium (Ca) per mL.

Assay preparation—Transfer 20.0 mL of Injection, equivalent to about 1.8 mg of calcium (Ca), to a 100-mL volumetric flask containing 5.0 mL of *Lathanum chloride solution*. Dilute the contents of the flask with water to volume, and mix.

Procedure—Concomitantly determine the absorbances of the *Standard preparations* and the *Assay preparation* at the calcium emission line at 422.7 nm, with a suitable atomic absorption spectrophotometer (see *Spectrophotometry and Light-scattering* ⟨851⟩) equipped with a calcium hollow-cathode lamp and an air–acetylene flame, using the *Blank solution* as the blank. Plot the absorbances of the *Standard preparations* versus concentration, in μg per mL, of calcium, and draw the straight line best fitting the three plotted points. From the graph so obtained, determine the concentration, C, in μg per mL, of calcium in the *Assay preparation*. Calculate the quantity, in mg, of calcium in each 100 mL of the Injection taken by the formula:

$$0.5(C).$$

Assay for potassium—

Standard stock solution—Dissolve 190.7 mg of potassium chloride, previously dried at 105° for 2 hours, in 50 mL of water, transfer to a 1000-mL volumetric flask, dilute with water to volume, and mix. Each mL of this solution contains 100 μg of potassium.

Standard preparations—Dissolve 1.093 g of sodium chloride in 100.0 mL of water, and transfer 10 mL of this solution to each of five 100-mL volumetric flasks containing 10.0 mL of a solution of a suitable nonionic wetting agent (1 in 500). Dilute the contents of one of the flasks with water to volume to provide a blank. To the remaining flasks add, respectively, 5.0, 10.0, 15.0, and 20.0 mL of *Standard stock solution*, dilute with water to volume, and mix.

Assay preparation—Pipet 10 mL of Injection into a 100-mL volumetric flask, add 10.0 mL of a solution of a suitable wetting agent (1 in 500), dilute with water to volume, and mix.

Standard graph—Set a suitable flame photometer for maximum transmittance at a wavelength of about 766 nm. Adjust the instrument to zero transmittance with the blank. Adjust the instrument to 100% transmittance with the most concentrated of the *Standard preparations*. Read the percentage transmittance of the other *Standard preparations*, and plot transmittances versus concentration of potassium.

Procedure—Adjust the instrument as directed under *Standard graph*, read the percentage transmittance of the *Assay preparation*, and calculate the potassium content, in mg per 100 mL, of Injection.

Assay for sodium—

Standard stock solution—Dissolve 254.2 mg of sodium chloride, previously dried at 105° for 2 hours, in 50 mL of water, transfer to a 1000-mL volumetric flask, dilute with water to volume, and mix. Each mL of this solution contains 100 μg of sodium.

Standard preparations—Transfer to each of five 100-mL volumetric flasks 10 mL of a solution of a suitable nonionic wetting agent (1 in 500). Dilute the contents of one of the flasks with water to volume to provide a blank. To the remaining flasks add, respectively, 5.0, 10.0, 15.0, and 20.0 mL of *Standard stock solution*, dilute with water to volume, and mix.

Assay preparation—Pipet 5 mL of Injection into a 1000-mL volumetric flask containing 100 mL of a solution of a suitable wetting agent (1 in 500), dilute with water to volume, and mix.

Procedure—Proceed as directed for *Standard graph* and for *Procedure* in the *Assay for potassium*, setting the flame photometer for maximum transmittance at a wavelength of about 589 nm, instead of about 766 nm. Calculate the sodium content, in mg per 100 mL, of Injection.

Assay for chloride—Pipet 10 mL of Injection into a conical flask, and add 10 mL of glacial acetic acid, 75 mL of methanol, and 3 drops of eosin Y TS. Titrate, with shaking, with 0.1 N silver nitrate VS to a pink endpoint. Each mL of 0.1 N silver nitrate is equivalent to 3.545 mg of Cl.

Ringer's and Dextrose Injection

» Ringer's and Dextrose Injection is a sterile solution of Sodium Chloride, Potassium Chloride, Calcium Chloride, and Dextrose in Water for Injection. It contains, in each 100 mL, not less than 323.0 mg and not more than 354.0 mg of sodium (Na, equivalent to not less than 820.0 mg and not more than 900.0 mg of NaCl), not less than 14.9 mg and not more than 16.5

mg of potassium (K, equivalent to not less than 28.5 mg and not more than 31.5 mg of KCl), not less than 8.20 mg and not more than 9.80 mg of calcium (Ca, equivalent to not less than 30.0 mg and not more than 36.0 mg of CaCl$_2$ · 2H$_2$O), and not less than 523.0 mg and not more than 608.5 mg of chloride (Cl, as NaCl, KCl, and CaCl$_2$ · 2H$_2$O). It contains not less than 95.0 percent and not more than 105.0 percent of the labeled amount of dextrose (C$_6$H$_{12}$O$_6$ · H$_2$O). It contains no antimicrobial agents.

NOTE—The calcium, chloride, potassium, and sodium ion contents of Ringer's and Dextrose Injection are approximately 4.5, 156, 4, and 147.5 milliequivalents per liter, respectively.

Packaging and storage—Preserve in single-dose glass or plastic containers. Glass containers are preferably of Type I or Type II glass.
Labeling—The label states the total osmolar concentration in mOsmol per L. Where the contents are less than 100 mL, the label alternatively may state the total osmolar concentration in mOsmol per mL.
USP Reference standards ⟨11⟩—*USP Endotoxin RS.*
Identification—
   A: It responds to the *Identification* test under *Dextrose.*
   B: It responds to the flame tests for *Sodium* ⟨191⟩ and for *Potassium* ⟨191⟩, to the test for *Chloride* ⟨191⟩, and to the ammonium oxalate test for *Calcium* ⟨191⟩.
Bacterial endotoxins ⟨85⟩—It contains not more than 0.5 USP Endotoxin Unit per mL.
pH ⟨791⟩: between 3.5 and 6.5.
Heavy metals ⟨231⟩—Transfer to a suitable vessel a volume, in mL, of Injection, calculated to two significant figures by the formula:

$$0.2 / [(G_S L_S) + (G_K L_K) + (G_C L_C) + (G_D L_D)]$$

in which G_S, G_K, G_C, and G_D are the labeled amounts, in g, of sodium chloride, potassium chloride, calcium chloride, and dextrose, respectively, in each 100 mL of Injection; and L_S, L_K, L_C, and L_D are the limits, in percentage, for *Heavy metals* specified under *Sodium Chloride, Potassium Chloride, Calcium Chloride,* and *Dextrose,* respectively. Adjust the volume by evaporation or addition of water to 25 mL, as necessary: it meets the requirements of the test.
Limit of 5-hydroxymethylfurfural and related substances—Dilute an accurately measured volume of Injection, equivalent to 1.0 g of C$_6$H$_{12}$O$_6$ · H$_2$O, with water to 500.0 mL. Determine the absorbance of this solution in a 1-cm cell at 284 nm, with a suitable spectrophotometer, using water as the blank: the absorbance is not more than 0.25.
Other requirements—It meets the requirements under *Injections* ⟨1⟩.
Assay for calcium—[NOTE—Concentrations of the *Standard preparations* and the *Assay preparation* may be modified to fit the linear or working range of the atomic absorption spectrophotometer.]
   Lanthanum chloride solution, Blank solution, Calcium stock solution, and *Standard preparations*—Prepare as directed in the *Assay for calcium* under *Ringer's Injection.*
   Assay preparation—Transfer 20.0 mL of Injection (equivalent to about 1.8 mg of calcium) to a 100-mL volumetric flask containing 5.0 mL of *Lanthanum chloride solution.* Dilute the contents of the flask with water to volume, and mix.
   Procedure—Proceed as directed in the *Assay for calcium* under *Ringer's Injection.* Calculate the quantity, in mg, of calcium in each 100 mL of the Injection taken by the formula:

$$0.5C$$

in which C is the concentration, in µg per mL, of calcium in the *Assay preparation,* as determined from the graph.
Assay for potassium—Proceed with Injection as directed in the *Assay for potassium* under *Ringer's Injection.*
Assay for sodium—Proceed with Injection as directed in the *Assay for sodium* under *Ringer's Injection.*

Assay for chloride—Proceed with Injection as directed in the *Assay for chloride* under *Ringer's Injection.*
Assay for dextrose—Transfer an accurately measured volume of Injection, containing 2 to 5 g of dextrose, to a 100-mL volumetric flask. Add 0.2 mL of 6 N ammonium hydroxide, dilute with water to volume, and mix. Determine the angular rotation in a suitable polarimeter tube (see *Optical Rotation* ⟨781⟩). Calculate the percentage (g per 100 mL) of dextrose (C$_6$H$_{12}$O$_6$ · H$_2$O) in the portion of Injection taken by the formula:

$$(100/52.9)(198.17/180.16)AR$$

in which 100 is the percentage; 52.9 is the midpoint of the specific rotation range for anhydrous dextrose, in degrees; 198.17 and 180.16 are the molecular weights for dextrose monohydrate and anhydrous dextrose, respectively; A is 100 mm divided by the length of the polarimeter tube, in mm; and R is the observed rotation, in degrees.

Lactated Ringer's Injection

» Lactated Ringer's Injection is a sterile solution of Calcium Chloride, Potassium Chloride, Sodium Chloride, and Sodium Lactate in Water for Injection. It contains, in each 100 mL, not less than 285.0 mg and not more than 315.0 mg of sodium (as NaCl and C$_3$H$_5$NaO$_3$), not less than 14.2 mg and not more than 17.3 mg of potassium (K, equivalent to not less than 27.0 mg and not more than 33.0 mg of KCl), not less than 4.90 mg and not more than 6.00 mg of calcium (Ca, equivalent to not less than 18.0 mg and not more than 22.0 mg of CaCl$_2$ · 2H$_2$O), not less than 368.0 mg and not more than 408.0 mg of chloride (Cl, as NaCl, KCl, and CaCl$_2$ · 2H$_2$O), and not less than 231.0 mg and not more than 261.0 mg of lactate (C$_3$H$_5$O$_3$, equivalent to not less than 290.0 mg and not more than 330.0 mg of C$_3$H$_5$NaO$_3$). Lactated Ringer's Injection contains no antimicrobial agents.

NOTE—The calcium, potassium, and sodium contents of Lactated Ringer's Injection are approximately 2.7, 4, and 130 milliequivalents per liter, respectively.

Packaging and storage—Preserve in single-dose glass or plastic containers. Glass containers are preferably of Type I or Type II glass.
Labeling—The label states the total osmolar concentration in mOsmol per L. Where the contents are less than 100 mL, the label alternatively may state the total osmolar concentration in mOsmol per mL. The label includes also the warning "Not for use in the treatment of lactic acidosis."
USP Reference standards ⟨11⟩—*USP Sodium Lactate RS. USP Endotoxin RS.*
Identification—
   A: It responds to the flame tests for *Sodium* ⟨191⟩ and for *Potassium* ⟨191⟩, to the ammonium oxalate test for *Calcium* ⟨191⟩, and to the tests for *Chloride* ⟨191⟩.
   B: The retention time of the lactate peak in the chromatogram of the *Assay preparation* corresponds to that of the *Standard preparation* as obtained in the *Assay for lactate.*
Bacterial endotoxins ⟨85⟩—It contains not more than 0.5 USP Endotoxin Unit per mL.
pH ⟨791⟩: between 6.0 and 7.5.
Heavy metals ⟨231⟩—Evaporate 67 mL to a volume of 20 mL, add 2 mL of 1 N acetic acid, then dilute with water to 25 mL: the limit is 0.3 ppm.
Other requirements—It meets the requirements under *Injections* ⟨1⟩.

Assay for calcium—Proceed with Injection as directed in the *Assay for calcium* under *Ringer's Injection*.
Assay for potassium—Proceed with Injection as directed in the *Assay for potassium* under *Ringer's Injection*.
Assay for sodium—Proceed with Injection as directed in the *Assay for sodium* under *Ringer's Injection*.
Assay for chloride—Proceed with Injection as directed in the *Assay for chloride* under *Ringer's Injection*.
Assay for lactate—

Mobile phase—Prepare a solution in water containing about 1 mL of formic acid and 1 mL of dicyclohexylamine per liter, filter, and degas. Make adjustments if necessary (see *System Suitability* under *Chromatography* ⟨621⟩).

Resolution solution—Prepare a solution in water containing about 3 mg of anhydrous sodium acetate and 3 mg of USP Sodium Lactate RS per mL.

Standard preparation—Dissolve an accurately weighed quantity of USP Sodium Lactate RS in water to obtain a solution having a known concentration of about 3 mg per mL.

Assay preparation—Use undiluted Injection.

Chromatographic system (see *Chromatography* ⟨621⟩)—The liquid chromatograph is equipped with a 210-nm detector and a 4.6-mm × 10-cm column that contains packing L1. The flow rate is about 1 mL per minute. Chromatograph the *Resolution solution*, and record the peak responses as directed for *Procedure*: the resolution, R, between the acetate peak and the lactate peak is not less than 2. Chromatograph the *Standard preparation*, and record the responses as directed for *Procedure*: the tailing factor for the analyte peak is not more than 2.0, and the relative standard deviation for replicate injections is not more than 2.0%.

Procedure—Separately inject equal volumes (about 20 µL) of the *Standard preparations* and the *Assay preparation* into the chromatograph, record the chromatograms, and measure the responses for the major peaks. Calculate the quantity, in mg, of lactate ($C_3H_5O_3$) in the Injection taken by the formula:

$$C(89.07 / 112.06)(r_U / r_S)$$

in which C is the concentration, in mg per mL, of USP Sodium Lactate RS in the *Standard preparation*, 89.07 and 112.06 are the molecular weights of lactate ($C_3H_5O_3$) and anhydrous sodium lactate ($C_3H_5NaO_3$), respectively, and r_U and r_S are the lactate peak responses obtained from the *Assay preparation* and the *Standard preparation*, respectively.

Lactated Ringer's and Dextrose Injection

» Lactated Ringer's and Dextrose Injection is a sterile solution of Calcium Chloride, Potassium Chloride, Sodium Chloride, Sodium Lactate, and Dextrose in Water for Injection. It contains, in each 100 mL, not less than 285.0 mg and not more than 315.0 mg of sodium (as NaCl and $C_3H_5NaO_3$), not less than 14.2 mg and not more than 17.3 mg of potassium (K, equivalent to not less than 27.0 mg and not more than 33.0 mg of KCl), not less than 4.90 mg and not more than 6.00 mg of calcium (Ca, equivalent to not less than 18.0 mg and not more than 22.0 mg of $CaCl_2 \cdot 2H_2O$), not less than 368.0 mg and not more than 428.0 mg of chloride (Cl, as NaCl, KCl, and $CaCl_2 \cdot 2H_2O$), and not less than 231.0 mg and not more than 261.0 mg of lactate ($C_3H_5O_3$, equivalent to not less than 290.0 mg and not more than 330.0 mg of $C_3H_5NaO_3$). It contains not less than 90.0 percent and not more than 105.0 percent of the labeled amount of dextrose ($C_6H_{12}O_6 \cdot H_2O$). It contains no antimicrobial agents.

NOTE—The calcium, potassium, and sodium contents of Lactated Ringer's and Dextrose Injection are approximately 2.7, 4, and 130 milliequivalents per liter, respectively.

Packaging and storage—Preserve in single-dose glass or plastic containers. Glass containers are preferably of Type I or Type II glass.

Labeling—The label states the total osmolar concentration in mOsmol per L. Where the contents are less than 100 mL, the label alternatively may state the total osmolar concentration in mOsmol per mL. The label includes also the warning: "Not for use in the treatment of lactic acidosis."

USP Reference standards ⟨11⟩—*USP Sodium Lactate RS. USP Endotoxin RS.*

Identification—

A: It responds to the *Identification* test under *Dextrose Injection*.

B: It responds to the flame tests for *Sodium* ⟨191⟩ and for *Potassium* ⟨191⟩, to the test for *Chloride* ⟨191⟩, and to the ammonium oxalate test for *Calcium* ⟨191⟩.

C: The retention time of the lactate peak in the chromatogram of the *Assay preparation* corresponds to that of the *Standard preparation* as obtained in the *Assay for lactate*.

Bacterial endotoxins ⟨85⟩—It contains not more than 0.5 USP Endotoxin Unit per mL.

pH ⟨791⟩: between 4.0 and 6.5.

Limit of 5-hydroxymethylfurfural and related substances—Dilute an accurately measured volume of Injection, equivalent to 1.0 g of $C_6H_{12}O_6 \cdot H_2O$, with water to 500.0 mL. Determine the absorbance of this solution in a 1-cm cell at 284 nm, with a suitable spectrophotometer, using water as the blank: the absorbance is not more than 0.25.

Heavy metals ⟨231⟩—Transfer to a suitable vessel a volume, in mL, of Injection, calculated to two significant figures by the formula:

$$0.2 / [(G_S L_S) + (G_K L_K) + (G_C L_C) + (G_L L_L) + (G_D L_D)]$$

in which G_S, G_K, G_C, G_L, and G_D are the labeled amounts, in g, of sodium chloride, potassium chloride, calcium chloride, sodium lactate, and dextrose, respectively, in each 100 mL of Injection, and L_S, L_K, L_C, L_L, and L_D are the limits, in percentage, for *Heavy metals* specified under *Sodium Chloride*, *Potassium Chloride*, *Calcium Chloride*, *Sodium Lactate*, and *Dextrose*, respectively. Adjust the volume by evaporation or addition of water to 25 mL, as necessary: it meets the requirements of the test.

Other requirements—It meets the requirements under *Injections* ⟨1⟩.

Assay for calcium—[NOTE—Concentrations of the *Standard preparations* and the *Assay preparation* may be modified to fit the linear or working range of the atomic absorption spectrophotometer.]

Lanthanum chloride solution, Blank solution, Calcium stock solution, and *Standard preparations*—Prepare as directed in the *Assay for calcium* under *Ringer's Injection*.

Assay preparation—Transfer 50.0 mL of Injection (equivalent to about 1.4 mg of calcium), to a 100-mL volumetric flask containing 5.0 mL of *Lanthanum chloride solution*. Dilute the contents of the flask with water to volume, and mix.

Procedure—Proceed as directed in the *Assay for calcium* under *Ringer's Injection*. Calculate the quantity, in mg, of calcium in each 100 mL of the Injection taken by the formula:

$$0.2C$$

in which C is the concentration, in µg per mL, of calcium in the *Assay preparation*, as determined from the graph.

Assay for potassium—Proceed with Injection as directed in the *Assay for potassium* under *Ringer's Injection*.

Assay for sodium—Proceed with Injection as directed in the *Assay for sodium* under *Ringer's Injection*.

Assay for chloride—Proceed with Injection as directed in the *Assay for chloride* under *Ringer's Injection*.

Assay for lactate—
Mobile phase, Resolution solution, Standard preparation, Chromatographic system, and *Procedure*—Proceed as directed in the *Assay for lactate* under *Lactated Ringer's Injection.*
Assay preparation—Use undiluted Injection.
Procedure—Proceed as directed in the *Assay for lactate* under *Lactated Ringer's Injection.* Calculate the concentration, in mg per mL, of lactate ($C_3H_5O_3$) in the *Assay preparation* taken by the formula:

$$C(89.07 / 112.06)(r_U / r_S)$$

in which the terms are as defined therein.
Assay for dextrose—Proceed with Injection as directed in the *Assay for dextrose* under *Ringer's and Dextrose Injection.*

Half-Strength Lactated Ringer's and Dextrose Injection

» Half-Strength Lactated Ringer's and Dextrose Injection is a sterile solution of Calcium Chloride, Potassium Chloride, Sodium Chloride, Sodium Lactate, and Dextrose in Water for Injection. It contains, in each 100 mL, not less than 142.5 mg and not more than 157.5 mg of sodium (as NaCl and $C_3H_5NaO_3$), not less than 7.08 mg and not more than 8.65 mg of potassium (K, equivalent to not less than 13.5 mg and not more than 16.5 mg of KCl), not less than 2.45 mg and not more than 3.00 mg of calcium (Ca, equivalent to not less than 9.0 mg and not more than 11.0 mg of $CaCl_2 \cdot 2H_2O$), not less than 184.0 mg and not more than 214.0 mg of chloride (Cl, as NaCl, KCl, and $CaCl_2 \cdot 2H_2O$), and not less than 115.5 mg and not more than 130.5 mg of lactate ($C_3H_5O_3$, equivalent to not less than 145.0 mg and not more than 165.0 mg of $C_3H_5NaO_3$). It contains not less than 90.0 percent and not more than 105.0 percent of the labeled amount of dextrose ($C_6H_{12}O_6 \cdot H_2O$). It contains no antimicrobial agents.

NOTE—The calcium, potassium, and sodium contents of Half-strength Lactated Ringer's and Dextrose Injection are approximately 1.4, 2, and 65 milliequivalents per liter, respectively.

Packaging and storage—Preserve in single-dose glass or plastic containers. Glass containers are preferably of Type I or Type II glass.
Labeling—The label states the total osmolar concentration in mOsmol per L. Where the contents are less than 100 mL, the label alternatively may state the total osmolar concentration in mOsmol per mL. The label includes also the warning: "Not for use in the treatment of lactic acidosis."
USP Reference standards ⟨11⟩—USP Sodium Lactate RS. USP Endotoxin RS.
Identification—
  A: It responds to the *Identification* test under *Dextrose.*
  B: It responds to the flame tests for *Sodium* ⟨191⟩ and for *Potassium* ⟨191⟩, to the test for *Chloride* ⟨191⟩, and to the ammonium oxalate test for *Calcium* ⟨191⟩.
  C: The retention time of the lactate peak in the chromatogram of the *Assay preparation* corresponds to that of the *Standard preparation* as obtained in the *Assay for lactate.*
Bacterial endotoxins ⟨85⟩—It contains not more than 0.5 USP Endotoxin Unit per mL.

pH ⟨791⟩: between 4.0 and 6.5.
Heavy metals ⟨231⟩—Transfer to a suitable vessel a volume, in mL, of Injection, calculated to two significant figures by the formula:

$$0.2 / [(G_S L_S) + (G_K L_K) + (G_C L_C) + (G_L L_L) + (G_D L_D)]$$

in which G_S, G_K, G_C, G_L, and G_D are the labeled amounts, in g, of sodium chloride, potassium chloride, calcium chloride, sodium lactate, and dextrose, respectively, in each 100 mL of Injection, and L_S, L_K, L_C, L_L, and L_D are the limits, in percentage, for *Heavy metals* specified under *Sodium Chloride, Potassium Chloride, Calcium Chloride, Sodium Lactate,* and *Dextrose,* respectively. Adjust the volume by evaporation or addition of water to 25 mL, as necessary: it meets the requirements of the test.
Limit of 5-hydroxymethylfurfural and related substances—Dilute an accurately measured volume of Injection, equivalent to 1.0 g of $C_6H_{12}O_6 \cdot H_2O$, with water to 500.0 mL. Determine the absorbance of this solution in a 1-cm cell at 284 nm, with a suitable spectrophotometer, using water as the blank: the absorbance is not more than 0.25.
Other requirements—It meets the requirements under *Injections* ⟨1⟩.
Assay for calcium—[NOTE—Concentrations of the *Standard preparations* and the *Assay preparation* may be modified to fit the linear or working range of the atomic absorption spectrophotometer.]
Lanthanum chloride solution, Blank solution, Calcium stock solution, and *Standard preparations*—Prepare as directed in the *Assay for calcium* under *Ringer's Injection.*
Assay preparation—Transfer 50.0 mL of Injection (equivalent to about 1.4 mg of calcium), to a 100-mL volumetric flask containing 5.0 mL of *Lanthanum chloride solution.* Dilute the contents of the flask with water to volume, and mix.
Procedure—Proceed as directed in the *Assay for calcium* under *Ringer's Injection.* Calculate the quantity, in mg, of calcium in each 100 mL of the Injection taken by the formula:

$$0.2C$$

in which C is the concentration, in μg per mL, of calcium in the *Assay preparation,* as determined from the graph.
Assay for potassium—
Standard stock solution, Standard preparations, and *Standard graph*—Proceed as directed in the *Assay for potassium* under *Ringer's Injection.*
Assay preparation—Transfer 20.0 mL of Injection to a 100-mL volumetric flask, add 10.0 mL of a solution of a suitable wetting agent (1 in 500), dilute with water to volume, and mix.
Procedure—Adjust the instrument as directed under *Standard graph,* read the percentage transmittance of the *Assay preparation,* and calculate the potassium content, in mg per mL, of Injection.
Assay for sodium—
Standard stock solution and *Standard preparations*—Proceed as directed in the *Assay for sodium* under *Ringer's Injection.*
Assay preparation—Transfer 10.0 mL of Injection to a 1000-mL volumetric flask containing 100 mL of a solution of a suitable wetting agent (1 in 500), dilute with water to volume, and mix.
Procedure—Proceed as directed for *Standard graph* and for *Procedure* in the *Assay for potassium* under *Ringer's Injection,* setting the flame photometer for maximum transmittance at a wavelength of about 589 nm, instead of about 766 nm. Calculate the sodium content, in mg per 100 mL, of Injection.
Assay for chloride—Proceed with Injection as directed in the *Assay for chloride* under *Ringer's Injection.*
Assay for lactate—
Mobile phase, Resolution solution, Chromatographic system, and *Procedure*—Proceed as directed in the *Assay for lactate* under *Lactated Ringer's Injection.*
Standard preparation—Dissolve an accurately weighed quantity of USP Sodium Lactate RS quantitatively in water to obtain a solution having a known concentration of about 1.6 mg per mL.
Assay preparation—Use undiluted Injection.
Procedure—Proceed as directed in the *Assay for lactate* under *Lactated Ringer's Injection.* Calculate the concentration, in mg per

mL, of lactate ($C_3H_5O_3$) in the *Assay preparation* taken by the formula:

$$C(89.07 / 112.06)(r_U / r_S)$$

in which the terms are as defined therein.
Assay for dextrose—Proceed with Injection as directed in the *Assay for dextrose* under *Ringer's and Dextrose Injection*.

Modified Lactated Ringer's and Dextrose Injection

» Modified Lactated Ringer's and Dextrose Injection is a sterile solution of Calcium Chloride, Potassium Chloride, Sodium Chloride, Sodium Lactate, and Dextrose in Water for Injection. It contains, in each 100 mL, not less than 57.0 mg and not more than 63.0 mg of sodium (as NaCl and $C_3H_5NaO_3$), not less than 2.82 mg and not more than 3.46 mg of potassium (K, equivalent to not less than 5.4 mg and not more than 6.6 mg of KCl), not less than 0.98 mg and not more than 1.20 mg of calcium (Ca, equivalent to not less than 3.6 mg and not more than 4.4 mg of $CaCl_2 \cdot 2H_2O$), not less than 73.6 mg and not more than 85.6 mg of chloride (Cl, as NaCl, KCl, and $CaCl_2 \cdot 2H_2O$), and not less than 46.2 mg and not more than 52.20 mg of lactate ($C_3H_5O_3$, equivalent to not less than 58.0 mg and not more than 66.0 mg of $C_3H_5NaO_3$). It contains not less than 90.0 percent and not more than 105.0 percent of the labeled amount of dextrose ($C_6H_{12}O_6 \cdot H_2O$). It contains no antimicrobial agents.

NOTE—The calcium, potassium, and sodium contents of Modified Lactated Ringer's and Dextrose Injection are approximately 0.5, 0.8, and 26 milliequivalents per liter, respectively.

Packaging and storage—Preserve in single-dose glass or plastic containers. Glass containers are preferably of Type I or Type II glass.
Labeling—The label states the total osmolar concentration in mOsmol per L. Where the contents are less than 100 mL, the label alternatively may state the total osmolar concentration in mOsmol per mL. The label includes also the warning: "Not for use in the treatment of lactic acidosis."
USP Reference standards ⟨11⟩—*USP Sodium Lactate RS. USP Endotoxin RS.*
Identification—
  A: It responds to the *Identification* test under *Dextrose*.
  B: It responds to the flame tests for *Sodium* ⟨191⟩ and for *Potassium* ⟨191⟩, to the test for *Chloride* ⟨191⟩, and to the ammonium oxalate test for *Calcium* ⟨191⟩.
  C: The retention time of the lactate peak in the chromatogram of the *Assay preparation* corresponds to that of the *Standard preparation* as obtained in the *Assay for lactate*.
Bacterial endotoxins ⟨85⟩—It contains not more than 0.5 USP Endotoxin Unit per mL.
pH ⟨791⟩: between 4.0 and 6.5.
Heavy metals ⟨231⟩—Transfer to a suitable vessel, a volume, in mL, of Injection, calculated to two significant figures by the formula:

$$0.2 / [(G_S L_S) + (G_K L_K) + (G_C L_C) + (G_L L_L) + (G_D L_D)]$$

in which G_S, G_K, G_C, G_L, and G_D are the labeled amounts, in g, of sodium chloride, potassium chloride, calcium chloride, sodium lactate, and dextrose, respectively, in each 100 mL of Injection; and L_S, L_K, L_C, L_L, and L_D are the limits, in percentage, for *Heavy metals* specified under *Sodium Chloride*, *Potassium Chloride*, *Calcium Chloride*, *Sodium Lactate*, and *Dextrose*, respectively. Adjust the volume by evaporation or addition of water to 25 mL, as necessary: it meets the requirements of the test.
Limit of 5-hydroxymethylfurfural and related substances—Dilute an accurately measured volume of Injection, equivalent to 1.0 g of $C_6H_{12}O_6 \cdot H_2O$, with water to 500.0 mL. Determine the absorbance of this solution in a 1-cm cell at 284 nm, with a suitable spectrophotometer, using water as the blank: the absorbance is not more than 0.25.
Other requirements—It meets the requirements under *Injections* ⟨1⟩.
Assay for calcium—[NOTE—Concentrations of the *Standard preparations* and the *Assay preparation* may be modified to fit the linear or working range of the atomic absorption spectrophotometer.]
  Lanthanum chloride solution, Dilute hydrochloric acid, Blank solution, Calcium stock solution, and *Standard preparations*—Prepare as directed in the *Assay for calcium* under *Ringer's Injection*.
  Assay preparation—Transfer 5.0 mL of *Lanthanum chloride solution* to a 100-mL volumetric flask, dilute with Injection to volume, and mix.
  Procedure—Proceed as directed in the *Assay for calcium* under *Ringer's Injection*. Calculate the quantity, in mg, of calcium in each 100 mL of the Injection taken by the formula:

$$0.105C$$

in which C is the concentration, in μg per mL, of calcium in the *Assay preparation*, as determined from the graph.
Assay for potassium—
  Standard stock solution, Standard preparations, and *Standard graph*—Proceed as directed in the *Assay for potassium* under *Ringer's Injection*.
  Assay preparation—Transfer 50.0 mL of Injection to a 100-mL volumetric flask, add 10.0 mL of a solution of a suitable wetting agent (1 in 500), dilute with water to volume, and mix.
  Procedure—Adjust the instrument as directed under *Standard graph*, read the percentage transmittance of the *Assay preparation*, and calculate the potassium content, in mg per 100 mL, of Injection.
Assay for sodium—
  Standard stock solution and *Standard preparations*—Proceed as directed in the *Assay for sodium* under *Ringer's Injection*.
  Assay preparation—Transfer 25.0 mL of Injection to a 1000-mL volumetric flask containing 100 mL of a solution of a suitable wetting agent (1 in 500), dilute with water to volume, and mix.
  Procedure—Proceed as directed for *Standard graph* and for *Procedure* in the *Assay for potassium* under *Ringer's Injection*, setting the flame photometer for maximum transmittance at a wavelength of about 589 nm, instead of about 766 nm. Calculate the sodium content, in mg per 100 mL, of Injection.
Assay for chloride—Proceed with Injection as directed in the *Assay for chloride* under *Ringer's Injection*.
Assay for lactate—
  Mobile phase, Resolution solution, Chromatographic system, and *Procedure*—Proceed as directed in the *Assay for lactate* under *Lactated Ringer's Injection*.
  Standard preparation—Dissolve an accurately weighed quantity of USP Sodium Lactate RS in water to obtain a solution having a known concentration of about 0.6 mg per mL.
  Assay preparation—Use undiluted Injection.
  Procedure—Proceed as directed in the *Assay for lactate* under *Lactated Ringer's Injection*. Calculate the concentration, in mg per mL, of lactate ($C_3H_5O_3$) in the *Assay preparation* taken by the formula:

$$C(89.07 / 112.06)(r_U / r_S)$$

in which the terms are as defined therein.
Assay for dextrose—Proceed with Injection as directed in the *Assay for dextrose* under *Ringer's and Dextrose Injection*.

Ringer's Irrigation

» Ringer's Irrigation is Ringer's Injection that has been suitably packaged, and it contains no antimicrobial agents.

Packaging and storage—Preserve in single-dose glass or plastic containers. Glass containers are preferably of Type I or Type II glass. The container may be designed to empty rapidly and may contain a volume of more than 1 L.
Labeling—The designation "not for injection" appears prominently on the label.
USP Reference standards ⟨11⟩—*USP Endotoxin RS.*
Bacterial endotoxins ⟨85⟩—It contains not more than 0.5 USP Endotoxin Unit per mL.
Sterility ⟨71⟩: meets the requirements.
Other requirements—It responds to the *Identification* tests, and meets the requirements for *pH*, *Heavy metals*, *Assay for calcium*, *Assay for potassium*, *Assay for sodium*, and *Assay for chloride* under *Ringer's Injection*.

Risperidone

$C_{23}H_{27}FN_4O_2$ 410.48
4*H*-Pyrido[1,2-*a*]pyrimidin-4-one, 3-[2-[4-(6-fluoro-1,2-benzisoxazol-3-yl)-1-piperidinyl]ethyl]-6,7,8,9-tetrahydro-2-methyl-.
3-[2-[4-(6-Fluoro-1,2-benzisoxazol-3-yl)piperidino]ethyl]-6,7,8,9-tetrahydro-2-methyl-4*H*-pyrido[1,2-*a*]pyrimidin-4-one [106266-06-2].

» Risperidone contains not less than 98.0 percent and not more than 102.0 percent of $C_{23}H_{27}FN_4O_2$, calculated on the dried basis.

Packaging and storage—Preserve in well-closed containers. Store at room temperature.
USP Reference standards ⟨11⟩—*USP Risperidone RS. USP Risperidone System Suitability Mixture RS.* [NOTE—This mixture contains risperidone, Z-oxime, 9-hydroxyrisperidone, and 6-methylrisperidone.]
Identification—
 A: *Infrared Absorption* ⟨197K⟩.
 B: The retention time of the major peak in the chromatogram of the *Assay preparation* corresponds to that in the chromatogram of the *Standard preparation*, as obtained in the *Assay*.
Loss on drying ⟨731⟩—Dry in vacuum at 80° for 4 hours: it loses not more than 0.5% of its weight.
Residue on ignition ⟨281⟩: not more than 0.1%, a 2.0-g test specimen being used.
Heavy metals, *Method II* ⟨231⟩: 0.001%.
Related compounds—
 Buffer solution, Solution A, Solution B, Mobile phase, Diluent, System suitability solution, and *Chromatographic system*—Prepare as directed in the *Assay*.
 Standard solution—Use the *Standard preparation*, prepared as directed in the *Assay.*
 Test solution—Use the *Assay preparation*.
 Procedure—Inject equal volumes (about 10 µL) of the *Standard solution* and the *Test solution* into the chromatograph, and record the chromatogram. Identify the impurities using the relative retention times given in *Table 1*, and measure the peak responses. Calculate the percentage of each risperidone related compound in the portion of Risperidone taken by the formula:

$$100(C_S/C_U)(r_U/r_S)(1/F)$$

in which C_S and C_U are the concentrations, in mg per mL, of risperidone in the *Standard solution* and the *Test solution* respectively; r_U is the peak area of each impurity obtained from the *Test solution*; r_S is the peak area of risperidone obtained from the *Standard solution*; and *F* is the relative response factor for each impurity relative to risperidone. In addition to not exceeding the limits in *Table 1*, not more than 0.10% of any unknown impurity (use *F* value of 1.0) is found and not more than 0.30% of the total impurities is found. Disregard the impurity peaks that are less than 0.05%.

Table 1

Related Compound	Relative Retention Time (RRT)	Relative Response Factor (*F*)	Limit (%)
E-oxime[1]	0.60	1.0	NMT 0.20
Z-oxime[2]	0.67	0.63	NMT 0.20
9-hydroxyrisperidone[3]	0.76	0.92	NMT 0.20
5-fluororisperidone[4]	0.94	1.0	NMT 0.20
Risperidone	1.0	1.0	—
6-methylrisperidone[5]	1.2	0.95	NMT 0.20

[1] 3-[2-[4-[(*E*)-(2,4-Difluorophenyl)(hydroxyimino)methyl]piperidin-1-yl]ethyl]-2-methyl-6,7,8,9-tetrahydro-4*H*-pyrido[1,2-*a*]pyrimidin-4-one
[2] 3-[2-[4-[(*Z*)-(2,4-Difluorophenyl)(hydroxyimino)methyl]piperidin-1-yl]ethyl]-2-methyl-6,7,8,9-tetrahydro-4*H*-pyrido[1,2-*a*]pyrimidin-4-one
[3] (9*RS*)-3-[2-[4-(6-Fluoro-1,2-benzisoxazol-3-yl)piperidin-1-yl]ethyl]-9-hydroxy-2-methyl-6,7,8,9-tetrahydro-4*H*-pyrido[1,2-*a*]pyrimidin-4-one
[4] 3-[2-[4-(5-Fluoro-1,2-benzisoxazol-3-yl)piperidin-1-yl]ethyl]-2-methyl-6,7,8,9-tetrahydro-4*H*-pyrido[1,2-*a*]pyrimidin-4-one
[5] (6*RS*)-3-[2-[4-(6-Fluoro-1,2-benzisoxazol-3-yl)piperidin-1-yl]ethyl]-2,6-dimethyl-6,7,8,9-tetrahydro-4*H*-pyrido[1,2-*a*]pyrimidin-4-one

Assay—
 Buffer solution—Dissolve 15.4 g of ammonium acetate in 1 L of water. Adjust with 10% acetic acid to a pH of 6.5, and mix.
 Solution A—Mix 100 mL of *Buffer solution* with 150 mL of methanol in a 1000-mL volumetric flask, and dilute with water to volume.
 Solution B—Mix 100 mL of *Buffer solution* with 850 mL of methanol in a 1000-mL volumetric flask, and dilute with water to volume.
 Mobile phase—Use variable mixtures of *Solution A* and *Solution B* as directed for *Chromatographic system*. Make adjustments if necessary (see *System Suitability* under *Chromatography* ⟨621⟩).
 Diluent—Mix 100 mL of *Buffer solution* with 900 mL of water and 1000 mL of methanol.
 System suitability solution—Prepare a 1 mg per mL solution of USP Risperidone System Suitability Mixture RS in *Diluent*.
 Standard preparation—Dissolve an accurately weighed quantity of USP Risperidone RS in *Diluent*, and dilute quantitatively, and stepwise if necessary, with *Diluent* to obtain a solution having a known concentration of about 1.0 mg per mL.
 Assay preparation—Dissolve an accurately weighed quantity of Risperidone in *Diluent*, and dilute quantitatively, and stepwise if necessary, with *Diluent* to obtain a solution having a concentration of about 1.0 mg per mL.
 Chromatographic system (see *Chromatography* ⟨621⟩)—The liquid chromatograph is equipped with a 275-nm detector and a 4.6-mm × 10-cm column that contains 3-µm packing L1. The flow rate is about 1.5 mL per minute. The column temperature is maintained at 35°. The chromatograph is programmed as follows.

Time (minutes)	Solution A (%)	Solution B (%)	Elution
0–1	70	30	isocratic
1–20	70→5	30→95	linear gradient
20–25	5	95	isocratic

Time (minutes)	Solution A (%)	Solution B (%)	Elution
25–27	5→70	95→30	linear gradient
27–35	70	30	re-equilbration

Inject the *System suitability solution*. Record the peak responses as directed for *Procedure*, and identify the peaks due to Z-oxime, 9-hydroxyrisperidone, 6-methylrisperidone, and risperidone using the relative retention times (RRT) from *Table 1*; the resolution, R, between Z-oxime and 9-hydroxyrisperidone is not less than 2.8; the tailing factor for risperidone is not more than 1.5; and the relative standard deviation for replicate injections is not more than 2.0% for the risperidone peak.

Procedure—Separately inject equal volumes (about 10 μL) of the *Standard preparation* and the *Assay preparation* into the chromatograph, and measure the responses for the risperidone peak. Calculate the quantity, in percent of $C_{23}H_{27}FN_4O_2$, in the portion of Risperidone taken by the formula:

$$100(C_S / C_U)(r_U / r_S)$$

in which C_S and C_U are the concentrations, in mg per mL, of risperidone in the *Standard preparation* and the *Assay preparation*, respectively; and r_U and r_S are the peak responses obtained from the *Assay preparation* and the *Standard preparation*, respectively.

Risperidone Tablets

» Risperidone Tablets contain not less than 90.0 percent and not more than 110.0 percent of the labeled amount of risperidone ($C_{23}H_{27}FN_4O_2$).

Packaging and storage—Preserve in tight, light-resistant containers. Store at controlled room temperature.

USP Reference standards ⟨11⟩—USP Risperidone RS.
Identification—
  A: *Infrared Absorption—*
  Test solution—Grind an appropriate number of Tablets to prepare a 550 ± 50 μg per mL solution of risperidone in ethyl acetate. Shake the solution for 30 minutes, and centrifuge for 20 minutes. Evaporate 5 mL of the supernatant with the aid of a stream of nitrogen to 2 mL on a warm water bath. Add 150 ± 50 mg of KBr powder, mix well, and evaporate to dryness. Grind the dried mixture, and press a small amount into a transparent pellet ⟨197K⟩.
  Standard solution—Grind about 2 mg of USP Risperidone RS with about 200 mg of KBr powder, and press into a transparent pellet.
  B: The retention time of the major peak in the chromatogram of the *Assay preparation* corresponds to that in the chromatogram of the *Standard preparation*, as obtained in the *Assay*.
Dissolution ⟨711⟩—
  Medium: 0.1 N hydrochloric acid; 500 mL.
  Apparatus 2: 50 rpm.
  Time: 45 minutes.
  Determine the amount of $C_{23}H_{27}FN_4O_2$ dissolved by employing the following method.
  Mobile phase—Prepare a filtered and degassed mixture of water and acetonitrile (65 : 35), and add 1 mL of trifluoroacetic acid to each 1 L of the mixture. Adjust with ammonium hydroxide to a pH of 3.0. Make adjustments if necessary (see *System Suitability* under *Chromatography* ⟨621⟩).
  Standard solution—Dissolve an accurately weighed quantity of USP Risperidone RS in *Medium,* and dilute quantitatively, and stepwise if necessary, with *Medium* to obtain a solution having a known concentration of about 0.006 mg per mL.
  Test solution—Use portions of the solution under test, and pass through a suitable filter having a porosity of 35 μm.
  Chromatographic system (see *Chromatography* ⟨621⟩)—The liquid chromatograph is equipped with a 237-nm detector and a 4.6-mm × 15-cm column that contains 5-μm packing L1. The flow rate is about 1.5 mL per minute. Chromatograph the *Standard solution* and the *Test solution* as directed for *Procedure:* the retention time of risperidone is about 2.1 minutes, and the relative standard deviation for replicate injections is not more than 2.0%.
  Procedure—Separately inject equal volumes (about 50 μL) of the *Standard solution* and the *Test solution* into the chromatograph, record the chromatograms, and measure the peak responses. Calculate the percentage of $C_{23}H_{27}FN_4O_2$ dissolved by the formula:

$$\frac{r_U \times C_S \times 500 \times 100}{r_S \times L}$$

in which r_U and r_S are the peak responses obtained from the *Test solution* and the *Standard solution*, respectively; C_S is the concentration, in mg per mL, of USP Risperidone RS in the *Standard solution;* 500 is the volume, in mL, of *Medium;* 100 is the conversion factor to percentage; and L is the Tablet label claim in mg.
  Tolerances—Not less than 75% (Q) of the labeled amount of $C_{23}H_{27}FN_4O_2$ is dissolved in 45 minutes.
Uniformity of dosage units ⟨905⟩—
  Mobile phase and *Chromatographic system*—Proceed as directed for *Dissolution*.
  Standard solution—Dissolve an accurately weighed quantity of USP Risperidone RS in a suitable volumetric flask, and dilute quantitatively with 0.1 N hydrochloric acid to obtain a solution having a known concentration of about 0.03 mg of risperidone per mL.
  Test solution—Transfer one Tablet into a 100-mL volumetric flask, add 50 mL of 0.1 N hydrochloric acid, and shake mechanically for about 30 minutes. Dilute with 0.1 N hydrochloric acid to volume, and mix. Pass a portion of this solution through a suitable filter having a 0.2-μm or finer porosity, and use the filtrate.
  Procedure—Separately inject equal volumes (about 20 μL) of the *Standard solution* and the *Test solution* into the chromatograph, record the chromatograms, and measure the areas for the risperidone peak. Calculate the quantitiy, in mg, of risperidone ($C_{23}H_{27}FN_4O_2$) in the portion of Tablets taken by the formula:

$$C(r_U / r_S)100$$

in which C is the concentration, in mg per mL, of USP Risperidone RS in the *Standard solution;* and r_U and r_S are the peak responses obtained from the *Test solution* and the *Standard solution,* respectively.

Add the following:
▲**Related compounds—**
  Mobile phase and *Diluent*—Proceed as directed in the *Assay*.
  Standard solution—Prepare as directed for the *Standard preparation* in the *Assay*.
  Diluted sodium hydroxide—To 1 L of water in a beaker, add 0.1 N sodium hydroxide dropwise to obtain a pH of about 8.5.
  Diluted hydrogen peroxide—Dilute 1 mL of hydrogen peroxide with water to 500 mL.
  Peak identification solution—Suspend 10 mg of USP Risperidone RS in 10 mL of *Diluted sodium hydroxide* in a 100-mL volumetric flask. Store the flask at 90° for 24 hours. Cool the solution to room temperature. Add 10 mL of aqueous *Diluted hydrogen peroxide* to the flask, and store at 90° for an additional two hours. Cool the mixture to room temperature, and dilute with methanol to volume.
  Test solution—Use the *Assay preparation*.
  Chromatographic system (see *Chromatography* ⟨621⟩)—Proceed as directed in the *Assay*. Chromatograph about 20 μL of the *Peak identification solution,* record the peak responses as directed for *Procedure*, and identify the peaks using the relative retention times given in *Table 1:* the resolution, R, between the *trans-N*-oxide and *cis-N*-oxide is not less than 1.2. [NOTE—The approximate relative retention times given in *Table 1* are for identification purposes only.]
  Procedure—Inject a volume (about 20 μL) of the *Test solution* into the chromatograph, record the chromatogram, and measure the

responses for all of the peaks. Calculate the percentage of each impurity in the portion of Tablets taken by the formula:

$$100(1/R)(r_i/r_S)$$

in which R is the appropriate relative response factor as listed in Table 1; r_i is the peak response for each impurity in the Test solution; and r_S is the peak response of risperidone in the Test solution: not more than 0.3% of any individual unidentified impurity is found, not more than 0.5% of any individual specified impurity is found, and not more than 1.0% of total impurities is found.▲USP31

Assay—
Diluent—Prepare a degassed mixture of methanol and water (80 : 20).

Solution A—Prepare a filtered and degassed mixture of water, acetonitrile, and trifluroacetic acid (80 : 19.5 : 0.1). Adjust with ammonium hydroxide to a pH of 3.0.

Solution B—Prepare a filtered and degassed mixture of water, methanol, and trifluoroacetic acid (61 : 39 : 0.1). Adjust with ammonium hydroxide to a pH of 3.0.

Mobile phase—Use variable mixtures of Solution A and Solution B as directed for Chromatographic system. Make adjustments if necessary (see System Suitability under Chromatography ⟨621⟩).

Standard preparation—Transfer an accurately weighed quantity of USP Risperidone RS to a suitable volumetric flask, and dissolve in and dilute quantitatively with Diluent to obtain a solution having a known concentration of about 0.1 mg per mL.

Assay preparation—Transfer an accurately weighed portion of not fewer than 10 Tablets to a volumetric flask that can accommodate a final concentration of 0.1 mg of risperidone per mL. Add an appropriate amount of water equivalent to 20% of the total volume of the volumetric flask, and mechanically shake for about 30 minutes. Add a volume of methanol equivalent to 60% of the total volume of the volumetric flask, and mechanically shake for about 30 minutes. Dilute with methanol to volume, and mix to obtain the final 0.1 mg per mL concentration. Pass a portion of this solution through a suitable filter having a 0.45-μm or finer porosity, and use the filtrate.

Chromatographic system (see Chromatography ⟨621⟩)—The liquid chromatograph is equipped with a 275-nm detector and a 4.6-mm × 15-cm column that contains 5-μm packing L1. The flow rate is about 2.5 mL per minute. The column is maintained at room temperature. The chromatograph is programmed as follows.

Time (minutes)	Solution A (%)	Solution B (%)	Elution
0–8	100	0	isocratic
8–16	100→0	0→100	linear gradient
16–20	0	100	isocratic
20–21	0→100	100→0	linear gradient
21–30	100	0	re-equilbration

Chromatograph the Standard preparation, and record the peak responses as directed for Procedure: the tailing factor of risperidone is not more than 2.5; and the relative standard deviation for replicate injections is not more than 2.0%.

Procedure—Separately inject equal volumes (about 20 μL) of the Standard preparation and the Assay preparation into the chromatograph, record the chromatograms, and measure the responses for the risperidone peak. Calculate the quantity, in mg, of risperidone ($C_{23}H_{27}FN_4O_2$) in the portion of Tablets taken by the formula:

$$100(C_S/C_U)(r_U/r_S)$$

in which C_S is the concentration, in mg per mL, of USP Risperidone RS in the Standard preparation; C_U is the concentration, in mg per mL, of risperidone in the Assay preparation; and r_U and r_S are the peak responses of risperidone obtained from the Assay preparation and the Standard preparation, respectively.

Table 1

Peak Identification	Approximate Relative Retention Time (RRT)	Relative Response Factor (R)	Limit of Impurity
Bicyclorisperidone[1]	0.68	0.81	Not more than 0.5%
Risperidone	1.0	1.0	—
Risperidone trans-N-oxide[2]	1.65	—	Not quantified. Used for identification and system suitability check only.
Risperidone cis-N-oxide[3]	1.81	0.95	Not more than 0.5%
Any other unspecified degradation product	—	1.0	Not more than 0.3%
Total impurities	—	—	Not more than 1.0%

[1] 3-(4-fluoro-2-hydroxyphenyl)-1-[2-(6,7,8,9-tetrahydro-2-methyl-4-oxo-4H-pyrido-[1,2-a]pyrimidin-3-yl)ethyl]-2-aza-1-azoniabicyclo[2.2.2]oct-2-ene iodide.
[2] trans-3-[2-[4-(6-fluoro-1,2-benzisoxazol-3-yl)-1-piperidinyl]ethyl]-6,7,8,9-tetrahydro-2-methyl-4H-pyrido[1,2-a]pyrimidin-4-one, N-oxide monohydrate.
[3] cis-3-[2-[4-(6-fluoro-1,2-benzisoxazol-3-yl)-1-piperidinyl]ethyl]-6,7,8,9-tetrahydro-2-methyl-4H-pyrido[1,2-a]pyrimidin-4-one, N-oxide monohydrate.

Ritodrine Hydrochloride

$C_{17}H_{21}NO_3 \cdot HCl$ 323.81

Benzenemethanol, 4-hydroxy-α-[1-[[2-(4-hydroxyphenyl)ethyl]amino]ethyl]-, hydrochloride, (R*, S*)-.
erythro-p-Hydroxy-α-[1-[(p-hydroxyphenethyl)amino]ethyl]benzyl alcohol hydrochloride   [23239-51-2].

» Ritodrine Hydrochloride contains not less than 97.0 percent and not more than 103.0 percent of $C_{17}H_{21}NO_3 \cdot HCl$, calculated on the dried basis.

Packaging and storage—Preserve in tight containers. Store at 25°, excursions permitted between 15° and 30°.

USP Reference standards ⟨11⟩—USP Ritodrine Hydrochloride RS.

Identification—
A: The IR absorption spectrum of a potassium bromide dispersion of it exhibits maxima only at the same wavelengths as that of a similar preparation of USP Ritodrine Hydrochloride RS.

B: The retention time of the ritodrine hydrochloride in the Assay preparation obtained in the Assay corresponds to that of the Standard preparation obtained in the Assay.

C: A solution (1 in 100) responds to the tests for Chloride ⟨191⟩.

pH ⟨791⟩:   between 4.5 and 6.0, in a solution (1 in 50).

Loss on drying ⟨731⟩:   Dry it at 105° for 2 hours: it loses not more than 1.0% of its weight.

Residue on ignition ⟨281⟩:   not more than 0.2%.

Heavy metals, Method II ⟨231⟩:   not more than 0.002%.

Related compounds—
Mobile phase and *Chromatographic system*—Prepare as directed in the Assay.

Test preparation—Prepare a solution containing about 1 mg of Ritodrine Hydrochloride in each mL of *Mobile phase*.

Diluted test preparation—Quantitatively dilute a suitable volume of the *Test preparation* with *Mobile phase* to obtain a solution having a known concentration of 0.01 mg per mL of ritodrine hydrochloride.

Procedure—Chromatograph the *Test preparation* and the *Diluted test preparation*, as directed in the *Assay*. The relative retention times are about 0.3 for tyramine, 0.65 for *erythro*-1-(4-ketocyclohexyl)-2-[(1-hydroxyphenethyl)amino]propanol-1, 0.85 for *erythro-p*-hydroxy-[1-(4-ketocyclohexylethyl)amino]ethyl benzyl alcohol, 1.0 for ritodrine, 1.15 for *threo* diastereomer of ritodrine, and 2.3 for *p*-hydroxy-β-(*p*-hydroxyphenethyl)amino]propiophenone. Determine the peak responses for ritodrine and for the related compounds from the chromatograms obtained from the *Diluted test preparation* and the *Test preparation*, respectively. Calculate the percentage of related compounds found: not more than 0.5% of any individual impurity and not more than 2.0% of total impurities is found.

Organic volatile impurities, *Method I* ⟨467⟩: meets the requirements.

(Official until July 1, 2008)

Assay—

Mobile phase—Dissolve 6.6 g of dibasic ammonium phosphate and 1.1 g of sodium 1-heptanesulfonate in 700 mL of water, and mix with 300 mL of methanol. Adjust by the addition of phosphoric acid to a pH of 3.0, mix, filter, and degas. Make adjustments if necessary (see *System Suitability* under *Chromatography* ⟨621⟩).

Standard preparation—Dissolve an accurately weighed quantity of USP Ritodrine Hydrochloride RS in *Mobile phase* to obtain a solution having a known concentration of about 0.2 mg per mL.

Assay preparation—Transfer about 200 mg of Ritodrine Hydrochloride, accurately weighed, to a 100-mL volumetric flask, dissolve in *Mobile phase*, dilute with *Mobile phase* to volume, and mix. Transfer 10.0 mL of this solution to a 100-mL volumetric flask, dilute with *Mobile phase* to volume, and mix.

System suitability preparation—Dissolve about 20 mg of Ritodrine Hydrochloride in about 50 mL of *Mobile phase*. Add 5.6 mL of sulfuric acid, dilute with *Mobile phase* to 100 mL, and mix. Heat a portion of this solution for about 2 hours at about 85°, and then cool to room temperature. Cautiously mix 10.0 mL of the cooled solution with 8.0 mL of sodium hydroxide solution (1 in 10), and allow to cool. This solution contains ritodrine and its *threo* diastereomer.

Chromatographic system—The chromatograph is equipped with a 4.6-mm × 25-cm stainless steel column that contains packing L7 and an UV detector that monitors absorption at 214 nm. Chromatograph about 50 μL of the *System suitability preparation*: the resolution between ritodrine and its *threo* diastereomer is not less than 1.0. [NOTE—Chromatograms obtained as directed for this test, exhibit relative retention times of 1.0 for ritodrine and approximately 1.2 for the *threo* diastereomer.]

Procedure—Separately inject equal volumes (20 to 50 μL) of the *Standard preparation* and the *Assay preparation* into the chromatograph (see *Chromatography* ⟨621⟩) by means of a suitable sampling valve. Record the chromatograms and measure the peak responses. Calculate the quantity, in mg, of $C_{17}H_{21}NO_3 \cdot HCl$ in the portion of Ritodrine Hydrochloride taken by the formula:

$$1000C(r_U/r_S)$$

in which *C* is the concentration, in mg per mL, of USP Ritodrine Hydrochloride RS in the *Standard preparation*; and r_U and r_S are the peak responses for Ritodrine Hydrochloride obtained from the *Assay preparation* and the *Standard preparation*, respectively.

Ritodrine Hydrochloride Injection

» Ritodrine Hydrochloride Injection is a sterile solution of Ritodrine Hydrochloride in Water for Injection. It contains not less than 90.0 percent and not more than 110.0 percent of the labeled amount of $C_{17}H_{21}NO_3 \cdot HCl$.

Packaging and storage—Preserve in single-dose containers, preferably of Type I glass. Store at room temperature, preferably below 30°.

USP Reference standards ⟨11⟩—USP Ritodrine Hydrochloride RS. USP Endotoxin RS.

Identification—The retention time of the ritodrine hydrochloride in the *Assay preparation* obtained in the *Assay* corresponds to that of the *Standard preparation* obtained in the *Assay*.

Bacterial endotoxins ⟨85⟩—It contains not more than 0.5 USP Endotoxin Unit per mg.

pH ⟨791⟩: between 4.8 and 5.5.

Other requirements—It meets the requirements under *Injections* ⟨1⟩.

Assay—

Mobile phase, Standard preparation, and *System suitability preparation*—Proceed as directed in the *Assay* under *Ritodrine Hydrochloride*.

Assay preparation—Dilute an accurately measured volume of Injection, equivalent to about 20 mg of ritodrine hydrochloride, with *Mobile phase* to 100.0 mL, and mix.

Chromatographic system—Proceed as directed in the *Assay* under *Ritodrine Hydrochloride* except that the liquid chromatograph is equipped with a 275-nm detector.

Procedure—Proceed as directed in the *Assay* under *Ritodrine Hydrochloride*. Calculate the quantity, in mg, of $C_{17}H_{21}NO_3 \cdot HCl$ in each mL of the Injection taken by the formula:

$$(100C/V)(r_U/r_S)$$

in which *V* is the volume, in mL, of Injection taken, and the other terms are as defined therein.

Ritodrine Hydrochloride Tablets

» Ritodrine Hydrochloride Tablets contain not less than 90.0 percent and not more than 110.0 percent of the labeled amount of $C_{17}H_{21}NO_3 \cdot HCl$.

Packaging and storage—Preserve in tight containers. Store at room temperature, preferably below 30°.

USP Reference standards ⟨11⟩—USP Ritodrine Hydrochloride RS.

Identification—The retention time of the Tablets in the *Assay preparation* obtained in the *Assay* corresponds to that of the *Standard preparation* obtained in the *Assay*.

Dissolution ⟨711⟩—

Medium: 0.01 N hydrochloric acid; 900 mL.
Apparatus 2: 50 rpm.
Time: 30 minutes.

Procedure—Determine the amount of $C_{17}H_{21}NO_3 \cdot HCl$ dissolved by employing the procedure set forth in the *Assay*, using a filtered portion of the solution under test as the *Assay preparation* in comparison with a Standard solution having a known concentration of USP Ritodrine Hydrochloride RS in the same *Medium*.

Tolerances—Not less than 80% (*Q*) of the labeled amount of $C_{17}H_{21}NO_3 \cdot HCl$ is dissolved in 30 minutes.

Uniformity of dosage units ⟨905⟩: meet the requirements.

Procedure for content uniformity—Transfer 1 Tablet to a 200-mL volumetric flask, add about 5 mL of water, and stir until disintegration is complete. Add about 150 mL of methanolic sulfuric acid solution (0.005 M sulfuric acid in methanol), continue stirring for an additional 15 minutes, dilute with methanolic sulfuric acid solution to volume, and mix. Filter a portion of the mixture, discarding the first 20 mL of the filtrate. Dissolve an accurately weighed quantity of USP Ritodrine Hydrochloride RS in methanolic sulfuric acid solution, and dilute quantitatively and stepwise with the same solvent to obtain a Standard solution having a known concentration of about 50 μg per mL. Concomitantly determine the absorbances of both solutions in 1-cm cells at the wavelength of maximum absorbance at about 276 nm, with a suitable spectrophotometer, using methanolic sulfuric acid solution as the blank. Calculate the quantity, in mg, of $C_{17}H_{21}NO_3 \cdot HCl$ in the Tablet taken by the formula:

$$(TC/D)(A_U/A_S)$$

in which T is the labeled quantity, in mg, of ritodrine hydrochloride in the Tablet, C is the concentration, in µg per mL, of USP Ritodrine Hydrochloride RS in the Standard solution, D is the concentration, in µg per mL, of ritodrine hydrochloride in the solution from the Tablet based upon the labeled quantity per Tablet and the extent of dilution, and A_U and A_S are the absorbances of the solution from the Tablet and the Standard solution, respectively.

Assay—
Mobile phase, Standard preparation, and *System suitability preparation*—Proceed as directed in the *Assay* under *Ritodrine Hydrochloride.*
Assay preparation—Weigh and finely powder not less than 20 Tablets. Transfer an accurately weighed portion of the powder, equivalent to about 20 mg of ritodrine hydrochloride, to a 100-mL volumetric flask. Add about 70 mL of *Mobile phase*, stir for about 15 minutes, dilute with *Mobile phase* to volume, mix, and filter a portion to remove any particulate matter.
Chromatographic system—Proceed as directed in the *Assay* under *Ritodrine Hydrochloride Injection.*
Procedure—Proceed as directed in the *Assay* under *Ritodrine Hydrochloride.* Calculate the quantity, in mg, of $C_{17}H_{21}NO_3 \cdot HCl$ in the portion of Tablets taken by the formula:

$$100C(r_U/r_S)$$

in which the terms are as defined therein.

Ritonavir

$C_{37}H_{48}N_6O_5S_2$ 720.94
2,4,7,12-Tetraazatridecan-13-oic acid, 10-hydroxy-2-methyl-5-(1-methylethyl)-1-[2-(1-methylethyl)-4-thiazolyl]-3,6-dioxo-8,11-bis(phenylmethyl)-5-thiazolylmethyl ester [5S-(5R*,8R*,10R*,11R*)]-.
5-Thiazolylmethyl [(αS)-α-[(1S,3S)-1-hydroxy-3-[(2S)-2-[3-[(2-isopropyl-4-thiazolyl)methyl]-3-methylureido]-3-methylbutyramido]-4-phenylbutyl]phenethyl]carbamate [155213-67-5].

» Ritonavir contains not less than 97.0 percent and not more than 102.0 percent of $C_{37}H_{48}N_6O_5S_2$, calculated on the anhydrous basis.

Packaging and storage—Preserve in tight, light-resistant containers. Store between 5° and 30°.
USP Reference standards ⟨11⟩—USP Ritonavir RS. USP Ritonavir Related Compounds Mixture RS.
Identification—
A: *Infrared Absorption* ⟨197⟩—
Test specimen—Dissolve 50 mg of Ritonavir in 1.0 mL of chloroform. Add 1 drop of this solution to the surface of a potassium bromide or a sodium chloride disk, and evaporate to dryness.
B: The retention time of the major peak in the chromatogram of the *Assay preparation* is within 2% of the retention time of the major peak in the chromatogram of the *Standard preparation*, as obtained in the *Assay*.
X-ray diffraction ⟨941⟩—The X-ray diffraction pattern conforms to that of USP Ritonavir RS if the drug substance is used for the solid dosage forms.

Heavy metals, *Method II* ⟨231⟩: not more than 0.002%, using 1.0 g of Ritonavir and 2 mL of *Standard Lead Solution* (10 ppm Pb) in the *Standard Preparation.*
Water, *Method I* ⟨921⟩: not more than 0.5%, determined on 0.500 g.
Residue on ignition ⟨281⟩: not more than 0.2%, determined on 1.0 g.
Organic volatile impurities ⟨467⟩: meets the requirements.
(Official until July 1, 2008)
Related compounds—[NOTE—Ritonavir is alkali sensitive. All glassware should be prerinsed with distilled water prior to use to remove residual detergent contamination.]
Monobasic potassium phosphate solution (0.03M), *Diluent, Solution A, Solution B,* and *Mobile phase*—Prepare as directed in the *Assay.*
Standard stock solution and *Intermediate stock solution*—Prepare as directed for *Standard stock preparation* and *Intermediate standard preparation* in the *Assay.*
Ritonavir identity standard solution—Transfer about 50 mg of USP Ritonavir Related Compounds Mixture RS, accurately weighed, to a 50-mL volumetric flask. Dissolve in and dilute with *Diluent* to volume, and mix.
Standard solution—Transfer 5.0 mL of the *Intermediate standard solution* to a 100-mL volumetric flask, dilute with *Diluent* to volume, and mix. [NOTE—This solution may be used for 48 hours if stored at room temperature.]
Test solution—Transfer about 50 mg of Ritonavir, accurately weighed, to a 50-mL volumetric flask. Dissolve in and dilute with *Diluent* to volume, and mix.
Chromatographic system (see *Chromatography* ⟨621⟩)—The liquid chromatograph is equipped with a 240-nm detector and a 4.6-mm × 15-cm column that contains 3-µm packing L26 and is maintained at a constant temperature of about 60°. The flow rate is about 1.0 mL per minute. The chromatograph is programmed as follows.

Time (minutes)	Solution A (%)	Solution B (%)	Elution
0	100	0	equilibrium
0–60	100	0	isocratic
60–120	100→0	0→100	gradient
120.1	0→100	100→0	step gradient
120.1–155	100	0	isocratic

The run time for the *Standard solution* is 40 minutes, and the run time for the *Test solution* is 155 minutes. Chromatograph the *Ritonavir identity standard solution* and the *Standard solution*, and record the responses as directed for *Procedure*: the retention time of ritonavir is between 30 and 35 minutes; the resolution, R, between impurity E and impurity F (see *Table 1*) in the *Ritonavir identity standard solution* is not less than 1.0; the ratio of peak (H_p) to valley (H_v) of Ritonavir and impurity N (regioisomer) is not less than 1; the capacity factor, k', using the main component peak of the first *Standard solution* injection, is not less than 13; the column efficiency, using the main component peak of the first *Standard solution* injection, is not less than 5000 theoretical plates; the tailing factor, using the main component peak of the first *Standard solution* injection, is between 0.8 and 1.2; and the relative standard deviation of the peak area response of the main component peak, for replicate injections of the *Standard solution*, is not more than 3.0%.
Procedure—Separately inject equal volumes (about 50 µL) of the *Diluent, Ritonavir identity standard solution, Standard solution,* and *Test solution* into the chromatograph, record the chromatograms, and measure the peak area responses. Calculate the percentage of each impurity in the portion of Ritonavir taken by the formula:

$$0.0025(W_S/W_T)(R_T/R_S)(1/F)P$$

in which W_S is the the weight, in mg, of USP Ritonavir RS taken to prepare the *Standard solution*; W_T is the weight, in mg, of Ritonavir taken to prepare the *Test solution*; R_T is the area of the impurity peak obtained from the *Test solution*; R_S is the average peak area of ritonavir obtained from the six injections of the *Standard solution*;

F is the response factor for the impurity (see values in *Table 1*); and P is the purity, in percentage, of USP Ritonavir RS taken to prepare the *Standard solution*. Not more than 0.3% of impurity E and O is found; not more than 0.2% of impurity T is found; not more than 0.1% of any other impurity is found; and not more than 1.0% of total impurities is found.

Assay—

Monobasic potassium phosphate solution (0.03M)—Dissolve about 8.2 of monobasic potassium phosphate in 2.0 L of water. Mix well, and filter through a 0.45-μm nylon membrane.

Diluent—Prepare a mixture of *Monobasic potassium phosphate solution (0.03M)* and acetonitrile (1 : 1). Mix well, and filter through a 0.45-μm nylon membrane.

Solution A—Prepare a mixture of the filtered *Monobasic potassium phosphate solution (0.03M)*, acetonitrile, tetrahydrofuran (inhibitor-free), and *n*-butanol (69 : 18 : 8 : 5).

Solution B—Prepare a mixture of acetonitrile, the filtered *Monobasic potassium phosphate solution (0.03M)*, tetrahydrofuran (inhibitor-free), and *n*-butanol (47 : 40 : 8 : 5).

Mobile phase—Use variable mixtures of *Solution A* and *Solution B* as directed for *Chromatographic system*. Make adjustments if necessary (see *System Suitability* under *Chromatography* ⟨621⟩). [NOTE—Because of the high dependence of retention time and selectivity on the *Mobile phase* composition, the volumes should be accurately measured. Excessive or continued helium sparging must be avoided. Store the *Mobile phase* in a tightly sealed container when not in use.]

Standard stock preparation—Transfer about 100 mg of USP Ritonavir RS, accurately weighed, to a 50-mL volumetric flask. Dissolve in and dilute with *Diluent* to volume, and mix. [NOTE—This solution may be kept for 5 days if refrigerated.]

Intermediate standard preparation—Transfer 5.0 mL of the *Standard stock preparation* to a 100-mL volumetric flask, dilute with *Diluent* to volume, and mix.

Standard preparation—Transfer 25.0 mL of the *Intermediate standard preparation* to a 100-mL volumetric flask, dilute with *Diluent* to volume, and mix.

Assay preparation—Transfer 5.0 mL of the *Test solution*, prepared as directed in the test for *Related compounds*, to a 50-mL volumetric flask, dilute with *Diluent* to volume, and mix. Dilute 25.0 mL of this solution with *Diluent* to 100-mL, and mix.

Chromatographic system—Proceed as directed in the test for *Related compounds*. The run time for the *Standard preparation* and *Assay preparation* is 40 minutes. Chromatograph the *Standard preparation*, and record the responses as directed for *Procedure*: the capacity factor, k', using the main component peak of the first *Standard preparation* injection, is not less than 13; the column efficiency, using the main component peak of the first *Standard preparation* injection, is not less than 5000 theoretical plates; the tailing factor, using the main component peak of the first *Standard preparation* injection, is between 0.8 and 1.2; and the relative standard deviation of the peak area response of the main component peak, for replicate injections of the *Standard preparation*, is not more than 2.0%.

Procedure—Separately inject equal volumes (about 50 μL) of the *Standard preparation* and the *Assay preparation* into the chromatograph, record the chromatograms, and measure the peak area responses. Calculate the percentage, on the as-is basis, of $C_{37}H_{48}N_6O_5S_2$ in the portion of Ritonavir taken by the formula:

$$0.5(W_S / W_T)(r_T / r_S)P$$

in which W_S is the weight, in mg, of USP Ritonavir RS taken to prepare the *Standard preparation*; W_T is the weight, in mg, of Ritonavir taken to prepare the *Assay preparation*; r_T is the peak area of the impurity obtained from the chromatogram of the *Assay preparation*; r_S is the average peak area of ritonavir obtained from the chromatograms of the five injections of the *Standard preparation*; and P is the purity, in percentage, of USP Ritonavir RS taken to prepare the *Standard preparation*.

Calculate the percentage, on the anhydrous basis, of $C_{37}H_{48}N_6O_5S_2$ in the portion of Ritonavir taken by the formula:

$$100A/(100 - B)$$

in which A is the percentage of $C_{37}H_{48}N_6O_5S_2$ on the as-is basis, as calculated above; and B is the percentage of water content.

Table 1. Approximate Relative Retention Time (RRT) for Known Related Impurities

Impurity Identity	Common Name	Response Factor	RRT
A + B	Mixture of 2,4-Wing acid and monoacyl valine	—	0.07
C	Monoacylacetamide	—	0.15
D	5-Wing diacyl	1.37	0.24
E	Oxidation impurity	—	0.36
F	Acid hydrolysis product	0.73	0.39
G	Ritonavir hydroperoxide	—	0.45
H	Acid/base by-product	0.76	0.47
I	Ethyl analog	—	0.64
J + K	Mixture of Boc-monoacyl and monoacyl isobutyl carbamate	0.74	0.81
L	Base cyclization product	0.53	0.87
M	2,4-Wing isobutyl ester	—	0.94
N	Regioisomer	—	1.05
O	Isomer #2	—	1.11
P	Di-monoacyl urea	—	1.14
Q	Isomer #4	—	1.23
R	Isomer #1	—	1.32
S	Di-monoacyl valine urea	—	1.62
T	2,4-Wing diacyl	0.73	2.87
U	Triacyl impurity	—	3.20

Ropivacaine Hydrochloride

$C_{17}H_{26}N_2O \cdot HCl \cdot H_2O$ 328.89

(S)-(−)-1-Propylpiperidine-2-carboxylic acid (2,6-dimethylphenyl)-amide hydrochloride monohydrate.
(S)-(−)-1-Propyl-2′,6′-pipecoloxylidine hydrochloride monohydrate [132112-35-7].

» Ropivacaine Hydrochloride contains not less than 98.5 percent and not more than 101.0 percent of $C_{17}H_{26}N_2O \cdot HCl$, calculated on the anhydrous basis.

Packaging and storage—Preserve in well-closed containers. Store at room temperature.

Labeling—Where it is intended for use in preparing injectable dosage forms, the label states that it is sterile or must be subjected to further processing during the preparation of injectable dosage forms.

USP Reference standards ⟨11⟩—*USP Bupivacaine Hydrochloride RS. USP Endotoxin RS. USP Ropivacaine Hydrochloride RS. USP Ropivacaine Related Compound A RS. USP Ropivacaine Related Compound B RS.*

Identification—
  A: *Infrared Absorption* ⟨197K⟩.
  B: A solution (1 in 100) responds to the test for *Chloride* ⟨191⟩.

Bacterial endotoxins ⟨85⟩—The level of bacterial endotoxins is such that the requirements under the relevant dosage form monograph(s) in which Ropivacaine Hydrochloride is used can be met. Where the label states that Ropivacaine Hydrochloride must be subjected to further processing during the preparation of injectable dosage forms, the level of bacterial endotoxins is such that the requirements under the relevant dosage form monograph(s) in which Ropivacaine Hydrochloride is used can be met.

Color—Transfer an accurately weighed aliquot of Ropivacaine Hydrochloride, about 480 to 500 mg, into a 25-mL volumetric flask, and dissolve in and dilute with water to volume. Pass the solution through a 5-μm polyvinylidene filter (PVDF). Immediately measure the absorbance at 405 nm and at 436 nm, using a suitable spectrophotometer and a path length of 5 cm, and using water as the reference: the absorbance at 405 nm is not more than 0.030, and the absorbance at 436 nm is not more than 0.025.

Clarity—
  Hydrazine sulfate solution—Dissolve 1.0 g of hydrazine sulfate in water, and dilute with water to 100 mL. Allow to stand 4 to 6 hours.
  Hexamethylenetetramine solution—Transfer 2.5 g of hexamethylenetetramine to a 100-mL glass-stoppered flask, and dissolve in 25 mL of water. Do not dilute to volume.
  Opalescence standard stock suspension—To the flask containing the *Hexamethylenetetramine solution,* add 25.0 mL of *Hydrazine sulfate solution,* mix, and allow to stand for 24 hours. This suspension is stable for up to 2 months when stored in a glass container free from surface defects. The suspension must not adhere to the flask and must be well mixed before use.
  Opalescence standard suspension—Dilute 15.0 mL of the *Opalescence standard stock suspension* with water to 1000 mL. This suspension should be freshly prepared and may be stored for not more than 24 hours.
  Reference suspension 1—Combine 5.0 mL of the *Opalescence standard suspension* and 95.0 mL of water. Shake before use.
  Reference suspension 2—Combine 10.0 mL of the *Opalescence standard suspension* and 90.0 mL of water. Shake before use.
  Test solution—Transfer about 480 to 500 mg of Ropivacaine Hydrochloride, accurately weighed, to a 25-mL volumetric flask, and dilute with water to volume.
  Procedure—Use identical tubes of colorless, transparent, neutral glass with a flat base and an internal diameter of 15 to 25 mm. The depth of the layer is 40 mm. Compare the solutions in diffused daylight 5 minutes after the preparation of *Reference suspension 1* and *Reference suspension 2,* viewing vertically against a black background. The diffusion of light must be such that *Reference suspension 1* can readily be distinguished from water, and *Reference suspension 2* can readily be distinguished from *Reference suspension 1.* The *Test solution* is considered clear if its clarity is the same as that of water or if its opalescence is not more pronounced than that of *Reference suspension 1.*

Specific rotation ⟨781S⟩:
  Solvent—Dissolve about 200 g of sodium hydroxide in water, and dilute with water to 1 L. Combine 20 mL of this solution and 300 mL of water in a 1-L volumetric flask. Dilute with alcohol to volume.
  Test solution: 10 mg per mL, in *Solvent.*
  Procedure—Obtain readings at 365 nm: between −210° and −255°.

pH ⟨791⟩: between 4.5 and 6.0, in a solution (1 in 100).

Water, *Method Ia* ⟨921⟩: between 5.0% and 6.0%. Perform the determination on 0.0900 to 0.1100 g of sample.

Heavy metals—
  pH 3.5 Acetate Buffer and Standard Lead Solution—Prepare as directed under *Heavy Metals* ⟨231⟩.
  Dilute lead standard solution—Dilute 10.0 mL of the *Standard Lead Solution* with water to 100 mL. Each mL of *Dilute lead standard solution* contains the equivalent of 1 μg of lead.
  0.25 M Sodium sulfide solution—Dissolve about 6.0 g of sodium sulfide in 40 g of glycerol, then dilute with water to 100 mL. Filter using a cotton pad, and store in a glass container protected from light.
  Test Preparation—Prepare as directed under *Heavy Metals, Method II* ⟨231⟩, using 3.97 to 4.00 g of ropivacaine hydrochloride.
  Standard solution—Combine 10.0 mL of the *Dilute lead standard solution* with 2 mL of the *Test Preparation* and 2 mL of *pH 3.5 Acetate Buffer,* and mix.
  Test solution—Combine 12 mL of the *Test Preparation* with 2 mL of *pH 3.5 Acetate Buffer,* and mix.
  Blank—Combine 10 mL of water, 2 mL of *pH 3.5 Acetate Buffer,* and 2 mL of the *Test Preparation.*
  Procedure—Transfer the *Blank* to a color-comparison tube. Transfer the *Standard solution* and the *Test solution* to individual color-comparison tubes each containing 1 drop of *0.25 M Sodium sulfide solution.* After 1 minute, compare the colors, viewing downward over a white surface: the *Standard solution* shows a slight brown color compared to the *Blank;* and the *Test solution* is not darker than the *Standard solution* (0.001%).

Limit of ropivacaine related compound A—
  Buffer solution, Mobile phase, System suitability solution, and Chromatographic system—Prepare as directed for *Related compounds.*
  Standard solution—Dissolve an accurately weighed quantity of USP Ropivacaine Related Compound A RS in *Mobile phase,* and dilute quantitatively, and stepwise if necessary, with *Mobile phase* to obtain a solution having a known concentration of about 0.13 μg per mL.
  Test solution—Transfer about 100 mg of Ropivacaine Hydrochloride, accurately weighed, to a 10-mL volumetric flask, dissolve in and dilute with *Mobile phase* to volume, and mix.
  Procedure—Separately inject equal volumes (about 20 μL) of the *Standard solution* and the *Test solution* into the chromatograph, record the chromatograms, and measure the responses for the major peaks: the signal-to-noise ratio of the principal peak in the *Standard solution* is at least 10; and the response for any peak corresponding to ropivacaine related compound A (2,6-dimethylaniline) in the chromatogram obtained from the *Test solution* is not greater than the response of the major peak in the chromatogram obtained from the *Standard solution* (10 μg per g).

Related compounds—
  Buffer solution—Combine 1.3 mL of sodium phosphate monobasic solution (138 g per L) and 32.5 mL of disodium hydrogen phosphate dihydrate solution (89 g per L), and dilute with water to 1 L. The pH of this solution is 8.0. Make adjustments if necessary.
  Mobile phase—Prepare a degassed mixture of *Buffer solution* and acetonitrile (50 : 50). Make adjustments if necessary (see *System suitability* under *Chromatography* ⟨621⟩).

System suitability solution—Dissolve accurately weighed quantities of USP Ropivacaine Hydrochloride RS and USP Bupivacaine Hydrochloride RS in *Mobile phase*, and dilute quantitatively, and stepwise if necessary, to obtain a solution having known concentrations of about 10 µg per mL of each compound.

Test solution—Transfer about 27.5 mg of Ropivacaine Hydrochloride, accurately weighed, to a 10-mL volumetric flask, dissolve in and dilute with *Mobile phase* to volume, and mix.

Dilute test solution—Dilute 1.0 mL of the *Test solution* with *Mobile phase* to 100 mL. Dilute 1.0 mL of this solution with *Mobile phase* to 10 mL.

Chromatographic system (see *Chromatography* ⟨621⟩)—The liquid chromatograph is equipped with a 240-nm detector and a 3.9-mm × 15-cm column that contains 4-µm packing L1. The flow rate is about 1 mL per minute. Check the stability of the baseline by injecting *Mobile phase*. Run the chromatogram for at least 15 minutes. Chromatograph the *System suitability solution* and the *Dilute test solution*, and record the peak responses as directed for *Procedure*: the relative retention times are 1.6 for bupivacaine and 1.0 for ropivacaine; the resolution, *R*, between ropivacaine and bupivacaine is not less than 6 (from the *System suitability solution*); and the signal-to-noise ratio of ropivacaine is at least 10 (from the *Dilute test solution*).

Procedure—Inject equal volumes (about 20 µL) of the *System suitability solution* and the *Test solution* into the chromatograph, record the chromatograms, and measure the responses for the major peaks. Calculate the percentage of each impurity in the portion of Ropivacaine Hydrochloride taken by the formula:

$$100(r_U / r_S)$$

in which r_U is the peak response for each impurity obtained from the *Test solution*; and r_S is the sum of all peak responses obtained from the *Test solution*: not more than 0.2% of bupivacaine is found, less than 0.1% for any other individual impurity is found, and not more than 0.5% of total impurities is found.

Enantiomeric purity—

Background electrolyte solution—Transfer 9.31 to 10.29 g of phosphoric acid to a 1-L volumetric flask, and dilute with water to volume. The pH is between 2.9 and 3.1. If necessary, adjust the pH with triethanolamine.

Run buffer—Prepare a solution containing approximately 13.3 mg of heptakis-(2,6-di-*O*-methyl)-β-cyclodextrin per mL of *Background electrolyte solution*. [NOTE—This solution is freshly prepared and passed through a 0.45-µm filter.]

System suitability solution—Dissolve accurately weighed quantities of USP Ropivacaine Hydrochloride RS and USP Ropivacaine Related Compound B RS in water, and dilute quantitatively, and stepwise if necessary, to obtain a solution having known concentrations of about 15 µg per mL of each compound.

Test solution—Transfer about 50 mg of Ropivacaine Hydrochloride, accurately weighed, to a 25-mL volumetric flask, and dissolve in and dilute with water.

Dilute test solution—Dilute 1.0 mL of the *Test solution* with water to 200 mL.

Capillary rinsing procedure—Use separate run buffer vials for capillary rinse and sample analysis. Rinse the capillary with water for 1 minute, with 0.1 N sodium hydroxide for 10 minutes, and with water for 3 minutes. If a new or dry capillary is being used, increase the sodium hydroxide rinse time to 30 minutes. Rinse the capillary between injections as follows: water for 1 minute, 0.1 N sodium hydroxide for 4 minutes, and water for 1 minute, then run buffer for 4 minutes. Rinse times are based on a pressure of 1 bar.

System setup (see *Capillary Electrophoresis* ⟨727⟩)—The system is equipped with a 206-nm detector and a 50-µm × 72-cm fused silica column. The temperature is maintained at 30°. A voltage of 375 V/cm is applied. The initial ramping is 500 V/s, positive polarity, and a resulting current of 40 to 45 µA. Inject the *Dilute test solution*: the signal-to-noise ratio is at least 10. Inject the *System suitability solution*, and record the peak responses as directed for *Procedure*: the relative migration times are about 0.96 for ropivacaine related compound B (*R* enantiomer) and 1.0 for ropivacaine (*S* enantiomer); the resolution, *R*, between ropivacaine related compound B and ropivacaine is not less than 3.7. The analysis run time is about 30 minutes. If needed, increase the resolution by increasing the concentration of heptakis-(2,6-di-*O*-methyl)-β-cyclodextrin or by lowering the system temperature.

Procedure—Separately inject equal volumes of the *Run buffer* and of water to ensure there are no interfering peaks (50 mbar for 5.0 seconds followed by injection of *Run buffer* at 50 mbar for 1.0 second). Inject the *Test solution* into the electrophoresis system, record the electropherograms, and measure the peak responses for ropivacaine and ropivacaine related compound B. Calculate the percentage of ropivacaine related compound B in the portion of Ropivacaine Hydrochloride taken by the formula:

$$100(r_R / M_R)/(r_S / M_S)$$

in which r_R is the peak response of ropivacaine related compound B obtained from the *Test solution*; r_S is the peak response of ropivacaine obtained from the *Test solution*; and M_R and M_S are the migration times, in minutes, of ropivacaine related compound B and ropivacaine, respectively: not more than 0.5% ropivacaine related compound B is found.

System shutdown—After the analysis, rinse the capillary for 10 minutes with 0.1 N sodium hydroxide, then for 10 minutes with water. Dry the capillary before storage.

Other requirements—Where the label states that Ropivacaine Hydrochloride is sterile, it meets the requirements for *Sterility Tests* ⟨71⟩ and *Labeling* under *Injections* ⟨1⟩.

Assay—Dissolve an accurately weighed quantity of Ropivacaine Hydrochloride, approximately 1000 mg, in 10 mL of water and 40 mL of alcohol. Add 1.0 mL of 1 N hydrochloric acid, and titrate with 1 N sodium hydroxide VS. Two equivalence points are obtained; the difference in titrant volume corresponds to the amount of ropivacaine hydrochloride. Each mL of 1 N sodium hydroxide is equivalent to 310.9 mg of anhydrous ropivacaine hydrochloride ($C_{17}H_{26}N_2O \cdot HCl$).

Ropivacaine Hydrochloride Injection

» Ropivacaine Hydrochloride Injection is a sterile solution of Ropivacaine Hydrochloride in Water for Injection. It contains not less than 90.0 percent and not more than 110.0 percent of the labeled amount of ropivacaine hydrochloride ($C_{17}H_{26}N_2O \cdot HCl$).

Packaging and storage—Preserve in single-dose or multiple-dose containers, preferably of Type 1 glass or of suitable plastic.

USP Reference standards ⟨11⟩—*USP Endotoxin RS. USP Ropivacaine Hydrochloride RS. USP Ropivacaine Related Compound A RS. USP Ropivacaine Related Compound B RS.*

Identification—

A: The retention time of the major peak in the chromatogram of the *Assay preparation* corresponds to that in the chromatogram of the *Standard preparation*, as obtained in the *Assay*.

B: The retention time of the major peak in the chromatogram of the *Test solution* corresponds to that in the chromatogram of the *System suitability solution*, as obtained in the test for *Enantiomeric purity*.

Bacterial endotoxins ⟨85⟩—It contains not more than 60 USP Endotoxin Units per g of ropivacaine hydrochloride.

Particulate matter ⟨788⟩: meets the requirements for injections.

Sterility ⟨71⟩—It meets the requirements when tested as directed for *Membrane Filtration* under *Test for Sterility of the Product to be Examined*.

pH ⟨791⟩: between 4.0 and 6.0.

Limit of 2,6-dimethylaniline (ropivacaine related compound A, base)—

pH 8.0 Buffer solution and *Mobile phase*—Prepare as directed in the *Assay*.

Standard solution—Prepare as directed for *Standard preparation* in the *Assay*.

Test solution—Dilute accurately the Injection with *Mobile phase* to obtain a concentration of 2.0 mg per mL.

Chromatographic system (see *Chromatography* ⟨621⟩)—The liquid chromatograph is equipped with a 240-nm detector and a 3.9-mm × 15-cm column that contains 5-μm packing L1. The flow rate is about 1.5 mL per minute. Chromatograph the *Standard solution*, and record the peak responses as directed for *Procedure*: the resolution, R, between ropivacaine related compound A and ropivacaine is not less than 5; and the signal-to-noise ratio for ropivacaine related compound A is not less than 10.

Procedure—Separately inject equal volumes (about 20 μL) of the *Standard solution* and the *Test solution* into the chromatograph, record the chromatograms, and measure the peak responses. The peak response of ropivacaine related compound A obtained from the *Test solution* is not greater than the corresponding response obtained from the *Standard solution* (not more than 0.01% of ropivacaine related compound A base is found).

Enantiomeric purity—

pH 7.2 Buffer solution—Transfer 7.5 mL of 1 M monobasic sodium phosphate solution and 28.5 mL of 0.5 M dibasic sodium phosphate dihydrate solution into a 1-L volumetric flask, and dilute with water to volume. Adjust the resulting solution to a pH of 7.2, if necessary.

Mobile phase—Transfer 35 mL of isopropyl alcohol into a 500-mL volumetric flask, dilute with *pH 7.2 Buffer solution* to volume, mix, and degas. Make adjustments if necessary (see *System Suitability* under *Chromatography* ⟨621⟩).

System suitability solution—Dissolve suitable quantities of USP Ropivacaine Hydrochloride RS and USP Ropivacaine Related Compound B RS in water, and dilute quantitatively, and stepwise, with water to obtain a solution containing about 75 μg per mL and 0.75 μg per mL, respectively.

Test solution—Dilute the Injection with *Mobile phase* to a concentration of about 75 μg per mL.

Chromatographic system (see *Chromatography* ⟨621⟩)—The liquid chromatograph is equipped with a 220-nm detector and a 4-mm × 10-cm column that contains packing L41. The flow rate is about 1 mL per minute. Chromatograph the *System suitability solution*, and record the peak responses as directed for *Procedure*: the resolution, R, between ropivacaine related compound B (R enantiomer) and ropivacaine (S enantiomer) is not less than 1.5. [NOTE—For the purpose of identification, the relative retention times are about 0.75 for ropivacaine related compound B and 1.0 for ropivacaine.]

Procedure—Inject about 20 μL of the *Test solution* into the chromatograph, record the chromatogram, and measure the peak responses. Calculate the percentage of ropivacaine related compound B (R enantiomer) in the portion of Injection taken by the formula:

$$100(r_i / r_s)$$

in which r_i is the peak response of ropivacaine related compound B (R enantiomer); and r_s is the sum of the peak responses of ropivacaine (S enantiomer) and ropivacaine related compound B (R enantiomer) obtained from the *Test solution*: not more than 2.0% of ropivacaine related compound B (R enantiomer) is found.

Other requirements—It meets the requirements under *Injections* ⟨1⟩.

Assay—

pH 8.0 Buffer solution—Transfer 1.3 mL of 1 M monobasic sodium phosphate solution and 32.5 mL of 0.5 M dibasic sodium phosphate dihydrate solution to a 1-L volumetric flask. Dilute with water to volume, and mix. Adjust the resulting solution to a pH of 8.0, if necessary.

Mobile phase—Prepare a filtered and degassed mixture of acetonitrile and *pH 8.0 Buffer solution* (60 : 40). Make adjustments if necessary (see *System Suitability* under *Chromatography* ⟨621⟩).

Standard preparation—Dissolve accurately weighed quantities of USP Ropivacaine Hydrochloride RS and USP Ropivacaine Related Compound A RS in *Mobile phase*, and dilute quantitatively, and stepwise, with *Mobile phase* to obtain a solution having known concentrations of about 0.25 mg per mL of USP Ropivacaine Hydrochloride RS and about 0.26 μg per mL of USP Ropivacaine Related Compound A RS.

Assay preparation—Dilute accurately the Injection with *Mobile phase* to obtain a concentration of about 0.25 mg per mL.

Chromatographic system (see *Chromatography* ⟨621⟩)—The liquid chromatograph is equipped with a 240-nm detector and a 3.9-mm × 15-cm column that contains 5- or 10-μm packing L1. The flow rate is about 1.2 mL per minute. Chromatograph the *Standard preparation*, and record the peak responses as directed for *Procedure*: the relative standard deviation for replicate injections, calculated for the ropivacaine peak, is not more than 1.0%; and the resolution, R, between ropivacaine related compound A and ropivacaine is not less than 5.

Procedure—Separately inject equal volumes (about 20 μL) of the *Standard preparation* and the *Assay preparation* into the chromatograph, record the chromatograms, and measure the responses for the major peaks. Calculate the quantity, in mg, of ropivacaine hydrochloride ($C_{17}H_{26}N_2O \cdot HCl$) in each mL of Injection taken by the formula:

$$CD(r_U / r_S)$$

in which C is the concentration, in mg per mL, of USP Ropivacaine Hydrochloride RS in the *Standard preparation*; D is the dilution factor, in mL, for the *Assay preparation*; and r_U and r_S are the peak responses obtained from the *Assay preparation* and the *Standard preparation*, respectively.

Rose Water Ointment

» Prepare Rose Water Ointment as follows:

Cetyl Esters Wax	125 g
White Wax	120 g
Almond Oil	560 g
Sodium Borate	5 g
Stronger Rose Water	25 mL
Purified Water	165 mL
Rose Oil	200 μL
To make about	1000 g

Reduce the cetyl esters wax and the white wax to small pieces, melt them on a steam bath, add the almond oil, and continue heating until the temperature of the mixture reaches 70°. Dissolve the sodium borate in the purified water and the stronger rose water, warmed to 70°, and gradually add the warm aqueous phase to the melted oil phase, stirring rapidly and continuously until it has cooled to about 45°. Then incorporate the rose oil.

NOTE—Rose Water Ointment is free from rancidity. If the Ointment has been chilled, warm it slightly before attempting to incorporate other ingredients (see *Ointments and Suppositories* in the section *Added Substances* under *Ingredients and Processes* in the *General Notices*).

Packaging and storage—Preserve in tight, light-resistant containers.

Roxarsone

$C_6H_6AsNO_6$ 263.04
Arsonic acid, (4-hydroxy-3-nitrophenyl)-.
4-Hydroxy-3-nitrobenzenearsonic acid   [121-19-7].

» Roxarsone contains not less than 98.0 percent and not more than 101.0 percent of $C_6H_6AsNO_6$, calculated on the dried basis.

Packaging and storage—Preserve in well-closed containers.
Labeling—Label it to indicate that it is for veterinary use only.
USP Reference standards ⟨11⟩—*USP Roxarsone RS*.
Identification—
  A: *Infrared Absorption* ⟨197K⟩.
  B: *Ultraviolet Absorption* ⟨197U⟩—
  Solution: 8 μg per mL.
  Medium: 0.1 N hydrochloric acid in methanol.
Loss on drying ⟨731⟩—Dry it at 100° for 6 hours: it loses not more than 1.0% of its weight.
Residue on ignition ⟨281⟩:   not more than 0.5%.
Limit of trivalent arsenic—Transfer 2.50 g of Roxarsone to a 250-mL conical flask, add 5.0 mL of a solution containing 0.1237 mg of anhydrous arsenic trioxide per mL, 10 mL of water, and 4.0 mL of 5 N sodium hydroxide, and swirl to dissolve. Add 5.0 mL of glacial acetic acid, and a stirring bar, and titrate with 0.0025 N iodine VS, determining the endpoint potentiometrically. Perform the same procedure on a second 2.50-g portion of Roxarsone, except to replace the 5.0 mL of arsenic trioxide solution with 5.0 mL of water. Calculate the percentage of trivalent arsenic (As^{+++}) in the Roxarsone taken by the formula:

$$(0.4623 / 25)[V_B / (V_A - V_B)]$$

in which 0.4623 is the arsenic equivalent of the 5.0 mL of arsenic trioxide solution, and V_A and V_B are the volumes, in mL, of 0.0025 N iodine consumed in the first and second titrations, respectively. Not more than 0.05% is found.
Content of total arsenic—Transfer about 200 mg of Roxarsone, accurately weighed, to a clean, dry 300-mL Kjeldahl flask, and clamp the flask at an angle of 45°. Add 5 mL of sulfuric acid, 10 mL of nitric acid, 5 mL of a saturated solution of sodium sulfate, and several glass beads. Heat to boiling, heat strongly until dense white fumes are produced, and continue heating until the volume is reduced to a few mL. Allow to cool, and cautiously rinse the neck of the flask with about 5 mL of water. Boil again, and continue heating for 30 minutes after the water has boiled away. Allow to cool, add 100 mL of water and 4 mL of 50% potassium iodide solution, and boil to expel the iodine vapors. Continue boiling until the solution becomes colorless, occasionally adding water to maintain the volume at about 60 mL. Add 60 mL of water, and immediately cool the solution. Add 2 drops of phenolphthalein TS, neutralize with 5 N sodium hydroxide, and then make slightly acidic (pH 6.5 to 7.0) by adding a small quantity of 18 N sulfuric acid. Transfer this solution to a beaker with the aid of a water rinse, add 4 g of sodium bicarbonate, and stir with a stirring bar. Titrate with 0.05 N iodine VS, determining the endpoint potentiometrically. Each mL of 0.05 N iodine is equivalent to 1.873 mg of arsenic (As): between 28.0% and 28.8% is found, calculated on the dried basis.
Assay—
  Mobile phase—Prepare a degassed mixture of water, methanol, and 0.17% (v/v) phosphoric acid (700 : 300 : 60). Make adjustments if necessary (see *System Suitability* under *Chromatography* ⟨621⟩).
  Standard preparation—Transfer about 50 mg of USP Roxarsone RS, accurately weighed, to a 50-mL volumetric flask. Dissolve in and dilute with 1.2 N sodium hydroxide to volume, and mix. Transfer 10.0 mL of this stock solution to a 100-mL volumetric flask, dilute with *Mobile phase* to volume, and mix. This solution contains about 0.1 mg of USP Roxarsone RS per mL.
  Assay preparation—Transfer about 50 mg of Roxarsone, accurately weighed, to a 50-mL volumetric flask. Dissolve in and dilute with 1.2 N sodium hydroxide to volume, and mix. Transfer 10.0 mL of this stock solution to a 100-mL volumetric flask, dilute with *Mobile phase* to volume, and mix.
  Chromatographic system (see *Chromatography* ⟨621⟩)—The liquid chromatograph is equipped with a 280-nm detector and a 4.6-mm × 15-cm column that contains 5-μm packing L1. The flow rate is about 1 mL per minute. Chromatograph the *Standard preparation*, and record the peak responses as directed for *Procedure*: the tailing factor is not more than 2.0, and the relative standard deviation for replicate injections is not more than 2.0%.
  Procedure—Separately inject equal volumes (about 20 μL) of the *Standard preparation* and the *Assay preparation* into the chromatograph, record the chromatograms, and measure the responses for the major peaks. Calculate the quantity, in mg, of $C_6H_6AsNO_6$ in the portion of Roxarsone taken by the formula:

$$500C(r_U / r_S)$$

in which C is the concentration, in mg per mL, of USP Roxarsone RS in the *Standard preparation*, and r_U and r_S are the roxarsone peak responses obtained from the *Assay preparation* and the *Standard preparation*, respectively.

Rubella Virus Vaccine Live

» Rubella Virus Vaccine Live conforms to the regulations of the FDA concerning biologics (630.60 to 630.67) (see *Biologics* ⟨1041⟩). It is a bacterially sterile preparation of live virus derived from a strain of rubella virus that has been tested for neurovirulence in monkeys, and for immunogenicity, that is free from all demonstrable viable microbial agents except unavoidable bacteriophage, and that has been found suitable for human immunization. The strain is grown, for purposes of vaccine production, on primary cell cultures of duck embryo tissue, derived from pathogen-free flocks, or on primary cell cultures of a designated strain of human tissue, provided that the same cell culture system is used as that in which the strain was tested. The strain meets the requirements of the specific safety tests in adult and suckling mice; and the requirements of the tests in monkey kidney, chicken embryo, and human tissue cell cultures and embryonated eggs. In the case of virus grown in duck embryo cell cultures, the strain meets the requirements of the test by inoculation of embryonated duck eggs, and of the tests for absence of *Mycobacterium tuberculosis* and of avian leucosis. In the case of virus grown in rabbit kidney cell cultures, the strain meets the requirements of the tests by inoculation of rabbits and guinea pigs, and of the tests for absence of *Mycobacterium tuberculosis* and of known adventitious agents of rabbits. In the case of virus grown in human tissue cell cultures, the strain meets the requirements of the specific safety tests and tests for absence of *Mycobacterium tuberculosis* or other adventitious agents tests by inoculation of rabbits and guinea pigs and the requirements for karyology and of the tests for absence of adventitious and other infective agents, including hemadsorption viruses and *Mycoplasma*, in human diploid cell cultures. The strain cultures are treated to remove all intact tissue cells. The Vaccine meets the requirements of the specific tissue culture test for live virus titer, in a single immunizing dose, of not less than the equivalent of 1000 TCID$_{50}$ (quantity of virus estimated to infect 50 percent of inoculated cultures × 1000) when tested in parallel with the U.S. Reference Rubella Virus, Live.

Packaging and storage—Preserve in single-dose containers, or in light-resistant, multiple-dose containers, at a temperature between 2° and 8°. Multiple-dose containers for 50 doses are adapted for use only in jet injectors, and those for 10 doses for use by jet or syringe injection.
Expiration date—The expiration date is 1 to 2 years, depending on the manufacturer's data, after date of issue from manufacturer's cold storage (−20°, 1 year).
Labeling—Label the Vaccine in multiple-dose containers to indicate that the contents are intended solely for use by jet injector or for use by either jet or syringe injection, whichever is applicable. Label the Vaccine in single-dose containers, if such containers are not light-resistant, to state that it should be protected from sunlight. Label it also to state that constituted Vaccine should be discarded if not used within 8 hours.

Rubidium Chloride Rb 82 Injection

» Rubidium Chloride Rb 82 Injection is a sterile solution, suitable for intravenous administration. It contains not less than 90.0 percent and not more than 110.0 percent of the labeled amount of ^{82}Rb expressed in megabecquerels (or in millicuries) per mL at the time indicated in the labeling. It is obtained by elution from a strontium 82-rubidium 82 generator system. ^{82}Rb, with a half-life of 76 seconds, is a short-lived positron-emitting radionuclide formed by the radioactive decay of the parent nuclide ^{82}Sr. Strontium Sr 82 with a half-life of 25.5 days is produced by the proton irradiation of rubidium or spallation of molybdenum. The chemical form of the Injection is ^{82}RbCl. [NOTE—Elute with additive-free Sodium Chloride Injection only. Discard the first 50 mL of the eluate each day the generator is eluted.]

Packaging, storage, and labeling—Requirements for packaging, storage, and labeling do not apply; Rubidium Chloride Rb 82 Injection is obtained by elution from the generator and is administered by direct infusion.
USP Reference standards ⟨11⟩—*USP Endotoxin RS*.
Bacterial endotoxins ⟨85⟩—It contains not more than 175/V USP Endotoxin Unit per mL of the Injection, when compared with the USP Endotoxin RS, in which V is the maximum recommended total dose, in mL, at the expiration date or time.
Radionuclide identification (see *Radioactivity* ⟨821⟩)—[NOTE—Perform this test quickly, because of the rapid decay of the ^{82}Rb.] The gamma-ray spectrum of eluted ^{82}Rb exhibits photopeaks at 511 and 777 keV.
pH ⟨791⟩: between 4.0 and 8.0.
Radionuclidic purity—Using a suitable counting assembly (see *Selection of a Counting Assembly* under *Radioactivity* ⟨821⟩), determine the radioactivity of each radionuclidic impurity, in kBq per MBq (or µCi per mCi), of Rb 82 in the generator eluate by use of a calibrated system as directed under *Radioactivity* ⟨821⟩. [NOTE—For the following tests, use the generator eluate containing ^{82}Rb that has been allowed to decay for 1 hour after the end of elution.]
  Sr 82 and Rb 83—Obtain a gamma-ray spectrum of the hour-old eluate, and measure the activities of the radionuclidic impurities directly from the spectrum. Sr 82 exhibits photopeaks at 511 and 777 keV and decays with a radioactive half-life of 25.5 days. Rb 83 exhibits a photopeak at 530 keV and decays with a radioactive half-life of 86.2 days. The activity levels of Sr 82 and Rb 83 are not more than 0.02 kBq per MBq (0.02 µCi per mCi) and not more than 0.05 kBq per MBq (0.05 µCi per mCi) of Rb 82 at the end of elution, respectively.
  Sr 85—Obtain a gamma spectrum of the hour-old eluate, and, using the same system and geometry, obtain a gamma spectrum of a pure Rb 82 specimen (generator eluate containing ^{82}Rb taken within 10 minutes of elution). Sr 85 exhibits a major photopeak at 514 keV and decays with a radioactive half-life of 64.8 days. Sr 85 may be determined by subtraction of the 511 and 777 keV peaks in the pure Rb 82, from the 511–514 keV and 777 keV peaks in the hour-old eluate. The activity level of Sr 85 is not more than 0.2 kBq per MBq (0.2 µCi per mCi) of Rb 82 at the end of elution.
  Other gamma-ray emitters—The total of other gamma-ray emitting radionuclidic impurities does not exceed 0.005 kBq per MBq (0.005 µCi per mCi) of Rb 82 at the end of elution.
Chemical purity—
  Electrolyte solution—Transfer 107 g of ammonium chloride, 25 g of gelatin, and 42 mL of hydrochloric acid to a 500-mL volumetric flask. Add about 450 mL of water, and sonicate until a clear solution is obtained. Dilute with water to volume, and mix.
  Tin stock standard solution—Dissolve 100 mg of metallic tin (Sn), accurately weighed, in 10 mL of dilute hydrochloric acid (1 in 2), and dilute with water to 100 mL.
  Tin standard solution A—Transfer 0.5 mL of *Tin stock standard solution* to a 50-mL volumetric flask and dilute with 0.1 N hydrochloric acid to volume.
  Tin standard solution B—Transfer 1.0 mL of *Tin standard solution A* to a 50-mL volumetric flask. Add 10.0 mL of 0.9% sodium chloride solution, dilute with *Electrolyte solution* to volume, and mix.
  Test solution—Obtain a 50-mL eluate from the generator, and allow to stand for at least 1 hour to allow for the complete decay of ^{82}Rb. Transfer 10.0 mL of the eluate to a 50-mL volumetric flask, dilute with the *Electrolyte solution* to volume, and mix.
  Procedure—Transfer a portion of the *Test solution* to a polarographic cell, and deaerate by bubbling nitrogen through the solution for 5 minutes. Insert the dropping mercury electrode of a suitable polarograph, and obtain the differential pulse polarogram from −0.15 to −0.75 volts, at a current range of 0.5 µA, using a saturated calomel electrode as the reference electrode and a platinum wire as the auxiliary electrode (see *Polarography* ⟨801⟩). Similarly, transfer a portion of the *Tin standard solution* to a polarographic cell and obtain the polarogram. A peak at −0.52 volts indicates the presence of tin. The peak height of the *Test solution* is not greater than that of the *Tin standard solution* (1 µg per mL).
Other requirements—It meets the requirements under *Injections* ⟨1⟩, except that the Injection may be distributed or dispensed prior to completion of the test for *Sterility*, the latter test being started on the day of final manufacture, and except that it is not subject to the recommendation for *Volume in Container* under *Injections* ⟨1⟩.
Assay for radioactivity—Using a suitable counting assembly (see *Selection of a Counting Assembly* under *Radioactivity* ⟨821⟩), determine the radioactivity, in MBq (or in µCi) per mL, of the Injection by use of a calibrated system as directed under *Radioactivity* ⟨821⟩.

Saccharin Calcium

$C_{14}H_8CaN_2O_6S_2 \cdot 3\frac{1}{2}H_2O$ 467.48
1,2-Benzisothiazol-3(2H)-one, 1,1-dioxide, calcium salt, hydrate (2 : 7).
1,2-Benzisothiazolin-3-one 1,1-dioxide calcium salt hydrate (2 : 7)   [6381-91-5].
Anhydrous   404.44   [6485-34-3].

» Saccharin Calcium contains not less than 99.0 percent and not more than 101.0 percent of $C_{14}H_8CaN_2O_6S_2$, calculated on the anhydrous basis.

Packaging and storage—Preserve in well-closed containers. Store at room temperature.

Labeling—Where the quantity of saccharin calcium is indicated in the labeling of any preparation containing Saccharin Calcium, this shall be expressed in terms of saccharin ($C_7H_5NO_3S$).

USP Reference standards ⟨11⟩—*USP Saccharin Calcium RS. USP o-Toluenesulfonamide RS. USP p-Toluenesulfonamide RS.*

Clarity of solution—[NOTE—The *Test solution* is to be compared to the *Reference suspension A* and to water in diffused daylight 5 minutes after preparation of *Reference suspension A*.]

Hydrazine solution—Transfer 1.0 g of hydrazine sulfate to a 100-mL volumetric flask, dissolve in and dilute with water to volume, and mix. Allow to stand for 4 to 6 hours.

Methenamine solution—Transfer 2.5 g of methenamine to a 100-mL glass-stoppered flask, add 25.0 mL of water, insert the glass stopper, and mix to dissolve.

Primary opalescent suspension—[NOTE—This suspension is stable for 2 months, provided it is stored in a glass container free from surface defects. The suspension must not adhere to the glass and must be well mixed before use.] Transfer 25.0 mL of *Hydrazine solution* to the *Methenamine solution* in the 100-mL glass-stoppered flask. Mix, and allow to stand for 24 hours.

Opalescence standard—[NOTE—This suspension should not be used beyond 24 hours after preparation.] Transfer 15.0 mL of the *Primary opalescent suspension* to a 1000-mL volumetric flask, dilute with water to volume, and mix.

Reference suspensions—Transfer 5.0 mL of the *Opalescence standard* to a 100-mL volumetric flask, dilute with water to volume, and mix to obtain *Reference suspension A*. Transfer 10.0 mL of the *Opalescence standard* to a second 100-mL volumetric flask, dilute with water to volume, and mix to obtain *Reference suspension B*.

Test solution—Dissolve 5.0 g of test material in about 20 mL of a 200 g per L solution of sodium acetate, dilute with the same solution to 25 mL, and mix.

Procedure—Transfer a sufficient portion of the *Test solution* to a test tube of colorless, transparent, neutral glass with a flat base and an internal diameter of 15 mm to 25 mm to obtain a depth of 40 mm. Similarly transfer portions of *Reference suspension A*, *Reference suspension B*, water, and a 200 g per L solution of sodium acetate to separate matching test tubes. Compare the *Test solution*, *Reference suspension A*, *Reference suspension B*, water, and a 200 g per L solution of sodium acetate in diffused daylight, viewing vertically against a black background (see *Visual Comparison* under *Spectrophotometry and Light-Scattering* ⟨851⟩). [NOTE—The diffusion of light must be such that *Reference suspension A* can readily be distinguished from water, and that *Reference suspension B* can readily be distinguished from *Reference suspension A*.] The *Test solution* shows the same clarity as that of water, or the 200 g per L solution of sodium acetate, or its opalescence is not more pronounced than that of *Reference suspension A*.

Color of solution—

Standard stock solution—Combine 3.0 mL of ferric chloride CS, 3.0 mL of cobaltous chloride CS, 2.4 mL of cupric sulfate CS, and 1.6 mL of dilute hydrochloric acid (10 g per L).

Standard solution—[NOTE—Prepare the *Standard solution* immediately before use.] Transfer 1.0 mL of *Standard stock solution* to a 100-mL volumetric flask, dilute with dilute hydrochloric acid (10 g per L) to volume, and mix.

Test solution—Use the *Test solution* from *Clarity of solution*.

Procedure—Transfer a sufficient portion of the *Test solution* to a test tube of colorless, transparent, neutral glass with a flat base and an internal diameter of 15 mm to 25 mm to obtain a depth of 40 mm. Similarly transfer portions of the *Standard solution*, a 200 g per L solution of sodium acetate, and water to separate matching test tubes. Compare the *Test solution*, the *Standard solution*, a 200 g per L solution of sodium acetate, and water in diffused daylight, viewing vertically against a white background (see *Visual Comparison* under *Spectrophotometry and Light-Scattering* ⟨851⟩). The *Test solution* has the appearance of water or the 200 g per L solution of sodium acetate, or is not more intensely colored than the *Standard solution*.

Identification—

A: *Infrared Absorption* ⟨197K⟩—

Test specimen—Dry the specimen at 105° to constant weight.

B: To a solution (1 in 10) add 2 drops of methyl red TS, and neutralize with 6 N ammonium hydroxide. Add 3 N hydrochloric acid, dropwise, until the solution is acid to the indicator. Upon the addition of ammonium oxalate TS, a white precipitate is formed. This precipitate is insoluble in 6 N acetic acid but dissolves in hydrochloric acid.

C: Calcium salts moistened with hydrochloric acid impart a transient yellowish-red color to a nonluminous flame.

Water, *Method I* ⟨921⟩: not more than 15.0%.

Readily carbonizable substances ⟨271⟩—Dissolve 200 mg in 5 mL of sulfuric acid (between 94.5% and 95.5% [w/w] of H_2SO_4), and maintain at a temperature of 48° to 50° for 10 minutes: the solution has no more color than *Matching Fluid A*, when viewed against a white background.

Heavy metals, *Method I* ⟨231⟩—Dissolve 4 g in 46 mL of water, add 4 mL of dilute hydrochloric acid (1 in 12), mix, and rub the inner wall of the vessel with a glass rod until crystallization begins. Allow the solution to stand for 1 hour, then pass through a dry filter, discarding the first 10 mL of the filtrate, and use 25 mL of the subsequent filtrate for the *Test Preparation*: the limit is 0.001%.

Limit of toluenesulfonamides—

Internal standard solution—Dissolve 25 mg of caffeine in methylene chloride, and dilute with the same solvent to 100 mL.

Reference solution—Dissolve 20.0 mg of USP o-Toluenesulfonamide RS and 20.0 mg of USP p-Toluenesulfonamide RS in methylene chloride, and dilute with the same solvent to 100.0 mL. Dilute 5.0 mL of the solution with methylene chloride to 50.0 mL. Evaporate 5.0 mL of the final solution to dryness in a stream of nitrogen. Dissolve the residue in 1.0 mL of the *Internal standard solution*.

Test solution—Dissolve 10.0 g of the substance to be examined in about 45 mL of water. If necessary, adjust the solution with 1 N sodium hydroxide or 1 N hydrochloric acid to a pH of 7 to 8, and dilute with water to 50 mL. Shake the solution with four quantities each of 50 mL of methylene chloride. Combine the lower layers, dry over anhydrous sodium sulfate, and filter. Wash the filter and the sodium sulfate with 10 mL of methylene chloride. Combine the solution and the washings, and evaporate almost to dryness in a water bath at a temperature not exceeding 40°. Using a small quantity of methylene chloride, quantitatively transfer the residue into a suitable 10-mL tube, evaporate to dryness in a stream of nitrogen, and dissolve the residue in 1.0 mL of the *Internal standard solution*.

Blank solution—Evaporate 200 mL of methylene chloride to dryness in a water bath at a temperature not exceeding 40°. Dissolve the residue in 1 mL of methylene chloride.

Chromatographic system (see *Chromatography* ⟨621⟩)—The gas chromatograph is equipped with a flame-ionization detector and contains a 0.53-mm × 10-m fused silica column, coated with G3 phase (film thickness 2 µm). The injection port, column, and detector temperatures are maintained at about 250°, 180°, and 250°, respectively; and nitrogen is used as the carrier gas at a flow rate of about 10 mL per minute. The injector employs a split ratio of 1 : 2.

Procedure—Inject about 1 µL of the *Reference solution*. Adjust the sensitivity of the detector so that the height of the peak due to caffeine is not less than 50% of the full scale of the recorder. The substances are eluted in the following order: o-toluenesulfonamide, p-toluenesulfonamide, and caffeine. The test is not valid unless the resolution between the peaks due to o-toluenesulfonamide and p-toluenesulfonamide is at least 1.5. Inject about 1 µL of the *Blank solution*. In the chromatogram obtained, verify that there are no peaks with the same retention times as the internal standard, o-toluenesulfonamide, and p-toluenesulfonamide. Inject about 1 µL of the *Test solution*, and 1 µL of the *Reference solution*. If any peaks due to o-toluenesulfonamide and p-toluenesulfonamide appear in the chromatogram obtained with the *Test solution*, the ratio of their areas to that of the internal standard is not greater than the corresponding ratio in the chromatogram obtained with the *Reference solution* (10 ppm of o-toluenesulfonamide and 10 ppm of p-toluenesulfonamide).

Limit of benzoate and salicylate—To 10 mL of a solution (1 in 20), previously acidified with 5 drops of 6 N acetic acid, add 3 drops of ferric chloride TS: no precipitate or violet color appears.
Organic volatile impurities, Method I ⟨467⟩: meets the requirements.

(Official until July 1, 2008)
Assay—Dissolve, with the aid of slight heating if necessary, about 150 mg of Saccharin Calcium, accurately weighed, in 50 mL of glacial acetic acid. Titrate with 0.1 N perchloric acid, determining the endpoint potentiometrically. Perform a blank titration, if necessary, and make the appropriate correction. Each mL of 0.1 N perchloric acid is equivalent to 20.22 mg of $C_{14}H_8CaN_2O_6S_2$.

Saccharin Sodium

$C_7H_4NNaO_3S \cdot 2H_2O$ 241.20
1,2-Benzisothiazol-3(2H)-one, 1,1-dioxide, sodium salt, dihydrate.
1,2-Benzisothiazolin-3-one 1,1-dioxide sodium salt dihydrate
[6155-57-3].
Anhydrous   205.17   [128-44-9].

» Saccharin Sodium contains not less than 99.0 percent and not more than 101.0 percent of $C_7H_4NNaO_3S \cdot 2H_2O$, calculated on the anhydrous basis.

Packaging and storage—Preserve in well-closed containers. Store at room temperature.
Labeling—Where the quantity of saccharin sodium is indicated in the labeling of any preparation containing Saccharin Sodium, this shall be expressed in terms of saccharin ($C_7H_5NO_3S$).
USP Reference standards ⟨11⟩—*USP Saccharin Sodium RS. USP o-Toluenesulfonamide RS. USP p-Toluenesulfonamide RS.*
Clarity of solution—[NOTE—The *Test solution* is to be compared to *Reference suspension A* and to water in diffused daylight 5 minutes after preparation of *Reference suspension A.*]
   Hydrazine solution—Transfer 1.0 g of hydrazine sulfate to a 100-mL volumetric flask, dissolve in and dilute with water to volume, and mix. Allow to stand for 4 to 6 hours.
   Methenamine solution—Transfer 2.5 g of methenamine to a 100-mL glass-stoppered flask, add 25.0 mL of water, insert the glass stopper, and mix to dissolve.
   Primary opalescent suspension—[NOTE—This suspension is stable for 2 months, provided it is stored in a glass container free from surface defects. The suspension must not adhere to the glass and must be well mixed before use.] Transfer 25.0 mL of *Hydrazine solution* to the *Methenamine solution* in the 100-mL glass-stoppered flask. Mix, and allow to stand for 24 hours.
   Opalescence standard—[NOTE—This suspension should not be used beyond 24 hours after preparation.] Transfer 15.0 mL of the *Primary opalescent suspension* to a 1000-mL volumetric flask, dilute with water to volume, and mix.
   Reference suspensions—Transfer 5.0 mL of the *Opalescence standard* to a 100-mL volumetric flask, dilute with water to volume, and mix to obtain *Reference suspension A*. Transfer 10.0 mL of the *Opalescence standard* to a second 100-mL volumetric flask, dilute with water to volume, and mix to obtain *Reference suspension B*.
   Test solution—Dissolve 5.0 g of test material in about 20 mL of a 200 g per L solution of sodium acetate, dilute with the same solution to 25 mL, and mix.
   Procedure—Transfer a sufficient portion of the *Test solution* to a test tube of colorless, transparent, neutral glass with a flat base and an internal diameter of 15 mm to 25 mm to obtain a depth of 40 mm. Similarly transfer portions of *Reference suspension A*, *Reference suspension B*, water, and a 200 g per L solution of sodium acetate to separate matching test tubes. Compare the *Test solution*, *Reference suspension A*, *Reference suspension B*, water, and a 200 g per L solution of sodium acetate in diffused daylight, viewing vertically against a black background (see *Visual Comparison* under *Spectrophotometry and Light-Scattering* ⟨851⟩). [NOTE—The diffusion of light must be such that *Reference suspension A* can readily be distinguished from water, and that *Reference suspension B* can readily be distinguished from *Reference suspension A*.] The *Test solution* shows the same clarity as that of water, or the 200 g per L solution of sodium acetate, or its opalescence is not more pronounced than that of *Reference suspension A*.
Color of solution—
   Standard stock solution—Combine 3.0 mL of ferric chloride CS, 3.0 mL of cobaltous chloride CS, 2.4 mL of cupric sulfate CS, and 1.6 mL of dilute hydrochloric acid (10 g per L).
   Standard solution—[NOTE—Prepare the *Standard solution* immediately before use.] Transfer 1.0 mL of the *Standard stock solution* to a 100-mL volumetric flask, dilute with dilute hydrochloric acid (10 g per L) to volume, and mix.
   Test solution—Use the *Test solution* from the test for *Clarity of solution*.
   Procedure—Transfer a sufficient portion of the *Test solution* to a test tube of colorless, transparent, neutral glass with a flat base and an internal diameter of 15 mm to 25 mm to obtain a depth of 40 mm. Similarly transfer portions of the *Standard solution*, a 200 g per L solution of sodium acetate, and water to separate matching test tubes. Compare the *Test solution*, the *Standard solution*, a 200 g per L solution of sodium acetate, and water in diffused daylight, viewing vertically against a white background (see *Visual Comparison* under *Spectrophotometry and Light-Scattering* ⟨851⟩). The *Test solution* has the appearance of water or of the 200 g per L solution of sodium acetate, or is not more intensely colored than the *Standard solution*.
Identification—
   A: *Infrared Absorption* ⟨197K⟩—
   Test specimen—Dry the specimen at 105° to constant weight.
   B: To a solution (1 in 10) add 2 mL of 15% potassium carbonate, and heat to boiling. No precipitate is formed. Add 4 mL of *Potassium pyroantimonate solution*, and heat to boiling. Allow to cool in ice water and, if necessary, rub the inside of the test tube with a glass rod. A dense precipitate is formed.
   Potassium pyroantimonate solution—Dissolve 2 g of potassium pyroantimonate in 95 mL of hot water. Cool quickly, and add a solution containing 2.5 g of potassium hydroxide in 50 mL of water and 1 mL of sodium hydroxide solution (8.5 in 100). Allow to stand for 24 hours, filter, and dilute with water to 150 mL.
   C: Sodium salts impart an intense yellow color to a nonluminous flame.
Acidity or alkalinity—To a solution of 1.0 g in 10 mL of carbon dioxide-free water add 1 drop of phenolphthalein TS: no pink color is produced. Then add 1 drop of 0.1 N sodium hydroxide: a pink color is produced.
Water, Method I ⟨921⟩:   not more than 15.0%.
Readily carbonizable substances ⟨271⟩—Dissolve 200 mg in 5 mL of sulfuric acid (between 94.5% and 95.5% [w/w] of H_2SO_4), and maintain at a temperature of 48° to 50° for 10 minutes: the solution has no more color than *Matching Fluid A*, when viewed against a white background.
Heavy metals, Method I ⟨231⟩—Dissolve 4 g in 46 mL of water, add 4 mL of dilute hydrochloric acid (1 in 12), mix, and rub the inner wall of the vessel with a glass rod until crystallization begins. Allow the solution to stand for 1 hour, then pass through a dry filter, discarding the first 10 mL of the filtrate, and use 25 mL of the subsequent filtrate for the *Test Preparation:* the limit is 0.001%.
Limit of toluenesulfonamides—
   Internal standard solution—Dissolve 25 mg of caffeine in methylene chloride, and dilute with the same solvent to 100 mL.
   Reference solution—Dissolve 20.0 mg of USP o-Toluenesulfonamide RS and 20.0 mg of USP p-Toluenesulfonamide RS in methylene chloride, and dilute with the same solvent to 100.0 mL. Dilute 5.0 mL of the solution with methylene chloride to 50.0 mL. Evaporate 5.0 mL of the final solution to dryness in a stream of nitrogen. Dissolve the residue in 1.0 mL of the *Internal standard solution*.
   Test solution—Dissolve 10.0 g of the substance to be examined in about 45 mL of water. If necessary, adjust the solution with 1 N sodium hydroxide or 1 N hydrochloric acid to a pH of 7 to 8, and dilute with water to 50 mL. Shake the solution with four quantities

each of 50 mL of methylene chloride. Combine the lower layers, dry over anhydrous sodium sulfate, and filter. Wash the filter and the sodium sulfate with 10 mL of methylene chloride. Combine the solution and the washings, and evaporate almost to dryness in a water bath at a temperature not exceeding 40°. Using a small quantity of methylene chloride, quantitatively transfer the residue into a suitable 10-mL tube, evaporate to dryness in a stream of nitrogen, and dissolve the residue in 1.0 mL of the *Internal standard solution*.

Blank solution—Evaporate 200 mL of methylene chloride to dryness in a water bath at a temperature not exceeding 40°. Dissolve the residue in 1 mL of methylene chloride.

Chromatographic system (see *Chromatography* ⟨621⟩)—The gas chromatograph is equipped with a flame-ionization detector and contains a 0.53-mm × 10-m fused silica column, coated with a 2-μm thickness of phase G3. The injection port, column, and detector temperatures are maintained at about 250°, 180°, and 250°, respectively; and nitrogen is used as the carrier gas at a flow rate of about 10 mL per minute. The injector employs a split ratio of 1 : 2.

Procedure—Inject about 1 μL of the *Reference solution*. Adjust the sensitivity of the detector so that the height of the peak due to caffeine is not less than 50% of the full scale of the recorder. The substances are eluted in the following order: *o*-toluenesulfonamide, *p*-toluenesulfonamide, and caffeine. The test is not valid unless the resolution between the peaks due to *o*-toluenesulfonamide and *p*-toluenesulfonamide is at least 1.5. Inject about 1 μL of the *Blank solution*. In the chromatogram obtained, verify that there are no peaks with the same retention times as the internal standard, *o*-toluenesulfonamide, and *p*-toluenesulfonamide. Inject about 1 μL of the *Test solution* and 1 μL of the *Reference solution*. If any peaks due to *o*-toluenesulfonamide and *p*-toluenesulfonamide appear in the chromatogram obtained with the *Test solution*, the ratio of their areas to that of the internal standard is not greater than the corresponding ratio in the chromatogram obtained with the *Reference solution* (10 ppm of *o*-toluenesulfonamide and 10 ppm of *p*-toluenesulfonamide).

Limit of benzoate and salicylate—To 10 mL of a solution (1 in 20), previously acidified with 5 drops of 6 N acetic acid, add 3 drops of ferric chloride TS: no precipitate or violet color appears.

Organic volatile impurities, Method IV ⟨467⟩: meets the requirements.

(Official until July 1, 2008)

Assay—Dissolve, with the aid of slight heating if necessary, about 150 mg of Saccharin Sodium, accurately weighed, in 50 mL of glacial acetic acid. Titrate with 0.1 N perchloric acid, determining the endpoint potentiometrically. Perform a blank titration, if necessary, and make the appropriate correction. Each mL of 0.1 N perchloric acid is equivalent to 20.52 mg of $C_7H_4NNaO_3S$.

Saccharin Sodium Oral Solution

» Saccharin Sodium Oral Solution contains the equivalent of not less than 95.0 percent and not more than 105.0 percent of the labeled amount of saccharin ($C_7H_5NO_3S$).

Packaging and storage—Preserve in tight containers.
USP Reference standards ⟨11⟩—*USP Saccharin RS*.
Identification—
 A: Transfer a volume of Oral Solution, equivalent to about 100 mg of saccharin, to a small dish, evaporate to dryness, and gently fuse the residue over a small flame until it no longer evolves ammonia. Allow the residue to cool, dissolve in 20 mL of water, neutralize the solution with 3 N hydrochloric acid, and filter: the addition of 1 drop of ferric chloride TS to the filtrate produces a violet color.
 B: It responds to the tests for *Sodium* ⟨191⟩.
pH ⟨791⟩: between 3.0 and 5.0.
Assay—
 Mobile phase—Mix 5 mL of 10 percent tetramethylammonium hydroxide solution and 400 mL of water in a 500-mL volumetric flask, adjust with phosphoric acid to a pH of 4.0, and mix. Add 50 mL of methanol to the solution, dilute with water to volume, mix, and degas the solution.

 Standard preparation—Add to an accurately weighed quantity of USP Saccharin RS an amount of 0.1 N sodium hydroxide sufficient to dissolve the solid, and dilute quantitatively with water to obtain a solution having a known concentration of about 1.2 mg of saccharin per mL.

 Assay preparation—Transfer an accurately measured volume of Oral Solution, equivalent to about 120 mg of saccharin, to a 100-mL volumetric flask, dilute with water to volume, and mix.

 Chromatographic system (see *Chromatography* ⟨621⟩)—The liquid chromatograph is equipped with a 257-nm detector and a 4.6-mm × 25-cm column that contains packing L1. The flow rate is about 2 mL per minute. Chromatograph three replicate injections of the *Standard preparation*, and record the peak responses as directed for *Procedure*: the relative standard deviation is not more than 2.0%.

 Procedure—Separately inject equal volumes (about 10 μL) of the *Standard preparation* and the *Assay preparation* into the chromatograph using a suitable microsyringe or sampling valve, record the chromatograms, and measure the responses for the major peaks. Calculate the quantity, in mg, of saccharin ($C_7H_5NO_3S$) in each mL of the Oral Solution taken by the formula:

$$(100C / V)(r_U / r_S)$$

in which *C* is the concentration, in mg per mL, of USP Saccharin RS in the *Standard preparation*, *V* is the volume, in mL, of Oral Solution taken, and r_U and r_S are the peak responses obtained from the *Assay preparation* and the *Standard preparation*, respectively.

Saccharin Sodium Tablets

» Saccharin Sodium Tablets contain the equivalent of not less than 95.0 percent and not more than 110.0 percent of the labeled amount of saccharin ($C_7H_5NO_3S$).

Packaging and storage—Preserve in well-closed containers.
USP Reference standards ⟨11⟩—*USP Saccharin RS*.
Completeness of solution—Place 5 Tablets in a 250-mL beaker containing 150 mL of water at 25°. Stir for 5 minutes: all of the Tablets dissolve to give a clear or practically clear solution.
Identification—
 A: Dissolve a quantity of Tablets, equivalent to about 1 g of saccharin, in 10 mL of water, filter if necessary, and to the solution add 5 mL of 3 N hydrochloric acid: a white precipitate of saccharin is formed. Collect the precipitate on a filter, wash with small portions of cold water until the last washing is practically free from chloride, and dry it at 105° for 2 hours: the saccharin so obtained melts between 226° and 230°, the procedure for *Class I* being used (see *Melting Range or Temperature* ⟨741⟩).
 [NOTE—Use the saccharin obtained in *Identification* test A for *Identification* tests B and C.]
 B: Dissolve about 100 mg in 5 mL of sodium hydroxide solution (1 in 20), evaporate to dryness, and gently fuse the residue over a small flame until it no longer evolves ammonia. Allow the residue to cool, dissolve in 20 mL of water, neutralize with 3 N hydrochloric acid, and filter: the addition of a drop of ferric chloride TS to the filtrate produces a violet color.
 C: Mix 20 mg with 40 mg of resorcinol, add 10 drops of sulfuric acid, and heat the mixture in a suitable liquid bath of 200° for 3 minutes. Allow it to cool, and add 10 mL of water and an excess of 1 N sodium hydroxide: a fluorescent green liquid results.
Limit of ammonium salts—Dissolve a quantity of powdered Tablets, equivalent to about 300 mg of saccharin, in 5 mL of water, and warm with 3 mL of 1 N sodium hydroxide: the odor of ammonia is not perceptible.
Assay—Weigh and finely powder not fewer than 20 Tablets. Transfer an accurately weighed portion of the powder, equivalent to about 100 mg of saccharin, to a 100-mL volumetric flask, add about 50 mL of water, agitate until the Tablet material is dissolved or evenly dispersed, dilute with water to volume, and mix. Transfer

10.0 mL to a separator, add 2 mL of 3 N hydrochloric acid, and extract with five 20-mL portions of a solvent composed of chloroform and alcohol (9:1). Collect the combined extracts in a beaker, and evaporate on a steam bath to dryness with the aid of a current of air. Dissolve the residue in 10 mL of sodium hydroxide solution (1 in 250), transfer the solution with the aid of water to a 200-mL volumetric flask, dilute with water to volume, and mix. Concomitantly determine the absorbances of this solution and a Standard solution of USP Saccharin RS in the same medium having a known concentration of about 50 μg per mL, in 1-cm cells at the wavelength of maximum absorbance at about 269 nm, with a suitable spectrophotometer, using water as the blank. Calculate the quantity, in mg, of saccharin ($C_7H_5NO_3S$) in the portion of Tablets taken by the formula:

$$(2C)(A_U / A_S)$$

in which C is the concentration, in μg per mL, of USP Saccharin RS in the Standard solution; and A_U and A_S are the absorbances of the solution from the Tablets and the Standard solution, respectively.

Safflower Oil

» Safflower Oil is the refined fixed oil yielded by the seed of *Carthamus tinctorius* Linné (Fam. Compositae).

Packaging and storage—Preserve in tight, light-resistant containers.
Fatty acid composition—Place about 1 g of Oil in a small conical flask fitted with a reflux attachment. Add 10 mL of methanol and 0.5 mL of 1 N methanolic potassium hydroxide solution prepared by dissolving 34 g of potassium hydroxide in sufficient methanol to produce 500 mL, allow to settle for 24 hours, and decant the clear solution. Reflux the mixture for 10 minutes, cool, transfer to a separator with the aid of 15 mL of *n*-heptane, shake with 10 mL of saturated sodium chloride solution, and allow to separate. Transfer the lower layer to another separator, and shake it with 10 mL of *n*-heptane. Wash the combined organic layers with 10 mL of water, dry over anhydrous sodium sulfate, and filter. Introduce a suitable portion of the filtrate into a gas chromatograph equipped with a flame-ionization detector and a column, preferably glass, 1.5 m in length and 4 mm in internal diameter packed with 10% liquid phase G4 on support S1A, maintained at a temperature of 175°. The carrier gas is nitrogen. Measure the 4 main peak areas of the methyl esters of the fatty acids. The order of elution is palmitate, stearate, oleate, and linoleate, and their relative areas, expressed as percentages of the total area of the 4 main peaks, are in the ranges 2 to 10, 1 to 10, 7 to 42, and 72 to 84, respectively.
Free fatty acids ⟨401⟩—The free fatty acids in 10 g require for neutralization not more than 2.5 mL of 0.020 N sodium hydroxide.
Iodine value, *Method II* ⟨401⟩: between 135 and 150.
Heavy metals, *Method II* ⟨231⟩: 0.001%.
Unsaponifiable matter ⟨401⟩: not more than 1.5%.
Peroxide—
 Mixed solvent—Mix 60 mL of glacial acetic acid with 40 mL of chloroform.
 Potassium iodide solution—Prepare a saturated solution of potassium iodide in freshly boiled and cooled water, and store it protected from light. Discard it if it gives a color on addition of *Mixed solvent* and starch TS.
 Procedure—Transfer about 10 g of Oil, accurately weighed, to a conical flask, add 30 mL of *Mixed solvent*, swirl to dissolve, add 0.5 mL of *Potassium iodide solution*, swirl the flask for 1 minute, accurately timed, add 30 mL of water, and titrate with 0.01 N sodium thiosulfate VS, with vigorous agitation, to a light yellow color. Add 0.5 mL of starch TS, and continue the titration until the blue color has disappeared. Perform a blank test, and make any necessary correction. Calculate the peroxide content, in mEq per kg, by the formula:

$$1000VN / W$$

in which V is the volume, in mL, of sodium thiosulfate required, N is its normality, and W is the weight, in g, of Oil taken. The limit is 10.0.

Salicylamide

$C_7H_7NO_2$ 137.14
Benzamide, 2-hydroxy-.
2-Hydroxybenzamide [65-45-2].

» Salicylamide contains not less than 98.0 percent and not more than 102.0 percent of $C_7H_7NO_2$, calculated on the anhydrous basis.

Packaging and storage—Preserve in well-closed containers.
USP Reference standards ⟨11⟩—*USP Salicylamide RS*.
Identification—
 A: *Infrared Absorption* ⟨197K⟩.
 B: *Ultraviolet Absorption* ⟨197U⟩—
 Solution: 16 μg per mL.
 Medium: methanol.
 Absorptivities at 302 nm, calculated on the anhydrous basis, do not differ by more than 3%.
 C: Dissolve about 100 mg in 5 mL of alcohol, and add a few drops of ferric chloride TS: a violet color develops.
Melting range ⟨741⟩: between 139° and 142°.
Water, *Method I* ⟨921⟩: not more than 0.5%.
Residue on ignition ⟨281⟩: not more than 0.1%.
Heavy metals, *Method II* ⟨231⟩: 0.001%.
Chromatographic purity—
 Standard preparations—Dissolve USP Salicylamide RS quantitatively in methanol, and mix to obtain a solution having a concentration of 1.0 mg per mL. Dilute quantitatively with methanol to obtain *Standard preparations*, designated by letter, having the following compositions:

Standard preparation	Dilution	Concentration (μg RS per mL)	Percentage (%, for comparison with test specimen)
A	(1 in 5)	200	1.0
B	(3 in 20)	150	0.75
C	(1 in 10)	100	0.5
D	(1 in 20)	50	0.25

 Test preparation—Dissolve 200 mg of Salicylamide in 10.0 mL of methanol, and mix.
 Developing solvent system—Prepare a mixture of normal butyl acetate, chloroform, and formic acid (6 : 4 : 2).
 Procedure—Apply separately 10 μL of the *Test preparation* and 10 μL of each of the *Standard preparations* to a suitable thin-layer chromatographic plate (see *Chromatography* ⟨621⟩) coated with a 0.25-mm layer of chromatographic silica gel mixture, and dry the spots with the aid of a current of air. Place the plate in a suitable chromatographic chamber, and develop the chromatograms with the *Developing solvent system* until the solvent front has moved about three-fourths of the length of the plate. Remove the plate from the developing chamber, mark the solvent front, allow the plate to dry, and locate the spots under short-wavelength UV light. Compare the

intensities of any secondary spots observed in the chromatogram of the *Test preparation* with those of the principal spots in the chromatograms of the *Standard preparations*: the total of the intensities of all secondary spots obtained from the *Test preparation* does not exceed that of the principal spot obtained from *Standard preparation B* (1%).

Organic volatile impurities, *Method V* ⟨467⟩: meets the requirements.

Solvent—Use dimethyl sulfoxide.

(Official until July 1, 2008)

Assay—Transfer about 500 mg of Salicylamide, accurately weighed, to a 100-mL beaker equipped with a mechanical stirrer and a suitable cover with a single hole for the buret tip. Add 30 mL of freshly neutralized dimethylformamide containing a few drops of thymol blue TS. Titrate with 0.1 N sodium methoxide VS in toluene to the same blue endpoint obtained in the standardization of the sodium methoxide solution. Perform a blank determination, and make any necessary correction. Each mL of 0.1 N sodium methoxide is equivalent to 13.71 mg of $C_7H_7NO_2$.

Salicylic Acid

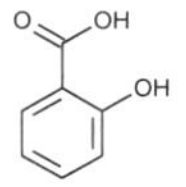

$C_7H_6O_3$ 138.12
Benzoic acid, 2-hydroxy-.
Salicylic acid   [69-72-7].

» Salicylic Acid contains not less than 99.5 percent and not more than 101.0 percent of $C_7H_6O_3$, calculated on the dried basis.

Packaging and storage—Preserve in well-closed containers.

Add the following:

▲USP **Reference standards** ⟨11⟩—USP Phenol RS. USP Salicylic Acid RS. USP Salicylic Acid Related Compound A RS. USP Salicylic Acid Related Compound B RS.▲USP31

Change to read:

Identification—▲In moderately dilute solutions of Salicylic Acid, ferric chloride TS produces a violet color.▲USP31

Melting range ⟨741⟩:   between 158° and 161°.

Loss on drying ⟨731⟩—Dry it over silica gel for 3 hours: it loses not more than 0.5% of its weight.

Residue on ignition ⟨281⟩:   not more than 0.05%.

Chloride ⟨221⟩—Heat 1.5 g with 75 mL of water until the acid is dissolved, cool, add water to restore the original volume, and filter: a 25-mL portion of the filtrate shows no more chloride than corresponds to 0.10 mL of 0.020 N hydrochloric acid (0.014%).

Change to read:

▲**Sulfate** ⟨221⟩—A 1.0-g portion dissolved in a mixture of alcohol and water (1 : 1) shows no more sulfate than corresponds to 0.2 mL of 0.020 N sulfuric acid (0.02%).▲USP31

Heavy metals—Dissolve 1 g in 25 mL of acetone, and add 2 mL of water. Add 1.2 mL of thioacetamide-glycerin base TS and 2 mL of *pH 3.5 Acetate Buffer*, and allow to stand for 5 minutes: any color produced is not darker than that of a control made with 25 mL of acetone and 2 mL of *Standard Lead Solution* (see *Heavy Metals* ⟨231⟩) and treated in the same manner. The limit is 20 µg per g.

Change to read:

Related compounds—
Mobile phase—Prepare a mixture of water, methanol, and glacial acetic acid (60 : 40 : 1). Make adjustments if necessary (see *System Suitability* under *Chromatography* ⟨621⟩).

Diluent—Prepare a mixture of methanol, water, and glacial acetic acid (70 : 30 : 4).
▲USP31

Standard solution—Dissolve accurately weighed quantities of ▲USP Salicylic Acid Related Compound A RS, USP Salicylic Acid Related Compound B RS, USP Phenol RS, and USP Salicylic Acid RS▲USP31in *Diluent* to obtain a solution having known concentrations of about 0.05 mg per mL, 0.025 mg per mL, 0.01 mg per mL, and ▲0.5 mg per mL,▲USP31respectively.

Test solution—Prepare a solution of Salicylic Acid in *Diluent* containing 50 mg per mL. Sonicate until completely dissolved.

Chromatographic system (see *Chromatography* ⟨621⟩)—The liquid chromatograph is equipped with a 270-nm detector and a 4.6-mm × 10-cm column containing 5-µm packing L1. The flow rate is about 0.5 mL per minute. Chromatograph the ▲*Standard solution,*▲USP31record the chromatograms, and ▲identify the peaks using the relative retention times given in *Table 1*. [NOTE—For the purpose of peak identification the approximate relative retention times are given in *Table 1*. The relative retention times are measured with respect to Salicylic Acid.]

Table 1

Name	Relative Retention Time	Limit (%)
Salicylic acid related compound A	0.35	NMT 0.1
Salicylic acid related compound B	0.45	NMT 0.05
Phenol	0.50	NMT 0.02
Other impurity	—	NMT 0.05
Total impurities	—	NMT 0.2▲USP31

Procedure—Separately inject equal volumes (about 2 µL) of the *Standard solution* and the *Test solution* into the chromatograph, record the chromatograms, and measure the areas for the major peaks. Calculate the percentage of each relevant related compound taken by the formula:

$$▲ 100(C_i / C_U)(r_i / r_{Si})▲USP31$$

in which C_i is the concentration, in mg per mL, of the relevant related compound in the *Standard solution*; ▲C_U is the concentration, in mg per mL, of the *Test solution*;▲USP31and r_i and $r_{Si}$are the peak responses for the relevant related compounds obtained from the *Test solution* and the *Standard solution*, respectively. ▲▲USP31Calculate the percentage of any other impurity, other than the solvent peak, observed in the chromatogram of the *Test solution* by the same formula, ▲using▲USP31the concentration of ▲salicylic acid related compound B▲USP31in the *Standard solution* as C_i;the response of the peak of ▲salicylic acid related compound B▲USP31in the chromatogram obtained from the *Standard solution* as r_{Si};and the response of any other impurity as r_i. ▲The limits are given in *Table 1*.▲USP31

Assay—Dissolve about 500 mg of Salicylic Acid, accurately weighed, in 25 mL of diluted alcohol that previously has been neutralized with 0.1 N sodium hydroxide, add phenolphthalein TS, and titrate with 0.1 N sodium hydroxide VS. Each mL of 0.1 N sodium hydroxide is equivalent to 13.81 mg of $C_7H_6O_3$.

Salicylic Acid Collodion

» Salicylic Acid Collodion contains not less than 9.5 percent and not more than 11.5 percent of $C_7H_6O_3$.

Salicylic Acid	100 g
Flexible Collodion, a sufficient quantity to make	1000 mL

Dissolve the Salicylic Acid in about 750 mL of Flexible Collodion, add sufficient of the latter to make the product measure 1000 mL, and mix.

Packaging and storage—Preserve in tight containers, at controlled room temperature, remote from fire.

Assay—Transfer to a 400-mL beaker 5 mL of Salicylic Acid Collodion, accurately measured, rinse the measuring device with three 10-mL portions of a mixture of ether and alcohol (3 : 1) that previously has been neutralized to bromothymol blue TS, and add the rinsings to the beaker. Add, with stirring, 5 mL of sodium lauryl sulfate solution (1 in 10) that previously has been neutralized with 0.1 N hydrochloric acid to the distinct yellow color of bromothymol blue TS, and finally add 20 mL of water. Mix, add 5 drops of bromothymol blue TS, and titrate the mixture with 0.1 N sodium hydroxide VS. Each mL of 0.1 N sodium hydroxide is equivalent to 13.81 mg of $C_7H_6O_3$.

Salicylic Acid Topical Foam

» Salicylic Acid Topical Foam contains not less than 90.0 percent and not more than 110.0 percent of the labeled amount of $C_7H_6O_3$.

Packaging and storage—Preserve in tight containers.

USP Reference standards ⟨11⟩—*USP Salicylic Acid RS*.

Identification—The retention time of the salicylic acid peak of the *Assay preparation* observed in the chromatogram obtained in the *Assay* corresponds to the retention time of the salicylic acid peak of the *Standard preparation*.

pH ⟨791⟩: between 5.0 and 6.0.

Assay—

Mobile phase—To 225 mg of tetramethylammonium hydroxide pentahydrate add 700 mL of water, 150 mL of methanol, 150 mL of acetonitrile, and 1.0 mL of glacial acetic acid, mix, filter, and degas.

Internal standard solution—Dissolve benzoic acid in methanol to obtain a solution having a concentration of about 8 mg per mL.

Standard preparation—Transfer about 20 mg of USP Salicylic Acid RS, accurately weighed, to a 100-mL volumetric flask, add 10.0 mL of *Internal standard solution*, dilute with *Mobile phase* to volume, and mix.

Assay preparation—Transfer an accurately weighed portion of Topical Foam, equivalent to about 20 mg of salicylic acid, to a 100-mL volumetric flask, add 10.0 mL of *Internal standard solution*, dilute with *Mobile phase* to volume, and mix. Cool in an ice bath to below room temperature and filter, discarding the first few mL of the filtrate.

Chromatographic system (see *Chromatography* ⟨621⟩)—The liquid chromatograph is equipped with a 280-nm detector and a 4-mm × 30-cm column that contains packing L1. The flow rate is about 2 mL per minute. Chromatograph four replicate injections of the *Standard preparation*, and record the peak responses as directed for *Procedure*: the relative standard deviation is not more than 3.0%, the resolution factor between salicylic acid and benzoic acid is not less than 3.0, and the tailing factors for the salicylic acid and benzoic acid peaks are not more than 2.0.

Procedure—Separately inject equal volumes (about 5 µL) of the *Standard preparation* and the *Assay preparation* into the chromatograph, record the chromatograms, and measure the responses for the major peaks. The retention times are about 2.5 minutes for salicylic acid and 5.5 minutes for benzoic acid. Calculate the quantity, in mg, of $C_7H_6O_3$ in the portion of Topical Foam taken by the formula:

$$(100C)(R_U / R_S)$$

in which C is the concentration, in mg per mL, of USP Salicylic Acid RS in the *Standard preparation*, and R_U and R_S are the ratios of the peak responses for salicylic acid to the peak responses for benzoic acid obtained from the *Assay preparation* and the *Standard preparation*, respectively.

Salicylic Acid Gel

» Salicylic Acid Gel is Salicylic Acid in a suitable viscous hydrophilic vehicle. It contains not less than 90.0 percent and not more than 110.0 percent of the labeled amount of $C_7H_6O_3$. It may contain alcohol.

Packaging and storage—Preserve in collapsible tubes or in tight containers, preferably at controlled room temperature.

Identification—Filter 5 mL of the solution obtained by titration in the *Assay*. Add 1 mL of ferric chloride TS to the filtrate: a violet color is produced. Add 1 mL of 6 N acetic acid: the violet color does not change. Add 1 mL of 6 N hydrochloric acid: the violet color is discharged. A small amount of white precipitate may appear.

Alcohol content (if present) ⟨611⟩: from 90.0% to 110.0% of the labeled amount of C_2H_5OH.

Assay—To 25 mL of diluted alcohol add 1 drop of phenolphthalein TS and sufficient 0.1 N sodium hydroxide to produce a faint pink color. Add 5.0 g of Gel, accurately weighed, and stir. Titrate the dispersion with 0.1 N sodium hydroxide VS until a pink color is produced. [NOTE—Reserve this solution for the *Identification* test.] Each mL of 0.1 N sodium hydroxide is equivalent to 13.81 mg of $C_7H_6O_3$.

Salicylic Acid Plaster

» Salicylic Acid Plaster is a uniform mixture of Salicylic Acid in a suitable base, spread on paper, cotton cloth, or other suitable backing material. The plaster mass contains not less than 90.0 percent and not more than 110.0 percent of the labeled amount of $C_7H_6O_3$.

Packaging and storage—Preserve in well-closed containers, preferably at controlled room temperature.

Assay—Weigh accurately an amount of Plaster, corresponding to about 500 mg of salicylic acid, cut the portion into small strips, place them in a small flask, add 50 mL of chloroform, and shake the mixture until the plaster mass is disintegrated. Decant the chloroform extract into a 250-mL beaker, and wash the plaster backing with two 25-mL portions of chloroform, receiving the washings in the same beaker. Then wash the backing with 50 mL of alcohol to which has been added 1 mL of 6 N ammonium hydroxide, and add the washing to the chloroform extract. Again wash the backing with 40 mL of alcohol, and add the washing to the chloroform extract. Dry the backing, weigh, and subtract the weight from the weight of Plaster taken for the assay to obtain the weight of plaster mass. Stir the chloroform extract until any coagulum has separated into a compact mass, and filter the extract through purified cotton into a separator. Knead the coagulum, if any, with a glass rod to expel the solvent, and rinse the coagulum and the beaker with 10 mL of alcohol. Pour the rinsing through the cotton, then press the cotton with a glass rod to expel the solvent. Extract the filtrate with three 10-mL portions of 1 N sodium hydroxide, drawing off each portion into a 500-mL volumetric flask, and finally wash with two 25-mL portions of water, receiving the washings in the same flask. Dilute with water to volume, and pipet a 25-mL aliquot into a 500-mL iodine flask. Add 30.0 mL of 0.1 N bromine VS, then add 5 mL of hydrochloric acid, and immediately insert the stopper. Shake the flask repeatedly during 30 minutes, allow it to stand for 15 minutes, add quickly 5 mL of potassium iodide solution (1 in 5), taking precautions against the escape of bromine vapor, and at once insert the stopper in the flask. Shake thoroughly, remove the stopper, and rinse it and the neck of the flask with a small quantity of water, so that the washing flows into the flask. Add 1 mL of chloroform, shake the mixture, and titrate the liberated iodine with 0.1 N sodium thiosulfate VS, adding 3 mL of starch TS as the endpoint is approached. Perform a blank determination (see *Residual Titrations* under *Titrimetry* ⟨541⟩). Each mL of 0.1 N bromine is equivalent to 2.302 mg of $C_7H_6O_3$.

Salsalate

$C_{14}H_{10}O_5$ 258.23
Benzoic acid, 2-hydroxy-, 2-carboxyphenyl ester.
Disalicylic acid.
Salicylsalicylic acid.
Salicylic acid, bimolecular ester   [552-94-3].

» Salsalate contains not less than 98.0 percent and not more than 102.0 percent of total salicylates, expressed as the sum of the percentages of salsalate, salicylic acid, and trisalicylic acid, calculated on the dried basis.

Packaging and storage—Preserve in tight containers.
USP Reference standards ⟨11⟩—*USP Salsalate RS. USP Salicylic Acid RS. USP Trisalicylic Acid RS.*
Identification, *Infrared Absorption* ⟨197M⟩.
Loss on drying ⟨731⟩—Dry it in vacuum at 60° for 3 hours: it loses not more than 0.5% of its weight.
Residue on ignition ⟨281⟩:   not more than 0.10%.
Chloride ⟨221⟩—Dissolve 1.4 g in 6 mL of methanol, warming if necessary to effect solution. Dilute with water to 50 mL to precipitate the salsalate, allow to stand for 5 minutes, and filter. A 25-mL portion of the filtrate shows no more chloride than corresponds to 0.20 mL of 0.010 N hydrochloric acid (0.01%).
Sulfate ⟨221⟩—A 17-mL portion of the filtrate prepared for the test for *Chloride* shows no more sulfate than corresponds to 0.50 mL of 0.010 N sulfuric acid (0.05%).
Heavy metals—Dissolve 2 g in 25 mL of methanol, and add 1 mL of water. Add 1.2 mL of thioacetamide-glycerin base TS and 2 mL of *pH 3.5 Acetate Buffer*, and allow to stand for 5 minutes: any color produced is not darker than that obtained from a standard prepared from 25 mL of methanol and 2 mL of *Standard Lead Solution* (see *Heavy metals* ⟨231⟩) and treated in the same manner. The limit is 10 µg per g.
Limit of dimethylaniline—
  Internal standard solution—Prepare a solution in methylene chloride containing 0.4 mg of indene per mL.
  Standard preparation—Transfer about 50 mg of *N,N*-dimethylaniline, accurately weighed, to a 100-mL volumetric flask, dilute with *Internal standard solution* to volume, insert the stopper securely, and mix.
  Test preparation—Transfer about 5 g of Salsalate, accurately weighed, to a 125-mL separator fitted with a cotton pledget in its stem. Add 50 mL of water and 6 mL of 6 N ammonium hydroxide, and swirl until dissolved. Add 5.0 mL of *Internal standard solution*, insert the stopper into the separator, and shake for 1 minute. Keep the separator stoppered, and allow the layers to separate. Loosen the stopper, and drain most of the lower phase into a screw-capped test tube. Use this solution as the *Test preparation*.
  Chromatographic system (see *Chromatography* ⟨621⟩)—The gas chromatograph is equipped with a flame-ionization detector, a split injector with a 10 : 1 split ratio, and a 30-m × 0.53-mm capillary column, the internal wall of which is coated with a 1.0-µm film of phase G42. Maintain the column at 105°, the injector at 250°, and the detector block at 250°, and use helium as the carrier gas, at a flow rate of about 13 mL per minute. Chromatograph the *Standard preparation*, and record the peak responses as directed for *Procedure:* the relative retention times are about 0.75 for indene and 1.0 for *N,N*-dimethylaniline, the resolution, *R*, between the indene peak and the *N,N*-dimethylaniline peak is not less than 2.0, and the relative standard deviation for replicate injections is not more than 3%.
  Procedure—[NOTE—Use peak areas where peak responses are indicated.] Inject equal volumes (about 1 µL) of the *Standard preparation* and the *Test preparation* into the chromatograph, record the chromatograms, and measure the responses for the major peaks. Indene elutes before *N,N*-dimethylaniline. Calculate the percentage of *N,N*-dimethylaniline in the portion of Salsalate taken by the formula:

$$0.5(C/W)(R_U/R_S)$$

in which *C* is the concentration, in mg per mL, of *N,N*-dimethylaniline in the *Standard preparation*, *W* is the weight, in g, of Salsalate taken to prepare the *Test preparation*, and R_U and R_S are the ratios of the response of the *N,N*-dimethylaniline peak to that of the indene peak obtained from the *Test preparation* and the *Standard preparation*, respectively. The limit is 0.05%.
Isopropyl, ethyl, and methyl salicylates—
  Standard stock solution—Prepare a solution in chromatographic *n*-heptane containing 0.20 mg of isopropyl salicylate, 0.50 mg of ethyl salicylate, and 0.50 mg of methyl salicylate per mL.
  Standard preparation—Transfer to a suitable screw-capped test tube 2.0 g of Salsalate, add 10 mL of 1 N sodium hydroxide and 2 mL of chromatographic *n*-heptane, shake until dissolved, and allow the layers to separate. Draw off and discard all of the upper layer. To the lower layer add 2.0 mL of *Standard stock solution*, shake for 1 minute, and allow the layers to separate. Use the upper layer as the *Standard preparation*.
  Test preparation—Transfer 2.0 g of Salsalate to a suitable screw-capped test tube, add 10 mL of 1 N sodium hydroxide and 2.0 mL of chromatographic *n*-heptane, shake until dissolved, and allow the layers to separate. Use the upper layer as the *Test preparation*.
  Chromatographic system (see *Chromatography* ⟨621⟩)—The gas chromatograph is equipped with a flame-ionization detector, a split injector with a 10 : 1 split ratio, and a 30-m × 0.53-mm capillary column, the internal wall of which is coated with a 1.0-µm film of phase G42. Maintain the column at 120° and the injector and detector block at about 250°. Helium is used as the carrier gas, flowing at the rate of about 13 mL per minute.
  Procedure—[NOTE—Use peak areas where peak responses are indicated.] Inject equal volumes (about 1 µL) of the *Standard preparation* and the *Test preparation* into the chromatograph, record the chromatograms, and measure the responses for the major peaks. The relative retention times are about 0.65 for methyl salicylate, 0.9 for ethyl salicylate, and 1.0 for isopropyl salicylate. The response of any isopropyl salicylate peak obtained from the *Test preparation* is not greater than that obtained from the *Standard preparation* (0.02%), the response of any ethyl salicylate peak obtained from the *Test preparation* is not greater than that obtained from the *Standard preparation* (0.05%), and the response of any methyl salicylate peak obtained from the *Test preparation* is not greater than that obtained from the *Standard preparation* (0.05%).
Chromatographic purity—Using the chromatograms obtained in the *Assay*, calculate the percentage of each impurity, other than salicylic acid and trisalicylic acid, in the portion of Salsalate taken by the formula:

$$10{,}000(C/W)(r_U/r_S)$$

in which *C* is the concentration, in mg per mL, of USP Salsalate RS in the *Salsalate standard preparation*, *W* is the weight, in mg, of Salsalate taken to prepare the *Assay stock solution*, r_U is the response of the particular impurity peak obtained from the *Assay stock solution*, and r_S is the salsalate peak response obtained from the *Salsalate standard preparation*: not more than 0.2% of each other impurity is found.

Related compounds—The percentages of salicylic acid and trisalicylic acid, determined as directed in the *Assay*, do not exceed 0.5% and 2.5%, respectively.

Organic volatile impurities, *Method V* ⟨467⟩: meets the requirements.

Solvent—Use dimethyl sulfoxide.

(Official until July 1, 2008)

Assay—

Mobile phase—Prepare a suitable filtered and degassed mixture of methanol, water, and phosphoric acid (650 : 350 : 1), and adjust with phosphoric acid or 1 N sodium hydroxide, if necessary, to a pH of 3.1. Make adjustments if necessary (see *System Suitability* under *Chromatography* ⟨621⟩).

Diluent—Prepare a mixture of water, acetonitrile, and phosphoric acid (540 : 460 : 1).

Salsalate standard preparation—Dissolve an accurately weighed quantity of USP Salsalate RS in *Diluent* to obtain a stock solution having a known concentration of about 1 mg per mL. Transfer 2.0 mL of this solution to a 100-mL volumetric flask, dilute with *Diluent* to volume, and mix. This solution contains about 0.02 mg per mL.

Salicylic acid standard preparation—Dissolve an accurately weighed quantity of USP Salicylic Acid RS in *Diluent* to obtain a stock solution having a known concentration of about 0.5 mg per mL. Transfer 1.0 mL of this solution to a 100-mL volumetric flask, dilute with *Diluent* to volume, and mix. This solution contains about 0.005 mg of USP Salicylic Acid RS per mL.

Trisalicylic acid standard preparation—Dissolve an accurately weighed quantity of USP Trisalicylic Acid RS in *Diluent* to obtain a stock solution having a known concentration of about 0.5 mg per mL. Transfer 5.0 mL of this solution to a 100-mL volumetric flask, dilute with *Diluent* to volume, and mix. This solution contains about 0.025 mg of USP Trisalicylic Acid RS per mL.

Resolution solution—Prepare a solution in *Diluent* containing about 0.02 mg of USP Salsalate RS per mL, 0.02 mg of USP Salicylic Acid RS per mL, and 0.04 mg of USP Trisalicylic Acid RS per mL.

Assay stock solution—Transfer about 100 mg of Salsalate, accurately weighed, to a 100-mL volumetric flask, dilute with *Diluent* to volume, and mix. Sonicate if necessary to effect the solution.

Assay preparation—Transfer 2.0 mL of the *Assay stock solution* to a 100-mL volumetric flask, dilute with *Diluent* to volume, and mix.

Chromatographic system (see *Chromatography* ⟨621⟩)—The liquid chromatograph is equipped with a 236-nm detector and a 4-mm × 15-cm column that contains 5-μm packing L7. The flow rate is about 1.5 mL per minute. Chromatograph the *Resolution solution*, and record the peak responses as directed for *Procedure*: the relative retention times are about 0.55 for salicylic acid, 1.0 for salsalate, and 1.5 for trisalicylic acid, and the resolution, *R*, between the salicylic acid and salsalate peaks and between the salsalate and trisalicylic acid peaks is not less than 2.0. Chromatograph the *Salicylic acid standard preparation*, and record the peak responses as directed for *Procedure*: the relative standard deviation of the salicylic acid peak responses for replicate injections is not more than 2.0%.

Procedure—Separately inject equal volumes (about 10 μL) of the *Salsalate standard preparation*, the *Salicylic acid standard preparation*, the *Trisalicylic acid standard preparation*, the *Assay stock solution*, and the *Assay preparation* into the chromatograph, record the chromatograms, and measure the responses for the major peaks. [NOTE—Continue chromatography after each injection for a period of time not less than the retention time of trisalicylic acid.] Calculate the percentage of salicylic acid ($C_7H_6O_3$) in the portion of Salsalate taken by the formula:

$$10{,}000(C/W)(r_U/r_S)$$

in which C is the concentration, in mg per mL, of USP Salicylic Acid RS in the *Salicylic acid standard preparation*, W is the weight, in mg, of the portion of Salsalate taken, and r_U and r_S are the responses of the salicylic acid peak obtained from the *Assay stock solution* and the *Salicylic acid standard preparation*, respectively. Calculate the percentage of trisalicylic acid ($C_{21}H_{14}O_7$) in the portion of Salsalate taken by the formula:

$$10{,}000(C/W)(r_U/r_S)$$

in which C is the concentration, in mg per mL, of USP Trisalicylic Acid RS in the *Trisalicylic acid standard preparation*, and r_U and r_S are the responses of the trisalicylic acid peaks obtained from the *Assay stock solution* and the *Trisalicylic acid standard preparation*, respectively. Calculate the percentage of salsalate ($C_{14}H_{10}O_5$) in the portion of Salsalate taken by the formula:

$$500{,}000(C/W)(r_U/r_S)$$

in which C is the concentration, in mg per mL, of USP Salsalate RS in the *Salsalate standard preparation*, and r_U and r_S are the salsalate peak responses obtained from the *Assay preparation* and the *Salsalate standard preparation*, respectively.

Salsalate Capsules

» Salsalate Capsules contain not less than 90.0 percent and not more than 110.0 percent of the labeled amount of $C_{14}H_{10}O_5$.

Packaging and storage—Preserve in tight containers.

USP Reference standards ⟨11⟩—*USP Salsalate RS. USP Salicylic Acid RS.*

Identification—Transfer a quantity of Capsule contents, equivalent to about 500 mg of salsalate, to a stoppered glass test tube. Add 20 mL of ether to the tube, close the tube tightly, shake by mechanical means for 10 minutes, and filter. Evaporate the filtrate to dryness using a stream of nitrogen: the IR absorption spectrum of a mineral oil dispersion of the residue thus obtained, exhibits maxima only at the same wavelengths as that of a similar preparation of USP Salsalate RS.

Disintegration ⟨701⟩: 30 minutes, simulated gastric fluid TS (without pepsin) being used.

Uniformity of dosage units ⟨905⟩: meet the requirements.

Limit of salicylic acid—

Mobile phase, Diluent, Resolution solution, and *Chromatographic system*—Proceed as directed in the *Assay*.

Standard preparation—Dissolve an accurately weighed quantity of USP Salicylic Acid RS in *Diluent* to obtain a stock solution having a known concentration of about 0.5 mg per mL. Transfer 3.0 mL of this solution to a 100-mL volumetric flask, dilute with *Diluent* to volume, and mix. This solution contains about 0.015 mg per mL.

Test preparation—Use the *Assay stock solution* prepared as directed in the *Assay*.

Procedure—Proceed as directed for *Procedure* in the *Assay*, except to inject equal volumes (about 10 μL) of the *Standard preparation* and the *Test preparation*. Calculate the percentage of salicylic acid ($C_7H_6O_3$) in the portion of Capsules taken by the formula:

$$10{,}000(C/O_T)(r_U/r_S)$$

in which C is the concentration, in mg per mL, of USP Salicylic Acid RS in the *Standard preparation*, O_T is the quantity, in mg, of salsalate in the portion of Capsules taken based on the labeled amount, and r_U and r_S are the salicylic acid peak responses obtained from the *Test preparation* and the *Standard preparation*, respectively: not more than 1.5% is found.

Assay—

Mobile phase, Diluent, Salsalate standard preparation, Resolution solution, and *Chromatographic system*—Proceed as directed in the *Assay* under *Salsalate*.

Assay preparation—Transfer as completely as possible the contents of not less than 20 Capsules to a suitable tared container, and weigh. Mix, and transfer an accurately weighed portion of the powder, equivalent to about 100 mg of salsalate, to a 100-mL volumetric flask, dilute with *Diluent* to volume, and mix. Sonicate for about 10 minutes, and mix. Filter a portion of this solution through a suitable filter of 0.5 μm or finer porosity. Use the clear filtrate as the *Assay stock solution*. Transfer 2.0 mL of the *Assay stock solution* to a 100-mL volumetric flask, dilute with *Diluent* to volume, and mix (*Assay preparation*).

Procedure—Separately inject equal volumes (about 10 μL) of the *Salsalate standard preparation* and the *Assay preparation* into the chromatograph, record the chromatograms, and measure the responses for the salsalate peaks. Calculate the quantity, in mg, of salsalate ($C_{14}H_{10}O_5$) in the portion of Capsules taken by the formula:

$$5000C(r_U / r_S)$$

in which C is the concentration, in mg per mL, of USP Salsalate RS in the *Salsalate standard preparation*, and r_U and r_S are the responses of the salsalate peaks obtained from the *Assay preparation* and the *Salsalate standard preparation*, respectively.

Salsalate Tablets

» Salsalate Tablets contain not less than 90.0 percent and not more than 110.0 percent of the labeled amount of $C_{14}H_{10}O_5$.

Packaging and storage—Preserve in tight containers.

USP Reference standards ⟨11⟩—*USP Salsalate RS. USP Salicylic Acid RS.*

Identification—Transfer a quantity of finely powdered Tablets, equivalent to about 500 mg of salsalate, to a stoppered glass test tube. Add 20 mL of ether to the tube, close the tube tightly, shake by mechanical means for 10 minutes, and filter. Evaporate the filtrate to dryness using a stream of nitrogen: the IR absorption spectrum of a mineral oil dispersion of the residue so obtained exhibits maxima only at the same wavelengths as that of a similar preparation of USP Salsalate RS.

Dissolution ⟨711⟩—

Test 1: If the product complies with this test, the labeling indicates that it meets USP *Dissolution Test 1*.

Medium: 0.25 M pH 7.4 phosphate buffer, prepared by mixing 5.175 g of monobasic sodium phosphate and 30.17 g of anhydrous dibasic sodium phosphate with water to obtain 1000 mL of solution, and adjusting by the dropwise addition of 50% sodium hydroxide solution to a pH of 7.40 ± 0.05; 900 mL.

Apparatus 2: 50 rpm.

Time: 60 minutes.

Procedure—Determine the amount of $C_{14}H_{10}O_5$ dissolved from UV absorbances at the wavelength of maximum absorbance at about 308 nm of filtered portions of the solution under test, suitably diluted with the *Dissolution Medium*, in comparison with a Standard solution having a known concentration of USP Salsalate RS in the same medium.

Tolerances—Not less than 70% (*Q*) of the labeled amount of $C_{14}H_{10}O_5$ is dissolved in 60 minutes.

Test 2: If the product complies with this test, the labeling indicates that it meets USP *Dissolution Test 2*.

Medium: 0.05 M, pH 7.5 phosphate buffer; prepared by mixing 40.83 g of monobasic potassium phosphate and 120 mL of 2 N sodium hydroxide with water to obtain 6 liters of solution, and adjusting by the dropwise addition of 2 N sodium hydroxide or phosphoric acid to a pH of 7.50 ± 0.05; 900 mL.

Apparatus 2: 100 rpm.

Time and *Procedure*—Proceed as directed for *Test 1*.

Tolerances—Not less than 70% (*Q*) of the labeled amount of $C_{14}H_{10}O_5$ is dissolved in 60 minutes.

Uniformity of dosage units ⟨905⟩: meet the requirements.

Limit of salicylic acid—

Mobile phase, Diluent, Resolution solution, and *Chromatographic system*—Proceed as directed in the *Assay*.

Standard preparation—Dissolve an accurately weighed quantity of USP Salicylic Acid RS in *Diluent* to obtain a stock solution having a known concentration of about 0.5 mg per mL. Transfer 3.0 mL of this solution to a 50-mL volumetric flask, dilute with *Diluent* to volume, and mix. This solution contains about 0.03 mg per mL.

Test preparation—Use the *Assay stock solution* prepared as directed in the *Assay*.

Procedure—Proceed as directed for *Procedure* in the *Assay*, except to inject equal volumes (about 10 μL) of the *Standard preparation* and the *Test preparation*. Calculate the percentage of salicylic acid ($C_7H_6O_3$) in the portion of Tablets taken by the formula:

$$10,000(C / O_T)(r_U / r_S)$$

in which C is the concentration, in mg per mL, of USP Salicylic Acid RS in the *Standard preparation*, O_T is the quantity, in mg, of salsalate in the portion of Tablets taken based on the labeled amount, and r_U and r_S are the salicylic acid peak responses obtained from the *Test preparation* and the *Standard preparation*, respectively: not more than 3.0% is found.

Assay—

Mobile phase, Diluent, Salsalate standard preparation, Resolution solution, and *Chromatographic system*—Proceed as directed in the *Assay* under *Salsalate*.

Assay preparation—Weigh and finely powder not less than 20 Tablets. Transfer an accurately weighed portion of the powder, equivalent to about 100 mg of salsalate, to a 100-mL volumetric flask, dilute with *Diluent* to volume, and mix. Sonicate for about 10 minutes, and mix. Filter a portion of this solution through a suitable filter of 0.5 μm or finer porosity. Use the clear filtrate as the *Assay stock solution*. Transfer 2.0 mL of the *Assay stock solution* to a 100-mL volumetric flask, dilute with *Diluent* to volume, and mix (*Assay preparation*).

Procedure—Proceed as directed for *Procedure* in the *Assay* under *Salsalate*. Calculate the quantity, in mg, of $C_{14}H_{10}O_5$ in the portion of Tablets taken by the formula:

$$5000C(r_U / r_S)$$

in which C is the concentration, in mg per mL, of USP Salsalate RS in the *Salsalate standard preparation*, and r_U and r_S are the responses of the salsalate peaks obtained from the *Assay preparation* and the *Salsalate standard preparation*, respectively.

Samarium Sm 153 Lexidronam Injection

» Samarium Sm 153 Lexidronam Injection is a sterile aqueous solution suitable for intravenous injection that contains ^{153}Sm in the form of a complex with ethylenediaminetetramethylenephosphonic acid (EDTMP). It contains not less than 90.0 percent and not more than 110.0 percent of the labeled amount of ^{153}Sm expressed in megabecquerels per mL (or in millicuries per mL) at the date and time indicated in the labeling. Not less than 99 percent of the Sm-153 is complexed by EDTMP. It contains no antimicrobial agents.

Packaging and storage—Preserve in adequately shielded single-dose containers in a freezer.

Labeling—Label it to include the following, in addition to the information specified for *Labeling* under *Injections* ⟨1⟩: the time and date of calibration; the amount of ^{153}Sm complexed with EDTMP expressed as total megabecquerels (or millicuries) and the concentration as megabecquerels per mL (or millicuries per mL) at the time of calibration; the expiration date and time; and the statement "Caution—Radioactive Material." The labeling indicates that in making dosage calculations, correction is to be made for radioactive decay, and also indicates that the radioactive half-life of ^{153}Sm is 46.3 hours. The labeling indicates that it should not be diluted or mixed with other solutions, that it is to be thawed at room temperature before administration, and that it is to be used within 8 hours of thawing.

Samarium / Official Monographs

USP Reference standards ⟨11⟩—*USP Endotoxin RS.*
Radionuclide identification ⟨821⟩—Samarium-153 decays by beta emission to stable Europium 153 as follows: 640 keV (30%), 710 keV (50%), and 810 keV (20%). The average emission energy is 233 keV. Its gamma-ray spectrum is identical to that of a specimen of known purity of ^{153}Sm that exhibits major photopeaks having energies of 70 keV and 103 keV.
Bacterial endotoxins ⟨85⟩—The limit of endotoxin content is not more than 175/*V* USP Endotoxin Unit per mL of Injection, in which *V* is the maximum recommended total dose, in mL, at the expiration time.
pH ⟨791⟩: between 7.0 and 8.5.
Radionuclidic purity ⟨821⟩—Using a gamma ray spectrophotometer, determine the radionuclidic purity of the Injection: not less than 99.8% of the total radioactivity is present as Sm 153 at the time of expiry. The Europium 154 radioactivity is not more than 3.44 kBq per 37 MBq of Samarium 153 (or 0.0093% of total Samarium 153 at expiry). The sum of all other radionuclidic impurities is less than or equal to 0.1907% of the total Sm 153 at expiry.
Radiochemical purity ⟨821⟩—
   Mobile phase—Transfer 8.0 g of sodium chloride, 0.2 g of monobasic potassium phosphate, 1.15 g of dibasic sodium phosphate, and 0.2 g of potassium chloride to a 1-liter volumetric flask, dilute with distilled water to volume, and mix. Make adjustments if necessary (see *System Suitability* under *Chromatography* ⟨621⟩).
   Chromatographic system (see *Chromatography* ⟨621⟩)—A 10-mm × 40-mm glass chromatographic column is packed using gravity flow with a strong cation-exchange resin* (prepared by mixing 5 g of resin with 25 mL of water in a suitable beaker) to a final resin volume of 0.5 mL.
   Procedure—Transfer the packed column to an ion-chamber dose counter to determine the background count for Sm 153. Apply about 10 μL of the Injection onto the column and place it in the ion-chamber counter, and record the total radioactivity. Elute the complexed radioactivity using about 20 mL of *Mobile phase*, and record the radioactivity retained on the column. Subtract the background radioactivity from all measured radioactivity values. Calculate the percentage of complexed radioactivity in the portion of Injection taken by the formula:

$$100(T - S/0.95)/T$$

in which *T* is the total amount of radioactivity; *S* is the quantity of free Sm-153 retained on the column; and 0.95 is the correction factor (5% of the uncomplexed Sm 153 passes through the column and into the Injection): not less than 99% of the Sm-153 is complexed by EDTMP.
Other requirements—It meets the requirements under *Injections* ⟨1⟩, except that it is not subject to the recommendation on *Volume in Container.*
Assay for radioactivity ⟨821⟩—Using a suitable counting assembly (see *Gamma-Emitting Radionuclides* under the *Assay*), determine the radioactivity in MBq (or mCi) per mL of Injection by use of a calibrated system: the activity is within ±10% of the labeled amount at the time of calibration.

---
*Sephadex-CM C-25 brand of ion exchange resin is available from Aldrich Chemical (No. 27, 124-1).

Saquinavir Mesylate

$C_{38}H_{50}N_6O_5 \cdot CH_4O_3S$ 766.96
Butanediamide, N^1-[3-[3-[[(1,1-dimethylethyl)amino]carbonyl]octahydro-2(1*H*)-isoquinolinyl]-2-hydroxy-1-(phenylmethyl)propyl]-2-[(2-quinolinylcarbonyl)amino]-, [3*S*-[2[1*R**(*R**),2*S**],3α,4aβ,8aβ]]-, monomethanesulfonate (salt).
(*S*)-*N*-[(α*S*)-α-[(1*R*)-2-[(3*S*,4a*S*,8a*S*)-3-(*tert*-Butylcarbamoyl)octahydro-2(1*H*)-isoquinolyl]-1-hydroxyethyl]phenethyl]-2-quinaldamidosuccinamide monomethanesulfonate (salt)   [*149845-06-7*].

» Saquinavir Mesylate contains not less than 98.5 percent and not more than 101.0 percent of $C_{38}H_{50}N_6O_5 \cdot CH_4O_3S$, calculated on the anhydrous basis.

Packaging and storage—Preserve in tight containers, and store at controlled room temperature.
USP Reference standards ⟨11⟩—*USP Saquinavir Mesylate RS. USP Saquinavir Related Compound A RS.*
Identification—
   A: *Infrared Absorption* ⟨197K⟩.
   B: *Ultraviolet Absorption* ⟨197U⟩—
   Solution: 12 μg per mL.
   Medium: methanol.
   The absorptivity of the sample preparation at 238 ± 2 nm, calculated on the anhydrous basis, is between 61.0 and 63.4.
   C: The retention time of the major peak in the chromatogram of the *Assay preparation* corresponds to that in the chromatogram of the *Standard preparation*, as obtained in the *Assay*.
Specific rotation ⟨781S⟩: between −66.8° and −69.6° (λ = 436 nm at 20°).
   Test solution: 5 mg per mL, in methanol.
Water, *Method I* ⟨921⟩: not more than 1.0%.
Residue on ignition ⟨281⟩: not more than 0.1%.
Heavy metals, *Method II* ⟨231⟩—Dissolve 2.5 g in 50 mL of a mixture of alcohol and water (7 : 1): the limit is 0.001%.
Chromatographic purity—
   Triethylamine phosphate solution, Mobile phase, System suitability solution, and *Chromatographic system*—Proceed as directed in the *Assay*.
   Standard solution—Use the *Standard preparation*, prepared as directed in the *Assay*.
   Test solution—Use the *Assay preparation*.
   Procedure—Separately inject equal volumes (about 20 μL) of the *Standard solution* and the *Test solution* into the chromatograph, record the chromatograms, and measure the peak responses. Calculate the percentage of each impurity in the portion of Saquinavir Mesylate taken by the formula:

$$100F(C_S/C_U)(r_i/r_S)$$

in which *F* is a response factor and is equal to 2 for peaks, if present, at a retention time of 0.32 relative to saquinavir, to 0.5 for peaks, if present, at retention times of about 0.38 and 0.53 relative to saquinavir, and to 1 for all other peaks; C_S is the concentration, in mg per mL, of USP Saquinavir Mesylate RS in the Standard solution; C_U is the concentration, in mg per mL, of Saquinavir Mesylate in the *Test solution*; r_i is the peak response for each impurity obtained from the *Test solution;* and r_S is the peak response for saquinavir obtained from the *Standard solution:* not more than 0.1% of any individual impurity is found; and not more than 0.5% of total impurities is found.

Assay—

Triethylamine phosphate solution—Transfer 10 mL of triethylamine to a 1-liter volumetric flask, dilute with water to volume, and mix. Adjust with phosphoric acid to a pH of 2.5, and filter.

Mobile phase—Prepare a filtered and degassed mixture of *Triethylamine phosphate solution*, tetrahydrofuran, and acetonitrile (14 : 5 : 1). [NOTE—Protect from light.] Make adjustments if necessary (see *System Suitability* under *Chromatography* ⟨621⟩).

System suitability solution—Dissolve suitable quantities of USP Saquinavir Related Compound A RS and USP Saquinavir Mesylate RS in *Mobile phase* to obtain a solution containing about 2 µg per mL and 0.25 mg per mL, respectively.

Standard preparation—Dissolve an accurately weighed quantity of USP Saquinavir Mesylate RS in *Mobile phase*, and dilute quantitatively, and stepwise if necessary, with *Mobile phase* to obtain a solution having a known concentration of about 0.25 mg per mL.

Assay preparation—Transfer about 12.5 mg of Saquinavir Mesylate, accurately weighed, to a 50-mL volumetric flask, dissolve in and dilute with *Mobile phase* to volume, and mix for about 20 minutes.

Chromatographic system (see *Chromatography* ⟨621⟩)—The liquid chromatograph is equipped with a 210-nm detector and a 4.6-mm × 25-cm column that contains packing L1. The column temperature is maintained at 20°, and the flow rate is about 1 mL per minute. Chromatograph the *System suitability solution,* and record the peak responses as directed for *Procedure:* the relative retention times are about 0.89 for saquinavir related compound A and 1.0 for saquinavir; and the resolution, *R,* between saquinavir related compound A and saquinavir is not less than 1.5. Chromatograph the *Standard preparation,* and record the peak responses as directed for *Procedure:* the column efficiency is not less than 500 theoretical plates; and the relative standard deviation for replicate injections is not more than 2.0%.

Procedure—Separately inject equal volumes (about 20 µL) of the *Standard preparation* and the *Assay preparation* into the chromatograph, record the chromatograms, and measure the responses for the major peaks. Calculate the quantity, in mg, of $C_{38}H_{50}N_6O_5 \cdot CH_4O_3S$ in the portion of Saquinavir Mesylate taken by the formula:

$$50C(r_U/r_S)$$

in which *C* is the concentration, in mg per mL, of USP Saquinavir Mesylate RS in the *Standard preparation;* and r_U and r_S are the peak responses obtained from the *Assay preparation* and the *Standard preparation,* respectively.

Saquinavir Capsules

» Saquinavir Capsules contain not less than 95.0 percent and not more than 105.0 percent of saquinavir ($C_{38}H_{50}N_6O_5$).

Packaging and storage—Preserve in tight containers, and store at controlled room temperature.

USP Reference standards ⟨11⟩—*USP Saquinavir Mesylate RS. USP Saquinavir Related Compound A RS.*

Identification—
A: *Infrared Absorption* ⟨197K⟩.
B: The retention time of the major peak in the chromatogram of the *Assay preparation* corresponds to that in the chromatogram of the *Standard preparation,* as obtained in the *Assay.*

Dissolution ⟨711⟩—
Citrate buffer—Transfer 5.82 g of anhydrous dibasic sodium phosphate and 16.7 g of citric acid monohydrate to a 1-L volumetric flask. Dissolve in and dilute with water to volume.
Medium: Citrate buffer; 900 mL.
Apparatus 2: 50 rpm.
Time: 45 minutes.
Procedure—Determine the amount of $C_{38}H_{50}N_6O_5$ dissolved by employing UV absorption at the wavelength of maximum absorbance at about 240 nm on filtered portions of the solution under test, suitably diluted with *Medium,* in comparison with a Standard solution having a known concentration of USP Saquinavir Mesylate RS in the same *Medium.*

Tolerances—Not less than 75% *(Q)* of the labeled amount of $C_{38}H_{50}N_6O_5$ is dissolved in 45 minutes.

Uniformity of dosage units ⟨905⟩: meet the requirements.

Water, *Method I* ⟨921⟩: not more than 3.0%.

Chromatographic purity—
Triethylamine phosphate solution, Mobile phase, System suitability solution, and *Chromatographic system*—Proceed as directed in the *Assay* under *Saquinavir Mesylate.*

Standard solution—Use the *Standard preparation,* prepared as directed in the *Assay* under *Saquinavir Mesylate.*

Test solution—Use the *Assay preparation.*

Procedure—Separately inject equal volumes (about 20 µL) of the *Test solution* and the *Standard solution* into the chromatograph, record the chromatograms, and measure the peak responses. Calculate the percentage of each impurity in the portion of Capsules taken by the formula:

$$10{,}000F(670.86/766.96)(C/W)(r_i/r_S)$$

in which *F* is a response factor, and is equal to 2 for a peak, if present, at a retention time of 0.32 relative to saquinavir, to 0.5 for peaks, if present, at relative retention times of about 0.38 and 0.53, and to 1 for all other peaks; 670.86 and 766.96 are the molecular weights of saquinavir and saquinavir mesylate, respectively; *C* is the concentration, in mg per mL, of USP Saquinavir Mesylate RS in the *Standard solution; W* is the weight, in mg, of Capsule contents taken for the *Test solution;* r_i is the peak response for each impurity obtained from the *Test solution;* and r_S is the peak response for saquinavir obtained from the *Standard solution:* not more than 0.2% of any individual impurity is found, and not more than 1.0% of total impurities is found.

Assay—
Triethylamine phosphate solution, Mobile phase, System suitability solution, Standard preparation, and *Chromatographic system*—Proceed as directed in the *Assay* under *Saquinavir Mesylate.*

Assay preparation—Empty and combine the contents of not fewer than 10 Capsules. Transfer an amount of Capsule contents, equivalent to about 22 mg of Saquinavir, accurately weighed, to a 100-mL volumetric flask, dissolve in and dilute with *Mobile phase* to volume, and mix.

Procedure—Separately inject equal volumes (about 20 µL) of the *Standard preparation* and the *Assay preparation* into the chromatograph, record the chromatograms, and measure the responses for the major peaks. Calculate the quantity, in mg, of saquinavir ($C_{38}H_{50}N_6O_5$) in the portion of Capsules taken by the formula:

$$(670.86/766.96)(100C)(r_U/r_S)$$

in which 670.86 and 766.96 are the molecular weights of saquinavir and saquinavir mesylate, respectively; *C* is the concentration, in mg per mL, of USP Saquinavir Mesylate RS in the *Standard preparation;* and r_U and r_S are the peaks obtained from the *Assay preparation* and the *Standard preparation,* respectively.

Sargramostim

```
APARSPSPST  QPWEHVNAIQ  EARRLLNLSR  DTAAEMNETV  EVISEMFDLG
EPTCLQTRLE  LYKQGLRGSL  TKLKGPLTMM  ASHYKQHCPP  TPETSCATQI
ITFESFKENL  KDFLLVIPFD  CWEPVQE
```

$C_{639}H_{1002}N_{168}O_{196}S_8$ 14,414   [*123774-72-1*].

» Sargramostim is a single chain, glycosylated polypeptide of 127 amino acid residues expressed from *Saccharomyces cerevisiae.* The glycoprotein primarily consists of three molecular species having relative molecular weights of approximately 19,500, 16,800, and 15,500 due to different levels of glycosylation. Sargramostim has the property of generating granulocyte, macrophage, and mixed granulocyte macrophage colonies from hematopoietic progenitor cells found in bone marrow. It possesses the primary sequence of the natural form of granulocyte-macrophage colony-stimulating factor with a substitution in the amino acid residue at position 23 (Leu_{23} in place of Arg_{23}). It has a biological potency of not less than 73.0 percent and not more than 146.0 percent of the potency stated on the label, the potency being 5.6 million USP Sargramostim Units per mg of protein. The presence of host cell DNA and host cell protein impurities in Sargramostim is process-specific; the limits of these impurities are determined by validated methods.

Packaging and storage—Preserve in sealed containers, and store at a temperature of −20° or below.

USP Reference standards ⟨11⟩—*USP Endotoxin RS. USP Sargramostim RS.*

Identification—The retention times of the peaks from the *Test solution* do not differ by more than 0.5 minutes from those of the *Standard solution*, as obtained in the test for *Chromatographic purity.*

Peptide mapping—

Mobile phase—Prepare separate filtered and degassed solutions consisting of a solution (1 in 1000) of trifluoroacetic acid in water *(Solution A)* and a 1 in 1000 solution of trifluoroacetic acid in acetonitrile*(Solution B).* Make adjustments if necessary (see *System Suitability* under *Chromatography* ⟨621⟩).

Digestion solution—Dissolve 29.4 mg of calcium chloride and 1.8 mg of β-alanine in 2 mL of water. Adjust with hydrochloric acid to a pH of 4.0. Add 0.4 mg of trypsin, and mix.

Standard solution—Dissolve an accurately weighed quantity of USP Sargramostim RS in water, and dilute quantitatively with water to obtain a solution having a known concentration of about 500 µg per mL. Transfer 100 µL of this solution to a clean test tube, and add 11 µL of pH 7.6 buffer solution (see *Buffer Solutions* in the section *Reagents, Indicators, and Solutions*) containing 0.1 M tris-(hydroxymethyl)aminomethane. Add 25 µL of *Digestion solution*, and incubate at 37° for 2 hours. Quench the reaction by adding 3 µL of 20% trifluoroacetic acid.

Test solution—Using an accurately weighed quantity of Sargramostim, proceed as directed for *Standard solution.*

Chromatographic system (see *Chromatography* ⟨621⟩)—The liquid chromatograph is equipped with a 220-nm detector and a 25-cm × 4.6-mm column that contains 10-µm packing L1. The column is maintained at ambient temperature, and the flow rate is about 1 mL per minute. The system is programmed to provide variable mixtures of *Mobile phase*. Equilibrate the system with a *Mobile phase* consisting of 100% *Solution A*. After injection of the solution under test, the composition is changed linearly at a rate of 1% per minute over the next 35 minutes so that it then consists of 65% *Solution A* and 35% *Solution B*, and then changed linearly at a rate of 2% per minute over the next 15 minutes to a mixture of 35% *Solution A* and 65% *Solution B*.

Procedure—Separately inject equal volumes (about 100 µL) of the *Standard solution* and the *Test solution* into the chromatograph, record the chromatograms, and measure the responses for the eight major peaks as defined in the USP Sargramostim RS Data Sheet. The retention times of the peak responses from the *Test solution* correspond to those from the *Standard solution* if the retention times of corresponding peaks do not differ by more than 0.3 minutes, the peak areas ratios for peaks 4, 8, and 10 are between 0.7 and 1.3, and no additional significant peaks or shoulders are found.

Bacterial endotoxins ⟨85⟩—It contains not more than 5 USP Endotoxin Units per mg.

Microbial limits ⟨61⟩—The total aerobic microbial count does not exceed 1 cfu per mL.

Chromatographic purity—

Mobile phase—Prepare separate filtered and degassed solutions consisting of a solution (1 in 1000) of trifluoroacetic acid in water *(Solution A),* a 1 in 1000 solution of trifluoroacetic acid in acetonitrile *(Solution B),* and a solution prepared by dissolving 116.9 g of sodium chloride in 2000 mL of water and adding 2 mL of trifluoroacetic acid *(Solution C).* Make adjustments if necessary (see *System Suitability* under *Chromatography* ⟨621⟩).

Standard solution—Dissolve an accurately weighed quantity of USP Sargramostim RS in water, and dilute quantitatively with water to obtain a solution having a known concentration of about 1.0 mg per mL.

Test solution—Using an accurately weighed quantity of Sargramostim, prepare as directed for *Standard solution.*

Chromatographic system (see *Chromatography* ⟨621⟩)—The liquid chromatograph is equipped with a 220-nm detector and a 4.6-mm × 25-cm column that contains packing L1. The flow rate is about 1 mL per minute. The system is programmed to provide a *Mobile phase* consisting of a mixture containing variable proportions of *Solution A* and *Solution B*, with a constant 20% of *Solution C*. Equilibrate the system with a mixture of 55% *Solution A*, 25% *Solution B*, and 20% *Solution C*. After injection of the *Test solution*, the proportion of *Solution A* is decreased linearly from 55% to 15% and the proportion of *Solution B* is increased linearly from 25% to 65% at a rate of 1% per minute.

Procedure—Separately inject equal volumes (about 50 µL) of the *Standard solution* and the *Test solution* into the chromatograph, record the chromatograms, and measure the responses for the major peaks. The major peaks are from hyperglycosylated sargramostim and from the three glycosylated forms of Sargramostim, as indicated in the USP Sargramostim RS Data Sheet. The peak responses from the *Test solution* correspond to those from the *Standard solution*, and no peaks or shoulders are present in the chromatogram of the *Test solution* that are not present in the chromatogram of the *Standard solution*. Calculate the percentage of hyperglycosylated sargramostim in the *Test solution* by the formula:

$$100(r_U / r_s)$$

in which r_U is the peak response for hyperglycosylated sargramostim, and r_s is the sum of the responses of all of the sargramostim peaks: not more than 5.6% is found. Calculate the percentage of each of the three glycosylated forms of Sargramostim in the *Test solution* by the formula:

$$100(r_i / r_s)$$

in which r_i is the peak response for each individual glycosylated form of Sargramostim, and r_s is the sum of the peak responses of all three glycosylated forms of Sargramostim. The percentages of each of the three glycosylated forms of Sargramostim, in order of elution, are between 25% and 42%, between 14% and 32%, and between 35% and 53%.

Protein content—

Standard solutions—Dissolve accurately weighed quantities of USP Sargramostim RS in water to obtain solutions having known concentrations of about 100, 200, 400, 600, 800, and 1000 µg per mL.

Test solution—Dissolve an accurately weighed quantity of Sargramostim in water to obtain a solution having a concentration of between 250 and 500 µg per mL.

BCA reagent—Dissolve 10 g of bicinchoninic acid, 20 g of sodium carbonate monohydrate, 1.6 g of sodium tartrate, 4 g of sodium hydroxide, and 9.5 g of sodium bicarbonate in water. Adjust, if necessary, with sodium hydroxide or sodium bicarbonate to a pH of 11.25. Dilute with water to 1 L, and mix.

Copper sulfate reagent—Dissolve 2 g of cupric sulfate in water, and dilute with water to 50 mL.

Copper-BCA reagent—Mix 1 mL of *Copper sulfate reagent* and 50 mL of *BCA reagent*. [NOTE—If a commercially available kit is used, follow the manufacturer's instructions for preparation of the *Copper-BCA reagent.*]

Procedure—Mix 0.1 mL of each *Standard solution*, the *Test solution*, and 0.1 mL of water to provide the blank with 2 mL of the *Copper-BCA reagent*. Incubate the solutions at 37° for 30 minutes, and allow to stand for 5 minutes at room temperature. Within 60 minutes following incubation, determine the absorbances of the *Standard solutions* and the *Test solution* in 1-cm cells at 562 nm, with a suitable spectrophotometer (see *Spectrophotometry and Light-scattering* ⟨851⟩), using the blank to set the instrument to zero. Plot the absorbances of the *Standard solutions* versus the concentrations, in µg per mL, of USP Sargramostim RS, and draw the straight line best fitting the plotted points. From the graph so obtained, determine the concentration, in µg per mL, of protein in the *Test solution*.

Assay—

Iscove's Modified Dulbecco's Medium—Prepare a mixture of the ingredients in the quantities shown in sufficient water to obtain 1 L of medium, and sterilize by filtration.

Calcium Chloride	165.00 mg
Potassium Chloride	330.00 mg
Potassium Nitrate	0.076 mg
Magnesium Sulfate	97.67 mg
Sodium Chloride	4505.00 mg
Sodium Bicarbonate	3024.00 mg
Monobasic Sodium Phosphate	125.00 mg
Sodium Selenite	0.0173 mg
Glucose	4500.00 mg
HEPES (4-[2-Hydroxyethyl]-1-piperazineethanesulfonic acid)	5958.00 mg
Phenol Red	15.00 mg
Sodium Pyruvate	110.00 mg
L-Alanine	25.00 mg
L-Arginine Hydrochloride	84.00 mg
L-Asparagine	28.40 mg
L-Aspartic Acid	30.00 mg
L-Cystine Dihydrochloride	91.24 mg
L-Glutamic Acid	75.00 mg
L-Glutamine	584.00 mg
Glycine	30.00 mg
L-Histidine Hydrochloride	42.00 mg
L-Isoleucine	105.00 mg
L-Leucine	105.00 mg
L-Lysine Hydrochloride	146.00 mg
L-Methionine	30.00 mg
L-Phenylalanine	66.00 mg
L-Proline	40.00 mg
L-Serine	42.00 mg
L-Threonine	95.00 mg
L-Tryptophan	16.00 mg
L-Tyrosine Disodium	103.79 mg
L-Valine	94.00 mg
Biotin	0.013 mg
Calcium Pantothenate	4.00 mg
Choline Chloride	4.00 mg
Cyanocobalamin	0.013 mg
Folic Acid	4.00 mg
Inositol	7.20 mg
Niacinamide	4.00 mg
Pyridoxal Hydrochloride	4.00 mg
Riboflavin	0.40 mg
Thiamine	4.00 mg

Medium A—Prepare a mixture of *Iscove's Modified Dulbecco's Medium* with 10% heat-inactivated fetal bovine serum as follows:

Iscove's Modified Dulbecco's Medium	500 mL
Fetal Bovine Serum (inactivated at 56° for 30 minutes)	50 mL
Penicillin, Streptomycin, and L-Glutamine mixture containing, in each mL, 5000 Units of penicillin G potassium, 5000 µg of streptomycin sulfate, and 29.2 mg of L-glutamine	5 mL
Gentamicin (50 mg per mL)	0.5 mL
2-Mercaptoethanol	0.5 mL

Prepare aseptically, sterilize by filtration, and store at 2° to 8°. Use within one month.

Medium B—Dissolve an accurately weighed quantity of USP Sargramostim RS in *Medium A*, and dilute quantitatively with *Medium A* to obtain a solution having a known concentration of about 1 µg per mL. Prepare aseptically, sterilize by filtration, and store at 2° to 8°. Use within one month.

Standard preparation—Dissolve an accurately weighed quantity of USP Sargramostim RS in *Medium A*, and dilute quantitatively with *Medium A* to obtain a solution having a known concentration of about 100 ng per mL. Dispense aseptically in equal portions, accurately measured, and store at −60° or below. Use within 24 months. Store thawed portions at a temperature between 2° and 8°, and use within one month. At the time of use, dilute with *Medium A* to obtain a solution having a known concentration of about 2 ng per mL.

Assay preparation—Dissolve an accurately weighed quantity of Sargramostim in *Medium A*, and dilute quantitatively with *Medium A* to obtain a solution containing about 2 ng per mL.

Cell culture preparation—Prepare cell cultures of [TF-1 cells (ATCC CRL-2003)]. Passage the cultures every 3 to 4 days, using a 1 : 10 subculture of the cells for up to 3 months. After 3 months, initiate a new culture. Use *Medium A* containing 0.5% *Medium B* for passage propagation and storage in the frozen state.

Cell suspension—Wash the cells three times in *Medium A*, and adjust the cell concentration to 5×10^4 cells per mL in *Medium A*.

Tritiated thymidine solution—Use a tritiated thymidine stock solution having a concentration of 20 Ci per mmol. Add 1.0 mL of the tritiated thymidine stock solution to 49 mL of *Medium A*, and store at 2° to 8°. Use within 2 weeks.

Procedure—Use a 96-well, flat-bottom microtitration plate with wells arranged in 8 rows (labeled A through H) with 12 wells (numbered 1 to 12) in each row. Place 50 µL of *Medium A* in wells 2 to 12. Place 100 µL of the *Standard preparation*, or each *Assay preparation* or *Medium A* (negative control) in well 1. Make serial dilutions by transferring 50 µL from well 1 to well 2, and so on through well 12 (serial twofold dilutions). Place 50 µL of the *Cell suspension* in each well, and incubate the microtitration plate for 72 hours at 37° in a 10% carbon dioxide incubator. Following incubation, add 25 µL of *Tritiated thymidine solution* to each well, and return the plate to the same incubator for an additional 4 to 5 hours. Before harvesting the cells on a filter mat, prewet the mat filter, using distilled water. [NOTE—The prewetting minimizes background radiation noise.] Using a multiple automated sample harvesting system, place the incubated plate under the harvesting system. Fill the wells to the top with deionized water. Aspirate the water, and pass it through the collecting filter mat. Repeat the procedure at least 5 times, or until all the cells have been fully harvested. When all wells have been fully harvested, pour 5 to 10 mL of alcohol on the plate tray, and aspirate the methanol. Repeat the procedure if further drying of the filter mat is desired. [NOTE—The alcohol helps to dry out the filter mat by carrying away the wash fluid.] Remove the filter mat, and repeat the procedure until all plates under test have been harvested.

Dry the filter mat in a drying oven for about 30 minutes. Place the completely dry filter mats in a beta counter, and determine the amount of radioactivity in each cell well.

Convert the amount of incorporated radioactivity in each well to a percentage of the maximum incorporated radioactivity. If fewer than 5 values are between 3% and 97% of the maximum revision, repeat the *Assay*. Using the least squares method of regression analysis, plot the slope of each test specimen versus the slope of the standard, excluding any values exceeding the maximum of each dilution set. Calculate the Sargramostim Units in each mL of the *Assay preparation* in terms of the dilution that gives half-maximal activity. To convert this value to units of protein per mg, divide the Sargramostim Units per mL by the weight, in mg per mL, of protein in the initial undiluted solution.

Sargramostim for Injection

» Sargramostim for Injection is a sterile, lyophilized preparation of Sargramostim. Its biological activity is not less than 73.0 percent and not more than 146.0 percent of that stated on the label in USP Sargramostim Units. It contains not less than 90.0 percent and not more than 110.0 percent of the total protein content stated on the label.

Packaging and storage—Preserve in hermetic containers at a temperature between 2° and 8°.
Labeling—Label it to state the biological activity in USP Sargramostim Units per vial and the amount of protein per vial.
USP Reference standards ⟨11⟩—*USP Sargramostim RS. USP Endotoxin RS.*
Constituted solution—At the time of use, it meets the requirements for *Constituted solutions* under *Injections* ⟨1⟩.
Identification—It responds to the tests for *Identification* and *Peptide mapping* under *Sargramostim*.
Bacterial endotoxins ⟨85⟩—It contains not more than 50 USP Endotoxin Units per mg.
Safety—It meets the requirements for biologics as set forth for *Safety Tests—General* under *Biological Reactivity Tests, In Vivo* ⟨88⟩.
Sterility ⟨71⟩—It meets the requirements when tested as directed for *Membrane Filtration* under *Test for Sterility of the Product to be Examined*.
Uniformity of dosage units ⟨905⟩: meets the requirements for *Content Uniformity*.
pH ⟨791⟩: between 7.1 and 7.7, in the solution constituted as directed in the labeling.
Water, *Method I* ⟨921⟩: not more than 2.0%.
Chromatographic purity—When constituted with water, it meets the requirements for *Chromatographic purity* under *Sargramostim*.
Assay—When constituted with water, Sargramostim for Injection meets the requirements of the *Assay* under *Sargramostim*.

Scopolamine Hydrobromide

$C_{17}H_{21}NO_4 \cdot HBr \cdot 3H_2O$ 438.31
Benzeneacetic acid, α-(hydroxymethyl)-, 9-methyl-3-oxa-9-azatricyclo[3.3.1.0.^{2,4}]non-[7-yl ester, hydrobromide, trihydrate, [7(S)-(1α,2β,4β,5α,7β)]-.
6β,7β-Epoxy-1αH,5αH-tropan-3α-ol (−)-tropate (ester) hydrobromide trihydrate [6533-68-2].
Anhydrous 384.27 [114-49-8].

» Scopolamine Hydrobromide contains not less than 98.5 percent and not more than 102.0 percent of $C_{17}H_{21}NO_4 \cdot HBr$, calculated on the anhydrous basis.

Caution—Handle Scopolamine Hydrobromide with exceptional care, since it is highly potent.

Packaging and storage—Preserve in tight, light-resistant containers.
USP Reference standards ⟨11⟩—*USP Scopolamine Hydrobromide RS.*
Identification—
  A: *Infrared Absorption* ⟨197K⟩—
  Test specimen—Dissolve 3 mg in 1 mL of alcohol, and evaporate the solution on a steam bath to dryness. Dissolve the residue in 0.5 mL of chloroform, add 200 mg of potassium bromide, previously dried at 105° for 30 minutes, and stir frequently for 5 minutes. Allow the chloroform to evaporate to dryness, and stir frequently to obtain a flowing powder residue. Dry the residue on a steam bath for 5 minutes, then immediately compress the residue to a disk.
  B: To 1 mL of a solution (1 in 20) add a few drops of chlorine TS, and shake the mixture with 1 mL of chloroform: the latter assumes a brownish color.
Specific rotation ⟨781S⟩: between −24° and −26°.
  Test solution: an amount equivalent to 50 mg of anhydrous Scopolamine Hydrobromide per mL, in water.
pH ⟨791⟩: between 4.0 and 5.5, in a solution (1 in 20).
Water, *Method III* ⟨921⟩—Dry it in two stages (see *Loss on drying* ⟨731⟩); first at 80° for 2 hours, and then at 105° for an additional 3 hours: it loses not more than 13.0% of its weight.
Residue on ignition ⟨281⟩: negligible, from 100 mg.
Limit of apoatropine—To 15 mL of a solution (1 in 100) add 0.05 mL of 0.1 N potassium permanganate VS: the solution is not completely decolorized within 5 minutes.
Other foreign alkaloids—To 1 mL of a solution (1 in 20) add a few drops of 6 N ammonium hydroxide: no turbidity is produced. Add 1 N potassium hydroxide to another 1-mL portion of the solution: only a transient whitish turbidity is produced.
Organic volatile impurities, *Method I* ⟨467⟩: meets the requirements.
            (Official until July 1, 2008)
Assay—Dissolve about 750 mg of Scopolamine Hydrobromide, accurately weighed, in a mixture of 30 mL of glacial acetic acid and 10 mL of mercuric acetate TS, warming slightly to effect solution. Cool the solution to room temperature, add 2 drops of crystal violet TS, and titrate with 0.1 N perchloric acid VS. Perform a blank determination, and make any necessary correction. Each mL of 0.1 N perchloric acid is equivalent to 38.43 mg of $C_{17}H_{21}NO_4 \cdot HBr$.

Scopolamine Hydrobromide Injection

» Scopolamine Hydrobromide Injection is a sterile solution of Scopolamine Hydrobromide in Water for Injection. It contains not less than 90.0 percent and not more than 110.0 percent of the labeled amount of $C_{17}H_{21}NO_4 \cdot HBr \cdot 3H_2O$.

Packaging and storage—Preserve in light-resistant, single-dose or multiple-dose containers, preferably of Type I glass.
USP Reference standards ⟨11⟩—*USP Scopolamine Hydrobromide RS. USP Endotoxin RS.*
Identification—
  A: Transfer a volume of Injection, equivalent to about 3 mg of scopolamine hydrobromide, to a 50-mL separator, dilute with water, if necessary, to 10 mL, add 0.2 mL of ammonium hydroxide, and extract with 25 mL of chloroform. Add 50 mL of ether to the chloroform solution, and pass the mixture through a 25- × 250-mm chromatographic tube fitted with a pledget of glass wool at the base and packed with 2 g of purified siliceous earth that previously has been mixed with 1 mL of 0.2 N phosphoric acid saturated with sodium bromide. Discard the eluate, and pass 25 mL of water-saturated ether through the column and discard. Elute with 100 mL of water-saturated chloroform, collect the eluate in a suitable receiver, and evaporate just to dryness. Dissolve the residue in 1 mL of alcohol, and proceed as directed in *Identification* test A under *Scopolamine Hydrobromide*, beginning with "and evaporate the solution on a steam bath to dryness."
  B: Add to the Injection silver nitrate TS: a yellowish white precipitate, insoluble in nitric acid but slightly soluble in 6 N ammonium hydroxide, is formed.
Bacterial endotoxins ⟨85⟩—It contains not more than 555.0 USP Endotoxin Units per mg of scopolamine hydrobromide.
pH ⟨791⟩: between 3.5 and 6.5.
Other requirements—It meets the requirements under *Injections* ⟨1⟩.

Assay—

pH 9.0 Buffer—Dissolve 34.8 g of dibasic potassium phosphate in 900 mL of water, and adjust with 3 N hydrochloric acid or 1 N sodium hydroxide, as necessary, to a pH of 9.0, determined electrometrically, and mix.

Internal standard solution—Transfer about 25 mg of homatropine hydrobromide to a 50-mL volumetric flask, dissolve in and dilute with water to volume, and mix. Prepare fresh daily.

Standard stock solution—Transfer about 10 mg of USP Scopolamine Hydrobromide RS, accurately weighed, to a 100-mL volumetric flask, dissolve in and dilute with water to volume, and mix. Prepare fresh daily.

Standard preparation—Pipet 10 mL of the *Standard stock solution* into a separator, add 2.0 mL of *Internal standard solution* and 5.0 mL of *pH 9.0 Buffer*, and carefully adjust the solution with 1 N sodium hydroxide to a pH of 9.0, avoiding any excess. Immediately extract with two 10-mL portions of methylene chloride, filter the methylene chloride extracts through 1 g of anhydrous sodium sulfate supported by a small cotton plug in a funnel into a 50-mL beaker, and evaporate under nitrogen to approximately 2.0 mL.

Assay solution—Transfer an accurately measured volume of Injection, equivalent to about 10 mg of scopolamine hydrobromide, to a 100-mL volumetric flask. Dilute with water to volume, and mix.

Assay preparation—Pipet 10 mL of the *Assay solution* into a separator, and proceed as directed for *Standard preparation*, beginning with "add 2.0 mL of *Internal standard solution*."

Chromatographic system (see *Chromatography* ⟨621⟩)—The gas chromatograph contains a 2-mm × 1.8-m glass column packed with 3% liquid phase G3 on support S1AB. The carrier gas is nitrogen, flowing at a rate of 25 mL per minute. The column temperature is maintained at 225°. Chromatograph the *Standard preparation*, and record the peak responses as directed for *Procedure*: the resolution factor, R, between homatropine and scopolamine is not less than 5; the tailing factor is not more than 2.0; and the relative standard deviation for replicate injections is not more than 2.0%.

Procedure—Separately inject equal volumes (about 1 μL) of the *Standard preparation* and the *Assay preparation* into the chromatograph, record the chromatograms, and measure the peak areas. Calculate the ratio, A_U, of the area of the scopolamine hydrobromide peak to the area of the internal standard peak in the chromatogram from the *Assay preparation*, and similarly calculate the ratio, A_S, in the chromatogram from the *Standard preparation*. Calculate the quantity, in mg, of scopolamine hydrobromide ($C_{17}H_{21}NO_4 \cdot HBr \cdot 3H_2O$) in the volume of Injection taken by the formula

$$1.141W(A_U / A_S)$$

in which 1.141 is the ratio of the molecular weight of scopolamine hydrobromide trihydrate to that of anhydrous scopolamine hydrobromide; W is the weight, in mg, of USP Scopolamine Hydrobromide RS in the *Standard preparation*; and A_U and A_S are as calculated above.

Scopolamine Hydrobromide Ophthalmic Ointment

» Scopolamine Hydrobromide Ophthalmic Ointment is Scopolamine Hydrobromide in a suitable ophthalmic ointment base. It contains not less than 90.0 percent and not more than 110.0 percent of the labeled amount of ($C_{17}H_{21}NO_4$) · HBr · $3H_2O$. It is sterile.

Packaging and storage—Preserve in collapsible ophthalmic ointment tubes.

USP Reference standards ⟨11⟩—*USP Scopolamine Hydrobromide RS.*

Identification—

A: Transfer a portion of Ophthalmic Ointment, equivalent to about 50 mg of scopolamine hydrobromide, to a suitable separator, and dissolve in 25 mL of ether. Add 25 mL of 0.01 N hydrochloric acid, shake vigorously, allow the layers to separate, and discard the organic phase. Proceed as directed under *Identification—Organic Nitrogenous Bases* ⟨181⟩, beginning with "In a second separator dissolve 50 mg."

B: Transfer about 5 g of Ophthalmic Ointment to a separator, dissolve in 50 mL of ether, and extract with 20 mL of water: the extracted solution so obtained responds to the tests for *Bromide* ⟨191⟩.

Sterility ⟨71⟩: meets the requirements.

Metal particles—It meets the requirements of the test for *Metal Particles in Ophthalmic Ointments* ⟨751⟩.

Assay—Proceed with Ophthalmic Ointment as directed in the *Assay* under *Scopolamine Hydrobromide Injection*, but to prepare the *Assay solution*, weigh accurately a portion of Ophthalmic Ointment equivalent to about 10 mg of scopolamine hydrobromide into a separator containing 50 mL of ether, shake to dissolve, extract with three 25-mL portions of 0.2 N sulfuric acid, collect the acid extracts in a 100-mL volumetric flask, dilute with 0.2 N sulfuric acid to volume, and mix. Calculate the quantity, in mg, of $C_{17}H_{21}NO_4 \cdot HBr \cdot 3H_2O$ in the portion of Ophthalmic Ointment taken by the formula given therein.

Scopolamine Hydrobromide Ophthalmic Solution

» Scopolamine Hydrobromide Ophthalmic Solution is a sterile, buffered, aqueous solution of Scopolamine Hydrobromide. It contains not less than 90.0 percent and not more than 110.0 percent of the labeled amount of $C_{17}H_{21}NO_4 \cdot HBr \cdot 3H_2O$. It may contain suitable antimicrobial agents and stabilizers, and may contain suitable additives for the purpose of increasing its viscosity.

Packaging and storage—Preserve in tight containers.

USP Reference standards ⟨11⟩—*USP Scopolamine Hydrobromide RS.*

Identification—

A: A volume of Ophthalmic Solution, equivalent to about 3 mg of scopolamine hydrobromide, responds to *Identification* test *A* under *Scopolamine Hydrobromide Injection*.

B: Add to the Ophthalmic Solution silver nitrate TS: a yellowish white precipitate, insoluble in nitric acid but slightly soluble in 6 N ammonium hydroxide, is formed.

Sterility ⟨71⟩: meets the requirements.

pH ⟨791⟩: between 4.0 and 6.0.

Assay—Transfer an accurately measured volume of Ophthalmic Solution, equivalent to about 10 mg of scopolamine hydrobromide, to a 100-mL volumetric flask, dilute with water to volume, and mix. Using this as the *Assay solution*, proceed as directed in the *Assay* under *Scopolamine Hydrobromide Injection*. Calculate the quantity, in mg, of $C_{17}H_{21}NO_4 \cdot HBr \cdot 3H_2O$ in the volume of Ophthalmic Solution taken by the formula given therein.

Scopolamine Hydrobromide Tablets

» Scopolamine Hydrobromide Tablets contain not less than 90.0 percent and not more than 110.0 percent of the labeled amount of $C_{17}H_{21}NO_4 \cdot HBr \cdot 3H_2O$.

Packaging and storage—Preserve in tight, light-resistant containers.

USP Reference standards ⟨11⟩—*USP Scopolamine Hydrobromide RS.*

Identification—Place an amount of powdered Tablets, equivalent to about 3 mg of scopolamine hydrobromide, in a 50-mL separator,

add 10 mL of water, and shake for 2 minutes. Proceed as directed in *Identification* test A under *Scopolamine Hydrobromide Injection*, beginning with "add 0.2 mL of ammonium hydroxide."
Disintegration ⟨701⟩: 15 minutes, the use of disks being omitted.
Uniformity of dosage units ⟨905⟩: meet the requirements.
Assay—Weigh and finely powder not less than 20 Tablets. Transfer an accurately weighed portion of the powder, equivalent to about 1.0 mg of scopolamine hydrobromide, to a separator containing 5 mL of *pH 9.0 buffer*, and add, by pipet, 2.0 mL of *Internal standard solution* (prepared as directed in the *Assay* under *Scopolamine Hydrobromide Injection*). Adjust with 1 N sodium hydroxide to a pH of 9.0, extract with two 10-mL portions of methylene chloride, filter the methylene chloride extracts through 1 g of anhydrous sodium sulfate supported by a small cotton plug in a funnel into a 50-mL beaker, and evaporate under nitrogen to approximately 2.0 mL. Using this as the *Assay preparation*, proceed as directed in the *Assay* under *Scopolamine Hydrobromide Injection*. Calculate the quantity, in mg, of $C_{17}H_{21}NO_4 \cdot HBr \cdot 3H_2O$ in the portion of Tablets taken by the formula:

$$1.141(W/10)(A_U/A_S)$$

in which W is the weight, in mg, of USP Scopolamine Hydrobromide RS in the *Standard solution*; and 1.141 is the ratio of the molecular weight of scopolamine hydrobromide trihydrate to that of anhydrous scopolamine hydrobromide and A_U and A_S are as defined therein.

Secobarbital

$C_{12}H_{18}N_2O_3$ 238.28
2,4,6(1*H*,3*H*,5*H*)-Pyrimidinetrione, 5-(1-methylbutyl)-5-(2-propenyl)-.
5-Allyl-5-(1-methylbutyl)barbituric acid   [76-73-3].

» Secobarbital contains not less than 97.5 percent and not more than 100.5 percent of $C_{12}H_{18}N_2O_3$, calculated on the dried basis.

Packaging and storage—Preserve in tight containers.

USP Reference standards ⟨11⟩—*USP Secobarbital RS*.
Identification, *Infrared Absorption* ⟨197M⟩.
Loss on drying ⟨731⟩—Dry it over silica gel for 18 hours: it loses not more than 1.0% of its weight.
Residue on ignition ⟨281⟩: not more than 0.1%.
Organic volatile impurities, *Method V* ⟨467⟩: meets the requirements.
  Solvent—Use dimethyl sulfoxide.
                                              (Official until July 1, 2008)
Isomer content—Dissolve about 300 ± 5 mg in 5 mL of sodium hydroxide solution (1 in 100), add a solution of 300 ± 5 mg of *p*-nitrobenzyl bromide in 10 mL of alcohol, reflux for 30 minutes, cool, collect the precipitate on a small filter, and wash with water: the precipitate, recrystallized from 25 mL of alcohol and dried at 105° for 30 minutes, melts between 156° and 161°.
Assay—Add about 450 mg of Secobarbital, accurately weighed, to 60 mL of dimethylformamide in a 125-mL conical flask. Add 4 drops of thymol blue TS, and titrate with 0.1 N sodium methoxide VS, using a magnetic stirrer and taking precautions against the absorption of atmospheric carbon dioxide. Perform a blank determination, and make any necessary correction. Each mL of 0.1 N sodium methoxide is equivalent to 23.83 mg of $C_{12}H_{18}N_2O_3$.

Secobarbital Oral Solution

» Secobarbital Oral Solution contains, in each 100 mL, not less than 417 mg and not more than 461 mg of secobarbital ($C_{12}H_{18}N_2O_3$), in a suitable, flavored vehicle.

Packaging and storage—Preserve in tight containers.

USP Reference standards ⟨11⟩—*USP Secobarbital RS*.
Identification—Place 10 mL of Oral Solution in a separator containing 20 mL of water, add 5 mL of 1 N sodium hydroxide, and extract with two 10-mL portions of chloroform, discarding the chloroform extracts. Add 5 mL of 3 N hydrochloric acid, and extract with two 25-mL portions of chloroform, filtering the extracts through paper into a beaker. Remove the chloroform by evaporation on a steam bath, and dry the residue at 105° for 2 hours: the residue so obtained meets the requirements of the *Identification* test under *Secobarbital*.
Alcohol content ⟨611⟩: between 10.0% and 14.0% of C_2H_5OH.
Assay—
  Internal standard—Butabarbital.
  Internal standard solution—Dissolve an accurately weighed quantity of Butabarbital in chloroform, and quantitatively dilute with chloroform to obtain a solution having a known concentration of about 0.7 mg per mL.
  Standard preparation—Dissolve accurately weighed quantities of USP Secobarbital RS and Butabarbital in chloroform, and quantitatively dilute with chloroform to obtain a solution that contains, in each mL, known amounts of about 1.2 mg of USP Secobarbital RS and about 0.9 mg of Butabarbital.
  Assay preparation—Transfer an accurately measured volume of Oral Solution, equivalent to about 22 mg of secobarbital, to a separator, add 1 mL of dilute hydrochloric acid (1 in 5), and extract with four 10-mL portions of chloroform. Filter the extracts through about 15 g of anhydrous sodium sulfate that is supported on a funnel by a small pledget of glass wool. Collect the combined filtrate in a 50-mL volumetric flask, wash the sodium sulfate with 5 mL of chloroform, dilute with chloroform to volume, and mix. Combine 4.0 mL of this solution with 2.0 mL of *Internal standard solution* in a suitable container, and reduce the volume to about 1.5 mL by evaporation, with the aid of a stream of dry nitrogen, at room temperature.
  Chromatographic system and *System suitability*—Proceed as directed for *Chromatographic System* and *System Suitability* under *Barbiturate Assay* ⟨361⟩, the resolution, *R*, between secobarbital and butabarbital being not less than 3.0. [NOTE—Relative retention times are, approximately, 0.6 for butabarbital and 1.0 for secobarbital.]
  Procedure—Proceed as directed for *Procedure* under *Barbiturate Assay* ⟨361⟩. Calculate the quantity, in mg, of secobarbital ($C_{12}H_{18}N_2O_3$) in each mL of the Oral Solution taken by the the formula:

$$25(R_U)(Q_S)(C_i)/V(R_S)$$

in which V is the volume, in mL, of Oral Solution taken; and the other terms are as defined therein.

Secobarbital Sodium

$C_{12}H_{17}N_2NaO_3$ 260.27
2,4,6(1*H*,3*H*,5*H*)-Pyrimidinetrione, 5-(1-methylbutyl)-5-(2-propenyl)-, monosodium salt.
Sodium 5-allyl-5-(1-methylbutyl)barbiturate   [309-43-3].

» Secobarbital Sodium contains not less than 98.5 percent and not more than 100.5 percent of $C_{12}H_{17}N_2NaO_3$, calculated on the dried basis.

Packaging and storage—Preserve in tight containers.
Labeling—Where it is intended for use in preparing injectable dosage forms, the label states that it is sterile or must be subjected to further processing during the preparation of injectable dosage forms.
USP Reference standards ⟨11⟩—*USP Secobarbital RS. USP Endotoxin RS.*
Completeness of solution—Mix 1.0 g with 10 mL of carbon dioxide-free water: after 1 minute, the solution is clear and free from undissolved solid.
Identification—
  A: The IR absorption spectrum of a chloroform solution of the residue of secobarbital obtained as directed in the *Assay* exhibits maxima only at the same wavelengths as that of a similar preparation of USP Secobarbital RS.
  B: Ignite about 500 mg: the residue effervesces with acids, and responds to the tests for *Sodium* ⟨191⟩.
pH ⟨791⟩: between 9.7 and 10.5, in the solution prepared in the test for *Completeness of solution*.
Loss on drying ⟨731⟩—Dry it at 80° for 5 hours: it loses not more than 3.0% of its weight.
Heavy metals, *Method II* ⟨231⟩: 0.003%.
Organic volatile impurities, *Method I* ⟨467⟩: meets the requirements.

(Official until July 1, 2008)
Isomer content—Dissolve about 300 ± 5 mg in 5 mL of sodium hydroxide solution (1 in 100), add a solution of 300 ± 5 mg of *p*-nitrobenzyl bromide in 10 mL of alcohol, reflux for 30 minutes, cool, collect the precipitate on a small filter, and wash with water: the precipitate, recrystallized from 25 mL of alcohol and dried at 105° for 30 minutes, melts between 156° and 161°.
Other requirements—Where the label states that Secobarbital Sodium is sterile, it meets the requirements for *Sterility Tests* ⟨71⟩ and for *Bacterial endotoxins* under *Secobarbital Sodium for Injection*. Where the label states that Secobarbital Sodium must be subjected to further processing during the preparation of injectable dosage forms, it meets the requirements for *Bacterial endotoxins* under *Secobarbital Sodium for Injection*.
Assay—Dissolve about 500 mg of Secobarbital Sodium, accurately weighed, in 15 mL of water in a separator. To the solution add 2 mL of hydrochloric acid, shake, and extract the liberated secobarbital with eight 25-mL portions of chloroform. Test for completeness of extraction by extracting with an additional 10-mL portion of chloroform and evaporating the solvent: not more than 0.5 mg of residue remains. Filter the extracts into a tared beaker, and finally rinse the separator and the filter with several small portions of chloroform. Evaporate the combined filtrate and washings on a steam bath with the aid of a current of air just to dryness. Dissolve the residue in 2 mL of dehydrated alcohol, and evaporate to dryness. Repeat the dissolution and evaporation with 2 mL of dehydrated alcohol, and dry the residue at 100° for 2 hours. The weight of the residue, multiplied by 1.092, represents the weight of $C_{12}H_{17}N_2NaO_3$.

Secobarbital Sodium Capsules

» Secobarbital Sodium Capsules contain not less than 92.5 percent and not more than 107.5 percent of the labeled amount of $C_{12}H_{17}N_2NaO_3$.

Packaging and storage—Preserve in tight containers.
USP Reference standards ⟨11⟩—*USP Secobarbital RS.*
Identification—
  A: Dissolve a portion of the contents of Capsules, equivalent to about 50 mg of secobarbital sodium, in 10 mL of water, and filter into a separator. Add 2 mL of 3 N hydrochloric acid, extract the liberated secobarbital with 20 mL of chloroform, and evaporate the extract to dryness: the IR absorption spectrum of a 1 in 20 solution of the residue in chloroform exhibits maxima only at the same wavelengths as that of a similar preparation of USP Secobarbital RS.
  B: Ignite a portion of the contents of Capsules, equivalent to about 500 mg of secobarbital sodium: the residue so obtained responds to the tests for *Sodium* ⟨191⟩.
Dissolution ⟨711⟩—
  Medium: water; 500 mL.
  Apparatus 1: 100 rpm.
  Time: 60 minutes.
  Procedure—Determine the amount of $C_{12}H_{17}N_2NaO_3$ dissolved from UV absorbances at the wavelength of maximum absorbance at about 243 nm of filtered portions of the solution under test, mixed with sufficient sodium hydroxide to provide a concentration of 0.1 N sodium hydroxide, and suitably diluted with *Dissolution Medium*, if necessary, in comparison with a Standard solution having a known concentration of USP Secobarbital RS in 0.1 N sodium hydroxide.
  Tolerances—Not less than 75% *(Q)* of the labeled amount of $C_{12}H_{17}N_2NaO_3$ is dissolved in 60 minutes.
Uniformity of dosage units ⟨905⟩: meet the requirements.
  Procedure for content uniformity—Transfer the contents of 1 Capsule to a 250-mL volumetric flask, with the aid of about 5 mL of alcohol. Add 10 mL of freshly prepared dilute ammonium hydroxide (1 in 200), and without delay dilute with the same solution to volume. Mix, filter if necessary, and discard the first 20 mL of filtrate. Dilute a portion of the clear solution with dilute ammonium hydroxide (1 in 200) to obtain a solution having a concentration of about 10 µg of secobarbital sodium per mL. Dissolve a suitable quantity of USP Secobarbital RS in dilute ammonium hydroxide (1 in 200) to obtain a Standard solution having a known concentration of about 10 µg per mL. Concomitantly determine the absorbances of both solutions in 1-cm cells at the wavelength of maximum absorbance at about 240 nm, with a suitable spectrophotometer, using dilute ammonium hydroxide (1 in 200) as the blank. Calculate the quantity, in mg, of $C_{12}H_{17}N_2NaO_3$ in the Capsule taken by the formula:

$$(260.27 / 238.28)(T / C_U)C_S(A_U / A_S)$$

in which 260.27 and 238.28 are the molecular weights of secobarbital sodium and secobarbital, respectively, *T* is the labeled quantity, in mg, of secobarbital sodium in the Capsule, C_U is the concentration, in µg per mL, of secobarbital sodium in the solution from the Capsule contents, on the basis of the labeled quantity per Capsule and the extent of dilution, C_S is the concentration, in µg per mL, of USP Secobarbital RS in the Standard solution, and A_U and A_S are the absorbances of the solution from the Capsule contents and the Standard solution, respectively.
Assay—
  Internal standard—Butabarbital.
  Internal standard solution—Dissolve an accurately weighed quantity of Butabarbital in chloroform, and dilute quantitatively with chloroform to obtain a solution having a known concentration of about 0.8 mg per mL.
  Standard preparation—Dissolve accurately weighed quantities of USP Secobarbital RS and Butabarbital in chloroform, and dilute quantitatively with chloroform to obtain a solution that contains, in each mL, known amounts of about 0.9 mg of USP Secobarbital RS and about 0.8 mg of Butabarbital.
  Assay preparation—Weigh not less than 20 Capsules, and transfer the contents as completely as possible to a suitable container. Remove any residual powder from the empty capsules with the aid of a current of air, and weigh the capsule shells, determining the weight of the contents by difference. Mix the contents of the Capsules, and transfer an accurately weighed portion of the powder, equivalent to about 100 mg of secobarbital sodium, to a separator. Add 15 mL of water, 1 mL of hydrochloric acid, and 100 mL of chloroform, and shake for 3 minutes. Filter a portion of the chloroform layer through about 15 g of anhydrous sodium sulfate that is supported on a funnel by a small pledget of glass wool, combine 2.0 mL of this solution with 2.0 mL internal standard solution in a suitable container, and reduce the volume to about 2 mL by evaporation, with the aid of a stream of dry nitrogen, at room temperature.
  Chromatographic system and *System suitability*—Proceed as directed for *Chromatographic System* and *System Suitability* under *Barbiturate Assay* ⟨361⟩, the resolution, *R*, between secobarbital and butabarbital being not less than 3.0. [NOTE—Relative retention

times are, approximately, 0.6 for butabarbital and 1.0 for secobarbital.]
Procedure—Proceed as directed for *Procedure* under *Barbiturate Assay* ⟨361⟩. Calculate the quantity, in mg, of $C_{12}H_{17}N_2NaO_3$ in the portion of Capsules taken by the formula:

$$(260.27 / 238.28)(100)(R_U)(Q_S)(C_i) / (R_S)$$

in which 260.27 and 238.28 are the molecular weights of secobarbital sodium and secobarbital, respectively, and the other terms are as defined therein.

Secobarbital Sodium Injection

» Secobarbital Sodium Injection is a sterile solution of Secobarbital Sodium in a suitable solvent. It contains not less than 90.0 percent and not more than 110.0 percent of the labeled amount of $C_{12}H_{17}N_2NaO_3$.

Packaging and storage—Preserve in single-dose or in multiple-dose containers, preferably of Type I glass, protected from light, in a refrigerator.
Labeling—The label indicates that the Injection is not to be used if it contains a precipitate.
USP Reference standards ⟨11⟩—*USP Secobarbital RS. USP Endotoxin RS.*
Identification—
  A: Transfer a volume of Injection, equivalent to about 100 mg of secobarbital sodium, to a separator containing 15 mL of water. Render the mixture distinctly acid to litmus with hydrochloric acid, extract the liberated secobarbital with 25 mL of ether, collect the ether extract in a separator, and wash with 10 mL of water. Discard the water solution. Filter the ether extract into a beaker, and evaporate on a steam bath with the aid of a current of air just to dryness. Dissolve the residue in 3 mL of alcohol, and evaporate to dryness. Repeat the dissolution and evaporation with 3 mL of alcohol, and dry the residue at 100° for 2 hours: the IR absorption spectrum of a solution prepared by dissolving the residue of secobarbital so obtained in chloroform to a concentration of about 50 mg per mL, 0.1-mm sodium chloride cells being used and chloroform being used as the blank, exhibits maxima only at the same wavelengths as that of a similar preparation of USP Secobarbital RS.
  B: It responds to the flame test for *Sodium* ⟨191⟩.
Bacterial endotoxins ⟨85⟩—It contains not more than 0.9 USP Endotoxin Unit per mg of secobarbital sodium.
pH ⟨791⟩: between 9.0 and 10.5.
Other requirements—It meets the requirements under *Injections* ⟨1⟩.
Assay—
  Buffer solution—Dissolve 6.19 g of boric acid and 14.91 g of potassium chloride in water, dilute with water to 200 mL, and mix. After 24 hours, filter if necessary to obtain a clear solution.
  Standard preparation 1—Dissolve a suitable quantity of USP Secobarbital RS, accurately weighed, in 0.5 N sodium hydroxide to obtain a solution having a known concentration of about 23 µg per mL.
  Standard preparation 2—Mix 5.0 mL of *Standard preparation 1* with 5.0 mL of *Buffer solution*.
  Assay preparation 1—Transfer an accurately measured volume of Injection, equivalent to about 50 mg of secobarbital sodium, to a 100-mL volumetric flask, dilute with 0.5 N sodium hydroxide to volume, and mix. Pipet 5 mL of this solution into a 100-mL volumetric flask, add 0.5 N sodium hydroxide to volume, and mix.
  Assay preparation 2—Mix 5.0 mL of *Assay preparation 1* with 5.0 mL of *Buffer solution*.
  Procedure—Concomitantly determine the absorbances of *Assay preparation 1* and *Standard preparation 1* in 1-cm cells at 260 nm, with a suitable spectrophotometer, using 0.5 N sodium hydroxide as the blank. Similarly determine the absorbances of *Assay preparation 2* and *Standard preparation 2*, using as the blank a mixture of equal volumes of 0.5 N sodium hydroxide and *Buffer solution*. Calculate the quantity, in mg, of $C_{12}H_{17}N_2NaO_3$ in the volume of Injection taken by the formula:

$$1.092(2C)(A_U - 2a_U) / (A_S - 2a_S)$$

in which 1.092 is the ratio of the molecular weight of sodium secobarbital to that of secobarbital, C is the concentration, in µg per mL, of USP Secobarbital RS in *Standard preparation 1*, A_U and A_S are the absorbances of *Assay preparation 1* and *Standard preparation 1*, respectively, and a_U and a_S are the absorbances of *Assay preparation 2* and *Standard preparation 2*, respectively.

Secobarbital Sodium for Injection

» Secobarbital Sodium for Injection is Secobarbital Sodium suitable for parenteral use. It contains not less than 90.0 percent and not more than 110.0 percent of the labeled amount of secobarbital sodium ($C_{12}H_{17}N_2NaO_3$).

Packaging and storage—Preserve in *Containers for Sterile Solids* as described under *Injections* ⟨1⟩.
USP Reference standards ⟨11⟩—*USP Secobarbital RS. USP Endotoxin RS.*
Constituted solution—At the time of use, it meets the requirements for *Constituted Solutions* under *Injections* ⟨1⟩.
Bacterial endotoxins ⟨85⟩—It contains not more than 0.9 USP Endotoxin Unit per mg of secobarbital sodium.
Other requirements—It conforms to the Definition, responds to the *Identification* tests, and meets the requirements for *pH, Completeness of solution, Loss on drying, Heavy metals*, and *Assay* under *Secobarbital Sodium*. It meets also the requirements for *Sterility Tests* ⟨71⟩, *Uniformity of Dosage Units* ⟨905⟩, and *Labeling* under *Injections* ⟨1⟩.

Secobarbital Sodium and Amobarbital Sodium Capsules

» Secobarbital Sodium and Amobarbital Sodium Capsules contain not less than 90.0 percent and not more than 110.0 percent of the labeled amounts of secobarbital sodium ($C_{12}H_{17}N_2NaO_3$) and amobarbital sodium ($C_{11}H_{17}N_2NaO_3$).

Packaging and storage—Preserve in well-closed containers.
USP Reference standards ⟨11⟩—*USP Amobarbital RS. USP Secobarbital RS.*
Identification—
  A: Suspend the contents of 1 Capsule in 10 mL of water, and filter: the filtrate responds to the flame test for *Sodium* ⟨191⟩.
  B: The retention times of the major peaks in the chromatogram of the *Assay preparation* correspond to those of the *Standard preparation* obtained in the *Assay*.
Dissolution ⟨711⟩—
  Medium: water; 500 mL.
  Apparatus 1: 100 rpm.
  Time: 60 minutes.
  Procedure—Determine the total amount of $C_{12}H_{17}N_2NaO_3$ and $C_{11}H_{17}N_2NaO_3$ dissolved from UV absorbances at the wavelength of maximum absorbance at about 239 nm of filtered portions of the solution under test, suitably diluted with 0.1 N sodium hydroxide, in comparison with a Standard solution having known concentrations of about 7.5 µg each per mL, of USP Secobarbital RS and USP Amobarbital RS in the same medium. An amount of alcohol not to exceed 1% of the total volume of the Standard solution may

be used to dissolve the Reference Standards prior to dilution with water and 0.1 N sodium hydroxide.

Tolerances—Not less than 60% (*Q*) of the labeled total amount of $C_{12}H_{17}N_2NaO_3$ and $C_{11}H_{17}N_2NaO_3$ is dissolved in 60 minutes.

Uniformity of dosage units ⟨905⟩: meet the requirements for *Content Uniformity* with respect to secobarbital sodium and to amobarbital.

Assay—

Internal standard solution—Dissolve aprobarbital in chloroform to obtain a solution having a concentration of about 0.75 mg per mL.

Standard preparation—Transfer about 92 mg of USP Secobarbital RS, and about 91 mg of USP Amobarbital RS, both accurately weighed, to a 100-mL volumetric flask, and dissolve in 50 mL of chloroform. Dilute with chloroform to volume, and mix.

Assay preparation—Remove, as completely as possible, the contents of not less than 20 Capsules. Transfer an accurately weighed portion of the powder, equivalent to about 100 mg of secobarbital sodium, to a separator, add 20 mL of water, 1 mL of hydrochloric acid, and 100.0 mL of chloroform, and shake for 3 minutes. Remove the chloroform layer, and use as directed in the *Procedure*.

Chromatographic system (see *Chromatography* ⟨621⟩)—The gas chromatograph is equipped with a flame-ionization detector and contains a 0.6-m × 3.5-mm glass column packed with 3 percent liquid phase G10 on 100- to 120-mesh support S1AB. The column is maintained at about 175°, the injection port at about 235°, the detector block at about 245°, and dry helium is used as the carrier gas at a flow rate of about 55 mL per minute. Chromatograph five replicate injections of the *Standard preparation*, and record the peak responses as directed for *Procedure*: the relative standard deviation is not more than 2%; the resolution factor between amobarbital and the internal standard is not less than 1.5; the resolution factor between amobarbital and secobarbital is not less than 2.5; and the tailing factor does not exceed 1.5 for any of the three peaks.

Procedure—Mix 5.0 mL of the *Standard preparation* with 5.0 mL of the *Internal standard solution*. Mix 5.0 mL of the *Assay preparation* with 5.0 mL of the *Internal standard solution*. Separately inject equal volumes (about 3 μL) of the resulting solutions into the chromatograph, and record the chromatograms. Measure the responses for the major peaks. The relative retention times with respect to the internal standard are about 1.3 for amobarbital and 1.8 for secobarbital. Calculate the quantity, in mg, of secobarbital sodium ($C_{12}H_{17}N_2NaO_3$) in the portion of Capsules taken by the formula:

$$(260.27 / 238.28)W(R_U / R_S)$$

in which 260.27 and 238.28 are the molecular weights of secobarbital sodium and secobarbital, respectively, *W* is the weight, in mg, of USP Secobarbital RS taken for the *Standard preparation*, and R_U and R_S are the ratios of the peak response of secobarbital to that of the internal standard in the *Assay preparation* and the *Standard preparation*, respectively. Similarly calculate the quantity, in mg, of amobarbital sodium ($C_{11}H_{17}N_2NaO_3$) in the portion of Capsules taken by the formula:

$$(248.26 / 226.28)W'(R'_U / R'_S)$$

in which 248.26 and 226.28 are the molecular weights of amobarbital sodium and amobarbital, respectively, *W'* is the weight, in mg, of USP Amobarbital RS taken for the *Standard preparation*, and R'_U and R'_S are the ratios of the peak response of amobarbital to that of the internal standard obtained from *Assay preparation* and the *Standard preparation*, respectively.

Selegiline Hydrochloride

$C_{13}H_{17}N \cdot HCl$ 223.74

Benzeneethanamine, *N*,α-dimethyl-*N*-2-propynyl-, hydrochloride, (*R*)-.

(−)-(*R*)-*N*,α-Dimethyl-*N*-2-propynylphenethylamine hydrochloride [14611-52-0].

» Selegiline Hydrochloride contains not less than 98.0 percent and not more than 101.0 percent of $C_{13}H_{17}N \cdot HCl$, calculated on the dried basis.

Packaging and storage—Preserve in tight, light-resistant containers.

USP Reference standards ⟨11⟩—*USP Selegiline Hydrochloride RS. USP Methamphetamine Hydrochloride RS.*

Identification—
 A: *Infrared Absorption* ⟨197K⟩.
 B: *Ultraviolet Absorption* ⟨197U⟩—
 Solution: 0.5 mg per mL.
 Medium: water.
 C: The retention time of the major peak in the chromatogram of the *Assay preparation* corresponds to that of the *Standard preparation* obtained as directed in the *Assay*.
 D: It responds to the tests for *Chloride* ⟨191⟩.

Melting range ⟨741⟩: not greater than 2°, within the limits of 141° and 145°.

Specific rotation ⟨781S⟩: between −10.0° and −12.0°.
 Test solution: 100 mg per mL, in water.

Loss on drying ⟨731⟩—Dry it in vacuum at 60° for 3 hours: it loses not more than 1.0% of its weight.

Residue on ignition ⟨281⟩: not more than 0.2%.

Heavy metals, *Method II* ⟨231⟩: not more than 0.002%.

Chromatographic purity—

Buffer solution, Mobile phase, and *System suitability solution*—Proceed as directed in the *Assay*.

Standard solution—Transfer 10.0 mL of the *System suitability solution* to a 100-mL volumetric flask, dilute with *Mobile phase* to volume, and mix. Transfer 10.0 mL of this solution to a 50 mL volumetric flask, dilute with *Mobile phase* to volume, and mix.

Test solution—Transfer 50 mg of Selegiline Hydrochloride to a 50-mL volumetric flask, dissolve in and dilute with *Mobile phase* to volume, and mix.

Chromatographic system—Proceed as directed in the *Assay*. Inject about 20 μL of the *Standard solution*, and record the peak responses as directed in the *Procedure*: the resolution, *R*, between the methamphetamine and selegiline peaks is not less than 3, and the relative standard deviation for replicate injections is not more than 5.0%.

Procedure—Separately inject equal volumes (about 20 μL) of the *Standard solution* and the *Test solution* into the chromatograph, and allow the *Test solution* to elute for not less than three times the retention time of selegiline. Record the chromatograms, and measure the peak responses. Calculate the percentage of each impurity in the portion of Selegiline Hydrochloride taken by the formula:

$$5000(C / W)(r_i / r_S)$$

in which *C* is the concentration, in mg per mL, of USP Selegiline Hydrochloride RS in the *Standard solution*, *W* is the weight, in mg, of Selegiline Hydrochloride taken to prepare the *Test solution*, r_i is the peak response for each impurity in the chromatogram of the *Test solution*, and r_S is the peak response for selegiline in the chromatogram of the *Standard solution*. Not more than 0.2% of any individual impurity is found, and the sum of all impurities is not more than 1.0%.

Assay—

Buffer solution—Prepare a solution of 0.1 M monobasic ammonium phosphate, adjust with phosphoric acid to a pH of 3.1, and mix.

Mobile phase—Prepare a filtered and degassed mixture of *Buffer solution* and acetonitrile (80 : 20). Make adjustments if necessary (see *System Suitability* under *Chromatography* ⟨621⟩).

Standard preparation—Dissolve an accurately weighed quantity of USP Selegiline Hydrochloride RS, and dilute quantitatively, and stepwise if necessary, with *Mobile phase* to obtain a solution having a known concentration of about 0.1 mg per mL.

System suitability solution—Dissolve accurately weighed quantities of USP Methamphetamine Hydrochloride RS and USP Selegiline Hydrochloride RS in *Mobile phase* to obtain a solution containing 0.1 mg per mL of each Reference Standard.

Assay preparation—Transfer an accurately weighed quantity, about 50 mg of Selegiline Hydrochloride, to a 50-mL volumetric flask, dissolve in and dilute with *Mobile phase* to volume, and mix. Transfer 10.0 mL of this solution to a 100-mL volumetric flask, dilute with *Mobile phase* to volume, and mix.

Chromatographic system (see *Chromatography* ⟨621⟩)—The liquid chromatograph is equipped with a 205-nm detector and a 3.9-mm × 30-cm column that contains packing L1. The flow rate is about 1 mL per minute. Chromatograph the *System suitability solution*, and record the peak responses as directed for *Procedure*: the resolution, R, between the methamphetamine and selegiline peaks is not less than 3, and the relative standard deviation for replicate injections is not more than 2.0%.

Procedure—Separately inject equal volumes (about 20 μL) of the *Standard preparation* and the *Assay preparation* into the chromatograph, record the chromatograms, and measure the responses for the major peaks. Calculate the quantity, in mg, of $C_{13}H_{17}N \cdot HCl$ in the portion of Selegiline Hydrochloride taken by the formula:

$$500C(r_U / r_S)$$

in which C is the concentration, in mg per mL, of USP Selegiline Hydrochloride RS in the *Standard preparation*, and r_U and r_S are the selegiline peak responses obtained from the *Assay preparation* and the *Standard preparation*, respectively.

Selegiline Hydrochloride Tablets

» Selegiline Hydrochloride Tablets contain not less than 90.0 percent and not more than 110.0 percent of the labeled amount of $C_{13}H_{17}N \cdot HCl$.

Packaging and storage—Preserve in tight, light-resistant containers.

USP Reference standards ⟨11⟩—*USP Selegiline Hydrochloride RS. USP Methamphetamine Hydrochloride RS.*

Identification—The retention time of the major peak in the chromatogram of the *Assay preparation* corresponds to that in the chromatogram of the *Standard preparation* as obtained in the *Assay*.

Dissolution ⟨711⟩—
  Medium: water; 500 mL.
  Apparatus 1: 50 rpm.
  Time: 20 minutes.
  Determine the amount of $C_{13}H_{17}N \cdot HCl$ dissolved using the following method.
  Monobasic ammonium phosphate solution—Dissolve 11.5 g of monobasic ammonium phosphate in 1000 mL of water. Adjust with 85% phosphoric acid to a pH of 3.1.
  Mobile phase—Prepare a filtered and degassed mixture of *Monobasic ammonium phosphate solution* and acetonitrile (4 : 1). Make adjustments if necessary (see *System Suitability* under *Chromatography* ⟨621⟩).
  Standard solution—Transfer 25.0 mg, accurately weighed, of USP Selegiline Hydrochloride RS to a 50-mL volumetric flask. Dissolve in and dilute with water to volume, and mix. Pipet 2.0 mL of this solution into a 100-mL volumetric flask, dilute with water to volume, and mix.
  Test solution—At 20 minutes withdraw a 10-mL portion of the solution under test and centrifuge for 10 minutes at 3500 rpm.
  Chromatographic system—The liquid chromatograph is equipped with a 205-nm detector and a 3.9-mm × 30-cm column that contains packing L1. Chromatograph the *Standard solution*, and record the peak responses. The relative standard deviation for replicate injections is not more than 2.0%.
  Procedure—Separately inject equal volumes (about 15 μL) of the *Standard solution* and the *Test solution* into the chromatograph, record the chromatograms, and measure the responses for the major peaks. Calculate the amount of $C_{13}H_{17}N \cdot HCl$ dissolved.
  Tolerances—Not less than 80% *(Q)* of the labeled amount of $C_{13}H_{17}N \cdot HCl$ is dissolved in 20 minutes.

Chromatographic purity—
  Buffer solution, Mobile phase, System suitability solution, and *Chromatographic system*—Proceed as directed in the test for *Chromatographic purity* under *Selegiline Hydrochloride*.
  Standard solution—Transfer 10.0 mL of the *System suitability solution* to a 100-mL volumetric flask, dilute with *Mobile phase* to volume, and mix. Transfer 10.0 mL of this solution to a 20-mL volumetric flask, dilute with *Mobile phase* to volume, and mix.
  Test solution—Use a portion of the supernatant obtained from the *Assay preparation*.
  Procedure—Proceed as directed in the test for *Chromatographic purity* under *Selegiline Hydrochloride*. Calculate the percentage of each impurity, excluding methamphetamine hydrochloride, in the portion of Tablets taken by the formula:

$$5000(C / W)(r_i / r_S)$$

in which W is the weight, in mg, of the labeled content of selegiline hydrochloride in the portion of Tablets taken to prepare the *Test solution*, and the other terms are as defined therein. Not more than 0.5% of any individual impurity is found, and the sum of all impurities, excluding methamphetamine hydrochloride, is not more than 2.0%.

Uniformity of dosage units ⟨905⟩: meet the requirements.

Limit of methamphetamine hydrochloride—
  Buffer solution, Mobile phase, System suitability solution, Test solution, and *Chromatographic system*—Proceed as directed in the test for *Chromatographic purity* under *Selegiline Hydrochloride*.
  Standard solution—Transfer 10.0 mL of the *System suitability solution* to a 50-mL volumetric flask, dilute with *Mobile phase* to volume, and mix.
  Procedure—Proceed as directed in the test for *Chromatographic purity* under *Selegiline Hydrochloride*. Calculate the percentage of methamphetamine hydrochloride in the portion of Tablets taken by the formula:

$$5000(C / W)(r_U / r_S)$$

in which C is the concentration, in mg per mL, of USP Methamphetamine Hydrochloride RS in the *Standard solution*, W is the weight, in mg, of the labeled content of selegiline hydrochloride in the portion of Tablets taken to prepare the *Test solution*, and r_U and r_S are the methamphetamine peak responses obtained from the *Test solution* and the *Standard solution*, respectively. Not more than 2.0% of methamphetamine hydrochloride is found.

Assay—
  Buffer solution, Mobile phase, Standard preparation, System suitability solution, and *Chromatographic system*—Proceed as directed in the test for *Assay* under *Selegiline Hydrochloride*.
  Assay preparation—Weigh and powder not less than 20 Tablets. Transfer an accurately weighed portion of the powder equivalent to about 50 mg of selegiline hydrochloride to a 50-mL volumetric flask. Add 40 mL of *Mobile phase*, sonicate for 10 minutes, dilute with *Mobile phase* to volume, and mix. Centrifuge a 25-mL aliquot of this solution at 3500 rpm for 10 minutes. [NOTE—Retain a portion of the supernatant for the *Chromatographic purity* and *Limit of methamphetamine hydrochloride* tests.] Transfer 10.0 mL of the supernatant to a 100-mL volumetric flask, dilute with *Mobile phase* to volume, and mix.
  Procedure—Proceed as directed for *Procedure* in the *Assay* under *Selegiline Hydrochloride*. Calculate the quantity, in mg, of $C_{13}H_{17}N \cdot HCl$ in the portion of Tablets taken by the formula:

$$500C(r_U / r_S)$$

in which the terms are as defined therein.

Selenious Acid

H$_2$SeO$_3$ 128.97
Selenium dioxide, monohydrated.
Selenious acid   [7783-00-8].

» Selenious Acid contains not less than 93.0 percent and not more than 101.0 percent of H$_2$SeO$_3$.

Packaging and storage—Preserve in tight containers.
Identification—
  A: Dissolve about 50 mg in 5 mL of water, add about 100 mg of sodium bicarbonate, and mix: gas bubbles develop.
  B: Dissolve about 50 mg in 5 mL of 0.1 N hydrochloric acid, and add about 50 mg of stannous chloride: a curdy tan-orange precipitate is formed.
Residue on ignition ⟨281⟩: not more than 1.0 mg, from 10.0 g (0.01%).
Insoluble matter—Dissolve 1 g in 5 mL of water: it dissolves completely and the solution is clear.
Selenate and sulfate—Dissolve about 0.5 g in 10 mL of water, add 0.1 mL of hydrochloric acid and 1 mL of barium chloride TS, and mix: no turbidity or precipitate is formed in 10 minutes.
Organic volatile impurities, *Method I* ⟨467⟩: meets the requirements.
(Official until July 1, 2008)
Assay—Transfer about 100 mg of Selenious Acid, accurately weighed, to a suitable glass-stoppered flask, and dissolve in 50 mL of water. Add 10 mL of potassium iodide solution (3 in 10) and 5 mL of hydrochloric acid, mix, insert the stopper in the flask, and allow to stand for 10 minutes. Add 50 mL of water and 3 mL of starch TS, and titrate with 0.1 N sodium thiosulfate VS until the solution is colorless, then titrate with 0.1 N iodine VS to a blue endpoint. Subtract the volume of 0.1 N iodine from the volume of 0.1 N sodium thiosulfate to obtain the volume of 0.1 N sodium thiosulfate equivalent to selenious acid. Each mL of 0.1 N sodium thiosulfate is equivalent to 3.225 mg of H$_2$SeO$_3$.

Selenious Acid Injection

» Selenious Acid Injection is a sterile solution in Water for Injection of Selenious Acid or of selenium dissolved in nitric acid. It contains not less than 95.0 percent and not more than 105.0 percent of the labeled amount of selenium (Se).

Packaging and storage—Preserve in single-dose or in multiple-dose containers, preferably of Type I or Type II glass.
Labeling—Label the Injection to indicate that it is to be diluted to the appropriate strength with Sterile Water for Injection or other suitable fluid prior to administration.
USP Reference standards ⟨11⟩—*USP Endotoxin RS*.
Identification—The *Assay preparation*, prepared as directed in the *Assay*, exhibits an absorption maximum at about 196 nm when tested as directed for *Procedure* in the *Assay*.
Bacterial endotoxins ⟨85⟩—It contains not more than 3.5 USP Endotoxin Units per µg of selenium.
pH ⟨791⟩: between 1.8 and 2.4.
Particulate matter ⟨788⟩: meets the requirements under small-volume injections.
Other requirements—It meets the requirements under *Injections* ⟨1⟩.
Assay—
  Selenium stock solution—Dissolve about 1 g of metallic selenium, accurately weighed, in a minimum volume of nitric acid. [*Caution*—*Selenium is toxic; handle it with care.*]Evaporate to dryness, add 2 mL of water, and evaporate to dryness. Repeat the addition of water and the evaporation to dryness three times. Dissolve the residue in 3 N hydrochloric acid, transfer to a 1000-mL volumetric flask, dilute with 3 N hydrochloric acid to volume, and mix. This solution contains about 1000 µg of selenium per mL.
  Standard preparations—Transfer 3.0, 4.0, and 5.0 mL, respectively, of *Selenium stock solution* to separate 100-mL volumetric flasks, dilute the contents of each flask with water to volume, and mix. These *Standard preparations* contain, respectively, about 30, 40, and 50 µg of selenium per mL.
  Assay preparation—Using water as the diluent, quantitatively dilute an accurately measured volume of Injection to obtain a solution containing about 40 µg of selenium per mL.
  Procedure—Concomitantly determine the absorbances of the *Standard preparations* and the *Assay preparation* at the selenium emission line of 196 nm, with a suitable atomic absorption spectrophotometer (see *Spectrophotometry and Light-scattering* ⟨851⟩) equipped with a selenium electrodeless discharge lamp and an air–acetylene flame, using water as the blank. Plot the absorbances of the *Standard preparations* versus concentration, in µg per mL, of selenium, and draw the straight line best fitting the three plotted points. From the graph so obtained, determine the concentration *C*, in µg per mL, of selenium in the *Assay preparation*. Calculate the quantity, in mg, of selenium in each mL of the Injection taken by the formula:

$$LC / D$$

in which *L* is the labeled quantity, in mg per mL, of selenium in the Injection taken, and *D* is the concentration, in µg of selenium per mL, of the *Assay preparation* on the basis of the labeled quantity in the Injection and the extent of dilution.

Selenium Sulfide

SeS$_2$ 143.09
Selenium sulfide (SeS$_2$).
Selenium sulfide (SeS$_2$)   [7488-56-4].

» Selenium Sulfide contains not less than 52.0 percent and not more than 55.5 percent of selenium (Se).

Packaging and storage—Preserve in well-closed containers.
Identification—
  A: Filter 20 mL of the solution of Selenium Sulfide prepared as directed in the *Assay*, and to 10 mL of the filtrate add 5 mL of water and 5 g of urea. Heat to boiling, cool, and add 2 mL of potassium iodide solution (1 in 10): a yellowish orange to orange color is produced, and it darkens rapidly (*presence of selenium*).
  B: Allow the solution obtained in *Identification* test A to stand for 10 minutes, filter, and to the filtrate add 10 mL of barium chloride TS: the solution becomes turbid (*presence of sulfur*).
Residue on ignition ⟨281⟩: not more than 0.2%.
Soluble selenium compounds—
  Test solution—Mix 10.0 g of Selenium Sulfide with 100.0 mL of water in a 250-mL flask, allow to stand for 1 hour, with frequent agitation, and filter. To 10.0 mL of the filtrate add 2 mL of 2.5 M formic acid, dilute with water to 50 mL, mix, and adjust, if necessary, to a pH of 2.5 ± 0.5. Add 2 mL of freshly prepared 3,3′-diaminobenzidine hydrochloride solution (1 in 200), mix, allow to stand for 45 minutes, and adjust with 6 N ammonium hydroxide to a pH of 6.5 ± 0.5. Transfer to a separator, add 10.0 mL of toluene, shake vigorously for 1 minute, allow the layers to separate, and discard the aqueous phase.
  Standard solution—Using 10.0 mL of a solution of selenious acid containing 0.5 µg of selenium per mL, prepare a solution as directed under *Test solution*, beginning with "add 2 mL of 2.5 M formic acid."
  Procedure—Concomitantly determine the absorbances of the toluene layers of the *Test solution* and the *Standard solution* in 1-cm cells at 420 nm, with a suitable spectrophotometer, using a blank consisting of the same quantities of the same reagents treated in the same manner as the *Test solution*: the absorbance of the *Test solution* is not greater than that of the *Standard solution* (5 ppm).
Assay—Place about 100 mg of Selenium Sulfide, accurately weighed, in a suitable container, add 25 mL of fuming nitric acid,

and digest over gentle heat until no further solution occurs. Cool, transfer the solution to a 250-mL volumetric flask containing 100 mL of water, cool again, dilute with water to volume, and mix. Pipet 50 mL of the solution into a suitable flask, add 25 mL of water and 10 g of urea, and heat to boiling. Cool, add 3 mL of starch TS, then add 10 mL of potassium iodide solution (1 in 10), and immediately titrate with 0.05 N sodium thiosulfate VS. Perform a blank determination, and make any necessary correction. Each mL of 0.05 N sodium thiosulfate is equivalent to 987.0 µg of Se.

Selenium Sulfide Topical Suspension

(Former monograph title is Selenium Sulfide Lotion)

» Selenium Sulfide Topical Suspension is an aqueous, stabilized suspension of Selenium Sulfide. It contains not less than 90.0 percent and not more than 110.0 percent of the labeled amount of SeS$_2$. It contains suitable buffering and dispersing agents.

NOTE—Where labeled for use as a shampoo, it contains a detergent. Where labeled for other uses, it may contain a detergent.

Packaging and storage—Preserve in tight containers.
Identification—Digest about 2 g with 5 mL of nitric acid over gentle heat for 1 hour, dilute with water to about 50 mL, and filter: the solution responds to *Identification* test A under *Selenium Sulfide,* when tested as directed, beginning with "to 10 mL of the filtrate add 5 mL of water."
pH ⟨791⟩: between 2.0 and 6.0.
Assay—Place a portion of well-mixed Topical Suspension, equivalent to about 100 mg of selenium sulfide and accurately weighed, in a suitable flask. Cautiously digest with 25 mL of fuming nitric acid over gentle heat for 2 hours, and proceed as directed in the *Assay* under *Selenium Sulfide,* beginning with "Cool, transfer the solution to a 250-mL volumetric flask." Each mL of 0.05 N sodium thiosulfate is equivalent to 1.789 mg of SeS$_2$. Where the Topical Suspension is labeled in terms of percentage (w/v) or of the amount of SeS$_2$ in a given volume of Topical Suspension, determine the density of the Topical Suspension as follows: Using a tared, 100-mL volumetric flask, weigh 100 mL of Topical Suspension that previously has been shaken to ensure homogeneity, allowed to stand until the entrapped air rises, and finally inverted carefully just prior to transfer to the volumetric flask. From the observed weight of 100 mL of the Topical Suspension, calculate the quantity of SeS$_2$ in each 100 mL.

Senna Leaf

» Senna Leaf consists of the dried leaflet of *Senna alexandrina* Mill also known as *Cassia acutifolia* Delile (Alexandrian senna) or *C. angustifolia* Vahl (Tinnevelly senna) (Fam. Fabaceae). Senna Leaf contains not less than 2.5 percent of anthraquinone glucosides, calculated as sennosides, on the dried basis.

Packaging and storage—Preserve against attack by insects and rodents (see *Vegetable and Animal Drugs—Preservation* in the *General Notices*). Store protected from light and moisture, at room temperature.
Labeling—The label states the Latin binomial and, following the official name, the part of the plant contained in the article.
USP Reference standards ⟨11⟩—USP Sennosides RS.
Botanic characteristics—
Unground Alexandrian senna leaf—Inequilaterally lanceolate or lance-ovate leaflets, frequently broken; from 1.5 cm to 3.5 cm in length and from 5 mm to 10 mm in width, unequal at the base, with very short, stout petiolules. The leaflets are acutely cuspidate, entire, brittle, and subcoriaceous, with short and somewhat appressed hairs, few on the upper surface, more numerous on the lower surface, where they occur spreading on the midrib, especially on its lower part. The color is weak yellow to light grayish-green to pale olive. The odor is characteristic.
Unground Tinnevelly senna leaf—Usually unbroken leaflets, from 2 cm to 5 cm in length and from 6 mm to 15 mm in width; acute at the apex; and slightly hairy. The color of the leaves is weak yellow to pale olive.
Histology—Senna leaf shows polygonal epidermal cells with straight walls and frequently containing mucilage; numerous, broadly elliptical stomata mostly from 20 to 35 µm in length, usually bordered by two neighbor-cells with their long axes parallel to that of the stoma, and rarely, though more frequently in Alexandrian senna leaf, a third epidermal cell at the end of the stoma. The hairs are nonglandular, one-celled, conical, often curved, with thick papillose walls, from 100 to 350 µm in length. Palisade cells in a single layer underlie both surfaces except in the midrib region where they occur only beneath the upper epidermis. A meristele occurs in the midrib composed of several radially arranged fibrovascular bundles, the latter separated by narrow vascular rays and supported above and below by arcs of lignified pericyclic fibers. Calcium oxalate occurs in rosette aggregates in the spongy parenchyma and in six- to eight-sided prisms in the crystal fibers, which lie on the outer surface of each group of pericyclic fibers.
Powdered senna leaf—Dusky greenish-yellow to light olive-brown, displaying fragments of veins bearing lignified vessels, tracheids, and crystal fibers, isolated hairs, masses of palisade and spongy parenchyma, fragments of epidermis with stomata, free calcium oxalate rosette aggregates, and prisms from 10 to 20 µm in length. In powdered Alexandrian senna leaf, the hairs are more numerous than in powdered Tinnevelly senna leaf.
Identification—Mix 500 mg of finely powdered Senna Leaf with 10 mL of a 1 in 10 solution of potassium hydroxide in alcohol, boil for about 2 minutes, dilute with 10 mL of water, and filter. Acidify the filtrate with hydrochloric acid, shake it with ether, remove the ether layer, and shake it with 5 mL of 6 N ammonium hydroxide: the latter is colored orange or bluish-red.
Microbial enumeration ⟨2021⟩—The total bacterial count does not exceed 10^5 cfu per g, the total combined molds and yeasts count does not exceed 10^3 cfu per g, the bile-tolerant Gram-negative bacteria does not exceed 10^3 cfu per g, and it meets the requirements of the tests for absence of *Salmonella* species and *Escherichia coli.*
Loss on drying ⟨731⟩—Dry 1.0 g of finely powdered Senna Leaf at 105° for 2 hours: it loses not more than 12.0% of its weight.
Senna stems, pods, or other foreign organic matter ⟨561⟩—The amount of senna stems does not exceed 8.0%, and the amount of senna pods or other foreign organic matter does not exceed 2.0%.
Total ash ⟨561⟩: not more than 12.0%.
Acid-insoluble ash ⟨561⟩: not more than 3.0%.
Assay—[NOTE—Conduct all sample preparations with minimal exposure to subdued light, and use low-actinic glassware to protect solutions from light.]
Ferric chloride solution—Dissolve 10.5 g of ferric chloride in 100 mL of water.
Methanolic magnesium acetate solution—Dissolve 5.0 g of magnesium acetate in 1 L of methanol.
Sodium bicarbonate solution—Dissolve 5.0 g of sodium bicarbonate in 1 L of water.
Standard preparation—Dissolve accurately weighed quantities of USP Sennosides RS in *Sodium bicarbonate solution* to obtain a solution having a known concentration of about 0.13 mg per mL.
Assay preparation—Weigh and pulverize about 10 g of Senna Leaf. Transfer about 0.15 g, accurately weighed, to a 100-mL round-bottom flask, add 30 mL of water, mix, weigh, attach a condenser, and reflux in a water bath for 15 minutes. Cool to room temperature, weigh, and adjust to the original weight with water. Centrifuge, and transfer 20.0 mL of the supernatant to a 150-mL separatory funnel. Add 0.1 mL of diluted hydrochloric acid, and shake with three quantities, each of 15 mL, of chloroform. Allow to separate, and discard the chloroform layer after each addition. Add about 0.1 g of sodium bicarbonate, shake for 3 minutes, and centrifuge. Use the supernatant as the *Assay preparation*.

Procedure—Transfer 10.0 mL each of the *Standard preparation* and the *Assay preparation* to separate 100-mL round-bottom flasks equipped with condensers, add 20 mL of *Ferric chloride solution*, and mix. Reflux in a water bath for 20 minutes. Add 1 mL of hydrochloric acid, and reflux for an additional 20 minutes, with frequent shaking, to dissolve the precipitates. Cool to room temperature, transfer the mixtures to separate 100-mL separatory funnels, and shake with three quantities, each of 25 mL, of ether previously used to rinse the flasks. Combine the ether extracts, mix, and wash with two quantities, each of 15 mL, of water. Tranfer the ether layers to separate 100-mL volumetric flasks, dilute with ether to volume, and mix. Evaporate 10.0 mL of the ether extracts to dryness, and dissolve the residue in 10.0 mL of *Methanolic magnesium acetate solution*. Determine the absorbance of the resulting solution from the *Standard preparation* and the *Assay preparation* at 515 nm, with a suitable spectrophotometer fitted with matched quartz cells, using methanol as the blank. Calculate the percentage of sennosides in the Senna Leaf by the formula:

$$3000(A_U / A_S)(C_S / W)$$

in which A_U and A_S are the absorbances of the solutions from the *Assay preparation* and the *Standard preparation*, respectively; C_S is the concentration, in mg per mL, of sennosides in the *Standard preparation*; and W is the weight, in mg, of powdered Senna Leaf used.

Senna Fluidextract

» Prepare Senna Fluidextract as follows.
Mix 1000 g of Senna, in coarse powder, with a sufficient quantity (600 mL to 800 mL) of menstruum consisting of a mixture of 1 volume of alcohol and 2 volumes of water to make it evenly and distinctly damp. After 15 minutes, pack the mixture firmly into a suitable percolator, and cover the drug with additional menstruum. Macerate for 24 hours, then percolate at a moderate rate, adding fresh menstruum, until the drug is practically exhausted of its active principles. Reserve the first 800 mL of percolate, and use it to dissolve the residue from the additional percolate that has been concentrated to a soft extract at a temperature not to exceed 60°. Add water and alcohol to make the product measure 1000 mL, and mix.

Packaging and storage—Preserve in tight, light-resistant containers, and avoid exposure to direct sunlight and to excessive heat.
Alcohol content, *Method I* ⟨611⟩: between 23.0% and 27.0% of C_2H_5OH.

Senna Pods

» Senna Pods are the dried ripe fruits of *Senna alexandrina* Mill also known as *Cassia acutifolia* Delile (Alexandrian senna) or *C. angustifolia* Vahl (Tinnevelly senna) (Fam. Fabaceae). Senna Pods contain not less than 3.4 percent (Alexandrian senna) and not less than 2.2 percent (Tinnevelly senna), of anthraquinone glucosides, calculated as sennosides, on the dried basis.

Packaging and storage—Preserve against attack by insects and rodents (see *Vegetable and Animal Drugs—Preservation* in the *General Notices*). Store protected from light and moisture, at room temperature.

Labeling—The label states the Latin binomial and, following the official name, the part of the plant contained in the article.

USP Reference standards ⟨11⟩—*USP Sennosides RS*.
Botanic characteristics—
Unground Alexandrian senna pods—Occur as flattened, reniform, membranous, leathery pods; green to greenish-brown with brown patches at the positions corresponding to the seeds; from 40 to 50 mm in length and at least 20 mm wide; at one end is a stylar point and at the other a short stalk. The pods contain six or seven flattened and obovate seeds, green to pale brown, with a continuous network of prominent ridges on the testa.
Unground Tinnevelly senna pods—Occur as flattened, slightly reniform, membranous, leathery pods; brown to yellowish-brown with brown patches at the positions corresponding to the seeds; slightly longer but narrower than Alexandrian senna pods, from 35 to 60 mm in length and 14 to 18 mm wide; at one end is a stylar point and at the other a short stalk. The pods contain five to eight flattened and obovate seeds, green to pale brown, with incomplete, wavy, transverse ridges on the testa.
Histology—Senna pods show epicarp with very thick cuticulized polygonal cells, occasional anomocytic or paracytic stomata, and very few nonglandular, one-celled, conical, often curved hairs, with thick papillose walls, from 100 to 350 μm in length; mesocarp consists of parenchymatous tissue containing a layer of calcium oxalate prisms and vascular bundles partially enclosed by fibers; endocarp with two crossed layers of fibers; seeds with a subepidermal layer of palisade cells with thick outer walls and endosperm of polyhedral cells with mucilaginous walls.
Powdered senna pods—Brown powder displaying polygonal cells with occasional small numbers of nonglandular hairs and anomocytic or paracytic stomata, fibers in two crossed layers accompanied by a crystal sheath of calcium oxalate prisms, isolated hairs, masses of palisade cells of the seeds, clusters, and prisms of calcium oxalate.
Identification—Proceed as directed in the *Identification* test under *Senna Leaf*, except to use 500 mg of finely powdered Senna Pods.
Microbial enumeration ⟨2021⟩—The total bacterial count does not exceed 10^5 cfu per g, the total combined molds and yeasts count does not exceed 10^3 cfu per g, the bile-tolerant Gram-negative bacteria does not exceed 10^3 cfu per g, and it meets the requirements of the tests for absence of *Salmonella* species and *Escherichia coli*.
Loss on drying ⟨731⟩—Dry 1.0 g of finely powdered Senna Pods at 105° for 2 hours: it loses not more than 12.0% of its weight.
Foreign organic matter ⟨561⟩: not more than 1.0%.
Total ash ⟨561⟩: not more than 9.0%.
Acid-insoluble ash ⟨561⟩: not more than 2.0%.
Assay—Proceed as directed in the *Assay* under *Senna Leaf*, using 0.15 g of finely powdered Senna Pods to prepare the *Assay preparation*.

Senna Oral Solution

» Prepare Senna Oral Solution as follows:

Senna Fluidextract	250 mL
Suitable essential oil(s)	
Sucrose	635 g
Purified Water, a sufficient quantity, to make	1000 mL

Mix the oil(s) with the Senna Fluidextract, and gradually add 330 mL of Purified Water. Allow the mixture to stand for 24 hours in a cool place, with occasional agitation, then filter, and pass enough Purified Water through the filter to obtain 580 mL of filtrate. Dissolve the Sucrose in this liquid, and add sufficient Purified

Water to make the product measure 1000 mL. Mix, and strain.

Packaging and storage—Preserve in tight containers, at a temperature not exceeding 25°.

Alcohol content, *Method I* ⟨611⟩: between 90.0% and 110.0% of the labeled amount of C₂H₅OH.

Sennosides

» Sennosides is a partially purified natural complex of anthraquinone glucosides, isolated from senna leaflets and/or senna pods, *Senna alexandrina* Mill (*Cassia acutifolia* or *C. angustifolia*), as calcium salts. It contains not less than 90.0 percent and not more than 110.0 percent of the labeled amount of sennosides. The labeled amount is not less than 60.0 percent (w/w), calculated on the dried basis.

Packaging and storage—Preserve in well-closed containers. Store protected from light and moisture, at controlled room temperature.

USP Reference standards ⟨11⟩—*USP Sennosides RS*.

Identification—Place equal volumes of ethyl acetate, *n*-propyl alcohol, and water in a separator, shake, and discard the upper layer. Add a sufficient quantity of Sennosides to obtain a solution having a concentration of 1 mg per mL. Prepare similarly a Standard solution of USP Sennosides RS. Apply 20-μL portions of each solution, as 1-cm streaks, on a line about 2.5 cm from the bottom edge of a thin-layer chromatographic plate (see *Chromatography* ⟨621⟩) coated with a 0.25-mm layer of chromatographic silica gel mixture. Develop the chromatogram in a solvent system consisting of a mixture of ethyl acetate, *n*-propyl alcohol, and water (4 : 4 : 3) until the solvent front has moved about 15 cm. Remove the plate from the developing chamber, air-dry, and examine under long-wavelength UV light. Expose the plate to ammonium hydroxide vapor until color develops (about 5 minutes). Cover the plate with a piece of glass, and heat at 120° for 5 minutes: the 2 most prominent spots from the test solution corresponds in color and mobility to those from the Standard solution.

pH ⟨791⟩: between 6.3 and 7.3, in a solution (1 in 10).

Loss on drying ⟨731⟩—Dry it in vacuum at 100° to constant weight: it loses not more than 5.0% of its weight.

Residue on ignition ⟨281⟩: between 5.0% and 8.0%, ignited at 800 ± 25°, the use of sulfuric acid being omitted.

Heavy metals, *Method II* ⟨231⟩: 0.006%.

Assay—

pH 7.0 phosphate buffer—Dissolve 4.54 g of monobasic potassium phosphate in water to make 500 mL of solution. Dissolve 4.73 g of anhydrous dibasic sodium phosphate in water to make 500 mL of solution. Mix 38.9 mL of the monobasic potassium phosphate solution with 61.1 mL of the dibasic sodium phosphate solution. Adjust dropwise, if necessary, with the dibasic sodium phosphate solution to a pH of 7.0.

Borate solution—Dissolve 75.80 g of sodium borate in water, dilute with water to 2000 mL, and mix.

Sodium dithionite solution—Prepare a 1.5 in 100 solution of sodium dithionite in water.

Standard preparation—Dissolve about 25 mg of USP Sennosides RS, accurately weighed, in *pH 7.0 phosphate buffer* in a 25-mL volumetric flask with the aid of an ultrasonic bath, dilute with *pH 7.0 phosphate buffer* to volume, and mix.

Assay preparation—Dissolve about 25 mg of Sennosides, accurately weighed, in *pH 7.0 phosphate buffer* in a 25-mL volumetric flask, with the aid of an ultrasonic bath, dilute with *pH 7.0 phosphate buffer* to volume, and mix.

Procedure—Pipet 1-mL portions of the *Standard preparation* and the *Assay preparation* into separate 100-mL volumetric flasks, dilute with *Borate solution* to volume, and mix. Transfer 5.0-mL portions of each of the resulting solutions to separate low-actinic glass, 50-mL volumetric flasks, and add 15 mL of *Borate solution* and 15.0 mL of *Sodium dithionite solution*. Pass nitrogen through the solutions, seal the flasks with nitrogen-filled balloons, and heat in a water bath for 30 minutes. Cool the flasks for 15 minutes in a water bath thermostatically controlled at 20°. Dilute the solutions with *Borate solution* to volume, and mix. Determine without delay the fluorescence intensities of the resulting solutions in a fluorometer at an excitation wavelength of 392 nm and an emission wavelength of 505 nm, the time elapsed between the addition of the *Sodium dithionite solution* and the measurement being the same for the two solutions. Calculate the quantity, in mg, of sennosides in the Sennosides taken by the formula:

$$25C(I_U / I_S)$$

in which C is the concentration, in mg per mL, of USP Sennosides RS, corrected for loss on drying, in the *Standard preparation*, and I_U and I_S are the fluorescence values observed for the solutions from the *Assay preparation* and the *Standard preparation*, respectively.

Sennosides Tablets

» Sennosides Tablets contain not less than 90.0 percent and not more than 110.0 percent of the labeled amount of Sennosides.

Packaging and storage—Preserve in well-closed containers.

USP Reference standards ⟨11⟩—*USP Sennosides RS*.

Identification—A portion of finely powdered Tablets, equivalent to about 20 mg of sennosides, responds to the *Identification* test under *Sennosides*.

Dissolution ⟨711⟩—

Medium: water; 900 mL.

Apparatus 1: 100 rpm.

Time: 120 minutes.

Procedure—Determine the amount of sennosides dissolved, employing the procedure set forth in the *Assay*, making any necessary volumetric adjustments.

Tolerances—Not less than 75% (*Q*) of the labeled amount of sennosides is dissolved in 120 minutes.

Uniformity of dosage units ⟨905⟩: meet the requirements.

Assay—

pH 7.0 phosphate buffer, Borate solution, Sodium dithionite solution, and *Standard preparation*—Prepare as directed in the *Assay* under *Sennosides*.

Assay preparation—Weigh and finely powder not less than 20 Tablets. Transfer an accurately weighed portion of the powder, equivalent to about 25 mg of sennosides, to a 25-mL volumetric flask. Add 20 mL of *pH 7.0 phosphate buffer*, sonicate to dissolve the sennosides, add *pH 7.0 phosphate buffer* to volume, and mix. Centrifuge the resulting suspension for 15 minutes at 3500 rpm. The supernatant is the *Assay preparation*.

Procedure—Proceed as directed for *Procedure* in the *Assay* under *Sennosides*. Calculate the quantity, in mg, of sennosides in the portion of Tablets taken by the formula:

$$25C(I_U / I_S)$$

in which C is the concentration, in mg per mL, of USP Sennosides RS, corrected for loss on drying, in the *Standard preparation*, and I_U and I_S are the fluorescence values observed for the solutions from the *Assay preparation* and the *Standard preparation,* respectively.

Serine

C₃H₇NO₃ 105.09
L-Serine
L-Serine [56-45-1].

» Serine contains not less than 98.5 percent and not more than 101.5 percent of C₃H₇NO₃, as L-serine, calculated on the dried basis.

Packaging and storage—Preserve in well-closed containers.
USP Reference standards ⟨11⟩—*USP L-Methionine RS. USP L-Serine RS.*
Identification, *Infrared Absorption* ⟨197K⟩.
Specific rotation ⟨781S⟩: between +14.0° and +15.6°.
  Test solution: 100 mg per mL, in 2 N hydrochloric acid.
Loss on drying ⟨731⟩—Dry it at 105° for 3 hours: it loses not more than 0.2% of its weight.
Residue on ignition ⟨281⟩: not more than 0.1%.
Chloride ⟨221⟩—A 0.73-g portion shows no more chloride than corresponds to 0.50 mL of 0.020 N hydrochloric acid (0.05%).
Sulfate ⟨221⟩—A 0.33-g portion shows no more sulfate than corresponds to 0.10 mL of 0.020 N sulfuric acid (0.03%).
Iron ⟨241⟩: 0.003%.
Heavy metals, *Method I* ⟨231⟩: 0.0015%.
Chromatographic purity—
  Adsorbent: 0.25-mm layer of chromatographic silica gel mixture.
  Test solution—Dissolve an accurately weighed quantity of Serine in 0.1 N hydrochloric acid to obtain a solution having a concentration of 10 mg per mL. Apply 5 µL.
  Standard solution—Dissolve an accurately weighed quantity of USP L-Serine RS in 0.1 N hydrochloric acid to obtain a solution having a known concentration of about 0.05 mg per mL. Apply 5 µL. [NOTE—This solution has a concentration equivalent to about 0.5% of that of the *Test solution.*]
  System suitability solution—Prepare a solution in 0.1 N hydrochloric acid containing 0.4 mg each of USP L-Serine RS and USP L-Methionine RS per mL. Apply 5 µL.
  Spray reagent—Dissolve 0.2 g of ninhydrin in 100 mL of a mixture of butyl alcohol and 2 N acetic acid (95 : 5).
  Developing solvent system—Prepare a mixture of butyl alcohol, glacial acetic acid, and water (60 : 20 : 20).
  Procedure—Proceed as directed for *Thin-Layer Chromatography* under *Chromatography* ⟨621⟩. After air-drying the plate, spray with *Spray reagent,* and heat between 100° and 105° for about 15 minutes. Examine the plate under white light. The chromatogram obtained from the *System suitability solution* exhibits two clearly separated spots. Any secondary spot in the chromatogram obtained from the *Test solution* is not larger or more intense than the principal spot in the chromatogram obtained from the *Standard solution:* not more than 0.5% of any individual impurity is found; and not more than 2.0% of total impurities is found.
Organic volatile impurities, *Method I* ⟨467⟩: meets the requirements.

(Official until July 1, 2008)

Assay—Transfer about 100 mg of Serine, accurately weighed, to a 125-mL flask, dissolve in a mixture of 3 mL of formic acid and 50 mL of glacial acetic acid, and titrate with 0.1 N perchloric acid VS, determining the endpoint potentiometrically. Perform a blank determination, and make any necessary correction. Each mL of 0.1 N perchloric acid is equivalent to 10.51 mg of C₃H₇NO₃.

Silver Nitrate

AgNO₃ 169.87
Nitric acid silver(1+) salt.
Silver(1+) nitrate [7761-88-8].

» Silver Nitrate, powdered and then dried in the dark over silica gel for 4 hours, contains not less than 99.8 percent and not more than 100.5 percent of AgNO₃.

Packaging and storage—Preserve in tight, light-resistant containers.
Clarity and color of solution—A solution of 2 g in 20 mL of water is clear and colorless.
Identification—
  A: A solution (1 in 50) responds to the tests for *Silver* ⟨191⟩.
  B: Mix a solution (1 in 10) in a test tube with 1 drop of diphenylamine TS, and then carefully superimpose it upon sulfuric acid: a deep blue color appears at the zone of contact.
Copper—To 5 mL of a solution (1 in 10) add 6 N ammonium hydroxide, dropwise, until a precipitate first formed is just dissolved: no blue color is produced.
Assay—Powder about 1 g of Silver Nitrate, and dry in the dark over silica gel for 4 hours. Weigh accurately about 700 mg of this dried salt, dissolve in 50 mL of water, add 2 mL of nitric acid and 2 mL of ferric ammonium sulfate TS, and titrate with 0.1 N ammonium thiocyanate VS. Each mL of 0.1 N ammonium thiocyanate is equivalent to 16.99 mg of AgNO₃.

Silver Nitrate Ophthalmic Solution

» Silver Nitrate Ophthalmic Solution is a solution of Silver Nitrate in a water medium. It contains not less than 0.95 percent and not more than 1.05 percent of AgNO₃. The solution may be buffered by the addition of Sodium Acetate.

Packaging and storage—Preserve it protected from light, in inert, collapsible capsules or in other suitable single-dose containers.
Clarity and color of solution—It is clear and colorless.
Identification—It responds to the tests for *Silver* ⟨191⟩ and for *Nitrate* ⟨191⟩.
Sterility ⟨71⟩: meets the requirements.
pH ⟨791⟩: between 4.5 and 6.0.
Assay—Place 5 mL of Ophthalmic Solution, accurately measured, in a conical flask, dilute with 20 mL of water, add 1 mL of nitric acid and 1 mL of ferric ammonium sulfate TS, and titrate with 0.02 N ammonium thiocyanate VS. Each mL of 0.02 N ammonium thiocyanate is equivalent to 3.397 mg of AgNO₃.

Toughened Silver Nitrate

» Toughened Silver Nitrate contains not less than 94.5 percent of AgNO₃, the remainder consisting of silver chloride (AgCl).

Packaging and storage—Preserve in tight, light-resistant containers.
Identification—
  A: A solution (1 in 50) responds to the tests for *Silver* ⟨191⟩.
  B: Mix a solution (1 in 10) in a test tube with 1 drop of diphenylamine TS, then carefully superimpose it upon sulfuric acid: a deep blue color appears at the zone of contact.
Copper—A solution (1 in 10) shows no trace of blue coloration when treated with an excess of 6 N ammonium hydroxide.

Assay—Add about 700 mg of Toughened Silver Nitrate, accurately weighed, to 50 mL of water, and when the silver nitrate has dissolved, filter the solution. Thoroughly wash the filter and sediment with water, add 2 mL of nitric acid and 2 mL of ferric ammonium sulfate TS to the combined filtrate and washings, and titrate with 0.1 N ammonium thiocyanate VS. Each mL of 0.1 N ammonium thiocyanate is equivalent to 16.99 mg of AgNO$_3$.

Simethicone

Simethicone.

α-(Trimethylsilyl)-ω-methylpoly[oxy(dimethylsilylene)], mixture with silicon dioxide [8050-81-5].

» Simethicone is a mixture of fully methylated linear siloxane polymers containing repeating units of the formula [–(CH$_3$)$_2$SiO–]$_n$, stabilized with trimethylsiloxy end-blocking units of the formula [(CH$_3$)$_3$SiO–], and silicon dioxide. It contains not less than 90.5 percent and not more than 99.0 percent of polydimethylsiloxane ([–(CH$_3$)$_2$SiO–]$_n$), and not less than 4.0 percent and not more than 7.0 percent of silicon dioxide.

Packaging and storage—Preserve in tight containers.
USP Reference standards ⟨11⟩—*USP Polydimethylsiloxane RS. USP Simethicone RS.*
Identification, *Infrared Absorption*⟨197F⟩.
Defoaming activity—
  Foaming solution—Dissolve 1 g of octoxynol 9 in 100 mL of water.
  Test preparation—Transfer 200 mg of Simethicone to a 60-mL bottle, add 50 mL of tertiary butyl alcohol, cap the bottle, and shake vigorously. [NOTE—Warm slightly, if necessary, to dissolve.]
  Procedure—[NOTE—For each test, employ a clean, unused, 250-mL glass jar.] Add, dropwise, 500 µL of the *Test preparation* to a clean, unused, cylindrical 250-mL glass jar, fitted with a 50-mm cap, containing 100 mL of the *Foaming solution*. Cap the jar, and clamp it in an upright position on a wrist-action shaker. Employing a radius of 13.3 ± 0.4 cm (measured from center of shaft to center of bottle), shake for 10 seconds through an arc of 10 degrees at a frequency of 300 ± 30 strokes per minute. Record the time required for the foam to collapse. The time, in seconds, for foam collapse is determined at the instant the first portion of foam-free liquid surface appears, measured from the end of the shaking period. The defoaming activity time does not exceed 15 seconds.
Loss on heating—Heat about 15 g, accurately weighed, in an open, tared vessel having a diameter of 5.5 ± 0.5 cm and a wall height of 2.5 ± 1.0 cm at 200° in a circulating air oven for 4 hours, and allow to come to room temperature in a desiccator before weighing: it loses not more than 18.0% of its weight.
Heavy metals—Mix 1.0 g of Simethicone with 10 mL of chloroform, and dilute with the same solvent to 20 mL. Add 1.0 mL of a freshly prepared 0.002% solution of dithizone in chloroform, 0.5 mL of water, and 0.5 mL of a mixture of 1 volume of ammonia TS and 9 volumes of a 0.2% solution of hydroxylamine hydrochloride. Concomitantly prepare a Standard solution as follows: to 20 mL of chloroform add 1.0 mL of a freshly prepared 0.002% solution of dithizone in chloroform, 0.5 mL of *Standard Lead Solution* (see *Heavy Metals* ⟨231⟩) (containing 10 µg of lead per mL) and 0.5 mL of a mixture of 1 volume of ammonia TS and 9 volumes of a 0.2% solution of hydroxylamine hydrochloride. Immediately shake both solutions vigorously for 1 minute. Any red color in the test solution is not more intense than that in the Standard solution (5 µg per g).
Organic volatile impurities, *Method IV* ⟨467⟩: meets the requirements.

(Official until July 1, 2008)

Content of silicon dioxide—Transfer 3.00 g of Simethicone to a screw-capped bottle, add 10.0 mL of *n*-hexane, cap, and mix by shaking (*Test solution*). Prepare a *Standard solution* by similarly treating a 3.00-g portion of USP Simethicone RS. Prepare a *Dimethicone preparation* by similarly treating a 3.00-g portion of dimethicone having a viscosity of 500 centistokes. Using an IR spectrophotometer and 0.1-mm cells, determine the absorbance spectra of well-mixed portions of the *Test solution*, the *Standard solution*, and the *Dimethicone preparation* between 7 and 9 µm, using *n*-hexane as the blank. Determine the absorbances of the *Test solution*, the *Standard solution*, and the *Dimethicone preparation* at the wavelength of minimum absorbance at about 8.2 µm observed in the spectrum obtained from the *Dimethicone preparation*. Calculate the percentage of silicon dioxide in the Simethicone taken by the formula:

$$C(A_U - A_D)/(A_S - A_D)$$

in which *C* is the designated percentage of silicon dioxide in USP Simethicone RS; A_U is the absorbance of the *Test solution*; A_D is the absorbance of the *Dimethicone preparation*; and A_S is the absorbance of the *Standard solution*.

Assay—Transfer about 50 mg of Simethicone, accurately weighed, to a round, narrow-mouth, screw-capped, 120-mL bottle, add 25.0 mL of toluene, and swirl to disperse. Add 50 mL of dilute hydrochloric acid (2 in 5), close the bottle securely with a cap having an inert liner, and shake for 5 minutes, accurately timed, on a reciprocating shaker at a suitable rate (e.g., about 200 oscillations per minute and a stroke of 38 ± 2 mm). Transfer the mixture to a 125-mL separator, and remove about 5 mL of the upper organic (toluene) layer to a 15-mL screw-capped test tube containing 0.5 g of anhydrous sodium sulfate. Close the tube with a screw-cap having an inert liner, agitate vigorously, and centrifuge the mixture until a clear supernatant (*Assay preparation*) is obtained. Prepare a *Standard preparation* by similarly treating a 25.0-mL portion of a solution of USP Polydimethylsiloxane RS in toluene having a known concentration of about 2 mg per mL. Prepare a procedural blank by similarly treating 25.0 mL of toluene. Concomitantly determine the absorbances of the solutions in 0.5-mm cells at the wavelength of maximum absorbance at about 7.9 µm, with an IR spectrophotometer, using the blank to set the instrument. Calculate the quantity, in mg, of [–(CH$_3$)$_2$SiO–]$_n$ in the Simethicone taken by the formula:

$$25C(A_U / A_S)$$

in which *C* is the concentration, in mg per mL, of USP Polydimethylsiloxane RS in the *Standard preparation*; and A_U and A_S are the absorbances of the *Assay preparation* and the *Standard preparation*, respectively.

Simethicone Capsules

» Simethicone Capsules contain an amount of polydimethylsiloxane ([–(CH$_3$)$_2$SiO–]$_n$) that is not less than 85.0 percent and not more than 115.0 percent of the labeled amount of simethicone.

Packaging and storage—Preserve in well-closed containers.
USP Reference standards ⟨11⟩—*USP Polydimethylsiloxane RS.*
Identification, *Infrared Absorption* ⟨197S⟩—[NOTE—Use the procedural blank, prepared as directed in the *Assay*, to set the instrument.]
  Test solution—Prepare as directed for the *Assay preparation* in the *Assay*.
  Standard solution—Prepare as directed for the *Standard preparation* in the *Assay*.
  Cell size: 0.5 mm.
Disintegration ⟨701⟩: 30 minutes.
Uniformity of dosage units ⟨905⟩: meet the requirements.
Defoaming activity—It meets the requirements of the test for *Defoaming activity* under *Simethicone Oral Suspension*, a quantity of Capsule contents equivalent to 20 mg of simethicone being used.

Assay—[NOTE—Perform this procedure on at least 3 individual Capsules. The mean of the assay values obtained is the assay value.] Transfer 1 Capsule to a round, narrow-mouth, screw-capped, 120-mL bottle, add about 20 mL of 6 N hydrochloric acid, and allow to stand, with frequent swirling, until the Capsule has dissolved. Add 10.0 mL of toluene, accurately measured, for each 25 mg of the labeled amount of simethicone in the Capsule, close the bottle securely with a cap having an inert liner, and shake by mechanical means for 5 minutes. Allow the phases to separate, draw off 10 mL of the upper organic (toluene) layer to a test tube containing 0.5 g of anhydrous sodium sulfate, agitate vigorously for 30 seconds, and allow the mixture to settle. If necessary, centrifuge the mixture to obtain a clear solution (*Assay preparation*). Prepare a *Standard preparation* by similarly treating a solution of USP Polydimethylsiloxane RS in toluene having a known concentration of about 2.5 mg per mL. Prepare a procedural blank by similarly treating 10.0 mL of toluene. Concomitantly determine the absorbances of the solutions in 0.5-mm cells at the wavelength of maximum absorbance at about 7.9 µm, with an IR spectrophotometer, using the blank to set the instrument. Calculate the quantity, in mg, of [–(CH$_3$)$_2$SiO–]$_n$ in the Capsule taken by the formula:

$$VC(A_U / A_S)$$

in which V is the volume, in mL, of toluene taken to prepare the *Assay preparation*; C is the concentration, in mg per mL, of USP Polydimethylsiloxane RS in the Standard solution; and A_U and A_S are the absorbances of the *Assay preparation* and the *Standard preparation*, respectively.

Simethicone Emulsion

» Simethicone Emulsion is a water-dispersible form of Simethicone composed of Simethicone, suitable emulsifiers, preservatives, and water. It may contain suitable viscosity-increasing agents. It contains an amount of polydimethylsiloxane ([–(CH$_3$)$_2$SiO–]$_n$) that is not less than 85.0 percent and not more than 110.0 percent of the labeled amount of simethicone.

Packaging and storage—Preserve in tight containers.

USP Reference standards ⟨11⟩—*USP Polydimethylsiloxane RS*.
Identification—The IR absorption spectrum, determined in a 0.5-mm cell, of the solution of Emulsion prepared as directed in the *Assay*, exhibits maxima only at the same wavelengths as that of a similar preparation of USP Polydimethylsiloxane RS. If necessary, the dilute hydrochloric acid may be omitted to improve separation. [NOTE—Prepare a procedural blank by similarly treating 25.0 mL of toluene, and use this blank to set the instrument.]
Microbial limits ⟨61⟩—Its total aerobic microbial count does not exceed 100 cfu per g.
Heavy metals—Using Simethicone Emulsion instead of Simethicone, proceed as directed for *Heavy metals* under *Simethicone*. The limit is 5 µg per g.
Defoaming activity—
Foaming solution—Dissolve 1 g of octoxynol 9 in 100 mL of water.
Test preparation—Transfer an accurately weighed quantity of Emulsion, equivalent to 300 mg of simethicone, to a 60-mL bottle, dilute with water to 30 g, cap the bottle, and shake vigorously.
Procedure—Proceed as directed for *Procedure* in the test for *Defoaming activity* under *Simethicone*. The defoaming activity time does not exceed 15 seconds.
Assay—Transfer an accurately weighed quantity of Emulsion, equivalent to about 50 mg of simethicone, to a round, narrow-mouth, screw-capped, 120-mL bottle, add 25.0 mL of toluene, and swirl to disperse. Proceed as directed in the *Assay* under *Simethicone*, beginning with "Add 50 mL of dilute hydrochloric acid." Calculate the quantity, in mg, of [–(CH$_3$)$_2$SiO–]$_n$ in each g of the Emulsion taken by the formula:

$$(25C/S)(A_U / A_S)$$

in which C is the concentration, in mg per mL, of USP Polydimethylsiloxane RS in the *Standard preparation*; S is the weight, in g, of Emulsion taken; and A_U and A_S are the absorbances of the *Assay preparation* and the *Standard preparation*, respectively.

Simethicone Oral Suspension

» Simethicone Oral Suspension is a suspension of Simethicone in Water. It contains an amount of polydimethylsiloxane ([–(CH$_3$)$_2$SiO–]$_n$) that is not less than 85.0 percent and not more than 115.0 percent of the labeled amount of simethicone.

Packaging and storage—Preserve in tight, light-resistant containers.

USP Reference standards ⟨11⟩—*USP Polydimethylsiloxane RS*.
Identification, *Infrared Absorption* ⟨197S⟩—[NOTE—Use the procedural blank, prepared as directed in the *Assay*, to set the instrument.]
Test solution—Prepare as directed for the *Assay preparation* in the *Assay*.
Standard solution—Prepare as directed for the *Standard preparation* in the *Assay*.
Cell size: 0.5 mm.
pH ⟨791⟩: between 3.5 and 4.6.
Defoaming activity—
Foaming solution—Dissolve 500 µg of FD&C Blue No. 1 and 1 g of octoxynol 9 in 100 mL of water.
Procedure—[NOTE—For each test, employ a clean, unused, 250-mL glass jar.] Transfer a volume of Oral Suspension, equivalent to 20 mg of simethicone, to a clean, unused, cylindrical 250-mL glass jar, fitted with a 50-mm cap, containing 100 mL of *Foaming solution* that has been warmed to 37°. Proceed as directed for *Procedure* in the test for *Defoaming activity* under *Simethicone*, beginning with "Cap the jar." The defoaming activity time does not exceed 45 seconds.
Assay—
Standard preparation—Transfer about 60 mg of USP Polydimethylsiloxane RS, accurately weighed, to a 25-mL volumetric flask, add 15 mL of hexanes, and sonicate for 3 minutes. Allow to cool, dilute with hexanes to volume, and mix. Transfer 10 mL of this solution to a capped test tube, add about 1 g of anhydrous sodium sulfate, mix for about 1 minute, and centrifuge. Use the clear supernatant as the *Standard preparation*. The *Standard preparation* has a concentration of about 2.4 mg of USP Polydimethylsiloxane RS per mL.
Assay preparation—Transfer an accurately measured quantity of Oral Suspension, equivalent to about 240 mg of simethicone, to a glass-stoppered centrifuge tube. Add 5 mL of methanol, and mix for about 15 seconds. Add 30.0 mL of hexanes, and mix for about 10 seconds. Loosen the stopper, and heat the tube for about 10 minutes in a water bath at 65 ± 1°. Mix for 1 minute, and centrifuge. Using a glass syringe, transfer the upper hexanes layer to a 100-mL volumetric flask. Repeat the extraction with two 30.0-mL portions of hexanes, combining the hexanes extracts in the 100-mL volumetric flask. [NOTE—If an emulsion forms during any of the extractions, as much as 2 mL of methanol may be added to disperse the emulsion.] Allow the combined extracts to cool, dilute with hexanes to volume, and mix. Transfer 10 mL of this solution to a capped test tube, add about 1 g of anhydrous sodium sulfate, mix for about 1 minute, and centrifuge. Use the clear supernatant as the *Assay preparation*.
Dry hexanes—Mix 100 mL of hexanes and 10 g of anhydrous sodium sulfate, allow to settle, and centrifuge. Use the clear supernatant.
Procedure—Concomitantly determine the absorbances of the *Standard preparation* and the *Assay preparation* at the wavelength of maximum absorption at about 7.9 µm, using *Dry hexanes* as the

blank to set the instrument. Calculate the quantity, in mg, of $[-(CH_3)_2SiO-]_n$ in each mL of the Oral Suspension taken by the formula:

$$(100C/V)(A_U/A_S)$$

in which C is the concentration, in mg per mL, of USP Polydimethylsiloxane RS in the *Standard preparation*; V is the volume, in mL, of Oral Suspension taken; and A_U and A_S are the absorbances of the *Assay preparation* and the *Standard preparation*, respectively.

Simethicone Tablets

» Simethicone Tablets contain an amount of polydimethylsiloxane ($[-(CH_3)_2SiO-]_n$) that is not less than 85.0 percent and not more than 115.0 percent of the labeled amount of simethicone.

Packaging and storage—Preserve in well-closed containers.

Labeling—Tablets that are gelatin-coated are so labeled.

USP Reference standards ⟨11⟩—*USP Polydimethylsiloxane RS*.

Identification, *Infrared Absorption* ⟨197S⟩—[NOTE—Use the procedural blank, prepared as directed in the *Assay*, to set the instrument.]

Test solution—Prepare as directed for the *Assay preparation* in the *Assay*.

Standard solution—Prepare as directed for the *Standard preparation* in the *Assay*.

Cell size: 0.5 mm.

Disintegration ⟨701⟩: 30 minutes; 60 minutes for plain-coated Tablets; and 45 minutes for Tablets labeled as gelatin-coated, simulated gastric fluid being used as the medium.

Uniformity of dosage units ⟨905⟩: meet the requirements.

Defoaming activity—

Foaming solution—Dissolve 500 μg of FD&C Blue No. 1 and 1 g of octoxynol 9 in 100 mL of water, except that where the Tablets are labeled as gelatin-coated, use 0.1 N hydrochloric acid instead of water.

Procedure—[NOTE—For each test, employ a clean, unused, 250-mL glass jar.] Transfer a quantity of finely powdered Tablets, equivalent to 20 mg of simethicone, to a clean, unused, cylindrical 250-mL glass jar, fitted with a 50-mm cap, containing 100 mL of *Foaming solution* that has been warmed to 37°. Proceed as directed for *Procedure* in the test for *Defoaming activity* under *Simethicone*, beginning with "Cap the jar." The defoaming activity time does not exceed 45 seconds.

Assay—Weigh and finely powder not fewer than 20 Tablets. Transfer an accurately weighed portion of the powder, equivalent to about 50 mg of simethicone, to a round, narrow-mouth, screw-capped, 120-mL bottle, and proceed as directed in the *Assay* under *Simethicone*, beginning with "add 25.0 mL of toluene," except that for Tablets labeled as gelatin-coated, shake for 30 minutes instead of 5 minutes. Calculate the quantity, in mg, of $[-(CH_3)_2SiO-]_n$ in the portion of Tablets taken by the formula:

$$25C(A_U/A_S)$$

in which C is the concentration, in mg per mL, of USP Polydimethylsiloxane RS in the Standard solution, and A_U and A_S are the absorbances of the solution from the Tablets and the Standard solution, respectively.

Simvastatin

$C_{25}H_{38}O_5$ 418.57

Butanoic acid, 2,2-dimethyl-, 1,2,3,7,8,8a-hexahydro-3,7-dimethyl-8-[2-(tetrahydro-4-hydroxy-6-oxo-2H-pyran-2-yl)ethyl]-1-naphthalenyl ester, [1S-[1α,3α,7β,8β(2S*,4S*),8aβ]].

2,2-Dimethylbutyric acid, 8-ester with (4R,6R)-6-2-[(1S,2S,6R,8S,8αR)-1,2,6,7,8,8a-hexahydro-8-hydroxy-2,6-dimethyl-1-naphthyl]ethyl]tetrahydro-4-hydroxy-2H-pyran-2-one   [79902-63-9].

» Simvastatin contains not less than 98.0 percent and not more than 101.0 percent of $C_{25}H_{38}O_5$, calculated on the dried basis. It may contain a suitable antioxidant.

Packaging and storage—Preserve in well-closed containers. Store between 15° and 30°, or under refrigeration.

USP Reference standards ⟨11⟩—*USP Lovastatin RS. USP Simvastatin RS*.

Identification—
 A: *Infrared Absorption* ⟨197M⟩.
 B: The retention time of the major peak in the chromatogram of the *Assay preparation* corresponds to that in the chromatogram of the *Standard preparation*, as obtained in the *Assay*.

Specific rotation ⟨781S⟩: between +285° and +298°.

Test solution: 5 mg per mL, in acetonitrile.

Loss on drying ⟨731⟩—Dry it in vacuum at 60° for 3 hours: it loses not more than 0.5% of its weight.

Residue on ignition ⟨281⟩: not more than 0.1%.

Heavy metals, *Method II* ⟨231⟩: 0.002%.

Chromatographic purity—[NOTE—The Simvastatin solutions are stable for up to 3 days when stored at 4°. Without refrigeration, they should be injected immediately after preparation.]

Mobile phase, Diluent, and *Chromatographic system*—Proceed as directed in the *Assay*.

Test solution—Use the *Assay preparation*.

Procedure—Inject about 5 μL of the *Test solution* into the chromatograph, record the chromatogram, and measure the areas for all the peaks. Calculate the percentage of each impurity in the portion of Simvastatin taken by the formula:

$$100(r_i/r_s)$$

in which r_i is the peak area for each impurity; and r_s is the sum of the areas of all the peaks. Not more than 1.0% of the sum of lovastatin and epilovastatin is found. [NOTE—If present, lovastatin and epilovastatin may not be completely resolved by the method. These peaks, appearing at a relative retention time of 0.6, are integrated together to determine conformance.] Not more than 0.4% of any individual impurity other than lovastatin and epilovastatin is found; and not more than 1.0% of total impurities other than lovastatin and epilovastatin is found.

Assay—[NOTE—The Simvastatin solutions are stable for up to 3 days when stored at 4°. Without refrigeration, they should be injected immediately after preparation.]

Dilute phosphoric acid—Transfer 1 mL of phosphoric acid to a 1-L volumetric flask, and dilute with water to volume.

Solution A—Prepare a mixture of acetonitrile and *Dilute phosphoric acid* (50 : 50).

Solution B—Transfer 1 mL of phosphoric acid to a 1-L volumetric flask, and dilute with acetonitrile to volume.

Mobile phase—Use variable mixtures of *Solution A* and *Solution B*, as directed for *Chromatographic system*. Make adjustments if necessary (see *System Suitability* under *Chromatography* ⟨621⟩).

Buffer solution—Prepare a solution containing 1.4 g of monobasic potassium phosphate per L, and adjust with phosphoric acid to a pH of 4.0.

Diluent—Prepare a mixture of acetonitrile and *Buffer solution* (3 : 2).

System suitability preparation—Dissolve accurately weighed quantities of USP Simvastatin RS and USP Lovastatin RS in *Diluent*, and dilute quantitatively, and stepwise if necessary, with *Diluent* to obtain a solution having known concentrations of about 1.5 mg per mL of USP Simvastatin RS and 0.015 mg per mL of USP Lovastatin RS.

Standard preparation—Dissolve an accurately weighed quantity of USP Simvastatin RS in *Diluent* to obtain a solution having a known concentration of about 1.5 mg per mL.

Assay preparation—Transfer about 75 mg of Simvastatin, accurately weighed, to a 50-mL volumetric flask, dissolve in and dilute with *Diluent* to volume, and mix.

Chromatographic system (see *Chromatography* ⟨621⟩)—The liquid chromatograph is equipped with a 238-nm detector and a 4.6- × 33-mm column that contains packing L1. The flow rate is about 3.0 mL per minute. The chromatograph is programmed as follows.

Time (minutes)	Solution A (%)	Solution B (%)	Elution
0–4.5	100	0	isocratic
4.5–4.6	100→95	0→5	linear gradient
4.6–8.0	95→25	5→75	linear gradient
8.0–11.5	25	75	isocratic
11.5–11.6	25→100	75→0	linear gradient
11.6–13	100	0	re-equilibration

Chromatograph the *System suitability preparation*, and record the peak responses as directed for *Procedure*: the relative retention times are about 0.60 for lovastatin and 1.0 for simvastatin; and the resolution, *R*, between simvastatin and lovastatin is greater than 3. Chromatograph the *Standard preparation*, and record the peak responses as directed for *Procedure*: the relative standard deviation for replicate injections is not more than 1.0%.

Procedure—Separately inject equal volumes (about 5 µL) of the *Standard preparation* and the *Assay preparation* into the chromatograph, record the chromatograms, and measure the areas for the major peaks. Calculate the quantity, in mg, of $C_{25}H_{38}O_5$ in the portion of Simvastatin taken by the formula:

$$VC(r_U / r_S)$$

in which V is the volume, in mL, of the *Assay preparation*; C is the concentration, in mg per mL, of USP Simvastatin RS in the *Standard preparation*; and r_U and r_S are the responses of the simvastatin peak obtained from the *Assay preparation* and the *Standard preparation*, respectively.

Simvastatin Tablets

» Simvastatin Tablets contain not less than 90.0 percent and not more than 110.0 percent of the labeled amount of simvastatin ($C_{25}H_{38}O_5$).

Packaging and storage—Preserve in tight containers.
USP Reference standards ⟨11⟩—*USP Simvastatin RS*.
Identification—The retention time of the major peak in the chromatogram of the *Assay preparation* corresponds to that in the chromatogram of the *Standard preparation*, as obtained in the *Assay*.
Dissolution ⟨711⟩—
Medium: pH 7.0 buffer solution containing 0.5% sodium dodecyl sulfate in 0.01 M sodium phosphate prepared by dissolving 30 g of sodium dodecyl sulfate and 8.28 g of monobasic sodium phosphate in 6000 mL of water, and adjusting with 50% (w/v) sodium hydroxide solution to a pH of 7.0; 900 mL.

Apparatus 2: 50 rpm.
Time: 30 minutes.
Prewashed manganese dioxide—Transfer 10 g of manganese dioxide to a suitable container, and treat as follows. Add 50 mL of *Dissolution Medium*, and shake vigorously for 5 minutes. Centrifuge, decant the supernatant layer, and discard. Repeat twice, first with *Dissolution Medium* and then with water. Dry the solid at 100° for 1 hour before use.

Test solution—Transfer a filtered portion of the solution under test to a centrifuge tube containing about 10 mg of *Prewashed manganese dioxide* per mL of transferred solution under test, and mix. Allow the mixture to stand for 30 minutes with occasional shaking, centrifuge, and use a portion of the clear supernatant as the *Test solution*.

Blank—Proceed as directed for *Test solution*, except to use the *Dissolution Medium*.

Procedure—Determine the amount of $C_{25}H_{38}O_5$ dissolved from the difference between the UV absorbances at the wavelengths of maximum and minimum absorbance at about 247 nm and 257 nm, respectively, on filtered portions of the *Test solution*, in comparison with a Standard solution having a known concentration of USP Simvastatin RS in the same *Medium* treated in the same way as the solution under test, each solution corrected for the *Blank*.

Tolerances—Not less than 75% (*Q*) of the labeled amount of $C_{25}H_{38}O_5$ is dissolved in 30 minutes.

Uniformity of dosage units ⟨905⟩: meet the requirements.
Assay—

Diluting solution—Add 3.0 mL of glacial acetic acid to 900 mL of water. Adjust with 5 N sodium hydroxide to a pH of 4.0, and dilute with water to 1000 mL. To 200 mL of this solution, add 800 mL of acetonitrile, and mix.

Buffer solution—Dissolve 3.9 g of monobasic sodium phosphate in 900 mL of water. Adjust, if necessary, with either 50% sodium hydroxide or 85% phosphoric acid to a pH of 4.5, dilute with water to 1000 mL, and mix.

Mobile phase—Prepare a filtered and degassed mixture of acetonitrile and *Buffer solution* (65 : 35). Make adjustments if necessary (see *System Suitability* under *Chromatography* ⟨621⟩).

Standard preparation—Dissolve an accurately weighed quantity of USP Simvastatin RS in *Diluting solution*, and dilute quantitatively, and stepwise if necessary, with *Diluting solution* to obtain a solution having a known concentration of about 0.1 mg per mL.

Assay preparation—Transfer 10 Tablets to a 250-mL volumetric flask. Add a small volume of water (not more than 10 mL), and swirl to disintegrate the Tablets. Dilute with *Diluting solution* to volume, sonicate for 15 minutes, and cool to room temperature. If necessary, dilute with *Diluting solution* to volume. Centrifuge a portion of the mixture, and dilute a portion of the clear supernatant with *Diluting solution* to obtain a solution having a concentration of about 0.1 mg of simvastatin per mL.

Chromatographic system (see *Chromatography* ⟨621⟩)—The liquid chromatograph is equipped with a 238-nm detector and a 4.6-mm × 25-cm column containing packing L1 and maintained at a temperature of 45°. The flow rate is about 1.5 mL per minute. Chromatograph the *Standard preparation*, and record the peak responses as directed for *Procedure*: the capacity factor, k', is not less than 3.0; the column efficiency is not less than 4500 theoretical plates; the tailing factor is not more than 2.0; and the relative standard deviation for replicate injections is not more than 2.0%.

Procedure—Separately inject equal volumes (about 10 µL) of the *Standard preparation* and the *Assay preparation* into the chromatograph, record the chromatograms, and measure the areas of the major peaks. Calculate the quantity, in mg, of simvastatin ($C_{25}H_{38}O_5$) in each Tablet taken by the formula:

$$(L / D)C(r_U / r_S)$$

in which L is the labeled quantity, in mg, of simvastatin in each Tablet; D is the concentration, in mg per mL, of simvastatin in the *Assay preparation*; C is the concentration, in mg per mL, of USP Simvastatin RS in the *Standard preparation*; and r_U and r_S are the peak areas of simvastatin obtained from the *Assay preparation* and the *Standard preparation*, respectively.

Sincalide for Injection

» Sincalide for Injection is a sterile, synthetically prepared C-terminal octapeptide of cholecystokinin and sodium chloride. It contains not less than 85.0 percent and not more than 125.0 percent of the labeled amount of sincalide ($C_{49}H_{62}N_{10}O_{16}S_3$).

Packaging and storage—Preserve in single-dose containers, preferably of Type I glass.

Labeling—Label it to state that it is to be used within 24 hours after constitution.

USP Reference standards ⟨11⟩—*USP Endotoxin RS. USP Sincalide RS.*

Constituted solution—At the time of use, it meets the requirements for *Constituted Solutions* under *Injections* ⟨1⟩.

Bacterial endotoxins ⟨85⟩—It contains not more than 83.3 USP Endotoxin Units per μg of sincalide.

pH ⟨791⟩: between 5.0 and 7.5, the contents of 1 vial being dissolved in 5 mL of water.

Particulate matter ⟨788⟩: meets the requirements for Small-volume injections.

Other requirements—It meets the requirements under *Injections* ⟨1⟩.

Assay—

Test animals—Select male guinea pigs, each weighing at least 500 g, but restrict selection so that no guinea pig is more than 30% heavier than the lightest. Withdraw food, but not water, from each animal.

Sodium chloride solution—Use Sodium Chloride Injection containing 0.9% of NaCl.

Standard preparations—Dissolve an accurately weighed quantity of USP Sincalide RS in *Sodium chloride solution* to obtain a stock solution having a known concentration of about 10 μg of sincalide per mL. Dilute an accurately measured volume of this solution quantitatively with *Sodium chloride solution* to obtain a solution containing 0.0624 μg of sincalide per kg of the animal's body weight in each 0.1 mL. Prepare a series of 1 in 2 dilutions of this solution with *Sodium chloride solution* to contain 0.0312, 0.0156, and 0.0078 μg of sincalide per kg of body weight. [NOTE—Other dose levels may be used if so indicated by the responses obtained in the *Procedure.*]

Assay preparations—Constitute 1 vial of Sincalide for Injection in a sufficient volume of Water for Injection, accurately measured, to obtain a solution having a concentration of about 1 μg of sincalide per mL. Proceed as directed for *Standard preparations*, beginning with "Dilute an accurately measured volume of this solution."

Procedure—Anesthetize each guinea pig by injecting it, subcutaneously, with 2.25 g of urethane per kg of body weight, administered as a 25% solution. Perform a tracheotomy, then expose a jugular vein, and cannulate with a polyethylene catheter. Tie a thin silk line to the free pole or fundus of the gallbladder, or attach a thin hook with connecting silk line to the wall of the fundus. Gallbladder contractile responses, transmitted through the silk line, cause a change in the line tension. Connect the free end of the silk line to a force transducer, and impose on the system an initial tension of about 2 g. Connect the force transducer to a polygraph, which records the contractile responses. Determine the sensitivity or the responsiveness of the guinea pig's gallbladder by making a few trial injections through the jugular vein catheter, then select two nonconsecutive dose levels (e.g., 0.0624 and 0.0156) for the assay. Use the same dose levels for the *Assay preparations* as for the *Standard preparations*. Administer the selected dose levels of the *Standard preparations* and the *Assay preparations* as 0.1-mL dose volumes in random order, taking 2 to 3 seconds to inject each dose volume and flushing each through the catheter with about 0.5 mL of *Sodium chloride solution*. Make injections at about 10-minute intervals or when the gallbladder has returned to approximately the initial 2 g of tension. [NOTE—Three injections of each dose level may be made. As many as 3 different samples can be tested on the same animal prior to retiring the animal.]

Calculation—Calculate the potency of each vial as directed under *Potencies Interpolated from a Standard Curve* (see *Design and Analysis of Biological Assays* ⟨111⟩), using a log transformation, straight-line method with a least-squares fitting procedure, and a test for linearity.

Sisomicin Sulfate

$(C_{19}H_{37}N_5O_7)_2 \cdot 5H_2SO_4$ 1385.45

D-Streptamine, (2S-cis)-4-O-[3-amino-6-(aminomethyl)-3,4-dihydro-2H-pyran-2-yl]-2-deoxy-6-O-[3-deoxy-4-C-methyl-3-(methylamino)-β-L-arabinopyranosyl]-, sulfate (2 : 5)(salt).
O-3-Deoxy-4-C-methyl-3-(methylamino)-β-L-arabinopyranosyl-(1 → 4)-O-[2,6-diamino-2,3,4,6-tetradeoxy-α-D-*glycero*-hex-4-enopyranosyl-(1 → 6)]-2-deoxy-L-streptamine sulfate (2 : 5)(salt)   [*53179-09-2*].

» Sisomicin Sulfate has a potency equivalent to not less than 580 μg of sisomicin ($C_{19}H_{37}N_5O_7$) per mg, calculated on the dried basis.

Packaging and storage—Preserve in tight containers.

USP Reference standards ⟨11⟩—*USP Sisomicin Sulfate RS.*

Identification—

A: Prepare a solution containing 10 mg of sisomicin per mL. Apply 5 μL of this solution, 5 μL of a solution of USP Sisomicin Sulfate RS containing 10 mg of sisomicin per mL, and 5 μL of a mixture of the two solutions (1 : 1) to a suitable thin-layer chromatographic plate (see *Chromatography* ⟨621⟩) coated with a 0.25-mm layer of chromatographic silica gel mixture. Allow the spots to dry, place the plate in a developing chamber fitted for continuous-flow thin-layer chromatography, and develop the chromatogram in a solvent system consisting of a mixture of methanol, ammonium hydroxide, and chloroform (60 : 30 : 25) for 3 hours. Remove the plate from the developing chamber, allow the solvent to evaporate, and heat the plate at 110° for 15 minutes. Spray the plate with a 1 in 100 solution of ninhydrin in butanol to which 1 mL of pyridine has been added: sisomicin appears as a brown spot, and the spots obtained from the test solution and from the mixture of test solution and Standard solution, respectively, correspond in distance from the origin to that of the spot from the Standard solution.

B: It responds to the tests for *Sulfate* ⟨191⟩.

Specific rotation ⟨781S⟩: between +100° and +110°.

Test solution: 10 mg per mL, in water.

pH ⟨791⟩: between 3.5 and 5.5, in a solution containing 40 mg of sisomicin per mL.

Loss on drying ⟨731⟩—Dry about 100 mg in vacuum at a pressure not exceeding 5 mm of mercury at 110° for 3 hours: it loses not more than 15.0% of its weight.

Residue on ignition ⟨281⟩: not more than 1.0%, the charred residue being moistened with 2 mL of nitric acid and 5 drops of sulfuric acid.

Assay—Proceed as directed under *Antibiotics—Microbial Assays* ⟨81⟩.

Sisomicin Sulfate Injection

» Sisomicin Sulfate Injection is a sterile solution of Sisomicin Sulfate in Water for Injection. It contains the equivalent of not less than 90.0 percent and not more than 120.0 percent of the labeled amount of sisomicin ($C_{19}H_{37}N_5O_7$). It may contain one or more suitable buffers, chelating agents, and preservatives.

Packaging and storage—Preserve in single-dose or in multiple-dose containers, preferably of Type I glass.
USP Reference standards ⟨11⟩—USP Sisomicin Sulfate RS. USP Endotoxin RS.
Identification—It responds to Identification test A under Sisomicin Sulfate.
Bacterial endotoxins ⟨85⟩—It contains not more than 0.5 USP Endotoxin Unit per mg of sisomicin.
pH ⟨791⟩: between 2.5 and 5.5.
Other requirements—It meets the requirements under Injections ⟨1⟩.
Assay—Proceed as directed under Antibiotics—Microbial Assays ⟨81⟩, using an accurately measured volume of Sisomicin Sulfate Injection diluted quantitatively and stepwise with Buffer No. 3 to yield a Test Dilution having a concentration assumed to be equal to the median dose level of the Standard (0.1 μg of sisomicin per mL).

Human Fibroblast-Derived Temporary Skin Substitute

» Human Fibroblast-Derived Temporary Skin Substitute is a nonliving monolayer skin substitute derived from neonatal foreskins. It is composed of fibroblasts, an extracellular matrix, and a nylon mesh bonded to a transparent, semi-permeable silicone membrane. Human fibroblasts are seeded onto the nylon mesh. The fibroblasts proliferate within the nylon mesh and secrete human dermal collagen, matrix proteins, growth factors, and cytokines. Following freezing, no cellular metabolic activity remains; however, the tissue matrix and bound growth factors remain. Human Fibroblast-Derived Temporary Skin Substitute does not contain macrophages, lymphocytes, blood vessels, hair follicles, muscle fibers, or keratin. The fibroblast-cell banks, from which Human Fibroblast-Derived Temporary Skin Substitute is derived, test negative for human and animal viruses and retroviruses and are also tested for normal cell morphology, human karyology, and isoenzymes. Maternal blood sera are tested for evidence of infection with human immunodeficiency virus types 1 and 2, hepatitis B and C viruses, syphilis, and human T-lymphotropic virus type 1 and is found negative for the purpose of donor selection. Reagents used in the manufacture of Human Fibroblast-Derived Temporary Skin Substitute are tested and found free from viruses, retroviruses, endotoxins, and mycoplasma before use. Human Fibroblast-Derived Temporary Skin Substitute is manufactured with sterile components under aseptic conditions within the final package. All materials derived from bovine sources originate from countries free of bovine spongiform encephalopathy. During subsequent screening of the fibroblast cell strain at various stages in the manufacturing process, testing for these same viruses, as well as Epstein-Barr virus and human T-lymphotropic virus type 2, is carried out and found to be negative. The final product tests negative for the presence of mycoplasma.

Packaging and storage—Human Fibroblast-Derived Temporary Skin Substitute is aseptically packaged and supplied frozen in a clear plastic cassette containing two, approximately 12.5- × 19-cm, units. The solution within the cassette is a phosphate-buffered cryoprotectant solution used to facilitate long-term storage. A clear plastic bag surrounds the cassette for its protection. Human Fibroblast-Derived Temporary Skin Substitute should be stored at a temperature of −70° to −20° for no longer than 18 months.
Labeling—The label indicates the dimensions of the Human Fibroblast-Derived Temporary Skin Substitute material enclosed. It contains the expiry date, required storage conditions, and the lot number. The label cautions that Human Fibroblast-Derived Temporary Skin Substitute is not to be used if the package shows signs of damage. Additional labeling requirements include instructions on the proper thawing and handling of Human Fibroblast-Derived Temporary Skin Substitute and the time frame for use after package opening.
USP Reference standards ⟨11⟩—USP Endotoxin RS.
USP Authentic Visual References ⟨11⟩—USP Human Fibroblast-Derived Skin Substitute Reference Photomicrographs. These three photomicrographs represent examples of passing units, prepared as directed in Hematoxylin–eosin staining, Collagen staining, and Distribution of fibronectin. They are specified to assist in ascertaining histological quality. The fibroblasts are embedded in an extracellular matrix that they have secreted (USP Human Fibroblast-Derived Skin Substitute Reference Photomicrograph 1). The collagen (USP Human Fibroblast-Derived Skin Substitute Reference Photomicrograph 2) and fibronectin (USP Human Fibroblast-Derived Skin Substitute Reference Photomicrograph 3) are to be found throughout the extracellular matrix. The nylon fibers (yellow in USP Human Fibroblast-Derived Skin Substitute Reference Photomicrograph 1) and the silicone backing (grey in USP Human Fibroblast-Derived Skin Substitute Reference Photomicrograph 1) are frequently visible although easily lost during processing. However, at this magnification, the presence of these components is the only visible difference between the Cryopreserved Human Fibroblast-Derived Dermal Substitute and the Human Fibroblast-Derived Temporary Skin Substitute.
Sterility tests ⟨71⟩: meets the requirements.
Test solution—Thaw Human Fibroblast-Derived Temporary Skin Substitute by placing the tissue, still in its polycarbonate cassette contained in a plastic covering bag, in a water bath heated to a maximum of 37° for 15 to 20 minutes until no visible ice remains in the cassette. The minimum amount of water in the water bath is 2 L per Human Fibroblast-Derived Temporary Skin Substitute unit. Perform the test on 20 mL of the cryopreservative.
Bacterial endotoxins ⟨85⟩—Thaw Human Fibroblast-Derived Temporary Skin Substitute by placing the tissue, still in its polycarbonate cassette contained in a plastic covering bag, in a water bath heated to a maximum of 37° for 15 to 20 minutes until no visible ice remains in the cassette. The minimum amount of water in the water bath is 2 L per Human Fibroblast-Derived Temporary Skin Substitute unit. Remove the unit from the polycarbonate cassette, and immerse in 25 mL of LAL Reagent Water. Extract for 60 minutes at 37° with shaking on an orbital shaker set at 125 revolutions per minute. Remove a 4-mL aliquot of the extract for testing: it contains not more than 0.5 USP Endotoxin Unit per mL.
Histological characterization—
Buffered formalin and *Preparation of tissue for staining*—Proceed as directed in the test for Histological characterization under Cryopreserved Human Fibroblast-Derived Dermal Substitute, substituting Human Fibroblast-Derived Temporary Skin Substitute for Cryopreserved Human Fibroblast-Derived Dermal Substitute. The fibroblasts appear elongated and spindle shaped. The tissue contains about 10^6 cells per cm^2 and about 500 cells per mm along the section.

HEMATOXYLIN–EOSIN STAINING—
Hematoxylin–alcohol solution, Hematoxylin staining solution, 10% Acid alcohol, Eosin solution, and *Procedure*—Proceed as directed for *Hematoxylin–eosin staining* in the test for *Histological characterization* under *Cryopreserved Human Fibroblast-Derived Dermal Substitute.* Using *USP Human Fibroblast-Derived Skin Substitute Reference Photomicrograph 1* (hematoxylin–eosin stained) for comparison, the nylon-scaffold mesh, silicone membrane, and secreted collagen-based matrix are present and the tissue contains normal human fibroblast distributed throughout the secreted matrix and resembles normal human papillary dermis.

COLLAGEN STAINING—
Bouins's solution, Weigert's iron hematoxylin working solution, Gomori's trichrome solution, 1% Acetic acid, and *Procedure*—Proceed as directed for *Collagen staining* in the test for *Histological characterization* under *Cryopreserved Human Fibroblast-Derived Dermal Substitute.* Using *USP Human Fibroblast-Derived Skin Reference Photomicrograph 2* for comparison, collagen is found throughout the extracellular matrix in a manner indistinguishable from Cryopreserved Human Fibroblast-Derived Dermal Substitute.

DISTRIBUTION OF FIBRONECTIN—
Tris-saline buffer, 3% Hydrogen peroxide, Diaminobenzidine solution, Hematoxylin staining solution, and *Procedure*—Proceed as directed for *Distribution of fibronectin* in the test for *Histological characterization* under *Cryopreserved Human Fibroblast-Derived Dermal Substitute.* Using *USP Human Fibroblast-Derived Skin Substitute Reference Photomicrograph 3* (diaminobenzidine–hematoxylin stained) for comparison, fibronectin binds to collagen and is found throughout the extracellular matrix in a manner indistinguishable from Cryopreserved Human Fibroblast-Derived Dermal Substitute.

Metabolic activity assessment—
DPBS working solution, Assay stock medium, MTT-assay solution, MTT formazan calibration solutions, and *Procedure*—Proceed as directed in the test for *Metabolic activity assessment* under *Cryopreserved Human Fibroblast-Derived Dermal Substitute,* substituting Human Fibroblast-Derived Temporary Skin Substitute for Cryopreserved Human Fibroblast-Derived Dermal Substitute: the absorbance value of individual Human Fibroblast-Derived Temporary Skin Substitute sections at 540 nm is less than 0.1.

DNA content—
Cell culture water, Working DNA extraction buffer, Dilution buffer, DPBS without Ca^{++}, Mg^{++} solution, Calf thymus DNA calibration solutions, DNA staining solution, and *Procedure*—Proceed as directed in the test for *DNA content* under *Cryopreserved Human Fibroblast-Derived Dermal Substitute,* substituting Human Fibroblast-Derived Temporary Skin Substitute for Cryopreserved Human Fibroblast-Derived Dermal Substitute. The amount of DNA in individual Human Fibroblast-Derived Temporary Skin Substitute 11- × 11-mm sections is between 6 and 14 µg.

Total collagen content—
DPBS without Ca^{++}, Mg^{++} solution, DPBS with Ca^{++}, Mg^{++} solution, Collagenase extraction solution, 2% Acetic acid solution, Collagen calibration standards, Sirius red solution, 1% (p-tert-Octylphenoxy)polyethoxyethanol solution, and *Procedure*—Proceed as directed in the test for *Total collagen content* under *Cryopreserved Human Fibroblast-Derived Dermal Substitute,* substituting Human Fibroblast-Derived Temporary Skin Substitute for Cryopreserved Human Fibroblast-Derived Dermal Substitute: the amount of collagen in individual Human Fibroblast-Derived Temporary Skin Substitute 11- × 11-mm samples is between 0.50 and 4.0 mg.

Smallpox Vaccine

» Smallpox Vaccine conforms to the regulations of the FDA concerning biologics (630.70 to 630.76) (see *Biologics* ⟨1041⟩). It is a suspension or solid containing the living virus of vaccinia of a strain of approved origin and manipulation, that has been grown in the skin of a vaccinated bovine calf. It meets the requirements of the specific potency test using embryonated chicken eggs in comparison with the U.S. Reference Smallpox Vaccine in the case of Vaccine intended for multiple-puncture administration or with such Reference Vaccine diluted (1 : 30) in the case of Vaccine intended for jet injection, and the requirements for the tests for absence of specific microorganisms. It may contain a suitable preservative.

Packaging and storage—Preserve and dispense in the containers in which it was placed by the manufacturer. Keep liquid Vaccine during storage and in shipment at a temperature below 0°. Keep dried Vaccine at a temperature between 2° and 8°.

Expiration date—The expiration date for liquid Vaccine is not later than 3 months after date of issue from manufacturer's cold storage (−10°, 9 months as glycerinated or equivalent preparation). The expiration date for dried Vaccine is not later than 18 months after date of issue from manufacturer's cold storage (5°, 6 months).

Labeling—Label it to state that it contains not more than 200 microorganisms per mL in the case of Vaccine intended for multiple-puncture administration, or that it contains not more than 1 microorganism per 100 doses in the case of Vaccine intended for jet injection, unless it meets the requirements for sterility. In the case of Vaccine intended for jet injection, so state on the label. In the case of dried Vaccine, label it to state that after constitution it is to be well shaken before use. Label it also to state that it was prepared in the bovine calf.

Sodium Acetate

$C_2H_3NaO_2 \cdot 3H_2O$ 136.08
Acetic acid, sodium salt, trihydrate.
Sodium acetate trihydrate   [6131-90-4].
Anhydrous   82.03   [127-09-3].

» Sodium Acetate contains three molecules of water of hydration, or is anhydrous. It contains not less than 99.0 percent and not more than 101.0 percent of $C_2H_3NaO_2$, calculated on the dried basis.

Packaging and storage—Preserve in tight containers.
Labeling—Label it to indicate whether it is the trihydrate or is anhydrous. Where Sodium Acetate is intended for use in hemodialysis, it is so labeled.
Identification—A solution responds to the tests for *Sodium* ⟨191⟩ and for *Acetate* ⟨191⟩.
pH ⟨791⟩: between 7.5 and 9.2, in a solution in carbon dioxide-free water containing the equivalent of 30 mg of anhydrous sodium acetate per mL.
Loss on drying ⟨731⟩—Dry at 120° to constant weight: the hydrous form loses between 38.0% and 41.0% of its weight, and the anhydrous form loses not more than 1.0% of its weight.
Insoluble matter—Dissolve the equivalent of 20 g of anhydrous sodium acetate in 150 mL of water, heat to boiling, and digest in a covered beaker on a steam bath for 1 hour. Filter through a tared filtering crucible, wash thoroughly, and dry at 105°: the weight of the residue does not exceed 10 mg (0.05%).
Chloride ⟨221⟩—A portion equivalent to 1.0 g of anhydrous sodium acetate shows no more chloride than corresponds to 0.50 mL of 0.020 N hydrochloric acid (0.035%).
Sulfate ⟨221⟩—A portion equivalent to 10 g of anhydrous sodium acetate shows no more sulfate than corresponds to 0.50 mL of 0.020 N sulfuric acid (0.005%).
Calcium and magnesium—To 20 mL of a solution containing the equivalent of 10 mg of anhydrous sodium acetate per mL add 2 mL

each of 6 N ammonium hydroxide, ammonium oxalate TS, and dibasic sodium phosphate TS: no turbidity is produced within 5 minutes.

Potassium—Dissolve the equivalent of 3 g of anhydrous sodium acetate in 5 mL of water, add 1 N acetic acid dropwise until the solution is slightly acidic, and then add 5 drops of sodium cobaltinitrite TS: no precipitate is formed.

Aluminum ⟨206⟩ (where it is labeled as intended for use in hemodialysis)—Proceed as directed using 10.0 g of Sodium Acetate to prepare the *Test Preparation*: the limit is 0.2 µg per g.

Heavy metals, *Method I* ⟨231⟩—Dissolve a portion equivalent to 4.2 g of $C_2H_3NaO_2$ in enough water to make 50 mL of stock solution. Transfer 12 mL of this stock solution to a 50-mL color-comparison tube (*Test Preparation*). Transfer 11 mL of the stock solution to a second color-comparison tube containing 1.0 mL of *Standard Lead Solution* (*Monitor Preparation*). Transfer 1.0 mL of *Standard Lead Solution* and 11 mL of water to a third color-comparison tube (*Standard Preparation*). Proceed as directed for *Procedure*, omitting the dilution to 50 mL: the limit is 0.001%.

Organic volatile impurities, *Method IV* ⟨467⟩: meets the requirements.

(Official until July 1, 2008)

Assay—Weigh accurately the equivalent of about 200 mg of anhydrous sodium acetate, and dissolve in 25 mL of glacial acetic acid, warming gently if necessary to effect complete solution. Add 2 drops of *p*-naphtholbenzein TS, and titrate with 0.1 N perchloric acid VS. Perform a blank determination, and make any necessary correction. Each mL of 0.1 N perchloric acid is equivalent to 8.203 mg of $C_2H_3NaO_2$.

Sodium Acetate Injection

» Sodium Acetate Injection is a sterile solution of Sodium Acetate in Water for Injection. It contains not less than 95.0 percent and not more than 105.0 percent of the labeled amount of CH_3COONa.

Packaging and storage—Preserve in single-dose containers, preferably of Type I glass.

Labeling—The label states the sodium acetate content in terms of weight and of milliequivalents in a given volume. Label the Injection to indicate that it is to be diluted to appropriate strength with water or other suitable fluid prior to administration. The label states also the total osmolar concentration in mOsmol per L. Where the contents are less than 100 mL, or where the label states that the Injection is not for direct injection but is to be diluted before use, the label alternatively may state the total osmolar concentration in mOsmol per mL.

USP Reference standards ⟨11⟩—*USP Endotoxin RS*.

Identification—It responds to the tests for *Sodium* ⟨191⟩ and for *Acetate* ⟨191⟩.

Bacterial endotoxins ⟨85⟩—It contains not more than 3.90 USP Endotoxin Units per mEq.

pH ⟨791⟩: between 6.0 and 7.0.

Particulate matter ⟨788⟩: meets the requirements under *Small-volume Injections*.

Other requirements—It meets the requirements under *Injections* ⟨1⟩.

Assay—

Standard stock solution—Dissolve 570.0 mg of sodium chloride, previously dried at 105° for 2 hours, in 100 mL of water, transfer to a 1000-mL volumetric flask, dilute with water to volume, and mix. Each mL of this solution contains 224 µg of sodium, equivalent to 800 µg of anhydrous sodium acetate.

Standard preparations—Transfer to each of four 100-mL volumetric flasks 10 mL of a nonionic wetting agent (1 in 500). Dilute the contents of one of the flasks with water to volume to provide a blank. To the remaining flasks add, respectively, 5.0, 10.0, and 15.0 mL of *Standard stock solution*, dilute with water to volume, and mix.

Assay preparation—Transfer an accurately measured volume of Injection, equivalent to about 800 mg of anhydrous sodium acetate, to a 1000-mL volumetric flask, dilute with water to volume, and mix. Pipet 10 mL of this solution into a 100-mL volumetric flask containing 10 mL of a nonionic wetting agent (1 in 500), dilute with water to volume, and mix.

Standard graph—Set a flame photometer for maximum transmittance at a wavelength of about 589 nm. Adjust the instrument to zero transmittance with the blank, and to 100% transmittance with the most concentrated of the *Standard preparations*. Read the transmittances of the other *Standard preparations*, and plot transmittances versus equivalent concentration of sodium acetate.

Procedure—Adjust the instrument as directed under *Standard graph*, read the transmittance of the *Assay preparation*, and calculate the sodium acetate content, in mg per mL, of Injection.

Sodium Acetate Solution

» Sodium Acetate Solution is an aqueous solution of Sodium Acetate. It contains not less than 97.0 percent and not more than 103.0 percent (w/w) of the labeled amount of $C_2H_3NaO_2$.

Packaging and storage—Preserve in tight containers.

Identification—It responds to the tests for *Sodium* ⟨191⟩ and for *Acetate* ⟨191⟩.

pH ⟨791⟩: between 7.5 and 9.2, when diluted with carbon dioxide-free water to contain 5% of solids.

Insoluble matter—Dilute a quantity of Solution, equivalent to 20 g of anhydrous sodium acetate, with water to 150 mL, heat to boiling, and digest in a covered beaker on a steam bath for 1 hour. Filter through a tared filtering crucible, wash thoroughly, and dry at 105°: the weight of the residue does not exceed 1 mg (0.005%).

Chloride ⟨221⟩—A quantity of Solution, equivalent to 1.0 g of anhydrous sodium acetate, shows no more chloride than corresponds to 0.50 mL of 0.020 N hydrochloric acid (0.035%).

Sulfate ⟨221⟩—A quantity of Solution, equivalent to 10 g of anhydrous sodium acetate, shows no more sulfate than corresponds to 0.50 mL of 0.020 N sulfuric acid (0.005%).

Calcium and magnesium—Dilute a quantity of Solution, equivalent to 1.0 g of anhydrous sodium acetate, to 100 mL with water. To 20 mL of this solution add 2 mL each of 6 N ammonium hydroxide, ammonium oxalate TS, and sodium phosphate TS: no turbidity is produced within 5 minutes.

Potassium—To a quantity of Solution, equivalent to 3.0 g of anhydrous sodium acetate, add 0.2 mL of sodium bitartrate TS: no turbidity is produced within 5 minutes.

Heavy metals, *Method I* ⟨231⟩—Dilute a quantity of Solution, equivalent to 2.0 g of anhydrous sodium acetate, with water to 25 mL, and use glacial acetic acid instead of 1 N acetic acid for adjustment of the pH: the limit is 0.001%.

Assay—Weigh accurately about 1 g of Solution into a 250-mL conical flask, cautiously add (in a fume hood) 2.6 mL of acetic anhydride, mix, and allow to stand for 5 minutes. Add 25 mL of glacial acetic acid and 2 drops of *p*-naphtholbenzein TS, and titrate with 0.1 N perchloric acid VS. Perform a blank determination, using 0.5 mL of water, and make any necessary correction. Each mL of 0.1 N perchloric acid is equivalent to 8.203 mg of $C_2H_3NaO_2$.

Sodium Ascorbate

$C_6H_7NaO_6$ 198.11
L-Ascorbic acid, monosodium salt.
Monosodium L-ascorbate   [134-03-2].

» Sodium Ascorbate contains not less than 99.0 percent and not more than 101.0 percent of $C_6H_7NaO_6$, calculated on the dried basis.

Packaging and storage—Preserve in tight, light-resistant containers.
USP Reference standards ⟨11⟩—*USP Sodium Ascorbate RS*.
Identification—
   A: *Infrared Absorption* ⟨197M⟩, on undried specimen.
   B: Add 1 mL of 0.1 N hydrochloric acid to 4 mL of a solution (1 in 50): the solution reduces alkaline cupric tartrate TS slowly at room temperature but more readily upon heating.
   C: A solution (1 in 50) responds to the tests for *Sodium* ⟨191⟩.
Specific rotation ⟨781S⟩: between +103° and +108°, determined immediately following the preparation of the solution.
   Test solution: 100 mg per mL, in carbon dioxide-free water.
pH ⟨791⟩: between 7.0 and 8.0, in a solution (1 in 10).
Loss on drying ⟨731⟩—Dry it in a suitable vacuum drying tube, phosphorus pentoxide being used as the desiccant, at 60° for 4 hours: it loses not more than 0.25% of its weight.
Heavy metals, *Method II* ⟨231⟩: 0.002%.
Organic volatile impurities, *Method I* ⟨467⟩: meets the requirements.
(Official until July 1, 2008)
Assay—Dissolve about 400 mg of Sodium Ascorbate, accurately weighed, in a mixture of 100 mL of carbon dioxide-free water and 25 mL of 2 N sulfuric acid. Titrate immediately with 0.1 N iodine VS, adding 3 mL of starch TS as the endpoint is approached. Each mL of 0.1 N iodine is equivalent to 9.905 mg of $C_6H_7NaO_6$.

Sodium Bicarbonate

$NaHCO_3$ 84.01
Carbonic acid monosodium salt.
Monosodium carbonate   [144-55-8].

» Sodium Bicarbonate contains not less than 99.0 percent and not more than 100.5 percent of $NaHCO_3$, calculated on the dried basis.

Packaging and storage—Preserve in well-closed containers.
Labeling—Where Sodium Bicarbonate is intended for use in hemodialysis, it is so labeled.
Identification—A solution of it meets the requirements of the tests for *Sodium* ⟨191⟩ and for *Bicarbonate* ⟨191⟩.
Loss on drying ⟨731⟩—Dry about 4 g, accurately weighed, over silica gel for 4 hours: it loses not more than 0.25% of its weight.
Insoluble substances—Dissolve 1 g in 20 mL of water: the resulting solution is complete and clear.
Carbonate (where it is labeled as intended for use in hemodialysis)—
   Apparatus—The apparatus (see illustration) consists of a 50-mL flask with a side arm connected to a source of carbon dioxide humidified by bubbling through a saturated solution of sodium bicarbonate and equipped with a top-mounted stopper fitted with an exit tube connected via a T-tube to a system vent and a leveling buret and reservoir.

   Reagents—
   SATURATED SODIUM BICARBONATE SOLUTION—Mix about 20 g of sodium bicarbonate and 100 mL of water, and allow any undissolved crystals to settle. Use the clear supernatant.
   DISPLACEMENT SOLUTION—Dissolve 100 g of sodium chloride in 350 mL of water, add about 1 g of sodium bicarbonate and 1 mL of methyl orange TS. After the sodium bicarbonate has dissolved, add

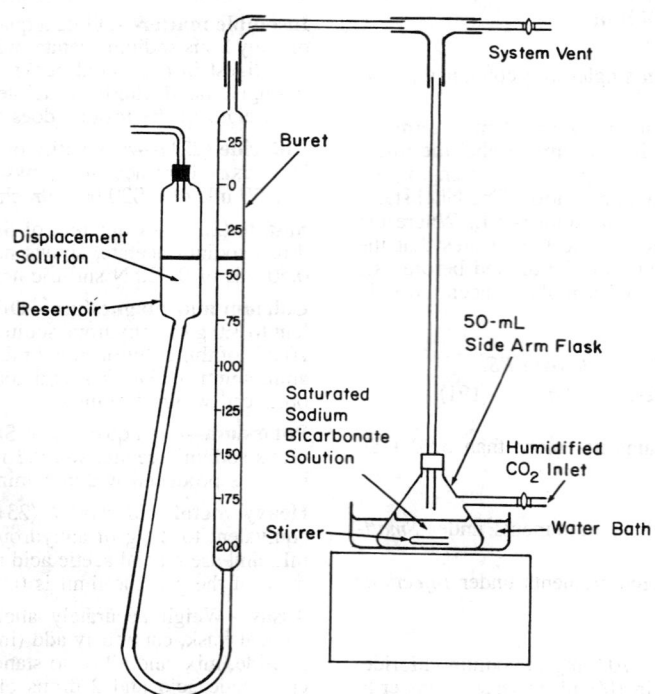

Carbonate Apparatus

6 N sulfuric acid until the solution turns pink. Use this solution to fill the reservoir of the apparatus.

Procedure—Add 25 mL of *Saturated sodium bicarbonate solution* to the 50-mL flask, and flush the system by allowing humidified carbon dioxide to enter through the side arm. Close the carbon dioxide inlet and the system vent, and stir the *Saturated sodium bicarbonate solution* until no further carbon dioxide absorption is noted from successive buret readings. Maintain atmospheric pressure in the apparatus by adjusting the *Displacement solution* to the same level in both the reservoir and the buret, noting the buret reading. Open the system vent, and reintroduce humidified carbon dioxide through the side arm of the flask. Close the carbon dioxide inlet and the system vent, and stir the *Saturated sodium bicarbonate solution* vigorously until no further carbon dioxide absorption is noted. Repeat the carbon dioxide absorption procedure starting with "Open the system vent" until no more than a 0.2-mL change in buret reading is noted. Discontinue stirring, reintroduce humidified carbon dioxide through the side arm of the flask, remove the top-mounted stopper from the flask briefly, and promptly add about 10 g of Sodium Bicarbonate, accurately weighed, to the flask. Replace the stopper, continue the flow of humidified carbon dioxide for about 30 seconds, and then close the carbon dioxide inlet and the system vent. Stir the solution in the flask vigorously until carbon dioxide absorption ceases, noting the volume absorbed from the buret reading. Restore atmospheric pressure in the apparatus by leveling the *Displacement solution* in the reservoir and the buret, and discontinue stirring. Open the system vent, and flush humidified carbon dioxide through the system. Close the carbon dioxide inlet and the system vent, and stir the solution in the flask vigorously until carbon dioxide absorption ceases. Determine the total volume, *V*, in mL, of carbon dioxide absorbed after the addition of the specimen to the flask, and calculate the percentage of carbonate in the portion of specimen tested by the formula:

$$273V(6001P)/[22400(273 + T)(760W)]$$

in which *P* is the ambient atmospheric pressure, in mm of mercury, *T* is the ambient temperature, and *W* is the quantity, in g, of specimen taken. [NOTE—Maintain a constant temperature during the measurement of the volume of carbon dioxide absorbed.] The limit of carbonate is not more than 0.23%.

Normal carbonate—Add 2.0 mL of 0.10 N hydrochloric acid and 2 drops of phenolphthalein TS to 1.0 g of Sodium Bicarbonate, previously dissolved with very gentle swirling in 20 mL of water at a temperature not exceeding 15°: the solution does not assume more than a faint pink color immediately.

Chloride ⟨221⟩: a 0.35-g portion shows no more chloride than corresponds to 1.48 mL of 0.0010 N hydrochloric acid (0.015%).

Limit of sulfur compounds—Dissolve 2.0 g of Sodium Bicarbonate in 20 mL of water, evaporate to 5 mL by boiling, add 1 mL of bromine TS, evaporate to dryness, and cool. Dissolve the residue in 10 mL of 3 N hydrochloric acid, evaporate to dryness, and cool. Dissolve the residue in 5 mL of 3 N hydrochloric acid, evaporate to dryness, and cool. Dissolve the residue in 10 mL of water, and adjust with 3 N hydrochloric acid or 6 N ammonium hydroxide to a pH of 2. If necessary to obtain a clear solution, filter the solution, washing the filter with two 2-mL portions of water. Dilute with water to 20 mL (test solution). To a 0.30 mL of 0.020 N sulfuric acid, add 1 mL of 0.06 N hydrochloric acid, and dilute with water to 20 mL (*Standard solution*). Add 1 mL of barium chloride TS to the test solution and the *Standard solution*, mix, and allow to stand for 30 minutes. Any turbidity produced in the test solution is not more intense than that produced in the *Standard solution*: not more than 0.015% is found.

Aluminum ⟨206⟩ (where it is labeled as intended for use in hemodialysis)—Proceed as directed except to prepare the *Test Preparation* as follows. Transfer 1.0 g of Sodium Bicarbonate to a 100-mL plastic volumetric flask, and carefully add 4 mL of nitric acid. Sonicate for 30 minutes, dilute with water to volume, and mix. The limit is 2 µg per g.

Arsenic, Method I ⟨211⟩—Prepare the *Test Preparation* by dissolving 1.5 g in 20 mL of 7 N sulfuric acid, and adding 35 mL of water: the resulting solution meets the requirements of the test, the addition of 20 mL of 7 N sulfuric acid specified under *Procedure* being omitted. The limit is 2 µg per g.

Calcium and magnesium (where it is labeled as intended for use in hemodialysis)—[NOTE—The *Standard preparations* and the *Test preparation* may be modified, if necessary, to obtain solutions, of suitable concentrations, adaptable to the linear or working range of the instrument.]

Potassium chloride solution—Dissolve 10 g of potassium chloride in 1000 mL of 0.36 N hydrochloric acid.

Calcium standard preparations—Transfer 249.7 mg of calcium carbonate, previously dried at 300° for 3 hours and cooled in a desiccator for 2 hours, to a 100-mL volumetric flask. Dissolve in 6 mL of 6 N hydrochloric acid, add 1 g of potassium chloride, dilute with water to volume, and mix. Transfer 10.0 mL of this solution to a second 100-mL volumetric flask, dilute with *Potassium chloride solution* to volume, and mix. This solution contains 100 µg of Ca per mL. Transfer 2.0-, 3.0-, 4.0-, and 5.0-mL portions of this solution to separate 100-mL volumetric flasks (each containing 6 mL of 6 N hydrochloric acid), dilute with *Potassium chloride solution* to volume, and mix. These *Calcium standard preparations* contain 2.0, 3.0, 4.0, and 5.0 µg of Ca per mL, respectively.

Magnesium standard preparations—Place 1.000 g of magnesium in a 250-mL beaker containing 20 mL of water, and carefully add 20 mL of hydrochloric acid, warming if necessary to complete the reaction. Transfer this solution to a 1000-mL volumetric flask containing 10 g of potassium chloride, dilute with water to volume, and mix. Transfer 10.0 mL of this solution to a 100-mL volumetric flask containing 1 g of potassium chloride, dilute with water to volume, and mix. Transfer 10.0 mL of this solution to a second 100-mL volumetric flask, dilute with *Potassium chloride solution* to volume, and mix. This solution contains 10.0 µg of Mg per mL. Transfer 2.0-, 3.0-, 4.0-, and 5.0-mL portions of this solution to separate 100-mL volumetric flasks (each containing 6 mL of 6 N hydrochloric acid), dilute with *Potassium chloride solution* to volume, and mix. These *Magnesium standard preparations* contain 0.2, 0.3, 0.4, and 0.5 µg of Mg per mL, respectively.

Test preparation—Transfer 3.0 g of Sodium Bicarbonate to a 100-mL volumetric flask, add 6 mL of 6 N hydrochloric acid and 1 g of potassium chloride, dilute with water to volume, and mix.

Procedure for calcium—Concomitantly determine the absorbances of the *Calcium standard preparations* and the *Test preparation* at the calcium emission line at 422.7 nm with a suitable atomic absorption spectrophotometer (see *Spectrophotometry and Light-Scattering* ⟨851⟩) equipped with a calcium hollow-cathode lamp and a nitrous oxide–acetylene flame, using *Potassium chloride solution* as the blank. Plot the absorbances of the *Calcium standard preparations* versus their contents of calcium, in µg per mL, by drawing a straight line best fitting the four plotted points. From the graph so obtained determine the quantity, in µg, of Ca in each mL of the *Test preparation*. Calculate the percentage of Ca in the specimen taken by dividing this value by 300: the limit is 0.01%.

Procedure for magnesium—Concomitantly determine the absorbances of the *Magnesium standard preparations* and the *Test preparation* at the magnesium emission line at 285.2 nm with a suitable atomic absorption spectrophotometer (see *Spectrophotometry and Light-Scattering* ⟨851⟩) equipped with a magnesium hollow-cathode lamp and a reducing air–acetylene flame, using *Potassium chloride solution* as the blank. Plot the absorbances of the *Magnesium standard preparations* versus their contents of magnesium, in µg per mL, by drawing a straight line best fitting the four plotted points. From the graph so obtained determine the quantity, in µg, of Mg in each mL of the *Test preparation*. Calculate the percentage of Mg in the specimen taken by dividing this value by 300: the limit is 0.004%.

Copper (where it is labeled as intended for use in hemodialysis)—[NOTE—The *Standard preparation* and the *Test preparation* may be modified, if necessary, to obtain solutions, of suitable concentrations, adaptable to the linear or working range of the instrument.]

Nitric acid diluent—Dilute 40 mL of nitric acid to 1000 mL with water.

Standard preparation—Transfer 1.000 g of copper to a 1000-mL volumetric flask, dissolve in 20 mL of nitric acid, dilute with 0.2 N nitric acid to volume, and mix. Transfer 10.0 mL of this solution to a second 1000-mL volumetric flask, dilute with 0.2 N nitric acid to volume, and mix. This solution contains 10.0 µg of copper per mL. Store in a polyethylene bottle.

Test preparation—Transfer 5.0 g of Sodium Bicarbonate to a 100-mL plastic volumetric flask, and carefully add 4 mL of nitric acid. Sonicate for 30 minutes, dilute with water to volume, and mix.

Procedure—To 10.0 mL of the *Test preparation* add 20 µL of *Standard preparation*, and mix. This *Spiked test preparation* contains 0.02 µg of added Cu per mL. Concomitantly determine the absorbances of the *Test preparation* and the *Spiked test preparation* at the copper emission line at 324.7 nm with a suitable atomic absorption spectrophotometer (see *Spectrophotometry and Light-Scattering* ⟨851⟩) equipped with a copper hollow-cathode lamp and a flameless electrically heated furnace, using *Nitric acid diluent* as the blank. Plot the absorbances of the *Test preparation* and the *Spiked test preparation* versus their contents of added Cu, in µg per mL, draw a line connecting the two points, and extrapolate the line until it intercepts the concentration axis. From the intercept determine the quantity, in µg, of Cu in each mL of the *Test preparation*. Calculate the quantity of Cu in the specimen tested by multiplying this value by 20: the limit is 1 µg per g.

Iron ⟨241⟩ (where it is labeled as intended for use in hemodialysis)—Place 2.0 g of Sodium Bicarbonate in a beaker, and neutralize with hydrochloric acid, noting the volume of acid consumed. Transfer this solution to a 25-mL volumetric flask with the aid of water (*Test preparation*). Prepare the *Standard preparation* by transferring 1.0 mL of *Standard Iron Solution* to a 25-mL volumetric flask and adding the same volume of hydrochloric acid as used to prepare the *Test preparation*. Prepare a *Blank* by adding the same volume of hydrochloric acid to a third 25-mL volumetric flask. To each of the flasks containing the *Standard preparation*, the *Test preparation*, and the *Blank* add 50 mg of ammonium peroxydisulfate crystals and 2 mL of *Ammonium Thiocyanate Solution*, dilute with water to volume, and mix. Concomitantly determine the absorbances of the solutions from the *Standard preparation* and the *Test preparation* at the wavelength of maximum absorbance at about 480 nm with a suitable spectrophotometer, using the solution from the *Blank* to set the instrument to zero. The absorbance of the solution from the *Test preparation* is not greater than that of the solution from the *Standard preparation*: not more than 5 µg per g is found.

Heavy metals, *Method I* ⟨231⟩—Mix 4.0 g with 5 mL of water and 19 mL of 3 N hydrochloric acid, heat to boiling, and maintain that temperature for 1 minute. Add 1 drop of phenolphthalein TS, then add sufficient 6 N ammonium hydroxide, dropwise, to give the solution a faint pink color. Cool, and dilute with water to 25 mL: the limit is 5 µg per g.

Limit of ammonia—

Sodium hypochlorite solution—Use a commercially available solution that contains 4.0% to 6.0% of sodium hypochlorite.

Oxidizing solution—[NOTE—Prepare on the day of use.] Prepare a mixture of alkaline sodium citrate TS and *Sodium hypochlorite solution* (4 : 1).

Diluted sodium nitroferricyanide solution—Prepare a mixture of water and sodium nitroferricyanide TS (10 : 1).

Test solution—Transfer 2.5 g of Sodium Bicarbonate to a 100-mL volumetric flask, dissolve in and dilute with water to volume, and mix.

Procedure—[NOTE—Carefully follow this order of addition stated below.] To 4.0 mL of the *Test solution*, add 0.4 mL of phenol TS, 0.4 mL of *Diluted sodium nitroferricyanide solution*, and 1.0 mL of *Oxidizing solution*. Dilute with water to 10 mL, mix, and allow to stand for 1 hour: no blue color develops.

Limit of organics—(where it is labeled as intended for use in hemodialysis)—

Silver sulfate solution—Dissolve 22 g of silver sulfate in 2000 mL of sulfuric acid.

Indicator solution—Dissolve 1.485 g of 1,10-phenanthroline and 695 mg of ferrous sulfate in water to make 100 mL of solution.

Standard preparation—Transfer 850.3 mg of potassium biphthalate, previously crushed lightly and dried at 120° for 2 hours, to a 1000-mL volumetric flask, dilute with water to volume, and mix. Transfer 6.0 mL of this solution to a 100-mL volumetric flask, dilute with water to volume, and mix. This solution contains the equivalent of 0.06 mg of organics equivalents per mL. Transfer 40.0 mL of this solution to a 500-mL reflux flask.

Test preparation—Transfer about 20 g of Sodium Bicarbonate, accurately weighed, to a 500-mL reflux flask. Add 20 mL of water, and swirl. Cautiously add 20 mL of sulfuric acid, and swirl. [*Caution—Perform this operation under a hood.*]

Blank—Add 40 mL of water to a 500-mL reflux flask.

Procedure—Concomitantly treat the *Standard preparation*, the *Test preparation*, and the *Blank* as follows. Add 1 g of mercuric sulfate and about 5 glass beads. Cool the flask in an ice bath, and add 5 mL of *Silver sulfate solution*. While gently swirling the flask in the ice bath, add 25.0 mL of 0.025 N potassium dichromate VS and, slowly, 70 mL of *Silver sulfate solution*. Fit a cold water condenser on the reflux flask, and reflux for 2 hours. Allow the contents of the flask to cool for 10 minutes, and wash the condenser with 50 mL of water, collecting the washings in the flask. Add water to the flask to obtain a volume of about 350 mL. Add 3 drops of *Indicator solution*, and titrate, at room temperature, with 0.07 N ferrous ammonium sulfate VS until the solution changes from greenish blue to reddish brown. Calculate the amount, in mg, of organics equivalent in the *Standard preparation* taken by the formula:

$$8N(V_B - V_S)$$

in which N is the normality of the ferrous ammonium sulfate VS; and V_B and V_S are the volumes, in mL, of 0.07 N ferrous ammonium sulfate VS consumed by the *Blank* and the *Standard preparation*, respectively. In a suitable system, between 2.328 and 2.424 mg is found. Calculate the amount, in mg, of organics equivalent in the portion of Sodium Bicarbonate taken by the formula:

$$8N(V_B - V_U)$$

in which V_U is the volume, in mL, of 0.07 N ferrous ammonium sulfate VS consumed by the *Test preparation*: the limit is 0.01%.

Organic volatile impurities, *Method IV* ⟨467⟩: meets the requirements.

(Official until July 1, 2008)

Assay—Weigh accurately about 3 g of Sodium Bicarbonate, mix with 100 mL of water, add methyl red TS, and titrate with 1 N hydrochloric acid VS. Add the acid slowly, with constant stirring, until the solution becomes faintly pink. Heat the solution to boiling, cool, and continue the titration until the faint pink color no longer fades after boiling. Each mL of 1 N hydrochloric acid is equivalent to 84.01 mg of $NaHCO_3$.

Sodium Bicarbonate Injection

» Sodium Bicarbonate Injection is a sterile solution of Sodium Bicarbonate in Water for Injection, the pH of which may be adjusted by means of added Carbon Dioxide. It contains not less than 95.0 percent and not more than 105.0 percent of the labeled amount of $NaHCO_3$.

NOTE—Do not use the Injection if it contains a precipitate.

Packaging and storage—Preserve in single-dose glass or plastic containers. Glass containers are preferably of Type I glass. Store at controlled room temperature.

Labeling—The label states the total osmolar concentration in mOsmol per L. Where the contents are less than 100 mL, or where the label states that the Injection is not for direct injection but is to be diluted before use, the label alternatively may state the total osmolar concentration in mOsmol per mL.

USP Reference standards ⟨11⟩—*USP Endotoxin RS*.

Identification—It responds to the tests for *Sodium* ⟨191⟩ and for *Bicarbonate* ⟨191⟩.

Bacterial endotoxins ⟨85⟩—It contains not more than 5.0 USP Endotoxin Units per mEq.

pH ⟨791⟩: between 7.0 and 8.5.

Particulate matter ⟨788⟩: meets the requirements under small-volume injections.

Other requirements—It meets the requirements under *Injections* ⟨1⟩.

Assay—Measure accurately a volume of Injection, equivalent to about 3 g of sodium bicarbonate, add methyl red TS, and titrate with 1 N hydrochloric acid VS. Add the acid slowly, with constant stirring, until the solution becomes faintly pink. Heat the solution to boiling, cool, and continue the titration until the faint pink color no longer fades after boiling. Each mL of 1 N hydrochloric acid is equivalent to 84.01 mg of NaHCO$_3$.

Sodium Bicarbonate Oral Powder

» Sodium Bicarbonate Oral Powder contains Sodium Bicarbonate and suitable added substances. It contains not less than 98.5 percent and not more than 100.5 percent of NaHCO$_3$, calculated on the dried basis.

Packaging and storage—Preserve in well-closed containers.
Labeling—Label Oral Powder to indicate that it is for oral use only.
Other requirements—It meets the requirements for *Identification* and *Loss on drying* under *Sodium Bicarbonate*.
Assay—Proceed with Oral Powder as directed in the *Assay* under *Sodium Bicarbonate*.

Sodium Bicarbonate Tablets

» Sodium Bicarbonate Tablets contain not less than 95.0 percent and not more than 105.0 percent of the labeled amount of NaHCO$_3$.

Packaging and storage—Preserve in well-closed containers.
Identification—A solution of Tablets responds to the tests for *Sodium* ⟨191⟩ and for *Bicarbonate* ⟨191⟩.
Disintegration ⟨701⟩: 30 minutes, simulated gastric fluid TS being substituted for water in the test.
Uniformity of dosage units ⟨905⟩: meet the requirements.
Assay—Weigh and finely powder not less than 20 Tablets. Weigh accurately a portion of the powder, equivalent to about 2 g of sodium bicarbonate, dissolve in 100 mL of water, add methyl red TS, and titrate with 1 N hydrochloric acid VS. Add the acid slowly, with constant stirring, until the solution becomes faintly pink. Heat the solution to boiling, cool, and continue the titration until the pink color no longer fades after boiling. Each mL of 1 N hydrochloric acid is equivalent to 84.01 mg of NaHCO$_3$.

Sodium Bromide

NaBr 102.89
Sodium bromide.
Sodium bromide [7647-15-6].

» Sodium Bromide contains not less than 98.0 percent and not more than 100.5 percent of NaBr, calculated on the dried basis. It contains no added substances.

Packaging and storage—Preserve in well-closed containers, and store at room temperature.
Appearance of solution: clear and colorless.
  Test solution—Dissolve 10.0 g in carbon dioxide-free water, and dilute with the same solvent to 100 mL.
Identification—
  A: A solution containing 4.0 mg of sodium bromide responds to the test for *Bromide* ⟨191⟩.
  B: It responds to the test for *Sodium* ⟨191⟩.
Acidity or alkalinity—To 10 mL of the solution prepared for the test for *Appearance of solution*, add 0.1 mL of bromothymol blue TS: not more than 0.5 mL of 0.01 N hydrochloric acid or 0.01 N sodium hydroxide is required to change the color of this solution.
Loss on drying ⟨731⟩—Dry it at 100° to 105° for 3 hours: it loses not more than 3.0% of its weight.
Bromates—
  Starch–mercuric iodide solution—Triturate 1.0 g of soluble starch with 5 mL of water, and pour the mixture into 100 mL of boiling water containing 10 mg of mercuric iodide.
  Procedure—To 10 mL of the solution prepared for the test for *Appearance of solution* add 1 mL of *Starch–mercuric iodide solution*, 0.1 mL of a 100 g per L solution of potassium iodide, and 0.25 mL of 0.5 M sulfuric acid. Allow to stand protected from light for 5 minutes. No blue or violet color develops.
Limit of chlorine: not more than 0.6%.
  Nitric acid solution and *Ferric ammonium sulfate solution*—Proceed as directed in the *Assay*.
  Procedure—Dissolve 1.000 g Sodium Bromide in 20 mL of *Nitric acid solution* in a conical flask, add and mix 5 mL of 30 percent hydrogen peroxide, and heat in a water bath until the solution is colorless. Rinse the sides of the flask with a small quantity of water, and heat in a water bath for 15 minutes. Allow to cool, dilute with water to 50 mL, and add 5.0 mL of silver nitrate VS and 1 mL of dibutyl phthalate. Mix, and back titrate the excess silver nitrate with ammonium thiocyanate VS (see *Titrimetry* ⟨541⟩), using 5 mL of *Ferric ammonium sulfate solution* as the indicator. Perform a blank titration. Not more than 1.7 mL of silver nitrate VS is used.
Iodides—To 5 mL of the solution prepared for the test for *Appearance of solution* add 0.15 mL of a 10.5 g per 100 mL ferric chloride solution, and 2 mL of dichloromethane. Shake, and allow to separate. The lower layer is colorless.
Sulfates ⟨221⟩—A 2.0-g portion shows no more sulfate than corresponds to 0.2 mL of 0.020 N sulfuric acid (0.01%).
Limit of iron: not more than 20 ppm.
  Citric acid solution—Prepare a 200 g citric acid per mL solution.
  Iron standard solution—Transfer 0.863 g of ferric ammonium sulfate to a 500-mL volumetric flask, and dissolve in 25 mL of dilute sulfuric acid. Dilute with water to volume. Transfer 1.0 mL of the resulting solution to a 10-mL volumetric flask, and dilute with water to volume. Transfer 2.5 mL of this resulting solution to a 50-mL volumetric flask, and dilute with water to volume. [NOTE—Prepare immediately before use.]
  Test solution—Transfer 5 mL of the solution prepared for the test for *Appearance of solution* to a 10-mL volumetric flask, and dilute with water to volume.
  Procedure—To 10 mL each of the *Iron standard solution* and the *Test solution* add 2.0 mL of the *Citric acid solution* and 0.1 mL of thioglycolic acid. Make alkaline to litmus with ammonia water, and dilute with water to 20 mL. After 5 minutes, any pink color in the *Test solution* is not more intense than that in the *Iron standard solution*.
Magnesium and alkaline-earth metals—To 200 mL of water add 0.1 g of hydroxylamine hydrochloride, 10 mL of pH 10.0 ammonia–ammonium chloride buffer (prepared by dissolving 5.4 g of ammonium chloride in 20 mL of water, adding 20 mL of ammonium hydroxide, and diluting to 100 mL), 1 mL of 0.1 M zinc sulfate, and about 0.2 g of eriochrome black T trituration. Heat to about 40°. Titrate this solution (see *Titrimetry* ⟨541⟩) with 0.01 M edetate disodium VS until the violet color changes to deep blue. To this solution add 10.0 g of Sodium Bromide dissolved in 100 mL of water. If the color changes to violet, titrate the solution with 0.01 M edetate disodium VS to a deep blue endpoint. The volume of 0.01 M edetate disodium consumed in the second titration does not exceed 5.0 mL (0.02%, calculated as Ca).
Heavy metals, *Method I* ⟨231⟩: not more than 10 ppm.
Assay—
  Nitric acid solution—Dilute 14 mL of nitric acid with water to 100 mL.
  Ferric ammonium sulfate solution—Transfer 10 g of ferric ammonium sulfate to a 100-mL volumetric flask. Dissolve in and dilute with water to volume.
  Procedure—Dissolve 2.000 g of Sodium Bromide in water, and dilute with water to 100.0 mL. To 10.0 mL of the solution add 50 mL of water, 5 mL of *Nitric acid solution*, 25.0 mL of silver nitrate VS, and 2 mL of dibutyl phthalate. Mix, and back titrate the excess silver nitrate with ammonium thiocyanate VS (see *Titrimetry*

⟨541⟩), using 2 mL of *Ferric ammonium sulfate solution* as the indicator, shaking vigorously towards the endpoint. Each mL of 0.1 M silver nitrate is equivalent to 10.29 mg of NaBr. Calculate the percent content of Sodium Bromide, corrected for the chloride content, by the formula:

$$a - 2.902b$$

in which a is the percent content of NaBr and NaCl obtained, calculated as NaBr; and b is the percent content of chlorides.

Sodium Butyrate

$C_4H_7NaO_2$ 110.10
Butyric acid, sodium salt.
Sodium butyrate [156-54-7].

» Sodium Butyrate contains not less than 98.0 percent and not more than 101.0 percent of $C_4H_7NaO_2$, calculated on the anhydrous basis.

Packaging and storage—Preserve in tight containers, and store at controlled room temperature.
Labeling—Label it to indicate that it is intended for use in compounding dosage forms for rectal use only.
USP Reference standards ⟨11⟩—USP Sodium Butyrate RS.
Identification—
 A: *Infrared Absorption* ⟨197K⟩, on the undried specimen.
 B: A solution (1 in 10) meets the requirements of the tests for *Sodium* ⟨191⟩.
Alkalinity—Dissolve 2.0 g in 20 mL of water, and add 1 drop of phenolphthalein TS: if a pink color is produced, it is discharged by 0.50 mL of 0.10 N sulfuric acid.
Water, *Method I* ⟨921⟩: not more than 1.0%.
Heavy metals, *Method II* ⟨231⟩: 0.001%.
Organic volatile impurities, *Method I* ⟨467⟩: meets the requirements.

(Official until July 1, 2008)

Assay—Dissolve about 200 mg of Sodium Butyrate, accurately weighed, in 50 mL of glacial acetic acid. Add 1 drop of crystal violet TS, and titrate with 0.1 N perchloric acid to a green endpoint. Perform a blank determination, and make any necessary correction. Each mL of 0.1 N perchloric acid is equivalent to 11.01 mg of $C_4H_7NaO_2$.

Sodium Chloride

NaCl 58.44
Sodium Chloride
Sodium Chloride [7647-14-5].

» Sodium Chloride contains not less than 99.0 percent and not more than 100.5 percent of NaCl, calculated on the dried basis.

Packaging and storage—Preserve in well-closed containers.
Labeling—Where Sodium Chloride is intended for use in the manufacture of injectable dosage forms, peritoneal dialysis solutions, hemodialysis solutions, or hemofiltration solutions, it is so labeled. Where Sodium Chloride must be subjected to further processing during the preparation of injectable dosage forms to ensure acceptable levels of *Bacterial endotoxins*, it is so labeled. Where Sodium Chloride is sterile, it is so labeled.
Appearance of solution—Dissolve 20.0 g of Sodium Chloride in carbon dioxide-free water, and dilute with the same solvent to 100.0 mL. This solution is clear and colorless.
Identification—It responds to the tests for *Sodium* ⟨191⟩ and for *Chloride*.
Chloride—Dissolve about 3 mg of Sodium Chloride in 2 mL of water. Acidify with diluted nitric acid and add 0.4 mL of silver nitrate TS. Shake, and allow to stand. A curdled, white precipitate is formed. Centrifuge, wash the precipitate with three 1-mL portions of water, and discard the washings. Carry out this operation rapidly in subdued light, disregarding the fact that the supernatant may not become perfectly clear. Suspend the precipitate in 2 mL of water and add 1.5 mL of 10 N ammonium hydroxide. The precipitate dissolves easily with the possible exception of a few large particles, which dissolve more slowly.
Bacterial endotoxins ⟨85⟩—The level of *Bacterial endotoxins* are such that the requirement under the relevant dosage form monograph(s) in which Sodium Chloride is used can be met. Where the label states that Sodium Chloride must be subjected to further processing during the preparation of injectable dosage forms, the level of *Bacterial endotoxins* are such that the requirement under the relevant dosage form monograph(s) in which Sodium Chloride is used can be met.
Sterility ⟨71⟩—Where the label states that Sodium Chloride is sterile, it meets the requirements for *Sterility* under the relevant dosage form monograph(s) in which Sodium Chloride is used.
Acidity or alkalinity—To 20 mL of the solution prepared for the test for *Appearance of solution*, add 0.1 mL of bromothymol blue TS: not more than 0.5 mL of 0.01 N hydrochloric acid or 0.01 N sodium hydroxide is required to change the color of this solution.
Loss on drying ⟨731⟩—Dry the test material at 105° for 2 hours: it loses not more than 0.5% of its weight, determined on a 1.000 g sample.
Limit of bromides—To 0.5 mL of the solution prepared for the test for *Appearance of solution*, add 4.0 mL of water, 2.0 mL of pH 4.7 phenol red TS, and 1.0 mL of chloramine T solution (0.1 mg per mL), and mix immediately. After 2 minutes, add 0.15 mL of 0.1 N sodium thiosulfate, mix, dilute with water to 10.0 mL, and mix. The absorbance of this solution measured at 590 nm, using water as the comparison liquid, is not greater than that of a *Standard solution*, concomitantly prepared, using 5.0 mL of a solution containing 3.0 mg of potassium bromide per L and proceeding as above, starting with the addition of 2.0 mL of pH 4.7 phenol red TS (0.010%).
Limit of phosphates—
 Phosphate stock standard solution—Dissolve an accurately weighed quantity of monobasic potassium phosphate in water to obtain a solution having a concentration of about 0.716 mg per mL.
 Phosphate standard solution—Dilute 1 mL of the *Phosphate stock standard solution* with water to 100 mL. Prepare this solution fresh.
 Standard solution—Dilute 2 mL of the *Phosphate standard solution* with water to 100 mL.
 Test solution—Dilute 2 mL of the solution prepared in the test for *Appearance of solution* with water to 100 mL.
 Procedure—To the *Standard solution* and the *Test solution*, add 4 mL of *Sulfomolybdic acid solution*, and add 0.1 mL of a mixture of 1 mL of stronger acid stannous chloride TS and 10 mL of 2 N hydrochloric acid. After 10 minutes, compare the colors of 20 mL of each solution: any color in the *Test solution* is not more intense than that in the *Standard solution* (0.0025%).
 Sulfomolybdic acid solution—Dissolve with heating 2.5 g of ammonium molybdate in 20 mL of water. Dilute 28 mL of sulfuric acid with 50 mL of water, then cool. Mix the two solutions, and dilute with water to 100 mL.
Limit of potassium (where it is labeled as intended for use in the manufacture of injectable dosage forms, peritoneal dialysis solutions, hemodialysis solutions, or hemofiltration solutions)—
 Test solution—Transfer 1.00 g of Sodium Chloride to a 100-mL volumetric flask, add water and swirl to dissolve, dilute with water to volume, and mix.
 Standard solution—[NOTE—The *Standard solution* and the *Test solution* may be modified, if necessary, to obtain solutions of suitable concentrations adaptable to the linear or working range of the instrument.] Dissolve 1.144 g of potassium chloride, previously dried at 105° for 3 hours, in water, dilute with water to 1000 mL, and mix. This solution contains the equivalent of 600 µg of potassium per mL. Dilute as required to obtain not fewer than three solu-

tions at concentrations that span the expected value in the *Test solution.*

Procedure—Using atomic absorption spectrophotometry (see *Spectrophotometry and Light-Scattering* ⟨851⟩), measure, at least three times, the emission intensity of the *Test solution* and the *Standard solution* using an air–acetylene flame and a wavelength of 766.5 nm. Prepare a calibration curve from the mean of the readings obtained with the *Standard solution,* and determine the concentration of potassium in the *Test solution.* The limit is 0.05%.

Iodides—Moisten 5 g of Sodium Chloride by the dropwise addition of a freshly prepared mixture of 0.15 mL of sodium nitrite solution (1 in 10), 2 mL of 1 N sulfuric acid, 25 mL of iodide-free starch TS, and 25 mL of water. After 5 minutes, examine the substance in natural light. No blue color is observed.

Aluminum (where it is labeled as intended for use in the manufacture of peritoneal dialysis solutions, hemodialysis solutions, or hemofiltration solutions)—

Standard aluminum solution—To 352 mg of aluminum potassium sulfate in a 100-mL volumetric flask, add a few mL of water, swirl to dissolve, add 20 mL of diluted sulfuric acid, dilute with water to volume, and mix. Immediately before use, transfer 1.0 mL of this solution to a 100-mL volumetric flask, dilute with water to volume, and mix.

pH 6.0 Acetate buffer—Dissolve 50 g of ammonium acetate in 150 mL of water, adjust with glacial acetic acid to a pH of 6.0, dilute with water to 250 mL, and mix.

Test solution—Dissolve 20.0 g of Sodium Chloride in 100 mL of water, and add 10 mL of *pH 6.0 Acetate buffer.* Extract this solution with successive portions of 20, 20, and 10 mL of a 0.5% solution of 8-hydroxyquinoline in chloroform, combining the chloroform extracts in a 50-mL volumetric flask. Dilute the combined extracts with chloroform to volume, and mix.

Standard solution—Prepare a mixture of 2.0 mL of *Standard aluminum solution,* 10 mL of *pH 6.0 Acetate buffer,* and 98 mL of water. Extract this mixture as described for the *Test solution,* dilute the combined extracts with chloroform to volume, and mix.

Blank solution—Prepare a mixture of 10 mL of *pH 6.0 Acetate buffer* and 100 mL of water. Extract this mixture as described for the *Test solution,* dilute the combined extracts with chloroform to volume, and mix.

Procedure—Determine the fluorescence intensities of the *Test solution* and the *Standard solution* in a fluorometer set at an excitation wavelength of 392 nm and an emission wavelength of 518 nm, using the *Blank solution* to set the instrument to zero. The fluorescence of the *Test solution* does not exceed that of the *Standard solution* (0.2 µg per g).

Magnesium and alkaline-earth metals—To 200 mL of water add 0.1 g of hydroxylamine hydrochloride, 10 mL of pH 10.0 ammonia–ammonium chloride buffer (prepared by dissolving 5.4 g of ammonium chloride in 20 mL of water, adding 20 mL of ammonium hydroxide and diluting to 100 mL), 1 mL of 0.1 M zinc sulfate, and about 0.2 g of eriochrome black T trituration. Heat to about 40°. Titrate this solution with 0.01 M edetate disodium VS until the violet color changes to deep blue. To this solution add 10.0 g of Sodium Chloride dissolved in 100 mL of water. If the color changes to violet, titrate the solution with 0.01 M edetate disodium VS to a deep blue endpoint. The volume of 0.01 M edetate disodium consumed in the second titration does not exceed 2.5 mL (0.01%, calculated as Ca).

Arsenic, *Method I* ⟨211⟩:   1 µg per g.

Iron—

Test solution—Use a 10-mL portion of the solution prepared for the test for *Appearance of solution.*

Standard solution—Immediately before use, dilute *Standard Iron Solution* (see *Iron* ⟨241⟩) 1 to 10 with water. This solution contains the equivalent of 1 µg of iron per mL. Combine 4 mL of this solution and 6 mL of water.

Procedure—To each of the solutions, add 2 mL of a 200 g per L solution of citric acid and 0.1 mL of thioglycolic acid. Mix, make alkaline with stronger ammonia water, and dilute with water to 20 mL. After 5 minutes, any pink color in the *Test solution* is not more intense than that from the *Standard solution.* The limit is 2 µg per g.

Barium—To 5 mL of the solution prepared for the test for *Appearance of solution,* add 2 mL of 2 N sulfuric acid and 5 mL of water. To another 5 mL of the solution prepared for the test for *Appearance of solution,* add 7 mL of water. The solutions are equally clear after standing for 2 hours.

Ferrocyanides—Dissolve 2.0 g in 6 mL of water. Add 0.5 mL of a mixture of 5 mL of ferric ammonium sulfate solution (1 g in 100 mL of 0.1 N sulfuric acid) and 95 mL of ferrous sulfate solution (1 in 100): no blue color develops in 10 minutes.

Sulfate—

Standard sulfate solution A—To 181 mg of potassium sulfate in a 100-mL volumetric flask, add a few mL of 30% alcohol, swirl to dissolve, dilute with 30% alcohol to volume, and mix. Immediately before use, transfer 10.0 mL of this solution to a 1000-mL volumetric flask, dilute with 30% alcohol to volume, and mix. This solution contains 10 µg of sulfate per mL.

Standard sulfate solution B—To 181 mg of potassium sulfate in a 100-mL volumetric flask, add a few mL of water, swirl to dissolve, dilute with water to volume, and mix. Immediately before use, transfer 10.0 mL of this solution to a 1000-mL volumetric flask, dilute with water to volume, and mix. This solution contains 10 µg of sulfate per mL.

Sodium chloride solution—Dissolve 2.5 g of Sodium Chloride in 50 mL of water.

Procedure—To 1.5 mL of *Standard sulfate solution A* add 1 mL of a barium chloride solution (1 in 4), shake, and allow to stand for 1 minute. To 2.5 mL of the resulting suspension, add 15 mL of the *Sodium chloride solution* and 0.5 mL of 5 N acetic acid, and mix (*Test solution*). Prepare the *Standard solution* in the same manner, except use 15 mL of *Standard sulfate solution B* instead of the *Sodium chloride solution:* any turbidity produced in the *Test solution* after 5 minutes standing is not greater than that produced in the *Standard solution* (0.020%).

Nitrites—To 10 mL of the solution prepared in the test for *Appearance of solution,* add 10 mL of water, and measure the absorbance of the solution in a 1-cm cell at 354 nm. The absorbance is not greater than 0.01.

Heavy metals, *Method I* ⟨231⟩:   5 ppm.

Assay—Dissolve 50 mg of Sodium Chloride, accurately weighed, in water, and dilute with water to 50 mL. Titrate with 0.1 N silver nitrate VS, determining the endpoint potentiometrically (see *Titrimetry* ⟨541⟩). Each mL of 0.1 N silver nitrate is equivalent to 5.844 mg of NaCl.

Sodium Chloride Injection

» Sodium Chloride Injection is a sterile solution of Sodium Chloride in Water for Injection. It contains no antimicrobial agents. It contains not less than 95.0 percent and not more than 105.0 percent of the labeled amount of NaCl.

Packaging and storage—Preserve in single-dose glass or plastic containers. Glass containers are preferably of Type I or Type II glass.

Labeling—The label states the total osmolar concentration in mOsmol per L. Where the contents are less than 100 mL, or where the label states that the Injection is not for direct injection but is to be diluted before use, the label alternatively may state the total osmolar concentration in mOsmol per mL.

USP Reference standards ⟨11⟩—*USP Endotoxin RS.*

Identification—It responds to the tests for *Sodium* ⟨191⟩ and for *Chloride* ⟨191⟩.

Bacterial endotoxins ⟨85⟩—It contains not more than 0.5 USP Endotoxin Unit per mL where the labeled amount of sodium chloride in the Injection is between 0.5% and 0.9%, and not more than 3.6 USP Endotoxin Units per mL where the labeled amount of sodium chloride in the Injection is between 3.0% and 24.3%.

pH ⟨791⟩:   between 4.5 and 7.0.

Particulate matter ⟨788⟩:   meets the requirements.

Iron ⟨241⟩—Dilute 5.0 mL of Injection with water to 45 mL, and add 2 mL of hydrochloric acid: the limit is 2 ppm.

Heavy metals, *Method I* ⟨231⟩—Place a volume of Injection, equivalent to 1.0 g of sodium chloride, in a suitable vessel, if neces-

sary evaporate to a volume of about 20 mL, add 2 mL of 1 N acetic acid, then dilute with water to 25 mL. Proceed as directed, except to use 1 mL of *Standard Lead Solution* (10 μg of Pb) in the *Standard Preparation* and in the *Monitor Preparation:* the limit is 0.001%, based on the amount of sodium chloride.
Other requirements—It meets the requirements under *Injections* ⟨1⟩.
Assay—Pipet a volume of Injection, equivalent to about 90 mg of sodium chloride, into a conical flask. Add water, if necessary, to bring the volume to about 10 mL, and add 10 mL of glacial acetic acid, 75 mL of methanol, and 3 drops of eosin Y TS. Titrate, with shaking, with 0.1 N silver nitrate VS to a pink endpoint. Each mL of 0.1 N silver nitrate is equivalent to 5.844 mg of NaCl.

Bacteriostatic Sodium Chloride Injection

» Bacteriostatic Sodium Chloride Injection is a sterile, isotonic solution of Sodium Chloride in Water for Injection, and it contains one or more suitable antimicrobial agents. It contains not less than 0.85 percent and not more than 0.95 percent of NaCl.

NOTE—Use Bacteriostatic Sodium Chloride Injection with due regard for the compatibility of the antimicrobial agent or agents it contains with the particular medicinal substance that is to be dissolved or diluted.

Packaging and storage—Preserve in single-dose or multiple-dose containers, of not larger than 30-mL size, preferably of Type I or Type II glass.
Labeling—Label it to indicate the name(s) and proportion(s) of the added antimicrobial agent(s). Label it also to include the statement "NOT FOR USE IN NEWBORNS" in boldface capital letters, on the label immediately under the official name, printed in a contrasting color, preferably red. Alternatively, the statement may be placed prominently elsewhere on the label if the statement is enclosed within a box. Label it also to include the statement "NOT FOR INHALATION."
USP Reference standards ⟨11⟩—*USP Endotoxin RS. USP Methylparaben RS. USP Propylparaben RS.*
Antimicrobial agent(s)—It meets the requirements under *Antimicrobial Preservatives—Effectiveness* ⟨51⟩, and meets the labeled claim for content of the antimicrobial agent(s) as determined by the method set forth under *Antimicrobial Agents—Content* ⟨341⟩, except to use the following procedure when methylparaben and propylparaben are used as the antimicrobial agents.
  Mobile phase—Prepare a filtered and degassed mixture of methanol and water (70 : 30). Make adjustments if necessary (see *System Suitability* under *Chromatography* ⟨621⟩).
  Standard preparation—Dissolve accurately weighed quantities of USP Methylparaben RS and USP Propylparaben RS in methanol, and dilute quantitatively, and stepwise if necessary, with methanol to obtain a solution having known concentrations of about 1.2 and 0.12 mg per mL, respectively. Pipet 5 mL of this solution into a 50-mL volumetric flask, add by pipet 30 mL of methanol, dilute with water to volume, and mix.
  Test preparation—Pipet 1 mL of Injection into a 10-mL volumetric flask, add by pipet 7 mL of methanol, dilute with water to volume, and mix.
  Chromatographic system (see *Chromatography* ⟨621⟩)—The liquid chromatograph is equipped with a 254-nm detector and a 4-mm × 30-cm column that contains packing L1. The flow rate is about 1.5 mL per minute. Chromatograph the *Standard preparation* as directed for *Procedure:* the capacity factor, k', is 0.52 for methylparaben and 1.05 for propylparaben, with a minimum separation factor (α) of about 2.0.
  Procedure—Separately inject equal volumes (about 12 μL) of the *Standard preparation* and the *Test preparation* into the chromatograph by means of a suitable microsyringe or sampling valve, adjusting the specimen size and other operating parameters such that the peak obtained with the *Standard preparation* is about 0.7 full scale. Record the chromatograms, and measure the height of the peaks, at identical retention times, obtained with the *Test preparation* and the *Standard preparation*, and calculate the concentration in mg per mL, in the portion of methylparaben or propylparaben taken by the formula:

$$C(H_U / H_S)$$

in which C is the concentration, in mg per mL, of USP Methylparaben RS or USP Propylparaben RS in the *Standard preparation;* and H_U and H_S are the peak heights obtained from the *Test preparation* and the *Standard preparation*, respectively.
Bacterial endotoxins ⟨85⟩—It contains not more than 1.0 USP Endotoxin Unit per mL.
Particulate matter ⟨788⟩: meets the requirements for small-volume injections.
Other requirements—It responds to the *Identification* test and meets the requirements for *pH, Iron, Heavy metals,* and *Assay* under *Sodium Chloride Injection*. It meets also the requirements under *Injections* ⟨1⟩.

Sodium Chloride Irrigation

» Sodium Chloride Irrigation is Sodium Chloride Injection that has been suitably packaged, and it contains no antimicrobial agents. It contains not less than 95.0 percent and not more than 105.0 percent of the labeled amount of NaCl.

Packaging and storage—Preserve in single-dose glass or plastic containers. Glass containers are preferably of Type I or Type II glass. The container may be designed to empty rapidly and may contain a volume of more than 1 L.
Labeling—The designation "not for injection" appears prominently on the label.
USP Reference standards⟨11⟩—*USP Endotoxin RS.*
Identification—It responds to the tests for *Sodium* ⟨191⟩ and for *Chloride* ⟨191⟩.
Bacterial endotoxins ⟨85⟩—It contains not more than 0.5 USP Endotoxin Unit per mL.
Sterility ⟨71⟩: meets the requirements.
Other requirements—It meets the requirements for *pH, Iron, Heavy metals,* and *Assay* under *Sodium Chloride Injection*.

Sodium Chloride Ophthalmic Ointment

» Sodium Chloride Ophthalmic Ointment is Sodium Chloride in a suitable ophthalmic ointment base. It contains not less than 90.0 percent and not more than 110.0 percent of the labeled amount of NaCl. It is sterile.

Packaging and storage—Preserve in collapsible ophthalmic ointment tubes.
Identification—Transfer a quantity of Ophthalmic Ointment, equivalent to about 200 mg of sodium chloride, to a separator containing about 25 mL of ether, and extract with 5 mL of water: the aqueous extract so obtained responds to the tests for *Sodium* ⟨191⟩, and for *Chloride* ⟨191⟩.
Sterility ⟨71⟩: meets the requirements.
Minimum fill ⟨755⟩: meets the requirements.
Metal particles ⟨751⟩: meets the requirements.
Assay—Transfer an accurately weighed quantity of Ophthalmic Ointment, equivalent to about 100 mg of sodium chloride, to a separator containing about 50 mL of ether, and extract with four 20-mL portions of water. Combine the aqueous extracts in a conical flask, evaporate to a volume of about 10 mL, and add 10 mL of glacial

acetic acid, 75 mL of methanol, and 0.5 mL of eosin Y TS. Titrate, with shaking, with 0.1 N silver nitrate VS to a pink endpoint. Each mL of 0.1 N silver nitrate is equivalent to 5.844 mg of NaCl.

Sodium Chloride Inhalation Solution

» Sodium Chloride Inhalation Solution is a sterile solution of Sodium Chloride in water purified by distillation or by reverse osmosis and rendered sterile. It contains not less than 90.0 percent and not more than 110.0 percent of the labeled amount of NaCl. It contains no antimicrobial agents or other added substances.

Packaging and storage—Preserve in single-dose containers.
Identification—It responds to the test for *Sodium* ⟨191⟩ and for *Chloride* ⟨191⟩.
Sterility ⟨71⟩: meets the requirements.
pH ⟨791⟩: between 4.5 and 7.0.
Assay—Pipet a volume of Inhalation Solution, equivalent to about 90 mg of sodium chloride, into a conical flask, and add 10 mL of glacial acetic acid, 75 mL of methanol, and 0.5 mL of eosin Y TS. Titrate, with shaking, with 0.1 N silver nitrate VS to a pink endpoint. Each mL of 0.1 N silver nitrate is equivalent to 5.844 mg of NaCl.

Sodium Chloride Ophthalmic Solution

» Sodium Chloride Ophthalmic Solution is a sterile solution of Sodium Chloride. It contains not less than 90.0 percent and not more than 110.0 percent of the labeled amount of sodium chloride. It may contain suitable antimicrobial and stabilizing agents. It contains a buffer.

Packaging and storage—Preserve in tight containers.
Identification—Heat a portion of Ophthalmic Solution to boiling, and filter while hot. After cooling, the filtrate responds to the tests for *Sodium* ⟨191⟩ and for *Chloride* ⟨191⟩.
Sterility ⟨71⟩: meets the requirements.
pH ⟨791⟩: between 6.0 and 8.0.
Assay—Transfer an accurately measured volume of Ophthalmic Solution, equivalent to about 90 mg of sodium chloride, to a conical flask, and add 10 mL of glacial acetic acid, 75 mL of methanol, and 0.5 mL of eosin Y TS. Titrate, with shaking, with 0.1 N silver nitrate VS to a pink endpoint. Each mL of 0.1 N silver nitrate is equivalent to 5.844 mg of NaCl.

Sodium Chloride Tablets

» Sodium Chloride Tablets contain not less than 95.0 percent and not more than 105.0 percent of the labeled amount of NaCl.

Packaging and storage—Preserve in well-closed containers.
Identification—A filtered extract of Tablets responds to the tests for *Sodium* ⟨191⟩ and for *Chloride* ⟨191⟩.
Disintegration ⟨701⟩: 30 minutes.
Uniformity of dosage units ⟨905⟩: meet the requirements.
Iodide or bromide—Digest 2.0 g of powdered Tablets with 25 mL of warm alcohol for 3 hours, cool, and filter. Evaporate the filtrate to dryness, dissolve the residue in 5 mL of water, filter if necessary, and add 1 mL of chloroform. Cautiously introduce, dropwise, with constant agitation, 5 drops of dilute chlorine TS (1 in 3): the chloroform does not acquire a violet, yellow, or orange color.
Barium—Digest 4.0 g of powdered Tablets with 20 mL of water, filter, and divide the solution into two equal portions. To one portion add 2 mL of 2 N sulfuric acid and to the other add 2 mL of water: the solutions are equally clear after standing for 2 hours.
Calcium and magnesium—Digest 1 g of powdered Tablets with 50 mL of water, and filter. Add 4 mL of 6 N ammonium hydroxide to the filtrate, and divide the mixture into two equal portions. Treat one portion with 1 mL of ammonium oxalate TS and the other portion with 1 mL of dibasic sodium phosphate TS: neither mixture becomes turbid within 5 minutes.
Assay—Dissolve a counted number of not less than 20 Tablets in about 100 mL of water, filter into a 500-mL volumetric flask, and wash the original container and the filter with 100 mL of water in divided portions, adding the washings to the original filtrate. Dilute with water to volume. Pipet a volume of the solution, equivalent to about 90 mg of sodium chloride, to a conical flask, and add 10 mL of glacial acetic acid, 75 mL of methanol, and 0.5 mL of eosin Y TS. Titrate, with shaking, with 0.1 N silver nitrate VS to a pink endpoint. Each mL of 0.1 N silver nitrate is equivalent to 5.844 mg of NaCl.

Sodium Chloride Tablets for Solution

» Sodium Chloride Tablets for Solution are composed of Sodium Chloride in compressed form, containing no added substance. Sodium Chloride Tablets for Solution contain not less than 95.0 percent and not more than 105.0 percent of the labeled amount of NaCl.

Other requirements—The Sodium Chloride Tablets for Solution respond to the *Identification* test and meet the requirements for *Packaging and storage*, *Iodide or bromide*, *Barium*, *Calcium and magnesium*, *Disintegration*, *Uniformity of dosage units*, and *Assay* under *Sodium Chloride Tablets*.

Sodium Chloride and Dextrose Tablets

» Sodium Chloride and Dextrose Tablets contain not less than 92.5 percent and not more than 107.5 percent of the labeled amount of sodium chloride (NaCl) and of dextrose ($C_6H_{12}O_6 \cdot H_2O$).

Packaging and storage—Preserve in well-closed containers.
Identification—
  A: A filtered solution of Tablets responds to the flame test for *Sodium* ⟨191⟩ and to the test for *Chloride* ⟨191⟩.
  B: Add a few drops of the filtered solution tablets to 5 mL of hot alkaline cupric tartrate TS: a copious red precipitate of cuprous oxide is formed.
Disintegration ⟨701⟩: 30 minutes.
Uniformity of dosage units ⟨905⟩: meet the requirements.
Assay for sodium chloride—Transfer 20.0 mL of the solution prepared for the *Assay for dextrose* to a 100-mL volumetric flask, dilute with water to volume, mix, and proceed as directed in the *Assay* under *Sodium Chloride Tablets*, beginning with "Pipet a volume of the solution."
Assay for dextrose—Dissolve not fewer than 10 Tablets, containing from 2 to 5 g of dextrose, in about 75 mL of water in a 100-mL volumetric flask, add several drops of 6 N ammonium hydroxide, dilute with water to volume, and mix. After 30 minutes, pass through a dry filter, and determine the angular rotation in a suitable polarimeter tube (see *Optical Rotation* ⟨781⟩), retaining the excess of the solution for the *Assay for sodium chloride*. Calculate the per-

centage (g per 100 mL) of dextrose ($C_6H_{12}O_6 \cdot H_2O$) in the portion of Injection taken by the formula:

$$(100/52.9)(198.17/180.16)AR$$

in which 100 is the percentage; 52.9 is the midpoint of the specific rotation range for anhydrous dextrose, in degrees; 198.17 and 180.16 are the molecular weights for dextrose monohydrate and anhydrous dextrose, respectively; A is 100 mm divided by the length of the polarimeter tube, in mm; and R is the observed rotation, in degrees.

Sodium Citrate

$C_6H_5Na_3O_7$ (anhydrous) 258.07
1,2,3-Propanetricarboxylic acid, 2-hydroxy-, trisodium salt.
Trisodium citrate (anhydrous)   [68-04-2].
Trisodium citrate dihydrate   294.10   [6132-04-3].

» Sodium Citrate is anhydrous or contains two molecules of water of hydration. It contains not less than 99.0 percent and not more than 100.5 percent of $C_6H_5Na_3O_7$, calculated on the anhydrous basis.

Packaging and storage—Preserve in tight containers.
Labeling—Label it to indicate whether it is anhydrous or hydrous.
Identification—
  A: A solution (1 in 20) responds to the tests for *Sodium* ⟨191⟩ and for *Citrate* ⟨191⟩.
  B: Upon ignition, it yields an alkaline residue which effervesces when treated with 3 N hydrochloric acid.
Alkalinity—A solution of 1.0 g in 20 mL of water is alkaline to litmus paper, but after the addition of 0.20 mL of 0.10 N sulfuric acid no pink color is produced by 1 drop of phenolphthalein TS.
Water, *Method III* ⟨921⟩—Dry it at 180° for 18 hours: the anhydrous form loses not more than 1.0%, and the hydrous form between 10.0 and 13.0%, of its weight.
Tartrate—To a solution of 1 g in 2 mL of water add 1 mL of potassium acetate TS and 1 mL of 6 N acetic acid. Rub the wall of the tube with a glass rod: no crystalline precipitate is formed.
Heavy metals ⟨231⟩—Dissolve a portion equivalent to 4.4 g of anhydrous sodium citrate in enough water to make 50 mL of stock solution. Transfer 12 mL of this stock solution to a 50-mL color-comparison tube (*Test Preparation*). Transfer 11 mL of the stock solution to a second 50-mL color-comparison tube containing 1.0 mL of *Standard Lead Solution* (*Monitor Preparation*). Transfer 1.0 mL of *Standard Lead Solution* and 11 mL of water to a third 50-mL color-comparison tube (*Standard Preparation*). Proceed as directed for *Procedure*, omitting the dilution to 50 mL: the limit is 0.001%.
Assay—Transfer about 350 mg of Sodium Citrate, previously dried at 180° for 18 hours and accurately weighed, to a 250-mL beaker. Add 100 mL of glacial acetic acid, stir until completely dissolved, and titrate with 0.1 N perchloric acid VS, determining the endpoint potentiometrically. Perform a blank determination, and make any necessary correction. Each mL of 0.1 N perchloric acid is equivalent to 8.602 mg of $C_6H_5Na_3O_7$.

Sodium Citrate and Citric Acid Oral Solution

» Sodium Citrate and Citric Acid Oral Solution is a solution of Sodium Citrate and Citric Acid in a suitable aqueous medium. It contains, in each 100 mL, not less than 2.23 g and not more than 2.46 g of sodium (Na), and not less than 6.11 g and not more than 6.75 g of citrate ($C_6H_5O_7$), equivalent to not less than 9.5 g and not more than 10.5 g of sodium citrate dihydrate ($C_6H_5Na_3O_7 \cdot 2H_2O$); and not less than 6.34 g and not more than 7.02 g of citric acid monohydrate ($C_6H_8O_7 \cdot H_2O$).

Packaging and storage—Preserve in tight containers.
Identification—
  A: It meets the requirements of the flame test for *Sodium* ⟨191⟩.
  B: Add 2 mL of 15% potassium carbonate TS to 2 mL of Oral Solution, boil, and cool. Add 4 mL of potassium pyroantimonate TS: a dense precipitate is formed (*presence of sodium*).
  C: To 2 mL of a dilution of Oral Solution (1 in 20) add 5 mL of sodium cobaltinitrite TS: a yellow precipitate is not formed immediately (*absence of potassium*).
  D: It meets the requirements of the tests for *Citrate* ⟨191⟩, 3 to 5 drops of Oral Solution and 20 mL of the mixture of pyridine and acetic anhydride being used.
Uniformity of dosage units ⟨905⟩—
  FOR ORAL SOLUTION PACKAGED IN SINGLE-UNIT CONTAINERS: meets the requirements.
Deliverable volume ⟨698⟩—
  FOR ORAL SOLUTION PACKAGED IN MULTIPLE-UNIT CONTAINERS: meets the requirements.
pH ⟨791⟩:   between 4.0 and 4.4.
Assay for sodium—
  Potassium stock solution, Sodium stock solution, Lithium diluent solution, and *Standard preparation*—Prepare as directed in the *Assay for sodium and potassium* under *Tricitrates Oral Solution*.
  Assay preparation—Transfer an accurately measured volume of Oral Solution, equivalent to about 1 g of sodium citrate dihydrate, to a 100-mL volumetric flask, dilute with water to volume, and mix. Transfer 50 µL of this solution to a 10-mL volumetric flask, dilute with *Lithium diluent solution* to volume, and mix.
  Procedure—Using a suitable flame photometer, adjusted to read zero with *Lithium diluent solution,* concomitantly determine the sodium flame emission readings for the *Standard preparation* and the *Assay preparation* at the wavelength of maximum emission at about 589 nm. Calculate the quantity, in g, of Na in each mL of Oral Solution taken by the formula:

$$(14.61/25V)(22.99/58.44)(R_{U,Na} / R_{S,Na})$$

in which 14.61 is the weight, in g, of sodium chloride in the *Sodium stock solution;* V is the volume, in mL, of Oral Solution taken, 22.99 is the atomic weight of sodium; 58.44 is the molecular weight of sodium chloride; and $R_{U,Na}$ and $R_{S,Na}$ are the sodium emission readings obtained for the *Assay preparation* and the *Standard preparation,* respectively.

Assay for sodium citrate—
  Cation-exchange column—Mix 10 g of styrene-divinylbenzene cation-exchange resin with 50 mL of water in a suitable beaker. Allow the resin to settle, and decant the supernatant until a slurry of resin remains. Pour the slurry into a 15-mm × 30-cm glass chromatographic tube (having a sealed-in, coarse-porosity fritted disk and fitted with a stopcock), and allow to settle as a homogeneous bed. Wash the resin bed with about 100 mL of water, closing the stopcock when the water level is about 2 mm above the resin bed.
  Procedure—Transfer an accurately measured volume of Oral Solution, equivalent to about 1 g of sodium citrate dihydrate, to a 100-mL volumetric flask; dilute with water to volume; and mix. Pipet 5 mL of this solution carefully onto the top of the resin bed in the *Cation-exchange column*. Place a 250-mL conical flask below the column, open the stopcock, and allow to flow until the solution has entered the resin bed. Elute the column with 60 mL of water at a flow rate of about 5 mL per minute, collecting about 65 mL of the eluate. Add 5 drops of phenolphthalein TS to the eluate, swirl the flask, and titrate with 0.02 N sodium hydroxide VS. Record the buret reading, and calculate the volume (B) of 0.02 N sodium hydroxide consumed. Calculate the quantity, in mg, of sodium citrate dihy-

drate (C₆H₅Na₃O₇ · 2H₂O) in each mL of the Oral Solution taken by the formula:

$$[1.961B(20/V)] - [(294.10/210.14)C]$$

in which 1.961 is the equivalent, in mg, of C₆H₅Na₃O₇ · 2H₂O, of each mL of 0.02 N sodium hydroxide; V is the volume, in mL, of Oral Solution taken; 294.10 and 210.14 are the molecular weights of sodium citrate dihydrate and citric acid monohydrate, respectively; and C is the concentration, in mg per mL, of citric acid monohydrate in the Oral Suspension, as obtained in the *Assay for citric acid*.

Assay for citric acid—Transfer an accurately measured volume of Oral Solution, equivalent to about 0.67 g of citric acid monohydrate, to a 100-mL volumetric flask; dilute with water to volume; and mix. Pipet 5 mL of this solution into a suitable flask, add 25 mL of water and 5 drops of phenolphthalein TS, and titrate with 0.02 N sodium hydroxide VS to a pink endpoint. Record the buret reading, and calculate the volume *(A)* of 0.02 N sodium hydroxide consumed. Calculate the quantity, in mg, of citric acid monohydrate (C₆H₈O₇ · H₂O) in each mL of the Oral Solution taken by the formula:

$$1.401A(20/V)$$

in which 1.401 is the equivalent, in mg, of C₆H₈O₇ · H₂O, of each mL of 0.02 N sodium hydroxide; and V is the volume, in mL, of Oral Solution taken.

Sodium Fluoride

NaF 41.99
Sodium fluoride.
Sodium fluoride [7681-49-4].

» Sodium Fluoride contains not less than 98.0 percent and not more than 102.0 percent of NaF, calculated on the dried basis.

Packaging and storage—Preserve in well-closed containers.
Identification—
  A: Place 1 g in a platinum crucible *in a well-ventilated hood*, add 15 mL of sulfuric acid, and cover the crucible with a piece of clear, polished glass. Heat the crucible on a steam bath for 1 hour, remove the glass cover, rinse it in water, and wipe dry: the surface of the glass is etched.
  B: A solution (1 in 25) responds to the tests for *Sodium* ⟨191⟩.
Acidity or alkalinity—Dissolve 2.0 g in 40 mL of water in a platinum dish, add 10 mL of a saturated solution of potassium nitrate, cool the solution to 0°, and add 3 drops of phenolphthalein TS. If no color appears, a pink color persisting for 15 seconds is produced by not more than 2.0 mL of 0.10 N sodium hydroxide. If the solution is colored pink by the addition of phenolphthalein TS, it is rendered colorless by not more than 0.50 mL of 0.10 N sulfuric acid. Save the neutralized solution for the test for *Fluosilicate*.
Loss on drying ⟨731⟩—Dry it at 150° for 4 hours: it loses not more than 1.0% of its weight.
Fluosilicate—After the solution from the test for *Acidity or alkalinity* has been neutralized, heat to boiling, and titrate while hot with 0.10 N sodium hydroxide until a permanent pink color is obtained: not more than 1.5 mL of 0.10 N sodium hydroxide is required.
Chloride—Dissolve 300 mg in 20 mL of water, and add 200 mg of boric acid, 1 mL of nitric acid, and 1 mL of 0.1 N silver nitrate: any turbidity produced is not greater than that of a blank to which has been added 1.0 mL of 0.0010 N hydrochloric acid (0.012%).
Heavy metals ⟨231⟩—To 1 g, in a platinum dish or crucible, under a hood, add 1 mL of water and 3 mL of sulfuric acid, and heat at as low a temperature as practicable until all of the sulfuric acid has been expelled. Dissolve the residue in 20 mL of water, neutralize the solution to phenolphthalein TS with ammonium hydroxide, add 1 mL of glacial acetic acid, dilute with water to 45 mL, filter, and use 30 mL of the filtrate for the test: the limit is 0.003%.

Organic volatile impurities, *Method I* ⟨467⟩: meets the requirements.

(Official until July 1, 2008)
Assay—To 80.0 mg of Sodium Fluoride add a mixture of 5 mL of acetic anhydride and 20 mL of glacial acetic acid, and heat to dissolve. Allow to cool, and add 20 mL of dioxane. Add 1 drop of crystal violet TS, and titrate with 0.1 N perchloric acid VS to a green endpoint. Perform a blank determination, and make any necessary correction. Each mL of 0.1 N perchloric acid is equivalent to 4.199 mg of NaF.

Sodium Fluoride Oral Solution

» Sodium Fluoride Oral Solution contains not less than 90.0 percent and not more than 110.0 percent of the labeled amount of NaF.

Packaging and storage—Preserve in tight containers, plastic containers being used for Oral Solution having a pH below 7.5.
Labeling—Label Oral Solution in terms of the content of sodium fluoride (NaF) and in terms of the content of fluoride ion.
USP Reference standards ⟨11⟩—*USP Sodium Fluoride RS*.
Identification—
  A: Transfer 0.1 mL of Oral Solution to a small test tube, and add 0.1 mL of a freshly prepared mixture (1 : 1) of sodium alizarinsulfonate solution (1 in 1000) and zirconyl nitrate solution (1 in 1000) in 7 N hydrochloric acid: a yellow color is produced.
  B: If necessary, reduce the volume of a portion of it by heating on a steam bath to a reduced volume containing about 10 mg of sodium per mL: the solution so obtained responds to the tests for *Sodium* ⟨191⟩.
Assay—[NOTE—Store all solutions, except *Buffer solution*, in plastic containers.]
  Buffer solution—Dissolve 57 mL of glacial acetic acid, 58 g of sodium chloride, and 4 g of (1,2-cyclohexylenedinitrilo)tetraacetic acid in 500 mL of water. Adjust with 5 N sodium hydroxide to a pH of 5.25 ± 0.25, dilute with water to 1000 mL, and mix.
  Standard preparations—Dissolve an accurately weighed quantity of USP Sodium Fluoride RS quantitatively in water to obtain a solution containing 420 µg per mL. Each mL of this solution (*Standard preparation A*) contains 190 µg of fluoride ion (10^{-2} M). Transfer 25.0 mL of *Standard preparation A* to a 250-mL volumetric flask, dilute with water to volume, and mix. This solution (*Standard preparation B*) contains 19 µg of fluoride ion per mL (10^{-3} M). Transfer 25.0 mL of *Standard preparation B* to a 250-mL volumetric flask, dilute with water to volume, and mix. This solution (*Standard preparation C*) contains 1.9 µg of fluoride ion per mL (10^{-4} M).
  Assay preparation—Transfer an accurately measured volume of Oral Solution, equivalent to about 10 mg of fluoride, to a 500-mL volumetric flask, dilute with water to volume, and mix.
  Procedure—Pipet 20 mL of each *Standard preparation* and of the *Assay preparation* into separate plastic beakers each containing a plastic-coated stirring bar. Pipet 20 mL of *Buffer solution* into each beaker. Concomitantly measure the potentials (see *pH* ⟨791⟩), in mV, of the solutions from the *Standard preparations* and of the solution from the *Assay preparation*, with a pH meter capable of a minimum reproducibility of ±0.2 mV and equipped with a fluoride-specific ion-indicating electrode and a suitable reference electrode. [NOTE—When taking measurements, immerse the electrodes in the solution, stir on a magnetic stirrer having an insulated top until equilibrium is attained (1 to 2 minutes), and record the potential. Rinse and dry the electrodes between measurements, taking care to avoid damaging the crystal of the specific-ion electrode.] Plot the logarithms of the fluoride-ion concentrations, in µg per mL, of the *Standard preparations* versus potential, in mV. From the measured potential of the *Assay preparation* and the standard response line, determine the concentration, C, in µg per mL, of fluoride ion in the

Assay preparation. Calculate the quantity, in mg, of fluoride ion in each mL of the Oral Solution taken by the formula:

$$0.5(C/V)$$

in which C is the determined concentration of fluoride, in µg per mL, in the *Assay preparation*, and V is the volume, in mL, of Oral Solution taken. Multiply the quantity of fluoride ion by 2.21 to obtain the quantity of NaF.

Sodium Fluoride Tablets

» Sodium Fluoride Tablets contain not less than 90.0 percent and not more than 110.0 percent of the labeled amount of NaF.

Packaging and storage—Preserve in tight containers.
Labeling—Label the Tablets in terms of the content of sodium fluoride (NaF) and in terms of the content of fluoride ion. The Tablets that are to be chewed may be labeled as Sodium Fluoride Chewable Tablets.
USP Reference standards ⟨11⟩—*USP Sodium Fluoride RS.*
Identification—
A: Disperse 20 finely powdered Tablets in 25 mL of water, shake, and filter: a portion of the filtrate responds to the tests for *Sodium* ⟨191⟩.
B: Evaporate a 10-mL portion of the filtrate obtained in *Identification* test A to dryness. To the residue add a mixture of 0.1 mL of freshly prepared sodium alizarinsulfonate solution (1 in 1000) and 0.1 mL of a 1 in 1000 solution of zirconyl nitrate in 7 N hydrochloric acid: a yellow color is produced.
Disintegration ⟨701⟩: 15 minutes.
Uniformity of dosage units ⟨905⟩: meet the requirements.
Assay—[NOTE—Store all solutions, except *Buffer solution*, in plastic containers.]
Buffer solution and *Standard preparations*—Prepare as directed in the *Assay* under *Sodium Fluoride Oral Solution*.
Assay preparation—Weigh and finely powder not less than 20 Tablets. Transfer an accurately weighed portion of the powder, equivalent to about 10 mg of fluoride, to a plastic 500-mL conical flask containing 400 mL of water. Heat on a steam bath for 25 minutes with occasional shaking, cool to room temperature, transfer to a 500-mL volumetric flask, dilute with water to volume, and mix.
Procedure—Proceed as directed for *Procedure* in the *Assay* under *Sodium Fluoride Oral Solution*. Calculate the quantity, in mg, of fluoride ion in the portion of Tablets taken by the formula:

$$0.5C$$

in which C is the determined concentration, in µg per mL, of fluoride ion in the *Assay preparation*. Multiply the quantity of fluoride ion by 2.21 to obtain the quantity of NaF.

Sodium Fluoride and Acidulated Phosphate Topical Solution

» Sodium Fluoride and Acidulated Phosphate Topical Solution contains not less than 90.0 percent and not more than 110.0 percent of the labeled amount of fluoride ion.

Packaging and storage—Preserve in tight plastic containers.
Labeling—Label Topical Solution in terms of the content of sodium fluoride (NaF) and in terms of the content of fluoride ion.
USP Reference standards ⟨11⟩—*USP Sodium Fluoride RS.*
pH ⟨791⟩—Place about 40 mL in a plastic beaker, add about 250 mg of quinhydrone, and stir for 1 minute, leaving some of the quinhydrone undissolved. Determine the pH using a hydrofluoric acid frit-junction calomel reference electrode and a hydrofluoric acid-resistant metallic electrode: the pH is between 3.0 and 4.5.
Other requirements—It responds to the *Identification* tests under *Sodium Fluoride and Phosphoric Acid Gel*.
Assay—
Buffer solution and *Standard preparations*—Prepare as directed in the *Assay* under *Sodium Fluoride Oral Solution*.
Assay preparation—Transfer an accurately measured volume of Topical Solution, equivalent to about 20 mg of fluoride ion, to a 1000-mL volumetric flask, add water to dissolve, dilute with water to volume, and mix.
Procedure—Proceed as directed for *Procedure* in the *Assay* under *Sodium Fluoride Oral Solution*. Calculate the quantity, in mg, of fluoride ion in each mL of the Topical Solution taken by the formula:

$$C/V$$

in which C is the determined concentration of fluoride ion, in µg per mL, in the *Assay preparation*, and V is the volume, in mL, of Topical Solution taken.

Sodium Fluoride and Phosphoric Acid Gel

» Sodium Fluoride and Phosphoric Acid Gel contains not less than 90.0 percent and not more than 110.0 percent of the labeled amount of fluoride ion, in an aqueous medium containing a suitable viscosity-inducing agent.

Packaging and storage—Preserve in tight, plastic containers.
Labeling—Label Gel in terms of the content of sodium fluoride (NaF) and in terms of the content of fluoride ion.
USP Reference standards ⟨11⟩—*USP Sodium Fluoride RS.*
Identification—
A: Place a quantity of Gel, equivalent to about 500 mg of fluoride ion, in a platinum crucible in a well-ventilated hood, and add 15 mL of sulfuric acid. Cover the crucible with a piece of clear, polished glass, and heat on a steam bath for 1 hour. Remove the glass cover, rinse it in water, and dry: the glass surface exposed to vapors from the crucible is etched.
B: It responds to the tests for *Phosphate* ⟨191⟩.
Viscosity ⟨911⟩—Place a quantity of Gel in a suitable plastic container, insert the stopper securely, and allow to stand until the gel is free from air bubbles. Place it in a water bath maintained at a temperature of 25 ± 0.5° until it adjusts to the temperature of the water bath (30 minutes or longer). Do not stir the gel while it is in the bath. Remove the sample from the bath, stir the gel gently for 5 seconds, and without delay, using a rotational viscosimeter, determine the viscosity using the appropriate spindle to obtain a scale reading between 10% and 90% of full scale at a speed of 60 rpm or of 30 rpm. Calculate the viscosity, in centipoises, by multiplying the scale reading by the constant for the spindle and speed used: the viscosity is between 7000 and 20,000 centipoises.
pH ⟨791⟩—Place about 40 mL in a plastic beaker, add about 250 mg of quinhydrone, and stir for 1 minute, leaving some of the quinhydrone undissolved. Determine the pH using a hydrofluoric acid frit-junction calomel reference electrode and a platinum electrode: the pH is between 3.0 and 4.0.
Assay—[NOTE—Store all solutions, except *Buffer solution*, in plastic containers.]
Buffer solution and *Standard preparations*—Prepare as directed in the *Assay* under *Sodium Fluoride Oral Solution*.
Assay preparation—Transfer a quantity of Gel, equivalent to about 20 mg of fluoride ion, accurately weighed, to a 1000-mL volumetric flask, add water to dissolve, dilute with water to volume, and mix.
Procedure—Proceed as directed for *Procedure* in the *Assay* under *Sodium Fluoride Oral Solution*. The quantity, in mg, of fluoride ion in the portion of Gel taken is equivalent to C, the determined

concentration of fluoride ion, in µg per mL, in the *Assay preparation*.

Sodium Gluconate

$C_6H_{11}NaO_7$ 218.14
D-Gluconic acid, monosodium salt.
Monosodium D-gluconate   [527-07-1].

» Sodium Gluconate contains not less than 98.0 percent and not more than 102.0 percent of $C_6H_{11}NaO_7$.

Packaging and storage—Preserve in well-closed containers.
USP Reference standards ⟨11⟩—*USP Potassium Gluconate RS*.
Identification—
  A: A solution (1 in 20) responds to the tests for *Sodium* ⟨191⟩.
  B: It responds to *Identification* test *B* under *Calcium Gluconate*.
Chloride ⟨221⟩—A 1.0-g portion shows no more chloride than corresponds to 1 mL of 0.020 N hydrochloric acid (0.07%).
Sulfate ⟨221⟩—A 2.0-g portion dissolved in boiling water shows no more sulfate than corresponds to 1 mL of 0.020 N sulfuric acid (0.05%).
Lead ⟨251⟩—Dissolve 1.0 g in 25 mL of water: the limit is 0.001%.
Heavy metals, *Method I* ⟨231⟩—Dissolve 1.0 g in 10 mL of water, add 6 mL of 3 N hydrochloric acid, and dilute with water to 25 mL: the limit is 0.002%.
Reducing substances—Transfer 1.0 g to a 250-mL conical flask, dissolve in 10 mL of water, and add 25 mL of alkaline cupric citrate TS. Cover the flask, boil gently for 5 minutes, accurately timed, and cool rapidly to room temperature. Add 25 mL of 0.6 N acetic acid, 10.0 mL of 0.1 N iodine VS, and 10 mL of 3 N hydrochloric acid, and titrate with 0.1 N sodium thiosulfate VS, adding 3 mL of starch TS as the endpoint is approached. Perform a blank determination, omitting the specimen, and note the difference in volumes required. Each mL of the difference in volume of 0.1 N sodium thiosulfate consumed is equivalent to 2.7 mg of reducing substances (as dextrose): the limit is 0.5%.
Assay—Transfer about 150 mg of Sodium Gluconate, accurately weighed, to a suitable conical flask, and dissolve in 75 mL of glacial acetic acid, warming if necessary to effect complete solution. Cool, add quinaldine red TS, and titrate with 0.1 N perchloric acid VS to a colorless endpoint. Each mL of 0.1 N perchloric acid is equivalent to 21.81 mg of $C_6H_{11}NaO_7$.

Sodium Hypochlorite Solution

NaClO   74.44
Hypochlorous acid, sodium salt.
Sodium hypochlorite   [7681-52-9].

» Sodium Hypochlorite Solution contains not less than 4.0 percent and not more than 6.0 percent, by weight, of NaClO.

Caution—This Solution is not suitable for application to wounds.

Packaging and storage—Preserve in tight, light-resistant containers, at a temperature not exceeding 25°.
Identification—
  A: The Solution at first colors red litmus blue and then bleaches it.
  B: The addition of 3 N hydrochloric acid to the Solution causes an evolution of chlorine.
  C: The solution obtained in *Identification* test *B* responds to the flame test for *Sodium* ⟨191⟩.
Assay—Weigh accurately, in a glass-stoppered flask, about 3 mL of Solution, and dilute it with 50 mL of water. Add 2 g of potassium iodide and 10 mL of 6 N acetic acid, and titrate the liberated iodine with 0.1 N sodium thiosulfate VS, adding 3 mL of starch TS as the endpoint is approached. Perform a blank determination, and make any necessary correction. Each mL of 0.1 N sodium thiosulfate is equivalent to 3.722 mg of NaClO.

Sodium Hypochlorite Topical Solution

» Sodium Hypochlorite Topical Solution contains not less than 0.20 g and not more than 0.32 g of Sodium Hypochlorite (NaClO) in 1000 mL of Topical Solution. Prepare Sodium Hypochlorite Topical Solution as follows (see *Pharmaceutical Compounding—Nonsterile Preparations* ⟨795⟩):

Sodium Hypochlorite Solution	5.0 mL
Monobasic Sodium Phosphate monohydrate	1.02 g
Dibasic Sodium Phosphate anhydrous	17.61 g
Purified Water, a sufficient quantity to make	1000 mL

Dissolve the Dibasic Sodium Phosphate anhydrous and the Monobasic Sodium Phosphate monohydrate in about 500 mL of Purified Water. Add the Sodium Hypochlorite Solution and sufficient Purified Water to make the product measure 1000 mL, and mix to produce the Topical Solution.

NOTE—The source of the Sodium Hypochlorite Solution may be commercial unscented laundry bleach (nominally 5.25% w/v) provided that the commercial laundry bleach was recently acquired.

Packaging and storage—Preserve in tight, light-resistant 1-liter plastic containers, and store at controlled room temperature.
Labeling—Label it to indicate that its strength is 0.025 percent, and to state the correct beyond-use date. [NOTE—For external use only; it may be applied to wounds and burns.]
pH ⟨791⟩:   between 7.8 and 8.2.
Beyond-use date—Seven days after the day on which it was compounded.
Assay—Transfer 50.0 mL of the Solution to a glass-stoppered flask, and add 0.5 g of potassium iodide and 10 mL of 6 N acetic acid. Titrate the liberated iodine with 0.1 N sodium thiosulfate VS, adding 2 mL of starch TS as the endpoint is approached. Perform a blank determination and make any necessary correction. Each mL of 0.1 N sodium thiosulfate is equivalent to 3.722 mg of NaClO.

Sodium Iodide

NaI   149.89
Sodium iodide.
Sodium iodide   [7681-82-5].

» Sodium Iodide contains not less than 99.0 percent and not more than 101.5 percent of NaI, calculated on the anhydrous basis.

Packaging and storage—Preserve in tight containers.
Identification—A solution (1 in 20) responds to the tests for *Sodium* ⟨191⟩ and for *Iodide* ⟨191⟩.
Alkalinity—Dissolve 1.0 g in 10 mL of water, and add 0.15 mL of 0.10 N sulfuric acid: no red color is produced by the addition of 1 drop of phenolphthalein TS.
Water, *Method I* ⟨921⟩: not more than 2.0%.
Iodate—It meets the requirements of the test for *Iodate* under *Potassium Iodide*, 100 mg of Sodium Iodide being used in the control.
Thiosulfate and barium—It meets the requirements of the test for *Thiosulfate and barium* under *Potassium Iodide*.
Potassium—A solution of 1.0 g in 2 mL of water yields no precipitate with 1.0 mL of sodium bitartrate TS.
Heavy metals ⟨231⟩—Dissolve 2.0 g in 25 mL of water: the limit is 0.001%.
Limit of nitrate, nitrite, and ammonia—Add 5 mL of 1 N sodium hydroxide and about 200 mg of aluminum wire to a solution of 1.0 g of Sodium Iodide in 5 mL of water, contained in a test tube of about 40-mL capacity. Insert a pledget of purified cotton in the upper portion of the test tube, and place a piece of moistened red litmus paper over the mouth of the tube. Heat in a steam bath for 15 minutes: no blue coloration of the paper is discernible.
Organic volatile impurities, *Method I* ⟨467⟩: meets the requirements.
(Official until July 1, 2008)
Assay—Weigh accurately about 500 mg of Sodium Iodide, and dissolve in about 10 mL of water. Add 35 mL of hydrochloric acid, and titrate with 0.05 M potassium iodate VS until the dark brown solution which is produced becomes pale brown. Add 1 mL of amaranth TS, and continue the titration slowly until the red color just changes to yellow. Each mL of 0.05 M potassium iodate is equivalent to 14.99 mg of NaI.

Sodium Lactate Injection

$C_3H_5NaO_3$ 112.06
Propanoic acid, 2-hydroxy-, monosodium salt.
Sodium lactate   [72-17-3].

» Sodium Lactate Injection is sterile Sodium Lactate Solution in Water for Injection, or a sterile solution of Lactic Acid in Water for Injection prepared with the aid of Sodium Hydroxide. It contains not less than 95.0 percent and not more than 110.0 percent of the labeled amount of $C_3H_5NaO_3$.

Packaging and storage—Preserve in single-dose glass or plastic containers. Glass containers are preferably of Type I or Type II glass.
Labeling—The label states the total osmolar concentration in mOsmol per L. Where the contents are less than 100 mL, or where the label states that the Injection is not for direct injection but is to be diluted before use, the label alternatively may state the total osmolar concentration in mOsmol per mL. The label includes also the warning: "Not for use in the treatment of lactic acidosis."
USP Reference standards ⟨11⟩—*USP Endotoxin RS*.
Identification—Overlay 2 mL of Injection on 5 mL of a 1 in 100 solution of catechol in sulfuric acid: a deep red color is produced at the zone of contact.
Bacterial endotoxins ⟨85⟩—It contains not more than 2.0 USP Endotoxin Units per mEq.
pH ⟨791⟩: between 6.0 and 7.3, the Injection being diluted with water, if necessary, to approximately 0.16 M (20 mg per mL).
Particulate matter ⟨788⟩: meets the requirements under small-volume injections.
Heavy metals ⟨231⟩—Evaporate a volume of Injection, equivalent to 2.0 g of sodium lactate, to 5 mL, and dilute with 1 N acetic acid to 25 mL: the limit is 0.001%.
Other requirements—It meets the requirements under *Injections* ⟨1⟩.
Assay—Pipet into a small beaker a volume of Injection, equivalent to about 300 mg of sodium lactate, and evaporate to dryness. Add to the residue 60 mL of a 1 in 5 mixture of acetic anhydride in glacial acetic acid, and stir until the residue is completely dissolved. Titrate with 0.1 N perchloric acid VS, determining the endpoint potentiometrically. Perform a blank determination, and make any necessary correction. Each mL of 0.1 N perchloric acid is equivalent to 11.21 mg of $C_3H_5NaO_3$.

Sodium Lactate Solution

» Sodium Lactate Solution is an aqueous solution containing not less than 50.0 percent, by weight, of monosodium lactate. It contains not less than 98.0 percent and not more than 102.0 percent of the labeled amount of $C_3H_5NaO_3$.

Packaging and storage—Preserve in tight containers.
Labeling—Label it to indicate its content of sodium lactate.
Identification—It responds to the tests for *Sodium* ⟨191⟩ and for *Lactate* ⟨191⟩.
pH ⟨791⟩: between 5.0 and 9.0.
Chloride ⟨221⟩—A portion, equivalent to 1 g of sodium lactate, shows no more chloride than corresponds to 0.7 mL of 0.020 N hydrochloric acid (0.05%).
Sulfate—To 10 mL of a solution (1 in 100) add 2 drops of hydrochloric acid and 1 mL of barium chloride TS: no turbidity is produced.
Heavy metals, *Method I* ⟨231⟩—Dilute a quantity of Solution, equivalent to 2.0 g of sodium lactate, with 1 N acetic acid to 25 mL: the limit is 0.001%.
Sugars—To 10 mL of hot alkaline cupric tartrate TS add 5 drops of Solution: no red precipitate is formed.
Limit of citrate, oxalate, phosphate, or tartrate—Dilute 5 mL with recently boiled and cooled water to 50 mL. To 4 mL of this solution add 6 N ammonium hydroxide or 3 N hydrochloric acid, if necessary, to bring the pH to between 7.3 and 7.7. Add 1 mL of calcium chloride TS, and heat in a boiling water bath for 5 minutes: the solution remains clear.
Limit of methanol and methyl esters—
Potassium permanganate and *phosphoric acid solution*—Dissolve 3 g of potassium permanganate in a mixture of 15 mL of phosphoric acid and 70 mL of water. Dilute with water to 100 mL.
Oxalic acid and *sulfuric acid solution*—Cautiously add 50 mL of sulfuric acid to 50 mL of water, mix, cool, add 5 g of oxalic acid, and mix to dissolve.
Standard preparation—Prepare a solution containing 10.0 mg of methanol in 100 mL of dilute alcohol (1 in 10).
Test preparation—Place 40.0 g in a glass-stoppered, round-bottom flask, add 10 mL of water, and add cautiously 30 mL of 5 N potassium hydroxide. Connect a condenser to the flask, and steam-distill, collecting the distillate in a suitable 100-mL graduated vessel containing 10 mL of alcohol. Continue the distillation until the volume in the receiver reaches approximately 95 mL, and dilute the distillate with water to 100.0 mL.
Procedure—Transfer 10.0 mL each of the *Standard preparation* and the *Test preparation* to 25-mL volumetric flasks, to each add 5.0 mL of *Potassium permanganate and phosphoric acid solution*, and mix. After 15 minutes, to each add 2.0 mL of *Oxalic acid and sulfuric acid solution*, stir with a glass rod until the solution is colorless, add 5.0 mL of fuchsin-sulfurous acid TS, and dilute with water to volume. After 2 hours, concomitantly determine the ab-

sorbances of both solutions in 1-cm cells at the wavelength of maximum absorbance at about 575 nm, with a suitable spectrophotometer, using water as the blank: the absorbance of the solution from the *Test preparation* is not greater than that from the *Standard preparation* (0.025%).

Assay—Weigh accurately into a suitable flask a volume of Solution, equivalent to about 300 mg of sodium lactate, add 60 mL of a 1 in 5 mixture of acetic anhydride in glacial acetic acid, mix, and allow to stand for 20 minutes. Titrate with 0.1 N perchloric acid VS, determining the endpoint potentiometrically. Perform a blank determination, and make any necessary correction. Each mL of 0.1 N perchloric acid is equivalent to 11.21 mg of $C_3H_5NaO_3$.

Sodium Monofluorophosphate

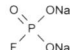

Na_2PFO_3 143.95
Phosphorofluoridic acid, disodium salt.
Disodium phosphorofluoridate   [10163-15-2].

» Sodium Monofluorophosphate contains not less than 91.7 percent and not more than 100.5 percent of Na_2PFO_3, calculated on the dried basis.

Packaging and storage—Preserve in well-closed containers.

USP Reference standards ⟨11⟩—*USP Sodium Fluoride RS.*

Identification—
 A: Place about 1 g in a platinum crucible in a well-ventilated hood, and add 15 mL of sulfuric acid. Cover the crucible with a piece of clear, polished glass, and heat on a steam bath for 1 hour. Remove the glass cover, rinse it in water, and dry: the glass surface exposed to vapors from the crucible is etched.
 B: A solution (1 in 10) with silver nitrate TS yields a white precipitate, which is soluble in diluted nitric acid and in dilute ammonium hydroxide (1 in 2).
 C: A solution responds to the tests for *Sodium* ⟨191⟩.

pH ⟨791⟩: between 6.5 and 8.0, in a solution (1 in 50).

Loss on drying ⟨731⟩—Dry it at 105° to constant weight: it loses not more than 0.2% of its weight.

Arsenic, *Method I* ⟨211⟩:   3 ppm.

Heavy metals, *Method I* ⟨231⟩—Dissolve 400 mg in 25 mL of water: the limit is 0.005%.

Limit of fluoride ion—[NOTE—Use plasticware throughout this test.]
 Buffer solution—To 55 g of sodium chloride in a 1000-mL volumetric flask add 500 mg of sodium citrate, 255 g of sodium acetate, and 300 mL of water. Shake to dissolve, and cautiously add 115 mL of glacial acetic acid with mixing. Cool to room temperature, add 300 mL of isopropyl alcohol, dilute with water to volume, and mix: the pH of this solution is between 5.0 and 5.5.
 Standard stock solution—Dissolve an accurately weighed quantity of USP Sodium Fluoride RS quantitatively in water to obtain a solution containing 1105 μg per mL. Each mL of this solution contains 500 μg of fluoride ion. Store in a tightly closed, plastic container.
 Standard preparations—To four 100-mL volumetric flasks transfer, respectively, 2.0-, 4.0-, 10.0-, and 20.0-mL portions of the *Standard stock solution*, dilute each with *Buffer solution* to volume, and mix to obtain solutions having fluoride ion concentrations of 10, 20, 50, and 100 μg per mL, respectively.
 Test preparation—Transfer about 1.8 g, accurately weighed, to a 100-mL volumetric flask, add water to dissolve, dilute with water to volume, and mix. Transfer 20.0 mL of this solution to a second 100-mL volumetric flask, dilute with *Buffer solution* to volume, and mix.
 Procedure—Concomitantly measure the potential (see *pH* ⟨791⟩), in mV, of the *Standard preparations* and of the *Test preparation* with a pH meter capable of a minimum reproducibility of ±0.2 mV,
equipped with a glass-sleeved calomel-fluoride specific-ion electrode system. [NOTE—When taking measurements, immerse the electrodes in the solution, which has been transferred to a 150-mL plastic beaker containing a plastic-coated stirring bar. Allow to stir on a magnetic stirrer having an insulated top until equilibrium is attained (1 to 2 minutes), and record the potential. Rinse and dry the electrodes between measurements, taking care to avoid damaging the crystal of the specific-ion electrode.] Plot the logarithm of the fluoride-ion concentrations, in μg per mL, of each *Standard preparation* versus potential, in mV. From the measured potential of the *Test preparation* and the standard curve, determine the concentration, in μg per mL, of fluoride ion in the *Test preparation*: not more than 1.2% is found.

Organic volatile impurities, *Method I* ⟨467⟩: meets the requirements.

(Official until July 1, 2008)

Assay—
 Monochloroacetate buffer—Dissolve 189 g of monochloroacetic acid and 55 g of sodium hydroxide in about 1500 mL of water. Cool, dilute with water to 2000 mL, and mix.
 0.025 M Thorium nitrate—Dissolve 13.8 g of thorium nitrate in about 800 mL of water, and filter the solution into a 1000-mL volumetric flask. Dilute with water to volume, and mix. Standardize this solution as follows. Transfer 20.0 mL of *Standard stock solution*, prepared as directed in the test for *Limit of fluoride ion*, to a 150-mL beaker containing 50 mL of water. Add 3 drops of sodium alizarinsulfonate TS, mix, and adjust the acidity by the careful addition, successively, of sodium hydroxide solution (1 in 50) and dilute hydrochloric acid (1 in 160), until the pink color has just been discharged. Add 1 mL of *Monochloroacetate buffer*, and titrate with *0.025 M Thorium nitrate* to a permanent pink color. Calculate the molarity of the thorium nitrate titrant taken by the equation:

$$M = (S) / [(4)(41.99V)]$$

in which S is the weight, in mg, of USP Sodium Fluoride RS in the portion of *Standard stock solution* taken, 41.99 is the molecular weight of sodium fluoride, and V is the volume, in mL, of titrant consumed.
 Procedure—Transfer about 1.8 g of Sodium Monofluorophosphate, accurately weighed, to a 100-mL volumetric flask. Add about 50 mL of water, mix to effect solution, dilute with water to volume, and mix. Transfer 20.0 mL of this solution to the reaction flask of a suitable fluoride steam distilling apparatus containing 10 lime-glass beads measuring 5 mm in diameter and 70 mL of dilute sulfuric acid (1 in 2). Distill, by passing steam through the solution in the reaction flask and applying heat to the flask, collecting the distillate in a 250-mL volumetric flask. Control the temperature of the solution in the reaction flask so that it does not exceed 140°. Change receivers when the flask is filled to volume with distillate, and continue distilling into a 400-mL beaker until an additional 150 mL to 200 mL of distillate tailing has been collected. Mix the solution in the 250-mL volumetric flask, and transfer 50.0 mL to a 150-mL beaker. To the 150-mL beaker add 50 mL of water and 3 drops of sodium alizarinsulfonate TS, and mix. Adjust the acidity of this solution by the careful addition, successively, of sodium hydroxide solution (1 in 50) and dilute hydrochloric acid (1 in 160), until the pink color has just been discharged. Add 1 mL of *Monochloroacetate buffer*, titrate with *0.025 M Thorium nitrate* to a permanent pink color, and record the volume, in mL, of titrant consumed as V_A. Add 3 drops of sodium alizarinsulfonate TS to the distillation tail in the 400-mL beaker, proceed as directed previously with the adjustment of the acidity, the addition of *Monochloroacetate buffer*, and the titration with *0.025 M Thorium nitrate*, and record the volume, in mL, of titrant consumed as V_B. Calculate the percentage of Na_2PFO_3 in the Sodium Monofluorophosphate taken by the formula:

$$[(2)(143.95)(5V_A + V_B)(M) / (W)] - (143.95 / 18.9984)(F)$$

in which M is the molarity of *0.025 M Thorium nitrate;* W is the weight, in g, of the Sodium Monofluorophosphate taken; F is the percentage of fluoride ions determined as directed in the test for *Limit of fluoride ion*; 143.95 is the molecular weight of sodium monofluorophosphate; 18.9984 is the atomic weight of fluorine; and the other terms are as defined therein.

Sodium Nitrite

NaNO₂   69.00
Nitrous acid, sodium salt.
Sodium nitrite   [7632-00-0].

» Sodium Nitrite contains not less than 97.0 percent and not more than 101.0 percent of NaNO₂, calculated on the dried basis.

Packaging and storage—Preserve in tight containers. Store at 25°, excursions permitted between 15° and 30°.
Identification—A solution of it responds to the tests for *Sodium* ⟨191⟩ and for *Nitrite* ⟨191⟩.
Loss on drying ⟨731⟩—Dry it over silica gel for 4 hours: it loses not more than 0.25% of its weight.
Heavy metals ⟨231⟩—Dissolve 1 g in 6 mL of 3 N hydrochloric acid, and evaporate on a steam bath to dryness. Reduce the residue to a coarse powder, and continue heating on the steam bath until the odor of hydrochloric acid no longer is perceptible. Dissolve the residue in 23 mL of water, and add 2 mL of 1 N acetic acid: the limit is 0.002%.
Assay—Dissolve about 1 g of Sodium Nitrite, accurately weighed, in water to make 100.0 mL. Pipet 10 mL of this solution into a mixture of 50.0 mL of 0.1 N potassium permanganate VS, 100 mL of water, and 5 mL of sulfuric acid. When adding the Sodium Nitrite solution, immerse the tip of the pipet beneath the surface of the permanganate mixture. Warm the liquid to 40°, allow it to stand for 5 minutes, and add 25.0 mL of 0.1 N oxalic acid VS. Heat the mixture to about 80°, and titrate with 0.1 N potassium permanganate VS. Each mL of 0.1 N potassium permanganate is equivalent to 3.450 mg of NaNO₂.

Sodium Nitrite Injection

» Sodium Nitrite Injection is a sterile solution of Sodium Nitrite in Water for Injection. It contains not less than 95.0 percent and not more than 105.0 percent of the labeled amount of NaNO₂.

Packaging and storage—Preserve in single-dose containers, of Type I glass.

USP Reference standards ⟨11⟩—*USP Endotoxin RS.*
Identification—It responds to the *Identification* tests under *Sodium Nitrite*.
Bacterial endotoxins ⟨85⟩—It contains not more than 0.33 USP Endotoxin Unit per mg of sodium nitrite.
pH ⟨791⟩: between 7.0 and 9.0.
Other requirements—It meets the requirements under *Injections* ⟨1⟩.
Assay—Pipet an accurately measured volume of Injection, containing about 150 mg of sodium nitrite into a mixture of 50.0 mL of 0.1 N potassium permanganate VS, 100 mL of water, and 5 mL of sulfuric acid, immersing the tip of the pipet beneath the surface of the mixture during the addition. Warm the liquid to 40°, allow it to stand for 5 minutes, and add 25.0 mL of 0.1 N oxalic acid VS. Heat the mixture to about 80°, and titrate with 0.1 N potassium permanganate VS. Each mL of 0.1 N potassium permanganate is equivalent to 3.450 mg of NaNO₂.

Sodium Nitroprusside

Na₂[Fe(CN)₅NO] · 2H₂O   297.95
Ferrate(2-), pentakis(cyano-*C*)nitrosyl-, disodium, dihydrate, (*OC*-6-22)-.
Disodium pentacyanonitrosylferrate(2-) dihydrate   [13755-38-9].
Sodium nitroferricyanide dihydrate.
Anhydrous   261.92   [14402-89-2].

» Sodium Nitroprusside contains not less than 99.0 percent of Na₂[Fe(CN)₅NO] · 2H₂O.

Packaging and storage—Preserve in tight, light-resistant containers. Store at 25°, excursions permitted between 15° and 30°.
Labeling—Where it is intended for use in preparing injectable dosage forms, the label states that it is sterile or must be subjected to further processing during the preparation of injectable dosage forms.
USP Reference standards ⟨11⟩—*USP Endotoxin RS. USP Sodium Nitroprusside RS.*
Identification—
  A: *Ultraviolet Absorption* ⟨197U⟩—[NOTE—Use low-actinic glassware.]
    Solution: 1 in 135.
    Medium: water.
    Wavelength range: 350 nm to 700 mm.
  B: Dissolve 5 mg in 2 mL of water, and add 2 drops of acetone and 0.5 mL of 2 N sodium hydroxide: an orange color is produced. Add 2 mL of acetic acid: the color changes to purple.
  C: A solution (1 in 4) responds to the flame test for *Sodium* ⟨191⟩.
Water, *Method I* ⟨921⟩:   between 9.0% and 15.0%.
Insoluble substances—Dissolve 10.0 g in 50 mL of water, heat the solution on a steam bath for 30 minutes, filter, wash the residue with water, and dry at 105° to constant weight: the weight of the residue is not greater than 1 mg (0.01%).
Chloride—
  Standard chloride solution—Dissolve 42.4 mg of potassium chloride in water to make 100.0 mL of solution. Each mL of this solution contains 0.2 mg of chloride.
  Procedure—Transfer 1.0 g of Sodium Nitroprusside to a 250-mL conical flask, transfer 1.0 mL of *Standard chloride solution* to a similar flask, and add to each flask 85 mL of water. To the flask containing the substance under test, add 15 mL of cupric sulfate solution (83 in 1000), mix, and allow any undissolved particles to settle. Carefully add cupric sulfate solution (83 in 1000) to the flask containing the diluted *Standard chloride solution*, with mixing, so that its color matches that of the test solution in the first flask. Filter the contents of each flask, and discard the first 25 mL of the filtrate. To 10 mL of the subsequent filtrate from each flask add 2 mL of nitric acid, and mix. Add 1 mL of 1 N silver nitrate to each, and again mix: the test solution so treated becomes no more turbid than the treated *Standard chloride solution* (0.02%).
Limit of ferricyanide—Dissolve 500 mg in 20 mL of ammonium acetate TS, previously adjusted with 1 N acetic acid to a pH of 4.62. Divide this solution into halves, and transfer each half to a separate 50-mL volumetric flask, identified as *A* and *B*, respectively. To flask *B* add 1.0 mL of a freshly prepared solution of potassium ferricyanide containing 78 µg per mL. To both flasks add 5 mL of ferrous ammonium sulfate solution (1 in 1000), dilute with water to volume, and mix. Allow the flasks to stand for 1 hour, and concomitantly determine the absorbance of the solutions at the wavelength of maximum absorbance at about 720 nm, using as a blank a solution prepared by dissolving 250 mg of the specimen in 10 mL of the pH 4.62 ammonium acetate TS and diluting with water to 50 mL. The absorbance of the solution in flask *A* is not greater than the absorbance of the solution in flask *B* minus the absorbance of the solution in flask *A* (0.02% of ferricyanide).
Limit of ferrocyanide—Dissolve 2.0 g in 40 mL of water, divide the solution into halves, and transfer each half to a separate 50-mL volumetric flask, identified as *A* and *B*, respectively. To flask *B* add 2 mL of a freshly prepared solution of potassium ferrocyanide containing 200 µg per mL. To both flasks add 0.2 mL of ferric chloride TS, dilute with water to volume, and mix. Allow to stand for 20

minutes, accurately timed, and concomitantly measure the absorbance of the solutions at the wavelength of maximum absorbance at about 695 nm, using as a blank a solution prepared by dissolving 1.0 g of the specimen in water to make 50 mL: the absorbance of the solution in flask *A* is not greater than the absorbance of the solution in flask *B* minus the absorbance of the solution in flask *A* (0.02% of ferrocyanide).

Sulfate—

Standard sulfate solution—Dissolve 15 mg of anhydrous sodium sulfate in water to make 100.0 mL of solution. Each mL of this solution contains 0.1 mg of sulfate.

Procedure—Dissolve 5.0 g of Sodium Nitroprusside in water to make 250.0 mL of solution, and filter the solution into a flat-bottom, 250-mL graduated flask. Transfer 5.0 mL of *Standard sulfate solution* to a similar flask, and dilute to the same volume as the test solution. To each flask add 10 drops of glacial acetic acid and 5 mL of 1 N barium chloride, and allow to stand for 10 minutes. Place both flasks over a fluorescent light source, and observe: the turbidity in the treated test solution is not more intense than that of the treated *Standard sulfate solution* (0.01%).

Other requirements—Where the label states that Sodium Nitroprusside is sterile, it meets the requirements for *Sterility Tests* ⟨71⟩ and for *Bacterial endotoxins* under Sodium Nitroprusside for Injection. Where the label states that Sodium Nitroprusside must be subjected to further processing during the preparation of injectable dosage forms, it meets the requirements for *Bacterial endotoxins* under Sodium Nitroprusside for Injection.

Assay—Dissolve about 500 mg of Sodium Nitroprusside, accurately weighed, in 130 mL of chloride-free water. Titrate with 0.1 N silver nitrate VS, determining the endpoint potentiometrically, using a silver-silver chloride electrode system. Each mL of 0.1 N silver nitrate is equivalent to 14.90 mg of $Na_2[Fe(CN)_5NO] \cdot 2H_2O$.

Sodium Nitroprusside for Injection

» Sodium Nitroprusside for Injection is Sodium Nitroprusside suitable for parenteral use. It contains not less than 90.0 percent and not more than 110.0 percent of the labeled amount of sodium nitroprusside ($Na_2[Fe(CN)_5NO] \cdot 2H_2O$).

Packaging and storage—Preserve protected from light in *Containers for Sterile Solids* as described under *Injections* ⟨1⟩.

USP Reference standards ⟨11⟩—*USP Endotoxin RS. USP Sodium Nitroprusside RS.*

Constituted solution—At the time of use, it meets the requirements for *Constituted Solutions* under *Injections* ⟨1⟩.

Identification—To 50 mg contained in a small test tube add 10 mL of ascorbic acid solution (1 in 50), and mix. Add 1 mL of dilute hydrochloric acid (1 in 10), mix, and add dropwise, while mixing, 1 to 2 mL of 1 N sodium hydroxide: a transient blue color is produced.

Bacterial endotoxins ⟨85⟩—It contains not more than 0.05 USP Endotoxin Unit per µg of sodium nitroprusside.

Water, *Method I* ⟨921⟩: not more than 15.0%.

Other requirements—It responds to the *Identification* test under Sodium Nitroprusside. It meets also the requirements for *Sterility Tests* ⟨71⟩, *Uniformity of Dosage Units* ⟨905⟩, and *Labeling* under *Injections* ⟨1⟩.

Assay—

pH 7.1 buffer—Dissolve 1.36 g of monobasic potassium phosphate and 5.2 mL of a 1 in 4 solution of tetrabutylammonium hydroxide in methanol in water to make 1000 mL, and adjust with phosphoric acid or with the tetrabutylammonium hydroxide solution to a pH of 7.1.

Mobile phase—Prepare a suitable filtered mixture of *pH 7.1 buffer* and acetonitrile (about 70 : 30).

NOTE—Use low-actinic glassware throughout the following sections.

Standard preparation—Dissolve an accurately weighed quantity of USP Sodium Nitroprusside RS, in *Mobile phase* to obtain a solution having a known concentration of about 0.05 mg per mL.

Assay preparation 1 (where the label states only the total contents of the container)—Transfer the contents of 1 container of Sodium Nitroprusside for Injection to a 100-mL volumetric flask with the aid of *Mobile phase*, dilute with *Mobile phase* to volume, and mix. Dilute an accurately measured volume of this solution quantitatively with *Mobile phase* to obtain a solution containing about 0.05 mg of $Na_2[Fe(CN)_5NO] \cdot 2H_2O$ per mL.

Assay preparation 2 (where the label states the quantity of $Na_2[Fe(CN)_5NO] \cdot 2H_2O$ in a given volume of constituted solution)—Constitute Sodium Nitroprusside for Injection as directed in the labeling. Dilute an accurately measured volume of the constituted solution thus obtained quantitatively and stepwise with *Mobile phase* to obtain a solution containing about 0.05 mg of $Na_2[Fe(CN)_5NO] \cdot 2H_2O$ per mL.

Chromatographic system (see *Chromatography* ⟨621⟩)—The liquid chromatograph is equipped with a 210-nm detector and a 3.9-mm × 30-cm column that contains 10-µm packing L11. The flow rate is about 2 mL per minute. Chromatograph the *Standard preparation*, and record the peak responses as directed for *Procedure*: the tailing factor for the analyte peak is not more than 2.0; and the relative standard deviation for replicate injections is not more than 1.5%.

Procedure—Separately inject equal volumes (about 25 µL) of the *Standard preparation* and the *Assay preparation* into the chromatograph, record the chromatograms, and measure the responses for the major peaks. Calculate the quantity, in mg, of $Na_2[Fe(CN)_5NO] \cdot 2H_2O$ in the container or in the portion of constituted solution taken by the formula:

$$L(C/D)(r_U/r_S)$$

in which L is the labeled quantity, in mg of $Na_2[Fe(CN)_5NO] \cdot 2H_2O$ in the container, or in the volume of constituted solution taken; C is the concentration, in mg per mL, of USP Sodium Nitroprusside RS in the *Standard preparation*; D is the concentration, in mg of $Na_2[Fe(CN)_5NO] \cdot 2H_2O$ per mL, of *Assay preparation 1* or of *Assay preparation 2*, on the basis of the labeled quantity in the container, or in the volume of constituted solution taken, respectively, and the extent of dilution; and r_U and r_S are the peak responses obtained from the *Assay preparation* and the *Standard preparation*, respectively.

Dibasic Sodium Phosphate

$Na_2HPO_4 \cdot xH_2O$ (anhydrous)   141.96
Phosphoric acid, disodium salt, dodecahydrate.
Disodium hydrogen phosphate, dodecahydrate   358.14   [10039-32-4].
Phosphoric acid, disodium salt, heptahydrate.
Disodium hydrogen phosphate heptahydrate   268.07   [7782-85-6].
Phosphoric acid, disodium salt, dihydrate.
Disodium hydrogen phosphate, dihydrate   177.99   [10028-24-7].
Phosphoric acid, sodium salt, monohydrate.
Disodium hydrogen phosphate, monohydrate   159.94   [118830-14-1].
Phosphoric acid, disodium salt, hydrate.
Disodium hydrogen phosphate hydrate   [10140-65-5].
Anhydrous   [7558-79-4].

» Dibasic Sodium Phosphate is dried or contains one, two, seven, or twelve molecules of water of hydration. It contains not less than 98.0 percent and not more than 100.5 percent of Na_2HPO_4, calculated on the dried basis.

Packaging and storage—Preserve in tight containers.
Labeling—Label it to indicate whether it is dried or is the monohydrate, the dihydrate, the heptahydrate, or the dodecahydrate.

Identification—A solution (the equivalent of 1 part of Na₂HPO₄ in 30) responds to the tests for *Sodium* ⟨191⟩ and for *Phosphate* ⟨191⟩.
Loss on drying ⟨731⟩—Dry it at 130° to constant weight: the dried form loses not more than 5.0% of its weight, the monohydrate loses between 10.3% and 12.0% of its weight, the dihydrate loses between 18.5% and 21.5% of its weight, the heptahydrate loses between 43.0% and 50.0% of its weight, and the dodecahydrate loses between 55.0% and 64.0% of its weight.
Insoluble substances—Dissolve the equivalent of 5.0 g of Na₂HPO₄ in 100 mL of hot water, filter through a tared filtering crucible, wash the insoluble residue with hot water, and dry at 105° for 2 hours: the weight of the residue so obtained does not exceed 20 mg (0.4%).
Chloride ⟨221⟩—A portion equivalent to 0.5 g of Na₂HPO₄ shows no more chloride than corresponds to 0.42 mL of 0.020 N hydrochloric acid (0.06%).
Sulfate ⟨221⟩—A portion equivalent to 0.1 g of Na₂HPO₄ shows no more sulfate than corresponds to 0.2 mL of 0.020 N sulfuric acid (0.2%).
Arsenic, *Method I* ⟨211⟩—Prepare a *Test Preparation* by dissolving a portion equivalent to 187.5 mg of Na₂HPO₄ in 35 mL of water: the limit is 16 ppm.
Heavy metals ⟨231⟩—Dissolve a portion equivalent to 2.1 g of Na₂HPO₄ in enough water to make 50 mL of stock solution. Transfer 12 mL of this stock solution to a 50-mL color-comparison tube *(Test Preparation)*. Transfer 11 mL of the stock solution to a second color-comparison tube containing 1.0 mL of *Standard Lead Solution (Monitor Preparation)*. Transfer 1.0 mL of *Standard Lead Solution* and 11 mL of water to a third color-comparison tube *(Standard Preparation)*. Proceed as directed for *Procedure*, omitting the dilution to 50 mL: the limit is 0.002%.
Assay—Transfer 40.0 mL of 1 N hydrochloric acid to a 250-mL beaker, add 50 mL of water, and titrate potentiometrically with 1 N sodium hydroxide VS to the endpoint. Record the volume of 1 N sodium hydroxide VS consumed as the blank. Transfer a portion of Dibasic Sodium Phosphate, accurately weighed, equivalent to about 2.5 g of Na₂HPO₄, to a 250-mL beaker, add 40.0 mL of 1 N hydrochloric acid and 50 mL of water, and stir until dissolved. Titrate the excess acid potentiometrically with 1 N sodium hydroxide VS to the inflection point at about pH 4, and record the buret reading. Subtract this buret reading from that of the blank, and designate the volume of 1 N sodium hydroxide VS resulting from this subtraction as *A*. Continue the titration with 1 N sodium hydroxide VS to the inflection point at about pH 8.8, record the buret reading, and calculate the volume *(B)* of 1 N sodium hydroxide required in the titration between the two inflection points (pH 4 to pH 8.8). Where *A* is equal to or less than *B*, each mL of the volume *A* of 1 N sodium hydroxide is equivalent to 142.0 mg of Na₂HPO₄. Where *A* is greater than *B*, each mL of the volume $2B - A$ of 1 N sodium hydroxide is equivalent to 142.0 mg of Na₂HPO₄.

Monobasic Sodium Phosphate

NaH₂PO₄ · xH₂O
(anhydrous)   119.98
Phosphoric acid, monosodium salt, monohydrate.
Monosodium phosphate monohydrate   137.99   [10049-21-5].
Phosphoric acid, monosodium salt, dihydrate.
Monosodium phosphate dihydrate   156.01   [13472-35-0].
Anhydrous   [7558-80-7].

» Monobasic Sodium Phosphate contains one or two molecules of water of hydration, or is anhydrous. It contains not less than 98.0 percent and not more than 103.0 percent of NaH₂PO₄, calculated on the anhydrous basis.

Packaging and storage—Preserve in well-closed containers.
Labeling—Label it to indicate whether it is anhydrous or is the monohydrate or the dihydrate.
Identification—A solution (1 in 20) responds to the tests for *Sodium* ⟨191⟩ and for *Phosphate* ⟨191⟩.
pH ⟨791⟩: between 4.1 and 4.5, in a solution containing the equivalent of 1.0 g of NaH₂PO₄ · H₂O in 20 mL of water.
Water, *Method I* ⟨921⟩: less than 2.0% (anhydrous form); between 10.0% and 15.0% (monohydrate); between 18.0% and 26.5% (dihydrate). For the monohydrate, the sample may be ground to a fine powder in an atmosphere of temperature and relative humidity known not to influence the results, prior to performing the test.
Insoluble substances—Dissolve a portion equivalent to 10.0 g of NaH₂PO₄ · H₂O in 100 mL of hot water, filter through a tared filtering crucible, wash the insoluble residue with hot water, and dry at 105° for 2 hours: the weight of the residue so obtained does not exceed 20 mg (0.2%).
Chloride ⟨221⟩—A portion equivalent to 1.0 g of NaH₂PO₄ · H₂O shows no more chloride than corresponds to 0.20 mL of 0.020 N hydrochloric acid (0.014%).
Sulfate ⟨221⟩—A portion equivalent to 0.20 g of NaH₂PO₄ · H₂O shows no more sulfate than corresponds to 0.30 mL of 0.020 N sulfuric acid (0.15%).
Aluminum, calcium, and related elements—A solution containing the equivalent of 1.0 g of NaH₂PO₄ · H₂O in 10 mL of water does not become turbid when rendered slightly alkaline to litmus paper with 6 N ammonium hydroxide.
Arsenic, *Method I* ⟨211⟩—Dissolve a portion equivalent to 0.375 g of NaH₂PO₄ · H₂O in 35 mL of water: the limit is 8 ppm.
Heavy metals ⟨231⟩—Dissolve a portion equivalent to 1.0 g of NaH₂PO₄ · H₂O in 20 mL of water, and add 1 mL of 3 N hydrochloric acid and water to make 25 mL: the limit is 0.002%.
Organic volatile impurities, *Method I* ⟨467⟩:   meets the requirements.

(Official until July 1, 2008)

Assay—Dissolve about 2.5 g of Monobasic Sodium Phosphate, accurately weighed, in 10 mL of cold water, add 20 mL of a cold, saturated solution of sodium chloride, then add phenolphthalein TS, and titrate with 1 N sodium hydroxide VS, keeping the temperature of the solution between 10° and 15° during the entire titration. Perform a blank determination, and make any necessary correction. Each mL of 1 N sodium hydroxide is equivalent to 120.0 mg of NaH₂PO₄.

Sodium Phosphates Injection

» Sodium Phosphates Injection is a sterile solution of Monobasic Sodium Phosphate and Dibasic Sodium Phosphate in Water for Injection. It contains not less than 95.0 percent and not more than 105.0 percent of the labeled amounts of monobasic sodium phosphate (NaH₂PO₄ · H₂O) and dibasic sodium phosphate (Na₂HPO₄ · 7H₂O). It contains no bacteriostat or other preservative.

Packaging and storage—Preserve in single-dose containers, preferably of Type I glass.
Labeling—The label states the sodium content in terms of milliequivalents in a given volume, and states also the phosphorus content in terms of millimoles in a given volume. Label the Injection to indicate that it is to be diluted to appropriate strength with water or other suitable fluid prior to administration and that once opened any unused portion is to be discarded. The label states also the total osmolar concentration in mOsmol per L. Where the contents are less than 100 mL, or where the label states that the Injection is not for direct injection but is to be diluted before use, the label alternatively may state the total osmolar concentration in mOsmol per mL.

USP Reference standards ⟨11⟩—*USP Endotoxin RS*.
Identification—It responds to the tests for *Sodium* ⟨191⟩ and for *Phosphate* ⟨191⟩.
Bacterial endotoxins ⟨85⟩—It contains not more than 1.10 USP Endotoxin Units per mg of sodium phosphates.
Particulate matter ⟨788⟩:   meets the requirements under small-volume injections.

Other requirements—It meets the requirements under *Injections* ⟨1⟩.
Assay for monobasic sodium phosphate—Transfer an accurately measured volume of Injection, equivalent to about 300 mg of anhydrous monobasic sodium phosphate, to a 100-mL beaker, and dilute with water to about 50 mL. Place the electrodes of a suitable pH meter in the solution, and titrate with 0.1 N sodium hydroxide VS to the inflection point to a pH of about 8.8. Each mL of 0.1 N sodium hydroxide is equivalent to 13.80 mg of $NaH_2PO_4 \cdot H_2O$.
Assay for dibasic sodium phosphate—Transfer an accurately measured volume of Injection, equivalent to about 300 mg of anhydrous dibasic sodium phosphate, to a 100-mL beaker, and dilute with water to about 50 mL. Place the electrodes of a suitable pH meter in the solution, and titrate with 0.1 N hydrochloric acid VS to the inflection point to a pH of about 4.0. Each mL of 0.1 N hydrochloric acid is equivalent to 26.81 mg of $Na_2HPO_4 \cdot 7H_2O$.

Sodium Phosphates Oral Solution

» Sodium Phosphates Oral Solution is a solution of Dibasic Sodium Phosphate and Monobasic Sodium Phosphate, or Dibasic Sodium Phosphate and Phosphoric Acid, in Purified Water. It contains, in each 100 mL, not less than 16.2 g and not more than 19.8 g of dibasic sodium phosphate ($Na_2HPO_4 \cdot 7H_2O$), and not less than 43.2 g and not more than 52.8 g of monobasic sodium phosphate ($NaH_2PO_4 \cdot H_2O$).

Packaging and storage—Preserve in tight containers.
Identification—It responds to the tests for *Sodium* ⟨191⟩ and for *Phosphate* ⟨191⟩.
Specific gravity ⟨841⟩: between 1.333 and 1.366.
pH ⟨791⟩: between 4.4 and 5.2.
Assay—Pipet 25.0 mL of Oral Solution into a 500-mL volumetric flask, dilute with water to volume, and mix. Transfer 25.0 mL of this stock solution to a 250-mL beaker, and add 15.0 mL of 0.5 N sodium hydroxide and 75 mL of water. Proceed as directed in the *Assay* under *Sodium Phosphates Rectal Solution*, beginning with "Titrate the excess base."

Sodium Phosphates Rectal Solution

» Sodium Phosphates Rectal Solution is a solution of Dibasic Sodium Phosphate and Monobasic Sodium Phosphate, or Dibasic Sodium Phosphate and Phosphoric Acid, in Purified Water. It contains, in each 100 mL, not less than 5.4 g and not more than 6.6 g of dibasic sodium phosphate ($Na_2HPO_4 \cdot 7H_2O$), and not less than 14.4 g and not more than 17.6 g of monobasic sodium phosphate ($NaH_2PO_4 \cdot H_2O$).

Packaging and storage—Preserve in tight, single-unit containers, at controlled room temperature.
Identification—It meets the requirements of the tests for *Sodium* ⟨191⟩ and for *Phosphate* ⟨191⟩.
Specific gravity ⟨841⟩: between 1.112 and 1.136.
pH ⟨791⟩: between 5.0 and 5.8.
Assay—Pipet 5.0 mL of Rectal Solution into a 250-mL beaker, and add 15.0 mL of 0.5 N sodium hydroxide VS and 95 mL of water. Titrate the excess base potentiometrically with 0.5 N hydrochloric acid VS to the first inflection point, at a pH of about 9.2. Record the volume, *A*, in mL, of 0.5 N hydrochloric acid consumed. Continue the titration to the second inflection point, at a pH of about 4.4, and record the total volume, *B*, in mL, of 0.5 N hydrochloric acid required in the titration. For a blank determination, transfer 15.0 mL of 0.5 N sodium hydroxide into a 250-mL beaker, add 100 mL of water, and immediately titrate potentiometrically with 0.5 N hydrochloric acid VS. Record the volume, *C*, in mL, of 0.5 N hydrochloric acid consumed. Each mL of the volume (*C − A*) of 0.5 N hydrochloric acid is equivalent to 69.0 mg of monobasic sodium phosphate ($NaH_2PO_4 \cdot H_2O$). Each mL of the volume (*B − C*) of 0.5 N hydrochloric acid is equivalent to 134.0 mg of dibasic sodium phosphate ($Na_2HPO_4 \cdot 7H_2O$).

Sodium Polystyrene Sulfonate

Benzene, diethenyl-, polymer with ethenylbenzene, sulfonated, sodium salt.
Divinylbenzene copolymer with styrene, sulfonated, sodium salt.

» Sodium Polystyrene Sulfonate is a cation-exchange resin prepared in the sodium form. Each g exchanges not less than 110 mg and not more than 135 mg of potassium, calculated on the anhydrous basis.

Packaging and storage—Preserve in well-closed containers.
Labeling—Sodium Polystyrene Sulfonate that is intended for preparing suspensions for oral or rectal administration may be labeled Sodium Polystyrene Sulfonate for Suspension.
Water, *Method I* ⟨921⟩: not more than 10.0%.
Limit of ammonium salts—Place 1 g in a 50-mL beaker, add 5 mL of 1 N sodium hydroxide, cover the beaker with a watch glass having a moistened strip of red litmus paper on the underside, and allow to stand for 15 minutes: the litmus paper shows no blue color.
Sodium content—
Sodium solution—Dissolve in water an accurately weighed quantity of sodium chloride to make a solution containing 5.00 mg of sodium per mL.
Standard graph—Into four 1-liter flasks pipet, respectively, 0, 1, 2, and 3 mL of *Sodium solution*. To each flask add 0.1 mL of nitric acid, 0.1 mL of sulfuric acid, and 10 mL of low-sodium, low-potassium, nonionic surfactant solution (1 in 50), dilute with water to volume, and mix. Adjust the scale of a suitable flame spectrophotometer to a reading of 100 at a wavelength of 588 nm with the solution containing 15 mg of sodium per L. Determine the instrument readings on the other three solutions, and plot the observed readings, on ruled coordinate paper, as the ordinate, and the concentration of sodium, in mg per liter, as the abscissa. The line intersects the ordinate at, or below, a scale reading of 25 ("blank reading").
Procedure—Ash the equivalent of 1 g of Sodium Polystyrene Sulfonate, accurately weighed, with a slight excess of sulfuric acid. Add 1 mL of nitric acid and a few mL of water to the residue. Warm to dissolve, and transfer with water to a 1-liter volumetric flask, dilute with water to volume, and mix. Pipet 10 mL of this solution into a 100-mL volumetric flask, add 1 mL of low-sodium, low-potassium, non-ionic surfactant solution (1 in 50), dilute with water to volume, and mix. Determine the instrument reading concomitantly with the readings obtained for plotting the *Standard graph*, and determine the sodium concentration, in mg per liter, by interpolation from the *Standard graph*. Calculate the percentage of sodium taken by the formula:

$$A / W$$

in which *A* is the weight, in mg, of sodium found per L and *W* is the weight, in g, of Sodium Polystyrene Sulfonate taken. The sodium content is not less than 9.4% and not more than 11.5%, calculated on the anhydrous basis.
Potassium exchange capacity—
Potassium solution—Dissolve an accurately weighed quantity of potassium chloride in water to make a solution containing 5.00 mg of potassium per mL.
Sodium solution—Dissolve an accurately weighed quantity of sodium chloride in water to make a solution containing 4.00 mg of sodium per mL.
Standard graph—Identify five 1-liter volumetric flasks by the numbers *1*, *2*, *3*, *4*, and *5*. In that order pipet into the flasks 4, 3, 2, 1, and 0 mL, respectively, of *Sodium solution*, and in the same order

0, 1, 2, 3, and 4 mL, respectively, of *Potassium solution.* To each flask add 10 mL of low-sodium, low-potassium, nonionic surfactant solution (1 in 50), dilute with water to volume, and mix. Adjust the scale of a suitable flame spectrophotometer to 100 with solution from flask *5* at 766 nm. Determine the instrument readings with solutions from flasks *4, 3, 2,* and *1.* On ruled coordinate paper, plot the observed instrument readings as the ordinate, and the concentrations, in mg per liter, of potassium as the abscissa.

Procedure—Pipet 100 mL of *Potassium solution* into a glass-stoppered flask containing about 1.6 g of Sodium Polystyrene Sulfonate, accurately weighed, shake by mechanical means for 15 minutes, filter, and discard the first 20 mL of the filtrate. Pipet 5 mL of the filtrate into a 1-liter volumetric flask, add 10 mL of low-sodium, low-potassium, nonionic surfactant solution (1 in 50), dilute with water to volume, and mix. Observe the flame spectrophotometer readings of the exchanged solution concomitantly with those obtained for plotting the *Standard graph,* and determine the potassium concentration, in mg per liter, by interpolation from the *Standard graph.* Calculate the quantity, in mg per g, of potassium adsorbed on the resin taken by the formula:

$$(X - 20Y) / W$$

in which *X* is the weight, in mg, of potassium in 100 mL of *Potassium solution* before exchange; *Y* is the weight, in mg, of potassium per L as interpolated from the *Standard graph;* and *W* is the weight, in g, of Sodium Polystyrene Sulfonate taken, expressed on the anhydrous basis.

Sodium Polystyrene Sulfonate Suspension

» Sodium Polystyrene Sulfonate Suspension is a suspension of Sodium Polystyrene Sulfonate in an aqueous vehicle that may contain suitable suspending or stabilizing agents. It exchanges not less than 110 mg and not more than 135 mg of potassium for each g of the labeled amount of sodium polystyrene sulfonate.

Packaging and storage—Preserve in well-closed containers, protected from freezing and from excessive heat.
Microbial limits ⟨61⟩—Its total aerobic microbial count does not exceed 100 cfu per mL, its total combined molds and yeasts count does not exceed 100 cfu per mL, and it meets the requirements of the test for absence of *Pseudomonas aeruginosa.*
Sodium content—
Sodium solution and *Standard graph*—Prepare as directed in the test for *Sodium content* under *Sodium Polystyrene Sulfonate.*
Procedure—Transfer an accurately measured quantity of Suspension, freshly mixed and free from air bubbles, equivalent to about 1 g of sodium polystyrene sulfonate, to a suitable crucible, heat at 80° until dry, and ash the residue with a slight excess of sulfuric acid. Proceed as directed for *Procedure* in the test for *Sodium content* under *Sodium Polystyrene Sulfonate,* beginning with "Add 1 mL of nitric acid." Calculate the percentage of sodium taken by the formula:

$$A / L$$

in which *A* is the quantity, in mg, of sodium found per liter, and *L* is the quantity, in g, of sodium polystyrene sulfonate in the portion of Suspension taken, based on the labeled amount: the sodium content is not less than 9.4% and not more than 11.5%.
Potassium exchange capacity—
Potassium solution, Sodium solution, and *Standard graph*—Prepare as directed in the test for *Potassium exchange capacity* under *Sodium Polystyrene Sulfonate.*
Procedure—Transfer an accurately measured quantity of Suspension, freshly mixed and free from air bubbles, equivalent to about 1.6 g of sodium polystyrene sulfonate, to a suitable glass-stoppered flask, add 100.0 mL of *Potassium solution,* shake by mechanical means for 15 minutes, filter, and discard the first 20 mL of the filtrate. Proceed as directed for *Procedure* in the test for *Potassium exchange capacity* under *Sodium Polystyrene Sulfonate,* beginning with "Pipet 5 mL of the filtrate." Calculate the quantity, in mg, of potassium adsorbed on each g of the sodium polystyrene sulfonate taken by the formula:

$$(X - 20Y) / L$$

in which *X* is the quantity, in mg, of potassium in 100 mL of *Potassium solution* before exchange; *Y* is the quantity, in mg, of potassium per L as interpolated from the *Standard graph;* and *L* is the labeled quantity, in g, of sodium polystyrene sulfonate in the portion of Suspension taken.

Sodium Salicylate

$C_7H_5NaO_3$ 160.10
Benzoic acid, 2-hydroxy-, monosodium salt.
Monosodium salicylate   [54-21-7].

» Sodium Salicylate contains not less than 99.5 percent and not more than 100.5 percent of $C_7H_5NaO_3$, calculated on the anhydrous basis.

Packaging and storage—Preserve in well-closed, light-resistant containers.
Identification—A solution (1 in 20) responds to the tests for *Sodium* ⟨191⟩ and for *Salicylate* ⟨191⟩.
Water, *Method I* ⟨921⟩: not more than 0.5%.
Sulfite or thiosulfate—Add 1 mL of hydrochloric acid to a solution of 1.0 g in 20 mL of water, and filter the liquid: not more than 0.15 mL of 0.10 N iodine is required to produce a yellow color in the filtrate.
Heavy metals, *Method I* ⟨231⟩—Dissolve 2 g in 46 mL of water. Add, with constant stirring, 4 mL of 3 N hydrochloric acid, filter, and use 25 mL of the filtrate: the limit is 0.002%.
Organic volatile impurities, *Method I* ⟨467⟩: meets the requirements.
(Official until July 1, 2008)
Assay—Transfer about 700 mg of Sodium Salicylate, accurately weighed, to a 250-mL beaker. Add 100 mL of glacial acetic acid, stir until the sample is completely dissolved, add crystal violet TS, and titrate with 0.1 N perchloric acid VS. Perform a blank determination, and make any necessary correction. Each mL of 0.1 N perchloric acid is equivalent to 16.01 mg of $C_7H_5NaO_3$.

Sodium Salicylate Tablets

» Sodium Salicylate Tablets contain not less than 95.0 percent and not more than 105.0 percent of the labeled amount of $C_7H_5NaO_3$.

Packaging and storage—Preserve in well-closed containers.
USP Reference standards ⟨11⟩—*USP Sodium Salicylate RS.*
Identification—
A: Digest a quantity of powdered Tablets, equivalent to about 1 g of sodium salicylate, with 20 mL of water, and filter: the filtrate responds to the flame test for *Sodium* ⟨191⟩ and to the tests for *Salicylate* ⟨191⟩.
B: To 10 mL of the filtrate obtained in *Identification* test A add a slight excess of 3 N hydrochloric acid, collect the precipitate on a filter, wash it with small portions of cold water until the last washing is free from chloride, and dry at about 105° for 1 hour: the sali-

cylic acid so obtained melts between 158° and 161° (see *Melting Range or Temperature* ⟨741⟩).
Dissolution ⟨711⟩—
  Medium: water; 900 mL.
  Apparatus 1: 100 rpm.
  Time: 45 minutes.
  Procedure—Determine the amount of $C_7H_5NaO_3$ dissolved from UV absorbances at the wavelength of maximum absorbance at about 230 nm, using filtered portions of the solution under test, diluted with water, if necessary, in comparison with a Standard solution having a known concentration of USP Sodium Salicylate RS in the same *Medium*.
  Tolerances—Not less than 75% (*Q*) of the labeled amount of $C_7H_5NaO_3$ is dissolved in 45 minutes.
Uniformity of dosage units ⟨905⟩: meet the requirements.
Assay—Place not less than 20 Tablets in a 200-mL volumetric flask, add 100 mL of water, and allow to stand, with frequent agitation, until the tablets disintegrate completely. Dilute with water to volume, and mix. Filter through a dry filter into a dry flask, discarding the first 10 mL of the filtrate. Transfer an accurately measured volume of the subsequent filtrate, equivalent to about 500 mg of sodium salicylate, to a separator, and dilute with water, if necessary, to make about 25 mL. Add 75 mL of ether and 10 drops of bromophenol blue TS, and titrate with 0.1 N hydrochloric acid VS, mixing the water and ether layers by vigorous shaking until a permanent, pale green color is produced in the water layer. Draw off the water layer into a small flask, wash the ether layer once with 5 mL of water, and add this to the water layer. Add 20 mL of ether to the combined water solutions, and mix. Continue the titration with vigorous shaking until a permanent, pale green color is produced in the water layer. Each mL of 0.1 N hydrochloric acid is equivalent to 16.01 mg of $C_7H_5NaO_3$.

Sodium Sulfate

$Na_2SO_4 \cdot 10H_2O$ 322.20
Sulfuric acid disodium salt, decahydrate.
Disodium sulfate decahydrate   [7727-73-3].
Anhydrous   142.04   [7757-82-6].

» Sodium Sulfate contains ten molecules of water of hydration, or is anhydrous. It contains not less than 99.0 percent of Na_2SO_4, calculated on the dried basis.

Packaging and storage—Preserve in tight containers, preferably at a temperature not exceeding 30°.
Labeling—Label it to indicate whether it is the decahydrate or is anhydrous.
Identification—A solution (1 in 20) responds to the tests for *Sodium* ⟨191⟩ and for *Sulfate* ⟨191⟩.
Acidity or alkalinity—To 10 mL of a solution, containing the equivalent of 1.0 g of $Na_2SO_4 \cdot 10H_2O$ in 20 mL of water, add 1 drop of bromothymol blue TS: not more than 0.50 mL of either 0.010 N hydrochloric acid or 0.010 N sodium hydroxide is required to change the color of the solution.
Loss on drying ⟨731⟩—Dry at 105° for 4 hours: the decahydrate loses between 51.0% and 57.0% of its weight, and the anhydrous form loses not more than 0.5% of its weight.
Chloride ⟨221⟩—A portion equivalent to 1.0 g of $Na_2SO_4 \cdot 10H_2O$ shows no more chloride than corresponds to 0.30 mL of 0.020 N hydrochloric acid (0.02%).
Heavy metals ⟨231⟩—Dissolve a portion containing the equivalent of 2.0 g of $Na_2SO_4 \cdot 10H_2O$ in 10 mL of water, add 2 mL of 0.1 N hydrochloric acid, then add water to make 25 mL: the limit is 0.001%.
Assay—Weigh accurately a portion of Sodium Sulfate, equivalent to about 400 mg of anhydrous sodium sulfate, dissolve in 200 mL of water, and add 1 mL of hydrochloric acid. Heat to boiling, and gradually add, in small portions and while constantly stirring, an excess of hot barium chloride TS (about 8 mL). Heat the mixture on a steam bath for 1 hour, collect the precipitate of barium sulfate on a tared filtering crucible, wash until free from chloride, dry, ignite, and weigh. The weight of the barium sulfate so obtained, multiplied by 0.6086, represents its equivalent of Na_2SO_4.

Sodium Sulfate Injection

» Sodium Sulfate Injection is a sterile, concentrated solution of Sodium Sulfate in Water for Injection, which upon dilution is suitable for parenteral use. It contains not less than 95.0 percent and not more than 105.0 percent of the labeled amount of $Na_2SO_4 \cdot 10H_2O$.

Packaging and storage—Preserve in single-dose containers, preferably of Type I glass.
Labeling—Label it to indicate that it is to be diluted before injection to render it isotonic (3.89% of $Na_2SO_4 \cdot 10H_2O$).
Identification—It responds to the tests for *Sodium* ⟨191⟩ and for *Sulfate* ⟨191⟩.
Pyrogen—When diluted with water for injection to contain 3.89% of $Na_2SO_4 \cdot 10H_2O$, it meets the requirements of the *Pyrogen Test* ⟨151⟩.
pH ⟨791⟩: between 5.0 and 6.5.
Other requirements—It meets the requirements under *Injections* ⟨1⟩.
Assay—Transfer an accurately measured volume of Injection, equivalent to about 400 mg of sodium sulfate ($Na_2SO_4 \cdot 10H_2O$), to a suitable vessel. Dilute if necessary, to 200 mL, and proceed as directed in the *Assay* under *Sodium Sulfate*, beginning with "add 1 mL of hydrochloric acid." The weight of the barium sulfate so obtained, multiplied by 1.3804, represents its equivalent of $Na_2SO_4 \cdot 10H_2O$.

Sodium Sulfide

$Na_2S \cdot 9H_2O$ 240.18
Sodium sulfide nonahydrate.
Disodium sulfide nonahydrate   [1313-84-4].

» Sodium Sulfide contains not less than 98.0 percent and not more than 103.0 percent of $Na_2S \cdot 9H_2O$.

Packaging and storage—Preserve in tight containers, and store in a cool place.
Identification—[NOTE—Conduct this test in a fume hood.] Transfer about 100 mg of Sodium Sulfide, to a suitable container, add 10 mL of 3 N hydrochloric acid, and cover the top of the container with filter paper saturated with a 0.2 M lead acetate solution: a brownish or silvery-black color forms on the paper.
Limit of iron—Dissolve about 5.0 g in 100 mL of water: the solution is clear and colorless.
Limit of sulfite and thiosulfate—Dissolve 3.0 g in 200.0 mL of filtered and degassed water. Add 100.0 mL of 0.2 N zinc sulfate, mix, and allow to stand for 30 minutes. Filter, add 1 mL of starch TS, and titrate 100.0 mL of the filtrate with 0.01 N iodine VS: not more than 3.0 mL is required.
Assay—Transfer about 275 mg of Sodium Sulfide, accurately weighed, to a 250-mL beaker, dissolve in 30 mL of filtered and degassed water, and mix. Add 50.0 mL of 0.1 N iodine while mixing, add 2 mL of hydrochloric acid, and allow to stand for 15 minutes in a dark place. Titrate with 0.1 N sodium thiosulfate VS to a pale yellow color. Add 5 mL of starch TS, and titrate with 0.1 N sodium thiosulfate VS to a clear endpoint. Perform a blank determination, and make any necessary correction. Each mL of 0.1 N sodium thiosulfate is equivalent to 12.01 mg of $Na_2S \cdot 9H_2O$.

Sodium Sulfide Topical Gel

» Sodium Sulfide Topical Gel contains not less than 90.0 percent and not more than 120.0 percent of the labeled amount of sodium sulfide (Na$_2$S · 9H$_2$O) in a suitable gel base.

Packaging and storage—Preserve in tight containers at controlled room temperature or in a cool place.
Identification—Proceed as directed for the *Identification* test under *Sodium Sulfide*.
pH ⟨791⟩: between 11.5 and 13.5.
Assay—
Diluent—Transfer 500.0 mL of a 4.0 M sodium hydroxide solution to a 1000-mL volumetric flask, and add about 67.0 g of edetate disodium and 36.0 g of ascorbic acid, each accurately weighed. Dilute with water to volume, and mix.
Assay preparation—Transfer an accurately weighed portion of the Topical Gel, equivalent to about 30 mg of sodium sulfide, to a 100-mL volumetric flask, add 50 mL of *Diluent*, and shake by mechanical means until the Topical Gel is dispersed. Dilute with *Diluent* to volume, and mix.
Procedure—Transfer 30.0 mL of the *Assay preparation* to a suitable beaker, and titrate with 0.01 M lead perchlorate VS, determining the endpoint potentiometrically. Perform a blank determination, and make any necessary correction. Each mL of 0.01 M lead perchlorate is equivalent to 2.4018 mg of sodium sulfide (Na$_2$S · 9H$_2$O).

Sodium Thiosulfate

Na$_2$S$_2$O$_3$ · 5H$_2$O   248.19
Thiosulfuric acid, disodium salt, pentahydrate.
Disodium thiosulfate pentahydrate.   [*10102-17-7*].
Anhydrous.   158.11   [*7772-98-7*].

» Sodium Thiosulfate contains not less than 99.0 percent and not more than 100.5 percent of Na$_2$S$_2$O$_3$, calculated on the anhydrous basis.

Packaging and storage—Preserve in tight containers.
Identification—
 A: To a solution (1 in 10) add a few drops of iodine TS: the color is discharged.
 B: A solution (1 in 10) responds to the tests for *Sodium* ⟨191⟩ and for *Thiosulfate* ⟨191⟩.
Water ⟨921⟩—Dry about 1.0 g, accurately weighed, in vacuum at 40° to 45° for 16 hours: it loses between 32.0% and 37.0% of its weight.
Calcium—Dissolve 1 g in 20 mL of water, and add a few mL of ammonium oxalate TS: no turbidity is produced.
Heavy metals ⟨231⟩—Dissolve 1 g in 10 mL of water, slowly add 5 mL of 3 N hydrochloric acid, evaporate on a steam bath nearly to dryness, and heat the residue at 150° for 1 hour. Add 15 mL of water to the residue, boil gently for 2 minutes, and filter. Heat the filtrate to boiling, and add sufficient bromine TS to produce a clear solution and provide a slight excess of bromine. Boil the solution to expel the excess bromine, cool to room temperature, add 1 drop of phenolphthalein TS, and neutralize with 1 N sodium hydroxide. Dilute with water to 25 mL: the limit is 0.002%.
Assay—Dissolve about 800 mg of Sodium Thiosulfate, accurately weighed, in 30 mL of water. If necessary, adjust by the addition of 3 N hydrochloric acid to a pH of between 6.2 and 6.7 and titrate with 0.1 N iodine VS, adding 3 mL of starch TS as the endpoint is approached. Each mL of 0.1 N iodine is equivalent to 15.81 mg of Na$_2$S$_2$O$_3$.

Sodium Thiosulfate Injection

» Sodium Thiosulfate Injection is a sterile solution of Sodium Thiosulfate in freshly boiled Water for Injection. It contains not less than 95.0 percent and not more than 105.0 percent of the labeled amount of Na$_2$S$_2$O$_3$ · 5H$_2$O.

Packaging and storage—Preserve in single-dose containers, of Type I glass.
USP Reference standards ⟨11⟩—*USP Endotoxin RS*.
Identification—It responds to the *Identification* tests under *Sodium Thiosulfate*.
Bacterial endotoxins ⟨85⟩—It contains not more than 0.03 USP Endotoxin Unit per mg of sodium thiosulfate.
pH ⟨791⟩: between 6.0 and 9.5.
Other requirements—It meets the requirements under *Injections* ⟨1⟩.
Assay—Transfer to a suitable container an accurately measured volume of Injection, containing about 1 g of sodium thiosulfate, and adjust by the addition of 3 N hydrochloric acid to a pH of between 6.2 and 6.7. Dilute with water to about 20 mL, and titrate with 0.1 N iodine VS, adding 3 mL of starch TS as the endpoint is approached. Each mL of 0.1 N iodine is equivalent to 24.82 mg of Na$_2$S$_2$O$_3$ · 5H$_2$O.

Somatropin

FPTIPLSRLF	DNAMLRAHRL	HQLAFDTYQE	FEEAYIPKEQ	KYSFLQNPQT
SLCFSESIPT	PSNREETQQK	SNLELLRISL	LLIQSWLEPV	QFLRSVFANS
LVYGASDSNV	YDLLKDLEEG	IQTLMGRLED	GSPRTGQIFK	QTYSKFDTNS
HNDDALLKNY	GLLYCFRKDM	DKVETFLRIV	QCRSVEGSCG	F

C$_{990}$H$_{1528}$N$_{262}$O$_{300}$S$_7$ 22,125   [*12629-01-5*].

» Somatropin is a protein hormone consisting of 191 amino acid residues, and its structure corresponds to the major component of the growth hormone extracted from human pituitary glands. It is produced as a lyophilized powder or bulk solution by methods based on recombinant DNA technology. When prepared as a lyophilized powder, it contains not less than 910 µg of somatropin per mg, calculated on the anhydrous basis. When prepared as a bulk solution, it contains not less than 910 µg of somatropin per mg of total protein. The presence of host-cell DNA and host-cell protein impurities in Somatropin is process specific—the limits of these impurities are determined by validated methods. Manufacturers must demonstrate a correlation between the *Assay* and a validated and approved growth-promotion based bioassay. It may contain excipients. [NOTE—One mg of anhydrous Somatropin is equivalent to 3.0 USP Somatropin Units.]

Packaging and storage—Preserve in tight containers, and store between −10° and −25°.
Labeling—The labeling states that the material is of recombinant DNA origin.
USP Reference standards ⟨11⟩—*USP Endotoxin RS. USP Somatropin RS.*
Identification—
 A: Proceed as directed in the test for *Chromatographic purity*, except to prepare a *Standard solution* by reconstituting a vial of USP Somatropin RS with the *Diluent* to obtain a solution having a known concentration of about 2.0 mg per mL. Chromatograph the *Standard solution* and the *Test solution* as directed for *Procedure:*

the retention time of the somatropin peak in the chromatogram of the *Test solution* corresponds to that in the chromatogram of the *Standard solution*.

B: *Peptide Mapping* (see *Biotechnology-Derived Articles—Tests* ⟨1047⟩)—

Solution A—Prepare a filtered and degassed solution of trifluoroacetic acid in water (1 in 1000, v/v).

Solution B—Transfer 100 mL of water to a 1000-mL volumetric flask, add 1 mL of trifluoroacetic acid, dilute with acetonitrile to volume, and mix.

Mobile phase—Use variable mixtures of *Solution A* and *Solution B* as directed for *Chromatographic system*. Make adjustments to either solution as necessary (see *System Suitability* under *Chromatography* ⟨621⟩).

Tris buffer—Prepare a 0.05 M solution of tris(hydroxymethyl)aminomethane (Tris), and adjust with hydrochloric acid to a pH of 7.5.

Trypsin solution—Prepare a solution containing 1 mg of trypsin per mL of *Tris buffer*, and mix. Store in a freezer, if necessary.

Standard solution—Prepare a solution containing 2.0 mg of USP Somatropin RS per mL of the *Tris buffer*, and mix. Add 1 mL of this solution to a suitable tube, and add 30 µL of *Trypsin solution*. Cap the tube, and place it in a water bath at 37° for 4 hours. [NOTE—If this solution is not injected immediately, store it in a freezer.]

Test solution—Prepare a solution containing 2.0 mg of Somatropin per mL of *Tris buffer*, and mix. Add 1 mL of this solution to a suitable tube, and add 30 µL of *Trypsin solution*. Cap the tube, and place it in a water bath at 37° for 4 hours. [NOTE—If this solution is not injected immediately, store it in a freezer.]

Chromatographic system (see *Chromatography* ⟨621⟩)—The liquid chromatograph is equipped with a 214-nm detector and a 4.6-mm × 25-cm column that contains packing L7. The flow rate is 1 mL per minute, and the column temperature is maintained at 30°. The chromatograph is programmed as follows.

Time (minutes)	Solution A (%)	Solution B (%)	Elution
0–20	100→80	0→20	linear gradient
20–40	80→75	20→25	linear gradient
40–65	75→50	25→50	linear gradient
65–70	50→20	50→80	linear gradient
70–71	20→100	80→0	linear gradient
71–86	100	0	isocratic, re-equilibration

Procedure—[NOTE—Condition the chromatographic system by running a blank gradient program prior to injecting the digests.] Separately inject equal volumes (about 100 µL) of the *Standard solution* and the *Test solution*, and record the chromatograms: the chromatographic profile of the *Test solution* is similar to that of the *Standard solution*.

Bioidentity—[NOTE—The *Bioidentity* test may be performed either on the Somatropin bulk drug substance or on the finished pharmaceutical product.]

Buffer solution—Prepare a solution of 0.1 M ammonium bicarbonate, and adjust with sodium hydroxide to a pH of 8.0.

Standard solutions—Reconstitute the USP Somatropin RS, and dissolve in and dilute quantitatively with *Buffer solution* to obtain solutions having known concentrations between 10 and 100 µg per mL.

Test solutions—Prepare a solution of Somatropin, and dissolve in and dilute quantitatively with *Buffer solution* to obtain solutions having concentrations similar to those of the *Standard solutions*. [NOTE—Do not agitate while mixing; swirl gently.]

Control solution—Use the *Buffer solution*.

Test animals—Select an appropriate number of only female or only male Sprague Dawley rats hypophysectomized at 25 to 30 days of age. After hypophysectomization, feed the rats on rat chow and 5% dextrose water for at least 72 hours. After 72 hours, feed the rats on rat chow and filtered and deionized water adjusted with 1 N hydrochloric acid to a pH of 3.0 ± 0.25. Weigh the rats when they are 37 to 44 days old, and retain only healthy rats. Reweigh the remaining rats 7 days later, and use only those rats that are in good health and have not gained or lost more than 10% of their body weight in the previous 7-day period.

Procedure—Randomly divide the rats into control, standard, and test groups, each group containing approximately 10 rats. Each day for 10 days inject subcutaneously 0.1 mL of the *Control solution*, *Standard solutions*, and *Test solutions* to the control, standard, and test groups, respectively. Record the body weight of each animal at the start of the test and at approximately 18 hours following the 10th injection. Determine the change in body weight for each rat during the 10-day period, and compute the potency of the *Test solution* relative to that of the *Standard solution* using appropriate statistical analysis. Calculate the mean potency in USP Somatropin Units per mg: not less than 2 USP Somatropin Units per mg is found. Using appropriate statistical methods, calculate the width, L, of a 95% confidence interval for the estimated logarithm of the relative potency: L is not more than 0.40, which corresponds to confidence limits between 63% and 158% of the calculated potency. If L is more than 0.40, repeat the test until the results from two or more tests, combined by appropriate statistical methods, meet this criterion.

Microbial limits ⟨61⟩—The total aerobic microbial count does not exceed 300 cfu per g, the test being performed on about 0.2 to 0.3 g of powder, accurately weighed.

Bacterial endotoxins ⟨85⟩—It contains not more than 10 USP Endotoxin Units per mg.

Water, *Method Ic* ⟨921⟩: not more than 10%, when prepared as a lyophilized powder.

Chromatographic purity—

Diluent—Prepare a solution of 0.05 M Tris in water, and adjust with hydrochloric acid to a pH of 7.5.

Mobile phase—Degas the *Diluent*, mix with *n*-propyl alcohol (71 : 29, v/v), and filter. Make adjustments if necessary (see *System Suitability* under *Chromatography* ⟨621⟩).

Resolution solution—Prepare a solution of 2.0 mg of Somatropin per mL of the *Diluent*, pass through a filter to sterilize or add sodium azide to a final concentration of 0.01%, and allow to stand at room temperature for 24 hours. [NOTE—Use within 48 hours after preparation, or store the solution in a refrigerator until ready to use.]

Test solution—Prepare a solution of 2.0 mg of Somatropin per mL of the *Diluent* immediately before use. [NOTE—Maintain the solutions between 2° and 8°, and use within 24 hours. If an automatic injector is used, maintain the temperature between 2° and 8°.]

Chromatographic system (see *Chromatography* ⟨621⟩)—The liquid chromatograph is equipped with a 220-nm detector and a 4.6-mm × 25-cm column that contains packing L26 and is maintained at 45°. The flow rate is about 0.5 mL per minute. Chromatograph the *Resolution solution*, and record the peak responses as directed for *Procedure*: the resolution, R, between somatropin and its adjacent peak is not less than 1.0; and the tailing factor of the somatropin peak (major peak) is between 0.9 and 1.8.

Procedure—Inject about 20 µL of the *Test solution*, record the chromatograms, and measure the peak responses. Calculate the percentage of impurities in the portion of Somatropin taken by the formula:

$$100A_I / (A_I + A_S)$$

in which A_I is the sum of the responses of all the peaks other than the somatropin peak (major peak) and disregarding any peak due to the solvent; and A_S is the response of the somatropin peak: not more than 6.0% of total impurities is found.

Limit of high molecular weight proteins—

Phosphate buffer, Mobile phase, Diluent, Resolution solution, and *Chromatographic system*—Proceed as directed in the *Assay*.

Test solution—Prepare as directed for the *Assay preparation*.

Procedure—Inject about 20 µL of the *Test solution*, record the chromatogram, and measure the areas of the main peak and of the peaks eluting prior to the main peak, excluding the solvent peaks. Calculate the percentage of high molecular weight proteins in the portion of Somatropin taken by the formula:

$$100A_H / (A_H + A_M)$$

in which A_H is the sum of the areas of the high molecular weight peaks, and A_M is the area of the monomer peak in the chromatogram

of the *Test solution:* not more than 4% of high molecular weight proteins is found.
Total protein (see *Spectrophotometry and Light-Scattering* ⟨851⟩)—
Phosphate buffer—Prepare a 0.025 M solution of monobasic potassium phosphate in water, and adjust with sodium hydroxide to a pH of 7.0.
Test solution—Dissolve an accurately weighed quantity of Somatropin in *Phosphate buffer* to obtain a solution having an absorbance value between 0.5 and 1.0 at the wavelength of maximum absorbance at about 280 nm.
Procedure—Determine the absorbance of the *Test solution* using a spectrophotometric cell of path length 1-cm, at the wavelength of maximum absorbance at around 280 nm and at 320 nm, using *Phosphate buffer* as the blank. Calculate the protein content, in mg, in the portion of Somatropin taken by the formula:

$$V(A_{max} - A_{320})/0.82$$

in which V is the volume of the *Test solution;* and A_{max} and A_{320} are the absorbance values of the *Test solution* at the wavelength of maximum absorbance and at 320 nm, respectively.
Assay—
Phosphate buffer—Dissolve 5.18 g of dibasic sodium phosphate and 3.65 g of monobasic sodium phosphate in 950 mL of water, adjust with phosphoric acid to a pH of 7.0, and dilute with water to 1000 mL.
Mobile phase—Prepare a filtered and degassed mixture of the *Phosphate buffer* and isopropyl alcohol (97 : 3, v/v). Make adjustments if necessary (see *System Suitability* under *Chromatography* ⟨621⟩).
Diluent—Prepare a mixture of water and *Phosphate buffer* (1.5 : 1).
Resolution solution—Place 1 vial of USP Somatropin RS in an oven at 50° for 12 to 24 hours. Remove from the oven, and dissolve the contents of the vial in *Diluent* to obtain a solution having a known concentration of about 1 mg per mL with the content of the dimer between 1% and 2%.
Standard preparation—Reconstitute a vial of USP Somatropin RS with the *Diluent* to obtain a solution having a known concentration of about 1.0 mg per mL.
Assay preparation—Dissolve an accurately weighed quantity of Somatropin in *Diluent*, or dilute a bulk solution of Somatropin with *Diluent*, to obtain a solution having a concentration of about 1 mg per mL. [NOTE—If necessary, the amount of protein in solution can be determined by the test for *Total protein*.]
Chromatographic system (see *Chromatography* ⟨621⟩)—The liquid chromatograph is equipped with a 214-nm detector and a 7.8-mm × 30-cm column that contains packing L33 and is maintained at ambient temperature. The flow rate is 0.6 mL per minute. Chromatograph the *Resolution solution* as directed for *Procedure:* the resolution, R, (determined as the ratio of the valley height, between the dimer and the monomer, and the dimer peak height) is not more than 0.4; and the tailing factor of the monomer peak (major peak) is not more than 1.7.
Procedure—Separately inject equal volumes (about 20 µL) of the the *Standard preparation* and the *Assay preparation,* record the chromatograms for not less than twice the retention time of the somatropin monomer peak (major peak), and measure the peak responses for the monomer. Calculate the concentration, in mg per mL, of somatropin in the *Assay preparation* by the formula:

$$C_S(r_U / r_S)$$

in which C_S is the concentration, in mg per mL, of USP Somatropin RS in the *Standard preparation;* and r_U and r_S are the peak responses of the monomer in the *Assay preparation* and the *Standard preparation*, respectively.

Somatropin for Injection

» Somatropin for Injection is a sterile, lyophilized mixture of Somatropin with one or more suitable buffering and stabilizing agents. It contains not less than 89.0 percent and not more than 110.0 percent of the amount of somatropin stated on the label. Manufacturers must demonstrate a corrrelation between the assay and a validated and approved growth-promotion based bioassay. [NOTE—One mg of anhydrous Somatropin is equivalent to 3.0 USP Somatropin Units.]

Packaging and storage—Preserve in tight containers, and store between 2° and 8°.
Labeling—The labeling states that the material is of recombinant DNA origin.
USP Reference standards ⟨11⟩—*USP Endotoxin RS. USP Somatropin RS.*
Identification—It meets the requirements for *Identification* test A under *Somatropin*.
Bioidentity—[NOTE—If the bulk material used to prepare Somatropin for Injection was tested and meets the requirements, it is not necessary to perform this test.] It meets the requirements for *Bioidentity* under *Somatropin*.
Bacterial endotoxins ⟨85⟩—It contains not more than 20 USP Endotoxin Units per mg of somatropin.
Sterility ⟨71⟩—It meets the requirements when tested as directed for *Membrane Filtration* under *Test for Sterility of the Product to be Examined*.
Chromatographic purity—Proceed as directed for the *Chromatographic purity* test under *Somatropin:* not more than 12% of total impurities is found.
Limit of high molecular weight proteins—Proceed as directed in the test for *Limit of high molecular weight proteins* under *Somatropin*, except to use the *Assay preparation* as the *Test solution:* not more than 6% of high molecular weight proteins is found.
Assay—
Phosphate buffer, Mobile phase, Diluent, Resolution solution, Standard preparation, and *Chromatographic system*—Proceed as directed in the *Assay* under *Somatropin*.
Assay preparation—Dissolve the contents of a suitable number of containers in *Diluent* to obtain a concentration of 1 mg of somatropin per mL.
Procedure—Proceed as directed under *Somatropin*. Calculate the quantity of somatropin, in mg of somatropin per container, by the formula:

$$C(V/N)(r_U / r_S)$$

in which C is the concentration, in mg per mL, of USP Somatropin RS in the *Standard preparation;* V is the total volume of the *Assay preparation; N* is the number of containers used to obtain the *Assay preparation;* and r_U and r_S are the peak responses of the monomer in the *Assay preparation* and the *Standard preparation,* respectively.

Sorbitol Solution

» Sorbitol Solution is an aqueous solution containing not less than 64.0 percent of D-sorbitol ($C_6H_{14}O_6$). The amounts of total sugars, other polyhydric alcohols, and any hexitol anhydrides, if detected, are not included in the requirements nor in the calculated amount under *Other Impurities*.

Packaging and storage—Preserve in well-closed containers. No storage requirements specified.
USP Reference standards ⟨11⟩—*USP Sorbitol RS.*
Identification—
A: Dissolve 1.4 g of Sorbitol Solution in 75 mL of water. Transfer 3 mL of this solution to a 15-cm test tube, add 3 mL of freshly prepared catechol solution (1 in 10), mix, add 6 mL of sulfuric acid, mix again, and gently heat the tube in a flame for about 30 seconds: a deep pink or wine color appears.

B: The retention time of the major peak in the chromatogram of the *Assay preparation* corresponds to that in the chromatogram of the *Standard preparation,* as obtained in the *Assay.*

pH ⟨791⟩: between 5.0 and 7.5, in a 14% (w/w) solution of Sorbitol Solution in carbon dioxide-free water.

Water, *Method I* ⟨921⟩: between 28.5% and 31.5%.

Residue on ignition ⟨281⟩: not more than 0.1%, calculated on the anhydrous basis, determined on a 2-g portion, accurately weighed.

Reducing sugars—To an amount of Sorbitol Solution, equivalent to 3.3 g on the anhydrous basis, add 3 mL of water, 20.0 mL of cupric citrate TS, and a few glass beads. Heat so that boiling begins after 4 minutes, and maintain boiling for 3 minutes. Cool rapidly, and add 40 mL of diluted acetic acid, 60 mL of water, and 20.0 mL of 0.05 N iodine VS. With continuous shaking, add 25 mL of a mixture of 6 mL of hydrochloric acid and 94 mL of water. When the precipitate has dissolved, titrate the excess of iodine with 0.05 N sodium thiosulfate VS using 2 mL of starch TS, added towards the end of the titration, as an indicator. Not less than 12.8 mL of 0.05 N sodium thiosulfate VS is required, corresponding to not more than 0.3% of reducing sugars, on the anhydrous basis, as glucose. The amount determined in this test is not included in the calculated amount under *Other Impurities.*

Limit of nickel—

Test solution—Dissolve 20.0 g of Sorbitol Solution in diluted acetic acid, and dilute with diluted acetic acid to 100.0 mL. Add 2.0 mL of a saturated ammonium pyrrolidine dithiocarbamate solution (containing about 10 g of ammonium pyrrolidine dithiocarbamate per L) and 10.0 mL of methyl isobutyl ketone, and shake for 30 seconds. Protect from bright light. Allow the two layers to separate, and use the methyl isobutyl ketone layer.

Blank solution—Prepare as directed for *Test solution,* except to omit the use of the Sorbitol Solution.

Standard solutions—Prepare as directed for *Test solution,* except to prepare three solutions by adding 0.5 mL, 1.0 mL, and 1.5 mL of nickel standard solution TS.

Procedure—Set the instrument to zero using the *Blank solution.* Concomitantly determine the absorbances of the *Standard solutions* and the *Test solution* at least three times each, at the wavelength of maximum absorbance at 232.0 nm, with a suitable atomic absorption spectrophotometer (see *Spectrophotometry and Light-Scattering* ⟨851⟩) equipped with a nickel hollow-cathode lamp and an air–acetylene flame. Record the average of the steady readings for each of the *Standard solutions* and the *Test solution.* Between each measurement, aspirate the *Blank solution,* and ascertain that the reading returns to zero. Plot the absorbances of the *Standard solutions* and the *Test solution* versus the added quantity of nickel. Extrapolate the line joining the points on the graph until it meets the concentration axis. The distance between this point and the intersection of the axes represents the concentration of nickel in the *Test solution.* Not more than 1 µg per g, calculated on the anhydrous basis, is found.

Assay—

Mobile phase, Resolution solution, Standard preparation, and *Chromatographic system*—Proceed as directed in the *Assay* under *Sorbitol.*

Assay preparation—Accurately weigh about 0.12 g of Sorbitol Solution, dissolve in and dilute with water to about 20 g. Accurately record the final solution weight, and mix thoroughly.

Procedure—Proceed as directed in the *Assay* under *Sorbitol.* Calculate the percentage of D-sorbitol ($C_6H_{14}O_6$) in the portion of Sorbitol Solution taken by the formula:

$$100(C_S / C_U)(r_U / r_S)$$

in which C_S is the concentration, in mg per g, of USP Sorbitol RS in the *Standard preparation;* C_U is the concentration, in mg per g, of Sorbitol Solution in the *Assay preparation;* and r_U and r_S are the peak responses obtained from the *Assay preparation* and the *Standard preparation,* respectively.

Sotalol Hydrochloride

$C_{12}H_{20}N_2O_3S \cdot HCl$ 308.83

Methanesulfonamide, *N*-[4-[1-hydroxy-2-[(1-methylethyl)amino]ethyl]phenyl]-, monohydrochloride.

4′-[1-Hydroxy-2-(isopropylamino)ethyl]methanesulfonanilide monohydrochloride   [959-24-0].

» Sotalol Hydrochloride contains not less than 98.5 percent and not more than 101.5 percent of $C_{12}H_{20}N_2O_3S \cdot HCl$.

Packaging and storage—Preserve in well-closed containers. Store at controlled room temperature.

USP Reference standards ⟨11⟩—*USP Sotalol Hydrochloride RS. USP Sotalol Related Compound A RS. USP Sotalol Related Compound B RS. USP Sotalol Related Compound C RS.*

Identification—

A: *Infrared Absorption* ⟨197K⟩.

B: *Thin-Layer Chromatographic Identification Test* ⟨201⟩—

Test solution—Dissolve a quantity of Sotalol Hydrochloride in methanol to obtain a solution having a concentration of about 2 mg per mL.

Developing solvent system: a mixture of chloroform and methanol (70 : 30).

Procedure—Proceed as directed in the chapter, except to place two 25-mL beakers, each containing about 10 mL of ammonium hydroxide, on the bottom of the chromatographic chamber that is lined with filter paper and contains the *Developing solvent system,* allow to equilibrate for 15 minutes, then place the plate in the chamber, and develop the chromatograms until the solvent front has moved about two-thirds of the length of the plate: meets the requirements.

Specific rotation ⟨781S⟩: between −0.7° and +0.7°.

Test solution: 125 mg per mL, in methanol.

Water, *Method I* ⟨921⟩: not more than 0.5%.

Residue on ignition ⟨281⟩: not more than 0.5%.

Heavy metals, *Method II* ⟨231⟩: 0.002%.

Limit of methanol, isopropyl alcohol, and acetone—

Standard solution—Transfer 10.0 µL each of methanol, isopropyl alcohol, and acetone to a 100-mL volumetric flask, dilute with *N,N*-dimethylacetamide to volume, and mix. Dilute 10.0 mL of this solution with 10.0 mL of *N,N*-dimethylacetamide to obtain a solution containing about 0.04 mg of each per mL.

Test solution—Transfer about 100 mg of Sotalol Hydrochloride, accurately weighed, to a 25-mL flask, dissolve in 10.0 mL of *N,N*-dimethylacetamide, and mix. [NOTE—Do not dilute to volume.]

Chromatographic system (see *Chromatography* ⟨621⟩)—The gas chromatograph is equipped with a flame-ionization detector and a 2.0-mm × 1.8-m glass column containing 5% phase G16 on 60-to 80-mesh support S12. The injection port temperature is maintained at 200°, and the detector temperature is maintained at 300°. The column temperature is maintained at 70° for 5 minutes, then increased at a rate of 30° per minute to 180°, and maintained at 180° for 3 minutes. Helium is used as the carrier gas, flowing at a rate of about 30 mL per minute. Chromatograph the *Standard solution,* and record the peak areas as directed for *Procedure*: the relative retention times are 1.0, 1.4, and 2.7 for methanol, acetone, and isopropyl alcohol, respectively; the resolution, *R,* between methanol and acetone and between acetone and isopropyl alcohol is not less than 2.0; and the relative standard deviation for replicate injections is not more than 2.0%.

Procedure—Separately inject equal volumes (about 1 µL) of the *Test solution* and the *Standard solution* into the chromatograph, record the chromatograms, and measure the methanol, isopropyl alcohol, and acetone peak areas. Calculate the percentages of methanol, isopropyl alcohol, and acetone in the portion of Sotalol Hydrochloride taken by the formula:

$$1000(C/W)(r_U/r_S)$$

in which C is the concentration, in mg per mL, of the appropriate analyte in the *Standard solution;* W is the quantity, in mg, of Sotalol Hydrochloride taken to prepare the *Test solution;* and r_U and r_S are the peak areas of the corresponding analyte obtained from the *Test solution* and the *Standard solution,* respectively: not more than 0.3% each of methanol, isopropyl alcohol, and acetone is found; and not more than 0.5% total of methanol, isopropyl alcohol, and acetone is found.

Related compounds—
Mobile phase—Proceed as directed in the *Assay.*
Standard solution—Dissolve accurately weighed quantities of USP Sotalol Hydrochloride RS, USP Sotalol Related Compound A RS, USP Sotalol Related Compound B RS, and USP Sotalol Related Compound C RS in *Mobile phase,* and dilute quantitatively, and stepwise if necessary, with *Mobile phase* to obtain a solution having known concentrations of about 6 µg of each per mL.
Test solution—Transfer about 200 mg of Sotalol Hydrochloride, accurately weighed, to a 100-mL volumetric flask, dissolve in and dilute with *Mobile phase* to volume, and mix.
Chromatographic system—Prepare as directed in the *Assay.* Chromatograph the *Standard solution,* and record the peak heights as directed for *Procedure:* the relative retention times are about 0.65 for sotalol hydrochloride related compound B, 1.0 for sotalol hydrochloride, 1.2 for sotalol hydrochloride related compound A, and 1.4 for sotalol hydrochloride related compound C; the resolution, *R*, between sotalol hydrochloride related compound A and sotalol hydrochloride is not less than 2.0; and the relative standard deviation for replicate injections is not more than 2.0%.
Procedure—Separately inject equal volumes (about 25 µL) of the *Standard solution* and the *Test solution* into the chromatograph, record the chromatograms, and measure the heights for the major peaks. Calculate the percentage of each sotalol hydrochloride related compound in the portion of Sotalol Hydrochloride taken by the formula:

$$10(C/W)(r_i/r_S)$$

in which C is the concentration, in µg per mL, of the appropriate USP Related Compound Reference Standard in the *Standard solution;* W is the weight, in mg, of Sotalol Hydrochloride taken to prepare the *Test solution;* and r_i and r_S are the peak heights for the corresponding related compound obtained from the *Test solution* and the *Standard solution,* respectively. Calculate the percentage of other impurities in the portion of Sotalol Hydrochloride taken by the formula:

$$10(C/W)(r_{si}/r_S)$$

in which C is the concentration, in µg per mL, of USP Sotalol Hydrochloride RS in the *Standard solution;* W is the weight, in mg, of Sotalol Hydrochloride taken to prepare the *Test solution;* r_{si} is the sum of the peak heights for all impurities, other than the related compounds, obtained from the *Test solution;* and r_S is the peak height of sotalol obtained from the *Standard solution.* Not more than 0.3% each of sotalol hydrochloride related compound A and sotalol hydrochloride related compound B is found; not more than 0.4% of sotalol hydrochloride related compound C is found; not more than 0.3% of other impurities is found; and not more than 0.5% of total impurities is found.

Organic volatile impurities, *Method IV* ⟨467⟩: meets the requirements.

(Official until July 1, 2008)

Content of chloride—Transfer about 310 mg of Sotalol Hydrochloride, accurately weighed, to a glass beaker, and dissolve in 100 mL of water and 10 mL of glacial acetic acid. Titrate with 0.1 N silver nitrate VS, and determine the endpoint potentiometrically. Each mL of 0.1 N silver nitrate is equivalent to 3.545 mg of chloride (Cl): between 11.1% and 11.9% of chloride is found.

Assay—
Diluent—Prepare a mixture of water and acetonitrile (4 : 1).
Mobile phase—Transfer about 1.08 g of sodium 1-octanesulfonate to a 1000-mL volumetric flask. Dissolve in 10 mL of glacial acetic acid and about 70 mL of water. Add 720 mL of water, dilute with acetonitrile to volume, and mix. Filter, and degas. Make adjustments if necessary (see *System Suitability* under *Chromatography* ⟨621⟩).
Internal standard solution—Transfer about 450 mg of caffeine to a 100-mL volumetric flask. Dissolve in and dilute with *Diluent* to volume, and mix.
Standard preparation—Transfer about 50 mg of USP Sotalol Hydrochloride RS, accurately weighed, to a 25-mL volumetric flask. Dissolve in and dilute with *Diluent* to volume, and mix. Transfer 10.0 mL of this solution and 5.0 mL of *Internal standard solution* to a 100-mL volumetric flask. Dilute with *Diluent* to volume, and mix.
Assay preparation—Transfer about 100 mg of Sotalol Hydrochloride, accurately weighed, to a 50-mL volumetric flask. Dissolve in and dilute with *Diluent* to volume, and mix. Pipet 10.0 mL of this solution and 5.0 mL of *Internal standard solution* into a 100-mL volumetric flask. Dilute with *Diluent* to volume, and mix.
Chromatographic system (see *Chromatography* ⟨621⟩)—The liquid chromatograph is equipped with a 238-nm detector and a 3.9-mm × 30-cm column that contains packing L1. The flow rate is about 1.5 mL per minute. Chromatograph the *Standard preparation,* and record the peak areas as directed for *Procedure:* the relative retention times are about 1.0 for sotalol and 0.39 for caffeine; the resolution, *R*, between caffeine and sotalol is not less than 8.5; and the relative standard deviation for replicate injections, determined from peak area ratios, is not more than 2.0%.
Procedure—Separately inject equal volumes (about 25 µL) of the *Standard preparation* and the *Assay preparation* into the chromatograph, record the chromatograms, and measure the areas for the major peaks. Calculate the quantity, in mg, of $C_{12}H_{20}N_2O_3S \cdot HCl$ in the portion of Sotalol Hydrochloride taken by the formula:

$$500C(R_U/R_S)$$

in which C is the concentration, in mg per mL, of USP Sotalol Hydrochloride RS in the *Standard preparation;* and R_U and R_S are the peak area ratios of sotalol to caffeine obtained from the *Assay preparation* and the *Standard preparation,* respectively.

Sotalol Hydrochloride Tablets

» Sotalol Hydrochloride Tablets contain not less than 95.0 percent and not more than 105.0 percent of the labeled amount of sotalol hydrochloride ($C_{12}H_{20}N_2O_3S \cdot HCl$).

Packaging and storage—Preserve in well-closed containers, and store at controlled room temperature.

USP Reference standards ⟨11⟩—*USP Sotalol Hydrochloride RS.*
Identification—Weigh and powder a quantity of the Tablets, equivalent to about 250 mg of sotalol hydrochloride, and transfer to a 50-mL volumetric flask. Add 25 mL of methanol, and shake for 10 minutes. Dilute with methanol to volume, mix, and filter: the filtrate so obtained meets the requirements for *Identification* test *B* under *Sotalol Hydrochloride.*

Dissolution ⟨711⟩—
Medium: water; 900 mL.
Apparatus 2: 50 rpm.
Time: 30 minutes.
Procedure—Determine the amount of $C_{12}H_{20}N_2O_3S \cdot HCl$ dissolved by employing UV absorption at the wavelength of maximum absorbance at about 230 nm on filtered portions of the solution under test, in comparison with a Standard solution having a known concentration of USP Sotalol Hydrochloride RS in the same *Medium.*
Tolerances—Not less than 80% (*Q*) of the labeled amount of $C_{12}H_{20}N_2O_3S \cdot HCl$ is dissolved in 30 minutes.

Uniformity of dosage units ⟨905⟩: meet the requirements.
Assay—
Phosphate buffer—Dissolve 6.8 g of monobasic potassium phosphate in about 800 mL of water. Dilute with water to 1000 mL, and mix.
Mobile phase—Prepare a filtered and degassed mixture of *Phosphate buffer* and acetonitrile (9 : 1).
Internal standard solution—Transfer about 1.8 g of caffeine, accurately weighed, to a 1000-mL volumetric flask. Dissolve in and dilute with water to volume, mix.
Standard preparation—Transfer about 80 mg of USP Sotalol Hydrochloride RS, accurately weighed, to a 25-mL volumetric flask. Add 2.5 mL of 1 N hydrochloric acid, dissolve in and dilute with water to volume, mix, and filter. Transfer 10.0 mL of the filtrate and 25.0 mL of the *Internal standard solution* to a 200-mL volumetric flask. Dilute with water to volume, and mix.
Assay preparation—Transfer an appropriate number of Tablets, equivalent to about 800 mg of sotalol hydrochloride, to a 250-mL volumetric flask. Add 25 mL of 1 N hydrochloric acid, and swirl. Dilute with water to about three-fourths of the volume of the flask, and shake for 15 minutes. Dilute with water to volume, mix, and filter. Transfer 10.0 mL of this solution and 25.0 mL of the *Internal standard solution* to a 200-mL volumetric flask. Dilute with water to volume, and mix.
Chromatographic system (see *Chromatography* ⟨621⟩)—The liquid chromatograph is equipped with a 238-nm detector and a 3.9-mm × 30-cm column that contains packing L1. The flow rate is about 1.5 mL per minute. Chromatograph the *Standard preparation,* and record the peak areas as directed for *Procedure:* the relative retention times for sotalol and caffeine are about 1.0 and 2.0, respectively; the resolution, *R,* between caffeine and sotalol is not less than 6.0; and the relative standard deviation for replicate injections, determined from peak area ratios, is not more than 2.0%.
Procedure—Separately inject equal volumes (about 25 µL) of the *Standard preparation* and the *Assay preparation* into the chromatograph, record the chromatograms, and measure the areas for the major peaks. Calculate the quantity, in mg, of sotalol hydrochloride ($C_{12}H_{20}N_2O_3S \cdot HCl$) in the portion of Tablets taken by the formula:

$$5000C(R_U/R_S)$$

in which *C* is the concentration, in mg per mL, of USP Sotalol Hydrochloride RS in the *Standard preparation;* and R_U and R_S are the peak area ratios of sotalol to caffeine obtained from the *Assay preparation* and the *Standard preparation,* respectively.

Soybean Oil

» Soybean Oil is the refined fixed oil obtained from the seeds of the soya plant *Glycine max* Merr. (Fabaceae). It may contain suitable antioxidants.

Packaging and storage—Preserve in tight, light-resistant containers, and avoid exposure to excessive heat.
Labeling—Label it to indicate the name and quantity of any added antioxidant.
Specific gravity ⟨841⟩: between 0.916 and 0.922.
Refractive index ⟨831⟩: between 1.465 and 1.475.
Heavy metals, *Method II* ⟨231⟩: 0.001%.
Free fatty acids ⟨401⟩—The free fatty acids in 10 g require for neutralization not more than 2.5 mL of 0.020 N sodium hydroxide.
Fatty acid composition—Place about 1 g of Oil in a small conical flask fitted with a reflux attachment. Add 10 mL of methanol and 0.5 mL of 1 N methanolic potassium hydroxide solution prepared by dissolving 34 g of potassium hydroxide in sufficient methanol to produce 500 mL, allowing to settle for 24 hours, and decanting the clear solution. Reflux the mixture for 10 minutes, cool, transfer to a separator with the aid of 15 mL of *n*-heptane, shake with 10 mL of saturated sodium chloride solution, and allow to separate. Transfer the lower layer to another separator, and shake it with 10 mL of *n*-heptane. Wash the combined organic layers with 10 mL of water, dry over anhydrous sodium sulfate, and filter. Introduce a suitable portion of the filtrate into a gas chromatograph equipped with a flame-ionization detector and a column, preferably glass, 1.5 m in length and 4 mm in internal diameter packed with 10% liquid phase G4 on support S1A, maintained at a temperature of 175°. The carrier gas is nitrogen. Measure the 5 main peak areas of the methyl esters of the fatty acids. The order of elution is palmitate, stearate, oleate, linoleate, and linolenate, and their relative areas, expressed as percentages of the total area of the 5 main peaks, are in the ranges 7 to 14, 1 to 6, 19 to 30, 44 to 62, and 4 to 11, respectively.
Iodine value, *Method II* ⟨401⟩: between 120 and 141.
Saponification value ⟨401⟩: between 180 and 200.
Unsaponifiable matter ⟨401⟩: not more than 1.0%.
Cottonseed oil—Mix 10 mL in a 250- × 25-mm test tube with 10 mL of a mixture of equal volumes of amyl alcohol and a 1 in 100 solution of sulfur in carbon disulfide. Warm the mixture carefully. *[Caution—Carbon disulfide vapors may be ignited with a hot bath or hot steam pipe.]* When the carbon disulfide has been expelled, immerse the tube to one-third of its length in a boiling, saturated solution of sodium chloride: no red color develops in the mixture within 15 minutes.
Peroxide—
Mixed solvent—Mix 60 mL of glacial acetic acid with 40 mL of chloroform.
Potassium iodide solution—Prepare a saturated solution of potassium iodide in freshly boiled and cooled water, and store it protected from light. Discard it if it gives a color on addition of *Mixed solvent* and starch TS.
Procedure—Transfer about 10 g of Oil, accurately weighed, to a conical flask, add 30 mL of *Mixed solvent,* swirl to dissolve, add 0.5 mL of *Potassium iodide solution,* swirl the flask for 1 minute, accurately timed, add 30 mL of water, and titrate with 0.01 N sodium thiosulfate VS, with vigorous agitation, to a light yellow color. Add 0.5 mL of starch TS, and continue the titration until the blue color has disappeared. Perform a blank test, and make any necessary correction. Calculate the peroxide content, in mEq per kg, taken by the formula:

$$1000VN/W$$

in which *V* is the volume, in mL, of sodium thiosulfate required and *N* is its normality; and *W* is the weight, in g, of Oil taken. The limit is 10.0.

Spectinomycin Hydrochloride

$C_{14}H_{24}N_2O_7 \cdot 2HCl \cdot 5H_2O$ 495.35
4*H*-Pyrano[2,3-*b*][1,4]benzodioxin-4-one, decahydro-4a,7,9-trihydroxy-2-methyl-6,8-bis(methylamino)-, dihydrochloride, pentahydrate, [2*R*-(2α,4a*β*,5a*β*,6*β*,7*β*,8*β*,9α,9a*α*,10a*β*)]-.
(2*R*,4a*R*,5a*R*,6*S*,7*S*,8*R*,9*S*,9a*R*,10a*S*)-Decahydro-4a,7,9-trihydroxy-2-methyl-6,8-bis(methylamino)-4*H*-pyrano[2,3-*b*]1,4]benzodioxin-4-one dihydrochloride pentahydrate   [22189-32-8].
Anhydrous   405.28   [21736-83-4].

» Spectinomycin Hydrochloride has a potency equivalent to not less than 603 µg of spectinomycin ($C_{14}H_{24}N_2O_7$) per mg.

Packaging and storage—Preserve in tight containers.
Labeling—Where it is intended for use in preparing injectable dosage forms, the label states that it is sterile or must be subjected to further processing during the preparation of injectable dosage forms.

USP Reference standards ⟨11⟩—*USP Spectinomycin Hydrochloride RS. USP Endotoxin RS.*

Identification, *Infrared Absorption* ⟨197M⟩—Do not dry specimen.
Crystallinity ⟨695⟩: meets the requirements.
Bacterial endotoxins ⟨85⟩—Where the label states that Spectinomycin Hydrochloride is sterile or that it must be subjected to further processing during the preparation of injectable dosage forms, it contains not more than 0.09 USP Endotoxin Unit per mg of spectinomycin.
Sterility ⟨71⟩—Where the label states that Spectinomycin Hydrochloride is sterile, it meets the requirements when tested as directed for *Membrane Filtration* under *Test for Sterility of the Product to be Examined.*
pH ⟨791⟩: between 3.8 and 5.6, in a solution containing 10 mg per mL.
Water, *Method I* ⟨921⟩: between 16.0% and 20.0%.
Residue on ignition ⟨281⟩: not more than 1.0%, the charred residue being moistened with 2 mL of nitric acid and 5 drops of sulfuric acid.
Assay—
Internal standard solution—Dissolve triphenylantimony in dimethylformamide to obtain a solution containing about 2 mg per mL.
Standard preparation—Transfer about 30 mg of USP Spectinomycin Hydrochloride RS, accurately weighed, to a glass-stoppered, 25-mL conical flask. Add 10.0 mL of *Internal standard solution* and 1.0 mL of hexamethyldisilazane, and shake intermittently for 1 hour.
Assay preparation—Proceed as directed under *Standard preparation* using Spectinomycin Hydrochloride.
Chromatographic system (see *Chromatography* ⟨621⟩)—The gas chromatograph is equipped with a flame-ionization detector and contains a 3-mm × 60-cm glass column packed with 5 percent phase G27 on 80- to 100-mesh support S1AB. The column and detector are maintained at about 190° and 220°, respectively, and the injection port is at about 215°, and dry helium is used as the carrier gas at a flow rate of about 45 mL per minute. Chromatograph the *Standard preparation,* and record the chromatogram as directed for *Procedure:* the resolution, R, between the major peaks is not less than 2.0; and the relative standard deviation of the peak response ratios, R_S, from replicate injections of the *Standard preparation* is not more than 3.5%.
Procedure—Separately inject equal volumes (about 1 μL) of the *Standard preparation* and the *Assay preparation* into the chromatograph, record the chromatograms, and measure the responses for the major peaks. Calculate the ratio, R_U, of the response of the spectinomycin peak to the response of the internal standard peak in the chromatogram from the *Assay preparation,* and similarly calculate the ratio, R_S, in the chromatogram from the *Standard preparation.* Calculate the quantity, in μg, of $C_{14}H_{24}N_2O_7$ in the portion of Spectinomycin Hydrochloride taken to prepare the *Assay preparation* by the formula:

$$P(W_S)(R_U / R_S)$$

in which P is the potency of USP Spectinomycin Hydrochloride RS, in μg of spectinomycin per mg; and W_S is the weight, in mg, of USP Spectinomycin Hydrochloride RS taken from the *Standard preparation;* and the other terms are as defined above.

Spectinomycin for Injectable Suspension

» Spectinomycin for Injectable Suspension contains an amount of Spectinomycin Hydrochloride equivalent to not less than 90.0 percent and not more than 120.0 percent of the labeled amount of spectinomycin ($C_{14}H_{24}N_2O_7$).

Packaging and storage—Preserve in *Containers for Sterile Solids* as described under *Injections* ⟨1⟩.
USP Reference standards ⟨11⟩—USP Endotoxin RS. USP Spectinomycin Hydrochloride RS.

pH ⟨791⟩: between 4.0 and 7.0, in the suspension constituted as directed in the labeling.
Other requirements—It conforms to the Definition, responds to the *Identification* test, and meets the requirements for *Crystallinity, Bacterial endotoxins, Sterility, Water,* and *Residue on ignition* under *Spectinomycin Hydrochloride.* It meets also the requirements for *Uniformity of Dosage Units* ⟨905⟩ and *Labeling* under *Injections* ⟨1⟩.
Assay—
Internal standard solution, Standard preparation, and *Chromatographic system*—Prepare as directed in the *Assay* under *Spectinomycin Hydrochloride.*
Assay preparation 1—Suspend the contents of 1 container of Spectinomycin for Injectable Suspension in water, and dilute quantitatively with water to obtain a stock solution containing about 20 mg of spectinomycin per mL. Transfer 1.0 mL of this solution to a glass-stoppered, 25-mL conical flask, and freeze-dry. Add 10.0 mL of *Internal standard solution* and 1.0 mL of hexamethyldisilazane, and shake intermittently for 1 hour.
Assay preparation 2 (where the label states the quantity of spectinomycin in a given volume of constituted suspension)—Constitute 1 container of Spectinomycin for Injectable Suspension in a volume of water, accurately measured, corresponding to the volume of diluent specified in the labeling. Dilute an accurately measured portion of the constituted suspension quantitatively with water to obtain a stock solution containing about 20 mg of spectinomycin per mL. Transfer 1.0 mL of this solution to a glass-stoppered, 25-mL conical flask, and freeze-dry. Add 10.0 mL of *Internal standard solution* and 1.0 mL of hexamethyldisilazane, and shake intermittently for 1 hour.
Procedure—Proceed as directed in the *Assay* under *Spectinomycin Hydrochloride.* Calculate the quantity, in g, of $C_{14}H_{24}N_2O_7$ in the container of Spectinomycin for Injectable Suspension taken to prepare *Assay preparation 1* taken by the formula:

$$(L_1 / D_1)(P / 1000)(W_S)(R_U / R_S)$$

in which L_1 is the labeled quantity, in g, of $C_{14}H_{24}N_2O_7$ in the container, and D_1 is the concentration, in mg per mL, of spectinomycin in the stock solution used to prepare *Assay preparation 1*, on the basis of the labeled quantity in the container and the extent of dilution, and the other terms are as defined therein. Calculate the quantity, in mg, of $C_{14}H_{24}N_2O_7$ in each mL of constituted Injectable Suspension taken to prepare *Assay preparation 2* taken by the formula:

$$(L_2 / D_2)(P / 1000)(W_S)(R_U / R_S)$$

in which L_2 is the labeled quantity, in mg, of $C_{14}H_{24}N_2O_7$ in each mL of constituted suspension of Spectinomycin for Injectable Suspension, and D_2 is the concentration, in mg per mL, of spectinomycin in the stock solution used to prepare *Assay preparation 2*, on the basis of the labeled quantity in each mL of constituted suspension and the extent of dilution.

Spironolactone

$C_{24}H_{32}O_4S$ 416.57

Pregn-4-ene-21-carboxylic acid, 7-(acetylthio)-17-hydroxy-3-oxo-, γ-lactone, (7α,17α)-.
17-Hydroxy-7α-mercapto-3-oxo-17α-pregn-4-ene-21-carboxylic acid γ-lactone acetate [52-01-7].

» Spironolactone contains not less than 97.0 percent and not more than 103.0 percent of $C_{24}H_{32}O_4S$, calculated on the dried basis.

Packaging and storage—Preserve in well-closed containers.

USP Reference standards ⟨11⟩—*USP Spironolactone RS*.

Identification—

A: *Infrared Absorption* ⟨197S⟩—
Solution: 1 in 20.
Medium: chloroform.

B: *Ultraviolet Absorption* ⟨197U⟩—
Solution: 10 μg per mL.
Medium: methanol.
Absorptivities at 238 nm, calculated on the dried basis, do not differ by more than 3.0%.

C: Add 100 mg to a mixture of 10 mL of water and 2 mL of 1 N sodium hydroxide, boil the mixture for 3 minutes, cool, and add 1 mL of glacial acetic acid and 1 mL of lead acetate TS: a brown to black precipitate of lead sulfide is formed.

Melting range ⟨741⟩: between 198° and 209°, with decomposition. Occasionally it may show preliminary melting at about 135°, followed by resolidification.

Specific rotation ⟨781S⟩: between −33° and −37°.
Test solution: 10 mg per mL, in chloroform.

Loss on drying ⟨731⟩—Dry it at 105° for 2 hours: it loses not more than 0.5% of its weight.

Limit of mercapto compounds—Shake 2.0 g with 30 mL of water, filter, then to 15 mL of the filtrate add 3 mL of starch TS, and titrate with 0.010 N iodine. Perform a blank determination, and make any necessary correction. Not more than 0.10 mL of 0.010 N iodine is consumed.

Ordinary impurities ⟨466⟩—
Test solution: chloroform.
Standard solution: chloroform.
Eluant: butyl acetate.
Visualization: 5.

Organic volatile impurities, *Method V* ⟨467⟩: meets the requirements.
Solvent—Use dimethyl sulfoxide.

(Official until July 1, 2008)

Assay—
Mobile phase—Prepare a filtered and degassed mixture of methanol and water (60 : 40).

Standard preparation—Dissolve an accurately weighed quantity of USP Spironolactone RS in a mixture of acetonitrile and water (50 : 50), and quantitatively dilute with the same mixture to obtain a solution having a known concentration of about 0.5 mg of USP Spironolactone RS per mL.

Assay preparation—Transfer about 50 mg of Spironolactone, accurately weighed, to a 100-mL volumetric flask, add a mixture of acetonitrile and water (50 : 50) to volume, and mix.

Chromatographic system (see *Chromatography* ⟨621⟩)—The liquid chromatograph is equipped with a 230-nm detector and a 4.6-mm × 15-cm column that contains packing L1. The flow rate is about 1 mL per minute. Chromatograph the *Standard preparation,* and record the peak responses as directed for *Procedure:* the tailing factor is not more than 2.0, and the relative standard deviation for replicate injections is not more than 1.5%.

Procedure—Separately inject equal volumes (about 20 μL) of the *Standard preparation* and the *Assay preparation* into the chromatograph, record the chromatograms, and measure the responses for the major peaks. Calculate the quantity, in mg, of $C_{24}H_{32}O_4S$ in the portion of Spironolactone taken by the formula:

$$100C(r_U / r_S)$$

in which *C* is the concentration, in mg per mL, of USP Spironolactone RS in the *Standard preparation;* and r_U and r_S are the spironolactone peak responses obtained from the *Assay preparation* and the *Standard preparation,* respectively.

Spironolactone Tablets

» Spironolactone Tablets contain not less than 95.0 percent and not more than 105.0 percent of the labeled amount of spironolactone ($C_{24}H_{32}O_4S$).

Packaging and storage—Preserve in tight, light-resistant containers.

USP Reference standards ⟨11⟩—*USP Spironolactone RS*.

Identification—Mix a quantity of finely powdered Tablets, equivalent to about 100 mg of spironolactone, with 25 mL of methanol, and filter. Apply 10 μL of this solution and 10 μL of a solution of USP Spironolactone RS in methanol containing 4 mg per mL to a suitable thin-layer chromatographic plate (see *Chromatography* ⟨621⟩) coated with a 0.25-mm layer of chromatographic silica gel mixture. Develop the chromatogram in a solvent system consisting of a mixture of chloroform, ethyl acetate, and methanol (2 : 2 : 1) until the solvent front has moved about three-fourths of the length of the plate. Remove the plate from the developing chamber, mark the solvent front, and allow the solvent to evaporate. Locate the spots on the plate by viewing under short-wavelength UV light: the R_F value of the principal spot obtained from the solution under test corresponds to that obtained from the Standard solution.

Dissolution ⟨711⟩—
Medium: 0.1 N hydrochloric acid containing 0.1% of sodium lauryl sulfate; 1000 mL.
Apparatus 2: 75 rpm.
Time: 60 minutes.
Procedure—Determine the amount of $C_{24}H_{32}O_4S$ dissolved using UV absorption at the wavelength of maximum absorbance at about 242 nm obtained on filtered portions of the solution under test, diluted with *Medium,* if necessary, in comparison with a Standard solution having a known concentration of USP Spironolactone RS in the same *Medium.* [NOTE—A volume of alcohol not exceeding 1% of the final volume of the solution may be used to prepare the Standard solution.]
Tolerances—Not less than 75% (*Q*) of the labeled amount of $C_{24}H_{32}O_4S$ is dissolved in 60 minutes.

Uniformity of dosage units ⟨905⟩: meet the requirements.

Assay—
Mobile phase, Standard preparation, and *Chromatographic system*—Prepare as directed in the *Assay* under *Spironolactone*.
Diluent—Prepare a mixture of acetonitrile and water (1 : 1).
Assay preparation—Accurately weigh not fewer than 10 Tablets, and transfer to a suitable volumetric flask. [NOTE—The target concentration is about 1 mg per mL.] Add a sufficient quantity of *Diluent,* shake for about 30 minutes, and sonicate for 30 minutes or until the Tablets are disintegrated. Cool the solution to room temperature, dilute with *Diluent* to volume, and centrifuge a suitable portion of the mixture. Quantitatively dilute a portion of this solution with *Diluent* to obtain a solution having a known concentration of about 0.5 mg of spironolactone per mL.
Procedure—Proceed as directed for *Procedure* in the *Assay* under *Spironolactone*. Calculate the quantity, in mg, of spironolactone ($C_{24}H_{32}O_4S$) in the portion of Tablets taken by the formula:

$$CD(r_U / r_S)$$

in which *C* is the concentration, in mg per mL, of USP Spironolactone RS in the *Standard preparation; D* is the dilution factor for the *Assay preparation;* and r_U and r_S are the peak responses for spironolactone obtained from the *Assay preparation* and the *Standard preparation,* respectively.

Spironolactone and Hydrochlorothiazide Tablets

» Spironolactone and Hydrochlorothiazide Tablets contain not less than 90.0 percent and not more than 110.0

percent of the labeled amounts of spironolactone ($C_{24}H_{32}O_4S$) and hydrochlorothiazide ($C_7H_8ClN_3O_4S_2$).

Packaging and storage—Preserve in tight, light-resistant containers.

USP Reference standards ⟨11⟩—*USP Hydrochlorothiazide RS. USP Spironolactone RS.*

Identification—The retention times of the major peaks in the chromatogram of the *Assay preparation* correspond to those in the chromatogram of the *Standard preparation,* as obtained in the *Assay.*

Dissolution ⟨711⟩—
Medium: 0.1 N hydrochloric acid containing 0.1% sodium lauryl sulfate; 900 mL.
Apparatus 2: 75 rpm.
Time: 60 minutes.

Determine the amounts of spironolactone and hydrochlorothiazide dissolved using the following method.

Standard solution—Prepare a solution of USP Spironolactone RS and USP Hydrochlorothiazide RS in a mixture of methanol and *Medium*(1 : 1) having accurately known concentrations of about 0.0125 mg of each per mL.

Test solution—Transfer a 5.0-mL portion of the solution under test to a 10-mL volumetric flask, dilute with methanol to volume, and mix.

Solution A—Use acetonitrile.

Solution B—Transfer about 4.5 g of monobasic potassium phosphate to a 1-L volumetric flask containing about 500 mL of water. Dissolve in and dilute with water to volume, and mix.

Mobile phase—Use variable amounts of *Solution A* and *Solution B* as directed for *Chromatographic system.* Make adjustments if necessary (see *System Suitability* under *Chromatography* ⟨621⟩).

Chromatographic system (see *Chromatography* ⟨621⟩)—The liquid chromatograph is equipped with a 254-nm detector and a 4.6-mm × 25-cm column that contains packing L1. The flow rate is about 1 mL per minute. The chromatograph is programmed as follows.

Time (minutes)	Solution A (%)	Solution B (%)	Elution
0	25	75	equilibration
0–10	25→75	75→25	linear gradient
10–18	75	25	isocratic
18–25	75→25	25→75	linear gradient

Chromatograph the *Standard solution,* and record the peak responses as directed for *Procedure:*the resolution, *R,* between hydrochlorothiazide and spironolactone is not less than 2.0; and the relative standard deviation for replicate injections is not more than 2.0%.

Procedure—Proceed as directed in the *Assay,* injecting 20 µL of each solution.

Tolerances—Not less than 75% (*Q*) of each of the labeled amounts of $C_{24}H_{32}O_4S$ and $C_7H_8ClN_3O_4S_2$ is dissolved in 60 minutes.

Uniformity of dosage units ⟨905⟩: meet the requirements for *Content uniformity* with respect to spironolactone and to hydrochlorothiazide.

Assay—
Mobile phase—Prepare a filtered and degassed mixture of methanol and water (7 : 3). Make adjustments if necessary (see *System Suitability* under *Chromatography* ⟨621⟩).

Standard preparation—Dissolve accurately weighed quantities of USP Spironolactone RS and USP Hydrochlorothiazide RS in methanol to obtain a solution having known concentrations of about 50 µg of each per mL.

Assay preparation—Weigh and finely powder not fewer than 20 Tablets. Transfer an accurately weighed portion of the powder, equivalent to about 25 mg of spironolactone, to a 100-mL volumetric flask, add about 70 mL of methanol, shake by mechanical means for 30 minutes, dilute with methanol to volume, mix, and centrifuge. Transfer 20.0 mL of the resultant clear liquid to a 100-mL volumetric flask, dilute with methanol to volume, and mix.

Chromatographic system (see *Chromatography* ⟨621⟩)—The liquid chromatograph is equipped with a 254-nm detector and a 4-mm × 30-cm column that contains packing L1. The flow rate is about 1 mL per minute. Chromatograph the *Standard preparation,* and record the peak responses as directed for *Procedure:* the resolution, *R,* between hydrochlorothiazide and spironolactone is not less than 2.0; and the relative standard deviation for replicate injections is not more than 2.0%.

Procedure—Separately inject equal volumes (about 10 µL) of the *Standard preparation* and the *Assay preparation* into the chromatograph, record the chromatograms, and measure the responses for the major peaks. The relative retention times are about 0.5 for hydrochlorothiazide and 1.0 for spironolactone. Calculate the quantity, in mg, of spironolactone ($C_{24}H_{32}O_4S$) in the portion of Tablets taken by the formula:

$$0.5C(r_U / r_S)$$

in which *C* is the concentration, in µg per mL, of USP Spironolactone RS in the *Standard preparation;* and r_U and r_S are the responses of the spironolactone peak obtained from the *Assay preparation* and the *Standard preparation,* respectively. Calculate the quantity, in mg, of hydrochlorothiazide ($C_7H_8ClN_3O_4S_2$) by the same formula, changing the terms to refer to hydrochlorothiazide.

Stannous Fluoride

SnF_2 156.71
Tin fluoride (SnF_2).
Tin fluoride (SnF_2)   [7783-47-3].

» Stannous Fluoride contains not less than 71.2 percent of stannous tin (Sn^{++}), and not less than 22.3 percent and not more than 25.5 percent of fluoride (F), calculated on the dried basis.

Packaging and storage—Preserve in well-closed containers.

USP Reference standards ⟨11⟩—*USP Sodium Fluoride RS.*

Identification—
A: To 5 mL of a solution (1 in 100) in a test tube add 2 mL of calcium chloride TS: a fine, white precipitate of calcium fluoride is formed.
B: Mix on a spot plate 2 drops of a solution (1 in 100) with 2 drops of silver nitrate TS: a brown-black precipitate is formed.
C: Add 1 drop of a solution (1 in 100) to 2 drops of mercuric chloride TS: a white, silky precipitate is formed. On further addition of the solution (1 in 100), a brown-black precipitate is formed.

pH ⟨791⟩: between 2.8 and 3.5, in a freshly prepared 0.4% solution.

Loss on drying ⟨731⟩—Dry it at 105° for 4 hours: it loses not more than 0.5% of its weight.

Water-insoluble substances—Transfer about 10 g, accurately weighed, to a 400-mL plastic beaker, add 200 mL of water, and stir with a plastic rod for 3 minutes, or until no more solid dissolves. Filter through a tared filtering crucible, and wash thoroughly, first with ammonium fluoride solution (1 in 100), then with water. [NOTE—Prepare and use the filtering crucible in a well-ventilated hood.] Dry the residue at 105° for 4 hours, cool, and weigh: the weight of the residue does not exceed 0.2%.

Antimony—
Rhodamine B solution—Dissolve 20 mg of rhodamine B in 200 mL of 0.5 N hydrochloric acid.

Standard preparation—Transfer 55.0 mg of antimony potassium tartrate, accurately weighed, to a 200-mL volumetric flask, dissolve in water, dilute with water to volume, and mix. Transfer 5.0 mL of this solution to a 500-mL volumetric flask, add 6 N hydrochloric acid to volume, and mix.

Test preparation—Transfer 1.0 g of Stannous Fluoride, accurately weighed, to a 50-mL volumetric flask, add 6 N hydrochloric acid to volume, and mix.

Procedure—Pipet 5 mL each of the *Standard preparation* and the *Test preparation* into separate 125-mL separators, add 15 mL of hydrochloric acid and 1 g of ceric sulfate, and allow to stand for 5 minutes, with occasional shaking. Add 500 mg of hydroxylamine hydrochloride, and shake for 1 minute. Pipet 15 mL of isopropyl ether into the mixture, shake for 30 seconds, add 7 mL of water, and mix. Cool in a water bath at room temperature for 10 minutes, shake for 30 seconds, allow the layers to separate, and discard the aqueous phase. Add 20 mL of *Rhodamine B solution*, shake for 30 seconds, and discard the aqueous layer. Decant the ether layer from the top of the separator, and centrifuge, if necessary, to obtain a clear solution. Concomitantly determine the absorbances of the ether solutions from the *Test preparation* and the *Standard preparation* at the wavelength of maximum absorbance at about 550 nm, with a suitable spectrophotometer, using water as the blank: the absorbance of the *Test preparation* does not exceed that of the *Standard preparation* (0.005%).

Assay for stannous ion—

0.1 N Potassium iodide-iodate—In a 1000-mL volumetric flask, dissolve 3.567 g of potassium iodate, previously dried at 110° to constant weight, in 200 mL of oxygen-free water containing 1 g of sodium hydroxide and 10 g of potassium iodide, dilute with oxygen-free water to volume, and mix. Standardize this solution by titrating a solution prepared from an accurately weighed quantity of reagent tin (Sn) and hydrochloric acid. Each mL of *0.1 N Potassium iodide-iodate* is equivalent to 5.935 mg of Sn.

Procedure—Transfer about 250 mg of Stannous Fluoride, accurately weighed, to a 500-mL conical flask, and add 300 mL of hot, recently boiled 3 N hydrochloric acid. While passing a stream of an oxygen-free inert gas over the surface of the liquid, swirl the flask to dissolve the Stannous Fluoride, and cool to room temperature. Add 5 mL of potassium iodide TS, and titrate in an inert atmosphere with *0.1 N Potassium iodide-iodate*, adding 3 mL of starch TS as the endpoint is approached. Each mL of *0.1 N Potassium iodide-iodate* is equivalent to 5.935 mg of Sn^{++}.

Assay for fluoride—[NOTE—Store all solutions, except *Buffer solution*, in plastic containers.]

Buffer solution—Dissolve 57 mL of glacial acetic acid, 58 g of sodium chloride, and 4 g of (1,2-cyclohexylenedinitrilo)tetraacetic acid in 500 mL of water. Adjust with 5 N sodium hydroxide to a pH of 5.25 ± 0.25, dilute with water to 1000 mL, and mix.

Standard preparations—Dissolve an accurately weighed quantity of USP Sodium Fluoride RS quantitatively in water to obtain a solution containing 420 µg per mL. Each mL of this solution *(Standard preparation A)* contains 190 µg of fluoride ion (10^{-2} M). Transfer 25.0 mL of *Standard preparation A* to a 250-mL volumetric flask, dilute with water to volume, and mix. This solution *(Standard preparation B)* contains 19 µg of fluoride ion per mL (10^{-3} M). Transfer 25.0 mL of *Standard preparation B* to a 250-mL volumetric flask, dilute with water to volume, and mix. This solution *(Standard preparation C)* contains 1.9 µg of fluoride ion per mL (10^{-4} M).

Assay preparation—Transfer to a 250-mL volumetric flask about 100 mg of Stannous Fluoride, accurately weighed. Add 50 mL of water, mix vigorously for 5 minutes, dilute with water to volume, and mix. Transfer 10.0 mL of this solution to a 50-mL volumetric flask, dilute with water to volume, and mix.

Procedure—Pipet 20 mL of each *Standard preparation* and of the *Assay preparation* into separate plastic beakers each containing a plastic-coated stirring bar. Pipet 20 mL of *Buffer solution* into each beaker. Concomitantly measure the potentials (see *pH ⟨791⟩*), in mV, of the solutions from the *Standard preparations* and of the solution from the *Assay preparation*, with a pH meter capable of a minimum reproducibility of ±0.2 mV and equipped with a fluoride-specific ion-indicating electrode and a calomel reference electrode. [NOTE—When taking measurements, immerse the electrodes in the solution, stir on a magnetic stirrer having an insulated top until equilibrium is attained (1 to 2 minutes), and record the potential. Rinse and dry the electrodes between measurements, taking care to avoid damaging the crystal of the specific-ion electrode.] Plot the logarithms of the fluoride-ion concentrations, in µg per mL, of the *Standard preparations* versus potential, in mV. From the measured potential of the *Assay preparation* and the standard reponse line, determine the concentration, *C*, in µg per mL, of fluoride ion in the *Assay preparation*. Calculate the percentage of fluoride (F) in the portion of Stannous Fluoride taken by the formula:

$$125C/W$$

in which *C* is the determined concentration of fluoride, in µg per mL, in the *Assay preparation*, and *W* is the weight, in mg, of Stannous Fluoride taken.

Stannous Fluoride Gel

» Stannous Fluoride Gel contains not less than 95.0 percent and not more than 115.0 percent of the labeled amount of SnF_2 in a suitable medium containing a suitable viscosity-inducing agent.

NOTE—If Glycerin is used as the medium in the preparation of this Gel, use Glycerin that has a low water content, that is, Glycerin having a specific gravity of not less than 1.2607, corresponding to a concentration of 99.5 percent.

Packaging and storage—Preserve in well-closed containers.
USP Reference standards ⟨11⟩—*USP Sodium Fluoride RS*.
Identification—It responds to the *Identification* tests under *Stannous Fluoride*, a solution of it in water containing about 1 mg of stannous fluoride per mL being used instead of a 1 in 100 solution.
Viscosity ⟨911⟩—Place a quantity of Gel in a suitable plastic container, insert the stopper securely, and allow to stand until the gel is free from air bubbles. Place it in a water bath maintained at a temperature of 25 ± 0.5° until it adjusts to the temperature of the water bath (4 hours or longer). Do not stir the gel while it is in the bath. Remove the specimen from the bath, stir the gel gently for 2 minutes, and without delay, using a rotational viscosimeter, determine the viscosity using a spindle having a cylinder 1.27 cm in diameter and 0.16 cm high attached to a shaft 0.32 cm in diameter, the distance from the top of the cylinder to the lower tip of the shaft being 2.54 cm and the immersion depth being 5.00 cm (No. 3 spindle). Operate the viscosimeter at 12 rpm, and record the scale reading at 1-minute intervals for 4 minutes. Calculate the viscosity, in centipoises, by multiplying the scale reading by 100: the viscosity is between 600 and 170,000 centipoises.
pH ⟨791⟩: between 2.8 and 4.0, in a freshly prepared mixture with water (1 : 1).
Stannous ion content—

0.1 N Potassium iodide-iodate—Prepare as directed in the *Assay for stannous ion* under *Stannous Fluoride*.

Procedure—Transfer an accurately weighed quantity of Gel, equivalent to about 80 mg of stannous fluoride, to a capped plastic vessel equipped for titration in an inert atmosphere. Add a plastic coated stirring bar, 20 mL of recently boiled 3 N hydrochloric acid, and 5 mL of potassium iodide TS. Close the vessel, purge the system with an oxygen-free inert gas, and titrate immediately with 0.1 *N Potassium iodide-iodate* adding 2 mL of starch TS as the endpoint is approached. Calculate the quantity, in mg, of stannous ion (Sn++) in each g of Gel by the formula:

$$5.935V/W$$

in which *V* is the volume, in mL, of 0.1 N potassium iodide-iodate consumed; 5.935 is the Sn++ equivalent, in mg, of each mL of 0.1 N potassium iodide-iodate; and *W* is the weight, in g, of Gel taken. The quantity, in mg, of stannous ion in each g of Gel is not less than 68.2% of the quantity, in mg, of stannous fluoride in each g of Gel as determined in the *Assay*, and is not less than 90.0% of the quantity, in mg, of total tin in each g of Gel as determined in the test for *Total tin content*.

Total tin content—

Potassium chloride solution—Dissolve 1.91 g of potassium chloride in water to make 100 mL of solution.

Tin stock standard solution—Transfer 1.000 g of tin, accurately weighed, to a 1000-mL volumetric flask, add 200 mL of hydrochloric acid, and swirl to dissolve. Add 200 mL of water, allow to cool, dilute with water to volume, and mix.

Standard preparations—Transfer 5.0, 10.0, and 15.0 mL of *Tin stock standard solution* to separate 100-mL volumetric flasks, add 1.0 mL of *Potassium chloride solution* to each flask, dilute with water to volume, and mix. The *Standard preparations* contain, respectively, 50.0, 100.0, and 150.0 µg of tin per mL.

Test preparation—Transfer an accurately weighed quantity of Gel, equivalent to about 132 mg of stannous fluoride, to a plastic beaker. Add 80 mL of water and 20 mL of hydrochloric acid, and mix. Transfer this mixture to a 1000-mL volumetric flask, add 10.0 mL of *Potassium chloride solution*, dilute with water to volume, and mix.

Blank—Add 2 mL of hydrochloric acid and 1.0 mL of *Potassium chloride solution* to a 100-mL volumetric flask, dilute with water to volume, and mix.

Procedure—Concomitantly determine the absorbance of the *Standard preparations*, the *Test preparation*, and the *Blank* at the tin emission line of 235.5 nm, with an atomic absorption spectrophotometer (see *Spectrophotometry and Light-scattering* ⟨851⟩) equipped with a tin hollow-cathode lamp and a nitrous oxide-acetylene oxidizing flame, using water to adjust the instrument to zero. Aspirate water into the spectrophotometer before and after each *Standard preparation*, the *Test preparation*, and the *Blank*. Correct the absorbances of the *Standard preparations* and the *Test preparation* by subtracting the absorbance of the *Blank*. Plot the corrected absorbances of the *Standard preparations* versus concentration, in µg per mL, of tin, and draw the straight line best fitting the three plotted points. From the graph so obtained, determine the concentration, in µg per mL, of tin in the *Test preparation*. Calculate the quantity, in mg, of tin in each g of Gel taken by the formula:

$$C/W$$

in which C is the concentration, in µg per mL, of tin in the *Test preparation*; and W is the quantity, in g, of Gel taken to prepare the *Test preparation*. Use this value to calculate the percentage of stannous ion in the test for *Stannous ion content*.

Assay—[NOTE—Store all solutions, except the *Buffer solution*, in plastic containers.]

Buffer solution and *Standard preparations*—Prepare as directed in the *Assay* under *Sodium Fluoride Oral Solution*.

Assay preparation—Transfer an accurately weighed quantity of Gel, equivalent to about 8 mg of stannous fluoride, to a 100-mL volumetric flask, dilute with water to volume, and mix.

Procedure—Proceed as directed for *Procedure* in the *Assay* under *Sodium Fluoride Oral Solution*. Calculate the quantity, in mg, of stannous fluoride (SnF$_2$) in each g of the Gel taken by the formula:

$$(156.71 / 38.0)(C / 10W)$$

in which 156.71 is the molecular weight of stannous fluoride, 38.0 is twice the atomic weight of fluorine; C is the determined concentration, in µg per mL, of fluoride in the *Assay preparation*; and W is the weight, in g, of the Gel taken.

Stanozolol

$C_{21}H_{32}N_2O$ 328.49
2′H-Androst-2-eno[3,2-c]pyrazol-17-ol, 17-methyl-, (5α,17β)-.
17-Methyl-2′H-5α-androst-2-eno[3,2-c]pyrazol-17β-ol   [10418-03-8].

» Stanozolol contains not less than 98.0 percent and not more than 100.5 percent of $C_{21}H_{32}N_2O$, calculated on the dried basis.

Packaging and storage—Preserve in tight, light-resistant containers.

USP Reference standards ⟨11⟩—*USP Stanozolol RS.*

Identification—
  A: *Infrared Absorption* ⟨197K⟩.
  B: *Ultraviolet Absorption* ⟨197U⟩—
  Solution: 50 µg per mL.
  Medium: alcohol.
  Absorptivities at 224 nm, calculated on the dried basis, do not differ by more than 3.0%.

Specific rotation ⟨781S⟩:   between +34° and +40°.
  Test solution: 10 mg per mL, in chloroform.

Loss on drying ⟨731⟩—Dry it at a pressure not exceeding 5 mm of mercury at 100° to constant weight: it loses not more than 1.0% of its weight.

Chromatographic purity—
  Standard dilutions—Dissolve an accurately weighed quantity of USP Stanozolol RS in a mixture of chloroform and methanol (9 : 1) to obtain a solution having a known concentration of about 20 mg per mL. Dilute this solution with the same medium to obtain *Standard dilutions* having known concentrations of about 50, 100, 200, and 400 µg per mL, respectively.
  Procedure—Score a 20- × 20-cm thin-layer chromatographic plate coated with a 0.25-mm layer of chromatographic silica gel mixture (binder-free) into channels 10 mm wide. Apply 10-µL portions, in two 5-µL increments, of a test solution prepared by dissolving Stanozolol in a mixture of chloroform and methanol (9 : 1) to obtain a solution containing about 20 mg per mL, and of each of the four *Standard dilutions* in the center of the channels at points about 2.5 cm from one edge of the plate. Develop the plate in a suitable chamber, lined with filter paper and previously equilibrated with 200 mL of a mixture of chloroform and methanol (188 : 12), for 15 minutes, taking care to ensure that the filter paper has been wetted completely with the solvent mixture. Allow the plate to develop until the solvent front has moved about 15 cm above the line of application. Remove the plate, and allow the solvent to evaporate completely. Spray it with 20% sulfuric acid, and heat in an oven at 100° for 15 minutes. Examine the plate under long-wavelength UV light: the channel for the test solution exhibits its principal spot at the same R_F value as the spots for the *Standard dilutions*. Estimate the concentration of any spots in the channel for the test solution, other than the principal spot, by comparison with the spots from the *Standard dilutions*. The spots from the 50-, 100-, 200-, and 400-µg-per-mL dilutions correspond to 0.25%, 0.5%, 1.0%, and 2.0% of chromatographic impurities, respectively, and the sum of the chromatographic impurities in the test solution is not greater than 2.0%.

Organic volatile impurities, Method V ⟨467⟩:   meets the requirements.
  Solvent—Use dimethyl sulfoxide.

(Official until July 1, 2008)

Assay—Dissolve about 700 mg of Stanozolol, accurately weighed, in 50 mL of glacial acetic acid, add 1 drop of crystal violet TS, and titrate with 0.1 N perchloric acid VS to a green endpoint. Perform a blank determination, and make any necessary correction. Each mL of 0.1 N perchloric acid is equivalent to 32.85 mg of $C_{21}H_{32}N_2O$.

Stanozolol Tablets

» Stanozolol Tablets contain not less than 90.0 percent and not more than 110.0 percent of the labeled amount of stanozolol ($C_{21}H_{32}N_2O$).

Packaging and storage—Preserve in tight, light-resistant containers.

USP Reference standards ⟨11⟩—*USP Stanozolol RS.*

Identification—Boil an amount of powdered Tablets, equivalent to about 2 mg of stanozolol, with 5 mL of benzene, filter, and evaporate on a steam bath to dryness. Add 3 mL of p-dimethylaminobenzaldehyde TS to the residue: a yellow color develops, which exhibits a green fluorescence under long-wavelength UV light.

Dissolution ⟨711⟩—
  Medium: 0.1 N hydrochloric acid; 500 mL.
  Apparatus 2: 50 rpm.
  Time: 45 minutes.
  Determine the amount of $C_{21}H_{32}N_2O$ dissolved by employing the following method.
  Bromocresol purple solution—Mix 1.0 g of bromocresol purple with 1000 mL of dilute glacial acetic acid (1 in 50), and filter if necessary to obtain a clear solution.
  Standard preparations—[NOTE—Prepare *Standard preparations* on the day of use.] Transfer about 50 mg of USP Stanozolol RS, accurately weighed, to a 50-mL volumetric flask, add 15.0 mL of methanol, and mix to dissolve. Add 5.0 mL of 1.0 N hydrochloric acid, dilute with water to volume, and mix. Transfer 5.0 mL of the resulting solution to a 200-mL volumetric flask, dilute with *Dissolution Medium* to volume, and mix. Separately pipet 2-mL, 4-mL, and 6-mL portions of the solution into three 60-mL separators, add accurately measured volumes of *Dissolution Medium* to adjust the volumes in each to 25.0 mL, and pipet 25 mL of *Dissolution Medium* into a fourth 60-mL separator.
  Procedure—Pipet 25 mL of a filtered portion of the solution under test into a 60-mL separator. To this separator and to each of the four separators containing *Standard preparations* add 1.0 mL of *Bromocresol purple solution* and 10.0 mL of chloroform. Insert the stopper in each, shake gently for 1 minute, allow the phases to separate, and swirl if necessary to break up emulsions. Transfer the lower chloroform layers to separate 50-mL centrifuge tubes, insert the glass stoppers, and centrifuge for 5 minutes to clarify the solutions. Concomitantly determine the absorbances of the solutions obtained from the solution under test and from the *Standard preparation* in 1-cm cells, at the wavelength of maximum absorbance at about 420 nm, with a suitable spectrophotometer, using chloroform as the blank. Construct a standard plot of absorbances versus the concentrations of the solutions from the *Standard preparations*. From the plot so obtained, determine the amount of $C_{21}H_{32}N_2O$ dissolved in the solution under test.
  Tolerances—Not less than 75% (*Q*) of the labeled amount of $C_{21}H_{32}N_2O$ is dissolved in 45 minutes.

Uniformity of dosage units ⟨905⟩—[NOTE—Maintain the acid concentration at a uniform level in the solutions being compared spectrophotometrically; the same acidic alcohol solution is to be used throughout this procedure. Also, take precautions throughout this procedure to minimize evaporation.] Transfer 1 Tablet to a 25-mL volumetric flask, add 0.5 mL of water, and shake to disintegrate. Add about 20 mL of alcohol, heat on a steam bath, with occasional swirling, for 10 to 15 minutes, then cool, dilute with alcohol to volume, and mix. Filter through medium-porosity filter paper, taking precautions to minimize evaporation, discard the first 5 mL of the filtrate, and proceed as directed for *Assay preparations* in the *Assay*, beginning with "Transfer 5.0 mL of the filtrate."

Assay—[NOTE—Maintain the acid concentration at a uniform level in the solutions being compared spectrophotometrically; the same acidic alcohol solution is to be used throughout this procedure.]
  Standard preparations—Dissolve a suitable quantity of USP Stanozolol RS, accurately weighed, in alcohol, and dilute quantitatively and stepwise with alcohol, if necessary, to obtain a stock solution having a known concentration of about 80 μg per mL. Transfer 5.0 mL of this stock solution to a 10-mL volumetric flask, dilute with alcohol to volume, and mix to prepare the *Neutral standard preparation*. Transfer another 5.0-mL portion of the stock solution to a second 10-mL volumetric flask, dilute with acidic alcohol (1.5 mL of hydrochloric acid in 100 mL of alcohol) to volume, and mix to prepare the *Acidic standard preparation*. The concentration of USP Stanozolol RS in the *Standard preparations* is about 40 μg per mL.
  Assay preparations—Weigh and finely powder not less than 20 Tablets. Transfer an accurately weighed portion of the powder, equivalent to about 4 mg of stanozolol, to a 50-mL volumetric flask, add about 25 mL of alcohol, and heat on a steam bath, with frequent swirling, for 15 minutes. Cool, dilute with alcohol to volume, mix, filter through medium-porosity filter paper, taking precautions to minimize evaporation, and discard the first 10 mL of the filtrate. Transfer 5.0 mL of the filtrate to a 10-mL volumetric flask, dilute with alcohol to volume, and mix to prepare the *Neutral assay preparation*. Transfer another 5.0-mL portion of the filtrate to a second 10-mL volumetric flask, dilute with acidic alcohol (1.5 mL of hydrochloric acid in 100 mL of alcohol) to volume, and mix to prepare the *Acidic assay preparation*.
  Procedure—Concomitantly determine the absorbances of the acidic alcohol solution, the *Acidic standard preparation*, and the *Acidic assay preparation* in 1-cm cells at the wavelength of maximum absorbance at about 235 nm, with a suitable spectrophotometer, using alcohol, the *Neutral standard preparation*, and the *Neutral assay preparation*, respectively, as the blanks. Calculate the quantity, in mg, of $C_{21}H_{32}N_2O$ in the portion of Tablets taken by the formula:

$$0.1C(A_U - A_O)/(A_S - A_O)$$

in which *C* is the concentration, in μg per mL, of USP Stanozolol RS in the *Standard preparations*; and A_U, A_S, and A_O are the absorbances of the *Acidic assay preparation*, the *Acidic standard preparation*, and the acidic alcohol solution, respectively.

Topical Starch

» Topical Starch consists of the granules separated from the mature grain of corn [*Zea mays* Linné (Fam. Gramineae)].

Packaging and storage—Preserve in well-closed containers.
Botanic characteristics—Polygonal, rounded or spheroidal granules up to about 35 μm in diameter and usually having a circular or several-rayed central cleft.
Identification—
  A: Prepare a smooth mixture of 1 g of it with 2 mL of cold water, stir it into 15 mL of boiling water, boil gently for 2 minutes, and cool: a translucent, whitish jelly is produced.
  B: A water slurry of it is colored reddish violet to deep blue by iodine TS.
Microbial limits ⟨61⟩—The total aerobic microbial count does not exceed 500 cfu per g and the total combined molds and yeasts count does not exceed 50 cfu per g.
pH ⟨791⟩—Prepare a slurry by weighing 20.0 g ± 100 mg of Topical Starch, transferring to a suitable nonmetallic container, and adding 100 mL of water. Agitate continuously at a moderate rate for 5 minutes, then stop agitation, and immediately determine the pH to the nearest 0.1 unit: the pH, determined potentiometrically, is between 4.5 and 7.0.
Loss on drying ⟨731⟩—Dry it at 120° for 4 hours: it loses not more than 14.0% of its weight.
Residue on ignition ⟨281⟩: not more than 0.5%, determined on a 2.0-g test specimen ignited at a temperature of 575 ± 25°.
Iron ⟨241⟩—Dissolve the residue obtained in the test for *Residue on ignition* in 4 mL of hydrochloric acid with the aid of gentle heating, dilute with water to 50 mL, and mix. Dilute 25 mL of the resulting solution with water to 47 mL: the limit is 0.001%.
Oxidizing substances—Transfer 4.0 g to a glass-stoppered, 125-mL conical flask, and add 50.0 mL of water. Insert the stopper, and swirl for 5 minutes. Decant into a glass-stoppered, 50-mL centrifuge tube, and spin to clarify. Transfer 30.0 mL of clear supernatant to a glass-stoppered, 125-mL conical flask. Add 1 mL of glacial acetic acid and 0.5 g to 1.0 g of potassium iodide. Insert the stopper, swirl, and allow to stand for 25 to 30 minutes in the dark. Add 1 mL of starch TS, and titrate with 0.002 N sodium thiosulfate VS to the disappearance of the starch-iodine color. Each mL of 0.002 N sodium thiosulfate is equivalent to 34 μg of oxidant, calculated as hydrogen peroxide. Not more than 12.6 mL of 0.002 N sodium thiosulfate is required (0.018%).
Sulfur dioxide—Mix 20 g with 200 mL of water to obtain a smooth suspension, and filter. To 100 mL of the clear filtrate add 3 mL of starch TS, and titrate with 0.01 N iodine VS to the first permanent blue color: not more than 2.7 mL is consumed (0.008%).

Stavudine

$C_{10}H_{12}N_2O_4$ 224.21
Thymidine, 2′,3′-didehydro-3′-deoxy-.
1-(2,3-Dideoxy-β-D-*glycero*-pent-2-enofuranosyl)thymine   [3056-17-5].

» Stavudine contains not less than 98.0 percent and not more than 102.0 percent of $C_{10}H_{12}N_2O_4$, calculated on an anhydrous and solvent-free basis.

Packaging and storage—Preserve in tight containers, protected from light and humidity. Store at 25°, excursions permitted between 15° and 30°.

USP Reference standards ⟨11⟩—*USP Stavudine RS. USP Stavudine System Suitability Mixture RS.*
Identification—
  A: *Infrared Absorption* ⟨197K⟩.
  B: The retention time of the major peak in the chromatogram of the *Assay preparation* corresponds to that in the chromatogram of the *Standard preparation*, as obtained in the *Assay*.
Specific rotation ⟨781⟩: between −45° and −40°, calculated on the anhydrous basis, determined in a solution in water containing 10 mg per mL.
Water, *Method 1* ⟨921⟩: not more than 0.5%.
Residue on ignition ⟨281⟩: not more than 0.3%.
Heavy metals, *Method I* ⟨231⟩: 0.002%.
Related compounds—[NOTE—All testing solutions must be prepared immediately prior to use and remain refrigerated until use.]
  0.01 M Ammonium acetate—Prepare as directed in the *Assay*.
  Solution A—Prepare a filtered and degassed mixture of *0.01 M Ammonium acetate* and acetonitrile (96.5 : 3.5).
  Solution B—Prepare a filtered and degassed mixture of *0.01 M Ammonium acetate* and acetonitrile (75 : 25).
  Mobile phase—Use variable mixtures of *Solution A* and *Solution B* as directed for *Chromatographic system*. Make adjustments if necessary (see *System Suitability* under *Chromatography* ⟨621⟩).
  System suitability solution—Prepare a 0.50 mg per mL solution of USP Stavudine System Suitability Mixture RS in water.
  Test solution—Prepare a solution of Stavudine, accurately weighed, in water, and having a concentration of about 0.5 mg per mL.
  Chromatographic system (see *Chromatography* ⟨621⟩)—The liquid chromatograph is equipped with a 254-nm detector and a 4.6-mm × 25-cm column that contains 5-μm packing L1. The flow rate is about 2.1 mL per minute. The chromatograph is programmed as follows.

Time (minutes)	Solution A (%)	Solution B (%)	Elution
0	100	0	equilibration
0–10	100	0	isocratic
10–20	100→0	0→100	linear gradient
20–30	0	100	isocratic
30–35	0→100	100→0	linear gradient
35–40	100	0	re-equilibration

Chromatograph the *System suitability solution*, and record the peak responses as directed for *Procedure:* the retention time of the main stavudine peak is 10.5 ± 2 minutes; the relative retention times are about 1.0 for stavudine and 0.28 for thymine; the resolution, *R*, between thymidine epimer and thymidine is greater than or equal to 1.15, and that between stavudine and α-stavudine is greater than or equal to 1.0; the capacity factor, *k′*, is greater than 4; and the column efficiency is greater than 9500 theoretical plates.

  Procedure—Inject equal volumes (about 10 μL) of the *System suitability solution* and the *Test solution* into the chromatograph, record the chromatograms for twice the retention time of the major peak, or at least until the last impurity has eluted, and measure the area of the responses for all the peaks. Determine the percentage of thymine in the portion of Stavudine taken by the formula:

$$(100)(F)(r_U / r_s)$$

in which *F* is the relative response factor and is equal to 0.69; r_U is the peak response of thymine obtained from the *Test solution;* and r_s is the sum of the responses of all the related peaks in the chromatogram of the *Test solution,* including that of the main stavudine peak: not more than 0.5% of thymine is found. Calculate the percentage of all other impurities in the portion of Stavudine taken by the formula:

$$100(r_U / r_s)$$

in which r_U is the peak area response of each impurity obtained from the *Test solution;* and r_s is the sum of the area responses of all the related peaks in the chromatogram of the *Test solution,* including that of the main stavudine peak and disregarding any peak observed in the blank: not more than 0.1% of any impurity is found; and not more than 1.0% of total impurities is found, including thymine. The quantitation limit is 0.03% of the total sample related peak areas.

Assay—[NOTE—All testing solutions must be prepared immediately prior to use and remain refrigerated until use.]
  0.01 M Ammonium acetate—Dissolve 0.77 g of ammonium acetate in about 900 mL of water in a 1000-mL volumetric flask. Dilute with water to volume, and mix.
  Mobile phase—Prepare a filtered and degassed mixture of *0.01 M Ammonium acetate* and acetonitrile (95 : 5).
  Standard preparation—Transfer about 10 mg of USP Stavudine RS, accurately weighed, to a 100-mL volumetric flask, and dissolve in and dilute with water to volume. Pipet 10.0 mL of this solution into a 50-mL volumetric flask, dilute with water to volume, and mix.
  Assay preparation—Transfer about 10 mg of the Stavudine to a 100-mL volumetric flask, dissolve in and dilute with water to volume, and mix. Pipet 10.0 mL of this solution into a 50-mL volumetric flask, dilute with water to volume, and mix.
  Chromatographic system (see *Chromatography* ⟨621⟩)—The liquid chromatograph is equipped with a 254-nm detector and a 4.6-mm × 3.3-cm column that contains 3-μm packing L1. The flow rate is about 0.7 mL per minute. Chromatograph the *Standard preparation,* and record the peak responses as directed for *Procedure:* the retention time of the stavudine peak is between 2.8 and 5.0 minutes; the column efficiency is not less than 800 theoretical plates; the tailing factor is less than or equal to 1.6; and the relative standard deviation for replicate injections is not more than 2.0%.
  Procedure—Separately inject equal volumes (about 25 μL) of the *Standard preparation* and the *Assay preparation* into the chromatograph, record the chromatograms, and measure the responses for the major peaks. Calculate the quantity, in mg, of $C_{10}H_{12}N_2O_4$ in the portion of Stavudine taken by the formula:

$$500C(r_U / r_s)$$

in which *C* is the concentration, in mg per mL, of USP Stavudine RS in the *Standard preparation;* and r_U and r_s are the peak responses obtained from the *Assay preparation* and the *Standard preparation*, respectively.

Stavudine Capsules

» Stavudine Capsules contain not less than 90.0 percent and not more than 105.0 percent of the labeled amount of stavudine ($C_{10}H_{12}N_2O_4$).

Packaging and storage—Preserve in tightly closed containers, and store at controlled room temperature.

USP Reference standards ⟨11⟩—USP Stavudine RS.
Identification—
  A: *Thin-Layer Chromatographic Identification Test* ⟨201⟩—
    Test solution—Using sonication, dissolve a portion of Capsule contents in enough water to obtain a solution having a concentration of 0.2 mg of stavudine per mL, filter, and mix. Use the filtrate as the *Test solution*.
    Application volume: 10 µL, applied in two 5-µL portions.
    Developing solvent system: a mixture of chloroform, alcohol, and water (100 : 50 : 2).
    Procedure—Proceed as directed in the chapter. Allow the spots to dry, and develop the chromatogram in the *Developing solvent system* until the solvent front has moved about 10 cm from the origin. Remove the plate from the developing chamber, mark the solvent front, and allow to air dry for 5 to 10 minutes.
  B: The retention time of the major peak in the chromatogram of the *Assay preparation* corresponds to that in the chromatogram of the *Standard preparation,* as obtained in the *Assay.*
Specific rotation ⟨781S⟩: between –40° and –45°, determined in a solution in water containing 10 mg of stavudine per mL. Disperse a sufficient quantity of Capsule content, equivalent to 200 mg of stavudine, in 50 mL of acetone. Bring to a boil, and pass through a fine-porosity filter. Precipitate the stavudine with 150 mL of heptane, filter the crystals, wash with heptane, and dry in air.
Dissolution ⟨711⟩—
  Medium: water; 900 mL.
  Apparatus 2: 75 rpm.
  Time: 30 minutes.
  Determine the amount of $C_{10}H_{12}N_2O_4$ dissolved by employing the following method.
  0.01 M Ammonium acetate and *Mobile phase*—Prepare as directed in the *Assay*.
  Standard solution—Dissolve an accurately weighed quantity of USP Stavudine RS in water, and dilute quantitatively, and stepwise if necessary, with water to obtain a solution having a known concentration corresponding to that of the solution under test.
  Chromatographic system (see *Chromatography* ⟨621⟩)—Proceed as directed in the *Assay* except that the liquid chromatograph is equipped with a 254-nm detector. Chromatograph the *Standard solution,* and record the peak responses as directed for *Procedure:* the column efficiency is not less than 800 theoretical plates; the tailing factor is not more than 2; and the relative standard deviation for replicate injections is not more than 2.0%.
  Procedure—Determine the amount of $C_{10}H_{12}N_2O_4$ dissolved, employing the procedure set forth in the *Assay,* making any necessary modifications. The injection volume is about 10 µL.
  Tolerances—Not less than 80% *(Q)* of the labeled amount of $C_{10}H_{12}N_2O_4$ is dissolved in 30 minutes.
Uniformity of dosage units ⟨905⟩: meet the requirements.
Water, *Method I* ⟨921⟩: not more than 3.5%.
Related compounds—
  0.01 M Ammonium acetate and *Mobile phase*—Prepare as directed in the *Assay*.
  Resolution solution—Proceed as directed in the *Assay*.
  Standard solution—Using sonication, dissolve an accurately weighed quantity of thymine in water, and dilute quantitatively, and stepwise if necessary, with water, to obtain a solution having a known concentration of about 1 µg per mL.
  Test solution—Use the *Assay preparation*.
  Chromatographic system—Proceed as directed in the *Assay*. The relative standard deviation for replicate injections of the *Standard solution* is not more than 3.0%.
  Procedure—Proceed as directed in the *Assay,* recording the chromatograms for a period of time that is 2.5 times the retention time of stavudine, and measure the responses of all the peaks. Calculate the quantity of thymine in each Capsule taken by the formula:

$$(CVD/N)(r_U / r_S)$$

in which *C* is the concentration, in mg per mL, of the *Standard solution; V* is the volume, in mL, used to prepare the *Test solution; D* is the dilution factor of the *Test solution; N* is the number of Capsules taken to prepare the *Test solution;* and r_U and r_S are the peak responses obtained from the *Test solution* and the *Standard solution,* respectively. Not more than 1.0% of thymine is found. Calculate the percentage of unknown impurities, not including thymine, in the portion of Capsules taken by the formula:

$$100(r_i / r_s)$$

in which r_i is the peak response for each impurity; and r_s is the sum of the responses of all the peaks: not more than 0.2% of any individual impurity is found; and not more than 2.0% of total impurities, including thymine, is found. The quantitation limit is 0.05% of the total sample related peak response.
Assay—[NOTE—All solutions must be prepared immediately prior to use and remain refrigerated until use.]
  0.01 M Ammonium acetate—Dissolve 0.77 g of ammonium acetate in about 900 mL of water in a 1000-mL volumetric flask. Dilute with water to volume, and mix.
  Mobile phase—Prepare a filtered and degassed mixture of *0.01 M Ammonium acetate* and acetonitrile (95 : 5).
  Resolution solution—Dissolve accurately weighed quantities of thymine and thymidine in water, and dilute quantitatively, and stepwise if necessary, with water to obtain a solution having a known concentration of 0.1 µg of each component per mL.
  Standard preparation—Using sonication, dissolve an accurately weighed quantity of USP Stavudine RS in water, and dilute quantitatively, and stepwise if necessary, with water to obtain a solution having a concentration of about 0.1 mg per mL.
  Assay preparation—Open not fewer than 3 Capsules, and dissolve the contents quantitatively in water. Dilute quantitatively, and stepwise if necessary, with water to obtain a solution having a concentration of about 0.1 mg of stavudine per mL.
  Chromatographic system (see *Chromatography* ⟨621⟩)—The liquid chromatograph is equipped with a 268-nm detector and a 4.6-mm × 3.3-cm column that contains packing L1. The flow rate is about 0.7 mL per minute. Chromatograph the *Resolution solution,* and record the peak responses as directed for *Procedure:* the resolution, *R,* between thymine and thymidine is not less than 2.0, and thymine is resolved from the void volume. Chromatograph the *Standard preparation,* and record the peak responses as directed for *Procedure:* the retention time for the stavudine peak is between 2.8 and 5.0 minutes; the column efficiency is not less than 800 theoretical plates; the tailing factor is not more than 1.8; and the relative standard deviation for replicate injections is not more than 2.0%.
  Procedure—Separately inject equal volumes (about 20 µL) of the *Standard preparation* and the *Assay preparation* into the chromatograph, record the chromatograms, and measure the responses for the major peaks. Calculate the quantity, in mg, of stavudine ($C_{10}H_{12}N_2O_4$) in each Capsule taken by the formula:

$$C(V/N)(r_U / r_S)$$

in which *C* is the concentration, in mg per mL, of USP Stavudine RS in the *Standard preparation; V* is the volume, in mL, used to prepare the *Assay preparation; N* is the number of Capsules taken to prepare the *Assay preparation;* and r_U and r_S are the peak responses obtained from the *Assay preparation* and the *Standard preparation,* respectively.

Stavudine for Oral Solution

» Stavudine for Oral Solution, when reconstituted as directed in the labeling, yields a 1 mg per mL solution that contains not less than 90.0 percent and not more than 110.0 percent of the labeled amount of stavudine ($C_{10}H_{12}N_2O_4$). It may contain suitable flavors, preservatives, sweeteners, and stabilizers.

Packaging and storage—Preserve in tightly closed containers, protected from excessive moisture. Store at controlled room temperature. After constitution, store the Stavudine for Oral Solution in tightly closed containers under refrigeration. Discard unused portion after 30 days.
Labeling—The label contains directions for constitution of the powder and states the equivalent amount of $C_{10}H_{12}N_2O_4$ in a given

volume of the Stavudine for Oral Solution obtained after constitution.

USP Reference standards ⟨11⟩—USP Stavudine RS.
Identification—The retention time of the major peak in the chromatogram of the *Assay preparation* corresponds to that in the chromatogram of the *Standard preparation*, as obtained in the *Assay*.
Deliverable volume ⟨698⟩: meets the requirements.
pH ⟨791⟩: between 5 and 7 when constituted as directed in the labeling.
Water, *Method I* ⟨921⟩: not more than 2.0%.
Related compounds—[NOTE—All testing solutions must be prepared immediately prior to use and remain refrigerated until use.]
Solution A, Solution B, Resolution solution, and *Chromatographic system*—Proceed as directed in the *Assay*.
Standard solution—Prepare as directed for *Standard preparation* in the *Assay*.
Test solution—Prepare as directed for *Assay preparation*.
Procedure—Noting the retention times of the impurities relative to that of stavudine, calculate the percentage of all other impurities in the portion of Stavudine for Oral Solution taken by the formula:

$$100(Fr_i / r_s)$$

in which F is the relative response factor and is equal to 0.69 for thymine (relative retention time of about 0.24) and equal to 1.0 for all other peaks; r_i is the peak area response of each impurity obtained from the *Test solution;* and r_s is the sum of the area responses of all the sample-related peaks in the chromatogram including that of the main stavudine peak: not more than 1.0% of thymine is found, not more than 0.2% of any other individual impurity is found, and not more than 1.5% of total impurities if found.
Assay—[NOTE—All testing solutions must be prepared immediately prior to use and remain refrigerated until use.]
25 mM Ammonium acetate—Dissolve 1.93 g of ammonium acetate in about 900 mL of water in a 1000-mL volumetric flask. Dilute with water to volume, and mix.
Solution A—Prepare a filtered and degassed mixture of *25 mM Ammonium acetate* and methanol (94 : 6).
Solution B—Prepare a filtered and degassed mixture of *25 mM Ammonium acetate* and methanol (1 : 1).
Resolution solution—Prepare a solution in water of thymidine and thymine containing 2.5 µg of each per mL.
Standard preparation—Prepare a solution of USP Stavudine RS in water having a concentration of 0.1 mg per mL.
Assay preparation—Transfer to a suitable volumetric flask an accurately measured volume of Stavudine for Oral Solution, constituted as directed in the labeling, and dilute quantitatively, and stepwise if necessary, with water to obtain a solution having a concentration of 0.1 mg of stavudine per mL.
Chromatographic system (see *Chromatography* ⟨621⟩)—The liquid chromatograph is equipped with a 268-nm detector and a 4.6-mm × 3.3-cm column that contains packing L1 and a 4-mm × 20-mm guard column (L1). The flow rate is about 1 mL per minute. The chromatograph is programmed as follows.

Time (minutes)	Solution A (%)	Solution B (%)	Elution
0	100	0	equilibration
0–12	100	0	isocratic
12.1	100→0	0→100	step gradient
12.1–17	0	100	isocratic
17.1	0→100	100→0	step gradient
17.1–35	100	0	re-equilibration

Chromatograph the *Resolution solution,* and record the peak responses as directed for *Procedure:* the resolution, *R*, between thymine and thymidine is not less than 8.4. Chromatograph the *Standard preparation,* and record the peak responses as directed for *Procedure:* the column efficiency is not less than 2000 theoretical plates; the tailing factor for the stavudine peak is not more than 2; and the relative standard deviation for replicate injections is not more than 2.0%.

Procedure—Separately inject equal volumes (about 20 µL) of the *Standard preparation* and the *Assay preparation* into the chromatograph, record the chromatograms, and measure the areas for the major peaks. Calculate the quantity, in mg, of stavudine ($C_{10}H_{12}N_2O_4$) in each mL of Stavudine for Oral Solution taken by the formula:

$$(L/D)(C)(r_U / r_S)$$

in which L is the labeled quantity, in mg, of stavudine ($C_{10}H_{12}N_2O_4$) in each mL of the Stavudine for Oral Solution; D is the concentration, in mg of stavudine per mL of the *Assay preparation*, based on the labeled quantity of stavudine in the portion of Stavudine for Oral Solution taken; C is the concentration, in mg per mL, of USP Stavudine RS in the *Standard preparation;* and r_U and r_S are the peak area responses obtained from the *Assay preparation* and the *Standard preparation,* respectively.

Storax

» Storax is a balsam obtained from the trunk of *Liquidambar orientalis* Miller, known in commerce as Levant Storax, or of *Liquidambar styraciflua* Linné, known in commerce as American Storax (Fam. Hamamelidaceae).

Packaging and storage—Preserve in well-closed containers.
Loss on drying ⟨731⟩—Dry about 2 g, accurately weighed, at 105° for 2 hours: it loses not more than 20.0% of its weight.
Alcohol-insoluble substances—Accurately weigh about 10 g of mixed Storax in a beaker, heat at 105° for 30 minutes, take up the residue in 100 mL of hot alcohol, filter through counter-balanced filters or a tared filter crucible, and wash the residue with small portions of hot alcohol until the last washing is colorless or practically so: the weight of the residue so obtained, after drying at 105° for 1 hour, does not exceed 5.0% of the weight of Storax taken.
Alcohol-soluble substances—Evaporate the combined alcohol filtrate and washings obtained in the test for *Alcohol-insoluble substances* at a temperature not exceeding 60°, and dry the residue at 105° for 1 hour: the weight of the yellow to brown residue of purified Storax so obtained is not less than 70.0% of the weight of the Storax taken.
Acid value, Saponification value, Cinnamic acid—The purified Storax obtained in the test for *Alcohol-soluble substances* meets the requirements of the following tests.
Acid value ⟨401⟩—Dissolve about 1 g of the purified Storax, accurately weighed, in 50 mL of neutralized alcohol, add 0.5 mL of phenolphthalein TS, and titrate with 0.5 N sodium hydroxide VS: the acid value is between 50 and 85 for Levant Storax and between 36 and 85 for American Storax.
Saponification value ⟨401⟩—Place about 2 g of the purified Storax, accurately weighed, in a 250-mL flask, mix it with 50 mL of solvent hexane, add 25.0 mL of 0.5 N alcoholic potassium hydroxide VS, and allow the mixture to stand for 24 hours with frequent agitation. Then add 0.5 mL of phenolphthalein TS, and titrate the excess alkali with 0.5 N hydrochloric acid VS: the saponification value thus determined is between 160 and 200.
Cinnamic acid—Add about 2 g of the purified Storax, accurately weighed, to 25 mL of 0.5 N alcoholic potassium hydroxide, and boil the mixture for 1 hour under a reflux condenser. Add 0.5 mL of phenolphthalein TS, neutralize with 0.5 N sulfuric acid, and evaporate the alcohol on a steam bath. Dissolve the residue in 50 mL of water, and shake the solution with 20 mL of ether. Shake the separated ether with 5 mL of water, adding the washing to the water solution, and reject the ether extract. Add to the water solution 10 mL of diluted sulfuric acid, and shake with four 20-mL portions of ether. Wash the combined ether extracts with 5 mL of water, rejecting the water washing, transfer to a flask, and distill off the ether. Add to the residue 100 mL of water, and boil the mixture vigorously for 15 minutes under a reflux condenser. Filter while hot, and allow the filtrate to cool to about 25°: white crystals of cinnamic acid separate. Collect and dry the cinnamic acid by vacuum filtration. Repeat the extraction of the residue twice by

boiling each time under a reflux condenser, as previously described, with the filtrate from the preceding crystallization, and collect the additional cinnamic acid in the same crucible. Finally wash the cinnamic acid with two 10-mL portions of ice-cold water, dry at 80°, and weigh. The weight of the cinnamic acid so obtained is not less than 25.0% of the weight of purified Storax taken. A portion of the acid recrystallized from hot water melts between 134° and 135°.

To about 50 mg of the cinnamic acid obtained as directed above add 5 mL of 2 N sulfuric acid, heat, and add potassium permanganate TS: the odor of benzaldehyde is perceptible.

Organic volatile impurities, *Method IV* ⟨467⟩: meets the requirements.

(Official until July 1, 2008)

Streptomycin Sulfate

$(C_{21}H_{39}N_7O_{12})_2 \cdot 3H_2SO_4$ 1457.41

D-Streptamine, *O*-2-deoxy-2-(methylamino)-α-L-glucopyranosyl-(1→2)-*O*-5-deoxy-3-*C*-formyl-α-L-lyxofuranosyl-(1→4)-*N,N'*-bis(aminoiminomethyl)-, sulfate (2 : 3) (salt).
Streptomycin sulfate (2 : 3) (salt)   [3810-74-0].

» Streptomycin Sulfate has a potency equivalent to not less than 650 μg and not more than 850 μg of streptomycin ($C_{21}H_{39}N_7O_{12}$) per mg.

Packaging and storage—Preserve in tight containers.
Labeling—Where it is intended for use in preparing injectable dosage forms, the label states that it is sterile or must be subjected to further processing during the preparation of injectable dosage forms.
USP Reference standards ⟨11⟩—*USP Endotoxin RS. USP Streptomycin Sulfate RS.*
Identification—
  A: Dissolve 5 g of ferric chloride in 50 mL of 0.1 N hydrochloric acid. Transfer 2.5 mL of this stock solution to a 100-mL volumetric flask, dilute with 0.01 N hydrochloric acid to volume, and mix. Prepare *Iron reagent* at the time of use. Dissolve the specimen in water, and dilute with water to obtain a solution containing about 1 mg of streptomycin per mL. To 5 mL of this solution add 2.0 mL of 1 N sodium hydroxide, and heat in a water bath for 10 minutes. Cool in ice water for 3 minutes, then add 2.0 mL of 1.2 N hydrochloric acid, and mix. Add 5 mL of *Iron reagent*, and mix: a violet color is produced.
  B: It responds to the tests for *Sulfate* ⟨191⟩.
pH ⟨791⟩: between 4.5 and 7.0, in a solution containing 200 mg of streptomycin per mL.
Loss on drying ⟨731⟩—Dry about 100 mg, accurately weighed, in a capillary-stoppered bottle in vacuum at a pressure not exceeding 5 mm of mercury at 60° for 3 hours: it loses not more than 5.0% of its weight.
Other requirements—Where the label states that Streptomycin Sulfate is sterile, it meets the requirements for *Sterility Tests* and *Bacterial endotoxins* under *Streptomycin for Injection*. Where the label states that Streptomycin Sulfate must be subjected to further processing during the preparation of injectable dosage forms, it meets the requirements for *Bacterial endotoxins* under *Streptomycin for Injection*. It meets also the requirements for *Uniformity of Dosage Units* ⟨905⟩ and *Labeling* under *Injections* ⟨1⟩.
Assay—
  Mobile phase—Use 70 mM sodium hydroxide. During use, store in a plastic bottle flushed with a blanket of helium above the liquid surface. Make adjustments if necessary (see *System Suitability* under *Chromatography* ⟨621⟩).
  Standard preparation—Dissolve an accurately weighed quantity of USP Streptomycin Sulfate RS in water, and quantitatively dilute with water to obtain a solution having a known concentration of about 0.03 mg per mL. Sonicate for 1 minute, and mix.
  Assay preparation—Transfer about 30 mg of Streptomycin Sulfate, accurately weighed, to a 100-mL volumetric flask, dilute with water to volume, sonicate for 1 minute, and mix. Transfer 10.0 mL of this solution to a second 100-mL volumetric flask, dilute with water to volume, and mix.
  System suitability solution—Heat about 10 mL of the *Standard preparation* at 75° for 1 hour. Allow to cool.
  Chromatographic system (see *Chromatography* ⟨621⟩)—The liquid chromatograph is equipped with an electrochemical detector, a gold working electrode, a pH silver–silver chloride reference electrode, a 4-mm × 5-cm guard column that contains packing L46, and a 4-mm × 25-cm analytical column that contains packing L46. The electrochemical detector is used in the integrated amperometric mode with a range of 300 nC, an output of 1 V full scale, and a rise time of 0.5 second, positive polarity. The potential is programmed as follows.

Step	Time (seconds)	Potential (V)	Integration
1	0.00	+0.1	
2	0.20	+0.1	begins
3	0.40	+0.1	ends
4	0.41	−2.0	
5	0.42	−2.0	
6	0.43	+0.6	
7	0.44	−0.1	
8	0.50	−0.1	

The flow rate is about 0.5 mL per minute. Chromatograph the *System suitability solution*, and measure the peak areas as directed for *Procedure*: the relative retention times are about 0.5 for the main degradation product and 1.0 for streptomycin; and the resolution, *R*, between the two peaks is not less than 3. Chromatograph the *Standard preparation*, and measure the peak areas as directed for *Procedure*: the tailing factor is not more than 2; the column efficiency is not less than 1000 theoretical plates; and the relative standard deviation for replicate injections is not more than 5%. [NOTE—If variation of retention time or increase of tailing occurs, clean the columns with 0.2 M sodium hydroxide. Carefully maintain the working and reference electrodes.]
  Procedure—Separately inject equal volumes (about 20 μL) of the *Standard preparation* and the *Assay preparation* into the chromatograph, record the chromatograms, and measure the areas for the major peaks. Calculate the quantity, in μg, of streptomycin ($C_{21}H_{39}N_7O_{12}$) in each mg of Streptomycin Sulfate taken by the formula:

$$1000(CP/W_U)(r_U / r_S)$$

in which *C* is the concentration, in mg per mL, of USP Streptomycin Sulfate RS in the *Standard preparation*; *P* is the designated streptomycin content, in μg per mg, of streptomycin ($C_{21}H_{39}N_7O_{12}$) in USP Streptomycin Sulfate RS; W_U is the weight, in mg, of Streptomycin Sulfate taken to prepare the *Assay preparation;* and r_U and r_S are the streptomycin peak areas obtained from the *Assay preparation* and the *Standard preparation*, respectively.

Streptomycin Injection

» Streptomycin Injection contains an amount of Streptomycin Sulfate equivalent to not less than 90.0 percent and not more than 115.0 percent of the labeled amount of streptomycin ($C_{21}H_{39}N_7O_{12}$).

Packaging and storage—Preserve in single-dose or in multiple-dose containers, preferably of Type I glass.
USP Reference standards ⟨11⟩—*USP Endotoxin RS. USP Streptomycin Sulfate RS.*
Bacterial endotoxins ⟨85⟩—It contains not more than 0.25 USP Endotoxin Unit per mg of streptomycin.
pH ⟨791⟩: between 5.0 and 8.0.
Other requirements—It responds to *Identification* test A and meets the requirements for *Sterility* under *Streptomycin for Injection*. It meets also the requirements under *Injections* ⟨1⟩.
Assay—
  Mobile phase, Standard preparation, System suitability solution, and *Chromatographic system*—Proceed as directed in the *Assay* under *Streptomycin Sulfate.*
  Assay preparation—Transfer an accurately measured volume of Injection, equivalent to about 500 mg of streptomycin, to a 500-mL volumetric flask, dilute with water to volume, and mix. Transfer 5.0 mL of this solution to a 200-mL volumetric flask, dilute with water to volume, and mix.
  Procedure—Proceed as directed in the *Assay* under *Streptomycin Sulfate*. Calculate the quantity, in mg, of streptomycin ($C_{21}H_{39}N_7O_{12}$) in each mL of the Injection taken by the formula:

$$20(CP/V)(r_U / r_S)$$

in which V is the volume, in mL, of Injection taken to prepare the *Assay preparation;* and the other terms are as defined therein.

Streptomycin for Injection

» Streptomycin for Injection contains an amount of Streptomycin Sulfate equivalent to not less than 90.0 percent and not more than 115.0 percent of the labeled amount of streptomycin ($C_{21}H_{39}N_7O_{12}$).

Packaging and storage—Preserve in *Containers for Sterile Solids* as described under *Injections* ⟨1⟩.
USP Reference standards ⟨11⟩—*USP Streptomycin Sulfate RS. USP Endotoxin RS.*
Constituted solution—At the time of use, it meets the requirements for *Constituted Solutions* under *Injections* ⟨1⟩.
Identification—
  A: Dissolve 5 g of ferric chloride in 50 mL of 0.1 N hydrochloric acid. Transfer 2.5 mL of this stock solution to a 100-mL volumetric flask, dilute with 0.01 N hydrochloric acid to volume, and mix. Prepare *Iron reagent* at the time of use. Dissolve the specimen in water, and dilute with water to obtain a solution containing about 1 mg of streptomycin per mL. To 5 mL of this solution add 2.0 mL of 1 N sodium hydroxide, and heat in a water bath for 10 minutes. Cool in ice water for 3 minutes, then add 2.0 mL of 1.2 N hydrochloric acid, and mix. Add 5 mL of *Iron reagent*, and mix: a violet color is produced.
  B: It responds to the tests for *Sulfate* ⟨191⟩.
Bacterial endotoxins ⟨85⟩—It contains not more than 0.25 USP Endotoxin Unit per mg of streptomycin.
Sterility ⟨71⟩—It meets the requirements when tested as directed for *Membrane Filtration* under *Test for Sterility of the Product to be Examined.*
pH ⟨791⟩: between 4.5 and 7.0, in a solution containing 200 mg of streptomycin per mL.
Loss on drying ⟨731⟩—Dry about 100 mg, accurately weighed, in a capillary-stoppered bottle in vacuum at a pressure not exceeding 5 mm of mercury at 60° for 3 hours: it loses not more than 5.0% of its weight.
Other requirements—It meets the requirements for *Uniformity of Dosage Units* ⟨905⟩ and *Labeling* under *Injections* ⟨1⟩.
Assay—
  Mobile phase, Standard preparation, System suitability solution, and *Chromatographic system*—Proceed as directed in the *Assay* under *Streptomycin Sulfate.*
  Assay preparation 1 (where it is represented as being in a single-dose container)—Constitute Streptomycin for Injection in a volume of water, accurately measured, corresponding to the volume of solvent specified in the labeling. Withdraw all of the withdrawable contents, using a suitable hypodermic needle and syringe, and dilute quantitatively, and stepwise if necessary, with water to obtain a solution containing about 0.025 mg of streptomycin per mL.
  Assay preparation 2 (where the label states the quantity of streptomycin in a given volume of constituted solution)—Constitute Streptomycin for Injection in a volume of water, accurately measured, corresponding to the volume of solvent specified in the labeling. Dilute an accurately measured volume of the constituted solution quantitatively, and stepwise if necessary, with water to obtain a solution containing about 0.025 mg of streptomycin per mL.
  Procedure—Proceed as directed in the *Assay* under *Streptomycin Sulfate*. Calculate the quantity, in mg, of streptomycin ($C_{21}H_{39}N_7O_{12}$) withdrawn from the container, or in the portion of constituted solution taken by the formula:

$$(CP/1000)(L/D)(r_U / r_S)$$

in which L is the labeled quantity, in mg, of streptomycin ($C_{21}H_{39}N_7O_{12}$) in the container, or in the volume of constituted solution taken; D is the concentration, in mg of streptomycin per mL, of *Assay preparation 1* or *Assay preparation 2*, based on the labeled quantity in the container, or in the volume of constituted solution taken, respectively; and the other terms are as defined therein.

Strontium Chloride Sr 89 Injection

$^{89}SrCl_2$ 159.9
Strontium chloride ($^{89}SrCl_2$) [38270-90-5].

» Strontium Chloride Sr 89 Injection is a sterile solution of radioactive strontium (^{89}Sr) processed in the form of strontium chloride in Water for Injection. Strontium Chloride Sr 89 Injection contains not less than 90.0 percent and not more than 110.0 percent of the labeled amount of ^{89}Sr as strontium chloride expressed in megabecquerels per mL (or in millicuries per mL) at the time indicated in the labeling. The strontium chloride content is not less than 90.0 percent and not more than 110.0 percent of the labeled amount.

Specific activity: not less than 2.96 MBq (80 µCi) per mg of strontium at the time indicated in the labeling.
Packaging and storage—Preserve in single-dose containers that are adequately shielded.
Labeling—Label it to include the following, in addition to the information specified for *Labeling* under *Injections* ⟨1⟩: the time and date of calibration; the amount of strontium chloride expressed as mg of strontium per mL; the amount of ^{89}Sr as labeled strontium chloride expressed as total megabecquerels (or millicuries) and concentration as megabecquerels per mL (or millicuries per mL) on the date and time of calibration; the expiration date; and the statement "Caution—Radioactive Material." The labeling indicates that in making dosage calculations, correction is to be made for radioactive decay, and also indicates that the radioactive half-life of ^{89}Sr is 50.5 days.
USP Reference standards ⟨11⟩—*USP Endotoxin RS.*
Radionuclide identification (see *Radioactivity* ⟨821⟩)—Strontium 89 decays by beta emission to stable Yttrium 89 with 0.01% of disintegrations going via the metastable daughter ^{89m}Y with a half-life

of 16 seconds, with which it rapidly establishes radioactive equilibrium. Its gamma-ray spectrum is identical to that of a specimen of strontium 89 in equilibrium with ^{89m}Y exhibiting bremsstrahlung and a gamma photopeak of 0.909 MeV. [NOTE—Use a plastic container to perform measurements.]

Bacterial endotoxins ⟨85⟩—It meets the requirements, the limit of endotoxin content being not more than 175/V USP Endotoxin Unit per mL of the Injection, when compared with the USP Endotoxin RS, in which V is the maximum recommended total dose, in mL, at the expiration date or time.

pH ⟨791⟩: between 4.0 and 7.5.

Radionuclidic purity—[NOTE—Use a plastic container to perform the following test.] Using a suitable counting assembly (see *Assay, Gamma-Emitting Radionuclides*, under *Radioactivity* ⟨821⟩), determine the radioactivity of each gamma-emitting radionuclidic impurity, in kBq per MBq (or µCi per mCi) of ^{89}Sr, in the Injection by use of a calibrated system as directed under *Radioactivity* ⟨821⟩. The total activity of all gamma-emitting impurities is not greater than 370 kBq per 37 MBq (or 10 µCi per mCi) of ^{89}Sr at the expiration date stated in the labeling.

Chemical purity (Limit of aluminum)—[NOTE—The *Standard preparations* and the *Test preparation* may be modified, if necessary, to obtain solutions of suitable concentrations adaptable to the linear or working range of the instrument.]

Nitric acid diluent—Dilute 40 mL of nitric acid with water to 1000 mL.

Standard preparations—Transfer 2000 mg of aluminum metal to a 1000-mL volumetric flask, add 50 mL of 6 N hydrochloric acid, swirl to ensure contact of the aluminum and the acid, and allow the reaction to proceed until all of the aluminum has dissolved. Dilute with water to volume, and mix. Transfer 5.0 mL of this solution to a 1000-mL volumetric flask, dilute with water to volume, and mix. Transfer 10.0 mL of this solution to a 100-mL volumetric flask, dilute with *Nitric acid diluent* to volume, and mix. Transfer 1.0-, 2.0-, and 4.0-mL portions of this solution to separate 100-mL volumetric flasks, dilute with *Nitric acid diluent* to volume, and mix. These solutions contain 0.01, 0.02, and 0.04 µg of Al per mL, respectively.

Test preparation—Transfer 1.0 mL of Injection to a 100-mL volumetric flask, and carefully add 4 mL of nitric acid. Dilute with water to volume, and mix.

Procedure—Determine the absorbances of the *Standard preparations* and the *Test preparation* at the aluminum emission line at 309.3 nm with an atomic absorption spectrophotometer (see *Spectrophotometry and Light-Scattering* ⟨851⟩) equipped with an aluminum hollow-cathode lamp and a flameless electrically heated furnace, using *Nitric acid diluent* as the blank. Plot the absorbances of the *Standard preparations* versus the contents of Al, in µg per mL, drawing the straight line best fitting the three points. From the graph so obtained, determine the quantity, in µg, of Al in each mL of the *Test preparation*. Calculate the quantity, in µg per g, of Al in the specimen taken by multiplying this value by 100: the limit is 2 µg per g.

Assay for radioactivity—Using a suitable counting assembly (see *Assay, Gamma-Emitting Radionuclides*, under *Radioactivity* ⟨821⟩), determine the radioactivity, in MBq (or mCi) per mL, of the Injection by use of a calibrated system as directed under *Radioactivity* ⟨821⟩.

Other requirements—It meets the requirements under *Injections* ⟨1⟩, except that it is not subject to the recommendation on *Volume in Container*.

Assay—

Potassium chloride solution—Dissolve 1.9 g of potassium chloride in water, dilute with water to 1000 mL, and mix. This solution contains 1000 µg of potassium per mL.

Strontium stock solution—Transfer 1.685 g of strontium carbonate, accurately weighed, to a 100-mL volumetric flask, and add water to dissolve. Add 10 mL of hydrochloric acid, dilute with water to volume, and mix to obtain a solution containing 10,000 µg of strontium per mL.

Standard preparations—Pipet 10 mL of *Strontium stock solution* into a 100-mL volumetric flask. Add 10 mL of hydrochloric acid, dilute with *Potassium chloride solution* to volume, and mix. Transfer 10 mL and 20 mL, respectively, of this solution into separate 100-mL volumetric flasks, dilute with *Potassium chloride solution* to volume, and mix. These *Standard preparations* contain 100 and 200 µg of strontium per mL.

Assay preparation—Pipet 0.1 mL of Injection into a small beaker. Add 5 mL of *Potassium chloride solution*, and mix.

Procedure—Concomitantly determine the absorbances of the *Standard preparations* and the *Assay preparation* at the strontium emission line of 407.8 nm with an atomic absorption spectrophotometer (see *Spectrophotometry and Light-Scattering* ⟨851⟩) equipped with a strontium hollow-cathode lamp and a nitrous oxide–acetylene flame, using *Potassium chloride solution* as the blank. Plot the absorbances of the *Standard preparations* versus concentration, in µg per mL, of strontium, and draw the straight line best fitting the four plotted points. From the graph so obtained, determine the concentration, in µg per mL, of strontium in the *Assay preparation*. Calculate the quantity, in µg, of strontium in each mL of the Injection taken by the formula:

$$51C$$

in which C is the concentration, in µg per mL, of strontium in the *Assay preparation*.

Succinylcholine Chloride

$C_{14}H_{30}Cl_2N_2O_4$(anhydrous)   361.30
Ethanaminium, 2,2'-[(1,4-dioxo-1,4-butanediyl)bis(oxy)]bis[N,N,N-trimethyl]-, dichloride.
Choline chloride succinate (2 : 1)   [71-27-2].
Dihydrate   397.34   [6101-15-1].

» Succinylcholine Chloride usually contains approximately two molecules of water of hydration. It contains not less than 96.0 percent and not more than 102.0 percent of $C_{14}H_{30}Cl_2N_2O_4$, calculated on the anhydrous basis.

Packaging and storage—Preserve in tight containers. Store at 25°, excursions permitted between 15° and 30°.

Labeling—Label it in terms of its anhydrous equivalent. Where it is intended for use in preparing injectable or other sterile dosage forms, the label states that it is sterile or must be subjected to further processing during the preparation of injectable dosage forms.

USP Reference standards ⟨11⟩—*USP Choline Chloride RS. USP Endotoxin RS. USP Succinylcholine Chloride RS. USP Succinylmonocholine Chloride RS.*

Identification—

A: *Infrared Absorption* ⟨197K⟩.

B: The retention time of the major peak in the chromatogram of the *Assay preparation* correspond to that in the chromatogram of the *Standard preparation,* as obtained in the *Assay.*

C: Dissolve a portion in water to obtain a solution containing 1 mg per mL. Applying 1-µL portions to a plate coated with a 0.25-mm layer of chromatographic silica gel (see *Chromatography* ⟨621⟩), and using a solvent system consisting of a mixture of acetone and 1 N hydrochloric acid (1 : 1), proceed as directed under *Thin-Layer Chromatographic Identification Test* ⟨201⟩. Use the following procedure to locate the spots. Heat the plate at 105° for 5 minutes, cool, and spray with potassium bismuth iodide TS, then heat again at 105° for 5 minutes.

Water, Method I ⟨921⟩: not more than 10.0%.
Residue on ignition ⟨281⟩: not more than 0.2%.

Change to read:
Chromatographic purity—
TEST 1—
  Buffer solution—Prepare a solution in water containing 3.85 g per L of 1-pentanesulfonic acid, 2.9 g per L of sodium chloride, and 1% (v/v) of 1 N sulfuric acid.
  Mobile phase—Prepare a filtered and degassed mixture of *Buffer solution* and acetonitrile (95 : 5).
  System suitability solution—Dissolve accurately weighed quantities of citric acid and succinic acid in *Mobile phase* to obtain a solution containing about 0.5 mg of each per mL.
  Standard solution—Dissolve an accurately weighed quantity of USP Succinylmonocholine Chloride RS in *Mobile phase*, and dilute quantitatively, and stepwise if necessary, with *Mobile phase* to obtain a solution having a known concentration of about 0.05 mg per mL.
  Test solution—Transfer about 100 mg of Succinylcholine Chloride, accurately weighed, to a 10-mL volumetric flask, and dissolve in and dilute with *Mobile phase* to volume.
  Chromatographic system (see *Chromatography* ⟨621⟩)—The chromatograph is equipped with a 214-nm detector and a 4.6-mm × 25-cm column that contains 5-μm packing L1. The flow rate is about 1 mL per minute. Samples are maintained at a temperature of about 4° during the analysis. Chromatograph the *System suitability solution*, and record the peak responses as directed for *Procedure*: the resolution, R, between citric acid and succinic acid is not less than 2.9. Chromatograph the *Standard solution*, and record the peak responses as directed for *Procedure*: the relative standard deviation for replicate injections is not more than 3.0%.
  Procedure—Separately inject equal volumes (about 50 μL) of the *Standard solution* and the *Test solution* into the chromatograph, record the chromatograms, and measure the peak responses. Begin integration after the edetate disodium peak, if present (retention time is about 3.5 minutes). The relative retention times are about 0.22 for succinic acid, 0.32 for the doublet of peaks quantitated as a single component, 0.49 for succinylmonocholine chloride, and 1.0 for succinylcholine chloride. Calculate the percentage of each impurity in the portion of Succinylcholine Chloride taken by the formula:

$$10C(r_i / r_S)F$$

in which C is the concentration, in mg per mL, of USP Succinylmonocholine Chloride RS in the *Standard solution*; r_i is the peak area for each impurity obtained from the *Test solution*; r_S is the succinylmonocholine chloride peak area obtained from the *Standard solution*; and F is the response factor (0.63 for succinic acid): not more than 0.1% of succinic acid is found; not more than 0.4% of the doublet of peaks quantitated as a single component is found; not more than 0.4% of succinylmonocholine chloride is found; and not more than 0.2% of any other individual impurity is found.
TEST 2 (LIMIT OF CHOLINE)—
  Solution A—Prepare a solution in water containing 5% (v/v) of acetonitrile and 5% (w/v) of 0.1 M 1-hexanesulfonic acid.
  Solution B—Prepare a solution of acetonitrile and water (1 : 1).
  Mobile phase—Use variable amounts of *Solution A* and *Solution B* as directed for *Chromatographic system*. Make adjustments if necessary (see *System Suitability* under *Chromatography* ⟨621⟩).
  System suitability solution—Dissolve an accurately weighed quantity of USP Choline Chloride RS and sodium chloride in water; and dilute quantitatively, and stepwise if necessary, with water to obtain a solution containing 0.05 mg per mL and 0.01 mg per mL, respectively.
  Standard stock solution—Dissolve an accurately weighed quantity of USP Choline Chloride RS in water; and dilute quantitatively, and stepwise if necessary, with water to obtain a solution containing 0.5 mg per mL.
  Standard solution—Dilute 1 mL of the *Standard stock solution* with water to 50 mL.
  Test solution—Transfer about 50 mg of Succinylcholine Chloride, accurately weighed, to a 25-mL flask, and dissolve in and dilute with water to volume.
  Chromatographic system (see *Chromatography* ⟨621⟩)—The ion chromatograph is equipped with a suitable device for chemical suppression, a conductivity detector at 30 μS, and a 4.6-mm × 25-cm column that contains 5-μm packing L1. ▲The eluent flow rate is about 1 mL per minute, and uses deionized water at a flow rate of 5–10 mL per minute as the regenerant for the chemical suppressor and a suppressor current setting of 50 mA.▲USP31

Time (minutes)	Solution A (%)	Solution B (%)	Elution
0–15	100	0	isocratic
15–16	100→0	0→100	linear gradient
16–25	0	100	isocratic
25–27	0→100	100→0	linear gradient
27–40	100	0	isocratic

Chromatograph the *System suitability solution*, and record the peak responses as directed for *Procedure*: the resolution, R, between sodium and choline is not less than 2.0; and the relative standard deviation for replicate injections is not more than 3.0%.
  Procedure—Separately inject equal volumes (about 50 μL) of the *Standard solution* and the *Test solution* into the chromatograph, record the chromatograms, and measure the peak responses. Calculate the percentage of choline in the portion of Succinylcholine Chloride taken by the formula:

$$37.5C(r_C / r_S)$$

in which C is the concentration, in mg per mL, of USP Choline Chloride RS in the *Standard solution*; and r_C and r_S are the choline peak areas obtained from the *Test solution* and the *Standard solution*, respectively: not more than 0.3% of choline is found; and not more than 1.5% of total impurities is found, the results for *Test 1* and *Test 2* being added.
Chloride content—Dissolve about 400 mg, accurately weighed, in 5 mL of water. Add 5 mL of glacial acetic acid, 50 mL of methanol, and 1 drop of eosin Y TS, and titrate with 0.1 N silver nitrate VS. Each mL of 0.1 N silver nitrate is equivalent to 3.545 mg of Cl. Not less than 19.3% and not more than 19.8% of Cl, calculated on the anhydrous basis, is found.
Other requirements—Where the label states that Succinylcholine Chloride is sterile, it meets the requirements for *Sterility Tests* ⟨71⟩ and for *Bacterial endotoxins* under *Succinylcholine Chloride for Injection*. Where the label states that Succinylcholine Chloride must be subjected to further processing during the preparation of injectable dosage forms, it meets the requirements for *Bacterial endotoxins* under *Succinylcholine Chloride for Injection*.
Assay—[NOTE—Since the *Mobile phase* employed in this procedure has a fairly high concentration of chloride ion and a low pH, it is advisable to rinse the entire system with water following the use of this *Mobile phase*.]
  Mobile phase—Prepare a 1 in 10 solution of 1 N aqueous tetramethylammonium chloride in methanol. Pass this solution through a 0.45-μm membrane filter, and adjust with hydrochloric acid to a pH of about 3.0.
  Standard preparation—Transfer about 88 mg of USP Succinylcholine Chloride RS, accurately weighed, to a 10-mL volumetric flask, add 4.0 mL of water, and dilute with *Mobile phase* to volume while mixing. Prepare the *Standard preparation* concurrently with the *Assay preparation*.
  Assay preparation—Transfer about 88 mg of Succinylcholine Chloride, accurately weighed, to a 10-mL volumetric flask, add 4.0 mL of water, and dilute with *Mobile phase* to volume while mixing.
  Chromatographic system (see *Chromatography* ⟨621⟩)—The liquid chromatograph is equipped with a 214-nm detector and a 4-mm × 25-cm column that contains packing L3. The flow rate is about 0.75 mL per minute. Chromatograph five replicate injections of the *Standard preparation*, and record the peak responses as directed for *Procedure*: the tailing factor is not greater than 2.5; and the relative standard deviation for replicate injections is not more than 1.5%.
  Procedure—Separately inject equal volumes (about 10 μL) of the *Standard preparation* and the *Assay preparation* into the chromatograph by means of a suitable microsyringe or sampling valve, record the chromatograms, and measure the responses for the major

peaks. Calculate the quantity, in mg, of $C_{14}H_{30}Cl_2N_2O_4$ in the Succinylcholine Chloride taken by the formula:

$$10C(r_U/r_S)$$

in which C is the concentration, in mg per mL, of anhydrous succinylcholine chloride in the *Standard preparation,* as determined from the concentration of USP Succinylcholine Chloride RS corrected for moisture content by a titrimetric water determination; r_U is the peak response obtained from the *Assay preparation;* and r_S is the average peak response obtained from the *Standard preparation.*

Succinylcholine Chloride Injection

» Succinylcholine Chloride Injection is a sterile solution of Succinylcholine Chloride in a suitable aqueous vehicle. It contains not less than 90.0 percent and not more than 110.0 percent of the labeled amount of anhydrous succinylcholine chloride ($C_{14}H_{30}Cl_2N_2O_4$).

Packaging and storage—Preserve in single-dose or in multiple-dose containers, preferably of Type I or Type II glass, in a refrigerator.
Labeling—Label it to indicate, as its expiration date, the month and year not more than 2 years from the month during which the Injection was last assayed and released by the manufacturer.
USP Reference standards ⟨11⟩—*USP Endotoxin RS. USP Succinylcholine Chloride RS.*
Identification—It responds to *Identification* tests B and C under *Succinylcholine Chloride.*
Bacterial endotoxins ⟨85⟩—It contains not more than 2.0 USP Endotoxin Units per mg of succinylcholine chloride.
pH ⟨791⟩: between 3.0 and 4.5.
Other requirements—It meets the requirements under *Injections* ⟨1⟩.
Assay—[NOTE—Since the *Mobile phase* employed in this procedure has a fairly high concentration of chloride ion and a low pH, it may be advisable to rinse the entire system with water following the use of this *Mobile phase.*]
  Mobile phase and *Chromatographic system*—Prepare as directed in the *Assay* under *Succinylcholine Chloride.*
  Standard preparation—Transfer about 88 mg of USP Succinylcholine Chloride RS, accurately weighed, to a 10-mL volumetric flask, add a volume of water to correspond to the solvent composition of the *Assay preparation,* and dilute with *Mobile phase* to volume while mixing. Prepare the *Standard preparation* concurrently with the *Assay preparation.*
  Assay preparation—Transfer a volume of Injection, equivalent to about 80 mg of anhydrous succinylcholine chloride, to a 10-mL volumetric flask, and dilute with *Mobile phase* to volume while mixing.
  Procedure—Proceed as directed for *Procedure* in the *Assay* under *Succinylcholine Chloride.* Calculate the quantity, in mg, of anhydrous succinylcholine chloride ($C_{14}H_{30}Cl_2N_2O_4$) in each mL of the Injection taken by the formula:

$$(10C/V)(r_U/r_S)$$

in which V is the volume, in mL, of Injection taken.

Succinylcholine Chloride for Injection

» Succinylcholine Chloride for Injection is Succinylcholine Chloride suitable for parenteral use.

Packaging and storage—Preserve in *Containers for Sterile Solids* as described under *Injections* ⟨1⟩.

USP Reference standards ⟨11⟩—*USP Endotoxin RS. USP Succinylcholine Chloride RS. USP Succinylmonocholine Chloride RS.*
Completeness of solution ⟨641⟩—A 500-mg portion dissolves in 10 mL of carbon dioxide-free water to yield a clear and colorless solution.
Constituted solution—At the time of use, it meets the requirements for *Constituted Solutions* under *Injections* ⟨1⟩.
Bacterial endotoxins ⟨85⟩—It contains not more than 2.0 USP Endotoxin Units per mg of succinylcholine chloride.
Chromatographic purity—
  Standard solution—Transfer 20 mg each of choline chloride and USP Succinylmonocholine Chloride RS, accurately weighed, to a 50-mL volumetric flask, dissolve in 40 mL of methanol, dilute with methanol to volume, and mix.
  Test solution—Prepare, immediately prior to use, a solution of Succinylcholine Chloride in methanol having a concentration of about 50 mg per mL.
  Procedure—Separately apply 2 μL of the *Test solution* and 5 μL of the *Standard solution* to a suitable high-performance 10- × 10-cm thin-layer chromatographic plate (see *Chromatography* ⟨621⟩) coated with a 0.10-mm layer of chromatographic cellulose. Allow the spots to dry, and immediately place the plate, its coated surface toward the nearer wall, in the dry trough of a twin-trough chromatographic chamber whose other trough contains a solvent system consisting of the upper layer of a mixture of butyl alcohol, water, and 96% formic acid (65 : 35 : 15) that has been shaken and allowed to stand for 24 hours until the phases have separated. Equilibrate the chromatographic chamber for 30 minutes, and tilt the chamber to introduce the developing solvent into the trough containing the plate. Develop the chromatogram until the solvent front has moved about three-fourths of the length of the plate, remove the plate from the developing chamber, quickly and thoroughly evaporate the solvent with the aid of a current of air, and dry at 105° for 15 minutes. [NOTE—During the drying, support the plate in such a manner that only the upper and lower edges of the plate, outside the chromatographic zone, are in direct contact with any heated surface.] Spray the plate with potassium iodoplatinate TS, dry at 105° for about 2 minutes, and allow to cool to room temperature: any spots from the *Test solution* are not greater in size or intensity than the spots, occurring at the respective R_F values (approximately 0.6 for succinylmonocholine chloride, and 0.5 for choline chloride), produced by 5 μL of the *Standard solution,* corresponding to 0.8% of each compound. Estimate the size and intensities of any other spots detected by comparison with the spot produced by succinylmonocholine chloride in the *Standard solution.* The total of any such spots detected is not more than 2.0%.

Other requirements—It conforms to the Definition, responds to the *Identification* tests, and meets the requirements for *Water, Residue on ignition, Chloride content,* and *Assay* under *Succinylcholine Chloride.* It meets also the requirements for *Sterility Tests* ⟨71⟩, *Uniformity of Dosage Units* ⟨905⟩, and *Labeling* under *Injections* ⟨1⟩.

Sucralfate

$Al_8(OH)_{16}(C_{12}H_{14}O_{35}S_8)[Al(OH)_3]_x[H_2O]_y$ in which x = 8 to 10, and y = 22 to 31.
α-D-Glucopyranoside, β-D-fructofuranosyl-, octakis(hydrogen sulfate), aluminum complex.
Sucrose octakis(hydrogen sulfate) aluminum complex [54182-58-0].

Sucralfate

» Sucralfate is the hydrous basic aluminum salt of sucrose octasulfate. It contains the equivalent of not less than 30.0 percent and not more than 38.0 percent of sucrose octasulfate ($C_{12}H_{14}O_{35}S_8$).

Packaging and storage—Preserve in tight containers.
USP Reference standards ⟨11⟩—*USP Potassium Sucrose Octasulfate RS.*
Clarity and color of solution—Dissolve 1.0 g in 10 mL of 2 N sulfuric acid: the solution is clear and practically colorless.
Identification—
  A: The retention time of the sucrose octasulfate peak in the chromatogram of the *Assay preparation* corresponds to that in the chromatogram of the *Standard preparation*, as obtained in the Assay.
  B: Add 0.1 N hydrochloric acid to a few g of Sucralfate, boil, and neutralize with 0.1 N sodium hydroxide. Add alkaline cupric tartrate TS. Boil a small amount of this solution: a red precipitate of cuprous oxide is produced.
  C: A solution in 3 N hydrochloric acid meets the requirements of the tests for *Aluminum* ⟨191⟩.
Acid-neutralizing capacity—Transfer about 250 mg, accurately weighed, to a 250-mL screw-capped bottle, add 100.0 mL of 0.1 N hydrochloric acid, previously heated to 37°, cap the bottle, place it in a 37° water bath, and stir the contents continuously for 1 hour. Cool to room temperature, and transfer 20.0 mL to a 100-mL beaker. Add 30 mL of water, and titrate with 0.1 N sodium hydroxide VS to a pH of 3.5. Perform a blank titration on a mixture of water and 0.1 N hydrochloric acid (30 : 20.0). Calculate the mEq of acid consumed per g of Sucralfate taken by the formula:

$$5N(V_B - V_T)/W$$

where N is the exact normality of the sodium hydroxide VS; V_B and V_T are the volumes, in mL, of sodium hydroxide VS consumed by the blank and the test solution, respectively; and W is the weight, in g, of Sucralfate taken: not less than 12 mEq of acid is consumed.
Chloride ⟨221⟩—Transfer 500 mg to a 100-mL volumetric flask, add 30 mL of 2 N nitric acid, dilute with water to volume, and mix. Transfer 10.0 mL of this solution to a 50-mL color comparison tube, add 3 mL of 2 N nitric acid and 2 mL of silver nitrate TS, dilute with water to 50 mL, and mix. Allow to stand, protected from direct sunlight, for 5 minutes. The sample shows no more turbidity than that produced in a solution containing 0.35 mL of 0.020 N hydrochloric acid: not more than 0.50% of chloride is found.
Arsenic, *Method II* ⟨211⟩: 4 ppm.
Heavy metals, *Method II* ⟨231⟩: 0.002%.
Limit of pyridine and 2-methylpyridine—
  Internal standard solution—Transfer 1.0 mL of 3-methylpyridine to a 50-mL volumetric flask, dilute with chloroform to volume, and mix. Transfer 1.0 mL of this solution to a 50-mL volumetric flask, dilute with chloroform to volume, and mix.
  Standard stock solution—Transfer about 0.5 g each of 2-methylpyridine and pyridine to a 50-mL volumetric flask, dissolve in chloroform, dilute with chloroform to volume, and mix. Quantitatively dilute 5.0 mL of this solution with chloroform to 50.0 mL. Transfer 5.0 mL of this solution to a 50.0 mL volumetric flask, dilute with chloroform to volume, and mix.
  Standard solution—Transfer 5.0 mL of *Standard stock solution* to a 20-mL volumetric flask, add 1.0 mL of the *Internal standard solution*, dilute with chloroform to volume, and mix.
  Test solution—Sonicate about 1 g of Sucralfate, accurately weighed, in 10.0 mL of 1 M sodium hydroxide until a uniformly cloudy mixture is obtained. Extract this solution with three 5-mL portions of chloroform, and collect the chloroform extracts in a 20-mL volumetric flask. Add 1.0 mL of the *Internal standard solution*, dilute with chloroform to volume, and mix.
  Chromatographic system (see *Chromatography* ⟨621⟩)—The gas chromatograph is equipped with a flame-ionization detector, a split injection system, and a 0.53-mm × 10-m capillary column coated with a 2.65-μm layer of phase G27. Helium is used as the carrier gas, at a pressure of 36-mm of mercury. The column temperature is maintained at 50°. The injection port temperature and the detector temperature are maintained at 150° and 200°, respectively. Chromatograph the *Standard solution*, and record the peak responses as directed for *Procedure:* the relative retention times of pyridine, 2-methylpyridine, and 3-methylpyridine are about 0.42, 0.72, and 1.0, respectively; the resolution, R, between pyridine and 2-methylpyridine is not less than 3.5; the resolution,R, between 2-methylpyridine and 3-methylpyridine is not less than 2.5; and the relative standard deviation for replicate injections is not more than 2.0%.
  Procedure—Separately inject equal volumes (about 1 μL) of the *Standard solution* and the *Test solution* into the chromatograph, record the chromatograms, and measure the peak responses. Separately calculate the quantities, in μg, of pyridine and 2-methylpyridine, if present, in the portion of Sucralfate taken by the formula:

$$20C(R_U / R_S)$$

in which C is the concentration, in μg per mL, of pyridine or 2-methylpyridine in the*Standard solution;* and R_U and R_S are the peak response ratios of the analyte to the internal standard obtained from the *Test solution* and the*Standard solution*, respectively: not more than 0.05% each of pyridine and 2-methylpyridine is found.
Limit of sucrose heptasulfate—
  Mobile phase—Dissolve 99.1 g of ammonium sulfate in 900 mL of water, dilute with water to 1000 mL, and mix. Adjust with phosphoric acid to a pH of 3.5 ± 0.1, filter, and degas. Make adjustments if necessary (see*System Suitability* under *Chromatography* ⟨621⟩).
  Standard solution—Prepare as directed for the *Standard preparation* in the*Assay.*
  Chromatographic system—Prepare as directed in the *Assay.*
  Test solution—Prepare as directed for *Assay preparation* in the*Assay.*
  Procedure—Inject about 50 μL of the *Test solution* into the chromatograph, record the chromatograms, and measure the responses for the major peaks. The relative retention times are about 0.6 for sucrose heptasulfate and 1.0 for sucrose octasulfate. The ratio of the peak response of the sucrose heptasulfate peak to that of the sucrose octasulfate peak is not more than 0.1.
Aluminum content—Transfer about 1.0 g, accurately weighed, to a 250-mL volumetric flask, add 10 mL of 6.0 N hydrochloric acid, mix, and heat with continuous stirring in a water bath at 70° for 5 minutes. Cool to room temperature, dilute with water to volume, and mix. Filter the solution, discarding the first portion of the filtrate. Transfer 25.0 mL of the filtrate to a 250-mL beaker, add 25.0 mL of 0.05 M edetate disodium VS, add 20 mL of acetic acid-ammonium acetate buffer TS, and mix. Heat in a water bath at 70° for 5 minutes. Cool to room temperature, add 50 mL of alcohol and 2 mL of dithizone TS, and mix. Titrate with 0.05 M zinc sulfate VS to a bright rose-pink color. Perform a blank determination and make any necessary correction. Each mL of 0.05 M edetate disodium consumed is equivalent to 1.349 mg of aluminum: between 15.5% and 18.5% of aluminum is found, calculated on an "as is" basis.
Organic volatile impurities, *Method IV* ⟨467⟩: meets the requirements.

(Official until July 1, 2008)

Assay—
  Mobile phase—Dissolve 132 g of ammonium sulfate in 900 mL of water, dilute with water to 1000 mL, and mix. Adjust with phosphoric acid to a pH of 3.5 ± 0.1, filter, and degas. Make adjustments if necessary (see*System Suitability* under *Chromatography* ⟨621⟩).
  Standard preparation—Dissolve an accurately weighed quantity of USP Potassium Sucrose Octasulfate RS in *Mobile phase*, and dilute quantitatively, and stepwise if necessary, with *Mobile phase* to obtain a solution having a known concentration of about 10 mg of anhydrous potassium sucrose octasulfate (as determined from the concentration of USP Potassium Sucrose Octasulfate RS corrected for water content by a titrimetric water determination) per mL.
  Assay preparation—Transfer about 450 mg of Sucralfate, accurately weighed, to a 35-mL centrifuge tube, and shake at a moderate rate on a vortex mixer. While shaking add 10.0 mL of a mixture of 4.0 N sulfuric acid and 2.2 N sodium hydroxide (1 : 1). Sonicate with swirling for 5 minutes, keeping the temperature of the mixture below 30°. Without delay transfer the tube to a vortex mixer and while shaking at moderate rate, add an accurately measured volume, V, in mL, of 0.1 N sodium hydroxide to bring the pH of the solution to approximately 2, and dilute the solution with

(15.0 − V) mL of water. Shake for 1 minute, and centrifuge for 5 minutes. Separate the clear supernatant layer, and allow it to stand at room temperature until the pH stabilizes. If the pH is not between 2.3 and 3.5, repeat the test using a different volume of 0.1 N sodium hydroxide. Use the clear supernatant layer.

Chromatographic system (see *Chromatography* ⟨621⟩)—The liquid chromatograph is equipped with a refractive index detector and a 3.9-mm × 30-cm column that contains packing L8. The detector and column temperatures are maintained at 30°. The flow rate is about 1 mL per minute. Chromatograph the *Standard preparation*, and record the peak responses as directed for *Procedure*: the column efficiency determined from the sucrose octasulfate peak is not less than 400 theoretical plates; the tailing factor for the sucrose octasulfate peak is not more than 4.0; and the relative standard deviation for replicate injections is not more than 2.0%.

Procedure—Separately inject equal volumes (about 50 μL) of the *Standard preparation* and the *Assay preparation* into the chromatograph, record the chromatograms, and measure the responses for the major peaks. Calculate the quantity, in mg, of sucrose octasulfate ($C_{12}H_{14}O_{35}S_8$) in the portion of Sucralfate taken by the formula:

$$(974.75/1287.53)(25C)(r_U / r_S)$$

in which 974.75 and 1287.53 are the molecular weights of sucrose octasulfate and anhydrous potassium sucrose octasulfate, respectively; *C* is the concentration, in mg per mL, of anhydrous potassium sucrose octasulfate in the *Standard preparation*; and r_U and r_S are the peak responses of sucrose octasulfate obtained from the *Assay preparation* and the *Standard preparation*, respectively.

Sucralfate Tablets

» Sucralfate Tablets contain not less than 90.0 percent and not more than 110.0 percent of the labeled amount of sucralfate ($Al_8(OH)_{16}(C_{12}H_{14}O_{35}S_8)[Al(OH)_3]_x[H_2O]_y$) corresponding to not less than 30.6 percent and not more than 37.4 percent of sucrose octasulfate ($C_{12}H_{14}O_{35}S_8$).

Packaging and storage—Preserve in tight containers.
USP Reference standards ⟨11⟩—*USP Potassium Sucrose Octasulfate RS*.
Identification—
 A: The retention time of the sucrose octasulfate peak in the chromatogram of the *Assay preparation* corresponds to that in the chromatogram of the *Standard preparation*, as obtained in the *Assay*.
 B: Shake a portion of finely powdered Tablets, equivalent to about 1 g of sucralfate, with 3 N hydrochloric acid, and filter: the solution so obtained meets the requirements of *Identification* test *C* under *Sucralfate*.
Disintegration ⟨701⟩: 15 minutes.
Uniformity of dosage units ⟨905⟩: meet the requirements.
Acid-neutralizing capacity—Weigh and finely powder not fewer than 20 Tablets. Transfer an accurately weighed portion of the powder, equivalent to about 250 mg of sucralfate, to a 250-mL screw-capped bottle, and proceed as directed in the test for *Acid-neutralizing capacity* under *Sucralfate*, beginning with "add 100.0 mL of 0.1 N hydrochloric acid": not less than 12 mEq of acid is consumed.
Assay—
 Mobile phase, *Standard preparation*, and *Chromatographic system*—Prepare as directed in the *Assay* under *Sucralfate*.
 Assay preparation—Weigh and finely powder not fewer than 20 Tablets. Transfer an accurately weighed portion of the powder, equivalent to about 450 mg of sucralfate, to a 35-mL centrifuge tube, and shake at a moderate rate on a vortex mixer. Proceed as directed for *Assay preparation* in the *Assay* under *Sucralfate* beginning with "While shaking, add 10.0 mL."

 Procedure—Proceed as directed for *Procedure* in the *Assay* under *Sucralfate*. Calculate the quantity, in mg, of sucrose octasulfate ($C_{12}H_{14}O_{35}S_8$) in the portion of Tablets taken by the formula:

$$(974.75/1287.53)(25C)(r_U / r_S)$$

in which the terms are as defined therein.

Sufentanil Citrate

» Sufentanil Citrate contains not less than 98.0 percent and not more than 101.0 percent of $C_{22}H_{30}N_2O_2S \cdot C_6H_8O_7$, calculated on the dried basis. [*Caution*—Handle Sufentanil Citrate with great care since it is a potent opioid analgesic. Great care should be taken to prevent inhaling particles of Sufentanil Citrate and exposing the skin to it.]

Packaging and storage—Preserve in well-closed containers. Store at 25°, excursions permitted between 15° and 30°.
USP Reference standards ⟨11⟩—*USP Sufentanil Citrate RS*.
Identification—
 A: *Infrared Absorption* ⟨197K⟩.
 B: *Ultraviolet Absorption* ⟨197U⟩—
 Solution: 50 μg per mL.
 Medium: Use *Mobile phase* prepared as directed in the *Assay*.
 C: Dissolve about 500 mg in 5 mL of water, and render the mixture alkaline with 1 N sodium hydroxide. Extract with three 5-mL portions of methylene chloride: the aqueous layer meets the requirements of the tests for *Citrate* ⟨191⟩.
 D: The retention time of the major peak in the chromatogram of the *Assay preparation* corresponds to that in the chromatogram of the *Standard preparation*, as obtained in the *Assay*.
Loss on drying ⟨731⟩—Dry it in vacuum at 60° for 2 hours: it loses not more than 0.5% of its weight. [NOTE—Retain the dried material for use in the *Heavy metals* test.]
Heavy metals, *Method II* ⟨231⟩: 0.002%. [NOTE—Use the dried material retained in the *Loss on drying* test.]
Limit of acetone—
 Standard solution—Pipet 25 μL of acetone into a 100-mL volumetric flask, dilute with dimethylformamide to volume, and mix.
 Test solution—Dissolve 100 mg of Sufentanil Citrate, accurately weighed, in 2.0 mL of dimethylformamide contained in a polytefined screw-cap vial.
 Chromatographic system (see *Chromatography* ⟨621⟩)—The gas chromatograph is equipped with a flame-ionization detector and a 4-mm × 1.83-m glass column containing support S2. The carrier gas is nitrogen with a flow rate of about 50 mL per minute. The injection port temperature and the detector temperature are both maintained at 230°. The column temperature is maintained at 175°. Inject the *Standard solution*, and record the peak responses as directed for *Procedure*: the relative standard deviation of the acetone peak responses for replicate injections is not more than 5%.
 Procedure—Separately inject equal volumes (about 2 μL) of the *Standard solution* and the *Test solution* into the chromatograph, record the chromatograms, and measure the peak responses. [NOTE—After injecting the *Test solution*, wait about 25 minutes to allow the sufentanil peak to completely elute from the column.] Calculate the percentage of acetone in the portion of Sufentanil Citrate taken by the formula:

$$100(C_S / C_U)(r_U / r_S)$$

in which C_S is the concentration, in mg per mL, of acetone in the *Standard solution*; C_U is the concentration, in mg per mL, of sufentanil citrate in the *Test solution*; and r_U and r_S are the peak responses obtained from the *Test solution* and the *Standard solution*, respectively. Not more than 0.5% of acetone is found.
Chromatographic purity—
 Mobile phase and *Chromatographic system*—Proceed as directed in the *Assay*.

Blank solution—Transfer 33.2 mg of citric acid, accurately weighed, to a 50-mL volumetric flask. Dilute with *Mobile phase* to volume, and mix.

Test solution—Transfer about 7.5 mg of Sufentanil Citrate to a 10-mL volumetric flask, dilute with *Mobile phase* to volume, and mix.

Procedure—Separately inject equal volumes (about 100 µL) of the *Blank solution* and the *Test solution* into the chromatograph, record the chromatograms, and measure the responses. Calculate the percentage of each impurity, disregarding any peaks corresponding to those found in the *Blank solution*, in the portion of Sufentanil Citrate taken by the formula:

$$100(r_i / r_s)$$

in which r_i is the peak response for each impurity; and r_s is the sum of the responses of all of the peaks: not more than 0.5% of any impurity is found, and the sum of all impurities is not more than 1.0%.

Assay—

Mobile phase—Prepare a filtered and degassed mixture of methanol, 0.13 M ammonium acetate, and acetonitrile (45 : 31 : 24). Adjust with glacial acetic acid or ammonium hydroxide to a pH of 7.2. Make adjustments if necessary (see *System Suitability* under *Chromatography* ⟨621⟩).

Standard preparation—Dissolve an accurately weighed quantity of USP Sufentanil Citrate RS in *Mobile phase*, and dilute quantitatively, and stepwise if necessary, with *Mobile phase* to obtain a solution having a known concentration of about 0.075 mg per mL.

Assay preparation—Transfer about 18.7 mg of Sufentanil Citrate, accurately weighed, to a 25-mL volumetric flask; dissolve in and dilute with *Mobile phase* to volume; and mix. Transfer 5.0 mL of this solution to a 50-mL volumetric flask, dilute with *Mobile phase* to volume, and mix.

Chromatographic system (see *Chromatography* ⟨621⟩)—The liquid chromatograph is equipped with a 228-nm detector and a 4.6-mm × 25-cm column that contains packing L1. The flow rate is about 1.5 mL per minute. Chromatograph the *Standard preparation*, and record the peak responses as directed for *Procedure*: the tailing factor is not more than 2, and the relative standard deviation for replicate injections is not more than 2.0%.

Procedure—Separately inject equal volumes (about 100 µL) of the *Standard preparation* and the *Assay preparation* into the chromatograph, record the chromatograms, and measure the responses for the major peaks. Calculate the quantity, in mg, of $C_{22}H_{30}N_2O_2S \cdot C_6H_8O_7$ in the portion of Sufentanil Citrate taken by the formula:

$$250C(r_U / r_S)$$

in which C is the concentration, in mg per mL, of USP Sufentanil Citrate RS in the *Standard preparation*; and r_U and r_S are the peak responses obtained from the *Assay preparation* and the *Standard preparation*, respectively.

Sufentanil Citrate Injection

» Sufentanil Citrate Injection is a sterile solution of Sufentanil Citrate in Water for Injection. It contains the equivalent of not less than 90.0 percent and not more than 110.0 percent of the labeled amount of sufentanil citrate ($C_{22}H_{30}N_2O_2S \cdot C_6H_8O_7$).

Caution—Handle Sufentanil Citrate Injection with great care, as it is a potent opioid analgesic.

Packaging and storage—Preserve in single-dose or multiple-dose containers, preferably of Type I glass.

USP Reference standards ⟨11⟩—USP Endotoxin RS. USP Sufentanil Citrate RS.

Identification—

A: *Ultraviolet Absorption* ⟨197U⟩—
  Solution: 50 µg per mL.
  Medium: Use *Mobile phase* prepared as directed in the *Assay*.
  [NOTE—For samples that do not require dilution to achieve 50 µg per mL, use Water for Injection as the medium for the Standard solution.]

B: The retention time of the major peak in the chromatogram of the *Assay preparation* corresponds to that in the chromatogram of the *Standard preparation*, as obtained in the *Assay*.

Bacterial endotoxins ⟨85⟩—It contains not more than 6.25 USP Endotoxin Units per mL.

pH ⟨791⟩: between 3.5 and 6.0.

Particulate matter ⟨788⟩: meets the requirements for small-volume injections.

Other requirements—It meets the requirements under *Injections* ⟨1⟩.

Assay—

Mobile phase and *Chromatographic system*—Prepare as directed in the test for *Chromatographic purity* under *Sufentanil Citrate*.

Standard preparation—Dissolve an accurately weighed quantity of USP Sufentanil Citrate RS in water, and dilute quantitatively, and stepwise if necessary, with water to obtain a solution having a known concentration of about 0.075 mg per mL.

Assay preparation—Use Sufentanil Citrate Injection.

Procedure—Separately inject equal volumes (about 100 µL) of the *Standard preparation* and the *Assay preparation* into the chromatograph, record the chromatograms, and measure the responses for the major peaks. Calculate the quantity, in mg, of sufentanil ($C_{22}H_{30}N_2O_2S$) in each mL of the Injection taken by the formula:

$$386.56 / 578.69 C(r_U / r_S)$$

in which 386.56 and 578.69 are the molecular weights of sufentanil and sufentanil citrate, respectively; C is the concentration, in mg per mL, of USP Sufentanil Citrate RS in the *Standard preparation*; and r_U and r_S are the peak responses obtained from the *Assay preparation* and the *Standard preparation*, respectively.

Invert Sugar Injection

» Invert Sugar Injection is a sterile solution of a mixture of equal amounts of Dextrose and Fructose in Water for Injection, or an equivalent sterile solution produced by the hydrolysis of Sucrose, in Water for Injection. It contains not less than 95.0 percent and not more than 105.0 percent of the labeled amount of $C_6H_{12}O_6$. It contains no antimicrobial agents.

NOTE—Invert Sugar Injection that is produced by mixing Dextrose and Fructose is exempt from the requirement of the test for *Completeness of inversion*.

Packaging and storage—Preserve in single-dose containers, preferably of Type I or Type II glass, or of a suitable plastic material.

Labeling—The label states the total osmolar concentration in mOsmol per L.

USP Reference standards ⟨11⟩—USP Endotoxin RS.

Identification—Add a few drops of Injection to 5 mL of hot alkaline cupric tartrate TS: a copious red precipitate of cupric oxide is formed.

Bacterial endotoxins ⟨85⟩—It contains not more than 0.5 USP Endotoxin Unit per mL.

pH ⟨791⟩: between 3.0 and 6.5.

Chloride ⟨221⟩—A 2.0-mL portion shows no more chloride than corresponds to 0.34 mL of 0.020 N hydrochloric acid (0.012%).

Heavy metals ⟨231⟩—Transfer a volume of Injection, equivalent to 4.0 g of invert sugar, to a suitable vessel, and adjust the volume to 25 mL by evaporation: the limit is 0.0005C%, in which C is the labeled amount, in g, of invert sugar per mL of Injection.

Limit of 5-hydroxymethylfurfural and related substances—Dilute an accurately measured volume of Injection, equivalent to 1.0 g of invert sugar, with water to 500.0 mL. Determine the absorbance of this solution in a 1-cm cell at 284 nm, with a suitable spectrophotometer, using water as the blank: the absorbance is not more than 0.25.

Completeness of inversion—

Mobile phase—Use filtered, degassed water.

Standard preparation—Prepare a solution in water containing known concentrations of about 0.25 mg of sucrose and about 12.5 mg of dextrose per mL.

Test preparation—Transfer a volume of Injection, equivalent to about 2.5 g of invert sugar, to a 100-mL volumetric flask, dilute with water to volume, and mix.

Chromatographic system (see *Chromatography* ⟨621⟩)—The liquid chromatograph is equipped with a refractive index detector and a 7.8-mm × 30-cm column that contains 9-μm packing L19, maintained at a constant temperature of about 40°. Chromatograph the *Standard preparation*, and record the peak responses as directed for *Procedure:* the sucrose elutes first, and the peak is baseline separated from the dextrose peak. The relative standard deviation for replicate injections is not more than 2.0%.

Procedure—Separately inject equal volumes (about 20 μL) of the *Standard preparation* and the *Test preparation* into the chromatograph, record the chromatograms, and measure the responses for the sucrose peaks. Calculate the quantity, in mg, of sucrose, in the volume of the Injection taken by the formula:

$$100C(r_U/r_S)$$

in which C is the concentration, in mg per mL, of sucrose in the *Standard preparation*, and r_U and r_S are the peak responses for sucrose obtained from the *Test preparation* and the *Standard preparation*, respectively: not more than 1.5% of the quantity of invert sugar in the volume of Injection taken, based on the value stated on the label, is found.

Other requirements—It meets the requirements under *Injections* ⟨1⟩.

Assay—Pipet 50 mL of alkaline cupric tartrate TS into a 400-mL beaker, add 48 mL of water, mix, and pipet into the mixture 2 mL of Injection that has been diluted quantitatively with water, if necessary, to a 5.0% concentration. Cover the beaker with a watch glass, heat the solution, regulating the heat so that boiling begins in 4 minutes, and continue boiling for 2.0 minutes. Filter the hot solution at once through a tared porcelain filtering crucible, wash the precipitate with water maintained at 60°, then with 10 mL of alcohol. Dry at 105° to constant weight. Perform a blank determination, and make any necessary correction. The corrected weight of the precipitate so obtained is not less than 204.0 mg and not more than 224.4 mg, corresponding to between 95.0 and 105.0 mg of $C_6H_{12}O_6$.

Sulbactam Sodium

$C_8H_{10}NNaO_5S$ 255.22

4-Thia-1-azabicyclo[3.2.0]heptane-2-carboxylic acid, 3,3-dimethyl-7-oxo-, 4,4-dioxide, sodium salt, (2S-cis)-.

Sodium (2S,5R)-3,3-dimethyl-7-oxo-4-thia-1-azabicyclo[3.2.0]heptane-2-carboxylate 4,4-dioxide   [69388-84-7].

» Sulbactam Sodium contains not less than 886 μg and not more than 941 μg of sulbactam ($C_8H_{11}NO_5S$) per mg, calculated on the anhydrous basis.

Packaging and storage—Preserve in tight containers.

Labeling—Where it is intended for use in preparing injectable dosage forms, the label states that it is sterile or must be subjected to further processing during the preparation of injectable dosage forms.

USP Reference standards ⟨11⟩—*USP Endotoxin RS. USP Sulbactam RS.*

Identification—

A: The retention time of the major peak in the chromatogram of the *Assay preparation* corresponds to that in the chromatogram of the *Standard preparation*, as obtained in the *Assay*.

B: It meets the requirements of the tests for *Sodium* ⟨191⟩.

Crystallinity ⟨695⟩:   meets the requirements.

Bacterial endotoxins ⟨85⟩—Where the label states that Sulbactam Sodium is sterile or must be subjected to further processing during the preparation of injectable dosage forms, it contains not more than 0.17 USP Endotoxin Unit per mg of sulbactam.

Sterility ⟨71⟩—Where the label states that Sulbactam Sodium is sterile, it meets the requirements when tested as directed for *Membrane Filtration* under *Test for Sterility of the Product to be Examined*.

Water, *Method I* ⟨921⟩:   not more than 1.0%.

Assay—

0.005 M Tetrabutylammonium hydroxide—Dilute 6.6 mL of a 40% solution of tetrabutylammonium hydroxide with water to obtain 1800 mL of solution. Adjust with 1 M phosphoric acid to a pH of 5.0 ± 0.1, dilute with water to 2000 mL, and mix.

Mobile phase—Prepare a filtered and degassed mixture of *0.005 M Tetrabutylammonium hydroxide* and acetonitrile (1650:350). Make adjustments if necessary (see *System Suitability* under *Chromatography* ⟨621⟩).

Standard preparation—Quantitatively dissolve an accurately weighed quantity of USP Sulbactam RS in *Mobile phase* to obtain a solution having a known concentration of about 1 mg per mL. [NOTE—Inject this solution promptly.]

Assay preparation—Transfer about 110 mg of Sulbactam Sodium, accurately weighed, to a 100-mL volumetric flask, dissolve in and dilute with *Mobile phase* to volume, and mix. [NOTE—Inject this solution promptly.]

Chromatographic system (see *Chromatography* ⟨621⟩)—The liquid chromatograph is equipped with a 230-nm detector and a 4-mm × 30-cm column that contains packing L1. The flow rate is about 2 mL per minute. Chromatograph the *Standard preparation*, and record the responses as directed for *Procedure:* the column efficiency is not less than 3500 theoretical plates; the tailing factor is not more than 1.5; and the relative standard deviation for replicate injections is not more than 2.0%.

Procedure—Separately inject equal volumes (about 10 μL) of the *Standard preparation* and the *Assay preparation* into the chromatograph, record the chromatograms, and measure the areas for the major peaks. Calculate the quantity, in μg, of sulbactam ($C_8H_{11}NO_5S$) in each mg of Sulbactam Sodium taken by the formula:

$$100(CP/W)(r_U/r_S)$$

in which C is the concentration, in mg per mL, of USP Sulbactam RS in the *Standard preparation*; P is the assigned sulbactam content, in μg per mg, of USP Sulbactam RS; W is the quantity, in mg, of Sulbactam Sodium taken to prepare the *Assay preparation*; and r_U and r_S are the peak areas for sulbactam obtained from the *Assay preparation* and the *Standard preparation*, respectively.

Sulconazole Nitrate

$C_{18}H_{15}Cl_3N_2S \cdot HNO_3$ 460.76

1*H*-Imidazole,   1-[2-[[(4-chlorophenyl)methyl]thio]-2-(2,4-dichlorophenyl)ethyl]-, mononitrate, (±)-.

(±)-1-[2,4-Dichloro-β-[(*p*-chlorobenzyl)thio]phenethyl]imidazole mononitrate   [61318-91-0].

» Sulconazole Nitrate contains not less than 98.0 percent and not more than 102.0 percent of $C_{18}H_{15}Cl_3N_2S \cdot HNO_3$, calculated on the dried basis.

Packaging and storage—Preserve in well-closed containers, protected from light.
USP Reference standards ⟨11⟩—*USP Sulconazole Nitrate RS*.
Identification—
A: *Infrared Absorption* ⟨197K⟩.
B: A solution of it responds to the ferrous sulfate-sulfuric acid test for *Nitrate* ⟨191⟩.
Loss on drying ⟨731⟩—Dry it in vacuum at 80° for 3 hours: it loses not more than 1.0% of its weight.
Residue on ignition ⟨281⟩: not more than 0.1%.
Ordinary impurities ⟨466⟩—
Test solution—Prepare a solution of it, in a mixture of dichloromethane and methanol (2 : 1), having an accurately known concentration of 20 mg per mL.
Standard solutions—Dissolve USP Sulconazole Nitrate RS in a mixture of dichloromethane and methanol (2 : 1), and dilute quantitatively with the same mixture to obtain separate solutions having accurately known concentrations of 0.02, 0.1, 0.2, and 0.4 mg per mL, respectively.
Eluant: a mixture of methylene chloride, cyclohexane, and diethylamine (50 : 45 : 5).
Visualization: 22.
Assay—
Mobile phase—Dissolve 1.9 g of sodium 1-pentanesulfonate in 300 mL of water, add 700 mL of methanol, and mix. Adjust with 2 N sulfuric acid to an apparent pH of 3.8 ± 0.1, filter, and degas. Make adjustments if necessary (see *System Suitability* under *Chromatography* ⟨621⟩).
Standard preparation—Dissolve an accurately weighed quantity of USP Sulconazole Nitrate RS in *Mobile phase*, and dilute quantitatively, and stepwise if necessary, with *Mobile phase* to obtain a solution having a known concentration of about 0.2 mg per mL.
Assay preparation—Transfer about 20 mg of Sulconazole Nitrate, accurately weighed, to a 100-mL volumetric flask, dissolve in *Mobile phase*, dilute with *Mobile phase* to volume, and mix.
Chromatographic system (see *Chromatography* ⟨621⟩)—The liquid chromatograph is equipped with a 230-nm detector and a 4.6-mm × 25-cm column that contains packing L1 and is maintained at 40 ± 1.0°. The flow rate is about 2 mL per minute. Chromatograph the *Standard preparation*, and record the peak responses as directed for *Procedure*: the column efficiency determined from the analyte peak is not less than 1500 theoretical plates, the tailing factor for the sulconazole nitrate peak is not more than 2.3, and the relative standard deviation for replicate injections is not more than 1.5%.
Procedure—Separately inject equal volumes (about 10 μL) of the *Standard preparation* and the *Assay preparation* into the chromatograph, record the chromatograms, and measure the responses for the major peaks. Calculate the quantity, in mg, of $C_{18}H_{15}Cl_3N_2S \cdot HNO_3$ in the portion of Sulconazole Nitrate taken by the formula:

$$100C(r_U / r_S)$$

in which C is the concentration, in mg per mL, of USP Sulconazole Nitrate RS in the *Standard preparation*, and r_U and r_S are the peak responses obtained from the *Assay preparation* and the *Standard preparation*, respectively.

Triple Sulfa Vaginal Cream

» Triple Sulfa Vaginal Cream contains not less than 90.0 percent and not more than 110.0 percent of the labeled amounts of sulfathiazole ($C_9H_9N_3O_2S_2$), sulfacetamide ($C_8H_{10}N_2O_3S$), and sulfabenzamide ($C_{13}H_{12}N_2O_3S$).

Packaging and storage—Preserve in well-closed, light-resistant containers, or in collapsible tubes.

USP Reference standards ⟨11⟩—*USP Sulfathiazole RS. USP Sulfacetamide RS. USP Sulfabenzamide RS.*
Identification—The retention times of the major peaks in the chromatogram of the *Assay preparation* correspond to those of the *Standard preparation*, as obtained in the *Assay*.
Minimum fill ⟨755⟩: meets the requirements.
pH ⟨791⟩: between 3.0 and 4.0.
Assay—
Mobile phase—Prepare a suitably degassed solution of water, acetonitrile, and 1 M tetrabutylammonium hydroxide (78 : 22 : 10). Adjust, dropwise with dilute phosphoric acid (1 in 10) to a pH of 7.7 ± 0.2, and mix for 5 minutes. If necessary, adjust to a pH of 7.7 ± 0.2, using dilute phosphoric acid (1 in 50) or 1 M tetrabutylammonium hydroxide.
Internal standard solution—Dissolve sulfapyridine in acetone to obtain a solution having a concentration of about 10 mg per mL.
Standard preparation—Weigh accurately about 29 mg of USP Sulfacetamide RS, 34 mg of USP Sulfathiazole RS, and 37 mg of USP Sulfabenzamide RS, and transfer to a 50-mL volumetric flask. Add 2.0 mL of *Internal standard solution* and 30 mL of acetone, and shake for 10 minutes. If necessary, sonicate to effect solution. Dilute with acetone to volume, and mix. Pipet 5 mL of this solution into a 50-mL volumetric flask, evaporate on a steam bath with the aid of a gentle stream of nitrogen to dryness, dissolve the residue in *Mobile phase*, dilute with *Mobile phase* to volume, and mix.
Assay preparation—Using a plastic syringe equipped with a suitable cannula, transfer an accurately weighed quantity of Vaginal Cream, equivalent to about 144 mg of sulfacetamide, 184 mg of sulfabenzamide, and 173 mg of sulfathiazole, to a 250-mL volumetric flask. Add 10.0 mL of *Internal standard solution* and 100 mL of acetone, and warm the flask on a steam bath while swirling the contents to dissolve the cream. Cool to room temperature, dilute with acetone to volume, and mix. Filter the solution through filter paper, discarding the first 10 mL of the filtrate. Pipet 5 mL of the filtrate so obtained into a 50-mL volumetric flask, and evaporate on a steam bath with the aid of a gentle stream of nitrogen to dryness. Dissolve the residue in *Mobile phase*, dilute with *Mobile phase* to volume, and mix. Cool the solution in an ice bath for 10 minutes, filter the cold solution through filter paper, discarding the first 10 mL to 15 mL of the filtrate, and collect 5 mL for analysis.
Chromatographic system (see *Chromatography* ⟨621⟩)—The liquid chromatograph is equipped with a 280-nm detector and a 3.9-mm × 30-cm column that contains packing L1. The flow rate is about 1.0 mL per minute. Chromatograph five replicate injections of the *Standard preparation*, and record the peak responses as directed for *Procedure*: the relative standard deviation is not more than 3.0%, and the resolution, R, between sulfacetamide and sulfapyridine is not less than 2.0.
Procedure—Separately inject equal volumes (about 10 μL) of the *Standard preparation* and the *Assay preparation* into the chromatograph, record the chromatograms, and measure the responses for the major peaks. Chromatograms exhibit relative retention times of about 0.8 for sulfacetamide, 1.0 for sulfapyridine, 1.8 for sulfathiazole, and 2.5 for sulfabenzamide. Calculate the quantity, in mg, of $C_8H_{10}N_2O_3S$, $C_9H_9N_3O_2S_2$, and $C_{13}H_{12}N_2O_3S$ in the portion of the Vaginal Cream taken by the formula:

$$2.5C(R_U / R_S)$$

in which C is the concentration, in μg per mL, of the appropriate USP Reference Standard in the *Standard preparation*, and R_U and R_S are the ratios of the peak responses of the corresponding sulfonamides to those of the internal standard obtained from the *Assay preparation* and the *Standard preparation*, respectively.

Triple Sulfa Vaginal Inserts

» Triple Sulfa Vaginal Inserts contain not less than 90.0 percent and not more than 110.0 percent of the labeled amounts of sulfathiazole ($C_9H_9N_3O_2S_2$), sulfacetamide ($C_8H_{10}N_2O_3S$), and sulfabenzamide ($C_{13}H_{12}N_2O_3S$).

Packaging and storage—Preserve in well-closed, light-resistant containers.

USP Reference standards ⟨11⟩—*USP Sulfabenzamide RS. USP Sulfacetamide RS. USP Sulfathiazole RS.*
Identification—The retention times of the major peaks in the chromatogram of the *Assay preparation* correspond to those in the chromatogram of the *Standard preparation,* as obtained in the *Assay.*
Disintegration ⟨701⟩: 30 minutes.
Uniformity of dosage units ⟨905⟩: meet the requirements for *Weight Variation* with respect to sulfathiazole, to sulfacetamide, and to sulfabenzamide.
Assay—
  Mobile phase, Internal standard solution, and *Standard preparation*—Prepare as directed in the *Assay* under *Triple Sulfa Vaginal Cream.*
  Assay preparation—Weigh and finely powder not fewer than 10 Vaginal Inserts. Transfer an accurately weighed portion of the powder, equivalent to about 144 mg of sulfacetamide, 184 mg of sulfabenzamide, and 173 mg of sulfathiazole, to a 250-mL volumetric flask. Add 10.0 mL of water, and shake for 10 minutes. Add 10.0 mL of *Internal standard solution* and 100 mL of acetone, and shake for 30 minutes at low speed on a mechanical shaker. Dilute with acetone to volume, mix, and allow to stand for 30 minutes. Pipet 5 mL of the clear supernatant into a 50-mL volumetric flask, and evaporate on a steam bath with the aid of a gentle stream of nitrogen to dryness. Dissolve the residue in *Mobile phase,* dilute with *Mobile phase* to volume, and mix.
  Chromatographic system and *Procedure*—Proceed with the Vaginal Inserts as directed in the *Assay* under *Triple Sulfa Vaginal Cream.*

Sulfabenzamide

C₁₃H₁₂N₂O₃S   276.31
Benzamide, *N*-[(4-aminophenyl)sulfonyl]-.
N-Sulfanilylbenzamide   [*127-71-9*].

» Sulfabenzamide contains not less than 99.0 percent and not more than 100.5 percent of C₁₃H₁₂N₂O₃S, calculated on the dried basis.

Packaging and storage—Preserve in well-closed, light-resistant containers.

USP Reference standards ⟨11⟩—*USP Sulfabenzamide RS.*
Clarity and color of solution—Dissolve 2.0 g in 15 mL of 1 N sodium hydroxide, with warming: a colorless to pale yellow solution having not more than a slight turbidity is produced.
Identification—
  A: *Infrared Absorption* ⟨197K⟩.
  B: To about 100 mg, suspended in 2 mL of water, add 100 mg of sodium bicarbonate: it dissolves with effervescence (*distinction from sulfanilamide, sulfapyridine, sulfathiazole, sulfadiazine, and sulfaguanidine*).
Melting range, *Class I* ⟨741⟩:   between 180° and 184°.
Loss on drying ⟨731⟩—Dry it at 105° for 2 hours: it loses not more than 0.5% of its weight.
Selenium ⟨291⟩:   0.001%, a 300-mg test specimen and 3 mL of *Stock Solution* being used.
Heavy metals, *Method II* ⟨231⟩:   0.002%.
Ordinary impurities ⟨466⟩—
  Test solution: methanol.
  Standard solution: methanol.
  Eluant: a mixture of chloroform, methanol, and glacial acetic acid (90 : 5 : 5).
  Visualization: 1.
Assay—Transfer about 800 mg of Sulfabenzamide, accurately weighed, to a 125-mL conical flask, and dissolve in 25 mL of dimethylformamide. Add 3 drops of thymol blue TS (prepared with methanol), and titrate with 0.1 N sodium methoxide VS to a blue endpoint. Perform a blank determination, and make any necessary correction. Each mL of 0.1 N sodium methoxide is equivalent to 27.63 mg of C₁₃H₁₂N₂O₃S.

Sulfacetamide

C₈H₁₀N₂O₃S   214.24
Acetamide, *N*-[(4-aminophenyl)sulfonyl]-.
N-Sulfanilylacetamide   [*144-80-9*].

» Sulfacetamide contains not less than 99.0 percent and not more than 100.5 percent of C₈H₁₀N₂O₃S, calculated on the dried basis.

Packaging and storage—Preserve in well-closed, light-resistant containers.

USP Reference standards ⟨11⟩—*USP Sulfacetamide RS.*
Clarity and color of solution—Dissolve about 200 mg in 5 mL of 1 N sodium hydroxide: a yellow to faintly yellow solution having not more than a trace of turbidity is produced.
Identification—
  A: *Infrared Absorption* ⟨197K⟩.
  B: Place about 500 mg in a test tube, heat gently until it boils, and cool: an oily liquid, which has the characteristic odor of acetamide, condenses on the walls of the test tube (*distinction from the sublimates of sulfadiazine, sulfamerazine, sulfamethazine, and sulfapyrazine, which are solids at room temperature*).
Melting range, *Class I* ⟨741⟩:   between 181° and 184°.
Reaction—A solution (1 in 150) is acid to litmus.
Loss on drying ⟨731⟩—Dry it at 105° for 2 hours: it loses not more than 0.5% of its weight.
Residue on ignition ⟨281⟩:   not more than 0.1%.
Sulfate ⟨221⟩—Digest 1 g with 50 mL of water at about 70° for 5 minutes. Cool immediately to room temperature, and filter. A 25-mL portion of the filtrate so obtained shows no more sulfate than corresponds to 0.2 mL of 0.02 N sulfuric acid (0.04%).
Selenium ⟨291⟩:   0.003%, a 200-mg test specimen being used.
Heavy metals, *Method II* ⟨231⟩:   0.002%.
Assay—Proceed with Sulfacetamide as directed under *Nitrite Titration* ⟨451⟩. Each mL of 0.1 M sodium nitrite is equivalent to 21.42 mg of C₈H₁₀N₂O₃S.

Sulfacetamide Sodium

C₈H₉N₂NaO₃S · H₂O   254.24
Acetamide, *N*-[(4-aminophenyl)sulfonyl]-, monosodium salt, monohydrate.
N-Sulfanilylacetamide monosodium salt monohydrate   [*6209-17-2*].
Anhydrous   236.23   [*127-56-0*].

» Sulfacetamide Sodium contains not less than 99.0 percent and not more than 100.5 percent of C₈H₉N₂NaO₃S, calculated on the anhydrous basis.

Packaging and storage—Preserve in tight, light-resistant containers.

USP Reference standards ⟨11⟩—*USP Sulfacetamide Sodium RS*.
Identification—
A: Dissolve about 1 g in 25 mL of water, adjust with 6 N acetic acid to a pH of between 4 and 5, and filter. Wash the precipitate with water, and dry at 105° for 2 hours: the sulfacetamide so obtained melts between 180° and 184°.
B: Place about 500 mg of the sulfacetamide obtained in *Identification* test *A* in a test tube, and heat gently until it boils: an oily liquid, which has the characteristic odor of acetamide, condenses on the walls of the test tube (*distinction from the sublimates of sulfadiazine, sulfamerazine, and sulfamethazine, which are solids at room temperature*).
C: The filtrate obtained in *Identification* test *A* responds to the tests for *Sodium* ⟨191⟩.
D: Dissolve about 100 mg in 5 mL of water, and add 5 drops of cupric sulfate TS: a light bluish green precipitate is formed, and it remains unchanged on standing.
E: Dissolve about 500 mg in 10 mL of dilute hydrochloric acid (1 in 10). To about one-half of the solution add 2 mL of trinitrophenol TS: a very heavy flocculent or almost gelatinous precipitate is formed. To the remainder of the solution add 3 drops of formaldehyde TS: a white precipitate is formed, and it changes to orange on standing (*distinction from sulfamethoxypyridazine*).
pH ⟨791⟩: between 8.0 and 9.5, in a solution (1 in 20).
Water, *Method I* ⟨921⟩: not more than 8.1%.
Selenium ⟨291⟩: 0.003%, a 200-mg test specimen being used.
Heavy metals—Dissolve 1.0 g in 25 mL of water, and add 5 drops of freshly prepared sodium sulfide TS: any color produced is not darker than that of a control made with 25 mL of water, 2.0 mL of *Standard Lead Solution* (see *Heavy Metals* ⟨231⟩), and 5 drops of sodium sulfide TS (0.002%).
Ordinary impurities ⟨466⟩—
Test solution: methanol.
Standard solution: methanol.
Eluant: a mixture of ethyl acetate, methanol, and ammonium hydroxide (17 : 6 : 5).
Visualization: 1.
Assay—Proceed with Sulfacetamide Sodium as directed under *Nitrite Titration* ⟨451⟩. Each mL of 0.1 M sodium nitrite is equivalent to 23.62 mg of $C_8H_9N_2NaO_3S$.

Sulfacetamide Sodium Ophthalmic Ointment

» Sulfacetamide Sodium Ophthalmic Ointment contains not less than 90.0 percent and not more than 110.0 percent of the labeled amount of $C_8H_9N_2NaO_3S \cdot H_2O$. It is sterile.

Packaging and storage—Preserve in collapsible ophthalmic ointment tubes.
USP Reference standards ⟨11⟩—*USP Sulfacetamide Sodium RS*.
Identification—Dissolve a quantity of Ophthalmic Ointment, equivalent to about 1 g of sulfacetamide sodium, in 100 mL of ether in a separator, and extract the mixture with 25 mL of water. Wash the extract with 25 mL of ether, and warm the water extract on a steam bath to remove the last traces of ether. Adjust with 6 N acetic acid to a pH of between 4 and 5, and filter. Wash the precipitate with water, and dry at 105° for 2 hours: the sulfacetamide so obtained melts between 180° and 184°, and responds to *Identification* tests *B*, *D*, and *E* under *Sulfacetamide Sodium*.
Sterility ⟨71⟩: meets the requirements.
Metal particles—It meets the requirements of the test for *Metal Particles in Ophthalmic Ointments* ⟨751⟩.
Assay—
Mobile phase—Prepare a filtered and degassed mixture of water, methanol, and glacial acetic acid (89 : 10 : 1). Make adjustments if necessary (see *System Suitability* under *Chromatography* ⟨621⟩).
Standard preparation—Transfer about 50 mg of USP Sulfacetamide Sodium RS, accurately weighed, to a 40-mL centrifuge tube. Add 10.0 mL of dilute methanol (1 in 5), insert the stopper, and mix, using a vortex mixer, for about 3 minutes to dissolve the Reference Standard. Add 7.5 mL of heptane, insert the stopper, and mix, using a vortex mixer, for another 3 minutes. Centrifuge to effect separation of the phases. Withdraw and discard the upper heptane layer. Transfer 3.0 mL of the bottom layer to a 500-mL volumetric flask, add dilute methanol (1 in 5) to volume, and mix.
Assay preparation—Transfer an accurately weighed quantity of Ophthalmic Ointment, equivalent to about 100 mg of sulfacetamide sodium, to a 40-mL centrifuge tube. Add 15.0 mL of heptane, insert the stopper, and mix, using a vortex mixer, for about 3 minutes to dissolve the Ophthalmic Ointment. Add 20.0 mL of dilute methanol (1 in 5), insert the stopper, and mix, using a vortex mixer, for 3 minutes. Centrifuge to effect separation of the phases. Withdraw and discard the upper heptane layer. Transfer 3.0 mL of the bottom layer to a 500-mL volumetric flask, add dilute methanol (1 in 5) to volume, and mix.
System suitability preparation—Dissolve 3 mg of sulfanilamide in 100 mL of the *Standard preparation*, and mix.
Chromatographic system (see *Chromatography* ⟨621⟩)—The liquid chromatograph is equipped with a 254-nm detector and a 4.6-mm × 25-cm column that contains packing L1. The flow rate is about 1.5 mL per minute. Chromatograph the *Standard preparation* and the *System suitability preparation*, and record the peak responses as directed for *Procedure:* the column efficiency determined from the analyte peak is not less than 1500 theoretical plates, the resolution, *R*, between the sulfacetamide and sulfanilamide peaks is not less than 3, and the relative standard deviation for replicate injections is not more than 2.0%.
Procedure—Separately inject equal volumes (about 90 µL) of the *Standard preparation* and the *Assay preparation* into the chromatograph, record the chromatograms, and measure the responses for the major peaks. Calculate the quantity, in mg, of $C_8H_9N_2NaO_3S \cdot H_2O$ sulfacetamide sodium in the portion of Ophthalmic Ointment taken by the formula:

$$3.33(254.24 / 236.23)C(r_U / r_S)$$

in which 254.24 and 236.23 are the molecular weights of sulfacetamide sodium monohydrate and anhydrous sulfacetamide sodium, respectively, *C* is the concentration, in µg per mL, of sulfacetamide sodium, calculated on the anhydrous basis, in the *Standard preparation*, and r_U and r_S are the peak responses obtained from the *Assay preparation* and the *Standard preparation*, respectively.

Sulfacetamide Sodium Ophthalmic Solution

» Sulfacetamide Sodium Ophthalmic Solution is a sterile solution containing not less than 90.0 percent and not more than 110.0 percent of the labeled amount of $C_8H_9N_2NaO_3S \cdot H_2O$. It may contain suitable buffers, stabilizers, and antimicrobial agents.

Packaging and storage—Preserve in tight, light-resistant containers, in a cool place.
USP Reference standards ⟨11⟩—*USP Sulfacetamide Sodium RS*.
Identification—Transfer to a beaker a volume of Solution, equivalent to about 1 g of sulfacetamide sodium, and dilute with water to 25 mL. Adjust with 6 N acetic acid to a pH of between 4 and 5, and filter. Wash the precipitate with water, and dry at 105° for 2 hours: the sulfacetamide so obtained melts between 180° and 184°, and responds to *Identification* tests *B* and *E* under *Sulfacetamide Sodium*.
Sterility ⟨71⟩: meets the requirements.
Assay—
Mobile phase, Standard preparation, System suitability preparation, and *Chromatographic system*—Proceed as directed in the *Assay* under *Sulfacetamide Sodium Ophthalmic Ointment*.
Assay preparation—Transfer an accurately measured volume of Ophthalmic Solution, freshly mixed and free from air bubbles,

equivalent to about 100 mg of sulfacetamide, to a 100-mL volumetric flask, dilute with a mixture of water and methanol (4 : 1) to volume, and mix. Dilute 3.0 mL of this solution with the same solvent mixture to 100.0 mL, and mix.

Procedure—Proceed as directed in the *Assay* under *Sulfacetamide Sodium Ophthalmic Ointment*. Calculate the quantity, in mg, of sulfacetamide sodium in the portion of Ophthalmic Solution taken by the formula:

$$3.33(254.24 / 236.23)C(r_U / r_S)$$

in which the terms are as defined therein.

Sulfacetamide Sodium Topical Suspension

» Sulfacetamide Sodium Topical Suspension contains not less than 90.0 percent and not more than 110.0 percent of the labeled amount of sulfacetamide sodium ($C_8H_9N_2NaO_3S$).

Packaging and storage—Preserve in well-closed containers, at controlled room temperature.

USP Reference standards ⟨11⟩—*USP Sulfacetamide Sodium RS*.

Identification—The retention time of the sulfacetamide peak in the chromatogram of the *Assay preparation* corresponds to that in the chromatogram of the *Standard preparation*, as obtained in the *Assay*.

Microbial limits ⟨61⟩—The total aerobic microbial count does not exceed 100 cfu per mL, the total combined molds and yeasts count does not exceed 50 cfu per mL, and it meets the requirements of the test for *Pseudomonas aeruginosa*.

Minimum fill ⟨755⟩: meets the requirements.

pH ⟨791⟩: between 6.5 and 7.5.

Assay—

Mobile phase—Prepare a filtered and degassed mixture of water, methanol, and glacial acetic acid (875 : 125 : 3). Make adjustments if necessary (see *System Suitability* under *Chromatography* ⟨621⟩).

Internal standard solution—Prepare a solution of sulfathiazole sodium in water containing about 5 mg per mL.

Standard preparation—Transfer about 25 mg of USP Sulfacetamide Sodium RS and 10 mg of *p*-hydroxybenzoic acid, each accurately weighed, to a 100-mL volumetric flask. Dissolve in water, add 5 mL of *Internal standard solution*, dilute with water to volume, and mix. Transfer 2 mL of this solution to a 25-mL volumetric flask, dilute with water to volume, and mix.

Assay preparation—Transfer about 250 mg of Topical Suspension, accurately weighed, to a 125-mL conical flask, add 5 mL of *Internal standard solution*, dilute with 95 mL of water, and mix. Transfer 2 mL of this solution to a 25-mL volumetric flask, dilute with water to volume, and mix. Centrifuge, and use the clear supernatant.

Chromatographic system (see *Chromatography* ⟨621⟩)—The liquid chromatograph is equipped with a 254-nm detector and a 3.9-mm × 30-cm column that contains packing L1. The flow rate is about 2.0 mL per minute. Chromatograph the *Standard preparation*, and record the peak responses as directed for *Procedure*: the relative retention times are about 0.2 for sulfanilamide, 0.5 for sulfacetamide, 1.0 for sulfathiazole, and 1.2 for *p*-hydroxybenzoic acid; the resolution, *R*, between sulfathiazole and *p*-hydroxybenzoic acid is not less than 2.0; the tailing factor is not more than 2; and the relative standard deviation for replicate injections is not more than 2.0%.

Procedure—Separately inject equal volumes (about 20 μL) of the *Standard preparation* and the *Assay preparation* into the chromatograph, record the chromatograms, and measure the areas for the major peaks. Calculate the quantity, in mg, of sulfacetamide sodium ($C_8H_9N_2NaO_3S$) in the portion of Topical Suspension taken by the formula:

$$1250C(R_U / R_S)$$

in which *C* is the concentration, in mg per mL, of USP Sulfacetamide Sodium RS in the *Standard preparation*; and R_U and R_S are the peak area ratios of sulfacetamide to sulfathiazole obtained from the *Assay preparation* and the *Standard preparation*, respectively.

Sulfacetamide Sodium and Prednisolone Acetate Ophthalmic Ointment

» Sulfacetamide Sodium and Prednisolone Acetate Ophthalmic Ointment is a sterile ointment containing not less than 90.0 percent and not more than 110.0 percent of the labeled amounts of sulfacetamide sodium ($C_8H_{92}NaO_3S \cdot H_2O$) and prednisolone acetate ($C_{23}H_{30}O_6$).

Packaging and storage—Preserve in collapsible ophthalmic ointment tubes that are tamper-proof so that sterility is assured at time of first use.

USP Reference standards ⟨11⟩—*USP Sulfacetamide Sodium RS. USP Prednisolone Acetate RS*.

Identification—Transfer the contents of 1 tube of Ophthalmic Ointment to a 100-mL beaker, add about 25 mL of alcohol, and stir by mechanical means for about 15 minutes. Filter, and use the clear solution as the *Test preparation*. Prepare Standard solutions in alcohol containing 0.7 mg per mL of USP Prednisolone Acetate RS and 14 mg per mL of USP Sulfacetamide Sodium RS. Apply separately 10 μL of the *Test preparation* and 10 μL of each Standard solution to a suitable thin-layer chromatographic plate (see *Chromatography* ⟨621⟩) coated with a 0.25-mm layer of chromatographic silica gel mixture. Position the plate in a chromatographic chamber, and develop the chromatograms in a solvent system consisting of a mixture of chloroform, heptane, alcohol, and water (50 : 50 : 50 : 2) until the solvent front has moved about three-fourths of the length of the plate. Remove the plate from the developing chamber, mark the solvent front, and allow the solvent to evaporate. Examine the plate under UV light: the *Test preparation* exhibits two spots whose R_F-values and intensities correspond to the respective spots from the Standard solutions.

Sterility ⟨71⟩: meets the requirements.

Minimum fill ⟨755⟩: meets the requirements.

Metal particles—It meets the requirements of the test for *Metal Particles in Ophthalmic Ointments* ⟨751⟩.

Assay for sulfacetamide sodium—

Mobile phase—Prepare a filtered and degassed mixture of water, methanol, and glacial acetic acid (890 : 100 : 10). Make adjustments if necessary (see *System Suitability* under *Chromatography* ⟨621⟩).

Standard preparation—Transfer about 50 mg of USP Sulfacetamide Sodium RS, accurately weighed, to a 40-mL centrifuge tube. Add 10.0 mL of dilute methanol (1 in 5), insert the stopper in the tube, and mix, using a vortex mixer for about 3 minutes to dissolve the standard. Add 7.5 mL of heptane, insert the stopper in the tube, and mix, using a vortex mixer for another 3 minutes. Centrifuge to effect separation of the phases. Withdraw and discard the upper, heptane layer. Transfer 3.0 mL of the bottom layer to a 500-mL volumetric flask, add dilute methanol (1 in 5) to volume, and mix.

Assay preparation—Transfer an accurately weighed quantity of Ophthalmic Ointment, equivalent to about 100 mg of sulfacetamide sodium, to a 40-mL centrifuge tube. Add 15.0 mL of heptane, insert the stopper in the tube, and mix, using a vortex mixer for about 3 minutes to dissolve the Ointment. Add 20.0 mL of dilute methanol (1 in 5), insert the stopper in the tube, and mix, using a vortex mixer for 3 minutes. Centrifuge to effect separation of the phases. Withdraw and discard the upper, heptane layer. Transfer 3.0 mL of the bottom layer into a 500-mL volumetric flask, add dilute methanol (1 in 5) to volume, and mix.

System suitability preparation—Dissolve 3 mg of sulfanilamide in 100 mL of the *Standard preparation*, and mix.

Chromatographic system (see *Chromatography* ⟨621⟩)—The liquid chromatograph is equipped with a 254-nm detector and a 4.6-mm × 25-cm column that contains packing L1. The flow rate is about 1.5 mL per minute. Chromatograph the *Standard preparation* and the *System suitability preparation*, and record the peak responses as directed for *Procedure*: the column efficiency determined for the analyte peak is not less than 1500 theoretical plates, the resolution, R, between the sulfacetamide and sulfanilamide peaks is not less than 3, and the relative standard deviation for replicate injections is not more than 2.0%.

Procedure—Separately inject equal volumes (about 90 μL) of the *Standard preparation* and the *Assay preparation* into the chromatograph, record the chromatograms, and measure the responses for the major peaks. Calculate the quantity, in mg, of $C_8H_9N_2NaO_3S \cdot H_2O$ in the portion of Ophthalmic Ointment taken by the formula:

$$3.33(254.24 / 236.23)C(r_U / r_S)$$

in which 254.24 and 236.23 are the molecular weights of sulfacetamide sodium monohydrate and anhydrous sulfacetamide sodium, respectively, C is the concentration, in μg per mL, calculated on the anhydrous basis, of USP Sulfacetamide Sodium RS in the *Standard preparation*, and r_U and r_S are the peak responses obtained from the *Assay preparation* and the *Standard preparation*, respectively.

Assay for prednisolone acetate—

Mobile phase—Prepare a filtered and degassed mixture of water and acetonitrile (60 : 40). Make adjustments if necessary (see *System Suitability* under *Chromatography* ⟨621⟩).

Internal standard solution—Transfer about 70 mg of norethindrone to a 100-mL volumetric flask, add dilute methanol (9 in 10) to volume, and mix.

Standard preparation—Transfer about 20 mg of USP Prednisolone Acetate RS, accurately weighed, to a 25-mL volumetric flask, add dilute methanol (9 in 10) to volume, and mix. Transfer 5.0 mL of this solution to a 100-mL volumetric flask, add 5.0 mL of *Internal standard solution*, add dilute methanol (9 in 10) to volume, and mix.

Assay preparation—Transfer an accurately weighed quantity of Ophthalmic Ointment, equivalent to about 4 mg of prednisolone acetate, to a 50-mL centrifuge tube. Add 10.0 mL of heptane, and mix, using a vortex mixer for about 2 minutes to dissolve the Ointment. Add 5.0 mL of *Internal standard solution* and 20.0 mL of dilute methanol (9 in 10), and mix, using a vortex mixer for 2 minutes. Centrifuge to effect separation of the phases. Withdraw and discard the upper, heptane layer. Transfer the lower layer to a 100-mL volumetric flask. Add dilute methanol (9 in 10) to volume, and mix to obtain the *Assay preparation*.

Chromatographic system (see *Chromatography* ⟨621⟩)—The liquid chromatograph is equipped with a 254-nm detector and a 3.9-mm × 30-cm column that contains packing L1. The flow rate is about 1.5 mL per minute. Chromatograph the *Standard preparation*, and record the peak responses as directed for *Procedure*: the column efficiency determined from the analyte peak is not less than 3000, the tailing factor for the analyte peak is not more than 2.5, the resolution, R, between the analyte and internal standard peaks is not less than 4.5, and the relative standard deviation for replicate injections is not more than 1.5%.

Procedure—Separately inject equal volumes (about 40 μL) of the *Standard preparation* and the *Assay preparation* into the chromatograph, record the chromatograms, and measure the responses for the major peaks. The relative retention times are about 1.0 for prednisolone acetate and 1.5 for norethindrone. Calculate the quantity, in mg, of $C_{23}H_{30}O_6$ in the portion of the Ophthalmic Ointment taken by the formula:

$$100C(R_U / R_S)$$

in which C is the concentration, in mg per mL, of USP Prednisolone Acetate RS in the *Standard preparation* taken; and R_U and R_S are the peak response ratios obtained from the *Assay preparation* and the *Standard preparation*, respectively.

Sulfacetamide Sodium and Prednisolone Acetate Ophthalmic Suspension

» Sulfacetamide Sodium and Prednisolone Acetate Ophthalmic Suspension is a sterile, aqueous suspension containing not less than 90.0 percent and not more than 110.0 percent of the labeled amounts of sulfacetamide sodium ($C_8H_9N_2NaO_3S.H_2O$) and prednisolone acetate ($C_{23}H_{30}O_6$). It may contain suitable preservatives, buffers, stabilizers, and suspending agents.

Packaging and storage—Preserve in tight containers. The containers or individual cartons are sealed and tamper-proof so that sterility is assured at time of first use.

USP Reference standards ⟨11⟩—*USP Prednisolone Acetate RS. USP Sulfacetamide Sodium RS.*

Identification—

A: Pass about 25 mL of the well-mixed Ophthalmic Suspension through a fine, sintered-glass filter, saving the filtrate. Wash the crystals in the funnel with a small amount of water. Dry the crystals at 105° for 3 hours: the IR absorption spectrum of a potassium bromide dispersion of the crystals exhibits maxima only at the same wavelengths as that of a similar preparation of USP Prednisolone Acetate RS.

B: To the filtrate saved from *Identification* test *A*, add 6 N acetic acid dropwise until the pH is between 4 and 5. Allow crystals of sulfacetamide to develop. Filter the crystals, wash with a small amount of water, and dry at 105° for 2 hours: the IR absorption spectrum of a potassium bromide dispersion of the crystals so obtained exhibits maxima only at the same wavelengths as a preparation of USP Sulfacetamide Sodium RS, similarly treated.

Sterility ⟨71⟩: meets the requirements.

pH ⟨791⟩: between 6.0 and 7.4.

Assay for sulfacetamide sodium—

Mobile phase—Prepare a filtered and degassed mixture of water, methanol, and glacial acetic acid (890 : 100 : 10). Make adjustments if necessary (see *System Suitability* under *Chromatography* ⟨621⟩).

Standard preparation—Dissolve an accurately weighed quantity of USP Sulfacetamide Sodium RS in a mixture of water and methanol (4 : 1), and dilute quantitatively, and stepwise if necessary, with the same solvent mixture to obtain a solution having a known concentration of about 30 μg per mL.

Assay preparation—Transfer an accurately measured volume of Ophthalmic Suspension, freshly mixed and free from air bubbles, equivalent to about 100 mg of sulfacetamide sodium, to a 100-mL volumetric flask, dilute with a mixture of water and methanol (4 : 1) to volume, and mix. Dilute 3.0 mL of this solution with the same solvent mixture to 100.0 mL, and mix.

System suitability preparation—Dissolve about 3 mg of sulfanilamide in 100 mL of the *Standard preparation*, and mix.

Chromatographic system (see *Chromatography* ⟨621⟩)—The liquid chromatograph is equipped with a 254-nm detector and a 4.6-mm × 25-cm column that contains packing L1. The flow rate is about 1.5 mL per minute. Chromatograph the *Standard preparation* and the *System suitability preparation*, and record the peak responses as directed for *Procedure*: the column efficiency determined for the analyte peak is not less than 1500 theoretical plates; the resolution, R, between the sulfacetamide and sulfanilamide peaks is not less than 3; and the relative standard deviation for replicate injections is not more than 2.0%.

Procedure—Separately inject equal volumes (about 90 μL) of the *Standard preparation* and the *Assay preparation* into the chromatograph, record the chromatograms, and measure the responses for the major peaks. Calculate the quantity, in mg, of sulfacetamide sodium ($C_8H_9N_2NaO_3S.H_2O$) in each mL of the Ophthalmic Suspension taken by the formula:

$$3.33(254.24 / 236.23)C(r_U / r_S)$$

in which 254.24 and 236.23 are the molecular weights of sulfacetamide sodium monohydrate and anhydrous sulfacetamide sodium, respectively; *C* is the concentration, in µg per mL, calculated on the anhydrous basis, of USP Sulfacetamide Sodium RS in the *Standard preparation;* and r_U and r_S are the peak responses obtained from the *Assay preparation* and the *Standard preparation*, respectively.

Assay for prednisolone acetate—

Mobile phase—Prepare a filtered and degassed mixture of water and acetonitrile (60 : 40). Make adjustments if necessary (see *System Suitability* under *Chromatography* ⟨621⟩).

Standard preparation—Dissolve an accurately weighed quantity of USP Prednisolone Acetate RS in methanol to obtain a solution containing about 2 mg per mL. Transfer 2.0 mL of this solution to a 100-mL volumetric flask, and dilute with a solvent mixture prepared by dissolving 2.72 g of monobasic potassium phosphate in 300 mL of water and 700 mL of methanol. The *Standard preparation* has a known concentration of about 0.04 mg per mL.

Assay preparation—Using a "To contain" pipet, transfer an accurately measured volume of Ophthalmic Suspension, freshly mixed and free from air bubbles, equivalent to about 10 mg of prednisolone acetate, to a 250-mL volumetric flask. Rinse the pipet with the solvent mixture described under *Standard preparation*, collecting the rinsings in the flask, dilute with the same solvent mixture to volume, and mix.

Chromatographic system (see *Chromatography* ⟨621⟩)—The liquid chromatograph is equipped with a 254-nm detector and a 4.0-mm × 30-cm column that contains packing L1. The flow rate is about 1.5 mL per minute. Chromatograph the *Standard preparation*, and record the peak responses as directed for *Procedure*: the column efficiency determined from the analyte peak is not less than 3000 theoretical plates; and the relative standard deviation for replicate injections is not more than 2.0%.

Procedure—Separately inject equal volumes (about 30 µL) of the *Standard preparation* and the *Assay preparation* into the chromatograph, record the chromatograms, and measure the responses for the major peaks. Calculate the quantity, in mg, of prednisolone acetate ($C_{23}H_{30}O_6$) in each mL of the Ophthalmic Suspension taken by the formula:

$$250(C/V)(r_U/r_S)$$

in which *C* is the concentration, in mg per mL, of USP Prednisolone Acetate RS in the *Standard preparation;* *V* is the volume, in mL, of Ophthalmic Suspension taken; and r_U and r_S are the peak responses obtained from the *Assay preparation* and the *Standard preparation*, respectively.

Sulfachlorpyridazine

$C_{10}H_9ClN_4O_2S$ 284.72
N^1-(6-Chloro-3-pyridazinyl)sulfanilamide   [80-32-0].

» Sulfachlorpyridazine contains not less than 97.0 percent and not more than 103.0 percent of $C_{10}H_9ClN_4O_2S$, calculated on the dried basis.

Packaging and storage—Preserve in well-closed, light-resistant containers.

Labeling—Label it to indicate that it is for veterinary use only.

USP Reference standards ⟨11⟩—*USP Sulfachlorpyridazine RS.*

Identification—

A: *Infrared Absorption* ⟨197M⟩.

B: The retention time of the main peak in the chromatogram of the *Assay preparation*, obtained as directed in the *Assay*, corresponds to that of the main peak observed in the chromatogram of the *Standard preparation*, obtained as directed in the *Assay*.

Clarity and color of solution—Dissolve 1.0 g of it in 50 mL of 0.1 N methanolic hydrochloric acid prepared by diluting 8.6 mL of hydrochloric acid with methanol to obtain 1000 mL of solvent: a clear solution is produced that is not deeper in color than pale yellow.

Acidity—Prepare a suspension of 3.0 g of it in 150.0 mL of carbon dioxide-free water, and heat at 70° for 5 minutes, maintaining the suspension. Cool rapidly in an ice bath to 20 ± 0.5°, stirring by mechanical means. Filter the suspension using vacuum, and collect the filtrate. Titrate 25.0 mL of the clear filtrate with 0.1 N sodium hydroxide VS, using 2 drops of thymolphthalein TS as the indicator. Transfer a second 25.0-mL portion of the clear filtrate to a 250-mL conical flask, add 10 mL of hydrochloric acid, and cool in an ice bath to 15°. Add about 25 g of crushed ice, prepared from frozen purified water, and titrate with 0.1 M sodium nitrite VS, stirring vigorously, until the titrated solution produces an immediate, stable, blue color on starch-iodide paper. The volume of 0.1 N sodium hydroxide consumed in the titration of the first 25.0-mL portion of the filtrate does not exceed the volume of 0.1 M sodium nitrite consumed in the titration of the second 25.0-mL portion of the filtrate by more than 0.5 mL.

Loss on drying ⟨731⟩:   Dry it at 105° for 3 hours: it loses not more than 0.5% of its weight.

Residue on ignition ⟨281⟩:   not more than 0.1%.

Heavy metals, *Method II* ⟨231⟩:   0.002%.

Assay—

pH 2.5 phosphate buffer—Dissolve 14 g of monobasic potassium phosphate in 1600 mL of water, adjust with phosphoric acid to a pH of 2.5 ± 0.1, dilute with water to 2000 mL, and mix.

Mobile phase—Prepare a filtered and degassed mixture of *pH 2.5 phosphate buffer* and methanol (700 : 300). Make adjustments if necessary (see *System Suitability* under *Chromatography* ⟨621⟩).

Standard preparation—Prepare a stock solution of USP Sulfachlorpyridazine RS in methanol having a known concentration of about 0.5 mg per mL. Transfer 3.0 mL of this stock solution to a 100-mL volumetric flask, dilute with *Mobile phase* to volume, and mix. Filter this solution through a nylon filter having a porosity of 0.5 µm or finer, and use the filtrate as the *Standard preparation*. The *Standard preparation* contains about 15 µg of USP Sulfachlorpyridazine RS per mL.

Assay preparation—Transfer about 50 mg of Sulfachlorpyridazine, accurately weighed, to a 100-mL volumetric flask. Dissolve in and dilute with methanol to volume, and mix. Transfer 3.0 mL of this solution to a second 100-mL volumetric flask, dilute with *Mobile phase* to volume, and mix. Filter this solution through a filter having a porosity of 0.5 µm or finer, and use the filtrate as the *Assay preparation*.

Chromatographic system (see *Chromatography* ⟨621⟩)—The liquid chromatograph is equipped with a 265-nm detector, a 4.6-mm × 25-cm analytical column containing 5-µm packing L1, and a guard column containing 5-µm packing L1, and is maintained at about 40°. The flow rate is about 1 mL per minute. Chromatograph the *Standard preparation*, and record the peak responses as directed for *Procedure:* the relative standard deviation for replicate injections is not more than 2.0%.

Procedure—Separately inject equal volumes (about 20 µL) of the *Standard preparation* and the *Assay preparation* into the chromatograph, record the chromatograms, and measure the responses for the major peaks. Calculate the quantity, in mg, of $C_{10}H_9ClN_4O_2S$ in the portion of Sulfachlorpyridazine taken by the formula:

$$(10/3)(C)(r_U/r_S)$$

in which *C* is the concentration, in µg per mL, of USP Sulfachlorpyridazine RS in the *Standard preparation;* and r_U and r_S are the sulfachlorpyridazine peak area responses obtained from the *Assay preparation* and the *Standard preparation*, respectively.

Sulfadiazine

$C_{10}H_{10}N_4O_2S$ 250.28
Benzenesulfonamide, 4-amino-N-2-pyrimidinyl-.
N^1-2-Pyrimidinylsulfanilamide   [68-35-9].

» Sulfadiazine contains not less than 98.0 percent and not more than 102.0 percent of $C_{10}H_{10}N_4O_2S$, calculated on the dried basis.

Packaging and storage—Preserve in well-closed, light-resistant containers.

USP Reference standards ⟨11⟩—*USP Sulfadiazine RS.*

Clarity and color of solution—Dissolve 1 g in a mixture of 20 mL of water and 5 mL of 1 N sodium hydroxide. The solution is clear and not more deeply colored than pale yellow.

Identification—
  A: *Infrared Absorption* ⟨197K⟩.
  B: Carefully melt about 50 mg in a small test tube: a reddish brown color develops. The fumes evolved during the decomposition do not discolor moistened lead acetate test paper (*distinction from sulfathiazole*).
  C: Gently heat about 1 g in a small test tube until a sublimate is formed. Collect a few mg of the sublimate with a glass rod, and mix in a test tube with 1 mL of a 1 in 20 solution of resorcinol in alcohol. Add 1 mL of sulfuric acid, and mix by shaking: a deep red color appears at once. Cautiously dilute the mixture with 25 mL of ice-cold water, and add an excess of 6 N ammonium hydroxide: a blue or reddish blue color is produced.

Acidity—Digest 2.00 g with 100 mL of water at about 70° for 5 minutes. Cool at once to room temperature, and filter. To 25.0 mL of the filtrate add 2 drops of phenolphthalein TS, and titrate with 0.10 N sodium hydroxide: not more than 0.20 mL is required to produce a pink color.

Loss on drying ⟨731⟩—Dry it at 105° for 2 hours: it loses not more than 0.5% of its weight.

Residue on ignition ⟨281⟩: not more than 0.1%.

Selenium ⟨291⟩: 0.003%, a 200-mg test specimen being used.

Heavy metals, *Method II* ⟨231⟩: 0.002%.

Ordinary impurities ⟨466⟩—
  Test solution: 8.3 mg per mL, in a mixture of toluene and dimethylformamide (2 : 1).
  Standard solutions: 0.008, 0.041, 0.08, and 0.17 mg per mL, in a mixture of toluene and dimethylformamide (2 : 1).
  Eluant: a mixture of chloroform, methanol, and ammonium hydroxide (30 : 12 : 1).
  Visualization: 11.

Assay—
  Mobile phase—Prepare a suitable degassed solution of water, acetonitrile, and glacial acetic acid (87 : 12 : 1).
  Standard preparation—Dissolve an accurately weighed quantity of USP Sulfadiazine RS in 0.025 N sodium hydroxide to obtain a solution having a known concentration of about 1 mg per mL.
  Assay preparation—Transfer about 100 mg of Sulfadiazine, accurately weighed, to a 100-mL volumetric flask, add 0.025 N sodium hydroxide to volume, and mix.
  Chromatographic system (see *Chromatography* ⟨621⟩)—The liquid chromatograph is equipped with a 254-nm detector and a 4-mm × 30-cm column that contains packing L1. The flow rate is about 2 mL per minute. Chromatograph five replicate injections of the *Standard preparation*, and record the peak responses as directed for *Procedure*: the relative standard deviation is not more than 2.0%, and the tailing factor for sulfadiazine is not more than 1.5.
  Procedure—Separately inject equal volumes (about 10 µL) of the *Standard preparation* and the *Assay preparation* into the chromatograph, record the chromatograms, and measure the responses for the major peaks. Calculate the quantity, in mg, of $C_{10}H_{10}N_4O_2S$ in the portion of Sulfadiazine taken by the formula:

$$100C(r_U/r_S)$$

in which C is the concentration, in mg per mL, of USP Sulfadiazine RS in the *Standard preparation;* and r_U and r_S are the peak responses for sulfadiazine obtained from the *Assay preparation* and the *Standard preparation*, respectively.

Sulfadiazine Tablets

» Sulfadiazine Tablets contain not less than 95.0 percent and not more than 105.0 percent of the labeled amount of $C_{10}H_{10}N_4O_2S$.

Packaging and storage—Preserve in well-closed, light-resistant containers.

USP Reference standards ⟨11⟩—*USP Sulfadiazine RS.*

Identification—Triturate a quantity of finely powdered Tablets, equivalent to about 500 mg of sulfadiazine, with 5 mL of chloroform, and transfer to a small filter. Wash with another 5-mL portion of chloroform, and discard the filtrate. Triturate the residue with 10 mL of 6 N ammonium hydroxide for 5 minutes, add 10 mL of water, and filter. Warm the filtrate until most of the ammonia is expelled, cool, and add 6 N acetic acid until the reaction is distinctly acid: a precipitate of sulfadiazine is formed. Collect the precipitate on a filter, wash it with cold water, and dry at 105° for 1 hour: the sulfadiazine so obtained melts between 250° and 254°, as determined by the method for *Class Ia* under *Melting Range or Temperature* ⟨741⟩ and responds to *Identification* test A under *Sulfadiazine*.

Dissolution ⟨711⟩—
  Medium: 0.1 N hydrochloric acid; 900 mL.
  Apparatus 2: 75 rpm.
  Time: 90 minutes.
  Procedure—Determine the amount of $C_{10}H_{10}N_4O_2S$ dissolved by employing UV absorption at the wavelength of maximum absorbance at about 254 nm on filtered portions of the solution under test, suitably diluted with 0.01 N sodium hydroxide, in comparison with a Standard solution having a known concentration of USP Sulfadiazine RS in the same media.
  Tolerances—Not less than 70% (*Q*) of the labeled amount of $C_{10}H_{10}N_4O_2S$ is dissolved in 90 minutes.

Uniformity of dosage units ⟨905⟩: meet the requirements.

Assay—
  Mobile phase and *Standard preparation*—Prepare as directed in the *Assay* under *Sulfadiazine*.
  Assay preparation—Weigh and finely powder not less than 20 Tablets. Transfer an accurately weighed portion of the powder, equivalent to about 100 mg of sulfadiazine, to a 100-mL volumetric flask, add 75 mL of 0.025 N sodium hydroxide, shake for 30 minutes, dilute with 0.025 N sodium hydroxide to volume, mix, and centrifuge.
  Chromatographic system and *Procedure*—Proceed as directed for *Chromatographic system* and for *Procedure* in the *Assay* under *Sulfadiazine*. Calculate the quantity, in mg, of $C_{10}H_{10}N_4O_2S$ in the portion of Tablets taken by the formula:

$$100C(r_U/r_S)$$

in which the terms are as defined therein.

Silver Sulfadiazine

$C_{10}H_9AgN_4O_2S$ 357.14

Benzenesulfonamide, 4-amino-*N*-2-pyrimidinyl-, monosilver(1+) salt.
N^1-2-Pyrimidinylsulfanilamide monosilver(1+) salt   [22199-08-2].

» Silver Sulfadiazine contains not less than 98.0 percent and not more than 102.0 percent of $C_{10}H_9AgN_4O_2S$, calculated on the dried basis.

Packaging and storage—Preserve in well-closed, light-resistant containers.

USP Reference standards ⟨11⟩—*USP Silver Sulfadiazine RS.*

Identification—
  A: *Infrared Absorption* ⟨197K⟩.
  B: The R_F value of the principal spot in the thin-layer chromatogram of the *Test solution* as obtained in the test for *Chromatographic purity* corresponds to that obtained from *Standard solution A*.
  C: Dissolve about 1 g in 15 mL of ammonium hydroxide and 15 mL of water in a 50-mL volumetric flask, dilute with water to volume, and mix: the solution so obtained responds to the tests for *Silver* ⟨191⟩.

Particle size—[NOTE—Perform in subdued light.] Wrap a 1-L flask in aluminum foil, add 0.5 g of Silver Sulfadiazine, add 1000 mL of a suitable isotonic solution, and mix for 2 hours. Add 5 or 6 drops of a suitable dispersant. Place the container in an ultrasonic bath, sonicate for 15 seconds, and immediately analyze, using a suitable electronic particle counter equipped with a population counter and 140- and 30-μm apertures. The average particle size is not greater than 10 μm and the size of not more than 10% of the particles is greater than 40 μm.

Loss on drying ⟨731⟩—Dry it at 105° for 1 hour: it loses not more than 0.5% of its weight.

Limit of nitrate—
Standard solution—Prepare a solution of potassium nitrate in water having a known concentration of about 200 μg of nitrate per mL.
Test solution—Transfer about 2 g of Silver Sulfadiazine, accurately weighed, to a beaker, add 30.0 mL of water, stir for 20 minutes, and filter through a suitable, nitrate-free filter.
Procedure—Pipet 3 mL of the *Test solution* and of deionized water to provide the blank into separate test tubes. Pipet 1 mL of the *Standard solution* and 2 mL of water into a third test tube. Cool the three test tubes in an ice bath. Slowly add 7.0 mL of cold chromotropic acid solution, prepared by dissolving 50 mg of chromotropic acid in 100 mL of cold sulfuric acid, to each test tube, while swirling, and allow the test tubes to remain in the ice bath for 3 minutes after the addition of the chromotropic acid solution. Remove the test tubes from the ice bath, and allow to stand for 30 minutes. Concomitantly determine the absorbances of the *Test solution* and the *Standard solution* at the wavelength of maximum absorbance at about 408 nm, with a suitable spectrophotometer, against the blank. Calculate the nitrate content, in mg, in the portion of Silver Sulfadiazine taken by the formula:

$$0.01C(A_U/A_S)$$

in which *C* is the concentration, in μg per mL, of nitrate in the *Standard solution;* and A_U and A_S are the absorbances obtained from the *Test solution* and the *Standard solution*, respectively: not more than 0.1% is found.

Chromatographic purity—
Standard solution A—Transfer about 50 mg of USP Silver Sulfadiazine RS to a 10-mL volumetric flask, and dissolve in 3.0 mL of ammonium hydroxide. Dilute with methanol to volume, and mix to obtain a solution having a known concentration of about 5 mg per mL.

Standard solution B—Dilute a volume of *Standard solution A* quantitatively, and stepwise if necessary, with a mixture of methanol and ammonium hydroxide (4 : 1) to obtain a solution having a known concentration of about 0.05 mg per mL.

Test solution—Transfer about 50 mg of Silver Sulfadiazine to a 10-mL volumetric flask, and dissolve in 3.0 mL of ammonium hydroxide. Dilute with methanol to volume, and mix to obtain a solution having a known concentration of about 5 mg per mL.

Procedure—Prepare a chromatographic chamber containing a mixture of chloroform, methanol, and ammonium hydroxide (7 : 4 : 1) as the developing solvent. [NOTE—Mix the chloroform and methanol, then add the ammonium hydroxide.] Separately apply 10-μL portions of *Standard solution A*, *Standard solution B*, and the *Test solution* to a suitable thin-layer chromatographic plate (see *Chromatography* ⟨621⟩) coated with a 0.25-mm layer of chromatographic silica gel mixture. Allow the spots to dry, and place the plate in the chromatographic chamber. When the solvent front has moved about three-fourths of the length of the plate, remove the plate from the chamber, mark the solvent front, and allow the solvent to evaporate. Examine the plate under short-wavelength UV light: no secondary spot in the chromatogram of the *Test solution* is larger or more intense than the principal spot obtained from *Standard solution B* (1.0%), and the sum of all secondary spots observed is not greater than 2.0%.

Silver content—Transfer about 500 mg, accurately weighed, to a beaker, add 150 mL of water and 50 mL of nitric acid, and stir for 15 minutes. Titrate with 0.1 N potassium thiocyanate VS to a potentiometric endpoint, using a silver-based indicator electrode and a double-junction reference electrode. Perform a blank determination (see *Titrimetry* ⟨541⟩), and make any necessary correction. Each mL of 0.1 N potassium thiocyanate is equivalent to 10.79 mg of silver: not less than 29.3% and not more than 30.5% of silver is found.

Assay—
Mobile phase—Prepare a degassed solution consisting of water, acetonitrile, and phosphoric acid (900 : 99 : 1). Make adjustments if necessary (see *System Suitability* under *Chromatography* ⟨621⟩).

Diluting solution—Transfer 100 mL of ammonium hydroxide to a 1-liter volumetric flask, dilute with water to volume, and mix.

Internal standard solution—Dissolve an accurately weighed quantity of sulfamerazine in *Diluting solution*, and dilute quantitatively, and stepwise if necessary, with *Diluting solution* to obtain a solution having a concentration of about 10 mg per mL.

Standard stock solution—Dissolve about 250 mg of USP Silver Sulfadiazine RS, accurately weighed, in 100 mL of *Diluting solution* in a 200-mL volumetric flask, and sonicate for five minutes. Add 25.0 mL of *Internal standard solution*, dilute with *Diluting solution* to volume, and mix.

Standard preparation—Pipet 2.0 mL of *Standard* into a 50-mL volumetric flask. Dilute with *Mobile phase* to volume, and mix.

Assay preparation—Transfer about 250 mg of Silver Sulfadiazine, accurately weighed, to a 50-mL round-bottom centrifuge tube. Add about 35 mL of methanol, tightly seal the tube with a cap containing an inert liner, and mix, using a vortex mixer, for about 15 seconds. Centrifuge for 15 minutes to separate the phases. Aspirate, and discard the methanol supernatant layer. [NOTE—Care should be taken to avoid aspirating any of the residue.] Pipet 25.0 mL of *Internal standard solution* into a 200-mL volumetric flask. Add about 30 mL of *Diluting solution* to the centrifuge tube, replace the cap, and mix, using a vortex mixer, for about 15 seconds. Quantitatively transfer the contents to the 200-mL volumetric flask, using the *Diluting solution* to rinse the tube. Repeat the addition of 30 mL of *Diluting solution*, mixing and quantitatively transferring three more times. Dilute with the *Diluting solution* to volume, and mix. Sonicate if necessary to obtain dissolution of the residue. Pipet 2.0 mL into a 50-mL volumetric flask, dilute with *Mobile phase* to volume, mix, and filter.

Chromatographic system (see *Chromatography* ⟨621⟩)—The liquid chromatograph is equipped with a 254-nm detector and a 3.9-mm × 30-cm column that contains packing L1. The flow rate is about 2.0 mL per minute. Chromatograph the *Standard preparation*, and record the responses as directed for *Procedure:* the resolution, *R*, between sulfadiazine and sulfamerazine is not less than 2.0, and the relative standard deviation for replicate injections is not more than 2.0%.

Procedure—Separately inject equal volumes (about 10 µL) of the *Standard preparation* and the *Assay preparation* into the chromatograph, record the chromatograms, and measure the responses for the major peaks. Calculate the quantity, in mg, of $C_{10}H_9AgN_4O_2S$ in the portion of Silver Sulfadiazine taken by the formula:

$$200C(R_U/R_S)$$

in which C is the concentration, in mg per mL, of Silver Sulfadiazine in the *Standard stock preparation*; and R_U and R_S are the relative peak ratios obtained from the *Assay preparation* and the *Standard preparation*, respectively.

Silver Sulfadiazine Cream

» Silver Sulfadiazine Cream contains not less than 90.0 percent and not more than 110.0 percent of the labeled amount of $C_{10}H_9AgN_4O_2S$.

Packaging and storage—Preserve in collapsible tubes or in tight, light-resistant containers.
USP Reference standards ⟨11⟩—*USP Silver Sulfadiazine RS. USP Sulfadiazine RS.*
Identification—Dissolve about 35 mg of USP Sulfadiazine RS in 4 mL of ammonium hydroxide, add 16 mL of methanol, and mix to obtain the Standard solution. Transfer a quantity of Cream, equivalent to about 50 mg of silver sulfadiazine, to a stoppered, 50-mL conical flask, add 4 mL of ammonium hydroxide, and mix until a smooth paste has been obtained. Add 16 mL of methanol, shake for 5 minutes, and filter to obtain the test solution: the test solution so obtained responds to the *Thin-layer Chromatographic Identification Test* ⟨201⟩, a mixture of chloroform, methanol, and ammonium hydroxide (7 : 4 : 1) being used as the developing solvent. [NOTE—Prepare the developing solvent by first mixing the chloroform and methanol, and then adding the ammonium hydroxide.]
Microbial limits ⟨61⟩—It meets the requirements of the tests for absence of *Staphylococcus aureus, Pseudomonas aeruginosa, Salmonella species,* and *Escherichia coli* and the total count does not exceed 23 cfu per g. It meets also the requirements for *Total Combined Molds and Yeasts Count,* fewer than 10 cfu per g being found.
Minimum fill ⟨755⟩: meets the requirements.
pH ⟨791⟩: between 4.0 and 7.0, determined in the supernatant obtained from a 1 in 20 mixture of the Cream in water.
Assay—
   Mobile phase and *Diluting solution*—Proceed as directed in the *Assay* under *Silver Sulfadiazine.*
   Internal standard solution—Dissolve an accurately weighed quantity of sulfamerazine in *Diluting solution,* and dilute quantitatively, and stepwise if necessary, with *Diluting solution* to obtain a solution having a known concentration of about 2 mg per mL.
   Standard stock solution—Dissolve an accurately weighed quantity of USP Silver Sulfadiazine RS in *Diluting solution* to obtain a solution having a known concentration of about 1 mg per mL.
   Standard preparation 1—Pipet 10.0 mL of the *Standard stock solution* into a 50-mL test tube. Add 20 mL of alcohol and 5.0 mL of the *Internal standard solution,* and mix.
   Standard preparation 2—Pipet 2.0 mL of *Standard preparation 1* into a 50-mL test tube. Add 40 mL of *Mobile phase,* and mix.
   Assay preparation—Transfer an accurately weighed portion of Cream, equivalent to about 10 mg of silver sulfadiazine, to a 50-mL round-bottom centrifuge tube. Add about 30 mL of methanol, tightly seal the tube with a cap containing an inert liner, and mix, using a vortex mixer, for about 15 seconds. Centrifuge for 15 minutes. Aspirate, and discard the methanol. [NOTE—Care should be taken to avoid aspirating any of the residue.] Transfer 5.0 mL of the *Internal standard solution* into the tube, and add 20 mL of alcohol. Replace the cap, and mix. Heat in a water bath at 60°, with periodic mixing, for 15 minutes to melt and disperse the Cream. While the mixture is still hot, transfer 10.0 mL of *Diluting solution* to the tube, mix, and cool to room temperature. Transfer 2.0 mL of this solution to another tube, add 40 mL of *Mobile phase,* mix, and filter.

Chromatographic system—Proceed as directed in the *Assay* under *Silver Sulfadiazine.* Chromatograph replicate injections of *Standard preparation 2,* and record the peak responses as directed for *Procedure:* the resolution, R, between sulfadiazine and sulfamerazine is not less than 2.0, and the relative standard deviation for replicate injections is not more than 2.0%.
   Procedure—Separately inject equal volumes (about 10 µL) of *Standard preparation 2* and the *Assay preparation* into the chromatograph, record the chromatograms, and measure the responses for the major peaks. Calculate the quantity, in mg, of silver sulfadiazine in the portion of Cream taken by the formula:

$$10C(R_U/R_S)$$

in which C is the concentration, in mg per mL, of USP Silver Sulfadiazine RS in the *Standard stock solution;* and R_U and R_S are the relative peak response ratios obtained from the *Assay preparation* and *Standard preparation 2,* respectively.

Sulfadiazine Sodium

$C_{10}H_9N_4NaO_2S$ 272.26
Benzenesulfonamide, 4-amino-*N*-2-pyrimidinyl-, monosodium salt.
N^1-2-Pyrimidinylsulfanilamide monosodium salt   [547-32-0].

» Sulfadiazine Sodium contains not less than 99.0 percent and not more than 100.5 percent of $C_{10}H_9N_4NaO_2S$, calculated on the dried basis.

Packaging and storage—Preserve in tight, light-resistant containers. Store at 25°, excursions permitted between 15° and 30°.
USP Reference standards ⟨11⟩—*USP Sulfadiazine RS.*
Identification—
   A: Dissolve about 1.5 g in 25 mL of water, and add 3 mL of 6 N acetic acid: a white precipitate of sulfadiazine is formed. Collect the precipitate on a filter, wash it well with cold water, and dry at 105° for 1 hour: the sulfadiazine so obtained melts between 250° and 254° as determined by the method for *Class Ia* under *Melting Range or Temperature* ⟨741⟩, and responds to *Identification* test *A* under *Sulfadiazine.*
   B: Ignite about 500 mg: the residue responds to the tests for *Sodium* ⟨191⟩.
Loss on drying ⟨731⟩—Dry it at 105° for 2 hours: it loses not more than 0.5% of its weight.
Selenium ⟨291⟩: 0.003%, a 200-mg test specimen being used.
Heavy metals—Dissolve 1.0 g in 25 mL of water, and add 5 drops of sodium sulfide TS: any dark color produced is not darker than that in a blank to which 2 mL of *Standard Lead Solution* (see *Heavy Metals* ⟨231⟩) has been added (0.002%).
Assay—Proceed with Sulfadiazine Sodium as directed under *Nitrite Titration* ⟨451⟩. Each mL of 0.1 M sodium nitrite is equivalent to 27.23 mg of $C_{10}H_9N_4NaO_2S$.

Sulfadiazine Sodium Injection

» Sulfadiazine Sodium Injection is a sterile solution of Sulfadiazine Sodium in Water for Injection. It contains, in each mL, not less than 237.5 mg and not more than 262.5 mg of $C_{10}H_9N_4NaO_2S$.

Packaging and storage—Preserve in single-dose, light-resistant containers, of Type I glass.
USP Reference standards ⟨11⟩—*USP Endotoxin RS. USP Sulfadiazine RS.*
Identification—It responds to *Identification* test A under *Sulfadiazine Sodium.*
Bacterial endotoxins ⟨85⟩—It contains not more than 0.1 USP Endotoxin Unit per mg of sulfadiazine sodium.

pH ⟨791⟩: between 8.5 and 10.5.
Particulate matter ⟨788⟩: meets the requirements under small-volume injections.
Other requirements—It meets the requirements under *Injections* ⟨1⟩.
Assay—Pipet a volume of *Injection*, equivalent to about 500 mg of sulfadiazine sodium, into a beaker or a casserole, and proceed as directed under *Nitrite Titration* ⟨451⟩, beginning with "Add 20 mL of hydrochloric acid." Each mL of 0.1 M sodium nitrite is equivalent to 27.23 mg of $C_{10}H_9N_4NaO_2S$.

Sulfadimethoxine

$C_{12}H_{14}N_4O_4S$ 310.34
Benzenesulfonamide, 4-amino-*N*-(2,6-dimethoxy-4-pyrimidinyl)-.
N^1-(2,6-Dimethoxy-4-pyrimidinyl)sulfanilamide   [122-11-2].

» Sulfadimethoxine contains not less than 98.0 percent and not more than 102.0 percent of $C_{12}H_{14}N_4O_4S$, calculated on the dried basis.

Packaging and storage—Preserve in tight, light-resistant containers, and store at controlled room temperature.
Labeling—Label it to indicate that it is for veterinary use only.
USP Reference standards ⟨11⟩—*USP Sulfadimethoxine RS*.
Identification—
  A: *Infrared Absorption* ⟨197K⟩.
  B: *Ultraviolet Absorption* ⟨197U⟩—
  Solution: 1 in 100,000.
  Medium: alcohol.
  Absorptivities, calculated on the dried basis, at 272 nm do not differ by more than 3.0%.
  C: To about 100 mg, add 3 mL of 2.5 N sodium hydroxide and 50 mL of water, mix until dissolved, and dilute with water to 100 mL. To about 5 mL of this solution, add 100 mg of phenol, and heat to boiling. Cool the solution, and add 0.5 mL of sodium hypochlorite TS and 3 drops of 2.5 N sodium hydroxide: a yellow color is produced.
  D: To about 10 mg dissolved in 2 mL of diluted hydrochloric acid, add 3 drops of sodium nitrite solution (1 in 100), and dilute with water to 4 mL: the solution turns yellow. Add 1 mL of 2.5 N sodium hydroxide containing 10 mg of 2-naphthol: a red-orange precipitate is formed.
Melting range ⟨741⟩: between 197° and 202°.
Loss on drying ⟨731⟩: Dry it at 105° for 3 hours: it loses not more than 0.5% of its weight.
Residue on ignition ⟨281⟩: not more than 0.1%.
Heavy metals, *Method II* ⟨231⟩: 0.002%.
Assay—
  Mobile phase—Dissolve 6 g of monobasic sodium phosphate in water to make 1000 mL. Adjust with 50% (w/v) sodium hydroxide solution to a pH of 7.0. Prepare a mixture of this solution and methanol (300 : 100). Make adjustments if necessary (see *System Suitability* under *Chromatography* ⟨621⟩).
  Standard preparation—Quantitatively dissolve an accurately weighed quantity of USP Sulfadimethoxine RS in *Mobile phase* to obtain a solution having a known concentration of about 0.2 mg per mL. Protect this solution from light.
  Assay preparation—Transfer about 20 mg of Sulfadimethoxine, accurately weighed, to a 100-mL volumetric flask, add about 75 mL of *Mobile phase*, and swirl to dissolve. Dilute this solution with *Mobile phase* to volume, and mix. Protect this solution from light.
  Chromatographic system (see *Chromatography* ⟨621⟩)—The liquid chromatograph is equipped with a 254-nm detector and a 4.6-mm × 25-cm column that contains packing L1. The flow rate is about 1 mL per minute. Chromatograph the *Standard preparation*, and record the peak responses as directed for *Procedure:* the tailing factor is not more than 1.5; and the relative standard deviation for replicate injections is not more than 1.0%.
  Procedure—Separately inject equal volumes (about 10 μL) of the *Standard preparation* and the *Assay preparation* into the chromatograph, record the chromatograms, and measure the responses for the major peaks. Calculate the quantity, in mg, of $C_{12}H_{14}N_4O_4S$ in the portion of Sulfadimethoxine taken by the formula:

$$100C(r_U/r_S)$$

in which *C* is the concentration, in mg per mL, of USP Sulfadimethoxine RS in the *Standard preparation;* and r_U and r_S are the peak responses obtained from the *Assay preparation* and the *Standard preparation*, respectively.

Sulfadimethoxine Soluble Powder

» Sulfadimethoxine Soluble Powder contains Sulfadimethoxine Sodium equivalent to not less than 90.0 percent and not more than 110.0 percent of the labeled amount of sulfadimethoxine ($C_{12}H_{14}N_4O_4S$).

Packaging and storage—Preserve in tight, light-resistant containers, and store at controlled room temperature.
Labeling—Label it to indicate that it is for veterinary use only.
USP Reference standards ⟨11⟩—*USP Sulfadimethoxine RS*.
Identification—Shake a quantity equivalent to about 1 g with 5 mL of diluted hydrochloric acid and 10 mL of water. Filter, and to the filtrate add 2.5 N sodium hydroxide dropwise until a precipitate forms and redissolves. Add diluted hydrochloric acid dropwise until a precipitate forms. Collect the precipitate on a very fine filter, and wash it with water and with ether: the sulfadimethoxine so obtained meets the requirements for the *Identification* tests under *Sulfadimethoxine*.
Minimum fill ⟨755⟩: meets the requirements.
pH ⟨791⟩: between 7.0 and 8.0, in a solution (1 in 20).
Assay—
  Mobile phase, Standard preparation, and *Chromatographic system*—Proceed as directed in the *Assay* under *Sulfadimethoxine*.
  Assay preparation—Transfer an accurately weighed portion of Powder, equivalent to about 50 mg of sulfadimethoxine, to a 250-mL volumetric flask, add about 200 mL of *Mobile phase*, and swirl to dissolve. Dilute with *Mobile phase* to volume, and mix. Protect this solution from light.
  Procedure—Proceed as directed in the *Assay* under *Sulfadimethoxine*. Calculate the quantity, in mg, of sulfadimethoxine ($C_{12}H_{14}N_4O_4S$) in the portion of Powder taken by the formula:

$$250C(r_U/r_S)$$

in which *C* is the concentration, in mg per mL, of USP Sulfadimethoxine RS in the *Standard preparation;* and r_U and r_S are the peak responses obtained from the *Assay preparation* and the *Standard preparation*, respectively.

Sulfadimethoxine Oral Suspension

» Sulfadimethoxine Oral Suspension contains not less than 90.0 percent and not more than 110.0 percent of the labeled amount of sulfadimethoxine ($C_{12}H_{14}N_4O_4S$).

Packaging and storage—Preserve in tight, light-resistant containers, and store at controlled room temperature.

Labeling—Label it to indicate that it is for veterinary use only.

USP Reference standards ⟨11⟩—*USP Sulfadimethoxine RS.*
Identification—Shake a quantity equivalent to about 50 mg with 50 mL of water, and add 2.5 N sodium hydroxide dropwise until the solution becomes clear. Add diluted hydrochloric acid dropwise until a precipitate forms. Collect the precipitate on a very fine filter, and wash it with water and with ether: the sulfadimethoxine so obtained meets the requirements for the *Identification* tests under *Sulfadimethoxine.*
pH ⟨791⟩: between 5.0 and 7.0.
Assay—
  Mobile phase, Standard preparation, and *Chromatographic system*—Proceed as directed in the *Assay* under *Sulfadimethoxine.*
  Assay preparation—Transfer an accurately measured volume of Suspension, previously mixed and free from air bubbles, equivalent to about 50 mg of sulfadimethoxine, to a 250-mL volumetric flask, add about 200 mL of *Mobile phase,* and swirl to dissolve. Dilute with *Mobile phase* to volume, and mix. Protect this solution from light.
  Procedure—Proceed as directed in the *Assay* under *Sulfadimethoxine.* Calculate the quantity, in mg, of sulfadimethoxine ($C_{12}H_{14}N_4O_4S$) in each mL of the Oral Suspension taken by the formula:

$$250(C/V)(r_U/r_S)$$

in which V is the volume, in mL, of Oral Suspension taken to prepare the *Assay preparation;* and the other terms are as defined therein.

Sulfadimethoxine Tablets

» Sulfadimethoxine Tablets contain not less than 90.0 percent and not more than 110.0 percent of the labeled amount of sulfadimethoxine ($C_{12}H_{14}N_4O_4S$).

Packaging and storage—Preserve in tight, light-resistant containers, and store at controlled room temperature.
Labeling—Label the Tablets to indicate that they are for veterinary use only.

USP Reference standards ⟨11⟩—*USP Sulfadimethoxine RS.*
Identification—Shake a quantity of finely powdered Tablets, equivalent to about 1 g of sulfadimethoxine, with 5 mL of diluted hydrochloric acid and 10 mL of water. Filter, and to the filtrate add 2.5 N sodium hydroxide dropwise until a precipitate forms and redissolves. Add diluted hydrochloric acid dropwise until a precipitate forms. Collect the filtrate on a very fine filter, and wash it with water and with ether: the sulfadimethoxine so obtained meets the requirements for the *Identification* tests under *Sulfadimethoxine.*
Disintegration ⟨701⟩: 30 minutes.
Uniformity of dosage units ⟨905⟩: meet the requirements.
Assay—
  Mobile phase, Standard preparation, and *Chromatographic system*—Proceed as directed in the *Assay* under *Sulfadimethoxine.*
  Assay preparation—Weigh and finely powder not fewer than 20 Tablets. Transfer an accurately weighed portion of the powder, equivalent to about 50 mg of sulfadimethoxine, to a 250-mL volumetric flask, add about 200 mL of *Mobile phase,* and swirl to dissolve. Dilute with *Mobile phase* to volume, and mix. Filter if necessary to obtain a clear solution. Protect this solution from light.
  Procedure—Proceed as directed in the *Assay* under *Sulfadimethoxine.* Calculate the quantity, in mg, of sulfadimethoxine ($C_{12}H_{14}N_4O_4S$) in the portion of Tablets taken by the formula:

$$250C(r_U/r_S)$$

in which the terms are as defined therein.

Sulfadimethoxine Sodium

$C_{12}H_{13}N_4NaO_4S$ 332.31
Benzenesulfonamide, 4-amino-*N*-(2,6-dimethoxy-4-pyrimidinyl)-, monosodium salt.
N^1-(2,6-Dimethoxy-4-pyrimidinyl)sulfanilamide   monosodium salt   [*1037-50-9*].

» Sulfadimethoxine Sodium contains not less than 98.0 percent and not more than 102.0 percent of $C_{12}H_{13}N_4NaO_4S$, calculated on the dried basis.

Packaging and storage—Preserve in tight, light-resistant containers, and store at controlled room temperature.
Labeling—Label it to indicate that it is for veterinary use only.
USP Reference standards ⟨11⟩—*USP Sulfadimethoxine RS.*
Identification—
  A: To about 100 mg, add 50 mL of water, mix until dissolved, and dilute with water to 100 mL. To about 5 mL of this solution add 100 mg of phenol, and heat to boiling. Cool the solution, and add 0.5 mL of sodium hypochlorite TS and 3 drops of 2.5 N sodium hydroxide: a yellow color is produced.
  B: The retention time of the major peak in the chromatogram of the *Assay preparation* corresponds to that in the chromatogram of the *Standard preparation,* as obtained in the *Assay.*
  C: Dissolve 10 mg in 2 mL of diluted hydrochloric acid, add 3 drops of sodium nitrite solution (1 in 100), and dilute with water to 4 mL: the solution turns yellow. Add 1 mL of 2.5 N sodium hydroxide containing 10 mg of 2-naphthol: a red-orange precipitate is formed.
pH ⟨791⟩: between 8.0 and 9.5, in a solution (1 in 20).
Loss on drying ⟨731⟩—Dry it at 105° for 3 hours: it loses not more than 5.0% of its weight.
Heavy metals—Dissolve 1.0 g in 25 mL of water, and add 5 drops of freshly prepared sodium sulfide TS: any color produced is not darker than that of a control made with 23 mL of water, 2.0 mL of *Standard Lead Solution* (see *Heavy Metals* ⟨231⟩), and 5 drops of freshly prepared sodium sulfide TS (0.002%).
Assay—
  Mobile phase, Standard preparation, and *Chromatographic system*—Proceed as directed in the *Assay* under *Sulfadimethoxine.*
  Assay preparation—Transfer about 60 mg of Sulfadimethoxine Sodium, accurately weighed, to a 250-mL volumetric flask, add about 200 mL of *Mobile phase,* and swirl to dissolve. Dilute with *Mobile phase* to volume, and mix. Protect this solution from light.
  Procedure—Proceed as directed in the *Assay* under *Sulfadimethoxine.* Calculate the quantity, in mg, of $C_{12}H_{13}N_4NaO_4S$ in the portion of Sulfadimethoxine Sodium taken by the formula:

$$(332.31/310.34)(250C)(r_U/r_S)$$

in which 332.31 and 310.34 are the molecular weights of sulfadimethoxine sodium and sulfadimethoxine, respectively; and the other terms are as defined therein.

Sulfadoxine

$C_{12}H_{14}N_4O_4S$ 310.33
Benzenesulfonamide, 4-amino-*N*-(5,6-dimethoxy-4-pyrimidinyl)-.
N^1-(5,6-Dimethoxy-4-pyrimidinyl)sulfanilamide   [*2447-57-6*].

» Sulfadoxine contains not less than 99.0 percent and not more than 101.0 percent of $C_{12}H_{14}N_4O_4S$, calculated on the dried basis.

Packaging and storage—Preserve in well-closed, light-resistant containers.

USP Reference standards⟨11⟩—*USP Sulfadoxine RS.*
Identification—
  A: *Infrared Absorption* ⟨197K⟩.
  B: *Ultraviolet Absorption* ⟨197U⟩—
  Solution: 6 μg per mL.
  Medium: 0.1 N sodium hydroxide.
Melting range ⟨741⟩: between 197° and 200°.
Loss on drying ⟨731⟩—Dry it at 105° for 4 hours: it loses not more than 0.5% of its weight.
Residue on ignition ⟨281⟩: not more than 0.1%.
Heavy metals, *Method II* ⟨231⟩: 0.002%.
Chromatographic purity—Prepare a solution in a mixture of alcohol and ammonium hydroxide (9 : 1) having a concentration of about 20 mg per mL. Prepare a Standard solution of USP Sulfadoxine RS having a concentration of about 0.10 mg per mL in a mixture of alcohol and ammonium hydroxide (9 : 1). Separately apply 10 μL each of the test solution and the Standard solution to a suitable chromatographic plate (see *Chromatography* ⟨621⟩) coated with a 0.25-mm layer of chromatographic silica gel. Develop the chromatogram in a solvent system consisting of a mixture of chloroform, methanol, and dimethylformamide (20 : 2 : 1) until the solvent front has moved about three-fourths of the length of the plate. Remove the plate from the chamber, and air-dry. Spray the dried plate with a 1 in 10 solution of sulfuric acid in alcohol, and expose to nitrous fumes generated by adding 7 M sulfuric acid dropwise to a solution containing 10% sodium nitrite and 3% potassium iodide. Dry the plate in a current of warm air for 15 minutes, and spray with a 1 in 200 solution of *N*-(1-naphthyl)ethylenediamine dihydrochloride in alcohol. No spot in the test solution, other than the principal spot, is greater in size and intensity than the spot obtained from the Standard solution.
Assay—Proceed with Sulfadoxine as directed under *Nitrite Titration* ⟨451⟩. Each mL of 0.1 M sodium nitrite is equivalent to 31.03 mg of $C_{12}H_{14}N_4O_4S$.

Sulfadoxine and Pyrimethamine Tablets

» Sulfadoxine and Pyrimethamine Tablets contain not less than 90.0 percent and not more than 110.0 percent of the labeled amount of sulfadoxine ($C_{12}H_{14}N_4O_4S$) and not less than 90.0 percent and not more than 110.0 percent of the labeled amount of pyrimethamine ($C_{12}H_{13}ClN_4$).

Packaging and storage—Preserve in well-closed, light-resistant containers.

USP Reference standards ⟨11⟩—*USP Sulfadoxine RS. USP Pyrimethamine RS.*
Identification—
  A: The retention times of the major peaks in the chromatogram of the *Assay preparation* correspond to those of the *Standard preparations* of sulfadoxine and pyrimethamine, relative to the internal standard, as obtained in the *Assay*.
  B: Vigorously shake 700 mg of finely ground Tablet powder with 50 mL of a 1 in 50 solution of ammonium hydroxide in methanol for 3 minutes, and filter. Separately apply 10 μL each of the test solution, a Standard solution of USP Sulfadoxine RS similarly prepared, containing 10 mg per mL, and a Standard solution of USP Pyrimethamine RS similarly prepared, containing 0.5 mg per mL, to a suitable thin-layer chromatographic plate (see *Chromatography* ⟨621⟩) coated with a 0.25-mm layer of chromatographic silica gel mixture. Dry the spots in a current of warm air, and develop the plate in a solvent system consisting of a mixture of heptane, chloroform, a 1 in 20 solution of methanol in alcohol, and glacial acetic acid (4 : 4 : 4 : 1). Allow the solvent front to move about two-thirds of the length of the plate, remove the plate, dry, and examine under short-wavelength UV light: the R_F values of the principal spots from the solution under test correspond to the R_F values of the principal spots from the corresponding Standard solutions.
Dissolution ⟨711⟩—
  Medium: pH 6.8 phosphate buffer, prepared as directed under *Buffer Solutions* in the section *Reagents, Indicators, and Solutions*; 1000 mL.
  Apparatus 2: 75 rpm.
  Time: 30 minutes.
  Procedure—Determine the amounts of $C_{12}H_{14}N_4O_4S$ and $C_{12}H_{13}ClN_4$ dissolved, employing the procedure set forth in the *Assay*, making any necessary modifications.
  Tolerances—Not less than 60% *(Q)* of the labeled amount of each of $C_{12}H_{14}N_4O_4S$ and $C_{12}H_{13}ClN_4$ is dissolved in 30 minutes.
Uniformity of dosage units ⟨905⟩: meet the requirements for *Content Uniformity* with respect to sulfadoxine and to pyrimethamine.
Assay—
  Mobile phase—Prepare a suitable degassed and filtered mixture of dilute glacial acetic acid (1 in 100) and acetonitrile (4 : 1).
  Internal standard solution—Prepare a solution of phenacetin in acetonitrile having a concentration of 1 mg per mL.
  Standard stock solution—Transfer about 500 mg, accurately weighed, of USP Sulfadoxine RS and 25 mg, accurately weighed, of USP Pyrimethamine RS to a 100-mL volumetric flask, dissolve in 35 mL of acetonitrile, dilute with *Mobile phase* to volume, and mix.
  Standard preparation 1—Pipet 25 mL of *Standard stock solution* and 2 mL of *Internal standard solution* into a 50-mL volumetric flask, dilute with *Mobile phase* to volume, and mix.
  Standard preparation 2—Pipet 2 mL of *Standard stock solution* and 10 mL of *Internal standard solution* into a 250-mL volumetric flask, dilute with *Mobile phase* to volume, and mix.
  Assay preparations—Weigh and finely powder not less than 20 Tablets. Transfer an accurately weighed portion of the finely ground powder, equivalent to about 500 mg of sulfadoxine and 25 mg of pyrimethamine, to a 100-mL volumetric flask, add 35 mL of acetonitrile, shake for 30 minutes, dilute with *Mobile phase* to volume, mix, and filter. Pipet 25 mL of the filtrate and 2 mL of *Internal standard solution* into a 50-mL volumetric flask, dilute with *Mobile phase* to volume, and mix (*Assay preparation 1*). Pipet 2 mL of the filtrate and 10 mL of the *Internal standard solution* into a 250-mL volumetric flask, dilute with *Mobile phase* to volume, and mix (*Assay preparation 2*).
  Chromatographic system (see *Chromatography* ⟨621⟩)—The liquid chromatograph is equipped with a 254-nm detector and a 3.9-mm × 30-cm column that contains packing L1. The flow rate is about 2.0 mL per minute. Chromatograph five replicate injections of the *Standard preparation*, and record the peak responses as directed for *Procedure:* the relative standard deviation is not more than 2.5%, and the resolution factor between sulfadoxine and phenacetin is not less than 1.0, and between pyrimethamine and phenacetin is not less than 1.0.
  Procedure—Separately inject equal volumes (about 10 μL) of the *Standard preparations* and the *Assay preparations* into the chromatograph, record the chromatograms, and measure the responses for the major peaks. The relative retention times are about 0.7 for sulfadoxine and 1.0 for phenacetin and 1.3 for pyrimethamine. Calculate the quantity, in mg, of sulfadoxine in the portion of Tablets taken by the formula:

$$12.5C(R_U/R_S)$$

in which C is the concentration, in μg per mL, of USP Sulfadoxine RS in *Standard preparation 2*, and R_U and R_S are the relative peak response ratios obtained from *Assay preparation 2* and *Standard preparation 2*, respectively. Calculate the quantity, in mg, of pyrimethamine in the portion of Tablets taken by the formula:

$$0.2C'(R'_U/R'_S)$$

in which C' is the concentration, in μg per mL, of USP Pyrimethamine RS in *Standard preparation 1*, and R'_U and R'_S are the relative peak response ratios obtained from *Assay preparation 1* and *Standard preparation 1*, respectively.

Sulfamethazine

$C_{12}H_{14}N_4O_2S$ 278.33
Benzenesulfonamide, 4-amino-N-(4,6-dimethyl-2-pyrimidinyl)-.
N^1-(4,6-Dimethyl-2-pyrimidinyl)sulfanilamide   [*57-68-1*].

» Sulfamethazine contains not less than 99.0 percent and not more than 100.5 percent of $C_{12}H_{14}N_4O_2S$, calculated on the dried basis.

Packaging and storage—Preserve in well-closed, light-resistant containers.

USP Reference standards ⟨11⟩—USP Sulfamethazine RS.

Clarity and color of solution—Dissolve 1.0 g in a mixture of 20 mL of water and 5 mL of 1 N sodium hydroxide: the solution is clear and not more deeply colored than pale yellow.

Identification—
 A: *Infrared Absorption* ⟨197K⟩.
 B: To 0.10 g add 10 mL of water and just sufficient sodium hydroxide solution (1 in 250) to give a faint pink spot on phenolphthalein paper. Add 5 drops of cupric sulfate TS: a yellow-green precipitate is formed, and it becomes brown on standing.

Melting range ⟨741⟩: between 197° and 200°.

Acidity—Digest 3.0 g with 150 mL of carbon dioxide-free water at 70° for about 5 minutes, stirring occasionally to maintain suspension of the test specimen. Cool the mixture rapidly in an ice bath to 20 ± 0.5°, with mechanical stirring. Filter immediately, with vacuum, omitting washing of the solid but drying it thoroughly by suction. Add 2 drops of thymolphthalein TS to 25.0 mL of the filtrate, and titrate with 0.1 N sodium hydroxide VS. To a second 25.0-mL portion of the filtrate add 10 mL of hydrochloric acid. Cool the mixture to 15°, and titrate with 0.1 M sodium nitrite VS as directed under *Nitrite Titration* ⟨451⟩: the volume of 0.1 N sodium hydroxide consumed does not exceed the volume of 0.1 M sodium nitrite consumed by more than 0.5 mL.

Loss on drying ⟨731⟩—Dry about 1 g, accurately weighed, at 105° for 2 hours: it loses not more than 0.5% of its weight.

Residue on ignition ⟨281⟩: not more than 0.1%.

Selenium ⟨291⟩: 0.003%, a 200-mg test specimen being used.

Heavy metals, *Method II* ⟨231⟩: 0.002%.

Ordinary impurities ⟨466⟩—
 Test solution: acetone.
 Standard solution: acetone.
 Eluant: a mixture of ethyl acetate, methanol, and ammonium hydroxide (17 : 6 : 5).
 Visualization: 11.

Assay—Proceed with Sulfamethazine as directed under *Nitrite Titration* ⟨451⟩. Each mL of 0.1 M sodium nitrite is equivalent to 27.83 mg of $C_{12}H_{14}N_4O_2S$.

Sulfamethazine Granulated

» Sulfamethazine Granulated contains Sulfamethazine mixed with suitable diluents, carriers, and inactive ingredients. It contains not less than 90.0 percent and not more than 110.0 percent of the labeled amount of sulfamethazine ($C_{12}H_{14}N_4O_2S$).

Packaging and storage—Preserve in well-closed containers. Avoid moisture and excessive heat.

Labeling—Label it to indicate that it is for veterinary use only. Label it also to indicate that it is for manufacturing, processing, or repackaging.

USP Reference standards ⟨11⟩—USP Sulfamethazine RS.

Identification—The chromatogram of the *Assay preparation* obtained as directed in the *Assay* exhibits a major peak for sulfamethazine, the retention time of which corresponds to that exhibited in the chromatogram of the *Standard preparation* obtained as directed in the *Assay*.

Loss on drying ⟨731⟩—Dry it in vacuum at 60° for 5 hours: it loses not more than 10% of its weight.

Powder fineness ⟨811⟩: not less than 95% passes a No. 20 sieve, and not more than 10% passes a No. 80 sieve.

Assay—
 Mobile phase—Prepare a mixture of water, methanol, and glacial acetic acid (68 : 30 : 2). Make adjustments if necessary (see *System Suitability* under *Chromatography* ⟨621⟩).
 Extractant—Prepare a mixture of 0.15 N hydrochloric acid and methanol (3 : 1).
 Standard preparation—Prepare a solution of USP Sulfamethazine RS in *Extractant* having a known concentration of about 0.01 mg per mL.
 Assay preparation—Transfer about 5 g of Sulfamethazine Granulated, accurately weighed, to a suitable container, add 250.0 mL of *Extractant*, and shake by mechanical means for 2 hours. Allow the mixture to settle, storing the mixture in a refrigerator if settling is allowed to continue overnight. Filter a portion of the supernatant, and transfer 10.0 mL of the clear filtrate to a 100-mL volumetric flask. Dilute with *Extractant* to volume, and mix. Transfer 5.0 mL of this solution to a 200-mL volumetric flask, dilute with *Extractant* to volume, and mix. Pass a portion of this solution through a filter having a 0.5-μm or finer porosity, and use the filtrate as the *Assay preparation*. This solution contains about 0.01 mg of sulfamethazine per mL.
 Derivatizing reagent—Dissolve 6.0 g of dimethylaminobenzaldehyde in 200 mL of glacial acetic acid, add 120 mL of methanol and 80 mL of water, mix, and degas. Prepare this reagent daily.
 Chromatographic system—The liquid chromatograph is equipped with a guard column that contains packing L1, a 4.6-mm × 25-cm analytical column that contains 10-μm packing L1, a separate pump to deliver the *Derivatizing reagent* via a T-junction installed immediately postcolumn, a postcolumn derivatization coil consisting of 3-m × 0.5-mm inside-diameter polytef tubing, a flow cell, and a 450-nm detector. The *Mobile phase* flow rate is about 2 mL per minute, and the *Derivatizing reagent* flow rate is about 1 mL per minute. Chromatograph the *Standard preparation,* and record the peak responses as directed for *Procedure:* the capacity factor, k', for the sulfamethazine peak is not less than 2.0; and the relative standard deviation for replicate injections is not more than 3.5%.
 Procedure—Separately inject equal volumes (about 100 μL) of the *Standard preparation* and the *Assay preparation* into the chromatograph, record the chromatograms, and measure the responses for the sulfamethazine peaks. Calculate the quantity, in mg, of sulfamethazine ($C_{12}H_{14}N_4O_2S$) in each g of the Sulfamethazine Granulated taken by the formula:

$$100{,}000(C/W)(r_U/r_S)$$

in which C is the concentration, in mg per mL, of USP Sulfamethazine RS in the *Standard preparation;* W is the quantity, in g, of Sulfamethazine Granulated taken to prepare the *Assay preparation;* and r_U and r_S are the sulfamethazine peak responses obtained from the *Assay preparation* and the *Standard preparation*, respectively.

Sulfamethizole

$C_9H_{10}N_4O_2S_2$ 270.33
Benzenesulfonamide, 4-amino-N-(5-methyl-1,3,4-thiadiazol-2-yl)-.
N^1-(5-Methyl-1,3,4-thiadiazol-2-yl)sulfanilamide   [*144-82-1*].

» Sulfamethizole contains not less than 98.0 percent and not more than 101.0 percent of $C_9H_{10}N_4O_2S_2$, calculated on the dried basis.

Packaging and storage—Preserve in well-closed, light-resistant containers.

USP Reference standards ⟨11⟩—*USP Sulfamethizole RS*.
Clarity and color of solution—Dissolve 1.0 g in 20 mL of water and 5 mL of 1 N sodium hydroxide: the solution is clear and not more than pale yellow.
Identification—
  A: *Infrared Absorption* ⟨197M⟩.
  B: To about 0.1 g add 5 mL of 3 N hydrochloric acid, and boil gently for about 5 minutes. Cool in an ice bath, then add 4 mL of a sodium nitrite solution (1 in 100), add water to make 10 mL, and place the mixture in an ice bath for 10 minutes. To 5 mL of the cooled mixture add a solution of 50 mg of 2-naphthol in 2 mL of sodium hydroxide solution (1 in 10): an orange-red precipitate is formed, and it darkens on standing.
  C: To about 20 mg suspended in 5 mL of water add, dropwise, 1 N sodium hydroxide until dissolved, then add 2 or 3 drops of cupric sulfate TS: a light green precipitate is formed, and it does not change on standing.
  D: The retention time of the major peak in the chromatogram of the *Assay preparation* corresponds to that of the *Standard preparation* as obtained in the *Assay*.
Melting range ⟨741⟩: between 208° and 212°.
Acidity—Digest 2.0 g with 100 mL of water at about 70° for 5 minutes, cool immediately to about 20°, and filter. To 25.0 mL of the filtrate add 2 drops of phenolphthalein TS, and titrate with 0.10 N sodium hydroxide: not more than 0.50 mL is required for neutralization. Save the remainder of the filtrate for the tests for *Chloride* and for *Sulfate*.
Loss on drying ⟨731⟩—Dry it at 105° for 2 hours: it loses not more than 0.5% of its weight.
Residue on ignition ⟨281⟩: not more than 0.1%.
Chloride ⟨221⟩—A 25.0-mL portion of the filtrate prepared in the test for *Acidity* shows no more chloride than corresponds to 0.10 mL of 0.020 N hydrochloric acid (0.014%).
Sulfate ⟨221⟩—A 25.0-mL portion of the filtrate prepared in the test for *Acidity* shows no more sulfate than corresponds to 0.20 mL of 0.020 N sulfuric acid (0.04%).
Selenium ⟨291⟩: 0.003%.
Heavy metals, *Method II* ⟨231⟩: 0.002%.
Ordinary impurities ⟨466⟩—
  Test solution: methanol.
  Standard solution: methanol.
  Eluant: acetone.
  Visualization: 1.
Assay—
  Mobile phase—Prepare a filtered and degassed mixture of water, methanol, and glacial acetic acid (69 : 30 : 1). Make adjustments if necessary (see *System Suitability* under *Chromatography* ⟨621⟩).
  Standard preparation—Dissolve an accurately weighed quantity of USP Sulfamethizole RS in methanol to obtain a solution having a known concentration of about 0.4 mg per mL. Quantitatively dilute a volume of this solution with *Mobile phase* to obtain the *Standard preparation* having a known concentration of about 8 µg per mL.
  Assay preparation—Transfer about 20 mg of sulfamethizole, accurately weighed, to a 50-mL volumetric flask, dilute with methanol to volume, and mix. Quantitatively dilute a volume of this solution with *Mobile phase* to obtain the *Assay preparation* having a concentration of about 8 µg per mL.
  Chromatographic system (see *Chromatography* ⟨621⟩)—The liquid chromatograph is equipped with a 254-nm detector and a 3.9-mm × 30-cm column that contains 10-µm packing L1. The flow rate is about 1.0 mL per minute. Chromatograph the *Standard preparation*, and record the peak responses as directed for *Procedure:* the column efficiency determined from the analyte peak is not less than 2000 theoretical plates, the tailing factor for the analyte peak is not more than 2.0, and the relative standard deviation for replicate injections is not more than 2.0%.
  Procedure—Separately inject equal volumes (about 50 µL) of the *Standard preparation* and the *Assay preparation* into the chromatograph, record the chromatograms, and measure the responses for the major peaks. Calculate the quantity, in mg, of $C_9H_{10}N_4O_2S_2$ in the portion of Sulfamethizole taken by the formula:

$$2.5C(r_U / r_S)$$

in which C is the concentration, in µg per mL, of USP Sulfamethizole RS in the *Standard preparation*, and r_U and r_S are the peak responses obtained from the *Assay preparation* and the *Standard preparation*, respectively.

Sulfamethizole Oral Suspension

» Sulfamethizole Oral Suspension contains not less than 90.0 percent and not more than 110.0 percent of the labeled amount of sulfamethizole ($C_9H_{10}N_4O_2S_2$), in a buffered aqueous suspension.

Packaging and storage—Preserve in tight, light-resistant containers.

USP Reference standards ⟨11⟩—*USP Sulfamethizole RS*.
Identification—Place a quantity of Oral Suspension, equivalent to about 500 mg of sulfamethizole, in a 50-mL centrifuge tube; add about 30 mL of water; mix; and centrifuge the mixture. Decant and discard the supernatant. Resuspend the residue in 15 mL of water, mix, and centrifuge the mixture. Decant and discard the clear supernatant. Repeat the washing procedure an additional two times. Dissolve the residue in a mixture of 10 mL of 6 N ammonium hydroxide and 10 mL of water, and filter. Warm the filtrate until most of the ammonia is expelled, cool, and add 6 N acetic acid until the mixture is distinctly acid: a precipitate of sulfamethizole is formed. Collect the precipitate on a filter, wash it well with cold water, and dry at 105° for 2 hours: the sulfamethizole so obtained responds to *Identification* test A under *Sulfamethizole*.
Uniformity of dosage units ⟨905⟩—
  FOR ORAL SUSPENSION PACKAGED IN SINGLE-UNIT CONTAINERS: meets the requirements.
Deliverable volume ⟨698⟩—
  FOR ORAL SUSPENSION PACKAGED IN MULTIPLE-UNIT CONTAINERS: meets the requirements.
Assay—Transfer an accurately measured volume of Oral Suspension, equivalent to about 500 mg of sulfamethizole, to a beaker. Add 50 mL of water and 20 mL of hydrochloric acid, stir until dissolved, cool to 15°, and slowly titrate with 0.1 M sodium nitrite VS, determining the endpoint potentiometrically, using suitable electrodes. Each mL of 0.1 M sodium nitrite is equivalent to 27.03 mg of sulfamethizole ($C_9H_{10}N_4O_2S_2$).

Sulfamethizole Tablets

» Sulfamethizole Tablets contain not less than 95.0 percent and not more than 105.0 percent of the labeled amount of $C_9H_{10}N_4O_2S_2$.

Packaging and storage—Preserve in well-closed containers.

USP Reference standards ⟨11⟩—*USP Sulfamethizole RS*.
Identification—
  A: Triturate a quantity of finely powdered Tablets, equivalent to about 500 mg of sulfamethizole, with 5 mL of chloroform, and transfer to a small filter. Wash with another 5-mL portion of chloroform, and discard the filtrate. Triturate the residue with 10 mL of 6 N ammonium hydroxide for 5 minutes, add 10 mL of water, filter, and proceed as directed in the *Identification* test under *Sulfamethizole Oral Suspension*, beginning with "Warm the filtrate."
  B: The retention time of the major peak in the chromatogram of the *Assay preparation* corresponds to that of the *Standard preparation* as obtained in the *Assay*.

Dissolution ⟨711⟩—
  Medium: 0.01 N hydrochloric acid; 900 mL.
  Apparatus 2: 50 rpm.
  Time: 30 minutes.
  Procedure—Determine the amount of $C_9H_{10}N_4O_2S_2$ dissolved by employing UV absorption at the wavelength of maximum absorbance at about 267 nm on filtered portions of the solution under test, suitably diluted with *Dissolution Medium*, if necessary, in comparison with a Standard solution having a known concentration of USP Sulfamethizole RS in the same *Medium*.
  Tolerances—Not less than 75% (*Q*) of the labeled amount of $C_9H_{10}N_4O_2S_2$ is dissolved in 30 minutes.
Uniformity of dosage units ⟨905⟩: meet the requirements.
Assay—
  Mobile phase, Standard preparation, and *Chromatographic system*—Prepare as directed in the *Assay* under *Sulfamethizole*.
  Assay preparation—Weigh and finely powder not less than 20 Tablets. Transfer an accurately weighed portion of the powder, equivalent to about 40 mg of sulfamethizole, to a 250-mL screw-capped bottle. Transfer 100.0 mL of methanol to the bottle, cap the bottle, shake by mechanical means for 30 minutes, and filter. Quantitatively dilute a portion of the filtered solution with *Mobile phase* to obtain the *Assay preparation* having a concentration of about 8 µg per mL.
  Procedure—Separately inject equal volumes (about 50 µL) of the *Standard preparation* and the *Assay preparation* into the chromatograph, record the chromatograms, and measure the responses for the major peaks. Calculate the quantity, in mg, of $C_9H_{10}N_4O_2S_2$ in the portion of Tablets taken by the formula:

$$5C(r_U / r_S)$$

in which *C* is the concentration, in µg per mL, of USP Sulfamethizole RS in the *Standard preparation*, and r_U and r_S are the peak responses obtained from the *Assay preparation* and the *Standard preparation*, respectively.

Sulfamethoxazole

$C_{10}H_{11}N_3O_3S$ 253.28
Benzenesulfonamide, 4-amino-*N*-(5-methyl-3-isoxazolyl)-.
N^1-(5-Methyl-3-isoxazolyl)sulfanilamide [723-46-6].

» Sulfamethoxazole contains not less than 99.0 percent and not more than 101.0 percent of $C_{10}H_{11}N_3O_3S$, calculated on the dried basis.

Packaging and storage—Preserve in well-closed, light-resistant containers. Store at 25°, excursions permitted between 15° and 30°.

USP Reference standards ⟨11⟩—*USP Sulfamethoxazole RS. USP Sulfanilamide RS.*
Identification—
  A: *Infrared Absorption* ⟨197K⟩.
  B: *Ultraviolet Absorption* ⟨197U⟩—
    Solution: 10 µg per mL.
    Medium: sodium hydroxide solution (1 in 250).
    Absorptivities at 257 nm, calculated on the dried basis, do not differ by more than 2.0%.
  C: Dissolve about 100 mg in 2 mL of hydrochloric acid, and add 3 mL of sodium nitrite solution (1 in 100) and 1 mL of sodium hydroxide solution (1 in 10) containing 10 mg of 2-naphthol: a red-orange precipitate is formed.
Melting range, *Class I* ⟨741⟩: between 168° and 172°.
Loss on drying ⟨731⟩—Dry it at 105° for 4 hours: it loses not more than 0.5% of its weight.

Residue on ignition ⟨281⟩: not more than 0.1%.
Selenium ⟨291⟩: 0.003%, a 200-mg test specimen being used.
Sulfanilamide and sulfanilic acid—
  Standard solution—Dissolve 100 mg of USP Sulfamethoxazole RS in 0.10 mL of ammonium hydroxide, dilute with methanol to 10.0 mL, and mix.
  Reference solution—Dissolve 20 mg of USP Sulfanilamide RS and 20 mg of sulfanilic acid in 10 mL of ammonium hydroxide, and dilute with methanol to 100 mL. Transfer 2.0 mL of the solution to a 50-mL volumetric flask, add 10 mL of ammonium hydroxide, dilute with methanol to volume, and mix.
  Test solution—Dissolve 100 mg in 0.10 mL of ammonium hydroxide, dilute with methanol to 10.0 mL, and mix.
  Procedure—Apply 10 µL of the *Standard solution*, 25 µL of the *Reference solution*, and 10 µL of the *Test solution* to a suitable thin-layer chromatographic plate (see *Chromatography* ⟨621⟩) coated with a 0.25-mm layer of chromatographic silica gel. Allow the spots to dry, and develop the chromatogram in a solvent system consisting of a mixture of alcohol, *n*-heptane, chloroform, and glacial acetic acid (25 : 25 : 25 : 7) until the solvent front has moved about three-fourths of the length of the plate. Remove the plate from the chamber, and allow it to air-dry. Spray the plate with a solution prepared by dissolving 0.10 g of *p*-dimethylaminobenzaldehyde in 1 mL of hydrochloric acid and diluting with alcohol to 100 mL. Sulfamethoxazole produces a spot at about R_F 0.7, sulfanilamide at about R_F 0.5, and sulfanilic acid at about R_F 0.1. Any spots produced by sulfanilamide or sulfanilic acid from the *Test solution* do not exceed in size or intensity similar spots, occurring at the respective R_F values, produced by sulfanilamide or sulfanilic acid from the *Reference preparation* (0.2%).
Organic volatile impurities, Method IV ⟨467⟩: meets the requirements.
                                                  (Official until July 1, 2008)
Assay—Dissolve about 500 mg of Sulfamethoxazole, accurately weighed, in a mixture of 20 mL of glacial acetic acid and 40 mL of water, and add 15 mL of hydrochloric acid. Cool to 15°, and immediately titrate with 0.1 M sodium nitrite VS, determining the endpoint potentiometrically using a calomel-platinum electrode system. Each mL of 0.1 M sodium nitrite is equivalent to 25.33 mg of $C_{10}H_{11}N_3O_3S$.

Sulfamethoxazole Oral Suspension

» Sulfamethoxazole Oral Suspension contains not less than 95.0 percent and not more than 110.0 percent of the labeled amount of sulfamethoxazole ($C_{10}H_{11}N_3O_3S$).

Packaging and storage—Preserve in tight, light-resistant containers.

USP Reference standards ⟨11⟩—*USP Sulfamethoxazole RS.*
Identification—
  A: Place a quantity of Oral Suspension, equivalent to about 100 mg of sulfamethoxazole, in a 50-mL centrifuge tube; add 5 mL of ammonium hydroxide; and shake gently. Add 25 mL of methanol, shake thoroughly for 3 minutes, centrifuge, decant the supernatant into a 50-mL volumetric flask, dilute with methanol to volume, and mix. Apply 50 µL of this solution and 50 µL of a solution prepared by dissolving 100 mg of USP Sulfamethoxazole RS in 5 mL of ammonium hydroxide and diluting with methanol to 50.0 mL to a suitable thin-layer chromatographic plate (see *Chromatography* ⟨621⟩) coated with a 0.25-mm layer of chromatographic silica gel. Allow the spots to dry, and develop the chromatogram in a solvent system consisting of a mixture of alcohol, *n*-heptane, chloroform, and glacial acetic acid (25 : 25 : 25 : 7) until the solvent front has moved about three-fourths of the length of the plate. Remove the plate from the developing chamber, mark the solvent front, and allow the solvent to evaporate. Locate the spots on the plate by lightly spraying with a solution prepared by dissolving 0.10 g of *p*-dimethylaminobenzaldehyde in 1 mL of hydrochloric acid and diluting with alcohol to 100 mL: the R_F value of the principal spot obtained from

the test solution corresponds to that obtained from the Standard solution.

B: Transfer a quantity of Oral Suspension, equivalent to about 500 mg of sulfamethoxazole, to a 50-mL centrifuge tube; add about 25 mL of water; mix; and centrifuge. Decant and discard the supernatant, resuspend the residue in 25 mL of water, mix, and centrifuge again. Decant and discard the clear supernatant. Repeat the washing procedure an additional two times. Dissolve the residue in 10 mL of hydrochloric acid, and add 15 mL of sodium nitrite solution (1 in 100) and 5 mL of sodium hydroxide solution (1 in 10) containing 10 mg of 2-naphthol: a red-orange precipitate is produced.

Uniformity of dosage units ⟨905⟩—
FOR ORAL SUSPENSION PACKAGED IN SINGLE-UNIT CONTAINERS: meets the requirements.

Deliverable volume ⟨698⟩—
FOR ORAL SUSPENSION PACKAGED IN MULTIPLE-UNIT CONTAINERS: meets the requirements.

Assay—Mix an accurately measured volume of Oral Suspension, equivalent to about 1 g of sulfamethoxazole, with 20 mL of glacial acetic acid and 40 mL of water; and add 15 mL of hydrochloric acid. Cool to 15°, and titrate immediately with 0.1 M sodium nitrite VS, determining the endpoint potentiometrically using a calomel-platinum electrode system. Each mL of 0.1 M sodium nitrite is equivalent to 25.33 mg of $C_{10}H_{11}N_3O_3S$.

Sulfamethoxazole Tablets

» Sulfamethoxazole Tablets contain not less than 95.0 percent and not more than 105.0 percent of the labeled amount of $C_{10}H_{11}N_3O_3S$.

Packaging and storage—Preserve in well-closed, light-resistant containers.

USP Reference standards ⟨11⟩—*USP Sulfamethoxazole RS.*

Identification—
A: Place a quantity of finely powdered Tablets, equivalent to about 100 mg of sulfamethoxazole, in a 50-mL centrifuge tube, and proceed as directed for *Identification* test A under *Sulfamethoxazole Oral Suspension*, beginning with "add 5 mL of ammonium hydroxide."

B: To a portion of finely powdered Tablets, equivalent to about 100 mg of sulfamethoxazole, add 2 mL of hydrochloric acid, 3 mL of sodium nitrite solution (1 in 100), and 1 mL of sodium hydroxide solution (1 in 10) containing 10 mg of 2-naphthol: a red-orange precipitate is formed.

Dissolution ⟨711⟩—
Medium: dilute hydrochloric acid (7 in 100); 900 mL.
Apparatus 1: 100 rpm.
Time: 30 minutes.
Procedure—Determine the amount of $C_{10}H_{11}N_3O_3S$ dissolved from UV absorbances at the wavelength of maximum absorbance at about 265 nm of filtered portions of the solution under test, suitably diluted with *Dissolution Medium*, if necessary, in comparison with a Standard solution having a known concentration of USP Sulfamethoxazole RS in the same medium.
Tolerances—Not less than 80% (*Q*) of the labeled amount of $C_{10}H_{11}N_3O_3S$ is dissolved in 30 minutes.

Uniformity of dosage units ⟨905⟩: meet the requirements.

Assay—Weigh and finely powder not less than 20 Tablets. Weigh accurately a portion of the powder, equivalent to about 500 mg of sulfamethoxazole, dissolve in a mixture of 20 mL of glacial acetic acid and 40 mL of water, and add 15 mL of hydrochloric acid. Cool to 15°, and titrate immediately with 0.1 M sodium nitrite VS, determining the endpoint potentiometrically using a calomel-platinum electrode system. Each mL of 0.1 M sodium nitrite is equivalent to 25.33 mg of $C_{10}H_{11}N_3O_3S$.

Sulfamethoxazole and Trimethoprim Injection

» Sulfamethoxazole and Trimethoprim Injection is a sterile solution of Sulfamethoxazole and Trimethoprim in Water for Injection, which, when diluted with Dextrose Injection, is suitable for intravenous infusion. It contains not less than 90.0 percent and not more than 110.0 percent of the labeled amounts of sulfamethoxazole ($C_{10}H_{11}N_3O_3S$) and trimethoprim ($C_{14}H_{18}N_4O_3$).

Packaging and storage—Preserve in single-dose, light-resistant containers, preferably of Type I glass. It may be packaged in 50-mL multiple-dose containers.

Labeling—Label it to indicate that it is to be diluted with 5% Dextrose Injection prior to administration.

USP Reference standards ⟨11⟩—*USP Sulfamethoxazole RS. USP Sulfanilamide RS. USP Sulfanilic Acid RS. USP Trimethoprim RS.*

Identification—In tests A and B under *Related compounds,* the respective *Test preparations* exhibit principal spots whose R_F values correspond to those spots produced by the *Standard preparations* of USP Trimethoprim RS (R_F about 0.5) and USP Sulfamethoxazole RS (R_F about 0.7).

Pyrogen—It meets the requirements of the *Pyrogen Test* ⟨151⟩, the test dose being 0.5 mL per kg.

pH ⟨791⟩: between 9.5 and 10.5.

Particulate matter ⟨788⟩: meets the requirements for small-volume injections.

Related compounds—
TEST A (FOR TRIMETHOPRIM DEGRADATION PRODUCT)—
Hydrochloric acid solution—Dilute 2 mL of 3 N hydrochloric acid with water to 100 mL.

Test preparation—Transfer an accurately measured volume of Injection, equivalent to about 48 mg of trimethoprim and 240 mg of sulfamethoxazole, to a glass-stoppered, 50-mL centrifuge tube. Add 15 mL of *Hydrochloric acid solution,* and mix. Add 15 mL of chloroform, shake for 30 seconds, and centrifuge at high speed for 3 minutes. Transfer the supernatant layer to a 125-mL separator. Extract the chloroform layer in the centrifuge tube with 15 mL of *Hydrochloric acid solution,* centrifuge at high speed, and add the extract to the separator. Add 2 mL of sodium hydroxide solution (1 in 10) to the solution in the separator, and extract with three 20-mL portions of chloroform, collecting the organic layer in a 125-mL conical flask. Evaporate the chloroform under a stream of nitrogen to dryness. Dissolve the residue in 1 mL of a mixture of chloroform and methanol (1 : 1).

Standard preparation A—Using an accurately weighed quantity of USP Trimethoprim RS, prepare a solution in chloroform and methanol (1 : 1) having a known concentration of 48 mg per mL.

Standard preparation B—Dilute an accurately measured volume of *Standard preparation A* with a mixture of chloroform and methanol (1 : 1) to obtain a solution having a known concentration of 240 µg per mL.

Procedure—Apply 10 µL each of the *Test preparation, Standard preparation A,* and *Standard preparation B* to separate points on a thin-layer chromatographic plate (see *Chromatography* ⟨621⟩) coated with a 0.25-mm layer of chromatographic silica gel. Develop the chromatogram in a solvent system consisting of a mixture of chloroform, methanol, and ammonium hydroxide (97 : 7.5 : 1) until the solvent front has moved at least 12 cm. Remove the plate from the developing chamber, and air-dry. Locate the bands by viewing under short-wavelength UV light and by spraying with a freshly prepared mixture of ferric chloride solution (1 in 10) and potassium ferricyanide solution (1 in 20) (1 : 1). Trimethoprim produces a spot at about R_F 0.5, and the trimethoprim degradation product produces a spot at about R_F 0.6 to 0.7. Any spot from the *Test preparation* at about R_F 0.6 to 0.7 is not greater in size and intensity than the spot produced by *Standard preparation B* at about R_F 0.5, corresponding to not more than 0.5%. [NOTE—There may be spots due to concentrate excipients at about R_F 0.1.]

TEST B (FOR SULFANILAMIDE AND SULFANILIC ACID)—
Alcohol–methanol mixture—Mix dehydrated alcohol and methanol (95 : 5).
Ammonium hydroxide solution—Dilute 1 mL of ammonium hydroxide with *Alcohol–methanol mixture* to 100 mL.
Modified Ehrlich's reagent—Dissolve 100 mg of p-dimethylaminobenzaldehyde in 1 mL of hydrochloric acid, dilute with alcohol to 100 mL, and mix.
Test preparation—Transfer an accurately measured volume of Injection, equivalent to about 32 mg of trimethoprim and 160 mg of sulfamethoxazole, to a 25-mL graduated cylinder, dilute with *Ammonium hydroxide solution* to 16 mL, and mix.
Standard preparation A—Transfer about 50 mg of USP Sulfamethoxazole RS, accurately weighed, to a 5-mL volumetric flask, dissolve in and dilute with *Ammonium hydroxide solution* to volume, and mix.
Standard preparation B—Transfer about 25 mg of USP Sulfanilamide RS, accurately weighed, to a 250-mL volumetric flask, dissolve in and dilute with *Ammonium hydroxide solution* to volume, and mix. Pipet 5 mL of this solution into a 10-mL volumetric flask, dilute with *Ammonium hydroxide solution* to volume, and mix.
Standard preparation C—Transfer about 25 mg of USP Sulfanilic Acid RS, accurately weighed, to a 250-mL volumetric flask, dissolve in and dilute with *Ammonium hydroxide solution*, and mix. Pipet 3 mL of this solution into a 10-mL volumetric flask, dilute with *Ammonium hydroxide solution* to volume, and mix.
Procedure—Apply 10 µL each of the *Test preparation* and *Standard preparations A, B,* and *C* to separate points on a thin-layer chromatographic plate (see *Chromatography* ⟨621⟩) coated with a 0.25-mm layer of chromatographic silica gel. Develop the chromatogram in a solvent system consisting of a mixture of *Alcohol-methanol mixture,* heptane, chloroform and glacial acetic acid (30: 30 : 30 : 10) until the solvent front has moved not less than 12 cm. Remove the plate from the developing chamber, air-dry, spray with *Modified Ehrlich's reagent,* and allow the plate to stand for 15 minutes: sulfamethoxazole produces a spot at about R_F 0.7. Any spots from the *Test preparation* at about R_F 0.5 or 0.1 are not greater in size or intensity than spots produced by *Standard preparations B* and *C,* respectively, corresponding to not more than 0.5% of sulfanilamide and 0.3% of sulfanilic acid.
Other requirements—It meets the requirements under *Injections* ⟨1⟩.
Assay—
Mobile phase, Standard preparation, and *Chromatographic system*—Proceed as directed in the *Assay* under *Sulfamethoxazole and Trimethoprim Oral Suspension.*
Assay preparation—Transfer an accurately measured volume of Injection, equivalent to about 80 mg of sulfamethoxazole, to a 50-mL volumetric flask. Add methanol to volume, and mix. Transfer 5.0 mL of this solution to a 50-mL volumetric flask, dilute with *Mobile phase* to volume, and mix.
Procedure—Separately inject equal volumes (about 20 µL) of the *Standard preparation* and the *Assay preparation* into the chromatograph, record the chromatograms, and measure the responses for the major peaks. Calculate the quantities, in mg, of trimethoprim ($C_{14}H_{18}N_4O_3$) and sulfamethoxazole ($C_{10}H_{11}N_3O_3S$) in each mL of the Injection taken by the formula:

$$(500C/V)(r_U/r_S)$$

in which *C* is the concentration, in mg per mL, of the appropriate USP Reference Standard in the *Standard preparation;* and r_U and r_S are the responses of the corresponding analyte obtained from the *Assay preparation* and the *Standard preparation,* respectively.

Sulfamethoxazole and Trimethoprim Oral Suspension

» Sulfamethoxazole and Trimethoprim Oral Suspension contains not less than 90.0 percent and not more than 110.0 percent of the labeled amounts of sulfamethoxazole ($C_{10}H_{11}N_3O_3S$) and trimethoprim ($C_{14}H_{18}N_4O_3$).

Packaging and storage—Preserve in tight, light-resistant containers.
USP Reference standards ⟨11⟩—*USP Sulfamethoxazole RS. USP Sulfamethoxazole N_4-Glucoside RS. USP Sulfanilamide RS. USP Sulfanilic Acid RS. USP Trimethoprim RS.*
Identification—In the *Chromatographic purity* test, the respective *Test solutions* exhibit spots whose R_F values correspond to those spots produced by the *Standard solutions* of USP Trimethoprim RS and USP Sulfamethoxazole RS.
Uniformity of dosage units ⟨905⟩—
  FOR ORAL SUSPENSION PACKAGED IN SINGLE-UNIT CONTAINERS: meets the requirements.
Deliverable volume ⟨698⟩—
  FOR ORAL SUSPENSION PACKAGED IN MULTIPLE-UNIT CONTAINERS: meets the requirements.
pH ⟨791⟩: between 5.0 and 6.5.
Chromatographic purity—
  LIMIT OF TRIMETHOPRIM DEGRADATION PRODUCT—
  Test solution—Transfer an accurately measured volume of Oral Suspension, equivalent to about 40 mg of trimethoprim, to a separatory funnel. Extract with three 25-mL portions of a mixture of chloroform and methanol (8 : 2), collecting the extracts in a 125-mL conical flask. Evaporate the combined extracts with the aid of a current of air to dryness on a steam bath. Dissolve the residue in 2.0 mL of the mixture of chloroform and methanol (8 : 2), then centrifuge.
  Standard solution A—Dissolve an accurately weighed quantity of USP Trimethoprim RS in a mixture of chloroform and methanol (8 : 2) to obtain a solution having a known concentration of about 20 mg per mL.
  Standard solution B—Dilute an accurately measured volume of *Standard solution A* with a mixture of chloroform and methanol (8 : 2) to obtain a solution having a known concentration of about 0.1 mg per mL.
  Procedure—Apply 5 µL each of the *Test solution, Standard solution A,* and *Standard solution B* to separate points on a thin-layer chromatographic plate (see *Chromatography* ⟨621⟩) coated with a 0.25-mm layer of chromatographic silica gel. Place the plate in a saturated chromatographic chamber, and develop the chromatogram in a solvent system consisting of a mixture of chloroform, methanol, and ammonium hydroxide (80 : 20 : 3) until the solvent front has moved at least 15 cm. Remove the plate from the chamber, air-dry, and view under short-wavelength UV light: trimethoprim produces a spot at about R_F 0.7, and the trimethoprim degradation product can be seen at R_F 0.3 to 0.5. Any spot from the *Test solution* at about R_F 0.3 to 0.5 is not greater in size and intensity than the spot produced by *Standard solution B* at about R_F 0.7, corresponding to not more than 0.5%.
  LIMIT OF SULFANILAMIDE, SULFANILIC ACID, AND SULFAMETHOXAZOLE N_4-GLUCOSIDE)—
  Alcohol–methanol mixture—Mix dehydrated alcohol and methanol (95 : 5).
  Modified Ehrlich's reagent—Dissolve 100 mg of p-dimethylaminobenzaldehyde in 1 mL of hydrochloric acid, and dilute with alcohol to 100 mL.
  Test solution—Using a syringe, transfer an accurately measured volume of Oral Suspension, equivalent to 200 mg of sulfamethoxazole, to a 100-mL volumetric flask containing 10 mL of ammonium hydroxide; and add 50 mL of methanol. Shake for 3 minutes, and dilute with methanol to volume. Centrifuge a portion of the solution for 3 minutes.
  Standard solution A—Weigh 20 mg of USP Sulfamethoxazole RS into a 10-mL volumetric flask, dissolve in 1 mL of ammonium hydroxide, dilute with methanol to volume, and mix.
  Standard solution B—Weigh 10 mg of USP Sulfanilamide RS into a 50-mL volumetric flask, dissolve in 5 mL of ammonium hydroxide, and dilute with methanol to volume. Pipet 5 mL of this solution into a 100-mL volumetric flask, add 10 mL of ammonium hydroxide, and dilute with methanol to volume.
  Standard solution C—Weigh 10 mg of USP Sulfanilic Acid RS into a 50-mL volumetric flask, dissolve in 5 mL of ammonium hydroxide, and dilute with methanol to volume. Pipet 3 mL of this

solution into a 100-mL volumetric flask, add 10 mL of ammonium hydroxide, and dilute with methanol to volume.

Standard solution D—Weigh 3.0 mg of USP Sulfamethoxazole N₄-Glucoside RS into a 50-mL volumetric flask, dissolve in 5 mL of ammonium hydroxide, and dilute with methanol to volume.

Procedure—Apply 50 µL each of the *Test solution* and *Standard solutions A, B, C,* and *D* to separate points on a thin-layer chromatographic plate (see *Chromatography* ⟨621⟩) coated with a 0.25-mm layer of chromatographic silica gel. Place the plate in an unsaturated chromatographic chamber, and develop the chromatogram in a solvent system consisting of a mixture of *Alcohol–methanol mixture,* heptane, chloroform, and glacial acetic acid (25 : 25 : 25 : 7) until the solvent front has moved at least 12 cm. Remove the plate from the developing chamber, air-dry, spray with *Modified Ehrlich's reagent,* and allow the plate to stand for 15 minutes: sulfamethoxazole produces a spot at about R_F 0.7. Any spots from the *Test solution* at about R_F 0.5, 0.1, and 0.3 are not greater in size and intensity than spots produced by *Standard solutions B, C,* and *D,* respectively, corresponding to not more than 0.5% of sulfanilamide, 0.3% of sulfanilic acid, and 3.0% of sulfamethoxazole N₄-glucoside.

Alcohol content, *Method II* ⟨611⟩: not more than 0.5% of C_2H_5OH.

Assay—

Mobile phase—Mix 1400 mL of water, 400 mL of acetonitrile, and 2.0 mL of triethylamine in a 2000-mL volumetric flask. Allow to equilibrate to room temperature, and adjust with 0.2 N sodium hydroxide or dilute glacial acetic acid (1 in 100) to a pH of 5.9 ± 0.1. Dilute with water to volume, and filter through a 0.45-µm membrane, making adjustments if necessary (see *System Suitability* under *Chromatography* ⟨621⟩).

Standard preparation—Dissolve accurately weighed quantities of USP Trimethoprim RS and USP Sulfamethoxazole RS in methanol, and quantitatively dilute with methanol to obtain a solution containing, in each mL, about 0.32 mg and 0.32J mg, respectively, J being the ratio of the labeled amount, in mg, of sulfamethoxazole to the labeled amount, in mg, of trimethoprim in the dosage form. Transfer 5.0 mL of this solution to a 50-mL volumetric flask, dilute with *Mobile phase* to volume, and mix to obtain a *Standard preparation* having known concentrations of about 0.032 mg of USP Trimethoprim RS per mL and 0.032J mg of USP Sulfamethoxazole RS per mL.

Assay preparation—Transfer an accurately measured volume of Oral Suspension, equivalent to about 80 mg of Sulfamethoxazole, to a 50-mL volumetric flask with the aid of about 30 mL of methanol. Sonicate the mixture for about 10 minutes with occasional shaking. Allow to equilibrate to room temperature, dilute with methanol to volume, mix, and centrifuge. Transfer 5.0 mL of the supernatant to a second 50-mL volumetric flask, dilute with *Mobile phase* to volume, mix, and filter.

Chromatographic system (see *Chromatography* ⟨621⟩)—The liquid chromatograph is equipped with a 254-nm detector and a 3.9-mm × 30-cm column that contains packing L1. The flow rate is about 2 mL per minute. Chromatograph the *Standard preparation,* and record the peak responses as directed for *Procedure:* the relative retention times are about 1.0 for trimethoprim and 1.8 for sulfamethoxazole; the resolution, *R,* between sulfamethoxazole and trimethoprim is not less than 5.0; the tailing factor for the trimethoprim and sulfamethoxazole peaks is not more than 2.0; and the relative standard deviation for replicate injections is not more than 2.0%.

Procedure—Separately inject equal volumes (about 20 µL) of the *Standard preparation* and the *Assay preparation* into the chromatograph, record the chromatograms, and measure the responses for the major peaks. Calculate the quantities, in mg, of trimethoprim ($C_{14}H_{18}N_4O_3$) and sulfamethoxazole ($C_{10}H_{11}N_3O_3S$) in each mL of the Oral Suspension taken by the formula:

$$(500C/V)(r_U / r_S)$$

in which *C* is the concentration, in mg per mL, of the appropriate USP Reference Standard in the *Standard preparation; V* is the volume, in mL, of Oral Suspension taken; and r_U and r_S are the peak responses of the corresponding analyte obtained from the *Assay preparation* and the *Standard preparation,* respectively.

Sulfamethoxazole and Trimethoprim Tablets

» Sulfamethoxazole and Trimethoprim Tablets contain not less than 93.0 percent and not more than 107.0 percent of the labeled amounts of sulfamethoxazole ($C_{10}H_{11}N_3O_3S$) and trimethoprim ($C_{14}H_{18}N_4O_3$).

Packaging and storage—Preserve in well-closed, light-resistant containers.

USP Reference standards ⟨11⟩—*USP Trimethoprim RS. USP Sulfamethoxazole RS.*

Identification—Transfer an amount of finely ground Tablets, equivalent to 4 mg of trimethoprim, to a 10-mL volumetric flask, add 8 mL of methanol, warm for several minutes on a steam bath with frequent shaking, cool, dilute with methanol to volume, mix, and centrifuge briefly. Apply 5 µL each of this solution, a Standard solution of USP Trimethoprim RS in methanol containing 0.4 mg per mL, and a Standard solution of USP Sulfamethoxazole RS in methanol containing 2 mg per mL to separate points about 3 cm from one end of a thin-layer chromatographic plate coated with chromatographic silica gel mixture. Dry the spots in a current of warm air, and develop the plate with a mixture of chloroform, isopropyl alcohol, and diethylamine (6 : 5 : 1) in a chamber lined with filter paper. Remove the plate, dry, and examine under short-wavelength UV light: the trimethoprim and sulfamethoxazole spots from the solution under test have the same R_F values as the spots from the corresponding Standard solutions.

Dissolution ⟨711⟩—

Medium: 0.1 N hydrochloric acid; 900 mL.

Apparatus 2: 75 rpm.

Time: 60 minutes.

Procedure—Determine the amounts of sulfamethoxazole ($C_{10}H_{11}N_3O_3S$) and trimethoprim ($C_{14}H_{18}N_4O_3$) dissolved, employing the procedure set forth in the *Assay,* making any necessary volumetric adjustments (see *Chromatography* ⟨621⟩). Calculate the percentage of each active component dissolved by comparison of the peak responses obtained from a filtered aliquot of the solution under test with the peak responses from the corresponding component obtained from the *Standard preparation.*

Tolerances—Not less than 70% *(Q)* of the labeled amounts of $C_{10}H_{11}N_3O_3S$ and $C_{14}H_{18}N_4O_3$ is dissolved in 60 minutes.

Uniformity of dosage units ⟨905⟩: meet the requirements.

Assay—

Mobile phase, Standard preparation, and *Chromatographic system*—Prepare as directed in the *Assay* under *Sulfamethoxazole and Trimethoprim Oral Suspension.*

Assay preparation—Weigh and finely powder not fewer than 20 Tablets. Transfer an accurately weighed portion of the powder, equivalent to about 160 mg of sulfamethoxazole, to a 100-mL volumetric flask. Add about 50 mL of methanol and sonicate, with intermittent shaking, for 5 minutes. Allow to equilibrate to room temperature, dilute with methanol to volume, mix, and filter. Transfer 5.0 mL of the clear filtrate to a 50-mL volumetric flask, dilute with *Mobile phase* to volume, and mix.

Procedure—Separately inject equal volumes (about 20 µL) of the *Standard preparation* and the *Assay preparation* into the chromatograph, record the chromatograms, and measure the responses for the major peaks. Calculate the quantities, in mg, of trimethoprim ($C_{14}H_{18}N_4O_3$) and sulfamethoxazole ($C_{10}H_{11}N_3O_3S$) in the portion of Tablets taken by the formula:

$$1000C(r_U / r_S)$$

in which *C* is the concentration, in mg per mL, of the appropriate USP Reference Standard in the *Standard preparation;* and r_U and r_S are the responses of the corresponding analyte obtained from the *Assay preparation* and the *Standard preparation,* respectively.

Sulfapyridine

$C_{11}H_{11}N_3O_2S$ 249.29
Benzenesulfonamide, 4-amino-*N*-2-pyridinyl-.
N^1-2-Pyridylsulfanilamide   [144-83-2].

» Sulfapyridine contains not less than 99.0 percent and not more than 100.5 percent of $C_{11}H_{11}N_3O_2S$, calculated on the dried basis.

Packaging and storage—Preserve in well-closed, light-resistant containers.
USP Reference standards ⟨11⟩—*USP Sulfapyridine RS.*
Clarity and color of solution—A solution of 1.0 g in a mixture of 20 mL of water and 5 mL of 1 N sodium hydroxide is clear and not more deeply colored than pale yellow.
Identification—
  A: *Infrared Absorption* ⟨197K⟩.
  B: Add 5 mL of 3 N hydrochloric acid to about 0.1 g of Sulfapyridine, and boil gently for about 5 minutes. Cool in an ice bath, add 4 mL of sodium nitrite solution (1 in 100), dilute with water to 10 mL, and place the mixture in the ice bath for 10 minutes. To 5 mL of the cooled mixture add a solution of 50 mg of 2-naphthol in 2 mL of sodium hydroxide solution (1 in 10): an orange-red precipitate is formed, and it darkens on standing.
Melting range ⟨741⟩: between 190° and 193°.
Acidity—Digest 2.0 g with 100 mL of water at about 70° for 5 minutes, cool at once to about 20°, and filter. To 25.0 mL of the filtrate add 2 drops of phenolphthalein TS, and titrate with 0.10 N sodium hydroxide: not more than 0.20 mL is required for neutralization.
Loss on drying ⟨731⟩—Dry it at 105° for 2 hours: it loses not more than 0.5% of its weight.
Residue on ignition ⟨281⟩: not more than 0.1%.
Selenium ⟨291⟩: 0.003%, a 200-mg test specimen being used.
Heavy metals, *Method II* ⟨231⟩: 0.002%.
Organic volatile impurities, *Method V* ⟨467⟩: meets the requirements.
  Solvent—Use dimethyl sulfoxide.
(Official until July 1, 2008)
Assay—Proceed with Sulfapyridine as directed under *Nitrite Titration* ⟨451⟩. Each mL of 0.1 N sodium nitrite is equivalent to 24.93 mg of $C_{11}H_{11}N_3O_2S$.

Sulfapyridine Tablets

» Sulfapyridine Tablets contain not less than 95.0 percent and not more than 105.0 percent of the labeled amount of $C_{11}H_{11}N_3O_2S$.

Packaging and storage—Preserve in well-closed, light-resistant containers.
USP Reference standards ⟨11⟩—*USP Sulfapyridine RS.*
Identification—Triturate a quantity of finely powdered Tablets, equivalent to about 500 mg of sulfapyridine, with 5 mL of chloroform, and transfer to a small filter. Wash with another 5-mL portion of chloroform, and discard the filtrate. Triturate the residue with 10 mL of 6 N ammonium hydroxide for 5 minutes, add 10 mL of water, and filter. Warm the filtrate until most of the ammonia is expelled, cool, and add 6 N acetic acid until the reaction is distinctly acid: a precipitate of sulfapyridine is formed. Collect the precipitate on a filter, wash it well with cold water, and dry at 105° for 1 hour: the sulfapyridine so obtained melts between 189° and 192° as determined by the method for *Class Ia* under *Melting Range or Temperature* ⟨741⟩, and responds to the *Identification* tests under *Sulfapyridine.*
Dissolution ⟨711⟩—
  Medium: 0.01 N hydrochloric acid; 900 mL.
  Apparatus 2: 50 rpm.
  Time: 60 minutes.
  Procedure—Determine the amount of $C_{11}H_{11}N_3O_2S$ dissolved by employing UV absorption at the wavelength of maximum absorbance at about 254 nm on filtered portions of the solution under test, suitably diluted with 0.01 N sodium hydroxide, in comparison with a Standard solution having a known concentration of USP Sulfapyridine RS in the same media.
  Tolerances—Not less than 70% (*Q*) of the labeled amount of $C_{11}H_{11}N_3O_2S$ is dissolved in 60 minutes.
Uniformity of dosage units ⟨905⟩: meet the requirements.
Assay—Weigh and finely powder not less than 20 Tablets. Weigh accurately a portion of the powder, equivalent to about 500 mg of sulfapyridine, and proceed as directed under *Nitrite Titration* ⟨451⟩, beginning with "and transfer to a suitable open vessel." Each mL of 0.1 M sodium nitrite is equivalent to 24.93 mg of $C_{11}H_{11}N_3O_2S$.

Sulfaquinoxaline

$C_{14}H_{12}N_4O_2S$ 300.34
N^1-2-Quinoxalinylsulfanilamide   [59-40-5].

» Sulfaquinoxaline contains not less than 98.0 percent and not more than 101.0 percent of $C_{14}H_{12}N_4O_2S$, calculated on the dried basis.

Packaging and storage—Preserve in well-closed containers, protected from light.
Labeling—Label it to indicate that it is for veterinary use only.
USP Reference standards ⟨11⟩—*USP Sulfaquinoxaline RS. USP Sulfaquinoxaline Related Compound A RS.*
Identification—
  A: *Infrared Absorption* ⟨197K⟩.
  B: *Ultraviolet Absorption* ⟨197U⟩—
  Solution: 10 µg per mL.
  Medium: 0.01 N sodium hydroxide.
  C: Dissolve 4 mg in 2 mL of 2 N hydrochloric acid, add 0.2 mL of sodium nitrite solution (1 in 100), and allow to stand for 2 minutes. Add the solution to 1 mL of 2-naphthol TS: an orange-red precipitate is formed.
Acidity—Digest 2 g of it with 100 mL of water at about 70° for 5 minutes, cool to about 20°, and filter. Titrate 50 mL of the filtrate with 0.1 N sodium hydroxide VS to a pH of 7.0: not more than 0.2 mL is required.
Loss on drying ⟨731⟩—Dry it at 105° for 4 hours: it loses not more than 1.0% of its weight.
Residue on ignition ⟨281⟩: not more than 0.1%.
Heavy metals, *Method II* ⟨231⟩: 0.002%.
Related compounds—Dissolve 400 mg of Sulfaquinoxaline in 4 mL of 1 N sodium hydroxide, add methanol to obtain 100 mL of solution, and mix (test solution). Prepare a solution of USP Sulfaquinoxaline Related Compound A RS in methanol containing 0.12 mg per mL (*Standard solution 1*). Prepare a solution of sulfanilamide in methanol containing 0.04 mg per mL (*Standard solution 2*). Separately apply 5 µL each of the test solution, *Standard solution 1*, and *Standard solution 2* to a thin-layer chromatographic plate (see *Chromatography* ⟨621⟩) coated with a 0.25-mm layer of chromatographic silica gel mixture. Allow the spots to dry, and develop the chromatogram in a solvent system consisting of a mixture of chloroform, methanol, and ammonium hydroxide (60 : 40 : 20) until the solvent front has moved about three-fourths of the length of the plate. Remove the plate from the chamber, mark the solvent

front, allow it to air-dry, and examine the plate under short-wavelength UV light: no spot corresponding to sulfaquinoxaline related compound A in the chromatogram obtained from the test solution is more intense than the principal spot in the chromatogram obtained from *Standard solution 1* (3.0%), and no spot, other than the principal spot and the sulfaquinoxaline related compound A spot, if any, in the chromatogram obtained from the test solution is more intense than the principal spot in the chromatogram obtained from *Standard solution 2* (1.0%).

Assay—
*Mobile phase—*Dissolve 2 g of monobasic ammonium phosphate in 1000 mL of a mixture of water, acetonitrile, glacial acetic acid, tetrahydrofuran, and ammonium hydroxide (583 : 400 : 10 : 5 : 2). Filter through a filter of 0.5 µm or finer porosity, and degas. Make adjustments if necessary (see *System suitability* under *Chromatography* ⟨621⟩).

*Standard preparation—*Dissolve an accurately weighed quantity of USP Sulfaquinoxaline RS in 0.01 N sodium hydroxide to obtain a solution having a known concentration of about 0.7 mg per mL.

*Assay preparation—*Transfer about 175 mg of Sulfaquinoxaline, accurately weighed, to a 250-mL volumetric flask, dilute with 0.01 N sodium hydroxide to volume, and mix.

Chromatographic system (see *Chromatography* ⟨621⟩)—The liquid chromatograph is equipped with a 254-nm detector and a 4-mm × 25-cm column that contains packing L1. The flow rate is about 1 mL per minute. Chromatograph the *Standard preparation*, and record the peak responses as directed for *Procedure:* the column efficiency is not less than 2500 theoretical plates, the tailing factor is not more than 1.2, and the relative standard deviation for replicate injections is not more than 2.0%.

*Procedure—*Separately inject equal volumes (about 15 µL) of the *Standard preparation* and the *Assay preparation* into the chromatograph, record the chromatograms, and measure the responses for the major peaks. Calculate the quantity, in mg, of $C_{14}H_{12}N_4O_2S$ in the portion of Sulfaquinoxaline taken by the formula:

$$250C(r_U / r_S)$$

in which *C* is the concentration, in µg per mL, of USP Sulfaquinoxaline RS in the *Standard preparation*, and r_U and r_S are the sulfaquinoxaline peak responses obtained from the *Assay preparation* and the *Standard preparation*, respectively.

Sulfaquinoxaline Oral Solution

» Sulfaquinoxaline Oral Solution contains the equivalent of not less than 90.0 percent and not more than 110.0 percent of the labeled concentration of sulfaquinoxaline ($C_{14}H_{12}N_4O_2S$).

Packaging and storage—Preserve in tight, light-resistant containers.

Labeling—Label it to indicate that it is for veterinary use only.

USP Reference standards ⟨11⟩—*USP Sulfaquinoxaline RS.*

Identification—The retention time of the major peak in the chromatogram of the *Assay preparation* corresponds to that in the chromatogram of the *Standard preparation*, as obtained in the *Assay*.

Deliverable volume ⟨698⟩: meets the requirements.

pH ⟨791⟩: not less than 12.

Assay—
Mobile phase and *Chromatographic system—*Proceed as directed in the *Assay* under *Sulfaquinoxaline*.

*Standard preparation—*Dissolve an accurately weighed quantity of USP Sulfaquinoxaline RS in 0.01 N sodium hydroxide to obtain a solution having a known concentration of about 0.7 mg per mL. Dilute an accurately measured volume of this solution quantitatively with water to obtain a solution having a known concentration of about 0.15 mg per mL.

*Assay preparation—*Transfer an accurately measured volume of Oral Solution, equivalent to about 300 mg of sulfaquinoxaline, to a 2000-mL volumetric flask, dilute with water to volume, and mix.

*Procedure—*Separately inject equal volumes (about 8 µL) of the *Standard preparation* and the *Assay preparation* into the chromatograph, record the chromatograms, and measure the responses for the major peaks. Calculate the quantity, in mg, of sulfaquinoxaline ($C_{14}H_{12}N_4O_2S$) in each mL of the Oral Solution taken by the formula:

$$2000(C / V)(r_U / r_S)$$

in which *C* is the concentration, in mg per mL, of USP Sulfaquinoxaline RS in the *Standard preparation*, *V* is the volume, in mL, of Oral Solution taken to prepare the *Assay preparation*, and r_U and r_S are the sulfaquinoxaline peak responses obtained from the *Assay preparation* and the *Standard preparation*, respectively.

Sulfasalazine

$C_{18}H_{14}N_4O_5S$ 398.39

Benzoic acid, 2-hydroxy-5-[[4-[(2-pyridinylamino)sulfonyl]phenyl]azo]-.
5-[[*p*-(2-Pyridylsulfamoyl)phenyl]azo]salicylic acid   [599-79-1].

» Sulfasalazine contains not less than 97.0 percent and not more than 101.5 percent of $C_{18}H_{14}N_4O_5S$, calculated on the dried basis.

Packaging and storage—Preserve in tight, light-resistant containers.

USP Reference standards ⟨11⟩—*USP Sulfasalazine RS.*

Identification—
A: *Infrared Absorption* ⟨197K⟩.
B: The visible absorption spectrum of the solution from the *Assay preparation*, prepared as directed in the *Assay*, exhibits maxima and minima at the same wavelengths as that of the solution from the *Standard preparation*, prepared as directed in the *Assay*, concomitantly measured.

Loss on drying ⟨731⟩—Dry it at 105° for 2 hours: it loses not more than 1.0% of its weight.

Residue on ignition ⟨281⟩: not more than 0.5%.

Chloride ⟨221⟩—Digest 2.0 g of Sulfasalazine with 100 mL of water at 70° for 5 minutes. Cool immediately to room temperature, and filter. Transfer a 25-mL portion of the filtrate to a 50-mL beaker (retain the remainder of this filtrate for the *Sulfate test*), add 1 mL of nitric acid, mix, and allow to stand for 5 minutes. Filter through a fine texture, retentive filter paper (Whatman No. 42, or equivalent): the filtrate shows no more chloride than corresponds to 0.10 mL of 0.020 N hydrochloric acid (0.014%).

Sulfate ⟨221⟩—Transfer a 25-mL portion of the filtrate from the *Chloride test* to a 50-mL beaker. Add 1 mL of 3 N hydrochloric acid, mix, and allow to stand for 5 minutes. Filter through a fine texture, retentive filter paper (Whatman No. 42, or equivalent): the filtrate shows no more sulfate than corresponds to 0.20 mL of 0.020 N sulfuric acid (0.04%).

Heavy metals, *Method II* ⟨231⟩: 0.002%.

Chromatographic purity—Prepare a solution of Sulfasalazine in a mixture of alcohol and 2 M ammonium hydroxide (4 : 1) having a concentration of 10 mg per mL. Similarly prepare a Standard solution of USP Sulfasalazine RS in the same medium having a concentration of 10 mg per mL. Dilute aliquots of the Standard solution quantitatively and stepwise with the same medium to obtain solutions having concentrations of 200, 150, 100, and 20 µg per mL, corresponding to 2.0%, 1.5%, 1.0%, and 0.2%, respectively (*Standard dilutions A*, *B*, *C*, and *D*). Separately apply 10-µL each of the test solution, the Standard solution, and the *Standard dilutions* to a suitable thin-layer chromatographic plate (see *Chromatography* ⟨621⟩) coated with a 0.25-mm layer of chromatographic silica gel mixture. Allow the spots to dry, and develop the chromatogram in an unequilibrated chamber with a solvent system consisting of a mixture of chloroform, acetone, and formic acid (60 : 30 : 5) until the solvent front has moved about three-fourths of the length of the plate. Remove the plate from the chamber, mark the solvent front, dry with the aid of a current of hot air, and examine the plate under short-wavelength UV light: the R_F value of the principal spot obtained from the test solution corresponds to that obtained from the Standard solution, and no spots, other than the principal spot, in the chromatogram of the test solution are larger or more intense than the principal spot obtained from *Standard dilution A* (2%), and the sum of the intensities of any secondary spots detected does not exceed 4%.

Organic volatile impurities, *Method V* ⟨467⟩: meets the requirements.

Solvent—Use dimethyl sulfoxide.

(Official until July 1, 2008)

Assay—Transfer about 150 mg of Sulfasalazine, accurately weighed, to a 100-mL volumetric flask. Dissolve in 0.1 N sodium hydroxide, dilute with 0.1 N sodium hydroxide to volume, and mix. Transfer 5.0 mL of this solution to a 1000-mL volumetric flask containing about 750 mL of water, mix, add 20.0 mL of 0.1 N acetic acid, dilute with water to volume, and mix. Concomitantly determine the absorbances of this solution and of a Standard solution of USP Sulfasalazine RS in the same medium having a known concentration of about 7.5 μg per mL, at the wavelength of maximum absorbance at about 359 nm, using water as the blank. Calculate the quantity, in mg, of $C_{18}H_{14}N_4O_5S$ in the Sulfasalazine taken by the formula:

$$20C(A_U / A_S)$$

in which C is the concentration, in μg per mL, of USP Sulfasalazine RS in the Standard solution, and A_U and A_S are the absorbances obtained from the assay solution and the Standard solution, respectively.

Sulfasalazine Tablets

» Sulfasalazine Tablets contain not less than 95.0 percent and not more than 105.0 percent of the labeled amount of sulfasalazine ($C_{18}H_{14}N_4O_5S$).

Packaging and storage—Preserve in well-closed containers.
USP Reference standards ⟨11⟩—*USP Sulfasalazine RS.*
Identification—The visible absorption spectrum of the solution from the *Assay preparation*, prepared as directed in the *Assay*, exhibits maxima and minima at the same wavelengths as that of the *Standard preparation*, prepared as directed in the *Assay* and concomitantly measured.
Dissolution ⟨711⟩—
Medium: pH 7.5 phosphate buffer (see under *Buffer Solutions* in the section *Reagents, Indicators, and Solutions*); 900 mL.
Apparatus 1: 100 rpm.
Time: 60 minutes.
Procedure—Determine the amount of $C_{18}H_{14}N_4O_5S$ dissolved from UV absorbances at the wavelength of maximum absorbance at about 358 nm of filtered portions of the solution under test, suitably diluted with *Dissolution Medium*, if necessary, in comparison with a Standard solution having a known concentration of USP Sulfasalazine RS in the same *Medium*.
Tolerances—Not less than 85% (Q) of the labeled amount of $C_{18}H_{14}N_4O_5S$ is dissolved in 60 minutes.
Uniformity of dosage units ⟨905⟩: meet the requirements.
Assay—Weigh and finely powder not less than 20 Tablets. Transfer an accurately weighed portion of the powder, equivalent to about 150 mg of sulfasalazine, to a 100-mL volumetric flask, add 50 mL of 0.1 N sodium hydroxide, and mix. Dilute with 0.1 N sodium hydroxide to volume, mix, and filter, discarding the first 20 mL of the filtrate. Transfer 5.0 mL of the filtrate to a 1000-mL volumetric flask containing about 750 mL of water, mix, add 20.0 mL of 0.1 N acetic acid, mix, dilute with water to volume, and mix. Concomitantly determine the absorbances of this solution and of a Standard solution of USP Sulfasalazine RS in the same medium having a known concentration of about 7.5 μg per mL, at the wavelength of maximum absorbance at about 359 nm, using water as the blank. Calculate the quantity, in mg, of sulfasalazine ($C_{18}H_{14}N_4O_5S$) in the portion of Tablets taken by the formula:

$$20C(A_U / A_S)$$

in which C is the concentration, in μg per mL, of USP Sulfasalazine RS in the Standard solution; and A_U and A_S are the absorbances of the solution from the Tablets and the Standard solution, respectively.

Sulfasalazine Delayed-Release Tablets

» Sulfasalazine Delayed-Release Tablets contain not less than 95.0 percent and not more than 105.0 percent of the labeled amount of sulfasalazine ($C_{18}H_{14}N_4O_5S$).

Packaging and storage—Preserve in well-closed containers.
USP Reference standards ⟨11⟩—*USP Sulfasalazine RS.*
Dissolution ⟨711⟩—Proceed as directed for *Procedure* for *Method B* under *Apparatus 1 and Apparatus 2, Delayed-Release Dosage Forms.*
ACID STAGE—
Medium: 0.1 N hydrochloric acid; 900 mL.
Apparatus 1: 100 rpm.
Time: 120 minutes.
At the end of 120 minutes, determine the amount of $C_{18}H_{14}N_4O_5S$ dissolved by employing the following method.
Mobile phase—Prepare a filtered and degassed mixture of water, isopropanol, acetonitrile, and glacial acetic acid (22 : 11 : 7 : 0.4). Make adjustments if necessary (see *System Suitability* under *Chromatography* ⟨621⟩).
Standard solution—Dissolve an accurately weighed quantity of USP Sulfasalazine RS in 0.1 N sodium hydroxide, and dilute quantitatively, and stepwise if necessary, with 0.1 N sodium hydroxide to obtain a solution having a known concentration of about 55.6 μg per mL.
Test solution—Pass about 7 mL of the solution under test through a membrane filter having a 0.45-μm porosity.
Chromatographic system (see *Chromatography* ⟨621⟩)—The liquid chromatograph is equipped with a 254-nm detector and a 4.6-mm × 25-cm column that contains packing L1. The flow rate is about 1 mL per minute. Chromatograph the *Standard solution*, and record the peak responses as directed for *Procedure:* the retention time for sulfasalazine is about 7.7 minutes; and the relative standard deviation for replicate injections is not more than 2.0%.
Procedure—Inject a volume (about 10 μL) of the *Standard solution* and the *Test solution* into the chromatograph, and measure the peak responses. Calculate the percentage of $C_{18}H_{14}N_4O_5S$ dissolved by the formula:

$$(900C_S / LC)(r_U / r_S)$$

in which C_S is the concentration, in mg per mL, of USP Sulfasalazine RS in the *Standard solution*; LC is the label claim, in mg; and r_U and r_S are the peak responses obtained from the *Test solution* and the *Standard solution*, respectively.
Tolerances—Not more than 10% of the labeled amount of $C_{18}H_{14}N_4O_5S$ is dissolved in 120 minutes.
BUFFER STAGE—
Medium: pH 7.5 phosphate buffer; 900 mL.
Apparatus 1: 100 rpm.
Time: 60 minutes.
At the end of 60 minutes, determine the amount of $C_{18}H_{14}N_4O_5S$ dissolved by employing the chromatographic method as described under *Acid stage.*
Tolerances—Not less than 85% (Q) of the labeled amount of $C_{18}H_{14}N_4O_5S$ is dissolved in 60 minutes.
Other requirements—Tablets respond to the *Identification* test and meet the requirements for *Uniformity of dosage units* and *Assay* under *Sulfasalazine Tablets.*

Sulfathiazole

$C_9H_9N_3O_2S_2$ 255.32
Benzenesulfonamide, 4-amino-*N*-2-thiazolyl-.
N¹-2-Thiazolylsulfanilamide   [72-14-0].

» Sulfathiazole contains not less than 99.0 percent and not more than 100.5 percent of $C_9H_9N_3O_2S_2$, calculated on the dried basis.

Packaging and storage—Preserve in well-closed, light-resistant containers.

USP Reference standards ⟨11⟩—*USP Sulfathiazole RS*.
Identification—
　A: *Infrared Absorption* ⟨197K⟩.
　B: To 100 mg add 5 mL of 3 N hydrochloric acid, and boil gently for about 5 minutes. Cool in an ice bath, add 4 mL of sodium nitrite solution (1 in 100), dilute with water to 10 mL, and place the mixture in an ice bath for 10 minutes. To 5 mL of the cooled mixture add a solution of 50 mg of 2-naphthol in 2 mL of sodium hydroxide solution (1 in 10): an orange-red precipitate is formed, and it darkens on standing.
Melting range, *Class I* ⟨741⟩:   between 200° and 204°.
Acidity—Digest 2 g with 100 mL of water at about 70° for 5 minutes, cool at once to about 20°, and filter. Titrate 25 mL of the filtrate with 0.10 N sodium hydroxide, using 2 drops of phenolphthalein TS as the indicator: not more than 0.5 mL is required to produce a pink color. (Retain the remainder of the filtrate for the tests for *Chloride* ⟨221⟩ and for *Sulfate* ⟨221⟩.)
Loss on drying ⟨731⟩—Dry it at 105° for 2 hours: it loses not more than 0.5% of its weight.
Residue on ignition ⟨281⟩:   not more than 0.1%.
Chloride ⟨221⟩—A 25-mL portion of the filtrate prepared as directed in the test for *Acidity* shows no more chloride than corresponds to 0.10 mL of 0.020 N hydrochloric acid (0.014%).
Sulfate ⟨221⟩—A 25-mL portion of the filtrate prepared as directed in the test for *Acidity* shows no more sulfate than corresponds to 0.2 mL of 0.02 N sulfuric acid (0.04%).
Heavy metals, *Method II* ⟨231⟩:   0.002%.
Ordinary impurities ⟨466⟩—
　Test solution: methanol.
　Standard solution: methanol.
　Eluant: a mixture of 1-propanol and 1 N ammonium hydroxide (22 : 3).
　Visualization: 1.
Assay—Proceed with Sulfathiazole as directed under *Nitrite Titration* ⟨451⟩. Each mL of 0.1 M sodium nitrite is equivalent to 25.53 mg of $C_9H_9N_3O_2S_2$.

Sulfinpyrazone

$C_{23}H_{20}N_2O_3S$ 404.48
3,5-Pyrazolidinedione, 1,2-diphenyl-4-[2-(phenylsulfinyl)ethyl]-.
1,2-Diphenyl-4-[2-(phenylsulfinyl)ethyl]-3,5-pyrazolidinedione [57-96-5].

» Sulfinpyrazone contains not less than 98.5 percent and not more than 101.5 percent of $C_{23}H_{20}N_2O_3S$, calculated on the dried basis.

Packaging and storage—Preserve in well-closed containers.
USP Reference standards ⟨11⟩—*USP Sulfinpyrazone RS*.
Solubility in acetone—A 250-mg portion dissolves in 5.0 mL of acetone to yield a clear, practically colorless solution.
Solubility in 0.50 N sodium hydroxide—A 0.50-g portion dissolves in 10.0 mL of 0.50 N sodium hydroxide to yield a clear, practically colorless solution.
Identification, *Infrared Absorption* ⟨197K⟩.
Melting range ⟨741⟩:   between 130.5° and 134.5°.
Loss on drying ⟨731⟩—Dry it at 105° for 2 hours: it loses not more than 0.5% of its weight.
Residue on ignition ⟨281⟩:   not more than 0.1%.
Heavy metals, *Method II* ⟨231⟩:   0.001%.
Chromatographic purity—
　Mobile phase—Proceed as directed in the *Assay* under *Sulfinpyrazone Capsules*.
　Acetate buffer—Transfer 240 mL of 0.1 N acetic acid to a 1-liter flask. Add 200 mL of 0.1 N potassium hydroxide, mix, and dilute with water to volume. Adjust to a pH of 5.0.
　Diluting solution—Prepare a mixture of acetonitrile and *Acetate buffer* (4 : 1).
　Standard preparation—Dissolve an accurately weighed quantity of USP Sulfinpyrazone RS in *Diluting solution*, and dilute quantitatively, and stepwise if necessary, with *Diluting solution* to obtain a solution having a known concentration of about 10 μg per mL.
　Test preparation—Prepare a solution of Sulfinpyrazone in *Diluting solution* having a known concentration of about 2 mg per mL.
　Chromatographic system (see *Chromatography* ⟨621⟩)—Proceed as directed in the *Assay* under *Sulfinpyrazone Capsules*. Chromatograph the *Standard preparation*, and record the peak responses as directed for *Procedure*: the retention time for sulfinpyrazone is between 4.0 and 4.6 minutes, the tailing factor is not more than 2.0, and the relative standard deviation for replicate injections is not more than 2.0%.
　Procedure—Separately inject equal volumes (about 10 μL) of the *Standard preparation* and the *Test preparation* into the chromatograph, record the chromatograms, and measure the responses for all of the peaks: the sum of the peak responses, other than that of the sulfinpyrazone peak, from the *Test preparation* is not more than four times the sulfinpyrazone peak response from the *Standard preparation* (2.0%), and no single peak response is greater than twice the sulfinpyrazone peak response from the *Standard preparation* (1.0%).
Organic volatile impurities, *Method V* ⟨467⟩: meets the requirements.
　Solvent—Use dimethyl sulfoxide.

(Official until July 1, 2008)

Assay—Dissolve about 600 mg of Sulfinpyrazone, accurately weighed, in 50 mL of neutralized alcohol, with slight heating. Add phenolphthalein TS, and titrate with 0.1 N sodium hydroxide VS. Each mL of 0.1 N sodium hydroxide is equivalent to 40.45 mg of $C_{23}H_{20}N_2O_3S$.

Sulfinpyrazone Capsules

» Sulfinpyrazone Capsules contain not less than 93.0 percent and not more than 107.0 percent of the labeled amount of $C_{23}H_{20}N_2O_3S$.

Packaging and storage—Preserve in well-closed containers.
USP Reference standards ⟨11⟩—*USP Sulfinpyrazone RS*.
Identification—To a quantity of the contents of Capsules, equivalent to about 400 mg of sulfinpyrazone, add 20 mL of a 1 in 20 solution of methanol in dehydrated alcohol, boil, and filter. Add water to the filtrate until the solution becomes turbid, allow to stand until crystals form (1 to 2 hours), remove the crystals by filtration, and dry at 105° for 1 hour: the sulfinpyrazone so obtained melts

between 128° and 134°, and responds to the *Identification* test under *Sulfinpyrazone*.
Dissolution ⟨711⟩—
Medium: pH 6.8 phosphate buffer (see under *Buffer Solutions* in the section *Reagents, Indicators, and Solutions*); 900 mL.
Apparatus 1: 100 rpm.
Time: 45 minutes.
Procedure—Determine the amount of $C_{23}H_{20}N_2O_3S$ dissolved from UV absorbances at the wavelength of maximum absorbance at about 259 nm of filtered portions of the solution under test, suitably diluted with *Dissolution Medium*, in comparison with a Standard solution having a known concentration of USP Sulfinpyrazone RS in the same *Medium*.
Tolerances—Not less than 75% (*Q*) of the labeled amount of $C_{23}H_{20}N_2O_3S$ is dissolved in 45 minutes.
Uniformity of dosage units ⟨905⟩: meet the requirements.
Assay—
Acetonitrile and *tetrahydrofuran mixture*—Prepare a mixture of acetonitrile and tetrahydrofuran (4 : 1).
Mobile phase—Prepare a degassed and filtered solution of dilute phosphoric acid (3 in 1000) and *Acetonitrile and tetrahydrofuran mixture* (65 : 35).
Internal standard solution—Prepare a solution of Benzoic Acid in acetonitrile having a concentration of about 2 mg per mL.
Standard preparation—Transfer about 100 mg, accurately weighed, of USP Sulfinpyrazone RS to a 200-mL volumetric flask, add 100 mL of acetonitrile, mix, add 10.0 mL of *Internal standard solution*, dilute with acetonitrile to volume, and mix. Filter, discarding the first 5 mL of the filtrate.
Assay preparation—Remove as completely as possible, and weigh, the contents of not less than 20 Capsules, and mix. Transfer an accurately weighed portion of the powder, equivalent to about 100 mg of sulfinpyrazone, to a 200-mL volumetric flask, add 100 mL of acetonitrile, mix, add 10.0 mL of *Internal standard solution*, dilute with acetonitrile to volume, and mix. Filter, discarding the first 5 mL of the filtrate.
Chromatographic system (see *Chromatography* ⟨621⟩)—The liquid chromatograph is equipped with a 235-nm detector and a 4.6-mm × 10-cm column that contains packing L1. The flow rate is about 3 mL per minute. Chromatograph the *Standard preparation*, and record the peak responses as directed under *Procedure*: the relative retention times are about 0.2 for benzoic acid and 1.0 for sulfinpyrazone; the resolution, *R*, between benzoic acid and sulfinpyrazone is not less than 13; and the relative standard deviation is not more than 2.0%.
Procedure—Separately inject equal volumes (about 10 µL) of the *Standard preparation* and the *Assay preparation* into the chromatograph, record the chromatograms, and measure the responses for the major peaks. The resolution, *R*, between benzoic acid and sulfinpyrazone is not less than 13. Calculate the quantity, in mg, of $C_{23}H_{20}N_2O_3S$ in the portion of Capsule contents taken by the formula:

$$200C(R_U / R_S)$$

in which *C* is the concentration, in mg per mL, of USP Sulfinpyrazone RS in the *Standard preparation*, and R_U and R_S are the relative peak response ratios obtained from the *Assay preparation* and the *Standard preparation*, respectively.

Sulfinpyrazone Tablets

» Sulfinpyrazone Tablets contain not less than 93.0 percent and not more than 107.0 percent of the labeled amount of sulfinpyrazone ($C_{23}H_{20}N_2O_3S$).

Packaging and storage—Preserve in well-closed containers.

USP Reference standards ⟨11⟩—*USP Sulfinpyrazone RS*.
Identification—Finely powder a quantity of Tablets, equivalent to about 400 mg of sulfinpyrazone, boil with 20 mL of alcohol, and filter. Add water to the filtrate until the solution becomes turbid, allow to stand until crystals form (1 to 2 hours), remove the crystals by filtration, and dry at 105° for 1 hour: the sulfinpyrazone so obtained melts between 128° and 134°, and responds to the *Identification* test under *Sulfinpyrazone*.
Dissolution ⟨711⟩—
Medium: pH 6.8 phosphate buffer (see under *Buffer Solutions* in the section *Reagents, Indicators, and Solutions*); 900 mL.
Apparatus 1: 100 rpm.
Time: 45 minutes.
Procedure—Determine the amount of $C_{23}H_{20}N_2O_3S$ dissolved from UV absorbances at the wavelength of maximum absorbance at about 259 nm of filtered portions of the solution under test, suitably diluted with *Dissolution Medium*, in comparison with a Standard solution having a known concentration of USP Sulfinpyrazone RS in the same *Medium*.
Tolerances—Not less than 75% (*Q*) of the labeled amount of $C_{23}H_{20}N_2O_3S$ is dissolved in 45 minutes.
Uniformity of dosage units ⟨905⟩: meet the requirements.
Assay—
Acetonitrile and *tetrahydrofuran mixture*, *Mobile phase*, *Internal standard solution*, *Standard preparation*, *Chromatographic system*, and *Procedure*—Proceed as directed in the *Assay* for *Sulfinpyrazone Capsules*.
Assay preparation—Weigh and finely powder not less than 20 Tablets. Transfer an accurately weighed portion of the powder, equivalent to about 100 mg of sulfinpyrazone, to a 200-mL volumetric flask, add 100 mL of acetonitrile, mix, add 10.0 mL of *Internal standard solution*, dilute with acetonitrile to volume, and mix. Filter, discarding the first 5 mL of the filtrate.

Sulfisoxazole

$C_{11}H_{13}N_3O_3S$ 267.31
Benzenesulfonamide, 4-amino-*N*-(3,4-dimethyl-5-isoxazolyl)-.
N^1-(3,4-Dimethyl-5-isoxazolyl)sulfanilamide   [*127-69-5*].

» Sulfisoxazole contains not less than 99.0 percent and not more than 101.0 percent of $C_{11}H_{13}N_3O_3S$, calculated on the dried basis.

Packaging and storage—Preserve in tight, light-resistant containers.

USP Reference standards ⟨11⟩—*USP Sulfisoxazole RS*.
Identification—
  A: *Infrared Absorption* ⟨197K⟩.
  B: The UV absorption spectrum of a 1 in 100,000 solution in pH 7.5 phosphate buffer (see *Buffer Solutions* in the section *Reagents, Indicators, and Solutions*), prepared by dissolving about 100 mg of Sulfisoxazole, accurately weighed, in 10 mL of sodium hydroxide solution (1 in 250) and adding sufficient amounts of the buffer solution to make 100 mL, then diluting 10 mL of the resulting solution with the buffer solution to 1000 mL, exhibits maxima and minima at the same wavelengths as that of a similar solution of USP Sulfisoxazole RS, concomitantly measured.
  C: Dissolve about 10 mg in 2 mL of 3 N hydrochloric acid with the aid of heat, cool for 5 minutes in an ice bath, add 3 drops of sodium nitrite solution (1 in 100), and dilute with water to 4 mL: a yellow solution is produced. Add 1 mL of sodium hydroxide solution (1 in 10) containing 10 mg of 2-naphthol: an orange-red precipitate is formed.
Melting range ⟨741⟩: between 194° and 199°.
Loss on drying ⟨731⟩—Dry it at 105° for 2 hours: it loses not more than 0.5% of its weight.

Residue on ignition ⟨281⟩: not more than 0.1%.
Selenium ⟨291⟩: 0.003%, a 200-mg test specimen being used.
Heavy metals, *Method II* ⟨231⟩: 0.002%.
Ordinary impurities ⟨466⟩—
  Test solution: ethyl acetate.
  Standard solution: ethyl acetate.
  Eluant: a mixture of acetone, cyclohexane, and glacial acetic acid (5 : 4 : 1).
  Visualization: 1.
Assay—Place about 800 mg of Sulfisoxazole, accurately weighed, in a 250-mL conical flask, add 50 mL of dimethylformamide, shake thoroughly to dissolve the solid, add 5 drops of a 1 in 100 solution of thymol blue in dimethylformamide, and titrate with 0.1 N lithium methoxide in toluene VS to a blue endpoint, taking precautions against absorption of atmospheric carbon dioxide. Perform a blank determination, and make any necessary correction. Each mL of 0.1 N lithium methoxide is equivalent to 26.73 mg of $C_{11}H_{13}N_3O_3S$.

Sulfisoxazole Tablets

» Sulfisoxazole Tablets contain not less than 95.0 percent and not more than 105.0 percent of the labeled amount of $C_{11}H_{13}N_3O_3S$.

Packaging and storage—Preserve in well-closed, light-resistant containers.
USP Reference standards ⟨11⟩—*USP Sulfisoxazole RS.*
Identification—Extract a quantity of powdered Tablets, equivalent to about 1 g of sulfisoxazole, with 50 mL of alcohol by boiling on a steam bath for 3 minutes, then immediately filter into a beaker. Allow to stand until a quantity of fine, needle-like crystals form. Cool, filter off the crystals, recrystallize from a small volume of alcohol, and dry at 105°: the crystals respond to *Identification* test *A* under *Sulfisoxazole*.
Dissolution ⟨711⟩—
  Medium: dilute hydrochloric acid (1 in 12.5); 900 mL.
  Apparatus 1: 100 rpm.
  Time: 30 minutes.
  Procedure—[NOTE—Because of the pH-dependent nature of the UV absorption spectrum, prepare the standard and specimen solutions in the same strength of acid at approximately equal concentrations.] Determine the amount of $C_{11}H_{13}N_3O_3S$ dissolved from UV absorbances at the wavelength of maximum absorbance at about 267 nm of filtered portions of the solution under test, suitably diluted with water, if necessary, in comparison with a Standard solution having a known concentration of USP Sulfisoxazole RS in the same medium.
  Tolerances—Not less than 70% (*Q*) of the labeled amount of $C_{11}H_{13}N_3O_3S$ is dissolved in 30 minutes.
Uniformity of dosage units ⟨905⟩: meet the requirements.
Assay—Weigh and finely powder not less than 20 Tablets. Weigh accurately a portion of the powder, equivalent to about 800 mg of sulfisoxazole, transfer to a 250-mL conical flask, and proceed as directed in the *Assay* under *Sulfisoxazole*, beginning with "add 50 mL of dimethylformamide."

Sulfisoxazole Acetyl

$C_{13}H_{15}N_3O_4S$ 309.34
Acetamide, *N*-[(4-aminophenyl)sulfonyl]-*N*-(3,4-dimethyl-5-isoxazolyl)-.
N-(3,4-Dimethyl-5-isoxazolyl)-*N*-sulfanilylacetamide [80-74-0].

» Sulfisoxazole Acetyl contains not less than 98.0 percent and not more than 100.5 percent of $C_{13}H_{15}N_3O_4S$, calculated on the dried basis.

Packaging and storage—Preserve in tight, light-resistant containers.
USP Reference standards ⟨11⟩—*USP Sulfisoxazole Acetyl RS.*
Identification—
  A: *Infrared Absorption* ⟨197K⟩.
  B: *Ultraviolet Absorption* ⟨197U⟩—
  Solution: 10 µg per mL.
  Medium: alcohol.
Absorptivities at 290 nm, calculated on the dried basis, do not differ by more than 3.0%.
Melting range ⟨741⟩: between 192° and 195°.
Loss on drying ⟨731⟩—Dry it at 105° for 3 hours: it loses not more than 0.5% of its weight.
Ordinary impurities ⟨466⟩—
  Test solution: methanol.
  Standard solution: methanol.
  Eluant: a mixture of toluene and acetone (1 : 1).
  Visualization: 1.
Organic volatile impurities, *Method IV* ⟨467⟩: meets the requirements.
(Official until July 1, 2008)
Other requirements—It meets the requirements for *Residue on ignition,* *Selenium,* and *Heavy metals* under *Sulfisoxazole.*
Assay—Transfer about 1 g of Sulfisoxazole Acetyl, accurately weighed, to a 250-mL beaker. Add 15 mL of glacial acetic acid, swirl to dissolve, then add 25 mL of hydrochloric acid and 80 mL of water. Proceed as directed under *Nitrite Titration* ⟨451⟩, beginning with "Cool to about 15°." Each mL of 0.1 M sodium nitrite is equivalent to 30.94 mg of $C_{13}H_{15}N_3O_4S$.

Sulfisoxazole Acetyl Oral Suspension

» Sulfisoxazole Acetyl Oral Suspension contains an amount of Sulfisoxazole Acetyl equivalent to not less than 93.0 percent and not more than 107.0 percent of the labeled amount of sulfisoxazole ($C_{11}H_{13}N_3O_3S$).

Packaging and storage—Preserve in tight, light-resistant containers.
USP Reference standards ⟨11⟩—*USP Sulfisoxazole Acetyl RS.*
Identification—Centrifuge a portion of it, wash the separated solid by centrifugation with several portions of water, and recrystallize from hot alcohol: the crystals so obtained respond to *Identification* tests *A* and *B* under *Sulfisoxazole Acetyl.*
Uniformity of dosage units ⟨905⟩—
  FOR ORAL SUSPENSION PACKAGED IN SINGLE-UNIT CONTAINERS: meets the requirements.
Deliverable volume ⟨698⟩—
  FOR ORAL SUSPENSION PACKAGED IN MULTIPLE-UNIT CONTAINERS: meets the requirements.
pH ⟨791⟩: between 5.0 and 5.5.
Assay—Transfer an accurately measured volume of Oral Suspension, previously mixed, equivalent to about 1 g of sulfisoxazole, to a 250-mL beaker. Add 40 mL of hydrochloric acid and 25 mL of glacial acetic acid, and swirl to dissolve. Cautiously add 100 mL of water, and proceed as directed under *Nitrite Titration* ⟨451⟩, beginning with "Cool to about 15°." Each mL of 0.1 M sodium nitrite is equivalent to 26.73 mg of sulfisoxazole ($C_{11}H_{13}N_3O_3S$).

Precipitated Sulfur

S 32.07
Sulfur.
Sulfur [7704-34-9].

» Precipitated Sulfur contains not less than 99.5 percent and not more than 100.5 percent of S, calculated on the anhydrous basis.

Packaging and storage—Preserve in well-closed containers.
Identification—It burns in the air, forming sulfur dioxide, which can be recognized by its characteristic odor.
Reaction—Agitate 2.0 g with 10 mL of water, and filter: the filtrate is neutral to litmus.
Water, *Method I* ⟨921⟩: not more than 0.5%.
Residue on ignition ⟨281⟩: not more than 0.3%.
Other forms of sulfur—Shake 1.0 g with 5 mL of carbon disulfide: it dissolves quickly, with the exception of a small amount of insoluble matter that is usually present.
Assay—Using about 60 mg of Precipitated Sulfur, accurately weighed, proceed as directed under *Oxygen Flask Combustion* ⟨471⟩, using a 1000-mL flask and using a mixture of 10 mL of water and 5.0 mL of hydrogen peroxide TS as the absorbing liquid. When the combustion is complete, fill the lip of the flask with water, loosen the stopper, then rinse the stopper, the sample holder, and the sides of the flask with water, and remove the stopper assembly. Heat the contents of the flask to boiling, and boil for about 2 minutes. Cool to room temperature, add phenolphthalein TS, and titrate with 0.1 N sodium hydroxide VS. Perform a blank determination, and make any necessary correction. Each mL of 0.1 N sodium hydroxide is equivalent to 1.603 mg of S.

Sulfur Ointment

» Sulfur Ointment contains not less than 9.5 percent and not more than 10.5 percent of S.

Precipitated Sulfur	100 g
Mineral Oil	100 g
White Ointment	800 g
To make	1000 g

Levigate the sulfur with the Mineral Oil to a smooth paste, and then incorporate with the White Ointment.

Packaging and storage—Preserve in well-closed containers, and avoid prolonged exposure to excessive heat.
Assay—Transfer about 500 mg of Ointment, accurately weighed, to a suitable conical flask, add 5 mL of nitric acid and 3 mL of bromine, warm slightly, and allow to stand overnight. Heat gently on a steam bath until the excess bromine has been dissipated. Add 30 mL of water and then 30 mL of ether, and swirl to dissolve most of the ointment base. Transfer the mixture to a separator, with the aid of a 20-mL and a 10-mL portion of ether, followed by two 10-mL portions of water. Shake the mixture, and draw off the water layer into a suitable beaker or flask. Extract the ether layer with two 40-mL portions of water each containing 1 mL of hydrochloric acid. Heat the combined water extracts on a steam bath to remove all traces of ether. Dilute the solution with water to about 200 mL, heat to boiling, and add slowly, with constant stirring, about 20 mL of hot barium chloride TS. Heat on a steam bath for 1 hour, then collect the precipitate on a filter, wash it well with hot water, dry, and ignite to constant weight. The weight of the barium sulfate so obtained, multiplied by 0.1374, represents the weight of S.

Sublimed Sulfur

S 32.07
Sulfur.
Sulfur [7704-34-9].

» Sublimed Sulfur, dried over phosphorus pentoxide for 4 hours, contains not less than 99.5 percent and not more than 100.5 percent of S.

Packaging and storage—Preserve in well-closed containers.
Solubility in carbon disulfide—One g dissolves slowly and usually incompletely in about 2 mL of carbon disulfide.
Identification—It burns in the air to sulfur dioxide, which can be recognized by its characteristic odor.
Residue on ignition ⟨281⟩: not more than 0.5%.
Arsenic, *Method I* ⟨211⟩—Prepare the *Test Preparation* as follows. Digest 750 mg of Sublimed Sulfur with 20 mL of 6 N ammonium hydroxide for 3 hours, filter, and evaporate the clear filtrate on a steam bath to dryness. Add 15 mL of 2 N sulfuric acid and 1 mL of 30 percent hydrogen peroxide solution, evaporate to strong fumes of sulfur trioxide, cool, add cautiously 10 mL of water, and again evaporate to strong fumes, repeating, if necessary, to remove any trace of hydrogen peroxide. Cool, and dilute cautiously with water to 35 mL. The limit is 4 ppm.
Assay—Proceed as directed under *Oxygen Flask Combustion* ⟨471⟩, using a 1000-mL flask and using about 60 mg of Sublimed Sulfur, previously dried over phosphorus pentoxide for 4 hours and accurately weighed, as the sample and a mixture of 10 mL of water and 5.0 mL of hydrogen peroxide TS as the absorbing liquid. When the combustion is complete, fill the lip of the flask with water, loosen the stopper, then rinse the stopper, sample holder, and sides of the flask with water, and remove the stopper assembly. Heat the contents of the flask to boiling, and boil for about 2 minutes. Cool to room temperature, add phenolphthalein TS, and titrate with 0.1 N sodium hydroxide VS. Perform a blank determination, and make any necessary correction. Each mL of 0.1 N sodium hydroxide is equivalent to 1.603 mg of S.

Sulindac

$C_{20}H_{17}FO_3S$ 356.41
1*H*-Indene-3-acetic acid, 5-fluoro-2-methyl-1-[[4-(methylsulfinyl)phenyl]methylene]-, (Z)-.
cis-5-Fluoro-2-methyl-1-[(*p*-methylsulfinyl)benzylidene]indene-3-acetic acid [38194-50-2].

» Sulindac contains not less than 99.0 percent and not more than 101.0 percent of $C_{20}H_{17}FO_3S$, calculated on the dried basis.

Packaging and storage—Preserve in well-closed containers.
USP Reference standards ⟨11⟩—*USP Sulindac RS.*
Identification—
  A: *Infrared Absorption* ⟨197M⟩.
  B: *Ultraviolet Absorption* ⟨197U⟩—
  Solution: 15 μg per mL.
  Medium: hydrochloric acid in methanol (1 in 120).
  Absorptivities at 284 nm, calculated on the dried basis, do not differ by more than 3.0%.
Loss on drying ⟨731⟩—Dry it in vacuum at 100° for 2 hours: it loses not more than 0.5% of its weight.
Residue on ignition ⟨281⟩: not more than 0.1%.
Heavy metals, *Method II* ⟨231⟩: 0.001%.
Chromatographic purity—
  Standard preparation—Prepare a solution of USP Sulindac RS in methanol having a concentration of 25 mg per mL (*Solution A*). Prepare a second solution by diluting 1.0 volume of *Solution A* with methanol to obtain 250 volumes of solution (*Solution B*).

Test preparation—Prepare a solution of the sample in methanol having a concentration of 25 mg per mL.

System suitability—From the chromatograms obtained as directed under *Procedure*, estimate the intensity of the origin spot, if any, in the chromatogram of *Solution A*. The system is satisfactory if any spot observed at the origin is less intense than that obtained from the principal spot in the chromatogram of 2 µL of *Solution B*.

Procedure—Apply 4-µL portions of *Solution A* and the *Test preparation* and 2-, 4-, 6-, 8-, and 10-µL portions of *Solution B* to a suitable thin-layer chromatographic plate (see *Chromatography* ⟨621⟩) coated with a 0.25-mm layer of chromatographic silica gel mixture. Allow the spots to dry, and develop the chromatogram in a solvent system consisting of a mixture of ethyl acetate and glacial acetic acid (97 : 3) until the solvent front has moved about three-fourths of the length of the plate. Remove the plate from the developing chamber, mark the solvent front, allow the solvent to evaporate, and examine the plate under short-wavelength UV light: the chromatograms show principal spots at about the same R_F value. Estimate the levels of any additional spots observed in the chromatogram of the *Test preparation* by comparison with the spots in the series of chromatograms of *Solution B*: the sum of the levels is not greater than that of the principal spot obtained from the 10-µL portion of *Solution B* (1%).

Organic volatile impurities, *Method V* ⟨467⟩: meets the requirements except that the limit for chloroform is 500 ppm.

Solvent—Use dimethyl sulfoxide.

(Official until July 1, 2008)

Assay—Dissolve about 700 mg of Sulindac, accurately weighed, in about 80 mL of methanol, and titrate with 0.1 N sodium hydroxide VS, determining the endpoint potentiometrically, using a glass-calomel electrode system (see *Titrimetry* ⟨541⟩). During the titration, and just prior to reaching the endpoint, wash down the walls of the titration vessel with small amounts of methanol. Each mL of 0.1 N sodium hydroxide is equivalent to 35.64 mg of $C_{20}H_{17}FO_3S$.

Sulindac Tablets

» Sulindac Tablets contain not less than 90.0 percent and not more than 110.0 percent of the labeled amount of $C_{20}H_{17}FO_3S$.

Packaging and storage—Preserve in well-closed containers.

USP Reference standards ⟨11⟩—*USP Sulindac RS*.

Identification—Compare the chromatograms obtained in the *Assay*: the *Assay preparation* exhibits a major peak for sulindac the retention time of which corresponds to that exhibited by the *Standard preparation*.

Dissolution ⟨711⟩—

Medium: 0.1 M pH 7.2 phosphate buffer prepared as directed under *Solutions* in the section *Reagents, Indicators, and Solutions*, except to use twice the stated quantities of the monobasic potassium phosphate solution and of the sodium hydroxide solution; 900 mL.

Apparatus 2: 50 rpm.

Time: 45 minutes.

Procedure—Filter 20 mL of the solution under test, and transfer 10.0 mL of the filtrate to a 100-mL volumetric flask. Dilute with *Dissolution Medium* to volume, and mix. Determine the absorbances of this solution and of a Standard solution prepared from USP Sulindac RS in the same medium, having a known concentration of about 20 µg per mL, in 1-cm cells at the wavelength of maximum absorbance at about 326 nm, using *Dissolution Medium* as the blank. Calculate the amount of $C_{20}H_{17}FO_3S$ dissolved by the formula:

$$10C(A_U / A_S)$$

in which C is the concentration, in mg per mL, of sulindac in the Standard solution, and A_U and A_S are the absorbances of the solutions obtained from the specimen under test and the Reference Standard, respectively.

Tolerances—Not less than 80% (*Q*) of the labeled amount of $C_{20}H_{17}FO_3S$ is dissolved in 45 minutes.

Uniformity of dosage units ⟨905⟩: meet the requirements.

Procedure for content uniformity—Using 1 finely powdered Tablet proceed as directed in the *Assay*, adjusting the degree of dilution used in preparing the *Assay preparation* to obtain a solution having a concentration of sulindac of about 0.5 mg per mL, and making appropriate corresponding changes in the calculation formula to account for the extent of dilution.

Related compounds—

Mobile phase—Prepare as directed in the *Assay*.

Standard preparation—Dilute the *Standard preparation* prepared as directed in the *Assay* with *Mobile phase* to obtain a solution having a known concentration of about 15 µg per mL.

Test preparation—Prepare as directed for *Assay preparation* in the *Assay*.

Procedure—Proceed as directed for *Procedure* in the *Assay*. Measure the responses of the sulindac peak of the *Standard preparation* and of all peaks other than that of sulindac in the *Test preparation*. Calculate the amount, in mg, of related compounds in the portion of Tablets taken by the formula:

$$0.1C(r_U / r_S)$$

in which C is the concentration, in µg per mL, of USP Sulindac RS in the *Standard preparation*, and r_U and r_S are the peak responses of the *Test preparation* and the *Standard preparation*, respectively: the limit is 3.0%, calculated on the basis of the *Assay* of sulindac in the portion of the Tablets taken.

Assay—

Mobile phase—Prepare a mixture of chloroform, ethyl acetate, and acetic acid (approximately 38 : 5 : 1). Make adjustments if necessary (see *System Suitability* under *Chromatography* ⟨621⟩). Degas the solution.

Standard preparation—Dissolve an accurately weighed quantity of USP Sulindac RS in *Mobile phase* to obtain a solution having a known concentration of about 0.5 mg per mL.

Assay preparation—Weigh and finely powder not less than 20 Tablets. Transfer an accurately weighed portion of the powder, equivalent to about 50 mg of sulindac, to a 100-mL volumetric flask. Add about 60 mL of *Mobile phase*, and shake by mechanical means for about 15 minutes. Dilute with *Mobile phase* to volume, mix, and centrifuge a portion of the mixture to obtain a clear supernatant.

Chromatographic system (see *Chromatography* ⟨621⟩)—The liquid chromatograph is equipped with a 332-nm detector and a 3.9-mm × 30-cm column that contains packing L3. The flow rate is about 2 mL per minute. Chromatograph the *Standard preparation*, and record the peak responses as directed for *Procedure*: the tailing factor is not more than 1.5, the column efficiency is not less than 1650 theoretical plates, and the relative standard deviation for replicate injections is not more than 1.0%.

Procedure—Separately inject equal volumes (about 10 µL) of the *Standard preparation* and the *Assay preparation* into the chromatograph, and record the chromatograms. Measure the sulindac peak responses. Calculate the quantity, in mg, of $C_{20}H_{17}FO_3S$ in the portion of Tablets taken by the formula:

$$100C(r_U / r_S)$$

in which C is the concentration, in mg per mL, of USP Sulindac RS in the *Standard preparation*, and r_U and r_S are the sulindac peak responses obtained from the *Assay preparation* and the *Standard preparation*, respectively.

Sulisobenzone

$C_{14}H_{12}O_6S$ 308.31
Benzenesulfonic acid, 5-benzoyl-4-hydroxy-2-methoxy-.
5-Benzoyl-4-hydroxy-2-methoxybenzenesulfonic acid   [4065-45-6].

» Sulisobenzone contains not less than 95.0 percent and not more than 105.0 percent of $C_{14}H_{12}O_6S$, calculated on the as-is basis.

Packaging and storage—Preserve in tight, light-resistant containers.

USP Reference standards ⟨11⟩—USP Sulisobenzone RS.
Identification, *Ultraviolet Absorption* ⟨197U⟩—
  Solution: 10 µg per mL.
  Medium: water.
  Absorptivities do not differ by more than 3.0%.

Assay—Accurately weigh about 1 g of Sulisobenzone, and dissolve in 20 mL of water in a conical flask. Add 200 mL of dehydrated isopropyl alcohol, titrate a portion with 0.1 N tetrabutylammonium hydroxide VS, and determine the two endpoints potentiometrically. Calculate the amount, in mg, of $C_{14}H_{12}O_6S$ in the portion of Sulisobenzone taken by the formula:

$$308.31 C(2V_1 - V_2)$$

in which 308.31 is the empirical weight of sulisobenzone; C is the concentration, in moles per liter, of the 0.1 N tetrabutylammonium hydroxide VS; and V_1 and V_2 are the volumes, in mL, of titrant needed to reach the first and second endpoints, respectively.

Sumatriptan

$C_{14}H_{21}N_3O_2S$ 295.40
1*H*-Indole-5-methanesulfonamide, 3-[2-(dimethylamino)ethyl]-*N*-methyl-.
3-[2-(Dimethylamino)ethyl]-*N*-methyl-1*H*-indole-5-methanesulfonamide   [103628-46-2].

» Sumatriptan contains not less than 98.0 percent and not more than 102.0 percent of $C_{14}H_{21}N_3O_2S$, calculated on the anhydrous and solvent-free basis.

Packaging and storage—Preserve in tight, light resistant containers. Protect from freezing, and store below 30°.

USP Reference standards ⟨11⟩—*USP Sumatriptan RS. USP Sumatriptan Succinate RS. USP Sumatriptan Succinate Related Compound A RS. USP Sumatriptan Succinate Related Compound C RS. USP Sumatriptan Succinate Related Impurities RS.*
Identification—
  A: *Infrared Absorption* ⟨197M⟩.
  B: The retention time of the major peak in the chromatogram of the *Assay preparation* corresponds to that in the chromatogram of the *Standard preparation*, as obtained in the *Assay*.

Water, *Method I* ⟨921⟩:   not more than 1.0%.
Limit of sumatriptan related compound A—
  10 M Ammonium acetate solution—Dissolve 77.1 g of ammonium acetate in 100 mL of water.
  Mobile phase—Prepare a filtered and degassed mixture of methanol and *10 M Ammonium acetate solution* (9 : 1). Make adjustments if necessary (see *System Suitability* under *Chromatography* ⟨621⟩).
  Standard solution—Dissolve an accurately weighed quantity of USP Sumatriptan Succinate Related Compound A RS in *Mobile phase*, and dilute quantitatively, and stepwise if necessary, with *Mobile phase* to obtain a solution having a known concentration of about 0.00625 mg per mL.
  Test solution—Transfer about 100 mg of Sumatriptan, accurately weighed, to a 50-mL volumetric flask, dissolve in and dilute with *Mobile phase* to volume, and mix.
  Chromatographic system (see *Chromatography* ⟨621⟩)—The liquid chromatograph is equipped with a 282-nm detector and a 4.6-mm × 25-cm column that contains 5-µm packing L3. The flow rate is about 2.0 mL per minute. Chromatograph the *Standard solution*, and record the peak responses as directed for *Procedure*: the relative standard deviation for replicate injections is not more than 5%.
  Procedure—Separately inject equal volumes (about 20 µL) of the *Standard solution* and the *Test solution* into the chromatograph, record the chromatograms, and measure the responses for the major peaks. Calculate the percentage of sumatriptan related compound A in the portion of Sumatriptan taken by the formula:

$$100(495.7/613.8)(C_S/C_U)(r_U/r_S)$$

in which 495.7 and 613.8 are the molecular weights of sumatriptan related compound A and sumatriptan succinate related compound A, respectively; C_S is the concentration, in mg per mL, of USP Sumatriptan Succinate Related Compound A RS in the *Standard solution*; C_U is the concentration, in mg per mL, of Sumatriptan in the *Test solution*; and r_U and r_S are the peak responses for sumatriptan related compound A obtained from the *Test solution* and the *Standard solution*, respectively: not more than 0.6% is found.

Related compounds—
  Diluent and *System suitability solution*—Proceed as directed in the *Assay*.
  Buffer solution—Dissolve about 1.7 mL of dibutylamine, about 0.6 mL of phosphoric acid, and about 3.9 g of monobasic sodium phosphate dihydrate in water. Adjust with a solution of 50 % (w/v) sodium hydroxide to a pH of about 7.5, dilute with water to 1000 mL, and mix.
  Mobile phase—Prepare a filtered and degassed mixture of *Buffer solution* and acetonitrile (3 : 1). Make adjustments if necessary (see *System Suitability* under *Chromatography* ⟨621⟩).
  Identification solution—Prepare a solution of USP Sumatriptan Succinate Related Impurities RS in *Mobile phase* having a concentration of about 3 mg per mL.
  Test solution—Dissolve an accurately weighed quantity of Sumatriptan in *Diluent* to obtain a solution having a concentration of about 2 mg per mL.
  Chromatographic system (see *Chromatography* ⟨621⟩)—The liquid chromatograph is equipped with a 282-nm detector and a 4.6-mm × 25-cm column that contains 5-µm packing L1. The flow rate is about 1.5 mL per minute. Chromatograph the *System suitability solution*, and record the peak responses as directed for *Procedure*: the relative retention times are about 0.9 for sumatriptan succinate related compound C and 1.0 for sumatriptan; the resolution, *R*, between sumatriptan succinate related compound C and sumatriptan is not less than 1.5. Chromatograph the *Identification solution*, and record the peak responses as directed for *Procedure*: identify the peaks according to *Table 1*.
  Procedure—Inject a volume (about 10 µL) of the *Test solution* into the chromatograph, record the chromatogram, and measure all of the peak responses. Calculate the percentage of each impurity in the portion of Sumatriptan taken by the formula:

$$100(r_i/r_s)$$

in which r_i is the peak response for each impurity, and r_s is the sum of the responses of all the peaks: meets the requirements given in *Table 1*.

Organic volatile impurities, *Method IV* ⟨467⟩: meets the requirements.

(Official until July 1, 2008)

Assay—

*Diluent—*Dissolve 3.9 g of monobasic sodium phosphate dihydrate in water. Adjust with a solution of 50 % (w/v) sodium hydroxide to a pH of about 6.5, and dilute with water to 1000 mL. Mix 750 mL of this solution with 250 mL of acetonitrile.

*Buffer solution—*Dissolve about 1.7 mL of dibutylamine, about 0.6 mL of phosphoric acid, and about 3.9 g of monobasic sodium phosphate dihydrate in water. Adjust with a solution of 50 % (w/v) sodium hydroxide to a pH of about 6.5, dilute with water to 1000 mL, and mix.

*Mobile phase—*Prepare a filtered and degassed mixture of *Buffer solution* and acetonitrile (3 : 1). Make adjustments if necessary (see *System Suitability* under *Chromatography* ⟨621⟩).

*System suitability solution—*Dissolve accurately weighed quantities of USP Sumatriptan Succinate RS and USP Sumatriptan Succinate Related Compound C RS in *Diluent* to obtain a solution having known concentrations of about 0.28 mg per mL and 0.14 mg per mL, respectively.

*Standard preparation—*Dissolve an accurately weighed quantity of USP Sumatriptan Succinate RS in *Diluent* to obtain a solution having a known concentration of about 0.14 mg per mL.

*Assay preparation—*Transfer about 10 mg of Sumatriptan, accurately weighed, to a 100-mL volumetric flask. Dissolve in and dilute with *Diluent* to volume, and mix.

Chromatographic system (see *Chromatography* ⟨621⟩)—The liquid chromatograph is equipped with a 282-nm detector and a 4.6-mm × 25-cm column that contains 5-µm packing L1. The flow rate is about 1.5 mL per minute. Chromatograph the *System suitability solution*, and record the peak responses as directed for *Procedure:* the relative retention times are about 0.9 for sumatriptan succinate related compound C and 1.0 for sumatriptan; and the resolution, *R*, between sumatriptan succinate related compound C and sumatriptan is not less than 1.5. Chromatograph the *Standard preparation*, and record the peak responses as directed for *Procedure:* the relative standard deviation for replicate injections is not more than 1.5%.

*Procedure—*Separately inject equal volumes (about 10 µL) of the *Standard preparation* and the *Assay preparation* into the chromatograph, record the chromatograms, and measure the areas for the major peaks. Calculate the amount, in mg, of $C_{14}H_{21}N_3O_2S$ in the portion of Sumatriptan taken by the formula:

$$(295.4/413.5)100C(r_U/r_S)$$

in which 295.4 and 413.5 are the molecular weights of sumatriptan and sumatriptan succinate, respectively; *C* is the concentration, in mg per mL, of USP Sumatriptan Succinate RS in the *Standard preparation;* and r_U and r_S are the peak responses for sumatriptan obtained from the *Assay preparation* and the *Standard preparation*, respectively.

Table 1

Compound Name	Relative Retention Time	Limit (%)
[3-[2-(Dimethylamino *N*-oxide)ethyl]-1*H*-indol-5-yl]-*N*-methylmethanesulfonamide	about 0.3	0.2
[3-[2-(Methylamino)ethyl]-1*H*-indol-5-yl]-*N*-methylmethanesulfonamide	about 0.6	0.5
Sumatriptan succinate related compound C	about 0.9	0.5
Sumatriptan	1.0	—
[3-[2-(Aminoethyl)-1*H*-indol-5-yl]-*N*-methylmethanesulfonamide	about 0.4	0.1
Unknown impurities	—	0.1
Total	—	1.5

[NOTE—The calculation of total impurities includes the amount of sumatriptan related compound A, determined in the test for *Limit of sumatriptan related compound A*.]

Sumatriptan Nasal Spray

» Sumatriptan Nasal Spray is an aqueous, buffered solution of Sumatriptan. It is supplied in a form suitable for nasal administration. It contains not less than 90.0 percent and not more than 110.0 percent of the labeled amount of sumatriptan ($C_{14}H_{21}N_3O_2S$).

Packaging and storage—Preserve in tight, light-resistant containers, and store between 2° and 30°.

USP Reference standards ⟨11⟩—*USP Sumatriptan Succinate RS. USP Sumatriptan Succinate Related Compound A RS. USP Sumatriptan Succinate Related Compound C RS. USP Sumatriptan Succinate Related Impurities RS.*

Identification, *Infrared Absorption* ⟨197M⟩—

*Test specimen—*To the contents of 1 vial of Nasal Spray add 1 mL of a saturated sodium chloride solution. Add 1 mL of a saturated solution of sodium carbonate, and shake vigorously for about 30 seconds. To the solution so obtained, add 2 mL of isopropyl alcohol, shake vigorously for about 30 seconds, and allow to stand until the phases separate. Transfer the organic phase to a suitable glass vial. Repeat the extraction with a second 2-mL portion of isopropyl alcohol, and transfer the organic phase to the same vial. Evaporate the solution under a stream of nitrogen. Dry the residue in an oven at 100° for 30 minutes, allow to cool to room temperature in a desiccator, and prepare a mull by the addition of 1 to 2 drops of mineral oil.

Microbial limits ⟨61⟩—The total aerobic microbial count does not exceed 100 cfu per mL, and it meets the requirements of the tests for absence of *Staphylococcus aureus* and *Pseudomonas aeruginosa* in 1 mL.

pH ⟨791⟩: between 5.0 and 6.0.

Deliverable volume—Test 10 vials separately. Weigh each vial before and after actuation, and calculate the individual volume delivered, in µL, by the formula:

$$(W_1 - W_2)/D$$

in which W_1 and W_2 are the weights, in mg, of the individual vials before and after actuation, respectively; and *D* is the density of the nasal solution. Calculate the mean volume delivered. The volume of each spray delivered is between 80 and 120 µL, and the mean volume is between 90 and 110 µL.

Limit of sumatriptan related compound A—

*10 M Ammonium acetate solution—*Dissolve 77.1 g of ammonium acetate in 100 mL of water.

*Mobile phase—*Prepare a filtered and degassed mixture of methanol and *10 M Ammonium acetate solution* (9 : 1). Make adjustments if necessary (see *System Suitability* under *Chromatography* ⟨621⟩).

*Diluent—*Proceed as described in the *Assay*.

*Standard solution—*Dissolve an accurately weighed quantity of USP Sumatriptan Succinate Related Compound A RS in *Diluent*, and dilute quantitatively, and stepwise if necessary, with *Diluent* to obtain a solution having a known concentration of about 0.007 mg per mL (equivalent to about 0.005 mg per mL of $C_{14}H_{21}N_3O_2S$).

*Test solution—*Dissolve an appropriate volume of Nasal Spray in *Diluent* to obtain a solution having a concentration of about 1.0 mg of sumatriptan per mL.

Chromatographic system (see *Chromatography* ⟨621⟩)—The liquid chromatograph is equipped with a 282-nm detector and a 4.6-mm × 20-cm column that contains packing L3. The flow rate is about 2.0 mL per minute. Chromatograph the *Standard solution*, and record the peak responses as directed for *Procedure:* the relative standard deviation for replicate injections is not more than 5%.

Procedure—Separately inject equal volumes (about 20 µL) of the *Standard solution* and the *Test solution* into the chromatograph, record the chromatograms, and measure the responses for the major peaks. Calculate the percentage of sumatriptan succinate related compound A in the portion of Nasal Spray taken by the formula:

$$100(495.7/613.8)(C_S/C_U)(r_U/r_S)$$

in which 495.7 and 613.8 are the molecular weights of sumatriptan related compound A and sumatriptan succinate related compound A, respectively; C_S is the concentration, in mg per mL, of USP Sumatriptan Succinate Related Compound A RS in the *Standard solution*; C_U is the concentration, in mg per mL, of sumatriptan in the *Test solution*; and r_U and r_S are the peak responses for sumatriptan related compound A from the *Test solution* and the *Standard solution*, respectively: Not more than 1.5% is found.

Related compounds—
Diluent—Proceed as directed in the *Assay*.
Buffer solution—Dissolve about 1.7 mL of dibutylamine, about 0.6 mL of phosphoric acid, and about 3.9 g of monobasic sodium phosphate dihydrate in water. Adjust with a solution of 50% (w/v) sodium hydroxide to a pH of about 7.5, dilute with water to 1000 mL, and mix.
Mobile phase—Prepare a filtered and degassed mixture of *Buffer solution* and acetonitrile (3 : 1). Make adjustments if necessary (see *System Suitability* under *Chromatography* 〈621〉).
System suitability solution—Dissolve accurately weighed quantities of USP Sumatriptan Succinate RS and USP Sumatriptan Succinate Related Compound C RS in *Diluent* to obtain a solution having known concentrations of about 1.4 mg per mL and 0.001 mg per mL, respectively.
Identification solution—Prepare a solution of USP Sumatriptan Succinate Related Impurities RS in *Diluent* having a concentration of about 3 mg per mL.
Test solution—Dissolve an appropriate volume of Nasal Spray in *Diluent* to obtain a solution having a concentration of about 1.0 mg of sumatriptan per mL.
Chromatographic system (see *Chromatography* 〈621〉)—The liquid chromatograph is equipped with a 282-nm detector and a 4.6-mm × 20-cm column that contains packing L1. The flow rate is about 1.5 mL per minute. Chromatograph the *System suitability solution*, and record the peak responses as directed for *Procedure*: the relative retention times are about 0.9 for sumatriptan succinate related compound C and 1.0 for sumatriptan; and the resolution, R, between sumatriptan succinate related compound C and sumatriptan is not less than 1.5. Chromatograph the *Identification solution*, and record the peak responses as directed for *Procedure*: identify the peaks according to *Table 1*.

Table 1

Compound Name	Relative Retention Time
[3-[2-(Dimethylamino-*N*-oxide)ethyl]-1*H*-indol-5-yl]-*N*-methylmethanesulfonamide	about 0.3
[3-[2-(Methylamino)ethyl]-1*H*-indol-5-yl]-*N*-methylmethanesulfonamide	about 0.6
Sumatriptan succinate related compound C	about 0.9
Sumatriptan	1.0
[3-[2-(Aminoethyl)-1*H*-indol-5-yl]-*N*-methylmethanesulfonamide	about 0.4

Procedure—Inject a volume (about 10 µL) of the *Test solution* into the chromatograph, record the chromatogram, and measure all of the peak responses. Calculate the percentage of each impurity in the portion of Nasal Spray taken by the formula:

$$100F(r_i/r_S)$$

in which F is the relative response factor, which is equal to 2.89 for 1-[3-[2-dimethylamino)ethyl]-3-hydroxy-2-oxo-2,3-dihydro-1*H*-indol-5-yl]-*N*-methylmethanesulfonamide that has a relative retention time of 0.46, 4.55 for 3a-hydroxy-1,1-dimethyl-5-{[(methylamino)sulfonyl]methyl}-1,2,3,3a,8,8a,hexahydropyrrolo[2,3-*b*]indol-1-ium that has a relative retention time of 0.64, and 1.0 for all other impurities; r_i is the peak response for each impurity; and r_S is the sum of the responses of all the peaks: not more than 1.5% of any impurity is found; and the total of all impurities, including the amount found in the test for *Limit of sumatriptan related compound A*, is not more than 4.0%.

Assay—
Diluent—Dissolve 3.9 g of monobasic sodium phosphate dihydrate in water. Adjust with a solution of 50% (w/v) sodium hydroxide to a pH of about 6.5, and dilute with water to 1000 mL. Mix 750 mL of this solution with 250 mL of acetonitrile.
Buffer solution—Dissolve about 1.7 mL of dibutylamine, about 0.6 mL of phosphoric acid, and about 3.9 g of monobasic sodium phosphate dihydrate in water. Adjust with a solution of 50% (w/v) sodium hydroxide to a pH of about 6.5, dilute with water to 1000 mL, and mix.
Mobile phase—Prepare a filtered and degassed mixture of *Buffer solution* and acetonitrile (3 : 1). Make adjustments if necessary (see *System Suitability* under *Chromatography* 〈621〉).
System suitability solution—Dissolve accurately weighed quantities of USP Sumatriptan Succinate RS and USP Sumatriptan Succinate Related Compound C RS in *Diluent* to obtain a solution having known concentrations of about 0.14 mg per mL and 0.07 mg per mL, respectively.
Standard preparation—Dissolve an accurately weighed quantity of USP Sumatriptan Succinate RS, and dissolve in *Diluent* to obtain a solution having a known concentration of about 0.14 mg per mL.
Assay preparation—Dissolve an appropriate volume of Nasal Spray in *Diluent* to obtain a solution having a known concentration of about 0.1 mg of sumatriptan per mL.
Chromatographic system (see *Chromatography* 〈621〉)—The liquid chromatograph is equipped with a 282-nm detector and a 4.6-mm × 20-cm column that contains packing L1. The flow rate is about 1.5 mL per minute. Chromatograph the *System suitability solution*, and record the peak responses as directed for *Procedure*: the relative retention times are about 0.9 for sumatriptan succinate related compound C and 1.0 for sumatriptan; and the resolution, R, between sumatriptan succinate related compound C and sumatriptan is not less than 1.5. Chromatograph the *Standard preparation*, and record the peak responses as directed for *Procedure*: the relative standard deviation for replicate injections is not more than 1.5%.
Procedure—Separately inject equal volumes (about 10 µL) of the *Standard preparation* and *Assay preparation* into the chromatograph, record the chromatograms, and measure the areas for the major peaks. Calculate the amount of sumatriptan ($C_{14}H_{21}N_3O_2S$), in mg, in the portion of Nasal Spray taken by the formula:

$$(295.4/413.5)C_S D(r_U/r_S)$$

in which C_S is the concentration, in mg per mL, of sumatriptan succinate in the *Standard preparation*; D is the dilution factor used in preparing the *Assay preparation*; and the other terms are as defined therein.

Add the following:

▲Sumatriptan Succinate Oral Suspension

» Sumatriptan Succinate Oral Suspension is a suspension of Sumatriptan Succinate. It contains not less than 90.0 percent and not more than 110.0 percent of the labeled amount of sumatriptan ($C_{14}H_{21}N_3O_2S$). Prepare Sumatriptan Succinate Oral Suspension 7 mg per mL of Sumatriptan Succinate equivalent to 5 mg of Sumatriptan per mL as follows (see *Pharmaceutical Compounding—Nonsterile Preparations* 〈795〉):

Sumatriptan (as the Succinate)   500 mg
Vehicle: a mixture of Vehicle for
  Oral Suspension, *NF,* and
  Vehicle for Oral Solution
  (regular or sugar-free), *NF* (1 : 1)
  a sufficient quantity to make   100 mL

If using Tablets, place the Sumatriptan Tablets in a suitable mortar, and comminute to a fine powder, or add Sumatriptan Succinate powder to the mortar. Add about 25 mL of Vehicle in portions, mixing thoroughly after each addition. Transfer the contents of the mortar, stepwise and quantitatively, to a calibrated bottle. Add sufficient Vehicle to bring to final volume, and mix well.

Packaging and storage—Preserve in tight, light-resistant containers. Store in a cold place.
Labeling—Label it to state that it is to be well shaken before use, and to state the beyond-use date. Label content as: Each mL of Sumatriptan Succinate Oral Suspension contains 7 mg of Sumatriptan Succinate equivalent to 5 mg of Sumatriptan.
USP Reference standards ⟨11⟩—*USP Sumatriptan Succinate RS.*
pH ⟨791⟩: between 3.6 and 4.6.
Beyond-use date: 14 days after the day on which it was compounded.
Assay—
  Mobile phase—Prepare a solution of 0.01 M dibutylamine in 0.025 M aqueous monobasic sodium phosphate dihydrate and acetonitrile (75 : 25). Adjust *Mobile phase* with 1 N sodium hydroxide to a pH of 8.0, filter, and degas. Make adjustments if necessary (see *System Suitability* under *Chromatography* ⟨621⟩).
  Internal standard solution—Dissolve an accurately weighed quantity of *N*-hydroxymethylsumatriptan succinate in *Mobile phase* to obtain a known concentration of about 3.0 mg per mL.
  Standard stock preparation—Dissolve an accurately weighed quantity of USP Sumatriptan Succinate RS in *Mobile phase* to obtain a known concentration of about 4.0 mg per mL.
  Standard preparation—Dilute the *Standard stock preparation* with *Mobile phase* to obtain a solution having a known concentration of about 120 μg per mL. Each solution contains 30 μg per mL of *Internal standard solution.*
  Assay preparation—Transfer about 1 mL of Oral Suspension from each bottle to a suitable container, and dilute with 0.1 M hydrochloric acid to obtain a concentration of about 0.15 mg per mL. Pass the solution through a 0.22-μm syringe filter into a 0.3-mL polypropylene sample vial for assay.
  Chromatographic system (see *Chromatography* ⟨621⟩)—The liquid chromatograph is equipped with a 282-nm detector and a 4.6-mm ×10-cm analytical column that contains 5-μm packing L1. The flow rate is about 1.5 mL per minute. Chromatograph the *Standard preparation,* and record the peak responses as directed for *Procedure:* the retention times for sumatriptan and *N*-hydroxymethylsumatriptan are 11 and 14 minutes, respectively; and the relative standard deviation for replicate injections is not more than 1.5%.
  Procedure—Separately inject equal volumes (about 10 μL) of the *Standard preparation* and the *Assay preparation* into the chromatograph, record the chromatograms, and measure the responses for the major peaks. Calculate the quantity, in mg, of sumatriptan succinate ($C_{14}H_{21}N_3O_2S \cdot C_4H_6O_4$) in the volume of Oral Suspension taken by the formula:

$$100(C/V)(r_U / r_S)$$

in which *C* is the concentration, in mg per mL, of USP Sumatriptan Succinate RS in the *Standard preparation; V* is the volume, in mL, of Oral Suspension taken; and r_U and r_S are the peak responses obtained from the *Assay preparation* and the *Standard preparation,* respectively.▲*USP31*

Suprofen

$C_{14}H_{12}O_3S$ 260.31
Benzeneacetic acid, α-methyl-4-(2-thienylcarbonyl)-.
p-2-Thenoylhydratropic acid   [40828-46-4].

» Suprofen contains not less than 98.0 percent and not more than 102.0 percent of $C_{14}H_{12}O_3S$, calculated on the dried basis.

Packaging and storage—Preserve in well-closed containers.
USP Reference standards ⟨11⟩—*USP Suprofen RS.*
Clarity of solution—Dissolve 50 mg in 10 mL of 0.1 N sodium hydroxide: the solution is clear and free of undissolved solid.
Identification—
  A: *Infrared Absorption* ⟨197K⟩.
  B: *Ultraviolet Absorption* ⟨197U⟩—
  Solution: 10 μg per mL.
  Medium: 0.1 N hydrochloric acid in isopropyl alcohol (10 in 100).
  Respective absorptivities at 267 nm and 297 nm, calculated on the dried basis, do not differ by more than 3.0%.
  Ratio: A_{267} / A_{297}, between 0.97 and 1.03.
Melting range ⟨741⟩: between 118° and 125°, within a range of less than 4°.
Loss on drying ⟨731⟩—Dry it in vacuum at 70° for 4 hours: it loses not more than 0.5% of its weight.
Residue on ignition ⟨281⟩—Add 1 mL of sulfuric acid to 500 mg of the test substance in the crucible, heat gently to char the substance, and ignite: the limit is 0.2%.
Heavy metals, *Method II* ⟨231⟩: 0.002%.
Ordinary impurities ⟨466⟩—
  Test solution: chloroform.
  Standard solution: chloroform.
  Eluant: a mixture of chloroform, methanol, and methyl ethyl ketone (40 : 30 : 30).
  Visualization: 1.
Assay—
  Buffer solution—Dissolve 7.1 g of anhydrous dibasic sodium phosphate in about 800 mL of water, adjust with phosphoric acid to a pH of 6.0 ± 0.1, dilute with water to make 1000 mL of solution, and mix.
  Mobile phase—Prepare a suitable degassed and filtered mixture of *Buffer solution* and methanol (60 : 40). Make adjustments if necessary (see *System Suitability* under *Chromatography* ⟨621⟩).
  Standard preparation—Transfer about 50 mg of USP Suprofen RS, accurately weighed, to a 50-mL volumetric flask, dilute with methanol to volume, and mix. Transfer 5.0 mL of this solution to a 25-mL volumetric flask, dilute with *Buffer solution* to volume, and mix. Transfer 2.0 mL of this solution to a 25-mL volumetric flask, dilute with *Buffer solution* to volume, and mix to obtain a solution having a known concentration of about 0.016 mg per mL.
  Assay preparation—Transfer about 50 mg of Suprofen, accurately weighed, to a 50-mL volumetric flask, dilute with methanol to volume, and mix. Transfer 5.0 mL of this solution to a 25-mL volumetric flask, dilute with *Buffer solution* to volume, and mix. Transfer 2.0 mL of this solution to a 25-mL volumetric flask, dilute with *Buffer solution* to volume, and mix.
  Chromatographic system—The liquid chromatograph is equipped with a 254-nm detector and a 4.6-mm × 25-cm column that contains packing L1. The flow rate is about 2 mL per minute. Chromatograph the *Standard preparation,* and record the peak responses as directed for *Procedure:* the column efficiency determined from the analyte peak is not less than 500 theoretical plates, the tailing factor for the peak is not more than 2.0, and the relative standard deviation for replicate injections is not more than 2%.

Procedure—[NOTE—Use peak areas where peak responses are indicated.] Separately inject equal volumes (about 20 µL) of the *Standard preparation* and the *Assay preparation* into the chromatograph, record the chromatograms, and measure the responses for the major peaks. Calculate the quantity, in mg, of $C_{14}H_{12}O_3S$ in the portion of Suprofen taken by the formula:

$$3125C(r_U/r_S)$$

in which C is the concentration, in mg per mL, of USP Suprofen RS in the *Standard preparation*, and r_U and r_S are the peak responses obtained from the *Assay preparation* and the *Standard preparation*, respectively.

Suprofen Ophthalmic Solution

» Suprofen Ophthalmic Solution is a sterile, buffered, aqueous solution of Suprofen adjusted to a suitable tonicity. It contains a suitable antimicrobial preservative. It contains not less than 90.0 percent and not more than 115.0 percent of the labeled amount of $C_{14}H_{12}O_3S$.

Packaging and storage—Preserve in tight containers.

USP Reference standards ⟨11⟩—*USP Suprofen RS.*
Identification—The retention time of the major peak in the chromatogram of the *Assay preparation* corresponds to that in the chromatogram of the *Standard preparation* as obtained in the *Assay.*
Sterility ⟨71⟩: meets the requirements when tested as directed for *Membrane Filtration* under *Test for Sterility of the Product to be Examined.*
pH ⟨791⟩: between 6.5 and 8.0.
Assay—
  Buffer solution, Mobile phase, Standard preparation, and *Chromatographic system*—Proceed as directed in the *Assay* under *Suprofen.*
  Assay preparation—Transfer an accurately measured volume of Ophthalmic Solution, equivalent to about 20 mg of suprofen, to a 100-mL volumetric flask. Dilute with *Buffer solution* to volume, and mix. Transfer 2.0 mL of this solution to a 25-mL volumetric flask, dilute with *Buffer solution* to volume, and mix.
  Procedure—Proceed as directed in the *Assay* under *Suprofen.* Calculate the quantity, in mg, of $C_{14}H_{12}O_3S$ in each mL of the Ophthalmic Solution taken by the formula:

$$1250(C/V)(r_U/r_S)$$

in which C is the concentration, in mg per mL, of USP Suprofen RS in the *Standard preparation,* V is the volume, in mL, of Ophthalmic Solution taken, and r_U and r_S are the peak responses obtained from the *Assay preparation* and the *Standard preparation,* respectively.

Absorbable Surgical Suture

» Absorbable Surgical Suture is a sterile, flexible strand prepared from collagen derived from healthy mammals, or from a synthetic polymer. Suture prepared from synthetic polymer may be in either monofilament or multifilament form. It is capable of being absorbed by living mammalian tissue, but may be treated to modify its resistance to absorption. Its diameter and tensile strength correspond to the size designation indicated on the label, within the limits prescribed herein. It may be modified with respect to body or texture. It may be impregnated or treated with a suitable coating, softening, or antimicrobial agent. It may be colored by a color additive approved by the FDA. The collagen suture is designated as either *Plain Suture* or *Chromic Suture.* Both types consist of processed strands of collagen, but *Chromic Suture* is processed by physical or chemical means so as to provide greater resistance to absorption in living mammalian tissue.

Packaging and storage—Preserve dry or in fluid, in containers (packets) so designed that sterility is maintained until the container is opened. A number of such containers may be placed in a box.
Labeling—The label of each individual container (packet) of Suture indicates the size, length, type of Suture, kind of needle (if a needle is included), number of sutures (if multiple), lot number, and name of the manufacturer or distributor. If removable needles are used, the labeling so indicates. Suture size is designated by the metric size (gauge number) and the corresponding USP size. The label of the box indicates also the address of the manufacturer, packer, or distributor, and the composition of any packaging fluids used.
  NOTE—If the Suture is packaged with a fluid, make the required measurements for the first four of the following tests within 2 minutes after removing it from the fluid.
Length—Determine the length of Suture without stretching: the length of each strand is not less than 95.0% of the length stated on the label.
Diameter—Determine the diameter of 10 strands of Suture as directed under *Sutures—Diameter* ⟨861⟩.
  Collagen suture—The average diameter, and not fewer than 20, of the 30 measurements on the 10-strand sample are within the limits on average diameter prescribed in *Table 1* for the respective size. None of the individual measurements is less than the midpoint of the range for the next smaller size or more than the midpoint of the range for the next larger size.
  Synthetic suture—The average diameter of the strands being measured is within the tolerances prescribed in *Table 2* for the respective size. None of the observed measurements is less than the midpoint of the range for the next smaller size or more than the midpoint of the range for the next larger size.

Table 1. Collagen Suture

USP Size	Metric Size (Gauge No.)	Limits on Average Diameter (mm) Min.	Limits on Average Diameter (mm) Max.	Knot-Pull Tensile Strength (kgf) Limit on Average Min.	Knot-Pull Tensile Strength (kgf) Limit on Individual Strand Min.	Knot-Pull Tensile Strength (in N) Limit on Average Min.	Knot-Pull Tensile Strength (in N) Limit on Individual Strand Min.
9-0	0.4	0.040	0.049	—	—	—	—
8-0	0.5	0.050	0.069	0.045	0.025	0.44	0.24
7-0	0.7	0.070	0.099	0.07	0.055	0.69	0.54
6-0	1	0.10	0.149	0.18	0.10	1.76	0.98
5-0	1.5	0.15	0.199	0.38	0.20	3.73	1.96

Table 1. Collagen Suture (Continued)

USP Size	Metric Size (Gauge No.)	Limits on Average Diameter (mm) Min.	Limits on Average Diameter (mm) Max.	Knot-Pull Tensile Strength (kgf) Limit on Average Min.	Knot-Pull Tensile Strength (kgf) Limit on Individual Strand Min.	Knot-Pull Tensile Strength (in N) Limit on Average Min.	Knot-Pull Tensile Strength (in N) Limit on Individual Strand Min.
4-0	2	0.20	0.249	0.77	0.40	7.55	3.92
3-0	3	0.30	0.339	1.25	0.68	12.2	6.67
2-0	3.5	0.35	0.399	2.00	1.04	19.6	10.2
0	4	0.40	0.499	2.77	1.45	27.2	14.2
1	5	0.50	0.599	3.80	1.95	37.3	19.1
2	6	0.60	0.699	4.51	2.40	44.2	25.5
3	7	0.70	0.799	5.90	2.99	57.8	29.3
4	8	0.80	0.899	7.00	3.49	68.6	34.2

Table 2. Synthetic Suture

USP Size Min.	Metric Size (Gauge No.) Max.	Limits on Average Diameter (mm) Min.	Limits on Average Diameter (mm) Max.	Knot-Pull Tensile Strength (in kgf) (except where otherwise specified)* Limit on Average Min.	Knot-Pull Tensile Strength (in N) (except where otherwise specified)
12-0	0.01	0.001	0.009	—	—
11-0	0.1	0.010	0.019	—	—
10-0	0.2	0.020	0.029	0.025*	0.24*
9-0	0.3	0.030	0.039	0.050*	0.49*
8-0	0.4	0.040	0.049	0.07	0.69
7-0	0.5	0.050	0.069	0.14	1.37
6-0	0.7	0.070	0.099	0.25	2.45
5-0	1	0.10	0.149	0.68	6.67
4-0	1.5	0.15	0.199	0.95	9.32
3-0	2	0.20	0.249	1.77	17.4
2-0	3	0.30	0.339	2.68	26.3
0	3.5	0.35	0.399	3.90	38.2
1	4	0.40	0.499	5.08	49.8
2	5	0.50	0.599	6.35	62.3
3 and 4	6	0.60	0.699	7.29	71.5
5	7	0.70	0.799	—	—

*The tensile strength of the specified USP size is measured by straight pull.

Tensile strength—Determine the tensile strength on not fewer than 10 strands of Suture as directed for *Surgical Sutures* under *Tensile Strength* ⟨881⟩.

Collagen suture—The tensile strength, determined as the minimum strength for each individual strand tested, and calculated as the average strength from any one lot, is as set forth in *Table 1*. If not more than one strand fails to meet the limit on individual strands, repeat the test with not fewer than 20 additional strands: the requirements of the test are met if none of the additional strands falls below the limit on individual strands, and if the average strength of all the strands tested does not fall below the stated limit in *Table 1*.

Synthetic suture—The minimum tensile strength of each size of synthetic suture, calculated as the average strength from any one lot, is as set forth in *Table 2*.

Needle attachment—Suture on which eyeless needles are swaged meets the requirements under *Sutures—Needle Attachment* ⟨871⟩.

Sterility ⟨71⟩: meets the requirements.

Extractable color (if Suture is dyed)—Prepare the *Matching Solution* that corresponds to the extractable color of the Suture by combining the Colorimetric Solutions in the proportions indicated in *Table 3*, and adding water, if necessary, to make 10.0 parts. [See under *Solutions* in the section *Reagents, Indicators, and Solutions*, for composition of the Colorimetric Solutions (CS).]

Table 3. Matching Solutions

Color of Suture (Extractable Color)	Cobaltous Chloride CS	Ferric Chloride CS	Cupric Sulfate CS
Yellow-brown	0.2	1.2	—
Pink-red	1.0	—	—
Green-blue	—	—	2.0
Violet	1.6	—	8.4

Weigh a quantity of Suture, equivalent to not less than 250 mg, and place in a conical flask containing 1.0 mL of water for each 10 mg of the sample. Close the flask, and allow it to stand at 37 ± 0.5° for 24 hours. Cool, decant the water from the Suture, and compare it with the *Matching Solution:* any color present is not more intense than that of the appropriate *Matching Solution.*

Soluble chromium compounds—Pipet 5 mL of the fluid prepared as directed in the test for *Extractable color* into a small test tube. Into a similar tube pipet 5 mL of a standard solution of potassium dichromate having a concentration of 2.83 µg per mL. To both tubes add 2 mL of a 1 in 100 solution of diphenylcarbazide in alcohol and 2 mL of 2 N sulfuric acid: any color that develops in the test solution is not more intense than that in the standard solution (0.0001% of Cr).

Nonabsorbable Surgical Suture

» Nonabsorbable Surgical Suture is a flexible strand of material that is suitably resistant to the action of living mammalian tissue. It may be in either monofilament or multifilament form. If it is a multifilament strand, the individual filaments may be combined by spinning, twisting, braiding, or any combination thereof. It may be either sterile or nonsterile. Its diameter and tensile strength correspond to the size designation indicated on the label, within the limits prescribed herein. It may be modified with respect to body or texture, or to reduce capillarity, and may be suitably bleached. It may be impregnated or treated with a suitable coating, softening, or antimicrobial agent. It may be colored by a color additive approved by the FDA.

Nonabsorbable Surgical Suture is classed and typed as follows. *Class I* Suture is composed of silk or synthetic fibers of monofilament, twisted, or braided construction where the coating, if any, does not significantly affect thickness (e.g., braided silk, polyester, or nylon; monofilament nylon or polypropylene). *Class II* Suture is composed of cotton or linen fibers or coated natural or synthetic fibers where the coating significantly affects thickness but does not contribute significantly to strength (e.g., virgin silk sutures). *Class III* Suture is composed of monofilament or multifilament metal wire.

Packaging and storage—Preserve nonsterilized Suture in well-closed containers. Preserve sterile Suture dry or in fluid, in containers (packets) so designed that sterility is maintained until the container is opened. A number of such containers may be placed in a box.

Labeling—The label of each individual container (packet) of Suture indicates the material from which the Suture is made, the size, construction, and length of the Suture, whether it is sterile or nonsterile, kind of needle (if a needle is included), number of sutures (if multiple), lot number, and name of the manufacturer or distributor. If removable needles are used, the labeling so indicates. Suture size is designated by the metric size (gauge number) and the corresponding USP size. The label of the box indicates also the address of the manufacturer, packer, or distributor, and the composition of any packaging fluids used.

NOTE—If the Suture is packaged with a fluid, make the required measurements for the first four of the following tests within 2 minutes after removing it from the fluid.

Length—Determine the length of Suture while the strand is laid out smooth, without tension, on a plane surface: the length of the strand is not less than 95.0% of the length stated on the label.

Diameter—Determine the diameter of 10 strands of Suture as directed under *Sutures—Diameter* ⟨861⟩. The average diameter of the strands being measured is within the tolerances prescribed in the accompanying table for the size stated on the label. In the case of braided or twisted Suture, none of the observed diameters is less than the midpoint of the range for the next smaller size or is greater than the midpoint of the range for the next larger size.

Tensile strength—Determine the tensile strength on not fewer than 10 strands of Suture as directed for *Surgical Sutures* under *Tensile Strength* ⟨881⟩. Average all observations obtained: the average tensile strength is not less than that set forth in the accompanying table for the class and the size stated on the label.

Needle attachment—Suture on which eyeless needles are swaged meets the requirements under *Sutures—Needle* ⟨871⟩.

Sterility ⟨71⟩: Suture that is claimed to be sterile meets the requirements.

Extractable color (if Suture is dyed)—Proceed as directed in the test for *Extractable color* under *Absorbable Surgical Suture*, but instead of allowing to stand at 37 ± 0.5° for 24 hours, cover the flask with a short-stemmed funnel, heat the contents of the flask at the boiling point for 15 minutes, cool, and restore the volume by the addition of water, if necessary, to replace that lost by evaporation.

Average Knot-Pull Limits of Various Sizes and Diameters of Sutures

USP Size	Metric Size (gauge no.)	Limits on Average Diameter (mm) Min.	Limits on Average Diameter (mm) Max.	Limits on Average Knot-Pull (except where otherwise specified)[a] Tensile Strength (in kgf)[b] Class I Min.	Class II Min.	Class III Min.	Limits on Average Knot-Pull (except where otherwise specified)[a] Tensile Strength (in N)[b] Class I Min.	Class II Min.	Class III Min.
12-0	0.01	0.001	0.009	0.001[a]	—	0.002[a]	0.01[a]	—	0.02[a]
11-0	0.1	0.010	0.019	0.006[a]	0.005[a]	0.02[a]	0.06[a]	0.05[a]	0.20[a]
10-0	0.2	0.020	0.029	0.019[a]	0.014[a]	0.06[a]	0.194[a]	0.14[a]	0.59[a]
9-0	0.3	0.030	0.039	0.043[a]	0.029[a]	0.07[a]	0.424[a]	0.28[a]	0.68[a]
8-0	0.4	0.040	0.049	0.06	0.04	0.11	0.59	0.39	1.08
7-0	0.5	0.050	0.069	0.11	0.06	0.16	1.08	0.59	1.57
6-0	0.7	0.070	0.099	0.20	0.11	0.27	1.96	1.08	2.65
5-0	1	0.10	0.149	0.40	0.23	0.54	3.92	2.26	5.30
4-0	1.5	0.15	0.199	0.60	0.46	0.82	5.88	4.51	8.04
3-0	2	0.20	0.249	0.96	0.66	1.36	9.41	6.47	13.3
2-0	3	0.30	0.339	1.44	1.02	1.80	14.1	10.0	17.6
0	3.5	0.35	0.399	2.16	1.45	3.40[a]	21.2	14.2	33.3[a]
1	4	0.40	0.499	2.72	1.81	4.76[a]	26.7	17.8	46.7[a]
2	5	0.50	0.599	3.52	2.54	5.90[a]	34.5	24.9	57.8[a]
3 and 4	6	0.60	0.699	4.88	3.68	9.11[a]	47.8	36.1	89.3[a]
5	7	0.70	0.799	6.16	—	11.4[a]	60.4	—	112[a]
6	8	0.80	0.899	7.28	—	13.6[a]	71.4	—	133[a]
7	9	0.90	0.999	9.04	—	15.9[a]	88.6	—	156[a]
8	10	1.00	1.099	—	—	18.2[a]	—	—	178[a]
9	11	1.100	1.199	—	—	20.5[a]	—	—	201[a]
10	12	1.200	1.299	—	—	22.8[a]	—	—	224[a]

[a] The tensile strength of sizes smaller than USP size 8-0 (metric size 0.4) is measured by straight pull. The tensile strength of sizes larger than USP size 2-0 (metric size 3) of monofilament *Class III* (metallic) Nonabsorbable Surgical Suture is measured by straight pull. Silver wire meets the tensile strength values of *Class I* Sutures but is tested in the same manner as *Class III* Sutures.

[b] The limits on knot-pull tensile strength apply to Nonabsorbable Surgical Suture that has been sterilized. For nonsterile Sutures of *Class I* and *Class II*, the limits are 25% higher.

Tacrine Hydrochloride

$C_{13}H_{14}N_2 \cdot HCl \cdot H_2O$ 252.74

9-Acridinamine, 1,2,3,4-tetrahydro-, monohydrochloride, monohydrate.

9-Amino-1,2,3,4-tetrahydroacridine monohydrochloride, monohydrate   [*1684-40-8*].

» Tacrine Hydrochloride contains not less than 98.5 percent and not more than 101.5 percent of $C_{13}H_{14}N_2 \cdot$ HCl, calculated on the anhydrous basis.

Packaging and storage—Preserve in well-closed containers.
USP Reference standards ⟨11⟩—*USP Tacrine Hydrochloride RS*.
Identification—
  A: *Infrared Absorption* ⟨197K⟩.
  B: The retention time of the major peak in the chromatogram of the *Assay preparation* corresponds to that in the chromatogram of the *Standard preparation*, as obtained in the *Assay*.
Water, *Method I* ⟨921⟩: between 6.0% and 8.0%.
Residue on ignition ⟨281⟩: not more than 0.1%.
Heavy metals, *Method II* ⟨231⟩: not more than 0.001%.
Chromatographic purity—
0.05 M Triethylamine solution, Mobile phase, System suitability solution, and *Chromatographic system*—Proceed as directed in the *Assay*.
Standard stock solution—Use the *Standard stock preparation* as prepared in the *Assay*.
Standard solution—Dilute 1.0 mL of the *Standard stock solution* quantitatively, and stepwise if necessary, with *Mobile phase* to obtain a solution having a known concentration of about 0.001 mg per mL.
Test solution—Use the *Assay stock preparation*.
Procedure—Separately inject equal volumes (about 10 µL) of the *Standard solution* and the *Test solution* into the chromatograph, record the chromatograms for not less than 20 minutes, and measure all of the peak areas. The area of any single peak obtained from the *Test solution* is not greater than the area of the tacrine hydrochloride peak obtained from the chromatogram of the *Standard solution*: not more than 0.1% of any individual impurity is found; and not more than 0.2% of total impurities is found.
Content of chloride—Transfer about 150 mg of Tacrine Hydrochloride, accurately weighed, to a 100-mL beaker. Dissolve in 40 mL of methanol and 10 mL of water, and acidify with 1 mL of nitric acid. Titrate with 0.1 N silver nitrate VS, determining the endpoint potentiometrically, using suitable electrodes (see *Titrimetry* ⟨541⟩). Each mL of 0.1 N silver nitrate is equivalent to 3.545 mg of chloride. Not less than 13.6% and not more than 14.4% is found.
Assay—
0.05 M Triethylamine solution—Dissolve 13.8 mL of triethylamine in 1900 mL of water. Adjust with formic acid to a pH of 3.0, dilute with water to 2000 mL, and mix.
Mobile phase—Prepare a filtered and degassed mixture of *0.05 M Triethylamine solution* and acetonitrile (87 : 13). Make adjustments if necessary (see *System Suitability* under *Chromatography* ⟨621⟩).
System suitability solution—Dissolve suitable quantities of USP Tacrine Hydrochloride RS and 2-aminobenzonitrile in *Mobile phase* to obtain a solution containing about 100 µg per mL and 25 µg per mL, respectively.
Standard stock preparation—Dissolve an accurately weighed quantity of USP Tacrine Hydrochloride RS in *Mobile phase* to obtain a solution containing about 1 mg per mL.

Standard preparation—Dilute 1.0 mL of the *Standard stock preparation* with *Mobile phase* to obtain a solution having a known concentration of about 0.1 mg per mL.

Assay stock preparation—Transfer about 100 mg of Tacrine Hydrochloride, accurately weighed, to a 100-mL volumetric flask, dissolve in and dilute with *Mobile phase* to volume, and mix.

Assay preparation—Transfer 1.0 mL of the *Assay stock preparation* to a 10-mL volumetric flask, and dilute with *Mobile phase* to volume to obtain a solution having a known concentration of about 0.1 mg per mL.

Chromatographic system (see *Chromatography* ⟨621⟩)—The liquid chromatograph is equipped with a 243-nm detector and a 4.6-mm × 25-cm column that contains 5-μm packing L11. The flow rate is about 1.5 mL per minute. Chromatograph the *System suitability solution*, and record the peak responses as directed for *Procedure*: the relative retention times are about 0.48 for 2-aminobenzonitrile and 1.0 for tacrine hydrochloride; the resolution, R, between 2-aminobenzonitrile and tacrine hydrochloride is not less than 10.0; and the column efficiency is not less than 5200 theoretical plates. Chromatograph the *Standard preparation*, and record the peak responses as directed for *Procedure*: the relative standard deviation for replicate injections is not more than 0.41%.

Procedure—Separately inject equal volumes (about 10 μL) of the *Standard preparation* and the *Assay preparation* into the chromatograph, record the chromatograms, and measure the areas for the major peaks. Calculate the quantity, in mg, of $C_{13}H_{14}N_2 \cdot HCl \cdot H_2O$, in the portion of Tacrine Hydrochloride taken by the formula:

$$1000C(r_U / r_S)$$

in which C is the concentration, in mg per mL, of USP Tacrine Hydrochloride RS in the *Standard preparation*; and r_U and r_S are the peak responses obtained from the *Assay preparation* and the *Standard preparation*, respectively.

Tacrine Capsules

» Tacrine Capsules contain an amount of Tacrine Hydrochloride equivalent to not less than 90.0 percent and not more than 110.0 percent of the labeled amount of tacrine ($C_{13}H_{14}N_2$).

Packaging and storage—Preserve in well-closed containers.

USP Reference standards ⟨11⟩—*USP Tacrine Hydrochloride RS*.

Identification—

A: *Infrared Absorption* ⟨197K⟩—

Test specimen—Transfer an amount of Capsules, equivalent to about 100 mg of tacrine, to a 250-mL separatory funnel containing 100 mL of water, and mix. Add 2 mL of 1 N sodium hydroxide, and shake. Add 30 mL of ether, and shake. Allow the layers to separate, transfer the top ether layer to a beaker, and evaporate in a hood under a stream of nitrogen. Allow the solid to air-dry, and then dry at 105° for 90 minutes. Prepare a mixture of about 0.5% to 1.0% of the isolated solid in potassium bromide.

B: The retention time of the major peak in the chromatogram of the *Assay preparation* corresponds to that in the chromatogram of the *Standard preparation*, as obtained in the *Assay*.

Dissolution ⟨711⟩—

Medium: 0.1 N hydrochloric acid; 900 mL.
Apparatus 2: 50 rpm.
Time: 30 minutes.

Procedure—Determine the amount of $C_{13}H_{14}N_2$ dissolved by employing UV absorption at the wavelength of maximum absorbance at about 240 nm on filtered portions of the solution under test, suitably diluted with *Dissolution Medium*, in comparison with a Standard solution having a known concentration of USP Tacrine Hydrochloride RS in the same *Medium*.

Tolerances—Not less than 85% (*Q*) of the labeled amount of $C_{13}H_{14}N_2$ is dissolved in 30 minutes.

Uniformity of dosage units ⟨905⟩: meet the requirements.

PROCEDURE FOR CONTENT UNIFORMITY—

Standard solution—Dissolve an accurately weighed quantity of USP Tacrine Hydrochloride RS in 0.1 N hydrochloric acid, and dilute quantitatively, and stepwise if necessary, with 0.1 N hydrochloric acid to obtain a solution having a known concentration of about 4.1 μg per mL.

Test solution—Place 1 intact Capsule in a 100-mL volumetric flask, add about 70 mL of 0.1 N hydrochloric acid, and sonicate until the gelatin capsule shell has dissolved completely (about 15 minutes). [NOTE—Periodically swirl the flask during the sonication to loosen the Capsule from the bottom of the flask and to dissolve a floating Capsule.] Shake mechanically for about 30 additional minutes, dilute with 0.1 N hydrochloric acid to volume, and mix. Pass a portion of the solution through a suitable filter, and dilute quantitatively with 0.1 N hydrochloric acid to obtain a solution having a concentration of about 4.1 μg of tacrine hydrochloride per mL. [NOTE—Do not use nylon filters.] Immediately prior to removing an aliquot for analysis, mix the solution vigorously.

Blank—Place an empty Capsule of each Capsule strength into a separate 100-mL volumetric flask and prepare as directed for *Test solution*.

Procedure—Concomitantly determine the absorbances at 240 nm of the *Blank*, the *Standard solution*, and the *Test solution* with a suitable spectrophotometer. Calculate the quantity, in mg, of tacrine ($C_{13}H_{14}N_2$) in the Capsule taken by the formula:

$$1000L(C_S / C_U)(198.27/234.73)(A_U / A_S)$$

in which L is the labeled quantity, in mg, of tacrine hydrochloride in the Capsule; C_S is the concentration, in μg per mL, of USP Tacrine Hydrochloride RS in the *Standard solution*; C_U is the concentration, in μg per mL, of tacrine hydrochloride in the *Test solution*, based on the labeled quantity per Capsule and the extent of dilution; 198.27 and 234.73 are the molecular weights of tacrine and tacrine hydrochloride, respectively; and A_U and A_S are the absorbances obtained from the *Test solution* and the *Standard solution*, respectively.

Assay—

0.1 M Triethylamine phosphate solution—Transfer 28 mL of triethylamine to a 2000-mL volumetric flask containing about 1800 mL of water, and mix. Adjust with phosphoric acid to a pH of 3.25, dilute with water to volume, and mix.

Mobile phase—Prepare a filtered and degassed mixture of *0.1 M Triethylamine phosphate solution* and methanol (85 : 15). Make adjustments if necessary (see *System Suitability* under *Chromatography* ⟨621⟩).

Standard preparation—Dissolve an accurately weighed quantity of USP Tacrine Hydrochloride RS in *Mobile phase*, and dilute quantitatively, and stepwise if necessary, with *Mobile phase* to obtain a solution having a known concentration of about 100 μg of tacrine per mL.

Assay preparation—Transfer 10 Capsules to a 1000-mL volumetric flask containing 500 mL of *Mobile phase*. Sonicate for about 45 minutes until the gelatin capsule shells have dissolved. Periodically swirl the flask during sonication to loosen any Capsules sticking to the bottom of the flask and to dissolve floating Capsules. Add an additional 300 mL of *Mobile phase*, shake for 30 minutes on a mechanical shaker, dilute with *Mobile phase* to volume, and mix. Pass an aliquot of this solution through an appropriate filter presaturated with the solution, and dilute, if necessary, with *Mobile phase* to obtain a solution containing about 100 μg of tacrine per mL.

Chromatographic system (see *Chromatography* ⟨621⟩)—The liquid chromatograph is equipped with a variable wavelength detector and a 4.6-mm × 15-cm column that contains 5-μm packing L1. The flow rate is about 2.5 mL per minute. Initially, the detector is maintained at a wavelength of 240 nm. At 7.0 minutes, the wavelength is changed to 260 nm. Chromatograph the *Standard preparation*, and record the peak responses as directed for *Procedure*: the column efficiency is not less than 3500 theoretical plates; the tailing factor is not more than 2.0; and the relative standard deviation for replicate injections is not more than 1.0%.

Procedure—Separately inject equal volumes (about 30 μL) of the *Standard preparation* and the *Assay preparation* into the chromatograph, record the chromatograms, and measure the areas for the ma-

jor peaks. Calculate the quantity, in mg, of tacrine ($C_{13}H_{14}N_2$) in the portion of Capsules taken by the formula:

$$1000C(198.27/234.73)(r_U / r_S)$$

in which C is the concentration, in mg per mL, of USP Tacrine Hydrochloride RS in the *Standard preparation;* 198.27 and 234.73 are the molecular weights of tacrine and tacrine hydrochloride, respectively; and r_U and r_S are the peak responses obtained from the *Assay preparation* and the *Standard preparation,* respectively.

Talc

» Talc is a powdered, selected, natural, hydrated magnesium silicate. Pure talc has the formula $Mg_3Si_4O_{10}(OH)_2$. It may contain variable amounts of associated minerals among which chlorites (hydrated aluminum and magnesium silicates), magnesite (magnesium carbonate), calcite (calcium carbonate), and dolomite (calcium and magnesium carbonate) are predominant.

Packaging and storage—Preserve in well-closed containers. No storage requirements specified.
Labeling—The label states, where applicable, that the substance is suitable for oral or topical administration. The certificate of analysis states the absence of asbestos. It also indicates which method specified under the test for*Absence of asbestos* was used for analysis.
Identification—
  A: The IR spectrum of a potassium bromide dispersion of it exhibits maxima at 3677 ± 2 cm^{-1}, at 1018 ± 2 cm^{-1}, and at 669 ± 2 cm^{-1}.
  B: Mix about 200 mg of anhydrous sodium carbonate with 2 g of anhydrous potassium carbonate, and melt in a platinum crucible. To the melt add 100 mg of the substance under test, and continue heating until fusion is complete. Cool, and transfer the fused mixture to a dish or beaker with the aid of about 50 mL of hot water. Add hydrochloric acid to the liquid until effervescence ceases, then add 10 mL more of the acid, and evaporate the mixture on a steam bath to dryness. Cool, add 20 mL of water, boil, and filter the mixture: [NOTE—Save the insoluble residue for use in*Identification* test C.] To 5 mL of the filtrate add 1 mL of 6 N ammonium hydroxide and 1 mL of ammonium chloride TS. Filter, if necessary, and add 1 mL of dibasic sodium phosphate TS to the filtrate: a white crystalline precipitate of magnesium ammonium phosphate is formed.
  C: In a lead or platinum crucible and using a copper wire, mix about 100 mg of the insoluble residue as obtained in *Identification* test B with about 10 mg of sodium fluoride and a few drops of sulfuric acid to give a thin slurry. Cover the crucible with a thin transparent plate of plastic under which a drop of water is suspended, and warm gently. Within a short time, a white ring is rapidly formed around the drop of water.
Microbial limits ⟨61⟩—If intended for topical administration, the total aerobic microbial count does not exceed 100 cfu per g, and the total combined molds and yeasts count does not exceed 50 cfu per g. If intended for oral administration, the total aerobic microbial count does not exceed 1000 cfu per g, and the total combined molds and yeasts count does not exceed 100 cfu per g.
Acidity and alkalinity—Boil 2.5 g of Talc with 50 mL of carbon dioxide-free water under reflux. Filter under vacuum. To 10 mL of the filtrate, add 0.1 mL of bromothymol blue TS. Not more than 0.4 mL of 0.01 N hydrochloric acid is required to change the color of the indicator. To 10 mL of the filtrate, add 0.1 mL of phenolphthalein TS: not more than 0.3 mL of 0.01 N sodium hydroxide is required to change the color of the indicator to pink.
Loss on ignition ⟨733⟩—Weigh accurately about 1 g, and ignite at $1075 \pm 25°$ to constant weight: it loses not more than 7.0% of its weight.
Water-soluble substances—To 10.0 g add 50 mL of carbon dioxide-free water, heat to boiling, and boil under a reflux condenser for 30 minutes. Allow to cool, filter, and dilute with carbon dioxide-free water to 50.0 mL: the filtrate is neutral to litmus paper. Evaporate 25.0 mL of the filtrate to dryness, and dry at 105° for 1 hour: the weight of the residue does not exceed 5 mg (0.1%).
Limit of iron—
  Test stock solution—Weigh 10.0 g of Talc into a conical flask fitted with a reflux condenser, gradually add 50 mL of 0.5 N hydrochloric acid while stirring, and heat on a water bath for 30 minutes. Allow to cool. Transfer the mixture to a beaker, and allow the undissolved material to settle. Filter the supernatant into a 100-mL volumetric flask, retaining as much as possible of the insoluble material in the beaker. Wash the residue and the beaker with three 10-mL portions of hot water. Wash the filter with 15 mL of hot water, allow the filtrate to cool, and dilute with water to 100.0 mL.
  Test solution—Transfer 2.5 mL of the *Test stock solution* to a 100-mL volumetric flask, add 50.0 mL of 0.5 N hydrochloric acid, and dilute with water to volume.
  Standard iron stock solution—Prepare a solution containing 4.840 g of ferric chloride in a 150 g per L solution of hydrochloric acid in water to obtain a concentration equivalent to 250 µg of iron per mL. Prepare immediately before use.
  Standard iron solutions—Into four 100-mL volumetric flasks, each containing 50.0 mL of 0.5 N hydrochloric acid, transfer respectively 2.0, 2.5, 3.0, and 4.0 mL of the *Standard iron stock solution,* and dilute each flask with water to volume.
  Procedure—Concomitantly determine the absorbance of the *Test solution* and the *Standard iron solutions* at the iron emission line of 248.3 nm with an atomic absorption spectrophotometer (see *Spectrophotometry and Light-Scattering* ⟨851⟩) equipped with an iron hollow-cathode lamp and an air–acetylene flame. Make any correction using a deuterium lamp: not more than 0.25% of iron is found.
Limit of lead—
  Test solution—Use the *Test stock solution,* prepared as directed in the test for *Limit of iron.*
  Lead standard stock solution—Dissolve 160 mg of lead nitrate in 100 mL water that contains 1 mL of nitric acid, and dilute with water to 1000 mL. Pipet 10 mL of this solution into a 100-mL volumetric flask, dilute with water to volume, and mix. This solution contains the equivalent of 10 µg of lead per mL.
  Standard lead solutions—Into four identical 100-mL volumetric flasks, each containing 50.0 mL of 0.5 N hydrochloric acid, transfer respectively 5.0, 7.5, 10.0, and 12.5 mL of *Lead standard stock solution,* and dilute with water to volume.
  Procedure—Concomitantly determine the absorbance of the *Test solution* and the *Standard lead solutions* at the lead emission line of 217.0 nm with an atomic absorption spectrophotometer (see *Spectrophotometry and Light-Scattering* ⟨851⟩) equipped with a lead hollow-cathode lamp and an air–acetylene flame: not more than 0.001% of lead is found.
Limit of calcium—
  Lanthanum chloride solution—To 5.9 g of lanthanum oxide slowly add 10 mL of hydrochloric acid, and heat to boiling. Allow to cool, and dilute with water to 100 mL.
  Test stock solution—[*Caution—Perchlorates mixed with heavy metals are known to be explosive. Take proper precautions while performing this procedure.*] Weigh 500 mg of Talc in a 100-mL polytetrafluoroethylene dish, add 5 mL of hydrochloric acid, 5 mL of lead-free nitric acid, and 5 mL of perchloric acid. Stir gently, then add 35 mL of hydrofluoric acid, and evaporate slowly on a hot plate to moist dryness (until about 0.5 mL remains). To the residue, add 5 mL of hydrochloric acid, cover with a watch glass, heat to boiling, and allow to cool. Rinse the watch glass and the dish with water, and transfer into a 50-mL volumetric flask, and dilute with water to volume.
  Test solution—Transfer 5.0 mL of the *Test stock solution* to a 100-mL volumetric flask, add 10.0 mL of hydrochloric acid and 10 mL of *Lanthanum chloride solution,* and dilute with water to volume.
  Calcium standard stock solution—Dissolve 3.67 g of calcium chloride dihydrate in diluted hydrochloric acid, and dilute with the same solvent to 1000 mL. Immediately before use, pipet 10 mL of this solution into a 100-mL volumetric flask, dilute with water to volume, and mix. This solution contains the equivalent of 100 µg of calcium per mL.
  Standard calcium solutions—Into four identical 100-mL volumetric flasks, each containing 10.0 mL of hydrochloric acid and 10

3320 Talc / Official Monographs

mL of *Lanthanum chloride solution,* transfer respectively 1.0, 2.0, 3.0, and 4.0 mL of *Calcium standard stock solution,* and dilute each flask with water to volume.

Procedure—Concomitantly determine the absorbance of the *Test solution* and the *Standard calcium solutions* at the calcium emission line of 422.7 nm with an atomic absorption spectrophotometer (see *Spectrophotometry and Light-Scattering* ⟨851⟩) equipped with a calcium hollow-cathode lamp and a nitrous oxide–acetylene flame: not more than 0.9% of calcium is found.

Limit of aluminum—
Cesium chloride solution—Dissolve 2.53 g of cesium chloride in 100 mL of water, and mix.
Test stock solution—Proceed as directed in the test for *Limit of calcium*. Transfer 5 mL of the *Cesium chloride solution* to the 50-mL volumetric flask, prior to transfer of residue, and dilute with water to volume.
Test solution—Transfer 5.0 mL of the *Test stock solution* to a 100-mL volumetric flask, add 10 mL of the *Cesium chloride solution* and 10.0 mL of hydrochloric acid, and dilute with water to volume.
Aluminum standard stock solution—Dissolve 8.947 g of aluminum chloride in water, and dilute with water to 1000 mL. Immediately before use, pipet 10 mL of this solution into a 100-mL volumetric flask, dilute with water to volume, and mix. This solution contains the equivalent of 100 µg of aluminum per mL.
Standard aluminum solutions—Into four identical 100-mL volumetric flasks, each containing 10.0 mL of hydrochloric acid and 10 mL of *Cesium chloride solution,* transfer respectively 5.0, 10.0, 15.0, and 20.0 mL of *Aluminum standard stock solution,* and dilute with water to volume.
Procedure—Concomitantly determine the absorbance of the *Test solution* and the *Standard aluminum solutions* at the aluminum emission line of 309.3 nm with an atomic absorption spectrophotometer (see *Spectrophotometry and Light-Scattering* ⟨851⟩) equipped with an aluminum hollow-cathode lamp and a nitrous oxide–acetylene flame: not more than 2.0% of aluminum is found.

Absence of asbestos—[NOTE—Suppliers of Talc may use one of the following methods to determine the absence of asbestos.] Proceed as directed for test A or testB. If either test is positive, perform test C.
A: The IR absorption spectrum of a potassium bromide dispersion of it at the absorption band 758 ± 1 cm^{-1}, using scale expansion, may indicate the presence of tremolite or of chlorite. If the absorption band remains after ignition of the substance at 850° for at least 30 minutes, it indicates the presence of the tremolite. In the range 600 cm^{-1} to 650 cm^{-1} using scale expansion, any absorption band or shoulder may indicate the presence of serpentines.
B: *X-ray diffraction* ⟨941⟩ employing the following conditions: Cu Kα monochromatic 40 kV radiation, 24 mA to 30 mA; the incident slit is set at 1°; the detection slit is set at 0.2°; the goniometer speed is 1/10° 2Θ per minute; the scanning range is 10° to 13° 2Θ and 24° to 26° 2Θ; the sample is not oriented. Prepare a random sample, and place on the sample holder. Pack and smooth its surface with a polished glass microscope slide. Record the diffractograms: the presence of amphiboles is detected by a diffraction peak at 10.5 ± 0.1° 2Θ, and the presence of serpentines is detected by diffraction peaks at 24.3 ± 0.1° 2Θ to 12.1 ± 0.1° 2Θ.
C: The presence of asbestos (see *Optical Microscopy* ⟨776⟩) is shown if there is a range of length to width ratios of 20 : 1 to 100 : 1, or higher for fibers longer than 5 µm; if there is a capability of splitting into very thin fibrils; and if there are two or more of the following four criteria: (1) parallel fibers occurring in bundles, (2) fiber bundles displaying frayed ends, (3) fibers in the form of thin needles, or (4) matted masses of individual fibers and/or fibers showing curvature.

Content of magnesium—
Lanthanum chloride solution and *Test stock solution*—Prepare as directed in the test for *Limit of calcium.*
Test solution—Dilute 0.5 mL of *Test stock solution* with water to 100.0 mL. Transfer 4.0 mL of this solution to a 100-mL volumetric flask, add 10.0 mL of hydrochloric acid and 10 mL of *Lanthanum chloride solution,* and dilute with water to volume.
Magnesium standard stock solution—Dissolve 8.365 g of magnesium chloride in diluted hydrochloric acid, and dilute with the same solvent to 1000 mL. Pipet 5 mL of this solution into a 500-mL volumetric flask, dilute with water to volume, and mix. This solution contains the equivalent of 10 µg of magnesium per mL.
Standard magnesium solutions—Into four identical 100-mL volumetric flasks, each containing 10.0 mL of hydrochloric acid and 10 mL of *Lanthanum chloride solution,* transfer respectively 2.5, 3.0, 4.0, and 5.0 mL of *Magnesium standard stock solution,* and dilute with water to volume.
Procedure—Concomitantly determine the absorbance of the *Test solution* and the *Standard magnesium solutions* at the magnesium emission line of 285.2 nm with an atomic absorption spectrophotometer (see *Spectrophotometry and Light-Scattering* ⟨851⟩) equipped with a magnesium hollow-cathode lamp and an air–acetylene flame: between 17.0% to 19.5% of magnesium is found.

Tamoxifen Citrate

$C_{26}H_{29}NO \cdot C_6H_8O_7$ 563.64
Ethanamine, 2-[4-(1,2-diphenyl-1-butenyl)phenoxy]-*N,N*-dimethyl, (Z)-, 2-hydroxy-1,2,3-propanetricarboxylate (1 : 1).
(Z)-2-[*p*-(1,2-Diphenyl-1-butenyl)phenoxy]-*N,N*-dimethylethylamine citrate (1 : 1) [54965-24-1].

» Tamoxifen Citrate contains not less than 99.0 percent and not more than 101.0 percent of $C_{26}H_{29}NO \cdot C_6H_8O_7$, calculated on the dried basis.

Packaging and storage—Preserve in well-closed, light-resistant containers.

USP Reference standards ⟨11⟩—*USP Tamoxifen Citrate RS.*
Identification—
A: *Infrared Absorption* ⟨197K⟩: a single band in the 1700 to 1740 cm^{-1} region of the spectrum.
B: *Ultraviolet Absorption* ⟨197U⟩—
Solution: 20 µg per mL.
Medium: methanol.
Loss on drying ⟨731⟩—Dry it at 105° for 4 hours: it loses not more than 0.5% of its weight.
Residue on ignition ⟨281⟩: not more than 0.2%.
Limit of *E*-isomer—
Mobile phase—Prepare a methanol solution containing, in each liter, 320 mL of water, 2 mL of glacial acetic acid, and 1.08 g of sodium 1-octanesulfonate.
Standard preparation—Dissolve a suitable quantity, accurately weighed, of USP Tamoxifen Citrate RS in *Mobile phase* to obtain a solution having a known concentration of about 600 µg per mL.
Test preparation—Using about 30 mg of Tamoxifen Citrate, accurately weighed, proceed as directed under *Standard preparation.*
Chromatographic system (see *Chromatography* ⟨621⟩)—The liquid chromatograph is equipped with a 254-nm detector and a 4-mm × 30-cm column that contains packing L11. The flow rate is about 0.7 mL per minute. Chromatograph five replicate injections of the *Standard preparation,* and record the responses of the major peak: the relative standard deviation is not more than 3.0%, and the relative retention time of the minor *E*-isomer peak to that of the Z-isomer peak is not greater than 0.93.
Procedure—Separately introduce equal volumes (about 20 µL) of the *Test preparation* and the *Standard preparation* into the liquid chromatograph by means of a suitable sampling valve. Measure the minor peak responses for the *E*-isomer obtained from the *Standard preparation* and the *Assay preparation.* Calculate the quantity, in

mg, of *E*-isomer (C$_{26}$H$_{29}$NO · C$_6$H$_8$O$_7$) in the portion of Tamoxifen Citrate taken by the formula:

$$0.05C(r_U / r_S)$$

in which *C* is the concentration, in μg per mL, of the *E*-isomer as the citrate, based on its declared content in USP Tamoxifen Citrate RS in the *Standard preparation*, and the r_U and r_S are the minor peak responses obtained from the *Assay preparation* and the *Standard preparation*, respectively. The *E*-isomer content is not more than 0.3% of tamoxifen citrate (C$_{26}$H$_{29}$NO · C$_6$H$_8$O$_7$).

Iron ⟨241⟩—Accurately weigh 1.0 g, and transfer to a suitable crucible. Add sufficient sulfuric acid to wet the substance, and carefully ignite at a low temperature until thoroughly charred. (The crucible may be loosely covered with a suitable lid during the charring.) Add to the carbonized mass 2 mL of nitric acid and 5 drops of sulfuric acid, and heat cautiously until white fumes no longer are evolved. Ignite, preferably in a muffle furnace, at 500° to 600°, until the carbon is completely burned off. Cool, add 10 mL of warm 0.1 N hydrochloric acid, and digest for about 5 minutes. Transfer the contents of the crucible with the aid of small portions of water to a 50-mL volumetric flask, dilute with water to volume, and mix. Pipet 10 mL from the volumetric flask into a color-comparison tube, dilute with water to 45 mL, add 2 mL of hydrochloric acid, and mix. The limit is 0.005%.

Heavy metals, *Method II* ⟨231⟩:   0.001%.

Related impurities—

Test preparation A—Disperse about 3 g in 100 mL of water in a separator. Over a 10-minute period add 50 mL of 0.5 N sodium hydroxide, with mixing. Extract with two 50-mL portions of ether, and combine the extracts. Wash with 20 mL of water, remove the water layer, and dry the ether layer over anhydrous sodium sulfate. Evaporate the ether layer under nitrogen, and dry in vacuum at room temperature for 2 hours. Accurately weigh 1.5 g of the residue into a 10-mL volumetric flask, add 5.0 mL of a mixture of 5 volumes of acetic anhydride and 95 volumes of pyridine, and heat at 60° for 10 to 15 minutes. Cool, dilute with the same solvent mixture to volume, and mix.

Test preparation B—Using the same acetic anhydride-pyridine mixture, prepare a 1 : 200 dilution of *Test preparation A*.

Chromatographic system (see *Chromatography* ⟨621⟩)—Typically, the gas chromatograph is equipped with a flame-ionization detector, and contains a 4-mm × 1-m glass column packed with 5% liquid phase G17 on 100- to 120-mesh support S1AB conditioned at 300° for 24 hours. The column and injection port temperatures are maintained at about 260° and the detector temperature at about 300°. Dry helium is used as the carrier gas at a flow rate of about 60 mL per minute. In a suitable chromatogram, five replicate injections of *Test preparation B* show a relative standard deviation of not more than 3.0%.

Procedure—Inject equal portions (about 2 μL), accurately measured, of *Test preparation A* and *Test preparation B* into the chromatograph, and record the chromatograms from 0.1 to 5.0, relative to the retention time of the major peak. Measure the individual areas of the peaks other than those produced by the solvent and the tamoxifen on the chromatograms obtained from *Test preparation A*, and calculate their sum. No single peak area is greater than the total area of the tamoxifen peak on the chromatogram obtained from *Test preparation B* (0.5%), and the sum of the peak areas is not greater than twice the total area of the tamoxifen peak on the chromatogram obtained from *Test preparation B* (1.0%).

Organic volatile impurities, *Method V* ⟨467⟩:   meets the requirements.

Solvent—Use dimethyl sulfoxide.

(Official until July 1, 2008)

Assay—Weigh accurately about 1 g of Tamoxifen Citrate, and dissolve in 150 mL of glacial acetic acid. Titrate the solution with 0.1 N perchloric acid VS, determining the endpoint potentiometrically, using a glass indicator electrode and a silver-silver chloride reference electrode. Each mL of 0.1 N perchloric acid is equivalent to 56.36 mg of C$_{26}$H$_{29}$NO · C$_6$H$_8$O$_7$.

Tamoxifen Citrate Tablets

» Tamoxifen Citrate Tablets contain not less than 90.0 percent and not more than 110.0 percent of the labeled amount of tamoxifen (C$_{26}$H$_{29}$NO).

Packaging and storage—Preserve in well-closed, light-resistant containers.

USP Reference standards ⟨11⟩—*USP Tamoxifen Citrate RS.*

Identification—

A: The UV absorption spectrum of the *Test preparation*, obtained as directed in the test for *Content uniformity*, exhibits maxima and minima at the same wavelengths as that of the *Standard preparation*, concomitantly measured.

B: To 1 Tablet contained in a 15-mL tube add 4 mL of pyridine and 2 mL of acetic anhydride: an immediate yellow color is produced on shaking. Then heat gently on a steam bath: a rose-pink to a deep red color develops, indicating the presence of citrate ion.

Dissolution ⟨711⟩—

Medium: 0.02 N hydrochloric acid; 1000 mL.
Apparatus 1:   100 rpm.
Time: 30 minutes.

Procedure—Determine the amount of tamoxifen (C$_{26}$H$_{29}$NO) dissolved from UV absorbances at the wavelength of maximum absorbance at about 275 nm of filtered portions of the solution under test, suitably diluted with *Medium*, if necessary, in comparison with a Standard solution having a known concentration of USP Tamoxifen Citrate RS in the same *Medium*.

Tolerances—Not less than 75% *(Q)* of the labeled amount of C$_{26}$H$_{29}$NO is dissolved in 30 minutes.

Uniformity of dosage units ⟨905⟩:   meet the requirements.

PROCEDURE FOR CONTENT UNIFORMITY—

Standard solution—Dissolve an accurately weighed quantity of USP Tamoxifen Citrate RS in methanol to obtain a solution having a known concentration of about 15 μg per mL.

Test solution—Place 1 Tablet in a 100-mL volumetric flask, and crush with a stirring rod. Add about 75 mL of methanol, and shake for about 5 minutes. Dilute with methanol to volume, mix, and filter the solution through paper. Pipet 10 mL of the filtrate into a 100-mL volumetric flask, dilute with methanol to volume, and mix.

Procedure—Determine the absorbances of the *Test solution* and the *Standard solution* in 1-cm cells at the wavelength of maximum absorbance at about 275 nm, with a suitable spectrophotometer, using methanol as the blank. Calculate the quantity, in mg, of tamoxifen (C$_{26}$H$_{29}$NO) in the Tablets taken by the formula:

$$(371.51 / 563.64)(TC / D)(A_U / A_S)$$

in which 371.51 and 563.64 are the molecular weights of tamoxifen and tamoxifen citrate, respectively; *T* is the labeled quantity, in mg, of tamoxifen in the Tablet; *C* is the concentration, in μg per mL, of USP Tamoxifen Citrate RS in the *Standard solution*; *D* is the concentration, in μg per mL, of tamoxifen in the solution from the Tablet, based upon the labeled quantity per Tablet and the extent of dilution; and A_U and A_S are the absorbances of the *Test solution* and the *Standard solution*, respectively.

Assay—

Mobile phase—Prepare a methanol solution containing, in each liter, 320 mL of water, 2 mL of glacial acetic acid, and 1.08 g of sodium 1-octanesulfonate.

Standard preparation—Dissolve a suitable quantity, accurately weighed, of USP Tamoxifen Citrate RS in *Mobile phase* to obtain a solution having a known concentration of about 200 μg per mL.

Assay preparation—Weigh and finely powder not fewer than 20 Tablets. Transfer an accurately weighed portion of the powder, equivalent to about 20 mg of tamoxifen, to a stoppered, 50-mL centrifuge tube. Pipet 30 mL of *Mobile phase* into the tube, and shake by mechanical means for not less than 15 minutes. Centrifuge at about 1000 rpm, pipet 5 mL of the clear supernatant into a 25-mL volumetric flask, dilute with *Mobile phase* to volume, and mix.

Chromatographic system (see *Chromatography* ⟨621⟩)—The liquid chromatograph is equipped with a 254-nm detector and a 4-mm × 30-cm column that contains packing L11. The flow rate is about

1.5 mL per minute. Chromatograph the *Standard preparation*, and record the peak areas as directed for *Procedure:* the relative standard deviation for replicate injections is not more than 3.0%.

Procedure—Separately inject equal volumes (about 25 µL) of the *Assay preparation* and the *Standard preparation* into the chromatograph by means of a suitable sampling valve, record the chromatograms, and measure the areas for the major peaks. Calculate the quantity, in mg, of tamoxifen ($C_{26}H_{29}NO$) in the portion of Tablets taken by the formula:

$$0.15C(371.51 / 563.64)(r_U / r_S)$$

in which 371.51 and 563.64 are the molecular weights of tamoxifen and tamoxifen citrate, respectively; C is the concentration, in µg per mL, of USP Tamoxifen Citrate RS in the *Standard preparation*; and r_U and r_S are the peak areas obtained from the *Assay preparation* and the *Standard preparation*, respectively.

Tannic Acid

Tannin.
Tannic acid; Tannin [1401-55-4].

» Tannic Acid is a tannin usually obtained from nutgalls, the excrescences produced on the young twigs of *Quercus infectoria* Oliver, and allied species of *Quercus* Linné (Fam. Fagaceae), from the seed pods of Tara (*Caesalpinia spinosa*), or from the nutgalls or leaves of sumac (any of a genus *Rhus*).

Packaging and storage—Preserve in tight, light-resistant containers.
Identification—
 A: To 2 mL of a solution (1 in 10) add 1 drop of ferric chloride TS: a bluish black color or precipitate results.
 B: To a solution (1 in 10) add an equal volume of gelatin solution (1 in 100): a precipitate is formed.
Loss on drying ⟨731⟩—Dry it at 105° for 2 hours: it loses not more than 12.0% of its weight.
Residue on ignition ⟨281⟩: not more than 1.0%.
Arsenic, *Method II* ⟨211⟩: 3 ppm.
Heavy metals, *Method II* ⟨231⟩: 0.004%.
Gum or dextrin—Dissolve 2 g in 10 mL of hot water: the solution is not more than slightly turbid. Cool, filter, and divide the filtrate into two equal portions. To one portion add 10 mL of alcohol: no turbidity is produced.
Resinous substances—To a portion of the filtrate obtained in the test for *Gum or dextrin* add 10 mL of water: no turbidity is produced.
Organic volatile impurities, *Method I* ⟨467⟩: meets the requirements.

(Official until July 1, 2008)

Adhesive Tape

» Adhesive Tape consists of fabric and/or film evenly coated on one side with a pressure-sensitive, adhesive mixture. Its length is not less than 98.0 percent of that declared on the label, and its average width is not less than 95.0 percent of the declared width. If Adhesive Tape has been rendered sterile, it is protected from contamination by appropriate packaging.

Packaging and storage—Preserve in well-closed containers, and prevent exposure to excessive heat and to sunlight. Tape that has been rendered sterile is so packaged that the sterility of the contents of the package is maintained until the package is opened for use.

Labeling—The package label of Tape that has been rendered sterile indicates that the contents may not be sterile if the package bears evidence of damage or previously has been opened. The package label indicates the length and width of the Tape, and the name of the manufacturer, packer, or distributor.
Dimensions—Measure its length: it is not less than 98.0% of the labeled length. Measure its width at 5 locations evenly spaced along the center line of the Tape: the average of 5 measurements is not less than 95% of the labeled width of the Tape.
Tensile strength—Determine the tensile strength of Tape, after previously unrolling and conditioning it for not less than 4 hours in a standard atmosphere of $65 \pm 2\%$ relative humidity, at $21 \pm 1.1°$ ($70 \pm 2°F$), with a pendulum-type testing machine, as described under *Tensile Strength* ⟨881⟩. The Tape made from fabric has a tensile strength, determined warpwise, of not less than 20.41 kg (45 pounds) per 2.54 cm of width. The Tape made from film has a tensile strength of not less than 3 kg per 2.54 cm of width.
Adhesive strength—Determine the adhesive strength of Tape that is made from fabric by cutting a strip of the Tape 2.54 cm wide and approximately 15 cm long, and applying 12.90 sq cm, 2.54 cm by 5.08 cm, of one end of the strip to a clean plastic or glass surface by means of a rubber roller under a pressure of 850 g, passing the roller twice over the Tape at a rate of 30 cm per minute. Adjust the temperature of the plastic or glass surface and the Tape to 37°, and conduct the test immediately thereafter as directed under *Tensile Strength* ⟨881⟩, using a pendulum-type testing machine, the pull being exerted parallel with the warp and the plastic or glass surface: the average of not less than 10 tests is not less than 18 kg.
Sterility ⟨71⟩—Tape that has been rendered sterile meets the requirements.

Taurine

$C_2H_7NO_3S$ 125.15
Taurine [107-35-7].

» Taurine contains not less than 98.5 percent and not more than 101.5 percent of $C_2H_7NO_3S$, calculated on the dried basis.

Packaging and storage—Preserve in well-closed containers.
USP Reference standards ⟨11⟩—USP Taurine RS.
Identification, *Infrared Absorption* ⟨197K⟩.
Loss on drying ⟨731⟩—Dry it at 105° for 3 hours: it loses not more than 0.3% of its weight.
Residue on ignition ⟨281⟩: not more than 0.3%.
Chloride ⟨221⟩—A 0.7-g portion shows no more chloride than corresponds to 0.50 mL of 0.020 N hydrochloric acid. Not more than 0.05% is found.
Sulfate ⟨221⟩—A 0.8-g portion shows no more sulfate than corresponds to 0.25 mL of 0.020 N sulfuric acid. Not more than 0.03% is found.
Iron ⟨241⟩: 0.003%.
Heavy metals, *Method I* ⟨231⟩: 0.0015%.
Chromatographic purity—
 Adsorbent: 0.25-mm layer of chromatographic silica gel mixture.
 Test solution—Dissolve an accurately weighed quantity of Taurine with water to obtain a solution having a concentration of about 10 mg per mL.
 Standard solution—Dissolve an accurately weighed quantity of USP Taurine RS with water to obtain a solution having a known concentration of about 0.05 mg per mL, equivalent concentration to about 0.5% of the *Test solution*.
 Application volume: 5 µL.
 Developing solvent system: a mixture of butyl alcohol, glacial acetic acid, and water (60 : 20 : 20).
 Spray reagent—Dissolve 0.2 g ninhydrin in 100 mL of a mixture of butyl alcohol and 2 N acetic acid (95 : 5).

Procedure—Proceed as directed for *Thin-Layer Chromatography* under *Chromatography* ⟨621⟩, except to dry the plate at 80° for 30 minutes. Spray the plate with *Spray reagent*, and heat at 80° for about 10 minutes. Examine the plate under white light: no secondary spot in the chromatogram of the *Test solution* is larger or more intense than the principal spot in the chromatogram of the *Standard solution*. Not more than 0.5% of individual impurities are found. [NOTE—The R_F value for the taurine spots should be about 0.2.]

Organic volatile impurities, *Method I* ⟨467⟩: meets the requirements.

(Official until July 1, 2008)

Assay—Proceed as directed for *Method II* under *Nitrogen Determination* ⟨461⟩. Each mL of 0.01 N sulfuric acid is equivalent to 1.25 mg of $C_2H_7NO_3S$.

Add the following:

▲Tazobactam

$C_{10}H_{12}N_4O_5S$ 300.29

4-Thia-1-azabicyclo[3.2.0]heptane-2-carboxylic acid, 3-methyl-7-oxo-3-(1*H*-1,2,3-triazol-1-ylmethyl)-, 4,4-dioxide, [2*S*-(2α,3β,5α)]-.

(2*S*,3*S*,5*R*)-3-Methyl-7-oxo-3-(1*H*-1,2,3-triazol-1-ylmethyl)-4-thia-1-azabicyclo[3.2.0]heptane-2-carboxylic acid, 4,4-dioxide [89786-04-9].

» Tazobactam contains not less than 98.0 percent and not more than 102.0 percent of $C_{10}H_{12}N_4O_5S$, calculated on the anhydrous basis.

Packaging and storage—Preserve in well-closed containers. Store at controlled room temperature.

USP Reference standards ⟨11⟩—*USP Endotoxin RS. USP Tazobactam RS. USP Tazobactam Related Compound A RS.*

Identification—
  A: *Infrared Absorption* ⟨197K⟩, on an undried specimen.
  B: The retention time of the major peak in the chromatogram of the *Assay preparation* corresponds to that in the chromatogram of the *Standard preparation*, as obtained in the *Assay*.

Bacterial endotoxins ⟨85⟩—The level of Bacterial Endotoxins are such that the requirements under the relevant dosage form monograph(s) in which Tazobactam is used can be met.

Specific rotation ⟨781S⟩: between 160° and 167° ($t = 20°$).
  Test solution: 10 mg per mL, in dimethylformamide.

Microbial limits ⟨61⟩—The total aerobic microbial count does not exceed 1000 cfu per g, and the total combined molds and yeasts count does not exceed 100 cfu per g.

pH ⟨791⟩: between 1.8 and 2.8, in a solution containing 2.5 mg per mL.

Water, *Method I* ⟨921⟩: not more than 0.6%.

Residue on ignition ⟨281⟩: not more than 0.1%.

Heavy metals, *Method II* ⟨231⟩: 0.002%.

Related compounds—
  Mobile phase, L-Phenylalanine solution, System suitability solution, and *Chromatographic system*—Prepare as directed in the *Assay*.
  Blank—Use water.
  Standard solution—Use the *Standard preparation*, prepared as directed in the *Assay*.
  Test solution—Use the *Assay preparation*.
  Procedure—Cool and maintain the *Standard solution*, the *System suitability solution*, the *Blank*, and the *Test solution* at 3° until injection. [NOTE—If an autosampler is used, replace the plastic tubing connected to the injection needle with a stainless steel assembly, and maintain at 3°. If a chilled autosampler is not used, then these solutions should be injected immediately after preparation.] Separately inject equal volumes (about 20 μL) of the *Standard solution*, the *System suitability solution*, the *Blank*, and the *Test solution* into the chromatograph; record the chromatograms; and measure the area responses for the peaks. Calculate the percentage of each related compound in the portion of Tazobactam taken by the formula:

$$100(r_i / r_s)$$

in which r_i is the response for each related compound in the chromatogram obtained from the *Test solution*, and r_s is the sum of the peak responses of all the peaks in the chromatogram obtained from the *Test solution*: not more than 1.0% of tazobactam related compound A is found; not more than 0.1% of any other individual impurity is found; and the sum of all impurities found, other than tazobactam related compound A, is not greater than 0.3%. [NOTE—Ignore any peaks in the chromatogram of the *Test solution* that correspond to any peaks in the chromatogram of the *Blank*.]

Organic volatile impurities, *Method IV* ⟨467⟩: meets the requirements.

(Official until July 1, 2008)

Assay—
  Mobile phase—Dissolve 1.32 g of dibasic ammonium phosphate in 750 mL of water. Adjust with 5% (v/v) phosphoric acid to a pH of 2.5, dilute with water to 1000 mL, and mix. Add 30 mL of acetonitrile, mix, and pass through a filter having a 0.2-μm porosity. Make adjustments if necessary (see *System Suitability* under *Chromatography* ⟨621⟩).
  Standard preparation—Dissolve accurately weighed quantities of USP Tazobactam RS and USP Tazobactam Related Compound A RS in water to obtain a solution having known concentrations of about 0.5 mg per mL and 0.08 mg per mL, respectively.
  L-Phenylalanine solution—Prepare an aqueous solution of L-phenylalanine containing 0.8 mg per mL.
  System suitability solution—Pipet 1.0 mL of *L-Phenylalanine solution* and 5.0 mL of the *Standard preparation* into a 50-mL volumetric flask. Dilute with water to volume, and mix. [NOTE—Maintain this solution at 3° until injection. Prepare fresh daily.]
  Assay preparation—Transfer about 25 mg of Tazobactam, accurately weighed, to a 50-mL volumetric flask, dissolve in and dilute with water to volume, and mix.
  Chromatographic system (see *Chromatography* ⟨621⟩)—The liquid chromatograph is equipped with a 210-nm detector and a 4.6-mm × 25-cm column that contains 5-μm packing L1. The flow rate is about 1.5 mL per minute. Chromatograph 20 μL of the *System suitability solution*, and record the peak responses as directed for *Procedure:* the resolution, *R*, between tazobactam and L-phenylalanine is not less than 6.0; the tailing factor is not more than 1.8; and the relative standard deviation for replicate injections is not more than 2.0%.
  Procedure—Cool and maintain the *Standard preparation*, the *System suitability solution*, and the *Assay preparation* at 3° until injection. [NOTE—If an autosampler is used, replace the plastic tubing connected to the injection needle with a stainless steel assembly, and maintain at 3°. If a chilled autosampler is not used, then these solutions should be injected immediately after preparation.] Separately inject equal volumes (about 20 μL) of the *Standard preparation* and the *Assay preparation* into the chromatograph, record the chromatograms, and measure the responses for the major peaks. Calculate the quantity, in mg, of $C_{10}H_{12}N_4O_5S$ in the portion of Tazobactam taken by the formula:

$$50C(r_U / r_S)$$

in which *C* is the concentration, in mg per mL, of USP Tazobactam RS in the *Standard preparation*; and r_U and r_S are the peak responses obtained from the *Assay preparation* and the *Standard preparation*, respectively.▲USP31

Technetium Tc 99m Albumin Injection

» Technetium Tc 99m Albumin Injection is a sterile, aqueous solution, suitable for intravenous administration, of Albumin Human that is labeled with ^{99m}Tc.

It contains not less than 90.0 percent and not more than 110.0 percent of the labeled amount of ^{99m}Tc as albumin expressed in megabecquerels (microcuries or millicuries) per mL at the time indicated in the labeling. It may contain antimicrobial agents, buffers, reducing agents, and stabilizers. Other chemical forms of radioactivity do not exceed 10.0 percent of the total radioactivity. Its production and distribution are subject to federal regulations (see *Biologics* ⟨1041⟩ and *Radioactivity* ⟨821⟩).

Packaging and storage—Preserve in single-dose or in multiple-dose containers, at a temperature between 2° and 8°.

Labeling—Label it to include the following in addition to the information specified for *Labeling* under *Injections* ⟨1⟩: the time and date of calibration; the amount of ^{99m}Tc as albumin expressed as total megabecquerels (microcuries or millicuries) and concentration as megabecquerels (microcuries or millicuries) per mL at the time of calibration; the expiration date; and the statement "Caution—Radioactive Material." The labeling indicates that in making dosage calculations, correction is to be made for radioactive decay, and also indicates that the radioactive half-life of ^{99m}Tc is 6.0 hours.

USP Reference standards ⟨11⟩—*USP Endotoxin RS*.

Bacterial endotoxins ⟨85⟩—The limit of endotoxin content is not more than 175/V USP Endotoxin Unit per mL of the Injection, when compared with the USP Endotoxin RS, in which V is the maximum recommended total dose, in mL, at the expiration date or time.

pH ⟨791⟩: between 2.5 and 5.0.

Radiochemical purity—Not more than 10.0% of unbound Tc 99m (free pertechnetate) and reduced Tc 99m is present, determined as follows.

System A—Place a measured volume of Injection, such that it provides a count rate of about 100,000 counts per minute, about 3 cm from the end of a 2- × 17-cm thin-layer chromatographic strip impregnated with silica gel (see *Chromatography* ⟨621⟩), and allow to dry. Develop the chromatogram over a suitable period (approximately 30 minutes) by ascending chromatography, using acetone, and air-dry. Determine the radioactivity distribution by scanning the chromatograph with a suitable collimated radiation detector. Reduced Tc 99m and Tc 99m labeled albumin are located at the origin (R_F 0 to 0.1). Not more than 5.0% of the total radioactivity is found as unbound Tc 99m (free pertechnetate) at the solvent front (R_F 0.9 to 1.0).

System B—Prepare a 4- × 30-cm strip of chromatographic paper by immersing in 1% human serum albumin for 30 minutes and air-drying for 2 to 4 hours. Place a measured volume of Injection (about 3 μL) on the strip, mark the origin, and allow to dry. Develop the chromatogram by descending chromatography (see *Chromatography* ⟨621⟩), using nitrogen-purged saline TS until the solvent front has moved approximately 15 cm from the origin, mark the solvent front, and air-dry. Determine the radioactivity distribution by scanning the chromatogram with a suitable collimated radiation detector. Unbound Tc 99m and Tc 99m labeled albumin are at the solvent front (R_F 0.7 to 1.0). Not more than 5.0% of the total radioactivity is found as reduced Tc 99m at the origin (R_F 0 to 0.1).

Biological distribution—Inject intravenously between 0.075 MBq and 185 MBq (2 μCi and 5 mCi) of the Injection in a volume not exceeding 0.2 mL into the caudal vein of each of two 20-to 25-g mice. Approximately 30 minutes after the injection, sacrifice the animals, and drain the blood into a suitable container. Dissect the animals, and place the liver, stomach, and a 1-g specimen of blood, accurately weighed, in separate, suitable counting containers, and discard the tail cut above the injection site. Determine the radioactivity, in counts per minute, in each container with an appropriate detector, using the same counting geometry. Determine the percentage of radioactivity in the liver and stomach taken by the formula:

$$100(A_i / A)$$

in which A_i is the net radioactivity, in counts per minute, in the organ, and A is the total radioactivity, in counts per minute, in the liver, stomach, blood, and carcass. Determine the percentage of radioactivity in the blood taken by the formula:

$$[100(B / W_S)0.078(W_R)] / A$$

in which B is the net radioactivity, in counts per minute, in the specimen of blood, W_S is the weight, in g, of the blood specimen, W_R is the weight, in g, of the mouse, and 0.078 is the assumption that the total blood weight of the mouse is 7.8% of the total body weight. Not more than 15.0% of the radioactivity is found in the liver, and not more than 1.0% of the radioactivity is found in the stomach. Not less than 30.0% of the radioactivity is found in the blood.

Other requirements—It meets the requirements of the tests for *Radionuclide identification* and *Radionuclidic purity* under *Sodium Pertechnetate Tc 99m Injection*. It meets also the requirements under *Injections* ⟨1⟩, except that it may be distributed or dispensed prior to completion of the test for *Sterility*, the latter test being started on the day of final manufacture, and except that it is not subject to the recommendation on *Volume in Container*.

Assay for radioactivity ⟨821⟩—Using a suitable counting assembly (see *Selection of a Counting Assembly*), determine the radioactivity, in MBq (μCi) per mL, of Technetium Tc 99m Albumin Injection by use of a calibrated system.

Technetium Tc 99m Albumin Aggregated Injection

Albumins, blood serum, metastable technetium-99 labeled.

» Technetium Tc 99m Albumin Aggregated Injection is a sterile, aqueous suspension of Albumin Human that has been denatured to produce aggregates of controlled particle size that are labeled with ^{99m}Tc. It is suitable for intravenous administration. It contains not less than 90.0 percent and not more than 110.0 percent of the labeled amount of ^{99m}Tc as aggregated albumin expressed in megabecquerels (microcuries or millicuries) per mL at the time indicated in the labeling. It may contain antimicrobial, reducing, chelating, and stabilizing agents, buffers, and nonaggregated albumin human. Other chemical forms of radioactivity do not exceed 10 percent of the total radioactivity. Its production and distribution are subject to federal regulations (see *Biologics* ⟨1041⟩ and *Radioactivity* ⟨821⟩).

Packaging and storage—Preserve in single-dose or in multiple-dose containers, at a temperature between 2° and 8°.

Labeling—Label it to include the following, in addition to the information specified for *Labeling* under *Injections* ⟨1⟩: the time and date of calibration; the amount of ^{99m}Tc as aggregated albumin expressed as total megabecquerels (millicuries or microcuries) and concentration as megabecquerels (microcuries or millicuries) per mL at the time of calibration; the expiration date; and the statement "Caution—Radioactive Material." The labeling indicates that in making dosage calculations, correction is to be made for radioactive decay, and also indicates that the radioactive half-life of ^{99m}Tc is 6.0 hours. In addition, the labeling states that it is not to be used if clumping of the albumin is observed and directs that the container be agitated before the contents are withdrawn into a syringe.

USP Reference standards ⟨11⟩—*USP Endotoxin RS*.

Particle size—Shake the Injection well, and determine the dimension of not less than 100 particles of a representative test specimen, using a suitable counting chamber, such as a hemacytometer grid, by optical microscopy. Not less than 90.0% of the observed aggregated particles have a diameter between 10 μm and 90 μm, and none of the observed particles have a diameter greater than 150 μm.

Bacterial endotoxins ⟨85⟩—The limit of endotoxin content is not more than 175/V USP Endotoxin Unit per mL of the Injection, when compared with the USP Endotoxin RS, in which V is the maximum recommended total dose, in mL, at the expiration date or time.

pH ⟨791⟩: between 3.8 and 8.0.

Radiochemical purity—Place a measured volume of Injection, appropriately diluted, such that it provides a count rate of about 20,000 counts per minute, about 25 mm from one end of a 25- × 300-mm strip of chromatographic paper (see *Chromatography* ⟨621⟩). Develop the chromatogram over a period of about 3 to 4 hours by ascending chromatography, using dilute methanol (7 in 10), and air-dry. Determine the radioactivity distribution by scanning the chromatogram with a suitable collimated radiation detector. Not less than 90% of the total radioactivity is found as aggregated albumin (at the point of application).

Place a measured volume of Injection in a centrifuge tube, and determine the net radioactivity in a suitable counting assembly. Centrifuge at approximately 2000 rpm for 5 to 10 minutes. Separate the supernatant by aspiration, and determine its net radioactivity in a suitable counting assembly. Determine the percentage of radioactivity in the supernatant taken by the formula:

$$100(A/B)$$

in which A is the net radioactivity, in counts per minute, in the supernatant aliquot, and B is the total radioactivity, in counts per minute, in the tube prior to centrifugation. Not more than 10.0% of the radioactivity is found in the supernatant, which contains soluble and dispersed radiochemical impurities, following centrifugation.

Protein concentration—

Test preparation—Transfer 2.0 mL of Injection to a suitable centrifuge tube, and centrifuge at about 2000 rpm for 5 to 10 minutes. Decant the supernatant, and add 2.0 mL of Sodium Chloride Injection to wash the centrifuged aggregate. Centrifuge again at 2000 rpm for 5 to 10 minutes, decant the supernatant, and add 2.0 mL of Sodium Chloride Injection.

Standard preparation—To a second test tube add 2.0 mL of a solution containing 2.0 mg of Albumin Human per mL in 0.9 percent sodium chloride solution.

Procedure—To a third test tube add 2.0 mL of Sodium Chloride Injection to provide a blank. To each of the three tubes containing the *Test preparation*, *Standard preparation*, and blank, add 4.0 mL of biuret reagent TS, mix, and allow to stand for 30 minutes, accurately timed, for maximum color development. Additional mixing or slight heating may be required to dissolve the aggregated albumin completely, but the *Test preparation*, *Standard preparation*, and blank are to be treated identically. Determine the absorbances of the solutions from the *Test preparation* and the *Standard preparation* in 1-cm cells at the wavelength of maximum absorbance at about 540 nm, with a suitable spectrophotometer, against the blank. Calculate the quantity, in mg, of aggregated albumin in each mL of the Injection taken by the formula:

$$2(A_U / A_S)$$

in which A_U and A_S are the absorbances of the solutions from the *Test preparation* and the *Standard preparation*, respectively. The protein concentration is not more than 1 mg, as aggregated albumin, per 37 MBq (1 mCi) of Tc 99m at the time of administration.

Biological distribution—Inject intravenously between 0.075 MBq and 0.75 MBq (2 μCi and 20 μCi) of Injection, in a volume not exceeding 0.2 mL, into the caudal vein of each of three 20- to 25-g mice. [NOTE—Other animal species, such as Sprague-Dawley rats (weighing 100 g to 175 g), may be used.] Five to 10 minutes after the injection, sacrifice the animals, and carefully remove the liver and lungs of each by dissection. Place each organ and the remaining carcass in separate, suitable counting containers, and determine the radioactivity, in counts per minute, in each container with an appropriate detector, using the same counting geometry. Determine the percentage of radioactivity in the liver and the lungs taken by the formula:

$$100(A/B)$$

in which A is the net radioactivity, in counts per minute, in the organ, and B is the total radioactivity, in counts per minute, in the lungs, liver, and carcass. Not less than 80.0% of the radioactivity is found in the lungs, and not more than 5.0% of the radioactivity is found in the liver, in not less than two of the animals.

Other requirements—It meets the requirements of the tests for *Radionuclide identification* and *Radionuclidic purity* under *Sodium Pertechnetate Tc 99m Injection*. It meets the requirements under *Injections* ⟨1⟩, except that it may be distributed or dispensed prior to completion of the test for *Sterility*, the latter test being started on the day of final manufacture, and except that it is not subject to the recommendation on *Volume in Container*.

Assay for radioactivity ⟨821⟩—Using a suitable counting assembly (see *Selection of a Counting Assembly*), determine the radioactivity, in MBq (μCi) per mL, of Injection by use of a calibrated system.

Technetium Tc 99m Albumin Colloid Injection

» Technetium Tc 99m Albumin Colloid Injection is a sterile, pyrogen-free, aqueous suspension of Albumin Human that has been denatured to produce colloids of controlled particle size and that are labeled with ^{99m}Tc. It contains not less than 90.0 percent and not more than 110.0 percent of the labeled amount of ^{99m}Tc as albumin colloid complex, expressed in megabecquerels (millicuries) per mL at the time indicated on the labeling. Other chemical forms of radioactivity do not exceed 10.0 percent of the total radioactivity. It may contain suitable reducing agents, buffers, stabilizers, and nonaggregated albumin human. The vials are sealed under a suitable inert atmosphere. Its production and distribution are subject to federal regulations (see *Biologics* ⟨1041⟩ and *Radioactivity* ⟨821⟩).

Packaging and storage—Preserve in single-dose or in multiple-dose containers, at a temperature between 2° and 8°.

Labeling—Label it to include the following, in addition to the information specified for *Labeling* under *Injections* ⟨1⟩: the time and date of calibration; the amount of ^{99m}Tc expressed as total megabecquerels (millicuries) and concentration as megabecquerels (millicuries) per mL at the time of calibration; the expiration date and time and a statement "Caution—Radioactive Material." The labeling indicates that in making dosage calculations, correction is to be made for radioactive decay, and also indicates that the radioactive half-life of ^{99m}Tc is 6.0 hours. In addition, the labeling states that it is not to be used if clumping of the albumin is observed, and directs that the container be agitated before the contents are withdrawn into a syringe.

USP Reference standards ⟨11⟩—*USP Endotoxin RS*.

Bacterial endotoxins ⟨85⟩—The limit of endotoxin content is not more than 175/V USP Endotoxin Unit per mL of the Injection, when compared with the USP Endotoxin RS, in which V is the maximum recommended total dose, in mL, at the expiration date or time.

pH ⟨791⟩: between 7.5 and 8.5.

Radiochemical purity—

A: *Unbound pertechnetate*—Apply a measured volume of Injection, appropriately diluted, such that it provides a count rate of about 20,000 counts per minute, about 10 mm from one end of a thin-layer chromatographic strip impregnated with silica gel (see *Chromatography* ⟨621⟩). Immediately develop the chromatogram over a suitable period by ascending chromatography, using methyl ethyl ketone as the solvent. Allow the chromatogram to dry. Determine the radioactivity distribution of the chromatogram by scanning with a suitable radiation detector. Not more than 10.0% of the total radioactivity is found at the solvent front as unbound pertechnetate.

B: *Soluble ^{99m}Tc species*—

Acetate buffer—Transfer 20.0 mL of 0.2 M acetic acid and 30.0 mL of 0.2 M sodium acetate to a 100-mL volumetric flask, dilute with water to volume, and mix.

Procedure—Transfer 1 mL of the Injection containing about 925 to 1110 MBq (25 to 30 mCi) to a 12-mL centrifuge tube, and add 4 mL of *Acetate buffer*. Determine the radioactivity with a suitable counting assembly. Centrifuge at a force of 34,600 g (gravity) for 15 minutes. Separate the supernatant, and determine its radioactivity. Correct both measurements for decay to the same reference time. Calculate the percentage of soluble ^{99m}Tc species taken by the formula:

$$100(S/I)$$

in which S is the radioactivity of the supernatant, and I is the radioactivity of the specimen before centrifuging. Not more than 10.0% of the total radioactivity is found in the supernatant.

Particle size distribution—

Albumin reagent—Transfer 3.3 g of Poloxamer 188, 56.6 g of dibasic sodium phosphate, and about 800 mL of Water for Injection to a 1-liter volumetric flask, and mix. Add 120 mL of 25% Albumin Human, dilute with Water for Injection to volume, and mix. The pH of the resulting solution is 8.2 ± 0.7. Store at 2° to 8°. Just prior to use, transfer 6.2 mL of this solution, measured at room temperature, to a 100-mL volumetric flask. Dilute with Sodium Chloride Injection to volume, and mix.

Procedure—Inject 0.5 mL of Injection into a 25-mL evacuated or nitrogen-filled vial. Inject 4.5 mL of *Albumin reagent*, and shake. Using a syringe, remove 0.2 mL of the resulting mixture, and attach the syringe by means of a locking-type connection to the top of a 25-mm filter housing assembly consisting of a 5.0-μm polycarbonate membrane filter on top followed by a distance of 3 cm by a 0.1-μm polycarbonate membrane filter. Pass the mixture through the filters, collecting the filtrate in a suitable container. Wash the filters by passing 12 mL of *Albumin reagent* through the filter housing assembly, adding the washing to the first filtrate. Using a suitable ionization chamber, measure the radioactivity in the filtrate and on each filter. Calculate the percentage of radioactivity retained on the 5.0-μm filter taken by the formula:

$$100F/T$$

in which F is the radioactivity on the filter, and T is the total radioactivity of each filter and filtrate: not more than 7.5% of the total radioactivity is retained on the 5.0-μm filter. Calculate the percentage of radioactivity retained on the 0.1-μm filter by the same formula: not less than 82.5% of the total radioactivity is retained, and not more than 10.0% of the total radioactivity passes through the 0.1-μm membrane.

Biological distribution—Inject intravenously between 55.5 and 111 MBq (1.5 and 3.0 mCi) of Injection, in a volume of 0.1 mL, into the caudal vein of each of three 20-g to 40-g mice. Fifteen minutes after injection, sacrifice the animals, and remove the tails, and discard. Carefully remove the liver and lungs of each. Place each organ and the remaining carcass in separate, suitable counting containers, and determine the radioactivity, in MBq (mCi), in each container in a calibrated ionization chamber, using the same counting geometry. Determine the percentage of radioactivity in the liver and the lungs taken by the formula:

$$100(A/B)$$

in which A is the radioactivity, in MBq (mCi), in the organ, and B is the total radioactivity, in MBq (mCi), in the lungs, liver, and carcass. Not less than 80% of the radioactivity is found in the liver and not more than 5% of the radioactivity is found in the lungs, in not less than two of the three mice.

Albumin content—Each container, prior to constitution with Sodium Pertechnetate Tc 99m Injection, contains not less than 0.8 mg and not more than 1.2 mg of aggregated (insoluble) albumin and not less than 8 mg and not more than 12 mg of nonaggregated (soluble) albumin.

Procedure—

Acetate buffer—Transfer 20.0 mL of 0.2 M acetic acid and 30.0 mL of 0.2 M sodium acetate to a 100-mL volumetric flask, dilute with water to volume, and mix. Adjust by the addition, if necessary, of 0.2 M acetic acid or 0.2 M sodium acetate to a pH of 4.9 ± 0.1.

Basic acetate buffer—Transfer 50 mL of 1 N sodium hydroxide to a 500-mL volumetric flask. Dilute with *Acetate buffer* to volume, and mix.

Standard preparation—Using a "To contain" pipet, transfer 2.0 mL of 7 Percent Bovine Serum Albumin Certified Standard (see under *Reagents* in the section *Reagents, Indicators, and Solutions*), to a 250-mL volumetric flask. Rinse the pipet with *Basic acetate buffer* collecting the rinse in the volumetric flask. Dilute with *Basic acetate buffer* to volume, and mix.

Standard solutions—Into 5 separate graduated test tubes pipet 1, 2, 3, 4, and 5 mL of the *Standard preparation*. Dilute the first four with *Basic acetate buffer* to a final volume of 5.0 mL. Pipet 5 mL of Biuret Reagent TS into each tube, and mix. Incubate each at 37 ± 1° for 30 minutes. Allow to cool to room temperature. Determine the absorbances of the solutions in 1-cm cells at the wavelength of maximum absorbance at about 555 nm using a mixture of *Basic acetate buffer* and Biuret Reagent TS (1 : 1) as the blank. Plot the concentration, in mg per mL, versus the absorbance of each *Standard solution* and draw the best straight line through the points to obtain the standard curve.

Test preparation—Constitute the contents of each of 2 containers with 2.0 mL of *Acetate buffer* and allow to stand for 30 minutes. Transfer the contents of both containers to a centrifuge tube rinsing the containers with four 1-mL portions of *Acetate buffer*. Collect all the washings in the same centrifuge tube. Centrifuge the tube for 15 minutes at 4° at a force of 86,400 g (gravity). Quantitatively transfer the supernatant to a 50-mL volumetric flask. Add 5.0 mL of 1 N sodium hydroxide, dilute with *Acetate buffer* to volume, and mix. Pipet 5 mL of this solution into a test tube to obtain the *Soluble albumin test solution*. Dissolve the residue from the centrifugation in 5.0 mL of *Basic acetate buffer* to obtain the *Insoluble albumin test solution*. Treat each solution in the same manner as described under *Standard solutions*, beginning with "Pipet 5 mL of Biuret Reagent TS" and determine the absorbance of each solution as directed for *Standard solutions*. From the observed absorbance of each *Test preparation*, determine the concentration of total albumin from the standard curve. Multiply the concentration obtained for the *Soluble albumin test solution* by 25 to obtain the mg of soluble albumin per container. Multiply the concentration obtained for the *Insoluble albumin test solution* by 2.5 to obtain the mg of insoluble albumin per container.

Other requirements—It meets the requirements of the tests for *Radionuclide identification* and *Radionuclidic purity* under *Sodium Pertechnetate Tc 99m Injection*. It meets also the requirements under *Injections* ⟨1⟩, except that it may be distributed or dispensed prior to completion of the test for *Sterility*, the latter test being started on the date of manufacture, and except that it is not subject to the recommendation on *Volume in Container*.

Assay for radioactivity ⟨821⟩—Using a suitable counting assembly (see *Selection of a Counting Assembly*), determine the radioactivity, in MBq (mCi) per mL, of Technetium Tc 99m Albumin Colloid by the use of a calibrated system.

Technetium Tc 99m Apcitide Injection

» Technetium Tc 99m Apcitide Injection is a sterile aqueous solution for intravenous injection that contains ^{99m}Tc in the form of an apcitide complex. It contains not less than 90.0 percent and not more than 110.0 percent of the labeled amount of ^{99m}Tc as the apcitide complex expressed in megabecquerels per mL (or in millicuries per mL) at the time indicated in the labeling. Other chemical forms of radioactivity do not exceed 10.0 percent of the total radioactivity. It may contain reducing agents, stabilizing agents, and buffers. It contains no antimicrobial agents.

Packaging and storage—Preserve in single-dose containers at controlled room temperature.

Labeling—Label it to include the following, in addition to the information specified for *Labeling* under *Injections* ⟨1⟩: the time and date of calibration; the amount of ^{99m}Tc as labeled apcitide complex expressed as total megabecquerels per mL (or millicuries per mL) at the time of calibration; the expiration date and time; the storage temperature; and the statement "Caution—Radioactive Material". The labeling indicates that in making dosage calculations, correction is to be made for radioactive decay, and also indicates that the radioactive half-life of ^{99m}Tc is 6.0 hours.

USP Reference standards ⟨11⟩—*USP Endotoxin RS.*
Bacterial endotoxins ⟨85⟩: not more than 175/V USP Endotoxin Unit per mL of the Injection, in which V is the maximum recommended total dose, in mL, at the expiration date or time.
pH ⟨791⟩: between 6.0 and 8.0.
Radiochemical purity—Separately apply equal volumes (about 10 µL) of Injection, accurately measured, about 1.0 cm from the bottom of each of two 2-cm × 10-cm instant chromatographic silica gel strips. (Do not allow to dry.) Immediately develop the chromatograms by ascending chromatography (see *Chromatography* ⟨621⟩), until the solvents reach the top of the strips, using saturated sodium chloride solution as the developing solvent for one strip (*Strip 1*) and water for the other strip (*Strip 2*). Remove the strips, and allow to air-dry. Cut *Strip 1* at an R_F value of about 0.75, and separately record the counts for each portion in a dose calibrator. Calculate the percentage of Tc 99m pertechnetate and Tc 99m glucoheptonate (hydrophilic impurities) in the portion of Injection taken by the formula:

$$100C_S / (C_S + P_S)$$

in which C_S is the count obtained from the top portion of *Strip 1*; and P_S is the count obtained from the bottom portion of *Strip 1*. Cut *Strip 2* at an R_F value of about 0.25, and separately record the counts for each portion in a dose calibrator. Calculate the percentage of Tc 99m immobile impurities in the portion of Injection taken by the formula:

$$100P_W / (C_W + P_W)$$

in which P_W is the count obtained from the bottom portion of *Strip 2*; and C_W is the count obtained from the top portion of *Strip 2*: the sum of hydrophilic and immobile impurities is not more than 10%.
Other requirements—It meets the requirements for *Radionuclide identification* and *Radionuclidic purity* under *Sodium Pertechnetate Tc 99m Injection*. It also meets the requirements under *Injections* ⟨1⟩, except that it is not subject to the recommendation on *Volume in Container* and that it may be distributed or dispensed prior to completion of the test for *Sterility*, the latter test being started on the date of manufacture.
Assay for radioactivity ⟨821⟩—Using a suitable counting assembly (see *Selection of a Counting Assembly*), determine the radioactivity, in MBq (or µCi) per mL, of Injection by use of a calibrated system.

Technetium Tc 99m Arcitumomab Injection

» Technetium Tc 99m Arcitumomab Injection is a sterile, nonpyrogenic preparation of the 50,000-dalton Fab′ fragment generated from the murine IgG monoclonal antibody Immu-4, suitable for intravenous administration that is labeled with ^{99m}Tc. It contains not less than 90.0 percent and not more than 110.0 percent of the labeled amount of ^{99m}Tc as an arcitumomab complex, expressed in MBq (or mCi) per mL at the time indicated in the labeling. Other chemical forms of radioactivity do not exceed 10.0 percent of the total radioactivity. The immunoreactive fraction determined by a validated method is not less than 75%. The Fab′ fragment content is not less than 90 percent as determined by size-exclusion HPLC.

Packaging and storage—Preserve in single-dose *Containers for Injections* that are adequately shielded as described under *Injections* ⟨1⟩, and store at controlled room temperature.
Labeling—Label it to include the following, in addition to the information specified for *Labeling* under *Injections* ⟨1⟩: the time and date of calibration; the amount of ^{99m}Tc as labeled arcitumomab expressed as total MBq (or mCi) per mL, at the time of calibration; the expiration date and time; the storage temperature; and the statement "Caution—Radioactive Material". The labeling indicates that, in making dosage calculations, correction is to be made for radioactive decay, and also indicates that the radioactive half-life of ^{99m}Tc is 6.0 hours. The labeling also states that it should be used within 4 hours following constitution.

USP Reference standards ⟨11⟩—*USP Endotoxin RS.*
Bacterial endotoxins ⟨85⟩—The limit of endotoxin content is not more than 175/V USP Endotoxin Unit per mL of the Injection, when compared with the USP Endotoxin RS, in which V is the maximum recommended total dose, in mL, at the expiration date and time.
pH ⟨791⟩: between 5.0 and 7.0.
Radiochemical purity—To determine the amount of free technetium, apply 1 µL of the Injection about 2.7 cm from the bottom of a 1-cm × 9-cm instant thin-layer chromatographic silica gel strip (see *Chromatography* ⟨621⟩). Immediately develop the chromatogram over a period of 4 minutes by ascending chromatography using acetone as the solvent. Allow the chromatogram to air-dry. Determine the radioactivity distribution of the chromatogram by scanning with a suitable radiation detector: not more than 5.0% of the total radioactivity is found at the solvent front as unbound pertechnetate.
Other requirements—It meets the requirements for *Radionuclide identification* and *Radionuclidic purity* under *Sodium Pertechnetate Tc 99m Injection*. It meets also the requirements under *Injections* ⟨1⟩, except that it may be distributed or dispensed prior to completion of the test for *Sterility*, the latter test being started on the date of manufacture.
Assay for radioactivity ⟨821⟩—Using a suitable counting assembly (see *Selection of a Counting Assembly*), determine the radioactivity, in MBq (or mCi) per mL, of Injection by use of a calibrated system.

Technetium Tc 99m Bicisate Injection

» Technetium Tc 99m Bicisate Injection is a sterile, clear, colorless solution, suitable for intravenous administration, of bicisate dihydrochloride complexed to radioactive technetium (^{99m}Tc). It contains not less than 90.0 percent and not more than 110.0 percent of the labeled amount of ^{99m}Tc as a complex with bicisate, expressed in megabecquerels (or in millicuries) per mL at the time indicated in the labeling. Other chemical forms of radioactivity do not exceed 10 percent of the total radioactivity.

Packaging and storage—Preserve in single-dose or multiple-dose containers, at controlled room temperature.
Labeling—Label it to include the following, in addition to the information specified for *Labeling* under *Injections* ⟨1⟩: the time and date of calibration; the amount of ^{99m}Tc as labeled bicisate expressed as total megabecquerels (or millicuries) per mL at the time of calibration; the expiration date and time; the lot number; and the statement "Caution—Radioactive Material." The labeling indicates that in making dosage calculations, correction is to be made for radioactive decay, and also indicates that the radioactive half-life of ^{99m}Tc is 6.0 hours.

USP Reference standards ⟨11⟩—*USP Endotoxin RS.*
Bacterial endotoxins ⟨85⟩—It contains not more than 175/V USP Endotoxin Units per mL, in which V is the maximum recommended total dose, in mL, at the expiration date or time.
Radiochemical purity—Prepare four vials of Injection and perform the test on each vial. Apply about 5 µL of Injection 2 cm from the bottom of a 2.5-cm × 7.5-cm thin-layer chromatographic silica gel sheet. Allow the spot to dry for 5 to 10 minutes. Position the plate in a pre-equilibrated chromatographic chamber containing HPLC grade ethyl acetate, and develop the chromatogram until the solvent front has moved 5 cm from the origin (see *Chromatography* ⟨621⟩). Remove the plate from the chamber, and allow to dry. Cut the chromatographic sheet 4.5 cm from the bottom. Separately count the activity on each piece in a dose calibrator or a gamma counter. The activity on the upper portion contains the ^{99m}Tc bicisate complex, and the activity on the lower section contains all radioimpurities. Calculate the percentage of radiochemical purity of the ^{99m}Tc Bicisate Injection by the formula:

$$100P/(P + C)$$

in which P is the count from the top part of the plate, and C is the count from the bottom part of the plate: not less than 90% of the total radioactivity is found as Tc^{99m} bicisate. Calculate the mean percent radiochemical purity of the four test vials.
Related radiochemical compounds—[NOTE—This test is performed on the same test specimen used to perform the *Radiochemical purity* test. Perform the tests in parallel with a minimal delay in spotting of the chromatographic media following the 30-minute Injection incubation period.] Apply about 2 µL of the Injection 1 cm from the bottom of a 2.5-cm × 7.5-cm reverse-phase thin-layer chromatographic plate (or equivalent), and allow the spot to air-dry thoroughly. Place the plate into a developing tank containing a mixture of acetone and 0.5 M ammonium acetate (60 : 40), develop to 7 cm, remove the plate, and air-dry (see *Chromatography* ⟨621⟩). Using a suitable calibrated scanner, determine the compounds present by calculating the retention factors for all peaks present. Compounds and approximate R_F values are as follows:

^{99m}Tc bicisate	0.15–0.44
^{99m}Tc(IV) bicisate	0.3–0.4
Tc99m Bicisate and Tc ^{99m}(IV) Bicisate	0.15–0.44
Hydrolyzed reduced Tc	0.00–0.14
Free pertechnetate and ^{99m}Tc ethylene cisteinate monomer	0.70–0.84
^{99m}Tc EDTA	0.95–1.0

Calculate the quantity of ^{99m}Tc(IV) ligand in the Injection by subtracting the Tc 99m Bicisate percentage obtained in the test for *Radiochemical purity* from the combined ^{99m}Tc Bicisate and ^{99m}Tc(IV) Bicisate Area percentage obtained in the *Related radiochemical compounds* test. The sum of the impurities is not greater than 10%.
Other requirements—It meets the requirements of the tests for *Radionuclide identification* and *Radionuclidic purity* under *Sodium Pertechnetate Tc 99m Injection*. It meets also the requirements for *Injections* ⟨1⟩, except that the Injection may be distributed or dispensed prior to the completion of the test for *Sterility*, the latter test being started on the day of manufacture.
Assay for radioactivity ⟨821⟩—Using a suitable counting assembly (see *Selection of a Counting Assembly*), determine the radioactivity, in Mbq (or in mCi) per mL, of the Injection by use of a calibrated system.

Technetium Tc 99m Depreotide Injection

» Technetium Tc 99m Depreotide Injection is a sterile, aqueous solution suitable for intravenous injection that contains ^{99m}Tc in the form of a depreotide complex. It contains not less than 90.0 percent and not more than 110.0 percent of the labeled amount of ^{99m}Tc as the depreotide complex expressed in megabecquerels (or in millicuries) per mL at the time indicated in the labeling. It may contain reducing agents, stabilizing agents, and buffers. It contains no antimicrobial agents. Other chemical forms of radioactivity do not exceed 10.0 percent of the total radioactivity.

Packaging and storage—Preserve in single-dose containers, at controlled room temperature.
Labeling—Label it to include the following, in addition to the information specified for *Labeling* under *Injections* ⟨1⟩: the time and date of calibration; the amount of ^{99m}Tc as labeled depreotide complex expressed as total MBq (or mCi) per mL at the time of calibration; the expiration date and time; the storage temperature; and the statement "Caution—Radioactive Material". The labeling indicates that, in making dosage calculations, correction is to be made for radioactive decay, and also indicates that the radioactive half-life of ^{99m}Tc is 6.0 hours.
USP Reference standards ⟨11⟩—*USP Endotoxin RS.*
Bacterial endotoxins ⟨85⟩: not more than 175/V USP Endotoxin Unit per mL of the Injection, in which V is the maximum recommended total dose, in mL, at the expiration date or time.
pH ⟨791⟩: between 6.0 and 8.0.
Radiochemical purity—Separately apply equal volumes (about 10 µL) of Injection, accurately measured, about 1.0 cm from the bottom of each of two 1.5-cm × 10-cm instant chromatographic silica gel strips. Do not allow the plates to dry. Immediately develop the chromatograms by ascending chromatography (see *Chromatography* ⟨621⟩), until the solvents reach the top of the strips, using saturated sodium chloride solution as the developing solvent for one strip (*Strip 1*), and a mixture of methanol and 1 M ammonium acetate (1 : 1) for the other strip (*Strip 2*). Remove the strips, and allow to air-dry. Cut *Strip 1* at an R_F value of about 0.75, and cut *Strip 2* at an R_F value of about 0.40. Separately record the counts for each portion in a dose calibrator. Calculate the percentage of nonmobile impurities in the portion of Injection taken by the formula:

$$100C_M / (C_M + P_M)$$

in which C_M is the count obtained from the bottom portion of *Strip 2*; and P_M is the count obtained from the top portion of *Strip 2*. Calculate the percentage of Tc 99m pertechnetate, Tc 99m glucoheptonate, and Tc 99m edetate in the portion of Injection taken by the formula:

$$100P_S / (C_S + P_S)$$

in which P_S is the count obtained from the top portion of *Strip 1*; and C_S is the count obtained from the bottom portion of *Strip 1*: not more than 10% of total impurities is found.
Other requirements—It meets the requirements for *Radionuclide identification* and *Radionuclidic purity* under *Sodium Pertechnetate Tc 99m Injection*. It also meets the requirements under *Injections* ⟨1⟩, except that the Injection is not subject to the recommendation on *Volume in Container*, and except that it may be distributed or dispensed prior to completion of the test for *Sterility*, the latter test being started on the date of manufacture.
Assay for radioactivity ⟨821⟩—Using a suitable counting assembly, determine the radioactivity, in MBq (or mCi) per mL, of Injection by use of a calibrated system.

Technetium Tc 99m Disofenin Injection

» Technetium Tc 99m Disofenin Injection is a sterile, aqueous solution, suitable for intravenous administration, of disofenin that is labeled with ^{99m}Tc. It contains not less than 90.0 percent and not more than 110.0 percent of the labeled amount of ^{99m}Tc as a disofenin complex, expressed in megabecquerels (microcuries or millicuries) per mL at the time indicated on the labeling. It contains a suitable reducing agent.

Packaging and storage—Preserve in single-dose or in multiple-dose containers sealed under a suitable inert atmosphere.

Labeling—Label it to include the following, in addition to the information specified for *Labeling* under *Injections* ⟨1⟩: the time and date of preparation; the amount of ^{99m}Tc as expressed as total megabecquerels (microcuries or millicuries) and concentration as megabecquerels (microcuries or millicuries) per mL at the time of preparation; the expiration date and time; and a statement "Caution—Radioactive Material." The labeling indicates that in making dosage calculations, correction is to be made for radioactive decay, and also indicates that the radioactive half-life of ^{99m}Tc is 6.0 hours.

pH ⟨791⟩: between 4.0 and 5.0.

Radiochemical purity—The determination of radiochemical purity for this Injection requires the use of two separate chromatography systems.

System A—Apply a measured volume of Injection, appropriately diluted, such that it provides a count rate of about 20,000 counts per minute, about 13 mm from one end of a 10- × 51-mm thin-layer chromatographic strip impregnated with silica gel (see *Chromatography* ⟨621⟩), and immediately develop the chromatogram over a suitable period by ascending chromatography, using methanol as the solvent. Allow the chromatogram to dry. Cut the chromatogram in two along a line about 13 mm from the top. Place the top and bottom strips into separate counting containers. Determine the radioactivity of each, using a suitable ionization chamber. Hydrolyzed Tc 99m and technetium-tin colloid are located at the origin of the bottom strip (R_F 0 to 0.1).

System B—Pretreat a 1.3- × 51-mm strip of chromatographic paper by soaking it for 1 minute in a 0.3 M carbonate-bicarbonate buffer, pH 9.0, prepared by dissolving 0.3 g of anhydrous sodium carbonate and 1.9 g of anhydrous sodium bicarbonate in 100 mL of water. Remove the paper strip, blot lightly with absorbent paper, and dry in an oven for about 45 minutes at 85°. Proceed as directed for *System A* using the pretreated chromatographic paper and a developing solvent of methyl ethyl ketone. Free pertechnetate is located at the solvent front (top strip). The sum of the percentage of radioactivity at the origin in *System A* and the percentage of radioactivity at the solvent front in *System B* is not greater than 10.0%.

Biological distribution—Inject between 75 MBq and 111 MBq (2 mCi and 3 mCi) of Injection, in a volume not exceeding 0.1 mL, into the caudal vein of each of three 25- to 40-g male albino mice. One hour after the injection, anesthetize and then decapitate the animals. Drain the blood of each separately into pre-weighed counting containers. Dissect the animals, and place the kidneys, liver, stomach (exclusive of duodenum), and gallbladder, and intestines, of each mouse into separate counting containers. Using a suitable counting assembly, determine the radioactivity of each container. Correct all radioactivity measurements for decay. Determine the percentage of radioactivity in the kidneys, liver, stomach, and gallbladder and intestines taken by the formula:

$$100(A / B)$$

in which A is the radioactivity, in counts per minute, in the organ, and B is the total radioactivity, in counts per minute, injected. Determine the percentage of radioactivity in the blood taken by the formula:

$$[100(C / W_S)0.07(W_R)] / B$$

in which C is the radioactivity, in counts per minute, in the specimen of blood, W_S is the weight, in g, of the blood specimen, 0.07 is the assumption that the total blood weight of the mouse is 7% of the total body weight, and W_R is the weight, in g, of the mouse. Not less than 70% of the injected radioactivity is present in the gallbladder and intestines, not more than 10.0% of the injected radioactivity is present in the liver, not more than 10.0% of the injected radioactivity is present in the kidneys, not more than 3.0% of the injected radioactivity is present in the stomach, and not more than 3.0% of the injected radioactivity is present in the blood, in not less than two mice.

Other requirements—It meets the requirements of the tests for *Radionuclide identification*, *Radionuclidic purity*, and *Bacterial endotoxins* under *Sodium Pertechnetate Tc 99m Injection*. It also meets the requirements under *Injections* ⟨1⟩, except that it may be distributed or dispensed prior to completion of the test for *Sterility*, the latter test being started on the date of preparation, and except that it is not subject to the recommendation on *Volume in Container*.

Assay for radioactivity ⟨821⟩—Using a suitable counting assembly (see *Selection of a Counting Assembly*), determine the radioactivity, in MBq (μCi or mCi) per mL, of Injection by the use of a calibrated system.

Technetium Tc 99m Etidronate Injection

» Technetium Tc 99m Etidronate Injection is a sterile, clear, colorless solution, suitable for intravenous administration, of radioactive technetium (^{99m}Tc) in the form of a chelate of etidronate sodium. It contains not less than 90.0 percent and not more than 110.0 percent of the labeled amount of ^{99m}Tc as chelate expressed in megabecquerels (microcuries or millicuries) per mL at the time indicated in the labeling. It may contain buffers, preservatives, reducing agents, and stabilizers. Other chemical forms of radioactivity do not exceed 10.0 percent of the total radioactivity.

Packaging and storage—Preserve in single-dose or multiple-dose containers.

Labeling—Label it to include the following, in addition to the information specified for *Labeling* under *Injections* ⟨1⟩: the time and date of calibration; the amount of ^{99m}Tc as labeled etidronate expressed as total megabecquerels (microcuries or millicuries) and concentration as megabecquerels (microcuries or millicuries) per mL at the time of calibration; the expiration date and time; and the statement "Caution—Radioactive Material." The labeling indicates that in making dosage calculations, correction is to be made for radioactive decay, and also indicates that the radioactive half-life of ^{99m}Tc is 6.0 hours.

USP Reference standards ⟨11⟩—*USP Endotoxin RS*.

pH ⟨791⟩: between 2.5 and 7.0.

Other requirements—It meets the requirements for *Bacterial endotoxins*, *Radiochemical purity*, *Biological distribution*, *Other requirements*, and *Assay for radioactivity* under *Technetium Tc 99m Pyrophosphate Injection*.

Technetium Tc 99m Exametazime Injection

2-Butanone, 3,3′-[(2,2-dimethyl-1,3-propanediyl)diimino]bis-dioxime-^{99m}Tc.
d,l-Hexamethylpropylene amine oxime-^{99m}Tc [105613-48-7].

» Technetium Tc 99m Exametazime Injection is a sterile, aqueous solution, suitable for intravenous administration, composed of the primary lipophilic complex of exametazime that is labeled with radioactive ^{99m}Tc. It contains not less than 90.0 percent and not more than 110.0 percent of the labeled amount of ^{99m}Tc as primary lipophilic exametazime complex expressed in megabecquerels (or in microcuries or millicuries) per mL at the date and time indicated in the labeling. It may contain antioxidants, reducing agents, and buffers. A stabilizing solution containing methylene blue and phosphate buffer may be added to the final radio labeled product to extend the expiration time. Other chemical forms of radioactivity (^{99m}Tc pertechnetate, ^{99m}Tc hydrolyzed reduced species, and ^{99m}Tc secondary exametazime complex) do not exceed 20.0 percent of the total radioactivity.

Packaging and storage—Preserve in single-dose or multiple-dose containers, at controlled room temperature.

Labeling—Label it to include the following, in addition to the information specified for *Labeling* under *Injections* ⟨1⟩: the time and date of calibration; the amount of ^{99m}Tc as labeled exametazime expressed as total megabecquerels (or as total microcuries or millicuries) and concentration as megabecquerels (or as microcuries or millicuries) per mL at the time of calibration; the expiration date and time; and a statement, "Caution—Radioactive Material." The labeling indicates that in making dosage calculations, correction is to be made for radioactive decay, and also indicates that the radioactive half-life of ^{99m}Tc is 6.0 hours. [NOTE—The label states that, upon constitution with Sodium Pertechnetate Tc 99m Injection, the beyond-use time is 30 minutes for the unstabilized Injection and between 4 hours and 6 hours for the stabilized Injection.]

USP Reference standards ⟨11⟩—*USP Endotoxin RS.*

pH ⟨791⟩: between 9.0 and 9.8 for unstabilized Injection, and between 6.5 and 7.5 for stabilized Injection.

Radiochemical purity—Prepare three 12- × 75-mm chromatographic tubes by packing with about 0.3 mL of fresh methyl ethyl ketone, 0.9% nonbacteriostatic sodium chloride solution, and a 50% acetonitrile solution, prepared with nonbacteriostatic water, respectively. To each of two 6- × 0.7-cm instant thin-layer chromatographic strips[1] and one 6- × 0.7-cm strip of chromatographic paper,[2] apply 5 μL of freshly prepared (within 2 minutes of reconstitution) Injection about 1 cm from the bottom of the strip. Do not allow to dry. Place one instant thin-layer chromatographic strip into the tube containing methyl ethyl ketone, the second instant thin-layer chromatographic strip into the tube containing the 0.9% sodium chloride solution, and the paper strip into the tube containing the 50% acetonitrile solution. The strips must not adhere to the sides of the tubes. Allow the chromatograms to develop until the solvent front has moved to the top of the strips. Remove the strips from the tubes, and allow the solvents to evaporate. Determine the radioactive distribution by scanning the strip sections, using a suitable collimated radiation detector. The difference between the radioactivity detected at the origin of the 0.9% sodium chloride strip and at the origin of the methyl ethyl ketone strip represents the primary lipophilic ^{99m}Tc exametazime complex. The radioactivity at the solvent front of the 0.9% sodium chloride strip represents the ^{99m}Tc pertechnetate radiochemical impurity. The radioactivity at the origin of the 50% acetonitrile strip represents the ^{99m}Tc hydrolyzed, reduced radiochemical impurity. The difference between the radioactivity detected at the origin of the methyl ethyl ketone strip and the origin of the 50% acetonitrile strip represents the secondary ^{99m}Tc exametazime complex radiochemical impurity. Not less than 80% of the total radioactivity is found as primary lipophilic ^{99m}Tc exametazime complex. [NOTE—Complete the measurement within 30 minutes after constitution of the unstabilized Injection and between 4 hours and 6 hours after constitution of the stabilized Injection.]

Biological distribution—Inject between 18.5 MBq and 37 MBq (between 0.5 mCi and 1 mCi) of Injection in a volume not exceeding 0.1 mL into the caudal vein of each of three 130- to 190-g Sprague-Dawley rats. Five to ten minutes after the injection, sacrifice the animals and carefully remove the brain, liver, and intestines (including gall bladder). Place each organ and the remaining carcass in separate, suitable counting containers, and determine the radioactivity, in counts per minute, in each container with an appropriate detector, using the same counting geometry. Determine the percentage of radioactivity in the brain, liver, intestines, and remaining carcass by the formula:

$$100(A/B)$$

in which A is the net radioactivity, in counts per minute, in the organ, and B is the total radioactivity, in counts per minute in the brain, liver, intestines, and carcass. Not less than 1.5% of the radioactivity is found in the brain. Not more than 20% of the radioactivity is found in the intestines, and not more than 15% of the radioactivity is found in the liver, in not less than two of the animals.

Other requirements—It meets the requirements of the tests for *Radionuclidic identification* and *Radionuclide purity* and *Bacterial endotoxins* under *Sodium Pertechnetate Tc 99m Injection*. It meets also the requirements under *Injections* ⟨1⟩, except that it may be distributed or dispensed prior to completion of the test for *Sterility*, the latter test being started on the day of manufacture, and except that it is not subject to the recommendation on *Volume in Container*.

Assay for radioactivity ⟨821⟩—Using a suitable counting assembly (see *Selection of a Counting Assembly*), determine the radioactivity, in MBq (or μCi) per mL, of Injection by use of a calibrated system.

Technetium ^{99m}Tc Fanolesomab Injection

» Technetium ^{99m}Tc Fanolesomab Injection is a sterile, nonpyrogenic preparation of anti-CD15 antibody, a partially reduced murine IgM monoclonal antibody that is labeled with ^{99m}Tc and is suitable for intravenous administration. It may contain reducing agents, buffers, and stabilizers. It contains no antimicrobial agents. Other chemical forms of radioactivity do not exceed 10 percent of the total radioactivity.

Caution—Components of the commercial kit that are used to prepare the Injection are not to be administered directly to the patient.

Packaging and storage—Preserve in single-dose containers. Store in a refrigerator. [NOTE—After radiolabeling, the Technetium Tc 99m Fanolesomab Injection can be kept at room temperature.]

Labeling—Label it to include the following, in addition to the information specified for *Labeling* under *Injections* ⟨1⟩: the time and date of calibration; the amount of ^{99m}Tc as labeled fanolesomab expressed in MBq (or mCi) per mL at the time of calibration; the expiration date and time; the storage temperature; and the statement "Caution—Radioactive Material". The labeling indicates that the radioactive half-life of ^{99m}Tc is 6.0 hours and that, in making dosage calculations, correction is to be made for radioactive decay. The labeling also states that the Injection is to be used within 6 hours following constitution.

USP Reference standards ⟨11⟩—*USP Endotoxin RS.*

Bacterial endotoxins ⟨85⟩: not more than 0.1 Endotoxin Unit per μg of fanolesomeb in the prepared Injection.

pH ⟨791⟩: between 5.8 and 6.6.

Particulate matter ⟨788⟩—It meets the requirements for particulate matter specified for small-volume injections.

Radiochemical purity—
SYSTEM 1 (*Free pertechnetate ^{99m}Tc*)—
Adsorbent: instant thin-layer chromatography (ITLC) strips,[1] heat-treated at 110° for 30 minutes.
Test solution—Use the Injection.
Application volume—Apply 3 μL of the *Test solution* to the origin.
Developing solvent system: methyl ethyl ketone (MEK).
Procedure—Apply the *Test solution* about 2 cm from the bottom of the *Adsorbent* strip. Immediately develop by ascending chromatography (see *Thin-Layer Chromatography* under *Chromatography*

---

[1] ITLC/SG, 6- × 0.7-cm strip available from Biodex Medical Systems, Shirley, NY.
[2] Whatman Grade 31ET Chr, available from Whatman LabSales, Hillsboro, OR.

[1] ITLC strips for free pertechnetate ^{99m}Tc may be obtained from Sunset Scientific Strips LLC (product number 10503), P.O. Box: 3895, Albuquerque, NM 87190-3895.

⟨621⟩) until the solvent front has moved about 7.5 cm from the origin. The radiochemical impurity, free pertechnetate ^{99m}Tc, migrates to the top section, while colloidal ^{99m}Tc and technetium ^{99m}Tc fanolesomab remains near the origin on the bottom section. Allow the chromatogram to air-dry. Determine the distribution of radioactivity on the chromatogram by cutting the developed strip at 4 cm from the bottom and then separately measuring and recording the net radioactivity in the top and bottom sections using a suitable radiation detector. Calculate the percentage of free pertechnetate ^{99m}Tc in the Injection by the formula:

$$100 A_T / (A_T + A_B)$$

in which A_T is the radioactivity measured on the top section; and A_B is the radioactivity measured on the bottom section.

SYSTEM 2 (Colloidal ^{99m}Tc)—
Adsorbent—Use affinity thin-layer chromatography (ATLC) strips[2] that have been soaked in a solution of 50% newborn calf serum (NBCS)[3] in water and allowed to air-dry overnight.
Test solution—Use the Injection.
Developing solvent system: 4% alcohol in 0.3 M sodium chloride.
Application volume—Prespot the point of origin with 3 µL of Developing solvent system followed immediately by 3 µL of the Test solution.
Procedure—Apply the Test solution about 2 cm from the bottom of the Adsorbent strip. Immediately develop the strip by ascending chromatography (see Thin-Layer Chromatography under Chromatography ⟨621⟩) until the solvent front has moved about 7.5 cm above the origin. The radiochemical impurity, colloidal ^{99m}Tc, will remain at the origin, while free pertechnetate ^{99m}Tc and technetium ^{99m}Tc fanolesomab migrate close to the solvent front. Remove the strip, and allow to air-dry. Cut the strip 4 cm from the bottom, and separately measure and record the background-corrected radioactivity found in the top and bottom sections, using a suitable radiation detector. Calculate the percentage of colloidal ^{99m}Tc by the formula:

$$100 A_B / (A_B + A_T)$$

in which A_B is the radioactivity measured in the bottom section; and A_T is the radioactivity measured in the top section. The sum of the result for free pertechnetate ^{99m}Tc in System 1 and for colloidal ^{99m}Tc measured in System 2 is not more than 10%.

Immunoreactivity—
Adsorbent—Use affinity thin-layer chromatography (ATLC) strips[2] that have been soaked in a solution of 50% newborn calf serum (NBCS)[3] in water and allowed to air-dry overnight.
Diluent—Prepare a mixture of NBCS and pH 7.4 phosphate-buffered saline (PBS) (1 : 1).
Test solution—Use the Injection diluted with Diluent (1 in 4).
REFERENCE MATERIALS—
Positive control: CD15 positive HL-60 (ATCC No. CCL240) formalin fixed-cell suspension (12×10^6 cells per mL).
Negative control: CD15 negative Raji (ATCC No. CCL86) formalin fixed-cell suspension (12×10^6 cells per mL).
Application volume—Thaw, and mix the HL-60 and Raji cell stock suspensions. Dispense 90-µL aliquots into individual incubation tubes. Add 3 µL of the Test solution to each incubation tube, and mix on a vortex mixer for 5 seconds. Incubate for 30 minutes with gentle rocking at 37 ± 2°.
Developing solvent system—Prepare a solution containing 0.05% sodium azide and 4% alcohol in 10 mM phosphate-buffered saline, pH 7.4 (PBS). Pass through a filter having a 0.22-µm porosity.
Procedure—Mix each incubation tube on a vortex mixer. Immediately remove, and apply 10 µL of sample to the origin of the Adsorbent ATLC strip (2 cm from bottom). Allow the sample to adsorb onto the strip, and immediately develop the strip by ascending chromatography (see Thin-Layer Chromatography under Chromatography ⟨621⟩) until the solvent front has moved about 7.5 cm from the origin. Remove the strips, and allow to air-dry. Cut both strips 4 cm above the origin. Separately measure and record the background-corrected radioactivity found on the top and bottom sections of each strip, using a suitable radiation detector. Immunoreactive technetium ^{99m}Tc fanolesomab, bound to the HL-60 cells, remains at the origin, while nonbound forms of ^{99m}Tc migrate away from the origin. Nonspecific binding is measured using the Raji negative control cells. Calculate the specific immunoreactive binding by the formula:

$$[100 A_{B(HL-60)} / (A_{B(HL-60)} + A_{T(HL-60)})] - [100 A_{B(Raji)} / (A_{B(Raji)} + A_{T(Raji)})]$$

in which $A_{B(HL-60)}$ and $A_{B(Raji)}$ are the radioactivity of the HL-60 positive control cells and Raji negative control cells, respectively, measured on the bottom section of each strip; and $A_{T(HL-60)}$ and $A_{T(Raji)}$ are the radioactivity of the HL-60 positive control cells and Raji negative control cells measured on the top section of each strip. A minimum specific immunoreactive binding of 40% is required for the CD15-positive HL-60 cells.

Other requirements—It meets the requirements for Radionuclide identification and Radionuclidic purity under Sodium Pertechnetate Tc 99m Injection. It also meets the requirements under Injections ⟨1⟩, except that it may be distributed or dispensed prior to completion of the test for Sterility, the latter test being started on the date of manufacture.

Assay for radioactivity ⟨821⟩—Using a suitable counting assembly (see Selection of a Counting Assembly), determine the radioactivity, in MBq (or mCi) per mL, of Injection by use of a calibrated system.

Technetium Tc 99m Gluceptate Injection

D-glycero-D-gulo-Heptonic acid, technetium-^{99m}Tc complex.
Technetium-^{99m}Tc D-glycero-D-gulo-heptonate complex.

» Technetium Tc 99m Gluceptate Injection is a sterile, aqueous solution, suitable for intravenous administration, of sodium gluceptate and stannous chloride that is labeled with ^{99m}Tc. It contains not less than 90.0 percent and not more than 110.0 percent of the labeled amount of ^{99m}Tc as stannous gluceptate complex expressed in megabecquerels (microcuries or millicuries) per mL at the time indicated in the labeling. It may contain antimicrobial agents and buffers. Other chemical forms of radioactivity do not exceed 10.0 percent of the total radioactivity.

Packaging and storage—Preserve in single-dose or in multiple-dose containers, at a temperature between 2° and 8°.
Labeling—Label it to include the following, in addition to the information specified for Labeling under Injections ⟨1⟩: the time and date of calibration; the amount of ^{99m}Tc as labeled stannous gluceptate expressed as total megabecquerels (microcuries or millicuries) and concentration as megabecquerels (microcuries or millicuries) per mL at the time of calibration; the expiration date and time; and the statement "Caution—Radioactive Material." The labeling indicates that in making dosage calculations, correction is to be made for radioactive decay, and also indicates that the radioactive half-life of ^{99m}Tc is 6.0 hours.
USP Reference standards ⟨11⟩—USP Endotoxin RS.
Bacterial endotoxins ⟨85⟩—The limit of endotoxin content is not more than 175/V USP Endotoxin Unit per mL of the Injection, when compared with the USP Endotoxin RS, in which V is the maximum recommended total dose, in mL, at the expiration date or time.
pH ⟨791⟩: between 4.0 and 8.0.
Radiochemical purity—Place a measured volume of Injection, appropriately diluted, such that it provides a count rate of about 20,000 counts per minute, about 25 mm from one end of a 25- × 300-mm strip of chromatographic paper (see Chromatography ⟨621⟩), and allow to air-dry. With no delay, develop the chromatogram over a suitable period of time by ascending chromatography, using acetone that has been purged with oxygen-free nitrogen for not less than 10 minutes. Allow the chromatogram to dry, and de-

---
[2] ATLC strips for colloidal ^{99m}Tc may be obtained from Sunset Scientific Strips LLC (product number 10506), P.O. Box: 3895, Albuquerque, NM 87190-3895.
[3] NBCS (heat inactivated) may be obtained from GIBCO/Invitrogen Corp. (catalog number 26010-074), 1600 Faraday Avenue, P.O. Box 6482, Carlsbad, CA 92008

termine the radioactivity distribution by scanning with a suitable collimated radiation detector. Not less than 90.0% of the total radioactivity is found as stannous gluceptate (at the point of application).

Biological distribution—Constitute 1 vial of Injection with 5 mL to 10 mL of Sodium Pertechnetate Tc 99m Injection. Inject intravenously 0.25 mL of the resulting undiluted Injection into the caudal vein of each of three 150- to 250-g rats. Discard any injections in which extravasation occurs. Approximately 1 hour after the injection, anesthetize the animals and exsanguinate, collecting the blood into a suitable container. Dissect the animals, and place the kidneys, liver, gastrointestinal tract, and a specimen of blood, accurately weighed, in separate, suitable counting containers, and determine the radioactivity, in counts per minute, in each container with an appropriate detector using the same counting geometry. Determine the percentage of radioactivity in the kidneys, liver, and gastrointestinal tract taken by the formula:

$$100A_i / A$$

in which A_i is the net radioactivity in the organ, and A is the total radioactivity, in MBq (µCi), injected, both corrected to injection time. Determine the percentage of radioactivity in the blood taken by the formula:

$$[100(B/W_S)0.07(W_R)]/A$$

in which B is the net radioactivity in the specimen of blood, and A is the total radioactivity, injected, both corrected to injection time, W_S is the weight, in g, of the blood specimen, W_R is the weight, in g, of the rat, and 0.07 is the assumption that the total blood weight of the rat is 7% of the total body weight. Not less than 15.0% of the radioactivity is found in the kidneys, not more than 5.0% of the radioactivity is found in the blood, not more than 15.0% of the radioactivity is found in the entire gastrointestinal tract and not more than 5.0% of the radioactivity is found in the liver, in not fewer than 2 of the rats.

Other requirements—It meets the requirements for *Radionuclide identification* and *Radionuclidic purity* under *Sodium Pertechnetate Tc 99m Injection*. It meets also the requirements under *Injections* ⟨1⟩, except that it may be distributed or dispensed prior to completion of the test for *Sterility*, the latter test being started on the date of manufacture, and except that it is not subject to the recommendation on *Volume in Container*.

Assay for radioactivity ⟨821⟩—Using a suitable counting assembly (see *Selection of a Counting Assembly*), determine the radioactivity, in MBq (µCi) per mL, of Technetium Tc 99m Gluceptate Injection by use of a calibrated system.

Technetium Tc 99m Lidofenin Injection

» Technetium Tc 99m Lidofenin Injection is a sterile, clear, colorless solution of lidofenin complexed to radioactive technetium (^{99m}Tc) in the form of a chelate. It is suitable for intravenous injection and may contain buffers. It contains not less than 90.0 percent and not more than 110.0 percent of the labeled amount of ^{99m}Tc as the lidofenin chelate expressed in megabecquerels (millicuries) per mL at the time indicated in the labeling. Other chemical forms of radioactivity do not exceed 10.0 percent of the total radioactivity.

Packaging and storage—Preserve in single-dose or multiple-dose containers at a temperature between 2° and 8°.

Labeling—Label it to include the following, in addition to the information specified for *Labeling* under *Injections* ⟨1⟩: the time and date of calibration; the amount of ^{99m}Tc as labeled lidofenin expressed as total megabecquerels (millicuries) per mL at the time of calibration; the expiration date and time; the storage temperature and the statement "Caution—Radioactive Material." The labeling indicates that, in making dosage calculations, correction is to be made for radioactive decay, and also indicates that the radioactive half-life of ^{99m}Tc is 6.0 hours.

USP Reference standards ⟨11⟩—*USP Endotoxin RS.*

Bacterial endotoxins ⟨85⟩—The limit of endotoxin content is not more than 175/V Endotoxin Units per mL of Injection, in which V is the maximum recommended total dose, in mL, at the expiration date or time.

pH ⟨791⟩: between 3.5 and 5.0.

Radiochemical purity—Not more than 10.0 percent of the total radioactivity is found as free ^{99m}Tc pertechnetate (TcO$_4$), hydrolysed ^{99m}Tc and ^{99m}Tc technetium tin colloid. The presence of these impurities is determined as follows:

Unbound pertechnetate—Apply a measured volume of Injection such that it provides a count rate of about 50,000 counts per minute, about 15 mm from the end of a 100-mm × 10-mm strip of silicic-acid impregnated fiberglass paper. Dry the spot using a gentle stream of nitrogen and develop immediately using a nitrogen-purged saturated solution of sodium chloride until the solvent front has moved four-fifths of the length of the strip. Determine the distribution of radioactivity on the strip by the use of a strip-scanner or other suitable method. Unbound pertechnetate is found at an R_F value between 0.5 and 1.0. Technetium Lidofenin, hydrolysed and colloidal ^{99m}Tc technetium remain at the origin.

Hydrolysed and *reduced* ^{99m}Tc *technetium*—Apply a measured volume of Injection such that it provides a count rate of about 50,000 counts per minute, about 15 mm from the end of a 100-mm × 10-mm strip of silica gel impregnated fiberglass paper. Dry the spot using a gentle stream of nitrogen and develop immediately using a solution consisting of a mixture of acetonitrile and water (3 : 1) until the solvent front has moved four-fifths of the length of the strip. Determine the distribution of radioactivity on the strip by the use of a strip-scanner or other suitable method. Unbound pertechnetate and Technetium Lidofenin are found at an R_F value between 0.5 and 1.0. Hydrolysed and colloidal ^{99m}Tc technetium remain at the origin.

Biological distribution—Inject intravenously between 0.75 and 1.85 MBq (20 µCi and 50 µCi) of the Injection into the lateral tail vein of each of three 20-g to 25-g mice. Maintain the injected animals in clean cages with free access to food and water for 1 hour. Sacrifice the animals by carbon dioxide or ether asphyxiation and withdraw approximately 1 mL of blood. Dissect the animals and remove the liver, gallbladder, and small and large intestines. Remove the tail. Weigh the blood sample. Place the blood sample, organs, and tail in separate counting tubes and determine the activity in each. Correct for decay to the time of injection. Determine the percentage of radioactivity in each organ and blood using the formula:

$$100B/A$$

in which B is the net radioactivity in the organ, and A is the total radioactivity injected. Assume that the total blood weight is 7.0% of total body weight. If more than 5% of the injected dose is found in the tail, disregard the results from that animal. If more than one animal is rejected on this basis, repeat the entire test with three more animals. Not less than 65% of the total radioactivity is found in the gallbladder and intestines, not more than 10% of the total radioactivity is found in the liver and not more than 2% of the total radioactivity is found in the blood in two out of three mice.

Other requirements—It meets the requirements of the tests for *Radionuclide identification* and *Radionuclide purity* under *Sodium Pertechnetate Tc 99m Injection*. It meets the requirements under *Injections* ⟨1⟩, except that it may be distributed or dispensed prior to completion of the test for *Sterility*, the latter test being started on the day of manufacture, and except that it is not subject to the recommendation on *Volume in Container*.

Assay for radioactivity ⟨821⟩—Using a suitable counting assembly (see *Selection of a Counting Assembly*), determine the radioactivity in MBq(µCi) per mL, of Injection by use of a calibrated system.

Technetium Tc 99m Mebrofenin Injection

» Technetium Tc 99m Mebrofenin Injection is a sterile aqueous solution of Stannous Fluoride and Mebrofenin labeled with radioactive technetium Tc 99m suitable for intravenous administration. It contains not less than 90.0 percent and not more than 110.0 percent of the labeled amount of ^{99m}Tc, as the complex with mebrofenin, expressed in megabecquerels (or in millicuries) per mL at the time indicated in the labeling. It may contain antimicrobial agents and buffers. Other chemical forms of radioactivity do not exceed 10.0 percent of the total radioactivity.

Packaging and storage—Preserve in single-dose or in multiple-dose containers, at controlled room temperature.

Labeling—Label it to include the following, in addition to the information specified for *Labeling* under *Injections* ⟨1⟩: the time and date of calibration; the amount of ^{99m}Tc as labeled mebrofenin expressed as total megabecquerels (or millicuries) and the concentration as megabecquerels per mL (or as millicuries per mL) on the date and time of calibration; the expiration date and time; and the statement, "Caution—Radioactive Material." The labeling indicates that in making dosage calculations, correction is to be made for radioactive decay, and also indicates that the radioactive half-life of ^{99m}Tc is 6.0 hours.

USP Reference standards ⟨11⟩—*USP Endotoxin RS*.

pH ⟨791⟩: between 4.2 and 5.7.

Radiochemical purity—[NOTE—The determination of radiochemical purity for this product requires the use of two separate chromatographic methods.]

Method 1—

pH 6.8 PHOSPHATE BUFFER—Mix 64 mL of 0.2 M monobasic sodium phosphate and 61 mL of 0.1 M dibasic sodium phosphate in a 1-liter volumetric flask, dilute with water to volume, and mix.

MOBILE PHASE—Prepare a filtered and degassed mixture of methanol and *pH 6.8 phosphate buffer* (625 : 375). Make adjustments if necessary (see *System Suitability* under *Chromatography* ⟨621⟩).

CHROMATOGRAPHIC SYSTEM (see *Chromatography* ⟨621⟩)—The liquid chromatograph is equipped with a 3.9-mm × 30-cm column that contains 10-µm packing L1. It is also equipped with a flow-through gamma ray detector having a cell volume of about 10 µL. A constant flow rate of about 1 mL per minute is maintained, and counts are recorded and charted at about 5-second intervals.

PROCEDURE—Constitute the Injection, and allow to stand for 15 minutes. Chromatograph a volume of Injection, with activity of 0.6 to 15 MBq (16 to 400 µCi), and record the chromatogram. The resolution between the secondary characteristic peak, eluting at about 3.5 minutes, and the principal peak, eluting at about 6 minutes, is not less than 1.5. The time interval between the elution of the Tc 99m pertechnetate peak, at about 2 minutes, and the principal peak is not less than 3.0 minutes. If the foregoing criteria are met, record the counts for the pertechnetate Tc 99m peak, the two complex peaks, a representative baseline segment, and the total counts for the chromatogram. Calculate the percentage of complexed radioactivity in the two characteristic peaks taken by the formula:

$$100C/(T - P)$$

in which *C* is the count of the complex peak of interest, *T* is the total count, and *P* is the pertechnetate peak count, each being corrected for the corresponding baseline count. The complexed radioactivity is not less than 90.0% in the principal peak and between 1% and 6% in the second characteristic peak. Calculate the percentage of all other complexed radioactivity (this excludes the main, secondary, and free pertechnetate peaks) taken by the formula:

$$100K/(T - P)$$

in which *K* is the sum of all other peaks, and *T* and *P* are as defined above. Record the result for use in the calculation as directed under *Method 2*.

Method 2—

CHROMATOGRAPHIC SYSTEM A (see *Chromatography* ⟨621⟩)—Prepare a 1.0- × 12.5-cm silicic acid-impregnated glass microfiber strip by dipping it in a 10% sodium chloride solution and removing the excess liquid by blotting. Dry the strip by heating in an oven at about 80°. Apply about 5 µL of the Injection with activity of about 3.7 MBq (100 µCi) about 1.5 cm from one end of the strip, and immediately develop the chromatogram in a chromatographic chamber containing saturated sodium chloride solution until the solvent front reaches a level about 1 cm from the top of the strip. Remove the strip from the chamber, and allow to air-dry. Separate the top and bottom portions of the chromatogram by cutting the strip in half, and record the counts separately for each portion. Calculate the percentage of unreduced pertechnetate taken by the formula:

$$100P/(P + C)$$

in which *P* is the count from the top half of the strip, and *C* is the count from the bottom half of the strip.

CHROMATOGRAPHIC SYSTEM B—Proceed as directed under *Chromatographic system A* except to use a 1.0- × 12.5-cm silica gel-impregnated glass microfiber strip, without preliminary treatment, and a mixture of acetonitrile and water (3 : 1) as the developing solvent. Calculate the percentage of reduced hydrolyzed Tc 99m taken by the formula:

$$100R/(R + D)$$

in which *R* is the count from the bottom half of the strip, and *D* is the count from the top half of the strip. The sum of the percentage of unreduced pertechnetate from *System A*, the percentage of reduced hydrolyzed Tc 99m from *System B*, and the percentage of other complexed radioactivity determined from *Method 1* is not greater than 10.0%.

Biological distribution—Inject 0.25 mL of Injection containing between 15 and 19 MBq (0.4 and 0.5 mCi) into the external jugular vein of each of three anesthetized male rats weighing between 150 and 350 g, and from which food has been withheld for 15 to 24 hours prior to the test. Thirty minutes after the injection, sacrifice the animals and carefully remove the liver, kidneys, and gastrointestinal tract of each rat. Place the organs in separate counting containers. Using a suitable counting assembly, determine the radioactivity in each container. Correct radioactivity measurements for decay. Determine the percentages of radioactivity in the liver, kidneys, and gastrointestinal tract taken by the formula:

$$100(A/B)$$

in which *A* is the radioactivity, in counts per minute, in the organ, and *B* is the average injected radioactivity, in counts per minute, in the corresponding standards. Not less than 75% of the injected radioactivity is found in the gastrointestinal tract, not more than 10% in the liver, and not more than 5% in the kidneys in not less than 2 of the rats.

Other requirements—It meets the requirements of the tests for *Radionuclide identification*, *Radionuclidic purity*, and *Bacterial endotoxins* under *Sodium Pertechnetate Tc 99m Injection*. It also meets the requirements for *Injections* ⟨1⟩, except that it may be distributed and dispensed prior to the completion of the test for *Sterility*, the latter being started on the day of manufacture, and except that it is not subject to the recommendation on *Volume in Container*.

Assay for radioactivity 821—Using a suitable counting assembly (see *Selection of a Counting Assembly*), determine the radioactivity, in MBq (or in mCi) per mL, of Injection by use of a calibrated system.

Technetium Tc 99m Medronate Injection

» Technetium Tc 99m Medronate Injection is a sterile, aqueous solution, suitable for intravenous administration, of sodium medronate and stannous chloride or stannous fluoride that is labeled with radioactive Tc 99m. It contains not less than 90.0 percent and not more than 110.0 percent of the labeled amount of Tc 99m as stannous medronate complex expressed in megabecquerels (microcuries or millicuries) per mL at the date and time indicated in the labeling. It may contain antimicrobial agents, antioxidants, and buffers. Other chemical forms of radioactivity do not exceed 10.0 percent of the total radioactivity.

Packaging and storage—Preserve in single-dose or multiple-dose containers at a temperature specified in the labeling.

USP Reference standards ⟨11⟩—*USP Endotoxin RS*.

Bacterial endotoxins ⟨85⟩—The limit of endotoxin content is not more than $175/V$ USP Endotoxin Unit per mL of the Injection, when compared with the USP Endotoxin RS, in which V is the maximum recommended total dose, in mL, at the expiration date or time.

pH ⟨791⟩: between 4.0 and 7.8.

Radiochemical purity—Not more than 10.0% of unbound Tc 99m (free pertechnetate), hydrolyzed Tc 99m, and technetium-tin colloid is present, determined as follows.

System A—Under an atmosphere of nitrogen, place a measured volume of Injection, such that it provides a count rate of about 20,000 counts per minute, about 25 mm from one end of a paper chromatographic strip (see *Chromatography* ⟨621⟩). Immediately develop the chromatogram over a suitable period by ascending chromatography, using sodium chloride solution (0.9 in 100), and dry it under nitrogen. Determine the radioactivity distribution by scanning the chromatogram with a suitable collimated radiation detector. Hydrolyzed Tc 99m and technetium-tin colloid are located at the origin (R_F 0 to 0.1).

System B—Proceed as directed for *System A*, except to develop the chromatogram in dilute methanol (85 in 100). Free pertechnetate is located at an R_F of 0.6 to 0.8. The sum of the percentage of radioactivity at the origin in *System A* plus the percentage of radioactivity at an R_F of 0.6 to 0.8 in *System B* is not greater than 10.0%.

Other requirements—It meets the requirements of the tests for *Radionuclide identification* and *Radionuclidic purity* under *Sodium Pertechnetate Tc 99m Injection*, and meets the requirements for *Labeling*, *Biological distribution*, and *Assay for radioactivity* under *Technetium Tc 99m Pyrophosphate Injection*. It meets also the requirements under *Injections* ⟨1⟩, except that it may be distributed or dispensed prior to completion of the test for *Sterility*, the latter test being started on the day of manufacture, and except that it is not subject to the recommendation on *Volume in Container*.

Technetium Tc 99m Mertiatide Injection

$C_8H_8N_3Na_2O_6S^{99m}Tc$

Technetate(2-)-^{99m}Tc,[*N*-[*N*-[*N*-(mercaptoacetyl)-glycyl]glycyl] glycinato(5-)-*N,N′,N″,S*]-oxo-, disodium, (*SP*-5-25)-.

Disodium [*N*-[*N*-[*N*-(mercaptoacetyl)glycyl]glycyl]glycinato(5-)-*N,N′,N″,S*]-oxo[^{99m}Tc]technetate(V)   [125224-05-7].

» Technetium Tc 99m Mertiatide Injection is a sterile aqueous solution, suitable for intravenous injection, that contains ^{99m}Tc in the form of a chelate of mertiatide. It contains not less than 90.0 percent and not more than 110.0 percent of the labeled amount of ^{99m}Tc as mertiatide complex expressed in megabecquerels (or in microcuries or millicuries) per mL at the date and time indicated in the labeling. It contains uncomplexed betiatide, a suitable ^{99m}Tc reducing agent, a transfer ligand, and stabilizers.

Packaging and storage—Preserve in single-dose or multiple-dose containers.

Labeling—Label it to include the following, in addition to the information specified for *Labeling* under *Injections* ⟨1⟩: the time and date of calibration; the amount of ^{99m}Tc as labeled mertiatide expressed as total megabecquerels (or millicuries) and the concentration as megabecquerels per mL (or as millicuries per mL) on the date and time of calibration; the expiration date and time; and a statement, "Caution—Radioactive Material." The labeling indicates that in making dosage calculations, correction is to be made for radioactive decay, and also indicates that the radioactive half-life of ^{99m}Tc is 6.0 hours.

USP Reference standards ⟨11⟩—*USP Endotoxin RS*.

Bacterial endotoxins ⟨85⟩—It contains not more than $175/V$ USP Endotoxin Unit per mL, in which V is the maximum recommended total dose, in mL, at the expiration date or time.

pH ⟨791⟩: between 5.0 and 6.0.

Radiochemical purity—

Method 1 (Determination of hydrolyzed reduced technetium)—Apply about 5 to 10 µL (100 to 250 µCi) 15 mm from the bottom of a 25-mm × 20-cm strip of chromatographic paper (see *Chromatography* ⟨621⟩). Immediately develop the chromatogram by ascending chromatography using a solvent system consisting of a mixture of acetonitrile and water (60 : 40) until the solvent front has moved about 13 cm from the origin. Remove the strip, and allow to dry. Determine the radioactivity distribution by scanning the chromatogram using a suitable collimated radiation detector. Calculate the percentage of hydrolyzed reduced technetium by the formula:

$$100(A_{ht} / B_s)$$

in which A_{ht} is the sum of all the peaks at or near the origin, where R_F is less than 0.25, and B_s is the sum of all of the peaks: not more than 2.0% of hydrolyzed reduced technetium is found.

Method 2 (Simultaneous determination of free pertechnetate and ^{99m}Tc mertiatide)—

SOLUTION A—Prepare a filtered and degassed solution of monobasic potassium phosphate in water to obtain a solution containing 1.36 mg per mL. To each L of this solution, add 1.0 mL of triethylamine, and adjust with 1.0 N hydrochloric acid to a pH of between 4.9 and 5.1. Make adjustments if necessary (see *System Suitability* under *Chromatography* ⟨621⟩).

SOLUTION B—Prepare a filtered and degassed solution of monobasic potassium phosphate in 900 mL of water, and add 100 mL of tetrahydrofuran to obtain a solution containing 1.36 mg per mL. To each L of this solution, add 1.0 mL of triethylamine, and adjust with 1.0 N hydrochloric acid to a pH of between 4.9 and 5.1. Make adjustments if necessary (see *System Suitability* under *Chromatography* ⟨621⟩).

MOBILE PHASE—Mix specified portions of freshly prepared and degassed *Solution A* and *Solution B*.

TEST SOLUTION—Immediately before testing, dilute a portion of the Injection with *Water for Injection* to obtain a concentration of between 400 to 600 µCi. [NOTE—The extent to which the sample is diluted is determined by the sensitivity of the radiometric detector.]

CHROMATOGRAPHIC SYSTEM (see *Chromatography* ⟨621⟩)—The liquid chromatograph is equipped with a 3.9-mm × 15-cm column that contains packing L1 and a flow-through gamma-ray detector and is programmed to provide a *Mobile phase* consisting of variable mixtures of *Solution A* and *Solution B*. The system is equilibrated for 15 minutes with a *Mobile phase* consisting of a mixture of 90% *Solution A* and 10% *Solution B*. After injecting the *Test solution*, change the composition of the *Mobile phase* linearly over the next 30 minutes so that the final *Mobile phase* composition consists of 20% *Solution A* and 80% *Solution B*. Hold with this composition for 5 minutes and then change in reverse to a composition of 90% *Solution A* and 10% *Solution B* over a 5-minute period. The flow rate is about 1 mL per minute.

PROCEDURE—Inject about 20 µL of the *Test solution* into the chromatograph, record the chromatograms by gradient elution (see the *Chromatographic system*). The retention time is between 1.8 and 2.2 minutes for ^{99m}Tc pertechnetate and between 10 and 14 minutes for ^{99m}Tc mertiatide. Calculate the percentage of ^{99m}Tc pertechnetate by the formula:

$$100(r_{pt}/r_s)$$

in which r_{pt} is the peak response of ^{99m}Tc pertechnetate, and r_s is the sum of all peak responses: not more than 6.0% of ^{99m}Tc pertechnetate is found.

Calculate the percentage of ^{99m}Tc mertiatide by the formula:

$$100(r_{mt}/r_s')$$

in which r_{mt} is the peak response of ^{99m}Tc mertiatide, and r_s' is the sum of all peak responses: not less than 90.0% of ^{99m}Tc mertiatide is found.

Other requirements—It meets the requirements of the tests for *Radionuclide identification* and *Radionuclidic purity* under *Sodium Pertechnetate Tc 99m Injection*. It also meets the requirement under *Injections* ⟨1⟩, except that it may be distributed or dispensed prior to completion of the test for *Sterility* ⟨71⟩, the latter test being started on the day of final manufacture, and except that it is not subject to the recommendation on *Volume in Container*.

Assay for radioactivity ⟨821⟩—Using a suitable counting assembly, determine the radioactivity, in Mbq (or millicuries) per mL, of the Injection by use of a calibrated system.

Technetium Tc 99m Nofetumomab Merpentan Injection

» Technetium Tc 99m Nofetumomab Merpentan Injection is a sterile, nonpyrogenic preparation of the Fab fragment of IgG2b murine monoclonal antibody NR-LU-10 that is labeled with ^{99m}Tc and is suitable for intravenous administration. It contains not less than 90.0 percent and not more than 110.0 percent of the labeled amount of ^{99m}Tc as the nofetumomab complex, expressed in megabecquerels (or millicuries) per mL at the time indicated in the labeling. It may contain reducing agents, buffers, and stabilizers. It contains no antimicrobial agents. Other chemical forms of radioactivity do not exceed 10 percent of the total radioactivity. The immunoreactive fraction, as determined by a validated method, is not less than 85 percent.

Caution—Components of the commercial kit that are used to prepare the Injection are not to be administered directly to the patient.

Packaging and storage—Preserve in single-dose containers.

Labeling—Label it to include the following, in addition to the information specified for *Labeling* under *Injections* ⟨1⟩: the time and date of calibration; the amount of ^{99m}Tc as labeled nofetumomab merpentan expressed in MBq (or mCi) per mL at the time of calibration; the expiration date and time; the storage temperature; and the statement "Caution—Radioactive Material". The labeling indicates that the radioactive half-life of ^{99m}Tc is 6.0 hours and that, in making dosage calculations, correction is to be made for radioactive decay. The labeling also states that the Injection is to be used within 6 hours following constitution.

USP Reference standards ⟨11⟩—*USP Endotoxin RS*.

Bacterial endotoxins ⟨85⟩: not more than 175/*V* USP Endotoxin Unit per mL of the Injection, in which *V* is the maximum recommended total dose, in mL, at the expiration date or time.

pH ⟨791⟩: between 7.0 and 8.0.

Radiochemical purity—

  Adsorbent: 1- × 10-cm instant silica gel strip.
  Test solution—Use the Injection.
  Application volume: 2 to 5 µL.
  Developing solvent system: 0.73 N trichloroacetic acid.
  Procedure—Apply the *Test solution* about 1.2 cm from the bottom of the silica gel strip. Immediately develop the chromatogram by ascending chromatography (see *Chromatography* ⟨621⟩) until the solvent front has moved 8 cm from the origin. Allow the chromatogram to air-dry. Determine the distribution of radioactivity on the chromatogram by scanning with a suitable collimated radiation detector. Technetium Tc 99m nofetumomab merpentan remains at the origin, and nonprotein bound Tc 99m labeled material travels with the solvent front. Not more than 5.0% of the total radioactivity is present as a band between R_F values of 0.4 and 0.7; and not less than 85% of the total radioactivity is found as ^{99m}Tc at the origin.

Other requirements—It meets the requirements for *Radionuclide identification* and *Radionuclidic purity* under *Sodium Pertechnetate Tc 99m Injection*. It also meets the requirements under *Injections* ⟨1⟩, except that it may be distributed or dispensed prior to completion of the test for *Sterility*, the latter test being started on the date of manufacture.

Assay for radioactivity ⟨821⟩—Using a suitable counting assembly (see *Selection of a Counting Assembly*), determine the radioactivity, in MBq (or µCi) per mL, of Injection by use of a calibrated system.

Technetium Tc 99m Oxidronate Injection

» Technetium Tc 99m Oxidronate Injection is a sterile, clear, colorless solution, suitable for intravenous administration, of radioactive technetium (^{99m}Tc) in the form of a chelate of oxidronate sodium. It contains not less than 90.0 percent and not more than 110.0 percent of the labeled amount of ^{99m}Tc as chelate expressed in megabecquerels (microcuries or millicuries) per mL at the time indicated in the labeling. It may contain buffers, preservatives, reducing agents, and stabilizers. Other chemical forms of radioactivity do not exceed 10.0 percent of the total radioactivity.

Packaging and storage—Preserve in single-dose or multiple-dose containers.

Labeling—Label it to include the following, in addition to the information specified for *Labeling* under *Injections* ⟨1⟩: the time and date of calibration; the amount of ^{99m}Tc as labeled oxidronate expressed as total megabecquerels (microcuries or millicuries) and concentration as megabecquerels (microcuries or millicuries) per mL at the time of calibration; the expiration date and time; and the statement "Caution—Radioactive Material." The labeling indicates that in making dosage calculations, correction is to be made for radioactive decay, and also indicates that the radioactive half-life of ^{99m}Tc is 6.0 hours.

USP Reference standards ⟨11⟩—*USP Endotoxin RS.*
pH ⟨791⟩: between 2.5 and 7.0.
Other requirements—It meets the requirements for *Bacterial endotoxins, Radiochemical purity, Biological distribution, Other requirements,* and *Assay for radioactivity* under *Technetium Tc 99m Pyrophosphate Injection.*

Technetium Tc 99m Pentetate Injection

$C_{14}H_{18}N_3NaO_{10}{}^{99m}Tc$
Technetate(1-)^{99m}Tc, [*N,N*-bis[2-[bis(carboxymethyl)amino]ethyl]glycinato(5-)]-, sodium.
Sodium [*N,N*-bis[2-[bis(carboxymethyl)amino]ethyl]glycinato(5-)]-technetate(1-)-^{99m}Tc [65454-61-7].

» Technetium Tc 99m Pentetate Injection is a sterile solution of pentetic acid that is complexed with ^{99m}Tc in Sodium Chloride Injection. It is suitable for intravenous administration and may contain buffers. It contains not less than 90.0 percent and not more than 110.0 percent of the labeled amount of ^{99m}Tc as the pentetic acid complex expressed in megabecquerels (microcuries or millicuries) per mL at the time indicated in the labeling. Other chemical forms of radioactivity do not exceed 10.0 percent of the total radioactivity.

Packaging and storage—Preserve in single-dose or in multiple-dose containers, at a temperature between 2° and 8°.
Labeling—Label it to include the following, in addition to the information specified for *Labeling* under *Injections* ⟨1⟩: the time and date of calibration; the amount of ^{99m}Tc as labeled pentetic acid complex expressed as total megabecquerels (millicuries or microcuries) and concentration as megabecquerels (microcuries or millicuries) per mL at the time of calibration; the expiration date; and the statement "Caution—Radioactive Material." The labeling indicates that in making dosage calculations, correction is to be made for radioactive decay and also indicates that the radioactive half-life of ^{99m}Tc is 6.0 hours.
USP Reference standards ⟨11⟩—*USP Endotoxin RS.*
Bacterial endotoxins ⟨85⟩—The limit of endotoxin content is not more than 175/*V* USP Endotoxin Unit per mL of the Injection, when compared with the USP Endotoxin RS, in which *V* is the maximum recommended total dose, in mL, at the expiration date or time.
pH ⟨791⟩: between 3.8 and 7.5.
Radiochemical purity—
  Phosphate buffer—Dissolve 2.6 g of monobasic sodium phosphate and 3.0 g of anhydrous dibasic sodium phosphate in water to make 1000 mL. Adjust, if necessary, by the addition of 0.2 M phosphoric acid or 0.2 M sodium hydroxide, to a pH of 6.8 ± 0.05.
  Procedure (see *Electrophoresis* ⟨726⟩)—Soak a 2.5- × 17.0-cm cellulose polyacetate strip in 100 mL of *Phosphate buffer* for 10 to 60 minutes. Remove the strip with forceps, taking care to handle the outer edges only. Place the strip between two absorbent pads, and blot to remove excess solution. Attach the strip to the support bridge of an electrophoresis chamber containing *Phosphate buffer* in each side of the chamber. Ensure that each end of the strip is in contact with *Phosphate buffer*. Mark the application line near the cathode end of the strip. Apply as a spot 1 µL of a 1 in 1000 solution of amaranth in *Phosphate buffer*. Adjacent to this, apply as a narrow streak 5 µL of Injection having an activity of about 1 mCi per mL, previously diluted with saline TS, if necessary. Attach the chamber cover, and perform the electrophoresis at 300 volts until the amaranth (red dye) has moved about four-fifths of the length of the strip. Remove the strip from the chamber, and blot the ends on paper towels. Using a suitable scanner and counting assembly, determine the radioactivity distribution. Labeled technetium pentetate migrates a distance that is 0.9 relative to that of amaranth. Hydrolyzed technetium Tc 99m is located at the origin and pertechnetate migrates a distance that is 0.7 relative to that of amaranth: the sum of the percentages of radioactivity of hydrolyzed technetium Tc 99m and pertechnetate is not greater than 10.0% of the total radioactivity on the strip.

Biological distribution—Inject intravenously between 0.075 MBq and 0.75 MBq (2 µCi and 20 µCi) of Injection, in a volume not exceeding 0.2 mL, into the caudal vein of each of three 20- to 25-g mice. Approximately 10 to 15 minutes after injection, place each animal in a suitable container and count the radioactivity of each with an appropriate radiation detector, using the same counting geometry, in order to determine the total activity injected. Approximately 24 hours after injection, repeat the radioactivity counting of each animal, as above. After correcting for decay, determine the percentage of radioactivity retained in each animal 24 hours after injection by the formula:

$$100(A/B)$$

in which *A* is the net radioactivity, in counts per minute (corrected for decay), in the animal at 24 hours, and *B* is the total radioactivity, in net counts per minute, at the time of injection. The percentage of injected radioactivity retained 24 hours after administration is not greater than 5.0% of the injected activity in any of the animals.
Other requirements—It meets the requirements of the tests for *Radionuclide identification* and *Radionuclidic purity* under *Sodium Pertechnetate Tc 99m Injection*. It meets the requirements under *Injections* ⟨1⟩, except that it may be distributed or dispensed prior to completion of the test for *Sterility*, the latter test being started on the day of manufacture, and except that it is not subject to the recommendation on *Volume in Container*.
Assay for radioactivity ⟨821⟩—Using a suitable counting assembly (see *Selection of a Counting Assembly*), determine the radioactivity, in MBq (µCi) per mL, of Injection by use of a calibrated system.

Sodium Pertechnetate Tc 99m Injection

Pertechnetic acid (H^{99m}TcO$_4$), sodium salt.
Sodium pertechnetate (Na^{99m}TcO$_4$) [23288-60-0].

» Sodium Pertechnetate Tc 99m Injection is a sterile solution, suitable for intravenous or oral administration, containing radioactive technetium (^{99m}Tc) in the form of sodium pertechnetate and sufficient Sodium Chloride to make the solution isotonic. Technetium 99m is a radioactive nuclide formed by the radioactive decay of molybdenum 99. Molybdenum 99 is a radioactive isotope of molybdenum and may be formed by the neutron bombardment of molybdenum 98 or as a product of uranium fission.

Sodium Pertechnetate Tc 99m Injection contains not less than 90.0 percent and not more than 110.0 percent of the labeled amount of ^{99m}Tc at the date and hour stated on the label. Other chemical forms of ^{99m}Tc do not exceed 5 percent of the total radioactivity.

Packaging and storage—Preserve in single-dose or multiple-dose containers.

Labeling—If intended for intravenous use, label it with the information specified for *Labeling* under *Injections* ⟨1⟩. Label it also to include the following: the time and date of calibration; the amount of ^{99m}Tc as sodium pertechnetate expressed as total megabecquerels (millicuries) and as megabecquerels (millicuries) per mL on the date and at the time of calibration; a statement of the intended use, whether oral or intravenous; the expiration date; and the statement "Caution—Radioactive Material." If the Injection has been prepared from molybdenum 99 produced from uranium fission, the label so states. The labeling indicates that in making dosage calculations, correction is to be made for radioactive decay, and also indicates that the radioactive half-life of ^{99m}Tc is 6.0 hours.

USP Reference standards ⟨11⟩—*USP Endotoxin RS*.

Radionuclide identification (see *Radioactivity* ⟨821⟩)—Its gamma-ray spectrum is identical to that of a specimen of ^{99m}Tc that exhibits a major photopeak having an energy of 0.140 MeV.

Bacterial endotoxins ⟨85⟩—The limit of endotoxin content is not more than 175/V USP Endotoxin Unit per mL of the Injection, when compared with the USP Endotoxin RS, in which V is the maximum recommended total dose, in mL, at the expiration date or time.

pH ⟨791⟩: between 4.5 and 7.5.

Radiochemical purity—Place a volume of Injection, appropriately diluted, such that it provides a count rate of about 20,000 counts per minute, about 25 mm from one end of a 25- × 300-mm strip of chromatographic paper (see *Chromatography* ⟨621⟩). Develop the chromatogram over a suitable period of time by ascending chromatography, using a mixture of acetone and 2 N hydrochloric acid (80 : 20). Allow the chromatogram to air-dry. Determine the radioactivity distribution by scanning the chromatogram with a suitable collimated radiation detector. The radioactivity of the pertechnetate band is not less than 95% of the total radioactivity in the test specimen. The R_F value for the pertechnetate band (approximately 0.9) falls within ±10.0% of the value found for a known sodium pertechnetate Tc 99m specimen when determined under identical conditions.

Radionuclidic purity—Using a suitable counting assembly (see *Selection of a Counting Assembly* under *Radioactivity* ⟨821⟩), determine the radioactivity of each radionuclidic impurity, in kBq per MBq (μCi per mCi) of technetium 99m, in the Injection by use of a calibrated system as directed under *Radioactivity* ⟨821⟩.

For Injection prepared from technetium 99m derived from parent molybdenum 99 formed as a result of neutron bombardment of stable molybdenum—

MOLYBDENUM 99—The presence of molybdenum 99 in the Injection is shown by its characteristic gamma-ray spectrum. The most prominent photopeaks of this radioactive nuclide have energies of 0.181, 0.740, and 0.780 MeV. Molybdenum 99 decays with a radioactive half-life of 66.0 hours. The amount of molybdenum 99 is not greater than 0.15 kBq per MBq (0.15 μCi per mCi) of technetium 99m per administered dose in the Injection, at the time of administration.

OTHER GAMMA-EMITTING RADIONUCLIDIC IMPURITIES—The total amount of other gamma-emitting radionuclidic impurities does not exceed 0.5 kBq per MBq (0.5 μCi per mCi) of technetium 99m, and does not exceed 92 kBq (2.5 μCi) per administered dose of the Injection, at the time of administration.

For Injection prepared from technetium 99m derived from parent molybdenum 99 formed as a result of uranium fission—Gamma-and beta-emitting impurities—

MOLYBDENUM 99—The Injection meets the requirements set forth for the Injection prepared by neutron irradiation of stable molybdenum (see foregoing).

IODINE 131—The most prominent photopeak of this radioactive nuclide has an energy of 0.364 MeV. Iodine 131 decays with a radioactive half-life of 8.08 days. The concentration of iodine 131 is not more than 0.05 kBq per MBq (0.05 μCi per mCi) of technetium 99m, at the time of administration.

RUTHENIUM 103—The most prominent photopeak of this radioactive nuclide has an energy of 0.497 MeV. Ruthenium 103 decays with a radioactive half-life of 39.5 days. The concentration of ruthenium 103 is not more than 0.05 kBq per MBq (0.05 μCi per mCi) of technetium 99m, at the time of administration.

STRONTIUM 89—Determine the presence of strontium 89 in the Injection by a counting system appropriate for the detection of particulate radiations. Strontium 89 decays by a beta emission with a maximum energy of 1.463 MeV, and a radioactive half-life of 52.7 days. Strontium 89 may be present in a concentration of not more than 0.0006 kBq per MBq (0.0006 μCi per mCi) of technetium 99m, at the time of administration.

STRONTIUM 90—Determine the presence of strontium 90 in the Injection by a counting system appropriate for the detection of particulate radiations. Strontium 90 decays by a beta emission with a maximum energy of 0.546 MeV, and a radioactive half-life of 27.7 years. Strontium 90 may be present in a concentration of not more than 0.00006 kBq per MBq (0.00006 μCi per mCi) of technetium 99m, at the time of administration.

ALL OTHER RADIONUCLIDIC IMPURITIES—Not more than 0.01% of all other beta and gamma emitters is present at the time of administration. Not more than 0.001 Bq of gross alpha impurity per 1 MBq (or 0.001 nCi of gross alpha impurity per 1 mCi) of technetium 99m is present at the time of administration.

Chemical purity—

Aluminum (To be determined if separation is accomplished by an alumina column in the preparation of the Injection)—

ALUMINUM STANDARD SOLUTION—Dissolve 35.17 mg, accurately weighed, of aluminum potassium sulfate dodecahydrate in water to make 1000.0 mL. Each mL of this solution contains 2 μg of Al.

PROCEDURE—Pipet 10 mL of *Aluminum standard solution* into each of two 50-mL volumetric flasks. To each flask add 3 drops of methyl orange TS and 2 drops of 6 N ammonium hydroxide, then add 0.5 N hydrochloric acid, dropwise, until the solution turns red. To one flask add 25 mL of sodium thioglycolate TS, and to the other flask add 1 mL of edetate disodium TS. To each flask add 5 mL of eriochrome cyanine TS and 5 mL of acetate buffer TS, and add water to volume. Immediately determine the absorbance of the solution containing sodium thioglycolate TS at the wavelength of maximum absorbance at about 535 nm, with a suitable spectrophotometer, using the solution containing the edetate disodium TS as a blank. Repeat the procedure using two 1.0-mL aliquots of Injection. Calculate the quantity, in μg per mL, of aluminum in the Injection taken by the formula:

$$20(T_U / T_S)$$

in which T_U and T_S are the absorbances of the solution from the Injection and the solution containing the aluminum standard, respectively. The concentration of aluminum ion in the Injection is not greater than 10 μg per mL.

Methyl ethyl ketone (To be determined if separation is accomplished by liquid-liquid extraction in the preparation of the Injection)—Place 1.0 mL of the Injection in a suitable container, and dilute with water to 20.0 mL. Add 2.0 mL of 1 N sodium hydroxide, mix, then add 2.0 mL of 0.1 N iodine, dropwise, and again mix. At the same time, prepare a standard by placing 1.0 mL of a solution of methyl ethyl ketone (1 in 1000) in a similar container and diluting with water to 20.0 mL. Add 2.0 mL of 1 N sodium hydroxide, mix, then add 2.0 mL of 0.1 N iodine, dropwise, and again mix. After 2 minutes, the turbidity of the test specimen does not exceed that of the standard (0.1%).

Other requirements—It meets the requirements under *Injections* ⟨1⟩, except that the Injection may be distributed or dispensed prior to the completion of the test for *Sterility*, the latter test being started on the day of manufacture, and except that it is not subject to the recommendation on *Volume in Container*.

Assay for radioactivity—Using a suitable counting assembly (see *Selection of a Counting Assembly*), determine the radioactivity, in MBq (mCi) per mL, in Injection by use of a calibrated system.

Technetium Tc 99m Pyrophosphate Injection

» Technetium Tc 99m Pyrophosphate Injection is a sterile, aqueous solution, suitable for intravenous administration, of pyrophosphate that is labeled with ^{99m}Tc. It contains not less than 90.0 percent and not more than 110.0 percent of the labeled amount of ^{99m}Tc as pyrophosphate expressed in megabecquerels (microcuries or millicuries) per mL at the time indicated in the labeling. It may contain antimicrobial agents, buffers, reducing agents, and stabilizers. Other chemical forms of radioactivity do not exceed 10.0 percent of the total radioactivity.

Packaging and storage—Preserve in single-dose or multiple-dose containers, at a temperature between 2° and 8°.
Labeling—Label it to include the following, in addition to the information specified for *Labeling* under *Injections* ⟨1⟩: the time and date of calibration; the amount of ^{99m}Tc as labeled tetrasodium pyrophosphate expressed as total megabecquerels (microcuries or millicuries) and concentration as megabecquerels (microcuries or millicuries) per mL at the time of calibration; the expiration date and time; and the statement "Caution—Radioactive Material." The labeling indicates that in making dosage calculations, correction is to be made for radioactive decay, and also indicates that the radioactive half-life of ^{99m}Tc is 6.0 hours.
USP Reference standards ⟨11⟩—*USP Endotoxin RS*.
Bacterial endotoxins ⟨85⟩—The limit of endotoxin content is not more than 175/*V* USP Endotoxin Unit per mL of the Injection, when compared with the USP Endotoxin RS, in which *V* is the maximum recommended total dose, in mL, at the expiration date or time.
pH ⟨791⟩: between 4.0 and 7.5.
Radiochemical purity—The determination of radiochemical purity for this product requires the use of two separate chromatography systems.
System A—Under an atmosphere of nitrogen, place a measured volume of Injection, appropriately diluted, such that it provides a count rate of about 20,000 counts per minute, about 20 mm from one end of a thin-layer chromatographic strip impregnated with silica gel (see *Chromatography* ⟨621⟩), and allow to dry. Develop the chromatogram over a suitable period by ascending chromatography, using saline TS, and dry it under nitrogen. Determine the radioactivity distribution by scanning the chromatogram with a suitable collimated radiation detector. Hydrolyzed Tc 99m and technetium-tin colloid are located at the origin (R_F 0 to 0.1).
System B—Proceed as directed for *System A*, except to develop the chromatogram in a mixture of methanol and acetone (1 : 1). Free pertechnetate is located at the solvent front. The sum of the percentage of radioactivity at the origin in *System A* plus the percentage of radioactivity at the solvent front in *System B* is not greater than 10.0%.
Biological distribution—Inject intravenously between 0.075 MBq and 75 MBq (2 μCi and 2 mCi) of Injection, in a volume not exceeding 0.2 mL, into the caudal or external jugular vein of each of three 175- to 250-g rats. Approximately 1 hour after the injection, sacrifice the animals, and carefully remove the liver, both kidneys, and one femur of each by dissection, freeing the femur from soft tissue. Remove the tail 20 to 30 mm above the injection site, and discard. Place each organ, both kidneys, and the remaining carcass in separate, suitable counting containers, and determine the radioactivity, in counts per minute, in each container with an appropriate detector, using the same counting geometry. Determine the percentage of radioactivity in the liver, kidneys, and femur taken by the formula:

$$100(A/B)$$

in which *A* is the net radioactivity, in counts per minute, in the organ, and *B* is the total radioactivity, in counts per minute, in the liver, kidneys, femur, and carcass. Not more than 5.0% of the total radioactivity is found in the liver or in the kidneys, and not less than 1.0% of the total radioactivity is found in the femur, in not fewer than 2 of the rats.
Other requirements—It meets the requirements of the tests for *Radionuclide identification* and *Radionuclidic purity* under *Sodium Pertechnetate Tc 99m Injection*. It meets also the requirements under *Injections* ⟨1⟩, except that it may be distributed or dispensed prior to completion of the test for *Sterility*, the latter test being started on the day of final manufacture, and except that it is not subject to the recommendation on *Volume in Container*.
Assay for radioactivity ⟨821⟩—Using a suitable counting assembly (see *Selection of a Counting Assembly*), determine the radioactivity, in MBq (μCi) per mL, of the Injection by use of a calibrated system.

Technetium Tc 99m (Pyro- and trimeta-) Phosphates Injection

» Technetium Tc 99m (Pyro- and trimeta-) Phosphates Injection is a sterile, aqueous solution, suitable for intravenous administration, composed of sodium pyrophosphate, sodium trimetaphosphate, and stannous chloride labeled with radioactive Tc 99m. It contains not less than 90.0 percent and not more than 110.0 percent of the labeled amount of ^{99m}Tc as phosphate expressed in megabecquerels (microcuries or millicuries) per mL at the time indicated in the labeling. Other chemical forms of radioactivity do not exceed 10.0 percent of the total radioactivity.

USP Reference standards ⟨11⟩—*USP Endotoxin RS*.
pH ⟨791⟩: between 4.0 and 7.0.
Radiochemical purity—Place a measured volume of Injection, appropriately diluted, such that it provides a count rate of about 20,000 counts per minute, about 10 mm from one end of a 10- × 50-mm strip of chromatographic paper (see *Chromatography* ⟨621⟩), and immediately develop the chromatogram over a period of 3 to 5 minutes by ascending chromatography, using saline TS, and air-dry. Determine the radioactivity distribution by scanning with a suitable collimated radiation detector. Not more than 10.0% of the total radioactivity is found at the point of application. Similarly prepare a second strip, and thoroughly dry the spot with nitrogen. Develop the chromatogram over a period of 35 to 45 seconds by ascending chromatography, using freshly distilled methyl ethyl ketone, and allow to dry. Determine the radioactivity distribution as previously directed. Not less than 90.0% of the total radioactivity is found at the point of application.
Other requirements—It meets the requirements of the tests for *Radionuclide identification* and *Radionuclidic purity* under *Sodium Pertechnetate Tc 99m Injection*, and the requirements of the tests for *Packaging and storage, Labeling, Bacterial endotoxins, Biological distribution,* and *Assay for radioactivity* under *Technetium Tc 99m Pyrophosphate Injection*. It meets the requirements under *Injections* ⟨1⟩, except that it may be distributed or dispensed prior to completion of the test for *Sterility*, the latter test being started on the day of manufacture, and except that it is not subject to the recommendation on *Volume in Container*.

Technetium Tc 99m Red Blood Cells Injection

» Technetium Tc 99m Red Blood Cells Injection is a preparation of anticoagulated whole blood that is labeled with ^{99m}Tc. The cells are prepared for labeling by collection of an autologous sample of whole blood, which is anticoagulated with Heparin Sodium or anticoagulant dextrose solution.

Technetium Tc 99m Red Blood Cells Injection contains not less than 90.0 percent and not more than 110.0

percent of the labeled concentration of ^{99m}Tc as labeled blood cells expressed in megabecquerels (or in microcuries or millicuries) per mL at the time indicated in the labeling. It may contain anticoagulants, such as heparin or anticoagulant citrate solution, chelating agents, stannous chloride, and sodium hypochlorite. Other chemical forms of radioactivity do not exceed 10.0 percent of the total radioactivity. When derived from donor blood, its production and distribution derived from donor blood are subject to federal regulations (see *Biologics* ⟨1041⟩ and *Radioactivity* ⟨821⟩).

Caution—A strict aseptic technique must be followed for collection of the blood sample, along with the processing steps required to label it with Technetium Tc 99m. The blood samples must be labeled with the name of the patient and patient's identification code to prevent administration of the sample to other than the intended patient. In the event that donor blood is used, it must first be tested for viral contaminants and carefully typed and cross-matched to ensure compatibility with that of the recipient.

Packaging and storage—Preserve in adequately shielded single-dose or multiple-dose containers, at controlled room temperature.

Labeling—Label it to include the following in addition to the information specified for *Labeling* under *Injections* ⟨1⟩: the patient's name and identification number; the type of anticoagulant used; the time and date of calibration; the amount expressed as total megabecquerels (or microcuries or millicuries) and concentration as megabecquerels (or microcuries or millicuries) per mL at the time of calibration; the expiration date; and the statement "Caution—Radioactive Material." The labeling indicates that in making dosage calculations, correction is to be made for radioactive decay, and also indicates that the radioactive half-life of ^{99m}Tc is 6.0 hours.

USP Reference standards ⟨11⟩—*USP Endotoxin RS*.

Clarity and color of solution—Observe the appearance and color of the supernatant diluted plasma obtained in the *Radiochemical purity* test procedure. The diluted plasma is clear and has a colorless to a very slight pink or yellow appearance. Samples that produce a distinctive red coloration are not acceptable for administration.

Bacterial endotoxins ⟨85⟩—It contains not more than $175/V$ USP Endotoxin Unit per mL of the Injection, when compared with the USP Endotoxin RS, in which V is the maximum recommended total dose, in mL, at the expiration date or time.

pH ⟨791⟩: between 5.5 and 8.0.

Radiochemical purity—Transfer 0.2 mL of the Injection to a centrifuge tube containing 2 mL of 0.9% sodium chloride solution. Centrifuge for five minutes, and carefully withdraw the diluted plasma by pipet. Measure the radioactivity in the plasma and red blood cells separately in a suitable counter. Calculate labeling efficiency by the formula:

$$100[A_{RBC} / (A_{RBC} + A_P)]$$

in which A_{RBC} is the activity in the red blood cells, and A_P is the activity in the plasma. Not less than 90% of the ^{99m}Tc present in the Injection is bound to the red blood cells.

Other requirements—It meets the requirements of the tests for *Radionuclide identification* and *Radionuclidic purity* under *Sodium Pertechnetate Tc 99m Injection*. It meets also the requirements under *Injections* ⟨1⟩, except that it may be distributed or dispensed prior to completion of the test for *Sterility*, the latter test being started on the day of final manufacture, and except that it is not subject to the recommendation on *Volume in Container*.

Assay for radioactivity ⟨821⟩—Using a suitable counting assembly (see *Selection of a Counting Assembly*), determine the radioactivity, in MBq (or µCi) per mL, of the Injection by use of a calibrated system.

Technetium Tc 99m Sestamibi Injection

$C_{36}H_{66}N_6O_6{}^{99m}Tc$

Technetium(1+)-^{99m}Tc,hexakis(1-isocyano-2-methoxy-2-methyl-propane)-, (*OC*-6-11)-.

Hexakis(2-methoxy-2methylpropyl isocyanide)[^{99m}Tc]technetium(1+) [*109581-73-9*].

» Technetium Tc 99m Sestamibi Injection is a sterile, aqueous solution of tetrakis(2–methoxy-isobutyl isonitrile) copper (I) tetrafluoroborate that is labeled with ^{99m}Tc suitable for intravenous administration. It contains not less than 90 percent and not more than 110 percent of the labeled amount of ^{99m}Tc as a complex with sestamibi, expressed in megabecquerels (or in milicuries) per mL at the time indicated in the labeling. It contains reducing agents, a buffer, and an inert filler. Other chemical forms of radioactivity do not exceed 10 percent of the total radioactivity.

Packaging and storage—Preserve in single-dose or multiple-dose containers.

Labeling—Label it to include the following, in addition to the information specified for *Labeling* under *Injections* ⟨1⟩: the time and date of constitution; the volume of constitution; the amount of ^{99m}Tc as labeled sestamibi expressed as total megabecquerels (or millicuries) per mL at the time of constitution; the expiration date and time; the lot number; and the statement "Caution—Radioactive Material." The labeling indicates that in making dosage calculations, correction is to be made for radioactive decay, and also indicates that the radioactive half-life of ^{99m}Tc is 6.0 hours.

USP Reference standards ⟨11⟩—*USP Endotoxin RS*.

Bacterial endotoxins ⟨85⟩—It contains not more than $175/V$ USP Endotoxin Units per mL, in which V is the maximum recommended total dose, in mL, at the expiration date or time.

pH ⟨791⟩: between 5.0 and 6.0.

Radiochemical purity—

Preparation of the test vials—Constitute each of 4 vials with 1 mL (1875 ± 187.5 MBq, or 50 ± 5 mCi) of *Sodium Pertechnetate Tc 99m Injection*. Heat the vials in boiling water for 10 minutes. After heating, allow the vials to cool to room temperature for 15 minutes.

Method 1 (Thin-layer chromatography)—Apply 1 to 2 µL of Injection about 1 cm from the bottom of a 25-mm × 7.75-cm reverse-phase chromatographic plate, and allow to dry (see *Chromatography* ⟨621⟩). Position the plate in a chromatographic chamber and develop the chromatograms in a freshly prepared (not more than 4 hours) solvent system consisting of a mixture of acetonitrile, methanol, 3.85% ammonium acetate, and tetrahydrofuran (4 : 3 : 2 : 1) until the solvent front has moved about 6 cm from the origin. Remove the plate and allow it to air-dry. Determine the radioactivity distribution by scanning the chromatogram with a suitable radiation detector. A mean of not less than 90% (area %) of the radioactivity is found at an R_F value between 0.3 and 0.6. Free pertechnetate is located at about the R_F 0.8 to 1.0, and radiocolloid is located at about R_F 0 to 0.1. The sum of the mean percentages of free pertechnetate and colloid does not exceed 10%.

Method 2 (High-pressure liquid chromatography)—

MOBILE PHASE—Prepare a filtered and degassed mixture of methanol, 0.05 M ammonium sulfate solution, and acetonitrile (45 : 35 :

20). Make adjustments if necessary (see *System Suitablity* under *Chromatography* ⟨621⟩).

CHROMATOGRAPHIC SYSTEM (see *Chromatography* ⟨621⟩)—The liquid chromatograph is equipped with a 3.9-mm × 30-cm column that contains 10-μm packing L1. It is also equipped with a flow-through gamma-ray detector. The flow rate is about 2 mL per minute. If ^{99m}Tc pentamibi dimethylvinyl isonitrile is present, the relative retention between the ^{99m}Tc sestamibi peak and the ^{99m}Tc pentamibi dimethylvinyl isonitrile peak is 1.3 to 1.5.

PROCEDURE—Inject about 5 μL (9.375 MBq or 250 μCi) of *Sodium Pertechnetate Tc 99m Injection* into the chromatograph, and adjust the integrator/recording device so that the peak is 25% to 100% of full scale. Separately inject equal volumes (about 5 μL, 9.375 MBq, or 250 μCi) of the injection under test into the chromatograph, record the chromatograms, and measure the area percentage for all of the peaks present. The retention time for ^{99m}Tc sestamibi is about 5 to 10 minutes. The retention time for ^{99m}Tc pentamibi dimethylvinyl isonitrile is about 6 to 13 minutes. Correct for the presence of colloid, which is not measured by this method, taken by the equation:

$$C_f = [(100\%) - (A_c)] / 100$$

in which C_f is the correction factor, and A_c is the mean area percentage for the colloid obtained from *Method 1*. Obtain corrected area percentage by multiplying the correction factor (C_f) by the area percentage of the peaks present in the chromatogram. A mean of not less than 90% (corrected area percentage) of the total radioactivity is represented by ^{99m}Tc sestamibi, and a mean of not more than 5% (corrected area percentage) of the total radioactivity is present as ^{99m}Tc pentamibi dimethylvinyl isonitrile.

Other requirements—It meets the requirements of the tests for *Radionuclide identification* and *Radionuclidic purity* under *Sodium Pertechnetate Tc 99m Injection*. It meets also the requirements for *Injections* ⟨1⟩, except that it may be distributed and dispensed prior to the completion of the test for *Sterility*, the latter being started on the day of manufacture, and except that it is not subject to the recommendation on *Volume in Container*.

Assay for radioactivity ⟨821⟩—Using a suitable counting assembly (see *Selection of a Counting Assembly*), determine the radioactivity, in MBq (or in mCi) per mL, of the Injection by use of a calibrated system.

Technetium Tc 99m Succimer Injection

meso-2,3-Dimercaptosuccinic acid, ^{99m}Tc complex.

» Technetium Tc 99m Succimer Injection is a sterile, clear, colorless, aqueous solution of succimer complexed with ^{99m}Tc. It is suitable for intravenous administration. It contains not less than 85.0 percent of the labeled amount of ^{99m}Tc as the succimer complex expressed in megabecquerels (microcuries or millicuries) per mL at the time indicated in the labeling. It may contain reducing agents. Other chemical forms of radioactivity do not exceed 15.0 percent of the total radioactivity.

Packaging and storage—Preserve in single-dose containers, at a temperature between 15° and 30°. Do not freeze or store above 30°. Protect from light.

Labeling—Label it to include the following, in addition to the information specified for *Labeling* under *Injections* ⟨1⟩: the time and date of calibration; the amount of ^{99m}Tc as labeled succimer expressed as total megabecquerels (microcuries or millicuries) and concentration as megabecquerels (microcuries or millicuries) per mL at the time of calibration; the expiration date and time; and the statement "Caution—Radioactive Material." The labeling indicates that in making dosage calculations, correction is to be made for radioactive decay, and also indicates that the radioactive half-life of ^{99m}Tc is 6.0 hours. In addition, the labeling states that it is not to be used if discoloration or particulate matter is observed. [NOTE—A beyond-use time of 30 minutes shall be stated on the label upon constitution with Sodium Pertechnetate Tc 99m Injection.]

USP Reference standards ⟨11⟩—*USP Endotoxin RS*.

Bacterial endotoxins ⟨85⟩—The limit of endotoxin content is not more than 175/V USP Endotoxin Unit per mL of the Injection, when compared with the USP Endotoxin RS, in which V is the maximum recommended total dose, in mL, at the expiration date or time.

pH ⟨791⟩: between 2.0 and 3.0.

Radiochemical purity—Activate a 65- × 95-mm silicic acid thin-layer chromatographic plate by heating at 100-110° for 30 minutes. Cool over silica gel and immediately apply 1 μL of Injection, appropriately diluted, if necessary, to a radioactive concentration of 18.5 to 370 MBq (0.5 to 10 mCi) per mL, about 17 mm from one end of the chromatographic plate, and allow to dry. Develop the chromatogram over a period of about 30 to 45 minutes by ascending chromatography, using *n*-butanol saturated with 0.3 N hydrochloric acid, and air-dry. Determine the radioactive distribution by scanning the chromatogram with a suitable collimated radiation detector. Not less than 85% of the total radioactivity is found as succimer at an R_F between 0.45 and 0.70. Hydrolyzed ^{99m}Tc is located at the origin (R_F 0 to 0.15) and the unbound ^{99m}Tc is located at the solvent front (R_F 1.0).

Biological distribution—Inject intravenously between 3.7 MBq and 92.5 MBq (100 μCi and 2500 μCi) of Injection, in a volume of 0.2 to 0.25 mL, into the caudal vein of each of three 125-g to 225-g anesthetized Sprague-Dawley female rats. Clamp the opening of the urethra with a hemostat. Sacrifice the animals 1 hour after the injection, and carefully remove the kidneys, bladder, and liver and spleen of each as *three* separate organs by dissections. Place each organ and the remaining carcass (excluding the tail) in separate, suitable counting containers, and determine the radioactivity, in counts per minute, in each container with an appropriate detector, using the same counting geometry. Determine the percentage of administered radioactive dose in each organ: not less than 40% of the administered radioactive dose is found in the kidneys and a ratio of not less than 6 : 1 of the administered dose is found in the ratio kidneys/(liver and spleen), in not fewer than two of the animals.

Other requirements—It meets the requirements of the tests for *Radionuclide identification* and *Radionuclidic purity* under *Sodium Pertechnetate Tc 99m Injection*. It meets also the requirements under *Injections* ⟨1⟩, except that it may be distributed or dispensed prior to completion of the test for *Sterility*, the latter test being started on the day of final manufacture, and except that it is not subject to the recommendation on *Volume in Container*.

Assay for radioactivity ⟨821⟩—Using a suitable counting assembly (see *Selection of a Counting Assembly*), determine the radioactivity, in MBq (μCi) per mL, of Injection by use of a calibrated system.

Technetium Tc 99m Sulfur Colloid Injection

Sulfur, colloidal, metastable technetium-99 labeled   [7704-34-9].

» Technetium Tc 99m Sulfur Colloid Injection is a sterile, colloidal dispersion of sulfur labeled with radioactive ^{99m}Tc, suitable for intravenous administration.

Technetium Tc 99m Sulfur Colloid Injection contains not less than 90.0 percent and not more than 110.0 percent of the labeled concentration of ^{99m}Tc as sulfur colloid expressed in megabecquerels (microcuries or millicuries) per mL at the time indicated in the labeling. It may contain chelating agents, buffers, and stabilizing agents. Other chemical forms of radioactivity do not exceed 8 percent of the total radioactivity.

NOTE—Agitate the container before withdrawing the Injection into a syringe.

Packaging and storage—Store in single-dose or multiple-dose containers.

Labeling—Label it to include the following, in addition to the information specified for *Labeling* under *Injections* ⟨1⟩: the time and date of calibration; the amount of ^{99m}Tc as sulfur colloid expressed as total megabecquerels (microcuries or millicuries) and concentration as megabecquerels (microcuries or millicuries) per mL at the time of calibration; the expiration date; and the statement "Caution—Radioactive Material." The labeling indicates that in making dosage calculations, correction is to be made for radioactive decay, and also indicates that the radioactive half-life of ^{99m}Tc is 6.0 hours; in addition, the labeling states that it is not to be used if flocculent material is visible and directs that the container be agitated before the Injection is withdrawn into a syringe.

USP Reference standards ⟨11⟩—*USP Endotoxin RS*.

Radionuclide identification (see *Radioactivity* ⟨821⟩)—It meets the requirements of the test for *Radionuclide identification* under *Sodium Pertechnetate Tc 99m Injection*.

Bacterial endotoxins ⟨85⟩—The limit of endotoxin content is not more than 175/*V* USP Endotoxin Unit per mL of the Injection, when compared with the USP Endotoxin RS, in which *V* is the maximum recommended total dose, in mL, at the expiration date or time.

pH ⟨791⟩: between 4.5 and 7.5.

Radionuclidic purity—It meets the requirements of the test for *Radionuclidic purity* under *Sodium Pertechnetate Tc 99m Injection*.

Radiochemical purity—Place a measured volume of Injection, appropriately diluted, such that it provides a count rate of about 20,000 counts per minute, about 25 mm from one end of a 25- × 300-mm strip of chromatographic paper (see *Chromatography* ⟨621⟩), and allow to dry. Develop the chromatogram over a suitable period by ascending chromatography, using dilute methanol (8.5 in 10), and air-dry. Determine the radioactivity distribution by scanning the chromatogram with a suitable collimated radiation detector. Not less than 92% of the total radioactivity is found as sulfur colloid (at the point of application).

Biological distribution—Inject intravenously between 0.075 MBq and 0.75 MBq (2 μCi and 20 μCi) of the Injection in a volume not exceeding 0.2 mL into the caudal vein of each of three 20-g to 25-g mice. Ten to 30 minutes after the injection, sacrifice the animals, and carefully remove the liver and lungs of each by dissection. Place each organ and remaining carcass in separate, suitable counting containers, and determine the radioactivity, in counts per minute, in each container in an appropriate scintillation well counter, using the same counting geometry. Determine the percentage of radioactivity in the liver and the lungs taken by the formula:

$$100(A/B)$$

in which *A* is the net radioactivity, in counts per minute, in the organ, and *B* is the total radioactivity, in counts per minute, in the lungs, liver, and carcass. Not less than 80% of the radioactivity is found in the liver and not more than 5% of the radioactivity is found in the lungs, in two of the mice.

Other requirements—It meets the requirements under *Injections* ⟨1⟩, except that the Injection may be distributed or dispensed prior to completion of the test for *Sterility*, the latter test being started on the day of final manufacture, and except that it is not subject to the recommendation on *Volume in Container*.

Assay for radioactivity ⟨821⟩—Using a suitable counting assembly (see *Selection of a Counting Assembly*), determine the radioactivity, in MBq (μCi) per mL, of Injection by use of a calibrated system.

Technetium Tc 99m Tetrofosmin Injection

» Technetium Tc 99m Tetrofosmin Injection is a sterile aqueous solution, suitable for intravenous injection, that contains ^{99m}Tc in the form of a complex of tetrofosmin. It contains not less than 90.0 percent and not more than 110.0 percent of the labeled amount of ^{99m}Tc as tetrofosmin complex expressed in MBq (or mCi) per mL at the date and time indicated in the labeling. It may contain reducing agents, stabilizers, and buffers. It contains no antimicrobial agents. Other chemical forms of radioactivity do not exceed 10.0 percent of the total.

Packaging and storage—Preserve in adequately shielded single-dose or in multiple-dose containers. Protect from light. Store at a temperature not exceeding 25°.

Labeling—Label it to include the following, in addition to the information specified for *Labeling* under *Injections* ⟨1⟩: the time and date of calibration; the amount of ^{99m}Tc as labeled tetrofosmin expressed as total MBq (or mCi) and the concentration as megabecquerels per mL (or as mCi per mL) on the date and time of calibration; the expiration date and time; and a statement, "Caution—Radioactive Material." The labeling indicates that in making dosage calculations, correction is to be made for radioactive decay, and also indicates that the radioactive half-life of ^{99m}Tc is 6.0 hours.

USP Reference standards ⟨11⟩—*USP Endotoxin RS*.

Bacterial endotoxins ⟨85⟩—The limit of endotoxin content is not more than 175/*V* USP Endotoxin Unit per mL of the Injection, when compared with USP Endotoxin RS, in which *V* is the maximum recommended total dose, in mL, at the expiration date or time.

pH ⟨791⟩: between 8.3 and 9.1.

Radiochemical purity—To determine the amount of free technetium, apply a 10- to 20-μL volume of Injection about 3.0 cm from the bottom of a 2- × 20-cm instant thin-layer chromatographic silica gel strip (see *Chromatography* ⟨621⟩). Immediately develop the chromatogram by ascending chromatography to a height of 15 cm using a solvent system consisting of a mixture of acetone and dichloromethane (35 : 65). Allow the chromatogram to air-dry. Determine the radioactivity distribution of the chromatogram by scanning with a suitable radiation detector. The R_F value of the technetium Tc 99m tetrofosmin spot is approximately 0.5: the sum of radioactivity at the solvent front (unbound pertechnetate) and the origin (reduced hydrolyzed technetium and hydrophilic impurities) is not more than 10%.

Other requirements—It meets the requirements for *Radionuclide identification* and *Radionuclidic purity* under *Sodium Pertechnetate Tc 99m Injection*. It meets also the requirements under *Injections* ⟨1⟩, except that it may be distributed or dispensed prior to completion of the test for *Sterility*, the latter test being started on the date of manufacture.

Assay for radioactivity ⟨821⟩—Using a suitable counting assembly (see *Selection of a Counting Assembly*), determine the radioactivity, in MBq (μCi) per mL, of the Injection by use of a calibrated system.

Temazepam

$C_{16}H_{13}ClN_2O_2$ 300.74

2*H*-1,4-Benzodiazepin-2-one, 7-chloro-1,3-dihydro-3-hydroxy-1-methyl-5-phenyl-.

7-Chloro-1,3-dihydro-3-hydroxy-1-methyl-5-phenyl-2*H*-1,4-benzodiazepin-2-one [*846-50-4*].

» Temazepam contains not less than 98.0 percent and not more than 102.0 percent of $C_{16}H_{13}ClN_2O_2$, calculated on the dried basis.

Caution—Temazepam is a potent sedative: its powder should not be inhaled.

Packaging and storage—Preserve in well-closed, light-resistant containers.

USP Reference standards ⟨11⟩—*USP Temazepam RS*.
Identification—
  A: *Infrared Absorption* ⟨197K⟩.
  B: The retention time of the major peak in the chromatogram of the *Assay preparation* corresponds to that in the chromatogram of the *Standard preparation*, as obtained in the *Assay*.
Loss on drying ⟨731⟩—Dry it at 105° for 2 hours; it loses not more than 0.5% of its weight.
Residue on ignition ⟨281⟩: not more than 0.1%.
Heavy metals, *Method II* ⟨231⟩: 20 ppm.
Chromatographic purity—
  Standard stock solution—Dissolve an accurately weighed quantity of USP Temazepam RS in chloroform, and dilute quantitatively and stepwise with chloroform to obtain a solution having a known concentration of about 10 mg per mL.
  Standard solutions A and B—Dilute accurately measured volumes of *Standard stock solution* quantitatively with chloroform to obtain *Standard solutions A* and *B* having known concentrations of about 0.1 and 0.05 mg per mL, respectively.
  Test solution—Transfer about 100 mg of Temazepam, accurately weighed, to a 10-mL volumetric flask, add chloroform to volume, and mix.
  Procedure—Separately apply 10 µL of the *Test solution* and 10 µL of each *Standard solution* to a thin-layer chromatographic plate (see *Chromatography* ⟨621⟩) coated with a 0.25-mm layer of chromatographic silica gel mixture. Position the plate in a chromatographic chamber, and develop the chromatograms in a solvent system consisting of cyclohexane, chloroform, methanol, and ammonium hydroxide (50 : 40 : 12 : 1) until the solvent front has moved about 10 cm above the point of application. Remove the plate from the developing chamber, mark the solvent front, and allow the solvent to evaporate. Examine the plate under short-wavelength UV light, and compare the intensities of any secondary spots observed in the chromatogram of the *Test solution* with those of the principal spots in the chromatograms of the *Standard solutions*: no secondary spot obtained from the *Test solution* is greater in intensity than 1.0%, and the sum of the intensities of secondary spots obtained from the *Test solution* corresponds to not more than 2.0%.
Assay—
  Buffer solution—Dissolve 5.444 g of monobasic potassium phosphate in 2000 mL of water. Adjust with phosphoric acid to a pH of 3.0.
  Mobile phase—Prepare a filtered and degassed mixture of *Buffer solution* and acetonitrile (53 : 47). Make adjustments if necessary (see *System Suitability* under *Chromatography* ⟨621⟩).
  Internal standard solution—Dissolve an accurately weighed quantity of benzophenone in a mixture of methanol and water (9 : 1), and dilute quantitatively and stepwise with the same solvent to obtain a solution having a concentration of 0.2 mg per mL.
  Standard preparation—Dissolve an accurately weighed quantity of USP Temazepam RS in *Internal standard solution* to obtain a solution having a known concentration of 0.2 mg per mL.
  Assay preparation—Transfer about 40.0 mg of temazepam, accurately weighed, to a 200-mL volumetric flask, add about 150 mL of *Internal standard solution*, mix, and dilute with *Internal standard solution* to volume.
  Chromatographic system (see *Chromatography* ⟨621⟩)—The liquid chromatograph is equipped with a 254-nm detector and a 4-mm × 25-cm column that contains packing L16. The flow rate is about 2 mL per minute. Chromatograph the *Standard preparation*, and record the peak responses as directed for *Procedure*: the column efficiency is not less than 800 theoretical plates; the tailing factor is not more than 2; the resolution, R, between the temazepam peak and any other peak is not less than 1, and the relative standard deviation for replicate injections is not more than 2.0%.
  Procedure—Separately inject equal volumes (about 10 µL) of the *Standard preparation* and the *Assay preparation* into the chromatograph, record the chromatograms, and measure the responses for the major peaks. The relative retention times are about 1.0 for temazepam and 2.0 for benzophenone. Calculate the quantity, in mg, of $C_{16}H_{13}ClN_2O_2$ in the portion of Temazepam taken by the formula:

$$200C(R_U / R_S)$$

in which C is the concentration, in mg per mL, of USP Temazepam RS in the *Standard preparation*; and R_U and R_S are the peak response ratios obtained from the *Assay preparation* and the *Standard preparation*, respectively.

Temazepam Capsules

» Temazepam Capsules contain not less than 90.0 percent and not more than 110.0 percent of the labeled amount of temazepam ($C_{16}H_{13}O_2N_2Cl$).

  Caution—Temazepam is a potent sedative: its powder should not be inhaled.

Packaging and storage—Preserve in well-closed, light-resistant containers.

USP Reference standards ⟨11⟩—*USP Temazepam RS*.
Identification—
  A: The retention time of the major peak in the chromatogram of the *Assay preparation* corresponds to that of the *Standard preparation*, both relative to the internal standard, as obtained in the *Assay*.
  B: Transfer a portion of the Capsule contents, equivalent to about 50 mg of temazepam, to a 25-mL volumetric flask, add 10 mL of methanol, shake by mechanical means, and allow to settle. Use the supernatant layer as the test solution. Separately apply 20 µL of the test solution and 20 µL of a Standard solution of USP Temazepam RS in methanol containing 5.0 mg per mL to a thin-layer chromatographic plate (see *Chromatography* ⟨621⟩) coated with a 0.25-mm layer of chromatographic silica gel mixture. Place the plate in a chromatographic chamber, and develop the chromatogram in a solvent system consisting of a mixture of toluene, dioxane, methanol, and ammonium hydroxide (65 : 30 : 5 : 1) until the solvent front has moved about three-fourths of the length of the plate. Remove the plate from the developing chamber, mark the solvent front, air-dry, and examine the plate under short-wavelength UV light: the R_F value of the principal spot obtained from the test solution corresponds to that obtained from the Standard solution.
Dissolution ⟨711⟩—
  Sodium acetate buffer—Dissolve 2 g of sodium hydroxide in 450 mL of water in a 1-liter volumetric flask. Adjust with acetic acid to a pH of 4.0, dilute with water to volume, mix, and deaerate.
  Medium: *Sodium acetate buffer* with 0.05% polysorbate 80; 900 mL.
  Apparatus 2: 75 rpm.
  Time: 30 minutes.
  Determine the amount of $C_{16}H_{13}O_2N_2Cl$ dissolved from UV absorbances, at the wavelength of maximum absorbance at about 310 nm of filtered portions of the solution under test, suitably diluted with *Sodium acetate buffer*, in comparison with a Standard solution having a known concentration of USP Temazepam RS in the same medium.
  Tolerances—Not less than 80% (*Q*) of the labeled amount of $C_{16}H_{13}O_2N_2Cl$ is dissolved in 30 minutes.
Uniformity of dosage units ⟨905⟩: meet the requirements.
Assay—
  Buffer solution, Mobile phase, Internal standard solution, Standard preparation, Chromatographic system, and *Procedure*—Proceed as directed in the *Assay* under *Temazepam*.
  Assay preparation—Weigh the contents of not less than 20 Capsules, and calculate the average weight per Capsule. Mix the combined contents, and transfer an accurately weighed portion of the Capsule contents, equivalent to about 40 mg of temazepam, to a 200-mL volumetric flask, add 150 mL of *Internal standard solution*, and shake the mixture by mechanical means for 30 minutes. Dilute with *Internal standard solution* to volume, and mix. Allow

the contents of the flask to settle, and filter, discarding the first 5 mL of the filtrate.

Terazosin Hydrochloride

$C_{19}H_{25}N_5O_4 \cdot HCl \cdot 2H_2O$ 459.92
Piperazine, 1-(4-amino-6,7-dimethoxy-2-quinazolinyl)-4-[(tetrahydro-2-furanyl)carbonyl]-, monohydrochloride, dihydrate.
1-(4-Amino-6,7-dimethoxy-2-quinazolinyl)-4-(tetrahydro-2-furoyl)piperazine monohydrochloride dihydrate   [70024-40-7].
Anhydrous   423.89   [63074-08-8].

» Terazosin Hydrochloride contains not less than 98.0 percent and not more than 102.0 percent of $C_{19}H_{25}N_5O_4 \cdot HCl$, calculated on the dried basis.

Packaging and storage—Preserve in tight containers, and store at a temperature between 20° and 25°.

USP Reference standards ⟨11⟩—*USP Terazosin Hydrochloride RS. USP Terazosin Related Compound A RS. USP Terazosin Related Compound B RS. USP Terazosin Related Compound C RS.*
Color and clarity of solution—Dissolve a quantity of Terazosin Hydrochloride in methanol solution (90 in 100) to obtain a 1 in 100 solution: this solution is clear and colorless to pale yellow, when compared to methanol solution (90 in 100).
Identification—
   A: *Infrared Absorption* ⟨197K⟩.
   B: The retention time of the major peak in the chromatogram of the *Assay preparation* corresponds to that in the chromatogram of the *Standard preparation,* as obtained in the *Assay.*
   C: It meets the requirements of the tests for *Chloride* ⟨191⟩, a solution prepared by dissolving 100 mg in 10 mL of methanol solution (90 in 100) being examined.
Loss on drying ⟨731⟩—Dry it in vacuum at 105° for 3 hours: it loses not more than 9.0% of its weight.
Residue on ignition ⟨281⟩:   not more than 0.2%, determined on a 1.0-g specimen.
Heavy metals, *Method II* ⟨231⟩:   0.002%.
Limit of tetrahydro-2-furancarboxylic acid—
   Blank solution—Transfer 2.0 mL of glacial acetic acid to a 100-mL volumetric flask, dilute with acetone to volume, and mix. Mix 5.0 mL of this solution and 5.0 mL of acetone; pass through a nylon membrane filter having a 0.45-μm or finer porosity, previously washed with acetone; and discard the first 1 mL of the filtrate.
   Internal standard solution—Transfer about 100 mg of capric acid, accurately weighed, to a 100-mL volumetric flask; dissolve in and dilute with acetone to volume; and mix. Transfer 10.0 mL of this solution and 2.0 mL of glacial acetic acid to a 100-mL volumetric flask, dilute with acetone to volume, and mix.
   Standard stock solution—Dissolve an accurately weighed amount of tetrahydro-2-furancarboxylic acid in acetone to obtain a solution having a known concentration of about 1.0 mg per mL. Dilute with acetone quantitatively, and stepwise if necessary, to obtain a solution having a known concentration of about 100 μg per mL.
   Standard solution—Transfer 5.0 mL of the *Standard stock solution* and 5.0 mL of *Internal standard solution* to a 50-mL centrifuge tube, and mix. Pass through a nylon membrane filter having a 0.45-μm or finer porosity, previously washed with acetone; and discard the first 1 mL of the filtrate.
   Test solution—Transfer about 100 mg of Terazosin Hydrochloride, accurately weighed, to a 50-mL centrifuge tube; add 5.0 mL of acetone and 5.0 mL of *Internal standard solution;* and shake for about 30 minutes. Centrifuge for about 10 minutes; pass through a nylon membrane filter having a 0.45-μm or finer porosity, previously washed with acetone; and discard the first 1 mL of the filtrate.
   Chromatographic system (see *Chromatography* ⟨621⟩)—The gas chromatograph is equipped with a flame-ionization detector and a 0.53-mm × 10-m fused-silica capillary column coated with a 1.2-μm film of liquid phase G25. The column temperature is maintained at about 170°. The injection port is configured for splitless injection, and its temperature is maintained at about 230°. The detector temperature is maintained at about 240°. The carrier gas is helium, flowing at a rate of about 9 mL per minute. Chromatograph the *Blank solution,* and measure the peak responses as directed for *Procedure:* ensure that there are no extraneous peaks. Chromatograph the *Standard solution,* and measure the peak responses as directed for *Procedure:* the relative retention times are 1.0 for tetrahydro-2-furancarboxylic acid and 1.2 for capric acid; the resolution, R, between tetrahydro-2-furancarboxylic acid and capric acid is not less than 2.3; and the relative standard deviation, determined from the peak response ratios of tetrahydro-2-furancarboxylic acid to capric acid for replicate injections is not more than 6.5%.
   Procedure—Separately inject equal volumes (about 0.2 μL) of the *Standard solution* and the *Test solution* into the chromatograph, record the chromatograms, and measure the peak responses. Calculate the percentage of tetrahydro-2-furancarboxylic acid in the portion of Terazosin Hydrochloride taken by the formula:

$$(C/W)(R_U / R_S)$$

in which C is the concentration, in μg per mL, of tetrahydro-2-furancarboxylic acid in the *Standard solution;* W is the weight, in mg, of Terazosin Hydrochloride taken to prepare the *Test solution;* and R_U and R_S are the peak response ratios obtained from the *Test solution* and the *Standard solution,* respectively: not more than 0.1% is found.
Limit of 1-[(tetrahydro-2-furanyl)carbonyl]piperazine—
   Derivatization solution—Dissolve about 2.0 g of 3,5-dinitrobenzoyl chloride in 250 mL of acetonitrile.
   Phosphate buffer solution—Transfer about 96.3 g of dibasic potassium phosphate and 3.85 g of monobasic potassium phosphate, each accurately weighed, to a 500-mL volumetric flask. Dissolve in and dilute with water to volume. Adjust with phosphoric acid solution (10 in 100) or sodium hydroxide solution (10 in 100) to a pH of 8.0 ± 0.1. Transfer 25.0 mL of this solution to a 100-mL volumetric flask, and dilute with water to volume. Adjust with phosphoric acid solution (10 in 100) or sodium hydroxide solution (10 in 100) to a pH of 8.0 ± 0.1.
   Solution A—Use filtered and degassed water.
   Solution B—Use filtered and degassed acetonitrile.
   Mobile phase—Use variable mixtures of *Solution A* and *Solution B* as directed for *Chromatographic system.* Make adjustments if necessary (see *System Suitability* under *Chromatography* ⟨621⟩).
   Blank solution—Use acetonitrile.
   Standard solution—Dissolve an accurately weighed quantity of 1-[(tetrahydro-2-furanyl)carbonyl]piperazine in acetonitrile to obtain a solution having a known concentration of about 1.0 mg per mL. Dilute quantitatively, and stepwise if necessary, with acetonitrile, to obtain a solution having a known concentration of about 5 μg per mL.
   Test solution—Transfer about 125 mg of Terazosin Hydrochloride, accurately weighed, to a 25-mL volumetric flask; dissolve in and dilute with a mixture of acetonitrile and water (1 : 1) to volume; and mix.
   Derivatization procedure—Transfer 5-mL portions of the *Blank solution,* the *Standard solution,* and the *Test solution,* each to a separate 100-mL volumetric flask, and proceed with each as follows. Add 5.0 mL of *Phosphate buffer solution,* and mix. Add 10.0 mL of *Derivatization solution* while swirling, allow to stand at room temperature for about 20 minutes, and mix. Dilute with a mixture of acetonitrile and water (1 : 1) to volume, and mix.
   Chromatographic system (see *Chromatography* ⟨621⟩)—The liquid chromatograph is equipped with a 254-nm detector and a 4.6-mm × 25-cm analytical column that contains packing L7. The flow rate is 1.5 mL per minute, except it is changed to 2.0 mL per minute during the period between 40 and 80 minutes. The chromatograph is programmed as follows.

Terazosin / Official Monographs

Time (minutes)	Solution A (%)	Solution B (%)	Elution
0–35	82	18	isocratic
35–40	82→10	18→90	linear gradient
40–75	10	90	isocratic
75–80	10→82	90→18	linear gradient
80–100	82	18	isocratic

Separately inject equal volumes (about 50 µL) of the derivatized *Blank solution* and the derivatized *Standard solution,* and measure the peak responses as directed for *Procedure,* ensuring that the peaks in the chromatogram of the derivatized *Standard solution* that correspond to those obtained from the derivatized *Blank solution* do not interfere with the determination: the retention time for 1-[(tetrahydro-2-furanyl)carbonyl]piperazine is more than 22 minutes; the column efficiency is not less than 3500 theoretical plates; and the relative standard deviation for replicate injections is not more than 3.0%.

Procedure—Separately inject equal volumes (about 50 µL) of the derivatized *Standard solution* and the derivatized *Test solution* into the chromatograph, record the chromatograms, and measure the peak areas. Calculate the percentage of 1-[(tetrahydro-2-furanyl)carbonyl]piperazine in the portion of Terazosin Hydrochloride taken by the formula:

$$2500(C/W)(r_U / r_S)$$

in which C is the concentration, in mg per mL, of 1-[(tetrahydro-2-furanyl)carbonyl]piperazine in the *Standard solution;* W is the weight, in mg, of Terazosin Hydrochloride taken to prepare the *Test solution;* and r_U and r_S are the peak areas for 1-[(tetrahydro-2-furanyl)carbonyl]piperazine derivative obtained from the derivatized *Test solution* and the derivatized *Standard solution,* respectively: not more than 0.1% is found.

Related compounds—

pH 3.2 Citrate buffer, Standard stock preparation, and *Mobile phase*—Proceed as directed in the *Assay.*

Diluent 1—Dissolve 6.0 g of sodium citrate and 4.0 g of anhydrous citric acid in water, dilute with water to 1.0 L, and mix.

Diluent 2—Prepare a mixture of water, acetonitrile, and methanol (60 : 30 : 10).

Standard stock solution 1—Dissolve an accurately weighed quantity of USP Terazosin Related Compound A RS in *Diluent 1,* and dilute with *Diluent 1* to obtain a solution having a known concentration of about 0.5 mg per mL.

Standard stock solution 2—Dissolve an accurately weighed quantity of USP Terazosin Related Compound B RS in methanol, and dilute with methanol to obtain a solution having a known concentration of about 0.5 mg per mL.

Standard stock solution 3—Dissolve an accurately weighed quantity of USP Terazosin Related Compound C RS in *Diluent 2,* and dilute with *Diluent 2* to obtain a solution having a known concentration of about 0.1 mg per mL.

Standard solution—Transfer 5.0 mL of *Standard stock preparation,* 4.0 mL of *Standard stock solution 1,* 4.0 mL of *Standard stock solution 2,* and 20 mL of *Standard stock solution 3* to a 100-mL volumetric flask containing about 60 mL of *Diluent 2.* Dilute with *Diluent 2* to volume, and mix. Transfer 10.0 mL of this solution to a 100-mL volumetric flask, dilute with *Mobile phase* to volume, and mix.

Test solution—Use the *Assay stock preparation* prepared as directed in the *Assay.*

Chromatographic system—Prepare as directed in the *Assay.* Chromatograph the *Mobile phase,* and record the peak responses as directed for *Procedure:* ensure that there are no significant interfering peaks. Chromatograph the *Standard solution,* and record the peak responses as directed for *Procedure:* the relative retention times are about 0.2 for terazosin related compound A, 1.0 for terazosin, 1.48 for terazosin related compound B, and 2.57 for terazosin related compound C; the resolution, R, between terazosin and terazosin related compound B is not less than 9.0; the column efficiency determined from the terazosin peak is not less than 12,000 theoretical plates; the tailing factor for the terazosin related compound C peak is not more than 3.0; and the relative standard deviation for replicate injections determined from the terazosin peak is not more than 2.0%, and not more than 5.0% determined from the terazosin related compound C peak.

Procedure—Separately inject equal volumes (about 20 µL) of the *Standard solution* and the *Test solution* into the chromatograph, record the chromatograms for about 60 minutes, and measure the peak responses. Separately calculate the quantities, in mg, of terazosin related compound A and terazosin related compound C in the portion of Terazosin Hydrochloride taken by the formula:

$$200C(r_U / r_S)$$

in which C is the concentration, in mg per mL, of the appropriate USP Reference Standard in the *Standard solution;* and r_U and r_S are the peak responses for the corresponding related compound obtained from the *Test solution* and the *Standard solution,* respectively: not more than 0.3% of terazosin related compound A is found; and not more than 0.4% of terazosin related compound C is found. Calculate the quantity, in mg, of each impurity in the portion of Terazosin Hydrochloride taken by the formula:

$$200C(r_i / r_T)$$

in which C is the concentration, in mg per mL, of USP Terazosin Hydrochloride RS in the *Standard solution;* r_i is the peak response for each impurity, other than terazosin related compound A and terazosin related compound C, obtained from the *Test solution;* and r_T is the terazosin peak response obtained from the *Standard solution:* not more than 0.3% of any impurity eluting prior to the terazosin peak is found; not more than 0.1% of any other impurity is found; and not more than 0.6% of total impurities is found.

Assay—

pH 3.2 Citrate buffer—Dissolve 12.0 g of sodium citrate dihydrate and 28.5 g of anhydrous citric acid in 1.95 L of water. Adjust with anhydrous citric acid or sodium citrate to a pH of 3.2 ± 0.1. Dilute with water to 2.0 L, and mix.

Mobile phase—Prepare a filtered and degassed mixture of *pH 3.2 Citrate buffer* and acetonitrile (1685 : 315). Make adjustments if necessary (see *System Suitability* under *Chromatography* ⟨621⟩).

Standard stock preparation—Dissolve an accurately weighed quantity of USP Terazosin Hydrochloride RS in *Mobile phase,* and dilute with *Mobile phase* to obtain a solution having a known concentration of about 0.5 mg per mL.

Standard preparation—Transfer 10.0 mL of *Standard stock preparation* to a 50-mL volumetric flask, and dilute with *Mobile phase* to volume. Transfer 10.0 mL of this solution to a 100-mL volumetric flask, dilute with *Mobile phase* to volume; and mix.

Assay stock preparation—Transfer about 100 mg of Terazosin Hydrochloride, accurately weighed, to a 200-mL volumetric flask; dissolve in and dilute with *Mobile phase* to volume; and mix.

Assay preparation—Transfer 10.0 mL of *Assay stock preparation* to a 50-mL volumetric flask, dilute with *Mobile phase* to volume, and mix. Transfer 10.0 mL of this solution to a 100-mL volumetric flask, dilute with *Mobile phase* to volume, and mix.

Chromatographic system (see *Chromatography* ⟨621⟩)—The liquid chromatograph is equipped with a 254-nm detector and a 4.6-mm × 25-cm column that contains packing L7. The column temperature is maintained at about 30°. The flow rate is about 1.0 mL per minute. Chromatograph the *Mobile phase,* and record the peak responses as directed for *Procedure:* ensure that there are no significant interfering peaks. Chromatograph the *Standard preparation,* and record the peak responses as directed for *Procedure:* the column efficiency is not less than 12,000 theoretical plates; the tailing factor is not less than 0.9 and not more than 1.3; and the relative standard deviation for replicate injections is not more than 0.9%.

Procedure—Separately inject equal volumes (about 20 µL) of the *Standard preparation* and the *Assay preparation* into the chromatograph, record the chromatograms for about 45 minutes, and measure the peak responses. Calculate the quantity, in mg, of $C_{19}H_{25}N_5O_4 \cdot HCl$ in the portion of Terazosin Hydrochloride taken by the formula:

$$10,000C(r_U / r_S)$$

in which C is the concentration, in mg per mL, of USP Terazosin Hydrochloride RS in the *Standard preparation;* and r_U and r_S are the peak responses obtained from the *Assay preparation* and the *Standard preparation*, respectively.

Terbutaline Sulfate

$(C_{12}H_{19}NO_3)_2 \cdot H_2SO_4$ 548.65
1,3-Benzenediol, 5-[2-[(1,1-dimethylethyl)amino]-1-hydroxyethyl]-, sulfate (2 : 1) (salt).
($\pm$)-α-[(*tert*-Butylamino)methyl]-3,5-dihydroxybenzyl alcohol sulfate (2 : 1) (salt)   [*23031-32-5*].

» Terbutaline Sulfate contains not less than 98.0 percent and not more than 101.0 percent of $(C_{12}H_{19}NO_3)_2 \cdot H_2SO_4$, calculated on the dried basis.

Packaging and storage—Preserve in well-closed, light-resistant containers, at controlled room temperature.
USP Reference standards ⟨11⟩—*USP Terbutaline Sulfate RS. USP Terbutaline Related Compound A RS.*
Identification—
  A: *Infrared Absorption* ⟨197K⟩.
  B: The retention time of the major peak in the chromatogram of the *Assay preparation* corresponds to that in the chromatogram of the *Standard preparation*, as obtained in the *Assay*.
Acidity—Dissolve 0.20 g in 10 mL of carbon dioxide-free water, and titrate with 0.020 N sodium hydroxide from a microburet to a pH of about 6, determining the endpoint potentiometrically, using a calomel-glass electrode system: not more than 0.50 mL of 0.020 N sodium hydroxide is required (0.3% as acetic acid).
Loss on drying ⟨731⟩—Dry it at 105° for 3 hours: it loses not more than 0.5% of its weight.
Residue on ignition ⟨281⟩: not more than 0.2%.
Heavy metals, *Method II* ⟨231⟩: 0.0025%.
Chromatographic purity—
  Ion-pair solution, Mobile phase, System suitability solution, and *Chromatographic system*—Proceed as directed in the *Assay*.
  Standard solution—Dissolve an accurately weighed quantity of USP Terbutaline Sulfate RS in *Mobile phase*, and dilute quantitatively, and stepwise if necessary, with *Mobile phase* to obtain a solution having a known concentration of about 3 µg per mL.
  Test solution—Use the *Assay preparation*.
  Procedure—Separately inject equal volumes (about 20 µL) of the *Standard solution* and the *Test solution* into the chromatograph, record the chromatograms, and measure the peak responses. Calculate the percentage of each impurity, if present, in the portion of Terbutaline Sulfate taken by the formula:

$$5000(C/W)(r_i / r_S)$$

in which *C* is the concentration, in mg per mL, of USP Terbutaline Sulfate RS in the *Standard solution; W* is the weight, in mg, of Terbutaline Sulfate taken to prepare the *Test solution; r_i* is the peak response for each impurity obtained from the *Test solution;* and r_S is the terbutaline peak response obtained from the *Standard solution:* the sum of all impurities is not more than 1.0%.
Organic volatile impurities, *Method I* ⟨467⟩: meets the requirements.

(Official until July 1, 2008)

Assay—
  Ion-pair solution—Transfer 3.15 g of ammonium formate to a 1000-mL volumetric flask, dissolve in about 900 mL of water, adjust the solution with formic acid to a pH of about 3.0, add 5.49 g of sodium 1-hexanesulfonate, dilute with water to volume, and mix.
  Mobile phase—Prepare a filtered and degassed mixture of *Ion-pair solution* and methanol (77 : 23). Make adjustments if necessary (see *System Suitability* under *Chromatography* ⟨621⟩).
  System suitability solution—Dissolve accurately weighed quantities of USP Terbutaline Sulfate RS and USP Terbutaline Related Compound A RS in *Mobile phase*, and dilute quantitatively, and stepwise if necessary, with *Mobile phase* to obtain a solution having known concentrations of 1.0 mg per mL and 0.4 mg per mL, respectively.
  Standard preparation—Dissolve an accurately weighed quantity of USP Terbutaline Sulfate RS in *Mobile phase*, and dilute quantitatively, and stepwise if necessary, with *Mobile phase* to obtain a solution having a known concentration of about 1.0 mg per mL.
  Assay preparation—Transfer about 50 mg of Terbutaline Sulfate, accurately weighed, to a 50-mL volumetric flask, dissolve in and dilute with *Mobile phase* to volume, and mix.
  Chromatographic system (see *Chromatography* ⟨621⟩)—The liquid chromatograph is equipped with a 276-nm detector and a 4.6-mm × 15-cm column that contains 5-µm packing L1. The flow rate is about 1 mL per minute. Chromatograph the *System suitability solution,* and record the peak responses as directed for *Procedure:* the relative retention times for terbutaline related compound A and terbutaline are 0.9 and 1.0, respectively; the resolution, *R,* between terbutaline related compound A and terbutaline is not less than 2.0; the column efficiency is not less than 1500 theoretical plates; the tailing factor for the terbutaline peak is not more than 2.0; and the relative standard deviation for replicate injections determined from the terbutaline peak is not more than 2.0%.
  Procedure—Separately inject equal volumes (about 20 µL) of the *Standard preparation* and the *Assay preparation* into the chromatograph, record the chromatograms, and measure the responses for the major peaks. Calculate the quantity, in mg, of $(C_{12}H_{19}NO_3)_2 \cdot H_2SO_4$ in the portion of Terbutaline Sulfate taken by the formula:

$$50C(r_U / r_S)$$

in which *C* is the concentration, in mg per mL, of USP Terbutaline Sulfate RS in the *Standard preparation;* and r_U and r_S are the peak responses obtained from the *Assay preparation* and the *Standard preparation,* respectively.

Terbutaline Sulfate Inhalation Aerosol

» Terbutaline Sulfate Inhalation Aerosol is a suspension of microfine Terbutaline Sulfate in suitable propellants in a pressurized container. It contains not less than 90.0 percent and not more than 110.0 percent of the labeled amount of $(C_{12}H_{19}NO_3)_2 \cdot H_2SO_4$.

Packaging and storage—Preserve in small, nonreactive, light-resistant aerosol containers equipped with metered-dose valves and provided with oral inhalation actuators. Store at controlled room temperature.
USP Reference standards ⟨11⟩—*USP Terbutaline Sulfate RS. USP Terbutaline Related Compound A RS.*
Identification—Chill 10 filled containers to about −75° in a dry ice-acetone mixture for 15 to 20 minutes. Carefully remove the top of each container with a tube cutter, allow to stand for 15 minutes, and pour the contents into a 100-mL beaker. Pour about 5 mL of the combined contents into a 100-mL beaker containing 50 mL of chloroform, shake, and filter through a medium-porosity sintered-glass funnel. Wash the residue with five 10-mL portions of chloroform. Allow the residue to dry by drawing air through the funnel: the IR absorption spectrum of a potassium bromide dispersion of the residue so obtained exhibits maxima only at the same wavelengths as that of a similar preparation of USP Terbutaline Sulfate RS.
Water, *Method I* ⟨921⟩—Transfer the contents of a weighed container to the titration vessel by attaching the valve stem to an inlet tube. Weigh the empty container, and determine the weight of the specimen taken. The *Water* content, determined by *Method I* ⟨921⟩, is not more than 0.02%.
Delivered dose uniformity over the entire contents: meets the requirements for *Metered-Dose Inhalers* under *Aerosols, Nasal Sprays, Metered-Dose Inhalers, and Dry Powder Inhalers* ⟨601⟩.

PROCEDURE FOR DOSE UNIFORMITY—
4-Aminoantipyrine solution—On the day of use, prepare a solution of 4-aminoantipyrine in water having a concentration of 20 mg per mL.

Potassium ferricyanide solution—On the day of use, prepare a solution of potassium ferricyanide in water having a concentration of 80 mg per mL.

Standard preparation—Dissolve an accurately weighed quantity of USP Terbutaline Sulfate RS in water, and dilute quantitatively and stepwise with water to obtain a solution having a known concentration of about 20 µg of terbutaline sulfate per mL.

Test preparation—Discharge the minimum recommended dose into the sampling apparatus and detach the inhaler as directed. Rinse the apparatus (filter and interior) with four 4.0-mL portions of 0.01 N sulfuric acid, and quantitatively transfer the resulting solutions to a 50-mL centrifuge tube. Wash the apparatus (filter and interior) with 10 mL of chloroform, and add the washing to the solution in the centrifuge tube. Wash the apparatus (filter and interior) with 4.0 mL of 0.01 N sulfuric acid, and quantitatively transfer the resulting liquid to the same centrifuge tube. Shake vigorously for 1 minute, and centrifuge for 10 minutes. Use the clear aqueous phase as the *Test preparation*.

Procedure—Pipet 2 mL of the *Test preparation*, 2 mL of the *Standard preparation*, and 2 mL of water to serve as a reagent blank, into separate 1-cm stoppered cells. To each cell add 0.5 mL of *4-Aminoantipyrine solution*, and mix. Add 0.5 mL of *Potassium ferricyanide solution* to each cell, and mix. Thirty seconds, accurately timed, after the addition of the *Potassium ferricyanide solution*, determine the absorbances of the solutions against the blank, at the wavelength of maximum absorbance at about 550 nm. Calculate the quantity, in µg, of $(C_{12}H_{19}NO_3)_2 \cdot H_2SO_4$ contained in the minimum dose taken by the formula:

$$10CN(A_U/A_S)$$

in which C is the concentration, in µg per mL, of USP Terbutaline Sulfate RS in the *Standard preparation*; N is the number of sprays discharged to obtain the minimum dose; and A_U and A_S are the absorbances of the solutions from the *Test preparation* and the *Standard preparation*, respectively, corrected for the absorbances of the reagent blank solution.

Particle size—Prime the valve of Aerosol container by alternately shaking and firing it several times, and actuate one measured spray onto a clean, dry microscope slide held 5 cm from the end of the oral inhalation actuator, perpendicular to the direction of the spray. Carefully rinse the slide with about 2 mL of carbon tetrachloride, and allow to dry. Prepare four additional slides in the same manner from four additional containers. Examine each slide under a microscope equipped with a calibrated ocular micrometer, using 450× magnification. Focus on the particles of 5 fields of view on each slide, near the center of the test specimen pattern, and note the size of the majority of individual particles. They are less than 5 µm along the longest axis. Record the number and size of all individual crystalline particles (not agglomerates) more than 10 µm in length, measured along the longest axis: not more than 10 such particles are observed.

Assay—
Mobile phase—Prepare a solution containing 750 mL of water, 140 mL of methanol, 110 mL of tetrahydrofuran, and 1.08 g of sodium 1-octanesulfonate. Filter and degas. Make adjustments if necessary (see *System Suitability* under *Chromatography* ⟨621⟩).

Resolution solution—Dissolve suitable quantities of USP Terbutaline Sulfate RS and USP Terbutaline Related Compound A RS in water to obtain a solution containing about 50 µg per mL and 20 µg per mL, respectively.

Standard preparation—Dissolve an accurately weighed quantity of USP Terbutaline Sulfate RS in water to obtain a solution having a known concentration of about 0.3 mg per mL.

Assay preparation—Accurately weigh not fewer than three containers, and separately perform the following procedure for each of the units. Chill in a dry ice–acetone mixture to about −75° for 15 to 20 minutes. Quickly and carefully remove the top of the container with a tube cutter. Allow the propellants to evaporate at room temperature for 10 to 15 minutes. [NOTE—Avoid complete evaporation of the propellants.] Quantitatively transfer the suspension to a 500-mL separatory funnel with the aid of chloroform. Wash all parts of the container alternately with several small portions of chloroform followed by small portions of 0.01 N sulfuric acid. Transfer the washings to the separatory funnel, and adjust the phase volumes to about 100 mL each with chloroform and 0.01 N sulfuric acid, respectively. Dry the container and all of its parts at 105° for 1 hour. Cool to room temperature, and weigh. Shake the separatory funnel for 1 minute, allow the phases to separate, and discard the chloroform layer. Pass the acidic aqueous phase through filter paper into a 250-mL volumetric flask. Wash the separatory funnel with two 10-mL portions of water, and transfer the washings to the volumetric flask. Dilute with water to volume, mix, and filter, discarding the first 2 mL of the filtrate.

Chromatographic system (see *Chromatography* ⟨621⟩)—The liquid chromatograph is equipped with a 280-nm detector, a 0.5-µm precolumn, and a 6.2-mm × 8-cm column that contains 3-µm packing L7. The column temperature is maintained at 40°. The flow rate is about 1.5 mL per minute. Chromatograph the *Resolution solution*, and record the peak responses as directed for *Procedure*: the relative retention times are about 1.0 and 0.83 for terbutaline and terbutaline related compound A, respectively; and the resolution, R, between terbutaline sulfate and terbutaline related compound A is not less than 1.6. Chromatograph the *Standard preparation*, and record the peak responses as directed for *Procedure*: the relative standard deviation for replicate injections is not more than 2.0%.

Procedure—Separately inject equal volumes (about 20 µL) of the *Standard preparation* and the *Assay preparation* into the chromatograph, record the chromatograms, and measure the responses for the major peaks. Calculate the quantity, in mg, of terbutaline sulfate $[(C_{12}H_{19}NO_3)_2 \cdot H_2SO_4]$ in each container taken by the formula:

$$250C(r_U/r_S)$$

in which C is the concentration, in mg per mL, of USP Terbutaline Sulfate RS in the *Standard preparation*; and r_U and r_S are the peak responses obtained from the *Assay preparation* and the *Standard preparation*, respectively.

Terbutaline Sulfate Injection

» Terbutaline Sulfate Injection is a sterile solution of Terbutaline Sulfate in Water for Injection. It contains not less than 90.0 percent and not more than 110.0 percent of the labeled amount of $(C_{12}H_{19}NO_3)_2 \cdot H_2SO_4$.

NOTE—Do not use the Injection if it is discolored.

Packaging and storage—Preserve in single-dose containers, preferably of Type I glass, protected from light, at controlled room temperature.

USP Reference standards ⟨11⟩—*USP Endotoxin RS. USP Terbutaline Sulfate RS.*

Identification—
A: Apply 2 µL of Injection and 2 µL of a solution of USP Terbutaline Sulfate RS in sodium chloride solution (0.9 in 100) containing 1 mg per mL to a suitable thin-layer chromatographic plate (see *Chromatography* ⟨621⟩) coated with a 0.25-mm layer of chromatographic silica gel. Develop the chromatogram in a solvent system consisting of a mixture of isopropyl alcohol, cyclohexane, and formic acid (13 : 5 : 1) until the solvent front has moved about three-fourths of the length of the plate. Remove the plate from the developing chamber, mark the solvent front, and dry with a current of air. Spray the plate with a 1 in 50 solution of 4-aminoantipyrine in methanol, allow to air-dry, and spray with a 2 in 25 solution of potassium ferricyanide in a solvent prepared by mixing ammonium hydroxide with water (4 : 1): the R_F value of the principal spot obtained from the Injection corresponds to that obtained from the Standard solution.

B: The retention time of the major peak in the chromatogram of the *Assay preparation* corresponds to that in the chromatogram of the *Standard preparation* as obtained in the *Assay*.

Bacterial endotoxins ⟨85⟩—It contains not more than 1250.0 USP Endotoxin Units per mg of terbutaline sulfate.

pH ⟨791⟩: between 3.0 and 5.0.
Other requirements—It meets the requirements under *Injections* ⟨1⟩.
Assay—
Mobile phase, Standard preparation, and *Chromatographic system*—Prepare as directed in the *Assay* under *Terbutaline Sulfate.*
Assay preparation—Use Injection. If necessary, quantitatively dilute an accurately measured volume of Injection with water to obtain a solution having a concentration of about 1 mg per mL.
Procedure—Separately inject equal volumes (about 20 µL) of the *Standard preparation* and the *Assay preparation* into the chromatograph, record the chromatograms, and measure the responses for the major peaks. Calculate the quantity, in mg, of $(C_{12}H_{19}NO_3)_2 \cdot H_2SO_4$ in each mL of the Injection taken by the formula:

$$(LC/D)(r_U/r_S)$$

in which L is the labeled quantity, in mg per mL, of terbutaline sulfate in the Injection, C is the concentration, in mg per mL, of USP Terbutaline Sulfate RS in the *Standard preparation*, D is the concentration, in mg per mL, of terbutaline sulfate in the *Assay preparation*, based upon the labeled quantity, in mg per mL, of terbutaline sulfate in the Injection and the extent of dilution, and r_U and r_S are the terbutaline peak responses obtained from the *Assay preparation* and the *Standard preparation*, respectively.

Terbutaline Sulfate Tablets

» Terbutaline Sulfate Tablets contain not less than 90.0 percent and not more than 110.0 percent of the labeled amount of $(C_{12}H_{19}NO_3)_2 \cdot H_2SO_4$.

Packaging and storage—Preserve in tight containers, at controlled room temperature.
USP Reference standards ⟨11⟩—*USP Terbutaline Sulfate RS. USP Terbutaline Related Compound A RS.*
Identification—The retention time of the major peak in the chromatogram of the *Assay preparation* corresponds to that in the chromatogram of the *Standard preparation*, as obtained in the *Assay.*
Dissolution, *Procedure for a Pooled Sample* ⟨711⟩—
Medium: water; 900 mL.
Apparatus 1: 100 rpm.
Time: 45 minutes.
Procedure—Determine the amount of $(C_{12}H_{19}NO_3)_2 \cdot H_2SO_4$ dissolved, employing the procedure set forth in the *Assay*, making any necessary modifications.
Tolerances—Not less than 75% (*Q*) of the labeled amount of $(C_{12}H_{19}NO_3)_2 \cdot H_2SO_4$ is dissolved in 45 minutes.
Uniformity of dosage units ⟨905⟩: meet the requirements.
Assay—
Ion-pair solution, Mobile phase, System suitability solution, and *Chromatographic system*—Proceed as directed in the *Assay* under *Terbutaline Sulfate.*
Standard preparation—Dissolve an accurately weighed quantity of USP Terbutaline Sulfate RS in *Mobile phase*, and dilute quantitatively, and stepwise if necessary, with *Mobile phase* to obtain a solution having a known concentration of about 1 mg per mL. Transfer 10.0 mL of the solution so obtained to a 100-mL volumetric flask, add 10 mL of 0.05 N sulfuric acid, dilute with water to volume, and mix.
Assay preparation—Weigh and finely powder not fewer than 20 Tablets. Transfer an accurately weighed portion of the powder, equivalent to about 10 mg of terbutaline sulfate, to a 100-mL volumetric flask. Add 10 mL of 0.05 N sulfuric acid and 20 mL of water, and shake for 15 minutes. Dilute with water to volume, mix, and filter.
Procedure—Separately inject equal volumes (about 20 µL) of the *Standard preparation* and the *Assay preparation* into the chromatograph, record the chromatograms, and measure the responses for the major peaks. Calculate the quantity, in mg, of terbutaline sulfate $[(C_{12}H_{19}NO_3)_2 \cdot H_2SO_4]$ in the portion of Tablets taken by the formula:

$$100C(r_U/r_S)$$

in which C is the concentration, in mg per mL, of USP Terbutaline Sulfate RS in the *Standard preparation*; and r_U and r_S are the terbutaline peak responses obtained from the *Assay preparation* and the *Standard preparation*, respectively.

Terpin Hydrate

$C_{10}H_{20}O_2 \cdot H_2O$ 190.28
Cyclohexanemethanol, 4-hydroxy-α,α,4-trimethyl-, monohydrate.
p-Menthane-1,8-diol monohydrate   [2451-01-6].
Anhydrous   172.27   [80-53-5].

» Terpin Hydrate contains not less than 98.0 percent and not more than 100.5 percent of $C_{10}H_{20}O_2$, calculated on the anhydrous basis.

Packaging and storage—Preserve in tight containers.
USP Reference standards ⟨11⟩—*USP Terpin Hydrate RS.*
Identification—
A: *Infrared Absorption* ⟨197K⟩: dried over a suitable desiccant for 4 hours.
B: Add a few drops of sulfuric acid to a hot solution: the liquid becomes turbid and develops a strongly aromatic odor.
Water, *Method I* ⟨921⟩: between 9.0% and 10.0%.
Residue on ignition ⟨281⟩: not more than 0.1%.
Residual turpentine—It has no odor of turpentine oil.
Assay—
Internal standard solution—Dissolve a quantity of biphenyl in chloroform to obtain a solution containing about 20 mg per mL.
Standard preparation—Transfer about 170 mg of USP Terpin Hydrate RS, accurately weighed, to a 100-mL volumetric flask, dissolve in 5 mL of alcohol, add 5.00 mL of *Internal standard solution*, dilute with chloroform to volume, and mix.
Assay preparation—Transfer about 170 mg of Terpin Hydrate, accurately weighed, to a 100-mL volumetric flask, and proceed as directed under *Standard preparation*, beginning with "dissolve in 5 mL of alcohol."
Chromatographic system—Under typical conditions, the gas chromatograph is equipped with a flame-ionization detector, and it contains a 3.5-mm × 1.2-m glass column packed with 6% G1 on support S1A; the injection port and the detector temperatures are maintained at 260°, and the column temperature at 120°; and nitrogen is used as the carrier gas, at a flow rate necessary to yield approximate retention times of 7 minutes for terpin and 11 minutes for biphenyl.
System suitability test—Chromatograph the *Standard preparation*, and record the chromatograms as directed for *Procedure*: the resolution, *R*, between the terpin and biphenyl peaks is not less than 2.0, and the relative standard deviation for replicate injections is not more than 2.0%.
Procedure—Inject about 1 µL of the *Standard preparation* into a suitable gas chromatograph, and record the chromatogram. Similarly, inject about 1 µL of the *Assay preparation*, and record the chromatogram. Calculate the quantity, in mg, of $C_{10}H_{20}O_2$ in the portion of Terpin Hydrate taken by the formula:

$$W_S(R_U/R_S)$$

in which W_S is the weight, in mg, of USP Terpin Hydrate RS, calculated on the anhydrous basis; and R_U and R_S are the area-ratios of terpin to the internal standard obtained from the chromatograms for the *Assay preparation* and the *Standard preparation*, respectively.

Terpin Hydrate Oral Solution

» Terpin Hydrate Oral Solution contains, in each 100 mL, not less than 1.53 g and not more than 1.87 g of terpin hydrate ($C_{10}H_{20}O_2 \cdot H_2O$).

Packaging and storage—Preserve in tight containers.
USP Reference standards ⟨11⟩—*USP Terpin Hydrate RS*.
Alcohol content, *Method II* ⟨611⟩: between 90.0% and 110.0% of the labeled amount of C_2H_5OH.
Assay—
Internal standard solution, *Standard preparation*, *Chromatographic system*, and *System suitability test*—Proceed as directed in the *Assay* under *Terpin Hydrate*.
Assay preparation—Pipet 10 mL of Oral Solution into a separator, add 20 mL of water and 10 mL of 5 N sodium hydroxide, and extract with three 25-mL portions of chloroform, filtering each, successively, through cotton. Rinse the cotton with chloroform. To the combined rinse and extracts add 5.00 mL of *Internal standard solution*, and mix.
Procedure—Inject about 1 µL of the *Standard preparation* into a suitable gas chromatograph, and record the chromatogram. Similarly, inject about 1 µL of the *Assay preparation*, and record the chromatogram. Calculate the quantity, in mg, of terpin hydrate ($C_{10}H_{20}O_2 \cdot H_2O$) in each mL of the Oral Solution taken by the formula:

$$0.1(190.28/172.27)W_S(R_U/R_S)$$

in which 190.28 and 172.27 are the molecular weights of terpin hydrate ($C_{10}H_{20}O_2 \cdot H_2O$) and anhydrous terpin ($C_{10}H_{20}O_2$), respectively; W_S is the weight, in mg, of USP Terpin Hydrate RS, calculated on the anhydrous basis; and R_U and R_S are the area-ratios of terpin to biphenyl obtained from the chromatograms for the *Assay preparation* and the *Standard preparation*, respectively.

Terpin Hydrate and Codeine Oral Solution

» Terpin Hydrate and Codeine Oral Solution contains, in each 100 mL, not less than 1.53 g and not more than 1.87 g of terpin hydrate ($C_{10}H_{20}O_2 \cdot H_2O$), and not less than 180 mg and not more than 220 mg of codeine ($C_{18}H_{21}NO_3 \cdot H_2O$).

Packaging and storage—Preserve in tight containers.
USP Reference standards ⟨11⟩—*USP Terpin Hydrate RS. USP Codeine Phosphate RS*.
Identification—
Developing solvent—Prepare a mixture of methylene chloride and methanol (9 : 1).
Standard solution A—Dissolve a suitable quantity of USP Terpin Hydrate RS in methylene chloride to obtain a solution having a concentration of about 3 mg per mL. [NOTE—A small volume of methanol may be used to aid dissolution of the terpin hydrate.]
Standard solution B—Transfer 20 mg of USP Codeine Phosphate RS to a suitable separator containing 10 mL of water, add 1 mL of 1 N sodium hydroxide, and mix. Add 10 mL of methylene chloride, and shake for 1 minute. Allow the layers to separate, and drain the lower organic layer into a suitable flask. Discard the aqueous layer.
Test solution—Transfer 10 mL of Oral Solution to a suitable separator containing 10 mL of water, and add 1 mL of 1 N sodium hydroxide. Add 10 mL of methylene chloride, shake for 1 minute, and allow the layers to separate. Use the clear lower organic layer as the *Test solution*.
Procedure—Apply separately 5 µL of *Standard solution A*, *Standard solution B*, and the *Test solution* to a suitable thin-layer chromatographic plate (see *Chromatography* ⟨621⟩) coated with a 0.25-mm layer of chromatographic silica gel mixture. Develop the chromatogram in a chromatographic chamber containing the *Developing solvent* until the solvent front has moved three-fourths of the length of the plate. Remove the plate from the chromatographic chamber, mark the solvent front, and allow the plate to dry. Examine the plate under short-wavelength UV light, and mark the location of the codeine spots. Spray the plate with phosphomolybdic acid TS, and heat at 105° for 5 minutes. The terpin hydrate spots appear blue on a yellow background. The R_F values of the spots due to terpin hydrate and codeine obtained from the *Test solution* correspond to those obtained from *Standard solutions A* and *B*, respectively.
Alcohol content, *Method II* ⟨611⟩: between 90.0% and 110.0% of the labeled amount of C_2H_5OH.
Assay for terpin hydrate—
Internal standard solution—Prepare a chloroform solution containing 20 mg of biphenyl and 2.6 mg of *N*-phenylcarbazole in each mL.
Standard preparation—Transfer about 26 mg of USP Codeine Phosphate RS and about 170 mg of USP Terpin Hydrate RS, both accurately weighed, to a separator, add 5 mL of alcohol, shake to dissolve the terpin hydrate, add 25 mL of water to dissolve the codeine phosphate, add 10 mL of 5 N sodium hydroxide, and extract with three 25-mL portions of chloroform, filtering each, successively, through cotton. Rinse the cotton with chloroform. To the combined rinse and extracts add 5.00 mL of *Internal standard solution*, and mix.
Assay preparation—Pipet 10 mL of Oral Solution into a separator, add 20 mL of water and 10 mL of 5 N sodium hydroxide, and extract with three 25-mL portions of chloroform, filtering each, successively, through cotton. Rinse the cotton with chloroform. To the combined rinse and extracts add 5.00 mL of *Internal standard solution*, and mix.
Chromatographic system and *System suitability*—Proceed as directed in the *Assay* under *Terpin Hydrate*. [NOTE—Heat the column to 230° to remove the *N*-phenylcarbazole and codeine from prior injections.]
Procedure—Inject about 1 µL of the *Standard preparation* into a suitable gas chromatograph, and record the chromatogram. Similarly, inject about 1 µL of the *Assay preparation*, and record the chromatogram. Calculate the quantity, in mg, of terpin hydrate ($C_{10}H_{20}O_2 \cdot H_2O$) in each mL of the Oral Solution taken by the formula:

$$0.1(190.28/172.27)W_S(R_U/R_S)$$

in which 190.28 and 172.27 are the molecular weights of terpin hydrate ($C_{10}H_{20}O_2 \cdot H_2O$) and anhydrous terpin ($C_{10}H_{20}O_2$); respectively; W_S is the weight, in mg, of USP Terpin Hydrate RS, calculated on the anhydrous basis; and R_U and R_S are the area-ratios of terpin to biphenyl obtained from the chromatograms for the *Assay preparation* and the *Standard preparation*, respectively.
Assay for codeine—
Internal standard solution—Prepare as directed under *Assay for terpin hydrate*.
Standard preparation—Evaporate the remaining *Standard preparation* for Oral Solution from the *Assay for terpin hydrate* nearly to dryness, and dissolve the residue in about 20 mL of chloroform.
Assay preparation—Evaporate the remaining *Assay preparation* for Oral Solution from the *Assay for terpin hydrate* nearly to dryness, and dissolve the residue in about 20 mL of chloroform.
Chromatographic system and *System suitability*—Proceed as directed in the *Assay* under *Terpin Hydrate*, except to maintain the temperature of the column at 230° instead of 120°.
Procedure—Proceed as directed under *Assay for terpin hydrate*, except to maintain the temperature of the column at 230° instead of 120°. The retention times for *N*-phenylcarbazole and codeine are about 7 minutes and 10 minutes, respectively. Calculate the quantity, in mg, of codeine ($C_{18}H_{21}NO_3 \cdot H_2O$) in each mL of the Oral Solution taken by the formula:

$$0.1(317.39/397.37)W_S(R_U/R_S)$$

in which 317.39 and 397.37 are the molecular weights of codeine ($C_{18}H_{21}NO_3 \cdot H_2O$) and codeine phosphate ($C_{18}H_{21}NO_3 \cdot H_3PO_4$), respectively; W_S is the weight, in mg, of USP Codeine Phosphate RS; and R_U and R_S are the area-ratios of codeine to *N*-phenylcarbazole

Testolactone

C₁₉H₂₄O₃   300.39
D-Homo-17a-oxaandrosta-1,4-diene-3,17-dione.
13-Hydroxy-3-oxo-13,17-secoandrosta-1,4-dien-17-oic acid δ-lactone [968-93-4].

» Testolactone contains not less than 95.0 percent and not more than 105.0 percent of C₁₉H₂₄O₃, calculated on the dried basis.

Packaging and storage—Preserve in tight containers.

USP Reference standards ⟨11⟩—*USP Testolactone RS*.
Identification—
  A: *Infrared Absorption* ⟨197K⟩.
  B: *Ultraviolet Absorption* ⟨197U⟩—
  Solution: 10 µg per mL.
  Medium: methanol.
Specific rotation ⟨781S⟩: between −44° and −52°.
  Test solution: 12.5 mg per mL, in chloroform.
Loss on drying ⟨731⟩—Dry it in vacuum at 100° for 3 hours: it loses not more than 1.0% of its weight.
Residue on ignition ⟨281⟩: not more than 0.1%.
Heavy metals, *Method II* ⟨231⟩: 0.003%.
Chromatographic purity—
  Standard preparation—Transfer 10 mg of USP Testolactone RS, accurately weighed, to a 50-mL volumetric flask, dissolve in acetone, dilute with acetone to volume, and mix.
  Test preparation—Transfer 250 mg of Testolactone, accurately weighed, to a 50-mL volumetric flask, dissolve in acetone, dilute with acetone to volume, and mix.
  Procedure—Coat a 20- × 20-cm thin-layer chromatographic plate (see *Chromatography* ⟨621⟩) with a 0.25-mm layer of chromatographic silica gel mixture, dry for 15 minutes at room temperature, heat at 105° for 1 hour, and cool in a desiccator. Divide the area of the plate into three approximately equal sections, the left and right sections to be used for the *Test preparation* and the *Standard preparation*, respectively, and the center section for the blank. Apply 10 µL of the *Standard preparation* and 20 µL of the *Test preparation* 2.5 cm from the bottom of the designated sections of the plate, and dry the spots with a current of air. Develop the chromatogram in a solvent system consisting of a mixture of butyl acetate and acetone (4 : 1) until the solvent front has moved to within about 1 cm of the top of the plate. Remove the plate from the developing chamber, mark the solvent front, and allow the solvent to evaporate. Locate the spots on the plate by viewing under short-wavelength UV light: the R_F value of the principal spot obtained from the *Test preparation* corresponds to that obtained from the *Standard preparation*, not more than two impurities are found in the chromatogram of the *Test preparation*, and the size and color of the spot representing any impurity obtained from the *Test preparation* are not greater or more intense than those of the principal spot obtained from the *Standard preparation*.
Ordinary impurities ⟨466⟩—
  Test solution: methanol.
  Standard solution: methanol.
  Eluant: a mixture of butyl acetate and acetone (4 : 1).
  Visualization: 6.
Organic volatile impurities, *Method V* ⟨467⟩: meets the requirements.
  Solvent—Use dimethyl sulfoxide.

(Official until July 1, 2008)

Assay—
  Isoniazid reagent—Dissolve 1.0 g of isoniazid in about 500 mL of methanol, add 1.25 mL of hydrochloric acid, dilute with methanol to 1000 mL, and mix.
  Standard preparation—Dissolve a suitable quantity of USP Testolactone RS, accurately weighed, in chloroform, and prepare, by quantitative, and stepwise dilution if necessary, a solution in chloroform having a known concentration of about 30 µg per mL.
  Assay preparation—Transfer about 60 mg of Testolactone, accurately weighed, to a 100-mL volumetric flask, dissolve in chloroform, dilute with chloroform to volume, and mix. Transfer 5.0 mL of this solution to a second 100-mL volumetric flask, dilute with chloroform to volume, and mix.
  Procedure—Transfer 5.0 mL each of the *Standard preparation*, the *Assay preparation*, and chloroform to provide the blank, to separate 25-mL volumetric flasks, add 10.0 mL of *Isoniazid reagent* to each flask, and mix. Place the flasks in a water bath maintained at a temperature of 55 ± 2°, and allow them to stand for 70 minutes. Cool, dilute each solution with chloroform to volume, and mix. Determine the absorbances of the solutions in 1-cm cells at the wavelength of maximum absorbance at about 415 nm, with a suitable spectrophotometer, against the blank. Calculate the quantity, in mg, of C₁₉H₂₄O₃ in the Testolactone taken by the formula:

$$2C(A_U / A_S)$$

in which C is the concentration, in µg per mL, of USP Testolactone RS in the *Standard preparation*, and A_U and A_S are the absorbances of the solutions from the *Assay preparation* and the *Standard preparation*, respectively.

Testolactone Tablets

» Testolactone Tablets contain not less than 90.0 percent and not more than 110.0 percent of the labeled amount of C₁₉H₂₄O₃.

Packaging and storage—Preserve in tight containers.
USP Reference standards ⟨11⟩—*USP Testolactone RS*.
Identification—
  A: *Hydroxylamine reagent*—Mix 5 mL of a solution of hydroxylamine hydrochloride in methanol (3.5 in 100) with 15 mL of a solution of potassium hydroxide in methanol (5.6 in 100), and use this reagent within 2 hours after mixing. [NOTE—Store the solution of hydroxylamine hydrochloride in methanol and the solution of potassium hydroxide in methanol in a refrigerator, and discard both after 1 month.]
  Iron reagent—Dissolve 1.5 g of ferric chloride in 30 mL of water, add 3 mL of perchloric acid and 15 mL of nitric acid, and heat the solution until dense, white fumes are produced. Cool, add 40 mL of water and 10 mL of nitric acid, and dilute with perchloric acid to 100 mL. [NOTE—This concentrate may be stored and used for several months.] Transfer 4.0 mL of this concentrate to a 100-mL volumetric flask, add 36 mL of alcohol, dilute with water to volume, and mix.
  Procedure—Place a portion of finely powdered Tablets, equivalent to about 250 mg of testolactone, in a 100-mL volumetric flask, add 85 mL of chloroform, and shake by mechanical means for 30 minutes. Add chloroform to volume, mix, and centrifuge the solution. Transfer 2 mL of the supernatant to a small test tube, and evaporate with the aid of a gentle current of air to dryness. Add 0.1 mL of *Hydroxylamine reagent*, heat in a water bath at about 60° for 1 minute, then add 1 mL of *Iron reagent*: a rose-violet color is produced.
  B: *Infrared Absorption* ⟨197K⟩—
  Test specimen—Place a portion of finely powdered Tablets, equivalent to about 100 mg of testolactone, in a glass-stoppered, 35-mL centrifuge tube. Add 20 mL of chloroform, insert the stopper, and shake by mechanical means for 10 minutes. Centrifuge the mixture, and filter the supernatant into a 50-mL beaker. Evaporate on a steam bath to dryness, and dry the residue in vacuum at 100° for 3 hours.

Dissolution ⟨711⟩—
Medium: 0.01 N hydrochloric acid; 900 mL.
Apparatus 2: 75 rpm.
Time: 120 minutes.
*Procedure—*Determine the amount of $C_{19}H_{24}O_3$ dissolved by employing UV absorption at the wavelength of maximum absorbance at about 247 nm on filtered portions of the solution under test, diluted with water if necessary, in comparison with a Standard solution having a known concentration of USP Testolactone RS in the same medium. An amount of methanol not to exceed 2% of the total volume of the Standard solution may be used to bring the testolactone standard into solution prior to dilution with water.
*Tolerances—*Not less than 80% (*Q*) of the labeled amount of $C_{19}H_{24}O_3$ is dissolved in 120 minutes.
Uniformity of dosage units ⟨905⟩: meet the requirements.
Assay—
Isoniazid reagent and *Standard preparation—*Prepare as directed in the *Assay* under *Testolactone*.
*Assay preparation—*Weigh and finely powder not fewer than 10 Tablets. Transfer an accurately weighed portion of the powder, equivalent to about 50 mg of testolactone, to a 100-mL volumetric flask, add 85 mL of chloroform, and shake by mechanical means for 30 minutes. Add chloroform to volume, mix, and centrifuge a portion of about 10 mL of the mixture. Transfer 3.0 mL of the clear supernatant to a 50-mL volumetric flask, dilute with chloroform to volume, and mix.
*Procedure—*Proceed as directed for *Procedure* in the *Assay* under *Testolactone*. Calculate the quantity, in mg, of $C_{19}H_{24}O_3$ in the portion of Tablets taken by the formula:

$$1.667C(A_U / A_S)$$

in which the terms are as defined therein.

Testosterone

$C_{19}H_{28}O_2$ 288.42
Androst-4-en-3-one, 17-hydroxy-, (17β)-.
17β-Hydroxyandrost-4-en-3-one [58-22-0].

» Testosterone contains not less than 97.0 percent and not more than 103.0 percent of $C_{19}H_{28}O_2$, calculated on the dried basis.

Packaging and storage—Preserve in well-closed containers. Store at 25°, excursions permitted between 15° and 30°.
USP Reference standards ⟨11⟩—*USP Testosterone RS.*
Identification—
  A: *Infrared Absorption* ⟨197K⟩.
  B: *Ultraviolet Absorption* ⟨197U⟩—
  Solution: 10 μg per mL.
  Medium: methanol.
Melting range ⟨741⟩: between 153° and 157°.
Specific rotation ⟨781S⟩: between +101° and +105°.
  Test solution: 10 mg per mL, in dioxane.
Loss on drying ⟨731⟩—Dry it in vacuum over phosphorus pentoxide for 4 hours: it loses not more than 1.0% of its weight.
Organic volatile impurities, *Method V* ⟨467⟩: meets the requirements.
  *Solvent—*Use dimethyl sulfoxide.

(Official until July 1, 2008)

Assay—
*Standard preparation—*Prepare as directed under *Single-Steroid Assay* ⟨511⟩, using USP Testosterone RS.
*Assay preparation—*Accurately weigh about 20 mg of Testosterone, previously dried; dissolve in a sufficient quantity of a mixture of equal volumes of alcohol and chloroform to make 10.0 mL; and mix.
*Procedure—*Proceed as directed for *Procedure* under *Single-Steroid Assay* ⟨511⟩, using a solvent system consisting of a mixture of benzene and ethyl acetate (1 : 1), through the fourth sentence of the second paragraph under *Procedure*. Then centrifuge the tubes for 5 minutes, and determine the absorbances of the supernatant in 1-cm cells at the wavelength of maximum absorbance at about 241 nm, with a suitable spectrophotometer, against the blank. Calculate the quantity, in mg, of $C_{19}H_{28}O_2$ in the portion of Testosterone taken by the formula:

$$10C(A_U / A_S)$$

in which *C* is the concentration, in mg per mL, of USP Testosterone RS in the *Standard preparation;* and A_U and A_S are the absorbances of the solutions from the *Assay preparation* and the *Standard preparation,* respectively.

Testosterone Injectable Suspension

» Testosterone Injectable Suspension is a sterile suspension of Testosterone in an aqueous medium. It contains not less than 90.0 percent and not more than 110.0 percent of the labeled amount of $C_{19}H_{28}O_2$.

Packaging and storage—Preserve in single-dose or multiple-dose containers, preferably of Type I glass.
USP Reference standards ⟨11⟩—*USP Endotoxin RS. USP Testosterone RS.*
Identification—The testosterone obtained by filtration and washing, as directed in the *Assay*, and dried at 105° to constant weight, meets the requirements for *Identification* tests *A* and *B* under *Testosterone*.
Bacterial endoxins ⟨85⟩—It contains not more than 3.5 USP Endotoxin Units per mg of testosterone.
Uniformity of dosage units ⟨905⟩: meets the requirements.
pH ⟨791⟩: between 4.0 and 7.5.
Other requirements—It meets the requirements under *Injections* ⟨1⟩.
Assay—Transfer an accurately measured volume of previously well-mixed Injectable Suspension, equivalent to about 100 mg of testosterone, to a fine-porosity, sintered-glass filtering crucible, previously dried at 105° for 1 hour, and filter with suction. If the filtrate is not clear, again pass it through the same filter into a second receiver. Wash the residue in the filter with several 5-mL portions of water until 2 mL of the last washing, when evaporated on a steam bath, leaves a negligible residue. [NOTE—If the Injectable Suspension is passed through the filter twice, rinse the first receiver with the portions of water before passing them through the filter.] Dry the crucible and the collected testosterone at 105° for 1 hour. Completely dissolve the testosterone with five 25-mL portions of methanol, passing each portion through the crucible under gentle suction, and transfer the combined methanol solution to a 200-mL volumetric flask. Rinse the crucible and receiver with two 25-mL portions of methanol, add the rinsings to the main solution, dilute with methanol to volume, and mix. Transfer 5.0 mL of this solution to a 250-mL volumetric flask, dilute with methanol to volume, and mix. Concomitantly determine the absorbances of this solution and a Standard solution of USP Testosterone RS, in the same medium having a known concentration of about 10 μg per mL in 1-cm cells at the wavelength of maximum absorbance at about 241 nm, with a suitable spectrophotometer, using methanol as the blank. Calculate the quantity, in mg, of $C_{19}H_{28}O_2$ in each mL of the Injectable Suspension taken by the formula:

$$(10C / V)(A_U / A_S)$$

in which *C* is the concentration, in μg per mL, of USP Testosterone RS in the Standard solution, *V* is the volume, in mL, of Injectable Suspension taken, and A_U and A_S are the absorbances of the solution

Testosterone Cypionate

$C_{27}H_{40}O_3$ 412.60

Androst-4-en-3-one, 17-(3-cyclopentyl-1-oxopropoxy)-, (17β)-.
Testosterone cyclopentanepropionate   [58-20-8].

» Testosterone Cypionate contains not less than 97.0 percent and not more than 103.0 percent of $C_{27}H_{40}O_3$, calculated on the dried basis.

Packaging and storage—Preserve in well-closed, light-resistant containers.

USP Reference standards ⟨11⟩—*USP Cholesteryl Caprylate RS. USP Testosterone Cypionate RS.*

Identification, *Infrared Absorption* ⟨197K⟩.

Melting range ⟨741⟩:   between 98° and 104°.

Specific rotation ⟨781S⟩:   between +85° and +92°.
  Test solution: 20 mg per mL, in chloroform.

Loss on drying ⟨731⟩—Dry it in vacuum over silica gel for 4 hours: it loses not more than 0.5% of its weight.

Residue on ignition ⟨281⟩:   not more than 0.2%.

Free cyclopentanepropionic acid—Dissolve 500 mg in 10 mL of alcohol that previously has been neutralized to a faint blue color following the addition of 2 or 3 drops of bromothymol blue TS, and promptly titrate with 0.01 N sodium hydroxide VS: not more than 0.70 mL of 0.01 N sodium hydroxide is required (0.20% of cyclopentanepropionic acid).

Organic volatile impurities, *Method V* ⟨467⟩:   meets the requirements.
  Solvent—Use dimethyl sulfoxide.

(Official until July 1, 2008)

Assay—

  Internal standard solution—Dissolve 80 mg of USP Cholesteryl Caprylate RS in a mixture of methanol and chloroform (4 : 1) in a 100-mL volumetric flask, then add the same solvent mixture to volume.

  Standard preparation—Weigh accurately about 10 mg of USP Testosterone Cypionate RS into a suitable vial, add by pipet 10 mL of *Internal standard solution*, and mix.

  Assay preparation—Prepare as directed for *Standard preparation*, using an accurately weighed portion of about 10 mg of Testosterone Cypionate instead of the Reference Standard.

  Procedure—Inject 1 μL of the *Assay preparation* and the *Standard preparation*, successively, into a suitable gas chromatograph fitted with a flame-ionization detector. Under typical conditions, the instrument contains a 3-mm × 1.2-m glass column packed with 1% (w/w) phase G6 on packing S1AB. The column temperature is maintained at 260° and the helium carrier gas flows at 50 mL per minute. In a suitable chromatogram, the resolution factor, *R* (see *Chromatography* ⟨621⟩), is not less than 3 between the internal standard and testosterone cypionate peaks, and five replicate injections of a single *Standard preparation* show a coefficient of variation of not more than 2% in the peak area ratio of testosterone cypionate to internal standard. Measure the areas under the peaks for testosterone cypionate and cholesteryl caprylate in each chromatogram. Calculate the ratio, R_U, of the area of the testosterone cypionate peak to the area of the internal standard peak in the chromatogram from the *Assay preparation*, and similarly calculate the ratio, R_S, in the chromatogram from the *Standard preparation*. Calculate the quantity, in mg, of $C_{27}H_{40}O_3$ in the portion of Testosterone Cypionate taken by the formula:

$$W(R_U / R_S)$$

in which *W* is the weight, in mg, of USP Testosterone Cypionate RS in the *Standard preparation*, and the other terms are as defined therein.

Testosterone Cypionate Injection

» Testosterone Cypionate Injection is a sterile solution of Testosterone Cypionate in a suitable vegetable oil. It contains not less than 90.0 percent and not more than 110.0 percent of the labeled amount of $C_{27}H_{40}O_3$. It may contain a suitable solubilizing agent.

Packaging and storage—Preserve in single-dose or multiple-dose containers, preferably of Type I glass, protected from light.

USP Reference standards ⟨11⟩—*USP Cholesteryl Caprylate RS. USP Testosterone Cypionate RS.*

Identification—Dilute a suitable volume of Injection with chloroform to obtain a solution having a concentration of about 400 μg of testosterone cypionate per mL. Prepare a 20- × 20-cm thin-layer chromatographic plate (see *Chromatography* ⟨621⟩), coated with a 0.25-mm layer of chromatographic siliceous earth, by placing it in a developing chamber containing and equilibrated with a mixture of chloroform and corn oil (90 : 10), and allowing the solvent front to move about three-fourths of the length of the plate. Remove the plate, and allow the chloroform to evaporate. Apply 10 μL each of the solution under test and of a solution of USP Testosterone Cypionate RS in chloroform containing about 400 μg per mL on the plate, on a line about 2.5 cm from the bottom edge and about 1.5 cm apart. Place the plate in a developing chamber that contains and has been equilibrated with a mixture of methanol and water (90 : 10) previously saturated with corn oil. Develop the chromatogram until the solvent front has moved to about 10 cm above the line of application. Remove the plate, and heat in an oven at 105° for a few minutes. Spray the plate with a mixture of alcohol and sulfuric acid (3 : 1), and heat in an oven at 105° for 1 to 2 minutes. Observe the plate under long-wavelength UV light: the R_F-value of the principal spot obtained from the solution under test corresponds to that obtained from the Standard solution.

Other requirements—It meets the requirements under *Injections* ⟨1⟩.

Assay—

  Internal standard solution and *Standard preparation*—Prepare as directed in the *Assay* under *Testosterone Cypionate*.

  Assay preparation—Transfer 1 mL of Injection, accurately measured, into a glass-stoppered, 50-mL centrifuge tube. Add 30 mL of a mixture of methanol and water (9 : 1), insert the stopper, and shake for 15 minutes. Centrifuge, remove the dilute methanol layer without disturbing the oil, and transfer it to a 200-mL volumetric flask. Repeat the extraction with three additional 30-mL portions of the dilute methanol, collecting the combined extracts in the volumetric flask. Dilute the combined extracts with the dilute methanol to volume, mix, and chill the contents of the flask to −8°. Remove the flask from the freezer, and immediately filter a portion of the contents. Allow the filtrate to reach room temperature, transfer a portion of it, equivalent to about 3 mg of testosterone cypionate, to a suitable vial, and evaporate to dryness. Add by pipet 3 mL of *Internal standard solution*, and shake vigorously to dissolve the residue.

  Procedure—Proceed as directed for *Procedure* in the *Assay* under *Testosterone Cypionate*. Calculate the quantity, in mg, of $C_{27}H_{40}O_3$ in the portion of Injection taken by the formula:

$$600(C / V)(R_U / R_S)$$

in which *C* is the concentration, in mg per mL, of USP Testosterone Cypionate RS in the *Standard preparation*; and *V* is the volume, in mL, of the filtrate used in the *Assay preparation*.

Testosterone Enanthate

$C_{26}H_{40}O_3$ 400.59
Androst-4-en-3-one, 17-(1-oxoheptyl)oxy-, (17β)-.
Testosterone heptanoate   [315-37-7].

» Testosterone Enanthate contains not less than 97.0 percent and not more than 103.0 percent of $C_{26}H_{40}O_3$.

Packaging and storage—Preserve in well-closed containers, and store in a cool place.
USP Reference standards ⟨11⟩—*USP Testosterone Enanthate RS*.
Identification—
   A: *Infrared Absorption* ⟨197K⟩.
   B: *Ultraviolet Absorption* ⟨197U⟩—
      Solution: 10 µg per mL.
      Medium: alcohol.
      Absorptivities at 240 nm, calculated on the anhydrous basis, do not differ by more than 3.0%.
   C: Reflux 25 mg with 2 mL of a 1 in 100 solution of potassium hydroxide in methanol for 1 hour. Cool the mixture, add 10 mL of water, filter, and wash the precipitate with water until the last washing is neutral to litmus. Dry the precipitate in vacuum at 60° for 3 hours: the testosterone so obtained melts between 151° and 157°.
Melting range ⟨741⟩: between 34° and 39°, the initial temperature of the bath not exceeding 20°.
Specific rotation ⟨781S⟩: between +77° and +82°.
   Test solution: 20 mg per mL, in dioxane.
Water, *Method I* ⟨921⟩: not more than 0.5%.
Free heptanoic acid—Dissolve 500 mg in 10 mL of alcohol that previously has been neutralized to a faint blue color following the addition of 2 or 3 drops of bromothymol blue TS, and promptly titrate with 0.01 N sodium hydroxide VS: not more than 0.6 mL of 0.01 N sodium hydroxide is required (0.16% of heptanoic acid).
Ordinary impurities ⟨466⟩—
   Test solution: methanol.
   Standard solution: methanol.
   Eluant: a mixture of cyclohexane and ethyl acetate (2 : 1).
   Visualization: 19.
   Limits—No individual impurity exceeds 1.0%, and the total of observed impurities does not exceed 2.0%.
Organic volatile impurities, *Method V* ⟨467⟩: meets the requirements.
   Solvent—Use dimethyl sulfoxide.
                                (Official until July 1, 2008)
Assay—Dissolve about 40 mg of Testosterone Enanthate, accurately weighed, in chloroform to make 100 mL, and mix. Pipet 10 mL of this solution into a 100-mL volumetric flask, add chloroform to volume, and mix. Dissolve a suitable quantity of USP Testosterone Enanthate RS, accurately weighed, in chloroform, and dilute quantitatively and stepwise with chloroform to obtain a Standard solution having a known concentration of about 40 µg per mL. Pipet 5 mL each of the solution of Testosterone Enanthate and the Standard solution into separate, glass-stoppered, 50-mL conical flasks, and place 5.0 mL of chloroform in a similar flask to provide a blank. Treat each flask as follows. Add 10.0 mL of a solution of 375 mg of isoniazid and 0.47 mL of hydrochloric acid in 500 mL of methanol, mix, and allow to stand for 45 minutes. Concomitantly determine the absorbances of the solutions at the wavelength of maximum absorbance at about 380 nm, with a suitable spectrophotometer, using the blank to set the instrument. Calculate the quantity, in mg, of $C_{26}H_{40}O_3$ in the Testosterone Enanthate taken by the formula:

$$C(A_U / A_S)$$

in which C is the concentration, in µg per mL, of USP Testosterone Enanthate RS in the Standard solution; and A_U and A_S are the absorbances of the solution of Testosterone Enanthate and the Standard solution, respectively.

Testosterone Enanthate Injection

» Testosterone Enanthate Injection is a sterile solution of Testosterone Enanthate in a suitable vegetable oil. It contains not less than 90.0 percent and not more than 110.0 percent of the labeled amount of $C_{26}H_{40}O_3$.

Packaging and storage—Preserve in single-dose or multiple-dose containers, preferably of Type I glass.
USP Reference standards ⟨11⟩—*USP Testosterone Enanthate RS*.
Identification—Dilute a suitable volume of Injection with chloroform to obtain a solution having a concentration of about 400 µg of testosterone enanthate per mL. Proceed as directed in the *Identification* test under *Testosterone Cypionate Injection*, beginning with "Prepare a 20- × 20-cm thin-layer chromatographic plate," but using USP Testosterone Enanthate RS. The R_F value of the principal spot obtained from the solution under test corresponds to that obtained from the Reference Standard solution.
Other requirements—It meets the requirements under *Injections* ⟨1⟩.
Assay—
   Chromatographic solvent—Equilibrate, by shaking in a separator, 95 mL of alcohol, 5 mL of water, and 50 mL of chromatographic *n*-heptane. Allow the layers to separate.
   Isoniazid reagent—Dissolve 375 mg of isoniazid and 0.47 mL of hydrochloric acid in 500 mL of methanol.
   Standard preparation—Dissolve a suitable quantity of USP Testosterone Enanthate RS, accurately weighed, in methanol, and dilute quantitatively and stepwise with methanol to obtain a solution having a known concentration of about 40 µg per mL.
   Assay preparation—Transfer to a 10-mL volumetric flask an accurately measured volume of Injection, equivalent to about 100 mg of testosterone enanthate, add chromatographic *n*-heptane to volume, and mix. Pipet 5 mL of this solution into a 100-mL volumetric flask, add chromatographic *n*-heptane to volume, and mix.
   Procedure—Mix in a beaker 3 g of silanized chromatographic siliceous earth and 3 mL of the upper layer of the *Chromatographic solvent*. Pack the mixture into a 250- × 25-mm chromatographic tube that contains a small pledget of glass wool above the stem constriction. Mix in a beaker 3 g of silanized chromatographic siliceous earth and 2.0 mL of *Assay preparation*, transfer the mixture to the tube, and pack. Dry-wash the beaker with 1 g of silanized chromatographic siliceous earth, and transfer to the tube. Place a small pad of glass wool above the column packing. Pass 35 mL of the lower layer of the *Chromatographic solvent* through the column, and collect the eluate in a 50-mL volumetric flask. Add alcohol to volume, and mix. Pipet 10 mL of the resulting solution into a glass-stoppered, 50-mL conical flask, and evaporate on a water bath to dryness. Pipet 5 mL of methanol into the flask, and swirl to dissolve the residue. Pipet 5 mL of *Standard preparation* into a similar flask. To each flask add 10.0 mL of *Isoniazid reagent*, mix, and allow to stand for about 45 minutes. Concomitantly determine the absorbances of both solutions at the wavelength of maximum absorbance at about 380 nm, with a suitable spectrophotometer, using as a blank 5 mL of methanol that has been treated similarly with *Isoniazid reagent*. Calculate the quantity, in mg, of $C_{26}H_{40}O_3$ in each mL of the Injection taken by the formula:

$$2.5(C / V)(A_U / A_S)$$

in which C is the concentration, in µg per mL, of USP Testosterone Enanthate RS in the *Standard preparation*; V is the volume, in mL, of Injection taken; and A_U and A_S are the absorbances of the solutions from the *Assay preparation* and the *Standard preparation*, respectively.

Testosterone Propionate

$C_{22}H_{32}O_3$ 344.49
Androst-4-en-3-one, 17-(1-oxopropoxy)-, (17β)-.
Testosterone propionate   [57-85-2].

» Testosterone Propionate contains not less than 97.0 percent and not more than 103.0 percent of $C_{22}H_{32}O_3$, calculated on the dried basis.

Packaging and storage—Preserve in well-closed, light-resistant containers.
USP Reference standards ⟨11⟩—*USP Testosterone Propionate RS*.
Identification—
   A: *Infrared Absorption* ⟨197K⟩.
   B: *Ultraviolet Absorption* ⟨197U⟩—
   Solution: 10 μg per mL.
   Medium: alcohol.
   Absorptivities at 241 nm, calculated on the dried basis, do not differ by more than 3.0%.
   C: It responds to *Identification* test C under *Testosterone Enanthate*.
Melting range ⟨741⟩: between 118° and 123°.
Specific rotation ⟨781S⟩: between +83° and +90°.
   Test solution: 20 mg, previously dried, per mL, in dioxane.
Loss on drying ⟨731⟩—Dry it in vacuum over silica gel for 4 hours: it loses not more than 0.5% of its weight.
Organic volatile impurities, Method IV ⟨467⟩: meets the requirements.
                                        (Official until July 1, 2008)
Assay—Proceed with Testosterone Propionate as directed in the *Assay* under *Testosterone Enanthate*, except to use USP Testosterone Propionate RS and otherwise substitute Testosterone Propionate throughout. Calculate the quantity, in mg, of $C_{22}H_{32}O_3$ in the Testosterone Propionate taken by the formula given therein.

Testosterone Propionate Injection

» Testosterone Propionate Injection is a sterile solution of Testosterone Propionate in a suitable vegetable oil. It contains not less than 88.0 percent and not more than 112.0 percent of the labeled amount of $C_{22}H_{32}O_3$.

Packaging and storage—Preserve in single-dose or multiple-dose containers, preferably of Type I glass.
USP Reference standards ⟨11⟩—*USP Testosterone Propionate RS*.
Identification—Dilute a suitable volume of Injection with chloroform to obtain a solution having a concentration of about 400 μg of testosterone propionate per mL. Proceed as directed in the *Identification* test under *Testosterone Cypionate Injection*, beginning with "Prepare a 20- × 20-cm thin-layer chromatographic plate," except to use USP Testosterone Propionate RS. The R_F value of the principal spot obtained from the solution under test corresponds to that obtained from the Standard solution.
Other requirements—It meets the requirements under *Injections* ⟨1⟩.
Assay—
   Chromatographic solvent and *Isoniazid reagent*—Prepare as directed in the *Assay* under *Testosterone Enanthate Injection*.
   Standard preparation—Prepare as directed in the *Assay* under *Testosterone Enanthate Injection*, using USP Testosterone Propionate RS.
   Assay preparation—Transfer to a 10-mL volumetric flask an accurately measured volume of Injection, equivalent to about 100 mg of testosterone propionate, add chromatographic *n*-heptane to volume, and mix. Pipet 5 mL of this solution into a 100-mL volumetric flask, add chromatographic *n*-heptane to volume, and mix.

   Procedure—Proceed as directed for *Procedure* in the *Assay* under *Testosterone Enanthate Injection*. Calculate the quantity, in mg, of $C_{22}H_{32}O_3$ in each mL of the Injection taken by the formula:

$$2.5(C / V)(A_U / A_S)$$

in which C is the concentration, in μg per mL, of USP Testosterone Propionate RS in the *Standard preparation*, V is the volume, in mL, of Injection taken, and A_U and A_S are the absorbances of the solutions from the *Assay preparation* and the *Standard preparation*, respectively.

Tetanus Immune Globulin

» Tetanus Immune Globulin conforms to the regulations of the FDA concerning biologics (see *Biologics* ⟨1041⟩). It is a sterile, nonpyrogenic solution of globulins derived from the blood plasma of adult human donors who have been immunized with tetanus toxoid. It has a potency of not less than 50 antitoxin units per mL based on the U.S. Standard Tetanus Antitoxin and the U.S. Control Tetanus Test Toxin, tested in guinea pigs. It contains not less than 10 g and not more than 18 g of protein per 100 mL, of which not less than 90 percent is gamma globulin. It contains 0.3 M glycine as a stabilizing agent, and it contains a suitable preservative.

Packaging and storage—Preserve at a temperature between 2° and 8°.
Expiration date—The expiration date for Tetanus Immune Globulin containing a 10% excess of potency is not later than 3 years after date of issue from manufacturer's cold storage (5°, 1 year).
Labeling—Label it to state that it is not for intravenous injection.

Tetanus Toxoid

» Tetanus Toxoid conforms to the regulations of the FDA concerning biologics (see *Biologics* ⟨1041⟩). It is a sterile solution of the formaldehyde-treated products of growth of the tetanus bacillus (*Clostridium tetani*). It meets the requirements of the specific guinea pig potency test of antitoxin production based on the U.S. Standard Tetanus Antitoxin and the U.S. Control Tetanus Test Toxin. It meets the requirements of the specific guinea pig detoxification test. It contains not more than 0.02 percent of residual free formaldehyde. It contains a preservative other than a phenoloid compound.

Packaging and storage—Preserve at a temperature between 2° and 8°.
Expiration date—The expiration date is not later than 2 years after date of issue from manufacturer's cold storage (5°, 1 year).
Labeling—Label it to state that it is not to be frozen.

Tetanus Toxoid Adsorbed

» Tetanus Toxoid Adsorbed conforms to the regulations of the FDA concerning biologics (see *Biologics* ⟨1041⟩). It is a sterile preparation of plain tetanus toxoid that meets all of the requirements for that product with the exception of those for potency, and that has been precipitated or adsorbed by alum, aluminum hydroxide, or aluminum phosphate adjuvants. It meets the requirements of the specific mouse or guinea pig potency test of antitoxin production based on the U.S. Standard Tetanus Antitoxin and the U.S. Control Test Tetanus Toxin. It meets the requirements of the specific guinea pig detoxification test.

Packaging and storage—Preserve at a temperature between 2° and 8°.
Expiration date—The expiration date is not later than 2 years after date of issue from manufacturer's cold storage (5°, 1 year).
Labeling—Label it to state that it is to be well-shaken before use and that it is not to be frozen.
Aluminum content—It contains not more than 0.85 mg per single injection, determined by analysis, or not more than 1.14 mg calculated on the basis of the amount of aluminum compound added.

Tetanus and Diphtheria Toxoids Adsorbed for Adult Use

» Tetanus and Diphtheria Toxoids Adsorbed for Adult Use conforms to the regulations of the FDA concerning biologics (see *Biologics* ⟨1041⟩). It is a sterile suspension prepared by mixing suitable quantities of adsorbed diphtheria toxoid and adsorbed tetanus toxoid using the same precipitating or adsorbing agent for both toxoids. The antigenicity or potency and the proportions of the toxoids are such as to provide, in each dose prescribed in the labeling, an immunizing dose of Tetanus Toxoid Adsorbed as defined for that product, and one-tenth of the immunizing dose of Diphtheria Toxoid Adsorbed as defined for that product for children, such that in the specific guinea pig antigenicity test it meets the requirement of production of not less than 0.5 unit of diphtheria antitoxin per mL and each immunizing dose has an antigen content of not more than 2 Lf (flocculating units) value as measured with the U.S. Reference Diphtheria Antitoxin for Flocculation Test. Each component meets the other requirements for those products. It contains not more than 0.02 percent of residual free formaldehyde.

Packaging and storage—Preserve at a temperature between 2° and 8°.
Expiration date—The expiration date is not later than 2 years after date of issue from manufacturer's cold storage (5°, 1 year).
Labeling—Label it to state that it is to be well-shaken before use and that it is not to be frozen.

Tetracaine

$C_{15}H_{24}N_2O_2$ 264.36
Benzoic acid, 4-(butylamino)-, 2-(dimethylamino)ethyl ester.
2-(Dimethylamino)ethyl *p*-(butylamino)benzoate [94-24-6].

» Tetracaine contains not less than 98.0 percent and not more than 101.0 percent of $C_{15}H_{24}N_2O_2$, calculated on the dried basis.

Packaging and storage—Preserve in tight, light-resistant containers.
USP Reference standards ⟨11⟩—*USP Tetracaine Hydrochloride RS.*
Identification—
  A: Dissolve 100 mg in 10 mL of dilute hydrochloric acid (1 in 120), and add 1 mL of potassium thiocyanate solution (1 in 4): a crystalline precipitate is formed. Recrystallize the precipitate from water, and dry at 80° for 2 hours: it melts between 130° and 132° (see *Melting Range or Temperature* ⟨741⟩).
  B: Dissolve about 90 mg, accurately weighed, in 10 mL of dilute hydrochloric acid (1 in 120) in a 500-mL volumetric flask, dilute with water to volume, and mix. Transfer 5.0 mL of this solution to a 100-mL volumetric flask, add 2 mL of *Buffer No. 6*, 10 percent, pH 6.0 (see *Phosphate Buffers* ⟨81⟩), dilute with water to volume, and mix: the UV absorption spectrum of the solution so obtained exhibits maxima and minima at the same wavelengths as that of a 1 in 100,000 solution of USP Tetracaine Hydrochloride RS in a mixture of water and *Buffer No. 6* (50:1), 10 percent, pH 6.0 (see *Phosphate Buffers* ⟨81⟩), and the respective molar absorptivities, calculated on the dried basis, at the wavelength of maximum absorbance at about 310 nm do not differ by more than 2.0%. [NOTE—The molecular weight of tetracaine hydrochloride ($C_{15}H_{24}N_2O_2 \cdot HCl$) is 300.82.]
Melting range, *Class I* ⟨741⟩: between 41° and 46°.
Loss on drying ⟨731⟩—Dry it in vacuum over phosphorus pentoxide for 18 hours: it loses not more than 0.5% of its weight.
Residue on ignition ⟨281⟩: not more than 0.1%.
Chromatographic purity—Dissolve an accurately weighed quantity of Tetracaine in chloroform to obtain a test solution containing 50 mg per mL. Prepare a Standard solution of 4-(butylamino) benzoic acid in methanol containing 0.2 mg per mL. Apply separate 5-µL portions of the test solution and the Standard solution to a suitable thin-layer chromatographic plate (see *Chromatography* ⟨621⟩) coated with a 0.25-mm layer of chromatographic silica gel mixture. Develop the plate in a suitable chromatographic chamber containing a solvent system consisting of a mixture of chloroform, methanol, and isopropylamine (98:7:2) until the solvent front has moved about three-fourths of the length of the plate. Remove the plate from the chamber, and dry in a current of warm air. Examine the plate under short-wavelength UV light: any spot obtained from the test solution, other than the principal spot, is not more intense than the principal spot obtained from the Standard solution (0.4%), and the sum of the intensities of any such spots is not greater than 0.8%.
Assay—Transfer about 500 mg of Tetracaine, accurately weighed, to a suitable vessel. Add 5 mL of hydrochloric acid and 50 mL of water, cool to 15°, and add about 25 g of crushed ice, and slowly titrate with 0.1 M sodium nitrite VS, stirring vigorously, until a glass rod dipped into the titrated solution produces an immediate blue ring when touched to starch iodide paper. When the titration is complete, the endpoint is reproducible after the mixture has been allowed to stand for 1 minute. Perform a blank determination, and make any necessary correction. Each mL of 0.1 M sodium nitrite is equivalent to 26.44 mg of $C_{15}H_{24}N_2O_2$.

Tetracaine Ointment

» Tetracaine Ointment contains not less than 90.0 percent and not more than 110.0 percent of the labeled amount of $C_{15}H_{24}N_2O_2$ in a suitable ointment base.

Packaging and storage—Preserve in collapsible ointment tubes.
USP Reference standards ⟨11⟩—*USP Tetracaine Hydrochloride RS.*
Identification—
  A: The solution employed for measurement of absorbance in the *Assay* exhibits a maximum at 310 ± 2 nm.

B: Dissolve 5 g in 50 mL of ether, extract the ether solution with 5 mL of 3 N hydrochloric acid, and filter the acid extract. Add 2 mL of potassium thiocyanate solution (1 in 2) to the filtrate: a crystalline precipitate is formed, and when recrystallized from water and dried at 80° for 2 hours, it melts between 130° and 132° (see *Melting Range or Temperature* ⟨741⟩).

Microbial limits ⟨61⟩—It meets the requirements of the tests for absence of *Staphylococcus aureus* and *Pseudomonas aeruginosa*.

Minimum fill ⟨755⟩: meets the requirements.

Assay—

Standard preparation—Transfer about 20 mg of USP Tetracaine Hydrochloride RS, accurately weighed, to a 100-mL volumetric flask, dissolve in water, add water to volume, and mix. Transfer 5.0 mL of this solution to a second 100-mL volumetric flask, add 5 mL of dilute hydrochloric acid (1 in 240) and 10 mL of *Buffer No. 6*, 10 percent, pH 6.0 (see *Phosphate Buffers* ⟨81⟩), dilute with water to volume, and mix. The concentration of USP Tetracaine Hydrochloride RS in the *Standard preparation* is about 10 μg per mL.

Assay preparation—Transfer an accurately weighed portion of Ointment, equivalent to about 9 mg of tetracaine, to a separator, and dissolve in 15 mL of ether. Extract with one 20-mL portion and two 10-mL portions of dilute hydrochloric acid (1 in 240), collecting the acid extracts in a second separator. Render the aqueous solution alkaline by the addition of 5 mL of sodium carbonate TS, and extract immediately with two 50-mL portions of ether, collecting the ether extracts in another separator. Wash the ether solution with 20 mL of water, discard the washing, and extract the ether solution with two 20-mL portions and one 5-mL portion of dilute hydrochloric acid (1 in 240), collecting the acid extracts in a 50-mL volumetric flask. Dilute with water to volume, and mix. Transfer 5.0 mL of this solution to a 100-mL volumetric flask, add 10 mL of *Buffer No. 6*, 10 percent, pH 6.0 (see *Phosphate Buffers* ⟨81⟩), dilute with water to volume, and mix.

Procedure—Concomitantly determine the absorbances of the *Assay preparation* and the *Standard preparation* in 1-cm cells at the wavelength of maximum absorbance at about 310 nm, with a suitable spectrophotometer, using water as the blank. Calculate the quantity, in mg, of $C_{15}H_{24}N_2O_2$ in the portion of Ointment taken by the formula:

$$(264.37/300.83)(C)(A_U/A_S)$$

in which 264.36 and 300.82 are the molecular weights of tetracaine and tetracaine hydrochloride, respectively; C is the concentration, in μg per mL, of USP Tetracaine Hydrochloride RS in the *Standard preparation*; and A_U and A_S are the absorbances of the *Assay preparation* and the *Standard preparation*, respectively.

Tetracaine Ophthalmic Ointment

» Tetracaine Ophthalmic Ointment is a sterile ointment containing not less than 0.45 percent and not more than 0.55 percent of $C_{15}H_{24}N_2O_2$ in White Petrolatum.

Packaging and storage—Preserve in collapsible ophthalmic ointment tubes.

USP Reference standards ⟨11⟩—*USP Tetracaine Hydrochloride RS*.

Identification—

A: The solution employed for measurement of absorbance in the *Assay* exhibits a maximum at 310 ± 2 nm.

B: Dissolve 5 g in 50 mL of ether, extract the ether solution with 5 mL of 3 N hydrochloric acid, and filter the extract. To the extract add 2 mL of potassium thiocyanate solution (1 in 2): a crystalline precipitate is formed, and when recrystallized from water and dried at 80° for 2 hours, it melts between 130° and 132° (see *Melting Range or Temperature* ⟨741⟩).

Sterility ⟨71⟩: meets the requirements.

Minimum fill ⟨755⟩: meets the requirements.

Metal particles—It meets the requirements of the test for *Metal Particles in Ophthalmic Ointments* ⟨751⟩.

Assay—

Standard preparation—Prepare as directed in the *Assay* under *Tetracaine Ointment*.

Assay preparation—Using an accurately weighed portion of Ophthalmic Ointment, prepare as directed in the *Assay* under *Tetracaine Ointment*.

Procedure—Proceed as directed for *Procedure* in the *Assay* under *Tetracaine Ointment*.

Tetracaine and Menthol Ointment

» Tetracaine and Menthol Ointment contains not less than 90.0 percent and not more than 110.0 percent of the labeled amounts of tetracaine ($C_{15}H_{24}N_2O_2$) and menthol ($C_{10}H_{20}O$) in a suitable ointment base.

Packaging and storage—Preserve in collapsible ointment tubes.

USP Reference standards ⟨11⟩—*USP Menthol RS. USP Tetracaine Hydrochloride RS*.

Identification—

A: The solution employed for measurement of absorbance in the *Assay for tetracaine* exhibits a maximum at 310 ± 2 nm (*presence of tetracaine*).

B: Dissolve 5 g in 50 mL of ether, extract the ether solution with 5 mL of 3 N hydrochloric acid, and filter the acid extract. Add 2 mL of potassium thiocyanate solution (1 in 2) to the filtrate: a crystalline precipitate is formed, and when recrystallized from water and dried at 80° for 2 hours, it melts between 130° and 132° (see *Melting Range or Temperature* ⟨741⟩) (*presence of tetracaine*).

C: When chromatographed as directed in the *Assay for menthol*, the *Assay preparation* exhibits a major peak for menthol, the retention time of which corresponds to that exhibited by menthol in the *Standard preparation*.

Minimum fill ⟨755⟩: meets the requirements.

Assay for tetracaine—

Standard preparation—Prepare as directed in the *Assay* under *Tetracaine Ointment*.

Assay preparation—Using Ointment, proceed as directed in the *Assay* under *Tetracaine Ointment*.

Procedure—Proceed as directed for *Procedure* in the *Assay* under *Tetracaine Ointment*.

Assay for menthol—

Internal standard solution—Dissolve decanol in *n*-hexane to obtain a solution having a concentration of about 1 mg per mL.

Standard preparation—Dissolve an accurately weighed quantity of USP Menthol RS in *n*-hexane to obtain a solution having a known concentration of about 1 mg per mL. Transfer 5.0 mL of this solution and 5.0 mL of *Internal standard solution* to a 50-mL volumetric flask, dilute with ether to volume, and mix. Combine 2.0 mL of this solution and 2.0 mL of ether in a suitable container, and mix. This *Standard preparation* has a known concentration of about 0.05 mg per mL.

Assay preparation—Transfer an accurately weighed quantity of Ointment, equivalent to about 5 mg of menthol, to a 50-mL volumetric flask, add 5.0 mL of *Internal standard solution*, dilute with *n*-hexane to volume, mix, and sonicate. Using a suitable syringe attached firmly to a 25- × 12.5-mm chromatographic cartridge containing packing L4, force 2.0 mL of the solution through the cartridge at a rate of 1 mL per 12 seconds. Wash the cartridge at the same rate with two 5-mL portions of *n*-hexane, and discard the washings. Force two 2.0-mL portions of ether through the cartridge, combine the ether eluates in a suitable container, and mix.

Chromatographic system (see *Chromatography* ⟨621⟩)—The gas chromatograph is equipped with a flame-ionization detector and contains a 2-mm × 1.8-m column packed with 10% phase G16 on support S1AB. The column temperature is maintained isothermally at about 170°, the injection port temperature is maintained at about 260°, and the detector block temperature is maintained at about 240°. Dry helium is used as the carrier gas at a flow rate of about 50 mL per minute.

System suitability—Chromatograph three injections of the *Standard preparation*, and record the peak responses as directed for *Procedure:* the retention time of menthol is about 0.7 relative to decanol; the resolution, *R*, between the 2 peaks is not less than 2.5; and the relative standard deviation of the ratio of the peak response obtained with menthol to that obtained with decanol is not more than 2%.

Procedure—Separately inject equal volumes (about 2 µL) of the *Assay preparation* and the *Standard preparation* into the gas chromatograph, and measure the peak responses for menthol and decanol in each chromatogram. Calculate the quantity, in mg, of $C_{10}H_{20}O$ in the portion of Ointment taken by the formula:

$$100C(R_U / R_S)$$

in which *C* is the concentration, in mg per mL, of USP Menthol RS in the *Standard preparation*; and R_U and R_S are the peak response ratios of menthol to decanol obtained from the *Assay preparation* and the *Standard preparation*, respectively.

Tetracaine Hydrochloride

$C_{15}H_{24}N_2O_2 \cdot HCl$ 300.82
Benzoic acid, 4-(butylamino)-, 2-(dimethylamino)ethyl ester, monohydrochloride.
2-(Dimethylamino)ethyl *p*-(butylamino)benzoate monohydrochloride [136-47-0].

» Tetracaine Hydrochloride contains not less than 98.5 percent and not more than 101.0 percent of $C_{15}H_{24}N_2O_2 \cdot HCl$, calculated on the anhydrous basis.

Packaging and storage—Preserve in tight, light-resistant containers.
Labeling—Where it is intended for use in preparing injectable dosage forms, the label states that it is sterile or must be subjected to further processing during the preparation of injectable or other sterile dosage forms.
USP Reference standards ⟨11⟩—*USP Endotoxin RS. USP Tetracaine Hydrochloride RS.*
Identification—
  A: *Ultraviolet Absorption* ⟨197U⟩—
  Solution—Prepare the test solution as follows. Dissolve about 50 mg, accurately weighed, in water to make 250.0 mL. Pipet 5 mL of this solution into a 100-mL volumetric flask, add 2 mL of *Buffer No. 6, 10 Percent, pH 6.0* (see *Antibiotics—Microbial Assays* ⟨81⟩), then dilute with water to volume, and mix. For the purposes of this test, *Buffer No. 6, 10 Percent, pH 6.0* does not have to be sterilized.
  Absorptivities at 310 nm, calculated on the anhydrous basis, do not differ by more than 2.0%.
  B: Dissolve 100 mg in 10 mL of water, and add 1 mL of potassium thiocyanate solution (1 in 4): a crystalline precipitate is formed. Recrystallize the precipitate from water, and dry at 80° for 2 hours: it melts between 130° and 132°.
  C: A solution of 100 mg in 5 mL of water meets the requirements of the tests for *Chloride* ⟨191⟩.
Water, *Method I* ⟨921⟩: not more than 2.0%.
Residue on ignition ⟨281⟩: not more than 0.1%.
Chromatographic purity—Dissolve an accurately weighed quantity in water to obtain a test solution containing 50 mg per mL, and proceed as directed in the test for *Chromatographic purity* under *Tetracaine*, beginning with "Prepare a Standard solution."
Other requirements—Where the label states that Tetracaine Hydrochloride is sterile, it meets the requirements for *Sterility Tests* ⟨71⟩ and for *Bacterial endotoxins* under *Tetracaine Hydrochloride for Injection*. Where the label states that Tetracaine Hydrochloride must be subjected to further processing during the preparation of injectable or other sterile dosage forms, it meets the requirements for *Bacterial endotoxins* under *Tetracaine Hydrochloride for Injection.*
Assay—Transfer about 500 mg of Tetracaine Hydrochloride, accurately weighed, to a suitable vessel, add 5 mL of hydrochloric acid and 50 mL of water, and proceed as directed under *Nitrite Titration* ⟨451⟩, beginning with "cool to 15°." Each mL of 0.1 M sodium nitrite is equivalent to 30.08 mg of $C_{15}H_{24}N_2O_2 \cdot HCl$.

Tetracaine Hydrochloride Cream

» Tetracaine Hydrochloride Cream contains Tetracaine Hydrochloride ($C_{15}H_{24}N_2O_2 \cdot HCl$) equivalent to not less than 90.0 percent and not more than 110.0 percent of the labeled amount of tetracaine ($C_{15}H_{24}N_2O_2$) in a suitable water-miscible base.

Packaging and storage—Preserve in collapsible, lined metal tubes.
USP Reference standards ⟨11⟩—*USP Tetracaine Hydrochloride RS.*
Identification, *Ultraviolet Absorption* ⟨197U⟩: *Assay preparation* compared to the *Standard preparation* from the *Assay*.
Microbial limits ⟨61⟩—It meets the requirements of the tests for absence of *Staphylococcus aureus* and *Pseudomonas aeruginosa*.
Minimum fill ⟨755⟩: meets the requirements.
pH ⟨791⟩: between 3.2 and 3.8.
Assay—
  pH 6 Acetate buffer—Dissolve 250 g of sodium acetate in about 500 mL of water in a 1000-mL volumetric flask, add 5.0 mL of glacial acetic acid, dilute with water to volume, and mix.
  Standard preparation—Transfer about 25 mg of USP Tetracaine Hydrochloride RS, accurately weighed, to a 100-mL volumetric flask, dissolve in isopropyl alcohol, add isopropyl alcohol to volume, and mix. Transfer 2.0 mL of this solution to another 100-mL volumetric flask, add 2.0 mL of *pH 6 Acetate buffer,* dilute with isopropyl alcohol to volume, and mix. The concentration of USP Tetracaine Hydrochloride RS in the *Standard preparation* is about 5 µg per mL.
  Assay preparation—Transfer an accurately weighed portion of Cream, equivalent to about 4.5 mg of tetracaine, to a 50-mL beaker, add 25 mL of isopropyl alcohol, and warm on a steam bath to dissolve the specimen completely. Transfer the solution with the aid of isopropyl alcohol to a 100-mL volumetric flask, dilute with isopropyl alcohol to volume, and mix. Transfer 10.0 mL of this solution to another 100-mL volumetric flask, add 2.0 mL of *pH 6 Acetate buffer*, dilute with isopropyl alcohol to volume, and mix.
  Procedure—Concomitantly determine the absorbances of the *Assay preparation* and the *Standard preparation* in 1-cm cells at the wavelength of maximum absorbance at about 310 nm, with a suitable spectrophotometer, using a 1 in 50 solution of *pH 6 Acetate buffer* in isopropyl alcohol as the blank. Calculate the quantity, in mg, of $C_{15}H_{24}N_2O_2$ in the portion of Cream taken by the formula:

$$(264.36/300.82)(C)(A_U / A_S)$$

in which 264.36 and 300.82 are the molecular weights of tetracaine and tetracaine hydrochloride, respectively; *C* is the concentration, in µg per mL, of USP Tetracaine Hydrochloride RS in the *Standard preparation;* and A_U and A_S are the absorbances of the *Assay preparation* and the *Standard preparation*, respectively.

Tetracaine Hydrochloride Injection

» Tetracaine Hydrochloride Injection is a sterile solution of Tetracaine Hydrochloride in Water for Injection. It contains not less than 95.0 percent and not more than 105.0 percent of the labeled amount of $C_{15}H_{24}N_2O_2 \cdot HCl$.

Packaging and storage—Preserve in single-dose or in multiple-dose containers, preferably of Type I glass, under refrigeration and protected from light. It may be packaged in 100-mL multiple-dose containers. Injection supplied as a component of spinal anesthesia trays may be stored at room temperature for 12 months.

Labeling—Label it to indicate that the Injection is not to be used if it contains crystals, or if it is cloudy or discolored.

USP Reference standards ⟨11⟩—*USP Endotoxin RS. USP Tetracaine Hydrochloride RS.*

Identification—
A: It responds to *Identification* test B under *Tetracaine Hydrochloride.*
B: The chromatogram of the *Assay preparation* obtained as directed in the *Assay* exhibits a major peak for tetracaine, the retention time of which corresponds to that in the chromatogram of the *Standard preparation* as obtained in the *Assay.*

Bacterial endotoxins ⟨85⟩—It contains not more than 0.7 USP Endotoxin Unit per mg of tetracaine hydrochloride.

pH ⟨791⟩: between 3.2 and 6.0.

Particulate matter ⟨788⟩: meets the requirements under small-volume injections.

Other requirements—It meets the requirements under *Injections* ⟨1⟩.

Assay—
Diluent—Prepare a mixture of water and methanol (1 : 1).
Mobile phase—Prepare a suitable mixture of water, acetonitrile, and methanol (60 : 20 : 20) containing 0.06% of sulfuric acid, 0.5% of sodium sulfate, and 0.02% of sodium 1-heptanesulfonate. The pH is about 2.6. Make adjustments if necessary (see *System Suitability* under *Chromatography* ⟨621⟩).
Standard preparation—Dissolve an accurately weighed quantity of USP Tetracaine Hydrochloride RS quantitatively in *Diluent* to obtain a solution having a known concentration of about 1 mg per mL.
Resolution solution—Dissolve a quantity of salicylic acid in a portion of the *Standard preparation* to obtain a solution containing about 4 mg of salicylic acid and 1 mg of tetracaine hydrochloride per mL.
Assay preparation—Transfer an accurately measured volume of Injection equivalent to about 50 mg of tetracaine hydrochloride, to a 50-mL volumetric flask, dilute with *Diluent* to volume, and mix.
Chromatographic system (see *Chromatography* ⟨621⟩)—The liquid chromatograph is equipped with a 305-nm detector and a 3.9-mm × 30-cm column containing packing L1. The flow rate is about 2 mL per minute. Chromatograph the *Resolution solution*, and record the responses as directed for *Procedure:* the relative retention times are about 0.8 for salicylic acid and 1.0 for tetracaine; and the resolution, R, between the salicylic acid peak and the tetracaine peak is not less than 2. Chromatograph the *Standard preparation*, and record the responses as directed for *Procedure:* the relative standard deviation for replicate injections is not more than 2.0%.
Procedure— Separately inject equal volumes (about 5 µL) of the *Standard preparation* and the *Assay preparation* into the chromatograph, record the chromatograms, and measure the areas for the major peaks. Calculate the quantity, in mg, of tetracaine hydrochloride ($C_{15}H_{24}N_2O_2 \cdot HCl$) in each mL of the Injection taken by the formula:

$$50(C / V)(r_U / r_S)$$

in which C is the concentration, in mg per mL, of USP Tetracaine Hydrochloride RS in the *Standard preparation;* V is the volume, in mL, of Injection taken; and r_U and r_S are the tetracaine peak responses obtained from the *Assay preparation* and the *Standard preparation*, respectively.

Tetracaine Hydrochloride for Injection

» Tetracaine Hydrochloride for Injection contains not less than 90.0 percent and not more than 110.0 percent of the labeled amount of tetracaine hydrochloride ($C_{15}H_{24}N_2O_2 \cdot HCl$).

Packaging and storage—Preserve in *Containers for Sterile Solids* as described under *Injections* ⟨1⟩, preferably of Type I glass.

USP Reference standards ⟨11⟩—*USP Endotoxin RS. USP Tetracaine Hydrochloride RS.*

Completeness of solution ⟨641⟩—A 10-mg portion dissolves in 1 mL of water in not more than 2 seconds to yield a colorless solution free from undissolved solid.

Constituted solution—At the time of use, it meets the requirements for *Constituted Solutions* under *Injections* ⟨1⟩.

Identification—
A: *Ultraviolet Absorption* ⟨197U⟩—
Solution: the solution employed for measurement of absorbance in the *Assay.*
B: It responds to *Identification* test B under *Tetracaine Hydrochloride.*

Bacterial endotoxins ⟨85⟩—It contains not more than 0.7 USP Endotoxin Unit per mg of tetracaine hydrochloride.

Uniformity of dosage units ⟨905⟩: it meets the requirements employing the following method.
Standard preparation—Prepare as directed in the *Assay* under *Tetracaine Hydrochloride in Dextrose Injection.*
Test preparation—Transfer the contents of one container, with the aid of water, to a 200-mL volumetric flask, add water to volume, and mix. Pipet a portion of this solution, equivalent to about 1 mg of tetracaine hydrochloride, to a 100-mL volumetric flask, add 5 mL of dilute hydrochloric acid (1 in 200) and 10 mL of *Buffer No. 6*, 10 percent, pH 6.0 (see *Phosphate Buffers and Other Solutions* under *Antibiotics— Microbial Assays* ⟨81⟩), add water to volume, and mix.
Procedure—Proceed as directed for *Procedure* in the *Assay*, except to use the *Test preparation* instead of the *Assay preparation.*
Calculate the quantity, in mg, of $C_{15}H_{24}N_2O_2 \cdot HCl$ in each container taken by the formula:

$$20(C / V)(A_U / A_S)$$

in which V is the volume, in mL, of the portion used in the *Test preparation*, A_U is the absorbance of the *Test preparation*, and C and A_S are as defined in the *Assay.*

pH ⟨791⟩: between 5.0 and 6.0, in a solution (1 in 100).

Water, *Method I* ⟨921⟩: not more than 2.0%.

Residue on ignition—Weigh accurately about 500 mg, transfer to a beaker, and dissolve in 10 mL of methanol. Filter through paper previously washed with methanol, collecting the filtrate in an ignited and tared crucible and washing the beaker and the filter paper with 25 mL to 30 mL of methanol. Evaporate with the aid of heat and a current of air to dryness, and proceed as directed under *Residue on Ignition* ⟨281⟩, beginning with "Heat, gently at first." Not more than 0.1% of residue is found.

Chromatographic purity—Dissolve an accurately weighed quantity of Tetracaine Hydrochloride for Injection in water to obtain a test solution containing 50 mg per mL, and proceed as directed in the test for *Chromatographic purity* under *Tetracaine*, beginning with "Prepare a Standard solution."

Other requirements—It meets the requirements for *Sterility Tests* ⟨71⟩ and *Labeling* under *Injections* ⟨1⟩.

Assay—
Standard preparation—Prepare as directed in the *Assay* under *Tetracaine Hydrochloride in Dextrose Injection.*
Assay preparation—Transfer to a tared 20-mL beaker the contents of a sufficient number of containers of Tetracaine Hydrochloride for Injection to yield about 100 mg of tetracaine hydrochloride. Weigh immediately, and transfer with the aid of water to a 500-mL volumetric flask. Add water to volume, and mix. Transfer 5.0 mL to a 100-mL volumetric flask, add 5 mL of dilute hydrochloric acid (1 in 200) and 10 mL of *Buffer No. 6*, 10 percent, pH 6.0 (see *Phosphate Buffers* ⟨81⟩), then add water to volume, and mix.
Procedure—Concomitantly determine the absorbances of the *Assay preparation* and the *Standard preparation* at the wavelength of maximum absorbance at about 310 nm, with a suitable spectrophotometer, using water as the blank. Calculate the quantity, in mg, of

$C_{15}H_{24}N_2O_2 \cdot HCl$ in the portion of Tetracaine Hydrochloride for Injection taken by the formula:

$$10C(A_U/A_S)$$

in which C is the concentration, in µg per mL, of USP Tetracaine Hydrochloride RS in the *Standard preparation*, and A_U and A_S are the absorbances of the *Assay preparation* and the *Standard preparation*, respectively.

Tetracaine Hydrochloride Ophthalmic Solution

» Tetracaine Hydrochloride Ophthalmic Solution is a sterile, aqueous solution of Tetracaine Hydrochloride. It contains not less than 90.0 percent and not more than 110.0 percent of the labeled amount of $C_{15}H_{24}N_2O_2 \cdot HCl$. It may contain suitable antimicrobial and thickening agents.

Packaging and storage—Preserve in tight, light-resistant containers.
Labeling—Label it to indicate that the Ophthalmic Solution is not to be used if it contains crystals, or if it is cloudy or discolored.
USP Reference standards ⟨11⟩—*USP Tetracaine Hydrochloride RS*.
Identification—Add 5 mL of Ophthalmic Solution to 5 mL of water in a test tube, then add 1 mL of potassium thiocyanate solution (1 in 4): a crystalline precipitate is formed. Recrystallize the precipitate from water, and dry at 80° for 2 hours: the crystals so obtained melt between 130° and 132°.
Sterility ⟨71⟩: meets the requirements.
pH ⟨791⟩: between 3.7 and 6.0.
Assay—
  Mobile phase—Prepare 0.01 M of dibasic ammonium phosphate in water, and adjust with phosphoric acid to a pH of 3.0. Prepare a filtered and degassed mixture of this solution and acetonitrile (70 : 30). Make adjustments if necessary (see *System Suitability* under *Chromatography* ⟨621⟩).
  Standard preparation—Dissolve an accurately weighed quantity of USP Tetracaine Hydrochloride RS in water to obtain a solution having a known concentration of about 0.1 mg per mL.
  Assay preparation—Transfer an accurately measured volume of Ophthalmic Solution, equivalent to about 10 mg of tetracaine hydrochloride, to a 100-mL volumetric flask, dilute with water to volume, and mix.
  Chromatographic system (see *Chromatography* ⟨621⟩)—The liquid chromatograph is equipped with a 280-nm detector and a 4.6-mm × 25-cm column containing packing L10. The flow rate is about 2 mL per minute. Chromatograph the *Standard preparation*, and record the peak responses as directed for *Procedure*: the column efficiency is not less than 500 theoretical plates; the tailing factor for the analyte peak is not more than 2.0; and the relative standard deviation for replicate injections is not more than 2.0%.
  Procedure—Separately inject equal volumes (about 10 µL) of the *Standard preparation* and the *Assay preparation* into the chromatograph, record the chromatograms, and measure the responses for the major peaks. Calculate the quantity, in mg, of $C_{15}H_{24}N_2O_2 \cdot HCl$ in each mL of the Ophthalmic Solution taken by the formula:

$$100(C/V)(r_U/r_S)$$

in which C is the concentration, in mg per mL, of USP Tetracaine Hydrochloride RS in the *Standard preparation*; V is the volume, in mL, of Ophthalmic Solution taken; and r_U and r_S are the tetracaine peak responses obtained from the *Assay preparation* and the *Standard preparation*, respectively.

Tetracaine Hydrochloride Topical Solution

» Tetracaine Hydrochloride Topical Solution is an aqueous solution of Tetracaine Hydrochloride. It contains not less than 95.0 percent and not more than 105.0 percent of the labeled amount of $C_{15}H_{24}N_2O_2 \cdot HCl$. It contains a suitable antimicrobial agent.

Packaging and storage—Preserve in tight, light-resistant containers.
Labeling—Label it to indicate that the Topical Solution is not to be used if it contains crystals, or if it is cloudy or discolored.
USP Reference standards ⟨11⟩—*USP Tetracaine Hydrochloride RS*.
Identification—
  A: *Ultraviolet Absorption* ⟨197U⟩—
  Solutions: solutions of the Topical Solution employed for measurement of absorbance in the *Assay*.
  B: It responds to the tests for *Chloride* ⟨191⟩.
pH ⟨791⟩: between 4.5 and 6.0.
Assay—
  Standard preparation—Prepare as directed in the *Assay* under *Tetracaine Hydrochloride in Dextrose Injection*.
  Assay preparation—Using an accurately measured volume of Topical Solution, prepare as directed in the *Assay* under *Tetracaine Hydrochloride in Dextrose Injection*.
  Procedure—Proceed as directed for *Procedure* in the *Assay* under *Tetracaine Hydrochloride in Dextrose Injection*. Calculate the quantity, in mg, of $C_{15}H_{24}N_2O_2 \cdot HCl$ in the volume of Topical Solution taken by the formula:

$$C(A_U/A_S)$$

in which C is the concentration, in µg per mL, of USP Tetracaine Hydrochloride RS in the *Standard preparation*, and A_U and A_S are the absorbances of the *Assay preparation* and the *Standard preparation*, respectively.

Tetracaine Hydrochloride in Dextrose Injection

» Tetracaine Hydrochloride in Dextrose Injection is a sterile solution of Tetracaine Hydrochloride and Dextrose in Water for Injection. It contains not less than 95.0 percent and not more than 105.0 percent of the labeled amounts of tetracaine hydrochloride ($C_{15}H_{24}N_2O_2 \cdot HCl$) and dextrose ($C_6H_{12}O_6$).

Packaging and storage—Preserve in single-dose or multiple-dose containers, preferably of Type I glass, under refrigeration and protected from light. It may be packaged in 100-mL multiple-dose containers. Injection supplied as a component of spinal anesthesia trays may be stored at room temperature for 12 months.
Labeling—Label it to indicate that the Injection is not to be used if it contains crystals, or if it is cloudy or discolored.
USP Reference standards ⟨11⟩—*USP Endotoxin RS. USP Tetracaine Hydrochloride RS*.
Identification—
  A: *Ultraviolet Absorption* ⟨197U⟩: *Assay preparation*, compared to the *Standard preparation* from the *Assay*.
  B: It responds to *Identification* test C under *Tetracaine Hydrochloride*.
  C: It responds to the *Identification* test under *Dextrose*.
Bacterial endotoxins ⟨85⟩—It contains not more than 1.0 USP Endotoxin Unit per mg of tetracaine hydrochloride.

pH ⟨791⟩: between 3.5 and 6.0
Particulate matter ⟨788⟩: meets the requirements under small-volume injections.
Other requirements—It meets the requirements under *Injections* ⟨1⟩.
Assay—

Standard preparation—Dissolve about 20 mg of USP Tetracaine Hydrochloride RS, accurately weighed, in water to make 100.0 mL, and mix. Pipet 5 mL of this solution into a 100-mL volumetric flask, add 5 mL of dilute hydrochloric acid (1 in 200) and 10 mL of *Buffer No. 6*, 10 percent, pH 6.0 (see *Phosphate Buffers* ⟨81⟩), dilute with water to volume, and mix.

Assay preparation—Transfer an accurately measured volume of Injection, equivalent to about 10 mg of tetracaine hydrochloride, to a separator, dilute with water to about 50 mL, and render alkaline by the addition of 5 mL of sodium carbonate TS. Extract immediately with two 50-mL portions of ether, collecting the extracts in a separator. Wash the ether extracts with 20 mL of water, discarding the wash solution, and extract the ether solution with two 20-mL portions and one 5-mL portion of dilute hydrochloric acid (1 in 200), collecting the extracts in a 50-mL volumetric flask. Dilute with water to volume, and mix. Transfer a 5.0-mL aliquot to a 100-mL volumetric flask, add 10 mL of *Buffer No. 6*, 10 percent, pH 6.0 (see *Phosphate Buffers and Other Solutions* under *Antibiotics—Microbial Assays* ⟨81⟩), dilute with water to volume, and mix.

Procedure—Concomitantly determine the absorbances of the *Assay preparation* and the *Standard preparation* at the wavelength of maximum absorbance at about 310 nm, with a suitable spectrophotometer, using water as the blank. Calculate the quantity, in mg, of tetracaine hydrochloride ($C_{15}H_{24}N_2O_2 \cdot HCl$) in the volume of Injection taken by the formula:

$$C(A_U / A_S)$$

in which C is the concentration, in µg per mL, of USP Tetracaine Hydrochloride RS in the *Standard preparation*; and A_U and A_S are the absorbances of the *Assay preparation* and the *Standard preparation*, respectively.

Assay for dextrose—Determine the angular rotation of the Injection in a suitable polarimeter tube (see *Optical Rotation* ⟨781⟩). Calculate the percentage (g per 100 mL) of dextrose ($C_6H_{12}O_6$) in the portion of Injection taken by the formula:

$$(100/52.9)AR$$

in which 100 is the percentage; 52.9 is the midpoint of the specific rotation range for anhydrous dextrose, in degrees; A is 100 mm divided by the length of the polarimeter tube, in mm; and R is the observed rotation, in degrees.

Tetracycline

$C_{22}H_{24}N_2O_8$ 444.43
2-Naphthacenecarboxamide, 4-(dimethylamino)-1,4,4a,5,5a, 6,11,12a-octahydro-3,6,10,12,12a-pentahydroxy-6-methyl-1,11-dioxo-, [4S-(4α,4aα,5aα,6β,12aα)]-.
(4S,4aS,5aS,12aS)-4-(Dimethylamino)-1,4,4a,5,5a,6,11,12a-octahydro-3,6,10,12,12a-pentahydroxy-6-methyl-1,11-dioxo-2-naphthacene-carboxamide   [*60-54-8*].
Trihydrate   498.49   [*6416-04-2*].

» Tetracycline has a potency equivalent to not less than 975 µg of tetracycline hydrochloride ($C_{22}H_{24}N_2O_8 \cdot HCl$) per mg, calculated on the anhydrous basis.

Packaging and storage—Preserve in tight, light-resistant containers.

Labeling—Label it to indicate that it is to be used in the manufacture of nonparenteral drugs only.
USP Reference standards ⟨11⟩—USP Tetracycline Hydrochloride RS. USP 4-Epianhydrotetracycline Hydrochloride RS.
Identification—
   A: *Ultraviolet Absorption* ⟨197U⟩—
   Solution: 20 µg per mL.
   Medium: 0.25 N sodium hydroxide.
   Absorptivity 6 minutes after preparation, calculated on the anhydrous basis, at 380 nm is between 104.5% and 111.95% of that of USP Tetracycline Hydrochloride RS, the potency of the Reference Standard being taken into account.
   B: The chromatogram of the *Assay* obtained as directed in the *Assay* exhibits a major peak for tetracycline, the retention time of which corresponds to that exhibited in the chromatogram of the *Standard preparation* obtained as directed in the *Assay*.
   C: To 0.5 mg add 2 mL of sulfuric acid: a purplish red color is produced. Add the solution to 1 mL of water: the color becomes yellow.
   D: Prepare a *Test Solution* in methanol containing the equivalent of 1 mg of tetracycline hydrochloride per mL, and proceed as directed for *Method II* under *Identification—Tetracyclines* ⟨193⟩.
Specific rotation ⟨781S⟩: between −260° and −280°, calculated on the anhydrous basis.
   Test solution: 5 mg per mL, in 0.1 N hydrochloric acid.
Crystallinity ⟨695⟩: meets the requirements.
pH ⟨791⟩: between 3.0 and 7.0, in an aqueous suspension containing 10 mg per mL.
Water, *Method I* ⟨921⟩: not more than 13.0%.
Heavy metals, *Method II* ⟨231⟩: 0.005%.
Limit of 4-epianhydrotetracycline—Using the *Diluting solvent*, *Chromatographic system*, and *Procedure* set forth in the *Assay*, chromatograph a Standard solution prepared by dissolving an accurately weighed quantity of USP 4-Epianhydrotetracycline Hydrochloride RS in *Diluting solvent* to obtain a solution having a known concentration of about 10 µg per mL. Using the chromatogram so obtained and the chromatogram of the *Assay preparation* obtained as directed in the *Assay*, calculate the percentage of 4-epianhydrotetracycline in the Tetracycline taken by the formula:

$$10(C_E / W)(r_U / r_S)$$

in which C_E is the concentration, in µg per mL, of USP 4-Epianhydrotetracycline Hydrochloride RS in the Standard solution, W is the weight, in mg, of Tetracycline taken to prepare the *Assay preparation*, and r_U and r_S are the 4-epianhydrotetracycline peak responses obtained from the *Assay preparation* and the Standard solution, respectively: not more than 2.0% is found.
Assay—

Diluting solvent, Mobile phase, Standard preparation, Resolution solution, and *Chromatographic system*—Prepare as directed in the *Assay* under *Tetracycline Hydrochloride*.

Assay preparation—Transfer about 45 mg of Tetracycline, accurately weighed, to a 100-mL volumetric flask, dissolve in *Diluting solvent*, dilute with the same solvent to volume, and mix.

Procedure—Proceed as directed in the *Assay* under *Tetracycline Hydrochloride*. Calculate the quantity, in µg, of tetracycline hydrochloride ($C_{22}H_{24}N_2O_8 \cdot HCl$) equivalent in each mg of Tetracycline taken by the formula:

$$100(CP / W)(r_U / r_S)$$

in which W is the weight, in mg, of Tetracycline taken to prepare the *Assay preparation*, and the other terms are as defined therein.

Tetracycline Boluses

» Tetracycline Boluses contain the equivalent of not less than 90.0 percent and not more than 120.0 percent of the labeled amount of tetracycline hydrochloride ($C_{22}H_{24}N_2O_8 \cdot HCl$).

Packaging and storage—Preserve in tight containers.
Labeling—Label Boluses to indicate that they are intended for veterinary use only.
USP Reference standards ⟨11⟩—*USP Tetracycline Hydrochloride RS.*
Identification—Shake a suitable quantity of finely powdered Boluses with methanol to obtain a solution containing the equivalent of 1 mg of tetracycline hydrochloride per mL, and filter. Using the filtrate as the *Test Solution*, proceed as directed under *Identification—Tetracyclines* ⟨193⟩.
Uniformity of dosage units ⟨905⟩: meet the requirements for *Weight Variation.*
Loss on drying ⟨731⟩—Dry about 100 mg of finely powdered Boluses, accurately weighed, in a capillary-stoppered bottle in vacuum at a pressure not exceeding 5 mm of mercury at 60° for 3 hours: it loses not more than 3.0% of its weight, or where the Boluses have a diameter of greater than 15 mm, it loses not more than 6.0% of its weight.
Assay—Transfer not less than 2 Boluses to a high-speed blender jar containing an accurately measured volume of 0.1 N hydrochloric acid, so that the solution so obtained contains not less than 150 µg of tetracycline hydrochloride per mL, and blend for about 3 to 5 minutes. Proceed as directed for tetracycline under *Antibiotics—Microbial Assays* ⟨81⟩, using an accurately measured volume of this solution diluted quantitatively and stepwise with water to obtain a *Test Dilution* having a concentration assumed to be equal to the median dose level of the Standard.

Tetracycline Oral Suspension

» Tetracycline Oral Suspension is Tetracycline with or without one or more suitable buffers, preservatives, stabilizers, and suspending agents. It contains the equivalent of not less than 90.0 percent and not more than 125.0 percent of the labeled amount of tetracycline hydrochloride ($C_{22}H_{24}N_2O_8 \cdot HCl$).

Packaging and storage—Preserve in tight, light-resistant containers.
USP Reference standards ⟨11⟩—*USP Tetracycline Hydrochloride RS. USP 4-Epianhydrotetracycline Hydrochloride RS.*
Identification—The chromatogram of the *Assay preparation* obtained as directed in the *Assay* exhibits a major peak for tetracycline, the retention time of which corresponds to that exhibited in the chromatogram of the *Standard preparation* obtained as directed in the *Assay.*
Uniformity of dosage units ⟨905⟩—
  For suspension packaged in single-unit containers: meets the requirements.
Deliverable volume ⟨698⟩: meets the requirements.
pH ⟨791⟩: between 3.5 and 6.0.
Limit of 4-epianhydrotetracycline—Using the *Diluting solvent*, *Chromatographic system*, and *Procedure* set forth in the *Assay*, chromatograph a Standard solution prepared by dissolving an accurately weighed quantity of USP 4-Epianhydrotetracycline Hydrochloride RS in *Diluting solvent* to obtain a solution having a known concentration of about 10 µg per mL. Using the chromatogram so obtained and the chromatogram of the *Assay preparation* obtained as directed in the *Assay*, calculate the percentage of 4-epianhydrotetracycline in the Oral Suspension taken by the formula:

$$(25C_E/T)(r_U/r_S)$$

in which C_E is the concentration, in µg per mL, of USP 4-Epianhydrotetracycline Hydrochloride RS in the Standard solution, T is the quantity, in mg, of tetracycline hydrochloride equivalent in the portion of Oral Suspension taken, based on the labeled quantity, and r_U and r_S are the 4-epianhydrotetracycline peak responses obtained from the *Assay preparation* and the Standard solution, respectively: not more than 5.0% is found.

Assay—
  Diluting solvent, Mobile phase, Standard preparation, Resolution solution, and *Chromatographic system*—Prepare as directed in the *Assay* under *Tetracycline Hydrochloride.*
  Assay preparation—Transfer an accurately measured volume of Oral Suspension, equivalent to about 125 mg of tetracycline hydrochloride, to a 250-mL volumetric flask, add 200 mL of *Diluting solvent*, and shake. Add *Diluting solvent* to volume, mix, and filter.
  Procedure—Proceed as directed in the *Assay* under *Tetracycline Hydrochloride*. Calculate the quantity, in mg per mL, of $C_{22}H_{24}N_2O_8 \cdot HCl$ equivalent in the Oral Suspension taken by the formula:

$$(CP/4V)(r_U/r_S)$$

in which V is the volume, in mL, of Oral Suspension taken, and the other terms are as defined therein.

Tetracycline Hydrochloride

$C_{22}H_{24}N_2O_8 \cdot HCl$ 480.90
2-Naphthacenecarboxamide, 4-(dimethylamino)-1,4,4a,5, 5a, 6, 11,12a-octahydro-3,6,10,12,12a-pentahydroxy-6-methyl-1, 11-dioxo-, monohydrochloride, [4S-(4α,4aα,5aα,6β,12aα)]-.
(4S, 4aS, 5aS, 6S,12aS)-4-(Dimethylamino)-1,4,4a,5,5a,6,11,12a-octahydro-3,6,10,12,12a-pentahydroxy-6-methyl-1,11-dioxo-2-naphthacenecarboxamide monohydrochloride   [64-75-5].

» Tetracycline Hydrochloride has a potency of not less than 900 µg of $C_{22}H_{24}N_2O_8 \cdot HCl$ per mg.

Packaging and storage—Preserve in tight, light-resistant containers.
Labeling—Where it is intended for use in preparing injectable or other sterile dosage forms, the label states that it is sterile or must be subjected to further processing during the preparation of injectable or other sterile dosage forms.
USP Reference standards ⟨11⟩—*USP Tetracycline Hydrochloride RS. USP 4-Epianhydrotetracycline Hydrochloride RS. USP Endotoxin RS.*
Identification—
  A: *Infrared Absorption* ⟨197K⟩—Do not dry specimen.
  B: *Ultraviolet Absorption* ⟨197U⟩—
    Solution: 20 µg per mL.
    Medium: 0.25 N sodium hydroxide.
  Absorptivity 6 minutes after preparation, calculated on the dried basis, at 380 nm is between 96.0% and 104.0% of that of USP Tetracycline Hydrochloride RS, the potency of the Reference Standard being taken into account.
  C: The chromatogram of the *Assay preparation* obtained as directed in the *Assay* exhibits a major peak for tetracycline, the retention time of which corresponds to that exhibited in the chromatogram of the *Standard preparation* obtained as directed in the *Assay.*
  D: To 0.5 mg add 2 mL of sulfuric acid: a purplish red color is produced. Add the solution to 1 mL of water: the color becomes yellow.
  E: Prepare a *Test Solution* in methanol containing 1 mg per mL, and proceed as directed for *Method II* under *Identification—Tetracyclines* ⟨193⟩.
  F: It responds to the silver nitrate test for *Chloride* ⟨191⟩.
Crystallinity ⟨695⟩: meets the requirements.
pH ⟨791⟩: between 1.8 and 2.8, in a solution containing 10 mg per mL.
Specific rotation ⟨781⟩: between −240° and −255°, calculated on the dried basis.
  Test solution: 5 mg per mL, in 0.1 N hydrochloric acid.
Loss on drying ⟨731⟩—Dry about 100 mg, accurately weighed, in a capillary-stoppered bottle in vacuum at a pressure not exceeding 5 mm of mercury at 60° for 3 hours: it loses not more than 2.0% of its weight.
Heavy metals, *Method II* ⟨231⟩:   0.005%.
Limit of 4-epianhydrotetracycline—Using the *Diluting solvent, Chromatographic system*, and *Procedure* set forth in the *Assay*,

chromatograph a Standard solution prepared by dissolving an accurately weighed quantity of USP 4-Epianhydrotetracycline Hydrochloride RS in *Diluting solvent* to obtain a solution having a known concentration of about 10 µg per mL. Using the chromatogram so obtained and the chromatogram of the *Assay preparation* obtained as directed in the *Assay*, calculate the percentage of 4-epianhydrotetracycline hydrochloride in the Tetracycline Hydrochloride taken by the formula:

$$10(C_E / W)(r_U / r_S)$$

in which C_E is the concentration, in µg per mL, of USP 4-Epianhydrotetracycline Hydrochloride RS in the Standard solution; W is the weight, in mg, of Tetracycline Hydrochloride taken to prepare the *Assay preparation*; and r_U and r_S are the 4-epianhydrotetracycline peak responses obtained from the *Assay preparation* and the Standard solution, respectively: not more than 2.0% is found.

Other requirements—Where the label states that Tetracycline Hydrochloride is sterile, it meets the requirements for *Sterility* and *Bacterial endotoxins* under *Tetracycline Hydrochloride for Injection*. Where the label states that Tetracycline Hydrochloride must be subjected to further processing during the preparation of injectable dosage forms, it meets the requirements for *Bacterial endotoxins* under *Tetracycline Hydrochloride for Injection*. Where it is intended for use in preparing nonparenteral sterile dosage forms, it is exempt from the requirements for *Bacterial endotoxins*.

Assay—

Diluting solvent—Mix 680 mL of 0.1 M ammonium oxalate and 270 mL of dimethylformamide.

Mobile phase—Mix 680 mL of 0.1 M ammonium oxalate, 270 mL of dimethylformamide, and 50 mL of 0.2 M dibasic ammonium phosphate. Adjust, if necessary, with 3 N ammonium hydroxide or 3 N phosphoric acid to a pH of 7.6 to 7.7. Make any other necessary adjustments (see *System Suitability* under *Chromatography* ⟨621⟩). Filter through a membrane filter of 0.5-µm or finer porosity.

Standard preparation—Dissolve an accurately weighed quantity of USP Tetracycline Hydrochloride RS in *Diluting solvent*, and dilute quantitatively with *Diluting solvent* to obtain a solution having a known concentration of about 0.5 mg per mL.

Assay preparation—Transfer about 50 mg of Tetracycline Hydrochloride, accurately weighed, to a 100-mL volumetric flask, dissolve in *Diluting solvent*, dilute with the same solvent to volume, and mix.

Resolution solution—Prepare a solution in *Diluting solvent* containing about 100 µg of tetracycline hydrochloride and 25 µg of USP 4-Epianhydrotetracycline Hydrochloride RS per mL.

Chromatographic system (see *Chromatography* ⟨621⟩)—The liquid chromatograph is equipped with a 280-nm detector, a 4.6-mm × 3-cm guard column that contains 10-µm packing L7, and a 4.6-mm × 25-cm analytical column that contains 5- to 10-µm packing L7. The flow rate is about 2 mL per minute. Chromatograph the *Resolution solution*, and record the peak responses as directed for *Procedure*: the relative retention times are about 0.9 for 4-epianhydrotetracycline and 1.0 for tetracycline; and the resolution, R, between the 4-epianhydrotetracycline and tetracycline peaks is not less than 1.2. Chromatograph the *Standard preparation*, and record the peak responses as directed for *Procedure*: the relative standard deviation for replicate injections is not more than 2.0%.

Procedure—Separately inject equal volumes (about 20 µL) of the *Standard preparation* and the *Assay preparation* into the chromatograph, record the chromatograms, and measure the responses for the major peaks. Calculate the quantity, in µg, of $C_{22}H_{24}N_2O_8 \cdot HCl$ in each mg of the Tetracycline Hydrochloride taken by the formula:

$$100(CP / W)(r_U / r_S)$$

in which C is the concentration, in mg per mL, of USP Tetracycline Hydrochloride RS in the *Standard preparation*; P is the potency, in µg per mg, of USP Tetracycline Hydrochloride RS; W is the weight, in mg, of Tetracycline Hydrochloride taken to prepare the *Assay preparation*; and r_U and r_S are the peak responses obtained from the *Assay preparation* and the *Standard preparation*, respectively.

Tetracycline Hydrochloride Capsules

» Tetracycline Hydrochloride Capsules contain not less than 90.0 percent and not more than 125.0 percent of the labeled amount of $C_{22}H_{24}N_2O_8 \cdot HCl$.

Packaging and storage—Preserve in tight, light-resistant containers.

USP Reference standards ⟨11⟩—*USP Tetracycline Hydrochloride RS. USP 4-Epianhydrotetracycline Hydrochloride RS.*

Identification—The chromatogram of the *Assay preparation* obtained as directed in the *Assay* exhibits a major peak for tetracycline, the retention time of which corresponds to that exhibited in the chromatogram of the *Standard preparation* obtained as directed in the *Assay*.

Dissolution ⟨711⟩—

Medium: water; 900 mL.

Apparatus 2: 75 rpm. Maintain a distance of 45 ± 5 mm between the blade and the inside bottom of the vessel.

Time: 60 minutes; 90 minutes for 500-mg capsules.

Procedure—Determine the amount of $C_{22}H_{24}N_2O_8 \cdot HCl$ dissolved from UV absorbances at the wavelength of maximum absorbance at about 276 nm of filtered portions of the solution under test, suitably diluted with *Dissolution Medium*, if necessary, in comparison with a Standard solution having a known concentration of USP Tetracycline Hydrochloride RS in the same *Medium*.

Tolerances—Not less than 80% (Q) of the labeled amount of $C_{22}H_{24}N_2O_8 \cdot HCl$ is dissolved in 60 minutes; 90 minutes for 500-mg capsules.

Uniformity of dosage units ⟨905⟩: meet the requirements.

Loss on drying ⟨731⟩—Dry about 100 mg of Capsule contents, accurately weighed, in a capillary-stoppered bottle in vacuum at a pressure not exceeding 5 mm of mercury at 60° for 3 hours: it loses not more than 4.0% of its weight.

Limit of 4-epianhydrotetracycline—Using the *Diluting solvent*, *Chromatographic system*, and *Procedure* set forth in the *Assay*, chromatograph a Standard solution prepared by dissolving an accurately weighed quantity of USP 4-Epianhydrotetracycline Hydrochloride RS in *Diluting solvent* to obtain a solution having a known concentration of about 10 µg per mL. Using the chromatogram so obtained and the chromatogram of the *Assay preparation* obtained as directed in the *Assay*, calculate the percentage of 4-epianhydrotetracycline hydrochloride in the Capsules taken by the formula:

$$(10C_E / T)(r_U / r_S)$$

in which C_E is the concentration, in µg per mL, of USP 4-Epianhydrotetracycline Hydrochloride RS in the Standard solution; T is the quantity, in mg, of tetracycline hydrochloride in the portion of Capsules taken to prepare the *Assay preparation*, based on the labeled quantity; and r_U and r_S are the 4-epianhydrotetracycline peak responses obtained from the *Assay preparation* and the Standard solution, respectively: not more than 3.0% is found.

Assay—

Diluting solvent, Mobile phase, Standard preparation, Resolution solution, and *Chromatographic system*—Prepare as directed in the *Assay* under *Tetracycline Hydrochloride*.

Assay preparation—Weigh accurately not fewer than 20 Capsules. Empty the Capsule contents into a mortar. Clean and accurately weigh the Capsule shells, and calculate the net weight of the Capsule contents. Mix the powder in the mortar, using a pestle, and transfer an accurately weighed quantity of the freshly mixed powder, equivalent to about 50 mg of tetracycline hydrochloride, to a 100-mL volumetric flask. Add about 50 mL of *Diluting solvent*, mix, and sonicate for about 5 minutes. Allow to cool, dilute with *Diluting solvent* to volume, mix, and filter.

Procedure—Proceed as directed in the *Assay* under *Tetracycline Hydrochloride*. Calculate the quantity, in mg, of $C_{22}H_{24}N_2O_8 \cdot HCl$ in the portion of Capsules taken by the formula:

$$(CP / 10)(r_U / r_S)$$

in which the terms are as defined therein.

Tetracycline Hydrochloride for Injection

» Tetracycline Hydrochloride for Injection is sterile Tetracycline Hydrochloride or a sterile, dry mixture of sterile Tetracycline Hydrochloride, one form of which contains Magnesium Chloride or magnesium ascorbate and one or more suitable buffers, and may contain one or more suitable preservatives, solubilizers, stabilizers, and anesthetic agents, and the other form of which contains one or more suitable stabilizing agents. It contains not less than 90.0 percent and not more than 115.0 percent of the labeled amount of $C_{22}H_{24}N_2O_8 \cdot HCl$.

Packaging and storage—Preserve in *Containers for Sterile Solids* as described under *Injections* ⟨1⟩, protected from light.
Labeling—Label Tetracycline Hydrochloride for Injection that contains an anesthetic agent to indicate that it is intended for intramuscular administration only.
USP Reference standards ⟨11⟩—*USP Tetracycline Hydrochloride RS. USP 4-Epianhydrotetracycline Hydrochloride RS. USP Endotoxin RS.*
Constituted solution—At the time of use, it meets the requirements for *Constituted Solutions* under *Injections* ⟨1⟩.
Identification—The chromatogram of the *Assay preparation* obtained as directed in the *Assay* exhibits a major peak for tetracycline, the retention time of which corresponds to that exhibited in the chromatogram of the *Standard preparation* obtained as directed in the *Assay*.
Bacterial endotoxins ⟨85⟩—It contains not more than 0.5 USP Endotoxin Unit per mg of tetracycline hydrochloride.
Sterility ⟨71⟩—It meets the requirements when tested as directed for *Membrane Filtration* under *Test for Sterility of the Product to be Examined*, *Fluid D* being used instead of *Fluid A*.
pH ⟨791⟩: between 2.0 and 3.0, in a solution containing 10 mg per mL.
Loss on drying ⟨731⟩—Dry about 100 mg, accurately weighed, in a capillary-stoppered bottle in vacuum at a pressure not exceeding 5 mm of mercury at 60° for 3 hours: it loses not more than 5.0% of its weight.
Particulate matter ⟨788⟩: meets the requirements for small-volume injections.
Limit of 4-epianhydrotetracycline—Using the *Diluting solvent*, *Chromatographic system*, and *Procedure* set forth in the *Assay*, chromatograph a Standard solution prepared by dissolving an accurately weighed quantity of USP 4-Epianhydrotetracycline Hydrochloride RS in *Diluting solvent* to obtain a solution having a known concentration of about 15 µg per mL. Using the chromatogram so obtained and the chromatogram of the *Assay preparation* obtained as directed in the *Assay*, calculate the percentage of 4-epianhydrotetracycline hydrochloride in the Tetracycline Hydrochloride for Injection taken by the formula:

$$(10C_E / T)(r_U / r_S)$$

in which C_E is the concentration, in µg per mL, of USP 4-Epianhydrotetracycline Hydrochloride RS in the Standard solution; T is the quantity, in mg, of tetracycline hydrochloride in the portion of Tetracycline Hydrochloride for Injection taken to prepare the *Assay preparation*, based on the labeled quantity; and r_U and r_S are the 4-epianhydrotetracycline peak responses obtained from the *Assay preparation* and the Standard solution, respectively: not more than 3.0% is found.
Other requirements—It meets the requirements for *Uniformity of Dosage Units* ⟨905⟩ and for *Labeling* under *Injections* ⟨1⟩.
Assay—
  Diluting solvent, Mobile phase, Standard preparation, Resolution solution, and *Chromatographic system*—Prepare as directed in the *Assay* under *Tetracycline Hydrochloride*.
  Assay preparation 1 (where it is represented as being in a single-dose container)—Constitute Tetracycline Hydrochloride for Injection as directed in the labeling. Withdraw all of the withdrawable contents, using a suitable hypodermic needle and syringe, and dilute quantitatively and stepwise with *Diluting solvent* to obtain a solution containing about 0.5 mg of tetracycline hydrochloride per mL.
  Assay preparation 2 (where the label states the quantity of tetracycline hydrochloride in a given volume of constituted solution)—Constitute Tetracycline Hydrochloride for Injection as directed in the labeling. Dilute an accurately measured volume of the constituted solution quantitatively with *Diluting solvent* to obtain a solution containing about 0.5 mg of tetracycline hydrochloride per mL.
  Procedure—Proceed as directed in the *Assay* under *Tetracycline Hydrochloride*. Calculate the quantity, in mg, of $C_{22}H_{24}N_2O_8 \cdot HCl$ withdrawn from the container, or in the portion of constituted solution taken by the formula:

$$(L / D)(CP / 1000)(r_U / r_S)$$

in which L is the labeled quantity, in mg, of $C_{22}H_{24}N_2O_8 \cdot HCl$ in the container, or in the volume of constituted solution taken; D is the concentration, in mg of tetracycline hydrochloride per mL, of *Assay preparation 1* or *Assay preparation 2*, based on the labeled quantity in the container or in the portion of constituted solution taken, respectively, and the extent of dilution; and the other terms are as defined therein.

Tetracycline Hydrochloride Ointment

» Tetracycline Hydrochloride Ointment contains not less than 90.0 percent and not more than 125.0 percent of the labeled amount of $C_{22}H_{24}N_2O_8 \cdot HCl$.

Packaging and storage—Preserve in well-closed containers, preferably at controlled room temperature.
USP Reference standards ⟨11⟩—*USP Tetracycline Hydrochloride RS. USP 4-Epianhydrotetracycline Hydrochloride RS.*
Identification—The chromatogram of the *Assay preparation* obtained as directed in the *Assay* exhibits a major peak for tetracycline, the retention time of which corresponds to that exhibited in the chromatogram of the *Standard preparation* obtained as directed in the *Assay*.
Minimum fill ⟨755⟩: meets the requirements.
Water, *Method I* ⟨921⟩: not more than 1.0%, 20 mL of a mixture of toluene and methanol (7 : 3) being used in place of methanol in the titration vessel.
Assay—
  Diluting solvent, Mobile phase, Resolution solution, and *Chromatographic system*—Prepare as directed in the *Assay* under *Tetracycline Hydrochloride*.
  Assay preparation—Transfer an accurately weighed portion of Ointment, equivalent to about 300 mg of tetracycline hydrochloride, to a glass-stoppered conical flask, add 20 mL of cyclohexane, and shake. Add 35 mL of methanol, and sonicate for about 20 minutes. Filter this solution into a 100-mL volumetric flask, and rinse the sides of the conical flask with 40 mL of methanol, filtering the rinsing through the filter into the volumetric flask. Dilute with methanol to volume, and mix. Transfer 2.0 mL of this solution to a 50-mL volumetric flask, dilute with *Diluting solvent* to volume, and mix.
  Standard preparation—Dissolve an accurately weighed quantity of USP Tetracycline Hydrochloride RS quantitatively in methanol to obtain a solution having a known concentration of about 1 mg per mL. Transfer 6.0 mL of this solution to a 50-mL volumetric flask, dilute with *Diluting solvent* to volume, and mix. This solution contains about 0.12 mg of USP Tetracycline Hydrochloride RS per mL.
  Procedure—Proceed as directed in the *Assay* under *Tetracycline Hydrochloride*. Calculate the quantity, in mg, of $C_{22}H_{24}N_2O_8 \cdot HCl$ in the portion of Ointment taken by the formula:

$$2.5CP(r_U / r_S)$$

in which the terms are as defined therein.

Tetracycline Hydrochloride Ophthalmic Ointment

» Tetracycline Hydrochloride Ophthalmic Ointment contains not less than 90.0 percent and not more than 125.0 percent of the labeled amount of $C_{22}H_{24}N_2O_8 \cdot HCl$.

Packaging and storage—Preserve in collapsible ophthalmic ointment tubes.
USP Reference standards ⟨11⟩—*USP Tetracycline Hydrochloride RS. USP 4-Epianhydrotetracycline Hydrochloride RS.*
Sterility ⟨71⟩: meets the requirements.
Minimum fill ⟨755⟩: meets the requirements.
Water, *Method I* ⟨921⟩: not more than 0.5%, 20 mL of a mixture of toluene and methanol (7 : 3) being used in place of methanol in the titration vessel.
Metal particles—It meets the requirements of the test for *Metal Particles in Ophthalmic Ointments* ⟨751⟩.
Assay—Proceed with Ophthalmic Ointment as directed in the *Assay* under *Tetracycline Hydrochloride Ointment*.

Tetracycline Hydrochloride Soluble Powder

» Tetracycline Hydrochloride Soluble Powder contains not less than 90.0 percent and not more than 125.0 percent of the labeled amount of $C_{22}H_{24}N_2O_8 \cdot HCl$.

Packaging and storage—Preserve in tight containers.
Labeling—Label it to indicate that it is intended for veterinary use only.
USP Reference standards ⟨11⟩—*USP Tetracycline Hydrochloride RS.*
Identification—Shake a suitable quantity of Powder with methanol to obtain a solution containing the equivalent of 1 mg of tetracycline hydrochloride per mL, and filter. Using the filtrate so obtained as the *Test Solution*, proceed as directed under *Identification—Tetracyclines* ⟨193⟩.
Loss on drying ⟨731⟩—Dry about 100 mg, accurately weighed, in a capillary-stoppered bottle in vacuum at a pressure not exceeding 5 mm of mercury at 60° for 3 hours: it loses not more than 2.0% of its weight.
Assay—Transfer an accurately weighed quantity of Powder to a high-speed blender jar containing an accurately measured volume of 0.1 N hydrochloric acid, so that the solution so obtained contains not less than 150 μg of tetracycline hydrochloride per mL, and blend for about 3 to 5 minutes. Proceed as directed for tetracycline under *Antibiotics—Microbial Assays* ⟨81⟩, diluting an accurately measured volume of this solution quantitatively and stepwise with water to yield a *Test Dilution* having a concentration assumed to be equal to the median dose level of the Standard.

Tetracycline Hydrochloride for Topical Solution

» Tetracycline Hydrochloride for Topical Solution is a dry mixture of Tetracycline Hydrochloride and Epitetracycline Hydrochloride with Sodium Metabisulfite packaged in conjunction with a suitable aqueous vehicle. It contains not less than 90.0 percent and not more than 130.0 percent of the labeled amount of tetracycline hydrochloride, when constituted as directed.

Packaging and storage—Preserve in tight, light-resistant containers.
USP Reference standards ⟨11⟩—*USP Tetracycline Hydrochloride RS.*
Identification—Dissolve a suitable quantity in methanol to obtain a solution containing 1 mg of tetracycline hydrochloride per mL, and filter, if necessary, to obtain a clear solution. Using the clear solution as the *Test Solution*, proceed as directed under *Identification—Tetracyclines* ⟨193⟩: the specified result is obtained.
pH ⟨791⟩: between 1.9 and 3.5, in the solution constituted as directed in the labeling.
Loss on drying ⟨731⟩—Dry the contents of 1 container, accurately weighed, in a capillary-stoppered bottle in vacuum at a pressure not exceeding 5 mm of mercury at 60° for 3 hours: it loses not more than 5.0% of its weight.
Content of epitetracycline hydrochloride—
Standard solution—Use the *Standard preparation* prepared as directed under the *Assay*.
Test solution—Open the column stopcock of the *Chromatographic column* remaining from the *Assay preparation* in the *Assay*, and collect the eluate in a low-actinic, 50-mL volumetric flask until the column runs dry. Use this as the *Test solution*.
Procedure—Proceed as directed for *Procedure* in the *Assay*. Calculate the quantity, in mg, of epitetracycline hydrochloride ($C_{22}H_{24}N_2O_8 \cdot HCl$) in each mL of the constituted Topical Solution taken by the formula:

$$0.002(WP/V)(A_U/A_S)$$

in which A_U is the absorbance of the solution from the *Test solution*, and the other terms are defined therein: the quantity of epitetracycline hydrochloride is between 115.0% and 140.0% of the quantity of tetracycline hydrochloride found as determined in the *Assay*.
Assay—
Edetate disodium solution—Dissolve 74.4 g of edetate disodium in about 1800 mL of water, adjust with ammonium hydroxide to a pH of 7.0, dilute with water to 2000 mL, and mix.
Stationary phase—Mix 95 mL of *Edetate disodium solution* and 5 mL of a mixture of glycerine and polyethylene glycol 400 (4 : 1).
Alkaline methanol solution—On the day of use, prepare a mixture of methanol and ammonium hydroxide (19 : 1).
Column support—Suspend 300 g of chromatographic siliceous earth in 2000 mL of 6 N hydrochloric acid in a suitable vessel, and mix for about 15 minutes. Filter, and wash the siliceous earth with water until the last washing is neutral to moistened litmus paper. Suspend the washed siliceous earth in 2000 mL of a mixture of ethyl acetate and methanol (1 : 1), and mix for about 15 minutes. Filter, and dry the siliceous earth in vacuum at 60° for about 16 hours. Weigh, add 0.5 mL of *Stationary phase* for each g of dried siliceous earth, and shake until the column packing is uniformly moist. Store in a tight container.
Chromatographic column—Prepare as directed under *Column Partition Chromatography* ⟨621⟩, using a 10- × 300-mm chromatographic tube equipped with a solvent reservoir on the top and a stopcock on the bottom and packed with 8 ± 0.1 g of *Column support*.
Standard preparation—Transfer about 22 mg of USP Tetracycline Hydrochloride RS, accurately weighed, to a 25-mL volumetric flask, add 1 mL of methanol, and swirl to dissolve. Dilute with *Stationary phase* to volume, and mix. Transfer 2.0 mL of this solution to a 10-mL volumetric flask, dilute with *Stationary phase* to volume, and mix. Pipet 2.0 mL of the resulting solution into the *Chromatographic column*, and allow it to permeate the *Column support*. Add 20 mL of benzene to the solvent reservoir, and collect the eluate at the rate of about 1 mL per minute, using a 50-mL graduated cylinder as a receiver. When the benzene level reaches the top of *Column support*, add 60 mL of chloroform to the solvent reservoir, and continue collecting the eluate until 30 mL has been collected. Discard this eluate, and continue collecting the eluate in a low-actinic, 50-mL volumetric flask. When the chloroform level reaches the top of the *Column support*, add 10 mL of a mixture of butyl alcohol and chloroform (1 : 1) to the solvent reservoir, and replace

the low-actinic, 50-mL volumetric flask with a 10-mL graduated cylinder. Collect 8 mL of the eluate, close the column stopcock, and transfer the eluate to the low-actinic, 50-mL volumetric flask. Rinse the graduated cylinder with 2 mL of chloroform, and add the rinsing to the volumetric flask. The eluate in the 50-mL volumetric flask is the *Standard preparation*.

Assay preparation—Constitute the Topical Solution as directed in the labeling. Transfer an accurately measured volume of the constituted Topical Solution, equivalent to about 4.4 mg of tetracycline hydrochloride, to a 25-mL volumetric flask, dilute with *Stationary phase* to volume, and mix. Pipet 2.0 mL of this solution into the *Chromatographic column*, and allow it to penetrate the *Column support*. Add 20 mL of benzene to the solvent reservoir, and collect the eluate at the rate of about 1 mL per minute, using a 50-mL graduated cylinder as a receiver. When the benzene level reaches the top of the *Column support*, add 60 mL of chloroform to the solvent reservoir, and continue collecting the eluate until 30 mL has been collected. Discard this eluate, and continue collecting the eluate in a low-actinic, 50-mL volumetric flask. When the chloroform level reaches the top of the *Column support*, add 50 mL of a mixture of butyl alcohol and chloroform (1 : 1) to the solvent reservoir, and replace the low-actinic, 50-mL volumetric flask with a 10-mL graduated cylinder. Collect 8 mL of the eluate, close the column stopcock, and transfer the eluate to the low-actinic, 50-mL volumetric flask. Rinse the graduated cylinder with 2 mL of chloroform, and add the rinsing to the volumetric flask. The eluate in the 50-mL volumetric flask is the *Assay preparation*. Retain the column for the test for *Content of epitetracycline hydrochloride*.

Procedure—Add 2.0 mL of *Alkaline methanol solution* to the *Standard preparation*, and the *Assay preparation*, dilute each with chloroform to volume, and mix. Concomitantly, within 10 minutes of preparation, determine the absorbances of these solutions at the wavelength of maximum absorbance at about 366 nm, with a suitable spectrophotometer, using chloroform as the blank. Calculate the quantity, in mg, of tetracycline hydrochloride in each mL of the constituted Topical Solution taken by the formula:

$$0.0002(WP / V)(A_U / A_S)$$

in which W is the weight, in mg, of USP Tetracycline Hydrochloride RS taken, P is the potency, in µg per mg, of USP Tetracycline Hydrochloride RS, V is the volume, in mL, of constituted Topical Solution taken, and A_U and A_S are the absorbances of the solutions from the *Assay preparation* and the *Standard preparation*, respectively.

Tetracycline Hydrochloride Ophthalmic Suspension

» Tetracycline Hydrochloride Ophthalmic Suspension is a sterile suspension of sterile Tetracycline Hydrochloride in a suitable oil. It contains not less than 90.0 percent and not more than 125.0 percent of the labeled amount of $C_{22}H_{24}N_2O_8 \cdot HCl$.

Packaging and storage—Preserve in tight, light-resistant containers of glass or plastic, containing not more than 15 mL. The containers or individual cartons are sealed and tamper-proof so that sterility is assured at time of first use.

USP Reference standards ⟨11⟩—*USP Tetracycline Hydrochloride RS. USP 4-Epianhydrotetracycline Hydrochloride RS.*
Identification—The chromatogram of the *Assay preparation* obtained as directed in the *Assay* exhibits a major peak for tetracycline, the retention time of which corresponds to that exhibited in the chromatogram of the *Standard preparation* obtained as directed in the *Assay*.
Sterility ⟨71⟩: meets the requirements.
Water, *Method I* ⟨921⟩: not more than 0.5%, 20 mL of a mixture of toluene and methanol (7 : 3) being used in place of methanol in the titration vessel.

Assay—
Diluting solvent, Mobile phase, Standard preparation, Resolution solution, and *Chromatographic system*—Prepare as directed in the *Assay* under *Tetracycline Hydrochloride*.
Assay preparation—Transfer an accurately measured volume of Ophthalmic Suspension, equivalent to about 50 mg of tetracycline hydrochloride, with the aid of 30 mL of cyclohexane to a 125-mL separator, add 30 mL of *Diluting solvent*, insert the stopper, and shake. Allow to separate, and collect the lower layer in a 100-mL volumetric flask. Repeat the extraction with two additional 30-mL portions of *Diluting solvent*, combining the extracts in the 100-mL volumetric flask. Add *Diluting solvent* to volume, mix, and filter.
Procedure—Proceed as directed for *Procedure* in the *Assay* under *Tetracycline Hydrochloride*. Calculate the quantity, in mg per mL, of $C_{22}H_{24}N_2O_8 \cdot HCl$ equivalent in the Ophthalmic Suspension taken by the formula:

$$(CP / 10V)(r_U / r_S)$$

in which V is the volume, in mL, of Ophthalmic Suspension taken, and the other terms are as defined therein.

Tetracycline Hydrochloride Oral Suspension

» Tetracycline Hydrochloride Oral Suspension contains not less than 2.25 g and not more than 2.75 g of Tetracycline Hydrochloride in 100 mL of Oral Suspension. Prepare Tetracycline Hydrochloride Oral Suspension as follows (see *Pharmaceutical Compounding—Nonsterile Preparations* ⟨795⟩):

Tetracycline Hydrochloride	2.50 g
Cetylpyridinium Chloride	10 mg
Xanthan Gum	0.15 g
Disbasic Sodium Phosphate	60 mg
Monobasic Sodium Phosphate	0.65 g
Sodium Hydroxide	0.30 g
Purified Water	35 mL
Suspension Structured Vehicle or Sugar-Free Suspension Structured Vehicle, a sufficient quantity to make	100 mL

Dissolve the Dibasic Sodium Phosphate and the Monobasic Sodium Phosphate in 25 mL of Purified Water. Separately dissolve an accurately weighed quantity of Cetylpyridinium Chloride in Purified Water and dilute quantitatively, and stepwise if necessary, with Purified Water to obtain 5 mL of a solution containing 10 mg of Cetylpyridinium Chloride. Mix this solution with 5 mL of the aqueous phosphate solution and add the resulting solution, in divided portions, with mixing, to the Tetracycline Hydrochloride in a glass mortar to completely wet the powder, and make a smooth paste.

Transfer the remaining 20 mL of the aqueous phosphate solution to a beaker. Using moderate heat, stir to form a vortex, and slowly sprinkle the Xanthan Gum into the vortex to produce a uniform dispersion. Add this dispersion to the paste in the glass mortar, and mix until smooth; then add 20 mL of the Suspension Structured Vehicle or Sugar-Free Suspension Vehicle to the mixture.

Dissolve the Sodium Hydroxide in 5 mL of Purified Water, and while mixing, slowly add this solution to the prepared mixture. Complete the suspension by adding a sufficient quantity of the Suspension Structured Vehicle or Sugar-Free Suspension Vehicle to make a final volume of 100 mL, and pass this final dispersion through a hand homogenizer prior to transferring it to the dispensing container.

Packaging and storage—Preserve in tight, light-resistant containers. Store at controlled room temperature, and protect from freezing.
Labeling—Label it to state that it should not be frozen and that it is to be well shaken before using.
pH $\langle 791 \rangle$: between 3.5 and 6.0.
Beyond-use date—Thirty days after the day on which it was compounded.
Assay—
Diluting solvent, Mobile phase, Standard preparation, Resolution solution, and *Chromatographic system*—Prepare as directed in the *Assay* under *Tetracycline Hydrochloride*.
Assay preparation—Transfer an accurately measured volume of Oral Suspension, equivalent to about 125 mg of tetracycline hydrochloride, to a 250-mL volumetric flask, add 200 mL of *Diluting solvent*, and shake. Add *Diluting solvent* to volume, mix, and filter.
Procedure—Proceed as directed in the *Assay* under *Tetracycline Hydrochloride*. Calculate the quantity, in mg per mL, of tetracycline hydrochloride ($C_{22}H_{24}N_2O_8 \cdot HCl$) in the Oral Suspension taken by the formula:

$$(CP/4V)(r_U / r_S)$$

in which V is the volume, in mL, of Oral Suspension taken; and the other terms are as defined therein.

Tetracycline Hydrochloride Tablets

» Tetracycline Hydrochloride Tablets contain not less than 90.0 percent and not more than 125.0 percent of the labeled amount of $C_{22}H_{24}N_2O_8 \cdot HCl$.

Packaging and storage—Preserve in tight, light-resistant containers.
USP Reference standards $\langle 11 \rangle$—*USP Tetracycline Hydrochloride RS. USP 4-Epianhydrotetracycline Hydrochloride RS.*
Identification—The chromatogram of the *Assay preparation* obtained as directed in the *Assay* exhibits a major peak for tetracycline, the retention time of which corresponds to that exhibited in the chromatogram of the *Standard preparation*, obtained as directed in the *Assay*.
Dissolution $\langle 711 \rangle$—
Medium: water; 900 mL.
Apparatus 2: 75 rpm. Maintain a distance of 45 ± 5 mm between the blade and the inside bottom of the vessel.
Time: 60 minutes.
Procedure—Determine the amount of $C_{22}H_{24}N_2O_8 \cdot HCl$ dissolved from UV absorbances at the wavelength of maximum absorbance at about 276 nm of filtered portions of the solution under test, suitably diluted with *Dissolution Medium*, if necessary, in comparison with a Standard solution having a known concentration of USP Tetracycline Hydrochloride RS in the same *Medium*.
Tolerances—Not less than 80% (*Q*) of the labeled amount of $C_{22}H_{24}N_2O_8 \cdot HCl$ is dissolved in 60 minutes.
Uniformity of dosage units $\langle 905 \rangle$: meet the requirements.
Loss on drying $\langle 731 \rangle$—Dry about 100 mg, accurately weighed, in vacuum at a pressure not exceeding 5 mm of mercury at 60° for 3 hours: it loses not more than 3.0% of its weight.

Limit of 4-epianhydrotetracycline—Using the *Diluting solvent, Chromatographic system,* and *Procedure* set forth in the *Assay*, chromatograph a Standard solution prepared by dissolving an accurately weighed quantity of USP 4-Epianhydrotetracycline Hydrochloride RS in *Diluting solvent* to obtain a solution having a known concentration of about 15 µg per mL. Using the chromatogram so obtained and the chromatogram of the *Assay preparation* obtained as directed in the *Assay*, calculate the percentage of 4-epianhydrotetracycline hydrochloride in the Tablets taken by the formula:

$$(10C_E / T)(r_U / r_S)$$

in which C_E is the concentration, in µg per mL, of USP 4-Epianhydrotetracycline Hydrochloride RS in the Standard solution; T is the quantity, in mg, of tetracycline hydrochloride in the portion of Tablets taken to prepare the *Assay preparation*, based on the labeled quantity; and r_U and r_S are the 4-epianhydrotetracycline peak responses obtained from the *Assay preparation* and the Standard solution, respectively: not more than 3.0% is found.
Assay—
Diluting solvent, Mobile phase, Standard preparation, Resolution solution, and *Chromatographic system*—Prepare as directed in the *Assay* under *Tetracycline Hydrochloride*.
Assay preparation—Weigh and finely powder not fewer than 20 Tablets. Transfer an accurately weighed portion of the powder, equivalent to about 50 mg of tetracycline hydrochloride, to a 100-mL volumetric flask, add 50 mL of *Diluting solvent*, mix, and sonicate for 5 minutes. Allow to cool, add *Diluting solvent* to volume, mix, and filter.
Procedure—Proceed as directed for *Procedure* in the *Assay* under *Tetracycline Hydrochloride*. Calculate the quantity, in mg, of $C_{22}H_{24}N_2O_8 \cdot HCl$ in the portion of Tablets taken by the formula:

$$(CP / 10)(r_U / r_S)$$

in which the terms are as defined therein.

Tetracycline Hydrochloride and Novobiocin Sodium Tablets

» Tetracycline Hydrochloride and Novobiocin Sodium Tablets contain the equivalent of not less than 90.0 percent and not more than 125.0 percent of the labeled amounts of tetracycline hydrochloride ($C_{22}H_{24}N_2O_8 \cdot HCl$) and novobiocin ($C_{31}H_{36}N_2O_{11}$).

Packaging and storage—Preserve in tight containers.
Labeling—Label the Tablets to indicate that they are intended for veterinary use only.
USP Reference standards $\langle 11 \rangle$—*USP Tetracycline Hydrochloride RS. USP Novobiocin RS.*
Identification—Shake a suitable quantity of finely powdered Tablets with methanol to obtain a solution containing 1 mg of tetracycline hydrochloride per mL, and filter. Using the filtrate as the *Test Solution*, proceed as directed under *Identification—Tetracyclines* $\langle 193 \rangle$.
Disintegration $\langle 701 \rangle$: 60 minutes, simulated gastric fluid TS being substituted for water in the test.
Uniformity of dosage units $\langle 905 \rangle$: meet the requirements for *Weight Variation* with respect to tetracycline hydrochloride and to novobiocin sodium.
Loss on drying $\langle 731 \rangle$—Dry about 100 mg, accurately weighed, of finely powdered Tablets in a capillary-stoppered bottle in vacuum at a pressure not exceeding 5 mm of mercury at 60° for 3 hours: it loses not more than 6.0% of its weight.
Limit of 4-epianhydrotetracycline $\langle 226 \rangle$—To an accurately weighed quantity of finely powdered Tablets, equivalent to about 250 mg of tetracycline hydrochloride, add 10 mL of 0.1 N hydrochloric acid, and adjust with 6 N ammonium hydroxide to a pH of 7.8. Transfer this solution with the aid of *EDTA Buffer* to a 50-mL volumetric flask, dilute with *EDTA Buffer* to volume, and mix. Use

this solution, without delay, as the *Test Solution:* not more than 2.0% is found.

Assay for tetracycline hydrochloride—Proceed as directed for tetracycline under *Antibiotics—Microbial Assays* ⟨81⟩, except to use *Escherichia coli* ATCC 10536 as the test organism instead of *Staphylococcus aureus* ATCC 29737 and an inoculum composition of about 0.2 mL of stock suspension in each 100 mL of *Medium 3*. Transfer not less than 5 Tablets to a high-speed blender jar containing an accurately measured volume of 0.1 N hydrochloric acid, so that, after blending for about 3 to 5 minutes, the solution so obtained contains not less than 150 μg of tetracycline hydrochloride per mL. Dilute an accurately measured volume of this solution quantitatively and stepwise with water to obtain a *Test Dilution* having a concentration of tetracycline hydrochloride assumed to be equal to the median dose level of the Standard.

Assay for novobiocin—Proceed as directed for novobiocin under *Antibiotics—Microbial Assays* ⟨81⟩, blending not less than 5 Tablets for 3 to 5 minutes in a high-speed glass blender jar containing 1.0 mL of polysorbate 80 and a sufficient accurately measured volume of *Buffer No. 3* to provide a stock solution of convenient concentration. Dilute an accurately measured volume of this stock solution quantitatively and stepwise with *Buffer No. 6* to obtain a *Test Dilution* having a concentration of novobiocin assumed to be equal to the median dose level of the Standard.

Tetracycline Hydrochloride, Novobiocin Sodium, and Prednisolone Tablets

» Tetracycline Hydrochloride, Novobiocin Sodium, and Prednisolone Tablets contain not less than 90.0 percent and not more than 125.0 percent of the labeled amounts of tetracycline hydrochloride ($C_{22}H_{24}N_2O_8 \cdot HCl$) and novobiocin ($C_{31}H_{36}N_2O_{11}$), and not less than 90.0 percent and not more than 110.0 percent of the labeled amount of prednisolone ($C_{21}H_{28}O_5$).

Packaging and storage—Preserve in tight containers.
Labeling—Label the Tablets to indicate that they are intended for veterinary use only.
USP Reference standards ⟨11⟩—*USP Tetracycline Hydrochloride RS. USP Novobiocin RS. USP Prednisolone RS.*
Disintegration ⟨701⟩: 60 minutes, simulated gastric fluid TS being substituted for water in the test.
Uniformity of dosage units ⟨905⟩: meet the requirements for *Weight Variation* with respect to tetracycline hydrochloride and to novobiocin sodium and for *Content Uniformity* with respect to prednisolone.

Procedure for content uniformity for prednisolone—

Mobile phase, Internal standard solution, and *Chromatographic system*—Prepare as directed in the *Assay* under *Prednisolone*.

Standard preparation—Prepare as directed in the *Assay for prednisolone*.

Test preparation—Transfer 1 Tablet to a suitable container, add 7 mL of diluted methanol (2 in 7) for each 1.5 mg of prednisolone in the Tablet, based on the labeled amount, and allow to stand for 90 minutes, occasionally agitating gently to ensure that the Tablet disintegrates. For each 1.5 mg of prednisolone, add 3.0 mL of *Internal standard solution,* 12 mL of water-saturated chloroform, and about 10 glass beads. Securely close the container, and shake by mechanical means for 30 minutes. Carefully open the container, add 0.5 mL of sodium carbonate solution (1 in 4), reclose the container, and shake by mechanical means for 5 minutes. Centrifuge, remove the upper layer by aspiration, discarding the aspirated liquid, and retain the clear chloroform layer (*Test preparation*).

Procedure—Proceed as directed for *Procedure* in the *Assay* under *Prednisolone*. Calculate the quantity, in mg, of prednisolone ($C_{21}H_{28}O_5$) in the Tablet taken by the formula:

$$0.015C(R_U / R_S)$$

in which the terms are as defined therein.

Limit of 4-epianhydrotetracycline ⟨226⟩—To an accurately weighed quantity of finely powdered Tablets, equivalent to about 250 mg of tetracycline hydrochloride, add 10 mL of 0.1 N hydrochloric acid, and adjust with 6 N ammonium hydroxide to a pH of 7.8. Transfer this solution with the aid of *EDTA Buffer* to a 50-mL volumetric flask, dilute with *EDTA Buffer* to volume, and mix. Use this solution, without delay, as the *Test Solution:* not more than 2.0% is found.

Other requirements—Tablets respond to the *Identification* test and meet the requirements of the test for *Loss on drying* under *Tetracycline Hydrochloride and Novobiocin Sodium Tablets*.

Assay for tetracycline hydrochloride and Assay for novobiocin—Using Tablets, proceed as directed in the *Assay for tetracycline hydrochloride* and the *Assay for novobiocin* under *Tetracycline Hydrochloride and Novobiocin Sodium Tablets*.

Assay for prednisolone—

Mobile phase, Internal standard solution, and *Chromatographic system*—Prepare as directed in the *Assay* under *Prednisolone*.

Standard preparation—Transfer about 10 mg of USP Prednisolone RS, accurately weighed, to a 100-mL volumetric flask, add 20.0 mL of *Internal standard solution,* and swirl to dissolve. Dilute with water-saturated chloroform to volume, and mix. Transfer 15.0 mL of this solution to a suitable container, add 7 mL of diluted methanol (2 in 7), securely close the container, and shake by mechanical means for 30 minutes. Carefully open the container, add 0.5 mL of sodium carbonate solution (1 in 4), reclose the container, and shake by mechanical means for 5 minutes. Centrifuge, remove the upper layer by aspiration, discarding the aspirated liquid, and retain the clear chloroform layer (*Standard preparation*).

Assay preparation—Weigh and finely powder not less than 20 Tablets. Transfer an accurately weighed portion of the powder, equivalent to about 1.5 mg of prednisolone, to a suitable container containing about 10 glass beads. Add 3.0 mL of *Internal standard solution,* 12 mL of water-saturated chloroform, and 7 mL of diluted methanol (2 in 7), securely close the container, and shake by mechanical means for 30 minutes. Carefully open the container, add 0.5 mL of sodium carbonate solution (1 in 4), reclose the container, and shake by mechanical means for 5 minutes. Centrifuge, remove the upper layer by aspiration, discarding the aspirated liquid, and retain the clear chloroform layer (*Assay preparation*).

Procedure—Proceed as directed for *Procedure* in the *Assay* under *Prednisolone*. Calculate the quantity, in mg, of prednisolone ($C_{21}H_{28}O_5$) in the portion of Tablets taken by the formula:

$$0.015C(R_U / R_S)$$

in which the terms are as defined therein.

Tetracycline Hydrochloride and Nystatin Capsules

» Tetracycline Hydrochloride and Nystatin Capsules contain not less than 90.0 percent and not more than 125.0 percent of the labeled amount of tetracycline hydrochloride ($C_{22}H_{24}N_2O_8 \cdot HCl$), and not less than 90.0 percent and not more than 135.0 percent of the labeled amount of USP Nystatin Units.

Packaging and storage—Preserve in tight, light-resistant containers.
USP Reference standards ⟨11⟩—*USP Tetracycline Hydrochloride RS. USP Nystatin RS.*
Identification—Shake a suitable quantity of Capsule contents with methanol to obtain a solution containing about 1 mg of tetracycline

hydrochloride per mL, and filter. Using the filtrate as the *Test Solution*, proceed as directed under *Identification—Tetracyclines* ⟨193⟩.
Dissolution ⟨711⟩—
  Medium: water; 900 mL.
  Apparatus 2: 75 rpm.
  Time: 60 minutes.
  Procedure—Determine the amount of tetracycline hydrochloride ($C_{22}H_{24}N_2O_8 \cdot HCl$) dissolved from UV absorbances at the wavelength of maximum absorbance at about 276 nm of filtered portions of the solution under test, suitably diluted with *Dissolution Medium*, if necessary, in comparison with a *Standard solution* having a known concentration of USP Tetracycline Hydrochloride RS in the same *Medium*.
  Tolerances—Not less than 70% (*Q*) of the labeled amount of $C_{22}H_{24}N_2O_8 \cdot HCl$ is dissolved in 60 minutes.
Loss on drying ⟨731⟩—Dry about 100 mg of Capsule contents, accurately weighed, in a capillary-stoppered bottle in vacuum at a pressure not exceeding 5 mm of mercury at 60° for 3 hours: it loses not more than 4.0% of its weight.
Limit of 4-epianhydrotetracycline ⟨226⟩—To a quantity of Capsule contents, equivalent to about 250 mg of tetracycline hydrochloride, add 10 mL of 0.1 N hydrochloric acid, and adjust with 6 N ammonium hydroxide to a pH of 7.8. Transfer this solution with the aid of *EDTA Buffer* to a 50-mL volumetric flask, dilute with *EDTA Buffer* to volume, and mix. Use this solution, without delay, as the *Test Solution:* not more than 3.0% is found.
Assay for tetracycline hydrochloride—Proceed with Capsules as directed in the *Assay* under *Tetracycline Hydrochloride Capsules*.
Assay for nystatin—Proceed as directed for Nystatin under *Antibiotics—Microbial Assays* ⟨81⟩, blending not less than 5 Capsules for 3 to 5 minutes in a high-speed blender with a sufficient, accurately measured, volume of dimethylformamide to obtain a solution of convenient concentration. Dilute an accurately measured portion of this solution quantitatively with dimethylformamide to obtain a stock solution containing about 400 USP Nystatin Units per mL. Dilute this stock solution quantitatively with *Buffer No. 6* to obtain a *Test Dilution* having a concentration of nystatin assumed to be equal to the median dose level of the Standard.

Tetrahydrozoline Hydrochloride

$C_{13}H_{16}N_2 \cdot HCl$ 236.74
1*H*-Imidazole, 4,5-dihydro-2-(1,2,3,4-tetrahydro-1-naphthalenyl)-, monohydrochloride.
2-(1,2,3,4-Tetrahydro-1-naphthyl)-2-imidazoline monohydrochloride [*522-48-5*].

» Tetrahydrozoline Hydrochloride contains not less than 98.0 percent and not more than 100.5 percent of $C_{13}H_{16}N_2 \cdot HCl$, calculated on the dried basis.

Packaging and storage—Preserve in tight containers.
USP Reference standards ⟨11⟩—*USP Tetrahydrozoline Hydrochloride RS*.
Identification—
  A: *Infrared Absorption* ⟨197K⟩.
  B: *Ultraviolet Absorption* ⟨197U⟩—
    Solution: 250 µg per mL.
    Medium: water.
  Absorptivities at 264 nm and 271 nm, calculated on the dried basis, do not differ by more than 4.0%.
  C: A solution (1 in 200) responds to the tests for *Chloride* ⟨191⟩.
Loss on drying ⟨731⟩—Dry it at 105° for 2 hours: it loses not more than 1.0% of its weight.

Residue on ignition ⟨281⟩: not more than 0.1%.
Heavy metals ⟨231⟩—Dissolve 0.40 g in 23 mL of water, and add 2 mL of 1 N acetic acid: the limit is 0.005%.
Ordinary impurities ⟨466⟩—
  Test solution: methanol.
  Standard solution: methanol.
  Eluant: a mixture of methanol, glacial acetic acid, and water (8 : 1 : 1).
  Visualization: 3, followed by overspraying with hydrogen peroxide TS. [NOTE—Cover the thin-layer chromatographic plate with a glass plate to slow fading of the spots.]
Assay—Transfer about 400 mg of Tetrahydrozoline Hydrochloride, accurately weighed, to a 250-mL beaker, and dissolve in 60 mL of glacial acetic acid, heating if necessary. Add 5 mL of acetic anhydride, 5 mL of mercuric acetate TS, and 3 drops of quinaldine red TS, and titrate with 0.1 N perchloric acid VS. Perform a blank determination, and make any necessary correction. Each mL of 0.1 N perchloric acid is equivalent to 23.67 mg of $C_{13}H_{16}N_2 \cdot HCl$.

Tetrahydrozoline Hydrochloride Nasal Solution

» Tetrahydrozoline Hydrochloride Nasal Solution is a solution of Tetrahydrozoline Hydrochloride in water adjusted to a suitable tonicity. It contains not less than 90.0 percent and not more than 110.0 percent of the labeled amount of $C_{13}H_{16}N_2 \cdot HCl$.

Packaging and storage—Preserve in tight containers.
USP Reference standards ⟨11⟩—*USP Tetrahydrozoline Hydrochloride RS*.
Identification—The UV absorption spectrum of the Nasal Solution, diluted with water, if necessary, to a concentration of about 1 in 4000, exhibits maxima and minima at the same wavelengths as that of a similar solution of USP Tetrahydrozoline Hydrochloride RS, concomitantly measured.
Microbial limits ⟨61⟩—It meets the requirements of the tests for absence of *Staphylococcus aureus* and *Pseudomonas aeruginosa*.
pH ⟨791⟩: between 5.3 and 6.5.
Assay—
  Oxidized nitroprusside reagent—Dissolve 1.0 g of sodium nitroferricyanide in water to make 10.0 mL (*Solution A*). Dissolve 1.0 g of potassium ferricyanide in water to make 10.0 mL (*Solution B*). Transfer 1.0 mL each of *Solution A* and *Solution B* to a 100-mL volumetric flask, add 1 mL of sodium hydroxide solution (1 in 10), and allow to stand until the solution changes to a light yellow color (about 20 to 30 minutes). Dilute with water to volume, and mix. Store in a refrigerator or keep in an ice bath, and use within 4 hours.
  Standard preparation—Dissolve a suitable quantity of USP Tetrahydrozoline Hydrochloride RS, accurately weighed, in water, and dilute with water to obtain a solution having a known concentration of about 100 µg per mL.
  Assay preparation—Transfer an accurately measured volume of Nasal Solution, equivalent to about 10 mg of tetrahydrozoline hydrochloride, to a 100-mL volumetric flask, dilute with water to volume, and mix.
  Procedure—Transfer 5.0 mL each of the *Standard preparation* and the *Assay preparation* to separate glass-stoppered test tubes. Pipet 5 mL of water into a third tube to provide a blank. To each tube add 4.0 mL of *Oxidized nitroprusside reagent*, mix, and allow to stand at 30° for 15 minutes. Concomitantly determine the absorbances of the solutions in 1-cm cells at the wavelength of maximum absorbance at about 570 nm, with a suitable spectrophotometer, using the blank to set the instrument. Calculate the quantity, in mg, of $C_{13}H_{16}N_2 \cdot HCl$ in each mL of the Nasal Solution taken by the formula:

$$0.1(C/V)(A_U/A_S)$$

in which *C* is the concentration, in µg per mL, of USP Tetrahydrozoline Hydrochloride RS in the *Standard preparation*, *V* is the volume, in mL, of Nasal Solution taken, and A_U and A_S are the absorbances of the solutions from the *Assay preparation* and the *Standard preparation*, respectively.

Tetrahydrozoline Hydrochloride Ophthalmic Solution

» Tetrahydrozoline Hydrochloride Ophthalmic Solution is a sterile, isotonic solution of Tetrahydrozoline Hydrochloride in water. It contains not less than 90.0 percent and not more than 110.0 percent of the labeled amount of $C_{13}H_{16}N_2 \cdot HCl$.

Packaging and storage—Preserve in tight containers.

USP Reference standards ⟨11⟩—*USP Tetrahydrozoline Hydrochloride RS.*

Identification—The UV absorption spectrum of the Ophthalmic Solution, diluted with dilute hydrochloric acid (1 in 100) to a concentration of about 1 in 4000, exhibits maxima and minima at the same wavelengths as that of a similar solution of USP Tetrahydrozoline Hydrochloride RS, concomitantly measured.

Sterility ⟨71⟩: meets the requirements.

pH ⟨791⟩: between 5.8 and 6.5.

Assay—

Standard preparation—Dissolve a suitable quantity of USP Tetrahydrozoline Hydrochloride RS, accurately weighed, in water, and dilute quantitatively with water to obtain a solution having a known concentration of about 500 μg per mL.

Procedure—Transfer 2.0 mL of *Standard preparation* to a 50-mL volumetric flask. Transfer an accurately measured volume of Ophthalmic Solution, equivalent to about 1 mg of tetrahydrozoline hydrochloride, to a second 50-mL flask, and transfer 2 mL of water to a third 50-mL volumetric flask to provide a blank. To each flask add 5.0 mL of bromophenol blue sodium salt solution (1 in 1000), dilute each flask with potassium biphthalate solution (1 in 100) to volume, and mix. Allow to stand for 20 minutes, and filter each mixture through a suitable filter paper (Whatman No. 42 or the equivalent) that does not absorb the dye, discarding the first 15 mL of the filtrate. Transfer 20.0 mL of the subsequent filtrate to separate 125-mL separators, and extract each solution with four 20-mL portions of chloroform, filtering each extract through a pledget of glass wool into a 100-mL volumetric flask. Dilute the combined extracts from each solution with chloroform to volume, and mix. Concomitantly determine the absorbances of the solutions in 1-cm cells at the wavelength of maximum absorbance at about 415 nm, with a suitable spectrophotometer, using the blank to set the instrument. Calculate the quantity, in μg, of $C_{13}H_{16}N_2 \cdot HCl$ in each mL of the Ophthalmic Solution taken by the formula:

$$2(C/V)(A_U/A_S)$$

in which C is the concentration, in μg per mL, of USP Tetrahydrozoline Hydrochloride RS in the *Standard preparation*, V is the volume, in mL, of Solution taken, and A_U and A_S are the absorbances of the solutions from the Ophthalmic Solution and the *Standard preparation*, respectively.

Thalidomide

$C_{13}H_{10}N_2O_4$ 258.23
1*H*-Isoindole-1,3(2*H*)-dione, 2-(2,6-dioxo-3-piperidinyl)-, (±)-.
(±)-*N*-(2,6-Dioxo-3-piperidyl)phthalimide.
α-(*N*-Phthalimido)glutarimide   [50-35-1].

» Thalidomide contains not less than 98.0 percent and not more than 101.5 percent of $C_{13}H_{10}N_2O_4$, calculated on the anhydrous basis.

Packaging and storage—Preserve in tight containers, protected from light, and store at controlled room temperature.
USP Reference standards ⟨11⟩—*USP Thalidomide RS.*
Identification, *Infrared Absorption* ⟨197K⟩.
Microbial limits ⟨61⟩—The total aerobic microbial count using the *Plate Method* is not more than 1000 cfu per g, and the total combined molds and yeasts count is not more than 100 cfu per g.
Water, *Method Ic* ⟨921⟩: not more than 0.5%.
   Solvent: anhydrous dimethyl sulfoxide.
Heavy metals, *Method II* ⟨231⟩: 0.002%.
Chromatographic purity—

Solution A—Prepare a filtered and degassed mixture of water, acetonitrile, and phosphoric acid (95 : 5 : 0.1).

Solution B—Prepare a filtered and degassed mixture of water, acetonitrile, and phosphoric acid (85 : 15 : 0.1).

Diluent—Prepare a mixture of water, acetonitrile, and phosphoric acid (50 : 50 : 0.1).

Mobile phase—Use variable mixtures of *Solution A* and *Solution B* as directed for *Chromatographic system*. Make adjustments if necessary (see *System Suitability* under *Chromatography* ⟨621⟩).

Phthalic acid stock solution—Transfer about 100 mg of phthalic acid to a 100-mL volumetric flask, dissolve in a mixture of acetonitrile and water (80 : 5), and dilute with acetonitrile to volume. Mix, and dilute quantitatively, and stepwise if necessary, with acetonitrile to obtain a solution having a concentration of about 0.1 mg per mL.

Standard stock solution—Dissolve, with the aid of sonication, an accurately weighed quantity of USP Thalidomide RS in acetonitrile to obtain a solution having a known concentration of about 1 mg per mL.

Standard solution—Pipet 2.0 mL of the *Standard stock solution* and 2.0 mL of the *Phthalic acid stock solution* into a 100-mL volumetric flask, dilute with *Diluent* to volume, and mix. Pipet 10.0 mL of this solution into a 100-mL volumetric flask, add 10.0 mL of phosphoric acid solution (1 in 100), dilute with water to volume, and mix to obtain a solution having a known concentration of about 0.0002 mg of phthalic acid per mL.

Test solution—Transfer about 100 mg of Thalidomide, accurately weighed, to a 50-mL volumetric flask, and dissolve, with the aid of sonication, in 40 mL of a mixture of water, acetonitrile, and phosphoric acid (50 : 50 : 0.1). Dilute with *Diluent* to volume, and mix. Pipet 10.0 mL of this solution into a 100-mL volumetric flask, add 10.0 mL of phosphoric acid solution (1 in 100), dilute with water to volume, and mix.

Chromatographic system (see *Chromatography* ⟨621⟩)—The liquid chromatograph is equipped with a 218-nm detector and a 3.9-mm × 15-cm column that contains 4-μm packing L1. The flow rate is about 2 mL per minute. The chromatograph is programmed as follows.

Time (minutes)	Solution A (%)	Solution B (%)	Elution
0	100	0	equilibration
0–15	100→50	0→50	linear gradient
15–20	50→100	50→0	linear gradient
20–30	100	0	isocratic

Chromatograph the *Standard solution*, and record the peak responses as directed for *Procedure*: the relative retention times are about 0.35 for phthalic acid and about 1.0 for thalidomide; the tailing factor for the phthalic acid and thalidomide peaks is not more than 2.0; and the relative standard deviation determined from the phthalic acid peak for replicate injections is not more than 2.0%.

Procedure—Separately inject equal volumes (about 200 µL) of the *Standard solution* and the *Test solution* into the chromatograph, record the chromatograms, and measure the areas for all the peaks. Calculate the percentage of each impurity in Thalidomide by the formula:

$$50{,}000(C_P / W)(r_i / r_P)$$

in which C_P is the concentration, in mg per mL, of phthalic acid in the *Standard solution*; W is the amount, in mg, of Thalidomide taken to prepare the *Test solution*; r_i is the peak response for each impurity obtained from the *Test solution*; and r_P is the phthalic acid peak response obtained from the *Standard solution*: not more than 0.1% of any individual impurity is found; and not more than 0.3% of total impurities is found.

Ordinary impurities ⟨466⟩—

Test solution—Dissolve an accurately weighed quantity of Thalidomide in acetonitrile to obtain a solution having a concentration of about 2 mg per mL.

Standard solution—Dissolve an accurately weighed quantity of glutamine in a mixture of acetonitrile and water (1 : 1) to obtain a solution having a concentration of about 0.1 mg per mL.

Eluant: a mixture of methylene chloride, methanol, and acetic acid (75 : 25 : 0.05).

Application volume: 2 µL (*Standard solution*) and 100 µL (*Test solution*).

Visualization: 4.

Limit: 0.1%.

Organic volatile impurities, *Method I* ⟨467⟩: meets the requirements.

(Official until July 1, 2008)

Assay—

Mobile phase—Prepare a filtered and degassed mixture of water, acetonitrile, and phosphoric acid (85 : 15 : 0.1). Make adjustments if necessary (see *System Suitability* under *Chromatography* ⟨621⟩).

Internal standard preparation—Transfer about 150 mg of phenacetin, accurately weighed, to a 100-mL volumetric flask, dissolve in about 80 mL of acetonitrile, dilute with acetonitrile to volume, and mix.

Standard preparation—Dissolve, with the aid of sonication, an accurately weighed quantity of USP Thalidomide RS in acetonitrile to obtain a solution having a known concentration of about 1 mg per mL. Transfer 10.0 mL of this solution and 5.0 mL of *Internal standard preparation* to a 100-mL volumetric flask, add 10.0 mL of phosphoric acid solution (1 in 100), dilute with water to volume, and mix.

Assay preparation—Transfer about 100 mg of Thalidomide, accurately weighed, to a 100-mL volumetric flask, and dissolve, with the aid of sonication, in 80 mL of acetonitrile. Dilute with acetonitrile to volume, and mix. Pipet 10.0 mL of this solution and 5.0 mL of *Internal standard preparation* into a 100-mL volumetric flask, add 10.0 mL of phosphoric acid solution (1 in 100), dilute with water to volume, and mix.

Chromatographic system (see *Chromatography* ⟨621⟩)—The liquid chromatograph is equipped with a 237-nm detector and a 3.9-mm × 15-cm column that contains 4-µm packing L1. The flow rate is about 1.0 mL per minute. Chromatograph the *Standard preparation*, and record the peak responses as directed for *Procedure*: the resolution, R, between thalidomide and phenacetin is not less than 3.0; the column efficiency determined from the thalidomide and phenacetin peaks is not less than 7000 and 9000 theoretical plates, respectively; the tailing factor is not more than 2.0; and the relative standard deviation for replicate injections is not more than 1.0%.

Procedure—Separately inject equal volumes (about 20 µL) of the *Standard preparation* and the *Assay preparation* into the chromatograph, record the chromatograms, and measure the areas for the major peaks. Calculate the quantity, in mg, of $C_{13}H_{10}N_2O_4$ in the portion of Thalidomide taken by the formula:

$$1000C(R_U / R_S)$$

in which C is the concentration, in mg per mL, of USP Thalidomide RS in the *Standard preparation*; and R_U and R_S are the peak area ratios obtained from the *Assay preparation* and the *Standard preparation*, respectively.

Thalidomide Capsules

» Thalidomide Capsules contain not less than 90.0 percent and not more than 110.0 percent of the labeled amount of thalidomide ($C_{13}H_{10}N_2O_4$).

Packaging and storage—Preserve in tight containers, protected from light, at controlled room temperature. Do not repackage.

USP Reference standards ⟨11⟩—*USP Thalidomide RS*.

Identification—

A: *Thin-Layer Chromatographic Identification Test* ⟨201⟩—

Test solution—Prepare a solution of it in acetonitrile containing about 3000 µg of thalidomide per mL.

Application volume: 5 µL.

Developing solvent system: a mixture of normal butyl acetate, glacial acetic acid, and butyl alcohol (50 : 25 : 5).

B: The relative retention time of the major peak in the chromatogram of the *Assay preparation* corresponds to that in the chromatogram of the *Standard preparation*, as obtained in the *Assay*.

Microbial limits ⟨61⟩—The total aerobic microbial count using the *Plate Method* is not more than 1000 cfu per g, and the total combined molds and yeasts count is not more than 100 cfu per g. It meets the requirements of the test for absence of *Escherichia coli*.

Dissolution ⟨711⟩—

Medium—Add 1.0 mL of polyoxyethylene (23) lauryl ether solution, prepared by dissolving 50 g in 100 mL of water, to 0.225 M hydrochloric acid; 4000 mL.

Apparatus 2: 75 rpm.

Time: 60 minutes.

Determine the amount of $C_{13}H_{10}N_2O_4$ dissolved by employing the following method.

Mobile phase—Prepare as directed in the *Assay* under *Thalidomide*.

Internal standard solution—Prepare a solution of phenacetin in acetonitrile containing about 375 µg per mL. Pipet 20.0 mL of this solution into a 100-mL volumetric flask, add 10.0 mL of phosphoric acid solution (1 in 100), dilute with water to volume, and mix.

Standard solution—Dissolve an accurately weighed quantity of USP Thalidomide RS in acetonitrile to obtain a solution having a known concentration of about 0.25 mg per mL. Pipet 10.0 mL of this solution into a 100-mL volumetric flask, add 10.0 mL of phosphoric acid solution (1 in 100), dilute with water to volume, and mix. Add 5.0 mL of *Internal standard solution* to 20.0 mL of this solution, and mix. This solution contains about 0.02 mg of USP Thalidomide RS per mL.

Test solution—Add 5.0 mL of *Internal standard solution* to each 20.0 mL of filtered solution under test, and mix.

Procedure—Separately inject equal volumes (about 20 µL) of the *Standard solution* and the *Test solution* into the chromatograph, record the chromatograms, and measure the areas for the major peaks. Calculate the quantity, in mg, of $C_{13}H_{10}N_2O_4$ dissolved by the formula:

$$2500C(R_U / R_S)$$

in which C is the concentration, in mg per mL, of USP Thalidomide RS in the *Standard solution*; and R_U and R_S are the peak area ratios of thalidomide to the internal standard obtained from the *Test solution* and the *Standard solution*, respectively.

Tolerances—Not less than 70% (*Q*) of the labeled amount of $C_{13}H_{10}N_2O_4$ is dissolved in 60 minutes.

Uniformity of dosage units ⟨905⟩: meet the requirements.

Assay—

Mobile phase, Internal standard preparation, Standard preparation, and *Chromatographic system*—Prepare as directed in the *Assay* under *Thalidomide*.

Assay preparation—Remove, as completely as possible, the contents of not fewer than 20 Capsules, and weigh accurately. Mix the combined contents, and transfer an accurately weighed portion of the powder, equivalent to about 50 mg of thalidomide, to a 100-mL volumetric flask, add 80 mL of acetonitrile to dissolve, and sonicate for about 20 minutes. Dilute with acetonitrile to volume, and mix. Transfer 20.0 mL of this solution and 5.0 mL of *Internal standard preparation* to a 100-mL volumetric flask, add 10.0 mL of phosphoric acid solution (1 in 100), dilute with water to volume, and mix.

Procedure—Separately inject equal volumes (about 20 µL) of the *Standard preparation* and the *Assay preparation* into the chromatograph, record the chromatograms, and measure the areas for the major peaks. Calculate the quantity, in mg, of thalidomide ($C_{13}H_{10}N_2O_4$) in the portion of Capsules taken by the formula:

$$1000C(R_U / R_S)$$

in which C is the concentration, in mg per mL, of USP Thalidomide RS in the *Standard preparation*; and R_U and R_S are the peak area ratios of thalidomide to the internal standard obtained from the *Assay preparation* and the *Standard preparation*, respectively.

Thallous Chloride Tl 201 Injection

» Thallous Chloride Tl 201 Injection is a sterile, isotonic, aqueous solution of radioactive thallium (^{201}Tl) in the form of thallous chloride suitable for intravenous administration. It contains not less than 90.0 percent and not more than 110.0 percent of the labeled amount of ^{201}Tl as chloride, expressed in megabecquerels (microcuries or millicuries) per mL, at the time indicated in the labeling. Other chemical forms of radioactivity do not exceed 5.0 percent of the total radioactivity. It may contain a preservative or stabilizer.

Packaging and storage—Preserve in single-dose or multiple-dose containers.

Labeling—Label it to include the following, in addition to the information specified for *Labeling* under *Injections* ⟨1⟩: the time and date of calibration; the amount of ^{201}Tl as labeled thallous chloride expressed as total megabecquerels (microcuries or millicuries) and concentration as megabecquerels (microcuries or millicuries) per mL at the time of calibration; the expiration date and time; and the statement "Caution—Radioactive Material." The labeling indicates that in making dosage calculations, correction is to be made for radioactive decay, and also indicates that the radioactive half-life of ^{201}Tl is 73.1 hours.

USP Reference standards ⟨11⟩—*USP Endotoxin RS.*

Radionuclide identification (see *Radioactivity* ⟨821⟩)—Its gamma-ray spectrum is identical to that of a specimen of ^{201}Tl of known purity that exhibits a major photopeak at an energy of 167 KeV and a minor photopeak of 135 KeV.

Bacterial endotoxins ⟨85⟩—The limit of endotoxin content is not more than 175/V USP Endotoxin Unit per mL of the Injection, when compared with the USP Endotoxin RS, in which V is the maximum recommended total dose, in mL, at the expiration date or time.

pH ⟨791⟩: between 4.5 and 7.5.

Radiochemical purity—Soak a 2.5- × 15.0-cm cellulose polyacetate strip in 0.05 M edetate disodium for 45 to 60 minutes. Remove the strip with forceps, taking care to handle the outer edges only. Place the strip between two absorbent pads, and blot to remove excess solution. Apply not less than 5 µL of a previously mixed solution consisting of equal volumes of Injection and 0.05 M edetate disodium to the center of the blotted strip, and mark the point of application. Attach the strip to the support bridge of an electrophoresis chamber containing equal portions of 0.05 M edetate disodium in each side of the chamber. Ensure that each end of the strip is in contact with the 0.05 M edetate disodium. Attach the chamber cover, and perform the electrophoresis at 250 volts for 30 minutes. Remove the strip from the chamber, and allow to air-dry without blotting. Using a suitable scanner and counting assembly, determine the radioactivity. Not less than 95.0% of the radioactivity on the strip migrates toward the cathode as a single peak.

Radionuclidic purity—Using a suitable counting assembly (see *Selection of a Counting Assembly* under *Radioactivity* ⟨821⟩), determine the radioactivity of each radionuclidic impurity in the Injection by use of a calibrated system. Not less than 95.0% of the total radioactivity is present as thallium 201. In addition, not more than 2.0% of thallium 200 (half-life is 26.1 hours), not more than 0.3% of lead 203 (half-life is 52.02 hours), and not more than 2.7% of thallium 202 (half-life is 12.23 days) are present.

Content of thallium—

Standard thallium solution—Transfer 235 mg of thallous chloride, accurately weighed, to a 1000-mL volumetric flask, dilute with water to volume, and mix. Transfer 1.0 mL of the resulting solution to a 100-mL volumetric flask, dilute with saline TS containing 0.9% benzyl alcohol to volume, and mix. This standard solution contains 2 µg of thallium per mL.

Procedure—Transfer 1.0-mL portions of the *Standard thallium solution* and the Injection to separate screw-cap test tubes. To each tube add 2 drops of a solution, prepared by carefully mixing 18 mL of nitric acid and 82 mL of hydrochloric acid, and mix. Then add to each tube 1.0 mL of sulfosalicylic acid solution (1 in 10), and mix. Add 2 drops of 12 N hydrochloric acid to each tube, and mix. To each tube add 4 drops of rhodamine B solution (50 mg of rhodamine B diluted with hydrochloric acid to 100.0 mL), and mix. Add 1.0 mL of diisopropyl ether. Screw the caps on tightly, shake the tubes by hand for 1 minute, accurately timed, releasing any pressure build-up by loosening the caps slightly. Recap the tubes and allow the phases to separate. Transfer 0.5 mL of the diisopropyl ether layer from each tube to clean tubes. Visually compare the ether layers: the color of the ether layer from the Injection is not darker than that from the *Standard thallium solution*.

Iron—Into separate cavities of a spot plate, place 0.1 mL of the Injection and 0.1 mL of *Standard Iron Solution* (see *Iron* ⟨241⟩) diluted with water to a concentration of 5 µg per mL. Add to each cavity 0.1 mL of hydroxylamine hydrochloride solution (1 in 10), 1 mL of sodium acetate solution (1 in 4), and 0.1 mL of 0.5% dipyridyl solution (0.5 g of 2,2'-dipyridyl dissolved in 100 mL of water containing 0.15 mL of hydrochloric acid), and mix. After 5 minutes, the color of the specimen of Injection is not darker than that of the *Standard Iron Solution*.

Copper—

Standard copper solution—Dissolve 0.982 g of $CuSO_4 \cdot 5H_2O$ in 1000 mL of 0.1 N hydrochloric acid. Transfer 2.0 mL of this solution to a 100-mL volumetric flask, dilute with 0.1 N hydrochloric acid to volume, and mix to obtain a Standard solution containing 5 µg of copper per mL.

Procedure—Into separate cavities of a spot plate, place 0.2 mL of the Injection and 0.2 mL of *Standard copper solution*. Add to each cavity 0.2 mL of water and 0.1 mL of iron thiocyanate solution (1.5 g ferric chloride and 2 g potassium thiocyanate dissolved in water and diluted with water to 100.0 mL). Mix, then add 0.1 mL of sodium thiosulfate solution (1 in 100), and again mix. The time required for the specimen of Thallous Chloride Tl 201 Injection to decolorize is equal to or longer than that observed for the *Standard copper solution*.

Other requirements—It meets the requirements under *Injections* ⟨1⟩, except that the Injection may be distributed or dispensed prior to the completion of the test for *Sterility*, the latter test being started on the day of final manufacture, and except that it is not subject to the recommendations on *Volume in Container*.

Assay for radioactivity ⟨821⟩—Using a suitable counting assembly (see *Selection of a Counting Assembly*), determine the radioactivity in MBq (µCi or mCi) per mL of Injection by use of a calibrated system.

Theophylline

$C_7H_8N_4O_2 \cdot H_2O$ 198.18
1*H*-Purine-2,6-dione, 3,7-dihydro-1,3-dimethyl-, monohydrate.
Theophylline monohydrate   [5967-84-0].
Anhydrous   180.17   [58-55-9].

» Theophylline contains one molecule of water of hydration or is anhydrous. It contains not less than 97.0 percent and not more than 102.0 percent of $C_7H_8N_4O_2$, calculated on the dried basis.

Packaging and storage—Preserve in well-closed containers.
Labeling—Label it to indicate whether it is hydrous or anhydrous.
USP Reference standards ⟨11⟩—*USP Theophylline RS*.
Identification—
   A: *Infrared Absorption* ⟨197K⟩.
   B: The retention time of the major peak in the chromatogram of the *Assay preparation* corresponds to that in the chromatogram of the *Standard preparation*, both relative to the internal standard, as obtained in the *Assay*.
Melting range ⟨741⟩: between 270° and 274°, but the range between beginning and end of melting does not exceed 3°.
Acidity—Dissolve 500 mg in 75 mL of water, and add 1 drop of methyl red TS: not more than 1.0 mL of 0.020 N sodium hydroxide is required to change the red color to yellow.
Loss on drying ⟨731⟩—Dry it at 105° for 4 hours: the hydrous form loses between 7.5% and 9.5% of its weight, and the anhydrous form loses not more than 0.5% of its weight.
Residue on ignition ⟨281⟩: not more than 0.15%.
Organic volatile impurities, *Method V* ⟨467⟩: meets the requirements.
   Solvent—Use dimethyl sulfoxide.

(Official until July 1, 2008)

Assay—
   Buffer solution—Transfer 2.72 g of sodium acetate trihydrate to a 2000-mL volumetric flask, add about 200 mL of water, and shake until dissolution is complete. Add 10.0 mL of glacial acetic acid, dilute with water to volume, and mix.
   Mobile phase—Transfer 70.0 mL of acetonitrile to a 1000-mL volumetric flask, dilute with *Buffer solution* to volume, and mix. Degas, and filter before using. Make adjustments if necessary (see *System Suitability* under *Chromatography* ⟨621⟩).
   Internal standard solution—Transfer about 50 mg of theobromine, accurately weighed, to a 100-mL volumetric flask, dissolve in 10.0 mL of 6 N ammonium hydroxide, dilute with *Mobile phase* to volume, and mix.
   Standard preparation—Dissolve an accurately weighed quantity of USP Theophylline RS in *Mobile phase*, and dilute quantitatively, and stepwise if necessary, with *Mobile phase* to obtain a solution having a known concentration of about 1 mg per mL. Transfer 10.0 mL of this solution to a 100-mL volumetric flask, add 20.0 mL of *Internal standard solution*, dilute with *Mobile phase* to volume, and mix to obtain a solution having a known concentration of about 0.1 mg of USP Theophylline RS per mL.
   Assay preparation—Transfer about 100 mg of Theophylline, accurately weighed, to a 100-mL volumetric flask, add about 50 mL of *Mobile phase*, shake by mechanical means until solution is complete, dilute with *Mobile phase* to volume, and mix. Transfer 10.0 mL of this solution to a second 100-mL volumetric flask, add 20.0 mL of *Internal standard solution*, dilute with *Mobile phase* to volume, and mix.
   Chromatographic system (see *Chromatography* ⟨621⟩)—The liquid chromatograph is equipped with a 280-nm detector and a 4-mm × 30-cm column that contains packing L1. The flow rate is about 1.0 mL per minute. Chromatograph the *Standard preparation*, and record the peak responses as directed for *Procedure*: the resolution, *R*, between the theophylline and theobromine peaks is not less than 2.0, the tailing factor for the theophylline peak is not more than 2.0, and the relative standard deviation for replicate injections is not more than 1.5%.
   Procedure—Separately inject equal volumes (between 10 µL and 25 µL) of the *Standard preparation* and the *Assay preparation* into the chromatograph, and measure the peak responses for the major peaks. The retention time of theophylline relative to that of theobromine is about 1.6. Calculate the quantity, in mg, of $C_7H_8N_4O_2$ in the portion of Theophylline taken by the formula:

$$1000C(R_U / R_S)$$

in which *C* is the concentration, in mg per mL, of USP Theophylline RS in the *Standard preparation*, and R_U and R_S are the response ratios of the theophylline peak to the internal standard peak obtained from the *Assay preparation* and the *Standard preparation*, respectively.

Theophylline Capsules

» Theophylline Capsules contain not less than 90.0 percent and not more than 110.0 percent of the labeled amount of anhydrous theophylline ($C_7H_8N_4O_2$).

Packaging and storage—Preserve in well-closed containers.
USP Reference standards ⟨11⟩—*USP Theophylline RS*.
Identification—
   A: The contents of the Capsules respond to *Identification* tests *A* and *B* under *Theophylline Tablets*.
   B: The retention time of the major peak in the chromatogram of the *Assay preparation* corresponds to that in the chromatogram of the *Standard preparation*, as obtained in the *Assay*.
Dissolution ⟨711⟩—
   Medium: water; 900 mL.
   Apparatus 2: 50 rpm.
   Time: 60 minutes.
   Procedure—Determine the amount of $C_7H_8N_4O_2$ dissolved from UV absorbances at the wavelength of maximum absorbance at about 268 nm of filtered portions of the solution under test, suitably diluted with 0.1 N hydrochloric acid, if necessary, in comparison with a Standard solution having a known concentration of USP Theophylline RS in the same medium.
   Tolerances—Not less than 80% (*Q*) of the labeled amount of $C_7H_8N_4O_2$ is dissolved in 60 minutes.
Uniformity of dosage units ⟨905⟩: meet the requirements.
Assay—
   Mobile phase—Prepare a solution containing a mixture of water, methanol, and glacial acetic acid (64 : 35 : 1).
   Standard preparation—Dissolve an accurately weighed quantity of USP Theophylline RS in methanol to obtain a solution having a known concentration of about 400 µg per mL.
   Assay preparation for hard Capsules—Remove, as completely as possible, the contents of not less than 20 Capsules, weigh, and mix. Transfer an accurately weighed portion of the powder, equivalent to about 100 mg of anhydrous theophylline, to a 250-mL volumetric flask, add about 150 mL of methanol, and shake to dissolve. Dilute with methanol to volume, mix, and filter, using a membrane filter.
   Assay preparation for soft Capsules—Cut open 20 Capsules, and place them in a 200-mL volumetric flask. Add 50 mL of 6 N ammonium hydroxide, shake to dissolve the contents, add water to volume, mix, and filter, discarding the first 20 mL of the filtrate. Transfer an accurately measured portion of the filtrate, equivalent to about 100 mg of anhydrous theophylline, to a 250-mL volumetric flask, add methanol to volume, mix, and filter through a membrane filter.
   Chromatographic system (see *Chromatography* ⟨621⟩)—The liquid chromatograph is equipped with a 254-nm detector and a 4-mm × 30-cm column that contains packing L1. The flow rate is about 2 mL per minute. Chromatograph three replicate injections of the *Standard preparation*, and record the peak responses as directed for *Procedure:* the relative standard deviation is not more than 2%.

Procedure—Separately inject equal volumes (about 20 µL) of the *Standard preparation* and the *Assay preparation* into the chromatograph, record the chromatograms, and measure the responses. Calculate the quantity, in mg, of anhydrous theophylline in the portion of Capsule contents taken by the formula:

$$0.25C(r_U / r_S)$$

in which C is the concentration, in µg per mL, of USP Theophylline RS in the *Standard preparation*, and r_U and r_S are the peak responses obtained from the *Assay preparation* and the *Standard preparation*, respectively.

Theophylline Extended-Release Capsules

» Theophylline Extended-Release Capsules contain not less than 90.0 percent and not more than 110.0 percent of the labeled amount of anhydrous theophylline ($C_7H_8N_4O_2$).

Packaging and storage—Preserve in well-closed containers.
Labeling—The labeling indicates whether the product is intended for dosing every 12 or 24 hours, and states with which in vitro *Dissolution Test* the product complies.
USP Reference standards ⟨11⟩—USP Theophylline RS.
Identification—
  A: Transfer a quantity of Capsule contents, equivalent to about 100 mg of anhydrous theophylline, to a suitable conical flask. Add 150 mL of methanol, and sonicate until the insoluble material is dispersed into fine particles. Shake by mechanical means for 15 minutes, and filter into a 250-mL volumetric flask. Dilute with water to volume, and mix. Pipet 5 mL of this solution into a 200-mL volumetric flask, dilute with 0.1 N hydrochloric acid to volume, and mix: the UV absorption spectrum of the solution so obtained exhibits maxima and minima at the same wavelengths as that of a similar solution of USP Theophylline RS, concomitantly measured.
  B: The retention time of the major peak in the chromatogram of the *Assay preparation* corresponds to that in the chromatogram of the *Standard preparation*, as obtained in the *Assay*.
Dissolution ⟨711⟩—[NOTE—The following tests, which were assigned numbers chronologically, are placed in groups corresponding to product dosing intervals. Thus, individual tests do not necessarily appear in numerical order.]
  FOR PRODUCTS LABELED FOR DOSING EVERY 12 HOURS—
  TEST 1—If the product complies with this test, the labeling indicates that it meets USP *Dissolution Test 1*. Proceed as directed for *Method B* under *Apparatus 1 and 2, Delayed-Release Dosage Forms*, except to use *Acceptance Table 2*.
  Medium: pH 1.2 simulated gastric fluid (without pepsin) for the first hour; pH 6.0 phosphate buffer (see *Buffer Solutions* in the section *Reagents, Indicators, and Solutions*); 900 mL.
  Apparatus 2: 50 rpm.
  Procedure—Determine the amount of $C_7H_8N_4O_2$ dissolved from UV absorbances at the wavelength of maximum absorbance at about 271 nm on filtered portions of the solution under test, diluted with *Medium*, if necessary, in comparison with a Standard solution having a known concentration of USP Theophylline RS in the same *Medium*.
  Times and *Tolerances*—The percentage of the labeled amount of $C_7H_8N_4O_2$ dissolved at the times given conforms to *Acceptance Table 2*.

Time (hours)	Amount dissolved
1	between 3% and 15%
2	between 20% and 40%
4	between 50% and 75%
6	between 65% and 100%
8	not less than 80%

  TEST 2—If the product complies with this test, the labeling indicates that it meets USP *Dissolution Test 2*.
  pH 4.5 Phosphate buffer—Dissolve 6.8 g of monobasic potassium phosphate in 750 mL of water, mix, and dilute with water to 1000 mL. Adjust with either 1 N hydrochloric acid or 1 N sodium hydroxide to a pH of 4.5 ± 0.05.
  Medium: pH 4.5 Phosphate buffer; 900 mL.
  Apparatus 2: 75 rpm.
  Procedure—Proceed as directed under *Test 1*.
  Times and *Tolerances*—The percentages of the labeled amount of $C_7H_8N_4O_2$ dissolved at the times specified conform to *Acceptance Table 2*.

Time (hours)	Amount dissolved
1	between 10% and 30%
2	between 30% and 55%
4	between 55% and 80%
8	not less than 80%

  TEST 3—If the product complies with this test, the labeling indicates that it meets USP *Dissolution Test 3*. Proceed as directed for *Method B* under *Apparatus 1 and 2, Delayed-Release Dosage Forms*, except to use *Acceptance Table 2*.
  Medium: pH 1.2 simulated gastric fluid (without pepsin) for 1 hour; pH 7.5 simulated intestinal fluid (without enzyme); 900 mL.
  Apparatus 2: 50 rpm.
  Procedure—Proceed as directed under *Test 1*.
  Times and *Tolerances*—The percentage of the labeled amount of $C_7H_8N_4O_2$ dissolved at the times given conforms to *Acceptance Table 2*.

Time (hours)	Amount dissolved
1	between 1% and 17%
2	between 30% and 60%
3	between 50% and 90%
4	not less than 65%
7	not less than 85%

  TEST 4—If the product complies with this test, the labeling indicates that it meets USP *Dissolution Test 4*. Proceed as directed for *Method A* under *Apparatus 1 and 2, Delayed-Release Dosage Forms*, except to use *Acceptance Table 2*.
  Medium: pH 3.0 phosphate buffer prepared by adjusting 0.05 M potassium phosphate buffer with phosphoric acid to a pH of 3.0 ± 0.05, for the first 3½ hours, followed by the addition of 5.3 M sodium hydroxide to adjust to a pH of 7.4 ± 0.05; 900 mL.
  Apparatus 2: 50 rpm.
  Procedure—Proceed as directed under *Test 1*.
  Times and *Tolerances*—The percentage of the labeled amount of $C_7H_8N_4O_2$ dissolved at the times given conforms to *Acceptance Table 2*.

Time (hours)	Amount dissolved
1	between 13% and 38%
2	between 25% and 50%
3.5	between 37% and 65%
5	between 85% and 115%

  TEST 5—If the product complies with this test, the labeling indicates that it meets USP *Dissolution Test 5*.
  Medium, Apparatus, and *Procedure*—Proceed as directed under *Test 4*.
  Times and *Tolerances*—The percentage of the labeled amount of $C_7H_8N_4O_2$ dissolved at the times given conforms to *Acceptance Table 2*.

Time (hours)	Amount dissolved
1	between 10% and 30%
3.5	between 30% and 60%

Time (hours)	Amount dissolved
5	between 50% and 80%
7	not less than 65%
10	not less than 80%

TEST 7—If the product complies with this test, the labeling indicates that it meets USP *Dissolution Test 7*.

Phosphate buffer—Dissolve 40.8 g of monobasic potassium phosphate in 6 L of water, add 667 mg of octoxynol 9, mix, and adjust with dilute hydrochloric acid or sodium hydroxide to a pH of 4.5.

Medium: Phosphate buffer; 900 mL.
Apparatus 2: 50 rpm.
Procedure—Proceed as directed under *Test 1*.
Times and *Tolerances*—The percentages of the labeled amount of $C_7H_8N_4O_2$ dissolved at the times specified conform to *Acceptance Table 2*.

Time (hours)	Amount dissolved
1	between 10% and 40%
2	between 35% and 70%
4	between 60% and 90%
8	not less than 85%

TEST 8—If the product complies with this test, the labeling indicates that it meets USP *Dissolution Test 8*.

Medium: pH 7.5 simulated intestinal fluid (without enzyme); 900 mL.
Apparatus 1: 100 rpm.
Procedure—Proceed as directed under *Test 1*.
Times and *Tolerances*—The percentages of labeled amount of $C_7H_8N_4O_2$ dissolved at the times specified conform to *Acceptance Table 2*.

Time (hours)	Amount dissolved
1	between 3% and 30%
2	between 15% and 50%
4	between 45% and 80%
6	not less than 70%
8	not less than 85%

TEST 9—If the product complies with this test, the labeling indicates that it meets USP *Dissolution Test 9*.

Medium 1: 0.1 N hydrochloric acid; 900 mL.
Medium 2: simulated intestinal fluid (without enzyme); 900 mL.
Apparatus 1: 50 rpm.
Determine the amount of theophylline dissolved at the times specified, using *Medium 1* for the first hour and *Medium 2* for the next five hours.
Procedure—Proceed as directed under *Test 1*.
Times and *Tolerances*—The percentage of the labeled amount of $C_7H_8N_4O_2$ dissolved at the times given conforms to *Acceptance Table 2*.

Time (hours)	Amount dissolved
1	between 5% and 15%
2	between 25% and 45%
3	between 50% and 65%
4	not less than 70%
6	not less than 85%

TEST 10—If the product complies with this test, the labeling indicates that it meets USP *Dissolution Test 10*. Proceed as directed for *Test 3*.
Times and *Tolerances*—The percentage of the labeled amount of $C_7H_8N_4O_2$ dissolved at the times given conforms to *Acceptance Table 2*.

Time (hours)	Amount dissolved
1	between 6% and 27%
2	between 25% and 50%
4	between 65% and 85%
8	not less than 80%

FOR PRODUCTS LABELED FOR DOSING EVERY 24 HOURS—

TEST 6—If the product complies with this test, the labeling indicates that it meets USP *Dissolution Test 6*.

Medium: 0.05 M pH 6.6 phosphate buffer (see *Buffer Solutions* in the section *Reagents, Indicators, and Solutions*); 1000 mL.
Apparatus 1: 100 rpm.
Procedure—Proceed as directed under *Test 1*.
Times and *Tolerances*—The percentages of the labeled amount of $C_7H_8N_4O_2$ dissolved at the times specified conform to *Acceptance Table 2*.

Time (hours)	Amount dissolved
1	between 5% and 15%
2	between 12% and 30%
4	between 25% and 50%
5	between 30% and 60%
8	between 55% and 75%

Uniformity of dosage units ⟨905⟩: meet the requirements.

Procedure for content uniformity—Using a mortar and pestle, triturate the contents of 1 Capsule with 20 mL of water. With the aid of water, transfer the mixture to a 100-mL volumetric flask. Add 25 mL of 6 N ammonium hydroxide, shake or sonicate for about 45 minutes, and cool to room temperature. Dilute with water to volume, and mix. Filter a portion of the mixture, discarding the first 20 mL of the filtrate. Dilute a portion of the filtrate quantitatively, and stepwise if necessary, with water to obtain a solution containing about 12 µg of theophylline per mL. Concomitantly determine the absorbances of this solution and a Standard solution of USP Theophylline RS, similarly prepared, having a known concentration of about 12 µg per mL, in 1-cm cells, at the wavelength of maximum absorbance at about 270 nm, with a suitable spectrophotometer, using water as the blank. Calculate the quantity, in mg, of $C_7H_8N_4O_2$ in the Capsule taken by the formula:

$$(TC/D)(A_U/A_S)$$

in which T is the labeled quantity, in mg, of theophylline in the Capsule; C is the concentration, in µg per mL, of USP Theophylline RS in the Standard solution; D is the concentration, in µg per mL, of theophylline in the solution from the Capsule, based on the labeled quantity per Capsule and the extent of dilution; and A_U and A_S are the absorbances of the solution from the Capsule and the Standard solution, respectively.

Assay—

Buffer solution, *Mobile phase*, *Internal standard solution*, and *Standard preparation*—Prepare as directed in the *Assay* under *Theophylline*.

Assay preparation—Quantitatively transfer the contents of 10 Capsules to a 500-mL volumetric flask, and add 100 mL of water and 50 mL of 6 N ammonium hydroxide. Heat on a hot plate, with occasional stirring, just to boiling. Remove from the hot plate, and sonicate for about 1 minute while still hot. Cool to room temperature, dilute with water to volume, mix, and centrifuge. Transfer an accurately measured aliquot portion of this concentrate, equivalent to about 10 mg of theophylline, to a 100-mL volumetric flask. Add 20.0 mL of *Internal standard solution*, dilute with *Mobile phase* to volume, and mix.

Chromatographic system—Proceed as directed in the *Assay* under *Theophylline*, except for flow rate, which may be 1.0 to 2.0 mL per minute.

Procedure—Proceed as directed for *Procedure* in the *Assay* under *Theophylline*. Calculate the quantity, in mg, of $C_7H_8N_4O_2$ per Capsule taken by the formula:

$$5000(C/V)(R_U/R_S)$$

in which C is the concentration, in mg per mL, of USP Theophylline RS in the *Standard preparation*; V is the volume, in mL, of concentrate taken for the *Assay preparation*; and R_U and R_S are the response ratios of the theophylline peak to the internal standard peak obtained from the *Assay preparation* and the *Standard preparation*, respectively.

Theophylline Oral Solution

» Theophylline Oral Solution contains not less than 95.0 percent and not more than 105.0 percent of theophylline ($C_7H_8N_4O_2$).

Packaging and storage—Preserve in tight, light-resistant containers, and avoid exposure to excessive heat.
Labeling—Label it to indicate the alcohol content (if present).
USP Reference standards ⟨11⟩—*USP Theophylline RS*.
Identification—
   A: *Thin-Layer Chromatographic Identification Test* ⟨201⟩—
   Test solution—Transfer a portion of Oral Solution, equivalent to about 100 mg of theophylline, to a separatory funnel. Extract with two 25-mL portions of chloroform, collecting the extracts in a 100-mL volumetric flask. Dilute with methanol to volume, and mix.
   Standard solution—Prepare a solution of USP Theophylline RS in methanol containing about 1 mg per mL.
   Application volume: 20 µL.
   Developing solvent system: a mixture of chloroform, methanol, and acetic acid (89 : 10 : 1).
   Procedure—Apply the *Standard solution* and the *Test solution* as directed in the chapter, and dry the plate in a current of cool air. Place the plate in a suitable chromatographic chamber lined with filter paper and previously equilibrated with the *Developing solvent system*. Upon removing the plate from the chamber, dry with a current of warm air in a suitable hood.
   B: The retention time of the major peak in the chromatogram of the *Assay preparation* corresponds to that in the chromatogram of the *Standard preparation*, as obtained in the *Assay*.
Microbial limits ⟨61⟩—It meets the requirements of the tests for absence of *Salmonella* species and *Escherichia coli*. The total aerobic microbial count does not exceed 100 cfu per mL, and the total combined molds and yeasts count does not exceed 50 cfu per mL.
pH ⟨791⟩: between 4.3 and 4.7.
Alcohol content, *Method II* ⟨611⟩ (*if present*): between 90.0% and 115.0% of the labeled amount of C_2H_5OH is found, using acetone as the internal standard.
Assay—
   Mobile phase—Prepare a filtered and degassed mixture of water, methanol, and acetic acid (76.5 : 22.5 : 1) containing 200 mg of sodium 1-octanesulfonate in each 1000 mL of solution. Make adjustments if necessary (see *System Suitability* under *Chromatography* ⟨621⟩).
   System suitability preparation—Dissolve accurately weighed quantities of USP Theophylline RS and caffeine in water to obtain a solution containing about 0.68 mg of each per mL.
   Standard preparation—Dissolve an accurately weighed quantity of USP Theophylline RS in water to obtain a solution having a known concentration of about 0.68 mg per mL.
   Assay preparation—Transfer an accurately measured volume of Oral Solution, equivalent to about 68 mg of theophylline, to a 100-mL volumetric flask. Dilute with water to volume, and mix.
   Chromatographic system (see *Chromatography* ⟨621⟩)—The liquid chromatograph is equipped with a 254-nm detector and a 4.0-mm × 30-cm column that contains packing L1. The flow rate is about 2.0 mL per minute. Chromatograph the *System suitability preparation*, and record the peak responses as directed for *Procedure*: the relative retention times are about 0.6 for theophylline and 1.0 for caffeine; the resolution, R, between theophylline and caffeine is not less than 2.0; the tailing factor is not more than 2; and the relative standard deviation for replicate injections is not more than 2.0%.
   Procedure—Separately inject equal volumes (about 10 µL) of the *Standard preparation* and the *Assay preparation* into the chromatograph, record the chromatograms, and measure the responses for the major peaks. Calculate the quantity, in mg, of theophylline ($C_7H_8N_4O_2$) in the portion of Oral Solution taken by the formula:

$$100C(r_U/r_S)$$

in which C is the concentration, in mg per mL, of USP Theophylline RS in the *Standard preparation*; and r_U and r_S are the peak responses obtained from the *Assay preparation* and the *Standard preparation*, respectively.

Theophylline Tablets

» Theophylline Tablets contain not less than 94.0 percent and not more than 106.0 percent of the labeled amount of anhydrous theophylline ($C_7H_8N_4O_2$).

Packaging and storage—Preserve in well-closed containers.
USP Reference standards ⟨11⟩—*USP Theophylline RS*.
Identification—
   A: Triturate a quantity of finely powdered Tablets, equivalent to about 500 mg of theophylline, with 10-mL and 5-mL portions of solvent hexane, and discard the solvent hexane. Triturate the residue with two 10-mL portions of a mixture of equal volumes of 6 N ammonium hydroxide and water, and filter each time. Evaporate the combined filtrates to about 5 mL, neutralize, if necessary, with 6 N acetic acid, using litmus, and then cool to about 15°, with stirring. Collect the precipitate on a filter, wash it with cold water, and dry at 105° for 2 hours: the theophylline so obtained melts between 270° and 274°, the procedure for *Class I* being used (see *Melting Range or Temperature* ⟨741⟩). Retain the remaining portion of the theophylline for use in *Identification* test B.
   B: The IR absorption spectrum of a potassium bromide dispersion of the residue obtained in *Identification* test A exhibits maxima only at the same wavelengths as that of a potassium bromide dispersion of USP Theophylline RS.
   C: The retention time of the major peak in the chromatogram of the *Assay preparation* corresponds to that in the chromatogram of the *Standard preparation*, both relative to the internal standard, as obtained in the *Assay*.
Dissolution ⟨711⟩—
   Medium: water; 900 mL.
   Apparatus 2: 50 rpm.
   Time: 45 minutes.
   Procedure—Determine the amount of $C_7H_8N_4O_2$ dissolved from UV absorbances at the wavelength of maximum absorbance at about 272 nm of filtered portions of the solution under test, suitably diluted with water, if necessary, in comparison with a Standard solution having a known concentration of USP Theophylline RS in the same medium.
   Tolerances—Not less than 80% (*Q*) of the labeled amount of $C_7H_8N_4O_2$ is dissolved in 45 minutes.
Uniformity of dosage units ⟨905⟩: meet the requirements.
Assay—
   Mobile phase, *Internal standard solution*, and *Standard preparation*—Prepare as directed in the *Assay* under *Theophylline*.
   Assay preparation—Place 10 Tablets in a 500-mL volumetric flask, add 50 mL of water, and when the Tablets have disintegrated add 50 mL of 6 N ammonium hydroxide. Shake until no more dissolves, dilute with water to volume, mix, and filter through a dry filter with the aid of suction, if necessary, into a dry flask, discarding the first 20 mL of the filtrate. Transfer an accurately measured aliquot portion of this concentrate, equivalent to about 10 mg of theophylline, to a 100-mL volumetric flask. Add 20.0 mL of *Internal standard solution*, dilute with *Mobile phase* to volume, and mix.

Chromatographic system—Proceed as directed in the *Assay* under *Theophylline*.

Procedure—Proceed as directed for *Procedure* in the *Assay* under *Theophylline*. Calculate the quantity, in mg, of $C_7H_8N_4O_2$ per Tablet taken by the formula:

$$5000(C/V)(R_U/R_S)$$

in which C is the concentration, in mg per mL, of USP Theophylline RS in the *Standard preparation*, V is the volume, in mL, of concentrate taken for the *Assay preparation*, and R_U and R_S are the response ratios of the theophylline peak to the internal standard peak obtained from the *Assay preparation* and the *Standard preparation*, respectively.

Theophylline in Dextrose Injection

» Theophylline in Dextrose Injection is a sterile solution of Theophylline and Dextrose in Water for Injection. It contains not less than 93.0 percent and not more than 107.0 percent of the labeled amount of anhydrous theophylline ($C_7H_8N_4O_2$) and not less than 95.0 percent and not more than 105.0 percent of the labeled amount of dextrose ($C_6H_{12}O_6 \cdot H_2O$).

Packaging and storage—Preserve in single-dose containers, preferably of Type I or Type II glass, or of a suitable plastic material.
USP Reference standards ⟨11⟩—*USP Endotoxin RS. USP Theophylline RS.*
Identification—
  A: The UV absorption spectrum of the Injection, diluted with 0.5 N sodium hydroxide to a concentration of about 8 µg of anhydrous theophylline per mL, exhibits maxima and minima at the same wavelengths as that of a similar solution of USP Theophylline RS, concomitantly measured.
  B: Add a few drops of the Injection to 5 mL of hot alkaline cupric tartrate TS: a red to orange precipitate of cuprous oxide is formed.
Bacterial endotoxins ⟨85⟩—It contains not more than 1.0 USP Endotoxin Unit per mg of anhydrous theophylline.
pH ⟨791⟩: between 3.5 and 6.5, determined on a portion diluted with water, if necessary, to a concentration of not more than 5% of dextrose.
Limit of 5-hydroxymethylfurfural and related substances—
  Cation-exchange column—Proceed as directed under *Column Partition Chromatography* (see *Chromatography* ⟨621⟩), using a chromatographic tube capable of providing a 0.8- × 4-cm bed volume (or about 2 mL) of 100- to 200-mesh, strongly acidic, styrene-divinylbenzene, cation-exchange resin. Condition the column by washing with about 30 mL of water, discarding the eluate.
  Procedure—Pass a volume of Injection containing about 100 mg of hydrous dextrose through the resin bed in the *Cation-exchange column*, allowing the specimen to flow down the wall of the column so as not to disturb the resin bed, and collect the eluate in a 50-mL volumetric flask. Wash the column with 25 mL of water, and collect the eluate in the same 50-mL volumetric flask. Dilute the eluate with water to volume, and mix to obtain the *Test solution*. In a similar manner, prepare a *Reference solution* by passing 27 mL of water through a freshly conditioned *Cation-exchange column*, collecting the eluate in a 50-mL volumetric flask. Dilute with water to volume, and mix. Determine the absorbance of the *Test solution* in a 1-cm cell at 284 nm, with a suitable spectrophotometer, using the *Reference solution* as the blank: the absorbance is not more than 0.25.
Other requirements—It meets the requirements under *Injections* ⟨1⟩.
Assay for theophylline—
  Buffer solution, Mobile phase, and *Internal standard solution*—Prepare as directed in the *Assay* under *Theophylline*.
  Standard preparation—Dissolve an accurately weighed quantity of USP Theophylline RS in *Mobile phase*, and dilute quantitatively, and stepwise if necessary, with *Mobile phase* to obtain a solution having a known concentration of about 1 mg per mL. Transfer 8.0 mL of this solution to a 50-mL volumetric flask, add 10.0 mL of *Internal standard solution*, dilute with *Mobile phase* to volume, and mix to obtain a solution having a known concentration of about 0.16 mg of USP Theophylline RS per mL.
  Assay preparation—Transfer an accurately measured volume of Injection, equivalent to about 16 mg of theophylline, to a 100-mL volumetric flask, add 20.0 mL of *Internal standard solution*, dilute with *Mobile phase* to volume, and mix.
  Chromatographic system—Proceed as directed in the *Assay* under *Theophylline*.
  Procedure—Proceed as directed for *Procedure* in the *Assay* under *Theophylline*. Calculate the quantity, in mg, of $C_7H_8N_4O_2$ in each mL of the Injection taken by the formula:

$$(100C/V)(R_U/R_S)$$

in which V is the volume, in mL, of Injection taken, and the other terms are as defined therein.
Assay for dextrose—Transfer an accurately measured volume of Injection, containing 2 to 5 g of dextrose, to a 100-mL volumetric flask. Add 0.2 mL of 6 N ammonium hydroxide, dilute with water to volume, and mix. Determine the angular rotation in a suitable polarimeter tube (see *Optical Rotation* ⟨781⟩). Calculate the percentage (g per 100 mL) of dextrose ($C_6H_{12}O_6 \cdot H_2O$) in the portion of Injection taken by the formula:

$$(100/52.9)(198.17/180.16)AR$$

in which 100 is the percentage; 52.9 is the midpoint of the specific rotation range for anhydrous dextrose, in degrees; 198.17 and 180.16 are the molecular weights for dextrose monohydrate and anhydrous dextrose, respectively; A is 100 mm divided by the length of the polarimeter tube, in mm; and R is the observed rotation, in degrees.

Theophylline, Ephedrine Hydrochloride, and Phenobarbital Tablets

» Theophylline, Ephedrine Hydrochloride, and Phenobarbital Tablets contain not less than 90.0 percent and not more than 110.0 percent of the labeled amounts of anhydrous theophylline ($C_7H_8N_4O_2$), ephedrine hydrochloride ($C_{10}H_{15}NO \cdot HCl$), and phenobarbital ($C_{12}H_{12}N_2O_3$).

Packaging and storage—Preserve in tight containers.
USP Reference standards ⟨11⟩—*USP Theophylline RS. USP Ephedrine Sulfate RS. USP Phenobarbital RS.*
Identification—Place a quantity of finely powdered Tablets, equivalent to about 24 mg of ephedrine hydrochloride, in a 15-mL centrifuge tube, add 4.0 mL of a mixture of chloroform and methanol (4 : 1), mix by sonication for 10 minutes, and filter to obtain the test solution. Prepare separate Standard solutions containing known concentrations of about 36 mg of USP Theophylline RS per mL, about 9.6 mg of USP Ephedrine Sulfate RS per mL, and about 5 mg of USP Phenobarbital RS per mL, respectively, in the mixture of chloroform and methanol (4 : 1). Apply 2 µL of the test solution and of each of the three Standard solutions at equidistant points about 2.5 cm above one edge of a suitable thin-layer chromatographic plate (see *Chromatography* ⟨621⟩) coated with a 0.25-mm layer of chromatographic silica gel mixture. Allow the spots to dry, and develop the chromatogram in a suitable chamber previously equilibrated with a solvent system consisting of a mixture of chloroform, acetone, methanol, and ammonium hydroxide (50 : 10 : 10 : 1) until the solvent front has moved about three-fourths of the length of the plate. Remove the plate from the developing chamber, mark the solvent front, air-dry, and locate the spots on the plate by viewing under short-wavelength UV light: the R_F values of the spots

obtained from the test solution correspond to those obtained from the Standard solutions.

Dissolution, *Procedure for a Pooled Sample* ⟨711⟩—
Medium: water; 900 mL.
Apparatus 1: 100 rpm.
Time: 30 minutes.
Determine the amounts of theophylline, ephedrine hydrochloride, and phenobarbital dissolved using the following procedure.

Mobile phase—Dissolve accurately weighed quantities of monobasic potassium phosphate and sodium 1-hexanesulfonate in water, and dilute quantitatively with water to obtain a solution having concentrations of 0.953 mg per mL (0.007 M monobasic potassium phosphate) and 0.564 mg per mL (0.003 M sodium 1-hexanesulfonate), respectively. Adjust, if necessary, with 0.3 M phosphoric acid or 0.2 M monobasic potassium phosphate to a pH of 3.0 ± 0.05, to obtain a *Phosphate buffer*. The *Mobile phase* is a mixture of *Phosphate buffer* and methanol (75 : 25).

Standard preparation—Dissolve accurately weighed quantities of USP Theophylline RS, USP Ephedrine Sulfate RS, and USP Phenobarbital RS in water, and dilute quantitatively and stepwise with water to obtain a solution having known concentrations of about 145 µg of anhydrous theophylline per mL, 28 µg of ephedrine sulfate per mL, and 9 µg of phenobarbital per mL.

Chromatographic system (see *Chromatography* ⟨621⟩)—The liquid chromatograph is equipped with a 215-nm detector and a 3.9-mm × 30-cm column that contains packing L1. The flow rate is about 3.0 mL per minute. Chromatograph the *Standard preparation*, and record the peak responses as directed for *Procedure:* the resolution, R, between the theophylline and phenobarbital peaks is not less than 4.0, the tailing factors for the ephedrine and phenobarbital peaks are not more than 3.0 and 2.0, respectively, and the relative standard deviation for replicate injections is not more than 2.0%.

Procedure—Inject an accurately measured volume (about 75 µL) of a filtered portion of the solution under test into the chromatograph, record the chromatogram, and measure the responses for the major peaks. The elution order is theophylline, ephedrine, and phenobarbital (last). Calculate the quantity, in mg, of $C_7H_8N_4O_2$ dissolved by the formula:

$$(0.9C)(r_U / r_S)$$

in which C is the concentration, in µg per mL, of USP Theophylline RS in the *Standard preparation*, and r_U and r_S are the peak responses for theophylline obtained from the solution under test and the similarly chromatographed *Standard preparation*, respectively. Calculate the quantity, in mg, of $C_{10}H_{15}NO \cdot HCl$ dissolved by the formula:

$$(201.69/214.27)(0.9C')(r'_U / r'_S)$$

in which 201.69 is the molecular weight of ephedrine hydrochloride, 214.27 is one-half the molecular weight of ephedrine sulfate, C' is the concentration, in µg per mL, of USP Ephedrine Sulfate RS in the *Standard preparation*, and r'_U and r'_S are the peak responses for ephedrine obtained from the solution under test and the similarly chromatographed *Standard preparation*, respectively. Calculate the quantity, in mg, of $C_{12}H_{12}N_2O_3$ dissolved by the formula:

$$(0.9C'')(r''_U / r''_S)$$

in which C'' is the concentration, in µg per mL, of USP Phenobarbital RS in the *Standard preparation*, and r''_U and r''_S are the peak responses for phenobarbital obtained from the solution under test and the similarly chromatographed *Standard preparation*, respectively.

Tolerances—Not less than 75% (*Q*) of the labeled amounts of $C_7H_8N_4O_2$, $C_{10}H_{15}NO \cdot HCl$, and $C_{12}H_{12}N_2O_3$ are dissolved in 30 minutes.

Uniformity of dosage units ⟨905⟩: meet the requirements.

Assay—
Mobile phase—Mix 240 mL of acetonitrile with 760 mL of 0.01 M, pH 7.8 phosphate buffer (see *Buffer Solutions* under *Solutions* in the section *Reagents, Indicators, and Solutions*).

Internal standard solution—Dissolve 25 mg of butabarbital sodium in 50 mL of dibasic potassium phosphate solution (17 in 1000). Mix 40 mL of this solution with 10 mL of sodium metaperiodate solution (1 in 100).

Standard preparation—Transfer about 120 mg of USP Theophylline RS, about 8 mg of USP Phenobarbital RS, and about 25 mg of USP Ephedrine Sulfate RS, each accurately weighed, to a 200-mL volumetric flask. Add 10 mL of methanol and 100 mL of chloroform, mix to dissolve, add chloroform to volume, and mix. Pipet 15 mL of this solution into a 50-mL volumetric flask, add chloroform to volume, and mix. The concentrations of anhydrous theophylline, phenobarbital, and ephedrine sulfate in the *Standard preparation* are about 180 µg per mL, 12 µg per mL, and 37.5 µg per mL, respectively.

Assay preparation—Weigh and finely powder not less than 20 Tablets. Transfer an accurately weighed portion of the powder, equivalent to about 120 mg of anhydrous theophylline, to a 200-mL volumetric flask, and shake by mechanical means for 20 minutes with a mixture of 10 mL of methanol and 100 mL of chloroform. Add chloroform to volume, mix, and filter. Pipet 15 mL of the clear filtrate into a 50-mL volumetric flask, dilute with chloroform to volume, and mix.

Standard solution and *Assay solution*—Pipet 10-mL portions of the *Standard preparation* and the *Assay preparation* into separate glass-stoppered, 25-mL conical flasks, and treat each as follows: Evaporate in a warm-water bath with the aid of a current of air to dryness. Add by pipet 4 mL of *Internal standard solution*, insert the stopper in the flask, mix to dissolve the residue, and allow to stand at room temperature for 30 minutes. Pipet 1 mL of propylene glycol solution (1 in 100) into the flask, insert the stopper, and mix.

Chromatographic system (see *Chromatography* ⟨621⟩)—The liquid chromatograph is equipped with a 241-nm detector and a 30-cm × 4-mm stainless steel column that contains packing L1. Set a flow rate of 1.0 mL per minute for the *Mobile phase*, and allow the system to equilibrate until a stable baseline is obtained on the recorder. Chromatograph a 10-µL portion of the *Standard preparation*, and record the peak responses as directed for *Procedure:* the peaks are completely resolved, and the resolution factors between each two neighboring peaks are not less than 1.5. Five replicate injections of the *Standard preparation* show a relative standard deviation of not more than 2.0%.

Procedure—Separately inject equal volumes (about 10 µL) of the *Standard preparation* and the *Assay solution* into the chromatograph, record the chromatograms, and measure the responses for the major peaks. In the order of increasing elution times, the five peaks correspond to the reagent (iodate), theophylline, phenobarbital, butabarbital, and benzaldehyde (from ephedrine). Designate the peak response ratio of each component to the internal standard in the *Standard solution* as R_S, and that of each component to the internal standard in the *Assay solution* as R_U.

Calculation for theophylline—Calculate the quantity, in mg, of anhydrous theophylline ($C_7H_8N_4O_2$) in the portion of Tablets taken by the formula:

$$0.667C(R_U / R_S)$$

in which C is the concentration, in µg per mL, of USP Theophylline RS in the *Standard preparation*.

Calculation for ephedrine hydrochloride—Calculate the quantity, in mg, of ephedrine hydrochloride ($C_{10}H_{15}NO \cdot HCl$) in the portion of Tablets taken by the formula:

$$(201.69/214.27)(0.667C)(R_U / R_S)$$

in which 201.69 is the molecular weight of ephedrine hydrochloride, 214.27 is one-half the molecular weight of ephedrine sulfate, and C is the concentration, in µg per mL, of USP Ephedrine Sulfate RS in the *Standard preparation*.

Calculation for phenobarbital—Calculate the quantity, in mg, of phenobarbital ($C_{12}H_{12}N_2O_3$) in the portion of Tablets taken by the formula:

$$0.667C(R_U / R_S)$$

in which C is the concentration, in mg per mL, of USP Phenobarbital RS in the *Standard preparation*.

Theophylline and Guaifenesin Capsules

» Theophylline and Guaifenesin Capsules contain not less than 90.0 percent and not more than 110.0 percent of the labeled amounts of anhydrous theophylline ($C_7H_8N_4O_2$) and guaifenesin ($C_{10}H_{14}O_4$).

Packaging and storage—Preserve in tight containers.

USP Reference standards ⟨11⟩—*USP Guaifenesin RS. USP Theophylline RS.*

Identification—Transfer a quantity of the contents of the Capsules, equivalent to about 150 mg of theophylline, to a separator, and add 15 mL of water. To a second separator transfer 15 mL of an aqueous Standard solution containing USP Theophylline RS and USP Guaifenesin RS corresponding, proportionately, to the amounts of theophylline and guaifenesin in the Capsules and having a known concentration of about 10 mg of theophylline per mL. Treat the contents of each separator as follows. Add 25 mL of chloroform, and shake vigorously for 0.5 minute. Allow the layers to separate, filter the lower chloroform layer through glass wool, and evaporate the filtrate to dryness. Dissolve the residue in 10 mL of chloroform. Apply separately 10 μL of each solution so obtained to a thin-layer chromatographic cellulose sheet with fluorescent indicator (see *Chromatography* ⟨621⟩), allow the spots to dry, and develop the chromatogram in a solvent system consisting of a mixture of methanol and water (95 : 5) until the solvent front has moved about 10 cm above the starting line. Remove the sheet from the developing chamber, mark the solvent front, and allow the solvent to evaporate. Expose the sheet to short-wavelength UV light: the R_F values of the spots obtained from the test preparation correspond to those obtained from the Standard solution.

Dissolution ⟨711⟩—
Medium: simulated gastric fluid; 900 mL.
Apparatus 1: 100 rpm.
Time: 45 minutes.
Procedure—Determine the amounts of theophylline ($C_7H_8N_4O_2$) and guaifenesin ($C_{10}H_{14}O_4$) dissolved in filtered portions of the solution under test and employing the procedure set forth in the *Assay*, making any necessary volumetric adjustments, in comparison with Standard solutions having known concentrations of USP Theophylline RS and USP Guaifenesin RS in the same medium.
Tolerances—Not less than 75% (*Q*) of the labeled amounts of $C_7H_8N_4O_2$ and $C_{10}H_{14}O_4$ are dissolved in 45 minutes.

Uniformity of dosage units ⟨905⟩: meet the requirements.

Assay—
pH 6.5 buffer solution—Dissolve 1.36 g of monobasic potassium phosphate in water to make 1000 mL. Carefully adjust with 2.5 N sodium hydroxide to a pH of 6.5, and filter.
Mobile phase—Prepare a degassed solution of *pH 6.5 buffer solution* and methanol (70 : 30).
Internal standard solution—Dissolve about 400 mg of caffeine in 1000 mL of a solution of methanol and water (90 : 10), and mix.
Standard preparation—Dissolve an accurately weighed quantity of USP Theophylline RS in *pH 6.5 buffer solution*, and dilute quantitatively with *pH 6.5 buffer solution* to obtain a solution (*Solution T*) having a known concentration of about 900*J* μg per mL, in which *J* is the ratio of the labeled amount of theophylline to that of guaifenesin. Transfer about 90 mg of USP Guaifenesin RS, accurately weighed, to a 200-mL volumetric flask, add about 150 mL of *pH 6.5 buffer solution*, shake to dissolve, dilute with *pH 6.5 buffer solution* to volume, and mix. Pipet 10 mL of this solution, 10 mL of *Internal standard solution*, and 5 mL of *Solution T* into a 50-mL volumetric flask, dilute with *Mobile phase* to volume, and mix to obtain a *Standard preparation* having known concentrations of about 90 μg of guaifenesin and about 90*J* μg of theophylline per mL.
Assay preparation—Transfer a number of Capsules, equivalent to about 900 mg of guaifenesin, to a 200-mL volumetric flask, add about 160 mL of *pH 6.5 buffer solution*, heat to dissolve completely, cool to room temperature, dilute with *pH 6.5 buffer solution* to volume, and mix. Dilute 10.0 mL of this solution with *pH 6.5 buffer solution* to 100.0 mL. Pipet 10 mL of the diluted solution and 10 mL of *Internal standard solution* into a 50-mL volumetric flask, dilute with *Mobile phase* to volume, and mix.
Chromatographic system (see *Chromatography* ⟨621⟩)—The liquid chromatograph is equipped with a 280-nm detector and a 3.9-mm × 30-cm column that contains packing L1. The flow rate is about 1.0 mL per minute. Chromatograph six replicate injections of the *Standard preparation*, and record the peak responses as directed for *Procedure*: the relative standard deviation of the ratio of peak responses (peak response of ingredient/peak response of internal standard) is not more than 2.0% for theophylline and not more than 2.5% for guaifenesin. The resolution, *R*, between theophylline and caffeine is not less than 3.0.
Procedure—Separately inject equal volumes (about 25 μL) of the *Standard preparation* and the *Assay preparation* into the chromatograph, record the chromatograms, and measure the responses for the major peaks. The relative retention times are about 0.7 for theophylline, 1.0 for caffeine, and 1.5 for guaifenesin. Calculate the quantities, in mg, of anhydrous theophylline ($C_7H_8N_4O_2$) and guaifenesin ($C_{10}H_{14}O_4$) in the portion of Capsules taken by the formula:

$$10C(R_U/R_S)$$

in which *C* is the concentration, in μg per mL, of the appropriate USP Reference Standard in the *Standard preparation*, and R_U and R_S are the ratios of the peak responses of the corresponding analyte to those of caffeine in the *Assay preparation* and the *Standard preparation*, respectively.

Theophylline and Guaifenesin Oral Solution

» Theophylline and Guaifenesin Oral Solution contains not less than 90.0 percent and not more than 110.0 percent of the labeled amount of anhydrous theophylline ($C_7H_8N_4O_2$) and not less than 86.7 percent and not more than 113.3 percent of the labeled amount of guaifenesin ($C_{10}H_{14}O_4$).

Packaging and storage—Preserve in tight containers.

USP Reference standards ⟨11⟩—*USP Guaifenesin RS. USP Theophylline RS.*

Identification—Transfer a volume of Oral Solution, equivalent to about 150 mg of theophylline, to a separator, add 15 mL of water, and proceed as directed in the *Identification* test under *Theophylline and Guaifenesin Capsules*, beginning with "To a second separator."

Alcohol content (if present), Method II ⟨611⟩: between 90.0% and 110.0% of the labeled amount of C_2H_5OH, determined by the gas-liquid chromatographic procedure, acetone being used as the internal standard.

Assay—
pH 6.5 buffer solution and *Mobile phase*—Prepare as directed in the *Assay* under *Theophylline and Guaifenesin Capsules*.
Caffeine solution—Dissolve about 400 mg of caffeine in 1000 mL of a mixture of methanol and water (90 : 10), and mix.
Standard preparation—Dissolve an accurately weighed quantity of USP Theophylline RS in *pH 6.5 buffer solution*, and dilute quantitatively with *pH 6.5 buffer solution* to obtain a solution (*Solution T*) having a known concentration of about 900*J* μg per mL, in which *J* is the ratio of the labeled amount of theophylline to that of guaifenesin. Transfer about 90 mg of USP Guaifenesin RS, accurately weighed, to a 200-mL volumetric flask, add about 150 mL of *pH 6.5 buffer solution*, shake to dissolve, dilute with *pH 6.5 buffer solution* to volume, and mix. Pipet 10 mL of this solution and 5 mL of *Solution T* into a 50-mL volumetric flask, dilute with *Mobile phase* to volume, and mix to obtain a *Standard preparation* having known concentrations of about 90 μg of guaifenesin and about 90*J* μg of theophylline per mL.
Assay preparation—Transfer an accurately measured volume of Oral Solution, equivalent to about 90 mg of guaifenesin, to a 200-mL volumetric flask, dilute with *pH 6.5 buffer solution* to volume,

and mix. Transfer 10.0 mL of this solution to a 50-mL volumetric flask, dilute with *Mobile phase* to volume, and mix.

Chromatographic system (see *Chromatography* ⟨621⟩)—The liquid chromatograph is equipped with a 280-nm detector and a 3.9-mm × 30-cm column that contains packing L1. The flow rate is about 1.0 mL per minute. Chromatograph a mixture of 4 mL of *Standard preparation* and 1 mL of *Caffeine solution*, and record the peak responses as directed for *Procedure*: the resolution, *R*, between the theophylline and caffeine peaks is not less than 3.0, and the relative standard deviation for replicate injections is not more than 2.0 for theophylline and not more than 2.5% for guaifenesin.

Procedure—Proceed as directed in the *Assay* under *Theophylline and Guaifenesin Capsules*. Calculate the quantities, in mg, of anhydrous theophylline ($C_7H_8N_4O_2$) and guaifenesin ($C_{10}H_{14}O_4$) per mL of the Oral Solution taken by the formula:

$$(C / V)(r_U / r_S)$$

in which *C* is the concentration, in µg per mL, of the appropriate USP Reference Standard in the *Standard preparation*, *V* is the volume, in mL, of Oral Solution taken, and r_U and r_S are the peak responses of the corresponding analyte in the *Assay preparation* and the *Standard preparation*, respectively.

Theophylline Sodium Glycinate

Glycine, mixture with 3,7-dihydro-1,3-dimethyl-1*H*-purine-2,6-dione, monosodium salt.
Theophylline sodium mixture with glycine   [8000-10-0].

» Theophylline Sodium Glycinate is an equilibrium mixture containing Theophylline Sodium ($C_7H_7N_4NaO_2$) and Glycine ($C_2H_5NO_2$) in approximately equimolecular proportions buffered with an additional mole of Glycine. Dried at 105° for 4 hours, it contains theophylline sodium glycinate equivalent to not less than 44.5 percent and not more than 47.3 percent of anhydrous theophylline ($C_7H_8N_4O_2$).

Packaging and storage—Preserve in tight containers.

USP Reference standards ⟨11⟩—*USP Glycine RS. USP Theophylline RS.*

Identification—
   A: Dissolve about 1 g in 20 mL of warm water, and neutralize the solution with 6 N acetic acid: a white, crystalline precipitate of theophylline is formed. Filter, wash the precipitate with small portions of cold water, and dry it at 105° for 1 hour: the theophylline so obtained melts between 270° and 274°, the procedure for *Class I* being used (see *Melting Range or Temperature* ⟨741⟩). Retain the remaining portion of the theophylline for use in *Identification* test *B*.
   B: *Infrared Absorption* ⟨197K⟩: residue obtained in *Identification* test *A*.
   C: Ignite it: the residue colors a nonluminous flame intensely yellow and effervesces with acids.

pH ⟨791⟩: between 8.5 and 9.5, in a saturated solution.

Loss on drying ⟨731⟩—Dry it at 105° for 4 hours: it loses not more than 2.0% of its weight.

Glycine content—
   Mobile phase—Prepare a solution containing 470 mg of sodium acetate trihydrate and 1 mL of glacial acetic acid in 2 liters of water. Adjust with 10 N sodium hydroxide to a pH of 4.3. Mix 3 volumes of the resulting solution with 7 volumes of acetonitrile. Make adjustments if necessary (see *System Suitability* under *Chromatography* ⟨621⟩).
   Standard preparation—Dissolve an accurately weighed quantity of USP Glycine RS in *Mobile phase*, and dilute quantitatively with *Mobile phase* to obtain a solution having a known concentration of about 1.3 mg per mL.
   Test preparation—Transfer about 153 mg of Theophylline Sodium Glycinate, accurately weighed, to a 50-mL volumetric flask, dissolve in *Mobile phase*, dilute with *Mobile phase* to volume, and mix.
   Chromatographic system (see *Chromatography* ⟨621⟩)—The liquid chromatograph is equipped with a 200-nm detector and a 3.9-mm × 30-cm column that contains packing L8. The flow rate is about 1.5 mL per minute. Chromatograph the *Standard preparation*, and record the peak responses as directed for *Procedure*: the column efficiency determined from the analyte peak is not less than 2000 theoretical plates, the tailing factor for the glycine peak is not more than 2.0, and the relative standard deviation for replicate injections is not more than 2.0%.
   Procedure—Separately inject equal volumes (about 20 µL) of the *Standard preparation* and the *Test preparation* into the chromatograph, record the chromatograms, and measure the responses for the glycine peaks. Calculate the quantity, in mg, of $C_2H_5NO_2$ in the portion of Theophylline Sodium Glycinate taken by the formula:

$$50C(r_U / r_S)$$

in which *C* is the concentration, in mg per mL, of USP Glycine RS in the *Standard preparation*, and r_U and r_S are the peak responses obtained from the *Test preparation* and the *Standard preparation*, respectively: not less than 42.0 percent and not more than 48.0 percent, on the dried basis, is found.

Organic volatile impurities, *Method I* ⟨467⟩: meets the requirements.

(Official until July 1, 2008)

Assay—
   Buffer solution, Mobile phase, Internal standard solution, Standard preparation, and *Chromatographic system*—Prepare as directed in the *Assay* under *Theophylline*.
   Assay preparation—Transfer about 550 mg of Theophylline Sodium Glycinate, previously dried and accurately weighed, to a 250-mL volumetric flask, add about 125 mL of *Mobile phase*, shake by mechanical means until solution is complete, dilute with *Mobile phase* to volume, and mix. Transfer 10.0 mL of this solution to a 100-mL volumetric flask, add 20.0 mL of *Internal standard solution*, dilute with *Mobile phase* to volume, and mix.
   Procedure—Proceed as directed for *Procedure* in the *Assay* under *Theophylline*. Calculate the quantity, in mg, of anhydrous theophylline ($C_7H_8N_4O_2$) in the portion of Theophylline Sodium Glycinate taken by the formula:

$$2500C(R_U / R_S)$$

in which the terms are as defined therein.

Theophylline Sodium Glycinate Oral Solution

» Theophylline Sodium Glycinate Oral Solution contains an amount of theophylline sodium glycinate equivalent to not less than 93.0 percent and not more than 107.0 percent of the labeled amount of anhydrous theophylline ($C_7H_8N_4O_2$).

Packaging and storage—Preserve in tight containers.

USP Reference standards ⟨11⟩—*USP Theophylline RS.*

Labeling—Label Oral Solution to state both the content of theophylline sodium glycinate and the content of anhydrous theophylline.

Identification—Mix a volume of Oral Solution, equivalent to about 500 mg of theophylline, with 10 mL of 6 N ammonium hydroxide, and evaporate on a steam bath to a volume of about 20 mL. Neutralize with 6 N acetic acid to litmus, and cool, with stirring, to about 15°. Collect the precipitate on a filter, wash with cold water, and dry at 105° for 4 hours: the theophylline so obtained melts between 270° and 274°, the procedure for *Class I* being used (see *Melting Range or Temperature* ⟨741⟩), and meets the requirements for *Identification* test *B* under *Theophylline Sodium Glycinate*.

pH ⟨791⟩: between 8.3 and 9.1.
Alcohol content, *Method II* ⟨611⟩: between 17.0% and 23.0% of C₂H₅OH.

Assay—
  Buffer solution, Mobile phase, Internal standard solution, Standard preparation, and *Chromatographic system*—Prepare as directed in the *Assay* under *Theophylline.*
  Assay preparation—Transfer an accurately measured volume of Oral Solution, equivalent to about 220 mg of theophylline sodium glycinate, to a 100-mL volumetric flask, dilute with water to volume, and mix. Transfer 10.0 mL of this solution to a 100-mL volumetric flask, add 20.0 mL of *Internal standard solution*, dilute with *Mobile phase* to volume, and mix.
  Procedure—Proceed as directed for *Procedure* in the *Assay* under *Theophylline.* Calculate the quantity, in mg, of anhydrous theophylline (C₇H₈N₄O₂) in each mL of the Oral Solution taken by the formula:

$$(1000C/V)(R_U/R_S)$$

in which V is the volume, in mL, of Oral Solution taken, and the other terms are as defined therein.

Theophylline Sodium Glycinate Tablets

» Theophylline Sodium Glycinate Tablets contain an amount of theophylline sodium glycinate equivalent to not less than 93.0 percent and not more than 107.0 percent of the labeled amount of anhydrous theophylline (C₇H₈N₄O₂).

Packaging and storage—Preserve in well-closed containers.
Labeling—Label the Tablets to state both the content of theophylline sodium glycinate and the content of anhydrous theophylline.
USP Reference standards ⟨11⟩—*USP Theophylline RS.*
Identification—Triturate a quantity of finely powdered Tablets, equivalent to about 500 mg of theophylline, with 10-mL and 15-mL portions of solvent hexane, and discard the solvent hexane. Triturate the residue with two 10-mL portions of a mixture of equal volumes of 6 N ammonium hydroxide and water, and filter each time. Evaporate the combined filtrates to about 5 mL, neutralize, if necessary, with 6 N acetic acid, using litmus, and cool to about 15°, with stirring. Collect the precipitate on a filter, wash it with cold water, and dry at 105° for 1 hour: the theophylline so obtained melts between 270° and 274°, the procedure for *Class I* being used (see *Melting Range or Temperature* ⟨741⟩), and responds to *Identification test B* under *Theophylline Sodium Glycinate.*

Dissolution ⟨711⟩—
  Medium: water; 900 mL.
  Apparatus 1: 100 rpm.
  Time: 45 minutes.
  Procedure—Determine the amount of anhydrous theophylline (C₇H₈N₄O₂) dissolved from UV absorbances at the wavelength of maximum absorbance at about 272 nm of filtered portions of the solution under test, suitably diluted with *Dissolution Medium,* if necessary, in comparison with a Standard solution having a known concentration of USP Theophylline RS in the same medium.
  Tolerances—Not less than 75% (Q) of the labeled amount of anhydrous C₇H₈N₄O₂ is dissolved in 45 minutes.

Uniformity of dosage units ⟨905⟩: meet the requirements.

Assay—Place 20 Tablets in a 200-mL volumetric flask, add 50 mL of water, and when the tablets have disintegrated add 50 mL of 6 N ammonium hydroxide. Shake until no more dissolves, then dilute with water to volume, mix, and filter through a dry filter into a dry flask, discarding the first 20 mL of the filtrate. Transfer an accurately measured aliquot of the subsequent filtrate, equivalent to about 250 mg of theophylline, to a 250-mL conical flask, add 20.0 mL of 0.1 N silver nitrate VS, and heat on a steam bath for 15 minutes. Filter through a filter crucible under reduced pressure, and wash the precipitate with three 10-mL portions of water. Acidify the combined filtrate and washings with nitric acid, and add an excess of 3 mL of the acid. Cool, add 2 mL of ferric ammonium sulfate TS, and titrate the excess silver nitrate with 0.1 N ammonium thiocyanate VS. Each mL of 0.1 N silver nitrate is equivalent to 18.02 mg of C₇H₈N₄O₂.

Thiabendazole

C₁₀H₇N₃S   201.25
1*H*-Benzimidazole, 2-(4-thiazolyl)-.
2-(4-Thiazolyl)benzimidazole   [*148-79-8*].

» Thiabendazole contains not less than 98.0 percent and not more than 101.0 percent of C₁₀H₇N₃S, calculated on the dried basis.
  NOTE—Thiabendazole labeled solely for veterinary use is exempt from the requirements of the tests for *Residue on ignition, Selenium, Heavy metals,* and *Chromatographic purity.*

Packaging and storage—Preserve in well-closed containers.
USP Reference standards ⟨11⟩—*USP Thiabendazole RS.*
Identification—
  A: *Infrared Absorption* ⟨197K⟩—Do not dry specimens.
  B: *Ultraviolet Absorption* ⟨197U⟩—
    Solution: 5 µg per mL.
    Medium: 0.1 N hydrochloric acid.
  C: Dissolve about 5 mg in 5 mL of 0.1 N hydrochloric acid, add 3 mg of *p*-phenylenediamine dihydrochloride, and shake to dissolve. Add about 0.1 g of zinc dust, mix, and allow to stand for 2 minutes. Add 5 mL of a solution prepared by dissolving 20 g of ferric ammonium sulfate in 75 mL of water, adding 10 mL of 1 N sulfuric acid, and diluting with water to 100 mL: a blue or blue-violet color develops.
  D: The R_F value of the principal spot in the chromatogram of the *Identification test preparation* corresponds to that of *Standard preparation A,* as obtained in the test for *Chromatographic purity.*

Loss on drying ⟨731⟩—Dry it in vacuum at 100° for 2 hours: it loses not more than 0.5% of its weight.
Melting range ⟨741⟩: between 296° and 303°.
Residue on ignition ⟨281⟩: not more than 0.1%.
Selenium ⟨291⟩: 0.003%, a 200-mg test specimen being used.
Heavy metals, *Method II* ⟨231⟩: 0.001%.
Chromatographic purity—
  Standard preparations—Dissolve USP Thiabendazole RS in glacial acetic acid, and mix to obtain a solution having a known concentration of 1.0 mg per mL. Dilute quantitatively with glacial acetic acid to obtain *Standard preparations A, B,* and *C* having the following compositions:

Standard preparation	Dilution	Concentration (µg RS per mL)	Percentage (%, for comparison with test specimen)
A	(1 in 4)	250	0.5
B	(3 in 20)	150	0.3
C	(1 in 20)	50	0.1

  Test preparation—Dissolve an accurately weighed quantity of Thiabendazole in glacial acetic acid to obtain a solution containing 50 mg per mL.
  Identification preparation—Dilute a portion of the *Test preparation* quantitatively with glacial acetic acid to obtain a solution containing 0.25 mg per mL.

Procedure—Apply separately 10 µL of the *Test preparation*, 10 µL of the *Identification preparation*, and 10 µL of each *Standard preparation* to a suitable thin-layer chromatographic plate (see *Chromatography* ⟨621⟩) coated with a 0.25-mm layer of chromatographic silica gel mixture. Position the plate in a chromatographic chamber, and develop the chromatograms in a solvent system consisting of a mixture of toluene, glacial acetic acid, acetone, and water (60 : 20 : 8 : 2) until the solvent front has moved about three-fourths of the length of the plate. Remove the plate from the developing chamber, mark the solvent front, and allow the solvent to evaporate. Examine the plate under short-wavelength UV light, and compare the intensities of any secondary spots observed in the chromatogram of the *Test preparation* with those of the principal spots in the chromatograms of the *Standard preparations*. No secondary spot from the chromatogram of the *Test preparation* is larger or more intense than the principal spot obtained from *Standard preparation* (0.5%), and the sum of the intensities of all secondary spots obtained from the *Test preparation* corresponds to not more than 1.0%.

Assay—Dissolve about 160 mg of Thiabendazole, accurately weighed, in 10 mL of glacial acetic acid. Add 50 mL of acetic anhydride, 1 mL of mercuric acetate TS, and 2 drops of crystal violet TS, and titrate with 0.1 N perchloric acid VS (the color change at the endpoint is from blue to blue-green). Perform a blank determination, and make any necessary correction. Each mL of 0.1 N perchloric acid is equivalent to 20.13 mg of $C_{10}H_7N_3S$.

Thiabendazole Oral Suspension

» Thiabendazole Oral Suspension contains not less than 90.0 percent and not more than 110.0 percent of the labeled amount of thiabendazole ($C_{10}H_7N_3S$).

Packaging and storage—Preserve in tight containers.

USP Reference standards ⟨11⟩—*USP Thiabendazole RS.*
Identification—
  A: Mix a portion of Oral Suspension, equivalent to about 0.5 g of thiabendazole, with about 20 mL of water, and filter. Wash the residue with 20 mL of water, discard the washing, dissolve the residue in 30 mL of 0.1 N hydrochloric acid, and filter. Collect the filtrate in a separator, render it alkaline with 1 N sodium hydroxide, and extract with 10 mL of carbon disulfide. Pass the carbon disulfide layer through a dry filter, collecting the filtrate in an evaporating dish. Evaporate the solvent with the aid of gentle heat and a stream of nitrogen. [*Caution*—*Do not overheat the residue.*] The residue so obtained responds to *Identification* test A under *Thiabendazole*.
  B: The retention time of the major peak in the chromatogram of the *Assay preparation* corresponds to that in the chromatogram of the *Standard preparation*, as obtained in the *Assay*.

Uniformity of dosage units ⟨905⟩—
  FOR ORAL SUSPENSION PACKAGED IN SINGLE-UNIT CONTAINERS: meets the requirements.

Deliverable volume ⟨698⟩—
  FOR ORAL SUSPENSION PACKAGED IN MULTIPLE-UNIT CONTAINERS: meets the requirements.

pH ⟨791⟩: between 3.4 and 4.2.

Assay—
  pH 3.1 Phosphate buffer—Dissolve 13.8 g of monobasic sodium phosphate in water to obtain 2000 mL of solution. Adjust this solution with phosphoric acid to a pH of 3.1 ± 0.05.
  Mobile phase—Prepare a filtered and degassed mixture of *pH 3.1 Phosphate buffer* and methanol (65 : 35). Make adjustments if necessary (see *System Suitability* under *Chromatography* ⟨621⟩).
  Standard preparation—Dissolve an accurately weighed quantity of USP Thiabendazole RS in 0.1 N hydrochloric acid, and dilute quantitatively, and stepwise if necessary, with 0.1 N hydrochloric acid to obtain a solution containing about 2 mg per mL. Transfer 5.0 mL of this solution to a 50-mL volumetric flask, dilute with water to volume, and mix to obtain a *Standard preparation* having a known concentration of about 0.2 mg of USP Thiabendazole RS per mL.
  Assay preparation—Transfer an accurately measured volume of Oral Suspension, equivalent to about 0.5 g of thiabendazole, to a 250-mL volumetric flask; dilute with 0.1 N hydrochloric acid to volume; and mix. Transfer 5.0 mL of this solution to a 50-mL volumetric flask, dilute with water to volume, and mix.
  Chromatographic system (see *Chromatography* ⟨621⟩)—The liquid chromatograph is equipped with a 254-nm detector and a 4-mm × 30-cm column that contains packing L1. The flow rate is about 2 mL per minute. Chromatograph the *Standard preparation*, and record the peak responses as directed for *Procedure*: the column efficiency determined from the analyte peak is not less than 960 theoretical plates, the tailing factor for the analyte peak is not more than 2.0, and the relative standard deviation for replicate injections is not more than 2%.
  Procedure—Separately inject equal volumes (about 20 µL) of the *Standard preparation* and the *Assay preparation* into the chromatograph, record the chromatograms, and measure the responses for the major peaks. Calculate the quantity, in g, of thiabendazole ($C_{10}H_7N_3S$) in each mL of the Oral Suspension taken by the formula:

$$2.5(C/V)(r_U / r_S)$$

in which C is the concentration, in mg per mL, of USP Thiabendazole RS in the *Standard preparation*; V is the volume, in mL, of Oral Suspension taken; and r_U and r_S are the peak responses obtained from the *Assay preparation* and the *Standard preparation*, respectively.

Thiabendazole Tablets

(Current title—not to change until February 1, 2010)
Monograph title change—to become official February 1, 2010
See **Thiabendazole Chewable Tablets**

» Thiabendazole Tablets contain not less than 90.0 percent and not more than 110.0 percent of the labeled amount of $C_{10}H_7N_3S$.

Packaging and storage—Preserve in tight containers.
Labeling—Label the Tablets to indicate that they are to be chewed before swallowing.
USP Reference standards ⟨11⟩—*USP Thiabendazole RS.*
Identification—
  A: Triturate a quantity of powdered Tablets, equivalent to about 0.5 g of thiabendazole, with about 20 mL of water, and filter. Wash the residue with 20 mL of water, discard the washing, dissolve the residue in 30 mL of 0.1 N hydrochloric acid, and filter. Collect the filtrate in a separator, render it alkaline with 1 N sodium hydroxide, and extract with 10 mL of carbon disulfide. Filter the carbon disulfide layer through a dry filter, collecting the filtrate in an evaporating dish. Evaporate the solvent with the aid of gentle heat and a stream of nitrogen. [*Caution*—*Do not overheat the residue.*] The residue so obtained responds to *Identification* test A under *Thiabendazole*.
  B: The retention time of the major peak in the chromatogram of the *Assay preparation* corresponds to that of the *Standard preparation* as obtained in the *Assay*.

Uniformity of dosage units ⟨905⟩: meet the requirements.
  Procedure for content uniformity—
  Standard preparation—Dissolve an accurately weighed quantity of USP Thiabendazole RS in 0.1 N hydrochloric acid, and dilute quantitatively and stepwise with 0.1 N hydrochloric acid to obtain a solution having a known concentration of about 5 µg per mL.
  Test preparation—Transfer 1 Tablet to a 1000-mL volumetric flask, add about 75 mL of 0.1 N hydrochloric acid, and heat on a steam bath for about 1 hour. Cool to room temperature, dilute with 0.1 N hydrochloric acid to volume, mix, and filter a portion of the solution, discarding the first 20 mL of the filtrate. Pipet 5 mL of the filtrate into a 500-mL volumetric flask, dilute with 0.1 N hydrochloric acid to volume, and mix.

Procedure—Concomitantly determine the absorbances of the *Standard preparation* and the *Test preparation* at the wavelength of maximum absorbance at about 302 nm, with a suitable spectrophotometer, using 0.1 N hydrochloric acid as the blank. Calculate the quantity, in mg, of $C_{10}H_7N_3S$ in the Tablet taken by the formula:

$$(TC/D)(A_U/A_S)$$

in which T is the labeled quantity, in mg, of thiabendazole in the Tablet, C is the concentration, in μg per mL, of USP Thiabendazole RS in the *Standard preparation*, D is the concentration, in μg per mL, of thiabendazole in the *Test preparation*, based upon the labeled quantity per Tablet and the extent of dilution, and A_U and A_S are the absorbances of the *Test preparation* and the *Standard preparation*, respectively.

Assay—
Standard preparation and *Chromatographic system*—Prepare as directed in the *Assay* under *Thiabendazole Oral Suspension*.
pH 3.5 phosphate buffer—Dissolve 13.8 g of monobasic sodium phosphate in water to obtain 2000 mL of solution. Adjust this solution with phosphoric acid to a pH of 3.5 ± 0.05.
Mobile phase—Prepare a filtered and degassed mixture of *pH 3.5 phosphate buffer* and methanol (54 : 46). Make adjustments if necessary (see *System Suitability* under *Chromatography* ⟨621⟩).
Assay preparation—Weigh and finely powder not less than 20 Tablets. Transfer an accurately weighed portion of the powder, equivalent to about 200 mg of thiabendazole, to a 1000-mL volumetric flask, add 100 mL of 0.1 N hydrochloric acid, mix, and warm the solution for a minimum of 30 minutes. Allow to cool to room temperature, dilute with water to volume, mix, and filter, discarding the first 20 mL of the filtrate.
Procedure—Proceed as directed for *Procedure* in the *Assay* under *Thiabendazole Oral Suspension*. Calculate the quantity, in mg, of $C_{10}H_7N_3S$ in the portion of Tablets taken by the formula:

$$1000C(r_U/r_S)$$

in which C is the concentration, in mg per mL, of USP Thiabendazole RS in the *Standard preparation*, and r_U and r_S are the peak responses obtained from the *Assay preparation* and the *Standard preparation*, respectively.

Thiabendazole Chewable Tablets

(Monograph under this new title—to become official February 1, 2010)
(Current monograph title is Thiabendazole Tablets)

» Thiabendazole Chewable Tablets contain not less than 90.0 percent and not more than 110.0 percent of the labeled amount of thiabendazole ($C_{10}H_7N_3S$).

Packaging and storage—Preserve in tight containers.
Labeling—Label the Chewable Tablets to indicate that they are to be chewed before swallowing.

USP Reference standards ⟨11⟩—*USP Thiabendazole RS*.
Identification—
  A: Triturate a quantity of powdered Chewable Tablets, equivalent to about 0.5 g of thiabendazole, with about 20 mL of water, and filter. Wash the residue with 20 mL of water, discard the washing, dissolve the residue in 30 mL of 0.1 N hydrochloric acid, and filter. Collect the filtrate in a separator, render it alkaline with 1 N sodium hydroxide, and extract with 10 mL of carbon disulfide. Pass the carbon disulfide layer through a dry filter, collecting the filtrate in an evaporating dish. Evaporate the solvent with the aid of gentle heat and a stream of nitrogen. *[Caution—Do not overheat the residue.]* The residue so obtained meets the requirements for *Identification test A* under *Thiabendazole*.
  B: The retention time of the major peak in the chromatogram of the *Assay preparation* corresponds to that in the chromatogram of the *Standard preparation*, as obtained in the *Assay*.

Uniformity of dosage units ⟨905⟩: meet the requirements.
PROCEDURE FOR CONTENT UNIFORMITY—
Standard preparation—Dissolve an accurately weighed quantity of USP Thiabendazole RS in 0.1 N hydrochloric acid, and dilute quantitatively and stepwise with 0.1 N hydrochloric acid to obtain a solution having a known concentration of about 5 μg per mL.
Test preparation—Transfer 1 Chewable Tablet to a 1000-mL volumetric flask, add about 75 mL of 0.1 N hydrochloric acid, and heat on a steam bath for about 1 hour. Cool to room temperature, dilute with 0.1 N hydrochloric acid to volume, mix, and filter a portion of the solution, discarding the first 20 mL of the filtrate. Pipet 5 mL of the filtrate into a 500-mL volumetric flask, dilute with 0.1 N hydrochloric acid to volume, and mix.
Procedure—Concomitantly determine the absorbances of the *Standard preparation* and the *Test preparation* at the wavelength of maximum absorbance at about 302 nm, with a suitable spectrophotometer, using 0.1 N hydrochloric acid as the blank. Calculate the quantity, in mg, of $C_{10}H_7N_3S$ in the Chewable Tablet taken by the formula:

$$(TC/D)(A_U/A_S)$$

in which T is the labeled quantity, in mg, of thiabendazole in the Chewable Tablet; C is the concentration, in μg per mL, of USP Thiabendazole RS in the *Standard preparation*; D is the concentration, in μg per mL, of thiabendazole in the *Test preparation*, based upon the labeled quantity per Chewable Tablet and the extent of dilution; and A_U and A_S are the absorbances of the *Test preparation* and the *Standard preparation*, respectively.

Assay—
Standard preparation and *Chromatographic system*—Prepare as directed in the *Assay* under *Thiabendazole Oral Suspension*.
pH 3.5 Phosphate buffer—Dissolve 13.8 g of monobasic sodium phosphate in water to obtain 2000 mL of solution. Adjust this solution with phosphoric acid to a pH of 3.5 ± 0.05.
Mobile phase—Prepare a filtered and degassed mixture of *pH 3.5 Phosphate buffer* and methanol (54 : 46). Make adjustments if necessary (see *System Suitability* under *Chromatography* ⟨621⟩).
Assay preparation—Weigh and finely powder not fewer than 20 Chewable Tablets. Transfer an accurately weighed portion of the powder, equivalent to about 200 mg of thiabendazole, to a 1000-mL volumetric flask, add 100 mL of 0.1 N hydrochloric acid, mix, and warm the solution for a minimum of 30 minutes. Allow to cool to room temperature, dilute with water to volume, mix, and filter, discarding the first 20 mL of the filtrate.
Procedure—Proceed as directed for *Procedure* in the *Assay* under *Thiabendazole Oral Suspension*. Calculate the quantity, in mg, of thiabendazole ($C_{10}H_7N_3S$) in the portion of Chewable Tablets taken by the formula:

$$1000C(r_U/r_S)$$

in which C is the concentration, in mg per mL, of USP Thiabendazole RS in the *Standard preparation*; and r_U and r_S are the peak responses obtained from the *Assay preparation* and the *Standard preparation*, respectively.

(Official February 1, 2010)

Thiamine Hydrochloride

$C_{12}H_{17}ClN_4OS \cdot HCl$ 337.27
Thiazolium, 3-[(4-amino-2-methyl-5-pyrimidinyl)methyl]-5-(2-hydroxyethyl)-4-methyl-, chloride, monohydrochloride.
Thiamine monohydrochloride   [67-03-8].

» Thiamine Hydrochloride contains not less than 98.0 percent and not more than 102.0 percent of

$C_{12}H_{17}ClN_4OS \cdot HCl$, calculated on the anhydrous basis.

Packaging and storage—Preserve in tight, light-resistant containers.

USP Reference standards ⟨11⟩—*USP Thiamine Hydrochloride RS.*

Identification—
  A: *Infrared Absorption* ⟨197K⟩—Dry specimens at 105° for 2 hours.
  B: A solution (1 in 50) responds to the tests for *Chloride* ⟨191⟩.

pH ⟨791⟩: between 2.7 and 3.4, in a solution (1 in 100).

Water, *Method I* ⟨921⟩: not more than 5.0%.

Residue on ignition ⟨281⟩: not more than 0.2%.

Absorbance of solution—Dissolve 1.0 g in water to make 10 mL. The absorbance of this solution, after filtration through a fine-porosity, sintered-glass funnel, determined in 1-cm cells at a wavelength of 400 nm, with a suitable spectrophotometer, water being used as the blank, does not exceed 0.025.

Limit of nitrate—To 2 mL of a solution (1 in 50) add 2 mL of sulfuric acid, cool, and superimpose 2 mL of ferrous sulfate TS: no brown ring is produced at the junction of the two layers.

Organic volatile impurities, *Method IV* ⟨467⟩: meets the requirements.

(Official until July 1, 2008)

Chromatographic purity—
  Solution A, Solution B, and *Mobile phase*—Prepare as directed in the *Assay.*
  Test solution—Dissolve quantitatively an accurately weighed quantity of Thiamine Hydrochloride in *Mobile phase* to obtain a solution having a concentration of about 1.0 mg per mL.
  Chromatographic system (see *Chromatography* ⟨621⟩)—The liquid chromatograph is equipped with a 254-nm detector and a 4.0-mm × 15-cm column that contains packing L1. The flow rate is about 0.75 mL per minute.
  Procedure—Inject about 10 μL of the *Test solution* into the chromatograph, and allow the *Test solution* to elute for not less than three times the retention time of the main peak. Record the chromatogram and measure the areas of the peak responses: the total of the responses of all secondary peaks is not greater than 1.0% of the total of the responses of all of the peaks.

Assay—
  Solution A—Prepare a 0.005 M solution of sodium 1-octanesulfonate in dilute glacial acetic acid (1 in 100).
  Solution B—Prepare a mixture of methanol and acetonitrile (3 : 2).
  Mobile phase—Prepare a mixture of *Solution A* and *Solution B* (60 : 40), filter, and degas. Make adjustments if necessary (see *System Suitability* under *Chromatography* ⟨621⟩).
  Internal standard solution—Transfer 2.0 mL of methylbenzoate to a 100-mL volumetric flask, dilute with methanol to volume, and mix.
  Standard preparation—Dissolve an accurately weighed quantity of USP Thiamine Hydrochloride RS in *Mobile phase* to obtain a solution having a known concentration of about 1 mg per mL. Transfer 20.0 mL of this solution to a 50-mL volumetric flask, add 5.0 mL of *Internal standard solution,* dilute with *Mobile phase* to volume, and mix to obtain a *Standard preparation* having a known concentration of about 400 μg per mL.
  Assay preparation—Transfer an accurately weighed quantity of about 200 mg of Thiamine Hydrochloride to a 100-mL volumetric flask, dissolve in and dilute with *Mobile phase* to volume, and mix. Transfer 10.0 mL of this solution to a 50-mL volumetric flask, add 5.0 mL of *Internal standard solution,* dilute with *Mobile phase* to volume, and mix.
  Chromatographic system (see *Chromatography* ⟨621⟩)—The liquid chromatograph is equipped with a 254-nm detector and a 4-mm × 30-cm column that contains packing L1. The flow rate is about 1 mL per minute. [NOTE—The flow rate may be adjusted as needed to obtain a retention time of about 12 minutes for thiamine hydrochloride.] Chromatograph the *Standard preparation,* and record the peak responses as directed for *Procedure:* the resolution, *R*, between the thiamine and methylbenzoate peaks is not less than 4.0; the tailing factor for the thiamine peak is not more than 2.0; the column efficiency determined from the thiamine peak is not less than 1500 theoretical plates; and the relative standard deviation for replicate injections is not more than 2.0%.
  Procedure—Separately inject equal volumes (about 10 μL) of the *Standard preparation* and the *Assay preparation* into the chromatograph, record the chromatograms, and measure the areas of the major peaks. Calculate the quantity, in mg, of $C_{12}H_{17}ClN_4OS \cdot HCl$ in the Thiamine Hydrochloride taken by the formula:

$$0.5C(R_U/R_S)$$

in which *C* is the concentration, in μg per mL, of USP Thiamine Hydrochloride RS in the *Standard preparation;* and R_U and R_S are the ratios of the peak areas of thiamine to methylbenzoate obtained from the *Assay preparation* and the *Standard preparation,* respectively.

Thiamine Hydrochloride Injection

» Thiamine Hydrochloride Injection is a sterile solution of Thiamine Hydrochloride in Water for Injection. It contains not less than 90.0 percent and not more than 110.0 percent of the labeled amount of thiamine hydrochloride ($C_{12}H_{17}ClN_4OS \cdot HCl$).

Packaging and storage—Preserve in single-dose or multiple-dose containers, preferably of Type I glass, protected from light.

USP Reference standards ⟨11⟩—*USP Endotoxin RS. USP Thiamine Hydrochloride RS.*

Identification—
  A: It yields a white precipitate with mercuric chloride TS, and a red-brown precipitate with iodine TS. It also yields a precipitate with mercuric-potassium iodide TS, and with trinitrophenol TS.
  B: Dilute a portion of Injection with water to a concentration of about 10 mg of thiamine hydrochloride per mL. To 0.5 mL of this solution add 5 mL of 0.5 N sodium hydroxide, then add 0.5 mL of potassium ferricyanide TS and 5 mL of isobutyl alcohol, shake the mixture vigorously for 2 minutes, and allow the liquid layers to separate: when illuminated from above by a vertical beam of UV light and viewed at a right angle to this beam, the air-liquid meniscus shows a vivid blue fluorescence, which disappears when the mixture is slightly acidified, but reappears when it is again made alkaline.
  C: It responds to the tests for *Chloride* ⟨191⟩.

Bacterial endotoxins ⟨85⟩—It contains not more than 3.5 USP Endotoxin Units per mg of thiamine hydrochloride.

pH ⟨791⟩: between 2.5 and 4.5.

Other requirements—It meets the requirements under *Injections* ⟨1⟩.

Assay—
  Mobile phase, Internal standard solution, Standard preparation, and *Chromatographic system*—Prepare as directed in the *Assay* under *Thiamine Hydrochloride Oral Solution.*
  Assay preparation—Quantitatively dilute an accurately measured volume of Injection with *Mobile phase* to obtain a solution containing about 500 μg of thiamine hydrochloride per mL. Pipet 10 mL of the resulting solution and 10 mL of *Internal standard solution* into a 100-mL volumetric flask, dilute with *Mobile phase* to volume, and mix.
  Procedure—Proceed as directed for *Procedure* in the *Assay* under *Thiamine Hydrochloride Oral Solution.* Calculate the quantity, in mg, of thiamine hydrochloride ($C_{12}H_{17}ClN_4OS \cdot HCl$) in each mL of the Injection taken by the formula:

$$C(L/D)(R_U/R_S)$$

in which *C* is the concentration, in mg per mL, of USP Thiamine Hydrochloride RS in the *Standard preparation;* *L* is the labeled quantity, in mg per mL, of thiamine hydrochloride in the Injection; *D* is the concentration, in mg per mL, of thiamine hydrochloride in the *Assay preparation* on the basis of the labeled quantity and the extent of dilution; and R_U and R_S are the ratios of the peak responses of thiamine to methylparaben obtained from the *Assay preparation* and the *Standard preparation*, respectively.

Thiamine Hydrochloride Oral Solution

» Thiamine Hydrochloride Oral Solution contains not less than 95.0 percent and not more than 135.0 percent of the labeled amount of thiamine hydrochloride ($C_{12}H_{17}ClN_4OS \cdot HCl$).

Packaging and storage—Preserve in tight, light-resistant containers.

USP Reference standards ⟨11⟩—*USP Thiamine Hydrochloride RS*.
Identification—It meets the requirements for *Identification* test B under *Thiamine Hydrochloride Injection*.
Alcohol content, *Method II* ⟨611⟩: between 90.0% and 110.0% of the labeled amount of C_2H_5OH, acetone being used as the internal standard.
Assay—
Mobile phase—Prepare a filtered and degassed mixture of 0.04 M aqueous monobasic potassium phosphate and methanol (55 : 45). Make adjustments if necessary (see *System Suitability* under *Chromatography* ⟨621⟩).
Internal standard solution—Prepare a solution of methylparaben in *Mobile phase* having a concentration of about 100 μg per mL.
Standard preparation—Prepare a solution of USP Thiamine Hydrochloride RS in *Mobile phase* having an accurately known concentration of about 500 μg per mL. Pipet 10 mL of this solution and 10 mL of *Internal standard solution* into a 100-mL volumetric flask, dilute with *Mobile phase* to volume, and mix to obtain a *Standard preparation* having a known concentration of about 50 μg per mL.
Assay preparation—Quantitatively dilute an accurately measured volume of Oral Solution with *Mobile phase* to obtain a solution containing about 500 μg of thiamine hydrochloride per mL. Pipet 10 mL of the resulting solution and 10 mL of *Internal standard solution* into a 100-mL volumetric flask, dilute with *Mobile phase* to volume, and mix.
Chromatographic system (see *Chromatography* ⟨621⟩)—The liquid chromatograph is equipped with a 254-nm detector and a 3.9-mm × 30-cm column that contains packing L1. The flow rate is about 1.0 mL per minute. Chromatograph the *Standard preparation,* and record the peak responses as directed for *Procedure:* the relative retention times are about 0.35 for thiamine and 1.0 for methylparaben; the resolution, *R*, between the thiamine and methylparaben peaks is not less than 6.0; and the relative standard deviation for replicate injections is not more than 2.0%.
Procedure—Separately inject equal volumes (about 25 μL) of the *Standard preparation* and the *Assay preparation* into the chromatograph, record the chromatograms, and measure the responses for the major peaks. Calculate the quantity, in mg, of thiamine hydrochloride ($C_{12}H_{17}ClN_4OS \cdot HCl$) in each mL of the Oral Solution taken by the formula:

$$C(L/D)(R_U / R_S)$$

in which *C* is the concentration, in mg per mL, of USP Thiamine Hydrochloride RS in the *Standard preparation;* *L* is the labeled quantity, in mg per mL, of thiamine hydrochloride in the Oral Solution; *D* is the concentration, in mg per mL, of thiamine hydrochloride in the *Assay preparation* on the basis of the labeled quantity and the extent of dilution; and R_U and R_S are the ratios of the peak responses of thiamine to methylparaben obtained from the *Assay preparation* and the *Standard preparation,* respectively.

Thiamine Hydrochloride Tablets

» Thiamine Hydrochloride Tablets contain not less than 90.0 percent and not more than 110.0 percent of the labeled amount of $C_{12}H_{17}ClN_4OS \cdot HCl$.

Packaging and storage—Preserve in tight, light-resistant containers.

USP Reference standards ⟨11⟩—*USP Thiamine Hydrochloride RS*.
Identification—
A: Triturate a quantity of powdered Tablets, equivalent to about 10 mg of thiamine hydrochloride, with 10 mL of 0.5 N sodium hydroxide, and filter. Using a 5-mL portion of the filtrate, proceed as directed in *Identification* test *B* under *Thiamine Hydrochloride Injection*, beginning with "then add 0.5 mL of potassium ferricyanide TS": the specified reaction is observed.
B: Triturate a quantity of powdered Tablets, equivalent to about 10 mg of thiamine hydrochloride, with 10 mL of water, and filter: treated separately, 2-mL portions of the filtrate yield a red-brown precipitate with iodine TS and a white precipitate with mercuric chloride TS, and respond to the tests for *Chloride* ⟨191⟩.
C: To the remainder of the filtrate prepared for the preceding test add 1 mL of lead acetate TS and 1 mL of 2.5 N sodium hydroxide: a yellow color is produced. Heat the mixture for several minutes on a steam bath: the color changes to brown, and, on standing, a precipitate of lead sulfide separates.
Dissolution, *Procedure for a Pooled Sample* ⟨711⟩—
Medium: water; 900 mL.
Apparatus 2: 50 rpm.
Time: 45 minutes.
Procedure—Determine the amount of $C_{12}H_{17}ClN_4OS \cdot HCl$ dissolved, employing the procedure set forth in the *Assay for niacin or niacinamide, pyridoxine hydrochloride, riboflavin, and thiamine* under *Water-Soluble Vitamins Tablets* using filtered portions of the solution under test, suitably diluted with *Dissolution Medium* if necessary, in comparison with a Standard solution having a known concentration of USP Thiamine Hydrochloride RS in the same *Medium*.
Tolerances—Not less than 75% (*Q*) of the labeled amount of $C_{12}H_{17}ClN_4OS \cdot HCl$ is dissolved in 45 minutes.
Uniformity of dosage units ⟨905⟩: meet the requirements.
Assay—
Standard preparation—Prepare as directed for *Standard Preparation* under *Thiamine Assay* ⟨531⟩.
Assay preparation—Place not fewer than 20 Tablets in a flask of suitable size, half fill the flask with 0.2 N hydrochloric acid, and heat on a steam bath, with frequent agitation, until the tablets have dissolved or have disintegrated so that a uniform dispersion is obtained. Cool, transfer the contents of the flask to a volumetric flask, and dilute with 0.2 N hydrochloric acid to volume. If the mixture is not clear, either centrifuge it or filter it through paper known not to adsorb thiamine. Dilute a portion of the clear solution quantitatively and stepwise with 0.2 N hydrochloric acid to obtain a solution containing about 0.2 μg of thiamine hydrochloride per mL. Using this as the *Assay Preparation,* proceed as directed for *Procedure* under *Thiamine Assay* ⟨531⟩.

Thiamine Mononitrate

$C_{12}H_{17}N_5O_4S$ 327.36
Thiazolium, 3-[(4-amino-2-methyl-5-pyrimidinyl)methyl]-5-(2-hydroxyethyl)-4-methyl-, nitrate (salt).
Thiamine nitrate (salt)   [532-43-4].

» Thiamine Mononitrate contains not less than 98.0 percent and not more than 102.0 percent of $C_{12}H_{17}N_5O_4S$, calculated on the dried basis.

Packaging and storage—Preserve in tight, light-resistant containers.

USP Reference standards ⟨11⟩—*USP Thiamine Hydrochloride RS.*

Identification—

A: To 2 mL of a solution (1 in 50) add 2 mL of sulfuric acid, cool, and superimpose 2 mL of ferrous sulfate TS: a brown ring is produced at the junction of the two liquids.

B: Dissolve about 5 mg in a mixture of 1 mL of lead acetate TS and 1 mL of 2.5 N sodium hydroxide: a yellow color is produced. Heat the mixture for several minutes on a steam bath: the color changes to brown, and, on standing, a precipitate of lead sulfide separates.

C: A solution of it responds to *Identification* test *A* under *Thiamine Hydrochloride Injection.*

D: Dissolve about 5 mg in 5 mL of 0.5 N sodium hydroxide, and proceed as directed in *Identification* test *B* under *Thiamine Hydrochloride Injection*, beginning with "then add 0.5 mL of potassium ferricyanide TS": the specified reaction is observed.

pH ⟨791⟩: between 6.0 and 7.5, in a solution (1 in 50).

Loss on drying ⟨731⟩—Dry about 500 mg, accurately weighed, at 105° for 2 hours: it loses not more than 1.0% of its weight.

Residue on ignition ⟨281⟩: not more than 0.2%.

Chloride ⟨221⟩—A 500-mg portion shows no more chloride than corresponds to 0.40 mL of 0.020 N hydrochloric acid (0.06%).

Organic volatile impurities, *Method IV* ⟨467⟩: meets the requirements.

(Official until July 1, 2008)

Chromatographic purity—

Solution A, *Solution B*, and *Mobile phase*—Prepare as directed in the *Assay* under *Thiamine Hydrochloride.*

Test solution—Dissolve quantitatively an accurately weighed quantity of Thiamine Mononitrate in *Mobile phase* to obtain a solution having a concentration of about 1.0 mg per mL.

Chromatographic system—Proceed as directed in the test for *Chromatographic purity* under *Thiamine Hydrochloride.*

Procedure—Proceed as directed in the test for *Chromatographic purity* under *Thiamine Hydrochloride*: the total of the responses of all secondary peaks is not greater than 1.0% of the total of the responses of all of the peaks.

Assay—

Solution A, *Solution B*, *Mobile phase*, *Internal standard solution*, *Standard preparation*, and *Chromatographic system*—Proceed as directed in the *Assay* under *Thiamine Hydrochloride.*

Assay preparation—Transfer an accurately weighed quantity of about 200 mg of Thiamine Mononitrate to a 100-mL volumetric flask, dissolve in *Mobile phase*, dilute with *Mobile phase* to volume, and mix. Transfer 10.0 mL of this solution to a 50-mL volumetric flask, add 5.0 mL of *Internal standard solution*, dilute with *Mobile phase* to volume, and mix.

Procedure—Separately inject equal volumes (about 10 μL) of the *Standard preparation* and the *Assay preparation* into the chromatograph, record the chromatograms, and measure the areas of the major peaks. Calculate the quantity, in mg, of $C_{12}H_{17}N_5O_4S$ in the Thiamine Mononitrate taken by the formula:

$$(327.36/337.27)0.5C(R_U/R_S)$$

in which 327.36 and 337.27 are the molecular weights of thiamine mononitrate and thiamine hydrochloride, respectively, *C* is the concentration, in μg per mL, of USP Thiamine Hydrochloride RS in the *Standard preparation*, and R_U and R_S are the ratios of the peak areas of thiamine to methylbenzoate obtained from the *Assay preparation* and the *Standard preparation*, respectively.

Thiamine Mononitrate Oral Solution

» Thiamine Mononitrate Oral Solution contains not less than 95.0 percent and not more than 115.0 percent of the labeled amount of thiamine mononitrate ($C_{12}H_{17}N_5O_4S$).

Packaging and storage—Preserve in tight, light-resistant containers.

USP Reference standards ⟨11⟩—*USP Thiamine Hydrochloride RS.*

Identification—

A: It meets the requirements for *Identification* test *B* under *Thiamine Hydrochloride Injection.*

B: To 5 mL of Oral Solution add 2 mL of sulfuric acid, cool, and superimpose 2 mL of ferrous sulfate TS: a brown ring is produced at the junction of the two liquids.

Alcohol content, *Method II* ⟨611⟩: between 90.0% and 110.0% of the labeled amount of C_2H_5OH, acetone being used as the internal standard.

Assay—

Mobile phase, *Internal standard solution*, *Standard preparation*, and *Chromatographic system*—Prepare as directed in the *Assay* under *Thiamine Hydrochloride Oral Solution.*

Assay preparation—Quantitatively dilute an accurately measured volume of Oral Solution with *Mobile phase* to obtain a solution containing about 500 μg of thiamine mononitrate per mL. Pipet 10 mL of the resulting solution and 10 mL of *Internal standard solution* into a 100-mL volumetric flask, dilute with *Mobile phase* to volume, and mix.

Procedure—Proceed as directed for *Procedure* in the *Assay* under *Thiamine Hydrochloride Oral Solution.* Calculate the quantity, in mg, of thiamine mononitrate ($C_{12}H_{17}N_5O_4S$) in each mL of the Oral Solution taken by the formula:

$$(327.36/337.27)C(L/D)(R_U/R_S)$$

in which 327.36 and 337.27 are the molecular weights of thiamine mononitrate and thiamine hydrochloride, respectively; *C* is the concentration, in mg per mL, of USP Thiamine Hydrochloride RS in the *Standard preparation*; *L* is the labeled quantity, in mg per mL, of thiamine mononitrate in the Oral Solution; *D* is the concentration, in mg per mL, of thiamine mononitrate in the *Assay preparation* on the basis of the labeled quantity and the extent of dilution; and R_U and R_S are the ratios of the peak responses of thiamine to methylparaben obtained from the *Assay preparation* and the *Standard preparation*, respectively.

Thiethylperazine Maleate

$C_{22}H_{29}N_3S_2 \cdot 2C_4H_4O_4$ 631.76

10*H*-Phenothiazine, 2-(ethylthio)-10-[3-(4-methyl-1-piperazinyl)propyl]-, (*Z*)-2-butenedioate (1 : 2).
2-(Ethylthio)-10-[3-(4-methyl-1-piperazinyl)propyl]pheno thiazine maleate (1 : 2) [*1179-69-7*].

» Thiethylperazine Maleate contains not less than 98.0 percent and not more than 101.5 percent of $C_{22}H_{29}N_3S_2 \cdot 2C_4H_4O_4$, calculated on the dried basis.

Packaging and storage—Preserve in tight, light-resistant containers.

USP Reference standards ⟨11⟩—*USP Thiethylperazine Maleate RS.*
  NOTE—Throughout the following procedures, protect test or assay specimens, the Reference Standard, and solutions containing them, by conducting the procedures without delay, under subdued light, or using low-actinic glassware.
Identification, *Infrared Absorption* ⟨197K⟩.
pH ⟨791⟩—Dissolve 100 mg in 100 mL of water, warming, if necessary, to effect solution: the pH of this solution is between 2.8 and 3.8.
Loss on drying ⟨731⟩—Dry it at 105° for 4 hours: it loses not more than 0.5% of its weight.
Residue on ignition ⟨281⟩: not more than 0.1%.
Selenium ⟨291⟩—The absorbance of the solution from the *Test Solution,* prepared with 100 mg of Thiethylperazine Maleate and 100 mg of magnesium oxide, is not greater than one-half that from the *Standard Solution* (0.003%).
Chromatographic purity—[NOTE—Conduct this test promptly without exposure to daylight and with minimum exposure to artificial light.]
  Diluting solution: a mixture of methanol and ammonium hydroxide (49 : 1).
  Test solution—Transfer 100 mg of Thiethylperazine Maleate, accurately weighed, to a 5-mL volumetric flask. Dissolve in and dilute with *Diluting solution* to volume, and mix.
  Standard solutions—Dissolve an accurately weighed quantity of USP Thiethylperazine Maleate RS in *Diluting solution,* and dilute quantitatively, and stepwise if necessary, with *Diluting solution* to obtain a solution having a known concentration of 20.0 mg per mL (*Standard solution A*). Dilute appropriate portions of this solution quantitatively with *Diluting solution* to obtain five *Standard solutions B* to *F* having known concentrations of 0.2, 0.1, 0.06, 0.04, and 0.02 mg per mL, respectively. The final concentrations of *Standard solutions B* to *F* represent 1%, 0.5%, 0.3%, 0.2%, and 0.1% concentration of *Standard solution A*, respectively.
  Application volume: 5 μL.
  Developing solvent system: a mixture of ether, cyclohexane, methanol, and ammonium hydroxide (25 : 10 : 5 : 1).
  Procedure—Apply equal spots of the *Test solution* and *Standard solutions A* to *F* as directed in *Ordinary Impurities* ⟨466⟩. Examine the plate under short- and long-wavelength UV light, then spray the plate with Dragendorff's TS, dry the plate with a stream of nitrogen, and then spray with hydrogen peroxide TS: any secondary spot in the *Test solution* is not more than 0.5%, and the sum of all secondary spots is not more than 2.0%.
Organic volatile impurities, *Method V* ⟨467⟩: meets the requirements.
  Solvent—Use dimethyl sulfoxide.
  (Official until July 1, 2008)
Assay—Dissolve about 250 mg of Thiethylperazine Maleate, accurately weighed, in 30 mL of glacial acetic acid, and warm on a steam bath to effect solution. Add 1 drop of crystal violet TS, and titrate with 0.1 N perchloric acid VS to a blue-green endpoint. Perform a blank determination, and make any necessary correction. Each mL of 0.1 N perchloric acid is equivalent to 31.59 mg of $C_{22}H_{29}N_3S_2 \cdot 2C_4H_4O_4$.

Thiethylperazine Maleate Suppositories

» Thiethylperazine Maleate Suppositories contain not less than 90.0 percent and not more than 110.0 percent of the labeled amount of $C_{22}H_{29}N_3S_2 \cdot 2C_4H_4O_4$.

Packaging and storage—Preserve in tight containers at temperatures below 25°. Do not expose unwrapped Suppositories to sunlight.
USP Reference standards ⟨11⟩—*USP Thiethylperazine Maleate RS.*
  NOTE—Throughout the following procedures, protect test or assay specimens, the Reference Standard, and solutions containing them, by conducting the procedures without delay, under subdued light, or using low-actinic glassware.
Identification—
  A: The retention time of the thiethylperazine peak in the chromatogram of the *Assay preparation* corresponds to that of the *Standard preparation* as obtained in the *Assay.*
  B: The R_F value of the principal spot and its color, as visualized by the spray reagents in the chromatogram of the *Test solution,* corresponds to that of *Standard solution A* as obtained in the test for *Chromatographic purity.*
Uniformity of dosage units ⟨905⟩: meet the requirements.
Chromatographic purity—
  Diluent—Prepare a mixture of methanol, chloroform (stabilized with 0.75% alcohol), and ammonium hydroxide (55 : 45 : 1).
  Standard solutions—Dissolve an accurately weighed quantity of USP Thiethylperazine Maleate RS in *Diluent,* and mix to obtain a solution having a known concentration of about 10 mg per mL. Dilute this solution quantitatively with *Diluent* to obtain *Standard solutions,* designated below by letter, having the following compositions:

Standard solution	Dilution	Concentration (μg RS per mL)	Percentage (%, for comparison with test specimen)
A	(1 in 20)	500	5
B	(1 in 33)	300	3
C	(1 in 50)	200	2
D	(1 in 100)	100	1
E	(1 in 200)	50	0.5

  Test solution—Transfer a number of Suppositories, equivalent to about 20 mg of thiethylperazine maleate, to a funnel having a fine porosity fritted disk. Add 50 mL of *n*-pentane, macerate, and mix with a glass stirring rod, collecting the filtrate in a filter flask under reduced pressure. Rinse the stirring rod and funnel with five 10-mL portions of *n*-pentane, and discard the filtrate. Transfer the funnel to a separate filter flask, add three 10-mL portions of *Diluent,* and collect the filtrate under reduced pressure. Evaporate the filtrate to dryness, add 2.0 mL of *Diluent,* and mix. Filter the resulting solution through a 0.45-μm filter, discarding the initial portion of the filtrate.
  Procedure—Equilibrate for 3 hours a thin-layer chromatographic plate (see *Chromatography* ⟨621⟩) coated with a 0.25-mm layer of chromatographic silica gel mixture in a solvent system consisting of methylene chloride, isopropyl alcohol, methanol, and ammonium hydroxide (85 : 15 : 2 : 1). Remove the plate from the chamber, and allow the solvent to evaporate. Separately apply 10 μL of the *Test solution* and 10 μL of each *Standard solution* to the plate, and develop the chromatogram in a separate lined chamber in the solvent system previously described until the solvent front has moved about three-fourths of the length of the plate. Remove the plate from the developing chamber, mark the solvent front, and allow to evaporate in a stream of nitrogen for about 10 minutes. Examine the plate under short- and long-wavelength UV light, and compare the intensities of any secondary spots observed in the chromatogram of the *Test solution* with those of the principal spots in the chromatograms of the *Standard solutions.* Spray the plate with Dragendorff's reagent followed by a 9% solution of hydrogen peroxide in water, and cover with a glass plate for 5 minutes. Remove the glass plate, and observe under white light. Record the R_F values and estimate the concentration of the secondary spots observed in the *Test solution.* No secondary spot from the chromatogram of the *Test solution* observed, using the visualization methods above, is larger or more intense than the principal spot obtained from *Standard solution E* (0.5%), and the sum of the intensities of the secondary spots obtained from the *Test solution* corresponds to not more than 5%.
Assay—
  Mobile phase—Prepare a filtered and degassed mixture of methanol and 10% ammonium carbonate (9 : 1). Make adjustments if necessary (see *System Suitability* under *Chromatography* ⟨621⟩).
  Diluent—Prepare a mixture of methanol, chloroform, and ammonium hydroxide (55 : 45 : 1).

Standard preparation—Dissolve an accurately weighed quantity of USP Thiethylperazine Maleate RS in *Diluent*, and dilute quantitatively, and stepwise if necessary, with *Diluent* to obtain a solution having a known concentration of about 0.1 mg per mL.

Assay preparation—Weigh not fewer than 20 Suppositories and freeze them at 0° for about 30 minutes. Grind the Suppositories into small particles, and transfer an accurately weighed portion of the mass, equivalent to about 10 mg of thiethylperazine maleate, to a 100-mL volumetric flask. Add about 30 mL of *Diluent*, and gently shake for about 10 minutes or until the mass dissolves. Dilute with *Diluent* to volume, mix, and filter through about 2 g of anhydrous sodium sulfate, discarding the first portion of the filtrate.

Chromatographic system (see *Chromatography* ⟨621⟩)—The liquid chromatograph is equipped with a 265-nm detector and a 4.6-mm × 25-cm column that contains 5-μm, base-deactivated packing L1. The flow rate is about 2 mL per minute, and the column temperature is maintained at 45°. Chromatograph the *Standard preparation*, and record the peak responses as directed for *Procedure*: the resolution, R, between the thiethylperazine peak and adjacent peaks is not less than 1.0; the column efficiency is not less than 1000 theoretical plates; the tailing factor for thiethylperazine is not more than 2.5; and the relative standard deviation for replicate injections is not more than 2.0%.

Procedure—Separately inject equal volumes (about 10 μL) of the *Standard preparation* and the *Assay preparation* into the chromatograph, record the chromatograms, and measure the responses for the major peaks. Calculate the quantity, in mg, of $C_{22}H_{29}N_3S_2 \cdot 2C_4H_4O_4$ in the portion of Suppositories taken by the formula:

$$100C(r_U / r_S)$$

in which C is the concentration, in mg per mL, of USP Thiethylperazine Maleate RS in the *Standard preparation*; and r_U and r_S are the peak responses obtained from the *Assay preparation* and the *Standard preparation*, respectively.

Thiethylperazine Maleate Tablets

» Thiethylperazine Maleate Tablets contain not less than 90.0 percent and not more than 110.0 percent of the labeled amount of $C_{22}H_{29}N_3S_2 \cdot 2C_4H_4O_4$.

Packaging and storage—Preserve in tight, light-resistant containers.

USP Reference standards ⟨11⟩—*USP Thiethylperazine Maleate RS*.

NOTE—Throughout the following procedures, protect test or assay specimens, the Reference Standard, and solutions containing them, by conducting the procedures without delay, under subdued light, or using low-actinic glassware.

Identification—The retention time of the thiethylperazine peak in the chromatogram of the *Assay preparation* corresponds to that of the *Standard preparation* as obtained in the *Assay*.

Dissolution ⟨711⟩—
 Medium: 0.01 N hydrochloric acid; 1000 mL.
 Apparatus 1: 120 rpm.
 Time: 30 minutes.
 Procedure—Determine the amount of $C_{22}H_{29}N_3S_2 \cdot 2C_4H_4O_4$ dissolved by employing UV absorption at the wavelength of maximum absorbance at about 263 nm on filtered portions of the solution under test, suitably diluted with *Dissolution Medium*, if necessary, in comparison with a Standard solution having a known concentration of USP Thiethylperazine Maleate RS in the same *Medium*.
 Tolerances—Not less than 75% (Q) of the labeled amount of $C_{22}H_{29}N_3S_2 \cdot 2C_4H_4O_4$ is dissolved in 30 minutes.

Uniformity of dosage units ⟨905⟩: meet the requirements.

Assay—
 Mobile phase—Proceed as directed under the *Assay* for *Thiethylperazine Maleate Suppositories*.
 Diluent—Prepare a mixture of acetonitrile and water (9 : 1).
 Standard preparation—Dissolve an accurately weighed quantity of USP Thiethylperazine Maleate RS in *Diluent* by sonicating for about 5 minutes, and dilute quantitatively, and stepwise if necessary, with *Diluent* to obtain a solution having a known concentration of about 0.2 mg per mL.

Assay preparation—Weigh and finely powder not less than 20 Tablets. Transfer an accurately weighed portion of the powder, equivalent to about 50 mg of thiethylperazine maleate, to a 250-mL volumetric flask. Add 150 mL of *Diluent*, and shake to disperse the powder. Sonicate the mixture for 10 minutes, then shake by mechanical means for 1 hour. Dilute with *Diluent* to volume, and mix. Filter through a 0.45-μm filter, discarding the first portion of the filtrate.

Chromatographic system (see *Chromatography* ⟨621⟩)—The liquid chromatograph is equipped with a 265-nm detector and a 4.6-mm × 25-cm column that contains 5-μm, base-deactivated packing L1. The flow rate is about 2 mL per minute, and the column temperature is maintained at 45°. Chromatograph the *Standard preparation*, and record the peak responses as directed for *Procedure*: the resolution, R, between the thiethylperazine peak and adjacent peaks is not less than 1.5, the column efficiency is not less than 1000 theoretical plates, the tailing factor for thiethylperazine is not more than 2.5, and the relative standard deviation for replicate injections is not more than 2.0%.

Procedure—Separately inject equal volumes (about 10 μL) of the *Standard preparation* and the *Assay preparation* into the chromatograph, record the chromatograms, and measure the responses for the major peaks. Calculate the quantity, in mg, of $C_{22}H_{29}N_3S_2 \cdot 2C_4H_4O_4$ in the portion of Tablets taken by the formula:

$$250C(r_U / r_S)$$

in which C is the concentration, in mg per mL, of USP Thiethylperazine Maleate RS in the *Standard preparation*, and r_U and r_S are the peak responses obtained from the *Assay preparation* and the *Standard preparation*, respectively.

Thimerosal

$C_9H_9HgNaO_2S$ 404.81
Mercury, ethyl(2-mercaptobenzoato-S)-, sodium salt.
Ethyl (sodium o-mercaptobenzoato)mercury   [54-64-8].

» Thimerosal contains not less than 97.0 percent and not more than 101.0 percent of $C_9H_9HgNaO_2S$, calculated on the dried basis.

Packaging and storage—Preserve in tight, light-resistant containers.

USP Reference standards ⟨11⟩—*USP Thimerosal RS*.

Identification—
 A: *Infrared Absorption* ⟨197K⟩.
 B: To a solution (1 in 100) add a few drops of silver nitrate TS: a pale yellow precipitate is formed.

Loss on drying ⟨731⟩—Dry it in vacuum over phosphorus pentoxide to constant weight: it loses not more than 0.5% of its weight.

Ether-soluble substances—Shake 500 mg, accurately weighed, with 20 mL of anhydrous ethyl ether for 10 minutes. Filter, evaporate the ether in a tared container, dry the residue in vacuum over phosphorus pentoxide, and weigh: the weight of residue does not exceed 4 mg (0.8%).

Mercury ions—
 Iodide reagent—[NOTE—Prepare fresh daily; keep the stopper in the flask and protect from light.] Dissolve 33.20 g of potassium iodide in 75 mL of water in a 100-mL volumetric flask, dilute with water to volume, and mix.
 Standard preparation—Transfer about 190 mg of mercuric chloride, accurately weighed, to a 200-mL volumetric flask, and dissolve in 100 mL of water. Dilute with water to volume, and mix.

Transfer 5.0 mL of this solution to a 50-mL volumetric flask, dilute with water to volume, and mix. The concentration of mercuric chloride in the *Standard preparation* is about 95 µg per mL.

Test solution—Transfer about 500 mg of Thimerosal, accurately weighed, to a 100-mL volumetric flask, add water to volume, and mix to dissolve.

Test preparation A—Transfer 10.0 mL of the *Test solution* to a 50-mL volumetric flask, dilute with water to volume, and mix.

Test preparation B—Transfer 10.0 mL of the *Test solution* to a 50-mL volumetric flask, add 5.0 mL of the *Standard preparation*, dilute with water to volume, and mix.

Procedure—[NOTE—Protect all solutions from light prior to determining their absorbances.] Label five 10-mL volumetric flasks *C*, *D*, *E*, *F*, and *R*. Transfer 5.0 mL of *Test preparation A* to flasks *C* and *D*, transfer 5.0 mL of *Test preparation B* to flasks *E* and *F*, and transfer 5.0 mL of water to flask *R*. Dilute flasks *C* and *E* with water to volume, and mix. Dilute flasks *D*, *F*, and *R* with the *Iodide reagent* to volume, and mix. Concomitantly determine the absorbances of the solutions in 1-cm cells at the wavelength of maximum absorbance for the tetraiodomercurate ion at about 323 nm (located from the similarly determined UV spectrum of a solution prepared by mixing 1.0 mL of the *Standard preparation* with 5.0 mL of *Iodide reagent* and diluting with water to 10.0 mL), with a suitable spectrophotometer, using water as the blank. Record the absorbances of the solutions in flasks *C*, *D*, *E*, *F*, and *R* as A_C, A_D, A_E, A_F, and A_R respectively. Calculate the percentage of mercury ions by the formula:

$$(200.59 / 271.50)(5C / W)(A_U / A_S)$$

in which 200.59 is the atomic weight of mercury, 271.50 is the molecular weight of mercuric chloride, A_U is the absorbance of the test specimen obtained by the equation:

$$A_U = (A_D - A_R - A_C)$$

A_S is the absorbance of the Standard obtained by the equation:

$$A_S = (A_F - A_R - A_E - A_U)$$

C is the concentration, in µg per mL, of mercuric chloride in the *Standard preparation;* and *W* is the weight, in mg, of Thimerosal taken: the limit is 0.70%.

Readily carbonizable substances ⟨271⟩—Dissolve about 200 mg in 5 mL of sulfuric acid TS: the solution has no more color than *Matching Fluid J*.

Assay—[NOTE—The *Standard preparation* and the *Assay preparation* may be diluted quantitatively with water, if necessary, to obtain solutions of suitable concentrations adaptable to the linear or working range of the instrument.]

Standard preparation—Dissolve an accurately weighed quantity of USP Thimerosal RS in water, and dilute quantitatively with water to obtain a solution having a known concentration of about 1 mg per mL.

Assay preparation—Transfer about 100 mg of Thimerosal, accurately weighed, to a 100-mL volumetric flask, add 25 mL of water, and mix to dissolve. Dilute with water to volume, and mix.

Procedure—Concomitantly determine the absorbances of the *Standard preparation* and the *Assay preparation*, at the mercury resonance line of 254 nm, with a suitable atomic absorption spectrophotometer (see *Spectrophotometry and Light-Scattering* ⟨851⟩), equipped with a mercury hollow-cathode lamp and an air–acetylene flame, using water as the blank. Calculate the quantity, in mg, of $C_9H_9HgNaO_2S$ in the portion of Thimerosal taken by the formula:

$$100C(A_U / A_S)$$

in which *C* is the concentration, in mg per mL, of USP Thimerosal RS in the *Standard preparation;* and A_U and A_S are the absorbances of the *Assay preparation* and the *Standard preparation*, respectively.

Thimerosal Topical Aerosol

» Thimerosal Topical Aerosol is an alcoholic solution of Thimerosal mixed with suitable propellants in a pressurized container. It contains not less than 85.0 percent and not more than 115.0 percent of the labeled amount of $C_9H_9HgNaO_2S$.

NOTE—Thimerosal Topical Aerosol is sensitive to some metals.

Packaging and storage—Preserve in tight, light-resistant, pressurized containers, and avoid exposure to excessive heat.

USP Reference standards ⟨11⟩—*USP Thimerosal RS*.

Identification—To about 10 mL of solution sprayed into a suitable container from Topical Aerosol add 10 mL of water, and heat on a steam bath until the odor of alcohol is no longer perceptible. Cool, and pass hydrogen sulfide through the solution: no black discoloration or black precipitate is formed. To 15 mL of solution sprayed into a suitable container from Topical Aerosol add 15 mL of water, heat on a steam bath until the odor of alcohol is no longer perceptible, and add 2 drops of bromine. Mix with 1.5 mL of 3 N hydrochloric acid, filter, evaporate the excess bromine with a current of air, and pass hydrogen sulfide through the filtrate: a black precipitate is formed.

Alcohol content—Weigh, chill, and open 1 Topical Aerosol container, and remove the propellant as directed for *Assay preparation* in the *Assay*, continuing until the bulk of the propellant has evaporated. Determine the alcohol content of the specimen thus prepared by the *Gas-Liquid Chromatographic Method* (see *Method II* under *Alcohol Determination* ⟨611⟩), using methyl ethyl ketone as the internal standard in place of acetone: between 18.7% and 25.3% (w/w) of C_2H_5OH is found.

Other requirements—It meets the requirements for *Pressure Test*, *Minimum Fill*, and *Leakage Test* under *Aerosols, Nasal Sprays, Metered-Dose Inhalers, and Dry Powder Inhalers* ⟨601⟩.

Assay—[NOTE—The *Standard preparations* and *Assay preparation* may be diluted quantitatively with water, if necessary, to yield solutions, of suitable concentration, adaptable to the linear or working range of the instrument.]

Stannous chloride solution—Dissolve 50 g of stannous chloride in 100 mL of hydrochloric acid on a steam bath, cool, dilute with water to 500 mL, and mix. Use within 3 months.

Standard solutions—Prepare aqueous solutions of USP Thimerosal RS of known concentrations of about 1.8, 2.0, and 2.2 µg per mL.

Standard preparations—Pipet 20 mL of each *Standard solution* into separate 100-mL volumetric flasks, and treat each flask as follows. Add 5 mL of sulfuric acid, cool, add 3 mL of nitric acid, and mix. Add potassium permanganate crystals, while mixing, until the purple color persists for not less than 15 minutes. Add about 200 mg of potassium persulfate, mix, and heat on a steam bath for 2 hours. Cool, dilute with water to volume, and mix.

Assay solution—Weigh accurately a filled Topical Aerosol container, and record the weight. Place the container in a dry ice-alcohol bath, and cool for 60 minutes. Remove the container from the bath, and carefully remove the spray cap with wire cutters, taking precautions to save all pieces of the spray head and cap. With the aid of three 5-mL portions of water, transfer the contents of the container to a beaker previously chilled in the bath. Dry the rinsed empty container and all of its parts in an oven at 105° for 2 hours, cool, and weigh. Calculate the weight of the container contents. Add a few boiling chips to the beaker, and carefully stir to help evaporate the propellant. After the bulk of the propellant has evaporated, place the beaker on a steam bath, evaporate the volatile solvents, and cool. Transfer the residual liquid with the aid of 35.0 mL of alcohol to a 50-mL volumetric flask, dilute with water to volume, and mix. Dilute quantitatively with water a volume, *v* mL, of this solution to *V* mL of *Assay solution* containing about 2 µg of thimerosal per mL.

Assay preparation—Pipet 20 mL of *Assay solution* into a 100-mL volumetric flask, and proceed as directed for *Standard preparations*, beginning with "Add 5 mL of sulfuric acid."

Blank preparation—Pipet 20 mL of water into a 100-mL volumetric flask, and proceed as directed for *Standard preparation*, beginning with "Add 5 mL of sulfuric acid."

Procedure—Proceed with each of the *Standard preparations*, the *Assay preparation*, and the *Blank preparation* as follows: Pipet 3 mL into the scrubbing chamber of a suitable system designed for determination of mercury by flameless atomic absorption, using a mercury hollow-cathode lamp, dilute with water to about 150 mL, and add hydroxylamine hydrochloride solution (1 in 10) just to reduce the excess permanganate. Add 5 mL of *Stannous chloride solution*, and immediately attach the scrubbing chamber to the system. Concomitantly determine the absorbance of the vapor from each solution at an integration time of 15 seconds. Use the absorbance of the *Blank preparation* to correct the absorbances of the *Standard preparations* and the *Assay preparation*. Plot the corrected absorbances of the standards versus the respective concentrations of the *Standard solutions*, in µg per mL, and from the curve so obtained determine the concentration, C, in µg per mL, of the *Assay solution*. Calculate the quantity, in mg, of $C_9H_9HgNaO_2S$ in the weight of the container contents taken by the formula:

$$50C(V/v)$$

in which the terms are as defined therein.

Thimerosal Topical Solution

» Thimerosal Topical Solution contains, in each 100 mL, not less than 95 mg and not more than 105 mg of $C_9H_9HgNaO_2S$.

NOTE—Thimerosal Topical Solution is sensitive to some metals.

Packaging and storage—Preserve in tight, light-resistant containers, and avoid exposure to excessive heat.

USP Reference standards ⟨11⟩—*USP Thimerosal RS*.
Identification—
A: Pass hydrogen sulfide through 50 mL of it: no black discoloration or black precipitate is formed. To 50 mL of Topical Solution add 3 or 4 drops of bromine, mix, and warm on a steam bath to expel the excess bromine. Add 5 mL of 3 N hydrochloric acid, filter, and pass hydrogen sulfide through the filtrate: a black precipitate is formed.
B: To 1 mL of Topical Solution add 9 mL of water, mix, and add 1 mL of cupric sulfate TS: a green color is produced immediately and is followed by the gradual precipitation of flocculent, greenish brown particles.
pH ⟨791⟩: between 9.6 and 10.2.
Assay—[NOTE—The *Standard preparations* and *Assay preparation* may be diluted quantitatively with water, if necessary, to yield solutions, of suitable concentration, adaptable to the linear or working range of the instrument.]
Stannous chloride solution—Dissolve 50 g of stannous chloride in 100 mL of hydrochloric acid on a steam bath, cool, dilute with water to 500 mL, and mix. Use within 3 months.
Standard solutions—Prepare aqueous solutions of USP Thimerosal RS of known concentrations of about 1.8, 2.0, and 2.2 µg per mL.
Standard preparations—Pipet 20 mL of each *Standard solution* into separate 100-mL volumetric flasks, and treat each flask as follows. Add 5 mL of sulfuric acid, cool, add 3 mL of nitric acid, and mix. Add potassium permanganate crystals, while mixing, until the purple color persists for not less than 15 minutes. Add about 200 mg of potassium persulfate, mix, and heat on a steam bath for 2 hours. Cool, dilute with water to volume, and mix.
Assay solution—Pipet 2 mL of Topical Solution into a 1000-mL volumetric flask, dilute with water to volume, and mix.
Assay preparation—Pipet 20 mL of *Assay solution* into a 100-mL volumetric flask, and proceed as directed for *Standard preparations*, beginning with "Add 5 mL of sulfuric acid."

Blank preparation—Pipet 20 mL of water into a 100-mL volumetric flask, and proceed as directed for *Standard preparation*, beginning with "Add 5 mL of sulfuric acid."

Procedure—Proceed with each of the *Standard preparations*, the *Assay preparation*, and the *Blank preparation* as follows: Pipet 3 mL into the scrubbing chamber of a suitable system designed for determination of mercury by flameless atomic absorption, using a mercury hollow-cathode lamp, dilute with water to about 150 mL, and add hydroxylamine hydrochloride solution (1 in 10) just to reduce the excess permanganate. Add 5 mL of *Stannous chloride solution*, and immediately attach the scrubbing chamber to the system. Concomitantly determine the absorbance of each solution at an integration time of 15 seconds. Use the absorbance of the *Blank preparation* to correct the absorbances of the *Standard preparations* and the *Assay preparation*. Plot the corrected absorbances of the standards versus the respective concentrations of the *Standard solutions*, in µg per mL, and from the curve so obtained determine the concentration, C, in µg per mL, of the *Assay solution*. Calculate the quantity, in mg, of $C_9H_9HgNaO_2S$ in each 100 mL of Topical Solution taken by the formula:

$$50C$$

in which the terms are defined above.

Thimerosal Tincture

» Thimerosal Tincture contains, in each 100 mL, not less than 90 mg and not more than 110 mg of $C_9H_9HgNaO_2S$.

NOTE—Thimerosal Tincture is sensitive to some metals.

Packaging and storage—Preserve in tight, light-resistant containers, and avoid exposure to excessive heat.

USP Reference standards ⟨11⟩—*USP Thimerosal RS*.
Identification—Heat 25 mL on a steam bath until the odors of alcohol and acetone are no longer perceptible. Cool and pass hydrogen sulfide through the solution: no black discoloration or black precipitate is formed. Evaporate 50 mL of Tincture on a steam bath to a volume of approximately 20 mL, cool, and add 3 or 4 drops of bromine. Add 5 mL of 3 N hydrochloric acid, filter, and pass hydrogen sulfide through the filtrate: a black precipitate is formed.
Alcohol content, *Method II* ⟨611⟩: between 45.0% and 55.0% of C_2H_5OH.
Assay—[NOTE—The *Standard preparations* and *Assay preparation* may be diluted quantitatively with water, if necessary, to yield solutions, of suitable concentration, adaptable to the linear or working range of the instrument.]
Stannous chloride solution—Dissolve 50 g of stannous chloride in 100 mL of hydrochloric acid on a steam bath, cool, dilute with water to 500 mL, and mix. Use within 3 months.
Standard solutions—Prepare aqueous solutions of USP Thimerosal RS of known concentrations of about 1.8, 2.0, and 2.2 µg per mL.
Standard preparations—Pipet 20 mL of each *Standard solution* into separate 100-mL volumetric flasks, and treat each flask as follows. Add 5 mL of sulfuric acid, cool, add 3 mL of nitric acid, and mix. Add potassium permanganate crystals, while mixing, until the purple color persists for not less than 15 minutes. Add about 200 mg of potassium persulfate, mix, and heat on a steam bath for 2 hours. Cool, dilute with water to volume, and mix.
Assay solution—Pipet 2 mL of Tincture into a 1000-mL volumetric flask, dilute with water to volume, and mix.
Assay preparation—Pipet 20 mL of *Assay solution* into a 100-mL volumetric flask, and proceed as directed for *Standard preparations*, beginning with "Add 5 mL of sulfuric acid."
Blank preparation—Pipet 20 mL of water into a 100-mL volumetric flask, and proceed as directed for *Standard preparation*, beginning with "Add 5 mL of sulfuric acid."

Procedure—Proceed with each of the *Standard preparations*, the *Assay preparation*, and the *Blank preparation* as follows: Pipet 3 mL into the scrubbing chamber of a suitable system designed for determination of mercury by flameless atomic absorption, using a mercury hollow-cathode lamp, dilute with water to about 150 mL, and add hydroxylamine hydrochloride solution (1 in 10) just to reduce the excess permanganate. Add 5 mL of *Stannous chloride solution*, and immediately attach the scrubbing chamber to the system. Concomitantly determine the absorbance of the vapor from each solution at an integration time of 15 seconds. Use the absorbance of the *Blank preparation* to correct the absorbances of the *Standard preparations* and the *Assay preparation*. Plot the corrected absorbances of the standards versus the respective concentrations of the *Standard solutions*, in μg per mL, and from the curve so obtained determine the concentration, C, in μg per mL, of the *Assay solution*. Calculate the quantity, in mg, of $C_9H_9HgNaO_2S$ in each 100 mL of Tincture taken by the formula:

$$50C$$

in which the terms are as defined therein.

Thioguanine

$C_5H_5N_5S \cdot xH_2O$ (anhydrous)   167.19
6*H*-Purine-6-thione, 2-amino-1,7-dihydro-.
2-Aminopurine-6(1*H*)-thione   [154-42-7].
Hemihydrate   176.20   [5580-03-0].

» Thioguanine is anhydrous or contains one-half molecule of water of hydration. It contains not less than 96.0 percent and not more than 100.5 percent of $C_5H_5N_5S$, calculated on the dried basis.

Packaging and storage—Preserve in tight containers.
Labeling—Label it to indicate its state of hydration.
USP Reference standards ⟨11⟩—*USP Thioguanine RS*.
Identification—
  A: *Infrared Absorption* ⟨197K⟩.
  B: The UV absorption spectrum of a 1 in 200,000 solution of it, prepared as directed in the *Assay*, exhibits maxima and minima at the same wavelengths as that of a similar solution of USP Thioguanine RS, concomitantly measured.
Loss on drying ⟨731⟩—Dry it in vacuum at 105° for 5 hours: it loses not more than 6.0% of its weight.
Selenium ⟨291⟩:   0.003%, 200 mg being used for the test.
Phosphorous-containing substances—
  Ammonium molybdate solution—Dissolve 8.3 g of ammonium molybdate in 40 mL of water, add 33 mL of dilute sulfuric acid (2 in 7), dilute with water to 100.0 mL, and mix. This solution is stable for about 2 weeks.
  Procedure—Transfer 50.0 mg, accurately weighed, to a large test tube, add 1 mL of dilute sulfuric acid (2 in 7), and heat in a boiling water bath for 5 minutes. Cautiously add nitric acid, dropwise, continue heating until the mixture becomes colorless, and then heat for 1 minute longer. Cool, dilute with water to about 10 mL, and transfer the solution to a 25-mL volumetric flask with the aid of a few mL of water. To the flask add 0.75 mL of *Ammonium molybdate solution* and 1.0 mL of aminonaphtholsulfonic acid TS, dilute with water to volume, and mix. Determine the absorbance of this solution in a 1-cm cell, with a suitable spectrophotometer, at a wavelength of about 620 nm, using a reagent blank to set the instrument: the absorbance is not greater than that produced by 1.5 mL of a similar solution of monobasic potassium phosphate in water having a known concentration of 10 μg of phosphate (PO_4) in each mL, concomitantly measured (0.03% as phosphate).

Free sulfur—Dissolve 50 mg in 5 mL of 1 N sodium hydroxide: the solution is clear.
Organic volatile impurities, Method V ⟨467⟩:   meets the requirements.
  Solvent—Use dimethyl sulfoxide.
                              (Official until July 1, 2008)
Nitrogen content—Determine the nitrogen content as directed under *Nitrogen Determination, Method II* ⟨461⟩, using about 100 mg, accurately weighed. Each mL of 0.1 N sulfuric acid is equivalent to 1.401 mg of N. Not less than 40.2% and not more than 43.1%, calculated on the dried basis, is found.
Limit of guanine—
  Mobile phase—Proceed as directed in the *Assay*.
  Standard solution—Dissolve an accurately weighed quantity of guanine in 0.01 N sodium hydroxide, and dilute quantitatively, and stepwise if necessary, to obtain a solution having a known concentration of about 0.04 mg per mL. Pipet 1.0 mL of this solution into a 100-mL volumetric flask, and dilute with *Mobile phase* to volume to obtain a solution having a known concentration of 0.4 μg per mL.
  Test solution—Transfer about 40 mg of Thioguanine, accurately weighed, to a 100-mL volumetric flask, dissolve in and dilute with 0.01 N sodium hydroxide to volume, and mix. Transfer 10.0 mL of this solution into a 100-mL volumetric flask, dilute with *Mobile phase* to volume, and mix.
  Chromatographic system (see *Chromatography* ⟨621⟩)—The liquid chromatograph is equipped with a 248-nm detector and a 4.6-mm × 5-cm column that contains packing L1. The flow rate is about 2.0 mL per minute. Chromatograph the *Standard solution*, and record the peak responses as directed for *Procedure*: the relative retention times are about 0.60 for guanine and 1.0 for thioguanine; the resolution, R, between guanine and thioguanine is not less than 3.0; the tailing factor is not more than 2.0; and the relative standard deviation for replicate injections is not more than 5.0% for the guanine peak.
  Procedure—Separately inject equal volumes (about 10 μL) of the *Standard solution* and the *Test solution* into the chromatograph, record the chromatograms, and measure the responses for the major peaks. Calculate the percentage of guanine in the portion of Thioguanine taken by the formula:

$$100(C/W)(r_U/r_S)$$

in which C is the concentration, in μg per mL, of guanine in the *Standard solution*; W is the weight, in mg, of Thioguanine taken to prepare the *Test solution*; and r_U and r_S are the peak responses of guanine obtained from the *Test solution* and the *Standard solution*, respectively: not more than 2.5% is found.
Assay—
  Phosphoric acid solution—Carefully add 1 mL of phosphoric acid to 99 mL of water, and mix.
  Mobile phase—Prepare a filtered and degassed solution of 0.05 M monobasic sodium phosphate. Adjust with phosphoric acid to a pH of 3.0. Make adjustments if necessary (see *System Suitability* under *Chromatography* ⟨621⟩).
  Standard preparation—Dissolve an accurately weighed quantity of USP Thioguanine RS in 0.01 N sodium hydroxide, and dilute quantitatively, and stepwise if necessary, to obtain a solution having a known concentration of about 0.4 mg per mL. Pipet 10.0 mL of this solution into a 100-mL volumetric flask, and dilute with *Phosphoric acid solution* to volume to obtain a solution having a known concentration of 0.04 mg per mL.
  Assay preparation—Transfer about 40 mg of Thioguanine, accurately weighed, to a 100-mL volumetric flask, dissolve in and dilute with 0.01 N sodium hydroxide to volume, and mix. Transfer 10.0 mL of this solution to a 100-mL volumetric flask, dilute with *Phosphoric acid solution* to volume, and mix.
  Chromatographic system (see *Chromatography* ⟨621⟩)—The liquid chromatograph is equipped with a 248-nm detector and a 4.6-mm × 5-cm column that contains packing L1. The flow rate is about 2.0 mL per minute. Chromatograph the *Standard preparation*, and record the peak responses as directed for *Procedure*: the relative retention times are about 0.60 for guanine and 1.0 for thioguanine, and the relative standard deviation for replicate injections is not more than 2.0%.

Procedure—Separately inject equal volumes (about 10 µL) of the *Standard preparation* and the *Assay preparation* into the chromatograph, record the chromatograms, and measure the responses for the major peaks. Calculate the quantity, in mg, of $C_5H_5N_5S$ in the portion of Thioguanine taken by the formula:

$$1000C(r_U/r_S)$$

in which C is the concentration, in mg per mL, of USP Thioguanine RS in the *Standard preparation*; and r_U and r_S are the peak responses obtained from the *Assay preparation* and the *Standard preparation*, respectively.

Thioguanine Tablets

» Thioguanine Tablets contain not less than 93.0 percent and not more than 107.0 percent of the labeled amount of $C_5H_5N_5S$.

Packaging and storage—Preserve in tight containers.

USP Reference standards ⟨11⟩—*USP Thioguanine RS*.

Identification—The UV absorption spectrum of the *Acidic assay preparation* employed for measurement of absorbance in the *Assay* exhibits maxima and minima at the same wavelengths as that of a similar solution of USP Thioguanine RS, concomitantly measured.

Dissolution ⟨711⟩—
Medium: water; 900 mL.
Apparatus 2: 50 rpm.
Time: 45 minutes.
Standard preparation—Dissolve an accurately weighed quantity of USP Thioguanine RS in 1 N sodium hydroxide to obtain a solution having a known concentration of about 4.5 µg per mL.
Procedure—Determine the amount of $C_5H_5N_5S$ dissolved from UV absorbances at the wavelength of maximum absorbance at about 348 nm of filtered portions of the solution under test, suitably diluted with 0.1 N hydrochloric acid, in comparison with the *Standard preparation*.
Tolerances—Not less than 75% (*Q*) of the labeled amount of $C_5H_5N_5S$ is dissolved in 45 minutes.

Uniformity of dosage units ⟨905⟩: meet the requirements.

Assay—
Standard preparations—Dissolve an accurately weighed quantity of USP Thioguanine RS in sodium hydroxide solution (1 in 250), and dilute quantitatively and stepwise with the sodium hydroxide solution to obtain a *Standard preparation* having a known concentration of 80 µg per mL. Transfer 5.0 mL of this solution to a 100-mL volumetric flask, add dilute hydrochloric acid (1 in 10) to volume, and mix, to obtain the *Acidic standard preparation*. Transfer another 5.0-mL portion of the solution to a second 100-mL volumetric flask, add 10.0 mL of 1 N sodium hydroxide, dilute with water to volume, and mix, to obtain the *Basic standard preparation*.
Assay preparations—Weigh and finely powder not less than 20 Tablets. Transfer an accurately weighed portion of the powder, equivalent to about 40 mg of thioguanine, to a 500-mL volumetric flask, add 50 mL of 1 N sodium hydroxide, and allow to stand for 10 minutes, with frequent swirling. Dilute with water to volume, mix, and filter a portion of the solution through a pledget of glass wool. Transfer 5.0 mL of the filtrate to a 100-mL volumetric flask, add dilute hydrochloric acid (1 in 10) to volume, and mix, to obtain the *Acidic assay preparation*. Transfer another 5.0-mL portion of the filtrate to a second 100-mL volumetric flask, add 10.0 mL of 1 N sodium hydroxide, dilute with water to volume, and mix, to obtain the *Basic assay preparation*.
Procedure—Concomitantly determine the absorbances of the *Acidic assay preparation* and the *Acidic standard preparation* in 1-cm cells at the wavelength of maximum absorbance at about 348 nm, with a suitable spectrophotometer, using the *Basic assay preparation* and the *Basic standard preparation*, respectively, as the blanks. Calculate the quantity, in mg, of $C_5H_5N_5S$ in the portion of Tablets taken by the formula:

$$10C(A_U/A_S)$$

in which C is the concentration, in µg per mL, of USP Thioguanine RS in the *Acidic standard preparation*, and A_U and A_S are the absorbances of the *Acidic assay preparation* and the *Acidic standard preparation*, respectively.

Thiopental Sodium

$C_{11}H_{17}N_2NaO_2S$ 264.32
4,6(1*H*,5*H*)-Pyrimidinedione, 5-ethyldihydro-5-(1-methylbutyl)-2-thioxo-, monosodium salt, (±)-.
Sodium (±)-5-ethyl-5-(1-methylbutyl)-2-thiobarbiturate   [71-73-8].

» Thiopental Sodium contains not less than 97.0 percent and not more than 102.0 percent of $C_{11}H_{17}N_2NaO_2S$, calculated on the dried basis.

Packaging and storage—Preserve in tight containers.

USP Reference standards ⟨11⟩—*USP Thiopental RS*.

Identification—
A: Dissolve about 500 mg in 10 mL of water in a separator, add 10 mL of 3 N hydrochloric acid, and extract the liberated thiopental with two 25-mL portions of chloroform. Evaporate the combined chloroform extracts to dryness. Add 10 mL of ether, evaporate again, and dry at 105° for 2 hours: the IR absorption spectrum of a potassium bromide dispersion of the residue so obtained exhibits maxima only at the same wavelengths as that of a similar preparation of USP Thiopental RS.
B: Ignite about 500 mg: the residue responds to the tests for *Sodium* ⟨191⟩.
C: Dissolve about 200 mg in 5 mL of 1 N sodium hydroxide, and add 2 mL of lead acetate TS: a white precipitate is formed, and it gradually darkens when the mixture is boiled. Acidify the darkened mixture with hydrochloric acid: hydrogen sulfide is evolved, and it is recognizable by its darkening of moistened lead acetate test paper held in the vapor.

Loss on drying ⟨731⟩—Dry it at 80° for 4 hours: it loses not more than 2.0% of its weight.

Heavy metals, *Method II* ⟨231⟩: 0.002%.

Ordinary impurities ⟨466⟩—
Test solution: 10 mg of Thiopental Sodium per mL of methanol.
Standard solution: 9.2 mg of USP Thiopental RS per mL of methanol.
Application volume: 40 µL.
Eluant: a mixture of toluene and methanol (85 : 15).
Visualization: 1.

Assay—Transfer about 100 mg of Thiopental Sodium, accurately weighed, to a 200-mL volumetric flask, add sodium hydroxide solution (1 in 250) to volume, and mix. Pipet 5 mL of the solution into a 500-mL volumetric flask, add sodium hydroxide solution (1 in 250) to volume, and mix. Dissolve an accurately weighed quantity of USP Thiopental RS in sodium hydroxide solution (1 in 250), and dilute quantitatively and stepwise with sodium hydroxide solution (1 in 250) to obtain a Standard solution having a known concentration of about 5 µg per mL. Concomitantly determine the absorbances of both solutions in 1-cm cells at the wavelength of maximum absorbance at about 304 nm, with a suitable spectrophotometer, using sodium hydroxide solution (1 in 250) as the blank. Calculate the quantity, in mg, of $C_{11}H_{17}N_2NaO_2S$ in the Thiopental Sodium taken by the formula:

$$20C(1.091A_U/A_S)$$

in which C is the concentration, in µg per mL, of USP Thiopental RS in the Standard solution, 1.091 is the ratio of the molecular weight of thiopental sodium to that of thiopental, and A_U and A_S are the absorbances of the solution of Thiopental Sodium and the Standard solution, respectively.

Thiopental Sodium for Injection

» Thiopental Sodium for Injection is a sterile mixture of Thiopental Sodium and anhydrous Sodium Carbonate as a buffer. It contains not less than 93.0 percent and not more than 107.0 percent of the labeled amount of $C_{11}H_{17}N_2NaO_2S$.

Packaging and storage—Preserve in *Containers for Sterile Solids* as described under *Injections* ⟨1⟩, preferably of Type III glass.

USP Reference standards ⟨11⟩—*USP Thiopental RS. USP Endotoxin RS.*

Completeness of solution ⟨641⟩—Mix 800 mg with 10 mL of carbon dioxide-free water: after 1 minute, the solution is clear and free from undissolved solid.

Constituted solution—At the time of use, it meets the requirements for *Constituted Solutions* under *Injections* ⟨1⟩.

Bacterial endotoxins ⟨85⟩—It contains not more than 1.0 USP Endotoxin Unit per mg of thiopental sodium.

pH ⟨791⟩: between 10.2 and 11.2, in the solution prepared in the test for *Completeness of solution*.

Other requirements—It responds to the *Identification* tests and meets the requirements of the test for *Heavy metals* under *Thiopental Sodium*. It meets also the requirements for *Sterility Tests* ⟨71⟩, *Uniformity of Dosage Units* ⟨905⟩, and for *Labeling* under *Injections* ⟨1⟩.

Assay—Dissolve the contents of 10 containers of Thiopental Sodium for Injection in sufficient water, diluting to an accurately measured volume, to obtain a solution containing about 50 mg of thiopental sodium per mL. Dilute this solution quantitatively and stepwise with sodium hydroxide solution (1 in 250) to obtain a solution having a concentration of about 5 µg of thiopental sodium per mL. Proceed as directed in the *Assay* under *Thiopental Sodium*, beginning with "Dissolve an accurately weighed quantity of USP Thiopental RS." Calculate the average quantity, in mg, of $C_{11}H_{17}N_2NaO_2S$ in each container of Thiopental Sodium for Injection taken by the formula:

$$VC(1.091A_U/A_S)$$

in which V is the volume, in mL, of the solution prepared to contain about 50 mg of thiopental sodium per mL, C is the concentration, in µg per mL, of USP Thiopental RS in the Standard solution, 1.091 is the ratio of the molecular weight of thiopental sodium to that of thiopental, and A_U and A_S are the absorbances of the solution of Thiopental Sodium for Injection and the Standard solution, respectively.

Thioridazine

$C_{21}H_{26}N_2S_2$ 370.58
10*H*-Phenothiazine, 10-[2-(1-methyl-2-piperidinyl)ethyl]-2-(methylthio)-.
10-[2-(1-Methyl-2-piperidyl)ethyl]-2-(methylthio)phenothiazine [*50-52-2*].

» Thioridazine contains not less than 99.0 percent and not more than 101.0 percent of $C_{21}H_{26}N_2S_2$, calculated on the dried basis.

Packaging and storage—Preserve in well-closed, light-resistant containers.

USP Reference standards ⟨11⟩—*USP Thioridazine RS.*
   NOTE—Throughout the following procedures, protect test, or assay specimens, the Reference Standard, and solutions containing them, by conducting the procedures without delay, under subdued light, or using low-actinic glassware.

Identification, *Infrared Absorption* ⟨197K⟩.

Loss on drying ⟨731⟩—Dry it in vacuum at 50° for 4 hours: it loses not more than 0.5% of its weight.

Residue on ignition ⟨281⟩: not more than 0.1%.

Chromatographic purity—[NOTE—Conduct this procedure without delay, under subdued light.] Transfer 100 mg of Thioridazine to a 10-mL volumetric flask, add a mixture of methanol and ammonium hydroxide (49 : 1) to volume, and mix to obtain the *Test solution*. Using an accurately weighed quantity of USP Thioridazine RS, prepare two solutions in the same solvent system containing 50 µg per mL (*Solution A*, equivalent to 0.5%) and 20 µg per mL (*Solution B*, equivalent to 0.2%). Apply 5-µL portions of the *Test solution* and each of the two Standard solutions to a thin-layer chromatographic plate (see *Chromatography* ⟨621⟩) coated with a 0.25-mm layer of chromatographic silica gel mixture. Immediately develop the chromatogram in a solvent system consisting of a mixture of chloroform, isopropyl alcohol, and ammonium hydroxide (74 : 25 : 1) until the solvent front has moved about three-fourths of the length of the plate. Remove the plate from the developing chamber, mark the solvent front, allow the solvent to evaporate, and examine the plate under short-wavelength UV light: the chromatograms show principal spots at about the same R_F value; no secondary spot, if present in the chromatogram from the *Test solution*, is more intense than the principal spot obtained from *Solution A* (0.5%); and the sum of the intensities of all secondary spots, if present in the chromatogram from the *Test solution*, is not greater than 0.5%.

Organic volatile impurities, *Method V* ⟨467⟩: meets the requirements.
   Solvent—Use dimethyl sulfoxide.
(Official until July 1, 2008)

Assay—Dissolve about 300 mg of Thioridazine, accurately weighed, in 60 mL of glacial acetic acid, and titrate with 0.1 N perchloric acid VS, determining the endpoint potentiometrically. Perform a blank determination, and make any necessary correction. Each mL of 0.1 N perchloric acid is equivalent to 37.06 mg of $C_{21}H_{26}N_2S_2$.

Thioridazine Oral Suspension

» Thioridazine Oral Suspension contains not less than 90.0 percent and not more than 110.0 percent of the labeled amount of thioridazine ($C_{21}H_{26}N_2S_2$).

Packaging and storage—Preserve in tight, light-resistant containers. Store at a temperature not exceeding 30°.
USP Reference standards ⟨11⟩—*USP Thioridazine RS*.
   NOTE—Throughout the following procedures, protect test or assay specimens, the USP Reference Standard, and solutions containing them, by conducting the procedures without delay, under subdued light, or using low-actinic glassware.
Identification—[NOTE—Conduct this test without exposure to daylight, and with a minimum of exposure to artificial light.] Transfer 40 mL of the combined chloroform extracts obtained for the *Assay* to a 50-mL beaker, and reduce the volume to 1 mL by evaporating the chloroform with the aid of a stream of nitrogen. Apply 25 µL of this test solution and 25 µL of a Standard solution of USP Thioridazine RS in chloroform containing 4 mg per mL to a thin-layer chromatographic plate (see *Chromatography* ⟨621⟩) coated with a 0.25-mm layer of chromatographic silica gel mixture. Allow the spots to dry, and develop the chromatogram in a solvent system consisting of a mixture of toluene, acetone, solvent hexane, and diethylamine (15 : 15 : 15 : 1) until the solvent front has moved about 10 cm from the origin. Remove the plate from the developing chamber, mark the solvent front, and locate the spots on the plate by viewing under short-wavelength and long-wavelength UV light: the R_F value of the principal spot obtained from the test solution corresponds to that obtained from the Standard solution.
Uniformity of dosage units ⟨905⟩—
   FOR ORAL SUSPENSION PACKAGED IN SINGLE-UNIT CONTAINERS: meets the requirements.
Deliverable volume ⟨698⟩—
   FOR ORAL SUSPENSION PACKAGED IN MULTIPLE-UNIT CONTAINERS: meets the requirements.
Specific gravity ⟨841⟩: between 1.180 and 1.310.
pH ⟨791⟩: between 8.0 and 10.0.
Assay—Transfer an accurately measured volume of Oral Suspension, freshly mixed but free from air bubbles, equivalent to about 100 mg of thioridazine, to a 125-mL separator, using a pipet calibrated to contain the required volume. Rinse the pipet with 10 to 15 mL of water, adding the rinsing to the separator. Render the mixture alkaline by adding several drops of ammonium hydroxide, and mix. Extract with six 30-mL portions of chloroform, and filter the extracts through anhydrous sodium sulfate, collecting the combined filtrates in a 200-mL volumetric flask. Dilute quantitatively and stepwise with chloroform to obtain a solution having a concentration of about 100 µg of thioridazine per mL. [NOTE—Reserve a 40-mL portion of this solution for the *Identification* test.] Transfer 5.0 mL of this solution to a 100-mL volumetric flask, dilute with chloroform to volume, and mix. Concomitantly determine the absorbances of this Assay solution and a Standard solution of USP Thioridazine RS in chloroform having a known concentration of about 5 µg per mL, in 1-cm cells at the wavelength of maximum absorbance at about 266 nm, with a suitable spectrophotometer, using chloroform as the blank. Calculate the quantity, in mg, of thioridazine ($C_{21}H_{26}N_2S_2$) in each mL of the Oral Suspension taken by the formula:

$$20(C/V)(A_U/A_S)$$

in which *C* is the concentration, in µg per mL, of USP Thioridazine RS in the Standard solution; *V* is the volume, in mL, of Oral Suspension taken; and A_U and A_S are the absorbances of the Assay solution and the Standard solution, respectively.

Thioridazine Hydrochloride

$C_{21}H_{26}N_2S_2 \cdot HCl$ 407.04
10*H*-Phenothiazine, 10-[2-(1-methyl-2-piperidinyl)ethyl]-2-(methylthio)-, monohydrochloride.
10-[2-(1-Methyl-2-piperidyl)ethyl]-2-(methylthio)phenothiazine monohydrochloride   [*130-61-0*].

» Thioridazine Hydrochloride contains not less than 99.0 percent and not more than 101.0 percent of $C_{21}H_{26}N_2S_2 \cdot HCl$, calculated on the dried basis.

Packaging and storage—Preserve in tight, light-resistant containers.
USP Reference standards ⟨11⟩—*USP Thioridazine Hydrochloride RS*.
   NOTE—Throughout the following procedures, protect test or assay specimens, the Reference Standard, and solutions containing them, by conducting the procedures without delay, under subdued light, or by using low-actinic glassware.
Identification—
   A: *Infrared Absorption* ⟨197K⟩.
   B: A solution (1 in 100) in a mixture of water and alcohol (1 : 1) responds to the test for *Chloride* ⟨191⟩ in amine hydrochlorides.
Melting range ⟨741⟩: between 159° and 165°, but the range between beginning and end of melting does not exceed 3°.
pH ⟨791⟩: between 4.2 and 5.2, in a solution (1 in 100).
Loss on drying ⟨731⟩—Dry it at 105° for 4 hours: it loses not more than 0.4% of its weight.
Residue on ignition ⟨281⟩: not more than 0.1%.
Selenium ⟨291⟩: 0.003%, a 100-mg specimen being used, 100 mg of magnesium oxide being added to the *Test Solution*.
Chromatographic purity—[NOTE—Conduct this procedure in subdued lighting without delay.]
   Diluting solution: a mixture of methanol and ammonium hydroxide (49 : 1).
   Test solution—Transfer 100 mg of Thioridazine Hydrochloride, accurately weighed, to a 5-mL volumetric flask. Dissolve in and dilute with *Diluting solution* to volume, and mix.
   Standard solutions—Dissolve an accurately weighed quantity of USP Thioridazine Hydrochloride RS in *Diluting solution*, and dilute quantitatively, and stepwise if necessary, with *Diluting solution* to obtain a solution having a known concentration of 20.0 mg per mL (*Standard solution A*). Dilute appropriate portions of this solution quantitatively with *Diluting solution* to obtain five *Standard solutions B* to *F* having known concentrations of 0.1, 0.067, 0.025, 0.02 and 0.01 mg per mL, respectively. The final concentrations of *Standard solutions B* to *F* represent 0.5%, 0.33%, 0.125%, 0.1% and 0.05% concentration of *Standard solution A*, respectively.
   Application volume: 5 µL.
   Developing solvent system: a mixture of chloroform, isopropyl alcohol, and ammonium hydroxide (74 : 25 : 1).
   Procedure—Apply equal spots of the *Test solution* and *Standard solutions A* to *F* as directed under *Ordinary Impurities* ⟨466⟩. Examine the plate under short- and long-wavelength UV light, then spray the plate with Dragendorff's TS, dry the plate with a stream of nitrogen, and then spray with hydrogen peroxide TS: any secondary spot in the *Test solution* is not more than 0.5%, and the sum of all secondary spots is not more than 0.5%.
Organic volatile impurities, *Method IV* ⟨467⟩: meets the requirements.
                                  (Official until July 1, 2008)
Assay—Dissolve about 350 mg of Thioridazine Hydrochloride, accurately weighed, in 80 mL of a solution of equal parts of glacial acetic acid and acetic anhydride, and titrate with 0.1 N perchloric acid VS, determining the endpoint potentiometrically. Perform a blank determination, and make any necessary correction. Each mL of 0.1 N perchloric acid is equivalent to 40.70 mg of $C_{21}H_{26}N_2S_2 \cdot HCl$.

Thioridazine Hydrochloride Oral Solution

» Thioridazine Hydrochloride Oral Solution contains not less than 90.0 percent and not more than 110.0 percent of the labeled amount of $C_{21}H_{26}N_2S_2 \cdot HCl$.

Packaging and storage—Preserve in tight, light-resistant containers, at controlled room temperature.
Labeling—Label it to indicate that it is to be diluted to appropriate strength with water or other suitable fluid prior to administration.

USP Reference standards ⟨11⟩—*USP Thioridazine Hydrochloride RS.*
NOTE—Throughout the following procedures, protect test or assay specimens, the Reference Standard, and solutions containing them, by conducting the procedures without delay, under subdued light, or using low-actinic glassware.
Identification—A volume of Oral Solution containing 50 mg of thioridazine hydrochloride, diluted with water to 25 mL, meets the requirements under *Identification—Organic Nitrogenous Bases* ⟨181⟩, 2 mL of sodium bicarbonate solution (1 in 12) being used in place of the 2 mL of 1 N sodium hydroxide specified in the test.
Alcohol content ⟨611⟩: not more than 4.75% of C_2H_5OH.
Assay—[NOTE—Conduct this procedure with a minimum of exposure to light.]
Ammoniacal chloroform—Shake 125 mL of chloroform with 5 mL of ammonium hydroxide in a separator, slowly filter the bottom layer through filter paper containing anhydrous sodium sulfate, and discard the top layer.
Standard preparation—Dissolve a suitable quantity of USP Thioridazine Hydrochloride RS, accurately weighed, in *Ammoniacal chloroform* to obtain a solution having a known concentration of about 6 µg per mL.
Assay preparation—Pipet a portion of Oral Solution, equivalent to about 120 mg of thioridazine hydrochloride, into a separator containing 15 mL of water. Render alkaline with ammonium hydroxide, and extract with three 25-mL portions of *Ammoniacal chloroform*. Filter the extracts through a pledget of glass wool into a 200-mL volumetric flask. Rinse the filter, add chloroform to volume, and mix. Dilute 2.0 mL of this solution with *Ammoniacal chloroform* to 200.0 mL, and mix.
Procedure—Concomitantly determine the absorbances of the *Standard preparation* and the *Assay preparation* in 1-cm cells at the wavelength of maximum absorbance at about 265 nm, with a suitable spectrophotometer, using *Ammoniacal chloroform* as the blank. Calculate the quantity, in mg, of $C_{21}H_{26}N_2S_2 \cdot HCl$ in each mL of the Oral Solution taken by the formula:

$$20(C/V)(A_U/A_S)$$

in which C is the concentration, in µg per mL, of USP Thioridazine Hydrochloride RS in the *Standard preparation*, V is the volume, in mL, of Oral Solution taken, and A_U and A_S are the absorbances of the *Assay preparation* and the *Standard preparation*, respectively.

Thioridazine Hydrochloride Tablets

» Thioridazine Hydrochloride Tablets contain not less than 90.0 percent and not more than 110.0 percent of the labeled amount of $C_{21}H_{26}N_2S_2 \cdot HCl$.

Packaging and storage—Preserve in tight, light-resistant containers.
USP Reference standards ⟨11⟩—*USP Thioridazine Hydrochloride RS.*
NOTE—Throughout the following procedures, protect test or assay specimens, the Reference Standard, and solutions containing them, by conducting the procedures without delay, under subdued light, or using low-actinic glassware.
Identification—Tablets meet the requirements under *Identification—Organic Nitrogenous Bases* ⟨181⟩, 2 mL of sodium bicarbonate solution (1 in 12) being used in place of the 2 mL of 1 N sodium hydroxide specified in the test.
Dissolution ⟨711⟩—
Medium: 0.01 N hydrochloric acid; 1000 mL.
Apparatus 2: 75 rpm.
Time: 60 minutes.
Procedure—Determine the amount of $C_{21}H_{26}N_2S_2 \cdot HCl$ dissolved by employing UV absorption at the wavelength of maximum absorbance at about 262 nm on filtered portions of the solution under test, suitably diluted with *Dissolution Medium*, if necessary, in comparison with a Standard solution having a known concentration of USP Thioridazine Hydrochloride RS in the same *Medium*.

Tolerances—Not less than 75% (Q) of the labeled amount of $C_{21}H_{26}N_2S_2 \cdot HCl$ is dissolved in 60 minutes.
Uniformity of dosage units ⟨905⟩: meet the requirements.
Assay—
Mobile phase—Prepare a filtered and degassed mixture of acetonitrile, water, and triethylamine (850 : 150 : 1). Make adjustments if necessary (see *System Suitability* under *Chromatography* ⟨621⟩).
Standard preparation—Dissolve an accurately weighed quantity of USP Thioridazine Hydrochloride RS in methanol with the aid of sonication, and dilute quantitatively and stepwise, if necessary, with methanol to obtain a solution having a known concentration of about 125 µg per mL.
Assay preparation—Weigh and finely powder not less than 20 Tablets. Transfer an accurately weighed portion of the powder, equivalent to about 100 mg of thioridazine hydrochloride, to a 100-mL volumetric flask. Add about 80 mL of methanol, and shake by mechanical means for 30 minutes. Dilute with methanol to volume, and sonicate for 45 minutes with intermittent shaking. Allow the undissolved solids to settle, and filter, discarding the first 20 mL of the filtrate. Transfer 25.0 mL of the clear filtrate to a 200-mL volumetric flask, dilute with methanol to volume, and mix. Filter through a 0.45-µm disk before injecting into the chromatograph.
System suitability preparation—Dissolve 100 mg of mesoridazine besylate in 100 mL of methanol. Mix 1.0 mL of this solution with 9.0 mL of the *Standard preparation*.
Chromatographic system (see *Chromatography* ⟨621⟩)—The liquid chromatograph is equipped with a 265-nm detector and a 4.6-mm × 25-cm column that contains packing L1. The flow rate is about 2.5 mL per minute. Chromatograph the *Standard preparation* and the *System suitability preparation*, and record the peak responses as directed for *Procedure:* the resolution, R, between the mesoridazine and thioridazine peaks is not less than 1.0, and the relative standard deviation for replicate injections of the *Standard preparation* is not more than 2.0%.
Procedure—Separately inject equal volumes (about 10 µL) of the *Standard preparation* and the *Assay preparation* into the chromatograph, record the chromatograms, and measure the responses for the major peaks. Calculate the quantity, in mg, of $C_{21}H_{26}N_2S_2 \cdot HCl$ in the portion of Tablets taken by the formula:

$$0.8C(r_U/r_S)$$

in which C is the concentration, in µg per mL, of USP Thioridazine Hydrochloride RS in the *Standard preparation*, and r_U and r_S are the peak responses obtained from the *Assay preparation* and the *Standard preparation*, respectively.

Thiostrepton

$C_{72}H_{85}N_{19}O_{18}S_5$ 1664.89   [1393-48-2].

» Thiostrepton is an antibacterial substance produced by the growth of strains of *Streptomyces azureus* (Fam. Streptomycetaceae). It has a potency of not less than 900 USP Thiostrepton Units per mg, calculated on the dried basis.

Packaging and storage—Preserve in tight containers.
Labeling—Label it to indicate that it is for veterinary use only.
USP Reference standards ⟨11⟩—*USP Thiostrepton RS*.
Identification, *Infrared Absorption* ⟨197K⟩.
Loss on drying ⟨731⟩—Dry about 1 g of sample in vacuum at 60° for 3 hours: it loses not more than 5.0% of its weight.
Residue on ignition ⟨281⟩: not more than 1.0%.
Assay—Proceed as directed under *Antibiotics—Microbial Assays* ⟨81⟩, preparing the *Test Dilution* as follows. Transfer about 60 mg of Thiostrepton, accurately weighed, to a beaker. Add about 125 mL of dimethyl sulfoxide, and stir with a magnetic stirrer until dissolved (about 5 minutes). Transfer this solution to a 200-mL volumetric flask, washing the beaker and the stirring bar with dimethyl sulfoxide. Add the washings to the volumetric flask, dilute with dimethyl sulfoxide to volume, and mix. Dilute this solution quantitatively with dimethyl sulfoxide to obtain a *Test Dilution* having a concentration of thiostrepton assumed to be equal to the median dose of the Standard.

Thiotepa

$C_6H_{12}N_3PS$ 189.22
Aziridine, 1,1′,1″-phosphinothioylidynetris-.
Tris(1-aziridinyl)phosphine sulfide   [52-24-4].

» Thiotepa contains not less than 97.0 percent and not more than 102.0 percent of $C_6H_{12}N_3PS$, calculated on the anhydrous basis.

Caution—Great care should be taken to prevent inhaling particles of Thiotepa or exposing the skin to it.

Packaging and storage—Preserve in tight, light-resistant containers, and store in a refrigerator.
USP Reference standards ⟨11⟩—*USP Thiotepa RS*.
Identification, *Infrared Absorption* ⟨197S⟩—
  Solution: 3 in 400.
  Medium: carbon disulfide.
Melting range ⟨741⟩: between 52° and 57°.
Water, *Method I* ⟨921⟩: not more than 2.0%.
Assay—
  Mobile phase—Prepare a suitable filtered and degassed mixture of water and acetonitrile (9 : 1). Make adjustments if necessary (see *System Suitability* under *Chromatography* ⟨621⟩).
  Standard preparation—Dissolve an accurately weighed quantity of USP Thiotepa RS in *Mobile phase* to obtain a solution having a known concentration of about 1.5 mg per mL.
  Assay preparation—Transfer about 75 mg of Thiotepa, accurately weighed, to a 50-mL volumetric flask, dissolve in *Mobile phase*, dilute with *Mobile phase* to volume, and mix.
  Resolution solution—Transfer about 10 mg of USP Thiotepa RS to a 4-mL vial, add 2 mL of methanol, and mix. Add 50 µL of 0.1% phosphoric acid solution. Place a cap on the vial, and heat at 65° for 50 seconds. Cool the solution, add 1 mL of methanol, and mix.
  Chromatographic system (see *Chromatography* ⟨621⟩)—The liquid chromatograph is equipped with a 215-nm detector and a 4-mm × 15-cm column that contains packing L1. The flow rate is about 0.8 mL per minute. Chromatograph the *Resolution solution*, and record the peak responses as directed for *Procedure:* the relative retention times are about 1.25 for methoxythiotepa and 1.0 for thiotepa, and the resolution, *R*, between the methoxythiotepa peak and the thiotepa peak is not less than 3.0. Chromatograph the *Standard preparation*, and record the responses as directed for *Procedure:* the tailing factor for the thiotepa peak is not more than 1.8, the column efficiency is not less than 2600 theoretical plates, and the relative standard deviation for replicate injections is not more than 2.0%.
  Procedure—Separately inject equal volumes (about 10 µL) of the *Standard preparation* and the *Assay preparation* into the chromatograph, record the chromatograms, and measure the responses for the major peaks. Calculate the quantity, in mg, of $C_6H_{12}N_3PS$ in the portion of Thiotepa taken by the formula:

$$50C(r_U / r_S)$$

in which *C* is the concentration, in mg per mL, of USP Thiotepa RS in the *Standard preparation*, and r_U and r_S are the thiotepa peak responses obtained from the *Assay preparation* and the *Standard preparation*, respectively.

Thiotepa for Injection

» Thiotepa for Injection is Thiotepa, with or without added substances, that is suitable for parenteral use. It contains not less than 95.0 percent and not more than 110.0 percent of the labeled amount of thiotepa ($C_6H_{12}N_3PS$).

Packaging and storage—Preserve in *Containers for Sterile Solids* as described under *Injections* ⟨1⟩, and store in a refrigerator, protected from light.
USP Reference standards ⟨11⟩—*USP Thiotepa RS*.
Completeness of solution ⟨641⟩—The contents of 1 container dissolved in Sterile Water for Injection or other diluent as directed in the labeling to obtain a solution containing 3.75 mg of thiotepa per mL yields a clear solution.
Identification, *Infrared Absorption* ⟨197S⟩—
  Test and *Standard solutions*—Use the *Assay solution* and *Standard solution* prepared as directed in the *Assay*.
pH ⟨791⟩: between 5.5 and 7.5, in a solution, constituted as directed in the labeling, containing 10 mg of thiotepa per mL.
Bacterial endotoxins ⟨85⟩: not more than 6.25 USP Endotoxin Units per mg of thiotepa.
Other requirements—It meets the requirements for *Sterility Tests* ⟨71⟩, *Uniformity of Dosage Units* ⟨905⟩, and *Labeling* under *Injections* ⟨1⟩.
Assay—Remove, as completely as possible, the contents of not less than 20 containers of Thiotepa for Injection, weigh, and mix. Transfer an accurately weighed portion of the powder, equivalent to about 75 mg of thiotepa, to a suitable container, extract with three 5-mL portions of carbon disulfide, and filter the carbon disulfide extract with the aid of vacuum. Concentrate the combined filtrates under vacuum to approximately 5 mL. Transfer the carbon disulfide solution to a 10-mL volumetric flask with the aid of a few mL of carbon disulfide, and dilute with carbon disulfide to volume (*Assay solution*). Concomitantly determine the absorbances of this solution and a Standard solution of USP Thiotepa RS in the same medium having a known concentration of about 7.5 mg per mL (*Standard solution*), in 0.1-mm cells, at the wavelength of maximum absorbance at about 10.75 µm, with a suitable IR spectrophotometer, using carbon disulfide as the blank. Calculate the quantity, in mg, of thiotepa ($C_6H_{12}N_3PS$) in the portion of Thiotepa for Injection taken by the formula:

$$10C(A_U / A_S)$$

in which *C* is the concentration, in mg per mL, of USP Thiotepa RS in the Standard solution; and A_U and A_S are the absorbances of the *Assay solution* and the *Standard solution*, respectively.

Thiothixene

C₂₃H₂₉N₃O₂S₂   443.63

9H-Thioxanthene-2-sulfonamide, N,N-dimethyl-9-[3-(4-methyl-1-piperazinyl)propylidene]-, (Z)-.
N,N-Dimethyl-9-[3-(4-methyl-1-piperazinyl)propylidene]thioxanthene-2-sulfonamide   [5591-45-7; 3313-26-6].

» Thiothixene contains not less than 96.0 percent and not more than 101.5 percent of C₂₃H₂₉N₃O₂S₂, calculated on the dried basis.

Packaging and storage—Preserve in tight, light-resistant containers.

USP Reference standards ⟨11⟩—*USP Thiothixene RS. USP (E)-Thiothixene RS.*

Identification—
  A: *Infrared Absorption* ⟨197S⟩—
  Solution: 1 in 20.
  Medium: chloroform.
  B: *Ultraviolet Absorption* ⟨197U⟩—
  Solution: 10 μg per mL.
  Medium: methanol.
  Absorptivities at about 230 nm and 307 nm, calculated on the dried basis, do not differ by more than 4.0%.

Melting range, *Class I* ⟨741⟩: between 147° and 153.5°.

Loss on drying ⟨731⟩—Dry it in vacuum at 100° for 3 hours: it loses not more than 2.0% of its weight.

Residue on ignition ⟨281⟩: not more than 0.2%.

Selenium ⟨291⟩: 0.003%.

Heavy metals, *Method II* ⟨231⟩: 0.0025%.

Limit of (E)-thiothixene—[NOTE—Prepare all solutions in low-actinic glassware.]
  Mobile phase—Transfer 6.9 g of monobasic sodium phosphate to a 1-liter volumetric flask, dissolve in and dilute with deionized water to volume, and mix. Filter through a suitable membrane filter. Mix 4 volumes of this solution with 6 volumes of methanol. The concentration of methanol may be adjusted to meet the system suitability requirements.
  Standard preparations—
  A—Using accurately weighed quantities of USP (E)-Thiothixene RS and USP Thiothixene RS, prepare a solution in methanol containing, in each mL, 0.4 mg and 1.2 mg, respectively.
  B—Transfer 5.0 mL of *Standard preparation A* to a 100-mL volumetric flask, dilute with methanol to volume, and mix.
  C—Transfer about 200 mg of thiothixene, accurately weighed, to a 100-mL volumetric flask. Transfer 5.0 mL of *Standard preparation A* to the same flask, dissolve in and dilute with methanol to volume, and mix.
  Test preparation—Transfer about 200 mg of Thiothixene, accurately weighed, to a 100-mL volumetric flask. Dissolve in methanol, dilute with methanol to volume, and mix.
  Procedure—Concomitantly introduce equal volumes (about 20 μL) of *Standard preparation C* and *Test preparation* into a high-pressure liquid chromatograph operated at room temperature and equipped with a suitable microsyringe or sampling valve, a column containing packing L9 (typically 25 cm × 4.6 mm), an UV detector capable of monitoring absorption at 254 nm, and a suitable recorder. The *Mobile phase* is maintained at a flow rate of about 1 to 1.5 mL per minute. In a suitable chromatographic system, three replicate injections of *Standard preparation B* show a resolution factor of not less than 2.2 between the thiothixene and (E)-thiothixene peaks, their retention times being 13 and 15 minutes, and between 16 and 18 minutes, respectively. Calculate the quantity, in mg, of (E)-thiothixene in the portion of Thiothixene taken by the formula:

$$5CH_U / (H_C - H_U)$$

in which C is the concentration of USP (E)-Thiothixene RS, in mg per mL, in *Standard preparation A*; and H_C and H_U are the peak responses of the (E)-thiothixene peaks corrected for the tailing of the main peak, obtained from *Standard preparation C* and the *Test preparation*, respectively: the limit of (E)-thiothixene is 1.0%.

Organic volatile impurities, *Method V* ⟨467⟩: meets the requirements.
  Solvent—Use dimethyl sulfoxide.
  (Official until July 1, 2008)

Assay—[NOTE—Perform the dilution operations in low-actinic glassware.]
  Mobile phase—Mix 0.5 mL of ethanolamine with 3780 mL of methanol, mix 1400 mL of this solution with 200 mL of water, filter, and degas. Make adjustments if necessary (see *System Suitability* under *Chromatography* ⟨621⟩).
  Standard preparation—Using an accurately weighed quantity of USP Thiothixene RS, prepare a solution in methanol having a known concentration of about 0.02 mg per mL.
  Assay preparation—Transfer about 100 mg of Thiothixene, accurately weighed, to a 100-mL volumetric flask, dissolve in and dilute with methanol to volume, and mix. Pipet 2 mL of the resulting solution into a 100-mL volumetric flask, dilute with methanol to volume, and mix.
  Chromatographic system (see *Chromatography* ⟨621⟩)—The liquid chromatograph is equipped with a 254-nm detector and a 3.9-mm × 30-cm column that contains packing L3. The flow rate is about 0.5 mL per minute. Chromatograph the *Standard preparation*, and record the peak responses as directed for *Procedure*: the column efficiency determined from the analyte peak is not less than 2000 theoretical plates, and the relative standard deviation for replicate injections is not more than 1.5%.
  Procedure—Separately inject equal volumes (about 20 μL) of the *Standard preparation* and the *Assay preparation* into the chromatograph, record the chromatograms, and measure the responses for the major peaks. Calculate the quantity, in mg, of C₂₃H₂₉N₃O₂S₂ in the portion of Thiothixene taken by the formula:

$$5000C(r_U / r_S)$$

in which C is the concentration, in mg per mL, of USP Thiothixene RS in the *Standard preparation*, and r_U and r_S are the peak responses obtained from the *Assay preparation* and the *Standard preparation*, respectively.

Thiothixene Capsules

» Thiothixene Capsules contain not less than 90.0 percent and not more than 110.0 percent of the labeled amount of C₂₃H₂₉N₃O₂S₂.

Packaging and storage—Preserve in well-closed, light-resistant containers.

USP Reference standards ⟨11⟩—*USP Thiothixene RS.*

Identification—Dissolve a portion of the contents of Capsules in a solvent consisting of equal volumes of chloroform and methanol to obtain a solution containing 1 mg of thiothixene per mL. Shake by mechanical means for 10 minutes, clarify a portion of the mixture by centrifugation, filter, if necessary, and use the clear supernatant or filtrate for the test. Apply 10 μL of this test solution, 10 μL of a Standard solution containing 1 mg of USP Thiothixene RS per mL in the same medium, and 10 μL of a mixture of equal volumes of the test solution and the Standard solution to a suitable thin-layer chromatographic plate (see *Chromatography* ⟨621⟩) coated with a 0.25-mm layer of chromatographic silica gel mixture. Allow the spots to dry, and develop the chromatogram in a solvent system consisting of a mixture of ethyl acetate, methanol, and diethylamine (65 : 35 : 5) until the solvent front has moved about three-fourths of the length of the plate. Remove the plate from the developing chamber, mark the solvent front, and locate the spots on the plate by viewing under short- and long-wavelength UV light. Spray the plate lightly with acidified iodoplatinate spray reagent (prepared by mixing 1 volume of hydrochloric acid with 50 volumes of potassium iodoplatinate TS): the R_F value of the principal spot obtained from the test solution corresponds to that obtained from the Standard solution and the mixed test-Standard solution.

Dissolution ⟨711⟩—
  Medium—Dissolve 2.0 g of sodium chloride and 7 mL of hydrochloric acid in water to make 1000 mL, and mix; 900 mL.
  Apparatus 1: 100 rpm.
  Time: 20 minutes.
  Buffer solution—On the day of use, prepare a mixture of 55 volumes of dibasic potassium phosphate solution (87 in 1000), 20 volumes of citric acid monohydrate solution (21 in 200), and 40 volumes of sodium hydroxide solution (1 in 25).
  Methyl orange solution—Transfer 15.5 g of boric acid and 2.0 g of methyl orange to a glass-stoppered, 1000-mL flask. Add 500 mL of water, insert the stopper, and shake by mechanical means for not less than 3 hours. Filter through retentive filter paper, and wash the filtrate with two 100-mL portions of chloroform, discarding the chloroform washings. Store the *Methyl orange solution* over 50 mL of chloroform in a glass-stoppered bottle.
  Procedure—Prepare a *Test preparation* by passing a 60-mL portion of the dissolution solution through a suitable filter, discarding the first 5 mL of the filtrate, and diluting the subsequent filtrate quantitatively, if necessary, to obtain a concentration of about 1 µg of thiothixene per mL. Prepare a *Standard preparation* of USP Thiothixene RS in *Dissolution Medium* having a known concentration of about 1 µg per mL. Transfer 40.0 mL each of the *Test preparation*, the *Standard preparation*, and *Dissolution Medium* to provide the blank, to individual separators, each containing 8.0 mL of *Buffer solution*, 10.0 mL of *Methyl orange solution*, and 50.0 mL of chloroform. Shake for 3 minutes, allow the layers to separate, transfer 40.0 mL of the chloroform layer, clarified by centrifugation, to a 60-mL separator containing 8.0 mL of dilute hydrochloric acid (1 in 120), shake for 1 minute, and allow the layers to separate. Concomitantly determine the absorbances of the aqueous layers in 1-cm cells, at the wavelength of maximum absorbance at about 508 nm, with a suitable spectrophotometer, using the blank to set the instrument. Calculate the quantity, in µg per mL, of $C_{23}H_{29}N_3O_2S_2$ in the *Test preparation* taken by the formula:

$$C(A_U / A_S)$$

in which C is the concentration, in µg per mL, of USP Thiothixene RS in the *Standard preparation*, and A_U and A_S are the absorbances of the solutions from the *Test preparation* and the *Standard preparation*, respectively, and, from the known extent of dilution, determine the amount of it in the dissolution solution.
  Tolerances—Not less than 80% (*Q*) of the labeled amount of $C_{23}H_{29}N_3O_2S_2$ is dissolved in 20 minutes.

Uniformity of dosage units ⟨905⟩: meet the requirements.
Assay—[NOTE—Perform the dilution operations in low-actinic glassware.]
  Mobile phase, Standard preparation, and *Chromatographic system*—Prepare as directed in the *Assay* under *Thiothixene*.
  Assay preparation—Transfer, as completely as possible, the contents of not less than 20 Capsules to a tared beaker, and weigh. Mix, and transfer an accurately weighed portion of the powder, equivalent to about 10 mg of thiothixene, to a 500-mL volumetric flask. Add about 400 mL of methanol, shake by mechanical means for 10 minutes, place in an ultrasonic bath for 5 minutes, dilute with methanol to volume, and filter the suspension through a 5-µm polytef membrane filter.
  Procedure—Proceed as directed for *Procedure* in the *Assay* under *Thiothixene*. Calculate the quantity, in mg, of $C_{23}H_{29}N_3O_2S_2$ in the portion of Capsules taken by the formula:

$$500C(r_U / r_S)$$

in which C is the concentration, in mg per mL, of USP Thiothixene RS in the *Standard preparation*, and r_U and r_S are the peak responses obtained from the *Assay preparation* and the *Standard preparation*, respectively.

Thiothixene Hydrochloride

$C_{23}H_{29}N_3O_2S_2 \cdot 2HCl \cdot 2H_2O$ 552.58
9*H*-Thioxanthene-2-sulfonamide, *N,N*-dimethyl-9-[3-(4-methyl-1-piperazinyl)propylidene]-, dihydrochloride, dihydrate, (*Z*)-.
N,N-Dimethyl-9-[3-(4-methyl-1-piperazinyl)propylidene]thioxanthene-2-sulfonamide dihydrochloride dihydrate   [22189-31-7; 49746-09-0].
Anhydrous   516.56   [58513-59-0; 49746-04-5].

» Thiothixene Hydrochloride contains two molecules of water of hydration or is anhydrous. It contains not less than 97.0 percent and not more than 102.5 percent of $C_{23}H_{29}N_3O_2S_2 \cdot 2HCl$, calculated on the anhydrous basis.

Packaging and storage—Preserve in tight, light-resistant containers.
USP Reference standards ⟨11⟩—*USP Thiothixene RS. USP (E)-Thiothixene RS.*
Identification—
  A: It meets the requirements under *Identification—Organic Nitrogenous Bases* ⟨181⟩, USP Thiothixene RS being used as the standard for comparison, chloroform being used instead of carbon disulfide, and a reagent blank being used in the matched reference cell.
  B: *Ultraviolet Absorption* ⟨197U⟩—
    Solution: 10 µg per mL.
    Medium: dilute methanolic hydrochloric acid (1 in 1200).
    Absorptivities at 307 nm, calculated on the anhydrous basis, do not differ by more than 3.0%.
  C: A solution (1 in 100) responds to the tests for *Chloride* ⟨191⟩.
Water, *Method I* ⟨921⟩: between 6.2% and 7.5% for the dihydrate; not more than 1.0% for the anhydrous form.
Residue on ignition ⟨281⟩: not more than 0.2%.
Heavy metals, *Method II* ⟨231⟩: 0.0025%.
Selenium ⟨291⟩: 0.003%.
Limit of (*E*)-thiothixene—[NOTE—Prepare all solutions in low-actinic glassware.]
  Mobile phase—Prepare as directed in the test for *Limit of (E)-thiothixene* under *Thiothixene*.
  Standard preparations and *Test preparation*—Prepare as directed in the test for *Limit of (E)-thiothixene* under *Thiothixene*, except to use 250 mg of Thiothixene Hydrochloride instead of 200 mg of Thiothixene.
  Procedure—Proceed as directed for *Procedure* in the test for *Limit of (E)-thiothixene* under *Thiothixene*. Calculate the quantity, in mg, of (*E*)-thiothixene hydrochloride in the portion of Thiothixene Hydrochloride taken by the formula:

$$5CH_U(516.56/443.63) / (H_C - H_U)$$

in which 516.56 and 443.63 are the molecular weights of anhydrous thiothixene hydrochloride and thiothixene, respectively; and the other terms are as previously defined. The limit of (*E*)-thiothixene, as the hydrochloride, is 1.0%.
Organic volatile impurities, *Method I* ⟨467⟩: meets the requirements.
(Official until July 1, 2008)
Assay—[NOTE—Perform the dilution operations in low-actinic glassware.]
  Mobile phase, Standard preparation, and *Chromatographic system*—Prepare as directed in the *Assay* under *Thiothixene*.
  Assay preparation—Transfer about 116 mg of Thiothixene Hydrochloride, accurately weighed, to a 100-mL volumetric flask, dissolve in and dilute with methanol to volume, and mix. Pipet 2 mL of this solution into a 100-mL volumetric flask, dilute with methanol to volume, and mix.
  Procedure—Proceed as directed for *Procedure* in the *Assay* under *Thiothixene*. Calculate the quantity, in mg, of $C_{23}H_{29}N_3O_2S_2 \cdot$

2HCl in the portion of Thiothixene Hydrochloride taken by the formula:

$$(516.56/443.64)(5000C)(r_U / r_S)$$

in which 516.56 and 443.64 are the molecular weights of anhydrous thiothixene hydrochloride and thiothixene, respectively; C is the concentration, in mg per mL, of USP Thiothixene RS in the *Standard preparation;* and r_U and r_S are the peak responses obtained from the *Assay preparation* and the *Standard preparation,* respectively.

Thiothixene Hydrochloride Injection

» Thiothixene Hydrochloride Injection is a sterile solution of Thiothixene Hydrochloride in Water for Injection. It contains an amount of thiothixene hydrochloride equivalent to not less than 90.0 percent and not more than 110.0 percent of the labeled amount of thiothixene ($C_{23}H_{29}N_3O_2S_2$).

Packaging and storage—Preserve in single-dose containers, preferably of Type I glass, protected from light.
USP Reference standards ⟨11⟩—*USP Endotoxin RS. USP Thiothixene RS.*
Identification—Transfer a volume of Injection, equivalent to about 20 mg of thiothixene hydrochloride, to a separator containing 20.0 mL of chloroform. Render the aqueous layer just basic with ammonium hydroxide, shake for 1 minute, and allow the layers to separate. Pass a portion of the chloroform layer through filter paper, previously washed with chloroform, and use the clear filtrate for the test. Proceed as directed in the *Identification* test under *Thiothixene Capsules,* beginning with "Apply 10 µL of this test solution."
Bacterial endotoxins ⟨85⟩—It contains not more than 88.0 USP Endotoxin Units per mg of thiothixene.
pH ⟨791⟩: between 2.5 and 3.5.
Other requirements—It meets the requirements under *Injections* ⟨1⟩.
Assay—[NOTE—Perform the dilution operations in low-actinic glassware.]

Mobile phase, Standard preparation, and *Chromatographic system*—Prepare as directed in the *Assay* under *Thiothixene.*

Assay preparation—Transfer an accurately measured volume of Injection, equivalent to about 2 mg of thiothixene, to a 100-mL volumetric flask, dilute with methanol to volume, and mix.

Procedure—Proceed as directed for *Procedure* in the *Assay* under *Thiothixene.* Calculate the quantity, in mg, of $C_{23}H_{29}N_3O_2S_2$ in each mL of the Injection taken by the formula:

$$(100C / V)(r_U / r_S)$$

in which C is the concentration, in mg per mL, of USP Thiothixene RS in the *Standard preparation,* V is the volume, in mL, of Injection taken, and r_U and r_S are the peak responses obtained from the *Assay preparation* and the *Standard preparation,* respectively.

Thiothixene Hydrochloride for Injection

» Thiothixene Hydrochloride for Injection is a sterile, dry mixture of Thiothixene Hydrochloride and Mannitol. It contains not less than 90.0 percent and not more than 110.0 percent of the labeled amount of $C_{23}H_{29}N_3O_2S_2$.

Packaging and storage—Preserve in light-resistant *Containers for Sterile Solids* as described under *Injections* ⟨1⟩.
USP Reference standards ⟨11⟩—*USP Endotoxin RS. USP Thiothixene RS.*

Identification—Constitute a vial of Thiothixene Hydrochloride for Injection with 2.2 mL of water. Further dilute one volume of the constituted solution with 4 volumes of methanol to obtain a test solution containing 1 mg of thiothixene per mL. Apply 10 µL of this test solution and 10 µL of a Standard solution containing 1 mg of USP Thiothixene RS per mL in the same medium to a suitable thin-layer chromatographic plate (see *Chromatography* ⟨621⟩) coated with a 0.25-mm layer of chromatographic silica gel mixture. Allow the spots to dry, and develop the chromatogram in a solvent system consisting of a mixture of isopropyl alcohol and diethylamine (25 : 1) until the solvent front has moved about three-fourths of the length of the plate. Remove the plate from the developing chamber, mark the solvent front, air-dry for 30 minutes, and then oven-dry at 110° for 30 minutes. Locate the spots on the plate by viewing under short-wavelength UV light. Spray the plate with alkaline permanganate spray reagent (prepared by dissolving 0.5 g of potassium permanganate and 2.0 g of sodium carbonate in 100 mL of water): the R_F value of the principal spot obtained from the test solution, under both detection conditions, corresponds to that obtained from the Standard solution.
Bacterial endotoxins ⟨85⟩—It contains not more than 88.0 USP Endotoxin Units per mg of thiothixene.
pH ⟨791⟩: between 2.3 and 3.7, in the solution constituted as directed in the labeling.
Water, *Method I* ⟨921⟩: not more than 4.0%.
Other requirements—It meets the requirements under *Injections* ⟨1⟩.
Assay—[NOTE—Perform the dilution operations in low-actinic glassware.]

Mobile phase, Standard preparation, and *Chromatographic system*—Prepare as directed in the *Assay* under *Thiothixene.*

Assay preparation—Constitute a vial of Thiothixene Hydrochloride for Injection with an accurately measured volume (V_L mL) of water as directed in the labeling. Transfer an accurately measured volume (V_F mL) of the constituted solution, equivalent to about 5 mg of thiothixene, to a 250-mL volumetric flask, dilute with methanol to volume, and mix.

Procedure—Proceed as directed for *Procedure* in the *Assay* under *Thiothixene.* Calculate the quantity, in mg, of $C_{23}H_{29}N_3O_2S_2$ in each mL of the constituted solution taken by the formula:

$$(250CV_L / V_F)(r_U / r_S)$$

in which C is the concentration, in mg per mL, of USP Thiothixene RS in the *Standard preparation,* and r_U and r_S are the peak responses obtained from the *Assay preparation* and the *Standard preparation,* respectively.

Thiothixene Hydrochloride Oral Solution

» Thiothixene Hydrochloride Oral Solution contains an amount of thiothixene hydrochloride equivalent to not less than 90.0 percent and not more than 110.0 percent of the labeled amount of thiothixene ($C_{23}H_{29}N_3O_2S_2$).

Packaging and storage—Preserve in tight, light-resistant containers.
USP Reference standards ⟨11⟩—*USP Thiothixene RS.*
Identification—Transfer a portion of Oral Solution, equivalent to about 20 mg of thiothixene hydrochloride, to a separator containing 20.0 mL of chloroform. Render the aqueous layer just basic with ammonium hydroxide, shake for 1 minute, and allow the layers to separate. Pass a portion of the chloroform layer through filter paper, previously washed with chloroform; and use the clear filtrate for the test. Proceed as directed in the *Identification* test under *Thiothixene Capsules,* beginning with "Apply 10 µL of this test solution."
Uniformity of dosage units ⟨905⟩—
FOR ORAL SOLUTION PACKAGED IN SINGLE-UNIT CONTAINERS: meets the requirements.

Deliverable volume ⟨698⟩—
FOR ORAL SOLUTION PACKAGED IN MULTIPLE-UNIT CONTAINERS: meets the requirements.
pH ⟨791⟩: between 2.0 and 3.0.
Alcohol content, *Method II* ⟨611⟩: if present, between 90.0% and 110.0% of the labeled amount, the labeled amount being not more than 7.0% of C_2H_5OH, determined by the gas-liquid chromatographic procedure, acetonitrile being used as the internal standard.
Assay—[NOTE—Perform the dilution operations in low-actinic glassware.]
Mobile phase, Standard preparation, and *Chromatographic system*—Prepare as directed in the *Assay* under *Thiothixene.*
Assay preparation—Transfer an accurately measured volume of Oral Solution, equivalent to about 25 mg of thiothixene, to a 25-mL volumetric flask; dissolve in and dilute with methanol to volume; and mix. Pipet 2 mL of this solution into a 100-mL volumetric flask, dilute with methanol to volume, and mix.
Procedure—Proceed as directed for *Procedure* in the *Assay* under *Thiothixene.* Calculate the quantity, in mg, of thiothixene ($C_{23}H_{29}N_3O_2S_2$) in each mL of the Oral Solution taken by the formula:

$$(1250C/V)(r_U/r_S)$$

in which C is the concentration, in mg per mL, of USP Thiothixene RS in the *Standard preparation; V* is the volume, in mL, of Oral Solution taken; and r_U and r_S are the peak responses obtained from the *Assay preparation* and the *Standard preparation,* respectively.

Threonine

$C_4H_9NO_3$ 119.12
L-Threonine.
L-Threonine   [72-19-5].

» Threonine contains not less than 98.5 percent and not more than 101.5 percent of $C_4H_9NO_3$, as L-threonine, calculated on the dried basis.

Packaging and storage—Preserve in well-closed containers.
USP Reference standards ⟨11⟩—USP L-Proline RS. USP L-Threonine RS.
Identification, *Infrared Absorption* ⟨197K⟩.
Specific rotation ⟨781S⟩: between −26.7° and −29.1°.
 Test solution: 60 mg per mL, in water.
pH ⟨791⟩: between 5.0 and 6.5 in a solution (1 in 20).
Loss on drying ⟨731⟩—Dry it at 105° for 3 hours: it loses not more than 0.2% of its weight.
Residue on ignition ⟨281⟩: not more than 0.4%.
Chloride ⟨221⟩—A 0.73-g portion shows no more chloride than corresponds to 0.50 mL of 0.020 N hydrochloric acid (0.05%).
Sulfate ⟨221⟩—A 0.33-g portion shows no more sulfate than corresponds to 0.10 mL of 0.020 N sulfuric acid (0.03%).
Iron ⟨241⟩: 0.003%.
Heavy metals, *Method I* ⟨231⟩: 0.0015%.
Chromatographic purity—
 Adsorbent: 0.25-mm layer of chromatographic silica gel mixture.
 Diluent—Prepare by mixing 10 mL of hydrochloric acid with sufficient water to make 1000 mL.
 Test solution—Dissolve an accurately weighed quantity of Threonine in 2 N hydrochloric acid to obtain a solution having a concentration of 10 mg per mL. Apply 5 µL.
 Standard solution—Dissolve an accurately weighed quantity of USP L-Threonine RS in *Diluent* to obtain a solution having a known concentration of about 0.05 mg per mL. Apply 5 µL. [NOTE—This solution has a concentration equivalent to about 0.5% of that of the *Test solution.*]
 System suitability solution—Prepare a solution in *Diluent* containing 0.4 mg each of USP L-Threonine RS and USP L-Proline RS per mL. Apply 5 µL.
 Spray reagent—Dissolve 0.2 g of ninhydrin in 100 mL of a mixture of butyl alcohol and 2 N acetic acid (95 : 5).
 Developing solvent system—Prepare a mixture of butyl alcohol, glacial acetic acid, and water (60 : 20 : 20).
 Procedure—Proceed as directed for *Thin-Layer Chromatography* under *Chromatography* ⟨621⟩. After air-drying the plate, spray with *Spray reagent,* and heat between 100° and 105° for about 15 minutes. Examine the plate under white light. The chromatogram obtained from the *System suitability solution* exhibits two clearly separated spots. Any secondary spot in the chromatogram obtained from the *Test solution* is not larger or more intense than the principal spot in the chromatogram obtained from the *Standard solution:* not more than 0.5% of any individual impurity is found; and not more than 2.0% of total impurities is found.
Organic volatile impurities, *Method V* ⟨467⟩: meets the requirements.

(Official until July 1, 2008)

Assay—Transfer about 110 mg of Threonine, accurately weighed, to a 125-mL flask, dissolve in a mixture of 3 mL of formic acid and 50 mL of glacial acetic acid, and titrate with 0.1 N perchloric acid VS, determining the endpoint potentiometrically. Perform a blank determination, and make any necessary correction. Each mL of 0.1 N perchloric acid is equivalent to 11.91 mg of $C_4H_9NO_3$.

Thrombin

» Thrombin conforms to the regulations of the FDA concerning biologics (see *Biologics* ⟨1041⟩). It is a sterile, freeze-dried powder derived from bovine plasma containing the protein substance prepared from prothrombin through interaction with added thromboplastin in the presence of calcium. It is capable, without the addition of other substances, of causing the clotting of whole blood, plasma, or a solution of fibrinogen. Its potency is determined in U.S. Units in terms of the U.S. Standard Thrombin in a test comparing clotting times of fibrinogen solution.

Packaging and storage—Preserve at a temperature between 2° and 8°. Dispense it in the unopened container in which it was placed by the manufacturer.
Expiration date—The expiration date is not more than 3 years after date of manufacture.
Labeling—Label it to indicate that solutions of Thrombin are to be used within a few hours after preparation and are not to be injected into or otherwise allowed to enter large blood vessels.

Thyroid

» Thyroid is the cleaned, dried, and powdered thyroid gland previously deprived of connective tissue and fat. It is obtained from domesticated animals that are used for food by humans.
 On hydrolysis it yields not less than 90.0 percent and not more than 110.0 percent each of the labeled amounts of levothyroxine ($C_{15}H_{11}I_4NO_4$) and liothyronine ($C_{15}H_{12}I_3NO_4$), calculated on the dried basis. It is free from iodine in inorganic or any form of combination other than that peculiar to the thyroid gland. It may

contain a suitable diluent such as Lactose, Sodium Chloride, Starch, Sucrose, or Dextrose.

Packaging and storage—Preserve in tight containers.

USP Reference standards ⟨11⟩—*USP Levothyroxine RS. USP Liothyronine RS.*

Identification—The retention times of the peaks for liothyronine and levothyroxine in the chromatogram of the *Assay preparation* correspond to those in the chromatogram of the *Standard preparation,* as obtained in the *Assay.*

Microbial limits ⟨61⟩—It meets the requirements of the tests for absence of *Salmonella* species and *Escherichia coli.*

Loss on drying ⟨731⟩—Dry it in vacuum at 60° for 4 hours: it loses not more than 6.0% of its weight.

Limit of inorganic iodides—

Extracting solution—Prepare a 1 in 100 solution of sulfuric acid in water.

Reference solution—Dissolve an accurately weighed quantity of potassium iodide in water to obtain a stock solution containing 0.131 mg, equivalent to 0.100 mg of iodide, per mL. Transfer 1.0 mL of this stock solution into a 100-mL volumetric flask, dilute with *Extracting solution* to volume, and mix. Each mL of the *Reference solution* contains 1.0 µg of iodide. [NOTE—Prepare this solution on the day of use.]

Test solution—Transfer 1.00 g, or proportionately less if the iodine content is greater than 0.2%, of Thyroid to a beaker, add 100.0 mL of *Extracting solution,* and sonicate for 5 minutes.

Electrode system—Use an iodide-specific, ion-indicating electrode and a silver-silver chloride reference electrode connected to a pH meter capable of measuring potentials with a minimum reproducibility of ±1 mV (see *pH* ⟨791⟩).

Procedure—Transfer the *Reference solution* to a beaker containing a magnetic stirring bar. Rinse and dry the electrodes, insert in the solution, stir for 5 minutes or until the reading stabilizes, and read the potential, in mV. Repeat this process using the *Test solution.* The requirements of the test are met if the *Test solution* has a higher potential, in mV, than the *Reference solution:* the limit is 0.01%.

Assay—

Mobile phase—Prepare a degassed and filtered mixture of water, acetonitrile, and phosphoric acid (650 : 350 : 5). Make adjustments if necessary (see *System Suitability* under *Chromatography* ⟨621⟩).

Reducing buffer solution—Freshly prepare a solution in 0.11 M sodium chloride that is 0.04 M with respect to tris(hydroxymethyl)aminomethane and 0.05 M with respect to methimazole. Adjust, if necessary, with 6 N hydrochloric acid or 0.1 N sodium hydroxide to a pH of 8.4 ± 0.05.

Proteolytic enzyme—Freshly prepare a solution containing 15 mg of bacterial protease[*] in each 5 mL of *Reducing buffer solution.*

Enzyme deactivating solution—Prepare a 1 in 100 mixture of phosphoric acid in acetonitrile.

Standard preparation—[NOTE—Protect solutions from light.] Transfer accurately weighed quantities of about 9 mg of USP Liothyronine RS and about 38 mg of USP Levothyroxine RS to a 100-mL volumetric flask, add 50 mL of a mixture of water, acetonitrile, and ammonium hydroxide (500 : 500 : 1), and swirl to dissolve. Dilute with a mixture of water and acetonitrile (1 : 1) to volume, and mix (stock solution). On the day of use, pipet 5 mL of the freshly prepared stock solution into a 250-mL volumetric flask, dilute with *Reducing buffer solution* to volume, and mix to obtain a solution having known concentrations of about 1.8 µg of liothyronine per mL and about 7.6 µg of levothyroxine per mL. Pipet 5 mL of this solution into a screw-capped 16- × 125-mm culture tube. Pipet 2 mL of *Enzyme deactivating solution* into the tube, place the cap on the tube, and shake the mixture vigorously.

Assay preparation—Transfer an accurately weighed portion of finely powdered Thyroid, equivalent to about 38 µg of levothyroxine, to a screw-capped 16- × 125-mm culture tube that previously has been flushed with nitrogen. Taking precautions to avoid unnecessary exposure to air, pipet 5 mL of *Proteolytic enzyme* into the tube. Allow nitrogen to flow gently over the mixture for 5 minutes. Place the cap on the tube, mix to disperse the contents, and place in a covered water bath maintained at a temperature of 37 ± 1° for 28 hours. Protect the contents of the tubes from light. Examine occasionally, and mix as necessary to ensure dispersion. At the end of the incubation period, pipet 2 mL of *Enzyme deactivating solution* into the tube, place the cap on the tube, mix vigorously, and centrifuge at about 2000 rpm for 5 minutes. Filter the supernatant through a 0.45-µm porosity filter, discarding the first 1 mL of the filtrate.

Chromatographic system (see *Chromatography* ⟨621⟩)—The liquid chromatograph is equipped with a 230-nm detector and a 4.6- × 25-cm column that contains packing L1. The flow rate is about 1.5 mL per minute. Chromatograph the *Standard preparation,* and record the peak responses as directed for *Procedure:* the tailing factors for the liothyronine and levothyroxine peaks are not more than 1.8, and the relative standard deviation for replicate injections is not more than 2.0%.

Procedure—Separately inject equal volumes (about 200 µL) of the *Assay preparation,* and the *Standard preparation,* record the chromatograms, and measure the responses for the major peaks. Calculate the quantity, in µg, of liothyronine ($C_{15}H_{12}I_3NO_4$) and levothyroxine ($C_{15}H_{11}I_4NO_4$) in the portion of Thyroid taken by the formula:

$$7C(r_U / r_S)$$

in which C is the concentration, in µg per mL, of the corresponding USP Reference Standard in the *Standard preparation,* and r_U and r_S are the peak responses for the corresponding analytes obtained from the *Assay preparation* and the *Standard preparation,* respectively.

Thyroid Tablets

» Thyroid Tablets contain not less than 90.0 percent and not more than 110.0 percent of the labeled amounts of levothyroxine and liothyronine, the labeled amounts being 38 µg of levothyroxine and 9 µg of liothyronine for each 65 mg of the labeled content of thyroid.

Packaging and storage—Preserve in tight containers.

USP Reference standards ⟨11⟩—*USP Liothyronine RS. USP Levothyroxine RS.*

Microbial limits ⟨61⟩—Tablets meet the requirements of the tests for absence of *Salmonella* species and *Escherichia coli.*

Disintegration ⟨701⟩: 15 minutes, with disks.

Uniformity of dosage units ⟨905⟩: meet the requirements, the following procedure being used where the test for *Content Uniformity* is required.

PROCEDURE FOR CONTENT UNIFORMITY—

Standard solution—Accurately weigh 1.69 g of potassium iodate, and transfer to a 1-liter volumetric flask. Dissolve in about 200 mL of water, dilute with water to volume, and mix. This is a stock solution having a concentration of about 1 mg per mL with respect to iodine. Pipet 8 mL of the stock solution into a 250-mL volumetric flask, dilute with water to volume, and mix. Transfer an appropriate aliquot, based on dosage being analyzed (i.e., ¼ gr, 1 mL; ½ gr, 2 mL; 1 gr, 4 mL; 1½ gr, 6 mL; 2 gr, 8 mL; 2½ gr, 10 mL; 3 gr, 12 mL; 4 gr, 16 mL; 5 gr, 20 mL), to a 100-mL volumetric flask containing 8 g of potassium carbonate dissolved in 70 mL of water. Add 1 mL of bromine TS, mix, add sufficient sodium sulfite (about 20 mg) until the solution becomes colorless, and mix. Dilute with water to volume, and mix.

Test solution—Crush 1 Tablet in a porcelain crucible with a glass rod. Remove any sample adhering to the glass rod with a spatula, and add it to the crucible. Add 4 g of anhydrous potassium carbonate, mix carefully, and gently tap the crucible several times to compact the mixture. Overlay with 4 g more of anhydrous potassium carbonate, and again compact the material thoroughly by tapping. Place the crucible in a preheated muffle furnace, and ignite at 675° to 700° for 25 minutes. Cool, add 30 mL of water, carefully heat on a hot plate to dissolve the residue, and filter through a funnel with a glass wool plug into a 100-mL volumetric flask. Repeat the heating and filtration with two additional 30-mL portions of water, and add

---

[*] A suitable grade is available as "Pronase" (Catalog number 53702) from Calbiochem-Behring, P. O. Box 12087, San Diego, CA 92112.

these filtrates to the volumetric flask. Add 1 mL of bromine TS, mix, add sufficient sodium sulfite (about 20 mg) until the solution becomes colorless, and mix. Dilute with water to volume, and mix.

Blank solution—Prepare a reagent blank by putting 8 g of anhydrous potassium carbonate into a 100-mL volumetric flask and dissolving it in 70 mL of water, add 1 mL of freshly prepared bromine TS, mix, add sufficient sodium sulfite (about 20 mg) until the solution becomes colorless, dilute with water to volume, and mix to obtain the *Blank solution*.

Procedure—Transfer 10 mL of the *Test solution* to a dry polarographic cell. Bubble nitrogen through the solution for 5 minutes, and then direct the stream of nitrogen above the solution. Use a suitable differential pulse polarograph equipped with a saturated calomel reference electrode and a dropping mercury electrode with a 1-second drop time. Scan from −0.8V to −1.5V at the rate of 5 mV per second, and 50-mV pulses. Record the polarogram of the *Test solution*, the *Standard solution*, and the *Blank solution*. At the peaks near −1.18V in the polarograms obtained from the *Standard solution* and the *Test solution* measure the heights from the baseline, as established by the *Blank solution*. Calculate the amount of iodine, in μg, in the Tablet taken by the formula:

$$(126.90 / 214.00)(54.08V)(PH_U / PH_S)$$

in which 126.90 and 214.00 are the atomic weight of iodine (I) and the molecular weight of potassium iodate (KIO$_3$), respectively; V is the volume, in mL, of the aliquot portion of potassium iodate solution used to prepare the *Standard Solution;* and PH_U and PH_S are the peak heights obtained from the *Test solution* and the *Standard solution*, respectively. Proceed as directed for *Content Uniformity* ⟨905⟩, using the results obtained by this procedure to determine the total iodine content of individual Tablets, and use the *Assay preparation* to perform the composite determination for iodine. The requirement is met if the amount of iodine in each Tablet is within the range of 85.0% to 115% of the composite assay for iodine with a relative standard deviation of not more than 6.0%.

Assay—
Mobile phase, Reducing buffer solution, Proteolytic enzyme, Enzyme deactivating solution, Standard preparation, Chromatographic system, and *Procedure*—Proceed as directed in the *Assay* under *Thyroid*.

Assay preparation—Weigh and finely powder not less than 20 Tablets. Using an accurately weighed portion of the powder, proceed as directed for *Assay preparation* in the *Assay* under *Thyroid*, beginning with "equivalent to about 38 μg of levothyroxine."

Tiagabine Hydrochloride

$C_{20}H_{25}NO_2S_2 \cdot HCl$ 412.02
3-Piperidinecarboxylic acid, 1-[4,4-bis(3-methyl-2-thienyl)-3-butenyl]-, hydrochloride, (R)-.
(−)-(R)-1-[4,4-Bis(3-methyl-2-thienyl)-3-butenyl]nipecotic acid, hydrochloride   [145821-59-6].

» Tiagabine Hydrochloride contains not less than 97.5 percent and not more than 102.5 percent of $C_{20}H_{25}NO_2S_2 \cdot HCl$, calculated on the anhydrous basis.

Packaging and storage—Preserve in tight, light-resistant containers. Store at a temperature not higher than 30°.

USP Reference standards ⟨11⟩—*USP Racemic Tiagabine Hydrochloride Mixture RS. USP Tiagabine Hydrochloride RS. USP Tiagabine Related Compound A RS.*

Identification—
    A: *Infrared Absorption* ⟨197K⟩.
    Test specimen—Transfer about 5 mg of Tiagabine Hydrochloride to a test tube, add 4 mL of 2-propanol, and sonicate if necessary for complete dissolution. Evaporate the solvent under inert atmosphere at 50° using a nitrogen evaporator for 2 hours.
    Standard specimen—A similar preparation of USP Tiagabine Hydrochloride RS.
    B: The retention time of the major peak in the chromatogram of the *Assay preparation* corresponds to that in the chromatogram of the *Standard preparation,* as obtained in the *Assay*.

Water, *Method I* ⟨921⟩:   not more than 6.0%.
Residue on ignition ⟨281⟩:   not more than 0.2%.
Heavy metals, *Method II* ⟨231⟩:   0.002%.

Limit of (S)-(+) isomer—
Mobile phase—Prepare a filtered and degassed mixture of solvent hexane, isopropyl alcohol, alcohol, and trifluoroacetic acid (80 : 14 : 6 : 0.5). Increase or decrease the percentage of hexane or alcohol, but keep the percentage of isopropyl alcohol constant. Make other adjustments if necessary (see *System Suitability* under *Chromatography* ⟨621⟩).

Standard solution—Transfer about 10 mg of USP Racemic Tiagabine Hydrochloride Mixture RS, accurately weighed, to a 100-mL volumetric flask. Add a few drops of methanol to dissolve, dilute with isopropyl alcohol to volume, and mix.

Test solution—Transfer about 50 mg of Tiagabine Hydrochloride, accurately weighed, to a 25-mL volumetric flask; add a few drops of methanol to dissolve; dilute with isopropyl alcohol to volume; and mix.

Chromatographic system (see *Chromatography* ⟨621⟩)—The liquid chromatograph is equipped with a 260-nm detector and a 4.6-mm × 25-cm column that contains packing L40. The flow rate is about 0.8 mL per minute. Chromatograph the *Standard solution*, and record the peak responses as directed for *Procedure:* the relative retention times are about 0.76 for the (S)-(+) isomer and 1.0 for the (R)-(−) isomer; and the resolution, R, between the (S)-(+) and (R)-(−) isomers is not less than 2.0.

Procedure—Inject about 10 μL of the *Test solution* into the chromatograph, record the chromatogram, and measure the responses for the major peaks obtained from the (S)-(+) and (R)-(−) isomers. Calculate the percentage of the (S)-(+) isomer in the portion of Tiagabine Hydrochloride taken by the formula:

$$100r_S / (r_S + r_R)$$

in which r_S and r_R are the peak responses of the (S)-(+) and (R)-(−) isomers, respectively: not more than 0.5% of the (S)-(+) isomer is found.

Chromatographic purity—
Solution A—Use a filtered and degassed solution of water adjusted with phosphoric acid to a pH of 2.3.
Solution B—Use filtered and degassed acetonitrile.
Mobile phase—Use variable mixtures of *Solution A* and *Solution B* as directed for *Chromatographic system*. Make adjustments if necessary (see *System Suitability* under *Chromatography* ⟨621⟩).

Standard stock solution—Dissolve an accurately weighed quantity of USP Tiagabine Hydrochloride RS in water to obtain a solution having a known concentration of about 1 mg per mL.

Standard solution—Dilute a portion of the *Standard stock solution* quantitatively, and stepwise if necessary, with water to obtain a solution having a known concentration of about 0.001 mg per mL.

Resolution solution—Dissolve an accurately weighed quantity of USP Tiagabine Related Compound A RS in water to obtain a solution having a known concentration of about 1 mg per mL. Transfer 1.0 mL of this solution and 1.0 mL of the *Standard stock solution* to a 10-mL volumetric flask, dilute with water to volume, and mix.

Test solution—Transfer about 100 mg of Tiagabine Hydrochloride, accurately weighed, to a 100-mL volumetric flask. Dissolve in and dilute with water to volume, and mix.

Chromatographic system (see *Chromatography* ⟨621⟩)—The liquid chromatograph is equipped with a 254-nm detector and a 4.6-mm × 15-cm column that contains 5-μm packing L1. The flow rate is about 1.0 mL per minute. The chromatograph is programmed as follows.

Time (minutes)	Solution A (%)	Solution B (%)	Elution
0	75	25	equilibration
0–30	75→45	25→55	linear gradient
30–40	45→10	55→90	linear gradient
40–45	10	90	isocratic

Chromatograph the *Resolution solution*, and record the peak responses as directed for *Procedure*: the resolution, R, between tiagabine hydrochloride and tiagabine related compound A is not less than 9.0. Chromatograph the *Standard solution*, and record the peak responses as directed for *Procedure*: the relative standard deviation for replicate injections is not more than 2.0%.

Interference check—Inject water as the blank: no interfering peaks are observed.

Procedure—Separately inject equal volumes (about 20 µL) of the *Standard solution* and the *Test solution* into the chromatograph, record the chromatograms, and measure all the peak responses. Calculate the percentage of each impurity in the portion of Tiagabine Hydrochloride taken by the formula:

$$100F(r_i / r_s)$$

in which F is the relative response factor (see the accompanying table for values) for each impurity; r_i is the peak response for each impurity obtained from the *Test solution*; and r_s is the sum of the responses of all the peaks, excluding the solvent peaks. (See the accompanying table for limits of individual impurities.) Not more than 1.0% of total impurities is found.

Relative Response Factors

Compound Name	Relative Retention Time (approximated)	F	Limit (%)
(R)-1-[4,4-Bis(3-methyl-2-thienyl)-3,4-dihydroxybutyl]-3-piperidinecarboxylic acid	0.51	0.75	0.2
(R)-1-[4,4-Bis(3-methyl-2-thienyl)-3-oxybutyl]-3-piperidinecarboxylic acid	0.79	0.63	0.1
(R)-1-[4-(3-Methyl-2-thienyl)-4-(2-thienyl)-3-butenyl]-3-piperidinecarboxylic acid	0.93	1.00	0.1
Tiagabine	1.0	—	—
(R)-Methyl 1-[[4-(x-methyl-2-thienyl)-4-(y-methyl-2-thienyl)]-3-butenyl]-3-piperidinecarboxylic acid *	1.13	1.00	0.6
(R)-Methyl 1-[4,4-bis(3-methyl-2-thienyl)-3-butenyl]-3-piperidinecarboxylate	1.32	1.01	0.2
Tiagabine related compound A	1.39	1.04	0.2
4,4-Bis(3-methyl-2-thienyl)-3-buten-1-ol	1.98	0.97	0.2
Bis(3-methyl-2-thienyl)methanone	2.27	0.39	0.1
4,4-Bis(3-methyl-2-thienyl)-3-buten-1-ol, methanesulfonate	2.33	0.96	0.1
2,2-Bis(3-methyl-2-thienyl)tetrahydrofuran	2.54	0.94	0.1
Any unknown impurity	—	1.00	0.1

*Where possible x,y combinations include (3,4), (4,3), (4,4), (5,5), (4,5), (5,4), (3,5), and (5,3).

Assay—

Diluent—Prepare a mixture of methanol and water (1 : 1).

Buffer solution—Dissolve 1.38 g of monobasic sodium phosphate in 1000 mL of water, and adjust with phosphoric acid to a pH of 2.0.

Mobile phase—Prepare a filtered and degassed mixture of *Buffer solution* and acetonitrile (65 : 35). Make adjustments if necessary (see *System Suitability* under *Chromatography* ⟨621⟩).

Internal standard preparation—Prepare a solution of butylparaben in *Diluent* having a concentration of about 0.4 mg per mL.

Standard stock preparation—Dissolve an accurately weighed quantity of USP Tiagabine Hydrochloride RS in *Diluent* to obtain a solution having a known concentration of about 1 mg per mL.

Standard preparation—Transfer 10.0 mL of the *Standard stock preparation* and 10.0 mL of the *Internal standard preparation* to a 100-mL volumetric flask, dilute with *Diluent* to volume, and mix.

Assay preparation—Transfer about 100 mg of Tiagabine Hydrochloride, accurately weighed, to a 100-mL volumetric flask; dilute with *Diluent* to volume; and mix. Transfer 10.0 mL of this solution and 10.0 mL of the *Internal standard preparation* to a 100-mL volumetric flask, dilute with *Diluent* to volume, and mix.

Chromatographic system (see *Chromatography* ⟨621⟩)—The liquid chromatograph is equipped with a 254-nm detector and a 4.6-mm × 15-cm column that contains 5-µm packing L1. The flow rate is about 1.0 mL per minute. Chromatograph the *Standard preparation*, and record the peak responses as directed for *Procedure*: the resolution, R, between tiagabine hydrochloride and butylparaben is not less than 5.5; and the relative standard deviation of the peak response ratios for replicate injections is not more than 1.5%.

Procedure—Separately inject equal volumes (about 20 µL) of the *Standard preparation* and the *Assay preparation* into the chromatograph, record the chromatograms, and measure the peak areas. Calculate the quantity, in mg, of $C_{20}H_{25}NO_2S_2 \cdot HCl$ in the portion of Tiagabine Hydrochloride taken by the formula:

$$1000C(R_U / R_S)$$

in which C is the concentration, in mg per mL, of USP Tiagabine Hydrochloride RS in the *Standard preparation*; and R_U and R_S are the peak area ratios of tiagabine hydrochloride to the internal standard obtained from the *Assay preparation* and the *Standard preparation*, respectively.

Tiamulin

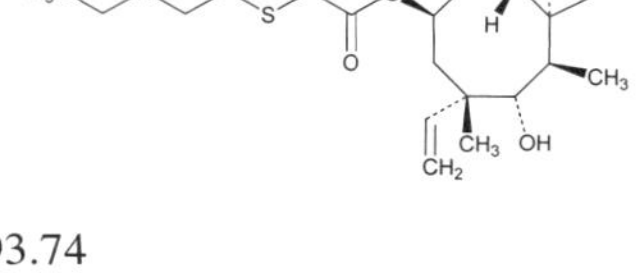

$C_{28}H_{47}NO_4S$ 493.74

Acetic acid, [[2-(diethylamino)ethyl]thio]-, 6-ethenyldecahydro-5-hydroxy-4,6,9,10-tetramethyl-1-oxo-3a,9-propano-3aH-cyclopentacyclooctsen-8-yl ester [3aS-(3aα,4β,5α,6α,8β,9α,9aβ,10S*)]-.

[[2-(Diethylamino)ethyl]thio]acetic acid 8-ester with (3aS,4R,5S,6S,8R,9R,9aR,10R)-octahydro-5,8-dihydroxy-4,6,9,10-tetramethyl-6-vinyl-3a,9-propano-3aH-cyclopentacyclooctsen-1(4H)-one   [55297-95-5].

Tiamulin

» Tiamulin contains not less than 96.5 percent and not more than 102.0 percent of $C_{28}H_{47}NO_4S$, calculated on the dried basis.

Packaging and storage—Preserve in well-closed, light-resistant containers, and store at room temperature.

Labeling—Label it to indicate that it is for veterinary use only.

USP Reference standards ⟨11⟩—*USP Endotoxin RS. USP Tiamulin RS. USP Tiamulin Fumarate RS.*

Clarity and color of solution—Dissolve 2.5 g in methanol, and dilute with methanol to 50.0 mL. The solution is clear, and its absorbance at 420 nm is not more than 0.050 (see *Spectrophotometry and Light-Scattering* ⟨851⟩).

Identification—
  A: *Infrared Absorption* ⟨197K⟩.
  B: The retention time of the tiamulin peak in the chromatogram of the *Assay preparation* corresponds to that in the chromatogram of the *Standard preparation*, as obtained in the *Assay*.

Bacterial endotoxins ⟨85⟩—It contains not more than 0.4 USP Endotoxin Unit per mg.

Loss on drying ⟨731⟩—Dry it at about 80° to constant weight: it loses not more than 1.0% of its weight.

Limit of alcohol and toluene—
  Internal standard solution—To a 100-mL volumetric flask add about 90 mL of dimethylformamide and 150 µL of dioxane, dilute with dimethylformamide to volume, and mix.
  Standard solution—To a 50-mL volumetric flask add about 40 mL of *Internal standard solution*, 100 µL of dehydrated alcohol, and 10 µL of toluene. Dilute with *Internal standard solution* to volume, and mix. Transfer 2 mL of this solution to a 20-mL headspace vial.
  Test solution—Transfer about 200 mg of Tiamulin, accurately weighed, to a 20-mL headspace vial. Add 2 mL of *Internal standard solution*, close the vial, and sonicate to dissolve.
  Chromatographic system (see *Chromatography* ⟨621⟩)—The gas chromatograph is equipped with a headspace injector, a flame-ionization detector, and a 0.530-mm × 30-m capillary column coated with a 1.0-µm film of phase G16 and operated in 1/10 split mode. The carrier gas is helium, flowing at a rate of about 30 mL per minute. The vial is heated to 100°, the injector syringe is heated to 130°, the injection port temperature is maintained at 200°, and the detector temperature is maintained at 250°. The column temperature is programmed to be isothermal at 50° for 8 minutes followed by a linear increase of 40° per minute until the temperature has reached 150°. Chromatograph the *Standard solution*, and record the peak areas as directed for *Procedure*: the relative retention times are about 0.5, 0.9, and 1.0 for alcohol, toluene, and dioxane, respectively; the resolution, R, between toluene and dioxane is not less than 2.0; the tailing factor of toluene and alcohol is not more than 2.0; and the relative standard deviation for triplicate injections, calculated from the ratio between the toluene or alcohol peak relative to the internal standard peak, is not more than 5.0%.
  Procedure—Separately inject equal volumes (about 1.0 mL) of the headspace of the *Standard solution* and the *Test solution* into the chromatograph, record the chromatograms, and measure the peak responses for alcohol, toluene, and dioxane. Calculate the percentages (w/w) of alcohol and toluene in the portion of Tiamulin taken by the formula:

$$0.04P(DV/W_U)(R_U/R_S)$$

in which P is the percent purity of the solvent of interest in the *Standard solution*; D is the density, in mg per mL, of the solvent of interest used to prepare the *Standard solution*; V is the volume, in mL, of the solvent of interest used to prepare the *Standard solution*; W_U is the weight, in mg, of Tiamulin taken to prepare the *Test solution*; and R_U and R_S are the peak response ratios of the solvents of interest obtained from the *Test solution* and the *Standard solution*, respectively: not more than 1.0% of alcohol is found, not more than 0.08% of toluene is found, and not more than 1.0% of alcohol plus toluene is found.

Related compounds—
  Ammonium carbonate buffer, Mobile phase, and *Diluent*—Proceed as directed in the *Assay*.
  Standard solution—Use the *Standard preparation*, prepared as directed in the *Assay*.
  Toluene solution—Transfer 0.1 mL of toluene to a 100-mL volumetric flask, dilute with acetonitrile to volume, and mix. Transfer 0.1 mL of this solution to another 100-mL volumetric flask, dilute with *Diluent* to volume, and mix.
  Test solution 1—Use the *Assay preparation*.
  Test solution 2—Add 1.0 mL of *Test solution 1* to a 100-mL volumetric flask, dilute with *Diluent* to volume, and mix.
  Chromatographic system—Proceed as directed in the *Assay*. Chromatograph the *Standard solution*, and record the peak areas as directed for *Procedure*: the relative retention times of possible tiamulin-related impurities relative to tiamulin are about 0.22 for mutilin, 0.50 for 2-(benzylsulfanyl)-N,N-diethylethanamine, 0.66 for 2,2'-(disulfane-1,2-diyl)bis(N,N-diethylethanamine), 1.1 for hydroxy-11-oxotiamulin, 1.6 for 1-hydroxy-11-oxotiamulin, and 2.4 for 11-oxotiamulin. [NOTE—Impurities are not limited to those listed above.]
  Procedure—Separately inject equal volumes (about 20 µL) of the *Standard solution*, *Toluene solution*, *Test solution 1*, and *Test solution 2* into the chromatograph, record the chromatograms, identify the peaks, and measure the areas for the major peaks. Disregarding the toluene peak and any peak in the chromatogram of *Test solution 1* less than 0.1 times the area of the principal peak in the chromatogram obtained with *Test solution 2*, calculate the area percentage of each impurity, relative to tiamulin, in the portion of Tiamulin taken by the formula:

$$(r_i / r_S)$$

in which r_i is the peak area of each individual impurity obtained from *Test solution 1;* and r_S is the peak area of Tiamulin obtained from *Test solution 2:* not more than 1.0% of any identified impurity is found; not more than 0.2% of any unidentified impurity is found; and not more than 3.0% of total impurities is found.

Assay—
  Ammonium carbonate buffer—Dissolve 10.0 g of ammonium carbonate in water, add 22 mL of perchloric acid TS, and dilute with water to 1000 mL. Adjust with ammonium hydroxide to a pH of 10.0.
  Mobile phase—Mix 490 mL of methanol, 300 mL of *Ammonium carbonate buffer*, and 210 mL of acetonitrile.
  Diluent—Mix 500 mL of *Ammonium carbonate buffer* and 500 mL of acetonitrile.
  Standard preparation—Dissolve an accurately weighed quantity of USP Tiamulin Fumarate RS in *Diluent* to obtain a solution having a known concentration of about 5.0 mg per mL.
  Assay preparation—Dissolve an accurately weighed quantity of Tiamulin in *Diluent* to obtain a solution having a known concentration of about 4.0 mg per mL.
  Chromatographic system (see *Chromatography* ⟨621⟩)—The liquid chromatograph is equipped with a 212-nm detector and a 4.6-mm × 15-cm column that contains 5-µm packing L1. The flow rate is about 1.0 mL per minute. Chromatograph the *Standard preparation*, and record the peak areas as directed for *Procedure*: the resolution, R, between tiamulin and its subsequent peak is not less than 2.
  Procedure—Separately inject equal volumes (about 20 µL) of the *Standard preparation* and the *Assay preparation* into the chromatograph, record the chromatograms, and measure the responses for the major peaks. Calculate the percentage of $C_{28}H_{47}NO_4S$ in the portion of Tiamulin taken by the formula:

$$P(C_S / C_U)(r_U / r_S)$$

in which P is the labeled percentage of tiamulin in USP Tiamulin Fumarate RS; C_S and C_U are the concentrations, in mg per mL, of the *Standard preparation* and the *Assay preparation*, respectively; and r_U and r_S are the peak areas of tiamulin obtained from the *Assay preparation* and *Standard preparation*, respectively.

Tiamulin Fumarate

$C_{28}H_{47}NO_4S \cdot C_4H_4O_4$ 609.82
Tiamulin Hydrogen Fumarate.
Acetic acid, [[2-(diethylaminoethyl]thio]-, 6-ethenyl-decahydro-5-hydroxy-4,6,9,10-tetramethyl-1-oxo-3a,9-propano-3a*H*-cyclopentacycloocten-8-yl   ester   [3a*S*-(3aα,4β,5α,6α,8β,9α,9aβ,10*S**)]-, (*E*)-2-butenedioate (1 : 1) (salt).
[[2-(Diethylamino)ethyl]thio]acetic acid 8-ester with (3a*S*,4*R*,5*S*,6*S*,8*R*,9*R*,9a*R*,10*R*)-octahydro-5,8-dihydroxy-4,6,9,10-tetramethyl-6-vinyl-3a,9-propano-3a*H*-cyclopentacycloocten-1(4*H*)-one fumarate (1 : 1) (salt)   [55297-96-6].

» Tiamulin Fumarate contains not less than 97.0 percent and not more than 102.0 percent of $C_{28}H_{47}NO_4S \cdot C_4H_4O_4$, calculated on the dried basis.

Packaging and storage—Preserve in tight, light-resistant containers, and store at room temperature.
Labeling—Label it to indicate that it is for veterinary use only.

USP Reference standards ⟨11⟩—*USP Tiamulin Fumarate RS. USP Tiamulin Related Compound A RS.*
Color and clarity of solution—Transfer about 5.0 g of Tiamulin Fumarate to a 100-mL volumetric flask, and dissolve in and dilute with water to volume: the solution is clear and colorless, and the absorbance of the solution, determined in a 1-cm cell at 400 and 650 nm, is not greater than 0.150 and 0.030 absorbance units, respectively.
Identification—
  A: *Infrared Absorption* ⟨197K⟩—[NOTE—Intimately mix Tiamulin Fumarate with potassium bromide, but do not grind.]
  B: The retention time of the tiamulin fumarate peak in the chromatogram of the *Assay preparation* corresponds to that in the chromatogram of the *Standard preparation*, as obtained in the *Assay*.
Melting temperature ⟨741⟩:   between 143° and 152°.
Specific rotation ⟨781S⟩:   between +24° and +28°, on the dried basis, measured at 20°.
  Test solution: 5.0 mg per mL, in dioxane.
pH ⟨791⟩:   between 3.1 and 4.1.
  Test solution: 1.0 g per 100 mL of water.
Loss on drying ⟨731⟩—Dry it in vacuum at 105° for 3 hours: it loses not more than 0.5% of its weight.
Residue on ignition ⟨281⟩:   not more than 0.1%.
Heavy metals, *Method II* ⟨231⟩:   not more than 0.001%.
Limit of residual solvents—
  Internal standard solution—Dilute 0.3 mL of *n*-butanol to 1000 mL.
  Standard solution—Transfer about 500 mg each of acetone, ethyl acetate, and isobutyl acetate, each accurately weighed, to a 250-mL volumetric flask, dilute with the *Internal standard solution* to volume, and mix. Transfer 2.5 mL of the solution so obtained to a 20-mL volumetric flask, dilute with the *Internal standard solution* to volume, and mix.
  Test solution—Transfer about 1 g of Tiamulin Fumarate, accurately weighed, to a 20-mL volumetric flask, dissolve in and dilute with the *Internal standard solution* to volume, and mix.
  Chromatographic system (see *Chromatography* ⟨621⟩)—The gas chromatograph is equipped with a flame-ionization detector and a 0.25-mm × 30-m capillary column coated with a 0.5-µm film of phase G16. The carrier gas is helium, flowing at a rate of 1.07 mL per minute, and the split flow ratio is 50 : 1. The column temperature is maintained at 75°, the injection port temperature is maintained at 250°, and the detector temperature is maintained at 300°. Chromatograph the *Standard solution*, and record the peak responses as directed for *Procedure:* the relative retention times are about 0.34, 0.38, 0.57, and 1.0 for acetone, ethyl acetate, isobutyl acetate, and *n*-butanol, respectively; the resolution, *R*, between acetone and ethyl acetate is not less than 2.0; the tailing factor for each of the analyte peaks is not more than 2; and the relative standard deviation for replicate injections is not more than 2%.
  Procedure—Separately inject equal volumes (about 1.0 µL) of the *Standard solution* and the *Test solution* into the chromatograph, record the chromatograms, and measure the peak responses for acetone, ethyl acetate, isobutyl acetate, and *n*-butanol. Calculate the percentages of acetone, ethyl acetate, and isobutyl acetate in the portion of Tiamulin Fumarate taken by the formula:

$$(W_S / W_U)(R_U / R_S)$$

in which W_S is the weight, in mg, of the solvent of interest taken to prepare the *Standard solution;* W_U is the weight, in mg, of Tiamulin Fumarate taken to prepare the *Test solution;* and R_U and R_S are the peak response ratios of the solvent of interest to the internal standard obtained from the *Test solution* and the *Standard solution*, respectively: not more than 0.5% each of acetone, ethyl acetate, and isobutyl acetate is found; and the sum of the percentages of acetone, ethyl acetate, and isobutyl acetate is not more than 0.5%.
Chromatographic purity—
  Dilute perchloric acid solution, Buffer solution, Mobile phase, System suitability solution, and *Chromatographic system*—Proceed as directed in the *Assay*.
  Standard solution—Use the *Standard preparation* prepared as directed in the *Assay*.
  Test solution—Use the *Assay preparation* prepared as directed in the *Assay*.
  Procedure—Separately inject equal volumes (about 20 µL) of the *Standard solution* and the *Test solution* into the chromatograph, record the chromatogram, identify the tiamulin fumarate peak, and measure all the peak responses. [NOTE—Possible tiamulin fumarate impurities include, but are not limited to, pleuromutilin, mutilin, 14-acetyl mutilin, 11-monoacetyl mutilin, tiamulin related compound A, 11,14-diacetyl mutilin, 8-dimethylderivative, bisdimethylthioderivative, and 11-ketoderivative, their retention times, relative to tiamulin fumarate, being about 0.25, 0.3, 0.5, 0.6, 0.8, 1.1, 1.3, 1.4, and 2.3, respectively.] Calculate the area percentage of each impurity, relative to tiamulin fumarate, in the portion of Tiamulin Fumarate taken by the formula:

$$100(r_i / r_U)$$

in which r_i and r_U are the peak responses of each impurity and tiamulin fumarate, respectively: not more than 1.0% of any identified impurity is found; not more than 0.5% of any unidentified impurity is found; and not more than 3.0% of total impurities is found.
Content of fumarate—Dissolve about 450 mg of Tiamulin Fumarate, accurately weighed, in 60 mL of a mixture of alcohol and water (1 : 1). Titrate with 0.1 N sodium hydroxide VS, determining the endpoint potentiometrically, using a glass–calomel electrode (see *Titrimetry* ⟨541⟩). Perform a blank determination, and make any necessary correction. Each mL of 0.1 N sodium hydroxide is equivalent to 5.8 mg of fumarate: between 83.7 and 87.3 mg of fumarate is found.
Assay—
  Dilute perchloric acid solution—Prepare a solution containing 6% of perchloric acid.
  Buffer solution—Transfer 10 g of ammonium carbonate to a 1000-mL volumetric flask, and dissolve in about 800 mL of water. Add 24 mL of *Dilute perchloric acid solution*, dilute with water to volume, mix, and filter.
  Mobile phase—Prepare a mixture of methanol, *Buffer solution,* and acetonitrile, (49 : 28 : 23), filter, and degas.
  System suitability solution—Dissolve accurately weighed quantities of USP Tiamulin Fumarate RS and USP Tiamulin Related Compound A RS in *Mobile phase* to obtain a solution having known concentrations of about 0.08 mg of each per mL.
  Standard preparation—Dissolve an accurately weighed quantity of USP Tiamulin Fumarate RS in *Mobile phase* to obtain a solution having a known concentration of about 4 mg per mL.

Assay preparation—Transfer about 200 mg of Tiamulin Fumarate, accurately weighed, to a 50-mL volumetric flask, dissolve in and dilute with *Mobile phase* to volume, and mix.

Chromatographic system (see *Chromatography* ⟨621⟩)—The liquid chromatograph is equipped with a 212-nm detector and a 4.6-mm × 25-cm column that contains 5-μm packing L1. The flow rate is about 1.2 mL per minute. The column temperature is maintained at 30 ± 3°. Chromatograph the *Standard preparation* and the *System suitability solution,* and record the peak responses as directed for *Procedure:* the tiamulin related compound A peak elutes prior to the tiamulin fumarate peak; the resolution, *R,* between tiamulin related compound A and tiamulin fumarate is not less than 2.0; the capacity factor, *k',* determined from the tiamulin fumarate peak, is not less than 2.0; the column efficiency is not less than 14,000 theoretical plates; the tailing factor is not more than 2.0; and the relative standard deviation for replicate injections is not more than 2.0%.

Procedure—Separately inject equal volumes (about 20 μL) of the *Standard preparation* and the *Assay preparation* into the chromatograph, record the chromatograms, and measure the responses for the major peaks. Calculate the quantity, in mg, of $C_{28}H_{47}NO_4S \cdot C_4H_4O_4$ in the portion of Tiamulin Fumarate taken by the formula:

$$50C(r_U / r_S)$$

in which *C* is the concentration, in mg per mL, of USP Tiamulin Fumarate RS in the *Standard preparation;* and r_U and r_S are the tiamulin fumarate peak responses obtained from the *Assay preparation* and the *Standard preparation,* respectively.

Ticarcillin Disodium

$C_{15}H_{14}N_2Na_2O_6S_2$ 428.40

4-Thia-1-azabicyclo[3.2.0]heptane-2-carboxylic acid, 6-(carboxy-3-thienylacetyl)amino-3,3-dimethyl-7-oxo-, disodium salt, [2*S*-2α,5α,6β(*S**)]-.

N-(2-Carboxy-3,3-dimethyl-7-oxo-4-thia-1-azabicyclo[3.2.0]hept-6-yl)-3-thiophenemalonamic acid disodium salt   [4697-14-7].

» Ticarcillin Disodium has a potency equivalent to not less than 800 μg of ticarcillin ($C_{15}H_{16}N_2O_6S_2$) per mg, calculated on the anhydrous basis.

Packaging and storage—Preserve in tight containers.
Labeling—Where it is intended for use in preparing injectable dosage forms, the label states that it is sterile or must be subjected to further processing during the preparation of injectable dosage forms.
USP Reference standards ⟨11⟩—*USP Endotoxin RS. USP Ticarcillin Monosodium Monohydrate RS.*
Identification—
  A: *Ultraviolet Absorption* ⟨197U⟩—
  Solution: 20 μg per mL. Use the solution prepared as directed in the test for *Ticarcillin content,* recording the spectrum between 200 and 300 nm.
  B: A solution (1 in 20) responds to the tests for *Sodium* ⟨191⟩.
Specific rotation ⟨781S⟩:   between +172° and +187°.
  Test solution: 10 mg per mL, in water.
pH ⟨791⟩:   between 6.0 and 8.0, in a solution containing 10 mg of ticarcillin per mL.
Water, *Method I* ⟨921⟩:   not more than 6.0%.
Dimethylaniline ⟨223⟩:   meets the requirement.
Ticarcillin content—Transfer about 40 mg, accurately weighed, to a 100-mL volumetric flask, dissolve in and dilute with water to volume, and mix. Transfer 5.0 mL of this solution to another 100-mL volumetric flask, dilute with 0.1 N methanolic hydrochloric acid (0.8 mL of hydrochloric acid diluted with methanol to 100 mL) to volume, and mix. Concomitantly determine the absorbances of this test solution with a similarly prepared Standard solution of USP Ticarcillin Monosodium Monohydrate RS, at the wavelength of maximum absorbance at about 230 nm, using a reagent blank. Calculate the percentage of ticarcillin ($C_{15}H_{16}N_2O_6S_2$) taken by the formula:

$$P(W_S / W_U)(A_U / A_S)$$

in which *P* is the percentage content of ticarcillin in USP Ticarcillin Monosodium Monohydrate RS; W_S and W_U are the amounts of USP Ticarcillin Monosodium Monohydrate RS and Ticarcillin Disodium taken, respectively; and A_U and A_S are the absorbances of the test solution and the Standard solution, respectively: between 80.0% and 94.0%, calculated on the anhydrous basis, is found.
Other requirements—Where the label states that Ticarcillin Disodium is sterile, it meets the requirements for *Sterility Tests* ⟨71⟩ and for *Bacterial endotoxins* under *Ticarcillin for Injection.* Where the label states that Ticarcillin Disodium must be subjected to further processing during the preparation of injectable dosage forms, it meets the requirements for *Bacterial endotoxins* under *Ticarcillin for Injection.*
Assay—
  pH 4.3 sodium phosphate buffer, Mobile phase, pH 6.4 sodium phosphate buffer, Standard preparation, Resolution solution, and *Chromatographic system*—Proceed as directed in the *Assay* under *Ticarcillin Monosodium.*
  Assay preparation—Transfer about 50 mg of Ticarcillin Disodium, accurately weighed, to a 50-mL volumetric flask, add *pH 6.4 sodium phosphate buffer* to volume, and mix.
  Procedure—Proceed as directed for *Procedure* in the *Assay* under *Ticarcillin Monosodium.* Calculate the quantity, in μg, of ticarcillin ($C_{15}H_{16}N_2O_6S_2$) per mg of the Ticarcillin Disodium taken by the formula:

$$50(CP / M)(r_U / r_S)$$

in which *C* is the concentration, in mg per mL, of USP Ticarcillin Monosodium Monohydrate RS in the *Standard preparation;* *P* is the designated potency, in μg of ticarcillin per mg, of USP Ticarcillin Monosodium Monohydrate RS; *M* is the quantity, in mg, of Ticarcillin Disodium taken to prepare the *Assay preparation;* and r_U and r_S are the ticarcillin peak responses obtained from the *Assay preparation* and the *Standard preparation,* respectively.

Ticarcillin for Injection

» Ticarcillin for Injection contains an amount of Ticarcillin Disodium equivalent to not less than 90.0 percent and not more than 115.0 percent of the labeled amount of ticarcillin ($C_{15}H_{16}N_2O_6S_2$).

Packaging and storage—Preserve in *Containers for Sterile Solids* as described under *Injections* ⟨1⟩.
USP Reference standards ⟨11⟩—*USP Endotoxin RS. USP Ticarcillin Monosodium Monohydrate RS.*
Constituted solution—At the time of use, it meets the requirements for *Constituted Solutions* under *Injections* ⟨1⟩.
Bacterial endotoxins ⟨85⟩—It contains not more than 0.05 USP Endotoxin Unit per mg of ticarcillin.
Sterility ⟨71⟩—It meets the requirements when tested as directed for *Membrane Filtration* under *Test for Sterility of the Product to be Examined.*
pH ⟨791⟩:   between 6.0 and 8.0, in the solution constituted as directed in the labeling.
Water, *Method I* ⟨921⟩:   not more than 6.0%.
Particulate matter ⟨788⟩:   meets the requirements for small-volume injections.
Other requirements—It responds to the *Identification* tests and meets the requirements for *Water* and *Dimethylaniline* under *Ticarcillin Disodium.* It meets also the requirements for *Uniformity of Dosage Units* ⟨905⟩ and *Labeling* under *Injections* ⟨1⟩. Ticarcillin

for Injection that contains no added substances meets also the requirements for *Specific rotation* and *Ticarcillin content* under *Ticarcillin Disodium*.

Assay—

pH 4.3 sodium phosphate buffer, Mobile phase, pH 6.4 sodium phosphate buffer, Standard preparation, Resolution solution, and *Chromatographic system*—Proceed as directed in the *Assay* under *Ticarcillin Monosodium*.

Assay preparation 1 (where it is represented as being in a single-dose container)—Constitute Ticarcillin for Injection as directed in the labeling. Withdraw all of the withdrawable contents, and dilute quantitatively with *pH 6.4 sodium phosphate buffer* to obtain a solution having a concentration of about 0.9 mg of ticarcillin ($C_{15}H_{16}N_2O_6S_2$) per mL.

Assay preparation 2 (where the label states the quantity of ticarcillin in a given volume of constituted solution)—Constitute Ticarcillin for Injection as directed in the labeling. Dilute an accurately measured volume of the constituted solution quantitatively with *pH 6.4 sodium phosphate buffer* to obtain a solution having a concentration of about 0.9 mg of ticarcillin ($C_{15}H_{16}N_2O_6S_2$) per mL.

Procedure—Proceed as directed for *Procedure* in the *Assay* under *Ticarcillin Monosodium*. Calculate the quantity, in mg, of ticarcillin ($C_{15}H_{16}N_2O_6S_2$) withdrawn from the container or in the volume of constituted solution taken by the formula:

$$(L / D)(CP / 1000)(r_U / r_S)$$

in which L is the labeled quantity, in mg per mL, of ticarcillin ($C_{15}H_{16}N_2O_6S_2$) in the container or in the volume of constituted solution taken; D is the concentration, in mg per mL, of ticarcillin in *Assay preparation 1* or *Assay preparation 2*, based on the labeled quantity in the container or in the portion of constituted solution taken, and the extent of dilution; C is the concentration, in mg per mL, of USP Ticarcillin Monosodium Monohydrate RS in the *Standard preparation*; P is the designated potency, in μg of ticarcillin per mg, of USP Ticarcillin Monosodium Monohydrate RS; and r_U and r_S are the ticarcillin peak responses obtained from the *Assay preparation* and the *Standard preparation*, respectively.

Ticarcillin and Clavulanic Acid Injection

» Ticarcillin and Clavulanic Acid Injection is a sterile isoosmotic solution of Ticarcillin Monosodium and Clavulanate Potassium in Water for Injection. It contains one or more suitable buffering agents and a tonicity-adjusting agent. It contains the equivalent of not less than 90.0 percent and not more than 115.0 percent of the labeled amount of ticarcillin ($C_{15}H_{16}N_2O_6S_2$) and the equivalent of not less than 85.0 percent and not more than 120.0 percent of the labeled amount of clavulanic acid ($C_8H_9NO_5$).

Packaging and storage—Preserve in *Containers for Injections* as described under *Injections* ⟨1⟩. Maintain in the frozen state.

Labeling—It meets the requirements for *Labeling* under *Injections* ⟨1⟩. The label states that it is to be thawed just prior to use, describes conditions for proper storage of the resultant solution, and directs that the solution is not to be refrozen.

USP Reference standards ⟨11⟩—*USP Clavulanate Lithium RS. USP Endotoxin RS. USP Ticarcillin Monosodium Monohydrate RS.*

Identification—The chromatogram of the *Assay preparation* obtained as directed in the *Assay* exhibits a major peak for ticarcillin, the retention time of which corresponds to that exhibited in the chromatogram of the *Standard preparation* obtained as directed in the *Assay*.

Bacterial endotoxins ⟨85⟩—It contains not more than 0.07 USP Endotoxin Unit per mg of ticarcillin.

Sterility ⟨71⟩—It meets the requirements when tested as directed for *Membrane Filtration* under *Test for Sterility of the Product to be Examined*.

pH ⟨791⟩: between 5.5 and 7.5.

Particulate matter ⟨788⟩: meets the requirements for small-volume injections.

Other requirements—It meets the requirements for *Uniformity of Dosage Units* ⟨905⟩ and for *Labeling* under *Injections* ⟨1⟩.

Assay—

pH 4.3 sodium phosphate buffer, Mobile phase, pH 6.4 phosphate buffer, Clavulanate lithium stock standard solution, Standard preparation, and *Chromatographic system*—Proceed as directed in the *Assay* under *Ticarcillin and Clavulanic Acid for Injection*.

Assay preparation—Allow a container of Injection to thaw, and mix the solution. Dilute an accurately measured volume of Injection quantitatively, and stepwise if necessary, with *pH 6.4 phosphate buffer* to obtain a solution having a concentration of about 0.9 mg of ticarcillin ($C_{15}H_{16}N_2O_6S_2$) per mL.

Procedure—Proceed as directed for *Procedure* in the *Assay* under *Ticarcillin and Clavulanic Acid for Injection*. Calculate the quantity, in mg, of ticarcillin ($C_{15}H_{16}N_2O_6S_2$) in each mL of the Injection taken by the formula:

$$(L / D)(CP / 1000)(r_U / r_S)$$

in which L is the labeled quantity, in mg per mL, of ticarcillin ($C_{15}H_{16}N_2O_6S_2$) in the Injection; D is the concentration, in mg per mL, of ticarcillin in the *Assay preparation*, based on the labeled quantity and the extent of dilution; C is the concentration, in mg per mL, of USP Ticarcillin Monosodium Monohydrate RS in the *Standard preparation*; P is the designated potency, in μg of ticarcillin per mg, of USP Ticarcillin Monosodium Monohydrate RS; and r_U and r_S are the ticarcillin peak responses obtained from the *Assay preparation* and the *Standard preparation*, respectively.

Calculate the quantity, in mg, of clavulanic acid ($C_8H_9NO_5$) in each mL of the Injection taken by the formula:

$$(L / D)(CP / 1000)(r_U / r_S)$$

in which L is the labeled quantity, in mg per mL, of clavulanic acid ($C_8H_9NO_5$) in the Injection; D is the concentration, in mg per mL, of clavulanic acid in the *Assay preparation*, based on the labeled quantity and the extent of dilution; C is the concentration, in mg per mL, of USP Clavulanate Lithium RS in the *Standard preparation*; P is the designated potency, in μg of clavulanic acid per mg, of USP Clavulanate Lithium RS; and r_U and r_S are the clavulanic acid peak responses obtained from the *Assay preparation* and the *Standard preparation*, respectively.

Ticarcillin and Clavulanic Acid for Injection

» Ticarcillin and Clavulanic Acid for Injection is a sterile, dry mixture of Ticarcillin Disodium and Clavulanate Potassium. It contains the equivalent of not less than 90.0 percent and not more than 115.0 percent of the labeled amount of ticarcillin ($C_{15}H_{16}N_2O_6S_2$) and the equivalent of not less than 85.0 percent and not more than 120.0 percent of the labeled amount of clavulanic acid ($C_8H_9NO_5$), the labeled amounts representing proportions of ticarcillin to clavulanic acid of 15 : 1 or 30 : 1.

Packaging and storage—Preserve in *Containers for Sterile Solids* as described under *Injections* ⟨1⟩.

USP Reference standards ⟨11⟩—*USP Clavulanate Lithium RS. USP Endotoxin RS. USP Ticarcillin Monosodium Monohydrate RS.*

Constituted solution—At the time of use, it meets the requirements for *Constituted Solutions* under *Injections* ⟨1⟩.

Identification—The retention times of the major peaks in the chromatogram of the *Assay preparation* correspond to those in the chromatogram of the *Standard preparation*, as obtained in the *Assay*.

Bacterial endotoxins ⟨85⟩—It contains not more than 0.07 USP Endotoxin Unit per mg of ticarcillin.

Sterility ⟨71⟩—It meets the requirements when tested as directed for *Membrane Filtration* under *Test for Sterility of the Product to be Examined*.

pH ⟨791⟩: between 5.5 and 7.5, in a solution (1 in 10).

Water, *Method I* ⟨921⟩: not more than 4.2%.

Particulate matter ⟨788⟩: meets the requirements for small-volume injections.

Other requirements—It meets the requirements for *Uniformity of Dosage Units* ⟨905⟩ and for *Labeling* under *Injections* ⟨1⟩.

Assay—
pH 4.3 sodium phosphate buffer—Dissolve 13.8 g of monobasic sodium phosphate in 900 mL of water, adjust with phosphoric acid or 10 N sodium hydroxide to a pH of 4.3 ± 0.1, dilute with water to make 1000 mL, and mix.

Mobile phase—Prepare a suitable mixture of *pH 4.3 sodium phosphate buffer* and acetonitrile (95 : 5), and pass through a membrane filter of 0.5-μm or finer porosity. Make adjustments if necessary (see *System Suitability* under *Chromatography* ⟨621⟩).

pH 6.4 sodium phosphate buffer—Dissolve 6.9 g of monobasic sodium phosphate in 900 mL of water, adjust with 10 N sodium hydroxide to a pH of 6.4 ± 0.1, dilute with water to make 1000 mL, and mix.

Clavulanate lithium stock standard solution—Dissolve an accurately weighed quantity of USP Clavulanate Lithium RS in *pH 6.4 sodium phosphate buffer* to obtain a solution having a known concentration of about 0.6 mg per mL.

Standard preparation—Transfer about 100 mg of USP Ticarcillin Monosodium Monohydrate RS, accurately weighed, to a 100-mL volumetric flask, add 150/*J* mL of *Clavulanate lithium stock standard solution*, accurately measured, *J* being the ratio of the labeled amount, in mg, of ticarcillin to the labeled amount, in mg, of clavulanic acid in the Ticarcillin Disodium and Clavulanic Acid for Injection, dilute with *pH 6.4 sodium phosphate buffer* to volume, and mix.

Assay preparation—Dissolve the contents of 1 container of Ticarcillin and Clavulanic Acid for Injection in a volume of water, accurately measured, corresponding to the volume of solvent specified in the labeling. Using a suitable hypodermic needle and syringe, remove all of the withdrawable contents from the container, and dilute quantitatively and stepwise with *pH 6.4 sodium phosphate buffer* to obtain a solution having a concentration of about 0.9 mg of ticarcillin ($C_{15}H_{16}N_2O_6S_2$) per mL.

Chromatographic system (see *Chromatography* ⟨621⟩)—The liquid chromatograph is equipped with a 220-nm detector and a 4-mm × 30-cm column that contains 3- to 10-μm packing L1. The flow rate is about 2 mL per minute. Chromatograph the *Standard preparation*, and record the peak responses as directed for *Procedure:* the relative retention times are about 0.2 for clavulanic acid and 1.0 for ticarcillin; the column efficiency determined from the analyte peaks is not less than 1000 theoretical plates; the tailing factors for the analyte peaks are not more than 2.0; the resolution, *R*, between the ticarcillin and clavulanic acid peaks is not less than 5.0; and the relative standard deviation for replicate injections is not more than 2.0%.

Procedure—Separately inject equal volumes (about 20 μL) of the *Standard preparation* and the *Assay preparations* into the chromatograph, record the chromatograms, and measure the responses for the major peaks. Calculate the quantity, in mg, of ticarcillin ($C_{15}H_{16}N_2O_6S_2$) in the container of Ticarcillin and Clavulanic Acid for Injection taken by the formula:

$$(L/D)(CP/1000)(r_U/r_S)$$

in which *L* is the labeled quantity, in mg, of ticarcillin in the container; *D* is the concentration, in mg per mL, of ticarcillin in the *Assay preparation* on the basis of the labeled quantity of ticarcillin in the container and the extent of dilution; *C* is the concentration, in mg per mL, of USP Ticarcillin Monosodium Monohydrate RS in the *Standard preparation*; *P* is the designated potency, in μg of ticarcillin per mg, of USP Ticarcillin Monosodium Monohydrate RS; and r_U and r_S are the ticarcillin peak responses obtained from the *Assay preparation* and the *Standard preparation*, respectively.

Calculate the quantity, in mg, of clavulanic acid ($C_8H_9NO_5$) in the container of Ticarcillin and Clavulanic Acid for Injection taken by the formula:

$$(L/D)(CP/1000)(r_U/r_S)$$

in which *L* is the labeled quantity, in mg, of clavulanic acid in the container; *D* is the concentration, in mg per mL, of clavulanic acid in the *Assay preparation* on the basis of the labeled quantity of clavulanic acid in the container and the extent of dilution; *C* is the concentration, in mg per mL, of USP Clavulanate Lithium RS in the *Standard preparation; P* is the designated potency, in μg of clavulanic acid per mg, of USP Clavulanate Lithium RS; and r_U and r_S are the clavulanic acid peak responses obtained from the *Assay preparation* and the *Standard preparation*, respectively.

Ticarcillin Monosodium

$C_{15}H_{15}N_2NaO_6S_2 \cdot H_2O$ 424.43

4-Thia-1-azabicyclo[3.2.0]heptane-2-carboxylic acid, 6-[(carboxy-3-thienylacetyl)amino]-3,3-dimethyl-7-oxo, monosodium salt, [2S-2α,5α,6β(S*)]-, monohydrate.

(*R*)-*N*-[(2S,5R,6R)-2-Carboxy-3,4-dimethyl-7-oxo-4-thia-1-azabicyclo[3.2.0]hept-6-yl-]3-thiophenemalonamic acid monosodium salt.

Anhydrous   406.42   [74682-62-5].

» Ticarcillin Monosodium contains the equivalent of not less than 890 μg of ticarcillin ($C_{15}H_{16}N_2O_6S_2$) per mg, calculated on the anhydrous basis.

Packaging and storage—Preserve in tight containers.

Labeling—Where it is intended for use in preparing injectable dosage forms, the label states that it is sterile or must be subjected to further processing during the preparation of injectable dosage forms.

USP Reference standards ⟨11⟩—*USP Clavulanate Lithium RS. USP Endotoxin RS. USP Ticarcillin Monosodium Monohydrate RS.*

Identification—
A: *Infrared Absorption* ⟨197K⟩.
B: *Ultraviolet Absorption* ⟨197U⟩—
Solution: 20 μg per mL, obtained as follows. Transfer about 40 mg, accurately weighed, to a 100-mL volumetric flask, dissolve in and dilute with water to volume, and mix. Transfer 5.0 mL of this solution to a second 100-mL volumetric flask, dilute with 0.1 N methanolic hydrochloric acid (0.8 mL of hydrochloric acid diluted with methanol to 100 mL) to volume, and mix. Record the spectrum between 200 and 300 nm.
C: A solution (1 in 20) responds to the tests for *Sodium* ⟨191⟩.

Specific rotation ⟨781S⟩: between +181° and +197°.
Test solution: 10 mg per mL, in *pH 6.4 sodium phosphate buffer*, prepared as directed in the *Assay*.

Crystallinity ⟨695⟩: meets the requirements.

pH ⟨791⟩: between 2.5 and 4.0, in a solution containing the equivalent of 10 mg of ticarcillin per mL.

Water, *Method I* ⟨921⟩: between 4.0% and 6.0%.

Dimethylaniline ⟨223⟩: meets the requirement.

Other requirements—Where the label states that Ticarcillin Monosodium is sterile, it meets the requirements for *Sterility* ⟨71⟩ and for *Bacterial endotoxins* under *Ticarcillin for Injection*. Where the label states that Ticarcillin Monosodium must be subjected to further processing during the preparation of injectable dosage forms, it meets the requirements for *Bacterial endotoxins* under *Ticarcillin for Injection*.

Assay—
pH 4.3 sodium phosphate buffer—Dissolve 13.8 g of monobasic sodium phosphate in 900 mL of water, adjust with phosphoric acid or 10 N sodium hydroxide to a pH of 4.3 ± 0.1, dilute with water to make 1000 mL, and mix.

Mobile phase—Prepare a suitable mixture of *pH 4.3 sodium phosphate buffer* and acetonitrile (95 : 5), and pass through a membrane filter of 0.5-μm or finer porosity. Make adjustments if necessary (see *System Suitability* under *Chromatography* ⟨621⟩).

pH 6.4 sodium phosphate buffer—Dissolve 6.9 g of monobasic sodium phosphate in 900 mL of water, adjust with 10 N sodium hydroxide to a pH of 6.4 ± 0.1, dilute with water to make 1000 mL, and mix.

Standard preparation—Transfer about 50 mg of USP Ticarcillin Monosodium Monohydrate RS, accurately weighed, to a 50-mL volumetric flask, dilute with *pH 6.4 sodium phosphate buffer* to volume, and mix.

Resolution solution—Transfer about 25 mg of USP Ticarcillin Monosodium Monohydrate RS, accurately weighed, to a 25-mL volumetric flask. Prepare a solution of USP Clavulanate Lithium RS in *pH 6.4 sodium phosphate buffer* containing the equivalent of about 0.15 mg of clavulanic acid per mL. Place 5 mL of this solution in the 25-mL volumetric flask, dilute with *pH 6.4 sodium phosphate buffer* to volume, and mix. [NOTE—Use this solution on the day prepared.]

Assay preparation—Transfer about 50 mg of Ticarcillin Monosodium, accurately weighed, to a 50-mL volumetric flask, dilute with *pH 6.4 sodium phosphate buffer* to volume, and mix.

Chromatographic system (see *Chromatography* ⟨621⟩)—The liquid chromatograph is equipped with a 220-nm detector and a 4-mm × 30-cm column that contains 3- to 10-μm packing L1. The flow rate is about 2 mL per minute. Chromatograph the *Resolution solution*, and record the peak responses as directed for *Procedure:* the relative retention times are about 0.2 for clavulanic acid and 1.0 for ticarcillin; and the resolution, *R*, between the clavulanic acid peak and the ticarcillin peak is not less than 5.0. Chromatograph the *Standard preparation*, and record the peak responses as directed for *Procedure:* the column efficiency is not less than 1000 theoretical plates; the tailing factor is not more than 2.0; and the relative standard deviation for replicate injections is not more than 2.0%.

Procedure—Separately inject equal volumes (about 20 μL) of the *Standard preparation* and the *Assay preparation* into the chromatograph, record the chromatograms, and measure the responses for the major peaks. Calculate the quantity, in μg, of ticarcillin ($C_{15}H_{16}N_2O_6S_2$) in each mg of the Ticarcillin Monosodium taken by the formula:

$$50(CP/W)(r_U/r_S)$$

in which *C* is the concentration, in mg per mL, of USP Ticarcillin Monosodium Monohydrate RS in the *Standard preparation; P* is the designated potency, in μg of ticarcillin ($C_{15}H_{16}N_2O_6S_2$) per mg, of USP Ticarcillin Monosodium Monohydrate RS; *W* is the weight, in mg, of Ticarcillin Monosodium taken to prepare the *Assay preparation;* and r_U and r_S are the ticarcillin peak responses obtained from the *Assay preparation* and the *Standard preparation*, respectively.

Tiletamine Hydrochloride

$C_{12}H_{17}NOS \cdot HCl$ 259.80
Cyclohexanone, 2-(ethylamino)-2-(2-thienyl)-.
2-(Ethylamino)-2-(2-thienyl)cyclohexanone   hydrochloride
[*14176-50-2*].

» Tiletamine Hydrochloride contains not less than 97.0 percent and not more than 103.0 percent of $C_{12}H_{17}NOS$ · HCl.

Packaging and storage—Preserve in tight containers.
Labeling—Label it to indicate that it is for veterinary use only. Where it is intended for use in preparing injectable dosage forms, the label states that it is sterile or must be subjected to further processing during the preparation of injectable dosage forms.

USP Reference standards ⟨11⟩—*USP Endotoxin RS. USP Tiletamine Hydrochloride RS.*
Clarity of solution—Dissolve 1.0 g of it in 10 mL of water: the solution is clear.
Identification—
  A: *Infrared Absorption* ⟨197K⟩.
  B: *Ultraviolet Absorption* ⟨197U⟩—
  Solution: 0.3 mg per mL.
  Medium: 0.1 N hydrochloric acid.
  Absorptivities at 234 nm do not differ by more than 3.0%.
  C: It meets the requirements of the tests for *Chloride* ⟨191⟩.
Melting range ⟨741⟩: between 190° and 195°, within a 2° range.
Bacterial endotoxins ⟨85⟩—Where the label states that Tiletamine Hydrochloride is sterile or must be subjected to further processing during the preparation of injectable dosage forms, it contains not more than 0.07 USP Endotoxin Unit per mg of tiletamine.
Sterility ⟨71⟩—Where the label states that Tiletamine Hydrochloride is sterile, it meets the requirements when tested as directed for *Membrane Filtration* under *Test for Sterility of the Product to be Examined*.
pH ⟨791⟩: between 3.0 and 5.0, in a solution (1 in 10).
Water, *Method I* ⟨921⟩: not more than 1.0%.
Residue on ignition ⟨281⟩: not more than 0.5%.
Heavy metals, *Method II* ⟨231⟩: 0.002%.
Chromatographic purity—Prepare a test solution of Tiletamine Hydrochloride in methanol containing 50.0 mg per mL. Prepare a Standard solution in methanol containing 1.0 mg of USP Tiletamine Hydrochloride RS per mL. Prepare a thin-layer chromatographic plate (see *Chromatography* ⟨621⟩) coated with a 0.25-mm layer of chromatographic silica gel mixture as follows. Prewash the plate by developing it in a mixture of methanol and ether (8 : 2) to the top of the plate, and allow the plate to dry. Separately apply 5 μL of the test solution and the Standard solution to the plate, and develop the chromatogram until the solvent front has moved about three-fourths of the length of the plate. Remove the plate from the chamber, mark the solvent front, allow the plate to air-dry, and examine under short- and long-wavelength UV light: no individual secondary spot observed in the chromatogram obtained from the test solution is greater in size or intensity than the principal spot observed in the chromatogram obtained from the Standard solution, corresponding to 2%, and the total of any such spots observed does not exceed 3%.
Chloride content—Transfer about 250 mg of it, accurately weighed, to a conical flask, add 5 mL of water, 5 mL of glacial acetic acid, and 50 mL of methanol, and swirl to dissolve. Add 1 drop of eosin Y TS, and titrate with 0.1 N silver nitrate VS to the endpoint when the granular precipitate first turns to a permanent pink color. Each mL of 0.1 N silver nitrate is equivalent to 3.545 mg of chloride: between 13.24% and 14.06% is found.
Assay—Transfer about 300 mg of Tiletamine Hydrochloride, accurately weighed, to a conical flask, add 70 mL of glacial acetic acid and 10 mL of mercuric acetate TS, and swirl to dissolve. Add 2 drops of crystal violet TS, and titrate with 0.1 N perchloric acid VS to a blue-green endpoint. Perform a blank determination, and make any necessary correction. Each mL of 0.1 N perchloric acid is equivalent to 25.98 mg of $C_{12}H_{17}NOS \cdot HCl$.

Tiletamine and Zolazepam for Injection

» Tiletamine and Zolazepam for Injection is a sterile dry mixture of Tiletamine Hydrochloride and Zolazepam Hydrochloride. It contains the equivalent of not less than 90.0 percent and not more than 110.0 percent of the labeled amounts of tiletamine ($C_{12}H_{17}NOS$) and zolazepam ($C_{15}H_{15}FN_4O$).

Packaging and storage—Preserve in *Containers for Sterile Solids* as described under *Injections* ⟨1⟩.
Labeling—Label it to indicate that it is for veterinary use only.

USP Reference standards ⟨11⟩—*USP Endotoxin RS. USP Tiletamine Hydrochloride RS. USP Zolazepam Hydrochloride RS.*

Identification—Constitute a container of Tiletamine and Zolazepam for Injection with a volume of water sufficient to yield a test solution containing the equivalent of about 10 mg of tiletamine and 10 mg of zolazepam per mL. Prepare two Standard solutions containing in each mL 10 mg of USP Tiletamine Hydrochloride RS and 10 mg of USP Zolazepam Hydrochloride RS, respectively. Separately apply 2 µL of the test solution and the Standard solutions to a thin-layer chromatographic plate (see *Chromatography* ⟨621⟩) coated with a 0.25-mm layer of chromatographic silica gel mixture, and allow the spots to dry. Place the plate in a saturated chamber containing ethyl acetate as the solvent system and lined with filter paper. Develop the chromatogram until the solvent front has moved about three-fourths of the length of the plate. Remove the plate from the chamber, mark the solvent front, allow the plate to air-dry, and examine under short-wavelength UV light: the R_F values of the principal spots obtained from the test solution correspond to those obtained from the Standard solutions.

Bacterial endotoxins ⟨85⟩—It contains not more than 0.07 USP Endotoxin Unit per mg of combined tiletamine and zolazepam equivalents.

Sterility ⟨71⟩—It meets the requirements when tested as directed for *Membrane Filtration* under *Test for Sterility of the Product to be Examined*.

pH ⟨791⟩: between 2.0 and 3.5, when constituted as directed in the labeling.

Water, *Method I* ⟨921⟩: not more than 20 mg in a container containing the equivalent of 250 mg of tiletamine and 250 mg of zolazepam.

Other requirements—It meets the requirements under *Injections* ⟨1⟩ and for *Uniformity of Dosage Units* ⟨905⟩.

Assay—

Internal standard solution—Prepare a solution of tetraphenylethylene in chloroform containing 10 mg per mL.

Standard preparation—Transfer accurately weighed quantities of about 116 mg of USP Tiletamine Hydrochloride RS and 113 mg of USP Zolazepam Hydrochloride RS to a 250-mL flask, add 2 mL of water, and swirl to dissolve. Add 30 mL of *Alkaline borate buffer, pH 10.0* (see *Buffer Solutions* in the section *Reagents, Indicators, and Solutions*), and swirl. Add 5.0 mL of *Internal standard solution* and 95.0 mL of chloroform, and shake by mechanical means for 30 minutes. Allow the phases to separate, and use the chloroform layer as the *Standard preparation*.

Assay preparation—Constitute a container of Tiletamine and Zolazepam for Injection with the volume of water specified in the labeling. Transfer an accurately measured volume of the resultant solution, equivalent to about 100 mg of tiletamine and 100 mg of zolazepam, to a 250-mL flask. Add 30.0 mL of *Alkaline borate buffer, pH 10.0* (see *Buffer Solutions* in the section *Reagents, Indicators, and Solutions*), and swirl. Add 5.0 mL of *Internal standard solution* and 95.0 mL of chloroform, and shake by mechanical means for 30 minutes. Allow the phases to separate, and use the chloroform layer as the *Assay preparation*.

Chromatographic system (see *Chromatography* ⟨621⟩)—The gas chromatograph is equipped with a flame-ionization detector and a 2-mm × 1.24-m column that contains 3% phase G2 on 100- to 120-mesh support S1AB. Helium is used as the carrier gas flowing at a rate of about 40 mL per minute. The column temperature is maintained at about 150° for 0.5 minute after injection and is programmed to rise to 230° at a rate of 10° per minute. The injector port is maintained at 160° and the detector at 250°. Chromatograph the *Standard preparation*, and record the peak responses as directed for *Procedure*: the relative retention times are about 0.4 for tiletamine, 0.8 for zolazepam, and 1.0 for tetraphenylethylene.

Procedure—Separately inject equal volumes (about 2 µL) of the *Standard preparation* and the *Assay preparation* into the chromatograph, record the chromatograms, and measure the area responses for the major peaks. Calculate the quantity, in mg, of tiletamine ($C_{12}H_{17}NOS$) in each mL of the constituted solution taken by the formula:

$$(223.33/259.79)(W/V)(R_U/R_S)$$

in which 223.33 and 259.79 are the molecular weights of tiletamine base and tiletamine hydrochloride, respectively; W is the weight, in mg, of USP Tiletamine Hydrochloride RS taken to prepare the *Standard preparation*; V is the volume, in mL, of the constituted solution taken to prepare the *Assay preparation*; and R_U and R_S are the peak area response ratios of the tiletamine peak to the tetraphenylethylene peak obtained from the *Assay preparation* and the *Standard preparation*, respectively. Calculate the quantity, in mg, of zolazepam ($C_{15}H_{15}FN_4O$) in each mL of the constituted solution taken by the formula:

$$(286.31/322.77)(W/V)(R_U/R_S)$$

in which 286.31 and 322.77 are the molecular weights of zolazepam base and zolazepam hydrochloride, respectively; W is the weight, in mg, of USP Zolazepam Hydrochloride RS taken to prepare the *Standard preparation*; V is the volume, in mL, of the constituted solution taken to prepare the *Assay preparation*; and R_U and R_S are the peak area response ratios of the zolazepam peak to the tetraphenylethylene peak obtained from the *Assay preparation* and the *Standard preparation*, respectively.

Tilmicosin

$C_{46}H_{80}N_2O_{13}$ 869.13

Tylosin, 4^A-*O*-de(2,6-dideoxy-3-*C*-methyl-α-L-*ribo*-hexopyranosyl)-20-deoxo-20-(3,5-dimethyl-1-piperidinyl)-, 20(*cis*)-.

4^A-*O*-de(2,6-Dideoxy-3-*C*-methyl-α-L-*ribo*-hexopyranosyl)-20-deoxo-20-(*cis*-3,5-dimethylpiperidino)-tylosin   [108050-54-0].

» Tilmicosin contains not less than 85.0 percent of $C_{46}H_{80}N_2O_{13}$, calculated on the anhydrous basis. The content of tilmicosin *cis*-isomers is between 82.0 percent and 88.0 percent, and the content of tilmicosin *trans*-isomers is between 12.0 percent and 18.0 percent of total $C_{46}H_{80}N_2O_{13}$.

Caution—Tilmicosin is irritating to the eyes and may cause allergic reaction. Avoid contact.

Packaging and storage—Preserve in well-closed, light-resistant containers. Avoid excessive heat.

Labeling—Label it to indicate that it is for veterinary use only.

USP Reference standards ⟨11⟩—*USP Tilmicosin RS*.

Identification—

A: *Infrared Absorption* ⟨197K⟩.

B: The chromatogram of the *Assay preparation* obtained as directed in the *Assay* exhibits peaks for the tilmicosin *trans*-isomer and the tilmicosin *cis*-isomer, the retention times of which correspond to those exhibited in the chromatogram of the *Standard preparation* obtained as directed in the *Assay*.

Water, *Method I* ⟨921⟩: not more than 5.0%, 20 mL of a mixture of methanol and pyridine (4:1) containing 10% of imidazole being used in place of methanol in the titration vessel.

Related compounds—

Dibutylammonium phosphate buffer and *Diluent*—Prepare as directed in the *Assay*.

Solution A—To 700 mL of water add 25 mL of *Dibutylammonium phosphate buffer*, dilute quantitatively with water to 1 L, and mix. Degas before use.

Solution B—Use degassed acetonitrile.

Mobile phase—Use variable mixtures of *Solution A* and *Solution B* as directed for *Chromatographic system*. Make adjustments if necessary (see *System Suitability* under *Chromatography* ⟨621⟩).

Standard solution—Dissolve an accurately weighed quantity of USP Tilmicosin RS in acetonitrile to obtain a solution having a known concentration of about 0.25 mg per mL, sonicating if necessary to dissolve. Transfer 5.0 mL of this solution to a 25-mL volumetric flask, dilute with *Diluent* to volume, and mix.

Test solution—Transfer about 200 mg of Tilmicosin, accurately weighed, to a 50-mL volumetric flask, add 10 mL of acetonitrile, and sonicate briefly to dissolve. Dilute with *Diluent* to volume, and mix. [NOTE—Use this solution within 24 hours.]

Chromatographic system (see *Chromatography* ⟨621⟩)—The liquid chromatograph is equipped with a 280-nm detector and a 4.6-mm × 25-cm column that contains 5-μm packing L1 and is programmed for gradient elution by delivering a mixture of *Solution A* and *Solution B* in a ratio of 82 : 18 initially, and by continuously varying the mixture linearly over a period of 30 minutes until the final ratio is 60 : 40. The flow rate is about 1.1 mL per minute. Chromatograph the *Standard solution,* and record the responses as directed for *Procedure:* the relative retention times are about 0.9 for the tilmicosin *trans*-isomers (two incompletely resolved peaks), 1.0 for the tilmicosin *cis*-isomer, and 1.1 for the tilmicosin *cis*-8-epimer.

Procedure—Separately inject equal volumes (about 10 μL) of the *Standard solution* and the *Test solution* into the chromatograph, record the chromatograms, and measure the area responses for the major peaks. Calculate the percentage of each related compound in the portion of Tilmicosin taken by the formula:

$$5(CP / W)(r_c / r_s)$$

in which C is the concentration, in mg per mL, of USP Tilmicosin RS in the *Standard solution;* P is the designated potency, in μg per mg, of tilmicosin in the USP Tilmicosin RS; W is the weight, in mg, of Tilmicosin taken to prepare the *Test solution;* r_c is the area response of the individual related compound peak, other than those obtained for tilmicosin *trans*-isomers, tilmicosin *cis*-isomer, and tilmicosin *cis*-8-epimer; and r_s is the sum of the peak area responses for the tilmicosin *trans*-isomers, the tilmicosin *cis*-isomer, and the tilmicosin *cis*-8-epimer obtained from the *Standard solution.* Not more than 3% of any individual related compound, calculated on the anhydrous basis, is found, and the sum of all the related compounds is not more than 10%, calculated on the anhydrous basis.

Assay—

Dibutylammonium phosphate buffer—Add, with stirring, 70 mL of dilute phosphoric acid (1 in 10) to 16.8 mL of dibutylamine (90 : 10). Allow to cool, and adjust with phosphoric acid to a pH of 2.5 ± 0.1. Dilute with water to 100 mL, and mix.

Mobile phase—To 700 mL of water, add 115 mL of acetonitrile, 55 mL of tetrahydrofuran, and 25 mL of *Dibutylammonium phosphate buffer*. Dilute with water to 1000 mL, and mix. Each component may be degassed before use, or the *Mobile phase* may be sparged with helium for 2 minutes before use. Store the *Mobile phase* in a sealed container when not in use. Make adjustments if necessary (see *System Suitability* under *Chromatography* ⟨621⟩). [NOTE—Decreasing the proportion of acetonitrile or tetrahydrofuran increases resolution.]

Diluent—To 900 mL of water, add 5.71 g of phosphoric acid, adjust with 12.5 N sodium hydroxide to a pH of 2.5 ± 0.1, dilute with water to 1000 mL, and mix.

Standard preparation—Transfer about 25 mg of USP Tilmicosin RS, accurately weighed, to a 50-mL volumetric flask, add 10 mL of acetonitrile, and sonicate to dissolve. Dilute with *Diluent* to volume, and mix. [NOTE—Use this solution on the day prepared.]

Assay preparation—Transfer about 25 mg of Tilmicosin, accurately weighed, to a 50-mL volumetric flask, add 10 mL of acetonitrile, and sonicate to dissolve. Dilute with *Diluent* to volume, and mix. [NOTE—Use this solution on the day prepared.]

Chromatographic system (see *Chromatography* ⟨621⟩)—The liquid chromatograph is equipped with a 280-nm detector and a 4.6-mm × 25-cm column that contains 5-μm packing L1. The flow rate is about 1 mL per minute. Chromatograph the *Standard preparation,* and record the responses as directed for *Procedure:* the relative retention times are about 0.8 for the tilmicosin *trans*-isomers and 1.0 for the tilmicosin *cis*-isomers [NOTE—Tilmicosin *cis*-isomer and tilmicosin *cis*-8-epimer co-elute in this chromatographic system]; the resolution, R, between the tilmicosin *trans*-isomers peak and the tilmicosin *cis*-isomers peak is not less than 1.25; the tailing factors for the peaks are not less than 0.7 and not more than 2; and the relative standard deviation for replicate injections is not more than 2.0%.

Procedure—Separately inject equal volumes (about 10 μL) of the *Standard preparation* and the *Assay preparation* into the chromatograph, record the chromatograms, and measure the area responses for the major peaks. Calculate the quantity, in μg, of tilmicosin *trans*- and *cis*-isomers in the portion of Tilmicosin taken by the formula:

$$50(CP / W)(r_i / r_S)$$

in which C is the concentration, in mg per mL, of USP Tilmicosin RS in the *Standard preparation;* P is the designated potency, in μg per mg, of the relevant (*trans* or *cis*) tilmicosin isomers in the USP Tilmicosin RS; W is the weight, in mg, of Tilmicosin taken to prepare the *Assay preparation;* r_i is the peak area response for the relevant (*trans* or *cis*) tilmicosin isomers obtained from the *Assay preparation;* and r_S is the peak area response for the relevant (*trans* or *cis*) tilmicosin isomers obtained from the *Standard preparation.* Calculate the percentage of tilmicosin ($C_{46}H_{80}N_2O_{13}$) in the portion of Tilmicosin taken by the formula:

$$0.1(trans + cis)$$

in which *trans* and *cis* are the quantities, in μg per mg, of tilmicosin *trans*-isomers and tilmicosin *cis*-isomers in the Tilmicosin, as determined above. Calculate the percentages of tilmicosin *trans*-isomers and tilmicosin *cis*-isomers taken by the formula:

$$100 \; isomer / (trans + cis)$$

in which *isomer* is the quantity, in μg per mg, of either the tilmicosin *trans*-isomers or the tilmicosin *cis*-isomers in the Tilmicosin, as determined above.

Tilmicosin Injection

» Tilmicosin Injection is a sterile solution of Tilmicosin in a mixture of Propylene Glycol and Water for Injection, and is solubilized with the aid of Phosphoric Acid. It contains not less than 90.0 percent and not more than 110.0 percent of the labeled amount of tilmicosin ($C_{46}H_{80}N_2O_{13}$).

Packaging and storage—Preserve in light-resistant *Containers for Injections* as described under *Injections* ⟨1⟩. Store at or below 30°.

Labeling—Label the Injection to indicate that it is for veterinary use only.

USP Reference standards ⟨11⟩—*USP Endotoxin RS. USP Tilmicosin RS.*

Identification—The chromatogram of the *Assay preparation* obtained as directed in the *Assay* exhibits major peaks for the tilmicosin *trans*-isomers and the tilmicosin *cis*-isomers, the retention times of which correspond to those exhibited in the chromatogram of the *Standard preparation* obtained as directed in the *Assay.*

Bacterial endoxtoxins ⟨85⟩—It contains not more than 0.5 USP Endotoxin Unit per mg of tilmicosin.

Sterility ⟨71⟩—It meets the requirements when tested as directed for *Membrane Filtration* under *Test for Sterility of the Product to be Examined,* except that the test mixture is prepared as follows. Transfer aseptically 1 mL from each of 20 containers to a vessel containing 200 mL of a mixture containing 2 mL of polysorbate 20 in pH 7 phosphate buffer prepared as directed for *Buffer No. 16* in the section *Phosphate Buffers and Other Solutions* under *Antimicrobial Assays—Antibiotics* ⟨81⟩. After that solution has been filtered, wash the filter with three 100-mL portions of the same solution, instead of *Diluting Fluid A.*

pH ⟨791⟩: between 5.5 and 6.5.

Particulate matter ⟨788⟩—Use the procedure under *Microscopic Particle Count Test:* not more than 50 particles per mL that are equal to or greater than 10 μm in effective spherical diameter, and not more than 5 particles per mL that are equal to or greater than 25 μm in effective spherical diameter are found.

Tilmicosin / Official Monographs

Content of propylene glycol—

Internal standard solution—Prepare a solution of pentadecane in acetone containing about 0.5 mg per mL.

Standard solution—Transfer about 125 mg of propylene glycol, accurately weighed, to a 100-mL volumetric flask, dilute with acetone to volume, and mix. Mix equal, accurately measured volumes of this solution and the *Internal standard solution*. This solution contains about 0.625 mg of propylene glycol per mL.

Test solution—Transfer an accurately measured volume of Injection, equivalent to about 250 mg of propylene glycol, to a 200-mL volumetric flask, dilute with acetone to volume, and mix. Mix equal, accurately measured volumes of this solution and the *Internal standard solution*.

Chromatographic system (see *Chromatography* ⟨621⟩)—The gas chromatograph is equipped with a flame-ionization detector and a 0.53-mm × 15-m fused silica column that has liquid phase G16 bonded to the inner surface at a thickness of 1 µm. The injection port and the detector block are maintained at about 250°, and the column is maintained at a temperature of about 100°. Helium is used as the carrier gas at a flow rate of about 15 mL per minute. Chromatograph the *Standard solution*, and record the peak responses as directed for *Procedure:* the relative retention times are about 0.6 for pentadecane and 1.0 for propylene glycol, the resolution, *R*, between the pentadecane peak and the propylene glycol peak is not less than 7.0, and the relative standard deviation for replicate injections is not more than 2.0%.

Procedure—Separately inject equal volumes (about 1 µL) of the *Standard solution* and the *Test solution* into the chromatograph, record the chromatograms, and measure the area responses for the major peaks. Calculate the quantity, in mg, of propylene glycol in each mL of the Injection taken by the formula:

$$400(C/V)(R_U/R_S)$$

in which *C* is the concentration, in mg per mL, of propylene glycol in the *Standard solution*, *V* is the volume, in mL, of Injection taken, and R_U and R_S are the ratios of the propylene glycol peak area response to the pentadecane peak area response obtained from the *Test solution* and the *Standard solution*, respectively. Between 80.0% and 120.0% of the labeled amount of propylene glycol is found.

Assay—

Dibutylammonium phosphate buffer—To 700 mL of water, add 168 mL of dibutylamine. Add phosphoric acid slowly until the dibutylamine is just dissolved, stirring vigorously during the addition. Allow to cool, and adjust with phosphoric acid to a pH of 2.55 ± 0.05. Dilute with water to 1000 mL, mix, and filter under vacuum.

Mobile phase—To 700 mL of water, add 115 mL of acetonitrile, 55 mL of tetrahydrofuran, and 25 mL of *Dibutylammonium phosphate buffer*. Dilute with water to 1000 mL, and mix. Each component may be filtered before mixing, or the *Mobile phase* may be filtered, minimizing solvent evaporation. Store the *Mobile phase* in a sealed container when not in use. Make adjustments if necessary (see *System Suitability* under *Chromatography* ⟨621⟩).

Diluent—To 700 mL of water add 200 mL of acetonitrile and 25 mL of *Dibutylammonium phosphate buffer*, dilute with water to 1000 mL, and mix.

Standard preparation—Quantitatively dissolve an accurately weighed quantity of USP Tilmicosin RS in acetonitrile to obtain a solution having a known concentration of about 2.5 mg per mL. Transfer 4.0 mL of this solution to a 20-mL volumetric flask, add 10 mL of water, and 0.5 mL of *Dibutylammonium phosphate buffer*, dilute with water to volume, and mix.

Assay preparation—Transfer an accurately measured volume of Injection, equivalent to about 300 mg of tilmicosin, to a 30-mL volumetric flask, dilute with *Diluent* to volume, and mix. Transfer 5.0 mL of this solution to a 100-mL volumetric flask, dilute with *Diluent* to volume, and mix.

Chromatographic system (see *Chromatography* ⟨621⟩)—The liquid chromatograph is equipped with a 280-nm detector and a 4.6-mm × 25-cm column that contains 5-µm packing L1. The flow rate is about 1.1 mL per minute. Chromatograph the *Standard preparation*, and record the responses as directed for *Procedure:* the relative retention times are about 0.8 for the tilmicosin *trans*-isomers and 1.0 for the tilmicosin *cis*-isomers, the resolution, *R*, between the tilmicosin *trans*-isomers peak and the tilmicosin *cis*-isomers peak is not less than 1.25, the tailing factors for the peaks are not less than 0.7 and not more than 2, and the relative standard deviation for replicate injections is not more than 1.5%.

Procedure—Separately inject equal volumes (about 10 µL) of the *Standard preparation* and the *Assay preparation* into the chromatograph, record the chromatograms, and measure the area responses for the major peaks. Calculate the quantity, in mg, of each of the tilmicosin isomers in each mL of the Injection taken by the formula:

$$0.6(CP/V)(r_I/r_S)$$

in which *C* is the concentration, in mg per mL, of USP Tilmicosin RS in the *Standard preparation*, *P* is the potency, in µg per mg, of the relevant (*trans* or *cis*) tilmicosin isomers in the USP Tilmicosin RS, *V* is the volume of Injection taken to prepare the *Assay preparation*, r_I is the peak response of the relevant tilmicosin isomers obtained from the *Assay preparation*, and r_S is the peak area response for the relevant (*trans* or *cis*) tilmicosin isomers obtained from the *Standard preparation*. Calculate the quantity, in mg, of $C_{46}H_{80}N_2O_{13}$ in each mL of the Injection taken by adding the quantities, in mg per mL, of *cis*- and *trans*-isomers found.

Timolol Maleate

$C_{13}H_{24}N_4O_3S \cdot C_4H_4O_4$ 432.49

2-Propanol, 1-(1,1-dimethylethyl)amino-3-[[4-(4-morpholinyl)-1,2,5-thiadiazol-3-yl]oxy]-, (*S*)-, (*Z*)-2-butenedioate (1 : 1) (salt).
(−)-1-(*tert*-Butylamino)-3-[(4-morpholino-1,2,5-thiadiazol-3-yl)oxy]-2-propanol maleate (1 : 1) (salt)   [26921-17-5].

» Timolol Maleate contains not less than 98.0 percent and not more than 101.0 percent of $C_{13}H_{24}N_4O_3S \cdot C_4H_4O_4$, calculated on the dried basis.

Packaging and storage—Preserve in well-closed containers.

USP Reference standards ⟨11⟩—*USP Timolol Maleate RS*.

Identification—

A: *Infrared Absorption* ⟨197M⟩.

B: *Ultraviolet Absorption* ⟨197U⟩—

Solution: 25 µg per mL.

Medium: 0.12 N hydrochloric acid.

Absorptivities at 294 nm, calculated on the dried basis, do not differ by more than 3.0%.

Specific rotation ⟨781S⟩: between −11.7° and −12.5° (λ= 405 nm).

Test solution: 50 mg per mL, in 1.0 N hydrochloric acid.

pH ⟨791⟩: between 3.8 and 4.3, in a solution containing 20 mg per mL.

Loss on drying ⟨731⟩—Dry it in vacuum at 100° to constant weight: it loses not more than 0.5% of its weight.

Residue on ignition ⟨281⟩: not more than 0.1%.

Heavy metals, *Method II* ⟨231⟩: 0.002%.

Chromatographic purity—Dissolve 500 mg in methanol to obtain 10.0 mL of test solution. Dissolve an accurately weighed quantity of USP Timolol Maleate RS in methanol, and dilute quantitatively and stepwise with methanol to obtain Standard solutions having the following compositions:

Standard solution	Concentration (µg RS per mL)	Percentage (%, for comparison with test specimen)
A	200	0.4
B	100	0.2
C	50	0.1

Separately apply 10-µL portions of the solutions to a suitable thin-layer chromatographic plate (see *Chromatography* ⟨621⟩) coated with a 0.25-mm layer of chromatographic silica gel mixture. Allow the spots to dry, and develop the chromatogram in a solvent system consisting of a mixture of chloroform, methanol, and ammonium hydroxide (80 : 20 : 1) until the solvent front has moved about three-fourths of the length of the plate. Remove the plate from the developing chamber, mark the solvent front, and allow the solvent to evaporate. Expose the plate to iodine vapors for 2 hours, and locate the spots on the plate by examination under short-wavelength UV light. Compare the intensities of any secondary spots observed in the chromatogram of the test solution, excluding the origin spot due to the maleate anion, with those of the principal spots in the chromatograms of the Standard solutions: no secondary spot is more intense than the principal spot obtained from Standard solution A (0.4%), and the sum of the intensities of all secondary spots, excluding any having intensities less than the principal spot obtained from Standard solution C, does not exceed 1.0%.

Organic volatile impurities, *Method I* ⟨467⟩: meets the requirements.

(Official until July 1, 2008)

Assay—Dissolve about 800 mg of Timolol Maleate, accurately weighed, in about 90 mL of glacial acetic acid, and titrate with 0.1 N perchloric acid VS, determining the endpoint potentiometrically, using a platinum electrode and a sleeve-type calomel electrode containing 0.1 N lithium perchlorate in acetic anhydride (see *Titrimetry* ⟨541⟩). Perform a blank determination, and make any necessary correction. Each mL of 0.1 N perchloric acid is equivalent to 43.25 mg of $C_{13}H_{24}N_4O_3S \cdot C_4H_4O_4$.

Timolol Maleate Ophthalmic Solution

» Timolol Maleate Ophthalmic Solution is a sterile, aqueous solution of Timolol Maleate. It contains an amount of $C_{13}H_{24}N_4O_3S \cdot C_4H_4O_4$ equivalent to not less than 90.0 percent and not more than 110.0 percent of the labeled amount of timolol ($C_{13}H_{24}N_4O_3S$).

Packaging and storage—Preserve in tight, light-resistant containers.

USP Reference standards ⟨11⟩—*USP Timolol Maleate RS*.

Identification—Dilute a suitable quantity of Ophthalmic Solution with water to obtain a solution having a concentration of about 20 µg of timolol per mL: the UV absorption spectrum of the solution so obtained exhibits maxima and minima at the same wavelengths as that of a similar preparation of USP Timolol Maleate RS, concomitantly measured.

Sterility ⟨71⟩: meets the requirements.

pH ⟨791⟩: between 6.5 and 7.5.

Assay—

pH 2.8 phosphate buffer—Dissolve 11.1 g of monobasic sodium phosphate in 1000 mL of water, adjust with phosphoric acid to a pH of 2.8 ± 0.05, filter, and degas.

Diluent—Prepare a mixture of acetonitrile and *pH 2.8 phosphate buffer* (2 : 1).

Mobile phase—Prepare a mixture of *pH 2.8 phosphate buffer* and methanol (65 : 35). Make adjustments if necessary (see *System Suitability* under *Chromatography* ⟨621⟩). [NOTE—Minimize the time the Reference Standard, the Ophthalmic Solution, the standard stock solution, the *Standard preparation*, and the *Assay preparation* are exposed to direct light.]

Standard preparation—Transfer about 34 mg of USP Timolol Maleate RS, accurately weighed, to a 25-mL volumetric flask, dissolve in and dilute with water to volume, and mix. Transfer 5.0 mL of this stock solution to a 50-mL volumetric flask, add 15 mL of *Diluent*, dilute with water to volume, and mix.

Assay preparation—Transfer an accurately measured volume of Ophthalmic Solution, equivalent to about 5 mg of timolol, to a 50-mL volumetric flask, add 15 mL of *Diluent*, dilute with water to volume, and mix.

Chromatographic system (see *Chromatography* ⟨621⟩)—The liquid chromatograph is equipped with a 295-nm detector and a 4.6-mm × 15-cm column that contains 5-µm packing L1. The column temperature is maintained at 40°, and the flow rate is about 1.2 mL per minute. Chromatograph the *Standard preparation*, and record the peak responses as directed for *Procedure*: the tailing factor is not more than 2.0, the column efficiency is not less than 3600 theoretical plates, and the relative standard deviation for replicate injections is not more than 2.0%.

Procedure—Separately inject equal volumes (about 10 µL) of the *Standard preparation* and the *Assay preparation* into the chromatograph, record the chromatograms, and measure the peak area responses for the major peaks. Calculate the quantity, in mg, of timolol ($C_{13}H_{24}N_4O_3S$) in each mL of Ophthalmic Solution taken by the formula:

$$(316.43 / 432.49)(50C / V)(r_U / r_S)$$

in which 316.43 and 432.49 are the molecular weights of timolol and timolol maleate, respectively, C is the concentration, in mg per mL, of USP Timolol Maleate RS in the *Standard preparation*, V is the volume, in mL, of Ophthalmic Solution taken, and r_U and r_S are the peak area responses of the timolol peaks obtained from the *Assay preparation* and the *Standard preparation*, respectively.

Timolol Maleate Tablets

» Timolol Maleate Tablets contain not less than 90.0 percent and not more than 110.0 percent of the labeled amount of $C_{13}H_{24}N_4O_3S \cdot C_4H_4O_4$.

Packaging and storage—Preserve in well-closed containers.

USP Reference standards ⟨11⟩—*USP Timolol Maleate RS*.

Identification—Transfer a portion of powdered Tablets, equivalent to about 30 mg of timolol maleate, to a 50-mL volumetric flask, add about 2 mL of 0.1 N hydrochloric acid, and shake gently. Add about 30 mL of methanol, agitate for 20 minutes, add methanol to volume, mix, and centrifuge. Similarly prepare a Standard solution containing 0.6 mg of USP Timolol Maleate RS per mL. Separately apply 10 µL of the test solution and 10 µL of the Standard solution to a thin-layer chromatographic plate (see *Chromatography* ⟨621⟩) coated with a 0.25-mm layer of chromatographic silica gel mixture. Develop the chromatogram using a solvent system consisting of a mixture of chloroform, methanol, and ammonium hydroxide (80 : 20 : 1) until the solvent front has moved about three-fourths of the length of the plate. Air-dry, and examine under short-wavelength UV light: the R_F values of the principal spots obtained from the test solution correspond to those obtained from the Standard solution.

Dissolution, *Procedure for a Pooled Sample* ⟨711⟩—

Medium: 0.1 N hydrochloric acid; 500 mL.

Apparatus 1: 100 rpm.

Time: 20 minutes.

Procedure—Determine the amount of timolol maleate in solution in filtered portions of the solution under test, in comparison with a Standard solution having a known concentration of USP Timolol Maleate RS in the same medium, employing the procedure set forth in the *Assay*, making any necessary modifications.

Tolerances—Not less than 80% (*Q*) of the labeled amount of timolol maleate ($C_{13}H_{24}N_4O_3S \cdot C_4H_4O_4$) is dissolved in 20 minutes.

Uniformity of dosage units 〈905〉: meet the requirements.

Assay—

pH 2.8 phosphate buffer—Transfer 22.08 g of monobasic sodium phosphate to a 2-liter volumetric flask, dilute with water to volume, adjust with phosphoric acid to a pH of 2.8 ± 0.05, and filter.

Mobile phase—Prepare a suitable degassed and filtered mixture of *pH 2.8 phosphate buffer* and methanol (3 : 2).

Standard preparation—Transfer about 50 mg of USP Timolol Maleate RS, accurately weighed, to a 500-mL volumetric flask. Add 50 mL of 0.05 M monobasic sodium phosphate. Sonicate until the standard is dissolved, add 100 mL of acetonitrile, shake, dilute with water to volume, and mix.

Assay preparation—Weigh and finely powder not less than 20 Tablets. Transfer an accurately weighed portion of the powder, equivalent to about 10 mg of timolol maleate, to a 100-mL volumetric flask, add 10 mL of 0.05 M monobasic sodium phosphate, sonicate for 5 minutes, and add 20 mL of acetonitrile. Sonicate for 5 minutes, add 20 mL of water, shake for 10 minutes, dilute with water to volume, and mix.

Chromatographic system (see *Chromatography* 〈621〉)—The liquid chromatograph is equipped with a 295-nm detector and a 3.9-mm × 30-cm column that contains packing L1. The flow rate is about 1.8 mL per minute. Chromatograph five replicate injections of the *Standard preparation*, and record the peak responses as directed for *Procedure*: the relative standard deviation is not more than 2.0%, and the tailing factor for the main peak is not greater than 2.0.

Procedure—Separately inject equal volumes (about 15 μL) of the *Standard preparation* and the *Assay preparation* into the chromatograph by means of a suitable microsyringe or sampling valve, record the chromatograms, and measure the responses for the major peaks. Calculate the quantity, in mg, of $C_{13}H_{24}N_4O_3S \cdot C_4H_4O_4$ in the portion of Tablets taken by the formula:

$$100C(r_U / r_S)$$

in which C is the concentration, in mg per mL, of USP Timolol Maleate RS in the *Standard preparation*, and r_U and r_S are the peak responses obtained for timolol maleate from the *Assay preparation* and the *Standard preparation*, respectively.

Timolol Maleate and Hydrochlorothiazide Tablets

» Timolol Maleate and Hydrochlorothiazide Tablets contain not less than 90.0 percent and not more than 110.0 percent of the labeled amounts of timolol maleate ($C_{17}H_{28}N_4O_7S$) and hydrochlorothiazide ($C_7H_8ClN_3O_4S_2$).

Packaging and storage—Preserve in well-closed, light-resistant containers.

USP Reference standards 〈11〉—*USP Timolol Maleate RS. USP Hydrochlorothiazide RS. USP Benzothiadiazine Related Compound A RS.*

Identification—Transfer a portion of powdered Tablets, equivalent to about 20 mg of timolol maleate, to a suitable centrifuge tube containing about 5 mL of methanol. Agitate for 20 minutes, and centrifuge. Separately dissolve suitable quantities of USP Timolol Maleate RS and USP Hydrochlorothiazide RS in methanol to obtain Standard solutions each having a concentration of 10 mg per mL. Separately apply 3 μL of the test solution and of each Standard solution to a thin-layer chromatographic plate (see *Chromatography* 〈621〉) coated with a 0.25-mm layer of chromatographic silica gel mixture. Develop the chromatogram using a solvent system consisting of a mixture of chloroform, methanol, and ammonium hydroxide (80 : 20 : 1) until the solvent front has moved about three-fourths of the length of the plate. Air-dry, and examine under short-wavelength UV light: the R_F values of the principal spots obtained from the Standard solutions correspond to those obtained from the test solution.

Dissolution 〈711〉—

Medium: 0.1 N hydrochloric acid; 900 mL.

Apparatus 2: 50 rpm.

Time: 20 minutes.

Procedure—Determine the amount of timolol maleate ($C_{13}H_{24}N_4O_3S \cdot C_4H_4O_4$) dissolved, employing the following procedure: Prepare a Standard solution of USP Timolol Maleate RS in 0.1 N hydrochloric acid having a known concentration of about 11 μg per mL. Filter a portion of the solution under test, and transfer 10.0 mL of the clear filtrate to a suitable separator. Transfer 10.0 mL each of the Standard solution and 0.1 N hydrochloric acid, to provide the blank, to individual separators, and treat each of three separators as follows: Add 20.0 mL of ethyl acetate, mix for 1 minute, allow the phases to separate, and filter the aqueous layer into a suitable vessel, retaining the ethyl acetate layer from the solution under test for the hydrochlorothiazide determination. Determine the amount of $C_{13}H_{24}N_4O_3S \cdot C_4H_4O_4$ dissolved from UV absorbances of the aqueous layer from the solution under test at the wavelength of maximum absorbance at about 293 nm in comparison with the aqueous layer from the Standard solution.

Determine the amount of hydrochlorothiazide ($C_7H_8ClN_3O_4S_2$) dissolved, employing the following procedure: Filter the ethyl acetate layer obtained previously from the solution under test through filter paper. Determine the amount of $C_7H_8ClN_3O_4S_2$ dissolved from UV absorbances at the wavelength of maximum absorbance at about 270 nm of the ethyl acetate layer from the solution under test in comparison with a Standard solution in ethyl acetate having a known concentration of USP Hydrochlorothiazide RS.

Tolerances—Not less than 80% (*Q*) of each of the labeled amounts of $C_{13}H_{24}N_4O_3S \cdot C_4H_4O_4$ and $C_7H_8ClN_3O_4S_2$, respectively, is dissolved in 20 minutes.

Uniformity of dosage units 〈905〉: meet the requirements for *Content Uniformity* with respect to timolol maleate and to hydrochlorothiazide.

Related compounds—

pH 3.0 Buffer and *Mobile phase*—Proceed as directed under *Assay*.

Standard solution—Dissolve an accurately weighed quantity of USP Benzothiadiazine Related Compound A RS in methanol to obtain a solution having a known concentration of about 0.5 mg per mL. Transfer an accurately measured volume of this solution, and dilute quantitatively, and stepwise if necessary, with *Mobile phase* to obtain a solution having a known concentration of about 0.5 μg per mL.

Test solution—Use the *Assay preparation* prepared as directed in the *Assay*.

Chromatographic system—Proceed as directed under *Assay*, except to chromatograph the *Standard solution:* the relative standard deviation for replicate injections is not more than 5.0%.

Procedure—Separately inject equal volumes (about 50 μL) of the *Standard solution* and the *Test solution* into the chromatograph, record the chromatograms, and measure the peak areas. Calculate the percentage of benzothiadiazine related compound A in the portion of Tablets taken by the formula:

$$100(C/L)(r_U / r_S)$$

in which C is the concentration in μg per mL, of USP Benzothiadiazine Related Compound A RS in the *Standard solution*; L is the amount, in mg, of hydrochlorothiazide in the portion of Tablets taken, based on the labeled amount; and r_U and r_S are the peak areas of benzothiadiazine related compound A obtained from the *Test solution* and *Standard solution*, respectively: not more than 1.0% is found.

Assay—

pH 3.0 phosphate buffer—Dissolve 13.6 g of monobasic potassium phosphate in 100 mL of water, adjust with phosphoric acid to a pH of 3.0 ± 0.05, and filter.

Mobile phase—Prepare a suitable filtered and degassed mixture of water, acetonitrile, methanol, and *pH 3.0 phosphate buffer* (38 : 8 : 2 : 2), making adjustments if necessary (see *System Suitability* under *Chromatography* 〈621〉).

Standard preparation—Transfer about 50 mg of USP Timolol Maleate RS, accurately weighed, to a 500-mL volumetric flask. Add 50*J* mg of USP Hydrochlorothiazide RS, accurately weighed, *J* being the ratio of the labeled amount, in mg, of hydrochlorothiazide to the labeled amount, in mg, of timolol maleate per Tablet. Add 50 mL of 0.05 M monobasic sodium phosphate, and 125 mL of acetonitrile, sonicate for 4 minutes, dilute with water to volume, and mix. Pipet 5 mL into a 25-mL volumetric flask, dilute with acetonitrile solution (1 in 10) to volume, and mix.

Assay preparation—Weigh and finely powder not fewer than 20 Tablets. Transfer an accurately weighed portion of the powder, equivalent to about 20 mg of timolol maleate, to a 1-liter volumetric flask, add about 100 mL of 0.05 M monobasic sodium phosphate, 125 mL of acetonitrile, and 100 mL of water, and mix by mechanical means. Allow to stand for 16 hours, dilute with water to volume, mix, and filter.

Chromatographic system (see *Chromatography* ⟨621⟩)—The liquid chromatograph is equipped with a 295-nm detector and a 4-mm × 30-cm column that contains packing L1. The flow rate is about 1.5 mL per minute. Chromatograph replicate injections of the *Standard preparation*, and record the peak responses as directed for *Procedure:* the relative standard deviation is not more than 1.5%; and the resolution, *R*, between hydrochlorothiazide and timolol maleate is not less than 4.0.

Procedure—Separately inject equal volumes (about 50 μL) of the *Standard preparation* and the *Assay preparation* into the chromatograph by means of a suitable microsyringe or sampling valve, record the chromatograms, and measure the responses for the major peaks. The relative retention times are about 0.5 for benzothiadiazine related compound A, 0.6 for hydrochlorothiazide, and 1.0 for timolol maleate. Calculate the quantity, in mg, of hydrochlorothiazide ($C_7H_8ClN_3O_4S_2$) in the portion of Tablets taken by the formula:

$$1000C(r_U / r_S)$$

in which *C* is the concentration, in mg per mL, of USP Hydrochlorothiazide RS in the *Standard preparation;* and r_U and r_S are the responses of the hydrochlorothiazide peak obtained from the *Assay preparation* and the *Standard preparation*, respectively. Calculate the quantity, in mg, of timolol maleate ($C_{17}H_{28}N_4O_7S$) by the same formula, changing the terms to refer to timolol maleate.

Tinidazole

$C_8H_{13}N_3O_4S$ 247.28

1*H*-Imidazole, 1-[2-(ethylsulfonyl)ethyl]-2-methyl-5-nitro-.
1-[2-(Ethylsulfonyl)ethyl]-2-methyl-5-nitroimidazole [*19387-91-8*].

» Tinidazole contains not less than 98.0 percent and not more than 101.0 percent of $C_8H_{13}N_3O_4S$, calculated on the dried basis.

Packaging and storage—Preserve in tight containers, protected from light, at controlled room temperature.

USP Reference standards ⟨11⟩—*USP Tinidazole RS. USP Tinidazole Related Compound A RS. USP Tinidazole Related Compound B RS.*

Identification—
  A: *Infrared Absorption* ⟨197K⟩.
  B: *Ultraviolet Absorption* ⟨197U⟩—
  Solution: 10 μg per mL.
  Medium: methanol.
  C: The R_F value and intensity of the principal spot obtained from the chromatogram of *Test solution 2* correspond to those obtained from the chromatogram of *Standard solution 1*, as obtained in the test for *Related compounds*.

Melting range ⟨741⟩:   between 125° and 128°.
Loss on drying ⟨731⟩—Dry it at a temperature between 100° and 105° to constant weight: it loses not more than 0.5% of its weight.

Residue on ignition ⟨281⟩:   not more than 0.1%.
Heavy metals, *Method II* ⟨231⟩:   0.002%.
Related compounds—
  Adsorbent: 0.25-mm layer of chromatographic silica gel mixture.
  Test solution 1—Dissolve about 200 mg of Tinidazole, accurately weighed, in 10 mL of methanol.
  Test solution 2—Transfer 1.0 mL of *Test solution 1* to a 10-mL volumetric flask, dilute with methanol to volume, and mix.
  Standard solution 1—Prepare a solution of USP Tinidazole RS in methanol containing 2.0 mg per mL.
  Standard solution 2—Dilute 1.0 mL of *Standard solution 1* with methanol to 20 mL.
  Standard solution 3—Dilute 4.0 mL of *Standard solution 2* with methanol to 10 mL.
  Standard solution 4—Prepare a solution of USP Tinidazole Related Compound A RS in methanol containing 0.1 mg per mL.
  Standard solution 5—Prepare a solution of USP Tinidazole Related Compound B RS in methanol containing 0.1 mg per mL.
  Application volume: 10 μL.
  Developing solvent system: a mixture of ethyl acetate and butyl alcohol (3 : 1).
  Procedure—Proceed as directed for *Thin-Layer Chromatography* under *Chromatography* ⟨621⟩. Activate the plate for at least 1 hour at 110°. Examine the plate under short-wavelength UV light: any spots due to tinidazole related compound A and tinidazole related compound B obtained from *Test solution 1* are no more intense than the corresponding spots obtained from *Standard solution 4* and *Standard solution 5*, respectively; any spot, other than the principal spot, obtained from *Test solution 1* is not more intense than the spot obtained from *Standard solution 2;* and not more than one such spot is more intense than the spot obtained from *Standard solution 3*.

Assay—Dissolve 150 mg of Tinidazole, accurately weighed, in 25.0 mL of glacial acetic acid, and titrate with 0.1 N perchloric acid VS, determining the endpoint potentiometrically with suitable electrodes (see *Titrimetry* ⟨541⟩). Perform a blank determination, and make any necessary correction. Each mL of 0.1 N perchloric acid is equivalent to 24.73 mg of $C_8H_{13}N_3O_4S$.

Tioconazole

$C_{16}H_{13}Cl_3N_2OS$ 387.71

1*H*-Imidazole,   1-[2-[(2-chloro-3-thienyl)methoxy]-2-(2,4-dichlorophenyl)ethyl]-.
1-[2,4-Dichloro-[β-(2-chloro-3-thenyl)-oxy]phenethyl]imidazole [*65899-73-2*].

» Tioconazole contains not less than 97.0 percent and not more than 103.0 percent of $C_{16}H_{13}Cl_3N_2OS$.

Packaging and storage—Preserve in tight containers.
USP Reference standards ⟨11⟩—*USP Tioconazole RS. USP Tioconazole Related Compound A RS. USP Tioconazole Related Compound B RS. USP Tioconazole Related Compound C RS.*
Identification—
  A: *Infrared Absorption* ⟨197M⟩.
  B: *Visualizing solution*—Dissolve 0.85 g of bismuth subnitrate in 10 mL of glacial acetic acid, dilute with water to 50 mL, and mix. Mix 10 mL of this solution, 50 mL of potassium iodide solution (2 in 25), and 20 mL of glacial acetic acid, dilute with water to 100 mL, and mix.
  Procedure—Prepare a test solution by dissolving 50 mg of Tioconazole in 1 mL of methanol. Separately apply 10 μL of the test solution and 10 μL of a Standard solution of USP Tioconazole RS,

similarly prepared, to a thin-layer chromatographic plate (see *Chromatography* ⟨621⟩), coated with a 0.25-mm layer of chromatographic silica gel mixture. Allow the spots to dry, and develop the chromatogram using a solvent system consisting of a mixture of chloroform, methanol, and glacial acetic acid (40 : 5 : 1) until the solvent front has moved three-fourths of the length of the plate. Remove the plate from the developing chamber, mark the solvent front, and locate the spots on the plate by viewing under short- and long-wavelength UV light after drying the plate at 80° for 5 minutes. Spray the plate with *Visualizing solution*, air-dry for 2 minutes, and overspray with sodium nitrite solution (1 in 20). Air-dry the plate for 5 minutes, and examine it for brown spots on a pale yellow background: the R_F value of the principal spot from the test solution corresponds to that obtained from the Standard solution.

C: The chromatogram of the *Assay preparation* obtained as directed in the *Assay* exhibits a major peak for tioconazole, the retention time of which corresponds to that exhibited in the chromatogram of the *Standard preparation* obtained as directed in the *Assay*.

Water, *Method I* ⟨921⟩: not more than 0.5%.
Residue on ignition ⟨281⟩: not more than 0.2%.
Chloride ⟨221⟩—A 0.7-g portion dissolved in methanol shows no more chloride than corresponds to 0.50 mL of 0.020 N hydrochloric acid (0.05%).
Heavy metals, *Method II* ⟨231⟩: 0.005%.
Related compounds—
  Mobile phase and *Chromatographic system*—Prepare as directed in the *Assay*.
  Standard preparation—Transfer about 1 mg each, accurately weighed, of USP Tioconazole Related Compound A RS, USP Tioconazole Related Compound B RS, and USP Tioconazole Related Compound C RS to a 25-mL flask. Add 15.0 mL of methanol, and shake until the contents are completely dissolved.
  Test preparation—Transfer about 100 mg of Tioconazole, accurately weighed, to a 25-mL flask, add 15.0 mL of methanol, and shake until the substance is completely dissolved.
  Procedure—Separately inject equal volumes (about 20 µL) of the *Standard preparation* and the *Test preparation* into the chromatograph, record the chromatograms, and measure the responses for the peaks. Calculate, in turn, the percentages of 1-[2,4-dichloro-β-[(3-thenyl)-oxy]phenethyl]imidazole hydrochloride (tioconazole related compound A), 1-[2,4-dichloro-β-[(2,5-dichloro-3-thenyl)-oxy]phenethyl]imidazole hydrochloride (tioconazole related compound B), and 1-[2,4-dichloro-β-[(5-bromo-2-chloro-3-thenyl)-oxy]phenethyl]imidazole hydrochloride (tioconazole related compound C) in the portion of Tioconazole taken by the same formula:

$$100(W_I / W_U)(r_U / r_S)$$

in which W_I is the weight, in mg, of the respective USP Reference Standard taken to prepare the *Standard preparation*, W_U is the weight, in mg, of Tioconazole taken to prepare the *Test preparation*, and r_U and r_S are the peak responses at corresponding retention times, obtained from the *Test preparation* and the *Standard preparation*, respectively. The limit of each related compound is 1.0%.

Assay—
  Mobile phase—[NOTE—Prepare the *Mobile phase* fresh daily.]
  Mix 440 mL of acetonitrile, 400 mL of methanol, and 280 mL of water. Degas the solution. Add 2.0 mL of ammonium hydroxide, and mix. Make adjustments if necessary (see *System Suitability* under *Chromatography* ⟨621⟩).
  Standard preparation—Dissolve an accurately weighed quantity of USP Tioconazole RS in methanol, and dilute quantitatively and stepwise, if necessary, with methanol to obtain a solution having a known concentration of about 200 µg per mL.
  Assay preparation—Transfer about 100 mg of Tioconazole, accurately weighed, to a 100-mL volumetric flask, dissolve in methanol, dilute with methanol to volume, and mix. Transfer 10.0 mL of the resulting solution to a 50-mL volumetric flask, dilute with methanol to volume, and mix.
  Chromatographic system (see *Chromatography* ⟨621⟩)—The liquid chromatograph is equipped with a 219-nm detector, a 4-mm × 10-cm precolumn that contains packing L4, installed between the pump and the injector, and a 5-mm × 25-cm analytical column that contains packing L1. [NOTE—Replace the precolumn daily.] The flow rate is adjusted to obtain a retention time of between 12 and 17 minutes for tioconazole. Chromatograph the *Standard preparation*, and record the peak responses as directed under *Procedure*. The column efficiency determined from the analyte peak is not less than 1000 theoretical plates, the tailing factor for the analyte peak is not more than 2.0, and the relative standard deviation for replicate injections is not more than 2.0%.
  Procedure—Separately inject equal volumes (about 20 µL) of the *Standard preparation* and the *Assay preparation* into the chromatograph, record the chromatograms, and measure the responses for the major peaks. Calculate the quantity, in mg, of $C_{16}H_{13}Cl_3N_2OS$ in the Tioconazole taken by the formula:

$$(0.5C)(r_U / r_S)$$

in which C is the concentration, in µg per mL, of USP Tioconazole RS, calculated on the anhydrous basis, in the *Standard preparation*, and r_U and r_S are the peak responses obtained from the *Assay preparation* and the *Standard preparation*, respectively.

Titanium Dioxide

TiO₂   79.87
Titanium oxide (TiO₂).
Titanium oxide (TiO₂)   [13463-67-7].

» Titanium Dioxide contains not less than 99.0 percent and not more than 100.5 percent of TiO_2, calculated on the dried basis. If labeled as attenuation grade, then Titanium Dioxide contains not less than 99.0 percent and not more than 100.5 percent of TiO_2, calculated on the ignited basis. Attenuation grade material may contain suitable coatings, stabilizers, and treatments to assist formulation.

NOTE—If labeled as attenuation grade, then all tests and assays are conducted on uncoated, untreated material. For UV attenuation grade, the test for *Loss on drying* does not apply. The FDA requires the content of lead to be not more than 10 ppm, that of antimony to be not more than 2 ppm, and that of mercury to be not more than 1 ppm (21 CFR 73.1575).

Packaging and storage—Preserve in well-closed containers.
Labeling—If intended for UV-attenuation, the material must be labeled as attenuation grade. If intended for UV-attenuation, and any added coatings, stabilizers, or treatments are used, the labeling shall include the name and amount of the additives.
Identification—To 500 mg add 5 mL of sulfuric acid, and heat gently. After fumes of sulfur trioxide appear, continue heating for a minimum of 10 seconds. Cool the suspension, and cautiously dilute with water to 100 mL. Filter, and to 5 mL of the clear filtrate add a few drops of hydrogen peroxide TS: a yellow-red to orange-red color develops immediately.
Loss on drying ⟨731⟩—Dry it at 105° for 3 hours: it loses not more than 0.5% of its weight.
Loss on ignition ⟨733⟩—Ignite 2 g, previously dried and accurately weighed, at 800 ± 25° to constant weight: it loses not more than 0.5% of its weight. If labeled as attenuation grade, ignite 4 g of titanium dioxide, accurately weighed, at 800 ± 25° to constant weight: it loses not more than 13% of its weight.
Water-soluble substances—Suspend 4.0 g in 50 mL of water, mix, and allow to stand overnight. Transfer to a 200-mL volumetric flask, add 2 mL of ammonium chloride TS, and mix. If the Titanium Dioxide does not settle, add another 2-mL portion of ammonium chloride TS. Allow the suspension to settle, dilute with water to volume, mix, and filter through a double thickness of fine-porosity filter paper, discarding the first 10 mL of the filtrate. Collect 100 mL of the clear filtrate, transfer to a tared platinum dish, evaporate on a hot plate to dryness, and ignite at a dull red heat to constant weight: the residue weighs not more than 5 mg (0.25%).

Acid-soluble substances—Suspend 5.0 g in 100 mL of 0.5 N hydrochloric acid, and heat on a steam bath for 30 minutes, with occasional stirring. Filter through an appropriate filter medium until clear. Wash with three 10-mL portions of 0.5 N hydrochloric acid. Evaporate the combined filtrate and washings to dryness, and ignite at a dull red heat to constant weight: the residue weighs not more than 25 mg (0.5%).

Arsenic, *Method I* ⟨211⟩—Prepare the *Test Preparation* as follows. Add 3.0 g to a 250-mL conical flask fitted with a thermometer and a vapor outlet. Add 50 mL of water, 500 mg of hydrazine sulfate, 500 mg of potassium bromide, 20 g of sodium chloride, and 25 mL of sulfuric acid. Arrange to collect the evolved vapors in 52 mL of water contained in the arsine generator flask, then heat the test specimen to 90°, and maintain the temperature at 90° to 100° for 15 minutes. Add 3 mL of hydrochloric acid to the solution in the generator flask: the resulting solution meets the requirements of the test, the addition of 20 mL of 7 N sulfuric acid specified for *Procedure* being omitted. The limit is 1 ppm.

Organic volatile impurities, *Method IV* ⟨467⟩: meets the requirements.

(Official until July 1, 2008)

Assay—Accurately weigh about 300 mg of Titanium Dioxide, transfer to a 250-mL beaker, and add 20 mL of sulfuric acid and 7 to 8 g of ammonium sulfate. Mix, heat on a hot plate until fumes of sulfur trioxide appear, and continue heating over a strong flame until solution is complete or it is apparent that the undissolved residue is siliceous matter. Cool, cautiously dilute with 100 mL of water, stir, heat carefully to boiling while stirring, and allow the insoluble matter to settle. Filter, transfer the entire residue to the filter, and wash thoroughly with cold 2 N sulfuric acid. Dilute the filtrate with water to 200 mL, and cautiously add about 10 mL of ammonium hydroxide.

Prepare a zinc amalgam column in a 25-cm Jones reductor tube, placing a pledget of glass wool in the bottom of the tube, and filling the constricted portion of the tube with zinc amalgam prepared as follows. Add 20- to 30-mesh zinc to mercuric chloride solution (1 in 50), using about 100 mL of the solution for each 100 g of zinc, and after about 10 minutes, decant the solution from the zinc, then wash the zinc by decantation. Wash the zinc amalgam column with 100-mL portions of 2 N sulfuric acid until 100 mL of the washing does not decolorize 1 drop of 0.1 N potassium permanganate.

Place 50 mL of ferric ammonium sulfate TS in a 1000-mL suction flask, and add 0.1 N potassium permanganate until a faint pink color persists for 5 minutes. Attach the Jones reductor tube to the neck of the flask, and pass 50 mL of 2 N sulfuric acid through the reductor at a rate of about 30 mL per minute. Pass the prepared titanium solution through the reductor at the same rate, and follow with 100 mL each of 2 N sulfuric acid and of water. During these operations, keep the reductor filled with solution or water above the upper level of the amalgam. Taking precautions against the admission of atmospheric oxygen, gradually release the suction, wash down the outlet tube of the reductor and the sides of the receiver, and titrate immediately with 0.1 N potassium permanganate VS. Perform a blank determination, substituting 200 mL of 2 N sulfuric acid for the assay solution, and make any necessary correction. Each mL of 0.1 N potassium permanganate is equivalent to 7.988 mg of TiO$_2$.

Tizanidine Hydrochloride

$C_9H_8ClN_5S \cdot HCl$ 290.17

2,1,3-Benzothiadiazol-4-amine, 5-chloro-*N*-(4,5-dihydro-1*H*-imidazol-2-yl)-, monohydrochloride.
5-Chloro-4-(2-imidazolin-2-ylamino)-2,1,3-benzothiadiazole monohydrochloride   [64461-82-1].

» Tizanidine Hydrochloride contains not less than 98.0 percent and not more than 102.0 percent of $C_9H_8ClN_5S \cdot HCl$, calculated on the dried basis.

Packaging and storage—Preserve in tight containers, and store at room temperature.

USP Reference standards ⟨11⟩—USP Tizanidine Hydrochloride RS. USP Tizanidine Related Compound A RS. USP Tizanidine Related Compound B RS. USP Tizanidine Related Compound C RS.

Change to read:
Identification—
  A: *Infrared Absorption* ⟨197K⟩.
  B: The retention time of the major peak in the chromatogram of the *Assay preparation* corresponds to that in the chromatogram of the *Standard preparation,* as obtained in the *Assay.*
  ▲**C:** A solution of 10 mg per mL in water meets the requirements of the silver nitrate precipitate test for *Chloride* ⟨191⟩.▲USP31
pH ⟨791⟩: between 4.3 and 5.3, in a 1% (w/v) solution.
Loss on drying ⟨731⟩—Dry about 0.5 g of sample at 105° for 3 hours: it loses not more than 0.5% of its weight.
Residue on ignition ⟨281⟩: not more than 0.1%.
Heavy metals ⟨231⟩: 0.002%.

Change to read:
Related compounds—
  Phosphoric acid solution—Transfer 6.0 mL of phosphoric acid to a 50-mL volumetric flask, and dilute with water to volume.
  Buffer solution—Dissolve about 3.5 g of sodium 1-pentanesulfonate in 1000 mL of water, and adjust with *Phosphoric acid solution* or 1 N sodium hydroxide to a pH of 3.0 ± 0.05.
  Mobile phase—Prepare a filtered and degassed mixture of *Buffer solution* and acetonitrile (80 : 20). Make adjustments if necessary (see *System Suitability* under *Chromatography* ⟨621⟩).
  Tizanidine related compound A solution—Dissolve an accurately weighed quantity of USP Tizanidine Related Compound A RS in methanol, and dilute quantitatively, and stepwise if necessary, with methanol to obtain a solution having a known concentration of about 0.1 mg per mL.
  Tizanidine related compound B solution—Dissolve an accurately weighed quantity of USP Tizanidine Related Compound B RS in methanol, and dilute quantitatively, and stepwise if necessary, with methanol to obtain a solution having a known concentration of about 0.1 mg per mL.
  Tizanidine related compound C solution—Dissolve an accurately weighed quantity of USP Tizanidine Related Compound C RS in methanol, and dilute quantitatively, and stepwise if necessary, with methanol to obtain a solution having a known concentration of about 0.1 mg per mL.
  Resolution solution—Transfer about 23 mg of USP Tizanidine Hydrochloride RS to a 100-mL volumetric flask, add 20 mL of *Mobile phase* and 10 mL each of *Tizanidine related compound A solution, Tizanidine related compound B solution,* and *Tizanidine related compound C solution.* Sonicate to dissolve the USP Tizanidine Hydrochloride RS, and dilute with *Mobile phase* to volume.
  Standard solution—Dissolve an accurately weighed quantity of USP Tizanidine Hydrochloride RS in *Mobile phase,* and dilute quantitatively, and stepwise if necessary, with *Mobile phase* to obtain a solution having a known concentration of about 0.046 mg per mL.
  Test solution—Transfer about 57 mg of Tizanidine Hydrochloride, accurately weighed, to a 50-mL volumetric flask, dissolve in and dilute with *Mobile phase* to volume, and mix.
  Chromatographic system (see *Chromatography* ⟨621⟩)—The liquid chromatograph is equipped with a 230-nm detector and a 4.6-mm × 25-cm column that contains packing L1. The flow rate is about 1.0 mL per minute. The column temperature is maintained at 50°. Chromatograph the *Resolution solution,* and record the peak responses as directed for *Procedure:* the relative retention times are given in *Table 1;* the resolution, *R,* between tizanidine and tizanidine related compound C is not less than 4.0; and the resolution, *R,* between tizanidine and tizanidine related compound B is not less than 4.0. Chromatograph the *Standard solution,* and record the peak

responses as directed for *Procedure:* the column efficiency is not less than 5000 theoretical plates; the tailing factor is not more than 2.0; and the relative standard deviation for replicate injections is not more than 2.0%.

Procedure—Inject equal volumes (about 10 µL) of the *Standard solution* and the *Test solution* into the chromatograph, record the chromatograms, and measure the responses for the major analyte peaks, disregarding the peaks due to the solvent. Calculate the percentage of each impurity in the portion of Tizanidine Hydrochloride taken by the formula:

$$\blacktriangle (253.71/290.17)100(C_S/C_T)(1/F)(r_I/r_S)$$

in which 253.71 and 290.17 are the molecular weights of tizanidine and tizanidine hydrochloride, respectively; C_S and C_T are the concentration, in mg per mL, of tizanidine hydrochloride in the *Standard solution* and the *Test solution; F* is the relative response factor for each impurity relative to tizanidine and is given in *Table 1*; r_I is the peak area for each impurity obtained from the *Test solution;*$_{\blacktriangle USP31}$ and r_S is the peak area of tizanidine obtained from the *Standard solution*. The limits for the impurities are specified in *Table 1*.

Table 1

Compound Name	Relative Retention Time	Relative Response Factor	Limit (%)
Tizanidine related compound C	about 0.8	1.0	0.1
Tizanidine	1.0	—	—
Tizanidine related compound B	about 1.4	▲1.1$_{\blacktriangle USP31}$	0.1
Tizanidine related compound A	about 10.2	▲1.1$_{\blacktriangle USP31}$	0.1
Individual unknown	—	1.0	0.1
Total	—	—	0.3

Organic volatile impurities ⟨467⟩: meets the requirements.
(Official until July 1, 2008)

Delete the following:
▲**Content of chloride**—Dissolve about 500 mg, accurately weighed, in 50 mL of water. Titrate with 0.1 N silver nitrate VS, determining the endpoint potentiometrically. Perform a blank determination, and make any necessary correction. Each mL of 0.1 N silver nitrate is equivalent to 3.545 mg of chloride. Not less than 11.9% and not more than 12.5%, calculated on the dried basis, is found.$_{\blacktriangle USP31}$

Change to read:
Assay—
Buffer solution—Dissolve 6.8 g of monobasic potassium phosphate in 1000 mL of water, and adjust with 5.3 N potassium hydroxide to a pH of 7.5 ± 0.05.

Mobile phase—Prepare a filtered and degassed mixture of *Buffer solution* and acetonitrile (80 : 20). Make adjustments if necessary (see *System Suitability* under *Chromatography* ⟨621⟩).

System suitability preparation—Dissolve suitable quantities of USP Tizanidine Hydrochloride RS and USP Tizanidine Related Compound C RS in *Mobile phase*, and dilute quantitatively, and stepwise if necessary, with *Mobile phase* ▲to obtain a solution containing about 46 µg per mL and 0.12 µg per mL, respectively.$_{\blacktriangle USP31}$

Standard preparation—Dissolve an accurately weighed quantity of USP Tizanidine Hydrochloride RS in *Mobile phase*, and dilute quantitatively, and stepwise if necessary, with *Mobile phase* to obtain a solution having a known concentration of about 0.046 mg per mL.

Assay preparation—Transfer about 23 mg of Tizanidine Hydrochloride, accurately weighed, to a 100-mL volumetric flask, dissolve in and dilute with *Mobile phase* to volume, and mix. Transfer 10.0 mL of this solution to a 50-mL volumetric flask, dilute with *Mobile phase* to volume, and mix.

Chromatographic system (see *Chromatography* ⟨621⟩)—The liquid chromatograph is equipped with a 230-nm detector and a 4.6-mm × 15-cm column that contains packing L7. The flow rate is about 1.0 mL per minute. The column temperature is maintained at 35°. Chromatograph the *System suitability preparation*, and record the peak responses as directed for *Procedure:* the relative retention times are about 0.5 for tizanidine related compound C and 1.0 for tizanidine; the resolution, *R*, between tizanidine and tizanidine related compound C is not less than ▲6; and the tailing factor for the tizanidine peak is not more than 2.0.$_{\blacktriangle USP31}$ Chromatograph the *Standard preparation*, and record the peak responses as directed for *Procedure:* the relative standard deviation for replicate injections is not more than 2.0%.

Procedure—Separately inject equal volumes (about 20 µL) of the *Standard preparation* and the *Assay preparation* into the chromatograph, record the chromatograms, and measure the responses for the major peaks. ▲Calculate the percentage of $C_9H_8ClN_5S \cdot HCl$ in the portion of Tizanidine Hydrochloride taken by the formula:

$$100(C_S/C_U)(r_U/r_S)$$

in which C_S and C_U are the concentrations of tizanidine hydrochloride, in mg per mL, in the *Standard preparation* and the *Assay preparation*, respectively;$_{\blacktriangle USP31}$ and r_U and r_S are the peak areas obtained from the *Assay preparation* and the *Standard preparation*, respectively.

Tizanidine Tablets

» Tizanidine Tablets contain Tizanidine Hydrochloride equivalent to not less than 90.0 percent and not more than 110.0 percent of the labeled amount of tizanidine ($C_9H_8ClN_5S$).

Packaging and storage—Preserve in tight containers, and store at controlled room temperature.

USP Reference standards ⟨11⟩—USP Tizanidine Hydrochloride RS. USP Tizanidine Related Compound A RS. USP Tizanidine Related Compound B RS. USP Tizanidine Related Compound C RS.

Identification—The retention time of the major peak in the chromatogram of the *Assay preparation* corresponds to that in the chromatogram of the *Standard preparation*, as obtained in the *Assay*.

Dissolution ⟨711⟩—
Medium: 0.1 N hydrochloric acid; 500 mL, degassed.
Apparatus 1: 100 rpm.
Time: 45 minutes.

Determine the amount of tizanidine hydrochloride ($C_9H_8ClN_5S \cdot HCl$) dissolved by employing the following method.

Phosphoric acid solution, Buffer solution, and *Mobile phase*—Proceed as directed in the *Assay*.

Standard stock solution—Dissolve an accurately weighed quantity of USP Tizanidine Hydrochloride RS, and dilute quantitatively, and stepwise if necessary, with *Medium* to obtain a solution having a concentration of about 201 µg per mL.

Working standard solution—For Tablets labeled to contain 2 mg, transfer 4.0 mL of the *Standard stock solution* to a 200-mL volumetric flask, dilute with *Medium* to volume, and mix. For Tablets labeled to contain 4 mg, transfer 4.0 mL of the *Standard stock solution* to a 100-mL volumetric flask, dilute with *Medium* to volume, and mix.

Test solution—Withdraw 10 mL of the solution under test. Pass through a suitable 0.45-µm filter, discarding the first 5 mL of the filtrate.

Chromatographic system (see *Chromatography* ⟨621⟩)—The liquid chromatograph is equipped with a 230-nm detector and a 4.6-mm × 25-cm column that contains packing L1. The flow rate is about 1.0 mL per minute. The column temperature is maintained at 50°. Chromatograph the *Working standard solution*, and record the peak responses as directed for *Procedure:* the column efficiency is not less than 2000 theoretical plates; the tailing factor is not more than 2.0; and the relative standard deviation for replicate injections is not more than 2.0%.

Procedure—Separately inject equal volumes (about 20 μL) of the *Working standard solution* and the *Test solution* into the chromatograph, record the chromatograms, and measure the responses for the major peaks. Calculate the quantity, in percentage, of $C_9H_8ClN_5S \cdot HCl$ dissolved by the formula:

$$\frac{r_U \times C_S \times 500 \times 100}{r_S \times LC} \times \frac{253.71}{290.17}$$

in which r_U and r_S are the peak responses for the *Test solution* and the *Working standard solution*, respectively; C_S is the concentration, in μg per mL, of the *Working standard solution*; 500 is the volume, in mL, of *Medium*; 100 is the conversion factor to percentage; *LC* is the Tablet label claim, in mg; 253.71 is the molecular weight of tizanidine; and 290.17 is the molecular weight of tizanidine hydrochloride.

Tolerances—Not less than 80% (*Q*) of the labeled amount of $C_9H_8ClN_5S \cdot HCl$ is dissolved in 45 minutes.

Related compounds—
Phosphoric acid solution, Buffer solution, Mobile phase, Tizanidine related compound A solution, Tizanidine related compound B solution, Tizanidine related compound C solution, Resolution solution, and *Chromatographic system*—Proceed as directed in the *Assay*.

Standard solution—Prepare as directed for the *Standard preparation* in the *Assay*.

Test solution—Weigh and finely powder not fewer than 20 Tablets. Transfer an accurately weighed portion of the powder, equivalent to about 20 mg of tizanidine, to a 100-mL volumetric flask, add about 50 mL of *Buffer solution*, sonicate for about 15 minutes with occasional shaking, and shake by mechanical means for 15 minutes. Add 20 mL of acetonitrile, and mix. Allow to cool, dilute with *Buffer solution* to volume, and mix. Centrifuge a portion of this solution at 2000 rpm or higher for 10 minutes. Pass a portion of this solution through a filter having a 45-μm or finer porosity, and use the filtrate.

Procedure—Inject equal volumes (about 10 μL) of the *Standard solution* and the *Test solution* into the chromatograph, record the chromatograms, and measure the responses for the major analyte peaks, disregarding the peaks due to the solvent. Calculate the percentage of each impurity in the portion of Tablets taken by the formula:

$$(253.71/290.17)10,000(C/W)(A/D)F(r_i/r_S)$$

in which 253.71 and 290.17 are the molecular weights of tizanidine and tizanidine hydrochloride, respectively; *C* is the concentration, in mg per mL, of USP Tizanidine Hydrochloride RS in the *Standard solution*; *A* is the average weight, in mg, of each Tablet; *D* is the labeled dose, in mg, of tizanidine per Tablet; *W* is the weight, in mg, of sample taken to prepare the *Test solution*; *F* is the relative response factor and is given in *Table 1*; r_i is the peak area for each impurity obtained from the *Test solution*; and r_S is the peak area of tizanidine in the *Standard solution*. The limits for the impurities are specified in *Table 1*.

Table 1

Compound Name	Relative Retention Time	Relative Response Factor	Limit (%)
Tizanidine related compound C	about 0.8	1.0	0.2
Tizanidine	1.0	—	—
Tizanidine related compound B	about 1.4	0.9	0.2
Tizanidine Related compound A	about 10.2	0.9	0.2
Individual unknown	—	1.0	0.2
Total	—	—	0.5

Assay—
Phosphoric acid solution—Dilute 6 mL of phosphoric acid with water to make 50 mL of solution.

Buffer solution—Dissolve about 3.5 g of sodium 1-pentanesulfonate in 1000 mL of water. Adjust with *Phosphoric acid solution* or 1 N sodium hydroxide to a pH of 3.0 ± 0.05.

Mobile phase—Prepare a filtered and degassed mixture of *Buffer solution* and acetonitrile (80 : 20). Make adjustments if necessary (see *System Suitability* under *Chromatography* ⟨621⟩).

Tizanidine related compound A solution—Dissolve an accurately weighed quantity of USP Tizanidine Related Compound A RS in methanol, and dilute quantitatively, and stepwise if necessary, with methanol to obtain a solution having a known concentration of about 0.1 mg per mL.

Tizanidine related compound B solution—Dissolve an accurately weighed quantity of USP Tizanidine Related Compound B RS in methanol, and dilute quantitatively, and stepwise if necessary, with methanol to obtain a solution having a known concentration of about 0.1 mg per mL.

Tizanidine related compound C solution—Dissolve an accurately weighed quantity of USP Tizanidine Related Compound C RS in methanol, and dilute quantitatively, and stepwise if necessary, with methanol to obtain a solution having a known concentration of about 0.1 mg per mL.

Resolution solution—Transfer about 23 mg of USP Tizanidine Hydrochloride RS to a 100-mL volumetric flask, add 20 mL of *Mobile phase* and 10 mL each of *Tizanidine related compound A solution, Tizanidine related compound B solution,* and *Tizanidine related compound C solution*. Sonicate to dissolve the USP Tizanidine Hydrochloride RS, and dilute with *Mobile phase* to volume.

Standard preparation—Dissolve an accurately weighed quantity of USP Tizanidine Hydrochloride RS in *Mobile phase*, and dilute quantitatively, and stepwise if necessary, with *Mobile phase* to obtain a solution having a known concentration of about 0.046 mg per mL.

Assay preparation—Weigh and finely powder not fewer than 20 Tablets. Transfer an accurately weighed portion of the powder, equivalent to about 20 mg of tizanidine, to a 500-mL volumetric flask, add about 250 mL of *Buffer solution*, sonicate for about 15 minutes with occasional shaking, and shake by mechanical means for 15 minutes. Add 100 mL of acetonitrile, and mix. Allow to cool, dilute with *Buffer solution* to volume, and mix. Centrifuge a portion of this solution at 2000 rpm or higher for 10 minutes. Pass a portion of this solution through a filter having a 45-μm or finer porosity, and use the filtrate.

Chromatographic system (see *Chromatography* ⟨621⟩)—The liquid chromatograph is equipped with a 230-nm detector and a 4.6-mm × 25-cm column that contains packing L1. The flow rate is about 1.0 mL per minute. The column temperature is maintained at 50°. Chromatograph the *Resolution solution*, and record the peak responses as directed for *Procedure*: the relative retention times are given in *Table 1*; the resolution, *R*, between tizanidine and tizanidine related compound C is not less than 4.0, and the resolution, *R*, between tizanidine and tizanidine related compound B is not less than 4.0. Chromatograph the *Standard preparation*, and record the peak responses as directed for *Procedure*: the column efficiency is not less than 5000 theoretical plates; the tailing factor is not more than 2.0; and the relative standard deviation for replicate injections is not more than 2.0%.

Procedure—Separately inject equal volumes (about 10 μL) of the *Standard preparation* and the *Assay preparation* into the chromatograph, record the chromatograms, and measure the responses for the

major peaks. Calculate the quantity, in mg, of tizanidine ($C_9H_8ClN_5S$) in the portion of Tablets taken by the formula:

$$(253.71/290.17)500C(r_U/r_S)$$

in which C is the concentration, in mg per mL, of USP Tizanidine Hydrochloride RS in the *Standard preparation;* and r_U and r_S are the peak areas obtained from the *Assay preparation* and the *Standard preparation,* respectively.

Tobramycin

$C_{18}H_{37}N_5O_9$ 467.52

D-Streptamine, *O*-3-amino-3-deoxy-α-D-glucopyranosyl-(1→ 6)-*O*-[2,6-diamino-2,3,6-trideoxy-α-D-*ribo*-hexopyranosyl-(1→4)]-2-deoxy-.
O-3-Amino-3-deoxy-α-D-glucopyranosyl-(1→4)-*O*-[2,6-diamino-2,3,6-trideoxy-α-D-*ribo*-hexopyranosyl-(1→6)]-2-deoxy-L-streptamine   [32986-56-4].

» Tobramycin has a potency of not less than 900 μg of $C_{18}H_{37}N_5O_9$ per mg, calculated on the anhydrous basis.

Packaging and storage—Preserve in tight containers.
Labeling—Where it is intended for use in preparing injectable or ophthalmic dosage forms, the label states that it is sterile or must be subjected to further processing during the preparation of injectable or ophthalmic dosage forms.

USP Reference standards ⟨11⟩—USP Endotoxin RS. USP Tobramycin RS.
Identification—
   A: Prepare a solution of it in water containing 6 mg per mL. Apply 3 μL of this test solution, 3 μL of a Standard solution of USP Tobramycin RS containing 6 mg per mL, and 3 μL of a mixture of equal volumes of the two solutions to a suitable thin-layer chromatographic plate (see *Chromatography* ⟨621⟩) coated with a 0.25-mm layer of chromatographic silica gel mixture. Place the plate in a suitable chromatographic chamber, and develop the chromatogram in a solvent system consisting of a mixture of methanol, ammonium hydroxide, and chloroform (60 : 30 : 25) until the solvent front has moved about three-fourths of the length of the plate. Remove the plate from the chamber, allow the solvent to evaporate, and heat the plate at 110° for 15 minutes. Immediately locate the spots on the plate by spraying with a 1 in 100 solution of ninhydrin in a mixture of butyl alcohol and pyridine (100 : 1): tobramycin appears as a pink spot, and the spots obtained from the test solution and from the mixture of test solution and Standard solution, respectively, correspond in distance from the origin to that obtained from the Standard solution.
   B: The chromatogram of the *Derivatized assay preparation* obtained as directed in the *Assay* exhibits a major peak for tobramycin, the retention time of which corresponds to that exhibited in the chromatogram of the *Derivatized standard preparation* obtained as directed in the *Assay.*
pH ⟨791⟩:   between 9 and 11, in a solution (1 in 10).
Water, *Method I* ⟨921⟩:   not more than 8.0%.
Residue on ignition ⟨281⟩:   not more than 1.0%, the charred residue being moistened with 2 mL of nitric acid and 5 drops of sulfuric acid.
Heavy metals, *Method II* ⟨231⟩:   0.003%.
Chromatographic purity—
   Diluted sodium hypochlorite solution—Dilute 20 mL of sodium hypochlorite solution with water to obtain 100 mL of solution.
   Starch-potassium iodide reagent—Dissolve 1.1 g of potassium iodide in 60 mL of water, boil for 15 minutes, and slowly add a suspension of 1.5 g of soluble starch in 10 mL of water. Add 25 mL of water, and boil for 10 minutes. Allow to cool, dilute with water to 100 mL, and mix.
   Procedure—Transfer 50 mg of Tobramycin to a 10-mL volumetric flask, add 7 mL of water to dissolve it, and adjust with 1 N sulfuric acid to a pH of 5.5 ± 0.4. Dilute with water to volume, and mix to obtain the test solution. Prepare a standard solution by diluting the test solution quantitatively with water to obtain a solution containing 0.05 mg per mL. Separately apply 1 μL of these solutions to a thin-layer chromatographic plate (see *Chromatography* ⟨621⟩) coated with a 0.25-mm layer of chromatographic silica gel, and allow to dry. Develop the chromatogram in a saturated chromatographic chamber containing a mixture of sodium chloride solution (29.2 in 100), alcohol, and water (50 : 30 : 20) until the solvent front has moved about three-fourths of the length of the plate. Remove the plate from the chromatographic chamber, evaporate the solvent in a current of hot air, then heat it at 110° for 10 minutes. Lightly spray the hot plate with *Diluted sodium hypochlorite solution.* Dry the plate in a current of cold air until a sprayed area of the plate below the origin gives at most a faint blue color with a drop of *Starch-potassium iodide reagent.* Then spray the plate with *Starch-potassium iodide reagent:* bluish-purple spots are immediately visible. Other than the principal tobramycin spot, no spot observed in the chromatogram obtained from the test solution is more intense than the principal spot obtained from the standard solution (1.0%).
Other requirements—Where the label states that Tobramycin is sterile, it meets the requirements for *Sterility* and *Bacterial endotoxins* under *Tobramycin for Injection.* Where the label states that Tobramycin must be subjected to further processing during the preparation of injectable dosage forms, it meets the requirements for *Bacterial endotoxins* under *Tobramycin for Injection.* Where it is intended for use in preparing ophthalmic dosage forms, it is exempt from the requirements for *Bacterial endotoxins.*
Assay—
   Mobile phase—Dissolve 2.0 g of tris(hydroxymethyl)aminomethane in about 800 mL of water. To this solution add 20 mL of 1 N sulfuric acid, dilute with acetonitrile to obtain 2000 mL of solution, and mix. Allow to cool, and pass through a filter of 0.2-μm or finer porosity. Make adjustments if necessary (see *System Suitability* under *Chromatography* ⟨621⟩).
   2,4-Dinitrofluorobenzene reagent—Prepare a solution of 2,4-dinitrofluorobenzene in alcohol containing 10 mg per mL. This solution may be used for 5 days if refrigerated when not in use.
   Tris(hydroxymethyl)aminomethane reagent—Prepare a stock solution of tris(hydroxymethyl)aminomethane in water containing 15 mg per mL. This stock solution may be used for 1 month if refrigerated when not in use. Transfer 40 mL of this stock solution to a 200-mL volumetric flask, add dimethyl sulfoxide with mixing, dilute with dimethyl sulfoxide to volume, and mix. Use this reagent within 4 hours. [NOTE—If kept immersed in an ice-water bath below 10°, the reagent may be used for up to 8 hours.]
   Standard preparation—Transfer about 55 mg of USP Tobramycin RS, accurately weighed, to a 50-mL volumetric flask, add 1 mL of 1 N sulfuric acid and enough water to dissolve it, dilute with water to volume, and mix. Transfer 10.0 mL of this solution to a second 50-mL volumetric flask, dilute with water to volume, and mix. This solution contains about 0.22 mg of USP Tobramycin RS per mL.
   Assay preparation—Transfer about 55 mg of Tobramycin, accurately weighed, to a 50-mL volumetric flask, add 1 mL of 1 N sulfuric acid and enough water to dissolve it, dilute with water to volume, and mix. Transfer 10.0 mL of this solution to a second 50-mL volumetric flask, dilute with water to volume, and mix.
   Derivatization procedure—[NOTE—Heat all solutions at the same temperature and for the same duration of time as indicated. Move all flasks to and from the 60° constant temperature bath at the same time.] To separate 50-mL volumetric flasks transfer 4.0 mL of the *Standard preparation,* 4.0 mL of the *Assay preparation,* and 4.0 mL of water. To each flask add 10 mL of *2,4-Dinitrofluorobenzene reagent* and 10 mL of *Tris(hydroxymethyl)aminomethane reagent,* shake, and insert the stopper. Place the flasks in a constant temperature bath at 60 ± 2°, and heat for 50 ± 5 minutes. Remove the flasks from the bath, and allow to stand for 10 minutes. Add acetonitrile to

about 2 mL below the 50-mL mark, allow to cool to room temperature, then dilute with acetonitrile to volume, and mix. The solutions thus obtained are the *Derivatized standard preparation*, the *Derivatized assay preparation*, and the *Blank preparation*, respectively.

Resolution solution—Prepare a fresh solution of *p*-naphtholbenzein in acetonitrile containing about 0.24 mg per mL. Transfer 2 mL of this solution to a 10-mL volumetric flask, dilute with *Derivatized standard preparation* to volume, and use promptly.

Chromatographic system (see *Chromatography* ⟨621⟩)—The liquid chromatograph is equipped with a 365-nm detector and a 3.9-mm × 30-cm column containing packing L1. The flow rate is about 1.2 mL per minute. Chromatograph the *Blank preparation*, and record the responses as directed for *Procedure*. Identify the solvent and reagent peaks. Chromatograph the *Resolution solution*, and record the responses as directed for *Procedure*: the relative retention times are about 0.6 for *p*-naphtholbenzein and 1.0 for tobramycin, and the resolution, *R*, between the two peaks is not less than 4.0. Chromatograph the *Derivatized standard preparation*, and record the responses as directed for *Procedure*: the relative standard deviation for replicate injections is not more than 2.0%.

Procedure—Separately inject equal volumes (about 20 µL) of the *Derivatized standard preparation* and the *Derivatized assay preparation* into the chromatograph, record the chromatograms, and measure the area responses for the major peaks. Calculate the quantity, in µg, of $C_{18}H_{37}N_5O_9$ in each mg of the Tobramycin taken by the formula:

$$250(CE/W)(r_U/r_S)$$

in which *C* is the concentration, in mg per mL, of USP Tobramycin RS in the *Standard preparation*; *E* is the tobramycin equivalent, in µg per mg, of USP Tobramycin RS; *W* is the weight, in mg, of the portion of Tobramycin taken; and r_U and r_S are the tobramycin peak area responses obtained from the *Derivatized assay preparation* and the *Derivatized standard preparation*, respectively.

Tobramycin Injection

» Tobramycin Injection is a sterile solution of Tobramycin Sulfate in Water for Injection, or of Tobramycin in Water for Injection prepared with the aid of Sulfuric Acid. It contains not less than 90.0 percent and not more than 120.0 percent of the labeled amount of tobramycin ($C_{18}H_{37}N_5O_9$).

Packaging and storage—Preserve in single-dose or multiple-dose glass or plastic containers. Glass containers are preferably of Type I glass.

USP Reference standards ⟨11⟩—*USP Endotoxin RS. USP Tobramycin RS.*

Identification—

A: Dilute the Injection with water to obtain a solution containing 6 mg of tobramycin per mL, and proceed as directed for *Identification* test *A* under *Tobramycin*, beginning with "Apply 3 µL of this test solution".

B: The retention time of the major peak for tobramycin in the chromatogram of the *Derivatized assay preparation* corresponds to that in the chromatogram of the *Derivatized standard preparation*, as obtained in the *Assay*.

Bacterial endotoxins ⟨85⟩—It contains not more than 2.00 USP Endotoxin Units per mg of tobramycin.

Sterility ⟨71⟩—It meets the requirements when tested as directed for *Membrane Filtration* under *Test for Sterility of the Product to be Examined*.

pH ⟨791⟩: between 3.0 and 6.5.

Particulate matter ⟨788⟩: meets the requirements for small-volume injections.

Other requirements—It meets the requirements under *Injections* ⟨1⟩.

Assay—

Mobile phase, 2,4-Dinitrofluorobenzene reagent, Tris(hydroxymethyl)aminomethane reagent, Standard preparation, Derivatization procedure, Resolution solution, and *Chromatographic system*—Proceed as directed in the *Assay* under *Tobramycin*.

Assay preparation—Dilute an accurately measured volume of Injection quantitatively, and stepwise if necessary, with water to obtain a solution containing the equivalent of about 0.2 mg of tobramycin per mL.

Procedure—Proceed as directed in the *Assay* under *Tobramycin*. Calculate the quantity, in mg, of tobramycin ($C_{18}H_{37}N_5O_9$) in each mL of the Injection taken by the formula:

$$(L/D)(CE/1000)(r_U/r_S)$$

in which *L* is the labeled quantity, in mg per mL, of tobramycin ($C_{18}H_{37}N_5O_9$) in the Injection; *D* is the concentration, in mg per mL, of tobramycin in the *Assay preparation*, on the basis of the labeled quantity, the volume taken, and the extent of dilution; and the other terms are as defined therein.

Tobramycin for Injection

» Tobramycin for Injection contains an amount of Tobramycin Sulfate equivalent to not less than 90.0 percent and not more than 115.0 percent of the labeled amount of tobramycin ($C_{18}H_{37}N_5O_9$).

Packaging and storage—Preserve in *Containers for Sterile Solids* as described under *Injections* ⟨1⟩.

USP Reference standards ⟨11⟩—*USP Endotoxin RS. USP Tobramycin RS.*

Constituted solution—At the time of use, it meets the requirements for *Constituted Solutions* under *Injections* ⟨1⟩.

Identification—

A: It responds to the *Identification* tests under *Tobramycin*.

B: It responds to the tests for *Sulfate* ⟨191⟩.

Bacterial endotoxins ⟨85⟩—It contains not more than 2.00 USP Endotoxin Units per mg of tobramycin.

Sterility ⟨71⟩—It meets the requirements when tested as directed for *Membrane Filtration* under *Test for Sterility of the Product to be Examined*, 6 g being used if it is not packaged for dispensing.

pH ⟨791⟩: between 6.0 and 8.0, in a solution containing 40 mg per mL (or, where packaged for dispensing, in the solution constituted as directed in the labeling).

Water, *Method I* ⟨921⟩: not more than 2.0%.

Particulate matter ⟨788⟩: meets the requirements for small-volume injections.

Other requirements—It meets the requirements for *Residue on ignition* and *Heavy metals* under *Tobramycin*. It meets also the requirements for *Uniformity of Dosage Units* ⟨905⟩ and *Labeling* under *Injections* ⟨1⟩.

Assay—

Mobile phase, 2,4-Dinitrofluorobenzene reagent, Tris(hydroxymethyl)aminomethane reagent, Standard preparation, Derivatization procedure, Resolution solution, and *Chromatographic system*—Proceed as directed in the *Assay* under *Tobramycin*.

Assay preparation 1 (where it is represented as being in a single-dose container)—Constitute a container of Tobramycin for Injection in a volume of water, accurately measured, corresponding to the volume of diluent specified in the labeling. Withdraw all of the withdrawable contents, using a suitable hypodermic needle and syringe, and dilute quantitatively with water to obtain a solution containing the equivalent of about 0.2 mg of tobramycin ($C_{18}H_{37}N_5O_9$) per mL.

Assay preparation 2 (where the label states the quantity of tobramycin in a given volume of constituted solution)—Constitute a container of Tobramycin for Injection in a volume of water, accurately measured, equivalent to the volume of diluent specified in the labeling. Dilute an accurately measured volume of the constituted solution quantitatively with water to obtain a solution containing about 0.2 mg of tobramycin ($C_{18}H_{37}N_5O_9$) per mL.

Procedure—Proceed as directed for *Procedure* in the *Assay* under *Tobramycin*. Calculate the quantity, in mg, of tobramycin ($C_{18}H_{37}N_5O_9$) withdrawn from the container, or in the portion of constituted solution taken by the formula:

$$(L/D)(CE/1000)(r_U/r_S)$$

in which L is the labeled quantity, in mg, of tobramycin ($C_{18}H_{37}N_5O_9$) in the container, or in the volume of constituted solution taken; D is the concentration, in mg of tobramycin per mL, of *Assay preparation 1* or *Assay preparation 2*, based on the labeled quantity in the container or in the volume of constituted solution taken, respectively, and the extent of dilution; and the other terms are as defined therein.

Tobramycin Ophthalmic Ointment

» Tobramycin Ophthalmic Ointment contains the equivalent of not less than 90.0 percent and not more than 120.0 percent of the labeled amount of tobramycin ($C_{18}H_{37}N_5O_9$).

Packaging and storage—Preserve in collapsible ophthalmic ointment tubes.
USP Reference standards ⟨11⟩—*USP Tobramycin RS*.
Identification—Vigorously shake by mechanical means a quantity of Ophthalmic Ointment, equivalent to about 3 mg of tobramycin, with 2 mL of chloroform. Add 1 mL of water, shake vigorously by mechanical means for 1 minute, and centrifuge for 15 minutes: the clear upper, aqueous layer so obtained meets the requirements of *Identification* test A under *Tobramycin*.
Sterility ⟨71⟩—It meets the requirements when tested as directed for *Membrane Filtration* under *Test for Sterility of the Product to be Examined*.
Minimum fill ⟨755⟩: meets the requirements.
Water, *Method I* ⟨921⟩: not more than 1.0%, 20 mL of a mixture of toluene and methanol (7 : 3) being used in place of methanol in the titration vessel.
Metal particles ⟨751⟩: meets the requirements.
Assay—
  Mobile phase, 2,4-Dinitrofluorobenzene reagent, Tris(hydroxymethyl)aminomethane reagent, Standard preparation, Resolution solution, and *Chromatographic system*—Proceed as directed in the *Assay* under *Tobramycin*.
  Assay preparation—Transfer an accurately weighed portion of Ophthalmic Ointment, equivalent to about 4.5 mg of tobramycin, to a separator, add 50 mL of ether, and extract with four 20- to 25-mL portions of water. Combine the water extracts in a 100-mL volumetric flask, dilute with water to volume, and mix.
  Derivatization procedure—Proceed as directed in the *Assay* under *Tobramycin*, except to use 15.0 mL of *Assay preparation* instead of 4.0 mL.
  Procedure—Proceed as directed in the *Assay* under *Tobramycin*. Calculate the quantity of tobramycin ($C_{18}H_{37}N_5O_9$), in mg, in the portion of Ophthalmic Ointment taken by the formula:

$$(4/150)(CE)(r_U/r_S)$$

in which the terms are as defined therein.

Tobramycin Inhalation Solution

» Tobramycin Inhalation Solution is a sterile, nonpyrogenic, preservative-free solution of Tobramycin in Water for Injection containing Sodium Chloride. It is prepared with the aid of Sulfuric Acid or Sodium Hydroxide and contains, in each mL, not less than 90.0 percent and not more than 110.0 percent of the labeled amount of tobramycin ($C_{18}H_{37}N_5O_9$).

Packaging and storage—Preserve in low-density, polyethylene, single-use ampules stored in light-resistant foil over-wrapped packaging, in a refrigerator.
USP Reference standards ⟨11⟩—*USP Endotoxin RS. USP Tobramycin RS*.
Absorbance—The absorbance of the Inhalation Solution determined at 410 nm in a 1-cm cell is not more than 0.24.
Bacterial endotoxins ⟨85⟩—It contains not more than 60 USP Endotoxin Units per mL.
Sterility ⟨71⟩—It meets the requirements when tested as directed for *Membrane Filtration* under *Test for Sterility of the Product to be Examined*.
Uniformity of dosage units ⟨905⟩: meets the requirements.
pH ⟨791⟩: between 5.5 and 6.5.
Particulate matter ⟨788⟩: meets the requirements for small-volume injections.
Osmolarity ⟨785⟩: the osmolality is between 135 and 200 mOsmol per kg.
Chromatographic purity—
  Solution A—Prepare a filtered and degassed mixture of water, acetonitrile, and phosphoric acid (95 : 5 : 0.08).
  Solution B—Prepare a filtered and degassed mixture of acetonitrile, water, and phosphoric acid (75 : 25 : 0.08).
  Mobile phase—Use variable mixtures of *Solution A* and *Solution B* as directed for *Chromatographic system*. Make adjustments if necessary (see *System Suitability* under *Chromatography* ⟨621⟩).
  Blank solution—Use water.
  2,4-Dinitrofluorobenzene reagent and *Tris(hydroxymethyl)aminomethane reagent*—Proceed as directed in the *Assay* under *Tobramycin*.
  System suitability stock solution—Dissolve an accurately weighed quantity of USP Tobramycin RS in water, and adjust with 1 N sulfuric acid to a pH of 6.0. Dilute with water to obtain a solution having a known concentration of about 1.1 mg per mL.
  System suitability solution 1—Dilute the *System suitability stock solution* quantitatively, and stepwise if necessary, with water to obtain a solution having a known concentration of about 0.22 mg per mL.
  System suitability solution 2—Heat a portion of the *System suitability stock solution* in a suitable sealed glass container at 100° for 8 to 9 hours. Cool to room temperature, and dilute with water to obtain a solution having a known concentration of about 0.22 mg per mL.
  Standard solution—Prepare a solution of about 55 mg of USP Tobramycin RS, accurately weighed, in a 50-mL volumetric flask. Dissolve in water, add 1.0 mL of 1.0 N sulfuric acid, dilute with water to volume, and mix. Dilute quantitatively, and stepwise if necessary, with water to obtain a solution having a concentration of 1.10 µg of tobramycin per mL.
  Test solution—Transfer an accurately measured volume of Inhalation Solution, equivalent to about 240 mg of tobramycin, to a 50-mL volumetric flask, dilute with water to volume, and mix. Dilute quantitatively, and stepwise if necessary, with water to obtain a solution having a concentration of 192 µg of tobramycin per mL.
  Derivatization procedure—[NOTE—Heat all solutions at the same temperature and for the same duration as indicated. Move all flasks to and from the 60° constant-temperature bath at the same time.] To separate 50-mL flasks transfer 15.0 mL of *System suitability solution 1*, 15.0 mL of *System suitability solution 2*, 15.0 mL of *Standard solution*, 15.0 mL of *Test solution*, and 15.0 mL of *Blank solution*. To each flask, add 10 mL of *2,4-Dinitrofluorobenzene reagent* and 10 mL of *Tris(hydroxymethyl)aminomethane reagent*, shake, and insert the stopper. Place the flasks in a constant-temperature bath at 60 ± 2°, and heat for 50 ± 5 minutes. Remove the flasks from the bath, and allow to stand for 10 minutes. Add acetonitrile to about 2 mL below the 50-mL mark, allow to cool to room temperature, dilute with acetonitrile to volume, and mix. Allow the solutions to stand for 16 hours. The solutions thus obtained are *Derivatized system suitability solution 1, Derivatized system suitability solution 2,* the *Derivatized standard solution*, the *Derivatized test solution*, and the *Derivatized blank solution*.

Chromatographic system (see *Chromatography* ⟨621⟩)—The liquid chromatograph is equipped with a 365-nm detector and a 4.6-mm × 25-cm column that contains packing L11. The flow rate is about 1.2 mL per minute. The chromatograph is programmed as follows.

Time (minutes)	Solution A (%)	Solution B (%)	Elution
0	79	21	equilibration
0–14	79→66	21→34	linear gradient
14–25	66→30	34→70	linear gradient
25–35	30	70	isocratic
35–40	30→20	70→80	linear gradient
40–50	20→5	80→95	linear gradient

Chromatograph *Derivatized system suitability solution 2*, and record the peak responses as directed for *Procedure:* the capacity factor, k', determined from tobramycin is not less than 15.5. Chromatograph *Derivatized system suitability solution 1*, and use the chromatogram to locate the degradation peaks from comparison to *Derivatized system suitability solution 2* (deoxystreptamine kanosaminide and nebramine will increase in response in *Derivatized system suitability solution 2* when viewed at a 0–10 mAbs unit or 0–5 mV unit full scale). Record the peak responses as directed for *Procedure:* the relative retention times are about 0.36 for an impurity, 0.66 for deoxystreptamine kanosaminide, 0.94 for nebramine, 0.96 for kanamycin B, and 1.00 for tobramycin. The resolution, R, between the nebramine and kanamycin peaks is not less than 1.0. The relative standard deviation for replicate injections of the *Derivatized standard solution* is not more than 2.0%.

Procedure—Separately inject equal volumes (about 45 μL) of *Derivatized system suitability solution 1*, *Derivatized system suitability solution 2*, the *Derivatized standard solution*, the *Derivatized test solution*, and the *Derivatized blank solution*, record the chromatograms, and measure the peak responses, disregarding any peak corresponding to those obtained from the *Derivatized blank solution*, and subtracting the quantities of any such peaks found at the relative retention times of 0.36, 0.66, and 0.94 from those found in the *Derivatized test solution*. For unknown peak determinations, disregard any peaks found in the chromatogram of the *Derivatized test solution* that correspond to those in the chromatogram of *Derivatized system suitability solution 1*. Calculate the percentage of each impurity in relation to the tobramycin content of the Inhalation Solution taken by the formula:

$$(110/192)(r_i / r_S)$$

in which r_i is the peak area of any impurity obtained from the *Derivatized test solution;* and r_S is the peak area for tobramycin obtained from the *Derivatized standard solution:* not more than 0.25% of the impurity noted at a relative retention time of 0.36 is found; not more than 0.3% of deoxystreptamine kanosaminide is found; not more than 0.4% of nebramine is found; not more than 0.1% of any unknown impurity is found; not more than 0.2% of total unknown impurities is found; and not more than 1.0% of total impurities is found.

Content of sodium chloride—Pipet 25 mL of Inhalation Solution into a suitable container. Add between 70 and 100 mL of water. Add 10 mL of an acidic gelatin solution, prepared by dissolving 2 g of gelatin and 50 mL of nitric acid in 1000 mL of water. Titrate potentiometrically with 0.1 N silver nitrate VS using a suitable silver electrode: not less than 90.0% and not more than 110.0% of the labeled amount of sodium chloride is found.

Other requirements—It meets the requirements for the *Identification* tests under *Tobramycin*.

Assay—
Mobile phase, 2,4-Dinitrofluorobenzene reagent, Tris(hydroxymethyl)aminomethane reagent, Standard preparation, Derivatization procedure, Resolution solution, and *Chromatographic system*—Proceed as directed in the *Assay* under *Tobramycin*.

Assay preparation—Transfer an accurately measured volume of Inhalation Solution to a suitable volumetric flask, and quantitatively dilute with water to obtain a solution having a concentration of about 192 μg of tobramycin per mL.

Procedure—Proceed as directed in the *Assay* under *Tobramycin*. Calculate the quantity, in mg, of tobramycin ($C_{18}H_{37}N_5O_9$) in each mL of Inhalation Solution taken by the formula:

$$(CE)(L/D)(r_U / r_S)$$

in which C, E, r_U, and r_S are as defined therein; L is the labeled quantity, in mg, of tobramycin per mL in the Inhalation Solution taken; and D is the concentration, in μg per mL, of tobramycin in the *Assay preparation*.

Tobramycin Ophthalmic Solution

» Tobramycin Ophthalmic Solution contains the equivalent of not less than 90.0 percent and not more than 120.0 percent of the labeled amount of tobramycin ($C_{18}H_{37}N_5O_9$). It may contain one or more suitable buffers, dispersants, preservatives, and tonicity agents.

Packaging and storage—Preserve in tight containers, and avoid exposure to excessive heat.

USP Reference standards ⟨11⟩—*USP Tobramycin RS*.

Identification—
A: Prepare a Standard solution of USP Tobramycin RS containing 3 mg per mL. Separately apply 6 μL of Ophthalmic Solution, 6 μL of the Standard solution, and 6 μL of a mixture consisting of equal volumes of the two solutions to a thin-layer chromatographic plate (see *Chromatography* ⟨621⟩) coated with a 0.25-mm layer of chromatographic silica gel mixture. Proceed as directed for *Identification* test A under *Tobramycin*, beginning with "Place the plate in a suitable chromatographic chamber." The specified results are obtained.

B: The retention time of the major peak for tobramycin in the chromatogram of the *Derivatized assay preparation* corresponds to that in the chromatogram of the *Derivatized standard preparation*, as obtained in the *Assay*.

Sterility ⟨71⟩—It meets the requirements when tested as directed for *Membrane Filtration* under *Test for Sterility of the Product to be Examined*.

pH ⟨791⟩: between 7.0 and 8.0.

Assay—
Mobile phase, 2,4-Dinitrofluorobenzene reagent, Tris(hydroxymethyl)aminomethane reagent, and *Resolution solution*—Prepare as directed in the *Assay* under *Tobramycin*.

Standard preparation—Transfer about 33 mg of USP Tobramycin RS, accurately weighed, to a 50-mL volumetric flask, add 20 mL of water and 1 mL of 1 N sulfuric acid, and swirl to dissolve. Dilute with water to volume, and mix. Transfer 10.0 mL of this solution to a second 50-mL volumetric flask, dilute with water to volume, and mix. This solution contains about 0.132 mg of USP Tobramycin RS per mL.

Assay preparation—Transfer an accurately measured volume of Ophthalmic Solution, equivalent to about 6 mg of tobramycin, to a 50-mL volumetric flask, dilute with water to volume, and mix.

Derivatization procedure—Proceed as directed in the *Assay* under *Tobramycin*, except to use 5.0 mL each of the *Standard preparation* and the *Assay preparation*, instead of 4.0 mL of each.

Chromatographic system—Proceed as directed in the *Assay* under *Tobramycin*, except to use a 4-mm × 15-cm column and to maintain the column temperature at 40°.

Procedure—Proceed as directed in the *Assay* under *Tobramycin*. Calculate the quantity, in mg, of tobramycin ($C_{18}H_{37}N_5O_9$) in each mL of the Ophthalmic Solution taken by the formula:

$$0.05(CE/V)(r_U / r_S)$$

in which V is the volume, in mL, of Ophthalmic Solution taken to prepare the *Assay preparation;* and the other terms are as defined therein.

Tobramycin and Dexamethasone Ophthalmic Ointment

» Tobramycin and Dexamethasone Ophthalmic Ointment contains not less than 90.0 percent and not more than 120.0 percent of the labeled amount of tobramycin ($C_{18}H_{37}N_5O_9$), and not less than 90.0 percent and not more than 110.0 percent of the labeled amount of dexamethasone ($C_{22}H_{29}FO_5$).

Packaging and storage—Preserve in collapsible ophthalmic ointment tubes.

USP Reference standards ⟨11⟩—*USP Dexamethasone RS. USP Tobramycin RS.*

Identification—
  A: To 1 g of Ophthalmic Ointment in a test tube add 2 mL of chloroform, and shake to dissolve. Add 0.5 mL of sodium sulfate solution (1 in 10), shake vigorously, and centrifuge: the clear supernatant aqueous liquid meets the requirements for *Identification* test A under *Tobramycin*. [NOTE—If, after centrifuging, an oily film remains on top of the supernatant aqueous liquid, transfer the supernatant aqueous liquid to a second test tube, and wash it with 2 mL of chloroform.]
  B: The retention time of the major peak for dexamethasone in the chromatogram of the *Assay preparation* corresponds to that in the chromatogram of the *Standard preparation*, as obtained in the *Assay for dexamethasone*.

Sterility ⟨71⟩—It meets the requirements when tested as directed for *Membrane Filtration* under *Test for Sterility of the Product to be Examined*.

Minimum fill ⟨755⟩: meets the requirements.

Water, *Method I* ⟨921⟩: not more than 1.0%, 20 mL of a mixture of toluene and methanol (7 : 3) being used in place of methanol in the titration vessel.

Metal particles ⟨751⟩: meets the requirements.

Assay for tobramycin—
  Mobile phase, 2,4-Dinitrofluorobenzene reagent, Tris(hydroxymethyl)aminomethane reagent, Standard preparation, Resolution solution, and *Chromatographic system*—Proceed as directed in the *Assay* under *Tobramycin*.
  Assay preparation—Transfer an accurately weighed portion of Ophthalmic Ointment, equivalent to about 4.5 mg of tobramycin, to a separator, add 50 mL of ether, and extract with four 20- to 25-mL portions of water. Combine the water extracts in a 100-mL volumetric flask, dilute with water to volume, and mix.
  Derivatization procedure—Proceed as directed in the *Assay* under *Tobramycin*, except to use 15.0 mL of *Assay preparation* instead of 4.0 mL.
  Procedure—Proceed as directed in the *Assay* under *Tobramycin*. Calculate the quantity of tobramycin ($C_{18}H_{37}N_5O_9$), in mg, in the portion of Ophthalmic Ointment taken by the formula:

$$(4 / 150)(CE)(r_U / r_S)$$

in which the terms are as defined therein.

Assay for dexamethasone—
  Diluent—Prepare a mixture of methanol and water (750 : 250).
  Mobile phase—Prepare a suitable mixture of methanol and water (55 : 45), pass through a suitable filter having a 1-μm or finer porosity, and degas. Make adjustments if necessary (see *System Suitability* under *Chromatography* ⟨621⟩).
  Standard preparation—Dissolve an accurately weighed quantity of USP Dexamethasone RS in *Diluent* to obtain a stock solution having a known concentration of about 0.2 mg per mL. Transfer 15.0 mL of this stock solution to a separator containing about 50 mL of *n*-hexane, and shake. Allow the layers to separate, and drain the lower phase into a 50-mL volumetric flask. Repeat the extraction with two 15-mL portions of *Diluent*, combining the lower phase from each extraction in the same 50-mL volumetric flask. Dilute with *Diluent* to volume, and mix. This solution contains about 0.06 mg of USP Dexamethasone RS per mL.
  Resolution solution—Prepare a stock solution of chlorobutanol and USP Dexamethasone RS in *Diluent* containing about 1 mg of anhydrous chlorobutanol and 0.2 mg of USP Dexamethasone RS per mL. Proceed as directed for *Standard preparation* beginning with "Transfer 15.0 mL of this stock solution to a separator." The solution so obtained contains about 0.3 mg of anhydrous chlorobutanol and 0.06 mg of USP Dexamethasone RS per mL.
  Assay preparation—Transfer an accurately weighed quantity of Ophthalmic Ointment, equivalent to about 3 mg of dexamethasone, to a separator containing about 50 mL of *n*-hexane, and shake. Add 15 mL of *Diluent*, and shake. Allow the layers to separate, and drain the lower phase into a 50-mL volumetric flask. Repeat the extraction with two 15-mL portions of *Diluent*, combining the lower phase from each extraction in the same 50-mL volumetric flask. Dilute with *Diluent* to volume, mix, and centrifuge. Use the clear solution.
  Chromatographic system (see *Chromatography* ⟨621⟩)—The liquid chromatograph is equipped with a 206-nm detector and an 8.0-mm × 10-cm column that contains packing L1. The flow rate is about 3 mL per minute. Chromatograph the *Resolution solution*, and measure the peak responses as directed for *Procedure*: the relative retention times are about 0.7 for chlorobutanol and 1.0 for dexamethasone; and the resolution, *R*, between chlorobutanol and dexamethasone is not less than 1.8. Chromatograph the *Standard preparation*, and measure the peak responses as directed for *Procedure*: the tailing factor is not more than 2; the column efficiency is not less than 350 theoretical plates; and the relative standard deviation for replicate injections is not more than 2.0%.
  Procedure—Separately inject equal volumes (about 100 μL) of the *Standard preparation* and the *Assay preparation* into the chromatograph, record the chromatograms, and measure the responses for the major peaks. Calculate the quantity, in mg, of dexamethasone ($C_{22}H_{29}FO_5$) in the portion of Ophthalmic Ointment taken by the formula:

$$50C(r_U / r_S)$$

in which *C* is the concentration, in mg per mL, of USP Dexamethasone RS in the *Standard preparation;* and r_U and r_S are the dexamethasone peak responses obtained from the *Assay preparation* and the *Standard preparation*, respectively.

Tobramycin and Dexamethasone Ophthalmic Suspension

» Tobramycin and Dexamethasone Ophthalmic Suspension is a sterile aqueous suspension containing Tobramycin and Dexamethasone. It contains not less than 90.0 percent and not more than 120.0 percent of the labeled amount of tobramycin ($C_{18}H_{37}N_5O_9$), and not less than 90.0 percent and not more than 110.0 percent of the labeled amount of dexamethasone ($C_{22}H_{29}FO_5$).

Packaging and storage—Preserve in tight containers.

USP Reference standards ⟨11⟩—*USP Dexamethasone RS. USP Tobramycin RS.*

Identification—
  A: To 1 mL of Ophthalmic Suspension in a test tube, add 100 mg of sodium sulfate, disperse by shaking, and centrifuge: the clear supernatant meets the requirements for *Identification* test A under *Tobramycin*.
  B: The retention time of the major peak for dexamethasone in the chromatogram of the *Assay preparation* corresponds to that in the chromatogram of the *Standard preparation*, as obtained in the *Assay for dexamethasone*.

Sterility ⟨71⟩—It meets the requirements when tested as directed for *Membrane Filtration* under *Test for Sterility of the Product to be Examined*.

pH ⟨791⟩: between 5.0 and 6.0.
Assay for tobramycin—
Mobile phase, 2,4-Dinitrofluorobenzene reagent, Tris(hydroxymethyl)*aminomethane reagent, Standard preparation, Resolution solution,* and *Chromatographic system*—Proceed as directed in the *Assay* under *Tobramycin.*

Assay preparation—Transfer an accurately weighed portion of Ophthalmic Suspension, equivalent to about 4.5 mg of tobramycin, to a 50-mL volumetric flask, dilute with water to volume, and mix.

Derivatization procedure—Proceed as directed in the *Assay* under *Tobramycin,* except to use 10.0 mL of the *Assay preparation* instead of 4.0 mL.

Procedure—Proceed as directed in the *Assay* under *Tobramycin.* Calculate the quantity, in mg, of tobramycin ($C_{18}H_{37}N_5O_9$) in the portion of Ophthalmic Suspension taken by the formula:

$$0.02CE(r_U/r_S)$$

in which the terms are as defined therein.
Assay for dexamethasone—
Mobile phase—Prepare a suitable mixture of water and acetonitrile (55 : 45), filter through a suitable filter having a porosity of 1 µm or less, and degas. Make adjustments if necessary (see *System Suitability* under *Chromatography* ⟨621⟩).

Standard preparation—Transfer about 25 mg of USP Dexamethasone RS, accurately weighed, to a 25-mL volumetric flask, dissolve in methanol, dilute with methanol to volume, and mix. Transfer 4.0 mL of this solution to a 100-mL volumetric flask, dilute with methanol to volume, and mix. This solution contains about 0.04 mg of USP Dexamethasone RS per mL.

Assay preparation—Transfer an accurately measured volume of Ophthalmic Suspension, freshly mixed and free from air bubbles, equivalent to about 4 mg of dexamethasone, to a 100-mL volumetric flask, dilute with methanol to volume, and mix.

Chromatographic system (see *Chromatography* ⟨621⟩)—The liquid chromatograph is equipped with a 254-nm detector and a 3.9-mm × 25-cm column that contains packing L1. The flow rate is about 1.5 mL per minute. Chromatograph the *Standard preparation,* and measure the peak responses as directed for *Procedure:* the tailing factor for the analyte peak is not more than 1.5, the column efficiency is not less than 1400 theoretical plates, and the relative standard deviation for replicate injections is not more than 2.0%.

Procedure—Separately inject equal volumes (about 20 µL) of the *Standard preparation* and the *Assay preparation* into the chromatograph, record the chromatograms, and measure the responses for the major peaks. Calculate the quantity, in mg, of dexamethasone ($C_{22}H_{29}FO_5$), in each mL of the Ophthalmic Suspension taken by the formula:

$$100(C/V)(r_U/r_S)$$

in which *C* is the concentration, in mg per mL, of USP Dexamethasone RS in the *Standard preparation, V* is the volume, in mL, of Ophthalmic Suspension taken, and r_U and r_S are the dexamethasone peak responses obtained from the *Assay preparation* and the *Standard preparation,* respectively.

Tobramycin and Fluorometholone Acetate Ophthalmic Suspension

» Tobramycin and Fluorometholone Acetate Ophthalmic Suspension is a sterile aqueous suspension of Tobramycin and Fluorometholone Acetate. It contains not less than 90.0 percent and not more than 120.0 percent of the labeled amount of tobramycin ($C_{18}H_{37}N_5O_9$) and not less than 90.0 percent and not more than 115.0 percent of the labeled amount of fluorometholone acetate ($C_{24}H_{31}FO_5$). It may contain suitable buffers, dispersants, tonicity-adjusting agents, and preservatives.

Packaging and storage—Preserve in tight containers.
USP Reference standards ⟨11⟩—*USP Fluorometholone RS. USP Fluorometholone Acetate RS. USP Tobramycin RS.*
Identification—
A: The relative retention time of the major peak in the chromatogram of the *Assay preparation* corresponds to that in the chromatogram of the *Standard preparation,* as obtained in the *Assay for fluorometholone acetate.*

B: Allow the Ophthalmic Suspension to settle, and decant 1 mL of the supernatant into a test tube. Add 0.1 g of sodium sulfate, mix, and centrifuge: the clear supernatant so obtained meets the requirements for *Identification* test A under *Tobramycin.*
Sterility ⟨71⟩—It meets the requirements when tested as directed for *Membrane Filtration* under *Test for Sterility of the Product to be Examined.*
pH ⟨791⟩: between 6.0 and 7.0.
Assay for tobramycin—
Mobile phase, 2,4-Dinitrofluorobenzene reagent, Tris(hydroxymethyl)*aminomethane reagent, Standard preparation, Resolution solution,* and *Chromatographic system*—Proceed as directed in the *Assay* under *Tobramycin.*

Assay preparation—Transfer an accurately weighed portion of Ophthalmic Suspension, equivalent to about 4.5 mg of tobramycin, to a 50-mL volumetric flask, dilute with water to volume, and mix.

Derivatization procedure—Proceed as directed in the *Assay* under *Tobramycin,* except to use 10.0 mL of *Assay preparation* instead of 4.0 mL.

Procedure—Proceed as directed in the *Assay* under *Tobramycin.* Calculate the quantity of tobramycin ($C_{18}H_{37}N_5O_9$), in mg, in the portion of Ophthalmic Suspension taken by the formula:

$$0.02CE(r_U/r_S)$$

in which the terms are as defined therein.
Assay for fluorometholone acetate—
Mobile phase—Prepare a suitable mixture of acetonitrile and water (50 : 50). Pass through a filter having a 1-µm or finer porosity, and degas. Make adjustments if necessary (see *System Suitability* under *Chromatography* ⟨621⟩). Reduce the proportion of acetonitrile to increase the retention time of fluorometholone acetate.

Resolution solution—Prepare a solution in acetonitrile containing 0.04 mg each of USP Fluorometholone RS and USP Fluorometholone Acetate RS per mL.

Standard preparation—Prepare a solution of USP Fluorometholone Acetate RS in acetonitrile having a known concentration of about 0.04 mg per mL.

Assay preparation—Transfer an accurately measured volume of Ophthalmic Suspension, freshly mixed and free from air bubbles, equivalent to about 2.5 mg of fluorometholone acetate, to a 25-mL volumetric flask, dilute with acetonitrile to volume, and mix. Transfer 4.0 mL of this solution to a 10-mL volumetric flask, dilute with acetonitrile to volume, and mix. Transfer a portion of this solution to a test tube, and centrifuge for about 15 minutes. Use the clear supernatant.

Chromatographic system (see *Chromatography* ⟨621⟩)—The liquid chromatograph is equipped with a 254-nm detector and a 4-mm × 25-cm column that contains packing L1. The flow rate is about 1.5 mL per minute. Chromatograph the *Resolution solution,* and record the peak areas as directed for *Procedure:* the relative retention times are about 0.7 for fluorometholone and 1.0 for fluorometholone acetate; and the resolution, *R,* between fluorometholone and fluorometholone acetate is not less than 2.0. Chromatograph the *Standard preparation,* and record the areas as directed for *Procedure:* the capacity factor, *k',* determined from fluorometholone acetate peak is between 1.0 and 5.0; the column efficiency is not less than 1000 theoretical plates; the tailing factor is not more than 1.35; and the relative standard deviation for replicate injections is not more than 2.0%.

Procedure—Separately inject equal volumes (about 10 µL) of the *Standard preparation* and the *Assay preparation* into the chromatograph, record the chromatograms, and measure the peak areas. Calculate the quantity, in mg, of fluorometholone acetate ($C_{24}H_{31}FO_5$) in each mL of Ophthalmic Suspension taken by the formula:

$$62.5(C/V)(r_U/r_S)$$

in which C is the concentration, in mg per mL, of USP Fluorometholone Acetate RS in the *Standard preparation*; V is the volume, in mL, of Ophthalmic Suspension taken; and r_U and r_S are the fluorometholone acetate peak areas obtained from the *Assay preparation* and the *Standard preparation*, respectively.

Tobramycin Sulfate

$(C_{18}H_{37}N_5O_9)_2 \cdot 5H_2SO_4$ 1425.45
D-Streptamine, O-3-amino-3-deoxy-α-D-glucopyranosyl-(1→6)-O-[2,6-diamino-2,3,6-tridoexy-α-D-*ribo*-hexopyranosyl-(1→4)]-2-deoxy-, sulfate (2 : 5) (salt).
O-3-Amino-3-deoxy-α-D-glucopyranosyl-(1→4)-O-[2,6-diamino-2,3,6-tridoexy-α-D-*ribo*-hexopyranosyl-(1→6)]-2-deoxy-L-streptamine, sulfate (2 : 5) (salt)   [79645-27-5].

» Tobramycin Sulfate has a potency of not less than 634 μg and not more than 739 μg of tobramycin ($C_{18}H_{37}N_5O_9$) per mg.

Packaging and storage—Preserve in tight containers.
Labeling—Where it is intended for use in preparing injectable dosage forms, the label states that it is sterile or must be subjected to further processing during the preparation of injectable dosage forms.

USP Reference standards ⟨11⟩—USP Endotoxin RS. USP Tobramycin RS.
Identification—
  A: It responds to the *Identification* tests under *Tobramycin*.
  B: It responds to the tests for *Sulfate* ⟨191⟩.
pH ⟨791⟩: between 6.0 and 8.0, in a solution containing 40 mg per mL.
Water, *Method I* ⟨921⟩: not more than 2.0%.
Other requirements—It meets the requirements for *Residue on ignition, Heavy metals,* and *Chromatographic purity* under *Tobramycin*. Where the label states that Tobramycin Sulfate is sterile, it meets the requirements for *Sterility Tests* ⟨71⟩ and for *Bacterial endotoxins* under *Tobramycin for Injection*. Where the label states that Tobramycin Sulfate must be subjected to further processing during the preparation of injectable dosage forms, it meets the requirements for *Bacterial endotoxins* under *Tobramycin for Injection*.
Assay—
  Mobile phase, 2,4-Dinitrofluorobenzene reagent, Tris(hydroxymethyl)aminomethane reagent, Standard preparation, Derivatization procedure, Resolution solution, and *Chromatographic system*—Proceed as directed in the *Assay* under *Tobramycin*.
  Assay preparation—Transfer an accurately weighed quantity of Tobramycin Sulfate, equivalent to about 50 mg of tobramycin ($C_{18}H_{37}N_5O_9$), to a 250-mL volumetric flask, dissolve in and dilute with water to volume, and mix.
  Procedure—Proceed as directed for *Procedure* in the *Assay* under *Tobramycin*. Calculate the quantity, in μg, of tobramycin ($C_{18}H_{37}N_5O_9$) in each mg of the Tobramycin Sulfate taken by the formula:

$$250(CE/W)(r_U/r_S)$$

in which the terms are as defined therein.

Tocainide Hydrochloride

$C_{11}H_{16}N_2O \cdot HCl$ 228.72
Propanamide, 2-amino-N-(2,6-dimethylphenyl)-, hydrochloride, (±)-.
(±)-2-Amino-2′,6′-propionoxylidide hydrochloride.

» Tocainide Hydrochloride contains not less than 98.0 percent and not more than 101.0 percent of $C_{11}H_{16}N_2O \cdot HCl$, calculated on the dried basis.

Packaging and storage—Preserve in well-closed containers.
USP Reference standards ⟨11⟩—*USP Tocainide Hydrochloride RS.*
Identification—
  A: *Infrared Absorption* ⟨197K⟩.
  B: It responds to the tests for *Chloride* ⟨191⟩.
Loss on drying ⟨731⟩—Dry it at 105° for 2 hours: it loses not more than 0.5% of its weight.
Residue on ignition ⟨281⟩: not more than 0.1%.
Heavy metals, *Method II* ⟨231⟩: 0.002%.
Chromatographic purity—
  Adsorbent: 0.25-mm layer of chromatographic silica gel mixture coating on a thin-layer chromatographic plate, previously washed with methanol.
  Test solution: 100 mg per mL, in methanol.
  Standard solutions: 1.0, 0.5, 0.25, and 0.1 mg per mL in methanol to obtain *Standard solutions A, B, C,* and *D*, respectively.
  Application volume: 20 μL.
  Developing solvent system: a freshly prepared mixture of toluene and alcohol (4 : 1) in a paper-lined equilibrated tank in an atmosphere of ammonia vapors.
  Procedure—Proceed as directed for *Thin-Layer Chromatography* under *Chromatography* ⟨621⟩. Examine the plate under short-wavelength UV light. Expose the plate to iodine vapors, and observe again under white light: the chromatograms show principal spots at about the same R_F value. Estimate the concentration of any spot observed in the chromatogram of the *Test solution*, other than the principal spot and that observed at the origin (which may appear because of the presence of ammonium chloride), by comparison with the principal spots in the chromatograms of *Standard solutions B, C,* and *D*: the intensity of any secondary spot is not greater than that of the principal spot obtained from *Standard solution B* (0.5%), and the sum of all secondary spots is not greater than the intensity of the principal spot obtained from *Standard solution A* (1.0%).
Organic volatile impurities, *Method I* ⟨467⟩: meets the requirements.
(Official until July 1, 2008)
Assay—Dissolve about 180 mg of Tocainide Hydrochloride, accurately weighed, in about 40 mL of glacial acetic acid and 15 mL of a 6 in 100 solution of mercuric acetate in glacial acetic acid, and titrate with 0.1 N perchloric acid VS, determining the endpoint potentiometrically, using a platinum ring electrode and a sleeve-type calomel electrode containing 0.1 N lithium perchlorate in acetic anhydride (see *Titrimetry* ⟨541⟩). Perform a blank determination, and make any necessary correction. Each mL of 0.1 N perchloric acid is equivalent to 22.87 mg of $C_{11}H_{16}N_2O \cdot HCl$.

Tocainide Hydrochloride Tablets

» Tocainide Hydrochloride Tablets contain not less than 95.0 percent and not more than 105.0 percent of the labeled amount of $C_{11}H_{16}N_2O \cdot HCl$.

Packaging and storage—Preserve in well-closed containers.
USP Reference standards ⟨11⟩—*USP Tocainide Hydrochloride RS.*
Identification—
  A: Transfer a quantity of finely powdered Tablets, equivalent to about 150 mg of tocainide hydrochloride, to a 100-mL volumetric flask, add 75 mL of water, shake for 15 minutes, dilute with water to volume, and mix. Filter a portion of this solution, and dilute 10 mL of the filtrate with water to 50 mL: the UV absorption spectrum of the solution so obtained exhibits a maximum at the same wavelength as that of a similar solution of USP Tocainide Hydrochloride RS, concomitantly measured.
  B: Transfer about 100 mg of finely powdered Tablets to a suitable separator, and add 10 mL of water and 2 mL of 2 M sodium carbonate. Extract with 20 mL of methylene chloride. Add 0.3 mL of filtered methylene chloride extract to 300 mg of potassium bromide, and grind in an agate mortar. Evaporate to dryness under a current of air: the IR absorption spectrum of the potassium bromide dispersion so obtained exhibits maxima only at the same wavelengths as that of a similar preparation of USP Tocainide Hydrochloride RS.
Dissolution ⟨711⟩—
  Medium: water; 750 mL.
  Apparatus 2: 50 rpm.
  Time: 30 minutes.
  Procedure—Determine the amount of $C_{11}H_{16}N_2O \cdot HCl$ dissolved from UV absorbances at the wavelength of maximum absorbance at about 263 nm of filtered portions of the solution under test, suitably diluted with *Dissolution Medium*, if necessary, in comparison with a Standard solution having a known concentration of USP Tocainide Hydrochloride RS in the same medium.
  Tolerances—Not less than 80% *(Q)* of the labeled amount of $C_{11}H_{16}N_2O \cdot HCl$ is dissolved in 30 minutes.
Uniformity of dosage units ⟨905⟩: meet the requirements.
  Procedure for content uniformity—Transfer 1 Tablet to a 100-mL volumetric flask, add 50 mL of water, place in an ultrasonic bath for 20 minutes, dilute with water to volume, and mix. Filter, discarding the first few mL of the filtrate. Transfer an accurately measured volume of the filtrate, equivalent to about 30 mg of tocainide hydrochloride, to a 100-mL volumetric flask, dilute with water to volume, and mix. Dissolve an accurately weighed quantity of USP Tocainide Hydrochloride RS in water, and dilute quantitatively and stepwise with water to obtain a Standard solution having a known concentration of about 300 μg per mL. Concomitantly determine the absorbances of both solutions at the wavelength of maximum absorbance at about 263 nm, with a suitable spectrophotometer, using water as the blank. Calculate the quantity, in mg, of $C_{11}H_{16}N_2O \cdot HCl$ in the Tablet taken by the formula:

$$(TC/D)(A_U/A_S)$$

in which *T* is the labeled quantity, in mg, of tocainide hydrochloride in the Tablet, *C* is the concentration, in μg per mL, of USP Tocainide Hydrochloride RS in the Standard solution, *D* is the concentration, in μg per mL, of tocainide hydrochloride in the solution from the Tablet on the basis of the labeled quantity per Tablet and the extent of dilution, and A_U and A_S are the absorbances of the solution from the Tablet and the Standard solution, respectively.
Assay—
  Mobile phase—Dissolve 2.16 g of sodium 1-octanesulfonate in 500 mL of 0.67 N acetic acid, add 500 mL of methanol, and mix. Degas, and filter the solution. Make adjustments if necessary (see *System Suitability* under *Chromatography* ⟨621⟩).
  Standard preparation—Dissolve an accurately weighed quantity of USP Tocainide Hydrochloride RS quantitatively in water to obtain a solution having a known concentration of about 0.5 mg per mL.
  Assay preparation—Weigh and finely powder not less than 20 Tablets. Transfer an accurately weighed portion of the powder, equivalent to about 100 mg of tocainide hydrochloride, to a 200-mL volumetric flask, add 100 mL of water, and place in an ultrasonic bath for 20 minutes. Dilute with water to volume, and mix. Filter the solution through a membrane filter, and use the filtrate as the *Assay preparation*.

  Chromatographic system (see *Chromatography* ⟨621⟩)—The liquid chromatograph is equipped with a 254-nm detector and a 3.9-mm × 30-cm column that contains packing L1. The flow rate is about 2 mL per minute. Chromatograph the *Standard preparation*, and record the peak responses as directed for *Procedure:*the capacity factor, *k′*, is greater than 1.6, the column efficiency determined from the analyte peak is not less than 1500 theoretical plates, the tailing factor for the analyte peak is not more than 2, and the relative standard deviation for replicate injections is not more than 2.0%.
  Procedure—Separately inject equal volumes (about 40 μL) of the *Standard preparation* and the *Assay preparation* into the chromatograph, record the chromatograms, and measure the responses for the major peaks. Calculate the quantity, in mg, of $C_{11}H_{16}N_2O \cdot HCl$ in the portion of Tablets taken by the formula:

$$200C(r_U/r_S)$$

in which *C* is the concentration, in mg per mL, of USP Tocainide Hydrochloride RS in the *Standard preparation*, and r_U and r_S are the peak responses obtained from the *Assay preparation* and the *Standard preparation*, respectively.

Tolazamide

$C_{14}H_{21}N_3O_3S$ 311.41
Benzenesulfonamide, *N*-[[(hexahydro-1*H*-azepin-1-yl)amino]carbonyl]-4-methyl-.
1-(Hexahydro-1*H*-azepin-1-yl)-3-(*p*-tolylsulfonyl)urea [*1156-19-0*].

» Tolazamide contains not less than 97.5 percent and not more than 102.5 percent of $C_{14}H_{21}N_3O_3S$, calculated on the dried basis.

Packaging and storage—Preserve in well-closed containers.
USP Reference standards ⟨11⟩—*USP Tolazamide RS.*
Identification—
  A: *Infrared Absorption* ⟨197K⟩.
  B: The relative retention time of the major peak for tolazamide in the chromatogram of the *Assay preparation* corresponds to that in the chromatogram of the *Standard preparation*, as obtained in the *Assay*.
Loss on drying ⟨731⟩—Dry it at a pressure not exceeding 5 mm of mercury at 60° for 3 hours: it loses not more than 0.5% of its weight.
Residue on ignition ⟨281⟩: not more than 0.2%.
Selenium ⟨291⟩: 0.003%, a 200-mg specimen being used.
Heavy metals, *Method II* ⟨231⟩: 0.002%.
Limit of *N*-aminohexamethyleneimine—
  Trisodium pentacyanoaminoferroate solution—Mix 1.0 g of sodium nitroferricyanide and 3.2 mL of ammonium hydroxide in a glass-stoppered flask, insert the stopper in the flask, and refrigerate the mixture overnight. Pour the solution into 10 mL of dehydrated alcohol, and collect the yellow precipitate that is formed on coarse filter paper in a Buchner-type funnel by filtration under reduced pressure. Wash the residue on the filter with anhydrous ether, and store the dry solid in a desiccator. Dissolve a portion of the dry solid in water to obtain a solution containing 1.0 mg per mL, store in a refrigerator, and use within 7 days.
  Buffer solution—Dissolve 0.96 g of anhydrous citric acid and 2.92 g of dibasic sodium phosphate in 200 mL of water. Adjust by adding phosphoric acid or 1 N sodium hydroxide, if necessary, to a pH of 5.4 ± 0.1.
  Standard solution—Transfer, with the aid of a syringe, 100 mg of *N*-aminohexamethyleneimine to a 200-mL volumetric flask, dilute

with acetone to volume, and mix. Dilute the resulting solution quantitatively with acetone to obtain a solution containing 12.5 µg per mL. Pipet 2 mL of this solution into a 25-mL glass-stoppered flask, add 8.0 mL of *Buffer solution*, shake the mixture, allow to stand for 15 minutes, and filter. Collect the filtrate in a suitable glass-stoppered tube, and use the filtrate as the *Standard solution*.

Test solution—Transfer 0.50 g of Tolazamide to a glass-stoppered, 25-mL flask, add 2.0 mL of acetone, insert the stopper in the flask, and shake the mixture vigorously for 15 minutes. Add 8.0 mL of *Buffer solution*, shake the mixture, allow to stand for 15 minutes, and filter. Collect the filtrate in a suitable glass-stoppered tube, and use the filtrate as the *Test solution*.

Procedure—Add 1.0 mL of *Trisodium pentacyanoaminoferroate solution* to the *Standard solution* and to the *Test solution*, and mix both solutions: the intensity of any pink color that may develop in the *Test solution* within 30 minutes does not exceed that produced in the *Standard solution* within 30 minutes (0.005%).

Chromatographic purity—
Mobile phase—Prepare a filtered and degassed mixture of water, acetonitrile, and glacial acetic acid (100 : 100 : 1). Make adjustments if necessary (see *System Suitability* under *Chromatography* ⟨621⟩).

System suitability solution—Dissolve an accurately weighed quantity of USP Tolazamide RS in *Mobile phase*, and dilute quantitatively, and stepwise if necessary, with *Mobile phase* to obtain a solution having a known concentration of about 0.014 mg per mL.

Test solution—[NOTE—Make solution fresh before each injection.] Transfer about 140 mg of Tolazamide, accurately weighed, to a 100-mL volumetric flask, dissolve in *Mobile phase*, sonicating if necessary, dilute with *Mobile phase* to volume, and mix.

Chromatographic system (see *Chromatography* ⟨621⟩)—The liquid chromatograph is equipped with a 254-nm detector and a 3.9-mm × 30-cm column that contains packing L1. The flow rate is about 1.0 mL per minute. Chromatograph the *System suitability solution*, and record the peak responses as directed for *Procedure*: the column efficiency is not less than 4000 theoretical plates; the tailing factor is not more than 3.0; and the relative standard deviation for replicate injections is not more than 5.0%.

Procedure—Inject a volume (about 50 µL) of the *Test solution* into the chromatograph, record the chromatogram, and measure all of the peak responses. Calculate the percentage of each impurity in the portion of Tolazamide taken by the formula:

$$100(1/F)(r_i / r_s)$$

in which F is the relative response factor, which is equal to 0.52 for the *p*-toluenesulfonic acid peak eluting at a relative retention time of 0.23 and equal to 1.0 for all other peaks; r_i is the peak response for each impurity; and r_s is the sum of the responses of all the peaks: not more than 0.5% of any individual impurity is found; and not more than 1.5% of total impurities is found.

Organic volatile impurities, *Method V* ⟨467⟩: meets the requirements.
Solvent—Use dimethyl sulfoxide.

(Official until July 1, 2008)

Assay—
Mobile phase—Prepare a filtered and degassed mixture of hexane, water-saturated hexane, tetrahydrofuran, alcohol, and glacial acetic acid (475 : 475 : 20 : 15 : 9). Make adjustments if necessary (see *System Suitability* under *Chromatography* ⟨621⟩).

Internal standard solution—Dissolve a suitable quantity of Tolbutamide in alcohol-free chloroform to obtain a solution having a known concentration of about 1.5 mg per mL.

Standard preparation—Dissolve an accurately weighed quantity of USP Tolazamide RS in *Internal standard solution* to obtain a solution having a known concentration of about 3 mg per mL.

Assay preparation—Transfer about 30 mg of Tolazamide, accurately weighed, to a 10-mL volumetric flask, dissolve in and dilute with *Internal standard solution* to volume, and mix.

Chromatographic system (see *Chromatography* ⟨621⟩)—The liquid chromatograph is equipped with a 254-nm detector and a 4-mm × 30-cm column that contains 10-µm packing L3. The flow rate is about 1.5 mL per minute. Chromatograph the *Standard preparation*, and record the peak responses as directed for *Procedure*: the resolution, R, between the analyte and internal standard peaks is not less than 2.0; and the relative standard deviation for four replicate injections is not more than 2.0%.

Procedure—Separately inject equal volumes (about 10 µL) of the *Standard preparation* and the *Assay preparation* into the chromatograph, record the chromatograms, and measure the responses for the major peaks. The relative retention times are about 0.6 for the internal standard and 1.0 for tolazamide. Calculate the quantity, in mg, of $C_{14}H_{21}N_3O_3S$ in the portion of Tolazamide taken by the formula:

$$10C(R_U / R_S)$$

in which C is the concentration, in mg per mL, of USP Tolazamide RS in the *Standard preparation*; and R_U and R_S are the ratios of the analyte peak response to the internal standard peak response obtained from the *Assay preparation* and the *Standard preparation*, respectively.

Tolazamide Tablets

» Tolazamide Tablets contain not less than 95.0 percent and not more than 105.0 percent of the labeled amount of $C_{14}H_{21}N_3O_3S$.

Packaging and storage—Preserve in tight containers.
USP Reference standards ⟨11⟩—*USP Tolazamide RS*.
Identification—Triturate a quantity of Tablets, equivalent to about 250 mg of tolazamide, with 50 mL of chloroform, and filter. Evaporate the filtrate to dryness, and dry in vacuum at 60° for 3 hours: the residue so obtained responds to *Identification* test A under *Tolazamide*.

Dissolution ⟨711⟩—
Medium: 0.05 M Tris(hydroxymethyl)aminomethane, pH 7.6, adjusted, if necessary, with hydrochloric acid to a pH of 7.6; 900 mL.
Apparatus 2: 75 rpm.
Time: 30 minutes.
Procedure—Determine the amount of $C_{14}H_{21}N_3O_3S$ dissolved from UV absorbances at the wavelength of maximum absorbance at about 224 nm of filtered portions of the solution under test, suitably diluted with *Dissolution Medium*, in comparison with a Standard solution having a known concentration of USP Tolazamide RS in the same medium. [NOTE—Sonicate the Standard solution until the Reference Standard is dissolved.]
Tolerances—Not less than 70% (*Q*) of the labeled amount of $C_{14}H_{21}N_3O_3S$ is dissolved in 30 minutes.

Uniformity of dosage units ⟨905⟩: meet the requirements.

Assay—
Internal standard preparation, *Mobile phase*, and *Standard preparation*—Prepare as directed in the *Assay* under *Tolazamide*.

Assay preparation—Weigh and finely powder not less than 10 Tablets. Weigh accurately a portion of the powder, equivalent to about 300 mg of tolazamide, and transfer to a suitable container. Add 100.0 mL of *Internal standard solution* and about 20 glass beads. Securely close the container, and shake vigorously for approximately 30 minutes. Centrifuge, and use the clear liquid as the *Assay preparation*.

Procedure—Proceed as directed for *Procedure* in the *Assay* under *Tolazamide*. Calculate the quantity, in mg, of $C_{14}H_{21}N_3O_3S$ in the portion of Tablets taken by the formula:

$$100C(R_U / R_S)$$

in which the terms are as defined therein.

Tolazoline Hydrochloride

$C_{10}H_{12}N_2 \cdot HCl$ 196.68
1*H*-Imidazole, 4,5-dihydro-2-(phenylmethyl)-, monohydrochloride.
2-Benzyl-2-imidazoline monohydrochloride   [59-97-2].

» Tolazoline Hydrochloride contains not less than 98.0 percent and not more than 101.0 percent of $C_{10}H_{12}N_2 \cdot$ HCl, calculated on the dried basis.

Packaging and storage—Preserve in well-closed containers. Store at 25°, excursions permitted between 15° and 30°.

USP Reference standards ⟨11⟩—*USP Tolazoline Hydrochloride RS.*

Identification—
  A: *Infrared Absorption* ⟨197M⟩.
  B: The R_F value of the principal spot in the chromatogram of the *Identification* corresponds to that of *Standard solution A*, as obtained in the test for *Chromatographic purity.*

Melting range ⟨741⟩:   between 172.0° and 176.0°.

Loss on drying ⟨731⟩—Dry it in vacuum over silica gel for 4 hours: it loses not more than 0.2% of its weight.

Residue on ignition ⟨281⟩:   not more than 0.1%.

Heavy metals, *Method II* ⟨231⟩:   0.001%.

Chromatographic purity—
  Standard solutions—Dissolve USP Tolazoline Hydrochloride RS in methanol, and mix to obtain *Standard solution A* having a known concentration of 100 μg per mL. Quantitatively dilute with methanol to obtain *Standard solutions,* designated below by letter, having the following compositions:

Standard solution	Dilution	Concentration (μg RS per mL)	Percentage (%, for comparison with test specimen)
A	undiluted	100	0.5
B	4 in 5	80	0.4
C	3 in 5	60	0.3
D	2 in 5	40	0.2
E	1 in 5	20	0.1

  Test solution—Dissolve an accurately weighed quantity of Tolazoline Hydrochloride in methanol to obtain a solution containing 20 mg per mL.
  Identification solution—Quantitatively dilute a portion of the *Test solution* with methanol to obtain a solution containing 100 μg per mL.
  Detection reagent—Prepare (1) a solution of 0.5 g of potassium iodide in 50 mL of water, and (2) a solution of 1.5 g of soluble starch in 50 mL of boiling water. Just prior to use, mix 10 mL of each solution with 3 mL of alcohol.
  Procedure—Apply separately 5 μL of the *Test solution,* 5 μL of the *Identification solution,* and 5 μL of each *Standard solution* to a suitable thin-layer chromatographic plate (see *Chromatography* ⟨621⟩) coated with a 0.25-mm layer of chromatographic silica gel. Position the plate in a chromatographic chamber, and develop the chromatograms in a solvent system consisting of a mixture of methanol and ammonium hydroxide (95 : 5) until the solvent front has moved about three-fourths of the length of the plate. Remove the plate from the developing chamber, mark the solvent front, and allow the plate to dry under a current of warm air for at least 30 minutes. Expose the plate to chlorine gas for not more than 5 minutes, and air-dry until the chlorine has dissipated (about 15 minutes). Spray the plate with *Detection reagent,* and immediately compare the intensities of any secondary spots observed in the chromatogram of the *Test solution* with those of the principal spots in the chromatograms of the *Standard solutions:* the sum of the intensities of all secondary spots obtained from the *Test solution* corresponds to not more than 1.0%.

Assay—Dissolve about 300 mg of Tolazoline Hydrochloride, accurately weighed, in 100 mL of glacial acetic acid; add 25 mL of mercuric acetate TS; and titrate with 0.1 N perchloric acid VS, determining the endpoint potentiometrically (see *Titrimetry* ⟨541⟩), using a calomel–glass electrode system. Perform a blank determination, and make any necessary correction. Each mL of 0.1 N perchloric acid is equivalent to 19.67 mg of $C_{10}H_{12}N_2 \cdot$ HCl.

Tolazoline Hydrochloride Injection

» Tolazoline Hydrochloride Injection is a sterile solution of Tolazoline Hydrochloride in Water for Injection. It contains not less than 95.0 percent and not more than 105.0 percent of the labeled amount of $C_{10}H_{12}N_2 \cdot$ HCl.

Packaging and storage—Preserve in single-dose or in multiple-dose containers, preferably of Type I glass.

USP Reference standards ⟨11⟩—*USP Endotoxin RS. USP Tolazoline Hydrochloride RS.*

Identification—
  A: *Infrared Absorption* ⟨197K⟩—Obtain the test specimen as follows. Steam-distill a volume of Injection, equivalent to about 250 mg of tolazoline hydrochloride, for 5 to 10 minutes, and discard the distillate. Transfer the remaining solution to a separator, add about 2 mL of 1 N sodium hydroxide, and extract with 20 mL of ether. Filter the ether extract through cotton into a beaker, evaporate to dryness, and dry the residue in vacuum over silica gel for 4 hours.
  B: It responds to *Identification* test B under *Tolazoline Hydrochloride.*
  C: To 1 mL of Injection add 1 mL of ammonium reineckate TS: a pink precipitate is formed.

Bacterial endotoxins ⟨85⟩—It contains not more than 0.8 USP Endotoxin Unit per mg of tolazoline hydrochloride.

pH ⟨791⟩:   between 3.0 and 4.0.

Other requirements—It meets the requirements under *Injections* ⟨1⟩.

Assay—
  Standard preparation—Transfer about 30 mg of USP Tolazoline Hydrochloride RS, accurately weighed, to a 100-mL volumetric flask, dissolve in and dilute with methanol to volume, and mix.
  Assay preparation—Transfer an accurately measured volume of Injection, equivalent to about 150 mg of tolazoline hydrochloride, to a 100-mL volumetric flask, dilute with methanol to volume, and mix. Transfer 20.0 mL of this solution to a second 100-mL volumetric flask, dilute with methanol to volume, and mix.
  Procedure—Transfer 3.0 mL each of the *Standard preparation,* the *Assay preparation,* and methanol to provide the blank, to separate 25-mL volumetric flasks. To each flask add 1 mL of 0.5 N sodium hydroxide and 1 mL of dilute sodium nitroferricyanide TS (1 in 2), mix, and allow to stand for 10 minutes. Add 3 mL of sodium bicarbonate solution (1 in 12) to each flask, dilute with water to volume, mix, and allow to stand for 10 minutes. Concomitantly determine the absorbances of the solutions in 1-cm cells at the wavelength of maximum absorbance at about 565 nm, with a suitable spectrophotometer, against the blank. Calculate the quantity, in mg, of $C_{10}H_{12}N_2 \cdot$ HCl in each mL of the Injection taken by the formula:

$$(0.5C/V)(A_U/A_S)$$

in which C is the concentration, in μg per mL, of USP Tolazoline Hydrochloride RS in the *Standard preparation,* V is the volume, in mL, of Injection taken, and A_U and A_S are the absorbances of the solutions from the *Assay preparation* and the *Standard preparation,* respectively.

Tolbutamide

$C_{12}H_{18}N_2O_3S$ 270.35
Benzenesulfonamide, N-[(butylamino)carbonyl]-4-methyl-.
1-Butyl-3-(p-tolylsulfonyl)urea   [64-77-7].

» Tolbutamide contains not less than 97.0 percent and not more than 103.0 percent of $C_{12}H_{18}N_2O_3S$, calculated on the dried basis.

Packaging and storage—Preserve in well-closed containers.
Labeling—Where it is intended for use in preparing injectable dosage forms, the label states that it is sterile or must be subjected to further processing during the preparation of injectable dosage forms.
USP Reference standards ⟨11⟩—*USP Tolbutamide RS. USP Endotoxin RS.*
Identification, *Infrared Absorption* ⟨197M⟩.
Melting range ⟨741⟩:   between 126° and 130°.
Loss on drying ⟨731⟩—Dry it at 105° for 3 hours: it loses not more than 0.5% of its weight.
Selenium ⟨291⟩:   0.003%, a 100-mg specimen, mixed with 100 mg of magnesium oxide, being used.
Heavy metals, *Method II* ⟨231⟩:   0.002%.
Limit of non-sulfonyl urea—Dissolve 500 mg in 10 mL of 0.5 N ammonium hydroxide: not more than a faint opalescence occurs.
Organic volatile impurities, *Method IV* ⟨467⟩:   meets the requirements.

(Official until July 1, 2008)

Other requirements—Where the label states that Tolbutamide is sterile, it meets the requirements for *Sterility Tests* ⟨71⟩ and for *Bacterial endotoxins* under *Tolbutamide for Injection*. Where the label states that Tolbutamide must be subjected to further processing during the preparation of injectable dosage forms, it meets the requirements for *Bacterial endotoxins* under *Tolbutamide for Injection*.

Assay—
  Mobile phase—Prepare a filtered and degassed mixture of hexane, water-saturated-hexane, tetrahydrofuran, alcohol, and glacial acetic acid (475 : 475 : 20 : 15 : 9). Make adjustments if necessary (see *System Suitability* under *Chromatography* ⟨621⟩).
  Internal standard solution—Dissolve a suitable quantity of tolazamide in alcohol-free chloroform to obtain a solution containing about 3 mg per mL.
  Standard preparation—Dissolve an accurately weighed quantity of USP Tolbutamide RS in *Internal standard solution* to obtain a solution having a known concentration of about 1.5 mg per mL.
  Assay preparation—Transfer about 15 mg of Tolbutamide, accurately weighed, to a 10-mL volumetric flask. Dissolve in and dilute with *Internal standard solution* to volume, and mix.
  Chromatographic system (see *Chromatography* ⟨621⟩)—The liquid chromatograph is equipped with a 254-nm detector and a 4.0-mm × 30-cm column that contains packing L3. The flow rate is about 1.5 mL per minute. Chromatograph the *Standard preparation*, and record the peak responses as directed for *Procedure*: the relative standard deviation for replicate injections is not more than 2.0%, and the resolution, *R*, between tolbutamide and tolazamide is not less than 2.0.
  Procedure—Separately inject equal volumes (about 10 μL) of the *Standard preparation* and the *Assay preparation* into the chromatograph, record the chromatograms, and measure the responses for the major peaks. The relative retention times are about 0.6 for tolbutamide and 1.0 for tolazamide. Calculate the quantity, in mg, of $C_{12}H_{18}N_2O_3S$ in the portion of Tolbutamide taken by the formula:

$$10C(R_U / R_S)$$

in which *C* is the concentration, in mg per mL, of USP Tolbutamide RS in the *Standard preparation*, and R_U and R_S are the peak response ratios obtained from the *Assay preparation* and the *Standard preparation*, respectively.

Tolbutamide for Injection

» Tolbutamide for Injection is prepared from Tolbutamide with the aid of Sodium Hydroxide. It contains an amount of tolbutamide sodium equivalent to not less than 95.0 percent and not more than 105.0 percent of the labeled amount of tolbutamide ($C_{12}H_{18}N_2O_3S$).

Packaging and storage—Preserve in *Containers for Sterile Solids* as described under *Injections* ⟨1⟩.
USP Reference standards ⟨11⟩—*USP Endotoxin RS. USP Tolbutamide RS.*
Constituted solution—At the time of use, it meets the requirements for *Constituted Solutions* under *Injections* ⟨1⟩.
Identification, *Infrared Absorption* ⟨197M⟩—Obtain the test specimen as follows. Place about 200 mg in a suitable container, dissolve in about 20 mL of water, add 2 mL of 2 N sulfuric acid, and extract with 10 mL of chloroform. Filter, and evaporate an aliquot of the chloroform layer. Dry the residue at 105° for 3 hours. Use USP Tolbutamide RS as the standard for comparison.
Bacterial endotoxins ⟨85⟩—It contains not more than 0.35 USP Endotoxin Unit per mg of tolbutamide sodium.
pH ⟨791⟩:   between 8.0 and 9.8, in a solution containing 50 mg per mL.
Loss on drying ⟨731⟩—Dry it at 105° for 4 hours: it loses not more than 1.0% of its weight.
Other requirements—It meets the requirements for *Sterility Tests* ⟨71⟩, *Uniformity of Dosage Units* ⟨905⟩, and *Labeling* under *Injections* ⟨1⟩.

Assay—
  Mobile phase and *Chromatographic system*—Prepare as directed in the *Assay* under *Tolbutamide*.
  Internal standard solution—Prepare a solution of tolazamide in alcohol-free chloroform containing about 15 mg per mL.
  Diluting solution—Prepare an alcohol-free chloroform solution containing 3% (v/v) of glacial acetic acid.
  Standard preparation—Dissolve an accurately weighed quantity of USP Tolbutamide RS in *Internal standard solution* to obtain a known concentration of about 7.5 mg per mL. Add *Diluting solution* to obtain a *Standard preparation* having a final known concentration of about 1.5 mg of tolbutamide per mL.
  Assay preparation—Add about 15 mL of water to 1 container of Tolbutamide for Injection, and shake vigorously to dissolve the contents. Transfer the contents, using adequate rinsing with water, to a 50-mL volumetric flask. Dilute with water to volume, and mix. Transfer an accurately measured portion of this solution, equivalent to about 75 mg of tolbutamide, to a 50-mL volumetric flask, add 10.0 mL of *Internal standard solution*, and dilute with *Diluting solution* to volume. Shake vigorously for about 15 minutes, and centrifuge or allow to stand for about 15 minutes. Use the lower, clear layer, as the *Assay preparation*.
  Procedure—Separately inject equal volumes (about 20 μL) of the *Standard preparation* and the *Assay preparation* into the chromatograph, record the chromatograms, and measure the responses for the major peaks. The relative retention times are about 0.6 for tolbutamide and 1.0 for tolazamide. Calculate the quantity, in mg, of $C_{12}H_{18}N_2O_3S$ in the portion of solution taken for the *Assay preparation* by the formula:

$$50C(R_U / R_S)$$

in which *C* is the concentration, in mg per mL, of USP Tolbutamide RS in the *Standard preparation*, and R_U and R_S are the peak response ratios of the tolbutamide and internal standard peaks obtained from the *Assay preparation* and the *Standard preparation*, respectively.

Tolbutamide Tablets

» Tolbutamide Tablets contain not less than 90.0 percent and not more than 110.0 percent of the labeled amount of $C_{12}H_{18}N_2O_3S$.

Packaging and storage—Preserve in well-closed containers.

USP Reference standards ⟨11⟩—*USP Tolbutamide RS*.

Identification—Triturate a quantity of finely powdered Tablets, equivalent to about 500 mg of tolbutamide, with 50 mL of chloroform, and filter. Evaporate the clear filtrate on a steam bath to dryness: the residue so obtained responds to *Identification* test A under *Tolbutamide*.

Dissolution ⟨711⟩—
  Medium: pH 7.4 phosphate buffer (see *Buffer Solutions* in the section *Reagents, Indicators, and Solutions*); 900 mL.
  Apparatus 2: 75 rpm.
  Time: 30 minutes.
  Procedure—Measure the amount in solution in filtered portions of the *Dissolution Medium*, suitably diluted with water, if necessary, at the wavelength of maximum absorbance at about 226 nm, with a suitable spectrophotometer, in comparison with a solution having a known concentration of USP Tolbutamide RS. An amount of alcohol not to exceed 1% of the total volume of the *Standard* solution may be used to bring the Reference Standard into solution prior to dilution with *Dissolution Medium*.
  Tolerances—Not less than 70% (*Q*) of the labeled amount of $C_{12}H_{18}N_2O_3S$ is dissolved in 30 minutes.

Uniformity of dosage units ⟨905⟩: meet the requirements.

Assay—
  Mobile phase, Internal standard solution, Standard preparation, and *Chromatographic system*—Prepare as directed in the *Assay* under *Tolbutamide*.
  Assay preparation—Weigh and finely powder not less than 10 Tablets. Transfer an accurately weighed portion of the powder, equivalent to about 150 mg of tolbutamide, to a suitable container. Add 100.0 mL of *Internal standard solution* and about 20 glass beads. Securely close the container, and shake vigorously by mechanical means for approximately 30 minutes. Centrifuge and use the clear supernatant.
  Procedure—Proceed as directed for *Procedure* in the *Assay* under *Tolbutamide*. Calculate the quantity, in mg, of $C_{12}H_{18}N_2O_3S$ in the portion of Tablets taken by the formula:

$$100C(R_U/R_S)$$

in which the terms are as defined therein.

Tolcapone

$C_{14}H_{11}NO_5$ 273.24
Methanone, (3,4-dihydroxy-5-nitrophenyl)(4-methylphenyl)-.
3,4-Dihydroxy-4′-methyl-5-nitrobenzophenone   [*134308-13-7*].

» Tolcapone contains not less than 98.5 percent and not more than 101.5 percent of $C_{14}H_{11}NO_5$, calculated on the anhydrous and solvent-free basis.

Packaging and storage—Preserve in tight, light-resistant containers, and store between 20° and 25°.

USP Reference standards ⟨11⟩—*USP Tolcapone RS. USP Tolcapone Related Compound A RS. USP Tolcapone Related Compound B RS.*

Identification—
  A: *Infrared Absorption* ⟨197K⟩.
  B: The retention time of the major peak in the chromatogram of the *Assay preparation* corresponds to that in the chromatogram of the *Standard preparation*, as obtained in the *Assay*.

Absorptivity—
  Diluent—Dilute 100 mL of 1 N hydrochloric acid with dehydrated alcohol to 1000 mL.
  Test preparation—Prepare a solution of Tolcapone having a concentration of 0.01 mg per mL in *Diluent*.
  Procedure—Proceed as directed under *Spectrophotometry and Light-Scattering* ⟨851⟩, and measure the absorbance: the maximum is between 265.2 and 269.3, and the absorptivity is between 75.29 and 79.93.

Water, *Method I* ⟨921⟩: not more than 0.1%.
Residue on ignition ⟨281⟩: not more than 0.1%.
Heavy metals, *Method II* ⟨231⟩: 0.002%.

Limit of residual solvents—
  Alcohol stock solution—Transfer 6.3 µL of absolute alcohol, using a microsyringe, to a 50-mL volumetric flask containing dimethylformamide, and mix.
  Methylene chloride stock solution—Transfer 3.8 µL of methylene chloride, using a microsyringe, to a 50-mL volumetric flask containing dimethylformamide, and mix.
  Standard solution—Transfer 10.0 mL of *Alcohol stock solution* and 1.0 mL of *Methylene chloride stock solution* to a 50-mL volumetric flask. Dilute with dimethylformamide to volume, and mix.
  Test solution—Transfer about 200 mg of Tolcapone, accurately weighed, to a 10-mL volumetric flask, add 7 mL of dimethylformamide, and sonicate to dissolve. Dilute with dimethylformamide to volume, and mix.
  Chromatographic system (see *Chromatography* ⟨621⟩)—The gas chromatograph is equipped with a flame-ionization detector, a 0.53-mm × 30-m fused silica column coated with 3.0-µm G43 stationary phase, and a 0.53-mm × 5-m fused silica column coated with 3.0-µm G3 stationary phase. The carrier gas is helium, flowing at a rate of 5 mL per minute. The column temperature is maintained at 35°. The temperatures of the injection port and the detector are maintained at 120° and 260°, respectively. Chromatograph the *Standard solution*, and record the peak responses as directed for *Procedure*: the relative retention time is about 0.7 for alcohol and 1.0 for methylene chloride; and the relative standard deviation for replicate injections is not more than 10.0%.
  Procedure—Separately inject equal volumes (about 1 µL) of the *Standard solution* and the *Test solution* into the chromatograph, record the chromatograms, and measure the peak responses. Calculate the percentages (w/w) of alcohol and methylene chloride in the portion of Tolcapone taken by the formula:

$$(1000D)(C/W)(r_U/r_S)$$

in which *C* is the concentration, in µL per mL, of each solvent in the *Standard solution; D* is the density, in mg per µL, of each solvent at 20°; *W* is the weight, in mg, of Tolcapone taken to prepare the *Test solution;* and r_U and r_S are the peak areas of the appropriate analyte obtained from the *Test solution* and the *Standard solution*, respectively: not more than 0.25% of alcohol is found; and not more than 0.01% of methylene chloride is found. [NOTE—Condition the column at 220° for 15 minutes after each injection.]

Related compounds—
  TEST 1—
  Adsorbent: 0.25-mm layer of chromatographic silica gel mixture with a suitable fluorescing substance (see *Chromatography* ⟨621⟩).
  Standard solution 1—Dissolve an accurately weighed portion of USP Tolcapone RS in chloroform, and dilute quantitatively, and stepwise if necessary, with chloroform to obtain a solution having a known concentration of 0.4 mg per mL.
  Standard solution 2—Transfer 2.0 mL of *Standard solution 1* to a 10-mL volumetric flask, dilute with chloroform to volume, and mix.
  Standard solution 3—Transfer 1.0 mL of *Standard solution 1* to a 10-mL volumetric flask, dilute with chloroform to volume, and mix.
  Standard solution 4—Transfer 5.0 mL of *Standard solution 3* to a 10-mL volumetric flask, dilute with chloroform to volume, and mix.
  Test solution—Transfer about 200 mg of Tolcapone, accurately weighed, to a 5-mL volumetric flask, dissolve in and dilute with

chloroform to volume, and mix. [NOTE—Prepare this solution last and chromatograph immediately.]

Application volume: 10 µL.

Developing solvent system: a mixture of chloroform, anhydrous formic acid, and ethyl acetate (83 : 15 : 2).

Procedure—Apply the *Test solution* and each of the *Standard solutions* as directed for *Thin-Layer Chromatography* under *Chromatography* ⟨621⟩ at about 4 cm from the lower edge of the plate. Dry the plate in a current of cold air, and view it under short-wavelength UV light. The R_F values of analytes are as follows.

Compound	R_F
Tolcapone related compound A	about 0.2
Tolcapone	about 0.5
Tolcapone related compound B	about 0.7

Compare any spot at R_F of 0.0 in the chromatogram obtained from the *Test solution* with the principal spot of *Standard solution 2*, *Standard solution 3*, and *Standard solution 4*, and obtain the approximate amount: not more than 0.1% of any impurity at R_F of 0.0 is found. [NOTE—The R_F of tolcapone related compound A and tolcapone related compound B are given just for reference. They are quantified in *Test 2*.]

TEST 2—

Diluent, System suitability solution, Mobile phase, and *Chromatographic system*—Proceed as directed in the *Assay*.

Standard solution—Use the *Standard preparation,* prepared as directed in the *Assay*.

Test solution—Use the *Assay preparation.*

Procedure—Separately inject equal volumes (about 20 µL) of the *Standard solution* and the *Test solution* into the chromatograph, record the chromatograms, and measure the peak areas. Calculate the percentage of each impurity in the portion of Tolcapone taken by the formula:

$$(50{,}000F)(C/W)(r_i / r_S)$$

in which C is the concentration, in mg per mL, of USP Tolcapone RS in the *Standard solution;* F is the relative response factor of the impurity according to the table below; W is the weight, in mg, of Tolcapone, calculated on the solvent- and water-free basis, used to prepare the *Test solution;* r_i is the peak area for any impurity in the *Test solution;* and r_S is the peak area for tolcapone in the *Standard solution:* the impurities meet the requirements given in the table below.

Compound Name	Relative Retention Time	Relative Response Factor	Limit (%)
Tolcapone related compound A	about 0.6	1.14	0.1
Tolcapone	1.0	—	—
Tolcapone related compound B	1.36	0.98	0.2
Unknown impurities	—	1.0	0.1 individual, 0.2 total unknown
Total impurities	—	—	0.5

Assay—

Diluent—Prepare a mixture of methanol and acetonitrile (24 : 15).

System suitability solution—Dissolve an accurately weighed quantity of USP Tolcapone Related Compound A RS, USP Tolcapone RS, and USP Tolcapone Related Compound B RS in *Diluent;* and dilute quantitatively, and stepwise if necessary, with *Diluent* to obtain a solution having a known concentration of about 5 µg per mL, 5 µg per mL, and 10 µg per mL, respectively. Transfer 2.0 mL of this solution to a 100-mL volumetric flask, add about 63 mL of *Diluent,* dilute with water to volume, and mix.

Mobile phase—Prepare a filtered and degassed mixture of methanol, 0.05 M monobasic potassium phosphate having a pH of 2.0 ± 0.1, and acetonitrile (8 : 7 : 5). Make adjustments if necessary (see *System Suitability* under *Chromatography* ⟨621⟩).

Standard preparation—Dissolve an accurately weighed quantity of USP Tolcapone RS in *Diluent;* and dilute quantitatively, and stepwise if necessary, with *Diluent* to obtain a solution having a known concentration of about 1.0 mg per mL. Transfer 5.0 mL of this solution to a 50-mL volumetric flask, add about 27.5 mL of *Diluent,* dilute with water to volume, and mix.

Assay preparation—Transfer about 50 mg of Tolcapone, accurately weighed, to a 50-mL volumetric flask, dissolve in and dilute with *Diluent* to volume, and mix. Transfer 5.0 mL of this solution to a 50-mL volumetric flask, add about 27.5 mL of *Diluent,* dilute with water to volume, and mix.

Chromatographic system (see *Chromatography* ⟨621⟩)—The liquid chromatograph is equipped with a 230-nm detector and a 4.0-mm × 25-cm column that contains packing L1. The flow rate is about 1 mL per minute. Chromatograph the *System suitability solution,* and record the peak responses as directed for *Procedure:* the relative retention times are about 0.6 for tolcapone related compound A, 1.0 for tolcapone, and about 1.4 for tolcapone related compound B; and the resolution, R, between tolcapone related compound B and tolcapone is not less than 4.0. Chromatograph the *Standard preparation,* and record the peak responses as directed for *Procedure:* the relative standard deviation for replicate injections is not more than 1.0%.

Procedure—Separately inject equal volumes (about 20 µL) of the *Standard preparation* and the *Assay preparation* into the chromatograph, record the chromatograms, and measure the areas for the major tolcapone peaks. Calculate the quantity, in mg, of $C_{14}H_{11}NO_5$ in the portion of Tolcapone taken by the formula:

$$500C(r_U / r_S)$$

in which C is the concentration, in mg per mL, of USP Tolcapone RS in the *Standard preparation;* and r_U and r_S are the peak responses obtained from the *Assay preparation* and the *Standard preparation,* respectively.

Tolcapone Tablets

» Tolcapone Tablets contain not less than 90.0 percent and not more than 110.0 percent of the labeled amount of tolcapone ($C_{14}H_{11}NO_5$).

Packaging and storage—Preserve in tight containers, and store between 20° and 25°.

USP Reference standards ⟨11⟩—*USP Tolcapone RS. USP Tolcapone Related Compound A RS. USP Tolcapone Related Compound B RS.*

Identification—

A: *Infrared Absorption*—Grind 10 Tablets to a fine powder. Transfer an amount of powder, equivalent to 3 mg of tolcapone, into a polystyrene vial containing two mixing beads. Add 300 mg of IR grade potassium bromide, and disperse the material in the matrix by agitating the capped vial in a grinding mill for 2 minutes. Transfer a portion of the sample to a sample cup. Record the diffuse reflectance IR spectrum between 2200 and 1090 cm^{-1} (see *Spectrophotometry and Light-Scattering* ⟨851⟩). The spectrum thus obtained exhibits maxima only at the same wavelengths as that of a similar preparation of USP Tolcapone RS, concomitantly measured.

B: The retention time of the major peak in the chromatogram of the *Assay preparation* corresponds to that in the chromatogram of the *Standard preparation,* as obtained in the *Assay*.

Dissolution ⟨711⟩—

Medium: pH 6.8 phosphate buffer containing 1% of sodium lauryl sulfate; 900 mL.

Apparatus 2: 75 rpm.

Time: 30 minutes.

Procedure—Determine the amount of $C_{14}H_{11}NO_5$ dissolved by employing UV absorption at the wavelength of maximum absorbance at about 271 nm on filtered portions of the solution under test, suitably diluted with *Medium,* if necessary, in comparison with a *Standard solution* having a known concentration of USP Tolcapone RS in the same *Medium.* Calculate the amount of $C_{14}H_{11}NO_5$ dissolved in each Tablet.

Tolerances—Not less than 75% (*Q*) of the labeled amount of $C_{14}H_{11}NO_5$ is dissolved in 30 minutes.

Uniformity of dosage units ⟨905⟩: meet the requirements.

Chromatographic purity—

Diluent 1, Diluent 2, System suitability solution, Mobile phase, and *Chromatographic system*—Proceed as directed in the *Assay.*

Standard solution—Use the *Standard preparation,* prepared as directed in the *Assay.*

Test solution—Use the *Assay preparation.*

Procedure—Separately inject equal volumes (about 20 μL) of the *Standard solution* and the *Test solution* into the chromatograph, record the chromatograms, and measure the areas for the major tolcapone peaks. Calculate the percentage of each impurity in the portion of Tablets taken by the formula:

$$(100{,}000A/D)(C/W)(r_i/r_S)$$

in which *C* is the concentration, in mg per mL, of USP Tolcapone RS in the *Standard solution*; *A* is the average weight, in mg, of the Tablets; *W* is the weight, in mg, of tablet powder taken to prepare the *Test solution*; *D* is the labeled quantity, in mg, of tolcapone per Tablet; r_i is the peak area for any impurity in the *Test solution*; and r_S is the peak area for tolcapone in the *Standard solution*: not more than 0.1% of any individual impurity is found, and not more than 0.5% of total impurities is found.

Assay—

Diluent 1—Prepare a mixture of methanol and acetonitrile (24 : 15).

Diluent 2—Prepare a mixture of methanol, water, and acetonitrile (8 : 7 : 5).

System suitability solution—Dissolve an accurately weighed quantity of USP Tolcapone RS, USP Tolcapone Related Compound A RS, and USP Tolcapone Related Compound B RS in *Diluent 2,* and dilute quantitatively, and stepwise if necessary, with *Diluent 2* to obtain a solution having a known concentration of about 104 μg per mL, 10.4 μg per mL, and 10.4 μg per mL, respectively.

Mobile phase—Prepare a filtered and degassed mixture of methanol, 0.05 M monobasic potassium phosphate having a pH of 2.0 ± 0.1, and acetonitrile (8 : 7 : 5). Make adjustments if necessary (see *System Suitability* under *Chromatography* ⟨621⟩).

Standard preparation—Dissolve an accurately weighed quantity of USP Tolcapone RS in *Diluent 1,* and dilute quantitatively, and stepwise if necessary, with *Diluent 1* to obtain a solution having a known concentration of about 1.0 mg per mL. Transfer 5.0 mL of this solution to a 50-mL volumetric flask, add about 27.5 mL of *Diluent 1,* dilute with water to volume, and mix.

Assay preparation—Weigh and finely powder not fewer than 20 Tablets. Transfer an accurately weighed portion of the powder, equivalent to about 100 mg of tolcapone, to a 100-mL volumetric flask, add 10 mL of water, and sonicate for about 10 minutes. Add 65 mL of *Diluent 1,* and sonicate for about 15 minutes. Allow the sample to settle. If the material is still undispersed, sonicate for an additional 5 minutes. Dilute with water to volume, and mix. Centrifuge a portion of this solution, and transfer 5.0 mL of the supernatant to a 50-mL volumetric flask. Dilute with *Diluent 2* to volume, and mix. Pass a portion of this solution through a 0.45-μm filter, and use the filtrate.

Chromatographic system (see *Chromatography* ⟨621⟩)—The liquid chromatograph is equipped with a 230-nm detector and a 4.0-mm × 25-cm column that contains packing L1. The flow rate is about 1 mL per minute. Chromatograph the *System suitability solution,* and record the peak responses as directed for *Procedure:* the relative retention times are about 0.6 for tolcapone related compound A, 1.0 for tolcapone, and about 1.4 for tolcapone related compound B; the resolution, *R,* between tolcapone related compound B and tolcapone is not less than 6.0; and the tailing factor for the tolcapone peak is not more than 1.5. Chromatograph the *Standard preparation,* and record the peak responses as directed for *Procedure:* the relative standard deviation for replicate injections is not more than 2.0%.

Procedure—Separately inject equal volumes (about 20 μL) of the *Standard preparation* and the *Assay preparation* into the chromatograph, record the chromatograms, and measure the areas for the major peaks. Calculate the quantity, in mg, of tolcapone ($C_{14}H_{11}NO_5$) in the portion of Tablets taken by the formula:

$$1000C(r_U/r_S)$$

in which *C* is the concentration, in mg per mL, of USP Tolcapone RS in the *Standard preparation;* and r_U and r_S are the peak responses obtained from the *Assay preparation* and the *Standard preparation,* respectively.

Tolmetin Sodium

$C_{15}H_{14}NNaO_3 \cdot 2H_2O$ 315.30

1*H*-Pyrrole-2-acetic acid, 1-methyl-5-(4-methylbenzoyl)-, sodium salt, dihydrate.

Sodium 1-methyl-5-*p*-toluoylpyrrole-2-acetate dihydrate [64490-92-2].

Anhydrous   279.27   [35711-34-3].

» Tolmetin Sodium contains not less than 98.0 percent and not more than 102.0 percent of $C_{15}H_{14}NNaO_3$, calculated on the dried basis.

Packaging and storage—Preserve in well-closed containers.

USP Reference standards ⟨11⟩—*USP Tolmetin Sodium RS.*

Identification—

A: *Infrared Absorption* ⟨197K⟩.

B: *Ultraviolet Absorption* ⟨197U⟩—

Solution: 10 μg per mL.

Medium: pH 7 phosphate buffer (see *Buffer solutions* in the section *Reagents, Indicators, and Solutions.*)

C: A solution (1 in 20) responds to the tests for *Sodium* ⟨191⟩.

Loss on drying ⟨731⟩—Dry it in vacuum at 60° for 4 hours: it loses between 10.4% and 12.4% of its weight.

Heavy metals, *Method II* ⟨231⟩:   0.002%.

Chromatographic purity—Dissolve 125 mg in 10 mL of methanol to obtain the *Test solution.* Dissolve USP Tolmetin Sodium RS in methanol to obtain a *Standard solution* having a concentration of 12.5 mg per mL. Dilute a portion of this *Standard solution* quantitatively with methanol to obtain a *Diluted standard solution* having a concentration of 62.5 μg per mL. Apply separate 20-μL portions of the three solutions on the starting line to a suitable thin-layer chromatographic plate (see *Chromatography* ⟨621⟩) coated with 0.25-mm layer of chromatographic silica gel mixture. Develop the chromatogram in a solvent system consisting of a mixture of chloroform and glacial acetic acid (95 : 5) until the solvent front has moved about three-fourths of the length of the plate. Remove the plate from the chamber, mark the solvent front, air-dry, and view under short-wavelength UV light: the R_F value of the principal spot from the *Test solution* corresponds to that from the *Standard solution.* Any other spot obtained from the *Test solution* does not exceed in size or intensity the principal spot obtained from the *Diluted standard solution* (0.5%), and the sum of the total impurities based on a comparison of the intensities of all such other spots with the *Diluted standard solution* does not exceed 2.0%.

Organic volatile impurities, *Method I* ⟨467⟩: meets the requirements.

(Official until July 1, 2008)

Assay—Dissolve, by warming, about 300 mg of Tolmetin Sodium, accurately weighed, in 150 mL of glacial acetic acid. Cool to room temperature, and titrate with 0.1 N perchloric acid VS, determining the endpoint electrometrically. Perform a blank determination, and make any necessary correction. Each mL of 0.1 N perchloric acid is equivalent to 27.93 mg of $C_{15}H_{14}NNaO_3$.

Tolmetin Sodium Capsules

» Tolmetin Sodium Capsules contain an amount of tolmetin sodium equivalent to not less than 93.0 percent and not more than 107.0 percent of the labeled amount of tolmetin ($C_{15}H_{15}NO_3$).

Packaging and storage—Preserve in tight containers.

USP Reference standards ⟨11⟩—*USP Tolmetin Sodium RS.*

Identification—
A: Transfer a quantity of Capsule contents, equivalent to about 10 mg of tolmetin, to a 100-mL volumetric flask. Add about 50 mL of methanol, shake for 2 minutes, dilute with methanol to volume, and mix. Filter a portion of this solution, transfer 10 mL of the filtrate to a second 100-mL volumetric flask, dilute with 0.1 N sodium hydroxide to volume, and mix: the UV absorption spectrum of the solution so obtained exhibits maxima and minima at the same wavelengths as that of a similar solution of USP Tolmetin Sodium RS, concomitantly measured.

B: The chromatogram of the *Assay preparation* obtained as directed in the *Assay* exhibits a major peak for tolmetin, the retention time of which corresponds to that exhibited in the chromatogram of the *Standard preparation* obtained as directed in the *Assay*.

Dissolution—
Medium—Dissolve 2.0 g of sodium chloride in 7.0 mL of hydrochloric acid, and add water to make 1000 mL (*Solution A*). Dissolve 6.8 g of monobasic potassium phosphate in 250 mL of water, mix, and add 190 mL of 0.2 N sodium hydroxide and 400 mL of water. Adjust the solution with 0.2 N sodium hydroxide to a pH of 7.4 to 7.6. Dilute with water to 1000 mL (*Solution B*). Add 336 mL of *Solution A* to 664 mL of *Solution B*, mix, and adjust the solution with small amounts of either solution to a pH of 4.5; 900 mL.
Apparatus 2: 50 rpm.
Time: 30 minutes.
Procedure—Determine the amount of $C_{15}H_{15}NO_3$ dissolved from UV absorbances at the wavelength of maximum absorbance at about 322 nm of filtered portions of the solution under test, suitably diluted with 0.1 N sodium hydroxide, in comparison with a Standard solution having a known concentration of USP Tolmetin Sodium RS in the same medium.
Tolerances—Not less than 85% (*Q*) of the labeled amount of $C_{15}H_{15}NO_3$ is dissolved in 30 minutes.

Uniformity of dosage units ⟨905⟩: meet the requirements.

Assay—
pH 2.7 buffer solution—Dissolve 1.7 g of tetrabutylammonium phosphate in 1000 mL of water, and adjust by the addition of phosphoric acid to a pH of 2.7 ± 0.1.
Mobile phase—Prepare a filtered and degassed mixture of 64 parts of *pH 2.7 buffer solution* and 36 parts of acetonitrile, making adjustments if necessary (see *System Suitability* under *Chromatography* ⟨621⟩).
Solvent mixture—Mix 400 mL of acetonitrile with 600 mL of 0.01 N sodium hydroxide.
Standard preparation—Dissolve an accurately weighed quantity of USP Tolmetin Sodium RS in *Solvent mixture* to obtain a solution having a known concentration of about 0.65 mg of anhydrous tolmetin sodium per mL.
Assay preparation—Remove, as completely as possible, the contents of not less than 20 Capsules, weigh, and mix. Transfer an accurately weighed portion of the powder, equivalent to about 60 mg of tolmetin, to a 100-mL volumetric flask. Add about 75 mL of *Solvent mixture*, and shake by mechanical means for 30 minutes. Dilute with *Solvent mixture* to volume, mix, and filter through a filter having a porosity of 0.45 μm or less.
Resolution solution—Dissolve suitable quantities of *p*-toluic acid and USP Tolmetin Sodium RS in *Solvent mixture* to obtain a solution containing 200 μg and 500 μg, respectively, in each mL.
Chromatographic system (see *Chromatography* ⟨621⟩)—The liquid chromatograph is equipped with a 254-nm detector and a 4.6-mm × 15-cm column that contains 5-μm packing L7, and is operated at a temperature of 40 ± 1.0°. The flow rate is about 3 mL per minute. Chromatograph the *Standard preparation* and the *Resolution solution*, and record the peak responses as directed for *Procedure:* the resolution, *R*, between the *p*-toluic acid and tolmetin sodium peaks is not less than 1.2, and the relative standard deviation for replicate injections of the *Standard preparation* is not more than 3.0%.
Procedure—Separately inject equal volumes (about 20 μL) of the *Standard preparation* and the *Assay preparation* into the chromatograph, record the chromatograms, and measure the responses for the major peaks. Calculate the quantity, in mg, of $C_{15}H_{15}NO_3$ in the portion of Capsule contents taken by the formula:

$$100C(257.29 / 279.27)(r_U / r_S)$$

in which *C* is the concentration, in mg per mL, of USP Tolmetin Sodium RS in the *Standard preparation*, 257.29 and 279.27 are the molecular weights of tolmetin and anhydrous tolmetin sodium, respectively, and r_U and r_S are the peak responses obtained from the *Assay preparation* and the *Standard preparation*, respectively.

Tolmetin Sodium Tablets

» Tolmetin Sodium Tablets contain an amount of tolmetin sodium equivalent to not less than 90.0 percent and not more than 110.0 percent of the labeled amount of tolmetin ($C_{15}H_{15}NO_3$).

Packaging and storage—Preserve in well-closed containers.

USP Reference standards ⟨11⟩—*USP Tolmetin Sodium RS.*

Identification—
A: A quantity of finely powdered Tablets, equivalent to about 10 mg of tolmetin, responds to *Identification* test A under *Tolmetin Sodium Capsules*.
B: The chromatogram of the *Assay preparation* obtained as directed in the *Assay* exhibits a major peak for tolmetin, the retention time of which corresponds to that exhibited in the chromatogram of the *Standard preparation* obtained as directed in the *Assay*.

Dissolution ⟨711⟩—
Medium, Apparatus, Time, and *Procedure*—Proceed as directed in the test for *Dissolution* under *Tolmetin Sodium Capsules*.
Tolerances—Not less than 75% (*Q*) of the labeled amount of $C_{15}H_{15}NO_3$ is dissolved in 30 minutes.

Uniformity of dosage units ⟨905⟩: meet the requirements.

Assay—
pH 2.7 buffer solution, Mobile phase, Solvent mixture, Standard preparation, Resolution solution, and *Chromatographic system*—Prepare as directed in the *Assay* under *Tolmetin Sodium Capsules*.
Assay preparation—Weigh and finely powder not less than 20 Tablets. Transfer an accurately weighed portion of the powder, equivalent to about 60 mg of tolmetin, to a 100-mL volumetric flask. Add about 75 mL of *Solvent mixture*, and shake by mechanical means for 30 minutes. Dilute with *Solvent mixture* to volume, mix, and filter through a filter having a porosity of 0.45 μm or less.
Procedure—Separately inject equal volumes (about 20 μL) of the *Standard preparation* and the *Assay preparation* into the chromatograph, record the chromatograms, and measure the responses for the major peaks. Calculate the quantity, in mg, of $C_{15}H_{15}NO_3$ in the portion of Tablets taken by the formula:

$$100C(257.29 / 279.27)(r_U / r_S)$$

in which *C* is the concentration, in mg per mL, of USP Tolmetin Sodium RS in the *Standard preparation*, 257.29 and 279.27 are the molecular weights of tolmetin and anhydrous tolmetin sodium, respectively, and r_U and r_S are the peak responses obtained from the *Assay preparation* and the *Standard preparation*, respectively.

Tolnaftate

C$_{19}$H$_{17}$NOS   307.41
Carbamothioic acid, methyl(3-methylphenyl)-, O-2-naphthalenyl ester.
O-2-Naphthyl m,N-dimethylthiocarbanilate   [2398-96-1].

» Tolnaftate contains not less than 98.0 percent and not more than 102.0 percent of C$_{19}$H$_{17}$NOS, calculated on the dried basis.

Packaging and storage—Preserve in tight containers.
USP Reference standards ⟨11⟩—*USP Tolnaftate RS.*
Identification—
  A: *Infrared Absorption* ⟨197K⟩.
  B: The UV absorption spectrum of the solution employed for measurement of absorbance in the *Assay* exhibits maxima and minima at the same wavelengths as that of a similar solution of USP Tolnaftate RS, concomitantly measured.
  C: Prepare a test solution by dissolving 10 mg in 10 mL of alcohol. Apply 10 µL of this test solution and 10 µL of a Standard solution of USP Tolnaftate RS in alcohol having a concentration of 1.0 mg per mL to a thin-layer chromatographic plate (see *Chromatography* ⟨621⟩) coated with a 0.25-mm layer of chromatographic silica gel mixture. Allow the spots to dry, and develop the chromatogram, using toluene as the solvent system, until the solvent front has moved about three-fourths of the length of the plate. Remove the plate from the developing chamber, allow the solvent to evaporate, and view under short-wavelength UV light: the R_F value of the principal spot obtained from the test solution corresponds to that obtained from the Standard solution.
Melting range ⟨741⟩: between 110° and 113°.
Loss on drying ⟨731⟩—Dry it in vacuum at 65° for 3 hours: it loses not more than 0.5% of its weight.
Residue on ignition ⟨281⟩: not more than 0.1%.
Heavy metals, *Method II* ⟨231⟩:   0.002%.
Assay—Dissolve about 50 mg of Tolnaftate, accurately weighed, in methanol, and dilute the solution quantitatively and stepwise with methanol to obtain a concentration of about 10 µg per mL. Dissolve an accurately weighed quantity of USP Tolnaftate RS in methanol, and dilute quantitatively and stepwise with methanol to obtain a Standard solution having a known concentration of about 10 µg per mL. Concomitantly determine the absorbances of both solutions in 1-cm cells at the wavelength of maximum absorbance at about 258 nm, with a suitable spectrophotometer, using methanol as the blank. Calculate the quantity, in mg, of C$_{19}$H$_{17}$NOS in the portion of Tolnaftate taken by the formula:

$$5C(A_U/A_S)$$

in which C is the concentration, in µg per mL, of USP Tolnaftate RS in the Standard solution, and A_U and A_S are the absorbances of the solution of Tolnaftate and the Standard solution, respectively.

Tolnaftate Topical Aerosol

» Tolnaftate Topical Aerosol is a suspension of powder in suitable propellants in a pressurized container. The powder contains not less than 90.0 percent and not more than 110.0 percent of the labeled amount of tolnaftate (C$_{19}$H$_{17}$NOS).

Packaging and storage—Preserve in tight, pressurized containers. Store at controlled room temperature, and avoid exposure to excessive heat.
USP Reference standards ⟨11⟩—*USP Tolnaftate RS.*
Identification—It meets the requirements of the *Identification* test under *Tolnaftate Topical Powder.*
Other requirements—It meets the requirements for *Pressure Test, Minimum Fill,* and *Leakage Test* under *Aerosols, Nasal Sprays, Metered-Dose Inhalers, and Dry Powder Inhalers* ⟨601⟩.
Assay—
  Mobile phase, Internal standard solution, Standard preparation, and *Chromatographic system*—Proceed as directed in the *Assay* under *Tolnaftate Topical Powder.*
  Assay preparation—Remove the actuator button, and replace it with an actuator button that has a small-diameter, stiff polyethylene tube about 15 cm in length fitted tightly into the orifice. Deliver the entire contents of the Topical Aerosol into a conical flask, and heat the flask gently to expel the liquid phase. Cool, mix, and transfer an accurately weighed portion of the powder, equivalent to about 5 mg of tolnaftate, to a screw-capped, 50-mL centrifuge tube. Proceed as directed in the *Assay* under *Tolnaftate Topical Powder,* beginning with "Add 25.0 mL of methanol."
  Procedure—Proceed as directed in the *Assay* under *Tolnaftate Topical Powder.*

Tolnaftate Cream

» Tolnaftate Cream contains not less than 90.0 percent and not more than 110.0 percent of the labeled amount of C$_{19}$H$_{17}$NOS.

Packaging and storage—Preserve in tight containers.
USP Reference standards ⟨11⟩—*USP Tolnaftate RS.*
Identification—Evaporate 10 mL of the next-to-final chloroform solution prepared in the *Assay* on a steam bath just to dryness, and dissolve the residue in 1 mL of alcohol. Using this as the test solution, proceed as directed in *Identification* test C under *Tolnaftate:* the specified result is observed.
Minimum fill ⟨755⟩: meets the requirements.
Assay—Transfer a portion of Cream, equivalent to about 10 mg of tolnaftate and accurately weighed, to a 250-mL separator containing about 75 mL of chloroform. Wash the chloroform solution successively with two 25-mL portions of 0.1 N sodium hydroxide, two 25-mL portions of 0.1 N hydrochloric acid, and 25 mL of water. Filter the chloroform layer through a chloroform-washed cotton pledget into a 100-mL volumetric flask. Add chloroform to volume, and mix. [NOTE—Reserve a 10-mL portion of this solution for the *Identification* test.] Dilute 5.0 mL of the solution with chloroform to 50.0 mL, and mix. Dissolve an accurately weighed quantity of USP Tolnaftate RS in chloroform, and dilute quantitatively and stepwise with chloroform to obtain a Standard solution having a known concentration of about 10 µg per mL. Concomitantly determine the absorbances of both solutions in 1-cm cells at the wavelength of maximum absorbance at about 258 nm, with a suitable spectrophotometer, using chloroform as the blank. Calculate the quantity, in mg, of C$_{19}$H$_{17}$NOS in the portion of Cream taken by the formula:

$$C(A_U/A_S)$$

in which C is the concentration, in µg per mL, of USP Tolnaftate RS in the Standard solution, and A_U and A_S are the absorbances of the solution from the Cream and the Standard solution, respectively.

Tolnaftate Gel

» Tolnaftate Gel contains not less than 90.0 percent and not more than 110.0 percent of the labeled amount of C$_{19}$H$_{17}$NOS.

Tolnaftate Topical Powder

» Tolnaftate Topical Powder contains not less than 90.0 percent and not more than 110.0 percent of the labeled amount of $C_{19}H_{17}NOS$.

Packaging and storage—Preserve in tight containers.

USP Reference standards ⟨11⟩—*USP Tolnaftate RS.*

Identification—Evaporate the 5-mL portion of the methanol solution, reserved from the *Assay preparation*, on a steam bath just to dryness, and dissolve the residue in 1 mL of alcohol. Using this as the test solution, proceed as directed in *Identification* test C under *Tolnaftate*: the specified result is observed.

Minimum fill ⟨755⟩: meets the requirements.

Assay—

Mobile phase—Prepare a filtered and degassed mixture of acetonitrile and water (2 : 1). Make adjustments if necessary (see *System Suitability* under *Chromatography* ⟨621⟩).

Internal standard solution—Dissolve progesterone in methanol to obtain a solution containing about 1 mg per mL.

Standard preparation—Dissolve an accurately weighed quantity of USP Tolnaftate RS in methanol to obtain a solution having a known concentration of about 0.22 mg per mL. Transfer 20.0 mL of this solution to a 50-mL volumetric flask, add 5.0 mL of *Internal standard solution*, dilute with methanol to volume, and mix to obtain a solution having a known concentration of about 0.088 mg of USP Tolnaftate RS per mL.

Assay preparation—Transfer an accurately weighed quantity of Topical Powder, equivalent to about 5 mg of tolnaftate, to a screw-capped, 50-mL centrifuge tube. Add 25.0 mL of methanol, place the cap on the tube, rotate on a rotating device for 10 minutes, and centrifuge at about 2000 rpm for 5 minutes. Pass the supernatant through a 0.45-μm porosity filter, and transfer 20.0 mL of the filtrate to a 50-mL volumetric flask, retaining the remaining portion of the filtrate (about 5 mL) for the *Identification* test. Add 5.0 mL of *Internal standard solution* to the volumetric flask, dilute with methanol to volume, and mix.

Chromatographic system (see *Chromatography* ⟨621⟩)—The liquid chromatograph is equipped with a 254-nm detector and a 4-mm × 30-cm column that contains 10-μm packing L1. The flow rate is about 1 mL per minute. Chromatograph the *Standard preparation*, and record the peak responses as directed for *Procedure*: the resolution, *R*, between the analyte and internal standard peaks is not less than 3.0, and the relative standard deviation for replicate injections is not more than 3.0%.

Procedure—Separately inject equal volumes (about 10 μL) of the *Standard preparation* and the *Assay preparation* into the chromatograph, record the chromatograms, and measure the responses for the major peaks. The relative retention times are about 0.7 for progesterone and 1.0 for tolnaftate. Calculate the quantity, in mg, of $C_{19}H_{17}NOS$ in the portion of Powder taken by the formula:

$$62.5C(R_U / R_S)$$

in which *C* is the concentration, in mg per mL, of USP Tolnaftate RS in the *Standard preparation*, and R_U and R_S are the peak response ratios obtained from the *Assay preparation* and the *Standard preparation*, respectively.

Tolnaftate Topical Solution

» Tolnaftate Topical Solution contains not less than 90.0 percent and not more than 115.0 percent of the labeled amount of $C_{19}H_{17}NOS$.

Packaging and storage—Preserve in tight containers.

USP Reference standards ⟨11⟩—*USP Tolnaftate RS.*

Identification—Evaporate 25 mL of the next-to-final chloroform solution prepared in the *Assay* on a steam bath just to dryness, and dissolve the residue in 1 mL of alcohol. Using this as the test solution, proceed as directed in *Identification* test C under *Tolnaftate*: the specified result is observed.

Assay—Pipet into a separator a volume of Topical Solution, equivalent to about 10 mg of tolnaftate, add 50 mL of chloroform, and extract with 50 mL of 0.1 N sodium hydroxide. Filter the chloroform layer through a chloroform-washed cotton pledget into a 250-mL volumetric flask, and extract the aqueous layer with two 45-mL portions of chloroform, filtering each portion into the flask. Add chloroform to volume, and mix. [NOTE—Reserve a 25-mL portion of this solution for the *Identification* test.] Dilute 25.0 mL of the solution with chloroform to 100.0 mL, and mix. Dissolve an accurately weighed quantity of USP Tolnaftate RS in chloroform, and dilute quantitatively and stepwise with chloroform to obtain a Standard solution having a known concentration of about 10 μg per mL. Concomitantly determine the absorbances of both solutions in 1-cm cells at the wavelength of maximum absorbance at about 258 nm, with a suitable spectrophotometer, using chloroform as the blank. Calculate the quantity, in mg, of $C_{19}H_{17}NOS$ in each mL of Topical Solution taken by the formula:

$$(C / V)(A_U / A_S)$$

in which *C* is the concentration, in μg per mL, of USP Tolnaftate RS in the Standard solution, *V* is the volume, in mL, of Topical Solution taken, and A_U and A_S are the absorbances of the solution from the Topical Solution and the Standard solution, respectively.

Tolu Balsam

» Tolu Balsam is a balsam obtained from *Myroxylon balsamum* (Linné) Harms (Fam. Leguminosae).

Packaging and storage—Preserve in tight containers, and avoid exposure to excessive heat.

Rosin, rosin oil, and copaiba—Place 1 g, powdered or crushed if necessary, in a small mortar, and add 10 mL of petroleum benzin. Triturate well for 1 to 2 minutes, filter into a test tube, and to the filtrate so obtained add 10 mL of freshly prepared cupric acetate solution (1 in 200). Shake, and allow the phases to separate: the petroleum benzin layer does not show a green color.

Acid value ⟨401⟩—Dissolve about 1 g, accurately weighed, in 50 mL of neutralized alcohol, add phenolphthalein TS, and titrate with 0.5 N alcoholic potassium hydroxide VS: the acid value is between 112 and 168.

Saponification value ⟨401⟩—Add sufficient 0.5 N alcoholic potassium hydroxide VS to the neutralized liquid obtained in the test for *Acid value* to make the total volume of the alkali solution added 20.0 mL, heat the liquid on a steam bath for 30 minutes under a reflux condenser, and cool. Add about 200 mL of water, or more if necessary, and titrate the excess potassium hydroxide with 0.5 N hydrochloric acid VS. Perform a blank determination (see *Residual Titrations* under *Titrimetry* ⟨541⟩). The total volume of 0.5 N alcoholic potassium hydroxide consumed, including that required to neutralize the free acid in the determination of *Acid value*, is equivalent to a saponification value of between 154 and 220.

Prior section (Tolnaftate Cream references):

Packaging and storage—Preserve in tight containers.

USP Reference standards ⟨11⟩—*USP Tolnaftate RS.*

Identification—It responds to the *Identification* test under *Tolnaftate Cream*.

Minimum fill ⟨755⟩: meets the requirements.

Assay—Proceed with Gel as directed in the *Assay* under *Tolnaftate Cream*., except to omit the filtration of the chloroform layer through a chloroform-washed cotton pledget.

Topiramate

C₁₂H₂₁NO₈S   339.36
β-D-Fructopyranose, 2,3 : 4,5-bis-*O*-(1-methylethylidene)-, sulfamate.
2,3 : 4,5-Di-*O*-isopropylidene-β-D-fructopyranose sulfamate [97240-79-4].

» Topiramate contains not less than 98.0 percent and not more than 102.0 percent of $C_{12}H_{21}NO_8S$, calculated on the anhydrous basis.

Packaging and storage—Preserve in tight, light-resistant containers, and store at controlled room temperature.

USP Reference standards ⟨11⟩—USP Topiramate RS. USP Topiramate Related Compound A RS.

Identification—
  A: *Infrared Absorption* ⟨197K⟩.
  B: The retention time of the major peak in the chromatogram of the *Assay preparation* corresponds to that in the chromatogram of the *Standard preparation*, as obtained in the *Assay*.

Specific rotation ⟨781S⟩: between −29° and −35°, measured at 20°.
  Test solution: 4 mg per mL, in methanol.

Water, *Method I* ⟨921⟩: not more than 0.5%.

Residue on ignition ⟨281⟩: not more than 0.2%.

Limit of sulfamate and sulfate—
  Diluent—Prepare a mixture of high-purity water and acetonitrile (80 : 20).
  Solution A—Transfer about 4 g of sodium hydroxide to a 1000-mL volumetric flask. Dissolve in and dilute with *High-Purity Water* (see *Reagents* in *Chemical Resistance—Glass Containers* under *Containers* ⟨661⟩) to volume, filter, and degas.
  Solution B—Use filtered and degassed *High-Purity Water*.
  Solution C—Dilute 50 mL of *Solution A* to 100-mL with *High-Purity Water*, filter, and degas.
  Mobile phase—Use variable mixtures of *Solution A*, *Solution B*, and *Solution C* as directed for *Chromatographic system*. Make adjustments if necessary (see *System Suitability* under *Chromatography* ⟨621⟩).
  Sulfamic acid stock solution—Transfer about 60 mg, accurately weighed, of sulfamic acid to a 100-mL volumetric flask. Dissolve in and dilute with *Diluent* to volume.
  Sulfate stock solution—Transfer about 90.7 mg, accurately weighed, of potassium sulfate to a 100-mL volumetric flask. Dissolve in and dilute with *Diluent* to volume.
  Standard solution—Transfer 3.0 mL each of *Sulfamic acid stock solution* and *Sulfate stock solution* to a 50-mL volumetric flask, dilute with *Diluent* to volume, and mix.
  Test solution—Transfer about 100 mg, accurately weighed, of Topiramate to a 10-mL volumetric flask. Dissolve in and dilute with *High-Purity Water* to volume.
  Chromatographic system (see *Chromatography* ⟨621⟩)—The liquid chromatograph is equipped with a conductivity detector, a 4.0-mm × 5-cm guard column that contains packing L46 and a 4.0-mm × 25-cm column that contains packing L46. The flow rate is about 2.0 mL per minute. The chromatograph is programmed as follows.

Time (minutes)	Solution A (%)	Solution B (%)	Solution C (%)	Elution
0	0	95	5	equilibration
0–7.0	0	95	5	isocratic
7.0–15.0	0→20	95→0	5→80	linear gradient
15.0–20.0	20	0	80	isocratic
20.0–20.1	20→0	0→95	80→5	linear gradient
20.1–25.0	0	95	5	re-equilibration

  Chromatograph the *Standard solution*, and record the peak areas as directed for *Procedure*: the relative retention time is 1.0 for the sulfate peak and about 0.27 for the sulfamate peak; and the relative standard deviation for replicate injections is not more than 2.0% for both the sulfate and sulfamate peaks.

  Procedure—Separately inject equal volumes (about 20 µL) of the *Standard solution* and the *Test solution* into the chromatograph, record the chromatograms, and measure the peak areas for the sulfate and sulfamate peaks. Calculate the percentage of sulfate and sulfamate in the portion of Topiramate taken by the formula:

$$1000F(C/W)(r_i / r_S)$$

in which C is the concentration, in mg per mL, of potassium sulfate or sulfamic acid in the *Standard solution*; F is the correction factor and is equal to 0.551 for sulfate and 0.989 for sulfamate; W is the weight, in mg, of Topiramate taken; and r_i and r_S are the peak areas of the sulfate or sulfamate ion obtained from the *Test solution* and the *Standard solution*, respectively: not more that 0.10% of sulfate ion is found; and not more than 0.10% of sulfamate ion is found.

Assay—
  Mobile phase—Prepare a filtered and degassed mixture of acetonitrile and water (1 : 1). Make adjustments if necessary (see *System Suitability* under *Chromatography* ⟨621⟩).
  Standard preparation—Dissolve an accurately weighed quantity of USP Topiramate RS in *Mobile phase*, and dilute quantitatively, and stepwise if necessary, with *Mobile phase* to obtain a solution having a known concentration of about 2.0 mg per mL.
  Assay preparation—Transfer about 50 mg of Topiramate, accurately weighed, to a 25-mL volumetric flask, and dissolve in and dilute with *Mobile phase* to volume.
  Chromatographic system (see *Chromatography* ⟨621⟩)—The liquid chromatograph is equipped with a refractive index detector and a 4.6-mm × 25-cm column that contains 5-µm packing L1. The flow rate is about 0.6 mL per minute. The detector and column temperatures are maintained at 50°. Chromatograph the *Standard preparation*, and record the peak responses as directed for *Procedure*: the column efficiency is not less than 1500 theoretical plates; the tailing factor is not more than 2.0; and the relative standard deviation for replicate injections is not more than 2.0%.
  Procedure—Separately inject equal volumes (about 20 µL) of the *Standard preparation* and the *Assay preparation* into the chromatograph, record the chromatograms, and measure the responses for the major peaks. Calculate the quantity, in mg, of $C_{12}H_{21}NO_8S$ in the portion of Topiramate taken by the formula:

$$25C(r_U / r_S)$$

in which C is the concentration, in mg per mL, of USP Topiramate RS in the *Standard preparation*; and r_U and r_S are the peak areas obtained from the *Assay preparation* and the *Standard preparation*, respectively.

Torsemide

$C_{16}H_{20}N_4O_3S$ 348.42

3-Pyridinesulfonamide, N-[[(1-methylethyl)amino]carbonyl]-4-[(3-methylphenyl)amino]-.

1-Isopropyl-3-[(4-m-toluidino-3-pyridyl)sulfonyl]urea   [56211-40-6].

» Torsemide contains not less than 98.0 percent and not more than 102.0 percent of $C_{16}H_{20}N_4O_3S$, calculated on the anhydrous basis.

Packaging and storage—Preserve in well-closed containers.

USP Reference standards ⟨11⟩—*USP Torsemide RS. USP Torsemide Related Compound A RS. USP Torsemide Related Compound B RS. USP Torsemide Related Compound C RS.*

Identification—
A: *Infrared Absorption* ⟨197K⟩.
B: The retention time of the major peak in the chromatogram of the *Assay preparation* corresponds to that in the chromatogram of the *Standard preparation*, as obtained in the *Assay*.

Water, *Method I* ⟨921⟩:   not more than 0.8%.

Residue on ignition ⟨281⟩:   not more than 0.1%.

Heavy metals, *Method II* ⟨231⟩:   0.001%.

Related compounds—
0.02 M Potassium phosphate buffer and *Mobile phase*—Prepare as directed in the *Assay*.

Resolution solution—Transfer about 3 mg each of USP Torsemide RS and USP Torsemide Related Compound A RS to a 10-mL volumetric flask, add 3 mL of methanol, mix, and sonicate for not less than 8 minutes. Add 4.5 mL of *0.02 M Potassium phosphate buffer*, cool to room temperature, dilute with *Mobile phase* to volume, and mix.

Standard solution—Transfer about 8 mg each of USP Torsemide Related Compound A RS, USP Torsemide Related Compound B RS, and USP Torsemide Related Compound C RS, accurately weighed, to a 100-mL volumetric flask, add 30 mL of methanol, mix, and sonicate for not less than 8 minutes. Add 45 mL of *0.02 M Potassium phosphate buffer*, cool to room temperature, dilute with *Mobile phase* to volume, and mix. Quantitatively dilute a portion of this solution with *Mobile phase* to obtain a solution having a known concentration of about 0.0019 mg per mL.

Test solution—Use the *Assay preparation*.

Chromatographic system—Prepare as directed in the *Assay*. Chromatograph the *Resolution solution* and the *Standard solution*, and record the peak responses over a period three times the retention time of torsemide as directed for *Procedure*: the resolution, R, between torsemide and torsemide related compound A is not less than 1.0; the tailing factors are not more than 2.0; and the relative standard deviation for replicate injections is not more than 10.0%.

Procedure—Separately inject equal volumes (about 20 µL) of the *Standard solution* and the *Test solution* into the chromatograph, record the chromatograms, and measure the peak areas for torsemide related compound A, torsemide related compound B, and torsemide related compound C. Calculate the percentage of each related compound, if present, in the portion of Torsemide taken by the formula:

$$100(C_S / C_U)(r_U / r_S)$$

in which C_S is the concentration, in mg per mL, of the relevant USP Reference Standard in the *Standard solution*; C_U is the concentration of Torsemide, in mg per mL, in the *Test solution*; and r_U and r_S are the peak areas for the relevant torsemide related compound obtained from the *Test solution* and the *Standard solution*, respectively: not more than 0.2% of torsemide related compound C, not more than 0.3% of torsemide related compound B, and not more than 0.5% of torsemide related compound A are found. Calculate the percentage of any other impurity in the portion of Torsemide taken by the formula:

$$100(r_i / r_s)$$

in which r_i is the peak response for each other impurity obtained from the *Test solution*; and r_s is the sum of the responses of all the peaks obtained from the *Test solution*: not more than 0.1% of any other impurity is found, not more than 0.2% of total other impurities is found, and not more than 1.0% of total impurities (including torsemide related compounds A, B, and C) is found.

Assay—
0.02 M Potassium phosphate buffer—Dissolve 2.7 g of monobasic potassium phosphate in about 900 mL of water. Adjust with phosphoric acid to a pH of 3.5, dilute with water to 1000 mL, and mix.

Mobile phase—Prepare a filtered and degassed mixture of *0.02 M Potassium phosphate buffer* and methanol (3 : 2). Make adjustments if necessary (see *System Suitability* under *Chromatography* ⟨621⟩).

Standard preparation—Transfer about 19 mg of USP Torsemide RS, accurately weighed, to a 50-mL volumetric flask, add 15 mL of methanol, mix, and sonicate for not less than 8 minutes. Add 22.5 mL of *0.02 M Potassium phosphate buffer*, cool to room temperature, dilute with *Mobile phase* to volume, and mix.

Assay preparation—Transfer about 38 mg of Torsemide, accurately weighed, to a 100-mL volumetric flask, add 30 mL of methanol, mix, and sonicate for not less than 8 minutes. Add 45 mL of *0.02 M Potassium phosphate buffer*, cool to room temperature, dilute with *Mobile phase* to volume, and mix.

Chromatographic system (see *Chromatography* ⟨621⟩)—The liquid chromatograph is equipped with a 288-nm detector and a 4.6-mm × 15-cm column that contains 7-µm packing L1. The flow rate is about 1.5 mL per minute. Chromatograph the *Standard preparation*, and record the peak responses as directed for *Procedure*: the tailing factor is not more than 2.0; and the relative standard deviation for replicate injections is not more than 2.0%.

Procedure—Separately inject equal volumes (about 20 µL) of the *Standard preparation* and the *Assay preparation* into the chromatograph, record the chromatograms, and measure the responses for the major peaks. Calculate the amount, in mg, of $C_{16}H_{20}N_4O_3S$ in the portion of Torsemide taken by the formula:

$$100C(r_U / r_S)$$

in which C is the concentration, in mg per mL, of USP Torsemide RS in the *Standard preparation*; and r_U and r_S are the peak responses obtained from the *Assay preparation* and the *Standard preparation*, respectively.

Trazodone Hydrochloride

$C_{19}H_{22}ClN_5O \cdot HCl$ 408.32

1,2,4-Triazolo[4,3-a]pyridin-3(2H)-one,2-[3-[4-(3-chlorophenyl)-1-piperazinyl]propyl]-, monohydrochloride.

2-[3-[4-(m-Chlorophenyl)-1-piperazinyl]propyl]s-triazolo[4,3-a]-pyridin-3(2H)-one monohydrochloride   [25332-39-2].

» Trazodone Hydrochloride contains not less than 97.0 percent and not more than 102.0 percent of $C_{19}H_{22}ClN_5O \cdot HCl$, calculated on the dried basis.

Packaging and storage—Preserve in tight, light-resistant containers.

USP Reference standards ⟨11⟩—*USP Trazodone Hydrochloride RS.*

Identification—
A: *Infrared Absorption* ⟨197K⟩.
B: The retention time of the major peak in the chromatogram of the *Assay preparation* corresponds to that of the *Standard preparation*, both relative to the internal standard, as obtained in the *Assay*.
Loss on drying ⟨731⟩—Dry it at a pressure of about 50 mm of mercury at 105° for 3 hours: it loses not more than 0.5% of its weight.
Residue on ignition ⟨281⟩: not more than 0.2%.
Chromatographic purity—
Mobile phase—Prepare a filtered and degassed mixture of 0.5% trifluoroacetic acid, tetrahydrofuran, acetonitrile, and methanol (13.5 : 3 : 3 : 1). Make adjustments if necessary (see *System Suitability* under *Chromatography* ⟨621⟩).
Standard solution—Dissolve an accurately weighed quantity of USP Trazodone Hydrochloride RS in *Mobile phase*, and dilute quantitatively, and stepwise if necessary, with *Mobile phase* to obtain a solution having a known concentration of about 2 µg per mL.
System suitability solution—Dissolve suitable quantities of 3-chloroaniline and USP Trazodone Hydrochloride RS in *Mobile phase* to obtain a solution containing about 0.1 mg per mL of 3-chloroaniline and 0.01 mg per mL of trazodone hydrochloride, respectively.
Test solution—Transfer about 50 mg of trazodone hydrochloride, accurately weighed, to a 50-mL volumetric flask, dissolve in and dilute with *Mobile phase* to volume, and filter.
Chromatographic system (see *Chromatography* ⟨621⟩)—The liquid chromatograph is equipped with a 248-nm detector and a 4.6-mm × 15-cm column that contains 3-µm packing L7. The flow rate is about 1.0 mL per minute. Chromatograph the *System suitability solution*, and record the peak responses as directed for *Procedure*: the relative retention times are about 0.6 for 3-chloroaniline and 1 for trazodone hydrochloride, and the resolution, *R*, between 3-chloroaniline and trazodone hydrochloride, is not less than 12. Chromatograph the *Standard solution*, and record the peak responses as directed for *Procedure*: the tailing factor for the analyte peak is not more than 2.0, and the relative standard deviation for replicate injections is not more than 5%.
Procedure—Separately inject equal volumes (about 10 µL) of the *Standard solution* and the *Test solution* into the chromatograph, record the chromatograms, and measure the responses for all of the peaks. Calculate the percentage of each peak, other than the trazodone hydrochloride peak, in the Trazodone Hydrochloride taken by the formula:

$$100(C_S/C_T)(r_U/r_S)$$

in which C_S is the concentration, in mg per mL, of USP Trazodone Hydrochloride RS in the *Standard solution*, C_T is the concentration, in mg per mL, of trazodone hydrochloride in the *Test solution*, r_U is the response of each peak, other than the trazodone hydrochloride peak, obtained from the *Test solution*, and r_S is the peak response for trazodone hydrochloride obtained from the *Standard solution*: not more than 0.4% for any single impurity and not more than 1.0% of total impurities are found.
Ordinary impurities ⟨466⟩—
Test solution: methanol.
Standard solution: methanol.
Eluant: a mixture of cyclohexane, acetone, and ammonium hydroxide (8 : 4.5 : 0.5).
Visualization: 1.
Assay—
0.01 M Ammonium phosphate buffer—Transfer 1.15 g of monobasic ammonium phosphate to a 1000-mL volumetric flask, and dissolve in water. Add 1.0 mL of 1 N sodium hydroxide, dilute with water to volume, and mix. Adjust this solution, if necessary, with either 10% phosphoric acid or 1 N sodium hydroxide to a pH of 6.0 ± 0.1, and filter.
Mobile phase—Prepare a filtered and degassed mixture of methanol and *0.01 M Ammonium phosphate buffer* (60 : 40). Make adjustments if necessary (see *System Suitability* under *Chromatography* ⟨621⟩).
Internal standard solution—Dissolve a suitable quantity of butylparaben in methanol to obtain a solution containing about 2 mg per mL.
Standard preparation—Dissolve an accurately weighed quantity of USP Trazodone Hydrochloride RS in *Mobile phase* to obtain a solution having a known concentration of about 2.5 mg per mL. Transfer 4.0 mL of this solution to a 100-mL volumetric flask, add 2.0 mL of *Internal standard solution*, dilute with *Mobile phase* to volume, and mix to obtain a solution having a known concentration of about 0.1 mg of USP Trazodone Hydrochloride RS per mL.
Assay preparation—Transfer an accurately weighed quantity of about 125 mg of Trazodone Hydrochloride to a 50-mL volumetric flask, dissolve in and dilute with *Mobile phase* to volume, and mix. Transfer 4.0 mL of this solution to a 100-mL volumetric flask, add 2.0 mL of the *Internal standard solution*, dilute with *Mobile phase* to volume, and mix.
Chromatographic system (see *Chromatography* ⟨621⟩)—The liquid chromatograph is equipped with a 254-nm detector and a 3.9-mm × 30-cm column that contains packing L1. The flow rate is about 1.5 mL per minute. Chromatograph the *Standard preparation*, and record the peak responses as directed for *Procedure*: the resolution, *R*, between the trazodone and butylparaben peaks is not less than 3.0, and the relative standard deviation for replicate injections is not more than 2.0%.
Procedure—Separately inject equal volumes (about 25 µL) of the *Standard preparation* and the *Assay preparation* into the chromatograph, record the chromatograms, and measure the responses for the major peaks. The relative retention times are about 0.6 for butylparaben and 1.0 for trazodone. Calculate the quantity, in mg, of $C_{19}H_{22}ClN_5O \cdot HCl$ in the portion of Trazodone Hydrochloride taken by the formula:

$$1250C(R_U/R_S)$$

in which C is the concentration, in mg per mL, of USP Trazodone Hydrochloride RS in the *Standard preparation*, and R_U and R_S are the ratios of the peak responses of the trazodone to the internal standard obtained from the *Assay preparation* and the *Standard preparation*, respectively.

Trazodone Hydrochloride Tablets

» Trazodone Hydrochloride Tablets contain not less than 90.0 percent and not more than 110.0 percent of the labeled amount of trazodone hydrochloride ($C_{19}H_{22}ClN_5O \cdot HCl$).

Packaging and storage—Preserve in tight, light-resistant containers.
USP Reference standards ⟨11⟩—*USP Trazodone Hydrochloride RS.*
Identification—
A: *Thin-Layer Chromatographic Identification Test* ⟨201⟩—
Test solution—Place a number of Tablets, equivalent to about 150 mg of trazodone hydrochloride, in a clean scintillation vial, add about 7.5 mL of methanol, and sonicate until the Tablets have disintegrated. Shake the vials, by hand, for a few seconds to mix, and filter to obtain the test solution.
Standard solution: 20 mg per mL, in methanol.
Application volume: 1 µL.
Developing solvent system: a mixture of cyclohexane, alcohol, toluene, and diethylamine (80 : 30 : 20 : 20).
Procedure: Proceed as directed in the chapter except locate the spots on the plate by examination under long-wavelength UV light.
B: The retention time of the major peak in the chromatogram of the *Assay preparation* corresponds to that in the chromatogram of the *Standard preparation*, as obtained in the *Assay*.
Dissolution ⟨711⟩—
Medium: 0.01 N hydrochloric acid; 900 mL.
Apparatus 2: 50 rpm.
Time: 60 minutes.
Determine the amount of $C_{19}H_{22}ClN_5O \cdot HCl$ dissolved by employing the following method.
Mobile phase, Standard preparation, and *Chromatographic system*—Proceed as directed in the *Assay*.
Procedure—Inject an appropriate volume (about 20 µL) of a portion of the solution under test, previously passed through a 0.45-µm

nylon filter, into the chromatograph, record the chromatogram, and measure the response for the major peak. Calculate the quantity of $C_{19}H_{22}ClN_5O \cdot HCl$ dissolved by comparing this peak response with the major peak response similarly obtained from the *Standard preparation*.

Tolerances—Not less than 80% (*Q*) of the labeled amount of $C_{19}H_{22}ClN_5O \cdot HCl$ is dissolved in 60 minutes.

Uniformity of dosage units ⟨905⟩: meet the requirements.

Assay—

Phosphate buffer—Dissolve about 1.15 g of monobasic ammonium phosphate in 1 L of water, and adjust with sodium hydroxide to a pH of 6.0.

Mobile phase—Prepare a filtered and degassed mixture of methanol and *Phosphate buffer* (3 : 1). Make adjustments if necessary (see *System Suitability* under *Chromatography* ⟨621⟩).

Standard preparation—Dissolve an accurately weighed quantity of USP Trazodone Hydrochloride RS in 0.01 N hydrochloric acid, and dilute quantitatively, and stepwise if necessary, with 0.01 N hydrochloric acid to obtain a solution having a known concentration of about 0.100 mg per mL.

Assay preparation—Weigh and finely powder not fewer than 20 Tablets. Transfer an accurately weighed portion of the powder, equivalent to about 10 mg of trazodone hydrochloride, to a 100-mL volumetric flask, dilute with 0.01 N hydrochloric acid to volume, and mix. Sonicate for about 30 minutes, and pass through a 0.45-μm nylon filter.

Chromatographic system (see *Chromatography* ⟨621⟩)—The liquid chromatograph is equipped with a 246-nm detector and a 5-mm × 10-cm column that contains packing L1. The flow rate is about 1.5 mL per minute. Chromatograph the *Standard preparation*, and record the peak responses as directed for *Procedure*: the capacity factor, k', is not less than 1.5; the column efficiency is not less than 900 theoretical plates; and the relative standard deviation for replicate injections is not more than 2.0%.

Procedure—Separately inject equal volumes (about 20 μL) of the *Standard preparation* and the *Assay preparation* into the chromatograph, record the chromatograms, and measure the responses for the major peaks. Calculate the quantity, in mg, of trazodone hydrochloride ($C_{19}H_{22}ClN_5O \cdot HCl$) in the portion of Tablets taken by the formula:

$$100C(r_U / r_S)$$

in which *C* is the concentration, in mg per mL, of USP Trazodone Hydrochloride RS in the *Standard preparation*; and r_U and r_S are the peak responses obtained from the *Assay preparation* and the *Standard preparation*, respectively.

Trenbolone Acetate

$C_{20}H_{24}O_3$ 312.40
Estra-4,9,11-trien-3-one, 17-(acetyloxy)-, (17β)-.
17β-Hydroxyestra-4,9,11-trien-3-one, acetate   [10161-34-9].

» Trenbolone Acetate contains not less than 97.0 percent and not more than 101.0 percent of $C_{20}H_{24}O_3$.

Packaging and storage—Preserve in tight containers, and store in a refrigerator.

Labeling—Label it to indicate that it is for veterinary use only.

USP Reference standards ⟨11⟩—USP Trenbolone RS. USP Trenbolone Acetate RS.

Identification—
  A: *Infrared Absorption* ⟨197K⟩.
  B: *Ultraviolet Absorption* ⟨197U⟩—
    Solution: 16 μg per mL.
    Medium: Alcohol.
  Absorption maxima at about 237 nm and 340 nm. Absorptivity at 340 nm is between 92.0 and 97.6.
  C: The chromatogram of the *Assay preparation* obtained as directed in the *Assay* exhibits a peak for trenbolone acetate, the retention time of which corresponds to that exhibited by the *Standard preparation*.

Absorbance—The absorbance of a 1 in 10 solution of it in dehydrated alcohol, determined in a 2-cm cell at 440 nm, is not more than 0.3, dehydrated alcohol being used as the blank.

Specific rotation ⟨781S⟩: between +39° and +43°.
  Test solution: 5 mg per mL, in methanol.

Loss on drying ⟨731⟩—Dry it in vacuum at 60° for 2 hours: it loses not more than 0.5% of its weight.

Residue on ignition ⟨281⟩: not more than 0.1%.

Chromatographic purity—
  Diluent—Prepare a mixture of chloroform and methanol (9 : 1).
  Standard solutions—Prepare four solutions in *Diluent* containing USP Trenbolone RS and USP Trenbolone Acetate RS containing in each mL 0.1 mg of each, 0.05 mg of each, 0.02 mg of each, and 0.01 mg of each, corresponding to 1.0%, 0.5%, 0.2%, and 0.1% of impurities, respectively.
  Test solution—Prepare a solution of Trenbolone Acetate in *Diluent* containing 10 mg per mL.
  Procedure—Separately apply 10 μL of each of the *Standard solutions* and the *Test solution* to a thin-layer chromatographic plate (see *Chromatography* ⟨621⟩) coated with a 0.25-mm layer of chromatographic silica gel mixture as follows. Develop the chromatograms in a solvent system consisting of a mixture of chloroform and acetone (98 : 2) in an unsaturated chromatographic chamber protected from light until the solvent front has moved about three-fourths of the length of the plate. Remove the plate from the chamber, dry it for about 15 seconds in a stream of dry nitrogen, and immediately develop the chromatograms a second time until the solvent front has moved about three-fourths of the length of the plate. Examine the plate under short-wavelength UV light. Spray the plate with phosphomolybdic acid TS, and heat the plate at 100° for about 10 minutes. Examine the plate under visible light, and compare the intensities of any secondary spots in the chromatogram of the *Test solution* with those of the principal spots in the chromatograms of the *Standard solutions*. No trenbolone spot from the chromatogram of the *Test solution* is larger or more intense than the trenbolone spots from the *Standard solution* containing 0.1 mg of USP Trenbolone RS per mL (1%). Estimate the percentage of each other impurity observed in the chromatogram of the *Test solution* by comparison with the trenbolone acetate spots in the chromatograms of the *Standard solutions*: No other impurity spot is greater than 0.5%, and the total of all other impurities, including that of the 17α-isomer obtained in the test for *Limit of trenbolone acetate 17α-isomer*, is not more than 1%.

Limit of trenbolone acetate 17α-isomer—
  Mobile phase, Resolution solution, and *Chromatographic system*—Proceed as directed in the *Assay*.
  Standard solution—Prepare a solution of USP Trenbolone Acetate RS in *Mobile phase* having a known concentration of 4 μg per mL.
  Test solution—Transfer about 20 mg of Trenbolone Acetate, accurately weighed, to a 20-mL volumetric flask, add about 10 mL of *Mobile phase*, swirl to dissolve, dilute with *Mobile phase* to volume, and mix.
  Procedure—Separately inject equal volumes (about 20 μL) of the *Standard solution* and the *Test solution* into the chromatograph, record the chromatograms, and measure the peak responses. Trenbolone acetate 17α-isomer, if present, has a retention time of about 0.8 relative to that of the trenbolone acetate peak. Calculate the percentage of 17α-isomer found in the Trenbolone Acetate taken by the formula:

$$2(C / W)(r_i / r_S)$$

in which *C* is the concentration, in μg per mL, of USP Trenbolone Acetate RS in the *Standard solution*, *W* is the weight, in mg, of

Trenbolone Acetate taken to prepare the *Test solution*, r_i is the response of any peak at a retention time of about 0.8 in relation to that of the main trenbolone acetate peak in the chromatogram obtained from the *Test solution*, and r_S is the peak area response of the trenbolone acetate peak in the chromatogram obtained from the *Standard solution*. Not more than 0.5% of the 17α-isomer is found.

Organic volatile impurities, Method IV ⟨467⟩: meets the requirements.

(Official until July 1, 2008)

Assay—
Mobile phase—Prepare a mixture of acetonitrile and 1% ammonium acetate solution (55 : 45). Make adjustments if necessary (see *System Suitability* under *Chromatography* ⟨621⟩).

Resolution solution—Prepare a solution in *Mobile phase* containing about 0.2 mg each of USP Trenbolone RS and USP Trenbolone Acetate RS per mL.

Standard preparation—Prepare a solution of USP Trenbolone Acetate RS in *Mobile phase* having a known concentration of about 0.2 mg per mL.

Assay preparation—Transfer about 20 mg of Trenbolone Acetate, accurately weighed, to a 100-mL volumetric flask, dissolve in and dilute with *Mobile phase* to volume, and mix.

Chromatographic system (see *Chromatography* ⟨621⟩)—The liquid chromatograph is equipped with a 344-nm detector and a 4.6-mm × 25-cm column that contains 5-μm packing L1. The flow rate is about 1 mL per minute. Chromatograph the *Resolution solution*, and record the peak responses as directed for *Procedure:* the relative retention times are about 0.4 for trenbolone and 1.0 for trenbolone acetate, and the resolution, *R*, between the trenbolone peak and the trenbolone acetate peak is not less than 25. Chromatograph the *Standard preparation*, and record the peak responses as directed for *Procedure:* the column efficiency is not less than 14,000 theoretical plates when calculated by the formula:

$$5.545(t_r / W_h / 2)^2$$

the tailing factor is not more than 1.2 when calculated by the formula:

$$W_{0.1} / 2f$$

in which $W_{0.1}$ is the width of the peak at 10% height, and the relative standard deviation for replicate injections is not more than 2%.

Procedure—Separately inject equal volumes (about 20 μL) of the *Standard preparation* and the *Assay preparation* into the chromatograph, record the chromatograms, and measure the responses for the major peaks. Calculate the quantity, in mg, of trenbolone acetate ($C_{20}H_{24}O_3$) in the portion of Trenbolone Acetate taken by the formula:

$$100C(r_U / r_S)$$

in which *C* is the concentration, in mg per mL, of USP Trenbolone Acetate RS in the *Standard preparation*, and r_U and r_S are the trenbolone acetate peak area responses obtained from the *Assay preparation* and the *Standard preparation*, respectively.

Tretinoin

$C_{20}H_{28}O_2$ 300.44
Retinoic acid.
all *trans*-Retinoic acid   [*302-79-4*].

» Tretinoin contains not less than 97.0 percent and not more than 103.0 percent of $C_{20}H_{28}O_2$, calculated on the dried basis.

Packaging and storage—Preserve in tight containers, preferably under an atmosphere of an inert gas, protected from light.

USP Reference standards ⟨11⟩—*USP Isotretinoin RS. USP Tretinoin RS.*

NOTE—Avoid exposure to strong light, and use low-actinic glassware in the performance of the following procedures.

Identification—
A: *Infrared Absorption* ⟨197M⟩.
B: *Ultraviolet Absorption* ⟨197U⟩—
Solution: 4 μg per mL.
Medium: acidified isopropyl alcohol (prepared by diluting 1 mL of 0.01 N hydrochloric acid with isopropyl alcohol to 1000 mL).

Absorptivities at 352 nm, calculated on the dried basis, do not differ by more than 3.0%.

Loss on drying ⟨731⟩—Dry it in vacuum at room temperature for 16 hours: it loses not more than 0.5% of its weight.

Residue on ignition ⟨281⟩: not more than 0.1%.

Heavy metals, Method II ⟨231⟩: 0.002%.

Limit of isotretinoin—
Mobile phase—Prepare a suitable filtered and degassed mixture of isooctane, isopropyl alcohol, and glacial acetic acid (99.65 : 0.25 : 0.1), making adjustments if necessary (see *System Suitability* under *Chromatography* ⟨621⟩).

System suitability solution—Dissolve a quantity of USP Tretinoin RS in a minimum amount of methylene chloride, add a suitable amount of isooctane to obtain a solution having a tretinoin concentration of about 250 μg per mL, and mix.

Standard solution—Dissolve an accurately weighed quantity of USP Isotretinoin RS in a minimum quantity of methylene chloride, and add isooctane to obtain a solution having a known concentration of about 250 μg per mL.

System suitability preparation—Pipet 5 mL of *Standard solution* into a 100-mL volumetric flask, add *System suitability solution* to volume, and mix.

Standard preparation—Pipet 5 mL of *Standard solution* into a 100-mL volumetric flask, add isooctane to volume, and mix.

Test preparation—Transfer about 25 mg of Tretinoin, accurately weighed, to a 100-mL volumetric flask, dissolve in a minimum quantity of methylene chloride, add isooctane to volume, and mix.

Chromatographic system (see *Chromatography* ⟨621⟩)—The liquid chromatograph is equipped with a 352-nm detector and a 4.0-mm × 25-cm column containing packing L3. The flow rate is about 1 mL per minute. Chromatograph about 20 μL of *System suitability preparation*, and record the peak responses. The relative retention times for isotretinoin and tretinoin are about 0.84 and 1.00, respectively. The relative standard deviation of the isotretinoin peak response in replicate injections is not more than 2.0%, and the resolution, *R*, of isotretinoin and tretinoin is not less than 2.0.

Procedure—Separately inject equal volumes (about 20 μL) of the *Standard preparation* and the *Test preparation* into the chromatograph, record the chromatograms, and measure the responses for the major peaks. Calculate the percentage of isotretinoin taken by the formula:

$$10(C / W)(r_U / r_S)$$

in which *C* is the concentration, in μg per mL, of USP Isotretinoin RS in the *Standard preparation*, *W* is the weight, in mg, of Tretinoin taken, and r_U and r_S are the peak responses of the isotretinoin peaks obtained from the *Test preparation* and the *Standard preparation*, respectively. The content of isotretinoin is not more than 5.0%.

Assay—Dissolve about 240 mg of Tretinoin, accurately weighed, in 50 mL of dimethylformamide, add 3 drops of a 1 in 100 solution of thymol blue in dimethylformamide, and titrate with 0.1 N sodium methoxide VS to a greenish endpoint. Perform a blank determination, and make any necessary correction. Each mL of 0.1 N sodium methoxide is equivalent to 30.04 mg of $C_{20}H_{28}O_2$.

Tretinoin Cream

» Tretinoin Cream contains not less than 90.0 percent and not more than 120.0 percent of the labeled amount of tretinoin.

Packaging and storage—Preserve in collapsible tubes or in tight, light-resistant containers.

USP Reference standards ⟨11⟩—*USP Tretinoin RS.*

Identification—The retention time of the major peak in the chromatogram of the *Assay preparation* corresponds to that in the chromatogram of the *Standard preparation* obtained as directed in the *Assay.*

Minimum fill ⟨755⟩: meets the requirements.

Assay—[NOTE—Avoid exposure to strong light, and use low-actinic glassware in the performance of the following procedure. Use stabilized tetrahydrofuran in the preparation of the *Standard preparation* and the *Assay preparation.*]

Dilute phosphoric acid—Dilute 10 mL of phosphoric acid with water to 100 mL.

Phosphate buffer—Dissolve 1.38 g of monobasic sodium phosphate in 1000 mL of water, adjust with *Dilute phosphoric acid* to a pH of 3.0, and mix.

Diluting solution—Prepare a mixture of water and *Dilute phosphoric acid* (9 : 1).

Mobile phase—[NOTE—*Phosphate buffer* and tetrahydrofuran may be filtered and degassed separately *before* mixing.] Prepare a filtered and degassed mixture of *Phosphate buffer* and tetrahydrofuran (58 : 42). Make adjustments if necessary (see *System Suitability* under *Chromatography* ⟨621⟩).

Standard preparation—Dissolve an accurately weighed quantity of USP Tretinoin RS in tetrahydrofuran to obtain a solution having a known concentration of about 0.4 mg per mL. Dilute a known volume of this solution, quantitatively and stepwise if necessary, with a mixture of tetrahydrofuran and *Diluting solution* (3 : 2) to obtain a solution having a known concentration of about 4 µg per mL.

Assay preparation—Transfer an accurately weighed quantity of Cream, equivalent to about 1.0 mg of tretinoin, to a 50-mL volumetric flask, and add 20.0 mL of tetrahydrofuran. Shake the flask to disperse the cream, dilute with tetrahydrofuran to volume, mix, and filter, if necessary. Transfer 5.0 mL of this solution to a 25-mL volumetric flask, dilute with a mixture of tetrahydrofuran and *Diluting solution* (3 : 2) to volume, mix, and filter.

Chromatographic system (see *Chromatography* ⟨621⟩)—The liquid chromatograph is equipped with a 365-nm detector and a 3.9-mm × 15-cm column that contains 4-µm packing L1. The flow rate is about 1 mL per minute. Chromatograph the *Standard preparation*, and record the peak responses as directed for *Procedure:* the relative standard deviation for replicate injections is not more than 2.0%.

Procedure—Separately inject equal volumes (about 25 µL) of the *Standard preparation* and the *Assay preparation* into the chromatograph, record the chromatograms, and measure the responses for the major peaks. Calculate the quantity, in mg, of tretinoin ($C_{20}H_{28}O_2$) in the portion of Cream taken by the formula:

$$0.250C(r_U / r_S)$$

in which C is the concentration, in µg per mL, of USP Tretinoin RS in the *Standard preparation*, and r_U and r_S are the peak responses obtained from the *Assay preparation* and the *Standard preparation*, respectively.

Tretinoin Gel

» Tretinoin Gel contains not less than 90.0 percent and not more than 130.0 percent of the labeled amount of $C_{20}H_{28}O_2$.

Packaging and storage—Preserve in tight containers, protected from light.

USP Reference standards ⟨11⟩—*USP Tretinoin RS.*

Identification—The absorption spectrum, obtained between wavelengths of 300 nm and 450 nm, of the solution employed for measurement of absorbance in the *Assay* exhibits maxima and minima at the same wavelengths as that of a similar solution of USP Tretinoin RS, concomitantly measured.

Minimum fill ⟨755⟩: meets the requirements.

Assay—[NOTE—Avoid exposure to strong light, and use low-actinic glassware in the performance of the following procedure.] Transfer to a 100-mL volumetric flask an accurately weighed quantity of Gel, equivalent to about 375 µg of tretinoin, and dissolve in about 70 mL of chloroform, dilute with chloroform to volume, and mix. Dissolve an accurately weighed quantity of USP Tretinoin RS in chloroform, and dilute quantitatively and stepwise with chloroform to obtain a Standard solution having a known concentration of about 3.75 µg per mL. Concomitantly determine the absorbances of both solutions in 1-cm cells at the wavelength of maximum absorbance at about 365 nm, with a suitable spectrophotometer, using chloroform as the blank. Calculate the quantity, in µg, of $C_{20}H_{28}O_2$ in the portion of Gel taken by the formula:

$$100C(A_U / A_S)$$

in which C is the concentration, in µg per mL, of USP Tretinoin RS in the Standard solution, and A_U and A_S are the absorbances of the solution from the Gel and the Standard solution, respectively.

Tretinoin Topical Solution

» Tretinoin Topical Solution is a solution of Tretinoin in a suitable nonaqueous, hydrophilic solvent. It contains not less than 90.0 percent and not more than 135.0 percent of the labeled amount of $C_{20}H_{28}O_2$ (w/w).

Packaging and storage—Preserve in tight, light-resistant containers.

USP Reference standards ⟨11⟩—*USP Tretinoin RS.*

Identification—

A: Mix 5 mL of Topical Solution with 5 mL of water: a voluminous yellow precipitate is formed.

B: The absorption spectrum, obtained between wavelengths of 300 nm and 450 nm, of the solution employed for measurement of absorbance in the *Assay* exhibits maxima and minima at the same wavelengths as that of a similar solution of USP Tretinoin RS, concomitantly measured.

Alcohol content ⟨611⟩: between 90.0% and 110.0% of the labeled amount of C_2H_5OH.

Assay—[NOTE—Avoid exposure to strong light, and use low-actinic glassware in the performance of the following procedure.] Transfer to a 100-mL volumetric flask an accurately weighed quantity of Topical Solution, equivalent to about 375 µg of tretinoin, dilute with acidified isopropyl alcohol (prepared by mixing 1 mL of 0.01 N hydrochloric acid with isopropyl alcohol to make 1000 mL of solution) to volume, and mix. Dissolve an accurately weighed quantity of USP Tretinoin RS in the acidified isopropyl alcohol, and dilute quantitatively and stepwise with the same solvent to obtain a Standard solution having a known concentration of about 3.75 µg per mL. Concomitantly determine the absorbances of both solutions in 1-cm cells at the wavelength of maximum absorbance at about 352 nm, with a suitable spectrophotometer, using the acidified isopropyl alcohol as the blank. Calculate the quantity, in µg, of $C_{20}H_{28}O_2$ in the portion of Topical Solution taken by the formula:

$$100C(A_U / A_S)$$

in which C is the concentration, in µg per mL, of USP Tretinoin RS in the Standard solution, and A_U and A_S are the absorbances of the solution from the Topical Solution and the Standard solution, respectively.

Triacetin

$C_9H_{14}O_6$ 218.21
1,2,3-Propanetriol triacetate.
Triacetin.
Glyceryl triacetate   [102-76-1].

» Triacetin contains not less than 97.0 percent and not more than 100.5 percent of $C_9H_{14}O_6$, calculated on the anhydrous basis.

Packaging and storage—Preserve in tight containers.
USP Reference standards ⟨11⟩—*USP Triacetin RS.*
Identification—
  A: *Infrared Absorption* ⟨197F⟩.
  B: The solution prepared as directed in the *Assay* responds to the tests for *Acetate* ⟨191⟩.
Specific gravity ⟨841⟩:   not less than 1.152 and not more than 1.158.
Refractive index ⟨831⟩:   not less than 1.429 and not more than 1.430.
Acidity—Dilute 25 g of Triacetin, accurately weighed, with 50 mL of neutralized alcohol, add 5 drops of phenolphthalein TS, and titrate with 0.020 N sodium hydroxide: not more than 1.0 mL of 0.020 N sodium hydroxide is required for neutralization.
Water, *Method I* ⟨921⟩:   not more than 0.2% is found.
Assay—Transfer about 1 g of Triacetin, accurately weighed, to a 250-mL boiling flask, add 50.0 mL of 0.5 N alcoholic potassium hydroxide VS, connect the flask to a water-jacketed condenser, and reflux on a steam bath for 45 minutes, swirling frequently. Cool, add 5 drops of phenolphthalein TS, and titrate the excess alkali with 0.5 N hydrochloric acid VS. Perform a blank determination (see *Residual Titrations* under *Titrimetry* ⟨541⟩). Each mL of 0.5 N alcoholic potassium hydroxide is equivalent to 36.37 mg of $C_9H_{14}O_6$.

Triamcinolone

$C_{21}H_{27}FO_6$ 394.43
Pregna-1,4-diene-3,20-dione, 9-fluoro-11,16,17,21-tetrahydroxy-, (11β,16α).
9-Fluoro-11β,16α,17,21-tetrahydroxypregna-1,4-diene-3,20-dione   [124-94-7].

» Triamcinolone contains not less than 97.0 percent and not more than 102.0 percent of $C_{21}H_{27}FO_6$, calculated on the dried basis.

Packaging and storage—Preserve in well-closed containers.
USP Reference standards ⟨11⟩—*USP Triamcinolone RS.*
Identification—
  A: *Infrared Absorption* ⟨197K⟩.
  B: *Ultraviolet Absorption* ⟨197U⟩—
    Solution: 20 μg per mL.
    Medium: methanol.
    Absorptivities at 238 nm, calculated on the dried basis, do not differ by more than 3.0%.
Specific rotation ⟨781S⟩:   between +65° and +72°.
  Test solution: 2 mg per mL, in dimethylformamide.
Loss on drying ⟨731⟩—Dry it in vacuum at 60° for 4 hours: it loses not more than 2.0% of its weight.
Residue on ignition ⟨281⟩:   0.5%.
Heavy metals, *Method II* ⟨231⟩:   0.0025%.
Assay—
  Mobile phase—Prepare a degassed solution containing about 60 volumes of methanol and 40 volumes of water such that the retention times for triamcinolone and hydrocortisone are about 5 and 10 minutes, respectively.
  Internal standard solution—Dissolve hydrocortisone in *Mobile phase* to obtain a solution having a concentration of about 0.3 mg per mL.
  Standard preparation—Transfer about 10 mg of USP Triamcinolone RS, accurately weighed, to a 50-mL volumetric flask, dissolve in *Internal standard solution*, dilute with the same solvent to volume, and mix.
  Assay preparation—Using about 10 mg of Triamcinolone, accurately weighed, prepare as directed under *Standard preparation*.
  Chromatographic system (see *Chromatography* ⟨621⟩)—The liquid chromatograph is equipped with a 254-nm detector and a 3.9-mm × 30-cm column that contains packing L1. The flow rate is about 1.5 mL per minute. Chromatograph the *Standard preparation*, and record the peak responses as directed for *Procedure*: the relative standard deviation for replicate injections is not more than 2.0%, and the resolution factor between triamcinolone and hydrocortisone is not less than 3.0.
  Procedure—Separately inject equal volumes (about 10 μL) of the *Standard preparation* and the *Assay preparation* into the chromatograph by means of a suitable microsyringe or sampling valve, record the chromatograms, and measure the responses for the major peaks. Calculate the quantity, in mg, of $C_{21}H_{27}FO_6$ in the portion of Triamcinolone taken by the formula:

$$50C(R_U/R_S)$$

in which C is the concentration, in mg per mL, of USP Triamcinolone RS in the *Standard preparation*, and R_U and R_S are the peak response ratios of triamcinolone to hydrocortisone obtained from the *Assay preparation* and the *Standard preparation*, respectively.

Triamcinolone Tablets

» Triamcinolone Tablets contain not less than 90.0 percent and not more than 110.0 percent of the labeled amount of $C_{21}H_{27}FO_6$.

Packaging and storage—Preserve in well-closed containers.
USP Reference standards ⟨11⟩—*USP Triamcinolone RS.*
Identification—Powder a number of Tablets, equivalent to about 25 mg of triamcinolone, and digest with 25 mL of acetone for 15 minutes. Filter through a fine-porosity, sintered-glass filtering funnel into about 100 mL of solvent hexane, swirl the liquid, and allow to stand for 30 minutes. Collect the crystals that form, wash the crystals with three 10-mL portions of water followed by 2 mL of acetone, and dry at 60° for 1 hour: the dried crystals so obtained respond to *Identification* test A under *Triamcinolone.*
Dissolution ⟨711⟩—
  Medium: 0.01 N hydrochloric acid; 900 mL.
  Apparatus 1:   100 rpm.
  Time: 45 minutes.
  Procedure—Determine the amount of $C_{21}H_{27}FO_6$ dissolved by employing UV absorption at the wavelength of maximum absorbance at about 238 nm on filtered portions of the solution under test, suitably diluted with *Dissolution Medium*, in comparison with a Standard solution having a known concentration of USP Triamcinolone RS in the same *Medium.*
  Tolerances—Not less than 75% (*Q*) of the labeled amount of $C_{21}H_{27}FO_6$ is dissolved in 45 minutes.

Uniformity of dosage units ⟨905⟩: meet the requirements.
Assay—
   Mobile phase, Internal standard solution, Standard preparation, and *Chromatographic system*—Prepare as directed in the *Assay* under *Triamcinolone.*
   Assay preparation—Weigh and finely powder not less than 20 Tablets. Transfer an accurately weighed portion of the powder, equivalent to about 10 mg of triamcinolone, to a suitable container. Add 50.0 mL of *Internal standard solution,* and shake vigorously by mechanical means for 10 minutes. Centrifuge for 10 minutes or until a clear supernatant is obtained.
   Procedure—Proceed as directed for *Procedure* in the *Assay* under *Triamcinolone.* The relative retention times are about 1.0 for triamcinolone and 1.9 for hydrocortisone. Calculate the quantity, in mg, of $C_{21}H_{27}FO_6$ in the portion of Tablets taken by the formula:

$$50C(R_U/R_S)$$

in which the terms are as defined therein.

Triamcinolone Acetonide

$C_{24}H_{31}FO_6$ 434.51
Pregna-1,4-diene-3,20-dione, 9-fluoro-11,21-dihydroxy-16,17-[(1-methylethylidene)bis(oxy)]-, (11β,16α)-.
9-Fluoro-11β,16α,17,21-tetrahydroxypregna-1,4-diene-3,20-dione cyclic 16,17-acetal with acetone   [76-25-5].

» Triamcinolone Acetonide contains not less than 97.0 percent and not more than 102.0 percent of $C_{24}H_{31}FO_6$, calculated on the dried basis.

Packaging and storage—Preserve in well-closed containers. Store at 25°, excursions permitted between 15° and 30°.
USP Reference standards ⟨11⟩—*USP Fluoxymesterone RS. USP Triamcinolone Acetonide RS.*
Identification—
   A: *Infrared Absorption* ⟨197K⟩: recrystallized from methanol.
   B: *Ultraviolet Absorption* ⟨197U⟩—
      Solution: 20 μg per mL.
      Medium: methanol.
Specific rotation ⟨781S⟩: between +118° and +130°.
   Test solution: 5 mg per mL, in dimethylformamide.
Loss on drying ⟨731⟩—Dry it in vacuum at 60° for 4 hours: it loses not more than 1.5% of its weight.
Heavy metals—Carefully ignite 1.0 g in a muffle furnace at about 550° until thoroughly charred. Cool, add to the contents of the crucible 5 drops of sulfuric acid and 2 mL of nitric acid, cautiously heat until reaction has ceased, then ignite in a muffle furnace at 500° to 600° until the carbon is entirely burned off. Cool, add 2 mL of hydrochloric acid, and slowly evaporate on a steam bath to dryness. Moisten the residue with 1 drop of hydrochloric acid and 5 mL of hot water, and digest for 2 minutes. Add 1 drop of phenolphthalein TS, then add 6 N ammonium hydroxide dropwise until the reaction is alkaline. Render the solution acid with 1 N acetic acid, then add 1 mL of excess, transfer to a beaker, and add water to make 10 mL. Pipet 2.5 mL (equivalent to 25 μg of lead) of *Standard Lead Solution* (see *Lead* ⟨231⟩) into a second beaker, add 3 mL of water and 1 drop of phenolphthalein TS, render just alkaline with 6 N ammonium hydroxide, then render acid with 1 N acetic acid, and add 1 mL in excess. Dilute with water to 10 mL. To each beaker add 5 mL of freshly prepared hydrogen sulfide TS, mix, and allow to stand for 5 minutes. Pass each solution through a separate, acid-resistant, white, plain membrane filter of 0.22-μm pore size and 25 mm in diameter, collecting the precipitates on the filter disks: the color of the precipitate from the solution under test is not darker than that from the control. The heavy metals limit is 0.0025%.
Chromatographic purity—
   Mobile phase—Prepare a filtered and degassed mixture of water and acetonitrile (17 : 8). Make adjustments if necessary (see *System Suitability* under *Chromatography* ⟨621⟩).
   Test solution—Transfer about 25 mg of Triamcinolone Acetonide, accurately weighed, to a 50-mL volumetric flask; dissolve in 25 mL of methanol, shake vigorously to aid dissolution; dilute with *Mobile phase* to volume; and mix.
   Chromatographic system (see *Chromatography* ⟨621⟩)—The liquid chromatograph is equipped with a 254-nm detector and a 3.9-mm × 30-cm column that contains packing L1. The flow rate is about 1.5 mL per minute. Chromatograph the *Test solution,* and record the peak responses as directed for *Procedure:* the resolution, *R*, between triamcinolone acetonide and any impurity peak is not less than 1.0.
   Procedure—Inject about 20 μL of the *Test solution* into the chromatograph, record the chromatogram for not less than four times the retention time of triamcinolone acetonide, and measure all of the peak responses. Calculate the percentage of each impurity in the portion of Triamcinolone Acetonide taken by the formula:

$$100(r_i/r_s)$$

in which r_i is the peak response for each impurity; and r_s is the sum of the responses of all the peaks: not more than 0.3% of any individual impurity is found, and not more than 0.8% of total impurities is found.
Assay—
   Mobile phase—Prepare a solution of acetonitrile in water containing approximately 30% (v/v) of acetonitrile.
   Internal standard solution—Dissolve USP Fluoxymesterone RS in methanol to obtain a solution having a concentration of about 50 μg per mL.
   Standard preparation—Dissolve an accurately weighed quantity of USP Triamcinolone Acetonide RS in *Internal standard solution* to obtain a solution having a known concentration of about 75 μg per mL. Mix an accurately measured volume of the resulting solution with an equal volume of *Mobile phase* to obtain a *Standard preparation* containing about 37.5 μg of USP Triamcinolone Acetonide RS per mL.
   Assay preparation—Using about 37 mg of Triamcinolone Acetonide, accurately weighed, proceed as directed for *Standard preparation.*
   Procedure—Introduce equal volumes (between 15 μL and 25 μL) of the *Assay preparation* and the *Standard preparation* into a high-pressure liquid chromatograph (see *Chromatography* ⟨621⟩) operated at room temperature, by means of a suitable microsyringe or sampling valve. Adjust the operating parameters with *Mobile phase* on the column so that the separation of triamcinolone acetonide and internal standard is optimized, with a retention time of about 14.5 minutes for triamcinolone acetonide. Typically, the apparatus is fitted with a 4-mm × 30-cm column containing packing L1 and is equipped with a UV detector capable of monitoring absorbance at 254 nm, and a suitable recorder. In a suitable chromatogram, the coefficient of variation for five replicate injections of a single specimen is not more than 3.0%; and the resolution factor, *R* (see *Chromatography* ⟨621⟩), between the peaks for triamcinolone acetonide and fluoxymesterone is not less than 2.0. Measure the heights of the internal standard and triamcinolone acetonide peaks at the same retention times obtained from the *Assay preparation* and the *Standard preparation.* Calculate the quantity, in mg, of $C_{24}H_{31}FO_6$ in the portion of Triamcinolone Acetonide taken by the formula:

$$1000C(R_U/R_S)$$

in which *C* is the concentration, in mg per mL, of USP Triamcinolone Acetonide RS in the *Standard preparation;* and R_U and R_S are the ratios of the peak heights of triamcinolone acetonide to the internal standard obtained from the *Assay preparation* and the *Standard preparation,* respectively.

Triamcinolone Acetonide Topical Aerosol

» Triamcinolone Acetonide Topical Aerosol is a solution of Triamcinolone Acetonide in a suitable propellant in a pressurized container. It contains not less than 90.0 percent and not more than 115.0 percent of the labeled amount of $C_{24}H_{31}FO_6$.

Packaging and storage—Preserve in pressurized containers, and avoid exposure to excessive heat.

USP Reference standards ⟨11⟩—*USP Triamcinolone Acetonide RS.*

Identification—Apply 20 μL of a solution prepared as directed for *Assay preparation* in the *Assay* but without the addition of the *Internal standard solution*, and 20 μL of a solution of USP Triamcinolone Acetonide RS in methanol containing 30 μg per mL, to a line parallel to and about 1.5 cm from the bottom edge of a thin-layer chromatographic plate (see *Chromatography* ⟨621⟩) coated with a 0.25-mm layer of chromatographic silica gel. Proceed as directed in the *Identification* test under *Triamcinolone Acetonide Cream*, beginning with "Place the plate in a developing chamber." The specified result is obtained.

Microbial limits ⟨61⟩—It meets the requirements of the tests for absence of *Staphylococcus aureus* and *Pseudomonas aeruginosa*.

Other requirements—It meets the requirements for *Pressure Test, Minimum Fill,* and *Leakage Test* under *Aerosols, Nasal Sprays, Metered-Dose Inhalers, and Dry Powder Inhalers* ⟨601⟩.

Assay—

Mobile phase—Prepare a degassed solution of water and acetonitrile (70 : 30).

Internal standard solution—Dissolve fluoxymesterone in methanol to obtain a solution having a concentration of about 25 μg per mL.

Standard preparation—Dissolve an accurately weighed quantity of USP Triamcinolone Acetonide RS in methanol to obtain a solution having a concentration of about 100 μg per mL. Transfer 15.0 mL of this solution to a 50-mL volumetric flask, add 25.0 mL of *Internal standard solution*, dilute with methanol to volume, and mix. This solution has a known concentration of about 30 μg per mL.

Assay preparation—Fit the valve of a previously weighed Triamcinolone Acetonide Aerosol container with a suitable tube assembly so that the contents can be sprayed directly into the bulb portion of a 100-mL volumetric flask containing 50.0 mL of *Internal standard solution* and 20 mL of methanol. Spray a portion of the contents, equivalent to about 3 mg of triamcinolone acetonide, into the flask, determining the exact amount sprayed by difference. Place in a sonic bath for about 5 minutes to expel the propellant. Dilute with methanol to volume, and mix. [NOTE—The propellant is extremely flammable. When evaporating, observe proper precautions and work under an explosion-proof hood.]

Procedure—Introduce equal volumes (between 15 μL and 25 μL) of the *Assay preparation* and the *Standard preparation* into a chromatograph (see *Chromatography* ⟨621⟩) operated at room temperature and fitted with a 3.9-mm × 30-cm column, packed with packing L1, and equipped with a 254-nm detector. Adjust the operating parameters and the *Mobile phase* composition such that the separation of triamcinolone acetonide and internal standard is optimized, with a retention time of about 14 minutes for triamcinolone acetonide. In a suitable system, the relative standard deviation for five replicate injections of the *Standard preparation* is not more than 3.0%. Measure the responses of the internal standard and triamcinolone acetonide peaks at the same retention times obtained from the *Assay preparation* and the *Standard preparation*. Calculate the quantity, in μg, of $C_{24}H_{31}FO_6$ in the portion of Topical Aerosol taken by the formula:

$$100C(R_U / R_S)$$

in which C is the concentration, in μg per mL, of USP Triamcinolone Acetonide RS in the *Standard preparation*, and R_U and R_S are the ratios of the peak responses of triamcinolone acetonide to internal standard obtained from the *Assay preparation* and the *Standard preparation*, respectively.

Triamcinolone Acetonide Cream

» Triamcinolone Acetonide Cream is Triamcinolone Acetonide in a suitable cream base. It contains not less than 90.0 percent and not more than 115.0 percent of the labeled amount of $C_{24}H_{31}FO_6$.

Packaging and storage—Preserve in tight containers.

USP Reference standards ⟨11⟩—*USP Triamcinolone Acetonide RS.*

Identification—Place a 2-g quantity of Cream in a conical flask, add 50 mL of chloroform and 15 g of anhydrous sodium sulfate, and swirl to dissolve the specimen. Filter the solution and clarify the filtrate, if necessary, by the further addition of anhydrous sodium sulfate and a second filtration. Evaporate the filtrate to near dryness, and dissolve the residue in chloroform to obtain a solution containing about 100 μg per mL. Apply 10 μL of this solution and 10 μL of a solution of USP Triamcinolone Acetonide RS in chloroform containing 100 μg per mL, on a line parallel to and about 1.5 cm from the bottom edge of a thin-layer chromatographic plate (see *Chromatography* ⟨621⟩) coated with a 0.25-mm layer of chromatographic silica gel. Place the plate in a developing chamber containing and equilibrated with a mixture of chloroform, benzene, and methanol (100 : 40 : 20). Develop the chromatogram until the solvent front has moved about 12 cm above the line of application. Remove the plate, allow the solvent to evaporate, and spray with a mixture of equal volumes of sodium hydroxide solution (1 in 5) and a 1 in 500 solution of blue tetrazolium in methanol: the intensity of the blue color and the R_F of the spot obtained with the solution under test are similar to those of the spot obtained with the Standard solution.

Microbial limits ⟨61⟩—It meets the requirements of the tests for absence of *Staphylococcus aureus* and *Pseudomonas aeruginosa*.

Minimum fill ⟨755⟩: meets the requirements.

Assay—

Mobile phase—Prepare a solution of acetonitrile in water containing approximately 30% (v/v) of acetonitrile.

Internal standard solution—Dissolve fluoxymesterone in isopropyl alcohol to obtain a solution having a concentration of about 50 μg per mL.

Standard preparation—Dissolve an accurately weighed quantity of USP Triamcinolone Acetonide RS in *Internal standard solution* to obtain a solution having a known concentration of about 75 μg per mL. Mix an accurately measured volume of the resulting solution with an equal volume of *Mobile phase* to obtain a *Standard preparation* containing about 37.5 μg of USP Triamcinolone Acetonide RS per mL.

Assay preparation—Transfer an accurately weighed quantity of Cream, equivalent to about 1.5 mg of triamcinolone acetonide, to a screw-cap tube. Add 20.0 mL of *Internal standard solution*, and cap securely. Heat for 5 minutes at 60°, then swirl vigorously for not less than 30 seconds. Repeat the heating and swirling sequence three times. Cool in a methanol-ice bath for 15 to 20 minutes, then centrifuge for 15 minutes at −5°. Dilute an accurately measured volume of the supernatant with an equal volume of *Mobile phase*. Cool in a methanol-ice bath for 10 to 15 minutes, with occasional agitation. Filter first through a pledget of glass wool or a prefilter disk and then through a 0.45-μm porosity membrane to obtain a clear solution.

Procedure—Introduce equal volumes (between 15 and 25 μL) of the *Assay preparation* and the *Standard preparation* into a high-pressure liquid chromatograph (see *Chromatography* ⟨621⟩), operated at room temperature, by means of a suitable microsyringe or sampling valve. Adjust the operating parameters with *Mobile phase* on the column, such that the separation of triamcinolone acetonide and internal standard is optimized, with a retention time of about 14.5 minutes for triamcinolone acetonide. Typically, the apparatus is fitted with a 30-cm × 4-mm column containing packing L1, and is equipped with a UV detector capable of monitoring absorbance at 254 nm, and a suitable recorder. In a suitable chromatograph, the coefficient of variation for five replicate injections of a single specimen is not more than 3.0%, and the resolution factor, R (see *Chromatography* ⟨621⟩), between the peaks for triamcinolone acetonide and fluoxymesterone is not less than 2.0. Measure the heights of the internal standard and triamcinolone acetonide peaks, at the same retention times obtained from the *Assay preparation* and the *Standard preparation*. Calculate the quantity, in mg, of $C_{24}H_{31}FO_6$ in the portion of Cream taken by the formula:

$$40C(R_U / R_S)$$

in which C is the concentration, in mg per mL, of USP Triamcinolone Acetonide RS in the *Standard preparation*, and R_U and R_S are the ratios of the peak heights of triamcinolone acetonide to the internal standard obtained from the *Assay preparation* and the *Standard preparation*, respectively.

Triamcinolone Acetonide Lotion

» Triamcinolone Acetonide Lotion is Triamcinolone Acetonide in a suitable lotion base. It contains not less than 90.0 percent and not more than 110.0 percent of the labeled amount of $C_{24}H_{31}FO_6$.

Packaging and storage—Preserve in tight containers.
USP Reference standards ⟨11⟩—*USP Triamcinolone Acetonide RS*.
Identification—It responds to the *Identification* test under *Triamcinolone Acetonide Cream*.
Microbial limits ⟨61⟩—It meets the requirements of the tests for absence of *Staphylococcus aureus* and *Pseudomonas aeruginosa*.
Minimum fill ⟨755⟩: meets the requirements.
Assay—Proceed with Lotion as directed in the *Assay* under *Triamcinolone Acetonide Cream*, except to read "Lotion" in place of "Cream" throughout.

Triamcinolone Acetonide Ointment

» Triamcinolone Acetonide Ointment is Triamcinolone Acetonide in a suitable ointment base. It contains not less than 90.0 percent and not more than 115.0 percent of the labeled amount of $C_{24}H_{31}FO_6$.

Packaging and storage—Preserve in well-closed containers.
USP Reference standards ⟨11⟩—*USP Triamcinolone Acetonide RS*.
Identification—Place 2 g of Ointment in a conical flask, add 5.0 mL of chloroform, and shake for 10 minutes. Add 15 mL of alcohol, and shake for an additional 10 minutes. Filter the solution into a centrifuge tube, and evaporate the filtrate to dryness. Dissolve the residue in alcohol to obtain a solution containing about 250 µg per mL. Apply 10 µL of this solution, and 10 µL of a solution of USP Triamcinolone Acetonide RS in alcohol containing 250 µg per mL, on a line parallel to and about 1.5 cm from the bottom edge of a thin-layer chromatographic plate (see *Chromatography* ⟨621⟩) coated with a 0.25-mm layer of chromatographic silica gel. Place the plate in a developing chamber containing and equilibrated with a mixture of chloroform, benzene, and methanol (100 : 40 : 20). Develop the chromatogram until the solvent front has moved about 12 cm above the line of application. Remove the plate, allow the solvent to evaporate, and spray with a mixture of equal volumes of sodium hydroxide solution (1 in 5) and a 1 in 500 solution of blue tetrazolium in methanol: the intensity of the blue color and the R_F of the spot obtained from the solution under test are similar to those of the spot obtained from the Standard solution.
Microbial limits ⟨61⟩—It meets the requirements of the tests for absence of *Staphylococcus aureus* and *Pseudomonas aeruginosa*.
Minimum fill ⟨755⟩: meets the requirements.
Assay—Proceed with Ointment as directed in the *Assay* under *Triamcinolone Acetonide Cream*, except to read "Ointment" in place of "Cream" throughout.

Triamcinolone Acetonide Dental Paste

» Triamcinolone Acetonide Dental Paste is Triamcinolone Acetonide in a suitable emollient paste. It contains not less than 90.0 percent and not more than 115.0 percent of the labeled amount of $C_{24}H_{31}FO_6$.

Packaging and storage—Preserve in tight containers.
USP Reference standards ⟨11⟩—*USP Triamcinolone Acetonide RS*.
Identification—It responds to the *Identification* test under *Triamcinolone Acetonide Cream*.
Microbial limits ⟨61⟩—It meets the requirements of the tests for absence of *Staphylococcus aureus* and *Pseudomonas aeruginosa*.
Minimum fill ⟨755⟩: meets the requirements.
Assay—
  Mobile phase—Prepare as directed in the *Assay* under *Triamcinolone Acetonide Cream*.
  Internal standard solution and *Standard preparation*—Prepare as directed in the *Assay* under *Triamcinolone Acetonide Cream*.
  Assay preparation—Transfer an accurately weighed quantity of Dental Paste, equivalent to about 1.5 mg of triamcinolone acetonide, to a screw-cap tube. Add 20.0 mL of *Internal standard solution*, cap, and place in a sonic bath for 15 to 20 minutes. Place in a water bath at 70° for 5 minutes, then swirl for 1 minute. Repeat the heating and swirling sequence once. Cool in an ice–methanol bath for 15 minutes, then centrifuge for 10 minutes at −5°. Mix an accurately measured volume of the supernatant with an equal volume of *Mobile phase*. Place in an ice–methanol bath for 15 minutes, then centrifuge for 15 minutes. Draw off and discard the upper phase. Filter the lower phase to obtain a clear solution.
  Procedure—Proceed as directed for *Procedure* in the *Assay* under *Triamcinolone Acetonide Cream*.

Triamcinolone Acetonide Injectable Suspension

» Triamcinolone Acetonide Injectable Suspension is a sterile suspension of Triamcinolone Acetonide in a suitable aqueous medium. It contains not less than 90.0 percent and not more than 115.0 percent of the labeled amount of $C_{24}H_{31}FO_6$.

Packaging and storage—Preserve in single-dose or in multiple-dose containers, preferably of Type I glass, protected from light.
USP Reference standards ⟨11⟩—*USP Triamcinolone Acetonide RS. USP Endotoxin RS*.
Identification—Extract a volume of Injectable Suspension, equivalent to about 50 mg of triamcinolone acetonide, with two 10-mL portions of peroxide-free ether, and discard the ether extracts. Filter with the aid of suction, wash with small portions of water, and dry the precipitate at 105° for 1 hour: the triamcinolone acetonide so obtained responds to the *Identification* tests under *Triamcinolone Acetonide*.
Bacterial endotoxins ⟨85⟩—It contains not more than 4.4 USP Endotoxin Units per mg of triamcinolone acetonide.

pH ⟨791⟩: between 5.0 and 7.5.
Other requirements—It meets the requirements under *Injections* ⟨1⟩.
Assay—
  Mobile phase: approximately 30% acetonitrile in water.
  Internal standard solution—Dissolve fluoxymesterone in methanol to obtain a solution having a concentration of about 84 µg per mL.
  Standard preparation—Dissolve an accurately weighed quantity of USP Triamcinolone Acetonide RS in methanol to obtain a solution having a known concentration of about 200 µg per mL. Pipet 20 mL of this solution into a 50-mL volumetric flask, dilute with *Internal standard solution* to volume, and mix. The *Standard preparation* has a known concentration of about 80 µg of USP Triamcinolone Acetonide RS per mL.
  Assay preparation—Dissolve an accurately measured volume of freshly mixed Injectable Suspension in methanol, and dilute quantitatively with methanol to obtain a solution having an expected concentration of about 200 µg of triamcinolone acetonide per mL. Pipet 20 mL of this solution into a 50-mL volumetric flask, dilute with *Internal standard solution* to volume, and mix.
  Procedure—Proceed as directed for *Procedure* in the *Assay* under *Triamcinolone Acetonide Cream*, except to use peak responses in the calculation. Calculate the quantity, in mg, of $C_{24}H_{31}FO_6$ in each mL of the Injectable Suspension taken by the formula:

$$(CD/V)(R_U/R_S)$$

in which C is the concentration, in mg per mL, of USP Triamcinolone Acetonide RS in the *Standard preparation*, D is the dilution factor used in the *Assay preparation*, V is the volume, in mL, of Injectable Suspension taken, and R_U and R_S are the ratios of the peak responses of triamcinolone acetonide to the internal standard, obtained from the *Assay preparation* and the *Standard preparation*, respectively.

Triamcinolone Diacetate

$C_{25}H_{31}FO_8$ 478.51
Pregna-1,4-diene-3,20-dione, 16,21-bis(acetyloxy)-9-fluoro-11,17-dihydroxy-, (11β,16α)-.
9-Fluoro-11β,16α,17,21-tetrahydroxypregna-1,4-diene-3,20-dione 16,21-diacetate [67-78-7].

» Triamcinolone Diacetate contains not less than 97.0 percent and not more than 103.0 percent of $C_{25}H_{31}FO_8$, calculated on the anhydrous basis.

Packaging and storage—Preserve in well-closed containers.
USP Reference standards ⟨11⟩—*USP Triamcinolone Diacetate RS*.
Identification—
  A: *Infrared Absorption* ⟨197K⟩.
  B: *Ultraviolet Absorption* ⟨197U⟩—
    Solution: 20 µg per mL.
    Medium: dehydrated alcohol.
  Absorptivities at 238 nm, calculated on the anhydrous basis, do not differ by more than 3.0%.
Specific rotation ⟨781S⟩: between +39° and +45°.
  Test solution: 5 mg per mL, in dimethylformamide.
Water, *Method I* ⟨921⟩: not more than 6.0%.
Residue on ignition ⟨281⟩: not more than 0.5%.
Heavy metals, *Method II* ⟨231⟩: 0.0025%.
Assay—
  0.005 M Monobasic sodium phosphate solution—Dissolve monobasic sodium phosphate in water to obtain a solution containing 690 µg per mL.
  Mobile phase—Prepare a mixture of *0.005 M Monobasic sodium phosphate solution*, acetonitrile, and tetrahydrofuran (62 : 37 : 1), filter through a 0.45-µm solvent-resistant filter, and degas. Make adjustments if necessary (see *System Suitability* under *Chromatography* ⟨621⟩).
  Standard preparation—Dissolve an accurately weighed quantity of USP Triamcinolone Diacetate RS in *Mobile phase*, and dilute quantitatively with *Mobile phase* to obtain a solution having a known concentration of about 40 µg per mL.
  Assay preparation—Transfer about 50 mg of Triamcinolone Diacetate, accurately weighed, to a 50-mL volumetric flask, dissolve in *Mobile phase*, dilute with *Mobile phase* to volume, and mix. Pipet 2 mL of this solution into a second 50-mL volumetric flask, dilute with *Mobile phase* to volume, and mix.
  System suitability preparation—Dissolve suitable quantities of USP Triamcinolone Diacetate RS and propylparaben in *Mobile phase* to obtain a solution containing about 40 µg per mL and 15 µg per mL, respectively.
  Chromatographic system (see *Chromatography* ⟨621⟩)—The liquid chromatograph is equipped with a 254-nm detector and a 3.9-mm × 30-cm column that contains packing L1. The flow rate is about 1 mL per minute. Chromatograph the *System suitability preparation*, and record the peak responses as directed for *Procedure:* the relative retention times are 1.0 for triamcinolone diacetate and about 1.1 for propylparaben, the resolution, R, between the triamcinolone diacetate and propylparaben peaks is not less than 1.7, and the tailing factor, T, for the analyte peak is not more than 1.5. Chromatograph replicate injections of the *Standard preparation*, and record the peak responses as directed for *Procedure:* the relative standard deviation is not more than 2.0%.
  Procedure—Separately inject equal volumes (about 10 µL) of the *Standard preparation* and the *Assay preparation* into the chromatograph, and measure the area responses for the major peaks. Calculate the quantity, in mg, of $C_{25}H_{31}FO_8$ in the portion of Triamcinolone Diacetate taken by the formula:

$$1.25C(r_U/r_S)$$

in which C is the concentration, in µg per mL, of USP Triamcinolone Diacetate RS in the *Standard preparation*, and r_U and r_S are the peak area responses obtained from the *Assay preparation* and the *Standard preparation*, respectively.

Triamcinolone Diacetate Oral Solution

» Triamcinolone Diacetate Oral Solution contains not less than 90.0 percent and not more than 110.0 percent of the labeled amount of triamcinolone diacetate ($C_{25}H_{31}FO_8$). It contains a suitable preservative.

Packaging and storage—Preserve in tight, light-resistant containers.
USP Reference standards ⟨11⟩—*USP Triamcinolone Diacetate RS*.
Identification—Transfer a quantity of Oral Solution, equivalent to about 10 mg of triamcinolone diacetate, to a separator, and extract with three 10-mL portions of chloroform. Evaporate the combined chloroform extracts on a steam bath to dryness, and dissolve the residue in 5.0 mL of chloroform. Apply 10 µL each of this solution and a solution of USP Triamcinolone Diacetate RS in chloroform containing 2 mg per mL to a suitable thin-layer chromatographic plate (see *Chromatography* ⟨621⟩) coated with a 0.25-mm layer of chromatographic silica gel. Allow the spots to dry, and develop the chromatogram in a solvent system consisting of a mixture of ethyl acetate and chloroform (9 : 1) until the solvent front has moved about three-fourths of the length of the plate. Remove the plate from the developing chamber, mark the solvent front, and allow the solvent to evaporate. Locate the spots on the plate by lightly spraying with dilute sulfuric acid (1 in 2) and heating on a hot plate or under a lamp until spots appear: the R_F value of the principal spot obtained from the test solution corresponds to that obtained from the Standard solution.
Assay—
  0.005 M Monobasic sodium phosphate solution, *Mobile phase*, *Standard preparation*, *System suitability preparation*, and *Chromatographic system*—Proceed as directed in the *Assay* under *Triamcinolone Diacetate*.

Assay preparation—Quantitatively transfer an accurately measured portion of Oral Solution, equivalent to about 50 mg of triamcinolone diacetate to a 100-mL volumetric flask. Dilute with *Mobile phase* to volume, and mix. Pipet 4 mL of this solution into a 50-mL volumetric flask, dilute with *Mobile phase* to volume, and mix. Transfer about 25 mL of this solution to a 50-mL, glass-stoppered centrifuge tube, and centrifuge at high speed for 10 minutes.

Procedure—Proceed as directed for *Procedure* in the *Assay* under *Triamcinolone Diacetate*. Calculate the quantity, in mg, of triamcinolone diacetate ($C_{25}H_{31}FO_8$) in the portion of Oral Solution taken by the formula:

$$1.25C(r_U/r_S)$$

in which C is the concentration, in µg per mL, of USP Triamcinolone Diacetate RS in the *Standard preparation*; and r_U and r_S are the peak responses obtained from the *Assay preparation* and the *Standard preparation*, respectively.

Triamcinolone Diacetate Injectable Suspension

» Triamcinolone Diacetate Injectable Suspension is a sterile suspension of Triamcinolone Diacetate in a suitable aqueous medium. It contains not less than 90.0 percent and not more than 115.0 percent of the labeled amount of $C_{25}H_{31}FO_8$.

Packaging and storage—Preserve in single-dose or in multiple-dose containers, preferably of Type I glass.

USP Reference standards ⟨11⟩—*USP Triamcinolone Diacetate RS. USP Endotoxin RS.*

Identification—Filter a volume of Injectable Suspension, equivalent to about 50 mg of triamcinolone diacetate, through a medium-porosity, sintered-glass funnel, wash with water, and dry the crystals in vacuum at 60° for 1 hour. Dissolve 2 mg of the dried crystals in 1 mL of methanol in a small mortar. Evaporate with the aid of gentle heat and a stream of nitrogen to dryness: the crystals so obtained respond to *Identification* test *A* under *Triamcinolone Diacetate*.

Bacterial endotoxins ⟨85⟩—It contains not more than 7.1 USP Endotoxin Units per mg of triamcinolone diacetate.

Uniformity of dosage units ⟨905⟩: meets the requirements.

pH ⟨791⟩: between 4.5 and 7.5.

Other requirements—It meets the requirements under *Injections* ⟨1⟩.

Assay—

0.005 M Monobasic sodium phosphate solution, Mobile phase, Standard preparation, System suitability preparation, and *Chromatographic system*—Proceed as directed in the *Assay* under *Triamcinolone Diacetate*.

Assay preparation—Quantitatively transfer an accurately measured portion of Injectable Suspension, equivalent to about 50 mg of triamcinolone diacetate, to a 100-mL volumetric flask. Dilute with *Mobile phase* to volume, and mix. Pipet 2 mL of this solution into a 25-mL volumetric flask, dilute with *Mobile phase* to volume, and mix.

Procedure—Proceed as directed for *Procedure* in the *Assay* under *Triamcinolone Diacetate*. Calculate the quantity, in mg, of $C_{25}H_{31}FO_8$ in the portion of Injectable Suspension taken by the formula:

$$1.25C(r_U/r_S)$$

in which C is the concentration, in µg per mL, of USP Triamcinolone Diacetate RS in the *Standard preparation*, and r_U and r_S are the peak responses obtained from the *Assay preparation* and the *Standard preparation*, respectively.

Triamcinolone Hexacetonide

$C_{30}H_{41}FO_7$ 532.64

Pregna-1,4-diene-3,20-dione, 21-(3,3-dimethyl-1-oxobutoxy)-9-fluoro-11-hydroxy-16,17-[(1-methylethylidene)bis(oxy)]-, (11β,16α)-.

9-Fluoro-11β,16α,17,21-tetrahydroxypregna-1,4-diene-3,20-dione cyclic 16,17-acetal with acetone 21-(3,3-dimethylbutyrate) [5611-51-8].

» Triamcinolone Hexacetonide contains not less than 97.0 percent and not more than 102.0 percent of $C_{30}H_{41}FO_7$, calculated on the dried basis.

Packaging and storage—Preserve in well-closed containers.

USP Reference standards ⟨11⟩—*USP Triamcinolone Hexacetonide RS.*

Identification, *Infrared Absorption* ⟨197K⟩.

Specific rotation ⟨781S⟩: between +85° and +95°.

Test solution: 10 mg per mL, in chloroform.

Loss on drying ⟨731⟩—Dry it in vacuum at 60° for 4 hours: it loses not more than 2.0% of its weight.

Heavy metals, *Method II* ⟨231⟩: 0.002%.

Limit of triamcinolone acetonide—

Mobile phase and *Chromatographic system*—Proceed as directed in the *Assay*.

Standard solution—Dissolve an accurately weighed quantity of triamcinolone acetonide in methanol, and dilute quantitatively, and stepwise if necessary, with methanol to obtain a solution having a known concentration of about 0.004 mg per mL.

Test solution—Use the *Assay preparation*.

Procedure—Separately inject equal volumes (about 10 µL) of the *Standard solution* and the *Test solution* into the chromatograph, record the chromatograms, and measure the responses for all of the peaks. Calculate the percentage of triamcinolone acetonide in the portion of Triamcinolone Hexacetonide taken by the formula:

$$100(C/D)(r_U/r_S)$$

in which C is the concentration, in mg per mL, of triamcinolone acetonide in the *Standard solution*, D is the concentration, in mg per mL, of triamcinolone hexacetonide in the *Test solution*, and r_U and r_S are the peak responses for triamcinolone acetonide obtained from the *Test solution* and the *Standard solution*, respectively: not more than 1.0% is found.

Assay—

Mobile phase—Prepare a filtered and degassed mixture of methanol and water (75 : 25). Make adjustments if necessary (see *System Suitability* under *Chromatography* ⟨621⟩).

Standard preparation—Dissolve an accurately weighed quantity of USP Triamcinolone Hexacetonide RS in methanol, and dilute quantitatively, and stepwise if necessary, with methanol to obtain a solution having a known concentration of about 0.4 mg per mL.

System suitability solution—Dissolve suitable quantities of triamcinolone acetonide and USP Triamcinolone Hexacetonide RS in methanol to obtain a solution containing about 0.4 mg per mL of each.

Assay preparation—Transfer about 40 mg of Triamcinolone Hexacetonide, accurately weighed, to a 100-mL volumetric flask. Dissolve in and dilute with methanol to volume, and mix.

Chromatographic system (see *Chromatography* ⟨621⟩)—The liquid chromatograph is equipped with a 254-nm detector and a 4.6-mm × 25-cm column that contains packing L1. The flow rate is about 2 mL per minute. Chromatograph the *System suitability solution*, and record the peak responses as directed for *Procedure*: the relative retention times are about 0.27 for triamcinolone acetonide and 1.0 for triamcinolone hexacetonide, the resolution, *R*, between triamcinolone acetonide and triamcinolone hexacetonide is not less than 7.5, the tailing factor for triamcinolone hexacetonide is not more than 1.3, and the relative standard deviation for replicate injections is not more than 2.0%.

Procedure—Separately inject equal volumes (about 10 µL) of the *Standard preparation* and the *Assay preparation* into the chromatograph, record the chromatograms, and measure the responses for the major peaks. Calculate the quantity, in mg, of $C_{30}H_{41}FO_7$ in the portion of Triamcinolone Hexacetonide taken by the formula:

$$100C(r_U / r_S)$$

in which *C* is the concentration, in mg per mL, of USP Triamcinolone Hexacetonide RS in the *Standard preparation*, and r_U and r_S are the peak responses obtained from the *Assay preparation* and the *Standard preparation*, respectively.

Triamcinolone Hexacetonide Injectable Suspension

» Triamcinolone Hexacetonide Injectable Suspension is a sterile suspension of Triamcinolone Hexacetonide in a suitable aqueous medium. It contains not less than 90.0 percent and not more than 115.0 percent of the labeled amount of $C_{30}H_{41}FO_7$.

Packaging and storage—Preserve in single-dose or in multiple-dose containers, preferably of Type I glass.
USP Reference standards ⟨11⟩—*USP Triamcinolone Hexacetonide RS. USP Endotoxin RS.*
Identification—Place a volume of Injectable Suspension, equivalent to about 25 mg of triamcinolone hexacetonide, and 2 mL of water in a membrane filter having a pore size of 0.20 µm. Apply vacuum to the filter, wash the residue with two 5-mL portions of water, and air-dry the filter and the precipitate. Place the dried filter and precipitate in a small beaker with 5 mL of alcohol, and dissolve the precipitate. Decant the alcohol solution into a small beaker, and evaporate, with the aid of low heat and a current of air, to dryness: the triamcinolone hexacetonide so obtained responds to the *Identification* test under *Triamcinolone Hexacetonide*.
Bacterial endotoxins ⟨85⟩—It contains not more than 17.2 USP Endotoxin Units per mg of triamcinolone hexacetonide.
pH ⟨791⟩: between 4.0 and 8.0.
Limit of triamcinolone acetonide—
Mobile phase, System suitability solution, and *Chromatographic system*—Proceed as directed in the *Assay*.
Standard solution and *Test solution*—Use the *Standard preparation* and the *Assay preparation*, respectively, and proceed as directed in the *Assay*.
Procedure—Separately inject equal volumes (about 10 µL) of the *Standard solution* and the *Test solution* into the chromatograph, record the chromatograms, and measure the responses for all of the peaks. The *Test solution* may exhibit a minor peak for triamcinolone acetonide whose retention time is 0.22 relative to triamcinolone hexacetonide. Calculate the percentage of triamcinolone acetonide in the portion of Injectable Suspension taken by the formula:

$$100(C / D)(r_U / r_S)$$

in which *C* is the concentration, in mg per mL, of USP Triamcinolone Hexacetonide RS in the *Standard solution*, *D* is the concentration, in mg per mL, of triamcinolone hexacetonide in the *Test solution*, and r_U and r_S are the peak responses for triamcinolone acetonide obtained from the *Test solution* and *Standard solution*, respectively: not more than 1.0% is found.
Other requirements—It meets the requirements under *Injections* ⟨1⟩.
Assay—
Mobile phase and *Standard preparation*—Proceed as directed in the *Assay* under *Triamcinolone Hexacetonide*.
System suitability solution—Dissolve suitable quantities of amcinonide and USP Triamcinolone Hexacetonide RS in methanol to obtain a solution containing about 0.3 mg per mL and 0.4 mg per mL, respectively.
Assay preparation—Using a "to contain" pipet, transfer an accurately measured volume of the Injectable Suspension, equivalent to about 40 mg of triamcinolone hexacetonide, to a 100-mL volumetric flask. Rinse the pipet with methanol, collecting the rinse in the volumetric flask. Dilute with methanol to volume, and mix.
Chromatographic system (see *Chromatography* ⟨621⟩)—The liquid chromatograph is equipped with a 254-nm detector and a 4.6-mm × 25-cm column that contains packing L1. The flow rate is about 1.4 mL per minute. Chromatograph the *System suitability solution*, and record the peak responses as directed for *Procedure*: the relative retention times are about 0.50 for amcinonide and 1.0 for triamcinolone hexacetonide, the resolution, *R*, between amcinonide and triamcinolone hexacetonide is not less than 10, the tailing factor for triamcinolone hexacetonide is not more than 1.2, and the relative standard deviation for replicate injections is not more than 2.0%.
Procedure—Separately inject equal volumes (about 10 µL) of the *Standard preparation* and the *Assay preparation* into the chromatograph, record the chromatograms, and measure the responses for the major peaks. Calculate the quantity, in mg, of $C_{30}H_{41}FO_7$ in the portion of Injectable Suspension taken by the formula:

$$100C(r_U / r_S)$$

in which *C* is the concentration, in mg per mL, of USP Triamcinolone Hexacetonide RS in the *Standard preparation*, and r_U and r_S are the peak responses obtained from the *Assay preparation* and the *Standard preparation*, respectively.

Triamterene

$C_{12}H_{11}N_7$ 253.26
2,4,7-Pteridinetriamine, 6-phenyl-.
2,4,7-Triamino-6-phenylpteridine   [396-01-0].

» Triamterene contains not less than 98.0 percent and not more than 102.0 percent of $C_{12}H_{11}N_7$, calculated on the dried basis.

Packaging and storage—Preserve in tight, light-resistant containers.
USP Reference standards ⟨11⟩—*USP Triamterene RS.*
Identification—
A: *Infrared Absorption* ⟨197M⟩.
B: A solution in formic acid solution (1 in 1000) shows an intense, bluish fluorescence.
Loss on drying ⟨731⟩—Dry it in vacuum at 105° for 2 hours: it loses not more than 1.0% of its weight.
Limit of 2,4,6-triamino-5-nitrosopyrimidine—
Mobile phase—Prepare a filtered and degassed mixture of 0.01 M potassium dihydrogen phosphate (adjusted to a pH of 3.0) and methanol (80 : 20). Make adjustments if necessary (see *System Suitability* under *Chromatography* ⟨621⟩).
Standard solution—[NOTE—Heating to 50° and sonication may be used to dissolve the 2,4,6-triamino-5-nitrosopyrimidine.] Dissolve an accurately weighed quantity of 2,4,6-triamino-5-nitrosopyrimidine in methanol, and dilute quantitatively if necessary with methanol to obtain a solution having a known concentration of about 10 µg per mL.
Test solution—Transfer about 1 g of Triamterene, accurately weighed, to a 250-mL conical flask. Add 100.0 mL of methanol, and stir for 30 minutes with heating to 50°, cool, and filter.

Chromatographic system—The liquid chromatograph is equipped with a 330-nm detector and a 3.9-mm × 30-cm column that contains 10-μm packing L10. The flow rate is about 1.5 mL per minute. Chromatograph the *Standard solution*, and record the peak responses as directed for *Procedure*: the relative retention times are about 0.4 for 2,4,6-triamino-5-nitrosopyrimidine and 1.0 for triamterene; the tailing factor is not more than 1.5; and the relative standard deviation for replicate injections is not more than 2.0%.

Procedure—Separately inject equal volumes (about 20 μL) of the *Standard solution* and the *Test solution* into the chromatograph, record the chromatograms, and measure the responses for the major peaks. Calculate the percentage of 2,4,6-triamino-5-nitrosopyrimidine in the portion of Triamterene taken by the formula:

$$10C / W(r_U / r_S)$$

in which the C is the concentration, in μg per mL, of 2,4,6-triamino-5-nitrosopyrimidine in the *Standard solution*; W is the weight, in mg of triamterene taken; and r_U and r_S are the peak responses for 2,4,6-triamino-5-nitrosopyrimidine obtained from the *Test solution* and the *Standard solution*, respectively: not more than 0.1% of 2,4,6-triamino-5-nitrosopyrimidine is found.

Organic volatile impurities, *Method IV* ⟨467⟩: meets the requirements.

(Official until July 1, 2008)

Ordinary impurities ⟨466⟩—

Test solution—Prepare a solution of Triamterene in dimethyl sulfoxide having a concentration of about 10 mg per mL. Quantitatively dilute with methanol to obtain a solution having a concentration of 0.25 mg per mL.

Standard solutions—Dissolve an accurately weighed quantity of USP Triamterene RS in dimethyl sulfoxide to obtain a solution having a known concentration of about 10 mg per mL. Dilute this solution with methanol to obtain solutions having known concentrations of about 0.00025, 0.00125, 0.0025, and 0.005 mg per mL.

Procedure—Separately apply 50 μL of each of the *Standard solutions* and the *Test solution* to a 0.5-mm thin-layer chromatographic plate that has been preconditioned by heating at 105° for 15 minutes and allowed to cool at room temperature in a closed chamber.

Eluant: a mixture of ethyl acetate, 15 M stronger ammonia water, and methanol (90 : 10 : 10).

Visualization: 1.

Assay—Transfer about 0.5 g of Triamterene, accurately weighed, to a 400-mL beaker, and dissolve in 250 mL of a solvent previously prepared by mixing, in the order named and with cooling prior to use, 1 volume of formic acid, 1 volume of acetic anhydride, and 2 volumes of glacial acetic acid. Titrate with 0.1 N perchloric acid VS, determining the endpoint potentiometrically. Perform a blank determination, and make any necessary correction. Each mL of 0.1 N perchloric acid is equivalent to 25.33 mg of $C_{12}H_{11}N_7$.

Triamterene Capsules

» Triamterene Capsules contain not less than 93.0 percent and not more than 107.0 percent of the labeled amount of triamterene ($C_{12}H_{11}N_7$).

Packaging and storage—Preserve in tight, light-resistant containers.

Labeling—When more than one *Dissolution* test is given, the labeling states the *Dissolution* test used only if *Test 1* is not used.

USP Reference standards ⟨11⟩—*USP Triamterene RS*.

Identification—

A: *Ultraviolet Absorption* ⟨197U⟩—Transfer a portion of the contents of the Capsules, equivalent to about 0.1 g of triamterene, to a 250-mL volumetric flask. Add 100 mL of methoxyethanol, shake until dissolved, dilute with water to volume, and mix. Transfer 5 mL of this solution to a 200-mL volumetric flask, add 5 mL of formic acid, and dilute with water to volume. Prepare a solution of USP Triamterene RS in the manner described above to obtain a Standard solution with a final concentration of about 10 μg per mL. Determine the UV spectrum from 280 nm to 420 nm.

B: The retention time of the major peak in the chromatogram of the *Assay preparation* corresponds to that in the chromatogram of the *Standard preparation*, as obtained in the *Assay*.

Dissolution ⟨711⟩—

TEST 1—

Medium: 1% w/v of polysorbate 20 in 0.1 N acetic acid; 900 mL.

Apparatus 2: 100 rpm.

Time: 120 minutes.

Procedure—Proceed as directed for *Test 2*.

Tolerances—Not less than 80% (*Q*) of the labeled amount of $C_{12}H_{11}N_7$ is dissolved in 120 minutes.

TEST 2—If the product complies with this test, the labeling indicates that it meets USP *Dissolution Test 2*.

Medium: 0.1 N hydrochloric acid; 900 mL.

Apparatus 1: 100 rpm.

Time: 45 minutes.

Procedure—Determine the amount of $C_{12}H_{11}N_7$ dissolved by employing UV absorption at the wavelength of maximum absorbance at about 357 nm on filtered portions of the solution under test, suitably diluted with *Medium*, if necessary, in comparison with a Standard solution having a known concentration of USP Triamterene RS in the same *Medium*.

Tolerances—Not less than 75% (*Q*) of the labeled amount of $C_{12}H_{11}N_7$ is dissolved in 45 minutes.

Uniformity of dosage units ⟨905⟩: meet the requirements.

Assay—

Buffer solution and *Mobile phase*—Proceed as directed in the *Assay* under *Triamterene and Hydrochlorothiazide Tablets*.

Standard preparation—Transfer about 50 mg of USP Triamterene RS, accurately weighed, to a 100-mL volumetric flask. Add 10 mL of acetonitrile, 10 mL of water, and 5 mL of glacial acetic acid, sonicating for 3 minutes after each addition. Cool to room temperature, dilute with water to volume, and mix.

Assay preparation—Remove, as completely as possible, the contents of 20 Capsules, combine the contents, and transfer an accurately weighed portion of powder, equivalent to about that which is in one dosage unit, to a 100-mL volumetric flask (*Flask 1*). To a separate 100-mL volumetric flask, add all 20 capsule shells (*Flask 2*). For each flask, add 10 mL of acetonitrile, and sonicate for 10 minutes. Add 10 mL of boiling water, sonicate for 5 minutes, and mix. Add 10 mL of glacial acetic acid, sonicate for 10 minutes, and mix. Add 60 mL of water, mix, and allow to cool to room temperature. Dilute the contents of *Flask 2* with water to volume, and add 5.0 mL of the solution from *Flask 2* to *Flask 1*. Dilute the contents of *Flask 1* with water to volume, and mix. If necessary, quantitatively dilute with a solution of acetonitrile, glacial acetic acid, and water (10 : 10 : 80) to obtain a final concentration of about 0.5 mg per mL. Filter a portion of this solution, discarding the first 3 mL of the filtrate.

Chromatographic system (see *Chromatography* ⟨621⟩)—The liquid chromatograph is equipped with a 280-nm detector and a 3.9-mm × 30-cm column that contains packing L1. The flow rate is about 1 mL per minute. Chromatograph the *Standard preparation*, and record the peak responses as directed for *Procedure*: the tailing factor is not more than 2.0; and the relative standard deviation for replicate injections is not more than 2.0%.

Procedure—Separately inject equal volumes (about 10 μL) of the *Standard preparation* and the *Assay preparation* into the chromatograph, record the chromatograms, and measure the responses of the major peaks. Calculate the quantity, in mg, of triamterene ($C_{12}H_{11}N_7$) in the portion of Capsules taken by the formula:

$$CV(r_U / r_S)$$

in which C is the concentration, in mg per mL, of USP Triamterene RS in the *Standard preparation*; V is the sample dilution volume, in mL, considering the 100-mL volume of the solution in *Flask 1* and any subsequent dilution factor, if used; and r_U and r_S are the peak responses obtained from the *Assay preparation* and the *Standard preparation*, respectively.

Triamterene and Hydrochlorothiazide Capsules

» Triamterene and Hydrochlorothiazide Capsules contain not less than 90.0 percent and not more than 110.0 percent of the labeled amounts of triamterene ($C_{12}H_{11}N_7$) and hydrochlorothiazide ($C_7H_8ClN_3O_4S_2$).

NOTE—The Capsules and Tablets dosage forms should not be considered bioequivalent. If patients are to be transferred from one dosage form to the other, retitration and appropriate changes in dosage may be necessary.

Packaging and storage—Preserve in tight, light-resistant containers.
Labeling—Label the Capsules to indicate the *Dissolution* test with which the product complies.
USP Reference standards ⟨11⟩—*USP Benzothiadiazine Related Compound A RS. USP Hydrochlorothiazide RS. USP Triamterene RS.*
Identification—
  A: *Thin-Layer Identification Test* ⟨201⟩—
  Test solution—Dissolve a portion of the Capsule contents, equivalent to about 50 mg of triamterene, in 25 mL of methoxyethanol, mix, and filter. Use the filtrate as the *Test solution*.
  Standard solution 1—Prepare a solution of USP Triamterene RS in methoxyethanol containing about 2 mg per mL.
  Standard solution 2: a sufficient quantity of USP Hydrochlorothiazide RS in methoxyethanol to obtain a solution having a concentration similar to that of the *Test solution*.
  Application volume: 2 µL.
  Developing solvent system: a mixture of ethyl acetate, glacial acetic acid, and water (8 : 1 : 1).
  Procedure—Locate the spots under short-wavelength and long-wavelength UV light: the intensity and R_F value correspond to that obtained from *Standard solution 1* and *Standard solution 2*.
  B: The retention times of the major peaks in the chromatogram of the *Assay preparation* correspond to those in the chromatogram of the *Standard preparation*, as obtained in the *Assay*.
Dissolution ⟨711⟩—
  TEST 1: If the product complies with this test, the labeling indicates that it meets USP *Dissolution Test 1*.
  Medium: 0.1 M acetic acid containing 1% polysorbate 20; 900 mL.
  Apparatus 2: 100 rpm.
  Time: 120 minutes.
  Procedure—Determine the amounts of triamterene ($C_{12}H_{11}N_7$) and hydrochlorothiazide ($C_7H_8ClN_3O_4S_2$) dissolved from UV absorption at the wavelength of maximum absorbance at about 357 nm for triamterene and 271 nm for hydrochlorothiazide (corrected for interference from triamterene on the basis of the absorbances of triamterene at 271 nm and 357 nm) on a filtered portion of the solution under test, suitably diluted with water, in comparison with a Standard solution having known concentrations of USP Triamterene RS and USP Hydrochlorothiazide RS in the same *Medium*.
  Tolerances—Not less than 80% *(Q)* of the labeled amounts of $C_{12}H_{11}N_7$ and $C_7H_8ClN_3O_4S_2$ is dissolved in 120 minutes.
  TEST 2: If the product complies with this test, the labeling indicates that it meets USP *Dissolution Test 2*.
  Medium: 4.0% tetrasodium ethylenediaminetetraacetate, 2.0% polysorbate 40, 0.05% pancreatin; 900 mL. Prepare a solution using the following procedure. Add the polysorbate 40 and the tetrasodium ethylenediaminetetraacetate to water, and mix thoroughly. Adjust with phosphoric acid to a pH of 8.0 ± 0.05. Heat to 37°, and add the pancreatin powder. Mix thoroughly, and transfer immediately to the dissolution vessel.
  Apparatus 1 (use 10-mesh baskets): 100 rpm.
  Time: 8 hours.
  Mobile phase—Prepare a filtered and degassed solution of 0.08 M monobasic sodium phosphate buffer and methanol (3 : 1). Make adjustments if necessary (see *System Suitability* under *Chromatography* ⟨621⟩).
  Standard preparation—Transfer about 110 mg of USP Triamterene RS and about 55 mg of USP Hydrochlorothiazide RS, each accurately weighed, to a 500-mL volumetric flask. Add 100 mL of methanol, sonicate for 10 minutes, and heat in a steam bath until completely dissolved. Dilute with *Medium* to volume, and mix. Transfer 25 mL of this solution into a 100-mL volumetric flask, dilute with *Medium* to volume, and mix gently to minimize foaming.
  Test preparation—Filter a portion of the solution under test. [NOTE—Do not use nylon filters.]
  Chromatographic system (see *Chromatography* ⟨621⟩)—The liquid chromatograph is equipped with a 254-nm detector, a guard column that contains packing L7, and an analytical 3.9-mm × 30-cm column that contains packing L11. The flow rate is about 2 mL per minute. Chromatograph the *Standard preparation*, and record the responses as directed for *Procedure*: the resolution, *R*, between the triamterene and hydrochlorothiazide peaks is not less than 2.0; and the relative standard deviation for replicate injections of each analyte is not more than 2.0%.
  Procedure—Separately inject equal volumes (about 50 µL) of the *Standard preparation* and the *Test preparation* in the chromatograph, record the chromatograms, and measure the responses for the major peaks. Calculate the quantities, in mg, of triamterene ($C_{12}H_{11}N_7$) and hydrochlorothiazide ($C_7H_8ClN_3O_4S_2$) dissolved by the formula:

$$900C(r_U / r_S)$$

in which *C* is the concentration, in mg per mL, of the appropriate USP Reference Standard in the *Standard preparation*; and r_U and r_S are the peak responses of the relevant analyte obtained from the *Test preparation* and the *Standard preparation*, respectively.
  Tolerances—Not less than 70% *(Q)* of the labeled amount of $C_{12}H_{11}N_7$ and not less than 80% *(Q)* of the labeled amount of $C_7H_8ClN_3O_4S_2$ are dissolved in 8 hours.
  TEST 3: If the product complies with this test, the labeling indicates that it meets USP *Dissolution Test 3*.
  Medium: 0.1 N hydrochloric acid; 900 mL.
  Apparatus 1: 100 rpm.
  Time: 45 minutes.
  Procedure—Proceed as directed for *Test 1*.
  Tolerances—Not less than 75% *(Q)* of the labeled amounts of $C_{12}H_{11}N_7$ and $C_7H_8ClN_3O_4S_2$ is dissolved in 45 minutes.
Uniformity of dosage units ⟨905⟩: meet the requirements for *Content Uniformity* with respect to triamterene and to hydrochlorothiazide.
Related compounds—
  Solution A, Solution B, Mobile phase, Standard solution, and *Chromatographic system*—Proceed as directed for the *Related compounds* test under *Triamterene and Hydrochlorothiazide Tablets*.
  Test solution—Remove, as completely as possible, the contents of not fewer than 20 Capsules, and weigh accurately. Mix the combined contents, and transfer an accurately weighed portion of the powder, equivalent to about 150 mg of hydrochlorothiazide, to a 100-mL volumetric flask. Add 60 mL of acetonitrile and 6 mL of glacial acetic acid, and sonicate for 10 minutes. Cool, dilute with water to volume, mix, and filter.
  Procedure—Proceed as directed for *Procedure* in the *Related compounds* test under *Triamterene and Hydrochlorothiazide Tablets*. Calculate the quantity, in mg, of benzothiadiazine related compound A in the hydrochlorothiazide contained in the portion of Capsules taken by the formula:

$$100C(r_U / r_S)$$

in which *C* is the concentration, in mg per mL, of USP Benzothiadiazine Related Compound A RS in the *Standard solution*; and r_U and r_S are the peak areas of benzothiadiazine related compound A obtained from the *Test solution* and the *Standard solution*, respectively: not more than 1.0% is present.
Assay—
  Buffer solution, Mobile phase, and *Standard preparation*—Proceed as directed in the *Assay* under *Triamterene and Hydrochlorothiazide Tablets*.

Assay preparation—Remove, as completely as possible, the contents of not fewer than 20 Capsules, combine the contents, and transfer an accurately weighed portion of powder, equivalent to about 50 mg of hydrochlorothiazide, to a 200-mL volumetric flask. Add 20 mL of acetonitrile, and sonicate for 10 minutes. Add 20 mL of boiling water, sonicate for 5 minutes, and mix. Add 10 mL of acetic acid, sonicate for 10 minutes, and mix. Add 140 mL of water, mix, and allow to cool to room temperature. Dilute with water to volume, mix, and filter, discarding the first 3 mL of the filtrate.

Chromatographic system (see *Chromatography* ⟨621⟩)—The liquid chromatograph is equipped with a 280-nm detector and a 3.9-mm × 30-cm column that contains packing L1. The flow rate is about 1 mL per minute. Chromatograph the *Standard preparation*, and record the peak responses as directed for *Procedure*: the relative retention times are 0.65 for hydrochlorothiazide and 1.0 for triamterene; the resolution, R, between hydrochlorothiazide and triamterene is not less than 3.0; and the relative standard deviation for replicate injections is not more than 2.0%.

Procedure—Separately inject equal volumes (about 10 μL) of the *Standard preparation* and the *Assay preparation* into the chromatograph, record the chromatograms, and measure the responses of the major peaks. Calculate the quantity, in mg, of triamterene ($C_{12}H_{11}N_7$) in the portion of Capsules taken by the formula:

$$200C(r_U / r_S)$$

in which C is the concentration, in mg per mL, of USP Triamterene RS in the *Standard preparation;* and r_U and r_S are the peak responses obtained from the *Assay preparation* and the *Standard preparation*, respectively. Calculate the quantity, in mg, of hydrochlorothiazide ($C_7H_8ClN_3O_4S_2$) in the portion of Capsules taken by the same formula, changing the terms to refer to hydrochlorothiazide.

Triamterene and Hydrochlorothiazide Tablets

» Triamterene and Hydrochlorothiazide Tablets contain not less than 90.0 percent and not more than 110.0 percent of the labeled amounts of triamterene ($C_{12}H_{11}N_7$) and hydrochlorothiazide ($C_7H_8ClN_3O_4S_2$).

NOTE—The Capsules and Tablets dosage forms should not be considered bioequivalent. If patients are to be transferred from one dosage form to the other, re-titration and appropriate changes in dosage may be necessary.

Packaging and storage—Preserve in tight, light-resistant containers.

USP Reference standards ⟨11⟩—USP Benzothiadiazine Related Compound A RS. USP Hydrochlorothiazide RS. USP Triamterene RS.

Identification—
A: The retention times of the major peaks in the chromatogram of the *Assay preparation* correspond to those in the chromatogram of the *Standard preparation*, as obtained in the *Assay*.

B: Dissolve a portion of finely ground Tablets, equivalent to about 50 mg of triamterene, in 25 mL of methoxyethanol, mix, and filter. Use the filtrate as the *Test solution*. Prepare Standard solutions containing 1.5 mg of USP Triamterene RS per mL of methoxyethanol (*Standard solution 1*) and containing 1 mg of USP Hydrochlorothiazide RS per mL of methoxyethanol (*Standard solution 2*). Separately apply 2 μL of the *Test solution* and 2 μL each of *Standard solution 1* and *Standard solution 2* to a suitable thin-layer chromatographic plate (see *Chromatography* ⟨621⟩) coated with a 0.25-mm layer of chromatographic silica gel mixture. Dry the spots with a current of air. Develop the plate in a solvent system consisting of a mixture of ethyl acetate, glacial acetic acid, and water (8 : 1 : 1) until the solvent front has moved about three-fourths of the length of the plate. Remove the plate from the developing chamber, mark the solvent front, and allow to dry. Locate the spots under short-wavelength and long-wavelength UV light: the intensity and the R_F value of the principal spots obtained from the *Test solution* correspond to those from *Standard solution 1* and *Standard solution 2*.

Dissolution ⟨711⟩—
Medium: 0.1 N hydrochloric acid; 900 mL.
Apparatus 2: 75 rpm.
Time: 30 minutes.
Determine the amount of triamterene and hydrochlorothiazide dissolved using the following method.

Buffer solution, Mobile phase, and *Chromatographic system*—Proceed as directed in the *Assay*.

Procedure—Inject a volume (about 10 μL) of a filtered portion of the solution under test into the chromatograph, record the chromatogram, and measure the responses for the major peaks. Calculate the amounts of triamterene ($C_{12}H_{11}N_7$) and hydrochlorothiazide ($C_7H_8ClN_3O_4S_2$) dissolved by comparison with a Standard solution having known concentrations of USP Triamterene RS and USP Hydrochlorothiazide RS in the same *Medium* and similarly chromatographed.

Tolerances—Not less than 80% (Q) each of the labeled amounts of $C_{12}H_{11}N_7$ and $C_7H_8ClN_3O_4S_2$ is dissolved in 30 minutes.

Uniformity of dosage units ⟨905⟩: meet the requirements for *Content Uniformity* with respect to triamterene and to hydrochlorothiazide.

Related compounds—
Solution A—Dissolve 0.68 g of sodium acetate trihydrate in 100.0 mL of water, adjust with glacial acetic acid to a pH of 5.0, and mix.

Solution B—Prepare a mixture of acetonitrile and methanol (75 : 25).

Mobile phase—Prepare a suitable filtered and degassed mixture of *Solution A* and *Solution B* (90 : 10). Make adjustments if necessary (see *System Suitability* under *Chromatography* ⟨621⟩).

Standard solution—Prepare a solution of USP Benzothiadiazine Related Compound A RS in acetonitrile having a known concentration of 0.15 mg per mL. Transfer 10.0 mL of this solution to a 100-mL volumetric flask, add 50 mL of acetonitrile and 6 mL of glacial acetic acid, dilute with water to volume, and mix.

Test solution—Weigh and finely powder not fewer than 20 Tablets. Transfer an accurately weighed portion of the powder, equivalent to about 150 mg of hydrochlorothiazide, to a 100-mL volumetric flask. Add 60 mL of acetonitrile and 6 mL of glacial acetic acid, and sonicate for 10 minutes. Cool, dilute with water to volume, mix, and filter.

Chromatographic system (see *Chromatography* ⟨621⟩)—The liquid chromatograph is equipped with a 273-nm detector and a 3.9-mm × 30-cm column that contains 10-μm packing L1. The flow rate is about 2 mL per minute. Chromatograph the *Standard solution*, and record the peak responses as directed for *Procedure*: the relative standard deviation for replicate injections is not more than 2.0%.

Procedure—Separately inject equal volumes (about 10 μL) of the *Standard solution* and the *Test solution* into the chromatograph, record the chromatograms, and measure the peak areas due to benzothiadiazine related compound A in the *Standard solution* and the *Test solution*. The retention times, relative to benzothiadiazine related compound A, are about 1.5 for hydrochlorothiazide and about 10 for triamterene. Calculate the quantity, in mg, of benzothiadiazine related compound A in the hydrochlorothiazide contained in the portion of Tablets taken by the formula:

$$100C(r_U / r_S)$$

in which C is the concentration, in mg per mL, of USP Benzothiadiazine Related Compound A RS in the *Standard solution;* and r_U and r_S are the peak areas of benzothiadiazine related compound A obtained from the *Test solution* and the *Standard solution*, respectively: not more than 1.0% is present.

Assay—
Buffer solution—Transfer 6.9 g of monobasic sodium phosphate and 1.43 g of propylamine hydrochloride to a 1000-mL volumetric flask, dissolve in about 900 mL of water, adjust with 1 N sodium hydroxide to a pH of 5.5, dilute with water to volume, and mix.

Mobile phase—Prepare a filtered and degassed mixture of *Buffer solution* and acetonitrile (80 : 20). Make adjustments if necessary (see *System Suitability* under *Chromatography* ⟨621⟩).

Solvent mixture—Prepare a mixture of water, acetonitrile, and glacial acetic acid (85 : 10 : 5).

Standard preparation—Transfer about 25 mg of USP Hydrochlorothiazide RS, accurately weighed, to a 100-mL volumetric flask. Add 25*J*mg of USP Triamterene RS, accurately weighed, *J* being the ratio of the labeled amount, in mg, of triamterene to the labeled amount, in mg, of hydrochlorothiazide per Tablet. Add 10 mL of acetonitrile, 10 mL of water, and 5 mL of glacial acetic acid, sonicating for 2 to 3 minutes after each addition. Cool to room temperature, dilute with water to volume, and mix.

Assay preparation—Weigh and finely powder not fewer than 20 Tablets. Transfer an accurately weighed portion of the powder, equivalent to about 50 mg of hydrochlorothiazide, to a 200-mL volumetric flask. Add about 100 mL of *Solvent mixture*, place the volumetric flask in a sonic bath heated to between 45° and 50°, and sonicate for about 30 minutes. Remove the flask from the bath, and carefully add 70 mL of *Solvent mixture*. Allow to cool to room temperature, and dilute with *Solvent mixture* to volume. Filter the solution, discarding the first few mL of the filtrate.

Chromatographic system (see *Chromatography* ⟨621⟩)—The liquid chromatograph is equipped with a 280-nm detector and a 4.0-mm × 25-cm column that contains packing L1. The flow rate is about 1.2 mL per minute. Chromatograph the *Standard preparation*, and record the peak responses as directed for *Procedure:* the relative retention times are about 0.65 for hydrochlorothiazide and 1.0 for triamterene; the resolution, *R*, between hydrochlorothiazide and triamterene is not less than 3.0; and the relative standard deviation for replicate injections is not more than 2.0%.

Procedure—Separately inject equal volumes (about 10 µL) of the *Standard preparation* and the *Assay preparation* into the chromatograph, record the chromatograms, and measure the responses for the major peaks. Separately calculate the quantities, in mg, of triamterene ($C_{12}H_{11}N_7$) and hydrochlorothiazide ($C_7H_8ClN_3O_4S_2$) in the portion of Tablets taken by the formula:

$$200C(r_U / r_S)$$

in which *C* is the concentration, in mg per mL, of the relevant USP Reference Standard in the *Standard preparation;* and r_U and r_S are the peak responses of the relevant analyte obtained from the *Assay preparation* and the *Standard preparation,* respectively.

Triazolam

$C_{17}H_{12}Cl_2N_4$ 343.21
4*H*-[1,2,4]Triazolo[4,3-*a*][1,4]benzodiazepine, 8-chloro-6-(2-chlorophenyl)-1-methyl-.
8-Chloro-6-(*o*-chlorophenyl)-1-methyl-4*H*-*s*-triazolo[4,3-*a*][1,4] benzodiazepine   [*28911-01-5*].

» Triazolam contains not less than 97.0 percent and not more than 103.0 percent of $C_{17}H_{12}Cl_2N_4$, calculated on the dried basis.

Caution—Exercise care to prevent inhaling particles of triazolam and to prevent its contacting any part of the body.

Packaging and storage—Preserve in well-closed containers.
USP Reference standards ⟨11⟩—*USP Triazolam RS.*
Identification—
  A: *Infrared Absorption* ⟨197M⟩.
  B: *Ultraviolet Absorption* ⟨197U⟩—
  Solution: 4 µg per mL.
  Medium: alcohol.
Absorptivities at 220 nm, calculated on the dried basis, do not differ by more than 3%.
Loss on drying ⟨731⟩—Dry it at 60° and at a pressure not exceeding 5 mm of mercury for 16 hours: it loses not more than 0.5% of its weight.
Residue on ignition ⟨281⟩:   not more than 0.5%.
Heavy metals, *Method II* ⟨231⟩:   0.002%.
Chromatographic purity—
  Test solution—Prepare a solution of Triazolam in chloroform containing about 2 mg per mL.
  Chromatographic system (see *Chromatography* ⟨621⟩)—The gas chromatograph is equipped with a flame-ionization detector, and contains a 3-mm × 120-cm glass column packed with 3% phase G6 on support S1AB. The column and injection port are maintained at a temperature of about 240°. The detector is maintained at a temperature of about 20° to 50° above column temperature. The carrier gas is helium.
  Procedure—[NOTE—Allow about three times the elution time of the major component before making another injection.] Chromatograph about 4 µL of the *Test solution*. Calculate the total percentage of impurities taken by the formula:

$$100S/(S + A)$$

in which *S* is the sum of the areas of each of the minor component peaks detected, and *A* is the area of the major component peak. The total amount of impurities present is not more than 1.5%.
Assay—
  Mobile phase—Prepare a filtered and degassed mixture of acetonitrile, chloroform, butyl alcohol, water, and glacial acetic acid (850 : 80 : 50 : 20 : 0.5). Make adjustments if necessary (see *System Suitability* under *Chromatography* ⟨621⟩).
  Internal standard solution—Dissolve an accurately weighed quantity of alprazolam in acetonitrile, and dilute with acetonitrile to obtain a solution having a known concentration of about 0.3 mg per mL.
  Standard stock solution—Dissolve an accurately weighed quantity of USP Triazolam RS in *Internal standard solution*, and dilute with *Internal standard solution* to obtain a solution having a known concentration of about 0.25 mg per mL.
  Assay stock solution—Transfer about 2.5 mg of Triazolam, accurately weighed, to a 10-mL volumetric flask, dissolve in and dilute with *Internal standard solution* to volume, and mix.
  Standard preparation—Dilute an accurately measured portion of the *Standard stock solution* with acetonitrile to obtain a solution having a known concentration of USP Triazolam RS of about 0.025 mg per mL.
  Assay preparation—Transfer about 5 mL of the *Assay stock solution*, accurately measured, to a 50-mL volumetric flask, dilute with acetonitrile to volume, and mix.
  Chromatographic system (see *Chromatography* ⟨621⟩)—The liquid chromatograph is equipped with a 254-nm detector and a 4.6-mm × 30-cm column that contains packing L3. The flow rate is about 2.0 mL per minute. Chromatograph the *Standard preparation*, and record the peak responses as directed under *Procedure:* the relative retention times are 1 for triazolam and about 1.4 for the internal standard, the resolution, *R*, between the internal standard and triazolam is not less than 2.0, and the relative standard deviation for replicate injections is not more than 2.0%.
  Procedure—Separately inject equal volumes (about 20 µL) of the *Standard preparation* and the *Assay preparation* into the chromatograph, record the chromatograms, and measure the area responses for the major peaks. Calculate the quantity, in mg, of $C_{17}H_{12}Cl_2N_4$ in the portion of Triazolam taken by the formula:

$$CV(R_U / R_S)$$

in which *C* is the concentration, in mg per mL, of USP Triazolam RS in the *Standard stock solution; V* is the volume of internal stan-

Triazolam Tablets

» Triazolam Tablets contain not less than 90.0 percent and not more than 110.0 percent of the labeled amount of $C_{17}H_{12}Cl_2N_4$.

Packaging and storage—Preserve in tight, light-resistant containers.

USP Reference standards ⟨11⟩—*USP Triazolam RS.*

Identification—The retention time of the major peak in the chromatogram of the *Assay preparation* obtained as directed in the *Assay* corresponds to that of the *Standard preparation*, relative to the internal standard.

Dissolution ⟨711⟩—
  Medium: water; 500 mL.
  Apparatus 2: 50 rpm.
  Time: 30 minutes.
  Stock standard solution—Weigh accurately about 5 mg of USP Triazolam RS, dissolve in and dilute with methanol to 200.0 mL, and mix.
  Working standard solution—For each 0.125 mg of the labeled amount of triazolam per Tablet, add 2.0 mL of *Stock standard solution* to a 200-mL volumetric flask. Dilute with water to volume, and mix.
  Procedure—After 30 minutes, withdraw a portion of the solution under test, and filter immediately. Inject equal volumes (about 200 μL) of this solution and the *Working standard solution* into a liquid chromatograph (see *Chromatography* ⟨621⟩) equipped with a detector capable of monitoring UV absorbance at 222 nm and a 4.6-mm × 10-cm stainless steel column containing packing L7. The mobile phase is a mixture of water and acetonitrile (60 : 40). The flow rate is about 1 mL per minute. The relative standard deviation of the peak response for the *Working standard solution* is not more than 3.0%, and the number of theoretical plates is not less than 500. Calculate the percentage of $C_{17}H_{12}Cl_2N_4$ dissolved by the formula:

$$50{,}000(r_U / r_S)(C / L)$$

in which r_U and r_S are the peak responses of the solution under test and the *Working standard solution*, respectively, *C* is the concentration, in mg per mL, of USP Triazolam RS in the *Working standard solution*, and *L* is the labeled amount, in mg, of triazolam in the Tablet.
  Tolerances—Not less than 70% (*Q*) of the labeled amount of $C_{17}H_{12}Cl_2N_4$ is dissolved in 30 minutes.

Uniformity of dosage units ⟨905⟩: meet the requirements.
  Procedure for content uniformity—
  Mobile phase and *Chromatographic system*—Proceed as directed in the *Assay* under *Triazolam*.
  Internal standard solution—Prepare a solution of alprazolam in acetonitrile having a concentration of about 0.025 mg per mL.
  Standard preparation—Dissolve about 3.2 mg of USP Triazolam RS, accurately weighed, in 100.0 mL of *Internal standard solution*, and mix.
  Test preparation—Transfer 1 Tablet to a container, add about 0.4 mL of water directly onto the Tablet, allow to stand for about 2 minutes, and swirl the container to disperse the Tablet. For each 0.25 mg of the labeled amount of triazolam in the Tablet, add 10.0 mL of *Internal standard solution* to the container. Shake, and centrifuge if necessary.
  Procedure—Proceed as directed for *Procedure* in the *Assay* under *Triazolam*. Calculate the quantity, in mg, of $C_{17}H_{12}Cl_2N_4$ in the Tablet taken by the formula:

$$CV(R_U / R_S)$$

in which *V* is the volume, in mL, of *Internal standard solution* in the *Test preparation*, *C* is the concentration, in mg per mL, of USP Triazolam RS in the *Standard preparation*; and R_U and R_S are the ratios of the internal standard peak area to the alprazolam peak area obtained from the *Assay preparation* and the *Standard preparation*, respectively.

Assay—
  Mobile phase and *Chromatographic system*—Proceed as directed in the *Assay* under *Triazolam*.
  Internal standard solution—Prepare a solution of alprazolam in acetonitrile, having a concentration of 0.1 mg per mL.
  Standard stock solution—Dissolve an accurately weighed quantity of USP Triazolam RS in acetonitrile, and dilute with acetonitrile to obtain a solution having a known concentration of about 0.1 mg per mL.
  Standard preparation—Transfer 8.0 mL of *Standard stock solution* to a 200-mL volumetric flask, add 8.0 mL of *Internal standard solution*, dilute with acetonitrile to volume, and mix.
  Assay preparation—Weigh and finely powder not less than 20 Tablets. Transfer an accurately weighed quantity of the powder, equivalent to about 0.8 mg of triazolam, to a 200-mL volumetric flask. Add 2 mL of water, mix, and allow to stand for 10 minutes. Mix vigorously for 10 seconds, and add 8.0 mL of *Internal standard solution*, shake vigorously for 10 minutes, dilute with acetonitrile to volume, and mix.
  Procedure—Separately inject equal volumes (about 20 μL) of the *Standard preparation* and the *Assay preparation* into the chromatograph, record the chromatograms, and measure the area responses for the major peaks. Calculate the quantity, in mg, of $C_{17}H_{12}Cl_2N_4$ in the portion of Triazolam taken by the formula:

$$200C(R_U / R_S)$$

in which *C* is the concentration, in mg per mL, of USP Triazolam RS in the *Standard preparation*, and R_U and R_S are the ratios of the internal standard peak area to the triazolam peak area obtained from the *Assay preparation* and the *Standard preparation*, respectively.

Trichlormethiazide

$C_8H_8Cl_3N_3O_4S_2$ 380.66
2*H*-1,2,4-Benzothiadiazine-7-sulfonamide, 6-chloro-3-(dichloromethyl)-3,4-dihydro-, 1,1-dioxide, (±)-.
(±)-6-Chloro-3-(dichloromethyl)-3,4-dihydro-2*H*-1,2,4-benzothiadiazine-7-sulfonamide 1,1-dioxide   [133-67-5].

» Trichlormethiazide, dried at 105° for 3 hours, contains not less than 98.0 percent and not more than 102.0 percent of $C_8H_8Cl_3N_3O_4S_2$.

Packaging and storage—Preserve in well-closed containers.

USP Reference standards ⟨11⟩—*USP Benzothiadiazine Related Compound A RS. USP Trichlormethiazide RS.*

Identification—
  A: *Infrared Absorption* ⟨197M⟩.
  B: Prepare a solution in a mixture of equal volumes of toluene and alcohol containing 1 mg per mL. Apply 10 μL of this solution and 10 μL of a Standard solution of USP Trichlormethiazide RS in the same medium having a known concentration of 1 mg per mL to a suitable thin-layer chromatographic plate (see *Thin-Layer Chromatography* under *Chromatography* ⟨621⟩) coated with a 0.25-mm layer of chromatographic silica gel mixture. Allow the spots to dry, and develop the chromatogram, using ethyl acetate as the solvent, until the solvent front has moved about three-fourths of the length of the plate. Remove the plate from the developing chamber, mark the solvent front, and allow the solvent to evaporate. Locate the spots using short-wavelength UV light: the R_F value of the principal spot obtained from the test solution corresponds to that obtained from the Standard solution.

Loss on drying ⟨731⟩—Dry it at 105° for 3 hours: it loses not more than 0.5% of its weight.

Residue on ignition ⟨281⟩: not more than 0.1%.
Selenium ⟨291⟩: 0.003%.
Heavy metals, *Method II* ⟨231⟩: 0.002%.
Diazotizable substances—
 Standard solution—Prepare a solution in a mixture of equal volumes of toluene and alcohol containing 250 µg of USP Benzothiadiazine Related Compound A RS in each mL.
 Test solution—Transfer 100.0 mg of Trichlormethiazide, accurately weighed, to a 10-mL volumetric flask, dissolve in 1 mL of acetone, dilute with a mixture of equal volumes of toluene and alcohol to volume, and mix.
 Procedure—Apply 5 µL each of the *Standard solution* and of the *Test solution* to a suitable thin-layer chromatographic plate (see *Thin-Layer Chromatography*, under *Chromatography* ⟨621⟩) coated with a 0.25-mm layer of chromatographic silica gel mixture. Allow the spots to dry, and develop the chromatogram in ethyl acetate until the solvent front has moved about three-fourths of the length of the plate. Remove the plate from the developing chamber, mark the solvent front, and locate the spots on the plate by spraying first with a 1 in 20 solution of sodium nitrite in dilute hydrochloric acid (1 in 12), and then with a 1 in 1000 solution of N-(1-naphthyl)ethylenediamine dihydrochloride in alcohol: after 3 minutes, any spot from the *Test solution*, occurring at the R_F value corresponding to that produced by the *Standard solution*, is not greater in size or intensity than the spot produced by the *Standard solution*, corresponding to not more than 2.5% of diazotizable substances.
Assay—
 Mobile phase—Prepare a filtered and degassed mixture of 0.05 M monobasic potassium phosphate and methanol (7 : 3). Make adjustments if necessary (see *System Suitability* under *Chromatography* ⟨621⟩).
 Internal standard solution—Transfer about 120 mg of methylparaben to a 50-mL volumetric flask, add methanol to volume, and mix.
 Standard preparation—Transfer about 25 mg of USP Trichlormethiazide RS, accurately weighed, to a 50-mL volumetric flask, add 4.0 mL of *Internal standard solution*, dilute with methanol to volume, and mix to obtain a solution having a known concentration of about 0.5 mg of USP Trichlormethiazide RS per mL.
 Assay preparation—Transfer about 50 mg of Trichlormethiazide, accurately weighed, to a 100-mL volumetric flask, add 8.0 mL of *Internal standard solution*, dilute with methanol to volume, and mix.
 Chromatographic system (see *Chromatography* ⟨621⟩)—The liquid chromatograph is equipped with a 254-nm detector and a 3.9-mm × 30-cm column that contains packing L1. The flow rate is about 2.3 mL per minute. Chromatograph the *Standard preparation*, and record the peak responses as directed for *Procedure*: the resolution, *R*, between the analyte and internal standard peaks is not less than 2.0, and the relative standard deviation for the response ratios calculated for replicate injections is not more than 2%.
 Procedure—Separately inject equal volumes (5 to 25 µL) of the *Standard preparation* and the *Assay preparation* into the chromatograph, record the chromatograms, and measure the responses for the major peaks. The relative retention times are about 0.56 for trichlormethiazide and 1.0 for methylparaben. Calculate the quantity, in mg, of $C_8H_8Cl_3N_3O_4S_2$ in the portion of Trichlormethiazide taken by the formula:

$$100C(R_U / R_S)$$

in which *C* is the concentration, in mg per mL, of USP Trichlormethiazide RS in the *Standard preparation*, and R_U and R_S are the peak response ratios obtained from the *Assay preparation* and the *Standard preparation*, respectively.

Trichlormethiazide Tablets

» Trichlormethiazide Tablets contain not less than 90.0 percent and not more than 110.0 percent of the labeled amount of $C_8H_8Cl_3N_3O_4S_2$.

Packaging and storage—Preserve in tight containers.
USP Reference standards ⟨11⟩—*USP Trichlormethiazide RS.*
Identification—Evaporate 25 mL of the combined ethyl acetate extracts obtained in the *Assay* on a steam bath to dryness, and dissolve the residue in 1 mL of a mixture of equal volumes of benzene and alcohol: a 10-µL portion of this solution responds to *Identification* test B under *Trichlormethiazide.*
Dissolution ⟨711⟩—
 Medium: water; 900 mL.
 Apparatus 2: 50 rpm.
 Time: 60 minutes.
 Procedure—[NOTE—Conduct the analysis of the specimen promptly after the specimen aliquot is withdrawn from the vessel, to minimize hydrolysis.] Determine the amount of $C_8H_8Cl_3N_3O_4S_2$ dissolved, employing the procedure set forth in the *Assay*, making any necessary volumetric adjustments.
 Tolerances—Not less than 65% (*Q*) of the labeled amount of $C_8H_8Cl_3N_3O_4S_2$ is dissolved in 60 minutes.
Uniformity of dosage units ⟨905⟩: meet the requirements.
Assay—
 Mobile phase and *Chromatographic system*—Prepare as directed in the *Assay* under *Trichlormethiazide.*
 Acidic methanol—Add 2.8 mL of sulfuric acid to 100 mL of water, mix, and cool. Dilute with methanol to 1000 mL, and mix.
 Internal standard solution—Transfer about 20 mg of methylparaben to a 200-mL volumetric flask, add *Acidic methanol* to volume, and mix.
 Standard preparation—Transfer about 20 mg of USP Trichlormethiazide RS, accurately weighed, to a 50-mL volumetric flask, add *Acidic methanol* to volume, and mix. Transfer 5.0 mL of this solution to a centrifuge tube, add 5.0 mL of *Internal standard solution*, and mix to obtain a solution having a known concentration of about 0.2 mg of USP Trichlormethiazide RS per mL.
 Assay preparation—Weigh and finely powder not less than 20 Tablets. Transfer an accurately weighed portion of the powder, equivalent to 2 mg of trichlormethiazide, to a centrifuge tube. Add 5.0 mL of *Acidic methanol* and 5.0 mL of *Internal standard solution*, and mix to disperse the powder. Insert the stopper in the tube, rotate by mechanical means for 20 minutes, and centrifuge to obtain a clear supernatant.
 Procedure—Separately inject equal volumes (5 µL to 25 µL) of the *Standard preparation* and the *Assay preparation* into the chromatograph, record the chromatograms, and measure the responses for the major peaks. The relative retention times are about 0.58 for trichlormethiazide and 1.0 for methylparaben. Calculate the quantity, in mg, of $C_8H_8Cl_3N_3O_4S_2$ in the portion of Tablets taken by the formula:

$$10C(R_U / R_S)$$

in which *C* is the concentration, in mg per mL, of USP Trichlormethiazide RS in the *Standard preparation*, and R_U and R_S are the peak response ratios obtained from the *Assay preparation* and the *Standard preparation*, respectively.

Tricitrates Oral Solution

» Tricitrates Oral Solution is a solution of Sodium Citrate, Potassium Citrate, and Citric Acid in a suitable aqueous medium. It contains, in each 100 mL, not less than 2.23 g and not more than 2.46 g of sodium (Na), equivalent to not less than 9.5 g and not more than 10.5 g of sodium citrate dihydrate ($C_6H_5Na_3O_7 \cdot 2H_2O$); not less than 3.78 g and not more than 4.18 g of potassium (K), equivalent to not less than 10.45 g and not more than 11.55 g of potassium citrate monohydrate ($C_6H_5K_3O_7 \cdot H_2O$); not less than 12.20 g and not more than 13.48 g of citrate ($C_6H_5O_7$) as sodium citrate and potassium citrate; and not less than 6.34 g and not more than 7.02 g of citric acid monohydrate ($C_6H_8O_7 \cdot H_2O$).

NOTE—The sodium and potassium ion contents of Tricitrates Oral Solution are each approximately 1 mEq per mL.

Packaging and storage—Preserve in tight containers.
USP Reference standards ⟨11⟩—*USP Citric Acid RS.*
(Official January 1, 2009)
Identification—
 A: It responds to the flame test for *Sodium* ⟨191⟩.
 B: Add 2 mL of a solution of anhydrous potassium carbonate (15 in 100) to 2 mL of Oral Solution, boil, and cool. Add 4 mL of potassium pyroantimonate TS: a dense precipitate is formed (*presence of sodium*).
 C: To 2 mL of a dilution of Oral Solution (1 in 20) add 5 mL of sodium cobaltinitrite TS: a yellow precipitate is formed immediately (*presence of potassium*).
 D: It responds to the tests for *Citrate* ⟨191⟩, 3 to 5 drops of Oral Solution and 20 mL of the mixture of pyridine and acetic anhydride being used.
pH ⟨791⟩: between 4.9 and 5.4.
Assay for sodium and potassium—
 Sodium stock solution—Transfer 14.61 g of sodium chloride, previously dried at 105° for 2 hours and accurately weighed, to a 250-mL volumetric flask, add water to volume, and mix.
 Potassium stock solution—Transfer 18.64 g of potassium chloride, previously dried at 105° for 2 hours and accurately weighed, to a 250-mL volumetric flask, add water to volume, and mix.
 Lithium diluent solution—Transfer 1.04 g of lithium nitrate to a 1000-mL volumetric flask, add a suitable nonionic surfactant, then add water to volume, and mix. This solution contains 15 mEq of Li per 1000 mL.
 Standard preparation—Pipet 50 mL of *Sodium stock solution* and 50 mL of *Potassium stock solution* into a 500-mL volumetric flask, dilute with water to volume, and mix. Each mL of this solution contains 0.1 mEq of Na and 0.1 mEq of K. Transfer 50 μL of this solution to a 10-mL volumetric flask, dilute with *Lithium diluent solution* to volume, and mix.
 Assay preparation—Transfer an accurately measured volume of Oral Solution, equivalent to about 2 g of combined citrates, to a 100-mL volumetric flask, dilute with water to volume, and mix. Transfer 50 μL of this solution to a 10-mL volumetric flask, dilute with *Lithium diluent solution* to volume, and mix.
 Procedure—Using a suitable flame photometer, adjusted to read zero with *Lithium diluent solution*, concomitantly determine the sodium flame emission readings for the *Standard preparation* and the *Assay preparation* at the wavelength of maximum emission at about 589 nm. Similarly determine the potassium flame emission readings for the same solutions at the wavelength of maximum emission at about 766 nm. Calculate the quantity, in g, of Na in the portion of Oral Solution taken by the formula:

$$(14.61/25)(22.99/58.44)(R_{U,Na} / R_{S,Na})$$

in which 14.61 is the weight, in g, of sodium chloride in the *Sodium stock solution;* 22.99 is the atomic weight of sodium; 58.44 is the molecular weight of sodium chloride; and $R_{U,Na}$ and $R_{S,Na}$ are the sodium emission readings obtained for the *Assay preparation* and the *Standard preparation*, respectively. Calculate the quantity, in g, of K in the portion of Oral Solution taken by the formula:

$$(18.64/25)(39.10/74.55)(R_{U,K} / R_{S,K})$$

in which 18.64 is the weight, in g, of potassium chloride in the *Potassium stock solution;* 39.10 is the atomic weight of potassium; 74.55 is the molecular weight of potassium chloride; and $R_{U,K}$ and $R_{S,K}$ are the potassium emission readings obtained from the *Assay preparation* and the *Standard preparation*, respectively.
Assay for citrate—
 Cation-exchange column—Mix 10 g of styrene-divinylbenzene cation-exchange resin with 50 mL of water in a suitable beaker. Allow the resin to settle, and decant the supernatant until a slurry of resin remains. Pour the slurry into a 15-mm × 30-cm glass chromatographic tube (having a sealed-in, coarse-porosity fritted disk and fitted with a stopcock), and allow to settle as a homogeneous bed. Wash the resin bed with about 100 mL of water, closing the stopcock when the water level is about 2 mm above the resin bed.
 Procedure—Pipet 15 mL of Oral Solution into a 250-mL volumetric flask, dilute with water to volume, and mix. Pipet 5 mL of this solution carefully onto the top of the resin bed in the *Cation-exchange column*. Place a 250-mL conical flask below the column, open the stopcock, and allow to flow until the solution has entered the resin bed. Elute the column with 60 mL of water at a flow rate of about 5 mL per minute, collecting about 65 mL of eluate. Add 5 drops of phenolphthalein TS to the eluate, swirl the flask, and titrate with 0.02 N sodium hydroxide VS. Record the buret reading, and calculate the volume (*B*) of 0.02 N sodium hydroxide consumed. Each mL of the difference between the volume (*B*) and the volume (*A*) of 0.02 N sodium hydroxide consumed in the *Assay for citric acid* is equivalent to 1.261 mg of $C_6H_5O_7$.

(Official until January 1, 2009)

Assay for citrate—
 Mobile phase, Standard Preparation 1, and *Chromatographic System*—Proceed as directed under *Assay for Citric Acid/Citrate and Phosphate* ⟨345⟩.
 Assay preparation—Pipet 15 mL of Oral Solution into a suitable volumetric flask, and proceed as directed for *Assay Preparation for Citric Acid/Citrate Assay* under *Assay for Citric Acid/Citrate and Phosphate* ⟨345⟩.
 Procedure—Proceed as directed for *Procedure* under ⟨345⟩, and calculate the concentration, in mg per mL, of citrate ($C_6H_5O_7$) in the Oral Solution taken by the formula:

$$0.001 C_S (D/V)(r_U / r_S) - A(189.10 / 210.14)$$

in which C_S is the concentration, in μg per mL, of citrate in *Standard Preparation 1; D* is the dilution factor; *V* is the volume of Oral Solution used in the preparation of the *Assay preparation;* r_U and r_S are the citrate peak areas obtained from the *Assay preparation* and *Standard Preparation 1,* respectively; 189.10 is the molecular weight of citrate ($C_6H_5O_7$); 210.14 is the molecular weight of citric acid monohydrate ($C_6H_8O_7 \cdot H_2O$); and *A* is the concentration of citric acid monohydrate, in mg per mL, determined in the *Assay for citric acid.*

(Official January 1, 2009)

Assay for citric acid—Transfer 15 mL of Oral Solution, accurately measured, to a 250-mL volumetric flask, dilute with water to volume, and mix. Pipet 5 mL of this solution into a suitable flask, add 25 mL of water and 5 drops of phenolphthalein TS, and titrate with 0.02 N sodium hydroxide VS to a pink endpoint. Record the buret reading, and calculate the volume (*A*) of 0.02 N sodium hydroxide consumed. Each mL of 0.02 N sodium hydroxide is equivalent to 1.401 mg of $C_6H_8O_7 \cdot H_2O$.

Triclosan

$C_{12}H_7Cl_3O_2$ 289.54
Phenol, 5-chloro-2-(2,4-dichlorophenoxy)-.
2,4,4′-Trichloro-2′-hydroxydiphenyl ether   [3380-34-5].

» Triclosan contains not less than 97.0 percent and not more than 103.0 percent of $C_{12}H_7Cl_3O_2$, calculated on the anhydrous basis.

Packaging and storage—Preserve in tight, light-resistant containers.

USP Reference standards ⟨11⟩—*USP 2,4-Dichlorophenol RS. USP Parachlorophenol RS. USP Triclosan RS. USP Triclosan Related Compounds Mixture A RS.*

Identification—
  A: *Infrared Absorption* ⟨197K⟩.
  B: The retention time of the major peak in the chromatogram of the *Assay preparation* corresponds to that in the chromatogram of the *Standard preparation*, as obtained in the *Assay*.
Water, *Method I* ⟨921⟩: not more than 0.1%.
Residue on ignition ⟨281⟩: not more than 0.1%.
Heavy metals, *Method II* ⟨231⟩: 0.002%.
Related compounds—
  Chromatographic system—Proceed as directed in the *Assay*.
  Test solution—Use the *Assay preparation*.
  Procedure—Inject a volume (about 0.5 µL) of the *Test solution* into the chromatograph, increase the column temperature by 20° per minute to 140°, then increase column temperature by 4° per minute to 240°, maintain this temperature for not less than 5 minutes, record the chromatogram, and measure the peak responses. Calculate the percentage of each impurity in the portion of Triclosan taken by the formula:

$$100(r_i / r_s)$$

in which r_i is the peak response for each impurity; and r_s is the sum of the responses of all of the peaks: not more than 0.1% of any individual impurity is found; and not more than 0.5% of total impurities is found.
Limit of monochlorophenols and 2,4-dichlorophenol—
  Phosphate buffer—Transfer about 1.38 g of anhydrous monobasic sodium phosphate and about 1.42 g of dibasic sodium phosphate to a 1-L volumetric flask, dissolve in and dilute with water to volume, and mix.
  Mobile phase—Prepare a filtered and degassed mixture of acetonitrile and *Phosphate buffer* (1 : 1). Make adjustments if necessary (see *System Suitability* under *Chromatography* ⟨621⟩).
  Standard solution—Quantitatively dissolve accurately weighed quantities of USP Parachlorophenol RS and USP 2,4-Dichlorophenol RS in acetonitrile, dilute with an equal volume of water, and mix. Transfer a portion of this solution to a suitable container, and dilute quantitatively, and stepwise if necessary, with a mixture of acetonitrile and water (1 : 1) to obtain a solution having known concentrations of about 0.5 µg of parachlorophenol and 0.1 µg of 2,4-dichlorophenol per mL.
  Test solution—Transfer about 250 mg of Triclosan, accurately weighed, to a 25-mL low-actinic volumetric flask, dissolve in 20 mL of acetonitrile, dilute with water to volume, and mix.
  Chromatographic system (see *Chromatography* ⟨621⟩)—The liquid chromatograph is equipped with a coulometric electrochemical detector with electrode 1 set at 0.45 V and electrode 2 set at 0.75 V, both having a positive (oxidative) polarity and a 4.6-mm × 25-cm column that contains packing L1. The flow rate is about 1 mL per minute. Chromatograph the *Standard solution,* and record the peak responses as directed for *Procedure*:the relative standard deviation for replicate injections is not more than 9.0% for 2,4-dichlorophenol.
  Procedure—Separately inject equal volumes (about 20 µL) of the *Standard solution* and the *Test solution* into the chromatograph, record the chromatograms, and measure the peak responses. The peak responses for parachlorophenol and 2,4-dichlorophenol in the chromatogram of the *Test solution* are not greater than the corresponding peaks in the chromatogram of the *Standard solution*.
Limit of 1,3,7-trichlorodibenzo-*p*-dioxin, 2,8-dichlorodibenzo-*p*-dioxin, 2,8-dichlorodibenzofuran, and 2,4,8-trichlorodibenzofuran—
  Mobile phase—Prepare a filtered and degassed mixture of acetonitrile, water, and glacial acetic acid (70 : 30 : 0.1). Make adjustments if necessary (see *System Suitability* under *Chromatography* ⟨621⟩).
  Test solution—Transfer about 2.0 g of Triclosan, accurately weighed, to a screw-capped centrifuge tube, add 5 mL of 2 N potassium hydroxide, and shake for 10 minutes to dissolve. Add 3 mL of *n*-hexane, shake for 10 minutes, and allow the phases to separate. Transfer the organic layer to a suitable container, add another 3 mL of *n*-hexane to the aqueous layer, shake for 10 minutes, and allow the phases to separate. Transfer the organic layer to the previous extract, discard the aqueous layer, add 3 mL of 2 N potassium hydroxide to the combined organic layers, shake for 10 minutes, and allow the phases to separate. Discard the aqueous layer, add another 3 mL of 2 N potassium hydroxide to the combined organic layers, shake for 10 minutes, and allow the phases to separate. Transfer the organic layer to a suitable container, and evaporate with the aid of a stream of nitrogen to dryness. Dissolve the residue in 1.0 mL of methanol, and mix.
  Chromatographic system (see *Chromatography* ⟨621⟩)—The liquid chromatograph is equipped with a 220-nm detector and a 4.6-mm × 25-cm column that contains packing L1. The flow rate is about 1.5 mL per minute. Chromatograph the USP Triclosan Related Compounds Mixture A RS, and record the peak responses as directed for *Procedure*:the relative retention times are about 0.59 for 2,8-dichlorodibenzofuran, 0.71 for 2,8-dichlorodibenzo-*p*-dioxin, 0.88 for 2,4,8-trichlorodibenzofuran, and 1.0 for 1,3,7-trichlorodibenzo-*p*-dioxin; and the relative standard deviation for replicate injections is not more than 15.0%, determined from the 2,8-dichlorodibenzo-*p*-dioxin peak.
  Procedure—Inject a volume (about 20 µL) of the *Test solution* into the chromatograph, record the chromatogram, and measure the peak responses. Calculate the concentration of each analyte in the portion of Triclosan taken by the formula:

$$(C / W)(r_i / r_S)$$

in which C is the concentration, in µg per mL, of the respective analyte in the USP Triclosan Related Compounds Mixture A RS; W is the weight, in g, of Triclosan taken; and r_i and r_S are the peak responses for the respective analyte obtained from the *Test solution* and the USP Triclosan Related Compounds Mixture A RS, respectively: not more than 0.25 ppm of 2,8-dichlorodibenzofuran is found; not more than 0.5 ppm of 2,4,8-trichlorodibenzofuran is found; not more than 0.25 ppm of 1,3,7-trichlorodibenzo-*p*-dioxin is found; and not more than 0.5 ppm of 2,8-dichlorodibenzo-*p*-dioxin is found.
Limit of 2,3,7,8-tetrachlorodibenzo-*p*-dioxin and 2,3,7,8-tetrachlorodibenzofuran—[*Caution—2,3,7,8-tetrachlorodibenzo-p-dioxin and 2,3,7,8-tetrachlorodibenzofuran are extremely toxic substances. Exercise all necessary precautions in the conduct of this procedure.*]
  Stationary phase A—Transfer about 10 g of silica gel to a suitable container, add about 3 mL of 1 N sodium hydroxide, and mix.
  Stationary phase B—Transfer about 60 g of silica gel to a suitable container, add about 74 mL of concentrated sulfuric acid, and mix.
  Chromatographic column A—Transfer 5.1 g of *Stationary phase A*, 0.5 g of silica gel, 6.2 g of *Stationary phase B*, and 3.2 g of sodium sulfate to a glass chromatographic column having an internal diameter of 10 mm. Wash the column with 50 mL of *n*-hexane, and discard the eluate.
  Chromatographic column B—Transfer 2.5 g of alumina and 2.5 g of sodium sulfate to a glass chromatographic column having an internal diameter of 6 mm. Wash the column with 30 mL of *n*-hexane, and discard the eluate.
  Internal standard solution—Transfer accurately measured quantities of 2,3,7,8-tetrachlorodibenzo-*p*-dioxin, ^{13}C-labeled, and 2,3,7,8-tetrachlorodibenzofuran, ^{13}C-labeled, in nonane, and dilute quantitatively, and stepwise if necessary, with 2,2,4-trimethylpentane to obtain a solution having known concentrations of about 1.0 pg of each per µL.
  Test solution—Transfer about 30 g of Triclosan, accurately weighed, to a separatory funnel, add 30 µL of *Internal standard solution*, dissolve in 200 mL of 1 N sodium hydroxide, extract with four 30-mL portions of *n*-hexane, and combine the extracts. Wash the combined extracts with 20 mL of water, extract the washing with 15 mL of *n*-hexane, and add the extract to the other combined extracts. Add about 3 g of anhydrous sodium sulfate to the combined extracts, allow to stand for 30 minutes, quantitatively transfer to an appropriate round-bottom flask, and distill, using a distillation apparatus with a vigreux column, until about 1 mL remains. Transfer this solution to the top of *Chromatographic column A*, and elute with 50 mL of *n*-hexane. Collect the eluate on top of *Chromatographic column B*, and elute with 30 mL of a mixture of *n*-hexane and methylene chloride (98 : 2), discarding the eluate. Elute with 40 mL of a mixture of *n*-hexane and methylene chloride (1 : 1), collecting the eluates in a round-bottom flask. Distill the combined eluates, using a distillation apparatus with a vigreux column, until about 1 mL remains. Further concentrate this solution with the aid

of a stream of nitrogen to about 50 µL, evaporate at room temperature to dryness, and dissolve in 10 µL of 2,2,4-trimethylpentane.

Chromatographic system (see *Chromatography* ⟨621⟩ and *Mass Spectrometry* ⟨736⟩)—The gas chromatograph is equipped with a high-resolution mass spectrograph with an electron-impact ionization source and a 0.25-mm × 60-m capillary column coated with phase G48. The carrier gas is helium. The chromatograph is programmed as follows. Initially the temperature of the column is equilibrated at 80°, then, 1 minute after the injection, the temperature is increased at a rate of 20° per minute to 220°, then increased at a rate of 2° per minute to 270°, and maintained at 270° for not less than 20 minutes. The injection port temperature is maintained at 280°. Chromatograph the *Internal standard solution*, and record the peak responses as directed for *Procedure*: the signal-to-noise ratio at a mass-to-charge ratio of 321.89 is not less than 50.

Procedure—Inject a volume (about 1 µL) of the *Test solution* into the chromatograph, record the chromatograms, and measure the peak responses at mass-to-charge ratios of 319.90, 321.89, 331.88, 333.93, 303.90, 305.90, 315.94, and 317.94. The peak response for 2,3,7,8-tetrachlorodibenzo-*p*-dioxin at a mass-to-charge ratio of 319.90 is not more than the peak response of the associated internal standard at a mass-to-charge ratio of 331.88; the peak response for 2,3,7,8-tetrachlorodibenzofuran at a mass-to-charge ratio of 303.90 is not more than the peak response of the associated internal standard at a mass-to-charge ratio of 315.94.

Assay—
Standard preparation—Dissolve an accurately weighed quantity of USP Triclosan RS in ethyl acetate, and dilute quantitatively, and stepwise if necessary, with ethyl acetate to obtain a solution having a known concentration of about 0.4 mg per mL.

Assay preparation—Transfer about 40 mg of Triclosan, accurately weighed, to a 100-mL volumetric flask, dissolve in and dilute with ethyl acetate to volume, and mix.

Chromatographic system (see *Chromatography* ⟨621⟩)—The gas chromatograph is equipped with a flame-ionization detector and a 0.53-mm × 15-m capillary column with phase G3. The carrier gas is helium maintained at about 6 psi. The injection port temperature is maintained at 34° and is increased rapidly to 200° immediately after the injection, the column temperature is maintained at 34°, and the detector temperature is maintained at 260°. Chromatograph the *Standard preparation*, and record the peak responses as directed for *Procedure*: the relative standard deviation for replicate injections is not more than 2.0%.

Procedure—Separately inject equal volumes (about 2.0 µL) of the *Standard preparation* and the *Assay preparation* into the chromatograph, increase the column temperature by 20° per minute to 140°, then increase the column temperature by 4° per minute to 240°, maintain this temperature for not less than 5 minutes, record the chromatograms, and measure the responses for the major peaks. Calculate the quantity, in mg, of $C_{12}H_7Cl_3O_2$ in the portion of Triclosan taken by the formula:

$$100C(r_U / r_S)$$

in which C is the concentration, in mg per mL, of USP Triclosan RS in the *Standard preparation*; and r_U and r_S are the peak responses obtained from the *Assay preparation* and the *Standard preparation*, respectively.

Trientine Hydrochloride

$C_6H_{18}N_4 \cdot 2HCl$ 219.16
1,2-Ethanediamine, *N,N'*-bis(2-aminoethyl)-, dihydrochloride.
Triethylenetetramine dihydrochloride   [38260-01-4].

» Trientine Hydrochloride contains not less than 97.0 percent and not more than 103.0 percent of $C_6H_{18}N_4 \cdot 2HCl$, calculated on the dried basis.

Packaging and storage—Preserve under an inert gas in tight, light-resistant containers, and store in a refrigerator.

USP Reference standards ⟨11⟩—*USP Trientine Hydrochloride RS.*
Identification, *Infrared Absorption* ⟨197M⟩.
pH ⟨791⟩: between 7.0 and 8.5, in a solution (1 in 100).
Loss on drying ⟨731⟩—Dry it in vacuum at a pressure not exceeding 5 mm of mercury at 40° for 4 hours: it loses not more than 2.0% of its weight.
Residue on ignition ⟨281⟩: not more than 0.15%.
Heavy metals, *Method II* ⟨231⟩: 0.001%.
Chromatographic purity—The sum of the intensities of all secondary spots obtained from the *Test preparation* in *Part I* and *Part II* corresponds to not more than 2.0%.

Part I—
Spray reagent—Dissolve 300 mg of ninhydrin in a mixture of 100 mL of butyl alcohol and 3 mL of glacial acetic acid.

Standard preparation A—[NOTE—Use low-actinic glassware.] Dissolve an accurately weighed quantity of USP Trientine Hydrochloride RS in methanol to obtain a solution containing 10 mg per mL.

Standard preparation B—[NOTE—Use low-actinic glassware.] Dissolve an accurately weighed quantity of diethylenetriamine in methanol to obtain a solution containing 1.0 mg per mL. Transfer 3.0 mL of this solution to a 100-mL volumetric flask, dilute with methanol to volume, and mix.

Standard preparation C—[NOTE—Use low-actinic glassware.] Dissolve an accurately weighed quantity of 1-(2-aminoethyl)piperazine in methanol to obtain a solution containing 1.0 mg per mL. Transfer 10.0 mL of this solution to a 100-mL volumetric flask, dilute with methanol to volume, and mix.

Standard preparation D—[NOTE—Use low-actinic glassware.] Transfer 5.0 mL of *Standard preparation C* to a 10-mL volumetric flask, dilute with methanol to volume, and mix.

Test preparation—[NOTE—Use low-actinic glassware.] Dissolve an accurately weighed quantity of Trientine Hydrochloride in methanol to obtain a solution containing 10 mg per mL.

Procedure—Apply separately 3 µL each of the *Test preparation*, of *Standard preparation B*, and of *Standard preparation C* to a suitable unwashed, high performance thin-layer chromatographic plate (see *Chromatography* ⟨621⟩) having a 1.5-cm preadsorbent zone and coated with a 0.15-mm layer of chromatographic silica gel mixture. To a fourth spot, apply 3 µL each of *Standard preparations A*, *B*, and *C*. To a fifth spot, apply 3 µL each of *Standard preparations A*, *B*, and *D*. Allow the spots to dry, place the plate in a chromatographic chamber, and develop the chromatograms in a solvent system consisting of a mixture of isopropyl alcohol and ammonium hydroxide (3 : 2) until the solvent front has moved about three-fourths of the length of the plate. Remove the plate from the developing chamber, mark the solvent front, and dry the plate with the aid of a current of air. Spray the plate with *Spray reagent*, dry at 105° for 5 minutes, and observe the plate under long-wavelength UV light. Determine the locus of the diethylenetriamine and the 1-(2-aminoethyl)piperazine spots from the chromatograms of *Standard preparations B* and *C*, respectively. Determine the concentration of diethylenetriamine in the *Test preparation* by comparing the size and intensity of any secondary spot from the chromatogram of the *Test preparation* having an R_F value corresponding to the R_F value of diethylenetriamine with the diethylenetriamine spots obtained from the chromatograms of the *Standard preparation* mixtures. Determine the concentration of any other observed impurities in the *Test preparation* by comparing the size and intensity of any other secondary spots from the chromatogram of the *Test preparation* with the 1-(2-aminoethyl)piperazine spots obtained from the chromatograms of the *Standard preparation* mixtures.

Part II—
Spray reagent—Dissolve 200 mg of ninhydrin in 100 mL of alcohol.

Tris(2-aminoethyl)amine stock solution—[NOTE—Use low-actinic glassware.] Dissolve an accurately weighed quantity of tris(2-aminoethyl)amine in methanol to obtain a solution containing 1.0 mg per mL.

Standard preparation A—[NOTE—Use low-actinic glassware.] Dissolve an accurately weighed quantity of USP Trientine Hydrochloride RS in methanol to obtain a solution containing 10 mg per mL.

Standard preparation B—[NOTE—Use low-actinic glassware.] Transfer 1.0 mL of *Tris(2-aminoethyl)amine stock solution* to a 10-mL volumetric flask, dilute with methanol to volume, and mix.

Standard preparation C—[NOTE—Use low-actinic glassware.] Transfer 0.5 mL of *Tris(2-aminoethyl)amine stock solution* to a 10-mL volumetric flask, dilute with methanol to volume, and mix.

Test preparation—[NOTE—Use low-actinic glassware.] Dissolve an accurately weighed quantity of Trientine Hydrochloride in methanol to obtain a solution containing 10 mg per mL.

Procedure—Apply separately 3 µL each of the *Test preparation* and of *Standard preparation A* to a suitable thin-layer chromatographic plate (see *Chromatography* ⟨621⟩) coated with a 0.25-mm layer of chromatographic silica gel mixture and previously washed with methanol. To a third spot apply 3 µL each of *Standard preparations A* and *B*. To a fourth spot, apply 3 µL each of *Standard preparations A* and *C*. Allow the spots to dry, place the plate in a chromatographic chamber, and develop the chromatograms in a solvent system consisting of a mixture of ammonium hydroxide and alcohol (2 : 1) at a temperature of 2° to 6° until the solvent front has moved about three-fourths of the length of the plate. Remove the plate from the developing chamber, mark the solvent front, and dry the plate with the aid of a current of air. Spray the plate with *Spray reagent*, dry at 105° for 5 minutes, and observe the plate under long-wavelength UV light. Determine the concentration of tris(2-aminoethyl)amine in the *Test preparation* by comparing the size and intensity of any secondary spot from the chromatogram of the *Test preparation* having an R_F value corresponding to the R_F value of tris(2-aminoethyl)amine with the tris(2-aminoethyl)amine spots obtained from the chromatograms of the *Standard preparation* mixtures.

Organic volatile impurities, *Method I* ⟨467⟩: meets the requirements.

(Official until July 1, 2008)
Assay—Dissolve about 220 mg of Trientine Hydrochloride, accurately weighed, in 150 mL of water in a 250-mL beaker. Adjust with hydrochloric acid to a pH of 2.0; then adjust with ammonium hydroxide to a pH of 9.5 ± 0.5; and then adjust with glacial acetic acid to a pH of 5.0. Heat the solution to 90°, and while hot, titrate with 0.1 N cupric nitrate VS, determining the endpoint potentiometrically, using an electrode system consisting of a cupric ion-selective electrode and a calomel reference electrode with an outer filling solution of 1 M potassium nitrate. Perform a blank determination (see *Titrimetry* ⟨541⟩), and make any necessary correction. Each mL of 0.1 N cupric nitrate is equivalent to 21.92 mg of $C_6H_{18}N_4 \cdot 2HCl$.

Trientine Hydrochloride Capsules

» Trientine Hydrochloride Capsules contain not less than 90.0 percent and not more than 110.0 percent of the labeled amount of $C_6H_{18}N_4 \cdot 2HCl$.

Packaging and storage—Preserve in tight containers, and store in a refrigerator.

USP Reference standards ⟨11⟩—*USP Trientine Hydrochloride RS*.

Identification—Triturate an amount of the contents of Capsules, equivalent to about 1.5 mg of trientine hydrochloride, with 0.5 mL of acetone in an agate or mullite mortar. Evaporate in a gentle current of air to dryness. Repeat the acetone addition, trituration, and drying steps: the IR absorption spectrum of a potassium bromide dispersion of the residue so obtained exhibits maxima only at the same wavelengths as that of a similar preparation of USP Trientine Hydrochloride RS.

Dissolution ⟨711⟩—
 Medium: water; 500 mL.
 Apparatus 2: 50 rpm.
 Time: 30 minutes.
 pH 8.2 buffer—Prepare as directed under *Assay*.
 Copper sulfate reagent—Mix 10 mL of copper sulfate solution (5 g copper sulfate pentahydrate in 100 mL of water) with 40 mL of *pH 8.2 buffer*. [NOTE—The solution must be clear.]

 Standard preparation—Dissolve an accurately weighed quantity of USP Trientine Hydrochloride RS in water to obtain a solution having a known concentration of about 0.5 mg per mL.

 Procedure—Pipet an aliquot of a filtered portion of the solution under test, estimated to contain about 5 mg of trientine hydrochloride, into a 50-mL centrifuge tube. Into a similar centrifuge tube, pipet an equivalent volume of water to provide a reagent blank, and into a third centrifuge tube pipet 10 mL of *Standard preparation*. Into each tube, pipet 5 mL of *Copper sulfate reagent*, stopper, and mix immediately using a vortex mixer. Determine the absorbances of the solutions from the *Standard preparation* and the test solution at 580 and 410 nm, with a suitable spectrophotometer, against the reagent blank. Calculate the quantity in mg of trientine hydrochloride dissolved by the formula:

$$5000(C/V)[(A_U - A_{UX})/(A_S - A_{SX})]$$

in which C is the concentration, in mg per mL, of USP Trientine Hydrochloride RS in the *Standard preparation*, V is the volume, in mL, of the aliquot of test solution used, A_U and A_S are the absorbances at 580 nm of test and standard solutions, respectively, and A_{UX} and A_{SX} are the absorbances at 410 nm of test and standard solutions, respectively.

 Tolerances—Not less than 80% (*Q*) of the labeled amount of $C_6H_{18}N_4 \cdot 2HCl$ is dissolved in 30 minutes.

Uniformity of dosage units ⟨905⟩: meet the requirements.

Assay—

 Copper reagent—Dissolve 5 g of copper sulfate pentahydrate in water to make 100 mL, and mix.

 pH 8.2 buffer—Dissolve 20.74 g of anhydrous dibasic sodium phosphate, 6.72 g of anhydrous citric acid, and 0.535 g of monobasic sodium phosphate in 400 mL of water, adjust with sodium hydroxide solution (1 in 2) to a pH of 8.2 ± 0.05, dilute with water to make 500 mL, and mix.

 Standard preparation—Dissolve an accurately weighed quantity of USP Trientine Hydrochloride RS in methanol to obtain a solution having a known concentration of about 2.5 mg per mL. Transfer 5.0 mL of this solution to a glass-stoppered, 50-mL conical flask.

 Assay preparation—Remove, as completely as possible, the contents of not less than 20 Capsules. Weigh the contents, and determine the average weight per capsule. Mix the combined contents, and transfer an accurately weighed quantity of the powder, equivalent to about 250 mg of trientine hydrochloride, to a 100-mL volumetric flask. Add about 70 mL of methanol, and shake or sonicate to dissolve. Dilute with methanol to volume, mix, and filter, discarding the first few mL of the filtrate. Transfer 5.0 mL of this solution to a glass-stoppered, 50-mL conical flask.

 Procedure—To each of the flasks containing the *Standard preparation* and the *Assay preparation* and to a similar flask containing 5.0 mL of methanol to provide the blank, add 10.0 mL of *pH 8.2 buffer* and 1.0 mL of *Copper reagent*, and mix. Concomitantly determine the absorbances of the solutions at the wavelength of maximum absorbance at about 580 nm, with a suitable spectrophotometer, against the blank. Calculate the quantity, in mg, of $C_6H_{18}N_4 \cdot 2HCl$ in the portion of Capsules taken by the formula:

$$100C(A_U/A_S)$$

in which C is the concentration, in mg per mL, of USP Trientine Hydrochloride RS in the *Standard preparation*, and A_U and A_S are the absorbances of the solutions from the *Assay preparation* and the *Standard preparation*, respectively.

Trifluoperazine Hydrochloride

$C_{21}H_{24}F_3N_3S \cdot 2HCl$ 480.42

10*H*-Phenothiazine, 10-[3-(4-methyl-1-piperazinyl)propyl-[2-(trifluoromethyl)-, dihydrochloride.
10-[3-(4-Methyl-1-piperazinyl)propyl-[2-(trifluoromethyl)phenothiazine dihydrochloride   [440-17-5].

» Trifluoperazine Hydrochloride, dried in vacuum at 60° for 4 hours, contains not less than 98.0 percent and not more than 101.0 percent of $C_{21}H_{24}F_3N_3S \cdot 2HCl$.

Packaging and storage—Preserve in tight, light-resistant containers. Store at 25°, excursions permitted between 15° and 30°.

USP Reference standards ⟨11⟩—*USP Trifluoperazine Hydrochloride RS.*

NOTE—Throughout the following procedures, protect test or assay specimens, the Reference Standard, and solutions containing them, by conducting the procedures without delay, under subdued light, or by using low-actinic glassware.

Identification—
   A: *Infrared Absorption* ⟨197M⟩.
   B: *Ultraviolet Absorption* ⟨197U⟩—
   Solution: 10 µg per mL.
   Medium: 0.1 N hydrochloric acid.
   Absorptivities at 255 nm, calculated on the dried basis, do not differ by more than 2.0%.
   C: A solution (1 in 100) responds to the tests for *Chloride* ⟨191⟩.
   D: Prepare a solution in methanol containing 1.2 mg per mL. Apply 5 µL each of this solution and a solution of USP Trifluoperazine Hydrochloride RS in methanol containing 1.2 mg per mL to a suitable thin-layer chromatographic plate (see *Chromatography* ⟨621⟩) coated with a 0.25-mm layer of chromatographic silica gel. Allow the spots to dry, and develop the chromatogram in a solvent system consisting of a mixture of acetone and ammonium hydroxide (200 : 1) until the solvent front has moved about three-fourths of the length of the plate. Remove the plate from the developing chamber, mark the solvent front, and allow the solvent to evaporate. Locate the spots on the plate by lightly spraying with a solution of iodoplatinic acid prepared by dissolving 100 mg of chloroplatinic acid in 1 mL of 1 N hydrochloric acid, adding 25 mL of potassium iodide solution (1 in 25), diluting with water to 100 mL, and then adding 0.5 mL of formic acid: the R_F value of the principal spot from the test solution corresponds to that from the Standard solution.

pH ⟨791⟩:   between 1.7 and 2.6, in a solution (1 in 20).

Loss on drying ⟨731⟩—Dry it in vacuum at 60° for 4 hours: it loses not more than 1.5% of its weight.

Residue on ignition ⟨281⟩:   not more than 0.1%.

Organic volatile impurities, *Method I* ⟨467⟩:   meets the requirements.

(Official until July 1, 2008)

Assay—Dissolve about 500 mg of Trifluoperazine Hydrochloride, previously dried and accurately weighed, in 50 mL of glacial acetic acid, and add crystal violet TS and 15 mL of mercuric acetate TS. Titrate with 0.1 N perchloric acid VS to a blue-green endpoint. Perform a blank determination, and make any necessary correction. Each mL of 0.1 N perchloric acid is equivalent to 24.02 mg of $C_{21}H_{24}F_3N_3S \cdot 2HCl$.

Trifluoperazine Hydrochloride Injection

» Trifluoperazine Hydrochloride Injection is a sterile solution of Trifluoperazine Hydrochloride in Water for Injection. It contains an amount of trifluoperazine hydrochloride ($C_{21}H_{24}F_3N_3S \cdot 2HCl$) equivalent to not less than 90.0 percent and not more than 110.0 percent of the labeled amount of trifluoperazine ($C_{21}H_{24}F_3N_3S$).

Packaging and storage—Preserve in multiple-dose containers, preferably of Type I glass, protected from light.

USP Reference standards ⟨11⟩—*USP Trifluoperazine Hydrochloride RS. USP Endotoxin RS.*

NOTE—Throughout the following procedures, protect test or assay specimens, the Reference Standard, and solutions containing them, by conducting the procedures without delay, under subdued light, or using low-actinic glassware.

Identification—
   A: The solution employed for measurement of absorbance in the *Assay* exhibits UV maxima and minima at the same wavelengths as that of a similar solution of USP Trifluoperazine Hydrochloride RS, concomitantly measured.
   B: Mix 5 mL of it with 5 mL of methanol: a 5-µL portion of this solution responds to *Identification* test D under *Trifluoperazine Hydrochloride*.

Bacterial endotoxins ⟨85⟩—It contains not more than 172.0 USP Endotoxin Units per mg of trifluoperazine.

pH ⟨791⟩:   between 4.0 and 5.0.

Other requirements—It meets the requirements under *Injections* ⟨1⟩.

Assay—[NOTE—Use low-actinic glassware.] Transfer an accurately measured volume of Injection, equivalent to about 20 mg of trifluoperazine, to a 250-mL separator. Add 10 mL of 4 N sulfuric acid, and extract with three 25-mL portions of carbon tetrachloride. Discard the carbon tetrachloride after each extraction. Add 10 mL of ammonium hydroxide, and extract with five 40-mL portions of cyclohexane. Extract the combined cyclohexane extracts with five 50-mL portions of 0.1 N hydrochloric acid, collecting the aqueous extracts in a 500-mL volumetric flask. Dilute with 0.1 N hydrochloric acid to volume, and mix. Transfer 25.0 mL of this solution to a 100-mL volumetric flask, dilute with 0.1 N hydrochloric acid to volume, and mix. Concomitantly determine the absorbances of this solution and of a Standard solution of USP Trifluoperazine Hydrochloride RS in the same medium having a known concentration of about 12 µg per mL in 1-cm cells at 278 nm and at the maximum at about 255 nm, with a suitable spectrophotometer, using 0.1 N hydrochloric acid as the blank. Calculate the quantity, in mg, of trifluoperazine ($C_{21}H_{24}F_3N_3S$) in each mL of the Injection taken by the formula:

$$(407.51/480.43)(2C/V)(A_{255} - A_{278})_U / (A_{255} - A_{278})_S$$

in which 407.51 and 480.43 are the molecular weights of trifluoperazine and trifluoperazine hydrochloride, respectively, *C* is the concentration, in µg per mL, of USP Trifluoperazine Hydrochloride RS in the Standard solution, *V* is the volume, in mL, of Injection taken, and the parenthetic expressions are the differences in the absorbances of the two solutions at the wavelengths indicated by the subscripts, for the assay solution (*U*) and the Standard solution (*S*), respectively.

Trifluoperazine Oral Solution

» Trifluoperazine Oral Solution contains an amount of trifluoperazine hydrochloride ($C_{21}H_{24}F_3N_3S \cdot 2HCl$) equivalent to not less than 93.0 percent and not more than 107.0 percent of the labeled amount of trifluoperazine ($C_{21}H_{24}F_3N_3S$).

Packaging and storage—Preserve in tight, light-resistant containers.

USP Reference standards ⟨11⟩—*USP Trifluoperazine Hydrochloride RS.*

NOTE—Throughout the following procedures, protect test or assay specimens, the Reference Standard, and solutions containing them, by conducting the procedures without delay, under subdued light, or using low-actinic glassware.

Identification—

A: *Ultraviolet Absorption* ⟨197U⟩—
  Solution: Prepared as directed in the *Assay.*
B: Mix 1 mL of Oral Solution with 5 mL of methanol: a 5-μL portion of this solution meets the requirements of *Identification* test D under *Trifluoperazine Hydrochloride.*

pH ⟨791⟩: between 2.0 and 3.2.

Assay—[NOTE—Use low-actinic glassware.] Transfer an accurately measured volume of Oral Solution, equivalent to about 50 mg of trifluoperazine, to a 250-mL separator with the aid of about 100 mL of water. Add 10 mL of sodium hydroxide solution (1 in 10), and extract with three 50-mL portions of cyclohexane. Wash the combined cyclohexane extracts with about 20 mL of water, and discard the water washing. Extract the combined cyclohexane extracts with four 50-mL portions of 0.1 N hydrochloric acid, collecting the aqueous extracts in a 500-mL volumetric flask. Dilute with 0.1 N hydrochloric acid to volume, and mix. Transfer 10.0 mL of this solution to a 100-mL volumetric flask, dilute with 0.1 N hydrochloric acid to volume, and mix. Concomitantly determine the absorbances of this solution and of a Standard solution of USP Trifluoperazine Hydrochloride RS in the same medium having a known concentration of about 12 μg per mL in 1-cm cells at 278 nm and at the wavelength of maximum absorbance at about 255 nm, with a suitable spectrophotometer, using 0.1 N hydrochloric acid as the blank. Calculate the quantity, in mg, of trifluoperazine ($C_{21}H_{24}F_3N_3S$) in each mL of the Oral Solution taken by the formula:

$$(407.51/480.43)(5C/V)(A_{255} - A_{278})_U / (A_{255} - A_{278})_S$$

in which 407.51 and 480.43 are the molecular weights of trifluoperazine and trifluoperazine hydrochloride, respectively; C is the concentration, in μg per mL, of USP Trifluoperazine Hydrochloride RS in the Standard solution; V is the volume, in mL, of Oral Solution taken; and the parenthetic expressions are the differences in the absorbances of the two solutions at the wavelengths indicated by the subscripts, for the assay solution (U) and the Standard solution (S), respectively.

Trifluoperazine Hydrochloride Tablets

» Trifluoperazine Hydrochloride Tablets contain an amount of trifluoperazine hydrochloride ($C_{21}H_{24}F_3N_3S \cdot 2HCl$) equivalent to not less than 93.0 percent and not more than 107.0 percent of the labeled amount of trifluoperazine ($C_{21}H_{24}F_3N_3S$).

Packaging and storage—Preserve in well-closed, light-resistant containers.

USP Reference standards ⟨11⟩—*USP Trifluoperazine Hydrochloride RS.*

NOTE—Throughout the following procedures, protect test or assay specimens, the Reference Standard, and solutions containing them, by conducting the procedures without delay, under subdued light, or using low-actinic glassware.

Identification—

A: The UV absorption spectrum of the solution employed for measurement of absorbance in the *Assay* exhibits maxima and minima at the same wavelengths as that of a similar solution of USP Trifluoperazine Hydrochloride RS, concomitantly measured.

B: Triturate a portion of powdered Tablets, equivalent to about 10 mg of trifluoperazine, with 10 mL of methanol, and centrifuge. A 5-μL portion of this solution responds to *Identification* test D under *Trifluoperazine Hydrochloride.*

Dissolution ⟨711⟩—
  Medium: 0.1 N hydrochloric acid; 900 mL.
  Apparatus 1: 50 rpm.
  Time: 30 minutes.
  Procedure—Determine the amount of trifluoperazine ($C_{21}H_{24}F_3N_3S$) dissolved from UV absorbances at the wavelength of maximum absorbance at about 255 nm (determine the analytical value to be used for the absorbance at 255 nm by subtracting the absorbance at 278 nm from the observed maximum absorbance at 255 nm), using filtered portions of the solution under test, suitably diluted with 0.1 N hydrochloric acid, in comparison with a Standard solution having a known concentration of USP Trifluoperazine Hydrochloride RS in the same medium.
  Tolerances—Not less than 75% (*Q*) of the labeled amount of $C_{21}H_{24}F_3N_3S$ is dissolved in 30 minutes.

Uniformity of dosage units ⟨905⟩: meet the requirements for *Content Uniformity.*

Assay—
  Mobile phase—To 2.9 g of *dl*-10-camphorsulfonic acid, add 200 mL of water and stir until solution is complete. Adjust with 1 N sodium hydroxide to a pH of 3.0, dilute with methanol to 1000 mL, mix, and filter through a 0.45-μm membrane filter.
  Standard preparation—Dissolve an accurately weighed quantity of USP Trifluoperazine Hydrochloride RS in methanol to obtain a solution having a known concentration of about 12 μg of trifluoperazine hydrochloride per mL (10 μg of trifluoperazine per mL).
  Assay preparation—Weigh and finely powder not less than 20 Tablets. Weigh accurately a portion of the powder, equivalent to about 20 mg of trifluoperazine, add to a 100-mL volumetric flask, dilute with methanol to volume, and mix. Transfer 5.0 mL of this solution to a second 100-mL volumetric flask, dilute with methanol to volume, and mix. Filter the solution through a 0.45-μm filter.
  Chromatographic system (see *Chromatography* ⟨621⟩)—The liquid chromatograph is equipped with a 262-nm detector and a 4.6-mm × 25-cm column that contains packing L1. The flow rate is about 1.5 mL per minute. Chromatograph replicate injections of the *Standard preparation*, and record the peak responses as directed for *Procedure*: the relative standard deviation for replicate injections is not more than 2.0%, and the tailing factor for the trifluoperazine peak is not more than 2.0.
  Procedure—Separately inject equal volumes (about 20 μL) of the *Standard preparation* and the *Assay preparation* into the chromatograph, record the chromatograms, and measure the responses for the major peaks. Calculate the quantity, in mg, of $C_{21}H_{24}F_3N_3S$, in the portion of Tablets taken by the formula:

$$2(407.51 / 480.43)C(r_U / r_S)$$

in which 407.51 and 480.43 are the molecular weights of trifluoperazine and trifluoperazine hydrochloride, respectively, C is the concentration, in mg per mL, of USP Trifluoperazine Hydrochloride RS in the *Standard preparation*, and r_U and r_S are the peak responses obtained from the *Assay preparation* and the *Standard preparation*, respectively.

Triflupromazine

$C_{18}H_{19}F_3N_2S$ 352.42

10*H*-Phenothiazine-10-propanamine, *N,N*-dimethyl-2-(trifluoromethyl)-.

10-3-(Dimethylamino)propyl-2-(trifluoromethyl)phenothiazine [146-54-3].

» Triflupromazine contains not less than 97.0 percent and not more than 103.0 percent of $C_{18}H_{19}F_3N_2S$.

Packaging and storage—Preserve in tight, light-resistant containers.

USP Reference standards ⟨11⟩—*USP Triflupromazine Hydrochloride RS*.
NOTE—Throughout the following procedures, protect test or assay specimens, the Reference Standard, and solutions containing them, by conducting the procedures without delay, under subdued light, or using low-actinic glassware.

Identification—
A: It meets the requirements under *Identification—Organic Nitrogenous Bases* ⟨181⟩, USP Triflupromazine Hydrochloride RS being used, and 0.01 N hydrochloric acid being used in place of water to dissolve the specimen.
B: *Ultraviolet Absorption* ⟨197U⟩—
Solution: 7 µg per mL.
Medium: 0.5 N sulfuric acid.
Absorptivities at 255 nm do not differ by more than 3.0%.

Residue on ignition ⟨281⟩: not more than 0.2%.

Ordinary impurities ⟨466⟩—
Test solution: acetone.
Standard solution: acetone.
Eluant: a mixture of chloroform and methanol (4 : 1).
Visualization: 1.

Organic volatile impurities, *Method V* ⟨467⟩: meets the requirements.
Solvent—Use dimethyl sulfoxide.
(Official until July 1, 2008)

Assay—Dissolve about 800 mg of Triflupromazine, accurately weighed, in 100 mL of glacial acetic acid. Add crystal violet TS, and titrate with 0.1 N perchloric acid VS to a blue endpoint. Perform a blank determination, and make any necessary correction. Each mL of 0.1 N perchloric acid is equivalent to 35.24 mg of $C_{18}H_{19}F_3N_2S$.

Triflupromazine Oral Suspension

» Triflupromazine Oral Suspension contains an amount of triflupromazine ($C_{18}H_{19}F_3N_2S$) equivalent to not less than 90.0 percent and not more than 110.0 percent of the labeled amount of triflupromazine hydrochloride ($C_{18}H_{19}F_3N_2S \cdot HCl$).

Packaging and storage—Preserve in tight, light-resistant glass containers.

USP Reference standards ⟨11⟩—*USP Triflupromazine Hydrochloride RS*.
NOTE—Throughout the following procedures, protect test or assay specimens, the USP Reference Standard, and solutions containing them, by conducting the procedures without delay, under subdued light, or using low-actinic glassware.

Identification—
A: Transfer about 1.0 mL of Oral Suspension, accurately weighed, to a glass-stoppered, low-actinic 35-mL centrifuge tube; add 10.0 mL of methanol; and shake vigorously by mechanical means for 3 minutes. Centrifuge for 5 minutes, and use the methanol layer for the test. Apply 50 µL of the test solution in streaks 4 to 5 cm in length and 0.2 cm in width and 50 µL of a Standard solution containing 1 mg of USP Triflupromazine Hydrochloride RS per mL of methanol to a suitable thin-layer chromatographic plate (see *Chromatography* ⟨621⟩) coated with a 0.25-mm layer of chromatographic silica gel. Allow the streaks to dry, and develop the chromatogram in a solvent system consisting of a mixture of chloroform and methanol (4 : 1) until the solvent front has moved about four-fifths of the length of the plate. Remove the plate from the developing chamber, mark the solvent front, and allow the solvent to evaporate. Locate the streaks by viewing the plate under short-wavelength and long-wavelength UV light: the R_F value and fluorescence of the streak obtained from the test solution correspond to those obtained from the Standard solution.
B: The UV absorption spectrum of the solution employed for measurement of absorbance in the *Assay* exhibits maxima and minima at the same wavelengths as that of a similar solution of USP Triflupromazine Hydrochloride RS, concomitantly measured.

Uniformity of dosage units ⟨905⟩—
FOR ORAL SUSPENSION PACKAGED IN SNGLE-UNIT CONTAINERS: meets the requirements.

Deliverable volume ⟨698⟩—
FOR ORAL SUSPENSION PACKAGED IN MULTIPLE-UNIT CONTAINERS: meets the requirements.

Assay—
Mixed solvent—Mix 25 mL of isoamyl alcohol with 10 mL of sodium hydroxide solution (1 in 25) in a separator, shake, and discard the aqueous washing. Add 10 mL of 0.1 N hydrochloric acid, shake, and discard the aqueous washing. Prepare 500 mL of a 3 in 100 solution of the washed isoamyl alcohol in *n*-heptane.
pH 5.6 Acetate buffer—Dissolve 1.4 g of sodium acetate in 100 mL of water, and adjust by the addition of glacial acetic acid to a pH of 5.6 ± 0.1.
Procedure—Transfer an accurately measured volume of well-mixed Oral Suspension, equivalent to about 20 mg of triflupromazine hydrochloride, to a glass-stoppered, 150-mL centrifuge bottle. In a second, similar bottle dissolve about 20 mg of USP Triflupromazine Hydrochloride RS, accurately weighed, in 1.0 mL of water; then add 1.0 mL of sodium hydroxide solution (1 in 25); and mix. To a third, similar bottle add 2 mL of water to provide the blank. Treat the two preparations and the blank as follows. Add 100.0 mL of ether, shake by mechanical means for 15 minutes, and allow the layers to separate. Transfer 50.0 mL of the ether layer to another glass-stoppered, 150-mL centrifuge bottle, and evaporate on a water bath maintained at about 35°, with the aid of a current of air, to dryness. Add 5.0 mL of sodium hydroxide solution (1 in 50), mix, add 100.0 mL of *Mixed solvent*, shake by mechanical means for 10 minutes, and centrifuge. Transfer 20.0 mL of the nonaqueous phase to a glass-stoppered centrifuge tube, add 10.0 mL of *pH 5.6 Acetate buffer*, shake by mechanical means for 5 minutes, and centrifuge. Transfer 2.0 mL of the nonaqueous phase to a glass-stoppered centrifuge tube containing 25.0 mL of 0.5 N sulfuric acid, shake by mechanical means for 5 minutes, and centrifuge. Concomitantly determine the absorbances of the aqueous solutions in 1-cm cells at the wavelength of maximum absorbance at about 255 nm, with a suitable spectrophotometer, using the blank to set the instrument. Calculate the quantity, in mg, of triflupromazine hydrochloride ($C_{18}H_{19}F_3N_2S \cdot HCl$) equivalent to the triflupromazine ($C_{18}H_{19}F_3N_2S$) in each mL of the Oral Suspension taken by the formula:

$$(W/V)(A_U/A_S)$$

in which W is the weight, in mg, of USP Triflupromazine Hydrochloride RS taken; V is the volume, in mL, of Oral Suspension taken; and A_U and A_S are the absorbances of the solution from the Oral Suspension and the Standard solution, respectively.

Triflupromazine Hydrochloride

$C_{18}H_{19}F_3N_2S \cdot HCl$ 388.88
10*H*-Phenothiazine-10-propanamine, *N,N*-dimethyl-2-(trifluoromethyl)-, monohydrochloride.
10-[3-(Dimethylamino)propyl]-2-(trifluoromethyl)phenothiazine monohydrochloride   [1098-60-8].

» Triflupromazine Hydrochloride contains not less than 97.0 percent and not more than 103.0 percent of $C_{18}H_{19}F_3N_2S \cdot HCl$, calculated on the dried basis.

Packaging and storage—Preserve in well-closed, light-resistant glass containers.

USP Reference standards ⟨11⟩—*USP Triflupromazine Hydrochloride RS*.

NOTE—Throughout the following procedures, protect test or assay specimens, the Reference Standard, and solutions containing them, by conducting the procedures without delay, under subdued light, or by using low-actinic glassware.

Identification—
A: *Infrared Absorption* ⟨197K⟩.
B: *Ultraviolet Absorption* ⟨197U⟩—
Solution: 10 µg per mL.
Medium: 0.5 N sulfuric acid.
Absorptivities at 255 nm, calculated on the dried basis, do not differ by more than 3.0%.
C: Prepare a solution of Triflupromazine Hydrochloride in methanol containing 10 mg per mL. Apply 10 µL each of this solution and a Standard solution of USP Triflupromazine Hydrochloride RS in methanol containing 10 mg per mL to a suitable thin-layer chromatographic plate (see *Chromatography* ⟨621⟩) coated with a 0.25-mm layer of chromatographic silica gel mixture. Allow the spots to dry, and develop the chromatogram in a solvent system consisting of a mixture of n-propyl alcohol, water, and ammonium hydroxide (88 : 11 : 1) until the solvent front has moved about three-fourths of the length of the plate. Remove the plate from the developing chamber, mark the solvent front, and allow the solvent to evaporate. Locate the spots on the plate by spraying lightly with dilute methanolic sulfuric acid (4 in 10) and then heating for 15 minutes: the R_F value and color (pink-orange) of the principal spot obtained from the test solution correspond to that obtained from the Standard solution.

Loss on drying ⟨731⟩—Dry it at 100° for 2 hours: it loses not more than 0.5% of its weight.
Residue on ignition ⟨281⟩: not more than 0.1%.
Ordinary impurities ⟨466⟩—
Test solution: acetone.
Standard solution: acetone.
Eluant: a mixture of chloroform and methanol (4 : 1).
Visualization: 1.
Organic volatile impurities, *Method I* ⟨467⟩: meets the requirements.

(Official until July 1, 2008)
Assay—Dissolve about 800 mg of Triflupromazine Hydrochloride, accurately weighed, in 100 mL of glacial acetic acid. Add 10 mL of mercuric acetate TS and 1 drop of crystal violet TS, and titrate with 0.1 N perchloric acid VS to a blue endpoint. Perform a blank determination, and make any necessary correction. Each mL of 0.1 N perchloric acid is equivalent to 38.89 mg of $C_{18}H_{19}F_3N_2S \cdot HCl$.

Triflupromazine Hydrochloride Injection

» Triflupromazine Hydrochloride Injection is a sterile solution of Triflupromazine Hydrochloride in Water for Injection. It contains not less than 90.0 percent and not more than 112.0 percent of the labeled amount of $C_{18}H_{19}F_3N_2S \cdot HCl$.

Packaging and storage—Preserve in single-dose or in multiple-dose containers, preferably of Type I glass, protected from light.
USP Reference standards ⟨11⟩—*USP Triflupromazine Hydrochloride RS. USP Endotoxin RS.*
NOTE—Throughout the following procedures, protect test or assay specimens, the Reference Standard, and solutions containing them, by conducting the procedures without delay, under subdued light, or using low-actinic glassware.
Identification—
A: Place a volume of Injection, equivalent to about 100 mg of triflupromazine hydrochloride, in a test tube, add 5 mL of 8 N nitric acid, and mix: a peach to amber color develops, quickly turns dark brown, and then changes to a clear solution having a yellow tint.
B: A volume of Injection, equivalent to about 50 mg of triflupromazine hydrochloride, meets the requirements under *Identification—Organic Nitrogenous Bases* ⟨181⟩.
C: The UV absorption spectrum of the *Assay preparation*, prepared as directed in the *Assay*, exhibits maxima and minima at the same wavelengths as that of the *Standard preparation*, prepared as directed in the *Assay*.
Bacterial endotoxins ⟨85⟩—It contains not more than 5.8 USP Endotoxin Units per mg of triflupromazine hydrochloride.
pH ⟨791⟩: between 3.5 and 5.2.
Other requirements—It meets the requirements under *Injections* ⟨1⟩.
Assay—
*Standard preparation—*Transfer about 50 mg of USP Triflupromazine Hydrochloride RS, accurately weighed, to a 50-mL volumetric flask, dissolve in 0.5 N sulfuric acid, dilute with 0.5 N sulfuric acid to volume, and mix. Proceed as directed under *Assay preparation*, beginning with "Transfer 10.0 mL of this solution to a 100-mL volumetric flask." The concentration of USP Triflupromazine Hydrochloride RS in the *Standard preparation* is about 5 µg per mL.

*Assay preparation—*Transfer an accurately measured volume of Injection, equivalent to about 50 mg of triflupromazine hydrochloride, to a 50-mL volumetric flask, dilute with 0.5 N sulfuric acid to volume, and mix. Transfer 10.0 mL of this solution to a 100-mL volumetric flask, dilute with the same acid to volume, and mix. Transfer 10.0 mL of this solution to a glass-stoppered, 50-mL centrifuge tube containing 10 mL of ether previously chilled in an ice bath, insert the stopper, shake for 3 minutes, and centrifuge at 1500 rpm for 5 minutes. Transfer 5.0 mL of the aqueous layer to a 100-mL volumetric flask, dilute with 0.5 N sulfuric acid to volume, and mix.

*Procedure—*Concomitantly determine the absorbances of the *Assay preparation* and the *Standard preparation* in 1-cm cells at the wavelength of maximum absorbance at about 255 nm, with a suitable spectrophotometer, using 0.5 N sulfuric acid as the blank. Calculate the quantity, in mg, of $C_{18}H_{19}F_3N_2S \cdot HCl$ in each mL of the Injection taken by the formula:

$$(10C/V)(A_U/A_S)$$

in which C is the concentration, in µg per mL, of USP Triflupromazine Hydrochloride RS in the *Standard preparation*, V is the volume, in mL, of Injection taken, and A_U and A_S are the absorbances of the *Assay preparation* and the *Standard preparation*, respectively.

Triflupromazine Hydrochloride Tablets

» Triflupromazine Hydrochloride Tablets contain not less than 90.0 percent and not more than 110.0 percent of the labeled amount of $C_{18}H_{19}F_3N_2S \cdot HCl$.

Packaging and storage—Preserve in well-closed, light-resistant containers.
USP Reference standards ⟨11⟩—*USP Triflupromazine Hydrochloride RS.*
NOTE—Throughout the following procedures, protect test or assay specimens, the Reference Standard, and solutions containing them, by conducting the procedures without delay, under subdued light, or using low-actinic glassware.
Identification—
A: Triturate a portion of powdered Tablets, equivalent to about 50 mg of triflupromazine hydrochloride, with 5 mL of methanol, and centrifuge. A 10-µL portion of the supernatant meets the requirements of *Identification* test C under *Triflupromazine Hydrochloride*.
B: The solution prepared from the Tablets for measurement of absorbance in the *Assay* exhibits an absorbance maximum at 255 ± 2 nm.

Dissolution ⟨711⟩—
  Medium: 0.01 N hydrochloric acid; 900 mL.
  Apparatus 1: 100 rpm.
  Time: 45 minutes.
  Procedure—Determine the amount of $C_{18}H_{19}F_3N_2S \cdot HCl$ dissolved by employing UV absorption at the wavelength of maximum absorbance at about 305 nm on filtered portions of the solution under test, suitably diluted with *Medium*, if necessary, in comparison with a Standard solution having a known concentration of USP Triflupromazine Hydrochloride RS in the same *Medium*.
  Tolerances—Not less than 75% (*Q*) of the labeled amount of $C_{18}H_{19}F_3N_2S \cdot HCl$ is dissolved in 45 minutes.
Uniformity of dosage units ⟨905⟩: meet the requirements.
Assay—Weigh and finely powder not less than 20 Tablets. Transfer an accurately weighed portion of the powder, equivalent to about 20 mg of triflupromazine hydrochloride, to a separator, add 10 mL of 0.1 N hydrochloric acid and 20 mL of water, and mix. Add 6 N ammonium hydroxide to render the mixture alkaline to litmus, add 1 mL in excess, and extract with five 50-mL portions of chloroform, passing each extract through anhydrous sodium sulfate into a 250-mL volumetric flask. Dilute with chloroform to volume, and mix. Evaporate 10.0 mL of this solution under reduced pressure to dryness, and dissolve the residue in 0.1 N hydrochloric acid to make 100.0 mL. Concomitantly determine the absorbances of this solution and of a Standard solution of USP Triflupromazine Hydrochloride RS in the same medium having a known concentration of about 8 µg per mL in 1-cm cells at the wavelength of maximum absorbance at about 255 nm, with a suitable spectrophotometer, using 0.1 N hydrochloric acid as the blank. Calculate the quantity, in mg, of $C_{18}H_{19}F_3N_2S \cdot HCl$ in the portion of Tablets taken by the formula:

$$2.5C(A_U/A_S)$$

in which *C* is the concentration, in µg per mL, of USP Triflupromazine Hydrochloride RS in the Standard solution, and A_U and A_S are the absorbances of the solution from the Tablets and the Standard solution, respectively.

Trifluridine

$C_{10}H_{11}F_3N_2O_5$ 296.20
Thymidine, α,α,α-trifluoro-.
2′-Deoxy-5-(trifluoromethyl)uridine [*70-00-8*].

» Trifluridine contains not less than 98.0 percent and not more than 102.0 percent of $C_{10}H_{11}F_3N_2O_5$, calculated on the dried basis.

Packaging and storage—Preserve in tight, light-resistant containers.
USP Reference standards ⟨11⟩—*USP Trifluridine RS. USP Trifluridine Related Compound A RS.*
Identification—
  A: *Infrared Absorption ⟨197K⟩.*
  B: *Ultraviolet Absorption ⟨197U⟩—*
    Solution: 25 µg per mL.
    Medium: 0.1 N hydrochloric acid.
  C: The retention time of the major peak in the chromatogram of the *Assay preparation* corresponds to that in the chromatogram of the *Standard preparation*, as obtained in the *Assay*.
Loss on drying ⟨731⟩—Dry it in vacuum at 105° for 4 hours: it loses not more than 1.0% of its weight.

Specific rotation ⟨781S⟩: between +47° and +51°.
  Test solution: 30 mg per mL, in water.
Related compounds—
  Mobile phase and *Chromatographic system*—Proceed as directed in the *Assay*.
  Standard solution—Use the *Standard preparation* prepared as directed in the *Assay*.
  Test solution—Use the *Assay preparation*.
  Procedure—Proceed as directed in the *Assay*. Calculate the percentages of trifluridine related compound A and 5-(trifluoromethyl)uracil in the portion of Trifluridine taken by the formula:

$$25{,}000(C/W)(r_U/r_S)$$

in which *C* is the concentration, in mg per mL, of USP Trifluridine Related Compound A RS and 5-(trifluoromethyl)uracil in the Standard solution; *W* is the weight, in mg, of Trifluridine taken; and r_U and r_S are the peak responses for the related compounds obtained from the *Test solution* and the *Standard solution*, respectively: not more than 1.0% of each related compound is found.
Assay—
  Mobile phase—Prepare a filtered and degassed 0.15% sodium citrate solution and adjust with 1 N hydrochloric acid to a pH of 6.8. Make adjustments if necessary (see *System Suitability* under *Chromatography ⟨621⟩*).
  Standard stock preparation—Dissolve accurately weighed quantities of USP Trifluridine RS, USP Trifluridine Related Compound A RS, and 5-(trifluoromethyl)uracil in water to obtain a solution having known concentrations of about 1 mg per mL, 0.01 mg per mL, and 0.01 mg per mL, respectively. [NOTE—This stock preparation may be stored at 0° to 5° for 3 months.]
  Standard preparation—Transfer 10.0 mL of the *Standard stock preparation* to a 50-mL volumetric flask, dilute with water to volume, and mix.
  Assay preparation—Transfer about 50 mg of Trifluridine, accurately weighed, to a 250-mL volumetric flask, dissolve in and dilute with water to volume, and mix.
  Chromatographic system (see *Chromatography ⟨621⟩*)—The liquid chromatograph is equipped with a 254-nm detector and a 4.2-mm × 25-cm column that contains packing L1. The flow rate is about 2 mL per minute. Chromatograph the *Standard preparation*, and record the peak responses as directed for *Procedure*: the resolution, *R*, between 5-(trifluoromethyl)uracil and trifluridine related compound A is not less than 3.0 and between trifluridine related compound A and trifluridine is not less than 4.0; and the relative standard deviation for replicate injections is not more than 2.0%.
  Procedure—Separately inject equal volumes (about 10 µL) of the *Standard preparation* and the *Assay preparation* into the chromatograph, record the chromatograms, and measure the areas for the major peaks. Calculate the quantity, in mg, of $C_{10}H_{11}F_3N_2O_5$ in the portion of Trifluridine taken by the formula:

$$250C(r_U/r_S)$$

in which *C* is the concentration, in mg per mL, of USP Trifluridine RS in the *Standard preparation*; and r_U and r_S are the peak responses obtained from the *Assay preparation* and the *Standard preparation*, respectively.

Trihexyphenidyl Hydrochloride

$C_{20}H_{31}NO \cdot HCl$ 337.93
1-Piperidinepropanol, α-cyclohexyl-α-phenyl-, hydrochloride, (±)-.
(±)-α-Cyclohexyl-α-phenyl-1-piperidinepropanol hydrochloride [*52-49-3*].

» Trihexyphenidyl Hydrochloride contains not less than 98.0 percent and not more than 102.0 percent of $C_{20}H_{31}NO \cdot HCl$, calculated on the dried basis.

Packaging and storage—Preserve in tight containers.

USP Reference standards ⟨11⟩—*USP Trihexyphenidyl Hydrochloride RS.*

Identification—
  A: *Infrared Absorption* ⟨197K⟩.
  B: It responds to the tests for *Chloride* ⟨191⟩.
  C: The retention time exhibited by trihexyphenidyl hydrochloride in the chromatogram of the *Assay preparation* corresponds to that of the *Standard preparation*, as obtained in the *Assay*.

Loss on drying ⟨731⟩—Dry it at 105° for 3 hours: it loses not more than 0.5% of its weight.

Residue on ignition ⟨281⟩: not more than 0.1%.

Heavy metals, *Method II* ⟨231⟩: 0.002%.

Chloride content—Dissolve about 1.2 g, accurately weighed, in a mixture consisting of 50 mL of methanol, 5 mL of glacial acetic acid, and 5 mL of water. Add 3 drops of eosin Y TS, and mix. Stir, preferably with a magnetic stirrer, and titrate with 0.1 N silver nitrate VS until the straw-orange suspension that forms during the titration changes sharply to red. Each mL of 0.1 N silver nitrate is equivalent to 3.545 mg of Cl. Not less than 10.3% and not more than 10.7% of Cl, calculated on the dried basis, is found.

Chromatographic purity—
  Standard preparations—Dissolve USP Trihexyphenidyl Hydrochloride RS in a mixture of chloroform and isopropylamine (98 : 2), and mix to obtain a solution having a known concentration of 2.5 mg per mL. Dilute quantitatively with a mixture of chloroform and isopropylamine (98 : 2) to obtain *Standard preparation A*, containing 500 µg of the Reference Standard per mL, and *Standard preparation B*, containing 250 µg of the Reference Standard per mL.
  Test preparation—Dissolve an accurately weighed quantity of Trihexyphenidyl Hydrochloride in a mixture of chloroform and isopropylamine (98 : 2) to obtain a solution containing 50 mg per mL.
  Spray reagent—Dissolve 0.8 g of bismuth subnitrate in a mixture of 40 mL of water and 10 mL of glacial acetic acid (*Solution A*). Dissolve 8 g of potassium iodide in 20 mL of water (*Solution B*). On the day of use, mix equal volumes of *Solution A* and *Solution B*.
  Procedure—Apply separately 10 µL of the *Test preparation* and 10 µL of each *Standard preparation* to a suitable thin-layer chromatographic plate (see *Chromatography* ⟨621⟩) coated with a 0.25-mm layer of chromatographic silica gel mixture. Position the plate in a chromatographic chamber, and develop the chromatograms in a solvent system consisting of a mixture of hexane and isopropylamine (98 : 2) until the solvent front has moved about three-fourths of the length of the plate. Remove the plate from the developing chamber, mark the solvent front, allow the solvent to evaporate, and spray the plate, first with the *Spray reagent*, and then with sodium nitrite solution (4 in 100). Compare the intensities of any secondary spots observed in the chromatogram of the *Test preparation* with those of the principal spots in the chromatograms of the *Standard preparations*. No secondary spot from the chromatogram of the *Test preparation* is larger or more intense than the principal spot obtained from *Standard preparation B* (0.5%), and the sum of the intensities of all secondary spots obtained from the *Test preparation* corresponds to not more than 1.0%.

Organic volatile impurities, *Method IV* ⟨467⟩: meets the requirements.

(Official until July 1, 2008)

Assay—
  Mobile phase—Prepare a mixture of acetonitrile, water, and triethylamine (920 : 80 : 0.2), adjust with phosphoric acid to a pH of 4.0, mix, filter, and degas. Make adjustments if necessary (see *System Suitability* under *Chromatography* ⟨621⟩).
  Standard preparation—Dissolve an accurately weighed quantity of USP Trihexyphenidyl Hydrochloride RS in acetonitrile, and dilute quantitatively, and stepwise if necessary, with acetonitrile to obtain a solution having a known concentration of about 0.2 mg per mL.
  Assay preparation—Transfer about 20 mg of Trihexyphenidyl Hydrochloride, accurately weighed, to a 100-mL volumetric flask, dissolve in acetonitrile, dilute with acetonitrile to volume, and mix.
  Chromatographic system (see *Chromatography* ⟨621⟩)—The liquid chromatograph is equipped with a 210-nm detector and a 4.6-mm × 8-cm column that contains 3-µm packing L1. The flow rate is about 2 mL per minute. Chromatograph the *Standard preparation*, and record the peak responses as directed for *Procedure*: the column efficiency determined from the analyte peak is not less than 1300 theoretical plates, the tailing factor for the analyte peak is not more than 3.0, and the relative standard deviation for replicate injections is not more than 1.0%.
  Procedure—Separately inject equal volumes (about 10 µL) of the *Standard preparation* and the *Assay preparation* into the chromatograph, record the chromatograms, and measure the responses for the major peaks. Calculate the quantity, in mg, of $C_{20}H_{31}NO \cdot HCl$ in the portion of Trihexyphenidyl Hydrochloride taken by the formula:

$$100C(r_U / r_S)$$

in which C is the concentration, in mg per mL, of USP Trihexyphenidyl Hydrochloride RS in the *Standard preparation*, and r_U and r_S are the trihexyphenidyl peak responses obtained from the *Assay preparation* and the *Standard preparation*, respectively.

Trihexyphenidyl Hydrochloride Extended-Release Capsules

» Trihexyphenidyl Hydrochloride Extended-Release Capsules contain not less than 90.0 percent and not more than 110.0 percent of the labeled amount of trihexyphenidyl hydrochloride ($C_{20}H_{31}NO \cdot HCl$).

Packaging and storage—Preserve in tight containers.

USP Reference standards ⟨11⟩—*USP Trihexyphenidyl Hydrochloride RS.*

Identification—
  A: Reduce the contents of a number of Capsules, equivalent to 20 mg of trihexyphenidyl hydrochloride, to a fine powder, and triturate with 25 mL of chloroform. Filter the mixture, and evaporate the filtrate, by gently heating, to about 10 mL. Add the solution to 100 mL of *n*-hexane: a white precipitate is formed. Allow the mixture to stand for 30 minutes, and collect the precipitate on a solvent-resistant membrane filter to 1-µm pore size. Wash the crystals with a small portion of *n*-hexane, and air-dry: the IR absorption spectrum of a potassium bromide dispersion of the crystals so obtained exhibits maxima only at the same wavelengths as that of a similar preparation of USP Trihexyphenidyl Hydrochloride RS.
  B: The precipitate obtained in *Identification* test A responds to the tests for *Chloride* ⟨191⟩.

Dissolution ⟨711⟩—
  Medium: water; 500 mL.
  Apparatus 1: 100 rpm.
  Times: 3, 6, and 12 hours.
  Determine the amount of $C_{20}H_{31}NO \cdot HCl$ dissolved, using the following method.
  Mobile phase—Prepare a filtered and degassed mixture of acetonitrile, water, and triethylamine (920 : 80 : 0.2), and adjust with phosphoric acid to a pH of 4.0.
  Standard solution—Dissolve an accurately weighed quantity of USP Trihexyphenidyl Hydrochloride RS in water, and dilute quantitatively and stepwise with water to obtain a solution having a known concentration of about 5 µg per mL.
  Chromatographic system (see *Chromatography* ⟨621⟩)—The liquid chromatograph is equipped with a 210-nm detector and a 4.6-mm × 8.3-cm column that contains packing L1. The flow rate is about 2 mL per minute. Chromatograph the *Standard solution,* and record the peak responses as directed for *Procedure*: the tailing factor for the trihexyphenidyl peak is not more than 2.8, and the relative standard deviation for replicate injections is not more than 2.0%.

Procedure—Dilute the *Standard solution* and the solution under test with acetonitrile (1 : 1). Separately inject equal volumes (about 20 µL) of these solutions into the chromatograph, record the chromatograms, and measure the peak responses for trihexyphenidyl. Calculate the percentage of the labeled amount of $C_{20}H_{31}NO \cdot HCl$ dissolved.

Tolerances—The percentages of the labeled amount of $C_{20}H_{31}NO \cdot HCl$ dissolved at the times specified conform to *Acceptance Table 2*.

Time (hours)	Amount dissolved
3	between 20% and 50%
6	between 40% and 70%
12	not less than 70%

Uniformity of dosage units ⟨905⟩: meet the requirements.

Assay—
Mobile phase and *Chromatographic system*—Prepare as directed in the *Assay* under *Trihexyphenidyl Hydrochloride*.

Standard preparation—Dissolve an accurately weighed quantity of USP Trihexyphenidyl Hydrochloride RS in *Mobile phase*, and dilute quantitatively, and stepwise if necessary, with *Mobile phase* to obtain a solution having a known concentration of about 0.2 mg per mL.

Assay preparation—Fill a 500-mL volumetric flask with *Mobile phase* to volume. Transfer to this flask the accurately weighed contents of a counted number of Capsules, equivalent to about 100 mg of trihexyphenidyl hydrochloride. Mix, sonicate, with occasional shaking for 45 minutes, allow to stand for 15 minutes, and filter, discarding the first 5 mL of the filtrate.

Procedure—Proceed as directed for *Procedure* in the *Assay* under *Trihexyphenidyl Hydrochloride*. Calculate the quantity, in mg, of trihexyphenidyl hydrochloride ($C_{20}H_{31}NO \cdot HCl$) in each of the Capsules taken by the formula:

$$(500C/N)(r_U/r_S)$$

in which N is the number of Capsules taken, and the other terms are as defined therein.

Trihexyphenidyl Hydrochloride Oral Solution

» Trihexyphenidyl Hydrochloride Oral Solution contains not less than 90.0 percent and not more than 110.0 percent of trihexyphenidyl hydrochloride ($C_{20}H_{31}NO \cdot HCl$).

Packaging and storage—Preserve in tight containers.
USP Reference standards ⟨11⟩—*USP Trihexyphenidyl Hydrochloride RS*.
Identification—
A: To 50 mL of Oral Solution add 50 mL of water and 50 mL of 1 N sodium hydroxide, and stir. Cool the mixture at 4° to 5° for 30 minutes: a white precipitate or cloudiness is observed. Add 100 mL of water to the cooled mixture, stir, and filter by means of vacuum through a 47-mm membrane filter of 1-µm pore size. Wash the crystals with about 100 mL of water, and allow to air-dry: the IR absorption spectrum of a potassium bromide dispersion of the crystals so obtained exhibits maxima only at the same wavelengths as that of the crystalline base obtained from about 20 mg of USP Trihexyphenidyl Hydrochloride RS, similarly prepared and measured.

B: The retention time exhibited by trihexyphenidyl hydrochloride in the chromatogram of the *Assay preparation* corresponds to that of the *Standard preparation*, both relative to the internal standard, as obtained in the *Assay*.

pH ⟨791⟩: between 2.0 and 3.0.
Alcohol content ⟨611⟩: between 90.0% and 110.0% of the labeled amount of C_2H_5OH.

Assay—
Mobile phase and *Chromatographic system*—Prepare as directed in the *Assay* under *Trihexyphenidyl Hydrochloride*.

Standard preparation—Dissolve an accurately weighed quantity of USP Trihexyphenidyl Hydrochloride RS in methanol, and dilute quantitatively, and stepwise if necessary, with methanol to obtain a solution having a known concentration of about 0.08 mg per mL.

Assay preparation—Transfer an accurately measured volume of Oral Solution, equivalent to about 2 mg of trihexyphenidyl hydrochloride, to a 25-mL volumetric flask, dilute with methanol to volume, and mix.

Procedure—Proceed as directed for *Procedure* in the *Assay* under *Trihexyphenidyl Hydrochloride*. Calculate the quantity, in mg, of trihexyphenidyl hydrochloride ($C_{20}H_{31}NO \cdot HCl$) in each mL of the Oral Solution taken by the formula:

$$(25C/V)(r_U/r_S)$$

in which V is the volume, in mL, of Oral Solution taken to prepare the *Assay preparation*, and the other terms are as defined therein.

Trihexyphenidyl Hydrochloride Tablets

» Trihexyphenidyl Hydrochloride Tablets contain not less than 90.0 percent and not more than 110.0 percent of the labeled amount of $C_{20}H_{31}NO \cdot HCl$.

Packaging and storage—Preserve in tight containers.
USP Reference standards ⟨11⟩—*USP Trihexyphenidyl Hydrochloride RS*.
Identification—
A: Reduce a number of Tablets, equivalent to 20 mg of trihexyphenidyl hydrochloride, to a fine powder, and triturate with 25 mL of chloroform. Filter the mixture, and evaporate the filtrate, by gently heating, to about 10 mL. Add the solution to 100 mL of *n*-hexane: a white precipitate is formed. Allow the mixture to stand for 30 minutes, and collect the precipitate on a solvent-resistant membrane filter of 1-µm pore size. Wash the crystals with a small portion of *n*-hexane, and allow them to air-dry: the IR absorption spectrum of a potassium bromide dispersion of the crystals so obtained exhibits maxima only at the same wavelengths as that of a similar preparation of USP Trihexyphenidyl Hydrochloride RS.

B: The precipitate obtained in *Identification* test A responds to the tests for *Chloride* ⟨191⟩.

C: The retention time exhibited by trihexyphenidyl hydrochloride in the chromatogram of the *Assay preparation* corresponds to that of the *Standard preparation*, both relative to the internal standard, as obtained in the *Assay*.

Dissolution ⟨711⟩—
Medium: pH 4.5 acetate buffer, prepared by mixing 2.99 g of sodium acetate trihydrate and 1.66 mL of glacial acetic acid with water to obtain 1000 mL of solution having a pH of 4.50 ± 0.05; 900 mL.
Apparatus 1: 100 rpm.
Time: 45 minutes.
Determination of dissolved trihexyphenidyl hydrochloride—
Bromocresol green solution—Dissolve 250 mg of bromocresol green in a mixture of 15 mL of water and 5 mL of 0.1 N sodium hydroxide, dilute with *Medium* to 500 mL, and mix. Extract 250-mL portions of this solution with two 100-mL portions of chloroform, and discard the chloroform extracts.

Procedure—Transfer an accurately measured, filtered portion of the solution under test, estimated to contain about 50 µg of trihexyphenidyl hydrochloride, to a 50-mL centrifuge tube. Transfer an equal, accurately measured volume of a Standard solution, having a known concentration of USP Trihexyphenidyl Hydrochloride RS in *Medium*, to a second 50-mL centrifuge tube, and transfer an equal, accurately measured volume of *Medium* to a third 50-mL centrifuge tube to provide a blank. Add 5 mL of *Bromocresol green solution* and 10.0 mL of chloroform to each tube, insert the stoppers into the tubes, and shake vigorously for not less than 20 seconds. Centrifuge the mixtures to separate the layers, and aspirate and discard the upper aqueous layers. Filter each chloroform layer through a separate phase-separating filter paper. Determine the amount of $C_{20}H_{31}NO \cdot HCl$ dissolved from absorbances, at the wavelength of maximum absorbance at about 415 nm, of the filtrate from the solution under test in comparison with that from the Standard solution, the filtrate from the blank being used to set the instrument.

Tolerances—Not less than 75% (*Q*) of the labeled amount of $C_{20}H_{31}NO \cdot HCl$ is dissolved in 45 minutes.

Uniformity of dosage units ⟨905⟩: meet the requirements.

Assay—

Mobile phase and *Chromatographic system*—Prepare as directed in the *Assay* under *Trihexyphenidyl Hydrochloride*.

Standard preparation—Dissolve an accurately weighed quantity of USP Trihexyphenidyl Hydrochloride RS in *Mobile phase*, and dilute quantitatively, and stepwise if necessary, with *Mobile phase* to obtain a solution having a known concentration of about 0.2 mg per mL.

Assay preparation—Transfer 20 Tablets, accurately counted, to a volumetric flask of sufficient capacity that when diluted to volume yields a concentration of about 0.2 mg of trihexyphenidyl hydrochloride per mL. Add a volume of 0.1 N hydrochloric acid equivalent to 10% of the capacity of the volumetric flask, and sonicate with occasional shaking until the Tablets have disintegrated. Add a volume of *Mobile phase* equivalent to about one-half of the capacity of the volumetric flask, sonicate with frequent shaking for 10 minutes, and shake by mechanical means for 10 minutes. Cool, dilute with *Mobile phase* to volume, mix, and filter.

Procedure—Proceed as directed for *Procedure* in the *Assay* under *Trihexyphenidyl Hydrochloride*. Calculate the quantity, in mg, of $C_{20}H_{31}NO \cdot HCl$ in each Tablet taken by the formula:

$$(V / 20)(C)(r_U / r_S)$$

in which *V* is the volume, in mL, of the *Assay preparation*, and the other terms are as defined therein.

Trikates Oral Solution

» Trikates Oral Solution is a solution of Potassium Acetate, Potassium Bicarbonate, and Potassium Citrate in Purified Water. It contains not less than 90.0 percent and not more than 110.0 percent of the labeled amount of potassium.

Packaging and storage—Preserve in tight, light-resistant containers.

Identification—

A: Two mL, diluted with water to 12 mL, responds to the ferric chloride test for *Acetate* ⟨191⟩.

B: It responds to the tests for *Bicarbonate* ⟨191⟩.

C: To 5 mL add 1 mL of hydrochloric acid, and heat to near boiling for 5 minutes to evolve carbon dioxide. Cool, add 1 mL of calcium chloride TS, and render just alkaline to bromothymol blue TS with 1 N sodium hydroxide. Boil for 3 minutes with gentle agitation: a white, crystalline precipitate appears that is insoluble in 1 N sodium hydroxide but dissolves in 3 N hydrochloric acid.

Assay—

Potassium stock solution—Dissolve, in water, 191 mg of potassium chloride, previously dried at 105° for 2 hours. Transfer to a 1000-mL volumetric flask, dilute with water to volume, and mix. Transfer 100.0 mL of this solution to a second 1000-mL volumetric flask, dilute with water to volume, and mix. This solution contains 10 μg of potassium per mL.

Standard preparations—To separate 100-mL volumetric flasks transfer 10.0 mL and 13.0 mL, respectively, of the *Potassium stock solution*. To each flask add 2.0 mL of sodium chloride solution (1 in 5) and 1.0 mL of hydrochloric acid, dilute with water to volume, and mix. The *Standard preparations* contain 1.0 μg and 1.3 μg of potassium per mL, respectively.

Assay preparation—Transfer 1.0 mL of Oral Solution to a 100-mL volumetric flask, dilute with water to volume, and mix. Transfer 1.0 mL of this solution to a second 100-mL volumetric flask, dilute with water to volume, and mix. Transfer 10.0 mL of this solution to a third 100-mL volumetric flask, add 2.0 mL of sodium chloride solution (1 in 5) and 1.0 mL of hydrochloric acid, dilute with water to volume, and mix.

Procedure—Concomitantly determine the absorbances of the *Standard preparations* and the *Assay preparation* at the resonance line of 766.5 nm, with a suitable atomic absorption spectrophotometer (see *Spectrophotometry and Light-scattering* ⟨851⟩) equipped with a potassium hollow-cathode lamp and an air–acetylene flame, using water as the blank. Plot the absorbances of the *Standard preparations* versus concentration, in μg per mL, of potassium. From the graph so obtained, determine the concentration, *C*, in μg per mL, of potassium in the *Assay preparation*. Calculate the quantity, in mEq, of potassium in the Oral Solution taken by the formula:

$$100C / 39.10$$

in which 39.10 is the atomic weight of potassium.

Trimeprazine Tartrate

$(C_{18}H_{22}N_2S)_2 \cdot C_4H_6O_6$ 746.98

10*H*-Phenothiazine-10-propanamine *N,N,β*-trimethyl-, [*R*-(*R**,*R**)]-2,3-dihydroxybutanedioate (2 : 1).

10-[3-(Dimethylamino)-2-methylpropyl]phenothiazine tartrate (2 : 1)   [4330-99-8; 41375-66-0].

» Trimeprazine Tartrate contains not less than 98.0 percent and not more than 101.0 percent of $(C_{18}H_{22}N_2S)_2 \cdot C_4H_6O_6$, calculated on the dried basis.

Packaging and storage—Preserve in tight, light-resistant containers.

USP Reference standards ⟨11⟩—*USP Trimeprazine Tartrate RS.*

NOTE—Throughout the following procedures, protect test or assay specimens, the Reference Standard, and solutions containing them, by conducting the procedures without delay, under subdued light, or using low-actinic glassware.

Identification—

A: *Infrared Absorption* ⟨197M⟩.

B: The retention time of the major peak in the chromatogram of the *Assay preparation* corresponds to that in the chromatogram of the *Standard preparation* obtained as directed in the *Assay*.

C: Prepare a solution of it in methanol containing 6 mg in each 5 mL. Proceed as directed under *Thin-layer Chromatographic Identification Test* ⟨201⟩, applying 5 μL of this solution and 5 μL of a similar solution of USP Trimeprazine Tartrate RS, using as the solvent system a mixture of 0.15 mL of ammonium hydroxide and 100 mL of acetone. Locate the spots on the plate by lightly spraying with iodoplatinic acid solution [prepared by dissolving 100 mg of chloroplatinic acid in 1 mL of 1 N hydrochloric acid, adding 25 mL of potassium iodide solution (1 in 25), diluting with water to 100 mL, and adding 0.5 mL of formic acid]: the R_F value of the principal spot obtained from the test solution corresponds to that obtained from the Standard solution.

Loss on drying ⟨731⟩—Dry it in vacuum at 60° for 4 hours: it loses not more than 0.5% of its weight.

Residue on ignition ⟨281⟩: not more than 0.1%.

Heavy metals, *Method II* ⟨231⟩: 0.002%.

Ordinary impurities ⟨466⟩—

Test solution: methanol.

Standard solution: methanol.

Eluant: a mixture of ethyl acetate saturated with ammonium hydroxide and ether (1 : 1).

Visualization: 1.

Assay—

Mobile phase—Prepare a filtered and degassed mixture of 0.005 M sodium 1-heptanesulfonate in methanol, water, and acetic acid (65 : 34 : 1). Make adjustments if necessary (see *System Suitability* under *Chromatography* ⟨621⟩).

Standard preparation—Dissolve an accurately weighed quantity of USP Trimeprazine Tartrate RS in *Mobile phase*, and dilute quantitatively, and stepwise if necessary, with *Mobile phase* to obtain a solution having a known concentration of about 0.031 mg per mL.

Assay preparation—Transfer about 62 mg of Trimeprazine Tartrate, accurately weighed, to a 100-mL volumetric flask, dissolve in and dilute with *Mobile phase* to volume. Transfer 5 mL of this solution into a 100-mL volumetric flask, dilute with *Mobile phase* to volume, and mix.

Chromatographic system (see *Chromatography* ⟨621⟩)—The liquid chromatograph is equipped with a 254-nm detector and a 3.9-mm × 30-cm column that contains packing L1. The flow rate is about 1.5 mL per minute. Chromatograph the *Standard preparation*, and record the peak responses as directed for *Procedure:* the capacity factor, k', is not less than 2.0 and not more than 5.0, the column efficiency is not less than 1200 theoretical plates, the tailing factor is not more than 3.5, and the relative standard deviation for replicate injections is not more than 0.6%.

Procedure—Separately inject equal volumes (about 25 µL) of the *Standard preparation* and the *Assay preparation* into the chromatograph, record the chromatograms, and measure the responses for the major peaks. Calculate the quantity, in mg, of $(C_{18}H_{22}N_2S)_2 \cdot C_4H_6O_6$ in the portion of Trimeprazine Tartrate taken by the formula:

$$2000C(r_U / r_S)$$

in which C is the concentration, in mg per mL, of USP Trimeprazine Tartrate RS in the *Standard preparation*, and r_U and r_S are the peak responses obtained from the *Assay preparation* and the *Standard preparation*, respectively.

Trimeprazine Oral Solution

» Trimeprazine Oral Solution contains an amount of trimeprazine tartrate [$(C_{18}H_{22}N_2S)_2 \cdot C_4H_6O_6$] equivalent to not less than 90.0 percent and not more than 110.0 percent of the labeled amount of trimeprazine ($C_{18}H_{22}N_2S$).

Packaging and storage—Preserve in tight, light-resistant containers.

USP Reference standards ⟨11⟩—*USP Trimeprazine Tartrate RS.*

NOTE—Throughout the following procedures, protect test or assay specimens, the Reference Standard, and solutions containing them, by conducting the procedures without delay, under subdued light, or using low-actinic glassware.

Identification—

A: The retention time of the major peak in the chromatogram of the *Assay preparation* corresponds to that in the chromatogram of the *Standard preparation,* as obtained in the *Assay*.

B: Mix 10 mL of Oral Solution with about 30 mL of water in a separator, render the solution alkaline with 1 N sodium hydroxide, and extract with two 30-mL portions of ether. Transfer the ether extracts to a beaker, evaporate the ether by warming, and dissolve the residue in 5 mL of methanol: 5 µL of this solution meets the requirements of *Identification* test C under *Trimeprazine Tartrate*.

Alcohol content ⟨611⟩: between 4.5% and 6.5% of C_2H_5OH.

Limit of trimeprazine sulfoxide—

Mobile phase and *Chromatographic system*—Proceed as directed in the *Assay*.

Standard solution—Transfer about 60.6 mg of USP Trimeprazine Tartrate RS, accurately weighed, to a 50-mL volumetric flask. Add 5 mL of dilute hydrochloric acid (1 in 100) followed by 2 mL of 30 percent hydrogen peroxide, and heat at 60° for 10 minutes. Cool, dilute with 1 M sodium bisulfite to volume, and mix. Transfer 10.0 mL to a 60-mL separator, add 2 mL of sodium hydroxide solution (1 in 2), and mix. Extract with three 30-mL portions of ether. Filter the extracts through ether-wetted anhydrous sodium sulfate into a 250-mL conical flask. Cautiously evaporate the flask to dryness. Dissolve the residue in 10.0 mL of methanol, and filter if necessary. Each mL of this solution contains about 1 mg of trimeprazine sulfoxide. Transfer 1.0 mL of this solution to a 500-mL volumetric flask, dilute with *Mobile phase* to volume, and mix to obtain a solution containing about 0.0024 mg per mL of trimeprazine sulfoxide, expressed as trimeprazine tartrate.

Test solution—Use the *Assay preparation* as directed in the *Assay*.

Procedure—Separately inject equal volumes (about 25 µL) of the *Standard solution* and the *Test solution* into the chromatograph, record the chromatograms, and measure the responses for the peaks. The *Test solution* may exhibit a minor peak whose retention time corresponds to the peak exhibited by the *Standard solution* and whose retention time is about 0.6 relative to the main peak. Calculate the concentration, in mg per mL, of trimeprazine sulfoxide, in the portion of Oral Solution taken by the formula:

$$100(C/V)(596.89/746.98)(r_U / r_S)$$

in which C is the concentration, in mg per mL, of trimeprazine tartrate in the *Standard solution;* V is the volume, in mL, of Oral Solution taken; 596.89 and 746.98 are the molecular weights of trimeprazine and trimeprazine tartrate, respectively, and r_U and r_S are the peak responses obtained from the *Test solution* and the *Standard solution*, respectively. Not more than 0.036 mg per mL is found.

Assay—

Mobile phase, Standard preparation, and *Chromatographic system*—Proceed as directed in the *Assay* under *Trimeprazine Tartrate*.

Assay preparation—Using a "to contain" pipet, transfer an accurately measured volume of Oral Solution, equivalent to about 2.5 mg of trimeprazine, to a 100-mL volumetric flask containing 50 mL of *Mobile phase*. Rinse the pipet with *Mobile phase*, collecting the rinses in the volumetric flask. Dilute with *Mobile phase* to volume, and mix.

Procedure—Separately inject equal volumes (about 25 µL) of the *Standard preparation* and the *Assay preparation* into the chromatograph, record the chromatograms, and measure the responses for the major peaks. Calculate the quantity, in mg, of trimeprazine ($C_{18}H_{22}N_2S$) in each mL of Oral Solution taken by the formula:

$$100(C/V)(596.89/746.98)(r_U / r_S)$$

in which C is the concentration, in mg per mL, of USP Trimeprazine Tartrate RS in the *Standard preparation;* V is the volume, in mL, of Oral Solution taken; 596.89 and 746.98 are the molecular weights of trimeprazine and trimeprazine tartrate, respectively; and r_U and r_S are the peak responses obtained from the *Assay preparation* and the *Standard preparation,* respectively.

Trimeprazine Tartrate Tablets

» Trimeprazine Tartrate Tablets contain an amount of trimeprazine tartrate [$(C_{18}H_{22}N_2S)_2 \cdot C_4H_6O_6$] equivalent to not less than 93.0 percent and not more than 107.0 percent of the labeled amount of trimeprazine ($C_{18}H_{22}N_2S$).

Packaging and storage—Preserve in well-closed, light-resistant containers.

USP Reference standards ⟨11⟩—*USP Trimeprazine Tartrate RS.*

NOTE—Throughout the following procedures, protect test or assay specimens, the Reference Standard, and solutions containing them, by conducting the procedures without delay, under subdued light, or using low-actinic glassware.

USP 31 / Official Monographs / Trimethobenzamide 3467

Identification—

A: The retention time of the major peak in the chromatogram of the *Assay preparation* corresponds to that in the chromatogram of the *Standard preparation* obtained as directed in the *Assay*.

B: Triturate a portion of powdered Tablets, equivalent to about 10 mg of trimeprazine, with 10 mL of methanol, and centrifuge: 5 µL of this solution meets the requirements of *Identification* test C under *Trimeprazine Tartrate*.

Dissolution ⟨711⟩—

Medium: 0.01 N hydrochloric acid; 500 mL.

Apparatus 1: 100 rpm.

Time: 45 minutes.

Procedure—Determine the amount of $C_{18}H_{22}N_2S$ dissolved by employing UV absorption at the wavelength of maximum absorbance at about 251 nm on filtered portions of the solution under test, suitably diluted with *Medium*, if necessary, in comparison with a Standard solution having a known concentration of USP Trimeprazine Tartrate RS in the same *Medium*.

Tolerances—Not less than 75% (Q) of the labeled amount of $C_{18}H_{22}N_2S$ is dissolved in 45 minutes.

Uniformity of dosage units ⟨905⟩: meet the requirements.

Procedure for content uniformity—Transfer 1 Tablet to a 100-mL volumetric flask, add about 50 mL of 0.1 N hydrochloric acid, and shake by mechanical means until the tablet is completely disintegrated. Add 0.1 N hydrochloric acid to volume, mix, and filter, discarding the first 20 mL of the filtrate. Dilute a portion of the subsequent filtrate, quantitatively and stepwise if necessary, with 0.1 N hydrochloric acid to obtain a solution having a known concentration of about 5 µg of trimeprazine per mL. Concomitantly determine the absorbances of this solution and a solution of USP Trimeprazine Tartrate RS in the same medium, having a known concentration of about 6 µg per mL, in 1-cm cells, at 276 nm and at the wavelength of maximum absorbance at about 251 nm, with a suitable spectrophotometer, using 0.1 N hydrochloric acid as the blank. Calculate the quantity, in mg, of trimeprazine in the Tablet by the formula:

$$(T/D)(0.7991C)(A_{251} - A_{276})_U / (A_{251} - A_{276})_S$$

in which T is the labeled quantity, in mg, of trimeprazine in the Tablet, D is the concentration, in µg per mL, of trimeprazine in the test solution, based on the labeled quantity per Tablet and the extent of dilution, C is the concentration, in µg per mL, of USP Trimeprazine Tartrate RS in the Standard solution, 0.7991 is the factor converting trimeprazine tartrate to trimeprazine, and the parenthetic expressions are the differences in the absorbances of the two solutions at the wavelengths indicated by the subscripts, for the solution from the Tablets (U) and the Standard solution (S), respectively.

Assay—

Mobile phase, Standard preparation, and *Chromatographic system*—Proceed as directed in the *Assay* under *Trimeprazine Tartrate*.

Assay preparation—Weigh and finely powder not less than 20 Tablets. Transfer an accurately weighed portion of the powder, equivalent to about 5 mg of trimeprazine, to a 100-mL volumetric flask, dissolve in and dilute with *Mobile phase* to volume, mix, and filter.

Procedure—Separately inject equal volumes (about 25 µL) of the *Standard preparation* and the *Assay preparation* into the chromatograph, record the chromatograms, and measure the responses for the major peaks. Calculate the quantity, in mg, of $C_{18}H_{22}N_2S$ in the portion of Tablets taken by the formula:

$$100C(596.89 / 746.98)(r_U / r_S)$$

in which C is the concentration, in mg per mL, of USP Trimeprazine Tartrate RS in the *Standard preparation*, 596.89 and 746.98 are the molecular weights of trimeprazine and trimeprazine tartrate, respectively, and r_U and r_S are the peak responses obtained from the *Assay preparation* and the *Standard preparation*, respectively.

Trimethobenzamide Hydrochloride

$C_{21}H_{28}N_2O_5 \cdot HCl$ 424.92

Benzamide, N-[[4-[2-(dimethylamino)ethoxy]phenyl]methyl]-3,4,5-trimethoxy-, monohydrochloride.

N-[p-[2-(Dimethylamino)ethoxy]benzyl]-3,4,5-trimethoxybenzamide monohydrochloride [554-92-7].

» Trimethobenzamide Hydrochloride, dried at 105° for 4 hours, contains not less than 98.5 percent and not more than 100.5 percent of $C_{21}H_{28}N_2O_5 \cdot HCl$.

Packaging and storage—Preserve in well-closed containers.

USP Reference standards ⟨11⟩—*USP Trimethobenzamide Hydrochloride RS*.

Identification—

A: *Infrared Absorption* ⟨197K⟩.

B: *Ultraviolet Absorption* ⟨197U⟩—

Solution: 20 µg per mL.

Medium: 0.1 N hydrochloric acid.

Absorptivities at 258 nm, calculated on the dried basis, do not differ by more than 3.0%.

C: It meets the requirements of the *Thin-layer Chromatographic Identification Test* ⟨201⟩. Prepare the test solution by dissolving 10 mg of Trimethobenzamide Hydrochloride in 10.0 mL of methanol. Apply 10-µL portions of the test solution and the Standard solution to the plate, and develop in a solvent system consisting of a mixture of ethyl acetate, alcohol, and ammonium hydroxide (90 : 10 : 5).

D: It meets the requirements of the tests for *Chloride* ⟨191⟩.

Melting range, Class I ⟨741⟩: between 186° and 190°.

Loss on drying ⟨731⟩—Dry it at 105° for 4 hours: it loses not more than 0.5% of its weight.

Residue on ignition ⟨281⟩: not more than 0.1%.

Heavy metals, *Method I* ⟨231⟩—Dissolve 1.0 g in 20 mL of water, add 2 mL of 1 N acetic acid, and dilute with water to 25 mL: the limit is 0.002%.

Assay—Dissolve about 1.3 g of Trimethobenzamide Hydrochloride, previously dried and accurately weighed, in 80 mL of glacial acetic acid and 15 mL of mercuric acetate TS. Titrate with 0.1 N perchloric acid VS, determining the endpoint potentiometrically using suitable electrodes. Perform a blank determination, and make any necessary correction. Each mL of 0.1 N perchloric acid is equivalent to 42.49 mg of $C_{21}H_{28}N_2O_5 \cdot HCl$.

Trimethobenzamide Hydrochloride Capsules

» Trimethobenzamide Hydrochloride Capsules contain not less than 90.0 percent and not more than 110.0 percent of the labeled amount of $C_{21}H_{28}N_2O_5 \cdot HCl$.

Packaging and storage—Preserve in well-closed containers.

USP Reference standards ⟨11⟩—*USP Trimethobenzamide Hydrochloride RS*.

Identification—

A: The UV absorption spectrum of the solution employed for measurement of absorbance in the *Assay* exhibits maxima and minima at the same wavelengths as that of the Standard solution.

B: Transfer a portion of the contents of Capsules, equivalent to about 20 mg of trimethobenzamide hydrochloride, to a suitable vessel, dissolve in 15 mL of 0.1 N hydrochloric acid, and filter. Transfer the filtrate to a separator, and add 5 mL of 1 N sodium hydroxide. Extract with 15 mL of chloroform, filtering the chloroform extract through anhydrous sodium sulfate into a suitable vessel, and evaporate to dryness. Allow to cool to room temperature, add a small portion of ether, and evaporate at room temperature to dryness. Dry the residue at 60° for 1 hour: the IR absorption spectrum of a potassium bromide dispersion of the residue so obtained exhibits maxima only at the same wavelengths as that of a similar preparation of USP Trimethobenzamide Hydrochloride RS.

C: Place a portion of the contents of Capsules, equivalent to about 25 mg of trimethobenzamide hydrochloride, in a 10-mL volumetric flask, add methanol to volume, mix, and filter: the filtrate so obtained responds to the *Thin-layer Chromatographic Identification Test* ⟨201⟩, a solvent system consisting of a mixture of ethyl acetate, alcohol, and ammonium hydroxide (90 : 10 : 5) being used.

Dissolution ⟨711⟩—
  Medium: water; 900 mL.
  Apparatus 1: 100 rpm.
  Time: 45 minutes.
  Procedure—Determine the amount of $C_{21}H_{28}N_2O_5 \cdot HCl$ dissolved from UV absorbances at the wavelength of maximum absorbance at about 258 nm of filtered portions of the solution under test, suitably diluted with *Medium*, if necessary, in comparison with a Standard solution having a known concentration of USP Trimethobenzamide Hydrochloride RS in the same *Medium*.
  Tolerances—Not less than 75% (*Q*) of the labeled amount of $C_{21}H_{28}N_2O_5 \cdot HCl$ is dissolved in 45 minutes.

Uniformity of dosage units ⟨905⟩: meet the requirements.

Assay—Transfer, as completely as possible, the contents of not less than 20 Capsules to a suitable tared container, and determine the average weight per Capsule. Mix the combined contents, and transfer an accurately weighed portion of the powder, equivalent to about 50 mg of trimethobenzamide hydrochloride, to a 100-mL volumetric flask. Add 50 mL of dilute hydrochloric acid (1 in 120), shake the mixture for several minutes, then add dilute hydrochloric acid (1 in 120) to volume, and mix. Filter through small retentive filter paper, discarding the first 20 mL of the filtrate. Transfer 4.0 mL of the subsequent filtrate to a 100-mL volumetric flask, add dilute hydrochloric acid (1 in 120) to volume, and mix. Concomitantly determine the absorbances of this solution and a Standard solution of USP Trimethobenzamide Hydrochloride RS in the same medium having a known concentration of about 20 µg per mL, in 1-cm cells at the wavelength of maximum absorbance at about 258 nm, with a suitable spectrophotometer, using dilute hydrochloric acid (1 in 120) as the blank. Calculate the quantity, in mg, of $C_{21}H_{28}N_2O_5 \cdot HCl$ in the portion of Capsules taken by the formula:

$$2.5C(A_U / A_S)$$

in which *C* is the concentration, in µg per mL, of USP Trimethobenzamide Hydrochloride RS in the Standard solution, and A_U and A_S are the absorbances of the solution from the Capsules and the Standard solution, respectively.

Trimethobenzamide Hydrochloride Injection

» Trimethobenzamide Hydrochloride Injection is a sterile solution of Trimethobenzamide Hydrochloride in Water for Injection. It contains not less than 95.0 percent and not more than 105.0 percent of the labeled amount of $C_{21}H_{28}N_2O_5 \cdot HCl$.

Packaging and storage—Preserve in single-dose or in multiple-dose containers, preferably of Type I glass.

USP Reference standards ⟨11⟩—*USP Endotoxin RS. USP Trimethobenzamide Hydrochloride RS.*

Identification—
  A: It meets the requirements of *Identification* test *A* under *Trimethobenzamide Hydrochloride Capsules*.

  B: Transfer a volume of Injection, equivalent to about 100 mg of trimethobenzamide hydrochloride, to a separator containing 20 mL of water. Add 2 mL of 1 N sodium hydroxide, and proceed as directed in *Identification* test *B* under *Trimethobenzamide Hydrochloride Capsules*, beginning with "Extract with 15 mL of chloroform."

  C: Dilute a portion of Injection quantitatively and stepwise with methanol to obtain a solution containing 2.5 mg of trimethobenzamide hydrochloride per mL: this solution meets the requirements of the *Thin-layer Chromatographic Identification Test* ⟨201⟩, a solvent system consisting of a mixture of ethyl acetate, alcohol, and ammonium hydroxide (90 : 10 : 5) being used.

Bacterial endotoxins ⟨85⟩—It contains not more than 1.80 USP Endotoxin Units per mg of trimethobenzamide hydrochloride.

pH ⟨791⟩: between 4.5 and 5.5.

Other requirements—It meets the requirements under *Injections* ⟨1⟩.

Assay—Transfer to a suitable separator an accurately measured volume of Injection, equivalent to about 200 mg of trimethobenzamide hydrochloride. Add 5 mL of water and 3 mL of dilute hydrochloric acid (1 in 12), and extract with four 20-mL portions of ether, collecting the ether extracts in a second separator, and transferring the aqueous layer to a 500-mL volumetric flask. Wash the combined ether extracts with one 20-mL portion of water, transfer the aqueous layer to the 500-mL volumetric flask, dilute with water to volume, and mix. Dilute 5.0 mL of the solution with dilute hydrochloric acid (1 in 120) to 100.0 mL, and mix. Concomitantly determine the absorbances of this solution and a Standard solution of USP Trimethobenzamide Hydrochloride RS in the same medium having a known concentration of about 20 µg per mL, in 1-cm cells at the wavelength of maximum absorbance at about 258 nm, with a suitable spectrophotometer, using dilute hydrochloric acid (1 in 120) as the blank. Calculate the quantity, in mg, of $C_{21}H_{28}N_2O_5 \cdot HCl$ in each mL of the Injection taken by the formula:

$$(10C / V)(A_U / A_S)$$

in which *C* is the concentration, in µg per mL, of USP Trimethobenzamide Hydrochloride RS in the Standard solution, *V* is the volume, in mL, of Injection taken, and A_U and A_S are the absorbances of the solution from the Injection and the Standard solution, respectively.

Trimethoprim

$C_{14}H_{18}N_4O_3$ 290.32
2,4-Pyrimidinediamine, 5-[(3,4,5-trimethoxyphenyl)methyl]-.
2,4-Diamino-5-(3,4,5-trimethoxybenzyl)pyrimidine   [738-70-5].

» Trimethoprim contains not less than 98.5 percent and not more than 101.0 percent of $C_{14}H_{18}N_4O_3$, calculated on the dried basis.

Packaging and storage—Preserve in tight, light-resistant containers. Store at room temperature.

USP Reference standards ⟨11⟩—*USP Trimethoprim RS.*

Identification—
  A: *Infrared Absorption* ⟨197S⟩—
    Solution: 1 in 100.
    Medium: chloroform.
  B: Transfer about 100 mg of it, accurately weighed, to a 100-mL volumetric flask, and dissolve in 25 mL of alcohol. Dilute quantitatively and stepwise with sodium hydroxide solution (1 in 250) to obtain a 1 in 50,000 solution: the UV absorption spectrum of this solution exhibits maxima and minima only at the same wavelengths as that of a similar solution of USP Trimethoprim RS, concomitantly measured; and the respective absorptivities, calcu-

lated on the dried basis for the test sample only, at the wavelength of maximum absorbance at about 287 nm do not differ by more than 3.0%.

Melting range ⟨741⟩: between 199° and 203°.

Loss on drying ⟨731⟩—Dry it in vacuum at 105° for 4 hours: it loses not more than 0.5% of its weight.

Residue on ignition ⟨281⟩: not more than 0.1%.

Chromatographic purity—

Buffer solution—Prepare a 10 mM sodium perchlorate solution in water, adjust with phosphoric acid to a pH of 3.6, and mix.

Mobile phase—Prepare a filtered and degassed mixture of *Buffer solution* and methanol (7 : 3). Make adjustments if necessary (see *System Suitability* under *Chromatography* ⟨621⟩).

Resolution solution—Dissolve accurately weighed quantities of USP Trimethoprim RS and diaveridine; and dilute quantitatively, and stepwise if necessary, with *Mobile phase* to obtain a solution having known concentrations of about 10 µg per mL and 5 µg per mL, respectively.

Test solution—Transfer about 25.0 mg of Trimethoprim, accurately weighed, to a 25-mL volumetric flask, dissolve in and dilute with *Mobile phase* to volume, and mix.

Chromatographic system (see *Chromatography* ⟨621⟩)—The liquid chromatograph is equipped with a 280-nm detector and a 4.6-mm × 25-cm column that contains base-deactivated packing L1. The flow rate is 1.3 mL per minute. Chromatograph the *Resolution solution,* and record the peak responses as directed for *Procedure:* the resolution, R, between the peaks for trimethoprim and diaveridine is not less than 2.5; and the relative standard deviation for replicate injections is not more than 2.0%.

Procedure—Inject a volume (about 20 µL) of the *Test solution* into the chromatograph, record the chromatogram for not less than 11 times the retention time of the trimethoprim peak, and measure all of the peak responses. Calculate the percentage of each impurity in the portion of Trimethoprim taken by the formula:

$$100\{Fr_i / [\Sigma(Fr_i) + Fr_T]\}$$

in which F is a relative response factor, and is equal to 0.5 for any peak having a relative retention time of 0.9, 2.3, 2.7, or 10.3, and is equal to 1.0 for all other peaks; r_i is the peak response for each impurity; and r_T is the peak response for trimethoprim obtained from the *Test solution*: not more than 0.1% of any individual impurity is found; and not more than 0.2% of total impurities is found.

Assay—Transfer about 300 mg of Trimethoprim, accurately weighed, to a conical flask, add 60 mL of glacial acetic acid, and titrate with 0.1 N perchloric acid VS, determining the endpoint potentiometrically. Perform a blank determination, and make any necessary correction. Each mL of 0.1 N perchloric acid is equivalent to 29.03 mg of $C_{14}H_{18}N_4O_3$.

Trimethoprim Tablets

» Trimethoprim Tablets contain not less than 90.0 percent and not more than 110.0 percent of the labeled amount of $C_{14}H_{18}N_4O_3$.

Packaging and storage—Preserve in tight, light-resistant containers.

USP Reference standards ⟨11⟩—*USP Trimethoprim RS.*

Identification—Triturate a quantity of finely powdered Tablets, equivalent to about 100 mg of trimethoprim, with 2.5 mL of methanol. Add 2.5 mL of chloroform, triturate again, and centrifuge. Apply 25 µL of this test solution and 25 µL of a Standard solution of USP Trimethoprim RS in a mixture of methanol and chloroform (1 : 1) containing 20 mg per mL to a suitable thin-layer chromatographic plate (see *Chromatography* ⟨621⟩) coated with a 0.25-mm layer of chromatographic silica gel mixture. Allow the spots to dry, and develop the chromatogram in an unsaturated chamber with a solvent system consisting of a mixture of chloroform, methanol, and ammonium hydroxide (95 : 7.5 : 1), until the solvent front has moved approximately 15 cm from the origin. Remove the plate from the developing chamber, mark the solvent front, and allow the solvent to evaporate. Locate the spots on the plate by viewing under short-wavelength UV light: the R_F value of the principal spot obtained from the test solution corresponds to that obtained from the Standard solution.

Dissolution ⟨711⟩—

Medium: 0.01 N hydrochloric acid; 900 mL.

Apparatus 2: 50 rpm.

Time: 45 minutes.

Procedure—Determine the amount of $C_{14}H_{18}N_4O_3$ dissolved from UV absorbances at the wavelength of maximum absorbance at about 271 nm of filtered portions of the solution under test, suitably diluted with 0.01 N hydrochloric acid to a concentration of about 20 µg per mL, in comparison with a Standard solution having a known concentration of USP Trimethoprim RS in the same *Medium*.

Tolerances—Not less than 75% (*Q*) of the labeled amount of $C_{14}H_{18}N_4O_3$ is dissolved in 45 minutes.

Uniformity of dosage units ⟨905⟩: meet the requirements.

Assay—

Mobile phase—Prepare a filtered and degassed mixture of 1% glacial acetic acid in water (v/v) and acetonitrile (21 : 4). Make adjustments if necessary (see *System Suitability* under *Chromatography* ⟨621⟩).

Standard preparation—Using an accurately weighed quantity of USP Trimethoprim RS, prepare a solution in methanol having a known concentration of about 0.2 mg per mL.

Assay preparation—Weigh and finely powder not less than 20 Tablets. Transfer an accurately weighed portion of the powder, equivalent to about 100 mg of trimethoprim, to a 100-mL volumetric flask, add 50 mL of methanol, and sonicate for 5 minutes, with intermittent swirling. Dilute with methanol to volume, and mix. Centrifuge, pipet 10 mL of the supernatant into a 50-mL volumetric flask, dilute with methanol to volume, and mix.

Chromatographic system (see *Chromatography* ⟨621⟩)—The liquid chromatograph is equipped with a 254-nm detector and a 4.2-mm × 25-cm column that contains packing L1. The flow rate is about 2 mL per minute. Chromatograph five replicate injections of the *Standard preparation,* and measure the peak responses as directed for *Procedure:* the relative standard deviation is not more than 2.0%.

Procedure—Separately inject equal volumes (about 10 µL) of the *Standard preparation* and the *Assay preparation* into the chromatograph, record the chromatograms, and measure the responses for the analyte peak. Calculate the quantity, in mg, of $C_{14}H_{18}N_4O_3$, in the portion of Tablets taken by the formula:

$$500C(r_U / r_S)$$

in which C is the concentration, in mg per mL, of USP Trimethoprim RS in the *Standard preparation,* and r_U and r_S are the peak responses obtained from the *Assay preparation* and the *Standard preparation*, respectively.

Trimethoprim Sulfate

$(C_{14}H_{18}N_4O_3)_2 \cdot H_2SO_4$ 678.73

2,4-Pyrimidinediamine, 5-[(3,4,5-trimethoxyphenyl)methyl]-, sulfate (2 : 1) (salt).

2,4-Diamino-5-[(3,4,5-trimethoxybenzyl)pyrimidine]-, sulfate (2 : 1) (salt)   [56585-33-2].

» Trimethoprim Sulfate contains not less than 98.5 percent and not more than 101.0 percent of $(C_{14}H_{18}N_4O_3)_2 \cdot H_2SO_4$, calculated on the anhydrous basis.

Packaging and storage—Preserve in well-closed containers. Store at 25°, excursions permitted between 15° and 30°.

3470 **Trimethoprim** / *Official Monographs*

USP Reference standards ⟨11⟩—*USP Trimethoprim RS.*
Identification—
  A: *Ultraviolet Absorption* ⟨197U⟩—
  Solution—Transfer about 100 mg of it, accurately weighed, to a 100-mL volumetric flask, dissolve in 25 mL of alcohol, dilute with 0.1 N sodium hydroxide to volume, and mix.
  Medium—Dilute the *Solution* quantitatively and stepwise with 0.1 N sodium hydroxide to obtain a solution containing a known concentration of about 20 µg per mL.
  Absorptivity, at about 287 nm, calculated on the anhydrous basis, is between 83.0% and 86.4% of USP Trimethoprim RS.
  B: It responds to the tests for *Sulfate* ⟨191⟩.
Melting range ⟨741⟩: between 210° and 215°.
pH ⟨791⟩: between 7.5 and 8.5, in a solution (0.5 mg per mL).
Water, *Method I* ⟨921⟩: not more than 3.0%.
Chromatographic purity—
  Adsorbent: 0.25-mm layer of chromatographic silica gel mixture.
  Diluent—Prepare a mixture of chloroform and methanol (9 : 1).
  Test solution—Transfer about 20 mg of Trimethoprim Sulfate, accurately weighed, to a 10-mL volumetric flask, add 4 mL of glacial acetic acid, and swirl to dissolve. Dilute with *Diluent* to volume, and mix.
  Standard solution—Dissolve an accurately weighed quantity of USP Trimethoprim RS in *Diluent*. Dilute an accurately measured volume of this solution quantitatively, and stepwise if necessary, with *Diluent* to obtain a solution having a known concentration of 0.02 mg per mL.
  Application volume: 10 µL.
  Developing solvent system: a mixture of chloroform, methanol, and 6 N ammonium hydroxide (95 : 7.5 : 1).
  Procedure—Proceed as directed for *Thin-Layer Chromatography* under *Chromatography* ⟨621⟩. Spray the plate with a freshly prepared mixture of 1.9 g of ferric chloride in 20 mL of water and 0.5 g of potassium ferricyanide in 10 mL of water. Compare the intensities of any secondary spots observed in the chromatogram of the *Test solution* with that of the principal spot in the chromatogram of the *Standard solution:* no secondary spot in the chromatogram obtained from the *Test solution* is larger or more intense than the principal spot obtained from the *Standard solution* (0.1%); and the sum of the intensities of the secondary spots obtained from the *Test solution* corresponds to not more than 0.5%.
Assay—Transfer about 800 mg of Trimethoprim Sulfate, accurately weighed, to a 50-mL conical flask, add about 60 mL of glacial acetic acid, and titrate with 0.1 N perchloric acid VS, determining the endpoint potentiometrically. Perform a blank determination, and make any necessary correction. Each mL of 0.1 N perchloric acid is equivalent to 67.87 mg of $(C_{14}H_{18}N_4O_3)_2 \cdot H_2SO_4$.

Add the following:

▲**Trimipramine Maleate**

$C_{20}H_{26}N_2 \cdot C_4H_4O_4$ 410.51
5*H*-Dibenz[*b,f*]azepine-5-propanamine, 10,11-dihydro-*N,N,β*-trimethyl-, (*Z*)-2-butenedioate (1 : 1).
5-[3-(Dimethylamino)-2-methylpropyl]-10,11-dihydro-5*H*-dibenz[*b,f*]azepine maleate (1 : 1)   [*521-78-8*].

» Trimipramine Maleate contains not less than 98.0 percent and not more than 102.0 percent of $C_{20}H_{26}N_2 \cdot C_4H_4O_4$, calculated on the dried basis.

Packaging and storage—Preserve in tight containers, and store at room temperature.
USP Reference standards ⟨11⟩—*USP Iminodibenzyl RS. USP Imipramine Hydrochloride RS. USP Trimipramine Maleate RS. USP Trimipramine Related Compound A RS.*
Identification—
  A: *Infrared Absorption* ⟨197K⟩.
  B: The retention time of the major peak in the chromatogram of the *Assay preparation* corresponds to that in the chromatogram of the *Standard preparation,* as obtained in the *Assay.*
Loss on drying ⟨731⟩—Dry it at 105° to constant weight: it loses not more than 0.5% of its weight.
Residue on ignition ⟨281⟩: not more than 0.1%.
Heavy metals, *Method II* ⟨231⟩: 0.002%.
Related compounds—
  Mobile phase and *Standard stock preparation*—Prepare as directed in the *Assay.*
  Impurity stock solution—Dissolve accurately weighed quantities of USP Imipramine Hydrochloride RS and USP Iminodibenzyl RS in a suitable volume of *Mobile phase* to obtain a solution having a known concentration of about 50 µg per mL of iminodibenzyl and 56.5 µg per mL of imipramine hydrochloride.
  Trimipramine related compound A solution—Dissolve a suitable quantity of USP Trimipramine Related Compound A RS in *Mobile phase* to obtain a solution having a concentration of about 50 µg per mL.
  Trimipramine stock solution—Quantitatively dilute the *Standard stock preparation* with *Mobile phase* to obtain a solution having a known concentration of about 70 µg per mL of trimipramine maleate.
  System suitability solution—Transfer about 7 mg of USP Trimipramine Maleate RS to a 10-mL volumetric flask, dissolve in a small amount of *Mobile phase,* add 0.1 mL each of the *Impurity stock solution* and the *Trimipramine related compound A solution,* and dilute with *Mobile phase* to volume.
  Standard solution—Transfer 5.0 mL each of the *Impurity stock solution* and the *Trimipramine stock solution* with *Mobile phase* to a 50-mL volumetric flask, and dilute with *Mobile phase* to volume. Dilute the resulting solution quantitatively, and stepwise if necessary, with *Mobile phase* to obtain a final solution having a known concentration of about 0.5 µg per mL each of iminodibenzyl, imipramine (free base), and trimipramine (free base). [NOTE—This solution is stable for one day at room temperature. The concentration of imipramine (free base), in µg per mL, can be calculated using the molecular weights of imipramine (282.41) and imipramine hydrochloride (318.88). The concentration of trimipramine (free base), in µg per mL, can be calculated using the molecular weights of trimipramine (294.43) and trimipramine maleate (410.51).]
  Test solution—Use the *Assay stock preparation.*
  Chromatographic system—Prepare as directed in the *Assay.* Chromatograph about 10 µL of the *System suitability solution,* and record the peak responses as directed for *Procedure:* the resolution, *R,* between trimipramine and trimipramine related compound A is not less than 1.5. [NOTE—For identification purposes, the approximate relative retention times of the specified impurities are given in Table 1.]
  Procedure—Separately inject about 10 µL of the *Standard solution* and the *Test solution* into the chromatograph, and record the chromatogram for three times the retention time for trimipramine. Identify the components based on their relative retention times in *Table 1.* Measure the peak areas of all the peaks in the *Test solution.* Calculate the percentage of imipramine and iminodibenzyl in the portion of Trimipramine Maleate taken by the formula:

$$100(C_S / C_T)(r_U / r_S)$$

in which C_S is the concentration, in mg per mL, of any given impurity (free base) in the *Standard solution;* C_T is the concentration of Trimipramine Maleate, in mg per mL, in the *Test solution;* r_U is the individual peak response of the given impurity obtained from the *Test solution;* and r_S is the corresponding response for the same impurity obtained from the *Standard solution.* Calculate the percentage of trimipramine related compound A in the portion of Trimipramine Maleate taken by the formula:

$$100(1/3.6)(C_S / C_T)(r_U / r_S)$$

in which 3.6 is the relative response factor for trimipramine related compound A; C_S is the concentration, in mg per mL, of trimipramine (free base) in the *Standard solution*; C_T is the concentration of Trimipramine Maleate, in mg per mL, in the *Test solution*; r_U is the peak response for trimipramine related compound A obtained from the *Test solution*; and r_S is the peak response of trimipramine obtained from the *Standard solution*. Calculate the percentage of each unknown impurity in the portion of Trimipramine Maleate taken by the formula:

$$100(C_S / C_T)(r_i / r_S)$$

in which C_S is the concentration, in mg per mL, of trimipramine (free base) in the *Standard solution*; C_T is the concentration of Trimipramine Maleate, in mg per mL, in the *Test solution*; r_i is the individual peak response of the given impurity obtained from the *Test solution*; and r_S is the response for trimipramine obtained from the *Standard solution*: the limits of the related compounds are given in *Table 1*. [NOTE—Disregard any peak due to the maleate counterion eluting at a relative retention time of about 0.13.]

Table 1

Peak Identification	Approximate Relative Retention Time (RRT)	Limit % (w/w)
Trimipramine N-oxide[1]	0.32	NMT 0.15
Iminodibenzyl[2]	0.49	NMT 0.20
Desmethyltrimipramine[3]	0.68	NMT 0.15
Imipramine[4]	0.72	NMT 0.20
Trimipramine related compound A[5]	0.80	NMT 0.10
Trimipramine diamine[6]	2.39	NMT 0.30
Any other individual impurity	—	NMT 0.10
Total impurites	—	NMT 1.0

[1] (2RS)-3-(10,11-Dihydro-5H-dibenzo[b,f]azepin-5-yl)-N,N,2-trimethylpropan-1-amine N-oxide.
[2] 10,11-Dihydro-5H-dibenzo[b,f]azepine.
[3] (2RS)-3-(10,11-Dihydro-5H-dibenzo[b,f]azepin-5-yl)-N,2-dimethylpropan-1-amine 6.
[4] (2RS)-3-(10,11-Dihydro-5H-dibenzo[b,f]azepin-5-yl)-N, N-dimethylpropan-1-amine.
[5] 5-[3-(Dimethylamino)-2-methylpropyl]-5H-dibenz[b,f]azepine.
[6] (2RS)-N1-((2RS)-3-(10,11-Dihydro-5H-dibenzo[b,f]azepin-5-yl)-2-methylpropyl)-N1,N3,N3,2-tetramethylpropane-1,3-diamine.

Assay—
Buffer solution—Dissolve about 1.4 g of anhydrous dibasic sodium phosphate in 1 L of water. Adjust with phosphoric acid to a pH of 7.7.
Mobile phase—Prepare a filtered and degassed mixture of acetonitrile, methanol, and *Buffer solution* (18 : 12 : 10). Make adjustments if necessary (see *System Suitability* under *Chromatography* ⟨621⟩).
Standard stock preparation—Dissolve an accurately weighed quantity of USP Trimipramine Maleate RS in a suitable volume of *Mobile phase* to obtain a solution having a known concentration of about 0.7 mg per mL.
Standard preparation—Transfer 3 mL of the *Standard stock preparation* to a 10-mL volumetric flask, and dilute with *Mobile phase* to volume to obtain a final solution having a known concentration of about 0.21 mg per mL of trimipramine maleate.
Assay stock preparation—Dissolve an accurately weighed quantity of Trimipramine Maleate in a suitable volume of *Mobile phase* to obtain a solution having a known concentration of about 0.7 mg per mL.
Assay preparation—Transfer 3 mL of the *Assay stock preparation* to a 10-mL volumetric flask, and dilute with *Mobile phase* to volume to obtain a final solution having a known concentration of about 0.21 mg per mL of trimipramine maleate.
Chromatographic system (see *Chromatography* ⟨621⟩)—The liquid chromatograph is equipped with a 254-nm detector and a 4.6-mm × 25-cm column that contains 5-μm packing L7. The flow rate is about 1.0 mL per minute. The column temperature is maintained at 30°. Chromatograph about 20 μL of the *Standard preparation*, and record the peak responses as directed for *Procedure*: the tailing factor for the rimipramine maleate peak is not more than 2.0; and the relative standard deviation for replicate injections of the *Standard preparation* is not more than 2.0%.
Procedure—Separately inject equal volumes (about 20 μL) of the *Standard preparation* and the *Assay preparation* into the chromatograph, record the chromatograms for up to 1.5 times the retention time of trimipramine maleate, and measure the responses for the trimipramine maleate peak. Calculate the percentage of $C_{20}H_{26}N_2 \cdot C_4H_4O_4$, in the portion of Trimipramine Maleate taken by the formula:

$$100(C_S / C_U)(r_U / r_S)$$

in which C_S is the concentration, in mg per mL, of USP Trimipramine Maleate RS in the *Standard preparation*; C_U is the concentration, in mg per mL, of Trimipramine Maleate in the *Assay preparation*; and r_U and r_S are the trimipramine peak responses obtained from the *Assay preparation* and the *Standard preparation*, respectively.▲USP31

Trioxsalen

$C_{14}H_{12}O_3$ 228.24
7H-Furo[3,2-g]1]benzopyran-7-one, 2,5,9-trimethyl-.
2,5,9-Trimethyl-7H-furo[3,2-g]1]benzopyran-7-one   [3902-71-4].

» Trioxsalen contains not less than 97.0 percent and not more than 103.0 percent of $C_{14}H_{12}O_3$, calculated on the dried basis.
Caution—Avoid exposing the skin to Trioxsalen.

Packaging and storage—Preserve in well-closed, light-resistant containers.
USP Reference standards ⟨11⟩—*USP Trioxsalen RS.*
Identification—
  A: *Infrared Absorption* ⟨197M⟩.
  B: *Ultraviolet Absorption* ⟨197U⟩—
  Solution: 5 μg per mL.
  Medium: chloroform.
  C: The retention time of the major peak in the chromatogram of the *Assay preparation* corresponds to that of the *Standard preparation* as obtained in the *Assay*.
Loss on drying ⟨731⟩—Dry it at 105° for 6 hours: it loses not more than 0.5% of its weight.
Residue on ignition ⟨281⟩: not more than 0.5%.
Related compounds—In the chromatogram obtained from the *Assay preparation* in the *Assay*, the sum of the responses of any peaks detected, other than the major peak due to trioxsalen, is not more than 2.0% of the total of all the peak responses and the response of the peak occurring at retention time relative to trioxsalen of about 0.75 is not more than 1.5% of the total of all responses.
Organic volatile impurities, *Method V* ⟨467⟩: meets the requirements.
  Solvent—Use dimethyl sulfoxide.

(Official until July 1, 2008)

Assay—

Mobile phase—Prepare a filtered and degassed mixture of methanol and water (70 : 30). Make adjustments if necessary (see *System Suitability* under *Chromatography* ⟨621⟩).

Standard preparation—Dissolve an accurately weighed quantity of USP Trioxsalen RS in tetrahydrofuran to obtain a solution having a known concentration of about 1 mg per mL. Transfer 5.0 mL of this solution to a 100-mL volumetric flask, dilute with *Mobile phase* to volume, and mix.

Assay preparation—Transfer about 100 mg of Trioxsalen, accurately weighed, to a 100-mL volumetric flask, dissolve in tetrahydrofuran, dilute with tetrahydrofuran to volume, mix, and filter. Transfer 5.0 mL of this solution to a 100-mL volumetric flask, dilute with *Mobile phase* to volume, and mix.

Chromatographic system (see *Chromatography* ⟨621⟩)—The liquid chromatograph is equipped with a 254-nm detector and a 4.6-nm × 25-cm column that contains packing L1. The flow rate is about 1 mL per minute. Chromatograph the *Standard preparation*, and record the peak responses as directed for *Procedure:* the tailing factor for the trioxsalen peak is not more than 2.0, and the relative standard deviation for replicate injections is not more than 2.0%.

Procedure—Separately inject equal volumes (about 20 µL) of the *Standard preparation* and the *Assay preparation* into the chromatograph, record the chromatograms, and measure the responses for the major peaks. Calculate the quantity, in mg, of $C_{14}H_{12}O_3$ in the portion of Trioxsalen taken by the formula:

$$2000C(r_U / r_S)$$

in which C is the concentration, in mg per mL, of USP Trioxsalen RS in the *Standard preparation*, and r_U and r_S are the peak responses obtained from the *Assay preparation* and the *Standard preparation*, respectively.

Trioxsalen Tablets

» Trioxsalen Tablets contain not less than 93.0 percent and not more than 107.0 percent of the labeled amount of $C_{14}H_{12}O_3$.

Packaging and storage—Preserve in well-closed, light-resistant containers.

USP Reference standards ⟨11⟩—*USP Trioxsalen RS.*

Identification—Triturate an amount of finely powdered Tablets, equivalent to about 10 mg of trioxsalen, with 100 mL of chloroform, and filter. Apply 5 µL each of this solution and a Standard solution of USP Trioxsalen RS in chloroform having a known concentration of 100 µg per mL to a suitable thin-layer chromatographic plate (see *Chromatography* ⟨621⟩) coated with a 0.25-mm layer of chromatographic silica gel. Allow the spots to dry, and develop the chromatogram, using methanol as the solvent, until the solvent front has moved about three-fourths of the length of the plate. Remove the plate from the developing chamber, mark the solvent front, and allow the solvent to evaporate. Locate the spots on the plate by viewing under an UV lamp: the R_F value of the principal spot obtained from the test solution corresponds to that obtained from the Standard solution.

Dissolution ⟨711⟩—

Apparatus 2: 100 rpm.

Time: 60 minutes.

Dilute simulated intestinal fluid—Prepare a 1 in 12 solution of simulated intestinal fluid TS and water.

Procedure—Assemble the apparatus, adding 225 mL of *Dilute simulated intestinal fluid* to each vessel, and operate the apparatus for 40 minutes. At the end of the 40 minutes, immediately add 675 mL of dehydrated alcohol to each of the vessels. Continue to operate the apparatus for an additional 20 minutes. Determine the amount of $C_{14}H_{12}O_3$ dissolved from UV absorbance determined at the wavelength of maximum absorbance at about 252 nm, filtered portions of the solution under test, in comparison with a Standard solution having a known concentration of USP Trioxsalen RS in the same medium.

Tolerances—Not less than 75% (*Q*) of the labeled amount of $C_{14}H_{12}O_3$ is dissolved in 60 minutes.

Uniformity of dosage units ⟨905⟩: meet the requirements.

Assay—Weigh and finely powder not less than 20 Tablets. Transfer an accurately weighed portion of the powder, equivalent to about 5 mg of trioxsalen, to a separator containing 25 mL of water. Extract with three 25-mL portions of chloroform, filtering each extract into a 100-mL volumetric flask. Wash the filter with chloroform, dilute with chloroform to volume, and mix. Transfer 10.0 mL of this solution to a second 100-mL volumetric flask, dilute with chloroform to volume, and mix. Concomitantly determine the absorbances of this solution and a solution of USP Trioxsalen RS in the same medium having a known concentration of about 5 µg per mL in 1-cm cells at the wavelength of maximum absorbance at about 252 nm, with a suitable spectrophotometer, using chloroform as the blank. Calculate the quantity, in mg, of $C_{14}H_{12}O_3$ in the portion of Tablets taken by the formula:

$$C(A_U / A_S)$$

in which C is the concentration, in µg per mL, of USP Trioxsalen RS in the Standard solution, and A_U and A_S are the absorbances of the solution from the Tablets and the Standard solution, respectively.

Tripelennamine Hydrochloride

$C_{16}H_{21}N_3 \cdot HCl$ 291.82

1,2-Ethanediamine, *N,N*-dimethyl-*N'*-(phenylmethyl)-*N'*-2-pyridinyl-, monohydrochloride.

2-[Benzyl[2-(dimethylamino)ethyl]amino]pyridine monohydrochloride [*154-69-8*].

» Tripelennamine Hydrochloride contains not less than 98.0 percent and not more than 102.0 percent of $C_{16}H_{21}N_3 \cdot HCl$, calculated on the dried basis.

Packaging and storage—Preserve in well-closed, light-resistant containers.

USP Reference standards ⟨11⟩—*USP Tripelennamine Hydrochloride RS.*

Identification—

  A: It meets the requirements under *Identification—Organic Nitrogenous Bases* ⟨181⟩.

  B: It meets the requirements of the tests for *Chloride* ⟨191⟩.

Melting range ⟨741⟩: between 188° and 192°.

Loss on drying ⟨731⟩—Dry it at 105° for 3 hours: it loses not more than 1.0% of its weight.

Residue on ignition ⟨281⟩: not more than 0.1%.

Chromatographic purity—

Ion-pair solution, Mobile phase, and *Benzaldehyde solution*—Proceed as directed in the *Assay.*

Chromatographic system—Proceed as directed in the *Assay.* To evaluate system suitability requirements, use the *System suitability preparation* and the *Standard preparation,* as prepared in the *Assay.*

Test solution—Use the *Assay preparation.*

Procedure—Inject a volume (about 10 µL) of the *Test solution* into the chromatograph, record the chromatogram, and measure all of the peak responses. Calculate the percentage of each impurity in the portion of Tripelennamine Hydrochloride taken by the formula:

$$100(r_i / r_S)$$

in which r_i is the peak response for each impurity, and r_S is the sum of the responses for all the peaks: not more than 0.1% of any individual impurity is found; and not more than 1.0% of total impurities is found.

Organic volatile impurities, *Method I* ⟨467⟩: meets the requirements.

(Official until July 1, 2008)

Assay—

Ion-pair solution—Prepare a 29-mM sodium 1-octanesulfonate solution.

Mobile phase—Transfer 530 mL of methanol to a suitable container, add 1.0 mL of *N,N*-dimethyloctylamine, and mix thoroughly. Add 430 mL of the *Ion-pair solution,* mix, and adjust with phosphoric acid to a pH of 3.0. Make adjustments if necessary (see *System Suitability* under *Chromatography* ⟨621⟩).

Benzaldehyde solution—Transfer 1.0 mL of benzaldehyde to a 100-mL volumetric flask, dilute with *Mobile phase* to volume, and mix. Transfer 5.0 mL of the solution so obtained to a 100-mL volumetric flask, dilute with *Mobile phase* to volume, and mix.

System suitability preparation—Transfer about 50 mg of 2-benzylaminopyridine, accurately weighed, to a 100-mL volumetric flask, add 10 mL of methanol, sonicate to dissolve, dilute with *Mobile phase* to volume, and mix. Transfer 5.0 mL of the solution so obtained to a 100-mL volumetric flask, add 5.0 mL of *Benzaldehyde solution,* dilute with *Mobile phase* to volume, and mix.

Standard preparation—Dissolve an accurately weighed quantity of USP Tripelennamine Hydrochloride RS in *Mobile phase,* and dilute quantitatively, and stepwise if necessary, with *Mobile phase* to obtain a solution having a known concentration of about 0.5 mg per mL.

Assay preparation—Transfer about 50 mg of Tripelennamine Hydrochloride, accurately weighed, to a 100-mL volumetric flask, dissolve in and dilute with *Mobile phase* to volume, and mix.

Chromatographic system (see *Chromatography* ⟨621⟩)—The liquid chromatograph is equipped with a 242-nm detector and a 4.6-mm × 25-cm column that contains packing L7. The flow rate is about 1 mL per minute. The column temperature is maintained at 35°. [NOTE—New columns are conditioned with *Mobile phase* overnight before the initial use and may be reconditioned, as necessary, thereafter.] Chromatograph the *System suitability preparation,* and record the peak responses as directed for *Procedure:* the relative retention times are about 0.75 for benzaldehyde and 1.0 for 2-benzylaminopyridine; and the resolution, *R,* between benzaldehyde and 2-benzylaminopyridine is not less than 3.5. Chromatograph the *Standard preparation,* and record the peak responses as directed for *Procedure:* the column efficiency is not less than 10,000 theoretical plates; and the relative standard deviation for replicate injections is not more than 1.0%.

Procedure—Separately inject equal volumes (about 10 µL) of the *Standard preparation* and the *Assay preparation* into the chromatograph, record the chromatograms, and measure the responses for the major peaks. Calculate the quantity, in percentage, of $C_{16}H_{21}N_3 \cdot HCl$ in the portion of Tripelennamine Hydrochloride taken by the formula:

$$100C_S(r_U/r_S)/C_U$$

in which C_U and C_S are the concentrations, in mg per mL, of the *Assay preparation* and of USP Tripelennamine Hydrochloride RS in the *Standard preparation,* respectively; and r_U and r_S are the peak responses obtained from the *Assay preparation* and the *Standard preparation,* respectively.

Tripelennamine Hydrochloride Injection

» Tripelennamine Hydrochloride Injection is a sterile solution of Tripelennamine Hydrochloride in Water for Injection. It contains not less than 90.0 percent and not more than 110.0 percent of the labeled amount of tripelennamine hydrochloride ($C_{16}H_{21}N_3 \cdot HCl$).

Packaging and storage—Preserve in tight, single-dose or multiple-dose *Containers for Injections,* as described under *Injections* ⟨1⟩. Store at a controlled room temperature, and protect from light.

Labeling—Label it to indicate that it is for veterinary use only.

USP Reference standards ⟨11⟩—*USP Endotoxin RS. USP Tripelennamine Hydrochloride RS.*

Identification—
   A: *Identification—Organic Nitrogenous Bases* ⟨181⟩.
   B: The retention time of the major peak in the chromatogram of the *Assay preparation* corresponds to that in the chromatogram of the *Standard preparation,* as obtained in the *Assay.*

Bacterial endotoxins ⟨85⟩—It contains not more than 4.6 USP Endotoxin Units per mg of tripelennamine hydrochloride.

Sterility ⟨71⟩—It meets the requirements when tested as directed for *Membrane Filtration* under *Test for Sterility of the Product to be Examined.*

pH ⟨791⟩:   between 6.0 and 7.0.

Particulate matter ⟨788⟩:   meets the requirements for small-volume injections.

Other requirements—It meets the requirements under *Injections* ⟨1⟩.

Assay—
Mobile phase—Dissolve 4.8 g of monobasic potassium phosphate in 880 mL of water in a 2-liter cylinder. Add 720 mL of methanol and 400 mL of acetonitrile, mix, filter, and degas. Make adjustments if necessary (see *System Suitability* under *Chromatography* ⟨621⟩).

Standard preparation—Dissolve an accurately weighed quantity of USP Tripelennamine Hydrochloride RS quantitatively in water to obtain a solution having a known concentration of about 0.02 mg per mL. Protect this solution from light.

Assay preparation—Transfer an accurately measured volume of Injection, equivalent to about 4 mg of tripelennamine hydrochloride, to a 200-mL volumetric flask, dilute with water to volume, and mix.

Chromatographic system (see *Chromatography* ⟨621⟩)—The liquid chromatograph is equipped with a 254-nm detector, a 3.9-mm × 30-mm guard column that contains packing L1, and a 3.9-mm × 30-cm analytical column that contains packing L1. The flow rate is about 1 mL per minute. Chromatograph the *Standard preparation,* and record the peak responses as directed for *Procedure:* the relative standard deviation for replicate injections is not more than 2.0%.

Procedure—Separately inject equal volumes (about 20 µL) of the *Standard preparation* and the *Assay preparation* into the chromatograph, record the chromatograms, and measure the responses for the tripelennamine peaks. Calculate the quantity, in mg, of tripelennamine hydrochloride ($C_{16}H_{21}N_3 \cdot HCl$) in each mL of the Injection taken by the formula:

$$200(C/V)(r_U/r_S)$$

in which *C* is the concentration, in mg per mL, of USP Tripelennamine Hydrochloride RS in the *Standard preparation; V* is the volume, in mL, of Injection taken to prepare the *Assay preparation;* and r_U and r_S are the peak responses obtained from the *Assay preparation* and the *Standard preparation,* respectively.

Tripelennamine Hydrochloride Tablets

» Tripelennamine Hydrochloride Tablets contain not less than 95.0 percent and not more than 105.0 percent of the labeled amount of $C_{16}H_{21}N_3 \cdot HCl$.

Packaging and storage—Preserve in well-closed containers.

USP Reference standards ⟨11⟩—*USP Tripelennamine Hydrochloride RS.*

Identification—Tablets meet the requirements under *Identification—Organic Nitrogenous Bases* ⟨181⟩.

Dissolution ⟨711⟩—
   Medium: water; 900 mL.
   Apparatus 1:   100 rpm.
   Time: 45 minutes.
   Procedure—Determine the amount of $C_{16}H_{21}N_3 \cdot HCl$ dissolved from UV absorbances at the wavelength of maximum absorbance at about 306 nm of filtered portions of the solution under test, suitably diluted with *Dissolution Medium,* if necessary, in comparison with

a Standard solution having a known concentration of USP Tripelennamine Hydrochloride RS in the same medium.

Tolerances—Not less than 75% (*Q*) of the labeled amount of $C_{16}H_{21}N_3 \cdot HCl$ is dissolved in 45 minutes.

Uniformity of dosage units ⟨905⟩: meet the requirements.

Assay—Proceed with Tablets as directed under *Salts of Organic Nitrogenous Bases* ⟨501⟩, determining the absorbance at 313 nm. Calculate the quantity, in mg, of $C_{16}H_{21}N_3 \cdot HCl$ in the portion of Tablets taken by the formula:

$$50C(A_U / A_S)$$

in which *C* is the concentration, in mg per mL, calculated on the dried basis, of USP Tripelennamine Hydrochloride RS in the *Standard Preparation*.

Triprolidine Hydrochloride

$C_{19}H_{22}N_2 \cdot HCl \cdot H_2O$ 332.87

Pyridine, 2-[1-(4-methylphenyl)-3-(1-pyrrolidinyl)-1-propenyl]-, monohydrochloride, monohydrate, (*E*)-.

(*E*)-2-[3-(1-Pyrrolidinyl)-1-*p*-tolylpropenyl]pyridine monohydrochloride monohydrate [6138-79-0].

Anhydrous 314.86 [550-70-9].

» Triprolidine Hydrochloride contains not less than 98.0 percent and not more than 101.0 percent of $C_{19}H_{22}N_2 \cdot HCl$, calculated on the anhydrous basis.

Packaging and storage—Preserve in tight, light-resistant containers.

USP Reference standards ⟨11⟩—*USP Triprolidine Hydrochloride RS. USP Triprolidine Hydrochloride Z-isomer RS.*

Identification—
  A: *Infrared Absorption* ⟨197K⟩.
  B: *Ultraviolet Absorption* ⟨197U⟩—
  Solution: 10 µg per mL.
  Medium: 0.1 N hydrochloric acid.
  Absorptivities at 290 nm, calculated on the anhydrous basis, do not differ by more than 3.0%.
  C: A solution of it responds to the tests for *Chloride* ⟨191⟩.

Water, *Method I* ⟨921⟩: between 4.0% and 6.0%.

Residue on ignition ⟨281⟩: not more than 0.1%.

Heavy metals, *Method II* ⟨231⟩: 0.002%.

Chromatographic purity—

Standard preparations—Dissolve USP Triprolidine Hydrochloride RS in chloroform, and mix to obtain a solution having a known concentration of 1.0 mg per mL. Dilute quantitatively with chloroform to obtain four diluted *Standard preparations*(A, B, C, and D) having the following compositions:

Standard preparation	Dilution	Concentration (µg RS per mL)	Percentage (%) for comparison with test specimen)
A	(1 in 5)	200	2.0
B	(15 in 100)	150	1.5
C	(1 in 10)	100	1.0
D	(5 in 100)	50	0.5

Standard Z-isomer preparations—Proceed as directed for *Standard preparations*, using USP Triprolidine Hydrochloride Z-isomer RS to obtain four diluted *Standard preparations* having the same compositions as in the table shown therein.

Test preparation—Dissolve an accurately weighed quantity of Triprolidine Hydrochloride in chloroform to obtain a solution containing 10 mg per mL.

Procedure—Apply separately 5 µL of the *Test preparation* and 5 µL of each of the eight diluted *Standard* to a suitable thin-layer chromatographic plate (see *Chromatography* ⟨621⟩) coated with a 0.25-mm layer of chromatographic silica gel mixture. Position the plate in a chromatographic chamber, and develop the chromatograms, protected from light, in a solvent system consisting of a mixture of chloroform and diethylamine (95 : 5) until the solvent front has moved about three-fourths of the length of the plate. Remove the plate from the developing chamber, mark the solvent front, and allow the solvent to evaporate. Examine the plate under long- and short-wavelength UV light. Compare the intensities of any secondary spots observed in the chromatogram of the *Test preparation* with those of the principal spots in the chromatograms of the *Standard preparations:* the intensity of the Z-isomer triprolidine hydrochloride spot (R_F value about 1.2 relative to the R_F value for triprolidine hydrochloride) obtained from the *Test preparation* corresponds to not more than 2.0%, and the sum of the intensities of all secondary spots obtained from the *Test preparation* corresponds to not more than 3.0%.

Organic volatile impurities, *Method V* ⟨467⟩: meets the requirements.

(Official until July 1, 2008)

Assay—Dissolve about 400 mg of Triprolidine Hydrochloride, accurately weighed, in 80 mL of glacial acetic acid, warming, if necessary, to effect solution. Add 15 mL of mercuric acetate TS, and titrate with 0.1 N perchloric acid VS, determining the endpoint potentiometrically. Perform a blank determination, and make any necessary correction. Each mL of 0.1 N perchloric acid is equivalent to 15.74 mg of $C_{19}H_{22}N_2 \cdot HCl$.

Triprolidine Hydrochloride Oral Solution

» Triprolidine Hydrochloride Oral Solution contains not less than 90.0 percent and not more than 110.0 percent of the labeled amount of triprolidine hydrochloride ($C_{19}H_{22}N_2 \cdot HCl \cdot H_2O$).

Packaging and storage—Preserve in tight, light-resistant containers.

USP Reference standards ⟨11⟩—*USP Triprolidine Hydrochloride RS.*

Identification—
  A: Transfer a volume of Oral Solution, equivalent to about 12 mg of triprolidine hydrochloride, to a 125-mL separator, add 25 mL of water, then add 4 mL of sodium hydroxide solution (1 in 2), and mix. Add 10 mL of cyclohexane, shake, allow the phases to separate completely, and discard the aqueous layer. Transfer 8 mL of the cyclohexane solution to a glass-stoppered, 25-mL conical flask, evaporate on a steam bath with the aid of a current of air to dryness, and continue to heat the flask for about 1 minute after the solvent has completely evaporated. Cool, add 2 mL of cyclohexane, and mix: the IR absorption spectrum of the cyclohexane solution so obtained exhibits maxima only at the same wavelengths as that of a similar preparation of USP Triprolidine Hydrochloride RS.
  B: The retention time of the major peak in the chromatogram of the *Assay preparation* corresponds to that in the chromatogram of the *Standard preparation*, as obtained in the *Assay*.

pH ⟨791⟩: between 5.6 and 6.6.

Alcohol content, *Method II* ⟨611⟩: between 3.0% and 5.0% of C_2H_5OH.

Assay—
  Mobile phase—Prepare a suitable degassed and filtered mixture of alcohol and ammonium acetate solution (1 in 250) (17 : 3).

Standard preparation—Dissolve an accurately weighed quantity of USP Triprolidine Hydrochloride RS in 0.01 N hydrochloric acid, and dilute quantitatively and stepwise with 0.01 N hydrochloric acid to obtain a solution having a known concentration of about 0.05 mg of anhydrous USP Triprolidine Hydrochloride RS per mL.

Assay preparation—Transfer an accurately measured volume of Oral Solution, equivalent to about 2.5 mg of triprolidine hydrochloride, to a 50-mL volumetric flask, dilute with 0.01 N hydrochloric acid to volume, and mix.

Chromatographic system (see *Chromatography* ⟨621⟩)—The liquid chromatograph is equipped with a 254-nm detector and a 4.2-mm × 25-cm column that contains packing L3. The flow rate is about 1.5 mL per minute. Chromatograph five replicate injections of the *Standard preparation,* and record the peak responses as directed for *Procedure:* the relative standard deviation is not more than 2.0%; and the tailing factor is not more than 1.5.

Procedure—Separately inject equal volumes (about 10 µL) of the *Standard preparation* and the *Assay preparation* into the chromatograph, record the chromatograms, and measure the responses for the major peaks. Calculate the quantity, in mg, of triprolidine hydrochloride ($C_{19}H_{22}N_2 \cdot HCl \cdot H_2O$) in the portion of Oral Solution taken by the formula:

$$(332.88/314.86)(50C)(r_U/r_S)$$

in which 332.88 and 314.86 are the molecular weights of triprolidine hydrochloride monohydrate and anhydrous triprolidine hydrochloride, respectively; C is the concentration, in mg per mL, calculated on the anhydrous basis, of USP Triprolidine Hydrochloride RS in the *Standard preparation;* and r_U and r_S are the peak responses obtained from the *Assay preparation* and the *Standard preparation,* respectively.

Triprolidine Hydrochloride Tablets

» Triprolidine Hydrochloride Tablets contain not less than 90.0 percent and not more than 110.0 percent of the labeled amount of $C_{19}H_{22}N_2 \cdot HCl \cdot H_2O$.

Packaging and storage—Preserve in tight, light-resistant containers.

USP Reference standards ⟨11⟩—*USP Triprolidine Hydrochloride RS.*

Identification—
  A: Weigh and finely powder not less than 20 Tablets. Transfer a portion of the powder, equivalent to about 20 mg of triprolidine hydrochloride, to a glass-stoppered test tube, add 20 mL of water, and shake for 3 minutes. Add 2 mL of 1 N sodium hydroxide, mix, then add 3 mL of cyclohexane, shake for 3 minutes, and centrifuge for 5 minutes: the IR absorption spectrum of the clear supernatant so obtained exhibits maxima only at the same wavelengths as that of a similar preparation of USP Triprolidine Hydrochloride RS.
  B: The retention time of the major peak in the chromatogram of the *Assay preparation* corresponds to that in the chromatogram of the *Standard preparation* as obtained in the *Assay.*

Dissolution ⟨711⟩—
  Medium: pH 4.0 ± 0.05 acetate buffer, prepared by mixing 4.9 g of glacial acetic acid and 2.45 g of sodium acetate trihydrate with water to obtain 1000 mL of solution; 500 mL.
  Apparatus 1: 50 rpm.
  Time: 30 minutes.
  Procedure—Determine the amount of $C_{19}H_{22}N_2 \cdot HCl \cdot H_2O$ dissolved from UV absorbances at the wavelength of maximum absorbance at about 277 nm of filtered portions of the solution under test, in comparison with a Standard solution having a known concentration of USP Triprolidine Hydrochloride RS in the same medium.
  Tolerances—Not less than 80% (*Q*) of the labeled amount of $C_{19}H_{22}N_2 \cdot HCl \cdot H_2O$ is dissolved in 30 minutes.

Uniformity of dosage units ⟨905⟩: meet the requirements.
  Procedure for content uniformity—Transfer 1 Tablet to a 100-mL volumetric flask, add 70 mL of water, and sonicate, swirling the flask intermittently, until the tablet is dissolved. Dilute with water to volume, mix, and filter, discarding the first 50 mL of the filtrate. Dilute a portion of the filtrate quantitatively and stepwise with 0.1 N sulfuric acid to obtain a solution having a concentration of about 1.25 µg of triprolidine hydrochloride per mL. Concomitantly determine the fluorescence intensities of this solution and a similarly prepared Standard solution having a known concentration of about 1.25 µg of USP Triprolidine Hydrochloride RS per mL, at the excitation wavelength of 300 nm with a slit width of 2 mm, and an emission wavelength of 460 nm with a slit width of 2 mm, with a suitable spectrophotometer, using 0.1 N sulfuric acid as the blank. Calculate the quantity, in mg, of $C_{19}H_{22}N_2 \cdot HCl \cdot H_2O$ in the Tablet taken by the formula:

$$(332.88/314.86)(TC/D)(I_U/I_S)$$

in which 332.88 and 314.86 are the molecular weights of the monohydrate and anhydrous forms of triprolidine hydrochloride, respectively; T is the labeled quantity, in mg, of triprolidine hydrochloride in the Tablet; C is the concentration, in µg per mL, of USP Triprolidine Hydrochloride RS in the Standard solution; D is the concentration, in µg per mL, of triprolidine hydrochloride in the solution from the Tablet, on the basis of the labeled quantity per Tablet and the extent of dilution, and I_U and I_S are the fluorescence intensities of the solution from the Tablet and the Standard solution, respectively.

Assay—
  Mobile phase and *Standard preparation*—Prepare as directed in the *Assay* under *Triprolidine Hydrochlorides Oral Solution.*
  Assay preparation—Weigh and finely powder not fewer than 20 Tablets. Transfer an accurately weighed portion of the powder, equivalent to about 5.0 mg of triprolidine hydrochloride, to a 100-mL volumetric flask. Add about 10 mL of 0.01 N hydrochloric acid, and sonicate for 10 minutes. Cool to room temperature. Dilute with 0.01 N hydrochloric acid to volume, mix, and filter.
  Chromatographic system and *Procedure*—Proceed as directed in the *Assay* under *Triprolidine Hydrochlorides Oral Solution,* except to calculate the quantity, in mg, of triprolidine hydrochloride ($C_{19}H_{22}N_2 \cdot HCl \cdot H_2O$) in the portion of Tablets taken by the formula:

$$(332.88/314.86)(100C)(r_U/r_S)$$

in which 332.88 and 314.86 are the molecular weights of triprolidine hydrochloride monohydrate and anhydrous triprolidine hydrochloride, respectively; C is the concentration, in mg per mL, calculated on the anhydrous basis, of USP Triprolidine Hydrochloride RS in the *Standard preparation;* and r_U and r_S are the peak responses obtained from the *Assay preparation* and the *Standard preparation,* respectively.

Triprolidine and Pseudoephedrine Hydrochlorides Oral Solution

» Triprolidine and Pseudoephedrine Hydrochlorides Oral Solution contains not less than 90.0 percent and not more than 110.0 percent of the labeled amounts of triprolidine hydrochloride ($C_{19}H_{22}N_2 \cdot HCl \cdot H_2O$) and pseudoephedrine hydrochloride ($C_{10}H_{15}NO \cdot HCl$).

Packaging and storage—Preserve in tight, light-resistant containers.

USP Reference standards ⟨11⟩—*USP Triprolidine Hydrochloride RS. USP Pseudoephedrine Hydrochloride RS.*

Identification—
  A: The retention times of the major peaks in the chromatogram of the *Assay preparation* correspond to those in the chromatogram of the *Standard preparation,* as obtained in the *Assay.*
  B: Transfer 10 mL of Oral Solution to a suitable glass-stoppered tube, add 10 mL of ether and 2 mL of 1 N sodium hydroxide, shake for 5 minutes, and allow the layers to separate. The ether layer is the test solution. Prepare a Standard solution in water of USP Pseudoephedrine Hydrochloride RS and USP Triprolidine

Hydrochloride RS having known concentrations of 6 mg per mL and 250 μg per mL, respectively. Separately apply 10-μL portions of the test solution and the Standard solution to a suitable thin-layer chromatographic plate (see *Chromatography* ⟨621⟩) coated with a 0.25-mm layer of chromatographic silica gel mixture. Allow the spots to dry, and develop the chromatogram in a solvent system consisting of a mixture of butyl alcohol, glacial acetic acid, and water (8 : 2 : 2) until the solvent front has moved about three-fourths of the length of the plate. Remove the plate, mark the solvent front, allow the solvent to evaporate, and examine the plate under short-wavelength and long-wavelength UV light: the R_F values of the principal spots obtained from the test solution correspond to those obtained from the Standard solution.

Assay—

Mobile phase—Prepare a filtered and degassed mixture of alcohol and 0.40% ammonium acetate solution (17 : 3). Make adjustments if necessary (see *System Suitability* under *Chromatography* ⟨621⟩).

Standard preparation—Dissolve accurately weighed quantities of USP Pseudoephedrine Hydrochloride RS and USP Triprolidine Hydrochloride RS in 0.01 N hydrochloric acid, and dilute quantitatively and stepwise with 0.01 N hydrochloric acid to obtain a solution having known concentrations of about 1.2 mg of USP Pseudoephedrine Hydrochloride RS per mL and about 0.05 mg of anhydrous USP Triprolidine Hydrochloride RS per mL, and filter.

Assay preparation—Transfer an accurately measured volume of Oral Solution, equivalent to about 60 mg of pseudoephedrine hydrochloride, to a 50-mL volumetric flask, dilute with 0.01 N hydrochloric acid to volume, and mix.

Chromatographic system (see *Chromatography* ⟨621⟩)—The liquid chromatograph is equipped with a 254-nm detector and a 4.6-mm × 25-cm column that contains packing L3. The flow rate is about 1.5 mL per minute. Chromatograph replicate injections of the *Standard preparation*, and record the peak responses as directed for *Procedure*: the relative standard deviation is not more than 2.0%; and the resolution factor between triprolidine and pseudoephedrine is not less than 2.0. The tailing factor for the triprolidine peak is not more than 2.0, and the pseudoephedrine peak is not more than 2.0.

Procedure—Separately inject equal volumes (about 10 μL) of the *Standard preparation* and the *Assay preparation* into the chromatograph, record the chromatograms, and measure the responses for the major peaks. The relative retention times are about 0.68 for pseudoephedrine hydrochloride and 1.0 for triprolidine hydrochloride. Calculate the quantity, in mg, of pseudoephedrine hydrochloride ($C_{10}H_{15}NO \cdot HCl$) in the portion of Oral Solution taken by the formula:

$$50C(r_U / r_S)$$

in which C is the concentration, in mg per mL, of USP Pseudoephedrine Hydrochloride RS in the *Standard preparation*; and r_U and r_S are the peak responses for pseudoephedrine hydrochloride obtained from the *Assay preparation* and the *Standard preparation*, respectively. Calculate the quantity, in mg, of triprolidine hydrochloride ($C_{19}H_{22}N_2 \cdot HCl \cdot H_2O$) in the portion of Oral Solution taken by the formula:

$$(332.88 / 314.86)(50C)(r_U / r_S)$$

in which 332.88 and 314.86 are the molecular weights of triprolidine hydrochloride monohydrate and anhydrous triprolidine hydrochloride, respectively; C is the concentration, in mg per mL, calculated on the anhydrous basis, of USP Triprolidine Hydrochloride RS in the *Standard preparation*; and r_U and r_S are the peak responses for triprolidine hydrochloride obtained from the *Assay preparation* and the *Standard preparation*, respectively.

Triprolidine and Pseudoephedrine Hydrochlorides Tablets

» Triprolidine and Pseudoephedrine Hydrochlorides Tablets contain not less than 90.0 percent and not more than 110.0 percent of the labeled amounts of triprolidine hydrochloride ($C_{19}H_{22}N_2 \cdot HCl \cdot H_2O$) and pseudoephedrine hydrochloride ($C_{10}H_{15}NO \cdot HCl$).

Packaging and storage—Preserve in tight, light-resistant containers.

USP Reference standards ⟨11⟩—*USP Triprolidine Hydrochloride RS. USP Pseudoephedrine Hydrochloride RS.*

Identification—

A: The retention times of the major peaks in the chromatogram of the *Assay preparation* correspond to those of the *Standard preparation* as obtained in the *Assay*.

B: Transfer 1 Tablet to a suitable glass-stoppered tube, add 10 mL of water, shake for 5 minutes, and allow the solids to settle. Prepare a Standard solution in water of USP Pseudoephedrine Hydrochloride RS and USP Triprolidine Hydrochloride RS having known concentrations of 6 mg per mL and 250 μg per mL, respectively. Separately apply 10-μL portions of the test solution and the Standard solution to a suitable thin-layer chromatographic plate (see *Chromatography* ⟨621⟩) coated with a 0.25-mm layer of chromatographic silica gel mixture. Allow the spots to dry, and develop the chromatogram in a solvent system consisting of a mixture of butyl alcohol, glacial acetic acid, and water (8 : 2 : 2) until the solvent front has moved about three-fourths of the length of the plate. Remove the plate, mark the solvent front, allow the solvent to evaporate, and examine the plate under short- and long-wavelength UV light: the R_F values of the principal spots obtained from the test solution correspond to those obtained from the Standard solution.

Dissolution, *Procedure for a Pooled Sample* ⟨711⟩—

Medium: water; 900 mL.
Apparatus 2: 50 rpm.
Time: 45 minutes.

Determine the amounts of pseudoephedrine hydrochloride and triprolidine hydrochloride dissolved using the following method.

Mobile phase and *Chromatographic system*—Proceed as directed in the *Assay* under *Triprolidine and Pseudoephedrine Hydrochlorides Oral Solution.*

Procedure—Inject an accurately measured volume (about 200 μL) of a filtered portion of the solution under test into the chromatograph by means of a microsyringe or a sampling valve, record the chromatogram, and measure the responses for the major peaks. Calculate the quantities of pseudoephedrine hydrochloride ($C_{10}H_{15}NO \cdot HCl$) and triprolidine hydrochloride ($C_{19}H_{22}N_2 \cdot HCl \cdot H_2O$) dissolved in comparison with a Standard solution having known concentrations of USP Pseudoephedrine Hydrochloride RS and USP Triprolidine Hydrochloride RS in the same medium and similarly chromatographed.

Tolerances—Not less than 75% (*Q*) of the labeled amounts of $C_{10}H_{15}NO \cdot HCl$ and $C_{19}H_{22}N_2 \cdot HCl \cdot H_2O$ is dissolved in 45 minutes.

Uniformity of dosage units ⟨905⟩: meet the requirements for *Content Uniformity* with respect to triprolidine hydrochloride and to pseudoephedrine hydrochloride.

Assay—

Mobile phase and *Standard preparation*—Prepare as directed in the *Assay* under *Triprolidine and Pseudoephedrine Hydrochlorides Oral Solution.*

Assay preparation—Weigh and finely powder not fewer than 20 Tablets. Transfer an accurately weighed portion of the powder, equivalent to about 120 mg of pseudoephedrine hydrochloride, to a 100-mL volumetric flask. Add about 10 mL of 0.01 N hydrochloric acid, and sonicate for 10 minutes. Cool to room temperature. Dilute with 0.01 N hydrochloric acid to volume, mix, and filter.

Chromatographic system (see *Chromatography* ⟨621⟩) and *Procedure*—Proceed as directed in the *Assay* under *Triprolidine and Pseudoephedrine Hydrochlorides Oral Solution*, except to calculate the quantity, in mg, of pseudoephedrine hydrochloride ($C_{10}H_{15}NO \cdot HCl$) in the portion of Tablets taken by the formula:

$$100C(r_U / r_S)$$

in which C is the concentration, in mg per mL, of USP Pseudoephedrine Hydrochloride RS in the *Standard preparation*; and r_U and r_S are the peak responses for pseudoephedrine hydrochloride obtained from the *Assay preparation* and the *Standard preparation*, respectively. Calculate the quantity, in mg, of triprolidine hydrochloride ($C_{19}H_{22}N_2 \cdot HCl \cdot H_2O$) in the portion of Tablets taken by the formula:

$$(332.88/314.86)(100C)(r_U / r_S)$$

in which 332.88 and 314.86 are the molecular weights of triprolidine hydrochloride monohydrate and anhydrous triprolidine hydrochloride, respectively; C is the concentration, in mg per mL, calculated on the anhydrous basis, of USP Triprolidine Hydrochloride RS in the *Standard preparation;* and r_U and r_S are the peak responses for triprolidine hydrochloride obtained from the *Assay preparation* and the *Standard preparation*, respectively.

Trisulfapyrimidines Oral Suspension

» Trisulfapyrimidines Oral Suspension contains, in each 100 mL, not less than 3.0 g and not more than 3.7 g of sulfadiazine ($C_{10}H_{10}N_4O_2S$), sulfamerazine ($C_{11}H_{12}N_4O_2S$), and sulfamethazine ($C_{12}H_{14}N_4O_2S$). It may contain either Sodium Citrate or Sodium Lactate, and it may contain a suitable antimicrobial agent.

Packaging and storage—Preserve in tight containers, at a temperature above freezing.
Labeling—Its label indicates the presence and proportion of any sodium citrate or sodium lactate and any antimicrobial agent.
USP Reference standards ⟨11⟩—*USP Sulfadiazine RS. USP Sulfamerazine RS. USP Sulfamethazine RS.*
Identification—The retention times of the three individual sulfapyrimidines obtained in the *Assay* correspond to the retention times of the respective USP Reference Standards.
Uniformity of dosage units ⟨905⟩—
  FOR ORAL SUSPENSION PACKAGED IN SINGLE-UNIT CONTAINERS: meets the requirements.
Deliverable volume ⟨698⟩—
  FOR ORAL SUSPENSION PACKAGED IN MULTIPLE-UNIT CONTAINERS: meets the requirements.
Assay—
  Mobile phase—Prepare a suitable degassed solution of water, acetonitrile, and glacial acetic acid (86 : 13 : 1) such that the relative retention times of sulfadiazine, sulfamerazine, and sulfamethazine are approximately 0.6, 0.8, and 1.0, respectively. (If the retention times are excessive, the concentration of acetonitrile may be increased.)
  Standard preparation—Transfer 33 mg each of USP Sulfadiazine RS, USP Sulfamerazine RS, and USP Sulfamethazine RS, accurately weighed, to a 100-mL volumetric flask, dissolve in 25 mL of 0.1 N sodium hydroxide, dilute with water to volume, and mix. Pipet 3 mL into a 25-mL volumetric flask, dilute with water to volume, and mix to obtain a *Standard preparation* having a known concentration of about 40 µg of each USP Reference Standard per mL.
  Assay preparation—Determine the specific gravity of the Oral Suspension, using a tared, 50-mL volumetric flask, by weighing 50 mL of Oral Suspension that previously has been shaken in the original container to ensure homogeneity, allowed to stand long enough for entrapped air to rise, and finally inverted carefully just prior to transfer to the volumetric flask. Transfer an accurately weighed quantity of Oral Suspension, well-shaken and free from entrapped air, equivalent to about 100 mg of total sulfapyrimidines, to a 100-mL volumetric flask, add 25 mL of 0.1 N sodium hydroxide, and swirl for several minutes to dissolve the sulfapyrimidines. Dilute with water to volume, and mix. Filter the mixture, discarding the first several mL of the filtrate. Pipet 3 mL of the clear filtrate into a 25-mL volumetric flask, dilute with water to volume, and mix.
  Chromatographic system (see *Chromatography* ⟨621⟩)—The liquid chromatograph is equipped with a 254-nm detector and a 3.9-mm × 30-cm column that contains packing L1. The flow rate is about 2 mL per minute. Chromatograph five replicate injections of the *Standard preparation*, and record the peak responses as directed for *Procedure:* the relative standard deviation is not more than 2.0%, and the resolution factors between sulfadiazine and sulfamerazine and between sulfamerazine and sulfamethazine are each not less than 3.0.
  Procedure—Separately inject equal volumes (about 20 µL) of the *Standard preparation* and the *Assay preparation* into the chromatograph, record the chromatograms, and measure the responses for the major peaks. The relative retention times for sulfadiazine, sulfamerazine, and sulfamethazine are approximately 0.6, 0.8, and 1.0, respectively. Calculate the quantity, in mg, of sulfadiazine in the portion of Oral Suspension taken by the formula:

$$0.833C(R_U / R_S)$$

in which C is the concentration, in µg per mL, of USP Sulfadiazine RS in the *Standard preparation;* and R_U and R_S are the peak responses obtained from the *Assay preparation* and the *Standard preparation*, respectively. Similarly measure the responses of the sulfamerazine and sulfamethazine peaks, and calculate the quantity, in mg, of each in the portion of Oral Suspension taken.

Trisulfapyrimidines Tablets

» Trisulfapyrimidines Tablets contain not less than 95.0 percent and not more than 105.0 percent of the labeled amount of each of the sulfapyrimidines, consisting of equal amounts of sulfadiazine ($C_{10}H_{10}N_4O_2S$), sulfamerazine ($C_{11}H_{12}N_4O_2S$), and sulfamethazine ($C_{12}H_{14}N_4O_2S$).

Packaging and storage—Preserve in well-closed containers.
USP Reference standards ⟨11⟩—*USP Sulfadiazine RS. USP Sulfamerazine RS. USP Sulfamethazine RS.*
Identification—The Tablets respond to the *Identification* test under *Trisulfapyrimidines Oral Suspension.*
Dissolution ⟨711⟩—
  Medium: 0.01 N hydrochloric acid; 900 mL.
  Apparatus 2: 50 rpm.
  Time: 60 minutes.
  Procedure—Determine the amount of total sulfapyrimidines dissolved by employing UV absorption at the wavelength of maximum absorbance at about 254 nm on filtered portions of the solution under test, suitably diluted with 0.01 N sodium hydroxide, in comparison with a Standard solution having approximately equal, known, concentrations of USP Sulfadiazine RS, USP Sulfamerazine RS, and USP Sulfamethazine RS in the same media.
  Tolerances—Not less than 70% (*Q*) of the labeled amount of total sulfapyrimidines is dissolved in 60 minutes.
Uniformity of dosage units ⟨905⟩: meet the requirements.
Assay—
  Mobile phase, Standard preparation, and *Chromatographic system*—Proceed as directed in the *Assay* under *Trisulfapyrimidines Oral Suspension.*
  Assay preparation—Weigh and finely powder not less than 20 Tablets. Transfer an accurately weighed portion of the powder, equivalent to about 250 mg of total sulfapyrimidines, to a 250-mL volumetric flask, add 50 mL of 0.1 N sodium hydroxide, swirl for several minutes to dissolve the sulfapyrimidines, dilute with water to volume, and mix. Filter the mixture, discarding the first several mL of the filtrate. Pipet 3 mL of the clear filtrate into a 25-mL volumetric flask, dilute with water to volume, and mix.
  Procedure—Proceed as directed for *Procedure* in the *Assay* under *Trisulfapyrimidines Oral Suspension.* Calculate the quantity, in mg, of sulfadiazine in the portion of Tablets taken by the formula:

$$2.08C(R_U / R_S)$$

in which C is the concentration, in µg per mL, of USP Sulfadiazine RS in the *Standard preparation,* and R_U and R_S are the peak responses obtained from the *Assay preparation* and the *Standard preparation*, respectively. Similarly measure the responses of the

Trolamine Salicylate

$C_{13}H_{21}NO_6$ 287.32
Triethanolamine salicylate   [2174-16-5].

» Trolamine Salicylate is a compounded mixture of Trolamine and Salicylic Acid in propylene glycol. It contains not less than 95.0 percent and not more than 105.0 percent of the labeled amount of $C_{13}H_{21}NO_6$.

Packaging and storage—Preserve in tight containers in a cool place.

USP Reference standards ⟨11⟩—*USP Salicylic Acid RS.*
Identification, *Ultraviolet Absorption* ⟨197U⟩—
  Solution: 1 mg per mL, in 0.1-cm cells. The test solution and the Standard solution contain the equivalent of 1 mg of salicylic acid per mL.
  Medium: methanol.
  Absorptivities do not differ by more than 1.0%.
Specific gravity ⟨841⟩: between 1.190 and 1.220.
Refractive index ⟨831⟩: between 1.505 and 1.535 at 20°.
pH ⟨791⟩: between 6.5 and 7.5, in a 50 mg per mL solution in water.
Limit of free salicylic acid—
  Adsorbent: 0.25-mm layer of chromatographic silica gel mixture.
  Test solution—Transfer about 48 mg of Trolamine Salicylate, accurately weighed, to a 50-mL volumetric flask, dilute with xylene to volume, and mix.
  Standard solution 1—Dissolve an accurately weighed quantity of USP Salicylic Acid RS in xylene, and dilute quantitatively, and stepwise if necessary, with xylene to obtain a solution having a known concentration of about 0.2 mg per mL.
  Standard solution 2—Dilute an accurately measured quantity of *Standard solution 1* in xylene to obtain a solution having a known concentration of about 0.1 mg per mL.
  Application volume: 5 μL of each solution.
  Developing solvent system: a mixture of toluene, acetone, and glacial acetic acid (17 : 8 : 0.2).
  Procedure—Proceed as directed for *Thin-Layer Chromatography* under *Chromatography* ⟨621⟩. Develop in a chamber previously equilibrated with *Developing solvent system*. Examine the plate under long-wavelength UV light. Any secondary spot obtained from the *Test solution* is not greater in size or intensity than the spot obtained from *Standard solution 1:* not more than 0.02% of free salicylic acid is found.

Chromatographic purity—
  Mobile phase, Standard preparation, and *Chromatographic system*—Proceed as directed in the *Assay*.
  Test preparation—Use the *Assay preparation*.
  Procedure—Inject a volume (about 10 μL) of the *Test preparation* into the chromatograph, record the chromatogram, and measure all of the peak responses. Calculate the percentage of each impurity in the portion of Trolamine Salicylate taken by the formula:

$$100(r_i / r_s)$$

in which r_i is the peak response for each impurity, and r_s is the sum of the responses of all the peaks: not more than 1.0% of any individual impurity is found, and not more than 2.0% of total impurities is found.

Assay—
  Mobile phase—Prepare a filtered and degassed mixture of water and acetonitrile (7 : 3). Make adjustments if necessary (see *System Suitability* under *Chromatography* ⟨621⟩).
  Standard preparation—Dissolve an accurately weighed quantity of USP Salicylic Acid RS in methanol, and dilute quantitatively, and stepwise if necessary, with methanol to obtain a solution having a known concentration of about 48 μg per mL.
  Assay preparation—Transfer a portion of Trolamine Salicylate, equivalent to about 300 mg of salicylic acid, accurately weighed, to a 250-mL volumetric flask, and dilute with methanol to volume. Transfer 2 mL of this solution to a 50-mL volumetric flask, dilute with methanol to volume, and mix.
  Chromatographic system (see *Chromatography* ⟨621⟩)—The liquid chromatograph is equipped with a 308-nm detector and a 4.0-mm × 12.5-cm column that contains packing L1. The flow rate is about 1 mL per minute. The column temperature is maintained at 30°. Chromatograph the *Standard preparation*, and record the peak responses as directed for *Procedure:* the column efficiency is not less than 8000 theoretical plates; the tailing factor is not more than 1.5; and the relative standard deviation for replicate injections is not more than 2.0%.
  Procedure—Separately inject equal volumes (about 10 μL) of the *Standard preparation* and the *Assay preparation* into the chromatograph, record the chromatograms, and measure the responses for the major peaks. Calculate the percentage of $C_{13}H_{21}NO_6$ in the portion of Trolamine Salicylate taken by the formula:

$$100(r_U / r_S)$$

in which r_U and r_S are the peak responses obtained from the *Assay preparation* and the *Standard preparation*, respectively.

Troleandomycin

$C_{41}H_{67}NO_{15}$ 813.97
Oleandomycin, triacetate (ester).
Triacetyloleandomycin   [2751-09-9].

» Troleandomycin contains the equivalent of not less than 750 μg of oleandomycin ($C_{35}H_{61}NO_{12}$) per mg.

Packaging and storage—Preserve in tight containers.

USP Reference standards ⟨11⟩—*USP Troleandomycin RS.*
Identification—
  A: Dissolve about 10 mg in 5 mL of hydrochloric acid, and heat in a water bath: a greenish yellow color is produced.
  B: Prepare a solution of it in methanol containing 10 mg per mL. Apply 5 μL of this test solution, 5 μL of a methanol solution of USP Troleandomycin RS containing 10 mg per mL (Standard solution), and 5 μL of a mixture of the two solutions (1 : 1) to a suitable thin-layer chromatographic plate (see *Chromatography* ⟨621⟩) coated with a 0.25-mm layer of chromatographic cellulose. Allow the spots to dry, and develop the chromatogram in a solvent system of ammonium carbonate solution (1 in 100) until the solvent front has moved three-fourths of the length of the plate. Remove the plate from the developing chamber, mark the solvent front, and allow the plate to dry. Expose the plate to iodine vapors in a closed chamber for about 20 minutes, and locate the spots: the R_F value of the principal spot obtained from the test solution and from the mixture of the

test solution and the Standard solution corresponds to that obtained from the Standard solution.
Crystallinity ⟨695⟩: meets the requirements.
pH ⟨791⟩: between 7.0 and 8.5, in a solution of alcohol and water (1 : 1) containing 100 mg per mL.
Loss on drying ⟨731⟩—Dry about 100 mg in vacuum at a pressure not exceeding 5 mm of mercury at 60° for 3 hours: it loses not more than 1.0% of its weight.
Residue on ignition ⟨281⟩: not more than 0.1%.
Content of acetyl—Transfer about 30 mg, accurately weighed, to a three-neck, ground-glass jointed 50-mL flask fitted with a glass-stoppered funnel in the center neck, and a condenser and a gas inlet with a bubble counter in the other two necks. Add 2 mL of methanol to the flask to dissolve the Troleandomycin, and, slowly with swirling, add 1 mL of 2 N sodium hydroxide and a boiling chip. Allow nitrogen to flow into the flask at a rate of about 2 bubbles per second. Add about 5 mL of water to the funnel, and heat the flask. Allow to reflux for 30 minutes. Allow the assembly to cool slightly, and rinse the condenser with about 3 mL of water, collecting the rinsings in the flask. Change the condenser to the distillation position, and add water from the funnel to make a total of 5 mL added to the flask. Heat the flask, and collect about 5 mL of distillate in about 10 minutes. Discard the distillate, and allow the flask to cool slightly. Add 1 mL of 12 N sulfuric acid to the flask through the funnel. Heat the flask, and collect about 20 mL of distillate in about 20 minutes, adding more water from time to time through the funnel to maintain the volume in the flask at about 2 to 3 mL. As the distillation proceeds, treat the first fraction as follows. Boil gently for about 20 seconds, and add a few drops of barium chloride TS: no turbidity is produced. Add 1 drop of phenolphthalein TS, and titrate the solution with 0.015 N sodium hydroxide VS until a permanent pale pink color is produced. Collect a second, 10-mL, fraction, and treat it as directed for the first fraction, beginning with "Boil gently for about 20 seconds." If the second fraction consumes more than 0.1 mL of 0.015 N sodium hydroxide, collect a third, 10-mL, fraction, and treat as directed for the first fraction, beginning with "Boil gently for about 20 seconds." Each mL of 0.015 N sodium hydroxide is equivalent to 0.6458 mg of CH_3CO: between 15.3% and 16.0% is found.
Assay—Proceed with Troleandomycin as directed for troleandomycin under *Antibiotics—Microbial Assays* ⟨81⟩.

Troleandomycin Capsules

» Troleandomycin Capsules contain the equivalent of not less than 90.0 percent and not more than 120.0 percent of the labeled amount of oleandomycin ($C_{35}H_{61}NO_{12}$).

Packaging and storage—Preserve in tight containers.

USP Reference standards ⟨11⟩—*USP Troleandomycin RS.*
Identification—Suspend mixed Capsule contents, equivalent to about 200 mg of oleandomycin ($C_{35}H_{61}NO_{12}$), in 20 mL of chloroform, allow to settle, and filter. Using the filtrate so obtained as the test solution, proceed as directed in *Identification* test B under *Troleandomycin*: the specified result is obtained.
Loss on drying ⟨731⟩—Dry about 100 mg, accurately weighed, of Capsule contents in a capillary-stoppered bottle in vacuum at 60° for 3 hours: it loses not more than 5.0% of its weight.
Assay—Place not less than 5 Capsules in a high-speed glass blender jar containing 500.0 mL of a mixture of isopropyl alcohol and water (4 : 1), and blend for 4 ± 1 minutes. Dilute this solution quantitatively with the same solvent to obtain a stock test solution containing the equivalent of about 1 mg of oleandomycin ($C_{35}H_{61}NO_{12}$) per mL. Proceed as directed for troleandomycin under *Antibiotics—Microbial Assays* ⟨81⟩, using an accurately measured volume of this stock test solution diluted quantitatively with water to yield a *Test Dilution* having a concentration assumed to be equal to the median dose level of the Standard.

Tromethamine

$C_4H_{11}NO_3$ 121.14
1,3-Propanediol, 2-amino-2-(hydroxymethyl)-.
2-Amino-2-(hydroxymethyl)-1,3-propanediol   [77-86-1].

» Tromethamine contains not less than 99.0 percent and not more than 101.0 percent of $C_4H_{11}NO_3$, calculated on the dried basis.

Packaging and storage—Preserve in tight containers.
USP Reference standards ⟨11⟩—*USP Tromethamine RS.*
Identification—
  A: *Infrared Absorption* ⟨197M⟩.
  B: To 4.5 mL of a saturated solution of salicylaldehyde add 0.5 mL of glacial acetic acid, and mix. Add 4.0 mL of a solution of Tromethamine (1 in 5), and mix: a yellow color is produced.
  C: To 0.5 mL of a 4 in 10 solution of ceric ammonium nitrate in 2 N nitric acid add 3 mL of water and 0.5 mL of a solution of Tromethamine (1 in 5), and mix: the color changes from light yellow to orange.
Melting range ⟨741⟩: between 168° and 172°.
pH ⟨791⟩: between 10.0 and 11.5, in a solution (1 in 20).
Loss on drying ⟨731⟩—Dry it at 105° for 3 hours: it loses not more than 1.0% of its weight.
Residue on ignition ⟨281⟩: not more than 0.1%.
Heavy metals, *Method II* ⟨231⟩: 0.001%.
Organic volatile impurities, *Method V* ⟨467⟩: meets the requirements.
(Official until July 1, 2008)
Assay—Dissolve about 250 mg of Tromethamine, accurately weighed, in 100 mL of water, add bromocresol purple TS, and titrate with 0.1 N hydrochloric acid VS to a yellow endpoint. Each mL of 0.1 N hydrochloric acid is equivalent to 12.11 mg of $C_4H_{11}NO_3$.

Tromethamine for Injection

» Tromethamine for Injection is a sterile, lyophilized mixture of tromethamine with Potassium Chloride and Sodium Chloride. It contains not less than 93.0 percent and not more than 107.0 percent of the labeled amount of tromethamine ($C_4H_{11}NO_3$), and not less than 90.0 percent and not more than 110.0 percent of the labeled amounts of potassium chloride (KCl) and of sodium chloride (NaCl).

Packaging and storage—Preserve in *Containers for Sterile Solids* as described under *Injections* ⟨1⟩.
USP Reference standards ⟨11⟩—*USP Tromethamine RS. USP Endotoxin RS.*
Constituted solution—At the time of use, it meets the requirements for *Constituted Solutions* under *Injections* ⟨1⟩.
Identification—
  A: The IR absorption spectrum of a mineral oil dispersion of it exhibits maxima only at the same wavelengths as that of a similar preparation of USP Tromethamine RS.
  B: A solution, prepared as directed in the labeling, responds to the tests for *Chloride* ⟨191⟩, for *Sodium* ⟨191⟩, and for *Potassium* ⟨191⟩.
Bacterial endotoxins ⟨85⟩—It contains not more than 0.03 USP Endotoxin Unit per mg of tromethamine.
pH ⟨791⟩: between 10.0 and 11.5, in a solution prepared as directed in the labeling.

Water, *Method I* ⟨921⟩—Add 5 mL of glacial acetic acid prior to the titration: the content is not more than 1.0%.
Particulate matter ⟨788⟩: meets the requirements for small-volume injections.
Potassium chloride content—
Standard solutions—Prepare five standard solutions (*1, 2, 3, 4,* and *5*) each containing 0.60 mEq of sodium (35 mg of sodium chloride) per liter, and to the solutions add, respectively, 0-, 2-, 4-, 6-, and 8-mg supplements of potassium, in the form of the chloride, per L. If necessary, because of changes in the sensitivity of the photometer, vary the levels of concentration of the potassium, keeping the ratios between solutions approximately as given.
Standard graph—Set a suitable flame photometer for maximum emittance at a wavelength of 766 nm to 767 nm. (The exact wavelength setting will vary slightly with the instrument.) Adjust the instrument to zero emittance with solution *1*. Then adjust the instrument to 100% emittance with solution *5*. Read the percentage emittance of solutions *2, 3,* and *4*. Plot the observed emittance of solutions *2, 3, 4,* and *5* as the ordinate and the concentration, in µg per mL, of potassium as the abscissa on arithmetic coordinate paper.
Procedure—Dissolve the entire contents of 1 container of Tromethamine for Injection in sufficient water, and dilute quantitatively and stepwise with water to obtain a solution containing about 4 µg of potassium per mL, or a quantity corresponding to the concentration of the *Standard solutions*. Adjust the instrument to zero emittance with solution *1* and to 100% emittance with solution *5*. Read the percentage emittance of the test solution. By reference to the *Standard graph*, determine the concentration, in µg per mL, of potassium in the test solution, apply the dilution factor, and calculate the quantity, in mg, of potassium in the container of Tromethamine for Injection. Each mg of potassium is equivalent to 1.907 mg of potassium chloride (KCl).
Sodium chloride content—Proceed as directed under *Potassium chloride content*, with the following modifications: (1) Prepare the *Standard solutions* to contain 0, 2, 4, 6, and 8 mg of sodium, in the form of the chloride, per 1000 mL, without added potassium; (2) prepare the *Standard graph* with the flame photometer set at 588 nm to 589 nm; and (3) under *Procedure* read "sodium" for "potassium" throughout. Each mg of sodium is equivalent to 2.542 mg of sodium chloride (NaCl).
Other requirements—It meets the requirements for *Sterility Tests* ⟨71⟩, *Uniformity of Dosage Units* ⟨905⟩, and *Labeling* under *Injections* ⟨1⟩.
Assay for tromethamine—Dissolve the entire contents of 1 container of Tromethamine for Injection in sufficient water, diluting with water to an accurately measured volume to obtain a solution containing about 36 mg of tromethamine per mL. Transfer to a beaker an accurately measured volume of the solution, equivalent to about 180 mg of tromethamine, dilute with water to about 100 mL, add bromocresol purple TS, and titrate with 0.1 N hydrochloric acid VS to a yellow endpoint. Each mL of 0.1 N hydrochloric acid is equivalent to 12.11 mg of $C_4H_{11}NO_3$.

Tropicamide

$C_{17}H_{20}N_2O_2$ 284.35
Benzeneacetamide, *N*-ethyl-α-(hydroxymethyl)-*N*-(4-pyridinylmethyl)-, (±)-.
(±)-*N*-Ethyl-2-phenyl-*N*-(4-pyridylmethyl)hydracrylamide   [1508-75-4].

» Tropicamide contains not less than 99.0 percent and not more than 101.0 percent of $C_{17}H_{20}N_2O_2$, calculated on the dried basis.

Packaging and storage—Preserve in tight, light-resistant containers.
USP Reference standards ⟨11⟩—*USP Tropicamide RS*.
Identification—
   A: *Infrared Absorption* ⟨197K⟩.
   B: *Ultraviolet Absorption* ⟨197U⟩—
   Solution: 25 µg per mL.
   Medium: 3 N hydrochloric acid.
Melting range, *Class I* ⟨741⟩: between 96° and 100°.
Loss on drying ⟨731⟩—Dry about 500 mg, accurately weighed, in vacuum over phosphorus pentoxide at 80° for 4 hours: it loses not more than 0.5% of its weight.
Heavy metals, *Method II* ⟨231⟩: 0.002%.
Assay—Dissolve about 750 mg of Tropicamide, accurately weighed, in 80 mL of glacial acetic acid, add 4 drops of crystal violet TS, and titrate with 0.1 N perchloric acid VS to a blue-green endpoint. Perform a blank determination, and make any necessary correction. Each mL of 0.1 N perchloric acid is equivalent to 28.44 mg of $C_{17}H_{20}N_2O_2$.

Tropicamide Ophthalmic Solution

» Tropicamide Ophthalmic Solution is a sterile, aqueous solution of Tropicamide. It contains not less than 95.0 percent and not more than 105.0 percent of the labeled amount of $C_{17}H_{20}N_2O_2$. It contains a suitable antimicrobial agent, and may contain suitable substances to increase its viscosity.

Packaging and storage—Preserve in tight containers, and avoid freezing.
USP Reference standards ⟨11⟩—*USP Tropicamide RS*.
Identification—
   A: Extract 10 mL of it with 25 mL of chloroform, filter the chloroform extract through dry, folded filter paper, and evaporate the filtrate to dryness: the residue so obtained responds to *Identification* test A under *Tropicamide*.
   B: The UV absorption spectrum of the solution employed for measurement of absorbance in the *Assay* exhibits maxima and minima at the same wavelengths as that of a similar solution of USP Tropicamide RS, concomitantly measured.
Sterility ⟨71⟩: meets the requirements.
pH ⟨791⟩: between 4.0 and 5.8.
Assay—Transfer an accurately measured volume of Ophthalmic Solution, equivalent to about 30 mg of tropicamide, to a 100-mL volumetric flask, add water to volume, and mix. Transfer 10.0 mL of this solution to a separator, add 2 mL of sodium carbonate solution (1 in 10), extract with four 20-mL portions of chloroform, and combine the extracts in a second separator. Wash the combined extracts with a 25-mL portion of pH 6.5 phosphate buffer (see *Buffer Solutions* in the section *Reagents, Indicators, and Solutions*), and transfer to another separator. Wash the aqueous layer with 10 mL of chloroform, and add it to the extracts. Extract the chloroform solution with four 20-mL portions of dilute sulfuric acid (1 in 6), combine the acid extracts in a 100-mL volumetric flask, and add the dilute acid to volume. Dissolve an accurately weighed quantity of USP Tropicamide RS in dilute sulfuric acid (1 in 6), and dilute quantitatively and stepwise with the same solvent to obtain a Standard solution having a known concentration of about 30 µg per mL. Concomitantly determine the absorbances of both solutions in 1-cm cells at the wavelength of maximum absorbance at about 253 nm, with a suitable spectrophotometer, using dilute sulfuric acid (1 in 6) as the blank. Calculate the quantity, in mg, of $C_{17}H_{20}N_2O_2$ in each mL of the Ophthalmic Solution taken by the formula:

$$(C/V)(A_U/A_S)$$

in which *C* is the concentration, in µg per mL, of USP Tropicamide RS in the Standard solution, *V* is the volume, in mL, of Ophthalmic Solution taken, and A_U and A_S are the absorbances of the solution from the Ophthalmic Solution and the Standard solution, respectively.

Crystallized Trypsin

» Crystallized Trypsin is a proteolytic enzyme crystallized from an extract of the pancreas of healthy bovine or porcine animals, or both. When assayed as directed herein, it contains not less than 2500 USP Trypsin Units in each mg, calculated on the dried basis, and not less than 90.0 percent and not more than 110.0 percent of the labeled potency.

NOTE—Determine the suitability of the substrates and check the adjustment of the spectrophotometer by performing the Assay using USP Crystallized Trypsin Reference Standard.

Packaging and storage—Preserve in tight containers, and avoid exposure to excessive heat.

USP Reference standards ⟨11⟩—*USP Trypsin Crystallized RS*.
Solubility test—An amount, equivalent to 500,000 USP Trypsin Units, is soluble in 10 mL of water and in 10 mL of saline TS.
Microbial limits ⟨61⟩—It meets the requirements of the tests for absence of *Staphylococcus aureus*, *Pseudomonas aeruginosa*, and *Salmonella* species.
Loss on drying ⟨731⟩—Dry it in vacuum at 60° for 4 hours: it loses not more than 5.0% of its weight.
Residue on ignition ⟨281⟩: not more than 2.5%.
Limit of chymotrypsin—
0.067 M Phosphate buffer, pH 7.0—Dissolve 4.54 g of monobasic potassium phosphate in water to make 500 mL of solution. Dissolve 4.73 g of anhydrous dibasic sodium phosphate in water to make 500 mL of solution. Mix 38.9 mL of the monobasic potassium phosphate solution with 61.1 mL of dibasic sodium phosphate solution. Adjust dropwise, if necessary, with dibasic sodium phosphate solution to a pH of 7.0.
Substrate solution—Dissolve 23.7 mg of N-acetyl-L-tyrosine ethyl ester, suitable for use in determining chymotrypsin, in about 50 mL of *0.067 M Phosphate buffer, pH 7.0* with warming. When cool, dilute with additional pH 7.0 buffer to 100 mL. (*Substrate solution* may be stored in the frozen state and used after thawing; it is important, however, to freeze immediately after preparation.)
Crystallized Trypsin solution—Dissolve a sufficient quantity of Crystallized Trypsin, accurately weighed, in 0.0010 N hydrochloric acid to obtain a solution containing 650 USP Trypsin Units per mL.
Procedure—Conduct the test in a suitable spectrophotometer equipped to maintain a temperature of 25 ± 0.1° in the cell compartment. Determine the temperature in the reaction cell before and after the measurement of absorbance to ensure that the temperature does not change by more than 0.5°. Pipet 200 µL of 0.0010 N hydrochloric acid and 3.0 mL of the *Substrate solution* into a 1-cm cell. Place this cell in the spectrophotometer, and adjust the instrument so that the absorbance reads 0.200 at 237 nm. Pipet 200 µL of *Crystallized Trypsin solution* into another 1-cm cell, add 3.0 mL of the *Substrate solution*, and place the cell in the spectrophotometer. [NOTE—This order of addition is to be followed.] At the time the *Substrate solution* is added, start a stopwatch, and read the absorbance at 30-second intervals for not less than 5 minutes. Repeat the procedure on the same dilution at least once. Absolute absorbance values are of less importance than the constancy of the rate of change of absorbance. If the rate of change does not remain constant for at least 3 minutes, repeat the run, and if necessary, use a lower concentration. The duplicate run at the same dilution should match the first run in rate of absorbance change. Determine the average absorbance change per minute, using only the values within the 3-minute portion of the curve where the rate of absorbance is constant. Plot a curve of absorbance against time. One USP Chymotrypsin Unit is the activity causing a change in absorbance of 0.0075 per minute under the conditions specified in this test. Calculate the number of USP Chymotrypsin Units per mg of Crystallized Trypsin taken by the formula:

$$(A_2 - A_1) / (0.0075TW)$$

in which A_2 is the absorbance straight-line initial reading, A_1 is the absorbance straight-line final reading, T is the elapsed time, in minutes, between the initial and final readings, and W is the weight, in mg, of Crystallized Trypsin in the volume of solution used in determining the absorbance. Not more than 50 USP Chymotrypsin Units per 2500 USP Trypsin Units is found, indicating the presence of not more than approximately 5% of chymotrypsin.

Assay—
0.067 M Phosphate buffer, pH 7.6—Dissolve 4.54 g of monobasic potassium phosphate in water to make 500 mL of solution. Dissolve 4.73 g of anhydrous dibasic sodium phosphate in water to make 500 mL of solution. Mix 13 mL of the monobasic potassium phosphate solution with 87 mL of the anhydrous dibasic sodium phosphate solution.
Substrate solution—Dissolve 85.7 mg of N-benzoyl-L-arginine ethyl ester hydrochloride, suitable for use in assaying Crystallized Trypsin (see NOTE), in water to make 100 mL. Dilute 10 mL of this solution with *0.067 M Phosphate buffer, pH 7.6* to 100 mL. Determine the absorbance of this solution, in a 1-cm cell, at 253 nm, in a suitable spectrophotometer equipped with thermospacers to maintain a temperature of 25 ± 0.1°, using water as the blank. By the addition of *0.067 M Phosphate buffer, pH 7.6*, or of the *Substrate solution* before dilution, adjust the absorbance so that it measures not less than 0.575 and not more than 0.585. Use this *Substrate solution* within 2 hours.
Crystallized Trypsin solution—Dissolve a sufficient quantity of Crystallized Trypsin, accurately weighed, in 0.0010 N hydrochloric acid to obtain a solution containing about 50 to 60 USP Trypsin Units per mL.
Procedure—Pipet 200 µL of 0.0010 N hydrochloric acid and 3.0 mL of the *Substrate solution* into a 1-cm cell. Place this cell in a spectrophotometer, and adjust the instrument so that the absorbance reads 0.050 at 253 nm. Pipet 200 µL of *Crystallized Trypsin solution*, containing 10 to 12 USP Trypsin Units, into another 1-cm cell, add 3.0 mL of *Substrate solution*, and place the cell in the spectrophotometer. At the time the *Substrate solution* is added, start a stopwatch, and read the absorbance at 30-second intervals for 5 minutes. Repeat the procedure on the same dilution at least once. Plot a curve of absorbance against time, and use only those values that form a straight line to determine the activity of the Crystallized Trypsin. If the rate of change does not remain constant for at least 3 minutes, repeat the run, and if necessary, use a lower concentration. One USP Trypsin Unit is the activity causing a change in absorbance of 0.003 per minute under the conditions specified in this *Assay*. Calculate the number of USP Trypsin Units per mg taken by the formula:

$$(A_1 - A_2) / (0.003TW)$$

in which A_1 is the absorbance straight-line final reading, A_2 is the absorbance straight-line initial reading, T is the elapsed time, in minutes, between the initial and final readings, and W is the weight, in mg, of Crystallized Trypsin in the volume of solution used in determining the absorbances.

Tryptophan

$C_{11}H_{12}N_2O_2$ 204.23
L-Tryptophan.
L-Tryptophan [*73-22-3*].

» Tryptophan contains not less than 98.5 percent and not more than 101.5 percent of $C_{11}H_{12}N_2O_2$, as L-tryptophan, calculated on the dried basis.

Packaging and storage—Preserve in well-closed containers.
USP Reference standards ⟨11⟩—*USP l-Tryptophan RS*.
Identification, *Infrared Absorption* ⟨197K⟩.
Specific rotation ⟨781S⟩: between −29.4° and −32.8°.
   Test solution: 10 mg per mL, in water (heat gently to dissolve, if necessary).
pH ⟨791⟩: between 5.5 and 7.0, in a solution (1 in 100).
Loss on drying ⟨731⟩—Dry it at 105° for 3 hours: it loses not more than 0.3% of its weight.
Residue on ignition ⟨281⟩: not more than 0.1%.
Chloride ⟨221⟩—A 0.73-g portion shows no more chloride than corresponds to 0.50 mL of 0.020 N hydrochloric acid (0.05%). [NOTE—Gently heat the sample preparation to dissolve, if necessary.]
Sulfate ⟨221⟩—A 0.33-g portion shows no more sulfate than corresponds to 0.10 mL of 0.020 N sulfuric acid (0.03%). [NOTE—Gently heat the sample preparation to dissolve, if necessary.]
Iron ⟨241⟩: 0.003%.
Heavy metals, *Method II* ⟨231⟩: 0.0015%.
Organic volatile impurities, *Method IV* ⟨467⟩: meets the requirements.

(Official until July 1, 2008)
Assay—Transfer about 200 mg of Tryptophan, accurately weighed, to a 125-mL flask, dissolve in a mixture of 3 mL of formic acid and 50 mL of glacial acetic acid, and titrate with 0.1 N perchloric acid VS, determining the endpoint potentiometrically. Perform a blank determination, and make any necessary correction. Each mL of 0.1 N perchloric acid is equivalent to 20.42 mg of $C_{11}H_{12}N_2O_2$.

Tuberculin

» Tuberculin conforms to the regulations of the FDA concerning biologics (650.10 to 650.15) (see *Biologics* ⟨1041⟩). It is a sterile solution derived from the concentrated, soluble products of growth of the tubercle bacillus (*Mycobacterium tuberculosis* or *Mycobacterium bovis*) prepared in a special medium. It is provided either as Old Tuberculin, a culture filtrate adjusted to the standard potency based on the U.S. Standard Tuberculin, Old, by addition of glycerin and isotonic sodium chloride solution, or as Purified Protein Derivative (PPD), a further purified protein fraction standardized with the U.S. Standard Tuberculin, Purified Protein Derivative. It has a potency, tested by comparison with the corresponding U.S. Standard Tuberculin, on intradermal injection of sensitized guinea pigs, of between 80 percent and 120 percent of that stated on the label. It is free from viable *Mycobacteria* as shown by injection into guinea pigs.

Packaging and storage—Preserve at a temperature between 2° and 8°. Multiple-puncture devices may be stored at a temperature not exceeding 30°.
Expiration date—The expiration date of concentrated Old Tuberculin containing 50% of glycerin is not later than 5 years after date of issue from manufacturer's cold storage (5°, 1 year; or 0°, 2 years). The expiration date of diluted Old Tuberculin is not later than 1 year after date of issue from manufacturer's cold storage (5°, 1 year; or 0°, 2 years). The expiration date of concentrated PPD containing 50% of glycerin is not later than 2 years after date of issue from manufacturer's cold storage (5°, 1 year). The expiration date of diluted PPD is not later than 1 year after date of issue by the manufacturer. The expiration date of Old Tuberculin and PPD dried on multiple-puncture devices is not later than 2 years after date of issue from manufacturer's cold storage (30°, 1 year), provided the recommended storage is at a temperature not exceeding 30°.

Tubocurarine Chloride

$C_{37}H_{41}ClN_2O_6 \cdot HCl \cdot 5H_2O$ 771.72
Tubocuraranium,   7′,12′-dihydroxy-6,6′-dimethoxy-2,2′,2′-trimethylchloride, hydrochloride, pentahydrate.
(+)-Tubocurarine chloride hydrochloride pentahydrate [6989-98-6].
Anhydrous   681.66   [57-94-3].

» Tubocurarine Chloride contains not less than 95.0 percent and not more than 105.0 percent of $C_{37}H_{41}ClN_2O_6 \cdot HCl$, calculated on the anhydrous basis.

Packaging and storage—Preserve in tight containers.
USP Reference standards ⟨11⟩—*USP Tubocurarine Chloride RS*.
Clarity of alcohol solution—A solution of 100 mg in 10 mL of alcohol is clear.
Identification—
   A: *Infrared Absorption* ⟨197K⟩.
   B: The chromatogram of the *Assay preparation* obtained as directed in the *Assay* exhibits a major peak, the retention time of which corresponds to that exhibited in the chromatogram of the *Standard preparation*.
   C: A solution (1 in 100) responds to the tests for *Chloride* ⟨191⟩.
Specific rotation ⟨781S⟩: between +210° and +224°.
   Test solution: 10 mg per mL, in water, allowed to stand for 3 hours.
Water, *Method I* ⟨921⟩: not more than 12.0%.
Residue on ignition ⟨281⟩: not more than 0.25%.
Related compounds—In the chromatogram obtained from the *Assay preparation* in the *Assay*, the sum of the responses of any peaks detected, other than the peak due to tubocurarine, is not more than 5.0% of the total of all peak responses.
Chloride content—Dissolve about 300 mg, accurately weighed, in 5 mL of water, warming slightly to effect solution. Add 5 mL of glacial acetic acid and 50 mL of methanol, and cool to room temperature. Add 1 drop of eosin Y TS, and titrate with 0.1 N silver nitrate VS. Each mL of 0.1 N silver nitrate is equivalent to 3.545 mg of Cl. Not less than 9.9% and not more than 10.7% of Cl is found, calculated on the anhydrous basis.
Assay—
   Mobile phase—Mix 3 volumes of acetonitrile and 2 volumes of methanol, and allow the mixture to attain room temperature. To 270 mL of this solution in a 1-liter graduated cylinder add 20.0 mL of 25% tetramethylammonium hydroxide solution in methanol, and add water to make 1 L. Adjust with phosphoric acid to a pH of 4.0, filter, and degas.
   Standard preparation—Dissolve an accurately weighed quantity of USP Tubocurarine Chloride RS in *Mobile phase* to obtain a solution having a known concentration of about 0.3 mg per mL.
   Assay preparation—Transfer 30 mg of Tubocurarine Chloride, accurately weighed, to a 100-mL volumetric flask. Dissolve in *Mobile phase*, dilute with *Mobile phase* to volume, and mix.
   System suitability preparation—Dissolve suitable quantities of tubocurarine chloride and phenol in *Mobile phase* to obtain a solution containing about 0.30 mg and 0.50 mg per mL, respectively.

Chromatographic system (see *Chromatography* ⟨621⟩)—The liquid chromatograph is equipped with a 220-nm detector, and a 4-mm × 25-cm column that contains packing L1. The flow rate is about 1 mL per minute. Chromatograph the *System suitability preparation*, and record the peak responses as directed for *Procedure*: the resolution, R, between the two major peaks is not less than 2.0, and the tailing factor, T, for tubocurarine chloride is not more than 2.0. The relative standard deviation for replicate injections of the *Standard preparation* is not more than 2.0%. The relative retention times are about 0.50 and 1.0 for tubocurarine chloride and phenol, respectively.

Procedure—Separately inject equal volumes (about 10 μL) of the *Standard preparation* and the *Assay preparation* into the chromatograph, record the chromatograms, and measure the responses for the major peaks. Calculate the quantity, in mg, of $C_{37}H_{41}ClN_2O_6 \cdot HCl$ in the portion of Tubocurarine Chloride taken by the formula:

$$100C(r_U / r_S)$$

in which C is the concentration, in mg per mL, of USP Tubocurarine Chloride RS in the *Standard preparation*, and r_U and r_S are the peak responses obtained from the *Assay preparation* and the *Standard preparation*, respectively.

Tubocurarine Chloride Injection

» Tubocurarine Chloride Injection is a sterile solution of Tubocurarine Chloride in Water for Injection. It contains not less than 93.0 percent and not more than 107.0 percent of the labeled amount of $C_{37}H_{41}ClN_2O_6 \cdot HCl \cdot 5H_2O$.

Packaging and storage—Preserve in single-dose or in multiple-dose containers.
USP Reference standards ⟨11⟩—*USP Tubocurarine Chloride RS. USP Endotoxin RS.*
Identification—
  A: It responds to *Identification* test C under *Tubocurarine Chloride*.
  B: The chromatogram of the *Assay preparation* obtained as directed in the *Assay* exhibits a major peak, the retention time of which corresponds to that exhibited in the chromatogram of the *Standard preparation*.
Angular rotation ⟨781⟩: between +0.32° and +0.48° for each mg of tubocurarine chloride per mL claimed on the label, determined in a suitable polarimeter tube and the observed reading being multiplied by the factor 200/L, in which L is the length, in mm, of the tube.
Bacterial endotoxins ⟨85⟩—It contains not more than 10.0 USP Endotoxin Units per mg of tubocurarine chloride.
pH ⟨791⟩: between 2.5 and 5.0.
Other requirements—It meets the requirements under *Injections* ⟨1⟩.
Assay—
Mobile phase, Standard preparation, System suitability preparation, and *Chromatographic system*—Prepare as directed in the *Assay* under *Tubocurarine Chloride*.
Assay preparation—Transfer an accurately measured volume of Injection, equivalent to about 15 mg of tubocurarine chloride, to a 50-mL volumetric flask, dilute with *Mobile phase* to volume, and mix.
Procedure—Separately inject equal volumes (about 10 μL) of the *Standard preparation* and the *Assay preparation* into the chromatograph, record the chromatograms, and measure the responses for the major peaks. Calculate the quantity, in mg, of $C_{37}H_{41}ClN_2O_6 \cdot HCl \cdot 5H_2O$ in each mL of the Injection taken by the formula:

$$50C(r_U / r_S)$$

in which C is the concentration, in mg per mL, of USP Tubocurarine Chloride RS in the *Standard preparation,* and r_U and r_S are the peak responses obtained from the *Assay preparation* and the *Standard preparation*, respectively.

Tylosin

$C_{46}H_{77}NO_{17}$ 916.1
(10E,12E)-(3R,4S,5S,6R,8R,14S,15R)-14-[(6-deoxy-2,3-di-O-methyl-β-D-allopyranosyl)oxymethyl]-5-[[3,6-dideoxy-4-O-(2,6-dideoxy-3-C-methyl-α-L-ribo-hexopyranosyl)-3-dimethylamino-β-D-glucopyranosyl]oxy]-6-formylmethyl-3-hydroxy-4,8,12-trimethyl-9-oxoheptadeca-10,12-dien-15-olide.
Tylosin A [*1401-69-0*].

» Tylosin is the macrolide antibiotic substance, or the mixture of such substances, produced by the growth of *Streptomyces fradiae*, or by any other means. Its potency is not less than 900 μg of tylosin per mg, calculated on the dried basis.

Packaging and storage—Preserve in well-closed containers, protected from light, moisture, and excessive heat.
Labeling—Label it to indicate that it is for use in animals only.
USP Reference standards ⟨11⟩—*USP Tylosin RS.*
Identification—
  A: *Ultraviolet Absorption* ⟨197U⟩.
  Acid solution—Transfer about 50 mg of Tylosin, accurately weighed, to a 100-mL volumetric flask, add 10 mL of 2 N hydrochloric acid, dilute with water to volume, and mix. Transfer 5.0 mL of this solution to a second 100-mL volumetric flask, dilute with water to volume, and mix. Absorptivity at 290 nm is 22.5 ± 2.5, calculated on the dried basis.
  Alkaline solution—To 10.0 mL of the final *Acid solution* add 1.0 mL of 2 N sodium hydroxide, and heat on a water bath for 20 minutes. Cool to room temperature: an absorption maximum is observed at about 332 nm.
  B: The retention time of the major peak for tylosin A in the chromatogram of the *Test solution* corresponds to that in the chromatogram of the *Standard solution*, as obtained in the test for *Content of tylosins*.
Loss on drying ⟨731⟩—Dry about 1 g, accurately weighed, in vacuum at a pressure of not more than 5 mm of mercury at 60° for 3 hours: it loses not more than 5% of its weight.
Residue on ignition ⟨281⟩: not more than 3.0%, the charred residue being moistened with 2 mL of nitric acid and 5 drops of sulfuric acid.
Heavy metals, *Method II* ⟨231⟩: 0.003%.
Limit of tyramine—Transfer 100 mg of it to a 25-mL volumetric flask, add 5.0 mL of 0.03 M phosphoric acid, and swirl to dissolve (*Test solution*). Transfer 5.0 mL of a solution containing 70 μg of tyramine per mL in 0.03 M phosphoric acid to a 25-mL volumetric flask (*Standard solution*). Transfer 5 mL of 0.03 M phosphoric acid to a 25-mL volumetric flask to provide the blank. Concurrently add to each flask 1.0 mL of a mixture of pyridine and 2.0 mL of filtered ninhydrin solution (1 in 25). Cover the flasks lightly with glass or aluminum foil caps, and heat in a water bath at 85° for not less than 20 minutes. Cool rapidly to room temperature, dilute with water to volume, and mix. Promptly determine the absorbances of the solutions from the *Test solution* and the *Standard solution* at the wavelength of maximum absorbance at about 570 nm, using the solution

from the blank to zero the instrument. The absorbance of the solution from the *Test solution* is not greater than that of the solution from the *Standard solution* (0.35% of tyramine). In a valid test the solution from the *Standard solution* exhibits a dark blue color.

Content of tylosins—
Mobile phase—Prepare a mixture of filtered 2 M sodium perchlorate, previously adjusted with 1 N hydrochloric acid to a pH of 2.5 ± 0.1, and acetonitrile (60 : 40). Make adjustments if necessary (see *System Suitability* under *Chromatography* ⟨621⟩).

Standard solution—Transfer about 30 mg of USP Tylosin RS, accurately weighed, to a 100-mL volumetric flask, add 10 mL of methanol, and swirl to dissolve. Dilute with water to volume, and mix.

Test solution—Transfer about 30 mg of Tylosin, accurately weighed, to a 100-mL volumetric flask, add 10 mL of methanol, and swirl to dissolve. Dilute with water to volume, and mix.

Chromatographic system (see *Chromatography* ⟨621⟩)—The liquid chromatograph is equipped with a 280-nm detector, a 4.6-mm × 20-cm column that contains 5-μm packing L1. The flow rate is about 0.7 mL per minute. Chromatograph the *Standard solution*, and record the peak responses as directed for *Procedure*: the resolution, R, between the tylosin D peak and the tylosin A peak is not less than 2, the tailing factor is not more than 1.5, and the relative standard deviation for replicate injections is not more than 2%.

Procedure—Separately inject equal volumes (about 20 μL) of the *Standard solution* and the *Test solution* into the chromatograph, record the chromatograms over a period of time 1.5 times the elution time of the main tylosin A peak, and measure the peak areas for all the peaks. The relative retention times are about 0.5 for tylosin C, 0.7 for tylosin B, 0.9 for tylosin D, and 1.0 for tylosin A. Calculate the percentages of tylosin A, tylosin B, tylosin C, and tylosin D in the Tylosin taken by the formula:

$$100(r_i / r_s)$$

in which r_i is the area of the tylosin A peak, the tylosin B peak, tylosin C peak, or the tylosin D peak, as appropriate, in the chromatogram obtained from the *Test solution*, and r_s is the sum of the areas of all of the peaks in the chromatogram obtained from the *Test solution*: the content of tylosin A is not less than 80% and the sum of the contents of tylosin A, tylosin B, tylosin C, and tylosin D is not less than 95%.

Assay—Proceed as directed for Tylosin under *Antibiotics—Microbial Assays* ⟨81⟩. Prepare the *Test Dilution* as follows. Transfer about 250 mg of Tylosin, accurately weighed, to a 500-mL volumetric flask, add 50 mL of methanol, and swirl to dissolve. Dilute with *Buffer No. 3* to volume, and mix. Transfer 4.0 mL of this solution to a second 500-mL volumetric flask, dilute with a mixture of *Buffer No. 3* and methanol (1 : 1), and mix. This solution contains about 4 μg of tylosin per mL.

Tylosin Granulated

» Tylosin Granulated contains tylosin phosphate mixed with suitable carriers and inactive ingredients. It contains not less than 80.0 percent and not more than 120.0 percent of the labeled amount of tylosin.

Packaging and storage—Preserve in well-closed, polyethylene-lined or polypropylene-lined containers, protected from moisture and excessive heat.
Labeling—Label it to indicate that it is for animal use only. Label it also to indicate that it is for manufacturing, processing, or repackaging.
USP Reference standards ⟨11⟩—*USP Tylosin RS*.
Identification—
A: The chromatogram of the *Test solution*, obtained as directed in the test for *Content of tylosins*, exhibits a major peak for tylosin A, the retention time of which corresponds to that exhibited in the chromatogram of the *Standard solution* obtained as directed in the test for *Content of tylosins*.

B: Transfer 2 g of Tylosin Granulated to a test tube, add 10 mL of water, and shake for 5 minutes. Filter the resulting suspension, and if necessary adjust the pH of the filtrate to a pH between 6 and 8 with 0.1 N sodium hydroxide or 0.1 N hydrochloric acid. This solution responds to the tests for *Phosphate* ⟨191⟩.
Loss on drying ⟨731⟩—Dry about 1 g of it, accurately weighed, in vacuum at a pressure of not more than 5 mm of mercury at 60° for 5 hours: it loses not more than 12.0% of its weight.
Powder fineness ⟨811⟩: not less than 99% passes a No. 20 sieve, and not more than 10% passes a No. 80 sieve.
Content of tylosins—
Mobile phase, *Standard solution*, and *Chromatographic system*—Proceed as directed in the test for *Content of tylosins* under *Tylosin*.

pH 7.0 buffer—Dissolve 13.6 g of monobasic potassium phosphate in 1000 mL of water, and adjust with 12 N sodium hydroxide to a pH of 7.0.

Test solution—Transfer about 1.4 g of Tylosin Granulated, accurately weighed, to a 250-mL volumetric flask, add 100 mL of *pH 7.0 buffer*, and shake by mechanical means for about 30 minutes. Dilute with water to volume, mix, and filter. Transfer 10.0 mL of the filtrate to a 50-mL volumetric flask, dilute with water to volume, and mix. Filter a portion of this solution through a filter having a porosity of 0.5 μm or finer, and use the filtrate as the *Test solution*.

Procedure—Separately inject equal volumes (about 20 μL) of the *Standard solutions* and the *Test solution* into the chromatograph, record the chromatograms over a period of time that is about twice the elution time of the main tylosin A peak, and measure the areas for all the major peaks: the relative retention times are about 0.5 for tylosin C, 0.7 for tylosin B, 0.9 for tylosin D, and 1.0 for tylosin A. Calculate the percentages of tylosin A, tylosin B, tylosin C, and tylosin D in the Tylosin taken by the formula:

$$100(r_i / r_s)$$

in which r_i is the area of the tylosin A peak, tylosin B peak, tylosin C peak, or tylosin D peak, as appropriate, in the chromatogram obtained from the *Test solution*, and r_s is the sum of the areas of all of the peaks in the chromatogram obtained from the *Test solution*: the content of tylosin A is not less than 80%, and the sum of the contents of tylosin A, tylosin B, tylosin C, and tylosin D is not less than 95%.

Assay—Proceed as directed for Tylosin under *Antibiotics—Microbial Assays* ⟨81⟩. Prepare the *Test Dilution* as follows. Transfer about 2 g of Tylosin Granulated, accurately weighed, to a suitable container, add 200.0 mL of a mixture of *Buffer No. 3* and methanol (1 : 1), seal to prevent evaporation, and shake by mechanical means for about 60 minutes. Filter the suspension so obtained, discarding the first 5 mL of the filtrate. Dilute an accurately measured portion of the filtrate quantitatively and stepwise with a mixture of *Buffer No. 3* and methanol (1 : 1) to obtain a *Test Dilution* having an estimated concentration of about 4 μg of tylosin per mL.

Tylosin Tartrate

(10*E*,12*E*)-(3*R*,4*S*,5*S*,6*R*,8*R*,14*S*,15*R*)-14-[(6-deoxy-2,3-di-*O*-methyl-*B*-D-allopyranosyl)oxymethyl]-5-[[3,6-dideoxy-4-*O*-(2,6-dideoxy-3-*C*-methyl-α-L-ribo-hexopyranosyl)-3-dimethylamino-*B*-D-glucopyranosyl]oxy]-6-formylmethyl-3-hydroxy-4,8,12-trimethyl-9-oxoheptadeca-10,12-dien-15-olide.
Tylosin A (Tylosin)   916.10   [1401-69-0].

» Tylosin Tartrate is a tartrate of a mixture of macrolide antibiotic substances, or the mixture of such substances, produced by the growth of *Streptomyces fradiae*, or by any other means. Its potency is not less than 800 μg of tylosin per mg, calculated on the dried basis.

Packaging and storage—Preserve in well-closed containers, protected from light, moisture, and excessive heat. Store at 25°, excursions permitted between 15° and 30°.

Labeling—Label it to indicate that it is for veterinary use only.

USP Reference standards ⟨11⟩—*USP Tylosin RS. USP Tylosin Tartrate RS.*

Identification—
  A: *Infrared Absorption* ⟨197K⟩.
  B: The retention time of the major peak for tylosin A in the chromatogram of the *Test solution* corresponds to that in the chromatogram of the *Standard solution,* as obtained in the test for *Content of tylosins.*
  C: It meets the requirements of the test for *Tartrate* ⟨191⟩.

pH ⟨791⟩: between 5.0 and 7.2 in a solution prepared by dissolving 0.25 g in 10 mL of carbon dioxide-free water.

Loss on drying ⟨731⟩—Dry about 1 g, accurately weighed, in vacuum at a pressure not exceeding 5 mm of mercury at 60° for 3 hours: it loses not more than 4.5% of its weight.

Residue on ignition ⟨281⟩: not more than 2.5%, the charred residue being moistened with 2 mL of nitric acid and 5 drops of sulfuric acid.

Limit of tyramine—In a 25-mL volumetric flask, dissolve 50.0 mg of tylosin in 5.0 mL of a 3.4 g per L solution of phosphoric acid. Add 1.0 mL of pyridine and 2.0 mL of a saturated solution of ninhydrin (about 40 g per L). Close the flask with aluminum foil, and heat in a water bath at 85° for 30 minutes. Cool the solution rapidly to room temperature, and dilute with water to volume. Mix, and measure immediately the absorbance (see *Spectrophotometry and Light-Scattering* ⟨851⟩) of the solution at 570 nm against a blank solution prepared in a similar manner. The absorbance is not greater than that of a standard prepared at the same time and in the same manner using 5.0 mL of a 35 mg per L solution of tyramine in a 3.4 g per L solution of phosphoric acid. If intended for use in the manufacture of parenteral dosage forms, the absorbance is not greater than that of a standard prepared at the same time and in the same manner using 5.0 mL of a 15 mg per L solution of tyramine in a 3.4 g per L solution of phosphoric acid.

Content of tylosins—
  Mobile phase—Prepare a mixture of filtered 200 g per L of sodium perchlorate, previously adjusted with 1 N hydrochloric acid to a pH of 2.5 ± 0.1, and acetonitrile (60 : 40). Make adjustments if necessary (see *System Suitability* under *Chromatography* ⟨621⟩).
  Standard solution—Dissolve an accurately weighed quantity of USP Tylosin RS in a mixture of acetonitrile and water (1 : 1) to obtain a solution having a known concentration of about 0.2 mg per mL. [NOTE—Prepare the *Standard solution* immediately before use.]
  Test solution—Dissolve an accurately weighed quantity of Tylosin in a mixture of acetonitrile and water (1 : 1) to obtain a solution having a known concentration of about 0.2 mg per mL. [NOTE—Prepare the *Test solution* immediately before use.]
  Chromatographic system (see *Chromatography* ⟨621⟩)—The liquid chromatograph is equipped with a 290-nm detector and a 4.6-mm × 20-cm column that contains 5-μm packing L1. The flow rate is about 1.0 mL per minute and the column temperature is maintained at 35°. Chromatograph the *Standard solution,* and record the peak responses as directed for *Procedure*: the order of elution is tylosin C, tylosin B, tylosin D, and tylosin A with relative retention times of about 0.5, 0.6, 0.8, and 1.0 minutes, respectively; the resolution of the peaks representing tylosin D and tylosin A is not less than 2.0; the tailing factors are not more than 1.5; and the relative standard deviation for replicate injections is not more than 2.0%.
  Procedure—Separately inject equal volumes (about 20 μL) of the *Standard solution* and the *Test solution* into the chromatograph, record the chromatograms over a period of time equivalent to 1.5 times the elution time of the main tylosin A peak, and measure the peak areas for all the peaks. Calculate the percentages of tylosin A, tylosin B, tylosin C, and tylosin D in the Tylosin taken by the formula:

$$100(r_I / r_s)$$

in which r_I is the area of the tylosin A peak, the tylosin B peak, the tylosin C peak, or the tylosin D peak, as appropriate, in the chromatogram obtained from the *Test solution;* and r_s is the sum of the areas of all the peaks in the chromatogram obtained from the *Test solution*: the content of tylosin A is not less than 80%; and the sum of the contents of tylosin A, tylosin B, tylosin C, and tylosin D is not less than 95%.

Assay—Proceed as directed for Tylosin under *Antibiotics—Microbial Assays* ⟨81⟩. Prepare the *Test Dilution* as follows. Transfer an accurately weighed quantity of Tylosin Tartrate, equivalent to about 250 mg of tylosin, to a 500-mL volumetric flask, add 50 mL of methanol, and swirl to dissolve. Dilute with *Buffer No. 3* to volume, and mix. Transfer 4.0 mL of this solution to a second 500-mL volumetric flask, dilute with a mixture of *Buffer No. 3* and methanol (1 : 1), and mix. This solution contains about 4 μg of tylosin per mL.

Tyloxapol

$R = CH_2CH_2O{-}[CH_2CH_2O]_n{-}OCH_2CH_2OH$
$m < 6$
$n = 6{-}8$

Phenol, 4-(1,1,3,3-tetramethylbutyl)-, polymer with formaldehyde and oxirane.
p-(1,1,3,3-Tetramethylbutyl)phenol polymer with ethylene oxide and formaldehyde [25301-02-4].

» Tyloxapol is a nonionic liquid polymer of the alkyl aryl polyether alcohol type.
  NOTE—Precautions should be exercised to prevent contact of Tyloxapol with metals.

Packaging and storage—Preserve in tight containers.
USP Reference standards ⟨11⟩—*USP Tyloxapol RS.*
Identification, *Infrared Absorption* ⟨197F⟩: on undried specimen.
Cloud point—Transfer 1.0 g of it, previously mixed, to a 150-mL beaker. Add 100.0 mL of water, and mix until solution is effected. Warm the solution while mixing: transient turbidity may be observed as the solution is warmed. Determine the temperature at which the mixture becomes completely turbid: the cloud point is between 92° and 97°.
pH ⟨791⟩: between 4.0 and 7.0, in a solution (1 in 20).
Residue on ignition ⟨281⟩: not more than 1.0%.
Free phenol—To 10 mL of a solution (1 in 100) add 1 mL of bromine TS, and mix: no cloudiness or precipitation is observed immediately.
Limit of anionic detergents—Mix 20 mL of a solution (1 in 100) with 30 mL of water in a 125-mL separator. In a second 125-mL separator mix 50 mL of water and 1 mL of a solution of sodium lauryl sulfate containing 150 μg per mL. To both separators add 2 drops of 3 N hydrochloric acid, 1 drop of methylene blue solution (1 in 25), and 25 mL of chloroform. Shake both separators gently for 2 minutes, allow to stand for 10 minutes, and transfer the chloroform layers to individual separators. Wash the chloroform extracts with separate 25-mL portions of water, transfer the chloroform solutions to matched 50-mL color-comparison tubes, and view downward over a white surface: the chloroform solution from the Tyloxapol preparation is not darker than that from the sodium lauryl sulfate preparation, corresponding to not more than 0.075% of anionic detergents (as sodium lauryl sulfate).

Limit of ethylene oxide—
  Standard preparation—[*Caution*—*Ethylene oxide is toxic and flammable. Prepare in a well-ventilated hood, using great care.*] Transfer 25 mL of dimethylformamide to a 50-mL volumetric flask, and weigh accurately. Add about 0.5 mL of ethylene oxide, and mix. Reweigh to obtain the weight of ethylene oxide by difference. Dilute with dimethylformamide to volume, and mix. Dilute a portion of this solution with dimethylformamide to obtain a *Standard preparation* having a known concentration of about 10 ppm of ethylene oxide.
  Test preparation—Transfer 1 g of Tyloxapol, accurately weighed, to a glass-stoppered, 5-mL graduated cylinder. Dilute with dimethylformamide to 2.0 mL, and mix.
  Chromatographic system (see *Chromatography* ⟨621⟩)—The gas chromatograph is equipped with a flame-ionization detector and a

1.8-m × 2-mm glass column containing 5% phase G16 on support S12. The injection port is maintained at about 200° and the detector at about 250°. The column temperature is programmed as follows. The temperature is maintained at 50° for 3 minutes, then increased to 200° at a rate of 25° per minute, and held at 200° for 5 minutes. Helium is used as the carrier gas at a flow rate of about 25 mL per minute. Chromatograph the *Standard preparation*, and record the peak responses as directed for *Procedure*: the relative standard deviation for replicate injections is not greater than 10%.

Procedure—Separately inject equal volumes (about 3 μL) of the *Standard preparation* and the *Test preparation* into the chromatograph, record the chromatograms, and measure the responses for the major peaks. Calculate the quantity, in ppm, of ethylene oxide in the portion of Tyloxapol taken by the formula:

$$2(C/W)(r_U/r_S)$$

in which C is the concentration, in μg per mL, of ethylene oxide in the *Standard preparation*, W is the weight, in g, of Tyloxapol taken in the *Test preparation*, and r_U and r_S are the ethylene oxide peak responses obtained from the *Test preparation* and the *Standard preparation*, respectively: not more than 10 ppm of ethylene oxide are found.

Limit of formaldehyde—

Standard preparations—Weigh 2.7 g of formaldehyde solution into a 100-mL volumetric flask, dilute with water to volume, and mix. Transfer 1.0 mL of this solution to a second 100-mL volumetric flask, dilute with water to volume, and mix. Transfer 10.0 mL of this second solution to a third 100-mL volumetric flask, dilute with water to volume, and mix. Transfer 750 μL of this solution to a 25-mL volumetric flask containing 5 mL of a solution of isopropyl alcohol (4 in 10).

Test preparation—Transfer 2.0 g of Tyloxapol to a 10-mL volumetric flask, and dissolve in a solution of isopropyl alcohol (4 in 10), then dilute with a solution of isopropyl alcohol (4 in 10) to volume, and mix. Transfer 500 μL of this solution to a 25-mL volumetric flask containing 5 mL of isopropyl alcohol solution (4 in 10).

Procedure—To the *Standard preparation*, the *Test preparation*, and a blank, prepared by placing 5 mL of isopropyl alcohol solution (4 in 10) in a 25-mL volumetric flask, add 500 μL of phenylhydrazine hydrochloride solution (7.5 in 100), mix, and allow to stand for 10 ± 1 minutes. Add 300 μL of potassium ferricyanide solution (1 in 20) to each flask, mix, and allow to stand for 5 minutes ± 30 seconds. Then add 2.0 mL of 2.5 N sodium hydroxide to each, mix, and allow to stand for 4 ± 1 minutes. Dilute each flask with isopropyl alcohol solution (4 in 10) to volume, mix, and after 10 ± 3 minutes determine the absorbances of the preparations, in 1-cm cells, at the wavelength of maximum absorbance at about 520 nm, with a suitable spectrophotometer, using the blank to set the instrument. The absorbance of the solution from the *Test preparation* does not exceed that of the solution from the *Standard preparation*, corresponding to not more than 0.0075% of formaldehyde.

Absence of cationic detergents—Place 10 mL of a solution (1 in 100) in a glass-stoppered, 50-mL graduated cylinder, and make distinctly alkaline to litmus with sodium carbonate TS (about 1 mL). Add 4 mL of aqueous bromophenol blue solution (1 in 2500), mix, and add 10 mL of a 1 in 10 solvent mixture of ethylene dichloride in toluene. Shake gently, and allow the layers to separate: no blue color is observed in the organic solvent layer.

Organic volatile impurities, *Method I* ⟨467⟩: meets the requirements.

(Official until July 1, 2008)

Tyrosine

$C_9H_{11}NO_3$ 181.19
L-Tyrosine.
L-Tyrosine [60-18-4].

» Tyrosine contains not less than 98.5 percent and not more than 101.5 percent of $C_9H_{11}NO_3$, as L-tyrosine, calculated on the dried basis.

Packaging and storage—Preserve in well-closed containers.
USP Reference standards ⟨11⟩—USP L-Phenylalanine RS. USP L-Tyrosine RS.
Identification, *Infrared Absorption* ⟨197K⟩.
Specific rotation ⟨781S⟩: between −9.8° and −11.2°.
 Test solution: 50 mg per mL, in 1 N hydrochloric acid.
Loss on drying ⟨731⟩—Dry it at 105° for 3 hours: it loses not more than 0.3% of its weight.
Residue on ignition ⟨281⟩: not more than 0.4%.
Chloride ⟨221⟩—A solution containing 0.35 g shows no more chloride than corresponds to 0.20 mL of 0.020 N hydrochloric acid (0.04%). [NOTE—If necessary, dissolve the test specimen by heating to near boiling and adding 1 mL of nitric acid.]

Change to read:
Sulfate ⟨221⟩—A solution containing 1.2 g shows no more sulfate than corresponds to 0.50 mL of 0.020 N sulfuric acid (0.04%). [NOTE—If necessary, dissolve the test specimen by ▲adding 6 mL of diluted▲*USP31* hydrochloric acid.]
Iron ⟨241⟩: 0.003%. [NOTE—If necessary, use 2 mL of hydrochloric acid to dissolve the test specimen.]
Heavy metals, *Method II* ⟨231⟩: 0.0015%.
Chromatographic purity—
 Adsorbent: 0.25-mm layer of chromatographic silica gel mixture.
 Diluted ammonia solution—Transfer 16 mL of concentrated ammonia to a 100-mL volumetric flask, and dilute with water to volume.
 Test solution—Transfer about 0.1 g of Tyrosine, accurately weighed, to a 10-mL volumetric flask, dissolve in *Diluted ammonia solution*, and dilute with water to volume. Apply 5 μL.
 Standard solution—In a suitable flask, dissolve an accurately weighed quantity of USP L-Tyrosine RS in 1 mL of *Diluted ammonia solution*, and dilute with water to volume to obtain a solution having a known concentration of about 0.05 mg per mL. Apply 5 μL. [NOTE—This solution has a concentration equivalent to about 0.5% of that of the *Test solution*.]
 System suitability solution—Dissolve about 10 mg of USP L-Tyrosine RS and about 10 mg of USP L-Phenylalanine RS in 1 mL of *Diluted ammonia solution*, dilute with water to 25.0 mL, and mix. Apply 5 μL.
 Spray reagent—Dissolve 0.2 g of ninhydrin in 100 mL of a mixture of butyl alcohol and 2 N acetic acid (95 : 5).
 Developing solvent system—Prepare a mixture of isopropyl alcohol and ammonium hydroxide (70 : 30).
 Procedure—Proceed as directed for *Thin-Layer Chromatography* under *Chromatography* ⟨621⟩. Dry the plate between 100° and 105° until the ammonia disappears completely. Spray with *Spray reagent*, and heat between 100° and 105° for about 15 minutes. Examine the plate under white light. The chromatogram obtained from the *System suitability solution* exhibits two clearly separated spots. Any secondary spot in the chromatogram obtained from the *Test solution* is not larger or more intense than the principal spot in the chromatogram obtained from the *Standard solution*: not more than 0.5% of any individual impurity is found; and not more than 2.0% of total impurities is found.

Organic volatile impurities, *Method IV* ⟨467⟩: meets the requirements.

(Official until July 1, 2008)

Assay—Transfer about 180 mg of Tyrosine, accurately weighed, to a 125-mL flask, dissolve in 6 mL of formic acid, add 50 mL of glacial acetic acid, and titrate with 0.1 N perchloric acid VS, determining the endpoint potentiometrically. Perform a blank determination, and make any necessary correction. Each mL of 0.1 N perchloric acid is equivalent to 18.12 mg of $C_9H_{11}NO_3$.

Tyrothricin

» Tyrothricin is an antibacterial substance produced by the growth of *Bacillus brevis* Dubos (Fam. *Bacteriaceae*). It consists principally of gramicidin and tyrocidine, the tyrocidine usually being present as the hydrochloride. It contains not less than 900 µg and not more than 1400 µg of tyrothricin per mg.

Packaging and storage—Preserve in tight containers.
USP Reference standards ⟨11⟩—*USP Gramicidin RS*.
Identification—Add about 5 mg to 5 mL of *p*-dimethylaminobenzaldehyde TS, and shake for 2 minutes. Add 2 drops of sodium nitrite solution (1 in 150) and 5 mL of water, and mix: a blue color is produced.
Loss on drying ⟨731⟩—Dry about 100 mg, accurately weighed, in a capillary-stoppered bottle in vacuum at a pressure not exceeding 5 mm of mercury at 60° for 3 hours: it loses not more than 5.0% of its weight.
Assay—Proceed as directed for gramicidin under *Antibiotics—Microbial Assays* ⟨81⟩, using a suitable, accurately weighed portion of Tyrothricin dissolved quantitatively in alcohol to yield a stock solution of convenient concentration. Dilute an accurately measured volume of this solution quantitatively and stepwise with alcohol to obtain a *Test Dilution* having a concentration of tyrothricin assumed to be 5.0 times the median dose level of the gramicidin Standard. Multiply the result of the gramicidin assay by 5.0 to obtain the amount of tyrothricin, in µg, in each mL of the *Test Dilution*.

Undecylenic Acid

$C_{11}H_{20}O_2$ 184.28
10-Undecenoic acid.
10-Undecenoic acid [112-38-9].

» Undecylenic Acid contains not less than 97.0 percent and not more than 100.5 percent of $C_{11}H_{20}O_2$.

Packaging and storage—Preserve in tight, light-resistant containers.
Identification—
 A: To 1 mL add potassium permanganate TS, dropwise: the permanganate color is discharged.
 B: Place 3 mL of it and 3 mL of freshly distilled aniline in a tall test tube, and heat for 10 minutes at a rate such that the ring of condensate remains just below the mouth of the tube. Cool, add 10 mL of alcohol and 10 mL of ether, and transfer to a separator. Wash the ether solution with four 20-mL portions of water, and discard the water washings. Heat on a steam bath until the odor of ether no longer is perceptible, then add a few mg of activated carbon, mix, and filter. Evaporate the filtrate nearly to dryness, and recrystallize the residue from 70 percent alcohol: the anilide so obtained melts between 66° and 67.5°.

Specific gravity ⟨841⟩: between 0.910 and 0.913.
Congealing range ⟨651⟩: not lower than 21°.
Refractive index ⟨831⟩: between 1.447 and 1.448.
Residue on ignition ⟨281⟩: not more than 0.15%.
Water-soluble acids—Shake 5 mL with 5 mL of water, and filter the water layer through a filter paper previously moistened with water. Add 1 drop of methyl orange TS, and titrate with 0.01 N sodium hydroxide VS: not more than 1.0 mL of 0.010 N sodium hydroxide is required to match the color produced by 1 drop of methyl orange TS in 5 mL of water.
Heavy metals, *Method II* ⟨231⟩: 0.001%.
Iodine value ⟨401⟩: between 131 and 138.
Assay—Dissolve about 750 mg of Undecylenic Acid, accurately weighed, in 50 mL of alcohol, add 3 drops of phenolphthalein TS, and titrate with 0.1 N sodium hydroxide VS to the first pink color that persists for not less than 30 seconds. Perform a blank determination, and make any necessary correction. Each mL of 0.1 N sodium hydroxide is equivalent to 18.43 mg of $C_{11}H_{20}O_2$.

Compound Undecylenic Acid Ointment

» Compound Undecylenic Acid Ointment contains undecylenic acid, calcium undecylenate, copper undecylenate, or zinc undecylenate, individually or in any combination, in a suitable ointment base. It contains not less than 90.0 percent and not more than 110.0 percent of the labeled amount of total undecylenic acid ($C_{11}H_{20}O_2$).

Packaging and storage—Preserve in tight containers, and avoid prolonged exposure to temperatures exceeding 30°.
USP Reference standards ⟨11⟩—*USP Undecylenic Acid RS*.
Assay for zinc undecylenate—
 Standard preparations—Prepare a solution of freshly ignited zinc oxide in dilute hydrochloric acid (1 in 60) to obtain the equivalent of 1.0 mg of zinc per mL. Dilute quantitatively with water to obtain separate solutions containing the equivalent of 15 and 30 µg of zinc per mL.
 Assay preparation—Transfer about 1.0 g of Ointment, accurately weighed, to a 100-mL beaker. Add 25 mL of dilute hydrochloric acid (1 in 20), swirl, and heat carefully until the mixture is liquefied. Cool, and transfer the mixture to a 250-mL separator. Complete the transfer of the waxy residue by thoroughly rinsing the beaker with 50 mL of water and two 50-mL portions of chloroform and adding the rinsings to the separator. Equilibrate the mixture, and transfer the chloroform extract to a 500-mL separator. Extract the aqueous phase with another 100-mL portion of chloroform, combine the second chloroform extract with the main extract in the 500-mL separator, and transfer the aqueous phase to a 200-mL volumetric flask. Wash the combined chloroform extracts with three 25-mL portions of water, add the aqueous washings to the 200-mL volumetric flask, dilute with water to volume, and mix to obtain a specimen stock solution. [NOTE—Retain the chloroform extract for the *Assay for undecylenic acid*.] Transfer 15.0 mL or other suitable volume (see *Procedure*) of this specimen stock solution to a 100-mL volumetric flask, dilute with water to volume, and mix.
 Procedure—Aspirate each *Standard preparation* and the *Assay preparation* into the flame of a suitable atomic absorption spectrophotometer, and determine the absorbances of the solutions at 214 nm. Typically, an acetylene–air mixture is adjusted to obtain a blue flame about 7 mm in height with a suitable burner that is rotated to a position perpendicular to the light path. [NOTE—If the absorbance of the *Assay preparation* is outside the central 70% of the range between the absorbances of the *Standard preparations*, discard the *Assay preparation* and prepare another by diluting the specimen stock solution quantitatively as necessary to obtain a suitable absor-

bance.] Calculate the percentage of zinc undecylenate in the Ointment taken by the formula:

$$(431.94/65.39)(0.2/W)C_L + \frac{(C_H - C_L)(A_U - A_L)}{(A_H - A_L)}$$

in which 431.94 is the molecular weight of zinc undecylenate; 65.39 is the atomic weight of zinc; W is the weight, in g, of Ointment taken; A_U, A_H, and A_L are the absorbances of the *Assay preparation* and the high- and low-concentration *Standard preparations*, respectively; and C_H and C_L are the concentrations, in µg per mL, of the high- and low-concentration *Standard preparations*, respectively.

Assay for undecylenic acid—
Internal standard solution—Prepare a solution in chloroform containing 10 mg of tridecanoic acid in each mL.

Standard preparation—Dissolve an accurately weighed quantity of USP Undecylenic Acid RS in chloroform to obtain a solution having a known concentration of about 3.8 mg per mL. Transfer 5.0 mL of this solution to a 50-mL volumetric flask, add 3.0 mL of *Internal standard solution*, dilute with chloroform to volume, and mix.

Assay preparation—Pass the chloroform extract prepared from the Ointment as directed in *Assay for zinc undecylenate* through phase-separating filter paper into a 250-mL volumetric flask. Rinse the separator with three 15-mL portions of chloroform, passing the rinsings through the filter and combining them with the main chloroform solution, add chloroform to volume, and mix. Transfer 20.0 mL of this solution to a 50-mL volumetric flask, add 3.0 mL of *Internal standard solution*, dilute with chloroform to volume, and mix.

Chromatographic system—Under typical conditions, the gas chromatograph is equipped with a flame-ionization detector and contains a 2-mm × 1.8-m glass column packed with 3% liquid phase G1 on 100- to 200-mesh support S1A. The column is maintained at a temperature of about 165°. Dry helium is used as the carrier gas at a flow rate of about 30 mL per minute.

System suitability—Chromatograph five injections of the silylated *Standard preparation*, and record the peak responses as directed for *Procedure*: the resolution, R (see *Chromatography* ⟨621⟩), is not less than 3.0.

Procedure—Transfer 1.0-mL portions of the *Standard preparation* and the *Assay preparation* to separate, stoppered test tubes. To each tube add 50 µL of bis(trimethylsilyl)trifluoroacetamide, insert the stopper, mix, and allow to stand for 30 minutes. Inject a suitable portion (2 to 5 µL) of the *Standard preparation* into a suitable gas chromatograph, and record the chromatogram so as to obtain not less than 50% of maximum recorder response. Similarly inject a suitable portion of the *Assay preparation*, and record the chromatogram. Measure the peak responses for the first (undecylenic acid) and second (tridecanoic acid) peaks of the chromatograms. [NOTE—Relative retention times are, approximately, 0.43 for undecylenic acid and 1.0 for tridecanoic acid.] Calculate the percentage of total undecylenic acid in the Ointment taken by the formula:

$$62.5(C/W)(R_U/R_S)$$

in which C is the concentration, in mg per mL, of USP Undecylenic Acid RS in the *Standard preparation*; W is the weight, in g, of Ointment taken; and R_U and R_S are the ratios of the peak responses of undecylenic acid to those of tridecanoic acid from the *Assay preparation* and the *Standard preparation*, respectively. The difference between the total undecylenic acid and the undecylenic acid equivalent to the determined zinc undecylenate (the weight of zinc undecylenate multiplied by 0.8533 gives the equivalent of undecylenic acid), both expressed as a percentage of the Ointment, gives the percentage of free undecylenic acid in the Ointment.

Urea

CH_4N_2O 60.06
Urea.
Carbamide   [57-13-6].

» Urea contains not less than 99.0 percent and not more than 100.5 percent of CH_4N_2O.

Packaging and storage—Preserve in well-closed containers. Store at 25°, excursions permitted between 15° and 30°.
Labeling—Where it is intended for use in preparing injectable dosage forms, the label states that it is sterile or must be subjected to further processing during the preparation of injectable dosage forms.
USP Reference standards ⟨11⟩—*USP Endotoxin RS*.
Identification—
   A: Heat about 500 mg in a test tube: it liquefies, and ammonia is evolved. Continue the heating until the liquid becomes turbid, then cool. Dissolve the fused mass in a mixture of 10 mL of water and 1 mL of sodium hydroxide solution (1 in 10), and add 1 drop of cupric sulfate TS: the solution acquires a reddish-violet color.
   B: Dissolve 100 mg in 1 mL of water, and add 1 mL of nitric acid: a white crystalline precipitate of urea nitrate is formed.
Melting range ⟨741⟩: between 132° and 135°.
Residue on ignition ⟨281⟩: not more than 0.1%.
Alcohol-insoluble matter—Dissolve 5.0 g in 50 mL of warm alcohol, and if any insoluble residue remains, filter the solution on a tared filter, wash the residue and the filter with 20 mL of warm alcohol, and dry at 105° for 1 hour: the weight of the residue does not exceed 2 mg (0.04%).
Chloride ⟨221⟩—A 2.0-g portion shows no more chloride than corresponds to 0.20 mL of 0.020 N hydrochloric acid (0.007%).
Sulfate ⟨221⟩—A 2.0-g portion shows no more sulfate than corresponds to 0.20 mL of 0.020 N sulfuric acid (0.010%).
Heavy metals ⟨231⟩—Dissolve 1.0 g in 20 mL of water, and add 5 mL of 0.1 N hydrochloric acid: the limit is 0.002%.
Other requirements—Where the label states that Urea is sterile, it meets the requirements for *Sterility Tests* ⟨71⟩ and for *Bacterial endotoxins* under *Urea for Injection*. Where the label states that Urea must be subjected to further processing during the preparation of injectable dosage forms, it meets the requirements for *Bacterial endotoxins* under *Urea for Injection*.
Assay—Transfer about 500 mg of Urea, accurately weighed, to a 200-mL volumetric flask, dissolve in and dilute with water to volume, and mix. Pipet 2 mL of this solution into a micro-Kjeldahl digestion flask, and proceed as directed under *Nitrogen Determination, Method II* ⟨461⟩, beginning with "Add 1 g of a powdered mixture." [NOTE—In this procedure, continue heating the flask until fuming begins, then heat for 1 additional hour.] Each mL of 0.01 N acid is equivalent to 0.3003 mg of CH_4N_2O.

Urea for Injection

» Urea for Injection is Urea suitable for parenteral use.

Packaging and storage—Preserve in *Containers for Sterile Solids* as described under *Injections* ⟨1⟩.
USP Reference standards ⟨11⟩—*USP Endotoxin RS*.
Completeness of solution ⟨641⟩—A 1.0-g portion dissolves in 10 mL of carbon dioxide-free water to yield a clear solution.
Constituted solution—At the time of use, it meets the requirements for *Constituted Solutions* under *Injections* ⟨1⟩.
Bacterial endotoxins ⟨85⟩—It contains not more than 0.003 USP Endotoxin Unit per mg of urea.

Other requirements—It responds to the *Identification* tests and meets the requirements for *Melting range*, *Residue on ignition*, *Alcohol-insoluble matter*, *Chloride*, *Sulfate*, *Heavy metals*, and *Assay* under *Urea*. It meets also the requirements for *Sterility Tests* ⟨71⟩, *Uniformity of Dosage Units* ⟨905⟩, and *Labeling* under *Injections* ⟨1⟩.

Ursodiol

$C_{24}H_{40}O_4$ 392.57
Cholan-24-oic acid, 3,7-dihydroxy-, (3α,5β,7β)-.
3α,7β-Dihydroxy-5β-cholan-24-oic acid   [128-13-2].

» Ursodiol contains not less than 98.5 percent and not more than 101.5 percent of $C_{24}H_{40}O_4$, calculated on the dried basis.

Packaging and storage—Preserve in tight containers.
USP Reference standards ⟨11⟩—*USP Ursodiol RS*.
Identification, *Infrared Absorption* ⟨197K⟩.
Melting range ⟨741⟩:   between 200° and 205°.
Specific rotation ⟨781S⟩:   between 57° and 62°.
    Test solution: 20 mg per mL, in alcohol.
Loss on drying ⟨731⟩—Dry it at 105° for 3 hours: it loses not more than 0.5% of its weight.
Residue on ignition ⟨281⟩:   not more than 0.1%.
Heavy metals, *Method II* ⟨231⟩:   0.001%.
Related compounds—
    Adsorbent: 0.25-mm layer of chromatographic silica gel.
    Solvent—Prepare a mixture of acetone and water (9 : 1).
    Standard solution 1—Prepare a solution of chenodiol in *Solvent* containing 600 µg per mL.
    Standard solution 2—Prepare a solution of lithocholic acid in *Solvent* containing 20 µg per mL.
    Test solution—Prepare a solution of Ursodiol in *Solvent* containing 40 mg per mL.
    Diluted test solution—Quantitatively dilute 1 mL of the *Test solution* with *Solvent* to obtain a solution having a concentration of 40 µg per mL.
    Developing solvent system: a mixture of chloroform, glacial acetic acid, and water (85 : 15 : 0.5)
    Spray reagent: phosphomolybdic acid TS.
    Procedure—Separately apply 10 µL each of *Standard solution 1*, *Standard solution 2*, the *Test solution*, and the *Diluted test solution* to a thin-layer chromatographic plate (see *Thin Layer Chromatography* under *Chromatography* ⟨621⟩), and proceed as directed in the chapter, allowing the solvent front to move about three-fourths of the length of the plate. Remove the plate from the developing chamber, mark the solvent front, and air-dry the plate. Spray the plate with phosphomolybdic acid TS, dry at 105° for 5 minutes, and examine the plate: any secondary spot in the chromatogram of the *Test solution* having the same R_F value as the principal spot from *Standard solution 1* is not greater in size or intensity than that obtained from *Standard solution 1*: not more than 1.5% of chenodiol is found. No secondary spot observed in the chromatogram of the *Test solution* having the same R_F value as the principal spot from *Standard solution 2* is greater in size or intensity than that obtained from *Standard solution 2*: not more than 0.05% of lithocholic acid is found. No other secondary spot observed in the chromatogram of the *Test solution* is greater in size or intensity than the principal spot obtained from the *Diluted test solution:* not more than 0.1% of any other impurity is found.

Assay—
    Mobile phase—Prepare a filtered and degassed mixture of acetonitrile and water (55 : 45). Adjust with 0.6 M phosphoric acid to a pH of 3.0. Make adjustments if necessary (see *System Suitability* under *Chromatography* ⟨621⟩).
    Internal standard solution—Dissolve an accurately weighed quantity of epiandrosterone in methanol to obtain a solution having a concentration of about 4 mg per mL. Dilute a portion of this solution quantitatively with *Mobile phase* to obtain a solution having a concentration of about 0.8 mg per mL.
    Standard preparation—Dissolve an accurately weighed quantity of USP Ursodiol RS in methanol, and dilute quantitatively, and stepwise if necessary, with methanol to obtain a solution having a known concentration of about 4 mg per mL. Transfer this solution to a suitable container, and dilute with *Mobile phase* to give a solution having a known concentration of about 0.8 mg of ursodiol per mL. Transfer equal volumes of this solution and the *Internal standard solution* to a suitable container, and mix.
    Assay preparation—Transfer about 100 mg of Ursodiol, accurately weighed, to a 25-mL volumetric flask, dissolve in and dilute with methanol to volume. Transfer 5.0 mL of this solution to a 25-mL volumetric flask, dilute with *Mobile phase* to volume, and mix. Transfer equal volumes of this solution and the *Internal standard solution* to a suitable container, and mix.
    Chromatographic system (see *Chromatography* ⟨621⟩)—The liquid chromatograph is equipped with a differential refractive index detector and a 3.9-mm × 30-cm column that contains packing L1. The flow rate is about 1.0 mL per minute. Both the detector temperature and the column temperature are maintained at 40°. Chromatograph the *Standard preparation*, and record the peak responses as directed for *Procedure:* the relative retention times are about 0.74 for ursodiol and 1.0 for epiandrosterone; the resolution, *R*, between ursodiol and epiandrosterone is not less than 3.8 (If the resolution specification is not met, increase the water content of the *Mobile phase*); and the relative standard deviation for replicate injections is not more than 1.0%.
    Procedure—Separately inject equal volumes (about 50 µL) of the *Standard preparation* and the *Assay preparation* into the chromatograph, record the chromatograms, and measure the responses for the major peaks. Calculate the quantity, in mg, of $C_{24}H_{40}O_4$ in the portion of Ursodiol taken by the formula:

$$250C(R_U / R_S)$$

in which *C* is the concentration, in mg per mL, of USP Ursodiol RS in the *Standard preparation;* and R_U and R_S are the ratios of the ursodiol peak to the internal standard peak obtained from the *Assay preparation* and the *Standard preparation*, respectively.

Ursodiol Capsules

» Ursodiol Capsules contain not less than 90.0 percent and not more than 110.0 percent of the labeled amount of ursodiol ($C_{24}H_{40}O_4$).

Packaging and storage—Preserve in well-closed containers.
USP Reference standards ⟨11⟩—*USP Ursodiol RS*.
Identification—The retention time of the major peak in the chromatogram of the *Assay preparation* corresponds to that in the chromatogram of the *Standard preparation*, both relative to the internal standard, as obtained in the *Assay*.
Dissolution ⟨711⟩—
    Medium: 0.05 M pH 8.4 phosphate buffer, prepared by mixing 250 mL of 0.2 M monobasic potassium phosphate, 280 mL of 0.2 M potassium hydroxide, and 5 mL of 2% sodium lauryl sulfate solution. Adjust with 0.2 M potassium hydroxide to a pH of 8.4, and dilute with water to 1000 mL; 1000 mL.
    Apparatus 2:   75 rpm.
    Time: 30 minutes.
    Determine the amount of ursodiol ($C_{24}H_{40}O_4$) dissolved by employing the following method.

Mobile phase—Prepare a filtered and degassed mixture of acetonitrile and 0.075 M monobasic potassium phosphate (50 : 50). Adjust with 85% phosphoric acid to a pH of 3.0. Make adjustments if necessary (see *System Suitability* under *Chromatography* ⟨621⟩).

Standard solution—Dissolve an accurately weighed quantity of USP Ursodiol RS, and dilute quantitatively, and stepwise if necessary, with *Medium* to obtain a solution having a known concentration equivalent to that expected in the solution under test.

Test solution—Use a filtered portion of the solution under test.

Chromatographic system—The liquid chromatograph is equipped with a refractive index detector, a guard column that contains packing L1, and a 3.9-mm × 30-cm column that contains packing L1. The flow rate is about 1 mL per minute, and the column and detector temperatures are maintained at 40°. Chromatograph the *Standard solution*, and record the peak responses as directed for *Procedure:* the tailing factor of the ursodiol peak is not more than 1.7; and the relative standard deviation for replicate injections is not more than 2%.

Procedure—Separately inject equal volumes (about 50 µL) of the *Standard solution* and the *Test solution* into the chromatograph, record the chromatograms, and measure the responses for the major peaks. Calculate the percentage of $C_{24}H_{40}O_4$ dissolved by the formula:

$$100{,}000(r_U / r_S)(C/W)$$

in which r_U and r_S are the peak responses obtained from the *Test solution* and the *Standard solution*, respectively; C is the concentration, in mg per mL, of USP Ursodiol RS in the *Standard solution;* and W is the labeled amount, in mg, of ursodiol in each Capsule.

Tolerances—Not less than 80% *(Q)* of the labeled amount of $C_{24}H_{40}O_4$ is dissolved in 30 minutes.

Uniformity of dosage units ⟨905⟩: meet the requirements for *Weight Variation*.

Assay—

Mobile phase, Internal standard solution, Standard preparation, and *Chromatographic system*—Proceed as directed in the *Assay* under *Ursodiol*.

Assay preparation—Accurately weigh the contents of not fewer than 20 Capsules, and mix. Transfer an accurately weighed portion of the powder, equivalent to about 200 mg of ursodiol, to a 50-mL volumetric flask. Add about 40 mL of methanol, and sonicate for about 15 minutes. Cool the mixture to room temperature, dilute with methanol to volume, and centrifuge a portion of this mixture. Transfer 5.0 mL of the clear supernatant to a 25-mL volumetric flask, and dilute with *Mobile phase* to volume. Transfer equal amounts of this solution and the *Internal standard solution* to a suitable container, mix, and filter.

Procedure—Separately inject equal volumes (about 50 µL) of the *Standard preparation* and the *Assay preparation* into the chromatograph, record the chromatograms, and measure the responses for the major peaks. Calculate the quantity, in mg, of ursodiol ($C_{24}H_{40}O_4$) in the portion of Capsules taken by the formula:

$$200(C_S / C_U)(R_U / R_S)$$

in which C_S and C_U are the concentrations, in mg per mL, of ursodiol in the *Standard preparation* and the *Assay preparation*, respectively; and R_U and R_S are the ratios of the ursodiol peak to the internal standard peak obtained from the *Assay preparation* and the *Standard preparation*, respectively.

Ursodiol Tablets

» Ursodiol Tablets contain not less than 90.0 percent and not more than 110.0 percent of the labeled amount of ursodiol ($C_{24}H_{40}O_4$).

Packaging and storage—Preserve in well-closed containers, and store at a temperature between 20° and 25°.

USP Reference standards ⟨11⟩—*USP Ursodiol RS*.

Identification—

Adsorbent, Developing solvent system, and *Spray reagent*—Proceed as directed for *Related compounds* test.

Application volume: 25 µL.

Standard solution—Prepare a solution of USP Ursodiol RS in methanol containing about 1 mg per mL.

Test solution—Transfer a quantity of finely powdered Tablets, equivalent to about 25 mg of ursodiol, to a conical flask. Add 25.0 mL of methanol, and mix for 20 minutes. Centrifuge this solution for 10 minutes at 4000 rpm, and use the clear supernatant.

Procedure—Proceed as directed for *Related compounds* test. The principal indigo-colored spot observed in the chromatogram of the *Test solution* corresponds in color and in R_F value to that in the chromatogram of the *Standard solution*.

Dissolution ⟨711⟩—

Medium: simulated intestinal fluid TS, prepared without pancreatin and adjusted with 0.1 N sodium hydroxide or 0.1 N hydrochloric acid to a pH of 8.0; 900 mL.

Apparatus 2: 75 rpm.

Time: 45 minutes.

Determine the amount of $C_{24}H_{40}O_4$ dissolved by employing the following method.

Mobile phase and *Chromatographic system*—Prepare as directed in the *Assay*.

Procedure—Inject a volume (about 25 µL) of a filtered portion of the solution under test into the chromatograph, record the chromatogram, and measure the heights of responses for the major peaks. Calculate the quantity of $C_{24}H_{40}O_4$ dissolved in comparison with a Standard solution having a known concentration of USP Ursodiol RS in the same *Medium* and similarly chromatographed.

Tolerances—Not less than 80% *(Q)* of the labeled amount of $C_{24}H_{40}O_4$ is dissolved in 45 minutes.

Uniformity of dosage units ⟨905⟩: meet the requirements.

Related compounds—

Adsorbent: 0.25-mm layer of chromatographic silica gel mixture (see *Chromatography* ⟨621⟩), activated for at least 4 hours at 105°.

Developing solvent system: a mixture of chloroform, acetone, and acetic acid (7 : 2 : 1).

Standard solution 1—Prepare a solution of USP Ursodiol RS in methanol containing 20 µg per mL.

Standard solution 2—Prepare a solution of lithocholic acid in methanol containing 10 µg per mL.

Standard solution 3—Prepare a solution of chenodeoxycholic acid in methanol containing 300 µg per mL.

Test solution—Transfer a quantity of finely powdered Tablets, equivalent to about 250 mg of ursodiol, to a conical flask. Add 25.0 mL of methanol, and mix for 20 minutes. Centrifuge this solution for 20 minutes at 4000 rpm, and use the clear supernatant.

Application volume: 25 µL each of *Standard solution 1, Standard solution 2,* and *Standard solution 3,* and 50 µL of the *Test solution*.

Spray reagent—Dissolve about 2.5 g of phosphomolybdic acid in 50 mL of glacial acetic acid, add 2.5 mL of concentrated sulfuric acid, and mix well.

Procedure—Proceed as directed for *Thin-Layer Chromatography* under *Chromatography* ⟨621⟩. Spray the plate lightly with *Spray reagent*. Dry the plate by heating at 105° for about 7 minutes. The spot due to lithocholic acid observed in the chromatogram of the *Test solution*, if present, is not greater in size and intensity than that obtained from *Standard solution 2* (0.05%). The spot due to chenodeoxycholic acid observed in the chromatogram of the *Test solution*, if present, is not greater in size and intensity than that obtained from *Standard solution 3* (1.5%). No other unidentified spot observed in the chromatogram of the *Test solution* is greater in size and intensity than the spot obtained from *Standard solution 1* (0.1%).

Assay—

Mobile phase—Prepare a filtered and degassed mixture of methanol, water, and phosphoric acid (77 : 23 : 0.6). Make adjustments if necessary (see *System Suitability* under *Chromatography* ⟨621⟩).

Internal standard solution—Dissolve an accurately weighed quantity of propylparaben in *Mobile phase* to obtain a solution having a known concentration of about 3.75 mg per mL.

Standard preparation—Dissolve an accurately weighed quantity of USP Ursodiol RS in *Internal standard solution* to obtain a solution having a known concentration of about 3.75 mg per mL.

Assay preparation—Weigh and finely powder 20 Tablets. Transfer an accurately weighed portion of the powder, equivalent to about 37.5 mg of ursodeoxycholic acid, to a glass-stoppered conical flask. Add 10.0 mL of *Internal standard solution*, and shake by mechanical means for 15 minutes. Sonicate at 40° for an additional 15 minutes, and filter.

Chromatographic system (see *Chromatography* ⟨621⟩)—The liquid chromatograph is equipped with a differential refractive index detector and a 4.6-mm × 25-cm column that contains packing L7. The flow rate is about 1.0 mL per minute. The detector temperature is maintained at 40°. Chromatograph the *Standard preparation*, and record the peak responses as directed for *Procedure*: the relative retention times are about 0.73 for propylparaben and 1.0 for ursodiol; the resolution, *R*, between ursodiol and propylparaben is not less than 3.0; the column efficiency is not less than 1600 theoretical plates; the tailing factor is not more than 2.0; and the relative standard deviation for replicate injections is not more than 2.0%.

Procedure—Separately inject equal volumes (about 10 µL) of the *Standard preparation* and the *Assay preparation* into the chromatograph, record the chromatograms, and measure the responses for the major peaks. Calculate the quantity, in mg, of ursodiol ($C_{24}H_{40}O_4$) in the portion of Tablets taken by the formula:

$$10C(R_U / R_S)$$

in which *C* is the concentration, in mg per mL, of USP Ursodiol RS in the *Standard preparation*; and R_U and R_S are the peak response ratios obtained from the *Assay preparation* and the *Standard preparation*, respectively.

Vaccinia Immune Globulin

» Vaccinia Immune Globulin conforms to the regulations of the FDA concerning biologics (see *Biologics* ⟨1041⟩). It is a sterile, nonpyrogenic solution of globulins derived from the blood plasma of adult human donors who have been immunized with vaccinia virus (Smallpox Vaccine). It is standardized for viral neutralizing activity in eggs or tissue culture with the U.S. Reference Vaccinia Immune Globulin and a specified vaccinia virus. It contains not less than 15 g and not more than 18 g of protein per 100 mL, not less than 90.0 percent of which is gamma globulin. It contains 0.3 M glycine as a stabilizing agent, and contains a suitable antimicrobial agent.

Packaging and storage—Preserve at a temperature between 2° and 8°.

Expiration date—The expiration date is not later than 3 years after date of issue.

Labeling—Label it to state that it is not intended for intravenous injection.

Valine

$C_5H_{11}NO_2$ 117.15
L-Valine.
L-Valine [*72-18-4*].

» Valine contains not less than 98.5 percent and not more than 101.5 percent of $C_5H_{11}NO_2$, as L-valine, calculated on the dried basis.

Packaging and storage—Preserve in well-closed containers.

USP Reference standards ⟨11⟩—*USP L-Phenylalanine RS. USP L-Valine RS.*

Identification, *Infrared Absorption* ⟨197K⟩.

Specific rotation ⟨781S⟩: between +26.6° and +28.8°.
  Test solution: 80 mg per mL, in 6 N hydrochloric acid.

pH ⟨791⟩: between 5.5 and 7.0, in a solution (1 in 20).

Loss on drying ⟨731⟩—Dry it at 105° for 3 hours: it loses not more than 0.3% of its weight.

Residue on ignition ⟨281⟩: not more than 0.1%.

Chloride ⟨221⟩—A 0.73-g portion shows no more chloride than corresponds to 0.50 mL of 0.020 N hydrochloric acid (0.05%).

Sulfate ⟨221⟩—A 0.33-g portion shows no more sulfate than corresponds to 0.10 mL of 0.020 N sulfuric acid (0.03%).

Iron ⟨241⟩: 0.003%.

Heavy metals, *Method I* ⟨231⟩ : 0.0015%.

Chromatographic purity—
  Adsorbent: 0.25-mm layer of chromatographic silica gel mixture.
  Test solution—Dissolve an accurately weighed quantity of Valine in 2 N hydrochloric acid to obtain a solution having a concentration of 10 mg per mL. Apply 5 µL.
  Standard solution—Dissolve an accurately weighed quantity of USP L-Valine RS in 0.1 N hydrochloric acid to obtain a solution having a known concentration of about 0.05 mg per mL. Apply 5 µL. [NOTE—This solution has a concentration equivalent to about 0.5% of that of the *Test solution*.]
  System suitability solution—Prepare a solution in 0.1 N hydrochloric acid containing 0.4 mg each of USP L-Valine RS and USP L-Phenylalanine RS per mL. Apply 5 µL.
  Spray reagent—Dissolve 0.2 g of ninhydrin in 100 mL of a mixture of butyl alcohol and 2 N acetic acid (95 : 5).
  Developing solvent system—Prepare a mixture of butyl alcohol, glacial acetic acid, and water (60 : 20 : 20).
  Procedure—Proceed as directed for *Thin-Layer Chromatography* under *Chromatography* ⟨621⟩. After air-drying the plate, spray with *Spray reagent*, and heat between 100° and 105° for about 15 minutes. Examine the plate under white light. The chromatogram obtained from the *System suitability solution* exhibits two clearly separated spots. Any secondary spot in the chromatogram obtained from the *Test solution* is not larger or more intense than the principal spot in the chromatogram obtained from the *Standard solution*: not more than 0.5% of any individual impurity is found; and not more than 2.0% of total impurities is found.

Organic volatile impurities, *Method I* ⟨467⟩ : meets the requirements.

(Official until July 1, 2008)

Assay—Transfer about 110 mg of Valine, accurately weighed, to a 125-mL flask, dissolve in a mixture of 3 mL of formic acid and 50 mL of glacial acetic acid, and titrate with 0.1 N perchloric acid VS, determining the endpoint potentiometrically. Perform a blank determination, and make any necessary correction. Each mL of 0.1 N perchloric acid is equivalent to 11.72 mg of $C_5H_{11}NO_2$.

Valproic Acid

$C_8H_{16}O_2$ 144.21
Pentanoic acid, 2-propyl-.
Propylvaleric acid [*99-66-1*].

» Valproic Acid contains not less than 98.0 percent and not more than 102.0 percent of $C_8H_{16}O_2$, calculated on the anhydrous basis.

Packaging and storage—Preserve in tight, glass, stainless steel or polyethylene (HDPE) containers.

USP Reference standards ⟨11⟩—*USP Valproic Acid RS. USP Valproic Acid Related Compound A RS.*

Identification—
  A: *Infrared Absorption* ⟨197F⟩.
  B: The retention time of the major peak in the chromatogram of the *Assay preparation* corresponds to that in the chromatogram of the *Standard preparation,* as obtained in the *Assay.*

Water, *Method I* ⟨921⟩: not more than 1.0%.
Residue on ignition ⟨281⟩: not more than 0.1%.
Heavy metals, *Method II* ⟨231⟩: 0.002%.

Chromatographic purity—
  System suitability solution—Mix suitable quantities of butyric acid, valeric acid, and USP Valproic Acid Related Compound A RS in Valproic Acid to obtain a solution containing about 1.0 µL per mL, 1.0 µL per mL, and 0.1 µL per mL, respectively.
  Test solution—Use Valproic Acid.
  Chromatographic system (see *Chromatography* ⟨621⟩)—The gas chromatograph is equipped with a flame-ionization detector and a 0.32-mm × 60-m column coated with a 0.3-µm film of phase G25. Helium is used as the carrier gas with a total flow rate of about 150 mL per minute with a split flow ratio of 100 : 1. The injection port and detector temperatures are maintained at 240° and 260°, respectively. The chromatograph is programmed as follows. Initially the temperature of the column is equilibrated at 145° for 48 minutes, then the temperature is linearly increased at a rate of 5° per minute to 190°, and maintained at 190°. Chromatograph the *System suitability solution,* and record the peak responses as directed for *Procedure:* the relative retention times are about 0.38 for butyric acid, 0.52 for valeric acid, 1.64 for related compound A, and 1.0 for valproic acid; the resolution, *R,* between butyric acid and valeric acid is not less than 23.0; the column efficiency determined from valeric acid is not less than 100,000 theoretical plates; and the tailing factor for the valeric acid peak is not more than 1.5. The related compound A peak must elute between 41 and 50 minutes and must have a peak area of not less than 0.01% relative to the valproic acid peak.
  Procedure—Inject a volume (about 0.5 µL) of the *Test solution* into the chromatograph, record the chromatogram, and measure the peak responses. Calculate the percentage of each impurity in the portion of Valproic Acid taken by the formula:

$$100(r_i / r_s)$$

in which r_i is the peak response for each impurity; and r_s is the sum of the responses for all the peaks: not more than 0.1% of any individual impurity is found; and not more than 0.3% of total impurities is found.

Organic volatile impurities, *Method V* ⟨467⟩: meets the requirements.
  Solvent—Use dimethyl sulfoxide.

(Official until July 1, 2008)

Assay—
  Internal standard solution—Transfer about 1.2 g of nonanoic acid to a 100-mL volumetric flask, and dissolve in and dilute with heptane to volume.
  Standard preparation—Dilute an accurately weighed quantity of USP Valproic Acid RS with heptane to obtain a solution having a known concentration of about 10.0 mg per mL. Transfer 5.0 mL of this solution to a 50-mL volumetric flask, add 5.0 mL of *Internal standard solution,* dilute with heptane to volume, and mix.
  Assay preparation—Transfer about 100 mg of Valproic Acid, accurately weighed, to a 10-mL volumetric flask, dilute with heptane to volume, and mix. Transfer 5.0 mL of this solution to a 50-mL volumetric flask, add 5.0 mL of *Internal standard solution,* dilute with heptane to volume, and mix.
  Chromatographic system (see *Chromatography* ⟨621⟩)—The gas chromatograph is equipped with a flame-ionization detector and a 2.0-mm × 1.8-m column packed with 10% phase G34 on 80- to 100-mesh support S1A. The carrier gas is helium. The flow rate is about 35 mL per minute. The column, injection port, and detector temperatures are maintained at 175°, 275°, and 300°, respectively. Chromatograph the *Standard preparation,* and record the peak responses as directed for *Procedure:* the relative retention times are about 1.0 for valproic acid and 2.0 for nonanoic acid; the resolution, *R,* between valproic acid and nonanoic acid is not less than 7.0; and the relative standard deviation for replicate injections is not more than 1.5%.
  Procedure—Separately inject equal volumes (about 3 µL) of the *Standard preparation* and the *Assay preparation* into the chromatograph, record the chromatograms, and measure the responses for the major peaks. Calculate the quantity, in mg, of $C_8H_{16}O_2$ in the portion of Valproic Acid taken by the formula:

$$100C(R_U / R_S)$$

in which *C* is the concentration, in mg per mL, of USP Valproic Acid RS in the *Standard preparation;* and R_U and R_S are the peak response ratios of valproic acid to the internal standard obtained from the *Assay preparation* and the *Standard preparation,* respectively.

Valproic Acid Capsules

» Valproic Acid Capsules contain not less than 90.0 percent and not more than 110.0 percent of the labeled amount of valproic acid ($C_8H_{16}O_2$).

Packaging and storage—Preserve in tight containers, at controlled room temperature.

USP Reference standards ⟨11⟩—*USP Valproic Acid RS.*

Identification—
  A: The retention time ratios of the valproic acid peak to the internal standard peak obtained from the *Standard preparation* and the *Assay preparation* as directed in the *Assay* do not differ by more than 2.0%.
  B: Place a portion of Capsule contents, equivalent to about 250 mg of valproic acid, in a separator. Add 20 mL of 1 N sodium hydroxide, shake, and allow the layers to separate. Transfer the aqueous layer to a second separator, add 4 mL of hydrochloric acid, mix, and extract with 40 mL of *n*-heptane. Filter the *n*-heptane layer through glass wool into a beaker, and evaporate the solvent completely on a steam bath with the aid of a current of air. Transfer 2 drops of the residue to a test tube containing 0.5 mL each of potassium iodide solution (1 in 50) and potassium iodate solution (1 in 25), and mix: a yellow color is produced.

Disintegration ⟨701⟩: 15 minutes, determined as directed for *Soft Gelatin Capsules.*

Dissolution ⟨711⟩—
  Medium: a solution containing 5 mg per mL of sodium lauryl sulfate in simulated intestinal fluid TS (prepared without the enzyme and with monobasic sodium phosphate instead of monobasic potassium phosphate), adjusted with 5 M sodium hydroxide to a pH of 7.5; 900 mL.
  Apparatus 2: 50 rpm.
  Time: 60 minutes.
  Internal standard solution and *Chromatographic system*—Proceed as directed in the *Assay.*
  Standard preparation—Prepare a solution of USP Valproic Acid RS having a concentration similar to that of the solution under test. Transfer 10.0 mL to a suitable container. Add about 3.0 g of sodium chloride, and mix on a vortex mixer for 5 minutes. Add about 1 mL of 6 N hydrochloric acid and 5.0 mL of *Internal standard solution,* and shake for 2 minutes. Allow the phases to separate, remove the *n*-heptane layer, and filter. Discard the aqueous layer.
  Test preparation—Transfer 10.0 mL of the solution under test to a suitable container. Proceed as directed for *Standard preparation,* beginning with "Add about 3.0 g".
  Procedure—Proceed as directed in the *Assay.*
  Tolerances—Not less than 85% (*Q*) of the labeled amount of $C_8H_{16}O_2$ is dissolved in 60 minutes.

Uniformity of dosage units ⟨905⟩: meet the requirements, chloroform being used as the solvent in the procedure for *Soft Capsules*.

Assay—

Internal standard solution—Dissolve a quantity of biphenyl in *n*-heptane to obtain a solution having a concentration of about 5 mg per mL.

Standard preparation—Dissolve an accurately weighed quantity of USP Valproic Acid RS in *n*-heptane to obtain a solution having a known concentration of about 2.5 mg per mL. Transfer 5.0 mL to a container equipped with a closure. Add 2.0 mL of *Internal standard solution*, close the container, and mix.

Assay preparation—Transfer not fewer than 20 Capsules to a blender jar or other container, add about 150 mL of methylene chloride, and cool in a solid carbon dioxide-acetone mixture until the contents have solidified. If necessary, transfer the mixture of Capsules and methylene chloride to a blender jar, and blend with a high-speed blender until all the solids are reduced to fine particles. Transfer the mixture to a 500-mL volumetric flask, add *n*-heptane to volume, mix, and allow solids to settle. Transfer an accurately measured volume of this solution, equivalent to 250 mg of valproic acid, to a 100-mL volumetric flask, dilute with *n*-heptane to volume, and mix. Transfer 5.0 mL to a container equipped with a closure. Add 2.0 mL of *Internal standard solution*, close the container, and mix.

Chromatographic system (see *Chromatography* ⟨621⟩)—The gas chromatograph is equipped with a flame-ionization detector and a 2-mm × 1.8-m glass column packed with 10% phase G34 on 80- to 100-mesh support S1A. The column temperature is maintained at about 150°, and the injection port and the detector block temperatures are maintained at about 250°. Dry helium is used as the carrier gas at a flow rate of about 40 mL per minute. Chromatograph the *Standard preparation*, measure the peak responses, and calculate the ratio, R_S, as directed for *Procedure*: the relative retention times are about 0.5 for valproic acid and 1.0 for biphenyl; the resolution, R, between valproic acid and biphenyl is not less than 3.0; the relative standard deviation for replicate injections is not more than 2.0%.

Procedure—Separately inject equal volumes (about 2 μL) of the *Standard preparation* and the *Assay preparation* into the chromatograph, record the chromatograms, and measure the peak responses for valproic acid and biphenyl. Calculate the quantity, in mg, of valproic acid ($C_8H_{16}O_2$) in the portion of Capsules taken by the formula:

$$100\ C(R_U / R_S)$$

in which C is the concentration, in mg per mL, of USP Valproic Acid RS in the *Standard preparation*; and R_U and R_S are the peak response ratios obtained from the *Assay preparation* and the *Standard preparation*, respectively.

Valproic Acid Injection

(Title for this new monograph—to become official October 1, 2008)

» Valproic Acid Injection is a sterile aqueous solution of sodium valproate, formed from the interaction of Valproic Acid and Sodium Hydroxide, in Water for Injection, and one or more suitable buffering or sequestering agents. It contains not less than 90.0 percent and not more than 110.0 percent of the labeled amount of valproic acid ($C_8H_{16}O_2$). It contains no antimicrobial agents.

Packaging and storage—Preserve in single-dose *Containers for Injection* as described under *Injections* ⟨1⟩, preferably of Type I glass. Store at controlled room temperature, excursions allowed between 15° and 30°.

Labeling—Label it to state the name and quantity of any buffering or sequestering agent used.

USP Reference standards ⟨11⟩—USP Endotoxin RS. USP Valproic Acid RS.

Identification—

A: The relative retention time of the major peak in the chromatogram of the *Assay preparation* corresponds to that in the chromatogram of the *Standard preparation*, as obtained in the *Assay*.

B: It meets the requirements of the tests for *Sodium* ⟨191⟩.

Bacterial endotoxins ⟨85⟩—It contains not more than 23 USP Endotoxin Units per mL of Injection.

Sterility ⟨71⟩—It meets the requirements when tested as directed for *Membrane Filtration* under *Test for Sterility of the Product to be Examined*.

pH ⟨791⟩: between 7.0 and 9.0.

Particulate matter ⟨788⟩—It meets the requirements for small-volume injections.

Other requirements—It meets the requirements under *Injections* ⟨1⟩.

Assay—

Internal standard solution—Dissolve a quantity of biphenyl in methylene chloride to obtain a solution containing 5 mg per mL.

Standard stock preparation—Prepare a solution of USP Valproic Acid RS in *Internal standard solution* having a concentration of about 8 mg per mL.

Standard preparation—Transfer 5.0 mL of the *Standard stock preparation* into a 50-mL volumetric flask, and dilute with methylene chloride to volume.

Assay preparation—Transfer an accurately measured volume of Injection, equivalent to 400 mg of valproic acid, into a suitable container; add about 20 mL of 5% (v/v) hydrochloric acid; shake by mechanical means for 2 minutes; add 50.0 mL of the *Internal standard solution;* and shake by mechanical means for 1 hour. Allow the phase to separate (approximately 1 hour). The bottom organic layer remains cloudy, and at times a slight emulsion may persist. If an emulsion forms, break it up by stirring it with a glass rod. Pipet 5 mL of the extract from the bottom organic layer into a 50-mL volumetric flask, and dilute with methylene chloride.

Chromatographic system (see *Chromatography* ⟨621⟩)—The gas chromatograph is equipped with a flame-ionization detector and a 2-mm × 1.8-m glass column packed with 10% phase G34 on 80-to 100-mesh support S1A. The column temperature is maintained at about 155°, the injection port temperature is maintained at about 275°, and the detector block temperature is maintained at about 300°. Dry helium is used as the carrier gas, at a flow rate of about 20 mL per minute. Chromatograph the *Standard preparation* as directed for *Procedure:* the resolution, R, between the valproic acid and biphenyl peaks is not less than 3.0; and the relative standard deviation of the peak area ratios for replicate injections is not more than 2.0%.

Procedure—Separately inject equal volumes (about 2 μL) of the *Standard preparation* and the *Assay preparation* into the chromatograph, record the chromatograms, and measure the peak areas for the valproic acid and biphenyl peaks. Calculate the quantity, in mg, of valproic acid in the volume of Injection taken by the formula:

$$C(R_U / R_S)\ D$$

in which C is the concentration, in mg per mL, of USP Valproic Acid RS in the *Standard preparation*; R_U and R_S are the peak area ratios obtained from the *Assay preparation* and the *Standard preparation*, respectively; and D is the appropriate dilution factor used to prepare the *Assay preparation*.

Valproic Acid Oral Solution

» Valproic Acid Oral Solution contains not less than 90.0 percent and not more than 110.0 percent of the labeled amount of valproic acid ($C_8H_{16}O_2$). It is prepared with the aid of Sodium Hydroxide.

Valproic / Official Monographs

Packaging and storage—Preserve in tight containers.

USP Reference standards ⟨11⟩—*USP Valproic Acid RS.*

Identification—
 A: The retention time ratios of the valproic acid peak to the internal standard peak obtained from the *Standard preparation* and the *Assay preparation* as directed in the *Assay* do not differ by more than 2.0%.
 B: Place a volume of Oral Solution, equivalent to about 250 mg of valproic acid, in a separator. Add 40 mL of water and 2 mL of hydrochloric acid, mix, and extract with 40 mL of *n*-heptane. Filter the *n*-heptane layer through glass wool into a beaker, and evaporate the solvent completely on a steam bath with the aid of a current of air. Transfer 2 drops of the residue to a test tube containing 0.5 mL each of potassium iodide solution (1 in 50) and potassium iodate solution (1 in 25), and mix: a yellow color is produced.

pH ⟨791⟩: between 7.0 and 8.0.

Assay—
 Internal standard solution, Standard preparation, and *Chromatographic system*—Prepare as directed in the *Assay* under *Valproic Acid Capsules.*
 Assay preparation—Transfer an accurately measured volume of Oral Solution, equivalent to about 250 mg of valproic acid, to a separator. Add 40 mL of water and 2 mL of hydrochloric acid, mix, and extract gently with 80 mL of *n*-heptane until the aqueous layer is clear (about 3 minutes). Filter the *n*-heptane layer through glass wool, collecting the filtrate in a 100-mL volumetric flask. Rinse the separator and the glass wool with small portions of *n*-heptane, add the rinsings to the flask, dilute with *n*-heptane to volume, and mix. Transfer 5.0 mL to a container equipped with a closure. Add 2.0 mL of *Internal standard solution*, close the container, and mix.
 Procedure—Separately inject equal volumes (about 2 μL) of the *Standard preparation* and the *Assay preparation* into the chromatograph, record the chromatograms, and measure the peak responses for valproic acid and biphenyl. Calculate the quantity, in mg, of valproic acid ($C_8H_{16}O_2$) in each mL of the Oral Solution taken by the formula:

$$100(C/V)(R_U/R_S)$$

in which C is the concentration, in mg per mL, of USP Valproic Acid RS in the *Standard preparation*; V is the volume, in mL, of Oral Solution taken; and R_U and R_S are the peak response ratios obtained from the *Assay preparation* and the *Standard preparation*, respectively.

Valrubicin

$C_{34}H_{36}F_3NO_{13}$ 723.65
(2*S-cis*)-2-[1,2,3,4,6,11-Hexahydro-2,5,12-trihydroxy-7-methoxy-6,11-dioxo-4-[[2,3,6-trideoxy-3-[(trifluoroacetyl)amino]-α-L-*lyxo*-hexopyranosyl]oxy]-2-naphthacenyl]-2-oxoethyl pentanoate.
(8*S*,10*S*)-8-Glycoloyl-7,8,9,10-tetrahydro-6,8,11-trihydroxy-1-methoxy-10-[[2,3,6-trideoxy-3-(2,2,2-trifluoroacetamido)-α-L-*lyxo*-hexopyranosyl]oxy]-5,12-naphthacenedione 8^2-valerate [56124-62-0].

» Valrubicin contains not less than 95.0 percent and not more than 103.0 percent of $C_{34}H_{36}F_3NO_{13}$, calculated on the dried basis.

Caution—*Great care should be taken to prevent inhaling particles of Valrubicin and exposing the skin to it.*

Packaging and storage—Preserve in tight, light-resistant containers, and store at controlled room temperature.

USP Reference standards ⟨11⟩—*USP Valrubicin RS. USP Valrubicin Related Compound A RS.*

Identification—
 A: *Infrared Absorption* ⟨197M⟩.
 B: *Ultraviolet Absorption* ⟨197U⟩—
  Solution: 10 mg per mL.
  Medium: methanol.
 Absorptivities, calculated on the dried basis, are 555 ± 20 at 233 nm and 382.5 ± 17.5 at 252 nm.
 C: The retention time of the major peak in the chromatogram of the *Assay preparation* corresponds to that in the chromatogram of the *Standard preparation*, as obtained in the *Assay*.

Loss on drying ⟨731⟩—Dry it in vacuum over phosphorus pentoxide at 80° for 4 hours: it loses not more than 3.0% of its weight.

Residue on ignition ⟨281⟩: not more than 0.2%.

Limit of residual solvents—
 Internal standard solution—Prepare a solution of *n*-propyl alcohol in dimethyl sulfoxide having a concentration of about 0.05 μL per mL.
 Standard solution—Prepare a solution in *Internal standard solution* having a concentration of 2.5 μg of chloroform, 5.0 μg of dehydrated alcohol, 5.0 μg of acetone, 5.0 μg of butyl alcohol, 5.0 μg of dioxane, 10.0 μg of methylene chloride, 15.0 μg of diisopropyl ether, 20.5 μg of acetonitrile, 50 μg of pentane, and 100 μg of methanol in each mL, and sonicate.
 Test solution—Dissolve about 200 mg of Valrubicin, accurately weighed, in 4.0 mL of *Internal standard solution,* and sonicate.
 Chromatographic system (see *Chromatography* ⟨621⟩)—The gas chromatograph is equipped with a flame-ionization detector and a 0.32-mm × 30-m fused-silica capillary column coated with a 5-μm film of G2 stationary phase. The carrier gas is helium, flowing at a rate of 30 mL per minute. The column temperature is maintained at 220°. The injection port temperature and the detector block temperature are maintained at 250°. Chromatograph the *Standard solution,* and record the responses as directed for *Procedure*: the relative retention times are about 0.48 for methanol, 0.66 for dehydrated alcohol, 0.71 for acetonitrile, 0.76 for acetone, 0.86 for pentane, 0.92 for methylene chloride, 1.0 for *n*-propyl alcohol, 1.19 for diisopropyl ether, 1.22 for chloroform, 1.35 for butyl alcohol, and 1.52 for dioxane; the component solvent peaks are resolved; and the relative standard deviation of the ratios of the peak area of each solvent to the peak area of *n*-propyl alcohol is not more than 10%.
 Procedure—Separately inject equal volumes (about 1 μL) of the *Standard solution* and the *Test solution* into the chromatograph, record the chromatograms, and measure the areas for the major peaks. Calculate the concentration, in μg per g, of each residual solvent in the portion of Valrubicin taken by the formula:

$$4000(C/W)(R_i/R_S)$$

in which C is the concentration, in μg per mL, of the respective individual solvent in the *Standard solution;* W is the quantity, in mg, of Valrubicin taken to prepare the *Test solution;* and R_i and R_S are the peak area ratios of the respective individual solvent to *n*-propyl alcohol obtained from the *Test solution* and the *Standard solution*, respectively: not more than 50 μg per g of chloroform, 100 μg per g of dehydrated alcohol, 100 μg per g of acetone, 100 μg per g of butyl alcohol, 100 μg per g of dioxane, 300 μg per g of methylene chloride, 410 μg per g of acetonitrile, 500 μg per g of diisopropyl ether, 1000 μg per g of pentane, and 2000 μg per g of methanol are found.

Related compounds—
 Mobile phase—Prepare as directed in the *Assay*.
 Resolution solution—Prepare a solution of USP Valrubicin Related Compound A RS and USP Valrubicin RS in acetonitrile having known concentrations of about 0.25 mg per mL and 1 mg per mL, respectively.

Test solution—Use the *Assay preparation*.

Chromatographic system (see *Chromatography* ⟨621⟩)—The liquid chromatograph is equipped with a 254-nm detector, a guard column, and a 5-mm × 10-cm analytical column that contains a 4-μm packing L1. The flow rate is about 3.5 mL per minute. Chromatograph the *Resolution solution*, and record the responses as directed for *Procedure*: the relative retention times are about 0.8 for valrubicin related compound A and 1.0 for valrubicin; and the resolution, R, between valrubicin related compound A and valrubicin is not less than 2.

Procedure—Inject a volume (about 10 μL) of the *Test solution* into the chromatograph, record the chromatogram, and measure the areas for the major peaks. Calculate the percentage of each impurity in the portion of Valrubicin taken by the formula:

$$100(r_i / r_s)$$

in which r_i is the peak area for each impurity; and r_s is the sum of the areas of all the peaks. Do not consider any peaks due to solvent or excipients. Not more than 0.3% of any individual impurity with a relative retention time of 0.06, 0.17, 0.27, or 0.52 is found; not more than 0.6% of any impurity with a relative retention time of about 0.14 is found; not more than 0.2% of any other individual impurity is found; not more than 1.0% of total other impurities that are not specified by relative retention time is found; and not more than 2.5% of total impurities that are not less than 0.1% is found.

Assay—

Mobile phase—Prepare a filtered and degassed mixture of 0.015 M phosphoric acid and acetonitrile (57 : 43). Make adjustments if necessary (see *System Suitability* under *Chromatography* ⟨621⟩).

Standard preparation—Dissolve an accurately weighed quantity of USP Valrubicin RS in acetonitrile, and dilute quantitatively with acetonitrile to obtain a solution having a known concentration of about 1 mg per mL.

Assay preparation—Transfer about 25 mg of Valrubicin, accurately weighed, to a 25-mL volumetric flask, dissolve in and dilute with acetonitrile to volume, and mix.

Chromatographic system (see *Chromatography* ⟨621⟩)—The liquid chromatograph is equipped with a 254-nm detector, a guard column, and a 5-mm × 10-cm analytical column that contains a 4-μm packing L1. The flow rate is about 3.5 mL per minute. Chromatograph the *Standard preparation*, and record the responses as directed for *Procedure*: the relative standard deviation for replicate injections is not more than 2%.

Procedure—Separately inject equal volumes (about 10 μL) of the *Standard preparation* and the *Assay preparation* into the chromatograph, record the chromatograms, and measure the areas for the major peaks. Calculate the quantity, in mg, of $C_{34}H_{36}F_3NO_{13}$ in the portion of Valrubicin taken by the formula:

$$0.25CP(r_U / r_S)$$

in which C is the concentration, in mg per mL, of USP Valrubicin RS in the *Standard preparation*; P is the specified percentage of valrubicin in USP Valrubicin RS; and r_U and r_S are the valrubicin peak areas obtained from the *Assay preparation* and the *Standard preparation*, respectively.

Valrubicin Intravesical Solution

» Valrubicin Intravesical Solution is a sterile solution of Valrubicin in a suitable vehicle. It contains not less than 95.0 percent and not more than 105.0 percent of the labeled amount of valrubicin ($C_{34}H_{36}F_3NO_{13}$).

Packaging and storage—Preserve in single-dose or multiple-dose containers, preferably of Type I glass. Store in a refrigerator.

Labeling—Label it to indicate that it is not intended for intravenous or intramuscular injection, but is to be used for intravesical instillation.

USP Reference standards ⟨11⟩—*USP Endotoxin RS. USP Valrubicin RS. USP Valrubicin Related Compound A RS.*

Identification—

A: *Thin-Layer Chromatographic Identification Test* ⟨201⟩—

Test solution—Use the *Assay preparation*, prepared as directed in the *Assay*, and suitably dilute with methanol.

Standard solution—Use the *Standard preparation*, prepared as directed in the *Assay*, and suitably dilute with methanol.

Developing solvent system—Use the *Mobile phase*, prepared as directed in the *Assay*.

B: The retention time of the major peak in the chromatogram of the *Assay preparation* corresponds to that in the chromatogram of the *Standard preparation*, as obtained in the *Assay*.

Bacterial endotoxins ⟨85⟩: not more than 0.14 USP Endotoxin Unit per mg of valrubicin.

pH ⟨791⟩: between 4.0 and 7.0, in a solution of 0.9% sodium chloride (1 in 15).

Related compounds—

Mobile phase—Prepare as directed in the *Assay*.

Resolution solution—Prepare a solution of USP Valrubicin RS and USP Valrubicin Related Compound A RS in methanol to obtain a solution having concentrations of about 0.2 mg per mL and 0.05 mg per mL, respectively.

Test solution—Use the *Assay preparation* as directed in the *Assay*.

Chromatographic system (see *Chromatography* ⟨621⟩)—The liquid chromatograph is equipped with a 254-nm detector, a guard column, and a 5-mm × 10-cm analytical column that contains 4-μm packing L1. The flow rate is about 2.5 mL per minute. Chromatograph the *Resolution solution*, and record the peak areas as directed for *Procedure*: the relative retention times are about 0.9 for valrubicin related compound A and 1.0 for valrubicin; and the resolution, R, between valrubicin related compound A and valrubicin is not less than 2.

Procedure—Inject a volume (about 10 μL) of the *Test solution* into the chromatograph, record the chromatogram, and measure the areas for the major peaks. Calculate the percentage of each impurity in the portion of Intravesical Solution taken by the formula:

$$100(r_i / r_s)$$

in which r_i is the peak area for each impurity; and r_s is the sum of the peak areas of all the peaks. Do not consider any peaks due to solvent or excipients. Not more than 0.5% of any impurity with a relative retention time of about 0.11 is found; not more than 0.8% of any individual impurity with a relative retention time of 0.16, 0.51 or 0.71 is found; not more than 0.5% of any other individual impurity is found; and the sum of all impurities is not more than 3.5%.

Other requirements—It meets the requirements under *Injections* ⟨1⟩.

Assay—

Mobile phase—Prepare a filtered and degassed mixture of 0.1 M ammonium formate, previously adjusted with formic acid and acetonitrile (55 : 45) to a pH of 4.0. Make adjustments if necessary (see *System Suitability* under *Chromatography* ⟨621⟩).

Standard preparation—Dissolve an accurately weighed quantity of USP Valrubicin RS in methanol, and quantitatively dilute with methanol to obtain a solution having a known concentration of about 0.2 mg per mL.

Assay preparation—Transfer an accurately measured volume of Intravesical Solution, equivalent to about 20 mg of valrubicin, to a 100-mL volumetric flask, dissolve in methanol, dilute with methanol to volume, and mix.

Chromatographic system (see *Chromatography* ⟨621⟩)—The liquid chromatograph is equipped with a 254-nm detector, a guard column, and a 5-mm × 10-cm analytical column that contains 4-μm packing L1. The flow rate is about 2.5 mL per minute. Chromatograph the *Standard preparation*, and record the peak responses as directed for *Procedure*: the relative standard deviation for replicate injections is not more than 2%.

Procedure—Separately inject equal volumes (about 10 μL) of the *Standard preparation* and the *Assay preparation* into the chromatograph, record the chromatograms, and measure the responses for the major peaks. Calculate the quantity, in mg, of valrubicin ($C_{34}H_{36}$

F_3NO_{13}) in each mL of the Intravesical Solution taken by the formula:

$$(CP/V)(r_U / r_S)$$

in which C is the concentration, in mg per mL, of USP Valrubicin RS in the *Standard preparation*; P is the specified percentage of valrubicin in USP Valrubicin RS; V is the volume, in mL, of Intravesical Solution taken to prepare the *Assay preparation*; and r_U and r_S are the valrubicin peak responses obtained from the *Assay preparation* and the *Standard preparation*, respectively.

Valsartan

$C_{24}H_{29}N_5O_3$ 435.52
L-Valine, N-(1-oxopentyl)-N-[[2'-(1H-tetrazol-5-yl)[1,1'-biphenyl]-4-yl]methyl]-.
N-[p-(o-1H-Tetrazol-5-ylphenyl)benzyl]-N-valeryl-L-valine [*137862-53-4*].

» Valsartan contains not less than 98.0 percent and not more than 102.0 percent of $C_{24}H_{29}N_5O_3$, calculated on the anhydrous basis.

Packaging and storage—Preserve in tight containers, and store at 25°, excursions permitted between 15° and 30°. Protect from moisture and heat.
USP Reference standards ⟨11⟩—*USP Valsartan RS. USP Valsartan Related Compound A RS. USP Valsartan Related Compound B RS. USP Valsartan Related Compound C RS.*
Identification—
  A: *Infrared Absorption* ⟨197M⟩.
  B: The retention time of the major peak in the chromatogram of the *Assay preparation* corresponds to that in the chromatogram of the *Standard preparation*, as obtained in the *Assay*.
Absorbance—Prepare a 1 in 20 solution in methanol, and determine the absorbance at 420 nm. The absorbance divided by the path length is not more than 0.02.
Water, *Method I* ⟨921⟩: not more than 2.0%.
Residue on ignition ⟨281⟩: not more than 0.1%.
Heavy metals, *Method II* ⟨231⟩: 0.001%.
Related compounds—
  TEST 1 (LIMIT OF VALSARTAN RELATED COMPOUND A)—
  Mobile phase—Prepare a mixture of *n*-hexane, 2-propanol, and trifluoroacetic acid (85 : 15 : 0.1). Make adjustments if necessary (see *System Suitability* under *Chromatography* ⟨621⟩).
  Standard solution—Dissolve an accurately weighed quantity of USP Valsartan Related Compound A RS in *Mobile phase*, and dilute quantitatively, and stepwise if necessary, to obtain a solution having a known concentration of about 0.01 mg per mL.
  System suitability solution—Dissolve accurately weighed quantities of USP Valsartan RS and USP Valsartan Related Compound A RS in *Mobile phase* to obtain a solution having known concentrations of about 0.04 mg per mL each of valsartan and valsartan related compound A.
  Test solution—Transfer about 50 mg of Valsartan, accurately weighed, to a 50-mL volumetric flask, add about 40 mL of *Mobile phase*, and sonicate for 5 minutes. Dilute with *Mobile phase* to volume, and mix.
  Chromatographic system (see *Chromatography* ⟨621⟩)—The liquid chromatograph is equipped with a 230-nm detector and a 4.6-mm × 25-cm column that contains 5-µm packing L40. The flow rate is about 0.8 mL per minute. Chromatograph the *System suitability solution*, and record the peak responses as directed for *Procedure*: the resolution, *R*, between valsartan related compound A and valsartan is not less than 2.0; and the relative standard deviation, determined from the valsartan related compound A peak, for replicate injections is not more than 5%.
  Procedure—Separately inject equal volumes (about 10 µL) of the *Standard solution* and the *Test solution* into the chromatograph, record the chromatograms, and measure the areas for the major peaks. Calculate the percentage of valsartan related compound A in the portion of Valsartan taken by the formula:

$$100(C_S / C_U)(r_U / r_S)$$

in which C_S is the concentration, in mg per mL, of USP Valsartan Related Compound A RS in the *Standard solution*; C_U is the concentration, in mg per mL, of valsartan in the *Test solution*; and r_U and r_S are the peak responses for valsartan related compound A obtained from the *Test solution* and the *Standard solution*, respectively: not more than 1.0% is found.
  TEST 2 (LIMIT OF VALSARTAN RELATED COMPOUND B, VALSARTAN RELATED COMPOUND C, AND OTHER RELATED COMPOUNDS)—
  Mobile phase—Proceed as directed in the *Assay*.
  Resolution solution—Dissolve accurately weighed quantities of USP Valsartan RS, USP Valsartan Related Compound B RS, and USP Valsartan Related Compound C RS in *Mobile phase*, and dilute quantitatively, and stepwise if necessary, with *Mobile phase* to obtain a solution having known concentrations of about 0.001 mg of valsartan per mL, 0.001 mg of valsartan related compound B per mL, and 0.001 mg of valsartan related compound C per mL.
  Standard solution— Dissolve an accurately weighed quantity of USP Valsartan RS in *Mobile phase*, and dilute quantitatively, and stepwise if necessary, with *Mobile Phase* to obtain a solution having a known concentration of about 0.001 mg of valsartan per mL.
  Test solution—Transfer about 50 mg of Valsartan, accurately weighed, to a 100-mL volumetric flask, dissolve in and dilute with *Mobile phase* to volume, and mix.
  Chromatographic system (see *Chromatography* ⟨621⟩)—Prepare as directed in the *Assay*, except to use a 225-nm detector. Chromatograph the *Resolution solution*, and record the peak responses as directed for *Procedure*: the resolution, *R*, between valsartan related compound B and valsartan is not less than 1.8; the relative standard deviation, determined from the valsartan related compound B peaks, for replicate injections is not more than 10.0%; and the relative standard deviation, determined from the valsartan peaks, for replicate injections is not more than 2.0%.
  Procedure—Separately inject equal volumes (about 10 µL) of the *Resolution solution*, the *Standard solution*, and the *Test solution* into the chromatograph, record the chromatograms, and measure the areas for the major peaks. Calculate the percentage of valsartan related compound B and valsartan related compound C in the portion of Valsartan taken by the formula:

$$100(C_S / C_U)(r_i / r_S)$$

in which C_S is the concentration, in mg per mL, of the appropriate USP Valsartan Related Compound RS in the *Resolution solution*; C_U is the concentration, in mg per mL, of valsartan in the *Test solution*; r_i is the peak response for the impurity obtained from the *Test solution*; and r_S is the peak response for the appropriate valsartan related compound obtained from the *Resolution solution*. Calculate the percentage of each other impurity in the portion of Valsartan taken by the formula:

$$100(C_S / C_U)(r_i / r_S)$$

in which C_S is the concentration, in mg per mL, of USP Valsartan RS in the *Standard solution*; r_S is the peak response for valsartan obtained from the *Standard solution*; and the other terms are as defined above: not more than 0.2% of valsartan related compound B is found; not more than 0.1% of valsartan related compound C is found; not more than 0.1% of any other individual impurity, excluding valsartan related compound A, is found; and not more than 0.3% of total impurities, excluding valsartan related compound A, is found.
Assay—
  Mobile phase—Prepare a filtered and degassed mixture of water, acetonitrile, and glacial acetic acid (500 : 500 : 1). Make adjustments if necessary (see *System Suitability* under *Chromatography* ⟨621⟩).

Standard preparation—Dissolve an accurately weighed quantity of USP Valsartan RS in *Mobile phase,* and dilute quantitatively, and stepwise if necessary, with *Mobile phase* to obtain a solution having a known concentration of about 0.5 mg per mL.

Assay preparation—Transfer about 50 mg of Valsartan, accurately weighed, to a 100-mL volumetric flask, dissolve in and dilute with *Mobile phase* to volume, and mix.

Chromatographic system (see *Chromatography* ⟨621⟩)—The liquid chromatograph is equipped with a 273-nm detector and a 3.0-mm × 12.5-cm column that contains 5-μm packing L1. The flow rate is about 0.4 mL per minute. Chromatograph the *Standard preparation*, and record the peak responses as directed for *Procedure*: the relative standard deviation for replicate injections is not more than 2.0%.

Procedure—Separately inject equal volumes (about 10 μL) of the *Standard preparation* and the *Assay preparation* into the chromatograph, record the chromatograms, and measure the areas for the major peaks. Calculate the quantity, in mg, of $C_{24}H_{29}N_5O_3$ in the portion of Valsartan taken by the formula:

$$100C(r_U / r_S)$$

in which C is the concentration, in mg per mL, of USP Valsartan RS in the *Standard preparation;* and r_U and r_S are the peak responses obtained from the *Assay preparation* and the *Standard preparation,* respectively.

Valsartan and Hydrochlorothiazide Tablets

» Valsartan and Hydrochlorothiazide Tablets contain not less than 90.0 percent and not more than 110.0 percent of the labeled amounts of valsartan ($C_{24}H_{29}N_{53}O_3$) and hydrochlorothiazide ($C_7H_8ClNO_4S_2$).

Packaging and storage—Preserve in tight containers, and store at 25°; excursions are permitted between 15° and 30°. Protect from moisture and heat.

USP Reference standards ⟨11⟩—*USP Benzothiadiazine Related Compound A RS. USP Hydrochlorothiazide RS. USP Valsartan RS. USP Valsartan Related Compound B RS.*

Identification—

A: *Thin-Layer Chromatographic Identification Test* ⟨201⟩—

Test solution—To a centrifuge tube transfer an amount of ground Tablets, equivalent in weight to a single Tablet, add 2.0 mL of acetone, sonicate for 15 minutes, and centrifuge.

Application volume: 2 μL.

Developing solvent system: a mixture of ethyl acetate, dehydrated alcohol, and a solution (25 in 100) of ammonium hydroxide (8 : 2 : 1).

Procedure—Proceed as directed in the chapter, except to develop the plate in a paper-lined chromatographic chamber equilibrated with *Developing solvent system* for about 15 minutes prior to use. Allow the chromatogram to develop until the solvent front has moved at least 7 cm. After removing the plate and marking the solvent front, dry the plate under a current of warm air until it is completely dry. The R_F values of the principal spots obtained from the *Test solution* correspond to those obtained from the Standard solution.

B: The retention times of the major peaks in the chromatogram of the *Assay preparation* correspond to those in the chromatogram of the *Standard preparation,* as obtained in the *Assay.*

Dissolution ⟨711⟩—

Medium: pH 6.8 phosphate buffer; 1000 mL.

Apparatus 2: 50 rpm.

Time: 30 minutes.

Procedure—Determine the amounts of valsartan ($C_{24}H_{29}N_5O_3$) and hydrochlorothiazide ($C_7H_8ClN_3O_4S_2$) dissolved by employing UV absorption at the wavelengths of maximum absorbance at about 250 nm for valsartan and at about 272 nm for hydrochlorothiazide on portions of the solution under test passed through a 1-μm glass fiber filter, diluted with *Medium* if necessary, using a 0.2-cm quartz cell. Calculate the amount of valsartan ($C_{24}H_{29}N_5O_3$) dissolved, in percentage, by the formula:

$$\frac{(AT2 \times A1\%H_{272nm}) - (AT1 \times A1\%H_{250nm})}{(A1\%V_{250nm} \times A1\%H_{272nm}) - (A1\%V_{272nm} \times A1\%H_{250nm})} \times 12{,}500$$

Calculate the amount of hydrochlorothiazide ($C_7H_8ClN_3O_4S_2$) dissolved, in percentage, by the formula:

$$\frac{(AT1 \times A1\%V_{250nm}) - (AT2 \times A1\%V_{272nm})}{(A1\%H_{272nm} \times A1\%V_{250nm}) - (A1\%H_{250nm} \times A1\%V_{272nm})} \times 80{,}000$$

in which $AT1$ is the absorbance of the solution under test at 272 nm; $AT2$ is the absorbance of the solution under test at 250 nm; $A1\%V_{272nm}$ is the absorptivity (1%, 0.2 cm, 272 nm) of valsartan in *Medium;* $A1\% V_{250nm}$ is the absorptivity (1%, 0.2 cm, 250 nm) of valsartan in *Medium;* $A1\%H_{272nm}$ is the absorptivity (1%, 0.2 cm, 272 nm) of hydrochlorothiazide in *Medium;* $A1\%H_{250nm}$ is the absorptivity (1%, 0.2 cm, 250 nm) of hydrochlorothiazide in *Medium.*

Tolerances—Not less than 80% (*Q*) of the labeled amounts of $C_{24}H_{29}N_5O_3$ and $C_7H_8ClN_3O_4S_2$ is dissolved in 30 minutes.

Uniformity of dosage units ⟨905⟩: meet the requirements.

PROCEDURE FOR CONTENT UNIFORMITY—

Diluent, Solution A, Solution B, Mobile phase, and *Chromatographic system*—Prepare as directed in the *Assay.*

Standard solution—Use the *Standard preparation,* as prepared in the *Assay.*

Test solution—Place 1 Tablet in a 200-mL volumetric flask, add 5 mL of water, and allow to stand for 5 minutes. Add about 100 mL of *Diluent,* and sonicate for 15 minutes. Dilute with *Diluent* to volume, mix, and centrifuge a portion of this solution at about 3000 rpm. Quantitatively dilute a volume of the clear supernatant with *Diluent* to obtain a solution having a concentration of about 0.2 mg of valsartan per mL.

Procedure—Separately inject equal volumes (about 10 μL) of the *Standard solution* and the *Test solution* into the chromatograph, record the chromatograms, and measure the areas for the major peaks. Separately calculate the quantities, in mg, of valsartan ($C_{24}H_{29}N_5O_3$) and hydrochlorothiazide ($C_7H_8ClN_3O_4S_2$) in the Tablet taken by the formula:

$$(LC_S / C_U)(r_U / r_S)$$

in which L is the labeled quantity, in mg, of the relevant analyte in the Tablet; C_S is the concentration, in mg per mL, of the appropriate USP Reference Standard in the *Standard solution; C_U* is the concentration, in mg per mL, of the corresponding analyte in the *Test solution,* based on the labeled quantity per Tablet and the extent of dilution; and r_U and r_S are the peak responses obtained from the *Test solution* and the *Standard solution,* respectively.

Related compounds—

Diluent, Solution A, Solution B, and *Mobile phase*—Prepare as directed in the *Assay.*

Standard stock solution—Dissolve accurately weighed quantities of USP Benzothiadiazine Related Compound A RS, USP Hydrochlorothiazide RS, USP Valsartan RS, and USP Valsartan Related Compound B RS in *Diluent* to obtain a solution having known concentrations of about 0.03 mg per mL, 0.06 mg per mL, 0.08 mg per mL, and 0.2 mg per mL, respectively.

Resolution solution—Dilute 5.0 mL of *Standard stock solution* with *Diluent* to 100.0 mL, and mix.

Standard solution—Dilute 10.0 mL of the *Resolution solution* with *Diluent* to 100.0 mL, and mix.

Test solution—Use the *Assay preparation* as specified.

Chromatographic system—Prepare as directed in the *Assay.* Chromatograph the *Resolution solution,* and record the peak responses as directed for *Procedure*: the resolution, *R,* between valsartan related compound B and valsartan, and between benzothiadiazine related compound A and hydrochlorothiazide is not less than 1.4. Chromatograph the *Standard solution,* and record the peak responses as directed for *Procedure*: the relative standard deviation, determined from the valsartan and hydrochlorothiazide peaks, for replicate injections is not more than 10.0%.

Procedure—Separately inject equal volumes (about 10 μL) of the *Standard solution* and the *Test solution* into the chromatograph, record the chromatograms, and measure the areas for the major peaks,

3498 **Valsartan** / *Official Monographs*

disregarding the peak, if any, with a retention time of about 22 minutes. Calculate the quantity, in mg, of each impurity in the portion of Tablets taken by the formula:

$$2000C(r_U / r_S)$$

in which C is the concentration, in mg per mL, of USP Benzothiadiazine Related Compound A RS, or the relevant USP Reference Standard (when determining the quantity of other impurities) in the *Standard solution;* and r_U and r_S are the corresponding peak responses obtained from the *Test solution* and the *Standard solution*, respectively: not more than 1.0% of benzothiadiazine related compound A is found; not more than 0.2% of any other impurity, excluding valsartan related compound A, is found; and not more than 1.3% of total impurities, excluding valsartan related compound A, is found. [NOTE—Valsartan related compound A is the enantiomer of valsartan and coelutes with valsartan in this test.]

Assay—
Diluent—Prepare a mixture of acetonitrile and water (1 : 1).
Solution A—Prepare a filtered and degassed mixture of water, acetonitrile, and trifluoroacetic acid (90 : 10 : 0.1).
Solution B—Prepare a filtered and degassed mixture of acetonitrile, water, and trifluoroacetic acid (90 : 10 : 0.1).
Mobile phase—Use variable mixtures of *Solution A* and *Solution B* as directed for *Chromatographic system*. Make adjustments if necessary (see *System Suitability* under *Chromatography* ⟨621⟩).
Standard preparation—Transfer about 12.5 mg of USP Hydrochlorothiazide RS, accurately weighed, to a 200-mL volumetric flask. Add about 12.5J mg of USP Valsartan RS, accurately weighed, J being the ratio of the labeled amount, in mg, of valsartan to the labeled amount, in mg, of hydrochlorothiazide per Tablet. Add about 100 mL of *Diluent*, sonicate for 15 minutes, dilute with *Diluent* to volume, and mix. Transfer 25.0 mL of this solution to a 50-mL volumetric flask, dilute with *Diluent* to volume, and mix. Quantitatively dilute a volume of this solution with *Diluent* to obtain a solution having a known concentration of about 0.2 mg of USP Valsartan RS per mL.
Assay preparation—Transfer a number of Tablets, equivalent to about 62.5 mg of hydrochlorothiazide, to a 250-mL volumetric flask. Add 5 mL of water, and allow to stand for 5 minutes. Then add about 100 mL of *Diluent*, sonicate for 15 minutes, and shake for 30 minutes. Dilute with *Diluent* to volume, mix, and centrifuge a portion of this solution at 3000 rpm. Dilute 25.0 mL of the clear supernatant with *Diluent* to 200.0 mL, and mix *(Solution 1)*. [NOTE—Retain a portion of *Solution 1* to use as the *Test solution* in the test for *Related compounds*.] Dilute an accurately measured volume of *Solution 1* with *Diluent* to obtain a solution containing about 0.2 mg of valsartan per mL.
Chromatographic system (see *Chromatography* ⟨621⟩)—The liquid chromatograph is equipped with a 265-nm detector and a 3.0-mm × 12.5-cm column that contains 5-μm packing L1. The flow rate is about 0.4 mL per minute. The chromatograph is programmed as follows.

Time (minutes)	Solution A (%)	Solution B (%)	Elution
0–25	90→10	10→90	linear gradient
25–27	10→90	90→10	linear gradient
27–40	90	10	isocratic

Chromatograph the *Standard preparation*, and record the peak responses as directed for *Procedure*: the relative standard deviation for replicate injections is not more than 2.0%.
Procedure—Separately inject equal volumes (about 10 μL) of the *Standard preparation* and the *Assay preparation* into the chromatograph, record the chromatograms, and measure the areas for the major peaks. Separately calculate the quantities, in mg, of valsartan ($C_{24}H_{29}N_5O_3$) and hydrochlorothiazide ($C_7H_8ClN_3O_4S_2$) in the portion of Tablets taken by the formula:

$$(LC_S / C_U)(r_U / r_S)$$

in which L is the labeled quantity, in mg, of the relevant analyte in each Tablet; C_S is the concentration, in mg per mL, of the appropriate USP Reference Standard in the *Standard preparation*; C_U is the concentration, in mg per mL, of the corresponding analyte in the *Assay preparation*, based on the labeled quantity per Tablet and the extent of dilution; and r_U and r_S are the peak responses obtained from the *Assay preparation* and the *Standard preparation*, respectively.

Vancomycin

$C_{66}H_{75}Cl_2N_9O_{24}$ 1449.25 Vancomycin. Vancomycin.
(S_a)-(3S,6R,7R,22R,23S,26S,36R,38aR)-44-[[2-O-(3-Amino-2,3,6-trideoxy-3-C-methyl-α-L-*lyxo*-hexopyranosyl)-β-D-glucopyranosyl]oxy]-3-(carbamoylmethyl)-10,19-dichloro-2,3,4,5,6,7,23,24,25,26,36,37,38,38a-tetradecahydro-7,22,28,30,32-pentahydroxy-6-[(2R)-4-methyl-2-(methylamino)valeramido]-2,5,24,38,39-pentaoxo-22H-8,11 : 18,21-dietheno-23,36-(iminomethano)-13,16 : 31,35-dimetheno-1H,16H-[1,6,9]oxadiazacyclohexadecino[4,5-m][10,2,16]-benzoxadiazacyclotetracosine-26-carboxylic acid.
[3S-[3R^*,6S^*(S^*),7S^*,22S^*,23R^*,26R^*,36S^*,38aS^*]]-3-(2-Amino-2-oxoethyl)-44-[[2-O-(3-amino-2,3,6-trideoxy-3-C-methyl-α-L-*lyxo*-hexopyranosyl)-β-D-glucopyranosyl]oxy]-10,19-dichloro-2,3,4,5,6,7,23,24,25,26,36,37,38,38a-tetra-decahydro-7,22,28,30,32-tahydroxy-6-[[4-methyl-2-(methylamino)-1-oxopentyl]amino]-2,5,24,38,39-pentaoxo-22H-8,11 : 18,21-dietheno-23,36-(iminomethano)-13,16 : 31,35-dimetheno-1H,16H-[1,6,9]oxadiazacyclohexadecino[4,5-m][10,2,16]-benzoxadiazacyclotetraine-26-carboxylic acid   [1404-90-6].

» Vancomycin has a potency equivalent to not less than 950 μg of vancomycin per mg, calculated on the anhydrous basis.

Packaging and storage—Preserve in tight containers.
USP Reference standards ⟨11⟩—*USP Vancomycin Hydrochloride RS.*
Identification—
  A: *Infrared Absorption* ⟨197K⟩.
  B: It does not respond to the test for *Chloride* ⟨191⟩.
Water, *Method I* ⟨921⟩: not more than 20%.
Heavy metals, *Method II* ⟨231⟩: 0.003%.
Chromatographic purity—
  Triethylamine buffer, Solution A, Solution B, Mobile Phase, Resolution solution, and *Chromatographic system*—Prepare as directed in the test for *Chromatographic purity* under *Vancomycin Hydrochloride*.
  Test preparation A—Transfer about 250 mg of Vancomycin to a 25-mL volumetric flask, add 5 mL of *Mobile phase A*, then add 0.1 N hydrochloric acid dropwise with swirling until dissolution is achieved. Dilute with *Mobile phase A* to volume, and mix.
  Test preparation B—Transfer 2.0 mL of *Test preparation A* to a 50-mL volumetric flask, dilute with *Mobile phase A* to volume, and mix.
  Procedure—Proceed as directed for *Procedure* in the test for *Chromatographic purity* under *Vancomycin Hydrochloride*. Calculate the percentage of vancomycin B in the specimen taken by the formula:

$$2500r_B / (25r_B + r_A)$$

in which the terms are as defined therein: not less than 92% of vancomycin B is found.
  Calculate the percentage of any individual peak, other than the main peak, by the formula:

$$100r_{Ai} / (25r_B + r_A)$$

in which the terms are as defined therein: not more than 3% of any peak other than the main peak is found.
Assay—Proceed as directed for Vancomycin under *Antibiotics—Microbial Assays* ⟨81⟩, preparing the *Test Dilution* as follows. Transfer about 100 mg of Vancomycin, accurately weighed, to a 100-mL volumetric flask. Add about 50 mL of water and 1 mL of 0.1 N hydrochloric acid, and swirl to dissolve, using sonication if necessary. Dilute with water to volume, and mix. Dilute an ac-

curately measured portion of this stock solution quantitatively with *Buffer No. 4* to yield a *Test Dilution* having a concentration assumed to be equal to that of the median dose of the Standard.

Vancomycin Hydrochloride

C₆₆H₇₅Cl₂N₉O₂₄ · HCl   1485.71
Vancomycin, monohydrochloride.
Vancomycin monohydrochloride.
(S_a)-(3S,6R,7R,22R,23S,26S,36R,38aR)-44-[[2-O-(3-Amino-2,3,6-trideoxy-3-C-methyl-α-L-*lyxo*-hexopyranosyl)-β-D-glucopyranosyl]oxy]-3-(carbamoylmethyl)-10,19-dichloro-2,3,4,5,6,7,23,24,25,26,36,37,38,38a-tetradecahydro-7,22,28,30,32-pentahydroxy-6-[(2R)-4-methyl-2-(methylamino)]valeramido]-2,5,24,38,39-pentaoxo-22H-8,11 : 18,21-dietheno-23,36-(iminomethano)-13,16 : 31,35-dimetheno-1H,16H-[1,6,9]oxadiazacyclohexadecino[4,5-m][10,2,16]benzoxadiazacyclotetracosine-26-carboxylic acid, monohydrochloride.
[3S-[3R*,6S*(S*),7S*,22S*,23R*,26R*,36S*,38aS*]]-3-(2-Amino-2-oxoethyl)-44-[[2-O-(3-amino-2,3,6-trideoxy-3-C-methyl-α-L-*lyxo*-hexopyranosyl)-β-D-glucopyranosyl]oxy]-10,19-dichloro-2,3,4,5,6,7,23,24,25,26,36,37,38,38a-tetradecahydro-7,22,28,30,32-pentahydroxy-6-[[4-methyl-2-(methylamino)-1-oxopentyl]amino]-2,5,24,38,39-pentaoxo-22H-8,11 : 18,21-dietheno-23,36-(iminomethano)-13,16 : 31,35-dimetheno-1H,16H-[1,6,9]oxadiazacyclohexadecino[4,5-m][10,2,16]-benzoxadiazacyclotetracosine-26-carboxylic acid, monohydrochloride [1404-93-9].

» Vancomycin Hydrochloride is the hydrochloride salt of a kind of vancomycin, a substance produced by the growth of *Streptomyces orientalis* (Fam. Streptomycetaceae), or a mixture of two or more such salts. It has a potency equivalent to not less than 900 μg of vancomycin per mg, calculated on the anhydrous basis.

Packaging and storage—Preserve in tight containers.
USP Reference standards ⟨11⟩—*USP Vancomycin Hydrochloride RS. USP Vancomycin B with Monodechlorovancomycin RS.*
Identification, *Infrared Absorption* ⟨197K⟩: undried.
pH ⟨791⟩:   between 2.5 and 4.5, in a solution containing 50 mg per mL.
Water, *Method I* ⟨921⟩:   not more than 5.0%.
Chromatographic purity—
  Triethylamine buffer—Mix 4 mL of triethylamine and 2000 mL of water, and adjust with phosphoric acid to a pH of 3.2.
  Solution A—Prepare a mixture of *Triethylamine buffer,* acetonitrile, and tetrahydrofuran (92 : 7 : 1), and degas briefly.
  Solution B—Prepare a suitable mixture of *Triethylamine buffer,* acetonitrile, and tetrahydrofuran (70 : 29 : 1), and degas briefly.
  Mobile phase—Use variable mixtures of *Solution A* and *Solution B* as directed for *Chromatographic system*. Make adjustments if necessary (see *System Suitability* under *Chromatography* ⟨621⟩), changing the acetonitrile proportion in *Solution A* to obtain a retention time of 7.5 to 10.5 minutes for the main vancomycin peak.
  Resolution solution—Prepare a solution of USP Vancomycin Hydrochloride RS in water containing 0.5 mg per mL, heat at 65° for 48 hours, and allow to cool.
  Test preparation A—Prepare a solution of Vancomycin Hydrochloride in *Solution A* containing 10 mg per mL.
  Test preparation B—Transfer 2.0 mL of *Test preparation A* to a 50-mL volumetric flask, dilute with *Solution A* to volume, and mix.
  Chromatographic system (see *Chromatography* ⟨621⟩)—The liquid chromatograph is equipped with a 280-nm detector and a 4.6-mm × 25-cm column that contains 5-μm packing L1. The flow rate is about 2 mL per minute. The chromatograph is programmed as follows.

Time (minutes)	Solution A (%)	Solution B (%)	Elution
0–12	100	0	isocratic
12–20	100→0	0→100	linear gradient
20–22	0	100	isocratic
22–23	0→100	100→0	linear gradient
23–30	100	0	isocratic

Chromatograph the *Resolution solution,* and record the peak responses as directed for *Procedure*: the elution order is resolution compound 1, vancomycin B, and resolution compound 2. The resolution, R, between resolution compound 1 and vancomycin B is not less than 3.0; and the column efficiency, calculated from the vancomycin B peak, is not less than 1500 theoretical plates. Resolution compound 2 is eluted at between 3 and 6 minutes after the start of the period when the percentage of *Solution B* is increasing from 0% to 100%.
  Procedure—[NOTE—Where baseline separation is not achieved, peak areas are defined by vertical lines extended from the valleys between peaks to the baseline. The main component peak may include a fronting shoulder, which is attributed to monodechlorovancomycin. This shoulder should not be integrated separately.] Separately inject equal volumes (about 20 μL) of *Test preparation A* and *Test preparation B* into the chromatograph, record the chromatograms, and measure the area responses for all of the peaks. [NOTE—Correct any peak observed in the chromatograms obtained from *Test preparation A* and *Test preparation B* by subtracting the area response of any peak observed in the chromatogram of *Solution A* at the corresponding elution time.] Calculate the percentage of vancomycin B in the specimen tested by the formula:

$$2500r_B / (25r_B + r_A)$$

in which r_B is the corrected area response of the main peak obtained in the chromatogram of *Test preparation B*; and r_A is the sum of the corrected area responses of all the peaks, other than the main peak, in the chromatogram obtained from *Test preparation A*: not less than 80.0% of vancomycin B is found. Calculate the percentage of each other peak taken by the formula:

$$100r_{Ai} / (25r_B + r_A)$$

in which r_{Ai} is the corrected area response of any individual peak, other than the main peak, obtained in the chromatogram of *Test preparation A*: not more than 9.0% of any peak other than the main peak is found.
Limit of monodechlorovancomycin—[NOTE—The *System suitability solution, Working standard solution,* and *Test solution* are to be refrigerated immediately after preparation and during analysis, using a refrigerated autosampler. The solutions are stable at refrigerated conditions for 4 days.]
  Mobile phase—Prepare a filtered and degassed mixture in a 1-L volumetric flask that is initially half filled with water. Dissolve 2.2 g of 1-heptanesulfonic acid sodium salt, add 125 mL of acetonitrile and 10 mL of acetic acid, and dilute with water to volume, making adjustments if necessary (see *System Suitability* under *Chromatography* ⟨621⟩).

Rinse solution—Prepare a solution containing approximately 10% (v/v) acetonitrile in water, to be used as the rinse solution for the needle and column.

System suitability solution—Dissolve an accurately weighed quantity of USP Vancomycin B with Monodechlorovancomycin RS that contains approximately 50 mg of vancomycin B in water in a 50-mL volumetric flask to obtain a solution having a known concentration of about 1 mg of vancomycin B per mL.

Working standard solution—Transfer 5.0 mL of the *System suitability solution* to a 100-mL volumetric flask, and dilute with water to volume. The final concentration is approximately 0.05 mg of vancomycin B per mL.

Test solution—Transfer about 100 mg of Vancomycin Hydrochloride, accurately weighed, to a 100-mL volumetric flask, dilute with water to volume, and mix.

Blank: water

Chromatographic system (see *Chromatography* ⟨621⟩)—The liquid chromatograph is equipped with a 280-nm detector and a 4.6-mm × 25-cm column that contains packing L1 and is maintained at a constant temperature of about 60°. The flow rate is about 1.5 mL per minute. The autosampler cooler temperature is maintained at 5°. The *Blank* and *Working standard solution* run time is 90 minutes, and the *System suitability solution* and *Test solution* run time is 120 minutes. [NOTE—This test is sensitive to temperature changes. To preheat the *Mobile phase*, *Working standard solution*, and *Test solution*, a length of tubing of at least 3 feet should be placed preceding the column within the column heater.] Chromatograph the *Blank* and the *System suitability solution*. There should be no peaks in the *Blank* chromatogram that interfere with the vancomycin B and monodechlorovancomycin peaks. The retention time of the vancomycin B peak is between 32 and 42 minutes. The monodechlorovancomycin elutes at a retention time ratio of approximately 1.1 compared to 1.0 for the main component, vancomycin B. The retention time of the monodechlorovancomycin peak in the *Test solution* chromatogram must be within ±3.0% of the mean retention time of the monodechlorovancomycin peaks in the chromatogram of the *Working standard solution*. The resolution, *R*, between vancomycin B and monodechlorovancomycin is not less than 1.9, using the chromatogram from the *System suitability solution;* and the relative standard deviation for replicate injections of the *Working standard solution* is not more than 2.0%.

Procedure—Separately inject equal volumes (about 50 µL) of the *Blank*, *System suitability solution*, *Working standard solution*, and *Test solution* into the chromatograph, record the chromatograms, and measure the peak area responses. Calculate the percentage of monodechlorovancomycin in the portion of Vancomycin Hydrochloride taken by the formula:

$$0.1 \, (W_S / W_U)(r_U / r_S) \, P$$

in which W_S is the weight, in mg, of USP Vancomycin B with Monodechlorovancomycin RS in the *Working standard solution*; W_U is the weight, in mg, of Vancomycin Hydrochloride taken to prepare the *Test solution*; r_U is the peak area response of the monodechlorovancomycin peak in the *Test solution*; r_S is the average peak area response of the vancomycin B peaks in the *Working standard solution*; and *P* is the vancomycin B purity of USP Vancomycin B with Monochlorovancomycin RS: not more than 4.7% of monodechlorovancomycin is found.

Assay—Proceed with Vancomycin Hydrochloride as directed under *Antibiotics—Microbial Assays* ⟨81⟩.

Vancomycin Hydrochloride Capsules

» Vancomycin Hydrochloride Capsules contain the equivalent of not less than 90.0 percent and not more than 115.0 percent of the labeled amount of vancomycin ($C_{66}H_{75}Cl_2N_9O_{24}$).

Packaging and storage—Preserve in tight containers.
USP Reference standards ⟨11⟩—*USP Vancomycin Hydrochloride RS.*
Identification—Place 1 or more Capsules in a high-speed glass blender jar containing a volume of water sufficient to yield a solution containing the equivalent of 1 mg of vancomycin per mL, and blend for 3 to 5 minutes. To a suitable sheet of chromatographic filter paper apply 5 µL of this solution and 5 µL of a solution of USP Vancomycin Hydrochloride RS containing the equivalent of 1 mg of vancomycin per mL. Develop by descending chromatography (see *Chromatography* ⟨621⟩) with a mixture of butyl alcohol, water, and pyridine (6 : 4 : 3) for 7 hours. Allow the paper to dry, and place it on an inoculated agar surface of sufficient area to accommodate the paper and prepared for vancomycin assay as directed under *Antibiotics—Microbial Assays* ⟨81⟩, except to use *Medium 2*. Remove the paper from the agar surface after 30 minutes, and incubate the agar medium at 37° for 18 hours: clear zones of inhibition are produced at corresponding positions on the two chromatograms.

Dissolution ⟨711⟩—
  Medium: water; 900 mL.
  Apparatus 1: 100 rpm.
  Time: 45 minutes.
  Procedure—Determine the amount of vancomycin dissolved by assaying a filtered portion of the solution under test as directed for vancomycin under *Antibiotics—Microbial Assays* ⟨81⟩.
  Tolerances—Not less than 85% (*Q*) of the labeled amount of vancomycin is dissolved in 45 minutes.

Uniformity of dosage units ⟨905⟩: meet the requirements.
Water, *Method I* ⟨921⟩: not more than 8.0%.
Assay—Proceed as directed for vancomycin under *Antibiotics—Microbial Assays* ⟨81⟩, using not less than 5 Capsules blended at high speed in a glass blender jar for 3 to 5 minutes with a sufficient, accurately measured, volume of *Buffer No. 4* to yield a stock solution having a convenient concentration of vancomycin. Dilute an accurately measured volume of this stock solution quantitatively and stepwise with *Buffer No. 4* to obtain a *Test Dilution* having a concentration assumed to be equal to the median dose level of the Standard.

Vancomycin Injection

» Vancomycin Injection is a sterile isoosmotic solution of Vancomycin Hydrochloride in Water for Injection. It contains not less than 90.0 percent and not more than 115.0 percent of the labeled amount of vancomycin. It contains a suitable tonicity-adjusting agent.

Packaging and storage—Preserve in *Containers for Injections* as described under *Injections* ⟨1⟩. Maintain in the frozen state.
Labeling—It meets the requirements for *Labeling* under *Injections* ⟨1⟩. The label states that it is to be thawed just prior to use, describes conditions for proper storage of the resultant solution, and directs that the solution is not to be refrozen.
USP Reference standards ⟨11⟩—*USP Endotoxin RS. USP Vancomycin Hydrochloride RS.*
Identification—The retention time of the main vancomycin peak in the chromatogram of *Test preparation A* obtained as directed in the test for *Chromatographic purity* corresponds to that in the chromatogram of a similar preparation of USP Vancomycin Hydrochloride RS similarly chromatographed.
Bacterial endotoxins ⟨85⟩—It contains not more than 0.33 USP Endotoxin Unit per mg of vancomycin.
Sterility ⟨71⟩—It meets the requirements when tested as directed for *Membrane Filtration* under *Test for Sterility of the Product to be Examined*, except to use water instead of *Diluting Fluid A*.
pH ⟨791⟩: between 3.0 and 5.0.
Particulate matter ⟨788⟩: meets the requirements under small-volume injections.
Chromatographic purity—
  Triethylamine buffer, Solution A, Solution B, Mobile phase, and *Chromatographic system*—Prepare as directed in the test for *Chromatographic purity* under *Vancomycin Hydrochloride*.

Resolution solution—Allow a container of Injection to thaw, and mix the solution. Dilute a portion of the solution with water to obtain a solution containing 0.5 mg of vancomycin per mL, heat at 65° for 24 hours, and allow to cool.

Test preparation A—Allow a container of Injection to thaw, and mix the solution.

Test preparation B—Transfer 2.0 mL of *Test preparation A* to a 50-mL volumetric flask, dilute with *Solution A* to volume, and mix.

Procedure—Proceed as directed for *Procedure* in the test for *Chromatographic purity* under *Vancomycin Hydrochloride*. Calculate the percentage of vancomycin B in the specimen taken by the formula:

$$2500 r_B / (25 r_B + r_A)$$

in which the terms are as defined therein: not less than 88% of vancomycin B is found.

Calculate the percentage of any individual peak, other than the main peak, by the formula:

$$100 r_{Ai} / (25 r_B + r_A)$$

in which the terms are as defined therein: not more than 4% of any peak other than the main peak is found.

Other requirements—It meets the requirements under *Injections* ⟨1⟩.

Assay—Proceed as directed for Vancomycin under *Antibiotics—Microbial Assays* ⟨81⟩, preparing the *Test Dilution* as follows. Allow a container of Injection to thaw, and mix the solution. Dilute an accurately measured portion of this solution quantitatively with *Buffer No. 4* to yield a *Test Dilution* having a concentration assumed to be equal to that of the median dose of the Standard.

and not more than 4.0% of any peak other than the main peak is found.

Other requirements—It responds to the *Identification* test and meets the requirements of the tests for *pH* and *Water* under *Vancomycin Hydrochloride*. It also meets the requirements for *Uniformity of Dosage Units* ⟨905⟩ and *Labeling* under *Injections* ⟨1⟩.

Assay—

Assay preparation 1 (for determining the µg of vancomycin equivalent per mg)—Dissolve a suitable quantity of Vancomycin Hydrochloride for Injection, accurately weighed, in water, and dilute quantitatively with water to obtain a solution containing about 1 mg of vancomycin per mL.

Assay preparation 2 (where it is represented as being in a single-dose container)—Constitute a container of Vancomycin Hydrochloride for Injection in a volume of water, accurately measured, corresponding to the volume of diluent specified in the labeling. Withdraw all of the withdrawable contents, using a suitable hypodermic needle and syringe, and dilute quantitatively with water to obtain a solution containing about 1 mg of vancomycin per mL.

Assay preparation 3 (where the label states the quantity of vancomycin in a given volume of constituted solution)—Constitute a container of Vancomycin Hydrochloride for Injection in a volume of water, accurately measured, equivalent to the volume of diluent specified in the labeling. Dilute an accurately measured volume of the constituted solution quantitatively with water to obtain a solution containing about 1 mg of vancomycin per mL.

Procedure—Proceed as directed under *Antibiotics—Microbial Assays* ⟨81⟩, using an accurately measured volume of the appropriate *Assay preparation* diluted quantitatively with *Buffer No. 4* to yield a *Test Dilution* having a concentration assumed to be equal to the median dose level of the Standard.

Vancomycin Hydrochloride for Injection

» Vancomycin Hydrochloride for Injection is a sterile dry mixture of Vancomycin Hydrochloride and a suitable stabilizing agent. It has a potency equivalent to not less than 925 µg of vancomycin per mg, calculated on the anhydrous basis. In addition, it contains not less than 90.0 percent and not more than 115.0 percent of the labeled amount of vancomycin.

Packaging and storage—Preserve in *Containers for Sterile Solids* as described under *Injections* ⟨1⟩.

USP Reference standards ⟨11⟩—*USP Endotoxin RS. USP Vancomycin Hydrochloride RS.*

Constituted solution—At the time of use, it meets the requirements for *Constituted Solutions* under *Injections* ⟨1⟩.

Bacterial endotoxins ⟨85⟩—It contains not more than 0.33 USP Endotoxin Unit per mg of vancomycin.

Sterility ⟨71⟩—It meets the requirements when tested as directed for *Membrane Filtration* under *Test for Sterility of the Product to be Examined*, except to dissolve the specimen in water, instead of in *Fluid A*.

Particulate matter ⟨788⟩: meets the requirements under small-volume injections.

Heavy metals, *Method II* ⟨231⟩: not more than 0.003%.

Chromatographic purity—

Triethylamine buffer, *Solution A*, *Solution B*, *Mobile phase*, *Resolution solution*, and *Chromatographic system*—Prepare as directed in the test for *Chromatographic purity* under *Vancomycin Hydrochloride*.

Test preparation A—Prepare a solution of Vancomycin Hydrochloride for Injection in *Solution A* containing 10 mg of vancomycin per mL.

Test preparation B—Transfer 2.0 mL of *Test preparation A* to a 50-mL flask, dilute with *Solution A* to volume, and mix.

Procedure—Proceed as directed for *Procedure* under *Vancomycin Hydrochloride*. Not less than 88.0% of vancomycin B is found,

Vancomycin Hydrochloride for Oral Solution

» Vancomycin Hydrochloride for Oral Solution contains the equivalent of not less than 90.0 percent and not more than 115.0 percent of the labeled amount of vancomycin.

Packaging and storage—Preserve in tight containers.

USP Reference standards ⟨11⟩—*USP Vancomycin Hydrochloride RS.*

Uniformity of dosage units ⟨905⟩—
FOR POWDER PACKAGED IN SINGLE-UNIT CONTAINERS: meets the requirements.

Deliverable volume ⟨698⟩—
FOR POWDER PACKAGED IN MULTIPLE-UNIT CONTAINERS: meets the requirements.

pH ⟨791⟩: between 2.5 and 4.5, for the solution constituted as directed in the labeling.

Water, *Method I* ⟨921⟩: not more than 5.0%.

Assay—Proceed as directed under *Antibiotics—Microbial Assays* ⟨81⟩, dissolving the contents of 1 container of Vancomycin Hydrochloride for Oral Solution in water as directed in the labeling. Dilute a portion of this solution quantitatively with *Buffer No. 4* to obtain a *Test Dilution* having a concentration assumed to be equal to the median dose level of the Standard.

Sterile Vancomycin Hydrochloride

» Sterile Vancomycin Hydrochloride has a potency equivalent to not less than 900 µg of vancomycin per mg, calculated on the anhydrous basis. In addition, where packaged for dispensing, it contains the equivalent of not less than 90.0 percent and not more than 115.0 percent of the labeled amount of vancomycin.

Packaging and storage—Preserve in *Containers for Sterile Solids* as described under *Injections* ⟨1⟩.
USP Reference standards ⟨11⟩—*USP Endotoxin RS. USP Vancomycin Hydrochloride RS.*
Constituted solution—At the time of use, it meets the requirements for *Constituted Solutions* under *Injections* ⟨1⟩.
Bacterial endotoxins ⟨85⟩—It contains not more than 0.33 USP Endotoxin Unit per mg of vancomycin hydrochloride.
Sterility ⟨71⟩—It meets the requirements when tested as directed for *Membrane Filtration* under *Test for Sterility of the Product to be Examined*, except to dissolve the specimen in water, instead of in *Fluid A*.
Particulate matter ⟨788⟩: meets the requirements under small-volume injections.
Heavy metals, *Method II* ⟨231⟩: not more than 0.003%.
Other requirements—It responds to the *Identification* test and meets the requirements of the tests for *pH*, *Water*, and *Chromatographic purity* under *Vancomycin Hydrochloride*. It meets also the requirements for *Uniformity of Dosage Units* ⟨905⟩ and for *Labeling* under *Injections* ⟨1⟩.
Assay—
Assay preparation 1—Dissolve a suitable quantity of Sterile Vancomycin Hydrochloride, accurately weighed, in water, and dilute quantitatively with water to obtain a solution containing about 1 mg of vancomycin per mL.
Assay preparation 2 (where it is packaged for dispensing)—Dissolve the contents of 1 container of Sterile Vancomycin Hydrochloride in water, and dilute quantitatively with water to obtain a solution having a concentration of about 1 mg of vancomycin per mL.
Assay preparation 3 (where the label states the quantity of vancomycin in a given volume of constituted solution)—Constitute 1 container of Sterile Vancomycin Hydrochloride in a volume of water, accurately measured, corresponding to the volume of solvent specified in the labeling. Dilute an accurately measured volume of the constituted solution quantitatively with water to obtain a solution having a concentration of about 1 mg of vancomycin per mL.
Procedure—Proceed as directed under *Antibiotics—Microbial Assays* ⟨81⟩, using an accurately measured volume of the appropriate *Assay preparation* diluted quantitatively with *Buffer No. 4* to yield a *Test Dilution* having a concentration assumed to be equal to the median dose level of the Standard.

Varicella-Zoster Immune Globulin

» Varicella-Zoster Immune Globulin conforms to the regulations of the FDA concerning biologics (see *Biologics* ⟨1041⟩). It is a sterile 15 percent to 18 percent solution of pH 7.0 containing the globulin fraction of human plasma consisting of not less than 99 percent of immunoglobulin G with traces of immunoglobulin A and immunoglobulin M, in 0.3 M glycine as a stabilizer and 1 : 10,000 thimerosal as a preservative. It is derived from adult human plasma selected for high titers of varicella-zoster antibodies. Each unit of blood or plasma has been found nonreactive for hepatitis B surface antigen by a suitable method. The proteins of the plasma pools are fractionated by the cold ethanol precipitation method. The content of specific antibody is not less than 125 units, deliverable from a vial containing not more than 2.5 mL solution. The unit is defined as equivalent to 0.01 mL of a Varicella-Zoster Immune Globulin lot found effective in clinical trials and used as a reference for potency determinations, based on a fluorescent-antibody membrane antigen (FAMA) method for antibody titration.

Packaging and storage—Preserve at a temperature between 2° and 8°.
Expiration date—The expiration date is not later than 2 years after date of issue from manufacturer's cold storage.
Labeling—Label it to state that it is to be administered by intramuscular injection, in the recommended dose based on body weight.

Vasopressin

CYFQNCPRG—NH$_2$

* in pig vasopressin, R is K

$C_{46}H_{65}N_{15}O_{12}S_2$ 1084.24
Vasopressin, 8-L-arginine-   [113-79-1].
$C_{46}H_{65}N_{13}O_{12}S_2$ 1056.22
Vasopressin, 8-L-lysine-   [50-57-7].

» Vasopressin is a polypeptide hormone having the properties of causing the contraction of vascular and other smooth muscles, and of antidiuresis. It is prepared by synthesis or obtained from the posterior lobe of the pituitary of healthy, domestic animals used for food by humans. Its vasopressor activity is not less than 300 USP Vasopressin Units per mg.

Packaging and storage—Preserve in tight containers, preferably of Type I glass, in a refrigerator.
USP Reference standards ⟨11⟩—*USP Oxytocin RS. USP Vasopressin RS.*
Microbial limits ⟨61⟩—The total bacterial count does not exceed 200 cfu per g. For products of animal origin, it meets also the requirements of the tests for absence of *Salmonella* species and *Escherichia coli*.
Identification—
A: The retention time of the vasopressin peak in the chromatogram of the *Assay preparation* corresponds to that in the chromatogram of the *Standard preparation*, as obtained in the *Assay*.
B: *Mass spectral analysis*—
Infusion solution—Prepare a mixture of acetonitrile, water, and trifluoroacetic acid (80 : 20 : 0.08).
Standard solution—Dissolve an accurately weighed quantity of USP Vasopressin RS in water to obtain a solution having a known concentration of about 1 mg per mL.
Test solution—Dissolve an accurately weighed quantity of Vasopressin in water to obtain a solution having a known concentration of about 1 mg per mL. [NOTE—The final concentrations of the *Standard solution* and the *Test solution* can be adjusted depending on the sensitivity of the mass spectrometer used in the testing.]
Mass spectrometric system (see *Mass Spectrometry* ⟨736⟩)—The LC/MS spectrometer is equipped with an infusion system connected to an electrospray interface. The mass spectrometer is operated in the positive ion mode. [NOTE—The infusion system flow rate can be adjusted, as needed. To assist in nebulization, the infusion system can contain a sheathing gas fluid.]
Procedure—Separately inject equal volumes of the *Standard solution* and the *Test solution* (about 10 µL) into the infusion system. The flow rate for the infusion system is approximately 0.3 mL per minute. Obtain an optimized mass spectra, following injection. The mass spectra of both the *Standard solution* and the *Test solution* should contain peaks with mass-to-charge ratios of 1084 and 543.
Oxytocic activity (for product labeled of animal origin)—Proceed as directed in the *Assay* under *Oxytocin*, except that a suitable dilution of the USP Oxytocin RS will contain approximately 1.2 USP Oxytocin Units per mL of *Standard preparation*. The oxytocic activity of the *Test preparation* is not more than 1.2 USP Oxytocin Units per mL.

Ordinary impurities—The sum of the responses of impurities in the chromatogram of the *Assay preparation* obtained in the *Assay* is not more than 5% of the area of the vasopressin peak.

Assay—

Mobile phase—Dissolve 6.6 g of dibasic ammonium phosphate in about 950 mL of water, and adjust with concentrated phosphoric acid to a pH of 3.0. Dilute with water to 1 L, and mix. To 870 mL of this solution add 130 mL of acetonitrile, and mix. Filter under vacuum through a 0.45-μm nylon membrane. [NOTE—The retention time of the vasopressin peak is very sensitive to small changes in acetonitrile concentration in the *Mobile phase*.]

Diluent—Dissolve 5.0 g of chlorobutanol in 5.0 mL of glacial acetic acid, add 5.0 g of alcohol, 1.1 g of sodium acetate, and 1000 mL of water, and mix.

Standard preparation—Dissolve the entire contents of a vial of USP Vasopressin RS in a known volume of *Diluent*. [NOTE—The solution may be diluted as necessary to a working concentration range for the assay.]

Assay preparation—Transfer about 10 mg of Vasopressin, accurately weighed, to a 100-mL volumetric flask. Dissolve in 0.25% glacial acetic acid, and dilute with the same solvent to volume. Mix, and pipet 5.0 mL of this solution into a 100-mL volumetric flask, and dilute with 0.25% glacial acetic acid to volume.

Chromatographic system (see *Chromatography* ⟨621⟩)—The liquid chromatograph is equipped with a variable wavelength detector set at 220 mm and a 4.6-mm × 25-cm column that contains packing L1. The flow rate is 1.0 mL per minute. The column is allowed to equilibrate for 1 hour before making the first injection. Determine the suitability of the system (see *System Suitability* under *Chromatography* ⟨621⟩) as follows. Inject 20 μL of the *Standard preparation* into the equilibrated liquid chromatograph, allow about 60 minutes for complete elution, and record the chromatogram as directed for *Procedure*: the retention time of the vasopressin peak is between 6 and 9 minutes, and is completely resolved from adjacent peaks; the resolution, R, between vasopressin and the nearest adjacent peak is not less than 1.5; and the relative standard deviation for replicate injections is not more than 2.0% for vasopressin.

Procedure—Separately inject equal volumes (about 20 μL) of the *Standard preparation* and the *Assay preparation* into the chromatograph, record the chromatograms, and measure the responses for the major peaks. Calculate the potency of Vasopressin, in USP Vasopressin Units per mg, by the formula:

$$20C(r_U/r_S)(V/W)$$

in which V is the volume of sample solution in which the sample was dissolved; and W is the amount, in mg, of vasopressin dissolved in the sample solution; C is the concentration in USP Vasopressin Units per mL in the *Standard preparation*; and r_U and r_S are the peak responses obtained from the *Assay preparation* and the *Standard preparation*, respectively.

Vasopressin Injection

» Vasopressin Injection is a sterile solution of Vasopressin in a suitable diluent. Each mL of Vasopressin Injection possesses an activity of not less than 90.0 percent and not more than 110.0 percent of that stated on the label in USP Vasopressin Units. It may contain a suitable preservative.

Packaging and storage—Preserve in single-dose or multiple-dose containers, preferably of Type I glass. Do not freeze.

Labeling—Label it to indicate its origin (animal or synthetic). Label it also to state the potency in USP Vasopressin Units per mL.

USP Reference standards ⟨11⟩—*USP Endotoxin RS. USP Vasopressin RS.*

Bacterial endotoxins ⟨85⟩—It contains not more than 17.0 Endotoxin Units per USP Vasopressin Unit.

pH ⟨791⟩: between 2.5 and 4.5.

Particulate matter ⟨788⟩—It meets the requirements under small-volume injections.

Other requirements—It meets the requirements under *Injections* ⟨1⟩.

Assay—

Mobile phase, Standard preparation, Chromatographic system, and *Procedure*—Proceed as directed in the *Assay* under *Vasopressin*.

Assay preparation—Pipet 2.0 mL of Injection into a 25-mL volumetric flask, dilute with 0.25% glacial acetic acid to volume, and mix. Calculate the potency, in USP Vasopressin Units per mL, by the formula:

$$C(r_U/r_S)$$

in which C is the concentration, in USP Vasopressin Units per mL, of the *Standard preparation*; and r_U and r_S are the mean values of the peak responses obtained from the *Assay preparation* and the *Standard preparation*, respectively.

Vecuronium Bromide

$C_{34}H_{57}BrN_2O_4$ 637.73

Piperidinium, 1-[(2β,3α,5α,16β,17β)-3,17-bis(acetyloxy)-2-(1-piperidinyl)androstan-16-yl]-1-methyl-, bromide.

1-(3α,17β-Dihydroxy-2β-piperidino-5α-androstan-16β,5α-yl)-1-methylpiperidinium bromide, diacetate   [50700-72-6].

» Vecuronium Bromide contains not less than 98.0 percent and not more than 102.0 percent of $C_{34}H_{57}BrN_2O_4$, calculated on the dried basis.

Packaging and storage—Preserve in tight containers, and store at room temperature.

USP Reference standards ⟨11⟩—*USP Endotoxin RS. USP Pancuronium Bromide RS. USP Vecuronium Bromide RS. USP Vecuronium Bromide Related Compound A RS. USP Vecuronium Bromide Related Compound B RS. USP Vecuronium Bromide Related Compound C RS. USP Vecuronium Bromide Related Compound F RS.*

Identification—

A: *Infrared Absorption* ⟨197K⟩.

B: The retention time of the major peak in the chromatogram of the *Assay preparation* corresponds to that in the chromatogram of the *Standard preparation*, as obtained in the *Assay*.

Specific rotation ⟨781S⟩: between −16° and −20°, at 20°.

Test solution: 10 mg per mL, in dehydrated alcohol.

Bacterial endotoxins ⟨85⟩: not more than 10 USP Endotoxin Units per mg of vecuronium bromide.

Loss on drying ⟨731⟩—Dry it at 105° for two hours: it loses not more than 2.5% of its weight.

Related compounds—

Cation suppressor regeneration solution: 0.02 M tetrabutylammonium hydroxide.

Mobile phase—Mix 1500 mL of filtered water, 250 mL of filtered methanol, 45 mL of filtered tetrahydrofuran, and 1 mL of hydrochloric acid in a 2000-mL volumetric flask. Leave at room temperature for few minutes, and dilute with water to volume. Mix, and degas. [NOTE—Avoid evaporation of tetrahydrofuran during degassing.]

Standard solution—Dissolve an accurately weighed quantity of USP Vecuronium Bromide RS, USP Pancuronium Bromide RS,

USP Vecuronium Bromide Related Compound A RS, USP Vecuronium Bromide Related Compound B RS, USP Vecuronium Bromide Related Compound C RS, and USP Vecuronium Bromide Related Compound F RS in 0.0025 N hydrochloric acid, and dilute quantitatively, and stepwise if necessary, to obtain a solution having a known concentration of about 0.005 mg of each compound per mL.

Test solution—Transfer about 25 mg of Vecuronium Bromide, accurately weighed, to a 25-mL volumetric flask. Add 0.5 mL of acetonitrile, dilute with 0.0025 N hydrochloric acid to volume, and mix.

Chromatographic system (see *Chromatography* ⟨621⟩)—The liquid-ion chromatograph is equipped with a conductivity detector, a 4-mm cation suppressor and a 4.6-mm × 25-cm column that contains packing L1. The flow rate is about 1.5 mL per minute. The flow rate for the cation suppressor is about 2 mL per minute. Chromatograph the *Standard solution,* and record the peak responses as directed for *Procedure:*the relative retention times are given in *Table 1*; the ratio of the height of the vecuronium bromide related compound F peak to the height of the valley between the vecuronium bromide related compound F peak and the pancuronium bromide peak is not less than 2.0; and the relative standard deviation for replicate injections is not more than 10.0% for each compound. [NOTE—The system may need equilibration for 4 hours.]

Procedure—Separately inject equal volumes (about 25 µL) of the *Standard solution* and the *Test solution* into the chromatograph, record the chromatograms, and measure the peak responses. Calculate the percentage of each vecuronium bromide related compound in the portion of Vecuronium Bromide taken by the formula:

$$2500(C/W)(r_U / r_S)$$

in which C is the concentration, in mg per mL, of the relevant USP Reference Standard in the *Standard solution;* W is the weight, in mg, of Vecuronium Bromide taken to prepare the *Test solution;* and r_U and r_S are the peak areas for the correspondent vecuronium bromide related compound obtained from the *Test solution* and *Standard solution,* respectively: the limits of impurities are specified in *Table 1.* [NOTE—Use the peak area of vecuronium bromide in the *Standard solution* as r_S to calculate any unknown impurity.]

Table 1

Compound Name	Relative Retention Time	Limit %
Pancuronium bromide	about 0.5	0.5
Vecuronium bromide related compound F[1]	about 0.6	0.5
Vecuronium bromide related compound C[2]	about 0.86	0.5
Vecuronium bromide	1.0	—
Vecuronium bromide related compound A[3]	about 2.0	0.3
Vecuronium bromide related compound B[4]	about 2.6	0.5
Unknown	—	0.1
Total	—	1.0

[1] 3-deacetyl vecuronium bromide, (Piperidinium, 1-[(2β,3α,5α,16β,17β)-17-acetyloxy-3-hydroxy-2-(1-piperidinyl)androstan-16-yl]-1-methyl bromide)
[2] 3,17-Bis deacetyl vecuronium bromide; (Piperidinium, 1-[(2β,3α,5α,16β,17β)-3,17-dihydroxy-2-(1-piperidinyl)androstan-16-yl]-1-methyl bromide)
[3] Dipiperidino diol diacetate; (3α,17β-diacetyl-oxy-2β,16β-bispiperidinyl-5α-androstan)
[4] 17-deacetyl vecuronium bromide; (Piperidinium, 1-[(2β,3α,5α,16β,17β)-3-acetyloxy-17-hydroxy-2-(1-piperidinyl)androstan-16-yl]-1-methyl bromide)

Assay—

Solution A—Transfer 8.0 g of sodium perchlorate to a 1000-mL volumetric flask, dissolve in 6.0 mL of water, dilute with acetonitrile to volume, mix, filter, and degas.

Solution B—Transfer 3.2 g of ammonium chloride to a 2000-mL volumetric flask, dissolve in 16 mL of ammonium hydroxide, dilute with methanol to volume, mix, filter, and degas. [NOTE—Avoid excessive degassing to prevent the loss of ammonium hydroxide.].

Mobile phase—Prepare a mixture of *Solution A* and *Solution B* (3 : 2). Make adjustments if necessary (see *System Suitability* under *Chromatography* ⟨621⟩).

Diluent—Pipet 1.0 mL of 1 N hydrochloric acid into a 1000-mL volumetric flask, dilute with acetonitrile to volume, and mix.

Standard preparation—Dissolve an accurately weighed quantity of USP Vecuronium Bromide RS in *Diluent* to obtain a solution having a known concentration of about 0.5 mg per mL.

Assay preparation—Transfer about 50 mg of Vecuronium Bromide, accurately weighed, to a 100-mL volumetric flask, dissolve in and dilute with *Diluent,* and mix.

Chromatographic system (see *Chromatography* ⟨621⟩)—The liquid chromatograph is equipped with a 215-nm detector and a 4.6-mm × 25-cm column that contains 5-µm packing L3. The flow rate is about 0.5 mL per minute. The column temperature is maintained at 40°. Chromatograph the *Standard preparation,* and record the peak responses as directed for *Procedure:* the column efficiency is not less than 5000 theoretical plates; and the relative standard deviation for replicate injections is not more than 2.0%.

Procedure—Separately inject equal volumes (about 20 µL) of the *Standard preparation* and the *Assay preparation* into the chromatograph, record the chromatograms, and measure the responses for the major peaks. Calculate the quantity, in mg, of $C_{34}H_{57}BrN_2O_4$ in the portion of Vecuronium Bromide taken by the formula:

$$100C(r_U / r_S)$$

in which C is the concentration, in mg per mL, of USP Vecuronium Bromide RS in the *Standard preparation;* and r_U and r_S are the peak responses obtained from the *Assay preparation* and the *Standard preparation,* respectively.

Verapamil Hydrochloride

$C_{27}H_{38}N_2O_4 \cdot HCl$ 491.06

Benzeneacetonitrile, α-[3-[[2-(3,4-dimethoxyphenyl)ethyl]methylamino]propyl]-3,4-dimethoxy-α-(1-methylethyl)-, monohydrochloride, (±)-.
(±)-5-[(3,4-Dimethoxyphenethyl)methylamino]-2-(3,4-dimethoxyphenyl)-2-isopropylvaleronitrile monohydrochloride [152-11-4].

» Verapamil Hydrochloride contains not less than 99.0 percent and not more than 100.5 percent of $C_{27}H_{38}N_2O_4 \cdot HCl$, calculated on the dried basis.

Packaging and storage—Preserve in tight, light-resistant containers. Store at 25°, excursions permitted between 15° and 30°.

USP Reference standards ⟨11⟩—*USP Verapamil Hydrochloride RS. USP Verapamil Related Compound B RS.*

Identification—
 A: *Infrared Absorption* ⟨197K⟩.
 B: The retention time of the major peak for verapamil in the chromatogram of the *Test preparation* corresponds to that exhibited in the chromatogram of *Standard preparation B,* as obtained in the test for *Chromatographic purity.*
 C: It responds to the tests for *Chloride* ⟨191⟩.

Melting range ⟨741⟩: between 140° and 144°.

pH ⟨791⟩: between 4.5 and 6.5, in a solution, prepared with gentle heating, containing 50 mg per mL.

Loss on drying ⟨731⟩—Dry it at 105° for 2 hours: it loses not more than 0.5% of its weight.

Residue on ignition ⟨281⟩: not more than 0.1%.
Chromatographic purity—
Aqueous solvent mixture—Prepare a 0.015 N sodium acetate solution containing about 33 mL of glacial acetic acid per L.
Mobile phase—Prepare a filtered and degassed mixture of *Aqueous solvent mixture*, acetonitrile, and 2-aminoheptane (70 : 30 : 0.5). Make adjustments if necessary (see *System Suitability* under *Chromatography* ⟨621⟩).
Standard preparations—Dissolve an accurately weighed quantity of USP Verapamil Hydrochloride RS in *Mobile phase*, and dilute quantitatively, and stepwise if necessary, with *Mobile phase* to obtain *Standard preparation A* and *Standard preparation B* having known concentrations of about 5.6 and 9.4 μg per mL, respectively.
Test preparation—Prepare a solution of Verapamil Hydrochloride in *Mobile phase* having a known concentration of about 1.9 mg per mL.
System suitability solution—Dissolve suitable quantities of USP Verapamil Hydrochloride RS and USP Verapamil Related Compound B RS in *Mobile phase* to obtain a *System suitability solution* having known concentrations of about 1.9 and 1.5 mg, respectively, in each mL.
Chromatographic system (see *Chromatography* ⟨621⟩)—The liquid chromatograph is equipped with a 278-nm detector and a 4.6-mm × 12.5- to 15-cm column that contains packing L1. The flow rate is about 0.9 mL per minute. Chromatograph the *System suitability solution*, and record the peak responses as directed for *Procedure*: the relative retention times are about 0.88 for verapamil related compound B and 1.0 for verapamil; the resolution, *R*, between the verapamil related compound B and verapamil peaks is not less than 1.5, and the relative standard deviation for replicate injections is not more than 2.0%.
Procedure—Separately inject equal volumes (about 10 μL) of *Standard preparations A* and *B* and the *Test preparation* into the chromatograph, and allow the *Test preparation* to elute for not less than four times the retention time for verapamil. Record the chromatograms, and measure all the peak responses. The sum of the peak responses, other than that of verapamil, from the *Test preparation* is not greater than the verapamil peak response obtained from *Standard preparation B* (0.5%); and no single peak response is greater than that of the verapamil peak response obtained from *Standard preparation A* (0.3%).
Organic volatile impurities, *Method V* ⟨467⟩: meets the requirements.
Solvent—Use 0.1% n-propanol in water.
(Official until July 1, 2008)
Assay—Dissolve about 400 mg of Verapamil Hydrochloride, accurately weighed, in 40 mL of glacial acetic acid; and add 10 mL of mercuric acetate TS and 5 mL of acetic anhydride. Titrate (see *Titrimetry* ⟨541⟩) with 0.10 N perchloric acid VS, determining the endpoint potentiometrically. Perform a blank determination, and make any necessary correction. Each mL of 0.10 N perchloric acid is equivalent to 49.11 mg of $C_{27}H_{38}N_2O_4 \cdot HCl$.

Verapamil Hydrochloride Injection

» Verapamil Hydrochloride Injection is a sterile solution of Verapamil Hydrochloride in Water for Injection. It contains not less than 90.0 percent and not more than 110.0 percent of the labeled amount of verapamil hydrochloride ($C_{27}H_{38}N_2O_4 \cdot HCl$).

Packaging and storage—Preserve in single-dose containers, preferably of Type I glass, protected from light.
USP Reference standards ⟨11⟩—*USP Endotoxin RS. USP Verapamil Hydrochloride RS. USP Verapamil Related Compound A RS. USP Verapamil Related Compound B RS. USP Verapamil Related Compound E RS. USP Verapamil Related Compound F RS.*
Identification—
A: It meets the requirements under *Identification—Organic Nitrogenous Bases* ⟨181⟩, a volume of Injection equivalent to 100 mg of verapamil hydrochloride being used, chloroform being used in place of carbon disulfide, and a 0.1-mm cell being used in place of a 1-mm cell.
B: The chromatogram of the *Assay preparation* obtained as directed in the *Assay* exhibits a major peak for verapamil hydrochloride, the retention time of which corresponds to that exhibited in the chromatogram of the *Standard preparation*, obtained as directed in the *Assay*.
C: It responds to the tests for *Chloride* ⟨191⟩.
Bacterial endotoxins ⟨85⟩—It contains not more than 16.7 USP Endotoxin Units per mg of verapamil hydrochloride.
pH ⟨791⟩: between 4.0 and 6.5.
Particulate matter ⟨788⟩: meets the requirements for small-volume injections.
Related compounds—
Aqueous solvent mixture, Mobile phase, System suitability solution, and *Chromatographic system*—Proceed as directed in the *Assay*.
Standard solution—Dissolve accurately weighed quantities of USP Verapamil Hydrochloride RS, USP Verapamil Related Compound A RS, USP Verapamil Related Compound E RS, and USP Verapamil Related Compound F RS in *Mobile phase* to obtain a solution having known concentrations of about 2.5 mg of USP Verapamil Hydrochloride RS per mL and 0.0075 mg each of USP Verapamil Related Compound A RS, USP Verapamil Related Compound E RS, and USP Verapamil Related Compound F RS per mL.
Test solution—Use the *Assay preparation*.
Procedure—Separately inject equal volumes (about 10 μL) of the *Standard solution* and the *Test solution* into the chromatograph, and allow the *Test solution* to elute for not less than four times the retention time for verapamil hydrochloride. Record the chromatograms, and measure all of the peak responses. The retention times are about 0.4 for verapamil related compound F, 0.5 for verapamil related compound A, 0.7 for verapamil related compound E, and 1.0 for verapamil. Calculate the quantity, in mg, of each individual impurity in each mL of the Injection taken by the formula:

$$C(L/D)(r_U / r_S)$$

in which *C* is the concentration, in mg per mL, verapamil related compound A, verapamil related compound E, or verapamil related compound F in the *Standard solution* [NOTE—For calculating any other unspecified impurity, *C* is the concentration, in mg per mL, of USP Verapamil Hydrochloride RS in the *Standard solution*.]; *L* is the labeled quantity, in mg per mL, of verapamil hydrochloride in the Injection; *D* is the concentration, in mg per mL, of verapamil hydrochloride in the *Test solution*, on the basis of the labeled quantity in each mL and the extent of dilution; and r_U and r_S are the peak responses of the appropriate impurity in the *Test solution* and the *Standard solution*, respectively: not more than 0.3% of any specified impurity is found, and the sum of all impurities is not greater than 1.0%.
Other requirements—It meets the requirements under *Injections* ⟨1⟩.
Assay—
Aqueous solvent mixture—Prepare a 0.015 N sodium acetate solution containing about 33 mL of glacial acetic acid per L.
Mobile phase—Prepare a filtered and degassed mixture of *Aqueous solvent mixture*, acetonitrile, and 2-aminoheptane (70 : 30 : 0.5). Make adjustments if necessary (see *System Suitability* under *Chromatography* ⟨621⟩).
Standard preparation—Dissolve an accurately weighed quantity of USP Verapamil Hydrochloride RS in *Mobile phase* to obtain a solution having a known concentration of about 2.5 mg per mL.
Assay preparation—Dilute the Injection quantitatively, if necessary, with *Mobile phase* to obtain a solution having a concentration of not more than 2.5 mg of verapamil hydrochloride per mL.
System suitability solution—Dissolve suitable quantities of USP Verapamil Hydrochloride RS and USP Verapamil Related Compound B RS in *Mobile phase* to obtain a solution having known concentrations of about 1.9 mg per mL and 1.5 mg per mL, respectively.
Chromatographic system (see *Chromatography* ⟨621⟩)—The liquid chromatograph is equipped with a 278-nm detector and a 4.6-mm × 12.5- to 15-cm column that contains packing L1. The flow rate is about 0.9 mL per minute. Chromatograph the *System suitability solution*, and record the peak responses as directed for

Procedure: the relative retention times are about 0.88 for verapamil related compound B and 1.0 for verapamil; the resolution, R, between the verapamil related compound B and verapamil peaks is not less than 1.5; and the relative standard deviation for replicate injections is not more than 2.0%.

Procedure—Separately inject equal volumes (about 10 μL) of the *Standard preparation* and the *Assay preparation* into the chromatograph, and allow the *Assay preparation* to elute for not less than four times the retention time for verapamil. Record the chromatograms, and measure the responses for all of the major peaks. Calculate the quantity, in mg, of verapamil hydrochloride ($C_{27}H_{38}N_2O_4 \cdot$ HCl) in each mL of the Injection taken by the formula:

$$C(L/D)(r_U / r_S)$$

in which C is the concentration, in mg per mL, of USP Verapamil Hydrochloride RS in the *Standard preparation*; L is the labeled quantity, in mg per mL, of verapamil hydrochloride in the Injection; D is the concentration, in mg per mL, of verapamil hydrochloride in the *Assay preparation,* on the basis of the labeled quantity in each mL and the extent of dilution; and r_U and r_S are the peak responses obtained from the *Assay preparation* and the *Standard preparation,* respectively.

Add the following:

▲Verapamil Hydrochloride Oral Solution

» Verapamil Hydrochloride Oral Solution contains not less than 90.0 percent and not more than 110.0 percent of the labeled amount of verapamil hydrochloride ($C_{27}H_{38}N_2O_4 \cdot$ HCl). Prepare Verapamil Hydrochloride Oral Solution 50 mg per mL as follows (see *Pharmaceutical Compounding—Nonsterile Preparations* ⟨795⟩. See also *Verapamil Hydrochloride Oral Suspension*):

Verapamil Hydrochloride powder	5 g
Vehicle for Oral Solution (regular or sugar-free), *NF,* a sufficient quantity to make	100 mL

Add Verapamil Hydrochloride powder and about 40 mL of Vehicle to a mortar, and mix. Add the Vehicle in small portions almost to volume, and mix thoroughly after each addition. Transfer the contents of the mortar, stepwise and quantitatively, to a calibrated bottle. Add enough Vehicle to bring to final volume, and mix well.

Packaging and storage—Preserve in tight, light-resistant containers. Store at controlled room temperature or in a cold place.
Labeling—Label it to indicate the beyond-use date.
USP Reference standards ⟨11⟩—*USP Verapamil Hydrochloride RS.*
pH ⟨791⟩: between 3.8 and 4.8.
Beyond-use date: 60 days after the day on which it was compounded.
Assay—
Sodium acetate solution—Dissolve an accurately weighed quantity of sodium acetate in acetic acid having a concentration of 33 mL per L to obtain a solution having a 0.01 M sodium acetate concentration.
Mobile phase—Prepare a mixture of *Sodium acetate solution,* acetonitrile, and 2-aminoheptane (50 : 50 : 0.5), filter, and degas. Make adjustments if necessary (see *System Suitability* under *Chromatography* ⟨621⟩).

Standard preparation—Dissolve an accurately weighed quantity of USP Verapamil Hydrochloride RS in *Mobile phase* to obtain a solution having a known concentration of about 500 μg per mL.
Assay preparation—Agitate containers of Oral Solution for 30 minutes on a rotating mixer, remove a 5-mL sample, and store in a clear glass vial at −70° until analyzed. At the time of analysis, remove the sample from the freezer, allow it to reach room temperature, and mix on a vortex mixer for 30 seconds. Pipet 1.0 mL into a 10-mL volumetric flask, and dilute with *Mobile phase* to volume.
Chromatographic system (see *Chromatography* ⟨621⟩)—The liquid chromatograph is equipped with a 278-nm detector and a 4.6-mm × 25-cm analytical column that contains 5-μm packing L1. The flow rate is about 0.5 mL per minute. Chromatograph the *Standard preparation,* and record the peak responses as directed for *Procedure:* the retention time for verapamil hydrochloride is about 4.8 minutes, and the relative standard deviation for replicate injections is not more than 0.7%.
Procedure—Separately inject equal volumes (about 20 μL) of the *Standard preparation* and the *Assay preparation* into the chromatograph, record the chromatograms, and measure the responses for the major peaks. Calculate the quantity, in mg, of verapamil hydrochloride ($C_{27}H_{38}N_2O_4 \cdot$ HCl) in the volume of Oral Solution taken by the formula:

$$100(C / V)(r_U / r_S)$$

in which C is the concentration, in μg per mL, of USP Verapamil Hydrochloride RS in the *Standard preparation;* V is the volume, in mL, of Oral Solution taken; and r_U and r_S are the peak responses obtained from the *Assay preparation* and the *Standard preparation,* respectively.▲USP31

Add the following:

▲Verapamil Hydrochloride Oral Suspension

» Verapamil Hydrochloride Oral Suspension contains not less than 90.0 percent and not more than 110.0 percent of the labeled amount of verapamil hydrochloride ($C_{27}H_{38}N_2O_4 \cdot$ HCl). Prepare Verapamil Hydrochloride Oral Suspension 50 mg per mL as follows (see *Pharmaceutical Compounding—Nonsterile Preparations* ⟨795⟩. See also *Verapamil Hydrochloride Oral Solution*):

Verapamil Hydrochloride	5 g
Vehicle: a mixture of Vehicle for Oral Solution, (regular or sugar-free), *NF* and Vehicle for Oral Suspension, *NF* (1 : 1), a sufficient quantity to make	100 mL

If using Verapamil Hydrochloride Tablets, comminute to a fine powder using a suitable mortar, or add Verapamil Hydrochloride powder. Add about 40 mL of the Vehicle in small portions, and mix to obtain a uniform paste. Transfer the mortar contents, stepwise and quantitatively, to a calibrated bottle. Add the Vehicle in portions to rinse the mortar, add sufficient Vehicle to final volume, and mix well.

Packaging and storage—Preserve in tight, light-resistant containers. Store at controlled room temperature, or in a cold place.

Labeling—Label it to state that it is to be well shaken before use, and to state the beyond-use date.
USP Reference standards ⟨11⟩—USP Verapamil Hydrochloride RS.
pH ⟨791⟩: between 3.8 and 4.8
Beyond-use date: 60 days after the day on which it was compounded.
Assay—
 Mobile phase—Prepare a suitable filtered and degassed mixture of 0.01 M sodium acetate with a mixture of acetic acid having a concentration of 33 mL per L, acetonitrile, and 2-aminoheptane (50 : 50 : 0.5). Make adjustments if necessary (see *System Suitability* under *Chromatography* ⟨621⟩).
 Standard preparation—Dissolve USP Verapamil Hydrochloride RS in *Mobile phase* to obtain a solution having a known concentration of 500 µg per mL.
 Assay preparation—Agitate the container of Oral Suspension for 30 minutes on a rotating mixer, remove a 5-mL sample, store in a clear glass vial at −70° until analyzed. At time of analysis, remove the sample from the freezer, allow it to reach room temperature, and mix on a vortex mixer for 30 seconds. Pipet 1.0 mL of the sample solution into a 10-mL volumetric flask, and dilute with *Mobile phase* to volume.
 Chromatographic system (see *Chromatography* ⟨621⟩)—The liquid chromatograph is equipped with a 278-nm detector and a 4.6-mm × 25-cm analytical column that contains 5-µm packing L1. The flow rate is about 0.5 mL per minute. Chromatograph the *Standard preparation*, and record the peak responses as directed for *Procedure*: the retention time for verapamil hydrochloride is about 4.8 minutes, and the relative standard deviation for replicate injections is not more than 0.7%.
 Procedure—Separately inject equal volumes (about 20 µL) of the *Standard preparation* and the *Assay preparation* into the chromatograph, record the chromatograms, and measure the responses for the major peaks. Calculate the quantity, in mg, of verapamil hydrochloride ($C_{27}H_{38}N_2O_4 \cdot HCl$) in the volume of Oral Suspension taken by the formula:

$$100(C/V)(r_U/r_S)$$

in which C is the concentration, in µg per mL, of USP Verapamil Hydrochloride RS in the *Standard preparation*; V is the volume, in mL, of Oral Suspension taken; and r_U and r_S are the peak responses obtained from the *Assay preparation* and the *Standard preparation*, respectively.▲USP31

Verapamil Hydrochloride Tablets

» Verapamil Hydrochloride Tablets contain not less than 90.0 percent and not more than 110.0 percent of the labeled amount of verapamil hydrochloride ($C_{27}H_{38}N_2O_4 \cdot HCl$).

Packaging and storage—Preserve in tight, light-resistant containers.
USP Reference standards ⟨11⟩—*USP Verapamil Hydrochloride RS. USP Verapamil Related Compound A RS. USP Verapamil Related Compound B RS. USP Verapamil Related Compound E RS. USP Verapamil Related Compound F RS.*
Identification—
 A: *Infrared Absorption* ⟨197K⟩—
 Test specimen—Transfer a portion of finely powdered Tablets, equivalent to about 25 mg of verapamil hydrochloride, to a separator. Add 25 mL of water, and shake by mechanical means for 30 minutes. Add 1 mL of 1 N sodium hydroxide, and extract with 25 mL of chloroform, shaking by mechanical means for 10 minutes. Pass the chloroform extract through a filter containing anhydrous sodium sulfate. Triturate the chloroform extract with 400 mg of potassium bromide and evaporate to dryness. Dry at 105° for 2 hours.

 B: The retention time of the major peak in the chromatogram of the *Assay preparation* corresponds to that in the chromatogram of the *Standard preparation*, as obtained in the *Assay*.
Dissolution ⟨711⟩—
 Medium: 0.01 N hydrochloric acid; 900 mL.
 Apparatus 2: 50 rpm.
 Time: 30 minutes.
 Procedure—Determine the amount of $C_{27}H_{38}N_2O_4 \cdot HCl$ dissolved from the difference between UV absorbances at the wavelengths of maximum absorbance at about 278 nm and 300 nm using filtered portions of the solution under test, suitably diluted with *Medium* if necessary, in comparison with a Standard solution having a known concentration of USP Verapamil Hydrochloride RS in the same *Medium*.
 Tolerances—Not less than 75% (*Q*) of the labeled amount of $C_{27}H_{38}N_2O_4 \cdot HCl$ is dissolved in 30 minutes.
Uniformity of dosage units ⟨905⟩: meet the requirements.
 Procedure for content uniformity—Transfer 1 Tablet to a 100-mL volumetric flask, add 50 mL of 0.01 N hydrochloric acid, and heat on a steam bath for 50 minutes. Sonicate the heated solution for about 10 minutes, cool, dilute with 0.01 N hydrochloric acid to volume, mix, and filter. Dilute an accurately measured portion of the filtrate quantitatively with 0.01 N hydrochloric acid to obtain a *Test preparation* containing about 48 µg of verapamil hydrochloride per mL. Dissolve an accurately weighed quantity of USP Verapamil Hydrochloride RS in 0.01 N hydrochloric acid to obtain a *Standard preparation* having a known concentration of about 48 µg per mL. Concomitantly determine the absorbances of the *Test preparation* and the *Standard preparation* in 1-cm cells at the wavelength of maximum absorbance at about 278 nm and the absorbance of the *Test preparation* at 300 nm, with a suitable spectrophotometer using 0.01 N hydrochloric acid as the blank. Calculate the quantity, in mg, of $C_{27}H_{38}N_2O_4 \cdot HCl$ in the Tablet taken by the formula:

$$(TC/D)(A_U/A_S)$$

in which T is the labeled quantity, in mg, of verapamil hydrochloride in the Tablet; C is the concentration, in µg per mL, of USP Verapamil Hydrochloride RS in the *Standard preparation*; D is the concentration, in µg per mL, of verapamil hydrochloride in the *Test preparation*, on the basis of the labeled quantity per Tablet and the extent of dilution; A_U is the difference between absorbances at 278 nm and 300 nm of the *Test preparation*; and A_S is the absorbance of the *Standard preparation* at 278 nm.
Related compounds—
 Aqueous solvent mixture, Mobile phase, System suitability solution, and *Chromatographic system*—Proceed as directed in the *Assay*.
 Standard solution—Dissolve accurately weighed quantities of USP Verapamil Hydrochloride RS, USP Verapamil Related Compound A RS, USP Verapamil Related Compound E RS, and USP Verapamil Related Compound F RS in *Mobile phase* to obtain a solution having known concentrations of about 1.6 mg of USP Verapamil Hydrochloride RS per mL and 0.0048 mg each of USP Verapamil Related Compound A RS, USP Verapamil Related Compound E RS, and USP Verapamil Related Compound F RS per mL.
 Test solution—Use the *Assay preparation*.
 Procedure—Separately inject equal volumes (about 10 µL) of the *Standard solution* and the *Test solution* into the chromatograph, and allow the *Test solution* to elute for not less than four times the retention time for verapamil. Record the chromatograms, and measure all of the peak responses. [NOTE—The retention times are about 0.4 for verapamil related compound F, 0.5 for verapamil related compound A, 0.7 for verapamil related compound E, and 1.0 for verapamil.] Calculate the quantity, in mg, of each individual impurity in each mL of the portion of Tablets taken by the formula:

$$25C(r_U/r_S)$$

in which C is the concentration, in mg per mL, of verapamil related compound A, verapamil related compound E, or verapamil related compound F in the *Standard solution* [NOTE—For calculating any other unspecified impurity, C is the concentration, in mg per mL, of USP Verapamil Hydrochloride RS in the *Standard solution*.]; and r_U and r_S are the peak responses of the appropriate impurity obtained from the *Test solution* and the *Standard solution*, respectively: not more than 0.3% of any specified impurity is found; and the sum of all impurities is not more than 1.0%.

Assay—
Aqueous solvent mixture—Prepare a 0.015 N sodium acetate solution containing about 33 mL of glacial acetic acid per L.

Mobile phase—Prepare a filtered and degassed mixture of *Aqueous solvent mixture*, acetonitrile, and 2-aminoheptane (70 : 30 : 0.5). Make adjustments if necessary (see *System Suitability* under *Chromatography* ⟨621⟩).

Standard preparation—Dissolve an accurately weighed quantity of USP Verapamil Hydrochloride RS in *Mobile phase* to obtain a solution having a known concentration of about 1.6 mg per mL.

Assay preparation—Weigh and finely powder not fewer than 20 Tablets. Transfer an accurately weighed portion of the powder, equivalent to about 40 mg of verapamil hydrochloride, to a stoppered centrifuge tube, and add 25 mL of *Mobile phase*. Shake by mechanical means for 15 minutes, centrifuge, and if necessary filter the supernatant.

System suitability solution—Dissolve suitable quantities of USP Verapamil Hydrochloride RS and USP Verapamil Related Compound B RS in *Mobile phase* to obtain a solution having known concentrations of about 1.9 mg per mL and 1.5 mg per mL, respectively.

Chromatographic system (see *Chromatography* ⟨621⟩)—The liquid chromatograph is equipped with a 278-nm detector and a 4.6-mm × 12.5- to 15-cm column that contains packing L1. The flow rate is about 0.9 mL per minute. Chromatograph the *System suitability solution*, and record the peak responses as directed for *Procedure*: the relative retention times are about 0.88 for verapamil related compound B and 1.0 for verapamil; the resolution, R, between the verapamil related compound B and verapamil peaks is not less than 1.5; and the relative standard deviation for replicate injections is not more than 2.0%.

Procedure—Separately inject equal volumes (about 10 μL) of the *Standard preparation* and the *Assay preparation* into the chromatograph, and allow the *Assay preparation* to elute for not less than four times the retention time for verapamil. Record the chromatograms, and measure the responses for all of the major peaks. Calculate the quantity, in mg, of verapamil hydrochloride ($C_{27}H_{38}N_2O_4 \cdot HCl$) in the portion of Tablets taken by the formula:

$$25C(r_U / r_S)$$

in which C is the concentration, in mg per mL, of USP Verapamil Hydrochloride RS in the *Standard preparation*; and r_U and r_S are the peak responses obtained from the *Assay preparation* and the *Standard preparation*, respectively.

Verapamil Hydrochloride Extended-Release Tablets

» Verapamil Hydrochloride Extended-Release Tablets contain not less than 90.0 percent and not more than 110.0 percent of the labeled amount of verapamil hydrochloride ($C_{27}H_{38}N_2O_4 \cdot HCl$).

Packaging and storage—Preserve in tight, light-resistant containers.

Labeling—The labeling indicates the *Dissolution Test* with which the product complies.

USP Reference standards ⟨11⟩—*USP Verapamil Hydrochloride RS. USP Verapamil Related Compound B RS.*

Identification, *Infrared Absorption* ⟨197F⟩—Prepare analytical specimens as follows.

Test specimen—Crush 1 Tablet, and transfer the powder to a volumetric flask of suitable size so that the final concentration is about 1.2 mg of verapamil hydrochloride per mL. Add 0.05 N hydrochloric acid to about 75% of the final volume, and dissolve by heating, with stirring, for 40 minutes. Cool, and dilute with 0.05 N hydrochloric acid to volume. Filter, and transfer 40 mL of the filtrate to a 125-mL separatory funnel. Add 4 mL of 1 N sodium hydroxide, and extract with 20 mL of chloroform, shaking for 2 minutes. Pass the chloroform extract through a filter containing anhydrous sodium sulfate, and collect the filtrate in a porcelain dish. Rinse with an additional 10 mL of chloroform, collecting the rinsing in the same porcelain dish. Evaporate on a steam bath with the aid of a current of air to dryness, and dry the oily residue at 105° for 30 minutes.

Standard specimen—Dissolve about 48 mg of USP Verapamil Hydrochloride RS, accurately weighed, in 25 mL of water. Transfer to a 125-mL separatory funnel, add 2 mL of 1 N sodium hydroxide, and extract with 25 mL of chloroform, shaking for two minutes. Proceed as directed for the *Test specimen*, beginning with "Pass the chloroform extract."

Dissolution ⟨711⟩—
TEST 1—If the product complies with this test, the labeling indicates that it meets USP *Dissolution Test 1*. Proceed as directed for *Procedure* for *Method B* under *Apparatus 1 and Apparatus 2, Delayed-Release Dosage Forms*.

Acid stage—Using 900 mL of simulated gastric fluid TS (without enzyme), conduct this stage of the test for 1 hour.

Buffer stage—Using 900 mL of simulated intestinal fluid TS (without enzyme), conduct this stage of the test for 7 hours.

Apparatus 2: 50 rpm.

Times: Acid stage—1 hour; *Buffer stage*—2, 3.5, 5, and 8 hours.

Procedure—Wrap each Tablet in a wire helix to prevent the Tablets from floating. After 1 hour in the *Acid stage*, withdraw a specimen for analysis, and carefully transfer the dosage form, including the wire helix, to a vessel containing the *Buffer stage* medium, which has been previously warmed to 37 ± 0.5°. Filter a portion of the solution under test at each time interval, using a suitable glass microfiber filter paper. [NOTE—Use only filters that have been shown not to absorb verapamil.] Dilute, if necessary, the filtered portions of the solutions under test with water at the 1-hour interval and with 0.1 N hydrochloric acid at the 2-, 3.5-, 5-, and 8-hour intervals. Determine the amounts of $C_{27}H_{38}N_2O_4 \cdot HCl$ dissolved by employing UV absorption at the wavelength of maximum absorbance at about 278 nm, using 0.01 N hydrochloric acid as the blank, by comparison with a Standard solution having a known concentration of USP Verapamil Hydrochloride RS in 0.01 N hydrochloric acid.

Tolerances—The percentage of the labeled amount of $C_{27}H_{38}N_2O_4 \cdot HCl$ dissolved at the times specified conforms to *Acceptance Table 2*.

FOR PRODUCTS LABELED TO CONTAIN 180 MG OR 240 MG:

Time (hours)	Amount dissolved
1	between 7% and 15%
2	between 16% and 30%
3.5	between 31% and 50%
5	between 51% and 75%
8	not less than 85%

FOR PRODUCTS LABELED TO CONTAIN 120 MG:

Time (hours)	Amount dissolved
1	between 10% and 21%
2	between 18% and 33%
3.5	between 35% and 60%
5	between 50% and 82%
8	not less than 85%

TEST 2—If the product complies with this test, the labeling indicates that it meets USP *Dissolution Test 2*. Proceed as directed for *Test 1*, except that under *Procedure*, the Tablet is not required to be wrapped in a wire helix.

Times and *Tolerances*—The percentage of the labeled amount of $C_{27}H_{38}N_2O_4 \cdot HCl$ dissolved at the times specified conforms to *Acceptance Table 2*.

FOR PRODUCTS LABELED TO CONTAIN 240 MG:

Time (hours)	Amount dissolved
1	between 8% and 20%
2	between 15% and 35%
3.5	between 35% and 65%
5	between 55% and 85%
8	not less than 80%

FOR PRODUCTS LABELED TO CONTAIN 180 MG:

Time (hours)	Amount dissolved
1	between 10% and 25%
2	between 20% and 40%
3.5	between 40% and 75%
8	not less than 80%

TEST 3—If the product complies with this test, the labeling indicates that it meets USP *Dissolution Test 3*. Proceed as directed for *Test 1*.

Times and *Tolerances*—The percentage of the labeled amount of $C_{27}H_{38}N_2O_4 \cdot HCl$ dissolved at the times specified conforms to *Acceptance Table 2*.

Time (hours)	Amount dissolved
1	between 8% and 20%
2	between 15% and 35%
3.5	between 27% and 57%
5	between 45% and 75%
8	not less than 80%

TEST 4—If the product complies with this test, the labeling indicates that it meets USP *Dissolution Test 4*.

Phosphate buffer solution—Dissolve 6.8 g of monobasic potassium phosphate in 250 mL of water. Add 190 mL of 0.2 N sodium hydroxide in 400 mL of water, adjust with 0.2 N sodium hydroxide to a pH of 7.5 ± 0.1, dilute with water to 1000 mL, and mix.

Medium: Phosphate buffer solution; 50 mL.

Apparatus 7 (see *Drug Release* ⟨724⟩): 20 cycles per minute.

Procedure—Scrape about 2 mm × 2 mm of the coating from the side edge of the Tablet under test. Glue the system to a plastic rod sample holder at the area where the color has been removed. Attach each plastic sample holder to an arm of the apparatus, which reciprocates at an amplitude of about 2 cm and 15 to 30 cycles per minute. The Tablet is continuously immersed in tubes containing 50 mL of *Medium* at 37°. At the end of each specified test interval, the systems are transferred to the next row of new test tubes containing 50 mL of fresh *Medium*. Remove the tubes after the last test interval, and allow them to cool to room temperature. Add 2.0 mL of 1.0 M phosphoric acid to each tube, and dilute with water to 50 mL. Stir and mix each tube thoroughly. Determine the amount of $C_{27}H_{38}N_2O_4 \cdot HCl$ dissolved by employing UV absorption at the wavelength of maximum absorbance at about 278 nm on filtered portions of the solution under test, suitably diluted with *Medium*, if necessary, in comparison with a Standard solution having a known concentration of USP Verapamil Hydrochloride RS in the same *Medium*.

Times and *Tolerances*—The percentages of the labeled amount of $C_{27}H_{38}N_2O_4 \cdot HCl$ dissolved at the times specified conform to *Acceptance Table 2*.

Time (hours)	Amount dissolved
3	not more than 10%
6	between 20% and 50%
9	between 52.5% and 82.5%
14	not less than 85%

TEST 5—If the product complies with this test, the labeling indicates that it meets USP *Dissolution Test 5*.

Phosphate buffer solution—Dissolve 6.8 g of monobasic potassium phosphate in 250 mL of water. Add 190 mL of 0.2 N sodium hydroxide in 400 mL of water, adjust with 0.2 N sodium hydroxide to a pH of 7.5 ± 0.1, dilute with water to 1000 mL, and mix.

Medium: Phosphate buffer solution; 900 mL.

Apparatus 2: 50 rpm.

Procedure—Determine the amount of $C_{27}H_{38}N_2O_4 \cdot HCl$ dissolved by employing UV absorption at the wavelength of maximum absorbance at about 278 nm on filtered portions of the solution under test, suitably diluted with *Medium*, if necessary, in comparison with a Standard solution having a known concentration of USP Verapamil Hydrochloride RS in the same *Medium*.

Times and *Tolerances*—The percentages of the labeled amount of $C_{27}H_{38}N_2O_4 \cdot HCl$ dissolved at the times specified conform to *Acceptance Table 2*.

Time (hours)	Amount dissolved
1	between 2% and 12%
2	between 10% and 25%
4	between 25% and 50%
8	not less than 80%

Uniformity of dosage units ⟨905⟩: meet the requirements.

Chromatographic purity—

Buffer solution, Mobile phase, Standard preparation, System suitability solution, and *Chromatographic system*—Proceed as directed in the *Assay*.

Test preparation—Prepare as directed for *Assay preparation* in the *Assay*.

Procedure—Proceed as directed for *Procedure* in the *Assay*. Calculate the percentage of each impurity in the portion of Tablets taken by the formula:

$$100(r_i / r_s)$$

in which r_i is the peak response for each impurity, and r_s is the sum of the responses of all of the peaks: not more than 0.5% of any individual impurity is found, and the sum of all impurities is not more than 1.0%.

Assay—

Buffer solution—Transfer 0.82 g of sodium acetate to a 1000-mL volumetric flask, add 33 mL of glacial acetic acid, dilute with water to volume, and mix.

Mobile phase—Prepare a filtered and degassed mixture of *Buffer solution*, acetonitrile, and 2-aminoheptane (70 : 30 : 0.5). Make adjustments if necessary (see *System Suitability* under *Chromatography* ⟨621⟩).

Standard preparation—Dissolve an accurately weighed quantity of USP Verapamil Hydrochloride RS in *Mobile phase*, and dilute quantitatively, and stepwise if necessary, with *Mobile phase* to obtain a solution having a known concentration of about 1.2 mg per mL.

System suitability solution—Dissolve suitable quantities of USP Verapamil Hydrochloride RS and USP Verapamil Related Compound B RS in *Mobile phase* to obtain a solution containing about 2.5 and 2.0 mg per mL, respectively.

Assay preparation—Weigh and finely powder not fewer than 20 Tablets. Transfer an accurately weighed portion of the powder, equivalent to about 240 mg of verapamil hydrochloride, to a 200-mL volumetric flask, and add about 160 mL of *Mobile phase*. Sonicate for 15 minutes, stir for 15 minutes, dilute with *Mobile phase* to volume, and mix. Centrifuge a portion for 20 minutes, and use as the *Assay preparation*.

Chromatographic system (see *Chromatography* ⟨621⟩)—The liquid chromatograph is equipped with a 278-nm detector and a 4.6-mm × 15-cm column that contains packing L1. The flow rate is about 1.0 mL per minute. Chromatograph the *System suitability solution*, and record the peak responses as directed for *Procedure:* the resolution, *R*, between verapamil and verapamil related compound B is not less than 1.5. Chromatograph the *Standard preparation*, and record the peak responses as directed for *Procedure:* the relative standard deviation for replicate injections is not more than 2.0%.

Procedure—Separately inject equal volumes (about 10 μL) of the *Standard preparation* and the *Assay preparation* into the chromatograph, record the chromatograms, and measure the responses for the major peaks. Calculate the quantity, in mg, of verapamil hydrochloride ($C_{27}H_{38}N_2O_4 \cdot HCl$) in the portion of Tablets taken by the formula:

$$200C(r_U / r_S)$$

in which C is the concentration, in mg per mL, of USP Verapamil Hydrochloride RS in the *Standard preparation;* and r_U and r_S are the peak responses obtained from the *Assay preparation* and the *Standard preparation,* respectively.

Verteporfin

$C_{41}H_{42}N_4O_8$ 718.79

23*H*,25*H*-Benzo[*b*]porphine-9,13-dipropanoic acid, 18-ethenyl-4,4a-dihydro-3,4-bis(methoxycarbonyl)-4a,8,14,19-tetramethyl-, monomethyl ester, *trans*-.
(±)-*trans*-3,4-Dicarboxy-4,4a-dihydro-4a,8,14,19-tetramethyl-18-vinyl-23*H*,25*H*-benzo[*b*]porphine-9,13-dipropanoic acid, 3,4,9-trimethyl ester mixture with (±)-*trans*-3,4-dicarboxy-4,4a-dihydro-4a,8,14,19-tetramethyl-18-vinyl-23*H*,25*H*-benzo[*b*]porphine-9,13-dipropionic acid, 3,4,13-trimethyl ester   [*129497-78-5*].

» Verteporfin contains not less than 94.0 percent and not more than 102.0 percent of $C_{41}H_{42}N_4O_8$, calculated on the anhydrous basis.

Caution—Verteporfin is a light-activated drug used in photodynamic therapy. Care should be taken to avoid contact with eyes and skin.

Packaging and storage—Preserve in tight containers, and store in a freezer.
USP Reference standards ⟨11⟩—USP Endotoxin RS. USP Verteporfin RS.
Identification—
  A: *Infrared Absorption* ⟨197M⟩.
  B: The retention times of the two major peaks in the chromatogram of the *Assay preparation* correspond to those in the chromatogram of the *Standard preparation,* as obtained in the *Assay.*
Microbial limits ⟨61⟩—The total aerobic microbial count does not exceed 100 cfu per g.
Bacterial endotoxins ⟨85⟩: not more than 0.5 USP Endotoxin Unit per mg of verteporfin.
Water, *Method Ic* ⟨921⟩: not more than 1.4%.
Residue on ignition ⟨281⟩: not more than 0.2%.
Heavy metals, *Method I* ⟨231⟩: not more than 0.002%.
Related compounds—
  Solution A, Solution B, and *Mobile phase*—Proceed as directed in the *Assay.*
  Standard solution—Prepare as directed for the *Standard preparation* in the *Assay.*
  Sensitivity check solution—Dilute the *Standard solution* with water to obtain a solution having a concentration of 0.25 µg per mL.
  Test solution—Prepare as directed for *Assay preparation* in the *Assay.*
  Chromatographic system—Chromatograph the *Sensitivity check solution* at 410 nm, and record the peak heights: the ratio of the verteporfin peak height to the noise height is not less than 10, the noise height being determined by a suitable procedure. Proceed as directed in the *Assay.* To evaluate the system suitability requirements, use the *Standard preparation* prepared as directed in the *Assay.*
  Procedure—Inject a volume (about 20 µL) of the *Test solution* into the chromatograph, record the chromatograms, and measure the peak responses. Calculate the percentage of each related compound in the portion of Verteporfin taken by the formula:

$$100(r_i / r_s)$$

in which r_i is the individual peak response of each related compound; and r_s is the sum of the responses of all the peaks. Not more than 0.6% of the peak having a retention time of about 0.56 relative to that of the first verteporfin isomer peak is found; not more than 0.8% of any other individual related compound is found; and the sum of all impurities is not more than 4.0%.
Organic volatile impurities *Method I* ⟨467⟩: meets the requirements.

(Official until July 1, 2008)

Assay—
  Solution A—Prepare a filtered and degassed mixture of 1% (w/v) aqueous ammonium sulfate, acetonitrile, glacial acetic acid, and 3.6 M sulfuric acid (10 : 10 : 1 : 0.027).
  Solution B—Prepare a filtered and degassed mixture of 1% (w/v) aqueous ammonium sulfate, tetrahydrofuran, glacial acetic acid, and 3.6 M sulfuric acid (10 : 10 : 1 : 0.034).
  Mobile phase—Use variable mixtures of *Solution A* and *Solution B* as directed for *Chromatographic system.* Make adjustments if necessary (see *System Suitability* under *Chromatography* ⟨621⟩).
  Standard preparation—To a suitable volumetric flask, transfer an accurately weighed quantity of USP Verteporfin RS sufficient to make a 0.25 mg per mL solution. Add a volume of a mixture of acetonitrile and tetrahydrofuran (1 : 1) equivalent to 60% of the flask volume, and dissolve. Dilute with water to volume, and mix. [NOTE—Protect the solution from light.]
  Assay preparation—Transfer about 25 mg of Verteporfin, accurately weighed, to a 100-mL volumetric flask. Add 60 mL of a mixture of acetonitrile and tetrahydrofuran (1 : 1), and dissolve. Dilute with water to volume, and mix. [NOTE—Protect the solution from light.]
  Chromatographic system (see *Chromatography* ⟨621⟩)—The liquid chromatograph is equipped with a 410-nm detector and a 4.6-mm × 25-cm column that contains packing L1. The flow rate is 1.5 mL per minute. The column temperature is maintained at 30°. The chromatograph is programmed as follows.

Time (minutes)	Solution A (%)	Solution B (%)	Elution
0–60	80	20	isocratic
60–90	80→60	20→40	linear gradient
90–91	60	40	isocratic
91–120	60→30	40→70	linear gradient
120–121	30	70	isocratic
121–125	30→0	70→100	linear gradient
125–137	0	100	isocratic
137–140	0→80	100→20	linear gradient
140–150	80	20	isocratic

Chromatograph the *Standard preparation,* and record the peak responses as directed for *Procedure:* the resolution, R, between the two verteporfin peaks is not less than 2.5; the tailing factor is not more than 1.3; and the relative standard deviation for replicate injections is not more than 2.0%.
  Procedure—Separately inject equal volumes (about 20 µL) of the *Standard preparation* and the *Assay preparation* into the chromatograph, record the chromatograms, and measure the responses for the verteporfin peaks. Calculate the quantity, in mg, of $C_{41}H_{42}N_4O_8$ in the portion of Verteporfin taken by the formula:

$$100C(r_U / r_S)$$

in which C is the concentration, in mg per mL, of USP Verteporfin RS in the *Standard preparation;* and r_U and r_S are the sums of the peak responses of the two verteporfin regioisomer peak responses obtained from the *Assay preparation* and the *Standard preparation*, respectively.

Calculate the ratio of the peak responses for the two peaks assigned to verteporfin: not less than 0.9 and not more than 1.1.

Verteporfin for Injection

» Verteporfin for Injection is a sterile mixture of Verteporfin and lipids. It contains not less than 91.0 percent and not more than 110.0 percent of the labeled amount of verteporfin ($C_{41}H_{42}N_4O_8$).

Packaging and storage—Preserve in tight *Containers for Sterile Solids* as described under *Injections* ⟨1⟩, and store at controlled room temperature, protected from light.

Labeling—The label states that it is to be protected from light after constitution. Label it to indicate that it is intended for intravenous use only; labeling indicates the name and amount of diluent for constitution.

USP Reference standards ⟨11⟩—*USP Verteporfin RS. USP Verteporfin Related Compound A RS.*

Identification—
  A: *Ultraviolet Absorption* ⟨197U⟩—
  Solution: 10 µg per mL.
  Medium: methanol.
  B: The retention times of the two major peaks in the chromatogram of the *Assay preparation* correspond to those in the chromatogram of the *Standard preparation*, as obtained in the *Assay*.

Pyrogen ⟨151⟩: meets the requirements, the test dose being 4 mg per kg.

Sterility ⟨71⟩—It meets the requirements when tested as directed for *Membrane Filtration* under *Test for Sterility of the Product to be Examined*.

Uniformity of dosage units ⟨905⟩: meets the requirements.

Water, *Method Ic* ⟨921⟩—Use a mixture of methanol and formamide (7 : 3) as the solvent: not more than 3.0%.

Particulate matter ⟨788⟩: meets the requirements for small-volume injections.

Limit of verteporfin related compound A—
  Mobile phase—Prepare as directed in the *Assay*.
  Standard stock solution—Dissolve accurately weighed quantities of USP Verteporfin RS and USP Verteporfin Related Compound A RS in a mixture of acetonitrile and tetrahydrofuran (1 : 1) to obtain a solution having known concentrations of about 0.167 mg per mL and 6.67 µg per mL, respectively.
  Standard solution— Dissolve 3 parts of the *Standard stock solution* with 2 parts water to obtain a solution having known concentrations of 0.1 mg per mL and 4 µg per mL, respectively. [NOTE—Protect solution from light.]
  Test solution—Use the *Assay preparation*.
  Chromatographic system—The liquid chromatograph is equipped with a 410-nm detector and a 4.6-mm × 25-cm column that contains 5-µm packing L1. The flow rate is 1.4 mL per minute. The column temperature is maintained at 30°. Chromatograph the *Standard solution*, and record the peak responses as directed for *Procedure*: the resolution, *R*, between the two verteporfin isomeric peaks is not less than 2.5; the tailing factor is not more than 1.3; and the relative standard deviation for replicate injections is not more than 2.0%.
  Procedure—Separately inject equal volumes of the *Standard solution* and the *Test solution* into the chromatograph, record the chromatograms, and measure the responses for the major peaks. Calculate the percentage of verteporfin related compound A in the portion of Verteporfin for Injection taken by the formula:

$$20(C_S / L)(r_U / r_S)$$

in which C_S is the concentration, in µg per mL, of USP Verteporfin Related Compound A RS in the *Standard solution*; *L* is the labeled quantity, in mg, of verteporfin in Verteporfin for Injection; and r_U and r_S are the peak responses for verteporfin related compound A in the *Test solution* and the *Standard solution*, respectively. Not more than 4.0% is found.

Assay—
  Mobile phase—Prepare a filtered and degassed mixture of 1% (w/v) ammonium sulfate solution, acetonitrile, tetrahydrofuran, and acetic acid (20 : 11 : 9 : 2), and adjust with 3.6 M sulfuric acid to a pH of 3.0.
  Standard preparation—Dissolve an accurately weighed quantity of USP Verteporfin RS in a mixture of acetonitrile and tetrahydrofuran (1 : 1) to obtain a solution containing 0.167 mg per mL. Quantitatively dilute this solution with water to obtain a solution having a known concentration of about 0.1 mg per mL. [NOTE—Protect solution from light.]
  Assay preparation—Reconstitute 1 vial of Verteporfin for Injection with deionized water to obtain an approximate concentration of 2 mg per mL, and mix. Quantitatively transfer the contents to a 200-mL volumetric flask, rinsing the vial with a mixture of water, tetrahydrofuran, and acetonitrile (4 : 3 : 3), and dilute with a mixture of water, tetrahydrofuran, and acetonitrile (4 : 3 : 3) to volume. [NOTE—Protect solution from light.]
  Chromatographic system (see *Chromatography* ⟨621⟩)—The liquid chromatograph is equipped with a 410-nm detector and a 4.6-mm × 25-cm column that contains 5-µm packing L1. The flow rate is 1.4 mL per minute. The column temperature is maintained at 30°. Chromatograph the *Standard preparation*, and record the peak responses as directed for *Procedure*: the resolution, *R*, between the peaks for the two verteporfin isomers is not less than 2.5; the tailing factor is not more than 1.3; and the relative standard deviation for replicate injections is not more than 2.0%.
  Procedure—Separately inject equal volumes (about 20 µL) of the *Standard preparation* and the *Assay preparation* into the chromatograph, record the chromatograms, and measure the peak responses for verteporfin. Calculate the quantity, in mg, of verteporfin ($C_{41}H_{42}N_4O_8$) in the portion of Verteporfin for Injection taken by the formula:

$$200C(r_U / r_S)$$

in which *C* is the concentration, in mg per mL, of USP Verteporfin RS in the *Standard preparation*; and r_U and r_S are the sums of the peak responses for the two verteporfin isomeric peaks in the *Assay preparation* and the *Standard preparation*, respectively.

Vidarabine

$C_{10}H_{13}N_5O_4 \cdot H_2O$ 285.26
9*H*-Purin-6-amine, 9-β-D-arabinofuranosyl-, monohydrate.
9-β-D-Arabinofuranosyladenine monohydrate   [24356-66-9].
Anhydrous   267.25   [5536-17-4].

» Vidarabine has a potency equivalent to not less than 845 µg and not more than 985 µg of $C_{10}H_{13}N_5O_4$ per mg.

Packaging and storage—Preserve in tight containers.
Labeling—Where it is intended for use in preparing injectable or other sterile dosage forms, the label states that it is sterile or must be subjected to further processing during the preparation of injectable or other sterile forms.
USP Reference standards ⟨11⟩—*USP Endotoxin RS. USP Vidarabine RS.*
Identification, *Infrared Absorption* ⟨197K⟩.
Specific rotation ⟨781S⟩: between −56.0° and −65.0° (λ = 365 nm).
  Test solution: 10 mg of anhydrous vidarabine per mL, in dimethylformamide.

Bacterial endotoxins ⟨85⟩—Where the label states that Vidarabine is sterile or must be subjected to further processing during the processing of injectable dosage forms, it contains not more than 0.5 USP Endotoxin Unit per mg of vidarabine. Where it is intended for use in preparing ophthalmic dosage forms, it is exempt from the requirements.

Sterility ⟨71⟩—Where the label states that Vidarabine is sterile, it meets the requirements when tested as directed for *Direct Inoculation of the Culture Medium* under *Test for Sterility of the Product to be Examined*, except to transfer 2 g of solid specimen to each test medium.

Loss on drying ⟨731⟩—Dry about 100 mg in vacuum at 100° and at a pressure not exceeding 5 mm of mercury for 4 hours: it loses between 5.0% and 7.0% of its weight.

Assay—

Mobile phase—Dissolve 2.2 g of docusate sodium in 10 mL of glacial acetic acid and 500 mL of methanol in a 1000-mL volumetric flask. Dilute with water to volume, and mix. Pass this solution through a membrane filter having a 1-μm or finer porosity.

Standard preparation—Dissolve about 24 mg of USP Vidarabine RS, accurately weighed, in 150 mL of water in a 200-mL volumetric flask by heating to 100° for 10 minutes. Cool, dilute with water to volume, and mix.

Assay preparation—Using Vidarabine, prepare as directed for *Standard preparation*.

Chromatographic system (see *Chromatography* ⟨621⟩)—The chromatograph is equipped with a 254-nm detector and a 4-mm × 30-cm column that contains packing L1. Chromatograph three replicate injections of the *Standard preparation*, and record the peak responses as directed for *Procedure*: the relative standard deviation is not more than 3.0%.

Procedure—Introduce equal volumes (approximately 10 μL) of the *Assay preparation* and the *Standard preparation* into the instrument, operated at room temperature, by means of a suitable microsyringe or sampling valve. Adjust the operating conditions so that satisfactory chromatography and peak responses are obtained. Use a detector sensitivity setting that gives a peak height for vidarabine that is at least 50% of scale. Measure peak responses at the same retention times obtained with the *Assay preparation* and the *Standard preparation*. Calculate the potency, in μg of $C_{10}H_{13}N_5O_4$ per mg, of the Vidarabine taken by the formula:

$$F(r_U / r_S)(W_S / W_U)$$

in which F is the potency of USP Vidarabine RS, in μg of vidarabine per mg; r_U and r_S are the peak responses obtained from the *Assay preparation* and the *Standard preparation*, respectively; and W_U and W_S are the amounts, in mg, of USP Vidarabine RS and Vidarabine taken, respectively.

Vidarabine Ophthalmic Ointment

» Vidarabine Ophthalmic Ointment contains not less than 90.0 percent and not more than 120.0 percent of the labeled amount of anhydrous vidarabine ($C_{10}H_{13}N_5O_4$).

Packaging and storage—Preserve in collapsible ophthalmic ointment tubes.

USP Reference standards ⟨11⟩—*USP Vidarabine RS.*

Sterility ⟨71⟩—It meets the requirements when tested as directed for *Membrane Filtration* under *Test for Sterility of the Product to be Examined*.

Minimum fill ⟨755⟩: meets the requirements.

Metal particles—It meets the requirements of the test for *Metal Particles in Ophthalmic Ointments* ⟨751⟩.

Assay—

Mobile phase, Standard preparation, and *Chromatographic system*—Proceed as directed in the *Assay* under *Vidarabine*.

Assay preparation—Transfer an accurately weighed portion of Ophthalmic Ointment, equivalent to about 12 mg of vidarabine, to a 100-mL volumetric flask, add 80 mL of water, and heat on a steam bath for 15 minutes. Shake, and add 10 mL of *n*-heptane to the hot suspension. Swirl, and cool to room temperature. Remove the *n*-heptane layer, and discard it. Dilute the aqueous phase with water to volume, and mix.

Procedure—Proceed as directed for *Procedure* in the *Assay* under *Vidarabine*. Calculate the potency, in mg, of $C_{10}H_{13}N_5O_4$ per g of the Ophthalmic Ointment taken by the formula:

$$0.5F(r_U / r_S)(W_S / W_U)$$

in which W_U is the amount, in mg, of Ophthalmic Ointment taken; and the other terms are as defined therein.

Vinblastine Sulfate

$C_{46}H_{58}N_4O_9 \cdot H_2SO_4$ 909.07

Vincaleukoblastine, sulfate (1 : 1) (salt).
Vincaleukoblastine sulfate (1 : 1) (salt)   [143-67-9].

» Vinblastine Sulfate contains not less than 96.0 percent and not more than 102.0 percent of $C_{46}H_{58}N_4O_9 \cdot H_2SO_4$, corrections being applied for loss in weight.

Caution—Handle Vinblastine Sulfate with great care, because it is a potent cytotoxic agent.

Packaging and storage—Preserve in tight, light-resistant containers, in a freezer.

Labeling—Where it is intended for use in preparing injectable dosage forms, the label states that it is sterile or must be subjected to further processing during the preparation of injectable dosage forms.

USP Reference standards ⟨11⟩—*USP Endotoxin RS. USP Vinblastine Sulfate RS. USP Vincristine Sulfate RS.* [NOTE—No *Loss on drying* determination is needed for USP Vincristine Sulfate RS.]

Identification—

A: *Infrared Absorption* ⟨197K⟩—The test specimen and Reference Standard are previously dried in vacuum at 60° for 16 hours.

B: A solution (1 in 10) responds to the test for *Sulfate* ⟨191⟩.

pH ⟨791⟩: between 3.5 and 5.0, in a solution prepared by dissolving 3 mg in 2 mL of water.

Loss on drying (see *Thermal Analysis* ⟨891⟩)—[NOTE—In this procedure, perform weighings rapidly with minimum exposure of the substances to air.] Determine the percentage of volatile substances by thermogravimetric analysis on an appropriately calibrated instrument, using about 10 mg of Vinblastine Sulfate, accurately weighed. Heat the specimen at the rate of 5° per minute between ambient temperature and 200° in an atmosphere of nitrogen at a flow rate of 40 mL per minute. From the thermogram, determine the accumulated loss in weight between ambient temperature and a point on the plateau before decomposition is indicated (at about 160°): it loses not more than 15.0% of its weight.

Related compounds—

Mobile phase, System suitability preparation, and *Chromatographic system*—Prepare as directed in the *Assay*.

High load test preparation—Prepare as directed for *Assay preparation* in the *Assay*.

Low load test preparation—Pipet 1 mL of *High load test preparation* into a 25-mL volumetric flask, dilute with water to volume, and mix.

Procedure—Separately inject 200 μL of the *Low load test preparation* and of the *High load test preparation* into the chromatograph, and record the chromatograms. Measure the peak responses, r_i, of any related substances appearing after the solvent peak in the chromatogram of the *High load test preparation*. Calculate the total percentage of responses due to related substances taken by the formula:

$$100r_t / (r_t + 25r_v)$$

in which r_t is the sum of the r_i responses; and r_v is the vinblastine peak response in the chromatogram of the *Low load test preparation*. Not more than 3.0% is found. Calculate the percentage response of each related substance taken by the formula:

$$100r_i / (r_t + 25r_v).$$

Not more than 1.0% of response due to any individual related substance is found.

Other requirements—Where the label states that Vinblastine Sulfate is sterile, it meets the requirements for *Sterility* and *Bacterial endotoxins* under *Vinblastine Sulfate for Injection*. Where the label states that Vinblastine Sulfate must be subjected to further processing during the preparation of injectable dosage forms, it meets the requirements for *Bacterial endotoxins* under *Vinblastine Sulfate for Injection*.

Assay—
Mobile phase—Mix 14 mL of diethylamine with 986 mL of water, and adjust with phosphoric acid to a pH of 7.5 (*Solution A*). Mix 200 mL of acetonitrile with 800 mL of methanol (*Solution B*). Mix 380 mL of *Solution A* with 620 mL of *Solution B*, pass through a 0.5-μm filter, and degas under vacuum. The ratio of *Solutions A* and *B* may be varied to meet system suitability requirements and to provide a suitable elution time for vinblastine sulfate.

Standard preparation—Dissolve an accurately weighed quantity of USP Vinblastine Sulfate RS in water to obtain a solution having a known concentration of about 0.4 mg per mL.

Assay preparation—Transfer about 4 mg of Vinblastine Sulfate, accurately weighed, to a 10-mL volumetric flask, dissolve in and dilute with water to volume, and mix.

System suitability preparation—Dissolve an amount of USP Vincristine Sulfate RS in a portion of *Standard preparation* to obtain a solution having concentrations of about 0.4 mg of each Reference Standard per mL.

Chromatographic system (see *Chromatography* ⟨621⟩)—The liquid chromatograph is equipped with a 262-nm detector, a pre-column packed with porous silica gel installed between the pump and the injector, and a 4.6-mm × 15-cm analytical column that contains packing L1. The *Mobile phase* is maintained at a pressure and flow rate (about 2 mL per minute) capable of producing the required resolution and a suitable elution time. Chromatograph replicate injections of the *Standard preparation*, and record the peak responses as directed for *Procedure*: the relative standard deviation is not more than 2.0%. Similarly chromatograph 20 μL of the *System suitability preparation*, and record the peak responses: the resolution, *R*, between the vincristine and vinblastine is not less than 4.0. [NOTE—For a particular column, the resolution may be increased by increasing the proportion of *Solution A* in the *Mobile phase*.]

Procedure—Separately inject equal volumes (about 20 μL) of the *Standard preparation* and the *Assay preparation* into the chromatograph, record the chromatograms, and measure the responses for the major peaks. Calculate the quantity, in mg, of $C_{46}H_{58}N_4O_9 \cdot H_2SO_4$ in the portion of Vinblastine Sulfate taken by the formula:

$$10C(r_U / r_S)$$

in which C is the concentration, in mg per mL, of USP Vinblastine Sulfate RS (corrected for loss in weight) in the *Standard preparation*; and r_U and r_S are the peak responses obtained from the *Assay preparation* and the *Standard preparation*, respectively.

Vinblastine Sulfate for Injection

» Vinblastine Sulfate for Injection is Vinblastine Sulfate suitable for parenteral use. It contains not less than 90.0 percent and not more than 110.0 percent of the labeled amount of vinblastine sulfate ($C_{46}H_{58}N_4O_9 \cdot H_2SO_4$).

Caution—Handle Vinblastine Sulfate for Injection with great care since it is a potent cytotoxic agent.

Packaging and storage—Preserve in *Containers for Sterile Solids* as described under *Injections* ⟨1⟩, in a refrigerator.

Labeling—The label states: "FATAL IF GIVEN INTRATHECALLY. FOR INTRAVENOUS USE ONLY."

When dispensed, the container or syringe (holding the individual dose prepared for administration to the patient) must be enclosed in an overwrap bearing the statement "DO NOT REMOVE COVERING UNTIL MOMENT OF INJECTION. FATAL IF GIVEN INTRATHECALLY. FOR INTRAVENOUS USE ONLY."

USP Reference standards ⟨11⟩—*USP Endotoxin RS. USP Vinblastine Sulfate RS. USP Vincristine Sulfate RS.* [NOTE—No *Loss on drying* determination is needed for USP Vincristine Sulfate RS.]

Completeness of solution ⟨641⟩—A 10-mg portion dissolves in 10 mL of *Water for Injection* to yield a clear solution.

Constituted solution—At the time of use, it meets the requirements for *Constituted Solutions* under *Injections* ⟨1⟩.

Bacterial endotoxins ⟨85⟩—It contains not more than 10.0 USP Endotoxin Units per mg of vinblastine sulfate.

Sterility ⟨71⟩: meets the requirements.

Uniformity of dosage units ⟨905⟩: meets the requirements.

PROCEDURE FOR CONTENT UNIFORMITY—
Buffer solution—Dissolve 13.61 g of sodium acetate in about 900 mL of water in a 1000-mL volumetric flask, adjust with glacial acetic acid to a pH of 5.0 while stirring, dilute with water to volume, and mix.

Standard preparation—Dissolve an accurately weighed quantity of USP Vinblastine Sulfate RS in *Buffer solution*, and dilute quantitatively and stepwise with *Buffer solution* to obtain a solution having a known concentration of about 40 μg per mL.

Test preparation—Dissolve the contents of 1 container of Vinblastine Sulfate for Injection in an accurately measured volume of *Buffer solution* to obtain a solution having a concentration between 40 μg per mL and 50 μg per mL.

Procedure—Concomitantly determine the absorbances of the *Test preparation* and the *Standard preparation* in 1-cm cells at the wavelength of maximum absorbance at about 269 nm versus the *Buffer solution* as the blank. Calculate the quantity, in mg, of $C_{46}H_{58}N_4O_9 \cdot H_2SO_4$ in the container taken by the formula:

$$0.001CV(A_U / A_S)$$

in which C is the concentration, in μg per mL, of USP Vinblastine Sulfate RS (corrected for loss on drying) in the *Standard preparation*; V is the volume, in mL, of *Buffer solution* taken for the *Test preparation*; and A_U and A_S are the absorbances of the *Test preparation* and the *Standard preparation*, respectively.

Related compounds—Proceed as directed in the test for *Related compounds* under *Vinblastine Sulfate*. The total of the responses due to related substances does not exceed 5.0%, and no single related substance response exceeds 2.0%.

Other requirements—It responds to the *Identification* tests under *Vinblastine Sulfate*. It meets the requirements for *Labeling* under *Injections* ⟨1⟩.

Assay—
Mobile phase, Standard preparation, System suitability preparation, and *Chromatographic system*—Prepare as directed in the *Assay* under *Vinblastine Sulfate*.

Assay preparation—Pipet a suitable volume of water into each of 5 containers of Vinblastine Sulfate for Injection to obtain a solution in each having a concentration of about 1 mg per mL. Insert the stopper, shake to mix, and combine the solutions from the 5 containers. Quantitatively dilute this solution with water to obtain a solution having a concentration of about 0.4 mg per mL, and mix.

Procedure—Separately inject equal volumes (about 20 μL) of the *Standard preparation* and the *Assay preparation* into the chromatograph, record the chromatograms, and measure the responses for the major peaks. Calculate the quantity, in mg, of vinablastine sulfate

($C_{46}H_{58}N_4O_9 \cdot H_2SO_4$) in each container of Vinblastine Sulfate for Injection taken by the formula:

$$0.2CV(r_U / r_S)$$

in which C is the concentration, in mg per mL, of USP Vinblastine Sulfate RS (corrected for loss in weight) in the *Standard preparation*; V is the volume, in mL, of the *Assay preparation*; and r_U and r_S are the peak responses obtained from the *Assay preparation* and the *Standard preparation*, respectively.

Vincristine Sulfate

$C_{46}H_{56}N_4O_{10} \cdot H_2SO_4$ 923.04
Vincaleukoblastine, 22-oxo-, sulfate (1 : 1) (salt).
Leurocristine sulfate (1 : 1) (salt)   [2068-78-2].

» Vincristine Sulfate contains not less than 95.0 percent and not more than 105.0 percent of $C_{46}H_{56}N_4O_{10} \cdot H_2SO_4$, corrections being applied for loss in weight.

Caution—Handle Vincristine Sulfate with great care since it is a potent cytotoxic agent.

Packaging and storage—Preserve in tight, light-resistant containers, and store in a freezer.

USP Reference standards ⟨11⟩—*USP Vincristine Sulfate RS. USP Vinblastine Sulfate RS.* [NOTE—No *Loss on drying* determination is needed for USP Vinblastine Sulfate RS.]

Identification—
  A: *Infrared Absorption* ⟨197K⟩.
  B: A solution (1 in 10) responds to the tests for *Sulfate* ⟨191⟩.

pH ⟨791⟩: between 3.5 and 4.5, in a solution (1 in 1000).

Loss on drying (see *Thermal Analysis* ⟨891⟩)—[NOTE—In this procedure, perform weighings rapidly with minimum exposure of the substances to air.] Determine the percentage of volatile substances by thermogravimetric analysis on an appropriately calibrated instrument, using about 10 mg of Vincristine Sulfate, accurately weighed. Heat the specimen at the rate of 5° per minute between ambient temperature and 200° in an atmosphere of nitrogen at a flow rate of 40 mL per minute. From the thermogram, determine the accumulated loss in weight between ambient temperature and a point on the plateau before decomposition is indicated (at about 160°): it loses not more than 12.0% of its weight.

Related compounds—
  Solvent A—Prepare a filtered and degassed mixture of water and diethylamine (985 : 15), adjusted with phosphoric acid to a pH of 7.5.
  Solvent B—Use methanol.
  High load test preparation—Prepare as directed for *Assay preparation* in the *Assay*.
  Low load test preparation—Pipet 1 mL of *High load test preparation* into a 25-mL volumetric flask, dilute with water to volume, and mix.
  Chromatographic system (see *Chromatography* ⟨621⟩)—Use the liquid chromatograph equipped as directed in the *Assay*. The mobile phase is maintained at a flow rate of about 2 mL per minute, with an initial gradient of 62% of *Solvent B* and 38% of *Solvent A* for 12 minutes, then changed to increase *Solvent B* at a rate of 2% per minute, so that after 15 minutes it will comprise 92% of the mixture, then changed to decrease *Solvent B* at a rate of 15% per minute, so that after 2 minutes it will again comprise 62% of the mixture, then maintained at this ratio for 5 minutes.
  Procedure—Separately inject equal volumes (about 200 µL) of the *Low load test preparation* and of the *High load test preparation* into the chromatograph, record the chromatograms, and measure the peak responses, r_i, of any related substances appearing after the solvent peak in the chromatogram of the *High load test preparation*. Calculate the total percentage of responses due to related substances taken by the formula:

$$100r_t / (r_t + 25r_v)$$

in which r_t is the sum of the r_i responses, and r_v is the vincristine peak response in the chromatogram of the *Low load test preparation*. Not more than 4.0% is found. Calculate the percentage response of each related substance taken by the formula:

$$100r_i / (r_t + 25r_v).$$

Not more than 1.0% of response due to any individual related substance is found.

Assay—
  Diethylamine solution—Mix 5 mL of diethylamine with 295 mL of water, and adjust with phosphoric acid to a pH of 7.5.
  Mobile phase—Prepare a filtered and degassed mixture of methanol and *Diethylamine solution* (70 : 30). Make adjustments if necessary (see *System Suitability* under *Chromatography* ⟨621⟩).
  Standard preparation—Dissolve an accurately weighed quantity of USP Vincristine Sulfate RS in water to obtain a solution having a known concentration of about 1 mg per mL.
  Assay preparation—Equilibrate a portion of Vincristine Sulfate for 30 minutes with the ambient humidity, transfer about 10 mg, accurately weighed, to a 10-mL volumetric flask, dissolve in and dilute with water to volume, and mix. Using another portion of the equilibrated specimen, determine the loss in weight as directed for USP Vincristine Sulfate RS.
  System suitability preparation—Transfer 5 mg of USP Vincristine Sulfate RS and 5 mg of Vinblastine Sulfate RS, each accurately weighed, to a 5-mL volumetric flask, dissolve in and dilute with water to volume, and mix.
  Chromatographic system (see *Chromatography* ⟨621⟩)—The liquid chromatograph is equipped with a 297-nm detector, a precolumn packed with porous silica gel, a 2- to 5-cm guard column containing packing L1, and a 4.6-mm × 25-cm analytical column that contains packing L7. The flow rate is about 1.5 mL per minute. Chromatograph the *Standard preparation*, and record the peak responses as directed for *Procedure*: the relative standard deviation for replicate injections is not more than 2.0%. Similarly chromatograph 10 µL of the *System suitability preparation*, and record the peak responses: the resolution, between vincristine sulfate and vinblastine sulfate is not less than 4.0. [NOTE—For a particular column, the resolution may be increased by increasing the proportion of water in the *Mobile phase*.]
  Procedure—Separately inject equal volumes (about 10 µL) of the *Standard preparation* and the *Assay preparation* into the chromatograph, record the chromatograms, and measure the responses for the major peaks. Calculate the quantity, in mg, of $C_{46}H_{56}N_4O_{10} \cdot H_2SO_4$ in the portion of Vincristine Sulfate taken, corrected for loss in weight in the *Assay preparation*, by the formula:

$$10C(r_U / r_S)$$

in which C is the concentration, in mg per mL, of USP Vincristine Sulfate RS, corrected for loss in weight in the *Standard preparation*; and r_U and r_S are the peak responses obtained from the *Assay preparation* and the *Standard preparation*, respectively.

Vincristine Sulfate Injection

» Vincristine Sulfate Injection is a sterile solution of Vincristine Sulfate in Water for Injection. It contains not less than 90.0 percent and not more than 110.0 percent of the labeled amount of vincristine sulfate ($C_{46}H_{56}N_4O_{10} \cdot H_2SO_4$).

Caution—Handle Vincristine Sulfate Injection with great care since it is a potent cytotoxic agent.

Packaging and storage—Preserve in light-resistant, glass containers, in a refrigerator.

Labeling—The label states: "FATAL IF GIVEN INTRATHECALLY. FOR INTRAVENOUS USE ONLY." Where labeled as containing more than 2 mg, it must also be labeled as a *Pharmacy Bulk Package*(see *Injections* ⟨1⟩). The labeling directs that the drug be dispensed only in containers enclosed in an overwrap labeled as directed below. When packaged in a *Pharmacy Bulk Package*, it is exempt from the requirement under *Injections* ⟨1⟩, that the closure be penetrated only one time after constitution with a suitable sterile transfer device or dispensing set, when it contains a suitable substance or mixture of substances to prevent the growth of microorganisms.

When dispensed, the container or syringe (holding the individual dose prepared for administration to the patient) must be enclosed in an overwrap bearing the statement "DO NOT REMOVE COVERING UNTIL MOMENT OF INJECTION. FATAL IF GIVEN INTRATHECALLY. FOR INTRAVENOUS USE ONLY."

USP Reference standards ⟨11⟩—*USP Endotoxin RS. USP Vinblastine Sulfate RS. USP Vincristine Sulfate RS.* [NOTE—No *Loss on drying* determination is needed for USP Vinblastine Sulfate RS.]

Identification—

Spray reagent—Dissolve 2.0 g of ceric ammonium sulfate in 100 mL of water with heating and stirring, and slowly add 100 mL of phosphoric acid. Filter if necessary.

Procedure—Transfer a volume of Injection, equivalent to 2 mg of vincristine sulfate, to a small centrifuge tube. For each mL of solution add 1 drop of ammonium hydroxide. Add 0.2 mL of dichloromethane. Place the cap on the tube, shake it vigorously for not less than 1 minute, and centrifuge for 1 minute. Carefully withdraw the dichloromethane layer, and transfer to a small stoppered vial. Proceed as directed for *Procedure* in the test for *Identification* under *Vincristine Sulfate for Injection*, beginning with "Also prepare a 10-mg-per-mL solution of USP Vincristine Sulfate RS."

Bacterial endotoxins ⟨85⟩—It contains not more than 62.5 USP Endotoxin Units per mg of vincristine sulfate.

pH ⟨791⟩: between 3.5 and 5.5.

Related compounds—Proceed as directed in the test for *Related compounds* under *Vincristine Sulfate*. Also inject into the chromatograph the same volume of a suitable dilution of any preservative present in the Injection, as identified in the labeling, and determine the retention time. The sum of the responses at retention times other than the retention time of vincristine and the retention times of preservatives does not exceed 6.0% of the total of all responses. The response due to *N*-desformylvincristine, eluting at 1.4 ± 0.1 of the retention time of vincristine, is not more than 3.0% of all responses, and the response due to any other related substance is not more than 2.0% of all responses.

Other requirements—It meets the requirements for *Sterility Tests* ⟨71⟩ and for *Labeling* under *Injections* ⟨1⟩.

Assay—

Mobile phase, Standard preparation, System suitability preparation, and *Chromatographic system*—Proceed as directed in the *Assay* under *Vincristine Sulfate*.

Assay preparation—Dilute, if necessary, an accurately measured volume of Injection quantitatively with water to obtain a solution having a concentration of about 1 mg per mL, insert the stopper, and shake to mix.

Procedure—Proceed as directed for *Procedure* in the *Assay* under *Vincristine Sulfate*. Calculate the quantity, in mg, of vincristine sulfate ($C_{46}H_{56}N_4O_{10} \cdot H_2SO_4$) in each mL of the Injection taken by the formula:

$$C(L/D)(r_U/r_S)$$

in which *C* is the concentration, in mg per mL, of USP Vincristine Sulfate RS corrected for loss in weight in the *Standard preparation*; *L* is the labeled quantity, in mg per mL, of vincristine sulfate in Injection; *D* is the concentration, in mg per mL, of vincristine sulfate in the *Assay preparation* on the basis of the labeled quantity and the extent of dilution, if any; and r_U and r_S are the peak responses obtained from the *Assay preparation* and the *Standard preparation,* respectively.

Vincristine Sulfate for Injection

» Vincristine Sulfate for Injection is a sterile mixture of Vincristine Sulfate with suitable diluents. It contains not less than 90.0 percent and not more than 110.0 percent of the labeled amount of vincristine sulfate ($C_{46}H_{56}N_4O_{10} \cdot H_2SO_4$).

Caution—Handle Vincristine Sulfate for Injection with great care since it is a potent cytotoxic agent.

Packaging and storage—Preserve in *Containers for Sterile Solids* as described under *Injections* ⟨1⟩, in a refrigerator.

Labeling—The label states: "FATAL IF GIVEN INTRATHECALLY. FOR INTRAVENOUS USE ONLY." Where labeled as containing more than 2 mg, it must also be labeled as a *Pharmacy Bulk Package* (see *Injections* ⟨1⟩). The labeling directs that the drug be dispensed only in containers enclosed in an overwrap labeled as directed below. When packaged in a *Pharmacy Bulk Package*, it is exempt from the requirement under *Injections* ⟨1⟩, that the closure be penetrated only one time after constitution with a suitable sterile transfer device or dispensing set, when it contains a suitable substance or mixture of substances to prevent the growth of microorganisms.

When dispensed, the container or syringe (holding the individual dose prepared for administration to the patient) must be enclosed in an overwrap bearing the statement "DO NOT REMOVE COVERING UNTIL MOMENT OF INJECTION. FATAL IF GIVEN INTRATHECALLY. FOR INTRAVENOUS USE ONLY."

USP Reference standards ⟨11⟩—*USP Endotoxin RS. USP Vinblastine Sulfate RS. USP Vincristine Sulfate RS.* [NOTE—No *Loss on drying* determination is needed for USP Vinblastine Sulfate RS.]

Constituted solution—At the time of use, it meets the requirements for *Constituted Solutions* under *Injections* ⟨1⟩.

Identification—

Spray reagent—Dissolve 2.0 g of ceric ammonium sulfate in 100 mL of water with heating and stirring, and slowly add 100 mL of phosphoric acid. Filter if necessary.

Procedure—Dissolve a sufficient quantity in water to obtain a solution containing 25 mg per mL. Further dilute the solution to 10 mg per mL with methanol, and mix. Also prepare a 10-mg-per-mL solution of USP Vincristine Sulfate RS in a mixture of dichloromethane and methanol (3:1), and mix. Use a thin-layer chromatographic plate coated with a 0.25-mm layer of chromatographic silica gel mixture (see *Chromatography* ⟨621⟩). Develop it in a methanol prewash tank, and dry it, for maximum sensitivity, not more than 2 hours before use. Score it about 15 cm above the points of application. Apply 20 μL of each solution at points about 2.5 cm from the lower edge of the plate, and dry thoroughly (a current of cool air may be used to help dry the spots). Prepare the developing solvent system consisting of a mixture of fresh ether, methanol, and methylamine solution (2 in 5) (95 : 10 : 5) immediately prior to development. Place the plate in the nonequilibrated developing chamber that contains a paper liner around the back and sides and developing solvent to a depth of about 2 cm. Remove the plate when the solvent moves to the scored line (about 80 minutes), and discard the solvent system. Dry the plate in a fume hood at room temperature, heat on a metal plate on a steam bath for about 15 minutes, and spray the plate while still hot with *Spray reagent.*Continue heating the plate for 15 minutes to stabilize the spots: the $R_F$value and the color of the principal spot obtained from the test specimen correspond to those obtained from the Reference Standard.

Bacterial endotoxins ⟨85⟩—It contains not more than 100.0 USP Endotoxin Units per mg of vincristine sulfate.

Uniformity of dosage units ⟨905⟩—It meets the requirements for solids.

PROCEDURE FOR CONTENT UNIFORMITY—

Buffer solution—Dissolve 6.3 g of ammonium formate in about 900 mL of water in a 1000-mL volumetric flask, adjust with formic acid to a pH of 5.0 while stirring, dilute with water to volume, and mix.

Standard preparation—Dissolve an accurately weighed quantity of USP Vincristine Sulfate RS in *Buffer solution*, and dilute quantitatively and stepwise with *Buffer solution* to obtain a solution having a known concentration of about 40 µg per mL.

Test preparation—Dissolve the contents of 1 container of Vincristine Sulfate for Injection in an accurately measured volume of *Buffer solution* to obtain a solution having a concentration between 40 and 50 µg per mL.

Procedure—Concomitantly determine the absorbances of the *Test preparation* and the *Standard preparation* in 1-cm cells at the wavelength of maximum absorbance at about 262 nm versus the *Buffer solution* as the blank. Calculate the quantity, in mg, of $C_{46}H_{56}N_4O_{10} \cdot H_2SO_4$ in the container taken by the formula:

$$0.001CV(A_U / A_S)$$

in which C is the concentration, in µg per mL, of USP Vincristine Sulfate RS (corrected for loss in weight) in the *Standard preparation*, V is the volume, in mL, to which the contents of the container are diluted, and A_U and A_S are the absorbances of the *Test preparation* and the *Standard preparation*, respectively.

Related compounds—Proceed as directed in the test for *Related compounds* under *Vincristine Sulfate*. The total of the responses due to related substances does not exceed 5.0%, and no single related substance response exceeds 2.0%.

Other requirements—It meets the requirements for *Sterility Tests* ⟨71⟩, and for *Labeling* under *Injections* ⟨1⟩.

Assay—

Mobile phase, Standard preparation, System suitability preparation, and *Chromatographic system*—Prepare as directed in the *Assay* under *Vincristine Sulfate*.

Assay preparation—Pipet a suitable volume of water into a container of Vincristine Sulfate for Injection to obtain a solution having a concentration of about 1 mg of vincristine sulfate per mL. Insert the stopper, and shake to mix.

Procedure—Proceed as directed for *Procedure* in the *Assay* under *Vincristine Sulfate*. Calculate the quantity, in mg, of vincristine sulfate ($C_{46}H_{56}N_4O_{10} \cdot H_2SO_4$) in the portion of Vincristine Sulfate for Injection taken by the formula:

$$10C(r_U / r_S)$$

in which C is the concentration, in mg per mL, of USP Vincristine Sulfate RS corrected for loss in weight in the *Standard preparation*; and r_U and r_S are the peak responses for vincristine sulfate obtained from the *Assay preparation* and the *Standard preparation*, respectively.

Vinorelbine Tartrate

$C_{45}H_{54}N_4O_8 \cdot 2C_4H_6O_6$ 1079.11

C'-Norvincaleukoblastine, 3′,4′-didehydro-4′-deoxy-, [R-(R*,R*)]-2,3-dihydroxybutanedioate (1 : 2) (salt).

3′,4′-Didehydro-4′-deoxy-8′-norvincaleukoblastine L-(+)-tartrate (1 : 2) (salt)   [125317-39-7].

» Vinorelbine Tartrate contains not less than 98.0 percent and not more than 102.0 percent of $C_{45}H_{54}N_4O_8 \cdot 2C_4H_6O_6$, calculated on the anhydrous basis.

Caution—Vinorelbine Tartrate is cytotoxic. Great care should be taken to prevent inhaling particles and exposing the skin to it.

Packaging and storage—Preserve in tight, light-resistant containers. Store in a freezer.

USP Reference standards ⟨11⟩—*USP Vinorelbine Tartrate RS. USP Vinorelbine Related Compound A RS.*

Clarity of solution—Dissolve an amount of Vinorelbine Tartrate, equivalent to 100.0 mg of anhydrous vinorelbine, in 10 mL of water: the solution is clear.

Color of solution—The absorbance of the solution prepared under *Clarity of solution*, determined in a 1-cm cell at 420 nm in a suitable spectrophotometer, using water as the blank, is not more than 0.03.

Identification—

A: *Infrared Absorption* ⟨197K⟩—

Test specimen—Dissolve 10 mg in 5 mL of water, add 0.5 mL of 5 N sodium hydroxide, and extract with 5 mL of methylene chloride. Filter the organic extract through anhydrous sodium sulfate, and evaporate the organic extract to a volume of about 0.5 mL.

B: The retention time of the major peak in the chromatogram of the *Test solution* corresponds to that in the chromatogram of the *Diluted standard solution*, as obtained in the test for *Related compounds*.

C: To 0.1 mL of a solution containing the equivalent of about 15 mg of tartaric acid per mL, add 0.1 mL of a 100 g per L solution of potassium bromide, 0.1 mL of a 20 g per L solution of resorcinol, and 3 mL of sulfuric acid. Heat on a hot water bath for 5 to 10 minutes until a dark blue color develops. Allow to cool, and pour the solution into water. The color changes to red (*presence of tartrate*).

pH ⟨791⟩: between 3.3 and 3.8, in a solution (10 mg per mL).

Water, *Method Ia* ⟨921⟩: not more than 4.0%.

Residue on ignition ⟨281⟩: not more than 0.1%.

Related compounds—

Phosphate buffer, Mobile phase, System suitability solution, and *Chromatographic system*—Proceed as directed in the *Assay*.

Standard solution—Use the *Standard preparation*, prepared as directed in the *Assay*.

Diluted standard solution—Transfer 1.0 mL of the *Standard solution* to a 50-mL volumetric flask, and dilute with *Mobile phase* to volume. Pipet 1.0 mL of this solution into a 100-mL volumetric flask, and dilute with *Mobile phase* to volume.

Test solution—Use the *Assay preparation*.

Procedure—Separately inject equal volumes (about 20 µL) of the *Test solution* and the *Diluted standard solution* into the chromatograph, record the chromatograms, and measure the areas for the major peaks. Record the chromatograms for three times the retention time of the vinorelbine peak. Disregard any peaks with an area less than or equal to one-half of the area of the peak obtained for vinorelbine in the *Diluted standard solution*. Calculate the percentage of each impurity in the portion of Vinorelbine Tartrate taken by the formula:

$$100(r_i / r_s)$$

in which r_i is the peak response for each impurity obtained from the *Test solution;* and r_s is the sum of the responses of all the peaks: not more than 0.3% of the photodegradation product is found; not more than 0.2% of any individual impurity or coeluted impurities comprising an individual peak is found; and not more than 0.7% of total impurities, excluding the photodegradation product, is found.

Assay—

Phosphate buffer—Dissolve 6.9 g of monobasic sodium phosphate in 900 mL of water. Adjust with phosphoric acid to a pH of 4.2, dilute with water to 1000 mL, and mix.

Mobile phase—Dissolve 1.22 g of sodium 1-decanesulfonate in 620 mL of methanol. Add 380 mL of *Phosphate buffer,* mix, filter, and degas. Make adjustments if necessary (see *System Suitability* under *Chromatography* ⟨621⟩).

System suitability solution—Dissolve accurately weighed quantities of USP Vinorelbine Tartrate RS and USP Vinorelbine Related Compound A RS in water, and dilute quantitatively, and stepwise if necessary, with water to obtain a solution having known concentrations of about 1.4 mg per mL and 0.01 mg per mL, respectively. Expose a portion of this solution in a suitable xenon lamp apparatus capable of supplying a dose of 1600 KJ/m² between 310 and 800 nm at a power of 500 W/m² for about 1 hour, in order to generate an additional degradation product (3',4',7,8-tetradehydro-3,4'-dideoxy-3,6-epoxy-6,7-dihydro-C'-norvincaleukoblastine) having a relative retention time of about 0.8.

Standard preparation—Dissolve an accurately weighed quantity of USP Vinorelbine Tartrate RS in *Mobile phase* to obtain a solution having a known concentration of about 1.4 mg per mL.

Assay preparation—Dissolve an accurately weighed quantity of Vinorelbine Tartrate in *Mobile phase* to obtain a solution having a known concentration of about 1.4 mg per mL.

Chromatographic system (see *Chromatography* ⟨621⟩)—The liquid chromatograph is equipped with a 267-nm detector and a 3.9-mm × 15-cm column that contains 5-µm packing L1. The column temperature is maintained at 40°. The flow rate is about 1.0 mL per minute. Chromatograph the *System suitability solution*, and record the peak responses as directed for *Procedure*: the relative retention, *r*, between vinorelbine tartrate and vinorelbine related compound A is not less than 1.1. Chromatograph the *Standard preparation*, and record the peak responses as directed for *Procedure*: the relative standard deviation for replicate injections is not more than 2.0%. [NOTE—For peak identification purposes, the relative retention times are about 0.8 for the photodegradation product, 1.0 for vinorelbine, and 1.2 for vinorelbine related compound A.]

Procedure—Separately inject equal volumes (about 20 µL) of the *Standard preparation* and the *Assay preparation* into the chromatograph, record the chromatograms, and measure the responses for the vinorelbine tartrate peaks. Calculate the quantity, in percentage, of $C_{45}H_{54}N_4O_8 \cdot 2C_4H_6O_6$ in the portion of Vinorelbine Tartrate taken by the formula:

$$100(C_S / C_U)(r_U/r_S)$$

in which C_S is the concentration, in mg per mL, of USP Vinorelbine Tartrate RS in the *Standard preparation*; C_U is the concentration of Vinorelbine Tartrate in the *Assay preparation*; and r_U and r_S are the peak responses obtained from the *Assay preparation* and the *Standard preparation*, respectively.

Vinorelbine Injection

» Vinorelbine Injection is a sterile solution of Vinorelbine Tartrate in Water for Injection. It contains not less than 90.0 percent and not more than 110.0 percent of the labeled amount of vinorelbine ($C_{45}H_{54}N_4O_8$).

Caution—Handle Vinorelbine Injection with great care because it is a potent cytotoxic agent.

Packaging and storage—Preserve in single-dose *Containers for Injections* as described under *Injections* ⟨1⟩, preferably of Type I glass, protected from light. Store in a refrigerator.

USP Reference standards ⟨11⟩—*USP Endotoxin RS. USP Vinorelbine Related Compound A RS. USP Vinorelbine Tartrate RS.*

Clarity and color of solution—The solution of Injection (10 mg per mL) is clear. The absorbance of a solution of Injection, determined in a 1-cm cell at 420 nm, with a suitable spectrophotometer, using water as the blank, is not greater than 0.060.

Identification—The retention time and the UV spectrum of the major peak in the chromatogram of the *Assay preparation* corresponds to that in the chromatogram of the *Standard preparation*, as obtained in the *Assay*.

Bacterial endotoxins ⟨85⟩—It contains not more than 3.0 USP Endotoxin units per mg of vinorelbine.

Sterility ⟨71⟩—It meets the requirements when tested as directed for *Membrane Filtration* under *Test for Sterility of the Product to be Examined*.

pH ⟨791⟩: between 3.3 and 3.8.

Particulate matter ⟨788⟩: meets the requirements for small-volume injections.

Related compounds—

Mobile phase and *System suitability solution*—Proceed as directed in the *Assay* under *Vinorelbine Tartrate*.

Standard solution and *Diluted standard solution*—Proceed as directed in the test for *Related compounds* under *Vinorelbine Tartrate*.

Chromatographic system—Proceed as directed in the *Assay*.

Test solution—Dilute a portion of Injection with *Mobile phase* to obtain a solution containing 1.0 mg of vinorelbine per mL.

Procedure—Proceed as directed for *Procedure* in the test for *Related compounds* under *Vinorelbine Tartrate*. Not more than 1.0% of the photodegradation product is found; not more than 0.3% of vinorelbine related compound A is found; not more than 0.2% of any other individual impurity is found; and the sum of all impurities, excluding any peaks that are below the limit of quantitation (0.02%), is not more than 2.0%.

Other requirements—It meets the requirements under *Injections* ⟨1⟩.

Assay—

Phosphate buffer, Mobile phase, and *System suitability solution*—Proceed as directed in the *Assay* under *Vinorelbine Tartrate*.

Standard preparation—Dissolve an accurately weighed quantity of USP Vinorelbine Tartrate RS in water to obtain a solution having a known concentration of about 0.14 mg per mL.

Assay preparation—Transfer an accurately measured volume of Injection, equivalent to about 10 mg of vinorelbine, to a 100-mL volumetric flask, dilute with water to volume, and mix.

Chromatographic system (see *Chromatography* ⟨621⟩)—The liquid chromatograph is equipped with a diode-array detector and a 3.9-mm × 15-cm column that contains packing L1. The column temperature is maintained at 40°. The flow rate is about 1.0 mL per minute. Chromatograph the *System suitability solution*, and record the peak responses as directed for *Procedure*: the relative retention, *r*, between vinorelbine tartrate and vinorelbine related compound A is not less than 1.1. [NOTE—For peak identification purposes, the relative retention times are about 0.8 for the photodegradation product, 1.0 for vinorelbine, and 1.2 for vinorelbine related compound A.]

Procedure—Separately inject equal volumes (about 20 µL) of the *Standard preparation* and the *Assay preparation* into the chromatograph, record the chromatograms, and measure the responses for the vinorelbine peaks, using a diode-array detector. Calculate the quantity, in mg, of vinorelbine ($C_{45}H_{54}N_4O_8$) in each mL of the Injection taken by the formula:

$$(778.93/1079.11)C(L/D)(r_U / r_S)$$

in which 778.93 and 1079.11 are the molecular weights of vinorelbine and vinorelbine tartrate, respectively; *C* is the concentration, in mg per mL, of USP Vinorelbine Tartrate RS in the *Standard preparation*; *L* is the labeled quantity, in mg, of vinorelbine in each mL of Injection taken; *D* is the concentration, in mg per mL, of vinorelbine in the *Assay preparation*; and r_U and r_S are the peak responses at 267 nm obtained from the *Assay preparation* and the *Standard preparation*, respectively.

Vitamin A

» Vitamin A contains a suitable form of retinol ($C_{20}H_{30}O$; vitamin A alcohol) and possesses vitamin A activity equivalent to not less than 95.0 percent of that declared on the label. It may consist of retinol or esters of retinol formed from edible fatty acids, principally acetic and palmitic acids. It may be diluted with edible oils; or it may be incorporated in solid, edible carriers or excipients; and it may contain suitable antimicrobial agents, dispersants, and antioxidants.

Packaging and storage—Preserve in tight containers, preferably under an atmosphere of an inert gas, protected from light.

Labeling—Label it to indicate the form in which the vitamin is present, and to indicate the presence of any antimicrobial agent, dispersant, antioxidant, or other added substance, and to indicate the vitamin A activity in terms of the equivalent amount of retinol, in mg per g. The vitamin A activity may be stated also in USP Units, on the basis that 1 USP Vitamin A Unit equals the biological activity of 0.3 μg of the all-*trans* isomer of retinol.

USP Reference standards ⟨11⟩—*USP Vitamin A RS.*
Identification—
  A: To 1 mL of a chloroform solution of it containing the equivalent of approximately 6 μg of retinol, add 10 mL of antimony trichloride TS: a transient blue color appears at once.
  B: *Thin-Layer Chromatographic Identification Test* ⟨201⟩—
  Test solution—
  FOR LIQUID FORM OF VITAMIN A—Dissolve a volume equivalent to about 15,000 USP Units in chloroform to obtain 10 mL of solution.
  FOR SOLID FORM OF VITAMIN A—Weigh a quantity equivalent to about 15,000 USP Units, place in a separator, add 75 mL of water, shake vigorously for 1 minute, extract with 10 mL of chloroform by shaking for 1 minute, and centrifuge to clarify the chloroform extract.
  *Standard solution—*Dissolve the contents of 1 ampul of USP Vitamin A RS in chloroform to obtain 25.0 mL.
  Developing solvent system: a mixture of cyclohexane and ether (4 : 1).
  *Procedure—*Apply at the starting point of the chromatogram 0.015 mL of the *Standard solution* and 0.01 mL of the *Test solution*, and proceed as directed for *Thin-Layer Chromatography* under *Chromatography* ⟨621⟩. Allow the solvent front to move a distance of 10 cm, remove the plate, and air-dry. Spray with phosphomolybdic acid TS: the blue-green spot formed is indicative of the presence of retinol. The approximate R_F values of the predominant spots, corresponding to the different forms of retinol, are 0.1 for the alcohol form, 0.45 for the acetate, and 0.7 for the palmitate.
Absorbance ratio—The ratio of the corrected absorbance (A_{325}) to the observed absorbance A_{325} determined as directed under *Vitamin A Assay* ⟨571⟩ is not less than 0.85.
Assay—Using a suitable quantity of Vitamin A, accurately weighed, proceed as directed under *Vitamin A Assay* ⟨571⟩.

Vitamin A Capsules

» Vitamin A Capsules contain not less than 95.0 percent and not more than 120.0 percent of the labeled amount of vitamin A.

Packaging and storage—Preserve in tight, light-resistant containers.
Labeling—Label the Capsules to indicate the form in which the vitamin is present, and to indicate the vitamin A activity in terms of the equivalent amount of retinol in mg. The vitamin A activity may be stated also in USP Units per Capsule, on the basis that 1 USP Vitamin A Unit equals the biological activity of 0.3 μg of the all-*trans*isomer of retinol.
USP Reference standards ⟨11⟩—*USP Vitamin A RS.*
Disintegration ⟨701⟩: 45 minutes, determined using 0.05 M acetate buffer, prepared by mixing 2.99 g of sodium acetate and 1.66 mL of glacial acetic acid with water to obtain 1000 mL of solution having a pH of 4.5 ± 0.05, maintained at 37 ± 2° as the immersion fluid.
Uniformity of dosage units ⟨905⟩: meet the requirements.
Other requirements—The contents of Capsules respond to the tests for *Identification*for vitamin A and meet the requirements of the test for *Absorbance ratio* under *Vitamin A*.
Assay—Using not less than 5 Capsules, proceed as directed under *Vitamin A Assay* ⟨571⟩. Calculate the content of retinol ($C_{20}H_{30}O$) in mg and in USP Vitamin A Units per Capsule.

Vitamin E

» Vitamin E is a form of alpha tocopherol ($C_{29}H_{50}O_2$). It includes the following: *d*- or *dl*-alpha tocopherol ($C_{29}H_{50}O_2$); *d*- or *dl*-alpha tocopheryl acetate ($C_{31}H_{52}O_3$); *d*- or *dl*-alpha tocopheryl acid succinate ($C_{33}H_{54}O_5$). It contains not less than 96.0 percent and not more than 102.0 percent of $C_{29}H_{50}O_2$, $C_{31}H_{52}O_3$, or $C_{33}H_{54}O_5$, respectively.

Packaging and storage—Preserve in tight containers, protected from light. Protect *d*- or *dl*-alpha tocopherol with a blanket of an inert gas.
Labeling—Label Vitamin E to indicate the chemical form and to indicate whether it is the *d*- or the *dl*-form. The Vitamin E activity may be expressed in terms of the equivalent amount of *d*-alpha tocopherol, in mg per g, based on the following relationship between the former USP Units (equal to the former International Units) and mass.[*]
USP Reference standards ⟨11⟩—*USP Alpha Tocopherol RS. USP Alpha Tocopheryl Acetate RS. USP Alpha Tocopheryl Acid Succinate RS.*
Identification—
  Test solution for alpha tocopheryl acetate—[NOTE—Use low-actinic glassware.] Transfer about 220 mg of *d*- or *dl*-alpha tocopheryl acetate, accurately weighed, to a round-bottom, glass-stoppered, 150-mL flask, and dissolve in 25 mL of dehydrated alcohol. Add 20 mL of dilute sulfuric acid in alcohol (1 in 7), and reflux in an all-glass apparatus for 3 hours, protected from sunlight. Cool, transfer to a 200-mL volumetric flask, add dilute sulfuric acid in alcohol (1 in 72) to volume, and mix.
  Test solution for alpha tocopheryl acid succinate—[NOTE—Use low-actinic glassware.] Transfer an accurately weighed amount of the sample, equivalent to about 200 mg of alpha tocopherol, to a round-bottom, glass-stoppered, 250-mL flask, dissolve in 50 mL of dehydrated alcohol, and reflux for 1 minute. While the solution is boiling, add, through the condenser, 1 g of potassium hydroxide pellets, one at a time to avoid overheating. *[Caution—Wear safety goggles.]* Continue refluxing for 20 minutes and, without cooling, add 2 mL of hydrochloric acid dropwise through the condenser. [NOTE—This technique is essential to prevent oxidative action by air while the sample is in an alkaline medium.] Cool, and transfer the contents of the flask to a 500-mL separator, rinsing the flask with 100 mL each of water and of ether, and adding the rinsings to the separator. Shake vigorously, allow the layers to separate, and collect each of the two layers in individual separators. Extract the aqueous layer with two 50-mL portions of ether, and add these extracts to the main ether extract. Wash the combined ether extracts with four 100-mL portions of water, then evaporate the ether solution on a water bath under reduced pressure or in an atmosphere of nitrogen until about 7 or 8 mL remain. Complete the evaporation, removing the last traces of ether without the application of heat. Immediately dissolve the residue in dilute sulfuric acid in alcohol (1 in 72), transfer to a 200-mL volumetric flask, dilute with the alcoholic sulfuric acid to volume, and mix.
  A: Prepare a solution in dehydrated alcohol containing 10 mg of unesterified alpha tocopherol in 10 mL, or use 10 mL of *Test solution for alpha tocopheryl acetate* or of *Test solution for alpha tocopheryl acid succinate*. Add, with swirling, 2 mL of nitric acid, and heat at about 75° for 15 minutes: a bright red or orange color develops.
  B: Prepare a solution of about 100 mg, accurately weighed, of unesterified alpha tocopherol in 50 mL of ether, or in the case of

---

[*] In terms of USP Units, 1 mg of *dl*-alpha tocopherol = 1.1 former USP Vitamin E Units; 1 mg of *dl*-alpha tocopheryl acetate = 1 former USP Vitamin E unit; 1 mg of >*dl*-alpha tocopheryl acid succinate = 0.89 former USP Vitamin E Unit; 1 mg of *d*-alpha tocopherol = 1.49 former USP Vitamin E Units; 1 mg of *d*-alpha tocopheryl acetate = 1.36 former USP Vitamin E Units; and 1 mg of *d*-alpha tocopheryl acid succinate = 1.21 former USP Vitamin E Units.
In terms of *d*-alpha tocopherol equivalents, 1 mg of *d*-alpha tocopheryl acetate = 0.91; 1 mg of *d*-alpha tocopheryl acid succinate = 0.81; 1 mg of *dl*-alpha tocopherol = 0.74; 1 mg of *dl*-alpha tocopheryl acetate = 0.67; and 1 mg of *dl*-alpha tocopheryl acid succinate = 0.60.

esterified *d*-tocopherols, transfer an accurately measured volume of *Test solution for alpha tocopheryl acetate* or of *Test solution for alpha tocopheryl acid succinate*, equivalent to about 100 mg of the test specimen, to a separator, and add 200 mL of water. Extract first with 75 mL, then with 25 mL, of ether, and combine the ether extracts in another separator. To the ether solution of unesterified or hydrolyzed alpha tocopherol, add 20 mL of a 1 in 10 solution of potassium ferricyanide in sodium hydroxide solution (1 in 125), and shake for 3 minutes. Wash the ether solution with four 50-mL portions of water, discard the washings, and dry over anhydrous sodium sulfate. Evaporate the dried ether solution on a water bath under reduced pressure or in an atmosphere of nitrogen until about 7 or 8 mL remain, then complete the evaporation, removing the last traces of ether without the application of heat. Immediately dissolve the residue in 5.0 mL of isooctane, and determine the optical rotation. Calculate the specific rotation (see *Optical Rotation* ⟨781⟩), using as *c* the number of g of total tocopherols, determined in the *Assay*, in each 100 mL of solution employed for the test: the *d*-isomers have a specific rotation of not less than +24°. The *dl*-forms show essentially no optical rotation.

C: The retention time of the major peak in the chromatogram of the *Assay preparation* is the same as that of the *Standard preparation*, both relative to the internal standard, as obtained in the *Assay*.

Acidity—Dissolve 1.0 g of the test specimen in 25 mL of a mixture of equal volumes of alcohol and ether (which has been neutralized to phenolphthalein with 0.1 N sodium hydroxide), add 0.5 mL of phenolphthalein TS, and titrate with 0.10 N sodium hydroxide until the solution remains faintly pink after shaking for 30 seconds: alpha tocopheryl acid succinate requires between 18.0 and 19.3 mL of 0.10 N sodium hydroxide; the other forms of Vitamin E require not more than 1.0 mL of 0.10 N sodium hydroxide.

Organic volatile impurities, *Method IV* ⟨467⟩: meets the requirements.

(Official until July 1, 2008)

Assay for alpha tocopherol—

Internal standard solution—Dissolve an accurately weighed quantity of hexadecyl hexadecanoate in *n*-hexane to obtain a solution having a known concentration of about 1 mg per mL.

Standard preparation—[NOTE—Use low-actinic glassware.] Dissolve in *Internal standard solution* a suitable quantity of USP Alpha Tocopherol RS, accurately weighed, to obtain a solution having a known concentration of about 1 mg of the Reference Standard in each mL.

Assay preparation—[NOTE—Use low-actinic glassware.] Transfer about 50 mg of Vitamin E (*d*- or *dl*-alpha tocopherol), accurately weighed, to a 50-mL volumetric flask, dissolve in *Internal standard solution*, dilute with *Internal standard solution* to volume, and mix.

Chromatographic system (see *Chromatography* ⟨621⟩)—Under typical conditions, the instrument is equipped with a flame-ionization detector and contains a 4-mm × 2-m borosilicate glass column packed with 2% to 5% liquid phase G2 on 80- to 100-mesh support S1AB utilizing either a glass-lined sample introduction system or on-column injection. The column is maintained isothermally at a temperature between 245° and 265°, and the injection port and detector block are maintained at about 10° higher than the column temperature; the flow rate of dry carrier gas is adjusted to obtain a hexadecyl hexadecanoate peak approximately 18 to 20 minutes after sample introduction when a 2% column is used, or 30 to 32 minutes when a 5% column is used. [NOTE—Cure and condition the column as necessary (see *Chromatography* ⟨621⟩).]

Interference check—Dissolve an accurately weighed quantity of the specimen in *n*-hexane to obtain a solution having a known concentration of about 1 mg per mL. Chromatograph an accurately measured volume of this solution to obtain a chromatogram in which the principal peak exhibits not less than 50% of maximum recorder response. Similarly chromatograph an accurately measured volume of *Internal standard solution*. If a peak observed in the chromatogram for the specimen has the same retention time as that for hexadecyl hexadecanoate, make any necessary correction for factors of dilution or attenuation, and determine the area due to the interfering component that must be subtracted from the area of the internal standard peak appearing in the chromatogram recorded for the *Assay preparation* as directed for *Procedure*.

System suitability—Chromatograph a sufficient number of injections of a mixture, in *n*-hexane, of 1 mg per mL each of USP Alpha Tocopherol RS and USP Alpha Tocopheryl Acetate RS as directed for *Procedure* to ensure that the resolution factor, *R* (see *Chromatography* ⟨621⟩), is not less than 1.0.

Calibration—Chromatograph a portion of the *Standard preparation*, and record peak areas as directed under *Procedure*. Calculate the relative response factor, *F*, for the *Standard preparation* taken by the formula:

$$(A_S / A_D)(C_D / C_S)$$

in which C_D and C_S are the concentrations, in mg per mL, of hexadecyl hexadecanoate and of USP Alpha Tocopherol RS, respectively, in the *Standard preparation*. Successively chromatograph a sufficient number of portions of the *Standard preparation* to ensure that the relative response factor, *F*, is constant within a range of 2.0%.

Procedure—Inject a suitable portion (2 to 5 µL) of the *Assay preparation* into a suitable gas chromatograph, and record the chromatogram so as to obtain at least 50% of maximum recorder response. Measure the areas under the first (alpha tocopherol) and second major (hexadecyl hexadecanoate) peaks, record the values as a_U and a_D, respectively. Calculate the quantity, in mg, of alpha tocopherol in the Vitamin E taken by the formula:

$$(50 C_D / F)(a_U / a_D)$$

in which C_D is the concentration, in mg per mL, of hexadecyl hexadecanoate in the *Standard preparation;* and *F* is the relative response factor (see *Calibration*).

Assay for alpha tocopheryl acetate—Proceed as directed in the *Assay for alpha tocopherol*, substituting alpha tocopheryl acetate for alpha tocopherol and USP Alpha Tocopheryl Acetate RS for USP Alpha Tocopherol RS.

Assay for alpha tocopheryl acid succinate—Proceed as directed in the *Assay for alpha tocopherol*, substituting alpha tocopheryl acid succinate for alpha tocopherol and USP Alpha Tocopheryl Acid Succinate RS for USP Alpha Tocopherol RS.

NOTE—Chromatograms obtained as directed in the foregoing *Assays* exhibit relative retention times of approximately 0.53 for alpha tocopherol, 0.62 for alpha tocopheryl acetate, 0.54 for alpha tocopheryl acid succinate, and 1.0 for hexadecyl hexadecanoate.

Vitamin E Preparation

» Vitamin E Preparation is a combination of a single form of Vitamin E with one or more inert substances. It may be in a liquid or solid form. It contains not less than 95.0 percent and not more than 120.0 percent of the labeled amount of Vitamin E. Vitamin E Preparation labeled to contain a *dl*-form of Vitamin E may contain also a small amount of a *d*-form occurring as a minor constituent of an added substance.

Packaging and storage—Preserve in tight containers, protected from light. Protect Preparation containing *d*- or *dl*-alpha tocopherol with a blanket of an inert gas.

Labeling—Label it to indicate the chemical form of Vitamin E present, and to indicate whether the *d*- or the *dl*-form is present, excluding any different forms that may be introduced as a minor constituent of the vehicle. Designate the quantity of Vitamin E present.

USP Reference standards ⟨11⟩—*USP Alpha Tocopherol RS. USP Alpha Tocopheryl Acetate RS. USP Alpha Tocopheryl Acid Succinate RS.*

Identification—

Test solution—Proceed with the extraction and isolation of the residue obtained by hydrolysis as directed for *Test solution for alpha tocopheryl acid succinate* in the *Identification* test under *Vitamin E*. Immediately dissolve the residue in dehydrated alcohol,

transfer to a 250-mL volumetric flask, dilute with dehydrated alcohol to volume, and mix.
A: To 10 mL of *Test solution* add, with swirling, 2 mL of nitric acid, and heat at about 75° for 15 minutes: a bright red or orange color develops.
B: Transfer an accurately measured volume of *Test solution*, equivalent to about 100 mg of the test specimen, to a separator, and add 200 mL of water. Proceed as directed in *Identification* test *B* under *Vitamin E*, beginning with "Extract first with 75 mL."
C: The retention time of the major peak in the chromatogram of the *Assay preparation* is the same as that of the *Standard preparation*, both relative to the internal standard, as obtained in the *Assay*.
Acidity—
Liquid forms of Vitamin E Preparation—Dissolve 1.0 g in 25 mL of a mixture of equal volumes of alcohol and ether (which has been neutralized to phenolphthalein with 0.1 N sodium hydroxide), add 0.5 mL of phenolphthalein TS, and titrate with 0.10 N sodium hydroxide until the solution remains faintly pink after shaking for 30 seconds: not more than 1.0 mL of 0.10 N sodium hydroxide is required.
Assay—Proceed with Vitamin E Preparation as directed for the appropriate *Assay* under *Vitamin E*, substituting the following for the *Assay preparation*.
Assay preparation—[NOTE—Use low-actinic glassware.]
If the Preparation is in the liquid form, transfer an accurately weighed portion of Vitamin E Preparation, equivalent to about 50 mg of the specified form, to a 50-mL volumetric flask, dissolve in *Internal standard solution*, dilute with *Internal standard solution* to volume, and mix.
If the Preparation is in the solid form, transfer an accurately weighed portion of Vitamin E Preparation, equivalent to about 50 mg of Vitamin E, into a flask suitable for refluxing. Add about 5 mL of water, and heat on a water bath at 60° for 10 minutes. Add about 25 mL of alcohol, and reflux for 30 minutes. Cool, and transfer to a separator with the aid of 50 mL of water and 50 mL of ether. Shake vigorously, allow the layers to separate, and collect each in individual separators. Extract the aqueous layer with two 25-mL portions of ether, combining the extracts with the original ether layer. Wash the combined ether extracts with one 25-mL portion of water, filter the ether solution through 1 g of granular anhydrous sodium sulfate, and evaporate the ether solution on a water bath, controlled at a temperature that will not cause the ether solution to boil over, with the aid of a stream of nitrogen. Remove the container from the water bath when 5 mL remains, and complete the evaporation without the application of heat. Dissolve the residue in 50.0 mL of *Internal standard solution*, and mix.

Vitamin E Capsules

» Vitamin E Capsules contain Vitamin E or Vitamin E Preparation. They contain not less than 95.0 percent and not more than 120.0 percent of the labeled amount of vitamin E.

Packaging and storage—Preserve in tight containers, and store at room temperature. Protect Capsules containing *d-* or *dl-*alpha tocopherol from light.
Labeling—The Capsules meet the requirements for *Labeling* under *Vitamin E Preparation*.
USP Reference standards ⟨11⟩—*USP Alpha Tocopherol RS. USP Alpha Tocopheryl Acetate RS. USP Alpha Tocopheryl Acid Succinate RS.*
Identification—The contents of Capsules respond to the *Identification* tests under *Vitamin E* or under *Vitamin E Preparation*.
Disintegration ⟨701⟩: 45 minutes, determined using 0.05 M acetate buffer prepared by mixing 2.99 g of sodium acetate and 1.66 mL of glacial acetic acid with water to obtain 1000 mL of solution having a pH of 4.5 ± 0.05, maintained at 37 ± 2° as the immersion fluid.

Uniformity of dosage units ⟨905⟩: meet the requirements.
Assay—Proceed as directed in the *Assay* for the labeled form under *Vitamin E*, substituting the following for the *Assay preparation*.
Assay preparation—Weigh accurately not fewer than 10 Capsules in a tared weighing bottle. With a sharp blade, or by other appropriate means, carefully open the capsules, without loss of shell material, and transfer the combined capsule contents to a 100-mL beaker. Remove any adhering substance from the emptied capsules by washing with several small portions of *n*-hexane. Discard the washings, and allow the empty capsules to dry in a current of dry air until the odor of *n*-hexane is no longer perceptible. Weigh the empty capsules in the original tared weighing bottle, and calculate the average net weight per capsule. Transfer an accurately weighed portion of the combined capsule contents, equivalent to the quantity of Vitamin E specified for the *Assay preparation* in the *Assay* for the labeled form under *Vitamin E*, dissolve in and dilute with *Internal standard solution* to volume, and mix.

Warfarin Sodium

$C_{19}H_{15}NaO_4$ 330.31
2*H*-1-Benzopyran-2-one, 4-hydroxy-3-(3-oxo-1-phenylbutyl)-, sodium salt.
3-(α-Acetonylbenzyl)-4-hydroxycoumarin sodium salt   [129-06-6].

» Warfarin Sodium is an amorphous solid or a crystalline clathrate. The clathrate form consists principally of warfarin sodium and isopropyl alcohol, in a 2 : 1 molecular ratio; it contains not less than 8.0 percent and not more than 8.5 percent of isopropyl alcohol. Warfarin Sodium contains not less than 97.0 percent and not more than 102.0 percent of $C_{19}H_{15}NaO_4$, calculated on the anhydrous basis for the amorphous form or on the anhydrous and isopropyl alcohol-free basis for the crystalline form.

Packaging and storage—Preserve in well-closed, light-resistant containers.
Labeling—Label it to indicate whether it is the amorphous or the crystalline form.
USP Reference standards ⟨11⟩—*USP Warfarin RS. USP Warfarin Related Compound A RS.*
Identification—
A: *Infrared Absorption* ⟨197K⟩—The test specimen is the residue of warfarin obtained in *Identification* test *B*.
B: Dissolve about 100 mg in 25 mL of water, and adjust with hydrochloric acid to a pH of less than 3, using short-range pH indicator paper. Stir the mixture and allow the precipitate to coagulate. Filter the mixture, wash the precipitate with four 5-mL portions of water, and dry in vacuum over phosphorus pentoxide for 4 hours: the warfarin so obtained melts between 157° and 167°, but the range between beginning and end of melting does not exceed 4°.
C: A solution of it responds to the tests for *Sodium* ⟨191⟩. The filtrate obtained in *Identification* test *B* responds to the flame test for *Sodium* ⟨191⟩.
pH ⟨791⟩: between 7.2 and 8.3, in a solution (1 in 100).
Water, *Method I* ⟨921⟩: not more than 4.5% for the amorphous form; not more than 0.3% for the crystalline clathrate form.
Heavy metals ⟨231⟩—Dissolve 4.0 g in 45 mL of water, add 5 mL of glacial acetic acid, stir until the precipitate agglomerates, filter, and use 25 mL of the filtrate, employing glacial acetic acid, if necessary, to make the pH adjustment: the limit is 0.001%.
Absorbance in alkaline solution—Dissolve 1.25 g, accurately weighed, in 10 mL of sodium hydroxide solution (1 in 20), filter through a membrane filter, and within 15 minutes determine the absorbance of the solution in a 1-cm cell at 385 nm, with a suitable spectrophotometer, using sodium hydroxide solution (1 in 20) as the blank: the absorbance does not exceed 0.1.

Chromatographic purity—

Solvent mixture—Prepare a mixture of water and methanol (75 : 25).

Mobile phase—Prepare a filtered and degassed mixture of water, acetonitrile, and glacial acetic acid (68 : 32 : 1). Make adjustments if necessary (see *System Suitability* under *Chromatography* ⟨621⟩).

Standard solution—Transfer an accurately weighed quantity of about 24 mg of USP Warfarin RS and 24 mg of USP Warfarin Related Compound A RS to a 200-mL volumetric flask, add 4.0 mL of 0.1 N sodium hydroxide, 50 mL of methanol, and dissolve. Dilute with water to volume, and mix. Transfer 10.0 mL of this solution to a 200-mL volumetric flask, dilute with *Solvent mixture* to volume, and mix. Transfer 20.0 mL of this solution to a 50-mL volumetric flask, dilute with *Solvent mixture* to volume, and mix.

Test solution—Transfer an accurately weighed quantity of about 80 mg of Warfarin Sodium to a 100-mL volumetric flask, dissolve in and dilute with *Solvent mixture* to volume, and mix.

Chromatographic system (see *Chromatography* ⟨621⟩)—The liquid chromatograph is equipped with a 260-nm detector and a 4.6-mm × 25-cm column that contains packing L10. The flow rate is about 1.5 mL per minute. Chromatograph the *Standard solution*, and record the chromatogram as directed for *Procedure*: the resolution, R, between warfarin and warfarin related compound A is not less than 3; and the relative standard deviation for replicate injections is not more than 5.0%.

Procedure—Separately inject equal volumes (about 50 µL) of the *Standard solution* and the *Test solution* into the chromatograph, record the chromatograms, and measure the responses for all of the peaks. The relative retention times of warfarin and warfarin related compound A are 1.0 and about 1.2, respectively. Calculate the percentage of each impurity in the portion of Warfarin Sodium taken by the formula:

$$10,000(C / M)(r_i / r_S)$$

in which C is the concentration, in mg per mL, of warfarin sodium in the *Standard solution*; M is the quantity, in mg, of warfarin sodium taken to prepare the *Test solution*; r_i is the peak response of the individual impurity; and r_S is the peak response due to warfarin in the *Standard solution*: not more than 0.3% of any individual impurity and not more than 1.0% of total impurities is found.

Isopropyl alcohol content (*crystalline clathrate form*)—

Internal standard solution—Dilute 2 mL of *n*-propyl alcohol with water to 100.0 mL in a volumetric flask.

Standard preparation—Transfer an accurately weighed quantity of about 1.6 g of isopropyl alcohol to a 100-mL volumetric flask, dilute with water to volume, and mix. Transfer 10.0 mL of this solution to a 100-mL volumetric flask, add 10.0 mL of the *Internal standard solution*, dilute with water to volume, and mix to obtain a *Standard preparation* having a known concentration of about 1.6 mg of isopropyl alcohol per mL.

Test preparation—Dissolve an accurately weighed quantity of about 1.85 g of Warfarin Sodium in about 50 mL of water in a 100-mL volumetric flask. Add 10.0 mL of the *Internal standard solution*, dilute with water to volume, and mix.

Chromatographic system (see *Chromatography* ⟨621⟩)—The gas chromatograph is equipped with a flame-ionization detector and a 4-mm × 1.8-m column packed with 80- to 100-mesh support S2. The temperatures of the column, injector, and the detector are maintained at about 140°, 200°, and 250°, respectively. The carrier gas is nitrogen, flowing at the rate of about 40 mL per minute. The column temperature may be varied so that the following system suitability criteria are met: the resolution, R, between *n*-propyl alcohol and isopropyl alcohol is not less than 2.0; the tailing factor, T, for the isopropyl alcohol peak is not more than 1.5; and the relative standard deviation of the ratio of isopropyl alcohol area to *n*-propyl alcohol area for five replicate injections of the *Standard preparation* is not more than 2.0%.

Procedure—Separately inject equal volumes (about 5 µL) of the *Standard preparation* and the *Test preparation* into the chromatograph, record the chromatograms, and measure the areas of the major peaks. Calculate the weight, in mg, of the major peaks. Calculate the weight, in mg, of isopropyl alcohol in the portion of Warfarin Sodium taken by the formula:

$$100C(R_U / R_S)$$

in which C is the concentration, in mg per mL, of isopropyl alcohol in the *Standard preparation*; and R_U and R_S are the peak area ratios of isopropyl alcohol to *n*-propyl alcohol obtained from the *Test preparation* and the *Standard preparation*, respectively.

Organic volatile impurities, *Method I* ⟨467⟩: meets the requirements.

(Official until July 1, 2008)

Assay—

pH 7.4 Buffer—Transfer 1.36 g of monobasic potassium phosphate to a 200-mL volumetric flask, and dissolve in 50 mL of water. Add 39.1 mL of 0.2 N sodium hydroxide, and dilute with water to volume. Adjust with sodium hydroxide or phosphoric acid to a pH of 7.4 ± 0.1.

Mobile phase—Prepare a degassed solution containing a mixture of methanol, water, and glacial acetic acid (64 : 36 : 1). Adjust the ratio as necessary.

Internal standard solution—Dissolve propylparaben in a mixed solvent consisting of acetonitrile and glacial acetic acid (988 : 12), to obtain a solution having a concentration of about 0.2 mg per mL.

Standard preparation—Transfer about 94 mg of USP Warfarin RS, accurately weighed, to a 250-mL volumetric flask, and dissolve in 97.8 mL of 0.1 N sodium hydroxide. Add 62.5 mL of 0.2 M monobasic potassium phosphate, dilute with water to volume, and mix. Pipet 5 mL of this solution, 5 mL of *pH 7.4 Buffer*, and 10 mL of *Internal standard solution* into a conical flask, and mix.

Assay preparation—Using about 100 mg of Warfarin Sodium, accurately weighed, prepare as directed under *Standard preparation*.

Chromatographic system (see *Chromatography* ⟨621⟩)—The liquid chromatograph is equipped with a 280-nm detector and a 4.6-mm × 25-cm column that contains packing L7. The flow rate is about 1.4 mL per minute. Chromatograph five replicate injections of the *Standard preparation*, and record the peak responses as directed for *Procedure*: the relative retention times of propylparaben and warfarin are about 0.75 and 1.0, respectively; the resolution of the two peaks is not less than 2.0; and the relative standard deviation of the warfarin responses is not more than 2.0%.

Procedure—Separately inject equal volumes (about 20 µL) of the *Standard preparation* and the *Assay preparation* into the chromatograph, record the chromatograms, and measure the responses for the major peaks. Calculate the quantity, in mg, of $C_{19}H_{15}NaO_4$ in the portion of Warfarin Sodium taken by the formula:

$$(330.32 / 308.34)C(R_U / R_S)$$

in which 330.32 and 308.34 are the molecular weights of warfarin sodium and warfarin, respectively; C is the concentration, in µg per mL, of USP Warfarin RS in the *Standard preparation*; and R_U and R_S are the peak response ratios of warfarin to propylparaben obtained from the *Assay preparation* and the *Standard preparation*, respectively.

Warfarin Sodium for Injection

» Warfarin Sodium for Injection is a sterile, freeze-dried mixture of Warfarin Sodium and suitable added substances. It contains not less than 95.0 percent and not more than 105.0 percent of the labeled amount of warfarin sodium ($C_{19}H_{15}NaO_4$). It may contain a suitable buffer.

Packaging and storage—Preserve in light-resistant *Containers for Sterile Solids* as described under *Injections* ⟨1⟩.

USP Reference standards ⟨11⟩—*USP Endotoxin RS. USP Warfarin RS.*

Completeness of solution ⟨641⟩—A 1.0-g portion dissolves in 10 mL of carbon dioxide-free water to yield a clear solution.

Constituted solution—At the time of use, it meets the requirements for *Constituted Solutions* under *Injections* ⟨1⟩.

Bacterial endotoxins ⟨85⟩—It contains not more than 24.0 USP Endotoxin Units per mg of warfarin sodium.

Water, *Method I* ⟨921⟩: not more than 4.5%.

Other requirements—It responds to *Identification* tests A and B, and meets the requirements for *pH* and *Heavy metals* under *Warfarin Sodium*. It meets also the requirements for *Sterility Tests* ⟨71⟩, *Uniformity of Dosage Units* ⟨905⟩, and *Labeling* under *Injections* ⟨1⟩.

Assay—

pH 7.4 Buffer, *Mobile phase*, and *Chromatographic system*—Prepare as directed in the *Assay* under *Warfarin Sodium*.

Internal standard solution—Dissolve propylparaben in a solvent consisting of a mixture of acetonitrile and glacial acetic acid (988 : 12) to obtain a solution having a concentration of about 1.0 mg per mL.

Standard preparation—Transfer about 94 mg of USP Warfarin RS, accurately weighed, to a 100-mL volumetric flask, and dissolve in 39.1 mL of 0.1 N sodium hydroxide. Add 25.0 mL of 0.2 M monobasic potassium phosphate, dilute with water to volume, and mix. Pipet 5 mL of this solution and 5 mL of *Internal standard solution* into a 50-mL volumetric flask, dilute with *pH 7.4 Buffer* to volume, and mix.

Assay preparation—Dissolve the contents of not fewer than 10 containers of Warfarin Sodium for Injection in a sufficient volume, accurately measured, of *pH 7.4 Buffer* to obtain a solution containing about 1 mg of warfarin sodium per mL. Pipet 5 mL of the resulting solution and 5 mL of *Internal standard solution* into a 50-mL volumetric flask, dilute with *pH 7.4 Buffer* to volume, and mix.

Procedure—Proceed as directed for *Procedure* in the *Assay* under *Warfarin Sodium*. Calculate the average quantity, in mg, of warfarin sodium ($C_{19}H_{15}NaO_4$) in each container of Warfarin Sodium for Injection taken by the formula:

$$10(330.32 / 308.34)(VC / N)(R_U / R_S)$$

in which 330.32 and 308.34 are the molecular weights of warfarin sodium and warfarin, respectively; V is the volume, in mL, of the solution prepared from the contents of the 10 or more containers; C is the concentration, in mg per mL, of USP Warfarin RS in the *Standard preparation*; N is the number of containers taken; and R_U and R_S are the peak response ratios of warfarin to propylparaben obtained from the *Assay preparation* and the *Standard preparation*, respectively.

Warfarin Sodium Tablets

» Warfarin Sodium Tablets contain not less than 95.0 percent and not more than 105.0 percent of the labeled amount of warfarin sodium ($C_{19}H_{15}NaO_4$).

Packaging and storage—Preserve in tight, light-resistant containers.

USP Reference standards ⟨11⟩—*USP Warfarin RS*.

Identification—

A: The retention time of the major peak obtained from the *Assay preparation* corresponds to that obtained from the *Standard preparation*, both relative to the internal standard, obtained as directed in the *Assay*.

B: *Infrared Absorption* ⟨197K⟩—Prepare the test specimen as follows. Triturate a quantity of finely powdered Tablets, equivalent to about 200 mg of warfarin sodium, with 50 mL of water, centrifuge, and filter the supernatant. Extract with 50 mL of ether, transfer the aqueous layer to a second separator, and discard the ether. Adjust with hydrochloric acid to a pH of less than 3, using short-range pH indicator paper, and extract with 50 mL of chloroform. Transfer the chloroform layer to another separator, extract with 50 mL of sodium hydroxide solution (1 in 250), and discard the chloroform. Transfer the aqueous layer to a beaker, and adjust with hydrochloric acid to a pH of less than 3 (using the pH indicator paper) to precipitate the warfarin. Stir the mixture and allow the precipitate to coagulate. Filter, and wash the precipitate with four 5-mL portions of water. If the precipitate is not white or practically white, dissolve it in a minimum volume of sodium hydroxide solution (1 in 250), dilute with water to 50 mL, and repeat the foregoing procedure, beginning with "Extract with 50 mL of ether." Dry the warfarin so obtained in vacuum over phosphorus pentoxide for 4 hours.

Dissolution ⟨711⟩—

Medium: water; 900 mL.

Apparatus 2: 50 rpm.

Time: 30 minutes.

Mobile phase and *Chromatographic system*—Proceed as directed in the *Assay*.

Internal standard solution—Prepare a solution of propylparaben in water containing, in each mL, an amount of propylparaben equivalent to 0.0025 times the labeled amount, in mg, of warfarin sodium in each Tablet. [NOTE—A small amount of methanol may be used, if necessary, to dissolve the propylparaben.]

Standard stock solution—Dissolve an accurately weighed quantity of USP Warfarin RS in water to obtain a solution having a known concentration of about $0.0011L$ mg per mL, L being the labeled amount, in mg, of warfarin sodium in the Tablets. [NOTE— Use a small amount of 0.1 N sodium hydroxide to aid in dissolution.]

Standard solution—To 3.0 mL of *Standard stock solution*, add 1.0 mL of *Internal standard solution*, and mix.

Test solution—To a filtered 3.0-mL aliquot of the solution under test, add 1.0 mL of *Internal standard solution*, and mix.

Procedure—Separately inject equal volumes (about 40 µL) of the *Standard solution* and the *Test solution* into the chromatograph, record the chromatograms, and measure the responses for the major peaks. Calculate the quantity, in mg, of warfarin sodium dissolved by the formula:

$$(330.32 / 308.34)(900C)(R_U / R_S)$$

in which C is the concentration, in mg per mL, of USP Warfarin RS in the *Standard stock solution*, 330.32 and 308.34 are the molecular weights of warfarin sodium and warfarin, respectively; and R_U and R_S are the ratios of the peak responses of warfarin to those of propylparaben obtained from the *Test solution* and the *Standard solution*, respectively.

Tolerances—Not less than 80% *(Q)* of the labeled amount of $C_{19}H_{15}NaO_4$ is dissolved in 30 minutes.

Uniformity of dosage units ⟨905⟩: meet the requirements.

Assay—

pH 7.4 Buffer and *Chromatographic system*—Proceed as directed in the *Assay* under *Warfarin Sodium*.

Solvent mixture—Prepare a mixture of *pH 7.4 Buffer* and acetonitrile (85 : 15).

Mobile phase—Prepare a filtered and degassed mixture of methanol, water, and glacial acetic acid (68 : 32 : 1). Make adjustments if necessary (see *System Suitability* under *Chromatography* ⟨621⟩).

Internal standard solution—Prepare a solution of propylparaben in acetonitrile having a concentration of 1 mg per mL.

Standard preparation—Transfer about 62.5 mg of USP Warfarin RS, accurately weighed, to a 200-mL volumetric flask, and dissolve in 78 mL of 0.1 N sodium hydroxide. Add 50 mL of 0.2 M monobasic potassium phosphate, dilute with water to volume, and mix. Transfer 15.0 mL of this solution to a 50-mL volumetric flask. Add 5.0 mL of *Internal standard solution*, and dilute with *Solvent mixture* to volume.

Assay preparation—Weigh and finely powder not fewer than 20 Tablets. Transfer an accurately weighed portion of the powder, equivalent to about 5 mg of warfarin sodium, to a 50-mL volumetric flask, and add 5 mL of *Internal standard solution* and about 30 mL of *Solvent mixture*. Sonicate for 10 minutes, and then shake by mechanical means for 60 minutes. Dilute with *Solvent* mixture to volume, and filter.

Procedure—Separately inject equal volumes (about 20 µL) of the *Standard preparation* and the *Assay preparation* into the chromatograph, record the chromatograms, and measure the responses for the

major peaks. Calculate the quantity, in mg, of $C_{19}H_{15}NaO_4$ in the portion of Tablets taken by the formula:

$$(330.32 / 308.34)C(R_U / R_S)$$

in which 330.32 and 308.34 are the molecular weights of warfarin sodium and warfarin, respectively; C is the concentration, in mg per mL, of USP Warfarin RS in the *Standard preparation*; and R_U and R_S are the ratios of the peak responses of warfarin to those of propylparaben obtained from the *Assay preparation* and the *Standard preparation*, respectively.

Water for Injection

NOTE—For microbiological guidance, see general information chapter *Water for Pharmaceutical Purposes* ⟨1231⟩.

» Water for Injection is water purified by distillation or a purification process that is equivalent or superior to distillation in the removal of chemicals and microorganisms. It is prepared from water complying with the U.S. Environmental Protection Agency National Primary Drinking Water Regulations or with the drinking water regulations of the European Union, Japan, or with the World Health Organization's Guidelines for Drinking Water Quality. It contains no added substance.

NOTE—Water for Injection is intended for use in the preparation of parenteral solutions. Where used for the preparation of parenteral solutions subject to final sterilization, use suitable means to minimize microbial growth, or first render the Water for Injection sterile and, thereafter, protect it from microbial contamination. For parenteral solutions that are prepared under aseptic conditions and are not sterilized by appropriate filtration or in the final container, first render the Water for Injection sterile and, thereafter, protect it from microbial contamination. The tests for *Total organic carbon* and *Water conductivity* apply to Water for Injection produced on site for use in manufacturing. Water for Injection packaged in bulk for commercial use elsewhere meets the requirement of the test for *Bacterial endotoxins* as indicated below and the requirements of all the tests under *Sterile Purified Water*, except *Labeling*.

USP Reference standards ⟨11⟩—*USP 1,4-Benzoquinone RS. USP Endotoxin RS. USP Sucrose RS.*
Bacterial endotoxins ⟨85⟩—It contains less than 0.25 USP Endotoxin Unit per mL.
Total organic carbon ⟨643⟩: meets the requirements.
Water conductivity ⟨645⟩: meets the requirements.

Bacteriostatic Water for Injection

NOTE—For microbiological guidance, see general information chapter *Water for Pharmaceutical Purposes* ⟨1231⟩.

» Bacteriostatic Water for Injection is prepared from Water for Injection that is sterilized and suitably packaged, containing one or more suitable antimicrobial agents.

NOTE—Use Bacteriostatic Water for Injection with due regard for the compatibility of the antimicrobial agent or agents it contains with the particular medicinal substance that is to be dissolved or diluted.

Packaging and storage—Preserve in single-dose or multiple-dose glass or plastic containers. Glass containers are preferably of Type I or Type II glass, of not larger than 30-mL size.
Labeling—Label it to indicate the name(s) and proportion(s) of the added antimicrobial agent(s). Label it also to include the statement "NOT FOR USE IN NEWBORNS" in boldface capital letters on the label immediately under the official name, printed in a contrasting color, preferably red. Alternatively, the statement may be placed prominently elsewhere on the label if the statement is enclosed within a box.
Sterility ⟨71⟩: meets the requirements.
USP Reference standards ⟨11⟩—*USP Endotoxin RS.*
Antimicrobial agent(s)—It meets the requirements under *Antimicrobial Effectiveness Testing* ⟨51⟩, and meets the labeled claim for content of the antimicrobial agent(s), as determined by the method set forth under *Antimicrobial Agents—Content* ⟨341⟩.
Bacterial endotoxins ⟨85⟩—It contains less than 0.5 USP Endotoxin Unit per mL.
Particulate matter ⟨788⟩: meets the requirements.
pH ⟨791⟩: between 4.5 and 7.0, in a solution containing 0.3 mL of saturated potassium chloride solution per 100 mL of test specimen.
Calcium—To 100 mL add 2 mL of ammonium oxalate TS: no turbidity is produced.
Carbon dioxide—To 25 mL add 25 mL of calcium hydroxide TS: the mixture remains clear.
Sulfate—To 100 mL add 1 mL of barium chloride TS: no turbidity is produced.

Sterile Water for Inhalation

NOTE—For microbiological guidance, see general information chapter *Water for Pharmaceutical Purposes* ⟨1231⟩.

» Sterile Water for Inhalation is prepared from Water for Injection that is sterilized and suitably packaged. It contains no antimicrobial agents, except where used in humidifiers or other similar devices and where liable to contamination over a period of time, or other added substances.

NOTE—Do not use Sterile Water for Inhalation for parenteral administration or for other sterile compendial dosage forms.

Packaging and storage—Preserve in glass or plastic containers. Glass containers are preferably of Type I or Type II glass.
Labeling—Label it to indicate that it is for inhalation therapy only and that it is not for parenteral administration.
USP Reference standards ⟨11⟩—*USP Endotoxin RS.*
Bacterial endotoxins ⟨85⟩—It contains less than 0.5 USP Endotoxin Unit per mL.
Sterility ⟨71⟩: meets the requirements.
Water conductivity ⟨645⟩—Perform *Stage 2, Step 4* using a sufficient amount of water to perform the test. The conductivity is not more than 25 µS/cm for containers with a nominal volume of 10 mL or less at 25 ± 1°; and not more than 5 µS/cm for containers with a nominal volume greater than 10 mL at 25 ± 1°.
Oxidizable substances—To 100 mL add 10 mL of 2 N sulfuric acid, and heat to boiling. For *Sterile Water for Inhalation* in containers having a fill volume of less than 50 mL, add 0.4 mL of 0.02 M potassium permanganate, and boil for 5 minutes; where the fill volume is 50 mL or more, add 0.2 mL of 0.02 M potassium permanganate, and boil for 5 minutes. If a precipitate forms, cool in an ice bath to room temperature, and pass through a sintered-glass filter: the pink color does not completely disappear.

Sterile Water for Injection

NOTE—For microbiological guidance, see general information chapter *Water for Pharmaceutical Purposes* ⟨1231⟩.

» Sterile Water for Injection is prepared from Water for Injection that is sterilized and suitably packaged. It contains no antimicrobial agent or other added substance.

Packaging and storage—Preserve in single-dose glass or plastic containers, of not larger than 1-L size. Glass containers are preferably of Type I or Type II glass.
Labeling—Label it to indicate that no antimicrobial or other substance has been added, and that it is not suitable for intravascular injection without first having been made approximately isotonic by the addition of a suitable solute.
USP Reference standards ⟨11⟩—*USP Endotoxin RS*.
Bacterial endotoxins ⟨85⟩—It contains less than 0.25 USP Endotoxin Unit per mL.
Sterility ⟨71⟩: meets the requirements.
pH ⟨791⟩: between 5.0 and 7.0 in a solution containing 0.3 mL of saturated potassium chloride solution per 100 mL of test specimen.
Particulate matter ⟨788⟩: meets the requirements.
Ammonia—For containers having a fill volume of less than 50 mL, dilute 50 mL of it with 50 mL of *High-Purity Water* (see *Reagents* under *Containers* ⟨661⟩), and use this dilution as the test solution; where the fill volume is 50 mL or more, use 100 mL of it as the test solution. To 100 mL of the test solution add 2 mL of alkaline mercuric-potassium iodide TS: any yellow color produced immediately is not darker than that of a control containing 30 µg of added ammonia (furnished by adding 1 mL of the final solution prepared by diluting 3.0 mL of ammonia TS with *High-Purity Water* to 100 mL; 1.0 mL of this solution is further diluted to 100 mL) in 100 mL of *High-Purity Water*. This corresponds to a limit of 0.6 mg per L for containers having a fill volume of less than 50 mL and 0.3 mg per L where the fill volume is 50 mL or more.
Calcium—To 100 mL add 2 mL of ammonium oxalate TS: no turbidity is produced.
Carbon dioxide—To 25 mL add 25 mL of calcium hydroxide TS: the mixture remains clear.
Chloride—To 20 mL in a color-comparison tube add 5 drops of nitric acid and 1 mL of silver nitrate TS, and gently mix: any turbidity formed within 10 minutes is not greater than that produced in a similarly treated control consisting of 20 mL of *High-Purity Water* (see *Reagents* under *Containers* ⟨661⟩) containing 10 µg of chloride (0.5 mg per L), viewed downward over a dark surface with light entering the tubes from the sides.
Sulfate—To 100 mL add 1 mL of barium chloride TS: no turbidity is produced.
Oxidizable substances—To 100 mL add 10 mL of 2 N sulfuric acid, and heat to boiling. For Sterile Water for Injection in containers having a fill volume of less than 50 mL, add 0.4 mL of 0.02 M potassium permanganate, and boil for 5 minutes; where the fill volume is 50 mL or more, add 0.2 mL of 0.02 M potassium permanganate, and boil for 5 minutes. If a precipitate forms, cool in an ice bath to room temperature, and pass through a sintered-glass filter: the pink color does not completely disappear.

Sterile Water for Irrigation

NOTE—For microbiological guidance, see general information chapter *Water for Pharmaceutical Purposes* ⟨1231⟩.

» Sterile Water for Irrigation is prepared from Water for Injection that is sterilized and suitably packaged. It contains no antimicrobial agent or other added substance.

Packaging and storage—Preserve in single-dose glass or plastic containers. Glass containers are preferably of Type I or Type II glass. The container may contain a volume of more than 1 L, and may be designed to empty rapidly.
Labeling—Label it to indicate that no antimicrobial or other substance has been added. The designations "For irrigation only" and "Not for injection" appear prominently on the label.
USP Reference standards ⟨11⟩—*USP Endotoxin RS*.
Bacterial endotoxins ⟨85⟩: not more than 0.25 Endotoxin Unit per mL.
Sterility ⟨71⟩: meets the requirements.
Water conductivity ⟨645⟩—Perform *Stage 2, Step 4* using a sufficient amount of water to perform the test. The conductivity is not more than 25 µS/cm for containers with a nominal volume of 10 mL or less at 25 ± 1°; and not more than 5 µS/cm for containers with a nominal volume greater than 10 mL at 25 ± 1°.
Oxidizable substances—To 100 mL add 10 mL of 2 N sulfuric acid, and heat to boiling. For Sterile Water for Irrigation in containers having a fill volume of less than 50 mL, add 0.4 mL of 0.02 M potassium permanganate, and boil for 5 minutes; where the fill volume is 50 mL or more, add 0.2 mL of 0.02 M potassium permanganate, and boil for 5 minutes. If a precipitate forms, cool in an ice bath to room temperature, and pass through a sintered-glass filter: the pink color does not completely disappear.

Purified Water

H_2O 18.02

NOTE—For microbiological guidance, see general information chapter *Water for Pharmaceutical Purposes* ⟨1231⟩.

» Purified Water is water obtained by a suitable process. It is prepared from water complying with the U.S. Environmental Protection Agency National Primary Drinking Water Regulations or with the drinking water regulations of the European Union, Japan, or with the World Health Organization's Guidelines for Drinking Water Quality. It contains no added substance.

NOTE—Purified Water is intended for use as an ingredient of official preparations and in tests and assays unless otherwise specified (see *Water* in *Ingredients and Processes* and in *Tests and Assays* under *General Notices and Requirements*). Where used for sterile dosage forms, other than for parenteral administration, process the article to meet the requirements under *Sterility Tests* ⟨71⟩, or first render the Purified Water sterile and thereafter protect it from microbial contamination. Do not use Purified Water in preparations intended for parenteral administration. For such purposes use Water for Injection, Bacteriostatic Water for Injection, or Sterile Water for Injection. The tests for *Total organic carbon* and *Conductivity* apply to Purified Water produced on site for use as an ingredient of official preparations and in tests and assays. Purified Water packaged in bulk for commercial use elsewhere meets the requirements of all of the tests under *Sterile Purified Water*, except *Labeling* and *Sterility* ⟨71⟩.

USP Reference standards ⟨11⟩—*USP 1,4-Benzoquinone RS. USP Sucrose RS.*
Total organic carbon ⟨643⟩: meets the requirements.
Water conductivity ⟨645⟩: meets the requirements.

Sterile Purified Water

H_2O 18.02

NOTE—For microbiological guidance, see general information chapter *Water for Pharmaceutical Purposes* ⟨1231⟩.

» **Sterile Purified Water** is Purified Water sterilized and suitably packaged. It contains no antimicrobial agent.

NOTE—Do not use Sterile Purified Water in preparations intended for parenteral administration. For such purposes use Water for Injection, Bacteriostatic Water for Injection, or Sterile Water for Injection.

Packaging and storage—Preserve in suitable, tight containers.
Labeling—Label it to indicate the method of preparation and that it is not for parenteral administration.
Sterility ⟨71⟩: meets the requirements.
Water conductivity ⟨645⟩—Perform *Stage 2, Step 4* using a sufficient amount of water to perform the test. The conductivity is not more than 25 µS/cm for containers with a nominal volume of 10 mL or less at 25 ± 1°; and not more than 5 µS/cm for containers with a nominal volume greater than 10 mL at 25 ± 1°.
Oxidizable substances—To 100 mL, add 10 mL of 2 N sulfuric acid, and heat to boiling. For Sterile Purified Water in containers having a fill volume of less than 50 mL, add 0.4 mL of 0.02 M potassium permanganate, and boil for 5 minutes; where the fill volume is 50 mL or more, add 0.2 mL of 0.02 M potassium permanganate, and boil for 5 minutes. If a precipitate forms, cool in an ice bath to room temperature, and pass through a sintered-glass filter: the pink color does not completely disappear.

Water for Hemodialysis

NOTE—See *Water for Health Applications* ⟨1230⟩ for guidelines on microbial and chemical testing.

» **Water for Hemodialysis** is water that complies with the U.S. Environmental Protection Agency National Primary Drinking Water Regulations and that has been subjected to further treatment, using a suitable process, to reduce chemical and microbiological components. It is produced and used onsite under the direction of qualified personnel. It contains no added antimicrobials and is not intended for injection.

Packaging and storage—Preserve in unreactive storage containers that are designed to prevent bacterial entry. Store at room temperature.
USP Reference standards ⟨11⟩—*USP Endotoxin RS.*
Microbial limits ⟨61⟩—The total viable count does not exceed 100 cfu per mL.
Bacterial endotoxins ⟨85⟩—It contains less than 2 USP Endotoxin Units per mL.
Water conductivity ⟨645⟩: meets the requirements.
Oxidizable substances—To 100 mL, add 10 mL of 2 N sulfuric acid, and heat to boiling. Add 0.2 mL of 0.02 M potassium permanganate, and boil for 5 minutes. The pink color does not completely disappear; or alternatively follow the test method for *Total Organic Carbon* ⟨643⟩.

Pure Steam

NOTE—For microbiological guidance, see general information chapter *Water for Pharmaceutical Purposes* ⟨1231⟩.

» **Pure Steam** is water that has been heated above 100° and vaporized in a manner that prevents source water entrainment. It is prepared from water complying with the U.S. Environmental Protection Agency National Primary Drinking Water Regulations, or with drinking water regulations of the European Union or Japan, or with WHO drinking water guidelines. It contains no added substance. The level of steam saturation or dryness, and the amount of noncondensable gases are to be determined by the Pure Steam application.

NOTE—Pure Steam is intended for use where the steam or its condensate comes in contact with the article or the preparation. Pure Steam quality is difficult to assess in its vapor state; therefore the attributes of its condensate are used to test its quality. The process used to create and collect the condensate for analysis must not adversely impact these quality attributes.

USP Reference standards ⟨11⟩—*USP 1,4-Benzoquinone RS. USP Endotoxin RS. USP Sucrose RS.*
Bacterial endotoxins ⟨85⟩—The condensate contains less than 0.25 USP Endotoxin Unit per mL (when used in the production of parenterals).
Total organic carbon ⟨643⟩: the condensate meets the requirement.
Water conductivity ⟨645⟩: the condensate meets the requirement.

Wheat Bran

» **Wheat Bran** is the outer fraction of the cereal grain, comprising the pericarp, seed coat (testa), nucellar tissue, and aleurone layer, and is derived from *Triticum aestivum* Linné, *T. compactum* Host, *T. durum* Desf., and other common einkorn and emmer wheat cultivars. It is obtained by the milling and processing of the whole wheat grain meeting U.S. Standards for Number 1 wheat (7 CFR 810.2201). It contains not less than 36.0 percent of dietary fiber.

Packaging and storage—Preserve in well-closed containers, secured against insect attack (see *Preservation* under *Vegetable and Animal Substances* in the *General Notices*).
Identification—When examined microscopically, the following components of Wheat Bran are visible. Fragments of aleurone and nucellar layers (about 60% of the components) and fragments of seed coat and pericarp (about 40%). Aleurone and nucellar tissues composed of a usually single layer of thick-walled, isodiametric, translucent cells having conspicuous protoplasm and a single, inconspicuous layer of thick-walled, nearly transparent cells. Inconspicuous seed coat, consisting of two layers of thin-walled cells crossing at roughly right angles to each other. Pericarp composed of an inconspicuous endocarp layer of elongated, thick-walled tube cells; a cross layer with cells longer than wide, arranged side-by-side in rows, having thick, highly pitted side and end walls; and epicarp and hypoderm layers with cells longer than wide, arranged alternately in rows and having thick, highly pitted side and end walls. Epicarp and hypoderm cells larger than and crossing at right angles to the cells of the cross layer. A few trichomes also present, with lumens narrower than the thickness of their cell walls and originating from isodiametric-polygonal epicarp cells. If micronized, the original structures are mostly destroyed.
Microbial limits ⟨61⟩—The total aerobic microbial count does not exceed 10,000 cfu per g, and it meets the requirements of the test for the absence of *Salmonella* species and *Escherichia coli*.
Water, *Method III, Procedure for Articles of Botanical Origin,* ⟨921⟩—It loses not more than 12% of its weight.
Total ash ⟨561⟩: not more than 8%.
Heavy metals, *Method II* ⟨231⟩: 0.004%.
Absence of peroxidase activity—Transfer about 1 g of Wheat Bran to a test tube, and add 50 mL of water. Add, in the order speci-

fied, 2 mL of 5.68 mM erythorbic acid, 3 mL of 0.69 mM dichloroindophenol, and 0.1 mL of 1.2% hydrogen peroxide, each freshly prepared. Stopper the test tube tightly, and shake until the sample is dissolved. Place into a water bath at 38° for 5 minutes: no color change is observed, indicating the absence of peroxidase activity.

Limit of fat—Transfer about 2 g of Wheat Bran, previously dried in a vacuum oven at 100° for 5 hours and accurately weighed, to an extraction thimble, and mix with an equivalent quantity of dry, clean sand. Place a fat-free cotton or glass wool plug on top of the thimble. Place the thimble in a continuous-extraction apparatus provided with a tared collection flask. Pour about 75 mL of solvent hexane through the sample into the collection flask. Extract at a condensation rate of 5 to 6 drops per second for 4 hours, then at a rate of 2 to 3 drops per second for the next 16 hours. Detach the collection flask, carefully evaporate the solvent, and dry the collection flask and its contents in a drying oven at 100° for 30 minutes to constant weight. Calculate the percentage of the extract (crude fat) in the portion of Wheat Bran taken: not more than 6% is found.

Limit of insect infestation—Prepare a smooth slurry by transferring about 50 g of Wheat Bran to a 1 L beaker and adding 500 mL of 1.5 N hydrochloric acid. Add 50 mL of light mineral oil, and carefully heat to boiling on a hot plate. Boil for 10 minutes to digest, stirring occasionally to prevent scorching. Remove from the hot plate, and stir for 5 minutes with a magnetic stirrer, increasing the stirring speed until a vortex is formed without visible splashing. Quantitatively transfer the contents of the beaker to a separatory funnel with the aid of hot water. Allow to stand for 30 minutes, stirring gently with a glass rod several times during the first 10 minutes. Drain the lower layer to about 2.5 cm from the layer interface. Wash the funnel with hot water, and allow 5 minutes for the layers to separate. Drain the lower layer and wash with cold water several times until the lower phase is clear. Filter the contents of the funnel through ruled filter paper with the aid of a Büchner funnel and suction. Thoroughly rinse the separatory funnel with water and a detergent solution, filtering each rinse through the same paper. Examine the ruled filter paper under a microscope at 30× magnification: not more than 25 insect fragments are seen.

Limit of protein—Place about 1 g of Wheat Bran, accurately weighed, in a 500-mL Kjeldahl flask, and proceed as directed for *Method I* under *Nitrogen Determination* ⟨461⟩. Multiply the percent of nitrogen found by 6.31: not more than 18.5% is found.

Content of total dietary fiber—

Phosphate buffer—Prepare a pH 6.0 phosphate buffer (see *Buffer Solutions* under *Solutions* in the section *Reagents, Indicators, and Solutions*).

Protease solution—Dissolve 5 mg of protease in 0.1 mL of *Phosphate buffer*.

Sample preparation—Prepare two samples in parallel. In order to correct for any contribution from reagents, also perform examinations of blanks, which are treated similarly to the samples. Proceed as directed for *Limit of fat*. Mill to a coarse powder, and store in a desiccator.

Procedure—Transfer about 1.0 g of each *Sample preparation*, accurately weighed, into separate 400-mL, tall-form beakers. Add 50 mL of *Phosphate buffer*, and adjust the pH, if necessary, to 6.0 ± 0.1. Add 0.2 mL of heat-stable α-amylase solution. Cover the beaker with aluminum foil, place in a boiling water bath for 15 minutes at 100°, shaking gently every 5 minutes, and cool to room temperature. Adjust with about 10 mL of 0.275 N sodium hydroxide solution to a pH of 7.5 ± 0.1. Add freshly prepared *Protease solution*, cover the beaker with aluminum foil, and incubate for 30 minutes at 60° with continuous agitation. Cool, and add about 10 mL of 0.325 N hydrochloric acid and adjust to a pH of 4.5 ± 0.2. Add 0.3 mL of amyloglucosidase, cover with aluminum foil, and incubate for 20 minutes at 60° with continuous agitation. Heat 280 mL of alcohol to 60°, add to the digest, and allow the precipitate to form at room temperature for 60 minutes. Place 0.5 g of chromatographic siliceous earth in a crucible with fritted disk, dry at 130° to constant weight, and weigh. Wet the chromatographic siliceous earth in the crucible by using a stream of 78% alcohol from a washing bottle, and apply suction to evenly distribute the chromatographic siliceous earth over the fritted disk. Maintain suction, and quantitatively transfer the enzyme digest precipitate to the crucible. Wash the residue successively with three 20-mL portions of 78% alcohol, two 10-mL portions of alcohol, and two 10-mL portions of acetone. In some cases, gums may form during filtration, trapping liquid in residue. If so, break the surface film with a spatula to improve filtration. Dry the crucible containing the residue at 105° in an air oven for 16 hours, cool in a desiccator, and determine the weight of the residue. Determine the percentage of protein in the first *Sample preparation* as directed for *Limit of protein*. Incinerate the residue from the second *Sample preparation* as directed for *Total Ash* under *Articles of Botanical Origin* ⟨561⟩. Calculate the corrected weight, W, of the sample residue by the formula:

$$W_U (1 - P_U / 100 - A_U / 100) - W_B (1 - P_B / 100 - A_B / 100)$$

in which W_U and W_B are the average weights of the sample residues and the blank residues, respectively; P_U and P_B are percentages of protein present in the sample and in the blank, respectively; and A_U and A_B are percentages of ash found in the sample and in the blank, respectively. Then calculate the percentage of the total dietary fiber in the portion of Wheat Bran taken by the formula:

$$100W / W_I$$

in which W_I is the weight of the *Sample preparation* taken. Correct the final percentage of the total dietary fiber for fat and for water: not less than 36.0% is found.

Witch Hazel

» Witch Hazel is a clear, colorless distillate prepared from recently cut and partially dried dormant twigs of *Hamamelis virginiana* Linné.

Prepare Witch Hazel as follows. Macerate a weighed amount of the twigs for about 24 hours in about twice their weight of water, then distill until not less than 800 mL and not more than 850 mL of clear, colorless distillate is obtained from each 1000 g of the twigs taken. Add 150 mL of Alcohol to each 850 mL of distillate, and mix thoroughly.

Packaging and storage—Preserve in tight containers, and avoid exposure to excessive heat.

Specific gravity ⟨841⟩: between 0.979 and 0.983.

pH ⟨791⟩: between 3.0 and 5.0.

Nonvolatile residue—Evaporate 100 mL to dryness in a tared dish on a hot plate at 60°: the weight of the residue does not exceed 25 mg (0.025%).

Limit of tannins—

Mobile phase A—Adjust 1000 mL of water with phosphoric acid to a pH of 2.5 ± 0.1. Filter and degas.

Mobile phase B—Use filtered and degassed acetonitrile.

Standard solution—Dissolve an accurately weighed quantity of tannic acid in water to obtain a solution having a known concentration of about 0.03 mg of tannic acid per mL.

Test solution—Use Witch Hazel.

Chromatographic system (see *Chromatography* ⟨621⟩)—The liquid chromatograph is equipped with a 280-nm detector and a 5.0-mm × 15-cm column that contains packing L1 and is programmed to provide variable mixtures of *Mobile phase A* and *Mobile phase B*. Initially, the system is held at a mixture consisting of 90% *Mobile phase A* and 10% *Mobile phase B* for 5.0 minutes. The proportion of *Solvent B* to *Solvent A* is increased linearly to 100% over the next 15 minutes. The flow rate is about 1 mL per minute.

Procedure—Separately inject equal volumes (about 25 µL) of the *Standard solution* and the *Test solution* into the chromatograph, record the chromatograms, and measure the responses for all peaks. If any peak corresponding to the retention time of tannic acid in the *Standard solution* is present in the chromatogram of the *Test solution*, its peak area is no more than that of the tannic acid in the *Standard solution*.

Alcohol content, *Method I* ⟨611⟩: between 14.0% and 15.0% of C_2H_5OH.

Small Intestinal Submucosa Wound Matrix

» Small Intestinal Submucosa Wound Matrix is a biologically derived, collagen-based wound care product, translucent and off-white in color. It is obtained from the small intestinal submucosa layer of the domestic pig (*Sus scrofa* L.). This layer has been mechanically separated from the adjoining layers of the intestine to remove the serosal, mucosal, and muscular elements. The isolated submucosa is chemically cleaned, decellularized, freeze-dried, and terminally sterilized. Small Intestinal Submucosa Wound Matrix also undergoes a viral inactivation; the inactivation method is validated using parvovirus, reovirus, pseudorabies virus, and leukemia retrovirus as the test viruses. By dried weight, Small Intestinal Submucosa Wound Matrix consists of about 70 percent protein, about 20 percent carbohydrate, and about 7 percent lipid. The protein component is primarily collagen type I (approximately 90 percent), with minor amounts of elastin and collagen type III, collagen type IV, and collagen type VI. In addition to these components, additional extracellular matrix components, such as glycosaminoglycans and basic fibroblast growth factor, are also retained.

Packaging and storage—Package in single-use, peel-open pouches that are gas permeable for sterilization purposes. Store under clean, dry conditions at 25°, excursions permitted between 15° and 30°.

Labeling—The package is labeled to indicate the dimensions of the enclosed Small Intestinal Submucosa Wound Matrix, the expiry date, required storage conditions, and the lot number. The label indicates that the Wound Matrix is sterile if the package is intact, and that the Wound Matrix is designed for single patient, one-time use.

USP Reference standards ⟨11⟩—*USP Endotoxin RS*.

USP Authentic visual references—*USP Cultured Rat Pheochromocytoma Reference Photomicrographs*. These photomicrographs represent examples of normal and differentiated rat pheochromocytoma cells and are used to assist in ascertaining bioactivity.

Bacterial endotoxins ⟨85⟩—Immerse 70 cm^2 of Small Intestinal Submucosa Wound Matrix in 40 mL of LAL Reagent Water. Extract for 60 minutes at 37° with shaking. Remove a 100-µL aliquot to measure the amount of bacterial endotoxins. It contains not more than 20.0 USP Endotoxin Units per 70 cm^2.

Sterility ⟨71⟩: meets the requirements.

Fibroblast growth factor-2 content—

Sterile PBS solution—Prepare a sterile solution that contains 8065.0 mg and 200.0 mg of sodium chloride and potassium chloride, respectively, per L of 0.01 M sodium phosphate buffer, pH 7.4.

Test solution—Obtain a 1-cm^2 sample of Small Intestinal Submucosa Wound Matrix, weigh, and submerge in 400 µL of *Sterile PBS solution*. Pulverize the tissue for 90 seconds using a tissue grinder, intermittently checking to be sure the tissue remains immersed in the *Sterile PBS solution* and becomes homogenized. Centrifuge at 12,000 × g for 5 minutes at 4°. Use immediately upon preparation. [NOTE—The *Test solution* may be stored for short periods at 4° or on ice.]

Procedure—Examine duplicate aliquots of the *Test solution* by a suitably sensitive ELISA method:[1] the analysis is considered valid if the ELISA kit generates a linear standard curve with the square of the correlation coefficient (r^2) not less than 0.95, and if the duplicate aliquots of the *Test solution* yield results that are within 20% of each other. The average content of fibroblast growth factor-2 is not less than 10,000 pg per g of Small Intestinal Submucosa Wound Matrix.

Glycosaminoglycan content—

1,9-Dimethylmethylene blue solution—Mix 95 mL of 0.1 M hydrochloric acid in 500 mL of water. Add 16 mg of 1,9-dimethylmethylene blue, 3.04 g of aminoacetic acid, and 2.37 g of sodium chloride. Dilute with water to 1 L, and adjust to a pH of 3.0 using sterile solutions of either 1.0 M sodium hydroxide or 1.0 M hydrochloric acid. Store in low-actinic glassware.

Sterile PBS solution—Prepare as directed under *Fibroblast growth factor-2 content*.

Proteinase K solution—Prepare a solution of *Tritirachium album* proteinase K in water having an activity of 600 units per mL.

Stock heparin standard solution—Prepare a solution containing 1 mg of heparin per mL of water.

Heparin standard curve solutions—Using the *Stock heparin standard solution*, prepare three solutions containing 20 µg per mL, 50 µg per mL, and 100 µg per mL of heparin, respectively.

Blank solution—Use water.

Test solution—Prepare test samples in duplicate. Accurately weigh about 25 mg of Small Intestinal Submucosa Wound Matrix and cut into small pieces (roughly 2 mm × 2 mm). Transfer to a 1.5-mL microcentrifuge tube, and add 180 µL of *Sterile PBS solution* and 20 µL of *Proteinase K solution*. Mix, and incubate the sample at 56° for 15 minutes; during the incubation mix intermittently on a vortex mixer. Cool the sample to room temperature. Dilute with water to obtain a concentration of 12.5 mg of digested Small Intestinal Submucosa Wound Matrix per mL.

Collagen control solution—Accurately weigh about 25 mg of a bovine collagen, type I, that contains less than 1 µg of glycosaminoglycan per mg. Transfer to a 1.5-mL microcentrifuge tube, and add 180 µL of *Sterile PBS solution* and 20 µL of *Proteinase K solution*. Mix, and incubate the sample at 56° for 15 minutes; during the incubation mix intermittently on a vortex mixer. Cool the sample to room temperature. Dilute with water to obtain a concentration of 12.5 mg of digested bovine collagen per mL.

Procedure (see *Spectrophotometry and Light-Scattering ⟨851⟩*)—To triplicate 100-µL aliquots each of *Heparin standard curve solutions*, *Blank solution*, *Test solution*, and *Collagen control solution*, add 2.5 mL of *1,9-Dimethylmethylene blue solution*. Mix on a vortex mixer for 1 second and immediately read the absorbance at 525 nm. Generate a standard curve of absorbance versus concentration using the averages of each *Heparin standard curve solution*, correcting for the blank, and calculate the regression line and regression coefficient. The concentration of glycosaminoglycan in the *Test solution* and the *Collagen control solution* is determined directly from the regression line. If the absorbance of the *Test solution* is greater than the highest *Heparin standard curve solution*, then dilute the *Test solution* appropriately, and repeat the *Procedure* beginning with "To triplicate 100-µL aliquots." The test is considered valid if the regression curve has a square of the correlation coefficient (r^2) not less than 0.95; the triplicate aliquots of the *Test solution* and *Collagen control solution* yield results that are within 20% of each other, respectively; and the average glycosaminoglycan content of the *Test solution* is statistically greater than the *Collagen control solution* using one-tailed, unequal variances, t-test at α = 0.05. The average glycosaminoglycan content of the *Test solution* is not less than 2 µg per mg.

Metabolic activity assessment—

Dulbecco's modified Eagle's tissue culture medium—Prepare a solution that contains the components included in the following *Table 1*:

Table 1

Component	Content (mg per L)
Calcium nitrate, tetrahydrate	100.0
Ferric nitrate, nonahydrate	0.10
Potassium chloride	400.0
Magnesium sulfate, anhydrous	48.840

---

[1] A suitably sensitive ELISA test kit for the quantitation can be obtained from R&D Systems Inc., 614 McKinley Place N.E., Minneapolis, MN (www.bioscience.org/company/r&d.htm); product number DFB50.

Table 1 *(Continued)*

Component	Content (mg per L)
Sodium chloride	6,000.0
Sodium bicarbonate	1,500.0
Sodium phosphate, dibasic (anhydrous)	800.0
Glucose	4,500.0
Glutathione (reduced)	1.0
Phenol red	5.0
Sodium pyruvate	110.0
L-Arginine (free base)	200.0
L-Asparagine, monohydrate	56.620
L-Aspartic Acid	20.0
L-Cystine dihydrochloride	65.20
Aminoacetic acid	10.0
L-Histidine (free base)	15.0
Hydroxy-L-proline	20.0
L-Isoleucine	50.0
L-Leucine	50.0
L-Lysine hydrochloride	40.0
L-Methionine	15.0
L-Phenylalanine	15.0
L-Proline	20.0
L-Serine	30.0
L-Threonine	20.0
L-Tryptophan	5.0
L-Tyrosine, disodium, dihydrate	28.830
L-Valine	20.0
D-Biotin	0.20
D-Calcium pantothenate	2.50
Choline chloride	3.0
Folic acid	1.0
Inositol	35.0
Nicotinamide	1.0
p-Aminobenzoic acid	1.0
Pyridoxine hydrochloride	1.0
Riboflavin	0.20
Thiamine hydrochloride	1.0
Cyanocobalamine	0.0050

MTT reagent—Use a suitable solution of 3-(4,5-dimethylthiazol-2yl)-2,5-diphenyl tetrazolium bromide.[2]

Detergent reagent—Use a suitable sodium dodecyl sulfate detergent solution.[3]

Procedure—Remove three 12-mm diameter circular sections of Small Intestinal Submucosa Wound Matrix, using the appropriate size biopsy punch. Immerse each section into individual wells of a 12-well cell culture plate (dimension of each well is about 22 to 23 mm in diameter and about 17 to 18 mm in depth), each containing 1 mL of *Dulbecco's modified Eagle's tissue culture medium*. Prepare a positive control by harvesting a full-thickness section of porcine jejunum immediately following slaughter. Rinse the section of jejunum in 37° isotonic sodium chloride solution for 5 minutes to remove intestinal debris. Using scissors, split open the section of jejunum to form a sheet. Remove three 12-mm diameter circular sections of jejunum, using the appropriate size biopsy punch. Immerse each section into individual wells of a 12-well cell culture plate, each well containing 1 mL of *Dulbecco's modified Eagle's tissue culture medium*. Treat these positive control wells in the same manner as the test wells. Prepare a blank solution using 1 mL of *Dulbecco's modified Eagle's tissue culture medium*. Allow sections to hydrate for 5 minutes, add 50 µL of *MTT reagent* to each of the sections and the blank, and mix. Incubate for 3 hours at 37° in an atmosphere containing 5% carbon dioxide. Add 100 µL of *Detergent reagent* to each well, and mix. Leave the samples at ambient temperature in the dark for 2 hours. Measure the absorbance of the resulting solution at 570 nm, adjusting for the blank. For the test to be valid, the average absorbance in the positive control wells is greater than 0.100. The average absorbance reading for the Small Intestinal Submucosa Wound Matrix wells is less than 0.100.

Bioactivity—[NOTE—Aseptic cell culture techniques should be employed throughout the performance of this test.]

Modified RPMI-1640 culture medium—Prepare a sterile solution that contains the components included in the following *Table 2*:

Table 2

Component	Content (mg per L)
Calcium chloride	264.9
Ferric nitrate, nonahydrate	0.10
Potassium chloride	400.0
Magnesium sulfate, heptahydrate	200.0
Sodium chloride	6,400.0
Sodium bicarbonate	3,700.0
Sodium phosphate, monobasic, monohydrate	125.0
Glucose	4,500.0
Phenol red	15.0
Sodium pyruvate	110.0
L-Arginine hydrochloride	84.0
L-Cystine	48.0
Aminoacetic acid	30.0
L-Histidine hydrochloride, monohydrate	42.0
L-Isoleucine	104.8
L-Leucine	104.8
L-Lysine hydrochloride	146.2
L-Methionine	30.0
L-Phenylalanine	66.0
L-Serine	42.0
L-Threonine	95.2
L-Tryptophan	16.0
L-Tyrosine	72.0
L-Valine	93.6
L-Calcium pantothenate	4.0
Choline chloride	4.0
Folic acid	4.0
Inositol	7.0
Nicotinamide	4.0
Pyridoxine hydrochloride	4.0
Riboflavin	0.40
Thiamine hydrochloride	4.0
Sodium 1-heptanesulfonic acid	2383.0

Penicillin–streptomycin solution—Prepare a suitable buffered solution containing 10,000 USP Penicillin Units of penicillin per mL and 10 mg of streptomycin per mL.[4]

PC12 cell line culture medium—Mix 420 mL of *Modified RPMI-1640 culture medium*, 50 mL of horse serum,[5] 25 mL of fetal bovine serum,[6] and 5 mL of *Penicillin–streptomycin solution*. Sterilize by passing through a 0.22-µm filter.

Sterile PBS solution—Prepare as directed under *Fibroblast growth factor-2 content*.

---

[2] A suitable solution of 3-(4,5-dimethylthiazol-2yl)-2,5-diphenyl tetrazolium bromide can be obtained from American Type Culture Collection, P.O. Box 1549, Manassas, VA (www.atcc.org).

[3] A suitable sodium dodecyl sulfate detergent reagent can be obtained from American Type Culture Collection, P.O. Box 1549, Manassas, VA (www.atcc.org).

[4] A suitable buffered solution containing 10,000 USP Penicillin Units of penicillin per mL and 10 mg streptomycin per mL can be obtained from Sigma-Aldrich Corp., St. Louis, MO (www.sigma-aldrich.com).

[5] A suitable horse serum can be obtained from American Type Culture Collection, P.O. Box 1549, Manassas, VA (www.atcc.org).

[6] A suitable fetal bovine serum can be obtained from American Type Culture Collection, P.O. Box 1549, Manassas, VA (www.atcc.org).

Rat tail collagen solution—Prepare a suspension containing 0.2 mg of rat tail collagen, type I, in sterile water.

Cell culture apparatus—Prepare by adding a sufficient volume of *Rat tail collagen solution* to completely cover the bottom of each well of a 12-well cell culture plate (dimension of each well is about 22 to 23 mm in diameter and about 17 to 18 mm in depth). Incubate under sterile conditions for 2 hours at 37° or overnight at room temperature. Remove the *Rat tail collagen solution* by aspiration. Rinse with *Sterile PBS solution* that has been preheated to 37°.

PC12 cells—Use cultured rat pheochromocytoma cells (ATCC CRL-1721).

Cultivation of PC12 cells—Starting from a frozen culture, prewarm *PC12 cell line culture medium* to 37°. Add 15 mL of prewarmed *PC12 cell line culture medium* to a T-75 culture flask. Place a single vial containing the frozen *PC12 cells* in a 37° water bath with gentle agitation until they start to thaw (about 1 minute). Complete the thawing procedure by slowly rotating the vial between the hands. Rinse the outside of the vial with 70 percent alcohol. Transfer the contents of the vial to the T-75 flask, and mix. Incubate the cells overnight at 37° in a 5% carbon dioxide atmosphere. Transfer the contents of the T-75 culture flask to a sterile centrifuge tube, centrifuge at $200 \times g$ for 5 minutes at 37°, and discard the supernatant. Resuspend the cells in 15 mL of *PC12 cell line culture medium,* and transfer the contents back into the T-75 culture flask. Incubate the cells at 37° in a 5% carbon dioxide atmosphere for 3 days.

Cell feeding—At the end of 3 days, the cells will need to be fed for optimal growth. To feed the cells, remove a flask of cells from the incubator, tightening the cap in the process. Examine the T-75 flask under the microscope and check for microbial contamination and confluency. If there is microbial contamination, then discard the flask. If the cells appear confluent, follow the instructions below for perpetuating the PC12 cell line (see *Culture perpetuation*). Otherwise, harvest the cells from the flask by pipeting the contents of the flask across the bottom of the flask several times. Transfer the cell suspension to a sterile 50-mL centrifuge tube. Centrifuge the cells at $200 \times g$ for 5 minutes at 37°, and discard the supernatant. Resuspend the cells in 13 mL of *PC12 cell line culture medium,* prewarmed to 37°. Transfer the cell suspension back to the T-75 flask, and mix. Loosen the cap of the flask, and return to the incubator; incubate the cells at 37° in a 5% carbon dioxide atmosphere for another 3 to 7 days.

Culture perpetuation—To perpetuate a line of *PC12 cells* for culture, examine under the microscope a T-75 flask containing cells and check for microbial contamination and confluency. If there is microbial contamination, discard the flask and use another. If the cells do not appear confluent, then follow the instructions above for feeding the PC12 cell line (see *Cell feeding*), beginning with "Otherwise, harvest the cells from the flask by pipeting the contents of the flask across the bottom of the flask several times." If the cells are confluent and there is no contamination, harvest the cells from the flask by pipeting the contents of the flask across the bottom of the flask several times to loosen up the cells from their attachment to the bottom of the flask and to break up cell clusters. Check under the microscope prior to proceeding to ensure that most of the cells have detached from the plastic. Transfer the cell suspension to a sterile 50-mL centrifuge tube, and centrifuge the cells at $200 \times g$ for 5 minutes at 37°. Discard the supernatant and resuspend the cells with 10 mL of *PC12 cell line culture medium,* prewarmed to 37°. Dispense an equal amount of the cell suspension into each of three to five T-75 flasks, each flask containing 10 mL of *PC12 cell line culture medium,* prewarmed to 37°, and mix. Return the passed cells to the incubator, being sure to loosen the cap of the flasks. Incubate the cells at 37° in a 5% carbon dioxide atmosphere. Feed the cells after 3 days as directed above, beginning with "To feed the cells, remove a flask of cells from the incubator, tightening the cap in the process." [NOTE—To perform the test for *Bioactivity,* cells that have undergone more than 15 passages after obtaining them from ATCC should not be used.]

Positive control solution—Prepare a solution containing about 10 ng of fibroblast growth factor-2 per mL of *PC12 cell line culture medium.*

Negative control solution—Use *PC12 cell line culture medium.*

Test solution—Immerse 70 cm^2 of Small Intestinal Submucosa Wound Matrix in sterile water for 5 minutes. Remove the Small Intestinal Submucosa Wound Matrix, and blot excess water using sterile gauze. Weigh the rehydrated Small Intestinal Submucosa Wound Matrix to the nearest 0.1 g and add *Modified RPMI-1640 culture medium* at a ratio of 7.5 mL of *Modified RPMI-1640 culture medium* for each 1.0 g of Small Intestinal Submucosa Wound Matrix. Incubate for 24 hours at 37° with constant shaking. Remove the Small Intestinal Submucosa Wound Matrix, and pass the solution through a 0.22-μm filter. Add sufficient quantities of sterile horse serum and sterile fetal bovine serum to concentrations of 10% and 5%, respectively, and add a sufficient quantity of *Penicillin–streptomycin solution* such that there are 100 USP Penicillin Units and 0.1 mg of streptomycin per mL. Adjust the pH of the *Test solution* to 7.4, using a sterile solution of either 1.0 M sodium hydroxide or 1.0 M hydrochloric acid.

Procedure—Harvest a flask of confluent *PC12 cells* by centrifuging at $200 \times g$ for 5 minutes. Remove the supernatant by aspiration, and resuspend the pellet to obtain a concentration of about 1×10^6 cells per mL of *PC12 cell line culture medium*. Add to each of three wells of the *Cell culture apparatus* 1.0 mL of *Negative control solution*. To a second set of three wells add to each 1.0 mL of *Positive control solution,* and to a third set of three wells add to each 1.0 mL of *Test solution*. Add to each well about 20,000 cells, mix by gentle rocking, and incubate for 48 hours at 37°. For each well, count three random microscopic fields of cells using a microscope with a 10× ocular lens and a 20× objective lens. Each field should have at least 20 cells; avoid large clumps of cells where individual cell bodies cannot be ascertained. Determine the total number of cells in the field and, using USP Cultured Rat Pheochromocytoma Reference Photomicrographs of normal and differentiated rat pheochromocytoma cells for comparison, determine the total number of cells that have formed at least one neurite-like extension at least twice the diameter of a normal, undifferentiated cell body. For each experimental group, record the total number of cells counted and the total number of cells differentiated across all three wells, and calculate the total percentage of cells that have differentiated. For a test to be valid, the following criteria must be met: (1) none of the wells are microbially contaminated; (2) the weighted percentage of differentiated cells across the *Negative control solution* wells is less than 5%; (3) the weighted percentage of differentiated cells across the *Positive control solution* wells is greater than 6%; and (4) the weighted percentage of differentiated cells across the *Negative control solution* wells is statistically less than the weighted percentage of differentiated cells across the *Positive control solution* wells, using a one-sided, two-sample test for proportions at α = 0.05. The weighted percentage of differentiated cells incubated in the *Test solution* wells is statistically greater than those incubated in the *Negative control solution* wells, using a one-sided, two-sample test for proportions at α = 0.05.

Xenon Xe 127

» Xenon Xe 127 is a gas suitable for inhalation in diagnostic studies. Xenon 127 is a radioactive nuclide that may be prepared from the bombardment of a cesium 133 target with high-energy protons. It contains not less than 85.0 percent and not more than 115.0 percent of the labeled amount of ^{127}Xe at the calibration date indicated on the labeling.

Packaging and storage—Preserve in single-dose vials having leak-proof stoppers, at room temperature. The vials are enclosed in appropriate lead radiation shields. The vial content may be diluted with air and is packaged at atmospheric pressure.

Labeling—Label it to include the following: the name of the preparation; the container volume, MBq (mCi) of ^{127}Xe per container; the amount of ^{127}Xe expressed as megabecquerels (millicuries) per mL; the intended route of administration; recommended storage conditions; the date of calibration; the expiration date; the name, address, and batch number of the manufacturer; the statement "Caution—Radioactive Material"; and a radioactive symbol. The labeling con-

tains a statement of radionuclide purity, identifies probable radionuclidic impurities, and indicates permissible quantities of each impurity. The labeling indicates that in making dosage calculations, correction is to be made for radioactive decay, and also indicates that the radioactive half-life of ^{127}Xe is 36.41 days.
Radionuclide identification (see *Radioactivity* ⟨821⟩)—Its gamma-ray spectrum is identical to that of a known specimen of xenon 127 that exhibits major photopeaks at 202.8 keV, and 172.1 keV, and 375.0 keV. Minor photopeaks from other xenon radioisotopes, namely Xe 129m (197 keV) and Xe 131m (164 keV) may also be present.
Radionuclidic purity—Using a suitable counting assembly (see *Selection of a Counting Assembly* under *Radioactivity* ⟨821⟩), determine the radioactivity of the Xe 127 in the gas by use of a calibrated system as directed under *Radioactivity* ⟨821⟩. Using the gamma-ray spectrum, determine the energy of each gamma photopeak. Identify each radionuclide present, and using the established detector efficiency and known gamma abundance, calculate the quantity of each radionuclide present in the specimen in MBq (mCi). The amount of Xe 127 present in the specimen is not less than 80%; the quantity of either Xe 131m or Xe 129m does not exceed 10%, and no other radioisotope exceeds 1%.
Assay for radioactivity—Using a suitable counting assembly (see *Selection of a Counting Assembly* under *Radioactivity* ⟨821⟩), determine the radioactivity, in MBq (mCi), of Xe 127 in each container by use of a calibrated system as directed under *Radioactivity* ⟨821⟩.

Xenon Xe 133

Xenon, isotope of mass 133.
Xenon, isotope of mass 133   [14932-42-4].

» Xenon Xe 133 is a gas suitable for inhalation in diagnostic studies. Xenon 133 is a radioactive nuclide that may be prepared from the fission of uranium 235. It contains not less than 85.0 percent and not more than 115.0 percent of the labeled amount of ^{133}Xe at the date and time indicated in the labeling.

Packaging and storage—Preserve in single-dose or in multiple-dose vials having leak-proof stoppers, at room temperature.
Other requirements—It meets the requirements for *Labeling*, except for the information specified for *Labeling* under *Injections;* for *Radionuclide identification;* and for *Radionuclidic purity* and *Assay for radioactivity* under *Xenon Xe 133 Injection*, except to determine the radioactivity in MBq (mCi) per container.

Xenon Xe 133 Injection

» Xenon Xe 133 Injection is a sterile, isotonic solution of Xenon 133 in Sodium Chloride Injection suitable for intravenous administration. Xenon 133 is a radioactive nuclide prepared from the fission of uranium 235. It contains not less than 90.0 percent and not more than 110.0 percent of the labeled amount of Xenon 133 at the date and time stated on the label.

Packaging and storage—Preserve in single-dose containers that are totally filled, so that any air present occupies not more than 0.5% of the total volume of the container. Store at a temperature between 2° and 8°. If there is free space above the solution, a significant amount of the xenon 133 is present in the gaseous phase. Glass containers may darken under the effects of radiation.
Labeling—Label it to include the following, in addition to the information specified for *Labeling* under *Injections* ⟨1⟩: the time and date of calibration; the amount of xenon 133 expressed as total megabecquerels (microcuries or millicuries), and concentration as megabecquerels (microcuries or millicuries), per mL at the time of calibration; the expiration date; the name and amount of any added bacteriostatic agent; and the statement "Caution—Radioactive Material." The labeling indicates that in making dosage calculations, correction is to be made for radioactive decay, and also indicates that the radioactive half-life of ^{133}Xe is 5.24 days.
USP Reference standards ⟨11⟩—*USP Endotoxin RS*.
Radionuclide identification (see *Radioactivity* ⟨821⟩)—Its gamma-ray and X-ray spectra are identical to those of a known specimen of xenon 133 that exhibits two major photopeaks having energies of 0.081 MeV and 0.031 MeV (X-ray peak).
Bacterial endotoxins ⟨85⟩—It contains not more than 175/V USP Endotoxin Unit per mL of the Injection, when compared with the USP Endotoxin RS, in which V is the maximum recommended total dose, in mL, at the expiration date or time.
pH ⟨791⟩:   between 4.5 and 8.0.
Radionuclidic purity—Using a suitable counting assembly (see *Selection of a Counting Assembly* under *Radioactivity* ⟨821⟩), determine the radioactivity of Xe 133 in the Injection by use of a calibrated system as directed under *Radioactivity* ⟨821⟩. The radioactivity exhibited at 0.081 MeV and 0.031 MeV is not less than 95.0% of the total radioactivity of the specimen.
Other requirements—It meets the requirements under *Injections* ⟨1⟩, except that the Injection may be distributed or dispensed prior to the completion of the test for *Sterility*, the latter test being started on the day of manufacture, and except that it is not subject to the recommendation on *Volume in Container*.
Assay for radioactivity—Using a suitable counting assembly (see *Selection of a Counting Assembly* under *Radioactivity* ⟨821⟩), determine the radioactivity, in MBq (mCi) per mL, of Injection by use of a calibrated system as directed under *Radioactivity* ⟨821⟩.

Xylazine

$C_{12}H_{16}N_2S$ 220.34
4H-1,3-Thiazin-2-amine, N-(2,6-dimethylphenyl)-5,6-dihydro-.
5,6-Dihydro-2-(2,6-xylidino)-4H-1,3-thiazine   [7361-61-7].

» Xylazine contains not less than 98.0 percent and not more than 102.0 percent of $C_{12}H_{16}N_2S$.

Packaging and storage—Preserve in tight containers. Store at 25°, excursions permitted between 15° and 30°.
Labeling—Where it is intended for veterinary use only, the label so states.
USP Reference standards ⟨11⟩—*USP Xylazine RS*.
Identification—
  A: *Infrared Absorption* ⟨197K⟩.
  B: *Ultraviolet Absorption* ⟨197U⟩—
  Solution: 5 µg per mL.
  Medium: 0.1 N hydrochloric acid.
  C: *Thin-Layer Chromatographic Identification Test* ⟨201⟩—
  Test solution: 2 mg per mL, in chloroform.
  Developing solvent system: acetone, chloroform, and methanol (2 : 1 : 1).
  Procedure—Prior to the applications of the *Test solution* and the *Standard solution*, dry the plate at 105° for not less than 30 minutes, and allow it to cool in a desiccator. Allow the applications to dry with the aid of a current of warm air, and develop. Examine under short-wavelength UV light: the size, intensity, and R_F value of the principal spot obtained from the *Test solution* correspond to those of the principal spot obtained from the *Standard solution*.
Melting range ⟨741⟩:   between 136° and 142°.
Loss on drying ⟨731⟩—Dry it in vacuum at 60° for 4 hours: it loses not more than 0.5% of its weight.

Residue on ignition ⟨281⟩: not more than 0.1%.
Heavy metals, *Method II* ⟨231⟩: 20 µg per g.
Limit of 3-amino-1-propanol—Prepare a test solution of Xylazine in methanol containing 100 mg per mL, using sonication to achieve dissolution. Prepare a Standard solution of 3-amino-1-propanol in methanol containing 0.5 mg per mL. Separately apply 5 µL of the test solution and the Standard solution to a thin-layer chromatographic plate (see *Chromatography* ⟨621⟩) coated with a 0.25-mm layer of chromatographic silica gel. Allow the applications to dry, and develop the chromatograms in a saturated chromatographic chamber, containing a solvent system consisting of a mixture of alcohol and ammonium hydroxide (80 : 20) until the solvent front has moved about three-fourths of the length of the plate. Remove the plate from the chromatographic chamber, mark the solvent front, and air-dry the plate. Spray the plate with an alcoholic solution of ninhydrin (1 in 500), and immediately heat the plate in an oven at 105°. When the spots are visible, remove the plate from the oven, and allow to cool. Examine the chromatograms, and compare the intensities of the spots corresponding to 3-amino-1-propanol: the intensity of the spot for 3-amino-1-propanol obtained from the test solution is not greater than that of the spot for 3-amino-1-propanol obtained from the Standard solution (0.5%).

Limit of acetone and isopropyl alcohol—
Diluent—Dilute 15 mL of glacial acetic acid with water to 1000 mL, and mix.
Standard solution—Transfer 10.0 µL each of acetone and isopropyl alcohol to a 500-mL volumetric flask, dilute with *Diluent* to volume, and mix. This solution contains 15.8 µg of acetone per mL and 15.7 µg of isopropyl alcohol per mL.
Test solution—Transfer about 100 mg of Xylazine, accurately weighed, to a 10-mL volumetric flask, dissolve in and dilute with *Diluent* to volume, and mix.
Chromatographic system (see *Chromatography* ⟨621⟩)—The gas chromatograph is equipped with a flame-ionization detector and a 2-mm × 1.8-m column packed with 0.1% phase G25 on 80- to 100-mesh support S7. Helium is used as the carrier gas with a flow rate of about 30 mL per minute. The injection port and detector temperatures are maintained at about 240° and 275°, respectively. The system is programmed according to the following steps. The column temperature is maintained at 30° for 6 minutes after each injection, then increased to 100° at a rate of 10° per minute, then increased further to 220° at a rate of 15° per minute, and maintained for 10 minutes. Chromatograph the *Standard solution*, and record the peak responses as directed for *Procedure*: the relative retention times are about 0.75 for acetone and 1.0 for isopropyl alcohol; the resolution, R, between acetone and isopropyl alcohol is not less than 2.0; the tailing factor determined from each analyte peak is not more than 2.0; and the relative standard deviation for replicate injections is not more than 2.0%.
Procedure—Separately inject equal volumes (about 2 µL) of the *Standard solution* and the *Test solution* into the chromatograph, record the chromatograms, and measure the areas for the major peaks. Calculate the percentages of acetone and isopropyl alcohol in the portion of Xylazine taken by the formula:

$$(C/W)(r_U/r_S)$$

in which C is the concentration, in µg per mL, of acetone or isopropyl alcohol in each mL of the *Standard solution*; W is the weight, in mg, of Xylazine taken to prepare the *Test solution*; and r_U and r_S are the responses for the relevant analyte peak obtained from the *Test solution* and the *Standard solution*, respectively: not more than 0.02% of acetone and not more than 0.2% of isopropyl alcohol are found.

Chromatographic purity—
Solution A, Solution B, Mobile phase, and *Diluent*—Proceed as directed in the *Assay*.
Standard solution—Quantitatively dilute an accurately measured volume of the *Standard preparation* prepared in the *Assay* with *Diluent* to obtain a solution having a concentration of 0.008 mg of USP Xylazine RS per mL.
Test solution—Transfer about 100 mg of Xylazine, accurately weighed, to a 10-mL volumetric flask, add 5.0 mL of *Solution B*, and swirl to dissolve. Add about 4 mL of *Solution A*, and swirl. Dilute with *Solution A* to volume, and mix.

Chromatographic system (see *Chromatography* ⟨621⟩)—The liquid chromatograph is equipped with a 205-nm detector and a 4.6-mm × 25-cm column that contains packing L7 and a guard column. The flow rate is about 1 mL per minute. Equilibrate the column with a mobile phase consisting of 75% *Solution A* and 25% *Solution B*. Maintain this composition for 8 minutes following each injection, after which the proportion of *Solution B* is increased linearly from 25% to 70% over a period of 27 minutes, and maintained at that composition for 5 minutes; then rapidly increase the proportion of *Solution A* to 75% before the next injection. Chromatograph the *Standard solution*, and record the peak responses as directed for *Procedure*: the tailing factor is not more than 1.5; and the relative standard deviation for replicate injections is not more than 5.0%.
Procedure—Separately inject equal volumes (about 10 µL) of the *Standard solution* and the *Test solution* into the chromatograph, record the chromatograms, and measure the areas for the major peaks. Calculate the percentage of each impurity in the Xylazine taken by the formula:

$$1000(C/W)(r_i F/r_S)$$

in which C is the concentration, in mg per mL, of USP Xylazine RS in the *Standard solution*; W is the weight, in mg, of Xylazine taken to prepare the *Test solution*; r_i is the response of any individual impurity peak in the chromatogram of the *Test solution* that is not present in the chromatogram of the *Diluent*; F is the response factor of 0.72 for the 2,6-dimethylaniline peak at a response time of about 0.8 relative to the retention time of xylazine, of 0.36 for an impurity at a relative retention time of about 1.3, 0.37 for 2,6-dimethylphenyl isothiocyanate at a relative retention time of about 2, and 1.0 for any other impurity; and r_S is the response of the xylazine peak in the chromatogram of the *Standard solution*: not more than 0.5% of any individual impurity is found; and the sum of all impurities found is not more than 1%.

Assay—
Solution A—Dissolve 3.03 g of sodium 1-heptanesulfonate in 800 mL of water, adjust with 2 N sulfuric acid to a pH of 3.0, dilute with water to 1000 mL, and mix. Pass through a filter having a 0.5-µm or finer porosity.
Solution B—Use acetonitrile.
Mobile phase—Use variable mixtures of *Solution A* and *Solution B* as directed for *Chromatographic system*.
Diluent—Prepare a mixture of *Solution A* and *Solution B* (50 : 50).
Standard preparation—Prepare a solution of USP Xylazine RS in *Diluent* having a known concentration of about 0.4 mg per mL.
Assay preparation—Transfer about 10 mg of Xylazine, accurately weighed, to a 25-mL volumetric flask, dilute with *Diluent* to volume, and mix.
Chromatographic system (see *Chromatography* ⟨621⟩)—The liquid chromatograph is equipped with a 226-nm detector and a 3.9-mm × 30-cm column that contains packing L1. The flow rate is about 1 mL per minute. Equilibrate the column with a mobile phase consisting of 70% *Solution A* and 30% *Solution B*. Maintain this composition for 5 minutes following each injection, after which the proportion of *Solution B* is increased linearly from 30% to 40% over a period of 5 minutes, and maintained at that composition for 5 minutes; then rapidly increase the proportion of *Solution A* to 70% before the next injection. Chromatograph the *Standard preparation*, and record the peak responses as directed for *Procedure*: the tailing factor is not more than 2.0; and the relative standard deviation for replicate injections is not more than 2.0%.
Procedure—Separately inject equal volumes (about 10 µL) of the *Standard preparation* and the *Assay preparation* into the chromatograph, record the chromatograms, and measure the areas for the major peaks. Calculate the quantity, in mg, of $C_{12}H_{16}N_2S$ in the portion of Xylazine taken by the formula:

$$25C(r_U/r_S)$$

in which C is the concentration, in mg per mL, of USP Xylazine RS in the *Standard preparation*; and r_U and r_S are the xylazine peak responses obtained from the *Assay preparation* and the *Standard preparation*, respectively.

Xylazine Hydrochloride

$C_{12}H_{16}N_2S \cdot HCl$ 256.80
4H-1,3-Thiazin-2-amine, N-(2,6-dimethylphenyl)-5,6-dihydro-, monohydrochloride.
5,6-Dihydro-2-(2,6-xylidino)-4H-1,3-thiazine hydrochloride [23076-35-9].

» Xylazine Hydrochloride contains not less than 98.0 percent and not more than 102.0 percent of $C_{12}H_{16}N_2S \cdot HCl$.

Packaging and storage—Preserve in tight containers. Store at 25°, excursions permitted between 15° and 30°.
Labeling—Where it is intended for veterinary use only, the label so states.
USP Reference standards ⟨11⟩—*USP Xylazine Hydrochloride RS.*
Identification—
  A: *Infrared Absorption* ⟨197K⟩.
  B: *Thin-Layer Chromatographic Identification Test* ⟨201⟩—
  Test solution: 5 mg per mL, in methanol.
  Developing solvent system: methanol and ammonium hydroxide (98.5 : 1.5).
  Procedure—Separately apply 1 µL of the *Test solution* and the *Standard solution*. Allow the applications to dry with the aid of a stream of nitrogen, develop in a saturated chromatographic chamber, and dry the plate in a current of air: the size, intensity, and R_F value of the principal spot obtained from the *Test solution* correspond to those of the principal spot obtained from the *Standard solution*.
Melting range ⟨741⟩: between 164° and 168°.
pH ⟨791⟩: between 4.0 and 6.0, in a solution (1 in 100).
Loss on drying ⟨731⟩—Dry it at 105° for 4 hours: it loses not more than 1.0% of its weight.
Residue on ignition ⟨281⟩: not more than 0.1%.
Heavy metals, *Method II* ⟨231⟩: 20 µg per g.
Chromatographic purity—Examine the chromatogram obtained from the *Assay preparation*. Calculate the percentage of impurities in the Xylazine Hydrochloride taken by the formula:

$$100 r_s / (r_U + r_s)$$

in which r_s is the sum of the areas of all the impurity peaks observed; and r_U is the area of the xylazine peak: the sum of the impurity responses is not greater than 2.0%.
Assay—
  Mobile phase—Dissolve 6.0 g of sodium 1-heptanesulfonate in 2500 mL of water, add 60 mL of glacial acetic acid, dilute with water to 3000 mL, and mix. Prepare a mixture of 2200 mL of this solution and 1800 mL of methanol, and pass through a filter having a 0.5-µm or finer porosity. Make adjustments if necessary (see *System Suitability* under *Chromatography* ⟨621⟩).
  Standard preparation—Prepare a solution of USP Xylazine Hydrochloride RS in *Mobile phase* having a known concentration of about 1 mg per mL.
  Assay preparation—Transfer about 25 mg of Xylazine Hydrochloride, accurately weighed, to a 25-mL volumetric flask, dissolve in and dilute with *Mobile phase* to volume, and mix.
  Chromatographic system (see *Chromatography* ⟨621⟩)—The liquid chromatograph is equipped with a 254-nm detector, a 2-mm × 2-cm guard column that contains packing L1, and a 3.9-mm × 30-cm analytical column that contains packing L1 and is maintained at a constant temperature of about 40°. The flow rate is about 2.5 mL per minute. Chromatograph the *Standard preparation*, and record the peak responses as directed for *Procedure*: the relative standard deviation for replicate injections is not more than 2.0%. [NOTE—After daily use, rinse the column with 100 mL of acetonitrile and with 100 mL of methanol, and store the column containing methanol.]
  Procedure—Separately inject equal volumes (about 20 µL) of the *Standard preparation* and the *Assay preparation* into the chromatograph, record the chromatograms, and measure the responses for the major peaks. Calculate the quantity, in mg, of $C_{12}H_{16}N_2S \cdot HCl$ in the portion of Xylazine Hydrochloride taken by the formula:

$$25C(r_U / r_S)$$

in which C is the concentration, in mg per mL, of USP Xylazine Hydrochloride RS in the *Standard preparation*; and r_U and r_S are the areas of the xylazine peak responses in the chromatograms obtained from the *Assay preparation* and the *Standard preparation*, respectively.

Xylazine Injection

» Xylazine Injection is a sterile solution of Xylazine in Water for Injection prepared with the aid of Hydrochloric Acid or a sterile solution of Xylazine Hydrochloride in Water for Injection. It contains the equivalent of not less than 90.0 percent and not more than 110.0 percent of the labeled amount of xylazine ($C_{12}H_{16}N_2S$).

Packaging and storage—Preserve in single-dose or multiple-dose containers.
Labeling—Where it is intended for veterinary use only, the label so states.
USP Reference standards ⟨11⟩—*USP Xylazine Hydrochloride RS. USP Endotoxin RS.*
Identification—
  A: *Ultraviolet Absorption* ⟨197U⟩—
  Solution: 5 µg per mL.
  Medium: 0.1 N hydrochloric acid.
  B: Transfer a volume of Injection equivalent to about 50 mg of xylazine to a separator, add 1 mL of sodium carbonate solution (1 in 20), and extract with four 10-mL portions of methylene chloride, combining the methylene chloride extracts in a beaker and evaporating to dryness. Add 10 mL of methanol to the beaker, and swirl to dissolve the residue. The test solution thus obtained responds to *Identification* test *B* under *Xylazine Hydrochloride*.
Bacterial endotoxins ⟨85⟩—It contains not more than 1.7 USP Endotoxin Units per mg of xylazine.
Sterility ⟨71⟩—It meets the requirements when tested as directed for *Membrane Filtration* under *Test for Sterility of the Product to be Examined*.
pH ⟨791⟩: between 4.5 and 5.5.
Other requirements—It meets the requirements under *Injections* ⟨1⟩.
Assay—
  Mobile phase—Dissolve 6.0 g of sodium 1-heptanesulfonate in 3000 mL of water, adjust to a pH of 3.0 by dropwise addition of phosphoric acid. Add 1000 mL of acetonitrile, mix, and pass through a filter having a 0.5-µm or finer porosity. Make adjustments if necessary (see *System Suitability* under *Chromatography* ⟨621⟩).
  Standard preparation—Dissolve an accurately weighed portion of USP Xylazine Hydrochloride RS quantitatively in *Mobile phase* to obtain a solution having a known concentration of about 1.2 mg per mL. Transfer 5.0 mL of this solution to a 50-mL volumetric flask, dilute with *Mobile phase* to volume, and mix. Pass a portion of this solution through a filter having a 0.5-µm or finer porosity, discarding the first 3 mL of the filtrate. Use the clear filtrate as the *Standard preparation*. This solution contains about 0.12 mg of USP Xylazine Hydrochloride RS per mL.
  Assay preparation—Transfer an accurately measured volume of Injection, equivalent to about 200 mg of xylazine, to a 100-mL volumetric flask, dilute with *Mobile phase* to volume, and mix. Transfer 5.0 mL of this solution to a second 100-mL volumetric flask, dilute with *Mobile phase* to volume, and mix. Pass a portion of this solution through a filter having a 0.5-µm or finer porosity, discarding the first 3 mL of the filtrate. Use the clear filtrate as the *Assay preparation*.

Chromatographic system (see *Chromatography* ⟨621⟩)—The liquid chromatograph is equipped with a 254-nm detector, a 2-mm × 2-cm guard column that contains packing L2, and a 4.6-mm × 25-cm analytical column that contains packing L1 and is maintained at a constant temperature of about 40°. The flow rate is about 1 mL per minute. Chromatograph the *Assay preparation*, and record the peak responses as directed for *Procedure*: the resolution, *R*, between the main xylazine peak and the closest eluting other peak, if any, is not less than 2.5; and the tailing factor for the xylazine peak is not more than 2.0. Chromatograph the *Standard preparation*, and record the peak responses as directed for *Procedure*: the relative standard deviation for replicate injections is not more than 2.0%. [NOTE—After daily use, rinse the column with 100 mL of water and with 100 mL of methanol, and store the column containing methanol.]

Procedure—Separately inject equal volumes (about 20 µL) of the *Standard preparation* and the *Assay preparation* into the chromatograph, record the chromatograms, and measure the responses for the major peaks. Calculate the quantity, in mg, of xylazine ($C_{12}H_{16}N_2S$) in each mL of the Injection taken by the formula:

$$(220.34 / 256.80)(2000C / V)(r_U / r_S)$$

in which 220.34 and 256.80 are the molecular weights of xylazine and xylazine hydrochloride, respectively; *C* is the concentration, in mg per mL, of USP Xylazine Hydrochloride RS in the *Standard preparation*; *V* is the volume, in mL, of Injection taken to prepare the *Assay preparation*; and r_U and r_S are the areas of the xylazine peak responses in the chromatograms obtained from the *Assay preparation* and the *Standard preparation*, respectively.

Xylometazoline Hydrochloride

$C_{16}H_{24}N_2 \cdot HCl$ 280.84

1*H*-Imidazole, 2-[[4-(1,1-dimethylethyl)-2,6-dimethylphenyl]methyl]-4,5-dihydro-, monohydrochloride.
2-(4-*tert*-Butyl-2,6-dimethylbenzyl)-2-imidazoline monohydrochloride [*1218-35-5*].

» Xylometazoline Hydrochloride contains not less than 99.0 percent and not more than 101.0 percent of $C_{16}H_{24}N_2 \cdot HCl$, calculated on the dried basis.

Packaging and storage—Preserve in tight, light-resistant containers.

USP Reference standards ⟨11⟩—*USP Xylometazoline Hydrochloride RS*.
Identification—
A: *Infrared Absorption* ⟨197M⟩.
B: The R_F value of the principal spot in the chromatogram of the *Identification preparation* corresponds to that of *Standard preparation A* as obtained in the test for *Chromatographic purity*.
pH ⟨791⟩: between 5.0 and 6.6, in a solution (1 in 20).
Loss on drying ⟨731⟩—Dry it at 105° for 4 hours: it loses not more than 0.5% of its weight.
Residue on ignition ⟨281⟩: not more than 0.1%.
Chromatographic purity—
Standard solutions—Dissolve USP Xylometazoline Hydrochloride RS in methanol, and mix to obtain *Standard preparation A* having a known concentration of 100 µg per mL. Dilute quantitatively with methanol to obtain *Standard solutions*, designated below by letter, having the following compositions:

Standard solution	Dilution	Concentration (µg RS per mL)	Percentage (%, for comparison with test specimen)
A	(undiluted)	100	0.5
B	(4 in 5)	80	0.4
C	(3 in 5)	60	0.3
D	(2 in 5)	40	0.2
E	(1 in 5)	20	0.1

Test solution—Dissolve an accurately weighed quantity of Xylometazoline Hydrochloride in methanol to obtain a solution containing 20 mg per mL.

Identification solution—Dilute a portion of the *Test solution* quantitatively with methanol to obtain a solution containing 100 µg per mL.

Detection reagent—Prepare (1) a solution of 0.5 g of potassium iodide in 50 mL of water, and (2) a solution of 1.5 g of soluble starch in 50 mL of boiling water. Just prior to use, mix 10 mL of each solution with 3 mL of alcohol.

Procedure—Apply separately 5 µL of the *Test solution*, 5 µL of the *Identification solution*, and 5 µL of each *Standard solution* to a suitable thin-layer chromatographic plate (see *Chromatography* ⟨621⟩) coated with a 0.25-mm layer of chromatographic silica gel. Position the plate in a chromatographic chamber, and develop the chromatograms in a solvent system consisting of a mixture of methanol and ammonium hydroxide (20 : 1) until the solvent front has moved about three-fourths of the length of the plate. Remove the plate from the developing chamber, mark the solvent front, and allow the plate to dry under a current of warm air for at least 30 minutes. Expose the plate to chlorine gas for not more than 5 minutes, and air-dry until the chlorine has dissipated (about 15 minutes). Spray the plate with *Detection reagent*, and immediately compare the intensities of any secondary spots observed in the chromatogram of the *Test solution* with those of the principal spots in the chromatograms of the *Standard solutions*: the sum of the intensities of all secondary spots obtained from the *Test solution* corresponds to not more than 1.0%.

Assay—Dissolve about 500 mg of Xylometazoline Hydrochloride, accurately weighed, in 70 mL of glacial acetic acid, add 10 mL of mercuric acetate TS, and titrate with 0.1 N perchloric acid VS, determining the endpoint potentiometrically (see *Titrimetry* ⟨541⟩), using a calomel-glass electrode system. Perform a blank determination, and make any necessary correction. Each mL of 0.1 N perchloric acid is equivalent to 28.08 mg of $C_{16}H_{24}N_2 \cdot HCl$.

Xylometazoline Hydrochloride Nasal Solution

» Xylometazoline Hydrochloride Nasal Solution is an isotonic solution of Xylometazoline Hydrochloride in Water. It contains not less than 90.0 percent and not more than 110.0 percent of the labeled amount of xylometazoline hydrochloride ($C_{16}H_{24}N_2 \cdot HCl$).

Packaging and storage—Preserve in tight, light-resistant containers.

USP Reference standards ⟨11⟩—*USP Xylometazoline Hydrochloride RS*.
Identification—
Standard solution—Dissolve an accurately weighed quantity of USP Xylometazoline Hydrochloride RS in water to obtain a solution having a known concentration of about 1 mg per mL, and proceed as directed for *Test solution*.

Test solution—Transfer 10 mL to a suitable separator, add 2 mL of sodium carbonate solution (1 in 10), and extract with 10 mL of chloroform, filtering the extract through anhydrous sodium sulfate. Evaporate the chloroform extract on a steam bath to dryness, and dissolve the residue in 1 mL of a mixture of chloroform and methanol (1 : 1).

Procedure—Apply separately 5-µL portions of the *Test solution* and the *Standard solution* to a suitable thin-layer chromatographic plate coated with a 0.25-mm layer of chromatographic silica gel mixture (see *Chromatography* ⟨621⟩). Allow the spots to dry, and develop the chromatogram in a solvent system consisting of a mixture of chloroform, methanol, and isopropylamine (92 : 3 : 3). Remove the plate from the developing chamber, mark the solvent front, and allow the solvent to evaporate. Spray the plate with *p*-nitrobenzenediazonium tetrafluoroborate solution, prepared by adding 250 mg to 5 mL of water, mixing, and filtering. Spray the plate with sodium carbonate solution (1 in 10): the R_F value of the principal spot obtained from the *Test solution* corresponds to that obtained from the *Standard solution*.

pH ⟨791⟩: between 5.0 and 7.5.

Assay—

Standard preparation—Dissolve an accurately weighed quantity of USP Xylometazoline Hydrochloride RS in water to obtain a solution having a known concentration of about 0.5 mg per mL. Transfer 10.0 mL of this solution to a 125-mL separator, and proceed as directed under *Assay preparation*, beginning with "add 10 mL each of water and dilute hydrochloric acid (1 in 6), respectively." The concentration of USP Xylometazoline Hydrochloride RS in the *Standard preparation* is about 100 µg per mL.

Assay preparation—Transfer an accurately measured volume of Nasal Solution, equivalent to about 5 mg of xylometazoline hydrochloride, to a 125-mL separator, add 10 mL each of water and dilute hydrochloric acid (1 in 6), respectively, and extract with three 10-mL portions of methylene chloride. Discard the methylene chloride extracts, add 10 mL of sodium hydroxide solution (1 in 5) to the separator, and extract with three 15-mL portions of methylene chloride. Filter the combined extracts through glass wool into a 50-mL volumetric flask, dilute with methylene chloride to volume, and mix.

Procedure—Transfer 5.0 mL each of the *Standard preparation* and the *Assay preparation*, respectively, to separate 10-mL volumetric flasks, and evaporate in a water bath maintained at 40°, with the aid of a stream of nitrogen, to dryness. Dissolve the residue in each flask in 0.50 mL of dehydrated alcohol, and add 0.50 mL of dehydrated alcohol to a third 10-mL volumetric flask to provide the blank. To each flask add 0.50 mL of sodium hydroxide solution (1 in 25), swirl, to each add 5.0 mL of sodium nitroferricyanide solution (1 in 200), and mix. After 10 minutes, accurately timed, add 1.0 mL of a saturated solution of sodium bicarbonate to each flask, swirl, and allow to stand for 10 minutes. Dilute each with water to volume, mix, and allow to stand for 15 minutes. Concomitantly determine the absorbances of the solutions in 1-cm cells at the wavelength of maximum absorbance at about 565 nm, with a suitable spectrophotometer, using the blank to set the instrument. Calculate the quantity, in mg, of xylometazoline hydrochloride ($C_{16}H_{24}N_2 \cdot HCl$) in each mL of the Nasal Solution taken by the formula:

$$(0.05C/V)(A_U/A_S)$$

in which C is the concentration, in µg per mL, of USP Xylometazoline Hydrochloride RS in the *Standard preparation*, V is the volume, in mL, of Nasal Solution taken, and A_U and A_S are the absorbances of the solutions from the *Assay preparation* and the *Standard preparation*, respectively.

Xylose

$C_5H_{10}O_5$ 150.13
D-Xylose.
D-Xylose   [58-86-6; 6763-34-4].

» Xylose contains not less than 98.0 percent and not more than 102.0 percent of $C_5H_{10}O_5$, calculated on the dried basis.

Packaging and storage—Preserve in tight containers at controlled room temperature.

USP Reference standards ⟨11⟩—*USP Xylose RS*.

Color of solution—A freshly prepared solution (1 in 10) is clear and colorless.

Identification—

A: *Solvent system*—Mix 60 mL of butyl alcohol with 40 mL of pyridine and 30 mL of water.

Standard preparation—Prepare a solution of USP Xylose RS in water to obtain a solution having a concentration of 100 mg per mL.

Test preparation—Dissolve 1 g of Xylose in water, and add water to make 10 mL.

Spray reagent—Dissolve 1.66 g of phthalic acid and 0.93 g of freshly distilled aniline in 100 mL of water-saturated butyl alcohol. The solution may be stored in a brown glass bottle in a cold place, but is to be discarded if darkening becomes marked.

Chromatographic sheet—Use filter paper (Whatman No. 1 or equivalent). Draw a spotting line 6 cm from one edge of the sheet.

Procedure—Line a suitable chromatographic chamber, prepared for descending chromatography (see *Chromatography* ⟨621⟩), with blotting paper. Fill the solvent trough with *Solvent system*, and place a sufficient amount of *Solvent system* in the bottom of the chamber to permit the lining to be in contact with it. Allow the chamber to equilibrate for not less than 16 hours. To the spotting line apply 2 µL of the *Standard preparation* stepwise so that the spot is not more than 3 mm in diameter. Similarly apply 2 µL of the *Test preparation* to the spotting line and 4 cm from the *Standard preparation* spot. Expose the sheet to the atmosphere of the *Solvent system* in the closed chamber for 4 hours, then dip the edge of the sheet into the *Solvent system* in the trough, and develop until the liquid front has reached about 2.5 cm from the end of the sheet. Remove the sheet from the chamber, dry it with the aid of a gentle current of air, apply the *Spray reagent*, and dry the sheet at 105° to 110° for 5 to 10 minutes. If the spots are faint, respray and redry, and if necessary view under UV light: the R_F value of the spot from the *Test preparation* corresponds to that from the *Standard preparation*.

B: *Standard preparation*—Transfer 10 mg of USP Xylose RS to a suitable vial, and add 1 mL of pyridine, 0.2 mL of hexamethyldisilazane, and 0.1 mL of chlorotrimethylsilane. Cap the vial, shake vigorously for 30 seconds, and allow to stand for 5 minutes.

Test preparation—Using 10 mg of Xylose, proceed as directed under *Standard preparation*.

Procedure—Use a gas chromatograph equipped with a flame-ionization detector and a 3-mm × 1.8-m stainless steel column packed with 10% phase G2 on support S1A. Under typical conditions, nitrogen being used as the carrier gas, the column temperature is operated at 170°, and the injector block and detector temperatures at 300°. Inject 0.5 µL each of the *Test preparation* and the *Standard preparation*: the retention times correspond.

Specific rotation ⟨781S⟩: between +18.2° and +19.4°.

Test solution: 100 mg per mL, in 0.012 N ammonium hydroxide.

Loss on drying ⟨731⟩—Dry 2 g to 5 g at a pressure not exceeding 50 mm of mercury at 60° to constant weight, a current of dried air

being passed through the oven during the drying period to remove water vapor: it loses not more than 0.1% of its weight.
Residue on ignition ⟨281⟩: not more than 0.05%.
Iron ⟨241⟩—Dissolve 2.0 g in 45 mL of water, and add 2 mL of hydrochloric acid: the limit is 5 ppm.
Heavy metals ⟨231⟩—Dissolve 2.0 g in water to make 25 mL of solution: the limit is 0.001%.
Chromatographic purity—The paper chromatogram of the *Test preparation* in *Identification* test *A* shows no foreign spot greater than any foreign spot from the *Standard preparation*, and the gas chromatogram of the *Test preparation* in *Identification* test *B* shows no foreign peak greater than any foreign peak from the *Standard preparation*.
Organic volatile impurities, *Method I* ⟨467⟩: meets the requirements.

(Official until July 1, 2008)
Assay—
p-Bromoaniline solution—Dissolve 2 g of *p*-bromoaniline in 100 mL of thiourea-saturated glacial acetic acid. Store in an amber glass bottle, and prepare weekly.
Standard preparation—Dissolve a suitable quantity of USP Xylose RS, accurately weighed, in saturated benzoic acid solution to obtain a solution having a known concentration of about 100 µg per mL.
Assay preparation—Dissolve about 1000 mg of Xylose, accurately weighed, in saturated benzoic acid solution in a 100-mL volumetric flask, and dilute with saturated benzoic acid solution to volume. Pipet 1 mL of this solution into a second 100-mL volumetric flask, dilute with saturated benzoic acid solution to volume, and mix.
Procedure—[NOTE—In this procedure, keep strict control of time between steps.] Pipet 1-mL portions of the *Standard preparation* into each of two test tubes, and pipet 1-mL portions of the *Assay preparation* into each of two other test tubes. Into each tube pipet 5 mL of *p-Bromoaniline solution*, and mix. Loosely stopper one tube from each pair, place in a water bath at 70° for 10 minutes, remove, cool rapidly to room temperature, and mix. Set the tubes in the dark for 70 minutes. Concomitantly determine the absorbances of the treated solutions at the wavelength of maximum absorbance at 520 nm, with a suitable spectrophotometer, using the respective untreated solutions as blanks. Calculate the quantity, in mg, of $C_5H_{10}O_5$ in the portion of Xylose taken by the formula:

$$10C(A_U / A_S)$$

in which *C* is the concentration, in µg per mL, of USP Xylose RS in the *Standard preparation*; and A_U and A_S are the absorbances of the solutions from the *Assay preparation* and the *Standard preparation*, respectively.

Yellow Fever Vaccine

» Yellow Fever Vaccine conforms to the regulations of the FDA concerning biologics (see *Biologics* ⟨1041⟩). It is the attenuated strain that has been tested in monkeys for viscerotropism, immunogenicity, and neurotropism of living yellow fever virus selected for high antigenic activity and safety. It is prepared by the culturing of the virus in the living embryos of chicken eggs, from which a suspension is prepared, processed with aseptic precautions, and finally dried from the frozen state. It meets the requirements of the specific mouse potency test in titer of mouse LD_{50} (quantity of virus estimated to produce fatal specific encephalitis in 50% of the mice) or the requirements for plaque-forming units in a suitable cell culture system, such as a Vero cell system for which the relationship between mouse LD_{50} and plaque-forming units has been established, in which cell monolayers in 35 mm petri dishes are inoculated for a specified time with dilutions of Vaccine, after which the dilutions are replaced with 0.5% agarose-containing medium. Following adsorption and incubation for five days an overlay is added of the 0.5% agarose medium containing 1 : 50,000 neutral red and the plaques are counted on the sixth day following inoculation. It is sterile, and contains no human serum and no antimicrobial agent.

Yellow Fever Vaccine is constituted, with Sodium Chloride Injection containing no antimicrobial agent, just prior to use.

Packaging and storage—Preserve in nitrogen-filled, flame-sealed ampuls or suitable stoppered vials at a temperature preferably below 0° but never above 5°, throughout the dating period. Preserve it during shipment in a suitable container adequately packed in solid carbon dioxide, or provided with other means of refrigeration, so as to ensure a temperature constantly below 0°.
Expiration date—The expiration date is not later than 1 year after date of issue from manufacturer's cold storage (−20°, 1 year).
Labeling—Label it to state that it is to be well shaken before use and that the constituted vaccine is to be used entirely or discarded within 1 hour of opening the container. Label it also to state that it is the living yellow fever vaccine virus prepared from chicken embryos and that the dose is the same for persons of all ages, but that it is not recommended for infants under six months of age.

Yohimbine Hydrochloride

$C_{21}H_{26}N_2O_3 \cdot HCl$ 390.91
17α-Hydroxy-20-α-yohimban-16-β-carboxylic acid, methyl ester, hydrochloride [65-19-0].

» Yohimbine Hydrochloride contains not less than 98.0 percent and not more than 102.0 percent of $C_{21}H_{26}N_2O_3 \cdot HCl$, calculated on the dried basis.

Packaging and storage—Preserve in tight containers, and store at controlled room temperature.
Labeling—Where it is intended for veterinary use only, it is so labeled.
USP Reference standards ⟨11⟩—*USP Yohimbine Hydrochloride RS*.
Identification—
  A: *Infrared Absorption* ⟨197K⟩.
  B: *Thin-Layer Chromatographic Identification Test* ⟨201⟩—
  Test solution—Dissolve 10 mg of it in 1 mL of methanol, add 1 drop of ammonium hydroxide, and mix.
  Application volume: 1 µL.
  Developing solvent system: methylene chloride, methanol, and ammonium hydroxide (90 : 14 : 1), in a saturated chamber.
  Procedure—Allow the plate to air-dry in a hood. Expose the dry plate for 30 minutes to short-wavelength UV light, then examine under long-wavelength UV light: the size, intensity, and R_F value of the principal spot in the chromatogram obtained from the *Test solution* correspond to those characteristics of the principal spot in the chromatogram obtained from the Standard solution.
  C: *Ultraviolet Absorption* ⟨197U⟩—
  Solution: 10 µg per mL.
  Medium: 0.1 N hydrochloric acid in methanol.
  D: To 10 mg of it add 3 drops of sulfuric acid. Mix, and add 50 mg of ammonium vanadate: a violet color is produced (differentia-

tion from *strychnine*, which produces a red color). Add 1 mL of water: no color change occurs.

Specific rotation ⟨781S⟩: between +100° and +105°.
Test solution: 10 mg per mL, in water, prepared by warming on a steam bath and allowing to cool.

Loss on drying ⟨731⟩—Dry it at 105° for 2 hours: it loses not more than 1.0% of its weight.

Chromatographic purity—Use the chromatogram of the *Assay preparation* obtained as directed in the *Assay*. Calculate the percentage of each impurity in the portion of Yohimbine Hydrochloride taken by the formula:

$$100(r_i / r_s)$$

in which r_i is the response of the individual impurity; and r_s is the sum of all the responses in the chromatogram: not more than 1.0% of any individual impurity is found, and the sum of all the impurities found is not more than 2.0%.

Assay—

Mobile phase—Prepare a mixture of water, dibasic sodium phosphate dihydrate solution (11.88 g per L), and monobasic potassium phosphate solution (9.08 g per L) (355 : 100 : 50). Add 4 g of sodium dodecyl sulfate, and mix. Add 285 mL of acetonitrile, and mix. Make adjustments if necessary (see *System Suitability* under *Chromatography* ⟨621⟩).

Standard preparation—Quantitatively dissolve an accurately weighed quantity of USP Yohimbine Hydrochloride RS in methanol to obtain a solution having a known concentration of about 0.2 mg per mL.

Assay preparation—Transfer about 50 mg of Yohimbine Hydrochloride, accurately weighed, to a 100-mL volumetric flask, dilute with methanol to volume, and mix. Transfer 10.0 mL of this solution to a 25-mL volumetric flask, dilute with methanol to volume, and mix.

System suitability solution—Quantitatively dilute an accurately measured volume of the *Standard preparation* with methanol to obtain a solution having a concentration of 0.40 μg of USP Yohimbine Hydrochloride RS per mL.

Chromatographic system (see *Chromatography* ⟨621⟩)—The liquid chromatograph is equipped with a 229-nm detector and a 4-mm × 12.5-cm column that contains 4-μm packing L7. The flow rate is about 2 mL per minute. Chromatograph the *System suitability solution*, and record the peak responses as directed for *Procedure*: the main yohimbine peak gives a measurable response. Chromatograph the *Standard preparation*, and record the peak responses as directed for *Procedure*: the tailing factor is not more than 2.5; and the relative standard deviation for replicate injections is not more than 1%.

Procedure—Separately inject equal volumes (about 10 μL) of the *Standard preparation* and the *Assay preparation* into the chromatograph, record the chromatograms, and measure the areas for the major peaks. Calculate the quantity, in mg, of $C_{21}H_{26}N_2O_3 \cdot HCl$ in the portion of Yohimbine Hydrochloride taken by the formula:

$$250C(r_U / r_S)$$

in which C is the concentration, in mg per mL, of USP Yohimbine Hydrochloride RS in the *Standard preparation*; and r_U and r_S are the yohimbine peak responses obtained from the *Assay preparation* and the *Standard preparation*, respectively.

Yohimbine Injection

» Yohimbine Injection is a sterile solution of Yohimbine Hydrochloride in Water for Injection. It contains not less than 90.0 percent and not more than 110.0 percent of the labeled amount of yohimbine ($C_{21}H_{26}N_2O_3$).

Packaging and storage—Preserve in single-dose or multiple-dose Containers for Injections as described under *Injections* ⟨1⟩, and store at controlled room temperature.

Labeling—Where it is intended for veterinary use only, it is so labeled.

USP Reference standards ⟨11⟩—USP Endotoxin RS. USP Yohimbine Hydrochloride RS.

Identification, *Thin-Layer Chromatographic Identification Test* ⟨201⟩—

Test solution—Transfer a volume of Injection, equivalent to about 40 mg of yohimbine, to a separator, add 5 mL of a sodium carbonate solution (1 in 20), and extract with four 10-mL portions of chloroform, combining the chloroform extracts in a beaker and evaporating to dryness. Add 20 mL of methanol to the beaker, and swirl to dissolve the residue.

Standard solution—Prepare a solution of USP Yohimbine Hydrochloride RS in methanol containing 2 mg per mL.

Mixed solution: a mixture of the *Test solution* and the *Standard solution* (1 : 1).

Application volume: 1 μL.

Developing solvent system: methylene chloride, methanol, and ammonium hydroxide (90 : 14 : 1), in a saturated chamber.

Procedure—Allow the plate to air-dry in a hood. Expose the dry plate for 30 minutes to short-wavelength UV light, then examine under long-wavelength UV light: the size, intensity, and R_F value of the principal spots in the chromatograms obtained from the *Test solution* and the *Mixed solution* correspond to those characteristics of the principal spot in the chromatogram obtained from the *Standard solution*.

Bacterial endotoxins ⟨85⟩—It contains not more than 45.5 USP Endotoxin Units per mg of yohimbine.

Sterility ⟨71⟩—It meets the requirements when tested as directed for *Membrane Filtration* under *Test for Sterility of the Product to be Examined*.

pH ⟨791⟩: between 3.7 and 4.3.

Other requirements—It meets the requirements under *Injections* ⟨1⟩.

Assay—

Diluent—Prepare a mixture of acetonitrile, water, and glacial acetic acid (49 : 49 : 2).

Mobile phase—Prepare a mixture of water, acetonitrile, and glacial acetic acid (603 : 377 : 20) containing 3.5 g of sodium 1-decanesulfonate in each 1000 mL. Make adjustments if necessary (see *System Suitability* under *Chromatography* ⟨621⟩).

Standard preparation—Transfer about 55 mg of USP Yohimbine Hydrochloride RS, accurately weighed, to a 25-mL volumetric flask, add 20 mL of water, warm, and swirl to dissolve. Add 84 mg of anhydrous citric acid, and swirl to dissolve. Allow the solution to cool, adjust with 1 N sodium hydroxide to a pH of 4.0, dilute with water to volume, and mix. Transfer 125.0 μL of this stock solution to a second 25-mL volumetric flask, dilute with *Diluent* to volume, and mix. This solution contains about 0.011 mg of USP Yohimbine Hydrochloride RS per mL.

Resolution solution—Prepare a solution in methanol containing about 0.56 mg of methylparaben and 0.06 mg of propylparaben per mL. Transfer 200 μL of this solution to a 25-mL volumetric flask, add 125.0 μL of the stock solution used to prepare the *Standard preparation*, dilute with *Diluent* to volume, and mix.

Assay preparation—Transfer an accurately measured volume of Injection, equivalent to about 0.25 mg of yohimbine, to a 25-mL volumetric flask, dilute with *Diluent* to volume, and mix.

Chromatographic system (see *Chromatography* ⟨621⟩)—The liquid chromatograph is equipped with a 254-nm detector and a 3.9-mm × 15-cm column that contains 5-μm packing L1. The flow rate is about 1 mL per minute. Chromatograph the *Resolution solution*, and record the peak responses as directed for *Procedure*: the relative retention times are about 0.4 for methylparaben, 0.7 for propylparaben, and 1.0 for yohimbine; and the resolution, R, between methylparaben and propylparaben and between propylparaben and yohimbine is not less than 2.0. Chromatograph the *Standard preparation*, and record the peak responses as directed for *Procedure*: the relative standard deviation for replicate injections is not more than 2.0%.

Procedure—Separately inject equal volumes (about 25 μL) of the *Standard preparation* and the *Assay preparation* into the chromatograph, record the chromatograms, and measure the areas for the ma-

jor peaks. Calculate the quantity, in mg, of yohimbine ($C_{21}H_{26}N_2O_3$) in each mL of the Injection taken by the formula:

$$(354.45/390.90)(25,000C/V)(r_U/r_S)$$

in which 354.45 and 390.90 are the molecular weights of yohimbine and yohimbine hydrochloride, respectively; C is the concentration, in mg per mL, of USP Yohimbine Hydrochloride RS in the *Standard preparation*; V is the volume, in μL, of Injection taken to prepare the *Assay preparation*; and r_U and r_S are the yohimbine peak responses obtained from the *Assay preparation* and the *Standard preparation*, respectively.

Yttrium Y 90 Ibritumomab Tiuxetan Injection

» Ibritumomab Tiuxetan is the immunoconjugate resulting from a stable thiourea covalent bond between the monoclonal antibody ibritumomab and the linker-chelator tiuxetan [*N*-[2-bis(carboxymethyl)amino]-3-(*p*-isothiocyanatophenyl)propyl]-[*N*-[2-bis(carboxymethyl)amino]-2-(methyl)ethyl)glycine. This chelate provides a high-affinity, conformationally restricted chelation site for ^{90}Y and ^{111}In. The approximate molecular weight of Ibritumomab Tiuxetan is 148 kD.

Ibritumomab is a murine IgG$_1$ kappa monoclonal antibody directed against the CD20 antigen, which is found on the surface of normal and malignant B lymphocytes. Ibritumomab is produced in Chinese hamster ovary cells and is composed of two murine gamma 1 heavy chains of 445 amino acids each and two kappa light chains of 213 amino acids each.

Yttrium Y 90 Ibritumomab Tiuxetan Injection is a sterile, nonpyrogenic preparation of the immunoconjugate of ibritumomab and tiuxetan that is labeled with ^{90}Y and is suitable for intravenous administration. It contains not less than 90.0 percent and not more than 110.0 percent of the labeled amount of ^{90}Y as the ibritumomab complex, expressed in megabecquerels (or millicuries) per mL at the time indicated in the labeling. It may contain buffers and stabilizers. It contains no antimicrobial agents. Other chemical forms of radioactivity do not exceed 5 percent of the total radioactivity. The immunoreactive fraction, as determined by a validated method, is not less than 90 percent.

Packaging and storage—Preserve in single-dose containers, and store in a refrigerator for not more than 8 hours. [NOTE—Translucent protein particles may develop, which are removed by filtration prior to administration using a 0.22-μm low-protein-binding filter.]
Labeling—Label it to include the following in addition to the information specified for *Labeling* under *Injections* ⟨1⟩: the time and date of calibration; the amount of Yttrium Y 90 ibritumomab tiuxetan as total MBq (or mCi) and concentration of yttrium ^{90}Y ibritumomab tiuxetan, in MBq (or mCi) per mL, at the time of calibration; the expiration date and time; the storage temperature; and the statement, "Caution—Radioactive Material." The labeling indicates that, in making dosage calculations, correction is to be made for radioactive decay, and also indicates that the radioactive half-life of ^{90}Y is 64.1 hours.
USP Reference standards ⟨11⟩—*USP Endotoxin RS*.
Radionuclide identification (see *Radioactivity* ⟨821⟩)—
  A: The beta radiation of the Injection shows a mass absorption coefficient within 5% of the value found for a known standard of the ^{90}Y when tested under the same counting conditions.

  B: The beta-ray spectrum, obtained on an energy calibrated beta spectrometer, is identical to that of the spectrum of ^{90}Y of known purity, showing a maximum beta particle energy (E_{max}) at about 2280 keV. [NOTE—Because of the inherent difficulty in measuring beta radiation, a second comparative test should be performed.]
Bacterial endotoxins ⟨85⟩—The limit of endotoxin content is not more than 175/V USP Endotoxin Units per mL of the Injection, when compared with the USP Endotoxin RS, in which V is the maximum recommended total dose, in mL, at the expiration date or time.
pH ⟨791⟩: between 5.5 and 7.5.
Radiochemical purity—
  Adsorbent: 1- × 8-cm instant silica gel strip.
  Test solution: the Injection.
  Application volume: 10 μL.
  Developing solvent system: 0.9% sodium chloride solution.
  Procedure—Proceed as directed for *Thin-Layer Chromatography* under *Chromatography* ⟨621⟩ by ascending chromatography. Determine the distribution of radioactivity on the chromatogram by scanning with a suitable collimated radiochromatogram strip scanner, and determine the percentage of radiochemical purity of the test specimen. Not less than 95% of the ^{90}Y activity is present as a band between the R_F values of 0.0 and 0.1.
Radionuclidic purity (Content of ^{90}Sr in an yttrium Y 90 chloride solution)—Prepare a strontium/yttrium carrier solution containing 0.34 mg of yttrium chloride (YCl$_3$ · 6H$_2$O) and 0.30 mg of strontium chloride (SrCl$_2$ · 6H$_2$O) per mL of 0.1 N hydrochloric acid. Apply about 50 μL of this solution at the origin of a 2- × 19-cm cellulose phosphate chromatographic strip (see *Chromatography* ⟨621⟩), and allow to dry. Apply about 5 μL of the yttrium Y 90 chloride radiolabeling solution at the origin, and develop the chromatogram by ascending chromatography over a period of about 1.25 hours, using 3 N hydrochloric acid as the developing solvent, until the solvent front migrates to the 15-cm mark. Allow to dry. Cut the strip at the 8-cm mark, and place the upper section (solvent front) in a suitable liquid scintillation solvent. Using a suitable counting assembly (see *Beta-Emitting Radionuclides* in the *Assay* section of *Identification and Assay of Radionuclides* under *Radioactivity* ⟨821⟩), determine the radioactivity, in KBq (or μCi) per mL of yttrium Y 90 chloride solution. The total radioactivity of ^{90}Sr is not greater than 740 KBq per 37 GBq (or 20 μCi per Ci) of ^{90}Y at the expiration date as stated on the labeling.
Other requirements—It meets the requirements under *Injections* ⟨1⟩, except that the radioactive component may be distributed or dispensed prior to completion of the test for *Sterility*, the latter test being started on the date of manufacture.
Assay for radioactivity ⟨821⟩—Using a suitable counting assembly (see *Scintillation and Semiconductor Detectors* in *Identification and Assay of Radionuclides*), determine the total radioactivity, in MBq (or μCi), of the unshielded Injection, using a calibrated system.

Zalcitabine

$C_9H_{13}N_3O_3$ 211.22
Cytidine, 2′,3′-dideoxy-.
2′,3′-Dideoxycytidine. [7481-89-2].

» Zalcitabine contains not less than 98.0 percent and not more than 102.0 percent of $C_9H_{13}N_3O_3$, calculated on the dried basis.

Zalcitabine / Official Monographs

Caution—*Great care should be taken to prevent inhaling particles of Zalcitabine and exposing it to the skin.*

Packaging and storage—Preserve in tight, light-resistant containers.

USP Reference standards ⟨11⟩—*USP Zalcitabine RS. USP Zalcitabine Related Compound A RS.*

Identification—
  A: *Infrared Absorption* ⟨197K⟩.
  B: The retention time of the major peak in the chromatogram of the *Assay preparation* corresponds to that of the *Standard preparation*, as obtained in the *Assay*.
  C: Prepare a test solution of it in a mixture of methanol and water (1 : 1) containing 50 mg per mL. Similarly prepare a Standard solution, using USP Zalcitabine RS. Separately apply 10 µL portions of the test solution and the Standard solution to a suitable thin-layer chromatographic plate (see *Chromatography* ⟨621⟩) coated with a 0.25-mm layer of chromatographic silica gel mixture. Place the plate in a paper-lined chromatographic chamber saturated with a solvent system consisting of the clear lower layer of a mixture of alcohol, dichloromethane, and water (3 : 2 : 2), and develop the chromatogram. When the solvent front has moved about three-fourths of the length of the plate, remove the plate from the chamber, mark the solvent front, and allow to dry. Locate the spots on the plate by examination under short-wavelength UV light: the R_F value of the principal spot obtained from the test solution corresponds to that obtained from the Standard solution.

Specific rotation ⟨781S⟩: between +73° and +77°.
  Test solution: 7 mg per mL, in water.
Water, *Method Ia* ⟨921⟩: not more than 0.3%.
Residue on ignition ⟨281⟩: not more than 0.1%.
Heavy metals, *Method II* ⟨231⟩: 0.002%.
Chromatographic purity—
  Phosphate buffer, Mobile phase, Resolution solution, Standard preparation, and *Assay preparation*—Prepare as directed in the *Assay*.
  Chromatographic system (see *Chromatography* ⟨621⟩)—The liquid chromatograph is equipped with a 270-nm detector and a 4.6-mm × 15-cm column that contains 5-µm packing L1. The flow rate is about 1 mL per minute. Chromatograph the *Resolution solution*, and record the peak responses as directed for *Procedure:* the resolution, R, between zalcitabine and zalcitabine related compound A is not less than 2.0, and the tailing factor for zalcitabine is not greater than 1.5. Chromatograph the *Standard preparation*, and record the peak responses as directed for *Procedure:* the relative standard deviation is not more than 2%.
  Procedure—Inject a volume (about 20 µL) of the *Assay preparation* into the chromatograph, record the chromatograms, and measure the responses of the major peaks. Inject a volume of acetonitrile in water (3 in 100) as a chromatographic blank. Calculate the percentage of each impurity in the portion of zalcitabine taken by the formula:

$$100(r_i / r_s)$$

in which r_i is the peak response for each impurity, and r_s is the sum of the responses of all of the peaks: not more than 0.3% of any individual impurity is found, and the sum of all impurities is not more than 2.0%.

Ordinary impurities ⟨466⟩—
  Test solution: 50 mg per mL, in a mixture of methanol and water (1 : 1).
  Standard solution: a mixture of methanol and water (1 : 1).
  Eluant: the lower layer of a mixture of alcohol, dichloromethane, and water (3 : 2 : 2).
  Visualization: 1.

Assay—
  Phosphate buffer—Dissolve 6.8 g of monobasic potassium phosphate and 8.7 g of dibasic potassium phosphate in 2000 mL of water. Adjust, if necessary, with dilute phosphoric acid or potassium hydroxide solution (1 in 10) to a pH of 6.8 ± 0.05.
  Mobile phase—Prepare a filtered and degassed mixture of *Phosphate buffer* and acetonitrile (97 : 3). Make adjustments if necessary (see *System Suitability* under *Chromatography* ⟨621⟩).
  Resolution solution—Dissolve USP Zalcitabine RS and USP Zalcitabine Related Compound A RS in a mixture of acetonitrile in water (3 in 100), and dilute quantitatively, and stepwise if necessary, with the same solvent to obtain a solution containing about 0.024 mg of each per mL.
  Standard preparation—Dissolve an accurately weighed quantity of USP Zalcitabine RS in a mixture of acetonitrile and water (3 in 100) to obtain a solution having a known concentration of about 0.5 mg per mL.
  Assay preparation—Transfer about 100 mg of Zalcitabine, accurately weighed, to a 200-mL volumetric flask. Dissolve in a mixture of acetonitrile and water (3 in 100), dilute with the same solvent to volume, and mix.
  Chromatographic system—The liquid chromatograph is equipped with a 270-nm detector and a 4.6-mm × 15-cm column that contains packing L1. The flow rate is about 1 mL per minute. Chromatograph the *Standard preparation*, and record the peak responses as directed for *Procedure:* the tailing factor for the zalcitabine peak is not greater than 1.5, and the relative standard deviation is not more than 2.0%. Chromatograph the *Resolution solution:* the resolution, R, between zalcitabine and zalcitabine related compound A is not less than 2.
  Procedure—Separately inject equal volumes (about 20 µL) of the *Standard preparation* and the *Assay preparation* into the chromatograph, record the chromatograms, and measure the responses for the major peaks. Calculate the quantity, in mg, of $C_9H_{13}N_3O_3$ in the portion of Zalcitabine taken by the formula:

$$200C(r_U / r_S)$$

in which C is the concentration, in mg per mL, of USP Zalcitabine RS in the *Standard preparation*; and r_U and r_S are the peak responses obtained from the *Assay preparation* and the *Standard preparation*, respectively.

Zalcitabine Tablets

» Zalcitabine Tablets contain not less than 90.0 percent and not more than 110.0 percent of the labeled amount of zalcitabine ($C_9H_{13}N_3O_3$).

Caution—*Great care should be taken to prevent inhaling particles of zalcitabine and exposing it to the skin.*

Packaging and storage—Preserve in tight, light-resistant containers.

USP Reference standards ⟨11⟩—*USP Zalcitabine RS. USP Zalcitabine Related Compound A RS.*

Identification—The retention time of the major peak in the chromatogram of the *Assay preparation* corresponds to that of the *Standard preparation*, as obtained in the *Assay*.

Dissolution ⟨711⟩—
  Medium: water; 900 mL.
  Apparatus 2: 50 rpm.
  Time: 20 minutes.
  Phosphate buffer—Transfer 8.7 g of dibasic potassium phosphate to a 1 L volumetric flask, dilute with water to volume, and adjust with phosphoric acid to a pH of 6.8.
  Mobile phase—Prepare a filtered and degassed mixture of *Phosphate buffer*, methanol, and acetonitrile (96 : 4 : 3). Make adjustments if necessary (see *System Suitability* under *Chromatography* ⟨621⟩).
  Standard preparation—Transfer about 10 mg of USP Zalcitabine RS, accurately weighed, to a 250-mL volumetric flask. Add about 200 mL of *Medium*, and sonicate until complete solution is effected. Dilute with *Medium* to volume, and mix.
  Chromatographic system (see *Chromatography* ⟨621⟩)—The liquid chromatograph is equipped with a 270-nm detector and a 3.9-mm × 15-cm column that contains 10-µm packing L1. The flow rate is about 1 mL per minute. Chromatograph the *Standard preparation*, and record the peak responses as described for

Procedure: the retention time is about 5 minutes; the tailing factor is not more than 2; and the relative standard deviation is not more than 2%.

Procedure—Separately inject equal volumes (about 150 µL) of the *Standard preparation* and a filtered portion of the solution under test into the chromatograph, record the chromatograms, and measure the responses of the major peaks. Calculate the quantity, in mg, of zalcitabine in the Tablets taken by the formula:

$$900C(r_U / r_S)$$

in which C is the concentration, in mg per mL, of USP Zalcitabine RS in the *Standard preparation*; and r_U and r_S are the zalcitabine peak responses obtained from the solution under test and the *Standard preparation*, respectively.

Tolerances—Not less than 80% (Q) of the labeled amount of $C_9H_{13}N_3O_3$ is dissolved in 20 minutes.

Uniformity of dosage units ⟨905⟩: meet the requirements.

Assay—

Buffer solution—Dissolve 3.4 g of monobasic potassium phosphate in sufficient water to make 1 L. Using a suitable pH meter, adjust with phosphoric acid to a pH of 2.2. [NOTE—If too much phosphoric acid is added, yielding a pH below 2.2, the pH may be adjusted to 2.2 with 0.025 M monobasic potassium phosphate.] Add 1.08 g of sodium 1-octanesulfonic acid, and mix.

Mobile phase—Prepare a filtered and degassed mixture of *Buffer solution* and acetonitrile (85 : 15).

Diluent—Prepare a mixture of water and acetonitrile (17 : 3).

Resolution solution—Dissolve weighed quantities of USP Zalcitabine RS and USP Zalcitabine Related Compound A RS in *Diluent*, and dilute quantitatively, and stepwise if necessary, with the same solvent to obtain a solution containing about 0.02 mg per mL of zalcitabine and 0.002 mg per mL of zalcitabine related compound A.

Standard preparation—Dissolve an accurately weighed quantity of USP Zalcitabine RS in *Diluent*, and dilute quantitatively, and stepwise if necessary, with the same solvent to obtain a solution having a known concentration of about 0.008 mg per mL.

Assay preparation—Transfer 5 Tablets to a volumetric flask suitable to obtain a solution containing about 0.008 mg zalcitabine per mL. Add a volume of *Diluent* that is about six-tenths of the volume of the flask, sonicate for 15 minutes, and shake by mechanical means for 10 minutes. Dilute with *Diluent* to volume, and mix. Filter before use.

Chromatographic system (see *Chromatography* ⟨621⟩)—The liquid chromatograph is equipped with a 280-nm detector, a precolumn cartridge that contains packing L1, and a 4.6-mm × 25-cm analytical column that contains 5-µm packing L1. The flow rate is about 1.5 mL per minute. Chromatograph the *Resolution solution*, and record the peak responses as directed for *Procedure:* the resolution, R, between the zalcitabine and zalcitabine related compound A peaks is not less than 1.1, and the tailing factor for the zalcitabine peak is not more than 1.5. Chromatograph the *Standard preparation*, and record the peak responses as directed for *Procedure:* the relative standard deviation for replicate injections is not more than 2%.

Procedure—Separately inject equal volumes (about 50 µL) of the *Standard preparation* and the *Assay preparation* into the chromatograph, record the chromatograms, and measure the responses of the major peaks. Calculate the quantity, in mg, of $C_9H_{13}N_3O_3$ in the portion of Tablets taken by the formula:

$$CV(r_U / r_S)$$

in which C is the concentration, in mg per mL, of USP Zalcitabine RS in the *Standard preparation*; V is the volume, in mL, of the volumetric flask used to prepare the *Assay preparation*; and r_U and r_S are the zalcitabine peak responses obtained from the *Assay preparation* and the *Standard preparation*, respectively.

Zidovudine

$C_{10}H_{13}N_5O_4$ 267.24
Thymidine, 3′-azido-3′-deoxy-.
3′-Azido-3′-deoxythymidine   [30516-87-1].

» Zidovudine contains not less than 97.0 percent and not more than 102.0 percent of $C_{10}H_{13}N_5O_4$, calculated on the anhydrous basis.

Packaging and storage—Preserve in tight, light-resistant containers. Store at 25°, excursions permitted between 15° and 30°.

USP Reference standards ⟨11⟩—*USP Zidovudine RS. USP Zidovudine Related Compound B RS. USP Zidovudine Related Compound C RS.*

Identification—

A: *Infrared Absorption* ⟨197K⟩.

B: The retention time of the major peak in the chromatogram of the *Assay preparation* corresponds to that in the chromatogram of the *Standard preparation,* as obtained in the *Assay.*

Specific rotation ⟨781S⟩: between +60.5° and +63°.

Test solution: 10 mg per mL, in alcohol.

Water, *Method I* ⟨921⟩: not more than 1.0%.

Residue on ignition ⟨281⟩: not more than 0.25%.

Chromatographic purity—

TEST A—

Standard solution—Dissolve accurately weighed quantities of USP Zidovudine RS, and triphenylmethanol in methanol, and mix to obtain a solution having known concentrations of about 0.1 mg of each per mL.

Test solution—Dissolve an accurately weighed quantity of Zidovudine in methanol to obtain a solution containing 20 mg per mL.

Procedure—Separately apply 10 µL of the *Test solution* and 10 µL of the *Standard solution* to a thin-layer chromatographic plate (see *Chromatography* ⟨621⟩) coated with a 0.25-mm layer of chromatographic silica gel mixture containing a fluorescent indicator having an optimal intensity at 254 nm. Develop the chromatogram in a solvent system consisting of chloroform and methanol (9 : 1) until the solvent front has moved about three-fourths of the length of the plate. Remove the plate from the chamber, mark the solvent front, and allow the solvent to evaporate. Examine the plate under short-wavelength UV light, and compare the intensities of any secondary spots observed in the chromatogram of the *Test solution* with those of the principal spot in the chromatogram of the *Standard solution:* no secondary spot from the chromatogram of the *Test solution* is larger or more intense than the principal spot obtained from the *Standard solution,* and the sum of the intensities of the secondary spots obtained from the *Test solution* corresponds to not more than 3.0%. Spray the plate with a mixture of 0.5 g of carbazole in 95 mL of alcohol and 5 mL of sulfuric acid, heat for 10 minutes at 120°, and compare the intensities of any secondary spots observed in the chromatogram of the *Test solution* with those of the principal spots in the chromatogram of the *Standard solution:* no spot corresponding to triphenylmethanol (R_F value about 2.3 relative to the R_F value of zidovudine) is more intense than the corresponding spot from the *Standard solution,* no secondary spot from the chromatogram of the *Test solution* is larger or more intense than the principal spot obtained from the *Standard solution,* and the sum of the intensities of the secondary spots obtained from the *Test solution* corresponds to not more than 3.0%.

Zidovudine / Official Monographs

TEST B—
Proceed as directed in the *Assay*, using the *Assay preparation* as the test solution. Calculate the percentage of each impurity in the portion of Zidovudine taken by the formula:

$$100(r_i / r_s)$$

in which r_i is the peak response for each impurity, and r_s is the sum of the responses of all of the peaks: not more than 1.0% of zidovudine related compound B and not more than 2.0% of zidovudine related compound C are found, and the sum of all impurities from *Test A* and *Test B* is not more than 3.0%.

Organic volatile impurities, *Method V* ⟨467⟩: meets the requirements.
  Solvent—Use dimethyl sulfoxide.

(Official until July 1, 2008)

Assay—
  Mobile phase—Prepare a filtered and degassed mixture of water and methanol (80 : 20). Make adjustments if necessary (see *System Suitability* under *Chromatography* ⟨621⟩).
  Standard stock solution—Dissolve an accurately weighed quantity of USP Zidovudine RS in methanol, and dilute quantitatively, and stepwise if necessary, with methanol to obtain a solution having a known concentration of about 1.0 mg per mL.
  Zidovudine related compound B standard stock solution—Dissolve an accurately weighed quantity of USP Zidovudine Related Compound B RS in methanol, and dilute quantitatively, and stepwise if necessary, with methanol to obtain a solution having a known concentration of about 0.1 mg per mL.
  Zidovudine related compound C standard stock solution—Transfer about 20 mg of USP Zidovudine Related Compound C RS, accurately weighed, to a 100-mL volumetric flask, add 75 mL of methanol, sonicate for 15 minutes, dilute with methanol to volume, and mix.
  Standard preparation—Transfer 10.0 mL of *Standard stock solution*, 1.0 mL of *Zidovudine related compound B standard stock solution*, and 1.0 mL of *Zidovudine related compound C standard stock solution* to a 100-mL volumetric flask, dilute with methanol to volume, and mix.
  Assay preparation—Transfer about 100 mg of Zidovudine, accurately weighed, to a 100-mL volumetric flask, dissolve in and dilute with methanol to volume, and mix. Transfer 10.0 mL of this solution to a 100-mL volumetric flask, dilute with methanol to volume, and mix.
  Chromatographic system (see *Chromatography* ⟨621⟩)—The liquid chromatograph is equipped with a 265-nm detector and a 4.0-mm × 25-cm column that contains packing L1 and a 3.2-mm × 1.5-cm guard column containing packing L1. The flow rate is about 1.0 mL per minute. Chromatograph the *Standard preparation*, and record the peak responses as directed for *Procedure*: the relative retention times are about 0.25 for zidovudine related compound C (thymine), 1.0 for zidovudine, and 1.17 for zidovudine related compound B (3'-chloro-3'-deoxythymidine); the resolution, R, between zidovudine and zidovudine related compound B is not less than 1.4; the tailing factor is not more than 1.5; and the relative standard deviation for replicate injections is not more than 2.0%.
  Procedure—Separately inject equal volumes (about 10 µL) of the *Standard preparation* and the *Assay preparation* into the chromatograph, record the chromatograms, and measure the responses for the major peaks. Calculate the quantity, in mg, of $C_{10}H_{13}N_5O_4$ in the portion of Zidovudine taken by the formula:

$$1000C(r_U / r_S)$$

in which C is the concentration, in mg per mL, of USP Zidovudine RS in the *Standard preparation*; and r_U and r_S are the peak responses obtained from the *Assay preparation* and the *Standard preparation*, respectively.

Zidovudine Capsules

» Zidovudine Capsules contain not less than 90.0 percent and not more than 110.0 percent of the labeled amount of zidovudine ($C_{10}H_{13}N_5O_4$).

Packaging and storage—Preserve in tight, light-resistant containers.
USP Reference standards ⟨11⟩—USP Zidovudine RS. USP Zidovudine Related Compound C RS.
Identification—
  A: *Ultraviolet Absorption* ⟨197U⟩—
  Medium: methanol and water (75 : 25).
  Solution: 15 µg per mL. Obtain the test solution as follows. Mix Capsule contents, equivalent to 300 mg of Zidovudine, with 50 mL of *Medium* in a 200-mL volumetric flask. Sonicate for 5 minutes, dilute with methanol to volume, and mix. Allow insoluble solids to settle, dilute the supernatant 100-fold with *Medium*, and mix.
  B: The retention time of the major peak in the chromatogram of the *Assay preparation* corresponds to that of the *Standard preparation*, as obtained in the *Assay*.
Dissolution ⟨711⟩—
  Medium: water; 900 mL.
  Apparatus 2: 50 rpm.
  Time: 45 minutes.
  Procedure—Determine the amount of $C_{10}H_{13}N_5O_4$ dissolved employing the procedure set forth in the *Assay*, making any necessary modifications.
  Tolerances—Not less than 75% (*Q*) of the labeled amount of $C_{10}H_{13}N_5O_4$ is dissolved in 45 minutes.
Uniformity of dosage units ⟨905⟩: meet the requirements.
Related compounds—
  Mobile phase, *Standard stock solution*, *Zidovudine related compound C standard stock solution*, and *Chromatographic system*—Proceed as directed in the *Assay* under *Zidovudine*.
  Standard solution—Proceed as directed for *Standard preparation* in the *Assay*.
  Test solution—Proceed as directed for *Assay preparation* in the *Assay*.
  Procedure—Separately inject equal volumes (about 10 µL) of the *Standard solution* and the *Test solution* into the chromatograph, record the chromatograms, and measure the peak responses. Calculate the quantity, in mg, of zidovudine related compound C (thymine) in the portion of Capsules taken by the formula:

$$1000C[(r_U / r_S)/Q]$$

in which C is the concentration, in mg per mL, of USP Zidovudine Related Compound C RS in the *Standard solution*; r_U and r_S are the peak responses of zidovudine related compound C (thymine) obtained from the *Test solution* and the *Standard solution*, respectively; and Q is the quantity, in mg, of zidovudine in the portion of Capsules taken, as determined in the *Assay*: not more than 3.0% is found.

Assay—
  Mobile phase, *Standard stock solution*, and *Zidovudine related compound C standard stock solution*—Prepare as directed in the *Assay* under *Zidovudine*.
  Standard preparation—Transfer 10.0 mL of *Standard stock solution* and 1.0 mL of *Zidovudine related compound C standard stock solution* to a 100-mL volumetric flask, add 25 mL of water, mix, dilute with methanol to volume, and mix.
  Assay preparation—Weigh the contents of not fewer than 20 Capsules, mix, and transfer an accurately weighed portion of the powder, equivalent to about 100 mg of zidovudine, to a 100-mL volumetric flask. Dissolve in a mixture of methanol and water (75 : 25), sonicate for 20 minutes, and dilute with a mixture of methanol and water (75 : 25) to volume. Allow the solids to settle, and transfer 10.0 mL of the supernatant layer to a 100-mL volumetric flask. Dilute with a mixture of methanol and water (75 : 25) to volume, and filter, discarding the first 4 mL of the filtrate.
  Chromatographic system (see *Chromatography* ⟨621⟩)—The liquid chromatograph is equipped with a 265-nm detector and a 4.0-

mm × 25-cm column that contains packing L1 and a 3.2-mm × 1.5-cm guard column containing packing L1. The flow rate is about 1.0 mL per minute. Chromatograph the *Standard preparation*, and record the peak responses as directed for *Procedure:* the relative retention times are about 0.2 for zidovudine related compound C (thymine) and 1.0 for zidovudine; the resolution, R, between zidovudine and zidovudine related compound C (thymine) is not less than 5.0; the tailing factor is not more than 2.0; and the relative standard deviation for replicate injections is not more than 2.0%.

Procedure—Separately inject equal volumes (about 10 µL) of the *Standard preparation* and the *Assay preparation* into the chromatograph, record the chromatograms, and measure the responses for the major peaks. Calculate the quantity, in mg, of zidovudine ($C_{10}H_{13}N_5O_4$) in the portion of Capsules taken by the formula:

$$1000C(r_U / r_S)$$

in which C is the concentration, in mg per mL, of USP Zidovudine RS in the *Standard preparation*; and r_U and r_S are the peak responses obtained from the *Assay preparation* and the *Standard preparation*, respectively.

Zidovudine Injection

» Zidovudine Injection is a sterile solution of Zidovudine in Water for Injection. It contains not less than 90.0 percent and not more than 110.0 percent of zidovudine ($C_{10}H_{13}N_5O_4$).

Packaging and storage—Preserve in tight, light-resistant containers.

USP Reference standards ⟨11⟩—*USP Endotoxin RS. USP Zidovudine RS. USP Zidovudine Related Compound C RS.*

Identification—
  A: *Ultraviolet Absorption* ⟨197U⟩—
    Medium: methanol and water (75 : 25).
    Solution: 15 µg per mL. Obtain the test solution as follows. Mix a volume of Injection, equivalent to 20 mg of zidovudine, with 50 mL of *Medium* in a 200-mL volumetric flask, and dilute with *Medium* to volume. Dilute the resulting solution 15 in 100 with *Medium*, and mix.
  B: The retention time of the major peak in the chromatogram of the *Assay preparation* corresponds to that of the *Standard preparation*, as obtained in the *Assay*.

Sterility ⟨71⟩—It meets the requirements when tested as directed for *Membrane Filtration* under *Test for Sterility of the Product to be Examined.*

pH ⟨791⟩: between 3.5 and 7.0, in a mixture containing a volume of Injection equivalent to 150 mg of zidovudine and 5 mL of 0.12 M potassium chloride.

Bacterial endotoxins ⟨85⟩—It contains not more than 1.0 USP Endotoxin Unit per mg of zidovudine.

Related compounds—
  Mobile phase, Standard stock solution, Zidovudine related compound C standard stock solution, and *Chromatographic system*—Proceed as directed in the *Assay* under *Zidovudine.*
  Standard solution—Transfer 10.0 mL of *Standard stock solution* and 1.0 mL of *Zidovudine related compound C standard stock solution* to a 100-mL volumetric flask, add 25 mL of water, mix, dilute with methanol to volume, and mix.
  Test solution—Proceed as directed for *Assay preparation* in the *Assay.*
  Procedure—Separately inject equal volumes (about 10 µL) of the *Standard solution* and the *Test solution* into the chromatograph, record the chromatograms, and measure the peak responses. Calculate the quantity, in mg, of zidovudine related compound C (thymine) in the volume of Injection taken by the formula:

$$1000C\,[(r_U / r_S) / Q]$$

in which C is the concentration, in mg per mL, of USP Zidovudine Related Compound C RS in the *Standard solution*; r_U and r_S are the peak responses of zidovudine related compound C (thymine) obtained from the *Test solution* and the *Standard solution*, respectively; and Q is the quantity, in mg, of zidovudine in the volume of Injection taken, as determined in the *Assay*: not more than 1.0% is found.

Other requirements—It meets the requirements under *Injections* ⟨1⟩.

Assay—
  Mobile phase, Standard stock solution, Zidovudine related compound C standard stock solution, and *Chromatographic system*—Proceed as directed in the *Assay* under *Zidovudine.*
  Standard preparation—Transfer 10.0 mL of *Standard stock solution* and 2.0 mL of *Zidovudine related compound C standard stock solution* to a 100-mL volumetric flask, add 25 mL of water, mix, dilute with methanol to volume, and mix.
  Assay preparation—Transfer an accurately measured volume of Injection, equivalent to about 25 mg of zidovudine, to a 250-mL volumetric flask, dissolve in and dilute with *Mobile phase* to volume, and mix.
  Procedure—Separately inject equal volumes (about 10 µL) of the *Standard preparation* and the *Assay preparation* into the chromatograph, record the chromatograms, and measure the responses for the major peaks. Calculate the quantity, in mg, of zidovudine ($C_{10}H_{13}N_5O_4$) in the volume of Injection taken by the formula:

$$1000C(r_U / r_S)$$

in which C is the concentration, in mg per mL, of USP Zidovudine RS in the *Standard preparation*; and r_U and r_S are the peak responses obtained from the *Assay preparation* and the *Standard preparation*, respectively.

Zidovudine Oral Solution

» Zidovudine Oral Solution contains not less than 90.0 percent and not more than 110.0 percent of the labeled amount of zidovudine ($C_{10}H_{13}N_5O_4$).

Packaging and storage—Preserve in tight, light-resistant containers.

USP Reference standards ⟨11⟩—*USP Zidovudine RS. USP Zidovudine Related Compound C RS.*

Identification—
  A: Prepare a test solution in methanol containing 5 mg per mL. Separately apply 5 µL of this solution and 5 µL of a Standard solution of USP Zidovudine RS in a mixture of methanol and water (75 : 25) containing 5 mg per mL to a thin-layer chromatographic plate (see *Chromatography* ⟨621⟩) coated with a 0.25-mm layer of chromatographic silica gel mixture containing a fluorescent indicator having an optimal intensity at 254 nm. Allow the applications to dry, and develop the chromatogram in a solvent system consisting of butyl alcohol, *n*-heptane, acetone, and ammonium hydroxide (40 : 30 : 30 : 10) until the solvent front has moved about three-fourths of the length of the plate. Remove the plate from the developing chamber, mark the solvent front, and allow the solvent to evaporate. Observe the plate under short-wavelength UV light: the R_F value of the principal spot obtained from the test solution corresponds to that of the principal spot obtained from the Standard solution.
  B: The retention time of the major peak in the chromatogram of the *Assay preparation* corresponds to that in the chromatogram of the *Standard preparation*, as obtained in the *Assay.*

Microbial limits ⟨61⟩—It meets the requirements of the tests for the absence of *Staphylococcus aureus* and *Pseudomonas aeruginosa* and for absence of *Salmonella* species and *Escherichia coli*.

Uniformity of dosage units ⟨905⟩—
  FOR ORAL SOLUTION PACKAGED IN SINGLE-UNIT CONTAINERS: meets the requirements.

Deliverable volume ⟨698⟩—
  FOR ORAL SOLUTION PACKAGED IN MULTIPLE-UNIT CONTAINERS: meets the requirements.

pH ⟨791⟩: between 3.0 and 4.0, in a mixture containing a volume of Oral Solution equivalent to 150 mg of zidovudine and 5 mL of 0.12 M potassium chloride (3 : 1).

Related compounds—

Mobile phase, Standard stock solution, Zidovudine related compound C standard stock solution, and *Chromatographic system—*Proceed as directed in the *Assay.*

*Standard solution—*Proceed as directed for *Standard preparation* in the *Assay.*

*Test solution—*Proceed as directed for *Assay preparation* in the *Assay.*

*Procedure—*Separately inject equal volumes (about 10 μL) of the *Standard solution* and the *Test solution* into the chromatograph, record the chromatograms, and measure the peak responses. Calculate the quantity, in mg, of zidovudine related compound C (thymine) in the volume of Oral Solution taken by the formula:

$$1000C[(r_U / r_S) / Q]$$

in which C is the concentration, in mg per mL, of USP Zidovudine Related Compound C RS in the *Standard solution;* r_U and r_S are the peak responses of zidovudine related compound C (thymine) obtained from the *Test solution* and the *Standard solution,* respectively; and Q is the quantity, in mg, of zidovudine in the volume of Oral Solution taken, as determined in the *Assay:* not more than 3.0% is found.

Assay—

*Mobile phase—*Prepare a filtered and degassed mixture of 0.040 M sodium acetate, methanol, acetonitrile, and glacial acetic acid (900 : 90 : 10 : 2). Make adjustments if necessary (see *System Suitability* under *Chromatography* ⟨621⟩).

*Standard stock solution—*Dissolve an accurately weighed quantity of USP Zidovudine RS in *Mobile phase,* and dilute quantitatively, and stepwise if necessary, with *Mobile phase* to obtain a solution having a known concentration of about 1.0 mg per mL.

*Zidovudine related compound C standard stock solution—*Transfer about 20 mg of USP Zidovudine Related Compound C RS, accurately weighed, to a 200-mL volumetric flask, add 150 mL of *Mobile phase,* sonicate for 10 minutes, dilute with *Mobile phase* to volume, and mix.

*Standard preparation—*Transfer 10.0 mL of the *Standard stock solution* and 2.0 mL of the *Zidovudine related compound C standard stock solution* to a 100-mL volumetric flask, dilute with *Mobile phase* to volume, and mix.

*Assay preparation—*Transfer an accurately measured volume of Oral Solution, equivalent to about 100 mg of zidovudine, to a 100-mL volumetric flask; dissolve in and dilute with *Mobile phase* to volume; and mix. Transfer 5.0 mL of this solution to a 50-mL volumetric flask, dilute with *Mobile phase* to volume, and mix.

Chromatographic system (see *Chromatography* ⟨621⟩)—The liquid chromatograph is equipped with a 240-nm detector and a 4.0-mm × 12.5-cm column that contains packing L1. The flow rate is about 1.0 mL per minute. Chromatograph the *Standard preparation,* and record the peak responses as directed for *Procedure:* the relative retention times are about 0.12 for zidovudine related compound C (thymine) and 1.0 for zidovudine; the resolution, *R*, between zidovudine and zidovudine related compound C (thymine) is not less than 4.0; the tailing factor is not more than 2.0; and the relative standard deviation for replicate injections is not more than 2.0%.

*Procedure—*Separately inject equal volumes (about 10 μL) of the *Standard preparation* and the *Assay preparation* into the chromatograph, record the chromatograms, and measure the responses for the major peaks. Calculate the quantity, in mg, of zidovudine ($C_{10}H_{13}N_5O_4$) in the portion of Oral Solution taken by the formula:

$$1000C(r_U / r_S)$$

in which C is the concentration, in mg per mL, of USP Zidovudine RS in the *Standard preparation;* and r_U and r_S are the peak responses obtained from the *Assay preparation* and the *Standard preparation,* respectively.

Zidovudine Tablets

» Zidovudine Tablets contain not less than 90.0 percent and not more than 110.0 percent of the labeled amount of zidovudine ($C_{10}H_{13}N_5O_4$).

Packaging and storage—Preserve in tight, light-resistant containers, and store at controlled room temperature.

USP Reference standards ⟨11⟩—*USP Zidovudine RS. USP Zidovudine Related Compound B RS. USP Zidovudine Related Compound C RS.*

Identification—

A: *Infrared Absorption* ⟨197K⟩—

*Test specimen—*Grind 1 Tablet in a mortar so that no large pieces remain, and remove the coating film so that about 5 mg of ground Tablet remain.

B: The retention time of the major peak in the chromatogram of the *Assay preparation* corresponds to that in the chromatogram of the *Standard preparation,* as obtained in the *Assay.*

Dissolution ⟨711⟩—

Medium: water; 900 mL.

Apparatus 2: 50 rpm.

Time: 30 minutes.

*Procedure—*Determine the amount of $C_{10}H_{13}N_5O_4$ dissolved by employing the procedure set forth in the *Assay,* using a filtered portion of the solution under test as the *Assay preparation* in comparison with a Standard solution having a known concentration of USP Zidovudine RS in the same *Medium.*

*Tolerances—*Not less than 80% (*Q*) of the labeled amount of $C_{10}H_{13}N_5O_4$ is dissolved in 30 minutes.

Uniformity of dosage units ⟨905⟩: meet the requirements.

PROCEDURE FOR CONTENT UNIFORMITY—

*Mobile phase—*Prepare a filtered and degassed mixture of water and methanol (4 : 1). Make adjustments if necessary (see *System Suitability* under *Chromatography* ⟨621⟩).

*Standard preparation—*Prepare as directed in the *Assay.*

*Test preparation—*Transfer 1 Tablet to a 100-mL volumetric flask, add about 20 mL of water, and shake by mechanical means to disperse the Tablet. Add about 30 mL of methanol, and sonicate for 10 minutes. Dilute with water to volume, and mix. Pipet 4.0 mL of the resulting solution into a 100-mL volumetric flask, and dilute with water to volume. Mix, and pass a portion of the solution through a suitable nylon filter, discarding the first 2 mL of the filtrate.

Chromatographic system (see *Chromatography* ⟨621⟩)—The liquid chromatograph is equipped with a 265-nm detector and a 4.6-mm × 15-cm column that contains base-deactivated packing L1. The flow rate is about 2.0 mL per minute. Chromatograph the *Standard preparation,* and record the peak responses as directed for *Procedure:* the tailing factor is not more than 2.0; and the relative standard deviation for replicate injections is not more than 2.0%.

*Procedure—*Separately inject equal volumes (about 10 μL) of the *Standard preparation* and the *Test preparation* into the chromatograph, record the chromatograms, and measure the responses for the major peaks. Calculate the quantity, in mg, of zidovudine ($C_{10}H_{13}N_5O_4$) in the Tablet taken by the formula:

$$2500C(r_U / r_S)$$

in which C is the concentration, in mg per mL, of USP Zidovudine RS in the *Standard preparation;* and r_U and r_S are the peak responses obtained from the *Test preparation* and the *Standard preparation,* respectively.

Related compounds—

Mobile phase and *Chromatographic system—*Proceed as directed in the *Assay.*

*Standard solution—*Use the *Standard preparation,* prepared as directed in the *Assay.*

*Test solution—*Use the *Assay preparation.*

*Procedure—*Separately inject equal volumes (about 20 μL) of the *Standard solution* and the *Test solution* into the chromatograph, record the chromatograms, and measure all of the peak responses. Calculate the percentage of each impurity in the portion of Tablets taken by the formula:

$$100/F \ (r_i / r_S)$$

in which F is the relative response factor and is equal to 1.7 for zidovudine related compound C, and is equal to 1.00 for all other peaks; r_i is the peak response for each impurity obtained from the *Test solution;* and r_S is the peak response for zidovudine obtained from the *Standard solution:* not more than 1.5% of zidovudine related compound C is found; not more than 0.2% of any other individual unidentified impurity is found; and not more than 2.0% of total impurities is found.

Assay—

*Mobile phase—*Dissolve 3.0 g of sodium acetate and 1.3 g of sodium 1-octanesulfonate in 900 mL of water. Add 90 mL of methanol and 40 mL of acetonitrile, and mix. Adjust with glacial acetic acid to a pH of 5.3, filter, and degas. Make adjustments if necessary (see *System Suitability* under *Chromatography* ⟨621⟩).

*Zidovudine related compound B standard stock solution—*Dissolve an accurately weighed quantity of USP Zidovudine Related Compound B RS in methanol, and dilute quantitatively, and stepwise if necessary, with methanol to obtain a solution having a known concentration of about 0.1 mg per mL.

*Zidovudine related compound C standard stock solution—*Dissolve by sonicating for about 15 minutes, an accurately weighed quantity of USP Zidovudine Related Compound C RS in methanol, and dilute quantitatively, and stepwise if necessary, with methanol to obtain a solution having a known concentration of about 0.2 mg per mL.

*Standard preparation—*Transfer about 30 mg of USP Zidovudine RS, accurately weighed, to a 250-mL volumetric flask, and dissolve in 3.0 mL of methanol. Add 2.5 mL of *Zidovudine related compound B standard stock solution,* 5.0 mL of *Zidovudine related compound C standard stock solution,* and dilute with water to volume. This solution contains zidovudine, zidovudine related compound B, and zidovudine related compound C at concentrations of about 0.12 mg per mL, 0.001 mg per mL, and 0.004 mg per mL, respectively.

*Assay preparation—*Transfer a counted number of Tablets, equivalent to 1500 mg of zidovudine, to a 500-mL volumetric flask. Add about 50 mL of water, and shake by mechanical means for 30 minutes to disperse the Tablets. Add about 150 mL of methanol, and sonicate for 10 minutes. Dilute with water to volume, and mix. Pipet 4.0 mL into a 100-mL volumetric flask, and dilute with water to volume. Mix, and pass a portion of the solution through a suitable nylon filter, discarding the first 2 mL of the filtrate.

Chromatographic system (see *Chromatography* ⟨621⟩)—The liquid chromatograph is equipped with a 265-nm detector and a 4.6-mm × 15-cm column that contains packing L1. The flow rate is about 1.3 mL per minute. Chromatograph the *Standard preparation,* and record the peak responses as directed for *Procedure:* the relative retention times are about 0.17 for zidovudine related compound C (thymine), 1.0 for zidovudine, and 1.2 for zidovudine related compound B; the resolution, R, between zidovudine and zidovudine related compound B is not less than 2.5; the tailing factor for the zidovudine peak is not more than 2.0; and the relative standard deviation for replicate injections is not more than 2.0%.

*Procedure—*Separately inject equal volumes (about 20 µL) of the *Standard preparation* and the *Assay preparation* into the chromatograph, record the chromatograms, and measure the responses for the major peaks. Calculate the quantity, in mg, of zidovudine ($C_{10}H_{13}N_5O_4$) in each Tablet taken by the formula:

$$12{,}500(C/N)(r_U / r_S)$$

in which C is the concentration, in mg per mL, of USP Zidovudine RS in the *Standard preparation;* N is the number of Tablets taken for the *Assay preparation;* and r_U and r_S are the peak responses obtained from the *Assay preparation* and the *Standard preparation,* respectively.

Zileuton

$C_{11}H_{12}N_2O_2S$ 236.29
Urea, *N*-(1-benzo[*b*]thien-2-ylethyl)-*N*-hydroxy-, (±)-.
(±)-1-(1-Benzo[*b*]thien-2-ylethyl)-1-hydroxyurea   [*111406-87-2*].

» Zileuton contains not less than 98.5 percent and not more than 101.5 percent of $C_{11}H_{12}N_2O_2S$, calculated on the anhydrous basis.

Packaging and storage—Preserve in tight, light-resistant containers, and store at room temperature.

USP Reference standards ⟨11⟩—*USP Zileuton RS. USP Zileuton Related Compound A RS. USP Zileuton Related Compound B RS. USP Zileuton Related Compound C RS.*

Identification—
A: *Infrared Absorption* ⟨197K⟩.
B: The retention time of the major peak in the chromatogram of the *Assay preparation* corresponds to that in the chromatogram of the *Standard preparation,* as obtained in the *Assay.*

Specific rotation ⟨781S⟩:   between –0.5° and +0.5°.
Test solution: 10 mg per mL, in methanol.

Water, *Method I* ⟨921⟩:   not more than 1.5%.

Residue on ignition ⟨281⟩:   not more than 0.2%.

Specific surface area, *Method I* ⟨846⟩—Outgas a portion of the test sample, about 100 mg, at 90° for 1 hour at ambient pressure using 0.001 mole fraction of krypton in helium as the adsorbate gas: between 0.9 and 3.1. m² per g.

Arsenic, *Method II* ⟨211⟩:   2 µg per g.

Heavy metals, *Method II* ⟨231⟩:   0.002%.

Limit of boron—

*Sulfuric acid solution—*Carefully add 50 mL of sulfuric acid to 450 mL of water, and mix.

*Standard solution—*Prepare a solution in *Sulfuric acid solution* having a concentration of about 2.0 µg of boron per mL. Use of a commercially prepared boron ICP standard solution is recommended.

*Test solution—*Accurately weigh approximately 1.0 g of Zileuton into a 125-mL conical flask. Add 1 to 1.5 mL of sulfuric acid, and digest in a fume hood on a hot plate until charring begins. Add 2 mL of nitric acid to the cooled sample to aid digestion, and heat until brown fumes are not evolved. Cautiously add 30 percent hydrogen peroxide, dropwise, allowing the reaction to subside, and heating between drops. Add the first few drops very slowly with sufficient mixing in order to prevent a rapid reaction. Discontinue heating if foaming becomes excessive. When the reaction has abated, heat cautiously, rotating the flask occasionally to prevent the sample from caking on glass exposed to the heating unit. Maintain oxidizing conditions at all times during the digestion by adding small quantities of the 30 percent hydrogen peroxide, whenever the mixture turns brown or darkens. Approximately 1 to 2 mL of nitric acid can be added, if necessary, which will create a refluxing effect to wash down any particles adhering to the neck of the flask. Continue the digestion until the organic matter is destroyed, gradually raising the temperature of the hot plate until fumes of sulfur trioxide are copiously evolved and the solution becomes colorless or retains only a light straw color. Transfer the solution to a 25-mL volumetric flask using about 7 mL of water. Repeat the washing twice more, and combine the washings in the volumetric flask. Dilute with water to volume, and mix.

*Procedure—*The inductively coupled plasma-atomic emission spectrometer is set up with wavelength of 249.7 nm, RF power of 1.25 KW, argon torch flow of about 13 L per minute, argon nebulizer flow of about 1 L per minute, and argon auxillary flow of about 0.5 L per minute. Analyze the *Standard solution* and the *Test solution,* using *Sulfuric acid solution* as the blank. Calculate the quantity, in μg of boron per g, in the portion of Zileuton taken by the formula:

$$25C/W,$$

where C is the concentration, in μg per mL, of boron in the *Test solution* determined from the instrument; and W is the weight, in g, of the Zileuton: not more than 10 μg per g is found.

Limit of pyridine—

Standard solution—Dissolve an accurately weighed quantity of pyridine, approximately 250 mg, in dimethyl sulfoxide, and dilute with dimethyl sulfoxide to 50 mL. Transfer 5 μL to a 100-mL sealed headspace vial.

Test solution—Transfer about 100 mg of Zileuton, accurately weighed, to a vial, add 5.0 mL of dimethyl sulfoxide and 1 g of anhydrous sodium sulfate, and seal with a septum and crimp cap. Heat the sealed vial at 80° for 60 minutes.

Chromatographic system (see *Chromatography* ⟨621⟩)—[NOTE—The use of a headspace apparatus is allowed.] The gas chromatograph is equipped with a flame-ionization detector, a 0.53-mm × 30-m fused silica analytical column coated with a 3.0-μm G43 stationary phase. The carrier gas is helium with a linear velocity of about 35 cm per second. The injection port and detector temperatures are maintained at 140° and 260°, respectively. The column temperature is programmed according to the following steps. It is maintained at 40° for 20 minutes, then increased rapidly to 240°, and maintained at 240° for 20 minutes. Inject the *Standard solution*, and record the peak responses as directed for *Procedure*: the relative standard deviation for replicate injections is not more than 15%.

Procedure—Using a heated gas-tight syringe separately inject equal volumes (about 1 mL) of the headspace of the *Standard solution* and the *Test solution* into the gas chromatograph, and record the peak responses. Calculate the quantity, in ppm, of pyridine in the portion of Zileuton taken by the formula:

$$100(r_U / r_S)(W_S / W_U)$$

in which r_U and r_S are the peak responses for pyridine in the *Test solution* and the *Standard solution*, respectively; W_S is the weight, in mg, of pyridine used to prepare the *Standard solution*; and W_U is the weight, in mg, of Zileuton: not more than 100 ppm is found.

Chromatographic purity—[NOTE—For *Test 1* and *Test 2*, the *System suitability solution*, the *Standard solution*, and the *Test solution* are to be refrigerated at or below 5° immediately after preparation and during analysis using a refrigerated autosampler. The solutions are stable at or below 5° for about 36 hours.]

TEST 1—

Buffer solution—Prepare as directed in the *Assay*.

Mobile phase—Prepare a filtered and degassed mixture of *Buffer solution* and acetonitrile (82 : 18). Make adjustments if necessary (see *System Suitability* under *Chromatography* ⟨621⟩).

System suitability solution—Dissolve accurately weighed quantities of USP Zileuton RS and USP Zileuton Related Compound A RS in acetonitrile, and dilute quantitatively, and stepwise if necessary, to obtain a solution having a known concentration of about 5 μg of each USP Reference Standard per mL.

Standard solution—Dissolve an accurately weighed quantity of USP Zileuton RS in acetonitrile to obtain a solution having a known concentration of about 10 μg per mL.

Test solution—Transfer about 125 mg of Zileuton, accurately weighed, to a 50-mL volumetric flask, dissolve in and dilute with acetonitrile to volume, and mix.

Chromatographic system—Prepare as directed in the *Assay*, except to use a flow rate of 2.2 mL per minute. Chromatograph the *System suitability solution*, and record the peak responses as directed for *Procedure*: the resolution, R, between zileuton and zileuton related compound A is not less than 1.5; and the relative standard deviation for replicate injections is not more than 5.0%.

Procedure—Separately inject equal volumes (about 20 μL) of the *Standard solution* and the *Test solution* into the chromatograph, and measure the areas for the major peaks. Calculate the percentage of each impurity in the portion of Zileuton taken by the formula:

$$100F(C_S / C_U)(r_i / r_S)$$

in which F is the relative response factor for each impurity, which is 1.0 for any peak with a relative retention time of 0.5, 0.7, 1.2, 1.6, 3.2, or 3.4, and is 1.2, 1.4, and 1.7 for peaks with relative retention times of 0.8, 2.1, and 2.8, respectively; C_S is the concentration, in mg per mL, of USP Zileuton RS in the *Standard solution*; C_U is the concentration, in mg per mL, of zileuton in the *Test solution*; r_i is the peak response for each impurity obtained from the *Test solution*; and r_S is the peak response for zileuton obtained from the *Standard solution*: not more than 0.1% of any individual impurity with a relative retention time of 0.8, 1.6, or 2.1 is found; not more than 0.10% of any individual impurity with a relative retention time of 0.7, 3.2, or 3.4 is found; not more than 0.20% of any individual impurity with a relative retention time of 0.5 or 1.2 is found; and not more than 0.07% of any individual impurity with a relative retention time of 2.8 is found.

TEST 2—

Perchloric acid solution—Dissolve 5.0 mL of perchloric acid in 1000 mL of water.

Mobile phase—Prepare a filtered and degassed mixture of *Perchloric acid solution* and acetonitrile (1 : 1). Make adjustments if necessary (see *System Suitability* under *Chromatography* ⟨621⟩).

Standard stock solution—Dissolve an accurately weighed quantity of USP Zileuton Related Compound B RS in acetonitrile to obtain a solution having a known concentration of about 0.25 mg per mL. Transfer 5.0 mL of this solution to a 50-mL volumetric flask, dilute with acetonitrile to volume, and mix.

System suitability solution—Dissolve an accurately weighed quantity of USP Zileuton Related Compound C RS in acetonitrile to obtain a solution having a known concentration of about 10 μg per mL. Transfer 5.0 mL of this solution and 5.0 mL of the *Standard stock solution* to a 50-mL volumetric flask, dilute with acetonitrile to volume, and mix.

Standard solution—Transfer 5.0 mL of the *Standard stock solution* to a 50-mL volumetric flask, dilute with acetonitrile to volume, and mix.

Test solution—Proceed as directed for *Test solution* under *Test 1*.

Chromatographic system—Prepare as directed in the *Assay*. Chromatograph the *System suitability solution*, and record the peak responses as directed for *Procedure*: the resolution, R, between zileuton related compound B and zileuton related compound C is not less than 20. Chromatograph the *Standard solution*, and record the peak responses as directed for *Procedure*: the relative standard deviation for replicate injections is not more than 5.0%.

Procedure—Separately inject equal volumes (about 50 μL) of the *Standard solution* and the *Test solution* into the chromatograph, record the chromatograms, and measure the areas for the major peaks. Calculate the percentage of each impurity in the portion of Zileuton taken by the formula:

$$100(C_S / C_U)(r_i / r_S)$$

in which C_S is the concentration, in mg per mL, of USP Zileuton Related Compound B RS in the *Standard solution*; C_U is the concentration, in mg per mL, of zileuton in the *Test solution*; r_i is the peak response for each impurity obtained from the *Test solution*; and r_S is the peak response for zileuton related compound B obtained from the *Standard solution*: not more than 0.1% of any individual impurity is found; and not more than 0.7% of total impurities is found, the results for *Test 1* and *Test 2* being added.

Organic volatile impurities, *Method IV* ⟨467⟩: meets the requirements.

(Official until July 1, 2008)

Assay—

NOTE—The *Standard preparation* and the *Assay preparation* are to be refrigerated at or below 5° immediately after preparation and during analysis using a refrigerated autosampler. The solutions are stable at or below 5° for about 36 hours.

Buffer solution—Dissolve 7.7 g of ammonium acetate and 0.25 g of acetohydroxamic acid in about 900 mL of water in a 1000-mL volumetric flask, adjust with perchloric acid to a pH of 2.0, dilute with water to volume, and mix.

Mobile phase—Prepare a filtered and degassed mixture of *Buffer solution* and acetonitrile (72 : 28). Make adjustments if necessary (see *System Suitability* under *Chromatography* ⟨621⟩).

Internal standard preparation—Transfer about 30 mg of methylparaben, accurately weighed, to a 100-mL volumetric flask, dissolve in and dilute with acetonitrile to volume, and mix.

Standard stock preparation—Dissolve an accurately weighed quantity of USP Zileuton RS in acetonitrile to obtain a solution having a known concentration of about 1 mg per mL.

Standard preparation—Transfer 5.0 mL of the *Standard stock preparation* and 4.0 mL of the *Internal standard preparation* to a 50-mL volumetric flask, dilute with acetonitrile to volume, and mix.

Assay preparation—Transfer about 100 mg of Zileuton, accurately weighed, to a 100-mL volumetric flask, dissolve in and dilute with acetonitrile to volume, and mix. Transfer 5.0 mL of this solution and 4.0 mL of the *Internal standard preparation* to a 50-mL volumetric flask, dilute with acetonitrile to volume, and mix.

Chromatographic system (see *Chromatography* ⟨621⟩)—The liquid chromatograph is equipped with a 260-nm detector and a 4.6-mm × 30-cm column that contains 10-μm packing L1. The flow rate is about 1.5 mL per minute. Chromatograph the *Standard preparation*, and record the peak responses as directed for *Procedure*: the resolution, *R*, between zileuton and methylparaben is not less than 5.0; the tailing factor is not more than 1.3; and the relative standard deviation for replicate injections is not more than 0.6%.

Procedure—Separately inject equal volumes (about 20 μL) of the *Assay preparation* and the *Standard preparation* into the chromatograph, record the chromatograms, and measure the peak areas. Calculate the quantity, in mg, of $C_{11}H_{12}N_2O_2S$ in the portion of Zileuton taken by the formula:

$$1000C(R_U / R_S)$$

in which *C* is the concentration, in mg per mL, of USP Zileuton RS in the *Standard preparation*; and R_U and R_S are the peak area ratios obtained from the *Assay preparation* and the *Standard preparation*, respectively.

Zinc Acetate

$C_4H_6O_4Zn \cdot 2H_2O$ 219.51
Acetic acid, zinc salt, dihydrate.
Zinc acetate dihydrate [5970-45-6].
Anhydrous 183.48 [557-34-6].

» Zinc Acetate contains not less than 98.0 percent and not more than 102.0 percent of $C_4H_6O_4Zn \cdot 2H_2O$.

Packaging and storage—Preserve in tight containers.
Identification—A solution (1 in 20) responds to the tests for *Zinc* ⟨191⟩ and for *Acetate* ⟨191⟩.
pH ⟨791⟩: between 6.0 and 8.0, in a solution (1 in 20).
Insoluble matter—A 20-g portion, dissolved in 150 mL of water containing 1 mL of glacial acetic acid, shows not more than 1.0 mg of insoluble matter (0.005%).
Arsenic, *Method I* ⟨211⟩: 3 ppm.
Lead ⟨251⟩—Dissolve 0.5 g in 1 mL of a mixture of equal parts, by volume, of nitric acid and water in a separator. Add 3 mL of *Ammonium Citrate Solution* and 0.5 mL of *Hydroxylamine Hydrochloride Solution*, and render alkaline, with ammonium hydroxide, to phenol red TS. Add 10 mL of *Potassium Cyanide Solution*, and immediately extract the solution with successive 5-mL portions of *Dithizone Extraction Solution*, draining off each extract into another separator, until the last portion of dithizone solution retains its green color. Shake the combined extracts for 30 seconds with 20 mL of dilute nitric acid (1 in 100), and discard the chloroform layer. Add to the acid solution 4.0 mL of *Ammonia-Cyanide Solution* and 2 drops of *Hydroxylamine Hydrochloride Solution*. Add 10.0 mL of *Standard Dithizone Solution*, and shake the mixture for 30 seconds. Filter the chloroform layer through acid-washed filter paper into a color-comparison tube, and compare the color with that of a standard prepared as follows: to 20 mL of dilute nitric acid (1 in 100) add 0.01 mg of lead, 4 mL of *Ammonia-Cyanide Solution*, and 2 drops of *Hydroxylamine Hydrochloride Solution*, and shake for 30 seconds with 10.0 mL of *Standard Dithizone Solution*. Filter through acid-washed filter paper into a color-comparison tube: the color of the sample solution does not exceed that of the control (0.002%).
Chloride ⟨221⟩—A 1.5-g portion shows no more chloride than corresponds to 0.10 mL of 0.020 N hydrochloric acid (0.005%).
Sulfate ⟨221⟩—A 1.0-g portion shows no more sulfate than corresponds to 0.10 mL of 0.020 N sulfuric acid (0.010%).
Alkalies and alkaline earths—Dissolve 2.0 g in about 150 mL of water contained in a 200-mL volumetric flask, add sufficient ammonium sulfide TS to precipitate the zinc completely, dilute with water to volume, and mix. Filter through a dry filter, rejecting the first portion of the filtrate. To 100 mL of the subsequent filtrate add 5 drops of sulfuric acid, evaporate to dryness, and ignite: the weight of the residue does not exceed 2 mg (0.2%).
Organic volatile impurities, *Method I* ⟨467⟩: meets the requirements.
(Official until July 1, 2008)
Assay—Dissolve about 400 mg of Zinc Acetate, accurately weighed, in 100 mL of water. Add 5 mL of ammonia–ammonium chloride buffer TS and 0.1 mL of eriochrome black TS, and titrate with 0.05 M edetate disodium VS until the solution is deep blue in color. Each mL of 0.05 M edetate disodium is equivalent to 10.98 mg of $C_4H_6O_4Zn \cdot 2H_2O$.

Zinc Carbonate

$3Zn(OH)_2 \cdot 2ZnCO_3$ 549.01
Basic zinc carbonate.
Zinc subcarbonate [3486-35-9].

» Zinc Carbonate contains the equivalent of not less than 70.0 percent of ZnO.

Packaging and storage—Preserve in tight containers.
Identification—A solution of it in a slight excess of hydrochloric acid responds to the tests for *Zinc* ⟨191⟩.
Insoluble matter—Dissolve a 10-g portion in a mixture of 100 mL of water and 7 mL of sulfuric acid, and heat on a steam bath for 1 hour. Filter the solution through a tared sintered-glass crucible, wash with hot water, dry the crucible at 105°, cool, and weigh: the residue weighs not more than 20 mg (0.02%).
Chloride ⟨221⟩—A 1.0-g portion dissolved in a mixture of 20 mL of water and 3 mL of nitric acid shows no more chloride than corresponds to 0.03 mL of 0.02 N hydrochloric acid (0.002%).
Sulfate—Dissolve a 10.0-g portion in a mixture of 75 mL of water and 10 mL of hydrochloric acid, and filter. Neutralize the filtrate with ammonium hydroxide, dilute with water to 100 mL, and mix. To 10.0 mL of this solution add 1 mL of 0.6 N hydrochloric acid and 1 mL of barium chloride TS, mix, and allow to stand for 10 minutes. This test solution shows no more turbidity, if any, than that produced in a solution containing 0.10 mL of 0.02 N sulfuric acid and the same quantities of reagents used to prepare the test solution (0.01%).
Iron ⟨241⟩—Dissolve a 1.0-g portion in 20 mL of water and 3 mL of hydrochloric acid: the limit is 0.002%.
Lead—Transfer a 10.0-g portion to a 100-mL volumetric flask, add 20 mL of nitric acid and 10 mL of water, swirl to dissolve, dilute with water to volume, and mix. Add 10.0 mL of this solution to each of three 25-mL volumetric flasks. To respective volumetric flasks add 0, 5.0, and 10.0 mL of *Standard Lead Solution*, prepared as directed in the test for *Heavy metals* ⟨231⟩, dilute with water to volume, and mix. These solutions contain 0 (*Test preparation*), 0.002, and 0.004 mg of added lead per mL, respectively. Concomitantly determine the absorbances of these three solutions at the lead emission line at 217.0 nm, with an atomic absorption spectrophotometer (see *Spectrophotometry and Light-scattering* ⟨851⟩)

equipped with a lead hollow-cathode lamp and an air–acetylene flame, using a 1 in 25 solution of nitric acid in water to set the instrument to zero. Plot the absorbances of the three solutions versus their contents of added lead, in mg per mL, as furnished by the *Standard Lead Solution*, draw the straight line best fitting the three points, and extrapolate the line until it intercepts the concentration axis. From the intercept determine the amount, in mg, in each mL of the *Test preparation*. Calculate the quantity, in ppm, of lead in the specimen by multiplying this value by 25,000: the limit is 5 ppm.

Substances not precipitated by ammonium sulfide—Dissolve a 1.0-g portion in 10 mL of water and 2 mL of sulfuric acid, dilute with water to 80 mL, add 10 mL of ammonium hydroxide, and pass hydrogen sulfide through the solution for about 30 minutes. Dilute with water to 100 mL, and allow the precipitate to settle. Decant the supernatant through a filter, and transfer 50 mL of the clear filtrate to a tared dish, evaporate to dryness, ignite, gently at first and finally at 800 ± 25°, cool, and weigh: the weight of the residue does not exceed 2 mg (0.4%).

Assay—Transfer about 2.0 g of Zinc Carbonate, accurately weighed, to a 125-mL conical flask, add 50.0 mL of 1 N sulfuric acid VS, and swirl to dissolve. Add 3 drops of methyl orange TS, and titrate with 1 N sodium hydroxide VS to a yellow endpoint. Each mL of 1 N sulfuric acid consumed is equivalent to 40.69 mg of ZnO.

Zinc Chloride

$ZnCl_2$ 136.30
Zinc chloride.
Zinc chloride   [7646-85-7].

» Zinc Chloride contains not less than 97.0 percent and not more than 100.5 percent of $ZnCl_2$.

Packaging and storage—Preserve in tight containers.
Identification—A solution of it responds to the tests for *Zinc* ⟨191⟩ and for *Chloride* ⟨191⟩.
Limit of oxychloride—Dissolve 1.0 g in 20 mL of water, add 20 mL of alcohol, and mix. To 10 mL of the mixture add 0.30 mL of 1.0 N hydrochloric acid: the solution becomes perfectly clear.
Sulfate ⟨221⟩—Dissolve 1.0 g in 30 mL of water: 20 mL of this solution shows no more sulfate than corresponds to 0.20 mL of 0.020 N sulfuric acid (0.03%).
Limit of ammonium salts—To 5 mL of a solution (1 in 10) add 1 N sodium hydroxide until the precipitate first formed is redissolved, and then warm the solution: no odor of ammonia is perceptible.
Lead ⟨251⟩—Dissolve 0.50 g in 5 mL of water, and transfer the solution to a color-comparison tube (A). Add 15 mL of *Potassium Cyanide Solution* (1 in 10), mix, and allow the mixture to become clear. In a similar, matched color-comparison tube (B) place 5 mL of water, and add 2.50 mL of *Standard Lead Solution* (see *Heavy Metals* ⟨231⟩) and 15 mL of *Potassium Cyanide Solution* (1 in 10). Add to the solution in each tube 0.1 mL of sodium sulfide TS. Mix the contents of each tube, and allow to stand for 5 minutes: viewed downward over a white surface, the solution in tube A is not darker than that in tube B (indicating not more than 0.005% of lead).
Alkalies and alkaline earths—Dissolve 2.0 g in about 150 mL of water contained in a 200-mL volumetric flask. Add sufficient ammonium sulfide TS to precipitate the zinc completely, dilute with water to volume, and mix. Filter through a dry filter, and reject the first portion of the filtrate. To 100 mL of the subsequent filtrate add 5 drops of sulfuric acid, evaporate to dryness, and ignite: the weight of the residue does not exceed 10 mg (1.0%).
Organic volatile impurities, *Method I* ⟨467⟩: meets the requirements.

(Official until July 1, 2008)

Assay—Dissolve about 12 g of Zinc Chloride, accurately weighed, in about 500 mL of water in a 1 L volumetric flask, add 12 g of ammonium chloride, dilute with water to volume, and mix. Pipet 25 mL of the solution into a 400-mL beaker, add 100 mL of water, 10 mL of ammonia–ammonium chloride buffer TS, and 1 mL of eriochrome black T solution (1 in 2000), and titrate with 0.05 M edetate disodium VS to a deep blue endpoint. Each mL of 0.05 M edetate disodium is equivalent to 6.815 mg of $ZnCl_2$.

Zinc Chloride Injection

» Zinc Chloride Injection is a sterile solution of Zinc Chloride in Water for Injection. It contains not less than 90.0 percent and not more than 110.0 percent of the labeled amount of zinc (Zn).

Packaging and storage—Preserve in single-dose or multiple-dose containers, preferably of Type I or Type II glass.
Labeling—Label the Injection to indicate that it is to be diluted with Water for Injection or other suitable fluid to appropriate strength prior to administration.
USP Reference standards ⟨11⟩—*USP Endotoxin RS*.
Identification—The *Assay preparation* prepared as directed in the *Assay* exhibits an absorption maximum at about 213.8 nm, when determined as directed in the *Assay*.
Bacterial endotoxins ⟨85⟩—It contains not more than 25.0 USP Endotoxin Units per mg of zinc.
pH ⟨791⟩:   between 1.5 and 2.5.
Particulate matter ⟨788⟩:   meets the requirements for small-volume injections.
Other requirements—It meets the requirements under *Injections* ⟨1⟩.
Assay—[NOTE—The *Standard preparations* and the *Assay preparation* may be diluted quantitatively with water, if necessary, to obtain solutions of suitable concentrations adaptable to the linear or working range of the instrument.]

Sodium chloride solution—Dissolve 450 mg of sodium chloride in water, dilute with water to 500 mL, and mix.

Standard preparations—Transfer 3.11 g of zinc oxide, accurately weighed, to a 250-mL volumetric flask, add 80 mL of 1 N sulfuric acid, warm to dissolve, cool, dilute with water to volume, and mix. This stock solution contains 10.0 mg of zinc per mL. Dilute an accurately measured volume of this solution quantitatively with water to obtain a solution containing 125 µg of zinc per mL. Transfer 2.0, 3.0, and 4.0 mL, respectively, of this solution to three separate 500-mL volumetric flasks, each containing 5 mL of *Sodium chloride solution*, dilute the contents of each flask with water to volume, and mix. These *Standard preparations* contain, respectively, 0.50, 0.75, and 1.0 µg of zinc per mL.

Assay preparation—Transfer an accurately measured volume of Injection, equivalent to about 5 mg of zinc, to a 500-mL volumetric flask, dilute with water to volume, and mix. Transfer 10.0 mL of this solution to a 100-mL volumetric flask. From the labeled amount of sodium chloride, if any, in the Injection, calculate the amount, in mg, of sodium chloride in the 10.0-mL portion and add sufficient *Sodium chloride solution* to bring the total sodium chloride content of the 100-mL volumetric flask to 0.9 mg. Dilute with water to volume, and mix.

Procedure—Concomitantly determine the absorbances of the *Standard preparations* and the *Assay preparation* at the zinc emission line at 213.8 nm, with a suitable atomic absorption spectrophotometer (see *Spectrophotometry and Light-scattering* ⟨851⟩) equipped with a zinc hollow-cathode lamp and an air–acetylene flame, using water as the blank. Plot the absorbances of the *Standard preparations* versus the concentration, in µg per mL, of zinc, and draw the straight line best fitting the three plotted points. From the graph so obtained, determine the concentration, in µg per mL, of zinc in the *Assay preparation*. Calculate the quantity, in mg, of zinc in each mL of the Injection taken by the formula:

$$5C/V$$

in which C is the concentration, in µg per mL, of zinc in the *Assay preparation*; and V is the volume, in mL, of Injection taken.

Zinc Gluconate

C$_{12}$H$_{22}$O$_{14}$Zn 455.68
Bis(D-gluconato-O^1,O^2) zinc.
Zinc D-gluconate (1 : 2) [4468-02-4].

» Zinc Gluconate contains not less than 97.0 percent and not more than 102.0 percent of C$_{12}$H$_{22}$O$_{14}$Zn, calculated on the anhydrous basis.

Packaging and storage—Preserve in well-closed containers.
USP Reference standards ⟨11⟩—*USP Potassium Gluconate RS.*
Identification—
  A: A solution (1 in 10) responds to the tests for *Zinc* ⟨191⟩.
  B: It responds to *Identification* test B under *Calcium Gluconate.*
pH ⟨791⟩: between 5.5 and 7.5, in a solution (1 in 100).
Water, *Method Ib* ⟨921⟩: not more than 11.6%.
Chloride ⟨221⟩—A 1.0-g portion shows no more chloride than corresponds to 0.70 mL of 0.020 N hydrochloric acid (0.05%).
Sulfate ⟨221⟩—A 2.0-g portion shows no more sulfate than corresponds to 1.0 mL of 0.020 N sulfuric acid (0.05%).
Arsenic, *Method I* ⟨211⟩—Dissolve 1.0 g in 35 mL of water: the limit is 3 ppm.
Reducing substances—Transfer 1.0 g to a 250-mL conical flask, dissolve in 10 mL of water, and add 25 mL of alkaline cupric citrate TS. Cover the flask, boil gently for 5 minutes, accurately timed, and cool rapidly to room temperature. Add 25 mL of 0.6 N acetic acid, 10.0 mL of 0.1 N iodine VS, and 10 mL of 3 N hydrochloric acid, and titrate with 0.1 N sodium thiosulfate VS, adding 3 mL of starch TS as the endpoint is approached. Perform a blank determination, omitting the specimen, and note the difference in volumes required. Each mL of the difference in volume of 0.1 N sodium thiosulfate consumed is equivalent to 2.7 mg of reducing substances (as dextrose): the limit is 1.0%.
Limit of cadmium—
  Standard preparation—Transfer 137.2 mg of cadmium nitrate to a 1000-mL volumetric flask, dissolve in water, dilute with water to volume, and mix. Pipet 25 mL of the resulting solution into a 100-mL volumetric flask, add 1 mL of hydrochloric acid, dilute with water to volume, and mix. Each mL of this *Standard preparation* contains 12.5 µg of Cd.
  Test preparation—Transfer 10.0 g of Zinc Gluconate to a 50-mL volumetric flask, dissolve in and dilute with water to volume, and mix.
  Procedure—To three separate 25-mL volumetric flasks add, respectively, 0, 2.0, and 4.0 mL of the *Standard preparation*. To each flask add 5.0 mL of the *Test preparation,* dilute with water to volume, and mix. These test solutions contain, respectively, 0, 1.0, and 2.0 µg per mL of cadmium from the *Standard preparation*. Concomitantly determine the absorbances of the test solutions at the cadmium emission line at 228.8 nm, with a suitable atomic absorption spectrophotometer (see *Spectrophotometry and Light-scattering* ⟨851⟩) equipped with a cadmium hollow-cathode lamp and an air–acetylene flame, using water as the blank. Plot the absorbances of the test solutions versus their contents of cadmium, in µg per mL, as furnished by the *Standard preparation*, draw the straight line best fitting the three points, and extrapolate the line until it intercepts the concentration axis. From the intercept determine the amount, in µg, of cadmium in each mL of the test solution containing 0 mL of the *Standard preparation*. Calculate the quantity, in ppm, of Cd in the specimen by multiplying this value by 25: the limit is 5 ppm.
Limit of lead—[NOTE—For the preparation of all aqueous solutions and for the rinsing of glassware before use, employ water that has been passed through a strong-acid, strong-base, mixed-bed ion-exchange resin before use. Select all reagents to have as low a content of lead as practicable, and store all reagent solutions in containers of borosilicate glass. Cleanse glassware before use by soaking in warm 8 N nitric acid for 30 minutes and by rinsing with deionized water.]
  Ascorbic acid–sodium iodide solution—Dissolve 20 g of ascorbic acid and 38.5 g of sodium iodide in water in a 200-mL volumetric flask, dilute with water to volume, and mix.
  Trioctylphosphine oxide solution—[*Caution*—This solution causes irritation. Avoid contact with eyes, skin, and clothing. Take special precautions in disposing of unused portions of solutions to which this reagent is added.] Dissolve 5.0 g of trioctylphosphine oxide in 4-methyl-2-pentanone in a 100-mL volumetric flask, dilute with the same solvent to volume, and mix.
  Standard solution and *Blank*—Transfer 5.0 mL of *Lead Nitrate Stock Solution*, prepared as directed in the test for *Heavy Metals* ⟨231⟩, to a 100-mL volumetric flask, dilute with water to volume, and mix. Transfer 2.0 mL of the resulting solution to a 50-mL volumetric flask. To this volumetric flask and to a second, empty 50-mL volumetric flask (*Blank*) add 10 mL of 9 N hydrochloric acid and about 10 mL of water. To each flask add 20 mL of *Ascorbic acid–sodium iodide solution* and 5.0 mL of *Trioctylphosphine oxide solution,* shake for 30 seconds, and allow to separate. Add water to bring the organic solvent layer into the neck of each flask, shake again, and allow to separate. The organic solvent layers are the *Blank* and the *Standard solution,* and they contain 0.0 µg and 2.0 µg of lead per mL, respectively.
  Test solution—Add 1.0 g of Zinc Gluconate, 10 mL of 9 N hydrochloric acid, about 10 mL of water, 20 mL of *Ascorbic acid–sodium iodide solution,* and 5.0 mL of *Trioctylphosphine oxide solution* to a 50-mL volumetric flask, shake for 30 seconds, and allow to separate. Add water to bring the organic solvent layer into the neck of the flask, shake again, and allow to separate. The organic solvent layer is the *Test solution*.
  Procedure—Concomitantly determine the absorbances of the *Blank, Standard solution,* and *Test solution* at the lead emission line at 283.3 nm, with a suitable atomic absorption spectrophotometer (see *Spectrophotometry and Light-Scattering* ⟨851⟩) equipped with a lead hollow-cathode lamp and an air–acetylene flame, using the *Blank* to set the instrument to zero. In a suitable analysis, the absorbance of the *Standard solution* and the absorbance of the *Blank* are significantly different: the absorbance of the *Test solution* does not exceed that of the *Standard solution* (0.001%).
Organic volatile impurities, *Method I* ⟨467⟩: meets the requirements.
                              (Official until July 1, 2008)
Assay—Dissolve about 700 mg of Zinc Gluconate, accurately weighed, in 100 mL of water. Add 5 mL of ammonia–ammonium chloride buffer TS and 0.1 mL of eriochrome black TS, and titrate with 0.05 M edetate disodium VS until the solution is deep blue in color. Each mL of 0.05 M edetate disodium is equivalent to 22.78 mg of C$_{12}$H$_{22}$O$_{14}$Zn.

Zinc Oxide

ZnO 81.39
Zinc oxide.
Zinc oxide [1314-13-2].

» Zinc Oxide, freshly ignited, contains not less than 99.0 percent and not more than 100.5 percent of ZnO.

Packaging and storage—Preserve in well-closed containers.
Identification—
  A: When strongly heated, it assumes a yellow color that disappears on cooling.
  B: A solution of it in a slight excess of 3 N hydrochloric acid responds to the tests for *Zinc* ⟨191⟩.
Alkalinity—Mix 1.0 g with 10 mL of hot water, add 2 drops of phenolphthalein TS, and filter: if a red color is produced, not more than 0.30 mL of 0.10 N hydrochloric acid is required to discharge it.
Loss on ignition ⟨733⟩—Weigh accurately about 2 g, and ignite at 500° to constant weight: it loses not more than 1.0% of its weight.

Carbonate and color of solution—Mix 2.0 g with 10 mL of water, add 30 mL of 2 N sulfuric acid, and heat on a steam bath, with constant stirring: no effervescence occurs and the resulting solution is clear and colorless.
Arsenic, *Method I* ⟨211⟩: 6 ppm.
Lead—Add 2 g to 20 mL of water, stir well, add 5 mL of glacial acetic acid, and warm on a steam bath until solution is effected: the addition of 5 drops of potassium chromate TS produces no turbidity or precipitate.
Iron and other heavy metals—Cool two separate 5-mL portions of the solution obtained in the test for *Carbonate and color of solution*. White precipitates are formed when potassium ferrocyanide TS is added to the first portion and when sodium sulfide TS is added to the second portion.
Assay—Dissolve about 1.5 g of freshly ignited Zinc Oxide, accurately weighed, and 2.5 g of ammonium chloride in 50.0 mL of 1 N sulfuric acid VS with the aid of gentle heat, if necessary. When solution is complete, add methyl orange TS, and titrate the excess sulfuric acid with 1 N sodium hydroxide VS. Each mL of 1 N sulfuric acid is equivalent to 40.69 mg of ZnO.

Zinc Oxide Neutral

ZnO 81.39

» Zinc Oxide Neutral, freshly ignited, contains not less than 95.0 percent and not more than 98.0 percent of ZnO.

Packaging and storage—Preserve in well-closed containers, and store at controlled room temperature.
Labeling—Label it to indicate that it is for use in sunscreen preparations only.
Identification—
  A: When strongly heated, it assumes a yellow color that disappears on cooling.
  B: A solution of it in a slight excess of 3 N hydrochloric acid responds to the tests for *Zinc* ⟨191⟩.
Alkalinity—Mix 1.0 g with 10 mL of hot water. The addition of two drops of phenolphthalein TS produces no color change.
Loss on ignition ⟨733⟩—Weigh accurately about 1 g, and ignite at 750° for 15 minutes: it loses not more than 5.0% of its weight.
Carbonate and color of solution—Mix 2.0 g with 10 mL of water, add 30 mL of 2 N sulfuric acid, and heat on a steam bath with constant stirring: no effervescence occurs and the resulting solution is clear and colorless. [NOTE—Use this solution in the test for *Iron and other heavy metals*.]
Sulfate ⟨221⟩—A 0.1 g portion shows no more sulfate than corresponds to 2.3 mL of 0.020 N sulfuric acid (2.2%).
Arsenic, *Method I* ⟨211⟩: 2 ppm.
Lead—Add 2 g to 20 mL of water, stir well, add 5 mL of glacial acetic acid, and warm on a steam bath until solution is effected: the addition of five drops of potassium chromate TS produces no turbidity or precipitate.
Mercury—
  Mercury Detection Instrument and *Aeration Apparatus*—Proceed as directed for the section *Method IIa and Method IIb* under *Mercury* ⟨261⟩.
  Nitric acid solution 1—Carefully add 50 mL of nitric acid to 450 mL of water, and mix.
  Nitric acid solution 2—Carefully add 10 mL of nitric acid to 490 mL of water, and mix.
  Hydrochloric acid–nitric acid solution—Carefully add three volumes of concentrated hydrochloric acid to one volume of concentrated nitric acid. [NOTE—Prepare immediately before use.]
  Stannous sulfate solution—Add 25 g of stannous sulfate to 250 mL of 0.5 N sulfuric acid. [NOTE—The mixture is a suspension and should be stirred continuously during use.]
  Sodium chloride–hydroxylamine sulfate solution—Dissolve 12 g of sodium chloride and 12 g of hydroxylamine sulfate in water, dilute with water to 100 mL, and mix.
  Potassium permanganate solution—Dissolve 5 g of potassium permanganate in 100 mL of water, and mix.
  Standard stock mercury solution—Dissolve 0.1354 g of mercuric chloride in *Nitric acid solution 1* to obtain a solution having a concentration of about 1.0 mg of mercury per mL. [NOTE—Use of a commercially prepared mercury standard is recommended.]
  Standard working mercury solution—Quantitatively dilute an accurately measured volume of the *Standard stock mercury solution* with *Nitric acid solution 2* to obtain a solution having a known concentration of about 0.5 µg of mercury per mL.
  Standard solutions—Transfer 1-, 2-, 3-, and 4-mL aliquots of *Standard stock mercury solution* to four separate 300-mL biological oxygen-demand (BOD) bottles. To each bottle, add 5 mL of water and 5 mL of *Hydrochloric acid–nitric acid solution*. Heat the sample for 2 minutes in a water bath at 95°. Cool, and add 50 mL of water and 15 mL of *Potassium permanganate solution*. Mix thoroughly, and place in a water bath for 30 minutes at 95°. Cool, add 5 mL of *Sodium chloride–hydroxylamine sulfate solution*, dilute with water to 200 mL, and mix. These solutions contain the equivalents of 2.5, 5, 7.5, and 10 ng of mercury per mL, respectively.
  Blank solution—To a 300-mL BOD bottle, add 5 mL of water and 5 mL of *Hydrochloric acid–nitric acid solution*. Heat the solution for 2 minutes in a water bath at 95°. Cool, and add 50 mL of water and 15 mL of *Potassium permanganate solution*. Mix thoroughly, and place in a water bath for 30 minutes at 95°. Cool, add 5 mL of *Sodium chloride–hydroxylamine sulfate solution*, dilute with water to 200 mL, and mix.
  Test solution—Transfer about 2.0 g of Zinc Oxide Neutral, accurately weighed, to a 300-mL BOD bottle. To the bottle, add 5 mL of water and 5 mL of *Hydrochloric acid–nitric acid solution*. Heat the sample in a water bath for 2 minutes at 95°. Cool, and add 50 mL of water and 15 mL of *Potassium permanganate solution*. Mix thoroughly, and place in a water bath for 30 minutes at 95°. Cool, add 5 mL of *Sodium chloride–hydroxylamine sulfate solution*, dilute with water to 200 mL, and mix.
  Procedure—Add 5 mL of *Stannous sulfate solution* to a *Standard solution*, and immediately insert the bottle into the *Aeration Apparatus*. Obtain the absorbance of the *Standard solution*. Repeat with the remaining *Standard solutions*, *Test solution*, and *Blank solution*. Perform a blank determination, and make any necessary corrections. Plot the absorbances of the *Standard solutions* versus concentrations, in µg per mL, and draw the straight line best fitting the plotted points. From the graph so obtained, determine the concentration, in µg per g of mercury, in the *Test solution*: not more than 1 µg per g is found.
Iron and other heavy metals—Cool two separate 5-mL portions of the solution obtained in the test for *Carbonate and color of solution*. White precipitates are formed when potassium ferrocyanide TS is added to the first portion and when sodium sulfide TS is added to the second portion.
Content of magnesium oxide—
  Nitric acid solution—Carefully add 10 mL of concentrated nitric acid to 490 mL of water, and mix.
  Standard solution—Prepare a solution in *Nitric acid solution* having a concentration of about 25 µg of magnesium per mL. [NOTE—Use of a commercially prepared magnesium–inductively coupled plasma standard solution is recommended.]
  Test solution—Transfer 200 mg of Zinc Oxide Neutral, accurately weighed, to a 50-mL volumetric flask. Dissolve in and dilute with *Nitric acid solution* to volume.
  Procedure—Set up an inductively coupled plasma–atomic emission spectrometer with a wavelength of 279.1 nm, RF power of about 1.2 KW, argon torch flow of about 17 L per minute, argon nebulizer flow of about 1.0 L per minute, and argon auxiliary flow of about 1.4 L per minute. Analyze the *Standard solution* and *Test solution*, using *Nitric acid solution* as the blank. Calculate the percentage of magnesium oxide in the portion of Zinc Oxide Neutral taken by the formula:

$$5F(C/W)$$

in which F is the conversion factor for conversion of magnesium to magnesium oxide (1.658); C is the concentration, in µg per mL, of magnesium found in the *Test solution*, determined from the instrument; and W is the weight, in mg, of the portion of Zinc Oxide Neutral taken to prepare the *Test solution*: not more than 0.7% is found.

Assay—Dissolve about 1.5 g of freshly ignited Zinc Oxide Neutral, accurately weighed, and 2.5 g of ammonium chloride in 50.0 mL of 1 N sulfuric acid VS, with the aid of gentle heat, if necessary. When dissolution is complete, add methyl orange TS, and titrate the excess sulfuric acid with 1 N sodium hydroxide VS. Each mL of 1 N sulfuric acid is equivalent to 40.69 mg of ZnO.

Zinc Oxide Ointment

» Zinc Oxide Ointment contains not less than 18.5 percent and not more than 21.5 percent of ZnO.

It may be prepared as follows:

Zinc Oxide	200 g
Mineral Oil	150 g
White Ointment	650 g
To make	1000 g

Levigate the Zinc Oxide with the Mineral Oil to a smooth paste, and then incorporate the White Ointment [see *Ointments and Suppositories* under *Added Substances* (*Ingredients and Processes*) in the *General Notices*].

Packaging and storage—Preserve in well-closed containers, and avoid prolonged exposure to temperatures exceeding 30°.
Identification—The residue obtained in the *Assay* is yellow when hot and white when cool.
Minimum fill ⟨755⟩: meets the requirements.
Calcium, magnesium, and other foreign substances—Heat about 2 g gently until melted, and continue the heating, gradually raising the temperature until the mass is thoroughly charred. Ignite the mass until the residue is uniformly yellow. To the residue add 6 mL of 3 N hydrochloric acid: no effervescence occurs. Heat the mixture on a steam bath for 10 to 15 minutes: not more than a trace of insoluble residue remains. Filter the solution, dilute with water to 10 mL, add 6 N ammonium hydroxide until the precipitate first formed redissolves, then add 2 mL each of ammonium oxalate TS and dibasic sodium phosphate TS: not more than a slight turbidity is produced in 5 minutes.
Assay—Weigh accurately in a porcelain crucible about 700 mg of Ointment, heat gently until melted, and continue the heating, gradually raising the temperature until the mass is thoroughly charred. Ignite the mass until the residue is uniformly yellow, and cool. Dissolve the residue in 10 mL of 2 N sulfuric acid, warming if necessary to effect complete solution, transfer the solution to a beaker, and rinse the crucible with small portions of water until the combined solution and rinsings measure 50 mL. Add 15 mL of ammonia–ammonium chloride buffer TS and 1 mL of eriochrome black TS, and titrate with 0.05 M edetate disodium VS until the solution is blue in color. Each mL of 0.05 M edetate disodium is equivalent to 4.069 mg of ZnO.

Zinc Oxide Paste

» Zinc Oxide Paste contains not less than 24.0 percent and not more than 26.0 percent of ZnO.

It may be prepared as follows:

Zinc Oxide	250 g
Starch	250 g
White Petrolatum	500 g
To make	1000 g

Mix the ingredients.

Packaging and storage—Preserve in well-closed containers, and avoid prolonged exposure to temperatures exceeding 30°.
Identification—The residue obtained in the *Assay* is yellow when hot and white when cool.
Minimum fill ⟨755⟩: meets the requirements.
Assay—Using about 600 mg of Paste, proceed as directed in the *Assay* under *Zinc Oxide Ointment*.

Zinc Oxide and Salicylic Acid Paste

» Zinc Oxide and Salicylic Acid Paste contains not less than 23.5 percent and not more than 25.5 percent of zinc oxide (ZnO), and not less than 1.9 percent and not more than 2.1 percent of salicylic acid ($C_7H_6O_3$).

It may be prepared as follows:

Salicylic Acid, in fine powder	20 g
Zinc Oxide Paste, a sufficient quantity to make	1000 g

Thoroughly triturate the Salicylic Acid with a portion of the paste, then add the remaining paste, and triturate until a smooth mixture is obtained.

Packaging and storage—Preserve in well-closed containers.
Identification—
  A: The residue obtained in the *Assay for zinc oxide* is yellow when hot and white when cool.
  B: Shake 1 g of it with 10 mL of water, and filter. To the filtrate add 1 mL of ferric chloride TS: an intense reddish violet color is produced. To this solution add 1 mL of acetic acid: the color is not dispersed. To this solution add 2 mL of 2 N hydrochloric acid: the color is dispersed and a white crystalline precipitate is formed.
Minimum fill ⟨755⟩: meets the requirements.
Assay for zinc oxide—Weigh accurately in a tared porcelain crucible about 500 mg of Paste, heat gently until melted, and continue the heating, gradually raising the temperature until the mass is thoroughly charred. Ignite the mass strongly until all of the carbonaceous material has been dissipated, the residue is uniformly yellow, and the weight of the cooled residue is constant. The weight of the residue represents the quantity of ZnO in the weight of the Paste taken for the assay.
Assay for salicylic acid—Transfer to a suitable beaker about 5 g of Paste, accurately weighed. Add 40 mL of alcohol, previously neutralized with 0.1 N sodium hydroxide to a phenol red endpoint, and heat on a water bath for 5 minutes, with frequent swirling. While still hot, add phenol red TS, and titrate with 0.1 N sodium hydroxide VS to a red endpoint. Each mL of 0.1 N sodium hydroxide is equivalent to 13.81 mg of salicylic acid ($C_7H_6O_3$).

Zinc Stearate

Octadecanoic acid, zinc salt.
Zinc stearate [*557-05-1*].

» Zinc Stearate is a compound of zinc with a mixture of solid organic acids obtained from fats, and consists chiefly of variable proportions of zinc stearate and zinc palmitate. It contains the equivalent of not less than 12.5 percent and not more than 14.0 percent of ZnO.

Packaging and storage—Preserve in well-closed containers.

Identification—

A: Mix 25 g with 200 mL of hot water, add 60 mL of 2 N sulfuric acid, and boil until the fatty acids separate as a transparent layer. Cool the mixture, and remove the solidified layer of fatty acids: a portion of the water layer responds to the tests for *Zinc* ⟨191⟩.

B: Place the separated fatty acids obtained in *Identification* test A in a filter wetted with water, and wash with boiling water until free from sulfate. Collect the fatty acids in a small beaker, allow to cool, pour off the separated water, then melt the acids, filter into a dry beaker while hot, and dry at 105° for 20 minutes: the fatty acids congeal (see *Congealing Temperature* ⟨651⟩) at a temperature not below 54°.

Arsenic, *Method I* ⟨211⟩—Prepare the *Test Preparation* as follows. Mix 5.0 g with 50 mL of water, cautiously add 5 mL of sulfuric acid, and boil gently until the fatty acids layer is clear and the volume is reduced to about 25 mL. Filter while hot, cool the filtrate, and dilute with water to 50 mL. Transfer a 20-mL aliquot to the arsine generator flask, and dilute with water to 35 mL. The limit is 1.5 ppm.

Lead—Ignite 0.50 g in a platinum crucible for 15 to 20 minutes in a muffle furnace at 475° to 500°. Cool, add 3 drops of nitric acid, evaporate over a low flame to dryness, and ignite again at 475° to 500° for 30 minutes. Dissolve the residue in 1 mL of 8 N nitric acid, and proceed as directed in the test for *Lead* under *Magnesium Stearate*. The limit is 0.001%.

Alkalies and alkaline earths—Mix 2.0 g with 50 mL of water, add 10 mL of hydrochloric acid, boil until the solution is clear, filter while hot, and wash the separated fatty acids with about 50 mL of hot water. Render the combined filtrate and washings alkaline with 6 N ammonium hydroxide, add ammonium sulfide TS to precipitate the zinc completely, dilute with water to 200 mL, mix, and filter. To 100 mL of the clear filtrate add 0.5 mL of sulfuric acid, evaporate to dryness, and ignite to constant weight: the weight of the residue does not exceed 10 mg (1.0%).

Organic volatile impurities, *Method IV* ⟨467⟩: meets the requirements.

(Official until July 1, 2008)

Assay—Boil about 1 g of Zinc Stearate, accurately weighed, with 50 mL of 0.1 N sulfuric acid for at least 10 minutes, or until the fatty acids layer is clear, adding more water as necessary to maintain the original volume, cool, and filter. Wash the filter and the flask thoroughly with water until the last washing is not acid to litmus paper. Add to the combined filtrate and washings 15 mL of ammonia–ammonium chloride buffer TS and 0.2 mL of eriochrome black TS, heat the solution to about 40°, and titrate with 0.05 M edetate disodium VS until the solution is deep blue in color. Each mL of 0.05 M edetate disodium is equivalent to 4.069 mg of ZnO.

Zinc Sulfate

$ZnSO_4 \cdot xH_2O$.
Sulfuric acid, zinc salt (1 : 1), hydrate.
Zinc sulfate (1:1) monohydrate   179.46
Zinc sulfate (1 : 1) heptahydrate   287.56   [7446-20-0].
Anhydrous   161.46   [7733-02-0].

» Zinc Sulfate contains one or seven molecules of water of hydration. The monohydrate contains not less than 89.0 percent and not more than 90.4 percent of $ZnSO_4$, corresponding to not less than 99.0 percent and not more than 100.5 percent of $ZnSO_4 \cdot H_2O$, and the heptahydrate contains not less than 55.6 percent and not more than 61.0 percent of $ZnSO_4$, corresponding to not less than 99.0 percent and not more than 108.7 percent of $ZnSO_4 \cdot 7H_2O$.

Packaging and storage—Preserve in tight containers.

Labeling—The label indicates whether it is the monohydrate or the heptahydrate. Label any oral or parenteral preparations containing Zinc Sulfate to state the content of elemental zinc.

Identification—A solution of it responds to the tests for *Zinc* ⟨191⟩ and for *Sulfate* ⟨191⟩.

Acidity—A solution containing the equivalent of 28 mg of $ZnSO_4$ per mL is not colored pink by methyl orange TS.

Arsenic, *Method I* ⟨211⟩—Prepare a *Test Preparation* by dissolving a portion equivalent to 215 mg of $ZnSO_4$ in 35 mL of water: the limit is 14 ppm.

Lead ⟨251⟩—Dissolve a portion equivalent to 0.25 g of $ZnSO_4$ in 5 mL of water, and transfer the solution to a color-comparison tube (A). Add 10 mL of *Potassium Cyanide Solution* (1 in 10), mix, and allow the mixture to become clear. In a similar, matched color-comparison tube (B) place 5 mL of water, and add 0.50 mL of *Standard Lead Solution* (see *Heavy Metals* ⟨231⟩) and 10 mL of *Potassium Cyanide Solution* (1 in 10). Add to the solution in each tube 0.1 mL of sodium sulfide TS. Mix the contents of each tube, and allow to stand for 5 minutes: viewed downward over a white surface, the solution in tube A is no darker than that in tube B. The lead limit is 0.002%.

Alkalies and alkaline earths—Dissolve the equivalent of 1.12 g of $ZnSO_4$ in about 150 mL of water contained in a 200-mL volumetric flask. Precipitate the zinc completely by means of ammonium sulfide TS, and dilute with water to volume. Mix, and filter through a dry filter, rejecting the first portion of the filtrate. To 100 mL of the subsequent filtrate add a few drops of sulfuric acid, evaporate to dryness in a tared dish, and ignite: the weight of the residue does not exceed 5 mg (0.9%).

Assay—Dissolve an accurately weighed quantity of Zinc Sulfate, equivalent to about 170 mg of $ZnSO_4$, in 100 mL of water. Add 5 mL of ammonia–ammonium chloride buffer TS and 0.1 mL of eriochrome black TS, and titrate with 0.05 M edetate disodium VS until the solution is deep blue in color. Each mL of 0.05 M edetate disodium is equivalent to 8.072 mg of $ZnSO_4$.

Zinc Sulfate Injection

» Zinc Sulfate Injection is a sterile solution of Zinc Sulfate in Water for Injection. It contains not less than 90.0 percent and not more than 110.0 percent of the labeled amount of zinc (Zn).

Packaging and storage—Preserve in single-dose or multiple-dose containers.

Labeling—Label the Injection in terms of its content of anhydrous zinc sulfate ($ZnSO_4$) and in terms of its content of elemental zinc. Label it to state that it is not intended for direct injection but is to be added to other intravenous solutions.

USP Reference standards ⟨11⟩—*USP Endotoxin RS*.

Identification—It responds to the tests for *Zinc* ⟨191⟩ and for *Sulfate* ⟨191⟩.

Bacterial endotoxins ⟨85⟩—It contains not more than 25.0 USP Endotoxin Units per mg of zinc.

pH ⟨791⟩: between 2.0 and 4.0.

Particulate matter ⟨788⟩: meets the requirements for small-volume injections.

Other requirements—It meets the requirements under *Injections* ⟨1⟩.

Assay—[NOTE—The *Standard preparations* and the *Assay preparation* may be diluted quantitatively with water, if necessary, to yield solutions of suitable concentrations adaptable to the linear or working range of the instrument.]

Standard preparations and *Assay preparation*—Proceed as directed in the *Assay* under *Zinc Chloride Injection*.

Procedure—Concomitantly determine the absorbances of the *Standard preparations* and the *Assay preparation* at the zinc emission line of 213.8 nm with a suitable atomic absorption spectrophotometer (see *Spectrophotometry and Light-scattering* ⟨851⟩) equipped with a zinc hollow-cathode lamp and an air–acetylene flame, using water as the blank. Plot the absorbances of the *Standard preparations* versus concentration, in μg per mL, of zinc, and draw the straight line best fitting the three plotted points. From the graph so obtained, determine the concentration, in μg per mL, of zinc in the *Assay preparation*. Determine the concentration, in mg per mL, of Zn in the Injection taken by the formula:

$$5C/V$$

in which C is the concentration, in μg per mL, of zinc in the *Assay preparation*; and V is the volume, in mL, of Injection taken.

Zinc Sulfate Ophthalmic Solution

» Zinc Sulfate Ophthalmic Solution is a sterile solution of Zinc Sulfate in Water rendered isotonic by the addition of suitable salts. It contains not less than 95.0 percent and not more than 105.0 percent of the labeled amount of $ZnSO_4$.

Packaging and storage—Preserve in tight containers.
Identification—It responds to the tests for *Zinc* ⟨191⟩ and for *Sulfate* ⟨191⟩.
Sterility ⟨71⟩: meets the requirements..
pH ⟨791⟩: between 5.8 and 6.2; or, if it contains sodium citrate, between 7.2 and 7.8.
Assay—Pipet into a beaker a volume of Ophthalmic Solution, equivalent to about 25 mg of zinc sulfate. Add 1 mL of glacial acetic acid, and adjust by the dropwise addition of 6 N ammonium hydroxide to a pH of between 5.0 and 5.5. Add 1 drop of copper ethylenediaminetetraacetate solution [prepared by mixing 1 mL of cupric sulfate solution (1 in 40) and 1 mL of 0.1 M edetate disodium] and 3 drops of a 1 in 1000 solution of 1-(2-pyridylazo)-2-naphthol in anhydrous methanol, and titrate with 0.01 M edetate disodium VS. Each mL of 0.01 M edetate disodium is equivalent to 1.614 mg of $ZnSO_4$.

Zinc Sulfate Oral Solution

» Zinc Sulfate Oral Solution contains not less than 90.0 percent and not more than 110.0 percent of the labeled amount of zinc sulfate ($ZnSO_4 \cdot H_2O$). It may contain one or more suitable flavors and sweeteners.

Packaging and storage—Preserve in well-closed containers protected from light, and store in a cool, dry place.
Labeling—Label the Oral Solution in terms of zinc sulfate ($ZnSO_4 \cdot H_2O$) and in terms of elemental zinc.
Identification—The Oral Solution responds to the tests for *Zinc* ⟨191⟩ and for *Sulfate* ⟨191⟩.
pH ⟨791⟩: between 2.5 and 4.5.
Specific gravity ⟨841⟩: between 1.18 and 1.24.
Assay—Transfer to a 250-mL flask an accurately measured volume of Oral Solution, equivalent to about 99 mg of $ZnSO_4 \cdot H_2O$. Add 50 mL of water and 10 mL of ammonia–ammonium chloride buffer TS and 0.3 mL of eriochrome black TS, and titrate with 0.05 M edetate disodium VS to a green endpoint. Each mL of 0.05 M edetate disodium is equivalent to 8.973 mg of zinc sulfate ($ZnSO_4 \cdot H_2O$).

Zinc Sulfate Tablets

» Zinc Sulfate Tablets contain not less than 95.0 percent and not more than 105.0 percent of the labeled amount of $ZnSO_4 \cdot H_2O$. It may contain one or more suitable flavors and sweeteners.

Packaging and storage—Preserve in well-closed containers, and store at controlled room temperature.
Labeling—Label the Tablets in terms of zinc sulfate ($ZnSO_4 \cdot H_2O$) and in terms of elemental zinc.
Identification—
  Test solution—Dissolve a portion of powdered Tablets in water to obtain a solution containing about 0.05 g of zinc sulfate per mL.
  Glycerin solution: a mixture of glycerin and water (85 : 15).
  Sodium sulfide solution—Dissolve 12 g of sodium sulfide with heating in a 45-mL mixture of *Glycerin solution* and water (29 : 10), allow to cool, and dilute with the same mixture of solvents to 100 mL. The solution should be colorless.
  Hydrochloric acid solution—Transfer 20 g of hydrochloric acid to a 100-mL volumetric flask, dilute with water to volume, and mix.
  Barium chloride solution—Transfer 61 g of barium chloride to a 1000-mL volumetric flask, dissolve in and dilute with water to volume, and mix.
  Sodium hydroxide solution—Transfer 42 g of sodium hydroxide to a 100-mL volumetric flask, dilute with water to volume, and mix.
  Ammonium chloride solution—Transfer 107 g of ammonium chloride to a 1000-mL volumetric flask, dilute with water to volume, and mix.
  A: To 5 mL of the *Test solution* add 1 mL of *Hydrochloric acid solution* and 1 mL of *Barium chloride solution*. A white precipitate is formed.
  B: To 5 mL of the *Test solution* add 0.2 mL of *Sodium hydroxide solution*. A white precipitate is formed. Add an additional 2 mL of *Sodium hydroxide solution* and the precipitate dissolves. Add 10 mL of *Ammonium chloride solution* and the solution remains clear. Add 0.1 mL of *Sodium sulfide solution* and a white precipitate is formed
Disintegration ⟨701⟩: 60 seconds.
Uniformity of dosage units ⟨905⟩: meet the requirements.
Assay—Weigh and finely powder not fewer than 20 Tablets. Transfer an accurately weighed portion of the powder, equivalent to about 90 mg of zinc, to a 200-mL volumetric flask. Dissolve in 15 mL of dilute acetic acid, and sonicate for 15 minutes. Dilute with water to volume, and mix. Add 50 mg of xylenol orange triturate to the solution, and mix. Neutralize the solution with about 2 g of methenamine until the solution is a violet-pink color. Titrate with 0.1 M edetate disodium VS until the solution is yellow. Each mL of 0.1 M edetate disodium VS is equivalent to 17.946 mg of $ZnSO_4 \cdot H_2O$.

Zinc Sulfide Topical Suspension

(Former monograph title is White Lotion)

» Prepare Zinc Sulfide Topical Suspension as follows:

Zinc Sulfate	40 g
Sulfurated Potash	40 g
Purified Water, a sufficient quantity to make	1000 mL

Dissolve the Zinc Sulfate and the Sulfurated Potash separately, each in 450 mL of Purified Water, and filter each solution. Add the sulfurated potash solution slowly to the zinc sulfate solution with constant stirring. Then add the required amount of Purified Water, and mix.

NOTE—Prepare the Topical Suspension fresh, and shake it thoroughly before dispensing.

Zinc Undecylenate

C$_{22}$H$_{38}$O$_4$Zn   431.92
10-Undecenoic acid, zinc(2+) salt.
Zinc 10-undecenoate   [557-08-4].

» Zinc Undecylenate contains not less than 98.0 percent and not more than 102.0 percent of C$_{22}$H$_{38}$O$_4$Zn, calculated on the dried basis.

Packaging and storage—Preserve in well-closed containers.
Identification—
    A: Acidify about 5 g with 25 mL of 2 N sulfuric acid, add 20 mL of water, and extract in a separator with two 25-mL portions of ether. Evaporate the ether solution until the odor of ether no longer is perceptible. Add potassium permanganate TS dropwise to a 1-mL portion of this residue: the permanganate color is discharged.
    B: A 3-mL portion of the residue of undecylenic acid obtained in *Identification* test A responds to *Identification* test B under *Undecylenic Acid*.
    C: Dissolve about 100 mg in a mixture of 10 mL of water and 1 mL of ammonium hydroxide, and add a few drops of sodium sulfide TS: a white, flocculent precipitate of zinc sulfide is formed.
Loss on drying ⟨731⟩—Dry it at 105° for 2 hours: it loses not more than 1.25% of its weight.
Alkalies and alkaline earths—Boil 1.50 g with a mixture of 50 mL of water and 10 mL of hydrochloric acid, filter while hot, and wash the separated acid with about 50 mL of hot water. Render the combined filtrate and washings alkaline with 6 N ammonium hydroxide, add ammonium sulfide TS to precipitate the zinc completely, dilute with water to 200 mL, mix, and filter. To 100 mL of the clear filtrate add 0.5 mL of sulfuric acid, evaporate to dryness, and ignite over a low flame to constant weight: the weight of the residue does not exceed 7.5 mg (1.0%).
Assay—Boil 50.0 mL of 0.1 N sulfuric acid VS with about 1 g of Zinc Undecylenate, accurately weighed, for 10 minutes, or until the undecylenic acid layer is clear, adding water, as necessary, to maintain the original volume. Cool, and transfer the mixture, with the aid of water, to a 500-mL separator. Dilute with water to about 250 mL, and extract with two 100-mL portions of solvent hexane. Wash the combined extracts with water until the last washing is neutral to litmus, add the washings to the original water layer, and evaporate on a steam bath to about 100 mL. Cool, add 3 drops of methyl orange TS, and titrate the excess sulfuric acid with 0.1 N sodium hydroxide VS. Perform a blank determination (see *Residual Titrations* under *Titrimetry* ⟨541⟩). Each mL of 0.1 N sulfuric acid is equivalent to 21.60 mg of C$_{22}$H$_{38}$O$_4$Zn.

Zolazepam Hydrochloride

C$_{15}$H$_{15}$FN$_4$O · HCl   322.77
Pyrazolo[3,4-*e*][1,4]diazepin-7(1*H*)-one, 4-(2-fluorophenyl)-6,8-dihydro-1,3,8-trimethyl-, monohydrochloride.
4-(*o*-Fluorophenyl)-6,8-dihydro-1,3,8-trimethylpyrazolo [3,4-*e*][1,4]diazepin-7(1*H*)-one monohydrochloride   [33754-49-3].

» Zolazepam Hydrochloride contains not less than 97.0 percent and not more than 103.0 percent of C$_{15}$H$_{15}$FN$_4$O · HCl.

Packaging and storage—Preserve in tight containers.
Labeling—Label it to indicate that it is for veterinary use only. Where it is intended for use in preparing injectable dosage forms, the label states that it is sterile or must be subjected to further processing during the preparation of injectable dosage forms.
USP Reference standards ⟨11⟩—*USP Endotoxin RS. USP Zolazepam Hydrochloride RS.*
Clarity of solution—Dissolve 2.0 g of it in 10 mL of water: the solution is clear.
Identification—
    A: *Infrared Absorption* ⟨197K⟩.
    B: *Ultraviolet Absorption* ⟨197U⟩—
    Solution: 0.015 mg per mL.
    Medium: 0.1 N hydrochloric acid.
    Absorptivities at 223 nm do not differ by more than 3.0%.
    C: It responds to the tests for *Chloride* ⟨191⟩.
Bacterial endotoxins ⟨85⟩—Where the label states that Zolazepam Hydrochloride is sterile or must be subjected to further processing during the preparation of injectable dosage forms, it contains not more than 0.07 USP Endotoxin Unit per mg of zolazepam.
Sterility ⟨71⟩—Where the label states that Zolazepam Hydrochloride is sterile, it meets the requirements when tested as directed for *Membrane Filtration* under *Test for Sterility of the Product to be Examined*.
pH ⟨791⟩: between 1.5 and 3.5, in a solution (1 in 10).
Loss on drying ⟨731⟩—Dry it at 105° for 4 hours: it loses not more than 1.0% of its weight.
Residue on ignition ⟨281⟩: not more than 0.5%.
Heavy metals, Method II ⟨231⟩: 0.002%.
Chromatographic purity—
    Modified Dragendorff's reagent—Dissolve 1.7 g of bismuth subnitrate in 80 mL of water and 20 mL of glacial acetic acid, warming, if necessary. Cool, add 100 mL of potassium iodide solution (1 in 2), and mix. Refrigerate this stock solution for prolonged storage. For use, dilute 10 mL of this stock solution with water to 100 mL, add 10 mL of glacial acetic acid, and mix. Then add 120 mg of iodine crystals, and shake until the iodine has completely dissolved. Store refrigerated, and discard after 2 weeks.
    Procedure—Prepare a test solution of Zolazepam Hydrochloride in methanol containing 100 mg per mL. Prepare a Standard solution in methanol containing 2.0 mg of USP Zolazepam Hydrochloride RS per mL. Prepare a thin-layer chromatographic plate (see *Chromatography* ⟨621⟩) coated with a 0.25-mm layer of chromatographic silica gel mixture. Separately apply 5 µL of the test solution and the Standard solution to the plate, and allow the spots to dry. Place the plate in a saturated chamber containing a solvent system consisting of a mixture of toluene, acetone, and ammonium hydroxide (75 : 18 : 7), and lined with filter paper. Develop the chromatogram until the solvent front has moved about three-fourths of the length of the plate. Remove the plate from the chamber, mark the solvent front, allow the plate to air-dry. Spray the plate with *Modified Dragendorff's reagent*, and examine the plate: no individual

secondary spot observed in the chromatogram obtained from the test solution is greater in size or intensity than the principal spot observed in the chromatogram obtained from the Standard solution, corresponding to 2%, and the total of any such spots observed does not exceed 3%.

Chloride content—Transfer about 400 mg of it, accurately weighed, to a conical flask, add 5 mL of water, 5 mL of glacial acetic acid, and 50 mL of methanol, and swirl to dissolve. Add 1 drop of eosin Y TS, and titrate with 0.1 N silver nitrate VS to the endpoint when the granular precipitate first turns to a permanent pink color. Each mL of 0.1 N silver nitrate is equivalent to 3.545 mg of chloride: between 10.5% and 11.5% is found.

Assay—Transfer about 480 mg of Zolazepam Hydrochloride, accurately weighed, to a conical flask, add 70 mL of glacial acetic acid, 10 mL of mercuric acetate TS, and swirl to dissolve. Titrate with 0.1 N perchloric acid VS, determining the endpoint potentiometrically. Perform a blank determination, and make any necessary correction (see *Titrimetry* ⟨541⟩). Each mL of 0.1 N perchloric acid is equivalent to 32.28 mg of $C_{15}H_{15}FN_4O \cdot HCl$.

Combined Index to USP 31 and NF 26, Volumes 1–3

Page citations refer to the pages of Volumes 1, 2, and 3 of the USP 31–NF 26. This index is repeated in its entirety in each Volume.

1–1263   Volume 1
1265–2559 Volume 2
2561–3553 Volume 3

Numbers in angle brackets such as ⟨421⟩ refer to chapter numbers in the General Chapters section.

A

Abbreviations, xii, 4
Absolute
  alcohol, 752
  ether, 751
Absorbable
  dusting powder, 2031
  gelatin film, 2259
  gelatin sponge, 2260
  surgical suture, 3314
Absorbent
  cotton, 751
  gauze, 2258
  odorless paper, 786
Acacia, 1063
  syrup, 1063
Acebutolol hydrochloride, 1265
  capsules, 1265
Acepromazine maleate, 1267
  injection, 1267
  tablets, 1268
Acesulfame potassium, 1063
Acetal, 751
Acetaldehyde, 751
  TS, 814
Acetaminophen, 1268
  aspirin and caffeine tablets, 1273
  and aspirin tablets, 1272
  butalbital and caffeine capsules, 1580
  butalbital and caffeine tablets, 1581
  and caffeine tablets, 1274
  capsules, 1269
  and (salts of) chlorpheniramine, dextromethorphan, and phenylpropanolamine, capsules containing at least three of the following, 1275
  and (salts of) chlorpheniramine, dextromethorphan, and phenylpropanolamine, oral solution containing at least three of the following, 1277
  and (salts of) chlorpheniramine, dextromethorphan, and phenylpropanolamine, tablets containing at least three of the following, 1278
  and (salts of) chlorpheniramine, dextromethorphan, and pseudoephedrine, capsules containing at least three of the following, 1280
  and (salts of) chlorpheniramine, dextromethorphan, and pseudoephedrine, oral powder containing at least three of the following, 1282
  and (salts of) chlorpheniramine, dextromethorphan, and pseudoephedrine, oral solution containing at least three of the following, 1283
  and (salts of) chlorpheniramine, dextromethorphan, and pseudoephedrine, tablets containing at least three of the following, 1285
  chlorpheniramine maleate, and dextromethorphan hydrobromide tablets, 1287
  and codeine phosphate capsules, 1288
  and codeine phosphate oral solution, 1289
  and codeine phosphate oral suspension, 1290
  and codeine phosphate tablets, 1291
  dextromethorphan hydrobromide, doxylamine succinate, and pseudoephedrine hydrochloride oral solution, 1292
  and diphenhydramine citrate tablets, 1293
  diphenhydramine hydrochloride, and pseudoephedrine hydrochloride tablets, 1294
  and hydrocodone bitartrate tablets, 2337
  isometheptene mucate and dichloralphenazone capsules, 2458
  oral solution, 1269
  for effervescent oral solution, 1270
  oral suspension, 1270
  and oxycodone capsules, 2882
  and oxycodone tablets, 2883
  and pentazocine tablets, 2948
  and propoxyphene hydrochloride tablets, 3106
  and propoxyphene napsylate tablets, 3111
  and pseudoephedrine hydrochloride tablets, 1295
  suppositories, 1270
  tablets, 1271
  extended-release tablets, 1271
Acetanilide, 751
Acetate
  methyl, 782
Acetate buffer, 814
  TS, 814
Acetazolamide, 1296
  for injection, 1297
  tablets, 1297
Acetic acid, 751, 1064
  ammonium acetate buffer TS, 815
  diluted, 751, 1064
  double-normal (2 N), 822
  glacial, 751, 1298
  glacial, TS, 814
  and hydrocortisone otic solution, 2343
  irrigation, 1298
  metaphosphoric, TS, 818
  otic solution, 1298
  strong, TS, 815
Acetic anhydride, 751
Acetohexamide, 1298
  tablets, 1299
Acetohydroxamic acid, 1299
  tablets, 1300
Acetone, 751, 1065
  anhydrous, 751
  buffered, TS, 751, 815
Acetonitrile, 751
  spectrophotometric, 751
Acetophenone, 751
p-Acetotoluidide, 751
Acetylacetone, 751
Acetyl chloride, 751
Acetylcholine chloride, 751, 1300
  for ophthalmic solution, 1300
Acetylcysteine, 1301
  and isoproterenol hydrochloride inhalation solution, 1302
  solution, 1302
3-Acetylthio-2-methylpropanoic acid, 752
Acetyltributyl citrate, 1065
Acetyltriethyl citrate, 1066
N-Acetyl-L-tyrosine ethyl ester, 752
Acid
  acrylic, 752
  alpha lipoic, 968
  ferric chloride TS, 815
  ferrous sulfate TS, 815

Acid *(continued)*
  phthalate buffer, 813
  stannous chloride TS, 815
  stannous chloride TS, stronger, 815
Acid-neutralizing capacity ⟨301⟩, 138
Acidulated phosphate and sodium fluoride topical solution, 3250
Acoustic emission ⟨1005⟩, 375
Acrylic acid, 752
Activated
  alumina, 752
  charcoal, 752, 1716
  magnesium silicate, 752
Acyclovir, 1303
  capsules, 1304
  for injection, 1304
  ointment, 1305
  oral suspension, 1306
  tablets, 1306
Adamantane, 752
Ademetionine disulfate tosylate, 907
Adenine, 1307
  sulfate, 752
Adenosine, 1308
  injection, 1308
Ad Hoc Advisory Panels (2005–2010), xv
Adipic acid, 752, 1066
Admissions
  to *NF 26*, 1056
  to *USP 31*, xxvii

Aerosol
Aerosols, nasal sprays, metered-dose inhalers, and dry powder inhalers ⟨601⟩, 209
Bacitracin and polymyxin B sulfate topical, 1484
Benzocaine, butamben, and tetracaine hydrochloride topical, 1503
Benzocaine and menthol topical, 1505
Benzocaine topical, 1501
Betamethasone dipropionate topical, 1520
Dexamethasone sodium phosphate inhalation, 1912
Dexamethasone topical, 1905
Epinephrine bitartrate inhalation, 2068
Epinephrine inhalation, 2065
Ergotamine tartrate inhalation, 2079
Isoetharine mesylate inhalation, 2453
Isoproterenol hydrochloride inhalation, 2463
Isoproterenol hydrochloride and phenylephrine bitartrate inhalation, 2465
Isoproterenol sulfate inhalation, 2467
Lidocaine topical, 2526
Metaproterenol sulfate inhalation, 2637
Polymyxin B sulfate and bacitracin zinc topical, 3024
Povidone-iodine topical, 3050
Terbutaline sulfate inhalation, 3345
Thimerosal topical, 3387
Tolnaftate topical, 3433
Triamcinolone acetonide topical, 3443

Agar, 752, 1067
Agarose, 752
Air, medical, 1309
Air-helium certified standard, 752
Alanine, 1309
Albendazole, 1310
  oral suspension, 1310
  tablets, 1311
Albumen TS, 815
Albumin
  bovine serum, 752
  human, 1311
Albuterol, 1312
  sulfate, 1312
    tablets, 1313
Alclometasone dipropionate, 1314
  cream, 1315
  ointment, 1315
Alcohol, 752, 1316
  70 percent, 80 percent, and 90 percent, 752
  absolute, 752
  aldehyde-free, 752
  alpha-(2-(methylamino)ethyl)benzyl, 753
  amyl, 752
  tert-amyl, 755
  butyl, 1085
  dehydrated, 752, 1317
  dehydrated isopropyl, 752
  determination ⟨611⟩, 230
  in dextrose injection, 1319
  diluted, 752, 1067
  injection, dehydrated, 1318
  isobutyl, 752
  isopropyl, 752
  methyl, 752
  neutralized, 752
  n-propyl, 752
  phenol TS, 815
  rubbing, 1319
  secondary butyl, 752
  tertiary butyl, 752
Alcoholic
  ammonia TS, 815
  mercuric bromide TS, 815
  potassium hydroxide TS, 815
Alcoholometric table, 900
Aldehyde dehydrogenase, 752
Alendronate sodium, 1320
Alendronic acid
  tablets, 1321
Alfadex, 1067
Alfentanil
  hydrochloride, 1322
  injection, 1323
Alginates assay ⟨311⟩, 139
Alginic acid, 1069
Alkaline
  borate buffer, 814
  cupric citrate TS, 815
  cupric iodide TS, 815
  cupric tartrate TS, 815
  mercuric-potassium iodide TS, 815
  phosphatase enzyme, 753
  picrate TS, 815
  pyrogallol TS, 820
  sodium hydrosulfite TS, 815
Alkyl (C12-15) benzoate, 1069
Alkylphenoxypolyethoxyethanol, 753
Allantoin, 1323
Allopurinol, 1324
  oral suspension, 1325
  tablets, 1325
Allyl isothiocyanate, 1326
Almond oil, 1069
Aloe, 1326
Alpha
  lipoic acid, 968
  tocopherol assay ⟨551⟩, 187
Alphanaphthol, 753
Alphazurine 2G, 809
Alpha-(2-(methylamino)ethyl)benzyl alcohol, 753
Alprazolam, 1327
  oral suspension, 1328
  tablets, 1328
Alprenolol hydrochloride, 753
Alprostadil, 1329
  injection, 1331
Alteplase, 1331
  for injection, 1334
Altretamine, 1334
  capsules, 1335

Alum, 753
  ammonium, 753, 1335
  potassium, 791, 1336
Alumina, 753
  activated, 753
  anhydrous, 753
  aspirin, codeine phosphate, and magnesia tablets, 1458
  aspirin, and magnesia tablets, 1454
  aspirin, and magnesium oxide tablets, 1455
  magnesia, and calcium carbonate chewable tablets, 1338
  magnesia, and calcium carbonate oral suspension, 1337
  magnesia, calcium carbonate, and simethicone tablets, 1339, 1341
  magnesia, and calcium carbonate tablets, 1338
  and magnesia oral suspension, 1336
  magnesia, and simethicone chewable tablets, 1344
  magnesia, and simethicone oral suspension, 1342
  magnesia, and simethicone tablets, 1344
  and magnesia tablets, 1337
  magnesium carbonate, and magnesium oxide tablets, 1347
  and magnesium carbonate oral suspension, 1345
  and magnesium carbonate tablets, 1346
  and magnesium trisilicate oral suspension, 1348
  and magnesium trisilicate tablets, 1348
Aluminon, 753
Aluminum, 753
  acetate topical solution, 1349
  chloride, 1350
  chlorohydrate, 1350
  chlorohydrate solution, 1351
  chlorohydrex polyethylene glycol, 1351
  chlorohydrex propylene glycol, 1352
  dichlorohydrate, 1352
  dichlorohydrate solution, 1353
  dichlorohydrex polyethylene glycol, 1353
  dichlorohydrex propylene glycol, 1354
  hydroxide gel, 1354
  hydroxide gel, dried, 1355
  hydroxide gel capsules, dried, 1355
  hydroxide gel tablets, dried, 1356
  monostearate, 1071
  oxide, acid-washed, 753
  phosphate gel, 1356
  potassium sulfate, 753
  sesquichlorohydrate, 1356
  sesquichlorohydrate solution, 1357
  sesquichlorohydrex polyethylene glycol, 1357
  sesquichlorohydrex propylene glycol, 1358
  subacetate topical solution, 1358
  sulfate, 1359
  sulfate and calcium acetate tablets for topical solution, 1360
  zirconium octachlorohydrate, 1360
  zirconium octachlorohydrate solution, 1361
  zirconium octachlorohydrex gly, 1362
  zirconium octachlorohydrex gly solution, 1363
  zirconium pentachlorohydrate, 1364
  zirconium pentachlorohydrate solution, 1364
  zirconium pentachlorohydrex gly, 1365
  zirconium pentachlorohydrex gly solution, 1366
  zirconium tetrachlorohydrate, 1367
  zirconium tetrachlorohydrate solution, 1368
  zirconium tetrachlorohydrex gly, 1369
  zirconium tetrachlorohydrex gly solution, 1369
  zirconium trichlorohydrate, 1370
  zirconium trichlorohydrate solution, 1371
  zirconium trichlorohydrex gly, 1372
  zirconium trichlorohydrex gly solution, 1373
Aluminum ⟨206⟩, 131

Aluminum sulfate
    and calcium acetate for topical solution, 1359
Amantadine hydrochloride, 1374
    capsules, 1374
    oral solution, 1375
Amaranth, 753
    TS, 815
Amcinonide, 1375
    cream, 1376
    ointment, 1376
American ginseng, 952
    capsules, 953
    extract, powdered, 953
    powdered, 952
    tablets, 954
Amifostine, 1377
    for injection, 1377
Amikacin, 1378
    sulfate, 1379
    sulfate injection, 1380
Amiloride hydrochloride, 1380
    and hydrochlorothiazide tablets, 1381
    tablets, 1380
Amiloxate, 1383
Aminoacetic acid, 753
4-Aminoantipyrine, 753
Aminobenzoate
    potassium, 1383
    potassium capsules, 1384
    potassium for oral solution, 1384
    potassium tablets, 1384
    sodium, 1384
Aminobenzoic acid, 1385
    gel, 1385
    topical solution, 1386
p-Aminobenzoic acid, 753
2-Aminobenzonitrile, 753
Aminocaproic acid, 1386
    injection, 1387
    oral solution, 1387
    tablets, 1387
4-Amino-6-chloro-1,3-benzenedisulfonamide, 753
4-Amino-2-chlorobenzoic acid, 753
2-Amino-5-chlorobenzophenone, 753
7-Aminodesacetoxycephalosporanic acid, 753
2-Aminoethyl diphenylborinate, 753
1-(2-Aminoethyl)piperazine, 753
Aminoglutethimide, 1388
    tablets, 1389
Aminoguanidine bicarbonate, 754
2-Aminoheptane, 754
N-Aminohexamethyleneimine, 754
Aminohippurate sodium injection, 1389
Aminohippuric acid, 1390
4-Amino-3-hydroxy-1-naphthalenesulfonic acid, 754
Amino methacrylate copolymer, 1072
1,2,4-Aminonaphtholsulfonic acid, 754
Aminonaphtholsulfonic acid TS, 815
Aminopentamide sulfate, 1390
    injection, 1390
    tablets, 1391
m-Aminophenol, 754
p-Aminophenol, 754
2-Aminophenol, 754
Aminophylline, 1391
    delayed-release tablets, 1394
    injection, 1392
    oral solution, 1392
    rectal solution, 1393
    suppositories, 1393
    tablets, 1394
3-Aminopropionic acid, 754
Aminosalicylate sodium, 1394
    tablets, 1395
Aminosalicylic acid, 1396
    tablets, 1397

3-Aminosalicylic acid, 754
3-Amino-1-propanol, 754
Amitraz, 1397
    concentrate for dip, 1398
Amitriptyline hydrochloride, 1398
    and chlordiazepoxide tablets, 1727
    injection, 1399
    and perphenazine tablets, 2965
    tablets, 1400
Amlodipine besylate, 1400
Ammonia
    alcoholic TS, 815
    detector tube, 754
    N 13 injection, 2816
    nitrate TS, silver, 820
    solution, diluted, 754
    solution, strong, 1072
    spirit, aromatic, 1401
    TS, 815
    TS alcoholic, 815
    TS stronger, 815
    water, stronger, 754
    water, 25 percent, 754
Ammonia-ammonium chloride buffer TS, 815
Ammoniacal potassium ferricyanide TS, 815
Ammonia-cyanide TS, 815
Ammoniated cupric oxide TS, 815
Ammonio methacrylate copolymer, 1073
    dispersion, 1073
Ammonium
    acetate, 754
    acetate TS, 815
    alum, 1335
    bisulfate, 754
    bromide, 754
    carbonate, 754, 1074
    carbonate TS, 815
    chloride, 754, 1402
    chloride–ammonium hydroxide TS, 815
    chloride delayed-release tablets, 1402
    chloride injection, 1402
    chloride, potassium gluconate, and potassium citrate oral solution, 3042
    chloride TS, 815
    citrate, dibasic, 754
    citrate, ferric, 1402
    citrate for oral solution, ferric, 1403
    dihydrogen phosphate, 754
    fluoride, 754
    formate, 754
    hydroxide, 754
    hydroxide 6 N, 754
    molybdate, 754, 1403
    molybdate injection, 1404
    molybdate TS, 815
    nitrate, 754
    nitrate, ceric TS, 816
    nitrate TS, silver, 820
    oxalate, 754
    oxalate TS, 815
    persulfate, 754
    phosphate, 1074
    phosphate, dibasic, 755
    phosphate, dibasic, TS, 815
    phosphate, monobasic, 755
    polysulfide TS, 815
    pyrrolidinedithiocarbamate, 755
    pyrrolidinedithiocarbamate, saturated, TS, 815
    reineckate, 755
    reineckate TS, 815
    sulfamate, 755
    sulfate, 755, 1074
    sulfate, cupric TS, 816
    sulfate, ferric TS, 817
    sulfide TS, 815
    thiocyanate, 755
    thiocyanate, tenth-normal (0.1 N), 822
    thiocyanate TS, 815

vanadate, 755
vanadate TS, 815
Amobarbital sodium, 1405
    for injection, 1405
    and secobarbital sodium capsules, 3224
Amodiaquine, 1405
    hydrochloride, 1406
    hydrochloride tablets, 1406
Amoxapine, 1407
    tablets, 1407
Amoxicillin, 1408
    boluses, 1408
    capsules, 1409
    and clavulanate potassium for oral suspension, 1412
    and clavulanate potassium tablets, 1412
    for injectable suspension, 1409
    intramammary infusion, 1409
    oral suspension, 1410
    for oral suspension, 1410
    tablets, 1410
    tablets for oral suspension, 1411
Amphetamine
    assay ⟨331⟩, 140
    sulfate, 1413
    sulfate tablets, 1414
Amphotericin B, 1414
    cream, 1415
    for injection, 1415
    lotion, 1415
    ointment, 1416
Ampicillin, 1416
    boluses, 1416
    capsules, 1417
    for injectable suspension, 1418
    for injection, 1417
    for oral suspension, 1419
    and probenecid for oral suspension, 1419
    sodium, 1420
    soluble powder, 1418
    and sulbactam for injection, 1421
    tablets, 1419
Amprolium, 1422
    oral solution, 1422
    soluble powder, 1422
Amyl
    acetate, 755
    alcohol, 755
    nitrite, 1423
    nitrite inhalant, 1423
α-Amylase, 755
Amylene hydrate, 1075
tert-Amyl alcohol, 755
Analytical data—interpretation and treatment ⟨1010⟩, 378
Ancillary materials for cell, gene, and tissue-engineered products ⟨1043⟩, 403
Anethole, 1075
(E)-Anethole, 755
Angustifolia
    extract, powdered echinacea, 930
    powdered echinacea, 930

Anhydrous
acetone, 751
alumina, 755
barium chloride, 755
calcium chloride, 755
calcium phosphate, dibasic, 1617
citric acid, 1781
cupric sulfate, 755
dibasic sodium phosphate, 755
magnesium perchlorate, 755
magnesium sulfate, 755
methanol, 755

Anhydrous *(continued)*
  potassium carbonate, 755
  sodium acetate, 755
  sodium carbonate, 755
  sodium sulfate, 755
  sodium sulfite, 755

Anileridine, 1424
  hydrochloride, 1425
  hydrochloride tablets, 1425
  injection, 1424
Aniline, 755
  blue, 755
  sulfate, 755
Anion-exchange resin
  chloromethylated polystyrene-divinylbenzene, 755
  strong, lightly cross-linked, in the chloride form, 755
  50- to 100-mesh, styrene-divinylbenzene, 755
p-Anisaldehyde, 756
Anise oil, 1076
p-Anisidine, 756
Anisole, 756
Antazoline phosphate, 1425
Anthracene, 756
Anthralin, 1426
  cream, 1427
  ointment, 1427
Anthrax vaccine adsorbed, 1427
Anthrone, 756
  TS, 815
Antibiotics—microbial assays $\langle 81 \rangle$, 91
Anticoagulant
  citrate dextrose solution, 1429
  citrate phosphate dextrose solution, 1430
  citrate phosphate dextrose adenine solution, 1431
  heparin solution, 1433
  sodium citrate solution, 1433
Anti-D reagent, 756
Anti-D (Rh₀) reagent, 756
Antifoam reagent, 756
Antihemophilic factor, 1433
  cryoprecipitated, 1434
Antihuman globulin reagent, 756
Antimicrobial
  agents—content $\langle 341 \rangle$, 140
  effectiveness testing $\langle 51 \rangle$, 67
Antimony
  pentachloride, 756
  potassium tartrate, 1434
  sodium tartrate, 1434
  trichloride, 757
  trichloride TS, 815
Antipyrine, 1435
  and benzocaine otic solution, 1435
  benzocaine, and phenylephrine hydrochloride otic solution, 1436
Antithrombin III, 757
  human, 1436
Antivenin
  (crotalidae) polyvalent, 1438
  (latrodectus mactans), 1438
  (micrurus fulvius), 1438
Apomorphine hydrochloride, 1438
  tablets, 1439
Application of water activity determination to nonsterile pharmaceutical products $\langle 1112 \rangle$, 580
Apraclonidine
  hydrochloride, 1439
  ophthalmic solution, 1440
Aprobarbital, 757
Aprotinin, 1441
  injection, 1442
Arcitumomab injection, technetium Tc 99m, 3327

Arginine, 1443
  hydrochloride, 1443
  hydrochloride injection, 1444
Aromatic
  castor oil, 1660
  elixir, 1076
Arsanilic acid, 1444
Arsenazo III acid, 757
Arsenic $\langle 211 \rangle$, 131
  in reagents, 748
  trioxide, 757
Articles
  of botanical origin $\langle 561 \rangle$, 188
  included in *USP 30* but not included in *USP 31*, xxx
  of Incorporation, xxiii
Ascorbic acid, 1445
  injection, 1445
  oral solution, 1446
  tablets, 1446
Ascorbyl palmitate, 1076
Asian ginseng, 955
  extract, powdered, 956
  powdered, 956
  tablets, 957
Asparagine, 1077
L-Asparagine, 757
Aspartame, 1077
  acesulfame, 1078
Aspartic acid, 1447
L-Aspartic acid, 757
Aspirin, 1447
  acetaminophen and caffeine tablets, 1273
  and acetaminophen tablets, 1272
  alumina and magnesia tablets, 1454
  alumina and magnesium oxide tablets, 1455
  boluses, 1448
  butalbital, and caffeine capsules, 1583
  butalbital, caffeine, and codeine phosphate capsules, 1585
  butalbital, and caffeine tablets, 1584
  and butalbital tablets, 1582
  caffeine, and dihydrocodeine bitartrate capsules, 1456
  capsules, 1448
  carisoprodol, and codeine phosphate tablets, 1650
  and carisoprodol tablets, 1649
  codeine phosphate, alumina, and magnesia tablets, 1458
  and codeine phosphate tablets, 1457
  delayed-release capsules, 1449
  delayed-release tablets, 1452
  effervescent tablets for oral solution, 1453
  extended-release tablets, 1453
  and oxycodone tablets, 2883
  and pentazocine tablets, 2949
  propoxyphene hydrochloride, and caffeine capsules, 3107
  and propoxyphene napsylate tablets, 3112
  suppositories, 1450
  tablets, 1450
  tablets, buffered, 1451
Assay
  alginates $\langle 311 \rangle$, 139
  alpha tocopherol $\langle 551 \rangle$, 187
  amphetamine $\langle 331 \rangle$, 140
  antibiotics, iodometric $\langle 425 \rangle$, 150
  barbituate $\langle 361 \rangle$, 143
  for citric acid/citrate and phosphate $\langle 345 \rangle$, 142
  cobalamin radiotracer $\langle 371 \rangle$, 143
  dexpanthenol $\langle 115 \rangle$, 120
  epinephrine $\langle 391 \rangle$, 145
  folic acid $\langle 411 \rangle$, 149
  niacin or niacinamide $\langle 441 \rangle$, 154
  riboflavin $\langle 481 \rangle$, 182
  single-steroid $\langle 511 \rangle$, 183
  for steroids $\langle 351 \rangle$, 143

  thiamine $\langle 531 \rangle$, 184
  vitamin A $\langle 571 \rangle$, 203
  vitamin B₁₂ activity $\langle 171 \rangle$, 125
  vitamin D $\langle 581 \rangle$, 204
Assays
  antibiotics—microbial $\langle 81 \rangle$, 91
  design and analysis of biological $\langle 111 \rangle$, 108
  insulin $\langle 121 \rangle$, 121
Astemizole, 1459
  tablets, 1460
Atenolol, 1460
  and chlorthalidone tablets, 1462
  injection, 1461
  oral solution, 1462
  tablets, 1462
Atomic masses, 898
Atomic weights, 895
  and chemical formulas, xi, 3
Atovaquone, 1464
  oral suspension, 1465
Atracurium besylate, 1465
  injection, 1467
Atropine, 1468
  sulfate, 1468
  sulfate and diphenoxylate hydrochloride oral solution, 1990
  sulfate and diphenoxylate hydrochloride tablets, 1991
  sulfate injection, 1469
  sulfate ophthalmic ointment, 1469
  sulfate ophthalmic solution, 1470
  sulfate tablets, 1470
Attapulgite, activated, 1470
  colloidal, 1471
Aurothioglucose, 1471
  injectable suspension, 1471
Automated
  methods of analysis $\langle 16 \rangle$, 59
  radiochemical synthesis apparatus $\langle 1015 \rangle$, 389
Avobenzone, 1472
Azaperone, 1472
  injection, 1473
Azatadine maleate, 1473
  tablets, 1474
Azathioprine, 1474
  oral suspension, 1475
  sodium for injection, 1476
  tablets, 1475
Azithromycin, 1476
  capsules, 1479
  for oral suspension, 1479
Azo violet, 809
Aztreonam, 1480
  injection, 1480
  for injection, 1481
Azure A, 757

B

Bacampicillin hydrochloride, 1482
  for oral suspension, 1482
  tablets, 1483
Bacitracin, 1483
  for injection, 1483
  methylene disalicylate, soluble, 1484
  methylene disalicylate soluble powder, 1485
  neomycin and polymyxin B sulfates and hydrocortisone acetate ointment, 2781
  neomycin and polymyxin B sulfates and hydrocortisone acetate ophthalmic ointment, 2781
  neomycin and polymyxin B sulfates and lidocaine ointment, 2781

Bacitracin *(continued)*
  and neomycin and polymyxin B sulfates ointment, 2780
  and neomycin and polymyxin B sulfates ophthalmic ointment, 2780
  and neomycin sulfate ointment, 2772
  ointment, 1484
  ophthalmic ointment, 1484
  and polymyxin B sulfate topical aerosol, 1484
  zinc, 1485
  zinc, neomycin and polymyxin B sulfates, and hydrocortisone ointment, 2782
  zinc, neomycin and polymyxin B sulfates, and hydrocortisone ophthalmic ointment, 2783
  zinc, neomycin and polymyxin B sulfates and hydrocortisone acetate ophthalmic ointment, 2783
  zinc, neomycin and polymyxin B sulfates, and lidocaine ointment, 2784
  zinc and neomycin and polymyxin B sulfates ointment, 2782
  zinc and neomycin and polymyxin B sulfates ophthalmic ointment, 2782
  zinc and neomycin sulfate ointment, 2772
  zinc ointment, 1485
  zinc and polymyxin B sulfate ointment, 1486
  zinc and polymyxin B sulfate ophthalmic ointment, 1486
  zinc and polymyxin B sulfate topical aerosol, 3024
  zinc and polymyxin B sulfate topical powder, 3024
  zinc soluble powder, 1485
Baclofen, 1486
  oral suspension, 1487
  tablets, 1487
Bacterial
  alkaline protease preparation, 757
  endotoxins test ⟨85⟩, 98
Bacteriostatic
  sodium chloride injection, 3246
  water for injection, 3523
Bandage
  adhesive, 1488
  gauze, 1488
Barbital sodium, 757
Barbiturate assay ⟨361⟩, 143
Barbituric acid, 757
Barium
  acetate, 757
  chloride, 757
  chloride, anhydrous, 757
  chloride dihydrate, 757
  chloride TS, 815
  hydroxide, 757
  hydroxide lime, 1489
  hydroxide TS, 815
  nitrate, 757
  nitrate TS, 815
  sulfate, 1489
  sulfate for suspension, 1490
  sulfate paste, 1490
  sulfate suspension, 1490
  sulfate tablets, 1491
Basic fuchsin, 757
BCG live, 1491
BCG vaccine, 1491
Beclomethasone dipropionate, 1492
Beef extract, 757
Belladonna
  leaf, 1492
  extract, 1493
  extract tablets, 1494
  tincture, 1494
Benazepril hydrochloride, 1495
  tablets, 1496
Bendroflumethiazide, 1497
  and nadolol tablets, 2746

  tablets, 1498
Benoxinate hydrochloride, 1498
  and fluorescein sodium ophthalmic solution, 2191
  ophthalmic solution, 1499
Bentonite, 1079
  magma, 1081
  purified, 1080
Benzaldehyde, 758, 1081
  elixir, compound, 1081
Benzalkonium chloride, 758, 1081
  solution, 1082
Benzamidine hydrochloride hydrate, 758
Benzanilide, 758
Benzene, 758
Benzenesulfonamide, 758
Benzenesulfonyl chloride, 758
Benzethonium chloride, 1499
  concentrate, 1499
  tincture, 1500
  topical solution, 1500
Benzhydrol, 758
Benzocaine, 1500
  and antipyrine otic solution, 1435
  antipyrine, and phenylephrine hydrochloride otic solution, 1436
  butamben, and tetracaine hydrochloride gel, 1503
  butamben, and tetracaine hydrochloride ointment, 1504
  butamben, and tetracaine hydrochloride topical aerosol, 1503
  butamben, and tetracaine hydrochloride topical solution, 1504
  cream, 1501
  gel, 1501
  lozenges, 1502
  and menthol topical aerosol, 1505
  ointment, 1502
  otic solution, 1503
  topical aerosol, 1501
  topical solution, 1503
Benzoic
  acid, 758, 1505
  and salicylic acids ointment, 1506
Benzoin, 1506
  tincture, compound, 1507
Benzonatate, 1507
  capsules, 1508
Benzophenone, 758
p-Benzoquinone, 758
Benzoyl
  chloride, 758
  peroxide and erythromycin topical gel, 2089
  peroxide gel, 1509
  peroxide, hydrous, 1508
  peroxide lotion, 1509
N-Benzoyl-L-arginine ethyl ester hydrochloride, 758
3-Benzoylbenzoic acid, 758
Benzoylformic acid, 758
Benzphetamine hydrochloride, 758
Benztropine mesylate, 1510
  injection, 1510
  tablets, 1511
Benzyl
  alcohol, 1083
  benzoate, 1511
  benzoate lotion, 1512
2-Benzylaminopyridine, 758
1-Benzylimidazole, 758
Benzylpenicilloyl polylysine
  concentrate, 1512
  injection, 1513
Benzyltrimethylammonium chloride, 758
Beta carotene, 1513
  capsules, 1513
Betadex, 1084

Betahistine hydrochloride, 1514
Betaine hydrochloride, 1515
Betamethasone, 1515
  acetate, 1517
  acetate and betamethasone sodium phosphate injectable suspension, 1523
  acetate and gentamicin sulfate ophthalmic solution, 2265
  benzoate, 1518
  benzoate gel, 1518
  cream, 1515
  dipropionate, 1519
  dipropionate and clotrimazole cream, 1829
  dipropionate cream, 1520
  dipropionate lotion, 1521
  dipropionate ointment, 1521
  dipropionate topical aerosol, 1520
  oral solution, 1516
  sodium phosphate, 1521
  sodium phosphate and betamethasone acetate injectable suspension, 1523
  sodium phosphate injection, 1522
  tablets, 1516
  valerate, 1524
  valerate cream, 1524
  valerate and gentamicin sulfate ointment, 2266
  valerate and gentamicin sulfate otic solution, 2267
  valerate and gentamicin sulfate topical solution, 2268
  valerate lotion, 1525
  valerate ointment, 1525
Betanaphthol, 759
  TS, 815
Betaxolol
  hydrochloride, 1526
  ophthalmic solution, 1526
  tablets, 1527
Bethanechol chloride, 1527
  injection, 1528
  oral solution, 1529
  oral suspension, 1529
  tablets, 1530
Beta-lactamase, 759
Bibenzyl, 759
Bile salts, 759
Biocompatibility of materials used in drug containers, medical devices, and implants, the ⟨1031⟩, 390
Biological
  indicator for dry-heat sterilization, paper carrier, 1531
  indicator for ethylene oxide sterilization, paper carrier, 1532
  indicator for steam sterilization, paper carrier, 1532
  indicator for steam sterilization, self-contained, 1533
  indicators—resistance performance tests ⟨55⟩, 69
  indicators for sterilization ⟨1035⟩, 399
  reactivity tests, in vitro ⟨87⟩, 102
  reactivity tests, in vivo ⟨88⟩, 104
Biologics ⟨1041⟩, 402
Biotechnological products: analysis of the expression construct in cells used for production of r-DNA derived protein products, quality of ⟨1048⟩, 449
Biotechnology products: stability testing of biotechnological/biological products, quality of ⟨1049⟩, 450
Biotechnology products derived from cell lines of human or animal origin, viral safety evaluation of ⟨1050⟩, 453
Biotechnology-derived articles
  ⟨1045⟩, 409
  —amino acid analysis ⟨1052⟩, 463
  —capillary electrophoresis ⟨1053⟩, 471

Biotechnologyerived articles *(continued)*
—isoelectric focusing ⟨1054⟩, 475
—peptide mapping ⟨1055⟩, 477
—polyacrylamide gel electrophoresis ⟨1056⟩, 481
—total protein assay ⟨1057⟩, 486
Biotin, 1534
Biperiden, 1534
  hydrochloride, 1535
  hydrochloride tablets, 1535
  lactate injection, 1536
Biphenyl, 759
2,2′-Bipyridine, 759
Bisacodyl, 1536
  delayed-release tablets, 1537
  rectal suspension, 1537
  suppositories, 1537
4,4′-Bis(4-amino-naphthylazo)-2,2′-stilbenedisulfonic acid, 759
Bis(2-ethylhexyl)
  maleate, 759
  (phosphoric acid), 759
  phthalate, 759
  sebacate, 759
Bismuth
  citrate, 1538
  iodide TS, potassium, 819
  milk of, 1538
  nitrate pentahydrate, 759
  nitrate, 0.01 mol/L, 822
  subcarbonate, 1539
  subgallate, 1540
  subnitrate, 1540
  subsalicylate, 1541
  subsalicylate magma, 1542
  subsalicylate oral suspension, 1542
  subsalicylate tablets, 1543
  sulfite, 809
  sulfite agar, 759
Bisoctrizole, 1543
Bisoprolol fumarate, 1544
  and hydrochlorothiazide tablets, 1546
  tablets, 1545
Bis(trimethylsilyl)
  acetamide, 759
  trifluoroacetamide, 759
  trifluoroacetamide with trimethylchlorosilane, 760
Biuret reagent TS, 815
Bleomycin
  for injection, 1548
  sulfate, 1547

Blood
Blood, 760
Cells, red, 1551
Group A₁ red blood cells and blood group B red blood cells, 760
Grouping reagent, anti-A, grouping reagent, anti-B, and grouping reagent, anti-AB, 760
Grouping serum, anti-A, 1548
Grouping serum, anti-B, 1548
Grouping serums, 1549
Grouping serums, anti-D, anti-C, anti-E, anti-c, anti-e, 1549
Platelets, 1554
Technetium Tc 99m red blood cells injection, 3338
Whole, 1550

Blue
B, oracet, 809
B TS, oracet, 819
G, brilliant TS, 815
tetrazolium, 760
tetrazolium TS, 815

Board of trustees
USP convention (2005–2010), xi
Boiling or distilling range for reagents, 748
Boluses
  amoxicillin, 1408
  ampicillin, 1416
  aspirin, 1448
  dihydrostreptomycin sulfate, 1968
  neomycin, 2770
  phenylbutazone, 2983
  tetracycline, 3359
Boric acid, 760, 1085
(−)-Bornyl acetate, 760
Boron trifluoride, 760
14% Boron trifluoride–methanol, 760
Botanical
  extracts ⟨565⟩, 201
  origin, identification of articles of ⟨563⟩, 195
Botulism antitoxin, 1555
Bovine collagen, 760
7 Percent bovine serum albumin certified standard, 760
Branched polymeric sucrose, 760
Bretylium tosylate, 1555
  in dextrose injection, 1556
  injection, 1556
Brilliant
  blue G TS, 815
  green, 760, 809
  yellow, 809
Brinzolamide, 1556
  ophthalmic suspension, 1557
Bromelain, 760
Bromine, 760
  sodium acetate TS, 815
  tenth-normal (0.1 N), 822
  TS, 815
α-Bromo-2′-acetonaphthone, 760
p-Bromoaniline, 760
  TS, 815
Bromocresol
  blue, 809
  blue TS, 816
  green, 809
  green-methyl red TS, 816
  green sodium salt, 809
  green TS, 816
  purple, 809
  purple sodium salt, 809
  purple TS, 816
Bromocriptine mesylate, 1558
  capsules, 1559
  tablets, 1560
Bromodiphenhydramine hydrochloride, 1561
  and codeine phosphate oral solution, 1562
  oral solution, 1561
Bromofluoromethane, 760
Bromophenol blue, 809
  sodium, 809
  TS, 816
N-Bromosuccinimide, 760
Bromothymol blue, 809
  TS, 816
Brompheniramine maleate, 1562
  injection, 1563
  oral solution, 1563
  and pseudoephedrine sulfate oral solution, 1564
  tablets, 1563
Brucine sulfate, 760
Budesonide, 1565

Buffer
Acetate, 814
Acetate TS, 814
Acetic acid–ammonium acetate TS, 815
Acetone buffered, TS, 815
Acid phthalate, 813

Alkaline borate, 814
Ammonia-ammonium chloride TS, 815
Hydrochloric acid, 813
Neutralized phthalate, 813
Phosphate, 814

Buffered acetone TS, 816
Buffers, 760
Buffer solutions, 813
  Acetate buffer, 814
  Acid phthalate buffer, 813
  Alkaline borate buffer, 814
  Hydrochloric acid buffer, 813
  Neutralized phthalate buffer, 813
  Phosphate buffer, 814
Bulk density and tapped density ⟨616⟩, 231
Bulk pharmaceutical excipients—certificate of analysis ⟨1080⟩, 517
Bumetanide, 1566
  injection, 1567
  tablets, 1568
Bupivacaine hydrochloride, 1568
  in dextrose injection, 1570
  and epinephrine injection, 1570
  injection, 1569
Buprenorphine hydrochloride, 1571
Bupropion hydrochloride, 1572
  extended-release tablets, 1573
  tablets, 1573
Buspirone hydrochloride, 1576
  tablets, 1576
Busulfan, 1577
  tablets, 1577
Butabarbital, 1577
  sodium, 1578
  sodium oral solution, 1578
  sodium tablets, 1579
Butalbital, 1580
  acetaminophen, and caffeine capsules, 1580
  acetaminophen, and caffeine tablets, 1581
  aspirin, and caffeine capsules, 1583
  aspirin, caffeine, and codeine phosphate capsules, 1585
  aspirin, and caffeine tablets, 1584
  and aspirin tablets, 1582
Butamben, 1586
  benzocaine, and tetracaine hydrochloride gel, 1503
  benzocaine, and tetracaine hydrochloride ointment, 1504
  benzocaine, and tetracaine hydrochloride topical aerosol, 1503
  benzocaine, and tetracaine hydrochloride topical solution, 1504
Butane, 1085
1,3-Butanediol, 760
2,3-Butanedione, 761
Butanol, 761
Butoconazole nitrate, 1586
  vaginal cream, 1587
Butorphanol tartrate, 1587
  injection, 1588
  nasal solution, 1589
Butyl
  acetate, normal, 761
  alcohol, 761, 1085
  alcohol, normal, 761
  alcohol, secondary, 761
  alcohol, tertiary, 761
  benzoate, 761
  ether, 761
  methacrylate, 761
n-Butyl chloride, 761
tert-Butyl methyl ether, 761
n-Butylamine, 761
tert-Butylamine, 761
4-(Butylamino)benzoic acid, 761

Butylated
  hydroxyanisole, 1086
  hydroxytoluene, 1086
n-Butylboronic acid, 761
tert-Butyldimethylchlorosilane in N-methyl-N-tert-butyldimethylsilyltrifluoroacetamide, (1 in 100), 761
Butylparaben, 1086
4-tert-Butylphenol, 761
Butyraldehyde, 761
Butyric acid, 761
Butyrolactone, 761

C

C 11
  carbon monoxide, 1638
  injection, flumazenil, 1639
  injection, mespiperone, 1640
  injection, methionine, 1640
  injection, raclopride, 1641
  injection, sodium acetate, 1642
C 13
  for oral solution, urea, 1643
  urea, 1643
C 14
  capsules, urea, 1643
Cadmium
  acetate, 761
  nitrate, 762
Caffeine, 1590
  acetaminophen and aspirin tablets, 1273
  and acetaminophen tablets, 1274
  aspirin and dihydrocodeine bitartrate capsules, 1456
  butalbital, and acetaminophen capsules, 1580
  butalbital, and acetaminophen tablets, 1581
  butalbital, and aspirin capsules, 1583
  butalbital, aspirin, and codeine phosphate capsules, 1585
  butalbital, and aspirin tablets, 1584
  citrate injection, 1590
  citrate oral solution, 1591
  and ergotamine tartrate suppositories, 2082
  and ergotamine tartrate tablets, 2083
  propoxyphene hydrochloride, and aspirin capsules, 3107
  and sodium benzoate injection, 1592
Calamine, 1592
  topical suspension, phenolated, 1593
  topical suspension, 1593
Calcifediol, 1593
  capsules, 1594
Calcitonin salmon, 1595
  injection, 1598
  nasal solution, 1598
Calcitriol, 1594
  injection, 1595
Calcium
  acetate, 762, 1599
  acetate and aluminum sulfate tablets for topical solution, 1360
  acetate tablets, 1600
  ascorbate, 1601
  carbonate, 762, 1601
  carbonate, alumina, and magnesia chewable tablets, 1338
  carbonate, alumina, and magnesia oral suspension, 1337
  carbonate, alumina, magnesia, and simethicone chewable tablets, 1341
  carbonate, alumina, magnesia, and simethicone tablets, 1339

carbonate, alumina, and magnesia tablets, 1338
carbonate, chelometric standard, 762
carbonate lozenges, 1602
carbonate, magnesia, and simethicone chewable tablets, 1605
carbonate, magnesia, and simethicone tablets, 1604
carbonate and magnesia tablets, 1603
carbonate oral suspension, 1602
carbonate tablets, 1603
caseinate, 762
chloride, 762, 1607
chloride, anhydrous, 762
chloride injection, 1608
chloride TS, 816
citrate, 762, 1608
glubionate syrup, 1609
gluceptate, 1609
gluceptate injection, 1610
gluconate, 1610
gluconate injection, 1611
gluconate tablets, 1612
glycerophosphate, 912
hydroxide, 762, 1612
hydroxide topical solution, 1612
hydroxide TS, 816
lactate, 762, 1613
lactate tablets, 1613
lactobionate, 1614
levulinate, 1614
levulinate injection, 1614
and magnesium carbonates oral suspension, 1607
and magnesium carbonates tablets, 1607
nitrate, 763
pantothenate, 1615
pantothenate assay ⟨91⟩, 107
pantothenate, dextro, 763
pantothenate, racemic, 1616
pantothenate tablets, 1615
phosphate, anhydrous dibasic, 1617
phosphate tablets, dibasic, 1618
phosphate, tribasic, 1087
phosphate dihydrate, dibasic, 1616
polycarbophil, 1618
saccharate, 1618
silicate, 1088
stearate, 1089
sulfate, 763, 1089
sulfate TS, 816
undecylenate, 1619
and vitamin D with minerals tablets, 914
with vitamin D tablets, 913
Calcium acetate
  and aluminum sulfate for topical solution, 1359
Calconcarboxylic acid, 763
  triturate, 763
Calf thymus DNA, 763
dl-Camphene, 763
Camphor, 1619
  spirit, 1620
dl-10-Camphorsulfonic acid, 763
Canada balsam, 763
Candelilla wax, 1090
Canola oil, 1090
Capecitabine, 1620
  tablets, 1621
Capillary electrophoresis ⟨727⟩, 281
Capreomycin
  for injection, 1623
  sulfate, 1623
Capric acid, 763
Caprylocaproyl polyoxylglycerides, 1091
Capsaicin, 1623
Capsicum, 1624
  oleoresin, 1625

Capsules
Acebutolol hydrochloride, 1265
Acetaminophen, 1269
Containing at least three of the following—acetaminophen and (salts of) chlorpheniramine, dextromethorphan, and phenylpropanolamine, 1275
Containing at least three of the following—acetaminophen and (salts of) chlorpheniramine, dextromethorphan, and pseudoephedrine, 1280
Acetaminophen and codeine phosphate, 1288
Acyclovir, 1304
Altretamine, 1335
Aluminum hydroxide gel, dried, 1355
Amantadine hydrochloride, 1374
Aminobenzoate potassium, 1384
Amoxicillin, 1409
Ampicillin, 1417
Aspirin, 1448
Aspirin, caffeine, and dihydrocodeine bitartrate, 1456
Aspirin delayed-release, 1449
Azithromycin, 1479
Benzonatate, 1508
Beta carotene, 1513
Bromocriptine mesylate, 1559
Butalbital, acetaminophen, and caffeine, 1580
Butalbital, aspirin, and caffeine, 1583
Butalbital, aspirin, caffeine, and codeine phosphate, 1585
Calcifediol, 1594
C 14, Urea, 1643
Castor oil, 1659
Cefaclor, 1661
Cefadroxil, 1663
Cephalexin, 1706
Cephradine, 1713
Chloral hydrate, 1717
Chloramphenicol, 1719
Chlordiazepoxide hydrochloride, 1729
Chlordiazepoxide hydrochloride and clidinium bromide, 1730
Chlorpheniramine maleate extended-release, 1740
Chlorpheniramine maleate and phenylpropanolamine hydrochloride extended-release, 1742
Chlorpheniramine maleate and pseudoephedrine hydrochloride extended-release, 1744
Cinoxacin, 1768
Clindamycin hydrochloride, 1796
Clofazimine, 1809
Clofibrate, 1810
Clomipramine hydrochloride, 1813
Cloxacillin sodium, 1832
Cod liver oil, 927
Cyanocobalamin Co 57, 1834
Cyanocobalamin Co 58, 1835
Cycloserine, 1867
Cyclosporine, 1869
Danazol, 1878
Dantrolene sodium, 1880
Demeclocycline hydrochloride, 1889
Dextroamphetamine sulfate, 1924
Diazepam, 1934
Diazepam extended-release, 1934
Diazoxide, 1936
Dicloxacillin sodium, 1945
Dicyclomine hydrochloride, 1946
Digitalis, 1961
Dihydrotachysterol, 1969
Diltiazem hydrochloride extended-release, 1976
Diphenhydramine hydrochloride, 1988

Capsules (continued)
Diphenhydramine and pseudoephedrine, 1989
Disopyramide phosphate, 1998
Disopyramide phosphate extended-release, 1998
Docusate calcium, 2005
Docusate potassium, 2006
Docusate sodium, 2007
Doxepin hydrochloride, 2019
Doxycycline, 2022
Doxycycline hyclate, 2024
Doxycycline hyclate delayed-release, 2025
Dronabinol, 2028
Ephedrine sulfate, 2063
Ergocalciferol, 2071
Ergoloid mesylates, 2074
Erythromycin delayed-release, 2085
Erythromycin estolate, 2090
Ethchlorvynol, 2117
Ethosuximide, 2122
Etodolac, 2130
Etoposide, 2133
Fenoprofen calcium, 2149
Ferrous gluconate, 2156
Fexofenadine hydrochloride, 2162
Flucytosine, 2173
Fluoxetine, 2201
Fluoxetine delayed-release, 2201
Flurazepam hydrochloride, 2213
Flutamide, 2217
Fluvastatin, 2223
Gabapentin, 2243
Gemfibrozil, 2262
Ginger, 946
Ginkgo, 950
Ginseng, American, 953
Griseofulvin, 2302
Guaifenesin, 2305
Guaifenesin and pseudoephedrine hydrochloride, 2307
Guaifenesin, pseudoephedrine hydrochloride, and dextromethorphan hydrobromide, 2308
Hydroxyurea, 2361
Hydroxyzine pamoate, 2365
Indomethacin, 2397
Indomethacin extended-release, 2397
Sodium iodide I 123, 2417
Sodium iodide I 131, 2421
Ipodate sodium, 2445
Isometheptene mucate, dichloralphenazone, and acetaminophen, 2458
Isosorbide dinitrate extended-release, 2471
Isotretinoin, 2479
Isradipine, 2482
Kanamycin sulfate, 2486
Lansoprazole delayed-release, 2503
Levodopa, 2519
Lincomycin hydrochloride, 2532
Alpha lipoic acid, 969
Lithium carbonate, 2540
Loperamide hydrochloride, 2543
Loracarbef, 2546
Loxapine, 2558
Magnesium oxide, 2576
Meclofenamate sodium, 2599
Mefenamic acid, 2602
Mesalamine extended-release, 2630
Methacycline hydrochloride, 2647
Methoxsalen, 2665
Methsuximide, 2669
Methyltestosterone, 2689
Metyrosine, 2707
Mexiletine hydrochloride, 2708
Milk thistle, 981
Minerals, 982
Minocycline hydrochloride, 2716
Morphine sulfate extended-release, 2736
Nafcillin sodium, 2747

Nifedipine, 2806
Nitrofurantoin, 2812
Nizatidine, 2821
Nortriptyline hydrochloride, 2838
Oil- and water-soluble vitamins with minerals, 1011
Oleovitamin A and D, 2850
Omeprazole delayed-release, 2851
Oxacillin sodium, 2862
Oxazepam, 2868
Oxycodone and acetaminophen, 2882
Oxytetracycline hydrochloride, 2894
Oxytetracycline and nystatin, 2892
Pancrelipase, 2909
Pancrelipase delayed-release, 2909
Paromomycin sulfate, 2919
Penicillamine, 2927
Pentobarbital sodium, 2955
Phendimetrazine tartrate, 2969
Phenoxybenzamine hydrochloride, 2977
Phensuximide, 2978
Phentermine hydrochloride, 2979
Phenylpropanolamine hydrochloride, 2990
Phenylpropanolamine hydrochloride extended-release, 2990
Phenytoin sodium, extended, 2996
Phenytoin sodium, prompt, 2999
Piroxicam, 3015
Potassium chloride extended-release, 3032
Potassium perchlorate, 3046
Prazosin hydrochloride, 3058
Procainamide hydrochloride, 3079
Procarbazine hydrochloride, 3084
Propoxyphene hydrochloride, 3106
Propoxyphene hydrochloride, aspirin, and caffeine, 3107
Propranolol hydrochloride extended-release, 3114
Propranolol hydrochloride and hydrochlorothiazide extended-release, 3116
Pseudoephedrine hydrochloride extended-release, 3125
Pygeum, 989
Quinidine sulfate, 3149
Quinine sulfate, 3152
Rifabutin, 3181
Rifampin, 3183
Rifampin and isoniazid, 3185
Salsalate, 3214
Saquinavir, 3217
Saw palmetto, 996
Secobarbital sodium, 3223
Secobarbital sodium and amobarbital sodium, 3224
Simethicone, 3232
Stavudine, 3272
Sulfinpyrazone, 3305
Tacrine, 3318
Temazepam, 3342
Tetracycline hydrochloride, 3361
Tetracycline hydrochloride and nystatin, 3366
Thalidomide, 3369
Theophylline, 3371
Theophylline extended-release, 3372
Theophylline and guaifenesin, 3377
Thiothixene, 3395
Tolmetin sodium, 3432
Triamterene, 3448
Triamterene and hydrochlorothiazide, 3449
Trientine hydrochloride, 3457
Trihexyphenidyl hydrochloride extended-release, 3463
Trimethobenzamide hydrochloride, 3467
Troleandomycin, 3479
Ubidecarenone, 999
Ursodiol, 3489
Valproic acid, 3492
Vancomycin hydrochloride, 3500

Vitamin A, 3518
Vitamin E, 3520
Vitamins, oil-soluble, 1003
Vitamins, oil- and water-soluble, 1005
Vitamins, water-soluble, 1041
Vitamins with minerals, oil- and water-soluble, 1011
Vitamins with minerals, water-soluble, 1046
Zidovudine, 3540

Captopril, 1625
and hydrochlorothiazide tablets, 1628
oral solution, 1626
oral suspension, 1626
tablets, 1627
Caramel, 1092
Caraway, 1092
oil, 1092
Carbachol, 1629
intraocular solution, 1629
ophthalmic solution, 1629
Carbamazepine, 1630
extended-release tablets, 1632
oral suspension, 1631
tablets, 1631
Carbamide peroxide, 1633
topical solution, 1633
Carbazole sulfate, 763
Carbenicillin
disodium, 1634
indanyl sodium, 1634
indanyl sodium tablets, 1635
for injection, 1634
Carbidopa, 1635
and levodopa tablets, 1636
Carbinoxamine maleate, 1637
pseudoephedrine hydrochloride, and dextromethorphan hydrobromide oral solution, 3128
tablets, 1637
Carbol-fuchsin topical solution, 1638
Carbomer
934, 1093
934P, 1093
940, 1094
941, 1094
1342, 1094
copolymer, 1095
homopolymer, 1096
interpolymer, 1098
Carbon
C 11, carbon monoxide, 1638
C 11 injection, flumazenil, 1639
C 11 injection, mespiperone, 1640
C 11 injection, methionine, 1640
C 11 injection, raclopride, 1641
C 11 injection, sodium acetate, 1642
C 13 for oral solution, urea, 1643
C 13, urea, 1643
C 14 capsules, urea, 1643
dioxide, 1638
dioxide detector tube, 763
disulfide, chromatographic, 763
disulfide, CS, 763
monoxide detector tube, 763
tetrachloride, 763
Carbonates
calcium and magnesium, oral suspension, 1607
calcium and magnesium, tablets, 1607
Carboplatin, 1644
for injection, 1645
Carboprost
tromethamine, 1646
tromethamine injection, 1646
Carboxylate (sodium form) cation-exchange resin (50- to 100-mesh), 763
Carboxymethoxylamine hemihydrochloride, 763

Carboxymethylcellulose
  calcium, 1099
  sodium, 1647
  sodium 12, 1101
  sodium, low-substituted, 1100
  sodium and microcrystalline cellulose, 1106
  sodium paste, 1647
  sodium tablets, 1648
Cardamom
  oil, 1102
  seed, 1102
  tincture, compound, 1102
Carisoprodol, 1648
  aspirin and codeine phosphate tablets, 1650
  and aspirin tablets, 1649
  tablets, 1648
Carmine, 763
Carprofen, 1651
  tablets, 1652
Carrageenan, 1102
Carteolol hydrochloride, 1653
  ophthalmic solution, 1654
  tablets, 1654
(R)-(−)-Carvone, 763
Casanthranol, 1655
Cascara
  fluidextract, aromatic, 1658
  sagrada, 1656
  sagrada extract, 1657
  sagrada fluidextract, 1658
  tablets, 1658
Casein, 763
  hammersten, 763
Castor oil, 1659
  aromatic, 1660
  capsules, 1659
  emulsion, 1659
  hydrogenated, 1103
  polyoxyl 35, 1205
Catechol, 763
Cation-exchange resin, 763
  carboxylate (sodium form) (50- to 100-mesh), 763
  polystyrene, 763
  styrene-divinylbenzene, 763
  styrene-divinylbenzene, strongly acidic, 764
  sulfonic acid, 764
Cedar oil, 764
Cefaclor, 1660
  capsules, 1661
  extended-release tablets, 1662
  for oral suspension, 1661
Cefadroxil, 1663
  capsules, 1663
  for oral suspension, 1664
  tablets, 1664
Cefamandole nafate, 1665
  for injection, 1665
Cefazolin, 1666
  injection, 1667
  for injection, 1667
  ophthalmic solution, 1668
  sodium, 1666
Cefepime
  hydrochloride, 1669
  for injection, 1670
Cefixime, 1671
  for oral suspension, 1672
  tablets, 1672
Cefmenoxime
  hydrochloride, 1672
  for injection, 1673
Cefmetazole, 1674
  injection, 1674
  for injection, 1675
  sodium, 1675
Cefonicid
  for injection, 1676

sodium, 1676
Cefoperazone
  injection, 1677
  for injection, 1678
  sodium, 1677
Ceforanide, 1678
  for injection, 1679
Cefotaxime
  injection, 1681
  for injection, 1681
  sodium, 1680
Cefotetan, 1682
  disodium, 1683
  injection, 1683
  for injection, 1683
Cefotiam
  hydrochloride, 1684
  for injection, 1685
Cefoxitin
  injection, 1686
  for injection, 1686
  sodium, 1685
Cefpiramide, 1687
  for injection, 1688
Cefpodoxime proxetil, 1688
  for oral suspension, 1690
  tablets, 1690
Cefprozil, 1691
  for oral suspension, 1691
  tablets, 1692
Ceftazidime, 1692
  injection, 1693
  for injection, 1693
Ceftizoxime
  injection, 1696
  for injection, 1696
  sodium, 1695
Ceftriaxone
  injection, 1697
  for injection, 1698
  sodium, 1697
Cefuroxime
  axetil, 1698
  axetil for oral suspension, 1699
  axetil tablets, 1700
  injection, 1701
  for injection, 1701
  sodium, 1700
Cell and gene therapy products ⟨1046⟩, 419
Cellaburate, 1104
Cellacefate, 1105
Cellulose
  acetate, 1107
  chromatographic, 764
  microcrystalline, 764, 1105
  microcrystalline and carboxymethylcellulose sodium, 1106
  mixture, chromatographic, 764
  oxidized, 1702
  oxidized regenerated, 1702
  powdered, 1107
  sodium phosphate, 1703
  sodium phosphate for oral suspension, 1704
Cephalexin, 1704
  capsules, 1706
  hydrochloride, 1705
  for oral suspension, 1706
  tablets, 1707
  tablets for oral suspension, 1707
Cephalothin
  injection, 1708
  for injection, 1709
  sodium, 1708
Cephapirin
  benzathine, 1709
  benzathine intramammary infusion, 1710
  for injection, 1711
  sodium, 1711

sodium intramammary infusion, 1712
Cephradine, 1712
  capsules, 1713
  for injection, 1713
  for oral suspension, 1714
  tablets, 1714
Ceric
  ammonium nitrate, 764
  ammonium nitrate TS, 816
  ammonium nitrate, twentieth-normal (0.05 N), 822
  ammonium sulfate, 764
  sulfate, 764
  sulfate, tenth-normal (0.1 N), 822
Cesium chloride, 764
Cetostearyl alcohol, 1108
Cetrimide, 764
Cetrimonium bromide, 1108
Cetyl
  alcohol, 1109
  esters wax, 1109
  palmitate, 1110
Cetylpyridinium chloride, 1715
  lozenges, 1715
  topical solution, 1716
Cetyltrimethylammonium chloride, 25 percent in water, 764
Chamomile, 916
Changes in official titles, xxviii
Chapters
  general, xiii, 5
Charcoal
  activated, 764, 1716
Chaste tree, 917
  powdered, 919
  powdered, extract, 919
Chenodeoxycholic acid, 765
Cherry
  juice, 1110
  syrup, 1111
Chloral hydrate, 1716
  capsules, 1717
  oral solution, 1717
  TS, 816
Chlorambucil, 1717
  tablets, 1717
Chloramine T, 765
Chloramphenicol, 1718
  capsules, 1719
  cream, 1719
  and hydrocortisone acetate for ophthalmic suspension, 1722
  injection, 1719
  ophthalmic ointment, 1720
  ophthalmic solution, 1720
  for ophthalmic solution, 1720
  oral solution, 1721
  otic solution, 1721
  palmitate, 1724
  palmitate oral suspension, 1724
  polymyxin B sulfate, and hydrocortisone acetate ophthalmic ointment, 1723
  and polymyxin B sulfate ophthalmic ointment, 1722
  and prednisolone ophthalmic ointment, 1723
  sodium succinate, 1725
  sodium succinate for injection, 1726
  tablets, 1721
Chlordiazepoxide, 1726
  and amitriptyline hydrochloride tablets, 1727
  hydrochloride, 1728
  hydrochloride capsules, 1729
  hydrochloride and clidinium bromide capsules, 1730
  hydrochloride for injection, 1729
  tablets, 1727
Chlorhexidine gluconate
  oral rinse, 1732

Chlorhexidine gluconate *(continued)*
  solution, 1731
Chloride
  cobaltous, TS, 816
  ferric, TS, 817
  gold, 777
  gold, TS, 817
  platinic, 790
  platinic, TS, 819
  in reagents, 749
Chloride and sulfate ⟨221⟩, 132
Chlorine, 765
  detector tube, 765
  TS, 816
m-Chloroacetanilide, 765
p-Chloroacetanilide, 765
1-Chloroadamantane, 765
2-Chloro-4-aminobenzoic acid, 765
5-Chloro-2-aminobenzophenone, 765
3-Chloroaniline, 765
p-Chloroaniline, 765
Chlorobenzene, 765
4-Chlorobenzoic acid, 765
m-Chlorobenzoic acid, 765
4-Chlorobenzophenone, 765
1-Chlorobutane, 765
Chlorobutanol, 1111
Chlorocresol, 1111
2-Chloroethylamine monohydrochloride, 765
Chloroform, 765
  alcohol-free, 765
  methyl, 765
Chlorogenic acid, 765
Chloromethylated polysterene-divinylbenzene
  anion-exchange resin, 765
1-Chloronaphthalene, 765
4-Chloro-1-naphthol, 765
2-Chloronicotinic acid, 765
2-Chloro-4-nitroaniline, 99%, 765
Chlorophyllin copper complex sodium, 1733
Chloroplatinic acid, 765
Chloroprocaine hydrochloride, 1734
  injection, 1735
Chloroquine, 1735
  hydrochloride injection, 1736
  phosphate, 1736
  phosphate tablets, 1736
5-Chlorosalicylic acid, 765
Chlorothiazide, 1737
  and methyldopa tablets, 2675
  oral suspension, 1738
  and reserpine tablets, 3170
  sodium for injection, 1738
  tablets, 1738
1-Chloro-2,2,2-
  trifluoroethylchlorodifluoromethyl ether, 766
Chlorotrimethylsilane, 766
Chloroxylenol, 1739
Chlorpheniramine
  dextromethorphan, phenylpropanolamine (salts
    of), and acetaminophen, capsules containing
    at least three of the following, 1275
  dextromethorphan, phenylpropanolamine (salts
    of), and acetaminophen, oral solution
    containing at least three of the following,
    1277
  dextromethorphan, phenylpropanolamine (salts
    of) and acetaminophen, tablets containing at
    least three of the following, 1278
  dextromethorphan, pseudoephedrine, (salts of),
    and acetaminophen, capsules containing at
    least three of the following, 1280
  dextromethorphan, pseudoephedrine (salts of),
    and acetaminophen, oral powder containing at
    least three of the following, 1282
  dextromethorphan, pseudoephedrine (salts of),
    and acetaminophen, oral solution containing
    at least three of the following, 1283
  dextromethorphan, pseudoephedrine (salts of),
    and acetaminophen, tablets containing at least
    three of the following, 1285
  maleate, 1740
  maleate extended-release capsules, 1740
  maleate injection, 1741
  maleate oral solution, 1741
  maleate, penicillin G procaine,
    dihydrostreptomycin sulfate, and
    dexamethasone injectable suspension, 2939
  maleate and phenylpropanolamine
    hydrochloride extended-release capsules,
    1742
  maleate and phenylpropanolamine
    hydrochlroride extended-release tablets, 1743
  maleate and pseudoephedrine hydrochloride
    extended-release capsules, 1744
  maleate and pseudoephedrine hydrochloride
    oral solution, 1745
  maleate tablets, 1742
  maleate, acetaminophen, and dextromethorphan
    hydrobromide tablets, 1287
Chlorpromazine, 1745
  hydrochloride, 1746
  hydrochloride injection, 1747
  hydrochloride oral concentrate, 1747
  hydrochloride syrup, 1748
  hydrochloride tablets, 1748
  suppositories, 1746
Chlorpropamide, 1749
  tablets, 1749
Chlortetracycline
  bisulfate, 1749
  hydrochloride, 766, 1750
  hydrochloride ointment, 1751
  hydrochloride ophthalmic ointment, 1751
  hydrochloride soluble powder, 1751
  hydrochloride tablets, 1752
  and sulfamethazine bisulfates soluble powder,
    1750
Chlorthalidone, 1752
  and atenolol tablets, 1462
  and clonidine hydrochloride tablets, 1818
  tablets, 1753
Chlorzoxazone, 1753
  tablets, 1754
Chocolate, 1112
  syrup, 1112
Cholecalciferol, 1754
  solution, 1755
Cholestane, 766
Cholesterol, 766, 1112
Cholesteryl
  benzoate, 766
  n-heptylate, 766
Cholestyramine
  for oral suspension, 1757
  resin, 1756
Choline
  bitartrate, 920
  chloride, 766, 920
Chondroitin sulfate
  sodium tablets, 923
Chondroitin sulfate sodium, 921
  and glucosamine tablets, 957
  glucosamine, and methylsulfonylmethane
    tablets, 961
Chromate, sodium, Cr 51 injection, 1758
Chromatographic
  fuller's earth, 766
  n-heptane, 766
  magnesium oxide, 766
  reagents, 766, 810
  silica gel, 766
  silica gel mixture, 766
  siliceous earth, 766
  siliceous earth, silanized, 766
  solvent hexane, 766
Chromatography ⟨621⟩, 232
Chromatography, ion ⟨1065⟩, 490
Chromic chloride, 1757
  injection, 1758
Chromium
  Cr 51 edetate injection, 1759
  Cr 51injection, sodium chromate, 1758
  picolinate, 923
  picolinate tablets, 924
  potassium sulfate dodecahydrate, 766
  trioxide, 766
Chromogenic
  substrate for amidolytic test, 766
Chromotrope 2R, 766
Chromotropic acid, 766
  disodium salt, 766
  TS, 816
Chymotrypsin, 1759
  for ophthalmic solution, 1760
Ciclopirox, 1761
  olamine, 1761
  olamine cream, 1762
  olamine topical suspension, 1763
Cilastatin
  and imipenem for injectable suspension, 2383
  and imipenem for injection, 2382
  sodium, 1763
Cilostazol, 1764
Cimetidine, 1765
  hydrochloride, 1766
  injection, 1767
  in sodium chloride injection, 1767
  tablets, 1766
Cinchonidine, 766
Cinchonine, 766
Cinoxacin, 1768
  capsules, 1768
Ciprofloxacin, 1769
  and dexamethasone otic suspension, 1771
  hydrochloride, 1770
  injection, 1772
  ophthalmic ointment, 1774
  ophthalmic solution, 1774
  tablets, 1775
Cisplatin, 1775
  for injection, 1777
Citalopram
  hydrobromide, 1778
  tablets, 1780
Citric acid
  magnesium carbonate, and potassium citrate for
    oral solution, 2569
Citric acid, 766
  anhydrous, 766, 1781
  and magnesium carbonate for oral solution,
    2569
  magnesium oxide, and sodium carbonate
    irrigation, 1784
  monohydrate, 1783
  and potassium citrate oral solution, 3039
  and potassium and sodium bicarbonates
    effervescent tablets for oral solution, 3029
  and sodium citrate oral solution, 3248
Cladribine, 1785
Clarithromycin, 1786
  for oral suspension, 1787
  tablets, 1788
  extended-release tablets, 1789
Clavulanate
  potassium, 1791
  potassium and amoxicillin for oral suspension,
    1412
  potassium and amoxicillin tablets, 1412
Clavulanic acid
  and ticarcillin injection, 3405
  and ticarcillin for injection, 3405
Cleaning glass apparatus ⟨1051⟩, 462

Clemastine fumarate, 1793
  tablets, 1794
Clidinium bromide, 1795
  and chlordiazepoxide hydrochloride capsules, 1730
Clindamycin
  hydrochloride, 1796
  hydrochloride capsules, 1796
  hydrochloride oral solution, 1797
  injection, 1800
  for injection, 1800
  palmitate hydrochloride, 1797
  palmitate hydrochloride for oral solution, 1798
  phosphate, 1798
  phosphate gel, 1799
  phosphate topical solution, 1800
  phosphate topical suspension, 1801
  phosphate vaginal cream, 1799
  phosphate vaginal inserts, 1801
Clioquinol, 1802
  cream, 1802
  and hydrocortisone cream, 1803
  and hydrocortisone ointment, 1804
  ointment, 1803
  topical powder, compound, 1803
Clobetasol propionate, 1805
  cream, 1805
  ointment, 1806
  topical solution, 1806
Clocortolone pivalate, 1807
  cream, 1808
Clofazimine, 1808
  capsules, 1809
Clofibrate, 1809
  capsules, 1810
Clomiphene citrate, 1811
  tablets, 1811
Clomipramine hydrochloride, 1812
  capsules, 1813
Clonazepam, 1814
  oral suspension, 1814
  tablets, 1815
Clonidine, 1816
  hydrochloride, 1817
  hydrochloride and chlorthalidone tablets, 1818
  hydrochloride tablets, 1817
  transdermal system, 1819
Clopidogrel
  bisulfate, 1820
  tablets, 1821
Clorazepate dipotassium, 1822
  tablets, 1823
Clorsulon, 1825
Clotrimazole, 1825
  and betamethasone dipropionate cream, 1829
  cream, 1826
  lotion, 1827
  lozenges, 1827
  topical solution, 1828
  vaginal inserts, 1829
Clove oil, 1113
Clover, red, 924
  extract, powdered, 926
  powdered, 925
  tablets, 926
Cloxacillin
  benzathine, 1830
  benzathine intramammary infusion, 1831
  sodium, 1831
  sodium capsules, 1832
  sodium intramammary infusion, 1832
  sodium for oral solution, 1832
Clozapine, 1833
  tablets, 1833
Co
  57 capsules, cyanocobalamin, 1834
  57 oral solution, cyanocobalamin, 1835
  58 capsules, cyanocobalamin, 1835

Coal tar, 1834
  ointment, 1834
  topical solution, 1834
Cobalamin radiotracer assay 〈371〉, 143
Cobalt
  chloride, 766
  Co 57 capsules, cyanocobalamin, 1834
  Co 57 oral solution, cyanocobalamin, 1835
  Co 58 capsules, cyanocobalamin, 1835
  nitrate, 766
  platinum, TS, 819
  uranyl acetate TS, 816
Cobaltous
  acetate, 766
  chloride, 766
  chloride CS, 814
  chloride TS, 816
Cocaine, 1836
  hydrochloride, 1837
  hydrochloride tablets for topical solution, 1837
  and tetracaine hydrochlorides and epinephrine topical solution, 1838
Coccidioidin, 1839
Cocoa butter, 1113
Coconut
  Oil, 1114
Codeine, 1841
  phosphate, 1841
  phosphate and acetaminophen capsules, 1288
  phosphate and acetaminophen oral solution, 1289
  phosphate and acetaminophen oral suspension, 1290
  phosphate and acetaminophen tablets, 1291
  phosphate, aspirin, alumina, and magnesia tablets, 1458
  phosphate and aspirin tablets, 1457
  phosphate and bromodiphenhydramine hydrochloride oral solution, 1562
  phosphate, butalbital, aspirin, and caffeine capsules, 1585
  phosphate, carisoprodol, and aspirin tablets, 1650
  phosphate and guaifenesin oral solution, 2306
  phosphate injection, 1841
  phosphate tablets, 1842
  sulfate, 1842
  sulfate tablets, 1843
  and terpin hydrate oral solution, 3348
Cod liver oil, 1839
  capsules, 927
Coenzyme Q9, 766
Cohosh
  black, 908
  black fluidextract, 910
  black, powdered, 910
  black, powdered extract, 911
  black tablets, 911
Colchicine, 1843
  injection, 1844
  and probenecid tablets, 3076
  tablets, 1844
Colestipol hydrochloride, 1845
  for oral suspension, 1846
Colistimethate
  for injection, 1847
  sodium, 1846
Colistin
  and neomycin sulfates and hydrocortisone acetate otic suspension, 1848
  sulfate, 1847
  sulfate for oral suspension, 1848
Collagen, 766
  rat tail, 766
Collagenase, 766
Collodion, 1848
  flexible, 1849
Colloidal oatmeal, 1849

Color
  and achromicity 〈631〉, 243
  instrumental measurement 〈1061〉, 489
Colorimetric solutions (CS), 814
Commentary for USP 31–NF 26, xxxi
Compactin, 766
Completeness of solution 〈641〉, 244
Compound cardamom tincture, 1102
Concentrations, xxi, 13
Congealing temperature 〈651〉, 247
Congo red, 767, 809
  TS, 816
Constitution and Bylaws, xxiv
Containers—glass 〈660〉, 248
Container specifications for capsules and tablets, 831
Containers—performance testing 〈671〉, 255
Containers—plastics 〈661〉, 251
Coomassie
  blue G-250, 767
  brilliant blue R-250, 767
Copovidone, 1114
Copper, 767
  gluconate, 1850
Coriander oil, 1115
Corn
  oil, 1115
  starch, 1240
  high fructose syrup, 1116
  syrup solids, 1117
Corticotropin
  injection, 1850
  for injection, 1851
  injection, repository, 1852
  zinc hydroxide injectable suspension, 1852
Cortisone, 767
  acetate, 1852
  acetate injectable suspension, 1853
  acetate tablets, 1854
Cotton 〈691〉, 259
  absorbent, 767
  purified, 1854
Cottonseed oil, 1118
  hydrogenated, 1119
Council of experts
  (2005–2010), xi
  executive committee (2005–2010), xii
Cr 51
  edetate injection, chromium, 1759
  injection, sodium chromate, 1758
Cranberry liquid preparation, 927

Cream

Alclometasone dipropionate, 1315
Amcinonide, 1376
Amphotericin B, 1415
Anthralin, 1427
Benzocaine, 1501
Betamethasone, 1515
Betamethasone dipropionate, 1520
Betamethasone valerate, 1524
Butoconazole nitrate, vaginal, 1587
Chloramphenicol, 1719
Ciclopirox olamine, 1762
Clindamycin phosphate, vaginal, 1799
Clioquinol, 1802
Clioquinol and hydrocortisone, 1803
Clobetasol propionate, 1805
Clocortolone pivalate, 1808
Clotrimazole, 1826
Clotrimazole and betamethasone dipropionate, 1829
Crotamiton, 1857
Desoximetasone, 1901
Dexamethasone sodium phosphate, 1912

Cream *(continued)*
  Dibucaine, 1938
  Dienestrol, 1950
  Diflorasone diacetate, 1957
  Dioxybenzone and oxybenzone, 1986
  Estradiol, vaginal, 2099
  Estropipate, vaginal, 2112
  Flumethasone pivalate, 2181
  Fluocinolone acetonide, 2185
  Fluocinonide, 2187
  Fluorometholone, 2197
  Fluorouracil, 2199
  Flurandrenolide, 2210
  Gentamicin sulfate, 2264
  Gentian violet, 2270
  Halcinonide, 2316
  Hydrocortisone, 2340
  Hydrocortisone acetate, 2344
  Hydrocortisone butyrate, 2347
  Hydrocortisone valerate, 2351
  Hydroquinone, 2356
  Lidocaine and prilocaine, 2530
  Lindane, 2534
  Mafenide acetate, 2561
  Meclocycline sulfosalicylate, 2598
  Methylprednisolone acetate, 2685
  Miconazole nitrate, 2712
  Mometasone furoate, 2727
  Monobenzone, 2732
  Mupirocin, 2741
  Naftifine hydrochloride, 2749
  Neomycin and polymyxin B sulfates, 2779
  Neomycin and polymyxin B sulfates and gramicidin, 2785
  Neomycin and polymyxin B sulfates, gramicidin, and hydrocortisone acetate, 2786
  Neomycin and polymyxin B sulfates and hydrocortisone acetate, 2787
  Neomycin and polymyxin B sulfates and lidocaine, 2788
  Neomycin and polymyxin B sulfates and pramoxine hydrochloride, 2788
  Neomycin sulfate, 2770
  Neomycin sulfate and dexamethasone sodium phosphate, 2772
  Neomycin sulfate and fluocinolone acetonide, 2773
  Neomycin sulfate and flurandrenolide, 2774
  Neomycin sulfate and hydrocortisone, 2775
  Neomycin sulfate and hydrocortisone acetate, 2776
  Neomycin sulfate and methylprednisolone acetate, 2779
  Neomycin sulfate and triamcinolone acetonide, 2792
  Nystatin, 2840
  Nystatin, neomycin sulfate, gramicidin, and triamcinolone acetonide, 2842
  Nystatin, neomycin sulfate, thiostrepton, and triamcinolone acetonide, 2843
  Nystatin and triamcinolone acetonide, 2844
  Piroxicam, 3015
  Pramoxine hydrochloride, 3052
  Prednicarbate, 3059
  Prednisolone, 3062
  Sulfadiazine, silver, 3292
  Sulfa, vaginal, triple, 3284
  Tetracaine hydrochloride, 3356
  Tolnaftate, 3433
  Tretinoin, 3440
  Triamcinolone acetonide, 3443

Creatinine, 1119
Cresol, 1119
  red, 809
  red-thymol blue TS, 816
  red TS, 816

m-Cresol purple, 767
  TS, 816
Cromolyn sodium, 1855
  inhalation powder, 1856
  inhalation solution, 1856
  nasal solution, 1857
  ophthalmic solution, 1857
Croscarmellose sodium, 1120
Crospovidone, 1121
Crotamiton, 1857
  cream, 1857
Crystallinity ⟨695⟩, 260
Crystallinity determination by solution calorimetry ⟨696⟩, 261
Crystal violet, 809
  TS, 816
Cupric
  acetate, 767
  acetate TS, 816
  acetate TS, stronger, 816
  ammonium sulfate TS, 816
  chloride, 767, 1858
  chloride injection, 1859
  citrate, 767
  citrate TS, 816
  citrate TS, alkaline, 816
  iodide TS, alkaline, 816
  nitrate, 767
  nitrate hydrate, 767
  nitrate, tenth-normal (0.1 N), 822
  oxide, ammoniated, TS, 816
  sulfate, 767, 1859
  sulfate, anhydrous, 767
  sulfate CS, 814
  sulfate injection, 1860
  sulfate test paper, 810
  sulfate TS, 816
  tartrate TS, alkaline, 816
Cupriethylenediamine hydroxide solution, 1.0 M, 767
Cyanoacetic acid, 767
Cyanocobalamin, 1860
  Co 57 capsules, 1834
  Co 57 oral solution, 1835
  Co 58 capsules, 1835
  injection, 1861
Cyanogen bromide, 767
4-Cyanophenol, 767
Cyclam, 767
Cyclandelate, 1861
Cyclizine hydrochloride, 1862
  tablets, 1862
Cyclobenzaprine hydrochloride, 1862
  tablets, 1863
Cyclohexane, 767
Cyclohexanol, 767
(1,2-Cyclohexylenedinitrilo)tetraacetic acid, 767
Cyclohexylmethanol, 767
Cyclomethicone, 1122
Cyclopentolate hydrochloride, 1863
  ophthalmic solution, 1864
Cyclophosphamide, 1864
  for injection, 1865
  tablets, 1865
Cyclopropane, 1866
Cycloserine, 1867
  capsules, 1867
Cyclosporine, 1868
  capsules, 1869
  injection, 1870
  oral solution, 1871
Cyproheptadine hydrochloride, 1871
  oral solution, 1872
  tablets, 1872
Cysteine hydrochloride, 1872
  injection, 1873
L-Cystine, 767

Cytarabine, 1873
  for injection, 1874

D

Dacarbazine, 1875
  for injection, 1875
Dactinomycin, 1876
  for injection, 1877
Danazol, 1877
  capsules, 1878
Dantrolene sodium, 1878
  capsules, 1880
  for injection, 1881
Dapsone, 1882
  tablets, 1882
Daunorubicin hydrochloride, 1883
  for injection, 1884
DEAE-Agarose, 767
Decanol, 767
Decoquinate, 1884
  premix, 1884
Decyl sodium sulfate, 767
Deferoxamine mesylate, 1885
  for injection, 1885
Dehydrated alcohol, 767
Dehydrocholic acid, 1886
  tablets, 1886
Delafield's hematoxylin TS, 816
Deliverable volume ⟨698⟩, 262
Demecarium bromide, 1886
  ophthalmic solution, 1887
Demeclocycline, 1887
  hydrochloride, 1888
  hydrochloride capsules, 1889
  hydrochloride tablets, 1889
  oral suspension, 1888
Denatonium benzoate, 1122
Denigès' reagent, 816
Density of solids ⟨699⟩, 265
Dental paste
  triamcinolone acetonide, 3444
Deoxyadenosine triphosphate, 767
Deoxycytidine triphosphate, 767
Deoxyguanosine triphosphate, 767
Deoxyribonucleic acid polymerase, 767
Deoxythymidine triphosphate, 768
Dermal substitute
  cryopreserved human fibroblast-derived, 1890
Description and relative solubility of USP and NF articles, 840
Desflurane, 1893
Design and analysis of biological assays ⟨111⟩, 108
Desipramine hydrochloride, 1895
  tablets, 1895
Deslanoside, 1896
  injection, 1896
Desmopressin acetate, 1897
  injection, 1899
Desogestrel
  and ethinyl estradiol tablets, 1899
Desoximetasone, 1900
  cream, 1901
  gel, 1901
  ointment, 1902
Desoxycorticosterone
  acetate, 1903
  acetate injection, 1903
  acetate pellets, 1903
  pivalate, 1904
  pivalate injectable suspension, 1904
Determination
  methoxy ⟨431⟩, 153

Determination (continued)
  nitrogen ⟨461⟩, 157
Deuterated water, 768
Deuterium oxide, 768
Deuterochloroform, 768
Devarda's alloy, 768
Dexamethasone, 1904
  acetate, 1909
  acetate injectable suspension, 1909
  and ciprofloxacin otic suspension, 1771
  elixir, 1906
  gel, 1906
  injection, 1906
  and neomycin and polymyxin B sulfates ophthalmic ointment, 2784
  and neomycin and polymyxin B sulfates ophthalmic suspension, 2785
  ophthalmic suspension, 1907
  oral solution, 1907
  penicillin G procaine, dihydrostreptomycin sulfate, and chlorpheniramine maleate injectable suspension, 2939
  sodium phosphate, 1910
  sodium phosphate cream, 1912
  sodium phosphate inhalation aerosol, 1912
  sodium phosphate injection, 1913
  sodium phosphate and neomycin sulfate cream, 2772
  sodium phosphate and neomycin sulfate ophthalmic ointment, 2772
  sodium phosphate and neomycin sulfate ophthalmic solution, 2773
  sodium phosphate ophthalmic ointment, 1913
  sodium phosphate ophthalmic solution, 1914
  tablets, 1908
  and tobramycin ophthalmic ointment, 3422
  and tobramycin ophthalmic suspension, 3422
  topical aerosol, 1905
Dexbrompheniramine maleate, 1914
  and pseudoephedrine sulfate oral solution, 1915
Dexchlorpheniramine maleate, 1915
  oral solution, 1916
  tablets, 1916
Dexpanthenol, 1917
  assay ⟨115⟩, 120
  preparation, 1917
Dextran
  1, 1918
  40, 1919
  40 in dextrose injection, 1921
  40 in sodium chloride injection, 1921
  70, 1922
  70 in dextrose injection, 1923
  70 in sodium chloride injection, 1923
  high molecular weight, 768
Dextrates, 1122
Dextrin, 768, 1123
Dextroamphetamine sulfate, 1923
  capsules, 1924
  tablets, 1925
Dextro calcium pantothenate, 768
Dextromethorphan, 1926
  chlorpheniramine, phenylpropanolamine (salts of) and acetaminophen, capsules containing at least three of the following, 1275
  chlorpheniramine, phenylpropanolamine (salts of), and acetaminophen, oral solution containing at least three of the following, 1277
  chlorpheniramine, phenylpropanolamine (salts of) and acetaminophen, tablets containing at least three of the following, 1278
  chlorpheniramine, pseudoephedrine (salts of), and acetaminophen, capsules containing at least three of the following, 1280
  chlorpheniramine, pseudoephedrine (salts of), and acetaminophen, oral powder containing at least three of the following, 1282
  chlorpheniramine, pseudoephedrine (salts of), and acetaminophen, oral solution containing at least three of the following, 1283
  chlorpheniramine, pseudoephedrine (salts of), and acetaminophen, tablets containing at least three of the following, 1285
  hydrobromide, 1926
  hydrobromide, acetaminophen, doxylamine succinate, and pseudoephedrine hydrochloride oral solution, 1292
  hydrobromide, guiafenesin, and pseudoephedrine hydrochloride capsules, 2308
  hydrobromide oral solution, 1927
  hydrobromide, pseudoephedrine hydrochloride, and carbinoxamine maleate oral solution, 3128
  hydrobromide, acetaminophen, and chlorpheniramine maleate tablets, 1287
Dextrose, 1927
  adenine solution, anticoagulant citrate phosphate, 1431
  anhydrous, 768
  and dopamine hydrochloride injection, 2013
  excipient, 1123
  and half-strength lactated Ringer's injection, 3194
  injection, 1927
  injection, alcohol in, 1319
  injection, bretylium tosylate in, 1556
  injection, bupivacaine hydrochloride in, 1570
  injection, dobutamine in, 2003
  injection, magnesium sulfate in, 2579
  injection, potassium chloride in, 3034
  injection and potassium chloride in lactated Ringer's, 3036
  injection and sodium chloride injection, potassium chloride in, 3035
  injection, tetracaine hydrochloride in, 3358
  injection, theophylline in, 3375
  injection type 1 and multiple electrolytes, 2044
  injection type 2 and multiple electrolytes, 2046
  injection type 3 and multiple electrolytes, 2047
  injection type 4 and multiple electrolytes, 2048
  and lactated Ringer's injection, 3193
  and lidocaine hydrochloride injection, 2529
  and modified lactated Ringer's injection, 3195
  and Ringer's injection, 3191
  and sodium chloride injection, 1928
  and sodium chloride tablets, 3247
  solution, anticoagulant citrate, 1429
  solution, anticoagulant citrate phosphate, 1430
Diacetyl, 768
Diacetylated monoglycerides, 1123
3,3′-Diaminobenzidine hydrochloride, 768
2,3-Diaminonaphthalene, 768
Diatomaceous earth
  flux-calcined, 768
  silanized, 768
Diatomaceous silica
  calcined, 768
Diatrizoate
  meglumine, 1928
  meglumine and diatrizoate sodium injection, 1930
  meglumine and diatrizoate sodium solution, 1931
  meglumine injection, 1929
  sodium, 1931
  sodium and diatrizoate meglumine injection, 1930
  sodium and diatrizoate meglumine solution, 1931
  sodium injection, 1932
  sodium solution, 1932
Diatrizoic acid, 1932
Diaveridine, 773
Diazepam, 1933
  capsules, 1934
  extended-release capsules, 1934
  injection, 1935
  tablets, 1935
Diazobenzenesulfonic acid TS, 816
Diazoxide, 1936
  capsules, 1936
  injection, 1937
  oral suspension, 1937
Dibasic
  ammonium citrate, 768
  ammonium phosphate, 768
  calcium phosphate, anhydrous, 1617
  calcium phosphate dihydrate, 1616
  calcium phosphate tablets, 1618
  potassium phosphate, 768, 3047
  sodium phosphate, 3255
Dibenzyl, 768
2,6-Dibromoquinone-chlorimide, 768
Dibucaine, 1938
  cream, 1938
  hydrochloride, 1939
  hydrochloride injection, 1939
  ointment, 1938
Dibutyl
  phthalate, 768, 1124
  sebacate, 1124
Dibutylamine, 768
Dibutylammonium phosphate, 769
Dichloralphenazone, 1940
  isometheptene mucate and acetaminophen capsules, 2458
Dichloroacetic acid, 769
2,5-Dichloroaniline, 769
2,6-Dichloroaniline, 769
o-Dichlorobenzene, 769
Dichlorodifluoromethane, 1125
1,2-Dichloroethane, 769
Dichlorofluorescein, 769
  TS, 816
Dichlorofluoromethane, 769
2,6-Dichloroindophenol sodium, 769
Dichloromethane, 769
2,4-Dichloro-1-naphthol, 769
2,6-Dichlorophenol-indophenol sodium, 769
Dichlorophenol-indophenol solution, standard, 823
2,6-Dichlorophenylacetic acid, 769
2,6-Dichloroquinone-chlorimide, 769
Dichlorotetrafluoroethane, 1125
Dichlorphenamide, 1940
  tablets, 1941
Diclofenac potassium, 1941
  tablets, 1942
Diclofenac sodium, 1943
  delayed-release tablets, 1944
Dicloxacillin sodium, 1945
  capsules, 1945
  for oral suspension, 1945
Dicyclohexyl, 769
Dicyclohexylamine, 769
  acetate TS, 816
Dicyclohexyl phthalate, 769
Dicyclomine hydrochloride, 1946
  capsules, 1946
  injection, 1947
  oral solution, 1947
  tablets, 1948
Didanosine, 1948
  for oral solution, 1949
Dienestrol, 1950
  cream, 1950

Dietary supplements
Ademetionine disulfate tosylate, 907
Calcium and vitamin D with minerals tablets, 914
Calcium with vitamin D tablets, 913
Chamomile, 916
Chaste tree, 917
Chaste tree, powdered, 919
Chaste tree extract, powdered, 919
Choline bitartrate, 920
Choline chloride, 920
Chondroitin sulfate sodium, 921
Chondroitin sulfate sodium tablets, 923
Chromium picolinate, 923
Chromium picolinate tablets, 924
Clover, red, 924
Clover, powdered red, 925
Clover extract, powdered red, 926
Clover tablets, red, 926
Cod liver oil capsules, 927
Black cohosh, 908
Black cohosh fluidextract, 910
Black cohosh, powdered, 910
Black cohosh powdered extract, 911
Black cohosh tablets, 911
Cranberry liquid preparation, 927
Echinacea angustifolia, 928
Echinacea angustifolia, powdered, 930
Echinacea angustifolia, powdered, extract, 930
Echinacea pallida, 931
Echinacea pallida, powdered, 932
Echinacea pallida, powdered, extract, 932
Echinacea purpurea aerial parts, 933
Echinacea purpurea, powdered, 936
Echinacea purpurea, powdered, extract, 936
Echinacea purpurea root, 934
Eleuthero, 937
Eleuthero, powdered, 938
Eleuthero, powdered, extract, 938
Feverfew, 938
Feverfew, powdered, 939
Garlic, 940
Garlic, powdered, 941
Garlic delayed-release tablets, 943
Garlic extract, powdered, 942
Garlic fluidextract, 942
Ginger, 944
Ginger, powdered, 945
Ginger capsules, 946
Ginger tincture, 946
Ginkgo, 947
Ginkgo extract, powdered, 949
Ginkgo capsules, 950
Ginkgo tablets, 951
Ginseng, American, 952
Ginseng, American, capsules, 953
Ginseng, American, powdered, 952
Ginseng, American, powdered, extract, 953
Ginseng, American, tablets, 954
Ginseng, Asian, 955
Ginseng, Asian, powdered, 956
Ginseng, Asian, powdered, extract, 956
Ginseng, Asian, tablets, 957
Glucosamine and chondroitin sulfate sodium tablets, 957
Glucosamine hydrochloride, 958
Glucosamine tablets, 959
Glucosamine sulfate potassium chloride, 959
Glucosamine sulfate sodium chloride, 960
Glucosamine and methylsulfonylmethane tablets, 960
Glucosamine, chondroitin sulfate sodium, and methylsulfonylmethane tablets, 961
Goldenseal, 962
Goldenseal, powdered, 962
Goldenseal, powdered, extract, 963

Hawthorn leaf with flower, 963
Hawthorn leaf with flower, powdered, 965
Horse chestnut, 965
Horse chestnut, powdered, 966
Horse chestnut, powdered, extract, 966
Licorice, 967
Licorice, powdered, 967
Licorice, powdered, extract, 967
Lipoic acid, alpha, 968
Lipoic acid capsules, alpha, 969
Lipoic acid tablets, alpha, 969
Lutein, 970
Lutein preparation, 971
Lycopene, 972
Lycopene preparation, 972
Lycopene, tomato extract containing, 973
Lysine hydrochloride tablets, 975
Maritime pine, 976
Maritime pine extract, 977
Methylsulfonylmethane, 978
Methylsulfonylmethane tablets, 979
Milk thistle, 979
Milk thistle, powdered, 980
Milk thistle, powdered, extract, 980
Milk thistle capsules, 981
Milk thistle tablets, 982
Minerals capsules, 982
Minerals tablets, 984
Nettle, stinging, 984
Nettle, stinging, powdered, 986
Nettle, stinging, powdered, extract, 986
Pygeum extract, 988
Saw palmetto, 993
Saw palmetto, powdered, 994
Saw palmetto capsules, 996
Saw palmetto extract, 994
Selenomethionine, 997
St. John's wort, 990
St. John's wort, powdered, 991
St. John's wort, powdered, extract, 992
Ubidecarenone, 998
Ubidecarenone capsules, 999
Ubidecarenone tablets, 1000
Valerian, 1000
Valerian, powdered, 1001
Valerian, powdered, extract, 1001
Valerian tablets, 1002
Vitamins tablets, oil-soluble, 1005
Vitamins capsules, oil-soluble, 1003
Vitamins capsules, oil- and water-soluble, 1005
Vitamins capsules, water-soluble, 1041
Vitamins with minerals capsules, oil- and water-soluble, 1011
Vitamins with minerals capsules, water-soluble, 1046
Vitamins with minerals oral solution, water-soluble, 1049
Vitamins with minerals tablets, oil- and water-soluble, 1022
Vitamins with minerals tablets, water-soluble, 1050
Vitamins tablets, oil- and water-soluble, 1010
Vitamins tablets, water-soluble, 1044
Vitamins with minerals oral solution, oil- and water-soluble, 1016
Vitamins oral solution, oil- and water-soluble, 1009

Diethanolamine, 1126
Diethylamine, 769
N,N-Diethylaniline, 769
Diethylcarbamazine citrate, 1951
 tablets, 1951
Diethylene glycol, 769
 monoethyl ether, 1126
 stearates, 1128
 succinate polyester, 769

Diethylenetriamine, 770
Di(2-ethylhexyl)phthalate, 770
Diethyl phthalate, 1126
Diethylpropion hydrochloride, 1952
 tablets, 1953
Diethylpyrocarbonate, 770
Diethylstilbestrol, 1953
 diphosphate, 1955
 diphosphate injection, 1956
 injection, 1954
 tablets, 1954
Diethyltoluamide, 1956
 topical solution, 1956
Diflorasone diacetate, 1957
 cream, 1957
 ointment, 1957
Diflunisal, 1958
 tablets, 1958
Digitalis, 1959
 capsules, 1961
 powdered, 1960
 tablets, 1961
Digitonin, 770
Digitoxin, 1961
 injection, 1962
 tablets, 1962
Digoxigenin, 770
 bisdigitoxoside, 770
Digoxin, 1963
 injection, 1964
 oral solution, 1964
 tablets, 1965
Dihydrocodeine bitartrate, 1966
 aspirin and caffeine capsules, 1456
Dihydroergotamine mesylate, 1966
 injection, 1967
Dihydroquinidine hydrochloride, 770
Dihydroquinine, 770
Dihydrostreptomycin
 injection, 1968
 sulfate, 1968
 sulfate boluses, 1968
 sulfate, penicillin G procaine, chlorpheniramine maleate, and dexamethasone injectable suspension, 2939
 sulfate and penicillin G procaine injectable suspension, 2939
 sulfate and penicillin G procaine intramammary infusion, 2938
 sulfate, penicillin G procaine, and prednisolone injectable suspension, 2941
Dihydrotachysterol, 1969
 capsules, 1969
 oral solution, 1970
 tablets, 1970
Dihydroxyacetone, 1970
Dihydroxyaluminum
 aminoacetate, 1971
 aminoacetate magma, 1971
 sodium carbonate, 1972
 sodium carbonate chewable tablets, 1973
 sodium carbonate tablets, 1973
2,5-Dihydroxybenzoic acid, 770
2,7-Dihydroxynaphthalene TS, 816
4,5-Dihydroxy-3-*p*-sulfophenylazo)-2,7-napthalenedisulfonic acid, trisodium salt, 809
Diiodofluorescein, 770
 TS, 816
Diisodecyl phthalate, 770
Diisopropanolamine, 1128
Diisopropyl ether, 770
Diisopropylamine, 770
Diisopropylethylamine, 770
1,2-Dilinoleoyl-3-oleoyl-rac-glycerol, 770
1,2-Dilinoleoyl-3-palmitoyl-rac-glycerol, 770
Diloxanide furoate, 1973
Diltiazem hydrochloride, 1974
 extended-release capsules, 1976

Diltiazem hydrochloride *(continued)*
  oral solution, 1974
  oral suspension, 1975
  tablets, 1978
Diluted
  acetic acid, 771, 1064
  alcohol, 771
  hydrochloric acid, 771
  lead subacetate TS, 816
  nitric acid, 771
  sulfuric acid, 771
Dimenhydrinate, 1979
  injection, 1979
  oral solution, 1980
  tablets, 1981
Dimercaprol, 1981
  injection, 1982
Dimethicone, 1129
  viscosity 500 centistokes, 771
2,5-Dimethoxybenzaldehyde, 771
1,2-Dimethoxyethane, 771
Dimethoxymethane, 771
(3,4-Dimethoxyphenyl)-acetonitrile, 771
Dimethyl
  phthalate, 771
  sulfone, 771
  sulfoxide, 771, 1982
  sulfoxide gel, 1983
  sulfoxide irrigation, 1983
  sulfoxide spectrophotometric grade, 771
  sulfoxide topical solution, 1984
N,N-Dimethylacetamide, 771
p-Dimethylaminoazobenzene, 771
p-Dimethylaminobenzaldehyde, 771
  TS, 816
p-Dimethylaminocinnamaldehyde, 771
2-Dimethylaminoethyl methacrylate, 771
Dimethylaminophenol, 771
Dimethylaniline ⟨223⟩, 132
2,6-Dimethylaniline, 771
N,N-Dimethylaniline, 771
3,4-Dimethylbenzophenone, 771
5,5-Dimethyl-1,3-cyclohexanedione, 771
1,5-Dimethyl-1,5-diazaundecamethylene polymethobromide, 771
N,N-Dimethyldodecylamine-N-oxide, 771
Dimethylethyl(3-hydroxyphenyl)ammonium chloride, 771
Dimethylformamide, 772
N,N-Dimethylformamide diethyl acetal, 772
1,3-Dimethyl-2-imidazolidinone, 772
1,9-Dimethyl-methylene blue, 772
N,N-Dimethyl-1-naphthylamine, 772
N,N-Dimethyloctylamine, 772
2,5-Dimethylphenol, 772
2,6-Dimethylphenol, 772
3,5-Dimethylphenol, 772
3-(4,5-Dimethylthiazol-2-yl)-2,5-diphenyl tetrazolium bromide, 772
N,N-Dimethyl-p-phenylenediamine dihydrochloride, 772
m-Dinitrobenzene, 772
3,5-Dinitrobenzoyl chloride, 772
2,4-Dinitrochlorobenzene, 772
2,4-Dinitrofluorobenzene, 772
2,4-Dinitrophenylhydrazine, 772
Dinitrophenylhydrazine TS, 817
Dinoprost tromethamine, 1984
Dinoprostone, 1985
Dioctyl sodium sulfosuccinate, 772
Dioxane, 772
Dioxybenzone, 1986
  and oxybenzone cream, 1986
Diphenhydramine
  citrate, 1987
  citrate and acetaminophen tablets, 1293
  hydrochloride, 1987

hydrochloride, acetaminophen, and pseudoephedrine hydrochloride tablets, 1294
hydrochloride capsules, 1988
hydrochloride injection, 1988
hydrochloride oral solution, 1989
and pseudoephedrine capsules, 1989
Diphenoxylate hydrochloride, 1990
  and atropine sulfate oral solution, 1990
  and atropine sulfate tablets, 1991
Diphenyl ether, 772
Diphenylamine, 772
  TS, 817
Diphenylborinic acid, ethanolamine ester, 772
Diphenylcarbazide, 772
Diphenylcarbazone, 772
  TS, 817
2,2-Diphenylglycine, 772
Diphtheria
  and tetanus toxoids adsorbed, 1992
  and tetanus toxoids adsorbed for adult use, 3354
Dipicrylamine, 772
Dipivefrin hydrochloride, 1992
  ophthalmic solution, 1993
Dipropyl phthalate, 772
Dipyridamole, 1993
  injection, 1994
  oral suspension, 1994
  tablets, 1995
α,α'-Dipyridyl, 772
4,4'-Dipyridyl dihydrochloride, 772
Direct red 80, 793
Dirithromycin, 1995
  delayed-release tablets, 1996
Disinfectants and Antiseptics ⟨1072⟩, 493
Disintegration
  ⟨701⟩, 266
  and dissolution of dietary supplements ⟨2040⟩, 732
Disodium
  chromotropate, 773
  ethylenediaminetetraacetate, 773
  phosphate, 773
Disopyramide phosphate, 1997
  capsules, 1998
  extended-release capsules, 1998
Dissolution ⟨711⟩, 267
The Dissolution procedure: development and validation ⟨1092⟩, 573
Distilling range ⟨721⟩, 274
Disulfiram, 1999
  tablets, 2000
5,5'-Dithiobis (2-nitrobenzoic acid), 773
Dithiothreitol, 773
Dithizone, 773
  TS, 817
Divalproex sodium, 2000
  delayed-release tablets, 2000
Dobutamine
  in dextrose injection, 2003
  hydrochloride, 2001
  injection, 2002
  for injection, 2003
Docusate
  calcium, 2004
  calcium capsules, 2005
  potassium, 2005
  potassium capsules, 2006
  sodium, 773, 2006
  sodium capsules, 2007
  sodium and ferrous fumarate extended-release tablets, 2154
  sodium solution, 2008
  sodium syrup, 2008
  sodium tablets, 2008
1-Dodecanol, 773
Dodecyl
  alcohol, 773
  lithium sulfate, 773

sodium sulfonate, 773
3-(Dodecyldimethylammonio)propanesulfonate, 773
Dodecyltriethylammonium phosphate, 0.5 M, 773
Dodecyltrimethylammonium bromide, 773
Dolasetron mesylate, 2009
  injection, 2010
  oral solution, 2010
  oral suspension, 2011
  tablets, 2012
Dopamine hydrochloride, 2012
  and dextrose injection, 2013
  injection, 2013
Dorzolamide hydrochloride, 2014
Doxapram hydrochloride, 2015
  injection, 2015
Doxazosin mesylate, 2016
  tablets, 2017
Doxepin hydrochloride, 2018
  capsules, 2019
  oral solution, 2019
Doxorubicin hydrochloride, 2020
  injection, 2021
  for injection, 2021
Doxycycline, 2022
  calcium oral suspension, 2023
  capsules, 2022
  hyclate, 2023
  hyclate capsules, 2024
  hyclate delayed-release capsules, 2025
  hyclate tablets, 2026
  for injection, 2025
  for oral suspension, 2023
Doxylamine succinate, 2026
  acetaminophen, dextromethorphan hydrobromide, and pseudoephedrine hydrochloride oral solution, 1292
  oral solution, 2027
  tablets, 2027
Drabkin's reagent, 773
Dragendorff's TS, 817
Dried peptone, 773
Dronabinol, 2028
  capsules, 2028
Droperidol, 2029
  injection, 2029
Drospirenone, 2030
Drug release ⟨724⟩, 275
Dulcitol, 773
Dusting powder, absorbable, 2031
Dyclonine hydrochloride, 2031
  gel, 2032
  topical solution, 2032
Dydrogesterone, 2032
  tablets, 2033
Dyphylline, 2033
  and guaifenesin oral solution, 2035
  and guaifenesin tablets, 2036
  injection, 2034
  oral solution, 2034
  tablets, 2035

E

Earth, chromatographic, silanized, acid-base washed, 773
Echinacea
  angustifolia, 928
  angustifolia extract, powdered, 930
  angustifolia, powdered, 930
  pallida, 931
  pallida extract, powdered, 932
  pallida, powdered, 932

Echinacea (continued)
  purpurea aerial parts, 933
  purpurea extract, powdered, 936
  purpurea, powdered, 936
  purpurea root, 934
Echothiophate
  iodide, 2036
  iodide for ophthalmic solution, 2037
Econazole nitrate, 2037
Edetate
  calcium disodium, 2038
  calcium disodium injection, 2039
  disodium, 773, 2039
  disodium injection, 2040
  disodium TS, 817
  disodium, twentieth-molar (0.05 M), 823
Edetic acid, 1130
Edrophonium
  chloride, 2040
  chloride injection, 2040
n-Eicosane, 773
Eicosanol, 773
Elastomeric closures for injections ⟨381⟩, 144
Electrolytes
  and dextrose injection type 1, multiple, 2044
  and dextrose injection type 2, multiple, 2046
  and dextrose injection type 3, multiple, 2047
  and dextrose injection type 4, multiple, 2048
  injection type 1, multiple, 2041
  injection type 2, multiple, 2042
  and invert sugar injection type 1, multiple, 2049
  and invert sugar injection type 2, multiple, 2050
  and invert sugar injection type 3, multiple, 2051
  and polyethylene glycol 3350 for oral solution, 3021
Electrophoresis ⟨726⟩, 278
Elements
  injection, trace, 2052
Eleuthero, 937
  extract, powdered, 938
  powdered, 938

Elixir
Aromatic, 1076
Benzaldehyde, compound, 1081
Dexamethasone, 1906
Fluphenazine hydrochloride, 2208
Hyoscyamine sulfate, 2368

Elm, 2053
Emedastine
  difumarate, 2054
  ophthalmic solution, 2054
Emergency medical services vehicles and ambulances—storage of preparations ⟨1070⟩, 493
Emetine hydrochloride, 2055
  injection, 2055
Enalapril maleate, 2056
  and hydrochlorothiazide tablets, 2058
  tablets, 2056
Enalaprilat, 2060
Enflurane, 2060
Ensulizole, 2061
Enzacamene, 2061
Eosin Y, 773, 809
  TS, 817
Ephedrine, 2062
  hydrochloride, 2062
  hydrochloride, theophylline, and phenobarbital tablets, 3375
  sulfate, 2063
  sulfate capsules, 2063
  sulfate injection, 2063
  sulfate nasal solution, 2064
  sulfate oral solution, 2064

Epiandrosterone, 773
4-Epianhydrotetracycline ⟨226⟩, 133
Epinephrine, 2064
  assay ⟨391⟩, 145
  bitartrate, 2067
  bitartrate inhalation aerosol, 2068
  bitartrate ophthalmic solution, 2069
  bitartrate for ophthalmic solution, 2069
  and bupivacaine hydrochloride injection, 1570
  and cocaine and tetracaine hydrochlorides topical solution, 1838
  inhalation aerosol, 2065
  inhalation solution, 2066
  injection, 2065
  and lidocaine hydrochloride injection, 2529
  nasal solution, 2066
  ophthalmic solution, 2067
  and prilocaine injection, 3072
  and procaine hydrochloride injection, 3083
Epinephryl borate ophthalmic solution, 2069
Epitetracycline hydrochloride, 2070
Equilenin, 773
Equilin, 2070
Ergocalciferol, 2071
  capsules, 2071
  oral solution, 2072
  tablets, 2073
α-Ergocryptine, 773
Ergoloid mesylates, 2073
  capsules, 2074
  oral solution, 2075
  sublingual tablets, 2076
  tablets, 2075
Ergonovine maleate, 2077
  injection, 2077
  tablets, 2078
Ergotamine tartrate, 2079
  and caffeine suppositories, 2082
  and caffeine tablets, 2083
  inhalation aerosol, 2079
  injection, 2080
  sublingual tablets, 2082
  tablets, 2081
Eriochrome
  black T, 809
  black TS, 817
  black T–sodium chloride indicator, 773
  black T trituration, 809
  cyanine R, 773
  cyanine TS, 817
Erythritol, 1130
Erythromycin, 2084
  and benzoyl peroxide topical gel, 2089
  delayed-release capsules, 2085
  delayed-release tablets, 2088
  estolate, 2089
  estolate capsules, 2090
  estolate oral suspension, 2090
  estolate for oral suspension, 2090
  estolate and sulfisoxazole acetyl oral suspension, 2091
  estolate tablets, 2091
  ethylsuccinate, 2092
  ethylsuccinate injection, 2093
  ethylsuccinate oral suspension, 2093
  ethylsuccinate for oral suspension, 2094
  ethylsuccinate, sterile, 2093
  ethylsuccinate and sulfisoxazole acetyl for oral suspension, 2095
  ethylsuccinate tablets, 2094
  gluceptate, sterile, 2096
  injection, 2086
  intramammary infusion, 2086
  lactobionate for injection, 2096
  lactobionate, sterile, 2096
  ointment, 2086
  ophthalmic ointment, 2087
  pledgets, 2087

  stearate, 2097
  stearate tablets, 2098
  tablets, 2088
  topical gel, 2085
  topical solution, 2088
Escin, 773
Estradiol, 2098
  vaginal cream, 2099
  pellets, 2100
  injectable suspension, 2100
  transdermal system, 2100
  tablets, 2101
  cypionate, 2102
  cypionate injection, 2102
  and norethindrone acetate tablets, 2102
  valerate, 2104
  valerate injection, 2105
Estriol, 2105
Estrogens
  conjugated, 2106
  esterified, 2109
  tablets, conjugated, 2107
  tablets, esterified, 2109
Estrone, 2110
  injectable suspension, 2111
  injection, 2110
Estropipate, 2111
  tablets, 2113
  vaginal cream, 2112
Ethacrynate sodium for injection, 2113
Ethacrynic acid, 2114
  tablets, 2114
Ethambutol hydrochloride, 2115
  rifampin, isoniazid, and pyrazinamide tablets, 3187
  tablets, 2116
Ethanesulfonic acid, 773
Ethchlorvynol, 2116
  capsules, 2117
Ether, 773, 2118
  absolute, 751, 773
  diphenyl, 773
  isopropyl, 773
  nonyl phenyl polyethylene glycol, 773
  peroxide-free, 773
Ethidium bromide, 774
Ethinyl estradiol, 2118
  and desogestrel tablets, 1899
  and ethynodiol diacetate tablets, 2127
  and levonorgestrel tablets, 2521
  and norethindrone acetate tablets, 2829
  and norethindrone tablets, 2826
  and norgestimate tablets, 2834
  and norgestrel tablets, 2836
  tablets, 2119
Ethiodized oil injection, 2120
Ethionamide, 2120
  tablets, 2120
Ethopabate, 2121
Ethosuximide, 2122
  capsules, 2122
  oral solution, 2123
Ethotoin, 2124
  tablets, 2125
4'-Ethoxyacetophenone, 774
2-Ethoxyethanol, 774
Ethyl
  acetate, 774, 1131
  acrylate, 774
  acrylate and methyl methacrylate copolymer dispersion, 1132
  alcohol, 774
  arachidate, 774
  benzoate, 774
  chloride, 2125
  cyanoacetate, 774
  ether, 774
  ether, anhydrous, 774

Ethyl *(continued)*
 oleate, 1132
 salicylate, 774
 vanillin, 1133
2-Ethylaminopropiophenone hydrochloride, 774
4-Ethylbenzaldehyde, 774
Ethylbenzene, 774
Ethylcellulose, 1133
 aqueous dispersion, 1134
Ethylene
 dichloride, 774
 glycol, 774
 glycol monoethyl ether, 774
 glycol stearates, 1134
Ethylenediamine, 2126
N-Ethylmaleimide, 774
2-Ethyl-2-methylsuccinic acid, 774
Ethylparaben, 1135
1-Ethylquinaldinium iodide, 774
Ethynodiol diacetate, 2126
 and ethinyl estradiol tablets, 2127
 and mestranol tablets, 2127
Etidronate disodium, 2128
 tablets, 2129
Etodolac, 2129
 capsules, 2130
 tablets, 2131
 extended-release tablets, 2131
Etoposide, 2132
 capsules, 2133
 injection, 2134
Eucalyptol, 2135
Eucatropine hydrochloride, 2135
 ophthalmic solution, 2136
Eugenol, 2136
Excipient biological safety evaluation guidelines ⟨1074⟩, 497
Excipients
 USP and NF, listed by category, 1057
Expert Committees (2005–2010), xii

Extract

Beef, 757
Belladonna, 1493
Belladonna tablets, 1494
Cascara fluidextract, aromatic, 1658
Cascara sagrada, 1657
Cascara sagrada fluidextract, 1658
Chaste tree, powdered, 919
Clover, red, powdered, 926
Echinacea angustifolia, powdered, 930
Echinacea pallida, powdered, 932
Echinacea purpurea, powdered, 936
Eleuthero, powdered, 938
Garlic, powdered, 942
Garlic fluidextract, 942
Ginkgo, powdered, 949
Ginseng, American, powdered, 953
Ginseng, Asian, powdered, 956
Goldenseal, powdered, 963
Horse chestnut, powdered, 966
Licorice, powdered, 967
Licorice fluidextract, 1162
Maritime pine, 977
Milk thistle, powdered, 980
Nettle, stinging, powdered, 986
Pygeum, 988
Pyrethrum, 3135
Saw palmetto, 994
Senna fluidextract, 3229
St. John's wort, powdered, 992
Tomato, containing lycopene, 973

Valerian, powdered, 1001
Yeast, 808

F

F 18
 injection, fludeoxyglucose, 2192
 injection, fluorodopa, 2193
 injection, sodium fluoride, 2195
Factor IX complex, 2136
Factor X$_a$ (Activated Factor X) for Anti-Factor X$_a$ Test, 774
Famotidine, 2137
 injection, 2137
 for oral suspension, 2138
 tablets, 2139
Fast
 blue BB salt, 775
 blue B salt, 775
 green FCF, 775
Fat, hard, 1136
Fats and fixed oils ⟨401⟩, 145
FD&C blue no. 1, 775
Fehling's solution, 817
Felodipine, 2141
 extended-release tablets, 2141
Fenbendazole, 2144
Fennel oil, 1136
Fenofibrate, 2145
Fenoldopam mesylate, 2146
 injection, 2148
Fenoprofen calcium, 2148
 capsules, 2149
 tablets, 2150
Fentanyl citrate, 2151
 injection, 2151
Ferric
 ammonium citrate, 775, 1402
 ammonium citrate for oral solution, 1403
 ammonium sulfate, 775
 ammonium sulfate, tenth-normal (0.1 N), 823
 ammonium sulfate TS, 817
 chloride, 775
 chloride CS, 814
 chloride TS, 817
 nitrate, 775
 oxide, 1136
 subsulfate solution, 2151
 sulfate, 775, 2152
Ferrocyphen, 775
Ferroin TS, 817
Ferrous
 ammonium sulfate, 775
 ammonium sulfate, tenth-normal (0.1 N), 823
 fumarate, 2152
 fumarate and docusate sodium extended-release tablets, 2154
 fumarate tablets, 2154
 gluconate, 2155
 gluconate capsules, 2156
 gluconate oral solution, 2156
 gluconate tablets, 2157
 sulfate, 775, 2157
 sulfate, dried, 2158
 sulfate oral solution, 2157
 sulfate syrup, 2157
 sulfate tablets, 2158
 sulfate, acid, TS, 817
 sulfate TS, 817
Ferulic acid, 775
Ferumoxides injection, 2158
Ferumoxsil oral suspension, 2160
Feverfew, 938
 powdered, 939

Fexofenadine hydrochloride, 2161
 capsules, 2162
 and pseudoephedrine hydrochloride extended-release tablets, 2164
 tablets, 2163
Fibroblast-derived
 dermal substitute, cryopreserved human, 1890
 temporary skin substitute, human, 3237
Fibroblast growth factor-2, 775
Filter paper, quantitative, 775
Finasteride, 2167
 tablets, 2167
Flame photometry for reagents, 749
Flecainide acetate, 2168
 tablets, 2169
Floxuridine, 2170
 for injection, 2170
Fluconazole, 2171
Flucytosine, 2172
 capsules, 2173
 oral suspension, 2173
Fludarabine phosphate, 2174
 for injection, 2176
Fludeoxyglucose F18 injection, 2192
Fludrocortisone acetate, 2177
 tablets, 2177
Flumazenil, 2178
 injection, 2179
Flumazenil C 11
 injection, 1639
Flumethasone pivalate, 2180
 cream, 2181
Flunisolide, 2181
 nasal solution, 2182
Flunixin meglumine, 2183
 granules, 2183
 injection, 2184
 paste, 2184
Fluocinolone acetonide, 2185
 cream, 2185
 and neomycin sulfate cream, 2773
 ointment, 2186
 topical solution, 2186
Fluocinonide, 2187
 cream, 2187
 gel, 2188
 ointment, 2188
 topical solution, 2188
Fluorene, 775
9-Fluorenylmethyl chloroformate, 775
Fluorescamine, 775
Fluorescein, 2189
 sodium, 2190
 injection, 2190
 sodium and benoxinate hydrochloride ophthalmic solution, 2191
 sodium ophthalmic strips, 2190
 sodium and proparacaine hydrochloride ophthalmic solution, 2191
Fluorine
 F 18 injection, fludeoxyglucose, 2192
 F 18 injection, fluorodopa, 2193
 F 18 injection, sodium fluoride, 2195
4'-Fluoroacetophenone, 776
Fluorodopa F18 injection, 2193
Fluorometholone, 2195
 acetate, 2196
 acetate and tobramycin ophthalmic suspension, 3423
 cream, 2197
 and neomycin sulfate ointment, 2774
 ophthalmic suspension, 2197
Fluorouracil, 2198
 cream, 2199
 injection, 2199
 topical solution, 2199
Fluoxetine
 capsules, 2201

Fluoxetine *(continued)*
  delayed-release capsules, 2201
  hydrochloride, 2200
  oral solution, 2202
  tablets, 2203
Fluoxymesterone, 2204
  tablets, 2205
Fluphenazine
  decanoate, 2206
  decanoate injection, 2206
  enanthate, 2207
  enanthate injection, 2208
  hydrochloride, 2208
  hydrochloride elixir, 2208
  hydrochloride injection, 2209
  hydrochloride oral solution, 2209
  hydrochloride tablets, 2209
Flurandrenolide, 2210
  cream, 2210
  lotion, 2211
  and neomycin sulfate cream, 2774
  and neomycin sulfate lotion, 2774
  and neomycin sulfate ointment, 2775
  ointment, 2211
  tape, 2212
Flurazepam hydrochloride, 2212
  capsules, 2213
Flurbiprofen, 2214
  sodium, 2215
  sodium ophthalmic solution, 2216
  tablets, 2214
Flutamide, 2216
  capsules, 2217
Fluticasone propionate, 2218
  nasal spray, 2219
Fluvastatin
  capsules, 2223
  sodium, 2222
Fluvoxamine maleate, 2225
  tablets, 2226
Folic acid, 2228
  assay ⟨411⟩, 149
  injection, 2228
  tablets, 2229
Folin-ciocalteu phenol TS, 817
Formaldehyde
  solution, 776, 2229
  TS, 817
Formamide, 776
  anhydrous, 776
Formic acid, 776
  96 percent, 776
  anhydrous, 776
Fosinopril sodium, 2230
  and hydrochlorothiazide tablets, 2232
  tablets, 2231
Fosphenytoin sodium, 2234
  injection, 2235
Fructose, 2236
  injection, 2236
  and sodium chloride injection, 2237
Fuchsin
  basic, 776, 2237
  pyrogallol TS, 817
  sulfurous acid TS, 817
Fuller's earth, chromatographic, 776
Fumaric acid, 1137
Fuming
  nitric acid, 776
  sulfuric acid, 776
Furazolidone, 2238
  oral suspension, 2238
  tablets, 2238
Furfural, 776
Furosemide, 2239
  injection, 2239
  oral solution, 2240
  tablets, 2241

G

G designations, 776
Ga 67 injection, gallium citrate, 2255
Gabapentin, 2241
  capsules, 2243
  tablets, 2244
Gadodiamide, 2245
  injection, 2247
Gadolinium (Gd III) acetate hydrate, 776
Gadopentetate dimeglumine injection, 2248
Gadoteridol, 2249
  injection, 2251
Gadoversetamide, 2252
  injection, 2254
Galactose, 1137
Galageenan, 1138
Gallamine triethiodide, 2255
  injection, 2255
Gallium citrate Ga 67 injection, 2255
Ganciclovir, 2256
  for injection, 2257
  oral suspension, 2257
Garlic, 940
  delayed-release tablets, 943
  extract, powdered, 942
  fluidextract, 942
  powdered, 941
Gastric fluid, simulated, TS, 817
Gauze
  absorbent, 2258
  petrolatum, 2259

Gel

Aluminum hydroxide, 1354
Aluminum hydroxide capsules, dried, 1355
Aluminum hydroxide, dried, 1355
Aluminum hydroxide tablets, dried, 1356
Aluminum phosphate, 1356
Aminobenzoic acid, 1385
Benzocaine, 1501
Benzocaine, butamben, and tetracaine hydrochloride, 1503
Benzoyl peroxide, 1509
Betamethasone benzoate, 1518
Chromatographic silica, 766
Chromatographic silica mixture, 766
Clindamycin phosphate, 1799
Desoximetasone, 1901
Dexamethasone, 1906
Dimethyl sulfoxide, 1983
Dyclonine hydrochloride, 2032
Erythromycin and benzoyl peroxide, topical, 2089
Erythromycin, topical, 2085
Fluocinonide, 2188
Gelatin, 1139
Gelatin film, absorbable, 2259
Gelatin sponge, absorbable, 2260
Gelatin TS, 817
Hydrocortisone, 2340
Indomethacin, topical, 2399
Metronidazole, 2703
Naftifine hydrochloride, 2750
Phenol topical, camphorated, 2976
Salicylic acid, 3212
Silica, 795
Silica, chromatographic, 795
Silica, impregnated glass microfiber sheet, 795
Silica, octadecylsilanized chromatographic, 795
Silica, porous, 795
Silica, binder-free, 795
Silica mixture, chromatographic, 795
Silica mixture, chromatographic, with chemically bound amino groups, 795
Silica mixture, dimethylsilanized, chromatographic, 795
Silica mixture, octadecylsilanized chromatographic, 795
Silica mixture, octylsilanized, chromatographic, 795
Sodium fluoride and phosphoric acid, 3250
Sodium sulfide topical, 3260
Stannous fluoride, 3269
Tolnaftate, 3433
Tretinoin, 3440

Gel strength of gelatin ⟨1081⟩, 523
Gelatin, 1139
  film, absorbable, 2259
  sponge, absorbable, 2260
  TS, 817
Gellan gum, 1140
Gemcitabine
  for injection, 2261
  hydrochloride, 2260
Gemfibrozil, 2262
  capsules, 2262
  tablets, 2263

General chapters, 29

⟨1⟩ Injections, 33
⟨11⟩ USP reference standards, 37
⟨16⟩ Automated methods of analysis, 59
⟨21⟩ Thermometers, 66
⟨31⟩ Volumetric apparatus, 66
⟨41⟩ Weights and balances, 67
⟨51⟩ Antimicrobial effectiveness testing, 67
⟨55⟩ Biological indicators—resistance performance tests, 69
⟨61⟩ Microbial limit tests, 71
⟨61⟩ Microbiological examination of nonsterile products: microbial enumeration tests, 76
⟨62⟩ Microbiological examination of nonsterile products: tests for specified organisms, 81
⟨71⟩ Sterility tests, 85
⟨81⟩ Antibiotics—microbial assays, 91
⟨85⟩ Bacterial endotoxins test, 98
⟨87⟩ Biological reactivity tests, in vitro, 102
⟨88⟩ Biological reactivity tests, in vivo, 104
⟨91⟩ Calcium pantothenate assay, 107
⟨111⟩ Design and analysis of biological assays, 108
⟨115⟩ Dexpanthenol assay, 120
⟨121⟩ Insulin assays, 121
⟨141⟩ Protein—biological adequacy test, 122
⟨151⟩ Pyrogen test, 123
⟨161⟩ Transfusion and infusion assemblies and similar medical devices, 124
⟨171⟩ Vitamin B_{12} activity assay, 125
⟨181⟩ Identification—organic nitrogenous bases, 126
⟨191⟩ Identification tests—general, 127
⟨193⟩ Identification—tetracyclines, 129
⟨197⟩ Spectrophotometric identification tests, 129
⟨201⟩ Thin-layer chromatographic identification test, 130
⟨206⟩ Aluminum, 131
⟨211⟩ Arsenic, 131
⟨221⟩ Chloride and sulfate, 132
⟨223⟩ Dimethylaniline, 132
⟨226⟩ 4-Epianhydrotetracycline, 133
⟨231⟩ Heavy metals, 133
⟨241⟩ Iron, 135
⟨251⟩ Lead, 135
⟨261⟩ Mercury, 136
⟨271⟩ Readily carbonizable substances test, 137
⟨281⟩ Residue on ignition, 137

General chapters (continued)
- ⟨291⟩ Selenium, 138
- ⟨301⟩ Acid-neutralizing capacity, 138
- ⟨311⟩ Alginates assay, 139
- ⟨331⟩ Amphetamine assay, 140
- ⟨341⟩ Antimicrobial agents—content, 140
- ⟨345⟩ Assay for citric acid/citrate and phosphate, 142
- ⟨351⟩ Assay for steroids, 143
- ⟨361⟩ Barbiturate assay, 143
- ⟨371⟩ Cobalamin radiotracer assay, 143
- ⟨381⟩ Elastomeric closures for injections, 144
- ⟨391⟩ Epinephrine assay, 145
- ⟨401⟩ Fats and fixed oils, 145
- ⟨411⟩ Folic acid assay, 149
- ⟨425⟩ Iodometric assay—antibiotics, 150
- ⟨429⟩ Light diffraction measurement of particle size, 150
- ⟨431⟩ Methoxy determination, 153
- ⟨441⟩ Niacin or niacinamide assay, 154
- ⟨451⟩ Nitrite titration, 156
- ⟨461⟩ Nitrogen determination, 157
- ⟨466⟩ Ordinary impurities, 157
- ⟨467⟩ Organic volatile impurities, 158
- ⟨467⟩ Residual solvents, 170
- ⟨471⟩ Oxygen flask combustion, 181
- ⟨481⟩ Riboflavin assay, 182
- ⟨501⟩ Salts of organic nitrogenous bases, 182
- ⟨511⟩ Single-steroid assay, 183
- ⟨521⟩ Sulfonamides, 183
- ⟨531⟩ Thiamine assay, 184
- ⟨541⟩ Titrimetry, 185
- ⟨551⟩ Alpha tocopherol assay, 187
- ⟨561⟩ Articles of botanical origin, 188
- ⟨563⟩ Identification of articles of botanical origin, 195
- ⟨565⟩ Botanical extracts, 201
- ⟨571⟩ Vitamin A assay, 203
- ⟨581⟩ Vitamin D assay, 204
- ⟨591⟩ Zinc determination, 208
- ⟨601⟩ Aerosols, nasal sprays, metered-dose inhalers, and dry powder inhalers, 209
- ⟨611⟩ Alcohol determination, 230
- ⟨616⟩ Bulk density and tapped density, 231
- ⟨621⟩ Chromatography, 232
- ⟨631⟩ Color and achromicity, 243
- ⟨641⟩ Completeness of solution, 244
- ⟨643⟩ Total organic carbon, 244
- ⟨645⟩ Water conductivity, 245
- ⟨651⟩ Congealing temperature, 247
- ⟨660⟩ Containers—glass, 248
- ⟨661⟩ Containers—plastics, 251
- ⟨671⟩ Containers—performance testing, 255
- ⟨681⟩ Repackaging into single-unit containers and unit-dose containers for nonsterile solid and liquid dosage forms, 258
- ⟨691⟩ Cotton, 259
- ⟨695⟩ Crystallinity, 260
- ⟨696⟩ Crystallinity determination by solution calorimetry, 261
- ⟨698⟩ Deliverable volume, 262
- ⟨699⟩ Density of solids, 265
- ⟨701⟩ Disintegration, 266
- ⟨711⟩ Dissolution, 267
- ⟨721⟩ Distilling range, 274
- ⟨724⟩ Drug release, 275
- ⟨726⟩ Electrophoresis, 278
- ⟨727⟩ Capillary electrophoresis, 281
- ⟨729⟩ Globule size distribution in lipid injectable emulsions, 285
- ⟨730⟩ Plasma spectrochemistry, 287
- ⟨731⟩ Loss on drying, 292
- ⟨733⟩ Loss on ignition, 293
- ⟨736⟩ Mass spectrometry, 293
- ⟨741⟩ Melting range or temperature, 297
- ⟨751⟩ Metal particles in ophthalmic ointments, 298
- ⟨755⟩ Minimum fill, 298
- ⟨761⟩ Nuclear magnetic resonance, 298
- ⟨771⟩ Ophthalmic ointments, 304
- ⟨776⟩ Optical microscopy, 304
- ⟨781⟩ Optical rotation, 306
- ⟨785⟩ Osmolality and osmolarity, 307
- ⟨786⟩ Particle size distribution estimation by analytical sieving, 308
- ⟨788⟩ Particulate matter in injections, 311
- ⟨789⟩ Particulate matter in ophthalmic solutions, 313
- ⟨791⟩ pH, 314
- ⟨795⟩ Pharmaceutical compounding—nonsterile preparations, 315
- ⟨797⟩ Pharmaceutical compounding—sterile preparations, 319
- ⟨801⟩ Polarography, 337
- ⟨811⟩ Powder fineness, 339
- ⟨821⟩ Radioactivity, 340
- ⟨823⟩ Radiopharmaceuticals for positron emission tomography—compounding, 347
- ⟨831⟩ Refractive index, 351
- ⟨841⟩ Specific gravity, 351
- ⟨846⟩ Specific surface area, 352
- ⟨851⟩ Spectrophotometry and light-scattering, 355
- ⟨861⟩ Sutures—diameter, 360
- ⟨871⟩ Sutures—needle attachment, 360
- ⟨881⟩ Tensile strength, 360
- ⟨891⟩ Thermal analysis, 362
- ⟨905⟩ Uniformity of dosage units, 363
- ⟨911⟩ Viscosity, 369
- ⟨921⟩ Water determination, 370
- ⟨941⟩ X-ray diffraction, 372
- ⟨1005⟩ Acoustic emission, 375
- ⟨1010⟩ Analytical data—interpretation and treatment, 378
- ⟨1015⟩ Automated radiochemical synthesis apparatus, 389
- ⟨1031⟩ The Biocompatibility of materials used in drug containers, medical devices, and implants, 390
- ⟨1035⟩ Biological indicators for sterilization, 399
- ⟨1041⟩ Biologics, 402
- ⟨1043⟩ Ancillary materials for cell, gene, and tissue-engineered products, 403
- ⟨1045⟩ Biotechnology-derived articles, 409
- ⟨1046⟩ Cell and gene therapy products, 419
- ⟨1048⟩ Quality of biotechnological products: analysis of the expression construct in cells used for production of r-DNA derived protein products, 449
- ⟨1049⟩ Quality of biotechnological products: stability testing of biotechnological/biological products, 450
- ⟨1050⟩ Viral safety evaluation of biotechnology products derived from cell lines of human or animal origin, 453
- ⟨1051⟩ Cleaning glass apparatus, 462
- ⟨1052⟩ Biotechnology-derived articles—amino acid analysis, 463
- ⟨1053⟩ Biotechnology-derived articles—capillary electrophoresis, 471
- ⟨1054⟩ Biotechnology-derived articles—isoelectric focusing, 475
- ⟨1055⟩ Biotechnology-derived articles—peptide mapping, 477
- ⟨1056⟩ Biotechnology-derived articles—polyacrylamide gel electrophoresis, 481
- ⟨1057⟩ Biotechnology-derived articles—total protein assay, 486
- ⟨1061⟩ Color—instrumental measurement, 489
- ⟨1065⟩ Ion chromatography, 490
- ⟨1070⟩ Emergency medical services vehicles and ambulances—storage of preparations, 493
- ⟨1072⟩ Disinfectants and Antiseptics, 493
- ⟨1074⟩ Excipient biological safety evaluation guidelines, 497
- ⟨1075⟩ Good compounding practices, 500
- ⟨1078⟩ Good manufacturing practices for bulk pharmaceutical excipients, 503
- ⟨1079⟩ Good storage and shipping practices, 512
- ⟨1080⟩ Bulk pharmaceutical excipients—certificate of analysis, 517
- ⟨1081⟩ Gel strength of gelatin, 523
- ⟨1086⟩ Impurities in official articles, 523
- ⟨1087⟩ Intrinsic dissolution, 526
- ⟨1088⟩ In vitro and in vivo evaluation of dosage forms, 527
- ⟨1090⟩ In vivo bioequivalence guidances, 532
- ⟨1091⟩ Labeling of inactive ingredients, 572
- ⟨1092⟩ The Dissolution procedure: development and validation, 573
- ⟨1101⟩ Medicine dropper, 578
- ⟨1111⟩ Microbiological attributes of nonsterile pharmaceutical products, 578
- ⟨1111⟩ Microbiological examination of nonsterile products: acceptance criteria for pharmaceutical preparations and substances for pharmaceutical use, 579
- ⟨1112⟩ Application of water activity determination to nonsterile pharmaceutical products, 580
- ⟨1116⟩ Microbiological evaluation of clean rooms and other controlled environments, 582
- ⟨1117⟩ Microbiological best laboratory practices, 589
- ⟨1118⟩ Monitoring devices—time, temperature, and humidity, 593
- ⟨1119⟩ Near-infrared spectrophotometry, 595
- ⟨1120⟩ Raman spectroscopy, 599
- ⟨1121⟩ Nomenclature, 605
- ⟨1136⟩ Packaging—unit-of-use, 607
- ⟨1146⟩ Packaging practice—repackaging a single solid oral drug product into a unit-dose container, 609
- ⟨1150⟩ Pharmaceutical stability, 613
- ⟨1151⟩ Pharmaceutical dosage forms, 615
- ⟨1160⟩ Pharmaceutical calculations in prescription compounding, 626
- ⟨1163⟩ Quality assurance in pharmaceutical compounding, 634
- ⟨1171⟩ Phase-solubility analysis, 638
- ⟨1174⟩ Powder flow, 639
- ⟨1176⟩ Prescription balances and volumetric apparatus, 642
- ⟨1177⟩ Good packaging practices, 643
- ⟨1178⟩ Good repackaging practices, 645
- ⟨1181⟩ Scanning electron microscopy, 646
- ⟨1184⟩ Sensitization testing, 650
- ⟨1191⟩ Stability considerations in dispensing practice, 656
- ⟨1196⟩ Pharmacopeial harmonization, 659
- ⟨1207⟩ Sterile product packaging—integrity evaluation, 664
- ⟨1208⟩ Sterility testing—validation of isolator systems, 665
- ⟨1209⟩ Sterilization—chemical and physicochemical indicators and integrators, 668
- ⟨1211⟩ Sterilization and sterility assurance of compendial articles, 670
- ⟨1216⟩ Tablet friability, 675
- ⟨1217⟩ Tablet breaking, 676
- ⟨1221⟩ Teaspoon, 678
- ⟨1222⟩ Terminally sterilized pharmaceutical products—parametric release, 678
- ⟨1223⟩ Validation of alternative microbiological methods, 681

General chapters (continued)
⟨1225⟩ Validation of compendial procedures, 683
⟨1226⟩ Verification of compendial procedures, 687
⟨1227⟩ Validation of microbial recovery from pharmacopeial articles, 687
⟨1230⟩ Water for health applications, 690
⟨1231⟩ Water for pharmaceutical purposes, 691
⟨1241⟩ Water–solid interactions in pharmaceutical systems, 710
⟨1251⟩ Weighing on an analytical balance, 712
⟨1265⟩ Written prescription drug information—guidelines, 714
⟨2021⟩ Microbial enumeration tests—nutritional and dietary supplements, 717
⟨2022⟩ Microbiological procedures for absence of specified microorganisms—nutritional and dietary supplements, 721
⟨2023⟩ Microbiological attributes of nonsterile nutritional and dietary supplements, 724
⟨2030⟩ Supplemental information for articles of botanical origin, 727
⟨2040⟩ Disintegration and dissolution of dietary supplements, 732
⟨2091⟩ Weight variation of dietary supplements, 736
⟨2750⟩ Manufacturing practices for dietary supplements, 736

General chapters, 29

Acid-neutralizing capacity ⟨301⟩, 138
Acoustic emission ⟨1005⟩, 375
Aerosols, nasal sprays, metered-dose inhalers, and dry powder inhalers ⟨601⟩, 209
Alcohol determination ⟨611⟩, 230
Alginates assay ⟨311⟩, 139
Alpha tocopherol assay ⟨551⟩, 187
Aluminum ⟨206⟩, 131
Amphetamine assay ⟨331⟩, 140
Analytical data—interpretation and treatment ⟨1010⟩, 378
Ancillary materials for cell, gene, and tissue-engineered products ⟨1043⟩, 403
Antibiotics—microbial assays ⟨81⟩, 91
Antimicrobial agents—content ⟨341⟩, 140
Antimicrobial effectiveness testing ⟨51⟩, 67
Application of water activity determination to nonsterile pharmaceutical products ⟨1112⟩, 580
Arsenic ⟨211⟩, 131
Articles of botanical origin ⟨561⟩, 188
Assay for citric acid/citrate and phosphate ⟨345⟩, 142
Assay for steroids ⟨351⟩, 143
Automated methods of analysis ⟨16⟩, 59
Automated radiochemical synthesis apparatus ⟨1015⟩, 389
Bacterial endotoxins test ⟨85⟩, 98
Barbiturate assay ⟨361⟩, 143
The Biocompatibility of materials used in drug containers, medical devices, and implants ⟨1031⟩, 390
Biological indicators—resistance performance tests ⟨55⟩, 69
Biological indicators for sterilization ⟨1035⟩, 399
Biological reactivity tests, in vitro ⟨87⟩, 102
Biological reactivity tests, in vivo ⟨88⟩, 104
Biologics ⟨1041⟩, 402
Biotechnology-derived articles ⟨1045⟩, 409
Biotechnology-derived articles—amino acid analysis ⟨1052⟩, 463
Biotechnology-derived articles—capillary electrophoresis ⟨1053⟩, 471
Biotechnology-derived articles—isoelectric focusing ⟨1054⟩, 475

Biotechnology-derived articles—peptide mapping ⟨1055⟩, 477
Biotechnology-derived articles—polyacrylamide gel electrophoresis ⟨1056⟩, 481
Biotechnology-derived articles—total protein assay ⟨1057⟩, 486
Botanical extracts ⟨565⟩, 201
Bulk density and tapped density ⟨616⟩, 231
Bulk pharmaceutical excipients—certificate of analysis ⟨1080⟩, 517
Calcium pantothenate assay ⟨91⟩, 107
Capillary electrophoresis ⟨727⟩, 281
Cell and gene therapy products ⟨1046⟩, 419
Chloride and sulfate ⟨221⟩, 132
Chromatography ⟨621⟩, 232
Cleaning glass apparatus ⟨1051⟩, 462
Cobalamin radiotracer assay ⟨371⟩, 143
Color and achromicity ⟨631⟩, 243
Color—instrumental measurement ⟨1061⟩, 489
Completeness of solution ⟨641⟩, 244
Congealing temperature ⟨651⟩, 247
Containers—glass ⟨660⟩, 248
Containers—performance testing ⟨671⟩, 255
Containers—plastics ⟨661⟩, 251
Cotton ⟨691⟩, 259
Crystallinity ⟨695⟩, 260
Crystallinity determination by solution calorimetry ⟨696⟩, 261
Deliverable volume ⟨698⟩, 262
Density of solids ⟨699⟩, 265
Design and analysis of biological assays ⟨111⟩, 108
Dexpanthenol assay ⟨115⟩, 120
Dimethylaniline ⟨223⟩, 132
Disinfectants and Antiseptics ⟨1072⟩, 493
Disintegration ⟨701⟩, 266
Disintegration and dissolution of dietary supplements ⟨2040⟩, 732
Dissolution ⟨711⟩, 267
The Dissolution procedure: development and validation ⟨1092⟩, 573
Distilling range ⟨721⟩, 274
Drug release ⟨724⟩, 275
Elastomeric closures for injections ⟨381⟩, 144
Electrophoresis ⟨726⟩, 278
Emergency medical services vehicles and ambulances—storage of preparations ⟨1070⟩, 493
4-Epianhydrotetracycline ⟨226⟩, 133
Epinephrine assay ⟨391⟩, 145
Excipient biological safety evaluation guidelines ⟨1074⟩, 497
Fats and fixed oils ⟨401⟩, 145
Folic acid assay ⟨411⟩, 149
Gel strength of gelatin ⟨1081⟩, 523
Globule size distribution in lipid injectable emulsions ⟨729⟩, 285
Good compounding practices ⟨1075⟩, 500
Good manufacturing practices for bulk pharmaceutical excipients ⟨1078⟩, 503
Good packaging practices ⟨1177⟩, 643
Good repackaging practices ⟨1178⟩, 645
Good storage and shipping practices ⟨1079⟩, 512
Heavy metals ⟨231⟩, 133
Identification of articles of botanical origin ⟨563⟩, 195
Identification—organic nitrogenous bases ⟨181⟩, 126
Identification tests—general ⟨191⟩, 127
Identification—tetracyclines ⟨193⟩, 129
Impurities in official articles ⟨1086⟩, 523
Injections ⟨1⟩, 33
Insulin assays ⟨121⟩, 121
Intrinsic dissolution ⟨1087⟩, 526
In vitro and in vivo evaluation of dosage forms ⟨1088⟩, 527

In vivo bioequivalence guidances ⟨1090⟩, 532
Iodometric assay—antibiotics ⟨425⟩, 150
Ion chromatography ⟨1065⟩, 490
Iron ⟨241⟩, 135
Labeling of inactive ingredients ⟨1091⟩, 572
Lead ⟨251⟩, 135
Light diffraction measurement of particle size ⟨429⟩, 150
Loss on drying ⟨731⟩, 292
Loss on ignition ⟨733⟩, 293
Manufacturing practices for dietary supplements ⟨2750⟩, 736
Mass spectrometry ⟨736⟩, 293
Medicine dropper ⟨1101⟩, 578
Melting range or temperature ⟨741⟩, 297
Mercury ⟨261⟩, 136
Metal particles in ophthalmic ointments ⟨751⟩, 298
Methoxy determination ⟨431⟩, 153
Microbial enumeration tests—nutritional and dietary supplements ⟨2021⟩, 717
Microbial limit tests ⟨61⟩, 71
Microbiological attributes of nonsterile nutritional and dietary supplements ⟨2023⟩, 724
Microbiological attributes of nonsterile pharmaceutical products ⟨1111⟩, 578
Microbiological best laboratory practices ⟨1117⟩, 589
Microbiological evaluation of clean rooms and other controlled environments ⟨1116⟩, 582
Microbiological examination of nonsterile products: acceptance criteria for pharmaceutical preparations and substances for pharmaceutical use ⟨1111⟩, 579
Microbiological examination of nonsterile products: microbial enumeration tests ⟨61⟩, 76
Microbiological examination of nonsterile products: tests for specified organisms ⟨62⟩, 81
Microbiological procedures for absence of specified microorganisms—nutritional and dietary supplements ⟨2022⟩, 721
Minimum fill ⟨755⟩, 298
Monitoring devices—time, temperature, and humidity ⟨1118⟩, 593
Near-infrared spectrophotometry ⟨1119⟩, 595
Niacin or niacinamide assay ⟨441⟩, 154
Nitrite titration ⟨451⟩, 156
Nitrogen determination ⟨461⟩, 157
Nomenclature ⟨1121⟩, 605
Nuclear magnetic resonance ⟨761⟩, 298
Ophthalmic ointments ⟨771⟩, 304
Optical microscopy ⟨776⟩, 304
Optical rotation ⟨781⟩, 306
Ordinary impurities ⟨466⟩, 157
Organic volatile impurities ⟨467⟩, 158
Osmolality and osmolarity ⟨785⟩, 307
Oxygen flask combustion ⟨471⟩, 181
Packaging practice—repackaging a single solid oral drug product into a unit-dose container ⟨1146⟩, 609
Packaging—unit-of-use ⟨1136⟩, 607
Particle size distribution estimation by analytical sieving ⟨786⟩, 308
Particulate matter in injections ⟨788⟩, 311
Particulate matter in ophthalmic solutions ⟨789⟩, 313
pH ⟨791⟩, 314
Pharmaceutical calculations in prescription compounding ⟨1160⟩, 626
Pharmaceutical compounding—nonsterile preparations ⟨795⟩, 315
Pharmaceutical compounding—sterile preparations ⟨797⟩, 319

General chapters (continued)
Pharmaceutical dosage forms ⟨1151⟩, 615
Pharmaceutical stability ⟨1150⟩, 613
Pharmacopeial harmonization ⟨1196⟩, 659
Phase-solubility analysis ⟨1171⟩, 638
Plasma spectrochemistry ⟨730⟩, 287
Polarography ⟨801⟩, 337
Powder flow ⟨1174⟩, 639
Powder fineness ⟨811⟩, 339
Prescription balances and volumetric apparatus ⟨1176⟩, 642
Protein—biological adequacy test ⟨141⟩, 122
Pyrogen test ⟨151⟩, 123
Quality assurance in pharmaceutical compounding ⟨1163⟩, 634
Quality of biotechnological products: analysis of the expression construct in cells used for production of r-DNA derived protein products ⟨1048⟩, 449
Quality of biotechnological products: stability testing of biotechnological/biological products ⟨1049⟩, 450
Radioactivity ⟨821⟩, 340
Radiopharmaceuticals for positron emission tomography—compounding ⟨823⟩, 347
Raman spectroscopy ⟨1120⟩, 599
Readily carbonizable substances test ⟨271⟩, 137
Refractive index ⟨831⟩, 351
Repackaging into single-unit containers and unit-dose containers for nonsterile solid and liquid dosage forms ⟨681⟩, 258
Residual solvents ⟨467⟩, 170
Residue on ignition ⟨281⟩, 137
Riboflavin assay ⟨481⟩, 182
Salts of organic nitrogenous bases ⟨501⟩, 182
Scanning electron microscopy ⟨1181⟩, 646
Selenium ⟨291⟩, 138
Sensitization testing ⟨1184⟩, 650
Single-steroid assay ⟨511⟩, 183
Specific gravity ⟨841⟩, 351
Specific surface area ⟨846⟩, 352
Spectrophotometric identification tests ⟨197⟩, 129
Spectrophotometry and light-scattering ⟨851⟩, 355
Stability considerations in dispensing practice ⟨1191⟩, 656
Sterile product packaging—integrity evaluation ⟨1207⟩, 664
Sterility testing—validation of isolator systems ⟨1208⟩, 665
Sterility tests ⟨71⟩, 85
Sterilization—chemical and physicochemical indicators and integrators ⟨1209⟩, 668
Sterilization and sterility assurance of compendial articles ⟨1211⟩, 670
Sulfonamides ⟨521⟩, 183
Supplemental information for articles of botanical origin ⟨2030⟩, 727
Sutures—diameter ⟨861⟩, 360
Sutures—needle attachment ⟨871⟩, 360
Tablet breaking ⟨1217⟩, 676
Tablet friability ⟨1216⟩, 675
Teaspoon ⟨1221⟩, 678
Tensile strength ⟨881⟩, 360
Terminally sterilized pharmaceutical products—parametric release ⟨1222⟩, 678
Thermal analysis ⟨891⟩, 362
Thermometers ⟨21⟩, 66
Thiamine assay ⟨531⟩, 184
Thin-layer chromatographic identification test ⟨201⟩, 130
Titrimetry ⟨541⟩, 185
Total organic carbon ⟨643⟩, 244
Transfusion and infusion assemblies and similar medical devices ⟨161⟩, 124
Uniformity of dosage units ⟨905⟩, 363
USP reference standards ⟨11⟩, 37
Validation of alternative microbiological methods ⟨1223⟩, 681
Validation of compendial procedures ⟨1225⟩, 683
Validation of microbial recovery from pharmacopeial articles ⟨1227⟩, 687
Verification of compendial procedures ⟨1226⟩, 687
Viral safety evaluation of biotechnology products derived from cell lines of human or animal origin ⟨1050⟩, 453
Viscosity ⟨911⟩, 369
Vitamin A assay ⟨571⟩, 203
Vitamin B$_{12}$ activity assay ⟨171⟩, 125
Vitamin D assay ⟨581⟩, 204
Volumetric apparatus ⟨31⟩, 66
Water conductivity ⟨645⟩, 245
Water determination ⟨921⟩, 370
Water for health applications ⟨1230⟩, 690
Water for pharmaceutical purposes ⟨1231⟩, 691
Water–solid interactions in pharmaceutical systems ⟨1241⟩, 710
Weighing on an analytical balance ⟨1251⟩, 712
Weight variation of dietary supplements ⟨2091⟩, 736
Weights and balances ⟨41⟩, 67
Written prescription drug information—guidelines ⟨1265⟩, 714
X-ray diffraction ⟨941⟩, 372
Zinc determination ⟨591⟩, 208

General notices and requirements
Abbreviations, xii, 4
Atomic weights and chemical formulas, xi, 3
Concentrations, xxi, 13
General chapters, xiii, 5
Ingredients and processes, xiii, 5
NF, 1062
"Official" and "Official articles", xi, 3
Pharmacopeial Forum, xiii, 5
Prescribing and dispensing, xvii, 9
Preservation, packaging, storage, and labeling, xvii, 9
reagent standards, xiii, 5
Reference reagents, xiii, 5
Significant figures and tolerances, xii, 4
Supplements, xiii, 5
Tests and assays, xiv, 6
Title, xi, 3
Units of potency, xiii, 5
USP, ix, 1
USP Reference standards, xiii, 5
Vegetable and animal substances, xx, 12
Weights and measures, xxi, 13
General tests for reagents, 748
Geneticin, 776
Gentamicin
injection, 2265
and prednisolone acetate ophthalmic ointment, 2268
and prednisolone acetate ophthalmic suspension, 2269
sulfate, 2263
sulfate and betamethasone acetate ophthalmic solution, 2265
sulfate and betamethasone valerate ointment, 2266
sulfate and betamethasone valerate otic solution, 2267
sulfate and betamethasone valerate topical solution, 2268
sulfate cream, 2264
sulfate ointment, 2265
sulfate ophthalmic ointment, 2265
sulfate ophthalmic solution, 2265
uterine infusion, 2264

Gentian violet, 2269
cream, 2270
topical solution, 2271
Ginger, 944
capsules, 946
powdered, 945
tincture, 946
Ginkgo, 947
capsules, 950
extract, powdered, 949
tablets, 951
Ginseng
American, 952
Asian, 955
capsules, American, 953
extract, powdered American, 953
extract, powdered Asian, 956
powdered, American, 952
powdered, Asian, 956
tablets, American, 954
tablets, Asian, 957
Girard reagent T, 776
Gitoxin, 776
Glacial acetic acid, 776, 1298
TS, 817
Glass wool, 776
Glaze, pharmaceutical, 1140
Glimepiride, 2271
Glipizide, 2272
tablets, 2273
and metformin hydrochloride tablets, 2274
Globule size distribution in lipid injectable emulsions ⟨729⟩, 285
Globulin
immune, 2276
reagent, anti-human, 756
RH$_o$ (D) immune, 2277
serum, anti-human, 2277
Glucagon, 2277
for injection, 2280
D-Gluconic acid, 50 percent in water, 776
Gluconolactone, 2280
Glucosamine
and chondroitin sulfate sodium tablets, 957
hydrochloride, 958
tablets, 959
sulfate potassium chloride, 959
sulfate sodium chloride, 960
and methylsulfonylmethane tablets, 960
chondroitin sulfate sodium, and methylsulfonylmethane tablets, 961
Glucose, 776
enzymatic test strip, 2281
liquid, 1140
oxidase-chromogen TS, 817
D-Glucuronolactone, 776
Glutamic acid, 776
L-Glutamic acid, 776
Glutamine, 2281
L-Glutamine, 776
Glutaral
concentrate, 2281
disinfectant solution, 1141
Glyburide, 2282
and metformin hydrochloride tablets, 2284
tablets, 2283
Glycerin, 776, 2286
base TS, 817
ophthalmic solution, 2287
oral solution, 2287
suppositories, 2287
Glyceryl
behenate, 1141
distearate, 1142
monolinoleate, 1143
monooleate, 1144
monostearate, 1145

Glycine, 2288
  irrigation, 2288
Glycolic acid, 776
Glycopyrrolate, 2288
  injection, 2289
  tablets, 2289
Gold
  chloride, 777
  chloride TS, 817
  sodium thiomalate, 2290
  sodium thiomalate injection, 2291
Goldenseal, 962
  extract, powdered, 963
  powdered, 962
Gonadorelin
  acetate, 2291
  hydrochloride, 2292
  for injection, 2294
Gonadotropin
  chorionic, 2294
  chorionic, for injection, 2295
Good compounding practices ⟨1075⟩, 500
Good manufacturing practices for bulk
    pharmaceutical excipients ⟨1078⟩, 503
Good packaging practices ⟨1177⟩, 643
Good repackaging practices ⟨1178⟩, 645
Good storage and shipping practices ⟨1079⟩, 512
Graftskin, 2295
Gramicidin, 2300
  and neomycin and polymyxin B sulfates cream, 2785
  and neomycin and polymyxin B sulfates and
    hydrocortisone acetate cream, 2786
  and neomycin and polymyxin B sulfates
    ophthalmic solution, 2785
  and neomycin sulfate ointment, 2775
  nystatin, neomycin sulfate, and triamcinolone
    acetonide cream, 2842
  nystatin, neomycin sulfate, and triamcinolone
    acetonide ointment, 2843
Gravity, specific ⟨841⟩, 351
Green
  brilliant, 760
  FCF, Fast, 775
  soap, 2300
  soap tincture, 2301
Griseofulvin, 2301
  capsules, 2302
  oral suspension, 2302
  tablets, 2303
  tablets, ultramicrosize, 2303
Guaiacol, 777
Guaifenesin, 2304
  capsules, 2305
  and codeine phosphate oral solution, 2306
  and dyphylline oral solution, 2035
  and dyphylline tablets, 2036
  for injection, 2305
  oral solution, 2305
  and pseudoephedrine hydrochloride capsules, 2307
  pseudoephedrine hydrochloride, and
    dextromethorphan hydrobromide capsules, 2308
  tablets, 2306
  and theophylline capsules, 3377
  and theophylline oral solution, 3377
Guanabenz acetate, 2309
  tablets, 2310
Guanadrel sulfate, 2311
  tablets, 2311
Guanethidine monosulfate, 2312
  tablets, 2312
Guanfacine
  hydrochloride, 2313
  tablets, 2314
Guanidine hydrochloride, 777
Guanidine isothiocyanate, 777

Guanine hydrochloride, 777
Guar gum, 1146
Guide to general chapters
  charts, 15
  table of contents, v, 29
Gutta percha, 2315

H

Halazone, 2315
  tablets for solution, 2315
Halcinonide, 2315
  cream, 2316
  ointment, 2316
  topical solution, 2317
Haloperidol, 2317
  injection, 2318
  oral solution, 2318
  tablets, 2318
Halothane, 2319
Hawthorn leaf
  with flower, 963
  with flower, powdered, 965
Heavy metals ⟨231⟩, 133
Heavy metals in reagents, 750
Helium, 2319
  oxygen certified standard, 786
Hematein, 777
Hematoxylin, 777
  TS, Delafield's, 816
Hemoglobin, bovine, 777
Heparin
  calcium, 2320
  calcium injection, 2321
  lock flush solution, 2320
  sodium, 2321
  sodium injection, 2322
Hepatitis B
  immune globulin, 2323
1-Heptadecanol, 777
Heptafluorobutyric acid, 777
Heptakis(2,6-di-O-methyl)-β-cyclodextrin, 777
n-Heptane, 777
  chromatographic, 777
Hexachlorophene, 2323
  cleansing emulsion, 2323
  liquid soap, 2324
Hexadecyl hexadecanoate, 777
Hexadimethrine bromide, 777
Hexamethyldisilazane, 777
Hexamethyleneimine, 777
n-Hexane, 777
Hexane, solvent, 777
  chromatographic, 777
Hexanes, 777
Hexanitrodiphenylamine, 777
Hexanophenone, 777
Hexylene glycol, 1146
Hexylresorcinol, 2325
  lozenges, 2325
Histamine
  dihydrochloride, 777
  phosphate, 2326
  phosphate injection, 2326
Histidine, 2326
L-Histidine hydrochloride monohydrate, 777
Histoplasmin, 2327
Homatropine
  hydrobromide, 2327
  hydrobromide ophthalmic solution, 2328
  methylbromide, 2328
  methylbromide tablets, 2329
Homatropine methylbromide
  and hydrocodone bitartrate tablets, 2338

Homosalate, 2330
Honey, purified, 1146
Horse chestnut, 965
  extract, powdered, 966
  powdered, 966
Horseradish peroxidase conjugated to goat anti-
    mouse IgG, 778
Hyaluronidase
  injection, 2330
  for injection, 2330
Hydralazine hydrochloride, 2331
  injection, 2332
  oral solution, 2333
  reserpine and hydrochlorothiazide tablets, 3172
  tablets, 2333
Hydrazine
  dihydrochloride, 778
  hydrate, 85% in water, 778
  sulfate, 778
Hydrindantin, 778
Hydriodic acid, 778
Hydrochloric acid, 778, 1146
  alcoholic, tenth-molar (0.1M), 823
  buffer, 813
  diluted, 778, 1147
  half-normal (0.5 N), 823
  half-normal (0.5 N) in methanol, 823
  normal (1 N), 823
Hydrochloride
  Nile blue, 809
Hydrochlorothiazide, 2334
  and amiloride hydrochloride tablets, 1381
  and bisoprolol fumarate tablets, 1546
  and captopril tablets, 1628
  and enalapril maleate tablets, 2058
  and fosinopril tablets, 2232
  and irbesartan tablets, 2447
  and methyldopa tablets, 2676
  and metoprolol tartrate tablets, 2699
  and propranolol hydrochloride extended-release
    capsules, 3116
  and propranolol hydrochloride tablets, 3117
  reserpine and hydralazine hydrochloride tablets, 3172
  and reserpine tablets, 3174
  and spironolactone tablets, 3267
  tablets, 2335
  and timolol maleate tablets, 3412
  and triamterene capsules, 3449
  and triamterene tablets, 3450
  and valsartan tablets, 3497
Hydrocodone bitartrate, 2336
  and acetaminophen tablets, 2337
  and homatropine methylbromide tablets, 2338
  tablets, 2336
Hydrocortisone, 2339
  acetate, 2344
  acetate and chloramphenicol for ophthalmic
    suspension, 1722
  acetate, chloramphenicol, and polymyxin B
    sulfate ophthalmic ointment, 1723
  acetate and colistin and neomycin sulfates otic
    suspension, 1848
  acetate cream, 2344
  acetate injectable suspension, 2346
  acetate lotion, 2345
  acetate, neomycin and polymyxin B sulfates,
    and bacitracin ointment, 2781
  acetate, neomycin and polymyxin B sulfates,
    and bacitracin ophthalmic ointment, 2781
  acetate, neomycin and polymyxin B sulfates,
    and bacitracin zinc ophthalmic ointment, 2783
  acetate and neomycin and polymyxin B sulfates
    cream, 2787
  acetate, neomycin and polymyxin B sulfates,
    and gramicidin cream, 2786

Hydrocortisone *(continued)*
  acetate and neomycin and polymyxin B sulfates ophthalmic suspension, 2787
  acetate and neomycin sulfate cream, 2776
  acetate and neomycin sulfate lotion, 2776
  acetate and neomycin sulfate ointment, 2776
  acetate and neomycin sulfate ophthalmic ointment, 2777
  acetate and neomycin sulfate ophthalmic suspension, 2777
  acetate ointment, 2345
  acetate ophthalmic ointment, 2345
  acetate ophthalmic suspension, 2346
  acetate and oxytetracycline hydrochloride ophthalmic suspension, 2895
  acetate, penicillin G, neomycin, polymyxin B, and hydrocortisone sodium succinate topical suspension, 2929
  acetate, penicillin G procaine, and neomycin and polymyxin B sulfates topical suspension, 2941
  and acetic acid otic solution, 2343
  butyrate, 2346
  butyrate cream, 2347
  and clioquinol cream, 1803
  and clioquinol ointment, 1804
  cream, 2340
  gel, 2340
  hemisuccinate, 2347
  injectable suspension, 2342
  lotion, 2341
  neomycin and polymyxin B sulfates and bacitracin zinc ointment, 2782
  neomycin and polymyxin B sulfates and bacitracin zinc ophthalmic ointment, 2783
  and neomycin and polymyxin B sulfates ophthalmic suspension, 2786
  and neomycin and polymyxin B sulfates otic solution, 2786
  and neomycin and polymyxin B sulfates otic suspension, 2787
  and neomycin sulfate cream, 2775
  and neomycin sulfate ointment, 2775
  and neomycin sulfate otic suspension, 2776
  ointment, 2341
  and oxytetracycline hydrochloride ointment, 2896
  and polymyxin B sulfate otic solution, 3025
  rectal suspension, 2342
  sodium phosphate, 2348
  sodium phosphate injection, 2349
  sodium succinate, 2350
  sodium succinate for injection, 2350
  sodium succinate, penicillin G, neomycin, polymyxin B, and hydrocortisone acetate topical suspension, 2929
  tablets, 2342
  valerate, 2351
  valerate cream, 2351
  valerate ointment, 2352
Hydroflumethiazide, 2352
  tablets, 2352
Hydrofluoric acid, 778
Hydrogen
  peroxide, 10 percent, 778
  peroxide, 30 percent, 778
  peroxide concentrate, 2353
  peroxide solution, 778
  peroxide topical solution, 2353
  peroxide TS, 817
  sulfide, 778
  sulfide detector tube, 778
  sulfide TS, 817
Hydrogenated vegetable oil, 1257
Hydromorphone hydrochloride, 2354
  injection, 2354
  tablets, 2355

Hydroquinone, 778, 2355
  cream, 2356
  topical solution, 2356
Hydroxocobalamin, 2356
  injection, 2357
3′-Hydroxyacetophenone, 778
4′-Hydroxyacetophenone, 778
Hydroxyamphetamine hydrobromide, 2358
  ophthalmic solution, 2358
Hydroxyanisole, butylated, 1086
p-Hydroxybenzoic acid, 778
4-Hydroxybenzoic acid isopropyl ester, 778
1-Hydroxybenzotriazole hydrate, 778
2-Hydroxybenzyl alcohol, 778
Hydroxychloroquine sulfate, 2358
  tablets, 2359
Hydroxyethyl cellulose, 1147
N-(2-Hydroxyethyl)piperazine-N′-(2-ethanesulfonic acid), 778
Hydroxylamine hydrochloride, 778
  TS, 817
Hydroxy naphthol blue, 778
10β-Hydroxynorandrostenedione, 778
2′-(4-Hydroxyphenyl)-5-(4-methyl-1-piperazinyl)-2,5′-bi-1H-benzimidazole trihydrochloride pentahydrate, 779
4-(4-Hydroxyphenyl)-2-butanone, 778
3-Hydroxyphenyldimethylethyl ammonium chloride, 778
D-α-4-Hydroxyphenylglycine, 779
Hydroxyprogesterone caproate, 2359
  injection, 2360
Hydroxypropyl
  betadex, 1147
  cellulose, 1149
  cellulose, low-substituted, 1151
  cellulose ocular system, 2360
Hydroxypropyl-β-cyclodextrin, 779
8-Hydroxyquinoline, 779
  TS, 817
Hydroxytoluene, butylated, 1086
Hydroxyurea, 2361
  capsules, 2361
Hydroxyzine
  hydrochloride, 2362
  hydrochloride injection, 2363
  hydrochloride oral solution, 2363
  hydrochloride tablets, 2363
  pamoate, 2364
  pamoate capsules, 2365
  pamoate oral suspension, 2366
Hymetellose, 1151
Hyoscyamine, 2366
  hydrobromide, 2367
  sulfate, 2367
  sulfate elixir, 2368
  sulfate injection, 2369
  sulfate oral solution, 2369
  sulfate tablets, 2370
  tablets, 2366
Hypophosphorous acid, 1152
  50 percent, 779
Hypoxanthine, 779
Hypromellose, 2370
  acetate succinate, 1152
  ophthalmic solution, 2372
  phthalate, 1154

I

I 123
  capsules, sodium iodide, 2417
  injection, iobenguane, 2415
  injection, iodohippurate sodium, 2416

  solution, sodium iodide, 2417
I 125
  albumin injection, iodinated, 2418
  injection, iothalamate sodium, 2418
I 131
  albumin aggregated injection, iodinated, 2419
  albumin injection, iodinated, 2419
  capsules, sodium iodide, 2421
  injection, iobenguane, 2416
  injection, iodohippurate sodium, 2420
  injection, rose bengal sodium, 2420
  solution, sodium iodide, 2421
Ibuprofen, 2372
  oral suspension, 2373
  and pseudoephedrine hydrochloride tablets, 2375
  tablets, 2374
Ichthammol, 2376
  ointment, 2377
Idarubicin hydrochloride, 2377
  for injection, 2378
Identification
  of articles of botanical origin ⟨563⟩, 195
  organic nitrogenous bases ⟨181⟩, 126
  test, thin-layer chromatographic ⟨201⟩, 130
  tests—general ⟨191⟩, 127
  tests, spectrophotometric ⟨197⟩, 129
  tetracyclines ⟨193⟩, 129
Idoxuridine, 2378
  ophthalmic ointment, 2378
  ophthalmic solution, 2379
Ifosfamide, 2379
  for injection, 2381
IgG-coated red cells, 779
Imidazole, 779
Imidurea, 1155
Imipenem, 2381
  and cilastatin for injectable suspension, 2383
  and cilastatin for injection, 2382
Imipramine hydrochloride, 2384
  injection, 2384
  tablets, 2385
Impurities
  in official articles ⟨1086⟩, 523
  ordinary ⟨466⟩, 157
  organic volatile ⟨467⟩, 158
Inamrinone, 2385
  injection, 2386
Indapamide, 2387
  tablets, 2388
Indene, 779
Indicator
  and test papers, 810
Indicators, 779, 808
  indicator test papers, 808
Indicators and indicator test papers, 808
Indigo carmine, 779
  TS, 817
Indigotindisulfonate sodium, 2389
  injection, 2389
Indinavir sulfate, 2390
Indium In 111
  capromab pendetide injection, 2391
  chloride solution, 2391
  ibritumomab tiuxetan injection, 2393
  oxyquinoline solution, 2393
  pentetate injection, 2394
  pentetreotide injection, 2394
  satumomab pendetide injection, 2395
Indocyanine green, 2395
  for injection, 2396
Indole, 779
Indole-3-carboxylic acid, 779
Indomethacin, 2396
  capsules, 2397
  extended-release capsules, 2397
  topical gel, 2399
  for injection, 2402

Indomethacin *(continued)*
  oral suspension, 2400
  sodium, 2401
  suppositories, 2399
Indophenol-acetate TS, 817
Influenza virus vaccine, 2403
Information Expert Committee, xiv
Ingredients and processes, xiii, 5
Inhalant
  amyl nitrite, 1423
  propylhexedrine, 3120

Inhalation
Acetylcysteine and isoproterenol hydrochloride solution, 1302
Cromolyn sodium powder, 1856
Cromolyn sodium solution, 1856
Dexamethasone sodium phosphate aerosol, 1912
Epinephrine aerosol, 2065
Epinephrine bitartrate aerosol, 2068
Epinephrine solution, 2066
Ergotamine tartrate aerosol, 2079
Isoetharine mesylate aerosol, 2453
Isoetharine solution, 2452
Isoproterenol hydrochloride aerosol, 2463
Isoproterenol hydrochloride and phenylephrine bitartrate aerosol, 2465
Isoproterenol solution, 2463
Isoproterenol sulfate aerosol, 2467
Isoproterenol sulfate solution, 2468
Metaproterenol sulfate aerosol, 2637
Metaproterenol sulfate solution, 2638
Racepinephrine solution, 3154
Ribavirin for solution, 3178
Sodium chloride, solution, 3247
Terbutaline sulfate aerosol, 3345
Tobramycin solution, 3420
Sterile water for, 3523

Injection
Acepromazine maleate, 1267
Acetazolamide for, 1297
Acyclovir for, 1304
Adenosine, 1308
Alcohol, dehydrated, 1318
Alcohol in dextrose, 1319
Alfentanil, 1323
Alprostadil, 1331
Alteplase for, 1334
Amifostine for, 1377
Amikacin sulfate, 1380
Aminocaproic acid, 1387
Aminohippurate sodium, 1389
Aminopentamide sulfate, 1390
Aminophylline, 1392
Amitriptyline hydrochloride, 1399
Ammonium chloride, 1402
Ammonium molybdate, 1404
Amobarbital sodium for, 1405
Amphotericin B for, 1415
Ampicillin for, 1417
Ampicillin and sulbactam for, 1421
Anileridine, 1424
Aprotinin, 1442
Arginine hydrochloride, 1444
Ascorbic acid, 1445
Atenolol, 1461
Atracurium besylate, 1467
Atropine sulfate, 1469
Azaperone, 1473
Azathioprine sodium for, 1476
Aztreonam, 1480
Aztreonam for, 1481
Bacitracin for, 1483

Bacteriostatic sodium chloride, 3246
Bacteriostatic water for, 3523
Benztropine mesylate, 1510
Benzylpenicilloyl polylysine, 1513
Betamethasone sodium phosphate, 1522
Bethanechol chloride, 1528
Biperiden lactate, 1536
Bleomycin for, 1548
Bretylium tosylate, 1556
Bretylium tosylate in dextrose, 1556
Brompheniramine maleate, 1563
Bumetanide, 1567
Bupivacaine hydrochloride, 1569
Bupivacaine hydrochloride in dextrose, 1570
Bupivacaine hydrochloride and epinephrine, 1570
Butorphanol tartrate, 1588
Caffeine citrate, 1590
Caffeine and sodium benzoate, 1592
Calcitonin salmon, 1598
Calcitriol, 1595
Calcium chloride, 1608
Calcium gluceptate, 1610
Calcium gluconate, 1611
Calcium levulinate, 1614
Capreomycin for, 1623
Carbenicillin for, 1634
C 11, flumazenil, 1639
C 11, mespiperone, 1640
C 11, methionine, 1640
C 11, raclopride, 1641
C 11, sodium acetate, 1642
Carboplatin for, 1645
Carboprost tromethamine, 1646
Cefamandole naftate for, 1665
Cefazolin, 1667
Cefazolin for, 1667
Cefepime for, 1670
Cefmenoxime for, 1673
Cefmetazole, 1674
Cefmetazole for, 1675
Cefonicid for, 1676
Cefoperazone, 1677
Cefoperazone for, 1678
Ceforanide for, 1679
Cefotaxime, 1681
Cefotaxime for, 1681
Cefotetan, 1683
Cefotetan for, 1683
Cefotiam for, 1685
Cefoxitin, 1686
Cefoxitin for, 1686
Cefpiramide for, 1688
Ceftazidime, 1693
Ceftazidime for, 1693
Ceftizoxime, 1696
Ceftizoxime for, 1696
Ceftriaxone, 1697
Ceftriaxone for, 1698
Cefuroxime, 1701
Cefuroxime for, 1701
Cephalothin, 1708
Cephalothin for, 1709
Cephapirin for, 1711
Cephradine for, 1713
Chloramphenicol, 1719
Chloramphenicol sodium succinate for, 1726
Chlordiazepoxide hydrochloride for, 1729
Chloroprocaine hydrochloride, 1735
Chloroquine hydrochloride, 1736
Chlorothiazide sodium for, 1738
Chlorpheniramine maleate, 1741
Chlorpromazine hydrochloride, 1747
Chorionic gonadotropin for, 2295
Chromic chloride, 1758
Cr 51, sodium chromate, 1758
Chromium Cr 51 edetate, 1759

Cimetidine, 1767
Cimetidine in sodium chloride, 1767
Ciprofloxacin, 1772
Cisplatin for, 1777
Clavulanic acid and ticarcillin, 3405
Clindamycin, 1800
Clindamycin for, 1800
Codeine phosphate, 1841
Colchicine, 1844
Colistimethate for, 1847
Corticotropin, 1850
Corticotropin for, 1851
Corticotropin, repository, 1852
Cupric chloride, 1859
Cupric sulfate, 1860
Cyanocobalamin, 1861
Cyclophosphamide for, 1865
Cyclosporine, 1870
Cysteine hydrochloride, 1873
Cytarabine for, 1874
Dacarbazine for, 1875
Dactinomycin for, 1877
Dantrolene sodium for, 1881
Daunorubicin hydrochloride for, 1884
Deferoxamine mesylate for, 1885
Dehydrated alcohol, 1318
Deslanoside, 1896
Desmopressin acetate, 1899
Desoxycorticosterone acetate, 1903
Dexamethasone, 1906
Dexamethasone sodium phosphate, 1913
Dextran 40 in dextrose, 1921
Dextran 40 in sodium chloride, 1921
Dextran 70 in dextrose, 1923
Dextran 70 in sodium chloride, 1923
Dextrose, 1927
Dextrose and sodium chloride, 1928
Diatrizoate meglumine, 1929
Diatrizoate meglumine and diatrizoate sodium, 1930
Diatrizoate sodium, 1932
Diazepam, 1935
Diazoxide, 1937
Dibucaine hydrochloride, 1939
Dicyclomine hydrochloride, 1947
Diethylstilbestrol, 1954
Diethylstilbestrol diphosphate, 1956
Digitoxin, 1962
Digoxin, 1964
Dihydroergotamine mesylate, 1967
Dihydrostreptomycin, 1968
Dimenhydrinate, 1979
Dimercaprol, 1982
Diphenhydramine hydrochloride, 1988
Dipyridamole, 1994
Dobutamine, 2002
Dobutamine in dextrose, 2003
Dobutamine for, 2003
Dolasetron mesylate, 2010
Dopamine hydrochloride, 2013
Dopamine hydrochloride and dextrose, 2013
Doxapram hydrochloride, 2015
Doxorubicin hydrochloride, 2021
Doxorubicin hydrochloride for, 2021
Doxycycline for, 2025
Droperidol, 2029
Dyphylline, 2034
Edetate calcium disodium, 2039
Edetate disodium, 2040
Edrophonium chloride, 2040
Electrolytes and dextrose type 1, multiple, 2044
Electrolytes and dextrose type 2, multiple, 2046
Electrolytes and dextrose type 3, multiple, 2047
Electrolytes and dextrose type 4, multiple, 2048

Injection (continued)
Electrolytes and invert sugar type 1, multiple, 2049
Electrolytes and invert sugar type 2, 2050
Electrolytes and invert sugar type 3, 2051
Electrolytes type 1, multiple, 2041
Electrolytes type 2, multiple, 2042
Elements, trace, 2052
Emetine hydrochloride, 2055
Ephedrine sulfate, 2063
Epinephrine, 2065
Ergonovine maleate, 2077
Ergotamine tartrate, 2080
Erythromycin, 2086
Erythromycin ethylsuccinate, 2093
Erythromycin lactobionate for, 2096
Estradiol cypionate, 2102
Estradiol valerate, 2105
Estrone, 2110
Ethacrynate sodium for, 2113
Ethiodized oil, 2120
Etoposide, 2134
Famotidine, 2137
Fenoldopam mesylate, 2148
Fentanyl citrate, 2151
Ferumoxides, 2158
Floxuridine for, 2170
Fludarabine phosphate for, 2176
Fludeoxyglucose F18, 2192
Flumazenil, 2179
Flunixin meglumine, 2184
Fluorescein, 2190
F 18, sodium fluoride, 2195
F 18, fluorodopa, 2193
Fluorouracil, 2199
Fluphenazine decanoate, 2206
Fluphenazine enanthate, 2208
Fluphenazine hydrochloride, 2209
Folic acid, 2228
Fosphenytoin sodium, 2235
Fructose, 2236
Fructose and sodium chloride, 2237
Furosemide, 2239
Gadodiamide, 2247
Gadopentetate dimeglumine, 2248
Gadoteridol, 2251
Gadoversetamide, 2254
Gallamine triethiodide, 2255
Gallium citrate Ga 67, 2255
Ganciclovir for, 2257
Gemcitabine for, 2261
Gentamicin, 2265
Glucagon for, 2280
Glycopyrrolate, 2289
Gold sodium thiomalate, 2291
Gonadorelin for, 2294
Gonadotropin, chorionic for, 2295
Guaifenesin for, 2305
Haloperidol, 2318
Heparin calcium, 2321
Heparin sodium, 2322
Histamine phosphate, 2326
Hyaluronidase, 2330
Hyaluronidase for, 2330
Hydralazine hydrochloride, 2332
Hydrocortisone sodium phosphate, 2349
Hydrocortisone sodium succinate for, 2350
Hydromorphone hydrochloride, 2354
Hydroxocobalamin, 2357
Hydroxyprogesterone caproate, 2360
Hydroxyzine hydrochloride, 2363
Hyoscyamine sulfate, 2369
Idarubicin hydrochloride for, 2378
Ifosfamide for, 2381
Imipenem and cilastatin for, 2382
Imipramine hydrochloride, 2384
Inamrinone, 2386
Indigotindisulfonate sodium, 2389

Indium In 111 capromab pendetide, 2391
Indium In 111 ibritumomab tiuxetan, 2393
Indium In 111 pentetate, 2394
Indium In 111 pentetreotide, 2394
Indium In 111 satumomab pendetide, 2395
Indocyanine green for, 2396
Indomethacin for, 2402
Insulin, 2405
Insulin human, 2406
Human insulin and human insulin isophane suspension, 2407
Insulin lispro, 2409
Inulin in sodium chloride, 2413
Invert sugar, 3282
I 123, iobenguane, 2415
I 123, iodohippurate sodium, 2416
I 125, iothalamate sodium, 2418
I 125 albumin, iodinated, 2418
I 131, iobenguane, 2416
I 131, iodohippurate sodium, 2420
I 131, Rose bengal sodium, 2420
I 131 albumin, iodinated, 2419
I 131 albumin aggregated, iodinated, 2419
Iodipamide meglumine, 2422
Iodixanol, 2426
Iohexol, 2430
Iopamidol, 2431
Iophendylate, 2433
Iopromide, 2435
Iothalamate meglumine, 2436
Iothalamate meglumine and iothalamate sodium, 2436
Iothalamate sodium, 2437
Ioversol, 2439
Ioxaglate meglumine and ioxaglate sodium, 2439
Ioxilan, 2442
Iron dextran, 2448
Iron sorbitex, 2449
Iron sucrose, 2449
Isoniazid, 2459
Isoproterenol hydrochloride, 2464
Isoxsuprine hydrochloride, 2480
Kanamycin, 2486
Ketamine hydrochloride, 2488
Ketorolac tromethamine, 2491
Labetalol hydrochloride, 2494
Leucovorin calcium, 2509
Levocarnitine, 2516
Levorphanol tartrate, 2522
Lidocaine hydrochloride, 2528
Lidocaine hydrochloride and dextrose, 2529
Lidocaine hydrochloride and epinephrine, 2529
Lincomycin, 2533
Lorazepam, 2551
Magnesium sulfate, 2579
Magnesium sulfate in dextrose, 2579
Mangafodipir trisodium, 2583
Manganese chloride, 2584
Manganese sulfate, 2586
Mannitol, 2587
Mannitol in sodium chloride, 2587
Mechlorethamine hydrochloride for, 2596
Menadiol sodium diphosphate, 2613
Menadione, 2614
Menotropins for, 2616
Meperidine hydrochloride, 2618
Mepivacaine hydrochloride, 2621
Mepivacaine hydrochloride and levonordefrin, 2622
Meropenem for, 2628
Mesoridazine besylate, 2634
Metaraminol bitartrate, 2640
Methadone hydrochloride, 2649
Methocarbamol, 2660
Methohexital sodium for, 2661
Methotrexate, 2663
Methotrexate for, 2663

Methotrimeprazine, 2664
Methyldopate hydrochloride, 2677
Methylene blue, 2679
Methylergonovine maleate, 2680
Methylprednisolone sodium succinate for, 2687
Metoclopramide, 2691
Metoprolol tartrate, 2697
Metronidazole, 2704
Mezlocillin for, 2709
Miconazole, 2711
Minocycline for, 2716
Mitomycin for, 2721
Mitoxantrone, 2723
Morphine sulfate, 2737
Morrhuate sodium, 2738
Nafcillin, 2747
Nafcillin for, 2748
Nalorphine hydrochloride, 2752
Naloxone hydrochloride, 2753
Nandrolone decanoate, 2756
Nandrolone phenpropionate, 2757
Neomycin for, 2771
Neostigmine methylsulfate, 2793
Netilmicin sulfate, 2794
Niacin, 2799
Niacinamide, 2800
N 13, ammonia, 2816
Nitroglycerin, 2817
Norepinephrine bitartrate, 2824
Ondansetron, 2856
Orphenadrine citrate, 2861
Oxacillin, 2863
Oxacillin for, 2864
O 15, water, 2887
Oxymorphone hydrochloride, 2890
Oxytetracycline, 2892
Oxytetracycline for, 2894
Oxytocin, 2898
Paclitaxel, 2901
Pamidronate disodium for, 2904
Papaverine hydrochloride, 2912
Paricalcitol, 2917
Particulate matter in injections ⟨788⟩, 311
Penicillin G potassium, 2934
Penicillin G potassium for, 2934
Penicillin G sodium for, 2943
Pentazocine, 2951
Pentobarbital sodium, 2955
Perphenazine, 2964
Phenobarbital sodium, 2975
Phentolamine mesylate for, 2981
Phenylbutazone, 2984
Phenylephrine hydrochloride, 2986
Phenytoin sodium, 2999
Physostigmine salicylate, 3002
Phytonadione injectable emulsion, 3004
Piperacillin for, 3013
Plicamycin for, 3018
Polymyxin B for, 3023
Potassium acetate, 3027
Potassium chloride concentrate for, 3033
Potassium chloride in dextrose, 3034
Potassium chloride in dextrose and sodium chloride, 3035
Potassium chloride in lactated Ringer's and dextrose, 3036
Potassium chloride in sodium chloride, 3037
Potassium phosphates, 3047
Pralidoxime chloride for, 3051
Prednisolone sodium phosphate, 3066
Prednisolone sodium succinate for, 3067
Prilocaine and epinephrine, 3072
Prilocaine hydrochloride, 3071
Procainamide hydrochloride, 3079
Procaine hydrochloride, 3082

Injection *(continued)*
  Procaine hydrochloride and epinephrine, 3083
  Procaine and tetracaine hydrochlorides and levonordefrin, 3083
  Prochlorperazine edisylate, 3087
  Progesterone, 3089
  Promazine hydrochloride, 3094
  Promethazine hydrochloride, 3095
  Propoxycaine and procaine hydrochlorides and levonordefrin, 3103
  Propoxycaine and procaine hydrochlorides and norepinephrine bitartrate, 3104
  Propranolol hydrochloride, 3115
  Protamine sulfate, 3122
  Protamine sulfate for, 3122
  Protein hydrolysate, 3123
  Pyridostigmine bromide, 3136
  Pyridoxine hydrochloride, 3137
  Quinidine gluconate, 3146
  Ranitidine, 3158
  Ranitidine in sodium chloride, 3160
  Repository corticotropin, 1852
  Reserpine, 3168
  Riboflavin, 3179
  Rifampin for, 3184
  Ringer's, 3190
  Ringer's and dextrose, 3191
  Ringer's and dextrose, half-strength lactated, 3194
  Ringer's and dextrose, lactated, 3193
  Ringer's and dextrose, modified, lactated, 3195
  Ringer's, lactated, 3192
  Ritodrine hydrochloride, 3199
  Ropivacaine hydrochloride, 3203
  Rose bengal sodium I 131, 2420
  Rubidium chloride Rb 82, 3206
  Sargramostim for, 3220
  Scopolamine hydrobromide, 3220
  Secobarbital sodium, 3224
  Secobarbital sodium for, 3224
  Selenious acid, 3227
  Sincalide for, 3236
  Sisomicin sulfate, 3237
  Sm 153 lexidronam, samarium, 3215
  Sodium acetate, 3239
  Sodium bicarbonate, 3242
  Sodium chloride, 3245
  Sodium chloride, bacteriostatic, 3246
  Sodium lactate, 3252
  Sodium nitrite, 3254
  Sodium nitroprusside for, 3255
  Sodium phosphates, 3256
  Sodium sulfate, 3259
  Sodium thiosulfate, 3260
  Somatropin for, 3262
  Strontium chloride Sr 89, 3276
  Streptomycin, 3276
  Streptomycin for, 3276
  Succinylcholine chloride, 3279
  Succinylcholine chloride for, 3279
  Sufentanil citrate, 3282
  Sugar, invert, 3282
  Sulfadiazine sodium, 3292
  Sulfamethoxazole and trimethoprim, 3299
  Technetium Tc 99m albumin, 3323
  Technetium Tc 99m albumin aggregated, 3324
  Technetium Tc 99m albumin colloid, 3325
  Technetium Tc 99m apcitide, 3326
  Technetium Tc 99m arcitumomab, 3327
  Technetium Tc 99m bicisate, 3327
  Technetium Tc 99m depreotide, 3328
  Technetium Tc 99m disofenin, 3328
  Technetium Tc 99m etidronate, 3329
  Technetium Tc 99m exametazime, 3329
  Technetium Tc 99m fanolesomab, 3330
  Technetium Tc 99m gluceptate, 3331
  Technetium Tc 99m lidofenin, 3332
  Technetium Tc 99m mebrofenin, 3333
  Technetium Tc 99m medronate, 3334
  Technetium Tc 99m mertiatide, 3334
  Technetium Tc 99m nofetumomab merpentan, 3335
  Technetium Tc 99m oxiseonate, 3335
  Technetium Tc 99m pentetate, 3336
  Technetium Tc 99m pertechnetate, sodium, 3336
  Technetium Tc 99m pyrophosphate, 3337
  Technetium Tc 99m (pyro- and trimeta-) phosphates, 3338
  Technetium Tc 99m red blood cells, 3338
  Technetium Tc 99m sestamibi, 3339
  Technetium Tc 99m succimer, 3340
  Technetium Tc 99m sulfur colloid, 3340
  Technetium Tc 99m tetrofosmin, 3341
  Terbutaline sulfate, 3346
  Testosterone cypionate, 3351
  Testosterone enanthate, 3352
  Testosterone propionate, 3353
  Tetracaine hydrochloride, 3356
  Tetracaine hydrochloride for, 3357
  Tetracaine hydrochloride in dextrose, 3358
  Tetracycline hydrochloride for, 3362
  Thallous chloride Tl 201, 3370
  Theophylline in dextrose, 3375
  Thiamine hydrochloride, 3382
  Thiopental sodium for, 3391
  Thiotepa for, 3394
  Thiothixene hydrochloride, 3397
  Thiothixene hydrochloride for, 3397
  Ticarcillin and clavulanic acid, 3405
  Ticarcillin and clavulanic acid for, 3405
  Ticarcillin for, 3404
  Tiletamine and zolazepam for, 3407
  Tilmicosin, 3409
  Thallous chloride Tl 201, 3370
  Tobramycin, 3419
  Tobramycin for, 3419
  Tolazoline hydrochloride, 3427
  Tolbutamide for, 3428
  Trifluoperazine hydrochloride, 3458
  Triflupromazine hydrochloride, 3461
  Trimethobenzamide hydrochloride, 3468
  Tripelennamine hydrochloride, 3473
  Tromethamine for, 3479
  Tubocurarine chloride, 3483
  Urea for, 3488
  Valproic acid, 3493
  Vancomycin, 3500
  Vancomycin hydrochloride for, 3501
  Vasopressin, 3503
  Verapamil hydrochloride, 3505
  Verteporfin for, 3511
  Vinblastine sulfate for, 3513
  Vincristine sulfate, 3514
  Vincristine sulfate for, 3515
  Vinorelbine, 3517
  Warfarin sodium for, 3521
  Water for, bacteriostatic, 3523
  Water for, sterile, 3524
  Water for, 3523
  Xenon Xe 133, 3530
  Xylazine, 3532
  Yohimbine, 3536
  Yttrium Y 90 ibritumomab tiuxetan, 3537
  Zidovudine, 3541
  Zinc chloride, 3546
  Zinc sulfate, 3550
  Zolazepam and tiletamine for injection, 3407

Injections ⟨1⟩, 33
Inosine, 779
Inositol, 779
Insoluble matter in reagents, 750
Insulin, 2403
  assays ⟨121⟩, 121
  human, 2405
  human injection, 2406
  human isophane suspension and human insulin injection, 2407
  human suspension, isophane, 2410
  human zinc suspension, 2411
  human zinc suspension, extended, 2411
  injection, 2405
  lispro, 2408
  lispro injection, 2409
  suspension, isophane, 2409
  zinc suspension, 2410
  zinc suspension, extended, 2410
  zinc suspension, prompt, 2411
Intestinal fluid, simulated, TS, 817
Intramammary infusion
  amoxicillin, 1409
  cloxacillin benzathine, 1831
Intrauterine contraceptive system
  progesterone, 3090
Intrinsic dissolution ⟨1087⟩, 526
Intrinsic viscosity table, 902
Inulin, 2412
  in sodium chloride injection, 2413
In vitro
  and in vivo evaluation of dosage forms ⟨1088⟩, 527
  reactivity tests ⟨87⟩, 102
In vivo
  bioequivalence guidances ⟨1090⟩, 532
  and in vitro evaluation of dosage forms ⟨1088⟩, 527
  biological reactivity tests ⟨88⟩, 104
Iobenguane
  I 123 injection, 2415
  I 131 injection, 2416
  sulfate, 779
Iodic acid, 779
Iodinated
  I 125 albumin injection, 2418
  I 131 albumin aggregated injection, 2419
  I 131 albumin injection, 2419
Iodine, 779, 2414
  diluted TS, 817
  hundredth-normal (0.01 N), 824
  I 123 capsules, sodium iodide, 2417
  I 123 injection, iobenguane, 2415
  I 123 injection, iodohippurate sodium, 2416
  I 123 solution, sodium iodide, 2417
  I 125 albumin injection, iodinated, 2418
  I 125 injection, iothalamate sodium, 2418
  I 131 albumin aggregated injection, iodinated, 2419
  I 131 albumin injection, iodinated, 2419
  I 131 capsules, sodium iodide, 2421
  I 131 injection, iobenguane, 2416
  I 131 injection, iodohippurate sodium, 2420
  I 131 injection, rose bengal sodium, 2420
  I 131 solution, sodium iodide, 2421
  monobromide, 779
  monochloride, 779
  monochloride TS, 817
  and potassium iodide TS 1, 818
  and potassium iodide TS 2, 818
  solution, strong, 2414
  tenth-normal (0.1 N), 824
  tincture, 2414
  tincture, strong, 2415
  topical solution, 2414
  TS, 817
Iodipamide, 2422
  meglumine injection, 2422
Iodixanol, 2423
  injection, 2426
Iodobromide TS, 818
Iodochloride TS, 818
Iodoethane, 779
Iodoform, 2427

Iodohippurate sodium
  I 123 injection, 2416
  I 131 injection, 2420
Iodometric assay—antibiotics ⟨425⟩, 150
p-Iodonitrotetrazolium violet, 779
Iodoplatinate TS, 818
Iodoquinol, 2427
  tablets, 2427
Iohexol, 2428
  injection, 2430
Ion chromatography ⟨1065⟩, 490
Ion-exchange resin, 779
Iopamidol, 2430
  injection, 2431
Iopanoic acid, 2432
  tablets, 2432
Iophendylate, 2432
  injection, 2433
Iopromide, 2433
  injection, 2435
Iothalamate
  meglumine injection, 2436
  meglumine and iothalamate sodium injection, 2436
  sodium I 125 injection, 2418
  sodium injection, 2437
  sodium and iothalamate meglumine injection, 2436
Iothalamic acid, 2437
Ioversol, 2438
  injection, 2439
Ioxaglate
  meglumine and ioxaglate sodium injection, 2439
  sodium and ioxaglate meglumine injection, 2439
Ioxaglic acid, 2440
Ioxilan, 2441
  injection, 2442
Ipecac, 2443
  oral solution, 2444
  powdered, 2444
Ipodate sodium, 2445
  capsules, 2445
Irbesartan, 2446
  and hydrochlorothiazide tablets, 2447
  tablets, 2447
Iron ⟨241⟩, 135
  dextran injection, 2448
  phenol TS, 818
  salicylate TS, 818
  sorbitex injection, 2449
  sucrose injection, 2449
  wire, 779
Isoamyl
  alcohol, 779
Isobutane, 1155
Isobutyl
  acetate, 779
  alcohol, 779
4-Isobutylacetophenone, 779
N-Isobutylpiperidone, 780
Isoetharine
  hydrochloride, 2451
  inhalation solution, 2452
  mesylate, 2452
  mesylate inhalation aerosol, 2453
Isoflupredone acetate, 780, 2453
  injectable suspension, 2454
  neomycin sulfate and tetracaine hydrochloride ointment, 2777
  neomycin sulfate and tetracaine hydrochloride topical powder, 2778
Isoflurane, 2455
Isoflurophate, 2456
  ophthalmic ointment, 2457
Isoleucine, 2457
Isomalt, 1156

Isomaltotriose, 780
Isometheptene mucate, 2458
  dichloralphenazone, and acetaminophen capsules, 2458
Isoniazid, 2459
  injection, 2459
  oral solution, 2459
  and rifampin capsules, 3185
  rifampin, pyrazinamide, and ethambutol hydrochloride tablets, 3187
  rifampin and pyrazinamide tablets, 3186
  tablets, 2460
Isonicotinic acid, 780
  hydrazide, 780
Isooctane, 780
Isopropamide iodide, 2460
  tablets, 2461
Isopropyl
  acetate, 780
  alcohol, 780, 2461
  alcohol, azeotropic, 2462
  alcohol, dehydrated, 780
  alcohol, rubbing, 2462
  ether, 780
  iodide, 780
  myristate, 780, 1157
  palmitate, 1158
  salicylate, 780
Isopropylamine, 780
Isoproterenol
  hydrochloride, 2462
  hydrochloride and acetylcysteine inhalation solution, 1302
  hydrochloride inhalation aerosol, 2463
  hydrochloride injection, 2464
  hydrochloride and phenylephrine bitartrate inhalation aerosol, 2465
  hydrochloride tablets, 2465
  inhalation solution, 2463
  sulfate, 2467
  sulfate inhalation aerosol, 2467
  sulfate inhalation solution, 2468
Isorhamnetin, 780
Isosorbide
  concentrate, 2469
  dinitrate chewable tablets, 2472
  dinitrate, diluted, 2470
  dinitrate extended-release capsules, 2471
  dinitrate extended-release tablets, 2472
  dinitrate sublingual tablets, 2473
  dinitrate tablets, 2471
  mononitrate, diluted, 2474
  mononitrate extended-release tablets, 2477
  mononitrate tablets, 2475
  oral solution, 2470
Isotretinoin, 2479
  capsules, 2479
Isovaleric acid, 780
Isoxsuprine hydrochloride, 2480
  injection, 2480
  tablets, 2481
Isradipine, 2482
  capsules, 2482
Ivermectin, 2483

J

Juniper tar, 2484

K

Kaempferol, 780
Kanamycin
  injection, 2486
  sulfate, 2485
  sulfate capsules, 2486
Kaolin, 2486
Kerosene, 780
Ketamine hydrochloride, 2487
  injection, 2488
Ketoconazole, 2488
  oral suspension, 2488
  tablets, 2489
Ketoprofen, 2490
Ketorolac tromethamine, 2490
  injection, 2491
  tablets, 2492
Kr 81m
  krypton, 2492
Krypton Kr 81m, 2492

L

L designations, 780
Labeling of inactive ingredients ⟨1091⟩, 572
Labetalol hydrochloride, 2493
  injection, 2494
  oral suspension, 2495
  tablets, 2495
Lactase, 2496
Lactic acid, 2496
Lactitol, 1158
Lactose, 780
  anhydrous, 1159
  beta, 780
  monohydrate, 1160
  monohydrate, alpha, 780
Lactulose
  concentrate, 2496
  solution, 2497
Lamivudine, 2498
Lanolin, 2499
  alcohols, 1161
  modified, 2501
Lansoprazole, 2502
  delayed-release capsules, 2503
Lanthanum
  alizarin complexan mixture, 780
  chloride, 780
  oxide, 780
Lauroyl polyoxylglycerides, 1161
Lauryl dimethyl amine oxide, 780
Lead
  acetate, 780
  acetate paper, 780
  acetate test paper, 810
  acetate TS, 818
  acetate TS, alcoholic, 818
  monoxide, 780
  nitrate, 781
  nitrate, hundredth-molar (0.01 M), 824
  perchlorate, 781
  perchlorate, hundredth-molar (0.01 M), 824
  perchlorate, tenth-molar (0.1 M), 824
  solution, standard, 820
  subacetate TS, 818
  subacetate TS, diluted, 818
  tetraacetate, 781
Lead ⟨251⟩, 135
Lecithin, 1161
Leflunomide, 2504
  tablets, 2505

Lemon
  oil, 1162
  tincture, 1162
Letrozole, 2506
  tablets, 2507
Leucine, 2508
Leucovorin calcium, 2509
  injection, 2509
  tablets, 2510
Leuprolide acetate, 2510
Levamisole hydrochloride, 2512
  tablets, 2512
Levmetamfetamine, 2513
Levobunolol hydrochloride, 2514
  ophthalmic solution, 2514
Levocabastine hydrochloride, 2515
Levocarnitine, 2516
  injection, 2516
  oral solution, 2517
  tablets, 2517
Levodopa, 2518
  capsules, 2519
  and carbidopa tablets, 1636
  tablets, 2519
Levonordefrin, 2520
  and mepivacaine hydrochloride injection, 2622
  and procaine and tetracaine hydrochlorides injection, 3083
  and propoxycaine and procaine hydrochlorides injection, 3103
Levonorgestrel, 2521
  and ethinyl estradiol tablets, 2521
Levorphanol tartrate, 2522
  injection, 2522
  tablets, 2523
Levothyroxine sodium, 2523
  oral powder, 2524
  tablets, 2525
Licorice, 967
  extract, powdered, 967
  fluidextract, 1162
  powdered, 967
Lidocaine, 2526
  hydrochloride, 2527
  hydrochloride and dextrose injection, 2529
  hydrochloride and epinephrine injection, 2529
  hydrochloride injection, 2528
  hydrochloride jelly, 2528
  hydrochloride oral topical solution, 2528
  hydrochloride topical solution, 2529
  neomycin and polymyxin B sulfates and bacitracin ointment, 2781
  neomycin and polymyxin B sulfates and bacitracin zinc ointment, 2784
  and neomycin and polymyxin B sulfates cream, 2788
  ointment, 2527
  oral topical solution, 2527
  and prilocaine cream, 2530
  topical aerosol, 2526
Light diffraction measurement of particle size ⟨429⟩, 150
Lime, 2531
Linalool, 781
Lincomycin
  hydrochloride, 2532
  hydrochloride capsules, 2532
  hydrochloride soluble powder, 2533
  injection, 2533
  oral solution, 2533
Lindane, 2534
  cream, 2534
  lotion, 2535
  shampoo, 2535
Linoleic acid, 781
Linoleoyl polyoxylglycerides, 1163
Liothyronine sodium, 2535
  tablets, 2536

Liotrix tablets, 2537
Lipoic acid
  alpha, 968
  capsules, alpha, 969
  tablets, alpha, 969
α-Lipoic acid, 781
Liquid petrolatum, 781
Lisinopril, 2538
  tablets, 2538
Lithium
  carbonate, 2539
  carbonate capsules, 2540
  carbonate extended-release tablets, 2540
  carbonate tablets, 2540
  chloride, 781
  citrate, 2541
  hydroxide, 781, 2542
  metaborate, 781
  methoxide, fiftieth-normal (0.02 N) in methanol, 824
  methoxide, tenth-normal (0.1 N) in chlorobenzene, 824
  methoxide, tenth-normal (0.1 N) in methanol, 824
  methoxide, tenth-normal (0.1 N) in toluene, 824
  nitrate, 781
  oral solution, 2542
  perchlorate, 781
  sulfate, 781
Lithocholic acid, 781
Litmus, 781, 809
  paper, blue, 810
  paper, red, 810
  TS, 818
Locke-Ringer's
  solution, 818
  TS, 818
Locust bean gum, 781
Loperamide hydrochloride, 2543
  capsules, 2543
  oral solution, 2544
  tablets, 2545
Loracarbef, 2545
  capsules, 2546
  for oral suspension, 2547
Loratadine, 2547
  oral solution, 2549
  tablets, 2550
Lorazepam, 2551
  injection, 2551
  oral concentrate, 2552
  tablets, 2553
Losartan potassium, 2554
Loss on drying ⟨731⟩, 292
Loss on drying for reagents, 750
Loss on ignition ⟨733⟩, 293

Lotion

Amphotericin B, 1415
Benzoyl peroxide, 1509
Benzyl benzoate, 1512
Betamethasone dipropionate, 1521
Betamethasone valerate, 1525
Clotrimazole, 1827
Flurandrenolide, 2211
Hydrocortisone, 2341
Hydrocortisone acetate, 2345
Lindane, 2535
Malathion, 2581
Methylbenzethonium chloride, 2671
Neomycin sulfate and flurandrenolide, 2774
Neomycin sulfate and hydrocortisone acetate, 2776

Nystatin, 2841
Padimate O, 2902
Triamcinolone acetonide, 3444

Lovastatin, 2555
  tablets, 2557
Loxapine
  capsules, 2558
  succinate, 2557
Lutein, 970
  preparation, 971
Lycopene, 972
  preparation, 972
  tomato extract containing, 973
Lypressin nasal solution, 2558
Lysine
  acetate, 2559
  hydrochloride, 2559
  hydrochloride tablets, 975
L-Lysine, 781

M

Mafenide acetate, 2561
  cream, 2561
  for topical solution, 2562
Magaldrate, 2563
  oral suspension, 2564
  and simethicone chewable tablets, 2566
  and simethicone oral suspension, 2565
  and simethicone tablets, 2566
  tablets, 2564
Magnesia
  alumina and calcium carbonate chewable tablets, 1338
  alumina and calcium carbonate oral suspension, 1337
  alumina, calcium carbonate, and simethicone chewable tablets, 1341
  alumina, calcium carbonate, and simethicone tablets, 1339
  alumina and calcium carbonate tablets, 1338
  and alumina oral suspension, 1336
  alumina and simethicone chewable tablets, 1344
  alumina and simethicone oral suspension, 1342
  alumina and simethicone tablets, 1344
  and alumina tablets, 1337
  aspirin and alumina tablets, 1454
  aspirin, codeine phosphate, and alumina tablets, 1458
  calcium carbonate and simethicone chewable tablets, 1605
  calcium carbonate and simethicone tablets, 1604
  and calcium carbonate tablets, 1603
  milk of, 2567
  mixture TS, 818
  tablets, 2568
Magnesium, 781
  acetate, 781
  aluminometasilicate, 1163
  aluminosilicate, 1164
  aluminum silicate, 1164
  and calcium carbonates oral suspension, 1607
  and calcium carbonates tablets, 1607
  carbonate, 2568
  carbonate and citric acid for oral solution, 2569
  carbonate, citric acid, and potassium citrate for oral solution, 2569
  carbonate and sodium bicarbonate for oral suspension, 2570

Magnesium *(continued)*
  carbonate, alumina, and magnesium oxide
    tablets, 1347
  carbonate and alumina oral suspension, 1345
  carbonate and alumina tablets, 1346
  chloride, 781, 2570
  chloride, 0.01 M, 825
  citrate, 2571
  citrate oral solution, 2571
  citrate for oral solution, 2572
  gluconate, 2573
  gluconate tablets, 2573
  hydroxide, 2574
  hydroxide paste, 2574
  nitrate, 781
  oxide, 781, 2575
  oxide, alumina, and magnesium carbonate
    tablets, 1347
  oxide, aspirin, and alumina tablets, 1455
  oxide, chromatographic, 781
  oxide, citric acid, and sodium carbonate
    irrigation, 1784
  oxide capsules, 2576
  oxide tablets, 2576
  perchlorate, anhydrous, 781
  phosphate, 2576
  salicylate, 2577
  salicylate tablets, 2577
  silicate, 1166
  silicate, activated, 781
  silicate, chromatographic, 781
  stearate, 1166
  sulfate, 781, 2578
  sulfate, anhydrous, 781
  sulfate in dextrose injection, 2579
  sulfate injection, 2579
  sulfate TS, 818
  trisilicate, 2579
  trisilicate and alumina oral suspension, 1348
  trisilicate and alumina tablets, 1348
  trisilicate tablets, 2580
Magnesium silicate
  activated, 752
Malachite green
  G, 781
  oxalate, 809
  TS, 818
Malathion, 2580
  lotion, 2581
Maleic acid, 781, 1168
Malic acid, 1168
Mallory's stain, 818
Maltitol, 1169
  solution, 1170
Maltodextrin, 1170
Maltol, 1172
Maltose, 1172
Mangafodipir trisodium, 2581
  injection, 2583
Manganese
  chloride, 2584
  chloride injection, 2584
  chloride for oral solution, 2585
  dioxide, 781
  dioxide, activated, 781
  gluconate, 2585
  sulfate, 2586
  sulfate injection, 2586
Mannitol, 2586
  injection, 2587
  in sodium chloride injection, 2587
Manufacturing practices for dietary supplements
  ⟨2750⟩, 736
Maprotiline hydrochloride, 2588
  tablets, 2588
Maritime pine, 976
  extract, 977
Mass spectrometry ⟨736⟩, 293

Mayer's reagent, 818
Mazindol, 2589
  tablets, 2590
Measles
  mumps, and rubella virus vaccine live, 2591
  and rubella virus vaccine live, 2591
  virus vaccine live, 2590
Mebendazole, 2591
  oral suspension, 2592
  tablets, 2592
Mebrofenin, 2593
Mecamylamine hydrochloride, 2594
  tablets, 2595
Mechlorethamine hydrochloride, 2596
  for injection, 2596
Meclizine hydrochloride, 2596
  tablets, 2597
Meclocycline sulfosalicylate, 2598
  cream, 2598
Meclofenamate sodium, 2599
  capsules, 2599
Medical air, 1309
Medicine dropper ⟨1101⟩, 578
Medium-chain triglycerides, 1254
Medroxyprogesterone acetate, 2600
  injectable suspension, 2601
  tablets, 2601
Mefenamic acid, 2602
  capsules, 2602
Mefloquine hydrochloride, 2603
Megestrol acetate, 2603
  oral suspension, 2604
  tablets, 2605
Meglumine, 2606
Melamine, 781
Melengestrol acetate, 2606
Meloxicam, 2607
  oral suspension, 2609
  tablets, 2610
Melphalan, 2611
  tablets, 2612
Melting range or temperature ⟨741⟩, 297
Members of the United States Pharmacopeial
  Convention as of June 30, 2005, xviii
Menadiol sodium diphosphate, 2613
  injection, 2613
  tablets, 2613
Menadione, 2614
  injection, 2614
Menotropins, 2615
  for injection, 2616
Menthol, 2616
  and benzocaine topical aerosol, 1505
  lozenges, 2617
  and tetracaine ointment, 3355
Meperidine hydrochloride, 2617
  injection, 2618
  oral solution, 2618
  tablets, 2619
Mephenytoin, 2619
  tablets, 2620
Mephobarbital, 2620
  tablets, 2621
Mepivacaine hydrochloride, 2621
  injection, 2621
  and levonordefrin injection, 2622
Meprednisone, 2623
Meprobamate, 2623
  oral suspension, 2624
  tablets, 2624
Meradimate, 2625
2-Mercaptoethanol, 781
Mercaptopurine, 2625
  tablets, 2626
Mercuric
  acetate, 781
  acetate TS, 818
  ammonium thiocyanate TS, 818

  bromide, 781
  bromide test paper, 810
  bromide TS, alcoholic, 818
  chloride, 781
  chloride TS, 818
  iodide, red, 781
  iodide, TS, 818
  nitrate, 781
  nitrate, tenth-molar (0.1 M), 825
  nitrate TS, 818
  oxide, yellow, 781
  potassium iodide TS, 818
  potassium iodide TS, alkaline, 818
  sulfate, 781
  sulfate TS, 818
  thiocyanate, 781
Mercurous nitrate
  dihydrate, 781
  TS, 818
Mercury, 781
  ammoniated, 2626
Mercury ⟨261⟩, 136
Meropenem, 2627
  for injection, 2628
Mesalamine, 2629
  delayed-release tablets, 2632
  extended-release capsules, 2630
  rectal suspension, 2631
Mesityl oxide, 781
Mesoridazine besylate, 2633
  injection, 2634
  oral solution, 2634
  tablets, 2635
Mespiperone C 11 injection, 1640
Mestranol, 2635
  and ethynodiol diacetate tablets, 2127
  and norethindrone tablets, 2826
Metacresol, 2636
Metal particles in ophthalmic ointments ⟨751⟩,
  298
Metaphenylenediamine hydrochloride, 782
  TS, 818
Metaphosphoric acid, 782
Metaphosphoric-acetic acid TS, 818
Metaproterenol sulfate, 2636
  inhalation aerosol, 2637
  inhalation solution, 2638
  oral solution, 2638
  tablets, 2639
Metaraminol bitartrate, 2639
  injection, 2640
Metformin hydrochloride, 2640
  and glipizide tablets, 2274
  and glyburide tablets, 2284
  tablets, 2641
  extended-release tablets, 2642
Methacholine chloride, 2646
Methacrylic
  acid, 782
  acid copolymer, 1173
  acid copolymer dispersion, 1174
Methacycline hydrochloride, 2647
  capsules, 2647
  oral suspension, 2648
Methadone hydrochloride, 2648
  injection, 2649
  oral concentrate, 2648
  oral solution, 2649
  tablets, 2650
  tablets for oral suspension, 2650
Methamphetamine hydrochloride, 2651
  tablets, 2651
Methanesulfonic acid, 782
Methanol, 782
  aldehyde-free, 782
  anhydrous, 782
  spectrophotometric, 782

Methazolamide, 2652
 tablets, 2652
Methdilazine hydrochloride, 2653
 oral solution, 2653
 tablets, 2654
Methenamine, 782, 2654
 hippurate, 2656
 hippurate tablets, 2656
 mandelate, 2656
 mandelate delayed-release tablets, 2658
 mandelate for oral solution, 2657
 mandelate oral suspension, 2657
 mandelate tablets, 2657
 oral solution, 2655
 tablets, 2655
Methimazole, 2658
 tablets, 2658
Methionine, 2659
 C 11 injection, 1640
Methocarbamol, 2659
 injection, 2660
 tablets, 2660
Methohexital, 2661
 sodium for injection, 2661
Methotrexate, 2662
 injection, 2663
 for injection, 2663
 tablets, 2663
Methotrimeprazine, 2664
 injection, 2664
Methoxsalen, 2665
 capsules, 2665
 topical solution, 2666
Methoxy determination ⟨431⟩, 153
Methoxyethanol, 782
2-Methoxyethanol, 782
Methoxyflurane, 2666
5-Methoxy-2-methyl-3-indoleacetic acid, 782
Methoxyphenylacetic acid, 782
Methscopolamine bromide, 2667
 tablets, 2667
Methsuximide, 2668
 capsules, 2669
Methyclothiazide, 2670
 tablets, 2670
Methyl
 acetate, 782
 alcohol, 1174
 4-aminobenzoate, 782
 arachidate, 782
 behenate, 782
 benzenesulfonate, 782
 caprate, 782
 caprylate, 782
 carbamate, 782
 chloroform, 782
 erucate, 782
 ethyl ketone, 782
 green, 782
 green—iodomercurate paper, 810
 heptadecanoate, 782
 iodide, 782
 isobutyl ketone, 783, 1175
 laurate, 783
 lignocerate, 783
 linoleate, 783
 linolenate, 783
 methacrylate, 783
 methacrylate and ethyl acrylate copolymer
  dispersion, 1132
 myristate, 783
 oleate, 783
 orange, 809
 orange TS, 818
 palmitate, 783
 purple TS, 819
 red, 783, 809
 red-methylene blue TS, 819
 red sodium, 809
 red TS, 819
 red TS, methanolic, 819
 salicylate, 1175
 stearate, 783
 sulfoxide, 783
 violet TS, 819
 yellow, 784, 809
 yellow-methylene blue TS, 819
 yellow paper, 810
 yellow TS, 819
3-Methyl-2-benzothiazolinone hydrazone
  hydrochloride TS, 818
Methylamine, 40 percent in water, 783
p-Methylaminophenol sulfate, 783
Methylbenzethonium chloride, 2671
 lotion, 2671
 ointment, 2672
 topical powder, 2672
4-Methylbenzophenone, 783
Methylbenzothiazolone hydrazone
  hydrochloride, 783
(S)-(−)-α-Methylbenzyl isocyanate, 783
Methylcellulose, 2672
 ophthalmic solution, 2673
 oral solution, 2673
 tablets, 2673
Methyldopa, 2674
 and chlorothiazide tablets, 2675
 and hydrochlorothiazide tablets, 2676
 oral suspension, 2674
 tablets, 2675
Methyldopate hydrochloride, 2677
 injection, 2677
Methylene
 blue, 783, 2678
 blue injection, 2679
 blue TS, 819
 chloride, 783, 1175
5,5′-Methylenedisalicylic acid, 783
Methylergonovine maleate, 2679
 injection, 2680
 tablets, 2681
3-O-Methylestrone, 783
2-Methyl-5-nitroimidazole, 783
N-Methyl-N-nitroso-p-toluenesulfonamide, 783
Methylparaben, 1176
 sodium, 1176
4-Methylpentan-2-ol, 783
4-Methyl-2-pentanone, 784
Methylphenidate hydrochloride, 2681
 extended-release tablets, 2683
 tablets, 2682
Methylprednisolone, 2683
 acetate, 2684
 acetate cream, 2685
 acetate injectable suspension, 2686
 acetate and neomycin sulfate cream, 2779
 hemisuccinate, 2686
 sodium succinate, 2687
 sodium succinate for injection, 2687
 tablets, 2684
2-Methyl-2-propyl-1,3-propanediol, 784
N-Methylpyrrolidine, 784
Methylsulfonylmethane, 978
 and glucosamine tablets, 960
 glucosamine, and chondroitin sulfate sodium
  tablets, 961
 tablets, 979
Methyltestosterone, 2688
 capsules, 2689
 tablets, 2689
Methylthionine perchlorate TS, 819
Methysergide maleate, 2690
 tablets, 2690
Metoclopramide
 hydrochloride, 2691
 injection, 2691
 oral solution, 2692
 tablets, 2692
Metolazone, 2693
 oral suspension, 2693
 tablets, 2694
Metoprolol
 fumarate, 2694
 succinate, 2695
 succinate extended-release tablets, 2696
 tartrate, 2697
 tartrate and hydrochlorothiazide tablets, 2699
 tartrate injection, 2697
 tartrate oral solution, 2698
 tartrate oral suspension, 2698
 tartrate tablets, 2699
Metrifonate, 2701
Metronidazole, 2702
 benzoate, 2703
 gel, 2703
 injection, 2704
 tablets, 2704
Metyrapone, 2705
 tablets, 2705
Metyrosine, 2706
 capsules, 2707
Mexiletine hydrochloride, 2707
 capsules, 2708
Mezlocillin
 for injection, 2709
 sodium, 2709
Mibolerone, 2710
 oral solution, 2710
Miconazole, 2711
 injection, 2711
 nitrate, 2712
 nitrate cream, 2712
 nitrate topical powder, 2713
 nitrate vaginal suppositories, 2713
Microbial enumeration tests—nutritional and
  dietary supplements ⟨2021⟩, 717
Microbial limit tests ⟨61⟩, 71
Microbiological attributes of nonsterile nutritional
  and dietary supplements ⟨2023⟩, 724
Microbiological attributes of nonsterile
  pharmaceutical products ⟨1111⟩, 578
Microbiological best laboratory practices ⟨1117⟩,
  589
Microbiological evaluation of clean rooms and
  other controlled environments ⟨1116⟩, 582
Microbiological examination of nonsterile
  products: acceptance criteria for
  pharmaceutical preparations and substances
  for pharmaceutical use ⟨1111⟩, 579
Microbiological examination of nonsterile
  products: microbial enumeration tests ⟨61⟩,
  76
Microbiological examination of nonsterile
  products: tests for specified organisms ⟨62⟩,
  81
Microbiological procedures for absence of
  specified microorganisms—nutritional and
  dietary supplements ⟨2022⟩, 721
Microscopy, optical ⟨776⟩, 304
Milk thistle, 979
 capsules, 981
 extract, powdered, 980
 powdered, 980
 tablets, 982
Millon's reagent, 819
Milrinone, 2714
Mineral
 acid, 784
 oil, 2714
 oil emulsion, 2715
 oil, light, 1177
 oil, rectal, 2715
 oil, topical light, 2715

Minerals
　with calcium and vitamin D tablets, 914
　capsules, 982
　oil and water-soluble vitamins with, capsules, 1011
　oil and water-soluble vitamins with, oral solution, 1016
　oil and water-soluble vitamins with, tablets, 1022
　tablets, 984
　water-soluble vitamins with, capsules, 1046
　water-soluble vitamins with, oral solution, 1049
　water-soluble vitamins with, tablets, 1050
Minimum fill ⟨755⟩, 298
Minocycline
　hydrochloride, 2715
　hydrochloride capsules, 2716
　hydrochloride oral suspension, 2717
　hydrochloride tablets, 2717
　for injection, 2716
Minoxidil, 2718
　tablets, 2718
　topical solution, 2718
Mirtazapine, 2719
　tablets, 2720
Mission
　and preface, v
　statement, v
Mitomycin, 2721
　for injection, 2721
Mitotane, 2722
　tablets, 2722
Mitoxantrone
　hydrochloride, 2722
　injection, 2723
Modafinil, 2724
　tablets, 2725
Molindone hydrochloride, 2725
　tablets, 2726
Molybdic acid, 784
Molybdo-phosphotungstate TS, 819
Mometasone furoate, 2727
　cream, 2727
　ointment, 2728
　topical solution, 2728
Monensin, 2729
　granulated, 2730
　premix, 2730
　sodium, 2731
Monitoring devices—time, temperature, and humidity ⟨1118⟩, 593
Monobasic
　potassium phosphate, 784, 1211
　sodium phosphate, 784, 3256
Monobenzone, 2731
　cream, 2732
Monochloroacetic acid, 784
Mono- and di-glycerides, 1177
Monoethanolamine, 784, 1178
Monoglyceride citrate, 1178
Monosodium glutamate, 1178
Monothioglycerol, 1179
Morantel tartrate, 2732
Moricizine hydrochloride, 2733
　tablets, 2734
Morphine sulfate, 2735
　extended-release capsules, 2736
　injection, 2737
　suppositories, 2737
Morpholine, 784
Morrhuate sodium injection, 2738
Mumps
　measles and rubella vaccine live, 2591
　skin test antigen, 2738
　virus vaccine live, 2739
Mupirocin, 2740
　calcium, 2740
　cream, 2741

　ointment, 2742
Myristic acid, 1179
Myristyl alcohol, 1180
Myrrh, 2742
　topical solution, 2743

N

N 13 injection, ammonia, 2816
Nabumetone, 2743
　tablets, 2744
Nadolol, 2745
　and bendroflumethiazide tablets, 2746
　tablets, 2745
Nafcillin
　injection, 2747
　for injection, 2748
　sodium, 2747
　sodium capsules, 2747
　sodium for oral solution, 2748
　sodium tablets, 2749
Naftifine hydrochloride, 2749
　cream, 2749
　gel, 2750
Nalidixic acid, 2750
　oral suspension, 2751
　tablets, 2751
Nalorphine hydrochloride, 2752
　injection, 2752
Naloxone
　hydrochloride, 2752
　hydrochloride injection, 2753
　and pentazocine tablets, 2950
Naltrexone hydrochloride, 2754
　tablets, 2755
Nandrolone
　decanoate, 2755
　decanoate injection, 2756
　phenpropionate, 2757
　phenpropionate injection, 2757
Naphazoline hydrochloride, 2757
　nasal solution, 2758
　ophthalmic solution, 2758
　and pheniramine maleate ophthalmic solution, 2759
Naphthalene, 784
1,3-Naphthalenediol, 784
2,7-Naphthalenediol, 784
2-Naphthalenesulfonic acid, 784
Naphthol
　dipotassium disulfonate, 784
　disodium disulfonate, 784
1-Naphthol, 784
　reagent, 819
　TS, 819
2-Naphthol, 784
　TS, 819
p-Naphtholbenzein, 784, 809
　TS, 819
β-Naphthoquinone-4-sodium sulfonate, 784
Naphthoresorcinol, 784
1-Naphthylamine, 784
1-Naphthylamine hydrochloride, 784
2-Naphthyl chloroformate, 784
N-(1-Naphthyl)ethylenediamine dihydrochloride, 784
　TS, 819
Naproxen, 2760
　delayed-release tablets, 2761
　oral suspension, 2760
　sodium, 2762
　sodium tablets, 2762
　tablets, 2761

Narasin
　granular, 2763
　premix, 2764
Naratriptan
　hydrochloride, 2764
　tablets, 2766

Nasal solution
　Butorphanol tartrate, 1589
　Calcitonin salmon, 1598
　Cromolyn sodium, 1857
　Ephedrine sulfate, 2064
　Epinephrine, 2066
　Flunisolide, 2182
　Lypressin, 2558
　Naphazoline hydrochloride, 2758
　Oxymetazoline hydrochloride, 2888
　Oxytocin, 2898
　Phenylephrine hydrochloride, 2987
　Tetrahydrozoline hydrochloride, 3367
　Xylometazoline hydrochloride, 3533

Nasal spray
　fluticasone propionate, 2219
Natamycin, 2767
　ophthalmic suspension, 2767
Near-infrared spectrophotometry ⟨1119⟩, 595
Nefazodone hydrochloride, 2768
　tablets, 2769
Neomycin
　boluses, 2770
　and colistin sulfates and hydrocortisone acetate otic suspension, 1848
　for injection, 2771
　penicillin G, polymyxin B, hydrocortisone acetate, and hydrocortisone sodium succinate topical suspension, 2929
　and polymyxin B sulfates, bacitracin, and hydrocortisone acetate ointment, 2781
　and polymyxin B sulfates, bacitracin, and hydrocortisone acetate ophthalmic ointment, 2781
　and polymyxin B sulfates, bacitracin, and lidocaine ointment, 2781
　and polymyxin B sulfates and bacitracin ointment, 2780
　and polymyxin B sulfates and bacitracin ophthalmic ointment, 2780
　and polymyxin B sulfates, bacitracin zinc, and hydrocortisone ointment, 2782
　and polymyxin B sulfates, bacitracin zinc, and hydrocortisone ophthalmic ointment, 2783
　and polymyxin B sulfates, bacitracin zinc, and hydrocortisone acetate ophthalmic ointment, 2783
　and polymyxin B sulfates, bacitracin zinc, and lidocaine ointment, 2784
　and polymyxin B sulfates and bacitracin zinc ointment, 2782
　and polymyxin B sulfates and bacitracin zinc ophthalmic ointment, 2782
　and polymyxin B sulfates cream, 2779
　and polymyxin B sulfates and dexamethasone ophthalmic ointment, 2784
　and polymyxin B sulfates and dexamethasone ophthalmic suspension, 2785
　and polymyxin B sulfates and gramicidin cream, 2785
　and polymyxin B sulfates, gramicidin, and hydrocortisone acetate cream, 2786
　and polymyxin B sulfates and gramicidin ophthalmic solution, 2785
　and polymyxin B sulfates and hydrocortisone ophthalmic suspension, 2786
　and polymyxin B sulfates and hydrocortisone otic solution, 2786

Neomycin *(continued)*
  and polymyxin B sulfates and hydrocortisone otic suspension, 2787
  and polymyxin B sulfates and hydrocortisone acetate cream, 2787
  and polymyxin B sulfates and hydrocortisone acetate ophthalmic suspension, 2787
  and polymyxin B sulfates and lidocaine cream, 2788
  and polymyxin B sulfates ophthalamic ointment, 2780
  and polymyxin B sulfates ophthalmic solution, 2780
  and polymyxin B sulfates, penicillin G procaine, and hydrocortisone acetate topical suspension, 2941
  and polymyxin B sulfates and pramoxine hydrochloride cream, 2788
  and polymyxin B sulfates and prednisolone acetate ophthalmic suspension, 2789
  and polymyxin B sulfates solution for irrigation, 2779
  sulfate, 2770
  sulfate and bacitracin ointment, 2772
  sulfate and bacitracin zinc ointment, 2772
  sulfate cream, 2770
  sulfate and dexamethasone sodium phosphate cream, 2772
  sulfate and dexamethasone sodium phosphate ophthalmic ointment, 2772
  sulfate and dexamethasone sodium phosphate ophthalmic solution, 2773
  sulfate and fluocinolone acetonide cream, 2773
  sulfate and fluorometholone ointment, 2774
  sulfate and flurandrenolide cream, 2774
  sulfate and flurandrenolide lotion, 2774
  sulfate and flurandrenolide ointment, 2775
  sulfate and gramicidin ointment, 2775
  sulfate and hydrocortisone cream, 2775
  sulfate and hydrocortisone ointment, 2775
  sulfate and hydrocortisone otic suspension, 2776
  sulfate and hydrocortisone acetate cream, 2776
  sulfate and hydrocortisone acetate lotion, 2776
  sulfate and hydrocortisone acetate ointment, 2776
  sulfate and hydrocortisone acetate ophthalmic ointment, 2777
  sulfate and hydrocortisone acetate ophthalmic suspension, 2777
  sulfate, isoflupredone acetate, and tetracaine hydrochloride ointment, 2777
  sulfate, isoflupredone acetate, and tetracaine hydrochloride topical powder, 2778
  sulfate and methylprednisolone acetate cream, 2779
  sulfate, nystatin, gramicidin, and triamcinolone acetonide cream, 2842
  sulfate, nystatin, gramicidin, and triamcinolone acetonide ointment, 2843
  sulfate, nystatin, thiostrepton, and triamcinolone acetonide cream, 2843
  sulfate, nystatin, thiostrepton, and triamcinolone acetonide ointment, 2844
  sulfate ointment, 2771
  sulfate ophthalmic ointment, 2771
  sulfate oral solution, 2771
  sulfate and prednisolone acetate ointment, 2789
  sulfate and prednisolone acetate ophthalmic ointment, 2789
  sulfate and prednisolone acetate ophthalmic suspension, 2790
  sulfate and prednisolone sodium phosphate ophthalmic ointment, 2790
  sulfate, sulfacetamide sodium, and prednisolone acetate ophthalmic ointment, 2791
  sulfate tablets, 2771
  sulfate and triamcinolone acetonide cream, 2792
  sulfate and triamcinolone acetonide ophthalmic ointment, 2792
Neostigmine
  bromide, 2792
  bromide tablets, 2793
  methylsulfate, 2793
  methylsulfate injection, 2793
Neotame, 1180
Nessler's reagent, 819
Netilmicin sulfate, 2794
  injection, 2794
Nettle
  stinging, 984
  stinging, powdered, 986
  stinging, powdered, extract, 986
Neutralized
  alcohol, 784
  phthalate buffer, 813
Neutral red, 809
  TS, 819
Nevirapine, 2795
  oral suspension, 2796
  tablets, 2797
Niacin, 2799
  injection, 2799
  or niacinamide assay ⟨441⟩, 154
  tablets, 2799
Niacinamide, 2800
  injection, 2800
  or niacin assay ⟨441⟩, 154
  tablets, 2801
Nickel-aluminum catalyst, 784
Nickel, 784
  standard solution TS, 819
  sulfate, 784
  (II) sulfate heptahydrate, 784
β-Nicotinamide adenine dinucleotide, 784
Nicotinamide adenine dinucleotide phosphate-adenosine-5′-triphosphate mixture, 785
Nicotine, 2801
  polacrilex, 2803
  polacrilex gum, 2804
  transdermal system, 2801
Nicotinic acid, 785
Nifedipine, 2805
  capsules, 2806
  extended-release tablets, 2807
Nile blue hydrochloride, 809
Nimodipine, 2810
Ninhydrin, 785
  TS, 819
Nitrate
  mercurous, dihydrate, 781
  mercurous, TS, 818
  ophthalmic solution, silver, 3231
  in reagents, 750
  silver, 796, 3231
  silver, TS, 820
  tenth-normal (0.1 N), silver, 826
  toughened silver, 3231
Nitric
  acid, 785, 1181
  acid, diluted, 785
  acid, fuming, 785
  acid, lead-free, 785
  oxide–nitrogen dioxide detector tube, 785
Nitrilotriacetic acid, 785
Nitrite titration ⟨451⟩, 156
4′-Nitroacetophenone, 785
o-Nitroaniline, 785
p-Nitroaniline, 785
  TS, 819
Nitrobenzene, 785
p-Nitrobenzenediazonium tetrafluoroborate, 785
p-Nitrobenzyl bromide, 785
4-(*p*-Nitrobenzyl) pyridine, 785
Nitrofurantoin, 2811
  capsules, 2812
  oral suspension, 2813
  tablets, 2814
Nitrofurazone, 2814
  ointment, 2815
  topical solution, 2815
Nitrogen, 1182
  97 percent, 1182
  compounds in reagents, 750
  determination ⟨461⟩, 157
  N 13 injection, ammonia, 2816
Nitroglycerin
  diluted, 2817
  injection, 2817
  ointment, 2818
  sublingual tablets, 2818
Nitromersol, 2819
  topical solution, 2819
Nitromethane, 785
5-Nitro-1,10-phenanthroline, 785
Nitrophenanthroline TS, 819
1-Nitroso-2-naphthol, 785
Nitroso R salt, 785
Nitrous
  oxide, 2819
  oxide certified standard, 785
Nizatidine, 2820
  capsules, 2821
Nomenclature ⟨1121⟩, 605
Nonadecane, 785
Nonanoic acid, 786
Nonionic wetting agent, 786
Nonoxynol 9, 2822
1-Nonyl Alcohol, 786
n-Nonylamine, 786
Nonylphenol polyoxyethylene ether, 786
Nonylphenoxypoly(ethyleneoxy)ethanol, 786
Norepinephrine bitartrate, 2824
  injection, 2824
  and propoxycaine and procaine hydrochlorides injection, 3104
Norethindrone, 2825
  acetate, 2827
  acetate and estradiol tablets, 2102
  acetate and ethinyl estradiol tablets, 2829
  acetate tablets, 2828
  and ethinyl estradiol tablets, 2826
  and mestranol tablets, 2826
  tablets, 2825
Norethynodrel, 2830
Norfloxacin, 2831
  ophthalmic solution, 2831
  tablets, 2832
Norgestimate, 2833
  and ethinyl estradiol tablets, 2834
Norgestrel, 2835
  and ethinyl estradiol tablets, 2836
  tablets, 2836
Normal
  butyl acetate, 761
  butyl alcohol, 786
  butylamine, 786
  butyl nitrite, 786
Nortriptyline hydrochloride, 2837
  capsules, 2838
  oral solution, 2838
Noscapine, 2839
Novobiocin
  sodium, 2839
  sodium intramammary infusion, 2839
  sodium and penicillin G procaine intramammary infusion, 2942
  sodium, tetracycline hydrochloride, and prednisolone tablets, 3366
  sodium and tetracycline hydrochloride tablets, 3365
Nuclear magnetic resonance ⟨761⟩, 298

Nystatin, 2840
  cream, 2840
  lotion, 2841
  lozenges, 2841
  neomycin sulfate, gramicidin, and triamcinolone acetonide cream, 2842
  neomycin sulfate, gramicidin, and triamcinolone acetonide ointment, 2843
  neomycin sulfate, thiostrepton, and triamcinolone acetonide cream, 2843
  neomycin sulfate, thiostrepton, and triamcinolone acetonide ointment, 2844
  ointment, 2841
  oral suspension, 2841
  for oral suspension, 2842
  and oxytetracycline capsules, 2892
  and oxytetracycline for oral suspension, 2893
  tablets, 2842
  and tetracycline hydrochloride capsules, 3366
  topical powder, 2841
  and triamcinolone acetonide cream, 2844
  and triamcinolone acetonide ointment, 2845
  vaginal inserts, 2842
  vaginal suppositories, 2841

O

O 15 injection, water, 2887
n-Octadecane, 786
Octadecyl silane, 786
Octanophenone, 786
Octinoxate, 2845
Octisalate, 2846
Octocrylene, 2846
Octoxynol 9, 786, 1182
Octyldodecanol, 1183
(p-tert-Octylphenoxy) nonaethoxyethanol, 786
(p-tert-Octylphenoxy)polyethoxyethanol, 786
Octyl sulfate, sodium salt, 786
Odorless absorbent paper, 786
Officers (2005–2010), xi
"Official" and "Official articles"
  General notices and requirements, xi, 3
Ofloxacin, 2847
  ophthalmic solution, 2848
  tablets, 2848

Oil

Almond, 1069
Anise, 1076
Canola, 1090
Caraway, 1092
Cardamom, 1102
Castor, 1659
Castor, aromatic, 1660
Castor, capsules, 1659
Castor, emulsion, 1659
Castor, hydrogenated, 1103
Cedar, 764
Clove, 1113
Coconut, 1114
Cod liver, 1839
Cod liver, capsules, 927
Coriander, 1115
Corn, 1115
Cottonseed, 1118
Cottonseed, hydrogenated, 1119
Ethiodized injection, 2120
Fats and fixed oils ⟨401⟩, 145
Fennel, 1136
Lemon, 1162
Mineral, 2714

Mineral emulsion, 2715
Mineral, light, 1177
Mineral, rectal, 2715
Mineral, topical light, 2715
Olive, 1184
Orange, 1185
Palm kernel, 1186
Peanut, 1188
Peppermint, 1189
Polyoxyl 35 castor, 1205
Polyoxyl 40 hydrogenated castor, 1205
Propyliodone injectable suspension, 3120
Fully hydrogenated rapeseed, 1217
Superglycerinated fully hydrogenated rapeseed, 1218
Rose, 1219
Safflower, 3210
Sesame, 1220
Soybean, 3265
Soybean, hydrogenated, 1237
sunflower, 1248
Vegetable, hydrogenated, 1257
Vitamins capsules, soluble, 1003
Vitamins capsules, and water-soluble, 1005
Vitamins with minerals capsules, and water-soluble, 1011
Vitamins with minerals oral solution, and water-soluble, 1016
Vitamins with minerals tablets, and water-soluble, 1022
Vitamins oral solution, and water-soluble, 1009
Vitamins tablets, soluble, 1005
Vitamins tablets, and water-soluble, 1010

Oil-soluble vitamins
  capsules, 1003
  tablets, 1005
Oil- and water-soluble vitamins
  capsules, 1005
  with minerals capsules, 1011
  with minerals oral solution, 1016
  with minerals tablets, 1022
  oral solution, 1009
  tablets, 1010

Ointment

Acyclovir, 1305
Alclometasone dipropionate, 1315
Amcinonide, 1376
Amphotericin B, 1416
Anthralin, 1427
Atropine sulfate ophthalmic, 1469
Bacitracin ophthalmic, 1484
Bacitracin zinc, 1485
Bacitracin zinc and polymyxin B sulfate, 1486
Bacitracin zinc and polymyxin B sulfate ophthalmic, 1486
Benzocaine, 1502
Benzocaine, butamben, and tetracaine hydrochloride, 1504
Benzoic and salicylic acids, 1506
Betamethasone dipropionate, 1521
Betamethasone valerate, 1525
Bland lubricating ophthalmic, 2859
Chloramphenicol, polymyxin B sulfate, and hydrocortisone acetate ophthalmic, 1723
Chloramphenicol and polymyxin B sulfate ophthalmic, 1722
Chloramphenicol and prednisolone ophthalmic, 1723
Chloramphenicol ophthalmic, 1720
Chlortetracycline hydrochloride, 1751
Chlortetracycline hydrochloride ophthalmic, 1751
Ciprofloxacin ophthalmic, 1774
Clioquinol, 1803

Clioquinol and hydrocortisone, 1804
Clobetasol propionate, 1806
Coal tar, 1834
Desoximetasone, 1902
Dexamethasone sodium phosphate ophthalmic, 1913
Dibucaine, 1938
Diflorasone diacetate, 1957
Erythromycin, 2086
Erythromycin ophthalmic, 2087
Fluocinolone acetonide, 2186
Fluocinonide, 2188
Flurandrenolide, 2211
Gentamicin and prednisolone acetate ophthalmic, 2268
Gentamicin sulfate, 2265
Gentamicin sulfate and betamethasone valerate, 2266
Gentamicin sulfate ophthalmic, 2265
Halcinonide, 2316
Hydrocortisone, 2341
Hydrocortisone acetate, 2345
Hydrocortisone acetate ophthalmic, 2345
Hydrocortisone valerate, 2352
Hydrophilic, 2849
Ichthammol, 2377
Idoxuridine ophthalmic, 2378
Isoflurophate ophthalmic, 2457
Lidocaine, 2527
Methylbenzethonium chloride, 2672
Mometasone furoate, 2728
Mupirocin, 2742
Neomycin and polymyxin B sulfates and bacitracin, 2780
Neomycin and polymyxin B sulfates, bacitracin, and hydrocortisone acetate, 2781
Neomycin and polymyxin B sulfates, bacitracin, and hydrocortisone acetate ophthalmic, 2781
Neomycin and polymyxin B sulfates, bacitracin, and lidocaine, 2781
Neomycin and polymyxin B sulfates and bacitracin ophthalmic, 2780
Neomycin and polymyxin B sulfates and bacitracin zinc, 2782
Neomycin and polymyxin B sulfates, bacitracin zinc, and hydrocortisone, 2782
Neomycin and polymyxin B sulfates, bacitracin zinc, and hydrocortisone acetate ophthalmic, 2783
Neomycin and polymyxin B sulfates, bacitracin zinc, and hydrocortisone ophthalmic, 2783
Neomycin and polymyxin B sulfates, bacitracin zinc, and lidocaine, 2784
Neomycin and polymyxin B sulfates and bacitracin zinc ophthalmic, 2782
Neomycin and polymyxin B sulfates and dexamethasone ophthalmic, 2784
Neomycin and polymyxin B sulfates ophthalmic, 2780
Neomycin sulfate, 2771
Neomycin sulfate and bacitracin, 2772
Neomycin sulfate and bacitracin zinc, 2772
Neomycin sulfate and dexamethasone sodium phosphate ophthalmic, 2772
Neomycin sulfate and fluorometholone, 2774
Neomycin sulfate and flurandrenolide, 2775
Neomycin sulfate and gramicidin, 2775
Neomycin sulfate and hydrocortisone, 2775
Neomycin sulfate and hydrocortisone acetate, 2776
Neomycin sulfate and hydrocortisone acetate ophthalmic, 2777
Neomycin sulfate, isoflupredone acetate, and tetracaine hydrochloride, 2777
Neomycin sulfate and prednisolone acetate, 2789

Ointment *(continued)*
  Neomycin sulfate and prednisolone acetate ophthalmic, 2789
  Neomycin sulfate and prednisolone sodium phosphate ophthalmic, 2790
  Neomycin sulfate, sulfacetamide sodium, and prednisolone acetate ophthalmic, 2791
  Neomycin sulfate and triamcinolone acetonide ophthalmic, 2792
  Neomycin sulfate ophthalmic, 2771
  Nitrofurazone, 2815
  Nitroglycerin, 2818
  Nystatin, 2841
  Nystatin, neomycin sulfate, gramicidin, and triamcinolone acetonide, 2843
  Nystatin, neomycin sulfate, thiostrepton, and triamcinolone acetonide, 2844
  Nystatin and triamcinolone acetonide, 2845
  Oxytetracycline hydrochloride and hydrocortisone, 2896
  Oxytetracycline hydrochloride and polymyxin B sulfate, 2896
  Oxytetracycline hydrochloride and polymyxin B sulfate ophthalmic, 2897
  Physostigmine sulfate ophthalmic, 3003
  Polyethylene glycol, 1199
  Povidone-iodine, 3050
  Prednicarbate, 3060
  Resorcinol ointment, compound, 3176
  Rose water, 3204
  Scopolamine hydrobromide ophthalmic, 3221
  Sodium chloride ophthalmic, 3246
  Sulfacetamide sodium ophthalmic, 3286
  Sulfacetamide sodium and prednisolone acetate ophthalmic, 3287
  Sulfur, 3308
  Tetracaine, 3354
  Tetracaine and menthol, 3355
  Tetracaine ophthalmic, 3355
  Tetracycline hydrochloride, 3362
  Tetracycline hydrochloride ophthalmic, 3363
  Tobramycin and dexamethasone ophthalmic, 3422
  Tobramycin ophthalmic, 3420
  Triamcinolone acetonide, 3444
  Undecylenic acid, compound, 3487
  Vidarabine ophthalmic, 3512
  White, 2849
  Yellow, 2849
  Zinc oxide, 3549

Ointments, ophthalmic ⟨771⟩, 304
Olefin detector tube, 786
Oleic acid, 1183
Oleoresin, capsicum, 1625
Oleovitamin A and D, 2850
  capsules, 2850
Oleoyl polyoxylglycerides, 1183
Oleyl
  alcohol, 1184
  oleate, 1184
Oligo-deoxythymidine, 786
Olive oil, 1184
Omeprazole, 2850
  delayed-release capsules, 2851
Ondansetron, 2853
  hydrochloride, 2854
  hydrochloride oral suspension, 2855
  injection, 2856
  oral solution, 2857
  orally disintegrating tablets, 2858
Ophthalmic
  ointment, bland lubricating, 2859
  ointments ⟨771⟩, 304

Ophthalmic ointment
Atropine sulfate, 1469
Bacitracin, 1484
Bacitracin zinc and polymyxin B sulfate, 1486
Bland lubricating, 2859
Chloramphenicol, 1720
Chloramphenicol and polymyxin B sulfate, 1722
Chloramphenicol, polymyxin B sulfate, and hydrocortisone acetate, 1723
Chloramphenicol and prednisolone, 1723
Chlortetracycline hydrochloride, 1751
Ciprofloxacin, 1774
Dexamethasone sodium phosphate, 1913
Erythromycin, 2087
Gentamicin and prednisolone acetate, 2268
Gentamicin sulfate, 2265
Hydrocortisone acetate, 2345
Idoxuridine, 2378
Isoflurophate, 2457
Neomycin and polymyxin B sulfates, 2780
Neomycin and polymyxin B sulfates and bacitracin, 2780
Neomycin and polymyxin B sulfates, bacitracin, and hydrocortisone acetate, 2781
Neomycin and polymyxin B sulfates and bacitracin zinc, 2782
Neomycin and polymyxin B sulfates, bacitracin zinc, and hydrocortisone, 2783
Neomycin and polymyxin B sulfates, bacitracin zinc, and hydrocortisone acetate, 2783
Neomycin and polymyxin B sulfates and dexamethasone, 2784
Neomycin sulfate, 2771
Neomycin sulfate and dexamethasone sodium phosphate, 2772
Neomycin sulfate and hydrocortisone acetate, 2777
Neomycin sulfate and prednisolone acetate, 2789
Neomycin sulfate and prednisolone sodium phosphate, 2790
Neomycin sulfate, sulfacetamide sodium, and prednisolone acetate, 2791
Neomycin sulfate and triamcinolone acetonide, 2792
Ophthalmic ointments ⟨771⟩, 304
Oxytetracycline hydrochloride and polymyxin B sulfate, 2897
Physostigmine sulfate, 3003
Scopolamine hydrobromide, 3221
Sodium chloride, 3246
Sulfacetamide sodium, 3286
Sulfacetamide sodium and prednisolone acetate, 3287
Tetracaine, 3355
Tetracycline hydrochloride, 3363
Tobramycin, 3420
Tobramycin and dexamethasone, 3422
Vidarabine, 3512

Ophthalmic solution
Acetylcholine chloride for, 1300
Apraclonidine, 1440
Atropine sulfate, 1470
Benoxinate hydrochloride, 1499
Betaxolol, 1526
Carbachol, 1629
Carteolol hydrochloride, 1654
Cefazolin, 1668
Chloramphenicol, 1720
Chloramphenicol for, 1720
Chymotrypsin for, 1760
Ciprofloxacin, 1774
Cromolyn sodium, 1857
Cyclopentolate hydrochloride, 1864
Demecarium bromide, 1887
Dexamethasone sodium phosphate, 1914
Dipivefrin hydrochloride, 1993
Echothiophate iodide for, 2037
Emedastine, 2054
Epinephrine, 2067
Epinephrine bitartrate, 2069
Epinephrine bitartrate for, 2069
Epinephryl borate, 2069
Eucatropine hydrochloride, 2136
Fluorescein sodium and benoxinate hydrochloride, 2191
Fluorescein sodium and proparacaine hydrochloride, 2191
Flurbiprofen sodium, 2216
Gentamicin sulfate, 2265
Gentamicin sulfate and betamethasone acetate, 2265
Glycerin, 2287
Homatropine hydrobromide, 2328
Hydroxyamphetamine hydrobromide, 2358
Hypromellose, 2372
Idoxuridine, 2379
Levobunolol hydrochloride, 2514
Methylcellulose, 2673
Naphazoline hydrochloride, 2758
Naphazoline hydrochloride and pheniramine maleate, 2759
Neomycin and polymyxin B sulfates, 2780
Neomycin and polymyxin B sulfates and gramicidin, 2785
Neomycin sulfate and dexamethasone sodium phosphate, 2773
Norfloxacin, 2831
Ofloxacin, 2848
Oxymetazoline hydrochloride, 2888
Phenylephrine hydrochloride, 2987
Physostigmine salicylate, 3002
Pilocarpine hydrochloride, 3007
Pilocarpine nitrate, 3007
Polymyxin B sulfate and trimethoprim, 3025
Prednisolone sodium phosphate, 3067
Proparacaine hydrochloride, 3100
Scopolamine hydrobromide, 3221
Silver nitrate, 3231
Sodium chloride, 3247
Sulfacetamide sodium, 3286
Suprofen, 3314
Tetracaine hydrochloride, 3358
Tetrahydrozoline hydrochloride, 3368
Timolol maleate, 3411
Tobramycin, 3421
Tropicamide, 3480
Zinc sulfate, 3551

Ophthalmic suspension
Brinzolamide, 1557
Chloramphenicol and hydrocortisone acetate for, 1722
Dexamethasone, 1907
Fluorometholone, 2197
Gentamicin and prednisolone acetate, 2269
Hydrocortisone acetate, 2346
Natamycin, 2767
Neomycin and polymyxin B sulfates and dexamethasone, 2785
Neomycin and polymyxin B sulfates and hydrocortisone, 2786
Neomycin and polymyxin B sulfates and hydrocortisone acetate, 2787
Neomycin and polymyxin B sulfates and prednisolone acetate, 2789
Neomycin sulfate and hydrocortisone acetate, 2777

Ophthalmic suspension *(continued)*
   Neomycin sulfate and prednisolone acetate, 2790
   Oxytetracycline hydrochloride and hydrocortisone acetate, 2895
   Prednisolone acetate, 3065
   Rimexolone, 3190
   Sulfacetamide sodium and prednisolone acetate, 3288
   Tetracycline hydrochloride, 3364
   Tobramycin and dexamethasone, 3422
   Tobramycin and fluorometholone acetate, 3423

Opium, 2860
   powdered, 2860
   tincture, 2860
Optical
   microscopy ⟨776⟩, 304
   rotation ⟨781⟩, 306
Oracet blue B, 809
   TS, 819

Oral powder
Containing at least three of the following—acetaminophen and (salts of) chlorpheniramine, dextromethorphan, and pseudoephedrine, 1282
Levothyroxine sodium, 2524
Sodium bicarbonate, 3243

Oral solution
Acacia syrup, 1063
Acetaminophen, 1269
Containing at least three of the following—acetaminophen and (salts of) chlorpheniramine, dextromethorphan, and phenylpropanolamine, 1277
Containing at least three of the following—acetaminophen and (salts of) chlorpheniramine, dextromethorphan, and pseudoephedrine, 1283
Acetaminophen and codeine phosphate, 1289
Acetaminophen, dextromethorphan hydrobromide, doxylamine succinate, and pseudoephedrine hydrochloride, 1292
Acetaminophen for effervescent, 1270
Amantadine hydrochloride, 1375
Aminobenzoate potassium for, 1384
Aminocaproic acid, 1387
Aminophylline, 1392
Amprolium, 1422
Aromatic elixir, 1076
Ascorbic acid, 1446
Aspirin effervescent tablets for, 1453
Atenolol, 1462
Benzaldehyde elixir, compound, 1081
Betamethasone, 1516
Bethanechol chloride, 1529
Bromodiphenhydramine hydrochloride, 1561
Bromodiphenhydramine hydrochloride and codeine phosphate, 1562
Brompheniramine maleate, 1563
Brompheniramine maleate and pseudoephedrine sulfate, 1564
Butabarbital sodium, 1578
Caffeine citrate, 1591
Calcium glubionate syrup, 1609
Captopril, 1626
C 13 for, urea, 1643
Cherry syrup, 1111
Chloral hydrate, 1717
Chloramphenicol, 1721
Chlorpheniramine maleate, 1741
Chlorpheniramine maleate and pseudoephedrine hydrochloride, 1745
Chlorpromazine hydrochloride syrup, 1748
Chocolate syrup, 1112
Clindamycin hydrochloride, 1797
Clindamycin palmitate hydrochloride for, 1798
Cloxacillin sodium for, 1832
Cyanocobalamin Co 57, 1835
Cyclosporine, 1871
Cyproheptadine hydrochloride, 1872
Dexamethasone, 1907
Dexamethasone elixir, 1906
Dexbrompheniramine maleate and pseudoephedrine sulfate, 1915
Dexchlorpheniramine maleate, 1916
Dextromethorphan hydrobromide, 1927
Dicyclomine hydrochloride, 1947
Didanosine for, 1949
Digoxin, 1964
Dihydrotachysterol, 1970
Diltiazem hydrochloride, 1974
Dimenhydrinate, 1980
Diphenhydramine hydrochloride, 1989
Diphenoxylate hydrochloride and atropine sulfate, 1990
Docusate sodium syrup, 2008
Dolasetron mesylate, 2010
Doxepin hydrochloride, 2019
Doxylamine succinate, 2027
Dyphylline, 2034
Dyphylline and guaifenesin, 2035
Ephedrine sulfate, 2064
Ergocalciferol, 2072
Ergoloid mesylates, 2075
Ethosuximide, 2123
Ferric ammonium citrate for, 1403
Ferrous gluconate, 2156
Ferrous sulfate, 2157
Ferrous sulfate syrup, 2157
Fluoxetine, 2202
Fluphenazine hydrochloride, 2209
Fluphenazine hydrochloride elixir, 2208
Furosemide, 2240
Glycerin, 2287
Guaifenesin, 2305
Guaifenesin and codeine phosphate, 2306
Haloperidol, 2318
Hydralazine hydrochloride, 2333
Hydroxyzine hydrochloride, 2363
Hyoscyamine sulfate, 2369
Hyoscyamine sulfate elixir, 2368
Ipecac, 2444
Isoniazid, 2459
Isosorbide, 2470
Levocarnitine, 2517
Lincomycin, 2533
Lithium, 2542
Loperamide hydrochloride, 2544
Loratadine, 2549
Magnesium carbonate, citric acid, and potassium citrate for, 2569
Magnesium carbonate and citric acid for, 2569
Manganese chloride for, 2585
Magnesium citrate, 2571
Magnesium citrate for, 2572
Meperidine hydrochloride, 2618
Mesoridazine besylate, 2634
Metaproterenol sulfate, 2638
Methadone hydrochloride, 2649
Methdilazine hydrochloride, 2653
Methenamine, 2655
Methenamine mandelate for, 2657
Methylcellulose, 2673
Metoclopramide, 2692
Metoprolol tartrate, 2698
Mibolerone, 2710
Nafcillin sodium for, 2748
Neomycin sulfate, 2771
Nortriptyline hydrochloride, 2838
Ondansetron, 2857
Orange syrup, 1186
Oxacillin sodium for, 2864
Oxtriphylline, 2872
Oxybutynin chloride, 2876
Oxycodone hydrochloride, 2879
Paromomycin, 2920
Penicillin G potassium for, 2935
Penicillin V potassium for, 2946
Pentobarbital, 2953
Perphenazine, 2964
Perphenazine syrup, 2965
Phenobarbital, 2973
Phenylpropanolamine hydrochloride, 2991
Piperazine citrate syrup, 3014
Polyethylene glycol 3350 and electrolytes for, 3021
Potassium bicarbonate effervescent tablets for, 3028
Potassium bicarbonate and potassium chloride for effervescent, 3028
Potassium bicarbonate and potassium chloride effervescent tablets for, 3029
Potassium bicarbonate, potassium chloride, and potassium citrate effervescent tablets for, 3036
Potassium chloride, 3033
Potassium chloride for, 3033
Potassium citrate and citric acid, 3039
Potassium gluconate, 3040
Potassium gluconate and potassium chloride, 3041
Potassium gluconate and potassium chloride for, 3041
Potassium gluconate and potassium citrate, 3042
Potassium gluconate, potassium citrate, and ammonium chloride, 3042
Potassium iodide, 3044
Potassium and sodium bicarbonates and citric acid effervescent tablets for, 3029
Prednisolone, 3062
Prednisone, 3069
Prochlorperazine, 3085
Promazine hydrochloride, 3094
Promazine hydrochloride syrup, 3094
Promethazine hydrochloride, 3096
Pseudoephedrine hydrochloride, 3126
Pseudoephedrine hydrochloride, carbinoxamine maleate, and dextromethorphan hydrobromide, 3128
Pyridostigmine bromide, 3136
Ranitidine, 3159
Reserpine, 3169
Saccharin sodium, 3209
Secobarbital, 3222
Senna, 3229
Sodium citrate and citric acid, 3248
Sodium fluoride, 3249
Sodium phosphates, 3257
Stavudine for, 3273
Sulfaquinoxaline, 3303
Syrup, 1249
Terpin hydrate, 3348
Terpin hydrate and codeine, 3348
Theophylline, 3374
Theophylline and guaifenesin, 3377
Theophylline sodium glycinate, 3378
Thiamine hydrochloride, 3383
Thiamine mononitrate, 3384
Thioridazine hydrochloride, 3392
Thiothixene hydrochloride, 3397
Tolu balsam syrup, 1252
Triamcinolone diacetate, 3445
Tricitrates, 3453
Trifluoperazine, 3458

Oral solution (continued)
  Trihexyphenidyl hydrochloride, 3464
  Trikates, 3465
  Trimeprazine, 3466
  Triprolidine hydrochloride, 3474
  Triprolidine and pseudoephedrine
    hydrochlorides, 3475
  Valproic acid, 3493
  Vancomycin hydrochloride for, 3501
  Vehicle for, 1257
  Vehicle for, sugar free, 1258
  Verapamil hydrochloride, 3506
  Vitamins with minerals, water-soluble, 1049
  Vitamins, oil- and water-soluble, 1009
  Vitamins with minerals, oil- and water-soluble,
    1016
  Zidovudine, 3541
  Zinc sulfate, 3551

Oral suspension
  Acetaminophen, 1270
  Acetaminophen and codeine phosphate, 1290
  Acyclovir, 1306
  Albendazole, 1310
  Allopurinol, 1325
  Alprazolam, 1328
  Alumina and magnesia, 1336
  Alumina, magnesia, and calcium carbonate,
    1337
  Alumina, magnesia, and simethicone, 1342
  Alumina and magnesium carbonate, 1345
  Alumina and magnesium trisilicate, 1348
  Amoxicillin, 1410
  Amoxicillin and clavulanate potassium for,
    1412
  Amoxicillin for, 1410
  Amoxicillin tablets for, 1411
  Ampicillin for, 1419
  Ampicillin and probenecid for, 1419
  Atovaquone, 1465
  Azathioprine, 1475
  Azithromycin for, 1479
  Bacampicillin hydrochloride for, 1482
  Baclofen, 1487
  Bethanechol chloride, 1529
  Bismuth subsalicylate, 1542
  Calcium carbonate, 1602
  Calcium and magnesium carbonates, 1607
  Captopril, 1626
  Carbamazepine, 1631
  Cefaclor for, 1661
  Cefadroxil for, 1664
  Cefixime for, 1672
  Cefpodoxime proxetil for, 1690
  Cefprozil for, 1691
  Cefuroxime axetil for, 1699
  Cellulose sodium phosphate for, 1704
  Cephalexin for, 1706
  Cephalexin tablets, 1707
  Cephradine for, 1714
  Chloramphenicol palmitate, 1724
  Chlorothiazide, 1738
  Cholestyramine for, 1757
  Clarithromycin for, 1787
  Clavulanate potassium and amoxicillin for,
    1412
  Clonazepam, 1814
  Colestipol hydrochloride for, 1846
  Colistin sulfate for, 1848
  Demeclocycline, 1888
  Diazoxide, 1937
  Dicloxacillin sodium for, 1945
  Diltiazem hydrochloride, 1975
  Dipyridamole, 1994
  Dolasetron mesylate, 2011
  Doxycycline for, 2023
  Doxycycline calcium, 2023

Erythromycin estolate, 2090
Erythromycin estolate for, 2090
Erythromycin estolate and sulfisoxazole acetyl,
  2091
Erythromycin ethylsuccinate, 2093
Erythromycin ethylsuccinate for, 2094
Erythromycin ethylsuccinate and sulfisoxazole
  acetyl for, 2095
Famotidine for, 2138
Ferumoxsil, 2160
Flucytosine, 2173
Furazolidone, 2238
Ganciclovir, 2257
Griseofulvin, 2302
Hydroxyzine pamoate, 2366
Ibuprofen, 2373
Indomethacin, 2400
Ketoconazole, 2488
Labetalol hydrochloride, 2495
Loracarbef for, 2547
Magaldrate, 2564
Magaldrate and simethicone, 2565
Magnesium carbonate and sodium bicarbonate
  for, 2570
Mebendazole, 2592
Megestrol acetate, 2604
Meloxicam, 2609
Meprobamate, 2624
Methacycline hydrochloride, 2648
Methadone hydrochloride tablets for, 2650
Methenamine mandelate, 2657
Methyldopa, 2674
Metolazone, 2693
Metoprolol tartrate, 2698
Minocycline hydrochloride, 2717
Nalidixic acid, 2751
Naproxen, 2760
Nevirapine, 2796
Nitrofurantoin, 2813
Nystatin, 2841
Nystatin for, 2842
Ondansetron hydrochloride, 2855
Oxfendazole, 2870
Oxytetracycline and nystatin for, 2893
Oxytetracycline calcium, 2893
Penicillin G benzathine, 2931
Penicillin V for, 2944
Penicillin V benzathine, 2945
Phenytoin, 2993
Primidone, 3074
Propoxyphene napsylate, 3110
Psyllium hydrophilic mucilloid for, 3132
Pyrantel pamoate, 3133
Pyrvinium pamoate, 3141
Quinidine sulfate, 3150
Rifampin, 3184
Simethicone, 3233
Sulfadimethoxine, 3293
Sulfamethizole, 3297
Sulfamethoxazole, 3298
Sulfamethoxazole and trimethoprim, 3300
Sulfisoxazole acetyl, 3307
Sumatriptan succinate, 3312
Tetracycline, 3360
Tetracycline hydrochloride, 3364
Thiabendazole, 3380
Thioridazine, 3391
Triflupromazine, 3460
Trisulfapyrimidines, 3477
Vehicle for, 1258
Verapamil hydrochloride, 3506

Orange
  G, 786
  oil, 1185
  peel tincture, sweet, 1185
  spirit, compound, 1185

  syrup, 1186
Orcinol, 786
Ordinary impurities ⟨466⟩, 157
Organic
  nitrogenous bases—identification ⟨181⟩, 126
  nitrogenous bases, salts of ⟨501⟩, 182
  volatile impurities ⟨467⟩, 158
Orphenadrine citrate, 2860
  injection, 2861
Orthophenanthroline, 786
  TS, 819
Osmium tetroxide, 786
Osmolality and osmolarity ⟨785⟩, 307
Otic solution
  acetic acid, 1298
  antipyrine and benzocaine, 1435
  antipyrine, benzocaine and phenylephrine
    hydrochloride, 1436
  benzocaine, 1503
  chloramphenicol, 1721
  gentamicin sulfate and betamethasone valerate,
    2267
  hydrocortisone and acetic acid, 2343
  neomycin and polymyxin B sulfates and
    hydrocortisone, 2786
  polymyxin B sulfate and hydrocortisone, 3025
Otic suspension
  Ciprofloxacin and dexamethasone, 1771
Oxacillin
  injection, 2863
  for injection, 2864
  sodium, 2862
  sodium capsules, 2862
  sodium for oral solution, 2864
Oxalic acid, 786
  tenth-normal (0.1 N), 825
  TS, 819
Oxandrolone, 2865
  tablets, 2865
Oxaprozin, 2867
  tablets, 2868
Oxazepam, 2868
  capsules, 2868
  tablets, 2869
Oxfendazole, 2869
  oral suspension, 2870
Oxidized cellulose, 1702
  regenerated, 1702
Oxprenolol hydrochloride, 2870
  extended-release tablets, 2871
  tablets, 2871
Oxtriphylline, 2872
  delayed-release tablets, 2873
  extended-release tablets, 2873
  oral solution, 2872
  tablets, 2872
Oxybenzone, 2874
  and dioxybenzone cream, 1986
Oxybutynin chloride, 2874
  oral solution, 2876
  tablets, 2876
  tablets, extended-release, 2876
Oxycodone
  terephthalate, 2884
  and acetaminophen capsules, 2882
  and acetaminophen tablets, 2883
  and aspirin tablets, 2883
Oxycodone hydrochloride, 2878
  oral solution, 2879
  tablets, 2879
  extended-release tablets, 2880
3,3′-Oxydipropionitrile, 786
Oxygen, 2886
  93 percent, 2886
  flask combustion ⟨471⟩, 181
  helium certified standard, 786
  O 15 injection, water, 2887

Oxymetazoline hydrochloride, 2887
　nasal solution, 2888
　ophthalmic solution, 2888
Oxymetholone, 2888
　tablets, 2889
Oxymorphone hydrochloride, 2889
　injection, 2890
　suppositories, 2890
Oxyquinoline sulfate, 1186
Oxytetracycline, 2891
　calcium, 2893
　calcium oral suspension, 2893
　for injection, 2894
　hydrochloride, 2894
　hydrochloride capsules, 2894
　hydrochloride and hydrocortisone acetate ophthalmic suspension, 2895
　hydrochloride and hydrocortisone ointment, 2896
　hydrochloride and polymyxin B sulfate ointment, 2896
　hydrochloride and polymyxin B sulfate ophthalmic ointment, 2897
　hydrochloride and polymyxin B sulfate topical powder, 2897
　hydrochloride and polymyxin B sulfate vaginal inserts, 2897
　hydrochloride soluble powder, 2895
　injection, 2892
　and nystatin capsules, 2892
　and nystatin for oral suspension, 2893
　tablets, 2892
Oxytocin, 2897
　injection, 2898
　nasal solution, 2898

P

P 32
　solution, sodium phosphate, 3001
　suspension, chromic phosphate, 3000
Packaging practice—repackaging a single solid oral drug product into a unit-dose container ⟨1146⟩, 609
Packaging—unit-of-use ⟨1136⟩, 607
Packings for high-pressure liquid chromatography, 786
Paclitaxel, 2899
　injection, 2901
Padimate O, 2902
　lotion, 2902
Palladium
　catalyst, 786
　chloride, 786
　chloride TS, buffered, 819
Palladous chloride, 787
Pallida
　echinacea, 931
　extract, powdered echinacea, 932
　powdered echinacea, 932
Palmitic acid, 1187
Palm kernel oil, 1186
Pamabrom, 2902
Pamidronate disodium, 2903
　for injection, 2904
Pancreatic digest of casein, 787
Pancreatin, 787, 2905
　tablets, 2907
Pancrelipase, 2907
　capsules, 2909
　delayed-release capsules, 2909
　tablets, 2909
Pancuronium bromide, 2909
Panthenol, 2910

Papaic digest of soybean meal, 787
Papain, 2911
　tablets for topical solution, 2911
Papaverine hydrochloride, 2912
　injection, 2912
　tablets, 2912
Paper
　lead acetate, 780
　odorless absorbent, 787
　quantitative filter, 793
Para-aminobenzoic acid, 787
Parachlorophenol, 2913
　camphorated, 2913
Paraffin, 1188
　synthetic, 1188
Paraformaldehyde, 787
Paraldehyde, 2914
Paramethasone acetate, 2914
　tablets, 2915
Paregoric, 2915
Paricalcitol, 2916
　injection, 2917
Paromomycin
　oral solution, 2920
　sulfate, 2919
　sulfate capsules, 2919
Paroxetine
　hydrochloride, 2920
　tablets, 2922
Particle size distribution estimation by analytical sieving ⟨786⟩, 308
Particulate matter in injections ⟨788⟩, 311
Particulate matter in ophthalmic solutions ⟨789⟩, 313
Peanut oil, 1188
Pectin, 2923
Pellets
　Estradiol, 2100
Penbutolol sulfate, 2924
　tablets, 2925
Penicillamine, 2925
　capsules, 2927
　tablets, 2928
Penicillin
　G benzathine, 2930
　G benzathine injectable suspension, 2930
　G benzathine oral suspension, 2931
　G benzathine and penicillin G procaine injectable suspension, 2932
　G benzathine tablets, 2931
　G, neomycin, polymyxin B, hydrocortisone acetate, and hydrocortisone sodium succinate topical suspension, 2929
　G potassium, 2933
　G potassium injection, 2934
　G potassium for injection, 2934
　G potassium for oral solution, 2935
　G potassium tablets, 2935
　G procaine, 2936
　G procaine, dihydrostreptomycin sulfate, chlorpheniramine maleate, and dexamethasone injectable suspension, 2939
　G procaine and dihydrostreptomycin sulfate injectable suspension, 2939
　G procaine and dihydrostreptomycin sulfate intramammary infusion, 2938
　G procaine, dihydrostreptomycin sulfate, and prednisolone injectable suspension, 2941
　G procaine injectable suspension, 2937
　G procaine for injectable suspension, 2938
　G procaine intramammary infusion, 2937
　G procaine, neomycin and polymyxin B sulfates, and hydrocortisone acetate topical suspension, 2941
　G procaine and novobiocin sodium intramammary infusion, 2942
　G procaine and penicillin G benzathine injectable suspension, 2932

　G sodium, 2942
　G sodium for injection, 2943
　V, 2943
　V benzathine, 2945
　V benzathine oral suspension, 2945
　V for oral suspension, 2944
　V potassium, 2946
　V potassium for oral solution, 2946
　V potassium tablets, 2947
　V tablets, 2944
Penicillinase, 788
Pentadecane, 788
Pentane, 788
1-Pentanesulfonic acid sodium salt, 788
2-Pentanone, 788
Pentazocine, 2947
　and acetaminophen tablets, 2948
　and aspirin tablets, 2949
　hydrochloride, 2947
　injection, 2951
　and naloxone tablets, 2950
Pentetic acid, 2952
Pentobarbital, 2952
　oral solution, 2953
　sodium, 2954
　sodium capsules, 2955
　sodium injection, 2955
Pentoxifylline, 2956
　extended-release tablets, 2957
People, xi
Peppermint, 1189
　oil, 1189
　spirit, 2957
　water, 1190
Pepsin, 788
　purified, 788
Peptic digest of animal tissue, 788
Peptone, dried, 788
Perchloric acid, 788
　tenth-normal (0.1 N) in dioxane, 825
　tenth-normal (0.1 N) (in glacial acetic acid), 825
　TS, 819
Perflubron, 2959
Perflutren protein-type A microspheres injectable suspension, 2959
Pergolide
　mesylate, 2961
　tablets, 2962
Periodic acid, 788
Perphenazine, 2963
　and amitriptyline hydrochloride tablets, 2965
　injection, 2964
　oral solution, 2964
　syrup, 2965
　tablets, 2965
Pertussis
　immune globulin, 2966
Petrolatum, 2966
　hydrophilic, 2967
　white, 2967
Petroleum benzin, 788
pH ⟨791⟩, 314
Pharmaceutical calculations in prescription compounding ⟨1160⟩, 626
Pharmaceutical compounding
　nonsterile preparations ⟨795⟩, 315
　sterile preparations ⟨797⟩, 319
Pharmaceutical dosage forms ⟨1151⟩, 615
Pharmaceutical stability ⟨1150⟩, 613
Pharmacopeial
　forum, xiii, 5
　harmonization ⟨1196⟩, 659
Phases for gas chromatography, 789
Phase-solubility analysis ⟨1171⟩, 638
Phenacetin, 789
1,10-Phenanthroline, 789
o-Phenanthroline monohydrochloride monohydrate, 789

Phenazopyridine hydrochloride, 2967
  tablets, 2968
Phendimetrazine tartrate, 2968
  capsules, 2969
  tablets, 2970
Phenelzine sulfate, 2970
  tablets, 2971
Pheniramine maleate, 2971
  and naphazoline hydrochloride ophthalmic solution, 2759
Phenmetrazine hydrochloride, 2972
  tablets, 2972
Phenobarbital, 2973
  oral solution, 2973
  sodium, 2974
  sodium injection, 2975
  sodium for injection, 2975
  tablets, 2974
  theophylline and ephedrine hydrochloride tablets, 3375
Phenol, 789, 2975
  alcohol TS, 815
  iron, TS, 818
  liquefied, 2976
  red, 809
  red, sodium, 789
  red TS, 819
  red TS, pH 4.7, 819
  camphorated, topical solution, 2976
  topical gel, camphorated, 2976
  TS, 819
Phenolated
  calamine topical suspension, 1593
Phenoldisulfonic acid TS, 819
Phenolphthalein, 809
  paper, 810
Phenolphthalein TS, 819
Phenolsulfonphthalein, 789, 1190
Phenoxybenzamine hydrochloride, 789, 2977
  capsules, 2977
3-Phenoxybenzoic acid, 789
2-Phenoxyethanol, 789
Phenoxyethanol, 1191
Phensuximide, 2978
  capsules, 2978
Phentermine hydrochloride, 2979
  capsules, 2979
  tablets, 2980
Phentolamine mesylate, 2981
  for injection, 2981
Phenyl
  ether, 789
  isocyanate, 789
2-Phenylacetamide, 789
Phenylalanine, 2982
dl-Phenylalanine, 789
Phenylbutazone, 2983
  boluses, 2983
  injection, 2984
  tablets, 2984
p-Phenylenediamine
  dihydrochloride, 789
  hydrochloride, 789
o-Phenylenediamine dihydrochloride, 789
Phenylephrine
  bitartrate, 2985
  bitartrate and isoproterenol hydrochloride inhalation aerosol, 2465
  hydrochloride, 2985
  hydrochloride, antipyrine, and benzocaine otic solution, 1436
  hydrochloride injection, 2986
  hydrochloride nasal jelly, 2987
  hydrochloride nasal solution, 2987
  hydrochloride ophthalmic solution, 2987
Phenylethyl alcohol, 2988
Phenylglycine, 789

Phenylhydrazine, 789
  acetate TS, 819
  hydrochloride, 789
  sulfuric acid TS, 819
Phenylmercuric
  acetate, 1191
  nitrate, 1192
Phenylmethylsulfonyl fluoride, 789
3-Phenylphenol, 789
Phenylpropanolamine
  bitartrate, 2988
  chlorpheniramine, dextromethorphan (salts of) and acetaminophen, capsules containing at least three of the following, 1275
  chlorpheniramine, dextromethorphan (salts of) and acetaminophen, oral solution containing at least three of the following, 1277
  chlorpheniramine, dextromethorphan (salts of) and acetaminophen, tablets containing at least three of the following, 1278
  hydrochloride, 2989
  hydrochloride capsules, 2990
  hydrochloride and chlorpheniramine maleate extended-release capsules, 1742
  hydrochloride and chlorpheniramine maleate extended-release tablets, 1743
  hydrochloride extended-release capsules, 2990
  hydrochloride extended-release tablets, 2992
  hydrochloride oral solution, 2991
  hydrochloride tablets, 2991
Phenyltoloxamine citrate, 2992
Phenytoin, 2993
  chewable tablets, 2995
  oral suspension, 2993
  sodium, 2995
  sodium capsules, extended, 2996
  sodium capsules, prompt, 2999
  sodium injection, 2999
  tablets, 2994
pH indicator paper, short-range, 810
Phloroglucinol, 789
  TS, 819
Phosphatase enzyme, alkaline, 789
Phosphate
  acidulated, and sodium fluoride topical solution, 3250
  buffer, 814
  P 32 solution, sodium, 3001
  P 32 suspension, chromic, 3000
  in reagents, 750
Phosphatic enzyme, 789
  TS, 819
Phosphomolybdic acid, 789
  TS, 819
Phosphoric acid, 789, 1192
  diluted, 1192
  and sodium fluoride gel, 3250
Phosphorus
  pentoxide, 790
  red, 790
Phosphotungstic acid, 790
  TS, 819
o-Phthalaldehyde, 790
Phthalazine, 790
Phthalic
  acid, 790
  anhydride, 790
Phthalimide, 790
Physostigmine, 3001
  salicylate, 3001
  salicylate injection, 3002
  salicylate ophthalmic solution, 3002
  sulfate, 3003
  sulfate ophthalmic ointment, 3003
Phytonadione, 3003
  injectable emulsion, 3004
  tablets, 3004
2-Picoline, 790

Picrate TS, alkaline, 819
Picric acid, 790
  TS, 819
Picrolonic acid, 790
Pilocarpine, 3005
  hydrochloride, 3006
  hydrochloride ophthalmic solution, 3007
  nitrate, 3007
  nitrate ophthalmic solution, 3007
  ocular system, 3006
Pimozide, 3008
  tablets, 3008
Pindolol, 3009
  tablets, 3010
Pipemidic acid, 790
Piperacillin, 3011
  for injection, 3013
  sodium, 3012
Piperazine, 790, 3013
  citrate, 3014
  citrate syrup, 3014
  citrate tablets, 3014
Piperidine, 790
Piroxicam, 3014
  capsules, 3015
  cream, 3015
Plantago seed, 3016
Plasma protein fraction, 3017
Plasma spectrochemistry ⟨730⟩, 287
Platelet concentrate, 3017
Platelets, 1554
Platinic
  chloride, 790
  chloride TS, 819
Platinum
  cobalt TS, 819
Plicamycin, 3018
  for injection, 3018
Podophyllum, 3019
  resin, 3019
  resin topical solution, 3019
Polacrilin potassium, 1193
Polarography ⟨801⟩, 337
Policy
  USP, xxiv
Poliovirus vaccine inactivated, 3020
Poloxalene, 3020
Poloxamer, 1194
Polycarbophil, 3021
  calcium, 1618
Polydextrose, 1195
Polydimethylsiloxane, viscosity 0.65 centistokes, 790
Polyethylene
  glycol, 1197
  glycol 200, 790
  glycol 600, 790
  glycol 20,000, 790
  glycol 3350 and electrolytes for oral solution, 3021
  glycol monomethyl ether, 1199
  glycol ointment, 1199
  oxide, 1201
Polyisobutylene, 1202
Polymyxin B
  for injection, 3023
  and neomycin sulfates, bacitracin, and hydrocortisone acetate ointment, 2781
  and neomycin sulfates, bacitracin, and hydrocortisone acetate ophthalmic ointment, 2781
  and neomycin sulfates, bacitracin, and lidocaine ointment, 2781
  and neomycin sulfates and bacitracin ointment, 2780
  and neomycin sulfates and bacitracin ophthalmic ointment, 2780

Polymyxin B *(continued)*
  and neomycin sulfates, bacitracin zinc, and hydrocortisone acetate ophthalmic ointment, 2783
  and neomycin sulfates, bacitracin zinc, and hydrocortisone ointment, 2782
  and neomycin sulfates, bacitracin zinc, and hydrocortisone ophthalmic ointment, 2783
  and neomycin sulfates, bacitracin zinc, and lidocaine ointment, 2784
  and neomycin sulfates and bacitracin zinc ointment, 2782
  and neomycin sulfates and bacitracin zinc ophthalmic ointment, 2782
  and neomycin sulfates and dexamethasone ophthalmic ointment, 2784
  and neomycin sulfates and dexamethasone ophthalmic suspension, 2785
  and neomycin sulfates, gramidicin, and hydrocortisone acetate cream, 2786
  and neomycin sulfates and gramidicin cream, 2785
  and neomycin sulfates and gramidicin ophthalmic solution, 2785
  and neomycin sulfates and hydrocortisone acetate cream, 2787
  and neomycin sulfates and hydrocortisone acetate ophthalmic suspension, 2787
  and neomycin sulfates and hydrocortisone ophthalmic suspension, 2786
  and neomycin sulfates and hydrocortisone otic solution, 2786
  and neomycin sulfates and hydrocortisone otic suspension, 2787
  and neomycin sulfates and lidocaine cream, 2788
  and neomycin sulfates ophthalmic ointment, 2780
  and neomycin sulfates ophthalmic solution, 2780
  and neomycin sulfates, penicillin G procaine, and hydrocortisone acetate topical suspension, 2941
  and neomycin sulfates and pramoxine hydrochloride cream, 2788
  and neomycin sulfates and prednisolone acetate ophthalmic suspension, 2789
  and neomycin sulfates solution for irrigation, 2779
  and neomycin sulfates cream, 2779
  penicillin G, neomycin, hydrocortisone acetate, and hydrocortisone sodium succinate topical suspension, 2929
  sulfate, 3023
  sulfate and bacitracin topical aerosol, 1484
  sulfate and bacitracin zinc ointment, 1486
  sulfate and bacitracin zinc ophthalmic ointment, 1486
  sulfate and bacitracin zinc topical aerosol, 3024
  sulfate and bacitracin zinc topical powder, 3024
  sulfate, chloramphenicol, and hydrocortisone acetate ophthalmic ointment chloramphenicol, 1723
  sulfate and chloramphenicol ophthalmic ointment, 1722
  sulfate and hydrocortisone otic solution, 3025
  sulfate and oxytetracycline hydrochloride ointment, 2896
  sulfate and oxytetracycline hydrochloride ophthalmic ointment, 2897
  sulfate and oxytetracycline hydrochloride topical powder, 2897
  sulfate and oxytetracycline hydrochloride vaginal inserts, 2897
  sulfate and trimethoprim ophthalmic solution, 3025
Polyoxyethylene (20) sorbitan monolaurate, 790
Polyoxyethylene (23) lauryl ether, 790

Polyoxyl
  10 oleyl ether, 1203
  20 cetostearyl ether, 1204
  35 castor oil, 1205
  40 hydrogenated castor oil, 1205
  40 stearate, 1205
  lauryl ether, 1206
  oleate, 1206
  stearyl ether, 1206
Polysacchloride molecular weight standards, 790
Polysorbate
  20, 1208
  40, 1208
  60, 1208
  80, 1208
Polystyrene
  cation-exchange resin, 790
Polytef, 790
Polyvinyl
  acetate phthalate, 1208
  alcohol, 791, 3026
Potash, sulfurated, 3026
Potassium
  acetate, 791, 3026
  acetate injection, 3027
  acetate TS, 819
  alginate, 1209
  alum, 791, 1336
  arsenite, tenth-normal (0.1 N), 825
  benzoate, 1210
  bicarbonate, 791, 3027
  bicarbonate effervescent tablets for oral solution, 3028
  bicarbonate, potassium chloride, and potassium citrate effervescent tablets for oral solution, 3036
  bicarbonate and potassium chloride for effervescent oral solution, 3028
  bicarbonate and potassium chloride effervescent tablets for oral solution, 3029
  biphosphate, 791
  biphthalate, 791
  bismuth iodide TS, 819
  bisulfate, 791
  bitartrate, 3030
  bromate, 791
  bromate, tenth-normal (0.1 N), 825
  bromide, 791, 3030
  bromide-bromate, tenth-normal (0.1 N), 826
  carbonate, 791, 3031
  carbonate, anhydrous, 791
  carbonate TS, 819
  chlorate, 791
  chloride, 791, 3031
  chloride in dextrose injection, 3034
  chloride in dextrose and sodium chloride injection, 3035
  chloride extended-release capsules, 3032
  chloride extended-release tablets, 3034
  chloride for injection concentrate, 3033
  chloride in lactated Ringer's and dextrose injection, 3036
  chloride oral solution, 3033
  chloride for oral solution, 3033
  chloride, potassium bicarbonate, and potassium citrate effervescent tablets for oral solution, 3036
  chloride and potassium bicarbonate for effervescent oral solution, 3028
  chloride and potassium bicarbonate effervescent tablets for oral solution, 3029
  chloride and potassium gluconate for oral solution, 3041
  chloride and potassium gluconate oral solution, 3041
  chloride in sodium chloride injection, 3037
  chloroplatinate, 791
  chromate, 791

  chromate TS, 819
  citrate, 3038
  citrate and citric acid oral solution, 3039
  citrate extended-release tablets, 3038
  citrate, magnesium carbonate, and citric acid for oral solution, 2569
  citrate, potassium chloride, and potassium bicarbonate effervescent tablets for oral solution, 3036
  citrate, potassium gluconate, and ammonium chloride oral solution, 3042
  citrate and potassium gluconate oral solution, 3042
  cyanide, 791
  dichromate, 791
  dichromate, tenth-normal (0.1 N), 826
  dichromate TS, 819
  ferricyanide, 791
  ferricyanide TS, 819
  ferricyanide, twentieth-molar (0.05 M), 826
  ferrocyanide, 791
  ferrocyanide TS, 819
  gluconate, 3040
  gluconate oral solution, 3040
  gluconate and potassium chloride oral solution, 3041
  gluconate and potassium chloride for oral solution, 3041
  gluconate, potassium citrate, and ammonium chloride oral solution, 3042
  gluconate and potassium citrate oral solution, 3042
  gluconate tablets, 3041
  guaiacolsulfonate, 3043
  hyaluronate, 791
  hydrogen sulfate, 791
  hydroxide, 791, 1210
  hydroxide, alcoholic, half-normal (0.5 N), 826
  hydroxide, alcoholic, tenth-molar (0.1 M), 826
  hydroxide methanolic, tenth-normal (0.1 N), 826
  hydroxide, normal (1 N), 826
  hydroxide TS, 819
  hydroxide TS, alcoholic, 820
  iodate, 791
  iodate, twentieth-molar (0.05 M), 826
  iodide, 791, 3043
  iodide delayed-release tablets, 3044
  iodide and iodine TS 1, 818
  iodide and iodine TS 2, 818
  iodide oral solution, 3044
  iodide and starch TS, 820
  iodide tablets, 3044
  iodide TS, 820
  iodoplatinate TS, 820
  metabisulfite, 1210
  metaphosphate, 1210
  nitrate, 791, 3044
  nitrate solution, 3045
  nitrite, 791
  perchlorate, 791, 3046
  perchlorate capsules, 3046
  periodate, 791
  permanganate, 791, 3046
  permanganate, tenth-normal (0.1 N), 826
  permanganate TS, 820
  persulfate, 791
  phosphate, dibasic, 791, 3047
  phosphate, monobasic, 791, 1211
  phosphate, tribasic, 792
  phosphates injection, 3047
  pyroantimonate, 792
  pyroantimonate TS, 820
  pyrophosphate, 792
  pyrosulfate, 792
  and sodium bicarbonates and citric acid effervescent tablets for oral solution, 3029
  sodium tartrate, 792, 3048

Potassium *(continued)*
  sorbate, 1211
  sulfate, 792
  sulfate TS, 820
  tellurite, 792
  thiocyanate, 792
  thiocyanate TS, 820
Potato starch, 792, 1240
Povidone, 3048
Povidone-iodine, 3049
  cleansing solution, 3050
  ointment, 3050
  topical aerosol, 3050
  topical solution, 3050

Powder

Absorbable dusting, 2031
Ampicillin soluble, 1418
Amprolium soluble, 1422
Bacitracin methylene disalicylate soluble, 1485
Bacitracin zinc soluble, 1485
Chlortetracycline and sulfamethazine bisulfates soluble, 1750
Chlortetracycline hydrochloride soluble, 1751
Compound clioquinol topical, 1803
Cromolyn sodium inhalation, 1856
Levothyroxine sodium oral, 2524
Lincomycin hydrochloride soluble, 2533
Methylbenzethonium chloride topical, 2672
Miconazole nitrate topical, 2713
Neomycin sulfate, isoflupredone acetate, and tetracaine hydrochloride topical, 2778
Nystatin topical, 2841
Oral, containing at least three of the following—acetaminophen and (salts of) chlorpheniramine, dextromethorphan, and pseudoephedrine, 1282
Oxytetracycline hydrochloride and polymyxin B sulfate topical, 2897
Oxytetracycline hydrochloride soluble, 2895
Polymyxin B sulfate and bacitracin zinc topical, 3024
Sodium bicarbonate oral, 3243
Sulfadimethoxine soluble, 3293
Tetracycline hydrochloride soluble, 3363
Tolnaftate topical, 3434

Powder flow ⟨1174⟩, 639
Powder fineness ⟨811⟩, 339
Powdered
  American ginseng, 952
  American ginseng extract, 953
  Asian ginseng, 956
  Asian ginseng extract, 956
  cellulose, 1107
  Black cohosh, 910
  Black cohosh extract, 911
  digitalis, 1960
  Echinacea angustifolia, 930
  Echinacea angustifolia extract, 930
  Echinacea pallida, 932
  Echinacea pallida extract, 932
  Echinacea purpurea, 936
  Echinacea purpurea extract, 936
  eleuthero, 938
  eleuthero extract, 938
  feverfew, 939
  garlic, 941
  garlic extract, 942
  ginger, 945
  Ginkgo extract, 949
  goldenseal, 962
  goldenseal extract, 963
  hawthorn leaf with flower, 965
  horse chestnut, 966
  horse chestnut, extract, 966
  ipecac, 2444
  licorice, 967
  licorice extract, 967
  milk thistle, 980
  milk thistle extract, 980
  stinging nettle, 986
  stinging nettle extract, 986
  opium, 2860
  rauwolfia serpentina, 3163
  saw palmetto, 994
  St. John's wort, 991
  St. John's wort extract, 992
  valerian, 1001
  valerian extract, 1001
  zinc chloride, anhydrous, 808
Pralidoxime
  chloride, 3051
  chloride for injection, 3051
Pramoxine
  hydrochloride, 3052
  hydrochloride cream, 3052
  hydrochloride jelly, 3053
  hydrochloride and neomycin and polymyxin B sulfates cream, 2788
Pravastatin sodium, 3053
  tablets, 3055
Praziquantel, 3056
  tablets, 3057
Prazosin hydrochloride, 3057
  capsules, 3058
Prednicarbate, 3059
  cream, 3059
  ointment, 3060
Prednisolone, 3061
  acetate, 3063
  acetate and gentamicin ophthalmic ointment, 2268
  acetate and gentamicin ophthalmic suspension, 2269
  acetate injectable suspension, 3064
  acetate and neomycin and polymyxin B sulfates ophthalmic suspension, 2789
  acetate, neomycin sulfate, and sulfacetamide sodium ophthalmic ointment, 2791
  acetate and neomycin sulfate ointment, 2789
  acetate and neomycin sulfate ophthalmic ointment, 2789
  acetate and neomycin sulfate ophthalmic suspension, 2790
  acetate ophthalmic suspension, 3065
  acetate and sulfacetamide sodium ophthalmic ointment, 3287
  acetate and sulfacetamide sodium ophthalmic suspension, 3288
  and chloramphenicol ophthalmic ointment, 1723
  cream, 3062
  hemisuccinate, 3065
  oral solution, 3062
  penicillin G procaine, and dihydrostreptomycin sulfate injectable suspension, 2941
  sodium phosphate, 3065
  sodium phosphate injection, 3066
  sodium phosphate and neomycin sulfate ophthalmic ointment, 2790
  sodium phosphate ophthalmic solution, 3067
  sodium succinate for injection, 3067
  tablets, 3063
  tebutate, 3067
  tebutate injectable suspension, 3068
  tetracycline hydrochloride and novobiocin sodium tablets, 3366
Prednisone, 3068
  injectable suspension, 3069
  oral solution, 3069
  tablets, 3070
Preface
  and mission, v

Prescribing and dispensing, xvii, 9
Prescription balances and volumetric apparatus ⟨1176⟩, 642
Preservation, packaging, storage, and labeling, xvii, 9
Prilocaine, 3070
  and epinephrine injection, 3072
  hydrochloride, 3071
  hydrochloride injection, 3071
  and lidocaine cream, 2530
Primaquine phosphate, 3073
  tablets, 3073
Primidone, 3073
  oral suspension, 3074
  tablets, 3074
Probenecid, 3075
  and ampicillin for oral suspension, 1419
  and colchicine tablets, 3076
  tablets, 3075
Probucol, 3077
  tablets, 3078
Procainamide hydrochloride, 3078
  capsules, 3079
  extended-release tablets, 3080
  injection, 3079
  tablets, 3080
Procaine
  hydrochloride, 3082
  hydrochloride and epinephrine injection, 3083
  hydrochloride injection, 3082
  and propoxycaine hydrochlorides and levonordefrin injection, 3103
  and propoxycaine hydrochlorides and norepinephrine bitartrate injection, 3104
  and tetracaine hydrochlorides and levonordefrin injection, 3083
Procarbazine hydrochloride, 3084
  capsules, 3084
Prochlorperazine, 3085
  edisylate, 3086
  edisylate injection, 3087
  maleate, 3087
  maleate tablets, 3087
  oral solution, 3085
  suppositories, 3086
Procyclidine hydrochloride, 3088
  tablets, 3088
Progesterone, 3089
  injectable suspension, 3091
  injection, 3089
  intrauterine contraceptive system, 3090
  vaginal suppositories, 3091
Proline, 3092
Promazine hydrochloride, 3093
  injection, 3094
  oral solution, 3094
  syrup, 3094
  tablets, 3095
Promethazine hydrochloride, 3095
  injection, 3095
  oral solution, 3096
  suppositories, 3096
  tablets, 3097
Propafenone hydrochloride, 3098
Propane, 1212
Propantheline bromide, 3098
  tablets, 3099
Proparacaine hydrochloride, 3100
  and fluorescein sodium ophthalmic solution, 2191
  ophthalmic solution, 3100
Propionaldehyde, 792
Propionic
  acid, 1212
  anhydride, 792
Propiophenone, 792
Propofol, 3101

Propoxycaine
  hydrochloride, 3103
  and procaine hydrochlorides and levonordefrin injection, 3103
  and procaine hydrochlorides and norepinephrine bitartrate injection, 3104
Propoxyphene
  hydrochloride, 3105
  hydrochloride and acetaminophen tablets, 3106
  hydrochloride, aspirin, and caffeine capsules, 3107
  hydrochloride capsules, 3106
  napsylate, 3109
  napsylate and acetaminophen tablets, 3111
  napsylate and aspirin tablets, 3112
  napsylate oral suspension, 3110
  napsylate tablets, 3110
Propranolol hydrochloride, 3113
  extended-release capsules, 3114
  and hydrochlorothiazide extended-release capsules, 3116
  and hydrochlorothiazide tablets, 3117
  injection, 3115
  tablets, 3115
iso-Propyl alcohol, 792
n-Propyl alcohol, 792
Propyl gallate, 1212
Propylamine hydrochloride, 792
Propylene
  carbonate, 1213
  glycol, 3119
  glycol alginate, 1213
  glycol dilaurate, 1214
  glycol monolaurate, 1214
  glycol monostearate, 1215
Propylhexedrine, 3119
  inhalant, 3120
Propyliodone, 3120
  injectable oil suspension, 3120
Propylparaben, 1216
  sodium, 1217
Propylthiouracil, 3121
  tablets, 3121
Protamine sulfate, 3122
  injection, 3122
  for injection, 3122
Protein
  biological adequacy test ⟨141⟩, 122
  hydrolysate injection, 3123
  molecular weight standard, 792
  standard solution (8 g/dL), 792
Protocatechuic acid, 792
Protriptyline hydrochloride, 3124
  tablets, 3124
Pseudoephedrine
  chlorpheniramine, dextromethorphan (salts of), and acetaminophen, capsules containing at least three of the following, 1280
  chlorpheniramine, dextromethorphan (salts of), and acetaminophen, oral powder containing at least three of the following, 1282
  chlorpheniramine, dextromethorphan (salts of), and acetaminophen, oral solution containing at least three of the following, 1283
  chlorpheniramine, dextromethorphan (salts of) and acetaminophen, tablets containing at least three of the following, 1285
  and diphenhydramine capsules, 1989
  hydrochloride, 3125
  hydrochloride, acetaminophen, dextromethorphan hydrobromide, and doxylamine succinate oral solution, 1292
  hydrochloride, acetaminophen, and diphenhydramine hydrochloride tablets, 1294
  hydrochloride and acetaminophen tablets, 1295
  hydrochloride, carbinoxamine maleate, and dextromethorphan hydrobromide oral solution, 3128

hydrochloride and chlorpheniramine maleate extended-release capsules, 1744
hydrochloride and chlorpheniramine maleate oral solution, 1745
hydrochloride extended-release capsules, 3125
hydrochloride extended-release tablets, 3127
hydrochloride, guaifenesin, and dextromethorphan hydrobromide capsules, 2308
hydrochloride and guaifenesin capsules, 2307
hydrochloride and ibuprofen tablets, 2375
hydrochloride oral solution, 3126
hydrochloride tablets, 3126
hydrochloride and fexofenadine hydrochloride extended-release tablets, 2164
sulfate, 3129
sulfate and brompheniramine maleate oral solution, 1564
sulfate and dexbrompheniramine maleate oral solution, 1915
and triprolidine hydrochlorides oral solution, 3475
and triprolidine hydrochlorides tablets, 3476
Psyllium
  hemicellulose, 3129
  husk, 3131
  hydrophilic mucilloid for oral suspension, 3132
5,800, 23,700, and 100,000 Molecular Weight (MW) Pullulan Standards, 784
Pumice, 792, 3132
Pure steam, 3525
Purine, 792
Purpurea
  extract, powdered echinacea, 936
  powdered echinacea, 936
  root, echinacea, 934
Putrescine dihydrochloride, 792
Pygeum, 987
  capsules, 989
  extract, 988
Pyrantel pamoate, 3132
  oral suspension, 3133
Pyrazinamide, 3134
  rifampin, isoniazid, and ethambutol hydrochloride tablets, 3187
  rifampin and isoniazid tablets, 3186
  tablets, 3134
Pyrazole, 792
Pyrene, 792
Pyrethrum extract, 3135
Pyridine, 792
  dried, 792
Pyridine-pyrazolone TS, 820
Pyridostigmine bromide, 3135
  injection, 3136
  oral solution, 3136
  tablets, 3136
Pyridoxal
  hydrochloride, 792
  5-phosphate, 792
Pyridoxamine dihydrochloride, 792
Pyridoxine hydrochloride, 3137
  injection, 3137
  tablets, 3138
1-(2-Pyridylazo)-2-naphthol, 792
3-(2-Pyridyl)-5,6-di(2-furyl)-1,2,4-triazine-5′,5″-disulfonic acid, disodium salt, 793
Pyrilamine maleate, 3138
  tablets, 3139
Pyrimethamine, 3140
  and sulfadoxine tablets, 3295
  tablets, 3140
Pyrogallol, 793
  TS, alkaline, 820
Pyrogen test ⟨151⟩, 123
Pyroxylin, 3140
Pyrrole, 793
Pyruvic acid, 793

Pyrvinium pamoate, 3141
  oral suspension, 3141
  tablets, 3142

Q

Quality assurance in pharmaceutical compounding ⟨1163⟩, 634
Quality of biotechnological products:
  analysis of the expression construct in cells used for production of r-DNA derived protein products ⟨1048⟩, 449
  stability testing of biotechnological/biological products ⟨1049⟩, 450
Quantitative filter paper, 793
Quazepam, 3142
  tablets, 3142
Quinaldine red, 809
  TS, 820
Quinapril
  hydrochloride, 3143
  tablets, 3144
Quinhydrone, 793
Quinidine gluconate, 3146
  extended-release tablets, 3147
  injection, 3146
Quinidine sulfate, 3148
  capsules, 3149
  oral suspension, 3150
  tablets, 3150
  extended-release tablets, 3151
Quinine sulfate, 3151
  capsules, 3152
  tablets, 3153
Quinone, 793
  TS, 820

R

Rabies
  immune globulin, 3153
  vaccine, 3154
Racemic
  calcium pantothenate, 1616
Racepinephrine, 3154
  hydrochloride, 3155
  inhalation solution, 3154
Raclopride
  C 11 injection, 1641
Radioactivity ⟨821⟩, 340

Radiopharmaceuticals
C 11, carbon monoxide, 1638
C 11, flumazenil injection, 1639
C 11, mespiperone injection, 1640
C 11, methionine injection, 1640
C 11, raclopride injection, 1641
C 11, sodium acetate injection, 1642
C 13, urea, 1643
C 13, urea for oral solution, 1643
C 14, urea capsules, 1643
Cr 51, sodium chromate injection, 1758
Cr 51, chromium edetate injection, 1759
Co 57, cyanocobalamin capsules, 1834
Co 57, cyanocobalamin oral solution, 1835
Co 58, cyanocobalamin capsules, 1835

Radiopharmaceuticals (continued)
F 18, fludeoxyglucose injection, 2192
F 18, fluorodopa injection, 2193
F 18, sodium fluoride injection, 2195
Ga 67 injection, gallium citrate, 2255
Indium In 111 capromab pendetide injection, 2391
Indium In 111 chloride solution, 2391
Indium In 111 ibritumomab tiuxetan injection, 2393
Indium In 111 oxyquinoline solution, 2393
Indium In 111 pentetate injection, 2394
Indium In 111 pentetreotide injection, 2394
Indium In 111 satumomab pendetide injection, 2395
I 123, iobenguane injection, 2415
I 123, iodohippurate sodium injection, 2416
I 123, sodium iodide capsules, 2417
I 123, sodium iodide solution, 2417
I 125, iodinated albumin injection, 2418
I 125, iothalamate sodium injection, 2418
I 131, iodinated albumin aggregated injection, 2419
I 131, iodinated albumin injection, 2419
I 131, iobenguane injection, 2416
I 131, iodohippurate sodium injection, 2420
I 131, rose bengal sodium injection, 2420
I 131, sodium iodide capsules, 2421
I 131, sodium iodide solution, 2421
Krypton Kr 81m, 2492
N 13, ammonia injection, 2816
O 15 injection, water, 2887
P 32, chromic phosphate suspension, 3000
P 32, sodium phosphate solution, 3001
Rubidium chloride Rb 82 injection, 3206
Samarium Sm 153 lexidronam injection, 3215
Sr 89 injection, strontium chloride, 3276
Technetium Tc 99m albumin aggregated injection, 3324
Technetium Tc 99m albumin colloid injection, 3325
Technetium Tc 99m albumin injection, 3323
Technetium Tc 99m apcitide injection, 3326
Technetium Tc 99m arcitumomab injection, 3327
Technetium Tc 99m bicisate injection, 3327
Technetium Tc 99m depreotide injection, 3328
Technetium Tc 99m disofenin injection, 3328
Technetium Tc 99m etidronate injection, 3329
Technetium Tc 99m exametazime injection, 3329
Technetium Tc 99m gluceptate injection, 3331
Technetium Tc 99m lidofenin injection, 3332
Technetium Tc 99m mebrofenin injection, 3333
Technetium Tc 99m medronate injection, 3334
Technetium Tc 99m mertiatide injection, 3334
Technetium Tc 99m nofetumomab merpentan injection, 3335
Technetium Tc 99m oxidronate injection, 3335
Technetium Tc 99m pentetate injection, 3336
Technetium Tc 99m pertechnetate injection, sodium, 3336
Technetium Tc 99m pyrophosphate injection, 3337
Technetium Tc 99m (pyro- and trimeta-) phosphates injection, 3338
Technetium Tc 99m red blood cells injection, 3338
Technetium Tc 99m sestamibi injection, 3339
Technetium Tc 99m succimer injection, 3340
Technetium Tc 99m sulfur colloid injection, 3340
Technetium Tc 99m tetrofosmin injection, 3341
Thallous chloride Tl 201 injection, 3370
Xenon Xe 127, 3529
Xenon Xe 133, 3530
Xenon Xe 133 injection, 3530

Yttrium Y 90 ibritumomab tiuxetan injection, 3537

Radiopharmaceuticals for positron emission tomography—compounding ⟨823⟩, 347
Raman spectroscopy ⟨1120⟩, 599
Ramipril, 3156
Ranitidine
  hydrochloride, 3157
  injection, 3158
  oral solution, 3159
  in sodium chloride injection, 3160
  tablets, 3160
Rapeseed oil
  Fully hydrogenated, 1217
  Superglycerinated fully hydrogenated, 1218
Rat tail collagen, 766
Rauwolfia serpentina, 3161
  powdered, 3163
  tablets, 3163
Rayon, 793
  purified, 3163
Rb 82
  injection, rubidium chloride, 3206
Readily carbonizable substances test ⟨271⟩, 137
Reagent
  specifications, 748
  standards, xiii, 5
Reagents
  arsenic in, 748
  boiling or distilling range for, 748
  chloride in, 749
  flame photometry for, 749
  general tests for, 748
  heavy metals in, 750
  insoluble matter in, 750
  loss on drying for, 750
  nitrate in, 750
  nitrogen compounds in, 750
  phosphate in, 750
  reference, xiii, 5
  residue on ignition in, 750
  sulfate in, 751
Rectal solution
  Aminophylline, 1393
  Sodium phosphates, 3257
Red
  80, direct, 793
  phosphorus, 793
Red-cell lysing agent, 793
Reference
  reagents, xiii, 5
  standards, USP, xiii, 5
  standards USP ⟨11⟩, 37
Reference tables, 831
  Alcoholometric, 900
  Atomic weights, 895
  Container specifications for capsules and tablets, 831
  Description and relative solubility of USP and NF articles, 840
  Intrinsic viscosity table, 902
  Relative atomic masses and half-lives of selected radionuclides, 898
  Solubilities, 886
  Thermometric equivalents, 905
Refractive index ⟨831⟩, 351
Rehydration salts, oral, 3163
Relative atomic masses and half-lives of selected radionuclides, 898
Repackaging into single-unit containers and unit-dose containers for nonsterile solid and liquid dosage forms ⟨681⟩, 258
Repaglinide, 3166
  tablets, 3166
Resazurin (sodium), 793

Reserpine, 3168
  and chlorothiazide tablets, 3170
  hydralazine hydrochloride and hydrochlorothiazide tablets, 3172
  and hydrochlorothiazide tablets, 3174
  injection, 3168
  oral solution, 3169
  tablets, 3169
Residual solvents ⟨467⟩, 170
Residue on ignition ⟨281⟩, 137
Residue on ignition in reagents, 750

Resin
Anion-exchange, chloromethylated polystyrene-divinylbenzene, 755
Anion-exchange, 50- to 100-mesh, styrene-divinylbenzene, 755
Anion-exchange, strong, lightly cross-linked, in the chloride form, 755
Capsicum oleoresin, 1625
Carboxylate (sodium form) cation-exchange (50- to 100-mesh), 763
Cation-exchange, 763
Cation-exchange, carboxylate (sodium form) 50- to 100-mesh, 763
Cation-exchange, polystyrene, 763
Cation-exchange, styrene-divinylbenzene, 763
Cation-exchange, styrene-divinylbenzene, strongly acidic, 764
Cation-exchange, sulfonic acid, 764
Chloromethylated polysterene-divinylbenzene anion-exchange, 765
Cholestyramine, 1756
Ion-exchange, 779
Podophyllum, 3019
Podophyllum topical solution, 3019
Polystyrene cation-exchange, 790
Styrene-divinylbenzene anion-exchange, 50- to 100-mesh, 801
Styrene-divinylbenzene cation-exchange, strongly acidic, 801
Sulfonic acid cation-exchange, 802

Resorcinol, 3176
  monoacetate, 3177
  ointment, compound, 3176
  and sulfur topical suspension, 3176
  TS, 820
Retinyl palmitate, 793
Reverse transcriptase, 793
Revisions appearing in *NF26* that were not included in *NF 25*, including supplements, 1056
Revisions appearing in *USP31* that were not included in *USP30*, including supplements, xxix
Rhodamine 6G, 793
Rhodamine B, 793
Ribavirin, 3177
  for inhalation solution, 3178
Riboflavin, 3178
  assay ⟨481⟩, 182
  injection, 3179
  5′-phosphate sodium, 3179
  tablets, 3179
Ribonuclease inhibitor, 793
Rifabutin, 3181
  capsules, 3181
Rifampin, 3182
  capsules, 3183
  for injection, 3184
  and isoniazid capsules, 3185
  isoniazid, pyrazinamide, and ethambutol hydrochloride tablets, 3187
  isoniazid, and pyrazinamide tablets, 3186
  oral suspension, 3184

Rimantadine hydrochloride, 3188
    tablets, 3189
Rimexolone, 3190
    ophthalmic suspension, 3190
Ringer's
    and dextrose injection, 3191
    and dextrose injection, half-strength lactated, 3194
    and dextrose injection, lactated, 3193
    and dextrose injection, modified lactated, 3195
    injection, 3190
    injection, lactated, 3192
    irrigation, 3196
    lactated, and dextrose injection, potassium chloride in, 3036
Risperidone, 3196
    tablets, 3197
Ritodrine hydrochloride, 3198
    injection, 3199
    tablets, 3199
Ritonavir, 3200
Ropivacaine hydrochloride, 3202
    injection, 3203
Rose
    bengal sodium, 793
    bengal sodium I 131 injection, 2420
    oil, 1219
    water ointment, 3204
    water, stronger, 1219
Roxarsone, 3205
Rubella
    measles and mumps virus vaccine live, 2591
    and measles virus vaccine live, 2591
    virus vaccine live, 3205
Rubidium chloride Rb 82 injection, 3206
Rules and Procedures, xxiv
Ruthenium red, 794
    TS, 820

S

Saccharin, 1219
    calcium, 3206
    sodium, 3208
    sodium oral solution, 3209
    sodium tablets, 3209
Saccharose, 794
Safflower oil, 3210
Safranin O, 794
Salicylaldazine, 794
Salicylaldehyde, 794
Salicylamide, 3210
Salicylic
    acid, 3211
    acid collodion, 3211
    acid gel, 3212
    acid plaster, 3212
    acid topical foam, 3212
    acid and zinc paste, 3549
    and benzoic acids ointment, 1506
Saline TS, 820
    pyrogen-free, 820
Salsalate, 3213
    capsules, 3214
    tablets, 3215
Salts of organic nitrogenous bases ⟨501⟩, 182
Samarium Sm 153 lexidronam injection, 3215
Sand
    standard 20- to 30-mesh, 794
    washed, 794
Saquinavir mesylate, 3216
    capsules, 3217
Sargramostim, 3217
    for injection, 3220

Sawdust, purified, 794
Saw palmetto, 993
    capsules, 996
    extract, 994
    powdered, 994
Scandium oxide, 794
Scanning electron microscopy ⟨1181⟩, 646
Schweitzer's reagent, 820
Scopolamine hydrobromide, 3220
    injection, 3220
    ophthalmic ointment, 3221
    ophthalmic solution, 3221
    tablets, 3221
S designations, 794
Secobarbital, 3222
    oral solution, 3222
    sodium, 3222
    sodium and amobarbital sodium capsules, 3224
    sodium capsules, 3223
    sodium injection, 3224
    sodium for injection, 3224
Secondary butyl alcohol, 794
Selegiline hydrochloride, 3225
    tablets, 3226
Selenious acid, 794, 3227
    injection, 3227
Selenium, 794
    sulfide, 3227
    sulfide topical suspension, 3228
Selenium ⟨291⟩, 138
Selenomethionine, 795, 997
Senna
    fluidextract, 3229
    leaf, 3228
    oral solution, 3229
    pods, 3229
Sennosides, 3230
    tablets, 3230
Sensitization testing ⟨1184⟩, 650
Serine, 3231
Sesame oil, 1220
Shellac, 1221
Significant figures and tolerances, xii, 4
Silica
    calcined diatomaceous, 795
    chromatographic, silanized, flux-calcined, acid-washed, 795
    dental-type, 1222
    gel, 795
    gel, binder-free, 795
    gel, chromatographic, 795
    gel-impregnated glass microfiber sheet, 795
    gel mixture, chromatographic, 795
    gel mixture, chromatographic, with chemically bound amino groups, 795
    gel mixture, dimethylsilanized, chromatographic, 795
    gel mixture, octadecylsilanized chromatographic, 795
    gel mixture, octylsilanized, chromatographic, 795
    gel, octadecylsilanized chromatographic, 795
    gel, porous, 795
    microspheres, 795
Siliceous earth
    chromatographic, 795
    chromatographic, silanized, 795
    purified, 1222
Silicic
    acid, 795
    acid—impregnated glass microfilament sheets with fluorescent indicator, 796
Silicon
    carbide, 796
    dioxide, 1222
    dioxide colloidal, 1123
Silicone
    75 percent phenyl, methyl, 796

Silicotungstic acid, n-hydrate, 796
Silver
    diethyldithiocarbamate, 796
    diethyldithiocarbamate TS, 820
    nitrate, 796, 3231
    nitrate ophthalmic solution, 3231
    nitrate, tenth-normal (0.1 N), 826
    nitrate, toughened, 3231
    nitrate TS, 820
    oxide, 796
Silver-ammonia-nitrate TS, 820
Silver-ammonium nitrate TS, 820
Simethicone, 3232
    alumina, magnesia, and calcium carbonate chewable tablets, 1341
    alumina, magnesia, and calcium carbonate tablets, 1339
    alumina and magnesia oral suspension, 1342
    alumina and magnesia chewable tablets, 1344
    alumina and magnesia tablets, 1344
    calcium carbonate and magnesia chewable tablets, 1605
    calcium carbonate and magnesia tablets, 1604
    capsules, 3232
    emulsion, 3233
    and magaldrate chewable tablets, 2566
    and magaldrate oral suspension, 2565
    and magaldrate tablets, 2566
    oral suspension, 3233
    tablets, 3234
Simulated gastric fluid TS, 820
Simulated intestinal fluid TS, 820
Simvastatin, 3234
    tablets, 3235
Sincalide for injection, 3236
Single-steroid assay ⟨511⟩, 183
Sisomicin sulfate, 3236
    injection, 3237
β-Sitosterol, 796
Skin substitute
    human fibroblast-derived temporary, 3237
Sm 153 lexidronam injection, samarium, 3215
Smallpox vaccine, 3238
Soda lime, 796, 1223
Sodium, 796
    acetate, 796, 3238
    acetate, anhydrous, 796
    acetate C 11 injection, 1642
    acetate injection, 3239
    acetate solution, 3239
    acetate TS, 820
    alginate, 1224
    alizarinsulfonate, 796
    alizarinsulfonate TS, 820
    aminoacetate TS, 820
    ammonium phosphate, 796
    arsenate, 796
    arsenite, 796
    arsenite, twentieth-molar (0.05 M), 827
    ascorbate, 3240
    azide, 796
    benzoate, 1224
    benzoate and caffeine injection, 1592
    bicarbonate, 797, 3240
    bicarbonate injection, 3242
    bicarbonate and magnesium carbonate for oral suspension, 2570
    bicarbonate oral powder, 3243
    bicarbonate tablets, 3243
    biphenyl, 797
    biphosphate, 797
    bisulfite, 797
    bisulfite TS, 820
    bitartrate, 797
    bitartrate TS, 820
    borate, 797, 1224
    borohydride, 797
    bromide, 797, 3243

Sodium (continued)
  butyrate, 3244
  caprylate, 1225
  carbonate, 797, 1225
  carbonate, anhydrous, 797
  carbonate, citric acid, and magnesium oxide irrigation, 1784
  carbonate, monohydrate, 797
  carbonate TS, 820
  carboxymethylcellulose, 1647
  carboxymethylcellulose, and microcrystalline cellulose, 1106
  carboxymethylcellulose, paste, 1647
  carboxymethylcellulose, tablets, 1648
  12, carboxymethylcellulose, 1101
  cefazolin, 1666
  cefmetazole, 1675
  cefoperazone, 1677
  cefotaxime, 1680
  cetostearyl sulfate, 1225
  chloride, 797, 3244
  chloride and dextrose injection, 1928
  chloride and dextrose tablets, 3247
  chloride and fructose injection, 2237
  chloride inhalation solution, 3247
  chloride injection, 3245
  chloride injection, bacteriostatic, 3246
  chloride injection, dextran 40 in, 1921
  chloride injection, dextran 70 in, 1923
  chloride injection, mannitol in, 2587
  chloride injection, potassium chloride in, 3037
  chloride injection, potassium chloride in dextrose injection and, 3035
  chloride injection, ranitidine in, 3160
  chloride irrigation, 3246
  chloride ophthalmic ointment, 3246
  chloride ophthalmic solution, 3247
  chloride solution, isotonic, 797
  chloride tablets, 3247
  chloride tablets for solution, 3247
  chloride TS, alkaline, 820
  chromate, Cr 51 injection, 1758
  chromate, 797
  chromotropate, 797
  cilastatin, 1763
  citrate, 3248
  citrate and citric acid oral solution, 3248
  citrate dihydrate, 797
  citrate TS, 820
  citrate TS, alkaline, 820
  cobaltinitrite, 797
  cobaltinitrite TS, 820
  cyanide, 797
  1-decanesulfonate, 797
  dehydroacetate, 1227
  desoxycholate, 797
  dichromate, 798
  diethyldithiocarbamate, 798
  2,2-dimethyl-2-silapentane-5-sulfonate, 798
  dithionite, 798
  dodecyl sulfate, 798
  ferrocyanide, 798
  fluorescein, 798
  fluoride, 798, 3249
  fluoride and acidulated phosphate topical solution, 3250
  fluoride F18 injection, 2195
  fluoride oral solution, 3249
  fluoride and phosphoric acid gel, 3250
  fluoride tablets, 3250
  fluoride TS, 820
  formaldehyde sulfoxylate, 1227
  gluconate, 3251
  glycocholate, 798
  1-heptanesulfonate, 798
  1-heptanesulfonate, monohydrate, 798
  1-hexanesulfonate, 798
  1-hexanesulfonate, monohydrate, 798

hydrogen sulfate, 798
hydrosulfite, 798
hydrosulfite TS, alkaline, 820
hydroxide, 798, 1228
hydroxide, alcoholic, tenth-normal (0.1 N), 827
hydroxide, normal (1 N), 827
hydroxide TS, 820
hypobromite TS, 820
hypochlorite solution, 798, 3251
hypochlorite topical solution, 3251
hypochlorite TS, 820
iodate, 798
iodide, 3251
iodide I 123 solution, 2417
iodide I 131 capsules, 2421
Iodide I 123 capsules, 2417
iodide I 131 solution, 2421
iodohydroxyquinolinesulfonate TS, 820
lactate injection, 3252
lactate solution, 3252
lauryl sulfate, 798, 1228
low-substituted carboxymethylcellulose, 1100
metabisulfite, 799, 1228
metaperiodate, 799
methoxide, 799
methoxide, half-normal (0.5 N) in methanol, 827
methoxide, tenth-normal (0.1 N) (in toluene), 827
molybdate, 799
monofluorophosphate, 3253
nitrate, 799
nitrite, 799, 3254
nitrite injection, 3254
nitrite, tenth-molar (0.1 M), 827
nitroferricyanide, 799
nitroferricyanide TS, 820
nitroprusside, 3254
nitroprusside for injection, 3255
1-octanesulfonate, 799
oxalate, 799
(tri) pentacyanoamino ferrate, 799
1-pentanesulfonate, 799
perchlorate, 799
peroxide, 799
pertechnetate Tc 99m injection, 3336
phosphate, dibasic, 799, 3255
phosphate, dibasic, anhydrous, 799
phosphate, dibasic, dodecahydrate, 799
phosphate, dibasic, TS, 820
phosphate, monobasic, 799, 3256
phosphate P 32 solution, 3001
phosphates injection, 3256
phosphates oral solution, 3257
phosphates rectal solution, 3257
phosphate, tribasic, 799, 1229
phosphotungstate TS, 820
polystyrene sulfonate, 3258
polystyrene sulfonate suspension, 3258
and potassium bicarbonates and citric acid effervescent tablets for oral solution, 3029
propionate, 1229
pyrophosphate, 799
pyruvate, 799
salicylate, 799, 3258
salicylate tablets, 3258
selenite, 799
starch glycolate, 1230
stearate, 1231
stearyl fumarate, 1231
sulfate, 799, 3259
sulfate, anhydrous, 799
sulfate decahydrate, 800
sulfate injection, 3259
sulfide, 800, 3259
sulfide topical gel, 3260
sulfide TS, 820
sulfite, 800, 1232

sulfite, anhydrous, 800
p-sulfophenylazochromotropate, 800
tartrate, 800, 1232
tartrate TS, 820
tetraphenylborate, 800
tetraphenylboron, 800
tetraphenylboron, fiftieth-molar (0.02 M), 827
tetraphenylboron TS, 820
thioglycolate, 800
thioglycolate TS, 820
thiosulfate, 800, 3260
thiosulfate injection, 3260
thiosulfate, tenth-normal (0.1 N), 828
thiosulfate TS, 820
L-thyroxine, 800
3-(trimethylsilyl)-1-propane sulfonate, 800
tungstate, 800
Solubilities, 886
Soluble starch, 800

Solution
  Oral, containing at least three of the following—acetaminophen and (salts of) chlorpheniramine, dextromethorphan, and phenylpropanolamine, 1277
  Oral, containing at least three of the following—acetaminophen and (salts of) chlorpheniramine, dextromethorphan, and pseudoephedrine, 1283
  Acetaminophen and codeine phosphate oral, 1289
  Acetaminophen, dextromethorphan hydrobromide, doxylamine succinate, and pseudoephedrine hydrochloride oral, 1292
  Acetaminophen for effervescent oral, 1270
  Acetaminophen oral, 1269
  Acetic acid otic, 1298
  Acetylcholine chloride for ophthalmic, 1300
  Acetylcysteine, 1302
  Acidulated phosphate and sodium fluoride topical, 3250
  Aluminum acetate topical, 1349
  Aluminum chlorohydrate, 1351
  Aluminum dichlorohydrate, 1353
  Aluminum sesquichlorohydrate, 1357
  Aluminum subacetate topical, 1358
  Aluminum sulfate and calcium acetate for topical, 1359
  Aluminum sulfate and calcium acetate tablets for topical, 1360
  Aluminum zirconium octachlorohydrate, 1361
  Aluminum zirconium octachlorohydrex gly, 1363
  Aluminum zirconium pentachlorohydrate, 1364
  Aluminum zirconium pentachlorohydrex gly, 1366
  Aluminum zirconium tetrachlorohydrate, 1368
  Aluminum zirconium tetrachlorohydrex gly, 1369
  Aluminum zirconium trichlorohydrate, 1371
  Aluminum zirconium trichlorohydrex gly, 1373
  Amantadine hydrochloride oral, 1375
  Aminobenzoate potassium for oral, 1384
  Aminobenzoic acid topical, 1386
  Aminocaproic acid oral, 1387
  Aminophylline oral, 1392
  Aminophylline rectal, 1393
  Ammonia, diluted, 754
  Ammonia, strong, 1072
  Amprolium oral, 1422
  Anticoagulant citrate dextrose, 1429
  Anticoagulant citrate phosphate dextrose, 1430
  Anticoagulant citrate phosphate dextrose adenine, 1431

Solution (continued)
  Anticoagulant heparin, 1433
  Anticoagulant sodium citrate, 1433
  Antipyrine and benzocaine otic, 1435
  Antipyrine, benzocaine, and phenylephrine hydrochloride otic, 1436
  Apraclonidine ophthalmic, 1440
  Aromatic elixir, 1076
  Ascorbic acid oral, 1446
  Aspirin effervescent tablets for oral, 1453
  Atenolol oral, 1462
  Atropine sulfate ophthalmic, 1470
  Benoxinate hydrochloride ophthalmic, 1499
  Benzaldehyde elixir, compound, 1081
  Benzalkonium chloride, 1082
  Benzethonium chloride topical, 1500
  Benzocaine, butamben, and tetracaine hydrochloride topical, 1504
  Benzocaine otic, 1503
  Benzocaine topical, 1503
  Betamethasone oral, 1516
  Betaxolol ophthalmic, 1526
  Bethanechol chloride oral, 1529
  Bromodiphenhydramine hydrochloride and codeine phosphate oral, 1562
  Bromodiphenhydramine hydrochloride oral, 1561
  Brompheniramine maleate and pseudoephedrine sulfate oral, 1564
  Brompheniramine maleate oral, 1563
  Butabarbital sodium oral, 1578
  Butorphanol tartrate nasal, 1589
  Caffeine citrate oral, 1591
  Calcitonin salmon nasal, 1598
  Calcium glubionate syrup, 1609
  Calcium hydroxide topical, 1612
  Captopril oral, 1626
  Carbachol intraocular, 1629
  Carbachol ophthalmic, 1629
  Carbamide peroxide topical, 1633
  Carbol-fuchsin topical, 1638
  C 13 for oral, urea, 1643
  Carteolol hydrochloride ophthalmic, 1654
  Cefazolin ophthalmic, 1668
  Cetylpyridinium chloride topical, 1716
  Cherry syrup, 1111
  Chloral hydrate oral, 1717
  Chloramphenicol for ophthalmic, 1720
  Chloramphenicol ophthalmic, 1720
  Chloramphenicol oral, 1721
  Chloramphenicol otic, 1721
  Chlorhexidine gluconate, 1731
  Chlorpheniramine maleate and pseudoephedrine hydrochloride oral, 1745
  Chlorpheniramine maleate oral, 1741
  Chlorpromazine hydrochloride syrup, 1748
  Chocolate syrup, 1112
  Cholecalciferol, 1755
  Chymotrypsin for ophthalmic, 1760
  Ciprofloxacin ophthalmic, 1774
  Clindamycin hydrochloride oral, 1797
  Clindamycin palmitate hydrochloride for oral, 1798
  Clindamycin phosphate topical, 1800
  Clobetasol propionate topical, 1806
  Clotrimazole topical, 1828
  Cloxacillin sodium for oral, 1832
  Coal tar topical, 1834
  Cyanocobalamin Co 57 oral, 1835
  Cocaine hydrochloride tablets for topical, 1837
  Cocaine and tetracaine hydrochlorides and epinephrine topical, 1838
  Cromolyn sodium ophthalmic, 1857
  Cupriethylenediamine hydroxide, 1.0 M, 767
  Cyclopentolate hydrochloride ophthalmic, 1864
  Cyclosporine oral, 1871
  Cyproheptadine hydrochloride oral, 1872
  Demecarium bromide ophthalmic, 1887

  Dexamethasone elixir, 1906
  Dexamethasone oral, 1907
  Dexamethasone sodium phosphate ophthalmic, 1914
  Dexbrompheniramine maleate and pseudoephedrine sulfate oral, 1915
  Dexchlorpheniramine maleate oral, 1916
  Dextromethorphan hydrobromide oral, 1927
  Diatrizoate meglumine and diatrizoate sodium, 1931
  Diatrizoate sodium, 1932
  Dichlorophenol-indophenol, standard, 823
  Dicyclomine hydrochloride oral, 1947
  Didanosine for oral, 1949
  Diethyltoluamide topical, 1956
  Digoxin oral, 1964
  Dihydrotachysterol oral, 1970
  Diltiazem hydrochloride oral, 1974
  Dimenhydrinate oral, 1980
  Dimethyl sulfoxide topical, 1984
  Diphenhydramine hydrochloride oral, 1989
  Diphenoxylate hydrochloride and atropine sulfate oral, 1990
  Dipivefrin hydrochloride ophthalmic, 1993
  Docusate sodium, 2008
  Docusate sodium syrup, 2008
  Dolasetron mesylate oral, 2010
  Doxepin hydrochloride oral, 2019
  Doxylamine succinate oral, 2027
  Dyclonine hydrochloride topical, 2032
  Dyphylline and guaifenesin oral, 2035
  Dyphylline oral, 2034
  Echothiophate iodide for ophthalmic, 2037
  Emedastine ophthalmic, 2054
  Ephedrine sulfate oral, 2064
  Epinephrine bitartrate for ophthalmic, 2069
  Epinephrine bitartrate ophthalmic, 2069
  Epinephrine ophthalmic, 2067
  Epinephryl borate ophthalmic, 2069
  Ergocalciferol oral, 2072
  Ergoloid mesylates oral, 2075
  Erythromycin topical, 2088
  Ethosuximide oral, 2123
  Eucatropine hydrochloride ophthalmic, 2136
  Fehling's, 817
  Ferric ammonium citrate for oral, 1403
  Ferric subsulfate, 2151
  Ferrous gluconate oral, 2156
  Ferrous sulfate oral, 2157
  Ferrous sulfate syrup, 2157
  Fluocinolone acetonide topical, 2186
  Fluocinonide topical, 2188
  Fluorescein sodium and benoxinate hydrochloride ophthalmic, 2191
  Fluorescein sodium and proparacaine hydrochloride ophthalmic, 2191
  Fluorouracil topical, 2199
  Fluoxetine oral, 2202
  Fluphenazine hydrochloride elixir, 2208
  Fluphenazine hydrochloride oral, 2209
  Flurbiprofen sodium ophthalmic, 2216
  Formaldehyde, 776, 2229
  Furosemide oral, 2240
  Gentamicin sulfate and betamethasone acetate ophthalmic, 2265
  Gentamicin sulfate and betamethasone valerate otic, 2267
  Gentamicin topical, 2268
  Gentamicin sulfate ophthalmic, 2265
  Gentian violet topical, 2271
  Glutaral disinfectant, 1141
  Glycerin ophthalmic, 2287
  Glycerin oral, 2287
  Guaifenesin and codeine phosphate oral, 2306
  Guaifenesin oral, 2305
  Halazone tablets for, 2315
  Halcinonide topical, 2317
  Haloperidol oral, 2318

  Heparin lock flush, 2320
  Homatropine hydrobromide ophthalmic, 2328
  Hydralazine hydrochloride oral, 2333
  Hydrocortisone and acetic acid otic, 2343
  Hydrogen peroxide, 778
  Hydrogen peroxide topical, 2353
  Hydroquinone topical, 2356
  Hydroxyamphetamine hydrobromide ophthalmic, 2358
  Hydroxyzine hydrochloride oral, 2363
  Hyoscyamine sulfate elixir, 2368
  Hyoscyamine sulfate oral, 2369
  Hypromellose ophthalmic, 2372
  Idoxuridine ophthalmic, 2379
  Indium In 111 chloride, 2391
  Indium In 111 oxyquinoline, 2393
  Iodine, strong, 2414
  Sodium iodide I 123, 2417
  Sodium iodide I 131, 2421
  Iodine topical, 2414
  Ipecac oral, 2444
  Isoniazid oral, 2459
  Isosorbide oral, 2470
  Lactulose, 2497
  Lead, standard, 820
  Levobunolol hydrochloride ophthalmic, 2514
  Levocarnitine oral, 2517
  Lidocaine hydrochloride topical, 2529
  Lincomycin oral, 2533
  Lithium oral, 2542
  Locke-Ringer's, 818
  Loperamide hydrochloride oral, 2544
  Loratadine oral, 2549
  Mafenide acetate for topical, 2562
  Magnesium carbonate and citric acid for oral, 2569
  Magnesium carbonate, citric acid, and potassium citrate for oral, 2569
  Manganese chloride for oral, 2585
  Magnesium citrate for oral, 2572
  Magnesium citrate oral, 2571
  Maltitol, 1170
  Meperidine hydrochloride oral, 2618
  Mesoridazine besylate oral, 2634
  Metaproterenol sulfate oral, 2638
  Methadone hydrochloride oral, 2649
  Methdilazine hydrochloride oral, 2653
  Methenamine mandelate for oral, 2657
  Methenamine oral, 2655
  Methoxsalen topical, 2666
  Methylcellulose ophthalmic, 2673
  Methylcellulose oral, 2673
  Metoclopramide oral, 2692
  Metoprolol tartrate oral, 2698
  Mibolerone oral, 2710
  Minoxidil topical, 2718
  Mometasone furoate topical, 2728
  Myrrh topical, 2743
  Nafcillin sodium for oral, 2748
  Naphazoline hydrochloride ophthalmic, 2758
  Naphazoline hydrochloride and pheniramine maleate ophthalmic, 2759
  Neomycin and polymyxin B sulfates and gramicidin ophthalmic, 2785
  Neomycin and polymyxin B sulfates and hydrocortisone otic, 2786
  Neomycin and polymyxin B sulfates for irrigation, 2779
  Neomycin and polymyxin B sulfates ophthalmic, 2780
  Neomycin sulfate and dexamethasone sodium phosphate ophthalmic, 2773
  Neomycin sulfate oral, 2771
  Nickel standard TS, 819
  Nitrofurazone topical, 2815
  Nitromersol topical, 2819

Solution *(continued)*
   Norfloxacin ophthalmic, 2831
   Nortriptyline hydrochloride oral, 2838
   Ofloxacin ophthalmic, 2848
   Ondansetron, oral, 2857
   Orange syrup, 1186
   Oxacillin sodium for oral, 2864
   Oxtriphylline oral, 2872
   Oxybutynin chloride oral, 2876
   Oxycodone hydrochloride oral, 2879
   Oxymetazoline hydrochloride ophthalmic, 2888
   Papain tablets for topical, 2911
   Paromomycin oral, 2920
   Penicillin G potassium for oral, 2935
   Penicillin V potassium for oral, 2946
   Pentobarbital oral, 2953
   Perphenazine oral, 2964
   Perphenazine syrup, 2965
   Phenobarbital oral, 2973
   Phenol, topical, camphorated, 2976
   Phenylephrine hydrochloride ophthalmic, 2987
   Phenylpropanolamine hydrochloride oral, 2991
   Phosphate P 32, sodium, 3001
   Physostigmine salicylate ophthalmic, 3002
   Pilocarpine hydrochloride ophthalmic, 3007
   Pilocarpine nitrate ophthalmic, 3007
   Piperazine citrate syrup, 3014
   Podophyllum resin topical, 3019
   polyethylene glycol 3350 and electrolytes for oral, 3021
   Polymyxin B sulfate and hydrocortisone otic, 3025
   Polymyxin B sulfate and trimethoprim ophthalmic, 3025
   Potassium bicarbonate effervescent tablets for oral, 3028
   Potassium bicarbonate and potassium chloride for effervescent oral, 3028
   Potassium bicarbonate and potassium chloride effervescent tablets for oral, 3029
   Potassium bicarbonate, potassium chloride, and potassium citrate effervescent tablets for oral, 3036
   Potassium chloride for oral, 3033
   Potassium chloride oral, 3033
   Potassium citrate and citric acid oral, 3039
   Potassium gluconate and potassium chloride for oral, 3041
   Potassium gluconate and potassium chloride oral, 3041
   Potassium gluconate, potassium citrate, and ammonium chloride oral, 3042
   Potassium gluconate and potassium citrate oral, 3042
   Potassium gluconate oral, 3040
   Potassium iodide oral, 3044
   Potassium nitrate, 3045
   Potassium and sodium bicarbonates and citric acid effervescent tablets for oral, 3029
   Povidone-iodine cleansing, 3050
   Povidone-iodine topical, 3050
   Prednisolone oral, 3062
   Prednisolone sodium phosphate ophthalmic, 3067
   Prednisone oral, 3069
   Prochlorperazine oral, 3085
   Promazine hydrochloride oral, 3094
   Promazine hydrochloride syrup, 3094
   Promethazine hydrochloride oral, 3096
   Proparacaine hydrochloride ophthalmic, 3100
   Protein standard (8 g/dL), 792
   Pseudoephedrine hydrochloride, carbinoxamine maleate, and dextromethorphan hydrobromide oral, 3128

   Pseudoephedrine hydrochloride oral, 3126
   Pyridostigmine bromide oral, 3136
   Ranitidine oral, 3159
   Reserpine oral, 3169
   Saccharin sodium oral, 3209
   Scopolamine hydrobromide ophthalmic, 3221
   Secobarbital oral, 3222
   Senna oral, 3229
   Silver nitrate ophthalmic, 3231
   Sodium acetate, 3239
   Sodium chloride, isotonic, 797
   Sodium chloride ophthalmic, 3247
   Sodium chloride tablets for, 3247
   Sodium citrate and citric acid oral, 3248
   Sodium fluoride and acidulated phosphate topical, 3250
   Sodium fluoride oral, 3249
   Sodium hypochlorite, 798, 3251
   Sodium hypochlorite topical, 3251
   Sodium lactate, 3252
   Sodium phosphate P 32, 3001
   Sodium phosphates oral, 3257
   Sodium phosphates rectal, 3257
   Sorbitol, 3262
   Sorbitol noncrystallizing, 1237
   Sorbitol sorbitan, 1236
   Stavudine for oral, 3273
   Sulfacetamide sodium ophthalmic, 3286
   Sulfaquinoxaline oral, 3303
   Suprofen ophthalmic, 3314
   Syrup, 1249
   Terpin hydrate and codeine oral, 3348
   Terpin hydrate oral, 3348
   Tetracaine hydrochloride ophthalmic, 3358
   Tetracaine hydrochloride topical, 3358
   Tetracycline hydrochloride for topical, 3363
   Tetrahydrozoline hydrochloride ophthalmic, 3368
   Tetramethylammonium hydroxide, in methanol, 803
   Theophylline and guaifenesin oral, 3377
   Theophylline oral, 3374
   Theophylline sodium glycinate oral, 3378
   Thiamine hydrochloride oral, 3383
   Thiamine mononitrate oral, 3384
   Thimerosal topical, 3388
   Thioridazine hydrochloride oral, 3392
   Thiothixene hydrochloride oral, 3397
   Timolol maleate ophthalmic, 3411
   Tobramycin ophthalmic, 3421
   Tolnaftate topical, 3434
   Tolu balsam syrup, 1252
   Tretinoin topical, 3440
   Triamcinolone diacetate oral, 3445
   Tricitrates oral, 3453
   Trifluoperazine oral, 3458
   Trihexyphenidyl hydrochloride oral, 3464
   Trikates oral, 3465
   Trimeprazine oral, 3466
   Triprolidine hydrochloride oral, 3474
   Triprolidine and pseudoephedrine hydrochlorides oral, 3475
   Tropicamide ophthalmic, 3480
   Valproic acid oral, 3493
   Valrubicin intravesical, 3495
   Vancomycin hydrochloride for oral, 3501
   Vehicle for oral, 1257
   Vehicle for oral, sugar free, 1258
   Verapamil hydrochloride oral, 3506
   Vitamins with minerals, water-soluble oral, 1049
   Vitamins, oil- and water-soluble oral, 1009
   Vitamins with minerals, oil- and water-soluble oral, 1016
   Xanthan gum, 1262
   Zidovudine oral, 3541

   Zinc sulfate ophthalmic, 3551
   Zinc sulfate oral, 3551

Solvent hexane, 800
Somatropin, 3260
   for injection, 3262
Sorbic acid, 1233
Sorbitan
   monolaurate, 1233
   monooleate, 1233
   monopalmitate, 1234
   monostearate, 1234
   sesquioleate, 1235
   sorbitol, solution, 1236
   trioleate, 1235
Sorbitol, 1235
   solution, 3262
   solution noncrystallizing, 1237
   sorbitan solution, 1236
Sotalol hydrochloride, 3263
   tablets, 3264
Soybean oil, 3265
   hydrogenated, 1237
Specific gravity ⟨841⟩, 351
Specific surface area ⟨846⟩, 352
Spectinomycin
   hydrochloride, 3265
   for injectable suspension, 3266
Spectrophotometric identification tests ⟨197⟩, 129
Spectrophotometry and light-scattering ⟨851⟩, 355
Spironolactone, 3266
   and hydrochlorothiazide tablets, 3267
   tablets, 3267
Squalane, 1238
Sr 89 injection, strontium chloride, 3276
Stability considerations in dispensing practice ⟨1191⟩, 656
Stachyose hydrate, 800
Standard sand, 20- to 30-mesh, 800
Stannous
   chloride, 800
   chloride acid, stronger, TS, 820
   chloride acid TS, 820
   fluoride, 3268
   fluoride gel, 3269
Stanozolol, 3270
   tablets, 3270
Starch
   corn, 1240
   iodate paper, 810
   iodide-free TS, 820
   iodide paper, 810
   iodide paste TS, 820
   modified, 1238
   potassium iodide and, TS, 820
   potassium iodide TS, 821
   potato, 800, 1240
   pregelatinized, 1239
   pregelatinized modified, 1239
   sodium, glycolate, 1230
   soluble, 800
   soluble, purified, 800
   tapioca, 1241
   topical, 3271
   TS, 821
   wheat, 1242
Stavudine, 3272
   capsules, 3272
   for oral solution, 3273
Steam, pure, 3525
Stearic acid, 800, 1243
   purified, 1243
Stearoyl polyoxylglycerides, 1244
Stearyl alcohol, 800, 1244

Combined Index to USP 31 and NF 26   Steri–Supro   I-47

Sterile
Erythromycin ethylsuccinate, 2093
Erythromycin gluceptate, 2096
Erythromycin lactobionate, 2096
Pharmaceutical compounding—sterile preparations ⟨797⟩, 319
Sterile product packaging—integrity evaluation ⟨1207⟩, 664
Sterility testing—validation of isolator systems ⟨1208⟩, 665
Sterilization—chemical and physicochemical indicators and integrators ⟨1209⟩, 668
Sterilization and sterility assurance of compendial articles ⟨1211⟩, 670
Vancomycin hydrochloride, 3501
Water for inhalation, 3523
Water for injection, 3524
Water for irrigation, 3524
Water, purified, 3524

Sterile product packaging—integrity evaluation ⟨1207⟩, 664
Sterility
  testing—validation of isolator systems ⟨1208⟩, 665
  tests ⟨71⟩, 85
Sterilization—chemical and physicochemical indicators and integrators ⟨1209⟩, 668
Sterilization and sterility assurance of compendial articles ⟨1211⟩, 670
Stinging nettle, 984
  powdered, 986
  powdered, extract, 986
St. John's wort, 990
  extract, powdered, 992
  powdered, 991
Storax, 3274
Streptomycin
  injection, 3276
  for injection, 3276
  sulfate, 3275
Stronger
  ammonia water, 800
  cupric acetate TS, 821
Strontium
  acetate, 801
  chloride Sr 89 injection, 3276
  hydroxide, 801
Strychnine sulfate, 801
Styrene-divinylbenzene
  anion-exchange resin, 50- to 100-mesh, 801
  cation-exchange resin, strongly acidic, 801
  copolymer beads, 801
Succinic acid, 801, 1245
Succinylcholine chloride, 3277
  injection, 3279
  for injection, 3279
Sucralfate, 3279
  tablets, 3281
Sucralose, 1245
Sucrose, 1246
  octaacetate, 1246
Sudan
  III, 801
  III TS, 821
  IV, 801
  IV TS, 821
Sufentanil citrate, 3281
  injection, 3282
Sugar
  compressible, 1246
  confectioner's, 1247
  free suspension structured vehicle, 1249
  injection, invert, 3282

  invert injection type 1, and multiple electrolytes, 2049
  invert injection type 2, and multiple electrolytes, 2050
  invert injection type 3, and multiple electrolytes, 2051
  spheres, 1247
Sulbactam
  and ampicillin for injection, 1421
  sodium, 3283
Sulconazole nitrate, 3283
Sulfa
  vaginal cream, triple, 3284
  vaginal inserts, triple, 3284
Sulfabenzamide, 3285
Sulfacetamide, 3285
  sodium, 3285
  sodium, neomycin sulfate, and prednisolone acetate ophthalmic ointment, 2791
  sodium ophthalmic ointment, 3286
  sodium ophthalmic solution, 3286
  sodium and prednisolone acetate ophthalmic ointment, 3287
  sodium and prednisolone acetate ophthalmic suspension, 3288
  sodium topical suspension, 3287
Sulfachlorpyridazine, 3289
Sulfadiazine, 3290
  cream, silver, 3292
  silver, 3291
  sodium, 3292
  sodium injection, 3292
  tablets, 3290
Sulfadimethoxine, 3293
  oral suspension, 3293
  sodium, 3294
  soluble powder, 3293
  tablets, 3294
Sulfadoxine, 3294
  and pyrimethamine tablets, 3295
Sulfamethazine, 3296
  and chlortetracycline bisulfates soluble powder, 1750
  granulated, 3296
Sulfamethizole, 3296
  oral suspension, 3297
  tablets, 3297
Sulfamethoxazole, 3298
  oral suspension, 3298
  tablets, 3299
  and trimethoprim injection, 3299
  and trimethoprim oral suspension, 3300
  and trimethoprim tablets, 3301
Sulfamic acid, 801
Sulfanilamide, 801
Sulfanilic
  acid, 801
  acid, diazotized TS, 821
  acid TS, 821
  α-naphthylamine TS, 821
  1-naphthylamine TS, 821
Sulfapyridine, 3302
  tablets, 3302
Sulfaquinoxaline, 3302
  oral solution, 3303
Sulfasalazine, 3303
  delayed-release tablets, 3304
  tablets, 3304
Sulfatase enzyme preparation, 801
Sulfate
  acid, ferrous, TS, 817
  and chloride ⟨221⟩, 132
  ferrous, TS, 817
  magnesium, TS, 818
  mercuric, TS, 818
  potassium, 792
  potassium, TS, 820
  in reagents, 751

  strychnine, 801
Sulfathiazole, 3305
  sodium, 801
Sulfinpyrazone, 3305
  capsules, 3305
  tablets, 3306
Sulfisoxazole, 3306
  acetyl, 3307
  acetyl and erythromycin estolate oral suspension, 2091
  acetyl and erythromycin ethylsuccinate for oral suspension, 2095
  acetyl oral suspension, 3307
  tablets, 3307
Sulfomolybdic acid TS, 821
Sulfonamides ⟨521⟩, 183
Sulfonic acid cation-exchange resin, 802
2-(4-Sulfophneylazo)-1,8-dihydroxy-3,6-naphthalenedisulfonic acid, trisodium salt, 810
Sulfosalicylic acid, 802
Sulfur, 802
  dioxide, 1247
  dioxide detector tube, 802
  ointment, 3308
  precipitated, 3307
  and resorcinol topical suspension, 3176
  sublimed, 3308
Sulfuric acid, 802, 1248
  diluted, 802
  fluorometric, 802
  fuming, 802
  half-normal (0.5 N) in alcohol, 828
  normal (1 N), 828
  phenylhydrazine, TS, 819
  TS, 821
Sulfuric acid-formaldehyde TS, 821
Sulfurous acid, 802
Sulindac, 3308
  tablets, 3309
Sulisobenzone, 3310
Sumatriptan, 3310
  nasal spray, 3311
Sumatriptan succinate
  oral suspension, 3312
Sunflower oil, 1248
Supplements, xiii, 5
Supplemental information for articles of botanical origin ⟨2030⟩, 727
Supports for gas chromatography, 802

Suppositories
Acetaminophen, 1270
Aminophylline, 1393
Aspirin, 1450
Bisacodyl, 1537
Chlorpromazine, 1746
Ergotamine tartrate and caffeine, 2082
Glycerin, 2287
Indomethacin, 2399
Miconazole nitrate vaginal, 2713
Morphine sulfate, 2737
Nystatin vaginal, 2841
Oxymorphone hydrochloride, 2890
Prochlorperazine, 3086
Progesterone vaginal, 3091
Promethazine hydrochloride, 3096
Thiethylperazine maleate, 3385

Suprofen, 3313
  ophthalmic solution, 3314

Suspension

Acetaminophen and codeine phosphate oral, 1290
Acetaminophen oral, 1270
Acyclovir oral, 1306
Albendazole oral, 1310
Allopurinol oral, 1325
Alprazolam oral, 1328
Alumina, magnesia, and calcium carbonate oral, 1337
Alumina and magnesia oral, 1336
Alumina, magnesia, and simethicone oral, 1342
Alumina and magnesium carbonate oral, 1345
Alumina and magnesium trisilicate oral, 1348
Amoxicillin and clavulanate potassium for oral, 1412
Amoxicillin for oral, 1410
Amoxicillin for injectable, 1409
Amoxicillin oral, 1410
Amoxicillin tablets for oral, 1411
Ampicillin for injectable, 1418
Ampicillin for oral, 1419
Ampicillin and probenecid for oral, 1419
Atovaquone oral, 1465
Aurothioglucose injectable, 1471
Azathioprine oral, 1475
Azithromycin for oral, 1479
Bacampicillin hydrochloride for oral, 1482
Baclofen oral, 1487
Barium sulfate, 1490
Barium sulfate for, 1490
Betamethasone sodium phosphate and betamethasone acetate injectable, 1523
Bethanechol chloride oral, 1529
Bisacodyl rectal, 1537
Bismuth subsalicylate oral, 1542
Brinzolamide ophthalmic, 1557
Calamine topical, 1593
Calamine topical, phenolated, 1593
Calcium carbonate oral, 1602
Calcium and magnesium carbonates oral, 1607
Captopril oral, 1626
Carbamazepine oral, 1631
Cefaclor for oral, 1661
Cefadroxil for oral, 1664
Cefixime for oral, 1672
Cefpodoxime proxetil for oral, 1690
Cefprozil for oral, 1691
Cefuroxime axetil for oral, 1699
Cellulose sodium phosphate for oral, 1704
Cephalexin for oral, 1706
Cephradine for oral, 1714
Chloramphenicol and hydrocortisone acetate for ophthalmic, 1722
Chloramphenicol palmitate oral, 1724
Chlorothiazide oral, 1738
Cholestyramine for oral, 1757
Chromic phosphate P 32, 3000
Ciclopirox olamine topical, 1763
Ciprofloxacin and dexamethasone otic, 1771
Clarithromycin for oral, 1787
Clavulanate potassium and amoxicillin for oral, 1412
Clindamycin phosphate topical, 1801
Clonazepam oral, 1814
Colestipol hydrochloride for oral, 1846
Colistin and neomycin sulfates and hydrocortisone acetate otic, 1848
Colistin sulfate for oral, 1848
Corticotropin zinc hydroxide injectable, 1852
Cortisone acetate injectable, 1853
Demeclocycline oral, 1888
Desoxycorticosterone pivalate injectable, 1904
Dexamethasone acetate injectable, 1909
Dexamethasone ophthalmic, 1907
Diazoxide oral, 1937

Dicloxacillin sodium for oral, 1945
Diltiazem hydrochloride oral, 1975
Dipyridamole oral, 1994
Dolasetron mesylate oral, 2011
Doxycycline calcium oral, 2023
Doxycycline for oral, 2023
Erythromycin estolate for oral, 2090
Erythromycin estolate oral, 2090
Erythromycin estolate and sulfisoxazole acetyl oral, 2091
Erythromycin ethylsuccinate for oral, 2094
Erythromycin ethylsuccinate oral, 2093
Erythromycin ethylsuccinate and sulfisoxazole acetyl for oral, 2095
Estradiol injectable, 2100
Estrone injectable, 2111
Famotidine for oral, 2138
Ferumoxsil oral, 2160
Flucytosine oral, 2173
Fluorometholone ophthalmic, 2197
Furazolidone oral, 2238
Ganciclovir oral, 2257
Gentamicin and prednisolone acetate ophthalmic, 2269
Griseofulvin oral, 2302
Hydrocortisone acetate injectable, 2346
Hydrocortisone acetate ophthalmic, 2346
Hydrocortisone injectable, 2342
Hydrocortisone rectal, 2342
Hydroxyzine pamoate oral, 2366
Ibuprofen oral, 2373
Imipenem and cilastatin for injectable, 2383
Indomethacin oral, 2400
Isophane insulin human, 2410
Human insulin isophane and human insulin injection, 2407
Insulin human zinc, 2411
Insulin human zinc, extended, 2411
Isophane insulin, 2409
Insulin zinc, 2410
Insulin zinc, extended, 2410
Insulin zinc, prompt, 2411
Isoflupredone acetate injectable, 2454
Ketoconazole oral, 2488
Labetalol hydrochloride oral, 2495
Loracarbef for oral, 2547
Magaldrate and simethicone oral, 2565
Magaldrate oral, 2564
Magnesium carbonate and sodium bicarbonate for oral, 2570
Mebendazole oral, 2592
Medroxyprogesterone acetate injectable, 2601
Megestrol acetate oral, 2604
Meloxicam oral, 2609
Meprobamate oral, 2624
Mesalamine rectal, 2631
Methacycline hydrochloride oral, 2648
Methadone hydrochloride tablets for oral, 2650
Methenamine mandelate oral, 2657
Methyldopa oral, 2674
Methylprednisolone acetate injectable, 2686
Metolazone oral, 2693
Metoprolol tartrate oral, 2698
Minocycline hydrochloride oral, 2717
Nalidixic acid oral, 2751
Naproxen oral, 2760
Natamycin ophthalmic, 2767
Neomycin and polymyxin B sulfates and dexamethasone ophthalmic, 2785
Neomycin and polymyxin B sulfates and hydrocortisone otic, 2787
Neomycin and polymyxin B sulfates and hydrocortisone acetate ophthalmic, 2787
Neomycin and polymyxin B sulfates and hydrocortisone ophthalmic, 2786
Neomycin and polymyxin B sulfates and prednisolone acetate ophthalmic, 2789

Neomycin sulfate and hydrocortisone otic, 2776
Neomycin sulfate and hydrocortisone acetate ophthalmic, 2777
Neomycin sulfate and prednisolone acetate ophthalmic, 2790
Nevirapine oral, 2796
Nitrofurantoin oral, 2813
Nystatin for oral, 2842
Nystatin oral, 2841
Ondansetron hydrochloride oral, 2855
Oxfendazole oral, 2870
Oxytetracycline and nystatin for oral, 2893
Oxytetracycline calcium oral, 2893
Oxytetracycline hydrochloride and hydrocortisone acetate ophthalmic, 2895
Penicillin G benzathine injectable, 2930
Penicillin G benzathine and penicillin G procaine injectable, 2932
Penicillin G benzathine oral, 2931
Penicillin G, neomycin, polymyxin B, hydrocortisone acetate, and hydrocortisone sodium succinate topical, 2929
Penicillin G procaine, dihydrostreptomycin sulfate, chlorpheniramine maleate, and dexamethasone injectable, 2939
Penicillin G procaine and dihydrostreptomycin sulfate injectable, 2939
Penicillin G procaine, dihydrostreptomycin sulfate, and prednisolone injectable, 2941
Penicillin G procaine, neomycin and polymyxin B sulfates, and hydrocortisone acetate topical, 2941
Penicillin G procaine injectable, 2937
Penicillin G procaine for injectable, 2938
Penicillin V benzathine oral, 2945
Penicillin V for oral, 2944
Perflutren protein-type A microspheres injectable, 2959
Phenytoin oral, 2993
Phosphate P 32, chromic, 3000
Prednisolone acetate injectable, 3064
Prednisolone acetate ophthalmic, 3065
Prednisone injectable, 3069
Prednisolone tebutate injectable, 3068
Primidone oral, 3074
Progesterone injectable, 3091
Propoxyphene napsylate oral, 3110
Propyliodone injectable oil, 3120
Psyllium hydrophilic mucilloid for oral, 3132
Pyrantel pamoate oral, 3133
Pyrvinium pamoate oral, 3141
Quinidine sulfate oral, 3150
Resorcinol and sulfur topical, 3176
Rifampin oral, 3184
Rimexolone ophthalmic, 3190
Selenium sulfide topical, 3228
Simethicone oral, 3233
Sodium polystyrene sulfonate, 3258
Spectinomycin for injectable, 3266
Structured vehicle, 1249
Structured vehicle, sugar-free, 1249
Sulfacetamide sodium and prednisolone acetate ophthalmic, 3288
Sulfacetamide sodium topical, 3287
Sulfadimethoxine oral, 3293
Sulfamethizole oral, 3297
Sulfamethoxazole oral, 3298
Sulfamethoxazole and trimethoprim oral, 3300
Sulfisoxazole acetyl oral, 3307
Sumatriptan succinate oral, 3312
Testosterone injectable, 3350
Tetracycline hydrochloride ophthalmic, 3364
Tetracycline hydrochloride oral, 3364
Tetracycline oral, 3360
Thiabendazole oral, 3380

Suspension (continued)
  Thioridazine oral, 3391
  Tobramycin and dexamethasone ophthalmic, 3422
  Tobramycin and fluorometholone acetate ophthalmic, 3423
  Triamcinolone acetonide injectable, 3444
  Triamcinolone diacetate injectable, 3446
  Triamcinolone hexacetonide injectable, 3447
  Triflupromazine oral, 3460
  Trisulfapyrimidines oral, 3477
  Vehicle for oral, 1258
  Verapamil hydrochloride oral, 3506
  Zinc sulfide topical, 3551

Suspension structured vehicle, 1249
  sugar-free, 1249
Suture
  absorbable surgical, 3314
  nonabsorbable surgical, 3316
Sutures—
  diameter ⟨861⟩, 360
  needle attachment ⟨871⟩, 360

Syrup, 1249
  Acacia, 1063
  Calcium glubionate, 1609
  Cherry, 1111
  Chlorpromazine hydrochloride, 1748
  Chocolate, 1112
  Corn, solids, 1117
  High fructose corn, 1116
  Docusate sodium, 2008
  Ferrous sulfate, 2157
  Orange, 1186
  Perphenazine, 2965
  Piperazine citrate, 3014
  Promazine hydrochloride, 3094
  Syrup, 1249
  Tolu balsam, 1252

T

Tablet breaking ⟨1217⟩, 676
Tablet friability ⟨1216⟩, 675

Tablets
  Acepromazine maleate, 1268
  Acetaminophen, 1271
  Containing at least three of the following—acetaminophen and (salts of) chlorpheniramine, dextromethorphan, and phenylpropanolamine, 1278
  Containing at least three of the following—acetaminophen and (salts of) chlorpheniramine, dextromethorphan, and pseudoephedrine, 1285
  Acetaminophen and aspirin, 1272
  Acetaminophen, aspirin, and caffeine, 1273
  Acetaminophen and caffeine, 1274
  Acetaminophen, chlorpheniramine maleate, and dextromethorphan hydrobromide, 1287
  Acetaminophen and codeine phosphate, 1291
  Acetaminophen and diphenhydramine citrate, 1293
  Acetaminophen, diphenhydramine hydrochloride, and pseudoephedrine hydrochloride, 1294
  Acetaminophen extended-release, 1271
  Acetaminophen and hydrocodone bitartrate, 2337
  Acetaminophen and pseudoephedrine hydrochloride, 1295
  Acetazolamide, 1297
  Acetohexamide, 1299
  Acetohydroxamic acid, 1300
  Acyclovir, 1306
  Albendazole, 1311
  Albuterol, 1313
  Alendronic acid, 1321
  Allopurinol, 1325
  Alprazolam, 1328
  Alumina and magnesia, 1337
  Alumina, magnesia, and calcium carbonate, 1338
  Alumina, magnesia, and calcium carbonate chewable, 1338
  Alumina, magnesia, calcium carbonate, and simethicone, 1339
  Alumina, magnesia, calcium carbonate, and simethicone chewable, 1341
  Alumina, magnesia, and simethicone, 1344
  Alumina, magnesia, and simethicone chewable, 1344
  Alumina and magnesium carbonate, 1346
  Alumina, magnesium carbonate, and magnesium oxide, 1347
  Alumina and magnesium trisilicate, 1348
  Aluminum hydroxide gel, dried, 1356
  Aluminum sulfate and calcium acetate for topical solution, 1360
  Amiloride hydrochloride, 1380
  Amiloride hydrochloride and hydrochlorothiazide, 1381
  Aminobenzoate potassium, 1384
  Aminocaproic acid, 1387
  Aminoglutethimide, 1389
  Aminopentamide sulfate, 1391
  Aminophylline, 1394
  Aminophylline delayed-release, 1394
  Aminosalicylate sodium, 1395
  Aminosalicylic acid, 1397
  Amitriptyline hydrochloride, 1400
  Ammonium chloride delayed-release, 1402
  Amodiaquine hydrochloride, 1406
  Amoxapine, 1407
  Amoxicillin, 1410
  Amoxicillin and clavulanate potassium, 1412
  Amphetamine sulfate, 1414
  Ampicillin, 1419
  Anileridine hydrochloride, 1425
  Apomorphine hydrochloride, 1439
  Ascorbic acid, 1446
  Aspirin, 1450
  Buffered aspirin, 1451
  Aspirin, alumina, and magnesia, 1454
  Aspirin, alumina, and magnesium oxide, 1455
  Aspirin and codeine phosphate, 1457
  Aspirin, codeine phosphate, alumina, and magnesia, 1458
  Aspirin delayed-release, 1452
  Aspirin effervescent for oral solution, 1453
  Aspirin extended-release, 1453
  Astemizole, 1460
  Atenolol, 1462
  Atenolol and chlorthalidone, 1462
  Atropine sulfate, 1470
  Azatadine maleate, 1474
  Azathioprine, 1475
  Bacampicillin hydrochloride, 1483
  Baclofen, 1487
  Barium sulfate, 1491
  Belladonna extract, 1494
  Benazepril hydrochloride, 1496
  Bendroflumethiazide, 1498
  Benztropine mesylate, 1511
  Betamethasone, 1516
  Betaxolol, 1527
  Bethanechol chloride, 1530
  Biperiden hydrochloride, 1535
  Bisacodyl delayed-release, 1537
  Bismuth subsalicylate, 1543
  Bisoprolol fumarate, 1545
  Bisoprolol fumarate and hydrochlorothiazide, 1546
  Bromocriptine mesylate, 1560
  Brompheniramine maleate, 1563
  Bumetanide, 1568
  Bupropion hydrochloride, 1573
  Bupropion hydrochloride extended-release, 1573
  Buspirone hydrochloride, 1576
  Busulfan, 1577
  Butabarbital sodium, 1579
  Butalbital, acetaminophen, and caffeine, 1581
  Butalbital and aspirin, 1582
  Butalbital, aspirin, and caffeine, 1584
  Calcium acetate, 1600
  Calcium carbonate, 1603
  Calcium carbonate and magnesia, 1603
  Calcium carbonate, magnesia, and simethicone, 1604
  Calcium carbonate, magnesia, and simethicone chewable, 1605
  Calcium gluconate, 1612
  Calcium lactate, 1613
  Calcium and magnesium carbonates, 1607
  Calcium pantothenate, 1615
  Calcium phosphate, dibasic, 1618
  Calcium with vitamin D, 913
  Calcium and vitamin D with minerals, 914
  Capecitabine, 1621
  Captopril, 1627
  Captopril and hydrochlorothiazide, 1628
  Carbamazepine, 1631
  Carbamazepine extended-release, 1632
  Carbenicillin indanyl sodium, 1635
  Carbidopa and levodopa, 1636
  Carbinoxamine maleate, 1637
  Carboxymethylcellulose sodium, 1648
  Carisoprodol, 1648
  Carisoprodol, aspirin, and codeine phosphate, 1650
  Carisoprodol and aspirin, 1649
  Carprofen, 1652
  Carteolol hydrochloride, 1654
  Cascara, 1658
  Cefaclor extended-release, 1662
  Cefadroxil, 1664
  Cefixime, 1672
  Cefpodoxime proxetil, 1690
  Cefprozil, 1692
  Cefuroxime axetil, 1700
  Cephalexin, 1707
  Cephalexin, for oral suspension, 1707
  Cephradine, 1714
  Chlorambucil, 1717
  Chloramphenicol, 1721
  Chlordiazepoxide, 1727
  Chlordiazepoxide and amitriptyline hydrochloride, 1727
  Chloroquine phosphate, 1736
  Chlorothiazide, 1738
  Chlorpheniramine maleate, 1742
  Chlorpheniramine maleate and phenylpropanolamine hydrochlroride extended-release, 1743
  Chlorpromazine hydrochloride, 1748
  Chlorpropamide, 1749
  Chlortetracycline hydrochloride, 1752
  Chlorthalidone, 1753
  Chlorzoxazone, 1754
  Chondroitin sulfate sodium, 923
  Chromium picolinate, 924
  Cimetidine, 1766
  Ciprofloxacin, 1775

Tablets *(continued)*
Citalopram, 1780
Clarithromycin, 1788
Clarithromycin extended-release, 1789
Clemastine fumarate, 1794
Clomiphene citrate, 1811
Clonazepam, 1815
Clonidine hydrochloride, 1817
Clonidine hydrochloride and chlorthalidone, 1818
Clopidogrel, 1821
Clorazepate dipotassium, 1823
Clover, red, 926
Clozapine, 1833
Cocaine hydrochloride for topical solution, 1837
Codeine phosphate, 1842
Codeine sulfate, 1843
Black cohosh, 911
Colchicine, 1844
Cortisone acetate, 1854
Cyclizine hydrochloride, 1862
Cyclobenzaprine hydrochloride, 1863
Cyclophosphamide, 1865
Cyproheptadine hydrochloride, 1872
Dapsone, 1882
Dehydrocholic acid, 1886
Demeclocycline hydrochloride, 1889
Desipramine hydrochloride, 1895
Desogestrel and ethinyl estradiol, 1899
Dexamethasone, 1908
Dexchlorpheniramine maleate, 1916
Dextroamphetamine sulfate, 1925
Diazepam, 1935
Dichlorphenamide, 1941
Diclofenac potassium, 1942
Diclofenac sodium delayed-release, 1944
Dicyclomine hydrochloride, 1948
Diethylcarbamazine citrate, 1951
Diethylpropion hydrochloride, 1953
Diethylstilbestrol, 1954
Diflunisal, 1958
Digitalis, 1961
Digitoxin, 1962
Digoxin, 1965
Dihydrotachysterol, 1970
Dihydroxyaluminum sodium carbonate chewable, 1973
Dihydroxyaluminum sodium carbonate, 1973
Diltiazem hydrochloride, 1978
Dimenhydrinate, 1981
Diphenoxylate hydrochloride and atropine sulfate, 1991
Dipyridamole, 1995
Dirithromycin delayed-release, 1996
Disulfiram, 2000
Divalproex sodium delayed-release, 2000
Docusate sodium, 2008
Dolasetron mesylate, 2012
Doxazosin, 2017
Doxycycline hyclate, 2026
Doxylamine succinate, 2027
Dydrogesterone, 2033
Dyphylline, 2035
Dyphylline and guaifenesin, 2036
Enalapril maleate, 2056
Enalapril maleate and hydrochlorothiazide, 2058
Ergocalciferol, 2073
Ergoloid mesylates, 2075
Ergoloid mesylates sublingual, 2076
Ergonovine maleate, 2078
Ergotamine tartrate, 2081
Ergotamine tartrate and caffeine, 2083
Ergotamine tartrate sublingual, 2082
Erythromycin, 2088
Erythromycin delayed-release, 2088
Erythromycin estolate, 2091

Erythromycin ethylsuccinate, 2094
Erythromycin stearate, 2098
Estradiol, 2101
Estradiol and norethindrone acetate, 2102
Estrogens, conjugated, 2107
Estrogens, esterified, 2109
Estropipate, 2113
Ethacrynic acid, 2114
Ethambutol hydrochloride, 2116
Ethinyl estradiol, 2119
Ethionamide, 2120
Ethotoin, 2125
Ethynodiol diacetate and ethinyl estradiol, 2127
Ethynodiol diacetate and mestranol, 2127
Etidronate disodium, 2129
Etodolac, 2131
Etodolac, extended-release, 2131
Famotidine, 2139
Felodipine extended-release, 2141
Fenoprofen calcium, 2150
Ferrous fumarate, 2154
Ferrous fumarate and docusate sodium extended-release, 2154
Ferrous gluconate, 2157
Ferrous sulfate, 2158
Fexofenadine hydrochloride, 2163
Fexofenadine hydrochloride and pseudoephedrine hydrochloride extended-release, 2164
Finasteride, 2167
Flecainide acetate, 2169
Fludrocortisone acetate, 2177
Fluoxetine, 2203
Fluoxymesterone, 2205
Flurbiprofen, 2214
Fluvoxamine maleate, 2226
Folic acid, 2229
Fosinopril sodium, 2231
Fosinopril sodium and hydrochlorothiazide, 2232
Furazolidone, 2238
Furosemide, 2241
Gabapentin, 2244
Garlic delayed-release, 943
Gemfibrozil, 2263
Ginkgo, 951
Ginseng, American, 954
Ginseng, Asian, 957
Glipizide, 2273
Glipizide and metformin hydrochloride, 2274
Glucosamine and chondroitin sodium sulfate, 957
Glucosamine, 959
Glucosamine and methylsulfonylmethane, 960
Glucosamine, chondroitin sulfate sodium, and methylsulfonylmethane tablets, 961
Glyburide, 2283
Glyburide and metformin hydrochloride, 2284
Glycopyrrolate, 2289
Griseofulvin, 2303
Griseofulvin, ultramicrosize, 2303
Guaifenesin, 2306
Guanabenz acetate, 2310
Guanadrel sulfate, 2311
Guanethidine monosulfate, 2312
Guanfacine, 2314
Halazone for solution, 2315
Haloperidol, 2318
Homatropine methylbromide, 2329
Hydralazine hydrochloride, 2333
Irbesartan and hydrochlorothiazide, 2335, 2447
Hydrochlorothiazide and amiloride hydrochloride, 1381
Hydrocodone bitartrate, 2336
Hydrocodone bitartrate and acetaminophen, 2337
Hydrocodone bitartrate and homatropine methylbromide, 2338

Hydrocortisone, 2342
Hydroflumethiazide, 2352
Hydromorphone hydrochloride, 2355
Hydroxychloroquine sulfate, 2359
Hydroxyzine hydrochloride, 2363
Hyoscyamine, 2366
Hyoscyamine sulfate, 2370
Ibuprofen, 2374
Ibuprofen and pseudoephedrine hydrochloride, 2375
Imipramine hydrochloride, 2385
Indapamide, 2388
Iodoquinol, 2427
Iopanoic acid, 2432
Irbesartan, 2447
Isoniazid, 2460
Isopropamide iodide, 2461
Isoproterenol hydrochloride, 2465
Isosorbide dinitrate, 2471
Isosorbide dinitrate chewable, 2472
Isosorbide dinitrate extended-release, 2472
Isosorbide dinitrate sublingual, 2473
Isosorbide mononitrate, 2475
Isosorbide mononitrate extended-release, 2477
Isoxsuprine hydrochloride, 2481
Ketoconazole, 2489
Ketorolac tromethamine, 2492
Labetalol hydrochloride, 2495
Leflunomide, 2505
Letrozole, 2507
Leucovorin calcium, 2510
Levamisole hydrochloride, 2512
Levocarnitine, 2517
Levodopa, 2519
Levonorgestrel and ethinyl estradiol, 2521
Levorphanol tartrate, 2523
Levothyroxine sodium, 2525
Liothyronine sodium, 2536
Liotrix, 2537
Lipoic acid, alpha, 969
Lisinopril, 2538
Lithium carbonate, 2540
Lithium carbonate extended-release, 2540
Loperamide hydrochloride, 2545
Loratadine, 2550
Lorazepam, 2553
Lovastatin, 2557
Lysine hydrochloride, 975
Magaldrate, 2564
Magaldrate and simethicone, 2566
Magaldrate and simethicone chewable, 2566
Magnesia, 2568
Magnesium gluconate, 2573
Magnesium oxide, 2576
Magnesium salicylate, 2577
Magnesium trisilicate, 2580
Maprotiline hydrochloride, 2588
Mazindol, 2590
Mebendazole, 2592
Mecamylamine hydrochloride, 2595
Meclizine hydrochloride, 2597
Medroxyprogesterone acetate, 2601
Megestrol acetate, 2605
Meloxicam, 2610
Melphalan, 2612
Menadiol sodium diphosphate, 2613
Meperidine hydrochloride, 2619
Mephenytoin, 2620
Mephobarbital, 2621
Meprobamate, 2624
Mercaptopurine, 2626
Mesalamine delayed-release, 2632
Mesoridazine besylate, 2635
Metaproterenol sulfate, 2639
Metformin hydrochloride, 2641

Tablets *(continued)*
  Metformin hydrochloride extended-release, 2642
  Methadone hydrochloride, 2650
  Methamphetamine hydrochloride, 2651
  Methazolamide, 2652
  Methdilazine hydrochloride, 2654
  Methenamine, 2655
  Methenamine hippurate, 2656
  Methenamine mandelate, 2657
  Methenamine mandelate delayed-release, 2658
  Methimazole, 2658
  Methocarbamol, 2660
  Methotrexate, 2663
  Methscopolamine bromide, 2667
  Methyclothiazide, 2670
  Methylcellulose, 2673
  Methyldopa, 2675
  Methyldopa and chlorothiazide, 2675
  Methyldopa and hydrochlorothiazide, 2676
  Methylergonovine maleate, 2681
  Methylphenidate hydrochloride, 2682
  Methylphenidate hydrochloride extended-release, 2683
  Methylprednisolone, 2684
  Methylsulfonylmethane, 979
  Methyltestosterone, 2689
  Methysergide maleate, 2690
  Metoclopramide, 2692
  Metolazone, 2694
  Metoprolol succinate extended-release, 2696
  Metoprolol tartrate, 2699
  Metoprolol tartrate and hydrochlorothiazide, 2699
  Metronidazole, 2704
  Metyrapone, 2705
  Milk thistle, 982
  Minerals, 984
  Minocycline hydrochloride, 2717
  Minoxidil, 2718
  Mirtazapine, 2720
  Mitotane, 2722
  Modafinil, 2725
  Molindone hydrochloride, 2726
  Moricizine hydrochloride, 2734
  Nabumetone, 2744
  Nadolol, 2745
  Nadolol and bendroflumethiazide, 2746
  Nafcillin sodium, 2749
  Nalidixic acid, 2751
  Naltrexone hydrochloride, 2755
  Naproxen, 2761
  Naproxen, delayed-release, 2761
  Naproxen sodium, 2762
  Naratriptan, 2766
  Nefazodone hydrochloride, 2769
  Neomycin sulfate, 2771
  Neostigmine bromide, 2793
  Nevirapine, 2797
  Niacin, 2799
  Niacinamide, 2801
  Nifedipine extended-release, 2807
  Nitrofurantoin, 2814
  Nitroglycerin, sublingual, 2818
  Norethindrone, 2825
  Norethindrone acetate, 2828
  Norethindrone acetate and ethinyl estradiol, 2829
  Norethindrone and ethinyl estradiol, 2826
  Norethindrone and mestranol, 2826
  Norfloxacin, 2832
  Norgestimate and ethinyl estradiol, 2834
  Norgestrel, 2836
  Norgestrel and ethinyl estradiol, 2836
  Nystatin, 2842
  Ofloxacin, 2848
  Ondansetron orally disintegrating, 2858
  Oxandrolone, 2865
  Oxaprozin, 2868
  Oxazepam, 2869
  Oxprenolol hydrochloride, 2871
  Oxprenolol hydrochloride extended-release, 2871
  Oxtriphylline, 2872
  Oxtriphylline delayed-release, 2873
  Oxtriphylline extended-release, 2873
  Oxybutynin chloride, 2876
  Oxybutynin chloride, extended-release, 2876
  Oxycodone hydrochloride, 2879
  Oxycodone hydrochloride extended-release, 2880
  Oxycodone and acetaminophen, 2883
  Oxycodone and aspirin, 2883
  Oxymetholone, 2889
  Oxytetracycline, 2892
  Pancreatin, 2907
  Pancrelipase, 2909
  Papain for topical solution, 2911
  Papaverine hydrochloride, 2912
  Paramethasone acetate, 2915
  Paroxetine, 2922
  Penbutolol sulfate, 2925
  Penicillamine, 2928
  Penicillin G benzathine, 2931
  Penicillin G potassium, 2935
  Penicillin V, 2944
  Penicillin V potassium, 2947
  Pentazocine and acetaminophen, 2948
  Pentazocine and aspirin, 2949
  Pentazocine and naloxone, 2950
  Pentoxifylline extended-release, 2957
  Pergolide, 2962
  Perphenazine, 2965
  Perphenazine and amitriptyline hydrochloride, 2965
  Phenazopyridine hydrochloride, 2968
  Phendimetrazine tartrate, 2970
  Phenelzine sulfate, 2971
  Phenmetrazine hydrochloride, 2972
  Phenobarbital, 2974
  Phentermine hydrochloride, 2980
  Phenylbutazone, 2984
  Phenylpropanolamine hydrochloride, 2991
  Phenylpropanolamine hydrochloride extended-release, 2992
  Phenytoin, 2994
  Phenytoin chewable, 2995
  Phytonadione, 3004
  Pimozide, 3008
  Pindolol, 3010
  Piperazine citrate, 3014
  Potassium bicarbonate effervescent for oral solution, 3028
  Potassium bicarbonate and potassium chloride effervescent for oral solution, 3029
  Potassium chloride extended-release, 3034
  Potassium chloride, potassium bicarbonate, and potassium citrate effervescent for oral solution, 3036
  Potassium citrate extended-release, 3038
  Potassium gluconate, 3041
  Potassium iodide, 3044
  Potassium iodide delayed-release, 3044
  Potassium and sodium bicarbonates and citric acid effervescent for oral solution, 3029
  Pravastatin sodium, 3055
  Praziquantel, 3057
  Prednisolone, 3063
  Prednisone, 3070
  Primaquine phosphate, 3073
  Primidone, 3074
  Probenecid, 3075
  Probenecid and colchicine, 3076
  Probucol, 3078
  Procainamide hydrochloride, 3080
  Procainamide hydrochloride extended-release, 3080
  Prochlorperazine maleate, 3087
  Procyclidine hydrochloride, 3088
  Promazine hydrochloride, 3095
  Promethazine hydrochloride, 3097
  Propantheline bromide, 3099
  Propoxyphene hydrochloride and acetaminophen, 3106
  Propoxyphene napsylate, 3110
  Propoxyphene napsylate and acetaminophen, 3111
  Propoxyphene napsylate and aspirin, 3112
  Propranolol hydrochloride, 3115
  Propranolol hydrochloride and hydrochlorothiazide, 3117
  Propylthiouracil, 3121
  Protriptyline hydrochloride, 3124
  Pseudoephedrine hydrochloride, 3126
  Pseudoephedrine hydrochloride extended-release, 3127
  Pyrazinamide, 3134
  Pyridostigmine bromide, 3136
  Pyridoxine hydrochloride, 3138
  Pyrilamine maleate, 3139
  Pyrimethamine, 3140
  Pyrvinium pamoate, 3142
  Quazepam, 3142
  Quinapril, 3144
  Quinidine gluconate extended-release, 3147
  Quinidine sulfate, 3150
  Quinidine sulfate extended-release, 3151
  Quinine sulfate, 3153
  Ranitidine, 3160
  Rauwolfia serpentina, 3163
  Repaglinide, 3166
  Reserpine, 3169
  Reserpine and chlorothiazide, 3170
  Reserpine hydralazine hydrochloride and hydrochlorothiazide, 3172
  Reserpine and hydrochlorothiazide, 3174
  Riboflavin, 3179
  Rifampin, isoniazid, and pyrazinamide, 3186
  Rifampin, isoniazid, pyrazinamide, and ethambutol hydrochloride, 3187
  Rimantadine hydrochloride, 3189
  Risperidone, 3197
  Ritodrine hydrochloride, 3199
  Saccharin sodium, 3209
  Salsalate, 3215
  Scopolamine hydrobromide, 3221
  Selegiline hydrochloride, 3226
  Sennosides, 3230
  Simethicone, 3234
  Simvastatin, 3235
  Sodium bicarbonate, 3243
  Sodium chloride, 3247
  Sodium chloride and dextrose, 3247
  Sodium chloride for solution, 3247
  Sodium fluoride, 3250
  Sodium salicylate, 3258
  Sotalol hydrochloride, 3264
  Spironolactone, 3267
  Spironolactone and hydrochlorothiazide, 3267
  Stanozolol, 3270
  Sucralfate, 3281
  Sulfadiazine, 3290
  Sulfadimethoxine, 3294
  Sulfadoxine and pyrimethamine, 3295
  Sulfamethizole, 3297
  Sulfamethoxazole, 3299
  Sulfamethoxazole and trimethoprim, 3301
  Sulfapyridine, 3302
  Sulfasalazine, 3304
  Sulfasalazine delayed-release, 3304
  Sulfinpyrazone, 3306

Tablets (continued)
Sulfisoxazole, 3307
Sulindac, 3309
Tamoxifen citrate, 3321
Terbutaline sulfate, 3347
Testolactone, 3349
Tetracycline hydrochloride, 3365
Tetracycline hydrochloride and novobiocin sodium, 3365
Tetracycline hydrochloride, novobiocin sodium, and prednisolone, 3366
Theophylline, 3374
Theophylline, ephedrine hydrochloride, and phenobarbital, 3375
Theophylline sodium glycinate, 3379
Thiabendazole, 3380
Thiabendazole chewable, 3381
Thiamine hydrochloride, 3383
Thiethylperazine maleate, 3386
Thioguanine, 3390
Thioridazine hydrochloride, 3393
Thyroid, 3399
Timolol maleate, 3411
Timolol maleate and hydrochlorothiazide, 3412
Tizanidine, 3416
Tocainide hydrochloride, 3424
Tolazamide, 3426
Tolbutamide, 3429
Tolcapone, 3430
Tolmetin sodium, 3432
Trazodone hydrochloride, 3437
Triamcinolone, 3441
Triamterene and hydrochlorothiazide, 3450
Triazolam, 3452
Trichlormethiazide, 3453
Trifluoperazine hydrochloride, 3459
Triflupromazine hydrochloride, 3461
Trihexyphenidyl hydrochloride, 3464
Trimeprazine tartrate, 3466
Trimethoprim, 3469
Trioxsalen, 3472
Tripelennamine hydrochloride, 3473
Triprolidine hydrochloride, 3475
Triprolidine and pseudoephedrine hydrochlorides, 3476
Trisulfapyrimidines, 3477
Ubidecarenone, 1000
Ursodiol, 3490
Valerian, 1002
Valsartan and hydrochlorothiazide, 3497
Verapamil hydrochloride, 3507
Verapamil hydrochloride extended-release, 3508
Vitamins with minerals, oil- and water-soluble, 1022
Vitamins with minerals, water-soluble, 1050
Vitamins, oil-soluble, 1005
Vitamins, oil- and water-soluble, 1010
Vitamins, water-soluble, 1044
Warfarin sodium, 3522
Zalcitabine, 3538
Zidovudine, 3542
Zinc sulfate, 3551

Tacrine
 capsules, 3318
 hydrochloride, 3317
Tagatose, 1250
Talc, 3319
Tamoxifen citrate, 3320
 tablets, 3321
Tannic acid, 802, 3322
 TS, 821
Tape, adhesive, 3322
Tapioca starch, 1241
Tartaric acid, 802, 1250
 TS, 821

Taurine, 3322
Tazobactam, 3323
Tc 99m
 albumin aggregated injection, technetium, 3324
 albumin colloid injection, technetium, 3325
 albumin injection, technetium, 3323
 apcitide injection, technetium, 3326
 arcitumomab injection, technetium, 3327
 bicisate injection, technetium, 3327
 depreotide injection, technetium, 3328
 disofenin injection, technetium, 3328
 etidronate injection, technetium, 3329
 exametazime injection, technetium, 3329
 fanolesomab injection, technetium, 3330
 gluceptate injection, technetium, 3331
 lidofenin injection, technetium, 3332
 mebrofenin injection, technetium, 3333
 medronate injection, technetium, 3334
 mertiatide injection, technetium, 3334
 nofetumomab merpentan injection, technetium, 3335
 oxidronate injection, technetium, 3335
 pentetate injection, technetium, 3336
 pertechnetate injection, sodium, 3336
 (pyro- and trimeta-) phosphates injection, technetium, 3338
 pyrophosphate injection, technetium, 3337
 red blood cells injection, technetium, 3338
 sestamibi injection, technetium, 3339
 succimer injection, technetium, 3340
 sulfur colloid injection, technetium, 3340
 tetrofosmin injection, technetium, 3341
Teaspoon ⟨1221⟩, 678
Technetium
 Tc 99m albumin aggregated injection, 3324
 Tc 99m albumin colloid injection, 3325
 Tc 99m albumin injection, 3323
 Tc 99m apcitide injection, 3326
 Tc 99m arcitumomab injection, 3327
 Tc 99m bicisate injection, 3327
 Tc 99m depreotide injection, 3328
 Tc 99m disofenin injection, 3328
 Tc 99m etidronate injection, 3329
 Tc 99m exametazime injection, 3329
 Tc 99m fanolesomab injection, 3330
 Tc 99m gluceptate injection, 3331
 Tc 99m lidofenin injection, 3332
 Tc 99m mebrofenin injection, 3333
 Tc 99m medronate injection, 3334
 Tc 99m mertiatide injection, 3334
 Tc 99m nofetumomab merpentan injection, 3335
 Tc 99m oxidronate injection, 3335
 Tc 99m pentetate injection, 3336
 Tc 99m pertechnetate injection, sodium, 3336
 Tc 99m pyrophosphate injection, 3337
 Tc 99m (pyro- and trimeta-) phosphates injection, 3338
 Tc 99m red blood cells injection, 3338
 Tc 99m sestamibi injection, 3339
 Tc 99m succimer injection, 3340
 Tc 99m sulfur colloid injection, 3340
 Tc 99m tetrofosmin injection, 3341
Temazepam, 3341
 capsules, 3342
Temperature, congealing ⟨651⟩, 247
Tensile strength ⟨881⟩, 360
Terazosin
 hydrochloride, 3343
Terbutaline sulfate, 3345
 inhalation aerosol, 3345
 injection, 3346
 tablets, 3347
Terminally sterilized pharmaceutical products— parametric release ⟨1222⟩, 678
Terpin hydrate, 3347
 and codeine oral solution, 3348
 oral solution, 3348

Tertiary butyl alcohol, 802
Test solutions, 814
Testolactone, 3349
 tablets, 3349
Testosterone, 3350
 benzoate, 802
 cypionate, 3351
 cypionate injection, 3351
 enanthate, 3352
 enanthate injection, 3352
 injectable suspension, 3350
 propionate, 3353
 propionate injection, 3353
Test papers
 and indicator, 810
 indicators and indicator, 808
Tests and assays, xiv, 6
Tetanus
 and diptheria toxoids adsorbed, 1992
 and diptheria toxoids adsorbed for adult use, 3354
 immune globulin, 3353
 toxoid, 3353
 toxoid adsorbed, 3353
2′,4′,5′,7′-Tetrabromofluorescein, 802
Tetrabromophenolphthalein ethyl ester, 802
 TS, 821
Tetrabutylammonium
 bromide, 802
 hydrogen sulfate, 802
 hydroxide, 1.0 M in methanol, 802
 hydroxide, 40 percent in water, 802
 hydroxide in methanol/isopropyl alcohol (0.1 N), 828
 hydroxide, tenth-normal (0.1 N), 828
 iodide, 802
 phosphate, 802
Tetracaine, 3354
 and cocaine hydrochlorides and epinephrine topical solution, 1838
 hydrochloride, 3356
 hydrochloride, benzocaine, and butamben gel, 1503
 hydrochloride, benzocaine, and butamben ointment, 1504
 hydrochloride, benzocaine, and butamben topical aerosol, 1503
 hydrochloride, benzocaine, and butamben topical solution, 1504
 hydrochloride cream, 3356
 hydrochloride in dextrose injection, 3358
 hydrochloride injection, 3356
 hydrochloride for injection, 3357
 hydrochloride, neomycin sulfate, and isoflupredone acetate ointment, 2777
 hydrochloride, neomycin sulfate, and isoflupredone acetate topical powder, 2778
 hydrochloride ophthalmic solution, 3358
 hydrochloride topical solution, 3358
 and menthol ointment, 3355
 ointment, 3354
 ophthalmic ointment, 3355
 and procaine hydrochlorides and levonordefrin injection, 3083
2,3,7,8-Tetrachlorodibenzo-p-dioxin, ^{13}C-labeled, 802
2,3,7,8-Tetrachlorodibenzofuran, ^{13}C-labeled, 802
1,1,2,2-Tetrachloroethane, 802
Tetracosane, 802
Tetracycline, 3359
 boluses, 3359
 hydrochloride, 3360
 hydrochloride capsules, 3361
 hydrochloride for injection, 3362
 hydrochloride, novobiocin sodium, and prednisolone tablets, 3366

Tetracycline (continued)
  hydrochloride and novobiocin sodium tablets, 3365
  hydrochloride and nystatin capsules, 3366
  hydrochloride ointment, 3362
  hydrochloride ophthalmic ointment, 3363
  hydrochloride ophthalmic suspension, 3364
  hydrochloride oral suspension, 3364
  hydrochloride soluble powder, 3363
  hydrochloride tablets, 3365
  hydrochloride for topical solution, 3363
  oral suspension, 3360
Tetradecane, 802
Tetraethylammonium perchlorate, 802
Tetraethylene glycol, 802
Tetraethylenepentamine, 802
Tetraheptylammonium bromide, 802
Tetrahydrofuran, 802
  peroxide-free, 803
  stabilizer-free, 803
Tetrahydro-2-furancarboxylic acid, 802
N-(2-Tetrahydrofuroyl)piperazine, 803
1,2,3,4-Tetrahydronaphthalene, 803
Tetrahydrozoline hydrochloride, 3367
  nasal solution, 3367
  ophthalmic solution, 3368
Tetramethylammonium
  bromide, 803
  bromide, tenth-molar (0.1 M), 828
  chloride, 803
  chloride, tenth-molar (0.1 M), 828
  hydroxide, 803
  hydroxide, pentahydrate, 803
  hydroxide solution in methanol, 803
  hydroxide TS, 821
  nitrate, 803
4,4′-Tetramethyldiaminodiphenylmethane, 803
Tetramethylsilane, 803
Tetrasodium ethylenediaminetetraacetate, 803
Thalidomide, 3368
  capsules, 3369
Thallous chloride, 803
  Tl 201 injection, 3370
Theobromine, 803
Theophylline, 3371
  capsules, 3371
  in dextrose injection, 3375
  ephedrine hydrochloride, and phenobarbital tablets, 3375
  extended-release capsules, 3372
  and guaifenesin capsules, 3377
  and guaifenesin oral solution, 3377
  oral solution, 3374
  sodium glycinate, 3378
  sodium glycinate oral solution, 3378
  sodium glycinate tablets, 3379
  tablets, 3374
Thermal analysis ⟨891⟩, 362
Thermometers ⟨21⟩, 66
Thermometric equivalents, 905
Thiabendazole, 3379
  chewable tablets, 3381
  oral suspension, 3380
  tablets, 3380
Thiamine
  hydrochloride, 3381
  hydrochloride injection, 3382
  hydrochloride oral solution, 3383
  hydrochloride tablets, 3383
  mononitrate, 3383
  mononitrate oral solution, 3384
Thiamine assay ⟨531⟩, 184
Thiazole yellow, 803
  paper, 810
Thiethylperazine maleate, 3384
  suppositories, 3385
  tablets, 3386

Thimerosal, 3386
  tincture, 3388
  topical aerosol, 3387
  topical solution, 3388
Thin-layer chromatographic identification test ⟨201⟩, 130
Thioacetamide, 803
  TS, 821
Thioacetamide-glycerin base TS, 821
2-Thiobarbituric acid, 803
2,2′-Thiodiethanol, 803
Thioglycolic acid, 804
Thioguanine, 3389
  tablets, 3390
Thionine acetate, 804
Thiopental sodium, 3390
  for injection, 3391
Thioridazine, 3391
  hydrochloride, 3392
  hydrochloride oral solution, 3392
  hydrochloride tablets, 3393
  oral suspension, 3391
Thiostrepton, 3393
  nystatin, neomycin sulfate, and triamcinolone acetonide cream, 2843
  nystatin, neomycin sulfate, and triamcinolone acetonide ointment, 2844
Thiotepa, 3394
  for injection, 3394
Thiothixene, 3395
  capsules, 3395
  hydrochloride, 3396
  hydrochloride injection, 3397
  hydrochloride for injection, 3397
  hydrochloride oral solution, 3397
Thiourea, 804
Thorium nitrate, 804
  TS, 821
Threonine, 3398
Thrombin, 3398
Thromboplastin, 804
Thymidine, 804
Thymol, 804, 1251
  blue, 810
  blue TS, 821
Thymolphthalein, 810
  TS, 821
Thyroglobulin, 804
Thyroid, 3398
  tablets, 3399
Tiagabine hydrochloride, 3400
Tiamulin, 3401
  fumarate, 3403
Ticarcillin
  and clavulanic acid injection, 3405
  and clavulanic acid for injection, 3405
  disodium, 3404
  for injection, 3404
  monosodium, 3406
Tiletamine
  hydrochloride, 3407
  and zolazepam for injection, 3407
Tilmicosin, 3408
  injection, 3409
Timolol
  maleate, 3410
  maleate and hydrochlorothiazide tablets, 3412
  maleate ophthalmic solution, 3411
  maleate tablets, 3411
Tin, 804

Tincture
Belladonna, 1494
Benzethonium chloride, 1500
Benzoin, compound, 1507
Cardamom, compound, 1102
Ginger, 946

Green soap, 2301
Iodine, 2414
Iodine, strong, 2415
Lemon, 1162
Opium, 2860
Orange peel, sweet, 1185
Thimerosal, 3388
Tolu balsam, 1252
Vanilla, 1256

Tinidazole, 3413
Tioconazole, 3413
Titanium
  dioxide, 3414
  tetrachloride, 804
  trichloride, 804
  trichloride-sulfuric acid TS, 821
  trichloride, tenth-normal (0.1 N), 829
  trichloride TS, 821
Title, xi, 3
Titles, changes in official, xxviii
Titration, nitrite ⟨451⟩, 156
Titrimetry ⟨541⟩, 185
Tizanidine
  hydrochloride, 3415
  tablets, 3416
Tl 201
  injection, thallous chloride, 3370
Tobramycin, 3418
  and dexamethasone ophthalmic ointment, 3422
  and dexamethasone ophthalmic suspension, 3422
  and fluorometholone acetate ophthalmic suspension, 3423
  inhalation solution, 3420
  injection, 3419
  for injection, 3419
  ophthalmic ointment, 3420
  ophthalmic solution, 3421
  sulfate, 3424
Tocainide hydrochloride, 3424
  tablets, 3424
tocopherol assay, alpha ⟨551⟩, 187
Tocopherols excipient, 1251
Tolazamide, 3425
  tablets, 3426
Tolazoline hydrochloride, 3427
  injection, 3427
Tolbutamide, 3428
  for injection, 3428
  tablets, 3429
Tolcapone, 3429
  tablets, 3430
o-Tolidine, 804
Tolmetin sodium, 3431
  capsules, 3432
  tablets, 3432
Tolnaftate, 3433
  cream, 3433
  gel, 3433
  topical aerosol, 3433
  topical powder, 3434
  topical solution, 3434
Tolualdehyde, 804
p-Tolualdehyde, 804
Tolu balsam, 3434
  syrup, 1252
  tincture, 1252
Toluene, 804
p-Toluenesulfonic acid, 804
  TS, 821
p-Toluenesulfonyl-L-arginine methyl ester hydrochloride, 804
p-Toluic acid, 804
Toluidine
  blue, 804
  blue O, 804

o-Toluidine, 804
p-Toluidine, 804
Tomato extract
  containing lycopene, 973

Topical solution
Aluminum acetate, 1349
Aluminum subacetate, 1358
Aluminum sulfate and calcium acetate for, 1359
Aluminum sulfate and calcium acetate tablets for, 1360
Aminobenzoic acid, 1386
Benzethonium chloride, 1500
Benzocaine, 1503
Benzocaine, butamben, and tetracaine hydrochloride, 1504
Calcium hydroxide, 1612
Carbamide peroxide, 1633
Carbol-fuchsin, 1638
Cetylpyridinium chloride, 1716
Clindamycin phosphate, 1800
Clobetasol propionate, 1806
Clotrimazole, 1828
Coal tar, 1834
Cocaine hydrochloride tablets for, 1837
Cocaine and tetracaine hydrochlorides and epinephrine, 1838
Diethyltoluamide, 1956
Dimethyl sulfoxide, 1984
Dyclonine hydrochloride, 2032
Erythromycin, 2088
Fluocinolone acetonide, 2186
Fluocinonide, 2188
Fluorouracil, 2199
Gentamicin sulfate and betamethasone valerate, 2268
Gentian violet, 2271
Halcinonide, 2317
Hydrogen peroxide, 2353
Hydroquinone, 2356
Iodine, 2414
Lidocaine hydrochloride, 2529
Mafenide acetate for, 2562
Methoxsalen, 2666
Minoxidil, 2718
Mometasone furoate, 2728
Myrrh, 2743
Nitrofurazone, 2815
Nitromersol, 2819
Papain tablets for, 2911
Phenol, camphorated, 2976
Podophyllum resin, 3019
Povidone-iodine, 3050
Sodium fluoride and acidulated phosphate, 3250
Sodium hypochlorite, 3251
Tetracaine hydrochloride, 3358
Tetracycline hydrochloride for, 3363
Thimerosal, 3388
Tolnaftate, 3434
Tretinoin, 3440

Topical suspension
Calamine, 1593
Calamine, phenolated, 1593
Ciclopirox olamine, 1763
Clindamycin phosphate, 1801
Penicillin G, neomycin, polymyxin B, hydrocortisone acetate, and hydrocortisone sodium succinate, 2929
Penicillin G procaine, neomycin and polymyxin B sulfates, and hydrocortisone acetate, 2941
Resorcinol and sulfur, 3176
Selenium sulfide, 3228

Sulfacetamide sodium, 3287
Zinc sulfide, 3551

Topiramate, 3435
Torsemide, 3436
Total organic carbon ⟨643⟩, 244
Tragacanth, 1252
Transdermal system
  clonidine, 1819
  nicotine, 2801
Transfusion and infusion assemblies and similar medical devices ⟨161⟩, 124
Trazodone hydrochloride, 3436
  tablets, 3437
Trenbolone acetate, 3438
Tretinoin, 3439
  cream, 3440
  gel, 3440
  topical solution, 3440
Triacetin, 3441
n-Triacontane, 804
Triamcinolone, 3441
  acetonide, 3442
  acetonide cream, 3443
  acetonide dental paste, 3444
  acetonide injectable suspension, 3444
  acetonide lotion, 3444
  acetonide and neomycin sulfate cream, 2792
  acetonide and neomycin sulfate ophthalmic ointment, 2792
  acetonide and nystatin cream, 2844
  acetonide, nystatin, neomycin sulfate, and gramicidin cream, 2842
  acetonide, nystatin, neomycin sulfate, and gramicidin ointment, 2843
  acetonide, nystatin, neomycin sulfate and thiostrepton cream, 2843
  acetonide, nystatin, neomycin sulfate, and thiostrepton ointment, 2844
  acetonide and nystatin ointment, 2845
  acetonide ointment, 2844
  acetonide topical aerosol, 3443
  diacetate, 3445
  diacetate injectable suspension, 3446
  diacetate oral solution, 3445
  hexacetonide, 3446
  hexacetonide injectable suspension, 3447
  tablets, 3441
2,4,6-Triamino-5-nitrosopyrimidine, 804
Triamterene, 3447
  capsules, 3448
  and hydrochlorothiazide capsules, 3449
  and hydrochlorothiazide tablets, 3450
Triazolam, 3451
  tablets, 3452
Tribasic calcium phosphate, 1087
Tribasic sodium phosphate, 1229
Tributyl
  citrate, 1253
  phosphate, 804
Tributylethylammonium hydroxide, 804
Tributyrin, 805
Trichlormethiazide, 3452
  tablets, 3453
Trichloroacetic acid, 805
Trichloroethane, 805
Trichlorofluoromethane, 805
Trichloromonofluoromethane, 1253
Trichlorotrifluoroethane, 805
Tricitrates oral solution, 3453
Triclosan, 3454
n-Tricosane, 805
Trientine hydrochloride, 3456
  capsules, 3457
Triethanolamine, 805
Triethylamine, 805
  hydrochloride, 805

Triethyl citrate, 1253
Triethylene glycol, 805
Trifluoperazine
  hydrochloride, 3458
  hydrochloride injection, 3458
  hydrochloride tablets, 3459
  oral solution, 3458
Trifluoroacetic
  acid, 805
  anhydride, 805
2,2,2-Trifluoroethanol, 805
2,2,2-Trifluoroethyldifluoromethyl ether, 805
(m-Trifluoromethylphenyl) trimethylammonium hydroxide in methanol, 805
5-(Trifluoromethyl)uracil, 805
α,α,α-Trifluoro-p-cresol, 806
Trifluorovinyl chloride polymer, 806
Triflupromazine, 3459
  hydrochloride, 3460
  hydrochloride injection, 3461
  hydrochloride tablets, 3461
  oral suspension, 3460
Trifluridine, 3462
Triglycerides
  medium-chain, 1254
Trihexyphenidyl hydrochloride, 3462
  extended-release capsules, 3463
  oral solution, 3464
  tablets, 3464
Trikates oral solution, 3465
Triketohydrindene hydrate
  TS, 821
Trimeprazine
  oral solution, 3466
  tartrate, 3465
  tartrate tablets, 3466
Trimethobenzamide hydrochloride, 3467
  capsules, 3467
  injection, 3468
Trimethoprim, 3468
  and polymyxin B sulfate ophthalmic solution, 3025
  and sulfamethoxazole injection, 3299
  and sulfamethoxazole oral suspension, 3300
  and sulfamethoxazole tablets, 3301
  sulfate, 3469
  tablets, 3469
Trimethylacethydrazide ammonium chloride, 806
Trimethylchlorosilane, 806
2,2,4-Trimethylpentane, 806
2,4,6-Trimethylpyridine, 806
N-(Trimethylsilyl)-imidazole, 806
Trimipramine maleate, 3470
2,4,6-Trinitrobenzenesulfonic acid, 806
Trinitrophenol, 806
  TS, 821
Trioctylphosphine oxide, 806
Trioxsalen, 3471
  tablets, 3472
Tripelennamine hydrochloride, 3472
  injection, 3473
  tablets, 3473
Triphenyltetrazolium
  chloride, 806
  chloride TS, 821
1,3,5-Triphenylbenzene, 806
Triphenylmethane, 806
Triphenylmethanol, 806
Triphenyltetrazolium chloride, 806
Triprolidine
  hydrochloride, 3474
  hydrochloride oral solution, 3474
  hydrochloride tablets, 3475
  and pseudoephedrine hydrochlorides oral solution, 3475
  and pseudoephedrine hydrochlorides tablets, 3476
Tris(2-aminoethyl)amine, 806

Tris(hydroxymethyl)aminomethane, 806
  acetate, 806
  hydrochloride, 806
N-Tris(hydroxymethyl)methylglycine, 806
Trisulfapyrimidines
  oral suspension, 3477
  tablets, 3477
Tritirachium album proteinase K, 806
Trolamine, 1256
  salicylate, 3478
Troleandomycin, 3478
  capsules, 3479
Tromethamine, 806, 3479
  carboprost, 1646
  carboprost, injection, 1646
  for injection, 3479
Tropaeolin OO, 806
Tropic acid, 806
Tropicamide, 3480
  ophthalmic solution, 3480
Tropine, 806
Trypan blue, 806
Trypsin, crystallized, 3481
Tryptone, 806
Tryptophan, 3481
L-Tryptophane, 806
Tuberculin, 3482
  purified protein derivative *(Tuberculin PPD)*, 806
Tubocurarine chloride, 807, 3482
  injection, 3483
Tungstic acid, 807
Turmeric paper, 810
Tylosin, 3483
  granulated, 3484
  tartrate, 3484
Tyloxapol, 3485
Tyrosine, 3486
L-Tyrosine disodium, 807
Tyrothricin, 3487

U

Ubidecarenone, 998
  capsules, 999
  tablets, 1000
Undecylenic acid, 3487
  ointment, compound, 3487
Uniformity of dosage units ⟨905⟩, 363
Units of potency, xiii, 5
Uracil, 807
Uranyl acetate, 807
  cobalt, TS, 816
  zinc, TS, 821
Urea, 807, 3488
  C 13, 1643
  C 13 for oral solution, 1643
  C 14 capsules, 1643
  for injection, 3488
Urethane, 807
Uridine, 807
Ursodiol, 3489
  capsules, 3489
  tablets, 3490
USP and NF excipients listed by category, 1057
USP policies, xxiv
USP reference standards, xiii, 5
USP reference standards ⟨11⟩, 37

V

Vaccine
Anthrax adsorbed, 1427
BCG, 1491
Influenza virus, 2403
Measles, mumps, and rubella virus live, 2591
Measles and rubella virus live, 2591
Measles virus live, 2590
Poliovirus inactivated, 3020
Rabies, 3154
Rubella virus live, 3205
Smallpox, 3238
Yellow fever, 3535

Vaccinia immune globulin, 3491
Valerian, 1000
  extract, powdered, 1001
  powdered, 1001
  tablets, 1002
Valeric acid, 807
Valerophenone, 807
Validation
  of alternative microbiological methods ⟨1223⟩, 681
  of compendial procedures ⟨1225⟩, 683
  of microbial recovery from pharmacopeial articles ⟨1227⟩, 687
Valine, 3491
Valproic acid, 3491
  capsules, 3492
  injection, 3493
  oral solution, 3493
Valrubicin, 3494
  intravesical solution, 3495
Valsartan, 3496
  and hydrochlorothiazide tablets, 3497
Vanadium pentoxide, 807
Vanadyl sulfate, 807
Vancomycin, 3498
  hydrochloride, 3499
  hydrochloride capsules, 3500
  hydrochloride for injection, 3501
  hydrochloride for oral solution, 3501
  hydrochloride, sterile, 3501
  injection, 3500
Vanilla, 1256
  tincture, 1256
Vanillin, 1257
Varicella-zoster immune globulin, 3502
Vasopressin, 3502
  injection, 3503
Vecuronium Bromide, 3503
Vegetable
  and animal substances, xx, 12
  oil, hydrogenated, 1257
Vehicle
  for oral solution, 1257
  for oral solution, sugar free, 1258
  for oral suspension, 1258
  suspension structured, 1249
  suspension structured, sugar-free, 1249
Verapamil hydrochloride, 3504
  extended-release tablets, 3508
  injection, 3505
  oral solution, 3506
  oral suspension, 3506
  tablets, 3507
Verification of compendial procedures ⟨1226⟩, 687
Verteporfin, 3510
  for injection, 3511
Vidarabine, 3511
  ophthalmic ointment, 3512

Vinblastine sulfate, 3512
  for injection, 3513
Vincristine sulfate, 3514
  injection, 3514
  for injection, 3515
Vinorelbine
  injection, 3517
  tartrate, 3516
Vinyl acetate, 807
2-Vinylpyridine, 807
Vinylpyrrolidinone, 807
Viral safety evaluation of biotechnology products derived from cell lines of human or animal origin ⟨1050⟩, 453
Viscosity ⟨911⟩, 369
Vitamin
  A, 3517
  A assay ⟨571⟩, 203
  A capsules, 3518
  B_{12} activity assay ⟨171⟩, 125
  D assay ⟨581⟩, 204
  D and calcium with minerals tablets, 914
  D with calcium tablets, 913
  E, 3518
  E capsules, 3520
  E polyethylene glycol succinate, 1258
  E preparation, 3519
Vitamins
  capsules, oil-soluble, 1003
  capsules, oil- and water-soluble, 1005
  capsules, water-soluble, 1041
  with minerals capsules, oil- and water-soluble, 1011
  with minerals capsules, water-soluble, 1046
  with minerals oral solution, oil- and water-soluble, 1016
  with minerals oral solution, water-soluble, 1049
  with minerals tablets, oil- and water-soluble, 1022
  with minerals tablets, water-soluble, 1050
  oral solution, oil- and water-soluble, 1009
  tablets, oil-soluble, 1005
  tablets, oil- and water-soluble, 1010
  tablets, water-soluble, 1044
Volumetric
  apparatus ⟨31⟩, 66
  solutions, 821

W

Warfarin sodium, 3520
  for injection, 3521
  tablets, 3522
Washed sand, 807

Water
Ammonia, stronger, 754
Ammonia, 25 percent, 754
Ammonia-free, 807
Carbon dioxide-free, 807
Cetyltrimethylammonium chloride, 25 percent in, 764
Deaerated, 807
Deuterated, 768
D-Gluconic acid, 50 percent in, 776
For hemodialysis, 3525
Hydrazine hydrate, 85% in, 778
For inhalation, sterile, 3523
For injection, 3523
For injection, bacteriostatic, 3523

Water *(continued)*
  For injection, sterile, 3524
  For irrigation, sterile, 3524
  Methylamine, 40 percent in, 783
  O 15 injection, 2887
  Peppermint, 1190
  Pure steam, 3525
  Purified, 3524
  Purified, sterile, 3524
  Rose ointment, 3204
  Rose, stronger, 1219
  Soluble vitamins capsules, 1041
  soluble vitamins with minerals capsules, 1046
  Soluble vitamins with minerals oral solution, 1049
  Soluble vitamins with minerals tablets, 1050
  soluble vitamins tablets, 1044
  Stronger ammonia, 800
  Tetrabutylammonium hydroxide, 40 percent in, 802
  Vapor detector tube, 808
  Vitamins capsules, and oil-soluble, 1005
  Vitamins with minerals capsules, oil-soluble, 1011
  Vitamins with minerals oral solution, oil-soluble, 1016
  Vitamins with minerals tablets, and oil-soluble, 1022
  Vitamins oral solution, oil-soluble, 1009
  Vitamins tablets, oil-soluble, 1010
  Water conductivity ⟨645⟩, 245
  Water determination ⟨921⟩, 370
  Water for health applications ⟨1230⟩, 690
  Water for pharmaceutical purposes ⟨1231⟩, 691
  Water–solid interactions in pharmaceutical systems ⟨1241⟩, 710

Water-soluble vitamins
  capsules, 1041
Wax
  carnauba, 1259
  emulsifying, 1260
  microcrystalline, 1260
  white, 1260
  yellow, 1261
Weighing on an analytical balance ⟨1251⟩, 712
Weight variation of dietary supplements ⟨2091⟩, 736
Weights
  and measures, xxi, 13
Weights and balances ⟨41⟩, 67

Wheat
  bran, 3525
  starch, 1242
Witch hazel, 3526
Wound matrix
  small intestinal submucosa, 3527
Wright's stain, 808
Written prescription drug information—
    guidelines ⟨1265⟩, 714

X

Xanthan gum, 1261
  solution, 1262
Xanthine, 808
Xanthydrol, 808
Xenon Xe 127, 3529
Xenon Xe 133, 3530
  injection, 3530
X-ray diffraction ⟨941⟩, 372
Xylazine, 3530
  hydrochloride, 3532
  injection, 3532
Xylene, 808
m-Xylene, 808
o-Xylene, 808
p-Xylene, 808
Xylene cyanole FF, 808
Xylenol orange, 810
  TS, 821
Xylitol, 1262
Xylometazoline hydrochloride, 3533
  nasal solution, 3533
Xylose, 808, 3534

Y

Yeast extract, 808
Yellow fever vaccine, 3535
Yellow mercuric oxide, 808
Yohimbine
  hydrochloride, 3535
  injection, 3536

Yttrium Y 90 ibritumomab tiuxetan
  injection, 3537

Z

Zalcitabine, 3537
  tablets, 3538
Zein, 1263
Zidovudine, 3539
  capsules, 3540
  injection, 3541
  oral solution, 3541
  tablets, 3542
Zileuton, 3543
Zinc, 808
  acetate, 808, 3545
  amalgam, 808
  carbonate, 3545
  chloride, 3546
  chloride, anhydrous, powdered, 808
  chloride injection, 3546
  determination ⟨591⟩, 208
  gluconate, 3547
  oxide, 3547
  oxide neutral, 3548
  oxide ointment, 3549
  oxide paste, 3549
  oxide and salicylic acid paste, 3549
  stearate, 3549
  sulfate, 3550
  sulfate heptahydrate, 808
  sulfate injection, 3550
  sulfate ophthalmic solution, 3551
  sulfate oral solution, 3551
  sulfate tablets, 3551
  sulfate, twentieth-molar (0.05 M), 829
  sulfide topical suspension, 3551
  undecylenate, 3552
  uranyl acetate TS, 821
Zirconyl
  chloride, octahydrate, basic, 808
  nitrate, 808
Zolazepam
  hydrochloride, 3552
  and tiletamine for injection, 3407